ICD·10·CM

International Classification of Diseases
10th Revision

Clinical Modification

Color Coded

2018

D1211462

Office, Hospital and Payer Edition

ISBN 978-1-946868-02-2 (Perfect bound)
ISBN 978-1-946868-05-3 (e-Book)

Home Health Edition

ISBN 978-1-946868-30-5 (Perfect bound)
ISBN 978-1-946868-31-2 (e-Book)

Practice Management Information Corporation (PMIC)
4727 Wilshire Boulevard
Los Angeles, California 90010
http://www.pmiconline.com

Preface

On October 1, 2015, a key element of the data foundation of the United States' health care system underwent a major transformation…the transition from the decades-old Ninth Edition of the International Classification of Diseases (ICD-9) set of diagnosis and inpatient procedure codes to the far more contemporary, vastly larger, and much more detailed Tenth Edition of those code sets—or ICD-10—used by most developed countries throughout the world. The transition had a major impact on any person or entity recording health care information containing a diagnosis and/or inpatient procedure code.

All "covered entities"—as defined by the Health Insurance Portability and Accountability Act of 1996 (HIPAA)—were required to adopt ICD-10 codes for use in all HIPAA transactions with dates of service on or after the October 1, 2015 compliance date. for HIPAA inpatient claims, ICD-10 diagnosis and procedure codes are required for all inpatient stays with discharge dates on or after October 1, 2015.

This Fiscal Year (FY) 2018 update of the International Statistical Classification of Diseases and Related Health Problems, 10th revision, Clinical Modification (ICD-10-CM) is being published by PMIC to promulgate this classification throughout the United States for morbidity coding. The International Statistical Classification of Diseases and Related Health Problems, 10th Revision (ICD-10), published by the World Health Organization (WHO), is the foundation of ICD-10-CM. ICD-10 continues to be the classification used in cause-of-death coding in the United States. The ICD-10-CM is comparable with the ICD-10.

The WHO Collaborating Center for the Family of International Classifications in North America, housed at the Centers for Disease Control and Prevention's National Center for Health Statistics (NCHS), has responsibility for the implementation of ICD and other WHO-FIC classifications and serves as a liaison with the WHO, fulfilling international obligations for comparable classifications and the national health data needs of the United States.

This edition of ICD-10-CM includes all official codes, descriptions, guidelines, tables and indexes. A new edition is available approximately mid-September of each year. New editions may be purchased from:

Practice Management Information Corporation
4727 Wilshire Boulevard, Suite 300
Los Angeles, CA 90010
1-800-MED-SHOP
http://pmiconline.com

Disclaimer

This publication includes all official ICD-10-CM codes, descriptions, annotations and guidelines. This publication is revised annually so that we may present the most current information possible. Though all of the information is carefully researched and checked for accuracy and completeness, the publisher accepts no responsibility with regard to errors, omissions, misuse or misinterpretation.

Table of Contents

Introduction to ICD-10-CM

On October 1, 2015, a key element of the data foundation of the United States' health care system underwent a major transformation…the transition from the decades-old Ninth Edition of the International Classification of Diseases (ICD-9) set of diagnosis and inpatient procedure codes to the far more contemporary, vastly larger, and much more detailed Tenth Edition of those code sets—or ICD-10—used by most developed countries throughout the world. The transition had a major impact on any person or entity recording health care information containing a diagnosis and/or inpatient procedure code.

HISTORY OF THE INTERNATIONAL CLASSIFICATION OF DISEASES

For students of medical nomenclature and coding systems, the following history of the International Classification of Diseases excerpted from Wikipedia may be interesting.

HISTORICAL SYNOPSIS

In 1893, a French physician, Jacques Bertillon, introduced the *Bertillon Classification of Causes of Death* at a congress of the International Statistical Institute in Chicago. a number of countries and cities adopted Dr. Bertillon's system, which was based on the principle of distinguishing between general diseases and those localized to a particular organ or anatomical site, as used by the City of Paris for classifying deaths. Subsequent revisions represented a synthesis of English, German and Swiss classifications, expanding from the original 44 titles to 161 titles. in 1898, the American Public Health Association (APHA) recommended that the registrars of Canada, Mexico, and the United States also adopt it. The APHA also recommended revising the system every ten years to ensure the system remained current with medical practice advances. As a result, the first international conference to revise the International Classification of Causes of Death convened in 1900; with revisions occurring every ten years thereafter. At that time the classification system was contained in one book, which included an Alphabetic Index as well as a Tabular List. The book was small compared with current coding texts.

The revisions that followed contained minor changes, until the sixth revision of the classification system. with the sixth revision, the classification system expanded to two volumes. The sixth revision included morbidity and mortality conditions, and its title was modified to reflect the changes: *International Statistical Classification of Diseases, Injuries and Causes of Death (ICD)*. Prior to the sixth revision, responsibility for ICD revisions fell to the Mixed Commission, a group composed of representatives from the International Statistical Institute and the Health Organization of the League of Nations. in 1948, the World Health Organization (WHO) assumed responsibility for preparing and publishing the revisions to the ICD every ten years. WHO sponsored the seventh and eighth revisions in 1957 and 1968, respectively. It later become clear that the established ten-year interval between revisions was too short.

The ICD is currently the most widely used statistical classification system for diseases in the world. International health statistics using this system are available at the WHO Statistical Information System (WHOSIS). in addition, some countries—including Australia, Canada and the United States—have developed their own adaptations of ICD, with more procedure for classification of operative or diagnostic procedures.

HISTORY AND USAGE IN THE UNITED STATES

In the United States, the U.S. Public Health Service published the *International Classification of Diseases, Adapted for Indexing of Hospital Records and Operation Classification (ICDA)*, completed in 1962 and expanding the ICD-7 in a number of areas to more completely meet the indexing needs of hospitals. The U.S. Public Health Service later published the *Eighth Revision, International Classification of Diseases, Adapted for Use in the United States*, commonly referred to as ICDA-8, for official national morbidity and mortality statistics. This was followed by the *ICD, 9th Revision, Clinical Modification*, known as ICD-9-CM, published by the U.S. Department of Health and Human Services and used by hospitals and other healthcare facilities to better describe the clinical picture of the patient. The diagnosis component of ICD-9-CM is completely consistent with ICD-9 codes, and remains the data standard for reporting morbidity. National adaptations of the ICD-10 progressed to incorporate both clinical code (ICD-10-CM) and procedure code (ICD-10-PCS) with the revisions completed in 2003. in 2009, the U.S. Centers for Medicare and Medicaid Services announced that it would begin using ICD-10 on April 1, 2010, with full compliance by all involved parties by 2013.

BRIEF HISTORY OF ICD-10

ICD-10 was first published by the World Health Organization (WHO) in 1992. The National Center for Health Statistics (NCHS), the Federal agency responsible for use of the International Statistical Classification of Diseases and Related Health Problems, 10th revision (ICD-10) in the United States, has developed a clinical modification of the classification for morbidity purposes. The ICD-10 is used to code and classify mortality data from death certificates, having replaced ICD-9 for this purpose as of January 1, 1999. ICD-10-CM is planned as the replacement for ICD-9-CM, volumes 1 and 2. ICD-10-PCS is the replacement for ICD-9-CM volume 3, Procedures.

ICD-10-CM was developed following a thorough evaluation by a Technical Advisory Panel and extensive additional consultation with physician groups, clinical coders, and others to assure clinical accuracy and utility. Notable improvements in the content and format include: the addition of information relevant to ambulatory and managed care encounters; expanded injury codes; the creation of combination diagnosis/symptom codes to reduce the number of codes needed to fully describe a condition; the addition of a sixth character; incorporation of common 4th and 5th digit subclassifications; laterality; and greater specificity in code assignment. After several delays, ICD-10 was officially implemented on October 1, 2015.

TERMINOLOGY

acute conditions	The medical conditions characterized by sudden onset, severe change, and/or short duration.
additional diagnosis	The secondary diagnosis code used, if available, to provide a more complete picture of the primary diagnosis.
alteration	Modifying the anatomic structure of a body part without affecting the function of the body part
applied mapping	Distillation of a reference mapping to conform to the needs of a particular application (e.g., data quality, research).
approach (5th character)	Defines the technique used to reach the site of the procedure.
backward mapping	mapping that proceeds from a newer code set to an older code set, for example from ICD-10-CM to ICD-9-CM.
bilateral	For bilateral sites, the final character of the codes in the ICD-10-CM indicates laterality. an unspecified side code is also provided should the side not be identified in the medical record. If no bilateral code is provided and the condition is bilateral, assign separate codes for both the left and right side.
body part or region (4th character)	Defines the specific anatomical site where the procedure is performed.
body system (2nd character)	Defines the general physiological system on which the procedure is performed or anatomical region where the procedure is performed.
bypass	Altering the route of passage of the contents of a tubular body part.
category	The three-digit diagnosis code classifications that broadly define each condition (e.g., 250 for diabetes mellitus).
Centers for Disease Control and Prevention (CDC)	A federal health data organization that helps maintain several code sets included in the HIPAA standards, including the ICD-9-CM codes. a division of the Department of Health and Human Services responsible for monitoring, researching and developing public health policies for the prevention of disease, injury and disability and the promotion of healthy behaviors. The National Center for Health Statistics is the part of the CDC that maintains health related statistics including the coordination with World Health Organization (WHO) on use of International Classification of Diseases (ICD) in North America.
Centers for Medicare & Medicaid Services (CMS)	The federal agency that runs the Medicare program. in addition, CMS works with the States to run the Medicaid program. CMS works to make sure that the beneficiaries in these programs are able to get high quality healthcare.
change	Taking out or off a device from a body part and putting back an identical or similar device in or on the same body part without cutting or puncturing the skin or a mucous membrane
character	One of the seven components that comprise an ICD-10-PCS procedure code.
chronic conditions	Medical conditions characterized by long duration, frequent recurrence over a long period of time, and/or slow progression over time.
cluster	in a combination entry, one instance where a code is chosen from each of the choice lists in the target system entry, that when combined satisfies the equivalent meaning of the corresponding code in the source system

combination codes — A single code used to classify any of the following: two diagnoses; a diagnosis with an associated secondary process (manifestation); or a diagnosis with an associated complication.

control — Stopping, or attempting to stop, postprocedural bleeding.

Conventions of ICD-10 — The general rules for use of the classification independent of guidelines. These conventions are incorporated within the Index and Tabular of the ICD-10-CM as instructional notes.

creation — Making a new genital structure that does not take over the function of a body part.

crosswalk/mapping — A new test is determined to be similar to an existing test, multiple existing test codes, or a portion of an existing test code. The new test code is then assigned to the related existing local fee schedule amounts and resulting national limitation amount. in some instances, a test may only equate to a portion of a test, and, in those instances, payment at an appropriate percentage of the payment for the existing test is assigned.

Current Procedural Terminology (CPT) Codes — This is the procedural coding system that is currently used in America primarily to report physician professional services. Frequently called "CPT", the Current Procedural Terminology, is a code set, developed in 1966 and maintained by the American Medical Association (AMA), used to describe what healthcare professional services were provided or utilized by healthcare professionals. CPT codes are also known as "Level I" codes. Additional codes to describe use of healthcare facilities and services provided by healthcare professionals are known as "Level II" or "Healthcare Common Procedure Coding System" (HCPCS). Level II codes were developed are maintained by CMS.

destruction — Physical eradication of all or a portion of a body part by the direct use of energy, force or a destructive agent.

detachment — Cutting off all or a portion of the upper or lower extremities.

dilation — Expanding an orifice or the lumen of a tubular body part.

division — Cutting into a body part without draining fluids and/or gases from the body part in order to separate or transect a body part.

drainage — Taking or letting out fluids and/or gases from a body part.

excision — Cutting out or off, without replacement, a portion of a body part.

external (approach) — Procedures performed directly on the skin or mucous membrane and procedures performed indirectly by the application of external force through the skin or mucous membrane.

extirpation — Taking or cutting out solid matter from a body part.

extraction — Pulling or stripping out or off all or a portion of a body part by the use of force.

Federal Register — The "Federal Register" is the official daily publication for rules, proposed rules and notices of federal agencies and organizations, as well as Executive Orders and other Presidential documents.

forward mapping — mapping that proceeds from an older code set to a newer code set, for example from ICD-9-CM Volume 3 to ICD-10-PCS.

fragmentation — Breaking solid matter in a body part into pieces.

GEMs — This reference mapping attempts to include all valid relationships between the codes in the ICD-9-CM diagnosis classification and the ICD-10-CM diagnosis classification.

General Equivalence Map (GEM) — reference mapping that attempts to include all valid relationships between the codes in the ICD-9- CM diagnosis classification and the ICD-10-CM diagnosis classification

Health Insurance Portability & Accountability Act (HIPAA) — A law passed in 1996 which is also sometimes called the "Kassebaum-Kennedy" law. This law expands healthcare coverage for patients who have lost or changed jobs, or have pre-existing conditions. HIPAA does not replace the states' roles as primary regulators of insurance. The HIPAA legislation has the following broad goals, to provide: 1) a way to uniquely identify providers, employers and health plans, 2) a uniform level of protection of health information, known as the "Security Rule," 3) a uniform level of protection of the privacy of health data associated with patients, known as the "Privacy Rule" and 4) a simpler healthcare electronic transaction process by describing standards by which all healthcare administrative entities would use, which is known as the "Transactions and Code Sets Rule".

Healthcare Common Procedure Coding System (HCPCS)

A medical code set that identifies healthcare procedures, equipment, and supplies for claim submission purposes. It has been selected for use in the HIPAA transactions. HCPCS Level I contains numeric CPT codes which are maintained by the AMA. HCPCS Level II contains alphanumeric codes used to identify various items and services that are not included in the CPT medical code set. These are maintained by Health Care Financing Administration (HCFA), Blue Cross and Blue Shield Association (BCBSA), and the Health Insurance Association of America (HIAA). HCPCS Level III contains alphanumeric codes that are assigned by Medicaid state agencies to identify additional items and services not included in levels I or II. These are usually called "local codes", and must have "W", "X", "Y", or "Z" in the first position. HCPCS Procedure Modifier Codes can be used with all three levels, with the WA - ZY range used for locally assigned procedure modifiers.

HIPAA 4010

The original healthcare transactions version of HIPAA (officially known as Version 004010 of the ASC X12 transaction implementation guides) named as part of HIPAA's Electronic Transaction Standards regulation. Version 4010 was required to be used by HIPAA covered healthcare entities by Oct. 16, 2003.

HIPAA 5010

Required by Jan. 1, 2012 to be the new version of the HIPAA healthcare transactions. Officially known as Version 005010 of the ASC X12 transaction Technical Report Type 3. This new version was required as a result of Department of Health and Human Services (HHS) final rules published on Jan. 6, 2009.

ICD-10

The mortality and morbidity classification coding system implemented by WHO in 1993 to replace ICD-9.

ICD-10-CM

The updated version of the clinical modification coding set defined by the National Center for Health Statistics that will replace ICD-9-CM on Oct. 1, 2013.

ICD-10-PCS

The updated procedural coding system defined by CMS that will replace Volume 3 of ICD-9-CM for hospital inpatient services.

ICD-9

The mortality and morbidity classification coding system used prior to ICD-10. Replaced by ICD-10 in October 2015.

ICD-9-CM

The "clinical modification" to the ICD-9 code used prior to ICD-10-CM in America to report medical diagnoses. Replaced by ICD-10 in October 2015.

index (to diseases)

The ICD-10-CM is divided into the Alphabetic Index, an alphabetical list of terms and their corresponding code, and the Tabular List, a chronological list of codes divided into chapters based on body system or condition. The Alphabetic Index consists of the following parts: the Index of Diseases and Injury, the Index of External Causes of Injury, the Table of Neoplasms and the Table of Drugs and Chemicals.

insertion

Putting in a nonbiological device that monitors, assists, performs or prevents a physiological function but does not physically take the place of a body part.

inspection

Visually and/or manually exploring a body part.

International Classification of Diseases (ICD)

A medical code set maintained by the World Health Organization (WHO). The primary purpose of this code set is to classify both causes of death or mortality and diseases or morbidity. A U.S. version, known as ICD-CM, "Clinical Modification," is maintained by the NCHS within the CDC to more precisely define ICD use in the U.S.

manifestation codes

Certain conditions have both an underlying etiology and multiple body system manifestations due to the underlying etiology. for such conditions, the ICD-10-CM has a coding convention that requires the underlying condition be sequenced first followed by the manifestation. Wherever such a combination exists, there is a "use additional code" note at the etiology code, and a "code first" note at the manifestation code. These instructional notes indicate the proper sequencing order of the codes, etiology followed by manifestation.

map

Locating the route of passage of electrical impulses and/or locating functional areas in a body part.

medical necessity	Services or supplies that: are proper and needed for the diagnosis or treatment of a medical condition; are provided for the diagnosis, direct care, and treatment of a medical condition; meet the standards of good medical practice in the local area; and are not mainly for the convenience of the patient or doctor.
morbidity	Term refers to the disease rate or number of cases of a particular disease in a given age range, gender, occupation, or other relevant population based grouping.
mortality	Term refers to the death rate reflected by the population in a given region, age range, or other relevant statistical grouping
National Center for Health Statistics (NCHS)	A federal organization within the CDC that collects, analyzes, and distributes healthcare statistics. The NCHS helps maintain the ICD-CM codes.
No Map Flag	attribute in a GEM that when turned on indicates that a code in the source system is not linked to any code in the target system .
occlusion	Completely closing an orifice or the lumen of a tubular body part.
open (approach)	Cutting through the skin or mucous membrane and any other body layers necessary to expose the site of the procedure.
percutaneous (approach)	Entry, by puncture or minor incision, of instrumentation through the skin or mucous membrane and any other body layers necessary to reach the site of the procedure.
percutaneous endoscopic (approach)	Entry, by puncture or minor incision, of instrumentation through the skin or mucous membrane and any other body layers necessary to reach and visualize the site of the procedure.
principle diagnosis	First-listed/primary diagnosis code. The code sequenced first on a medical record defines the primary reason for the encounter as determined at the end of the encounter.
procedure	The complete specification of the ICD-10-PCS seven characters.
reattachment	Putting back in or on all or a portion of a separated body part to its normal location or other suitable location.
release	Freeing a body part from an abnormal physical constraint by cutting or by use of force.
removal	Taking out or off a device from a body part.
repair	Restoring, to the extent possible, a body part to its normal anatomic structure and function.
replacement	Putting in or on biological or synthetic material that physically takes the place and/or function of all or a portion of a body part.
reposition	Moving to its normal location, or other suitable location, all or a portion of a body part.
resection	Cutting out or off, without replacement, all of a body part.
restriction	Partially closing an orifice or the lumen of a tubular body part.
reverse lookup	using a GEM by looking up a target system code to see all the codes in the source system that translate to it.
revision	Correcting, to the extent possible, a portion of a malfunctioning device or the position of a displaced device.
root operation/type (3rd character)	Defines the objective of the procedure.
section (1st character)	Defines the general type of procedure.
sequelae	A late effect is the residual effect (condition produced) after the acute phase of an illness or injury has terminated. There is no time limit on when a late effect code can be used. The residual may be apparent early, such as in cerebral infarction, or it may occur months or years later, such as that due to a previous injury.
signs/symptoms	Codes that describe symptoms and signs, as opposed to diagnoses, are acceptable for reporting purposes when a related definitive diagnosis has not been established (confirmed) by the provider.
source system	code set of origin in the mapping; the set being mapped 'from'

supplement	Putting in or on biological or synthetic material that physically reinforces and/or augments the function of a portion of a body part
Tabular List	It is essential to use both the Alphabetic Index and Tabular List when locating and assigning a code. The Alphabetic Index does not always provide the full code. Selection of the full code, including laterality and any applicable 7th character can only be done in the Tabular List. a dash (-) at the end of an Alphabetic Index entry indicates that additional characters are required. Even if a dash is not included at the Alphabetic Index entry, it is necessary to refer to the Tabular List to verify that no 7th character is required.
target system	destination code set in the mapping; the set being mapped 'to'.
transfer	Moving, without taking out, all or a portion of a body part to another location to take over the function of all or a portion of a body part.
transplantation	Putting in or on all or a portion of a living body part taken from another individual or animal to physically take the place and/or function of all or a portion of a similar body part.
Uniform Hospital Discharge Data Set (UHDDS)	The UHDDS definitions are used by hospitals to report inpatient data elements in a standardized manner. These data elements and their definitions can be found in the July 31, 1985, Federal Register (Vol. 50, No, 147), pp. 31038-40.
value	Individual units defined for each character of ICD-10-PCS and represented by a number or letter.
via natural or artificial opening (approach)	Entry of instrumentation through a natural or artificial external opening to reach the site of the procedure.
via natural or artificial opening endoscopic (approach)	Entry of instrumentation through a natural or artificial external opening to reach and visualize the site of the procedure.
via natural or artificial opening with percutaneous endoscopic assistance (approach)	Entry of instrumentation through a natural or artificial external opening and entry, by puncture or minor incision, of instrumentation through the skin or mucous membrane and any other body layers necessary to aid in the performance of the procedure.
Volume I	The detailed, tabular list of diagnosis codes in the ICD-9-CM manual.
Volume II	The alphabetical index to diseases in the ICD-9-CM diagnosis coding manual.
Volume III	The ICD-9/ICD-10 list of procedure codes, used in inpatient settings.
World Health Organization (WHO)	An organization that maintains the International Classification of Diseases (ICD) medical code set.

ICD-10-CM OVERVIEW

WHAT IS ICD-10-CM?

ICD-10-CM is an acronym for ***International Classification of Diseases, 10th Revision, Clinical Modification***, published under different names since 1900. ICD-10-CM is a statistical classification system that arranges diseases and injuries into groups according to established criteria. Most ICD-9-CM codes are numeric and consist of three seven digits and a description. The codes are revised approximately every 10 years by the World Health Organization and annual updates are published by Center for Medicare and Medicaid Services (CMS).

ICD-10-CM is the United States' clinical modification of the World Health Organization's ICD-10. The term "clinical" is used to emphasize the modification's intent: to serve as a useful tool in the area of classification of morbidity data for indexing of health records, medical care review, and ambulatory and other health care programs, as well as for basic health statistics. To describe the clinical picture of the patient the codes must be more precise than those needed only for statistical groupings and trend analysis.

ICD-10-CM far exceeds its predecessors in the number of concepts and codes provided. The disease classification has been expanded to include health-related conditions and to provide greater specificity at the sixth and seventh character level. The sixth and seventh characters are not optional and are intended for use in recording the information documented in the clinical record.

KEY POINTS REGARDING ICD-10-CM

1. ICD-10-CM codes are three (3) to seven (7) digit alphanumeric codes.

2. ICD-10-CM codes describe illnesses, injuries, signs and symptoms, and procedures.

3. ICD-10-CM codes must be used on all health insurance claims as of October 1, 2014 (subject to extension by CMS).

4. Most ICD-10-CM codes have a specific definition; however, some ICD-10-CM codes have more than one definition.

5. Correct ICD-10-CM coding can make a significant difference in your reimbursement.

6. Accurate ICD-10-CM coding puts you in control of the reimbursement process.

STRUCTURE OF AN ICD-10-CM CODE

S32.010A   Wedge compression fracture of first lumbar vertebra, initial encounter for closed fracture

Letter	Number or Letter					
1ST Digit	2nd Digit	3rd Digit	4th Digit	5th Digit	6th Digit	7th Digit
S	**3**	**2 .**	**0**	**1**	**0**	**A**
Category			Etiology, anatomic site, severity			Added code extensions for obstetrics, injuries and external causes of injury

ITEM	DESCRIPTION
Length:	ICD-10-CM codes are from 3-7 digits
First character Error! Bookmark not defined.**:**	The first character of all ICD-10-CM codes is a Letter only (all letters except U are used)
Character 2:	The second character of all ICD-10-CM codes is a Number only
Characters 3-7:	The 3rd through 7th characters of an ICD-10-CM codes may be Numbers or letter
Decimal:	The decimal for all ICD-10-CM codes occurs after the 3rd character**Error! Bookmark not defined.**
Placeholder:	In cases where a 7th digit is required on an ICD-10-CM codes of less than 6 digits, the character "X" is used as a dummy placeholder
Letter format:	Letters are case-sensitive

SIMILARITY OF ICD-10-CM TO ICD-9-CM

While there are more codes in the ICD-10-CM coding system than the ICD-9-CM coding system and the coding is a bit more complex, there are many similarities between the two systems. Experienced coders should be able to use the ICD-10-CM system relatively quickly due in part to these similarities.

1. Format – Both ICD-10-CM and ICD-9-CM have a Tabular List and Index.

2. Chapters in the ICD-10-CM Tabular list are structured similarly to ICD-9-CM, with minor exceptions.

   - A few chapters have been restructured
   - Sense organs (eye and ear) separated from Nervous System chapter and moved to their own Chapters

3. Index of ICD-10-CM is structured the same as ICD-9-CM.

- Alphabetic Index of Diseases and Injuries
- Alphabetic Index of External Causes
- Table of Neoplasms
- Table of Drugs and Chemicals

4. Divided into Alphabetic Index and Tabular List.

    - Structure and format are the same
    - Index is alphabetical list of terms and their corresponding codes

5. Alphabetic Index lists main terms in alphabetical order with indented subterms under main terms.

6. The Alphabetic Index is divided into 2 parts: Index to Diseases and Injuries and Index to External Causes.

7. The Tabular List is a chronological list of codes divided into chapters based on body system or condition.

8. The Tabular List is presented in code number order.
9. ICD-10-CM and ICD-9-CM have the same hierarchical structure.

10. Codes are invalid in both ICD-10-CM and ICD-9-CM if they are missing an applicable character.

11. ICD-10-CM and ICD-9-CM codes are looked up the same way.

    - Look up diagnostic terms in Alphabetic Index
    - Then verify code number in Tabular List

12. Many conventions have same meaning in ICD-10-CM and ICD-9-CM.

    - Abbreviations, punctuation, symbols, notes such as "code first" and "use additional code"

13. Nonspecific codes ("unspecified" or "not otherwise specified") are available to use when detailed documentation to support more specific code is not available.

14. ICD-10-CM Official Guidelines for Coding and Reporting accompany and complement ICD-10-CM conventions and instructions.

15. Adherence to the official coding guidelines in all healthcare settings is required under the Health Insurance Portability and Accountability Act.

DIFFERENCES BETWEEN ICD-10-CM AND ICD-9-CM

While there are more similarities than differences between the ICD-10-CM and ICD-9-CM, the differences are significant. Understanding the differences will be the key to a successful transition to the new coding system.

1. All ICD-10-CM codes are alphanumeric (letter and numbers).

    - 1st character is always alpha and alpha characters may appear elsewhere in the code as well

2. ICD-10-CM codes can be up to 7 characters in length.

3. ICD-10-CM codes are more specific than ICD-9-CM codes.

4. ICD-10-CM code titles are more complete (no need to refer back to a category, subcategory, or subclassification level to determine complete meaning of code).

5. Laterality (side of the body affected) has been added to relevant ICD-10-CM codes.

6. ICD-10-CM features an expanded use of combination codes.

   - Certain conditions and associated common symptoms or manifestations
   - Poisonings and associated external cause

7. Injuries grouped by anatomical site rather than type of injury.

8. Codes reflect modern medicine and updated medical terminology.

9. Addition of 7th character

   - Used in certain chapters to provide information about the characteristic of the encounter
   - Must always be used in the 7th character position
   - If a code has an applicable 7th character, the code must be reported with an appropriate 7th character value in order to be valid

   Valid 7th Digit Character for Injuries and External Causes

   A   Initial encounter
   D   Subsequent encounter S Sequela

   Note: for aftercare of an injury, assign acute injury code with 7th character "D"

   Valid 7th Digit Character for Fractures

   A   Initial encounter for closed fracture

   B   Initial encounter for open fracture

   D   Subsequent encounter for fracture with routine healing

   G   Subsequent encounter for fracture with delayed healing

   K   Subsequent encounter for fracture with nonunion

   P   Subsequent encounter for fracture with malunion

   S   Sequela

10. Addition of dummy placeholder "X" is used in certain codes to:

    - Allow for future expansion
    - Fill out empty characters when a code contains fewer than 6 characters and a 7th character applies

    When placeholder character applies, it must be used in order for the code to be considered valid.

11. ICD-10-CM includes two types of Excludes Notes.

    - **Excludes 1 Note**

      Indicates that code identified in the note and code where the note appears cannot be reported together because the 2 conditions cannot occur together.

      Examples:

      E10   Type 1 Diabetes mellitus

            diabetes mellitus due to underlying condition (E08.-)

drug or chemical induced diabetes mellitus (E09.-)
gestational diabetes (O24.4-)
hyperglycemia NOS (R73.9)
neonatal diabetes mellitus (P70.2)
type 2 diabetes mellitus (E11.-)

M21   Other acquired deformities of limbs

acquired absence of limb (Z89.-)
congenital absence of limbs (Q71-Q73)

- **Excludes 2 Note**

  Indicates that condition identified in the note is not part of the condition represented by the code where the note appears, so both codes may be reported together if the patient has both conditions.

  Examples:

  L89   Pressure ulcer

  diabetic ulcers (E08.621, E08.622, E09.621, E09.622, E10.621, E10.622, E11.621, E11.622, E13.621, E13.622)
  non-pressure chronic ulcer of skin (L97.-)
  skin infections (L00-L08)
  varicose ulcer (I83.0, I83.2)

  I70.2   Atherosclerosis of native arteries of the extremities
  atherosclerosis of bypass graft of extremities (I70.30-I70.79)

12. ICD-10-CM provides for increased specificity in comparison to ICD-9-CM.

    Examples

    S72.044G   Nondisplaced fracture of base of neck of right femur, subsequent encounter for closed fracture with delayed healing

    I69.351   Sequelae of cerebral infarction, Hemiplegia and hemiparesis following cerebral infarction affecting right dominant side

    Z47.81   Encounter for orthopedic aftercare following surgical amputation

    Z48.21   Encounter for aftercare following heart transplant

13. ICD-10-CM provides specific codes to identify laterality, i.e. left, right, unspecified. This applies to extremities as well as many organ systems; i.e. eyes, ears, shoulders, arms, hands, hips, legs, feet, lungs, kidneys, ovaries, testicles, etc.

    Examples

    C50.511   Malignant neoplasm of lower-outer quadrant of <u>right</u> female breast

    C50.512   Malignant neoplasm of lower-outer quadrant of <u>left</u> female breast

    C50.519   Malignant neoplasm of lower-outer quadrant of <u>unspecified</u> female breast

FORMAT OF ICD-10-CM

The Tabular List (Volume 1)

The ICD-10-CM Tabular List contains categories, subcategories and codes. Characters for categories, subcategories and codes may be either a letter or a number. All categories are 3 characters. a three-character category that has no further subdivision is equivalent to a code. Subcategories are either 4 or 5 characters. Codes may be 3, 4, 5, 6 or 7 characters. That is, each level of subdivision after a category is a subcategory. The final level of subdivision is a code. Codes that have applicable 7th characters are still referred to as codes, not subcategories. a code that has an applicable 7th character is considered invalid without the 7th character.

The Alphabetic Index (Volume 2)

The Alphabetic Index consists of the following parts: the Index of Diseases and Injury, the Index of External Causes of Injury, the Table of Neoplasms and the Table of Drugs and Chemicals.

CONVENTIONS USED IN THE TABULAR LIST

The ICD-10-CM Tabular List (Volume 1) makes use of certain abbreviations, punctuation, symbols, and other conventions that must be clearly understood. The purpose of these conventions is to provide special coding instructions and conserve space. Most of the conventions are defined in the ICD-10-CM Official Guidelines to Coding and Reporting following this chapter. There are sym

SYMBOLS AND COLOR CODING

All PMIC versions of ICD-10-CM include color-coding to alert the user to special coding situations or conditions that require additional attention. The use of color-coding is found in the Tabular List (Volume 1). The color is applied as solid rectangular bars over the codes only so that the descriptions remain clear and legible. The color codes and definitions are printed at the bottom of all right-sided pages of the Tabular List (Volume 1)

Color Coding

Three digit code that requires the addition of 4th – 7th digits. Coding to higher level of specificity is required.

Unspecified code. Descriptions include the term "unspecified." Use only if a more specific diagnosis is not known or available.

Nonspecific code. Descriptions include the term "nonspecific, unspecified, other specified or other." A report *may* be required by insurance carriers.

Manifestation codes. Used only to code the manifestation of an underlying disease. Code the underlying disease first.

Symbols

- A filled BLACK CIRCLE preceding a code indicates that the code is new to this revision of ICD-9-CM. A symbol key appears on all left-hand pages of the Tabular List, Volume 1.

- ▲ A filled BLACK TRIANGLE preceding a code indicates that there is a revision to the text of an existing code. A symbol key appears on all left-hand pages of the Tabular List, Volume 1.

- ⑦ A red circle containing the number 7 preceding a code indicates that a seventh digit is required for coding to the highest level of specificity. The appropriate 7th character is to be added to each code from category. Definitions of valid seventh digits are found under the major category. If a code that requires a 7th character is not 6 characters, a placeholder X must be used to fill in the empty characters.

- ⊗ A red circle containing the letter P preceding a code indicates that a placeholder character "X" is required for the code to be complete. An example of this is at the poisoning, adverse effect and underdosing codes, categories T36-T50. Where a place holder exists, the X must be used in order for the code to be considered a valid code.

Sex Specific Diagnosis Codes

Some ICD-10-CM codes apply only to female or male patients. Some ICD-10-CM codes include the word "male" or "female" in the diagnosis description, while others are known to apply to female or male because of sex specific terms such as ovary, vagina, prostate, testes, etc. For chapters or sections where all of the diagnosis codes are sex specific, the following alerts appear at the beginning of the section:

> **NOTE: ALL DIAGNOSIS CODES IN THIS SECTION APPLY TO FEMALE PATIENTS ONLY**

> **NOTE: ALL DIAGNOSIS CODES IN THIS SECTION APPLY TO MALE PATIENTS ONLY**

Age Specific Diagnosis Codes

Some ICD-10-CM codes apply to patients of general age ranges. These codes are identified by the inclusion of the following terms within the diagnosis description: "adult", "child", "infant", "juvenile", or "newborn".

ICD-10-CM Official Guidelines for Coding and Reporting

NOTE: The following ICD-10-CM Official Guidelines for Coding and Reporting are from the official August 9, 2017 Final Version release from the National Center for Health Statistics (NCHS) dated August 9, 2017. Changes are highlighted in red.

The Centers for Medicare and Medicaid Services (CMS) and the National Center for Health Statistics (NCHS), two departments within the U.S. Federal Government's Department of Health and Human Services (DHHS) provide the following guidelines for coding and reporting using the International Classification of Diseases, 10th Revision, Clinical Modification (ICD-10-CM). These guidelines should be used as a companion document to the official version of the ICD-10-CM as published on the NCHS website. The ICD-10-CM is a morbidity classification published by the United States for classifying diagnoses and reason for visits in all health care settings. The ICD-10-CM is based on the ICD-10, the statistical classification of disease published by the World Health Organization (WHO).

These guidelines have been approved by the four organizations that make up the Cooperating Parties for the ICD-10-CM: the American Hospital Association (AHA), the American Health Information Management Association (AHIMA), CMS, and NCHS.

These guidelines are a set of rules that have been developed to accompany and complement the official conventions and instructions provided within the ICD-10-CM itself. The instructions and conventions of the classification take precedence over guidelines. These guidelines are based on the coding and sequencing instructions in the Tabular List and Alphabetic Index of ICD-10-CM, but provide additional instruction. Adherence to these guidelines when assigning ICD-10-CM diagnosis codes is required under the Health Insurance Portability and Accountability Act (HIPAA). The diagnosis codes (Tabular List and Alphabetic Index) have been adopted under HIPAA for all healthcare settings. A joint effort between the healthcare provider and the coder is essential to achieve complete and accurate documentation, code assignment, and reporting of diagnoses and procedures. These guidelines have been developed to assist both the healthcare provider and the coder in identifying those diagnoses that are to be reported. The importance of consistent, complete documentation in the medical record cannot be overemphasized. Without such documentation accurate coding cannot be achieved. The entire record should be reviewed to determine the specific reason for the encounter and the conditions treated.

The term encounter is used for all settings, including hospital admissions. In the context of these guidelines, the term provider is used throughout the guidelines to mean physician or any qualified health care practitioner who is legally accountable for establishing the patient's diagnosis. Only this set of guidelines, approved by the Cooperating Parties, is official.

The guidelines are organized into sections. Section I includes the structure and conventions of the classification and general guidelines that apply to the entire classification, and chapter-specific guidelines that correspond to the chapters as they are arranged in the classification. Section II includes guidelines for selection of principal diagnosis for non-outpatient settings. Section III includes guidelines for reporting additional diagnoses in non-outpatient settings. Section IV is for outpatient coding and reporting. It is necessary to review all sections of the guidelines to fully understand all of the rules and instructions needed to code properly.

SECTION I. CONVENTIONS, GENERAL CODING GUIDELINES AND CHAPTER SPECIFIC GUIDELINES

The conventions, general guidelines and chapter-specific guidelines are applicable to all health care settings unless otherwise indicated. The conventions and instructions of the classification take precedence over guidelines.

A. Conventions for the ICD-10-CM

The conventions for the ICD-10-CM are the general rules for use of the classification independent of the guidelines. These conventions are incorporated within the Alphabetic Index and Tabular List of the ICD-10-CM as instructional notes.

1. The Alphabetic Index and Tabular List

The ICD-10-CM is divided into the Alphabetic Index, an alphabetical list of terms and their corresponding code, and the Tabular List, a structured list of codes divided into chapters based on body system or condition. The Alphabetic Index consists of the following parts: the Index of Diseases and Injury, the Index of External Causes of Injury, the Table of Neoplasms and the Table of Drugs and Chemicals.
See Section I.C2. General guidelines

See Section I.C.19. Adverse effects, poisoning, underdosing and toxic effects

2. Format and Structure:

The ICD-10-CM Tabular List contains categories, subcategories and codes. Characters for categories, subcategories and codes may be either a letter or a number. All categories are 3 characters. A three-character category that has no further subdivision is equivalent to a code. Subcategories are either 4 or 5 characters. Codes may be 3, 4, 5, 6 or 7 characters. That is, each level of subdivision after a category is a subcategory. The final level of subdivision is a code. Codes that have applicable 7th characters are still referred to as codes, not subcategories. A code that has an applicable 7th character is considered invalid without the 7th character.

The ICD-10-CM uses an indented format for ease in reference.

3. Use of codes for reporting purposes

For reporting purposes only codes are permissible, not categories or subcategories, and any applicable 7th character is required.

4. Placeholder character

The ICD-10-CM utilizes a placeholder character "X". The "X" is used as a placeholder at certain codes to allow for future expansion. An example of this is at the poisoning, adverse effect and underdosing codes, categories T36-T50.

Where a placeholder exists, the X must be used in order for the code to be considered a valid code.

5. 7th Characters

Certain ICD-10-CM categories have applicable 7th characters. The applicable 7th character is required for all codes within the category, or as the notes in the Tabular List instruct. The 7th character must always be the 7th character in the data field. If a code that requires a 7th character is not 6 characters, a placeholder X must be used to fill in the empty characters.

6. Abbreviations

a. Alphabetic Index abbreviations

NEC "Not elsewhere classifiable"

This abbreviation in the Alphabetic Index represents "other specified." When a specific code is not available for a condition, the Alphabetic Index directs the coder to the "other specified" code in the Tabular List.

NOS "Not otherwise specified"

This abbreviation is the equivalent of unspecified.

b. Tabular List abbreviations

NEC "Not elsewhere classifiable"

This abbreviation in the Tabular List represents "other specified". When a specific code is not available for a condition, the Tabular List includes an NEC entry under a code to identify the code as the "other specified" code.
NOS "Not otherwise specified"

This abbreviation is the equivalent of unspecified.

7. Punctuation

[ ] Brackets are used in the Tabular List to enclose synonyms, alternative wording or explanatory phrases. Brackets are used in the Alphabetic Index to identify manifestation codes.

( )   Parentheses are used in both the Alphabetic Index and Tabular List to enclose supplementary words that may be present or absent in the statement of a disease or procedure without affecting the code number to which it is assigned. The terms within the parentheses are referred to as nonessential modifiers. The nonessential modifiers in the Alphabetic Index to Diseases apply to subterms following a main term except when a nonessential modifier and a subentry are mutually exclusive, the subentry takes precedence. For example, in the ICD-10-CM Alphabetic Index under the main term Enteritis, "acute" is a nonessential modifier and "chronic" is a subentry. In this case, the nonessential modifier "acute" does not apply to the subentry "chronic".

:   Colons are used in the Tabular List after an incomplete term which needs one or more of the modifiers following the colon to make it assignable to a given category.

8. Use of "and".

See Section I.A.14. Use of the term "And"

9. Other and Unspecified codes

a. "Other" codes

Codes titled "other" or "other specified" are for use when the information in the medical record provides detail for which a specific code does not exist. Alphabetic Index entries with NEC in the line designate "other" codes in the Tabular List. These Alphabetic Index entries represent specific disease entities for which no specific code exists so the term is included within an "other" code.

b. "Unspecified" codes

Codes titled "unspecified" are for use when the information in the medical record is insufficient to assign a more specific code. For those categories for which an unspecified code is not provided, the "other specified" code may represent both other and unspecified.

See Section I.B.18 Use of Signs/Symptom/Unspecified Codes

10. Includes Notes

This note appears immediately under a three character code title to further define, or give examples of, the content of the category.

11. Inclusion terms

List of terms is included under some codes. These terms are the conditions for which that code is to be used. The terms may be synonyms of the code title, or, in the case of "other specified" codes, the terms are a list of the various conditions assigned to that code. The inclusion terms are not necessarily exhaustive. Additional terms found only in the Alphabetic Index may also be assigned to a code.

12. Excludes Notes

The ICD-10-CM has two types of excludes notes. Each type of note has a different definition for use but they are all similar in that they indicate that codes excluded from each other are independent of each other.

a. Excludes1

A type 1 Excludes note is a pure excludes note. It means "NOT CODED HERE!" An Excludes1 note indicates that the code excluded should never be used at the same time as the code above the Excludes1 note. An Excludes1 is used when two conditions cannot occur together, such as a congenital form versus an acquired form of the same condition.

An exception to the Excludes1 definition is the circumstance when the two conditions are unrelated to each other. If it is not clear whether the two conditions involving an Excludes1 note are related or not, query the provider. For example, code F45.8, Other somatoform disorders, has an Excludes1 note for "sleep related teeth grinding (G47.63)," because "teeth grinding" is an inclusion term under F45.8.

Only one of these two codes should be assigned for teeth grinding. However psychogenic dysmenorrhea is also an inclusion term under F45.8, and a patient could have both this condition and sleep related teeth grinding. In this case, the two conditions are clearly unrelated to each other, and so it would be appropriate to report F45.8 and G47.63 together.

b. Excludes2

A type 2 Excludes note represents "Not included here." An excludes2 note indicates that the condition excluded is not part of the condition represented by the code, but a patient may have both conditions at the same time. When an Excludes2 note appears under a code, it is acceptable to use both the code and the excluded code together, when appropriate.

13. Etiology/manifestation convention ("code first", "use additional code" and "in diseases classified elsewhere" notes)

Certain conditions have both an underlying etiology and multiple body system manifestations due to the underlying etiology. For such conditions, the ICD-10-CM has a coding convention that requires the underlying condition be sequenced first, **if** applicable, followed by the manifestation. Wherever such a combination exists, there is a "use additional code" note at the etiology code, and a "code first" note at the manifestation code. These instructional notes indicate the proper sequencing order of the codes, etiology followed by manifestation.

In most cases the manifestation codes will have in the code title, "in diseases classified elsewhere." Codes with this title are a component of the etiology/ manifestation convention. The code title indicates that it is a manifestation code. "In diseases classified elsewhere" codes are never permitted to be used as first-listed or principal diagnosis codes. They must be used in conjunction with an underlying condition code and they must be listed following the underlying condition. See category F02, Dementia in other diseases classified elsewhere, for an example of this convention.

There are manifestation codes that do not have "in diseases classified elsewhere" in the title. For such codes, there is a "use additional code" note at the etiology code and a "code first" note at the manifestation code, and the rules for sequencing apply.

In addition to the notes in the Tabular List, these conditions also have a specific Alphabetic Index entry structure. In the Alphabetic Index both conditions are listed together with the etiology code first followed by the manifestation codes in brackets. The code in brackets is always to be sequenced second.

An example of the etiology/manifestation convention is dementia in Parkinson's disease. In the Alphabetic Index, code G20 is listed first, followed by code F02.80 or F02.81 in brackets. Code G20 represents the underlying etiology, Parkinson's disease, and must be sequenced first, whereas codes F02.80 and F02.81 represent the manifestation of dementia in diseases classified elsewhere, with or without behavioral disturbance.

"Code first" and "Use additional code" notes are also used as sequencing rules in the classification for certain codes that are not part of an etiology/ manifestation combination.

See Section I.B.7. Multiple coding for a single condition.

14. "And"

The word "and" should be interpreted to mean either "and" or "or" when it appears in a title.

For example, cases of "tuberculosis of bones", "tuberculosis of joints" and "tuberculosis of bones and joints" are classified to subcategory A18.0, Tuberculosis of bones and joints.

15. "With"

The word "with" should be interpreted to mean "associated with" or "due to" when it appears in a code title, the Alphabetic Index, or an instructional note in the Tabular List. The classification presumes a causal relationship between the two conditions linked by these terms in the Alphabetic Index or Tabular List.

These conditions should be coded as related even in the absence of provider documentation explicitly linking them, unless the documentation clearly states the conditions are unrelated or when another guideline exists that specifically requires a documented linkage between two conditions (e.g., sepsis guideline for "acute organ dysfunction that is not clearly associated with the sepsis").

For conditions not specifically linked by these relational terms in the classification or when a guideline requires that a linkage between two conditions be explicitly documented, provider documentation must link the conditions in order to code them as related.

The word "with" in the Alphabetic Index is sequenced immediately following the main term, not in alphabetical order.

16. "See" and "See Also"

The "see" instruction following a main term in the Alphabetic Index indicates that another term should be referenced. It is necessary to go to the main term referenced with the "see" note to locate the correct code.

A "see also" instruction following a main term in the Alphabetic Index instructs that there is another main term that may also be referenced that may provide additional Alphabetic Index entries that may be useful. It is not necessary to follow the "see also" note when the original main term provides the necessary code.

17. "Code also" note

A "code also" note instructs that two codes may be required to fully describe a condition, but this note does not provide sequencing direction. The sequencing depends on the circumstances of the encounter.

18. Default codes

A code listed next to a main term in the ICD-10-CM Alphabetic Index is referred to as a default code. The default code represents that condition that is most commonly associated with the main term, or is the unspecified code for the condition. If a condition is documented in a medical record (for example, appendicitis) without any additional information, such as acute or chronic, the default code should be assigned.

19. Code assignment and Clinical Criteria

The assignment of a diagnosis code is based on the provider's diagnostic statement that the condition exists. The provider's statement that the patient has a particular condition is sufficient. Code assignment is not based on clinical criteria used by the provider to establish the diagnosis.

B. General Coding Guidelines

1. Locating a code in the ICD-10-CM

To select a code in the classification that corresponds to a diagnosis or reason for visit documented in a medical record, first locate the term in the Alphabetic Index, and then verify the code in the Tabular List. Read and be guided by instructional notations that appear in both the Alphabetic Index and the Tabular List.

It is essential to use both the Alphabetic Index and Tabular List when locating and assigning a code. The Alphabetic Index does not always provide the full code. Selection of the full code, including laterality and any applicable 7th character can only be done in the Tabular List. A dash (-) at the end of an Alphabetic Index entry indicates that additional characters are required. Even if a dash is not included at the Alphabetic Index entry, it is necessary to refer to the Tabular List to verify that no 7th character is required.

2. **Level of Detail in Coding**

   Diagnosis codes are to be used and reported at their highest number of characters available.

   ICD-10-CM diagnosis codes are composed of codes with 3, 4, 5, 6 or 7 characters. Codes with three characters are included in ICD-10-CM as the heading of a category of codes that may be further subdivided by the use of fourth and/or fifth characters and/or sixth characters, which provide greater detail.

   A three-character code is to be used only if it is not further subdivided. A code is invalid if it has not been coded to the full number of characters required for that code, including the 7th character, if applicable.

3. **Code or codes from A00.0 through T88.9, Z00-Z99.8**

   The appropriate code or codes from A00.0 through T88.9, Z00-Z99.8 must be used to identify diagnoses, symptoms, conditions, problems, complaints or other reason(s) for the encounter/visit.

4. **Signs and symptoms**

   Codes that describe symptoms and signs, as opposed to diagnoses, are acceptable for reporting purposes when a related definitive diagnosis has not been established (confirmed) by the provider. Chapter 18 of ICD-10-CM, Symptoms, Signs, and Abnormal Clinical and Laboratory Findings, Not Elsewhere Classified (codes R00.0 - R99) contains many, but not all, codes for symptoms.

   See Section I.B.18 Use of Signs/Symptom/Unspecified Codes

5. **Conditions that are an integral part of a disease process**

   Signs and symptoms that are associated routinely with a disease process should not be assigned as additional codes, unless otherwise instructed by the classification.

6. **Conditions that are not an integral part of a disease process**

   Additional signs and symptoms that may not be associated routinely with a disease process should be coded when present.

7. **Multiple coding for a single condition**

   In addition to the etiology/manifestation convention that requires two codes to fully describe a single condition that affects multiple body systems, there are other single conditions that also require more than one code. "Use additional code" notes are found in the Tabular List at codes that are not part of an etiology/manifestation pair where a secondary code is useful to fully describe a condition. The sequencing rule is the same as the etiology/manifestation pair, "use additional code" indicates that a secondary code should be added, if known.

   For example, for bacterial infections that are not included in chapter 1, a secondary code from category B95, Streptococcus, Staphylococcus, and Enterococcus, as the cause of diseases classified elsewhere, or B96, Other bacterial agents as the cause of diseases classified elsewhere, may be required to identify the bacterial organism causing the infection. A "use additional code" note will normally be found at the infectious disease code, indicating a need for the organism code to be added as a secondary code.

   "Code first" notes are also under certain codes that are not specifically manifestation codes but may be due to an underlying cause. When there is a "code first" note and an underlying condition is present, the underlying condition should be sequenced first, if known.

   "Code, if applicable, any causal condition first" notes indicate that this code may be assigned as a principal diagnosis when the causal condition is unknown or not applicable. If a causal condition is known, then the code for that condition should be sequenced as the principal or first-listed diagnosis.

   Multiple codes may be needed for sequela, complication codes and obstetric codes to more fully describe a condition. See the specific guidelines for these conditions for further instruction.

8. **Acute and Chronic Conditions**

    If the same condition is described as both acute (subacute) and chronic, and separate subentries exist in the Alphabetic Index at the same indentation level, code both and sequence the acute (subacute) code first.

9. **Combination Code**

    A combination code is a single code used to classify: Two diagnoses, or

    A diagnosis with an associated secondary process (manifestation) A diagnosis with an associated complication

    Combination codes are identified by referring to subterm entries in the Alphabetic Index and by reading the inclusion and exclusion notes in the Tabular List.

    Assign only the combination code when that code fully identifies the diagnostic conditions involved or when the Alphabetic Index so directs. Multiple coding should not be used when the classification provides a combination code that clearly identifies all of the elements documented in the diagnosis. When the combination code lacks necessary specificity in describing the manifestation or complication, an additional code should be used as a secondary code.

10. **Sequela (Late Effects)**

    A sequela is the residual effect (condition produced) after the acute phase of an illness or injury has terminated. There is no time limit on when a sequela code can be used. The residual may be apparent early, such as in cerebral infarction, or it may occur months or years later, such as that due to a previous injury. Examples of sequela include: scar formation resulting from a burn, deviated septum due to a nasal fracture, and infertility due to tubal occlusion from old tuberculosis. Coding of sequela generally requires two codes sequenced in the following order: the condition or nature of the sequela is sequenced first. The sequela code is sequenced second.

    An exception to the above guidelines are those instances where the code for the sequela is followed by a manifestation code identified in the Tabular List and title, or the sequela code has been expanded (at the fourth, fifth or sixth character levels) to include the manifestation(s). The code for the acute phase of an illness or injury that led to the sequela is never used with a code for the late effect.

    See Section I.C.9. Sequelae of cerebrovascular disease
    See Section I.C.15. Sequelae of complication of pregnancy, childbirth and the puerperium
    See Section I.C.19. Application of 7th characters for Chapter 19

11. **Impending or Threatened Condition**

    Code any condition described at the time of discharge as "impending" or "threatened" as follows:

    If it did occur, code as confirmed diagnosis.

    If it did not occur, reference the Alphabetic Index to determine if the condition has a subentry term for "impending" or "threatened" and also reference main term entries for "Impending" and for "Threatened."
    If the subterms are listed, assign the given code.

    If the subterms are not listed, code the existing underlying condition(s) and not the condition described as impending or threatened.

12. **Reporting Same Diagnosis Code More than Once**

    Each unique ICD-10-CM diagnosis code may be reported only once for an encounter. This applies to bilateral conditions when there are no distinct codes identifying laterality or two different conditions classified to the same ICD-10-CM diagnosis code.

13. Laterality

Some ICD-10-CM codes indicate laterality, specifying whether the condition occurs on the left, right or is bilateral. If no bilateral code is provided and the condition is bilateral, assign separate codes for both the left and right side. If the side is not identified in the medical record, assign the code for the unspecified side.
When a patient has a bilateral condition and each side is treated during separate encounters, assign the "bilateral" code (as the condition still exists on both sides), including for the encounter to treat the first side.

For the second encounter for treatment after one side has previously been treated and the condition no longer exists on that side, assign the appropriate unilateral code for the side where the condition still exists (e.g., cataract surgery performed on each eye in separate encounters). The bilateral code would not be assigned for the subsequent encounter, as the patient no longer has the condition in the previously-treated site. If the treatment on the first side did not completely resolve the condition, then the bilateral code would still be appropriate.

14. Documentation for BMI, *Depth of* Non-pressure ulcers, Pressure Ulcer Stages, Coma Scale, *and NIH Stroke Scale*

For the Body Mass Index (BMI), depth of non-pressure chronic ulcers, pressure ulcer stage, coma scale, and NIH stroke scale (NIHSS) codes, code assignment may be based on medical record documentation from clinicians who are not the patient's provider (i.e., physician or other qualified healthcare practitioner legally accountable for establishing the patient's diagnosis), since this information is typically documented by other clinicians involved in the care of the patient (e.g., a dietitian often documents the BMI, a nurse often documents the pressure ulcer stages, and an emergency medical technician often documents the coma scale). However, the associated diagnosis (such as overweight, obesity, acute stroke, or pressure ulcer) must be documented by the patient's provider. If there is conflicting medical record documentation, either from the same clinician or different clinicians, the patient's attending provider should be queried for clarification.

The BMI, coma scale, and NIHSS codes should only be reported as secondary diagnoses.

15. Syndromes

Follow the Alphabetic Index guidance when coding syndromes. In the absence of Alphabetic Index guidance, assign codes for the documented manifestations of the syndrome. Additional codes for manifestations that are not an integral part of the disease process may also be assigned when the condition does not have a unique code.

16. Documentation of Complications of Care

Code assignment is based on the provider's documentation of the relationship between the condition and the care or procedure, unless otherwise instructed by the classification. The guideline extends to any complications of care, regardless of the chapter the code is located in. It is important to note that not all conditions that occur during or following medical care or surgery are classified as complications. There must be a cause-and-effect relationship between the care provided and the condition, and an indication in the documentation that it is a complication. Query the provider for clarification, if the complication is not clearly documented.

17. Borderline Diagnosis

If the provider documents a "borderline" diagnosis at the time of discharge, the diagnosis is coded as confirmed, unless the classification provides a specific entry (e.g., borderline diabetes). If a borderline condition has a specific index entry in ICD-10-CM, it should be coded as such. Since borderline conditions are not uncertain diagnoses, no distinction is made between the care setting (inpatient versus outpatient). Whenever the documentation is unclear regarding a borderline condition, coders are encouraged to query for clarification.

18. Use of Sign/Symptom/Unspecified Codes

Sign/symptom and "unspecified" codes have acceptable, even necessary, uses. While specific diagnosis codes should be reported when they are supported by the available medical record documentation and clinical knowledge of the patient's health condition, there are instances when signs/symptoms or unspecified codes are the best choices for accurately reflecting the healthcare encounter. Each healthcare encounter should be coded to the level of certainty known for that encounter.

If a definitive diagnosis has not been established by the end of the encounter, it is appropriate to report codes for sign(s) and/or symptom(s) in lieu of a definitive diagnosis. When sufficient clinical information isn't known or available about a particular health condition to assign a more specific code, it is acceptable to report the appropriate "unspecified" code (e.g., a diagnosis of pneumonia has been determined, but not the specific type). Unspecified codes should be reported when they are the codes that most accurately reflect what is known about the patient's condition at the time of that particular encounter. It would be inappropriate to select a specific code that is not supported by the medical record documentation or conduct medically unnecessary diagnostic testing in order to determine a more specific code.

C. Chapter-Specific Coding Guidelines

In addition to general coding guidelines, there are guidelines for specific diagnoses and/or conditions in the classification. Unless otherwise indicated, these guidelines apply to all health care settings. Please refer to Section II for guidelines on the selection of principal diagnosis.

1. **Chapter 1: Certain Infectious and Parasitic Diseases (A00-B99)**

   a. **Human Immunodeficiency Virus (HIV) Infections**

      1) **Code only confirmed cases**

         Code only confirmed cases of HIV infection/illness. This is an exception to the hospital inpatient guideline Section II, H.

         In this context, "confirmation" does not require documentation of positive serology or culture for HIV; the provider's diagnostic statement that the patient is HIV positive, or has an HIV-related illness is sufficient.

      2) **Selection and sequencing of HIV codes**

         (a) **Patient admitted for HIV-related condition**

            If a patient is admitted for an HIV-related condition, the principal diagnosis should be B20, Human immunodeficiency virus [HIV] disease followed by additional diagnosis codes for all reported HIV-related conditions.

         (b) **Patient with HIV disease admitted for unrelated condition**

            If a patient with HIV disease is admitted for an unrelated condition (such as a traumatic injury), the code for the unrelated condition (e.g., the nature of injury code) should be the principal diagnosis. Other diagnoses would be B20 followed by additional diagnosis codes for all reported HIV-related conditions.

         (c) **Whether the patient is newly diagnosed**

            Whether the patient is newly diagnosed or has had previous admissions/encounters for HIV conditions is irrelevant to the sequencing decision.

         (d) **Asymptomatic human immunodeficiency virus**

            Z21, Asymptomatic human immunodeficiency virus [HIV] infection status, is to be applied when the patient without any documentation of symptoms is listed as being "HIV positive," "known HIV," "HIV test positive," or similar terminology. Do not use this code if the term "AIDS" is used or if the patient is treated for any HIV-related illness or is described as having any condition(s) resulting from his/her HIV positive status; use B20 in these cases.

         (e) **Patients with inconclusive HIV serology**

            Patients with inconclusive HIV serology, but no definitive diagnosis or manifestations of the illness, may be assigned code R75, Inconclusive laboratory evidence of human immunodeficiency virus [HIV].

(f) **Previously diagnosed HIV-related illness**

Patients with any known prior diagnosis of an HIV-related illness should be coded to B20. Once a patient has developed an HIV-related illness, the patient should always be assigned code B20 on every subsequent admission/encounter. Patients previously diagnosed with any HIV illness (B20) should never be assigned to R75 or Z21, Asymptomatic human immunodeficiency virus [HIV] infection status.

(g) **HIV Infection in Pregnancy, Childbirth and the Puerperium**

During pregnancy, childbirth or the puerperium, a patient admitted (or presenting for a health care encounter) because of an HIV-related illness should receive a principal diagnosis code of O98.7-, Human immunodeficiency [HIV] disease complicating pregnancy, childbirth and the puerperium, followed by B20 and the code(s) for the HIV-related illness(es). Codes from Chapter 15 always take sequencing priority.

Patients with asymptomatic HIV infection status admitted (or presenting for a health care encounter) during pregnancy, childbirth, or the puerperium should receive codes of O98.7- and Z21.

(h) **Encounters for testing for HIV**

If a patient is being seen to determine his/her HIV status, use code Z11.4, Encounter for screening for human immunodeficiency virus [HIV]. Use additional codes for any associated high risk behavior.

If a patient with signs or symptoms is being seen for HIV testing, code the signs and symptoms. An additional counseling code Z71.7, Human immunodeficiency virus [HIV] counseling, may be used if counseling is provided during the encounter for the test.

When a patient returns to be informed of his/her HIV test results and the test result is negative, use code Z71.7, Human immunodeficiency virus [HIV] counseling.

If the results are positive, see previous guidelines and assign codes as appropriate.

b. **Infectious agents as the cause of diseases classified to other chapters**

Certain infections are classified in chapters other than Chapter 1 and no organism is identified as part of the infection code. In these instances, it is necessary to use an additional code from Chapter 1 to identify the organism. A code from category B95, Streptococcus, Staphylococcus, and Enterococcus as the cause of diseases classified to other chapters, B96, Other bacterial agents as the cause of diseases classified to other chapters, or B97, Viral agents as the cause of diseases classified to other chapters, is to be used as an additional code to identify the organism. An instructional note will be found at the infection code advising that an additional organism code is required.

c. **Infections resistant to antibiotics**

Many bacterial infections are resistant to current antibiotics. It is necessary to identify all infections documented as antibiotic resistant. Assign a code from category Z16, Resistance to antimicrobial drugs, following the infection code only if the infection code does not identify drug resistance.

d. **Sepsis, Severe Sepsis, and Septic Shock**

1) **Coding of Sepsis and Severe Sepsis**

(a) **Sepsis**

For a diagnosis of sepsis, assign the appropriate code for the underlying systemic infection. If the type of infection or causal organism is not further specified, assign code A41.9, Sepsis, unspecified organism.

A code from subcategory R65.2, Severe sepsis, should not be assigned unless severe sepsis or an associated acute organ dysfunction is documented.

(i) Negative or inconclusive blood cultures and sepsis
Negative or inconclusive blood cultures do not preclude a diagnosis of sepsis in patients with clinical evidence of the condition; however, the provider should be queried.

(ii) Urosepsis

The term urosepsis is a nonspecific term. It is not to be considered synonymous with sepsis. It has no default code in the Alphabetic Index. Should a provider use this term, he/she must be queried for clarification.

(iii) Sepsis with organ dysfunction

If a patient has sepsis and associated acute organ dysfunction or multiple organ dysfunction (MOD), follow the instructions for coding severe sepsis.

(iv) Acute organ dysfunction that is not clearly associated with the sepsis

If a patient has sepsis and an acute organ dysfunction, but the medical record documentation indicates that the acute organ dysfunction is related to a medical condition other than the sepsis, do not assign a code from subcategory R65.2, Severe sepsis. An acute organ dysfunction must be associated with the sepsis in order to assign the severe sepsis code.

If the documentation is not clear as to whether an acute organ dysfunction is related to the sepsis or another medical condition, query the provider.

(b) **Severe sepsis**

The coding of severe sepsis requires a minimum of 2 codes: first a code for the underlying systemic infection, followed by a code from subcategory R65.2, Severe sepsis. If the causal organism is not documented, assign code A41.9, Sepsis, unspecified organism, for the infection. Additional code(s) for the associated acute organ dysfunction are also required.

Due to the complex nature of severe sepsis, some cases may require querying the provider prior to assignment of the codes.

2) **Septic shock**

(a) Septic shock generally refers to circulatory failure associated with severe sepsis, and therefore, it represents a type of acute organ dysfunction.

For cases of septic shock, the code for the systemic infection should be sequenced first, followed by code R65.21, Severe sepsis with septic shock or code T81.12, Postprocedural septic shock. Any additional codes for the other acute organ dysfunctions should also be assigned. As noted in the sequencing instructions in the Tabular List, the code for septic shock cannot be assigned as a principal diagnosis.

3) **Sequencing of severe sepsis**

If severe sepsis is present on admission, and meets the definition of principal diagnosis, the underlying systemic infection should be assigned as principal diagnosis followed by the appropriate code from subcategory R65.2 as required by the sequencing rules in the Tabular List. A code from subcategory R65.2 can never be assigned as a principal diagnosis.

When severe sepsis develops during an encounter (it was not present on admission), the underlying systemic infection and the appropriate code from subcategory R65.2 should be assigned as secondary diagnoses.

Severe sepsis may be present on admission, but the diagnosis may not be confirmed until sometime after admission. If the documentation is not clear whether severe sepsis was present on admission, the provider should be queried.

4) Sepsis and severe sepsis with a localized infection

If the reason for admission is both sepsis or severe sepsis and a localized infection, such as pneumonia or cellulitis, a code(s) for the underlying systemic infection should be assigned first and the code for the localized infection should be assigned as a secondary diagnosis. If the patient has severe sepsis, a code from subcategory R65.2 should also be assigned as a secondary diagnosis. If the patient is admitted with a localized infection, such as pneumonia, and sepsis/severe sepsis doesn't develop until after admission, the localized infection should be assigned first, followed by the appropriate sepsis/severe sepsis codes.

5) Sepsis due to a postprocedural infection

(a) **Documentation of causal relationship**

As with all postprocedural complications, code assignment is based on the provider's documentation of the relationship between the infection and the procedure.

(b) **Sepsis due to a postprocedural infection**

For such cases, the postprocedural infection code, such as T80.2, Infections following infusion, transfusion, and therapeutic injection, T81.4, Infection following a procedure, T88.0, Infection following immunization, or O86.0, Infection of obstetric surgical wound, should be coded first, followed by the code for the specific infection. If the patient has severe sepsis, the appropriate code from subcategory R65.2 should also be assigned with the additional code(s) for any acute organ dysfunction.

(c) **Postprocedural infection and postprocedural septic shock**

In cases where a postprocedural infection has occurred and has resulted in severe sepsis the code for the precipitating complication such as code T81.4, Infection following a procedure, or O86.0, Infection of obstetrical surgical wound should be coded first followed by code R65.20, Severe sepsis without septic shock. A code for the systemic infection should also be assigned.

If a postprocedural infection has resulted in postprocedural septic shock, the code for the precipitating complication such as code T81.4, Infection following a procedure, or O86.0, Infection of obstetrical surgical wound should be coded first followed by code T81.12-, Postprocedural septic shock. A code for the systemic infection should also be assigned.

6) Sepsis and severe sepsis associated with a noninfectious process (condition)

In some cases a noninfectious process (condition), such as trauma, may lead to an infection which can result in sepsis or severe sepsis. If sepsis or severe sepsis is documented as associated with a noninfectious condition, such as a burn or serious injury, and this condition meets the definition for principal diagnosis, the code for the noninfectious condition should be sequenced first, followed by the code for the resulting infection. If severe sepsis is present, a code from subcategory

R65.2 should also be assigned with any associated organ dysfunction(s) codes. It is not necessary to assign a code from subcategory R65.1, Systemic inflammatory response syndrome (SIRS) of non-infectious origin, for these cases.

If the infection meets the definition of principal diagnosis, it should be sequenced before the non-infectious condition. When both the associated non-infectious condition and the infection meet the definition of principal diagnosis, either may be assigned as principal diagnosis.

Only one code from category R65, Symptoms and signs specifically associated with systemic inflammation and infection, should be assigned. Therefore, when a non-infectious condition leads to an infection resulting in severe sepsis, assign the appropriate code from subcategory R65.2, Severe sepsis. Do not additionally assign a code from subcategory R65.1, Systemic inflammatory response syndrome (SIRS) of non-infectious origin.

See Section I.C.18. SIRS due to non-infectious process

7) Sepsis and septic shock complicating abortion, pregnancy, childbirth, and the puerperium

See Section I.C.15. Sepsis and septic shock complicating abortion, pregnancy, childbirth and the puerperium

8) Newborn sepsis

See Section I.C.16. f. Bacterial sepsis of Newborn

e. Methicillin Resistant *Staphylococcus aureus* (MRSA) Conditions

1) Selection and sequencing of MRSA codes

(a) Combination codes for MRSA infection

When a patient is diagnosed with an infection that is due to methicillin resistant *Staphylococcus aureus* (MRSA), and that infection has a combination code that includes the causal organism (e.g., sepsis, pneumonia) assign the appropriate combination code for the condition (e.g., code A41.02, Sepsis due to Methicillin resistant Staphylococcus aureus or code J15.212, Pneumonia due to Methicillin resistant Staphylococcus aureus). Do not assign code B95.62, Methicillin resistant Staphylococcus aureus infection as the cause of diseases classified elsewhere, as an additional code, because the combination code includes the type of infection and the MRSA organism. Do not assign a code from subcategory Z16.11, Resistance to penicillins, as an additional diagnosis.

See Section C.1. for instructions on coding and sequencing of sepsis and severe sepsis.

(b) Other codes for MRSA infection

When there is documentation of a current infection (e.g., wound infection, stitch abscess, urinary tract infection) due to MRSA, and that infection does not have a combination code that includes the causal organism, assign the appropriate code to identify the condition along with code B95.62, Methicillin resistant Staphylococcus aureus infection as the cause of diseases classified elsewhere for the MRSA infection. Do not assign a code from subcategory Z16.11, Resistance to penicillins.

(c) Methicillin susceptible Staphylococcus aureus (MSSA) and MRSA colonization

The condition or state of being colonized or carrying MSSA or MRSA is called colonization or carriage, while an individual person is described as being colonized or being a carrier. Colonization means that MSSA or MSRA is present on or in the body without necessarily causing illness. A positive MRSA colonization test might be documented by the provider as "MRSA screen positive" or "MRSA nasal swab positive".

Assign code Z22.322, Carrier or suspected carrier of Methicillin resistant Staphylococcus aureus, for patients documented as having MRSA colonization. Assign code Z22.321, Carrier or suspected carrier of Methicillin susceptible Staphylococcus aureus, for patient documented as having MSSA colonization. Colonization is not necessarily indicative of a disease process or as the cause of a specific condition the patient may have unless documented as such by the provider.

(d) MRSA colonization and infection

If a patient is documented as having both MRSA colonization and infection during a hospital admission, code Z22.322, Carrier or suspected carrier of Methicillin resistant Staphylococcus aureus, and a code for the MRSA infection may both be assigned.

f. Zika virus infections

1) Code only confirmed cases

Code only a confirmed diagnosis of Zika virus (A92.5, Zika virus disease) as documented by the provider. This is an exception to the hospital inpatient guideline Section II, H.

In this context, "confirmation" does not require documentation of the type of test performed; the physician's diagnostic statement that the condition is confirmed is sufficient. This code should be assigned regardless of the stated mode of transmission.

If the provider documents "suspected", "possible" or "probable" Zika, do not assign code A92.5. Assign a code(s) explaining the reason for encounter (such as fever, rash, or joint pain) or Z20.828, Contact with and (suspected) exposure to other viral communicable diseases.

2. **Chapter 2: Neoplasms (C00-D49)**

General guidelines

Chapter 2 of the ICD-10-CM contains the codes for most benign and all malignant neoplasms. Certain benign neoplasms, such as prostatic adenomas, may be found in the specific body system chapters. To properly code a neoplasm it is necessary to determine from the record if the neoplasm is benign, in-situ, malignant, or of uncertain histologic behavior. If malignant, any secondary (metastatic) sites should also be determined.

Primary malignant neoplasms overlapping site boundaries

A primary malignant neoplasm that overlaps two or more contiguous (next to each other) sites should be classified to the subcategory/code .8 ('overlapping lesion'), unless the combination is specifically indexed elsewhere. For multiple neoplasms of the same site that are not contiguous such as tumors in different quadrants of the same breast, codes for each site should be assigned.

Malignant neoplasm of ectopic tissue

Malignant neoplasms of ectopic tissue are to be coded to the site of origin mentioned, e.g., ectopic pancreatic malignant neoplasms involving the stomach are coded to malignant neoplasm of pancreas, unspecified (C25.9).

The neoplasm table in the Alphabetic Index should be referenced first. However, if the histological term is documented, that term should be referenced first, rather than going immediately to the Neoplasm Table, in order to determine which column in the Neoplasm Table is appropriate. For example, if the documentation indicates "adenoma," refer to the term in the Alphabetic Index to review the entries under this term and the instructional note to "see also neoplasm, by site, benign." The table provides the proper code based on the type of neoplasm and the site. It is important to select the proper column in the table that corresponds to the type of neoplasm. The Tabular List should then be referenced to verify that the correct code has been selected from the table and that a more specific site code does not exist.

See Section I.C.21. Factors influencing health status and contact with health services, Status, for information regarding Z15.0, codes for genetic susceptibility to cancer.

a. **Treatment directed at the malignancy**

If the treatment is directed at the malignancy, designate the malignancy as the principal diagnosis.

The only exception to this guideline is if a patient admission/encounter is solely for the administration of chemotherapy, immunotherapy or external beam radiation therapy, assign the appropriate Z51.-- code as the first-listed or principal diagnosis, and the diagnosis or problem for which the service is being performed as a secondary diagnosis.

b. **Treatment of secondary site**

When a patient is admitted because of a primary neoplasm with metastasis and treatment is directed toward the secondary site only, the secondary neoplasm is designated as the principal diagnosis even though the primary malignancy is still present.

c. Coding and sequencing of complications

Coding and sequencing of complications associated with the malignancies or with the therapy thereof are subject to the following guidelines:

1) Anemia associated with malignancy

When admission/encounter is for management of an anemia associated with the malignancy, and the treatment is only for anemia, the appropriate code for the malignancy is sequenced as the principal or first-listed diagnosis followed by the appropriate code for the anemia (such as code D63.0, Anemia in neoplastic disease).

2) Anemia associated with chemotherapy, immunotherapy and radiation therapy

When the admission/encounter is for management of an anemia associated with an adverse effect of the administration of chemotherapy or immunotherapy and the only treatment is for the anemia, the anemia code is sequenced first followed by the appropriate codes for the neoplasm and the adverse effect (T45.1X5, Adverse effect of antineoplastic and immunosuppressive drugs).

When the admission/encounter is for management of an anemia associated with an adverse effect of radiotherapy, the anemia code should be sequenced first, followed by the appropriate neoplasm code and code Y84.2, Radiological procedure and radiotherapy as the cause of abnormal reaction of the patient, or of later complication, without mention of misadventure at the time of the procedure.

3) Management of dehydration due to the malignancy

When the admission/encounter is for management of dehydration due to the malignancy and only the dehydration is being treated (intravenous rehydration), the dehydration is sequenced first, followed by the code(s) for the malignancy.

4) Treatment of a complication resulting from a surgical procedure

When the admission/encounter is for treatment of a complication resulting from a surgical procedure, designate the complication as the principal or first-listed diagnosis if treatment is directed at resolving the complication.

d. Primary malignancy previously excised

When a primary malignancy has been previously excised or eradicated from its site and there is no further treatment directed to that site and there is no evidence of any existing primary malignancy, a code from category Z85, Personal history of malignant neoplasm, should be used to indicate the former site of the malignancy. Any mention of extension, invasion, or metastasis to another site is coded as a secondary malignant neoplasm to that site. The secondary site may be the principal or first-listed with the Z85 code used as a secondary code.

e. Admissions/Encounters involving chemotherapy, immunotherapy and radiation therapy

1) Episode of care involves surgical removal of neoplasm

When an episode of care involves the surgical removal of a neoplasm, primary or secondary site, followed by adjunct chemotherapy or radiation treatment during the same episode of care, the code for the neoplasm should be assigned as principal or first-listed diagnosis.

2) Patient admission/encounter solely for administration of chemotherapy, immunotherapy and radiation therapy

If a patient admission/encounter is solely for the administration of chemotherapy, immunotherapy or external beam radiation therapy assign code Z51.0, Encounter for antineoplastic radiation therapy, or Z51.11, Encounter for antineoplastic chemotherapy, or Z51.12, Encounter for antineoplastic immunotherapy as the first-listed or principal diagnosis. If a patient receives more than one of these therapies during the same admission more than one of these codes may be assigned, in any sequence.

The malignancy for which the therapy is being administered should be assigned as a secondary diagnosis.

If a patient admission/encounter is for the insertion or implantation of radioactive elements (e.g., brachytherapy) the appropriate code for the malignancy is sequenced as the principal or first-listed diagnosis. Code Z51.0 should not be assigned.

3) **Patient admitted for radiation therapy, chemotherapy or immunotherapy and develops complications**

When a patient is admitted for the purpose of radiotherapy, immunotherapy or chemotherapy and develops complications such as uncontrolled nausea and vomiting or dehydration, the principal or first-listed diagnosis is Z51.0, Encounter for antineoplastic radiation therapy, or Z51.11, Encounter for antineoplastic chemotherapy, or Z51.12, Encounter for antineoplastic immunotherapy followed by any codes for the complications.

When a patient is admitted for the purpose of insertion or implantation of radioactive elements (e.g., brachytherapy) and develops complications such as uncontrolled nausea and vomiting or dehydration, the principal or first-listed diagnosis is the appropriate code for the malignancy followed by any codes for the complications.

f. **Admission/encounter to determine extent of malignancy**

When the reason for admission/encounter is to determine the extent of the malignancy, or for a procedure such as paracentesis or thoracentesis, the primary malignancy or appropriate metastatic site is designated as the principal or first-listed diagnosis, even though chemotherapy or radiotherapy is administered.

g. **Symptoms, signs, and abnormal findings listed in Chapter 18 associated with neoplasms**

Symptoms, signs, and ill-defined conditions listed in Chapter 18 characteristic of, or associated with, an existing primary or secondary site malignancy cannot be used to replace the malignancy as principal or first-listed diagnosis, regardless of the number of admissions or encounters for treatment and care of the neoplasm.

See section I.C.21. Factors influencing health status and contact with health services, Encounter for prophylactic organ removal.

h. **Admission/encounter for pain control/management**

See Section I.C.6. for information on coding admission/encounter for pain control/management.

i. **Malignancy in two or more noncontiguous sites**

A patient may have more than one malignant tumor in the same organ. These tumors may represent different primaries or metastatic disease, depending on the site. Should the documentation be unclear, the provider should be queried as to the status of each tumor so that the correct codes can be assigned.

j. **Disseminated malignant neoplasm, unspecified**

Code C80.0, Disseminated malignant neoplasm, unspecified, is for use only in those cases where the patient has advanced metastatic disease and no known primary or secondary sites are specified. It should not be used in place of assigning codes for the primary site and all known secondary sites.

k. **Malignant neoplasm without specification of site**

Code C80.1, Malignant (primary) neoplasm, unspecified, equates to Cancer, unspecified. This code should only be used when no determination can be made as to the primary site of a malignancy. This code should rarely be used in the inpatient setting.

l. **Sequencing of neoplasm codes**

1) **Encounter for treatment of primary malignancy**

If the reason for the encounter is for treatment of a primary malignancy, assign the malignancy as the principal/first-listed diagnosis. The primary site is to be sequenced first, followed by any metastatic sites.

2) **Encounter for treatment of secondary malignancy**

When an encounter is for a primary malignancy with metastasis and treatment is directed toward the metastatic (secondary) site(s) only, the metastatic site(s) is designated as the principal/first-listed diagnosis. The primary malignancy is coded as an additional code.

3) **Malignant neoplasm in a pregnant patient**

When a pregnant woman has a malignant neoplasm, a code from subcategory O9A.1-, Malignant neoplasm complicating pregnancy, childbirth, and the puerperium, should be sequenced first, followed by the appropriate code from Chapter 2 to indicate the type of neoplasm.

4) **Encounter for complication associated with a neoplasm**

When an encounter is for management of a complication associated with a neoplasm, such as dehydration, and the treatment is only for the complication, the complication is coded first, followed by the appropriate code(s) for the neoplasm.

The exception to this guideline is anemia. When the admission/encounter is for management of an anemia associated with the malignancy, and the treatment is only for anemia, the appropriate code for the malignancy is sequenced as the principal or first-listed diagnosis followed by code D63.0, Anemia in neoplastic disease.

5) **Complication from surgical procedure for treatment of a neoplasm**

When an encounter is for treatment of a complication resulting from a surgical procedure performed for the treatment of the neoplasm, designate the complication as the principal/first-listed diagnosis. See guideline regarding the coding of a current malignancy versus personal history to determine if the code for the neoplasm should also be assigned.

6) **Pathologic fracture due to a neoplasm**

When an encounter is for a pathological fracture due to a neoplasm, and the focus of treatment is the fracture, a code from subcategory M84.5, Pathological fracture in neoplastic disease, should be sequenced first, followed by the code for the neoplasm.

If the focus of treatment is the neoplasm with an associated pathological fracture, the neoplasm code should be sequenced first, followed by a code from M84.5 for the pathological fracture.

m. **Current malignancy versus personal history of malignancy**

When a primary malignancy has been excised but further treatment, such as an additional surgery for the malignancy, radiation therapy or chemotherapy is directed to that site, the primary malignancy code should be used until treatment is completed.

When a primary malignancy has been previously excised or eradicated from its site, there is no further treatment (of the malignancy) directed to that site, and there is no evidence of any existing primary malignancy, a code from category Z85, Personal history of malignant neoplasm, should be used to indicate the former site of the malignancy.

See Section I.C.21. Factors influencing health status and contact with health services, History (of)

n. **Leukemia, Multiple Myeloma, and Malignant Plasma Cell Neoplasms in remission versus personal history**

The categories for leukemia, and category C90, Multiple myeloma and malignant plasma cell neoplasms, have codes indicating whether or not the leukemia has achieved remission. There are also codes Z85.6, Personal history of leukemia, and Z85.79, Personal history of other malignant neoplasms of lymphoid, hematopoietic and related tissues. If the documentation is unclear as to whether the leukemia has achieved remission, the provider should be queried.

See Section I.C.21. Factors influencing health status and contact with health services, History (of)

o. **Aftercare following surgery for neoplasm**

See Section I.C.21. Factors influencing health status and contact with health services, Aftercare

p. **Follow-up care for completed treatment of a malignancy**

See Section I.C.21. Factors influencing health status and contact with health services, Follow-up

q. **Prophylactic organ removal for prevention of malignancy**

See Section I.C. 21, Factors influencing health status and contact with health services, Prophylactic organ removal

r. **Malignant neoplasm associated with transplanted organ**

A malignant neoplasm of a transplanted organ should be coded as a transplant complication. Assign first the appropriate code from category T86.-, Complications of transplanted organs and tissue, followed by code C80.2, Malignant neoplasm associated with transplanted organ. Use an additional code for the specific malignancy.

3. **Chapter 3: Disease of the blood and blood-forming organs and certain disorders involving the immune mechanism (D50-D89)**

Reserved for future guideline expansion

4. **Chapter 4: Endocrine, Nutritional, and Metabolic Diseases (E00-E89)**

a. **Diabetes mellitus**

The diabetes mellitus codes are combination codes that include the type of diabetes mellitus, the body system affected, and the complications affecting that body system. As many codes within a particular category

as are necessary to describe all of the complications of the disease may be used. They should be sequenced based on the reason for a particular encounter. Assign as many codes from categories E08 – E13 as needed to identify all of the associated conditions that the patient has.

1) **Type of diabetes**

The age of a patient is not the sole determining factor, though most type 1 diabetics develop the condition before reaching puberty. For this reason type 1 diabetes mellitus is also referred to as juvenile diabetes.

2) **Type of diabetes mellitus not documented**

If the type of diabetes mellitus is not documented in the medical record the default is E11.-, Type 2 diabetes mellitus.

3) **Diabetes mellitus and the use of insulin and oral hypoglycemics**

If the documentation in a medical record does not indicate the type of diabetes but does indicate that the patient uses insulin, code E11, Type 2 diabetes mellitus, should be assigned. An additional code should be assigned from category Z79 to identify the long-term (current) use of insulin or oral hypoglycemic drugs. If the patient is treated with both oral medications and insulin, only the code for long-term (current) use of insulin should be assigned. Code Z79.4 should not be assigned if insulin is given temporarily to bring a type 2 patient's blood sugar under control during an encounter.

4) Diabetes mellitus in pregnancy and gestational diabetes

See Section I.C.15. Diabetes mellitus in pregnancy.
See Section I.C.15. Gestational (pregnancy induced) diabetes

5) Complications due to insulin pump malfunction

(a) Underdose of insulin due to insulin pump failure

An underdose of insulin due to an insulin pump failure should be assigned to a code from subcategory T85.6, Mechanical complication of other specified internal and external prosthetic devices, implants and grafts, that specifies the type of pump malfunction, as the principal or first-listed code, followed by code T38.3X6-, Underdosing of insulin and oral hypoglycemic [antidiabetic] drugs. Additional codes for the type of diabetes mellitus and any associated complications due to the underdosing should also be assigned.

(b) Overdose of insulin due to insulin pump failure

The principal or first-listed code for an encounter due to an insulin pump malfunction resulting in an overdose of insulin, should also be T85.6-, Mechanical complication of other specified internal and external prosthetic devices, implants and grafts, followed by code T38.3X1-, Poisoning by insulin and oral hypoglycemic [antidiabetic] drugs, accidental (unintentional).

6) Secondary diabetes mellitus

Codes under categories E08, Diabetes mellitus due to underlying condition, E09, Drug or chemical induced diabetes mellitus, and E13, Other specified diabetes mellitus, identify complications/manifestations associated with secondary diabetes mellitus. Secondary diabetes is always caused by another condition or event (e.g., cystic fibrosis, malignant neoplasm of pancreas, pancreatectomy, adverse effect of drug, or poisoning).

(a) Secondary diabetes mellitus and the use of insulin or oral hypoglycemic drugs

For patients with secondary diabetes mellitus who routinely use insulin or oral hypoglycemic drugs, an additional code from category Z79 should be assigned to identify the long-term (current) use of insulin or oral hypoglycemic drugs. If the patient is treated with both oral medications and insulin, only the code for long-term (current) use of insulin should be assigned. Code Z79.4 should not be assigned if insulin is given temporarily to bring a type 2 patient's blood sugar under control during an encounter.

(b) Assigning and sequencing secondary diabetes codes and its causes

The sequencing of the secondary diabetes codes in relationship to codes for the cause of the diabetes is based on the Tabular List instructions for categories E08, E09 and E13.

(i) Secondary diabetes mellitus due to pancreatectomy

For postpancreatectomy diabetes mellitus (lack of insulin due to the surgical removal of all or part of the pancreas), assign code E89.1, Postprocedural hypoinsulinemia. Assign a code from category E13 and a code from subcategory Z90.41-, Acquired absence of pancreas, as additional codes.

(ii) Secondary diabetes due to drugs

Secondary diabetes may be caused by an adverse effect of correctly administered medications, poisoning or sequela of poisoning.

See section I.C.19.e for coding of adverse effects and poisoning, and section I.C.20 for external cause code reporting.

5. **Chapter 5: Mental, Behavioral and Neurodevelopmental disorders (F01 – F99)**

   a. **Pain disorders related to psychological factors**

   Assign code F45.41, for pain that is exclusively related to psychological disorders. As indicated by the Excludes 1 note under category G89, a code from category G89 should not be assigned with code F45.41.

   Code F45.42, Pain disorders with related psychological factors, should be used with a code from category G89, Pain, not elsewhere classified, if there is documentation of a psychological component for a patient with acute or chronic pain.

   See Section I.C.6. Pain

   b. **Mental and behavioral disorders due to psychoactive substance use**

   1) **In Remission**

   Selection of codes for "in remission" for categories F10-F19, Mental and behavioral disorders due to psychoactive substance use (categories F10-F19 with -11, -.21) requires the provider's clinical judgment. The appropriate codes for "in remission" are assigned only on the basis of provider documentation (as defined in the Official Guidelines for Coding and Reporting) unless otherwise instructed by the classification. Mild substance use disorders in early or sustained remission are classified to the appropriate codes for substance abuse in remission, and moderate or severe substance use disorders in early or sustained remission are classified to the appropriate codes for substance dependence in remission.

   2) **Psychoactive Substance Use, Abuse And Dependence**

   When the provider documentation refers to use, abuse and dependence of the same substance (e.g. alcohol, opioid, cannabis, etc.), only one code should be assigned to identify the pattern of use based on the following hierarchy:

   - If both use and abuse are documented, assign only the code for abuse

   - If both abuse and dependence are documented, assign only the code for dependence

   - If use, abuse and dependence are all documented, assign only the code for dependence

   - If both use and dependence are documented, assign only the code for dependence.

   3) **Psychoactive Substance Use Disorders**

   As with all other diagnoses, the codes for psychoactive substance use disorders (F10.9-, F11.9-, F12.9-, F13.9-, F14.9-, F15.9-, F16.9-) should only be assigned based on provider documentation and when they meet the definition of a reportable diagnosis (see Section III, Reporting Additional Diagnoses). The codes are to be used only when the psychoactive substance use is associated with a physical, mental or behavioral disorder, and such a relationship is documented by the provider.

6. **Chapter 6: Diseases of the Nervous System (G00-G99)**

   a. **Dominant/nondominant side**

   Codes from category G81, Hemiplegia and hemiparesis, and subcategories G83.1, Monoplegia of lower limb, G83.2, Monoplegia of upper limb, and G83.3, Monoplegia, unspecified, identify whether the dominant or nondominant side is affected. Should the affected side be documented, but not specified as dominant or nondominant, and the classification system does not indicate a default, code selection is as follows:

- For ambidextrous patients, the default should be dominant.

- If the left side is affected, the default is non-dominant.

- If the right side is affected, the default is dominant.

b. Pain - Category G89

1) General coding information

Codes in category G89, Pain, not elsewhere classified, may be used in conjunction with codes from other categories and chapters to provide more detail about acute or chronic pain and neoplasm-related pain, unless otherwise indicated below.

If the pain is not specified as acute or chronic, post-thoracotomy, postprocedural, or neoplasm-related, do not assign codes from category G89.

A code from category G89 should not be assigned if the underlying (definitive) diagnosis is known, unless the reason for the encounter is pain control/ management and not management of the underlying condition.

When an admission or encounter is for a procedure aimed at treating the underlying condition (e.g., spinal fusion, kyphoplasty), a code for the underlying condition (e.g., vertebral fracture, spinal stenosis) should be assigned as the principal diagnosis. No code from category G89 should be assigned.

(a) Category G89 Codes as Principal or First-Listed Diagnosis

Category G89 codes are acceptable as principal diagnosis or the first-listed code:

- When pain control or pain management is the reason for the admission/encounter (e.g., a patient with displaced intervertebral disc, nerve impingement and severe back pain presents for injection of steroid into the spinal canal). The underlying cause of the pain should be reported as an additional diagnosis, if known.

- When a patient is admitted for the insertion of a neurostimulator for pain control, assign the appropriate pain code as the principal or first-listed diagnosis. When an admission or encounter is for a procedure aimed at treating the underlying condition and a neurostimulator is inserted for pain control during the same admission/encounter, a code for the underlying condition should be assigned as the principal diagnosis and the appropriate pain code should be assigned as a secondary diagnosis.

(b) Use of Category G89 Codes in Conjunction with Site Specific Pain Codes

(i) Assigning Category G89 and Site-Specific Pain Codes

Codes from category G89 may be used in conjunction with codes that identify the site of pain (including codes from chapter 18) if the category G89 code provides additional information. For example, if the code describes the site of the pain, but does not fully describe whether the pain is acute or chronic, then both codes should be assigned.

(ii) Sequencing of Category G89 Codes with Site-Specific Pain Codes

The sequencing of category G89 codes with site-specific pain codes (including chapter 18 codes), is dependent on the circumstances of the encounter/admission as follows:

- If the encounter is for pain control or pain management, assign the code from category G89 followed by the code identifying the specific site of pain (e.g., encounter for pain management for acute neck pain from trauma is assigned code G89.11, Acute pain due to trauma, followed by code M54.2, Cervicalgia, to identify the site of pain).

- If the encounter is for any other reason except pain control or pain management, and a related definitive diagnosis has not been established (confirmed) by the provider, assign the code for the specific site of pain first, followed by the appropriate code from category G89.

2) **Pain due to devices, implants and grafts**

   See Section I.C.19. Pain due to medical devices

3) **Postoperative Pain**

   The provider's documentation should be used to guide the coding of postoperative pain, as well as *Section III. Reporting Additional Diagnoses* and *Section IV. Diagnostic Coding and Reporting in the Outpatient Setting.*
   The default for post-thoracotomy and other postoperative pain not specified as acute or chronic is the code for the acute form.

   Routine or expected postoperative pain immediately after surgery should not be coded.

   (a) **Postoperative pain not associated with specific postoperative complication**

   Postoperative pain not associated with a specific postoperative complication is assigned to the appropriate postoperative pain code in category G89.

   (b) **Postoperative pain associated with specific postoperative complication**

   Postoperative pain associated with a specific postoperative complication (such as painful wire sutures) is assigned to the appropriate code(s) found in Chapter 19, Injury, poisoning, and certain other consequences of external causes. If appropriate, use additional code(s) from category G89 to identify acute or chronic pain (G89.18 or G89.28).

4) **Chronic pain**

   Chronic pain is classified to subcategory G89.2. There is no time frame defining when pain becomes chronic pain. The provider's documentation should be used to guide use of these codes.

5) **Neoplasm Related Pain**

   Code G89.3 is assigned to pain documented as being related, associated or due to cancer, primary or secondary malignancy, or tumor. This code is assigned regardless of whether the pain is acute or chronic.

   This code may be assigned as the principal or first-listed code when the stated reason for the admission/encounter is documented as pain control/pain management. The underlying neoplasm should be reported as an additional diagnosis.

   When the reason for the admission/encounter is management of the neoplasm and the pain associated with the neoplasm is also documented, code G89.3 may be assigned as an additional diagnosis. It is not necessary to assign an additional code for the site of the pain.

   See Section I.C.2 for instructions on the sequencing of neoplasms for all other stated reasons for the admission/encounter (except for pain control/pain management).

6) **Chronic pain syndrome**

   Central pain syndrome (G89.0) and chronic pain syndrome (G89.4) are different than the term "chronic pain," and therefore codes should only be used when the provider has specifically documented this condition.

See Section I.C.5. Pain disorders related to psychological factors

7. **Chapter 7: Diseases of the Eye and Adnexa (H00-H59)**

   a. **Glaucoma**

      1) **Assigning Glaucoma Codes**

         Assign as many codes from category H40, Glaucoma, as needed to identify the type of glaucoma, the affected eye, and the glaucoma stage.

      2) **Bilateral glaucoma with same type and stage**

         When a patient has bilateral glaucoma and both eyes are documented as being the same type and stage, and there is a code for bilateral glaucoma, report only the code for the type of glaucoma, bilateral, with the seventh character for the stage.

         When a patient has bilateral glaucoma and both eyes are documented as being the same type and stage, and the classification does not provide a code for bilateral glaucoma (i.e. subcategories H40.10, H40.11 and H40.20) report only one code for the type of glaucoma with the appropriate seventh character for the stage.

      3) **Bilateral glaucoma stage with different types or stages**

         When a patient has bilateral glaucoma and each eye is documented as having a different type or stage, and the classification distinguishes laterality, assign the appropriate code for each eye rather than the code for bilateral glaucoma.

         When a patient has bilateral glaucoma and each eye is documented as having a different type, and the classification does not distinguish laterality (i.e. subcategories H40.10, H40.11 and H40.20), assign one code for each type of glaucoma with the appropriate seventh character for the stage.

         When a patient has bilateral glaucoma and each eye is documented as having the same type, but different stage, and the classification does not distinguish laterality (i.e. subcategories H40.10, H40.11 and H40.20), assign a code for

         the type of glaucoma for each eye with the seventh character for the specific glaucoma stage documented for each eye.

      4) **Patient admitted with glaucoma and stage evolves during the admission**

         If a patient is admitted with glaucoma and the stage progresses during the admission, assign the code for highest stage documented.

      5) **Indeterminate stage glaucoma**

         Assignment of the seventh character "4" for "indeterminate stage" should be based on the clinical documentation. The seventh character "4" is used for glaucomas whose stage cannot be clinically determined. This seventh character should not be confused with the seventh character "0", unspecified, which should be assigned when there is no documentation regarding the stage of the glaucoma.

   b. **Blindness**

      If "blindness" or "low vision" of both eyes is documented but the visual impairment category is not documented, assign code H54.3, Unqualified visual loss, both eyes. If "blindness" or "low vision" in one eye is documented but the visual impairment category is not documented, assign a code from H54.6-, Unqualified visual loss, one eye. If "blindness" or "visual loss" is documented without any information about whether one or both eyes are affected, assign code H54.7, Unspecified visual loss.

8. **Chapter 8: Diseases of the Ear and Mastoid Process (H60-H95)**

   Reserved for future guideline expansion

9. **Chapter 9: Diseases of the Circulatory System (I00-I99)**

   a. **Hypertension**

   The classification presumes a causal relationship between hypertension and heart involvement and between hypertension and kidney involvement, as the two conditions are linked by the term "with" in the Alphabetic Index. These conditions should be coded as related even in the absence of provider documentation explicitly linking them, unless the documentation clearly states the conditions are unrelated.

   For hypertension and conditions not specifically linked by relational terms such as "with," "associated with" or "due to" in the classification, provider documentation must link the conditions in order to code them as related.

   1) **Hypertension with Heart Disease**

   Hypertension with heart conditions classified to I50.- or I51.4-I51.9, are assigned to a code from category I11, Hypertensive heart disease. Use an additional code from category I50, Heart failure, to identify the type of heart failure in those patients with heart failure.

   The same heart conditions (I50.-, I51.4-I51.9) with hypertension are coded separately if the provider has specifically documented a different cause. Sequence according to the circumstances of the admission/encounter.

   2) **Hypertensive Chronic Kidney Disease**

   Assign codes from category I12, Hypertensive chronic kidney disease, when both hypertension and a condition classifiable to category N18, Chronic kidney disease (CKD), are present. CKD should not be coded as hypertensive if the physician has specifically documented a different cause.

   The appropriate code from category N18 should be used as a secondary code with a code from category I12 to identify the stage of chronic kidney disease.

   See Section I.C.14. Chronic kidney disease.

   If a patient has hypertensive chronic kidney disease and acute renal failure, an additional code for the acute renal failure is required.

   3) **Hypertensive Heart and Chronic Kidney Disease**

   Assign codes from combination category I13, Hypertensive heart and chronic kidney disease, when there is hypertension with both heart and kidney involvement. If heart failure is present, assign an additional code from category I50 to identify the type of heart failure.

   The appropriate code from category N18, Chronic kidney disease, should be used as a secondary code with a code from category I13 to identify the stage of chronic kidney disease.

   See Section I.C.14. Chronic kidney disease.

   The codes in category I13, Hypertensive heart and chronic kidney disease, are combination codes that include hypertension, heart disease and chronic kidney disease. The Includes note at I13 specifies that the conditions included at I11 and I12 are included together in I13. If a patient has hypertension, heart disease and chronic kidney disease, then a code from I13 should be used, not individual codes for hypertension, heart disease and chronic kidney disease, or codes from I11 or I12.

For patients with both acute renal failure and chronic kidney disease, an additional code for acute renal failure is required.

4) Hypertensive Cerebrovascular Disease

For hypertensive cerebrovascular disease, first assign the appropriate code from categories I60-I69, followed by the appropriate hypertension code.

5) Hypertensive Retinopathy

Subcategory H35.0, Background retinopathy and retinal vascular changes, should be used with a code from category I10 – I15, Hypertensive disease to include the systemic hypertension. The sequencing is based on the reason for the encounter.

6) Hypertension, Secondary

Secondary hypertension is due to an underlying condition. Two codes are required: one to identify the underlying etiology and one from category I15 to identify the hypertension. Sequencing of codes is determined by the reason for admission/encounter.

7) Hypertension, Transient

Assign code R03.0, Elevated blood pressure reading without diagnosis of hypertension, unless patient has an established diagnosis of hypertension. Assign code O13.-, Gestational [pregnancy-induced] hypertension without significant proteinuria, or O14.-, Pre-eclampsia, for transient hypertension of pregnancy.

8) Hypertension, Controlled

This diagnostic statement usually refers to an existing state of hypertension under control by therapy. Assign the appropriate code from categories I10-I15, Hypertensive diseases.

9) Hypertension, Uncontrolled

Uncontrolled hypertension may refer to untreated hypertension or hypertension not responding to current therapeutic regimen. In either case, assign the appropriate code from categories I10-I15, Hypertensive diseases.

10) Hypertensive Crisis

Assign a code from category I16, Hypertensive crisis, for documented hypertensive urgency, hypertensive emergency or unspecified hypertensive crisis. Code also any identified hypertensive disease (I10-I15). The sequencing is based on the reason for the encounter.

11) Pulmonary Hypertension

Pulmonary hypertension is classified to category I27, Other pulmonary heart diseases. For secondary pulmonary hypertension (I27.1, I27.2-), code also any associated conditions or adverse effects of drugs or toxins. The sequencing is based on the reason for the encounter.

b. Atherosclerotic Coronary Artery Disease and Angina

ICD-10-CM has combination codes for atherosclerotic heart disease with angina pectoris. The subcategories for these codes are I25.11, Atherosclerotic heart disease of native coronary artery with angina pectoris and I25.7, Atherosclerosis of coronary artery bypass graft(s) and coronary artery of transplanted heart with angina pectoris.

When using one of these combination codes it is not necessary to use an additional code for angina pectoris. A causal relationship can be assumed in a patient with both atherosclerosis and angina pectoris, unless the documentation indicates the angina is due to something other than the atherosclerosis.

If a patient with coronary artery disease is admitted due to an acute myocardial infarction (AMI), the AMI should be sequenced before the coronary artery disease.

See Section I.C.9. Acute myocardial infarction (AMI)

c. **Intraoperative and Postprocedural Cerebrovascular Accident**

Medical record documentation should clearly specify the cause- and-effect relationship between the medical intervention and the cerebrovascular accident in order to assign a code for intraoperative or postprocedural cerebrovascular accident.

Proper code assignment depends on whether it was an infarction or hemorrhage and whether it occurred intraoperatively or postoperatively. If it was a cerebral hemorrhage, code assignment depends on the type of procedure performed.

d. **Sequelae of Cerebrovascular Disease**

1) **Category I69, Sequelae of Cerebrovascular disease**

Category I69 is used to indicate conditions classifiable to categories I60-I67 as the causes of sequela (neurologic deficits), themselves classified elsewhere. These "late effects" include neurologic deficits that persist after initial onset of conditions classifiable to categories I60-I67. The neurologic deficits caused by cerebrovascular disease may be present from the onset or may arise at any time after the onset of the condition classifiable to categories I60-I67.
Codes from category I69, Sequelae of cerebrovascular disease, that specify hemiplegia, hemiparesis and monoplegia identify whether the dominant or nondominant side is affected. Should the affected side be documented, but not specified as dominant or nondominant, and the classification system does not indicate a default, code selection is as follows:

- For ambidextrous patients, the default should be dominant.

- If the left side is affected, the default is non-dominant.

- If the right side is affected, the default is dominant.

2) **Codes from category I69 with codes from I60-I67**

Codes from category I69 may be assigned on a health care record with codes from I60-I67, if the patient has a current cerebrovascular disease and deficits from an old cerebrovascular disease.

3) **Codes from category I69 and Personal history of transient ischemic attack (TIA) and cerebral infarction (Z86.73)**

Codes from category I69 should not be assigned if the patient does not have neurologic deficits.

See Section I.C.21. 4. History (of) for use of personal history codes

e. **Acute myocardial infarction (AMI)**

1) **Type 1 ST elevation myocardial infarction (STEMI) and non-ST elevation myocardial infarction (NSTEMI)**

The ICD-10-CM codes for type 1 acute myocardial infarction (AMI) identify the site, such as anterolateral wall or true posterior wall. Subcategories I21.0-I21.2 and code I21.3 are used for type 1 ST elevation myocardial infarction (STEMI).

Code I21.4, Non-ST elevation (NSTEMI) myocardial infarction, is used for type 1 non ST elevation myocardial infarction (NSTEMI) and nontransmural MIs. If a type 1 NSTEMI evolves to STEMI, assign the STEMI code. If a type 1 STEMI converts to NSTEMI due to thrombolytic therapy, it is still coded as STEMI.

For encounters occurring while the myocardial infarction is equal to, or less than, four weeks old, including transfers to another acute setting or a postacute setting, and the myocardial infarction **meets** the definition for "other diagnoses" (see Section III, Reporting Additional Diagnoses), codes from category I21 may continue to be reported. For encounters after the 4 week time frame and the patient is still receiving care related to the myocardial infarction, the appropriate aftercare code should be assigned, rather than a code from category I21. For old or healed myocardial infarctions not requiring further care, code I25.2, Old myocardial infarction, may be assigned.

2) Acute myocardial infarction, unspecified

Code I21.9, Acute myocardial infarction, unspecified, is the default for unspecified acute myocardial infarction or unspecified type. If only type 1 STEMI or transmural MI without the site is documented, assign code I21.3, ST elevation (STEMI) myocardial infarction of unspecified site.

3) AMI documented as nontransmural or subendocardial but site provided

If an AMI is documented as nontransmural or subendocardial, but the site is provided, it is still coded as a subendocardial AMI.

See Section I.C.21.3 for information on coding status post administration of tPA in a different facility within the last 24 hours.

4) Subsequent acute myocardial infarction

A code from category I22, Subsequent ST elevation (STEMI) and non-ST elevation (NSTEMI) myocardial infarction, is to be used when a patient who has suffered a type 1 or unspecified AMI has a new AMI within the 4 week time frame of the initial AMI. A code from category I22 must be used in conjunction with a code from category I21. The sequencing of the I22 and I21 codes depends on the circumstances of the encounter. Do not assign code I22 for subsequent myocardial infarctions other than type 1 or unspecified. For subsequent type 2 AMI assign only code I21.A1. For subsequent type 4 or type 5 AMI, assign only code I21.A9.

5) Other Types of Myocardial Infarction

The ICD-10-CM provides codes for different types of myocardial infarction. Type 1 myocardial infarctions are assigned to codes I21.0-I21.4. Type 2 myocardial infarction, and myocardial infarction due to demand ischemia or secondary to ischemic balance, is assigned to code I21.A1, Myocardial infarction type 2 with a code for the underlying cause. Do not assign code I24.8, Other forms of acute ischemic heart disease for the demand ischemia. Sequencing of type 2 AMI or the underlying cause is dependent on the circumstances of admission. When a type 2 AMI code is described as NSTEMI or STEMI, only assign code I21.A1. Codes I21.01-I21.4 should only be assigned for type 1 AMIs. Acute myocardial infarctions type 3, 4a, 4b, 4c and 5 are assigned to code I21.A9, Other myocardial infarction type. The "Code also" and "Code first" notes should be followed related to complications, and for coding of postprocedural myocardial infarctions during or following cardiac surgery.

10. Chapter 10: Diseases of the Respiratory System (J00-J99)

a. Chronic Obstructive Pulmonary Disease [COPD] and Asthma

1) Acute exacerbation of chronic obstructive bronchitis and asthma

The codes in categories J44 and J45 distinguish between uncomplicated cases and those in acute exacerbation. An acute exacerbation is a worsening or a decompensation of a chronic condition. An acute exacerbation is not equivalent to an infection superimposed on a chronic condition, though an exacerbation may be triggered by an infection.

b. Acute Respiratory Failure

1) Acute respiratory failure as principal diagnosis

A code from subcategory J96.0, Acute respiratory failure, or subcategory J96.2, Acute and chronic respiratory failure, may be assigned as a principal diagnosis when it is the condition established after study to be chiefly responsible for occasioning the admission to the hospital, and the selection is supported by the Alphabetic Index and Tabular List. However, chapter-specific coding guidelines (such as obstetrics, poisoning, HIV, newborn) that provide sequencing direction take precedence.

2) Acute respiratory failure as secondary diagnosis

Respiratory failure may be listed as a secondary diagnosis if it occurs after admission, or if it is present on admission, but does not meet the definition of principal diagnosis.

3) Sequencing of acute respiratory failure and another acute condition

When a patient is admitted with respiratory failure and another acute condition, (e.g., myocardial infarction, cerebrovascular accident, aspiration pneumonia), the principal diagnosis will not be the same in every situation. This applies whether the other acute condition is a respiratory or nonrespiratory condition. Selection of the principal diagnosis will be dependent on the circumstances of admission. If both the respiratory failure and the other acute condition are equally responsible for occasioning the admission to the hospital, and there are no chapter-specific sequencing rules, the guideline regarding two or more diagnoses that equally meet the definition for principal diagnosis *(Section II, C.)* may be applied in these situations.

If the documentation is not clear as to whether acute respiratory failure and another condition are equally responsible for occasioning the admission, query the provider for clarification.

c. Influenza due to certain identified influenza viruses

Code only confirmed cases of influenza due to certain identified influenza viruses (category J09), and due to other identified influenza virus (category J10). This is an exception to the hospital inpatient guideline Section II, H. (Uncertain Diagnosis).

In this context, "confirmation" does not require documentation of positive laboratory testing specific for avian or other novel influenza A or other identified influenza virus. However, coding should be based on the provider's diagnostic statement that the patient has avian influenza, or other novel influenza A, for category J09, or has another particular identified strain of influenza, such as H1N1 or H3N2, but not identified as novel or variant, for category J10.

If the provider records "suspected" or "possible" or "probable" avian influenza, or novel influenza, or other identified influenza, then the appropriate influenza code from category J11, Influenza due to unidentified influenza virus, should be assigned. A code from category J09, Influenza due to certain identified influenza viruses, should not be assigned nor should a code from category J10, Influenza due to other identified influenza virus.

d. Ventilator associated Pneumonia

1) Documentation of Ventilator associated Pneumonia

As with all procedural or postprocedural complications, code assignment is based on the provider's documentation of the relationship between the condition and the procedure.

Code J95.851, Ventilator associated pneumonia, should be assigned only when the provider has documented ventilator associated pneumonia (VAP). An additional code to identify the organism (e.g., Pseudomonas aeruginosa, code B96.5) should also be assigned. Do not assign an additional code from categories J12-J18 to identify the type of pneumonia.

Code J95.851 should not be assigned for cases where the patient has pneumonia and is on a mechanical ventilator and the provider has not specifically stated that the pneumonia is ventilator-associated pneumonia. If the documentation is unclear as to whether the patient has a pneumonia that is a complication attributable to the mechanical ventilator, query the provider.

2) Ventilator associated Pneumonia Develops after Admission

A patient may be admitted with one type of pneumonia (e.g., code J13, Pneumonia due to Streptococcus pneumonia) and subsequently develop VAP. In this instance, the principal diagnosis would be the appropriate code from categories J12-

J18 for the pneumonia diagnosed at the time of admission. Code J95.851, Ventilator associated pneumonia, would be assigned as an additional diagnosis when the provider has also documented the presence of ventilator associated pneumonia.

11. Chapter 11: Diseases of the Digestive System (K00-K95)

Reserved for future guideline expansion

12. Chapter 12: Diseases of the Skin and Subcutaneous Tissue (L00-L99)

a. Pressure ulcer stage codes

1) Pressure ulcer stages

Codes from category L89, Pressure ulcer, identify the site of the pressure ulcer as well as the stage of the ulcer.

The ICD-10-CM classifies pressure ulcer stages based on severity, which is designated by stages 1-4, unspecified stage and unstageable.

Assign as many codes from category L89 as needed to identify all the pressure ulcers the patient has, if applicable.

2) Unstageable pressure ulcers

Assignment of the code for unstageable pressure ulcer (L89.--0) should be based on the clinical documentation. These codes are used for pressure ulcers whose stage cannot be clinically determined (e.g., the ulcer is covered by eschar or has been treated with a skin or muscle graft) and pressure ulcers that are documented as deep tissue injury but not documented as due to trauma. This code should not be confused with the codes for unspecified stage (L89.--9). When there is no documentation regarding the stage of the pressure ulcer, assign the appropriate code for unspecified stage (L89.--9).

3) Documented pressure ulcer stage

Assignment of the pressure ulcer stage code should be guided by clinical documentation of the stage or documentation of the terms found in the Alphabetic Index. For clinical terms describing the stage that are not found in the Alphabetic Index, and there is no documentation of the stage, the provider should be queried.

4) Patients admitted with pressure ulcers documented as healed

No code is assigned if the documentation states that the pressure ulcer is completely healed.

5) Patients admitted with pressure ulcers documented as healing

Pressure ulcers described as healing should be assigned the appropriate pressure ulcer stage code based on the documentation in the medical record. If the documentation does not provide information about the stage of the healing pressure ulcer, assign the appropriate code for unspecified stage.

If the documentation is unclear as to whether the patient has a current (new) pressure ulcer or if the patient is being treated for a healing pressure ulcer, query the provider.

For ulcers that were present on admission but healed at the time of discharge, assign the code for the site and stage of the pressure ulcer at the time of admission.

6) **Patient admitted with pressure ulcer evolving into another stage during the admission**

If a patient is admitted with a pressure ulcer at one stage and it progresses to a higher stage, two separate codes should be assigned: one code for the site and stage of the ulcer on admission and a second code for the same ulcer site and the highest stage reported during the stay.

b. **Non-Pressure Chronic Ulcers**

1) Patients admitted with non-pressure ulcers documented as healed

No code is assigned if the documentation states that the nonpressure ulcer is completely healed.

2) Patients admitted with non-pressure ulcers documented as healing

Non-pressure ulcers described as healing should be assigned the appropriate non-pressure ulcer code based on the documentation in the medical record. If the documentation does not provide information about the severity of the healing non-pressure ulcer, assign the appropriate code for unspecified severity.

If the documentation is unclear as to whether the patient has a current (new) non-pressure ulcer or if the patient is being treated for a healing non-pressure ulcer, query the provider.

For ulcers that were present on admission but healed at the time of discharge, assign the code for the site and severity of the non-pressure ulcer at the time of admission.

3) Patient admitted with non-pressure ulcer that progresses to another severity level during the Admission

If a patient is admitted to an inpatient hospital with a nonpressure ulcer at one severity level and it progresses to a higher severity level, two separate codes should be assigned:

one code for the site and severity level of the ulcer on admission and a second code for the same ulcer site and the highest severity level reported during the stay.

13. **Chapter 13: Diseases of the Musculoskeletal System and Connective Tissue (M00-M99)**

a. **Site and laterality**

Most of the codes within Chapter 13 have site and laterality designations. The site represents the bone, joint or the muscle involved. For some conditions where more than one bone, joint or muscle is usually involved, such as osteoarthritis, there is a "multiple sites" code available. For categories where no multiple site code is provided and more than one bone, joint or muscle is involved, multiple codes should be used to indicate the different sites involved.

1) **Bone versus joint**

For certain conditions, the bone may be affected at the upper or lower end, (e.g., avascular necrosis of bone, M87, Osteoporosis, M80, M81). Though the portion of the bone affected may be at the joint, the site designation will be the bone, not the joint.

b. **Acute traumatic versus chronic or recurrent musculoskeletal conditions**

Many musculoskeletal conditions are a result of previous injury or trauma to a site, or are recurrent conditions. Bone, joint or muscle conditions that are the result of a healed injury are usually found in chapter 13. Recurrent bone, joint or muscle conditions are also usually found in chapter 13. Any current, acute injury should be coded to the appropriate injury code from chapter 19. Chronic or recurrent conditions should generally be coded with a code from chapter 13. If it is difficult to determine from the documentation in the record which code is best to describe a condition, query the provider.

c. Coding of Pathologic Fractures

7th character A is for use as long as the patient is receiving active treatment for the fracture. While the patient may be seen by a new or different provider over the course of treatment for a pathological fracture, assignment of the 7th character is based on whether the patient is undergoing active treatment and not whether the provider is seeing the patient for the first time.

7th character D is to be used for encounters after the patient has completed active treatment for the fracture and is receiving routine care for the fracture during the healing or recovery phase. The other 7th characters, listed under each subcategory in the Tabular List, are to be used for subsequent encounters for treatment of problems associated with the healing, such as malunions, nonunions, and sequelae.

Care for complications of surgical treatment for fracture repairs during the healing or recovery phase should be coded with the appropriate complication codes.

See Section I.C.19. Coding of traumatic fractures.

d. Osteoporosis

Osteoporosis is a systemic condition, meaning that all bones of the musculoskeletal system are affected. Therefore, site is not a component of the codes under category M81, Osteoporosis without current pathological fracture. The site codes under category M80, Osteoporosis with current pathological fracture, identify the site of the fracture, not the osteoporosis.

1) Osteoporosis without pathological fracture

Category M81, Osteoporosis without current pathological fracture, is for use for patients with osteoporosis who do not currently have a pathologic fracture due to the osteoporosis, even if they have had a fracture in the past. For patients with a history of osteoporosis fractures, status code Z87.310, Personal history of (healed) osteoporosis fracture, should follow the code from M81.

2) Osteoporosis with current pathological fracture

Category M80, Osteoporosis with current pathological fracture, is for patients who have a current pathologic fracture at the time of an encounter. The codes under M80 identify the site of the fracture. A code from category M80, not a traumatic fracture code, should be used for any patient with known osteoporosis who suffers a fracture, even if the patient had a minor fall or trauma, if that fall or trauma would not usually break a normal, healthy bone.

14. Chapter 14: Diseases of Genitourinary System (N00-N99)

a. Chronic kidney disease

1) Stages of chronic kidney disease (CKD)

The ICD-10-CM classifies CKD based on severity. The severity of CKD is designated by stages 1-5. Stage 2, code N18.2, equates to mild CKD; stage 3, code N18.3, equates to moderate CKD; and stage 4, code N18.4, equates to severe CKD. Code N18.6, End stage renal disease (ESRD), is assigned when the provider has documented end-stage-renal disease (ESRD).

If both a stage of CKD and ESRD are documented, assign code N18.6 only.

2) Chronic kidney disease and kidney transplant status

Patients who have undergone kidney transplant may still have some form of chronic kidney disease (CKD) because the kidney transplant may not fully restore kidney function. Therefore, the presence of CKD alone does not constitute a transplant complication. Assign the appropriate N18 code for the patient's stage of CKD and code Z94.0, Kidney transplant status. If a transplant complication such as failure or rejection or other transplant complication is documented, see section I.C.19.g for information on coding complications of a kidney transplant. If the documentation is unclear as to whether the patient has a complication of the transplant, query the provider.

3) Chronic kidney disease with other conditions

Patients with CKD may also suffer from other serious conditions, most commonly diabetes mellitus and hypertension. The sequencing of the CKD code in relationship to codes for other contributing conditions is based on the conventions in the Tabular List.

See I.C.9. Hypertensive chronic kidney disease.
See I.C.19. Chronic kidney disease and kidney transplant complications.

15. Chapter 15: Pregnancy, Childbirth, and the Puerperium (O00-O9A)

a. General Rules for Obstetric Cases

1) Codes from chapter 15 and sequencing priority

Obstetric cases require codes from chapter 15, codes in the range O00-O9A, Pregnancy, Childbirth, and the Puerperium. Chapter 15 codes have sequencing priority over codes from other chapters. Additional codes from other chapters may be used in conjunction with chapter 15 codes to further specify conditions. Should the provider document that the pregnancy is incidental to the encounter, then code Z33.1, Pregnant state, incidental, should be used in place of any chapter 15 codes. It is the provider's responsibility to state that the condition being treated is not affecting the pregnancy.

2) Chapter 15 codes used only on the maternal record

Chapter 15 codes are to be used only on the maternal record, never on the record of the newborn.

3) Final character for trimester

The majority of codes in Chapter 15 have a final character indicating the trimester of pregnancy. The timeframes for the trimesters are indicated at the beginning of the chapter. If trimester is not a component of a code, it is because the condition always occurs in a specific trimester, or the concept of trimester of pregnancy is not applicable. Certain codes have characters for only certain trimesters because the condition does not occur in all trimesters, but it may occur in more than just one.

Assignment of the final character for trimester should be based on the provider's documentation of the trimester (or number of weeks) for the current admission/encounter. This applies to the assignment of trimester for pre-existing conditions as well as those that develop during or are due to the pregnancy. The provider's documentation of the number of weeks may be used to assign the appropriate code identifying the trimester.

Whenever delivery occurs during the current admission, and there is an "in childbirth" option for the obstetric complication being coded, the "in childbirth" code should be assigned.

4) Selection of trimester for inpatient admissions that encompass more than one trimester

In instances when a patient is admitted to a hospital for complications of pregnancy during one trimester and remains in the hospital into a subsequent trimester, the trimester character for the antepartum complication code should be assigned on the basis of the trimester when the complication developed, not the trimester of the discharge. If the condition developed prior to the current admission/encounter or represents a pre-existing condition, the trimester character for the trimester at the time of the admission/encounter should be assigned.

5) Unspecified trimester

Each category that includes codes for trimester has a code for "unspecified trimester." The "unspecified trimester" code should rarely be used, such as when the documentation in the record is insufficient to determine the trimester and it is not possible to obtain clarification.

6) 7th character for Fetus Identification

Where applicable, a 7th character is to be assigned for certain categories (O31, O32, O33.3 - O33.6, O35, O36, O40, O41, O60.1, O60.2, O64, and O69) to identify the fetus for which the complication code applies.

Assign 7th character "0":

- For single gestations

- When the documentation in the record is insufficient to determine the fetus affected and it is not possible to obtain clarification.

- When it is not possible to clinically determine which fetus is affected.

b. Selection of OB Principal or First-listed Diagnosis

1) Routine outpatient prenatal visits

For routine outpatient prenatal visits when no complications are present, a code from category Z34, Encounter for supervision of normal pregnancy, should be used as the first-listed diagnosis. These codes should not be used in conjunction with chapter 15 codes.

2) *Supervision of High-Risk Pregnancy*

Codes from category O09, Supervision of high-risk pregnancy, are intended for use only during the prenatal period. For complications during the labor or delivery episode as a result of a high-risk pregnancy, assign the applicable complication codes from Chapter 15. If there are no complications during the labor or delivery episode, assign code O80, Encounter for full-term uncomplicated delivery.

For routine prenatal outpatient visits for patients with high-risk pregnancies, a code from category O09, Supervision of high-risk pregnancy, should be used as the first-listed diagnosis. Secondary chapter 15 codes may be used in conjunction with these codes if appropriate.

3) Episodes when no delivery occurs

In episodes when no delivery occurs, the principal diagnosis should correspond to the principal complication of the pregnancy which necessitated the encounter. Should more than one complication exist, all of which are treated or monitored, any of the complications codes may be sequenced first.

4) When a delivery occurs

When an obstetric patient is admitted and delivers during that admission, the condition that prompted the admission should be sequenced as the principal diagnosis. If multiple conditions prompted the admission, sequence the one most related to the delivery as the principal diagnosis. A code for any complication of the delivery should be assigned as an additional diagnosis. In cases of cesarean delivery, if the patient was admitted with a condition that resulted in the performance of a cesarean procedure, that condition should be selected as the principal diagnosis. If the reason for the admission was unrelated to the condition resulting in the cesarean delivery, the condition related to the reason for the admission should be selected as the principal diagnosis.

5) Outcome of delivery

A code from category Z37, Outcome of delivery, should be included on every maternal record when a delivery has occurred. These codes are not to be used on subsequent records or on the newborn record.

c. Pre-existing conditions versus conditions due to the pregnancy

Certain categories in Chapter 15 distinguish between conditions of the mother that existed prior to pregnancy (pre-existing) and those that are a direct result of pregnancy. When assigning codes from Chapter 15, it is important to assess if a condition was pre-existing prior to pregnancy or developed during or due to the pregnancy in order to assign the correct code.

Categories that do not distinguish between pre-existing and pregnancy-related conditions may be used for either. It is acceptable to use codes specifically for the puerperium with codes complicating pregnancy and childbirth if a condition arises postpartum during the delivery encounter.

d. Pre-existing hypertension in pregnancy

Category O10, Pre-existing hypertension complicating pregnancy, childbirth and the puerperium, includes codes for hypertensive heart and hypertensive chronic kidney disease. When assigning one of the O10 codes that includes hypertensive heart disease or hypertensive chronic kidney disease, it is necessary to add a secondary code from the appropriate hypertension category to specify the type of heart failure or chronic kidney disease.

See Section I.C.9. Hypertension.

e. Fetal Conditions Affecting the Management of the Mother

1) Codes from categories O35 and O36

Codes from categories O35, Maternal care for known or suspected fetal abnormality and damage, and O36, Maternal care for other fetal problems, are assigned only when the fetal condition is actually responsible for modifying the management of the mother, i.e., by requiring diagnostic studies, additional observation, special care, or termination of pregnancy. The fact that the fetal condition exists does not justify assigning a code from this series to the mother's record.

2) In utero surgery

In cases when surgery is performed on the fetus, a diagnosis code from category O35, Maternal care for known or suspected fetal abnormality and damage, should be assigned identifying the fetal condition. Assign the appropriate procedure code for the procedure performed.

No code from Chapter 16, the perinatal codes, should be used on the mother's record to identify fetal conditions. Surgery performed in utero on a fetus is still to be coded as an obstetric encounter.

f. HIV Infection in Pregnancy, Childbirth and the Puerperium

During pregnancy, childbirth or the puerperium, a patient admitted because of an HIV-related illness should receive a principal diagnosis from subcategory O98.7-, Human immunodeficiency [HIV] disease complicating pregnancy, childbirth and the puerperium, followed by the code(s) for the HIV-related illness(es).

Patients with asymptomatic HIV infection status admitted during pregnancy, childbirth, or the puerperium should receive codes of O98.7- and Z21, Asymptomatic human immunodeficiency virus [HIV] infection status.

g. Diabetes mellitus in pregnancy

Diabetes mellitus is a significant complicating factor in pregnancy. Pregnant women who are diabetic should be assigned a code from category O24, Diabetes mellitus in pregnancy, childbirth, and the puerperium, first, followed by the appropriate diabetes code(s) (E08-E13) from Chapter 4.

h.   Long term use of insulin and oral hypoglycemics

Code Z79.4, Long-term (current) use of insulin, or code Z79.84, Long-term (current) use of oral hypoglycemic drugs, should also be assigned if the diabetes mellitus is being treated with insulin or oral medications. If the patient is treated with both oral medications and insulin, only the code for insulin-controlled should be assigned.

i.   Gestational (pregnancy induced) diabetes

Gestational (pregnancy induced) diabetes can occur during the second and third trimester of pregnancy in women who were not diabetic prior to pregnancy. Gestational diabetes can cause complications in the pregnancy similar to those of pre-existing diabetes mellitus. It also puts the woman at greater risk of developing diabetes after the pregnancy. Codes for gestational diabetes are in subcategory O24.4, Gestational diabetes mellitus. No other code from category O24, Diabetes mellitus in pregnancy, childbirth, and the puerperium, should be used with a code from O24.4.

The codes under subcategory O24.4 include diet controlled, insulin controlled, and controlled by oral hypoglycemic drugs. If a patient with gestational diabetes is treated with both diet and insulin, only the code for insulin-controlled is required. If a patient with gestational diabetes is treated with both diet and oral hypoglycemic medications, only the code for "controlled by oral hypoglycemic drugs" is required. Code Z79.4, Long-term (current) use of insulin or code Z79.84, Long-term (current) use of oral hypoglycemic drugs, should not be assigned with codes from subcategory O24.4.

An abnormal glucose tolerance in pregnancy is assigned a code from subcategory O99.81, Abnormal glucose complicating pregnancy, childbirth, and the puerperium.

j.   Sepsis and septic shock complicating abortion, pregnancy, childbirth and the puerperium

When assigning a chapter 15 code for sepsis complicating abortion, pregnancy, childbirth, and the puerperium, a code for the specific type of infection should be assigned as an additional diagnosis. If severe sepsis is present, a code from subcategory R65.2, Severe sepsis, and code(s) for associated organ dysfunction(s) should also be assigned as additional diagnoses.

k.   Puerperal sepsis

Code O85, Puerperal sepsis, should be assigned with a secondary code to identify the causal organism (e.g., for a bacterial infection, assign a code from category B95-B96, Bacterial infections in conditions classified elsewhere). A code from category A40, Streptococcal sepsis, or A41, Other sepsis, should not be used for puerperal sepsis. If applicable, use additional codes to identify severe sepsis (R65.2-) and any associated acute organ dysfunction.

l.   Alcohol and tobacco use during pregnancy, childbirth and the puerperium

1)   Alcohol use during pregnancy, childbirth and the puerperium

Codes under subcategory O99.31, Alcohol use complicating pregnancy, childbirth, and the puerperium, should be assigned for any pregnancy case when a mother uses alcohol during the pregnancy or postpartum. A secondary code from category F10, Alcohol related disorders, should also be assigned to identify manifestations of the alcohol use.

2)   Tobacco use during pregnancy, childbirth and the puerperium

Codes under subcategory O99.33, Smoking (tobacco) complicating pregnancy, childbirth, and the puerperium, should be assigned for any pregnancy case when a mother uses any type of tobacco product during the pregnancy or postpartum. A secondary code from category F17, Nicotine dependence, should also be assigned to identify the type of nicotine dependence.

m. Poisoning, toxic effects, adverse effects and underdosing in a pregnant patient

A code from subcategory O9A.2, Injury, poisoning and certain other consequences of external causes complicating pregnancy, childbirth, and the puerperium, should be sequenced first, followed by the appropriate injury, poisoning, toxic effect, adverse effect or underdosing code, and then the additional code(s) that specifies the condition caused by the poisoning, toxic effect, adverse effect or underdosing.

See Section I.C.19. Adverse effects, poisoning, underdosing and toxic effects.

n. Normal Delivery, Code O80

1) Encounter for full term uncomplicated delivery

Code O80 should be assigned when a woman is admitted for a full-term normal delivery and delivers a single, healthy infant without any complications antepartum, during the delivery, or postpartum during the delivery episode. Code O80 is always a principal diagnosis. It is not to be used if any other code from chapter 15 is needed to describe a current complication of the antenatal, delivery, or perinatal period. Additional codes from other chapters may be used with code O80 if they are not related to or are in any way complicating the pregnancy.

2) Uncomplicated delivery with resolved antepartum complication

Code O80 may be used if the patient had a complication at some point during the pregnancy, but the complication is not present at the time of the admission for delivery.

3) Outcome of delivery for O80

Z37.0, Single live birth, is the only outcome of delivery code appropriate for use with O80.

o. The Peripartum and Postpartum Periods

1) Peripartum and Postpartum periods

The postpartum period begins immediately after delivery and continues for six weeks following delivery. The peripartum period is defined as the last month of pregnancy to five months postpartum.

2) Peripartum and postpartum complication

A postpartum complication is any complication occurring within the six-week period.

3) Pregnancy-related complications after 6 week period

Chapter 15 codes may also be used to describe pregnancy-related complications after the peripartum or postpartum period if the provider documents that a condition is pregnancy related.

4) Admission for routine postpartum care following delivery outside hospital

When the mother delivers outside the hospital prior to admission and is admitted for routine postpartum care and no complications are noted, code Z39.0, Encounter for care and examination of mother immediately after delivery, should be assigned as the principal diagnosis.

5) Pregnancy associated cardiomyopathy

Pregnancy associated cardiomyopathy, code O90.3, is unique in that it may be diagnosed in the third trimester of pregnancy but may continue to progress months after delivery. For this reason, it is referred to as peripartum cardiomyopathy. Code O90.3 is only for use when the cardiomyopathy develops as a result of pregnancy in a woman who did not have pre-existing heart disease.

p. Code O94, Sequelae of complication of pregnancy, childbirth, and the puerperium

1) Code O94

Code O94, Sequelae of complication of pregnancy, childbirth, and the puerperium, is for use in those cases when an initial complication of a pregnancy develops a sequelae requiring care or treatment at a future date.

2) After the initial postpartum period

This code may be used at any time after the initial postpartum period.

3) Sequencing of Code O94

This code, like all sequela codes, is to be sequenced following the code describing the sequelae of the complication.

q. *Termination of Pregnancy and Spontaneous abortions*

1) Abortion with Liveborn Fetus

When an attempted termination of pregnancy results in a liveborn fetus, assign code Z33.2, Encounter for elective termination of pregnancy and a code from category Z37, Outcome of Delivery.

2) Retained Products of Conception following an abortion

Subsequent encounters for retained products of conception following a spontaneous abortion or elective termination of pregnancy, without complications are assigned O03.4, Incomplete spontaneous, abortion without complication, or codes O07.4, Failed attempted termination of pregnancy without complication. This advice is appropriate even when the patient was discharged previously with a discharge diagnosis of complete abortion. If the patient has a specific complication associated with the spontaneous abortion or elective termination of pregnancy in addition to retained products of conception, assign the appropriate complication in category O03 or O07 instead of code O03.4 or O07.4

3) Complications leading to abortion

Codes from Chapter 15 may be used as additional codes to identify any documented complications of the pregnancy in conjunction with codes in categories in O07 and O08.

r. Abuse in a pregnant patient

For suspected or confirmed cases of abuse of a pregnant patient, a code(s) from subcategories O9A.3, Physical abuse complicating pregnancy, childbirth, and the puerperium, O9A.4, Sexual abuse complicating pregnancy, childbirth, and the puerperium, and O9A.5, Psychological abuse complicating pregnancy, childbirth, and the puerperium, should be sequenced first, followed by the appropriate codes (if applicable) to identify any associated current injury due to physical abuse, sexual abuse, and the perpetrator of abuse.

See Section I.C.19. Adult and child abuse, neglect and other maltreatment.

16. Chapter 16: Certain Conditions Originating in the Perinatal Period (P00-P96)

For coding and reporting purposes the perinatal period is defined as before birth through the 28th day following birth. The following guidelines are provided for reporting purposes.

a. General Perinatal Rules

1) Use of Chapter 16 Codes
Codes in this chapter are <u>never</u> for use on the maternal record. Codes from Chapter 15, the obstetric chapter, are never permitted on the newborn record. Chapter 16 codes may be used throughout the life of the patient if the condition is still present.

2) Principal Diagnosis for Birth Record

When coding the birth episode in a newborn record, assign a code from category Z38, Liveborn infants according to place of birth and type of delivery, as the principal diagnosis. A code from category Z38 is assigned only once, to a newborn at the time of birth. If a newborn is transferred to another institution, a code from category Z38 should not be used at the receiving hospital.

A code from category Z38 is used only on the newborn record, not on the mother's record.

3) Use of Codes from other Chapters with Codes from Chapter 16

Codes from other chapters may be used with codes from chapter 16 if the codes from the other chapters provide more specific detail. Codes for signs and symptoms may be assigned when a definitive diagnosis has not been established. If the reason for the encounter is a perinatal condition, the code from chapter 16 should be sequenced first.

4) Use of Chapter 16 Codes after the Perinatal Period

Should a condition originate in the perinatal period, and continue throughout the life of the patient, the perinatal code should continue to be used regardless of the patient's age.

5) Birth process or community acquired conditions

If a newborn has a condition that may be either due to the birth process or community acquired and the documentation does not indicate which it is, the default is due to the birth process and the code from Chapter 16 should be used. If the condition is community-acquired, a code from Chapter 16 should not be assigned.

6) Code all clinically significant conditions

All clinically significant conditions noted on routine newborn examination should be coded. A condition is clinically significant if it requires:

§ clinical evaluation; or

§ therapeutic treatment; or

§ diagnostic procedures; or

§ extended length of hospital stay; or

§ increased nursing care and/or monitoring; or

§ has implications for future health care needs

Note: The perinatal guidelines listed above are the same as the general coding guidelines for "additional diagnoses", except for the final point regarding implications for future health care needs. Codes should be assigned for conditions that have been specified by the provider as having implications for future health care needs.

b. Observation and Evaluation of Newborns for Suspected Conditions not Found

1) Assign a code from category Z05, Observation and evaluation of newborns and infants for suspected conditions ruled out, to identify those instances when a healthy newborn is evaluated for a suspected condition that is determined after study not to be present. Do not use a code from category Z05 when the patient has identified signs or symptoms of a suspected problem; in such cases code the sign or symptom.

2) A code from category Z05 may also be assigned as a principal or first-listed code for readmissions or encounters when the code from category Z38 code no longer applies. Codes from category Z05 are for use only for healthy newborns and infants for which no condition after study is found to be present.

3) Z05 on a birth record

A code from category Z05 is to be used as a secondary code after the code from category Z38, liveborn infants according to place of birth and type of delivery.

c. **Coding Additional Perinatal Diagnoses**

1) **Assigning codes for conditions that require treatment**

Assign codes for conditions that require treatment or further investigation, prolong the length of stay, or require resource utilization.

2) **Codes for conditions specified as having implications for future health care needs**

Assign codes for conditions that have been specified by the provider as having implications for future health care needs.

Note: This guideline should not be used for adult patients.

d. **Prematurity and Fetal Growth Retardation**

Providers utilize different criteria in determining prematurity. A code for prematurity should not be assigned unless it is documented. Assignment of codes in categories P05, Disorders of newborn related to slow fetal growth and fetal malnutrition, and P07, Disorders of newborn related to short gestation and low birth weight, not elsewhere classified, should be based on the recorded birth weight and estimated gestational age. Codes from category P05 should not be assigned with codes from category P07.

When both birth weight and gestational age are available, two codes from category P07 should be assigned, with the code for birth weight sequenced before the code for gestational age.

e. **Low birth weight and immaturity status**

Codes from category P07, Disorders of newborn related to short gestation and low birth weight, not elsewhere classified, are for use for a child or adult who was premature or had a low birth weight as a newborn and this is affecting the patient's current health status.

See Section I.C.21. Factors influencing health status and contact with health services, Status.

f. **Bacterial Sepsis of Newborn**

Category P36, Bacterial sepsis of newborn, includes congenital sepsis. If a perinate is documented as having sepsis without documentation of congenital or community acquired, the default is congenital and a code from category P36 should be assigned. If the P36 code includes the causal organism, an additional code from category B95, Streptococcus, Staphylococcus, and Enterococcus as the cause of diseases classified elsewhere, or B96, Other bacterial agents as the cause of diseases classified elsewhere, should not be assigned. If the P36 code does not include the causal organism, assign an additional code from category B96. If applicable, use additional codes to identify severe sepsis (R65.2-) and any associated acute organ dysfunction.

g. **Stillbirth**

Code P95, Stillbirth, is only for use in institutions that maintain separate records for stillbirths. No other code should be used with P95. Code P95 should not be used on the mother's record.

17. Chapter 17: Congenital malformations, deformations, and chromosomal abnormalities (Q00-Q99)

Assign an appropriate code(s) from categories Q00-Q99, Congenital malformations, deformations, and chromosomal abnormalities when a malformation/deformation or chromosomal abnormality is documented. A malformation/deformation/or chromosomal abnormality may be the principal/first-listed diagnosis on a record or a secondary diagnosis.

When a malformation/deformation or chromosomal abnormality does not have a unique code assignment, assign additional code(s) for any manifestations that may be present.

When the code assignment specifically identifies the malformation/deformation or chromosomal abnormality, manifestations that are an inherent component of the anomaly should not be coded separately. Additional codes should be assigned for manifestations that are not an inherent component.

Codes from Chapter 17 may be used throughout the life of the patient. If a congenital malformation or deformity has been corrected, a personal history code should be used to identify the history of the malformation or deformity. Although present at birth, malformation/deformation/or chromosomal abnormality may not be identified until later in life. Whenever the condition is diagnosed by the physician, it is appropriate to assign a code from codes Q00-Q99.For the birth admission, the appropriate code from category Z38, Liveborn infants, according to place of birth and type of delivery, should be sequenced as the principal diagnosis, followed by any congenital anomaly codes, Q00-Q99.

18. Chapter 18: Symptoms, signs, and abnormal clinical and laboratory findings, not elsewhere classified (R00-R99)

Chapter 18 includes symptoms, signs, abnormal results of clinical or other investigative procedures, and ill-defined conditions regarding which no diagnosis classifiable elsewhere is recorded. Signs and symptoms that point to a specific diagnosis have been assigned to a category in other chapters of the classification.

a. Use of symptom codes

Codes that describe symptoms and signs are acceptable for reporting purposes when a related definitive diagnosis has not been established (confirmed) by the provider.

b. Use of a symptom code with a definitive diagnosis code

Codes for signs and symptoms may be reported in addition to a related definitive diagnosis when the sign or symptom is not routinely associated with that diagnosis, such as the various signs and symptoms associated with complex syndromes. The definitive diagnosis code should be sequenced before the symptom code.

Signs or symptoms that are associated routinely with a disease process should not be assigned as additional codes, unless otherwise instructed by the classification.

c. Combination codes that include symptoms

ICD-10-CM contains a number of combination codes that identify both the definitive diagnosis and common symptoms of that diagnosis. When using one of these combination codes, an additional code should not be assigned for the symptom.

d. Repeated falls

Code R29.6, Repeated falls, is for use for encounters when a patient has recently fallen and the reason for the fall is being investigated.

Code Z91.81, History of falling, is for use when a patient has fallen in the past and is at risk for future falls. When appropriate, both codes R29.6 and Z91.81 may be assigned together.

e. Coma scale

The coma scale codes (R40.2-) can be used in conjunction with traumatic brain injury codes, acute cerebrovascular disease or sequelae of cerebrovascular disease codes. These codes are primarily for use by trauma registries, but they may be used in any setting where this information is collected. The coma scale may also be used to assess the status of the central nervous system for other non-trauma conditions, such as monitoring patients in the intensive care unit regardless of medical condition. The coma scale codes should be sequenced after the diagnosis code(s).

These codes, one from each subcategory, are needed to complete the scale. The 7th character indicates when the scale was recorded. The 7th character should match for all three codes.

At a minimum, report the initial score documented on presentation at your facility. This may be a score from the emergency medicine technician (EMT) or in the emergency department. If desired, a facility may choose to capture multiple coma scale scores.

Assign code R40.24, Glasgow coma scale, total score, when only the total score is documented in the medical record and not the individual score(s).

f. Functional quadriplegia

GUIDELINE HAS BEEN DELETED EFFECTIVE OCTOBER 1, 2017

g. SIRS due to Non-Infectious Process

The systemic inflammatory response syndrome (SIRS) can develop as a result of certain non-infectious disease processes, such as trauma, malignant neoplasm, or pancreatitis. When SIRS is documented with a noninfectious condition, and no subsequent infection is documented, the code for the underlying condition, such as an injury, should be assigned, followed by code R65.10, Systemic inflammatory response syndrome (SIRS) of non-infectious origin without acute organ dysfunction, or code R65.11, Systemic inflammatory response syndrome (SIRS) of non-infectious origin with acute organ dysfunction. If an associated acute organ dysfunction is documented, the appropriate code(s) for the specific type of organ dysfunction(s) should be assigned in addition to code R65.11. If acute organ dysfunction is documented, but it cannot be determined if the acute organ dysfunction is associated with SIRS or due to another condition (e.g., directly due to the trauma), the provider should be queried.

h. Death NOS

Code R99, Ill-defined and unknown cause of mortality, is only for use in the very limited circumstance when a patient who has already died is brought into an emergency department or other healthcare facility and is pronounced dead upon arrival. It does not represent the discharge disposition of death.

i. NIHSS Stroke Scale

The NIH stroke scale (NIHSS) codes (R29.7- -) can be used in conjunction with acute stroke codes (I63) to identify the patient's neurological status and the severity of the stroke. The stroke scale codes should be sequenced after the acute stroke diagnosis code(s).

At a minimum, report the initial score documented. If desired, a facility may choose to capture multiple stroke scale scores.

See Section I.B.14.for information concerning the medical record documentation that may be used for assignment of the NIHSS codes.

19. Chapter 19: Injury, poisoning, and certain other consequences of external causes (S00-T88)

a. Application of 7th Characters in Chapter 19

Most categories in chapter 19 have a 7th character requirement for each applicable code. Most categories in this chapter have three 7th character values (with the exception of fractures): A, initial encounter, D, subsequent encounter and S, sequela. Categories for traumatic fractures have additional 7th character values. While the patient may be seen by a new or different provider over the course of treatment for an injury, assignment of the 7th character is based on whether the patient is undergoing active treatment and not whether the provider is seeing the patient for the first time.

For complication codes, active treatment refers to treatment for the condition described by the code, even though it may be related to an earlier precipitating problem. For example, code T84.50XA, Infection and inflammatory reaction due to unspecified internal joint prosthesis, initial encounter, is used when active treatment is provided for the infection, even though the condition relates to the prosthetic device, implant or graft that was placed at a previous encounter.

7th character "A", initial encounter is used for each encounter where the patient is receiving active treatment for the condition.

7th character "D" subsequent encounter is used for encounters after the patient has completed active treatment of the condition and is receiving routine care for the condition during the healing or recovery phase.

The aftercare Z codes should not be used for aftercare for conditions such as injuries or poisonings, where 7th characters are provided to identify subsequent care. For example, for aftercare of an injury, assign the acute injury code with the 7th character "D" (subsequent encounter).

7th character "S", sequela, is for use for complications or conditions that arise as a direct result of a condition, such as scar formation after a burn. The scars are sequelae of the burn. When using 7th character "S", it is necessary to use both the injury code that precipitated the sequela and the code for the sequela itself. The "S" is added only to the injury code, not the sequela code. The 7th character "S" identifies the injury responsible for the sequela. The specific type of sequela (e.g. scar) is sequenced first, followed by the injury code.

See Section I.B.10 Sequelae, (Late Effects)

b. Coding of Injuries

When coding injuries, assign separate codes for each injury unless a combination code is provided, in which case the combination code is assigned. Codes from category T07, Unspecified multiple injuries should not be assigned in the inpatient setting unless information for a more specific code is not available. Traumatic injury codes (S00-T14.9) are not to be used for normal, healing surgical wounds or to identify complications of surgical wounds.

The code for the most serious injury, as determined by the provider and the focus of treatment, is sequenced first.

1) Superficial injuries

Superficial injuries such as abrasions or contusions are not coded when associated with more severe injuries of the same site.

2) Primary injury with damage to nerves/blood vessels

When a primary injury results in minor damage to peripheral nerves or blood vessels, the primary injury is sequenced first with additional code(s) for injuries to nerves and spinal cord (such as category S04), and/or injury to blood vessels (such as category S15). When the primary injury is to the blood vessels or nerves, that injury should be sequenced first.

c. Coding of Traumatic Fractures

The principles of multiple coding of injuries should be followed in coding fractures. Fractures of specified sites are coded individually by site in accordance with both the provisions within categories S02, S12, S22,

S32, S42, S49, S52, S59, S62, S72, S79, S82, S89, S92 and the level of detail furnished by medical record content.

A fracture not indicated as open or closed should be coded to closed. A fracture not indicated whether displaced or not displaced should be coded to displaced.

More specific guidelines are as follows:

1) **Initial vs. Subsequent Encounter for Fractures**

Traumatic fractures are coded using the appropriate 7th character for initial encounter (A, B, C) for each encounter where the patient is receiving active treatment for the fracture. The appropriate 7th character for initial encounter should also be assigned for a patient who delayed seeking treatment for the fracture or nonunion.

Fractures are coded using the appropriate 7th character for subsequent care for encounters after the patient has completed active treatment of the fracture and is receiving routine care for the fracture during the healing or recovery phase.

Care for complications of surgical treatment for fracture repairs during the healing or recovery phase should be coded with the appropriate complication codes.

Care of complications of fractures, such as malunion and nonunion, should be reported with the appropriate 7th character for subsequent care with nonunion (K, M, N,) or subsequent care with malunion (P, Q, R).

Malunion/nonunion: The appropriate 7th character for initial encounter should also be assigned for a patient who delayed seeking treatment for the fracture or nonunion.

The open fracture designations in the assignment of the 7th character for fractures of the forearm, femur and lower leg, including ankle are based on the Gustilo open fracture classification. When the Gustilo classification type is not specified for an open fracture, the 7th character for open fracture type I or II should be assigned (B, E, H, M, Q).

A code from category M80, not a traumatic fracture code, should be used for any patient with known osteoporosis who suffers a fracture, even if the patient had a minor fall or trauma, if that fall or trauma would not usually break a normal, healthy bone.

See Section I.C.13. Osteoporosis.

The aftercare Z codes should not be used for aftercare for traumatic fractures. For aftercare of a traumatic fracture, assign the acute fracture code with the appropriate 7th character.

2) **Multiple fractures sequencing**

Multiple fractures are sequenced in accordance with the severity of the fracture.

d. **Coding of Burns and Corrosions**

The ICD-10-CM makes a distinction between burns and corrosions. The burn codes are for thermal burns, except sunburns, that come from a heat source, such as a fire or hot appliance. The burn codes are also for burns resulting from electricity and radiation. Corrosions are burns due to chemicals. The guidelines are the same for burns and corrosions.

Current burns (T20-T25) are classified by depth, extent and by agent (X code). Burns are classified by depth as first degree (erythema), second degree (blistering), and third degree (full-thickness involvement). Burns of the eye and internal organs (T26-T28) are classified by site, but not by degree.

1) Sequencing of burn and related condition codes

Sequence first the code that reflects the highest degree of burn when more than one burn is present.

    a. When the reason for the admission or encounter is for treatment of external multiple burns, sequence first the code that reflects the burn of the highest degree.

    b. When a patient has both internal and external burns, the circumstances of admission govern the selection of the principal diagnosis or first-listed diagnosis.

    c. When a patient is admitted for burn injuries and other related conditions such as smoke inhalation and/or respiratory failure, the circumstances of admission govern the selection of the principal or first-listed diagnosis.

2) Burns of the same local site

Classify burns of the same local site (three-character category level, T20-T28) but of different degrees to the subcategory identifying the highest degree recorded in the diagnosis.

3) Non-healing burns

Non-healing burns are coded as acute burns.

Necrosis of burned skin should be coded as a non-healed burn.

4) Infected Burn

For any documented infected burn site, use an additional code for the infection.

5) Assign separate codes for each burn site

When coding burns, assign separate codes for each burn site. Category T30, Burn and corrosion, body region unspecified is extremely vague and should rarely be used.

6) Burns and Corrosions Classified According to Extent of Body Surface Involved

Assign codes from category T31, Burns classified according to extent of body surface involved, or T32, Corrosions classified according to extent of body surface involved, when the site of the burn is not specified or when there is a need for additional data. It is advisable to use category T31 as additional coding when needed to provide data for evaluating burn mortality, such as that needed by burn units. It is also advisable to use category T31 as an additional code for reporting purposes when there is mention of a third-degree burn involving 20 percent or more of the body surface.

Categories T31 and T32 are based on the classic "rule of nines" in estimating body surface involved: head and neck are assigned nine percent, each arm nine percent, each leg 18 percent, the anterior trunk 18 percent, posterior trunk 18 percent, and genitalia one percent. Providers may change these percentage assignments where necessary to accommodate infants and children who have proportionally larger heads than adults, and patients who have large buttocks, thighs, or abdomen that involve burns.

7) Encounters for treatment of sequela of burns

Encounters for the treatment of the late effects of burns or corrosions (i.e., scars or joint contractures) should be coded with a burn or corrosion code with the 7th character "S" for sequela.

8) Sequelae with a late effect code and current burn

When appropriate, both a code for a current burn or corrosion with 7th character "A" or "D" and a burn or corrosion code with 7th character "S" may be assigned on the same record (when both a current burn and sequelae of an old burn exist). Burns and corrosions do not heal at the same rate and a current healing wound may still exist with sequela of a healed burn or corrosion.

See Section I.B.10 Sequela (Late Effects)

9) Use of an external cause code with burns and corrosions

An external cause code should be used with burns and corrosions to identify the source and intent of the burn, as well as the place where it occurred.

e. Adverse Effects, Poisoning, Underdosing and Toxic Effects

Codes in categories T36-T65 are combination codes that include the substance that was taken as well as the intent. No additional external cause code is required for poisonings, toxic effects, adverse effects and underdosing codes.

1) Do not code directly from the Table of Drugs

Do not code directly from the Table of Drugs and Chemicals. Always refer back to the Tabular List.

2) Use as many codes as necessary to describe

Use as many codes as necessary to describe completely all drugs, medicinal or biological substances.

3) If the same code would describe the causative agent

If the same code would describe the causative agent for more than one adverse reaction, poisoning, toxic effect or underdosing, assign the code only once.

4) If two or more drugs, medicinal or biological substances

If two or more drugs, medicinal or biological substances are reported, code each individually unless a combination code is listed in the Table of Drugs and Chemicals.

5) The occurrence of drug toxicity is classified in ICD-10-CM as follows:

(a) Adverse Effect

When coding an adverse effect of a drug that has been correctly prescribed and properly administered, assign the appropriate code for the nature of the adverse effect followed by the appropriate code for the adverse effect of the drug (T36-T50). The code for the drug should have a 5th or 6th character "5" (for example T36.0X5-) Examples of the nature of an adverse effect are tachycardia, delirium, gastrointestinal hemorrhaging, vomiting, hypokalemia, hepatitis, renal failure, or respiratory failure.

(b) Poisoning

When coding a poisoning or reaction to the improper use of a medication (e.g., overdose, wrong substance given or taken in error, wrong route of administration), first assign the appropriate code from categories T36-T50. The poisoning codes have an associated intent as their 5th or 6th character (accidental, intentional self-harm, assault and undetermined. If the intent of the poisoning is unknown or unspecified, code the intent as accidental intent. The undetermined intent is only for use if the documentation in the record specifies that the intent cannot be determined. Use additional code(s) for all manifestations of poisonings.

If there is also a diagnosis of abuse or dependence of the substance, the abuse or dependence is assigned as an additional code.

Examples of poisoning include:

(i) Error was made in drug prescription Errors made in drug prescription or in the administration of the drug by provider, nurse, patient, or other person.

(ii) Overdose of a drug intentionally taken

If an overdose of a drug was intentionally taken or administered and resulted in drug toxicity, it would be coded as a poisoning.

(iii) Nonprescribed drug taken with correctly prescribed and properly administered drug

If a nonprescribed drug or medicinal agent was taken in combination with a correctly prescribed and properly administered drug, any drug toxicity or other reaction resulting from the interaction of the two drugs would be classified as a poisoning.

(iv) Interaction of drug(s) and alcohol

When a reaction results from the interaction of a drug(s) and alcohol, this would be classified as poisoning.

See Section I.C.4. if poisoning is the result of insulin pump malfunctions.

(c) **Underdosing**

Underdosing refers to taking less of a medication than is prescribed by a provider or a manufacturer's instruction. For underdosing, assign the code from categories T36-T50 (fifth or sixth character "6").

Codes for underdosing should never be assigned as principal or first-listed codes. If a patient has a relapse or exacerbation of the medical condition for which the drug is prescribed because of the reduction in dose, then the medical condition itself should be coded.

Noncompliance (Z91.12-, Z91.13-) or complication of care (Y63.6-Y63.9) codes are to be used with an underdosing code to indicate intent, if known.

(d) **Toxic Effects**

When a harmful substance is ingested or comes in contact with a person, this is classified as a toxic effect. The toxic effect codes are in categories T51-T65.

Toxic effect codes have an associated intent: accidental, intentional self-harm, assault and undetermined.

f. Adult and child abuse, neglect and other maltreatment

Sequence first the appropriate code from categories T74.- (Adult and child abuse, neglect and other maltreatment, confirmed) or T76.-(Adult and child abuse, neglect and other maltreatment, suspected) for abuse, neglect and other maltreatment, followed by any accompanying mental health or injury code(s).

If the documentation in the medical record states abuse or neglect it is coded as confirmed (T74.-). It is coded as suspected if it is documented as suspected (T76.-).

For cases of confirmed abuse or neglect an external cause code from the assault section (X92-Y09) should be added to identify the cause of any physical injuries. A perpetrator code (Y07) should be added when the perpetrator of the abuse is known. For suspected cases of abuse or neglect, do not report external cause or perpetrator code.

If a suspected case of abuse, neglect or mistreatment is ruled out during an encounter code Z04.71, Encounter for examination and observation following alleged physical adult abuse, ruled out, or code Z04.72, Encounter for examination and observation following alleged child physical abuse, ruled out, should be used, not a code from T76.

If a suspected case of alleged rape or sexual abuse is ruled out during an encounter code Z04.41, Encounter for examination and observation following alleged adult rape or code Z04.42, Encounter for examination and observation following alleged child rape, should be used, not a code from T76.

See Section I.C.15. Abuse in a pregnant patient.

g. Complications of care

1) General guidelines for complications of care

(a) Documentation of complications of care

See Section I.B.16. for information on documentation of complications of care.

2) Pain due to medical devices

Pain associated with devices, implants or grafts left in a surgical site (for example painful hip prosthesis) is assigned to the appropriate code(s) found in Chapter 19, Injury, poisoning, and certain other consequences of external causes. Specific codes for pain due to medical devices are found in the T code section of the ICD-10-CM. Use additional code(s) from category G89 to identify acute or chronic pain due to presence of the device, implant or graft (G89.18 or G89.28).

3) Transplant complications

(a) Transplant complications other than kidney

Codes under category T86, Complications of transplanted organs and tissues, are for use for both complications and rejection of transplanted organs. A transplant complication code is only assigned if the complication affects the function of the transplanted organ. Two codes are required to fully describe a transplant complication: the appropriate code from category T86 and a secondary code that identifies the complication.

Pre-existing conditions or conditions that develop after the transplant are not coded as complications unless they affect the function of the transplanted organs.

See I.C.21. for transplant organ removal status See I.C.2. for malignant neoplasm associated with transplanted organ.

(b) Kidney transplant complications

Patients who have undergone kidney transplant may still have some form of chronic kidney disease (CKD) because the kidney transplant may not fully restore kidney function. Code T86.1- should be assigned for documented complications of a kidney transplant, such as transplant failure or rejection or other transplant complication. Code T86.1- should not be assigned for post kidney transplant patients who have chronic kidney (CKD) unless a transplant complication such as transplant failure or rejection is documented. If the documentation is unclear as to whether the patient has a complication of the transplant, query the provider.

Conditions that affect the function of the transplanted kidney, other than CKD, should be assigned a code from subcategory T86.1, Complications of transplanted organ, Kidney, and a secondary code that identifies the complication.

For patients with CKD following a kidney transplant, but who do not have a complication such as failure or rejection, *see section I.C.14. Chronic kidney disease and kidney transplant status.*

4) Complication codes that include the external cause

As with certain other T codes, some of the complications of care codes have the external cause included in the code. The code includes the nature of the complication as well as the type of procedure that caused the complication. No external cause code indicating the type of procedure is necessary for these codes.

5) Complications of care codes within the body system chapters

Intraoperative and postprocedural complication codes are found within the body system chapters with codes specific to the organs and structures of that body system. These codes should be sequenced first, followed by a code(s) for the specific complication, if applicable.

20. Chapter 20: External Causes of Morbidity (V00-Y99)

The external causes of morbidity codes should never be sequenced as the first-listed or principal diagnosis.

External cause codes are intended to provide data for injury research and evaluation of injury prevention strategies. These codes capture how the injury or health condition happened (cause), the intent (unintentional or accidental; or intentional, such as suicide or assault), the place where the event occurred the activity of the patient at the time of the event, and the person's status (e.g., civilian, military).

There is no national requirement for mandatory ICD-10-CM external cause code reporting. Unless a provider is subject to a state-based external cause code reporting mandate or these codes are required by a particular payer, reporting of ICD-10-CM codes in Chapter 20, External Causes of Morbidity, is not required. In the absence of a mandatory reporting requirement, providers are encouraged to voluntarily report external cause codes, as they provide valuable data for injury research and evaluation of injury prevention strategies.

a. General External Cause Coding Guidelines

1) Used with any code in the range of A00.0-T88.9, Z00-Z99

An external cause code may be used with any code in the range of A00.0-T88.9, Z00-Z99, classification that represents a health condition due to an external cause. Though they are most applicable to injuries, they are also valid for use with such things as infections or diseases due to an external source, and other health conditions, such as a heart attack that occurs during strenuous physical activity.

2) External cause code used for length of treatment

Assign the external cause code, with the appropriate 7th character (initial encounter, subsequent encounter or sequela) for each encounter for which the injury or condition is being treated.
Most categories in chapter 20 have a 7th character requirement for each applicable code. Most categories in this chapter have three 7th character values: A, initial encounter, D, subsequent encounter and S, sequela. While the patient may be seen by a new or different provider over the course of treatment for an injury or condition, assignment of the 7th character for external cause should match the 7th character of the code assigned for the associated injury or condition for the encounter.

3) Use the full range of external cause codes

Use the full range of external cause codes to completely describe the cause, the intent, the place of occurrence, and if applicable, the activity of the patient at the time of the event, and the patient's status, for all injuries, and other health conditions due to an external cause.

4) Assign as many external cause codes as necessary

Assign as many external cause codes as necessary to fully explain each cause. If only one external code can be recorded, assign the code most related to the principal diagnosis.

5) The selection of the appropriate external cause code

The selection of the appropriate external cause code is guided by the Alphabetic Index of External Causes and by Inclusion and Exclusion notes in the Tabular List.

6) External cause code can never be a principal diagnosis

An external cause code can never be a principal (first-listed) diagnosis.

7) Combination external cause codes

Certain of the external cause codes are combination codes that identify sequential events that result in an injury, such as a fall which results in striking against an object. The injury may be due to either event or both. The combination external cause code used should correspond to the sequence of events regardless of which caused the most serious injury.

8) No external cause code needed in certain circumstances

No external cause code from Chapter 20 is needed if the external cause and intent are included in a code from another chapter (e.g. T36.0X1- Poisoning by penicillins, accidental (unintentional)).

b. Place of Occurrence Guideline

Codes from category Y92, Place of occurrence of the external cause, are secondary codes for use after other external cause codes to identify the location of the patient at the time of injury or other condition.

Generally, a place of occurrence code is assigned only once, at the initial encounter for treatment. However, in the rare instance that a new injury occurs during hospitalization, an additional place of occurrence code may be assigned. No 7th characters are used for Y92.

Do not use place of occurrence code Y92.9 if the place is not stated or is not applicable.

c. Activity Code

Assign a code from category Y93, Activity code, to describe the activity of the patient at the time the injury or other health condition occurred.

An activity code is used only once, at the initial encounter for treatment. Only one code from Y93 should be recorded on a medical record.

The activity codes are not applicable to poisonings, adverse effects, misadventures or sequela.

Do not assign Y93.9, Unspecified activity, if the activity is not stated.

A code from category Y93 is appropriate for use with external cause and intent codes if identifying the activity provides additional information about the event.

d. Place of Occurrence, Activity, and Status Codes Used with other External Cause Code

When applicable, place of occurrence, activity, and external cause status codes are sequenced after the main external cause code(s). Regardless of the number of external cause codes assigned, generally there should be only one place of occurrence code, one activity code, and one external cause status code assigned to an encounter. However, in the rare instance that a new injury occurs during hospitalization, an additional place of occurrence code may be assigned.

e. If the Reporting Format Limits the Number of External Cause Codes

If the reporting format limits the number of external cause codes that can be used in reporting clinical data, report the code for the cause/intent most related to the principal diagnosis. If the format permits capture of additional external cause codes, the cause/intent, including medical misadventures, of the additional events should be reported rather than the codes for place, activity, or external status.

f. Multiple External Cause Coding Guidelines

More than one external cause code is required to fully describe the external cause of an illness or injury. The assignment of external cause codes should be sequenced in the following priority:

If two or more events cause separate injuries, an external cause code should be assigned for each cause. The first-listed external cause code will be selected in the following order:

External codes for child and adult abuse take priority over all other external cause codes.

See Section I.C.19., Child and Adult abuse guidelines.

External cause codes for terrorism events take priority over all other external cause codes except child and adult abuse.

External cause codes for cataclysmic events take priority over all other external cause codes except child and adult abuse and terrorism.

External cause codes for transport accidents take priority over all other external cause codes except cataclysmic events, child and adult abuse and terrorism.

Activity and external cause status codes are assigned following all causal (intent) external cause codes.

The first-listed external cause code should correspond to the cause of the most serious diagnosis due to an assault, accident, or self-harm, following the order of hierarchy listed above.

g. Child and Adult Abuse Guideline

Adult and child abuse, neglect and maltreatment are classified as assault. Any of the assault codes may be used to indicate the external cause of any injury resulting from the confirmed abuse.

For confirmed cases of abuse, neglect and maltreatment, when the perpetrator is known, a code from Y07, Perpetrator of maltreatment and neglect, should accompany any other assault codes.

See Section I.C.19. Adult and child abuse, neglect and other maltreatment

h. Unknown or Undetermined Intent Guideline

If the intent (accident, self-harm, assault) of the cause of an injury or other condition is unknown or unspecified, code the intent as accidental intent. All transport accident categories assume accidental intent.

1) Use of undetermined intent

External cause codes for events of undetermined intent are only for use if the documentation in the record specifies that the intent cannot be determined.

i. Sequelae (Late Effects) of External Cause Guidelines

1) Sequelae external cause codes

Sequela are reported using the external cause code with the 7th character "S" for sequela. These codes should be used with any report of a late effect or sequela resulting from a previous injury.

See Section I.B.10 Sequela (Late Effects)

2) Sequela external cause code with a related current injury

A sequela external cause code should never be used with a related current nature of injury code.

3) Use of sequela external cause codes for subsequent visits

Use a late effect external cause code for subsequent visits when a late effect of the initial injury is being treated. Do not use a late effect external cause code for subsequent visits for follow-up care (e.g., to assess healing, to receive rehabilitative therapy) of the injury when no late effect of the injury has been documented.

j. Terrorism Guidelines

1) Cause of injury identified by the Federal Government (FBI) as terrorism

When the cause of an injury is identified by the Federal Government (FBI) as terrorism, the first-listed external cause code should be a code from category Y38, Terrorism. The definition of terrorism employed by the FBI is found at the inclusion note at the beginning of category Y38. Use additional code for place of occurrence (Y92.-). More than one Y38 code may be assigned if the injury is the result of more than one mechanism of terrorism.

2) Cause of an injury is suspected to be the result of terrorism

When the cause of an injury is suspected to be the result of terrorism a code from category Y38 should not be assigned. Suspected cases should be classified as assault.

3) Code Y38.9, Terrorism, secondary effects

Assign code Y38.9, Terrorism, secondary effects, for conditions occurring subsequent to the terrorist event. This code should not be assigned for conditions that are due to the initial terrorist act.

It is acceptable to assign code Y38.9 with another code from Y38 if there is an injury due to the initial terrorist event and an injury that is a subsequent result of the terrorist event.

k. External cause status

A code from category Y99, External cause status, should be assigned whenever any other external cause code is assigned for an encounter, including an Activity code, except for the events noted below. Assign a code from category Y99, External cause status, to indicate the work status of the person at the time the event occurred. The status code indicates whether the event occurred during military activity, whether a non-military person was at work, whether an individual including a student or volunteer was involved in a non-work activity at the time of the causal event.

A code from Y99, External cause status, should be assigned, when applicable, with other external cause codes, such as transport accidents and falls. The external cause status codes are not applicable to poisonings, adverse effects, misadventures or late effects.

Do not assign a code from category Y99 if no other external cause codes (cause, activity) are applicable for the encounter.

An external cause status code is used only once, at the initial encounter for treatment. Only one code from Y99 should be recorded on a medical record.

Do not assign code Y99.9, Unspecified external cause status, if the status is not stated.

21. Chapter 21: Factors influencing health status and contact with health services (Z00-Z99)

Note: The chapter specific guidelines provide additional information about the use of Z codes for specified encounters.

a. Use of Z codes in any healthcare setting

Z codes are for use in any healthcare setting. Z codes may be used as either a first-listed (principal diagnosis code in the inpatient setting) or secondary code, depending on the circumstances of the encounter. Certain Z codes may only be used as first-listed or principal diagnosis.

b. Z Codes indicate a reason for an encounter

Z codes are not procedure codes. A corresponding procedure code must accompany a Z code to describe any procedure performed.

c. Categories of Z Codes

1) Contact/Exposure

Category Z20 indicates contact with, and suspected exposure to, communicable diseases. These codes are for patients who do not show any sign or symptom of a disease but are suspected to have been exposed to it by close personal contact with an infected individual or are in an area where a disease is epidemic.

Category Z77, Other contact with and (suspected) exposures hazardous to health, indicates contact with and suspected exposures hazardous to health.
Contact/exposure codes may be used as a first-listed code to explain an encounter for testing, or, more commonly, as a secondary code to identify a potential risk.

2) Inoculations and vaccinations

Code Z23 is for encounters for inoculations and vaccinations. It indicates that a patient is being seen to receive a prophylactic inoculation against a disease. Procedure codes are required to identify the actual administration of the injection and the type(s) of immunizations given. Code Z23 may be used as a secondary code if the inoculation is given as a routine part of preventive health care, such as a well-baby visit.

3) Status

Status codes indicate that a patient is either a carrier of a disease or has the sequelae or residual of a past disease or condition. This includes such things as the presence of prosthetic or mechanical devices resulting from past treatment. A status code is informative, because the status may affect the course of treatment and its outcome. A status code is distinct from a history code. The history code indicates that the patient no longer has the condition.

A status code should not be used with a diagnosis code from one of the body system chapters, if the diagnosis code includes the information provided by the status code. For example, code Z94.1, Heart transplant status, should not be used with a code from subcategory T86.2, Complications of heart transplant. The status code does not provide additional information. The complication code indicates that the patient is a heart transplant patient.

For encounters for weaning from a mechanical ventilator, assign a code from subcategory J96.1, Chronic respiratory failure, followed by code Z99.11, Dependence on respirator [ventilator] status.
The status Z codes/categories are: Z14 Genetic carrier

Genetic carrier status indicates that a person carries a gene, associated with a particular disease, which may be passed to offspring who may develop that disease. The person does not have the disease and is not at risk of developing the disease.

Z15   Genetic susceptibility to disease

Genetic susceptibility indicates that a person has a gene that increases the risk of that person developing the disease.

Codes from category Z15 should not be used as principal or first-listed codes. If the patient has the condition to which he/she is susceptible, and that condition is the reason for the encounter, the code for the current condition should be sequenced first. If the patient is being seen for follow-up after completed treatment for this condition, and the condition no longer exists, a follow-up code should be sequenced first, followed by the appropriate personal history and genetic susceptibility codes. If the purpose of the encounter is genetic counseling associated with procreative management, code Z31.5, Encounter for genetic counseling, should be assigned as the first-listed code, followed by a code from category Z15. Additional codes should be assigned for any applicable family or personal history.

Z16   Resistance to antimicrobial drugs

This code indicates that a patient has a condition that is resistant to antimicrobial drug treatment. Sequence the infection code first.

Z17   Estrogen receptor status

Z18   Retained foreign body fragments

Z19   Hormone sensitivity malignancy status

Z21   Asymptomatic HIV infection status

This code indicates that a patient has tested positive for HIV but has manifested no signs or symptoms of the disease.

Z22   Carrier of infectious disease

Carrier status indicates that a person harbors the specific organisms of a disease without manifest symptoms and is capable of transmitting the infection.

Z28.3   Underimmunization status

Z33.1   Pregnant state, incidental

This code is a secondary code only for use when the pregnancy is in no way complicating the reason for visit. Otherwise, a code from the obstetric chapter is required.

Z66   Do not resuscitate

This code may be used when it is documented by the provider that a patient is on do not resuscitate status at any time during the stay.

Z67   Blood type

Z68   Body mass index (BMI)

As with all other secondary diagnosis codes, the BMI codes should only be assigned when they meet the definition of a reportable diagnosis (see Section III, Reporting Additional Diagnoses).

Z74.01   Bed confinement status

Z76.82   Awaiting organ transplant status

Z78   Other specified health status

Code Z78.1, Physical restraint status, may be used when it is documented by the provider that a patient has been put in restraints during the current encounter. Please note that this code should not be reported when it is documented by the provider that a patient is temporarily restrained during a procedure.

Z79   Long-term (current) drug therapy

Codes from this category indicate a patient's continuous use of a prescribed drug (including such things as aspirin therapy) for the long-term treatment of a condition or for prophylactic use. It is not for use for patients who have addictions to drugs. This subcategory is not for use of medications for detoxification or maintenance programs to prevent withdrawal symptoms in patients with drug dependence (e.g., methadone maintenance for opiate dependence). Assign the appropriate code for the drug dependence instead.

Assign a code from Z79 if the patient is receiving a medication for an extended period as a prophylactic measure (such as for the prevention of deep vein thrombosis) or as treatment of a chronic condition (such as arthritis) or a disease requiring a lengthy course of treatment (such as cancer). Do not assign a code from category Z79 for medication being administered for a brief period of time to treat an acute illness or injury (such as a course of antibiotics to treat acute bronchitis).

Z88	Allergy status to drugs, medicaments and biological substances

Except: Z88.9, Allergy status to unspecified drugs, medicaments and biological substances status

Z89	Acquired absence of limb
Z90	Acquired absence of organs, not elsewhere classified
Z91.0-	Allergy status, other than to drugs and biological substances
Z92.82	Status post administration of tPA (rtPA) in a different facility within the last 24 hours prior to admission to a current facility

Assign code Z92.82, Status post administration of tPA (rtPA) in a different facility within the last 24 hours prior to admission to current facility, as a secondary diagnosis when a patient is received by transfer into a facility and documentation indicates they were administered tissue plasminogen activator (tPA) within the last 24 hours prior to admission to the current facility.

This guideline applies even if the patient is still receiving the tPA at the time they are received into the current facility.

The appropriate code for the condition for which the tPA was administered (such as cerebrovascular disease or myocardial infarction) should be assigned first.

Code Z92.82 is only applicable to the receiving facility record and not to the transferring facility record.

Z93	Artificial opening status
Z94	Transplanted organ and tissue status
Z95	Presence of cardiac and vascular implants and grafts Z96 Presence of other functional implants
Z97	Presence of other devices Z98 Other postprocedural states

Assign code Z98.85, Transplanted organ removal status, to indicate that a transplanted organ has been previously removed. This code should not be assigned for the encounter in which the transplanted organ is removed. The complication necessitating removal of the transplant organ should be assigned for that encounter.

See section I.C19. for information on the coding of organ transplant complications.

Z99	Dependence on enabling machines and devices, not elsewhere classified

Note: Categories Z89-Z90 and Z93-Z99 are for use only if there are no complications or malfunctions of the organ or tissue replaced, the amputation site or the equipment on which the patient is dependent.

4) **History (of)**

There are two types of history Z codes, personal and family. Personal history codes explain a patient's past medical condition that no longer exists and is not receiving any treatment, but that has the potential for recurrence, and therefore may require continued monitoring.

Family history codes are for use when a patient has a family member(s) who has had a particular disease that causes the patient to be at higher risk of also contracting the disease.

Personal history codes may be used in conjunction with follow-up codes and family history codes may be used in conjunction with screening codes to explain the need for a test or procedure. History codes are also acceptable on any medical record regardless of the reason for visit. A history of an illness, even if no longer present, is important information that may alter the type of treatment ordered.

The history Z code categories are:

Z80	Family history of primary malignant neoplasm
Z81	Family history of mental and behavioral disorders
Z82	Family history of certain disabilities and chronic diseases (leading to disablement)
Z83	Family history of other specific disorders
Z84	Family history of other conditions

Z85	Personal history of malignant neoplasm
Z86	Personal history of certain other diseases
Z87	Personal history of other diseases and conditions
Z91.4-	Personal history of psychological trauma, not elsewhere classified
Z91.5	Personal history of self-harm
Z91.81	History of falling
Z91.82	Personal history of military deployment
Z92	Personal history of medical treatment
	Except: Z92.0, Personal history of contraception
	Except: Z92.82, Status post administration of tPA (rtPA) in a different facility within the last 24 hours prior to admission to a current facility

5) Screening

Screening is the testing for disease or disease precursors in seemingly well individuals so that early detection and treatment can be provided for those who test positive for the disease (e.g., screening mammogram).

The testing of a person to rule out or confirm a suspected diagnosis because the patient has some sign or symptom is a diagnostic examination, not a screening. In these cases, the sign or symptom is used to explain the reason for the test.

A screening code may be a first-listed code if the reason for the visit is specifically the screening exam. It may also be used as an additional code if the screening is done during an office visit for other health problems. A screening code is not necessary if the screening is inherent to a routine examination, such as a pap smear done during a routine pelvic examination.

Should a condition be discovered during the screening then the code for the condition may be assigned as an additional diagnosis.

The Z code indicates that a screening exam is planned. A procedure code is required to confirm that the screening was performed.

The screening Z codes/categories:

Z11	Encounter for screening for infectious and parasitic diseases
Z12	Encounter for screening for malignant neoplasms
Z13	Encounter for screening for other diseases and disorders
	Except: Z13.9, Encounter for screening, unspecified
Z36	Encounter for antenatal screening for mother

6) Observation

There are three observation Z code categories. They are for use in very limited circumstances when a person is being observed for a suspected condition that is ruled out. The observation codes are not for use if an injury or illness or any signs or symptoms related to the suspected condition are present. In such cases the diagnosis/symptom code is used with the corresponding external cause code.

The observation codes are to be used as principal diagnosis only. The only exception to this is when the principal diagnosis is required to be a code from category Z38, Liveborn infants according to place of birth and type of delivery. Then a code from category Z05, Encounter for observation and evaluation of newborn for suspected diseases and conditions ruled out, is sequenced after the Z38 code. Additional codes may be used in addition to the observation code, but only if they are unrelated to the suspected condition being observed.

Codes from subcategory Z03.7, Encounter for suspected maternal and fetal conditions ruled out, may either be used as a first-listed or as an additional code assignment depending on the case. They are for use in very limited circumstances on a maternal record when an encounter is for a suspected maternal or fetal condition that is ruled out during that encounter (for example, a maternal or fetal condition may be suspected due to an abnormal test result). These codes should not be used when the condition is confirmed. In those cases, the confirmed condition should be coded. In addition, these codes are not for use if an illness or any signs or symptoms related to the suspected condition or problem are present. In such cases the diagnosis/symptom code is used.

Additional codes may be used in addition to the code from subcategory Z03.7, but only if they are unrelated to the suspected condition being evaluated.

Codes from subcategory Z03.7 may not be used for encounters for antenatal screening of mother. *See Section I.C.21. Screening.*

For encounters for suspected fetal condition that are inconclusive following testing and evaluation, assign the appropriate code from category O35, O36, O40 or O41.

The observation Z code categories:

Z03	Encounter for medical observation for suspected diseases and conditions ruled out
Z04	Encounter for examination and observation for other reasons
	Except: Z04.9, Encounter for examination and observation for unspecified reason
Z05	Encounter for observation and evaluation of newborn for suspected diseases and conditions ruled out

7) Aftercare

Aftercare visit codes cover situations when the initial treatment of a disease has been performed and the patient requires continued care during the healing or recovery phase, or for the long-term consequences of the disease. The aftercare Z code should not be used if treatment is directed at a current, acute disease. The diagnosis code is to be used in these cases. Exceptions to this rule are codes Z51.0, Encounter for antineoplastic radiation therapy, and codes from subcategory Z51.1, Encounter for antineoplastic chemotherapy and immunotherapy. These codes are to be first-listed, followed by the diagnosis code when a patient's encounter is solely to receive radiation therapy, chemotherapy, or immunotherapy for the treatment of a neoplasm. If the reason for the encounter is more than one type of antineoplastic therapy, code Z51.0 and a code from subcategory Z51.1 may be assigned together, in which case one of these codes would be reported as a secondary diagnosis.

The aftercare Z codes should also not be used for aftercare for injuries. For aftercare of an injury, assign the acute injury code with the appropriate 7th character (for subsequent encounter).

The aftercare codes are generally first-listed to explain the specific reason for the encounter. An aftercare code may be used as an additional code when some type of aftercare is provided in addition to the reason for admission and no diagnosis code is applicable. An example of this would be the closure of a colostomy during an encounter for treatment of another condition.

Aftercare codes should be used in conjunction with other aftercare codes or diagnosis codes to provide better detail on the specifics of an aftercare encounter visit, unless otherwise directed by the classification. Should a patient receive multiple types of antineoplastic therapy during the same encounter, code Z51.0, Encounter for antineoplastic radiation therapy, and codes from subcategory Z51.1, Encounter for antineoplastic chemotherapy and immunotherapy, may be used together on a record. The sequencing of multiple aftercare codes depends on the circumstances of the encounter.

Certain aftercare Z code categories need a secondary diagnosis code to describe the resolving condition or sequelae. For others, the condition is included in the code title.

Additional Z code aftercare category terms include fitting and adjustment, and attention to artificial openings.

Status Z codes may be used with aftercare Z codes to indicate the nature of the aftercare. For example code Z95.1, Presence of aortocoronary bypass graft, may be used with code Z48.812, Encounter for surgical aftercare following surgery on the circulatory system, to indicate the surgery for which the aftercare is being performed. A status code should not be used when the aftercare code indicates the type of status, such as using Z43.0, Encounter for attention to tracheostomy, with Z93.0, Tracheostomy status.

The aftercare Z category/codes:

Z42	Encounter for plastic and reconstructive surgery following medical procedure or healed injury
Z43	Encounter for attention to artificial openings
Z44	Encounter for fitting and adjustment of external prosthetic device
Z45	Encounter for adjustment and management of implanted device
Z46	Encounter for fitting and adjustment of other devices
Z47	Orthopedic aftercare
Z48	Encounter for other postprocedural aftercare
Z49	Encounter for care involving renal dialysis
Z51	Encounter for other aftercare and medical care

8) Follow-up

The follow-up codes are used to explain continuing surveillance following completed treatment of a disease, condition, or injury. They imply that the condition has been fully treated and no longer exists. They should not be confused with aftercare codes, or injury codes with a 7th character for subsequent encounter, that explain ongoing care of a healing condition or its sequelae. Follow-up codes may be used in conjunction with history codes to provide the full picture of the healed condition and its treatment. The follow-up code is sequenced first, followed by the history code.

A follow-up code may be used to explain multiple visits. Should a condition be found to have recurred on the follow-up visit, then the diagnosis code for the condition should be assigned in place of the follow-up code.

The follow-up Z code categories:

Z08	Encounter for follow-up examination after completed treatment for malignant neoplasm
Z09	Encounter for follow-up examination after completed treatment for conditions other than malignant neoplasm
Z39	Encounter for maternal postpartum care and examination

9) Donor

Codes in category Z52, Donors of organs and tissues, are used for living individuals who are donating blood or other body tissue. These codes are only for individuals donating for others, not for self-donations. They are not used to identify cadaveric donations.

10) Counseling

Counseling Z codes are used when a patient or family member receives assistance in the aftermath of an illness or injury, or when support is required in coping with family or social problems. They are not used in conjunction with a diagnosis code when the counseling component of care is considered integral to standard treatment.

The counseling Z codes/categories:

Z30.0- Encounter for general counseling and advice on contraception
Z31.5   Encounter for procreative genetic counseling
Z31.6- Encounter for general counseling and advice on procreation
Z32.2   Encounter for childbirth instruction
Z32.3   Encounter for childcare instruction
Z69   Encounter for mental health services for victim and perpetrator of abuse
Z70   Counseling related to sexual attitude, behavior and orientation
Z71   Persons encountering health services for other counseling and medical advice, not elsewhere classified
Z76.81 Expectant mother prebirth pediatrician visit

11) Encounters for Obstetrical and Reproductive Services

See Section I.C.15. Pregnancy, Childbirth, and the Puerperium, for further instruction on the use of these codes.

Z codes for pregnancy are for use in those circumstances when none of the problems or complications included in the codes from the Obstetrics chapter exist (a routine prenatal visit or postpartum care). Codes in category Z34, Encounter for supervision of normal pregnancy, are always first-listed and are not to be used with any other code from the OB chapter.

Codes in category Z3A, Weeks of gestation, may be assigned to provide additional information about the pregnancy. Category Z3A codes should not be assigned for pregnancies with abortive outcomes (categories O00-O08), elective termination of pregnancy (code Z33.2), nor for postpartum conditions, as category Z3A is not applicable to these conditions. The date of the admission should be used to determine weeks of gestation for inpatient admissions that encompass more than one gestational week.

The outcome of delivery, category Z37, should be included on all maternal delivery records. It is always a secondary code. Codes in category Z37 should not be used on the newborn record.

Z codes for family planning (contraceptive) or procreative management and counseling should be included on an obstetric record either during the pregnancy or the postpartum stage, if applicable.

Z codes/categories for obstetrical and reproductive services:

Z30   Encounter for contraceptive management
Z31   Encounter for procreative management
Z32.2   Encounter for childbirth instruction
Z32.3   Encounter for childcare instruction
Z33   Pregnant state
Z34   Encounter for supervision of normal pregnancy
Z36   Encounter for antenatal screening of mother
Z3A   Weeks of gestation
Z37   Outcome of delivery
Z39   Encounter for maternal postpartum care and examination
Z76.81 Expectant mother prebirth pediatrician visit

12) Newborns and Infants

See Section I.C.16. Newborn (Perinatal) Guidelines, for further instruction on the use of these codes.

Newborn Z codes/categories:

Z76.1	Encounter for health supervision and care of foundling
Z00.1-	Encounter for routine child health examination
Z38	Liveborn infants according to place of birth and type of delivery

13) Routine and administrative examinations

The Z codes allow for the description of encounters for routine examinations, such as, a general check-up, or, examinations for administrative purposes, such as, a pre-employment physical. The codes are not to be used if the examination is for diagnosis of a suspected condition or for treatment purposes. In such cases the diagnosis code is used. During a routine exam, should a diagnosis or condition be discovered, it should be coded as an additional code. Pre-existing and chronic conditions and history codes may also be included as additional codes as long as the examination is for administrative purposes and not focused on any particular condition.

Some of the codes for routine health examinations distinguish between "with" and "without" abnormal findings. Code assignment depends on the information that is known at the time the encounter is being coded. For example, if no abnormal findings were found during the examination, but the encounter is being coded before test results are back, it is acceptable to assign the code for "without abnormal findings." When assigning a code for "with abnormal findings," additional code(s) should be assigned to identify the specific abnormal finding(s).

Pre-operative examination and pre-procedural laboratory examination Z codes are for use only in those situations when a patient is being cleared for a procedure or surgery and no treatment is given.

The Z codes/categories for routine and administrative examinations:

Z00	Encounter for general examination without complaint, suspected or reported diagnosis
Z01	Encounter for other special examination without complaint, suspected or reported diagnosis
Z02	Encounter for administrative examination
	Except: Z02.9, Encounter for administrative examinations, unspecified
Z32.0-	Encounter for pregnancy test

14) Miscellaneous Z codes

The miscellaneous Z codes capture a number of other health care encounters that do not fall into one of the other categories. Certain of these codes identify the reason for the encounter; others are for use as additional codes that provide useful information on circumstances that may affect a patient's care and treatment.

Prophylactic Organ Removal

For encounters specifically for prophylactic removal of an organ (such as prophylactic removal of breasts due to a genetic susceptibility to cancer or a family history of cancer), the principal or first-listed code should be a code from category Z40, Encounter for prophylactic surgery, followed by the appropriate codes to identify the associated risk factor (such as genetic susceptibility or family history).

If the patient has a malignancy of one site and is having prophylactic removal at another site to prevent either a new primary malignancy or metastatic disease, a code for the malignancy should also be assigned in addition to a code from subcategory Z40.0, Encounter for prophylactic surgery for risk factors related to malignant neoplasms. A Z40.0 code should not be assigned if the patient is having organ removal for treatment of a malignancy, such as the removal of the testes for the treatment of prostate cancer.

Miscellaneous Z codes/categories:

Z28	Immunization not carried out
	Except: Z28.3, Underimmunization status
Z29	Encounter for other prophylactic measures
Z40	Encounter for prophylactic surgery
Z41	Encounter for procedures for purposes other than remedying health state
	Except: Z41.9, Encounter for procedure for purposes other than remedying health state, unspecified
Z53	Persons encountering health services for specific procedures and treatment, not carried out
Z55	Problems related to education and literacy
Z56	Problems related to employment and unemployment
Z57	Occupational exposure to risk factors
Z58	Problems related to physical environment
Z59	Problems related to housing and economic circumstances
Z60	Problems related to social environment
Z62	Problems related to upbringing
Z63	Other problems related to primary support group, including family circumstances
Z64	Problems related to certain psychosocial circumstances
Z65	Problems related to other psychosocial circumstances
Z72	Problems related to lifestyle
	Note: These codes should be assigned only when the documentation specifies that the patient has an associated problem
Z73	Problems related to life management difficulty
Z74	Problems related to care provider dependency
	Except: Z74.01, Bed confinement status
Z75	Problems related to medical facilities and other health care
Z76.0	Encounter for issue of repeat prescription
Z76.3	Healthy person accompanying sick person
Z76.4	Other boarder to healthcare facility
Z76.5	Malingerer [conscious simulation]
Z91.1-	Patient's noncompliance with medical treatment and regimen
Z91.83	Wandering in diseases classified elsewhere
Z91.84 -	Oral health risk factors
Z91.89	Other specified personal risk factors, not elsewhere classified

15) Nonspecific Z codes

Certain Z codes are so non-specific, or potentially redundant with other codes in the classification, that there can be little justification for their use in the inpatient setting. Their use in the outpatient setting should be limited to those instances when there is no further documentation to permit more precise coding. Otherwise, any sign or symptom or any other reason for visit that is captured in another code should be used.

Nonspecific Z codes/categories:

Z02.9	Encounter for administrative examinations, unspecified
Z04.9	Encounter for examination and observation for unspecified reason
Z13.9	Encounter for screening, unspecified
Z41.9	Encounter for procedure for purposes other than remedying health state, unspecified

Z52.9	Donor of unspecified organ or tissue
Z86.59	Personal history of other mental and behavioral disorders
Z88.9	Allergy status to unspecified drugs, medicaments and biological substances status
Z92.0	Personal history of contraception

16) Z Codes That May Only be Principal/First-Listed Diagnosis

The following Z codes/categories may only be reported as the principal/first-listed diagnosis, except when there are multiple encounters on the same day and the medical records for the encounters are combined:

Z00	Encounter for general examination without complaint, suspected or reported diagnosis
	Except: Z00.6
Z01	Encounter for other special examination without complaint, suspected or reported diagnosis
Z02	Encounter for administrative examination
Z03	Encounter for medical observation for suspected diseases and conditions ruled out
Z04	Encounter for examination and observation for other reasons
Z33.2	Encounter for elective termination of pregnancy
Z31.81	Encounter for male factor infertility in female patient
Z31.83	Encounter for assisted reproductive fertility procedure cycle
Z31.84	Encounter for fertility preservation procedure
Z34	Encounter for supervision of normal pregnancy
Z39	Encounter for maternal postpartum care and examination
Z38	Liveborn infants according to place of birth and type of delivery
Z40	Encounter for prophylactic surgery
Z42	Encounter for plastic and reconstructive surgery following medical procedure or healed injury
Z51.0	Encounter for antineoplastic radiation therapy
Z51.1-	Encounter for antineoplastic chemotherapy and immunotherapy
Z52	Donors of organs and tissues
	Except: Z52.9, Donor of unspecified organ or tissue
Z76.1	Encounter for health supervision and care of foundling
Z76.2	Encounter for health supervision and care of other healthy infant and child
Z99.12	Encounter for respirator [ventilator] dependence during power failure

SECTION II. SELECTION OF PRINCIPAL DIAGNOSIS

The circumstances of inpatient admission always govern the selection of principal diagnosis. The principal diagnosis is defined in the Uniform Hospital Discharge Data Set (UHDDS) as "that condition established after study to be chiefly responsible for occasioning the admission of the patient to the hospital for care."

The UHDDS definitions are used by hospitals to report inpatient data elements in a standardized manner. These data elements and their definitions can be found in the July 31, 1985, Federal Register (Vol. 50, No, 147), pp. 31038-40.

Since that time the application of the UHDDS definitions has been expanded to include all non-outpatient settings (acute care, short term, long term care and psychiatric hospitals; home health agencies; rehab facilities; nursing homes, etc). The UHDDS definitions also apply to hospice services (all levels of care).

In determining principal diagnosis, coding conventions in the ICD-10-CM, the Tabular List and Alphabetic Index take precedence over these official coding guidelines.

(See Section I.A., Conventions for the ICD-10-CM)

The importance of consistent, complete documentation in the medical record cannot be overemphasized. Without such documentation the application of all coding guidelines is a difficult, if not impossible, task.

A. Codes for symptoms, signs, and ill-defined conditions

Codes for symptoms, signs, and ill-defined conditions from Chapter 18 are not to be used as principal diagnosis when a related definitive diagnosis has been established.

B. Two or more interrelated conditions, each potentially meeting the definition for principal diagnosis.

When there are two or more interrelated conditions (such as diseases in the same ICD-10-CM chapter or manifestations characteristically associated with a certain disease) potentially meeting the definition of principal diagnosis, either condition may be sequenced first, unless the circumstances of the admission, the therapy provided, the Tabular List, or the Alphabetic Index indicate otherwise.

C. Two or more diagnoses that equally meet the definition for principal diagnosis

In the unusual instance when two or more diagnoses equally meet the criteria for principal diagnosis as determined by the circumstances of admission, diagnostic workup and/or therapy provided, and the Alphabetic Index, Tabular List, or another coding guidelines does not provide sequencing direction, any one of the diagnoses may be sequenced first.

D. Two or more comparative or contrasting conditions

In those rare instances when two or more contrasting or comparative diagnoses are documented as "either/or" (or similar terminology), they are coded as if the diagnoses were confirmed and the diagnoses are sequenced according to the circumstances of the admission. If no further determination can be made as to which diagnosis should be principal, either diagnosis may be sequenced first.

E. A symptom(s) followed by contrasting/comparative diagnoses

GUIDELINE DELETED EFFECTIVE OCTOBER 1, 2014

F. Original treatment plan not carried out

Sequence as the principal diagnosis the condition, which after study occasioned the admission to the hospital, even though treatment may not have been carried out due to unforeseen circumstances.

G. Complications of surgery and other medical care

When the admission is for treatment of a complication resulting from surgery or other medical care, the complication code is sequenced as the principal diagnosis. If the complication is classified to the T80-T88 series and the code lacks the necessary specificity in describing the complication, an additional code for the specific complication should be assigned.

H. Uncertain Diagnosis

If the diagnosis documented at the time of discharge is qualified as "probable", "suspected", "likely", "questionable", "possible", or "still to be ruled out", or other similar terms indicating uncertainty, code the condition as if it existed or was established. The bases for these guidelines are the diagnostic workup, arrangements for further workup or observation, and initial therapeutic approach that correspond most closely with the established diagnosis.

Note: This guideline is applicable only to inpatient admissions to short-term, acute, long-term care and psychiatric hospitals.

I. Admission from Observation Unit

1. Admission Following Medical Observation

When a patient is admitted to an observation unit for a medical condition, which either worsens or does not improve, and is subsequently admitted as an inpatient of the same hospital for this same medical condition, the principal diagnosis would be the medical condition which led to the hospital admission.

2. **Admission Following Post-Operative Observation**

When a patient is admitted to an observation unit to monitor a condition (or complication) that develops following outpatient surgery, and then is subsequently admitted as an inpatient of the same hospital, hospitals should apply the Uniform Hospital Discharge Data Set (UHDDS) definition of principal diagnosis as "that condition established after study to be chiefly responsible for occasioning the admission of the patient to the hospital for care."

J. Admission from Outpatient Surgery

When a patient receives surgery in the hospital's outpatient surgery department and is subsequently admitted for continuing inpatient care at the same hospital, the following guidelines should be followed in selecting the principal diagnosis for the inpatient admission:

- If the reason for the inpatient admission is a complication, assign the complication as the principal diagnosis.

- If no complication, or other condition, is documented as the reason for the inpatient admission, assign the reason for the outpatient surgery as the principal diagnosis.

- If the reason for the inpatient admission is another condition unrelated to the surgery, assign the unrelated condition as the principal diagnosis.

K. Admissions/Encounters for Rehabilitation

When the purpose for the admission/encounter is rehabilitation, sequence first the code for the condition for which the service is being performed. For example, for an admission/encounter for rehabilitation for right-sided dominant hemiplegia following a cerebrovascular infarction, report code I69.351, Hemiplegia and hemiparesis following cerebral infarction affecting right dominant side, as the first-listed or principal diagnosis.

If the condition for which the rehabilitation service is no longer present, report the appropriate aftercare code as the first-listed or principal diagnosis, unless the rehabilitation service is being provided following an injury. For rehabilitation services following active treatment of an injury, assign the injury code with the appropriate seventh character for subsequent encounter as the first-listed or principal diagnosis. For example, if a patient with severe degenerative osteoarthritis of the hip, underwent hip replacement and the current encounter/admission is for rehabilitation, report code Z47.1, Aftercare following joint replacement surgery, as the first-listed or principal diagnosis. If the patient requires rehabilitation post hip replacement for right intertrochanteric femur fracture, report code S72.141D, Displaced intertrochanteric fracture of right femur, subsequent encounter for closed fracture with routine healing, as the first-listed or principal diagnosis.

See Section I.C.21.c.7, Factors influencing health states and contact with health services, Aftercare.
See Section I.C.19.a for additional information about the use of 7th characters for injury codes.

SECTION III. REPORTING ADDITIONAL DIAGNOSES

GENERAL RULES FOR OTHER (ADDITIONAL) DIAGNOSES

For reporting purposes the definition for "other diagnoses" is interpreted as additional conditions that affect patient care in terms of requiring:

- clinical evaluation; or therapeutic treatment; or diagnostic procedures; or

- extended length of hospital stay; or increased nursing care and/or monitoring.

The UHDDS item #11-b defines Other Diagnoses as "all conditions that coexist at the time of admission, that develop subsequently, or that affect the treatment received and/or the length of stay. Diagnoses that relate to an earlier episode which have no bearing on the current hospital stay are to be excluded." UHDDS definitions apply to inpatients in acute care, short-term, long term care and psychiatric hospital setting. The UHDDS definitions are used by acute care short-term hospitals to report inpatient data elements in a standardized manner. These data elements and their definitions can be found in the July 31, 1985, Federal Register (Vol. 50, No, 147), pp. 31038-40.

Since that time the application of the UHDDS definitions has been expanded to include all non-outpatient settings (acute care, short term, long term care and psychiatric hospitals; home health agencies; rehab facilities; nursing homes, etc). The UHDDS definitions also apply to hospice services (all levels of care).

The following guidelines are to be applied in designating "other diagnoses" when neither the Alphabetic Index nor the Tabular List in ICD-10-CM provide direction. The listing of the diagnoses in the patient record is the responsibility of the attending provider.

A. Previous conditions

If the provider has included a diagnosis in the final diagnostic statement, such as the discharge summary or the face sheet, it should ordinarily be coded. Some providers include in the diagnostic statement resolved conditions or diagnoses and status-post procedures from previous admission that have no bearing on the current stay. Such conditions are not to be reported and are coded only if required by hospital policy.

However, history codes (categories Z80-Z87) may be used as secondary codes if the historical condition or family history has an impact on current care or influences treatment.

B. Abnormal findings

Abnormal findings (laboratory, x-ray, pathologic, and other diagnostic results) are not coded and reported unless the provider indicates their clinical significance. If the findings are outside the normal range and the attending provider has ordered other tests to evaluate the condition or prescribed treatment, it is appropriate to ask the provider whether the abnormal finding should be added.

Please note: This differs from the coding practices in the outpatient setting for coding encounters for diagnostic tests that have been interpreted by a provider.

C. Uncertain Diagnosis

If the diagnosis documented at the time of discharge is qualified as "probable", "suspected", "likely", "questionable", "possible", or "still to be ruled out" or other similar terms indicating uncertainty, code the condition as if it existed or was established. The bases for these guidelines are the diagnostic workup, arrangements for further workup or observation, and initial therapeutic approach that correspond most closely with the established diagnosis.

Note: This guideline is applicable only to inpatient admissions to short-term, acute, long-term care and psychiatric hospitals.

SECTION IV. DIAGNOSTIC CODING AND REPORTING GUIDELINES FOR OUTPATIENT SERVICES

These coding guidelines for outpatient diagnoses have been approved for use by hospitals/ providers in coding and reporting hospital-based outpatient services and provider-based office visits. Guidelines in Section I, Conventions, general coding guidelines and chapter-specific guidelines, should also be applied for outpatient services and office visits.

Information about the use of certain abbreviations, punctuation, symbols, and other conventions used in the ICD-10-CM Tabular List (code numbers and titles), can be found in Section IA of these guidelines, under "Conventions Used in the Tabular List." Section I.B. contains general guidelines that apply to the entire classification. Section I.C. contains chapter-specific guidelines that correspond to the chapters as they are arranged in the classification. Information about the correct sequence to use in finding a code is also described in Section I.

The terms encounter and visit are often used interchangeably in describing outpatient service contacts and, therefore, appear together in these guidelines without distinguishing one from the other.

Though the conventions and general guidelines apply to all settings, coding guidelines for outpatient and provider reporting of diagnoses will vary in a number of instances from those for inpatient diagnoses, recognizing that:

The Uniform Hospital Discharge Data Set (UHDDS) definition of principal diagnosis does not apply to hospital-based outpatient services and provider-based office visits.

Coding guidelines for inconclusive diagnoses (probable, suspected, rule out, etc.) were developed for inpatient reporting and do not apply to outpatients.

A. Selection of first-listed condition

In the outpatient setting, the term first-listed diagnosis is used in lieu of principal diagnosis.

In determining the first-listed diagnosis the coding conventions of ICD-10-CM, as well as the general and disease specific guidelines take precedence over the outpatient guidelines.

Diagnoses often are not established at the time of the initial encounter/visit. It may take two or more visits before the diagnosis is confirmed.

The most critical rule involves beginning the search for the correct code assignment through the Alphabetic Index. Never begin searching initially in the Tabular List as this will lead to coding errors.

1. Outpatient Surgery

When a patient presents for outpatient surgery (same day surgery), code the reason for the surgery as the first-listed diagnosis (reason for the encounter), even if the surgery is not performed due to a contraindication.

2. Observation Stay

When a patient is admitted for observation for a medical condition, assign a code for the medical condition as the first-listed diagnosis.

When a patient presents for outpatient surgery and develops complications requiring admission to observation, code the reason for the surgery as the first reported diagnosis (reason for the encounter), followed by codes for the complications as secondary diagnoses.

B. Codes from A00.0 through T88.9, Z00-Z99

The appropriate code(s) from A00.0 through T88.9, Z00-Z99 must be used to identify diagnoses, symptoms, conditions, problems, complaints, or other reason(s) for the encounter/visit.

C. Accurate reporting of ICD-10-CM diagnosis codes

For accurate reporting of ICD-10-CM diagnosis codes, the documentation should describe the patient's condition, using terminology which includes specific diagnoses as well as symptoms, problems, or reasons for the encounter. There are ICD-10-CM codes to describe all of these.

D. Codes that describe symptoms and signs

Codes that describe symptoms and signs, as opposed to diagnoses, are acceptable for reporting purposes when a diagnosis has not been established (confirmed) by the provider. Chapter 18 of ICD-10-CM, Symptoms, Signs, and Abnormal Clinical and Laboratory Findings Not Elsewhere Classified (codes R00-R99) contain many, but not all codes for symptoms.

E. Encounters for circumstances other than a disease or injury

ICD-10-CM provides codes to deal with encounters for circumstances other than a disease or injury. The Factors Influencing Health Status and Contact with Health Services codes (Z00-Z99) are provided to deal with occasions when circumstances other than a disease or injury are recorded as diagnosis or problems.

See Section I.C.21. Factors influencing health status and contact with health services.

F. Level of Detail in Coding

1. ICD-10-CM codes with 3, 4, 5, 6 or 7 characters

ICD-10-CM is composed of codes with 3, 4, 5, 6 or 7 characters. Codes with three characters are included in ICD-10-CM as the heading of a category of codes that may be further subdivided by the use of fourth, fifth, sixth or seventh characters to provide greater specificity.

2. Use of full number of characters required for a code

A three-character code is to be used only if it is not further subdivided. A code is invalid if it has not been coded to the full number of characters required for that code, including the 7th character, if applicable.

G. ICD-10-CM code for the diagnosis, condition, problem, or other reason for encounter/visit

List first the ICD-10-CM code for the diagnosis, condition, problem, or other reason for encounter/visit shown in the medical record to be chiefly responsible for the services provided. List additional codes that describe any coexisting conditions. In some cases the first-listed diagnosis may be a symptom when a diagnosis has not been established (confirmed) by the physician.

H. Uncertain diagnosis

Do not code diagnoses documented as "probable", "suspected," "questionable," "rule out," or "working diagnosis" or other similar terms indicating uncertainty. Rather, code the condition(s) to the highest degree of certainty for that encounter/visit, such as symptoms, signs, abnormal test results, or other reason for the visit.

Please note: This differs from the coding practices used by short-term, acute care, long-term care and psychiatric hospitals.

I. Chronic diseases

Chronic diseases treated on an ongoing basis may be coded and reported as many times as the patient receives treatment and care for the condition(s)

J. Code all documented conditions that coexist

Code all documented conditions that coexist at the time of the encounter/visit, and require or affect patient care treatment or management. Do not code conditions that were previously treated and no longer exist. However, history codes (categories Z80-Z87) may be used as secondary codes if the historical condition or family history has an impact on current care or influences treatment.

K. Patients receiving diagnostic services only

For patients receiving diagnostic services only during an encounter/visit, sequence first the diagnosis, condition, problem, or other reason for encounter/visit shown in the medical record to be chiefly responsible for the outpatient services provided during the encounter/visit. Codes for other diagnoses (e.g., chronic conditions) may be sequenced as additional diagnoses.

For encounters for routine laboratory/radiology testing in the absence of any signs, symptoms, or associated diagnosis, assign Z01.89, Encounter for other specified special examinations. If routine testing is performed during the same encounter as a test to evaluate a sign, symptom, or diagnosis, it is appropriate to assign both the Z code and the code describing the reason for the non-routine test.

For outpatient encounters for diagnostic tests that have been interpreted by a physician, and the final report is available at the time of coding, code any confirmed or definitive diagnosis(es) documented in the interpretation. Do not code related signs and symptoms as additional diagnoses.

Please note: This differs from the coding practice in the hospital inpatient setting regarding abnormal findings on test results.

L. Patients receiving therapeutic services only

For patients receiving therapeutic services only during an encounter/visit, sequence first the diagnosis, condition, problem, or other reason for encounter/visit shown in the medical record to be chiefly responsible for the outpatient services provided during the encounter/visit. Codes for other diagnoses (e.g., chronic conditions) may be sequenced as additional diagnoses.

The only exception to this rule is that when the primary reason for the admission/encounter is chemotherapy or radiation therapy, the appropriate Z code for the service is listed first, and the diagnosis or problem for which the service is being performed listed second.

M. Patients receiving preoperative evaluations only

For patients receiving preoperative evaluations only, sequence first a code from subcategory Z01.81, Encounter for pre-procedural examinations, to describe the pre-op consultations. Assign a code for the condition to describe the reason for the surgery as an additional diagnosis. Code also any findings related to the pre-op evaluation.

N. Ambulatory surgery

For ambulatory surgery, code the diagnosis for which the surgery was performed. If the postoperative diagnosis is known to be different from the preoperative diagnosis at the time the diagnosis is confirmed, select the postoperative diagnosis for coding, since it is the most definitive.

O. Routine outpatient prenatal visits

See Section I.C.15. Routine outpatient prenatal visits.

P. Encounters for general medical examinations with abnormal findings

The subcategories for encounters for general medical examinations, Z00.0-, provide codes for with and without abnormal findings. Should a general medical examination result in an abnormal finding, the code for general medical examination with abnormal finding should be assigned as the first-listed diagnosis. An examination with abnormal findings refers to a condition/diagnosis that is newly identified or a change in severity of a chronic condition (such as uncontrolled hypertension, or an acute exacerbation of chronic obstructive pulmonary disease) during a routine physical examination. A secondary code for the abnormal finding should also be coded.

Q. Encounters for routine health screenings

See Section I.C.21. Factors influencing health status and contact with health services, Screening

APPENDIX I

PRESENT ON ADMISSION REPORTING GUIDELINES

INTRODUCTION

These guidelines are to be used as a supplement to the *ICD-10-CM Official Guidelines for Coding and Reporting* to facilitate the assignment of the Present on Admission (POA) indicator for each diagnosis and external cause of injury code reported on claim forms (UB-04 and 837 Institutional).

These guidelines are not intended to replace any guidelines in the main body of the *ICD-10-CM Official Guidelines for Coding and Reporting*. The POA guidelines are not intended to provide guidance on when a condition should be coded, but rather, how to apply the POA indicator to the final set of diagnosis codes that have been assigned in accordance with Sections I, II, and III of the official coding guidelines. Subsequent to the assignment of the ICD-10-CM codes, the POA indicator should then be assigned to those conditions that have been coded.

As stated in the Introduction to the ICD-10-CM Official Guidelines for Coding and Reporting, a joint effort between the healthcare provider and the coder is essential to achieve complete and accurate documentation, code assignment, and reporting of diagnoses and procedures. The importance of consistent, complete documentation in the medical record cannot be overemphasized. Medical record documentation from any provider involved in the care and treatment of the patient may be used to support the determination of whether a condition was present on admission or not. In the context of the official coding guidelines, the term "provider" means a physician or any qualified healthcare practitioner who is legally accountable for establishing the patient's diagnosis.

These guidelines are not a substitute for the provider's clinical judgment as to the determination of whether a condition was/was not present on admission. The provider should be queried regarding issues related to the linking of signs/symptoms, timing of test results, and the timing of findings.

Please see the CDC website for the detailed list of ICD-10-CM codes that do not require the use of a POA indicator (https://www.cdc.gov/nchs/icd/icd10cm.htm) (https://www.cms.gov/Medicare/Coding/ICD10/2018-ICD-10-CM-and-GEMs.html). The codes and categories on this exempt list are for circumstances regarding the healthcare encounter or factors influencing health status that do not represent a current disease or injury or that describe conditions that are always present on admission.

General Reporting Requirements

All claims involving inpatient admissions to general acute care hospitals or other facilities that are subject to a law or regulation mandating collection of present on admission information.

Present on admission is defined as present at the time the order for inpatient admission occurs -- conditions that develop during an outpatient encounter, including emergency department, observation, or outpatient surgery, are considered as present on admission.

POA indicator is assigned to principal and secondary diagnoses (as defined in Section II of the Official Guidelines for Coding and Reporting) and the external cause of injury codes.
Issues related to inconsistent, missing, conflicting or unclear documentation must still be resolved by the provider.

If a condition would not be coded and reported based on UHDDS definitions and current official coding guidelines, then the POA indicator would not be reported.

Reporting Options

Y - Yes

N - No

U - Unknown

W - Clinically undetermined

Unreported/Not used – (Exempt from POA reporting)

Reporting Definitions

Y =   present at the time of inpatient admission

N =   not present at the time of inpatient admission

U =   documentation is insufficient to determine if condition is present on admission

W =   provider is unable to clinically determine whether condition was present on admission or not

Timeframe for POA Identification and Documentation

There is no required timeframe as to when a provider (per the definition of "provider" used in these guidelines) must identify or document a condition to be present on admission. In some clinical situations, it may not be possible for a provider to make a definitive diagnosis (or a condition may not be recognized or reported by the patient) for a period of time after admission. In some cases it may be several days before the provider arrives at a definitive diagnosis. This does not mean that the condition was not present on admission. Determination of whether the condition was present on admission or not will be based on the applicable POA guideline as identified in this document, or on the provider's best clinical judgment.

If at the time of code assignment the documentation is unclear as to whether a condition was present on admission or not, it is appropriate to query the provider for clarification.

Assigning the POA Indicator

Condition is on the "Exempt from Reporting" list

Leave the "present on admission" field blank if the condition is on the list of ICD-10-CM codes for which this field is not applicable. This is the only circumstance in which the field may be left blank.

POA Explicitly Documented

Assign Y for any condition the provider explicitly documents as being present on admission.

Assign N for any condition the provider explicitly documents as not present at the time of admission.

Conditions diagnosed prior to inpatient admission

Assign "Y" for conditions that were diagnosed prior to admission (example: hypertension, diabetes mellitus, asthma)

Conditions diagnosed during the admission but clearly present before admission

Assign "Y" for conditions diagnosed during the admission that were clearly present but not diagnosed until after admission occurred.

Diagnoses subsequently confirmed after admission are considered present on admission if at the time of admission they are documented as suspected, possible, rule out, differential diagnosis, or constitute an underlying cause of a symptom that is present at the time of admission.

Condition develops during outpatient encounter prior to inpatient admission

Assign Y for any condition that develops during an outpatient encounter prior to a written order for inpatient admission.

Documentation does not indicate whether condition was present on admission

Assign "U" when the medical record documentation is unclear as to whether the condition was present on admission. "U" should not be routinely assigned and used only in very limited circumstances. Coders are encouraged to query the providers when the documentation is unclear.

Documentation states that it cannot be determined whether the condition was or was not present on admission

Assign "W" when the medical record documentation indicates that it cannot be clinically determined whether or not the condition was present on admission.

Chronic condition with acute exacerbation during the admission

If a single code identifies both the chronic condition and the acute exacerbation, see POA guidelines pertaining to codes that contain multiple clinical concepts.

If a single code only identifies the chronic condition and not the acute exacerbation (e.g., acute exacerbation of chronic leukemia), assign "Y."

Conditions documented as possible, probable, suspected, or rule out at the time of discharge

If the final diagnosis contains a possible, probable, suspected, or rule out diagnosis, and this diagnosis was based on signs, symptoms or clinical findings suspected at the time of inpatient admission, assign "Y."

If the final diagnosis contains a possible, probable, suspected, or rule out diagnosis, and this diagnosis was based on signs, symptoms or clinical findings that were not present on admission, assign "N".

Conditions documented as impending or threatened at the time of discharge

If the final diagnosis contains an impending or threatened diagnosis, and this diagnosis is based on symptoms or clinical findings that were present on admission, assign "Y".
If the final diagnosis contains an impending or threatened diagnosis, and this diagnosis is based on symptoms or clinical findings that were not present on admission, assign "N".

Acute and Chronic Conditions

Assign "Y" for acute conditions that are present at time of admission and N for acute conditions that are not present at time of admission.

Assign "Y" for chronic conditions, even though the condition may not be diagnosed until after admission.

If a single code identifies both an acute and chronic condition, see the POA guidelines for codes that contain multiple clinical concepts.

Codes That Contain Multiple Clinical Concepts

Assign "N" if at least one of the clinical concepts included in the code was not present on admission (e.g., COPD with acute exacerbation and the exacerbation was not present on admission; gastric ulcer that does not start bleeding until after admission; asthma patient develops status asthmaticus after admission).

Assign "Y" if all of the clinical concepts included in the code were present on admission (e.g., duodenal ulcer that perforates prior to admission).

For infection codes that include the causal organism, assign "Y" if the infection (or signs of the infection) **were** present on admission, even though the culture results may not be known until after admission (e.g., patient is admitted with pneumonia and the provider documents Pseudomonas as the causal organism a few days later).

Same Diagnosis Code for Two or More Conditions

When the same ICD-10-CM diagnosis code applies to two or more conditions during the same encounter (e.g. two separate conditions classified to the same ICD-10-CM diagnosis code):

Assign "Y" if all conditions represented by the single ICD-10-CM code were present on admission (e.g. bilateral unspecified age-related cataracts).

Assign "N" if any of the conditions represented by the single ICD-10-CM code was not present on admission (e.g. traumatic secondary and recurrent hemorrhage and seroma is assigned to a single code T79.2, but only one of the conditions was present on admission).

Obstetrical conditions

Whether or not the patient delivers during the current hospitalization does not affect assignment of the POA indicator. The determining factor for POA assignment is whether the pregnancy complication or obstetrical condition described by the code was present at the time of admission or not.

If the pregnancy complication or obstetrical condition was present on admission (e.g., patient admitted in preterm labor), assign "Y".

If the pregnancy complication or obstetrical condition was not present on admission (e.g., 2nd degree laceration during delivery, postpartum hemorrhage that occurred during current hospitalization, fetal distress develops after admission), assign "N".

If the obstetrical code includes more than one diagnosis and any of the diagnoses identified by the code were not present on admission assign "N".

(e.g., Category O11, Pre-existing hypertension with pre-eclampsia)

Perinatal conditions

Newborns are not considered to be admitted until after birth. Therefore, any condition present at birth or that developed in utero is considered present at admission and should be assigned "Y". This includes conditions that occur during delivery (e.g., injury during delivery, meconium aspiration, exposure to streptococcus B in the vaginal canal).

Congenital conditions and anomalies

Assign "Y" for congenital conditions and anomalies except for categories Q00-Q99, Congenital anomalies, which are on the exempt list. Congenital conditions are always considered present on admission.

External cause of injury codes

Assign "Y" for any external cause code representing an external cause of morbidity that occurred prior to inpatient admission (e.g., patient fell out of bed at home, patient fell out of bed in emergency room prior to admission)

Assign "N" for any external cause code representing an external cause of morbidity that occurred during inpatient hospitalization (e.g., patient fell out of hospital bed during hospital stay, patient experienced an adverse reaction to a medication administered after inpatient admission)

Anatomical Illustrations

A fundamental knowledge and understanding of basic human anatomy and physiology is a prerequisite for accurate diagnosis coding. While a comprehensive treatment of anatomy and physiology is beyond the scope of this text, the large scale, full color anatomical illustrations on the following pages are designed to facilitate the procedure coding process for both beginning and experienced coders.

The illustrations provide an anatomical perspective of procedure coding by providing a side-by-side view of the major systems of the human body and a corresponding list of the most common ICD-10-CM categories used to report medical, surgical and diagnostic services performed on the illustrated system.

The ICD-10-CM categories listed on the left facing page of each anatomical illustration are code ranges only and should not be used for coding. These categories are provided as "pointers" to the appropriate section of ICD-10-CM, where the definitive code may be found.

PLATE 1. SKIN AND SUBCUTANEOUS TISSUE – MALE

Viral infections characterized by skin and mucous membrane lesions	**B00-B09**
Bacterial and viral infectious agents	**B95-B97**
Melanoma and other malignant neoplasms of skin	**C43-C44**
Malignant neoplasms of mesothelial and soft tissue	**C45-C49**
Malignant neoplasms of ill-defined, other secondary and unspecified sites	**C76-C80**
In situ neoplasms	**D00-D09**
Benign neoplasms, except benign neuroendocrine tumors	**D10-D36**
Neoplasms of uncertain behavior, polycythemia vera and myelodysplastic syndromes	**D37-D48**
Neoplasms of unspecified behavior	**D49**
Infections of the skin and subcutaneous tissue	**L00-L08**
Bullous disorders	**L10-L14**
Dermatitis and eczema	**L20-L30**
Papulosquamous disorders	**L40-L45**
Urticaria and erythema	**L49-L54**
Radiation-related disorders of the skin and subcutaneous tissue	**L55-L59**
Disorders of skin appendages	**L60-L75**
Intraoperative and postprocedural complications of skin and subcutaneous tissue	**L76**
Other disorders of the skin and subcutaneous tissue	**L80-L99**
Symptoms and signs involving the skin and subcutaneous tissue	**R20-R23**
General symptoms and signs	**R50-R69**
Abnormal findings on diagnostic imaging and in function studies, without diagnosis	**R90-R94**
Burns and corrosions of external body surface, specified by site	**T20-T25**
Burns and corrosions	**T20-T32**
Burns and corrosions of multiple and unspecified body regions	**T30-T32**
Persons encountering health services for examinations	**Z00-Z13**
Encounters for other specific health care	**Z40-Z53**

Male Figure
(Anterior View)

Parietal region

Temporal region

Nasal region

Frontal region

Orbital region

Oral region

Mental region

Anterior neck region

Lateral neck region

Infraclavicular region

Deltoid region

Sternal region

Pectoral region

Brachial region

Axillary region

Hypochondriac region

Epigastric region

Cubital region

Antebrachial region

Umbilical region

Lateral abdominal region

Inguinal region

Pubic region

Femoral region

Knee region

Crural region

PLATE 2. SKIN AND SUBCUTANEOUS TISSUE - FEMALE

Viral infections characterized by skin and mucous membrane lesions	**B00-B09**
Bacterial and viral infectious agents	**B95-B97**
Melanoma and other malignant neoplasms of skin	**C43-C44**
Malignant neoplasms of mesothelial and soft tissue	**C45-C49**
Malignant neoplasms of ill-defined, other secondary and unspecified sites	**C76-C80**
In situ neoplasms	**D00-D09**
Benign neoplasms, except benign neuroendocrine tumors	**D10-D36**
Neoplasms of uncertain behavior, polycythemia vera and myelodysplastic syndromes	**D37-D48**
Neoplasms of unspecified behavior	**D49**
Infections of the skin and subcutaneous tissue	**L00-L08**
Bullous disorders	**L10-L14**
Dermatitis and eczema	**L20-L30**
Papulosquamous disorders	**L40-L45**
Urticaria and erythema	**L49-L54**
Radiation-related disorders of the skin and subcutaneous tissue	**L55-L59**
Disorders of skin appendages	**L60-L75**
Intraoperative and postprocedural complications of skin and subcutaneous tissue	**L76**
Other disorders of the skin and subcutaneous tissue	**L80-L99**
Symptoms and signs involving the skin and subcutaneous tissue	**R20-R23**
General symptoms and signs	**R50-R69**
Abnormal findings on diagnostic imaging and in function studies, without diagnosis	**R90-R94**
Burns and corrosions of external body surface, specified by site	**T20-T25**
Burns and corrosions	**T20-T32**
Burns and corrosions of multiple and unspecified body regions	**T30-T32**
Persons encountering health services for examinations	**Z00-Z13**
Encounters for other specific health care	**Z40-Z53**

Female Figure
(Anterior View)

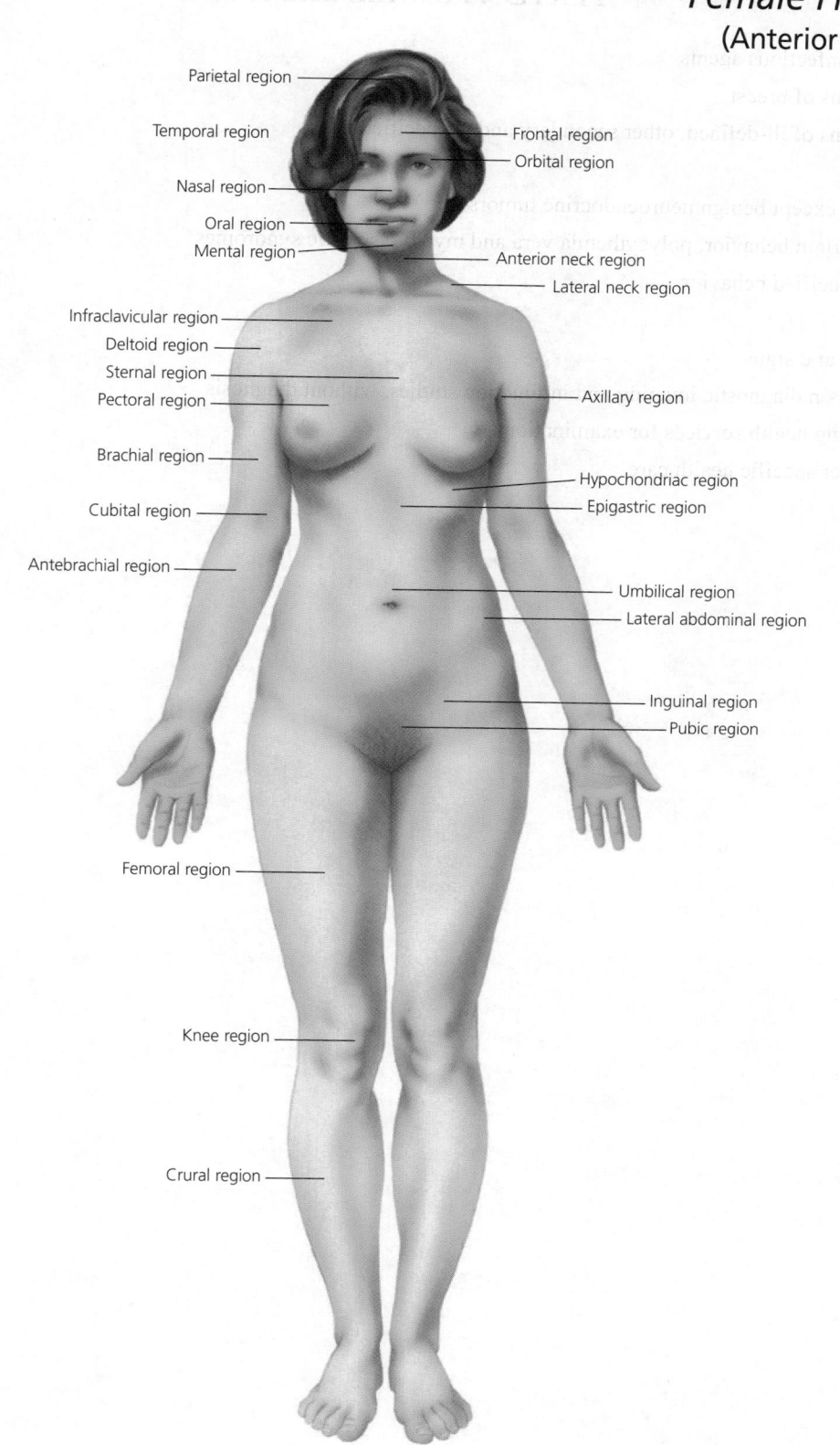

Parietal region

Temporal region

Frontal region

Orbital region

Nasal region

Oral region

Mental region

Anterior neck region

Lateral neck region

Infraclavicular region

Deltoid region

Sternal region

Pectoral region

Axillary region

Brachial region

Cubital region

Hypochondriac region

Epigastric region

Antebrachial region

Umbilical region

Lateral abdominal region

Inguinal region

Pubic region

Femoral region

Knee region

Crural region

PLATE 3. FEMALE BREAST

Bacterial and viral infectious agents	**B95-B97**
Malignant neoplasms of breast	**C50**
Malignant neoplasms of ill-defined, other secondary and unspecified sites	**C76-C80**
In situ neoplasms	**D00-D09**
Benign neoplasms, except benign neuroendocrine tumors	**D10-D36**
Neoplasms of uncertain behavior, polycythemia vera and myelodysplastic syndromes	**D37-D48**
Neoplasms of unspecified behavior	**D49**
Disorders of breast	**N60-N65**
General symptoms and signs	**R50-R69**
Abnormal findings on diagnostic imaging and in function studies, without diagnosis	**R90-R94**
Persons encountering health services for examinations	**Z00-Z13**
Encounters for other specific health care	**Z40-Z53**

Female Breast

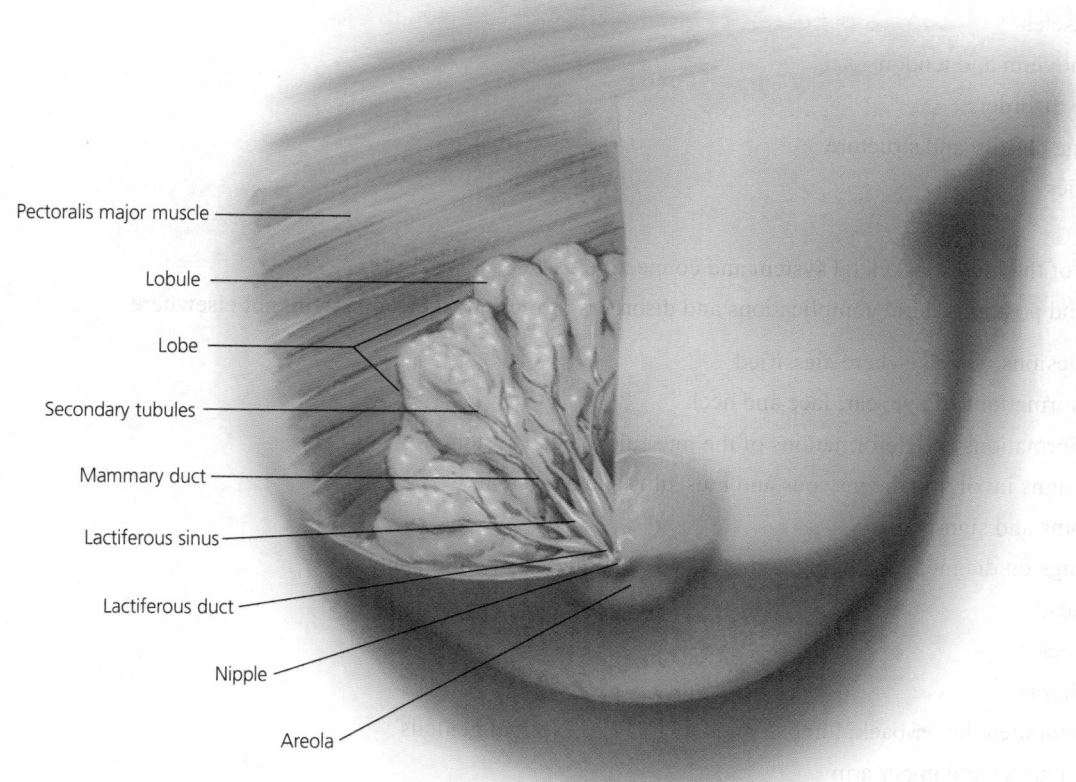

Pectoralis major muscle

Lobule

Lobe

Secondary tubules

Mammary duct

Lactiferous sinus

Lactiferous duct

Nipple

Areola

PLATE 4. MUSCULAR SYSTEM AND CONNECTIVE TISSUE – ANTERIOR VIEW

Malignant neoplasms of bone and articular cartilage	**C40-C41**
Infectious arthropathies	**M00-M02**
Inflammatory polyarthropathies	**M05-M14**
Osteoarthritis	**M15-M19**
Other joint disorders	**M20-M25**
Dentofacial anomalies [including malocclusion] and other disorders of jaw	**M26-M27**
Systemic connective tissue disorders	**M30-M36**
Deforming dorsopathies	**M40-M43**
Spondylopathies	**M45-M49**
Other dorsopathies	**M50-M54**
Disorders of muscles	**M60-M63**
Disorders of synovium and tendon	**M65-M67**
Other soft tissue disorders	**M70-M79**
Disorders of bone density and structure	**M80-M85**
Other osteopathies	**M86-M90**
Chondropathies	**M91-M94**
Other disorders of the musculoskeletal system and connective tissue	**M95**
Intraoperative and postprocedural complications and disorders of musculoskeletal system, not elsewhere classified	**M96**
Biomechanical lesions, not elsewhere classified	**M99**
Congenital malformations of eye, ear, face and neck	**Q10-Q18**
Congenital malformations and deformations of the musculoskeletal system	**Q65-Q79**
Symptoms and signs involving the nervous and musculoskeletal systems	**R25-R29**
General symptoms and signs	**R50-R69**
Abnormal findings on diagnostic imaging and in function studies, without diagnosis	**R90-R94**
Injuries to the head	**S00-S09**
Injuries to the neck	**S10-S19**
Injuries to the thorax	**S20-S29**
Injuries to the abdomen, lower back, lumbar spine, pelvis and external genitals	**S30-S39**
Injuries to the shoulder and upper arm	**S40-S49**
Injuries to the elbow and forearm	**S50-S59**
Injuries to the wrist, hand and fingers	**S60-S69**
Injuries to the hip and thigh	**S70-S79**
Injuries to the knee and lower leg	**S80-S89**
Injuries to the ankle and foot	**S90-S99**
Injuries involving multiple body regions	**T07**
Certain early complications of trauma	**T79**
Accidents	**V00-X58**
Persons encountering health services for examinations	**Z00-Z13**
Encounters for other specific health care	**Z40-Z53**

Muscular System
(Anterior View)

Temporalis m.
Orbicularis oculi m.
Masseter m.
Sternocleidomastoid m.
Trapezius m.
Levator scapulae m.

Frontalis m.
Buccinator
Orbicularis oris m.
Depressor anguli oris m.

Deltoid m.
Pectoralis major m.
Serratus anterior m.
Biceps m.
External abdominal oblique m.
Brachialis m.
Brachioradialis m.
Extensor carpi radialis longus m.
Palmaris longus m.
Flexor carpi radialis m.
Superficial inguinal ring
Tensor fasciae latae m.
Sartorius m.
Rectus femoris m.
Adductor longus m.
Vastus lateralis m.

Pectoralis minor m.
Internal intercostal m.
Coracobrachialis m.
Brachialis m.
Rectus sheath
Rectus abdominis m.
Linea alba
Internal abdominal oblique m.
Transversus abdominis m.
Flexor digitorum superficialis m.
Flexor pollicis longus m.
Abductor digiti minimi m.
Abductor pollicis brevis m.
Flexor pollicis brevis m.
Iliopsoas m.
Pectineus m.
Adductor brevis m.
Gracilis m.
Adductor magnus m.
Vastus medialis m.
Vastus lateralis m.

Iliotibial tract
Vastus medialis m.

Sartorius m.

Lateral patellar retinaculum

Patella
Patellar ligament
Medial patellar retinaculum

Tibialis anterior m.
Gastrocnemius m.
Extensor digitorum longus m.
Peroneus longus m.
Soleus m.
Peroneus brevis m.
Extensor hallucis longus m.
Extensor hallucis brevis m.
Extensor digitorum brevis m.

Gastrocnemius m.
Soleus m.
Tibia
Flexor digitorum longus m.
Extensor hallucis brevis m.
Abductor hallucis m.

PLATE 5. MUSCULAR SYSTEM AND CONNECTIVE TISSUE – POSTERIOR VIEW

Malignant neoplasms of bone and articular cartilage	**C40-C41**
Infectious arthropathies	**M00-M02**
Inflammatory polyarthropathies	**M05-M14**
Osteoarthritis	**M15-M19**
Other joint disorders	**M20-M25**
Dentofacial anomalies [including malocclusion] and other disorders of jaw	**M26-M27**
Systemic connective tissue disorders	**M30-M36**
Deforming dorsopathies	**M40-M43**
Spondylopathies	**M45-M49**
Other dorsopathies	**M50-M54**
Disorders of muscles	**M60-M63**
Disorders of synovium and tendon	**M65-M67**
Other soft tissue disorders	**M70-M79**
Disorders of bone density and structure	**M80-M85**
Other osteopathies	**M86-M90**
Chondropathies	**M91-M94**
Other disorders of the musculoskeletal system and connective tissue	**M95**
Intraoperative and postprocedural complications and disorders of musculoskeletal system, not elsewhere classified	**M96**
Biomechanical lesions, not elsewhere classified	**M99**
Congenital malformations of eye, ear, face and neck	**Q10-Q18**
Congenital malformations and deformations of the musculoskeletal system	**Q65-Q79**
Symptoms and signs involving the nervous and musculoskeletal systems	**R25-R29**
General symptoms and signs	**R50-R69**
Abnormal findings on diagnostic imaging and in function studies, without diagnosis	**R90-R94**
Injuries to the head	**S00-S09**
Injuries to the neck	**S10-S19**
Injuries to the thorax	**S20-S29**
Injuries to the abdomen, lower back, lumbar spine, pelvis and external genitals	**S30-S39**
Injuries to the shoulder and upper arm	**S40-S49**
Injuries to the elbow and forearm	**S50-S59**
Injuries to the wrist, hand and fingers	**S60-S69**
Injuries to the hip and thigh	**S70-S79**
Injuries to the knee and lower leg	**S80-S89**
Injuries to the ankle and foot	**S90-S99**
Injuries involving multiple body regions	**T07**
Certain early complications of trauma	**T79**
Accidents	**V00-X58**
Persons encountering health services for examinations	**Z00-Z13**
Encounters for other specific health care	**Z40-Z53**

Muscular System
(Posterior View)

Frontalis m.

Temporoparietalis m.

Zygomaticus major m.

Masseter m.

Risorius m.

Trapezius m.

Deltoid m.

Infraspinatus m.

Teres minor m.

Teres major m.

Triceps m.

Latissimus dorsi m.

Brachialis m.

Brachioradialis m.

Extensor carpi radialis longus m.

Flexor carpi ulnaris m.

Extensor digitorum m.

Extensor carpi radialis brevis m.

Extensor carpi ulnaris m.

Abductor pollicis longus m.

Extensor pollicis brevis m.

Gluteus medius m.

Gluteus maximus m.

Biceps femoris m.

Adductor magnus m.

Iliotibial tract

Vastus lateralis m.

Semimembranosus m.

Semitendinosus m.

Gastrocnemius m.

Peroneus longus m.

Soleus m.

Calcaneal t. (Achilles)

Galea aponeurotica

Occipitalis m.

Sternocleidomastoid m.

Splenius capitis m.

Splenius cervicis m.

Levator scapulae m.

Supraspinatus m.

Rhomboid minor m.

Rhomboid major m.

Spinalis thoracis m.

Iliocostalis thoracis m.

Longissimus thoracis m.

Serratus posterior inferior m.

Brachioradialis m.

Extensor carpi radialis longus m.

External abdominal oblique m.

Supinator m.

Gluteus medius m.

Extensor pollicis longus m.

Gluteus minimus m.

Piriformis m.

Superior gemellus m.

Obturator internus m.

Inferior gemellus m.

Quadratus femoris m.

Adductor magnus m.

Gracilis m.

Biceps femoris m.

Semimembranosus m.

Plantaris m.

Popliteus m.

Soleus m.

Flexor digitorum longus m.

Peroneus longus m.

Flexor hallucis longus m.

Peroneus brevis m.

PLATE 6. MUSCULAR SYSTEM - SHOULDER AND ELBOW

Malignant neoplasms of bone and articular cartilage	**C40-C41**
Infectious arthropathies	**M00-M02**
Inflammatory polyarthropathies	**M05-M14**
Osteoarthritis	**M15-M19**
Other joint disorders	**M20-M25**
Dentofacial anomalies [including malocclusion] and other disorders of jaw	**M26-M27**
Systemic connective tissue disorders	**M30-M36**
Deforming dorsopathies	**M40-M43**
Spondylopathies	**M45-M49**
Other dorsopathies	**M50-M54**
Disorders of muscles	**M60-M63**
Disorders of synovium and tendon	**M65-M67**
Other soft tissue disorders	**M70-M79**
Disorders of bone density and structure	**M80-M85**
Other osteopathies	**M86-M90**
Chondropathies	**M91-M94**
Other disorders of the musculoskeletal system and connective tissue	**M95**
Intraoperative and postprocedural complications and disorders of musculoskeletal system, not elsewhere classified	**M96**
Biomechanical lesions, not elsewhere classified	**M99**
Congenital malformations and deformations of the musculoskeletal system	**Q65-Q79**
Symptoms and signs involving the nervous and musculoskeletal systems	**R25-R29**
General symptoms and signs	**R50-R69**
Abnormal findings on diagnostic imaging and in function studies, without diagnosis	**R90-R94**
Injuries to the shoulder and upper arm	**S40-S49**
Injuries to the elbow and forearm	**S50-S59**
Injuries involving multiple body regions	**T07**
Certain early complications of trauma	**T79**
Accidents	**V00-X58**
Persons encountering health services for examinations	**Z00-Z13**
Encounters for other specific health care	**Z40-Z53**

Shoulder and Elbow
(Anterior View)

Coracoclavicular ligament

Acromioclavicular ligament

Coracoacromial ligament

Supraspinatus tendon

Coracohumeral ligament

Transverse humeral ligament

Tendon of long head of biceps muscle

Subscapularis tendon

Articular capsule

Acromion

Clavicle

Coracoid process

Scapular notch

Subscapular fossa

Head of humerus

Lesser tubercle

Greater tubercle

Scapula

Nutrient foramen

Humerus

Deltoid tuberosity

Articular capsule

Radial collateral ligament

Annular ligament

Ulnar collateral ligament

Interosseous membrane

Radius

Ulna

Lateral epicondyle

Capitulum

Coronoid fossa

Medial epicondyle

Trochlea

Coronoid process

Head of radius

Ulnar tuberosity

Radial tuberosity

PLATE 7. MUSCULAR SYSTEM - HAND AND WRIST

Malignant neoplasms of bone and articular cartilage	**C40-C41**
Infectious arthropathies	**M00-M02**
Inflammatory polyarthropathies	**M05-M14**
Osteoarthritis	**M15-M19**
Other joint disorders	**M20-M25**
Dentofacial anomalies [including malocclusion] and other disorders of jaw	**M26-M27**
Systemic connective tissue disorders	**M30-M36**
Deforming dorsopathies	**M40-M43**
Spondylopathies	**M45-M49**
Other dorsopathies	**M50-M54**
Disorders of muscles	**M60-M63**
Disorders of synovium and tendon	**M65-M67**
Other soft tissue disorders	**M70-M79**
Disorders of bone density and structure	**M80-M85**
Other osteopathies	**M86-M90**
Chondropathies	**M91-M94**
Other disorders of the musculoskeletal system and connective tissue	**M95**
Intraoperative and postprocedural complications and disorders of musculoskeletal system, not elsewhere classified	**M96**
Biomechanical lesions, not elsewhere classified	**M99**
Congenital malformations and deformations of the musculoskeletal system	**Q65-Q79**
Symptoms and signs involving the nervous and musculoskeletal systems	**R25-R29**
General symptoms and signs	**R50-R69**
Abnormal findings on diagnostic imaging and in function studies, without diagnosis	**R90-R94**
Injuries to the wrist, hand and fingers	**S60-S69**
Injuries involving multiple body regions	**T07**
Certain early complications of trauma	**T79**
Accidents	**V00-X58**
Persons encountering health services for examinations	**Z00-Z13**
Encounters for other specific health care	**Z40-Z53**

Hand and Wrist

Abductor pollicis longus muscle

Extensor pollicis brevis muscle

Extensor digitorum tendons

Extensor pollicis brevis tendon

Extensor pollicis longus tendon

Extensor carpi radialis brevis tendon

Extensor carpi radialis longus tendon

1st dorsal interosseous muscle

Extensor digiti minimi muscle

Extensor carpi ulnaris muscle

Extensor retinaculum

Extensor digiti minimi tendons

Extensor digitorum tendons

2nd, 3rd, 4th dorsal interosseous muscles

Brachioradialis tendon

Flexor carpi radialis tendon

Flexor pollicis longus muscle

Abductor pollicis longus tendon

Opponens pollicis muscle

Abductor pollicis brevis muscle

Flexor pollicis brevis muscle

Flexor digitorum superficialis muscle & tendons

Flexor carpi ulnaris tendon

Palmaris longus tendon

Opponens digiti minimi muscle

Flexor digiti minimi brevis muscle

Abductor digiti minimi muscle

Flexor digitorum superficialis tendons

Palmar interosseous muscles

Fibrous digital sheath:
anular part
cruciform part

Adductor pollicis muscle

Lumbrical muscles

Flexor digitorum profundus tendon

PLATE 8. MUSCULOSKELETAL SYSTEM - HIP AND KNEE

Malignant neoplasms of bone and articular cartilage	**C40-C41**
Infectious arthropathies	**M00-M02**
Inflammatory polyarthropathies	**M05-M14**
Osteoarthritis	**M15-M19**
Other joint disorders	**M20-M25**
Dentofacial anomalies [including malocclusion] and other disorders of jaw	**M26-M27**
Systemic connective tissue disorders	**M30-M36**
Deforming dorsopathies	**M40-M43**
Spondylopathies	**M45-M49**
Other dorsopathies	**M50-M54**
Disorders of muscles	**M60-M63**
Disorders of synovium and tendon	**M65-M67**
Other soft tissue disorders	**M70-M79**
Disorders of bone density and structure	**M80-M85**
Other osteopathies	**M86-M90**
Chondropathies	**M91-M94**
Other disorders of the musculoskeletal system and connective tissue	**M95**
Intraoperative and postprocedural complications and disorders of musculoskeletal system, not elsewhere classified	**M96**
Biomechanical lesions, not elsewhere classified	**M99**
Congenital malformations and deformations of the musculoskeletal system	**Q65-Q79**
Symptoms and signs involving the nervous and musculoskeletal systems	**R25-R29**
General symptoms and signs	**R50-R69**
Abnormal findings on diagnostic imaging and in function studies, without diagnosis	**R90-R94**
Injuries to the hip and thigh	**S70-S79**
Injuries to the knee and lower leg	**S80-S89**
Injuries involving multiple body regions	**T07**
Certain early complications of trauma	**T79**
Accidents	**V00-X58**
Persons encountering health services for examinations	**Z00-Z13**
Encounters for other specific health care	**Z40-Z53**

Hip and Knee
(Anterior View)

Sacral promontory
Sacrum
Iliac crest
Ilium
Anterior superior iliac spine
Spine of ischium
Anterior inferior iliac spine
Head of femur
Greater trochanter
Obturator foramen
Pubis
Lesser trochanter

Anterior longitudinal ligament
Iliolumbar ligament
Anterior sacroiliac ligament
Coccyx
Sacrotuberous ligament
Sacrospinous ligament
Inguinal ligament
Iliofemoral ligament
Pubofemoral ligament
Obturator membrane
Pubic symphysis
Femur

Medial epicondyle
Lateral epicondyle
Patella
Lateral condyles
Head of fibula
Tibial tuberosity
Medial condyles
Tibia
Fibula

Quadriceps femoris tendon
Medial patellar retinaculum
Fibular collateral ligament
Tibial collateral ligament
Lateral patellar retinaculum
Patellar ligament
Interosseous membrane

PLATE 9. MUSCULOSKELETAL SYSTEM – FOOT AND ANKLE

Malignant neoplasms of bone and articular cartilage	**C40-C41**
Infectious arthropathies	**M00-M02**
Inflammatory polyarthropathies	**M05-M14**
Osteoarthritis	**M15-M19**
Other joint disorders	**M20-M25**
Dentofacial anomalies [including malocclusion] and other disorders of jaw	**M26-M27**
Systemic connective tissue disorders	**M30-M36**
Deforming dorsopathies	**M40-M43**
Spondylopathies	**M45-M49**
Other dorsopathies	**M50-M54**
Disorders of muscles	**M60-M63**
Disorders of synovium and tendon	**M65-M67**
Other soft tissue disorders	**M70-M79**
Disorders of bone density and structure	**M80-M85**
Other osteopathies	**M86-M90**
Chondropathies	**M91-M94**
Other disorders of the musculoskeletal system and connective tissue	**M95**
Intraoperative and postprocedural complications and disorders of musculoskeletal system, not elsewhere classified	**M96**
Biomechanical lesions, not elsewhere classified	**M99**
Congenital malformations of eye, ear, face and neck	**Q10-Q18**
Congenital malformations and deformations of the musculoskeletal system	**Q65-Q79**
Symptoms and signs involving the nervous and musculoskeletal systems	**R25-R29**
General symptoms and signs	**R50-R69**
Abnormal findings on diagnostic imaging and in function studies, without diagnosis	**R90-R94**
Injuries to the ankle and foot	**S90-S99**
Injuries involving multiple body regions	**T07**
Certain early complications of trauma	**T79**
Accidents	**V00-X58**
Persons encountering health services for examinations	**Z00-Z13**
Encounters for other specific health care	**Z40-Z53**

Foot and Ankle

Soleus muscle

Tibia

Flexor digitorum longus muscle

Flexor hallucis tendon

Achilles tendon

Medial malleolus

Tibialis posterior tendon

Retinaculum

Tibialis posterior tendon

Tibialis anterior tendon

Extensor hallucis brevis muscle

Abductor hallucis muscle

Tibialis anterior muscle

Peroneus brevis muscle

Peroneus longus tendon

Extensor digitorum longus muscle

Tibia

Fibula

Extensor hallucis longus muscle

Lateral malleous

Retinaculum

Peroneus longus tendon

Extensor digitorum brevis muscle

Calcaneus

Peroneus brevis tendon

Peroneus tertius tendon

Opponens digiti minimi muscle

Dorsal interosseous muscles

Extensor hallucis longus tendon

Extensor hallucis brevis muscle

Extensor digitorum longus tendons

PLATE 10. SKELETAL SYSTEM - ANTERIOR VIEW

Malignant neoplasms of bone and articular cartilage	**C40-C41**
Infectious arthropathies	**M00-M02**
Inflammatory polyarthropathies	**M05-M14**
Osteoarthritis	**M15-M19**
Other joint disorders	**M20-M25**
Dentofacial anomalies [including malocclusion] and other disorders of jaw	**M26-M27**
Systemic connective tissue disorders	**M30-M36**
Deforming dorsopathies	**M40-M43**
Spondylopathies	**M45-M49**
Other dorsopathies	**M50-M54**
Disorders of muscles	**M60-M63**
Disorders of synovium and tendon	**M65-M67**
Other soft tissue disorders	**M70-M79**
Disorders of bone density and structure	**M80-M85**
Other osteopathies	**M86-M90**
Chondropathies	**M91-M94**
Other disorders of the musculoskeletal system and connective tissue	**M95**
Intraoperative and postprocedural complications and disorders of musculoskeletal system, not elsewhere classified	**M96**
Biomechanical lesions, not elsewhere classified	**M99**
Congenital malformations of eye, ear, face and neck	**Q10-Q18**
Congenital malformations and deformations of the musculoskeletal system	**Q65-Q79**
Symptoms and signs involving the nervous and musculoskeletal systems	**R25-R29**
General symptoms and signs	**R50-R69**
Abnormal findings on diagnostic imaging and in function studies, without diagnosis	**R90-R94**
Injuries to the head	**S00-S09**
Injuries to the neck	**S10-S19**
Injuries to the thorax	**S20-S29**
Injuries to the abdomen, lower back, lumbar spine, pelvis and external genitals	**S30-S39**
Injuries to the shoulder and upper arm	**S40-S49**
Injuries to the elbow and forearm	**S50-S59**
Injuries to the wrist, hand and fingers	**S60-S69**
Injuries to the hip and thigh	**S70-S79**
Injuries to the knee and lower leg	**S80-S89**
Injuries to the ankle and foot	**S90-S99**
Injuries involving multiple body regions	**T07**
Certain early complications of trauma	**T79**
Accidents	**V00-X58**
Persons encountering health services for examinations	**Z00-Z13**
Encounters for other specific health care	**Z40-Z53**

Skeletal System
(Anterior View)

Frontal bone
Temporal bone
Nasal conchae
Maxilla
Manubrium of sternum
Coracoid process
Acromion
Greater tubercle
Head of humerus
Scapula
Humerus
True ribs (1–7)
False ribs (8–12)
Medial epicondyle
Lateral epicondyle
Radius
Ulna
Sacrum
Anterior superior iliac spine
Head of femur
Greater trochanter

Parietal bone
Orbit
Zygomatic bone
Nasal septum
Mandible
Hyoid bone
Clavicle
Coracoclavicular ligament
Supraspinatus tendon
Subscapularis tendon
Body of sternum
Xiphoid process
Costal cartilages
Anterior longitudinal ligament
Ulnar collateral ligament
Radial collateral ligament
Annular ligament
Iliac crest
Anterior sacroiliac ligament
Interosseous membrane
Inguinal ligament
Coccyx
Iliofemoral ligament

L3
Pubic symphysis
Femur

Metacarpals
Proximal phalanges
Middle phalanges
Distal phalanges

Key to Carpal Bones

A Scaphoid
B Trapezium
C Trapezoid
D Capitate
E Lunate
F Pisiform
G Triquetral
H Hamate

Medial epicondyle
Lateral epicondyle
Patella
Head of fibula
Tibial tuberosity

Quadriceps femoris tendon
Tibial collateral ligament
Fibular collateral ligament
Patellar ligament
Tibia
Fibula
Interosseous membrane

Key to Tarsal Bones

J Intermediate cuneiform
K Lateral cuneiform
L Cuboid
M Talus
N Navicular
O Calcaneus
P Medial cuneiform

Medial malleolus
Lateral malleolus

PLATE 11. SKELETAL SYSTEM - POSTERIOR VIEW

Malignant neoplasms of bone and articular cartilage	**C40-C41**
Infectious arthropathies	**M00-M02**
Inflammatory polyarthropathies	**M05-M14**
Osteoarthritis	**M15-M19**
Other joint disorders	**M20-M25**
Dentofacial anomalies [including malocclusion] and other disorders of jaw	**M26-M27**
Systemic connective tissue disorders	**M30-M36**
Deforming dorsopathies	**M40-M43**
Spondylopathies	**M45-M49**
Other dorsopathies	**M50-M54**
Disorders of muscles	**M60-M63**
Disorders of synovium and tendon	**M65-M67**
Other soft tissue disorders	**M70-M79**
Disorders of bone density and structure	**M80-M85**
Other osteopathies	**M86-M90**
Chondropathies	**M91-M94**
Other disorders of the musculoskeletal system and connective tissue	**M95**
Intraoperative and postprocedural complications and disorders of musculoskeletal system, not elsewhere classified	**M96**
Biomechanical lesions, not elsewhere classified	**M99**
Congenital malformations of eye, ear, face and neck	**Q10-Q18**
Congenital malformations and deformations of the musculoskeletal system	**Q65-Q79**
Symptoms and signs involving the nervous and musculoskeletal systems	**R25-R29**
General symptoms and signs	**R50-R69**
Abnormal findings on diagnostic imaging and in function studies, without diagnosis	**R90-R94**
Injuries to the head	**S00-S09**
Injuries to the neck	**S10-S19**
Injuries to the thorax	**S20-S29**
Injuries to the abdomen, lower back, lumbar spine, pelvis and external genitals	**S30-S39**
Injuries to the shoulder and upper arm	**S40-S49**
Injuries to the elbow and forearm	**S50-S59**
Injuries to the wrist, hand and fingers	**S60-S69**
Injuries to the hip and thigh	**S70-S79**
Injuries to the knee and lower leg	**S80-S89**
Injuries to the ankle and foot	**S90-S99**
Injuries involving multiple body regions	**T07**
Certain early complications of trauma	**T79**
Accidents	**V00-X58**
Persons encountering health services for examinations	**Z00-Z13**
Encounters for other specific health care	**Z40-Z53**

Skeletal System
(Posterior View)

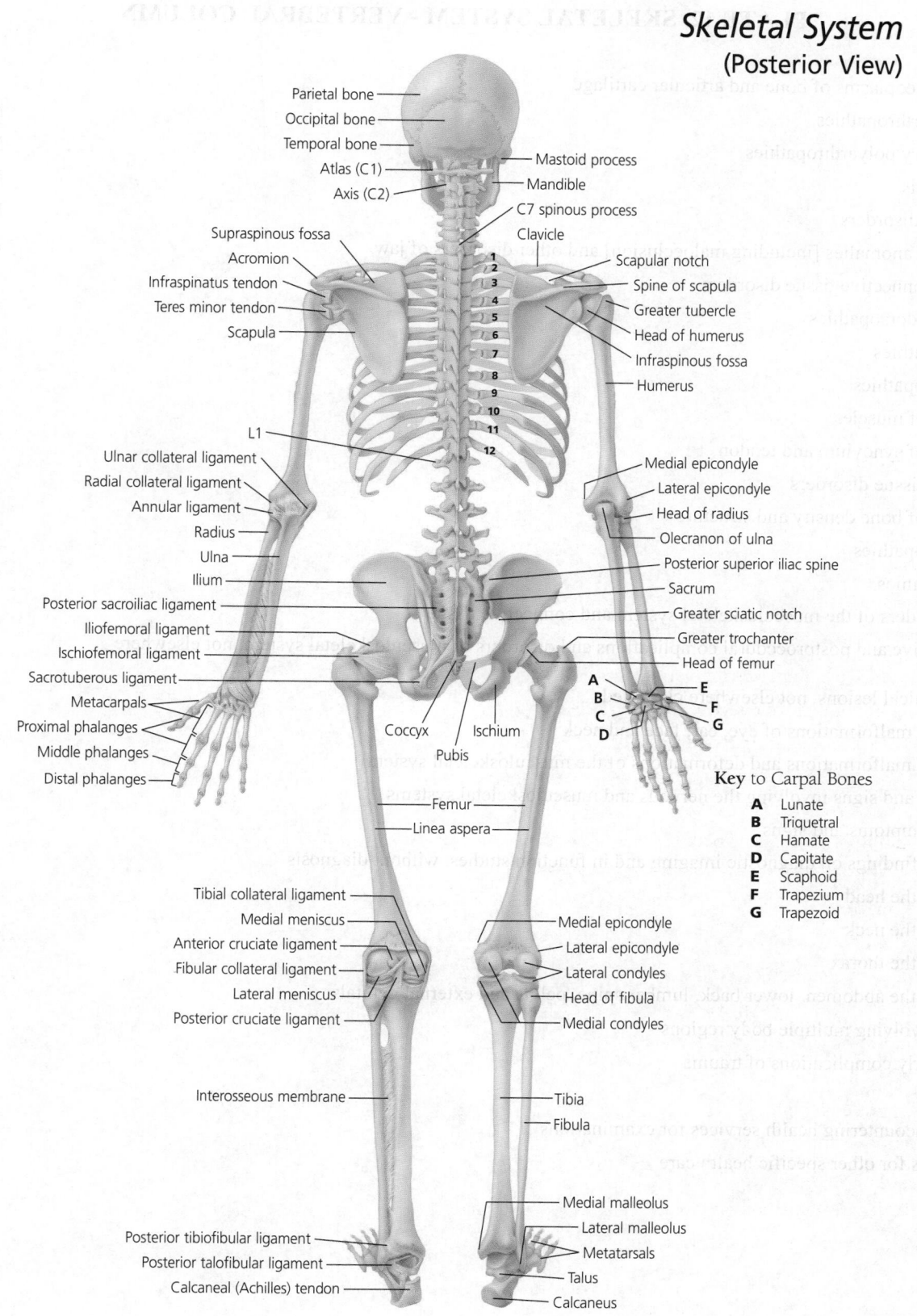

Parietal bone
Occipital bone
Temporal bone
Atlas (C1)
Axis (C2)
Mastoid process
Mandible
C7 spinous process
Clavicle
Supraspinous fossa
Acromion
Infraspinatus tendon
Teres minor tendon
Scapula
Scapular notch
Spine of scapula
Greater tubercle
Head of humerus
Infraspinous fossa
Humerus
L1
Ulnar collateral ligament
Radial collateral ligament
Annular ligament
Radius
Ulna
Ilium
Posterior sacroiliac ligament
Iliofemoral ligament
Ischiofemoral ligament
Sacrotuberous ligament
Medial epicondyle
Lateral epicondyle
Head of radius
Olecranon of ulna
Posterior superior iliac spine
Sacrum
Greater sciatic notch
Greater trochanter
Head of femur
Metacarpals
Proximal phalanges
Middle phalanges
Distal phalanges
Coccyx
Pubis
Ischium

A
B
C
D
E
F
G

Femur
Linea aspera

Key to Carpal Bones
A Lunate
B Triquetral
C Hamate
D Capitate
E Scaphoid
F Trapezium
G Trapezoid

Tibial collateral ligament
Medial meniscus
Anterior cruciate ligament
Fibular collateral ligament
Lateral meniscus
Posterior cruciate ligament
Medial epicondyle
Lateral epicondyle
Lateral condyles
Head of fibula
Medial condyles

Interosseous membrane
Tibia
Fibula

Posterior tibiofibular ligament
Posterior talofibular ligament
Calcaneal (Achilles) tendon
Medial malleolus
Lateral malleolus
Metatarsals
Talus
Calcaneus

PLATE 12. SKELETAL SYSTEM - VERTEBRAL COLUMN

Malignant neoplasms of bone and articular cartilage	**C40-C41**
Infectious arthropathies	**M00-M02**
Inflammatory polyarthropathies	**M05-M14**
Osteoarthritis	**M15-M19**
Other joint disorders	**M20-M25**
Dentofacial anomalies [including malocclusion] and other disorders of jaw	**M26-M27**
Systemic connective tissue disorders	**M30-M36**
Deforming dorsopathies	**M40-M43**
Spondylopathies	**M45-M49**
Other dorsopathies	**M50-M54**
Disorders of muscles	**M60-M63**
Disorders of synovium and tendon	**M65-M67**
Other soft tissue disorders	**M70-M79**
Disorders of bone density and structure	**M80-M85**
Other osteopathies	**M86-M90**
Chondropathies	**M91-M94**
Other disorders of the musculoskeletal system and connective tissue	**M95**
Intraoperative and postprocedural complications and disorders of musculoskeletal system, not elsewhere classified	**M96**
Biomechanical lesions, not elsewhere classified	**M99**
Congenital malformations of eye, ear, face and neck	**Q10-Q18**
Congenital malformations and deformations of the musculoskeletal system	**Q65-Q79**
Symptoms and signs involving the nervous and musculoskeletal systems	**R25-R29**
General symptoms and signs	**R50-R69**
Abnormal findings on diagnostic imaging and in function studies, without diagnosis	**R90-R94**
Injuries to the head	**S00-S09**
Injuries to the neck	**S10-S19**
Injuries to the thorax	**S20-S29**
Injuries to the abdomen, lower back, lumbar spine, pelvis and external genitals	**S30-S39**
Injuries involving multiple body regions	**T07**
Certain early complications of trauma	**T79**
Accidents	**V00-X58**
Persons encountering health services for examinations	**Z00-Z13**
Encounters for other specific health care	**Z40-Z53**

Vertebral Column
(Lateral View)

Atlas (C1)

Axis (C2)

Cervical
vertebrae
(C1–C7)

Cervical
curve

C7

T1

Intervertebral
discs

Thoracic
vertebrae
(T1–T12)

Thoracic
curve

Foveae for
ribs

T12

L1

Lumbar
curve

Lumbar
vertebrae
(L1–L5)

Intervertebral
foramina

L5

Sacrum

Pelvic
curve

Coccyx

PLATE 13. RESPIRATORY SYSTEM

Tuberculosis	**A15-A19**
Bacterial and viral infectious agents	**B95-B97**
Malignant neoplasms of respiratory and intrathoracic organs	**C30-C39**
Malignant neoplasms of ill-defined, other secondary and unspecified sites	**C76-C80**
In situ neoplasms	**D00-D09**
Benign neoplasms, except benign neuroendocrine tumors	**D10-D36**
Neoplasms of uncertain behavior, polycythemia vera and myelodysplastic syndromes	**D37-D48**
Neoplasms of unspecified behavior	**D49**
Acute upper respiratory infections	**J00-J06**
Influenza and pneumonia	**J09-J18**
Other acute lower respiratory infections	**J20-J22**
Other diseases of upper respiratory tract	**J30-J39**
Chronic lower respiratory diseases	**J40-J47**
Lung diseases due to external agents	**J60-J70**
Other respiratory diseases principally affecting the interstitium	**J80-J84**
Suppurative and necrotic conditions of the lower respiratory tract	**J85-J86**
Other diseases of the pleura	**J90-J94**
Intraoperative and postprocedural complications and disorders of respiratory system, not elsewhere classified	**J95**
Other diseases of the respiratory system	**J96-J99**
Congenital malformations of the respiratory system	**Q30-Q34**
Symptoms and signs involving the circulatory and respiratory systems	**R00-R09**
General symptoms and signs	**R50-R69**
Abnormal findings on diagnostic imaging and in function studies, without diagnosis	**R90-R94**
Persons encountering health services for examinations	**Z00-Z13**
Encounters for other specific health care	**Z40-Z53**

Respiratory System

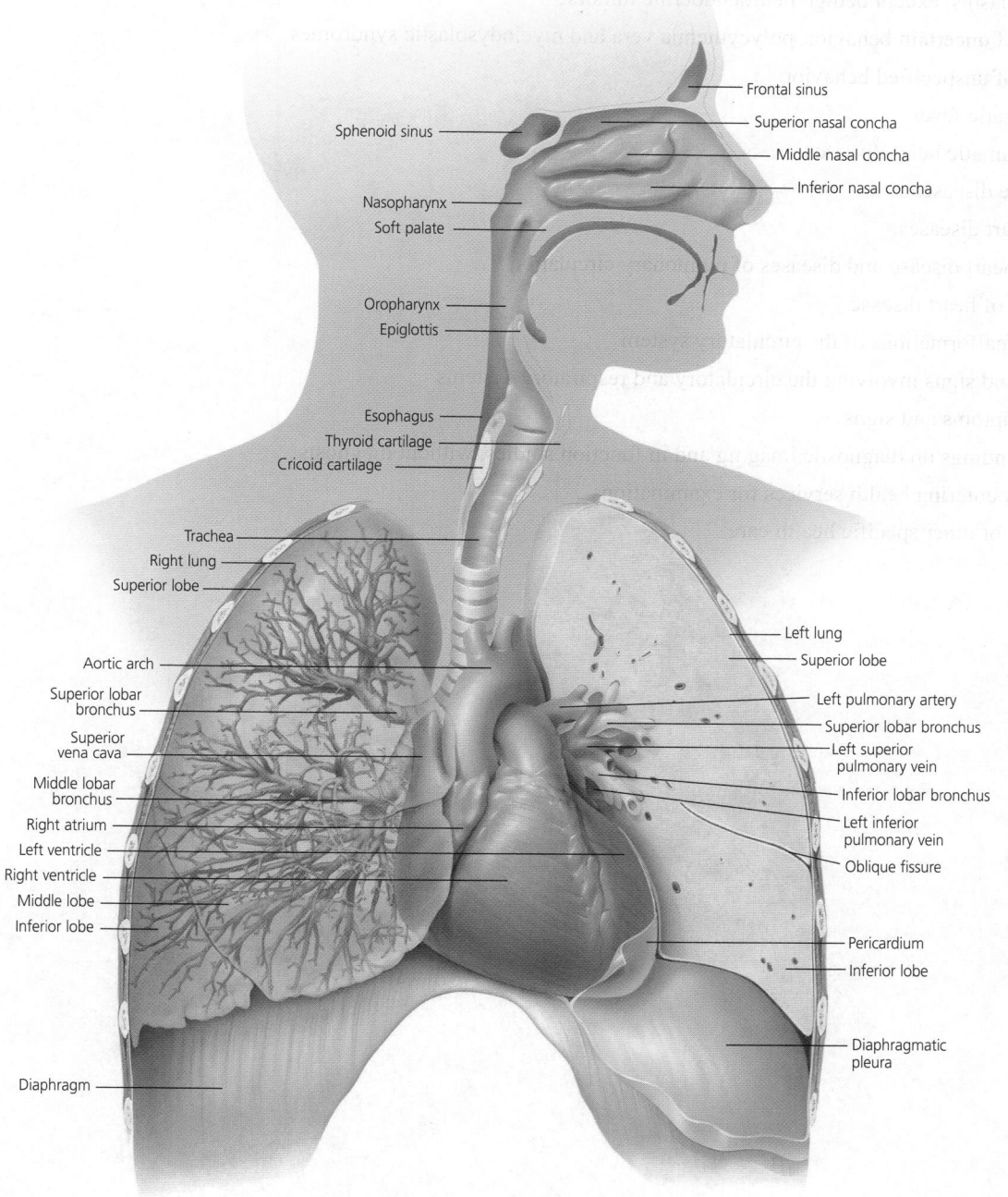

Frontal sinus

Sphenoid sinus

Superior nasal concha

Middle nasal concha

Inferior nasal concha

Nasopharynx

Soft palate

Oropharynx

Epiglottis

Esophagus

Thyroid cartilage

Cricoid cartilage

Trachea

Right lung

Superior lobe

Aortic arch

Superior lobar bronchus

Superior vena cava

Middle lobar bronchus

Right atrium

Left ventricle

Right ventricle

Middle lobe

Inferior lobe

Diaphragm

Left lung

Superior lobe

Left pulmonary artery

Superior lobar bronchus

Left superior pulmonary vein

Inferior lobar bronchus

Left inferior pulmonary vein

Oblique fissure

Pericardium

Inferior lobe

Diaphragmatic pleura

PLATE 14. HEART AND PERICARDIUM

Bacterial and viral infectious agents	**B95-B97**
Malignant neoplasms of ill-defined, other secondary and unspecified sites	**C76-C80**
In situ neoplasms	**D00-D09**
Benign neoplasms, except benign neuroendocrine tumors	**D10-D36**
Neoplasms of uncertain behavior, polycythemia vera and myelodysplastic syndromes	**D37-D48**
Neoplasms of unspecified behavior	**D49**
Acute rheumatic fever	**I00-I02**
Chronic rheumatic heart diseases	**I05-I09**
Hypertensive diseases	**I10-I15**
Ischemic heart diseases	**I20-I25**
Pulmonary heart disease and diseases of pulmonary circulation	**I26-I28**
Other forms of heart disease	**I30-I52**
Congenital malformations of the circulatory system	**Q20-Q28**
Symptoms and signs involving the circulatory and respiratory systems	**R00-R09**
General symptoms and signs	**R50-R69**
Abnormal findings on diagnostic imaging and in function studies, without diagnosis	**R90-R94**
Persons encountering health services for examinations	**Z00-Z13**
Encounters for other specific health care	**Z40-Z53**

Heart
(External View)

Left common carotid artery

Brachiocephalic artery

Left subclavian artery

Aortic arch

Ligamentum arteriosum

Left pulmonary artery

Superior vena cava

Ascending aorta

Pulmonary trunk

Left auricle

Right coronary artery

Circumflex artery

Right atrium

Great cardiac vein

Right ventricle

Anterior descending (interventricular) artery

Anterior cardiac vein

Left ventricle

Right marginal artery

Small cardiac vein

Apex

Heart
(Internal View)

Superior vena cava

Right pulmonary artery branches

Left pulmonary artery

Aorta

Pulmonary trunk

Left pulmonary veins

Right pulmonary veins

Left atrium

Pulmonary semilunar valve

Aortic semilunar valve

Right atrium

Bicuspid (left AV) valve

Left ventricle

Tricuspid (right AV) valve

Papillary muscle

Interventricular septum

Chordae tendineae

Inferior vena cava

Myocardium

Right ventricle

Trabeculae carneae

PLATE 15. VASCULAR SYSTEM

Bacterial and viral infectious agents	**B95-B97**
Malignant neoplasms of ill-defined, other secondary and unspecified sites	**C76-C80**
In situ neoplasms	**D00-D09**
Benign neoplasms, except benign neuroendocrine tumors	**D10-D36**
Neoplasms of uncertain behavior, polycythemia vera and myelodysplastic syndromes	**D37-D48**
Neoplasms of unspecified behavior	**D49**
Cerebrovascular diseases	**I60-I69**
Diseases of arteries, arterioles and capillaries	**I70-I79**
Diseases of veins, lymphatic vessels and lymph nodes, not elsewhere classified	**I80-I89**
Other and unspecified disorders of the circulatory system	**I95-I99**
General symptoms and signs	**R50-R69**
Abnormal findings on diagnostic imaging and in function studies, without diagnosis	**R90-R94**
Persons encountering health services for examinations	**Z00-Z13**
Encounters for other specific health care	**Z40-Z53**

Vascular System

Internal carotid a.

Common carotid a.

Vertebral a.

External jugular v.

Internal jugular v.

Subclavian a. & v.

Brachiocephalic trunk

Superior vena cava

Brachiocephalic v.

Aortic arch

Axillary a. & v.

Pulmonary a.

Cephalic v.

Pulmonary veins

Cardiac a.

Brachial a. & v.

Hepatic v.

Aorta

Celiac trunk

Basilic v.

Superior mesenteric a.

Renal a. & v.

Median cubital v.

Gonadal a. & v.

Radial a.

Inferior mesenteric a.

Ulnar a.

Inferior vena cava

Medial antebrachial v.

Common iliac a. & v.

Internal iliac a. & v.

External iliac a. & v.

Deep palmar arch

Superficial palmar arch

Superficial venous
palmar arch

Deep femoral a. & v.

Femoral a. & v.

Saphenous v.

Descending genicular a.

Popliteal a. & v.

Small saphenous v.

Anterior tibial a. & v.

Peroneal a.

Posterior tibial a. & v.

Lateral tarsal a.

Dorsal pedis a.

Arcuate a.

Dorsal venous arch

PLATE 16. DIGESTIVE SYSTEM

Intestinal infectious diseases	**A00-A09**
Bacterial and viral infectious agents	**B95-B97**
Malignant neoplasms of lip, oral cavity and pharynx	**C00-C14**
Malignant neoplasms of digestive organs	**C15-C26**
Malignant neoplasms of ill-defined, other secondary and unspecified sites	**C76-C80**
In situ neoplasms	**D00-D09**
Benign neoplasms, except benign neuroendocrine tumors	**D10-D36**
Neoplasms of uncertain behavior, polycythemia vera and myelodysplastic syndromes	**D37-D48**
Neoplasms of unspecified behavior	**D49**
Diseases of oral cavity and salivary glands	**K00-K14**
Diseases of esophagus, stomach and duodenum	**K20-K31**
Diseases of appendix	**K35-K38**
Hernia	**K40-K46**
Noninfective enteritis and colitis	**K50-K52**
Other diseases of intestines	**K55-K64**
Diseases of peritoneum and retroperitoneum	**K65-K68**
Diseases of liver	**K70-K77**
Disorders of gallbladder, biliary tract and pancreas	**K80-K87**
Other diseases of the digestive system	**K90-K95**
Cleft lip and cleft palate	**Q35-Q37**
Other congenital malformations of the digestive system	**Q38-Q45**
Symptoms and signs involving the digestive system and abdomen	**R10-R19**
General symptoms and signs	**R50-R69**
Abnormal findings on diagnostic imaging and in function studies, without diagnosis	**R90-R94**
Persons encountering health services for examinations	**Z00-Z13**
Encounters for other specific health care	**Z40-Z53**

Digestive System

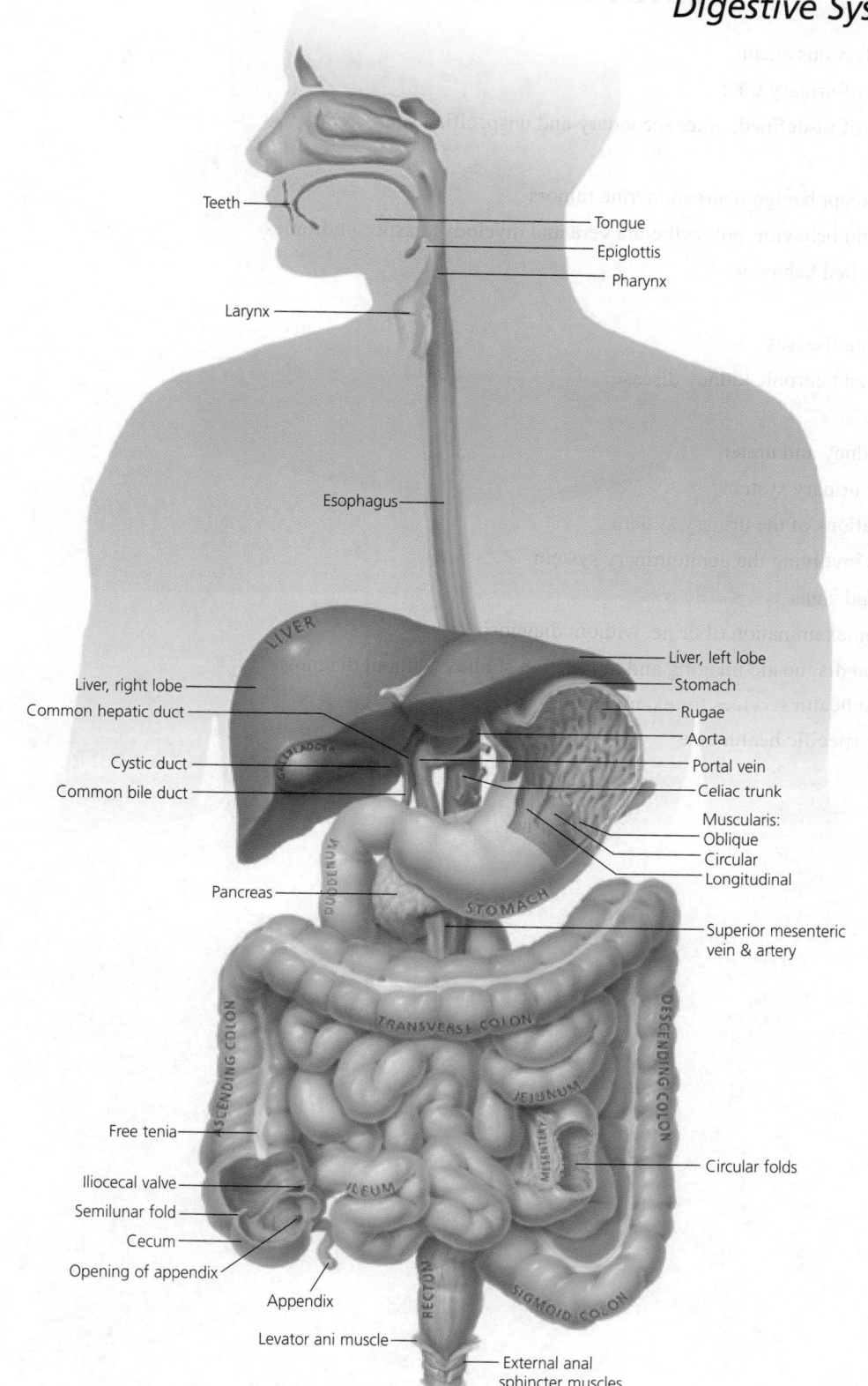

Teeth

Tongue

Epiglottis

Pharynx

Larynx

Esophagus

LIVER

Liver, left lobe

Stomach

Rugae

Liver, right lobe

Common hepatic duct

Aorta

Cystic duct

Portal vein

Common bile duct

Celiac trunk

Muscularis:
Oblique
Circular
Longitudinal

Pancreas

DUODENUM

STOMACH

Superior mesenteric
vein & artery

ASCENDING COLON

TRANSVERSE COLON

DESCENDING COLON

JEJUNUM

MESENTERY

Free tenia

Circular folds

Iliocecal valve

ILEUM

Semilunar fold

Cecum

Opening of appendix

Appendix

RECTUM

SIGMOID COLON

Levator ani muscle

External anal
sphincter muscles

PLATE 17. GENITOURINARY SYSTEM

Bacterial and viral infectious agents	**B95-B97**
Malignant neoplasms of urinary tract	**C64-C68**
Malignant neoplasms of ill-defined, other secondary and unspecified sites	**C76-C80**
In situ neoplasms	**D00-D09**
Benign neoplasms, except benign neuroendocrine tumors	**D10-D36**
Neoplasms of uncertain behavior, polycythemia vera and myelodysplastic syndromes	**D37-D48**
Neoplasms of unspecified behavior	**D49**
Glomerular diseases	**N00-N08**
Renal tubulointerstitial diseases	**N10-N16**
Acute kidney failure and chronic kidney disease	**N17-N19**
Urolithiasis	**N20-N23**
Other disorders of kidney and ureter	**N25-N29**
Other diseases of the urinary system	**N30-N39**
Congenital malformations of the urinary system	**Q60-Q64**
Symptoms and signs involving the genitourinary system	**R30-R39**
General symptoms and signs	**R50-R69**
Abnormal findings on examination of urine, without diagnosis	**R80-R82**
Abnormal findings on diagnostic imaging and in function studies, without diagnosis	**R90-R94**
Persons encountering health services for examinations	**Z00-Z13**
Encounters for other specific health care	**Z40-Z53**

Urinary System

Inferior vena cava

Adrenal gland

Kidney

Renal artery

Renal vein

Renal pelvis

Cortex

Medulla

Fibrous capsule

Major calyx

Minor calyx

Cortex

Renal pyramid

Renal column

Ureter

Abdominal aorta

Right common iliac vein

Right common iliac artery

Left common iliac artery

Left common iliac vein

Urinary bladder

Opening of ureter

Trigone

Urethra

PLATE 18. MALE REPRODUCTIVE SYSTEM

Infections with a predominantly sexual mode of transmission	A50-A64
Bacterial and viral infectious agents	B95-B97
Malignant neoplasms of male genital organs	C60-C63
Malignant neoplasms of ill-defined, other secondary and unspecified sites	C76-C80
In situ neoplasms	D00-D09
Benign neoplasms, except benign neuroendocrine tumors	D10-D36
Neoplasms of uncertain behavior, polycythemia vera and myelodysplastic syndromes	D37-D48
Neoplasms of unspecified behavior	D49
Diseases of male genital organs	N40-N53
Congenital malformations of genital organs	Q50-Q56
General symptoms and signs	R50-R69
Abnormal findings on diagnostic imaging and in function studies, without diagnosis	R90-R94
Persons encountering health services for examinations	Z00-Z13
Persons encountering health services in circumstances related to reproduction	Z30-Z39
Encounters for other specific health care	Z40-Z53

Male Reproductive System

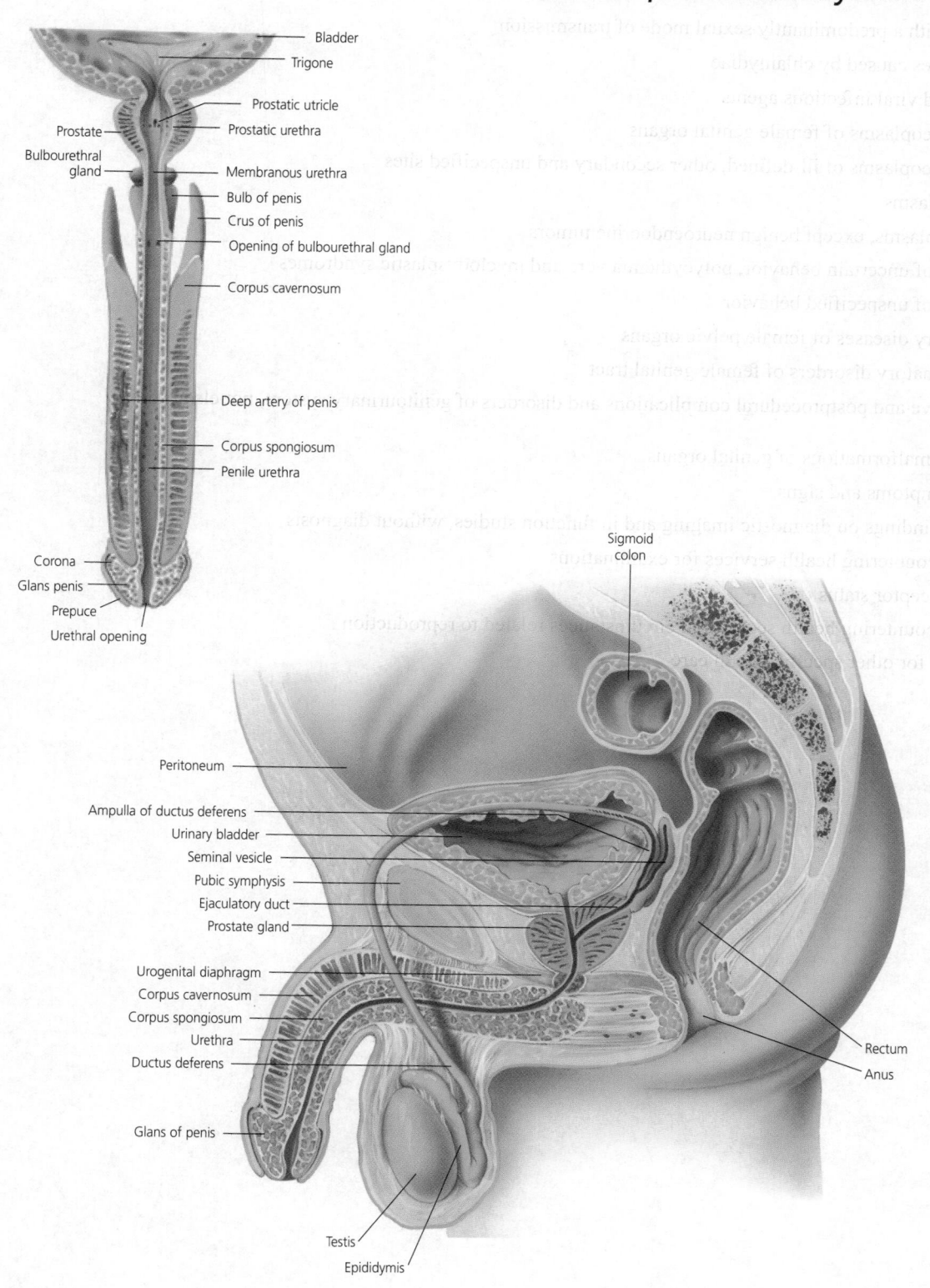

Bladder

Trigone

Prostatic utricle

Prostate

Prostatic urethra

Bulbourethral gland

Membranous urethra

Bulb of penis

Crus of penis

Opening of bulbourethral gland

Corpus cavernosum

Deep artery of penis

Corpus spongiosum

Penile urethra

Corona

Glans penis

Prepuce

Urethral opening

Sigmoid colon

Peritoneum

Ampulla of ductus deferens

Urinary bladder

Seminal vesicle

Pubic symphysis

Ejaculatory duct

Prostate gland

Urogenital diaphragm

Corpus cavernosum

Corpus spongiosum

Urethra

Ductus deferens

Glans of penis

Testis

Epididymis

Rectum

Anus

PLATE 19. FEMALE REPRODUCTIVE SYSTEM

Infections with a predominantly sexual mode of transmission	**A50-A64**
Other diseases caused by chlamydiae	**A70-A74**
Bacterial and viral infectious agents	**B95-B97**
Malignant neoplasms of female genital organs	**C51-C58**
Malignant neoplasms of ill-defined, other secondary and unspecified sites	**C76-C80**
In situ neoplasms	**D00-D09**
Benign neoplasms, except benign neuroendocrine tumors	**D10-D36**
Neoplasms of uncertain behavior, polycythemia vera and myelodysplastic syndromes	**D37-D48**
Neoplasms of unspecified behavior	**D49**
Inflammatory diseases of female pelvic organs	**N70-N77**
Noninflammatory disorders of female genital tract	**N80-N98**
Intraoperative and postprocedural complications and disorders of genitourinary system, not elsewhere classified	**N99**
Congenital malformations of genital organs	**Q50-Q56**
General symptoms and signs	**R50-R69**
Abnormal findings on diagnostic imaging and in function studies, without diagnosis	**R90-R94**
Persons encountering health services for examinations	**Z00-Z13**
Estrogen receptor status	**Z17**
Persons encountering health services in circumstances related to reproduction	**Z30-Z39**
Encounters for other specific health care	**Z40-Z53**

Female Reproductive System

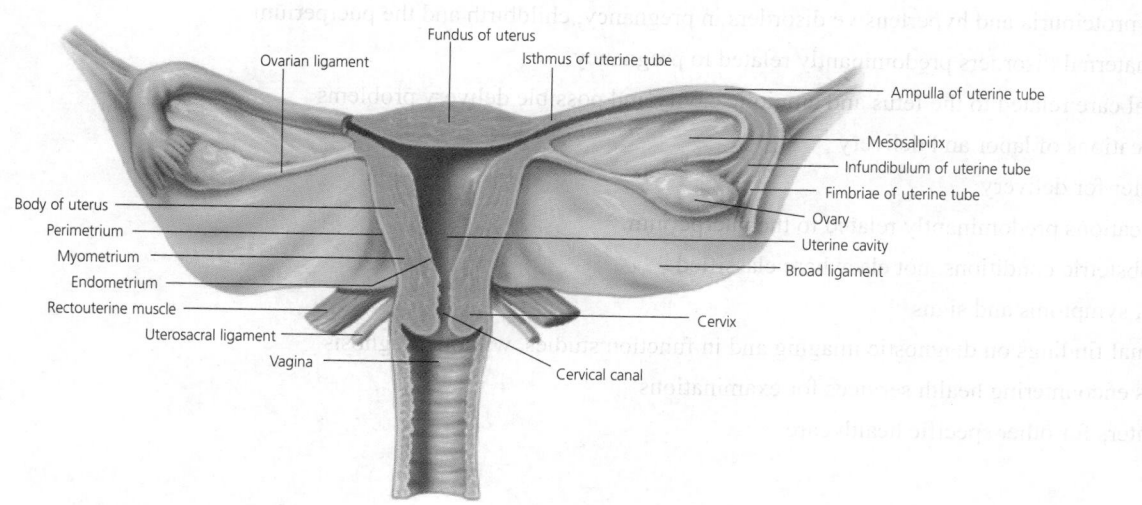

Ovarian ligament
Fundus of uterus
Isthmus of uterine tube
Ampulla of uterine tube
Mesosalpinx
Infundibulum of uterine tube
Fimbriae of uterine tube
Body of uterus
Ovary
Perimetrium
Uterine cavity
Myometrium
Broad ligament
Endometrium
Rectouterine muscle
Uterosacral ligament
Cervix
Vagina
Cervical canal

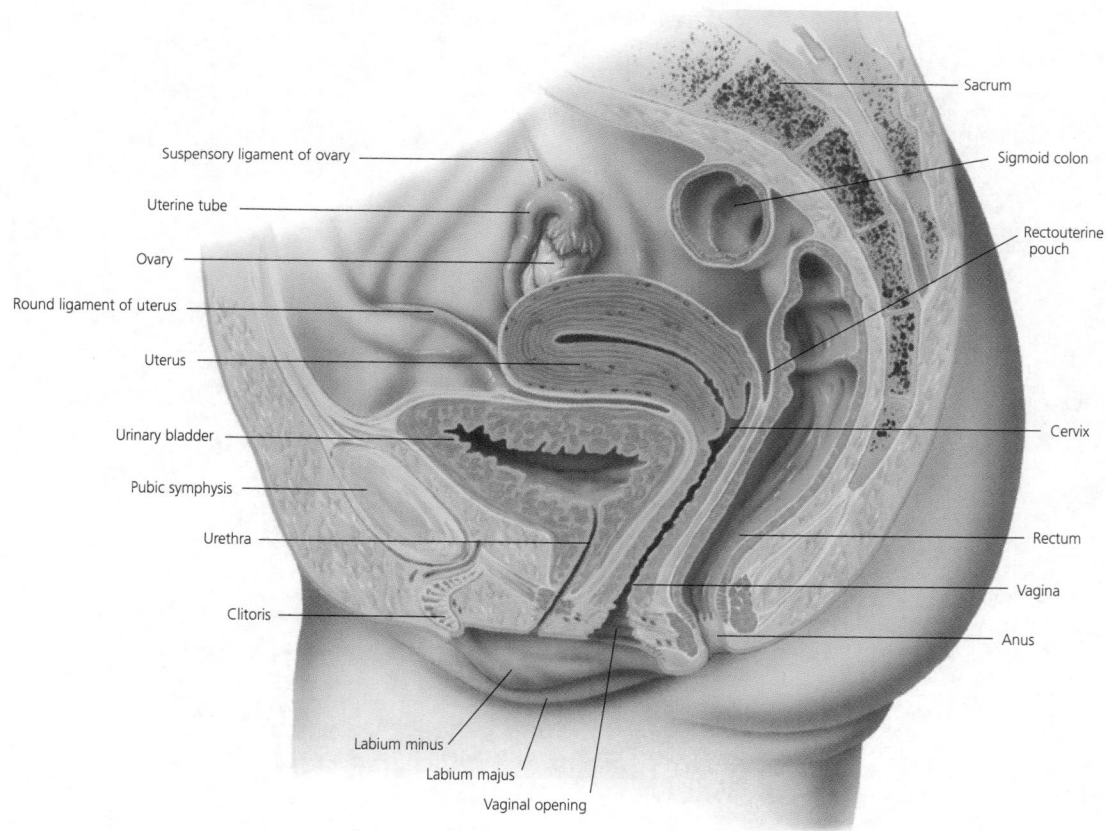

Suspensory ligament of ovary
Sacrum
Sigmoid colon
Uterine tube
Rectouterine pouch
Ovary
Round ligament of uterus
Uterus
Urinary bladder
Cervix
Pubic symphysis
Urethra
Rectum
Clitoris
Vagina
Anus
Labium minus
Labium majus
Vaginal opening

PLATE 20. PREGNANCY, CHILDBIRTH AND THE PUERPERIUM

Pregnancy with abortive outcome	**O00-O08**
Supervision of high risk pregnancy	**O09**
Edema, proteinuria and hypertensive disorders in pregnancy, childbirth and the puerperium	**O10-O16**
Other maternal disorders predominantly related to pregnancy	**O20-O29**
Maternal care related to the fetus and amniotic cavity and possible delivery problems	**O30-O48**
Complications of labor and delivery	**O60-O77**
Encounter for delivery	**O80-O82**
Complications predominantly related to the puerperium	**O85-O92**
Other obstetric conditions, not elsewhere classified	**O94-O9A**
General symptoms and signs	**R50-R69**
Abnormal findings on diagnostic imaging and in function studies, without diagnosis	**R90-R94**
Persons encountering health services for examinations	**Z00-Z13**
Encounters for other specific health care	**Z40-Z53**

Female Reproductive System: Pregnancy
(Lateral View)

Vertebral column

Intervertebral disks

Spinous processes

Vertebral bodies

Spinal cord

Superior vena cava

Aorta

Pulmonary trunk

Lung

Heart

Right atrium

Inferior vena cava

Diaphragm

Right ventricle

Liver

Stomach

Transverse colon

Pancreas

Placenta

Uterus

Umbilical cord

Small intestine

Sacrum

Rectum

Cervix

Coccyx

Vagina

Bladder

Pubic symphysis

Urethra

PLATE 21. NERVOUS SYSTEM – BRAIN

Viral and prion infections of the central nervous system	**A80-A89**
Bacterial and viral infectious agents	**B95-B97**
Malignant neoplasms of eye, brain and other parts of central nervous system	**C69-C72**
Malignant neoplasms of ill-defined, other secondary and unspecified sites	**C76-C80**
In situ neoplasms	**D00-D09**
Benign neoplasms, except benign neuroendocrine tumors	**D10-D36**
Neoplasms of uncertain behavior, polycythemia vera and myelodysplastic syndromes	**D37-D48**
Neoplasms of unspecified behavior	**D49**
Inflammatory diseases of the central nervous system	**G00-G09**
Systemic atrophies primarily affecting the central nervous system	**G10-G14**
Extrapyramidal and movement disorders	**G20-G26**
Other degenerative diseases of the nervous system	**G30-G32**
Demyelinating diseases of the central nervous system	**G35-G37**
Episodic and paroxysmal disorders	**G40-G47**
Nerve, nerve root and plexus disorders	**G50-G59**
Polyneuropathies and other disorders of the peripheral nervous system	**G60-G65**
Diseases of myoneural junction and muscle	**G70-G73**
Cerebral palsy and other paralytic syndromes	**G80-G83**
Other disorders of the nervous system	**G89-G99**
Congenital malformations of the nervous system	**Q00-Q07**
Symptoms and signs involving the nervous and musculoskeletal systems	**R25-R29**
General symptoms and signs	**R50-R69**
Abnormal findings on diagnostic imaging and in function studies, without diagnosis	**R90-R94**
Persons encountering health services for examinations	**Z00-Z13**
Encounters for other specific health care	**Z40-Z53**

Brain
(Base View)

Olfactory bulb

Cerebrum

Olfactory tract (I)

Anterior communicating artery

Anterior cerebral artery

Optic nerve (II)

Optic chiasm

Middle cerebral artery

Internal carotid artery

Posterior communicating artery

Pituitary gland

Posterior cerebral artery

Oculomotor nerve (III)

Superior cerebellar artery

Troclear nerve (IV)

Basilar artery

Trigeminal nerve (V)

Abducens nerve

Pons

Abducens nerve (VI)

Facial nerve (VII)

Vestibulocochlear nerve (VIII)

Hypoglossal nerve (XII)

Glossopharyngeal nerve (IX)

Accessory nerve (XI)

Vagus nerve (X)

Anterior inferior cerebellar artery

Vertebral artery

Medulla oblongata

Anterior spinal artery

Cerebellum

Spinal cord

Posterior inferior cerebellar artery

PLATE 22. NERVOUS SYSTEM

Viral and prion infections of the central nervous system	**A80-A89**
Bacterial and viral infectious agents	**B95-B97**
Malignant neoplasms of eye, brain and other parts of central nervous system	**C69-C72**
Malignant neoplasms of ill-defined, other secondary and unspecified sites	**C76-C80**
In situ neoplasms	**D00-D09**
Benign neoplasms, except benign neuroendocrine tumors	**D10-D36**
Neoplasms of uncertain behavior, polycythemia vera and myelodysplastic syndromes	**D37-D48**
Neoplasms of unspecified behavior	**D49**
Inflammatory diseases of the central nervous system	**G00-G09**
Systemic atrophies primarily affecting the central nervous system	**G10-G14**
Extrapyramidal and movement disorders	**G20-G26**
Other degenerative diseases of the nervous system	**G30-G32**
Demyelinating diseases of the central nervous system	**G35-G37**
Episodic and paroxysmal disorders	**G40-G47**
Nerve, nerve root and plexus disorders	**G50-G59**
Polyneuropathies and other disorders of the peripheral nervous system	**G60-G65**
Diseases of myoneural junction and muscle	**G70-G73**
Cerebral palsy and other paralytic syndromes	**G80-G83**
Other disorders of the nervous system	**G89-G99**
Congenital malformations of the nervous system	**Q00-Q07**
Symptoms and signs involving the nervous and musculoskeletal systems	**R25-R29**
General symptoms and signs	**R50-R69**
Abnormal findings on diagnostic imaging and in function studies, without diagnosis	**R90-R94**
Persons encountering health services for examinations	**Z00-Z13**
Encounters for other specific health care	**Z40-Z53**

Nervous System

Brain

Cerebrum

Brain stem

Cerebellum

Cervical plexus

Lateral cord

Spinal cord

Medial cord

Brachial plexus

Posterior cord

Phrenic nerve

Musculocutaneous
nerve

Intercostal nerves

Ulnar nerve

Median nerve

Subcostal nerve

Radial nerve

Iliohypogastric nerve

Lumbar plexus

Ilioinguinal nerve

Genitofemoral nerve

Deep branch of radial nerve

Sacral plexus

Lateral femoral
cutaneous nerve

Coccygeal plexus

Superficial branch
of radial nerve

Femoral nerve

Obturator nerve

Pudendal nerve

Sciatic nerve

Muscular branches
of femoral nerve

Saphenous nerve

Common peroneal nerve

Deep peroneal nerve

Superficial peroneal nerve

Tibial nerve

PLATE 23. EYE AND OCULAR ADNEXA

Bacterial and viral infectious agents	**B95-B97**
Malignant neoplasms of eye, brain and other parts of central nervous system	**C69-C72**
Malignant neoplasms of ill-defined, other secondary and unspecified sites	**C76-C80**
In situ neoplasms	**D00-D09**
Benign neoplasms, except benign neuroendocrine tumors	**D10-D36**
Neoplasms of uncertain behavior, polycythemia vera and myelodysplastic syndromes	**D37-D48**
Neoplasms of unspecified behavior	**D49**
Disorders of eyelid, lacrimal system and orbit	**H00-H05**
Disorders of conjunctiva	**H10-H11**
Disorders of sclera, cornea, iris and ciliary body	**H15-H22**
Disorders of lens	**H25-H28**
Disorders of choroid and retina	**H30-H36**
Glaucoma	**H40-H42**
Disorders of vitreous body and globe	**H43-H44**
Disorders of optic nerve and visual pathways	**H46-H47**
Disorders of ocular muscles, binocular movement, accommodation and refraction	**H49-H52**
Visual disturbances and blindness	**H53-H54**
Other disorders of eye and adnexa	**H55-H57**
Intraoperative and postprocedural complications and disorders of eye and adnexa, not elsewhere classified	**H59**
Congenital malformations of eye, ear, face and neck	**Q10-Q18**
General symptoms and signs	**R50-R69**
Abnormal findings on diagnostic imaging and in function studies, without diagnosis	**R90-R94**
Burns and corrosions confined to eye and internal organs	**T26-T28**
Persons encountering health services for examinations	**Z00-Z13**
Encounters for other specific health care	**Z40-Z53**

Right Eye
(Horizontal Section)

Lateral rectus muscle

Conjunctiva

Canal of Schlemm

Zonular fibers

Iris

Lens

Cornea

Pupil

Aqueous humor

Anterior chamber

Posterior chamber

Ciliary body

Sclera

Ora serrata

Choroid

Medial rectus muscle

Vitreous body

Hyaloid canal

Macula lutea

Optic disc

Retinal vessels

Optic nerve

Nerve sheath

Retina

PLATE 24. AUDITORY SYSTEM

Bacterial and viral infectious agents	**B95-B97**
Malignant neoplasms of ill-defined, other secondary and unspecified sites	**C76-C80**
In situ neoplasms	**D00-D09**
Benign neoplasms, except benign neuroendocrine tumors	**D10-D36**
Neoplasms of uncertain behavior, polycythemia vera and myelodysplastic syndromes	**D37-D48**
Neoplasms of unspecified behavior	**D49**
Diseases of external ear	**H60-H62**
Diseases of middle ear and mastoid	**H65-H75**
Diseases of inner ear	**H80-H83**
Other disorders of ear	**H90-H94**
Intraoperative and postprocedural complications and disorders of ear and mastoid process, not elsewhere classified	**H95**
Congenital malformations of eye, ear, face and neck	**Q10-Q18**
General symptoms and signs	**R50-R69**
Abnormal findings on diagnostic imaging and in function studies, without diagnosis	**R90-R94**
Persons encountering health services for examinations	**Z00-Z13**
Encounters for other specific health care	**Z40-Z53**

The Ear

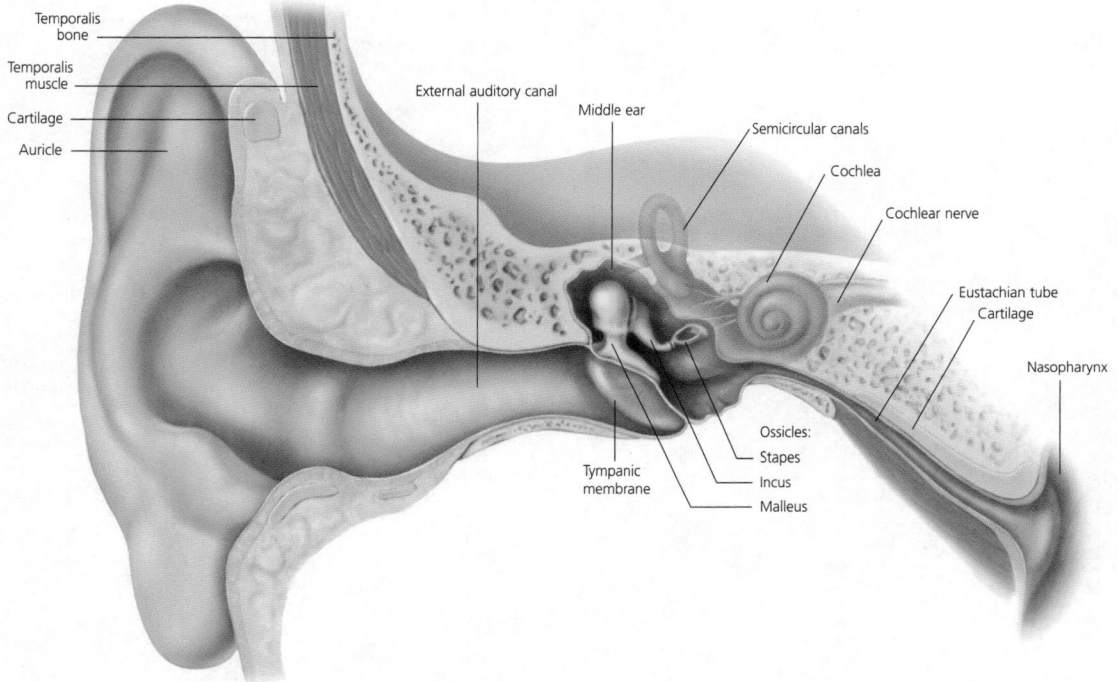

Chapter 1: Certain Infectious And Parasitic Diseases (A00-B99)

DEFINITIONS

This chapter includes definitions of selected key words, terms and phrases and coding alerts for adding points to the clinical domain, and references to coding late effects where appropriate. An example from this chapter is as follows:

A01   Typhoid and paratyphoid fevers

Definition: Typhoid fever, aka enteric fever, salmonella typhi is an illness caused by the bacterium salmonella enterica serovar typhi.

MULTIPLE CODING FOR A SINGLE CONDITION

In addition to the etiology/manifestation convention that requires two codes to fully describe a single condition that affects multiple body systems, there are other single conditions that also require more than one code. "Use additional code" notes are found in the Tabular List at codes that are not part of an etiology/manifestation pair where a secondary code is useful to fully describe a condition. The sequencing rule is the same as the etiology/manifestation pair, "use additional code" indicates that a secondary code should be added.

For example, for bacterial infections that are not included in chapter 1, a secondary code from category B95, Streptococcus, Staphylococcus, and Enterococcus, as the cause of diseases classified elsewhere, or B96, Other bacterial agents as the cause of diseases classified elsewhere, may be required to identify the bacterial organism causing the infection. A "use additional code" note will normally be found at the infectious disease code, indicating a need for the organism code to be added as a secondary code.

"Code first" notes are also under certain codes that are not specifically manifestation codes but may be due to an underlying cause. When there is a "code first" note and an underlying condition is present, the underlying condition should be sequenced first.

"Code, if applicable, any causal condition first", notes indicate that this code may be assigned as a principal diagnosis when the causal condition is unknown or not applicable. If a causal condition is known, then the code for that condition should be sequenced as the principal or first-listed diagnosis.

Multiple codes may be needed for sequela, complication codes and obstetric codes to more fully describe a condition. See the specific guidelines for these conditions for further instruction.

COMBINATION CODE

A combination code is a single code used to classify: Two diagnoses, or a diagnosis with an associated secondary process (manifestation) A diagnosis with an associated complication

Combination codes are identified by referring to subterm entries in the Alphabetic Index and by reading the inclusion and exclusion notes in the Tabular List.

Assign only the combination code when that code fully identifies the diagnostic conditions involved or when the Alphabetic Index so directs. Multiple coding should not be used when the classification provides a combination code that clearly identifies all of the elements documented in the diagnosis. When the combination code lacks necessary specificity in describing the manifestation or complication, an additional code should be used as a secondary code.

SEQUELA (LATE EFFECTS)

A sequela is the residual effect (condition produced) after the acute phase of an illness or injury has terminated. There is no time limit on when a sequela code can be used. The residual may be apparent early, such as in cerebral infarction, or it may occur months or years later, such as that due to a previous injury. Coding of sequela generally requires two codes sequenced in the following order: The condition or nature of the sequela is sequenced first.

The sequela code is sequenced second.

An exception to the above guidelines are those instances where the code for the sequela is followed by a manifestation code identified in the Tabular List and title, or the sequela code has been expanded (at the fourth, fifth or sixth character levels) to include the manifestation(s). The code for the acute phase of an illness or injury that led to the sequela is never used with a code for the late effect.

HUMAN IMMUNODEFICIENCY VIRUS (HIV) INFECTIONS

1)   **Code only confirmed cases**

Code only confirmed cases of HIV infection/illness. This is an exception to the hospital inpatient guideline Section II, H.

In this context, "confirmation" does not require documentation of positive serology or culture for HIV; the provider's diagnostic statement that the patient is HIV positive, or has an HIV-related illness is sufficient.

2)   **Selection and sequencing of HIV codes**

(a)   **Patient admitted for HIV-related condition**

If a patient is admitted for an HIV-related condition, the principal diagnosis should be B20, Human immunodeficiency virus [HIV] disease followed by additional diagnosis codes for all reported HIV-related conditions.

(b)   **Patient with HIV disease admitted for unrelated condition**

If a patient with HIV disease is admitted for an unrelated condition (such as a traumatic injury), the code for the unrelated condition (e.g., the nature of injury code) should be the principal diagnosis. Other diagnoses would be B20 followed by additional diagnosis codes for all reported HIV-related conditions.

(c) **Whether the patient is newly diagnosed**

Whether the patient is newly diagnosed or has had previous admissions/encounters for HIV conditions is irrelevant to the sequencing decision.

(d) **Asymptomatic human immunodeficiency virus**

Z21, Asymptomatic human immunodeficiency virus [HIV] infection status, is to be applied when the patient without any documentation of symptoms is listed as being "HIV positive," "known HIV," "HIV test positive," or similar terminology. Do not use this code if the term "AIDS" is used or if the patient is treated for any HIV-related illness or is described as having any condition(s) resulting from his/her HIV positive status; use B20 in these cases.

(e) **Patients with inconclusive HIV serology**

Patients with inconclusive HIV serology, but no definitive diagnosis or manifestations of the illness, may be assigned code R75, Inconclusive laboratory evidence of human immunodeficiency virus [HIV].

(f) **Previously diagnosed HIV-related illness**

Patients with any known prior diagnosis of an HIV-related illness should be coded to B20. Once a patient has developed an HIV-related illness, the patient should always be assigned code B20 on every subsequent admission/encounter. Patients previously diagnosed with any HIV illness (B20) should never be assigned to R75 or Z21, Asymptomatic human immunodeficiency virus [HIV] infection status.

(g) **HIV Infection in Pregnancy, Childbirth and the Puerperium**

During pregnancy, childbirth or the puerperium, a patient admitted (or presenting for a health care encounter) because of an HIV-related illness should receive a principal diagnosis code of O98.7-, Human immunodeficiency [HIV] disease complicating pregnancy, childbirth and the puerperium, followed by B20 and the code(s) for the HIV-related illness(es). Codes from Chapter 15 always take sequencing priority.

Patients with asymptomatic HIV infection status admitted (or presenting for a health care encounter) during pregnancy, childbirth, or the puerperium should receive codes of O98.7- and Z21.

(h) **Encounters for testing for HIV**

If a patient is being seen to determine his/her HIV status, use code Z11.4, Encounter for screening for human immunodeficiency virus [HIV]. Use additional codes for any associated high risk behavior.

If a patient with signs or symptoms is being seen for HIV testing, code the signs and symptoms. An additional counseling code Z71.7, Human immunodeficiency virus [HIV] counseling, may be used if counseling is provided during the encounter for the test.

When a patient returns to be informed of his/her HIV test results and the test result is negative, use code Z71.7, Human immunodeficiency virus [HIV] counseling.

If the results are positive, see previous guidelines and assign codes as appropriate.

INFECTIOUS AGENTS AS THE CAUSE OF DISEASES CLASSIFIED TO OTHER CHAPTERS

Certain infections are classified in chapters other than Chapter 1 and no organism is identified as part of the infection code. In these instances, it is necessary to use an additional code from Chapter 1 to identify the organism. A code from category B95, Streptococcus, Staphylococcus, and Enterococcus as the cause of diseases classified to other chapters, B96, Other bacterial agents as the cause of diseases classified to other chapters, or B97, Viral agents as the cause of diseases classified to other chapters, is to be used as an additional code to identify the organism. An instructional note will be found at the infection code advising that an additional organism code is required.

INFECTIONS RESISTANT TO ANTIBIOTICS

Many bacterial infections are resistant to current antibiotics. It is necessary to identify all infections documented as antibiotic resistant. Assign a code from category Z16, Resistance to antimicrobial drugs, following the infection code only if the infection code does not identify drug resistance.

SEPSIS, SEVERE SEPSIS, AND SEPTIC SHOCK

1) **Coding of Sepsis and Severe Sepsis**

(a) **Sepsis**

For a diagnosis of sepsis, assign the appropriate code for the underlying systemic infection. If the type of infection or causal organism is not further specified, assign code A41.9, Sepsis, unspecified organism.

A code from subcategory R65.2, Severe sepsis, should not be assigned unless severe sepsis or an associated acute organ dysfunction is documented.

(i) Negative or inconclusive blood cultures and sepsis

Negative or inconclusive blood cultures do not preclude a diagnosis of sepsis in patients with clinical evidence of the condition; however, the provider should be queried.

 (ii) Urosepsis

  The term urosepsis is a nonspecific term. It is not to be considered synonymous with sepsis. It has no default code in the Alphabetic Index. Should a provider use this term, he/she must be queried for clarification.

 (iii) Sepsis with organ dysfunction

  If a patient has sepsis and associated acute organ dysfunction or multiple organ dysfunction (MOD), follow the instructions for coding severe sepsis.

 (iv) Acute organ dysfunction that is not clearly associated with the sepsis

  If a patient has sepsis and an acute organ dysfunction, but the medical record documentation indicates that the acute organ dysfunction is related to a medical condition other than the sepsis, do not assign a code from subcategory R65.2, Severe sepsis. An acute organ dysfunction must be associated with the sepsis in order to assign the severe sepsis code.

  If the documentation is not clear as to whether an acute organ dysfunction is related to the sepsis or another medical condition, query the provider.

 (b) **Severe sepsis**

  The coding of severe sepsis requires a minimum of 2 codes: first a code for the underlying systemic infection, followed by a code from subcategory R65.2, Severe sepsis. If the causal organism is not documented, assign code A41.9, Sepsis, unspecified organism, for the infection. Additional code(s) for the associated acute organ dysfunction are also required.

  Due to the complex nature of severe sepsis, some cases may require querying the provider prior to assignment of the codes.

2) Septic shock

 (a) Septic shock generally refers to circulatory failure associated with severe sepsis, and therefore, it represents a type of acute organ dysfunction.

  For cases of septic shock, the code for the systemic infection should be sequenced first, followed by code R65.21, Severe sepsis with septic shock or code T81.12, Postprocedural septic shock. Any additional codes for the other acute organ dysfunctions should also be assigned. As noted in the sequencing instructions in the Tabular List, the code for septic shock cannot be assigned as a principal diagnosis.

3) Sequencing of severe sepsis

 If severe sepsis is present on admission, and meets the definition of principal diagnosis, the underlying systemic infection should be assigned as principal diagnosis followed by the appropriate code from subcategory R65.2 as required by the sequencing rules in the Tabular List. A code from subcategory R65.2 can never be assigned as a principal diagnosis.

 When severe sepsis develops during an encounter (it was not present on admission), the underlying systemic infection and the appropriate code from subcategory R65.2 should be assigned as secondary diagnoses.

 Severe sepsis may be present on admission, but the diagnosis may not be confirmed until sometime after admission. If the documentation is not clear whether severe sepsis was present on admission, the provider should be queried.

4) Sepsis and severe sepsis with a localized infection

 If the reason for admission is both sepsis or severe sepsis and a localized infection, such as pneumonia or cellulitis, a code(s) for the underlying systemic infection should be assigned first and the code for the localized infection should be assigned as a secondary diagnosis. If the patient has severe sepsis, a code from subcategory R65.2 should also be assigned as a secondary diagnosis. If the patient is admitted with a localized infection, such as pneumonia, and sepsis/severe sepsis doesn't develop until after admission, the localized infection should be assigned first, followed by the appropriate sepsis/severe sepsis codes.

5) Sepsis due to a postprocedural infection

 (a) **Documentation of causal relationship**

  As with all postprocedural complications, code assignment is based on the provider's documentation of the relationship between the infection and the procedure.

 (b) **Sepsis due to a postprocedural infection**

  For such cases, the postprocedural infection code, such as T80.2, Infections following infusion, transfusion, and therapeutic injection, T81.4, Infection following a procedure, T88.0, Infection following immunization, or O86.0, Infection of obstetric surgical wound, should be coded first, followed by the code for the specific infection. If the patient has severe sepsis, the appropriate code from subcategory R65.2 should also be assigned with the additional code(s) for any acute organ dysfunction.

 (c) **Postprocedural infection and postprocedural septic shock**

In cases where a postprocedural infection has occurred and has resulted in severe sepsis the code for the precipitating complication such as code T81.4, Infection following a procedure, or O86.0, Infection of obstetrical surgical wound should be coded first followed by code R65.20, Severe sepsis without septic shock. A code for the systemic infection should also be assigned.

If a postprocedural infection has resulted in postprocedural septic shock, the code for the precipitating complication such as code T81.4, Infection following a procedure, or O86.0, Infection of obstetrical surgical wound should be coded first followed by code T81.12-, Postprocedural septic shock. A code for the systemic infection should also be assigned.

6) **Sepsis and severe sepsis associated with a noninfectious process (condition)**

In some cases a noninfectious process (condition), such as trauma, may lead to an infection which can result in sepsis or severe sepsis. If sepsis or severe sepsis is documented as associated with a noninfectious condition, such as a burn or serious injury, and this condition meets the definition for principal diagnosis, the code for the noninfectious condition should be sequenced first, followed by the code for the resulting infection. If severe sepsis is present, a code from subcategory

R65.2 should also be assigned with any associated organ dysfunction(s) codes. It is not necessary to assign a code from subcategory R65.1, Systemic inflammatory response syndrome (SIRS) of non-infectious origin, for these cases.

If the infection meets the definition of principal diagnosis, it should be sequenced before the non-infectious condition. When both the associated non-infectious condition and the infection meet the definition of principal diagnosis, either may be assigned as principal diagnosis.

Only one code from category R65, Symptoms and signs specifically associated with systemic inflammation and infection, should be assigned. Therefore, when a non-infectious condition leads to an infection resulting in severe sepsis, assign the appropriate code from subcategory R65.2, Severe sepsis. Do not additionally assign a code from subcategory R65.1, Systemic inflammatory response syndrome (SIRS) of non-infectious origin.

See Section I.C.18. SIRS due to non-infectious process

7) **Sepsis and septic shock complicating abortion, pregnancy, childbirth, and the puerperium**

See Section I.C.15. Sepsis and septic shock complicating abortion, pregnancy, childbirth and the puerperium

8) **Newborn sepsis**

See Section I.C.16. f. Bacterial sepsis of Newborn

METHICILLIN RESISTANT *STAPHYLOCOCCUS AUREUS* (MRSA) CONDITIONS

1) **Selection and sequencing of MRSA codes**

   (a) **Combination codes for MRSA infection**

   When a patient is diagnosed with an infection that is due to methicillin resistant *Staphylococcus aureus* (MRSA), and that infection has a combination code that includes the causal organism (e.g., sepsis, pneumonia) assign the appropriate combination code for the condition (e.g., code A41.02, Sepsis due to Methicillin resistant Staphylococcus aureus or code J15.212, Pneumonia due to Methicillin resistant Staphylococcus aureus). Do not assign code B95.62, Methicillin resistant Staphylococcus aureus infection as the cause of diseases classified elsewhere, as an additional code, because the combination code includes the type of infection and the MRSA organism. Do not assign a code from subcategory Z16.11, Resistance to penicillins, as an additional diagnosis.

   See Section C.1. for instructions on coding and sequencing of sepsis and severe sepsis.

   (b) **Other codes for MRSA infection**

   When there is documentation of a current infection (e.g., wound infection, stitch abscess, urinary tract infection) due to MRSA, and that infection does not have a combination code that includes the causal organism, assign the appropriate code to identify the condition along with code B95.62, Methicillin resistant Staphylococcus aureus infection as the cause of diseases classified elsewhere for the MRSA infection. Do not assign a code from subcategory Z16.11, Resistance to penicillins.

   (c) **Methicillin susceptible Staphylococcus aureus (MSSA) and MRSA colonization**

   The condition or state of being colonized or carrying MSSA or MRSA is called colonization or carriage, while an individual person is described as being colonized or being a carrier. Colonization means that MSSA or MSRA is present on or in the body without necessarily causing illness. A positive MRSA colonization test might be documented by the provider as "MRSA screen positive" or "MRSA nasal swab positive".

   Assign code Z22.322, Carrier or suspected carrier of Methicillin resistant Staphylococcus aureus, for patients documented as having MRSA colonization. Assign code Z22.321, Carrier or suspected carrier of Methicillin susceptible Staphylococcus aureus, for patient documented as having MSSA colonization. Colonization is not necessarily indicative of a disease process or as the cause of a specific condition the patient may have unless documented as such by the provider.

   (d) **MRSA colonization and infection**

   If a patient is documented as having both MRSA colonization and infection during a hospital admission, code Z22.322, Carrier or suspected carrier of Methicillin resistant Staphylococcus aureus, and a code for the MRSA infection may both be assigned.

● New code   ▲ Revised code   **Excludes1:** Not coded here   **Excludes2:** Not included here   ⊗ Placeholder required   ⑦7ᵗʰ digit required

ZIKA VIRUS INFECTIONS

1) **Code only confirmed cases**

Code only a confirmed diagnosis of Zika virus (A92.5, Zika virus disease) as documented by the provider. This is an exception to the hospital inpatient guideline Section II, H.

In this context, "confirmation" does not require documentation of the type of test performed; the physician's diagnostic statement that the condition is confirmed is sufficient. This code should be assigned regardless of the stated mode of transmission.

If the provider documents "suspected", "possible" or "probable" Zika, do not assign code A92.5. Assign a code(s) explaining the reason for encounter (such as fever, rash, or joint pain) or Z20.828, Contact with and (suspected) exposure to other viral communicable diseases.

Chapter 1

Certain Infectious and Parasitic Diseases (A00-B99)

Includes: diseases generally recognized as communicable or transmissible

Use additional code to identify resistance to antimicrobial drugs (Z16.-)

Excludes1: certain localized infections - see body system-related chapters

Excludes2: carrier or suspected carrier of infectious disease (Z22.-)

infectious and parasitic diseases complicating pregnancy, childbirth and the puerperium (O98.-)

infectious and parasitic diseases specific to the perinatal period (P35-P39)

influenza and other acute respiratory infections (J00-J22)

This chapter contains the following blocks:

A00-A09 Intestinal infectious diseases
A15-A19 Tuberculosis
A20-A28 Certain zoonotic bacterial diseases
A30-A49 Other bacterial diseases
A50-A64 Infections with a predominantly sexual mode of transmission
A65-A69 Other spirochetal diseases
A70-A74 Other diseases caused by chlamydiae
A75-A79 Rickettsioses
A80-A89 Viral and prion infections of the central nervous system
A90-A99 Arthropod-borne viral fevers and viral hemorrhagic fevers
B00-B09 Viral infections characterized by skin and mucous membrane lesions
B10 Other human herpesviruses
B15-B19 Viral hepatitis
B20 Human immunodeficiency virus [HIV] disease
B25-B34 Other viral diseases
B35-B49 Mycoses
B50-B64 Protozoal diseases
B65-B83 Helminthiases
B85-B89 Pediculosis, acariasis and other infestations
B90-B94 Sequelae of infectious and parasitic diseases
B95-B97 Bacterial and viral infectious agents
B99 Other infectious diseases

INTESTINAL INFECTIOUS DISEASES (A00-A09)

A00 Cholera

Definition: Cholera, aka Asiatic or epidemic cholera, is an infectious gastroenteritis caused by enterotoxin-producing strains of the bacterium vibrio cholerae.

A00.0 Cholera due to Vibrio cholerae 01, biovar cholerae
Classical cholera

A00.1 Cholera due to Vibrio cholerae 01, biovar eltor
Cholera eltor

A00.9 Cholera, unspecified

A01 Typhoid and paratyphoid fevers

A01.0 Typhoid fever

Definition: Typhoid fever, aka enteric fever, salmonella typhi is an illness caused by the bacterium salmonella enterica serovar typhi.

Infection due to Salmonella typhi

A01.00 Typhoid fever, unspecified
A01.01 Typhoid meningitis
A01.02 Typhoid fever with heart involvement

Typhoid endocarditis
Typhoid myocarditis
A01.03 Typhoid pneumonia
A01.04 Typhoid arthritis
A01.05 Typhoid osteomyelitis
A01.09 Typhoid fever with other complications
A01.1 Paratyphoid fever A
A01.2 Paratyphoid fever B
A01.3 Paratyphoid fever C
A01.4 Paratyphoid fever, unspecified
Infection due to Salmonella paratyphi NOS

A02 Other salmonella infections

Definition: Salmonellosis is an infection with salmonella bacteria. Most persons infected with salmonella develop diarrhea, fever, vomiting, and abdominal cramps.

Includes: infection or foodborne intoxication due to any Salmonella species other than S. typhi and S. paratyphi

A02.0 Salmonella enteritis
Salmonellosis

A02.1 Salmonella sepsis

A02.2 Localized salmonella infections
A02.20 Localized salmonella infection, unspecified
A02.21 Salmonella meningitis
A02.22 Salmonella pneumonia
A02.23 Salmonella arthritis
A02.24 Salmonella osteomyelitis
A02.25 Salmonella pyelonephritis
Salmonella tubulo-interstitial nephropathy
A02.29 Salmonella with other localized infection

A02.8 Other specified salmonella infections
A02.9 Salmonella infection, unspecified

A03 Shigellosis

Definition: Shigellosis, aka bacillary dysentery, is a food borne illness caused by infection by bacteria of the genus shigella.

A03.0 Shigellosis due to Shigella dysenteriae
Group A shigellosis [Shiga-Kruse dysentery]

A03.1 Shigellosis due to Shigella flexneri
Group B shigellosis

A03.2 Shigellosis due to Shigella boydii
Group C shigellosis

A03.3 Shigellosis due to Shigella sonnei
Group D shigellosis

A03.8 Other shigellosis

A03.9 Shigellosis, unspecified
Bacillary dysentery NOS

A04 Other bacterial intestinal infections

Excludes1: bacterial foodborne intoxications, NEC (A05.-)
tuberculous enteritis (A18.32)

A04.0 Enteropathogenic Escherichia coli infection
A04.1 Enterotoxigenic Escherichia coli infection
A04.2 Enteroinvasive Escherichia coli infection
A04.3 Enterohemorrhagic Escherichia coli infection
A04.4 Other intestinal Escherichia coli infections
Escherichia coli enteritis NOS
A04.5 Campylobacter enteritis
A04.6 Enteritis due to Yersinia enterocolitica
Excludes1: extraintestinal yersiniosis (A28.2)

Add 4th-7th digits   Nonspecific code   Unspecified code   Manifestation code

A04.7 Enterocolitis due to Clostridium difficile

Foodborne intoxication by Clostridium difficile

Pseudomembranous colitis

- **A04.71 Enterocolitis due to Clostridium difficile, recurrent**

- **A04.72 Enterocolitis due to Clostridium difficile, not specified as recurrent**

A04.8 Other specified bacterial intestinal infections

A04.9 Bacterial intestinal infection, unspecified

Bacterial enteritis NOS

A05 Other bacterial foodborne intoxications, not elsewhere classified

Excludes1: Clostridium difficile foodborne intoxication and infection (A04.7-)

Escherichia coli infection (A04.0-A04.4)

listeriosis (A32.-)

salmonella foodborne intoxication and infection (A02.-)

toxic effect of noxious foodstuffs (T61-T62)

A05.0 Foodborne staphylococcal intoxication

A05.1 Botulism food poisoning

Botulism NOS

Classical foodborne intoxication due to Clostridium botulinum

Excludes1: infant botulism (A48.51)

wound botulism (A48.52)

A05.2 Foodborne Clostridium perfringens [Clostridium welchii] intoxication

Enteritis necroticans

Pig-bel

A05.3 Foodborne Vibrio parahaemolyticus intoxication

A05.4 Foodborne Bacillus cereus intoxication

A05.5 Foodborne Vibrio vulnificus intoxication

A05.8 Other specified bacterial foodborne intoxications

A05.9 Bacterial foodborne intoxication, unspecified

A06 Amebiasis

Definition: Amebiasis is an inflammation of the intestines caused by infection with entamoeba histolytica characterized by frequent, loose stools flecked with blood and mucus.

Includes: infection due to Entamoeba histolytica

Excludes1: Other protozoal intestinal diseases (A07.-)

Excludes2: acanthamebiasis (B60.1-)

Naegleriasis (B60.2)

A06.0 Acute amebic dysentery

Acute amebiasis

Intestinal amebiasis NOS

A06.1 Chronic intestinal amebiasis

A06.2 Amebic nondysenteric colitis

A06.3 Ameboma of intestine

Ameboma NOS

A06.4 Amebic liver abscess

Hepatic amebiasis

A06.5 Amebic lung abscess

Amebic abscess of lung (and liver)

A06.6 Amebic brain abscess

Amebic abscess of brain (and liver) (and lung)

A06.7 Cutaneous amebiasis

A06.8 Amebic infection of other sites

A06.81 Amebic cystitis

A06.82 Other amebic genitourinary infections

Amebic balanitis

Amebic vesiculitis

Amebic vulvovaginitis

A06.89 Other amebic infections

Amebic appendicitis

Amebic splenic abscess

A06.9 Amebiasis, unspecified

A07 Other protozoal intestinal diseases

Definition: Protozoal intestinal diseases refers to diseases of the intestinal system caused by protozoa, which are single-cell organisms that can only divide within a host organism. Malaria , Giardia and toxoplasmosis are examples of diseases caused by protozoa.

A07.0 Balantidiasis

Balantidial dysentery

A07.1 Giardiasis [lambliasis]

A07.2 Cryptosporidiosis

A07.3 Isosporiasis

Infection due to Isospora belli and Isospora hominis

Intestinal coccidiosis

Isosporosis

A07.4 Cyclosporiasis

A07.8 Other specified protozoal intestinal diseases

Intestinal microsporidiosis

Intestinal trichomoniasis

Sarcocystosis

Sarcosporidiosis

A07.9 Protozoal intestinal disease, unspecified

Flagellate diarrhea

Protozoal colitis

Protozoal diarrhea

Protozoal dysentery

A08 Viral and other specified intestinal infections

Excludes1: influenza with involvement of gastrointestinal tract (J09.X3, J10.2, J11.2)

A08.0 Rotaviral enteritis

A08.1 Acute gastroenteropathy due to Norwalk agent and other small round viruses

A08.11 Acute gastroenteropathy due to Norwalk agent

Acute gastroenteropathy due to Norovirus

Acute gastroenteropathy due to Norwalk-like agent

A08.19 Acute gastroenteropathy due to other small round viruses

Acute gastroenteropathy due to small round virus [SRV] NOS

A08.2 Adenoviral enteritis

A08.3 Other viral enteritis

A08.31 Calicivirus enteritis

A08.32 Astrovirus enteritis

A08.39 Other viral enteritis

Coxsackie virus enteritis

Echovirus enteritis

Enterovirus enteritis NEC

Torovirus enteritis

A08.4 Viral intestinal infection, unspecified

Viral enteritis NOS

Viral gastroenteritis NOS

Viral gastroenteropathy NOS

A08.8   **Other specified intestinal infections**

A09   **Infectious gastroenteritis and colitis, unspecified**

Infectious colitis NOS

Infectious enteritis NOS

Infectious gastroenteritis NOS

Excludes1: colitis NOS (K52.9)

    diarrhea NOS (R19.7)

    enteritis NOS (K52.9)

    gastroenteritis NOS (K52.9)

    noninfective gastroenteritis and colitis, unspecified (K52.9)

TUBERCULOSIS (A15-A19)

Definition: Tuberculosis is a common and often deadly infectious disease caused by mycobacteria, in humans mainly mycobacterium tuberculosis. Tuberculosis usually attacks the lungs but can also affect the central nervous system, the lymphatic system, the circulatory system, the genitourinary system, the gastrointestinal system, bones, joints, and even the skin.

Includes: infections due to Mycobacterium tuberculosis and Mycobacterium bovis

Excludes1: congenital tuberculosis (P37.0)

nonspecific reaction to test for tuberculosis without active tuberculosis (R76.1-)

pneumoconiosis associated with tuberculosis, any type in A15 (J65)

positive PPD (R76.11)

positive tuberculin skin test without active tuberculosis (R76.11)

sequelae of tuberculosis (B90.-)

silicotuberculosis (J65)

A15   **Respiratory tuberculosis**

  A15.0   **Tuberculosis of lung**

    Tuberculous bronchiectasis

    Tuberculous fibrosis of lung

    Tuberculous pneumonia

    Tuberculous pneumothorax

  A15.4   **Tuberculosis of intrathoracic lymph nodes**

    Tuberculosis of hilar lymph nodes

    Tuberculosis of mediastinal lymph nodes

    Tuberculosis of tracheobronchial lymph nodes

    Excludes1: tuberculosis specified as primary (A15.7)

  A15.5   **Tuberculosis of larynx, trachea and bronchus**

    Tuberculosis of bronchus

    Tuberculosis of glottis

    Tuberculosis of larynx

    Tuberculosis of trachea

  A15.6   **Tuberculous pleurisy**

    Tuberculosis of pleura

    Tuberculous empyema

    Excludes1: primary respiratory tuberculosis (A15.7)

  A15.7   **Primary respiratory tuberculosis**

  A15.8   **Other respiratory tuberculosis**

    Mediastinal tuberculosis

    Nasopharyngeal tuberculosis

    Tuberculosis of nose

    Tuberculosis of sinus [any nasal]

  A15.9   **Respiratory tuberculosis unspecified**

A17   **Tuberculosis of nervous system**

  A17.0   **Tuberculous meningitis**

Tuberculosis of meninges (cerebral)(spinal)

Tuberculous leptomeningitis

Excludes1: tuberculous meningoencephalitis (A17.82)

  A17.1   **Meningeal tuberculoma**

    Tuberculoma of meninges (cerebral) (spinal)

    Excludes2: tuberculoma of brain and spinal cord (A17.81)

  A17.8   **Other tuberculosis of nervous system**

    A17.81   **Tuberculoma of brain and spinal cord**

      Tuberculous abscess of brain and spinal cord

    A17.82   **Tuberculous meningoencephalitis**

      Tuberculous myelitis

    A17.83   **Tuberculous neuritis**

      Tuberculous mononeuropathy

    A17.89   **Other tuberculosis of nervous system**

      Tuberculous polyneuropathy

  A17.9   **Tuberculosis of nervous system, unspecified**

A18   **Tuberculosis of other organs**

  A18.0   **Tuberculosis of bones and joints**

    A18.01   **Tuberculosis of spine**

      Pott's disease or curvature of spine

      Tuberculous arthritis

      Tuberculous osteomyelitis of spine

      Tuberculous spondylitis

    A18.02   **Tuberculous arthritis of other joints**

      Tuberculosis of hip (joint)

      Tuberculosis of knee (joint)

    A18.03   **Tuberculosis of other bones**

      Tuberculous mastoiditis

      Tuberculous osteomyelitis

    A18.09   **Other musculoskeletal tuberculosis**

      Tuberculous myositis

      Tuberculous synovitis

      Tuberculous tenosynovitis

  A18.1   **Tuberculosis of genitourinary system**

    A18.10   **Tuberculosis of genitourinary system, unspecified**

    A18.11   **Tuberculosis of kidney and ureter**

    A18.12   **Tuberculosis of bladder**

    A18.13   **Tuberculosis of other urinary organs**

      Tuberculous urethritis

    A18.14   **Tuberculosis of prostate**

    A18.15   **Tuberculosis of other male genital organs**

    A18.16   **Tuberculosis of cervix**

    A18.17   **Tuberculous female pelvic inflammatory disease**

      Tuberculous endometritis

      Tuberculous oophoritis and salpingitis

    A18.18   **Tuberculosis of other female genital organs**

      Tuberculous ulceration of vulva

  A18.2   **Tuberculous peripheral lymphadenopathy**

    Tuberculous adenitis

    Excludes2: tuberculosis of bronchial and mediastinal lymph nodes (A15.4)

      tuberculosis of mesenteric and retroperitoneal lymph nodes (A18.39)

      tuberculous tracheobronchial adenopathy (A15.4)

  A18.3   **Tuberculosis of intestines, peritoneum and mesenteric glands**

Add 4th-7th digits	Nonspecific code	Unspecified code	Manifestation code	143

A18.31 **Tuberculous peritonitis**

Tuberculous ascites

A18.32 **Tuberculous enteritis**

Tuberculosis of anus and rectum

Tuberculosis of intestine (large) (small)

A18.39 **Retroperitoneal tuberculosis**

Tuberculosis of mesenteric glands

Tuberculosis of retroperitoneal (lymph glands)

A18.4 **Tuberculosis of skin and subcutaneous tissue**

Erythema induratum, tuberculous

Lupus exedens

Lupus vulgaris NOS

Lupus vulgaris of eyelid

Scrofuloderma

Tuberculosis of external ear

Excludes2: lupus erythematosus (L93.-)

lupus NOS (M32.9) systemic (M32.-)

A18.5 **Tuberculosis of eye**

Excludes2: lupus vulgaris of eyelid (A18.4)

A18.50 **Tuberculosis of eye, unspecified**

A18.51 **Tuberculous episcleritis**

A18.52 **Tuberculous keratitis**

Tuberculous interstitial keratitis

Tuberculous keratoconjunctivitis (interstitial) (phlyctenular)

A18.53 **Tuberculous chorioretinitis**

A18.54 **Tuberculous iridocyclitis**

A18.59 **Other tuberculosis of eye**

Tuberculous conjunctivitis

A18.6 **Tuberculosis of (inner) (middle) ear**

Tuberculous otitis media

Excludes2: tuberculosis of external ear (A18.4)

tuberculous mastoiditis (A18.03)

A18.7 **Tuberculosis of adrenal glands**

Tuberculous Addison's disease

A18.8 **Tuberculosis of other specified organs**

A18.81 **Tuberculosis of thyroid gland**

A18.82 **Tuberculosis of other endocrine glands**

Tuberculosis of pituitary gland

Tuberculosis of thymus gland

A18.83 **Tuberculosis of digestive tract organs, not elsewhere classified**

Excludes1: tuberculosis of intestine (A18.32)

A18.84 **Tuberculosis of heart**

Tuberculous cardiomyopathy

Tuberculous endocarditis

Tuberculous myocarditis

Tuberculous pericarditis

A18.85 **Tuberculosis of spleen**

A18.89 **Tuberculosis of other sites**

Tuberculosis of muscle

Tuberculous cerebral arteritis

A19 **Miliary tuberculosis**

Definition: Miliary tuberculosis acute tuberculosis characterized by the appearance of tiny tubercles on one or more organs of the body.

Includes: disseminated tuberculosis

generalized tuberculosis tuberculous polyserositis

A19.0 **Acute miliary tuberculosis of a single specified site**

A19.1 **Acute miliary tuberculosis of multiple sites**

A19.2 **Acute miliary tuberculosis, unspecified**

A19.8 **Other miliary tuberculosis**

A19.9 **Miliary tuberculosis, unspecified**

CERTAIN ZOONOTIC BACTERIAL DISEASES (A20-A28)

A20 **Plague**

Definition: Plague is a deadly infectious disease caused by the enterobacteria yersinia pestis (pasteurella pestis).

Includes: infection due to Yersinia pestis

A20.0 **Bubonic plague**

A20.1 **Cellulocutaneous plague**

A20.2 **Pneumonic plague**

A20.3 **Plague meningitis**

A20.7 **Septicemic plague**

A20.8 **Other forms of plague**

Abortive plague

Asymptomatic plague

Pestis minor

A20.9 **Plague, unspecified**

A21 **Tularemia**

Definition: Tularemia, aka rabbit fever, deer fly fever, O'Hara's fever is a serious infectious disease caused by the bacterium Francisella tularensis.

Includes: deer-fly fever

infection due to Francisella tularensis rabbit fever

A21.0 **Ulceroglandular tularemia**

A21.1 **Oculoglandular tularemia**

Ophthalmic tularemia

A21.2 **Pulmonary tularemia**

A21.3 **Gastrointestinal tularemia**

Abdominal tularemia

A21.7 **Generalized tularemia**

A21.8 **Other forms of tularemia**

A21.9 **Tularemia, unspecified**

A22 **Anthrax**

Definition: Anthrax is an acute disease in humans and animals caused by the bacterium bacillus anthracis which is highly lethal in some forms.

Includes: infection due to Bacillus anthracis

A22.0 **Cutaneous anthrax**

Malignant carbuncle

Malignant pustule

A22.1 **Pulmonary anthrax**

Inhalation anthrax

Ragpicker's disease

Woolsorter's disease

A22.2 **Gastrointestinal anthrax**

A22.7 **Anthrax sepsis**

A22.8 **Other forms of anthrax**

Anthrax meningitis

A22.9 **Anthrax, unspecified**

A23 **Brucellosis**

Definition: Brucellosis, aka undulant fever, or Malta fever is a highly contagious zoonosis caused by ingestion of unsterilized milk or meat from infected animals, or close contact with their secretions.

Includes: Malta fever

Mediterranean fever undulant fever

A23.0 **Brucellosis due to Brucella melitensis**

A23.1 **Brucellosis due to Brucella abortus**

A23.2 **Brucellosis due to Brucella suis**

A23.3 **Brucellosis due to Brucella canis**

A23.8 **Other brucellosis**

A23.9 **Brucellosis, unspecified**

A24 **Glanders and melioidosis**

Definition: Glanders is an infectious disease that occurs primarily in horses, mules, and donkeys and other animals such as dogs, cats and goats that can be transmitted to humans. It is caused by infection with the bacterium Burkholderia mallei.

A24.0 **Glanders**

Infection due to Pseudomonas mallei

Malleus

A24.1 **Acute and fulminating melioidosis**

Melioidosis pneumonia

Melioidosis sepsis

A24.2 **Subacute and chronic melioidosis**

A24.3 **Other melioidosis**

A24.9 **Melioidosis, unspecified**

Infection due to Pseudomonas pseudomallei NOS

Whitmore's disease

A25 **Rat-bite fevers**

A25.0 **Spirillosis**

Sodoku

A25.1 **Streptobacillosis**

Epidemic arthritic erythema

Haverhill fever

Streptobacillary rat-bite fever

A25.9 **Rat-bite fever, unspecified**

A26 **Erysipeloid**

A26.0 **Cutaneous erysipeloid**

Erythema migrans

A26.7 **Erysipelothrix sepsis**

A26.8 **Other forms of erysipeloid**

A26.9 **Erysipeloid, unspecified**

A27 **Leptospirosis**

A27.0 **Leptospirosis icterohemorrhagica**

Leptospiral or spirochetal jaundice (hemorrhagic) Weil's disease

A27.8 **Other forms of leptospirosis**

A27.81 **Aseptic meningitis in leptospirosis**

A27.89 **Other forms of leptospirosis**

A27.9 **Leptospirosis, unspecified**

A28 **Other zoonotic bacterial diseases, not elsewhere classified**

Definition: Zoonotic refers to other diseases that can be passed from animals, whether wild or domesticated, to humans.

A28.0 **Pasteurellosis**

A28.1 **Cat-scratch disease**

Cat-scratch fever

A28.2 **Extraintestinal yersiniosis**

Excludes1: enteritis due to Yersinia

enterocolitica (A04.6)

plague (A20.-)

A28.8 **Other specified zoonotic bacterial diseases, not elsewhere classified**

A28.9 **Zoonotic bacterial disease, unspecified**

OTHER BACTERIAL DISEASES (A30-A49)

A30 **Leprosy [Hansen's disease]**

Definition: Leprosy is an infectious disease characterized by disfiguring skin sores, nerve damage, and progressive debilitation. Leprosy is caused by the organism mycobacterium leprae.

Includes: infection due to Mycobacterium leprae

Excludes1: sequelae of leprosy (B92)

A30.0 **Indeterminate leprosy**

I leprosy

A30.1 **Tuberculoid leprosy**

TT leprosy

A30.2 **Borderline tuberculoid leprosy**

BT leprosy

A30.3 **Borderline leprosy**

BB leprosy

A30.4 **Borderline lepromatous leprosy**

BL leprosy

A30.5 **Lepromatous leprosy**

LL leprosy

A30.8 **Other forms of leprosy**

A30.9 **Leprosy, unspecified**

A31 **Infection due to other mycobacteria**

Excludes2: leprosy (A30.-)

tuberculosis (A15-A19)

A31.0 **Pulmonary mycobacterial infection**

Infection due to Mycobacterium avium

Infection due to Mycobacterium intracellulare [Battey bacillus]

Infection due to Mycobacterium kansasii

A31.1 **Cutaneous mycobacterial infection**

Buruli ulcer

Infection due to Mycobacterium marinum

Infection due to Mycobacterium ulcerans

A31.2 **Disseminated mycobacterium avium-intracellulare complex (DMAC)**

MAC sepsis

A31.8 **Other mycobacterial infections**

A31.9 **Mycobacterial infection, unspecified**

Atypical mycobacterial infection NOS

Mycobacteriosis NOS

A32 **Listeriosis**

Includes: listerial foodborne infection

Excludes1: neonatal (disseminated) listeriosis (P37.2)

A32.0 **Cutaneous listeriosis**

A32.1 **Listerial meningitis and meningoencephalitis**

A32.11 **Listerial meningitis**

A32.12 **Listerial meningoencephalitis**

A32.7 **Listerial sepsis**

A32.8 **Other forms of listeriosis**

A32.81 **Oculoglandular listeriosis**

A32.82 **Listerial endocarditis**

A32.89   **Other forms of listeriosis**
     Listerial cerebral arteritis

A32.9   **Listeriosis, unspecified**

A33   **Tetanus neonatorum**

A34   **Obstetrical tetanus**

A35   **Other tetanus**
     Tetanus NOS

     Excludes1: obstetrical tetanus (A34)

               tetanus neonatorum (A33)

A36   **Diphtheria**

     Definition: Diphtheria is a highly infectious disease of the upper respiratory tract characterized by a sore throat, fever and causing difficulty in breathing.

A36.0   **Pharyngeal diphtheria**
     Diphtheritic membranous angina
     Tonsillar diphtheria

A36.1   **Nasopharyngeal diphtheria**

A36.2   **Laryngeal diphtheria**
     Diphtheritic laryngotracheitis

A36.3   **Cutaneous diphtheria**

     Excludes2: erythrasma (L08.1)

A36.8   **Other diphtheria**

     A36.81   **Diphtheritic cardiomyopathy**
           Diphtheritic myocarditis

     A36.82   **Diphtheritic radiculomyelitis**

     A36.83   **Diphtheritic polyneuritis**

     A36.84   **Diphtheritic tubulo-interstitial nephropathy**

     A36.85   **Diphtheritic cystitis**

     A36.86   **Diphtheritic conjunctivitis**

     A36.89   **Other diphtheritic complications**
           Diphtheritic peritonitis

A36.9   **Diphtheria, unspecified**

A37   **Whooping cough**

     Definition: Whooping cough, aka pertussis, is a highly contagious disease caused by bacteria. The most prominent symptom of whooping cough is a distinctive, uncontrollable cough, followed by a sharp, high-pitched intake of air.

A37.0   **Whooping cough due to Bordetella pertussis**

     A37.00   **Whooping cough due to Bordetella pertussis without pneumonia**

     A37.01   **Whooping cough due to Bordetella pertussis with pneumonia**

A37.1   **Whooping cough due to Bordetella parapertussis**

     A37.10   **Whooping cough due to Bordetella parapertussis without pneumonia**

     A37.11   **Whooping cough due to Bordetella parapertussis with pneumonia**

A37.8   **Whooping cough due to other Bordetella species**

     A37.80   **Whooping cough due to other Bordetella species without pneumonia**

     A37.81   **Whooping cough due to other Bordetella species with pneumonia**

A37.9   **Whooping cough, unspecified species**

     A37.90   **Whooping cough, unspecified species without pneumonia**

     A37.91   **Whooping cough, unspecified species with pneumonia**

A38   **Scarlet fever**

     Includes: scarlatina

     Excludes2: streptococcal sore throat (J02.0)

A38.0   **Scarlet fever with otitis media**

A38.1   **Scarlet fever with myocarditis**

A38.8   **Scarlet fever with other complications**

A38.9   **Scarlet fever, uncomplicated**
     Scarlet fever, NOS

A39   **Meningococcal infection**

A39.0   **Meningococcal meningitis**

A39.1   **Waterhouse-Friderichsen syndrome**
     Meningococcal hemorrhagic adrenalitis
     Meningococcic adrenal syndrome

A39.2   **Acute meningococcemia**

A39.3   **Chronic meningococcemia**

A39.4   **Meningococcemia, unspecified**

A39.5   **Meningococcal heart disease**

     A39.50   **Meningococcal carditis, unspecified**

     A39.51   **Meningococcal endocarditis**

     A39.52   **Meningococcal myocarditis**

     A39.53   **Meningococcal pericarditis**

A39.8   **Other meningococcal infections**

     A39.81   **Meningococcal encephalitis**

     A39.82   **Meningococcal retrobulbar neuritis**

     A39.83   **Meningococcal arthritis**

     A39.84   **Postmeningococcal arthritis**

     A39.89   **Other meningococcal infections**
           Meningococcal conjunctivitis

A39.9   **Meningococcal infection, unspecified**
     Meningococcal disease NOS

A40   **Streptococcal sepsis**

     Code first postprocedural streptococcal sepsis (T81.4-)
     streptococcal sepsis during labor (O75.3)
     streptococcal sepsis following abortion or ectopic or molar pregnancy (O03-O07, O08.0)
     streptococcal sepsis following immunization (T88.0)
     streptococcal sepsis following infusion, transfusion or therapeutic injection (T80.2-)

     Excludes1: neonatal (P36.0-P36.1)

            puerperal sepsis (O85)

            sepsis due to Streptococcus, group D (A41.81)

A40.0   **Sepsis due to streptococcus, group A**

A40.1   **Sepsis due to streptococcus, group B**

A40.3   **Sepsis due to Streptococcus pneumoniae**
     Pneumococcal sepsis

A40.8   **Other streptococcal sepsis**

A40.9   **Streptococcal sepsis, unspecified**

A41   **Other sepsis**

     Code first postprocedural sepsis (T81.4-)
     sepsis during labor (O75.3)
     sepsis following abortion, ectopic or molar pregnancy (O03-O07, O08.0)
     sepsis following immunization (T88.0)
     sepsis following infusion, transfusion or therapeutic injection (T80.2-)

     Excludes1: bacteremia NOS (R78.81)

            neonatal (P36.-) puerperal sepsis (O85)

   ● New code   ▲ Revised code   **Excludes1:** Not coded here   **Excludes2:** Not included here   ⊗ Placeholder required   ⑦7th digit required

streptococcal sepsis (A40.-)

Excludes2: sepsis (due to) (in) actinomycotic (A42.7)

sepsis (due to) (in) anthrax (A22.7)

sepsis (due to) (in) candidal (B37.7)

sepsis (due to) (in) Erysipelothrix (A26.7)

sepsis (due to) (in) extraintestinal yersiniosis (A28.2)

sepsis (due to) (in) gonococcal (A54.86)

sepsis (due to) (in) herpesviral (B00.7)

sepsis (due to) (in) listerial (A32.7)

sepsis (due to) (in) melioidosis (A24.1)

sepsis (due to) (in) meningococcal (A39.2-A39.4)

sepsis (due to) (in) plague (A20.7)

sepsis (due to) (in) tularemia (A21.7)

toxic shock syndrome (A48.3)

A41.0   **Sepsis due to Staphylococcus aureus**

    A41.01   **Sepsis due to Methicillin susceptible Staphylococcus aureus**

      MSSA sepsis

      Staphylococcus aureus sepsis NOS

    A41.02   **Sepsis due to Methicillin resistant Staphylococcus aureus**

A41.1   **Sepsis due to other specified staphylococcus**

  Coagulase negative staphylococcus sepsis

A41.2   **Sepsis due to unspecified staphylococcus**

A41.3   **Sepsis due to Hemophilus influenzae**

A41.4   **Sepsis due to anaerobes**

    Excludes1: gas gangrene (A48.0)

A41.5   **Sepsis due to other Gram-negative organisms**

    A41.50   **Gram-negative sepsis, unspecified**

      Gram-negative sepsis NOS

    A41.51   **Sepsis due to Escherichia coli [E. coli]**

    A41.52   **Sepsis due to Pseudomonas**

      Pseudomonas aeruginosa

    A41.53   **Sepsis due to Serratia**

    A41.59   **Other Gram-negative sepsis**

A41.8   **Other specified sepsis**

    A41.81   **Sepsis due to Enterococcus**

    A41.89   **Other specified sepsis**

A41.9   **Sepsis, unspecified organism**

  Septicemia NOS

A42   **Actinomycosis**

  Definition: Actinomycosis is an infection primarily caused by the bacterium actinomyces israelii. Infection most often occurs in the face and neck region and is characterized by the presence of a slowly enlarging, hard, red lump.

  Excludes1: actinomycetoma (B47.1)

A42.0   **Pulmonary actinomycosis**

A42.1   **Abdominal actinomycosis**

A42.2   **Cervicofacial actinomycosis**

A42.7   **Actinomycotic sepsis**

A42.8   **Other forms of actinomycosis**

    A42.81   **Actinomycotic meningitis**

    A42.82   **Actinomycotic encephalitis**

    A42.89   **Other forms of actinomycosis**

A42.9   **Actinomycosis, unspecified**

A43   **Nocardiosis**

A43.0   **Pulmonary nocardiosis**

A43.1   **Cutaneous nocardiosis**

A43.8   **Other forms of nocardiosis**

A43.9   **Nocardiosis, unspecified**

A44   **Bartonellosis**

A44.0   **Systemic bartonellosis**

  Oroya fever

A44.1   **Cutaneous and mucocutaneous bartonellosis**

  Verruga peruana

A44.8   **Other forms of bartonellosis**

A44.9   **Bartonellosis, unspecified**

A46   **Erysipelas**

  Definition: Erysipelas is an acute febrile disease that is associated with intense often vesicular and edematous local inflammation of the skin and subcutaneous tissues and that is caused by a hemolytic streptococcus.

  Excludes1: postpartum or puerperal erysipelas (O86.89)

A48   **Other bacterial diseases, not elsewhere classified**

  Excludes1: actinomycetoma (B47.1)

A48.0   **Gas gangrene**

  Clostridial cellulitis

  Clostridial myonecrosis

A48.1   **Legionnaires' disease**

A48.2   **Nonpneumonic Legionnaires' disease [Pontiac fever]**

A48.3   **Toxic shock syndrome**

  Use additional code to identify the organism (B95, B96)

  Excludes1: endotoxic shock NOS (R57.8)

    sepsis NOS (A41.9)

A48.4   **Brazilian purpuric fever**

  Systemic Hemophilus aegyptius infection

A48.5   **Other specified botulism**

  Non-foodborne intoxication due to toxins of Clostridium botulinum [C. botulinum]

  Excludes1: food poisoning due to toxins of Clostridium botulinum (A05.1)

    A48.51   **Infant botulism**

    A48.52   **Wound botulism**

      Non-foodborne botulism NOS

      Use additional code for associated wound

A48.8   **Other specified bacterial diseases**

A49   **Bacterial infection of unspecified site**

  Excludes1: bacterial agents as the cause of diseases classified elsewhere (B95-B96)

  chlamydial infection NOS (A74.9)

  meningococcal infection NOS (A39.9)

  rickettsial infection NOS (A79.9)

  spirochetal infection NOS (A69.9)

A49.0   **Staphylococcal infection, unspecified site**

    A49.01   **Methicillin susceptible Staphylococcus aureus infection, unspecified site**

      Methicillin susceptible Staphylococcus aureus (MSSA) infection

      Staphylococcus aureus infection NOS

    A49.02   **Methicillin resistant Staphylococcus aureus infection, unspecified site**

      Methicillin resistant Staphylococcus aureus (MRSA) infection

A49.1   **Streptococcal infection, unspecified site**

A49.2   **Hemophilus influenzae infection, unspecified site**

A49.3 **Mycoplasma infection, unspecified site**

A49.8 **Other bacterial infections of unspecified site**

A49.9 **Bacterial infection, unspecified**

Excludes1: bacteremia NOS (R78.81)

INFECTIONS WITH A PREDOMINANTLY SEXUAL MODE OF TRANSMISSION (A50-A64)

Excludes1: human immunodeficiency virus [HIV] disease (B20)

nonspecific and nongonococcal urethritis (N34.1)

Reiter's disease (M02.3-)

A50 **Congenital syphilis**

Definition: Congenital syphilis is syphilis present in utero and at birth, and occurs when a child is born to a mother with secondary or tertiary syphilis.

A50.0 **Early congenital syphilis, symptomatic**

Any congenital syphilitic condition specified as early or manifest less than two years after birth.

A50.01 **Early congenital syphilitic oculopathy**

A50.02 **Early congenital syphilitic osteochondropathy**

A50.03 **Early congenital syphilitic pharyngitis**

Early congenital syphilitic laryngitis

A50.04 **Early congenital syphilitic pneumonia**

A50.05 **Early congenital syphilitic rhinitis**

A50.06 **Early cutaneous congenital syphilis**

A50.07 **Early mucocutaneous congenital syphilis**

A50.08 **Early visceral congenital syphilis**

A50.09 **Other early congenital syphilis, symptomatic**

A50.1 **Early congenital syphilis, latent**

Congenital syphilis without clinical manifestations, with positive serological reaction and negative spinal fluid test, less than two years after birth.

A50.2 **Early congenital syphilis, unspecified**

Congenital syphilis NOS less than two years after birth.

A50.3 **Late congenital syphilitic oculopathy**

Excludes1: Hutchinson's triad (A50.53)

A50.30 **Late congenital syphilitic oculopathy, unspecified**

A50.31 **Late congenital syphilitic interstitial keratitis**

A50.32 **Late congenital syphilitic chorioretinitis**

A50.39 **Other late congenital syphilitic oculopathy**

A50.4 **Late congenital neurosyphilis [juvenile neurosyphilis]**

Use additional code to identify any associated mental disorder

Excludes1: Hutchinson's triad (A50.53)

A50.40 **Late congenital neurosyphilis, unspecified**

Juvenile neurosyphilis NOS

A50.41 **Late congenital syphilitic meningitis**

A50.42 **Late congenital syphilitic encephalitis**

A50.43 **Late congenital syphilitic polyneuropathy**

A50.44 **Late congenital syphilitic optic nerve atrophy**

A50.45 **Juvenile general paresis**

Dementia paralytica juvenilis

Juvenile tabetoparetic neurosyphilis

A50.49 **Other late congenital neurosyphilis**

Juvenile tabes dorsalis

A50.5 **Other late congenital syphilis, symptomatic**

Any congenital syphilitic condition specified as late or manifest two years or more after birth.

A50.51 **Clutton's joints**

A50.52 **Hutchinson's teeth**

A50.53 **Hutchinson's triad**

A50.54 **Late congenital cardiovascular syphilis**

A50.55 **Late congenital syphilitic arthropathy**

A50.56 **Late congenital syphilitic osteochondropathy**

A50.57 **Syphilitic saddle nose**

A50.59 **Other late congenital syphilis, symptomatic**

A50.6 **Late congenital syphilis, latent**

Congenital syphilis without clinical manifestations, with positive serological reaction and negative spinal fluid test, two years or more after birth.

A50.7 **Late congenital syphilis, unspecified**

Congenital syphilis NOS two years or more after birth.

A50.9 **Congenital syphilis, unspecified**

A51 **Early syphilis**

Definition: Early syphilis is defined as the stages of syphilis (primary, secondary, and early latent syphilis) that typically occur within the first year after acquisition of the infection.

A51.0 **Primary genital syphilis**

Syphilitic chancre NOS

A51.1 **Primary anal syphilis**

A51.2 **Primary syphilis of other sites**

A51.3 **Secondary syphilis of skin and mucous membranes**

A51.31 **Condyloma latum**

A51.32 **Syphilitic alopecia**

A51.39 **Other secondary syphilis of skin**

Syphilitic leukoderma

Syphilitic mucous patch

Excludes1: late syphilitic leukoderma (A52.79)

A51.4 **Other secondary syphilis**

A51.41 **Secondary syphilitic meningitis**

A51.42 **Secondary syphilitic female pelvic disease**

A51.43 **Secondary syphilitic oculopathy**

Secondary syphilitic chorioretinitis

Secondary syphilitic iridocyclitis, iritis

Secondary syphilitic uveitis

A51.44 **Secondary syphilitic nephritis**

A51.45 **Secondary syphilitic hepatitis**

A51.46 **Secondary syphilitic osteopathy**

A51.49 **Other secondary syphilitic conditions**

Secondary syphilitic lymphadenopathy

Secondary syphilitic myositis

A51.5 **Early syphilis, latent**

Syphilis (acquired) without clinical manifestations, with positive serological reaction and negative spinal fluid test, less than two years after infection.

A51.9 **Early syphilis, unspecified**

A52 **Late syphilis**

A52.0 **Cardiovascular and cerebrovascular syphilis**

Definition: Cardiovascular syphilis refers to the involvement of the cardiovascular system in late syphilis usually resulting in aortitis aneurysm formation, and aortic valvular insufficiency.

A52.00 **Cardiovascular syphilis, unspecified**

A52.01 **Syphilitic aneurysm of aorta**

A52.02 **Syphilitic aortitis**

A52.03 **Syphilitic endocarditis**

Syphilitic aortic valve incompetence or stenosis

Syphilitic mitral valve stenosis

Syphilitic pulmonary valve regurgitation

A52.04 Syphilitic cerebral arteritis

A52.05 Other cerebrovascular syphilis

Syphilitic cerebral aneurysm (ruptured) (non-ruptured)

Syphilitic cerebral thrombosis

A52.06 Other syphilitic heart involvement

Syphilitic coronary artery disease

Syphilitic myocarditis

Syphilitic pericarditis

A52.09 Other cardiovascular syphilis

A52.1 Symptomatic neurosyphilis

Definition: Neurosyphilis, aka tabes dorsalis, is the slowly progressive degeneration of the spinal cord that occurs in the late (tertiary) phase of syphilis a decade or more after contracting the infection.

A52.10 Symptomatic neurosyphilis, unspecified

A52.11 Tabes dorsalis

Locomotor ataxia (progressive)

Tabetic neurosyphilis

A52.12 Other cerebrospinal syphilis

A52.13 Late syphilitic meningitis

A52.14 Late syphilitic encephalitis

A52.15 Late syphilitic neuropathy

Late syphilitic acoustic neuritis

Late syphilitic optic (nerve) atrophy

Late syphilitic polyneuropathy

Late syphilitic retrobulbar neuritis

A52.16 Charcôt's arthropathy (tabetic)

A52.17 General paresis

Dementia paralytica

A52.19 Other symptomatic neurosyphilis

Syphilitic parkinsonism

A52.2 Asymptomatic neurosyphilis

A52.3 Neurosyphilis, unspecified

Gumma (syphilitic)

Syphilis (late)

Syphiloma

A52.7 Other symptomatic late syphilis

Definition: Late syphilis is defined as involvement of the cardiovascular or central nervous system, or the development of a gumma in any organ, due to infection with treponema pallidum; usually several years to 2-3 decades after the initial infection. Also known as tertiary syphilis.

A52.71 Late syphilitic oculopathy

Late syphilitic chorioretinitis

Late syphilitic episcleritis

A52.72 Syphilis of lung and bronchus

A52.73 Symptomatic late syphilis of other respiratory organs

A52.74 Syphilis of liver and other viscera

Late syphilitic peritonitis

A52.75 Syphilis of kidney and ureter

Syphilitic glomerular disease

A52.76 Other genitourinary symptomatic late syphilis

Late syphilitic female pelvic inflammatory disease

A52.77 Syphilis of bone and joint

A52.78 Syphilis of other musculoskeletal tissue

Late syphilitic bursitis

Syphilis [stage unspecified] of bursa

Syphilis [stage unspecified] of muscle

Syphilis [stage unspecified] of synovium

Syphilis [stage unspecified] of tendon

A52.79 Other symptomatic late syphilis

Late syphilitic leukoderma

Syphilis of adrenal gland

Syphilis of pituitary gland

Syphilis of thyroid gland

Syphilitic splenomegaly

Excludes1: syphilitic leukoderma (secondary) (A51.39)

A52.8 Late syphilis, latent

Syphilis (acquired) without clinical manifestations, with positive serological reaction and negative spinal fluid test, two years or more after infection

A52.9 Late syphilis, unspecified

A53 Other and unspecified syphilis

A53.0 Latent syphilis, unspecified as early or late

Latent syphilis NOS

Positive serological reaction for syphilis

A53.9 Syphilis, unspecified

Infection due to Treponema pallidum NOS

Syphilis (acquired) NOS

Excludes1: syphilis NOS under two years of age (A50.2)

A54 Gonococcal infection

Definition: Gonococcal infection is a sexually transmitted disease caused by gonococcal bacteria that affects the mucous membrane chiefly of the genital and urinary tracts and is characterized by an acute purulent discharge and painful or difficult urination, though women often have no symptoms.

A54.0 Gonococcal infection of lower genitourinary tract without periurethral or accessory gland abscess

Excludes1: gonococcal infection with genitourinary gland abscess (A54.1)

gonococcal infection with periurethral abscess (A54.1)

A54.00 Gonococcal infection of lower genitourinary tract, unspecified

A54.01 Gonococcal cystitis and urethritis, unspecified

A54.02 Gonococcal vulvovaginitis, unspecified

A54.03 Gonococcal cervicitis, unspecified

A54.09 Other gonococcal infection of lower genitourinary tract

A54.1 Gonococcal infection of lower genitourinary tract with periurethral and accessory gland abscess

Gonococcal Bartholin's gland abscess

A54.2 Gonococcal pelviperitonitis and other gonococcal genitourinary infection

A54.21 Gonococcal infection of kidney and ureter

A54.22 Gonococcal prostatitis

A54.23 Gonococcal infection of other male genital organs

Gonococcal epididymitis

Gonococcal orchitis

A54.24 **Gonococcal female pelvic inflammatory disease**

Gonococcal pelviperitonitis

Excludes1: gonococcal peritonitis (A54.85)

A54.29 **Other gonococcal genitourinary infections**

A54.3 **Gonococcal infection of eye**

A54.30 **Gonococcal infection of eye, unspecified**

A54.31 **Gonococcal conjunctivitis**

Ophthalmia neonatorum due to gonococcus

A54.32 **Gonococcal iridocyclitis**

A54.33 **Gonococcal keratitis**

A54.39 **Other gonococcal eye infection**

Gonococcal endophthalmia

A54.4 **Gonococcal infection of musculoskeletal system**

A54.40 **Gonococcal infection of musculoskeletal system, unspecified**

A54.41 **Gonococcal spondylopathy**

A54.42 **Gonococcal arthritis**

Excludes2: gonococcal infection of spine (A54.41)

A54.43 **Gonococcal osteomyelitis**

Excludes2: gonococcal infection of spine (A54.41)

A54.49 **Gonococcal infection of other musculoskeletal tissue**

Gonococcal bursitis

Gonococcal myositis

Gonococcal synovitis

Gonococcal tenosynovitis

A54.5 **Gonococcal pharyngitis**

A54.6 **Gonococcal infection of anus and rectum**

A54.8 **Other gonococcal infections**

A54.81 **Gonococcal meningitis**

A54.82 **Gonococcal brain abscess**

A54.83 **Gonococcal heart infection**

Gonococcal endocarditis

Gonococcal myocarditis

Gonococcal pericarditis

A54.84 **Gonococcal pneumonia**

A54.85 **Gonococcal peritonitis**

Excludes1: gonococcal pelviperitonitis (A54.24)

A54.86 **Gonococcal sepsis**

A54.89 **Other gonococcal infections**

Gonococcal keratoderma

Gonococcal lymphadenitis

A54.9 **Gonococcal infection, unspecified**

A55 **Chlamydial lymphogranuloma (venereum)**

Climatic or tropical bubo

Durand-Nicolas-Favre disease

Esthiomene

Lymphogranuloma inguinale

A56 **Other sexually transmitted chlamydial diseases**

Includes: sexually transmitted diseases due to Chlamydia trachomatis

Excludes1: neonatal chlamydial conjunctivitis (P39.1)

neonatal chlamydial pneumonia (P23.1)

Excludes2: chlamydial lymphogranuloma (A55)

conditions classified to A74.-

A56.0 **Chlamydial infection of lower genitourinary tract**

A56.00 **Chlamydial infection of lower genitourinary tract, unspecified**

A56.01 **Chlamydial cystitis and urethritis**

A56.02 **Chlamydial vulvovaginitis**

A56.09 **Other chlamydial infection of lower genitourinary tract**

Chlamydial cervicitis

A56.1 **Chlamydial infection of pelviperitoneum and other genitourinary organs**

A56.11 **Chlamydial female pelvic inflammatory disease**

A56.19 **Other chlamydial genitourinary infection**

Chlamydial epididymitis

Chlamydial orchitis

A56.2 **Chlamydial infection of genitourinary tract, unspecified**

A56.3 **Chlamydial infection of anus and rectum**

A56.4 **Chlamydial infection of pharynx**

A56.8 **Sexually transmitted chlamydial infection of other sites**

A57 **Chancroid**

Ulcus molle

A58 **Granuloma inguinale**

Donovanosis

A59 **Trichomoniasis**

Definition: Trichomoniasis is a common sexually transmitted disease caused by the parasite trichomonas vaginalis and infecting the urinary tract or vagina.

Excludes2: intestinal trichomoniasis (A07.8)

A59.0 **Urogenital trichomoniasis**

A59.00 **Urogenital trichomoniasis, unspecified**

Fluor (vaginalis) due to Trichomonas

Leukorrhea (vaginalis) due to Trichomonas

A59.01 **Trichomonal vulvovaginitis**

A59.02 **Trichomonal prostatitis**

A59.03 **Trichomonal cystitis and urethritis**

A59.09 **Other urogenital trichomoniasis**

Trichomonas cervicitis

A59.8 **Trichomoniasis of other sites**

A59.9 **Trichomoniasis, unspecified**

A60 **Anogenital herpesviral [herpes simplex] infections**

A60.0 **Herpesviral infection of genitalia and urogenital tract**

A60.00 **Herpesviral infection of urogenital system, unspecified**

A60.01 **Herpesviral infection of penis**

A60.02 **Herpesviral infection of other male genital organs**

A60.03 **Herpesviral cervicitis**

A60.04 **Herpesviral vulvovaginitis**

Herpesviral [herpes simplex] ulceration

Herpesviral [herpes simplex] vaginitis

Herpesviral [herpes simplex] vulvitis

A60.09 **Herpesviral infection of other urogenital tract**

A60.1 **Herpesviral infection of perianal skin and rectum**

A60.9 **Anogenital herpesviral infection, unspecified**

A63 **Other predominantly sexually transmitted diseases, not elsewhere classified**

Excludes2: molluscum contagiosum (B08.1)

papilloma of cervix (D26.0)

A63.0 Anogenital (venereal) warts

Anogenital warts due to (human) papillomavirus [HPV]

Condyloma acuminatum

A63.8 Other specified predominantly sexually transmitted diseases

A64 Unspecified sexually transmitted disease

OTHER SPIROCHETAL DISEASES (A65-A69)

Excludes2: leptospirosis (A27.-)

syphilis (A50-A53)

A65 Nonvenereal syphilis

Bejel

Endemic syphilis

Njovera

A66 Yaws

Definition: Yaws is a contagious tropical disease caused by the spirochete treponema pertenue, characterized by yellowish or reddish tumors, which often resemble currants, strawberries, or raspberries.

Includes: bouba

frambesia (tropica) pian

A66.0 Initial lesions of yaws

Chancre of yaws

Frambesia, initial or primary

Initial frambesial ulcer

Mother yaw

A66.1 Multiple papillomata and wet crab yaws

Frambesioma

Pianoma

Plantar or palmar papilloma of yaws

A66.2 Other early skin lesions of yaws

Cutaneous yaws, less than five years after infection

Early yaws (cutaneous)(macular)(maculopapular)(micropapular)(papular)

Frambeside of early yaws

A66.3 Hyperkeratosis of yaws

Ghoul hand

Hyperkeratosis, palmar or plantar (early) (late) due to yaws

Worm-eaten soles

A66.4 Gummata and ulcers of yaws

Gummatous frambeside

Nodular late yaws (ulcerated)

A66.5 Gangosa

Rhinopharyngitis mutilans

A66.6 Bone and joint lesions of yaws

Yaws ganglion

Yaws goundou

Yaws gumma, bone

Yaws gummatous osteitis or periostitis

Yaws hydrarthrosis

Yaws osteitis

Yaws periostitis (hypertrophic)

A66.7 Other manifestations of yaws

Juxta-articular nodules of yaws

Mucosal yaws

A66.8 Latent yaws

Yaws without clinical manifestations, with positive serology

A66.9 Yaws, unspecified

A67 Pinta [carate]

A67.0 Primary lesions of pinta

Chancre (primary) of pinta

Papule (primary) of pinta

A67.1 Intermediate lesions of pinta

Erythematous plaques of pinta

Hyperchromic lesions of pinta

Hyperkeratosis of pinta

Pintids

A67.2 Late lesions of pinta

Achromic skin lesions of pinta

Cicatricial skin lesions of pinta

Dyschromic skin lesions of pinta

A67.3 Mixed lesions of pinta

Achromic with hyperchromic skin lesions of pinta [carate]

A67.9 Pinta, unspecified

A68 Relapsing fevers

Definition: Relapsing fever is an infection caused by certain bacteria in the genus Borrelia. It is a vector-borne disease that is transmitted through louse or soft-bodied tick bites.

Includes: recurrent fever

Excludes2: Lyme disease (A69.2-)

A68.0 Louse-borne relapsing fever

Relapsing fever due to Borrelia recurrentis

A68.1 Tick-borne relapsing fever

Relapsing fever due to any Borrelia species other than Borrelia recurrentis

A68.9 Relapsing fever, unspecified

A69 Other spirochetal infections

A69.0 Necrotizing ulcerative stomatitis

Cancrum oris

Fusospirochetal gangrene Noma

Stomatitis gangrenosa

A69.1 Other Vincent's infections

Fusospirochetal pharyngitis

Necrotizing ulcerative (acute) gingivitis

Necrotizing ulcerative (acute) gingivostomatitis

Spirochetal stomatitis

Trench mouth

Vincent's angina

Vincent's gingivitis

A69.2 Lyme disease

Erythema chronicum migrans due to Borrelia burgdorferi

A69.20 Lyme disease, unspecified

A69.21 Meningitis due to Lyme disease

A69.22 Other neurologic disorders in Lyme disease

Cranial neuritis

Meningoencephalitis

Polyneuropathy

A69.23 Arthritis due to Lyme disease

A69.29 Other conditions associated with Lyme disease

Myopericarditis due to Lyme disease

A69.8 Other specified spirochetal infections

A69.9 Spirochetal infection, unspecified

OTHER DISEASES CAUSED BY CHLAMYDIAE (A70-A74)

Excludes1: sexually transmitted chlamydial diseases (A55-A56)

A70 **Chlamydia psittaci infections**
Ornithosis
Parrot fever
Psittacosis

A71 **Trachoma**
Excludes1: sequelae of trachoma (B94.0)
- **A71.0** **Initial stage of trachoma**
  Trachoma dubium
- **A71.1** **Active stage of trachoma**
  Granular conjunctivitis (trachomatous)
  Trachomatous follicular conjunctivitis
  Trachomatous pannus
- **A71.9** **Trachoma, unspecified**

A74 **Other diseases caused by chlamydiae**
Excludes1: neonatal chlamydial conjunctivitis (P39.1)
neonatal chlamydial pneumonia (P23.1)
Reiter's disease (M02.3-)
sexually transmitted chlamydial diseases (A55-A56)
Excludes2: chlamydial pneumonia (J16.0)
- **A74.0** **Chlamydial conjunctivitis**
  Paratrachoma
- **A74.8** **Other chlamydial diseases**
  - **A74.81** **Chlamydial peritonitis**
  - **A74.89** **Other chlamydial diseases**
- **A74.9** **Chlamydial infection, unspecified**
  Chlamydiosis NOS

RICKETTSIOSES (A75-A79)

Definition: Rickettsioses is a disease caused by intracellular bacteria. Examples of rickettsioses include typhus, Rocky Mountain spotted fever, and Rickettsialpox.

A75 **Typhus fever**
Excludes1: rickettsiosis due to Ehrlichia sennetsu (A79.81)
- **A75.0** **Epidemic louse-borne typhus fever due to Rickettsia prowazekii**
  Classical typhus (fever)
  Epidemic (louse-borne) typhus
- **A75.1** **Recrudescent typhus [Brill's disease]**
  Brill-Zinsser disease
- **A75.2** **Typhus fever due to Rickettsia typhi**
  Murine (flea-borne) typhus
- **A75.3** **Typhus fever due to Rickettsia tsutsugamushi**
  Scrub (mite-borne) typhus
  Tsutsugamushi fever
- **A75.9** **Typhus fever, unspecified**
  Typhus (fever) NOS

A77 **Spotted fever [tick-borne rickettsioses]**
- **A77.0** **Spotted fever due to Rickettsia rickettsii**
  Rocky Mountain spotted fever
  Sao Paulo fever
- **A77.1** **Spotted fever due to Rickettsia conorii**
  African tick typhus
  Boutonneuse fever
  India tick typhus
  Kenya tick typhus

Marseilles fever
Mediterranean tick fever
- **A77.2** **Spotted fever due to Rickettsia siberica**
  North Asian tick fever
  Siberian tick typhus
- **A77.3** **Spotted fever due to Rickettsia australis**
  Queensland tick typhus
- **A77.4** **Ehrlichiosis**
  Excludes1: Rickettsiosis due to Ehrlichia sennetsu (A79.81)
  - **A77.40** **Ehrlichiosis, unspecified**
  - **A77.41** **Ehrlichiosis chafeensis [E. chafeensis]**
  - **A77.49** **Other ehrlichiosis**
- **A77.8** **Other spotted fevers**
- **A77.9** **Spotted fever, unspecified**
  Tick-borne typhus NOS

A78 **Q fever**
Infection due to Coxiella burnetii
Nine Mile fever
Quadrilateral fever

A79 **Other rickettsioses**
- **A79.0** **Trench fever**
  Quintan fever
  Wolhynian fever
- **A79.1** **Rickettsialpox due to Rickettsia akari**
  Kew Garden fever
  Vesicular rickettsiosis
- **A79.8** **Other specified rickettsioses**
  - **A79.81** **Rickettsiosis due to Ehrlichia sennetsu**
  - **A79.89** **Other specified rickettsioses**
- **A79.9** **Rickettsiosis, unspecified**
  Rickettsial infection NOS

VIRAL AND PRION INFECTIONS OF THE CENTRAL NERVOUS SYSTEM (A80-A89)

Excludes1: postpolio syndrome (G14)
sequelae of poliomyelitis (B91)
sequelae of viral encephalitis (B94.1)

A80 **Acute poliomyelitis**
- **A80.0** **Acute paralytic poliomyelitis, vaccine-associated**
- **A80.1** **Acute paralytic poliomyelitis, wild virus, imported**
- **A80.2** **Acute paralytic poliomyelitis, wild virus, indigenous**
- **A80.3** **Acute paralytic poliomyelitis, other and unspecified**
  - **A80.30** **Acute paralytic poliomyelitis, unspecified**
  - **A80.39** **Other acute paralytic poliomyelitis**
- **A80.4** **Acute nonparalytic poliomyelitis**
- **A80.9** **Acute poliomyelitis, unspecified**

A81 **Atypical virus infections of central nervous system**
Includes: diseases of the central nervous system caused by prions
Use additional code to identify:
dementia with behavioral disturbance (F02.81)
dementia without behavioral disturbance (F02.80)
- **A81.0** **Creutzfeldt-Jakob disease**
  - **A81.00** **Creutzfeldt-Jakob disease, unspecified**
    Jakob-Creutzfeldt disease, unspecified
  - **A81.01** **Variant Creutzfeldt-Jakob disease**
    vCJD
  - **A81.09** **Other Creutzfeldt-Jakob disease**

● New code ▲ Revised code Excludes1: Not coded here Excludes2: Not included here ⊗ Placeholder required ⑦7th digit required

CJD

Familial Creutzfeldt-Jakob disease

Iatrogenic Creutzfeldt-Jakob disease

Sporadic Creutzfeldt-Jakob disease

Subacute spongiform encephalopathy (with dementia)

A81.1   Subacute sclerosing panencephalitis

Dawson's inclusion body encephalitis

Van Bogaert's sclerosing leukoencephalopathy

A81.2   Progressive multifocal leukoencephalopathy

Multifocal leukoencephalopathy NOS

A81.8   Other atypical virus infections of central nervous system

A81.81   Kuru

A81.82   Gerstmann-Sträussler-Scheinker syndrome

GSS syndrome

A81.83   Fatal familial insomnia

FFI

A81.89   Other atypical virus infections of central nervous system

A81.9   Atypical virus infection of central nervous system, unspecified

Prion diseases of the central nervous system NOS

A82   Rabies

Definition: Rabies is a viral disease that causes acute encephalitis in warm-blooded animals and people, characterized by abnormal behavior such as excitement, aggressiveness, and dementia, followed by paralysis and death.

A82.0   Sylvatic rabies

A82.1   Urban rabies

A82.9   Rabies, unspecified

A83   Mosquito-borne viral encephalitis

Includes: mosquito-borne viral meningoencephalitis

Excludes2: Venezuelan equine encephalitis (A92.2)

West Nile fever (A92.3-) West Nile virus (A92.3-)

A83.0   Japanese encephalitis

A83.1   Western equine encephalitis

A83.2   Eastern equine encephalitis

A83.3   St Louis encephalitis

A83.4   Australian encephalitis

Kunjin virus disease

A83.5   California encephalitis

California meningoencephalitis

La Crosse encephalitis

A83.6   Rocio virus disease

A83.8   Other mosquito-borne viral encephalitis

A83.9   Mosquito-borne viral encephalitis, unspecified

A84   Tick-borne viral encephalitis

Includes: tick-borne viral meningoencephalitis

A84.0   Far Eastern tick-borne encephalitis [Russian spring-summer encephalitis]

A84.1   Central European tick-borne encephalitis

A84.8   Other tick-borne viral encephalitis

Louping ill

Powassan virus disease

A84.9   Tick-borne viral encephalitis, unspecified

A85   Other viral encephalitis, not elsewhere classified

Includes: specified viral encephalomyelitis NEC

specified viral meningoencephalitis NEC

Excludes1: benign myalgic encephalomyelitis (G93.3)

encephalitis due to cytomegalovirus (B25.8)

encephalitis due to herpesvirus NEC (B10.0-)

encephalitis due to herpesvirus [herpes simplex] (B00.4)

encephalitis due to measles virus (B05.0)

encephalitis due to mumps virus (B26.2)

encephalitis due to poliomyelitis virus (A80.-)

encephalitis due to zoster (B02.0)

lymphocytic choriomeningitis (A87.2)

A85.0   Enteroviral encephalitis

Enteroviral encephalomyelitis

A85.1   Adenoviral encephalitis

Adenoviral meningoencephalitis

A85.2   Arthropod-borne viral encephalitis, unspecified

Excludes1: West Nile virus with encephalitis (A92.31)

A85.8   Other specified viral encephalitis

Encephalitis lethargica

Von Economo-Cruchet disease

A86   Unspecified viral encephalitis

Viral encephalomyelitis NOS

Viral meningoencephalitis NOS

A87   Viral meningitis

Definition: Meningitis due to enterovirus refers to any of a subgroup of picornaviruses, including polioviruses, coxsackie viruses, and echoviruses, that infect the gastrointestinal tract and often spread to other areas of the body, especially the nervous system

Excludes1: meningitis due to herpesvirus [herpes simplex] (B00.3)

meningitis due to herpesvirus [herpes simplex] (B00.3)

meningitis due to measles virus (B05.1)

meningitis due to mumps virus (B26.1)

meningitis due to poliomyelitis virus (A80.-)

meningitis due to zoster (B02.1)

A87.0   Enteroviral meningitis

Coxsackievirus meningitis

Echovirus meningitis

A87.1   Adenoviral meningitis

A87.2   Lymphocytic choriomeningitis

Lymphocytic meningoencephalitis

A87.8   Other viral meningitis

A87.9   Viral meningitis, unspecified

A88   Other viral infections of central nervous system, not elsewhere classified

Excludes1: viral encephalitis NOS (A86)

viral meningitis NOS (A87.9)

A88.0   Enteroviral exanthematous fever [Boston exanthem]

A88.1   Epidemic vertigo

A88.8   Other specified viral infections of central nervous system

A89   Unspecified viral infection of central nervous system

ARTHROPOD-BORNE VIRAL FEVERS AND VIRAL HEMORRHAGIC FEVERS (A90-A99)

Definition: Hemorrhagic fever is a group of viral infections characterized by fever, chills, headache, malaise, and respiratory or gastrointestinal symptoms, followed by capillary hemorrhages and, in severe infection, by oliguria, kidney failure, hypotension, and possibly death.

A90 **Dengue fever [classical dengue]**
> **Excludes1:** dengue hemorrhagic fever (A91)

A91 **Dengue hemorrhagic fever**

A92 **Other mosquito-borne viral fevers**
> **Excludes1:** Ross River disease (B33.1)

A92.0 **Chikungunya virus disease**
Chikungunya (hemorrhagic) fever

A92.1 **O'nyong-nyong fever**

A92.2 **Venezuelan equine fever**
Venezuelan equine encephalitis
Venezuelan equine encephalomyelitis virus disease

A92.3 **West Nile virus infection**
West Nile fever

> **A92.30** **West Nile virus infection, unspecified**
> West Nile fever NOS
> West Nile fever without complications
> West Nile virus NOS

> **A92.31** **West Nile virus infection with encephalitis**
> West Nile encephalitis
> West Nile encephalomyelitis

> **A92.32** **West Nile virus infection with other neurologic manifestation**
> **Use additional code** to specify the neurologic manifestation

> **A92.39** **West Nile virus infection with other complications**
> **Use additional code** to specify the other conditions

A92.4 **Rift Valley fever**

A92.5 **Zika virus disease**
Zika virus fever
Zika virus infection
Zika NOS

A92.8 **Other specified mosquito-borne viral fevers**

A92.9 **Mosquito-borne viral fever, unspecified**

A93 **Other arthropod-borne viral fevers, not elsewhere classified**

A93.0 **Oropouche virus disease**
Oropouche fever

A93.1 **Sandfly fever**
Pappataci fever
Phlebotomus fever

A93.2 **Colorado tick fever**

A93.8 **Other specified arthropod-borne viral fevers**
Piry virus disease
Vesicular stomatitis virus disease [Indiana fever]

A94 **Unspecified arthropod-borne viral fever**
Arboviral fever NOS
Arbovirus infection NOS

A95 **Yellow fever**
> **Definition:** Yellow fever is an acute systemic (body wide) illness caused by a virus called a flavivirus. In severe cases, the viral

infection causes a high fever, bleeding into the skin, and necrosis (death) of cells in the kidney and liver.

A95.0 **Sylvatic yellow fever**
Jungle yellow fever

A95.1 **Urban yellow fever**

A95.9 **Yellow fever, unspecified**

A96 **Arenaviral hemorrhagic fever**

A96.0 **Junin hemorrhagic fever**
Argentinian hemorrhagic fever

A96.1 **Machupo hemorrhagic fever**
Bolivian hemorrhagic fever

A96.2 **Lassa fever**

A96.8 **Other arenaviral hemorrhagic fevers**

A96.9 **Arenaviral hemorrhagic fever, unspecified**

A98 **Other viral hemorrhagic fevers, not elsewhere classified**
> **Excludes1:** chikungunya hemorrhagic fever (A92.0)
> dengue hemorrhagic fever (A91)

A98.0 **Crimean-Congo hemorrhagic fever**
Central Asian hemorrhagic fever

A98.1 **Omsk hemorrhagic fever**

A98.2 **Kyasanur Forest disease**

A98.3 **Marburg virus disease**

A98.4 **Ebola virus disease**

A98.5 **Hemorrhagic fever with renal syndrome**
Epidemic hemorrhagic fever
Korean hemorrhagic fever
Russian hemorrhagic fever
Hantaan virus disease
Hantavirus disease with renal manifestations
Nephropathia epidemica
Songo fever
> **Excludes1:** hantavirus (cardio)-pulmonary syndrome (B33.4)

A98.8 **Other specified viral hemorrhagic fevers**

A99 **Unspecified viral hemorrhagic fever**

VIRAL INFECTIONS CHARACTERIZED BY SKIN AND MUCOUS MEMBRANE LESIONS (B00-B09)

B00 **Herpesviral [herpes simplex] infections**
> **Definition:** Herpes simplex is an infection caused by the herpes simplex virus; affects the skin and nervous system; produces small temporary blisters on the skin and mucous membranes.
> **Excludes1:** congenital herpesviral infections (P35.2)
> **Excludes2:** anogenital herpesviral infection (A60.-)
> gammaherpesviral mononucleosis (B27.0-)
> herpangina (B08.5)

B00.0 **Eczema herpeticum**
Kaposi's varicelliform eruption

B00.1 **Herpesviral vesicular dermatitis**
Herpes simplex facialis
Herpes simplex labialis
Herpes simplex otitis externa
Vesicular dermatitis of ear
Vesicular dermatitis of lip

B00.2 **Herpesviral gingivostomatitis and pharyngotonsillitis**
Herpesviral pharyngitis

B00.3 **Herpesviral meningitis**

B00.4**Herpesviral encephalitis**

Herpesviral meningoencephalitis

Simian B disease

Excludes1: herpesviral encephalitis due to herpesvirus 6
and 7 (B10.01, B10.09)

non-simplex herpesviral encephalitis (B10.0-)

B00.5**Herpesviral ocular disease**

B00.50**Herpesviral ocular disease, unspecified**

B00.51**Herpesviral iridocyclitis**

Herpesviral iritis

Herpesviral uveitis, anterior

B00.52**Herpesviral keratitis**

Herpesviral keratoconjunctivitis

B00.53**Herpesviral conjunctivitis**

B00.59**Other herpesviral disease of eye**

Herpesviral dermatitis of eyelid

B00.7**Disseminated herpesviral disease**

Herpesviral sepsis

B00.8**Other forms of herpesviral infections**

B00.81**Herpesviral hepatitis**

B00.82**Herpes simplex myelitis**

B00.89**Other herpesviral infection**

Herpesviral whitlow

B00.9**Herpesviral infection, unspecified**

Herpes simplex infection NOS

B01**Varicella [chickenpox]**

Definition: Chickenpox is an acute contagious disease caused by
herpes varicella zoster virus; causes a rash of vesicles on the face
and body.

B01.0**Varicella meningitis**

B01.1**Varicella encephalitis, myelitis and encephalomyelitis**

Post chickenpox encephalitis, myelitis and
encephalomyelitis

B01.11**Varicella encephalitis and encephalomyelitis**

Post chickenpox encephalitis and
encephalomyelitis

B01.12**Varicella myelitis**

Post chickenpox myelitis

B01.2**Varicella pneumonia**

B01.8**Varicella with other complications**

B01.81**Varicella keratitis**

B01.89**Other varicella complications**

B01.9**Varicella without complication**

Varicella NOS

B02**Zoster [herpes zoster]**

Definition: Herpes zoster is a viral disease characterized by a
painful skin rash with blisters in a limited area on one side of the
body, often in a stripe.

Includes: shingles

zona

B02.0**Zoster encephalitis**

Zoster meningoencephalitis

B02.1**Zoster meningitis**

B02.2**Zoster with other nervous system involvement**

B02.21**Postherpetic geniculate ganglionitis**

B02.22**Postherpetic trigeminal neuralgia**

B02.23**Postherpetic polyneuropathy**

B02.24**Postherpetic myelitis**

Herpes zoster myelitis

B02.29**Other postherpetic nervous system involvement**

Postherpetic radiculopathy

B02.3**Zoster ocular disease**

B02.30**Zoster ocular disease, unspecified**

B02.31**Zoster conjunctivitis**

B02.32**Zoster iridocyclitis**

B02.33**Zoster keratitis**

Herpes zoster keratoconjunctivitis

B02.34**Zoster scleritis**

B02.39**Other herpes zoster eye disease**

Zoster blepharitis

B02.7**Disseminated zoster**

B02.8**Zoster with other complications**

Herpes zoster otitis externa

B02.9**Zoster without complications**

Zoster NOS

B03**Smallpox**

Note: In 1980 the 33rd World Health Assembly declared that
smallpox had been eradicated.

The classification is maintained for surveillance purposes.

B04**Monkeypox**

B05**Measles**

Definition: Measles is a viral infection which causes an illness
displaying a characteristic skin rash. Measles is also sometimes
called rubeola, 5-day measles, or hard measles.

Includes: morbilli

Excludes1: subacute sclerosing panencephalitis (A81.1)

B05.0**Measles complicated by encephalitis**

Postmeasles encephalitis

B05.1**Measles complicated by meningitis**

Postmeasles meningitis

B05.2**Measles complicated by pneumonia**

Postmeasles pneumonia

B05.3**Measles complicated by otitis media**

Postmeasles otitis media

B05.4**Measles with intestinal complications**

B05.8**Measles with other complications**

B05.81**Measles keratitis and keratoconjunctivitis**

B05.89**Other measles complications**

B05.9**Measles without complication**

Measles NOS

B06**Rubella [German measles]**

Definition: Rubella is a highly contagious viral disease, aka
german measles. The symptoms include swollen glands, joint pain,
low fever, and a fine red rash.

Excludes1: congenital rubella (P35.0)

B06.0**Rubella with neurological complications**

B06.00**Rubella with neurological complication, unspecified**

B06.01**Rubella encephalitis**

Rubella meningoencephalitis

B06.02**Rubella meningitis**

B06.09**Other neurological complications of rubella**

B06.8**Rubella with other complications**

B06.81**Rubella pneumonia**

Add 4th-7th digits   Nonspecific code   Unspecified code   Manifestation code

B06.82   **Rubella arthritis**

B06.89   **Other rubella complications**

B06.9   **Rubella without complication**

Rubella NOS

B07   **Viral warts**

Includes: verruca simplex

verruca vulgaris

viral warts due to human papillomavirus

Excludes2: anogenital (venereal) warts (A63.0)

papilloma of bladder (D41.4)

papilloma of cervix (D26.0)

papilloma larynx (D14.1)

B07.0   **Plantar wart**

Verruca plantaris

B07.8   **Other viral warts**

Common wart

Flat wart

Verruca plana

B07.9   **Viral wart, unspecified**

B08   **Other viral infections characterized by skin and mucous membrane lesions, not elsewhere classified**

Excludes1: vesicular stomatitis virus disease (A93.8)

B08.0   **Other orthopoxvirus infections**

Excludes2: monkeypox (B04)

B08.01   **Cowpox and vaccinia not from vaccine**

B08.010   **Cowpox**

B08.011   **Vaccinia not from vaccine**

Excludes1: vaccinia (from vaccination) (generalized) (T88.1)

B08.02   **ORF virus disease**

Contagious pustular dermatitis

Ecthyma contagiosum

B08.03   **Pseudocowpox [milker's node]**

B08.04   **Paravaccinia, unspecified**

B08.09   **Other orthopoxvirus infections**

Orthopoxvirus infection NOS

B08.1   **Molluscum contagiosum**

B08.2   **Exanthema subitum [sixth disease]**

Roseola infantum

B08.20   **Exanthema subitum [sixth disease], unspecified**

Roseola infantum, unspecified

B08.21   **Exanthema subitum [sixth disease] due to human herpesvirus 6**

Roseola infantum due to human herpesvirus 6

B08.22   **Exanthema subitum [sixth disease] due to human herpesvirus 7**

Roseola infantum due to human herpesvirus 7

B08.3   **Erythema infectiosum [fifth disease]**

B08.4   **Enteroviral vesicular stomatitis with exanthem**

Hand, foot and mouth disease

B08.5   **Enteroviral vesicular pharyngitis**

Herpangina

B08.6   **Parapoxvirus infections**

B08.60   **Parapoxvirus infection, unspecified**

B08.61   **Bovine stomatitis**

B08.62   **Sealpox**

B08.69   **Other parapoxvirus infections**

B08.7   **Yatapoxvirus infections**

B08.70   **Yatapoxvirus infection, unspecified**

B08.71   **Tanapox virus disease**

B08.72   **Yaba pox virus disease**

Yaba monkey tumor disease

B08.79   **Other yatapoxvirus infections**

B08.8   **Other specified viral infections characterized by skin and mucous membrane lesions**

Enteroviral lymphonodular pharyngitis

Foot-and-mouth disease

Poxvirus NEC

B09   **Unspecified viral infection characterized by skin and mucous membrane lesions**

Viral enanthema NOS

Viral exanthema NOS

OTHER HUMAN HERPESVIRUSES (B10)

Definition: Human herpes viruses, refers to a family of viruses including herpes simplex, varicella zoster, and Epstein-Barr.

B10   **Other human herpesviruses**

Excludes2: cytomegalovirus (B25.9)

Epstein-Barr virus (B27.0-)

herpes NOS (B00.9)

herpes simplex (B00.-)

herpes zoster (B02.-)

human herpesvirus NOS (B00.-)

human herpesvirus 1 and 2 (B00.-)

human herpesvirus 3 (B01.-, B02.-)

human herpesvirus 4 (B27.0-)

human herpesvirus 5 (B25.-)

varicella (B01.-)

zoster (B02.-)

B10.0   **Other human herpesvirus encephalitis**

Excludes2: herpes encephalitis NOS (B00.4)

herpes simplex encephalitis (B00.4)

human herpesvirus encephalitis (B00.4)

simian B herpes virus encephalitis (B00.4)

B10.01   **Human herpesvirus 6 encephalitis**

B10.09   **Other human herpesvirus encephalitis**

Human herpesvirus 7 encephalitis

B10.8   **Other human herpesvirus infection**

B10.81   **Human herpesvirus 6 infection**

B10.82   **Human herpesvirus 7 infection**

B10.89   **Other human herpesvirus infection**

Human herpesvirus 8 infection

Kaposi's sarcoma-associated herpesvirus infection

VIRAL HEPATITIS (B15-B19)

Definition: Viral hepatitis is a liver inflammation due to a viral infection. It may present in acute or chronic forms. The most common causes of viral hepatitis are the five unrelated hepatotropic viruses hepatitis A, hepatitis B, hepatitis C, hepatitis D, and hepatitis E.

Excludes1: sequelae of viral hepatitis (B94.2)

Excludes2: cytomegaloviral hepatitis (B25.1)

herpesviral [herpes simplex] hepatitis (B00.81)

B15   **Acute hepatitis A**

B15.0   **Hepatitis A with hepatic coma**

B15.9 **Hepatitis A without hepatic coma**

Hepatitis A (acute)(viral) NOS

B16 **Acute hepatitis B**

B16.0 **Acute hepatitis B with delta-agent with hepatic coma**

B16.1 **Acute hepatitis B with delta-agent without hepatic coma**

B16.2 **Acute hepatitis B without delta-agent with hepatic coma**

B16.9 **Acute hepatitis B without delta-agent and without hepatic coma**

Hepatitis B (acute) (viral) NOS

B17 **Other acute viral hepatitis**

B17.0 **Acute delta-(super) infection of hepatitis B carrier**

B17.1 **Acute hepatitis C**

B17.10 **Acute hepatitis C without hepatic coma**

Acute hepatitis C NOS

B17.11 **Acute hepatitis C with hepatic coma**

B17.2 **Acute hepatitis E**

B17.8 **Other specified acute viral hepatitis**

Hepatitis non-A non-B (acute) (viral) NEC

B17.9 **Acute viral hepatitis, unspecified**

Acute hepatitis NOS

Acute infectious hepatitis NOS

B18 **Chronic viral hepatitis**

Includes: Carrier of viral hepatitis

B18.0 **Chronic viral hepatitis B with delta-agent**

B18.1 **Chronic viral hepatitis B without delta-agent**

Carrier of viral hepatitis B

Chronic (viral) hepatitis B

B18.2 **Chronic viral hepatitis C**

Carrier of viral hepatitis C

B18.8 **Other chronic viral hepatitis**

Carrier of other viral hepatitis

B18.9 **Chronic viral hepatitis, unspecified**

Carrier of unspecified viral hepatitis

B19 **Unspecified viral hepatitis**

B19.0 **Unspecified viral hepatitis with hepatic coma**

B19.1 **Unspecified viral hepatitis B**

B19.10 **Unspecified viral hepatitis B without hepatic coma**

Unspecified viral hepatitis B NOS

B19.11 **Unspecified viral hepatitis B with hepatic coma**

B19.2 **Unspecified viral hepatitis C**

B19.20 **Unspecified viral hepatitis C without hepatic coma**

Viral hepatitis C NOS

B19.21 **Unspecified viral hepatitis C with hepatic coma**

B19.9 **Unspecified viral hepatitis without hepatic coma**

Viral hepatitis NOS

HUMAN IMMUNODEFICIENCY VIRUS [HIV] DISEASE (B20)

Definition: Human immunodeficiency virus (HIV) disease is a virus that can lead to acquired immunodeficiency syndrome (AIDS), a condition in humans in which the immune system begins to fail, leading to life-threatening opportunistic infections.

B20 **Human immunodeficiency virus [HIV] disease**

Includes: acquired immune deficiency syndrome [AIDS]

AIDS-related complex [ARC]

HIV infection, symptomatic

Code first Human immunodeficiency virus [HIV] disease complicating pregnancy, childbirth and the puerperium, if applicable (O98.7-)

Use additional code(s) to identify all manifestations of HIV infection

Excludes1: asymptomatic human immunodeficiency virus [HIV] infection status (Z21)

exposure to HIV virus (Z20.6)

inconclusive serologic evidence of HIV (R75)

OTHER VIRAL DISEASES (B25-B34)

B25 **Cytomegaloviral disease**

Excludes1: congenital cytomegalovirus infection (P35.1)

cytomegaloviral mononucleosis (B27.1-)

B25.0 **Cytomegaloviral pneumonitis**

B25.1 **Cytomegaloviral hepatitis**

B25.2 **Cytomegaloviral pancreatitis**

B25.8 **Other cytomegaloviral diseases**

Cytomegaloviral encephalitis

B25.9 **Cytomegaloviral disease, unspecified**

B26 **Mumps**

Includes: epidemic parotitis

infectious parotitis

B26.0 **Mumps orchitis**

B26.1 **Mumps meningitis**

B26.2 **Mumps encephalitis**

B26.3 **Mumps pancreatitis**

B26.8 **Mumps with other complications**

B26.81 **Mumps hepatitis**

B26.82 **Mumps myocarditis**

B26.83 **Mumps nephritis**

B26.84 **Mumps polyneuropathy**

B26.85 **Mumps arthritis**

B26.89 **Other mumps complications**

B26.9 **Mumps without complication**

Mumps NOS

Mumps parotitis NOS

B27 **Infectious mononucleosis**

Definition: Infectious mononucleosis, aka mono, glandular fever, kissing disease is an acute disease characterized by fever and swollen lymph nodes and an abnormal increase of mononuclear leucocytes or monocytes in the bloodstream.

Includes: glandular fever

monocytic angina

Pfeiffer's disease

B27.0 **Gammaherpesviral mononucleosis**

Mononucleosis due to Epstein-Barr virus

B27.00 **Gammaherpesviral mononucleosis without complication**

B27.01 **Gammaherpesviral mononucleosis with polyneuropathy**

B27.02 **Gammaherpesviral mononucleosis with meningitis**

B27.09 **Gammaherpesviral mononucleosis with other complications**

Hepatomegaly in gammaherpesviral mononucleosis

B27.1 **Cytomegaloviral mononucleosis**

B27.10 Cytomegaloviral mononucleosis without complications

B27.11 Cytomegaloviral mononucleosis with polyneuropathy

B27.12 Cytomegaloviral mononucleosis with meningitis

B27.19 Cytomegaloviral mononucleosis with other complication

Hepatomegaly in cytomegaloviral mononucleosis

B27.8 Other infectious mononucleosis

B27.80 Other infectious mononucleosis without complication

B27.81 Other infectious mononucleosis with polyneuropathy

B27.82 Other infectious mononucleosis with meningitis

B27.89 Other infectious mononucleosis with other complication

Hepatomegaly in other infectious mononucleosis

B27.9 Infectious mononucleosis, unspecified

B27.90 Infectious mononucleosis, unspecified without complication

B27.91 Infectious mononucleosis, unspecified with polyneuropathy

B27.92 Infectious mononucleosis, unspecified with meningitis

B27.99 Infectious mononucleosis, unspecified with other complication

Hepatomegaly in unspecified infectious mononucleosis

B30 Viral conjunctivitis

Excludes1: herpesviral [herpes simplex] ocular disease (B00.5)

ocular zoster (B02.3)

B30.0 Keratoconjunctivitis due to adenovirus

Epidemic keratoconjunctivitis

Shipyard eye

B30.1 Conjunctivitis due to adenovirus

Acute adenoviral follicular conjunctivitis

Swimming-pool conjunctivitis

B30.2 Viral pharyngoconjunctivitis

B30.3 Acute epidemic hemorrhagic conjunctivitis (enteroviral)

Conjunctivitis due to coxsackievirus 24

Conjunctivitis due to enterovirus 70

Hemorrhagic conjunctivitis (acute)(epidemic)

B30.8 Other viral conjunctivitis

Newcastle conjunctivitis

B30.9 Viral conjunctivitis, unspecified

B33 Other viral diseases, not elsewhere classified

B33.0 Epidemic myalgia

Bornholm disease

B33.1 Ross River disease

Epidemic polyarthritis and exanthema

Ross River fever

B33.2 Viral carditis

Coxsackie (virus) carditis

B33.20 Viral carditis, unspecified

B33.21 Viral endocarditis

B33.22 Viral myocarditis

B33.23 Viral pericarditis

B33.24 Viral cardiomyopathy

B33.3 Retrovirus infections, not elsewhere classified

Retrovirus infection NOS

B33.4 Hantavirus (cardio)-pulmonary syndrome [HPS] [HCPS]

Hantavirus disease with pulmonary manifestations

Sin nombre virus disease

Use additional code to identify any associated acute kidney failure (N17.9)

Excludes1: hantavirus disease with renal manifestations (A98.5)

hemorrhagic fever with renal manifestations (A98.5)

B33.8 Other specified viral diseases

Excludes1: anogenital human papillomavirus infection (A63.0)

viral warts due to human papillomavirus infection (B07)

B34 Viral infection of unspecified site

Excludes1: anogenital human papillomavirus infection (A63.0)

cytomegaloviral disease NOS (B25.9)

herpesvirus [herpes simplex] infection NOS (B00.9)

retrovirus infection NOS (B33.3)

viral agents as the cause of diseases classified elsewhere (B97.-)

viral warts due to human papillomavirus infection (B07)

B34.0 Adenovirus infection, unspecified

B34.1 Enterovirus infection, unspecified

Coxsackievirus infection NOS

Echovirus infection NOS

B34.2 Coronavirus infection, unspecified

Excludes1: pneumonia due to SARS-associated coronavirus (J12.81)

B34.3 Parvovirus infection, unspecified

B34.4 Papovavirus infection, unspecified

B34.8 Other viral infections of unspecified site

B34.9 Viral infection, unspecified

Viremia NOS

MYCOSES (B35-B49)

Excludes2: hypersensitivity pneumonitis due to organic dust (J67.-)

mycosis fungoides (C84.0-)

B35 Dermatophytosis

Definition: Dermatophytosis, aka tinea or ringworm, is a disease that can affect the scalp (tinea capitis), body (tinea corporis), nails (tinea unguium), feet (tinea pedis), groin (tinea cruris), and bearded skin (tinea hebrae).

Includes: favus infections due to species of Epidermophyton, Microsporum and Trichophyton tinea, any type except those in B36.-

B35.0 Tinea barbae and tinea capitis

Beard ringworm

Kerion

Scalp ringworm

Sycosis, mycotic

B35.1 Tinea unguium

Dermatophytic onychia

Dermatophytosis of nail

Onychomycosis

Ringworm of nails

B35.2 Tinea manuum

Dermatophytosis of hand ringworm

● New code ▲ Revised code **Excludes1:** Not coded here **Excludes2:** Not included here ⊗ Placeholder required ⑦ 7th digit required

B35.3 Tinea pedis
Athlete's foot
Dermatophytosis of foot ringworm

B35.4 Tinea corporis
Ringworm of the body

B35.5 Tinea imbricata
Tokelau

B35.6 Tinea cruris
Dhobi itch Groin ringworm Jock itch

B35.8 Other dermatophytoses
Disseminated dermatophytosis
Granulomatous dermatophytosis

B35.9 Dermatophytosis, unspecified
Ringworm NOS

B36 Other superficial mycoses

B36.0 Pityriasis versicolor
Tinea flava
Tinea versicolor

B36.1 Tinea nigra
Keratomycosis nigricans palmaris
Microsporosis nigra
Pityriasis nigra

B36.2 White piedra
Tinea blanca

B36.3 Black piedra

B36.8 Other specified superficial mycoses

B36.9 Superficial mycosis, unspecified

B37 Candidiasis

Definition: Candidiasis is an infection caused by a species of the yeast candida, usually candida albicans. Candidiasis is a common cause of vaginal infections in women.

Includes: candidosis
moniliasis

Excludes1: neonatal candidiasis (P37.5)

B37.0 Candidal stomatitis
Oral thrush

B37.1 Pulmonary candidiasis
Candidal bronchitis
Candidal pneumonia

B37.2 Candidiasis of skin and nail
Candidal onychia
Candidal paronychia

Excludes2: diaper dermatitis (L22)

B37.3 Candidiasis of vulva and vagina
Candidal vulvovaginitis
Monilial vulvovaginitis
Vaginal thrush

B37.4 Candidiasis of other urogenital sites
B37.41 Candidal cystitis and urethritis
B37.42 Candidal balanitis
B37.49 Other urogenital candidiasis
Candidal pyelonephritis

B37.5 Candidal meningitis

B37.6 Candidal endocarditis

B37.7 Candidal sepsis
Disseminated candidiasis

Systemic candidiasis

B37.8 Candidiasis of other sites
B37.81 Candidal esophagitis
B37.82 Candidal enteritis
Candidal proctitis
B37.83 Candidal cheilitis
B37.84 Candidal otitis externa
B37.89 Other sites of candidiasis
Candidal osteomyelitis

B37.9 Candidiasis, unspecified
Thrush NOS

B38 Coccidioidomycosis
B38.0 Acute pulmonary coccidioidomycosis
B38.1 Chronic pulmonary coccidioidomycosis
B38.2 Pulmonary coccidioidomycosis, unspecified
B38.3 Cutaneous coccidioidomycosis
B38.4 Coccidioidomycosis meningitis
B38.7 Disseminated coccidioidomycosis
Generalized coccidioidomycosis
B38.8 Other forms of coccidioidomycosis
B38.81 Prostatic coccidioidomycosis
B38.89 Other forms of coccidioidomycosis
B38.9 Coccidioidomycosis, unspecified

B39 Histoplasmosis

Definition: Histoplasmosis, aka Darling's disease, is a disease caused by the fungus histoplasma capsulatum. Symptoms vary greatly, but the disease primarily affects the lungs. Histoplasmosis is common among aids patients because of their lowered immune system.

Code first associated AIDS (B20)

Use additional code for any associated manifestations, such as:
endocarditis (I39)
meningitis (G02)
pericarditis (I32)
retinitis (H32)

B39.0 Acute pulmonary histoplasmosis capsulati
B39.1 Chronic pulmonary histoplasmosis capsulati
B39.2 Pulmonary histoplasmosis capsulati, unspecified
B39.3 Disseminated histoplasmosis capsulati
Generalized histoplasmosis capsulati
B39.4 Histoplasmosis capsulati, unspecified
American histoplasmosis
B39.5 Histoplasmosis duboisii
African histoplasmosis
B39.9 Histoplasmosis, unspecified

B40 Blastomycosis

Definition: Blastomycotic infection, aka North American blastomycosis, blastomycetic dermatitis, and Gilchrist's disease, is a fungal infection caused by the organism Blastomyces dermatitidis. Endemic to portions of north America, blastomycosis causes clinical symptoms similar to histoplasmosis.

Excludes1: Brazilian blastomycosis (B41.-)
keloidal blastomycosis (B48.0)

B40.0 Acute pulmonary blastomycosis
B40.1 Chronic pulmonary blastomycosis
B40.2 Pulmonary blastomycosis, unspecified

Add 4th-7th digits   Nonspecific code   Unspecified code   Manifestation code   159

B40.3	**Cutaneous blastomycosis**
B40.7	**Disseminated blastomycosis**
	Generalized blastomycosis
B40.8	**Other forms of blastomycosis**
B40.81	**Blastomycotic meningoencephalitis**
	Meningomyelitis due to blastomycosis
B40.89	**Other forms of blastomycosis**
B40.9	**Blastomycosis, unspecified**

B41 **Paracoccidioidomycosis**

Includes: Brazilian blastomycosis
Lutz' disease

B41.0	**Pulmonary paracoccidioidomycosis**
B41.7	**Disseminated paracoccidioidomycosis**
	Generalized paracoccidioidomycosis
B41.8	**Other forms of paracoccidioidomycosis**
B41.9	**Paracoccidioidomycosis, unspecified**

B42 **Sporotrichosis**

B42.0	**Pulmonary sporotrichosis**
B42.1	**Lymphocutaneous sporotrichosis**
B42.7	**Disseminated sporotrichosis**
	Generalized sporotrichosis
B42.8	**Other forms of sporotrichosis**
B42.81	**Cerebral sporotrichosis**
	Meningitis due to sporotrichosis
B42.82	**Sporotrichosis arthritis**
B42.89	**Other forms of sporotrichosis**
B42.9	**Sporotrichosis, unspecified**

B43 **Chromomycosis and pheomycotic abscess**

B43.0	**Cutaneous chromomycosis**
	Dermatitis verrucosa
B43.1	**Pheomycotic brain abscess**
	Cerebral chromomycosis
B43.2	**Subcutaneous pheomycotic abscess and cyst**
B43.8	**Other forms of chromomycosis**
B43.9	**Chromomycosis, unspecified**

B44 **Aspergillosis**

Includes: aspergilloma

B44.0	**Invasive pulmonary aspergillosis**
B44.1	**Other pulmonary aspergillosis**
B44.2	**Tonsillar aspergillosis**
B44.7	**Disseminated aspergillosis**
	Generalized aspergillosis
B44.8	**Other forms of aspergillosis**
B44.81	**Allergic bronchopulmonary aspergillosis**
B44.89	**Other forms of aspergillosis**
B44.9	**Aspergillosis, unspecified**

B45 **Cryptococcosis**

B45.0	**Pulmonary cryptococcosis**
B45.1	**Cerebral cryptococcosis**
	Cryptococcal meningitis
	Cryptococcosis meningocerebralis
B45.2	**Cutaneous cryptococcosis**
B45.3	**Osseous cryptococcosis**
B45.7	**Disseminated cryptococcosis**
	Generalized cryptococcosis
B45.8	**Other forms of cryptococcosis**

B45.9	**Cryptococcosis, unspecified**

B46 **Zygomycosis**

B46.0	**Pulmonary mucormycosis**
B46.1	**Rhinocerebral mucormycosis**
B46.2	**Gastrointestinal mucormycosis**
B46.3	**Cutaneous mucormycosis**
	Subcutaneous mucormycosis
B46.4	**Disseminated mucormycosis**
	Generalized mucormycosis
B46.5	**Mucormycosis, unspecified**
B46.8	**Other zygomycoses**
	Entomophthoromycosis
B46.9	**Zygomycosis, unspecified**
	Phycomycosis NOS

B47 **Mycetoma**

B47.0	**Eumycetoma**
	Madura foot, mycotic
	Maduromycosis
B47.1	**Actinomycetoma**
B47.9	**Mycetoma, unspecified**
	Madura foot NOS

B48 **Other mycoses, not elsewhere classified**

B48.0	**Lobomycosis**
	Keloidal blastomycosis Lobo's disease
B48.1	**Rhinosporidiosis**
B48.2	**Allescheriasis**
	Infection due to Pseudallescheria boydii
	Excludes1: eumycetoma (B47.0)
B48.3	**Geotrichosis**
	Geotrichum stomatitis
B48.4	**Penicillosis**
B48.8	**Other specified mycoses**
	Adiaspiromycosis
	Infection of tissue and organs by Alternaria
	Infection of tissue and organs by Drechslera
	Infection of tissue and organs by Fusarium
	Infection of tissue and organs by saprophytic fungi NEC

B49 **Unspecified mycosis**

Fungemia NOS

PROTOZOAL DISEASES (B50-B64)

Excludes1: amebiasis (A06.-)

Other protozoal intestinal diseases (A07.-)

B50 **Plasmodium falciparum malaria**

Includes: mixed infections of Plasmodium falciparum with any other Plasmodium species

B50.0	**Plasmodium falciparum malaria with cerebral complications**
	Cerebral malaria NOS
B50.8	**Other severe and complicated Plasmodium falciparum malaria**
	Severe or complicated Plasmodium falciparum malaria NOS
B50.9	**Plasmodium falciparum malaria, unspecified**

B51 **Plasmodium vivax malaria**

Includes: mixed infections of Plasmodium vivax with other Plasmodium species, except Plasmodium falciparum

Excludes1: plasmodium vivax with Plasmodium falciparum (B50.-)

● New code ▲ Revised code **Excludes1:** Not coded here **Excludes2:** Not included here ⊗ Placeholder required ⑦ 7th digit required

B51.0 **Plasmodium vivax malaria with rupture of spleen**

B51.8 **Plasmodium vivax malaria with other complications**

B51.9 **Plasmodium vivax malaria without complication**

Plasmodium vivax malaria NOS

B52 **Plasmodium malariae malaria**

Includes: mixed infections of Plasmodium malariae with other Plasmodium species, except Plasmodium falciparum and Plasmodium vivax

Excludes1: Plasmodium falciparum (B50.-)

Plasmodium vivax (B51.-)

B52.0 **Plasmodium malariae malaria with nephropathy**

B52.8 **Plasmodium malariae malaria with other complications**

B52.9 **Plasmodium malariae malaria without complication**

Plasmodium malariae malaria NOS

B53 **Other specified malaria**

B53.0 **Plasmodium ovale malaria**

Excludes1: Plasmodium ovale with Plasmodium falciparum (B50.-)

Plasmodium ovale with Plasmodium malariae (B52.-)

Plasmodium ovale with Plasmodium vivax (B51.-)

B53.1 **Malaria due to simian plasmodia**

Excludes1: Malaria due to simian plasmodia with Plasmodium falciparum (B50.-)

Malaria due to simian plasmodia with Plasmodium malariae (B52.-)

Malaria due to simian plasmodia with Plasmodium ovale (B53.0)

Malaria due to simian plasmodia with Plasmodium vivax (B51.-)

B53.8 **Other malaria, not elsewhere classified**

B54 **Unspecified malaria**

B55 **Leishmaniasis**

B55.0 **Visceral leishmaniasis**

Kala-azar

Post-kala-azar dermal leishmaniasis

B55.1 **Cutaneous leishmaniasis**

B55.2 **Mucocutaneous leishmaniasis**

B55.9 **Leishmaniasis, unspecified**

B56 **African trypanosomiasis**

B56.0 **Gambiense trypanosomiasis**

Infection due to Trypanosoma brucei gambiense

West African sleeping sickness

B56.1 **Rhodesiense trypanosomiasis**

East African sleeping sickness

Infection due to Trypanosoma brucei rhodesiense

B56.9 **African trypanosomiasis, unspecified**

Sleeping sickness NOS

B57 **Chagas' disease**

Includes: American trypanosomiasis

infection due to Trypanosoma cruzi

B57.0 **Acute Chagas' disease with heart involvement**

Acute Chagas' disease with myocarditis

B57.1 **Acute Chagas' disease without heart involvement**

Acute Chagas' disease NOS

B57.2 **Chagas' disease (chronic) with heart involvement**

American trypanosomiasis NOS

Chagas' disease (chronic) NOS

Chagas' disease (chronic) with myocarditis

Trypanosomiasis NOS

B57.3 **Chagas' disease (chronic) with digestive system involvement**

B57.30 **Chagas' disease with digestive system involvement, unspecified**

B57.31 **Megaesophagus in Chagas' disease**

B57.32 **Megacolon in Chagas' disease**

B57.39 **Other digestive system involvement in Chagas' disease**

B57.4 **Chagas' disease (chronic) with nervous system involvement**

B57.40 **Chagas' disease with nervous system involvement, unspecified**

B57.41 **Meningitis in Chagas' disease**

B57.42 **Meningoencephalitis in Chagas' disease**

B57.49 **Other nervous system involvement in Chagas' disease**

B57.5 **Chagas' disease (chronic) with other organ involvement**

B58 **Toxoplasmosis**

Definition: Toxoplasmosis is an infection caused by the parasite named toxoplasma gondii that can invade tissues and damage the brain, especially in a fetus and in a newborn baby. Symptoms include fever, fatigue, headache, swollen lymph glands, and muscle aches and pains.

Includes: infection due to Toxoplasma gondii

Excludes1: congenital toxoplasmosis (P37.1)

B58.0 **Toxoplasma oculopathy**

B58.00 **Toxoplasma oculopathy, unspecified**

B58.01 **Toxoplasma chorioretinitis**

B58.09 **Other toxoplasma oculopathy**

Toxoplasma uveitis

B58.1 **Toxoplasma hepatitis**

B58.2 **Toxoplasma meningoencephalitis**

B58.3 **Pulmonary toxoplasmosis**

B58.8 **Toxoplasmosis with other organ involvement**

B58.81 **Toxoplasma myocarditis**

B58.82 **Toxoplasma myositis**

B58.83 **Toxoplasma tubulo-interstitial nephropathy**

Toxoplasma pyelonephritis

B58.89 **Toxoplasmosis with other organ involvement**

B58.9 **Toxoplasmosis, unspecified**

B59 **Pneumocystosis**

Pneumonia due to Pneumocystis carinii

Pneumonia due to Pneumocystis jiroveci

B60 **Other protozoal diseases, not elsewhere classified**

Excludes1: cryptosporidiosis (A07.2)

intestinal microsporidiosis (A07.8)

isosporiasis (A07.3)

B60.0 **Babesiosis**

Piroplasmosis

B60.1 **Acanthamebiasis**

B60.10 **Acanthamebiasis, unspecified**

B60.11 **Meningoencephalitis due to Acanthamoeba (culbertsoni)**

B60.12 **Conjunctivitis due to Acanthamoeba**

B60.13 **Keratoconjunctivitis due to Acanthamoeba**

B60.19   Other acanthamebic disease

B60.2   Naegleriasis

Primary amebic meningoencephalitis

B60.8   Other specified protozoal diseases

Microsporidiosis

B64   Unspecified protozoal disease

HELMINTHIASES (B65-B83)

B65   Schistosomiasis [bilharziasis]

Definition: Schistosomiasis [bilharziasis], aka bilharzia, bilharziosis or snail fever, is a parasitic disease caused by several species of fluke of the genus Schistosoma. Schistosomiasis often is a chronic illness that can damage internal organs and, in children, impair growth and cognitive development.

Includes: snail fever

B65.0   Schistosomiasis due to Schistosoma haematobium [urinary schistosomiasis]

B65.1   Schistosomiasis due to Schistosoma mansoni [intestinal schistosomiasis]

B65.2   Schistosomiasis due to Schistosoma japonicum

Asiatic schistosomiasis

B65.3   Cercarial dermatitis

Swimmer's itch

B65.8   Other schistosomiasis

Infection due to Schistosoma intercalatum

Infection due to Schistosoma mattheei

Infection due to Schistosoma mekongi

B65.9   Schistosomiasis, unspecified

B66   Other fluke infections

B66.0   Opisthorchiasis

Infection due to cat liver fluke

Infection due to Opisthorchis (felineus)(viverrini)

B66.1   Clonorchiasis

Chinese liver fluke disease

Infection due to Clonorchis sinensis

Oriental liver fluke disease

B66.2   Dicroceliasis

Infection due to Dicrocoelium dendriticum

Lancet fluke infection

B66.3   Fascioliasis

Infection due to Fasciola gigantica

Infection due to Fasciola hepatica

Infection due to Fasciola indica

Sheep liver fluke disease

B66.4   Paragonimiasis

Infection due to Paragonimus species

Lung fluke disease

Pulmonary distomiasis

B66.5   Fasciolopsiasis

Infection due to Fasciolopsis buski

Intestinal distomiasis

B66.8   Other specified fluke infections

Echinostomiasis

Heterophyiasis

Metagonimiasis Nanophyetiasis Watsoniasis

B66.9   Fluke infection, unspecified

B67   Echinococcosis

Includes: hydatidosis

B67.0   Echinococcus granulosus infection of liver

B67.1   Echinococcus granulosus infection of lung

B67.2   Echinococcus granulosus infection of bone

B67.3   Echinococcus granulosus infection, other and multiple sites

B67.31   Echinococcus granulosus infection, thyroid gland

B67.32   Echinococcus granulosus infection, multiple sites

B67.39   Echinococcus granulosus infection, other sites

B67.4   Echinococcus granulosus infection, unspecified

Dog tapeworm (infection)

B67.5   Echinococcus multilocularis infection of liver

B67.6   Echinococcus multilocularis infection, other and multiple sites

B67.61   Echinococcus multilocularis infection, multiple sites

B67.69   Echinococcus multilocularis infection, other sites

B67.7   Echinococcus multilocularis infection, unspecified

B67.8   Echinococcosis, unspecified, of liver

B67.9   Echinococcosis, other and unspecified

B67.90   Echinococcosis, unspecified

Echinococcosis NOS

B67.99   Other echinococcosis

B68   Taeniasis

Excludes1: cysticercosis (B69.-)

B68.0   Taenia solium taeniasis

Pork tapeworm (infection)

B68.1   Taenia saginata taeniasis

Beef tapeworm (infection)

Infection due to adult tapeworm

Taenia saginata

B68.9   Taeniasis, unspecified

B69   Cysticercosis

Includes: cysticerciasis infection due to larval form of Taenia solium

B69.0   Cysticercosis of central nervous system

B69.1   Cysticercosis of eye

B69.8   Cysticercosis of other sites

B69.81   Myositis in cysticercosis

B69.89   Cysticercosis of other sites

B69.9   Cysticercosis, unspecified

B70   Diphyllobothriasis and sparganosis

B70.0   Diphyllobothriasis

Diphyllobothrium (adult) (latum) (pacificum) infection

Fish tapeworm (infection)

Excludes2: larval diphyllobothriasis (B70.1)

B70.1   Sparganosis

Infection due to Sparganum (mansoni) (proliferum)

Infection due to Spirometra larva

Larval diphyllobothriasis

Spirometrosis

B71   Other cestode infections

B71.0   Hymenolepiasis

Dwarf tapeworm infection

Rat tapeworm (infection)

B71.1   Dipylidiasis

B71.8   Other specified cestode infections

Coenurosis

B71.9   Cestode infection, unspecified

Tapeworm (infection) NOS

B72   Dracunculiasis

Includes: guinea worm infection

infection due to Dracunculus medinensis

B73   Onchocerciasis

Includes: onchocerca volvulus infection

onchocercosis river blindness

B73.0   Onchocerciasis with eye disease

B73.00   Onchocerciasis with eye involvement, unspecified

B73.01   Onchocerciasis with endophthalmitis

B73.02   Onchocerciasis with glaucoma

B73.09   Onchocerciasis with other eye involvement

Infestation of eyelid due to onchocerciasis

B73.1   Onchocerciasis without eye disease

B74   Filariasis

Excludes2: onchocerciasis (B73)

tropical (pulmonary) eosinophilia NOS (J82)

B74.0   Filariasis due to Wuchereria bancrofti

Bancroftian elephantiasis

Bancroftian filariasis

B74.1   Filariasis due to Brugia malayi

B74.2   Filariasis due to Brugia timori

B74.3   Loiasis

Calabar swelling

Eyeworm disease of Africa

Loa Loa infection

B74.4   Mansonelliasis

Infection due to Mansonella ozzardi

Infection due to Mansonella perstans

Infection due to Mansonella streptocerca

B74.8   Other filariases

Dirofilariasis

B74.9   Filariasis, unspecified

B75   Trichinellosis

Includes: infection due to Trichinella species

trichiniasis

B76   Hookworm diseases

Includes: uncinariasis

B76.0   Ancylostomiasis

Infection due to Ancylostoma species

B76.1   Necatoriasis

Infection due to Necator americanus

B76.8   Other hookworm diseases

B76.9   Hookworm disease, unspecified

Cutaneous larva migrans NOS

B77   Ascariasis

Includes: ascaridiasis

roundworm infection

B77.0   Ascariasis with intestinal complications

B77.8   Ascariasis with other complications

B77.81   Ascariasis pneumonia

B77.89   Ascariasis with other complications

B77.9   Ascariasis, unspecified

B78   Strongyloidiasis

Excludes1: trichostrongyliasis (B81.2)

B78.0   Intestinal strongyloidiasis

B78.1   Cutaneous strongyloidiasis

B78.7   Disseminated strongyloidiasis

B78.9   Strongyloidiasis, unspecified

B79   Trichuriasis

Includes: trichocephaliasis

whipworm (disease)(infection)

B80   Enterobiasis

Includes: oxyuriasis

pinworm infection threadworm infection

B81   Other intestinal helminthiases, not elsewhere classified

Definition: Helminthiases is a disease in which a part of the body is infested with worms such as pinworm, roundworm or tapeworm.

Excludes1: angiostrongyliasis due to:

Angiostrongylus cantonensis (B83.2)

Parastrongylus cantonensis (B83.2)

B81.0   Anisakiasis

Infection due to Anisakis larva

B81.1   Intestinal capillariasis

Capillariasis NOS

Infection due to Capillaria philippinensis

Excludes2: hepatic capillariasis (B83.8)

B81.2   Trichostrongyliasis

B81.3   Intestinal angiostrongyliasis

Angiostrongyliasis due to:

Angiostrongylus costaricensis

Parastrongylus costaricensis

B81.4   Mixed intestinal helminthiases

Infection due to intestinal helminths classified to more than one of the categories B65.0-B81.3 and B81.8

Mixed helminthiasis NOS

B81.8   Other specified intestinal helminthiases

Infection due to Oesophagostomum species [esophagostomiasis]

Infection due to Ternidens diminutus [Ternidensiasis]

B82   Unspecified intestinal parasitism

B82.0   Intestinal helminthiasis, unspecified

B82.9   Intestinal parasitism, unspecified

B83   Other helminthiases

Excludes1: capillariasis NOS (B81.1)

Excludes2: intestinal capillariasis (B81.1)

B83.0   Visceral larva migrans

Toxocariasis

B83.1   Gnathostomiasis

Wandering swelling

B83.2   Angiostrongyliasis due to Parastrongylus cantonensis

Eosinophilic meningoencephalitis due to Parastrongylus cantonensis

Excludes2: intestinal angiostrongyliasis (B81.3)

B83.3   Syngamiasis

Syngamosis

B83.4   Internal hirudiniasis

Excludes2: external hirudiniasis (B88.3)

B83.8   Other specified helminthiases

Acanthocephaliasis

| | Add 4th-7th digits | Nonspecific code | Unspecified code | Manifestation code | 163 |

Gongylonemiasis

Hepatic capillariasis

Metastrongyliasis

Thelaziasis

B83.9 **Helminthiasis, unspecified**

Worms NOS

Excludes1: intestinal helminthiasis NOS (B82.0)

PEDICULOSIS, ACARIASIS AND OTHER INFESTATIONS (B85-B89)

Definition: Pediculosis and Phthirus infestation is an infestation with lice (pediculus humanus) or true lice or crab lice (Phthirus) resulting in severe itching.

Definition: Acariasis is an infestation with arthropod parasites of the order Acarina including the ticks and mites.

B85 **Pediculosis and phthiriasis**

B85.0 **Pediculosis due to Pediculus humanus capitis**

Head-louse infestation

B85.1 **Pediculosis due to Pediculus humanus corporis**

Body-louse infestation

B85.2 **Pediculosis, unspecified**

B85.3 **Phthiriasis**

Infestation by crab-louse

Infestation by Phthirus pubis

B85.4 **Mixed pediculosis and phthiriasis**

Infestation classifiable to more than one of the categories B85.0-B85.3

B86 **Scabies**

Sarcoptic itch

B87 **Myiasis**

Includes: infestation by larva of flies

B87.0 **Cutaneous myiasis**

Creeping myiasis

B87.1 **Wound myiasis**

Traumatic myiasis

B87.2 **Ocular myiasis**

B87.3 **Nasopharyngeal myiasis**

Laryngeal myiasis

B87.4 **Aural myiasis**

B87.8 **Myiasis of other sites**

B87.81 **Genitourinary myiasis**

B87.82 **Intestinal myiasis**

B87.89 **Myiasis of other sites**

B87.9 **Myiasis, unspecified**

B88 **Other infestations**

B88.0 **Other acariasis**

Acarine dermatitis

Dermatitis due to Demodex species

Dermatitis due to Dermanyssus gallinae

Dermatitis due to Liponyssoides sanguineus

Trombiculosis

Excludes2: scabies (B86)

B88.1 **Tungiasis [sandflea infestation]**

B88.2 **Other arthropod infestations**

Scarabiasis

B88.3 **External hirudiniasis**

Leech infestation NOS

Excludes2: internal hirudiniasis (B83.4)

B88.8 **Other specified infestations**

Ichthyoparasitism due to Vandellia cirrhosa

Linguatulosis

Porocephaliasis

B88.9 **Infestation, unspecified**

Infestation (skin) NOS

Infestation by mites NOS

Skin parasites NOS

B89 **Unspecified parasitic disease**

SEQUELAE OF INFECTIOUS AND PARASITIC DISEASES (B90-B94)

Note: Categories B90-B94 are to be used to indicate conditions in categories A00-B89 as the cause of sequelae, which are themselves classified elsewhere. The 'sequelae' include conditions specified as such; they also include residuals of diseases classifiable to the above categories if there is evidence that the disease itself is no longer present. Codes from these categories are not to be used for chronic infections. Code chronic current infections to active infectious disease as appropriate.

Code first condition resulting from (sequela) the infectious or parasitic disease

B90 **Sequelae of tuberculosis**

B90.0 **Sequelae of central nervous system tuberculosis**

B90.1 **Sequelae of genitourinary tuberculosis**

B90.2 **Sequelae of tuberculosis of bones and joints**

B90.8 **Sequelae of tuberculosis of other organs**

Excludes2: sequelae of respiratory tuberculosis (B90.9)

B90.9 **Sequelae of respiratory and unspecified tuberculosis**

Sequelae of tuberculosis NOS

B91 **Sequelae of poliomyelitis**

Excludes1: postpolio syndrome (G14)

B92 **Sequelae of leprosy**

B94 **Sequelae of other and unspecified infectious and parasitic diseases**

B94.0 **Sequelae of trachoma**

B94.1 **Sequelae of viral encephalitis**

B94.2 **Sequelae of viral hepatitis**

B94.8 **Sequelae of other specified infectious and parasitic diseases**

B94.9 **Sequelae of unspecified infectious and parasitic disease**

BACTERIAL AND VIRAL INFECTIOUS AGENTS (B95-B97)

Note: These categories are provided for use as supplementary or additional codes to identify the infectious agent(s) in diseases classified elsewhere.

B95 **Streptococcus, Staphylococcus, and Enterococcus as the cause of diseases classified elsewhere**

B95.0 **Streptococcus, group A, as the cause of diseases classified elsewhere**

B95.1 **Streptococcus, group B, as the cause of diseases classified elsewhere**

B95.2 **Enterococcus as the cause of diseases classified elsewhere**

B95.3 **Streptococcus pneumoniae as the cause of diseases classified elsewhere**

B95.4 **Other streptococcus as the cause of diseases classified elsewhere**

B95.5 **Unspecified streptococcus as the cause of diseases classified elsewhere**

B95.6 **Staphylococcus aureus as the cause of diseases classified elsewhere**

B95.61 **Methicillin susceptible Staphylococcus aureus infection as the cause of diseases classified elsewhere**

Methicillin susceptible Staphylococcus aureus (MSSA) infection as the cause of diseases classified elsewhere

Staphylococcus aureus infection NOS as the cause of diseases classified elsewhere

B95.62 **Methicillin resistant Staphylococcus aureus infection as the cause of diseases classified elsewhere**

Methicillin resistant staphylococcus aureus (MRSA) infection as the cause of diseases classified elsewhere

B95.7 **Other staphylococcus as the cause of diseases classified elsewhere**

B95.8 **Unspecified staphylococcus as the cause of diseases classified elsewhere**

B96 **Other bacterial agents as the cause of diseases classified elsewhere**

B96.0 **Mycoplasma pneumoniae [M. pneumoniae] as the cause of diseases classified elsewhere**

Pleuro-pneumonia-like-organism [PPLO]

B96.1 **Klebsiella pneumoniae [K. pneumoniae] as the cause of diseases classified elsewhere**

B96.2 **Escherichia coli [E. coli] as the cause of diseases classified elsewhere**

B96.20 **Unspecified Escherichia coli [E. coli] as the cause of diseases classified elsewhere**

Escherichia coli [E. coli] NOS

B96.21 **Shiga toxin-producing Escherichia coli [E. coli] (STEC) O157 as the cause of diseases classified elsewhere**

E. coli O157:H- (nonmotile) with confirmation of Shiga toxin

E. coli O157 with confirmation of Shiga toxin when H antigen is unknown, or is not H7 O157:H7

Escherichia coli [E. coli] with or without confirmation of Shiga toxin-production

Shiga toxin-producing Escherichia coli [E. coli] O157:H7 with or without confirmation of Shiga toxin-production

STEC O157:H7 with or without confirmation of Shiga toxin-production

B96.22 **Other specified Shiga toxin-producing Escherichia coli [E. coli] (STEC) as the cause of diseases classified elsewhere**

Non-O157 Shiga toxin-producing Escherichia coli [E. coli]

Non-O157 Shiga toxin-producing Escherichia coli [E. coli] with known O group

B96.23 **Unspecified Shiga toxin-producing Escherichia coli [E. coli] (STEC) as the cause of diseases classified elsewhere**

Shiga toxin-producing Escherichia coli [E. coli] with unspecified O group STEC NOS

B96.29 **Other Escherichia coli [E. coli] as the cause of diseases classified elsewhere**

Non-Shiga toxin-producing E. coli

B96.3 **Hemophilus influenzae [H. influenzae] as the cause of diseases classified elsewhere**

B96.4 **Proteus (mirabilis) (morganii) as the cause of diseases classified elsewhere**

B96.5 **Pseudomonas (aeruginosa) (mallei) (pseudomallei) as the cause of diseases classified elsewhere**

B96.6 **Bacteroides fragilis [B. fragilis] as the cause of diseases classified elsewhere**

B96.7 **Clostridium perfringens [C. perfringens] as the cause of diseases classified elsewhere**

B96.8 **Other specified bacterial agents as the cause of diseases classified elsewhere**

B96.81 **Helicobacter pylori [H. pylori] as the cause of diseases classified elsewhere**

B96.82 **Vibrio vulnificus as the cause of diseases classified elsewhere**

B96.89 **Other specified bacterial agents as the cause of diseases classified elsewhere**

B97 **Viral agents as the cause of diseases classified elsewhere**

B97.0 **Adenovirus as the cause of diseases classified elsewhere**

B97.1 **Enterovirus as the cause of diseases classified elsewhere**

B97.10 **Unspecified enterovirus as the cause of diseases classified elsewhere**

B97.11 **Coxsackievirus as the cause of diseases classified elsewhere**

B97.12 **Echovirus as the cause of diseases classified elsewhere**

B97.19 **Other enterovirus as the cause of diseases classified elsewhere**

B97.2 **Coronavirus as the cause of diseases classified elsewhere**

B97.21 **SARS-associated coronavirus as the cause of diseases classified elsewhere**

Excludes1: pneumonia due to SARS-associated coronavirus (J12.81)

B97.29 **Other coronavirus as the cause of diseases classified elsewhere**

B97.3 **Retrovirus as the cause of diseases classified elsewhere**

Excludes1: Human immunodeficiency virus [HIV] disease (B20)

B97.30 **Unspecified retrovirus as the cause of diseases classified elsewhere**

B97.31 **Lentivirus as the cause of diseases classified elsewhere**

B97.32 **Oncovirus as the cause of diseases classified elsewhere**

B97.33 **Human T-cell lymphotrophic virus, type I [HTLV-I] as the cause of diseases classified elsewhere**

B97.34 **Human T-cell lymphotrophic virus, type II [HTLV-II] as the cause of diseases classified elsewhere**

B97.35 **Human immunodeficiency virus, type 2[HIV 2] as the cause of diseases classified elsewhere**

B97.39 **Other retrovirus as the cause of diseases classified elsewhere**

B97.4 **Respiratory syncytial virus as the cause of diseases classified elsewhere**

B97.5 **Reovirus as the cause of diseases classified elsewhere**

B97.6 **Parvovirus as the cause of diseases classified elsewhere**

B97.7 **Papillomavirus as the cause of diseases classified elsewhere**

B97.8 **Other viral agents as the cause of diseases classified elsewhere**

B97.81 **Human metapneumovirus as the cause of diseases classified elsewhere**

B97.89 **Other viral agents as the cause of diseases classified elsewhere**

OTHER INFECTIOUS DISEASES (B99)

B99 **Other and unspecified infectious diseases**

Add 4th-7th digits   Nonspecific code   Unspecified code   Manifestation code

B99.8   Other infectious disease

B99.9   Unspecified infectious disease

Chapter 2: Neoplasms (C00-D49)

DEFINITIONS

This chapter includes definitions of selected key words, terms and phrases and coding alerts for adding points to the clinical domain, and references to coding late effects where appropriate. An example from this chapter is as follows:

C46 Kaposi's sarcoma

Definition: Kaposi's sarcoma is a form of skin cancer that can involve internal organs. It is most often found in patients with acquired immunodeficiency syndrome (AIDS), and can be fatal.

MULTIPLE CODING FOR A SINGLE CONDITION

In addition to the etiology/manifestation convention that requires two codes to fully describe a single condition that affects multiple body systems, there are other single conditions that also require more than one code. "Use additional code" notes are found in the Tabular List at codes that are not part of an etiology/manifestation pair where a secondary code is useful to fully describe a condition. The sequencing rule is the same as the etiology/manifestation pair, "use additional code" indicates that a secondary code should be added.

For example, for bacterial infections that are not included in chapter 1, a secondary code from category B95, Streptococcus, Staphylococcus, and Enterococcus, as the cause of diseases classified elsewhere, or B96, Other bacterial agents as the cause of diseases classified elsewhere, may be required to identify the bacterial organism causing the infection. A "use additional code" note will normally be found at the infectious disease code, indicating a need for the organism code to be added as a secondary code.

"Code first" notes are also under certain codes that are not specifically manifestation codes but may be due to an underlying cause. When there is a "code first" note and an underlying condition is present, the underlying condition should be sequenced first.

"Code, if applicable, any causal condition first", notes indicate that this code may be assigned as a principal diagnosis when the causal condition is unknown or not applicable. If a causal condition is known, then the code for that condition should be sequenced as the principal or first-listed diagnosis.

Multiple codes may be needed for sequela, complication codes and obstetric codes to more fully describe a condition. See the specific guidelines for these conditions for further instruction.

COMBINATION CODE

A combination code is a single code used to classify: Two diagnoses, or a diagnosis with an associated secondary process (manifestation) A diagnosis with an associated complication

Combination codes are identified by referring to subterm entries in the Alphabetic Index and by reading the inclusion and exclusion notes in the Tabular List.

Assign only the combination code when that code fully identifies the diagnostic conditions involved or when the Alphabetic Index so directs. Multiple coding should not be used when the classification provides a combination code that clearly identifies all of the elements documented in the diagnosis. When the combination code lacks necessary specificity in describing the manifestation or complication, an additional code should be used as a secondary code.

SEQUELA (LATE EFFECTS)

A sequela is the residual effect (condition produced) after the acute phase of an illness or injury has terminated. There is no time limit on when a sequela code can be used. The residual may be apparent early, such as in cerebral infarction, or it may occur months or years later, such as that due to a previous injury. Coding of sequela generally requires two codes sequenced in the following order: The condition or nature of the sequela is sequenced first.

The sequela code is sequenced second.

An exception to the above guidelines are those instances where the code for the sequela is followed by a manifestation code identified in the Tabular List and title, or the sequela code has been expanded (at the fourth, fifth or sixth character levels) to include the manifestation(s). The code for the acute phase of an illness or injury that led to the sequela is never used with a code for the late effect.

GENERAL GUIDELINES

Chapter 2 of the ICD-10-CM contains the codes for most benign and all malignant neoplasms. Certain benign neoplasms, such as prostatic adenomas, may be found in the specific body system chapters. To properly code a neoplasm it is necessary to determine from the record if the neoplasm is benign, in-situ, malignant, or of uncertain histologic behavior. If malignant, any secondary (metastatic) sites should also be determined.

Primary malignant neoplasms overlapping site boundaries

A primary malignant neoplasm that overlaps two or more contiguous (next to each other) sites should be classified to the subcategory/code .8 ('overlapping lesion'), unless the combination is specifically indexed elsewhere. For multiple neoplasms of the same site that are not contiguous such as tumors in different quadrants of the same breast, codes for each site should be assigned.

Malignant neoplasm of ectopic tissue

Malignant neoplasms of ectopic tissue are to be coded to the site of origin mentioned, e.g., ectopic pancreatic malignant neoplasms involving the stomach are coded to pancreas, unspecified (C25.9).

 Add 4th-7th digits   Nonspecific code   Unspecified code   Manifestation code

The neoplasm table in the Alphabetic Index should be referenced first. However, if the histological term is documented, that term should be referenced first, rather than going immediately to the Neoplasm Table, in order to determine which column in the Neoplasm Table is appropriate. For example, if the documentation indicates "adenoma," refer to the term in the Alphabetic Index to review the entries under this term and the instructional note to "see also neoplasm, by site, benign." The table provides the proper code based on the type of neoplasm and the site. It is important to select the proper column in the table that corresponds to the type of neoplasm. The Tabular List should then be referenced to verify that the correct code has been selected from the table and that a more specific site code does not exist.

See Section I.C.21. Factors influencing health status and contact with health services, Status, for information regarding Z15.0, codes for genetic susceptibility to cancer.

TREATMENT DIRECTED AT THE MALIGNANCY

If the treatment is directed at the malignancy, designate the malignancy as the principal diagnosis.

The only exception to this guideline is if a patient admission/encounter is solely for the administration of chemotherapy, immunotherapy or radiation therapy, assign the appropriate Z51.-- code as the first-listed or principal diagnosis, and the diagnosis or problem for which the service is being performed as a secondary diagnosis.

TREATMENT OF SECONDARY SITE

When a patient is admitted because of a primary neoplasm with metastasis and treatment is directed toward the secondary site only, the secondary neoplasm is designated as the principal diagnosis even though the primary malignancy is still present.

CODING AND SEQUENCING OF COMPLICATIONS

Coding and sequencing of complications associated with the malignancies or with the therapy thereof are subject to the following guidelines:

1) **Anemia associated with malignancy**

   When admission/encounter is for management of an anemia associated with the malignancy, and the treatment is only for anemia, the appropriate code for the malignancy is sequenced as the principal or first-listed diagnosis followed by the appropriate code for the anemia (such as code D63.0, Anemia in neoplastic disease).

2) **Anemia associated with chemotherapy, immunotherapy and radiation therapy**

   When the admission/encounter is for management of an anemia associated with an adverse effect of the administration of chemotherapy or immunotherapy and the only treatment is for the anemia, the anemia code is sequenced first followed by the appropriate codes for the neoplasm and the adverse effect (T45.1X5, Adverse effect of antineoplastic and immunosuppressive drugs).

   When the admission/encounter is for management of an anemia associated with an adverse effect of radiotherapy, the anemia code should be sequenced first, followed by the appropriate neoplasm code and code Y84.2, Radiological procedure and radiotherapy as the cause of abnormal reaction of the patient, or of later complication, without mention of misadventure at the time of the procedure.

3) **Management of dehydration due to the malignancy**

   When the admission/encounter is for management of dehydration due to the malignancy and only the dehydration is being treated (intravenous rehydration), the dehydration is sequenced first, followed by the code(s) for the malignancy.

4) **Treatment of a complication resulting from a surgical procedure**

   When the admission/encounter is for treatment of a complication resulting from a surgical procedure, designate the complication as the principal or first-listed diagnosis if treatment is directed at resolving the complication.

PRIMARY MALIGNANCY PREVIOUSLY EXCISED

When a primary malignancy has been previously excised or eradicated from its site and there is no further treatment directed to that site and there is no evidence of any existing primary malignancy, a code from category Z85, Personal history of malignant neoplasm, should be used to indicate the former site of the malignancy. Any mention of extension, invasion, or metastasis to another site is coded as a secondary malignant neoplasm to that site. The secondary site may be the principal or first-listed with the Z85 code used as a secondary code.

ADMISSIONS/ENCOUNTERS INVOLVING CHEMOTHERAPY, IMMUNOTHERAPY AND RADIATION THERAPY

1) **Episode of care involves surgical removal of neoplasm**

   When an episode of care involves the surgical removal of a neoplasm, primary or secondary site, followed by adjunct chemotherapy or radiation treatment during the same episode of care, the code for the neoplasm should be assigned as principal or first-listed diagnosis.

2) **Patient admission/encounter solely for administration of chemotherapy, immunotherapy and radiation therapy**

   If a patient admission/encounter is solely for the administration of chemotherapy, immunotherapy or radiation therapy assign code Z51.0, Encounter for antineoplastic radiation therapy, or Z51.11, Encounter for antineoplastic chemotherapy, or Z51.12, Encounter for antineoplastic immunotherapy as the first-listed or principal diagnosis. If a patient receives more than one of these therapies during the same admission more than one of these codes may be assigned, in any sequence.

   The malignancy for which the therapy is being administered should be assigned as a secondary diagnosis.

3) **Patient admitted for radiation therapy, chemotherapy or immunotherapy and develops complications**

When a patient is admitted for the purpose of radiotherapy, immunotherapy or chemotherapy and develops complications such as uncontrolled nausea and vomiting or dehydration, the principal or first-listed diagnosis is Z51.0, Encounter for antineoplastic radiation therapy, or Z51.11, Encounter for antineoplastic chemotherapy, or Z51.12, Encounter for antineoplastic immunotherapy followed by any codes for the complications.

ADMISSION/ENCOUNTER TO DETERMINE EXTENT OF MALIGNANCY

When the reason for admission/encounter is to determine the extent of the malignancy, or for a procedure such as paracentesis or thoracentesis, the primary malignancy or appropriate metastatic site is designated as the principal or first-listed diagnosis, even though chemotherapy or radiotherapy is administered.

SYMPTOMS, SIGNS, AND ABNORMAL FINDINGS LISTED IN CHAPTER 18 ASSOCIATED WITH NEOPLASMS

Symptoms, signs, and ill-defined conditions listed in Chapter 18 characteristic of, or associated with, an existing primary or secondary site malignancy cannot be used to replace the malignancy as principal or first-listed diagnosis, regardless of the number of admissions or encounters for treatment and care of the neoplasm.

See section I.C.21. Factors influencing health status and contact with health services, Encounter for prophylactic organ removal.

ADMISSION/ENCOUNTER FOR PAIN CONTROL/MANAGEMENT

See Section I.C.6. for information on coding admission/encounter for pain control/management.

MALIGNANCY IN TWO OR MORE NONCONTIGUOUS SITES

A patient may have more than one malignant tumor in the same organ. These tumors may represent different primaries or metastatic disease, depending on the site. Should the documentation be unclear, the provider should be queried as to the status of each tumor so that the correct codes can be assigned.

DISSEMINATED MALIGNANT NEOPLASM, UNSPECIFIED

Code C80.0, Disseminated malignant neoplasm, unspecified, is for use only in those cases where the patient has advanced metastatic disease and no known primary or secondary sites are specified. It should not be used in place of assigning codes for the primary site and all known secondary sites.

MALIGNANT NEOPLASM WITHOUT SPECIFICATION OF SITE

Code C80.1, Malignant (primary) neoplasm, unspecified, equates to Cancer, unspecified. This code should only be used when no determination can be made as to the primary site of a malignancy. This code should rarely be used in the inpatient setting.

SEQUENCING OF NEOPLASM CODES

1) **Encounter for treatment of primary malignancy**

If the reason for the encounter is for treatment of a primary malignancy, assign the malignancy as the principal/first-listed diagnosis. The primary site is to be sequenced first, followed by any metastatic sites.

2) **Encounter for treatment of secondary malignancy**

When an encounter is for a primary malignancy with metastasis and treatment is directed toward the metastatic (secondary) site(s) only, the metastatic site(s) is designated as the principal/first-listed diagnosis. The primary malignancy is coded as an additional code.

3) **Malignant neoplasm in a pregnant patient**

When a pregnant woman has a malignant neoplasm, a code from subcategory O9A.1-, Malignant neoplasm complicating pregnancy, childbirth, and the puerperium, should be sequenced first, followed by the appropriate code from Chapter 2 to indicate the type of neoplasm.

4) **Encounter for complication associated with a neoplasm**

When an encounter is for management of a complication associated with a neoplasm, such as dehydration, and the treatment is only for the complication, the complication is coded first, followed by the appropriate code(s) for the neoplasm.

The exception to this guideline is anemia. When the admission/encounter is for management of an anemia associated with the malignancy, and the treatment is only for anemia, the appropriate code for the malignancy is sequenced as the principal or first-listed diagnosis followed by code D63.0, Anemia in neoplastic disease.

5) **Complication from surgical procedure for treatment of a neoplasm**

When an encounter is for treatment of a complication resulting from a surgical procedure performed for the treatment of the neoplasm, designate the complication as the principal/first-listed diagnosis. See guideline regarding the coding of a current malignancy versus personal history to determine if the code for the neoplasm should also be assigned.

6) **Pathologic fracture due to a neoplasm**

When an encounter is for a pathological fracture due to a neoplasm, and the focus of treatment is the fracture, a code from subcategory M84.5, Pathological fracture in neoplastic disease, should be sequenced first, followed by the code for the neoplasm.

If the focus of treatment is the neoplasm with an associated pathological fracture, the neoplasm code should be sequenced first, followed by a code from M84.5 for the pathological fracture.

CURRENT MALIGNANCY VERSUS PERSONAL HISTORY OF MALIGNANCY

When a primary malignancy has been excised but further treatment, such as an additional surgery for the malignancy, radiation therapy or chemotherapy is directed to that site, the primary malignancy code should be used until treatment is completed.

When a primary malignancy has been previously excised or eradicated from its site, there is no further treatment (of the malignancy) directed to that site, and there is no evidence of any existing primary malignancy, a code from category Z85, Personal history of malignant neoplasm, should be used to indicate the former site of the malignancy.

See Section I.C.21. Factors influencing health status and contact with health services, History (of)

LEUKEMIA, MULTIPLE MYELOMA, AND MALIGNANT PLASMA CELL NEOPLASMS IN REMISSION VERSUS PERSONAL HISTORY

The categories for leukemia, and category C90, Multiple myeloma and malignant plasma cell neoplasms, have codes indicating whether or not the leukemia has achieved remission. There are also codes Z85.6, Personal history of leukemia, and Z85.79, Personal history of other malignant neoplasms of lymphoid, hematopoietic and related tissues. If the documentation is unclear as to whether the leukemia has achieved remission, the provider should be queried.

See Section I.C.21. Factors influencing health status and contact with health services, History (of)

AFTERCARE FOLLOWING SURGERY FOR NEOPLASM

See Section I.C.21. Factors influencing health status and contact with health services, Aftercare

FOLLOW-UP CARE FOR COMPLETED TREATMENT OF A MALIGNANCY

See Section I.C.21. Factors influencing health status and contact with health services, Follow-up

PROPHYLACTIC ORGAN REMOVAL FOR PREVENTION OF MALIGNANCY

See Section I.C. 21, Factors influencing health status and contact with health services, Prophylactic organ removal

MALIGNANT NEOPLASM ASSOCIATED WITH TRANSPLANTED ORGAN

A malignant neoplasm of a transplanted organ should be coded as a transplant complication. Assign first the appropriate code from category T86.-, Complications of transplanted organs and tissue, followed by code C80.2, Malignant neoplasm associated with transplanted organ. Use an additional code for the specific malignancy.

Chapter 2

Neoplasms (C00-D49)

This chapter contains the following blocks:

Note: Functional activity

All neoplasms are classified in this chapter, whether they are functionally active or not. An additional code from Chapter 4 may be used, to identify functional activity associated with any neoplasm. Morphology [Histology]

Chapter 2 classifies neoplasms primarily by site (topography), with broad groupings for behavior, malignant, in situ, benign, etc. The Table of Neoplasms should be used to identify the correct topography code. In a few cases, such as for malignant melanoma and certain neuroendocrine tumors, the morphology (histologic type) is included in the category and codes.

Primary malignant neoplasms overlapping site boundaries

A primary malignant neoplasm that overlaps two or more contiguous (next to each Other) sites should be classified to the subcategory/code .8 ('overlapping lesion'), unless the combination is specifically indexed elsewhere. For multiple neoplasms of the same site that are not contiguous, such as tumors in different quadrants of the same breast, codes for each site should be assigned.

Malignant neoplasm of ectopic tissue

Malignant neoplasms of ectopic tissue are to be coded to the site mentioned, e.g., ectopic pancreatic malignant neoplasms are coded to pancreas, unspecified (C25.9).

MALIGNANT NEOPLASMS (C00-C96)

Definition: Malignant neoplasm refers to a tumor that tends to grow, invade, and metastasize. The tumor usually has an irregular shape and is composed of poorly differentiated cells. If untreated, it may result in death.

MALIGNANT NEOPLASMS, STATED OR PRESUMED TO BE PRIMARY (OF SPECIFIED SITES), AND CERTAIN SPECIFIED HISTOLOGIES, EXCEPT NEUROENDOCRINE, AND OF LYMPHOID, HEMATOPOIETIC AND RELATED TISSUE (C00-C75)

MALIGNANT NEOPLASMS OF LIP, ORAL CAVITY AND PHARYNX (C00-C14)

C00 Malignant neoplasm of lip

Use additional code to identify:

alcohol abuse and dependence (F10.-)

history of tobacco dependence (Z87.891)

tobacco dependence (F17.-)

tobacco use (Z72.0)

Excludes1: malignant melanoma of lip (C43.0)

Merkel cell carcinoma of lip (C4A.0)

Other and unspecified malignant neoplasm of skin of lip (C44.0-)

C00.0 Malignant neoplasm of external upper lip

Malignant neoplasm of lipstick area of upper lip

Malignant neoplasm of upper lip NOS

Malignant neoplasm of vermilion border of upper lip

C00.1 Malignant neoplasm of external lower lip

Malignant neoplasm of lower lip NOS

Malignant neoplasm of lipstick area of lower lip

Malignant neoplasm of vermilion border of lower lip

C00.2 Malignant neoplasm of external lip, unspecified

Malignant neoplasm of vermilion border of lip NOS

C00.3 Malignant neoplasm of upper lip, inner aspect

Malignant neoplasm of buccal aspect of upper lip

Malignant neoplasm of frenulum of upper lip

Malignant neoplasm of mucosa of upper lip

Malignant neoplasm of oral aspect of upper lip

C00.4 Malignant neoplasm of lower lip, inner aspect

Malignant neoplasm of buccal aspect of lower lip

Malignant neoplasm of frenulum of lower lip

Malignant neoplasm of mucosa of lower lip

Malignant neoplasm of oral aspect of lower lip

C00.5 Malignant neoplasm of lip, unspecified, inner aspect

Malignant neoplasm of buccal aspect of lip, unspecified

Malignant neoplasm of frenulum of lip, unspecified

Malignant neoplasm of mucosa of lip, unspecified

Malignant neoplasm of oral aspect of lip, unspecified

C00.6 Malignant neoplasm of commissure of lip, unspecified

C00.8 Malignant neoplasm of overlapping sites of lip

C00.9 Malignant neoplasm of lip, unspecified

C01 Malignant neoplasm of base of tongue

Malignant neoplasm of dorsal surface of base of tongue

Malignant neoplasm of fixed part of tongue NOS

Malignant neoplasm of posterior third of tongue

Use additional code to identify:

alcohol abuse and dependence (F10.-)

history of tobacco dependence (Z87.891)

tobacco dependence (F17.-)

tobacco use (Z72.0)

C02 Malignant neoplasm of other and unspecified parts of tongue

Use additional code to identify:

alcohol abuse and dependence (F10.-)

history of tobacco dependence (Z87.891)

tobacco dependence (F17.-)

tobacco use (Z72.0)

C02.0 Malignant neoplasm of dorsal surface of tongue

Malignant neoplasm of anterior two-thirds of tongue, dorsal surface

> **Excludes2:** malignant neoplasm of dorsal surface of base of tongue (C01)

C02.1 Malignant neoplasm of border of tongue

Malignant neoplasm of tip of tongue

C02.2 Malignant neoplasm of ventral surface of tongue

Malignant neoplasm of anterior two-thirds of tongue, ventral surface

Malignant neoplasm of frenulum linguae

C02.3 Malignant neoplasm of anterior two-thirds of tongue, part unspecified

Malignant neoplasm of middle third of tongue NOS

Malignant neoplasm of mobile part of tongue NOS

C02.4 Malignant neoplasm of lingual tonsil

> **Excludes2:** malignant neoplasm of tonsil NOS (C09.9)

C02.8 Malignant neoplasm of overlapping sites of tongue

Malignant neoplasm of two or more contiguous sites of tongue

C02.9 Malignant neoplasm of tongue, unspecified

C03 Malignant neoplasm of gum

> **Includes:** malignant neoplasm of alveolar (ridge) mucosa
>
> malignant neoplasm of gingiva

Use additional code to identify:

alcohol abuse and dependence (F10.-)

history of tobacco dependence (Z87.891)

tobacco dependence (F17.-)

tobacco use (Z72.0)

> **Excludes2:** malignant odontogenic neoplasms (C41.0-C41.1)

C03.0 Malignant neoplasm of upper gum

C03.1 Malignant neoplasm of lower gum

C03.9 Malignant neoplasm of gum, unspecified

C04 Malignant neoplasm of floor of mouth

Use additional code to identify:

alcohol abuse and dependence (F10.-)

history of tobacco dependence (Z87.891)

tobacco dependence (F17.-)

tobacco use (Z72.0)

C04.0 Malignant neoplasm of anterior floor of mouth

Malignant neoplasm of anterior to the premolar-canine junction

C04.1 Malignant neoplasm of lateral floor of mouth

C04.8 Malignant neoplasm of overlapping sites of floor of mouth

C04.9 Malignant neoplasm of floor of mouth, unspecified

C05 Malignant neoplasm of palate

Use additional code to identify:

alcohol abuse and dependence (F10.-)

history of tobacco dependence (Z87.891)

tobacco dependence (F17.-)

tobacco use (Z72.0)

> **Excludes1:** Kaposi's sarcoma of palate (C46.2)

C05.0 Malignant neoplasm of hard palate

C05.1 Malignant neoplasm of soft palate

> **Excludes2:** malignant neoplasm of nasopharyngeal surface of soft palate (C11.3)

C05.2 Malignant neoplasm of uvula

C05.8 Malignant neoplasm of overlapping sites of palate

C05.9 Malignant neoplasm of palate, unspecified

Malignant neoplasm of roof of mouth

C06 Malignant neoplasm of other and unspecified parts of mouth

Use additional code to identify:

alcohol abuse and dependence (F10.-)

history of tobacco dependence (Z87.891)

tobacco dependence (F17.-)

tobacco use (Z72.0)

C06.0 Malignant neoplasm of cheek mucosa

Malignant neoplasm of buccal mucosa NOS

Malignant neoplasm of internal cheek

C06.1 Malignant neoplasm of vestibule of mouth

Malignant neoplasm of buccal sulcus (upper) (lower)

Malignant neoplasm of labial sulcus (upper) (lower)

C06.2 Malignant neoplasm of retromolar area

C06.8 Malignant neoplasm of overlapping sites of other and unspecified parts of mouth

C06.80 Malignant neoplasm of overlapping sites of unspecified parts of mouth

C06.89 Malignant neoplasm of overlapping sites of other parts of mouth

'book leaf' neoplasm [ventral surface of tongue and floor of mouth]

C06.9 Malignant neoplasm of mouth, unspecified

Malignant neoplasm of minor salivary gland, unspecified site

Malignant neoplasm of oral cavity NOS

C07 Malignant neoplasm of parotid gland

Use additional code to identify:

alcohol abuse and dependence (F10.-)

exposure to environmental tobacco smoke (Z77.22)

exposure to tobacco smoke in the perinatal period (P96.81)

history of tobacco dependence (Z87.891)

occupational exposure to environmental tobacco smoke (Z57.31)

tobacco dependence (F17.-)

tobacco use (Z72.0)

C08 Malignant neoplasm of other and unspecified major salivary glands

> **Includes:** malignant neoplasm of salivary ducts

Use additional code to identify:

alcohol abuse and dependence (F10.-)

exposure to environmental tobacco smoke (Z77.22)

exposure to tobacco smoke in the perinatal period (P96.81)

history of tobacco dependence (Z87.891)

occupational exposure to environmental tobacco smoke (Z57.31)

tobacco dependence (F17.-)

tobacco use (Z72.0)

> **Excludes1:** malignant neoplasms of specified minor salivary glands which are classified according to their anatomical location

> **Excludes2:** malignant neoplasms of minor salivary glands NOS (C06.9)

malignant neoplasm of parotid gland (C07)

C08.0 Malignant neoplasm of submandibular gland

Malignant neoplasm of submaxillary gland

C08.1 Malignant neoplasm of sublingual gland

C08.9 Malignant neoplasm of major salivary gland, unspecified

Malignant neoplasm of salivary gland (major) NOS

C09 Malignant neoplasm of tonsil

● New code ▲ Revised code **Excludes1:** Not coded here **Excludes2:** Not included here ⊗ Placeholder required ⑦ 7th digit required

<u>Use additional code</u> to identify:

alcohol abuse and dependence (F10.-)

exposure to environmental tobacco smoke (Z77.22)

exposure to tobacco smoke in the perinatal period (P96.81)

history of tobacco dependence (Z87.891)

occupational exposure to environmental tobacco smoke (Z57.31)

tobacco dependence (F17.-)

tobacco use (Z72.0)

Excludes2: malignant neoplasm of lingual tonsil (C02.4)

malignant neoplasm of pharyngeal tonsil (C11.1)

C09.0   **Malignant neoplasm of tonsillar fossa**

C09.1   **Malignant neoplasm of tonsillar pillar (anterior) (posterior)**

C09.8   **Malignant neoplasm of overlapping sites of tonsil**

C09.9   **Malignant neoplasm of tonsil, unspecified**

Malignant neoplasm of tonsil NOS

Malignant neoplasm of faucial tonsils

Malignant neoplasm of palatine tonsils

C10   **Malignant neoplasm of oropharynx**

<u>Use additional code</u> to identify:

alcohol abuse and dependence (F10.-)

exposure to environmental tobacco smoke (Z77.22)

exposure to tobacco smoke in the perinatal period (P96.81)

history of tobacco dependence (Z87.891)

occupational exposure to environmental tobacco smoke (Z57.31)

tobacco dependence (F17.-)

tobacco use (Z72.0)

Excludes2: malignant neoplasm of tonsil (C09.-)

C10.0   **Malignant neoplasm of vallecula**

C10.1   **Malignant neoplasm of anterior surface of epiglottis**

Malignant neoplasm of epiglottis, free border [margin]

Malignant neoplasm of glossoepiglottic fold(s)

Excludes2: malignant neoplasm of epiglottis (suprahyoid portion) NOS (C32.1)

C10.2   **Malignant neoplasm of lateral wall of oropharynx**

C10.3   **Malignant neoplasm of posterior wall of oropharynx**

     C10.4   **Malignant neoplasm of branchial cleft**

Malignant neoplasm of branchial cyst [site of neoplasm]

C10.8   **Malignant neoplasm of overlapping sites of oropharynx**

Malignant neoplasm of junctional region of oropharynx

C10.9   **Malignant neoplasm of oropharynx, unspecified**

C11   **Malignant neoplasm of nasopharynx**

<u>Use additional code</u> to identify:

exposure to environmental tobacco smoke (Z77.22)

exposure to tobacco smoke in the perinatal period (P96.81)

history of tobacco dependence (Z87.891)

occupational exposure to environmental tobacco smoke (Z57.31)

tobacco dependence (F17.-)

tobacco use (Z72.0)

C11.0   **Malignant neoplasm of superior wall of nasopharynx**

Malignant neoplasm of roof of nasopharynx

C11.1   **Malignant neoplasm of posterior wall of nasopharynx**

Malignant neoplasm of adenoid

Malignant neoplasm of pharyngeal tonsil

C11.2   **Malignant neoplasm of lateral wall of nasopharynx**

Malignant neoplasm of fossa of Rosenmüller

Malignant neoplasm of opening of auditory tube

Malignant neoplasm of pharyngeal recess

C11.3   **Malignant neoplasm of anterior wall of nasopharynx**

Malignant neoplasm of floor of nasopharynx

Malignant neoplasm of nasopharyngeal (anterior) (posterior) surface of soft palate

Malignant neoplasm of posterior margin of nasal choana

Malignant neoplasm of posterior margin of nasal septum

C11.8   **Malignant neoplasm of overlapping sites of nasopharynx**

C11.9   **Malignant neoplasm of nasopharynx, unspecified**

Malignant neoplasm of nasopharyngeal wall NOS

C12   **Malignant neoplasm of pyriform sinus**

Malignant neoplasm of pyriform fossa

<u>Use additional code</u> to identify:

exposure to environmental tobacco smoke (Z77.22)

exposure to tobacco smoke in the perinatal period (P96.81)

history of tobacco dependence (Z87.891)

occupational exposure to environmental tobacco smoke (Z57.31)

tobacco dependence (F17.-)

tobacco use (Z72.0)

C13   **Malignant neoplasm of hypopharynx**

<u>Use additional code</u> to identify:

exposure to environmental tobacco smoke (Z77.22)

exposure to tobacco smoke in the perinatal period (P96.81)

history of tobacco dependence (Z87.891)

occupational exposure to environmental tobacco smoke (Z57.31)

tobacco dependence (F17.-)

tobacco use (Z72.0)

Excludes2: malignant neoplasm of pyriform sinus (C12)

C13.0   **Malignant neoplasm of postcricoid region**

C13.1   **Malignant neoplasm of aryepiglottic fold, hypopharyngeal aspect**

Malignant neoplasm of aryepiglottic fold, marginal zone

Malignant neoplasm of aryepiglottic fold NOS

Malignant neoplasm of interarytenoid fold, marginal zone

Malignant neoplasm of interarytenoid fold NOS

Excludes2: malignant neoplasm of aryepiglottic fold or interarytenoid fold, laryngeal aspect (C32.1)

C13.2   **Malignant neoplasm of posterior wall of hypopharynx**

C13.8   **Malignant neoplasm of overlapping sites of hypopharynx**

C13.9   **Malignant neoplasm of hypopharynx, unspecified**

Malignant neoplasm of hypopharyngeal wall NOS

C14   **Malignant neoplasm of other and ill-defined sites in the lip, oral cavity and pharynx**

<u>Use additional code</u> to identify:

alcohol abuse and dependence (F10.-)

exposure to environmental tobacco smoke (Z77.22)

exposure to tobacco smoke in the perinatal period (P96.81)

history of tobacco dependence (Z87.891)

occupational exposure to environmental tobacco smoke (Z57.31)

tobacco dependence (F17.-)

tobacco use (Z72.0)

Excludes1: malignant neoplasm of oral cavity NOS (C06.9)

C14.0   **Malignant neoplasm of pharynx, unspecified**

C14.2   **Malignant neoplasm of Waldeyer's ring**

C14.8   **Malignant neoplasm of overlapping sites of lip, oral cavity and pharynx**

Primary malignant neoplasm of two or more contiguous sites of lip, oral cavity and pharynx

> **Excludes1:** 'book leaf' neoplasm [ventral surface of tongue and floor of mouth] (C06.89)

MALIGNANT NEOPLASMS OF DIGESTIVE ORGANS (C15-C26)

Excludes1: Kaposi's sarcoma of gastrointestinal sites (C46.4)

Excludes2: gastrointestinal stromal tumors (C49.A-)

C15 **Malignant neoplasm of esophagus**

Use additional code to identify:

alcohol abuse and dependence (F10.-)

C15.3 **Malignant neoplasm of upper third of esophagus**

C15.4 **Malignant neoplasm of middle third of esophagus**

C15.5 **Malignant neoplasm of lower third of esophagus**

> **Excludes1:** malignant neoplasm of cardio-esophageal junction (C16.0)

C15.8 **Malignant neoplasm of overlapping sites of esophagus**

C15.9 **Malignant neoplasm of esophagus, unspecified**

C16 **Malignant neoplasm of stomach**

Use additional code to identify:

alcohol abuse and dependence (F10.-)

Excludes2: malignant carcinoid tumor of the stomach (C7A.092)

C16.0 **Malignant neoplasm of cardia**

Malignant neoplasm of cardiac orifice

Malignant neoplasm of cardio-esophageal junction

Malignant neoplasm of esophagus and stomach

Malignant neoplasm of gastro-esophageal junction

C16.1 **Malignant neoplasm of fundus of stomach**

C16.2 **Malignant neoplasm of body of stomach**

C16.3 **Malignant neoplasm of pyloric antrum**

Malignant neoplasm of gastric antrum

C16.4 **Malignant neoplasm of pylorus**

Malignant neoplasm of prepylorus

Malignant neoplasm of pyloric canal

C16.5 **Malignant neoplasm of lesser curvature of stomach, unspecified**

Malignant neoplasm of lesser curvature of stomach, not classifiable to C16.1-C16.4

C16.6 **Malignant neoplasm of greater curvature of stomach, unspecified**

Malignant neoplasm of greater curvature of stomach, not classifiable to C16.0-C16.4

C16.8 **Malignant neoplasm of overlapping sites of stomach**

C16.9 **Malignant neoplasm of stomach, unspecified**

Gastric cancer NOS

C17 **Malignant neoplasm of small intestine**

Excludes1: malignant carcinoid tumors of the small intestine (C7A.01)

C17.0 **Malignant neoplasm of duodenum**

C17.1 **Malignant neoplasm of jejunum**

C17.2 **Malignant neoplasm of ileum**

> **Excludes1:** malignant neoplasm of ileocecal valve (C18.0)

C17.3 **Meckel's diverticulum, malignant**

> **Excludes1:** Meckel's diverticulum, congenital (Q43.0)

C17.8 **Malignant neoplasm of overlapping sites of small intestine**

C17.9 **Malignant neoplasm of small intestine, unspecified**

C18 **Malignant neoplasm of colon**

Excludes1: malignant carcinoid tumors of the colon (C7A.02-)

C18.0 **Malignant neoplasm of cecum**

Malignant neoplasm of ileocecal valve

C18.1 **Malignant neoplasm of appendix**

C18.2 **Malignant neoplasm of ascending colon**

C18.3 **Malignant neoplasm of hepatic flexure**

C18.4 **Malignant neoplasm of transverse colon**

C18.5 **Malignant neoplasm of splenic flexure**

C18.6 **Malignant neoplasm of descending colon**

C18.7 **Malignant neoplasm of sigmoid colon**

Malignant neoplasm of sigmoid (flexure)

> **Excludes1:** malignant neoplasm of rectosigmoid junction (C19)

C18.8 **Malignant neoplasm of overlapping sites of colon**

C18.9 **Malignant neoplasm of colon, unspecified**

Malignant neoplasm of large intestine NOS

C19 **Malignant neoplasm of rectosigmoid junction**

Malignant neoplasm of colon with rectum

Malignant neoplasm of rectosigmoid (colon)

Excludes1: malignant carcinoid tumors of the colon (C7A.02-)

C20 **Malignant neoplasm of rectum**

Malignant neoplasm of rectal ampulla

Excludes1: malignant carcinoid tumor of the rectum (C7A.026)

C21 **Malignant neoplasm of anus and anal canal**

Excludes2: malignant carcinoid tumors of the colon (C7A.02-)

malignant melanoma of anal margin (C43.51)

malignant melanoma of anal skin (C43.51)

malignant melanoma of perianal skin (C43.51)

Other and unspecified malignant neoplasm of anal margin (C44.500, C44.510, C44.520, C44.590)

Other and unspecified malignant neoplasm of anal skin (C44.500, C44.510, C44.520, C44.590)

Other and unspecified malignant neoplasm of perianal skin (C44.500, C44.510, C44.520, C44.590)

C21.0 **Malignant neoplasm of anus, unspecified**

C21.1 **Malignant neoplasm of anal canal**

Malignant neoplasm of anal sphincter

C21.2 **Malignant neoplasm of cloacogenic zone**

C21.8 **Malignant neoplasm of overlapping sites of rectum, anus and anal canal**

Malignant neoplasm of anorectal junction

Malignant neoplasm of anorectum

Primary malignant neoplasm of two or more contiguous sites of rectum, anus and anal canal

C22 **Malignant neoplasm of liver and intrahepatic bile ducts**

Excludes1: malignant neoplasm of biliary tract NOS (C24.9)

secondary malignant neoplasm of liver and intrahepatic bile duct (C78.7)

Use additional code to identify:

alcohol abuse and dependence (F10.-)

hepatitis B (B16.-, B18.0-B18.1)

hepatitis C (B17.1-, B18.2)

C22.0 **Liver cell carcinoma**

Hepatocellular carcinoma

Hepatoma

C22.1 **Intrahepatic bile duct carcinoma**

Cholangiocarcinoma

> **Excludes1:** malignant neoplasm of hepatic duct (C24.0)

C22.2 **Hepatoblastoma**

● New code ▲ Revised code **Excludes1:** Not coded here **Excludes2:** Not included here ⊗ Placeholder required ⑦7th digit required

C22.3 **Angiosarcoma of liver**

Kupffer cell sarcoma

C22.4 **Other sarcomas of liver**

C22.7 **Other specified carcinomas of liver**

C22.8 **Malignant neoplasm of liver, primary, unspecified as to type**

C22.9 **Malignant neoplasm of liver, not specified as primary or secondary**

C23 **Malignant neoplasm of gallbladder**

C24 **Malignant neoplasm of other and unspecified parts of biliary tract**

> **Excludes1:** malignant neoplasm of intrahepatic bile duct (C22.1)

C24.0 **Malignant neoplasm of extrahepatic bile duct**

Malignant neoplasm of biliary duct or passage NOS

Malignant neoplasm of common bile duct

Malignant neoplasm of cystic duct

Malignant neoplasm of hepatic duct

C24.1 **Malignant neoplasm of ampulla of Vater**

C24.8 **Malignant neoplasm of overlapping sites of biliary tract**

Malignant neoplasm involving both intrahepatic and extrahepatic bile ducts

Primary malignant neoplasm of two or more contiguous sites of biliary tract

C24.9 **Malignant neoplasm of biliary tract, unspecified**

C25 **Malignant neoplasm of pancreas**

Code also exocrine pancreatic insufficiency (K86.81)

Use additional code to identify:

alcohol abuse and dependence (F10.-)

C25.0 **Malignant neoplasm of head of pancreas**

C25.1 **Malignant neoplasm of body of pancreas**

C25.2 **Malignant neoplasm of tail of pancreas**

C25.3 **Malignant neoplasm of pancreatic duct**

C25.4 **Malignant neoplasm of endocrine pancreas**

Malignant neoplasm of islets of Langerhans

Use additional code to identify any functional activity.

C25.7 **Malignant neoplasm of other parts of pancreas**

Malignant neoplasm of neck of pancreas

C25.8 **Malignant neoplasm of overlapping sites of pancreas**

C25.9 **Malignant neoplasm of pancreas, unspecified**

C26 **Malignant neoplasm of other and ill-defined digestive organs**

> **Excludes1:** malignant neoplasm of peritoneum and retroperitoneum (C48.-)

C26.0 **Malignant neoplasm of intestinal tract, part unspecified**

Malignant neoplasm of intestine NOS

C26.1 **Malignant neoplasm of spleen**

> **Excludes1:** Hodgkin lymphoma (C81.-)
>
> non-Hodgkin lymphoma (C82-C85)

C26.9 **Malignant neoplasm of ill-defined sites within the digestive system**

Malignant neoplasm of alimentary canal or tract NOS

Malignant neoplasm of gastrointestinal tract NOS

> **Excludes1:** malignant neoplasm of abdominal NOS (C76.2)
>
> malignant neoplasm of intra-abdominal NOS (C76.2)

MALIGNANT NEOPLASMS OF RESPIRATORY AND INTRATHORACIC ORGANS (C30-C39)

Includes: malignant neoplasm of middle ear

Excludes1: mesothelioma (C45.-)

C30 **Malignant neoplasm of nasal cavity and middle ear**

C30.0 **Malignant neoplasm of nasal cavity**

Malignant neoplasm of cartilage of nose

Malignant neoplasm of nasal concha

Malignant neoplasm of internal nose

Malignant neoplasm of septum of nose

Malignant neoplasm of vestibule of nose

> **Excludes1:** malignant neoplasm of nasal bone (C41.0)
>
> malignant neoplasm of nose NOS (C76.0)
>
> malignant neoplasm of olfactory bulb (C72.2-)
>
> malignant neoplasm of posterior margin of nasal septum and choana (C11.3)
>
> malignant melanoma of skin of nose (C43.31)
>
> malignant neoplasm of turbinates (C41.0)
>
> Other and unspecified malignant neoplasm of skin of nose C44.301, C44.311, C44.321, C44.391)

C30.1 **Malignant neoplasm of middle ear**

Malignant neoplasm of antrum tympanicum

Malignant neoplasm of auditory tube

Malignant neoplasm of eustachian tube

Malignant neoplasm of inner ear

Malignant neoplasm of mastoid air cells

Malignant neoplasm of tympanic cavity

> **Excludes1:** malignant neoplasm of auricular canal (external) (C43.2-,C44.2-)
>
> malignant neoplasm of bone of ear (meatus) (C41.0)
>
> malignant neoplasm of cartilage of ear (C49.0)
>
> malignant melanoma of skin of (external) ear (C43.2-)
>
> Other and unspecified malignant neoplasm of skin of (external) ear (C44.2-)

C31 **Malignant neoplasm of accessory sinuses**

C31.0 **Malignant neoplasm of maxillary sinus**

Malignant neoplasm of antrum (Highmore) (maxillary)

C31.1 **Malignant neoplasm of ethmoidal sinus**

C31.2 **Malignant neoplasm of frontal sinus**

C31.3 **Malignant neoplasm of sphenoid sinus**

C31.8 **Malignant neoplasm of overlapping sites of accessory sinuses**

C31.9 **Malignant neoplasm of accessory sinus, unspecified**

C32 **Malignant neoplasm of larynx**

Use additional code to identify:

alcohol abuse and dependence (F10.-)

exposure to environmental tobacco smoke (Z77.22)

exposure to tobacco smoke in the perinatal period (P96.81)

history of tobacco dependence (Z87.891)

occupational exposure to environmental tobacco smoke (Z57.31)

tobacco dependence (F17.-)

tobacco use (Z72.0)

C32.0 **Malignant neoplasm of glottis**

Malignant neoplasm of intrinsic larynx

Malignant neoplasm of laryngeal commissure (anterior)(posterior)

Malignant neoplasm of vocal cord (true) NOS

C32.1 **Malignant neoplasm of supraglottis**

Malignant neoplasm of aryepiglottic fold or interarytenoid fold, laryngeal aspect

Malignant neoplasm of epiglottis (suprahyoid portion) NOS

Add 4th-7th digits   Nonspecific code   Unspecified code   Manifestation code

Malignant neoplasm of extrinsic larynx

Malignant neoplasm of false vocal cord

Malignant neoplasm of posterior (laryngeal) surface of epiglottis

Malignant neoplasm of ventricular bands

Excludes2: malignant neoplasm of anterior surface of epiglottis (C10.1)

malignant neoplasm of aryepiglottic fold or interarytenoid fold, hypopharyngeal aspect (C13.1)

malignant neoplasm of aryepiglottic fold or interarytenoid fold, marginal zone (C13.1)

malignant neoplasm of aryepiglottic fold or interarytenoid fold NOS (C13.1)

C32.2 **Malignant neoplasm of subglottis**

C32.3 **Malignant neoplasm of laryngeal cartilage**

C32.8 **Malignant neoplasm of overlapping sites of larynx**

C32.9 **Malignant neoplasm of larynx, unspecified**

C33 **Malignant neoplasm of trachea**

Use additional code to identify:

exposure to environmental tobacco smoke (Z77.22)

exposure to tobacco smoke in the perinatal period (P96.81)

history of tobacco dependence (Z87.891)

occupational exposure to environmental tobacco smoke (Z57.31)

tobacco dependence (F17.-)

tobacco use (Z72.0)

C34 **Malignant neoplasm of bronchus and lung**

Use additional code to identify:

exposure to environmental tobacco smoke (Z77.22)

exposure to tobacco smoke in the perinatal period (P96.81)

history of tobacco dependence (Z87.891)

occupational exposure to environmental tobacco smoke (Z57.31)

tobacco dependence (F17.-)

tobacco use (Z72.0)

Excludes1: Kaposi's sarcoma of lung (C46.5-)

malignant carcinoid tumor of the bronchus and lung (C7A.090)

C34.0 **Malignant neoplasm of main bronchus**

Malignant neoplasm of carina

Malignant neoplasm of hilus (of lung)

C34.00 **Malignant neoplasm of unspecified main bronchus**

C34.01 **Malignant neoplasm of right main bronchus**

C34.02 **Malignant neoplasm of left main bronchus**

C34.1 **Malignant neoplasm of upper lobe, bronchus or lung**

C34.10 **Malignant neoplasm of upper lobe, unspecified bronchus or lung**

C34.11 **Malignant neoplasm of upper lobe, right bronchus or lung**

C34.12 **Malignant neoplasm of upper lobe, left bronchus or lung**

C34.2 **Malignant neoplasm of middle lobe, bronchus or lung**

C34.3 **Malignant neoplasm of lower lobe, bronchus or lung**

C34.30 **Malignant neoplasm of lower lobe, unspecified bronchus or lung**

C34.31 **Malignant neoplasm of lower lobe, right bronchus or lung**

C34.32 **Malignant neoplasm of lower lobe, left bronchus or lung**

C34.8 **Malignant neoplasm of overlapping sites of bronchus and lung**

C34.80 **Malignant neoplasm of overlapping sites of unspecified bronchus and lung**

C34.81 **Malignant neoplasm of overlapping sites of right bronchus and lung**

C34.82 **Malignant neoplasm of overlapping sites of left bronchus and lung**

C34.9 **Malignant neoplasm of unspecified part of bronchus or lung**

C34.90 **Malignant neoplasm of unspecified part of unspecified bronchus or lung**

Lung cancer NOS

C34.91 **Malignant neoplasm of unspecified part of right bronchus or lung**

C34.92 **Malignant neoplasm of unspecified part of left bronchus or lung**

C37 **Malignant neoplasm of thymus**

Excludes1: malignant carcinoid tumor of the thymus (C7A.091)

C38 **Malignant neoplasm of heart, mediastinum and pleura**

Excludes1: mesothelioma (C45.-)

C38.0 **Malignant neoplasm of heart**

Malignant neoplasm of pericardium

Excludes1: malignant neoplasm of great vessels (C49.3)

C38.1 **Malignant neoplasm of anterior mediastinum**

C38.2 **Malignant neoplasm of posterior mediastinum**

C38.3 **Malignant neoplasm of mediastinum, part unspecified**

C38.4 **Malignant neoplasm of pleura**

C38.8 **Malignant neoplasm of overlapping sites of heart, mediastinum and pleura**

C39 **Malignant neoplasm of other and ill-defined sites in the respiratory system and intrathoracic organs**

Use additional code to identify:

exposure to environmental tobacco smoke (Z77.22)

exposure to tobacco smoke in the perinatal period (P96.81)

history of tobacco dependence (Z87.891)

occupational exposure to environmental tobacco smoke (Z57.31)

tobacco dependence (F17.-)

tobacco use (Z72.0)

Excludes1: intrathoracic malignant neoplasm NOS (C76.1)

thoracic malignant neoplasm NOS (C76.1)

C39.0 **Malignant neoplasm of upper respiratory tract, part unspecified**

C39.9 **Malignant neoplasm of lower respiratory tract, part unspecified**

Malignant neoplasm of respiratory tract NOS

MALIGNANT NEOPLASMS OF BONE AND ARTICULAR CARTILAGE (C40-C41)

Includes: malignant neoplasm of cartilage (articular) (joint)

malignant neoplasm of periosteum

Excludes1: malignant neoplasm of bone marrow NOS (C96.9)

malignant neoplasm of synovia (C49.-)

C40 **Malignant neoplasm of bone and articular cartilage of limbs**

Use additional code to identify major osseous defect, if applicable (M89.7-)

C40.0 **Malignant neoplasm of scapula and long bones of upper limb**

C40.00 **Malignant neoplasm of scapula and long bones of unspecified upper limb**

● New code ▲ Revised code **Excludes1:** Not coded here **Excludes2:** Not included here ⊗ Placeholder required ⑦7th digit required

C40.01   Malignant neoplasm of scapula and long bones of right upper limb

C40.02   Malignant neoplasm of scapula and long bones of left upper limb

C40.1   **Malignant neoplasm of short bones of upper limb**

     C40.10   Malignant neoplasm of short bones of unspecified upper limb

     C40.11   Malignant neoplasm of short bones of right upper limb

     C40.12   Malignant neoplasm of short bones of left upper limb

C40.2   **Malignant neoplasm of long bones of lower limb**

     C40.20   Malignant neoplasm of long bones of unspecified lower limb

     C40.21   Malignant neoplasm of long bones of right lower limb

     C40.22   Malignant neoplasm of long bones of left lower limb

C40.3   **Malignant neoplasm of short bones of lower limb**

     C40.30   Malignant neoplasm of short bones of unspecified lower limb

     C40.31   Malignant neoplasm of short bones of right lower limb

     C40.32   Malignant neoplasm of short bones of left lower limb

C40.8   **Malignant neoplasm of overlapping sites of bone and articular cartilage of limb**

     C40.80   Malignant neoplasm of overlapping sites of bone and articular cartilage of unspecified limb

     C40.81   Malignant neoplasm of overlapping sites of bone and articular cartilage of right limb

     C40.82   Malignant neoplasm of overlapping sites of bone and articular cartilage of left limb

C40.9   **Malignant neoplasm of unspecified bones and articular cartilage of limb**

     C40.90   Malignant neoplasm of unspecified bones and articular cartilage of unspecified limb

     C40.91   Malignant neoplasm of unspecified bones and articular cartilage of right limb

     C40.92   Malignant neoplasm of unspecified bones and articular cartilage of left limb

C41   **Malignant neoplasm of bone and articular cartilage of other and unspecified sites**

     Excludes1: malignant neoplasm of bones of limbs (C40.-)

     malignant neoplasm of cartilage of ear (C49.0)

     malignant neoplasm of cartilage of eyelid (C49.0)

     malignant neoplasm of cartilage of larynx (C32.3)

     malignant neoplasm of cartilage of limbs (C40.-)

     malignant neoplasm of cartilage of nose (C30.0)

C41.0   **Malignant neoplasm of bones of skull and face**

     Malignant neoplasm of maxilla (superior)

     Malignant neoplasm of orbital bone

     Excludes2: carcinoma, any type except intraosseous or odontogenic of:

       maxillary sinus (C31.0)

       upper jaw (C03.0)

     malignant neoplasm of jaw bone (lower) (C41.1)

C41.1   **Malignant neoplasm of mandible**

     Malignant neoplasm of inferior maxilla

     Malignant neoplasm of lower jaw bone

     Excludes2: carcinoma, any type except intraosseous or odontogenic of:

       jaw NOS (C03.9)

       lower (C03.1)

     malignant neoplasm of upper jaw bone (C41.0)

C41.2   **Malignant neoplasm of vertebral column**

     Excludes1: malignant neoplasm of sacrum and coccyx (C41.4)

C41.3   **Malignant neoplasm of ribs, sternum and clavicle**

C41.4   **Malignant neoplasm of pelvic bones, sacrum and coccyx**

C41.9   **Malignant neoplasm of bone and articular cartilage, unspecified**

MELANOMA AND OTHER MALIGNANT NEOPLASMS OF SKIN (C43-C44)

C43   **Malignant melanoma of skin**

     Excludes1: melanoma in situ (D03.-)

     Excludes2: malignant melanoma of skin of genital organs (C51-C52, C60.-, C63.-)

     Merkel cell carcinoma (C4A.-)

     sites other than skin-code to malignant neoplasm of the site

C43.0   **Malignant melanoma of lip**

     Excludes1: malignant neoplasm of vermilion border of lip (C00.0-C00.2)

C43.1   **Malignant melanoma of eyelid, including canthus**

     C43.10   Malignant melanoma of unspecified eyelid, including canthus

     C43.11   Malignant melanoma of right eyelid, including canthus

     C43.12   Malignant melanoma of left eyelid, including canthus

C43.2   **Malignant melanoma of ear and external auricular canal**

     C43.20   Malignant melanoma of unspecified ear and external auricular canal

     C43.21   Malignant melanoma of right ear and external auricular canal

     C43.22   Malignant melanoma of left ear and external auricular canal

C43.3   **Malignant melanoma of other and unspecified parts of face**

     C43.30   Malignant melanoma of unspecified part of face

     C43.31   Malignant melanoma of nose

     C43.39   Malignant melanoma of other parts of face

C43.4   **Malignant melanoma of scalp and neck**

C43.5   **Malignant melanoma of trunk**

     Excludes2: malignant neoplasm of anus NOS (C21.0)

       malignant neoplasm of scrotum (C63.2)

     C43.51   Malignant melanoma of anal skin

       Malignant melanoma of anal margin

       Malignant melanoma of perianal skin

     C43.52   Malignant melanoma of skin of breast

     C43.59   Malignant melanoma of other part of trunk

C43.6   **Malignant melanoma of upper limb, including shoulder**

     C43.60   Malignant melanoma of unspecified upper limb, including shoulder

     C43.61   Malignant melanoma of right upper limb, including shoulder

     C43.62   Malignant melanoma of left upper limb, including shoulder

C43.7   **Malignant melanoma of lower limb, including hip**

     C43.70   Malignant melanoma of unspecified lower limb, including hip

---

C43.71 **Malignant melanoma of right lower limb, including hip**

C43.72 **Malignant melanoma of left lower limb, including hip**

C43.8 **Malignant melanoma of overlapping sites of skin**

C43.9 **Malignant melanoma of skin, unspecified**

Malignant melanoma of unspecified site of skin

Melanoma (malignant) NOS

C4A **Merkel cell carcinoma**

C4A.0 **Merkel cell carcinoma of lip**

Excludes1: malignant neoplasm of vermilion border of lip (C00.0-C00.2)

C4A.1 **Merkel cell carcinoma of eyelid, including canthus**

C4A.10 **Merkel cell carcinoma of unspecified eyelid, including canthus**

C4A.11 **Merkel cell carcinoma of right eyelid, including canthus**

C4A.12 **Merkel cell carcinoma of left eyelid, including canthus**

C4A.2 **Merkel cell carcinoma of ear and external auricular canal**

C4A.20 **Merkel cell carcinoma of unspecified ear and external auricular canal**

C4A.21 **Merkel cell carcinoma of right ear and external auricular canal**

C4A.22 **Merkel cell carcinoma of left ear and external auricular canal**

C4A.3 **Merkel cell carcinoma of other and unspecified parts of face**

C4A.30 **Merkel cell carcinoma of unspecified part of face**

C4A.31 **Merkel cell carcinoma of nose**

C4A.39 **Merkel cell carcinoma of other parts of face**

C4A.4 **Merkel cell carcinoma of scalp and neck**

C4A.5 **Merkel cell carcinoma of trunk**

Excludes2: malignant neoplasm of anus NOS (C21.0)

malignant neoplasm of scrotum (C63.2)

C4A.51 **Merkel cell carcinoma of anal skin**

Merkel cell carcinoma of anal margin

Merkel cell carcinoma of perianal skin

C4A.52 **Merkel cell carcinoma of skin of breast**

C4A.59 **Merkel cell carcinoma of other part of trunk**

C4A.6 **Merkel cell carcinoma of upper limb, including shoulder**

C4A.60 **Merkel cell carcinoma of unspecified upper limb, including shoulder**

C4A.61 **Merkel cell carcinoma of right upper limb, including shoulder**

C4A.62 **Merkel cell carcinoma of left upper limb, including shoulder**

C4A.7 **Merkel cell carcinoma of lower limb, including hip**

C4A.70 **Merkel cell carcinoma of unspecified lower limb, including hip**

C4A.71 **Merkel cell carcinoma of right lower limb, including hip**

C4A.72 **Merkel cell carcinoma of left lower limb, including hip**

C4A.8 **Merkel cell carcinoma of overlapping sites**

C4A.9 **Merkel cell carcinoma, unspecified**

Merkel cell carcinoma of unspecified site

Merkel cell carcinoma NOS

C44 **Other and unspecified malignant neoplasm of skin**

Includes: malignant neoplasm of sebaceous glands

malignant neoplasm of sweat glands

Excludes1: Kaposi's sarcoma of skin (C46.0)

malignant melanoma of skin (C43.-)

malignant neoplasm of skin of genital organs (C51-C52, C60.-, C63.2)

Merkel cell carcinoma (C4A.-)

C44.0 **Other and unspecified malignant neoplasm of skin of lip**

Excludes1: malignant neoplasm of lip (C00.-)

C44.00 **Unspecified malignant neoplasm of skin of lip**

C44.01 **Basal cell carcinoma of skin of lip**

C44.02 **Squamous cell carcinoma of skin of lip**

C44.09 **Other specified malignant neoplasm of skin of lip**

C44.1 **Other and unspecified malignant neoplasm of skin of eyelid, including canthus**

Excludes1: connective tissue of eyelid (C49.0)

C44.10 **Unspecified malignant neoplasm of skin of eyelid, including canthus**

C44.101 **Unspecified malignant neoplasm of skin of unspecified eyelid, including canthus**

C44.102 **Unspecified malignant neoplasm of skin of right eyelid, including canthus**

C44.109 **Unspecified malignant neoplasm of skin of left eyelid, including canthus**

C44.11 **Basal cell carcinoma of skin of eyelid, including canthus**

C44.111 **Basal cell carcinoma of skin of unspecified eyelid, including canthus**

C44.112 **Basal cell carcinoma of skin of right eyelid, including canthus**

C44.119 **Basal cell carcinoma of skin of left eyelid, including canthus**

C44.12 **Squamous cell carcinoma of skin of eyelid, including canthus**

C44.121 **Squamous cell carcinoma of skin of unspecified eyelid, including canthus**

C44.122 **Squamous cell carcinoma of skin of right eyelid, including canthus**

C44.129 **Squamous cell carcinoma of skin of left eyelid, including canthus**

C44.19 **Other specified malignant neoplasm of skin of eyelid, including canthus**

C44.191 **Other specified malignant neoplasm of skin of unspecified eyelid, including canthus**

C44.192 **Other specified malignant neoplasm of skin of right eyelid, including canthus**

C44.199 **Other specified malignant neoplasm of skin of left eyelid, including canthus**

C44.2 **Other and unspecified malignant neoplasm of skin of ear and external auricular canal**

Excludes1: connective tissue of ear (C49.0)

C44.20 **Unspecified malignant neoplasm of skin of ear and external auricular canal**

C44.201 **Unspecified malignant neoplasm of skin of unspecified ear and external auricular canal**

● New code ▲ Revised code **Excludes1:** Not coded here **Excludes2:** Not included here ⊗ Placeholder required ⑦7th digit required

C44.202 Unspecified malignant neoplasm of skin of right ear and external auricular canal

C44.209 Unspecified malignant neoplasm of skin of left ear and external auricular canal

C44.21 Basal cell carcinoma of skin of ear and external auricular canal

    C44.211 Basal cell carcinoma of skin of unspecified ear and external auricular canal

    C44.212 Basal cell carcinoma of skin of right ear and external auricular canal

    C44.219 Basal cell carcinoma of skin of left ear and external auricular canal

C44.22 Squamous cell carcinoma of skin of ear and external auricular canal

    C44.221 Squamous cell carcinoma of skin of unspecified ear and external auricular canal

    C44.222 Squamous cell carcinoma of skin of right ear and external auricular canal

    C44.229 Squamous cell carcinoma of skin of left ear and external auricular canal

C44.29 Other specified malignant neoplasm of skin of ear and external auricular canal

    C44.291 Other specified malignant neoplasm of skin of unspecified ear and external auricular canal

    C44.292 Other specified malignant neoplasm of skin of right ear and external auricular canal

    C44.299 Other specified malignant neoplasm of skin of left ear and external auricular canal

C44.3 Other and unspecified malignant neoplasm of skin of other and unspecified parts of face

C44.30 Unspecified malignant neoplasm of skin of other and unspecified parts of face

    C44.300 Unspecified malignant neoplasm of skin of unspecified part of face

    C44.301 Unspecified malignant neoplasm of skin of nose

    C44.309 Unspecified malignant neoplasm of skin of other parts of face

C44.31 Basal cell carcinoma of skin of other and unspecified parts of face

    C44.310 Basal cell carcinoma of skin of unspecified parts of face

    C44.311 Basal cell carcinoma of skin of nose

    C44.319 Basal cell carcinoma of skin of other parts of face

C44.32 Squamous cell carcinoma of skin of other and unspecified parts of face

    C44.320 Squamous cell carcinoma of skin of unspecified parts of face

    C44.321 Squamous cell carcinoma of skin of nose

    C44.329 Squamous cell carcinoma of skin of other parts of face

C44.39 Other specified malignant neoplasm of skin of other and unspecified parts of face

    C44.390 Other specified malignant neoplasm of skin of unspecified parts of face

C44.391 Other specified malignant neoplasm of skin of nose

C44.399 Other specified malignant neoplasm of skin of other parts of face

C44.4 Other and unspecified malignant neoplasm of skin of scalp and neck

C44.40 Unspecified malignant neoplasm of skin of scalp and neck

C44.41 Basal cell carcinoma of skin of scalp and neck

C44.42 Squamous cell carcinoma of skin of scalp and neck

C44.49 Other specified malignant neoplasm of skin of scalp and neck

C44.5 Other and unspecified malignant neoplasm of skin of trunk

Excludes1: anus NOS (C21.0)

    scrotum (C63.2)

C44.50 Unspecified malignant neoplasm of skin of trunk

    C44.500 Unspecified malignant neoplasm of anal skin

        Unspecified malignant neoplasm of anal margin

        Unspecified malignant neoplasm of perianal skin

    C44.501 Unspecified malignant neoplasm of skin of breast

    C44.509 Unspecified malignant neoplasm of skin of other part of trunk

C44.51 Basal cell carcinoma of skin of trunk

    C44.510 Basal cell carcinoma of anal skin

        Basal cell carcinoma of anal margin

        Basal cell carcinoma of perianal skin

    C44.511 Basal cell carcinoma of skin of breast

    C44.519 Basal cell carcinoma of skin of other part of trunk

C44.52 Squamous cell carcinoma of skin of trunk

    C44.520 Squamous cell carcinoma of anal skin

        Squamous cell carcinoma of anal margin

        Squamous cell carcinoma of perianal skin

    C44.521 Squamous cell carcinoma of skin of breast

    C44.529 Squamous cell carcinoma of skin of other part of trunk

C44.59 Other specified malignant neoplasm of skin of trunk

    C44.590 Other specified malignant neoplasm of anal skin

        Other specified malignant neoplasm of anal margin

        Other specified malignant neoplasm of perianal skin

    C44.591 Other specified malignant neoplasm of skin of breast

    C44.599 Other specified malignant neoplasm of skin of other part of trunk

C44.6 Other and unspecified malignant neoplasm of skin of upper limb, including shoulder

C44.60 Unspecified malignant neoplasm of skin of upper limb, including shoulder

---

C44.601 Unspecified malignant neoplasm of skin of unspecified upper limb, including shoulder

C44.602 Unspecified malignant neoplasm of skin of right upper limb, including shoulder

C44.609 Unspecified malignant neoplasm of skin of left upper limb, including shoulder

C44.61 Basal cell carcinoma of skin of upper limb, including shoulder

C44.611 Basal cell carcinoma of skin of unspecified upper limb, including shoulder

C44.612 Basal cell carcinoma of skin of right upper limb, including shoulder

C44.619 Basal cell carcinoma of skin of left upper limb, including shoulder

C44.62 Squamous cell carcinoma of skin of upper limb, including shoulder

C44.621 Squamous cell carcinoma of skin of unspecified upper limb, including shoulder

C44.622 Squamous cell carcinoma of skin of right upper limb, including shoulder

C44.629 Squamous cell carcinoma of skin of left upper limb, including shoulder

C44.69 Other specified malignant neoplasm of skin of upper limb, including shoulder

C44.691 Other specified malignant neoplasm of skin of unspecified upper limb, including shoulder

C44.692 Other specified malignant neoplasm of skin of right upper limb, including shoulder

C44.699 Other specified malignant neoplasm of skin of left upper limb, including shoulder

C44.7 Other and unspecified malignant neoplasm of skin of lower limb, including hip

C44.70 Unspecified malignant neoplasm of skin of lower limb, including hip

C44.701 Unspecified malignant neoplasm of skin of unspecified lower limb, including hip

C44.702 Unspecified malignant neoplasm of skin of right lower limb, including hip

C44.709 Unspecified malignant neoplasm of skin of left lower limb, including hip

C44.71 Basal cell carcinoma of skin of lower limb, including hip

C44.711 Basal cell carcinoma of skin of unspecified lower limb, including hip

C44.712 Basal cell carcinoma of skin of right lower limb, including hip

C44.719 Basal cell carcinoma of skin of left lower limb, including hip

C44.72 Squamous cell carcinoma of skin of lower limb, including hip

C44.721 Squamous cell carcinoma of skin of unspecified lower limb, including hip

C44.722 Squamous cell carcinoma of skin of right lower limb, including hi

C44.729 Squamous cell carcinoma of skin of left lower limb, including hip

C44.79 Other specified malignant neoplasm of skin of lower limb, including hip

C44.791 Other specified malignant neoplasm of skin of unspecified lower limb, including hip

C44.792 Other specified malignant neoplasm of skin of right lower limb, including hip

C44.799 Other specified malignant neoplasm of skin of left lower limb, including hip

C44.8 Other and unspecified malignant neoplasm of overlapping sites of skin

C44.80 Unspecified malignant neoplasm of overlapping sites of skin

C44.81 Basal cell carcinoma of overlapping sites of skin

C44.82 Squamous cell carcinoma of overlapping sites of skin

C44.89 Other specified malignant neoplasm of overlapping sites of skin

C44.9 Other and unspecified malignant neoplasm of skin, unspecified

C44.90 Unspecified malignant neoplasm of skin, unspecified

Malignant neoplasm of unspecified site of skin

C44.91 Basal cell carcinoma of skin, unspecified

C44.92 Squamous cell carcinoma of skin, unspecified

C44.99 Other specified malignant neoplasm of skin, unspecified

MALIGNANT NEOPLASMS OF MESOTHELIAL AND SOFT TISSUE (C45-C49)

C45 Mesothelioma

C45.0 Mesothelioma of pleura

Excludes1: Other malignant neoplasm of pleura (C38.4)

C45.1 Mesothelioma of peritoneum

Mesothelioma of cul-de-sac

Mesothelioma of mesentery

Mesothelioma of mesocolon

Mesothelioma of omentum

Mesothelioma of peritoneum (parietal) (pelvic)

Excludes1: Other malignant neoplasm of soft tissue of peritoneum (C48.-)

C45.2 Mesothelioma of pericardium

Excludes1: Other malignant neoplasm of pericardium (C38.0)

C45.7 Mesothelioma of other sites

C45.9 Mesothelioma, unspecified

C46 Kaposi's sarcoma

Definition: Kaposi's sarcoma is a form of skin cancer that can involve internal organs. It is most often found in patients with acquired immunodeficiency syndrome (AIDS), and can be fatal.

Code first any human immunodeficiency virus [HIV] disease (B20)

C46.0 Kaposi's sarcoma of skin

C46.1 Kaposi's sarcoma of soft tissue

Kaposi's sarcoma of blood vessel

Kaposi's sarcoma of connective tissue

Kaposi's sarcoma of fascia

Kaposi's sarcoma of ligament

Kaposi's sarcoma of lymphatic(s) NEC

Kaposi's sarcoma of muscle

Excludes2: Kaposi's sarcoma of lymph glands and nodes (C46.3)

C46.2 **Kaposi's sarcoma of palate**

C46.3 **Kaposi's sarcoma of lymph nodes**

C46.4 **Kaposi's sarcoma of gastrointestinal sites**

C46.5 **Kaposi's sarcoma of lung**

    C46.50 **Kaposi's sarcoma of unspecified lung**

    C46.51 **Kaposi's sarcoma of right lung**

    C46.52 **Kaposi's sarcoma of left lung**

C46.7 **Kaposi's sarcoma of other sites**

C46.9 **Kaposi's sarcoma, unspecified**

    Kaposi's sarcoma of unspecified site

C47 **Malignant neoplasm of peripheral nerves and autonomic nervous system**

Includes: malignant neoplasm of sympathetic and parasympathetic nerves and ganglia

Excludes1: Kaposi's sarcoma of soft tissue (C46.1)

C47.0 **Malignant neoplasm of peripheral nerves of head, face and neck**

    Excludes1: malignant neoplasm of peripheral nerves of orbit (C69.6-)

C47.1 **Malignant neoplasm of peripheral nerves of upper limb, including shoulder**

    C47.10 **Malignant neoplasm of peripheral nerves of unspecified upper limb, including shoulder**

    C47.11 **Malignant neoplasm of peripheral nerves of right upper limb, including shoulder**

    C47.12 **Malignant neoplasm of peripheral nerves of left upper limb, including shoulder**

C47.2 **Malignant neoplasm of peripheral nerves of lower limb, including hip**

    C47.20 **Malignant neoplasm of peripheral nerves of unspecified lower limb, including hip**

    C47.21 **Malignant neoplasm of peripheral nerves of right lower limb, including hip**

    C47.22 **Malignant neoplasm of peripheral nerves of left lower limb, including hip**

C47.3 **Malignant neoplasm of peripheral nerves of thorax**

C47.4 **Malignant neoplasm of peripheral nerves of abdomen**

C47.5 **Malignant neoplasm of peripheral nerves of pelvis**

C47.6 **Malignant neoplasm of peripheral nerves of trunk, unspecified**

    Malignant neoplasm of peripheral nerves of unspecified part of trunk

C47.8 **Malignant neoplasm of overlapping sites of peripheral nerves and autonomic nervous system**

C47.9 **Malignant neoplasm of peripheral nerves and autonomic nervous system, unspecified**

    Malignant neoplasm of unspecified site of peripheral nerves and autonomic nervous system

C48 **Malignant neoplasm of retroperitoneum and peritoneum**

Excludes1: Kaposi's sarcoma of connective tissue (C46.1)

    mesothelioma (C45.-)

C48.0 **Malignant neoplasm of retroperitoneum**

C48.1 **Malignant neoplasm of specified parts of peritoneum**

    Malignant neoplasm of cul-de-sac

    Malignant neoplasm of mesentery

    Malignant neoplasm of mesocolon

    Malignant neoplasm of omentum

    Malignant neoplasm of parietal peritoneum

    Malignant neoplasm of pelvic peritoneum

C48.2 **Malignant neoplasm of peritoneum, unspecified**

C48.8 **Malignant neoplasm of overlapping sites of retroperitoneum and peritoneum**

C49 **Malignant neoplasm of other connective and soft tissue**

Includes: malignant neoplasm of blood vessel

    malignant neoplasm of bursa

    malignant neoplasm of cartilage

    malignant neoplasm of fascia

    malignant neoplasm of fat

    malignant neoplasm of ligament, except uterine

    malignant neoplasm of lymphatic vessel

    malignant neoplasm of muscle

    malignant neoplasm of synovia

    malignant neoplasm of tendon (sheath)

Excludes1: malignant neoplasm of cartilage (of):

    articular (C40-C41)

    larynx (C32.3)

    nose (C30.0)

    malignant neoplasm of connective tissue of breast (C50.-)

Excludes2: Kaposi's sarcoma of soft tissue (C46.1)

    malignant neoplasm of heart (C38.0)

    malignant neoplasm of peripheral nerves and autonomic nervous system (C47.-)

    malignant neoplasm of peritoneum (C48.2)

    malignant neoplasm of retroperitoneum (C48.0)

    malignant neoplasm of uterine ligament (C57.3)

    mesothelioma (C45.-)

C49.0 **Malignant neoplasm of connective and soft tissue of head, face and neck**

    Malignant neoplasm of connective tissue of ear

    Malignant neoplasm of connective tissue of eyelid

    Excludes1: connective tissue of orbit (C69.6-)

C49.1 **Malignant neoplasm of connective and soft tissue of upper limb, including shoulder**

    C49.10 **Malignant neoplasm of connective and soft tissue of unspecified upper limb, including shoulder**

    C49.11 **Malignant neoplasm of connective and soft tissue of right upper limb, including shoulder**

    C49.12 **Malignant neoplasm of connective and soft tissue of left upper limb, including shoulder**

C49.2 **Malignant neoplasm of connective and soft tissue of lower limb, including hip**

    C49.20 **Malignant neoplasm of connective and soft tissue of unspecified lower limb, including hip**

    C49.21 **Malignant neoplasm of connective and soft tissue of right lower limb, including hip**

    C49.22 **Malignant neoplasm of connective and soft tissue of left lower limb, including hip**

C49.3 **Malignant neoplasm of connective and soft tissue of thorax**

    Malignant neoplasm of axilla

    Malignant neoplasm of diaphragm

    Malignant neoplasm of great vessels

    Excludes1: malignant neoplasm of breast (C50.-)

    malignant neoplasm of heart (C38.0)

    malignant neoplasm of mediastinum (C38.1-C38.3)

    malignant neoplasm of thymus (C37)

C49.4 **Malignant neoplasm of connective and soft tissue of abdomen**

Malignant neoplasm of abdominal wall

Malignant neoplasm of hypochondrium

C49.5 **Malignant neoplasm of connective and soft tissue of pelvis**

Malignant neoplasm of buttock

Malignant neoplasm of groin

Malignant neoplasm of perineum

C49.6 **Malignant neoplasm of connective and soft tissue of trunk, unspecified**

Malignant neoplasm of back NOS

C49.8 **Malignant neoplasm of overlapping sites of connective and soft tissue**

Primary malignant neoplasm of two or more contiguous sites of connective and soft tissue

C49.9 **Malignant neoplasm of connective and soft tissue, unspecified**

C49.A **Gastrointestinal stromal tumor**

C49.A0 **Gastrointestinal stromal tumor, unspecified site**

C49.A1 **Gastrointestinal stromal tumor of esophagus**

C49.A2 **Gastrointestinal stromal tumor of stomach**

C49.A3 **Gastrointestinal stromal tumor of small intestine**

C49.A4 **Gastrointestinal stromal tumor of large intestine**

C49.A5 **Gastrointestinal stromal tumor of rectum**

C49.A9 **Gastrointestinal stromal tumor of other sites**

MALIGNANT NEOPLASMS OF BREAST (C50)

C50 **Malignant neoplasm of breast**

Includes: connective tissue of breast

Paget's disease of breast

Paget's disease of nipple

Use additional code to identify estrogen receptor status (Z17.0, Z17.1)

Excludes1: skin of breast (C44.501, C44.511, C44.521, C44.591)

C50.0 **Malignant neoplasm of nipple and areola**

C50.01 **Malignant neoplasm of nipple and areola, female**

C50.011 **Malignant neoplasm of nipple and areola, right female breast**

C50.012 **Malignant neoplasm of nipple and areola, left female breast**

C50.019 **Malignant neoplasm of nipple and areola, unspecified female breast**

C50.02 **Malignant neoplasm of nipple and areola, male**

C50.021 **Malignant neoplasm of nipple and areola, right male breast**

C50.022 **Malignant neoplasm of nipple and areola, left male breast**

C50.029 **Malignant neoplasm of nipple and areola, unspecified male breast**

C50.1 **Malignant neoplasm of central portion of breast**

C50.11 **Malignant neoplasm of central portion of breast, female**

C50.111 **Malignant neoplasm of central portion of right female breast**

C50.112 **Malignant neoplasm of central portion of left female breast**

C50.119 **Malignant neoplasm of central portion of unspecified female breast**

C50.12 **Malignant neoplasm of central portion of breast, male**

C50.121 **Malignant neoplasm of central portion of right male breast**

C50.122 **Malignant neoplasm of central portion of left male breast**

C50.129 **Malignant neoplasm of central portion of unspecified male breast**

C50.2 **Malignant neoplasm of upper-inner quadrant of breast**

C50.21 **Malignant neoplasm of upper-inner quadrant of breast, female**

C50.211 **Malignant neoplasm of upper-inner quadrant of right female breast**

C50.212 **Malignant neoplasm of upper-inner quadrant of left female breast**

C50.219 **Malignant neoplasm of upper-inner quadrant of unspecified female breast**

C50.22 **Malignant neoplasm of upper-inner quadrant of breast, male**

C50.221 **Malignant neoplasm of upper-inner quadrant of right male breast**

C50.222 **Malignant neoplasm of upper-inner quadrant of left male breast**

C50.229 **Malignant neoplasm of upper-inner quadrant of unspecified male breast**

C50.3 **Malignant neoplasm of lower-inner quadrant of breast**

C50.31 **Malignant neoplasm of lower-inner quadrant of breast, female**

C50.311 **Malignant neoplasm of lower-inner quadrant of right female breast**

C50.312 **Malignant neoplasm of lower-inner quadrant of left female breast**

C50.319 **Malignant neoplasm of lower-inner quadrant of unspecified female breast**

C50.32 **Malignant neoplasm of lower-inner quadrant of breast, male**

C50.321 **Malignant neoplasm of lower-inner quadrant of right male breast**

C50.322 **Malignant neoplasm of lower-inner quadrant of left male breast**

C50.329 **Malignant neoplasm of lower-inner quadrant of unspecified male breast**

C50.4 **Malignant neoplasm of upper-outer quadrant of breast**

C50.41 **Malignant neoplasm of upper-outer quadrant of breast, female**

C50.411 **Malignant neoplasm of upper-outer quadrant of right female breast**

C50.412 **Malignant neoplasm of upper-outer quadrant of left female breast**

C50.419 **Malignant neoplasm of upper-outer quadrant of unspecified female breast**

C50.42 **Malignant neoplasm of upper-outer quadrant of breast, male**

C50.421 **Malignant neoplasm of upper-outer quadrant of right male breast**

C50.422 **Malignant neoplasm of upper-outer quadrant of left male breast**

C50.429 **Malignant neoplasm of upper-outer quadrant of unspecified male breast**

C50.5   **Malignant neoplasm of lower-outer quadrant of breast**

    C50.51   **Malignant neoplasm of lower-outer quadrant of breast, female**

      C50.511   **Malignant neoplasm of lower-outer quadrant of right female breast**

      C50.512   **Malignant neoplasm of lower-outer quadrant of left female breast**

      C50.519   **Malignant neoplasm of lower-outer quadrant of unspecified female breast**

    C50.52   **Malignant neoplasm of lower-outer quadrant of breast, male**

      C50.521   **Malignant neoplasm of lower-outer quadrant of right male breast**

      C50.522   **Malignant neoplasm of lower-outer quadrant of left male breast**

      C50.529   **Malignant neoplasm of lower-outer quadrant of unspecified male breast**

C50.6   **Malignant neoplasm of axillary tail of breast**

    C50.61   **Malignant neoplasm of axillary tail of breast, female**

      C50.611   **Malignant neoplasm of axillary tail of right female breast**

      C50.612   **Malignant neoplasm of axillary tail of left female breast**

      C50.619   **Malignant neoplasm of axillary tail of unspecified female breast**

    C50.62   **Malignant neoplasm of axillary tail of breast, male**

      C50.621   **Malignant neoplasm of axillary tail of right male breast**

      C50.622   **Malignant neoplasm of axillary tail of left male breast**

      C50.629   **Malignant neoplasm of axillary tail of unspecified male breast**

C50.8   **Malignant neoplasm of overlapping sites of breast**

    C50.81   **Malignant neoplasm of overlapping sites of breast, female**

      C50.811   **Malignant neoplasm of overlapping sites of right female breast**

      C50.812   **Malignant neoplasm of overlapping sites of left female breast**

      C50.819   **Malignant neoplasm of overlapping sites of unspecified female breast**

    C50.82   **Malignant neoplasm of overlapping sites of breast, male**

      C50.821   **Malignant neoplasm of overlapping sites of right male breast**

      C50.822   **Malignant neoplasm of overlapping sites of left male breast**

      C50.829   **Malignant neoplasm of overlapping sites of unspecified male breast**

C50.9   **Malignant neoplasm of breast of unspecified site**

    C50.91   **Malignant neoplasm of breast of unspecified site, female**

      C50.911   **Malignant neoplasm of unspecified site of right female breast**

      C50.912   **Malignant neoplasm of unspecified site of left female breast**

      C50.919   **Malignant neoplasm of unspecified site of unspecified female breast**

    C50.92   **Malignant neoplasm of breast of unspecified site, male**

      C50.921   **Malignant neoplasm of unspecified site of right male breast**

      C50.922   **Malignant neoplasm of unspecified site of left male breast**

      C50.929   **Malignant neoplasm of unspecified site of unspecified male breast**

MALIGNANT NEOPLASMS OF FEMALE GENITAL ORGANS (C51-C58)

NOTE: ALL DIAGNOSIS CODES IN THIS SECTION APPLY TO FEMALE PATIENTS ONLY

Includes: malignant neoplasm of skin of female genital organs

C51   **Malignant neoplasm of vulva**

  Excludes1: carcinoma in situ of vulva (D07.1)

    C51.0   **Malignant neoplasm of labium majus**

      Malignant neoplasm of Bartholin's [greater vestibular] gland

    C51.1   **Malignant neoplasm of labium minus**

    C51.2   **Malignant neoplasm of clitoris**

    C51.8   **Malignant neoplasm of overlapping sites of vulva**

    C51.9   **Malignant neoplasm of vulva, unspecified**

      Malignant neoplasm of external female genitalia NOS

      Malignant neoplasm of pudendum

C52   **Malignant neoplasm of vagina**

  Excludes1: carcinoma in situ of vagina (D07.2)

C53   **Malignant neoplasm of cervix uteri**

  Excludes1: carcinoma in situ of cervix uteri (D06.-)

    C53.0   **Malignant neoplasm of endocervix**

    C53.1   **Malignant neoplasm of exocervix**

    C53.8   **Malignant neoplasm of overlapping sites of cervix uteri**

    C53.9   **Malignant neoplasm of cervix uteri, unspecified**

C54   **Malignant neoplasm of corpus uteri**

    C54.0   **Malignant neoplasm of isthmus uteri**

      Malignant neoplasm of lower uterine segment

    C54.1   **Malignant neoplasm of endometrium**

    C54.2   **Malignant neoplasm of myometrium**

    C54.3   **Malignant neoplasm of fundus uteri**

    C54.8   **Malignant neoplasm of overlapping sites of corpus uteri**

    C54.9   **Malignant neoplasm of corpus uteri, unspecified**

C55   **Malignant neoplasm of uterus, part unspecified**

C56   **Malignant neoplasm of ovary**

  Use additional code to identify any functional activity

    C56.1   **Malignant neoplasm of right ovary**

    C56.2   **Malignant neoplasm of left ovary**

    C56.9   **Malignant neoplasm of unspecified ovary**

C57   **Malignant neoplasm of other and unspecified female genital organs**

    C57.0   **Malignant neoplasm of fallopian tube**

      Malignant neoplasm of oviduct

      Malignant neoplasm of uterine tube

      C57.00   **Malignant neoplasm of unspecified fallopian tube**

      C57.01   **Malignant neoplasm of right fallopian tube**

      C57.02   **Malignant neoplasm of left fallopian tube**

    C57.1   **Malignant neoplasm of broad ligament**

      C57.10   **Malignant neoplasm of unspecified broad ligament**

      C57.11   **Malignant neoplasm of right broad ligament**

      C57.12   **Malignant neoplasm of left broad ligament**

    C57.2   **Malignant neoplasm of round ligament**

C57.20   **Malignant neoplasm of unspecified round ligament**

C57.21   **Malignant neoplasm of right round ligament**

C57.22   **Malignant neoplasm of left round ligament**

C57.3   **Malignant neoplasm of parametrium**

Malignant neoplasm of uterine ligament NOS

C57.4   **Malignant neoplasm of uterine adnexa, unspecified**

C57.7   **Malignant neoplasm of other specified female genital organs**

Malignant neoplasm of wolffian body or duct

C57.8   **Malignant neoplasm of overlapping sites of female genital organs**

Primary malignant neoplasm of two or more contiguous sites of the female genital organs whose point of origin cannot be determined

Primary tubo-ovarian malignant neoplasm whose point of origin cannot be determined Primary utero-ovarian malignant neoplasm whose point of origin cannot be determined

C57.9   **Malignant neoplasm of female genital organ, unspecified**

Malignant neoplasm of female genitourinary tract NOS

C58   **Malignant neoplasm of placenta**

Includes: choriocarcinoma NOS

chorionepithelioma NOS

Excludes1: chorioadenoma (destruens) (D39.2)

hydatidiform mole NOS (O01.9)

invasive hydatidiform mole (D39.2)

male choriocarcinoma NOS (C62.9-)

malignant hydatidiform mole (D39.2)

MALIGNANT NEOPLASMS OF MALE GENITAL ORGANS (C60-C63)

NOTE: ALL DIAGNOSIS CODES IN THIS SECTION APPLY TO MALE PATIENTS ONLY

Includes: malignant neoplasm of skin of male genital organs

C60   **Malignant neoplasm of penis**

C60.0   **Malignant neoplasm of prepuce**

Malignant neoplasm of foreskin

C60.1   **Malignant neoplasm of glans penis**

C60.2   **Malignant neoplasm of body of penis**

Malignant neoplasm of corpus cavernosum

C60.8   **Malignant neoplasm of overlapping sites of penis**

C60.9   **Malignant neoplasm of penis, unspecified**

Malignant neoplasm of skin of penis NOS

C61   **Malignant neoplasm of prostate**

Use additional code to identify:

hormone sensitivity status (Z19.1-Z19.2)

rising PSA following treatment for malignant neoplasm of prostate (R97.21)

Excludes1: malignant neoplasm of seminal vesicle (C63.7)

C62   **Malignant neoplasm of testis**

Use additional code to identify any functional activity

C62.0   **Malignant neoplasm of undescended testis**

Malignant neoplasm of ectopic testis

Malignant neoplasm of retained testis

C62.00   **Malignant neoplasm of unspecified undescended testis**

C62.01   **Malignant neoplasm of undescended right testis**

C62.02   **Malignant neoplasm of undescended left testis**

C62.1   **Malignant neoplasm of descended testis**

Malignant neoplasm of scrotal testis

C62.10   **Malignant neoplasm of unspecified descended testis**

C62.11   **Malignant neoplasm of descended right testis**

C62.12   **Malignant neoplasm of descended left testis**

C62.9   **Malignant neoplasm of testis, unspecified whether descended or undescended**

C62.90   **Malignant neoplasm of unspecified testis, unspecified whether descended or undescended**

Malignant neoplasm of testis NOS

C62.91   **Malignant neoplasm of right testis, unspecified whether descended or undescended**

C62.92   **Malignant neoplasm of left testis, unspecified whether descended or undescended**

C63   **Malignant neoplasm of other and unspecified male genital organs**

C63.0   **Malignant neoplasm of epididymis**

C63.00   **Malignant neoplasm of unspecified epididymis**

C63.01   **Malignant neoplasm of right epididymis**

C63.02   **Malignant neoplasm of left epididymis**

C63.1   **Malignant neoplasm of spermatic cord**

C63.10   **Malignant neoplasm of unspecified spermatic cord**

C63.11   **Malignant neoplasm of right spermatic cord**

C63.12   **Malignant neoplasm of left spermatic cord**

C63.2   **Malignant neoplasm of scrotum**

Malignant neoplasm of skin of scrotum

C63.7   **Malignant neoplasm of other specified male genital organs**

Malignant neoplasm of seminal vesicle

Malignant neoplasm of tunica vaginalis

C63.8   **Malignant neoplasm of overlapping sites of male genital organs**

Primary malignant neoplasm of two or more contiguous sites of male genital organs whose point of origin cannot be determined

C63.9   **Malignant neoplasm of male genital organ, unspecified**

Malignant neoplasm of male genitourinary tract NOS

MALIGNANT NEOPLASMS OF URINARY TRACT (C64-C68)

C64   **Malignant neoplasm of kidney, except renal pelvis**

Excludes1: malignant carcinoid tumor of the kidney (C7A.093)

malignant neoplasm of renal calyces (C65.-)

malignant neoplasm of renal pelvis (C65.-)

C64.1   **Malignant neoplasm of right kidney, except renal pelvis**

C64.2   **Malignant neoplasm of left kidney, except renal pelvis**

C64.9   **Malignant neoplasm of unspecified kidney, except renal pelvis**

C65   **Malignant neoplasm of renal pelvis**

Includes: malignant neoplasm of pelviureteric junction

malignant neoplasm of renal calyces

C65.1   **Malignant neoplasm of right renal pelvis**

C65.2   **Malignant neoplasm of left renal pelvis**

C65.9   **Malignant neoplasm of unspecified renal pelvis**

C66   **Malignant neoplasm of ureter**

Excludes1: malignant neoplasm of ureteric orifice of bladder (C67.6)

C66.1   **Malignant neoplasm of right ureter**

C66.2   **Malignant neoplasm of left ureter**

C66.9   **Malignant neoplasm of unspecified ureter**

C67 **Malignant neoplasm of bladder**

   C67.0   **Malignant neoplasm of trigone of bladder**

   C67.1   **Malignant neoplasm of dome of bladder**

   C67.2   **Malignant neoplasm of lateral wall of bladder**

   C67.3   **Malignant neoplasm of anterior wall of bladder**

   C67.4   **Malignant neoplasm of posterior wall of bladder**

   C67.5   **Malignant neoplasm of bladder neck**

      Malignant neoplasm of internal urethral orifice

   C67.6   **Malignant neoplasm of ureteric orifice**

   C67.7   **Malignant neoplasm of urachus**

   C67.8   **Malignant neoplasm of overlapping sites of bladder**

   C67.9   **Malignant neoplasm of bladder, unspecified**

C68 **Malignant neoplasm of other and unspecified urinary organs**

   Excludes1: malignant neoplasm of female genitourinary tract NOS (C57.9)

   malignant neoplasm of male genitourinary tract NOS (C63.9)

   C68.0   **Malignant neoplasm of urethra**

      Excludes1: malignant neoplasm of urethral orifice of bladder (C67.5)

   C68.1   **Malignant neoplasm of paraurethral glands**

   C68.8   **Malignant neoplasm of overlapping sites of urinary organs**

      Primary malignant neoplasm of two or more contiguous sites of urinary organs whose point of origin cannot be determined

   C68.9   **Malignant neoplasm of urinary organ, unspecified**

      Malignant neoplasm of urinary system NOS

MALIGNANT NEOPLASMS OF EYE, BRAIN AND OTHER PARTS OF CENTRAL NERVOUS SYSTEM (C69-C72)

C69 **Malignant neoplasm of eye and adnexa**

   Excludes1: malignant neoplasm of connective tissue of eyelid (C49.0)

      malignant neoplasm of eyelid (skin) (C43.1-, C44.1-)

      malignant neoplasm of optic nerve (C72.3-)

   C69.0   **Malignant neoplasm of conjunctiva**

      C69.00   **Malignant neoplasm of unspecified conjunctiva**

      C69.01   **Malignant neoplasm of right conjunctiva**

      C69.02   **Malignant neoplasm of left conjunctiva**

   C69.1   **Malignant neoplasm of cornea**

      C69.10   **Malignant neoplasm of unspecified cornea**

      C69.11   **Malignant neoplasm of right cornea**

      C69.12   **Malignant neoplasm of left cornea**

   C69.2   **Malignant neoplasm of retina**

      Excludes1: dark area on retina (D49.81)

         neoplasm of unspecified behavior of retina and choroid (D49.81)

         retinal freckle (D49.81)

      C69.20   **Malignant neoplasm of unspecified retina**

      C69.21   **Malignant neoplasm of right retina**

      C69.22   **Malignant neoplasm of left retina**

   C69.3   **Malignant neoplasm of choroid**

      C69.30   **Malignant neoplasm of unspecified choroid**

      C69.31   **Malignant neoplasm of right choroid**

      C69.32   **Malignant neoplasm of left choroid**

   C69.4   **Malignant neoplasm of ciliary body**

      C69.40   **Malignant neoplasm of unspecified ciliary body**

      C69.41   **Malignant neoplasm of right ciliary body**

      C69.42   **Malignant neoplasm of left ciliary body**

   C69.5   **Malignant neoplasm of lacrimal gland and duct**

      Malignant neoplasm of lacrimal sac

      Malignant neoplasm of nasolacrimal duct

      C69.50   **Malignant neoplasm of unspecified lacrimal gland and duct**

      C69.51   **Malignant neoplasm of right lacrimal gland and duct**

      C69.52   **Malignant neoplasm of left lacrimal gland and duct**

   C69.6   **Malignant neoplasm of orbit**

      Malignant neoplasm of connective tissue of orbit

      Malignant neoplasm of extraocular muscle

      Malignant neoplasm of peripheral nerves of orbit

      Malignant neoplasm of retrobulbar tissue

      Malignant neoplasm of retro-ocular tissue

      Excludes1: malignant neoplasm of orbital bone (C41.0)

      C69.60   **Malignant neoplasm of unspecified orbit**

      C69.61   **Malignant neoplasm of right orbit**

      C69.62   **Malignant neoplasm of left orbit**

   C69.8   **Malignant neoplasm of overlapping sites of eye and adnexa**

      C69.80   **Malignant neoplasm of overlapping sites of unspecified eye and adnexa**

      C69.81   **Malignant neoplasm of overlapping sites of right eye and adnexa**

      C69.82   **Malignant neoplasm of overlapping sites of left eye and adnexa**

   C69.9   **Malignant neoplasm of unspecified site of eye**

      Malignant neoplasm of eyeball

      C69.90   **Malignant neoplasm of unspecified site of unspecified eye**

      C69.91   **Malignant neoplasm of unspecified site of right eye**

      C69.92   **Malignant neoplasm of unspecified site of left eye**

C70 **Malignant neoplasm of meninges**

   C70.0   **Malignant neoplasm of cerebral meninges**

   C70.1   **Malignant neoplasm of spinal meninges**

   C70.9   **Malignant neoplasm of meninges, unspecified**

C71 **Malignant neoplasm of brain**

   Excludes1: malignant neoplasm of cranial nerves (C72.2-C72.5)

      retrobulbar malignant neoplasm (C69.6-)

   C71.0   **Malignant neoplasm of cerebrum, except lobes and ventricles**

      Malignant neoplasm of supratentorial NOS

   C71.1   **Malignant neoplasm of frontal lobe**

   C71.2   **Malignant neoplasm of temporal lobe**

   C71.3   **Malignant neoplasm of parietal lobe**

   C71.4   **Malignant neoplasm of occipital lobe**

   C71.5   **Malignant neoplasm of cerebral ventricle**

      Excludes1: malignant neoplasm of fourth cerebral ventricle (C71.7)

   C71.6   **Malignant neoplasm of cerebellum**

   C71.7   **Malignant neoplasm of brain stem**

      Malignant neoplasm of fourth cerebral ventricle

      Infratentorial malignant neoplasm NOS

   C71.8   **Malignant neoplasm of overlapping sites of brain**

   C71.9   **Malignant neoplasm of brain, unspecified**

C72 Malignant neoplasm of spinal cord, cranial nerves and other parts of central nervous system

Excludes1: malignant neoplasm of meninges (C70.-)

malignant neoplasm of peripheral nerves and autonomic nervous system (C47.-)

C72.0 **Malignant neoplasm of spinal cord**

C72.1 **Malignant neoplasm of cauda equina**

C72.2 **Malignant neoplasm of olfactory nerve**

Malignant neoplasm of olfactory bulb

C72.20 **Malignant neoplasm of unspecified olfactory nerve**

C72.21 **Malignant neoplasm of right olfactory nerve**

C72.22 **Malignant neoplasm of left olfactory nerve**

C72.3 **Malignant neoplasm of optic nerve**

C72.30 **Malignant neoplasm of unspecified optic nerve**

C72.31 **Malignant neoplasm of right optic nerve**

C72.32 **Malignant neoplasm of left optic nerve**

C72.4 **Malignant neoplasm of acoustic nerve**

C72.40 **Malignant neoplasm of unspecified acoustic nerve**

C72.41 **Malignant neoplasm of right acoustic nerve**

C72.42 **Malignant neoplasm of left acoustic nerve**

C72.5 **Malignant neoplasm of other and unspecified cranial nerves**

C72.50 **Malignant neoplasm of unspecified cranial nerve**

Malignant neoplasm of cranial nerve NOS

C72.59 **Malignant neoplasm of other cranial nerves**

C72.9 **Malignant neoplasm of central nervous system, unspecified**

Malignant neoplasm of unspecified site of central nervous system

Malignant neoplasm of nervous system NOS

MALIGNANT NEOPLASMS OF THYROID AND OTHER ENDOCRINE GLANDS (C73-C75)

C73 Malignant neoplasm of thyroid gland

Use additional code to identify any functional activity

C74 Malignant neoplasm of adrenal gland

C74.0 **Malignant neoplasm of cortex of adrenal gland**

C74.00 **Malignant neoplasm of cortex of unspecified adrenal gland**

C74.01 **Malignant neoplasm of cortex of right adrenal gland**

C74.02 **Malignant neoplasm of cortex of left adrenal gland**

C74.1 **Malignant neoplasm of medulla of adrenal gland**

C74.10 **Malignant neoplasm of medulla of unspecified adrenal gland**

C74.11 **Malignant neoplasm of medulla of right adrenal gland**

C74.12 **Malignant neoplasm of medulla of left adrenal gland**

C74.9 **Malignant neoplasm of unspecified part of adrenal gland**

C74.90 **Malignant neoplasm of unspecified part of unspecified adrenal gland**

C74.91 **Malignant neoplasm of unspecified part of right adrenal gland**

C74.92 **Malignant neoplasm of unspecified part of left adrenal gland**

C75 Malignant neoplasm of other endocrine glands and related structures

Excludes1: malignant carcinoid tumors (C7A.0-)

malignant neoplasm of adrenal gland (C74.-)

malignant neoplasm of endocrine pancreas (C25.4)

malignant neoplasm of islets of Langerhans (C25.4)

malignant neoplasm of ovary (C56.-)

malignant neoplasm of testis (C62.-)

malignant neoplasm of thymus (C37)

malignant neoplasm of thyroid gland (C73)

malignant neuroendocrine tumors (C7A.-)

C75.0 **Malignant neoplasm of parathyroid gland**

C75.1 **Malignant neoplasm of pituitary gland**

C75.2 **Malignant neoplasm of craniopharyngeal duct**

C75.3 **Malignant neoplasm of pineal gland**

C75.4 **Malignant neoplasm of carotid body**

C75.5 **Malignant neoplasm of aortic body and other paraganglia**

C75.8 **Malignant neoplasm with pluriglandular involvement, unspecified**

C75.9 **Malignant neoplasm of endocrine gland, unspecified**

MALIGNANT NEUROENDOCRINE TUMORS (C7A)

C7A Malignant neuroendocrine tumors

Code also any associated multiple endocrine neoplasia [MEN] syndromes (E31.2-)

Use additional code to identify any associated endocrine syndrome, such as:

carcinoid syndrome (E34.0)

Excludes2: malignant pancreatic islet cell tumors (C25.4)

Merkel cell carcinoma (C4A.-)

C7A.0 **Malignant carcinoid tumors**

C7A.00 **Malignant carcinoid tumor of unspecified site**

C7A.01 **Malignant carcinoid tumors of the small intestine**

C7A.010 **Malignant carcinoid tumor of the duodenum**

C7A.011 **Malignant carcinoid tumor of the jejunum**

C7A.012 **Malignant carcinoid tumor of the ileum**

C7A.019 **Malignant carcinoid tumor of the small intestine, unspecified portion**

C7A.02 **Malignant carcinoid tumors of the appendix, large intestine, and rectum**

C7A.020 **Malignant carcinoid tumor of the appendix**

C7A.021 **Malignant carcinoid tumor of the cecum**

C7A.022 **Malignant carcinoid tumor of the ascending colon**

C7A.023 **Malignant carcinoid tumor of the transverse colon**

C7A.024 **Malignant carcinoid tumor of the descending colon**

C7A.025 **Malignant carcinoid tumor of the sigmoid colon**

C7A.026 **Malignant carcinoid tumor of the rectum**

C7A.029 **Malignant carcinoid tumor of the large intestine, unspecified portion**

Malignant carcinoid tumor of the colon NOS

C7A.09 **Malignant carcinoid tumors of other sites**

C7A.090 **Malignant carcinoid tumor of the bronchus and lung**

C7A.091 **Malignant carcinoid tumor of the thymus**

C7A.092 **Malignant carcinoid tumor of the stomach**

C7A.093 **Malignant carcinoid tumor of the kidney**

C7A.094 **Malignant carcinoid tumor of the foregut, unspecified**

C7A.095 **Malignant carcinoid tumor of the midgut, unspecified**

C7A.096 **Malignant carcinoid tumor of the hindgut, unspecified**

C7A.098 **Malignant carcinoid tumors of other sites**

C7A.1 **Malignant poorly differentiated neuroendocrine tumors**

Malignant poorly differentiated neuroendocrine tumor NOS

Malignant poorly differentiated neuroendocrine carcinoma, any site

High grade neuroendocrine carcinoma, any site

C7A.8 **Other malignant neuroendocrine tumors**

SECONDARY NEUROENDOCRINE TUMORS (C7B)

C7B **Secondary neuroendocrine tumors**

Use additional code to identify any functional activity

C7B.0 **Secondary carcinoid tumors**

C7B.00 **Secondary carcinoid tumors, unspecified site**

C7B.01 **Secondary carcinoid tumors of distant lymph nodes**

C7B.02 **Secondary carcinoid tumors of liver**

C7B.03 **Secondary carcinoid tumors of bone**

C7B.04 **Secondary carcinoid tumors of peritoneum**

Mesentery metastasis of carcinoid tumor

C7B.09 **Secondary carcinoid tumors of other sites**

C7B.1 **Secondary Merkel cell carcinoma**

Merkel cell carcinoma nodal presentation

Merkel cell carcinoma visceral metastatic presentation

C7B.8 **Other secondary neuroendocrine tumors**

MALIGNANT NEOPLASMS OF ILL-DEFINED, OTHER SECONDARY AND UNSPECIFIED SITES (C76-C80)

C76 **Malignant neoplasm of other and ill-defined sites**

Excludes1: malignant neoplasm of female genitourinary tract NOS (C57.9)

malignant neoplasm of male genitourinary tract NOS (C63.9)

malignant neoplasm of lymphoid, hematopoietic and related tissue (C81-C96)

malignant neoplasm of skin (C44.-)

malignant neoplasm of unspecified site NOS (C80.1)

C76.0 **Malignant neoplasm of head, face and neck**

Malignant neoplasm of cheek NOS

Malignant neoplasm of nose NOS

C76.1 **Malignant neoplasm of thorax**

Intrathoracic malignant neoplasm NOS

Malignant neoplasm of axilla NOS

Thoracic malignant neoplasm NOS

C76.2 **Malignant neoplasm of abdomen**

C76.3 **Malignant neoplasm of pelvis**

Malignant neoplasm of groin NOS

Malignant neoplasm of sites overlapping systems within the pelvis

Rectovaginal (septum) malignant neoplasm

Rectovesical (septum) malignant neoplasm

C76.4 **Malignant neoplasm of upper limb**

C76.40 **Malignant neoplasm of unspecified upper limb**

C76.41 **Malignant neoplasm of right upper limb**

C76.42 **Malignant neoplasm of left upper limb**

C76.5 **Malignant neoplasm of lower limb**

C76.50 **Malignant neoplasm of unspecified lower limb**

C76.51 **Malignant neoplasm of right lower limb**

C76.52 **Malignant neoplasm of left lower limb**

C76.8 **Malignant neoplasm of other specified ill-defined sites**

Malignant neoplasm of overlapping ill-defined sites

C77 **Secondary and unspecified malignant neoplasm of lymph nodes**

Excludes1: malignant neoplasm of lymph nodes, specified as primary (C81-C86, C88, C96.-)

mesentery metastasis of carcinoid tumor (C7B.04)

secondary carcinoid tumors of distant lymph nodes (C7B.01)

C77.0 **Secondary and unspecified malignant neoplasm of lymph nodes of head, face and neck**

Secondary and unspecified malignant neoplasm of supraclavicular lymph nodes

C77.1 **Secondary and unspecified malignant neoplasm of intrathoracic lymph nodes**

C77.2 **Secondary and unspecified malignant neoplasm of intra-abdominal lymph nodes**

C77.3 **Secondary and unspecified malignant neoplasm of axilla and upper limb lymph nodes**

Secondary and unspecified malignant neoplasm of pectoral lymph nodes

C77.4 **Secondary and unspecified malignant neoplasm of inguinal and lower limb lymph nodes**

C77.5 **Secondary and unspecified malignant neoplasm of intrapelvic lymph nodes**

C77.8 **Secondary and unspecified malignant neoplasm of lymph nodes of multiple regions**

C77.9 **Secondary and unspecified malignant neoplasm of lymph node, unspecified**

C78 **Secondary malignant neoplasm of respiratory and digestive organs**

Excludes1: secondary carcinoid tumors of liver (C7B.02)

secondary carcinoid tumors of peritoneum (C7B.04)

Excludes2: lymph node metastases (C77.0)

C78.0 **Secondary malignant neoplasm of lung**

C78.00 **Secondary malignant neoplasm of unspecified lung**

C78.01 **Secondary malignant neoplasm of right lung**

C78.02 **Secondary malignant neoplasm of left lung**

C78.1 **Secondary malignant neoplasm of mediastinum**

C78.2 **Secondary malignant neoplasm of pleura**

C78.3 **Secondary malignant neoplasm of other and unspecified respiratory organs**

C78.30 **Secondary malignant neoplasm of unspecified respiratory organ**

C78.39 Secondary malignant neoplasm of other respiratory organs

C78.4 Secondary malignant neoplasm of small intestine

C78.5 Secondary malignant neoplasm of large intestine and rectum

C78.6 Secondary malignant neoplasm of retroperitoneum and peritoneum

C78.7 Secondary malignant neoplasm of liver and intrahepatic bile duct

C78.8 Secondary malignant neoplasm of other and unspecified digestive organs

    C78.80 Secondary malignant neoplasm of unspecified digestive organ

    C78.89 Secondary malignant neoplasm of other digestive organs

        Code also exocrine pancreatic insufficiency (K86.81)

C79 Secondary malignant neoplasm of other and unspecified sites

    Excludes1: secondary carcinoid tumors (C7B.-)

        secondary neuroendocrine tumors (C7B.-)

C79.0 Secondary malignant neoplasm of kidney and renal pelvis

    C79.00 Secondary malignant neoplasm of unspecified kidney and renal pelvis

    C79.01 Secondary malignant neoplasm of right kidney and renal pelvis

    C79.02 Secondary malignant neoplasm of left kidney and renal pelvis

    C79.1 Secondary malignant neoplasm of bladder and other and unspecified urinary organs

    C79.10 Secondary malignant neoplasm of unspecified urinary organs

    C79.11 Secondary malignant neoplasm of bladder

        Excludes2: lymph node metastases (C77.0)

    C79.19 Secondary malignant neoplasm of other urinary organs

C79.2 Secondary malignant neoplasm of skin

    Excludes1: secondary Merkel cell carcinoma (C7B.1)

C79.3 Secondary malignant neoplasm of brain and cerebral meninges

    C79.31 Secondary malignant neoplasm of brain

    C79.32 Secondary malignant neoplasm of cerebral meninges

C79.4 Secondary malignant neoplasm of other and unspecified parts of nervous system

    C79.40 Secondary malignant neoplasm of unspecified part of nervous system

    C79.49 Secondary malignant neoplasm of other parts of nervous system

C79.5 Secondary malignant neoplasm of bone and bone marrow

    Excludes1: secondary carcinoid tumors of bone (C7B.03)

    C79.51 Secondary malignant neoplasm of bone

    C79.52 Secondary malignant neoplasm of bone marrow

C79.6 Secondary malignant neoplasm of ovary

    C79.60 Secondary malignant neoplasm of unspecified ovary

    C79.61 Secondary malignant neoplasm of right ovary

    C79.62 Secondary malignant neoplasm of left ovary

C79.7 Secondary malignant neoplasm of adrenal gland

    C79.70 Secondary malignant neoplasm of unspecified adrenal gland

    C79.71 Secondary malignant neoplasm of right adrenal gland

    C79.72 Secondary malignant neoplasm of left adrenal gland

C79.8 Secondary malignant neoplasm of other specified sites

    C79.81 Secondary malignant neoplasm of breast

    C79.82 Secondary malignant neoplasm of genital organs

    C79.89 Secondary malignant neoplasm of other specified sites

C79.9 Secondary malignant neoplasm of unspecified site

    Metastatic cancer NOS

    Metastatic disease NOS

    Excludes1: carcinomatosis NOS (C80.0)

        generalized cancer NOS (C80.0)

        malignant (primary) neoplasm of unspecified site (C80.1)

C80 Malignant neoplasm without specification of site

    Excludes1: malignant carcinoid tumor of unspecified site (C7A.00)

        malignant neoplasm of specified multiple sites- code to each site

C80.0 Disseminated malignant neoplasm, unspecified

    Carcinomatosis NOS

    Generalized cancer, unspecified site (primary) (secondary)

    Generalized malignancy, unspecified site (primary) (secondary)

C80.1 Malignant (primary) neoplasm, unspecified

    Cancer NOS

    Cancer unspecified site (primary)

    Carcinoma unspecified site (primary)

    Malignancy unspecified site (primary)

    Excludes1: secondary malignant neoplasm of unspecified site (C79.9)

C80.2 Malignant neoplasm associated with transplanted organ

    Code first complication of transplanted organ (T86.-)

    Use additional code to identify the specific malignancy

MALIGNANT NEOPLASMS OF LYMPHOID, HEMATOPOIETIC AND RELATED TISSUE (C81-C96)

Excludes2: Kaposi's sarcoma of lymph nodes (C46.3)

    secondary and unspecified neoplasm of lymph nodes (C77.-)

    secondary neoplasm of bone marrow (C79.52)

    secondary neoplasm of spleen (C78.89)

C81 Hodgkin lymphoma

    Definition: Hodgkin's disease is a malignant disease of the lymphatic system is characterized by painless enlargement of lymph nodes, the spleen, or other lymphatic tissue. It is sometimes accompanied by symptoms such as fever, weight loss, fatigue and night sweats.

    Excludes1: personal history of Hodgkin lymphoma (Z85.71)

C81.0 Nodular lymphocyte predominant Hodgkin lymphoma

    C81.00 Nodular lymphocyte predominant Hodgkin lymphoma, unspecified site

    C81.01 Nodular lymphocyte predominant Hodgkin lymphoma, lymph nodes of head, face, and neck

    C81.02 Nodular lymphocyte predominant Hodgkin lymphoma, intrathoracic lymph nodes

    C81.03 Nodular lymphocyte predominant Hodgkin lymphoma, intra-abdominal lymph nodes

C81.04 Nodular lymphocyte predominant Hodgkin lymphoma, lymph nodes of axilla and upper limb

C81.05 Nodular lymphocyte predominant Hodgkin lymphoma, lymph nodes of inguinal region and lower limb

C81.06 Nodular lymphocyte predominant Hodgkin lymphoma, intrapelvic lymph nodes

C81.07 Nodular lymphocyte predominant Hodgkin lymphoma, spleen

C81.08 Nodular lymphocyte predominant Hodgkin lymphoma, lymph nodes of multiple sites

C81.09 Nodular lymphocyte predominant Hodgkin lymphoma, extranodal and solid organ sites

C81.1 Nodular sclerosis Hodgkin lymphoma

Nodular sclerosis classical Hodgkin lymphoma

C81.10 Nodular sclerosis Hodgkin lymphoma, unspecified site

C81.11 Nodular sclerosis Hodgkin lymphoma, lymph nodes of head, face, and neck

C81.12 Nodular sclerosis Hodgkin lymphoma, intrathoracic lymph nodes

C81.13 Nodular sclerosis Hodgkin lymphoma, intra-abdominal lymph nodes

C81.14 Nodular sclerosis Hodgkin lymphoma, lymph nodes of axilla and upper limb

C81.15 Nodular sclerosis Hodgkin lymphoma, lymph nodes of inguinal region and lower limb

C81.16 Nodular sclerosis Hodgkin lymphoma, intrapelvic lymph nodes

C81.17 Nodular sclerosis Hodgkin lymphoma, spleen

C81.18 Nodular sclerosis Hodgkin lymphoma, lymph nodes of multiple sites

C81.19 Nodular sclerosis Hodgkin lymphoma, extranodal and solid organ sites

C81.2 Mixed cellularity Hodgkin lymphoma

Mixed cellularity classical Hodgkin lymphoma

C81.20 Mixed cellularity Hodgkin lymphoma, unspecified site

C81.21 Mixed cellularity Hodgkin lymphoma, lymph nodes of head, face, and neck

C81.22 Mixed cellularity Hodgkin lymphoma, intrathoracic lymph nodes

C81.23 Mixed cellularity Hodgkin lymphoma, intra-abdominal lymph nodes

C81.24 Mixed cellularity Hodgkin lymphoma, lymph nodes of axilla and upper limb

C81.25 Mixed cellularity Hodgkin lymphoma, lymph nodes of inguinal region and lower limb

C81.26 Mixed cellularity Hodgkin lymphoma, intrapelvic lymph nodes

C81.27 Mixed cellularity Hodgkin lymphoma, spleen

C81.28 Mixed cellularity Hodgkin lymphoma, lymph nodes of multiple sites

C81.29 Mixed cellularity Hodgkin lymphoma, extranodal and solid organ sites

C81.3 Lymphocyte depleted Hodgkin lymphoma

Lymphocyte depleted classical Hodgkin lymphoma

C81.30 Lymphocyte depleted Hodgkin lymphoma, unspecified site

C81.31 Lymphocyte depleted Hodgkin lymphoma, lymph nodes of head, face, and neck

C81.32 Lymphocyte depleted Hodgkin lymphoma, intrathoracic lymph nodes

C81.33 Lymphocyte depleted Hodgkin lymphoma, intra-abdominal lymph nodes

C81.34 Lymphocyte depleted Hodgkin lymphoma, lymph nodes of axilla and upper limb

C81.35 Lymphocyte depleted Hodgkin lymphoma, lymph nodes of inguinal region and lower limb

C81.36 Lymphocyte depleted Hodgkin lymphoma, intrapelvic lymph nodes

C81.37 Lymphocyte depleted Hodgkin lymphoma, spleen

C81.38 Lymphocyte depleted Hodgkin lymphoma, lymph nodes of multiple sites

C81.39 Lymphocyte depleted Hodgkin lymphoma, extranodal and solid organ sites

C81.4 Lymphocyte-rich Hodgkin lymphoma

Lymphocyte-rich classical Hodgkin lymphoma

Excludes1: nodular lymphocyte predominant Hodgkin lymphoma (C81.0-)

C81.40 Lymphocyte-rich Hodgkin lymphoma, unspecified site

C81.41 Lymphocyte-rich Hodgkin lymphoma, lymph nodes of head, face, and neck

C81.42 Lymphocyte-rich Hodgkin lymphoma, intrathoracic lymph nodes

C81.43 Lymphocyte-rich Hodgkin lymphoma, intra-abdominal lymph nodes

C81.44 Lymphocyte-rich Hodgkin lymphoma, lymph nodes of axilla and upper limb

C81.45 Lymphocyte-rich Hodgkin lymphoma, lymph nodes of inguinal region and lower limb

C81.46 Lymphocyte-rich Hodgkin lymphoma, intrapelvic lymph nodes

C81.47 Lymphocyte-rich Hodgkin lymphoma, spleen

C81.48 Lymphocyte-rich Hodgkin lymphoma, lymph nodes of multiple sites

C81.49 Lymphocyte-rich Hodgkin lymphoma, extranodal and solid organ sites

C81.7 Other Hodgkin lymphoma

Classical Hodgkin lymphoma NOS

Other classical Hodgkin lymphoma

C81.70 Other Hodgkin lymphoma, unspecified site

C81.71 Other Hodgkin lymphoma, lymph nodes of head, face, and neck

C81.72 Other Hodgkin lymphoma, intrathoracic lymph nodes

C81.73 Other Hodgkin lymphoma, intra-abdominal lymph nodes

C81.74 Other Hodgkin lymphoma, lymph nodes of axilla and upper limb

C81.75 Other Hodgkin lymphoma, lymph nodes of inguinal region and lower limb

C81.76 Other Hodgkin lymphoma, intrapelvic lymph nodes

C81.77 Other Hodgkin lymphoma, spleen

C81.78 Other Hodgkin lymphoma, lymph nodes of multiple sites

C81.79 Other Hodgkin lymphoma, extranodal and solid organ sites

C81.9 Hodgkin lymphoma, unspecified

C81.90 Hodgkin lymphoma, unspecified, unspecified site

C81.91 Hodgkin lymphoma, unspecified, lymph nodes of head, face, and neck

C81.92 Hodgkin lymphoma, unspecified, intrathoracic lymph nodes

C81.93 Hodgkin lymphoma, unspecified, intra-abdominal lymph nodes

C81.94 Hodgkin lymphoma, unspecified, lymph nodes of axilla and upper limb

C81.95 Hodgkin lymphoma, unspecified, lymph nodes of inguinal region and lower limb

C81.96 Hodgkin lymphoma, unspecified, intrapelvic lymph nodes

C81.97 Hodgkin lymphoma, unspecified, spleen

C81.98 Hodgkin lymphoma, unspecified, lymph nodes of multiple sites

C81.99 Hodgkin lymphoma, unspecified, extranodal and solid organ sites

C82 Follicular lymphoma

Includes: follicular lymphoma with or without diffuse areas

Excludes1: mature T/NK-cell lymphomas (C84.-)

personal history of non-Hodgkin lymphoma (Z85.72)

C82.0 Follicular lymphoma grade I

C82.00 Follicular lymphoma grade I, unspecified site

C82.01 Follicular lymphoma grade I, lymph nodes of head, face, and neck

C82.02 Follicular lymphoma grade I, intrathoracic lymph nodes

C82.03 Follicular lymphoma grade I, intra-abdominal lymph nodes

C82.04 Follicular lymphoma grade I, lymph nodes of axilla and upper limb

C82.05 Follicular lymphoma grade I, lymph nodes of inguinal region and lower limb

C82.06 Follicular lymphoma grade I, intrapelvic lymph nodes

C82.07 Follicular lymphoma grade I, spleen

C82.08 Follicular lymphoma grade I, lymph nodes of multiple sites

C82.09 Follicular lymphoma grade I, extranodal and solid organ sites

C82.1 Follicular lymphoma grade II

C82.10 Follicular lymphoma grade II, unspecified site

C82.11 Follicular lymphoma grade II, lymph nodes of head, face, and neck

C82.12 Follicular lymphoma grade II, intrathoracic lymph nodes

C82.13 Follicular lymphoma grade II, intra-abdominal lymph nodes

C82.14 Follicular lymphoma grade II, lymph nodes of axilla and upper limb

C82.15 Follicular lymphoma grade II, lymph nodes of inguinal region and lower limb

C82.16 Follicular lymphoma grade II, intrapelvic lymph nodes

C82.17 Follicular lymphoma grade II, spleen

C82.18 Follicular lymphoma grade II, lymph nodes of multiple sites

C82.19 Follicular lymphoma grade II, extranodal and solid organ sites

C82.2 Follicular lymphoma grade III, unspecified

C82.20 Follicular lymphoma grade III, unspecified, unspecified site

C82.21 Follicular lymphoma grade III, unspecified, lymph nodes of head, face, and neck

C82.22 Follicular lymphoma grade III, unspecified, intrathoracic lymph nodes

C82.23 Follicular lymphoma grade III, unspecified, intra-abdominal lymph nodes

C82.24 Follicular lymphoma grade III, unspecified, lymph nodes of axilla and upper limb

C82.25 Follicular lymphoma grade III, unspecified, lymph nodes of inguinal region and lower limb

C82.26 Follicular lymphoma grade III, unspecified, intrapelvic lymph nodes

C82.27 Follicular lymphoma grade III, unspecified, spleen

C82.28 Follicular lymphoma grade III, unspecified, lymph nodes of multiple sites

C82.29 Follicular lymphoma grade III, unspecified, extranodal and solid organ sites

C82.3 Follicular lymphoma grade IIIa

C82.30 Follicular lymphoma grade IIIa, unspecified site

C82.31 Follicular lymphoma grade IIIa, lymph nodes of head, face, and neck

C82.32 Follicular lymphoma grade IIIa, intrathoracic lymph nodes

C82.33 Follicular lymphoma grade IIIa, intra-abdominal lymph nodes

C82.34 Follicular lymphoma grade IIIa, lymph nodes of axilla and upper limb

C82.35 Follicular lymphoma grade IIIa, lymph nodes of inguinal region and lower limb

C82.36 Follicular lymphoma grade IIIa, intrapelvic lymph nodes

C82.37 Follicular lymphoma grade IIIa, spleen

C82.38 Follicular lymphoma grade IIIa, lymph nodes of multiple sites

C82.39 Follicular lymphoma grade IIIa, extranodal and solid organ sites

C82.4 Follicular lymphoma grade IIIb

C82.40 Follicular lymphoma grade IIIb, unspecified site

C82.41 Follicular lymphoma grade IIIb, lymph nodes of head, face, and neck

C82.42 Follicular lymphoma grade IIIb, intrathoracic lymph nodes

C82.43 Follicular lymphoma grade IIIb, intra-abdominal lymph nodes

C82.44 Follicular lymphoma grade IIIb, lymph nodes of axilla and upper limb

C82.45 Follicular lymphoma grade IIIb, lymph nodes of inguinal region and lower limb

C82.46 Follicular lymphoma grade IIIb, intrapelvic lymph nodes

C82.47 Follicular lymphoma grade IIIb, spleen

C82.48 Follicular lymphoma grade IIIb, lymph nodes of multiple sites

C82.49 Follicular lymphoma grade IIIb, extranodal and solid organ sites

C82.5 Diffuse follicle center lymphoma

C82.50 Diffuse follicle center lymphoma, unspecified site

C82.51 Diffuse follicle center lymphoma, lymph nodes of head, face, and neck

C82.52 Diffuse follicle center lymphoma, intrathoracic lymph nodes

● New code ▲ Revised code **Excludes1:** Not coded here **Excludes2:** Not included here ⊗ Placeholder required ⑦ 7th digit required

C82.53   Diffuse follicle center lymphoma, intra-abdominal lymph nodes

C82.54   Diffuse follicle center lymphoma, lymph nodes of axilla and upper limb

C82.55   Diffuse follicle center lymphoma, lymph nodes of inguinal region and lower limb

C82.56   Diffuse follicle center lymphoma, intrapelvic lymph nodes

C82.57   Diffuse follicle center lymphoma, spleen

C82.58   Diffuse follicle center lymphoma, lymph nodes of multiple sites

C82.59   Diffuse follicle center lymphoma, extranodal and solid organ sites

C82.6   Cutaneous follicle center lymphoma

C82.60   Cutaneous follicle center lymphoma, unspecified site

C82.61   Cutaneous follicle center lymphoma, lymph nodes of head, face, and neck

C82.62   Cutaneous follicle center lymphoma, intrathoracic lymph nodes

C82.63   Cutaneous follicle center lymphoma, intra-abdominal lymph nodes

C82.64   Cutaneous follicle center lymphoma, lymph nodes of axilla and upper limb

C82.65   Cutaneous follicle center lymphoma, lymph nodes of inguinal region and lower limb

C82.66   Cutaneous follicle center lymphoma, intrapelvic lymph nodes

C82.67   Cutaneous follicle center lymphoma, spleen

C82.68   Cutaneous follicle center lymphoma, lymph nodes of multiple sites

C82.69   Cutaneous follicle center lymphoma, extranodal and solid organ sites

C82.8   Other types of follicular lymphoma

C82.80   Other types of follicular lymphoma, unspecified site

C82.81   Other types of follicular lymphoma, lymph nodes of head, face, and neck

C82.82   Other types of follicular lymphoma, intrathoracic lymph nodes

C82.83   Other types of follicular lymphoma, intra-abdominal lymph nodes

C82.84   Other types of follicular lymphoma, lymph nodes of axilla and upper limb

C82.85   Other types of follicular lymphoma, lymph nodes of inguinal region and lower limb

C82.86   Other types of follicular lymphoma, intrapelvic lymph nodes

C82.87   Other types of follicular lymphoma, spleen

C82.88   Other types of follicular lymphoma, lymph nodes of multiple sites

C82.89   Other types of follicular lymphoma, extranodal and solid organ sites

C82.9   Follicular lymphoma, unspecified

C82.90   Follicular lymphoma, unspecified, unspecified site

C82.91   Follicular lymphoma, unspecified, lymph nodes of head, face, and neck

C82.92   Follicular lymphoma, unspecified, intrathoracic lymph nodes

C82.93   Follicular lymphoma, unspecified, intra-abdominal lymph nodes

C82.94   Follicular lymphoma, unspecified, lymph nodes of axilla and upper limb

C82.95   Follicular lymphoma, unspecified, lymph nodes of inguinal region and lower limb

C82.96   Follicular lymphoma, unspecified, intrapelvic lymph nodes

C82.97   Follicular lymphoma, unspecified, spleen

C82.98   Follicular lymphoma, unspecified, lymph nodes of multiple sites

C82.99   Follicular lymphoma, unspecified, extranodal and solid organ sites

C83   Non-follicular lymphoma

Excludes1: personal history of non-Hodgkin lymphoma (Z85.72)

C83.0   Small cell B-cell lymphoma

Lymphoplasmacytic lymphoma

Nodal marginal zone lymphoma

Non-leukemic variant of B-CLL

Splenic marginal zone lymphoma

Excludes1: chronic lymphocytic leukemia (C91.1)

mature T/NK-cell lymphomas (C84.-)

Waldenström macroglobulinemia (C88.0)

C83.00   Small cell B-cell lymphoma, unspecified site

C83.01   Small cell B-cell lymphoma, lymph nodes of head, face, and neck

C83.02   Small cell B-cell lymphoma, intrathoracic lymph nodes

C83.03   Small cell B-cell lymphoma, intra-abdominal lymph nodes

C83.04   Small cell B-cell lymphoma, lymph nodes of axilla and upper limb

C83.05   Small cell B-cell lymphoma, lymph nodes of inguinal region and lower limb

C83.06   Small cell B-cell lymphoma, intrapelvic lymph nodes

C83.07   Small cell B-cell lymphoma, spleen

C83.08   Small cell B-cell lymphoma, lymph nodes of multiple sites

C83.09   Small cell B-cell lymphoma, extranodal and solid organ sites

C83.1   Mantle cell lymphoma

Centrocytic lymphoma

Malignant lymphomatous polyposis

C83.10   Mantle cell lymphoma, unspecified site

C83.11   Mantle cell lymphoma, lymph nodes of head, face, and neck

C83.12   Mantle cell lymphoma, intrathoracic lymph nodes

C83.13   Mantle cell lymphoma, intra-abdominal lymph nodes

C83.14   Mantle cell lymphoma, lymph nodes of axilla and upper limb

C83.15   Mantle cell lymphoma, lymph nodes of inguinal region and lower limb

C83.16   Mantle cell lymphoma, intrapelvic lymph nodes

C83.17   Mantle cell lymphoma, spleen

C83.18   Mantle cell lymphoma, lymph nodes of multiple sites

C83.19   Mantle cell lymphoma, extranodal and solid organ sites

C83.3   Diffuse large B-cell lymphoma

Anaplastic diffuse large B-cell lymphoma

CD30-positive diffuse large B-cell lymphoma

Centroblastic diffuse large B-cell lymphoma

Diffuse large B-cell lymphoma, subtype not specified

Immunoblastic diffuse large B-cell lymphoma

Plasmablastic diffuse large B-cell lymphoma

Diffuse large B-cell lymphoma, subtype not specified

T-cell rich diffuse large B-cell lymphoma

Excludes1: mediastinal (thymic) large B-cell lymphoma (C85.2-)

mature T/NK-cell lymphomas (C84.-)

C83.30 Diffuse large B-cell lymphoma, unspecified site

C83.31 Diffuse large B-cell lymphoma, lymph nodes of head, face, and neck

C83.32 Diffuse large B-cell lymphoma, intrathoracic lymph nodes

C83.33 Diffuse large B-cell lymphoma, intra-abdominal lymph nodes

C83.34 Diffuse large B-cell lymphoma, lymph nodes of axilla and upper limb

C83.35 Diffuse large B-cell lymphoma, lymph nodes of inguinal region and lower limb

C83.36 Diffuse large B-cell lymphoma, intrapelvic lymph nodes

C83.37 Diffuse large B-cell lymphoma, spleen

C83.38 Diffuse large B-cell lymphoma, lymph nodes of multiple sites

C83.39 Diffuse large B-cell lymphoma, extranodal and solid organ sites

C83.5 **Lymphoblastic (diffuse) lymphoma**

B-precursor lymphoma

Lymphoblastic B-cell lymphoma

Lymphoblastic lymphoma NOS

Lymphoblastic T-cell lymphoma

T-precursor lymphoma

C83.50 Lymphoblastic (diffuse) lymphoma, unspecified site

C83.51 Lymphoblastic (diffuse) lymphoma, lymph nodes of head, face, and neck

C83.52 Lymphoblastic (diffuse) lymphoma, intrathoracic lymph nodes

C83.53 Lymphoblastic (diffuse) lymphoma, intra-abdominal lymph nodes

C83.54 Lymphoblastic (diffuse) lymphoma, lymph nodes of axilla and upper limb

C83.55 Lymphoblastic (diffuse) lymphoma, lymph nodes of inguinal region and lower limb

C83.56 Lymphoblastic (diffuse) lymphoma, intrapelvic lymph nodes

C83.57 Lymphoblastic (diffuse) lymphoma, spleen

C83.58 Lymphoblastic (diffuse) lymphoma, lymph nodes of multiple sites

C83.59 Lymphoblastic (diffuse) lymphoma, extranodal and solid organ sites

C83.7 **Burkitt lymphoma**

Atypical Burkitt lymphoma Burkitt-like lymphoma

Excludes1: mature B-cell leukemia Burkitt type (C91.A-)

C83.70 Burkitt lymphoma, unspecified site

C83.71 Burkitt lymphoma, lymph nodes of head, face, and neck

C83.72 Burkitt lymphoma, intrathoracic lymph nodes

C83.73 Burkitt lymphoma, intra-abdominal lymph nodes

C83.74 Burkitt lymphoma, lymph nodes of axilla and upper limb

C83.75 Burkitt lymphoma, lymph nodes of inguinal region and lower limb

C83.76 Burkitt lymphoma, intrapelvic lymph nodes

C83.77 Burkitt lymphoma, spleen

C83.78 Burkitt lymphoma, lymph nodes of multiple sites

C83.79 Burkitt lymphoma, extranodal and solid organ sites

C83.8 **Other non-follicular lymphoma**

Intravascular large B-cell lymphoma Lymphoid granulomatosis

Primary effusion B-cell lymphoma

Excludes1: mediastinal (thymic) large B-cell lymphoma (C85.2-)

T-cell rich B-cell lymphoma (C83.3-)

C83.80 Other non-follicular lymphoma, unspecified site

C83.81 Other non-follicular lymphoma, lymph nodes of head, face, and neck

C83.82 Other non-follicular lymphoma, intrathoracic lymph nodes

C83.83 Other non-follicular lymphoma, intra-abdominal lymph nodes

C83.84 Other non-follicular lymphoma, lymph nodes of axilla and upper limb

C83.85 Other non-follicular lymphoma, lymph nodes of inguinal region and lower limb

C83.86 Other non-follicular lymphoma, intrapelvic lymph nodes

C83.87 Other non-follicular lymphoma, spleen

C83.88 Other non-follicular lymphoma, lymph nodes of multiple sites

C83.89 Other non-follicular lymphoma, extranodal and solid organ sites

C83.9 **Non-follicular (diffuse) lymphoma, unspecified**

C83.90 Non-follicular (diffuse) lymphoma, unspecified, unspecified site

C83.91 Non-follicular (diffuse) lymphoma, unspecified, lymph nodes of head, face, and neck

C83.92 Non-follicular (diffuse) lymphoma, unspecified, intrathoracic lymph nodes

C83.93 Non-follicular (diffuse) lymphoma, unspecified, intra-abdominal lymph nodes

C83.94 Non-follicular (diffuse) lymphoma, unspecified, lymph nodes of axilla and upper limb

C83.95 Non-follicular (diffuse) lymphoma, unspecified, lymph nodes of inguinal region and lower limb

C83.96 Non-follicular (diffuse) lymphoma, unspecified, intrapelvic lymph nodes

C83.97 Non-follicular (diffuse) lymphoma, unspecified, spleen

C83.98 Non-follicular (diffuse) lymphoma, unspecified, lymph nodes of multiple sites

C83.99 Non-follicular (diffuse) lymphoma, unspecified, extranodal and solid organ sites

C84 **Mature T/NK-cell lymphomas**

Excludes1: personal history of non-Hodgkin lymphoma (Z85.72)

C84.0 **Mycosis fungoides**

Excludes1: peripheral T-cell lymphoma, not classified (C84.4-)

C84.00 Mycosis fungoides, unspecified site

C84.01 Mycosis fungoides, lymph nodes of head, face, and neck

C84.02 Mycosis fungoides, intrathoracic lymph nodes

● New code   ▲ Revised code   **Excludes1:** Not coded here   **Excludes2:** Not included here   ⊗ Placeholder required   ⑦ 7th digit required

C84.03 **Mycosis fungoides, intra-abdominal lymph nodes**

C84.04 **Mycosis fungoides, lymph nodes of axilla and upper limb**

C84.05 **Mycosis fungoides, lymph nodes of inguinal region and lower limb**

C84.06 **Mycosis fungoides, intrapelvic lymph nodes**

C84.07 **Mycosis fungoides, spleen**

C84.08 **Mycosis fungoides, lymph nodes of multiple sites**

C84.09 **Mycosis fungoides, extranodal and solid organ sites**

C84.1 **Sézary disease**

C84.10 **Sézary disease, unspecified site**

C84.11 **Sézary disease, lymph nodes of head, face, and neck**

C84.12 **Sézary disease, intrathoracic lymph nodes**

C84.13 **Sézary disease, intra-abdominal lymph nodes**

C84.14 **Sézary disease, lymph nodes of axilla and upper limb**

C84.15 **Sézary disease, lymph nodes of inguinal region and lower limb**

C84.16 **Sézary disease, intrapelvic lymph nodes**

C84.17 **Sézary disease, spleen**

C84.18 **Sézary disease, lymph nodes of multiple sites**

C84.19 **Sézary disease, extranodal and solid organ sites**

C84.4 **Peripheral T-cell lymphoma, not classified**

Lennert's lymphoma Lymphoepithelioid lymphoma

Mature T-cell lymphoma, not elsewhere classified

C84.40 **Peripheral T-cell lymphoma, not classified, unspecified site**

C84.41 **Peripheral T-cell lymphoma, not classified, lymph nodes of head, face, and neck**

C84.42 **Peripheral T-cell lymphoma, not classified, intrathoracic lymph nodes**

C84.43 **Peripheral T-cell lymphoma, not classified, intra-abdominal lymph nodes**

C84.44 **Peripheral T-cell lymphoma, not classified, lymph nodes of axilla and upper limb**

C84.45 **Peripheral T-cell lymphoma, not classified, lymph nodes of inguinal region and lower limb**

C84.46 **Peripheral T-cell lymphoma, not classified, intrapelvic lymph nodes**

C84.47 **Peripheral T-cell lymphoma, not classified, spleen**

C84.48 **Peripheral T-cell lymphoma, not classified, lymph nodes of multiple sites**

C84.49 **Peripheral T-cell lymphoma, not classified, extranodal and solid organ sites**

C84.6 **Anaplastic large cell lymphoma, ALK-positive**

Anaplastic large cell lymphoma, CD30-positive

C84.60 **Anaplastic large cell lymphoma, ALK-positive, unspecified site**

C84.61 **Anaplastic large cell lymphoma, ALK-positive, lymph nodes of head, face, and neck**

C84.62 **Anaplastic large cell lymphoma, ALK-positive, intrathoracic lymph nodes**

C84.63 **Anaplastic large cell lymphoma, ALK-positive, intra-abdominal lymph nodes**

C84.64 **Anaplastic large cell lymphoma, ALK-positive, lymph nodes of axilla and upper limb**

C84.65 **Anaplastic large cell lymphoma, ALK-positive, lymph nodes of inguinal region and lower limb**

C84.66 **Anaplastic large cell lymphoma, ALK-positive, intrapelvic lymph nodes**

C84.67 **Anaplastic large cell lymphoma, ALK-positive, spleen**

C84.68 **Anaplastic large cell lymphoma, ALK-positive, lymph nodes of multiple sites**

C84.69 **Anaplastic large cell lymphoma, ALK-positive, extranodal and solid organ sites**

C84.7 **Anaplastic large cell lymphoma, ALK-negative**

Excludes1: primary cutaneous CD30-positive T-cell proliferations (C86.6-)

C84.70 **Anaplastic large cell lymphoma, ALK-negative, unspecified site**

C84.71 **Anaplastic large cell lymphoma, ALK-negative, lymph nodes of head, face, and neck**

C84.72 **Anaplastic large cell lymphoma, ALK-negative, intrathoracic lymph nodes**

C84.73 **Anaplastic large cell lymphoma, ALK-negative, intra-abdominal lymph nodes**

C84.74 **Anaplastic large cell lymphoma, ALK-negative, lymph nodes of axilla and upper limb**

C84.75 **Anaplastic large cell lymphoma, ALK-negative, lymph nodes of inguinal region and lower limb**

C84.76 **Anaplastic large cell lymphoma, ALK-negative, intrapelvic lymph nodes**

C84.77 **Anaplastic large cell lymphoma, ALK-negative, spleen**

C84.78 **Anaplastic large cell lymphoma, ALK-negative, lymph nodes of multiple sites**

C84.79 **Anaplastic large cell lymphoma, ALK-negative, extranodal and solid organ sites**

C84.A **Cutaneous T-cell lymphoma, unspecified**

C84.A0 **Cutaneous T-cell lymphoma, unspecified, unspecified site**

C84.A1 **Cutaneous T-cell lymphoma, unspecified lymph nodes of head, face, and neck**

C84.A2 **Cutaneous T-cell lymphoma, unspecified, intrathoracic lymph nodes**

C84.A3 **Cutaneous T-cell lymphoma, unspecified, intra-abdominal lymph nodes**

C84.A4 **Cutaneous T-cell lymphoma, unspecified, lymph nodes of axilla and upper limb**

C84.A5 **Cutaneous T-cell lymphoma, unspecified, lymph nodes of inguinal region and lower limb**

C84.A6 **Cutaneous T-cell lymphoma, unspecified, intrapelvic lymph nodes**

C84.A7 **Cutaneous T-cell lymphoma, unspecified, spleen**

C84.A8 **Cutaneous T-cell lymphoma, unspecified, lymph nodes of multiple sites**

C84.A9 **Cutaneous T-cell lymphoma, unspecified, extranodal and solid organ sites**

C84.Z **Other mature T/NK-cell lymphomas**

Note: If T-cell lineage or involvement is mentioned in conjunction with a specific lymphoma, code to the more specific description.

Excludes1: angioimmunoblastic T-cell lymphoma (C86.5)

blastic NK-cell lymphoma (C86.4)

enteropathy-type T-cell lymphoma (C86.2)

extranodal NK-cell lymphoma, nasal type (C86.0)

hepatosplenic T-cell lymphoma (C86.1)

primary cutaneous CD30-positive T-cell
proliferations (C86.6)

subcutaneous panniculitis-like T-cell lymphoma
(C86.3)

T-cell leukemia (C91.1-)

C84.Z0   **Other mature T/NK-cell lymphomas,
unspecified site**

C84.Z1   **Other mature T/NK-cell lymphomas, lymph
nodes of head, face, and neck**

C84.Z2   **Other mature T/NK-cell lymphomas,
intrathoracic lymph nodes**

C84.Z3   **Other mature T/NK-cell lymphomas, intra-
abdominal lymph nodes**

C84.Z4   **Other mature T/NK-cell lymphomas, lymph
nodes of axilla and upper limb**

C84.Z5   **Other mature T/NK-cell lymphomas, lymph
nodes of inguinal region and lower limb**

C84.Z6   **Other mature T/NK-cell lymphomas,
intrapelvic lymph nodes**

C84.Z7   **Other mature T/NK-cell lymphomas, spleen**

C84.Z8   **Other mature T/NK-cell lymphomas, lymph
nodes of multiple sites**

C84.Z9   **Other mature T/NK-cell lymphomas,
extranodal and solid organ sites**

C84.9   **Mature T/NK-cell lymphomas, unspecified**

NK/T cell lymphoma NOS

Excludes1: mature T-cell lymphoma, not elsewhere
classified (C84.4-)

C84.90   **Mature T/NK-cell lymphomas, unspecified,
unspecified site**

C84.91   **Mature T/NK-cell lymphomas, unspecified,
lymph nodes of head, face, and neck**

C84.92   **Mature T/NK-cell lymphomas, unspecified,
intrathoracic lymph nodes**

C84.93   **Mature T/NK-cell lymphomas, unspecified,
intra-abdominal lymph nodes**

C84.94   **Mature T/NK-cell lymphomas, unspecified,
lymph nodes of axilla and upper limb**

C84.95   **Mature T/NK-cell lymphomas, unspecified,
lymph nodes of inguinal region and lower limb**

C84.96   **Mature T/NK-cell lymphomas, unspecified,
intrapelvic lymph nodes**

C84.97   **Mature T/NK-cell lymphomas, unspecified,
spleen**

C84.98   **Mature T/NK-cell lymphomas, unspecified,
lymph nodes of multiple sites**

C84.99   **Mature T/NK-cell lymphomas, unspecified,
extranodal and solid organ sites**

C85   **Other specified and unspecified types of non-Hodgkin lymphoma**

Excludes1: Other specified types of T/NK-cell lymphoma (C86.-)

personal history of non-Hodgkin lymphoma (Z85.72)

C85.1   **Unspecified B-cell lymphoma**

Note: If B-cell lineage or involvement is mentioned in
conjunction with a specific lymphoma, code to the more
specific description.

C85.10   **Unspecified B-cell lymphoma, unspecified site**

C85.11   **Unspecified B-cell lymphoma, lymph nodes of
head, face, and neck**

C85.12   **Unspecified B-cell lymphoma, intrathoracic
lymph nodes**

C85.13   **Unspecified B-cell lymphoma, intra-abdominal
lymph nodes**

C85.14   **Unspecified B-cell lymphoma, lymph nodes of
axilla and upper limb**

C85.15   **Unspecified B-cell lymphoma, lymph nodes of
inguinal region and lower limb**

C85.16   **Unspecified B-cell lymphoma, intrapelvic
lymph nodes**

C85.17   **Unspecified B-cell lymphoma, spleen**

C85.18   **Unspecified B-cell lymphoma, lymph nodes of
multiple sites**

C85.19   **Unspecified B-cell lymphoma, extranodal and
solid organ sites**

C85.2   **Mediastinal (thymic) large B-cell lymphoma**

C85.20   **Mediastinal (thymic) large B-cell lymphoma,
unspecified site**

C85.21   **Mediastinal (thymic) large B-cell lymphoma,
lymph nodes of head, face, and neck**

C85.22   **Mediastinal (thymic) large B-cell lymphoma,
intrathoracic lymph nodes**

C85.23   **Mediastinal (thymic) large B-cell lymphoma,
intra-abdominal lymph nodes**

C85.24   **Mediastinal (thymic) large B-cell lymphoma,
lymph nodes of axilla and upper limb**

C85.25   **Mediastinal (thymic) large B-cell lymphoma,
lymph nodes of inguinal region and lower limb**

C85.26   **Mediastinal (thymic) large B-cell lymphoma,
intrapelvic lymph nodes**

C85.27   **Mediastinal (thymic) large B-cell lymphoma,
spleen**

C85.28   **Mediastinal (thymic) large B-cell lymphoma,
lymph nodes of multiple sites**

C85.29   **Mediastinal (thymic) large B-cell lymphoma,
extranodal and solid organ sites**

C85.8   **Other specified types of non-Hodgkin lymphoma**

C85.80   **Other specified types of non-Hodgkin
lymphoma, unspecified site**

C85.81   **Other specified types of non-Hodgkin
lymphoma, lymph nodes of head, face, and neck**

C85.82   **Other specified types of non-Hodgkin
lymphoma, intrathoracic lymph nodes**

C85.83   **Other specified types of non-Hodgkin
lymphoma, intra-abdominal lymph nodes**

C85.84   **Other specified types of non-Hodgkin
lymphoma, lymph nodes of axilla and upper
limb**

C85.85   **Other specified types of non-Hodgkin
lymphoma, lymph nodes of inguinal region and
lower limb**

C85.86   **Other specified types of non-Hodgkin
lymphoma, intrapelvic lymph nodes**

C85.87   **Other specified types of non-Hodgkin
lymphoma, spleen**

C85.88   **Other specified types of non-Hodgkin
lymphoma, lymph nodes of multiple sites**

C85.89   **Other specified types of non-Hodgkin
lymphoma, extranodal and solid organ sites**

C85.9   **Non-Hodgkin lymphoma, unspecified**

Lymphoma NOS

Malignant lymphoma NOS

Non-Hodgkin lymphoma NOS

C85.90   **Non-Hodgkin lymphoma, unspecified,
unspecified site**

C85.91   **Non-Hodgkin lymphoma, unspecified, lymph
nodes of head, face, and neck**

● New code   ▲ Revised code   **Excludes1:** Not coded here   **Excludes2:** Not included here   ⊗ Placeholder required   ⑦7ᵗʰ digit required

C85.92   Non-Hodgkin lymphoma, unspecified, intrathoracic lymph nodes

C85.93   Non-Hodgkin lymphoma, unspecified, intra-abdominal lymph nodes

C85.94   Non-Hodgkin lymphoma, unspecified, lymph nodes of axilla and upper limb

C85.95   Non-Hodgkin lymphoma, unspecified, lymph nodes of inguinal region and lower limb

C85.96   Non-Hodgkin lymphoma, unspecified, intrapelvic lymph nodes

C85.97   Non-Hodgkin lymphoma, unspecified, spleen

C85.98   Non-Hodgkin lymphoma, unspecified, lymph nodes of multiple sites

C85.99   Non-Hodgkin lymphoma, unspecified, extranodal and solid organ sites

C86   **Other specified types of T/NK-cell lymphoma**

Excludes1: anaplastic large cell lymphoma, ALK negative (C84.7-)

anaplastic large cell lymphoma, ALK positive (C84.6-)

mature T/NK-cell lymphomas (C84.-)

Other specified types of non-Hodgkin lymphoma (C85.8-)

C86.0   **Extranodal NK/T-cell lymphoma, nasal type**

C86.1   **Hepatosplenic T-cell lymphoma**

Alpha-beta and gamma delta types

C86.2   **Enteropathy-type (intestinal) T-cell lymphoma**

Enteropathy associated T-cell lymphoma

C86.3   **Subcutaneous panniculitis-like T-cell lymphoma**

C86.4   **Blastic NK-cell lymphoma**

Blastic plasmacytoid dendritic cell neoplasm (BPDCN)

C86.5   **Angioimmunoblastic T-cell lymphoma**

Angioimmunoblastic lymphadenopathy with dysproteinemia (AILD)

C86.6   **Primary cutaneous CD30-positive T-cell proliferations**

Lymphomatoid papulosis

Primary cutaneous anaplastic large cell lymphoma

Primary cutaneous CD30-positive large T-cell lymphoma

C88   **Malignant immunoproliferative diseases and certain other B-cell lymphomas**

Excludes1: B-cell lymphoma, unspecified (C85.1-)

personal history of other malignant neoplasms of lymphoid, hematopoietic and related tissues (Z85.79)

C88.0   **Waldenström macroglobulinemia**

Lymphoplasmacytic lymphoma with IgM-production

Macroglobulinemia (idiopathic) (primary)

Excludes1: small cell B-cell lymphoma (C83.0)

C88.2   **Heavy chain disease**

Franklin disease

Gamma heavy chain disease

Mu heavy chain disease

C88.3   **Immunoproliferative small intestinal disease**

Alpha heavy chain disease

Mediterranean lymphoma

C88.4   **Extranodal marginal zone B-cell lymphoma of mucosa-associated lymphoid tissue [MALT-lymphoma]**

Lymphoma of skin-associated lymphoid tissue [SALT-lymphoma]

Lymphoma of bronchial-associated lymphoid tissue [BALT-lymphoma]

Excludes1: high malignant (diffuse large B-cell) lymphoma (C83.3-)

C88.8   **Other malignant immunoproliferative diseases**

C88.9   **Malignant immunoproliferative disease, unspecified**

Immunoproliferative disease NOS

C90   **Multiple myeloma and malignant plasma cell neoplasms**

Definition: Multiple myeloma and immunoproliferative neoplasms is a cancer in which there is a uncontrolled proliferation and disordered function of cells called plasma cells in the bone marrow., aka a plasma cell neoplasm.

Excludes1: personal history of other malignant neoplasms of lymphoid, hematopoietic and related tissues (Z85.79)

C90.0   **Multiple myeloma**

Kahler's disease

Medullary plasmacytoma

Myelomatosis

Plasma cell myeloma

Excludes1: solitary myeloma (C90.3-)

solitary plasmacytoma (C90.3-)

C90.00   **Multiple myeloma not having achieved remission**

Multiple myeloma with failed remission

Multiple myeloma NOS

C90.01   **Multiple myeloma in remission**

C90.02   **Multiple myeloma in relapse**

C90.1   **Plasma cell leukemia**

Plasmacytic leukemia

C90.10   **Plasma cell leukemia not having achieved remission**

Plasma cell leukemia with failed remission

Plasma cell leukemia NOS

C90.11   **Plasma cell leukemia in remission**

C90.12   **Plasma cell leukemia in relapse**

C90.2   **Extramedullary plasmacytoma**

C90.20   **Extramedullary plasmacytoma not having achieved remission**

Extramedullary plasmacytoma with failed remission

Extramedullary plasmacytoma NOS

C90.21   **Extramedullary plasmacytoma in remission**

C90.22   **Extramedullary plasmacytoma in relapse**

C90.3   **Solitary plasmacytoma**

Localized malignant plasma cell tumor NOS

Plasmacytoma NOS

Solitary myeloma

C90.30   **Solitary plasmacytoma not having achieved remission**

Solitary plasmacytoma with failed remission

Solitary plasmacytoma NOS

C90.31   **Solitary plasmacytoma in remission**

C90.32   **Solitary plasmacytoma in relapse**

C91   **Lymphoid leukemia**

Excludes1: personal history of leukemia (Z85.6)

C91.0   **Acute lymphoblastic leukemia [ALL]**

Note: Code C91.0 should only be used for T-cell and B-cell precursor leukemia

C91.00   **Acute lymphoblastic leukemia not having achieved remission**

Acute lymphoblastic leukemia with failed remission

Acute lymphoblastic leukemia NOS

C91.01   **Acute lymphoblastic leukemia, in remission**

C91.02   Acute lymphoblastic leukemia, in relapse

C91.1   Chronic lymphocytic leukemia of B-cell type

Lymphoplasmacytic leukemia

Richter syndrome

Excludes1: lymphoplasmacytic lymphoma (C83.0-)

C91.10   Chronic lymphocytic leukemia of B-cell type not having achieved remission

Chronic lymphocytic leukemia of B-cell type with failed remission

Chronic lymphocytic leukemia of B-cell type NOS

C91.11   Chronic lymphocytic leukemia of B-cell type in remission

C91.12   Chronic lymphocytic leukemia of B-cell type in relapse

C91.3   Prolymphocytic leukemia of B-cell type

C91.30   Prolymphocytic leukemia of B-cell type not having achieved remission

Prolymphocytic leukemia of B-cell type with failed remission

Prolymphocytic leukemia of B-cell type NOS

C91.31   Prolymphocytic leukemia of B-cell type, in remission

C91.32   Prolymphocytic leukemia of B-cell type, in relapse

C91.4   Hairy cell leukemia

Leukemic reticuloendotheliosis

C91.40   Hairy cell leukemia not having achieved remission

Hairy cell leukemia with failed remission

Hairy cell leukemia NOS

C91.41   Hairy cell leukemia, in remission

C91.42   Hairy cell leukemia, in relapse

C91.5   Adult T-cell lymphoma/leukemia (HTLV-1-associated)

Acute variant of adult T-cell lymphoma/leukemia (HTLV-1-associated)

Chronic variant of adult T-cell lymphoma/leukemia (HTLV-1-associated)

Lymphomatoid variant of adult T-cell lymphoma/leukemia (HTLV-1-associated)

Smouldering variant of adult T-cell lymphoma/leukemia (HTLV-1-associated)

C91.50   Adult T-cell lymphoma/leukemia (HTLV-1-associated) not having achieved remission

Adult T-cell lymphoma/leukemia (HTLV-1-associated) with failed remission

Adult T-cell lymphoma/leukemia (HTLV-1-associated) NOS

C91.51   Adult T-cell lymphoma/leukemia (HTLV-1-associated), in remission

C91.52   Adult T-cell lymphoma/leukemia (HTLV-1-associated), in relapse

C91.6   Prolymphocytic leukemia of T-cell type

C91.60   Prolymphocytic leukemia of T-cell type not having achieved remission

Prolymphocytic leukemia of T-cell type with failed remission

Prolymphocytic leukemia of T-cell type NOS

C91.61   Prolymphocytic leukemia of T-cell type, in remission

C91.62   Prolymphocytic leukemia of T-cell type, in relapse

C91.A   Mature B-cell leukemia Burkitt-type

Excludes1: Burkitt lymphoma (C83.7-)

C91.A0   Mature B-cell leukemia Burkitt-type not having achieved remission

Mature B-cell leukemia Burkitt-type with failed remission

Mature B-cell leukemia Burkitt-type NOS

C91.A1   Mature B-cell leukemia Burkitt-type, in remission

C91.A2   Mature B-cell leukemia Burkitt-type, in relapse

C91.Z   Other lymphoid leukemia

T-cell large granular lymphocytic leukemia (associated with rheumatoid arthritis)

C91.Z0   Other lymphoid leukemia not having achieved remission

Other lymphoid leukemia with failed remission

Other lymphoid leukemia NOS

C91.Z1   Other lymphoid leukemia, in remission

C91.Z2   Other lymphoid leukemia, in relapse

C91.9   Lymphoid leukemia, unspecified

C91.90   Lymphoid leukemia, unspecified not having achieved remission

Lymphoid leukemia with failed remission

Lymphoid leukemia NOS

C91.91   Lymphoid leukemia, unspecified, in remission

C91.92   Lymphoid leukemia, unspecified, in relapse

C92   Myeloid leukemia

Includes: granulocytic leukemia

myelogenous leukemia

Excludes1: personal history of leukemia (Z85.6)

C92.0   Acute myeloblastic leukemia

Acute myeloblastic leukemia, minimal differentiation

Acute myeloblastic leukemia (with maturation)

Acute myeloblastic leukemia 1/ETO

Acute myeloblastic leukemia M0

Acute myeloblastic leukemia M1

Acute myeloblastic leukemia M2

Acute myeloblastic leukemia with t(8;21)

Acute myeloblastic leukemia (without a FAB classification) NOS

Refractory anemia with excess blasts in transformation [RAEB T]

Excludes1: acute exacerbation of chronic myeloid leukemia (C92.10)

refractory anemia with excess of blasts not in transformation (D46.2-)

C92.00   Acute myeloblastic leukemia, not having achieved remission

Acute myeloblastic leukemia with failed remission

Acute myeloblastic leukemia NOS

C92.01   Acute myeloblastic leukemia, in remission

C92.02   Acute myeloblastic leukemia, in relapse

C92.1   Chronic myeloid leukemia, BCR/ABL-positive

Chronic myelogenous leukemia, Philadelphia chromosome (Ph1) positive

Chronic myelogenous leukemia, t(9;22) (q34;q11)

Chronic myelogenous leukemia with crisis of blast cells

Excludes1: atypical chronic myeloid leukemia BCR/ABL-negative (C92.2-)

chronic myelomonocytic leukemia (C93.1-)

chronic myeloproliferative disease (D47.1)

● New code   ▲ Revised code   **Excludes1:** Not coded here   **Excludes2:** Not included here   ⊗ Placeholder required   ⑦ 7th digit required

C92.10 **Chronic myeloid leukemia, BCR/ABL-positive, not having achieved remission**

Chronic myeloid leukemia, BCR/ABL-positive with failed remission

Chronic myeloid leukemia, BCR/ABL-positive NOS

C92.11 **Chronic myeloid leukemia, BCR/ABL-positive, in remission**

C92.12 **Chronic myeloid leukemia, BCR/ABL-positive, in relapse**

C92.2 **Atypical chronic myeloid leukemia, BCR/ABL-negative**

C92.20 **Atypical chronic myeloid leukemia, BCR/ABL-negative, not having achieved remission**

Atypical chronic myeloid leukemia, BCR/ABL-negative with failed remission

Atypical chronic myeloid leukemia, BCR/ABL-negative NOS

C92.21 **Atypical chronic myeloid leukemia, BCR/ABL-negative, in remission**

C92.22 **Atypical chronic myeloid leukemia, BCR/ABL-negative, in relapse**

C92.3 **Myeloid sarcoma**

A malignant tumor of immature myeloid cells

Chloroma

Granulocytic sarcoma

C92.30 **Myeloid sarcoma, not having achieved remission**

Myeloid sarcoma with failed remission

Myeloid sarcoma NOS

C92.31 **Myeloid sarcoma, in remission**

C92.32 **Myeloid sarcoma, in relapse**

C92.4 **Acute promyelocytic leukemia**

AML M3

AML Me with t(15;17) and variants

C92.40 **Acute promyelocytic leukemia, not having achieved remission**

Acute promyelocytic leukemia with failed remission

Acute promyelocytic leukemia NOS

C92.41 **Acute promyelocytic leukemia, in remission**

C92.42 **Acute promyelocytic leukemia, in relapse**

C92.5 **Acute myelomonocytic leukemia**

AML M4

AML M4 EO with inv(16) or t(16;16)

C92.50 **Acute myelomonocytic leukemia, not having achieved remission**

Acute myelomonocytic leukemia with failed remission

Acute myelomonocytic leukemia NOS

C92.51 **Acute myelomonocytic leukemia, in remission**

C92.52 **Acute myelomonocytic leukemia, in relapse**

C92.6 **Acute myeloid leukemia with 11q23-abnormality**

Acute myeloid leukemia with variation of MLL-gene

C92.60 **Acute myeloid leukemia with 11q23-abnormality not having achieved remission**

Acute myeloid leukemia with 11q23-abnormality with failed remission

Acute myeloid leukemia with 11q23-abnormality NOS

C92.61 **Acute myeloid leukemia with 11q23-abnormality in remission**

C92.62 **Acute myeloid leukemia with 11q23-abnormality in relapse**

C92.A **Acute myeloid leukemia with multilineage dysplasia**

Acute myeloid leukemia with dysplasia of remaining hematopoesis and/or myelodysplastic disease in its history

C92.A0 **Acute myeloid leukemia with multilineage dysplasia, not having achieved remission**

Acute myeloid leukemia with multilineage dysplasia with failed remission

Acute myeloid leukemia with multilineage dysplasia NOS

C92.A1 **Acute myeloid leukemia with multilineage dysplasia, in remission**

C92.A2 **Acute myeloid leukemia with multilineage dysplasia, in relapse**

C92.Z **Other myeloid leukemia**

C92.Z0 **Other myeloid leukemia not having achieved remission**

Myeloid leukemia NEC with failed remission

Myeloid leukemia NEC

C92.Z1 **Other myeloid leukemia, in remission**

C92.Z2 **Other myeloid leukemia, in relapse**

C92.9 **Myeloid leukemia, unspecified**

C92.90 **Myeloid leukemia, unspecified, not having achieved remission**

Myeloid leukemia, unspecified with failed remission

Myeloid leukemia, unspecified NOS

C92.91 **Myeloid leukemia, unspecified in remission**

C92.92 **Myeloid leukemia, unspecified in relapse**

C93 **Monocytic leukemia**

Includes: monocytoid leukemia

Excludes1: personal history of leukemia (Z85.6)

C93.0 **Acute monoblastic/monocytic leukemia**

AML M5 AML M5a AML M5b

C93.00 **Acute monoblastic/monocytic leukemia, not having achieved remission**

Acute monoblastic/monocytic leukemia with failed remission

Acute monoblastic/monocytic leukemia NOS

C93.01 **Acute monoblastic/monocytic leukemia, in remission**

C93.02 **Acute monoblastic/monocytic leukemia, in relapse**

C93.1 **Chronic myelomonocytic leukemia**

Chronic monocytic leukemia CMML-1

CMML-2

CMML with eosinophilia

C93.10 **Chronic myelomonocytic leukemia not having achieved remission**

Chronic myelomonocytic leukemia with failed remission

Chronic myelomonocytic leukemia NOS

C93.11 **Chronic myelomonocytic leukemia, in remission**

C93.12 **Chronic myelomonocytic leukemia, in relapse**

C93.3 **Juvenile myelomonocytic leukemia**

C93.30 **Juvenile myelomonocytic leukemia, not having achieved remission**

| | Add 4th-7th digits | | Nonspecific code | | Unspecified code | | Manifestation code | **197** |

Juvenile myelomonocytic leukemia with failed remission Juvenile myelomonocytic leukemia NOS

    C93.31 **Juvenile myelomonocytic leukemia, in remission**

    C93.32 **Juvenile myelomonocytic leukemia, in relapse**

C93.Z **Other monocytic leukemia**

    C93.Z0 **Other monocytic leukemia, not having achieved remission**

    Other monocytic leukemia NOS

    C93.Z1 **Other monocytic leukemia, in remission**

    C93.Z2 **Other monocytic leukemia, in relapse**

C93.9 **Monocytic leukemia, unspecified**

    C93.90 **Monocytic leukemia, unspecified, not having achieved remission**

    Monocytic leukemia, unspecified with failed remission

    Monocytic leukemia, unspecified NOS

    C93.91 **Monocytic leukemia, unspecified in remission**

    C93.92 **Monocytic leukemia, unspecified in relapse**

C94 **Other leukemias of specified cell type**

    Excludes1: leukemic reticuloendotheliosis (C91.4-)

    myelodysplastic syndromes (D46.-)

    personal history of leukemia (Z85.6)

    plasma cell leukemia (C90.1-)

C94.0 **Acute erythroid leukemia**

    Acute myeloid leukemia M6(a)(b)

    Erythroleukemia

    C94.00 **Acute erythroid leukemia, not having achieved remission**

    Acute erythroid leukemia with failed remission

    Acute erythroid leukemia NOS

    C94.01 **Acute erythroid leukemia, in remission**

    C94.02 **Acute erythroid leukemia, in relapse**

C94.2 **Acute megakaryoblastic leukemia**

    Acute myeloid leukemia M7

    Acute megakaryocytic leukemia

    C94.20 **Acute megakaryoblastic leukemia not having achieved remission**

    Acute megakaryoblastic leukemia with failed remission

    Acute megakaryoblastic leukemia NOS

    C94.21 **Acute megakaryoblastic leukemia, in remission**

    C94.22 **Acute megakaryoblastic leukemia, in relapse**

C94.3 **Mast cell leukemia**

    C94.30 **Mast cell leukemia not having achieved remission**

    Mast cell leukemia with failed remission

    Mast cell leukemia NOS

    C94.31 **Mast cell leukemia, in remission**

    C94.32 **Mast cell leukemia, in relapse**

C94.4 **Acute panmyelosis with myelofibrosis**

    Acute myelofibrosis

    Excludes1: myelofibrosis NOS (D75.81)

    secondary myelofibrosis NOS (D75.81)

    C94.40 **Acute panmyelosis with myelofibrosis not having achieved remission**

    Acute myelofibrosis NOS

Acute panmyelosis with myelofibrosis with failed remission

Acute panmyelosis NOS

    C94.41 **Acute panmyelosis with myelofibrosis, in remission**

    C94.42 **Acute panmyelosis with myelofibrosis, in relapse**

C94.6 **Myelodysplastic disease, not classified**

    Myeloproliferative disease, not classified

C94.8 **Other specified leukemias**

    Aggressive NK-cell leukemia

    Acute basophilic leukemia

    C94.80 **Other specified leukemias not having achieved remission**

    Other specified leukemia with failed remission

    Other specified leukemias NOS

    C94.81 **Other specified leukemias, in remission**

    C94.82 **Other specified leukemias, in relapse**

C95 **Leukemia of unspecified cell type**

    Excludes1: personal history of leukemia (Z85.6)

C95.0 **Acute leukemia of unspecified cell type**

    Acute bilineal leukemia

    Acute mixed lineage leukemia

    Biphenotypic acute leukemia

    Stem cell leukemia of unclear lineage

    Excludes1: acute exacerbation of unspecified chronic leukemia (C95.10)

    C95.00 **Acute leukemia of unspecified cell type not having achieved remission**

    Acute leukemia of unspecified cell type with failed remission

    Acute leukemia NOS

    C95.01 **Acute leukemia of unspecified cell type, in remission**

    C95.02 **Acute leukemia of unspecified cell type, in relapse**

C95.1 **Chronic leukemia of unspecified cell type**

    C95.10 **Chronic leukemia of unspecified cell type not having achieved remission**

    Chronic leukemia of unspecified cell type with failed remission

    Chronic leukemia NOS

    C95.11 **Chronic leukemia of unspecified cell type, in remission**

    C95.12 **Chronic leukemia of unspecified cell type, in relapse**

C95.9 **Leukemia, unspecified**

    C95.90 **Leukemia, unspecified not having achieved remission**

    Leukemia, unspecified with failed remission

    Leukemia NOS

    C95.91 **Leukemia, unspecified, in remission**

    C95.92 **Leukemia, unspecified, in relapse**

C96 **Other and unspecified malignant neoplasms of lymphoid, hematopoietic and related tissue**

    Excludes1: personal history of other malignant neoplasms of lymphoid, hematopoietic and related tissues (Z85.79)

C96.0 **Multifocal and multisystemic (disseminated) Langerhans-cell histiocytosis**

    Histiocytosis X, multisystemic Letterer-Siwe disease

Excludes1: adult pulmonary Langerhans cell histiocytosis J84.82)

multifocal and unisystemic Langerhans-cell histiocytosis (C96.5)

unifocal Langerhans-cell histiocytosis (C96.6)

C96.2 **Malignant mast cell neoplasm**

Excludes1: indolent mastocytosis (D47.02)

mast cell leukemia (C94.30)

mastocytosis (congenital) (cutaneous) (Q82.2)

- C96.20 **Malignant mast cell neoplasm, unspecified**
- C96.21 **Aggressive systemic mastocytosis**
- C96.22 **Mast cell sarcoma**
- C96.29 **Other malignant mast cell neoplasm**

C96.4 **Sarcoma of dendritic cells (accessory cells)**

Follicular dendritic cell sarcoma

Interdigitating dendritic cell sarcoma Langerhans cell sarcoma

C96.5 **Multifocal and unisystemic Langerhans-cell histiocytosis**

Hand-Schüller-Christian disease

Histiocytosis X, multifocal

Excludes1: multifocal and multisystemic (disseminated) Langerhans-cell histiocytosis (C96.0)

unifocal Langerhans-cell histiocytosis (C96.6)

C96.6 **Unifocal Langerhans-cell histiocytosis**

Eosinophilic granuloma

Histiocytosis X, unifocal

Histiocytosis X NOS

Langerhans-cell histiocytosis NOS

Excludes1: multifocal and multisystemic (disseminated) Langerhans-cell histiocytosis (C96.0)

multifocal and unisystemic Langerhans-cell histiocytosis (C96.5)

C96.A **Histiocytic sarcoma**

Malignant histiocytosis

C96.Z **Other specified malignant neoplasms of lymphoid, hematopoietic and related tissue**

C96.9 **Malignant neoplasm of lymphoid, hematopoietic and related tissue, unspecified**

IN SITU NEOPLASMS (D00-D09)

Definition: Carcinoma in situ is a cluster of malignant cells that has not yet invaded the deeper epithelial tissue or spread to other parts of the body.

Includes: Bowen's disease

erythroplasia

grade III intraepithelial neoplasia

Queyrat's erythroplasia

D00 **Carcinoma in situ of oral cavity, esophagus and stomach**

Excludes1: melanoma in situ (D03.-)

D00.0 **Carcinoma in situ of lip, oral cavity and pharynx**

Use additional code to identify:

exposure to environmental tobacco smoke (Z77.22)

exposure to tobacco smoke in the perinatal period (P96.81)

history of tobacco dependence (Z87.891)

occupational exposure to environmental tobacco smoke (Z57.31)

tobacco dependence (F17.-)

tobacco use (Z72.0)

Excludes1: carcinoma in situ of aryepiglottic fold or interarytenoid fold, laryngeal aspect (D02.0)

carcinoma in situ of epiglottis NOS (D02.0)

carcinoma in situ of epiglottis suprahyoid portion (D02.0)

carcinoma in situ of skin of lip (D03.0, D04.0)

D00.00 **Carcinoma in situ of oral cavity, unspecified site**

D00.01 **Carcinoma in situ of labial mucosa and vermilion border**

D00.02 **Carcinoma in situ of buccal mucosa**

D00.03 **Carcinoma in situ of gingiva and edentulous alveolar ridge**

D00.04 **Carcinoma in situ of soft palate**

D00.05 **Carcinoma in situ of hard palate**

D00.06 **Carcinoma in situ of floor of mouth**

D00.07 **Carcinoma in situ of tongue**

D00.08 **Carcinoma in situ of pharynx**

Carcinoma in situ of aryepiglottic fold NOS

Carcinoma in situ of hypopharyngeal aspect of aryepiglottic fold

Carcinoma in situ of marginal zone of aryepiglottic fold

D00.1 **Carcinoma in situ of esophagus**

D00.2 **Carcinoma in situ of stomach**

D01 **Carcinoma in situ of other and unspecified digestive organs**

Excludes1: melanoma in situ (D03.-)

D01.0 **Carcinoma in situ of colon**

Excludes1: carcinoma in situ of rectosigmoid junction (D01.1)

D01.1 **Carcinoma in situ of rectosigmoid junction**

D01.2 **Carcinoma in situ of rectum**

D01.3 **Carcinoma in situ of anus and anal canal**

Anal intraepithelial neoplasia III [AIN III]

Severe dysplasia of anus

Excludes1: anal intraepithelial neoplasia I and II [AIN I and AIN II] (K62.82)

carcinoma in situ of anal margin (D04.5)

carcinoma in situ of anal skin (D04.5)

carcinoma in situ of perianal skin (D04.5)

D01.4 **Carcinoma in situ of other and unspecified parts of intestine**

Excludes1: carcinoma in situ of ampulla of Vater (D01.5)

D01.40 **Carcinoma in situ of unspecified part of intestine**

D01.49 **Carcinoma in situ of other parts of intestine**

D01.5 **Carcinoma in situ of liver, gallbladder and bile ducts**

Carcinoma in situ of ampulla of Vater

D01.7 **Carcinoma in situ of other specified digestive organs**

Carcinoma in situ of pancreas

D01.9 **Carcinoma in situ of digestive organ, unspecified**

D02 **Carcinoma in situ of middle ear and respiratory system**

Use additional code to identify:

exposure to environmental tobacco smoke (Z77.22)

exposure to tobacco smoke in the perinatal period (P96.81)

history of tobacco dependence (Z87.891)

occupational exposure to environmental tobacco smoke (Z57.31)

tobacco dependence (F17.-)

tobacco use (Z72.0)

Excludes1: melanoma in situ (D03.-)

D02.0 Carcinoma in situ of larynx

Carcinoma in situ of aryepiglottic fold or interarytenoid fold, laryngeal aspect

Carcinoma in situ of epiglottis (suprahyoid portion)

Excludes1: carcinoma in situ of aryepiglottic fold or interarytenoid fold NOS (D00.08)

carcinoma in situ of hypopharyngeal aspect (D00.08)

carcinoma in situ of marginal zone (D00.08)

D02.1 Carcinoma in situ of trachea

D02.2 Carcinoma in situ of bronchus and lung

D02.20 Carcinoma in situ of unspecified bronchus and lung

D02.21 Carcinoma in situ of right bronchus and lung

D02.22 Carcinoma in situ of left bronchus and lung

D02.3 Carcinoma in situ of other parts of respiratory system

Carcinoma in situ of accessory sinuses

Carcinoma in situ of middle ear

Carcinoma in situ of nasal cavities

Excludes1: carcinoma in situ of ear (external) (skin) (D04.2-)

carcinoma in situ of nose NOS D09.8

carcinoma in situ of skin of nose (D04.3)

D02.4 Carcinoma in situ of respiratory system, unspecified

D03 Melanoma in situ

D03.0 Melanoma in situ of lip

D03.1 Melanoma in situ of eyelid, including canthus

D03.10 Melanoma in situ of unspecified eyelid, including canthus

D03.11 Melanoma in situ of right eyelid, including canthus

D03.12 Melanoma in situ of left eyelid, including canthus

D03.2 Melanoma in situ of ear and external auricular canal

D03.20 Melanoma in situ of unspecified ear and external auricular canal

D03.21 Melanoma in situ of right ear and external auricular canal

D03.22 Melanoma in situ of left ear and external auricular canal

D03.3 Melanoma in situ of other and unspecified parts of face

D03.30 Melanoma in situ of unspecified part of face

D03.39 Melanoma in situ of other parts of face

D03.4 Melanoma in situ of scalp and neck

D03.5 Melanoma in situ of trunk

D03.51 Melanoma in situ of anal skin

Melanoma in situ of anal margin

Melanoma in situ of perianal skin

D03.52 Melanoma in situ of breast (skin) (soft tissue)

D03.59 Melanoma in situ of other part of trunk

D03.6 Melanoma in situ of upper limb, including shoulder

D03.60 Melanoma in situ of unspecified upper limb, including shoulder

D03.61 Melanoma in situ of right upper limb, including shoulder

D03.62 Melanoma in situ of left upper limb, including shoulder

D03.7 Melanoma in situ of lower limb, including hip

D03.70 Melanoma in situ of unspecified lower limb, including hip

D03.71 Melanoma in situ of right lower limb, including hip

D03.72 Melanoma in situ of left lower limb, including hip

D03.8 Melanoma in situ of other sites

Melanoma in situ of scrotum

Excludes1: carcinoma in situ of scrotum (D07.61)

D03.9 Melanoma in situ, unspecified

D04 Carcinoma in situ of skin

Excludes1: erythroplasia of Queyrat (penis) NOS (D07.4)

melanoma in situ (D03.-)

D04.0 Carcinoma in situ of skin of lip

Excludes1: carcinoma in situ of vermilion border of lip (D00.01)

D04.1 Carcinoma in situ of skin of eyelid, including canthus

D04.10 Carcinoma in situ of skin of unspecified eyelid, including canthus

D04.11 Carcinoma in situ of skin of right eyelid, including canthus

D04.12 Carcinoma in situ of skin of left eyelid, including canthus

D04.2 Carcinoma in situ of skin of ear and external auricular canal

D04.20 Carcinoma in situ of skin of unspecified ear and external auricular canal

D04.21 Carcinoma in situ of skin of right ear and external auricular canal

D04.22 Carcinoma in situ of skin of left ear and external auricular canal

D04.3 Carcinoma in situ of skin of other and unspecified parts of face

D04.30 Carcinoma in situ of skin of unspecified part of face

D04.39 Carcinoma in situ of skin of other parts of face

D04.4 Carcinoma in situ of skin of scalp and neck

D04.5 Carcinoma in situ of skin of trunk

Carcinoma in situ of anal margin

Carcinoma in situ of anal skin

Carcinoma in situ of perianal skin

Carcinoma in situ of skin of breast

Excludes1: carcinoma in situ of anus NOS (D01.3)

carcinoma in situ of scrotum (D07.61)

carcinoma in situ of skin of genital organs (D07.-)

D04.6 Carcinoma in situ of skin of upper limb, including shoulder

D04.60 Carcinoma in situ of skin of unspecified upper limb, including shoulder

D04.61 Carcinoma in situ of skin of right upper limb, including shoulder

D04.62 Carcinoma in situ of skin of left upper limb, including shoulder

D04.7 Carcinoma in situ of skin of lower limb, including hip

D04.70 Carcinoma in situ of skin of unspecified lower limb, including hip

D04.71 Carcinoma in situ of skin of right lower limb, including hip

D04.72 Carcinoma in situ of skin of left lower limb, including hip

D04.8   Carcinoma in situ of skin of other sites

D04.9   Carcinoma in situ of skin, unspecified

D05   Carcinoma in situ of breast

> **Excludes1:** carcinoma in situ of skin of breast (D04.5)
>
> melanoma in situ of breast (skin) (D03.5)
>
> Paget's disease of breast or nipple (C50.-)

D05.0   Lobular carcinoma in situ of breast

   D05.00   Lobular carcinoma in situ of unspecified breast

   D05.01   Lobular carcinoma in situ of right breast

   D05.02   Lobular carcinoma in situ of left breast

D05.1   Intraductal carcinoma in situ of breast

   D05.10   Intraductal carcinoma in situ of unspecified breast

   D05.11   Intraductal carcinoma in situ of right breast

   D05.12   Intraductal carcinoma in situ of left breast

D05.8   Other specified type of carcinoma in situ of breast

   D05.80   Other specified type of carcinoma in situ of unspecified breast

   D05.81   Other specified type of carcinoma in situ of right breast

   D05.82   Other specified type of carcinoma in situ of left breast

D05.9   Unspecified type of carcinoma in situ of breast

   D05.90   Unspecified type of carcinoma in situ of unspecified breast

   D05.91   Unspecified type of carcinoma in situ of right breast

   D05.92   Unspecified type of carcinoma in situ of left breast

D06   Carcinoma in situ of cervix uteri

> **Includes:** cervical adenocarcinoma in situ
>
> cervical intraepithelial glandular neoplasia
>
> cervical intraepithelial neoplasia III [CIN III]
>
> severe dysplasia of cervix uteri

> **Excludes1:** cervical intraepithelial neoplasia II [CIN II] (N87.1)
>
> cytologic evidence of malignancy of cervix without histologic confirmation (R87.614)
>
> high grade squamous intraepithelial lesion (HGSIL) of cervix (R87.613)
>
> melanoma in situ of cervix (D03.5)
>
> moderate cervical dysplasia (N87.1)

D06.0   Carcinoma in situ of endocervix

D06.1   Carcinoma in situ of exocervix

D06.7   Carcinoma in situ of other parts of cervix

D06.9   Carcinoma in situ of cervix, unspecified

D07   Carcinoma in situ of other and unspecified genital organs

> **Excludes1:** melanoma in situ of trunk (D03.5)

D07.0   Carcinoma in situ of endometrium

D07.1   Carcinoma in situ of vulva

Severe dysplasia of vulva

Vulvar intraepithelial neoplasia III [VIN III]

> **Excludes1:** moderate dysplasia of vulva (N90.1)
>
> vulvar intraepithelial neoplasia II [VIN II] (N90.1)

D07.2   Carcinoma in situ of vagina

Severe dysplasia of vagina

Vaginal intraepithelial neoplasia III [VAIN III]

> **Excludes1:** moderate dysplasia of vagina (N89.1)
>
> vaginal intraepithelial neoplasia II [VIN II] (N89.1)

D07.3   Carcinoma in situ of other and unspecified female genital organs

   D07.30   Carcinoma in situ of unspecified female genital organs

   D07.39   Carcinoma in situ of other female genital organs

D07.4   Carcinoma in situ of penis

Erythroplasia of Queyrat NOS

D07.5   Carcinoma in situ of prostate

Prostatic intraepithelial neoplasia III (PIN III)

Severe dysplasia of prostate

> **Excludes1:** dysplasia (mild) (moderate) of prostate (N42.3-)
>
> prostatic intraepithelial neoplasia II [PIN II] (N42.3-)

D07.6   Carcinoma in situ of other and unspecified male genital organs

   D07.60   Carcinoma in situ of unspecified male genital organs

   D07.61   Carcinoma in situ of scrotum

   D07.69   Carcinoma in situ of other male genital organs

D09   Carcinoma in situ of other and unspecified sites

> **Excludes1:** melanoma in situ (D03.-)

D09.0   Carcinoma in situ of bladder

D09.1   Carcinoma in situ of other and unspecified urinary organs

   D09.10   Carcinoma in situ of unspecified urinary organ

   D09.19   Carcinoma in situ of other urinary organs

D09.2   Carcinoma in situ of eye

> **Excludes1:** carcinoma in situ of skin of eyelid (D04.1-)

   D09.20   Carcinoma in situ of unspecified eye

   D09.21   Carcinoma in situ of right eye

   D09.22   Carcinoma in situ of left eye

D09.3   Carcinoma in situ of thyroid and other endocrine glands

> **Excludes1:** carcinoma in situ of endocrine pancreas (D01.7)
>
> carcinoma in situ of ovary (D07.39)
>
> carcinoma in situ of testis (D07.69)

D09.8   Carcinoma in situ of other specified sites

D09.9   Carcinoma in situ, unspecified

BENIGN NEOPLASMS, EXCEPT BENIGN NEUROENDOCRINE TUMORS (D10-D36)

Definition: A benign neoplasm is a localized tumor that has a fibrous capsule, limited potential for growth, a regular shape, and cells that are well differentiated. A benign neoplasm does not invade surrounding tissue or metastasize to distant sites. Some kinds of benign neoplasms are adenoma, fibroma, hemangioma, and lipoma.

D10 Benign neoplasm of mouth and pharynx

D10   Benign neoplasm of mouth and pharynx

D10.0   Benign neoplasm of lip

Benign neoplasm of lip (frenulum) (inner aspect) (mucosa) (vermilion border)

> **Excludes1:** benign neoplasm of skin of lip (D22.0, D23.0)

D10.1   Benign neoplasm of tongue

Benign neoplasm of lingual tonsil

D10.2   Benign neoplasm of floor of mouth

D10.3   Benign neoplasm of other and unspecified parts of mouth

   D10.30   Benign neoplasm of unspecified part of mouth

   D10.39   Benign neoplasm of other parts of mouth

Benign neoplasm of minor salivary gland NOS

Excludes1: benign odontogenic neoplasms
(D16.4-D16.5)

benign neoplasm of mucosa of lip
(D10.0)

benign neoplasm of nasopharyngeal
surface of soft palate (D10.6)

D10.4 **Benign neoplasm of tonsil**

Benign neoplasm of tonsil (faucial) (palatine)

Excludes1: benign neoplasm of lingual tonsil (D10.1)

benign neoplasm of pharyngeal tonsil (D10.6)

benign neoplasm of tonsillar fossa (D10.5)

benign neoplasm of tonsillar pillars (D10.5)

D10.5 **Benign neoplasm of other parts of oropharynx**

Benign neoplasm of epiglottis, anterior aspect

Benign neoplasm of tonsillar fossa

Benign neoplasm of tonsillar pillars

Benign neoplasm of vallecula

Excludes1: benign neoplasm of epiglottis NOS (D14.1)

benign neoplasm of epiglottis, suprahyoid portion
(D14.1)

D10.6 **Benign neoplasm of nasopharynx**

Benign neoplasm of pharyngeal tonsil

Benign neoplasm of posterior margin of septum and
choanae

D10.7 **Benign neoplasm of hypopharynx**

D10.9 **Benign neoplasm of pharynx, unspecified**

D11 **Benign neoplasm of major salivary glands**

Excludes1: benign neoplasms of specified minor salivary glands
which are classified according to their anatomical location

benign neoplasms of minor salivary glands NOS (D10.39)

D11.0 **Benign neoplasm of parotid gland**

D11.7 **Benign neoplasm of other major salivary glands**

Benign neoplasm of sublingual salivary gland

Benign neoplasm of submandibular salivary gland

D11.9 **Benign neoplasm of major salivary gland, unspecified**

D12 **Benign neoplasm of colon, rectum, anus and anal canal**

Excludes1: benign carcinoid tumors of the large intestine, and
rectum (D3A.02-)

D12.0 **Benign neoplasm of cecum**

Benign neoplasm of ileocecal valve

D12.1 **Benign neoplasm of appendix**

Excludes1: benign carcinoid tumor of the appendix
(D3A.020)

D12.2 **Benign neoplasm of ascending colon**

D12.3 **Benign neoplasm of transverse colon**

Benign neoplasm of hepatic flexure

Benign neoplasm of splenic flexure

D12.4 **Benign neoplasm of descending colon**

D12.5 **Benign neoplasm of sigmoid colon**

D12.6 **Benign neoplasm of colon, unspecified**

Adenomatosis of colon

Benign neoplasm of large intestine NOS

Polyposis (hereditary) of colon

Excludes1: inflammatory polyp of colon (K51.4-)

polyp of colon NOS (K63.5)

D12.7 **Benign neoplasm of rectosigmoid junction**

D12.8 **Benign neoplasm of rectum**

Excludes1: benign carcinoid tumor of the rectum
(D3A.026)

D12.9 **Benign neoplasm of anus and anal canal**

Benign neoplasm of anus NOS

Excludes1: benign neoplasm of anal margin (D22.5, D23.5)

benign neoplasm of anal skin (D22.5, D23.5)

benign neoplasm of perianal skin (D22.5, D23.5)

D13 **Benign neoplasm of other and ill-defined parts of digestive
system**

Excludes1: benign stromal tumors of digestive system (D21.4)

D13.0 **Benign neoplasm of esophagus**

D13.1 **Benign neoplasm of stomach**

Excludes1: benign carcinoid tumor of the stomach
(D3A.092)

D13.2 **Benign neoplasm of duodenum**

Excludes1: benign carcinoid tumor of the duodenum
(D3A.010)

D13.3 **Benign neoplasm of other and unspecified parts of small
intestine**

Excludes1: benign carcinoid tumors of the small
intestine(D3A.01-)

benign neoplasm of ileocecal valve (D12.0)

D13.30 **Benign neoplasm of unspecified part of small
intestine**

D13.39 **Benign neoplasm of other parts of small
intestine**

D13.4 **Benign neoplasm of liver**

Benign neoplasm of intrahepatic bile ducts

D13.5 **Benign neoplasm of extrahepatic bile ducts**

D13.6 **Benign neoplasm of pancreas**

Excludes1: benign neoplasm of endocrine pancreas (D13.7)

D13.7 **Benign neoplasm of endocrine pancreas**

Islet cell tumor Benign neoplasm of islets of Langerhans

Use additional code to identify any functional activity.

D13.9 **Benign neoplasm of ill-defined sites within the digestive
system**

Benign neoplasm of digestive system NOS

Benign neoplasm of intestine NOS

Benign neoplasm of spleen

D14 **Benign neoplasm of middle ear and respiratory system**

D14.0 **Benign neoplasm of middle ear, nasal cavity and
accessory sinuses**

Benign neoplasm of cartilage of nose

Excludes1: benign neoplasm of auricular canal (external)
(D22.2-, D23.2-)

benign neoplasm of bone of ear (D16.4)

benign neoplasm of bone of nose (D16.4)

benign neoplasm of cartilage of ear (D21.0)

benign neoplasm of ear (external)(skin) (D22.2-,
D23.2-)

benign neoplasm of nose NOS (D36.7)

benign neoplasm of skin of nose (D22.39, D23.39)

benign neoplasm of olfactory bulb (D33.3)

benign neoplasm of posterior margin of septum
and choanae (D10.6)

polyp of accessory sinus (J33.8)

polyp of ear (middle) (H74.4)

polyp of nasal (cavity) (J33.-)

D14.1 **Benign neoplasm of larynx**

Adenomatous polyp of larynx

Benign neoplasm of epiglottis (suprahyoid portion)

Excludes1: benign neoplasm of epiglottis, anterior aspect (D10.5)

polyp (nonadenomatous) of vocal cord or larynx (J38.1)

D14.2 **Benign neoplasm of trachea**

D14.3 **Benign neoplasm of bronchus and lung**

Excludes1: benign carcinoid tumor of the bronchus and lung (D3A.090)

D14.30 **Benign neoplasm of unspecified bronchus and lung**

D14.31 **Benign neoplasm of right bronchus and lung**

D14.32 **Benign neoplasm of left bronchus and lung**

D14.4 **Benign neoplasm of respiratory system, unspecified**

D15 **Benign neoplasm of other and unspecified intrathoracic organs**

Excludes1: benign neoplasm of mesothelial tissue (D19.-)

D15.0 **Benign neoplasm of thymus**

Excludes1: benign carcinoid tumor of the thymus (D3A.091)

D15.1 **Benign neoplasm of heart**

Excludes1: benign neoplasm of great vessels (D21.3)

D15.2 **Benign neoplasm of mediastinum**

D15.7 **Benign neoplasm of other specified intrathoracic organs**

D15.9 **Benign neoplasm of intrathoracic organ, unspecified**

D16 **Benign neoplasm of bone and articular cartilage**

Excludes1: benign neoplasm of connective tissue of ear (D21.0)

benign neoplasm of connective tissue of eyelid (D21.0)

benign neoplasm of connective tissue of larynx (D14.1)

benign neoplasm of connective tissue of nose (D14.0)

benign neoplasm of synovia (D21.-)

D16.0 **Benign neoplasm of scapula and long bones of upper limb**

D16.00 **Benign neoplasm of scapula and long bones of unspecified upper limb**

D16.01 **Benign neoplasm of scapula and long bones of right upper limb**

D16.02 **Benign neoplasm of scapula and long bones of left upper limb**

D16.1 **Benign neoplasm of short bones of upper limb**

D16.10 **Benign neoplasm of short bones of unspecified upper limb**

D16.11 **Benign neoplasm of short bones of right upper limb**

D16.12 **Benign neoplasm of short bones of left upper limb**

D16.2 **Benign neoplasm of long bones of lower limb**

D16.20 **Benign neoplasm of long bones of unspecified lower limb**

D16.21 **Benign neoplasm of long bones of right lower limb**

D16.22 **Benign neoplasm of long bones of left lower limb**

D16.3 **Benign neoplasm of short bones of lower limb**

D16.30 **Benign neoplasm of short bones of unspecified lower limb**

D16.31 **Benign neoplasm of short bones of right lower limb**

D16.32 **Benign neoplasm of short bones of left lower limb**

D16.4 **Benign neoplasm of bones of skull and face**

Benign neoplasm of maxilla (superior)

Benign neoplasm of orbital bone

Keratocyst of maxilla

Keratocystic odontogenic tumor of maxilla

Excludes2: benign neoplasm of lower jaw bone (D16.5)

D16.5 **Benign neoplasm of lower jaw bone**

Keratocyst of mandible

Keratocystic odontogenic tumor of mandible

D16.6 **Benign neoplasm of vertebral column**

Excludes1: benign neoplasm of sacrum and coccyx (D16.8)

D16.7 **Benign neoplasm of ribs, sternum and clavicle**

D16.8 **Benign neoplasm of pelvic bones, sacrum and coccyx**

D16.9 **Benign neoplasm of bone and articular cartilage, unspecified**

D17 **Benign lipomatous neoplasm**

D17.0 **Benign lipomatous neoplasm of skin and subcutaneous tissue of head, face and neck**

D17.1 **Benign lipomatous neoplasm of skin and subcutaneous tissue of trunk**

D17.2 **Benign lipomatous neoplasm of skin and subcutaneous tissue of limb**

D17.20 **Benign lipomatous neoplasm of skin and subcutaneous tissue of unspecified limb**

D17.21 **Benign lipomatous neoplasm of skin and subcutaneous tissue of right arm**

D17.22 **Benign lipomatous neoplasm of skin and subcutaneous tissue of left arm**

D17.23 **Benign lipomatous neoplasm of skin and subcutaneous tissue of right leg**

D17.24 **Benign lipomatous neoplasm of skin and subcutaneous tissue of left leg**

D17.3 **Benign lipomatous neoplasm of skin and subcutaneous tissue of other and unspecified sites**

D17.30 **Benign lipomatous neoplasm of skin and subcutaneous tissue of unspecified sites**

D17.39 **Benign lipomatous neoplasm of skin and subcutaneous tissue of other sites**

D17.4 **Benign lipomatous neoplasm of intrathoracic organs**

D17.5 **Benign lipomatous neoplasm of intra-abdominal organs**

Excludes1: benign lipomatous neoplasm of peritoneum and retroperitoneum (D17.79)

D17.6 **Benign lipomatous neoplasm of spermatic cord**

D17.7 **Benign lipomatous neoplasm of other sites**

D17.71 **Benign lipomatous neoplasm of kidney**

D17.72 **Benign lipomatous neoplasm of other genitourinary organ**

D17.79 **Benign lipomatous neoplasm of other sites**

Benign lipomatous neoplasm of peritoneum

Benign lipomatous neoplasm of retroperitoneum

D17.9 **Benign lipomatous neoplasm, unspecified**

Lipoma NOS

D18 **Hemangioma and lymphangioma, any site**

Definition: Hemangioma is a benign skin lesion consisting of dense, usually elevated masses of dilated blood vessels. Lymphangioma is a benign neoplasm characterized by lymph vessel proliferation.

Excludes1: benign neoplasm of glomus jugulare (D35.6)

blue or pigmented nevus (D22.-) nevus NOS (D22.-)

vascular nevus (Q82.5)

D18.0 **Hemangioma**

Angioma NOS

Cavernous nevus

D18.00 Hemangioma unspecified site

D18.01 Hemangioma of skin and subcutaneous tissue

D18.02 Hemangioma of intracranial structures

D18.03 Hemangioma of intra-abdominal structures

D18.09 Hemangioma of other sites

D18.1 Lymphangioma, any site

D19 Benign neoplasm of mesothelial tissue

D19.0 Benign neoplasm of mesothelial tissue of pleura

D19.1 Benign neoplasm of mesothelial tissue of peritoneum

D19.7 Benign neoplasm of mesothelial tissue of other sites

D19.9 Benign neoplasm of mesothelial tissue, unspecified

Benign mesothelioma NOS

D20 Benign neoplasm of soft tissue of retroperitoneum and peritoneum

Excludes1: benign lipomatous neoplasm of peritoneum and retroperitoneum (D17.79)

benign neoplasm of mesothelial tissue (D19.-)

D20.0 Benign neoplasm of soft tissue of retroperitoneum

D20.1 Benign neoplasm of soft tissue of peritoneum

D21 Other benign neoplasms of connective and other soft tissue

Includes: benign neoplasm of blood vessel

benign neoplasm of bursa

benign neoplasm of cartilage

benign neoplasm of fascia

benign neoplasm of fat

benign neoplasm of ligament, except uterine

benign neoplasm of lymphatic channel

benign neoplasm of muscle

benign neoplasm of synovia

benign neoplasm of tendon (sheath)

benign stromal tumors

Excludes1: benign neoplasm of articular cartilage (D16.-)

benign neoplasm of cartilage of larynx (D14.1)

benign neoplasm of cartilage of nose (D14.0)

benign neoplasm of connective tissue of breast (D24.-)

benign neoplasm of peripheral nerves and autonomic nervous system (D36.1-)

benign neoplasm of peritoneum (D20.1)

benign neoplasm of retroperitoneum (D20.0)

benign neoplasm of uterine ligament, any (D28.2)

benign neoplasm of vascular tissue (D18.-)

hemangioma (D18.0-)

lipomatous neoplasm (D17.-)

lymphangioma (D18.1)

uterine leiomyoma (D25.-)

D21.0 Benign neoplasm of connective and other soft tissue of head, face and neck

Benign neoplasm of connective tissue of ear

Benign neoplasm of connective tissue of eyelid

Excludes1: benign neoplasm of connective tissue of orbit (D31.6-)

D21.1 Benign neoplasm of connective and other soft tissue of upper limb, including shoulder

D21.10 Benign neoplasm of connective and other soft tissue of unspecified upper limb, including shoulder

D21.11 Benign neoplasm of connective and other soft tissue of right upper limb, including shoulder

D21.12 Benign neoplasm of connective and other soft tissue of left upper limb, including shoulder

D21.2 Benign neoplasm of connective and other soft tissue of lower limb, including hip

D21.20 Benign neoplasm of connective and other soft tissue of unspecified lower limb, including hip

D21.21 Benign neoplasm of connective and other soft tissue of right lower limb, including hip

D21.22 Benign neoplasm of connective and other soft tissue of left lower limb, including hip

D21.3 Benign neoplasm of connective and other soft tissue of thorax

Benign neoplasm of axilla

Benign neoplasm of diaphragm

Benign neoplasm of great vessels

Excludes1: benign neoplasm of heart (D15.1)

benign neoplasm of mediastinum (D15.2)

benign neoplasm of thymus (D15.0)

D21.4 Benign neoplasm of connective and other soft tissue of abdomen

Benign stromal tumors of abdomen

D21.5 Benign neoplasm of connective and other soft tissue of pelvis

Excludes1: benign neoplasm of any uterine ligament (D28.2)

uterine leiomyoma (D25.-)

D21.6 Benign neoplasm of connective and other soft tissue of trunk, unspecified

Benign neoplasm of back NOS

D21.9 Benign neoplasm of connective and other soft tissue, unspecified

D22 Melanocytic nevi

Includes: atypical nevus

blue hairy pigmented nevus NOS

D22.0 Melanocytic nevi of lip

D22.1 Melanocytic nevi of eyelid, including canthus

D22.10 Melanocytic nevi of unspecified eyelid, including canthus

D22.11 Melanocytic nevi of right eyelid, including canthus

D22.12 Melanocytic nevi of left eyelid, including canthus

D22.2 Melanocytic nevi of ear and external auricular canal

D22.20 Melanocytic nevi of unspecified ear and external auricular canal

D22.21 Melanocytic nevi of right ear and external auricular canal

D22.22 Melanocytic nevi of left ear and external auricular canal

D22.3 Melanocytic nevi of other and unspecified parts of face

D22.30 Melanocytic nevi of unspecified part of face

D22.39 Melanocytic nevi of other parts of face

D22.4 Melanocytic nevi of scalp and neck

D22.5 Melanocytic nevi of trunk

Melanocytic nevi of anal margin

Melanocytic nevi of anal skin

Melanocytic nevi of perianal skin

Melanocytic nevi of skin of breast

D22.6 Melanocytic nevi of upper limb, including shoulder

D22.60 Melanocytic nevi of unspecified upper limb, including shoulder

● New code ▲ Revised code **Excludes1:** Not coded here **Excludes2:** Not included here ⊗ Placeholder required ⑦ 7th digit required

D22.61   Melanocytic nevi of right upper limb, including shoulder

D22.62   Melanocytic nevi of left upper limb, including shoulder

D22.7   Melanocytic nevi of lower limb, including hip

     D22.70   Melanocytic nevi of unspecified lower limb, including hip

     D22.71   Melanocytic nevi of right lower limb, including hip

     D22.72   Melanocytic nevi of left lower limb, including hip

D22.9   Melanocytic nevi, unspecified

D23   Other benign neoplasms of skin

Includes: benign neoplasm of hair follicles

         benign neoplasm of sebaceous glands

         benign neoplasm of sweat glands

Excludes1: benign lipomatous neoplasms of skin (D17.0-D17.3)

         melanocytic nevi (D22.-)

D23.0   Other benign neoplasm of skin of lip

     Excludes1: benign neoplasm of vermilion border of lip (D10.0)

D23.1   Other benign neoplasm of skin of eyelid, including canthus

     D23.10   Other benign neoplasm of skin of unspecified eyelid, including canthus

     D23.11   Other benign neoplasm of skin of right eyelid, including canthus

     D23.12   Other benign neoplasm of skin of left eyelid, including canthus

D23.2   Other benign neoplasm of skin of ear and external auricular canal

     D23.20   Other benign neoplasm of skin of unspecified ear and external auricular canal

     D23.21   Other benign neoplasm of skin of right ear and external auricular canal

     D23.22   Other benign neoplasm of skin of left ear and external auricular canal

D23.3   Other benign neoplasm of skin of other and unspecified parts of face

     D23.30   Other benign neoplasm of skin of unspecified part of face

     D23.39   Other benign neoplasm of skin of other parts of face

D23.4   Other benign neoplasm of skin of scalp and neck

D23.5   Other benign neoplasm of skin of trunk

     Other benign neoplasm of anal margin

     Other benign neoplasm of anal skin

     Other benign neoplasm of perianal skin

     Other benign neoplasm of skin of breast

     Excludes1: benign neoplasm of anus NOS (D12.9)

D23.6   Other benign neoplasm of skin of upper limb, including shoulder

     D23.60   Other benign neoplasm of skin of unspecified upper limb, including shoulder

     D23.61   Other benign neoplasm of skin of right upper limb, including shoulder

     D23.62   Other benign neoplasm of skin of left upper limb, including shoulder

D23.7   Other benign neoplasm of skin of lower limb, including hip

     D23.70   Other benign neoplasm of skin of unspecified lower limb, including hip

     D23.71   Other benign neoplasm of skin of right lower limb, including hip

     D23.72   Other benign neoplasm of skin of left lower limb, including hip

D23.9   Other benign neoplasm of skin, unspecified

D24   Benign neoplasm of breast

Includes: benign neoplasm of connective tissue of breast

         benign neoplasm of soft parts of breast

         fibroadenoma of breast

Excludes2: adenofibrosis of breast (N60.2)

         benign cyst of breast (N60.-)

         benign mammary dysplasia (N60.-)

         benign neoplasm of skin of breast (D22.5, D23.5)

         fibrocystic disease of breast (N60.-)

D24.1   Benign neoplasm of right breast

D24.2   Benign neoplasm of left breast

D24.9   Benign neoplasm of unspecified breast

D25   Leiomyoma of uterus

Includes: uterine fibroid

         uterine fibromyoma

         uterine myoma

D25.0   Submucous leiomyoma of uterus

D25.1   Intramural leiomyoma of uterus

     Interstitial leiomyoma of uterus

D25.2   Subserosal leiomyoma of uterus

     Subperitoneal leiomyoma of uterus

D25.9   Leiomyoma of uterus, unspecified

D26   Other benign neoplasms of uterus

D26.0   Other benign neoplasm of cervix uteri

D26.1   Other benign neoplasm of corpus uteri

D26.7   Other benign neoplasm of other parts of uterus

D26.9   Other benign neoplasm of uterus, unspecified

D27   Benign neoplasm of ovary

Use additional code to identify any functional activity.

Excludes2: corpus albicans cyst (N83.2-)

         corpus luteum cyst (N83.1-)

         endometrial cyst (N80.1)

         follicular (atretic) cyst (N83.0-)

         graafian follicle cyst (N83.0-)

         ovarian cyst NEC (N83.2-)

         ovarian retention cyst (N83.2-)

D27.0   Benign neoplasm of right ovary

D27.1   Benign neoplasm of left ovary

D27.9   Benign neoplasm of unspecified ovary

D28   Benign neoplasm of other and unspecified female genital organs

Includes: adenomatous polyp

         benign neoplasm of skin of female genital organs

         benign teratoma

Excludes1: epoophoron cyst (Q50.5)

         fimbrial cyst (Q50.4)

         Gartner's duct cyst (Q52.4)

         parovarian cyst (Q50.5)

D28.0   Benign neoplasm of vulva

D28.1   Benign neoplasm of vagina

D28.2   Benign neoplasm of uterine tubes and ligaments

     Benign neoplasm of fallopian tube

     Benign neoplasm of uterine ligament (broad) (round)

D28.7   Benign neoplasm of other specified female genital organs

D28.9   Benign neoplasm of female genital organ, unspecified

D29   Benign neoplasm of male genital organs

Includes: benign neoplasm of skin of male genital organs

D29.0   Benign neoplasm of penis

D29.1   Benign neoplasm of prostate

Excludes1: enlarged prostate (N40.-)

D29.2   Benign neoplasm of testis

Use additional code to identify any functional activity.

    D29.20   Benign neoplasm of unspecified testis

    D29.21   Benign neoplasm of right testis

    D29.22   Benign neoplasm of left testis

D29.3   Benign neoplasm of epididymis

    D29.30   Benign neoplasm of unspecified epididymis

    D29.31   Benign neoplasm of right epididymis

    D29.32   Benign neoplasm of left epididymis

D29.4   Benign neoplasm of scrotum

Benign neoplasm of skin of scrotum

D29.8   Benign neoplasm of other specified male genital organs

Benign neoplasm of seminal vesicle

Benign neoplasm of spermatic cord

Benign neoplasm of tunica vaginalis

D29.9   Benign neoplasm of male genital organ, unspecified

D30   Benign neoplasm of urinary organs

D30.0   Benign neoplasm of kidney

Excludes1: benign carcinoid tumor of the kidney (D3A.093)

benign neoplasm of renal calyces (D30.1-)

benign neoplasm of renal pelvis (D30.1-)

    D30.00   Benign neoplasm of unspecified kidney

    D30.01   Benign neoplasm of right kidney

    D30.02   Benign neoplasm of left kidney

D30.1   Benign neoplasm of renal pelvis

    D30.10   Benign neoplasm of unspecified renal pelvis

    D30.11   Benign neoplasm of right renal pelvis

    D30.12   Benign neoplasm of left renal pelvis

D30.2   Benign neoplasm of ureter

Excludes1: benign neoplasm of ureteric orifice of bladder (D30.3)

    D30.20   Benign neoplasm of unspecified ureter

    D30.21   Benign neoplasm of right ureter

    D30.22   Benign neoplasm of left ureter

D30.3   Benign neoplasm of bladder

Benign neoplasm of ureteric orifice of bladder

Benign neoplasm of urethral orifice of bladder

D30.4   Benign neoplasm of urethra

Excludes1: benign neoplasm of urethral orifice of bladder (D30.3)

D30.8   Benign neoplasm of other specified urinary organs

Benign neoplasm of paraurethral glands

D30.9   Benign neoplasm of urinary organ, unspecified

Benign neoplasm of urinary system NOS

D31   Benign neoplasm of eye and adnexa

Excludes1: benign neoplasm of connective tissue of eyelid (D21.0)

benign neoplasm of optic nerve (D33.3)

benign neoplasm of skin of eyelid (D22.1-, D23.1-)

D31.0   Benign neoplasm of conjunctiva

    D31.00   Benign neoplasm of unspecified conjunctiva

    D31.01   Benign neoplasm of right conjunctiva

    D31.02   Benign neoplasm of left conjunctiva

D31.1   Benign neoplasm of cornea

    D31.10   Benign neoplasm of unspecified cornea

    D31.11   Benign neoplasm of right cornea

    D31.12   Benign neoplasm of left cornea

D31.2   Benign neoplasm of retina

Excludes1: dark area on retina (D49.81)

hemangioma of retina (D49.81)

neoplasm of unspecified behavior of retina and choroid (D49.81)

retinal freckle (D49.81)

    D31.20   Benign neoplasm of unspecified retina

    D31.21   Benign neoplasm of right retina

    D31.22   Benign neoplasm of left retina

D31.3   Benign neoplasm of choroid

    D31.30   Benign neoplasm of unspecified choroid

    D31.31   Benign neoplasm of right choroid

    D31.32   Benign neoplasm of left choroid

D31.4   Benign neoplasm of ciliary body

    D31.40   Benign neoplasm of unspecified ciliary body

    D31.41   Benign neoplasm of right ciliary body

    D31.42   Benign neoplasm of left ciliary body

D31.5   Benign neoplasm of lacrimal gland and duct

Benign neoplasm of lacrimal sac

Benign neoplasm of nasolacrimal duct

    D31.50   Benign neoplasm of unspecified lacrimal gland and duct

    D31.51   Benign neoplasm of right lacrimal gland and duct

    D31.52   Benign neoplasm of left lacrimal gland and duct

D31.6   Benign neoplasm of unspecified site of orbit

Benign neoplasm of connective tissue of orbit

Benign neoplasm of extraocular muscle

Benign neoplasm of peripheral nerves of orbit

Benign neoplasm of retrobulbar tissue

Benign neoplasm of retro-ocular tissue

Excludes1: benign neoplasm of orbital bone (D16.4)

    D31.60   Benign neoplasm of unspecified site of unspecified orbit

    D31.61   Benign neoplasm of unspecified site of right orbit

    D31.62   Benign neoplasm of unspecified site of left orbit

D31.9   Benign neoplasm of unspecified part of eye

Benign neoplasm of eyeball

    D31.90   Benign neoplasm of unspecified part of unspecified eye

    D31.91   Benign neoplasm of unspecified part of right eye

    D31.92   Benign neoplasm of unspecified part of left eye

D32   Benign neoplasm of meninges

D32.0   Benign neoplasm of cerebral meninges

D32.1   Benign neoplasm of spinal meninges

D32.9   Benign neoplasm of meninges, unspecified

Meningioma NOS

D33 **Benign neoplasm of brain and other parts of central nervous system**

> Excludes1: angioma (D18.0-)
>
> benign neoplasm of meninges (D32.-)
>
> benign neoplasm of peripheral nerves and autonomic nervous system (D36.1-)
>
> hemangioma (D18.0-)
>
> neurofibromatosis (Q85.0-)
>
> retro-ocular benign neoplasm (D31.6-)

D33.0 **Benign neoplasm of brain, supratentorial**

Benign neoplasm of cerebral ventricle

Benign neoplasm of cerebrum

Benign neoplasm of frontal lobe

Benign neoplasm of occipital lobe

Benign neoplasm of parietal lobe

Benign neoplasm of temporal lobe

> Excludes1: benign neoplasm of fourth ventricle (D33.1)

D33.1 **Benign neoplasm of brain, infratentorial**

Benign neoplasm of brain stem

Benign neoplasm of cerebellum

Benign neoplasm of fourth ventricle

D33.2 **Benign neoplasm of brain, unspecified**

D33.3 **Benign neoplasm of cranial nerves**

Benign neoplasm of olfactory bulb

D33.4 **Benign neoplasm of spinal cord**

D33.7 **Benign neoplasm of other specified parts of central nervous system**

D33.9 **Benign neoplasm of central nervous system, unspecified**

Benign neoplasm of nervous system (central) NOS

D34 **Benign neoplasm of thyroid gland**

Use additional code to identify any functional activity

D35 **Benign neoplasm of other and unspecified endocrine glands**

Use additional code to identify any functional activity

> Excludes1: benign neoplasm of endocrine pancreas (D13.7)
>
> benign neoplasm of ovary (D27.-)
>
> benign neoplasm of testis (D29.2.-)
>
> benign neoplasm of thymus (D15.0)

D35.0 **Benign neoplasm of adrenal gland**

D35.00 **Benign neoplasm of unspecified adrenal gland**

D35.01 **Benign neoplasm of right adrenal gland**

D35.02 **Benign neoplasm of left adrenal gland**

D35.1 **Benign neoplasm of parathyroid gland**

D35.2 **Benign neoplasm of pituitary gland**

D35.3 **Benign neoplasm of craniopharyngeal duct**

D35.4 **Benign neoplasm of pineal gland**

D35.5 **Benign neoplasm of carotid body**

D35.6 **Benign neoplasm of aortic body and other paraganglia**

Benign tumor of glomus jugulare

D35.7 **Benign neoplasm of other specified endocrine glands**

D35.9 **Benign neoplasm of endocrine gland, unspecified**

Benign neoplasm of unspecified endocrine gland

D36 **Benign neoplasm of other and unspecified sites**

D36.0 **Benign neoplasm of lymph nodes**

> Excludes1: lymphangioma (D18.1)

D36.1 **Benign neoplasm of peripheral nerves and autonomic nervous system**

> Excludes1: benign neoplasm of peripheral nerves of orbit (D31.6-)

neurofibromatosis (Q85.0-)

D36.10 **Benign neoplasm of peripheral nerves and autonomic nervous system, unspecified**

D36.11 **Benign neoplasm of peripheral nerves and autonomic nervous system of face, head, and neck**

D36.12 **Benign neoplasm of peripheral nerves and autonomic nervous system, upper limb, including shoulder**

D36.13 **Benign neoplasm of peripheral nerves and autonomic nervous system of lower limb, including hip**

D36.14 **Benign neoplasm of peripheral nerves and autonomic nervous system of thorax**

D36.15 **Benign neoplasm of peripheral nerves and autonomic nervous system of abdomen**

D36.16 **Benign neoplasm of peripheral nerves and autonomic nervous system of pelvis**

D36.17 **Benign neoplasm of peripheral nerves and autonomic nervous system of trunk, unspecified**

D36.7 **Benign neoplasm of other specified sites**

Benign neoplasm of nose NOS

D36.9 **Benign neoplasm, unspecified site**

BENIGN NEUROENDOCRINE TUMORS (D3A)

Definition: Neuroendocrine tumor is a tumor derived from cells that release a hormone in response to a signal from the nervous system. Examples of neuroendocrine tumors include carcinoid tumors islet cell tumors, medullary thyroid carcinoma, and pheochromocytoma.

D3A **Benign neuroendocrine tumors**

Code also any associated multiple endocrine neoplasia [MEN] syndromes (E31.2-)

Use additional code to identify any associated endocrine syndrome, such as:

carcinoid syndrome (E34.0)

> Excludes2: benign pancreatic islet cell tumors (D13.7)

D3A.0 **Benign carcinoid tumors**

D3A.00 **Benign carcinoid tumor of unspecified site**

Carcinoid tumor NOS

D3A.01 **Benign carcinoid tumors of the small intestine**

D3A.010 **Benign carcinoid tumor of the duodenum**

D3A.011 **Benign carcinoid tumor of the jejunum**

D3A.012 **Benign carcinoid tumor of the ileum**

D3A.019 **Benign carcinoid tumor of the small intestine, unspecified portion**

D3A.020 **Benign carcinoid tumor of the appendix**

D3A.021 **Benign carcinoid tumor of the cecum**

D3A.022 **Benign carcinoid tumor of the ascending colon**

D3A.023 **Benign carcinoid tumor of the transverse colon**

D3A.024 **Benign carcinoid tumor of the descending colon**

D3A.025 **Benign carcinoid tumor of the sigmoid colon**

D3A.026 **Benign carcinoid tumor of the rectum**

D3A.029 **Benign carcinoid tumor of the large intestine, unspecified portion**

Benign carcinoid tumor of the colon NOS

D3A.09 **Benign carcinoid tumors of other sites**

D3A.090 **Benign carcinoid tumor of the bronchus and lung**

D3A.091 **Benign carcinoid tumor of the thymus**

D3A.092 **Benign carcinoid tumor of the stomach**

D3A.093 **Benign carcinoid tumor of the kidney**

D3A.094 **Benign carcinoid tumor of the foregut, unspecified**

D3A.095 **Benign carcinoid tumor of the midgut, unspecified**

D3A.096 **Benign carcinoid tumor of the hindgut, unspecified**

D3A.098 **Benign carcinoid tumors of other sites**

D3A.8 **Other benign neuroendocrine tumors**

Neuroendocrine tumor NOS

NEOPLASMS OF UNCERTAIN BEHAVIOR, POLYCYTHEMIA VERA AND MYELODYSPLASTIC SYNDROMES (D37-D48)

Note: Categories D37-D44, and D48 classify by site neoplasms of uncertain behavior, i.e., histologic confirmation whether the neoplasm is malignant or benign cannot be made.

Excludes1: neoplasms of unspecified behavior (D49.-)

D37 **Neoplasm of uncertain behavior of oral cavity and digestive organs**

Excludes1: stromal tumors of uncertain behavior of digestive system (D48.1)

D37.0 **Neoplasm of uncertain behavior of lip, oral cavity and pharynx**

Excludes1: neoplasm of uncertain behavior of aryepiglottic fold or interarytenoid fold, laryngeal aspect (D38.0)

neoplasm of uncertain behavior of epiglottis NOS (D38.0)

neoplasm of uncertain behavior of skin of lip (D48.5)

neoplasm of uncertain behavior of suprahyoid portion of epiglottis (D38.0)

D37.01 **Neoplasm of uncertain behavior of lip**

Neoplasm of uncertain behavior of vermilion border of lip

D37.02 **Neoplasm of uncertain behavior of tongue**

D37.03 **Neoplasm of uncertain behavior of the major salivary glands**

D37.030 **Neoplasm of uncertain behavior of the parotid salivary glands**

D37.031 **Neoplasm of uncertain behavior of the sublingual salivary glands**

D37.032 **Neoplasm of uncertain behavior of the submandibular salivary glands**

D37.039 **Neoplasm of uncertain behavior of the major salivary glands, unspecified**

D37.04 **Neoplasm of uncertain behavior of the minor salivary glands**

Neoplasm of uncertain behavior of submucosal salivary glands of lip

Neoplasm of uncertain behavior of submucosal salivary glands of cheek

Neoplasm of uncertain behavior of submucosal salivary glands of hard palate

Neoplasm of uncertain behavior of submucosal salivary glands of soft palate

D37.05 **Neoplasm of uncertain behavior of pharynx**

Neoplasm of uncertain behavior of aryepiglottic fold of pharynx NOS

Neoplasm of uncertain behavior of hypopharyngeal aspect of aryepiglottic fold of pharynx

Neoplasm of uncertain behavior of marginal zone of aryepiglottic fold of pharynx

D37.09 **Neoplasm of uncertain behavior of other specified sites of the oral cavity**

D37.1 **Neoplasm of uncertain behavior of stomach**

D37.2 **Neoplasm of uncertain behavior of small intestine**

D37.3 **Neoplasm of uncertain behavior of appendix**

D37.4 **Neoplasm of uncertain behavior of colon**

D37.5 **Neoplasm of uncertain behavior of rectum**

Neoplasm of uncertain behavior of rectosigmoid junction

D37.6 **Neoplasm of uncertain behavior of liver, gallbladder and bile ducts**

Neoplasm of uncertain behavior of ampulla of Vater

D37.8 **Neoplasm of uncertain behavior of other specified digestive organs**

Neoplasm of uncertain behavior of anal canal

Neoplasm of uncertain behavior of anal sphincter

Neoplasm of uncertain behavior of anus NOS

Neoplasm of uncertain behavior of esophagus

Neoplasm of uncertain behavior of intestine NOS

Neoplasm of uncertain behavior of pancreas

Excludes1: neoplasm of uncertain behavior of anal margin (D48.5)

neoplasm of uncertain behavior of anal skin (D48.5)

neoplasm of uncertain behavior of perianal skin (D48.5)

D37.9 **Neoplasm of uncertain behavior of digestive organ, unspecified**

D38 **Neoplasm of uncertain behavior of middle ear and respiratory and intrathoracic organs**

Excludes1: neoplasm of uncertain behavior of heart (D48.7)

D38.0 **Neoplasm of uncertain behavior of larynx**

Neoplasm of uncertain behavior of aryepiglottic fold or interarytenoid fold, laryngeal aspect

Neoplasm of uncertain behavior of epiglottis (suprahyoid portion)

Excludes1: neoplasm of uncertain behavior of aryepiglottic fold or interarytenoid fold NOS (D37.05)

neoplasm of uncertain behavior of hypopharyngeal aspect of aryepiglottic fold (D37.05)

neoplasm of uncertain behavior of marginal zone of aryepiglottic fold (D37.05)

D38.1 **Neoplasm of uncertain behavior of trachea, bronchus and lung**

D38.2 **Neoplasm of uncertain behavior of pleura**

D38.3 **Neoplasm of uncertain behavior of mediastinum**

D38.4 **Neoplasm of uncertain behavior of thymus**

D38.5 **Neoplasm of uncertain behavior of other respiratory organs**

Neoplasm of uncertain behavior of accessory sinuses

Neoplasm of uncertain behavior of cartilage of nose

Neoplasm of uncertain behavior of middle ear

Neoplasm of uncertain behavior of nasal cavities

Excludes1: neoplasm of uncertain behavior of ear (external) (skin) (D48.5)

neoplasm of uncertain behavior of nose NOS (D48.7)

neoplasm of uncertain behavior of skin of nose (D48.5)

D38.6 **Neoplasm of uncertain behavior of respiratory organ, unspecified**

D39 **Neoplasm of uncertain behavior of female genital organs**

D39.0 **Neoplasm of uncertain behavior of uterus**

D39.1 **Neoplasm of uncertain behavior of ovary**

Use additional code to identify any functional activity.

D39.10 **Neoplasm of uncertain behavior of unspecified ovary**

D39.11 **Neoplasm of uncertain behavior of right ovary**

D39.12 **Neoplasm of uncertain behavior of left ovary**

D39.2 **Neoplasm of uncertain behavior of placenta**

Chorioadenoma destruens

Invasive hydatidiform mole

Malignant hydatidiform mole

Excludes1: hydatidiform mole NOS (O01.9)

D39.8 **Neoplasm of uncertain behavior of other specified female genital organs**

Neoplasm of uncertain behavior of skin of female genital organs

D39.9 **Neoplasm of uncertain behavior of female genital organ, unspecified**

D40 **Neoplasm of uncertain behavior of male genital organs**

D40.0 **Neoplasm of uncertain behavior of prostate**

D40.1 **Neoplasm of uncertain behavior of testis**

D40.10 **Neoplasm of uncertain behavior of unspecified testis**

D40.11 **Neoplasm of uncertain behavior of right testis**

D40.12 **Neoplasm of uncertain behavior of left testis**

D40.8 **Neoplasm of uncertain behavior of other specified male genital organs**

Neoplasm of uncertain behavior of skin of male genital organs

D40.9 **Neoplasm of uncertain behavior of male genital organ, unspecified**

D41 **Neoplasm of uncertain behavior of urinary organs**

D41.0 **Neoplasm of uncertain behavior of kidney**

Excludes1: neoplasm of uncertain behavior of renal pelvis (D41.1-)

D41.00 **Neoplasm of uncertain behavior of unspecified kidney**

D41.01 **Neoplasm of uncertain behavior of right kidney**

D41.02 **Neoplasm of uncertain behavior of left kidney**

D41.1 **Neoplasm of uncertain behavior of renal pelvis**

D41.10 **Neoplasm of uncertain behavior of unspecified renal pelvis**

D41.11 **Neoplasm of uncertain behavior of right renal pelvis**

D41.12 **Neoplasm of uncertain behavior of left renal pelvis**

D41.2 **Neoplasm of uncertain behavior of ureter**

D41.20 **Neoplasm of uncertain behavior of unspecified ureter**

D41.21 **Neoplasm of uncertain behavior of right ureter**

D41.22 **Neoplasm of uncertain behavior of left ureter**

D41.3 **Neoplasm of uncertain behavior of urethra**

D41.4 **Neoplasm of uncertain behavior of bladder**

D41.8 **Neoplasm of uncertain behavior of other specified urinary organs**

D41.9 **Neoplasm of uncertain behavior of unspecified urinary organ**

D42 **Neoplasm of uncertain behavior of meninges**

D42.0 **Neoplasm of uncertain behavior of cerebral meninges**

D42.1 **Neoplasm of uncertain behavior of spinal meninges**

D42.9 **Neoplasm of uncertain behavior of meninges, unspecified**

D43 **Neoplasm of uncertain behavior of brain and central nervous system**

Excludes1: neoplasm of uncertain behavior of peripheral nerves and autonomic nervous system (D48.2)

D43.0 **Neoplasm of uncertain behavior of brain, supratentorial**

Neoplasm of uncertain behavior of cerebral ventricle

Neoplasm of uncertain behavior of cerebrum

Neoplasm of uncertain behavior of frontal lobe

Neoplasm of uncertain behavior of occipital lobe

Neoplasm of uncertain behavior of parietal lobe

Neoplasm of uncertain behavior of temporal lobe

Excludes1: neoplasm of uncertain behavior of fourth ventricle (D43.1)

D43.1 **Neoplasm of uncertain behavior of brain, infratentorial**

Neoplasm of uncertain behavior of brain stem Neoplasm of uncertain behavior of cerebellum Neoplasm of uncertain behavior of fourth ventricle

D43.2 **Neoplasm of uncertain behavior of brain, unspecified**

D43.3 **Neoplasm of uncertain behavior of cranial nerves**

D43.4 **Neoplasm of uncertain behavior of spinal cord**

D43.8 **Neoplasm of uncertain behavior of other specified parts of central nervous system**

D43.9 **Neoplasm of uncertain behavior of central nervous system, unspecified**

Neoplasm of uncertain behavior of nervous system (central) NOS

D44 **Neoplasm of uncertain behavior of endocrine glands**

Excludes1: multiple endocrine adenomatosis (E31.2-)

multiple endocrine neoplasia (E31.2-)

neoplasm of uncertain behavior of endocrine pancreas (D37.8)

neoplasm of uncertain behavior of ovary (D39.1-)

neoplasm of uncertain behavior of testis (D40.1-)

neoplasm of uncertain behavior of thymus (D38.4)

D44.0 **Neoplasm of uncertain behavior of thyroid gland**

D44.1 **Neoplasm of uncertain behavior of adrenal gland**

Use additional code to identify any functional activity.

D44.10 **Neoplasm of uncertain behavior of unspecified adrenal gland**

D44.11 **Neoplasm of uncertain behavior of right adrenal gland**

D44.12 **Neoplasm of uncertain behavior of left adrenal gland**

D44.2 **Neoplasm of uncertain behavior of parathyroid gland**

D44.3 **Neoplasm of uncertain behavior of pituitary gland**

Use additional code to identify any functional activity.

D44.4 **Neoplasm of uncertain behavior of craniopharyngeal duct**

D44.5 Neoplasm of uncertain behavior of pineal gland

D44.6 Neoplasm of uncertain behavior of carotid body

D44.7 Neoplasm of uncertain behavior of aortic body and other paraganglia

D44.9 Neoplasm of uncertain behavior of unspecified endocrine gland

D45 Polycythemia vera
Excludes1: familial polycythemia (D75.0)
secondary polycythemia (D75.1)

D46 Myelodysplastic syndromes
Use additional code for adverse effect, if applicable, to identify drug (T36-T50 with fifth or sixth character 5)
Excludes2: drug-induced aplastic anemia (D61.1)

D46.0 Refractory anemia without ring sideroblasts, so stated
Refractory anemia without sideroblasts, without excess of blasts

D46.1 Refractory anemia with ring sideroblasts
RARS

D46.2 Refractory anemia with excess of blasts [RAEB]

D46.20 Refractory anemia with excess of blasts, unspecified
RAEB NOS

D46.21 Refractory anemia with excess of blasts 1
RAEB 1

D46.22 Refractory anemia with excess of blasts 2
RAEB 2

D46.A Refractory cytopenia with multilineage dysplasia

D46.B Refractory cytopenia with multilineage dysplasia and ring sideroblasts
RCMD RS

D46.C Myelodysplastic syndrome with isolated del(5q) chromosomal abnormality
Myelodysplastic syndrome with 5q deletion 5q minus syndrome NOS

D46.4 Refractory anemia, unspecified

D46.Z Other myelodysplastic syndromes
Excludes1: chronic myelomonocytic leukemia (C93.1-)

D46.9 Myelodysplastic syndrome, unspecified
Myelodysplasia NOS

D47 Other neoplasms of uncertain behavior of lymphoid, hematopoietic and related tissue

▲D47.0 Mast cell neoplasms of uncertain behavior
Excludes1: congenital cutaneous mastocytosis (Q82.2-)
histiocytic neoplasms of uncertain behavior (D47.Z9)
malignant mast cell neoplasm (C96.2-)

•D47.01 Cutaneous mastocytosis
Diffuse cutaneous mastocytosis
Maculopapular cutaneous mastocytosis
Solitary mastocytoma
Telangiectasia macularis eruptiva perstans
Urticaria pigmentosa
Excludes1: congenital (diffuse) (maculopapular) cutaneous mastocytosis (Q82.2)
congenital urticaria pigmentosa (Q82.2)
extracutaneous mastocytoma (D47.09)

•D47.02 Systemic mastocytosis
Indolent systemic mastocytosis
Isolated bone marrow mastocytosis
Smoldering systemic mastocytosis

Systemic mastocytosis, with an associated hematological non-mast cell lineage disease (SM-AHNMD)
Code also, if applicable, any associated hematological non-mast cell lineage disease, such as:
acute myeloid leukemia (C92.6-, C92.A-)
chronic myelomonocytic leukemia (C93.1-)
essential thrombocytosis (D47.3)
hypereosinophilic syndrome (D72.1)
myelodysplastic syndrome (D46.9)
myeloproliferative syndrome (D47.1)
non-Hodgkin lymphoma (C82-C85)
plasma cell myeloma (C90.0-)
polycythemia vera (D45)
Excludes1: aggressive systemic mastocytosis (C96.21)
mast cell leukemia (C94.3-)

•D47.09 Other mast cell neoplasms of uncertain behavior
Extracutaneous mastocytoma
Mast cell tumor NOS
Mastocytoma NOS
Mastocytosis NOS Monoclonal gammopathy of undetermined significance [MGUS]

D47.3 Essential (hemorrhagic) thrombocythemia
Essential thrombocytosis
Idiopathic hemorrhagic thrombocythemia

D47.4 Osteomyelofibrosis
Chronic idiopathic myelofibrosis
Myelofibrosis (idiopathic) (with myeloid metaplasia)
Myelosclerosis (megakaryocytic) with myeloid metaplasia
Secondary myelofibrosis in myeloproliferative disease
Excludes1: acute myelofibrosis (C94.4-)

D47.1 Chronic myeloproliferative disease
Chronic neutrophilic leukemia
Myeloproliferative disease, unspecified
Excludes1: atypical chronic myeloid leukemia BCR/ABL-negative (C92.2-)
chronic myeloid leukemia BCR/ABL-positive (C92.1-)
myelofibrosis NOS (D75.81)
myelophthisic anemia (D61.82)
myelophthisis (D61.82)
secondary myelofibrosis NOS (D75.81)

D47.2 Monoclonal gammopathy

D47.Z Other specified neoplasms of uncertain behavior of lymphoid, hematopoietic and related tissue

D47.Z1 Post-transplant lymphoproliferative disorder (PTLD)
Code first complications of transplanted organs and tissue (T86.-)

D47.Z2 Castleman disease
Code also if applicable human herpesvirus 8 infection (B10.89)
Excludes2: Kaposi's sarcoma (C46-)

D47.Z9 Other specified neoplasms of uncertain behavior of lymphoid, hematopoietic and related tissue
Histiocytic tumors of uncertain behavior

D47.9 **Neoplasm of uncertain behavior of lymphoid, hematopoietic and related tissue, unspecified**

Lymphoproliferative disease NOS

D48 **Neoplasm of uncertain behavior of other and unspecified sites**

Excludes1: neurofibromatosis (nonmalignant) (Q85.0-)

D48.0 **Neoplasm of uncertain behavior of bone and articular cartilage**

Excludes1: neoplasm of uncertain behavior of cartilage of ear (D48.1)

neoplasm of uncertain behavior of cartilage of larynx (D38.0)

neoplasm of uncertain behavior of cartilage of nose (D38.5)

neoplasm of uncertain behavior of connective tissue of eyelid (D48.1)

neoplasm of uncertain behavior of synovia (D48.1)

D48.1 **Neoplasm of uncertain behavior of connective and other soft tissue**

Neoplasm of uncertain behavior of connective tissue of ear

Neoplasm of uncertain behavior of connective tissue of eyelid

Stromal tumors of uncertain behavior of digestive system

Excludes1: neoplasm of uncertain behavior of articular cartilage (D48.0)

neoplasm of uncertain behavior of cartilage of larynx (D38.0)

neoplasm of uncertain behavior of cartilage of nose (D38.5)

neoplasm of uncertain behavior of connective tissue of breast (D48.6-)

D48.2 **Neoplasm of uncertain behavior of peripheral nerves and autonomic nervous system**

Excludes1: neoplasm of uncertain behavior of peripheral nerves of orbit (D48.7)

D48.3 **Neoplasm of uncertain behavior of retroperitoneum**

D48.4 **Neoplasm of uncertain behavior of peritoneum**

D48.5 **Neoplasm of uncertain behavior of skin**

Neoplasm of uncertain behavior of anal margin

Neoplasm of uncertain behavior of anal skin

Neoplasm of uncertain behavior of perianal skin

Neoplasm of uncertain behavior of skin of breast

Excludes1: neoplasm of uncertain behavior of anus NOS (D37.8)

neoplasm of uncertain behavior of skin of genital organs (D39.8, D40.8)

neoplasm of uncertain behavior of vermilion border of lip (D37.0)

D48.6 **Neoplasm of uncertain behavior of breast**

Neoplasm of uncertain behavior of connective tissue of breast

Cystosarcoma phyllodes

Excludes1: neoplasm of uncertain behavior of skin of breast (D48.5)

D48.60 **Neoplasm of uncertain behavior of unspecified breast**

D48.61 **Neoplasm of uncertain behavior of right breast**

D48.62 **Neoplasm of uncertain behavior of left breast**

D48.7 **Neoplasm of uncertain behavior of other specified sites**

Neoplasm of uncertain behavior of eye Neoplasm of uncertain behavior of heart

Neoplasm of uncertain behavior of peripheral nerves of orbit

Excludes1: neoplasm of uncertain behavior of connective tissue (D48.1)

neoplasm of uncertain behavior of skin of eyelid (D48.5)

D48.9 **Neoplasm of uncertain behavior, unspecified**

NEOPLASMS OF UNSPECIFIED BEHAVIOR (D49)

D49 **Neoplasms of unspecified behavior Note:**

Category D49 classifies by site neoplasms of unspecified morphology and behavior. The term 'mass', unless otherwise stated, is not to be regarded as a neoplastic growth.

Includes: 'growth' NOS

neoplasm NOS

new growth NOS

tumor NOS

Excludes1: neoplasms of uncertain behavior (D37-D44, D48)

D49.0 **Neoplasm of unspecified behavior of digestive system**

Excludes1: neoplasm of unspecified behavior of margin of anus (D49.2)

neoplasm of unspecified behavior of perianal skin (D49.2)

neoplasm of unspecified behavior of skin of anus (D49.2)

D49.1 **Neoplasm of unspecified behavior of respiratory system**

D49.2 **Neoplasm of unspecified behavior of bone, soft tissue, and skin**

Excludes1: neoplasm of unspecified behavior of anal canal (D49.0)

neoplasm of unspecified behavior of anus NOS (D49.0)

neoplasm of unspecified behavior of bone marrow (D49.89)

neoplasm of unspecified behavior of cartilage of larynx (D49.1)

neoplasm of unspecified behavior of cartilage of nose (D49.1)

neoplasm of unspecified behavior of connective tissue of breast (D49.3)

neoplasm of unspecified behavior of skin of genital organs (D49.59)

neoplasm of unspecified behavior of vermilion border of lip (D49.0)

D49.3 **Neoplasm of unspecified behavior of breast**

Excludes1: neoplasm of unspecified behavior of skin of breast (D49.2)

D49.4 **Neoplasm of unspecified behavior of bladder**

D49.5 **Neoplasm of unspecified behavior of other genitourinary organs**

D49.51 **Neoplasm of unspecified behavior of kidney**

D49.511 **Neoplasm of unspecified behavior of right kidney**

D49.512 **Neoplasm of unspecified behavior of left kidney**

D49.519 **Neoplasm of unspecified behavior of unspecified kidney**

D49.59 **Neoplasm of unspecified behavior of other genitourinary organ**

D49.6 **Neoplasm of unspecified behavior of brain**

Excludes1: neoplasm of unspecified behavior of cerebral meninges (D49.7)

neoplasm of unspecified behavior of cranial nerves (D49.7)

D49.7 **Neoplasm of unspecified behavior of endocrine glands and other parts of nervous system**

Excludes1: neoplasm of unspecified behavior of peripheral, sympathetic, and parasympathetic nerves and ganglia (D49.2)

D49.8 **Neoplasm of unspecified behavior of other specified sites**

Excludes1: neoplasm of unspecified behavior of eyelid (skin) (D49.2)

neoplasm of unspecified behavior of eyelid cartilage (D49.2)

neoplasm of unspecified behavior of great vessels (D49.2)

neoplasm of unspecified behavior of optic nerve (D49.7)

D49.81 **Neoplasm of unspecified behavior of retina and choroid**

Dark area on retina

Retinal freckle

D49.89 **Neoplasm of unspecified behavior of other specified sites**

D49.9 **Neoplasm of unspecified behavior of unspecified site**

Chapter 3: Diseases Of The Blood And Blood-Forming Organs and Certain Disorders Involving The Immune Mechanism (D50-D89)

DEFINITIONS AND CODING ALERTS

This chapter includes definitions of selected key words, terms and phrases and coding alerts for adding points to the clinical domain, and references to coding late effects where appropriate. An example from this chapter is as follows:

D50   Iron deficiency anemia

     Definition: Iron deficiency anemia is a form of anemia due to lack of iron in the diet or to iron loss as a result of chronic bleeding.

MULTIPLE CODING FOR A SINGLE CONDITION

In addition to the etiology/manifestation convention that requires two codes to fully describe a single condition that affects multiple body systems, there are other single conditions that also require more than one code. "Use additional code" notes are found in the Tabular List at codes that are not part of an etiology/manifestation pair where a secondary code is useful to fully describe a condition. The sequencing rule is the same as the etiology/manifestation pair, "use additional code" indicates that a secondary code should be added.

For example, for bacterial infections that are not included in chapter 1, a secondary code from category B95, Streptococcus, Staphylococcus, and Enterococcus, as the cause of diseases classified elsewhere, or B96, Other bacterial agents as the cause of diseases classified elsewhere, may be required to identify the bacterial organism causing the infection. A "use additional code" note will normally be found at the infectious disease code, indicating a need for the organism code to be added as a secondary code.

"Code first" notes are also under certain codes that are not specifically manifestation codes but may be due to an underlying cause. When there is a "code first" note and an underlying condition is present, the underlying condition should be sequenced first.

"Code, if applicable, any causal condition first", notes indicate that this code may be assigned as a principal diagnosis when the causal condition is unknown or not applicable. If a causal condition is known, then the code for that condition should be sequenced as the principal or first-listed diagnosis.

Multiple codes may be needed for sequela, complication codes and obstetric codes to more fully describe a condition. See the specific guidelines for these conditions for further instruction.

COMBINATION CODE

A combination code is a single code used to classify: Two diagnoses, or a diagnosis with an associated secondary process (manifestation) A diagnosis with an associated complication

Combination codes are identified by referring to subterm entries in the Alphabetic Index and by reading the inclusion and exclusion notes in the Tabular List.

Assign only the combination code when that code fully identifies the diagnostic conditions involved or when the Alphabetic Index so directs. Multiple coding should not be used when the classification provides a combination code that clearly identifies all of the elements documented in the diagnosis. When the combination code lacks necessary specificity in describing the manifestation or complication, an additional code should be used as a secondary code.

SEQUELA (LATE EFFECTS)

A sequela is the residual effect (condition produced) after the acute phase of an illness or injury has terminated. There is no time limit on when a sequela code can be used. The residual may be apparent early, such as in cerebral infarction, or it may occur months or years later, such as that due to a previous injury. Coding of sequela generally requires two codes sequenced in the following order: The condition or nature of the sequela is sequenced first.

The sequela code is sequenced second.

An exception to the above guidelines are those instances where the code for the sequela is followed by a manifestation code identified in the Tabular List and title, or the sequela code has been expanded (at the fourth, fifth or sixth character levels) to include the manifestation(s). The code for the acute phase of an illness or injury that led to the sequela is never used with a code for the late effect.

Chapter 3

Diseases of the Blood and Blood-Forming Organs and Certain Disorders Involving the Immune Mechanism (D50-D89)

Excludes2: autoimmune disease (systemic) NOS (M35.9)

certain conditions originating in the perinatal period (P00-P96)

complications of pregnancy, childbirth and the puerperium (O00-O9A)

congenital malformations, deformations and chromosomal abnormalities (Q00-Q99)

endocrine, nutritional and metabolic diseases (E00-E88)

human immunodeficiency virus [HIV] disease (B20)

injury, poisoning and certain other consequences of external causes (S00-T88)

neoplasms (C00-D49)

symptoms, signs and abnormal clinical and laboratory findings, not elsewhere classified (R00-R94)

This chapter contains the following blocks:

D50-D53	Nutritional anemias
D55-D59	Hemolytic anemias
D60-D64	Aplastic and other anemias and other bone marrow failure syndromes
D65-D69	Coagulation defects, purpura and other hemorrhagic conditions
D70-D77	Other disorders of blood and blood-forming organs
D78	Intraoperative and postprocedural complications of the spleen
D80-D89	Certain disorders involving the immune mechanism

NUTRITIONAL ANEMIAS (D50-D53)

D50 Iron deficiency anemia

Includes: asiderotic anemia

hypochromic anemia

D50.0 Iron deficiency anemia secondary to blood loss (chronic)

Posthemorrhagic anemia (chronic)

Excludes1: acute posthemorrhagic anemia (D62)

congenital anemia from fetal blood loss (P61.3)

D50.1 Sideropenic dysphagia

Kelly-Paterson syndrome

Plummer-Vinson syndrome

D50.8 Other iron deficiency anemias

Iron deficiency anemia due to inadequate dietary iron intake

D50.9 Iron deficiency anemia, unspecified

D51 Vitamin B12 deficiency anemia

Excludes1: vitamin B12 deficiency (E53.8)

D51.0 Vitamin B12 deficiency anemia due to intrinsic factor deficiency

Addison anemia

Biermer anemia

Pernicious (congenital) anemia

Congenital intrinsic factor deficiency

D51.1 Vitamin B12 deficiency anemia due to selective vitamin B12 malabsorption with proteinuria

Imerslund (Gräsbeck) syndrome

Megaloblastic hereditary anemia

D51.2 Transcobalamin II deficiency

D51.3 Other dietary vitamin B12 deficiency anemia

Vegan anemia

D51.8 Other vitamin B12 deficiency anemias

D51.9 Vitamin B12 deficiency anemia, unspecified

D52 Folate deficiency anemia

Excludes1: folate deficiency without anemia (E53.8)

D52.0 Dietary folate deficiency anemia

Nutritional megaloblastic anemia

D52.1 Drug-induced folate deficiency anemia

Use additional code for adverse effect, if applicable, to identify drug (T36-T50 with fifth or sixth

character 5)

D52.8 Other folate deficiency anemias

D52.9 Folate deficiency anemia, unspecified

Folic acid deficiency anemia NOS

D53 Other nutritional anemias

Includes: megaloblastic anemia unresponsive to vitamin B12 or folate therapy

D53.0 Protein deficiency anemia

Amino-acid deficiency anemia

Orotaciduric anemia

Excludes1: Lesch-Nyhan syndrome (E79.1)

D53.1 Other megaloblastic anemias, not elsewhere classified

Megaloblastic anemia NOS

Excludes1: Di Guglielmo's disease (C94.0)

D53.2 Scorbutic anemia

Excludes1: scurvy (E54)

D53.8 Other specified nutritional anemias

Anemia associated with deficiency of copper

Anemia associated with deficiency of molybdenum

Anemia associated with deficiency of zinc

Excludes1: nutritional deficiencies without anemia, such as:

copper deficiency NOS (E61.0)

molybdenum deficiency NOS (E61.5)

zinc deficiency NOS (E60)

D53.9 Nutritional anemia, unspecified

Simple chronic anemia

Excludes1: anemia NOS (D64.9)

HEMOLYTIC ANEMIAS (D55-D59)

D55 Anemia due to enzyme disorders

Excludes1: drug-induced enzyme deficiency anemia (D59.2)

D55.0 Anemia due to glucose-6-phosphate dehydrogenase [G6PD] deficiency

Favism

G6PD deficiency anemia

D55.1 Anemia due to other disorders of glutathione metabolism

Anemia (due to) enzyme deficiencies, except G6PD, related to the hexose monophosphate [HMP] shunt pathway

Anemia (due to) hemolytic nonspherocytic (hereditary), type I

D55.2 Anemia due to disorders of glycolytic enzymes

Hemolytic nonspherocytic (hereditary) anemia, type II

Hexokinase deficiency anemia

Pyruvate kinase [PK] deficiency anemia

Triose-phosphate isomerase deficiency anemia

Excludes1: disorders of glycolysis not associated with anemia (E74.8)

D55.3 Anemia due to disorders of nucleotide metabolism

D55.8 Other anemias due to enzyme disorders

D55.9 Anemia due to enzyme disorder, unspecified

D56 **Thalassemia**

Excludes1: sickle-cell thalassemia (D57.4-)

D56.0 **Alpha thalassemia**

Alpha thalassemia major

Hemoglobin H Constant Spring

Hemoglobin H disease

Hydrops fetalis due to alpha thalassemia

Severe alpha thalassemia

Triple gene defect alpha thalassemia

Use additional code, if applicable, for hydrops fetalis due to alpha thalassemia (P56.99)

Excludes1: alpha thalassemia trait or minor (D56.3)

asymptomatic alpha thalassemia (D56.3)

hydrops fetalis due to isoimmunization (P56.0)

hydrops fetalis not due to immune hemolysis (P83.2)

D56.1 **Beta thalassemia**

Beta thalassemia major Cooley's anemia

Homozygous beta thalassemia

Severe beta thalassemia

Thalassemia intermedia

Thalassemia major

Excludes1: beta thalassemia minor (D56.3)

beta thalassemia trait (D56.3)

delta-beta thalassemia (D56.2)

hemoglobin E-beta thalassemia (D56.5)

sickle-cell beta thalassemia (D57.4-)

D56.2 **Delta-beta thalassemia**

Homozygous delta-beta thalassemia

Excludes1: delta-beta thalassemia minor (D56.3)

delta-beta thalassemia trait (D56.3)

D56.3 **Thalassemia minor** Alpha thalassemia minor

Alpha thalassemia silent carrier

Alpha thalassemia trait

Beta thalassemia minor Beta thalassemia trait

Delta-beta thalassemia minor

Delta-beta thalassemia trait

Thalassemia trait NOS

Excludes1: alpha thalassemia (D56.0)

beta thalassemia (D56.1)

delta-beta thalassemia (D56.2)

hemoglobin E-beta thalassemia (D56.5)

sickle-cell trait (D57.3)

D56.4 **Hereditary persistence of fetal hemoglobin [HPFH]**

D56.5 **Hemoglobin E-beta thalassemia**

Excludes1: beta thalassemia (D56.1)

beta thalassemia minor (D56.3)

beta thalassemia trait (D56.3)

delta-beta thalassemia (D56.2)

delta-beta thalassemia trait (D56.3)

hemoglobin E disease (D58.2)

Other hemoglobinopathies (D58.2)

sickle-cell beta thalassemia (D57.4-)

D56.8 **Other thalassemias**

Dominant thalassemia

Hemoglobin C thalassemia

Mixed thalassemia

Thalassemia with other hemoglobinopathy

Excludes1: hemoglobin C disease (D58.2)

hemoglobin E disease (D58.2)

Other hemoglobinopathies (D58.2)

sickle-cell anemia (D57.-)

sickle-cell thalassemia (D57.4)

D56.9 **Thalassemia, unspecified**

Mediterranean anemia (with other hemoglobinopathy)

D57 **Sickle-cell disorders**

Use additional code for any associated fever (R50.81)

Excludes1: Other hemoglobinopathies (D58.-)

D57.0 **Hb-SS disease with crisis**

Sickle-cell disease NOS with crisis

Hb-SS disease with vasoocclusive pain

D57.00 **Hb-SS disease with crisis, unspecified**

D57.01 **Hb-SS disease with acute chest syndrome**

D57.02 **Hb-SS disease with splenic sequestration**

D57.1 **Sickle-cell disease without crisis**

Hb-SS disease without crisis

Sickle-cell anemia NOS

Sickle-cell disease NOS

Sickle-cell disorder NOS

D57.2 **Sickle-cell/Hb-C disease**

Hb-SC disease

Hb-S/Hb-C disease

D57.20 **Sickle-cell/Hb-C disease without crisis**

D57.21 **Sickle-cell/Hb-C disease with crisis**

D57.211 **Sickle-cell/Hb-C disease with acute chest syndrome**

D57.212 **Sickle-cell/Hb-C disease with splenic sequestration**

D57.219 **Sickle-cell/Hb-C disease with crisis, unspecified**

Sickle-cell/Hb-C disease with crisis NOS

D57.3 **Sickle-cell trait**

Hb-S trait

Heterozygous hemoglobin S

D57.4 **Sickle-cell thalassemia**

Sickle-cell beta thalassemia

Thalassemia Hb-S disease

D57.40 **Sickle-cell thalassemia without crisis**

Microdrepanocytosis

Sickle-cell thalassemia NOS

D57.41 **Sickle-cell thalassemia with crisis**

Sickle-cell thalassemia with vasoocclusive pain

D57.411 **Sickle-cell thalassemia with acute chest syndrome**

D57.412 **Sickle-cell thalassemia with splenic sequestration**

D57.419 **Sickle-cell thalassemia with crisis, unspecified**

Sickle-cell thalassemia with crisis NOS

D57.8 **Other sickle-cell disorders**

Hb-SD disease Hb-SE disease

D57.80 **Other sickle-cell disorders without crisis**

D57.81 **Other sickle-cell disorders with crisis**

● New code ▲ Revised code **Excludes1:** Not coded here **Excludes2:** Not included here ⊗ Placeholder required ⑦7th digit required

> **D57.811** **Other sickle-cell disorders with acute chest syndrome**
>
> **D57.812** **Other sickle-cell disorders with splenic sequestration**
>
> **D57.819** **Other sickle-cell disorders with crisis, unspecified**
>
> Other sickle-cell disorders with crisis NOS

D58 **Other hereditary hemolytic anemias**

Excludes1: hemolytic anemia of the newborn (P55.-)

D58.0 **Hereditary spherocytosis**

Acholuric (familial) jaundice

Congenital (spherocytic) hemolytic icterus

Minkowski-Chauffard syndrome

D58.1 **Hereditary elliptocytosis**

Elliptocytosis (congenital)

Ovalocytosis (congenital) (hereditary)

D58.2 **Other hemoglobinopathies**

Abnormal hemoglobin NOS

Congenital Heinz body anemia

Hb-C disease

Hb-D disease

Hb-E disease

Hemoglobinopathy NOS

Unstable hemoglobin hemolytic disease

Excludes1: familial polycythemia (D75.0)

Hb-M disease (D74.0)

hemoglobin E-beta thalassemia (D56.5)

hereditary persistence of fetal hemoglobin [HPFH] (D56.4)

high-altitude polycythemia (D75.1)

methemoglobinemia (D74.-)

Other hemoglobinopathies with thalassemia (D56.8)

D58.8 **Other specified hereditary hemolytic anemias**

Stomatocytosis

D58.9 **Hereditary hemolytic anemia, unspecified**

D59 **Acquired hemolytic anemia**

D59.0 **Drug-induced autoimmune hemolytic anemia**

Use additional code for adverse effect, if applicable, to identify drug (T36-T50 with fifth or sixth character 5)

D59.1 **Other autoimmune hemolytic anemias**

Autoimmune hemolytic disease (cold type) (warm type)

Chronic cold hemagglutinin disease

Cold agglutinin disease

Cold agglutinin hemoglobinuria

Cold type (secondary) (symptomatic) hemolytic anemia

Warm type (secondary) (symptomatic) hemolytic anemia

Excludes1: Evans syndrome (D69.41)

hemolytic disease of newborn (P55.-)

paroxysmal cold hemoglobinuria (D59.6)

D59.2 **Drug-induced nonautoimmune hemolytic anemia**

Drug-induced enzyme deficiency anemia

Use additional code for adverse effect, if applicable, to identify drug (T36-T50 with fifth or sixth character 5)

D59.3 **Hemolytic-uremic syndrome**

Use additional code to identify associated:

E. coli infection (B96.2-)

Pneumococcal pneumonia (J13)

Shigella dysenteriae (A03.9)

D59.4 **Other nonautoimmune hemolytic anemias**

Mechanical hemolytic anemia

Microangiopathic hemolytic anemia

Toxic hemolytic anemia

D59.5 **Paroxysmal nocturnal hemoglobinuria [Marchiafava-Micheli]**

Excludes1: hemoglobinuria NOS (R82.3)

D59.6 **Hemoglobinuria due to hemolysis from other external causes**

Hemoglobinuria from exertion

March hemoglobinuria

Paroxysmal cold hemoglobinuria

Use additional code (Chapter 20) to identify external cause

Excludes1: hemoglobinuria NOS (R82.3)

D59.8 **Other acquired hemolytic anemias**

D59.9 **Acquired hemolytic anemia, unspecified**

Idiopathic hemolytic anemia, chronic

APLASTIC AND OTHER ANEMIAS AND OTHER BONE MARROW FAILURE SYNDROMES (D60-D64)

D60 **Acquired pure red cell aplasia [erythroblastopenia]**

Includes: red cell aplasia (acquired) (adult) (with thymoma)

Excludes1: congenital red cell aplasia (D61.01)

D60.0 **Chronic acquired pure red cell aplasia**

D60.1 **Transient acquired pure red cell aplasia**

D60.8 **Other acquired pure red cell aplasias**

D60.9 **Acquired pure red cell aplasia, unspecified**

D61 **Other aplastic anemias and other bone marrow failure syndromes**

Excludes1: neutropenia (D70.-)

D61.0 **Constitutional aplastic anemia**

D61.01 **Constitutional (pure) red blood cell aplasia**

Blackfan-Diamond syndrome

Congenital (pure) red cell aplasia

Familial hypoplastic anemia

Primary (pure) red cell aplasia

Red cell (pure) aplasia of infants

Excludes1: acquired red cell aplasia (D60.9)

D61.09 **Other constitutional aplastic anemia**

Fanconi's anemia

Pancytopenia with malformations

D61.1 **Drug-induced aplastic anemia**

Use additional code for adverse effect, if applicable, to identify drug (T36-T50 with fifth or sixth character 5)

D61.2 **Aplastic anemia due to other external agents**

Code first, if applicable, toxic effects of substances chiefly nonmedicinal as to source (T51-T65)

D61.3 **Idiopathic aplastic anemia**

D61.8 **Other specified aplastic anemias and other bone marrow failure syndromes**

D61.81 **Pancytopenia**

Excludes1: pancytopenia (due to) (with) aplastic anemia (D61.9)

pancytopenia (due to) (with) bone marrow infiltration (D61.82)

pancytopenia (due to) (with) congenital (pure) red cell aplasia (D61.01) pancytopenia (due to) (with) hairy cell leukemia (C91.4-)

pancytopenia (due to) (with) human immunodeficiency virus disease (B20.-)

pancytopenia (due to) (with) leukoerythroblastic anemia (D61.82)

pancytopenia (due to) (with) myeloproliferative disease (D47.1)

Excludes2: pancytopenia (due to) (with) myelodysplastic syndromes (D46.-)

D61.810 Antineoplastic chemotherapy induced pancytopenia

Excludes2: aplastic anemia due to antineoplastic chemotherapy (D61.1)

D61.811 Other drug-induced pancytopenia

Excludes2: aplastic anemia due to drugs (D61.1)

D61.818 Other pancytopenia

D61.82 Myelophthisis

Leukoerythroblastic anemia

Myelophthisic anemia

Panmyelophthisis

Code also the underlying disorder, such as:

malignant neoplasm of breast (C50.-)

tuberculosis (A15.-)

Excludes1: idiopathic myelofibrosis (D47.1)

myelofibrosis NOS (D75.81)

myelofibrosis with myeloid metaplasia (D47.4)

primary myelofibrosis (D47.1)

secondary myelofibrosis (D75.81)

D61.89 Other specified aplastic anemias and other bone marrow failure syndromes

D61.9 Aplastic anemia, unspecified

Hypoplastic anemia NOS

Medullary hypoplasia

D62 Acute posthemorrhagic anemia

Excludes1: anemia due to chronic blood loss (D50.0)

blood loss anemia NOS (D50.0)

congenital anemia from fetal blood loss (P61.3)

D63 Anemia in chronic diseases classified elsewhere

D63.0 Anemia in neoplastic disease

Code first neoplasm (C00-D49)

Excludes2: anemia due to antineoplastic chemotherapy (D64.81)

aplastic anemia due to antineoplastic chemotherapy (D61.1)

D63.1 Anemia in chronic kidney disease

Erythropoietin resistant anemia (EPO resistant anemia)

Code first underlying chronic kidney disease (CKD) (N18.-)

D63.8 Anemia in other chronic diseases classified elsewhere

Code first underlying disease, such as:

diphyllobothriasis (B70.0)

hookworm disease (B76.0-B76.9)

hypothyroidism (E00.0-E03.9)

malaria (B50.0-B54)

symptomatic late syphilis (A52.79)

tuberculosis (A18.89)

D64 Other anemias

Excludes1: refractory anemia (D46.-)

refractory anemia with excess blasts in transformation [RAEB T] (C92.0-)

D64.0 Hereditary sideroblastic anemia

Sex-linked hypochromic sideroblastic anemia

D64.1 Secondary sideroblastic anemia due to disease

Code first underlying disease

D64.2 Secondary sideroblastic anemia due to drugs and toxins

Code first poisoning due to drug or toxin, if applicable (T36-T65 with fifth or sixth character 1-4 or 6)

Use additional code for adverse effect, if applicable, to identify drug (T36-T50 with fifth or sixth character 5)

D64.3 Other sideroblastic anemias

Sideroblastic anemia NOS

Pyridoxine-responsive sideroblastic anemia NEC

D64.4 Congenital dyserythropoietic anemia

Dyshematopoietic anemia (congenital)

Excludes1: Blackfan-Diamond syndrome (D61.01)

Di Guglielmo's disease (C94.0)

D64.8 Other specified anemias

D64.81 Anemia due to antineoplastic chemotherapy

Antineoplastic chemotherapy induced anemia

Excludes1: aplastic anemia due to antineoplastic chemotherapy (D61.1)

Excludes2: anemia in neoplastic disease (D63.0)

D64.89 Other specified anemias

Infantile pseudoleukemia

D64.9 Anemia, unspecified

COAGULATION DEFECTS, PURPURA AND OTHER HEMORRHAGIC CONDITIONS (D65-D69)

D65 Disseminated intravascular coagulation [defibrination syndrome]

Afibrinogenemia, acquired

Consumption coagulopathy

Diffuse or disseminated intravascular coagulation [DIC]

Fibrinolytic hemorrhage, acquired

Fibrinolytic purpura

Purpura fulminans

Excludes1: disseminated intravascular coagulation (complicating):

abortion or ectopic or molar pregnancy (O00-O07, O08.1)

in newborn (P60)

pregnancy, childbirth and the puerperium (O45.0, O46.0, O67.0, O72.3)

D66 Hereditary factor VIII deficiency

Classical hemophilia

Deficiency factor VIII (with functional defect)

Hemophilia NOS

Hemophilia A

Excludes1: factor VIII deficiency with vascular defect (D68.0)

D67 Hereditary factor IX deficiency

Christmas disease

Factor IX deficiency (with functional defect)

Hemophilia B

Plasma thromboplastin component [PTC] deficiency

D68 Other coagulation defects

Excludes1: abnormal coagulation profile (R79.1)

coagulation defects complicating abortion or ectopic or molar pregnancy (O00-O07, O08.1) coagulation defects complicating pregnancy, childbirth and the puerperium (O45.0, O46.0, O67.0, O72.3)

D68.0 **Von Willebrand's disease**

Angiohemophilia

Factor VIII deficiency with vascular defect

Vascular hemophilia

Excludes1: capillary fragility (hereditary) (D69.8)

factor VIII deficiency NOS (D66)

factor VIII deficiency with functional defect (D66)

D68.1 **Hereditary factor XI deficiency**

Hemophilia C

Plasma thromboplastin antecedent [PTA] deficiency

Rosenthal's disease

D68.2 **Hereditary deficiency of other clotting factors**

AC globulin deficiency

Congenital afibrinogenemia

Deficiency of factor I [fibrinogen]

Deficiency of factor II [prothrombin]

Deficiency of factor V [labile]

Deficiency of factor VII [stable]

Deficiency of factor X [Stuart-Prower]

Deficiency of factor XII [Hageman]

Deficiency of factor XIII [fibrin stabilizing]

Dysfibrinogenemia (congenital)

Hypoproconvertinemia

Owren's disease

Proaccelerin deficiency

D68.3 **Hemorrhagic disorder due to circulating anticoagulants**

D68.31 **Hemorrhagic disorder due to intrinsic circulating anticogulants, antibodies, or inhibitors**

D68.311 **Acquired hemophilia**

Autoimmune hemophilia

Autoimmune inhibitors to clotting factors

Secondary hemophilia

D68.312 **Antiphospholipid antibody with hemorrhagic disorder**

Lupus anticoagulant (LAC) with hemorrhagic disorder

Systemic lupus erythematosus [SLE] inhibitor with hemorrhagic disorder

Excludes1: antiphospholipid antibody, finding without diagnosis (R76.0)

antiphospholipid antibody syndrome (D68.61)

antiphospholipid antibody with hypercoagulable state (D68.61)

lupus anticoagulant (LAC) finding without diagnosis (R76.0)

lupus anticoagulant (LAC) with hypercoagulable state (D68.62)

systemic lupus erythematosus [SLE] inhibitor finding without diagnosis (R76.0)

systemic lupus erythematosus [SLE] inhibitor with hypercoagulable state (D68.62)

D68.318 **Other hemorrhagic disorder due to intrinsic circulating anticoagulants, antibodies, or inhibitors**

Antithromboplastinemia

Antithromboplastinogenemia

Hemorrhagic disorder due to intrinsic increase in antithrombin

Hemorrhagic disorder due to intrinsic increase in anti-VIIIa

Hemorrhagic disorder due to intrinsic increase in anti-IXa

Hemorrhagic disorder due to intrinsic increase in anti-XIa

D68.32 **Hemorrhagic disorder due to extrinsic circulating anticoagulants**

Drug-induced hemorrhagic disorder

Hemorrhagic disorder due to increase in anti-IIa

Hemorrhagic disorder due to increase in anti-Xa

Hyperheparinemia

Use additional code for adverse effect, if applicable, to identify drug (T45.515, T45.525)

D68.4 **Acquired coagulation factor deficiency**

Deficiency of coagulation factor due to liver disease

Deficiency of coagulation factor due to vitamin K deficiency

Excludes1: vitamin K deficiency of newborn (P53)

D68.5 **Primary thrombophilia**

Primary hypercoagulable states

Excludes1: antiphospholipid syndrome (D68.61)

lupus anticoagulant (D68.62)

secondary activated protein C resistance (D68.69)

secondary antiphospholipid antibody syndrome (D68.69)

secondary lupus anticoagulant with hypercoagulable state (D68.69)

secondary systemic lupus erythematosus [SLE] inhibitor with hypercoagulable state (D68.69)

systemic lupus erythematosus [SLE] inhibitor finding without diagnosis (R76.0)

systemic lupus erythematosus [SLE] inhibitor with hemorrhagic disorder (D68.312)

thrombotic thrombocytopenic purpura (M31.1)

D68.51 **Activated protein C resistance**

Factor V Leiden mutation

D68.52 **Prothrombin gene mutation**

D68.59 **Other primary thrombophilia**

Antithrombin III deficiency

Hypercoagulable state NOS

Primary hypercoagulable state NEC

Primary thrombophilia NEC

Protein C deficiency

Protein S deficiency

Thrombophilia NOS

D68.6 **Other thrombophilia**

Other hypercoagulable states

Excludes1: diffuse or disseminated intravascular coagulation [DIC] (D65)

heparin induced thrombocytopenia (HIT) (D75.82)

hyperhomocysteinemia (E72.11)

D68.61 **Antiphospholipid syndrome**

Anticardiolipin syndrome

Antiphospholipid antibody syndrome

Excludes1: anti-phospholipid antibody, finding without diagnosis (R76.0)

anti-phospholipid antibody with hemorrhagic disorder (D68.312)

lupus anticoagulant syndrome (D68.62)

D68.62 Lupus anticoagulant syndrome

Lupus anticoagulant

Presence of systemic lupus erythematosus [SLE] inhibitor

Excludes1: anticardiolipin syndrome (D68.61)

antiphospholipid syndrome (D68.61)

lupus anticoagulant (LAC) finding without diagnosis (R76.0)

lupus anticoagulant (LAC) with hemorrhagic disorder (D68.312)

D68.69 Other thrombophilia

Hypercoagulable states NEC

Secondary hypercoagulable state NOS

D68.8 Other specified coagulation defects

Excludes1: hemorrhagic disease of newborn (P53)

D68.9 Coagulation defect, unspecified

D69 Purpura and other hemorrhagic conditions

Excludes1: benign hypergammaglobulinemic purpura (D89.0)

cryoglobulinemic purpura (D89.1)

essential (hemorrhagic) thrombocythemia (D47.3)

hemorrhagic thrombocythemia (D47.3)

purpura fulminans (D65)

thrombotic thrombocytopenic purpura (M31.1)

Waldenström hypergammaglobulinemic purpura (D89.0)

D69.0 Allergic purpura

Allergic vasculitis

Nonthrombocytopenic hemorrhagic purpura

Nonthrombocytopenic idiopathic purpura

Purpura anaphylactoid

Purpura Henoch(-Schönlein)

Purpura rheumatica

Vascular purpura

Excludes1: thrombocytopenic hemorrhagic purpura (D69.3)

D69.1 Qualitative platelet defects

Bernard-Soulier [giant platelet] syndrome Glanzmann's disease

Grey platelet syndrome

Thromboasthenia (hemorrhagic) (hereditary)

Thrombocytopathy

Excludes1: von Willebrand's disease (D68.0)

D69.2 Other nonthrombocytopenic purpura

Purpura NOS

Purpura simplex

Senile purpura

D69.3 Immune thrombocytopenic purpura

Hemorrhagic (thrombocytopenic) purpura

Idiopathic thrombocytopenic purpura

Tidal platelet dysgenesis

D69.4 Other primary thrombocytopenia

Excludes1: transient neonatal thrombocytopenia (P61.0)

Wiskott-Aldrich syndrome (D82.0)

D69.41 Evans syndrome

D69.42 Congenital and hereditary thrombocytopenia purpura

Congenital thrombocytopenia

Hereditary thrombocytopenia

Code first congenital or hereditary disorder, such as:

thrombocytopenia with absent radius (TAR syndrome) (Q87.2)

D69.49 Other primary thrombocytopenia

Megakaryocytic hypoplasia

Primary thrombocytopenia NOS

D69.5 Secondary thrombocytopenia

Excludes1: heparin induced thrombocytopenia (HIT) (D75.82)

transient thrombocytopenia of newborn (P61.0)

D69.51 Posttransfusion purpura

Posttransfusion purpura from whole blood (fresh) or blood products PTP

D69.59 Other secondary thrombocytopenia

D69.6 Thrombocytopenia, unspecified

D69.8 Other specified hemorrhagic conditions

Capillary fragility (hereditary)

Vascular pseudohemophilia

D69.9 Hemorrhagic condition, unspecified

OTHER DISORDERS OF BLOOD AND BLOOD-FORMING ORGANS (D70-D77)

D70 Neutropenia

Includes: agranulocytosis

decreased absolute neutrophile count (ANC)

Use additional code for any associated:

fever (R50.81)

mucositis (J34.81, K12.3-, K92.81, N76.81)

Excludes1: neutropenic splenomegaly (D73.81)

transient neonatal neutropenia (P61.5)

D70.0 Congenital agranulocytosis

Congenital neutropenia

Infantile genetic agranulocytosis

Kostmann's disease

D70.1 Agranulocytosis secondary to cancer chemotherapy

Code also underlying neoplasm

Use additional code for adverse effect, if applicable, to identify drug (T45.1X5)

D70.2 Other drug-induced agranulocytosis

Use additional code for adverse effect, if applicable, to identify drug (T36-T50 with fifth or sixth character 5)

D70.3 Neutropenia due to infection

D70.4 Cyclic neutropenia

Cyclic hematopoiesis

Periodic neutropenia

D70.8 Other neutropenia

D70.9 Neutropenia, unspecified

D71 Functional disorders of polymorphonuclear neutrophils

Cell membrane receptor complex [CR3] defect

Chronic (childhood) granulomatous disease

Congenital dysphagocytosis

Progressive septic granulomatosis

D72 Other disorders of white blood cells

● New code ▲ Revised code **Excludes1:** Not coded here **Excludes2:** Not included here ⊗ Placeholder required ⑦7th digit required

Definition: White blood cells, aka leukocyte, refers to any of various blood cells that help protect the body from infection and disease. White blood cells include neutrophils, eosinophils, basophils, lymphocytes, and monocytes

Excludes1: basophilia (D72.824)

immunity disorders (D80-D89)

neutropenia (D70)

preleukemia (syndrome) (D46.9)

D72.0 Genetic anomalies of leukocytes

Alder (granulation) (granulocyte) anomaly

Alder syndrome

Hereditary leukocytic hypersegmentation

Hereditary leukocytic hyposegmentation

Hereditary Leukomelanopathy

May-Hegglin (granulation) (granulocyte) anomaly

May-Hegglin syndrome

Pelger-Huët (granulation) (granulocyte anomaly

Pelger-Huët syndrome

Excludes1: Chédiak (-Steinbrinck)-Higashi syndrome(E70.330)

D72.1 Eosinophilia

Allergic eosinophilia

Hereditary eosinophilia

Excludes1: Löffler's syndrome (J82)

pulmonary eosinophilia (J82)

D72.8 Other specified disorders of white blood cells

Excludes1: leukemia (C91-C95)

D72.81 Decreased white blood cell count

Excludes1: neutropenia (D70.-)

D72.810 Lymphocytopenia

Decreased lymphocytes

D72.818 Other decreased white blood cell count

Basophilic leukopenia Eosinophilic leukopenia

Monocytopenia

Other decreased leukocytes

Plasmacytopenia

D72.819 Decreased white blood cell count, unspecified

Decreased leukocytes, unspecified

Leukocytopenia, unspecified

Leukopenia

Excludes1: malignant leukopenia (D70.9)

D72.82 Elevated white blood cell count

Excludes1: eosinophilia (D72.1)

D72.820 Lymphocytosis (symptomatic)

Elevated lymphocytes

D72.821 Monocytosis (symptomatic)

Excludes1: infectious mononucleosis (B27.-)

D72.822 Plasmacytosis

D72.823 Leukemoid reaction

Basophilic leukemoid reaction

Leukemoid reaction NOS

Lymphocytic leukemoid reaction

Monocytic leukemoid reaction

Myelocytic leukemoid reaction

Neutrophilic leukemoid reaction

D72.824 Basophilia

D72.825 Bandemia

Bandemia without diagnosis of specific infection

Excludes1: confirmed infection - code to infection

leukemia (C91.-, C92.-, C93.-, C94.-, C95.-)

D72.828 Other elevated white blood cell count

D72.829 Elevated white blood cell count, unspecified

Elevated leukocytes, unspecified

Leukocytosis, unspecified

D72.89 Other specified disorders of white blood cells

Abnormality of white blood cells NEC

D72.9 Disorder of white blood cells, unspecified

Abnormal leukocyte differential NOS

D73 Diseases of spleen

D73.0 Hyposplenism

Atrophy of spleen

Excludes1: asplenia (congenital) (Q89.01)

postsurgical absence of spleen (Z90.81)

D73.1 Hypersplenism

Excludes1: neutropenic splenomegaly (D73.81)

primary splenic neutropenia (D73.81)

splenitis, splenomegaly in late syphilis (A52.79)

splenitis, splenomegaly in tuberculosis (A18.85)

splenomegaly NOS (R16.1)

splenomegaly congenital (Q89.0)

D73.2 Chronic congestive splenomegaly

D73.3 Abscess of spleen

D73.4 Cyst of spleen

D73.5 Infarction of spleen

Splenic rupture, nontraumatic

Torsion of spleen

Excludes1: rupture of spleen due to Plasmodium vivax malaria (B51.0)

traumatic rupture of spleen (S36.03-)

D73.8 Other diseases of spleen

D73.81 Neutropenic splenomegaly

Werner-Schultz disease

D73.89 Other diseases of spleen

Fibrosis of spleen NOS

Perisplenitis

Splenitis NOS

D73.9 Disease of spleen, unspecified

D74 Methemoglobinemia

D74.0 Congenital methemoglobinemia

Congenital NADH-methemoglobin reductase deficiency

Hemoglobin-M [Hb-M] disease

Methemoglobinemia, hereditary

D74.8 Other methemoglobinemias

Acquired methemoglobinemia (with sulfhemoglobinemia)

Toxic methemoglobinemia

D74.9 Methemoglobinemia, unspecified

D75 **Other and unspecified diseases of blood and blood-forming organs**

Excludes2: acute lymphadenitis (L04.-)

chronic lymphadenitis (I88.1)

enlarged lymph nodes (R59.-)

hypergammaglobulinemia NOS (D89.2)

lymphadenitis NOS (I88.9)

mesenteric lymphadenitis (acute) (chronic) (I88.0)

D75.0 **Familial erythrocytosis**

Benign polycythemia

Familial polycythemia

Excludes1: hereditary ovalocytosis (D58.1)

D75.1 **Secondary polycythemia**

Acquired polycythemia

Emotional polycythemia

Erythrocytosis NOS

Hypoxemic polycythemia

Nephrogenous polycythemia

Polycythemia due to erythropoietin

Polycythemia due to fall in plasma volume

Polycythemia due to high altitude

Polycythemia due to stress

Polycythemia NOS

Relative polycythemia

Excludes1: polycythemia neonatorum (P61.1)

polycythemia vera (D45)

D75.8 **Other specified diseases of blood and blood-forming organs**

D75.81 **Myelofibrosis**

Myelofibrosis NOS

Secondary myelofibrosis NOS

Code first the underlying disorder, such as:

malignant neoplasm of breast (C50.-)

Use additional code, if applicable, for associated therapy-related myelodysplastic syndrome (D46.-)

Use additional code for adverse effect, if applicable, to identify drug (T45.1X5)

Excludes1: acute myelofibrosis (C94.4-)

idiopathic myelofibrosis (D47.1)

leukoerythroblastic anemia (D61.82)

myelofibrosis with myeloid metaplasia (D47.4)

myelophthisic anemia (D61.82)

myelophthisis (D61.82)

primary myelofibrosis (D47.1)

D75.82 **Heparin induced thrombocytopenia (HIT)**

D75.89 **Other specified diseases of blood and blood-forming organs**

D75.9 **Disease of blood and blood-forming organs, unspecified**

D76 **Other specified diseases with participation of lymphoreticular and reticulohistiocytic tissue**

Excludes1: (Abt-) Letterer-Siwe disease (C96.0)

eosinophilic granuloma (C96.6)

Hand-Schüller-Christian disease (C96.5)

histiocytic medullary reticulosis (C96.9)

histiocytic sarcoma (C96.A)

histiocytosis X, multifocal (C96.5)

histiocytosis X, unifocal (C96.6)

Langerhans-cell histiocytosis, multifocal (C96.5)

Langerhans-cell histiocytosis NOS (C96.6)

Langerhans-cell histiocytosis, unifocal (C96.6)

leukemic reticuloendotheliosis (C91.4-)

lipomelanotic reticulosis (I89.8)

malignant histiocytosis (C96.A)

malignant reticulosis (C86.0)

nonlipid reticuloendotheliosis (C96.0)

D76.1 **Hemophagocytic lymphohistiocytosis**

Familial hemophagocytic reticulosis

Histiocytoses of mononuclear phagocytes

D76.2 **Hemophagocytic syndrome, infection-associated**

Use additional code to identify infectious agent or disease.

D76.3 **Other histiocytosis syndromes**

Reticulohistiocytoma (giant-cell)

Sinus histiocytosis with massive lymphadenopathy Xanthogranuloma

D77 **Other disorders of blood and blood-forming organs in diseases classified elsewhere**

Code first underlying disease, such as:

amyloidosis (E85.-)

congenital early syphilis (A50.0)

echinococcosis (B67.0-B67.9)

malaria (B50.0-B54)

schistosomiasis [bilharziasis] (B65.0-B65.9)

vitamin C deficiency (E54)

Excludes1: rupture of spleen due to Plasmodium vivax malaria (B51.0)

splenitis, splenomegaly in late syphilis (A52.79)

splenitis, splenomegaly in tuberculosis (A18.85)

INTRAOPERATIVE AND POSTPROCEDURAL COMPLICATIONS OF THE SPLEEN (D78)

D78 **Intraoperative and postprocedural complications of the spleen**

D78.0 **Intraoperative hemorrhage and hematoma of the spleen complicating a procedure**

Excludes1: intraoperative hemorrhage and hematoma of the spleen due to accidental puncture or laceration during a procedure (D78.1-)

D78.01 **Intraoperative hemorrhage and hematoma of the spleen complicating a procedure on the spleen**

D78.02 **Intraoperative hemorrhage and hematoma of the spleen complicating other procedure**

D78.1 **Accidental puncture and laceration of the spleen during a procedure**

D78.11 **Accidental puncture and laceration of the spleen during a procedure on the spleen**

D78.12 **Accidental puncture and laceration of the spleen during other procedure**

D78.2 **Postprocedural hemorrhage of the spleen following a procedure**

D78.21 **Postprocedural hemorrhage of the spleen following a procedure on the spleen**

D78.22 **Postprocedural hemorrhage of the spleen following other procedure**

D78.3 **Postprocedural hematoma and seroma of the spleen following a procedure**

D78.31 **Postprocedural hematoma of the spleen following a procedure on the spleen**

D78.32 **Postprocedural hematoma of the spleen following other procedure**

D78.33 **Postprocedural seroma of the spleen following a procedure on the spleen**

D78.34 **Postprocedural seroma of the spleen following other procedure**

D78.8 **Other intraoperative and postprocedural complications of the spleen**

Use additional code, if applicable, to further specify disorder

D78.81 **Other intraoperative complications of the spleen**

D78.89 **Other postprocedural complications of the spleen**

CERTAIN DISORDERS INVOLVING THE IMMUNE MECHANISM (D80-D89)

Includes: defects in the complement system

immunodeficiency disorders, except human

immunodeficiency virus [HIV] disease sarcoidosis

Excludes1: autoimmune disease (systemic) NOS (M35.9)

functional disorders of polymorphonuclear neutrophils (D71)

human immunodeficiency virus [HIV] disease (B20)

D80 Immunodeficiency with predominantly antibody defects

D80.0 **Hereditary hypogammaglobulinemia**

Autosomal recessive agammaglobulinemia (Swiss type)

X-linked agammaglobulinemia [Bruton] (with growth hormone deficiency)

D80.1 **Nonfamilial hypogammaglobulinemia**

Agammaglobulinemia with immunoglobulin-bearing B-lymphocytes

Common variable agammaglobulinemia [CVA gamma]

Hypogammaglobulinemia NOS

D80.2 **Selective deficiency of immunoglobulin A [IgA]**

D80.3 **Selective deficiency of immunoglobulin G [IgG] subclasses**

D80.4 **Selective deficiency of immunoglobulin M [IgM]**

D80.5 **Immunodeficiency with increased immunoglobulin M [IgM]**

D80.6 **Antibody deficiency with near-normal immunoglobulins or with hyperimmunoglobulinemia**

D80.7 **Transient hypogammaglobulinemia of infancy**

D80.8 **Other immunodeficiencies with predominantly antibody defects**

Kappa light chain deficiency

D80.9 **Immunodeficiency with predominantly antibody defects, unspecified**

D81 Combined immunodeficiencies

Excludes1: autosomal recessive agammaglobulinemia (Swiss type) (D80.0)

D81.0 **Severe combined immunodeficiency [SCID] with reticular dysgenesis**

D81.1 **Severe combined immunodeficiency [SCID] with low T- and B-cell numbers**

D81.2 **Severe combined immunodeficiency [SCID] with low or normal B-cell numbers**

D81.3 **Adenosine deaminase [ADA] deficiency**

D81.4 **Nezelof's syndrome**

D81.5 **Purine nucleoside phosphorylase [PNP] deficiency**

D81.6 **Major histocompatibility complex class I deficiency**

Bare lymphocyte syndrome

D81.7 **Major histocompatibility complex class II deficiency**

D81.8 **Other combined immunodeficiencies**

D81.81 **Biotin-dependent carboxylase deficiency**

Multiple carboxylase deficiency

Excludes1: biotin-dependent carboxylase deficiency due to dietary deficiency of biotin (E53.8)

D81.810 **Biotinidase deficiency**

D81.818 **Other biotin-dependent carboxylase deficiency**

Holocarboxylase synthetase deficiency

Other multiple carboxylase deficiency

D81.819 **Biotin-dependent carboxylase deficiency, unspecified**

Multiple carboxylase deficiency, unspecified

D81.89 **Other combined immunodeficiencies**

D81.9 **Combined immunodeficiency, unspecified**

Severe combined immunodeficiency disorder [SCID] NOS

D82 Immunodeficiency associated with other major defects

Excludes1: ataxia telangiectasia [Louis-Bar] (G11.3)

D82.0 **Wiskott-Aldrich syndrome**

Immunodeficiency with thrombocytopenia and eczema

D82.1 **Di George's syndrome**

Pharyngeal pouch syndrome

Thymic alymphoplasia

Thymic aplasia or hypoplasia with immunodeficiency

D82.2 **Immunodeficiency with short-limbed stature**

D82.3 **Immunodeficiency following hereditary defective response to Epstein-Barr virus**

X-linked lymphoproliferative disease

D82.4 **Hyperimmunoglobulin E [IgE] syndrome**

D82.8 **Immunodeficiency associated with other specified major defects**

D82.9 **Immunodeficiency associated with major defect, unspecified**

D83 Common variable immunodeficiency

D83.0 **Common variable immunodeficiency with predominant abnormalities of B-cell numbers and function**

D83.1 **Common variable immunodeficiency with predominant immunoregulatory T-cell disorders**

D83.2 **Common variable immunodeficiency with autoantibodies to B- or T-cells**

D83.8 **Other common variable immunodeficiencies**

D83.9 **Common variable immunodeficiency, unspecified**

D84 Other immunodeficiencies

D84.0 **Lymphocyte function antigen-1[LFA-1] defect**

D84.1 **Defects in the complement system**

C1 esterase inhibitor [C1-INH] deficiency

D84.8 **Other specified immunodeficiencies**

D84.9 **Immunodeficiency, unspecified**

D86 Sarcoidosis

D86.0 **Sarcoidosis of lung**

D86.1 **Sarcoidosis of lymph nodes**

D86.2 **Sarcoidosis of lung with sarcoidosis of lymph nodes**

D86.3 **Sarcoidosis of skin**

D86.8 **Sarcoidosis of other sites**

D86.81 **Sarcoid meningitis**

D86.82 **Multiple cranial nerve palsies in sarcoidosis**

D86.83 **Sarcoid iridocyclitis**

D86.84 **Sarcoid pyelonephritis**

Tubulo-interstitial nephropathy in sarcoidosis

D86.85 Sarcoid myocarditis

D86.86 Sarcoid arthropathy

Polyarthritis in sarcoidosis

D86.87 Sarcoid myositis

D86.89 Sarcoidosis of other sites

Hepatic granuloma

Uveoparotid fever [Heerfordt]

D86.9 Sarcoidosis, unspecified

D89 Other disorders involving the immune mechanism, not elsewhere classified

Excludes1: hyperglobulinemia NOS (R77.1)

monoclonal gammopathy (of undetermined significance) (D47.2)

Excludes2: transplant failure and rejection (T86.-)

D89.0 Polyclonal hypergammaglobulinemia

Benign hypergammaglobulinemic purpura

Polyclonal gammopathy NOS

D89.1 Cryoglobulinemia

Cryoglobulinemic purpura

Cryoglobulinemic vasculitis

Essential cryoglobulinemia

Idiopathic cryoglobulinemia

Mixed cryoglobulinemia

Primary cryoglobulinemia

Secondary cryoglobulinemia

D89.2 Hypergammaglobulinemia, unspecified

D89.3 Immune reconstitution syndrome

Immune reconstitution inflammatory syndrome [IRIS]

Use additional code for adverse effect, if applicable, to identify drug (T36-T50 with fifth or sixth character 5)

D89.4 Mast cell activation syndrome and related disorders

Excludes1: aggressive systemic mastocytosis (C96.21)

congenital cutaneous mastocytosis (Q82.2)

(non-congenital) cutaneous mastocytosis (D47.01)

(indolent) systemic mastocytosis (D47.02)

malignant mast cell neoplasm (C96.2-)

malignant mastocytoma (C96.29)

mast cell leukemia (C94.3-)

mast cell sarcoma (C96.22)

mastocytoma NOS (D47.09)

other mast cell neoplasms of uncertain behavior (D47.09)

systemic mastocytosis associated with a clonal hematologic non-mast cell lineage disease (SM-AHNMD) (D47.02)

D89.40 Mast cell activation, unspecified

Mast cell activation disorder, unspecified

Mast cell activation syndrome, NOS

D89.41 Monoclonal mast cell activation syndrome

D89.42 Idiopathic mast cell activation syndrome

D89.43 Secondary mast cell activation

Secondary mast cell activation syndrome

Code also underlying etiology, if known

D89.49 Other mast cell activation disorder

Other mast cell activation syndrome

D89.8 Other specified disorders involving the immune mechanism, not elsewhere classified

D89.81 Graft-versus-host disease

Code first underlying cause, such as:

complications of transplanted organs and tissue (T86.-)

complications of blood transfusion (T80.89)

Use additional code to identify associated manifestations, such as:

desquamative dermatitis (L30.8)

diarrhea (R19.7)

elevated bilirubin (R17)

hair loss (L65.9)

D89.810 Acute graft-versus-host disease

D89.811 Chronic graft-versus-host disease

D89.812 Acute on chronic graft-versus-host disease

D89.813 Graft-versus-host disease, unspecified

D89.82 Autoimmune lymphoproliferative syndrome [ALPS]

D89.89 Other specified disorders involving the immune mechanism, not elsewhere classified

Excludes1: human immunodeficiency virus disease (B20)

D89.9 Disorder involving the immune mechanism, unspecified

Immune disease NOS

Chapter 4: Endocrine, Nutritional And Metabolic Diseases (E00-E89)

DEFINITIONS

This chapter includes definitions of selected key words, terms and phrases and coding alerts for adding points to the clinical domain, and references to coding late effects where appropriate. An example from this chapter is as follows:

E20 Hypoparathyroidism

Definition: Parathyroid glands are small endocrine glands in the neck that produce parathyroid hormone. Humans have four parathyroid glands, which are usually located behind the thyroid gland.

MULTIPLE CODING FOR A SINGLE CONDITION

In addition to the etiology/manifestation convention that requires two codes to fully describe a single condition that affects multiple body systems, there are other single conditions that also require more than one code. "Use additional code" notes are found in the Tabular List at codes that are not part of an etiology/manifestation pair where a secondary code is useful to fully describe a condition. The sequencing rule is the same as the etiology/manifestation pair, "use additional code" indicates that a secondary code should be added.

For example, for bacterial infections that are not included in chapter 1, a secondary code from category B95, Streptococcus, Staphylococcus, and Enterococcus, as the cause of diseases classified elsewhere, or B96, Other bacterial agents as the cause of diseases classified elsewhere, may be required to identify the bacterial organism causing the infection. A "use additional code" note will normally be found at the infectious disease code, indicating a need for the organism code to be added as a secondary code.

"Code first" notes are also under certain codes that are not specifically manifestation codes but may be due to an underlying cause. When there is a "code first" note and an underlying condition is present, the underlying condition should be sequenced first.

"Code, if applicable, any causal condition first", notes indicate that this code may be assigned as a principal diagnosis when the causal condition is unknown or not applicable. If a causal condition is known, then the code for that condition should be sequenced as the principal or first-listed diagnosis.

Multiple codes may be needed for sequela, complication codes and obstetric codes to more fully describe a condition. See the specific guidelines for these conditions for further instruction.

COMBINATION CODE

A combination code is a single code used to classify: Two diagnoses, or a diagnosis with an associated secondary process (manifestation) A diagnosis with an associated complication

Combination codes are identified by referring to subterm entries in the Alphabetic Index and by reading the inclusion and exclusion notes in the Tabular List.

Assign only the combination code when that code fully identifies the diagnostic conditions involved or when the Alphabetic Index so directs. Multiple coding should not be used when the classification provides a combination code that clearly identifies all of the elements documented in the diagnosis. When the combination code lacks necessary specificity in describing the manifestation or complication, an additional code should be used as a secondary code.

SEQUELA (LATE EFFECTS)

A sequela is the residual effect (condition produced) after the acute phase of an illness or injury has terminated. There is no time limit on when a sequela code can be used. The residual may be apparent early, such as in cerebral infarction, or it may occur months or years later, such as that due to a previous injury. Coding of sequela generally requires two codes sequenced in the following order: The condition or nature of the sequela is sequenced first.

The sequela code is sequenced second.

An exception to the above guidelines are those instances where the code for the sequela is followed by a manifestation code identified in the Tabular List and title, or the sequela code has been expanded (at the fourth, fifth or sixth character levels) to include the manifestation(s). The code for the acute phase of an illness or injury that led to the sequela is never used with a code for the late effect.

DIABETES MELLITUS

The diabetes mellitus codes are combination codes that include the type of diabetes mellitus, the body system affected, and the complications affecting that body system. As many codes within a particular category

as are necessary to describe all of the complications of the disease may be used. They should be sequenced based on the reason for a particular encounter. Assign as many codes from categories E08 – E13 as needed to identify all of the associated conditions that the patient has.

1) **Type of diabetes**

   The age of a patient is not the sole determining factor, though most type 1 diabetics develop the condition before reaching puberty. For this reason type 1 diabetes mellitus is also referred to as juvenile diabetes.

2) **Type of diabetes mellitus not documented**

   If the type of diabetes mellitus is not documented in the medical record the default is E11.-, Type 2 diabetes mellitus.

3) Diabetes mellitus and the use of insulin and oral hypoglycemics

If the documentation in a medical record does not indicate the type of diabetes but does indicate that the patient uses insulin, code E11, Type 2 diabetes mellitus, should be assigned. Code Z79.4, Long-term (current) use of insulin, or Z79.84, Long term (current) use of oral hypoglycemic drugs, should also be assigned to indicate that the patient uses insulin or hypoglycemic drugs. Code Z79.4 should not be assigned if insulin is given temporarily to bring a type 2 patient's blood sugar under control during an encounter.

4) Diabetes mellitus in pregnancy and gestational diabetes

See Section I.C.15. Diabetes mellitus in pregnancy.

See Section I.C.15. Gestational (pregnancy induced) diabetes

5) Complications due to insulin pump malfunction

(a) Underdose of insulin due to insulin pump failure

An underdose of insulin due to an insulin pump failure should be assigned to a code from subcategory T85.6, Mechanical complication of other specified internal and external prosthetic devices, implants and grafts, that specifies the type of pump malfunction, as the principal or first-listed code, followed by code T38.3X6-, Underdosing of insulin and oral hypoglycemic [antidiabetic] drugs. Additional codes for the type of diabetes mellitus and any associated complications due to the underdosing should also be assigned.

(b) Overdose of insulin due to insulin pump failure

The principal or first-listed code for an encounter due to an insulin pump malfunction resulting in an overdose of insulin, should also be T85.6-, Mechanical complication of other specified internal and external prosthetic devices, implants and grafts, followed by code T38.3X1-, Poisoning by insulin and oral hypoglycemic [antidiabetic] drugs, accidental (unintentional).

6) Secondary diabetes mellitus

Codes under categories E08, Diabetes mellitus due to underlying condition, E09, Drug or chemical induced diabetes mellitus, and E13, Other specified diabetes mellitus, identify complications/manifestations associated with secondary diabetes mellitus. Secondary diabetes is always caused by another condition or event (e.g., cystic fibrosis, malignant neoplasm of pancreas, pancreatectomy, adverse effect of drug, or poisoning).

(a) Secondary diabetes mellitus and the use of insulin or hypoglycemic drugs

For patients who routinely use insulin or hypoglycemic drugs, code Z79.4, Long-term (current) use of insulin, or Z79.84, Long term (current) use of oral hypoglycemic drugs should also be assigned. Code Z79.4 should not be assigned if insulin is given temporarily to bring a patient's blood sugar under control during an encounter.

(b) Assigning and sequencing secondary diabetes codes and its causes

The sequencing of the secondary diabetes codes in relationship to codes for the cause of the diabetes is based on the Tabular List instructions for categories E08, E09 and E13.

(i) Secondary diabetes mellitus due to pancreatectomy

For postpancreatectomy diabetes mellitus (lack of insulin due to the surgical removal of all or part of the pancreas), assign code E89.1, Postprocedural hypoinsulinemia. Assign a code from category E13 and a code from subcategory Z90.41-, Acquired absence of pancreas, as additional codes.

(ii) Secondary diabetes due to drugs

Secondary diabetes may be caused by an adverse effect of correctly administered medications, poisoning or sequela of poisoning.

See section I.C.19.e for coding of adverse effects and poisoning, and section I.C.20 for external cause code reporting.

Chapter 4

Endocrine, Nutritional and Metabolic Diseases (E00-E89)

Note: All neoplasms, whether functionally active or not, are classified in Chapter 2. Appropriate codes in this chapter (i.e. E05.8, E07.0, E16-E31, E34.-) may be used as additional codes to indicate either functional activity by neoplasms and ectopic endocrine tissue or hyperfunction and hypofunction of endocrine glands associated with neoplasms and other conditions classified elsewhere.

Excludes1: transitory endocrine and metabolic disorders specific to newborn (P70-P74)

This chapter contains the following blocks:

E00-E07	Disorders of thyroid gland
E08-E13	Diabetes mellitus
E15-E16	Other disorders of glucose regulation and pancreatic internal secretion
E20-E35	Disorders of other endocrine glands
E36	Intraoperative complications of endocrine system
E40-E46	Malnutrition
E50-E64	Other nutritional deficiencies
E65-E68	Overweight, obesity and other hyperalimentation
E70-E88	Metabolic disorders
E89	Postprocedural endocrine and metabolic complications and disorders, not elsewhere classified

DISORDERS OF THYROID GLAND (E00-E07)

E00 Congenital iodine-deficiency syndrome

Use additional code (F70-F79) to identify associated intellectual disabilities.

Excludes1: subclinical iodine-deficiency hypothyroidism (E02)

E00.0 Congenital iodine-deficiency syndrome, neurological type

Endemic cretinism, neurological type

E00.1 Congenital iodine-deficiency syndrome, myxedematous type

Endemic hypothyroid cretinism

Endemic cretinism, myxedematous type

E00.2 Congenital iodine-deficiency syndrome, mixed type

Endemic cretinism, mixed type

E00.9 Congenital iodine-deficiency syndrome, unspecified

Congenital iodine-deficiency hypothyroidism NOS

Endemic cretinism NOS

E01 Iodine-deficiency related thyroid disorders and allied conditions

Excludes1: congenital iodine-deficiency syndrome (E00.-)

subclinical iodine-deficiency hypothyroidism (E02)

E01.0 Iodine-deficiency related diffuse (endemic) goiter

E01.1 Iodine-deficiency related multinodular (endemic) goiter

Iodine-deficiency related nodular goiter

E01.2 Iodine-deficiency related (endemic) goiter, unspecified

Endemic goiter NOS

E01.8 Other iodine-deficiency related thyroid disorders and allied conditions

Acquired iodine-deficiency hypothyroidism NOS

E02 Subclinical iodine-deficiency hypothyroidism

E03 Other hypothyroidism

Excludes1: iodine-deficiency related hypothyroidism (E00-E02)

postprocedural hypothyroidism (E89.0)

E03.0 Congenital hypothyroidism with diffuse goiter

Congenital parenchymatous goiter (nontoxic)

Congenital goiter (nontoxic) NOS

Excludes1: transitory congenital goiter with normal function (P72.0)

E03.1 Congenital hypothyroidism without goiter

Aplasia of thyroid (with myxedema)

Congenital atrophy of thyroid

Congenital hypothyroidism NOS

E03.2 Hypothyroidism due to medicaments and other exogenous substances

Code first poisoning due to drug or toxin, if applicable (T36-T65 with fifth or sixth character 1-4 or 6)

Use additional code for adverse effect, if applicable, to identify drug (T36-T50 with fifth or sixth character 5)

E03.3 Postinfectious hypothyroidism

E03.4 Atrophy of thyroid (acquired)

Excludes1: congenital atrophy of thyroid (E03.1)

E03.5 Myxedema coma

E03.8 Other specified hypothyroidism

E03.9 Hypothyroidism, unspecified

Myxedema NOS

E04 Other nontoxic goiter

Definition: Nontoxic nodular goiter is a type of simple goiter with enlargement caused by nodules, or lumps, on the thyroid.

Excludes1: congenital goiter (NOS) (diffuse) (parenchymatous) (E03.0)

iodine-deficiency related goiter (E00-E02)

E04.0 Nontoxic diffuse goiter

Diffuse (colloid) nontoxic goiter

Simple nontoxic goiter

E04.1 Nontoxic single thyroid nodule

Colloid nodule (cystic) (thyroid)

Nontoxic uninodular goiter

Thyroid (cystic) nodule NOS

E04.2 Nontoxic multinodular goiter

Cystic goiter NOS

Multinodular (cystic) goiter NOS

E04.8 Other specified nontoxic goiter

E04.9 Nontoxic goiter, unspecified

Goiter NOS

Nodular goiter (nontoxic) NOS

E05 Thyrotoxicosis [hyperthyroidism]

Definition: Thyrotoxicosis with or without goiter is a condition resulting from excessive concentrations of thyroid hormones in the body, as in hyperthyroidism.

Excludes1: chronic thyroiditis with transient thyrotoxicosis (E06.2)

neonatal thyrotoxicosis (P72.1)

E05.0 Thyrotoxicosis with diffuse goiter

Exophthalmic or toxic goiter NOS Graves' disease

Toxic diffuse goiter

  E05.00 Thyrotoxicosis with diffuse goiter without thyrotoxic crisis or storm

  E05.01 Thyrotoxicosis with diffuse goiter with thyrotoxic crisis or storm

E05.1 Thyrotoxicosis with toxic single thyroid nodule

Thyrotoxicosis with toxic uninodular goiter

  E05.10 Thyrotoxicosis with toxic single thyroid nodule without thyrotoxic crisis or storm

---

Add 4th-7th digits	Nonspecific code	Unspecified code	Manifestation code

E05.11   **Thyrotoxicosis with toxic single thyroid nodule with thyrotoxic crisis or storm**

E05.2   **Thyrotoxicosis with toxic multinodular goiter**

Toxic nodular goiter NOS

E05.20   **Thyrotoxicosis with toxic multinodular goiter without thyrotoxic crisis or storm**

E05.21   **Thyrotoxicosis with toxic multinodular goiter with thyrotoxic crisis or storm**

E05.3   **Thyrotoxicosis from ectopic thyroid tissue**

E05.30   **Thyrotoxicosis from ectopic thyroid tissue without thyrotoxic crisis or storm**

E05.31   **Thyrotoxicosis from ectopic thyroid tissue with thyrotoxic crisis or storm**

E05.4   **Thyrotoxicosis factitia**

E05.40   **Thyrotoxicosis factitia without thyrotoxic crisis or storm**

E05.41   **Thyrotoxicosis factitia with thyrotoxic crisis or storm**

E05.8   **Other thyrotoxicosis**

Overproduction of thyroid-stimulating hormone

E05.80   **Other thyrotoxicosis without thyrotoxic crisis or storm**

E05.81   **Other thyrotoxicosis with thyrotoxic crisis or storm**

E05.9   **Thyrotoxicosis, unspecified**

Hyperthyroidism NOS

E05.90   **Thyrotoxicosis, unspecified without thyrotoxic crisis or storm**

E05.91   **Thyrotoxicosis, unspecified with thyrotoxic crisis or storm**

E06   **Thyroiditis**

Excludes1: postpartum thyroiditis (O90.5)

E06.0   **Acute thyroiditis**

Abscess of thyroid

Pyogenic thyroiditis

Suppurative thyroiditis

Use additional code (B95-B97) to identify infectious agent.

E06.1   **Subacute thyroiditis**

de Quervain thyroiditis

Giant-cell thyroiditis

Granulomatous thyroiditis

Nonsuppurative thyroiditis

Viral thyroiditis

Excludes1: autoimmune thyroiditis (E06.3)

E06.2   **Chronic thyroiditis with transient thyrotoxicosis**

Excludes1: autoimmune thyroiditis (E06.3)

E06.3   **Autoimmune thyroiditis**

Hashimoto's thyroiditis

Hashitoxicosis (transient)

Lymphadenoid goiter

Lymphocytic thyroiditis

Struma lymphomatosa

E06.4   **Drug-induced thyroiditis**

Use additional code for adverse effect, if applicable, to identify drug (T36-T50 with fifth or sixth character 5)

E06.5   **Other chronic thyroiditis**

Chronic fibrous thyroiditis

Chronic thyroiditis NOS

Ligneous thyroiditis

Riedel thyroiditis

E06.9   **Thyroiditis, unspecified**

E07   **Other disorders of thyroid**

E07.0   **Hypersecretion of calcitonin**

C-cell hyperplasia of thyroid

Hypersecretion of thyrocalcitonin

E07.1   **Dyshormogenetic goiter**

Familial Dyshormogenetic goiter

Pendred's syndrome

Excludes1: transitory congenital goiter with normal function (P72.0)

E07.8   **Other specified disorders of thyroid**

E07.81   **Sick-euthyroid syndrome**

Euthyroid sick-syndrome

E07.89   **Other specified disorders of thyroid**

Abnormality of thyroid-binding globulin

Hemorrhage of thyroid

Infarction of thyroid

E07.9   **Disorder of thyroid, unspecified**

DIABETES MELLITUS (E08-E13)

Definition: Diabetes mellitus is a condition in which the pancreas no longer produces enough insulin or cells stop responding to the insulin that is produced, so that glucose in the blood cannot be absorbed into the cells of the body. Symptoms include frequent urination, lethargy, excessive thirst, and hunger.

E08   **Diabetes mellitus due to underlying condition**

Code first the underlying condition, such as:

congenital rubella (P35.0)

Cushing's syndrome (E24.-)

cystic fibrosis (E84.-)

malignant neoplasm (C00-C96)

malnutrition (E40-E46)

pancreatitis **and other** diseases of the pancreas (K85-K86.-)

Use additional code to identify control using:

insulin (Z79.4)

oral antidiabetic drugs (Z79.84)

oral hypoglycemic drugs (Z79.84)

Excludes1: drug or chemical induced diabetes mellitus (E09.-)

gestational diabetes (O24.4-)

neonatal diabetes mellitus (P70.2)

postpancreatectomy diabetes mellitus (E13.-)

postprocedural diabetes mellitus (E13.-)

secondary diabetes mellitus NEC (E13.-)

type 1 diabetes mellitus (E10.-)

type 2 diabetes mellitus (E11.-)

E08.0   **Diabetes mellitus due to underlying condition with hyperosmolarity**

E08.00   **Diabetes mellitus due to underlying condition with hyperosmolarity without nonketotic hyperglycemic-hyperosmolar coma (NKHHC)**

E08.01   **Diabetes mellitus due to underlying condition with hyperosmolarity with coma**

E08.1   **Diabetes mellitus due to underlying condition with ketoacidosis**

E08.10   **Diabetes mellitus due to underlying condition with ketoacidosis without coma**

● New code   ▲ Revised code   **Excludes1:** Not coded here   **Excludes2:** Not included here   ⊗ Placeholder required   ⑦7th digit required

E08.11   **Diabetes mellitus due to underlying condition with ketoacidosis with coma**

E08.2   **Diabetes mellitus due to underlying condition with kidney complications**

E08.21   **Diabetes mellitus due to underlying condition with diabetic nephropathy**

Diabetes mellitus due to underlying condition with intercapillary glomerulosclerosis

Diabetes mellitus due to underlying condition with intracapillary glomerulonephrosis

Diabetes mellitus due to underlying condition with Kimmelstiel-Wilson disease

E08.22   **Diabetes mellitus due to underlying condition with diabetic chronic kidney disease**

<u>Use additional code</u> to identify stage of chronic kidney disease (N18.1-N18.6)

E08.29   **Diabetes mellitus due to underlying condition with other diabetic kidney complication**

Renal tubular degeneration in diabetes mellitus due to underlying condition

E08.3   **Diabetes mellitus due to underlying condition with ophthalmic complications**

E08.31   **Diabetes mellitus due to underlying condition with unspecified diabetic retinopathy**

E08.311   **Diabetes mellitus due to underlying condition with unspecified diabetic retinopathy with macular edema**

E08.319   **Diabetes mellitus due to underlying condition with unspecified diabetic retinopathy without macular edema**

E08.32   **Diabetes mellitus due to underlying condition with mild nonproliferative diabetic retinopathy**

Diabetes mellitus due to underlying condition with nonproliferative diabetic retinopathy NOS

One of the following 7th characters is to be assigned to codes in subcategory E08.32 to designate laterality of the disease:

1 - right eye

2 - left eye

3 – bilateral

9 - unspecified eye

⑦ **E08.321**   **Diabetes mellitus due to underlying condition with mild nonproliferative diabetic retinopathy with macular edema**

⑦ **E08.329**   **Diabetes mellitus due to underlying condition with mild nonproliferative diabetic retinopathy without macular edema**

E08.33   **Diabetes mellitus due to underlying condition with moderate nonproliferative diabetic retinopathy**

One of the following 7th characters is to be assigned to codes in subcategory E08.33 to designate laterality of the disease:

1 - right eye

2 - left eye

3 - bilateral

9 - unspecified eye

⑦ **E08.331**   **Diabetes mellitus due to underlying condition with moderate nonproliferative diabetic retinopathy with macular edema**

⑦ **E08.339**   **Diabetes mellitus due to underlying condition with moderate**

nonproliferative diabetic retinopathy without macular edema

E08.34   **Diabetes mellitus due to underlying condition with severe nonproliferative diabetic retinopathy**

One of the following 7th characters is to be assigned to codes in subcategory E08.34 to designate laterality of the disease:

1 - right eye

2 - left eye

3 - bilateral

9 - unspecified eye

⑦ **E08.341**   **Diabetes mellitus due to underlying condition with severe nonproliferative diabetic retinopathy with macular edema**

⑦ **E08.349**   **Diabetes mellitus due to underlying condition with severe nonproliferative diabetic retinopathy without macular edema**

E08.35   **Diabetes mellitus due to underlying condition with proliferative diabetic retinopathy**

One of the following 7th characters is to be assigned to codes in subcategory E08.35 to designate laterality of the disease:

1 - right eye

2 - left eye

3 - bilateral

9 - unspecified eye

⑦ **E08.351**   **Diabetes mellitus due to underlying condition with proliferative diabetic retinopathy with macular edema**

⑦ **E08.352**   **Diabetes mellitus due to underlying condition with proliferative diabetic retinopathy with traction retinal detachment involving the macula**

⑦ **E08.353**   **Diabetes mellitus due to underlying condition with proliferative diabetic retinopathy with traction retinal detachment not involving the macula**

⑦ **E08.354**   **Diabetes mellitus due to underlying condition with proliferative diabetic retinopathy with combined traction retinal detachment and rhegmatogenous retinal detachment**

⑦ **E08.355**   **Diabetes mellitus due to underlying condition with stable proliferative diabetic retinopathy**

⑦ **E08.359**   **Diabetes mellitus due to underlying condition with proliferative diabetic retinopathy without macular edema**

E08.36   **Diabetes mellitus due to underlying condition with diabetic cataract**

⊗⑦ **E08.37**   **Diabetes mellitus due to underlying condition with diabetic macular edema, resolved following treatment**

One of the following 7th characters is to be assigned to code E08.37 to designate laterality of the disease:

1 - right eye

2 - left eye

3 - bilateral

9 - unspecified eye

E08.39   **Diabetes mellitus due to underlying condition with other diabetic ophthalmic complication**

Use additional code to identify manifestation, such as:

diabetic glaucoma (H40-H42)

E08.4 Diabetes mellitus due to underlying condition with neurological complications

   E08.40 Diabetes mellitus due to underlying condition with diabetic neuropathy, unspecified

   E08.41 Diabetes mellitus due to underlying condition with diabetic mononeuropathy

   E08.42 Diabetes mellitus due to underlying condition with diabetic polyneuropathy

   Diabetes mellitus due to underlying condition with diabetic neuralgia

   E08.43 Diabetes mellitus due to underlying condition with diabetic autonomic (poly)neuropathy

   Diabetes mellitus due to underlying condition with diabetic gastroparesis

   E08.44 Diabetes mellitus due to underlying condition with diabetic amyotrophy

   E08.49 Diabetes mellitus due to underlying condition with other diabetic neurological complication

E08.5 Diabetes mellitus due to underlying condition with circulatory complications

   E08.51 Diabetes mellitus due to underlying condition with diabetic peripheral angiopathy without gangrene

   E08.52 Diabetes mellitus due to underlying condition with diabetic peripheral angiopathy with gangrene

   Diabetes mellitus due to underlying condition with diabetic gangrene

   E08.59 Diabetes mellitus due to underlying condition with other circulatory complications

E08.6 Diabetes mellitus due to underlying condition with other specified complications

   E08.61 Diabetes mellitus due to underlying condition with diabetic arthropathy

      E08.610 Diabetes mellitus due to underlying condition with diabetic neuropathic arthropathy

      Diabetes mellitus due to underlying condition with Charcôt's joints

      E08.618 Diabetes mellitus due to underlying condition with other diabetic arthropathy

   E08.62 Diabetes mellitus due to underlying condition with skin complications

      E08.620 Diabetes mellitus due to underlying condition with diabetic dermatitis

      Diabetes mellitus due to underlying condition with diabetic necrobiosis lipoidica

      E08.621 Diabetes mellitus due to underlying condition with foot ulcer

      Use additional code to identify site of ulcer (L97.4-, L97.5-)

      E08.622 Diabetes mellitus due to underlying condition with other skin ulcer

      Use additional code to identify site of ulcer (L97.1-L97.9, L98.41-L98.49)

      E08.628 Diabetes mellitus due to underlying condition with other skin complications

   E08.63 Diabetes mellitus due to underlying condition with oral complications

      E08.630 Diabetes mellitus due to underlying condition with periodontal disease

      E08.638 Diabetes mellitus due to underlying condition with other oral complications

   E08.64 Diabetes mellitus due to underlying condition with hypoglycemia

      E08.641 Diabetes mellitus due to underlying condition with hypoglycemia with coma

      E08.649 Diabetes mellitus due to underlying condition with hypoglycemia without coma

   E08.65 Diabetes mellitus due to underlying condition with hyperglycemia

   E08.69 Diabetes mellitus due to underlying condition with other specified complication

      Use additional code to identify complication

E08.8 Diabetes mellitus due to underlying condition with unspecified complications

E08.9 Diabetes mellitus due to underlying condition without complications

E09 Drug or chemical induced diabetes mellitus

   Code first poisoning due to drug or toxin, if applicable (T36-T65 with fifth or sixth character 1-4 or 6)

   Use additional code for adverse effect, if applicable, to identify drug (T36-T50 with fifth or sixth character 5)

   Use additional code to identify control using:

   insulin (Z79.4)

      oral antidiabetic drugs (Z79.84)

      oral hypoglycemic drugs (Z79.84)

   Excludes1: diabetes mellitus due to underlying condition (E08.-)

      gestational diabetes (O24.4-)

      neonatal diabetes mellitus (P70.2)

      postpancreatectomy diabetes mellitus (E13.-)

      postprocedural diabetes mellitus (E13.-)

      secondary diabetes mellitus NEC (E13.-)

      type 1 diabetes mellitus (E10.-)

      type 2 diabetes mellitus (E11.-)

   E09.0 Drug or chemical induced diabetes mellitus with hyperosmolarity

      E09.00 Drug or chemical induced diabetes mellitus with hyperosmolarity without nonketotic hyperglycemic-hyperosmolar coma (NKHHC)

      E09.01 Drug or chemical induced diabetes mellitus with hyperosmolarity with coma

   E09.1 Drug or chemical induced diabetes mellitus with ketoacidosis

      E09.10 Drug or chemical induced diabetes mellitus with ketoacidosis without coma

      E09.11 Drug or chemical induced diabetes mellitus with ketoacidosis with coma

   E09.2 Drug or chemical induced diabetes mellitus with kidney complications

      E09.21 Drug or chemical induced diabetes mellitus with diabetic nephropathy

      Drug or chemical induced diabetes mellitus with intercapillary glomerulosclerosis

      Drug or chemical induced diabetes mellitus with intracapillary glomerulonephrosis

      Drug or chemical induced diabetes mellitus with Kimmelstiel-Wilson disease

E09.22 **Drug or chemical induced diabetes mellitus with diabetic chronic kidney disease**

<u>Use additional code</u> to identify stage of chronic kidney disease (N18.1-N18.6)

E09.29 **Drug or chemical induced diabetes mellitus with other diabetic kidney complication**

Drug or chemical induced diabetes mellitus with renal tubular degeneration

E09.3 **Drug or chemical induced diabetes mellitus with ophthalmic complications**

E09.31 **Drug or chemical induced diabetes mellitus with unspecified diabetic retinopathy**

E09.311 **Drug or chemical induced diabetes mellitus with unspecified diabetic retinopathy with macular edema**

E09.319 **Drug or chemical induced diabetes mellitus with unspecified diabetic retinopathy without macular edema**

E09.32 **Drug or chemical induced diabetes mellitus with mild nonproliferative diabetic retinopathy**

Drug or chemical induced diabetes mellitus with nonproliferative diabetic retinopathy NOS

One of the following 7th characters is to be assigned to codes in subcategory E09.32 to designate laterality of the disease:

1 - right eye 2 - left eye

3 - bilateral

9 - unspecified eye

⑦ **E09.321** **Drug or chemical induced diabetes mellitus with mild nonproliferative diabetic retinopathy with macular edema**

⑦ **E09.329** **Drug or chemical induced diabetes mellitus with mild nonproliferative diabetic retinopathy without macular edema**

E09.33 **Drug or chemical induced diabetes mellitus with moderate nonproliferative diabetic retinopathy**

One of the following 7th characters is to be assigned to codes in subcategory E09.33 to designate laterality of the disease:

1 - right eye

2 - left eye

3 - bilateral

9 - unspecified eye

⑦ **E09.331** **Drug or chemical induced diabetes mellitus with moderate nonproliferative diabetic retinopathy with macular edema**

⑦ **E09.339** **Drug or chemical induced diabetes mellitus with moderate nonproliferative diabetic retinopathy without macular edema**

E09.34 **Drug or chemical induced diabetes mellitus with severe nonproliferative diabetic retinopathy**

One of the following 7th characters is to be assigned to codes in subcategory E09.34 to designate laterality of the disease:

1 - right eye

2 - left eye

3 - bilateral

9 - unspecified eye

⑦ **E09.341** **Drug or chemical induced diabetes mellitus with severe nonproliferative diabetic retinopathy with macular edema**

⑦ **E09.349** **Drug or chemical induced diabetes mellitus with severe nonproliferative diabetic retinopathy without macular edema**

E09.35 **Drug or chemical induced diabetes mellitus with proliferative diabetic retinopathy**

One of the following 7th characters is to be assigned to codes in subcategory E09.35 to designate laterality of the disease:

1 - right eye

2 - left eye

3 - bilateral

9 - unspecified eye

⑦ **E09.351** **Drug or chemical induced diabetes mellitus with proliferative diabetic retinopathy with macular edema**

⑦ **E09.352** **Drug or chemical induced diabetes mellitus with proliferative diabetic retinopathy with traction retinal detachment involving the macula**

⑦ **E09.353** **Drug or chemical induced diabetes mellitus with proliferative diabetic retinopathy with traction retinal detachment not involving the macula**

⑦ **E09.354** **Drug or chemical induced diabetes mellitus with proliferative diabetic retinopathy with combined traction retinal detachment and rhegmatogenous retinal detachment**

⑦ **E09.355** **Drug or chemical induced diabetes mellitus with stable proliferative diabetic retinopathy**

⑦ **E09.359** **Drug or chemical induced diabetes mellitus with proliferative diabetic retinopathy without macular edema**

E09.36 **Drug or chemical induced diabetes mellitus with diabetic cataract**

⊗⑦ **E09.37** **Drug or chemical induced diabetes mellitus with diabetic macular edema, resolved following treatment**

One of the following 7th characters is to be assigned to code E09.37 to designate laterality of the disease:

1 - right eye

2 - left eye

3 - bilateral

9 - unspecified eye

E09.39 **Drug or chemical induced diabetes mellitus with other diabetic ophthalmic complication**

<u>Use additional code</u> to identify manifestation, such as: diabetic glaucoma (H40-H42)

E09.4 **Drug or chemical induced diabetes mellitus with neurological complications**

E09.40 **Drug or chemical induced diabetes mellitus with neurological complications with diabetic neuropathy, unspecified**

E09.41 **Drug or chemical induced diabetes mellitus with neurological complications with diabetic mononeuropathy**

E09.42 **Drug or chemical induced diabetes mellitus with neurological complications with diabetic polyneuropathy**

Drug or chemical induced diabetes mellitus with diabetic neuralgia

E09.43 **Drug or chemical induced diabetes mellitus with neurological complications with diabetic autonomic (poly)neuropathy**

Drug or chemical induced diabetes mellitus with diabetic gastroparesis

E09.44 **Drug or chemical induced diabetes mellitus with neurological complications with diabetic amyotrophy**

E09.49 **Drug or chemical induced diabetes mellitus with neurological complications with other diabetic neurological complication**

E09.5 **Drug or chemical induced diabetes mellitus with circulatory complications**

E09.51 **Drug or chemical induced diabetes mellitus with diabetic peripheral angiopathy without gangrene**

E09.52 **Drug or chemical induced diabetes mellitus with diabetic peripheral angiopathy with gangrene**

Drug or chemical induced diabetes mellitus with diabetic gangrene

E09.59 **Drug or chemical induced diabetes mellitus with other circulatory complications**

E09.6 **Drug or chemical induced diabetes mellitus with other specified complications**

E09.61 **Drug or chemical induced diabetes mellitus with diabetic arthropathy**

E09.610 **Drug or chemical induced diabetes mellitus with diabetic neuropathic arthropathy**

Drug or chemical induced diabetes mellitus with Charcôt's joints

E09.618 **Drug or chemical induced diabetes mellitus with other diabetic arthropathy**

E09.62 **Drug or chemical induced diabetes mellitus with skin complications**

E09.620 **Drug or chemical induced diabetes mellitus with diabetic dermatitis**

Drug or chemical induced diabetes mellitus with diabetic necrobiosis lipoidica

E09.621 **Drug or chemical induced diabetes mellitus with foot ulcer**

Use additional code to identify site of ulcer (L97.4-, L97.5-)

E09.622 **Drug or chemical induced diabetes mellitus with other skin ulcer**

Use additional code to identify site of ulcer (L97.1-L97.9, L98.41-L98.49)

E09.628 **Drug or chemical induced diabetes mellitus with other skin complications**

E09.63 **Drug or chemical induced diabetes mellitus with oral complications**

E09.630 **Drug or chemical induced diabetes mellitus with periodontal disease**

E09.638 **Drug or chemical induced diabetes mellitus with other oral complications**

E09.64 **Drug or chemical induced diabetes mellitus with hypoglycemia**

E09.641 **Drug or chemical induced diabetes mellitus with hypoglycemia with coma**

E09.649 **Drug or chemical induced diabetes mellitus with hypoglycemia without coma**

E09.65 **Drug or chemical induced diabetes mellitus with hyperglycemia**

E09.69 **Drug or chemical induced diabetes mellitus with other specified complication**

Use additional code to identify complication

E09.8 **Drug or chemical induced diabetes mellitus with unspecified complications**

E09.9 **Drug or chemical induced diabetes mellitus without complications**

E10 **Type 1 diabetes mellitus**

Includes: brittle diabetes (mellitus)

diabetes (mellitus) due to autoimmune process

diabetes (mellitus) due to immune mediated pancreatic islet beta-cell destruction idiopathic diabetes (mellitus)

juvenile onset diabetes (mellitus)

ketosis-prone diabetes (mellitus)

Excludes1: diabetes mellitus due to underlying condition (E08.-)

drug or chemical induced diabetes mellitus (E09.-)

gestational diabetes (O24.4-)

hyperglycemia NOS (R73.9)

neonatal diabetes mellitus (P70.2)

postpancreatectomy diabetes mellitus (E13.-)

postprocedural diabetes mellitus (E13.-)

secondary diabetes mellitus NEC (E13.-)

type 2 diabetes mellitus (E11.-)

E10.1 **Type 1 diabetes mellitus with ketoacidosis**

E10.10 **Type 1diabetes mellitus with ketoacidosis without coma**

E10.11 **Type 1diabetes mellitus with ketoacidosis with coma**

E10.2 **Type 1 diabetes mellitus with kidney complications**

E10.21 **Type 1diabetes mellitus with diabetic nephropathy**

Type 1 diabetes mellitus with intercapillary glomerulosclerosis

Type 1 diabetes mellitus with intracapillary glomerulonephrosis

Type 1 diabetes mellitus with Kimmelstiel-Wilson disease

E10.22 **Type 1diabetes mellitus with diabetic chronic kidney disease**

Use additional code to identify stage of chronic kidney disease (N18.1-N18.6)

E10.29 **Type 1diabetes mellitus with other diabetic kidney complication**

Type 1 diabetes mellitus with renal tubular degeneration

E10.3 **Type 1 Diabetes mellitus with ophthalmic complications**

E10.31 **Type 1diabetes mellitus with unspecified diabetic retinopathy**

E10.311 **Type 1 diabetes mellitus with unspecified diabetic retinopathy with macular edema**

E10.319 **Type 1 diabetes mellitus with unspecified diabetic retinopathy without macular edema**

● New code   ▲ Revised code   **Excludes1:** Not coded here   **Excludes2:** Not included here   ⊗ Placeholder required   ⑦7th digit required

E10.32 **Type 1 diabetes mellitus with mild nonproliferative diabetic retinopathy**

Type 1 diabetes mellitus with nonproliferative diabetic retinopathy NOS

One of the following 7th characters is to be assigned to codes in subcategory E10.32 to designate laterality of the disease:

1 - right eye

2 - left eye

3 - bilateral

9 - unspecified eye

⑦**E10.321** **Type 1 diabetes mellitus with mild nonproliferative diabetic retinopathy with macular edema**

⑦**E10.329** **Type 1 diabetes mellitus with mild nonproliferative diabetic retinopathy without macular edema**

E10.33 **Type 1 diabetes mellitus with moderate nonproliferative diabetic retinopathy**

One of the following 7th characters is to be assigned to codes in subcategory E10.33 to designate laterality of the disease:

1 - right eye

2 - left eye

3 - bilateral

9 - unspecified eye

⑦**E10.331** **Type 1 diabetes mellitus with moderate nonproliferative diabetic retinopathy with macular edema**

⑦**E10.339** **Type 1 diabetes mellitus with moderate nonproliferative diabetic retinopathy without macular edema**

E10.34 **Type 1 diabetes mellitus with severe nonproliferative diabetic retinopathy**

One of the following 7th characters is to be assigned to codes in subcategory E10.34 to designate laterality of the disease:

1 - right eye

2 - left eye

3 - bilateral

9 - unspecified eye

⑦**E10.341** **Type 1 diabetes mellitus with severe nonproliferative diabetic retinopathy with macular edema**

⑦**E10.349** **Type 1 diabetes mellitus with severe nonproliferative diabetic retinopathy without macular edema**

E10.35 **Type 1 diabetes mellitus with proliferative diabetic retinopathy**

One of the following 7th characters is to be assigned to codes in subcategory E10.35 to designate laterality of the disease:

1 - right eye

2 - left eye

3 - bilateral

9 - unspecified eye

⑦**E10.351** **Type 1 diabetes mellitus with proliferative diabetic retinopathy with macular edema**

⑦**E10.352** **Type 1 diabetes mellitus with proliferative diabetic retinopathy with traction retinal detachment involving the macula**

⑦**E10.353** **Type 1 diabetes mellitus with proliferative diabetic retinopathy with traction retinal detachment not involving the macula**

⑦**E10.354** **Type 1 diabetes mellitus with proliferative diabetic retinopathy with combined traction retinal detachment and rhegmatogenous retinal detachment**

⑦**E10.355** **Type 1 diabetes mellitus with stable proliferative diabetic retinopathy**

⑦**E10.359** **Type 1 diabetes mellitus with proliferative diabetic retinopathy without macular edema**

⊗⑦**E10.36** **Type 1 diabetes mellitus with diabetic cataract**

⊗⑦**E10.37** **Type 1 diabetes mellitus with diabetic macular edema, resolved following treatment**

One of the following 7th characters is to be assigned to code E10.37 to designate laterality of the disease:

1 - right eye

2 - left eye

3 - bilateral

9 - unspecified eye

E10.39 **Type 1 diabetes mellitus with other diabetic ophthalmic complication**

<u>Use additional code</u> to identify manifestation, such as:

diabetic glaucoma (H40-H42)

E10.4 **Type 1 diabetes mellitus with neurological complications**

E10.40 **Type 1 diabetes mellitus with diabetic neuropathy, unspecified**

E10.41 **Type 1 diabetes mellitus with diabetic mononeuropathy**

E10.42 **Type 1 diabetes mellitus with diabetic polyneuropathy**

Type 1 diabetes mellitus with diabetic neuralgia

E10.43 **Type 1 diabetes mellitus with diabetic autonomic (poly)neuropathy**

Type 1 diabetes mellitus with diabetic gastroparesis

E10.44 **Type 1 diabetes mellitus with diabetic amyotrophy**

E10.49 **Type 1 diabetes mellitus with other diabetic neurological complication**

E10.5 **Type 1 diabetes mellitus with circulatory complications**

E10.51 **Type 1 diabetes mellitus with diabetic peripheral angiopathy without gangrene**

E10.52 **Type 1 diabetes mellitus with diabetic peripheral angiopathy with gangrene**

Type 1 diabetes mellitus with diabetic gangrene

E10.59 **Type 1 diabetes mellitus with other circulatory complications**

E10.6 **Type 1 diabetes mellitus with other specified complications**

E10.61 **Type 1 diabetes mellitus with diabetic arthropathy**

E10.610 **Type 1 diabetes mellitus with diabetic neuropathic arthropathy**

Type 1 diabetes mellitus with Charcôt's joints

E10.618 **Type 1 diabetes mellitus with other diabetic arthropathy**

E10.62 Type 1 diabetes mellitus with skin complications

    E10.620 Type 1 diabetes mellitus with diabetic dermatitis

        Type 1 diabetes mellitus with diabetic necrobiosis lipoidica

    E10.621 Type 1 diabetes mellitus with foot ulcer

        <u>Use additional code</u> to identify site of ulcer (L97.4-, L97.5-)

    E10.622 Type 1 diabetes mellitus with other skin ulcer

        <u>Use additional code</u> to identify site of ulcer (L97.1-L97.9, L98.41-L98.49)

    E10.628 Type 1 diabetes mellitus with other skin complications

E10.63 Type 1 diabetes mellitus with oral complications

    E10.630 Type 1 diabetes mellitus with periodontal disease

    E10.638 Type 1 diabetes mellitus with other oral complications

E10.64 Type 1 diabetes mellitus with hypoglycemia

    E10.641 Type 1 diabetes mellitus with hypoglycemia with coma

    E10.649 Type 1 diabetes mellitus with hypoglycemia without coma

E10.65 Type 1 diabetes mellitus with hyperglycemia

E10.69 Type 1 diabetes mellitus with other specified complication

    <u>Use additional code</u> to identify complication

E10.8 Type 1 diabetes mellitus with unspecified complications

E10.9 Type 1 diabetes mellitus without complications

E11 Type 2 diabetes mellitus

Includes: diabetes (mellitus) due to insulin secretory defect

diabetes NOS

insulin resistant diabetes (mellitus)

<u>Use additional code</u> to identify control using:

insulin (Z79.4)

oral antidiabetic drugs (Z79.84)

oral hypoglycemic drugs (Z79.84)

Excludes1: diabetes mellitus due to underlying condition (E08.-)

    drug or chemical induced diabetes mellitus (E09.-)

    gestational diabetes (O24.4-)

    neonatal diabetes mellitus (P70.2)

    postpancreatectomy diabetes mellitus (E13.-)

    postprocedural diabetes mellitus (E13.-)

    secondary diabetes mellitus NEC (E13.-)

    type 1 diabetes mellitus (E10.-)

E11.0 Type 2 diabetes mellitus with hyperosmolarity

    E11.00 Type 2 diabetes mellitus with hyperosmolarity without nonketotic hyperglycemic-hyperosmolar coma (NKHHC)

    E11.01 Type 2 diabetes mellitus with hyperosmolarity with coma

●**E11.1** Type 2 diabetes mellitus with ketoacidosis

    ●**E11.10** Type 2 diabetes mellitus with ketoacidosis without coma

    ●**E11.11** Type 2 diabetes mellitus with ketoacidosis with coma

E11.2 Type 2 diabetes mellitus with kidney complications

E11.21 Type 2 diabetes mellitus with diabetic nephropathy

    Type 2 diabetes mellitus with intercapillary glomerulosclerosis

    Type 2 diabetes mellitus with intracapillary glomerulonephrosis

    Type 2 diabetes mellitus with Kimmelstiel-Wilson disease

E11.22 Type 2 diabetes mellitus with diabetic chronic kidney disease

    <u>Use additional code</u> to identify stage of chronic kidney disease (N18.1-N18.6)

E11.29 Type 2 diabetes mellitus with other diabetic kidney complication

    Type 2 diabetes mellitus with renal tubular degeneration

E11.3 Type 2 diabetes mellitus with ophthalmic complications

E11.31 Type 2 diabetes mellitus with unspecified diabetic retinopathy

    E11.311 Type 2 diabetes mellitus with unspecified diabetic retinopathy with macular edema

    E11.319 Type 2 diabetes mellitus with unspecified diabetic retinopathy without macular edema

E11.32 Type 2 diabetes mellitus with mild nonproliferative diabetic retinopathy

    Type 2 diabetes mellitus with nonproliferative diabetic retinopathy NOS

    One of the following 7th characters is to be assigned to codes in subcategory E11.32 to designate laterality of the disease:

    1 - right eye

    2 - left eye

    3 – bilateral

    9 - unspecified eye

    ⑦**E11.321** Type 2 diabetes mellitus with mild nonproliferative diabetic retinopathy with macular edema

    ⑦**E11.329** Type 2 diabetes mellitus with mild nonproliferative diabetic retinopathy without macular edema

E11.33 Type 2 diabetes mellitus with moderate nonproliferative diabetic retinopathy

    One of the following 7th characters is to be assigned to codes in subcategory E11.33 to designate laterality of the disease:

    1 - right eye

    2 - left eye

    3 - bilateral

    9 - unspecified eye

    ⑦**E11.331** Type 2 diabetes mellitus with moderate nonproliferative diabetic retinopathy with macular edema

    ⑦**E11.339** Type 2 diabetes mellitus with moderate nonproliferative diabetic retinopathy without macular edema

E11.34 Type 2 diabetes mellitus with severe nonproliferative diabetic retinopathy

    One of the following 7th characters is to be assigned to codes in subcategory E11.34 to designate laterality of the disease:

    1 - right eye

2 - left eye

3 - bilateral

9 - unspecified eye

⑦**E11.341**   Type 2 diabetes mellitus with severe nonproliferative diabetic retinopathy with macular edema

⑦**E11.349**   Type 2 diabetes mellitus with severe nonproliferative diabetic retinopathy without macular edema

E11.35   Type 2 diabetes mellitus with proliferative diabetic retinopathy

One of the following 7th characters is to be assigned to codes in subcategory E11.35 to designate laterality of the disease:

1 - right eye

2 - left eye

3 - bilateral

9 - unspecified eye

⑦**E11.351**   Type 2 diabetes mellitus with proliferative diabetic retinopathy with macular edema

⑦**E11.352**   Type 2 diabetes mellitus with proliferative diabetic retinopathy with traction retinal detachment involving the macula

⑦**E11.353**   Type 2 diabetes mellitus with proliferative diabetic retinopathy with traction retinal detachment not involving the macula

⑦**E11.354**   Type 2 diabetes mellitus with proliferative diabetic retinopathy with combined traction retinal detachment and rhegmatogenous retinal detachment

⑦**E11.355**   Type 2 diabetes mellitus with stable proliferative diabetic retinopathy

⑦**E11.359**   Type 2 diabetes mellitus with proliferative diabetic retinopathy without macular edema

E11.36   Type 2 diabetes mellitus with diabetic cataract

⊗⑦**E11.37**   Type 2 diabetes mellitus with diabetic macular edema, resolved following treatment

One of the following 7th characters is to be assigned to code E11.37 to designate laterality of the disease:

1 - right eye

2 - left eye

3 - bilateral

9 - unspecified eye

E11.39   Type 2 diabetes mellitus with other diabetic ophthalmic complication

Use additional code to identify manifestation, such as: diabetic glaucoma (H40-H42)

E11.4   Type 2 diabetes mellitus with neurological complications

E11.40   Type 2 diabetes mellitus with diabetic neuropathy, unspecified

E11.41   Type 2 diabetes mellitus with diabetic mononeuropathy

E11.42   Type 2 diabetes mellitus with diabetic polyneuropathy

Type 2 diabetes mellitus with diabetic neuralgia

E11.43   Type 2 diabetes mellitus with diabetic autonomic (poly)neuropathy

Type 2 diabetes mellitus with diabetic gastroparesis

E11.44   Type 2 diabetes mellitus with diabetic amyotrophy

E11.49   Type 2 diabetes mellitus with other diabetic neurological complication

E11.5   Type 2 diabetes mellitus with circulatory complications

E11.51   Type 2 diabetes mellitus with diabetic peripheral angiopathy without gangrene

E11.52   Type 2 diabetes mellitus with diabetic peripheral angiopathy with gangrene

Type 2 diabetes mellitus with diabetic gangrene

E11.59   Type 2 diabetes mellitus with other circulatory complications

E11.6   Type 2 diabetes mellitus with other specified complications

E11.61   Type 2 diabetes mellitus with diabetic arthropathy

E11.610   Type 2 diabetes mellitus with diabetic neuropathic arthropathy

Type 2 diabetes mellitus with Charcôt's joints

E11.618   Type 2 diabetes mellitus with other diabetic arthropathy

E11.62   Type 2 diabetes mellitus with skin complications

E11.620   Type 2 diabetes mellitus with diabetic dermatitis

Type 2 diabetes mellitus with diabetic necrobiosis lipoidica

E11.621   Type 2 diabetes mellitus with foot ulcer

Use additional code to identify site of ulcer (L97.4-, L97.5-)

E11.622   Type 2 diabetes mellitus with other skin ulcer

Use additional code to identify site of ulcer (L97.1-L97.9, L98.41-L98.49)

E11.628   Type 2 diabetes mellitus with other skin complications

E11.63   Type 2 diabetes mellitus with oral complications

E11.630   Type 2 diabetes mellitus with periodontal disease

E11.638   Type 2 diabetes mellitus with other oral complications

E11.64   Type 2 diabetes mellitus with hypoglycemia

E11.641   Type 2 diabetes mellitus with hypoglycemia with coma

E11.649   Type 2 diabetes mellitus with hypoglycemia without coma

E11.65   Type 2 diabetes mellitus with hyperglycemia

E11.69   Type 2 diabetes mellitus with other specified complication

Use additional code to identify complication

E11.8   Type 2 diabetes mellitus with unspecified complications

E11.9   Type 2 diabetes mellitus without complications

E13   **Other specified diabetes mellitus**

Includes: diabetes mellitus due to genetic defects of beta-cell function

diabetes mellitus due to genetic defects in insulin action

postpancreatectomy diabetes mellitus

postprocedural diabetes mellitus secondary diabetes mellitus NEC

Use additional code to identify control using:

insulin (Z79.4)

oral antidiabetic drugs (Z79.84)

oral hypoglycemic drugs (Z79.84)

Excludes1: diabetes (mellitus) due to autoimmune process (E10.-)

diabetes (mellitus) due to immune mediated pancreatic islet beta-cell destruction (E10.-)

diabetes mellitus due to underlying condition (E08.-)

drug or chemical induced diabetes mellitus (E09.-)

gestational diabetes (O24.4-)

neonatal diabetes mellitus (P70.2)

type 1 diabetes mellitus (E10.-)

E13.0   Other specified diabetes mellitus with hyperosmolarity

E13.00   Other specified diabetes mellitus with hyperosmolarity without nonketotic hyperglycemic-hyperosmolar coma (NKHHC)

Excludes2: type 2 diabetes mellitus (E11.-)

E13.01   Other specified diabetes mellitus with hyperosmolarity with coma

E13.1   Other specified diabetes mellitus with ketoacidosis

E13.10   Other specified diabetes mellitus with ketoacidosis without coma

E13.11   Other specified diabetes mellitus with ketoacidosis with coma

E13.2   Other specified diabetes mellitus with kidney complications

E13.21   Other specified diabetes mellitus with diabetic nephropathy

Other specified diabetes mellitus with intercapillary glomerulosclerosis

Other specified diabetes mellitus with intracapillary glomerulonephrosis

Other specified diabetes mellitus with Kimmelstiel-Wilson disease

E13.22   Other specified diabetes mellitus with diabetic chronic kidney disease

Use additional code to identify stage of chronic kidney disease (N18.1-N18.6)

E13.29   Other specified diabetes mellitus with other diabetic kidney complication

Other specified diabetes mellitus with renal tubular degeneration

E13.3   Other specified diabetes mellitus with ophthalmic complications

E13.31   Other specified diabetes mellitus with unspecified diabetic retinopathy

E13.311   Other specified diabetes mellitus with unspecified diabetic retinopathy with macular edema

E13.319   Other specified diabetes mellitus with unspecified diabetic retinopathy without macular edema

E13.32   Other specified diabetes mellitus with mild nonproliferative diabetic retinopathy

Other specified diabetes mellitus with nonproliferative diabetic retinopathy NOS

One of the following 7th characters is to be assigned to codes in subcategory E13.32 to designate laterality of the disease:

1 - right eye

2 - left eye

3 - bilateral

9 - unspecified eye

⑦ **E13.321   Other specified diabetes mellitus with mild nonproliferative diabetic retinopathy with macular edema**

⑦ **E13.329   Other specified diabetes mellitus with mild nonproliferative diabetic retinopathy without macular edema**

E13.33   Other specified diabetes mellitus with moderate nonproliferative diabetic retinopathy

One of the following 7th characters is to be assigned to codes in subcategory E13.33 to designate laterality of the disease:

1 - right eye

2 - left eye

3 - bilateral

9 - unspecified eye

⑦ **E13.331   Other specified diabetes mellitus with moderate nonproliferative diabetic retinopathy with macular edema**

⑦ **E13.339   Other specified diabetes mellitus with moderate nonproliferative diabetic retinopathy without macular edema**

E13.34   Other specified diabetes mellitus with severe nonproliferative diabetic retinopathy

One of the following 7th characters is to be assigned to codes in subcategory E13.34 to designate laterality of the disease:

1 - right eye

2 - left eye

3 - bilateral

9 - unspecified eye

⑦ **E13.341   Other specified diabetes mellitus with severe nonproliferative diabetic retinopathy with macular edema**

⑦ **E13.349   Other specified diabetes mellitus with severe nonproliferative diabetic retinopathy without macular edema**

E13.35   Other specified diabetes mellitus with proliferative diabetic retinopathy

One of the following 7th characters is to be assigned to codes in subcategory E13.35 to designate laterality of the disease:

1 - right eye

2 - left eye

3 - bilateral

9 - unspecified eye

⑦ **E13.351   Other specified diabetes mellitus with proliferative diabetic retinopathy with macular edema**

⑦ **E13.352   Other specified diabetes mellitus with proliferative diabetic retinopathy with traction retinal detachment involving the macula**

⑦ **E13.353   Other specified diabetes mellitus with proliferative diabetic retinopathy with traction retinal detachment not involving the macula**

⑦ **E13.354   Other specified diabetes mellitus with proliferative diabetic retinopathy with combined traction retinal detachment and rhegmatogenous retinal detachment**

⑦**E13.355** Other specified diabetes mellitus with stable proliferative diabetic retinopathy

⑦**E13.359** Other specified diabetes mellitus with proliferative diabetic retinopathy without macular edema

E13.36 Other specified diabetes mellitus with diabetic cataract

⊗⑦**E13.37** Other specified diabetes mellitus with diabetic macular edema, resolved following treatment

One of the following 7th characters is to be assigned to code E13.37 to designate laterality of the disease:

1 - right eye

2 - left eye

3 - bilateral

9 - unspecified eye

E13.39 Other specified diabetes mellitus with other diabetic ophthalmic complication

Use additional code to identify manifestation, such as:

diabetic glaucoma (H40-H42)

E13.4 Other specified diabetes mellitus with neurological complications

E13.40 Other specified diabetes mellitus with diabetic neuropathy, unspecified

E13.41 Other specified diabetes mellitus with diabetic mononeuropathy

E13.42 Other specified diabetes mellitus with diabetic polyneuropathy

Other specified diabetes mellitus with diabetic neuralgia

E13.43 Other specified diabetes mellitus with diabetic autonomic (poly)neuropathy

Other specified diabetes mellitus with diabetic gastroparesis

E13.44 Other specified diabetes mellitus with diabetic amyotrophy

E13.49 Other specified diabetes mellitus with other diabetic neurological complication

E13.5 Other specified diabetes mellitus with circulatory complications

E13.51 Other specified diabetes mellitus with diabetic peripheral angiopathy without gangrene

E13.52 Other specified diabetes mellitus with diabetic peripheral angiopathy with gangrene

Other specified diabetes mellitus with diabetic gangrene

E13.59 Other specified diabetes mellitus with other circulatory complications

E13.6 Other specified diabetes mellitus with other specified complications

E13.61 Other specified diabetes mellitus with diabetic arthropathy

E13.610 Other specified diabetes mellitus with diabetic neuropathic arthropathy

Other specified diabetes mellitus with Charcôt's joints

E13.618 Other specified diabetes mellitus with other diabetic arthropathy

E13.62 Other specified diabetes mellitus with skin complications

E13.620 Other specified diabetes mellitus with diabetic dermatitis

Other specified diabetes mellitus with diabetic necrobiosis lipoidica

E13.621 Other specified diabetes mellitus with foot ulcer

Use additional code to identify site of ulcer (L97.4-, L97.5-)

E13.622 Other specified diabetes mellitus with other skin ulcer

Use additional code to identify site of ulcer (L97.1-L97.9, L98.41-L98.49)

E13.628 Other specified diabetes mellitus with other skin complications

E13.63 Other specified diabetes mellitus with oral complications

E13.630 Other specified diabetes mellitus with periodontal disease

E13.638 Other specified diabetes mellitus with other oral complications

E13.64 Other specified diabetes mellitus with hypoglycemia

E13.641 Other specified diabetes mellitus with hypoglycemia with coma

E13.649 Other specified diabetes mellitus with hypoglycemia without coma

E13.65 Other specified diabetes mellitus with hyperglycemia

E13.69 Other specified diabetes mellitus with other specified complication

Use additional code to identify complication

E13.8 Other specified diabetes mellitus with unspecified complications

E13.9 Other specified diabetes mellitus without complications

OTHER DISORDERS OF GLUCOSE REGULATION AND PANCREATIC INTERNAL SECRETION (E15-E16)

E15 Nondiabetic hypoglycemic coma

Includes: drug-induced insulin coma in nondiabetic

hyperinsulinism with hypoglycemic coma hypoglycemic coma NOS

E16 Other disorders of pancreatic internal secretion

E16.0 Drug-induced hypoglycemia without coma

Excludes1: diabetes with hypoglycemia without coma (E09.649)

Use additional code for adverse effect, if applicable, to identify drug (T36-T50 with fifth or sixth character 5)

E16.1 Other hypoglycemia

Functional hyperinsulinism

Functional nonhyperinsulinemic hypoglycemia

Hyperinsulinism NOS

Hyperplasia of pancreatic islet beta cells NOS

Excludes1: diabetes with hypoglycemia (E08.649, E10.649, E11.649, E13.649)

hypoglycemia in infant of diabetic mother (P70.1)

neonatal hypoglycemia (P70.4)

E16.2 Hypoglycemia, unspecified

Definition: Hypoglycemia is the medical term for abnormally low blood sugar usually resulting from excessive insulin or a poor diet.

Excludes1: diabetes with hypoglycemia (E08.649, E10.649, E11.649, E13.649)

E16.3 **Increased secretion of glucagon**

Hyperplasia of pancreatic endocrine cells with glucagon excess

E16.4 **Increased secretion of gastrin**

Hypergastrinemia

Hyperplasia of pancreatic endocrine cells with gastrin excess

Zollinger-Ellison syndrome

E16.8 **Other specified disorders of pancreatic internal secretion**

Increased secretion from endocrine pancreas of growth hormone-releasing hormone

Increased secretion from endocrine pancreas of pancreatic polypeptide

Increased secretion from endocrine pancreas of somatostatin

Increased secretion from endocrine pancreas of vasoactive-intestinal polypeptide

E16.9 **Disorder of pancreatic internal secretion, unspecified**

Islet-cell hyperplasia NOS

Pancreatic endocrine cell hyperplasia NOS

DISORDERS OF OTHER ENDOCRINE GLANDS (E20-E35)

Excludes1: galactorrhea (N64.3)

gynecomastia (N62)

E20 **Hypoparathyroidism**

Excludes1: Di George's syndrome (D82.1)

postprocedural hypoparathyroidism (E89.2)

tetany NOS (R29.0)

transitory neonatal hypoparathyroidism (P71.4)

E20.0 **Idiopathic hypoparathyroidism**

E20.1 **Pseudohypoparathyroidism**

E20.8 **Other hypoparathyroidism**

E20.9 **Hypoparathyroidism, unspecified**

Parathyroid tetany

E21 **Hyperparathyroidism and other disorders of parathyroid gland**

Excludes1: adult osteomalacia (M83.-)

ectopic hyperparathyroidism (E34.2)

familial hypocalciuric hypercalcemia (E83.52)

hungry bone syndrome (E83.81)

infantile and juvenile osteomalacia (E55.0)

E21.0 **Primary hyperparathyroidism**

Hyperplasia of parathyroid

Osteitis fibrosa cystica generalisata [von Recklinghausen's disease of bone]

E21.1 **Secondary hyperparathyroidism, not elsewhere classified**

Excludes1: secondary hyperparathyroidism of renal origin (N25.81)

E21.2 **Other hyperparathyroidism**

Tertiary hyperparathyroidism

Excludes1: familial hypocalciuric hypercalcemia (E83.52)

E21.3 **Hyperparathyroidism, unspecified**

E21.4 **Other specified disorders of parathyroid gland**

E21.5 **Disorder of parathyroid gland, unspecified**

E22 **Hyperfunction of pituitary gland**

Excludes1: Cushing's syndrome (E24.-)

Nelson's syndrome (E24.1)

overproduction of ACTH not associated with Cushing's disease (E27.0)

overproduction of pituitary ACTH (E24.0)

overproduction of thyroid-stimulating hormone (E05.8-)

E22.0 **Acromegaly and pituitary gigantism**

Overproduction of growth hormone

Excludes1: constitutional gigantism (E34.4)

constitutional tall stature (E34.4)

increased secretion from endocrine pancreas of growth hormone-releasing hormone (E16.8)

E22.1 **Hyperprolactinemia**

Use additional code for adverse effect, if applicable, to identify drug (T36-T50 with fifth or sixth character 5)

E22.2 **Syndrome of inappropriate secretion of antidiuretic hormone**

E22.8 **Other hyperfunction of pituitary gland**

Central precocious puberty

E22.9 **Hyperfunction of pituitary gland, unspecified**

E23 **Hypofunction and other disorders of the pituitary gland**

Includes: the listed conditions whether the disorder is in the pituitary or the hypothalamus

Excludes1: postprocedural hypopituitarism (E89.3)

E23.0 **Hypopituitarism**

Fertile eunuch syndrome

Hypogonadotropic hypogonadism

Idiopathic growth hormone deficiency

Isolated deficiency of gonadotropin

Isolated deficiency of growth hormone

Isolated deficiency of pituitary hormone

Kallmann's syndrome

Lorain-Levi short stature

Necrosis of pituitary gland (postpartum)

Panhypopituitarism

Pituitary cachexia

Pituitary insufficiency NOS

Pituitary short stature

Sheehan's syndrome

Simmonds' disease

E23.1 **Drug-induced hypopituitarism**

Use additional code for adverse effect, if applicable, to identify drug (T36-T50 with fifth or sixth character 5)

E23.2 **Diabetes insipidus**

Excludes1: nephrogenic diabetes insipidus (N25.1)

E23.3 **Hypothalamic dysfunction, not elsewhere classified**

Excludes1: Prader-Willi syndrome (Q87.1)

Russell-Silver syndrome (Q87.1)

E23.6 **Other disorders of pituitary gland**

Abscess of pituitary

Adiposogenital dystrophy

E23.7 **Disorder of pituitary gland, unspecified**

E24 **Cushing's syndrome**

Definition: Cushing's syndrome is a condition due to tumors of the adrenal cortex or the anterior lobe of the pituitary gland.

Excludes1: congenital adrenal hyperplasia (E25.0)

E24.0 **Pituitary-dependent Cushing's disease**

Overproduction of pituitary ACTH

Pituitary-dependent hypercorticalism

E24.1 **Nelson's syndrome**

E24.2 **Drug-induced Cushing's syndrome**

Use additional code for adverse effect, if applicable, to identify drug (T36-T50 with fifth or sixth character 5)

E24.3 **Ectopic ACTH syndrome**

E24.4   Alcohol-induced pseudo-Cushing's syndrome

E24.8   Other Cushing's syndrome

E24.9   Cushing's syndrome, unspecified

E25   **Adrenogenital disorders**

Includes: adrenogenital syndromes, virilizing or feminizing, whether acquired or due to adrenal hyperplasia consequent on inborn enzyme defects in hormone synthesis

Female adrenal pseudohermaphroditism

Female heterosexual precocious pseudopuberty

Male isosexual precocious pseudopuberty

Male macrogenitosomia praecox

Male sexual precocity with adrenal hyperplasia

Male virilization (female)

Excludes1: indeterminate sex and pseudohermaphroditism (Q56)

chromosomal abnormalities (Q90-Q99)

E25.0   **Congenital adrenogenital disorders associated with enzyme deficiency**

Congenital adrenal hyperplasia 21-Hydroxylase deficiency

Salt-losing congenital adrenal hyperplasia

E25.8   **Other adrenogenital disorders**

Idiopathic adrenogenital disorder

Use additional code for adverse effect, if applicable, to identify drug (T36-T50 with fifth or sixth character 5)

E25.9   **Adrenogenital disorder, unspecified**

Adrenogenital syndrome NOS

E26   **Hyperaldosteronism**

E26.0   **Primary hyperaldosteronism**

    E26.01   **Conn's syndrome**

       Code also adrenal adenoma (D35.0-)

    E26.02   **Glucocorticoid-remediable aldosteronism**

       Familial aldosteronism type I

    E26.09   **Other primary hyperaldosteronism**

       Primary aldosteronism due to adrenal hyperplasia (bilateral)

E26.1   **Secondary hyperaldosteronism**

E26.8   **Other hyperaldosteronism**

    E26.81   **Bartter's syndrome**

    E26.89   **Other hyperaldosteronism**

E26.9   **Hyperaldosteronism, unspecified**

Aldosteronism NOS

Hyperaldosteronism NOS

E27   **Other disorders of adrenal gland**

E27.0   **Other adrenocortical overactivity**

Overproduction of ACTH, not associated with Cushing's disease

Premature adrenarche

Excludes1: Cushing's syndrome (E24.-)

E27.1   **Primary adrenocortical insufficiency**

Addison's disease

Autoimmune adrenalitis

Excludes1: Addison only phenotype adrenoleukodystrophy (E71.528)

amyloidosis (E85.-)

tuberculous Addison's disease (A18.7)

Waterhouse-Friderichsen syndrome (A39.1)

E27.2   **Addisonian crisis**

Adrenal crisis

Adrenocortical crisis

E27.3   **Drug-induced adrenocortical insufficiency**

Use additional code for adverse effect, if applicable, to identify drug (T36-T50 with fifth or sixth character 5)

E27.4   **Other and unspecified adrenocortical insufficiency**

Excludes1: adrenoleukodystrophy [Addison-Schilder] (E71.528)

Waterhouse-Friderichsen syndrome (A39.1)

    E27.40   **Unspecified adrenocortical insufficiency**

       Adrenocortical insufficiency NOS

       Hypoaldosteronism

    E27.49   **Other adrenocortical insufficiency**

       Adrenal hemorrhage

       Adrenal infarction

E27.5   **Adrenomedullary hyperfunction**

Adrenomedullary hyperplasia

Catecholamine hypersecretion

E27.8   **Other specified disorders of adrenal gland**

Abnormality of cortisol-binding globulin

E27.9   **Disorder of adrenal gland, unspecified**

E28   **Ovarian dysfunction**

Excludes1: isolated gonadotropin deficiency (E23.0)

postprocedural ovarian failure (E89.4-)

E28.0   **Estrogen excess**

Use additional code for adverse effect, if applicable, to identify drug (T36-T50 with fifth or sixth character 5)

E28.1   **Androgen excess**

Hypersecretion of ovarian androgens

Use additional code for adverse effect, if applicable, to identify drug (T36-T50 with fifth or sixth character 5)

E28.2   **Polycystic ovarian syndrome**

Sclerocystic ovary syndrome

Stein-Leventhal syndrome

E28.3   **Primary ovarian failure**

Excludes1: pure gonadal dysgenesis (Q99.1)

Turner's syndrome (Q96.-)

    E28.31   **Premature menopause**

       E28.310   **Symptomatic premature menopause**

          Symptoms such as flushing, sleeplessness, headache, lack of concentration, associated with premature menopause

       E28.319   **Asymptomatic premature menopause**

          Premature menopause NOS

    E28.39   **Other primary ovarian failure**

       Decreased estrogen

       Resistant ovary syndrome

E28.8   **Other ovarian dysfunction**

Ovarian hyperfunction NOS

Excludes1: postprocedural ovarian failure (E89.4-)

E28.9   **Ovarian dysfunction, unspecified**

E29   **Testicular dysfunction**

Excludes1: androgen insensitivity syndrome (E34.5-)

azoospermia or oligospermia NOS (N46.0-N46.1)

isolated gonadotropin deficiency (E23.0)

Klinefelter's syndrome (Q98.0-Q98.1, Q98.4)

E29.0   **Testicular hyperfunction**

Hypersecretion of testicular hormones

E29.1 Testicular hypofunction

Defective biosynthesis of testicular androgen NOS

5-delta-Reductase deficiency (with male pseudohermaphroditism)

Testicular hypogonadism NOS

<u>Use additional code</u> for adverse effect, if applicable, to identify drug (T36-T50 with fifth or sixth character 5)

Excludes1: postprocedural testicular hypofunction (E89.5)

E29.8 Other testicular dysfunction

E29.9 Testicular dysfunction, unspecified

E30 Disorders of puberty, not elsewhere classified

E30.0 Delayed puberty

Constitutional delay of puberty

Delayed sexual development

E30.1 Precocious puberty

Precocious menstruation

Excludes1: Albright (-McCune) (-Sternberg) syndrome (Q78.1)

central precocious puberty (E22.8)

congenital adrenal hyperplasia (E25.0)

female heterosexual precocious pseudopuberty (E25.-)

male isosexual precocious pseudopuberty (E25.-)

E30.8 Other disorders of puberty

Premature thelarche

E30.9 Disorder of puberty, unspecified

E31 Polyglandular dysfunction

Excludes1: ataxia telangiectasia [Louis-Bar] (G11.3)

dystrophia myotonica [Steinert] (G71.11)

pseudohypoparathyroidism (E20.1)

E31.0 Autoimmune polyglandular failure

Schmidt's syndrome

E31.1 Polyglandular hyperfunction

Excludes1: multiple endocrine adenomatosis (E31.2-)

multiple endocrine neoplasia (E31.2-)

E31.2 Multiple endocrine neoplasia [MEN] syndromes

Multiple endocrine adenomatosis

Code also any associated malignancies **and other** conditions associated with the syndromes

E31.20 Multiple endocrine neoplasia [MEN] syndrome, unspecified

Multiple endocrine adenomatosis NOS

Multiple endocrine neoplasia [MEN] syndrome NOS

E31.21 Multiple endocrine neoplasia [MEN] type I

Wermer's syndrome

E31.22 Multiple endocrine neoplasia [MEN] type IIA

Sipple's syndrome

E31.23 Multiple endocrine neoplasia [MEN] type IIB

E31.8 Other polyglandular dysfunction

E31.9 Polyglandular dysfunction, unspecified

E32 Diseases of thymus

Definition: The thymus is a gland located behind the breastbone that functions in the development of the immune system. The thymus is large in infancy and early childhood but begins to atrophy between ages eight and ten.

Excludes1: aplasia or hypoplasia of thymus with immunodeficiency (D82.1)

E32.0 Persistent hyperplasia of thymus

Hypertrophy of thymus

E32.1 Abscess of thymus

E32.8 Other diseases of thymus

Excludes1: aplasia or hypoplasia with immunodeficiency (D82.1)

thymoma (D15.0)

E32.9 Disease of thymus, unspecified

E34 Other endocrine disorders

Definition: Endocrine disorders refers to disorders which involve the over-production or under-production of hormone substances from an endocrine gland. Examples include diabetes, hypothyroidism, hyperthyroidism, hyperparathyroidism, Cushing's disease, Cushing's syndrome and acromegaly.

Excludes1: pseudohypoparathyroidism (E20.1)

E34.0 Carcinoid syndrome

Note: May be used as an additional code to identify functional activity associated with a carcinoid tumor.

E34.1 Other hypersecretion of intestinal hormones

E34.2 Ectopic hormone secretion, not elsewhere classified

Excludes1: ectopic ACTH syndrome (E24.3)

E34.3 Short stature due to endocrine disorder

Constitutional short stature

Laron-type short stature

Excludes1: achondroplastic short stature (Q77.4)

hypochondroplastic short stature (Q77.4)

nutritional short stature (E45)

pituitary short stature (E23.0)

progeria (E34.8)

renal short stature (N25.0)

Russell-Silver syndrome (Q87.1)

short-limbed stature with immunodeficiency (D82.2)

short stature in specific dysmorphic syndromes - code to syndrome - see Alphabetical Index short stature NOS (R62.52)

E34.4 Constitutional tall stature

Constitutional gigantism

E34.5 Androgen insensitivity syndrome

E34.50 Androgen insensitivity syndrome, unspecified

Androgen insensitivity NOS

E34.51 Complete androgen insensitivity syndrome

Complete androgen insensitivity de Quervain syndrome

Goldberg-Maxwell syndrome

E34.52 Partial androgen insensitivity syndrome

Partial androgen insensitivity

Reifenstein syndrome

E34.8 Other specified endocrine disorders

Pineal gland dysfunction

Progeria

Excludes2: pseudohypoparathyroidism (E20.1)

E34.9 Endocrine disorder, unspecified

Endocrine disturbance NOS

Hormone disturbance NOS

E35 Disorders of endocrine glands in diseases classified elsewhere

Code first underlying disease, such as:

late congenital syphilis of thymus gland [Dubois disease] (A50.5)

Use additional code , if applicable, to identify:

sequelae of tuberculosis **of other** organs (B90.8)

> **Excludes1:** Echinococcus granulosus infection of thyroid gland (B67.3)
>
> meningococcal hemorrhagic adrenalitis (A39.1)
>
> syphilis of endocrine gland (A52.79)
>
> tuberculosis of adrenal gland, except calcification (A18.7)
>
> tuberculosis of endocrine gland NEC (A18.82)
>
> tuberculosis of thyroid gland (A18.81)
>
> Waterhouse-Friderichsen syndrome (A39.1)

INTRAOPERATIVE COMPLICATIONS OF ENDOCRINE SYSTEM (E36)

E36 **Intraoperative complications of endocrine system**

> **Excludes2:** postprocedural endocrine and metabolic complications and disorders, not elsewhere classified (E89.-)

E36.0 **Intraoperative hemorrhage and hematoma of an endocrine system organ or structure complicating a procedure**

> **Excludes1:** intraoperative hemorrhage and hematoma of an endocrine system organ or structure due to accidental puncture or laceration during a procedure (E36.1-)

E36.01 **Intraoperative hemorrhage and hematoma of an endocrine system organ or structure complicating an endocrine system procedure**

E36.02 **Intraoperative hemorrhage and hematoma of an endocrine system organ or structure complicating other procedure**

E36.1 **Accidental puncture and laceration of an endocrine system organ or structure during a procedure**

E36.11 **Accidental puncture and laceration of an endocrine system organ or structure during an endocrine system procedure**

E36.12 **Accidental puncture and laceration of an endocrine system organ or structure during other procedure**

E36.8 **Other intraoperative complications of endocrine system**

> **Use additional code**, if applicable, to further specify disorder

MALNUTRITION (E40-E46)

Excludes1: intestinal malabsorption (K90.-)

sequelae of protein-calorie malnutrition (E64.0)

Excludes2: nutritional anemias (D50-D53)

starvation (T73.0)

E40 **Kwashiorkor**

Severe malnutrition with nutritional edema with dyspigmentation of skin and hair

> **Excludes1:** marasmic kwashiorkor (E42)

E41 **Nutritional marasmus**

Severe malnutrition with marasmus

> **Excludes1:** marasmic kwashiorkor (E42)

E42 **Marasmic kwashiorkor**

Intermediate form severe protein-calorie malnutrition

Severe protein-calorie malnutrition with signs of both kwashiorkor and marasmus

E43 **Unspecified severe protein-calorie malnutrition**

Starvation edema

E44 **Protein-calorie malnutrition of moderate and mild degree**

E44.0 **Moderate protein-calorie malnutrition**

E44.1 **Mild protein-calorie malnutrition**

E45 **Retarded development following protein-calorie malnutrition**

Nutritional short stature

Nutritional stunting

Physical retardation due to malnutrition

E46 **Unspecified protein-calorie malnutrition**

Malnutrition NOS

Protein-calorie imbalance NOS

> **Excludes1:** nutritional deficiency NOS (E63.9)

OTHER NUTRITIONAL DEFICIENCIES (E50-E64)

Excludes2: nutritional anemias (D50-D53)

E50 **Vitamin A deficiency**

> **Definition:** Vitamin A deficiency (VAD) occurs where diets contain insufficient vitamin A for meeting the needs associated with growth and development, physiological functions, and periods of added stress due to illness.

> **Excludes1:** sequelae of vitamin A deficiency (E64.1)

E50.0 **Vitamin A deficiency with conjunctival xerosis**

E50.1 **Vitamin A deficiency with Bitot's spot and conjunctival xerosis**

Bitot's spot in the young child

E50.2 **Vitamin A deficiency with corneal xerosis**

E50.3 **Vitamin A deficiency with corneal ulceration and xerosis**

E50.4 **Vitamin A deficiency with keratomalacia**

E50.5 **Vitamin A deficiency with night blindness**

E50.6 **Vitamin A deficiency with xerophthalmic scars of cornea**

E50.7 **Other ocular manifestations of vitamin A deficiency**

Xerophthalmia NOS

E50.8 **Other manifestations of vitamin A deficiency**

Follicular keratosis Xeroderma

E50.9 **Vitamin A deficiency, unspecified**

Hypovitaminosis A NOS

E51 **Thiamine deficiency**

> **Excludes1:** sequelae of thiamine deficiency (E64.8)

E51.1 **Beriberi**

E51.11 **Dry beriberi**

Beriberi NOS

Beriberi with polyneuropathy

E51.12 **Wet beriberi**

Beriberi with cardiovascular manifestations

Cardiovascular beriberi

Shoshin disease

E51.2 **Wernicke's encephalopathy**

E51.8 **Other manifestations of thiamine deficiency**

E51.9 **Thiamine deficiency, unspecified**

E52 **Niacin deficiency [pellagra]**

Niacin (-tryptophan) deficiency

Nicotinamide deficiency

Pellagra (alcoholic)

> **Excludes1:** sequelae of niacin deficiency (E64.8)

E53 **Deficiency of other B group vitamins**

> **Excludes1:** sequelae of vitamin B deficiency (E64.8)

E53.0 **Riboflavin deficiency**

Ariboflavinosis

Vitamin B2 deficiency

E53.1 Pyridoxine deficiency

Vitamin B6 deficiency

Excludes1: pyridoxine-responsive sideroblastic anemia (D64.3)

E53.8 Deficiency of other specified B group vitamins

Biotin deficiency

Cyanocobalamin deficiency

Folate deficiency

Folic acid deficiency

Pantothenic acid deficiency

Vitamin B12 deficiency

Excludes1: folate deficiency anemia (D52.-)

vitamin B12 deficiency anemia (D51.-)

E53.9 Vitamin B deficiency, unspecified

E54 Ascorbic acid deficiency

Deficiency of vitamin C

Scurvy

Excludes1: scorbutic anemia (D53.2)

sequelae of vitamin C deficiency (E64.2)

E55 Vitamin D deficiency

Excludes1: adult osteomalacia (M83.-)

osteoporosis (M80.-)

sequelae of rickets (E64.3)

E55.0 Rickets, active

Infantile osteomalacia Juvenile osteomalacia

Excludes1: celiac rickets (K90.0)

Crohn's rickets (K50.-)

hereditary vitamin D-dependent rickets (E83.32)

inactive rickets (E64.3)

renal rickets (N25.0)

sequelae of rickets (E64.3)

vitamin D-resistant rickets (E83.31)

E55.9 Vitamin D deficiency, unspecified

Avitaminosis D

E56 Other vitamin deficiencies

Excludes1: sequelae of other vitamin deficiencies (E64.8)

E56.0 Deficiency of vitamin E

E56.1 Deficiency of vitamin K

Excludes1: deficiency of coagulation factor due to vitamin K deficiency (D68.4)

vitamin K deficiency of newborn (P53)

E56.8 Deficiency of other vitamins

E56.9 Vitamin deficiency, unspecified

E58 Dietary calcium deficiency

Excludes1: disorders of calcium metabolism (E83.5-)

sequelae of calcium deficiency (E64.8)

E59 Dietary selenium deficiency

Keshan disease

Excludes1: sequelae of selenium deficiency (E64.8)

E60 Dietary zinc deficiency

E61 Deficiency of other nutrient elements

Use additional code for adverse effect, if applicable, to identify drug (T36-T50 with fifth or sixth character 5)

Excludes1: disorders of mineral metabolism (E83.-)

iodine deficiency related thyroid disorders (E00-E02)

sequelae of malnutrition and other nutritional deficiencies (E64.-)

E61.0 Copper deficiency

E61.1 Iron deficiency

Excludes1: iron deficiency anemia (D50.-)

E61.2 Magnesium deficiency

E61.3 Manganese deficiency

E61.4 Chromium deficiency

E61.5 Molybdenum deficiency

E61.6 Vanadium deficiency

E61.7 Deficiency of multiple nutrient elements

E61.8 Deficiency of other specified nutrient elements

E61.9 Deficiency of nutrient element, unspecified

E63 Other nutritional deficiencies

Excludes1: dehydration (E86.0)

failure to thrive, adult (R62.7)

failure to thrive, child (R62.51)

feeding problems in newborn (P92.-)

sequelae of malnutrition and other nutritional deficiencies (E64.-)

E63.0 Essential fatty acid [EFA] deficiency

E63.1 Imbalance of constituents of food intake

E63.8 Other specified nutritional deficiencies

E63.9 Nutritional deficiency, unspecified

E64 Sequelae of malnutrition and other nutritional deficiencies

Note: This category is to be used to indicate conditions in categories E43, E44, E46, E50-E63 as the cause of sequelae, which are themselves classified elsewhere. The 'sequelae' include conditions specified as such; they also include the late effects of diseases classifiable to the above categories if the disease itself is no longer present

Code first condition resulting from (sequela) of malnutrition and other nutritional deficiencies

E64.0 Sequelae of protein-calorie malnutrition

Excludes2: retarded development following protein-calorie malnutrition (E45)

E64.1 Sequelae of vitamin A deficiency

E64.2 Sequelae of vitamin C deficiency

E64.3 Sequelae of rickets

E64.8 Sequelae of other nutritional deficiencies

E64.9 Sequelae of unspecified nutritional deficiency

OVERWEIGHT, OBESITY AND OTHER HYPERALIMENTATION (E65-E68)

E65 Localized adiposity

Fat pad

E66 Overweight and obesity

Code first obesity complicating pregnancy, childbirth and the puerperium, if applicable (O99.21-)

Use additional code to identify body mass index (BMI), if known (Z68.-)

Excludes1: adiposogenital dystrophy (E23.6)

lipomatosis NOS (E88.2)

lipomatosis dolorosa [Dercum] (E88.2)

Prader-Willi syndrome (Q87.1)

E66.0 Obesity due to excess calories

E66.01 Morbid (severe) obesity due to excess calories

Excludes1: morbid (severe) obesity with alveolar hypoventilation (E66.2)

E66.09 Other obesity due to excess calories

E66.1 Drug-induced obesity

Use additional code for adverse effect, if applicable, to identify drug (T36-T50 with fifth or sixth character 5)

E66.2 **Morbid (severe) obesity with alveolar hypoventilation**

Obesity hypoventilation syndrome (OHS)

Pickwickian syndrome

E66.3 **Overweight**

E66.8 **Other obesity**

E66.9 **Obesity, unspecified**

Obesity NOS

E67 **Other hyperalimentation**

Excludes1: hyperalimentation NOS (R63.2)

sequelae of hyperalimentation (E68)

E67.0 **Hypervitaminosis A**

E67.1 **Hypercarotenemia**

E67.2 **Megavitamin-B6 syndrome**

E67.3 **Hypervitaminosis D**

E67.8 **Other specified hyperalimentation**

E68 **Sequelae of hyperalimentation**

Code first condition resulting from (sequela) of hyperalimentation

METABOLIC DISORDERS (E70-E88)

Excludes1: androgen insensitivity syndrome (E34.5-)

congenital adrenal hyperplasia (E25.0)

Ehlers-Danlos syndrome (Q79.6)

hemolytic anemias attributable to enzyme disorders (D55.-)

Marfan's syndrome (Q87.4)

5-alpha-reductase deficiency (E29.1)

E70 **Disorders of aromatic amino-acid metabolism**

E70.0 **Classical phenylketonuria**

E70.1 **Other hyperphenylalaninemias**

E70.2 **Disorders of tyrosine metabolism**

Excludes1: transitory tyrosinemia of newborn (P74.5)

E70.20 **Disorder of tyrosine metabolism, unspecified**

E70.21 **Tyrosinemia**

Hypertyrosinemia

E70.29 **Other disorders of tyrosine metabolism**

Alkaptonuria

Ochronosis

E70.3 **Albinism**

E70.30 **Albinism, unspecified**

E70.31 **Ocular albinism**

E70.310 **X-linked ocular albinism**

E70.311 **Autosomal recessive ocular albinism**

E70.318 **Other ocular albinism**

E70.319 **Ocular albinism, unspecified**

E70.32 **Oculocutaneous albinism**

Excludes1: Chediak-Higashi syndrome (E70.330)

Hermansky-Pudlak syndrome (E70.331)

E70.320 **Tyrosinase negative oculocutaneous albinism**

Albinism I

Oculocutaneous albinism ty-neg

E70.321 **Tyrosinase positive oculocutaneous albinism**

Albinism II

Oculocutaneous albinism ty-pos

E70.328 **Other oculocutaneous albinism**

Cross syndrome

E70.329 **Oculocutaneous albinism, unspecified**

E70.33 **Albinism with hematologic abnormality**

E70.330 **Chediak-Higashi syndrome**

E70.331 **Hermansky-Pudlak syndrome**

E70.338 **Other albinism with hematologic abnormality**

E70.339 **Albinism with hematologic abnormality, unspecified**

E70.39 **Other specified albinism**

Piebaldism

E70.4 **Disorders of histidine metabolism**

E70.40 Disorders of histidine metabolism, unspecified

E70.41 **Histidinemia**

E70.49 **Other disorders of histidine metabolism**

E70.5 **Disorders of tryptophan metabolism**

E70.8 **Other disorders of aromatic amino-acid metabolism**

E70.9 **Disorder of aromatic amino-acid metabolism, unspecified**

E71 **Disorders of branched-chain amino-acid metabolism and fatty-acid metabolism**

E71.0 **Maple-syrup-urine disease**

E71.1 **Other disorders of branched-chain amino-acid metabolism**

E71.11 **Branched-chain organic acidurias**

E71.110 **Isovaleric acidemia**

E71.111 **3-methylglutaconic aciduria**

E71.118 **Other branched-chain organic acidurias**

E71.12 **Disorders of propionate metabolism**

E71.120 **Methylmalonic acidemia**

E71.121 **Propionic acidemia**

E71.128 **Other disorders of propionate metabolism**

E71.19 **Other disorders of branched-chain amino-acid metabolism**

Hyperleucine-isoleucinemia

Hypervalinemia

E71.2 **Disorder of branched-chain amino-acid metabolism, unspecified**

E71.3 **Disorders of fatty-acid metabolism**

Excludes1: peroxisomal disorders (E71.5)

Refsum's disease (G60.1)

Schilder's disease (G37.0)

Excludes2: carnitine deficiency due to inborn error of metabolism (E71.42)

E71.30 **Disorder of fatty-acid metabolism, unspecified**

E71.31 **Disorders of fatty-acid oxidation**

E71.310 **Long chain/very long chain acyl CoA dehydrogenase deficiency**

LCAD

VLCAD

E71.311 **Medium chain acyl CoA dehydrogenase deficiency**

MCAD

E71.312 **Short chain acyl CoA dehydrogenase deficiency**

SCAD

| | Add 4th-7th digits | | Nonspecific code | | Unspecified code | | Manifestation code | 243 |

E71.313 Glutaric aciduria type II

Glutaric aciduria type II A

Glutaric aciduria type II B

Glutaric aciduria type II C

Excludes1: glutaric aciduria (type 1) NOS (E72.3)

E71.314 Muscle carnitine palmitoyltransferase deficiency

E71.318 Other disorders of fatty-acid oxidation

E71.32 Disorders of ketone metabolism

E71.39 Other disorders of fatty-acid metabolism

E71.4 Disorders of carnitine metabolism

Excludes1: Muscle carnitine palmitoyltransferase deficiency (E71.314)

E71.40 Disorder of carnitine metabolism, unspecified

E71.41 Primary carnitine deficiency

E71.42 Carnitine deficiency due to inborn errors of metabolism

Code also associated inborn error or metabolism

E71.43 Iatrogenic carnitine deficiency

Carnitine deficiency due to hemodialysis

Carnitine deficiency due to Valproic acid therapy

E71.44 Other secondary carnitine deficiency

E71.440 Ruvalcaba-Myhre-Smith syndrome

E71.448 Other secondary carnitine deficiency

E71.5 Peroxisomal disorders

Excludes1: Schilder's disease (G37.0)

E71.50 Peroxisomal disorder, unspecified

E71.51 Disorders of peroxisome biogenesis

Group 1 peroxisomal disorders

Excludes1: Refsum's disease (G60.1)

E71.510 Zellweger syndrome

E71.511 Neonatal adrenoleukodystrophy

Excludes1: X-linked adrenoleukodystrophy (E71.42-)

E71.518 Other disorders of peroxisome biogenesis

E71.52 X-linked adrenoleukodystrophy

E71.520 Childhood cerebral X-linked adrenoleukodystrophy

E71.521 Adolescent X-linked adrenoleukodystrophy

E71.522 Adrenomyeloneuropathy

E71.528 Other X-linked adrenoleukodystrophy

Addison only phenotype adrenoleukodystrophy

Addison-Schilder adrenoleukodystrophy

E71.529 X-linked adrenoleukodystrophy, unspecified type

E71.53 Other group 2 peroxisomal disorders

E71.54 Other peroxisomal disorders

E71.540 Rhizomelic chondrodysplasia punctata

Excludes1: chondrodysplasia punctata NOS (Q77.3)

E71.541 Zellweger-like syndrome

E71.542 Other group 3 peroxisomal disorders

E71.548 Other peroxisomal disorders

E72 Other disorders of amino-acid metabolism

Excludes1: disorders of:

aromatic amino-acid metabolism (E70.-)

branched-chain amino-acid metabolism (E71.0-E71.2)

fatty-acid metabolism (E71.3)

purine and pyrimidine metabolism (E79.-)

gout (M1A.-, M10.-)

E72.0 Disorders of amino-acid transport

Excludes1: disorders of tryptophan metabolism (E70.5)

E72.00 Disorders of amino-acid transport, unspecified

E72.01 Cystinuria

E72.02 Hartnup's disease

E72.03 Lowe's syndrome

Use additional code for associated glaucoma (H42)

E72.04 Cystinosis

Fanconi (-de Toni) (-Debré) syndrome with cystinosis

Excludes1: Fanconi (-de Toni) (-Debré) syndrome without cystinosis (E72.09)

E72.09 Other disorders of amino-acid transport

Fanconi (-de Toni) (-Debré) syndrome, unspecified

E72.1 Disorders of sulfur-bearing amino-acid metabolism

Excludes1: cystinosis (E72.04)

cystinuria (E72.01)

transcobalamin II deficiency (D51.2)

E72.10 Disorders of sulfur-bearing amino-acid metabolism, unspecified

E72.11 Homocystinuria

Cystathionine synthase deficiency

E72.12 Methylenetetrahydrofolate reductase deficiency

E72.19 Other disorders of sulfur-bearing amino-acid metabolism

Cystathioninuria

Methioninemia

Sulfite oxidase deficiency

E72.2 Disorders of urea cycle metabolism

Excludes1: disorders of ornithine metabolism (E72.4)

E72.20 Disorder of urea cycle metabolism, unspecified

Hyperammonemia

Excludes1: hyperammonemia-hyperornithinemia-homocitrullinemia syndrome E72.4

transient hyperammonemia of newborn (P74.6)

E72.21 Argininemia

E72.22 Arginosuccinic aciduria

E72.23 Citrullinemia

E72.29 Other disorders of urea cycle metabolism

E72.3 Disorders of lysine and hydroxylysine metabolism

Glutaric aciduria NOS Glutaric aciduria (type I)

Hydroxylysinemia

Hyperlysinemia

Excludes1: glutaric aciduria type II (E71.313)

Refsum's disease (G60.1)

Zellweger syndrome (E71.510)

● New code ▲ Revised code **Excludes1:** Not coded here **Excludes2:** Not included here ⊗ Placeholder required ⑦ 7th digit required

E72.4 **Disorders of ornithine metabolism**

Hyperammonemia-Hyperornithinemia-Homocitrullinemia syndrome

Ornithinemia (types I, II)

Ornithine transcarbamylase deficiency

Excludes1: hereditary choroidal dystrophy (H31.2-)

E72.5 **Disorders of glycine metabolism**

E72.50 **Disorder of glycine metabolism, unspecified**

E72.51 **Non-ketotic hyperglycinemia**

E72.52 **Trimethylaminuria**

E72.53 **Hyperoxaluria**

Oxalosis

Oxaluria

E72.59 **Other disorders of glycine metabolism**

D-glycericacidemia

Hyperhydroxyprolinemia

Hyperprolinemia (types I, II)

Sarcosinemia

E72.8 **Other specified disorders of amino-acid metabolism**

Disorders of beta-amino-acid metabolism

Disorders of gamma-glutamyl cycle

E72.9 **Disorder of amino-acid metabolism, unspecified**

E73 **Lactose intolerance**

E73.0 **Congenital lactase deficiency**

E73.1 **Secondary lactase deficiency**

E73.8 **Other lactose intolerance**

E73.9 **Lactose intolerance, unspecified**

E74 **Other disorders of carbohydrate metabolism**

Excludes1: diabetes mellitus (E08-E13)

hypoglycemia NOS (E16.2)

increased secretion of glucagon (E16.3)

mucopolysaccharidosis (E76.0-E76.3)

E74.0 **Glycogen storage disease**

E74.00 **Glycogen storage disease, unspecified**

E74.01 **von Gierke disease**

Type I glycogen storage disease

E74.02 **Pompe disease**

Cardiac glycogenosis

Type II glycogen storage disease

E74.03 **Cori disease**

Forbes disease

Type III glycogen storage disease

E74.04 **McArdle disease**

Type V glycogen storage disease

E74.09 **Other glycogen storage disease**

Andersen disease

Hers disease

Tarui disease

Glycogen storage disease, types 0, IV, VI-XI

Liver phosphorylase deficiency

Muscle phosphofructokinase deficiency

E74.1 **Disorders of fructose metabolism**

Excludes1: muscle phosphofructokinase deficiency (E74.09)

E74.10 **Disorder of fructose metabolism, unspecified**

E74.11 **Essential fructosuria**

Fructokinase deficiency

E74.12 **Hereditary fructose intolerance**

Fructosemia

E74.19 **Other disorders of fructose metabolism**

Fructose-1, 6-diphosphatase deficiency

E74.2 **Disorders of galactose metabolism**

E74.20 **Disorders of galactose metabolism, unspecified**

E74.21 **Galactosemia**

E74.29 **Other disorders of galactose metabolism**

Galactokinase deficiency

E74.3 **Other disorders of intestinal carbohydrate absorption**

Excludes2: lactose intolerance (E73.-)

E74.31 **Sucrase-isomaltase deficiency**

E74.39 **Other disorders of intestinal carbohydrate absorption**

Disorder of intestinal carbohydrate absorption NOS

Glucose-galactose malabsorption

Sucrase deficiency

E74.4 **Disorders of pyruvate metabolism and gluconeogenesis**

Deficiency of phosphoenolpyruvate carboxykinase

Deficiency of pyruvate carboxylase

Deficiency of pyruvate dehydrogenase

Excludes1: disorders of pyruvate metabolism and gluconeogenesis with anemia (D55.-)

Leigh's syndrome (G31.82)

E74.8 **Other specified disorders of carbohydrate metabolism**

Essential pentosuria

Renal glycosuria

E74.9 **Disorder of carbohydrate metabolism, unspecified**

E75 **Disorders of sphingolipid metabolism and other lipid storage disorders**

Excludes1: mucolipidosis, types I-III (E77.0-E77.1)

Refsum's disease (G60.1)

E75.0 **GM2 gangliosidosis**

E75.00 **GM2 gangliosidosis, unspecified**

E75.01 **Sandhoff disease**

E75.02 **Tay-Sachs disease**

E75.09 **Other GM2 gangliosidosis**

Adult GM2 gangliosidosis

Juvenile GM2 gangliosidosis

E75.1 **Other and unspecified gangliosidosis**

E75.10 **Unspecified gangliosidosis**

Gangliosidosis NOS

E75.11 **Mucolipidosis IV**

E75.19 **Other gangliosidosis**

GM1 gangliosidosis

GM3 gangliosidosis

E75.2 **Other sphingolipidosis**

Excludes1: adrenoleukodystrophy [Addison-Schilder] (E71.528)

E75.21 **Fabry (-Anderson) disease**

E75.22 **Gaucher disease**

E75.23 **Krabbe disease**

E75.24 **Niemann-Pick disease**

E75.240 **Niemann-Pick disease type A**

E75.241 **Niemann-Pick disease type B**

E75.242 **Niemann-Pick disease type C**

E75.243 **Niemann-Pick disease type D**

E75.248 **Other Niemann-Pick disease**

E75.249 Niemann-Pick disease, unspecified

E75.25 **Metachromatic leukodystrophy**

E75.29 **Other sphingolipidosis**

Farber's syndrome

Sulfatase deficiency

Sulfatide lipidosis

E75.3 **Sphingolipidosis, unspecified**

E75.4 **Neuronal ceroid lipofuscinosis**

Batten disease

Bielschowsky-Jansky disease

Kufs disease

Spielmeyer-Vogt disease

E75.5 **Other lipid storage disorders**

Cerebrotendinous cholesterosis [van Bogaert-Scherer-Epstein]

Wolman's disease

E75.6 **Lipid storage disorder, unspecified**

E76 **Disorders of glycosaminoglycan metabolism**

E76.0 **Mucopolysaccharidosis, type I**

E76.01 **Hurler's syndrome**

E76.02 **Hurler-Scheie syndrome**

E76.03 **Scheie's syndrome**

E76.1 **Mucopolysaccharidosis, type II**

Hunter's syndrome

E76.2 **Other mucopolysaccharidoses**

E76.21 **Morquio mucopolysaccharidoses**

E76.210 **Morquio A mucopolysaccharidoses**

Classic Morquio syndrome

Morquio syndrome A

Mucopolysaccharidosis, type IVA

E76.211 **Morquio B mucopolysaccharidoses**

Morquio-like mucopolysaccharidoses

Morquio-like syndrome

Morquio syndrome B

Mucopolysaccharidosis, type IVB

E76.219 **Morquio mucopolysaccharidoses, unspecified**

Morquio syndrome

Mucopolysaccharidosis, type IV

E76.22 **Sanfilippo mucopolysaccharidoses**

Mucopolysaccharidosis, type III (A) (B) (C) (D)

Sanfilippo A syndrome

Sanfilippo B syndrome

Sanfilippo C syndrome

Sanfilippo D syndrome

E76.29 **Other mucopolysaccharidoses**

beta-Glucuronidase deficiency

Maroteaux-Lamy (mild) (severe) syndrome

Mucopolysaccharidosis, types VI, VII

E76.3 **Mucopolysaccharidosis, unspecified**

E76.8 **Other disorders of glucosaminoglycan metabolism**

E76.9 **Glucosaminoglycan metabolism disorder, unspecified**

E77 **Disorders of glycoprotein metabolism**

E77.0 **Defects in post-translational modification of lysosomal enzymes**

Mucolipidosis II [I-cell disease]

Mucolipidosis III [pseudo-Hurler polydystrophy]

E77.1 **Defects in glycoprotein degradation**

Aspartylglucosaminuria

Fucosidosis

Mannosidosis

Sialidosis [mucolipidosis I]

E77.8 **Other disorders of glycoprotein metabolism**

E77.9 **Disorder of glycoprotein metabolism, unspecified**

E78 **Disorders of lipoprotein metabolism and other lipidemias**

Excludes1: sphingolipidosis (E75.0-E75.3)

E78.0 **Pure hypercholesterolemia**

E78.00 **Pure hypercholesterolemia, unspecified**

(Pure) hypercholesterolemia NOS

Fredrickson's hyperlipoproteinemia, type IIa

Hyperbetalipoproteinemia

Low-density-lipoprotein-type [LDL] hyperlipoproteinemia

E78.01 **Familial hypercholesterolemia**

E78.1 **Pure hyperglyceridemia**

Elevated fasting triglycerides

Endogenous hyperglyceridemia

Fredrickson's hyperlipoproteinemia, type IV

Hyperlipidemia, group B

Hyperprebetalipoproteinemia

Very-low-density-lipoprotein-type [VLDL] hyperlipoproteinemia

E78.2 **Mixed hyperlipidemia**

Broad- or floating-betalipoproteinemia

Combined hyperlipidemia NOS

Elevated cholesterol with elevated triglycerides NEC

Fredrickson's hyperlipoproteinemia, type IIb or III

Hyperbetalipoproteinemia with prebetalipoproteinemia

Hypercholesteremia with endogenous hyperglyceridemia

Hyperlipidemia, group C

Tubo-eruptive xanthoma Xanthoma tuberosum

Excludes1: cerebrotendinous cholesterosis [van Bogaert-Scherer- Epstein] (E75.5)

familial combined hyperlipidemia (E78.4)

E78.3 **Hyperchylomicronemia**

Chylomicron retention disease

Fredrickson's hyperlipoproteinemia, type I or V

Hyperlipidemia, group D

Mixed hyperglyceridemia

E78.4 **Other hyperlipidemia**

Familial combined hyperlipidemia

E78.5 **Hyperlipidemia, unspecified**

E78.6 **Lipoprotein deficiency**

Abetalipoproteinemia

Depressed HDL cholesterol

High-density lipoprotein deficiency

Hypoalphalipoproteinemia

Hypobetalipoproteinemia (familial)

Lecithin cholesterol acyltransferase deficiency

Tangier disease

E78.7 **Disorders of bile acid and cholesterol metabolism**

Excludes1: Niemann-Pick disease type C (E75.242)

E78.70 **Disorder of bile acid and cholesterol metabolism, unspecified**

● New code   ▲ Revised code   **Excludes1:** Not coded here   **Excludes2:** Not included here   ⊗ Placeholder required   ⑦ 7th digit required

E78.71   **Barth syndrome**

E78.72   **Smith-Lemli-Opitz syndrome**

E78.79   **Other disorders of bile acid and cholesterol metabolism**

E78.8   **Other disorders of lipoprotein metabolism**

E78.81   **Lipoid dermatoarthritis**

E78.89   **Other lipoprotein metabolism disorders**

E78.9   **Disorder of lipoprotein metabolism, unspecified**

E79   Disorders of purine and pyrimidine metabolism

   Excludes1: Ataxia-telangiectasia (Q87.1)

      Bloom's syndrome (Q82.8)

      Cockayne's syndrome (Q87.1)

      calculus of kidney (N20.0)

      combined immunodeficiency disorders (D81.-)

      Fanconi's anemia (D61.09)

      gout (M1A.-, M10.-)

      orotaciduric anemia (D53.0)

      progeria (E34.8)

      Werner's syndrome (E34.8)

      xeroderma pigmentosum (Q82.1)

E79.0   **Hyperuricemia without signs of inflammatory arthritis and tophaceous disease**

      Asymptomatic hyperuricemia

E79.1   **Lesch-Nyhan syndrome**

      HGPRT deficiency

E79.2   **Myoadenylate deaminase deficiency**

E79.8   **Other disorders of purine and pyrimidine metabolism**

      Hereditary xanthinuria

E79.9   **Disorder of purine and pyrimidine metabolism, unspecified**

E80   Disorders of porphyrin and bilirubin metabolism

   Includes: defects of catalase and peroxidase

E80.0   **Hereditary erythropoietic porphyria**

      Congenital erythropoietic porphyria

      Erythropoietic protoporphyria

E80.1   **Porphyria cutanea tarda**

E80.2   **Other and unspecified porphyria**

E80.20   **Unspecified porphyria**

      Porphyria NOS

E80.21   **Acute intermittent (hepatic) porphyria**

E80.29   **Other porphyria**

      Hereditary coproporphyria

E80.3   **Defects of catalase and peroxidase**

      Acatalasia [Takahara]

E80.4   **Gilbert syndrome**

E80.5   **Crigler-Najjar syndrome**

E80.6   **Other disorders of bilirubin metabolism**

      Dubin-Johnson syndrome

      Rotor's syndrome

E80.7   **Disorder of bilirubin metabolism, unspecified**

E83   Disorders of mineral metabolism

   Excludes1: dietary mineral deficiency (E58-E61)

      parathyroid disorders (E20-E21)

      vitamin D deficiency (E55.-)

E83.0   **Disorders of copper metabolism**

E83.00   **Disorder of copper metabolism, unspecified**

E83.01   **Wilson's disease**

   Code also associated Kayser Fleischer ring (H18.04-)

E83.09   **Other disorders of copper metabolism**

      Menkes' (kinky hair) (steely hair) disease

E83.1   **Disorders of iron metabolism**

   Excludes1: iron deficiency anemia (D50.-)

      sideroblastic anemia (D64.0-D64.3)

E83.10   **Disorder of iron metabolism, unspecified**

E83.11   **Hemochromatosis**

      Excludes1: GALD (P78.84)

         Gestational alloimmune liver disease (P78.84)

         Neonatal hemochromatosis (P78.84)

E83.110   **Hereditary hemochromatosis**

      Bronzed diabetes

      Pigmentary cirrhosis (of liver)

      Primary (hereditary) hemochromatosis

E83.111   **Hemochromatosis due to repeated red blood cell transfusions**

      Iron overload due to repeated red blood cell transfusions

      Transfusion (red blood cell) associated hemochromatosis

E83.118   **Other hemochromatosis**

E83.119   **Hemochromatosis, unspecified**

E83.19   **Other disorders of iron metabolism**

      Use additional code, if applicable, for idiopathic pulmonary hemosiderosis (J84.03)

E83.2   **Disorders of zinc metabolism**

      Acrodermatitis enteropathica

E83.3   **Disorders of phosphorus metabolism and phosphatases**

   Excludes1: adult osteomalacia (M83.-)

      osteoporosis (M80.-)

E83.30   **Disorder of phosphorus metabolism, unspecified**

E83.31   **Familial hypophosphatemia**

      Vitamin D-resistant osteomalacia

      Vitamin D-resistant rickets

      Excludes1: vitamin D-deficiency rickets (E55.0)

E83.32   **Hereditary vitamin D-dependent rickets (type 1) (type 2)**

      25-hydroxyvitamin D 1-alpha-hydroxylase deficiency

      Pseudovitamin D deficiency

      Vitamin D receptor defect

E83.39   **Other disorders of phosphorus metabolism**

      Acid phosphatase deficiency

      Hypophosphatasia

E83.4   **Disorders of magnesium metabolism**

E83.40   **Disorders of magnesium metabolism, unspecified**

E83.41   **Hypermagnesemia**

E83.42   **Hypomagnesemia**

E83.49   **Other disorders of magnesium metabolism**

E83.5   **Disorders of calcium metabolism**

   Excludes1: chondrocalcinosis (M11.1-M11.2)

      hungry bone syndrome (E83.81)

---

hyperparathyroidism (E21.0-E21.3)

E83.50   **Unspecified disorder of calcium metabolism**

E83.51   **Hypocalcemia**

E83.52   **Hypercalcemia**

     Familial hypocalciuric hypercalcemia

E83.59   **Other disorders of calcium metabolism**

     Idiopathic hypercalciuria

E83.8   **Other disorders of mineral metabolism**

E83.81   **Hungry bone syndrome**

E83.89   **Other disorders of mineral metabolism**

E83.9   **Disorder of mineral metabolism, unspecified**

E84   **Cystic fibrosis**

Includes: mucoviscidosis

Code also exocrine pancreatic insufficiency (K86.81)

E84.0   **Cystic fibrosis with pulmonary manifestations**

     Use additional code to identify any infectious organism present, such as:

     Pseudomonas (B96.5)

E84.1   **Cystic fibrosis with intestinal manifestations**

E84.11   **Meconium ileus in cystic fibrosis**

     Excludes1: meconium ileus not due to cystic fibrosis (P76.0)

E84.19   **Cystic fibrosis with other intestinal manifestations**

     Distal intestinal obstruction syndrome

E84.8   **Cystic fibrosis with other manifestations**

E84.9   **Cystic fibrosis, unspecified**

E85   **Amyloidosis**

Excludes2: Alzheimer's disease (G30.0-)

E85.0   **Non-neuropathic heredofamilial amyloidosis**

     Hereditary amyloid nephropathy

     Code also associated disorders, such as:

     Autoinflammatory syndromes (M04.-)

     Transthyretin-related (ATTR) familial amyloid cardiomyopathy (E85.4)

E85.1   **Neuropathic heredofamilial amyloidosis**

     Amyloid polyneuropathy (Portuguese)

     Transthyretin-related (ATTR) familial amyloid polyneuropathy

E85.2   **Heredofamilial amyloidosis, unspecified**

E85.3   **Secondary systemic amyloidosis**

     Hemodialysis-associated amyloidosis

E85.4   **Organ-limited amyloidosis**

     Localized amyloidosis

     Transthyretin-related (ATTR) familial amyloid cardiomyopathy

E85.8   **Other amyloidosis**

 • **E85.81**   **Light chain (AL) amyloidosis**

 • **E85.82**   **Wild-type transthyretin-related (ATTR) amyloidosis**

     Senile systemic amyloidosis (SSA)

 • **E85.89**   **Other amyloidosis**

E85.9   **Amyloidosis, unspecified**

E86   **Volume depletion**

Use additional code(s) for any associated disorders of electrolyte and acid-base balance (E87.-)

Excludes1: dehydration of newborn (P74.1)

     hypovolemic shock NOS (R57.1)

postprocedural hypovolemic shock (T81.19)

traumatic hypovolemic shock (T79.4)

E86.0   **Dehydration**

E86.1   **Hypovolemia**

     Depletion of volume of plasma

E86.9   **Volume depletion, unspecified**

E87   **Other disorders of fluid, electrolyte and acid-base balance**

Excludes1: diabetes insipidus (E23.2)

     electrolyte imbalance associated with hyperemesis gravidarum (O21.1)

     electrolyte imbalance following ectopic or molar pregnancy (O08.5)

     familial periodic paralysis (G72.3)

E87.0   **Hyperosmolality and hypernatremia**

     Sodium [Na] excess

     Sodium [Na] overload

E87.1   **Hypo-osmolality and hyponatremia**

     Sodium [Na] deficiency

     Excludes1: syndrome of inappropriate secretion of antidiuretic hormone (E22.2)

E87.2   **Acidosis**

     Acidosis NOS

     Lactic acidosis

     Metabolic acidosis

     Respiratory acidosis

     Excludes1: diabetic acidosis - see categories E08-E10, E13 with ketoacidosis

E87.3   **Alkalosis**

     Alkalosis NOS

     Metabolic alkalosis

     Respiratory alkalosis

E87.4   **Mixed disorder of acid-base balance**

E87.5   **Hyperkalemia**

     Potassium [K] excess

     Potassium [K] overload

E87.6   **Hypokalemia**

     Potassium [K] deficiency

E87.7   **Fluid overload**

     Excludes1: edema NOS (R60.9)

     fluid retention (R60.9)

E87.70   **Fluid overload, unspecified**

E87.71   **Transfusion associated circulatory overload**

     Fluid overload due to transfusion (blood) (blood components) TACO

E87.79   **Other fluid overload**

E87.8   **Other disorders of electrolyte and fluid balance, not elsewhere classified**

     Electrolyte imbalance NOS

     Hyperchloremia

     Hypochloremia

E88   **Other and unspecified metabolic disorders**

Use additional codes for associated conditions

Excludes1: histiocytosis X (chronic) (C96.6)

E88.0   **Disorders of plasma-protein metabolism, not elsewhere classified**

     Excludes1: disorder of lipoprotein metabolism (E78.-)

     monoclonal gammopathy (of undetermined significance) (D47.2) polyclonal hypergammaglobulinemia (D89.0)

Waldenström macroglobulinemia (C88.0)

E88.01 Alpha-1-antitrypsin deficiency

AAT deficiency

E88.09 Other disorders of plasma-protein metabolism, not elsewhere classified

Bisalbuminemia

E88.1 Lipodystrophy, not elsewhere classified

Lipodystrophy NOS

Excludes1: Whipple's disease (K90.81)

E88.2 Lipomatosis, not elsewhere classified

Lipomatosis NOS

Lipomatosis (Check) dolorosa [Dercum]

E88.3 Tumor lysis syndrome

Tumor lysis syndrome (spontaneous)

Tumor lysis syndrome following antineoplastic drug chemotherapy

Use additional code for adverse effect, if applicable, to identify drug (T45.1X5)

E88.4 Mitochondrial metabolism disorders

Excludes1: disorders of pyruvate metabolism (E74.4)

Kearns-Sayre syndrome (H49.81)

Leber's disease (H47.22)

Leigh's encephalopathy (G31.82)

Mitochondrial myopathy, NEC (G71.3)

Reye's syndrome (G93.7)

E88.40 Mitochondrial metabolism disorder, unspecified

E88.41 MELAS syndrome

Mitochondrial myopathy, encephalopathy, lactic acidosis and stroke-like episodes

E88.42 MERRF syndrome

Myoclonic epilepsy associated with ragged-red fibers

Code also progressive myoclonic epilepsy (G40.3-)

E88.49 Other mitochondrial metabolism disorders

E88.8 Other specified metabolic disorders

E88.81 Metabolic syndrome

Dysmetabolic syndrome X

Use additional codes for associated manifestations, such as:

obesity (E66.-)

E88.89 Other specified metabolic disorders

Launois-Bensaude adenolipomatosis

Excludes1: adult pulmonary Langerhans cell histiocytosis (J84.82)

E88.9 Metabolic disorder, unspecified

POSTPROCEDURAL ENDOCRINE AND METABOLIC COMPLICATIONS AND DISORDERS, NOT ELSEWHERE CLASSIFIED (E89)

E89 Postprocedural endocrine and metabolic complications and disorders, not elsewhere classified

Excludes2: intraoperative complications of endocrine system organ or structure (E36.0-, E36.1-, E36.8)

E89.0 Postprocedural hypothyroidism

Postirradiation hypothyroidism

Postsurgical hypothyroidism

E89.1 Postprocedural hypoinsulinemia

Postpancreatectomy hyperglycemia

Postsurgical hypoinsulinemia

Use additional code, if applicable, to identify:

acquired absence of pancreas (Z90.41-)

diabetes mellitus (postpancreatectomy) (postprocedural) (E13.-)

insulin use (Z79.4)

Excludes1: transient postprocedural hyperglycemia (R73.9)

transient postprocedural hypoglycemia (E16.2)

E89.2 Postprocedural hypoparathyroidism

Parathyroprival tetany

E89.3 Postprocedural hypopituitarism

Postirradiation hypopituitarism

E89.4 Postprocedural ovarian failure

E89.40 Asymptomatic postprocedural ovarian failure

Postprocedural ovarian failure NOS

E89.41 Symptomatic postprocedural ovarian failure

Symptoms such as flushing, sleeplessness, headache, lack of concentration, associated with postprocedural menopause

E89.5 Postprocedural testicular hypofunction

E89.6 Postprocedural adrenocortical (-medullary) hypofunction

E89.8 Other postprocedural endocrine and metabolic complications and disorders

E89.81 Postprocedural hemorrhage of an endocrine system organ or structure following a procedure

E89.810 Postprocedural hemorrhage of an endocrine system organ or structure following an endocrine system procedure

E89.811 Postprocedural hemorrhage of an endocrine system organ or structure following other procedure

E89.82 Postprocedural hematoma and seroma of an endocrine system organ or structure

E89.820 Postprocedural hematoma of an endocrine system organ or structure following an endocrine system procedure

E89.821 Postprocedural hematoma of an endocrine system organ or structure following other procedure

E89.822 Postprocedural seroma of an endocrine system organ or structure following an endocrine system procedure

E89.823 Postprocedural seroma of an endocrine system organ or structure following other procedure

E89.89 Other postprocedural endocrine and metabolic complications and disorders

Use additional code, if applicable, to further specify disorder

Chapter 5: Mental, Behavioral And Neurodevelopmental Disorders (F01-F99)

DEFINITIONS

This chapter includes definitions of selected key words, terms and phrases and coding alerts for adding points to the clinical domain, and references to coding late effects where appropriate. An example from this chapter is as follows:

F02   Dementia in other diseases classified elsewhere
Definition: Dementia refers to a group of symptoms caused by disorders that affect the brain. It is not a specific disease.

MULTIPLE CODING FOR A SINGLE CONDITION

In addition to the etiology/manifestation convention that requires two codes to fully describe a single condition that affects multiple body systems, there are other single conditions that also require more than one code. "Use additional code" notes are found in the Tabular List at codes that are not part of an etiology/manifestation pair where a secondary code is useful to fully describe a condition. The sequencing rule is the same as the etiology/manifestation pair, "use additional code" indicates that a secondary code should be added.

For example, for bacterial infections that are not included in chapter 1, a secondary code from category B95, Streptococcus, Staphylococcus, and Enterococcus, as the cause of diseases classified elsewhere, or B96, Other bacterial agents as the cause of diseases classified elsewhere, may be required to identify the bacterial organism causing the infection. A "use additional code" note will normally be found at the infectious disease code, indicating a need for the organism code to be added as a secondary code.

"Code first" notes are also under certain codes that are not specifically manifestation codes but may be due to an underlying cause. When there is a "code first" note and an underlying condition is present, the underlying condition should be sequenced first.

"Code, if applicable, any causal condition first", notes indicate that this code may be assigned as a principal diagnosis when the causal condition is unknown or not applicable. If a causal condition is known, then the code for that condition should be sequenced as the principal or first-listed diagnosis.

Multiple codes may be needed for sequela, complication codes and obstetric codes to more fully describe a condition. See the specific guidelines for these conditions for further instruction.

COMBINATION CODE

A combination code is a single code used to classify: Two diagnoses, or a diagnosis with an associated secondary process (manifestation) A diagnosis with an associated complication

Combination codes are identified by referring to subterm entries in the Alphabetic Index and by reading the inclusion and exclusion notes in the Tabular List.

Assign only the combination code when that code fully identifies the diagnostic conditions involved or when the Alphabetic Index so directs. Multiple coding should not be used when the classification provides a combination code that clearly identifies all of the elements documented in the diagnosis. When the combination code lacks necessary specificity in describing the manifestation or complication, an additional code should be used as a secondary code.

SEQUELA (LATE EFFECTS)

A sequela is the residual effect (condition produced) after the acute phase of an illness or injury has terminated. There is no time limit on when a sequela code can be used. The residual may be apparent early, such as in cerebral infarction, or it may occur months or years later, such as that due to a previous injury. Coding of sequela generally requires two codes sequenced in the following order: The condition or nature of the sequela is sequenced first.

The sequela code is sequenced second.

An exception to the above guidelines are those instances where the code for the sequela is followed by a manifestation code identified in the Tabular List and title, or the sequela code has been expanded (at the fourth, fifth or sixth character levels) to include the manifestation(s). The code for the acute phase of an illness or injury that led to the sequela is never used with a code for the late effect.

PAIN DISORDERS RELATED TO PSYCHOLOGICAL FACTORS

Assign code F45.41, for pain that is exclusively related to psychological disorders. As indicated by the Excludes 1 note under category G89, a code from category G89 should not be assigned with code F45.41.

Code F45.42, Pain disorders with related psychological factors, should be used with a code from category G89, Pain, not elsewhere classified, if there is documentation of a psychological component for a patient with acute or chronic pain.

See Section I.C.6. Pain

MENTAL AND BEHAVIORAL DISORDERS DUE TO PSYCHOACTIVE SUBSTANCE USE

1)   **In Remission**

Selection of codes for "in remission" for categories F10-F19, Mental and behavioral disorders due to psychoactive substance use (categories F10-F19 with -.21) requires the provider's clinical judgment. The appropriate codes for "in remission" are assigned only on the basis of provider documentation (as defined in the Official Guidelines for Coding and Reporting).

	Add 4th-7th digits		Nonspecific code		Unspecified code		Manifestation code	

2) **Psychoactive Substance Use, Abuse And Dependence**

When the provider documentation refers to use, abuse and dependence of the same substance (e.g. alcohol, opioid, cannabis, etc.), only one code should be assigned to identify the pattern of use based on the following hierarchy:

- If both use and abuse are documented, assign only the code for abuse

- If both abuse and dependence are documented, assign only the code for dependence

- If use, abuse and dependence are all documented, assign only the code for dependence

- If both use and dependence are documented, assign only the code for dependence.

3) **Psychoactive Substance Use**

As with all other diagnoses, the codes for psychoactive substance use (F10.9-, F11.9-, F12.9-, F13.9-, F14.9-, F15.9-, F16.9-) should only be assigned based on provider documentation and when they meet the definition of a reportable diagnosis (see Section III, Reporting Additional Diagnoses). The codes are to be used only when the psychoactive substance use is associated with a mental or behavioral disorder, and such a relationship is documented by the provider.

● New code ▲ Revised code **Excludes1:** Not coded here **Excludes2:** Not included here ⊗ Placeholder required ⑦ 7th digit required

Chapter 5

Mental, Behavioral and Neurodevelopmental Disorders (F01-F99)

Includes: disorders of psychological development

Excludes2: symptoms, signs and abnormal clinical laboratory findings, not elsewhere classified (R00-R99)

This chapter contains the following blocks:

F01-F09	Mental disorders due to known physiological conditions
F10-F19	Mental and behavioral disorders due to psychoactive substance use
F20-F29	Schizophrenia, schizotypal, delusional, and other non-mood psychotic disorders
F30-F39	Mood [affective] disorders
F40-F48	Anxiety, dissociative, stress-related, somatoform and other nonpsychotic mental disorders
F50-F59	Behavioral syndromes associated with physiological disturbances and physical factors
F60-F69	Disorders of adult personality and behavior
F70-F79	Intellectual disabilities
F80-F89	Pervasive and specific developmental disorders
F90-F98	Behavioral and emotional disorders with onset usually occurring in childhood and adolescence
F99	Unspecified mental disorder

MENTAL DISORDERS DUE TO KNOWN PHYSIOLOGICAL CONDITIONS (F01-F09)

Note: This block comprises a range of mental disorders grouped together on the basis of their having in common a demonstrable etiology in cerebral disease, brain injury, or other insult leading to cerebral dysfunction. The dysfunction may be primary, as in diseases, injuries, and insults that affect the brain directly and selectively; or secondary, as in systemic diseases and disorders that attack the brain only as one of the multiple organs or systems of the body that are involved.

F01 Vascular dementia

Vascular dementia as a result of infarction of the brain due to vascular disease, including hypertensive cerebrovascular disease.

Includes: arteriosclerotic dementia

Code first the underlying physiological condition or sequelae of cerebrovascular disease.

F01.5 Vascular dementia

F01.50 Vascular dementia without behavioral disturbance

Major neurocognitive disorder without behavioral disturbance

F01.51 Vascular dementia with behavioral disturbance

Major neurocognitive disorder due to vascular disease, with behavioral disturbance

Major neurocognitive disorder with aggressive behavior

Major neurocognitive disorder with combative behavior

Major neurocognitive disorder with violent behavior

Vascular dementia with aggressive behavior

Vascular dementia with combative behavior

Vascular dementia with violent behavior

Use additional code, if applicable, to identify wandering in vascular dementia (Z91.83)

F02 Dementia in other diseases classified elsewhere

Definition: Dementia refers to a group of symptoms caused by

disorders that affect the brain. It is not a specific disease.

Includes: Major neurocognitive disorder **in other** diseases classified elsewhere

Code first the underlying physiological condition, such as:

Alzheimer's (G30.-)

cerebral lipidosis (E75.4)

Creutzfeldt-Jakob disease (A81.0-)

dementia with Lewy bodies (G31.83)

dementia with Parkinsonism (G31.83)

epilepsy and recurrent seizures (G40.-)

frontotemporal dementia (G31.09)

hepatolenticular degeneration (E83.0)

human immunodeficiency virus [HIV] disease (B20)

Huntington's disease (G10)

hypercalcemia (E83.52)

hypothyroidism, acquired (E00-E03.-)

intoxications (T36-T65)

Jakob-Creutzfeldt disease (A81.0-)

multiple sclerosis (G35)

neurosyphilis (A52.17)

niacin deficiency [pellagra] (E52)

Parkinson's disease (G20)

Pick's disease (G31.01)

polyarteritis nodosa (M30.0)

prion disease (A81.9)

systemic lupus erythematosus (M32.-)

traumatic brain injury (S06.-)

trypanosomiasis (B56.-, B57.-)

vitamin B deficiency (E53.8)

Excludes2: dementia in alcohol and psychoactive substance disorders (F10-F19, with .17, .27, .97)

vascular dementia (F01.5-)

F02.8 Dementia in other diseases classified elsewhere

F02.80 Dementia in other diseases classified elsewhere without behavioral disturbance

Dementia **in other** diseases classified elsewhere NOS

Major neurocognitive disorder **in other** diseases classified elsewhere

F02.81 Dementia in other diseases classified elsewhere with behavioral disturbance

Dementia **in other** diseases classified elsewhere with aggressive behavior

Dementia **in other** diseases classified elsewhere with combative behavior

Dementia **in other** diseases classified elsewhere with violent behavior

Major neurocognitive disorder **in other** diseases classified elsewhere with aggressive behavior

Major neurocognitive disorder **in other** diseases classified elsewhere with combative behavior

Major neurocognitive disorder **in other** diseases classified elsewhere with violent behavior

Use additional code, if applicable, to identify wandering in dementia in conditions classified elsewhere (Z91.83)

F03 Unspecified dementia

Presenile dementia NOS

Presenile psychosis NOS

Primary degenerative dementia NOS

Senile dementia NOS

Senile dementia depressed or paranoid type

Senile psychosis NOS

Excludes1: senility NOS (R41.81)

Excludes2: mild memory disturbance due to known physiological condition (F06.8)

senile dementia with delirium or acute confusional state (F05)

F03.9 Unspecified dementia

> **F03.90 Unspecified dementia without behavioral disturbance**
>
> Dementia NOS
>
> **F03.91 Unspecified dementia with behavioral disturbance**
>
> Unspecified dementia with aggressive behavior
>
> Unspecified dementia with combative behavior
>
> Unspecified dementia with violent behavior
>
> **Use additional code**, if applicable, to identify wandering in unspecified dementia (Z91.83)

F04 Amnestic disorder due to known physiological condition

Korsakov's psychosis or syndrome, nonalcoholic

Code first the underlying physiological condition

Excludes1: amnesia NOS (R41.3)

anterograde amnesia (R41.1)

dissociative amnesia (F44.0)

retrograde amnesia (R41.2)

Excludes2: alcohol-induced or unspecified Korsakov's syndrome (F10.26, F10.96)

Korsakov's syndrome induced by other psychoactive substances (F13.26, F13.96, F19.16, F19.26,F19.96)

F05 Delirium due to known physiological condition

Acute or subacute brain syndrome

Acute or subacute confusional state (nonalcoholic)

Acute or subacute infective psychosis

Acute or subacute organic reaction

Acute or subacute psycho-organic syndrome

Delirium of mixed etiology

Delirium superimposed on dementia

Sundowning

Code first the underlying physiological condition

Excludes1: delirium NOS (R41.0)

Excludes2: delirium tremens alcohol-induced or unspecified (F10.231, F10.921)

F06 Other mental disorders due to known physiological condition

Includes: mental disorders due to endocrine disorder

mental disorders due to exogenous hormone

mental disorders due to exogenous toxic substance

mental disorders due to primary cerebral disease

mental disorders due to somatic illness

mental disorders due to systemic disease affecting the brain

Code first the underlying physiological condition

Excludes1: unspecified dementia (F03)

Excludes2: delirium due to known physiological condition (F05)

dementia as classified in F01-F02

Other mental disorders associated with alcohol and other psychoactive substances (F10-F19)

F06.0 Psychotic disorder with hallucinations due to known physiological condition

Organic hallucinatory state (nonalcoholic)

Excludes2: hallucinations and perceptual disturbance induced by alcohol and other psychoactive substances (F10-F19 with .151, .251, .951)

schizophrenia (F20.-)

F06.1 Catatonic disorder due to known physiological condition

Catatonia associated with another mental disorder

Catatonia NOS

Excludes1: catatonic stupor (R40.1)

stupor NOS (R40.1)

Excludes2: catatonic schizophrenia (F20.2)

dissociative stupor (F44.2)

F06.2 Psychotic disorder with delusions due to known physiological condition

Paranoid and paranoid-hallucinatory organic states

Schizophrenia-like psychosis in epilepsy

Excludes2: alcohol and drug-induced psychotic disorder (F10-F19 with .150, .250, .950)

brief psychotic disorder (F23)

delusional disorder (F22)

schizophrenia (F20.-)

F06.3 Mood disorder due to known physiological condition

Excludes2: mood disorders due to alcohol and other psychoactive substances (F10-F19 with .14, .24, .94)

mood disorders, not due to known physiological condition or unspecified (F30-F39)

> **F06.30 Mood disorder due to known physiological condition, unspecified**
>
> **F06.31 Mood disorder due to known physiological condition with depressive features**
>
> Depressive disorder due to known physiological condition, with depressive features
>
> **F06.32 Mood disorder due to known physiological condition with major depressive-like episode**
>
> Depressive disorder due to known physiological condition, with major depressive-like episode
>
> **F06.33 Mood disorder due to known physiological condition with manic features**
>
> Bipolar and related disorder due to a known physiological condition, with manic features
>
> Bipolar and related disorder due to known physiological condition, with manic- or hypomanic-like episodes
>
> **F06.34 Mood disorder due to known physiological condition with mixed features**
>
> Bipolar and related disorder due to known physiological condition, with mixed features
>
> Depressive disorder due to known physiological condition, with mixed features

F06.4 Anxiety disorder due to known physiological condition

Excludes2: anxiety disorders due to alcohol and other psychoactive substances (F10-F19 with .180, .280, .980)

anxiety disorders, not due to known physiological condition or unspecified (F40.-, F41.-)

F06.8 Other specified mental disorders due to known physiological condition

Epileptic psychosis NOS

Obsessive-compulsive and related disorder due to a known physiological condition

Organic dissociative disorder

● New code ▲ Revised code **Excludes1:** Not coded here **Excludes2:** Not included here ⊗ Placeholder required ⑦ 7th digit required

Organic emotionally labile [asthenic] disorder

F07 **Personality and behavioral disorders due to known physiological condition**

Code first the underlying physiological condition

F07.0 **Personality change due to known physiological condition**

Frontal lobe syndrome

Limbic epilepsy personality syndrome

Lobotomy syndrome

Organic personality disorder

Organic pseudopsychopathic personality

Organic pseudoretarded personality

Postleucotomy syndrome

Code first underlying physiological condition

Excludes1: mild cognitive impairment (G31.84)

postconcussional syndrome (F07.81)

postencephalitic syndrome (F07.89)

signs and symptoms involving emotional state (R45.-)

Excludes2: specific personality disorder (F60.-)

F07.8 **Other personality and behavioral disorders due to known physiological condition**

F07.81 **Postconcussional syndrome**

Postcontusional syndrome (encephalopathy)

Post-traumatic brain syndrome, nonpsychotic

Use additional code to identify associated post-traumatic headache, if applicable (G44.3-)

Excludes1: current concussion (brain) (S06.0-)

postencephalitic syndrome (F07.89)

F07.89 **Other personality and behavioral disorders due to known physiological condition**

Postencephalitic syndrome

Right hemispheric organic affective disorder

F07.9 **Unspecified personality and behavioral disorder due to known physiological condition**

Organic psychosyndrome

F09 **Unspecified mental disorder due to known physiological condition**

Mental disorder NOS due to known physiological condition

Organic brain syndrome NOS

Organic mental disorder NOS

Organic psychosis NOS

Symptomatic psychosis NOS

Code first the underlying physiological condition

Excludes1: psychosis NOS (F29)

MENTAL AND BEHAVIORAL DISORDERS DUE TO PSYCHOACTIVE SUBSTANCE USE (F10-F19)

F10 **Alcohol related disorders**

Definition: Alcohol-induced mental disorders is an alcohol-induced psychological or behavioral pattern that occurs in an individual and is thought to cause distress or disability that is not expected as part of normal development or culture.

Use additional code for blood alcohol level, if applicable (Y90.-)

F10.1 **Alcohol abuse**

Excludes1: alcohol dependence (F10.2-)

alcohol use, unspecified (F10.9-)

F10.10 **Alcohol abuse, uncomplicated**

Alcohol use disorder, mild

●**F10.11** **Alcohol abuse, in remission**

Alcohol use disorder, mild, in early remission

Alcohol use disorder, mild, in sustained remission

F10.12 **Alcohol abuse with intoxication**

F10.120 **Alcohol abuse with intoxication, uncomplicated**

F10.121 **Alcohol abuse with intoxication delirium**

F10.129 **Alcohol abuse with intoxication, unspecified**

F10.14 **Alcohol abuse with alcohol-induced mood disorder**

Alcohol use disorder, mild, with alcohol-induced bipolar or related disorder

Alcohol use disorder, mild, with alcohol-induced depressive disorder

F10.15 **Alcohol abuse with alcohol-induced psychotic disorder**

F10.150 **Alcohol abuse with alcohol-induced psychotic disorder with delusions**

F10.151 **Alcohol abuse with alcohol-induced psychotic disorder with hallucinations**

F10.159 **Alcohol abuse with alcohol-induced psychotic disorder, unspecified**

F10.18 **Alcohol abuse with other alcohol-induced disorders**

F10.180 **Alcohol abuse with alcohol-induced anxiety disorder**

F10.181 **Alcohol abuse with alcohol-induced sexual dysfunction**

F10.182 **Alcohol abuse with alcohol-induced sleep disorder**

F10.188 **Alcohol abuse with other alcohol-induced disorder**

F10.19 **Alcohol abuse with unspecified alcohol-induced disorder**

F10.2 **Alcohol dependence**

Excludes1: alcohol abuse (F10.1-)

alcohol use, unspecified (F10.9-)

Excludes2: toxic effect of alcohol (T51.0-)

F10.20 **Alcohol dependence, uncomplicated**

Alcohol use disorder, moderate

Alcohol use disorder, severe

F10.21 **Alcohol dependence, in remission**

Alcohol use disorder, moderate, in early remission

Alcohol use disorder, moderate, in sustained remission

Alcohol use disorder, severe, in early remission

Alcohol use disorder, severe, in sustained remission

F10.22 **Alcohol dependence with intoxication**

Acute drunkenness (in alcoholism)

Excludes2: alcohol dependence with withdrawal (F10.23-)

F10.220 **Alcohol dependence with intoxication, uncomplicated**

F10.221 **Alcohol dependence with intoxication delirium**

F10.229 **Alcohol dependence with intoxication, unspecified**

F10.23 **Alcohol dependence with withdrawal**

Excludes2: Alcohol dependence with intoxication (F10.22-)

F10.230 Alcohol dependence with withdrawal, uncomplicated

F10.231 Alcohol dependence with withdrawal delirium

F10.232 Alcohol dependence with withdrawal with perceptual disturbance

F10.239 Alcohol dependence with withdrawal, unspecified

F10.24 Alcohol dependence with alcohol-induced mood disorder

Alcohol use disorder, moderate, with alcohol-induced bipolar or related disorder

Alcohol use disorder, moderate, with alcohol-induced depressive disorder

Alcohol use disorder, severe, with alcohol-induced bipolar or related disorder

Alcohol use disorder, severe, with alcohol-induced depressive disorder

F10.25 Alcohol dependence with alcohol-induced psychotic disorder

F10.250 Alcohol dependence with alcohol-induced psychotic disorder with delusions

F10.251 Alcohol dependence with alcohol-induced psychotic disorder with hallucinations

F10.259 Alcohol dependence with alcohol-induced psychotic disorder, unspecified

F10.26 Alcohol dependence with alcohol-induced persisting amnestic disorder

Alcohol use disorder, moderate, with alcohol-induced major neurocognitive disorder, amnestic-confabulatory type

Alcohol use disorder, severe, with alcohol-induced major neurocognitive disorder, amnestic-confabulatory type

F10.27 Alcohol dependence with alcohol-induced persisting dementia

Alcohol use disorder, moderate, with alcohol-induced major neurocognitive disorder, non amnestic-confabulatory type

Alcohol use disorder, severe, with alcohol-induced major neurocognitive disorder, non amnestic-confabulatory type

F10.28 Alcohol dependence with other alcohol-induced disorders

F10.280 Alcohol dependence with alcohol-induced anxiety disorder

F10.281 Alcohol dependence with alcohol-induced sexual dysfunction

F10.282 Alcohol dependence with alcohol-induced sleep disorder

F10.288 Alcohol dependence with other alcohol-induced disorder

Alcohol use disorder, moderate, with alcohol-induced mild neurocognitive disorder

Alcohol use disorder, severe, with alcohol-induced mild neurocognitive disorder

F10.29 Alcohol dependence with unspecified alcohol-induced disorder

F10.9 Alcohol use, unspecified

Excludes1: alcohol abuse (F10.1-)

alcohol dependence (F10.2-)

F10.92 Alcohol use, unspecified with intoxication

F10.920 Alcohol use, unspecified with intoxication, uncomplicated

F10.921 Alcohol use, unspecified with intoxication delirium

F10.929 Alcohol use, unspecified with intoxication, unspecified

F10.94 Alcohol use, unspecified with alcohol-induced mood disorder

Alcohol induced bipolar or related disorder, without use disorder

Alcohol induced depressive disorder, without use disorder

F10.95 Alcohol use, unspecified with alcohol-induced psychotic disorder

F10.950 Alcohol use, unspecified with alcohol-induced psychotic disorder with delusions

F10.951 Alcohol use, unspecified with alcohol-induced psychotic disorder with hallucinations

F10.959 Alcohol use, unspecified with alcohol-induced psychotic disorder, unspecified

Alcohol-induced psychotic disorder without use disorder

F10.96 Alcohol use, unspecified with alcohol-induced persisting amnestic disorder

Alcohol-induced major neurocognitive disorder, amnestic-confabulatory type, without use disorder

F10.97 Alcohol use, unspecified with alcohol-induced persisting dementia

Alcohol-induced major neurocognitive disorder, non amnestic-confabulatory type, without use disorder

F10.98 Alcohol use, unspecified with other alcohol-induced disorders

F10.980 Alcohol use, unspecified with alcohol-induced anxiety disorder

Alcohol induced anxiety disorder, without use disorder

F10.981 Alcohol use, unspecified with alcohol-induced sexual dysfunction

Alcohol induced sexual dysfunction, without use disorder

F10.982 Alcohol use, unspecified with alcohol-induced sleep disorder

Alcohol induced sleep disorder, without use disorder

F10.988 Alcohol use, unspecified with other alcohol-induced disorder

Alcohol induced mild neurocognitive disorder, without use disorder

F10.99 Alcohol use, unspecified with unspecified alcohol-induced disorder

F11 **Opioid related disorders**

Definition: Opioids are medications that relieve pain. They reduce the intensity of pain signals reaching the brain and affect those brain areas controlling emotion, which diminishes the effects of a painful stimulus. Medications that fall within this class include hydrocodone (e.g., Vicodin), oxycodone (e.g., OxyContin,

Percocet), morphine (e.g., Kadian, Avinza), codeine, and related drugs.

F11.1 Opioid abuse

Excludes1: opioid dependence (F11.2-)

opioid use, unspecified (F11.9-)

F11.10 Opioid abuse, uncomplicated

Opioid use disorder, mild

●**F11.11 Opioid abuse, in remission**

Opioid use disorder, mild, in early remission

Opioid use disorder, mild, in sustained remission

F11.12 Opioid abuse with intoxication

F11.120 Opioid abuse with intoxication, uncomplicated

F11.121 Opioid abuse with intoxication delirium

F11.122 Opioid abuse with intoxication with perceptual disturbance

F11.129 Opioid abuse with intoxication, unspecified

F11.14 Opioid abuse with opioid-induced mood disorder

Opioid use disorder, mild, with opioid-induced depressive disorder

F11.15 Opioid abuse with opioid-induced psychotic disorder

F11.150 Opioid abuse with opioid-induced psychotic disorder with delusions

F11.151 Opioid abuse with opioid-induced psychotic disorder with hallucinations

F11.159 Opioid abuse with opioid-induced psychotic disorder, unspecified

F11.18 Opioid abuse with other opioid-induced disorder

F11.181 Opioid abuse with opioid-induced sexual dysfunction

F11.182 Opioid abuse with opioid-induced sleep disorder

F11.188 Opioid abuse with other opioid-induced disorder

F11.19 Opioid abuse with unspecified opioid-induced disorder

F11.2 Opioid dependence

Excludes1: opioid abuse (F11.1-)

opioid use, unspecified (F11.9-)

Excludes2: opioid poisoning (T40.0-T40.2-)

F11.20 Opioid dependence, uncomplicated

Opioid use disorder, moderate

Opioid use disorder, severe

F11.21 Opioid dependence, in remission

Opioid use disorder, moderate, in early remission

Opioid use disorder, moderate, in sustained remission

Opioid use disorder, severe, in early remission

Opioid use disorder, severe, in sustained remission

F11.22 Opioid dependence with intoxication

Excludes1: opioid dependence with withdrawal (F11.23)

F11.220 Opioid dependence with intoxication, uncomplicated

F11.221 Opioid dependence with intoxication delirium

F11.222 Opioid dependence with intoxication with perceptual disturbance

F11.229 Opioid dependence with intoxication, unspecified

F11.23 Opioid dependence with withdrawal

Excludes1: opioid dependence with intoxication (F11.22-)

F11.24 Opioid dependence with opioid-induced mood disorder

Opioid use disorder, moderate, with opioid induced depressive disorder

F11.25 Opioid dependence with opioid-induced psychotic disorder

F11.250 Opioid dependence with opioid-induced psychotic disorder with delusions

F11.251 Opioid dependence with opioid-induced psychotic disorder with hallucinations

F11.259 Opioid dependence with opioid-induced psychotic disorder, unspecified

F11.28 Opioid dependence with other opioid-induced disorder

F11.281 Opioid dependence with opioid-induced sexual dysfunction

F11.282 Opioid dependence with opioid-induced sleep disorder

F11.288 Opioid dependence with other opioid-induced disorder

F11.29 Opioid dependence with unspecified opioid-induced disorder

F11.9 Opioid use, unspecified

Excludes1: opioid abuse (F11.1-)

opioid dependence (F11.2-)

F11.90 Opioid use, unspecified, uncomplicated

F11.92 Opioid use, unspecified with intoxication

Excludes1: opioid use, unspecified with withdrawal (F11.93)

F11.920 Opioid use, unspecified with intoxication, uncomplicated

F11.921 Opioid use, unspecified with intoxication delirium

Opioid-induced delirium

F11.922 Opioid use, unspecified with intoxication with perceptual disturbance

F11.929 Opioid use, unspecified with intoxication, unspecified

F11.93 Opioid use, unspecified with withdrawal

Excludes1: opioid use, unspecified with intoxication (F11.92-)

F11.94 Opioid use, unspecified with opioid-induced mood disorder

Opioid induced depressive disorder, without use disorder

F11.95 Opioid use, unspecified with opioid-induced psychotic disorder

F11.950 Opioid use, unspecified with opioid-induced psychotic disorder with delusions

F11.951 Opioid use, unspecified with opioid-induced psychotic disorder with hallucinations

F11.959 Opioid use, unspecified with opioid-induced psychotic disorder, unspecified

F11.98 Opioid use, unspecified with other specified opioid-induced disorder

F11.981 Opioid use, unspecified with opioid-induced sexual dysfunction

Opioid induced sexual dysfunction, without use disorder

F11.982 Opioid use, unspecified with opioid-induced sleep disorder

Opioid induced sleep disorder, without use disorder

F11.988 Opioid use, unspecified with other opioid-induced disorder

Opioid induced anxiety disorder, without use disorder

F11.99 Opioid use, unspecified with unspecified opioid-induced disorder

F12 **Cannabis related disorders**

Includes: marijuana

F12.1 **Cannabis abuse**

Excludes1: cannabis dependence (F12.2-)

cannabis use, unspecified (F12.9-)

F12.10 Cannabis abuse, uncomplicated

Cannabis use disorder, mild

●**F12.11** Cannabis abuse, in remission

Cannabis use disorder, mild, in early remission

Cannabis use disorder, mild, in sustained remission

F12.12 Cannabis abuse with intoxication

F12.120 Cannabis abuse with intoxication, uncomplicated

F12.121 Cannabis abuse with intoxication delirium

F12.122 Cannabis abuse with intoxication with perceptual disturbance

F12.129 Cannabis abuse with intoxication, unspecified

F12.15 Cannabis abuse with psychotic disorder

F12.150 Cannabis abuse with psychotic disorder with delusions

F12.151 Cannabis abuse with psychotic disorder with hallucinations

F12.159 Cannabis abuse with psychotic disorder, unspecified

F12.18 Cannabis abuse with other cannabis-induced disorder

F12.180 Cannabis abuse with cannabis-induced anxiety disorder

F12.188 Cannabis abuse with other cannabis-induced disorder

Cannabis use disorder, mild, with cannabis-induced sleep disorder

F12.19 Cannabis abuse with unspecified cannabis-induced disorder

F12.2 **Cannabis dependence**

Excludes1: cannabis abuse (F12.1-)

cannabis use, unspecified (F12.9-)

Excludes2: cannabis poisoning (T40.7-)

F12.20 Cannabis dependence, uncomplicated

Cannabis use disorder, moderate

Cannabis use disorder, severe

F12.21 Cannabis dependence, in remission

Cannabis use disorder, moderate, in early remission

Cannabis use disorder, moderate, in sustained remission

Cannabis use disorder, severe, in early remission

Cannabis use disorder, severe, in sustained remission

F12.22 Cannabis dependence with intoxication

F12.220 Cannabis dependence with intoxication, uncomplicated

F12.221 Cannabis dependence with intoxication delirium

F12.222 Cannabis dependence with intoxication with perceptual disturbance

F12.229 Cannabis dependence with intoxication, unspecified

F12.25 Cannabis dependence with psychotic disorder

F12.250 Cannabis dependence with psychotic disorder with delusions

F12.251 Cannabis dependence with psychotic disorder with hallucinations

F12.259 Cannabis dependence with psychotic disorder, unspecified

F12.28 Cannabis dependence with other cannabis-induced disorder

F12.280 Cannabis dependence with cannabis-induced anxiety disorder

F12.288 Cannabis dependence with other cannabis-induced disorder

Cannabis use disorder, moderate, with cannabis-induced sleep disorder

Cannabis use disorder, severe, with cannabis-induced sleep disorder

Cannabis withdrawal

F12.29 Cannabis dependence with unspecified cannabis-induced disorder

F12.9 **Cannabis use, unspecified**

Excludes1: cannabis abuse (F12.1-)

cannabis dependence (F12.2-)

F12.90 Cannabis use, unspecified, uncomplicated

F12.92 Cannabis use, unspecified with intoxication

F12.920 Cannabis use, unspecified with intoxication, uncomplicated

F12.921 Cannabis use, unspecified with intoxication delirium

F12.922 Cannabis use, unspecified with intoxication with perceptual disturbance

F12.929 Cannabis use, unspecified with intoxication, unspecified

F12.95 Cannabis use, unspecified with psychotic disorder

F12.950 Cannabis use, unspecified with psychotic disorder with delusions

F12.951 Cannabis use, unspecified with psychotic disorder with hallucinations

● New code ▲ Revised code **Excludes1:** Not coded here **Excludes2:** Not included here ⊗ Placeholder required ⑦7th digit required

F12.959 **Cannabis use, unspecified with psychotic disorder, unspecified**

Cannabis induced psychotic disorder, without use disorder

F12.98 **Cannabis use, unspecified with other cannabis-induced disorder**

F12.980 **Cannabis use, unspecified with anxiety disorder**

Cannabis induced anxiety disorder, without use disorder

F12.988 **Cannabis use, unspecified with other cannabis-induced disorder**

Cannabis induced sleep disorder, without use disorder

F12.99 **Cannabis use, unspecified with unspecified cannabis-induced disorder**

F13 **Sedative, hypnotic, or anxiolytic related disorders**

F13.1 **Sedative, hypnotic or anxiolytic-related abuse**

Excludes1: sedative, hypnotic or anxiolytic-related dependence (F13.2-)

sedative, hypnotic, or anxiolytic use, unspecified (F13.9-)

F13.10 **Sedative, hypnotic or anxiolytic abuse, uncomplicated**

Sedative, hypnotic, or anxiolytic use disorder, mild

• **F13.11** **Sedative, hypnotic or anxiolytic abuse, in remission**

Sedative, hypnotic or anxiolytic use disorder, mild, in early remission

Sedative, hypnotic or anxiolytic use disorder, mild, in sustained remission

F13.12 **Sedative, hypnotic or anxiolytic abuse with intoxication**

F13.120 **Sedative, hypnotic or anxiolytic abuse with intoxication, uncomplicated**

F13.121 **Sedative, hypnotic or anxiolytic abuse with intoxication delirium**

F13.129 **Sedative, hypnotic or anxiolytic abuse with intoxication, unspecified**

F13.14 **Sedative, hypnotic or anxiolytic abuse with sedative, hypnotic or anxiolytic-induced mood disorder**

Sedative, hypnotic, or anxiolytic use disorder, mild, with sedative, hypnotic, or anxiolytic-induced bipolar or related disorder

Sedative, hypnotic, or anxiolytic use disorder, mild, with sedative, hypnotic, or anxiolytic-induced depressive disorder

F13.15 **Sedative, hypnotic or anxiolytic abuse with sedative, hypnotic or anxiolytic-induced psychotic disorder**

F13.150 **Sedative, hypnotic or anxiolytic abuse with sedative, hypnotic or anxiolytic-induced psychotic disorder with delusions**

F13.151 **Sedative, hypnotic or anxiolytic abuse with sedative, hypnotic or anxiolytic-induced psychotic disorder with hallucinations**

F13.159 **Sedative, hypnotic or anxiolytic abuse with sedative, hypnotic or anxiolytic-induced psychotic disorder, unspecified**

F13.18 **Sedative, hypnotic or anxiolytic abuse with other sedative, hypnotic or anxiolytic-induced disorders**

F13.180 **Sedative, hypnotic or anxiolytic abuse with sedative, hypnotic or anxiolytic-induced anxiety disorder**

F13.181 **Sedative, hypnotic or anxiolytic abuse with sedative, hypnotic or anxiolytic-induced sexual dysfunction**

F13.182 **Sedative, hypnotic or anxiolytic abuse with sedative, hypnotic or anxiolytic-induced sleep disorder**

F13.188 **Sedative, hypnotic or anxiolytic abuse with other sedative, hypnotic or anxiolytic-induced disorder**

F13.19 **Sedative, hypnotic or anxiolytic abuse with unspecified sedative, hypnotic or anxiolytic-induced disorder**

F13.2 **Sedative, hypnotic or anxiolytic-related dependence**

Excludes1: sedative, hypnotic or anxiolytic-related abuse (F13.1-)

sedative, hypnotic, or anxiolytic use, unspecified (F13.9-)

Excludes2: sedative, hypnotic, or anxiolytic poisoning (T42.-)

F13.20 **Sedative, hypnotic or anxiolytic dependence, uncomplicated**

F13.21 **Sedative, hypnotic or anxiolytic dependence, in remission**

Sedative, hypnotic or anxiolytic use disorder, moderate, in early remission

Sedative, hypnotic or anxiolytic use disorder, moderate, in sustained remission

Sedative, hypnotic or anxiolytic use disorder, severe, in early remission

Sedative, hypnotic or anxiolytic use disorder, severe, in sustained remission

F13.22 **Sedative, hypnotic or anxiolytic dependence with intoxication**

Excludes1: sedative, hypnotic or anxiolytic dependence with withdrawal (F13.23-)

F13.220 **Sedative, hypnotic or anxiolytic dependence with intoxication, uncomplicated**

F13.221 **Sedative, hypnotic or anxiolytic dependence with intoxication delirium**

F13.229 **Sedative, hypnotic or anxiolytic dependence with intoxication, unspecified**

F13.23 **Sedative, hypnotic or anxiolytic dependence with withdrawal**

Sedative, hypnotic, or anxiolytic use disorder, moderate

Sedative, hypnotic, or anxiolytic use disorder, severe

Excludes1: sedative, hypnotic or anxiolytic dependence with intoxication (F13.22-)

F13.230 **Sedative, hypnotic or anxiolytic dependence with withdrawal, uncomplicated**

F13.231 **Sedative, hypnotic or anxiolytic dependence with withdrawal delirium**

F13.232 Sedative, hypnotic or anxiolytic dependence with withdrawal with perceptual disturbance

Sedative, hypnotic, or anxiolytic withdrawal with perceptual disturbances

F13.239 Sedative, hypnotic or anxiolytic dependence with withdrawal, unspecified

Sedative, hypnotic, or anxiolytic withdrawal without perceptual disturbances

F13.24 Sedative, hypnotic or anxiolytic dependence with sedative, hypnotic or anxiolytic-induced mood disorder

Sedative, hypnotic, or anxiolytic use disorder, moderate, with sedative, hypnotic, or anxiolytic-induced bipolar or related disorder

Sedative, hypnotic, or anxiolytic use disorder, moderate, with sedative, hypnotic, or anxiolytic-induced depressive disorder

Sedative, hypnotic, or anxiolytic use disorder, severe, with sedative, hypnotic, or anxiolytic-induced depressive disorder

F13.25 Sedative, hypnotic or anxiolytic dependence with sedative, hypnotic or anxiolytic-induced psychotic disorder

F13.250 Sedative, hypnotic or anxiolytic dependence with sedative, hypnotic or anxiolytic-induced psychotic disorder with delusions

F13.251 Sedative, hypnotic or anxiolytic dependence with sedative, hypnotic or anxiolytic-induced psychotic disorder with hallucinations

F13.259 Sedative, hypnotic or anxiolytic dependence with sedative, hypnotic or anxiolytic-induced psychotic disorder, unspecified

F13.26 Sedative, hypnotic or anxiolytic dependence with sedative, hypnotic or anxiolytic-induced persisting amnestic disorder

F13.27 Sedative, hypnotic or anxiolytic dependence with sedative, hypnotic or anxiolytic-induced persisting dementia

Sedative, hypnotic, or anxiolytic use disorder, moderate, with sedative, hypnotic, or anxiolytic-induced major neurocognitive disorder

Sedative, hypnotic, or anxiolytic use disorder, severe, with sedative, hypnotic, or anxiolytic-induced major neurocognitive disorder

F13.28 Sedative, hypnotic or anxiolytic dependence with other sedative, hypnotic or anxiolytic-induced disorders

F13.280 Sedative, hypnotic or anxiolytic dependence with sedative, hypnotic or anxiolytic-induced anxiety disorder

F13.281 Sedative, hypnotic or anxiolytic dependence with sedative, hypnotic or anxiolytic-induced sexual dysfunction

F13.282 Sedative, hypnotic or anxiolytic dependence with sedative, hypnotic or anxiolytic-induced sleep disorder

F13.288 Sedative, hypnotic or anxiolytic dependence with other sedative,

hypnotic or anxiolytic-induced disorder

Sedative, hypnotic, or anxiolytic use disorder, moderate, with sedative, hypnotic, or anxiolytic-induced mild neurocognitive disorder

Sedative, hypnotic, or anxiolytic use disorder, severe, with sedative, hypnotic, or anxiolytic-induced mild neurocognitive disorder

F13.29 Sedative, hypnotic or anxiolytic dependence with unspecified sedative, hypnotic or anxiolytic-induced disorder

F13.9 Sedative, hypnotic or anxiolytic-related use, unspecified

Excludes1: sedative, hypnotic or anxiolytic-related abuse (F13.1-)

sedative, hypnotic or anxiolytic-related dependence (F13.2-)

F13.90 Sedative, hypnotic, or anxiolytic use, unspecified, uncomplicated

F13.92 Sedative, hypnotic or anxiolytic use, unspecified with intoxication

Excludes1: sedative, hypnotic or anxiolytic use, unspecified with withdrawal (F13.93-)

F13.920 Sedative, hypnotic or anxiolytic use, unspecified with intoxication, uncomplicated

F13.921 Sedative, hypnotic or anxiolytic use, unspecified with intoxication delirium

Sedative, hypnotic, or anxiolytic-induced delirium

F13.929 Sedative, hypnotic or anxiolytic use, unspecified with intoxication, unspecified

F13.93 Sedative, hypnotic or anxiolytic use, unspecified with withdrawal

Excludes1: sedative, hypnotic or anxiolytic use, unspecified with intoxication (F13.92-)

F13.930 Sedative, hypnotic or anxiolytic use, unspecified with withdrawal, uncomplicated

F13.931 Sedative, hypnotic or anxiolytic use, unspecified with withdrawal delirium

F13.932 Sedative, hypnotic or anxiolytic use, unspecified with withdrawal with perceptual disturbances

F13.939 Sedative, hypnotic or anxiolytic use, unspecified with withdrawal, unspecified

F13.94 Sedative, hypnotic or anxiolytic use, unspecified with sedative, hypnotic or anxiolytic-induced mood disorder

Sedative, hypnotic, or anxiolytic-induced bipolar or related disorder, without use disorder

Sedative, hypnotic, or anxiolytic-induced depressive disorder, without use disorder

F13.95 Sedative, hypnotic or anxiolytic use, unspecified with sedative, hypnotic or anxiolytic-induced psychotic disorder

F13.950 Sedative, hypnotic or anxiolytic use, unspecified with sedative, hypnotic or anxiolytic-induced psychotic disorder with delusions

F13.951   **Sedative, hypnotic or anxiolytic use, unspecified with sedative, hypnotic or anxiolytic-induced psychotic disorder with hallucinations**

F13.959   **Sedative, hypnotic or anxiolytic use, unspecified with sedative, hypnotic or anxiolytic-induced psychotic disorder, unspecified**

Sedative, hypnotic, or anxiolytic-induced psychotic disorder, without use disorder

F13.96   **Sedative, hypnotic or anxiolytic use, unspecified with sedative, hypnotic or anxiolytic-induced persisting amnestic disorder**

F13.97   **Sedative, hypnotic or anxiolytic use, unspecified with sedative, hypnotic or anxiolytic-induced persisting dementia**

Sedative, hypnotic, or anxiolytic-induced major neurocognitive disorder, without use disorder

F13.98   **Sedative, hypnotic or anxiolytic use, unspecified with other sedative, hypnotic or anxiolytic-induced disorders**

F13.980   **Sedative, hypnotic or anxiolytic use, unspecified with sedative, hypnotic or anxiolytic-induced anxiety disorder**

Sedative, hypnotic, or anxiolytic-induced anxiety disorder, without use disorder

F13.981   **Sedative, hypnotic or anxiolytic use, unspecified with sedative, hypnotic or anxiolytic-induced sexual dysfunction**

Sedative, hypnotic, or anxiolytic-induced sexual dysfunction disorder, without use disorder

F13.982   **Sedative, hypnotic or anxiolytic use, unspecified with sedative, hypnotic or anxiolytic-induced sleep disorder**

Sedative, hypnotic, or anxiolytic-induced sleep disorder, without use disorder

F13.988   **Sedative, hypnotic or anxiolytic use, unspecified with other sedative, hypnotic or anxiolytic-induced disorder**

Sedative, hypnotic, or anxiolytic-induced mild neurocognitive disorder

F13.99   **Sedative, hypnotic or anxiolytic use, unspecified with unspecified sedative, hypnotic or anxiolytic-induced disorder**

F14   **Cocaine related disorders**

Excludes2: Other stimulant-related disorders (F15.-)

F14.1   **Cocaine abuse**

Excludes1: cocaine dependence (F14.2-)

cocaine use, unspecified (F14.9-)

F14.10   **Cocaine abuse, uncomplicated**

Cocaine use disorder, mild

●**F14.11**   **Cocaine abuse, in remission**

Cocaine use disorder, mild, in early remission

Cocaine use disorder, mild, in sustained remission

F14.12   **Cocaine abuse with intoxication**

F14.120   **Cocaine abuse with intoxication, uncomplicated**

F14.121   **Cocaine abuse with intoxication with delirium**

F14.122   **Cocaine abuse with intoxication with perceptual disturbance**

F14.129   **Cocaine abuse with intoxication, unspecified**

F14.14   **Cocaine abuse with cocaine-induced mood disorder**

Cocaine use disorder, mild, with cocaine-induced bipolar or related disorder

Cocaine use disorder, mild, with cocaine-induced depressive disorder

F14.15   **Cocaine abuse with cocaine-induced psychotic disorder**

F14.150   **Cocaine abuse with cocaine-induced psychotic disorder with delusions**

F14.151   **Cocaine abuse with cocaine-induced psychotic disorder with hallucinations**

F14.159   **Cocaine abuse with cocaine-induced psychotic disorder, unspecified**

F14.18   **Cocaine abuse with other cocaine-induced disorder**

F14.180   **Cocaine abuse with cocaine-induced anxiety disorder**

F14.181   **Cocaine abuse with cocaine-induced sexual dysfunction**

F14.182   **Cocaine abuse with cocaine-induced sleep disorder**

F14.188   **Cocaine abuse with other cocaine-induced disorder**

Cocaine use disorder, mild, with cocaine-induced obsessive compulsive or related disorder

F14.19   **Cocaine abuse with unspecified cocaine-induced disorder**

F14.2   **Cocaine dependence**

Excludes1: cocaine abuse (F14.1-)

cocaine use, unspecified (F14.9-)

Excludes2: cocaine poisoning (T40.5-)

F14.20   **Cocaine dependence, uncomplicated**

Cocaine use disorder, moderate

Cocaine use disorder, severe

F14.21   **Cocaine dependence, in remission**

Cocaine use disorder, moderate, in early remission

Cocaine use disorder, moderate, in sustained remission

Cocaine use disorder, severe, in early remission

Cocaine use disorder, severe, in sustained remission

F14.22   **Cocaine dependence with intoxication**

Excludes1: cocaine dependence with withdrawal (F14.23)

F14.220   **Cocaine dependence with intoxication, uncomplicated**

F14.221   **Cocaine dependence with intoxication delirium**

F14.222   **Cocaine dependence with intoxication with perceptual disturbance**

F14.229   **Cocaine dependence with intoxication, unspecified**

F14.23   **Cocaine dependence with withdrawal**

Excludes1: cocaine dependence with intoxication (F14.22-)

F14.24 **Cocaine dependence with cocaine-induced mood disorder**

Cocaine use disorder, moderate, with cocaine-induced bipolar or related disorder

Cocaine use disorder, moderate, with cocaine-induced depressive disorder

Cocaine use disorder, severe, with cocaine-induced bipolar or related disorder

Cocaine use disorder, severe, with cocaine-induced depressive disorder

F14.25 **Cocaine dependence with cocaine-induced psychotic disorder**

F14.250 **Cocaine dependence with cocaine-induced psychotic disorder with delusions**

F14.251 **Cocaine dependence with cocaine-induced psychotic disorder with hallucinations**

F14.259 **Cocaine dependence with cocaine-induced psychotic disorder, unspecified**

F14.28 **Cocaine dependence with other cocaine-induced disorder**

F14.280 **Cocaine dependence with cocaine-induced anxiety disorder**

F14.281 **Cocaine dependence with cocaine-induced sexual dysfunction**

F14.282 **Cocaine dependence with cocaine-induced sleep disorder**

F14.288 **Cocaine dependence with other cocaine-induced disorder**

Cocaine use disorder, moderate, with cocaine-induced obsessive compulsive or related disorder

Cocaine use disorder, severe, with cocaine-induced obsessive compulsive or related disorder

F14.29 **Cocaine dependence with unspecified cocaine-induced disorder**

F14.9 **Cocaine use, unspecified**

Excludes1: cocaine abuse (F14.1-)

cocaine dependence (F14.2-)

F14.90 **Cocaine use, unspecified, uncomplicated**

F14.92 **Cocaine use, unspecified with intoxication**

F14.920 **Cocaine use, unspecified with intoxication, uncomplicated**

F14.921 **Cocaine use, unspecified with intoxication delirium**

F14.922 **Cocaine use, unspecified with intoxication with perceptual disturbance**

F14.929 **Cocaine use, unspecified with intoxication, unspecified**

F14.94 **Cocaine use, unspecified with cocaine-induced mood disorder**

Cocaine induced bipolar or related disorder, without use disorder

Cocaine induced depressive disorder, without use disorder

F14.95 **Cocaine use, unspecified with cocaine-induced psychotic disorder**

F14.950 **Cocaine use, unspecified with cocaine-induced psychotic disorder with delusions**

F14.951 **Cocaine use, unspecified with cocaine-induced psychotic disorder with hallucinations**

F14.959 **Cocaine use, unspecified with cocaine-induced psychotic disorder, unspecified**

Cocaine induced psychotic disorder, without use disorder

F14.98 **Cocaine use, unspecified with other specified cocaine-induced disorder**

F14.980 **Cocaine use, unspecified with cocaine-induced anxiety disorder**

Cocaine induced anxiety disorder, without use disorder

F14.981 **Cocaine use, unspecified with cocaine-induced sexual dysfunction**

Cocaine induced sexual dysfunction, without use disorder

F14.982 **Cocaine use, unspecified with cocaine-induced sleep disorder**

Cocaine induced sleep disorder, without use disorder

F14.988 **Cocaine use, unspecified with other cocaine-induced disorder**

Cocaine induced obsessive compulsive or related disorder

F14.99 **Cocaine use, unspecified with unspecified cocaine-induced disorder**

F15 **Other stimulant related disorders**

Includes: amphetamine-related disorders

caffeine

Excludes2: cocaine-related disorders (F14.-)

F15.1 **Other stimulant abuse**

Excludes1: Other stimulant dependence (F15.2-)

Other stimulant use, unspecified (F15.9-)

F15.10 **Other stimulant abuse, uncomplicated**

Amphetamine type substance use disorder, mild

Other or unspecified stimulant use disorder, mild

● **F15.11** **Other stimulant abuse, in remission**

Amphetamine type substance use disorder, mild, in early remission

Amphetamine type substance use disorder, mild, in sustained remission

Other or unspecified stimulant use disorder, mild, in early remission

Other or unspecified stimulant use disorder, mild, in sustained remission

F15.12 **Other stimulant abuse with intoxication**

F15.120 **Other stimulant abuse with intoxication, uncomplicated**

F15.121 **Other stimulant abuse with intoxication delirium**

F15.122 **Other stimulant abuse with intoxication with perceptual disturbance**

Amphetamine or other stimulant use disorder, mild, with amphetamine or other stimulant intoxication, with perceptual disturbances

F15.129 **Other stimulant abuse with intoxication, unspecified**

Amphetamine or other stimulant use disorder, mild, with amphetamine or other stimulant intoxication, without perceptual disturbances

F15.14 **Other stimulant abuse with stimulant-induced mood disorder**

Amphetamine or other stimulant use disorder, mild, with amphetamine or other stimulant induced bipolar or related disorder

Amphetamine or other stimulant use disorder, mild, with amphetamine or other stimulant induced depressive disorder

F15.15 **Other stimulant abuse with stimulant-induced psychotic disorder**

F15.150 **Other stimulant abuse with stimulant-induced psychotic disorder with delusions**

F15.151 **Other stimulant abuse with stimulant-induced psychotic disorder with hallucinations**

F15.159 **Other stimulant abuse with stimulant-induced psychotic disorder, unspecified**

F15.18 **Other stimulant abuse with other stimulant-induced disorder**

F15.180 **Other stimulant abuse with stimulant-induced anxiety disorder**

F15.181 **Other stimulant abuse with stimulant-induced sexual dysfunction**

F15.182 **Other stimulant abuse with stimulant-induced sleep disorder**

F15.188 **Other stimulant abuse with other stimulant-induced disorder**

Amphetamine or other stimulant use disorder, mild, with amphetamine or other stimulant induced obsessive-compulsive or related disorder

F15.19 **Other stimulant abuse with unspecified stimulant-induced disorder**

F15.2 **Other stimulant dependence**

Excludes1: Other stimulant abuse (F15.1-)

Other stimulant use, unspecified (F15.9-)

F15.20 **Other stimulant dependence, uncomplicated**

Amphetamine type substance use disorder, moderate

Amphetamine type substance use disorder, severe

Other or unspecified stimulant use disorder, moderate

Other or unspecified stimulant use disorder, severe

F15.21 **Other stimulant dependence, in remission**

Amphetamine type substance use disorder, moderate, in early remission

Amphetamine type substance use disorder, moderate, in sustained remission

Amphetamine type substance use disorder, severe, in early remission

Amphetamine type substance use disorder, severe, in sustained remission

Other or unspecified stimulant use disorder, moderate, in early remission

Other or unspecified stimulant use disorder, moderate, in sustained remission

Other or unspecified stimulant use disorder, severe, in early remission

Other or unspecified stimulant use disorder, severe, in sustained remission

F15.22 **Other stimulant dependence with intoxication**

Excludes1: Other stimulant dependence with withdrawal (F15.23)

F15.220 **Other stimulant dependence with intoxication, uncomplicated**

F15.221 **Other stimulant dependence with intoxication delirium**

F15.222 **Other stimulant dependence with intoxication with perceptual disturbance**

Amphetamine or other stimulant use disorder, moderate, with amphetamine or other stimulant intoxication, with perceptual disturbances

Amphetamine or other stimulant use disorder, severe, with amphetamine or other stimulant intoxication, with perceptual disturbances

F15.229 **Other stimulant dependence with intoxication, unspecified**

Amphetamine **or other** stimulant use disorder, moderate, with amphetamine or other stimulant intoxication, without perceptual disturbances

Amphetamine **or other** stimulant use disorder, severe, with amphetamine **or other** stimulant intoxication, without perceptual disturbances

F15.23 **Other stimulant dependence with withdrawal**

Amphetamine **or other** stimulant withdrawal

Excludes1: Other stimulant dependence with intoxication (F15.22-)

F15.24 **Other stimulant dependence with stimulant-induced mood disorder**

Amphetamine or other stimulant use disorder, moderate, with amphetamine or other stimulant-induced bipolar or related disorder

Amphetamine or other stimulant use disorder, moderate, with amphetamine or other stimulant induced depressive disorder

Amphetamine or other stimulant use disorder, severe, with amphetamine or other stimulant-induced bipolar or related disorder

Amphetamine or other stimulant use disorder, severe, with amphetamine or other stimulant-induced depressive disorder

F15.25 **Other stimulant dependence with stimulant-induced psychotic disorder**

F15.250 **Other stimulant dependence with stimulant-induced psychotic disorder with delusions**

F15.251 **Other stimulant dependence with stimulant-induced psychotic disorder with hallucinations**

F15.259 **Other stimulant dependence with stimulant-induced psychotic disorder, unspecified**

F15.28 **Other stimulant dependence with other stimulant-induced disorder**

F15.280 **Other stimulant dependence with stimulant-induced anxiety disorder**

F15.281 **Other stimulant dependence with stimulant-induced sexual dysfunction**

F15.282   **Other stimulant dependence with stimulant-induced sleep disorder**

F15.288   **Other stimulant dependence with other stimulant-induced disorder**

Amphetamine or other stimulant use disorder, moderate, with amphetamine or other stimulant induced obsessive compulsive or related disorder

Amphetamine or other stimulant use disorder, severe, with amphetamine or other stimulant induced obsessive compulsive or related disorder

F15.29   **Other stimulant dependence with unspecified stimulant-induced disorder**

F15.9   **Other stimulant use, unspecified**

> **Excludes1:** Other stimulant abuse (F15.1-)
>
> Other stimulant dependence (F15.2-)

F15.90   **Other stimulant use, unspecified, uncomplicated**

F15.92   **Other stimulant use, unspecified with intoxication**

> **Excludes1:** Other stimulant use, unspecified with withdrawal (F15.93)

F15.920   **Other stimulant use, unspecified with intoxication, uncomplicated**

F15.921   **Other stimulant use, unspecified with intoxication delirium**

Amphetamine or other stimulant-induced delirium

F15.922   **Other stimulant use, unspecified with intoxication with perceptual disturbance**

F15.929   **Other stimulant use, unspecified with intoxication, unspecified**

Caffeine intoxication

F15.93   **Other stimulant use, unspecified with withdrawal**

Caffeine withdrawal

> **Excludes1:** Other stimulant use, unspecified with ntoxication (F15.92-)

F15.94   **Other stimulant use, unspecified with stimulant-induced mood disorder**

Amphetamine or other stimulant-induced bipolar or related disorder, without use disorder

Amphetamine or other stimulant-induced depressive disorder, without use disorder

F15.95   **Other stimulant use, unspecified with stimulant-induced psychotic disorder**

F15.950   **Other stimulant use, unspecified with stimulant-induced psychotic disorder with delusions**

F15.951   **Other stimulant use, unspecified with stimulant-induced psychotic disorder with hallucinations**

F15.959   **Other stimulant use, unspecified with stimulant-induced psychotic disorder, unspecified**

Amphetamine or other stimulant-induced psychotic disorder, without use disorder

F15.98   **Other stimulant use, unspecified with other stimulant-induced disorder**

F15.980   **Other stimulant use, unspecified with stimulant-induced anxiety disorder**

Amphetamine or other stimulant-induced anxiety disorder, without use disorder

Caffeine induced anxiety disorder, without use disorder

F15.981   **Other stimulant use, unspecified with stimulant-induced sexual dysfunction**

Amphetamine or other stimulant-induced sexual dysfunction, without use disorder

F15.982   **Other stimulant use, unspecified with stimulant-induced sleep disorder**

Amphetamine or other stimulant-induced sleep disorder, without use disorder

Caffeine induced sleep disorder, without use disorder

F15.988   **Other stimulant use, unspecified with other stimulant-induced disorder**

Amphetamine or other stimulant-induced obsessive compulsive or related disorder, without use disorder

F15.99   **Other stimulant use, unspecified with unspecified stimulant-induced disorder**

F16   **Hallucinogen related disorders**

> **Includes:** ecstasy
>
> PCP phencyclidine

F16.1   **Hallucinogen abuse**

> **Excludes1:** hallucinogen dependence (F16.2-)
>
> hallucinogen use, unspecified (F16.9-)

F16.10   **Hallucinogen abuse, uncomplicated**

Other hallucinogen use disorder, mild

Phencyclidine use disorder, mild

● **F16.11**   **Hallucinogen abuse, in remission**

Other hallucinogen use disorder, mild, in early remission

Other hallucinogen use disorder, mild, in sustained remission

Phencyclidine use disorder, mild, in early remission

Phencyclidine use disorder, mild, in sustained remission

F16.12   **Hallucinogen abuse with intoxication**

F16.120   **Hallucinogen abuse with intoxication, uncomplicated**

F16.121   **Hallucinogen abuse with intoxication with delirium**

F16.122   **Hallucinogen abuse with intoxication with perceptual disturbance**

F16.129   **Hallucinogen abuse with intoxication, unspecified**

F16.14   **Hallucinogen abuse with hallucinogen-induced mood disorder**

Other hallucinogen use disorder, mild, with other hallucinogen induced bipolar or related disorder

Other hallucinogen use disorder, mild, with other hallucinogen induced depressive disorder

Phencyclidine use disorder, mild, with phencyclidine induced bipolar or related disorder

Phencyclidine use disorder, mild, with phencyclidine induced depressive disorder

F16.15   **Hallucinogen abuse with hallucinogen-induced psychotic disorder**

F16.150 **Hallucinogen abuse with hallucinogen-induced psychotic disorder with delusions**

F16.151 **Hallucinogen abuse with hallucinogen-induced psychotic disorder with hallucinations**

F16.159 **Hallucinogen abuse with hallucinogen-induced psychotic disorder, unspecified**

F16.18 **Hallucinogen abuse with other hallucinogen-induced disorder**

F16.180 **Hallucinogen abuse with hallucinogen-induced anxiety disorder**

F16.183 **Hallucinogen abuse with hallucinogen persisting perception disorder (flashbacks)**

F16.188 **Hallucinogen abuse with other hallucinogen-induced disorder**

F16.19 **Hallucinogen abuse with unspecified hallucinogen-induced disorder**

F16.2 **Hallucinogen dependence**

Excludes1: hallucinogen abuse (F16.1-)

hallucinogen use, unspecified (F16.9-)

F16.20 **Hallucinogen dependence, uncomplicated**

Other hallucinogen use disorder, moderate

Other hallucinogen use disorder, severe

Phencyclidine use disorder, moderate

Phencyclidine use disorder, severe

F16.21 **Hallucinogen dependence, in remission**

Other hallucinogen use disorder, moderate, in early remission

Other hallucinogen use disorder, moderate, in sustained remission

Other hallucinogen use disorder, severe, in early remission

Other hallucinogen use disorder, severe, in sustained remission

Phencyclidine use disorder, moderate, in early remission

Phencyclidine use disorder, moderate, in sustained remission

Phencyclidine use disorder, severe, in early remission

Phencyclidine use disorder, severe, in sustained remission

F16.22 **Hallucinogen dependence with intoxication**

F16.220 **Hallucinogen dependence with intoxication, uncomplicated**

F16.221 **Hallucinogen dependence with intoxication with delirium**

F16.229 **Hallucinogen dependence with intoxication, unspecified**

F16.24 **Hallucinogen dependence with hallucinogen-induced mood disorder**

Other hallucinogen use disorder, moderate, with other hallucinogen induced bipolar or related disorder

Other hallucinogen use disorder, moderate, with other hallucinogen induced depressive disorder

Other hallucinogen use disorder, severe, with other hallucinogen-induced bipolar or related disorder

Other hallucinogen use disorder, severe, with other hallucinogen-induced depressive disorder

Phencyclidine use disorder, moderate, with phencyclidine induced bipolar or related disorder

Phencyclidine use disorder, moderate, with phencyclidine induced depressive disorder

Phencyclidine use disorder, severe, with phencyclidine induced bipolar or related disorder

Phencyclidine use disorder, severe, with phencyclidine-induced depressive disorder

F16.25 **Hallucinogen dependence with hallucinogen-induced psychotic disorder**

F16.250 **Hallucinogen dependence with hallucinogen-induced psychotic disorder with delusions**

F16.251 **Hallucinogen dependence with hallucinogen-induced psychotic disorder with hallucinations**

F16.259 **Hallucinogen dependence with hallucinogen-induced psychotic disorder, unspecified**

F16.28 **Hallucinogen dependence with other hallucinogen-induced disorder**

F16.280 **Hallucinogen dependence with hallucinogen-induced anxiety disorder**

F16.283 **Hallucinogen dependence with hallucinogen persisting perception disorder (flashbacks)**

F16.288 **Hallucinogen dependence with other hallucinogen-induced disorder**

F16.29 **Hallucinogen dependence with unspecified hallucinogen-induced disorder**

F16.9 **Hallucinogen use, unspecified**

Excludes1: hallucinogen abuse (F16.1-)

hallucinogen dependence (F16.2-)

F16.90 **Hallucinogen use, unspecified, uncomplicated**

F16.92 **Hallucinogen use, unspecified with intoxication**

F16.920 **Hallucinogen use, unspecified with intoxication, uncomplicated**

F16.921 **Hallucinogen use, unspecified with intoxication with delirium**

Other hallucinogen intoxication delirium

F16.929 **Hallucinogen use, unspecified with intoxication, unspecified**

F16.94 **Hallucinogen use, unspecified with hallucinogen-induced mood disorder**

Other hallucinogen induced bipolar or related disorder, without use disorder

Other hallucinogen induced depressive disorder, without use disorder

Phencyclidine induced bipolar or related disorder, without use disorder

Phencyclidine induced depressive disorder, without use disorder

F16.95 **Hallucinogen use, unspecified with hallucinogen-induced psychotic disorder**

F16.950 **Hallucinogen use, unspecified with hallucinogen-induced psychotic disorder with delusions**

F16.951 **Hallucinogen use, unspecified with hallucinogen-induced psychotic disorder with hallucinations**

F16.959 **Hallucinogen use, unspecified with hallucinogen-induced psychotic disorder, unspecified**

Other hallucinogen induced psychotic disorder, without use disorder

Phencyclidine induced psychotic disorder, without use disorder

F16.98 **Hallucinogen use, unspecified with other specified hallucinogen-induced disorder**

F16.980 **Hallucinogen use, unspecified with hallucinogen-induced anxiety disorder**

Other hallucinogen-induced anxiety disorder, without use disorder

Phencyclidine induced anxiety disorder, without use disorder

F16.983 **Hallucinogen use, unspecified with hallucinogen persisting perception disorder (flashbacks)**

F16.988 **Hallucinogen use, unspecified with other hallucinogen-induced disorder**

F16.99 **Hallucinogen use, unspecified with unspecified hallucinogen-induced disorder**

F17 **Nicotine dependence**

Excludes1: history of tobacco dependence (Z87.891)
tobacco use NOS (Z72.0)

Excludes2: tobacco use (smoking) during pregnancy, childbirth and the puerperium (O99.33-)
toxic effect of nicotine (T65.2-)

F17.2 **Nicotine dependence**

F17.20 **Nicotine dependence, unspecified**

F17.200 **Nicotine dependence, unspecified, uncomplicated**

Tobacco use disorder, mild

Tobacco use disorder, moderate

Tobacco use disorder, severe

F17.201 **Nicotine dependence, unspecified, in remission**

Tobacco use disorder, mild, in early remission

Tobacco use disorder, mild, in sustained remission

Tobacco use disorder, moderate, in early remission

Tobacco use disorder, moderate, in sustained remission

Tobacco use disorder, severe, in early remission

Tobacco use disorder, severe, in sustained remission

F17.203 **Nicotine dependence unspecified, with withdrawal**

Tobacco withdrawal

F17.208 **Nicotine dependence, unspecified, with other nicotine-induced disorders**

F17.209 **Nicotine dependence, unspecified, with unspecified nicotine-induced disorders**

F17.21 **Nicotine dependence, cigarettes**

F17.210 **Nicotine dependence, cigarettes, uncomplicated**

F17.211 **Nicotine dependence, cigarettes, in remission**

Tobacco use disorder, cigarettes, mild, in early remission

Tobacco use disorder, cigarettes, mild, in sustained remission

Tobacco use disorder, cigarettes, moderate, in early remission

Tobacco use disorder, cigarettes, moderate, in sustained remission

Tobacco use disorder, cigarettes, severe, in early remission

Tobacco use disorder, cigarettes, severe, in sustained remission

F17.213 **Nicotine dependence, cigarettes, with withdrawal**

F17.218 **Nicotine dependence, cigarettes, with other nicotine-induced disorders**

F17.219 **Nicotine dependence, cigarettes, with unspecified nicotine-induced disorders**

F17.22 **Nicotine dependence, chewing tobacco**

F17.220 **Nicotine dependence, chewing tobacco, uncomplicated**

F17.221 **Nicotine dependence, chewing tobacco, in remission**

Tobacco use disorder, chewing tobacco, mild, in early remission

Tobacco use disorder, chewing tobacco, mild, in sustained remission

Tobacco use disorder, chewing tobacco, moderate, in early remission

Tobacco use disorder, chewing tobacco, moderate, in sustained remission

Tobacco use disorder, chewing tobacco, severe, in early remission

Tobacco use disorder, chewing tobacco, severe, in sustained remission

F17.223 **Nicotine dependence, chewing tobacco, with withdrawal**

F17.228 **Nicotine dependence, chewing tobacco, with other nicotine-induced disorders**

F17.229 **Nicotine dependence, chewing tobacco, with unspecified nicotine-induced disorders**

F17.29 **Nicotine dependence, other tobacco product**

F17.290 **Nicotine dependence, other tobacco product, uncomplicated**

F17.291 **Nicotine dependence, other tobacco product, in remission**

Tobacco use disorder, other tobacco product, mild, in early remission

Tobacco use disorder, other tobacco product, mild, in sustained remission

Tobacco use disorder, other tobacco product, moderate, in early remission

Tobacco use disorder, other tobacco product, moderate, in sustained remission

Tobacco use disorder, other tobacco product, severe, in early remission

Tobacco use disorder, other tobacco product, severe, in sustained remission

F17.293 **Nicotine dependence, other tobacco product, with withdrawal**

● New code   ▲ Revised code   **Excludes1:** Not coded here   **Excludes2:** Not included here   ⊗ Placeholder required   ⑦7th digit required

F17.298 Nicotine dependence, other tobacco product, with other nicotine-induced disorders

F17.299 Nicotine dependence, other tobacco product, with unspecified nicotine-induced disorders

F18 **Inhalant related disorders**

Includes: volatile solvents

F18.1 **Inhalant abuse**

Excludes1: inhalant dependence (F18.2-)

inhalant use, unspecified (F18.9-)

F18.10 **Inhalant abuse, uncomplicated**

Inhalant use disorder, mild

●**F18.11** **Inhalant abuse, in remission**

Inhalant use disorder, mild, in early remission

Inhalant use disorder, mild, in sustained remission

F18.12 **Inhalant abuse with intoxication**

F18.120 **Inhalant abuse with intoxication, uncomplicated**

F18.121 **Inhalant abuse with intoxication delirium**

F18.129 **Inhalant abuse with intoxication, unspecified**

F18.14 **Inhalant abuse with inhalant-induced mood disorder**

Inhalant use disorder, mild, with inhalant induced depressive disorder

F18.15 **Inhalant abuse with inhalant-induced psychotic disorder**

F18.150 **Inhalant abuse with inhalant-induced psychotic disorder with delusions**

F18.151 **Inhalant abuse with inhalant-induced psychotic disorder with hallucinations**

F18.159 **Inhalant abuse with inhalant-induced psychotic disorder, unspecified**

F18.17 **Inhalant abuse with inhalant-induced dementia**

Inhalant use disorder, mild, with inhalant induced major neurocognitive disorder

F18.18 **Inhalant abuse with other inhalant-induced disorders**

F18.180 **Inhalant abuse with inhalant-induced anxiety disorder**

F18.188 **Inhalant abuse with other inhalant-induced disorder**

Inhalant use disorder, mild, with inhalant induced mild neurocognitive disorder

F18.19 **Inhalant abuse with unspecified inhalant-induced disorder**

F18.2 **Inhalant dependence**

Excludes1: inhalant abuse (F18.1-)

inhalant use, unspecified (F18.9-)

F18.20 **Inhalant dependence, uncomplicated**

Inhalant use disorder, moderate

Inhalant use disorder, severe

F18.21 **Inhalant dependence, in remission**

Inhalant use disorder, moderate, in early remission

Inhalant use disorder, moderate, in sustained remission

Inhalant use disorder, severe, in early remission

Inhalant use disorder, severe, in sustained remission

F18.22 **Inhalant dependence with intoxication**

F18.220 **Inhalant dependence with intoxication, uncomplicated**

F18.221 **Inhalant dependence with intoxication delirium**

F18.229 **Inhalant dependence with intoxication, unspecified**

F18.24 **Inhalant dependence with inhalant-induced mood disorder**

Inhalant use disorder, moderate, with inhalant induced depressive disorder

Inhalant use disorder, severe, with inhalant induced depressive disorder

F18.25 **Inhalant dependence with inhalant-induced psychotic disorder**

F18.250 **Inhalant dependence with inhalant-induced psychotic disorder with delusions**

F18.251 **Inhalant dependence with inhalant-induced psychotic disorder with hallucinations**

F18.259 **Inhalant dependence with inhalant-induced psychotic disorder, unspecified**

F18.27 **Inhalant dependence with inhalant-induced dementia**

Inhalant use disorder, moderate, with inhalant induced major neurocognitive disorder

Inhalant use disorder, severe, with inhalant induced major neurocognitive disorder

F18.28 **Inhalant dependence with other inhalant-induced disorders**

F18.280 **Inhalant dependence with inhalant-induced anxiety disorder**

F18.288 **Inhalant dependence with other inhalant-induced disorder**

Inhalant use disorder, moderate, with inhalant-induced mild neurocognitive disorder

Inhalant use disorder, severe, with inhalant-induced mild neurocognitive disorder

F18.29 **Inhalant dependence with unspecified inhalant-induced disorder**

F18.9 **Inhalant use, unspecified**

Excludes1: inhalant abuse (F18.1-)

inhalant dependence (F18.2-)

F18.90 **Inhalant use, unspecified, uncomplicated**

F18.92 **Inhalant use, unspecified with intoxication**

F18.920 **Inhalant use, unspecified with intoxication, uncomplicated**

F18.921 **Inhalant use, unspecified with intoxication with delirium**

F18.929 **Inhalant use, unspecified with intoxication, unspecified**

F18.94 **Inhalant use, unspecified with inhalant-induced mood disorder**

Inhalant induced depressive disorder

F18.95 **Inhalant use, unspecified with inhalant-induced psychotic disorder**

▨ Add 4th-7th digits	▨ Nonspecific code	▨ Unspecified code	▨ Manifestation code

F18.950   **Inhalant use, unspecified with inhalant-induced psychotic disorder with delusions**

F18.951   **Inhalant use, unspecified with inhalant-induced psychotic disorder with hallucinations**

F18.959   **Inhalant use, unspecified with inhalant-induced psychotic disorder, unspecified**

F18.97   **Inhalant use, unspecified with inhalant-induced persisting dementia**

Inhalant-induced major neurocognitive disorder

F18.98   **Inhalant use, unspecified with other inhalant-induced disorders**

F18.980   **Inhalant use, unspecified with inhalant-induced anxiety disorder**

F18.988   **Inhalant use, unspecified with other inhalant-induced disorder**

Inhalant-induced mild neurocognitive disorder

F18.99   **Inhalant use, unspecified with unspecified inhalant-induced disorder**

F19   **Other psychoactive substance related disorders**

Includes: polysubstance drug use (indiscriminate drug use)

F19.1   **Other psychoactive substance abuse**

Excludes1: Other psychoactive substance dependence (F19.2-)

Other psychoactive substance use, unspecified (F19.9-)

F19.10   **Other psychoactive substance abuse, uncomplicated**

Other (or unknown) substance use disorder, mild

•F19.11   **Other psychoactive substance abuse, in remission**

Other (or unknown) substance use disorder, mild, in early remission

Other (or unknown) substance use disorder, mild, in sustained remission

F19.12   **Other psychoactive substance abuse with intoxication**

F19.120   **Other psychoactive substance abuse with intoxication, uncomplicated**

F19.121   **Other psychoactive substance abuse with intoxication delirium**

F19.122   **Other psychoactive substance abuse with intoxication with perceptual disturbances**

F19.129   **Other psychoactive substance abuse with intoxication, unspecified**

F19.14   **Other psychoactive substance abuse with psychoactive substance-induced mood disorder**

Other (or unknown) substance use disorder, mild, with other (or unknown) substance-induced bipolar or related disorder

Other (or unknown) substance use disorder, mild, with other (or unknown) substance-induced depressive disorder

F19.15   **Other psychoactive substance abuse with psychoactive substance-induced psychotic disorder**

F19.150   **Other psychoactive substance abuse with psychoactive substance-induced psychotic disorder with delusions**

F19.151   **Other psychoactive substance abuse with psychoactive substance-induced psychotic disorder with hallucinations**

F19.159   **Other psychoactive substance abuse with psychoactive substance-induced psychotic disorder, unspecified**

F19.16   **Other psychoactive substance abuse with psychoactive substance-induced persisting amnestic disorder**

F19.17   **Other psychoactive substance abuse with psychoactive substance-induced persisting dementia**

Other (or unknown) substance use disorder, mild, with other (or unknown) substance-induced major neurocognitive disorder

F19.18   **Other psychoactive substance abuse with other psychoactive substance-induced disorders**

F19.180   **Other psychoactive substance abuse with psychoactive substance-induced anxiety disorder**

F19.181   **Other psychoactive substance abuse with psychoactive substance-induced sexual dysfunction**

F19.182   **Other psychoactive substance abuse with psychoactive substance-induced sleep disorder**

F19.188   **Other psychoactive substance abuse with other psychoactive substance-induced disorder**

Other (or unknown) substance use disorder, mild, with other (or unknown) substance induced mild neurocognitive disorder

Other (or unknown) substance use disorder, mild, with other (or unknown) substance induced obsessive-compulsive or elated disorder

F19.19   **Other psychoactive substance abuse with unspecified psychoactive substance-induced disorder**

F19.2   **Other psychoactive substance dependence**

Excludes1: Other psychoactive substance abuse (F19.1-)

Other psychoactive substance use, unspecified (F19.9-)

F19.20   **Other psychoactive substance dependence, uncomplicated**

Other (or unknown) substance use disorder, moderate **Other** (or unknown) substance use disorder, severe

F19.21   **Other psychoactive substance dependence, in remission**

Other (or unknown) substance use disorder, moderate, in early remission

Other (or unknown) substance use disorder, moderate, in sustained remission

Other (or unknown) substance use disorder, severe, in early remission

Other (or unknown) substance use, severe, in sustained remission

F19.22   **Other psychoactive substance dependence with intoxication**

Excludes1: Other psychoactive substance dependence with withdrawal (F19.23-)

   ● New code   ▲ Revised code   **Excludes1:** Not coded here   **Excludes2:** Not included here   ⊗ Placeholder required   ⑦ 7th digit required

F19.220 **Other psychoactive substance dependence with intoxication, uncomplicated**

F19.221 **Other psychoactive substance dependence with intoxication delirium**

F9.2122 **Other psychoactive substance dependence with intoxication with perceptual disturbance**

F19.229 **Other psychoactive substance dependence with intoxication, unspecified**

F19.23 **Other psychoactive substance dependence with withdrawal**

Excludes1: Other psychoactive substance dependence with intoxication (F19.22-)

F19.230 **Other psychoactive substance dependence with withdrawal, uncomplicated**

F19.231 **Other psychoactive substance dependence with withdrawal delirium**

F19.232 **Other psychoactive substance dependence with withdrawal with perceptual disturbance**

F19.239 **Other psychoactive substance dependence with withdrawal, unspecified**

F19.24 **Other psychoactive substance dependence with psychoactive substance-induced mood disorder**

Other (or unknown) substance use disorder, moderate, with other (or unknown) substance induced bipolar or related disorder

Other (or unknown) substance use disorder, moderate, with other (or unknown) substance induced depressive disorder

Other (or unknown) substance use disorder, severe, with other (or unknown) substance induced bipolar or related disorder

Other (or unknown) substance use disorder, severe, with other (or unknown) substance induced depressive disorder

F19.25 **Other psychoactive substance dependence with psychoactive substance-induced psychotic disorder**

F19.250 **Other psychoactive substance dependence with psychoactive substance-induced psychotic disorder with delusions**

F19.251 **Other psychoactive substance dependence with psychoactive substance-induced psychotic disorder with hallucinations**

F19.259 **Other psychoactive substance dependence with psychoactive substance-induced psychotic disorder, unspecified**

F19.26 **Other psychoactive substance dependence with psychoactive substance-induced persisting amnestic disorder**

F19.27 **Other psychoactive substance dependence with psychoactive substance-induced persisting dementia**

Other (or unknown) substance use disorder, moderate, with other (or unknown) substance induced major neurocognitive disorder

Other (or unknown) substance use disorder, severe, with other (or unknown) substance induced major neurocognitive disorder

F19.28 **Other psychoactive substance dependence with other psychoactive substance-induced disorders**

F19.280 **Other psychoactive substance dependence with psychoactive substance-induced anxiety disorder**

F19.281 **Other psychoactive substance dependence with psychoactive substance-induced sexual dysfunction**

F19.282 **Other psychoactive substance dependence with psychoactive substance-induced sleep disorder**

F19.288 **Other psychoactive substance dependence with other psychoactive substance-induced disorder**

Other (or unknown) substance use disorder, moderate, with other (or unknown) substance induced mild neurocognitive disorder

Other (or unknown) substance use disorder, severe, with other (or unknown) substance induced mild neurocognitive disorder

Other (or unknown) substance use disorder, moderate, with other (or unknown) substance induced obsessive compulsive or related disorder

Other (or unknown) substance use disorder, severe, with other (or unknown) substance induced obsessive-compulsive or related disorder

F19.29 **Other psychoactive substance dependence with unspecified psychoactive substance-induced disorder**

F19.9 **Other psychoactive substance use, unspecified**

Excludes1: Other psychoactive substance abuse (F19.1-)

Other psychoactive substance dependence (F19.2-)

F19.90 **Other psychoactive substance use, unspecified, uncomplicated**

F19.92 **Other psychoactive substance use, unspecified with intoxication**

Excludes1: Other psychoactive substance use, unspecified with withdrawal (F19.93)

F19.920 **Other psychoactive substance use, unspecified with intoxication, uncomplicated**

F19.921 **Other psychoactive substance use, unspecified with intoxication with delirium**

Other (or unknown) substance-induced delirium

F19.922 **Other psychoactive substance use, unspecified with intoxication with perceptual disturbance**

F19.929 **Other psychoactive substance use, unspecified with intoxication, unspecified**

F19.93 **Other psychoactive substance use, unspecified with withdrawal**

Excludes1: Other psychoactive substance use, unspecified with intoxication (F19.92-)

F19.930   **Other psychoactive substance use, unspecified with withdrawal, uncomplicated**

F19.931   **Other psychoactive substance use, unspecified with withdrawal delirium**

F19.932   **Other psychoactive substance use, unspecified with withdrawal with perceptual disturbance**

F19.939   **Other psychoactive substance use, unspecified with withdrawal, unspecified**

F19.94   **Other psychoactive substance use, unspecified with psychoactive substance-induced mood disorder**

Other (or unknown) substance-induced bipolar or related disorder, without use disorder

Other (or unknown) substance-induced depressive disorder, without use disorder

F19.95   **Other psychoactive substance use, unspecified with psychoactive substance-induced psychotic disorder**

F19.950   **Other psychoactive substance use, unspecified with psychoactive substance-induced psychotic disorder with delusions**

F19.951   **Other psychoactive substance use, unspecified with psychoactive substance-induced psychotic disorder with hallucinations**

F19.959   **Other psychoactive substance use, unspecified with psychoactive substance-induced psychotic disorder, unspecified**

Other or unknown substance-induced psychotic disorder, without use disorder

F19.96   **Other psychoactive substance use, unspecified with psychoactive substance-induced persisting amnestic disorder**

F19.97   **Other psychoactive substance use, unspecified with psychoactive substance-induced persisting dementia**

Other (or unknown) substance-induced major neurocognitive disorder, without use disorder

F19.98   **Other psychoactive substance use, unspecified with other psychoactive substance-induced disorders**

F19.980   **Other psychoactive substance use, unspecified with psychoactive substance-induced anxiety disorder**

Other (or unknown) substance-induced anxiety disorder, without use disorder

F19.981   **Other psychoactive substance use, unspecified with psychoactive substance-induced sexual dysfunction**

Other (or unknown) substance-induced sexual dysfunction, without use disorder

F19.982   **Other psychoactive substance use, unspecified with psychoactive substance-induced sleep disorder**

Other (or unknown) substance-induced sleep disorder, without use disorder

F19.988   **Other psychoactive substance use, unspecified with other psychoactive substance-induced disorder**

Other (or unknown) substance-induced mild neurocognitive disorder, without use disorder

Other (or unknown) substance-induced obsessive-compulsive or related disorder, without use disorder

F19.99   **Other psychoactive substance use, unspecified with unspecified psychoactive substance-induced disorder**

SCHIZOPHRENIA, SCHIZOTYPAL, DELUSIONAL, AND OTHER NON-MOOD PSYCHOTIC DISORDERS (F20-F29)

F20   **Schizophrenia**

Definition: Schizophrenia is a psychotic disorder marked by severely impaired thinking, emotions, and behaviors. Schizophrenic patients are typically unable to filter sensory stimuli and may have enhanced perceptions of sounds, colors, and other features of their environment.

Excludes1: brief psychotic disorder (F23)

cyclic schizophrenia (F25.0)

mood [affective] disorders with psychotic symptoms (F30.2, F31.2, F31.5, F31.64, F32.3, F33.3)

schizoaffective disorder (F25.-)

schizophrenic reaction NOS (F23)

Excludes2: schizophrenic reaction in:

alcoholism (F10.15-, F10.25-, F10.95-)

brain disease (F06.2)

epilepsy (F06.2)

psychoactive drug use (F11-F19 with .15. .25, .95)

schizotypal disorder (F21)

F20.0   **Paranoid schizophrenia**

Paraphrenic schizophrenia

Excludes1: involutional paranoid state (F22)

paranoia (F22)

F20.1   **Disorganized schizophrenia**

Hebephrenic schizophrenia

Hebephrenia

F20.2   **Catatonic schizophrenia**

Schizophrenic catalepsy

Schizophrenic catatonia

Schizophrenic flexibilitas cerea

Excludes1: catatonic stupor (R40.1)

F20.3   **Undifferentiated schizophrenia**

Atypical schizophrenia

Excludes1: acute schizophrenia-like psychotic disorder (F23)

Excludes2: post-schizophrenic depression (F32.89)

F20.5   **Residual schizophrenia**

Restzustand (schizophrenic)

Schizophrenic residual state

F20.8   **Other schizophrenia**

F20.81   **Schizophreniform disorder**

Schizophreniform psychosis NOS

F20.89   **Other schizophrenia**

Cenesthopathic schizophrenia

Simple schizophrenia

F20.9   **Schizophrenia, unspecified**

F21   **Schizotypal disorder**

Borderline schizophrenia

Latent schizophrenia

Latent schizophrenic reaction

Prepsychotic schizophrenia

Prodromal schizophrenia

Pseudoneurotic schizophrenia

Pseudopsychopathic schizophrenia

Schizotypal personality disorder

Excludes2: Asperger's syndrome (F84.5)

    schizoid personality disorder (F60.1)

F22 **Delusional disorders**

Delusional dysmorphophobia

Involutional paranoid state

Paranoia

Paranoia querulans

Paranoid psychosis

Paranoid state

Paraphrenia (late)

Sensitiver Beziehungswahn

Excludes1: mood [affective] disorders with psychotic symptoms
    (F30.2, F31.2, F31.5, F31.64, F32.3, F33.3)

    paranoid schizophrenia (F20.0)

Excludes2: paranoid personality disorder (F60.0)

    paranoid psychosis, psychogenic (F23)

    paranoid reaction (F23)

F23 **Brief psychotic disorder**

Paranoid reaction

Psychogenic paranoid psychosis

Excludes2: mood [affective] disorders with psychotic symptoms
    (F30.2, F31.2, F31.5, F31.64, F32.3, F33.3)

F24 **Shared psychotic disorder**

Folie à deux

Induced paranoid disorder

Induced psychotic disorder

F25 **Schizoaffective disorders**

Excludes1: mood [affective] disorders with psychotic symptoms
    (F30.2, F31.2, F31.5, F31.64, F32.3, F33.3)

    schizophrenia (F20.-)

F25.0 **Schizoaffective disorder, bipolar type**
Cyclic schizophrenia

Schizoaffective disorder, mixed type

Schizoaffective psychosis, bipolar type

Schizophreniform psychosis, manic type

F25.1 **Schizoaffective disorder, depressive type**

Schizophreniform psychosis, depressive type

F25.8 **Other schizoaffective disorders**

F25.9 **Schizoaffective disorder, unspecified**

Schizoaffective psychosis NOS

F28 **Other psychotic disorder not due to a substance or known physiological condition**

Chronic hallucinatory psychosis

F29 **Unspecified psychosis not due to a substance or known physiological condition**

Psychosis NOS

Excludes1: mental disorder NOS (F99)

    unspecified mental disorder due to known physiological condition (F09)

MOOD [AFFECTIVE] DISORDERS (F30-F39)

Definition: A mood disorder, also referred to as an affective disorder, is a condition impacting mood and related functions. In a mood disorder,

moods range from extremely low (depressed) to extremely high or irritable (manic).

F30 **Manic episode**

Includes: bipolar disorder, single manic episode

    mixed affective episode

Excludes1: bipolar disorder (F31.-)

    major depressive disorder, single episode (F32.-)

    major depressive disorder, recurrent (F33.-)

F30.1 **Manic episode without psychotic symptoms**

F30.10 **Manic episode without psychotic symptoms, unspecified**

F30.11 **Manic episode without psychotic symptoms, mild**

F30.12 **Manic episode without psychotic symptoms, moderate**

F30.13 **Manic episode, severe, without psychotic symptoms**

F30.2 **Manic episode, severe with psychotic symptoms**

Manic stupor

Mania with mood-congruent psychotic symptoms

Mania with mood-incongruent psychotic symptoms

F30.3 **Manic episode in partial remission**

F30.4 **Manic episode in full remission**

F30.8 **Other manic episodes**

Hypomania

F30.9 **Manic episode, unspecified**

Mania NOS

F31 **Bipolar disorder**

Definition: Bipolar disorder, formerly called manic depression, is a mental illness that brings severe high and low moods and changes in sleep, energy, thinking, and behavior.

Includes: bipolar I disorder

    bipolar type I disorder

    manic-depressive illness

    manic-depressive psychosis manic-depressive reaction

Excludes1: bipolar disorder, single manic episode (F30.-)

    major depressive disorder, single episode (F32.-)

    major depressive disorder, recurrent (F33.-)

Excludes2: cyclothymia (F34.0)

F31.0 **Bipolar disorder, current episode hypomanic**

F31.1 **Bipolar disorder, current episode manic without psychotic features**

F31.10 **Bipolar disorder, current episode manic without psychotic features, unspecified**

F31.11 **Bipolar disorder, current episode manic without psychotic features, mild**

F31.12 **Bipolar disorder, current episode manic without psychotic features, moderate**

F31.13 **Bipolar disorder, current episode manic without psychotic features, severe**

F31.2 **Bipolar disorder, current episode manic severe with psychotic features**

Bipolar disorder, current episode manic with mood-congruent psychotic symptoms

Bipolar disorder, current episode manic with mood-incongruent psychotic symptoms

F31.3 **Bipolar disorder, current episode depressed, mild or moderate severity**

F31.30 **Bipolar disorder, current episode depressed, mild or moderate severity, unspecified**

F31.31 **Bipolar disorder, current episode depressed, mild**

F31.32 **Bipolar disorder, current episode depressed, moderate**

F31.4 **Bipolar disorder, current episode depressed, severe, without psychotic features**

F31.5 **Bipolar disorder, current episode depressed, severe, with psychotic features**

Bipolar disorder, current episode depressed with mood-incongruent psychotic symptoms

Bipolar disorder, current episode depressed with mood-congruent psychotic symptoms

Bipolar I disorder, current or most recent episode depressed, with psychotic features

F31.6 **Bipolar disorder, current episode mixed**

    F31.60 **Bipolar disorder, current episode mixed, unspecified**

    F31.61 **Bipolar disorder, current episode mixed, mild**

    F31.62 **Bipolar disorder, current episode mixed, moderate**

    F31.63 **Bipolar disorder, current episode mixed, severe, without psychotic features**

    F31.64 **Bipolar disorder, current episode mixed, severe, with psychotic features**

Bipolar disorder, current episode mixed with mood-congruent psychotic symptoms

Bipolar disorder, current episode mixed with mood-incongruent psychotic symptoms

F31.7 **Bipolar disorder, currently in remission**

    F31.70 **Bipolar disorder, currently in remission, most recent episode unspecified**

    F31.71 **Bipolar disorder, in partial remission, most recent episode hypomanic**

    F31.72 **Bipolar disorder, in full remission, most recent episode hypomanic**

    F31.73 **Bipolar disorder, in partial remission, most recent episode manic**

    F31.74 **Bipolar disorder, in full remission, most recent episode manic**

    F31.75 **Bipolar disorder, in partial remission, most recent episode depressed**

    F31.76 **Bipolar disorder, in full remission, most recent episode depressed**

    F31.77 **Bipolar disorder, in partial remission, most recent episode mixed**

    F31.78 **Bipolar disorder, in full remission, most recent episode mixed**

F31.8 **Other bipolar disorders**

    F31.81 **Bipolar II disorder**

Bipolar disorder, type 2

    F31.89 **Other bipolar disorder**

Recurrent manic episodes NOS

F31.9 **Bipolar disorder, unspecified**

Manic depression

F32 **Major depressive disorder, single episode**

Includes: single episode of agitated depression

single episode of depressive reaction single episode of major depression

single episode of psychogenic depression single episode of reactive depression single episode of vital depression

Excludes1: bipolar disorder (F31.-)

manic episode (F30.-)

recurrent depressive disorder (F33.-)

Excludes2: adjustment disorder (F43.2)

F32.0 **Major depressive disorder, single episode, mild**

F32.1 **Major depressive disorder, single episode, moderate**

F32.2 **Major depressive disorder, single episode, severe without psychotic features**

F32.3 **Major depressive disorder, single episode, severe with psychotic features**

Single episode of major depression with mood-congruent psychotic symptoms

Single episode of major depression with mood-incongruent psychotic symptoms

Single episode of major depression with psychotic symptoms

Single episode of psychogenic depressive psychosis

Single episode of psychotic depression

Single episode of reactive depressive psychosis

F32.4 **Major depressive disorder, single episode, in partial remission**

F32.5 **Major depressive disorder, single episode, in full remission**

F32.8 **Other depressive episodes**

    F32.81 **Premenstrual dysphoric disorder**

        Excludes1: premenstrual tension syndrome (N94.3)

    F32.89 **Other specified depressive episodes**

Atypical depression

Post-schizophrenic depression

Single episode of 'masked' depression NOS

F32.9 **Major depressive disorder, single episode, unspecified**

Depression NOS

Depressive disorder NOS

Major depression NOS

F33 **Major depressive disorder, recurrent**

Includes: recurrent episodes of depressive reaction

recurrent episodes of endogenous depression recurrent episodes of major depression

recurrent episodes of psychogenic depression recurrent episodes of reactive depression

recurrent episodes of seasonal depressive disorder recurrent episodes of vital depression

Excludes1: bipolar disorder (F31.-)

manic episode (F30.-)

F33.0 **Major depressive disorder, recurrent, mild**

F33.1 **Major depressive disorder, recurrent, moderate**

F33.2 **Major depressive disorder, recurrent severe without psychotic features**

F33.3 **Major depressive disorder, recurrent, severe with psychotic symptoms**

Endogenous depression with psychotic symptoms

Major depressive disorder, recurrent, with psychotic features

Recurrent severe episodes of major depression with mood-congruent psychotic symptoms

Recurrent severe episodes of major depression with mood-incongruent psychotic symptoms

Recurrent severe episodes of major depression with psychotic symptoms

Recurrent severe episodes of psychogenic depressive psychosis

Recurrent severe episodes of psychotic depression

Recurrent severe episodes of reactive depressive psychosis

F33.4 **Major depressive disorder, recurrent, in remission**

  ● New code ▲ Revised code **Excludes1:** Not coded here **Excludes2:** Not included here ⊗ Placeholder required ⑦7th digit required

F33.40   Major depressive disorder, recurrent, in remission, unspecified

F33.41   Major depressive disorder, recurrent, in partial remission

F33.42   Major depressive disorder, recurrent, in full remission

F33.8   Other recurrent depressive disorders

Recurrent brief depressive episodes

F33.9   Major depressive disorder, recurrent, unspecified

Monopolar depression NOS

F34   Persistent mood [affective] disorders

F34.0   Cyclothymic disorder

Affective personality disorder

Cycloid personality

Cyclothymia

Cyclothymic personality

F34.1   Dysthymic disorder

Depressive neurosis

Depressive personality disorder

Dysthymia

Neurotic depression

Persistent anxiety depression

Persistent depressive disorder

Excludes2:   anxiety depression (mild or not persistent) (F41.8)

F34.8   Other persistent mood [affective] disorders

F34.81   Disruptive mood dysregulation disorder

F34.89   Other specified persistent mood disorders

F34.9   Persistent mood [affective] disorder, unspecified

F39   Unspecified mood [affective] disorder

Affective psychosis NOS

ANXIETY, DISSOCIATIVE, STRESS-RELATED, SOMATOFORM AND OTHER NONPSYCHOTIC MENTAL DISORDERS (F40-F48)

Definition: Anxiety disorders are a group of mental disorders characterized by feelings of anxiety and fear, where anxiety is a worry about future events and fear is a reaction to current events.

F40   Phobic anxiety disorders

F40.0   Agoraphobia

F40.00   Agoraphobia, unspecified

F40.01   Agoraphobia with panic disorder

Panic disorder with agoraphobia

Excludes1:   panic disorder without agoraphobia (F41.0)

F40.02   Agoraphobia without panic disorder

F40.1   Social phobias

Anthropophobia

Social anxiety disorder

Social anxiety disorder of childhood

Social neurosis

F40.10   Social phobia, unspecified

F40.11   Social phobia, generalized

F40.2   Specific (isolated) phobias

Excludes2:   dysmorphophobia (nondelusional) (F45.22)

nosophobia (F45.22)

F40.21   Animal type phobia

F40.210   Arachnophobia

Fear of spiders

F40.218   Other animal type phobia

F40.22   Natural environment type phobia

F40.220   Fear of thunderstorms

F40.228   Other natural environment type phobia

F40.23   Blood, injection, injury type phobia

F40.230   Fear of blood

F40.231   Fear of injections and transfusions

F40.232   Fear of other medical care

F40.233   Fear of injury

F40.24   Situational type phobia

F40.240   Claustrophobia

F40.241   Acrophobia

F40.242   Fear of bridges

F40.243   Fear of flying

F40.248   Other situational type phobia

F40.29   Other specified phobia

F40.290   Androphobia

Fear of men

F40.291   Gynephobia

Fear of women

F40.298   Other specified phobia

F40.8   Other phobic anxiety disorders

Phobic anxiety disorder of childhood

F40.9   Phobic anxiety disorder, unspecified

Phobia NOS

Phobic state NOS

F41   Other anxiety disorders

Excludes2:   anxiety in:

acute stress reaction (F43.0)

transient adjustment reaction (F43.2)

neurasthenia (F48.8)

psychophysiologic disorders (F45.-)

separation anxiety (F93.0)

▲ F41.0   Panic disorder [episodic paroxysmal anxiety]

Panic attack

Panic state

Excludes1:   panic disorder with agoraphobia (F40.01)

F41.1   Generalized anxiety disorder

Anxiety neurosis

Anxiety reaction

Anxiety state

Overanxious disorder

Excludes2:   neurasthenia (F48.8)

F41.3   Other mixed anxiety disorders

F41.8   Other specified anxiety disorders

Anxiety depression (mild or not persistent)

Anxiety hysteria

Mixed anxiety and depressive disorder

F41.9   Anxiety disorder, unspecified

Anxiety NOS

F42   Obsessive-compulsive disorder

Excludes2:   obsessive-compulsive personality (disorder) (F60.5)

obsessive-compulsive symptoms occurring in depression (F32-F33)

obsessive-compulsive symptoms occurring in schizophrenia (F20.-)

F42.2 **Mixed obsessional thoughts and acts**

F42.3 **Hoarding disorder**

F42.4 **Excoriation (skin-picking) disorder**

Excludes1: factitial dermatitis (L98.1)

Other specified behavioral and emotional disorders with onset usually occurring in early childhood and adolescence (F98.8)

F42.8 **Other obsessive-compulsive disorder**

Anancastic neurosis

Obsessive-compulsive neurosis

F42.9 **Obsessive-compulsive disorder, unspecified**

F43 **Reaction to severe stress, and adjustment disorders**

F43.0 **Acute stress reaction**

Acute crisis reaction

Acute reaction to stress

Combat and operational stress reaction

Combat fatigue

Crisis state

Psychic shock

F43.1 **Post-traumatic stress disorder (PTSD)**

Traumatic neurosis

F43.10 **Post-traumatic stress disorder, unspecified**

F43.11 **Post-traumatic stress disorder, acute**

F43.12 **Post-traumatic stress disorder, chronic**

F43.2 **Adjustment disorders**

Culture shock Grief reaction

Hospitalism in children

Excludes2: separation anxiety disorder of childhood (F93.0)

F43.20 **Adjustment disorder, unspecified**

F43.21 **Adjustment disorder with depressed mood**

F43.22 **Adjustment disorder with anxiety**

F43.23 **Adjustment disorder with mixed anxiety and depressed mood**

F43.24 **Adjustment disorder with disturbance of conduct**

F43.25 **Adjustment disorder with mixed disturbance of emotions and conduct**

F43.29 **Adjustment disorder with other symptoms**

F43.8 **Other reactions to severe stress**

Other specified trauma and stressor-related disorder

F43.9 **Reaction to severe stress, unspecified**

Trauma and stressor-related disorder, NOS

F44 **Dissociative and conversion disorders**

Includes: conversion hysteria

conversion reaction hysteria

hysterical psychosis

Excludes2: malingering [conscious simulation] (Z76.5)

F44.0 **Dissociative amnesia**

Excludes1: amnesia NOS (R41.3)

anterograde amnesia (R41.1)

dissociative amnesia with dissociative fugue (F44.1)

retrograde amnesia (R41.2)

Excludes2: alcohol-**or other** psychoactive substance-induced amnestic disorder (F10, F13, F19 with .26, .96)

amnestic disorder due to known physiological condition (F04)

postictal amnesia in epilepsy (G40.-)

F44.1 **Dissociative fugue**

Dissociative amnesia with dissociative fugue

Excludes2: postictal fugue in epilepsy (G40.-)

F44.2 **Dissociative stupor**

Excludes1: catatonic stupor (R40.1)

stupor NOS (R40.1)

Excludes2: catatonic disorder due to known physiological condition (F06.1)

depressive stupor (F32, F33)

manic stupor (F30, F31)

F44.4 **Conversion disorder with motor symptom or deficit**

Conversion disorder with abnormal movement

Conversion disorder with speech symptoms

Conversion disorder with swallowing symptoms

Conversion disorder with weakness/paralysis

Dissociative motor disorders

Psychogenic aphonia

Psychogenic dysphonia

F44.5 **Conversion disorder with seizures or convulsions**

Conversion disorder with attacks or seizures

Dissociative convulsions

F44.6 **Conversion disorder with sensory symptom or deficit**

Conversion disorder with anesthesia or sensory loss

Conversion disorder with special sensory symptoms

Dissociative anesthesia and sensory loss

Psychogenic deafness

F44.7 **Conversion disorder with mixed symptom presentation**

F44.8 **Other dissociative and conversion disorders**

F44.81 **Dissociative identity disorder**

Multiple personality disorder

F44.89 **Other dissociative and conversion disorders**

Ganser's syndrome

Psychogenic confusion

Psychogenic twilight state

Trance and possession disorders

F44.9 **Dissociative and conversion disorder, unspecified**

Dissociative disorder NOS

F45 **Somatoform disorders**

Definition: **Somatoform disorder** is the name for a group of conditions in which the physical pain and symptoms a person feels are related to psychological factors. These symptoms can't be traced to a specific physical cause.

Excludes2: dissociative and conversion disorders (F44.-)

factitious disorders (F68.1-)

hair-plucking (F63.3)

lalling (F80.0)

lisping (F80.0)

malingering [conscious simulation] (Z76.5)

nail-biting (F98.8)

psychological or behavioral factors associated with disorders or diseases classified elsewhere (F54)

sexual dysfunction, not due to a substance or known physiological condition (F52.-)

thumb-sucking (F98.8)

tic disorders (in childhood and adolescence) (F95.-)

Tourette's syndrome (F95.2)

trichotillomania (F63.3)

F45.0   **Somatization disorder**

Briquet's disorder

Multiple psychosomatic disorder

F45.1   **Undifferentiated somatoform disorder**

Somatic symptom disorder

Undifferentiated psychosomatic disorder

F45.2   **Hypochondriacal disorders**

Excludes2: delusional dysmorphophobia (F22)

fixed delusions about bodily functions or shape (F22)

F45.20   **Hypochondriacal disorder, unspecified**

F45.21   **Hypochondriasis**

Hypochondriacal neurosis

Illness anxiety disorder

F45.22   **Body dysmorphic disorder**

Dysmorphophobia (nondelusional)

Nosophobia

F45.29   **Other hypochondriacal disorders**

F45.4   **Pain disorders related to psychological factors**

Excludes1: pain NOS (R52)

F45.41   **Pain disorder exclusively related to psychological factors**

Somatoform pain disorder (persistent)

F45.42   **Pain disorder with related psychological factors**

Code also associated acute or chronic pain (G89.-)

F45.8   **Other somatoform disorders**

Psychogenic dysmenorrhea

Psychogenic dysphagia, including 'globus hystericus'

Psychogenic pruritus

Psychogenic torticollis

Somatoform autonomic dysfunction

Teeth grinding

Excludes1: sleep related teeth grinding (G47.63)

F45.9   **Somatoform disorder, unspecified**

Psychosomatic disorder NOS

F48   **Other nonpsychotic mental disorders**

F48.1   **Depersonalization-derealization syndrome**

F48.2   **Pseudobulbar affect**

Involuntary emotional expression disorder

Code first underlying cause, if known, such as:

amyotrophic lateral sclerosis (G12.21)

multiple sclerosis (G35)

sequelae of cerebrovascular disease (I69.-)

sequelae of traumatic intracranial injury (S06.-)

F48.8   **Other specified nonpsychotic mental disorders**

Dhat syndrome Neurasthenia

Occupational neurosis, including writer's cramp

Psychasthenia

Psychasthenic neurosis

Psychogenic syncope

F48.9   **Nonpsychotic mental disorder, unspecified**

Neurosis NOS

BEHAVIORAL SYNDROMES ASSOCIATED WITH PHYSIOLOGICAL DISTURBANCES AND PHYSICAL FACTORS (F50-F59)

F50   **Eating disorders**

Excludes1: anorexia NOS (R63.0)

feeding difficulties (R63.3)

feeding problems of newborn (P92.-)

polyphagia (R63.2)

Excludes2: feeding disorder in infancy or childhood (F98.2-)

F50.0   **Anorexia nervosa**

Excludes1: loss of appetite (R63.0)

psychogenic loss of appetite (F50.89)

F50.00   **Anorexia nervosa, unspecified**

F50.01   **Anorexia nervosa, restricting type**

F50.02   **Anorexia nervosa, binge eating/purging type**

Excludes1: bulimia nervosa (F50.2)

F50.2   **Bulimia nervosa**

Bulimia NOS

Hyperorexia nervosa

Excludes1: anorexia nervosa, binge eating/purging type (F50.02)

F50.8   **Other eating disorders**

Excludes2: pica of infancy and childhood (F98.3)

F50.81   **Binge eating disorder**

● **F50.82**   **Avoidant/restrictive food intake disorder**

F50.89   **Other specified eating disorder**

Pica in adults

Psychogenic loss of appetite

F50.9   **Eating disorder, unspecified**

Atypical anorexia nervosa

Atypical bulimia nervosa

Feeding or eating disorder, unspecified

Other specified feeding disorder

F51   **Sleep disorders not due to a substance or known physiological condition**

Excludes2: organic sleep disorders (G47.-)

F51.0   **Insomnia not due to a substance or known physiological condition**

Excludes2: alcohol related insomnia (F10.182, F10.282, F10.982)

drug-related insomnia (F11.182, F11.282, F11.982, F13.182, F13.282, F13.982, F14.182, F14.282, F14.982, F15.182, F15.282, F15.982, F19.182, F19.282, F19.982)

insomnia NOS (G47.0-)

insomnia due to known physiological condition (G47.0-)

organic insomnia (G47.0-)

sleep deprivation (Z72.820)

F51.01   **Primary insomnia**

Idiopathic insomnia

F51.02   **Adjustment insomnia**

F51.03   **Paradoxical insomnia**

F51.04   **Psychophysiologic insomnia**

F51.05   **Insomnia due to other mental disorder**

Code also associated mental disorder

F51.09   **Other insomnia not due to a substance or known physiological condition**

F51.1   **Hypersomnia not due to a substance or known physiological condition**

Excludes2: alcohol related hypersomnia (F10.182, F10.282, F10.982)

drug-related hypersomnia (F11.182, F11.282, F11.982, F13.182, F13.282, F13.982,

---

| | Add 4th-7th digits | | Nonspecific code | | Unspecified code | | Manifestation code | 275 |

F14.182, F14.282, F14.982, F15.182, F15.282, F15.982, F19.182, F19.282, F19.982)

hypersomnia NOS (G47.10)

hypersomnia due to known physiological condition (G47.10)

idiopathic hypersomnia (G47.11, G47.12)

narcolepsy (G47.4-)

F51.11   Primary hypersomnia

F51.12   Insufficient sleep syndrome

> Excludes1: sleep deprivation (Z72.820)

F51.13   Hypersomnia due to other mental disorder

> **Code also** associated mental disorder

F51.19   Other hypersomnia not due to a substance or known physiological condition

F51.3   Sleepwalking [somnambulism]

Non-rapid eye movement sleep arousal disorders, sleepwalking type

Non-rapid eye movement sleep arousal disorders, sleep terror type

F51.4   Sleep terrors [night terrors]

Non-rapid eye movement sleep arousal disorders, sleep terror type

F51.5   Nightmare disorder

Dream anxiety disorder

F51.8   Other sleep disorders not due to a substance or known physiological condition

F51.9   Sleep disorder not due to a substance or known physiological condition, unspecified

Emotional sleep disorder NOS

F52   Sexual dysfunction not due to a substance or known physiological condition

> Excludes2: Dhat syndrome (F48.8)

F52.0   Hypoactive sexual desire disorder

Lack or loss of sexual desire

Male hypoactive sexual desire disorder

Sexual anhedonia

> Excludes1: decreased libido (R68.82)

F52.1   Sexual aversion disorder

Sexual aversion and lack of sexual enjoyment

F52.2   Sexual arousal disorders

Failure of genital response

F52.21   Male erectile disorder

Erectile disorder
Psychogenic impotence

> Excludes1: impotence of organic origin (N52.-)
> impotence NOS (N52.-)

F52.22   Female sexual arousal disorder

Female sexual interest/arousal disorder

F52.3   Orgasmic disorder

Inhibited orgasm

Psychogenic anorgasmy

F52.31   Female orgasmic disorder

F52.32   Male orgasmic disorder

Delayed ejaculation

F52.4   Premature ejaculation

F52.5   Vaginismus not due to a substance or known physiological condition

Psychogenic vaginismus

> Excludes2: vaginismus (due to a known physiological condition) (N94.2)

F52.6   Dyspareunia not due to a substance or known physiological condition

Genito-pelvic pain penetration disorder

Psychogenic dyspareunia

> Excludes2: dyspareunia (due to a known physiological condition) (N94.1-)

F52.8   Other sexual dysfunction not due to a substance or known physiological condition

Excessive sexual drive

Nymphomania

Satyriasis

F52.9   Unspecified sexual dysfunction not due to a substance or known physiological condition

Sexual dysfunction NOS

F53   Puerperal psychosis

Postpartum depression

> Excludes1: mood disorders with psychotic features (F30.2, F31.2, F31.5, F31.64, F32.3, F33.3)
> postpartum dysphoria (O90.6)
> psychosis in schizophrenia, schizotypal, delusional, and other psychotic disorders (F20-F29)

F54   Psychological and behavioral factors associated with disorders or diseases classified elsewhere

Psychological factors affecting physical conditions

> **Code first** the associated physical disorder, such as:

asthma (J45.-)

dermatitis (L23-L25)

gastric ulcer (K25.-)

mucous colitis (K58.-)

ulcerative colitis (K51.-)

urticaria (L50.-)

> Excludes2: tension-type headache (G44.2)

F55   Abuse of non-psychoactive substances

> Excludes2: abuse of psychoactive substances (F10-F19)

F55.0   Abuse of antacids

F55.1   Abuse of herbal or folk remedies

F55.2   Abuse of laxatives

F55.3   Abuse of steroids or hormones

F55.4   Abuse of vitamins

F55.8   Abuse of other non-psychoactive substances

F59   Unspecified behavioral syndromes associated with physiological disturbances and physical factors

Psychogenic physiological dysfunction NOS

DISORDERS OF ADULT PERSONALITY AND BEHAVIOR (F60-F69)

F60   Specific personality disorders

F60.0   Paranoid personality disorder

Expansive paranoid personality (disorder)

Fanatic personality (disorder)

Querulant personality (disorder)

Paranoid personality (disorder)

Sensitive paranoid personality (disorder)

> Excludes2: paranoia (F22)
> paranoia querulans (F22)
> paranoid psychosis (F22)
> paranoid schizophrenia (F20.0)

paranoid state (F22)

F60.1 Schizoid personality disorder

Excludes2: Asperger's syndrome (F84.5)

delusional disorder (F22)

schizoid disorder of childhood (F84.5)

schizophrenia (F20.-)

schizotypal disorder (F21)

F60.2 Antisocial personality disorder

Amoral personality (disorder)

Asocial personality (disorder)

Dissocial personality disorder

Psychopathic personality (disorder)

Sociopathic personality (disorder)

Excludes1: conduct disorders (F91.-)

Excludes2: borderline personality disorder (F60.3)

F60.3 Borderline personality disorder

Aggressive personality (disorder)

Emotionally unstable personality disorder

Explosive personality (disorder)

Excludes2: antisocial personality disorder (F60.2)

F60.4 Histrionic personality disorder

Hysterical personality (disorder)

Psychoinfantile personality (disorder)

F60.5 Obsessive-compulsive personality disorder

Anankastic personality (disorder)

Compulsive personality (disorder)

Obsessional personality (disorder)

Excludes2: obsessive-compulsive disorder (F42-)

F60.6 Avoidant personality disorder

Anxious personality disorder

F60.7 Dependent personality disorder

Asthenic personality (disorder)

Inadequate personality (disorder)

Passive personality (disorder)

F60.8 Other specific personality disorders

    F60.81 Narcissistic personality disorder

    F60.89 Other specific personality disorders

      Eccentric personality disorder

      'Haltlose' type personality disorder

      Immature personality disorder

      Passive-aggressive personality disorder

      Psychoneurotic personality disorder

      Self-defeating personality disorder

F60.9 Personality disorder, unspecified

Character disorder NOS

Character neurosis NOS

Pathological personality NOS

F63 Impulse disorders

Excludes2: habitual excessive use of alcohol or psychoactive substances (F10-F19)

impulse disorders involving sexual behavior (F65.-)

F63.0 Pathological gambling

Compulsive gambling

Gambling disorder

Excludes1: gambling and betting NOS (Z72.6)

Excludes2: excessive gambling by manic patients (F30, F31)

gambling in antisocial personality disorder (F60.2)

F63.1 Pyromania

Pathological fire-setting

Excludes2: fire-setting (by) (in):

adult with antisocial personality disorder (F60.2)

alcohol or psychoactive substance intoxication (F10-F19)

conduct disorders (F91.-)

mental disorders due to known physiological condition (F01-F09)

schizophrenia (F20.-)

F63.2 Kleptomania

Pathological stealing

Excludes1: shoplifting as the reason for observation for suspected mental disorder (Z03.8)

Excludes2: depressive disorder with stealing (F31-F33)

stealing due to underlying mental condition-code to mental condition stealing in mental disorders due to known physiological condition (F01-F09)

F63.3 Trichotillomania

Hair plucking

Excludes2: Other stereotyped movement disorder (F98.4)

F63.8 Other impulse disorders

    F63.81 Intermittent explosive disorder

    F63.89 Other impulse disorders

F63.9 Impulse disorder, unspecified

Impulse control disorder NOS

F64 Gender identity disorders

F64.0 Transsexualism

Gender identity disorder in adolescence and adulthood

Gender dysphoria in adolescents and adults

F64.1 Dual role transvestism

Use additional code to identify sex reassignment status (Z87.890)

Excludes1: gender identity disorder in childhood (F64.2)

Excludes2: fetishistic transvestism (F65.1)

F64.2 Gender identity disorder of childhood

Gender dysphoria in children

Excludes1: gender identity disorder in adolescence and adulthood (F64.0)

Excludes2: sexual maturation disorder (F66)

F64.8 Other gender identity disorders

Other specified gender dysphoria

F64.9 Gender identity disorder, unspecified

Gender dysphoria, unspecified

Gender-role disorder NOS

F65 Paraphilias

F65.0 Fetishism

Fetishistic disorder

F65.1 Transvestic fetishism

Transvestic disorder

Fetishistic transvestism

F65.2 Exhibitionism

Exhibitionistic disorder

F65.3 Voyeurism

Voyeuristic disorder

F65.4 Pedophilia

Pedophilic disorder

F65.5 **Sadomasochism**

   F65.50 **Sadomasochism, unspecified**

   F65.51 **Sexual masochism**

     Sexual masochism disorder

   F65.52 **Sexual sadism**

     Sexual sadism disorder

F65.8 **Other paraphilias**

   F65.81 **Frotteurism**

     Frotteuristic disorder

   F65.89 **Other paraphilias**

     Necrophilia

     Other specified paraphilic disorder

F65.9 **Paraphilia, unspecified**

   Paraphilic disorder, unspecified

   Sexual deviation NOS

F66 **Other sexual disorders**

   Sexual maturation disorder

   Sexual relationship disorder

F68 **Other disorders of adult personality and behavior**

F68.1 **Factitious disorder**

   Compensation neurosis

   Elaboration of physical symptoms for psychological reasons

   Hospital hopper syndrome

   Munchausen's syndrome

   Peregrinating patient

   Excludes2: factitial dermatitis (L98.1)

     person feigning illness (with obvious motivation) (Z76.5)

   F68.10 **Factitious disorder, unspecified**

   F68.11 **Factitious disorder with predominantly psychological signs and symptoms**

   F68.12 **Factitious disorder with predominantly physical signs and symptoms**

   F68.13 **Factitious disorder with combined psychological and physical signs and symptoms**

F68.8 **Other specified disorders of adult personality and behavior**

F69 **Unspecified disorder of adult personality and behavior**

INTELLECTUAL DISABILITIES (F70-F79)

Code first any associated physical or developmental disorders

Excludes1: borderline intellectual functioning, IQ above 70 to 84 (R41.83)

F70 **Mild intellectual disabilities**

   IQ level 50-55 to approximately 70

   Mild mental subnormality

F71 **Moderate intellectual disabilities**

   IQ level 35-40 to 50-55

   Moderate mental subnormality

F72 **Severe intellectual disabilities**

   IQ 20-25 to 35-40

   Severe mental subnormality

F73 **Profound intellectual disabilities**

   IQ level below 20-25 Profound mental subnormality

F78 **Other intellectual disabilities**

F79 **Unspecified intellectual disabilities**

   Mental deficiency NOS

   Mental subnormality NOS

PERVASIVE AND SPECIFIC DEVELOPMENTAL DISORDERS (F80-F89)

F80 **Specific developmental disorders of speech and language**

F80.0 **Phonological disorder**

   Dyslalia

   Functional speech articulation disorder

   Lalling

   Lisping

   Phonological developmental disorder

   Speech articulation developmental disorder

   Speech-sound disorder

   Excludes1: speech articulation impairment due to aphasia NOS (R47.01)

     speech articulation impairment due to apraxia (R48.2)

   Excludes2: speech articulation impairment due to hearing loss (F80.4)

     speech articulation impairment due to intellectual disabilities (F70-F79)

     speech articulation impairment with expressive language developmental disorder (F80.1)

     speech articulation impairment with mixed receptive expressive language developmental disorder (F80.2)

F80.1 **Expressive language disorder**

   Developmental dysphasia or aphasia, expressive type

   Excludes1: mixed receptive-expressive language disorder (F80.2)

     dysphasia and aphasia NOS (R47.-)

   Excludes2: acquired aphasia with epilepsy [Landau-Kleffner] (G40.80-)

     selective mutism (F94.0)

     intellectual disabilities (F70-F79)

     pervasive developmental disorders (F84.-)

F80.2 **Mixed receptive-expressive language disorder**

   Developmental dysphasia or aphasia, receptive type

   Developmental Wernicke's aphasia

   Excludes1: central auditory processing disorder (H93.25)

     dysphasia or aphasia NOS (R47.-)

     expressive language disorder (F80.1)

     expressive type dysphasia or aphasia (F80.1)

     word deafness (H93.25)

   Excludes2: acquired aphasia with epilepsy [Landau-Kleffner] (G40.80-)

     pervasive developmental disorders (F84.-)

     selective mutism (F94.0)

     intellectual disabilities (F70-F79)

F80.4 **Speech and language development delay due to hearing loss**

   Code also type of hearing loss (H90.-, H91.-)

F80.8 **Other developmental disorders of speech and language**

   F80.81 **Childhood onset fluency disorder**

     Cluttering NOS

     Stuttering NOS

     Excludes1: adult onset fluency disorder (F98.5)

       fluency disorder in conditions classified elsewhere (R47.82)

       fluency disorder (stuttering) following cerebrovascular disease (I69. with final characters - 23)

● New code ▲ Revised code **Excludes1:** Not coded here **Excludes2:** Not included here ⊗ Placeholder required ⑦7th digit required

F80.82 **Social pragmatic communication disorder**

Excludes1: Asperger's syndrome (F84.5)

autistic disorder (F84.0)

F80.89 **Other developmental disorders of speech and language**

F80.9 **Developmental disorder of speech and language, unspecified**

Communication disorder NOS

Language disorder NOS

F81 **Specific developmental disorders of scholastic skills**

F81.0 **Specific reading disorder**

Backward reading'

Developmental dyslexia

Specific learning disorder, with impairment in reading

Specific reading retardation

Excludes1: alexia NOS (R48.0)

dyslexia NOS (R48.0)

F81.2 **Mathematics disorder**

Developmental acalculia

Developmental arithmetical disorder

Developmental Gerstmann's syndrome

Specific learning disorder, with impairment in mathematics

Excludes1: acalculia NOS (R48.8)

Excludes2: arithmetical difficulties associated with a reading disorder (F81.0)

arithmetical difficulties associated with a spelling disorder (F81.81)

arithmetical difficulties due to inadequate teaching (Z55.8)

F81.8 **Other developmental disorders of scholastic skills**

F81.81 **Disorder of written expression**

Specific learning disorder, with impairment in written expression

Specific spelling disorder

F81.89 **Other developmental disorders of scholastic skills**

F81.9 **Developmental disorder of scholastic skills, unspecified**

Knowledge acquisition disability NOS

Learning disability NOS

Learning disorder NOS

F82 **Specific developmental disorder of motor function**

Clumsy child syndrome

Developmental coordination disorder

Developmental dyspraxia

Excludes1: abnormalities of gait and mobility (R26.-)

lack of coordination (R27.-)

Excludes2: lack of coordination secondary to intellectual disabilities (F70-F79)

F84 **Pervasive developmental disorders**

Use additional code to identify any associated medical condition and intellectual disabilities.

F84.0 **Autistic disorder**

Autism spectrum disorder

Infantile autism

Infantile psychosis

Kanner's syndrome

Excludes1: Asperger's syndrome (F84.5)

F84.2 **Rett's syndrome**

Excludes1: Asperger's syndrome (F84.5)

Autistic disorder (F84.0)

Other childhood disintegrative disorder (F84.3)

F84.3 **Other childhood disintegrative disorder**

Dementia infantilis

Disintegrative psychosis

Heller's syndrome

Symbiotic psychosis

Use additional code to identify any associated neurological condition.

Excludes1: Asperger's syndrome (F84.5)

Autistic disorder (F84.0)

Rett's syndrome (F84.2)

F84.5 **Asperger's syndrome**

Asperger's disorder

Autistic psychopathy

Schizoid disorder of childhood

F84.8 **Other pervasive developmental disorders**

Overactive disorder associated with intellectual disabilities and stereotyped movements

F84.9 **Pervasive developmental disorder, unspecified**

Atypical autism

F88 **Other disorders of psychological development**

Developmental agnosia Global developmental delay

Other specified neurodevelopmental disorder

F89 **Unspecified disorder of psychological development**

Developmental disorder NOS

Neurodevelopmental disorder NOS

BEHAVIORAL AND EMOTIONAL DISORDERS WITH ONSET USUALLY OCCURRING IN CHILDHOOD AND ADOLESCENCE (F90-F98)

Note: Codes within categories F90-F98 may be used regardless of the age of a patient. These disorders generally have onset within the childhood or adolescent years, but may continue throughout life or not be diagnosed until adulthood

F90 **Attention-deficit hyperactivity disorders**

Definition: Attention deficit hyperactivity disorder refers to any of a range of behavioral disorders occurring primarily in children, including such symptoms as poor concentration, hyperactivity, and impulsivity.

Includes: attention deficit disorder with hyperactivity

attention deficit syndrome with hyperactivity

Excludes2: anxiety disorders (F40.-, F41.-)

mood [affective] disorders (F30-F39)

pervasive developmental disorders (F84.-)

schizophrenia (F20.-)

F90.0 **Attention-deficit hyperactivity disorder, predominantly inattentive type**

F90.1 **Attention-deficit hyperactivity disorder, predominantly hyperactive type**

Attention-deficit/hyperactivity disorder, predominantly hyperactive impulsive presentation

F90.2 **Attention-deficit hyperactivity disorder, combined type**

Attention-deficit/hyperactivity disorder, combined presentation

F90.8 **Attention-deficit hyperactivity disorder, other type**

F90.9 **Attention-deficit hyperactivity disorder, unspecified type**

Attention-deficit hyperactivity disorder of childhood or adolescence NOS

Attention-deficit hyperactivity disorder NOS

F91   Conduct disorders
Excludes1: antisocial behavior (Z72.81-)
antisocial personality disorder (F60.2)
Excludes2: conduct problems associated with attention-deficit hyperactivity disorder (F90.-)
mood [affective] disorders (F30-F39)
pervasive developmental disorders (F84.-)
schizophrenia (F20.-)

F91.0   Conduct disorder confined to family context

F91.1   Conduct disorder, childhood-onset type
Unsocialized conduct disorder
Conduct disorder, solitary aggressive type
Unsocialized aggressive disorder

F91.2   Conduct disorder, adolescent-onset type
Socialized conduct disorder
Conduct disorder, group type

F91.3   Oppositional defiant disorder

F91.8   Other conduct disorders
Other specified conduct disorder
Other specified disruptive disorder

F91.9   Conduct disorder, unspecified
Behavioral disorder NOS
Conduct disorder NOS
Disruptive behavior disorder NOS
Disruptive disorder NOS

F93   Emotional disorders with onset specific to childhood

F93.0   Separation anxiety disorder of childhood
Excludes2: mood [affective] disorders (F30-F39)
nonpsychotic mental disorders (F40-F48)
phobic anxiety disorder of childhood (F40.8)
social phobia (F40.1)

F93.8   Other childhood emotional disorders
Identity disorder
Excludes2: gender identity disorder of childhood (F64.2)

F93.9   Childhood emotional disorder, unspecified

F94   Disorders of social functioning with onset specific to childhood and adolescence

F94.0   Selective mutism
Elective mutism
Excludes2: pervasive developmental disorders (F84.-)
schizophrenia (F20.-)
specific developmental disorders of speech and language (F80.-)
transient mutism as part of separation anxiety in young children (F93.0)

F94.1   Reactive attachment disorder of childhood
Use additional code to identify any associated failure to thrive or growth retardation
Excludes1: disinhibited attachment disorder of childhood (F94.2)
normal variation in pattern of selective attachment
Excludes2: Asperger's syndrome (F84.5)
maltreatment syndromes (T74.-)
sexual or physical abuse in childhood, resulting in psychosocial problems (Z62.81-)

F94.2   Disinhibited attachment disorder of childhood
Affectionless psychopathy

Institutional syndrome
Excludes1: reactive attachment disorder of childhood (F94.1)
Excludes2: Asperger's syndrome (F84.5)
attention-deficit hyperactivity disorders (F90.-)
hospitalism in children (F43.2-)

F94.8   Other childhood disorders of social functioning
F94.9   Childhood disorder of social functioning, unspecified

F95   Tic disorder
F95.0   Transient tic disorder
Provisional tic disorder
F95.1   Chronic motor or vocal tic disorder
F95.2   Tourette's disorder
Combined vocal and multiple motor tic disorder [de la Tourette]
Tourette's syndrome
F95.8   Other tic disorders
F95.9   Tic disorder, unspecified
Tic NOS

F98   Other behavioral and emotional disorders with onset usually occurring in childhood and adolescence
Excludes2: breath-holding spells (R06.89)
gender identity disorder of childhood (F64.2)
Kleine-Levin syndrome (G47.13)
obsessive-compulsive disorder (F42-)
sleep disorders not due to a substance or known physiological condition (F51.-)

F98.0   Enuresis not due to a substance or known physiological condition
Enuresis (primary) (secondary) of nonorganic origin
Functional enuresis
Psychogenic enuresis
Urinary incontinence of nonorganic origin
Excludes1: enuresis NOS (R32)

F98.1   Encopresis not due to a substance or known physiological condition
Functional encopresis
Incontinence of feces of nonorganic origin
Psychogenic encopresis
Use additional code to identify the cause of any coexisting constipation.
Excludes1: encopresis NOS (R15.-)

F98.2   Other feeding disorders of infancy and childhood
Excludes1: feeding difficulties (R63.3)
Excludes2: anorexia nervosa **and other** eating disorders (F50.-)
feeding problems of newborn (P92.-)
pica of infancy or childhood (F98.3)
F98.21   Rumination disorder of infancy
F98.29   Other feeding disorders of infancy and early childhood

F98.3   Pica of infancy and childhood

F98.4   Stereotyped movement disorders
Stereotype/habit disorder
Excludes1: abnormal involuntary movements (R25.-)
Excludes2: compulsions in obsessive-compulsive disorder (F42-)
hair plucking (F63.3)
movement disorders of organic origin (G20-G25)

nail-biting (F98.8)

nose-picking (F98.8)

stereotypies that are part of a broader psychiatric condition (F01-F95)

thumb-sucking (F98.8)

tic disorders (F95.-)

trichotillomania (F63.3)

F98.5   Adult onset fluency disorder

Excludes1: childhood onset fluency disorder (F80.81)

dysphasia (R47.02)

fluency disorder in conditions classified elsewhere (R47.82)

fluency disorder (stuttering)

following cerebrovascular disease (I69. with final characters -23)

tic disorders (F95.-)

F98.8   Other specified behavioral and emotional disorders with onset usually occurring in childhood and adolescence

Excessive masturbation Nail-biting

Nose-picking

Thumb-sucking

F98.9   Unspecified behavioral and emotional disorders with onset usually occurring in childhood and adolescence

UNSPECIFIED MENTAL DISORDER (F99)

F99   Mental disorder, not otherwise specified

Mental illness NOS

Excludes1: **unspecified** mental disorder due to known physiological condition (F09)

Chapter 6: Diseases Of The Nervous System (G00-G99)

DEFINITIONS

This chapter includes definitions of selected key words, terms and phrases and coding alerts for adding points to the clinical domain, and references to coding late effects where appropriate. An example from this chapter is as follows:

G00   Bacterial meningitis, not elsewhere classified

> **Definition:** Meningitis is an infectious disease characterized by inflammation of the meninges (the tissues that surround the brain or spinal cord) usually caused by a bacterial infection; symptoms include headache and stiff neck and fever and nausea.

MULTIPLE CODING FOR A SINGLE CONDITION

In addition to the etiology/manifestation convention that requires two codes to fully describe a single condition that affects multiple body systems, there are other single conditions that also require more than one code. "Use additional code" notes are found in the Tabular List at codes that are not part of an etiology/manifestation pair where a secondary code is useful to fully describe a condition. The sequencing rule is the same as the etiology/manifestation pair, "use additional code" indicates that a secondary code should be added.

For example, for bacterial infections that are not included in chapter 1, a secondary code from category B95, Streptococcus, Staphylococcus, and Enterococcus, as the cause of diseases classified elsewhere, or B96, Other bacterial agents as the cause of diseases classified elsewhere, may be required to identify the bacterial organism causing the infection. A "use additional code" note will normally be found at the infectious disease code, indicating a need for the organism code to be added as a secondary code.

"Code first" notes are also under certain codes that are not specifically manifestation codes but may be due to an underlying cause. When there is a "code first" note and an underlying condition is present, the underlying condition should be sequenced first.

"Code, if applicable, any causal condition first", notes indicate that this code may be assigned as a principal diagnosis when the causal condition is unknown or not applicable. If a causal condition is known, then the code for that condition should be sequenced as the principal or first-listed diagnosis.

Multiple codes may be needed for sequela, complication codes and obstetric codes to more fully describe a condition. See the specific guidelines for these conditions for further instruction.

COMBINATION CODE

A combination code is a single code used to classify: Two diagnoses, or a diagnosis with an associated secondary process (manifestation) A diagnosis with an associated complication

Combination codes are identified by referring to subterm entries in the Alphabetic Index and by reading the inclusion and exclusion notes in the Tabular List.

Assign only the combination code when that code fully identifies the diagnostic conditions involved or when the Alphabetic Index so directs. Multiple coding should not be used when the classification provides a combination code that clearly identifies all of the elements documented in the diagnosis. When the combination code lacks necessary specificity in describing the manifestation or complication, an additional code should be used as a secondary code.

SEQUELA (LATE EFFECTS)

A sequela is the residual effect (condition produced) after the acute phase of an illness or injury has terminated. There is no time limit on when a sequela code can be used. The residual may be apparent early, such as in cerebral infarction, or it may occur months or years later, such as that due to a previous injury. Coding of sequela generally requires two codes sequenced in the following order: The condition or nature of the sequela is sequenced first.

The sequela code is sequenced second.

An exception to the above guidelines are those instances where the code for the sequela is followed by a manifestation code identified in the Tabular List and title, or the sequela code has been expanded (at the fourth, fifth or sixth character levels) to include the manifestation(s). The code for the acute phase of an illness or injury that led to the sequela is never used with a code for the late effect.

DOMINANT/NONDOMINANT SIDE

Codes from category G81, Hemiplegia and hemiparesis, and subcategories G83.1, Monoplegia of lower limb, G83.2, Monoplegia of upper limb, and G83.3, Monoplegia, unspecified, identify whether the dominant or nondominant side is affected. Should the affected side be documented, but not specified as dominant or nondominant, and the classification system does not indicate a default, code selection is as follows:

- For ambidextrous patients, the default should be dominant.

- If the left side is affected, the default is non-dominant.

- If the right side is affected, the default is dominant.

PAIN - CATEGORY G89

1)   **General coding information**

	Add 4th-7th digits		Nonspecific code		Unspecified code		Manifestation code

Codes in category G89, Pain, not elsewhere classified, may be used in conjunction with codes from other categories and chapters to provide more detail about acute or chronic pain and neoplasm-related pain, unless otherwise indicated below.

If the pain is not specified as acute or chronic, post-thoracotomy, postprocedural, or neoplasm-related, do not assign codes from category G89.

A code from category G89 should not be assigned if the underlying (definitive) diagnosis is known, unless the reason for the encounter is pain control/management and not management of the underlying condition.

When an admission or encounter is for a procedure aimed at treating the underlying condition (e.g., spinal fusion, kyphoplasty), a code for the underlying condition (e.g., vertebral fracture, spinal stenosis) should be assigned as the principal diagnosis. No code from category G89 should be assigned.

(a) **Category G89 Codes as Principal or First-Listed Diagnosis**

Category G89 codes are acceptable as principal diagnosis or the first-listed code:

- When pain control or pain management is the reason for the admission/encounter (e.g., a patient with displaced intervertebral disc, nerve impingement and severe back pain presents for injection of steroid into the spinal canal). The underlying cause of the pain should be reported as an additional diagnosis, if known.

- When a patient is admitted for the insertion of a neurostimulator for pain control, assign the appropriate pain code as the principal or first-listed diagnosis. When an admission or encounter is for a procedure aimed at treating the underlying condition and a neurostimulator is inserted for pain control during the same admission/encounter, a code for the underlying condition should be assigned as the principal diagnosis and the appropriate pain code should be assigned as a secondary diagnosis.

(b) **Use of Category G89 Codes in Conjunction with Site Specific Pain Codes**

(i) **Assigning Category G89 and Site-Specific Pain Codes**

Codes from category G89 may be used in conjunction with codes that identify the site of pain (including codes from chapter 18) if the category G89 code provides additional information. For example, if the code describes the site of the pain, but does not fully describe whether the pain is acute or chronic, then both codes should be assigned.

(ii) **Sequencing of Category G89 Codes with Site-Specific Pain Codes**

The sequencing of category G89 codes with site-specific pain codes (including chapter 18 codes), is dependent on the circumstances of the encounter/admission as follows:

- If the encounter is for pain control or pain management, assign the code from category G89 followed by the code identifying the specific site of pain (e.g., encounter for pain management for acute neck pain from trauma is assigned code G89.11, Acute pain due to trauma, followed by code M54.2, Cervicalgia, to identify the site of pain).

- If the encounter is for any other reason except pain control or pain management, and a related definitive diagnosis has not been established (confirmed) by the provider, assign the code for the specific site of pain first, followed by the appropriate code from category G89.

2) **Pain due to devices, implants and grafts**

See Section I.C.19. Pain due to medical devices

3) **Postoperative Pain**

The provider's documentation should be used to guide the coding of postoperative pain, as well as *Section III. Reporting Additional Diagnoses* and *Section IV. Diagnostic Coding and Reporting in the Outpatient Setting.*

The default for post-thoracotomy and other postoperative pain not specified as acute or chronic is the code for the acute form.

Routine or expected postoperative pain immediately after surgery should not be coded.

(a) **Postoperative pain not associated with specific postoperative complication**

Postoperative pain not associated with a specific postoperative complication is assigned to the appropriate postoperative pain code in category G89.

(b) **Postoperative pain associated with specific postoperative complication**

Postoperative pain associated with a specific postoperative complication (such as painful wire sutures) is assigned to the appropriate code(s) found in Chapter 19, Injury, poisoning, and certain other consequences of external causes. If appropriate, use additional code(s) from category G89 to identify acute or chronic pain (G89.18 or G89.28).

4) **Chronic pain**

Chronic pain is classified to subcategory G89.2. There is no time frame defining when pain becomes chronic pain. The provider's documentation should be used to guide use of these codes.

5) **Neoplasm Related Pain**

Code G89.3 is assigned to pain documented as being related, associated or due to cancer, primary or secondary malignancy, or tumor. This code is assigned regardless of whether the pain is acute or chronic.

This code may be assigned as the principal or first-listed code when the stated reason for the admission/encounter is documented as pain control/pain management. The underlying neoplasm should be reported as an additional diagnosis.

When the reason for the admission/encounter is management of the neoplasm and the pain associated with the neoplasm is also documented, code G89.3 may be assigned as an additional diagnosis. It is not necessary to assign an additional code for the site of the pain.

See Section I.C.2 for instructions on the sequencing of neoplasms for all other stated reasons for the admission/encounter (except for pain control/pain management).

6) **Chronic pain syndrome**

Central pain syndrome (G89.0) and chronic pain syndrome (G89.4) are different than the term "chronic pain," and therefore codes should only be used when the provider has specifically documented this condition.

See Section I.C.5. Pain disorders related to psychological factors

● New code   ▲ Revised code   **Excludes1:** Not coded here   **Excludes2:** Not included here   ⊗ Placeholder required   ⑦ 7th digit required

Chapter 6
Diseases of the Nervous System (G00-G99)

Excludes2: certain conditions originating in the perinatal period (P04-P96)

certain infectious and parasitic diseases (A00-B99)

complications of pregnancy, childbirth and the puerperium (O00-O9A)

congenital malformations, deformations, and chromosomal abnormalities (Q00-Q99)

endocrine, nutritional and metabolic diseases (E00-E88)

injury, poisoning and certain other consequences of external causes (S00-T88)

neoplasms (C00-D49)

symptoms, signs and abnormal clinical and laboratory findings, not elsewhere classified (R00-R94)

This chapter contains the following blocks:

G00-G09	Inflammatory diseases of the central nervous system
G10-G14	Systemic atrophies primarily affecting the central nervous system
G20-G26	Extrapyramidal and movement disorders
G30-G32	Other degenerative diseases of the nervous system
G35-G37	Demyelinating diseases of the central nervous system
G40-G47	Episodic and paroxysmal disorders
G50-G59	Nerve, nerve root and plexus disorders
G60-G65	Polyneuropathies and other disorders of the peripheral nervous system
G70-G73	Diseases of myoneural junction and muscle
G80-G83	Cerebral palsy and other paralytic syndromes
G89-G99	Other disorders of the nervous system

INFLAMMATORY DISEASES OF THE CENTRAL NERVOUS SYSTEM (G00-G09)

G00 **Bacterial meningitis, not elsewhere classified**

Definition: Meningitis is an infectious disease characterized by inflammation of the meninges (the tissues that surround the brain or spinal cord) usually caused by a bacterial infection; symptoms include headache and stiff neck and fever and nausea.

Includes: bacterial arachnoiditis

bacterial leptomeningitis

bacterial meningitis

bacterial pachymeningitis

Excludes1: bacterial meningoencephalitis (G04.2)

bacterial meningomyelitis (G04.2)

G00.0 **Hemophilus meningitis**

Meningitis due to Hemophilus influenzae

G00.1 **Pneumococcal meningitis**

Meningitis due to

Streptococcal pneumoniae

G00.2 **Streptococcal meningitis**

Use additional code to further identify organism (B95.0-B95.5)

G00.3 **Staphylococcal meningitis**

Use additional code to further identify organism (B95.61-B95.8)

G00.8 **Other bacterial meningitis**

Meningitis due to Escherichia coli

Meningitis due to Friedländer's bacillus

Meningitis due to Klebsiella

Use additional code to further identify organism (B96.-)

G00.9 **Bacterial meningitis, unspecified**

Meningitis due to gram-negative bacteria, unspecified

Purulent meningitis NOS

Pyogenic meningitis NOS

Suppurative meningitis NOS

G01 **Meningitis in bacterial diseases classified elsewhere**

Code first underlying disease

Excludes1: meningitis (in):

gonococcal (A54.81)

leptospirosis (A27.81)

listeriosis (A32.11)

Lyme disease (A69.21)

meningococcal (A39.0)

neurosyphilis (A52.13)

tuberculosis (A17.0)

meningoencephalitis and meningomyelitis in bacterial diseases classified elsewhere (G05)

G02 **Meningitis in other infectious and parasitic diseases classified elsewhere**

Code first underlying disease, such as:

African trypanosomiasis (B56.-)

poliovirus infection (A80.-)

Excludes1: candidal meningitis (B37.5)

coccidioidomycosis meningitis (B38.4)

cryptococcal meningitis (B45.1)

herpesviral [herpes simplex] meningitis (B00.3)

infectious mononucleosis complicated by meningitis (B27.- with fourth character 2)

measles complicated by meningitis (B05.1)

meningoencephalitis and meningomyelitis in other infectious and parasitic diseases classified elsewhere (G05)

mumps meningitis (B26.1)

rubella meningitis (B06.02)

varicella [chickenpox] meningitis (B01.0)

zoster meningitis (B02.1)

G03 **Meningitis due to other and unspecified causes**

Includes: arachnoiditis NOS

leptomeningitis NOS

meningitis NOS

pachymeningitis NOS

Excludes1: meningoencephalitis (G04.-)

meningomyelitis (G04.-)

G03.0 **Nonpyogenic meningitis**

Aseptic meningitis Nonbacterial meningitis

G03.1 **Chronic meningitis**

G03.2 **Benign recurrent meningitis [Mollaret]**

G03.8 **Meningitis due to other specified causes**

G03.9 **Meningitis, unspecified**

Arachnoiditis (spinal) NOS

G04 **Encephalitis, myelitis and encephalomyelitis**

Definition: Encephalitis is an inflammation of the brain, usually caused by a direct viral infection or a hypersensitivity reaction to a virus or foreign protein. Myelitis is an inflammation of the spinal column. Encephalomyelitis is an inflammation of the brain and spinal cord.

Includes: acute ascending myelitis

meningoencephalitis meningomyelitis

Excludes1: encephalopathy NOS (G93.40)

Excludes2: acute transverse myelitis (G37.3-)

alcoholic encephalopathy (G31.2)

benign myalgic encephalomyelitis (G93.3)

multiple sclerosis (G35)

subacute necrotizing myelitis (G37.4)

toxic encephalitis (G92)

toxic encephalopathy (G92)

G04.0 Acute disseminated encephalitis and encephalomyelitis (ADEM)

Excludes1: acute necrotizing hemorrhagic encephalopathy (G04.3-)

Other noninfectious acute disseminated encephalomyelitis (noninfectious ADEM) (G04.81)

G04.00 Acute disseminated encephalitis and encephalomyelitis, unspecified

G04.01 Postinfectious acute disseminated encephalitis and encephalomyelitis (postinfectious ADEM)

Excludes1: post chickenpox encephalitis (B01.1)

post measles encephalitis (B05.0)

post measles myelitis (B05.1)

G04.02 Postimmunization acute disseminated encephalitis, myelitis and encephalomyelitis

Encephalitis, post immunization

Encephalomyelitis, post immunization

Use additional code to identify the vaccine (T50.A-, T50.B-, T50.Z-)

G04.1 Tropical spastic paraplegia

G04.2 Bacterial meningoencephalitis and meningomyelitis, not elsewhere classified

G04.3 Acute necrotizing hemorrhagic encephalopathy

Excludes1: acute disseminated encephalitis and encephalomyelitis (G04.0-)

G04.30 Acute necrotizing hemorrhagic encephalopathy, unspecified

G04.31 Postinfectious acute necrotizing hemorrhagic encephalopathy

G04.32 Postimmunization acute necrotizing hemorrhagic encephalopathy

Use additional code to identify the vaccine (T50.A-, T50.B-, T50.Z-)

G04.39 Other acute necrotizing hemorrhagic encephalopathy

Code also underlying etiology, if applicable

G04.8 Other encephalitis, myelitis and encephalomyelitis

Code also any associated seizure (G40.-, R56.9)

G04.81 Other encephalitis and encephalomyelitis

Noninfectious acute disseminated encephalomyelitis (noninfectious ADEM)

G04.89 Other myelitis

G04.9 Encephalitis, myelitis and encephalomyelitis, unspecified

G04.90 Encephalitis and encephalomyelitis, unspecified

Ventriculitis (cerebral) NOS

G04.91 Myelitis, unspecified

G05 Encephalitis, myelitis and encephalomyelitis in diseases classified elsewhere

Code first underlying disease, such as:

human immunodeficiency virus [HIV] disease (B20)

poliovirus (A80.-)

suppurative otitis media (H66.01-H66.4)

trichinellosis (B75)

Excludes1: adenoviral encephalitis, myelitis and encephalomyelitis (A85.1)

congenital toxoplasmosis encephalitis, myelitis and encephalomyelitis (P37.1)

cytomegaloviral encephalitis, myelitis and encephalomyelitis (B25.8)

encephalitis, myelitis and encephalomyelitis (in) measles (B05.0)

encephalitis, myelitis and encephalomyelitis (in) systemic lupus erythematosus (M32.19)

enteroviral encephalitis, myelitis and encephalomyelitis (A85.0)

eosinophilic meningoencephalitis (B83.2)

herpesviral [herpes simplex] encephalitis, myelitis and encephalomyelitis (B00.4)

listerial encephalitis, myelitis and encephalomyelitis (A32.12)

meningococcal encephalitis, myelitis and encephalomyelitis (A39.81)

mumps encephalitis, myelitis and encephalomyelitis (B26.2)

post chickenpox encephalitis, myelitis and encephalomyelitis (B01.1-)

rubella encephalitis, myelitis and encephalomyelitis (B06.01)

toxoplasmosis encephalitis, myelitis and encephalomyelitis (B58.2)

zoster encephalitis, myelitis and encephalomyelitis (B02.0)

G05.3 Encephalitis and encephalomyelitis in diseases classified elsewhere

Meningoencephalitis in diseases classified elsewhere

G05.4 Myelitis in diseases classified elsewhere

Meningomyelitis in diseases classified elsewhere

G06 Intracranial and intraspinal abscess and granuloma

Use additional code (B95-B97) to identify infectious agent.

G06.0 Intracranial abscess and granuloma

Brain [any part] abscess (embolic)

Cerebellar abscess (embolic)

Cerebral abscess (embolic)

Intracranial epidural abscess or granuloma

Intracranial extradural abscess or granuloma

Intracranial subdural abscess or granuloma

Otogenic abscess (embolic)

Excludes1: tuberculous intracranial abscess and granuloma (A17.81)

G06.1 Intraspinal abscess and granuloma

Abscess (embolic) of spinal cord [any part]

Intraspinal epidural abscess or granuloma

Intraspinal extradural abscess or granuloma

Intraspinal subdural abscess or granuloma

Excludes1: tuberculous intraspinal abscess and granuloma (A17.81)

G06.2 Extradural and subdural abscess, unspecified

G07 Intracranial and intraspinal abscess and granuloma in diseases classified elsewhere

Code first underlying disease, such as:

schistosomiasis granuloma of brain (B65.-)

Excludes1: abscess of brain:

amebic (A06.6)

chromomycotic (B43.1)

gonococcal (A54.82)

tuberculous (A17.81)

tuberculoma of meninges (A17.1)

G08 **Intracranial and intraspinal phlebitis and thrombophlebitis**

Septic embolism of intracranial or intraspinal venous sinuses and veins

Septic endophlebitis of intracranial or intraspinal venous sinuses and veins

Septic phlebitis of intracranial or intraspinal venous sinuses and veins

Septic thrombophlebitis of intracranial or intraspinal venous sinuses and veins

Septic thrombosis of intracranial or intraspinal venous sinuses and veins

Excludes1: intracranial phlebitis and thrombophlebitis complicating:

abortion, ectopic or molar pregnancy (O00-O07, O08.7)

pregnancy, childbirth and the puerperium (O22.5, O87.3)

nonpyogenic intracranial phlebitis and thrombophlebitis (I67.6)

Excludes2: intracranial phlebitis and thrombophlebitis complicating nonpyogenic intraspinal phlebitis and thrombophlebitis (G95.1)

G09 **Sequelae of inflammatory diseases of central nervous system**

Note: Category G09 is to be used to indicate conditions whose primary classification is to G00-G08 as the cause of sequelae, themselves classifiable elsewhere. The 'sequelae' include conditions specified as residuals.

Code first condition resulting from (sequela) of inflammatory diseases of central nervous system

SYSTEMIC ATROPHIES PRIMARILY AFFECTING THE CENTRAL NERVOUS SYSTEM (G10-G14)

G10 **Huntington's disease**

Huntington's chorea

Huntington's dementia

Code also dementia in other diseases classified elsewhere without behavioral disturbance (F02.80)

G11 **Hereditary ataxia**

Excludes2: cerebral palsy (G80.-)

hereditary and idiopathic neuropathy (G60.-)

metabolic disorders (E70-E88)

G11.0 **Congenital nonprogressive ataxia**

G11.1 **Early-onset cerebellar ataxia**

Early-onset cerebellar ataxia with essential tremor

Early-onset cerebellar ataxia with myoclonus [Hunt's ataxia]

Early-onset cerebellar ataxia with retained tendon reflexes

Friedreich's ataxia (autosomal recessive)

X-linked recessive spinocerebellar ataxia

G11.2 **Late-onset cerebellar ataxia**

G11.3 **Cerebellar ataxia with defective DNA repair**

Ataxia telangiectasia [Louis-Bar]

Excludes2: Cockayne's syndrome (Q87.1)

Other disorders of purine and pyrimidine metabolism (E79.-)

xeroderma pigmentosum (Q82.1)

G11.4 **Hereditary spastic paraplegia**

G11.8 **Other hereditary ataxias**

G11.9 **Hereditary ataxia, unspecified**

Hereditary cerebellar ataxia NOS

Hereditary cerebellar degeneration

Hereditary cerebellar disease

Hereditary cerebellar syndrome

G12 **Spinal muscular atrophy and related syndromes**

G12.0 **Infantile spinal muscular atrophy, type I [Werdnig-Hoffman]**

G12.1 **Other inherited spinal muscular atrophy**

Adult form spinal muscular atrophy

Childhood form, type II spinal muscular atrophy

Distal spinal muscular atrophy

Juvenile form, type III spinal muscular atrophy [Kugelberg-Welander]

Progressive bulbar palsy of childhood [Fazio-Londe]

Scapuloperoneal form spinal muscular atrophy

G12.2 **Motor neuron disease**

G12.20 **Motor neuron disease, unspecified**

G12.21 **Amyotrophic lateral sclerosis**

G12.22 **Progressive bulbar palsy**

•**G12.23** **Primary lateral sclerosis**

•**G12.24** **Familial motor neuron disease**

•**G12.25** **Progressive spinal muscle atrophy**

G12.29 **Other motor neuron disease**

G12.8 **Other spinal muscular atrophies and related syndromes**

G12.9 **Spinal muscular atrophy, unspecified**

G13 **Systemic atrophies primarily affecting central nervous system in diseases classified elsewhere**

G13.0 **Paraneoplastic neuromyopathy and neuropathy**

Carcinomatous neuromyopathy

Sensorial paraneoplastic neuropathy [Denny Brown]

Code first underlying neoplasm (C00-D49)

G13.1 **Other systemic atrophy primarily affecting central nervous system in neoplastic disease**

Paraneoplastic limbic encephalopathy

Code first underlying neoplasm (C00-D49)

G13.2 **Systemic atrophy primarily affecting the central nervous system in myxedema**

Code first underlying disease, such as:

hypothyroidism (E03.-)

myxedematous congenital iodine deficiency (E00.1)

G13.8 **Systemic atrophy primarily affecting central nervous system in other diseases classified elsewhere**

Code first underlying disease

G14 **Postpolio syndrome**

Includes: postpolio myelitic syndrome

Excludes1: sequelae of poliomyelitis (B91)

EXTRAPYRAMIDAL AND MOVEMENT DISORDERS (G20-G26)

Definition: Extrapyramidal symptoms (EPS) are various movement disorders such as acute dystonic reactions, pseudoparkinsonism, Tardive dyskinesia or akathisia suffered as a result of taking dopamine antagonists, usually antipsychotic (neuroleptic) drugs, which are often used to control psychosis.

G20 **Parkinson's disease**

Hemiparkinsonism

Idiopathic Parkinsonism or Parkinson's disease

Paralysis agitans

Parkinsonism or Parkinson's disease NOS

Primary Parkinsonism or Parkinson's disease

Excludes1: dementia with Parkinsonism (G31.83)

G21 **Secondary parkinsonism**

Excludes1: dementia with Parkinsonism (G31.83)

Huntington's disease (G10)

Shy-Drager syndrome (G90.3)

syphilitic Parkinsonism (A52.19)

G21.0 **Malignant neuroleptic syndrome**

Use additional code for adverse effect, if applicable, to identify drug (T43.3X5, T43.4X5, T43.505, T43.595)

Excludes1: neuroleptic induced parkinsonism (G21.11)

G21.1 **Other drug-induced secondary parkinsonism**

G21.11 **Neuroleptic induced parkinsonism**

Use additional code for adverse effect, if applicable, to identify drug (T43.3X5, T43.4X5, T43.505, T43.595)

Excludes1: malignant neuroleptic syndrome (G21.0)

G21.19 **Other drug induced secondary parkinsonism**

Other medication-induced parkinsonism

Use additional code for adverse effect, if applicable, to identify drug (T36-T50 with fifth or sixth character 5)

G21.2 **Secondary parkinsonism due to other external agents**

Code first (T51-T65) to identify external agent

G21.3 **Postencephalitic parkinsonism**

G21.4 **Vascular parkinsonism**

G21.8 **Other secondary parkinsonism**

G21.9 **Secondary parkinsonism, unspecified**

G23 **Other degenerative diseases of basal ganglia**

Excludes2: multi-system degeneration of the autonomic nervous system (G90.3)

G23.0 **Hallervorden-Spatz disease**

Pigmentary pallidal degeneration

G23.1 **Progressive supranuclear ophthalmoplegia [Steele-Richardson-Olszewski]**

Progressive supranuclear palsy

G23.2 **Striatonigral degeneration**

G23.8 **Other specified degenerative diseases of basal ganglia**

Calcification of basal ganglia

G23.9 **Degenerative disease of basal ganglia, unspecified**

G24 **Dystonia**

Includes: dyskinesia

Excludes2: athetoid cerebral palsy (G80.3)

G24.0 **Drug induced dystonia**

Use additional code for adverse effect, if applicable, to identify drug (T36-T50 with fifth or sixth character 5)

G24.01 **Drug induced subacute dyskinesia**

Drug induced blepharospasm

Drug induced orofacial dyskinesia

Neuroleptic induced tardive dyskinesia

Tardive dyskinesia

G24.02 **Drug induced acute dystonia**

Acute dystonic reaction to drugs

Neuroleptic induced acute dystonia

G24.09 **Other drug induced dystonia**

G24.1 **Genetic torsion dystonia**

Dystonia deformans progressiva

Dystonia musculorum deformans

Familial torsion dystonia

Idiopathic familial dystonia

Idiopathic (torsion) dystonia NOS (Schwalbe-) Ziehen-Oppenheim disease

G24.2 **Idiopathic nonfamilial dystonia**

G24.3 **Spasmodic torticollis**

Excludes1: congenital torticollis (Q68.0)

hysterical torticollis (F44.4)

ocular torticollis (R29.891)

psychogenic torticollis (F45.8)

torticollis NOS (M43.6)

traumatic recurrent torticollis (S13.4)

G24.4 **Idiopathic orofacial dystonia**

Orofacial dyskinesia

Excludes1: drug induced orofacial dyskinesia (G24.01)

G24.5 **Blepharospasm**

Excludes1: drug induced blepharospasm (G24.01)

G24.8 **Other dystonia**

Acquired torsion dystonia NOS

G24.9 **Dystonia, unspecified**

Dyskinesia NOS

G25 **Other extrapyramidal and movement disorders**

Definition: Extrapyramidal disease is a general term for a number of disorders caused by abnormalities of the basal ganglia or certain brain stem or thalamic nuclei; characterized by motor deficits, loss of postural reflexes, bradykinesia, tremor, rigidity, and various involuntary movements.

Excludes2: sleep related movement disorders (G47.6-)

G25.0 **Essential tremor** Familial tremor

Excludes1: tremor NOS (R25.1)

G25.1 **Drug-induced tremor**

Use additional code for adverse effect, if applicable, to identify drug (T36-T50 with fifth or sixth character 5)

G25.2 **Other specified forms of tremor**

Intention tremor

G25.3 **Myoclonus**

Drug-induced myoclonus

Palatal myoclonus

Use additional code for adverse effect, if applicable, to identify drug (T36-T50 with fifth or sixth character 5)

Excludes1: facial myokymia (G51.4)

myoclonic epilepsy (G40.-)

G25.4 **Drug-induced chorea**

Use additional code for adverse effect, if applicable, to identify drug (T36-T50 with fifth or sixth character 5)

G25.5 **Other chorea**

Chorea NOS

Excludes1: chorea NOS with heart involvement (I02.0)

Huntington's chorea (G10)

rheumatic chorea (I02.-)

Sydenham's chorea (I02.-)

G25.6 **Drug induced tics and other tics of organic origin**

G25.61 **Drug induced tics**

Use additional code for adverse effect, if applicable, to identify drug (T36-T50 with fifth or sixth character 5)

G25.69 **Other tics of organic origin**

Excludes1: habit spasm (F95.9)

tic NOS (F95.9)

Tourette's syndrome (F95.2)

● New code ▲ Revised code **Excludes1:** Not coded here **Excludes2:** Not included here ⊗ Placeholder required ⑦7th digit required

G25.7 **Other and unspecified drug induced movement disorders**

<u>Use additional code</u> for adverse effect, if applicable, to identify drug (T36-T50 with fifth or sixth character 5)

G25.70 **Drug induced movement disorder, unspecified**

G25.71 **Drug induced akathisia**

Drug induced acathisia

Neuroleptic induced acute akathisia

Tardive akathisia

G25.79 **Other drug induced movement disorders**

G25.8 **Other specified extrapyramidal and movement disorders**

G25.81 **Restless legs syndrome**

G25.82 **Stiff-man syndrome**

G25.83 **Benign shuddering attacks**

G25.89 **Other specified extrapyramidal and movement disorders**

G25.9 **Extrapyramidal and movement disorder, unspecified**

G26 **Extrapyramidal and movement disorders in diseases classified elsewhere**

<u>Code first</u> underlying disease

OTHER DEGENERATIVE DISEASES OF THE NERVOUS SYSTEM (G30-G32)

G30 **Alzheimer's disease**

<u>Includes:</u> Alzheimer's dementia senile and presenile forms

<u>Use additional code</u> to identify:

delirium, if applicable (F05)

dementia with behavioral disturbance (F02.81)

dementia without behavioral disturbance (F02.80)

<u>Excludes1:</u> senile degeneration of brain NEC (G31.1)

senile dementia NOS (F03)

senility NOS (R41.81)

G30.0 **Alzheimer's disease with early onset**

G30.1 **Alzheimer's disease with late onset**

G30.8 **Other Alzheimer's disease**

G30.9 **Alzheimer's disease, unspecified**

G31 **Other degenerative diseases of nervous system, not elsewhere classified**

<u>Use additional code</u> to identify:

dementia with behavioral disturbance (F02.81)

dementia without behavioral disturbance (F02.80)

<u>Excludes2:</u> Reye's syndrome (G93.7)

G31.0 **Frontotemporal dementia**

G31.01 **Pick's disease**

Primary progressive aphasia

Progressive isolated aphasia

G31.09 **Other frontotemporal dementia**

Frontal dementia

G31.1 **Senile degeneration of brain, not elsewhere classified**

<u>Excludes1:</u> Alzheimer's disease (G30.-)

senility NOS (R41.81)

G31.2 **Degeneration of nervous system due to alcohol**

Alcoholic cerebellar ataxia

Alcoholic cerebellar degeneration

Alcoholic cerebral degeneration

Alcoholic encephalopathy

Dysfunction of the autonomic nervous system due to alcohol

<u>Code also</u> associated alcoholism (F10.-)

G31.8 **Other specified degenerative diseases of nervous system**

G31.81 **Alpers disease**

Grey-matter degeneration

G31.82 **Leigh's disease**

Subacute necrotizing encephalopathy

G31.83 **Dementia with Lewy bodies**

Dementia with Parkinsonism

Lewy body dementia

Lewy body disease

G31.84 **Mild cognitive impairment, so stated**

Mild neurocognitive disorder

<u>Excludes1:</u> age related cognitive decline (R41.81)

altered mental status (R41.82)

cerebral degeneration (G31.9)

change in mental status (R41.82)

cognitive deficits following (sequelae of) cerebral hemorrhage or infarction (I69.01-, I69.11-, I69.21-, I69.31-, I69.81-, I69.91-)

cognitive impairment due to intracranial or head injury (S06.-)

dementia (F01.-, F02.-, F03)

mild memory disturbance (F06.8)

neurologic neglect syndrome (R41.4)

personality change, nonpsychotic (F68.8)

G31.85 **Corticobasal degeneration**

G31.89 **Other specified degenerative diseases of nervous system**

G31.9 **Degenerative disease of nervous system, unspecified**

G32 **Other degenerative disorders of nervous system in diseases classified elsewhere**

G32.0 **Subacute combined degeneration of spinal cord in diseases classified elsewhere**

Dana-Putnam syndrome

Sclerosis of spinal cord (combined) (dorsolateral) (posterolateral)

<u>Code first</u> underlying disease, such as:

anemia (D51.9)

dietary (D51.3)

pernicious (D51.0)

vitamin B12 deficiency (E53.8)

<u>Excludes1:</u> syphilitic combined degeneration of spinal cord (A52.11)

G32.8 **Other specified degenerative disorders of nervous system in diseases classified elsewhere**

<u>Code first</u> underlying disease, such as:

amyloidosis cerebral degeneration (E85.-)

cerebral degeneration (due to) hypothyroidism (E00.0-E03.9)

cerebral degeneration (due to) neoplasm (C00-D49)

cerebral degeneration (due to) vitamin B deficiency, except thiamine (E52-E53.-)

<u>Excludes1:</u> superior hemorrhagic polioencephalitis [Wernicke's encephalopathy] (E51.2)

G32.81 **Cerebellar ataxia in diseases classified elsewhere**

<u>Code first</u> underlying disease, such as:

celiac disease (with gluten ataxia) (K90.0)

cerebellar ataxia (in) neoplastic disease (paraneoplastic cerebellar degeneration) (C00-D49)

non-celiac gluten ataxia (M35.9)

Add 4th-7th digits   Nonspecific code   Unspecified code   Manifestation code

Excludes1: systemic atrophy primarily affecting the central nervous system in alcoholic cerebellar ataxia (G31.2)

systemic atrophy primarily affecting the central nervous system in myxedema (G13.2)

G32.89 **Other specified degenerative disorders of nervous system in diseases classified elsewhere**

Degenerative encephalopathy in diseases classified elsewhere

DEMYELINATING DISEASES OF THE CENTRAL NERVOUS SYSTEM (G35-G37)

Definition: A demyelinating disease is any condition that results in damage to the protective covering (myelin sheath) that surrounds nerve fibers in your brain and spinal cord. When the myelin sheath is damaged, nerve impulses slow or even stop, causing neurological problems.

G35 **Multiple sclerosis**

Definition: Multiple sclerosis is a chronic autoimmune disorder affecting movement, sensation, and bodily functions. It is caused by destruction of the myelin insulation covering nerve fibers in the central nervous system.

Disseminated multiple sclerosis Generalized multiple sclerosis

Multiple sclerosis NOS

Multiple sclerosis of brain stem

Multiple sclerosis of cord

G36 **Other acute disseminated demyelination**

Excludes1: postinfectious encephalitis and encephalomyelitis NOS (G04.01)

G36.0 **Neuromyelitis optica [Devic]**

Demyelination in optic neuritis

Excludes1: optic neuritis NOS (H46)

G36.1 **Acute and subacute hemorrhagic leukoencephalitis [Hurst]**

G36.8 **Other specified acute disseminated demyelination**

G36.9 **Acute disseminated demyelination, unspecified**

G37 **Other demyelinating diseases of central nervous system**

Definition: Demyelinating diseases of the central nervous system is any disease of the nervous system in which the myelin sheath of neurons is damaged.

G37.0 **Diffuse sclerosis of central nervous system**

Periaxial encephalitis

Schilder's disease

Excludes1: X linked adrenoleukodystrophy (E71.52-)

G37.1 **Central demyelination of corpus callosum**

G37.2 **Central pontine myelinolysis**

G37.3 **Acute transverse myelitis in demyelinating disease of central nervous system**

Acute transverse myelitis NOS

Acute transverse myelopathy

Excludes1: multiple sclerosis (G35)

neuromyelitis optica [Devic] (G36.0)

G37.4 **Subacute necrotizing myelitis of central nervous system**

G37.5 **Concentric sclerosis [Balo] of central nervous system**

G37.8 **Other specified demyelinating diseases of central nervous system**

G37.9 **Demyelinating disease of central nervous system, unspecified**

EPISODIC AND PAROXYSMAL DISORDERS (G40-G47)

G40 **Epilepsy and recurrent seizures**

Definition: Epilepsy and recurrent seizures is a common chronic neurological disorder characterized by recurrent unprovoked seizures. These seizures are transient signs and/or symptoms of abnormal, excessive or synchronous neuronal activity in the brain.

Note: the following terms are to be considered equivalent to intractable: pharmacoresistent (pharmacologically resistant), treatment resistant, refractory (medically) and poorly controlled

Excludes1: conversion disorder with seizures (F44.5)

convulsions NOS (R56.9)

post traumatic seizures (R56.1)

seizure (convulsive) NOS (R56.9)

seizure of newborn (P90)

Excludes2: hippocampal sclerosis (G93.81)

mesial temporal sclerosis (G93.81)

temporal sclerosis (G93.81)

Todd's paralysis (G83.84)

G40.0 **Localization-related (focal) (partial) idiopathic epilepsy and epileptic syndromes with seizures of localized onset**

Benign childhood epilepsy with centrotemporal EEG spikes

Childhood epilepsy with occipital EEG paroxysms

Excludes1: adult onset localization-related epilepsy (G40.1-, G40.2-)

G40.00 **Localization-related (focal) (partial) idiopathic epilepsy and epileptic syndromes with seizures of localized onset, not intractable**

Localization-related (focal) (partial) idiopathic epilepsy and epileptic syndromes with seizures of localized onset without intractability

G40.001 **Localization-related (focal) (partial) idiopathic epilepsy and epileptic syndromes with seizures of localized onset, not intractable, with status epilepticus**

G40.009 **Localization-related (focal) (partial) idiopathic epilepsy and epileptic syndromes with seizures of localized onset, not intractable, without status epilepticus**

Localization-related (focal) (partial) idiopathic epilepsy and epileptic syndromes with seizures of localized onset NOS

G40.01 **Localization-related (focal) (partial) idiopathic epilepsy and epileptic syndromes with seizures of localized onset, intractable**

G40.011 **Localization-related (focal) (partial) idiopathic epilepsy and epileptic syndromes with seizures of localized onset, intractable, with status epilepticus**

G40.019 **Localization-related (focal) (partial) idiopathic epilepsy and epileptic syndromes with seizures of localized onset, intractable, without status epilepticus**

G40.1 **Localization-related (focal) (partial) symptomatic epilepsy and epileptic syndromes with simple partial seizures**

Attacks without alteration of consciousness

Epilepsia partialis continua [Koshevnikoff]

Simple partial seizures developing into secondarily generalized seizures

● New code ▲ Revised code **Excludes1:** Not coded here **Excludes2:** Not included here ⊗ Placeholder required ⑦ 7th digit required

G40.10 **Localization-related (focal) (partial) symptomatic epilepsy and epileptic syndromes with simple partial seizures, not intractable**

Localization-related (focal) (partial) symptomatic epilepsy and epileptic syndromes with simple partial seizures without intractability

G40.101 **Localization-related (focal) (partial) symptomatic epilepsy and epileptic syndromes with simple partial seizures, not intractable, with status epilepticus**

G40.109 **Localization-related (focal) (partial) symptomatic epilepsy and epileptic syndromes with simple partial seizures, not intractable, without status epilepticus**

Localization-related (focal) (partial) symptomatic epilepsy and epileptic syndromes with simple partial seizures NOS

G40.11 **Localization-related (focal) (partial) symptomatic epilepsy and epileptic syndromes with simple partial seizures, intractable**

G40.111 **Localization-related (focal) (partial) symptomatic epilepsy and epileptic syndromes with simple partial seizures, intractable, with status epilepticus**

G40.119 **Localization-related (focal) (partial) symptomatic epilepsy and epileptic syndromes with simple partial seizures, intractable, without status epilepticus**

G40.2 **Localization-related (focal) (partial) symptomatic epilepsy and epileptic syndromes with complex partial seizures**

Attacks with alteration of consciousness, often with automatisms

Complex partial seizures developing into secondarily generalized seizures

G40.20 **Localization-related (focal) (partial) symptomatic epilepsy and epileptic syndromes with complex partial seizures, not intractable**

Localization-related (focal) (partial) symptomatic epilepsy and epileptic syndromes with complex partial seizures without intractability

G40.201 **Localization-related (focal) (partial) symptomatic epilepsy and epileptic syndromes with complex partial seizures, not intractable, with status epilepticus**

G40.209 **Localization-related (focal) (partial) symptomatic epilepsy and epileptic syndromes with complex partial seizures, not intractable, without status epilepticus**

Localization-related (focal) (partial) symptomatic epilepsy and epileptic syndromes with complex partial seizures NOS

G40.21 **Localization-related (focal) (partial) symptomatic epilepsy and epileptic syndromes with complex partial seizures, intractable**

G40.211 **Localization-related (focal) (partial) symptomatic epilepsy and epileptic syndromes with complex partial**

seizures, intractable, with status epilepticus

G40.219 **Localization-related (focal) (partial) symptomatic epilepsy and epileptic syndromes with complex partial seizures, intractable, without status epilepticus**

G40.3 **Generalized idiopathic epilepsy and epileptic syndromes**

Code also MERRF syndrome, if applicable (E88.42)

G40.30 **Generalized idiopathic epilepsy and epileptic syndromes, not intractable**

Generalized idiopathic epilepsy and epileptic syndromes without intractability

G40.301 **Generalized idiopathic epilepsy and epileptic syndromes, not intractable, with status epilepticus**

G40.309 **Generalized idiopathic epilepsy and epileptic syndromes, not intractable, without status epilepticus**

Generalized idiopathic epilepsy and epileptic syndromes NOS

G40.31 **Generalized idiopathic epilepsy and epileptic syndromes, intractable**

G40.311 **Generalized idiopathic epilepsy and epileptic syndromes, intractable, with status epilepticus**

G40.319 **Generalized idiopathic epilepsy and epileptic syndromes, intractable, without status epilepticus**

G40.A **Absence epileptic syndrome**

Childhood absence epilepsy [pyknolepsy]

Juvenile absence epilepsy

Absence epileptic syndrome, NOS

G40.A0 **Absence epileptic syndrome, not intractable**

G40.A01 **Absence epileptic syndrome, not intractable, with status epilepticus**

G40.A09 **Absence epileptic syndrome, not intractable, without status epilepticus**

G40.A1 **Absence epileptic syndrome, intractable**

G40.A11 **Absence epileptic syndrome, intractable, with status epilepticus**

G40.A19 **Absence epileptic syndrome, intractable, without status epilepticus**

G40.B **Juvenile myoclonic epilepsy [impulsive petit mal]**

G40.B0 **Juvenile myoclonic epilepsy, not intractable**

G40.B01 **Juvenile myoclonic epilepsy, not intractable, with status epilepticus**

G40.B09 **Juvenile myoclonic epilepsy, not intractable, without status epilepticus**

G40.B1 **Juvenile myoclonic epilepsy, intractable**

G40.B11 **Juvenile myoclonic epilepsy, intractable, with status epilepticus**

G40.B19 **Juvenile myoclonic epilepsy, intractable, without status epilepticus**

G40.4 **Other generalized epilepsy and epileptic syndromes**

Epilepsy with grand mal seizures on awakening

Epilepsy with myoclonic absences

Epilepsy with myoclonic-astatic seizures

Grand mal seizure NOS

Nonspecific atonic epileptic seizures

Nonspecific clonic epileptic seizures

Nonspecific myoclonic epileptic seizures

Nonspecific tonic epileptic seizures

Nonspecific tonic-clonic epileptic seizures

Symptomatic early myoclonic encephalopathy

G40.40 **Other generalized epilepsy and epileptic syndromes, not intractable**

Other generalized epilepsy and epileptic syndromes without intractability

Other generalized epilepsy and epileptic syndromes NOS

G40.401 **Other generalized epilepsy and epileptic syndromes, not intractable, with status epilepticus**

G40.409 **Other generalized epilepsy and epileptic syndromes, not intractable, without status epilepticus**

G40.41 **Other generalized epilepsy and epileptic syndromes, intractable**

G40.411 **Other generalized epilepsy and epileptic syndromes, intractable, with status epilepticus**

G40.419 **Other generalized epilepsy and epileptic syndromes, intractable, without status epilepticus**

G40.5 **Epileptic seizures related to external causes**

Epileptic seizures related to alcohol

Epileptic seizures related to drugs

Epileptic seizures related to hormonal changes

Epileptic seizures related to sleep deprivation

Epileptic seizures related to stress

Code also, if applicable, associated epilepsy and recurrent seizures (G40.-)

Use additional code for adverse effect, if applicable, to identify drug (T36-T50 with fifth or sixth character 5)

G40.50 **Epileptic seizures related to external causes, not intractable**

G40.501 **Epileptic seizures related to external causes, not intractable, with status epilepticus**

G40.509 **Epileptic seizures related to external causes, not intractable, without status epilepticus**

Epileptic seizures related to external causes, NOS

G40.8 **Other epilepsy and recurrent seizures**

Epilepsies and epileptic syndromes undetermined as to whether they are focal or generalized Landau-Kleffner syndrome

G40.80 **Other epilepsy**

G40.801 **Other epilepsy, not intractable, with status epilepticus**

Other epilepsy without intractability with status epilepticus

G40.802 **Other epilepsy, not intractable, without status epilepticus**

Other epilepsy NOS

Other epilepsy without intractability without status epilepticus

G40.803 **Other epilepsy, intractable, with status epilepticus**

G40.804 **Other epilepsy, intractable, without status epilepticus**

G40.81 **Lennox-Gastaut syndrome**

G40.811 **Lennox-Gastaut syndrome, not intractable, with status epilepticus**

G40.812 **Lennox-Gastaut syndrome, not intractable, without status epilepticus**

G40.813 **Lennox-Gastaut syndrome, intractable, with status epilepticus**

G40.814 **Lennox-Gastaut syndrome, intractable, without status epilepticus**

G40.82 **Epileptic spasms**

Infantile spasms

Salaam attacks West's syndrome

G40.821 **Epileptic spasms, not intractable, with status epilepticus**

G40.822 **Epileptic spasms, not intractable, without status epilepticus**

G40.823 **Epileptic spasms, intractable, with status epilepticus**

G40.824 **Epileptic spasms, intractable, without status epilepticus**

G40.89 **Other seizures**

Excludes1: post traumatic seizures (R56.1)

recurrent seizures NOS (G40.909)

seizure NOS (R56.9)

G40.9 **Epilepsy, unspecified**

G40.90 **Epilepsy, unspecified, not intractable**

Epilepsy, unspecified, without intractability

G40.901 **Epilepsy, unspecified, not intractable, with status epilepticus**

G40.909 **Epilepsy, unspecified, not intractable, without status epilepticus**

Epilepsy NOS

Epileptic convulsions NOS

Epileptic fits NOS

Epileptic seizures NOS

Recurrent seizures NOS

Seizure disorder NOS

G40.91 **Epilepsy, unspecified, intractable**

Intractable seizure disorder NOS

G40.911 **Epilepsy, unspecified, intractable, with status epilepticus**

G40.919 **Epilepsy, unspecified, intractable, without status epilepticus**

G43 **Migraine**

Definition: Migraine is a severe, disabling headache, usually affecting only one side of the head, and often accompanied by nausea, vomiting, photophobia and visual disturbances.

Note: the following terms are to be considered equivalent to intractable: pharmacoresistant (pharmacologically resistant), treatment resistant, refractory (medically) and poorly controlled

Use additional code for adverse effect, if applicable, to identify drug (T36-T50 with fifth or sixth character 5)

Excludes1: headache NOS (R51)

lower half migraine (G44.00)

Excludes2: headache syndromes (G44.-)

G43.0 **Migraine without aura**

Common migraine

Excludes1: chronic migraine without aura (G43.7-)

G43.00 **Migraine without aura, not intractable**

● New code ▲ Revised code **Excludes1:** Not coded here **Excludes2:** Not included here ⊗ Placeholder required ⑦ 7th digit required

Migraine without aura without mention of refractory migraine

G43.001 **Migraine without aura, not intractable, with status migrainosus**

G43.009 **Migraine without aura, not intractable, without status migrainosus**

Migraine without aura NOS

G43.01 **Migraine without aura, intractable**

Migraine without aura with refractory migraine

G43.011 **Migraine without aura, intractable, with status migrainosus**

G43.019 **Migraine without aura, intractable, without status migrainosus**

G43.1 **Migraine with aura**

Basilar migraine

Classical migraine

Migraine equivalents

Migraine preceded or accompanied by transient focal neurological phenomena

Migraine triggered seizures

Migraine with acute-onset aura

Migraine with aura without headache (migraine equivalents)

Migraine with prolonged aura

Migraine with typical aura

Retinal migraine

Code also any associated seizure (G40.-, R56.9)

Excludes1: persistent migraine aura (G43.5-, G43.6-)

G43.10 **Migraine with aura, not intractable**

Migraine with aura without mention of refractory migraine

G43.101 **Migraine with aura, not intractable, with status migrainosus**

G43.109 **Migraine with aura, not intractable, without status migrainosus**

Migraine with aura NOS

G43.11 **Migraine with aura, intractable**

Migraine with aura with refractory migraine

G43.111 **Migraine with aura, intractable, with status migrainosus**

G43.119 **Migraine with aura, intractable, without status migrainosus**

G43.4 **Hemiplegic migraine**

Familial migraine

Sporadic migraine

G43.40 **Hemiplegic migraine, not intractable**

Hemiplegic migraine without refractory migraine

G43.401 **Hemiplegic migraine, not intractable, with status migrainosus**

G43.409 **Hemiplegic migraine, not intractable, without status migrainosus**

Hemiplegic migraine NOS

G43.41 **Hemiplegic migraine, intractable**

Hemiplegic migraine with refractory migraine

G43.411 **Hemiplegic migraine, intractable, with status migrainosus**

G43.419 **Hemiplegic migraine, intractable, without status migrainosus**

G43.5 **Persistent migraine aura without cerebral infarction**

G43.50 **Persistent migraine aura without cerebral infarction, not intractable**

Persistent migraine aura without cerebral infarction, without refractory migraine

G43.501 **Persistent migraine aura without cerebral infarction, not intractable, with status migrainosus**

G43.509 **Persistent migraine aura without cerebral infarction, not intractable, without status migrainosus**

Persistent migraine aura NOS

G43.51 **Persistent migraine aura without cerebral infarction, intractable**

Persistent migraine aura without cerebral infarction, with refractory migraine

G43.511 **Persistent migraine aura without cerebral infarction, intractable, with status migrainosus**

G43.519 **Persistent migraine aura without cerebral infarction, intractable, without status migrainosus**

G43.6 **Persistent migraine aura with cerebral infarction**

Code also the type of cerebral infarction (I63.-)

G43.60 **Persistent migraine aura with cerebral infarction, not intractable**

Persistent migraine aura with cerebral infarction, without refractory migraine

G43.601 **Persistent migraine aura with cerebral infarction, not intractable, with status migrainosus**

G43.609 **Persistent migraine aura with cerebral infarction, not intractable, without status migrainosus**

G43.61 **Persistent migraine aura with cerebral infarction, intractable**

Persistent migraine aura with cerebral infarction, with refractory migraine

G43.611 **Persistent migraine aura with cerebral infarction, intractable, with status migrainosus**

G43.619 **Persistent migraine aura with cerebral infarction, intractable, without status migrainosus**

G43.7 **Chronic migraine without aura**

Transformed migraine

Excludes1: migraine without aura (G43.0-)

G43.70 **Chronic migraine without aura, not intractable**

Chronic migraine without aura, without refractory migraine

G43.701 **Chronic migraine without aura, not intractable, with status migrainosus**

G43.709 **Chronic migraine without aura, not intractable, without status migrainosus**

Chronic migraine without aura NOS

G43.71 **Chronic migraine without aura, intractable**

Chronic migraine without aura, with refractory migraine

G43.711 **Chronic migraine without aura, intractable, with status migrainosus**

G43.719 **Chronic migraine without aura, intractable, without status migrainosus**

G43.A **Cyclical vomiting**

G43.A0 **Cyclical vomiting, not intractable**

Cyclical vomiting, without refractory migraine

G43.A1 **Cyclical vomiting, intractable**

Cyclical vomiting, with refractory migraine

G43.B **Ophthalmoplegic migraine**

G43.B0 **Ophthalmoplegic migraine, not intractable**

Ophthalmoplegic migraine, without refractory migraine

G43.B1 **Ophthalmoplegic migraine, intractable**

Ophthalmoplegic migraine, with refractory migraine

G43.C **Periodic headache syndromes in child or adult**

G43.C0 **Periodic headache syndromes in child or adult, not intractable**

Periodic headache syndromes in child or adult, without refractory migraine

G43.C1 **Periodic headache syndromes in child or adult, intractable**

Periodic headache syndromes in child or adult, with refractory migraine

G43.D **Abdominal migraine**

G43.D0 **Abdominal migraine, not intractable**

Abdominal migraine, without refractory migraine

G43.D1 **Abdominal migraine, intractable**

Abdominal migraine, with refractory migraine

G43.8 **Other migraine**

G43.80 **Other migraine, not intractable**

Other migraine, without refractory migraine

G43.801 **Other migraine, not intractable, with status migrainosus**

G43.809 **Other migraine, not intractable, without status migrainosus**

G43.81 **Other migraine, intractable**

Other migraine, with refractory migraine

G43.811 **Other migraine, intractable, with status migrainosus**

G43.819 **Other migraine, intractable, without status migrainosus**

G43.82 **Menstrual migraine, not intractable**

Menstrual headache, not intractable

Menstrual migraine, without refractory migraine

Menstrually related migraine, not intractable

Pre-menstrual headache, not intractable

Pre-menstrual migraine, not intractable

Pure menstrual migraine, not intractable

Code also associated premenstrual tension syndrome (N94.3)

G43.821 **Menstrual migraine, not intractable, with status migrainosus**

G43.829 **Menstrual migraine, not intractable, without status migrainosus**

Menstrual migraine NOS

G43.83 **Menstrual migraine, intractable**

Menstrual headache, intractable

Menstrual migraine, with refractory migraine

Menstrually related migraine, intractable

Pre-menstrual headache, intractable

Pre-menstrual migraine, intractable

Pure menstrual migraine, intractable

Code also associated premenstrual tension syndrome (N94.3)

G43.831 **Menstrual migraine, intractable, with status migrainosus**

G43.839 **Menstrual migraine, intractable, without status migrainosus**

G43.9 **Migraine, unspecified**

G43.90 **Migraine, unspecified, not intractable**

Migraine, unspecified, without refractory migraine

G43.901 **Migraine, unspecified, not intractable, with status migrainosus**

Status migrainosus NOS

G43.909 **Migraine, unspecified, not intractable, without status migrainosus**

Migraine NOS

G43.91 **Migraine, unspecified, intractable**

Migraine, unspecified, with refractory migraine

G43.911 **Migraine, unspecified, intractable, with status migrainosus**

G43.919 **Migraine, unspecified, intractable, without status migrainosus**

G44 **Other headache syndromes**

Excludes1: headache NOS (R51)

Excludes2: atypical facial pain (G50.1)

headache due to lumbar puncture (G97.1)

migraines (G43.-)

trigeminal neuralgia (G50.0)

G44.0 **Cluster headaches and other trigeminal autonomic cephalgias (TAC)**

G44.00 **Cluster headache syndrome, unspecified**

Ciliary neuralgia

Cluster headache NOS

Histamine cephalgia

Lower half migraine

Migrainous neuralgia

G44.001 **Cluster headache syndrome, unspecified, intractable**

G44.009 **Cluster headache syndrome, unspecified, not intractable**

Cluster headache syndrome NOS

G44.01 **Episodic cluster headache**

G44.011 **Episodic cluster headache, intractable**

G44.019 **Episodic cluster headache, not intractable**

Episodic cluster headache NOS

G44.02 **Chronic cluster headache**

G44.021 **Chronic cluster headache, intractable**

G44.029 **Chronic cluster headache, not intractable**

Chronic cluster headache NOS

G44.03 **Episodic paroxysmal hemicrania**

Paroxysmal hemicrania NOS

G44.031 **Episodic paroxysmal hemicrania, intractable**

G44.039 **Episodic paroxysmal hemicrania, not intractable**

Episodic paroxysmal hemicrania NOS

G44.04 **Chronic paroxysmal hemicrania**

G44.041 **Chronic paroxysmal hemicrania, intractable**

● New code ▲ Revised code **Excludes1:** Not coded here **Excludes2:** Not included here ⊗ Placeholder required ⑦ 7th digit required

G44.049 **Chronic paroxysmal hemicrania, not intractable**

Chronic paroxysmal hemicrania NOS

G44.05 **Short lasting unilateral neuralgiform headache with conjunctival injection and tearing (SUNCT)**

G44.051 **Short lasting unilateral neuralgiform headache with conjunctival injection and tearing (SUNCT), intractable**

G44.059 **Short lasting unilateral neuralgiform headache with conjunctival injection and tearing (SUNCT), not intractable**

Short lasting unilateral neuralgiform headache with conjunctival injection and tearing (SUNCT) NOS

G44.09 **Other trigeminal autonomic cephalgias (TAC)**

G44.091 **Other trigeminal autonomic cephalgias (TAC), intractable**

G44.099 **Other trigeminal autonomic cephalgias (TAC), not intractable**

G44.1 **Vascular headache, not elsewhere classified**

Excludes2: cluster headache (G44.0)

complicated headache syndromes (G44.5-)

drug-induced headache (G44.4-)

migraine (G43.-)

Other specified headache syndromes (G44.8-)

post-traumatic headache (G44.3-)

tension-type headache (G44.2-)

G44.2 **Tension-type headache**

G44.20 **Tension-type headache, unspecified**

G44.201 **Tension-type headache, unspecified, intractable**

G44.209 **Tension-type headache, unspecified, not intractable**

Tension headache NOS

G44.21 **Episodic tension-type headache**

G44.211 **Episodic tension-type headache, intractable**

G44.219 **Episodic tension-type headache, not intractable**

Episodic tension-type headache NOS

G44.22 **Chronic tension-type headache**

G44.221 **Chronic tension-type headache, intractable**

G44.229 **Chronic tension-type headache, not intractable**

Chronic tension-type headache NOS

G44.3 **Post-traumatic headache**

G44.30 **Post-traumatic headache, unspecified**

G44.301 **Post-traumatic headache, unspecified, intractable**

G44.309 **Post-traumatic headache, unspecified, not intractable**

Post-traumatic headache NOS

G44.31 **Acute post-traumatic headache**

G44.311 **Acute post-traumatic headache, intractable**

G44.319 **Acute post-traumatic headache, not intractable**

Acute post-traumatic headache NOS

G44.32 **Chronic post-traumatic headache**

G44.321 **Chronic post-traumatic headache, intractable**

G44.329 **Chronic post-traumatic headache, not intractable**

Chronic post-traumatic headache NOS

G44.4 **Drug-induced headache, not elsewhere classified**

Medication overuse headache

Use additional code for adverse effect, if applicable, to identify drug (T36-T50 with fifth or sixth character 5)

G44.40 **Drug-induced headache, not elsewhere classified, not intractable**

G44.41 **Drug-induced headache, not elsewhere classified, intractable**

G44.5 **Complicated headache syndromes**

G44.51 **Hemicrania continua**

G44.52 **New daily persistent headache (NDPH)**

G44.53 **Primary thunderclap headache**

G44.59 **Other complicated headache syndrome**

G44.8 **Other specified headache syndromes**

G44.81 **Hypnic headache**

G44.82 **Headache associated with sexual activity**

Orgasmic headache

Preorgasmic headache

G44.83 **Primary cough headache**

G44.84 **Primary exertional headache**

G44.85 **Primary stabbing headache**

G44.89 **Other headache syndrome**

G45 **Transient cerebral ischemic attacks and related syndromes**

Definition: Transient cerebral ischemic attack is a brief episode of neurological dysfunction resulting from an interruption in the blood supply to the brain or the eye, sometimes as a precursor to a stroke.

Excludes1: neonatal cerebral ischemia (P91.0)

transient retinal artery occlusion (H34.0-)

G45.0 **Vertebro-basilar artery syndrome**

G45.1 **Carotid artery syndrome (hemispheric)**

G45.2 **Multiple and bilateral precerebral artery syndromes**

G45.3 **Amaurosis fugax**

G45.4 **Transient global amnesia**

Excludes1: amnesia NOS (R41.3)

G45.8 **Other transient cerebral ischemic attacks and related syndromes**

G45.9 **Transient cerebral ischemic attack, unspecified**

Spasm of cerebral artery TIA

Transient cerebral ischemia NOS

G46 **Vascular syndromes of brain in cerebrovascular diseases**

Code first underlying cerebrovascular disease (I60-I69)

G46.0 **Middle cerebral artery syndrome**

G46.1 **Anterior cerebral artery syndrome**

G46.2 **Posterior cerebral artery syndrome**

G46.3 **Brain stem stroke syndrome**

Benedikt syndrome

Claude syndrome

Foville syndrome

Millard-Gubler syndrome

Wallenberg syndrome

Weber syndrome

G46.4 **Cerebellar stroke syndrome**

G46.5 **Pure motor lacunar syndrome**

G46.6 **Pure sensory lacunar syndrome**

G46.7 **Other lacunar syndromes**

G46.8 **Other vascular syndromes of brain in cerebrovascular diseases**

G47 **Sleep disorders**

Excludes2: nightmares (F51.5)

nonorganic sleep disorders (F51.-)

sleep terrors (F51.4)

sleepwalking (F51.3)

G47.0 **Insomnia**

Excludes2: alcohol related insomnia (F10.182, F10.282, F10.982)

drug-related insomnia (F11.182, F11.282, F11.982, F13.182, F13.282, F13.982, F14.182, F14.282, F14.982, F15.182, F15.282, F15.982, F19.182, F19.282, F19.982)

idiopathic insomnia (F51.01)

insomnia due to a mental disorder (F51.05)

insomnia not due to a substance or known physiological condition (F51.0-)

nonorganic insomnia (F51.0-)

primary insomnia (F51.01)

sleep apnea (G47.3-)

G47.00 **Insomnia, unspecified**

Insomnia NOS

G47.01 **Insomnia due to medical condition**

Code also associated medical condition

G47.09 **Other insomnia**

G47.1 **Hypersomnia**

Excludes2: alcohol-related hypersomnia (F10.182, F10.282, F10.982)

drug-related hypersomnia (F11.182, F11.282, F11.982, F13.182, F13.282, F13.982, F14.182, F14.282, F14.982, F15.182, F15.282, F15.982, F19.182, F19.282, F19.982)

hypersomnia due to a mental disorder (F51.13)

hypersomnia not due to a substance or known physiological condition (F51.1-)

primary hypersomnia (F51.11)

sleep apnea (G47.3-)

G47.10 **Hypersomnia, unspecified**

Hypersomnia NOS

G47.11 **Idiopathic hypersomnia with long sleep time**

Idiopathic hypersomnia NOS

G47.12 **Idiopathic hypersomnia without long sleep time**

G47.13 **Recurrent hypersomnia**

Kleine-Levin syndrome

Menstrual related hypersomnia

G47.14 **Hypersomnia due to medical condition**

Code also associated medical condition

G47.19 **Other hypersomnia**

G47.2 **Circadian rhythm sleep disorders**

Disorders of the sleep wake schedule

Inversion of nyctohemeral rhythm

Inversion of sleep rhythm

G47.20 **Circadian rhythm sleep disorder, unspecified type**

Sleep wake schedule disorder NOS

G47.21 **Circadian rhythm sleep disorder, delayed sleep phase type**

Delayed sleep phase syndrome

G47.22 **Circadian rhythm sleep disorder, advanced sleep phase type**

G47.23 **Circadian rhythm sleep disorder, irregular sleep wake type**

Irregular sleep-wake pattern

G47.24 **Circadian rhythm sleep disorder, free running type**

Circadian rhythm sleep disorder, non-24-hour sleep-wake type

G47.25 **Circadian rhythm sleep disorder, jet lag type**

G47.26 **Circadian rhythm sleep disorder, shift work type**

G47.27 **Circadian rhythm sleep disorder in conditions classified elsewhere**

Code first underlying condition

G47.29 **Other circadian rhythm sleep disorder**

G47.3 **Sleep apnea**

Definition: Sleep apnea is a potentially serious sleep disorder in which breathing repeatedly stops and starts.

Code also any associated underlying condition

Excludes1: apnea NOS (R06.81)

Cheyne-Stokes breathing (R06.3)

pickwickian syndrome (E66.2)

sleep apnea of newborn (P28.3)

G47.30 **Sleep apnea, unspecified**

Sleep apnea NOS

G47.31 **Primary central sleep apnea**

Idiopathic central sleep apnea

G47.32 **High altitude periodic breathing**

G47.33 **Obstructive sleep apnea (adult) (pediatric)**

Obstructive sleep apnea hypopnea

Excludes1: obstructive sleep apnea of newborn (P28.3)

G47.34 **Idiopathic sleep related nonobstructive alveolar hypoventilation**

Sleep related hypoxia

G47.35 **Congenital central alveolar hypoventilation syndrome**

G47.36 **Sleep related hypoventilation in conditions classified elsewhere**

Sleep related hypoxemia in conditions classified elsewhere

Code first underlying condition

G47.37 **Central sleep apnea in conditions classified elsewhere**

Code first underlying condition

G47.39 **Other sleep apnea**

G47.4 **Narcolepsy and cataplexy**

G47.41 **Narcolepsy**

G47.411 **Narcolepsy with cataplexy**

G47.419 **Narcolepsy without cataplexy**

Narcolepsy NOS

G47.42 **Narcolepsy in conditions classified elsewhere**

Code first underlying condition

G47.421 **Narcolepsy in conditions classified elsewhere with cataplexy**

G47.429 **Narcolepsy in conditions classified elsewhere without cataplexy**

G47.5 **Parasomnia**

Excludes1: alcohol induced parasomnia (F10.182, F10.282, F10.982)

drug induced parasomnia (F11.182, F11.282, F11.982, F13.182, F13.282, F13.982, F14.182, F14.282, F14.982, F15.182, F15.282, F15.982, F19.182, F19.282, F19.982)

parasomnia not due to a substance or known physiological condition (F51.8)

G47.50 Parasomnia, unspecified
Parasomnia NOS

G47.51 Confusional arousals

G47.52 REM sleep behavior disorder

G47.53 Recurrent isolated sleep paralysis

G47.54 Parasomnia in conditions classified elsewhere
Code first underlying condition

G47.59 Other parasomnia

G47.6 Sleep related movement disorders
Excludes2: restless legs syndrome (G25.81)

G47.61 Periodic limb movement disorder

G47.62 Sleep related leg cramps

G47.63 Sleep related bruxism
Excludes1: psychogenic bruxism (F45.8)

G47.69 Other sleep related movement disorders

G47.8 Other sleep disorders
Other specified sleep-wake disorder

G47.9 Sleep disorder, unspecified
Sleep disorder NOS
Unspecified sleep-wake disorder

NERVE, NERVE ROOT AND PLEXUS DISORDERS (G50-G59)

Excludes1: current traumatic nerve, nerve root and plexus disorders - see Injury, nerve by body region
neuralgia NOS (M79.2)
neuritis NOS (M79.2)
peripheral neuritis in pregnancy (O26.82-)
radiculitis NOS (M54.1-)

G50 Disorders of trigeminal nerve
Includes: disorders of 5th cranial nerve

G50.0 Trigeminal neuralgia
Syndrome of paroxysmal facial pain
Tic douloureux

G50.1 Atypical facial pain

G50.8 Other disorders of trigeminal nerve

G50.9 Disorder of trigeminal nerve, unspecified

G51 Facial nerve disorders
Definition: Facial nerve disorders refers to a disorder resulting from a weakness of the facial nerve. Bell's palsy is an example of a facial nerve disorder.
Includes: disorders of 7th cranial nerve

G51.0 Bell's palsy
Facial palsy

G51.1 Geniculate ganglionitis
Excludes1: postherpetic geniculate ganglionitis (B02.21)

G51.2 Melkersson's syndrome
Melkersson-Rosenthal syndrome

G51.3 Clonic hemifacial spasm

G51.4 Facial myokymia

G51.8 Other disorders of facial nerve

G51.9 Disorder of facial nerve, unspecified

G52 Disorders of other cranial nerves
Excludes2: disorders of acoustic [8th] nerve (H93.3)
disorders of optic [2nd] nerve (H46, H47.0)
paralytic strabismus due to nerve palsy (H49.0-H49.2)

G52.0 Disorders of olfactory nerve
Disorders of 1st cranial nerve

G52.1 Disorders of glossopharyngeal nerve
Disorder of 9th cranial nerve
Glossopharyngeal neuralgia

G52.2 Disorders of vagus nerve
Disorders of pneumogastric [10th] nerve

G52.3 Disorders of hypoglossal nerve
Disorders of 12th cranial nerve

G52.7 Disorders of multiple cranial nerves
Polyneuritis cranialis

G52.8 Disorders of other specified cranial nerves

G52.9 Cranial nerve disorder, unspecified

G53 Cranial nerve disorders in diseases classified elsewhere
Code first underlying disease, such as:
neoplasm (C00-D49)
Excludes1: multiple cranial nerve palsy in sarcoidosis (D86.82)
multiple cranial nerve palsy in syphilis (A52.15)
postherpetic geniculate ganglionitis (B02.21)
postherpetic trigeminal neuralgia (B02.22)

G54 Nerve root and plexus disorders
Definition: A nerve root is the initial segment of a nerve leaving the central nervous system. Plexus refers to a network of intersecting nerves and blood vessels or of lymphatic vessels. The body contains many plexuses, such as the brachial plexus, the cardiac plexus, the cervical plexus, and the lumbar plexus.
Excludes1: current traumatic nerve root and plexus disorders - see nerve injury by body region
intervertebral disc disorders (M50-M51)
neuralgia or neuritis NOS (M79.2)
neuritis or radiculitis brachial NOS (M54.13)
neuritis or radiculitis lumbar NOS (M54.16)
neuritis or radiculitis lumbosacral NOS (M54.17)
neuritis or radiculitis thoracic NOS (M54.14)
radiculitis NOS (M54.10)
radiculopathy NOS (M54.10)
spondylosis (M47.-)

G54.0 Brachial plexus disorders
Thoracic outlet syndrome

G54.1 Lumbosacral plexus disorders

G54.2 Cervical root disorders, not elsewhere classified

G54.3 Thoracic root disorders, not elsewhere classified

G54.4 Lumbosacral root disorders, not elsewhere classified

G54.5 Neuralgic amyotrophy
Parsonage-Aldren-Turner syndrome
Shoulder-girdle neuritis
Excludes1: neuralgic amyotrophy in diabetes mellitus (E08-E13 with .44)

G54.6 Phantom limb syndrome with pain

G54.7 Phantom limb syndrome without pain
Phantom limb syndrome NOS

G54.8 Other nerve root and plexus disorders

Add 4th-7th digits	Nonspecific code	Unspecified code	Manifestation code

G54.9   Nerve root and plexus disorder, unspecified

G55   Nerve root and plexus compressions in diseases classified elsewhere

Code first underlying disease, such as:

neoplasm (C00-D49)

Excludes1: nerve root compression (due to) (in) ankylosing spondylitis (M45.-)

nerve root compression (due to) (in) dorsopathies (M53.-, M54.-)

nerve root compression (due to) (in) intervertebral disc disorders (M50.1.-, M51.1.-)

nerve root compression (due to) (in) spondylopathies (M46.-, M48.-)

nerve root compression (due to) (in) spondylosis (M47.0-M47.2.-)

G56   Mononeuropathies of upper limb

Definition: Mononeuropathy: A disorder of a single nerve or nerve trunk. Mononeuropathies may be due to entrapment, compression, stretch injury, ischemia, infection, or inflammation of a nerve.

Excludes1: current traumatic nerve disorder - see nerve injury by body region

G56.0   Carpal tunnel syndrome

G56.00   Carpal tunnel syndrome, unspecified upper limb

G56.01   Carpal tunnel syndrome, right upper limb

G56.02   Carpal tunnel syndrome, left upper limb

G56.03   Carpal tunnel syndrome, bilateral upper limbs

G56.1   Other lesions of median nerve

G56.10   Other lesions of median nerve, unspecified upper limb

G56.11   Other lesions of median nerve, right upper limb

G56.12   Other lesions of median nerve, left upper limb

G56.13   Other lesions of median nerve, bilateral upper limbs

G56.2   Lesion of ulnar nerve

Tardy ulnar nerve palsy

G56.20   Lesion of ulnar nerve, unspecified upper limb

G56.21   Lesion of ulnar nerve, right upper limb

G56.22   Lesion of ulnar nerve, left upper limb

G56.23   Lesion of ulnar nerve, bilateral upper limbs

G56.3   Lesion of radial nerve

G56.30   Lesion of radial nerve, unspecified upper limb

G56.31   Lesion of radial nerve, right upper limb

G56.32   Lesion of radial nerve, left upper limb

G56.33   Lesion of radial nerve, bilateral upper limbs

G56.4   Causalgia of upper limb

Complex regional pain syndrome II of upper limb

Excludes1: complex regional pain syndrome I of lower limb (G90.52-)

complex regional pain syndrome I of upper limb (G90.51-)

complex regional pain syndrome II of lower limb (G57.7-)

reflex sympathetic dystrophy of lower limb (G90.52-)

reflex sympathetic dystrophy of upper limb (G90.51-)

G56.40   Causalgia of unspecified upper limb

G56.41   Causalgia of right upper limb

G56.42   Causalgia of left upper limb

G56.43   Causalgia of bilateral upper limbs

G56.8   Other specified mononeuropathies of upper limb

Interdigital neuroma of upper limb

G56.80   Other specified mononeuropathies of unspecified upper limb

G56.81   Other specified mononeuropathies of right upper limb

G56.82   Other specified mononeuropathies of left upper limb

G56.83   Other specified mononeuropathies of bilateral upper limbs

G56.9   Unspecified mononeuropathy of upper limb

G56.90   Unspecified mononeuropathy of unspecified upper limb

G56.91   Unspecified mononeuropathy of right upper limb

G56.92   Unspecified mononeuropathy of left upper limb

G56.93   Unspecified mononeuropathy of bilateral upper limbs

G57   Mononeuropathies of lower limb

Excludes1: current traumatic nerve disorder - see nerve injury by body region

G57.0   Lesion of sciatic nerve

Excludes1: sciatica NOS (M54.3-)

Excludes2: sciatica attributed to intervertebral disc disorder (M51.1.-)

G57.00   Lesion of sciatic nerve, unspecified lower limb

G57.01   Lesion of sciatic nerve, right lower limb

G57.02   Lesion of sciatic nerve, left lower limb

G57.03   Lesion of sciatic nerve, bilateral lower limbs

G57.1   Meralgia paresthetica

Lateral cutaneous nerve of thigh syndrome

G57.10   Meralgia paresthetica, unspecified lower limb

G57.11   Meralgia paresthetica, right lower limb

G57.12   Meralgia paresthetica, left lower limb

G57.13   Meralgia paresthetica, bilateral lower limbs

G57.2   Lesion of femoral nerve

G57.20   Lesion of femoral nerve, unspecified lower limb

G57.21   Lesion of femoral nerve, right lower limb

G57.22   Lesion of femoral nerve, left lower limb

G57.23   Lesion of femoral nerve, bilateral lower limbs

G57.3   Lesion of lateral popliteal nerve

Peroneal nerve palsy

G57.30   Lesion of lateral popliteal nerve, unspecified lower limb

G57.31   Lesion of lateral popliteal nerve, right lower limb

G57.32   Lesion of lateral popliteal nerve, left lower limb

G57.33   Lesion of lateral popliteal nerve, bilateral lower limbs

G57.4   Lesion of medial popliteal nerve

G57.40   Lesion of medial popliteal nerve, unspecified lower limb

G57.41   Lesion of medial popliteal nerve, right lower limb

G57.42   Lesion of medial popliteal nerve, left lower limb

G57.43   Lesion of medial popliteal nerve, bilateral lower limbs

G57.5   Tarsal tunnel syndrome

● New code   ▲ Revised code   **Excludes1:** Not coded here   **Excludes2:** Not included here   ⊗ Placeholder required   ⑦ 7th digit required

G57.50 **Tarsal tunnel syndrome, unspecified lower limb**

G57.51 **Tarsal tunnel syndrome, right lower limb**

G57.52 **Tarsal tunnel syndrome, left lower limb**

G57.53 **Tarsal tunnel syndrome, bilateral lower limbs**

G57.6 **Lesion of plantar nerve**

Morton's metatarsalgia

G57.60 **Lesion of plantar nerve, unspecified lower limb**

G57.61 **Lesion of plantar nerve, right lower limb**

G57.62 **Lesion of plantar nerve, left lower limb**

G57.63 **Lesion of plantar nerve, bilateral lower limbs**

G57.7 **Causalgia of lower limb**

Complex regional pain syndrome II of lower limb

Excludes1: complex regional pain syndrome I of lower limb (G90.52-)

complex regional pain syndrome I of upper limb (G90.51-)

complex regional pain syndrome II of upper limb (G56.4-)

reflex sympathetic dystrophy of lower limb (G90.52-)

reflex sympathetic dystrophy of upper limb (G90.51-)

G57.70 **Causalgia of unspecified lower limb**

G57.71 **Causalgia of right lower limb**

G57.72 **Causalgia of left lower limb**

G57.73 **Causalgia of bilateral lower limbs**

G57.8 **Other specified mononeuropathies of lower limb**

Interdigital neuroma of lower limb

G57.80 **Other specified mononeuropathies of unspecified lower limb**

G57.81 **Other specified mononeuropathies of right lower limb**

G57.82 **Other specified mononeuropathies of left lower limb**

G57.83 **Other specified mononeuropathies of bilateral lower limbs**

G57.9 **Unspecified mononeuropathy of lower limb**

G57.90 **Unspecified mononeuropathy of unspecified lower limb**

G57.91 **Unspecified mononeuropathy of right lower limb**

G57.92 **Unspecified mononeuropathy of left lower limb**

G57.93 **Unspecified mononeuropathy of bilateral lower limbs**

G58 **Other mononeuropathies**

G58.0 **Intercostal neuropathy**

G58.7 **Mononeuritis multiplex**

G58.8 **Other specified mononeuropathies**

G58.9 **Mononeuropathy, unspecified**

G59 **Mononeuropathy in diseases classified elsewhere**

Code first underlying disease

Excludes1: diabetic mononeuropathy (E08-E13 with .41)

syphilitic nerve paralysis (A52.19)

syphilitic neuritis (A52.15)

tuberculous mononeuropathy (A17.83)

POLYNEUROPATHIES AND OTHER DISORDERS OF THE PERIPHERAL NERVOUS SYSTEM (G60-G65)

Definition: Polyneuropathy is damage or disease affecting peripheral nerves (peripheral neuropathy) in roughly the same areas on both sides of the body, featuring weakness, numbness, pins-and-needles and burning pain.

Excludes1: neuralgia NOS (M79.2)

neuritis NOS (M79.2)

peripheral neuritis in pregnancy (O26.82-)

radiculitis NOS (M54.10)

G60 **Hereditary and idiopathic neuropathy**

G60.0 **Hereditary motor and sensory neuropathy**

Charcot-Marie-Tooth disease

Déjérine-Sottas disease

Hereditary motor and sensory neuropathy, types I-IV

Hypertrophic neuropathy of infancy

Peroneal muscular atrophy (axonal type) (hypertrophic type)

Roussy-Levy syndrome

G60.1 **Refsum's disease**

Infantile Refsum disease

G60.2 **Neuropathy in association with hereditary ataxia**

G60.3 **Idiopathic progressive neuropathy**

G60.8 **Other hereditary and idiopathic neuropathies**

Dominantly inherited sensory neuropathy

Morvan's disease

Nélaton's syndrome

Recessively inherited sensory neuropathy

G60.9 **Hereditary and idiopathic neuropathy, unspecified**

G61 **Inflammatory polyneuropathy**

G61.0 **Guillain-Barre syndrome**

Acute (post-)infective polyneuritis

Miller Fisher Syndrome

G61.1 **Serum neuropathy**

Use additional code for adverse effect, if applicable, to identify serum (T50.-)

G61.8 **Other inflammatory polyneuropathies**

G61.81 **Chronic inflammatory demyelinating polyneuritis**

G61.82 **Multifocal motor neuropathy**

MMN

G61.89 **Other inflammatory polyneuropathies**

G61.9 **Inflammatory polyneuropathy, unspecified**

G62 **Other and unspecified polyneuropathies**

G62.0 **Drug-induced polyneuropathy**

Use additional code for adverse effect, if applicable, to identify drug (T36-T50 with fifth or sixth character 5)

G62.1 **Alcoholic polyneuropathy**

G62.2 **Polyneuropathy due to other toxic agents**

Code first (T51-T65) to identify toxic agent

G62.8 **Other specified polyneuropathies**

G62.81 **Critical illness polyneuropathy**

Acute motor neuropathy

G62.82 **Radiation-induced polyneuropathy**

Use additional external cause code (W88-W90, X39.0-) to identify cause

G62.89 **Other specified polyneuropathies**

G62.9 **Polyneuropathy, unspecified**

Neuropathy NOS

G63 **Polyneuropathy in diseases classified elsewhere**

Code first underlying disease, such as:

amyloidosis (E85.-)

---

endocrine disease, except diabetes (E00-E07, E15-E16, E20-E34)

metabolic diseases (E70-E88)

neoplasm (C00-D49)

nutritional deficiency (E40-E64)

Excludes1: polyneuropathy (in):

  diabetes mellitus (E08-E13 with .42)

  diphtheria (A36.83)

  infectious mononucleosis (B27.0-B27.9 with 1)

  Lyme disease (A69.22)

  mumps (B26.84)

  postherpetic (B02.23)

  rheumatoid arthritis (M05.33)

  scleroderma (M34.83)

  systemic lupus erythematosus (M32.19)

G64   Other disorders of peripheral nervous system

Disorder of peripheral nervous system NOS

G65   Sequelae of inflammatory and toxic polyneuropathies

Code first condition resulting from (sequela) of inflammatory and toxic polyneuropathies

G65.0   Sequelae of Guillain-Barré syndrome

G65.1   Sequelae of other inflammatory polyneuropathy

G65.2   Sequelae of toxic polyneuropathy

DISEASES OF MYONEURAL JUNCTION AND MUSCLE (G70-G73)

G70   Myasthenia gravis and other myoneural disorders

Excludes1: botulism (A05.1, A48.51-A48.52)

  transient neonatal myasthenia gravis (P94.0)

G70.0   Myasthenia gravis

G70.00   Myasthenia gravis without (acute) exacerbation

Myasthenia gravis NOS

G70.01   Myasthenia gravis with (acute) exacerbation

Myasthenia gravis in crisis

G70.1   Toxic myoneural disorders

Code first (T51-T65) to identify toxic agent

G70.2   Congenital and developmental myasthenia

G70.8   Other specified myoneural disorders

G70.80   Lambert-Eaton syndrome, unspecified

Lambert-Eaton syndrome NOS

G70.81   Lambert-Eaton syndrome in disease classified elsewhere

Code first underlying disease

Excludes1: Lambert-Eaton syndrome in neoplastic disease (G73.1)

G70.89   Other specified myoneural disorders

G70.9   Myoneural disorder, unspecified

G71   Primary disorders of muscles

Excludes2: arthrogryposis multiplex congenita (Q74.3)

  metabolic disorders (E70-E88)

  myositis (M60.-)

G71.0   Muscular dystrophy

Definition: Muscular dystrophy refers to a group of genetic, hereditary muscle diseases that weaken the muscles that move the human body. Muscular dystrophies are characterized by progressive skeletal muscle weakness, defects in muscle proteins, and the death of muscle cells and tissue.

Autosomal recessive, childhood type, muscular dystrophy resembling Duchenne or Becker muscular dystrophy

Benign [Becker] muscular dystrophy

Benign scapuloperoneal muscular dystrophy with early contractures [Emery-Dreifuss]

Congenital muscular dystrophy NOS

Congenital muscular dystrophy with specific morphological abnormalities of the muscle fiber

Distal muscular dystrophy

Facioscapulohumeral muscular dystrophy

Limb-girdle muscular dystrophy

Ocular muscular dystrophy

Oculopharyngeal muscular dystrophy

Scapuloperoneal muscular dystrophy

Severe [Duchenne] muscular dystrophy

G71.1   Myotonic disorders

G71.11   Myotonic muscular dystrophy

Dystrophia myotonica [Steinert]

Myotonia atrophica

Myotonic dystrophy

Proximal myotonic myopathy (PROMM)

Steinert disease

G71.12   Myotonia congenita

Acetazolamide responsive myotonia congenita

Dominant myotonia congenita [Thomsen disease]

Myotonia levior

Recessive myotonia congenita [Becker disease]

G71.13   Myotonic chondrodystrophy

Chondrodystrophic myotonia

Congenital myotonic chondrodystrophy

Schwartz-Jampel disease

G71.14   Drug induced myotonia

Use additional code for adverse effect, if applicable, to identify drug (T36-T50 with fifth or sixth

character 5)

G71.19   Other specified myotonic disorders

Myotonia fluctuans

Myotonia permanens Neuromyotonia [Isaacs]

Paramyotonia congenita (of von Eulenburg)

Pseudomyotonia

Symptomatic myotonia

G71.2   Congenital myopathies

Central core disease

Fiber-type disproportion

Minicore disease

Multicore disease

Myotubular (centronuclear) myopathy Nemaline myopathy

Excludes1: arthrogryposis multiplex congenita (Q74.3)

G71.3   Mitochondrial myopathy, not elsewhere classified

Excludes1: Kearns-Sayre syndrome (H49.81)

  Leber's disease (H47.21)

  Leigh's encephalopathy (G31.82)

  mitochondrial metabolism disorders (E88.4.-)

  Reye's syndrome (G93.7)

G71.8   Other primary disorders of muscles

G71.9   Primary disorder of muscle, unspecified

Hereditary myopathy NOS

G72 **Other and unspecified myopathies**

Excludes1: arthrogryposis multiplex congenita (Q74.3)

dermatopolymyositis (M33.-)

ischemic infarction of muscle (M62.2-)

myositis (M60.-)

polymyositis (M33.2.-)

G72.0 **Drug-induced myopathy**

Use additional code for adverse effect, if applicable, to identify drug (T36-T50 with fifth or sixth character 5)

G72.1 **Alcoholic myopathy**

Use additional code to identify alcoholism (F10.-)

G72.2 **Myopathy due to other toxic agents**

Code first (T51-T65) to identify toxic agent

G72.3 **Periodic paralysis**

Familial periodic paralysis

Hyperkalemic periodic paralysis (familial)

Hypokalemic periodic paralysis (familial)

Myotonic periodic paralysis (familial)

Normokalemic paralysis (familial)

Potassium sensitive periodic paralysis

Excludes1: paramyotonia congenita (of von Eulenburg) (G71.19)

G72.4 **Inflammatory and immune myopathies, not elsewhere classified**

G72.41 **Inclusion body myositis [IBM]**

G72.49 **Other inflammatory and immune myopathies, not elsewhere classified**

Inflammatory myopathy NOS

G72.8 **Other specified myopathies**

G72.81 **Critical illness myopathy**

Acute necrotizing myopathy

Acute quadriplegic myopathy

Intensive care (ICU) myopathy

Myopathy of critical illness

G72.89 **Other specified myopathies**

G72.9 **Myopathy, unspecified**

G73 **Disorders of myoneural junction and muscle in diseases classified elsewhere**

G73.1 **Lambert-Eaton syndrome in neoplastic disease**

Code first underlying neoplasm (C00-D49)

Excludes1: Lambert-Eaton syndrome not associated with neoplasm (G70.80-G70.81)

G73.3 **Myasthenic syndromes in other diseases classified elsewhere**

Code first underlying disease, such as:

neoplasm (C00-D49)

thyrotoxicosis (E05.-)

G73.7 **Myopathy in diseases classified elsewhere**

Code first underlying disease, such as:

hyperparathyroidism (E21.0, E21.3)

hypoparathyroidism (E20.-)

glycogen storage disease (E74.0)

lipid storage disorders (E75.-)

Excludes1: myopathy in:

rheumatoid arthritis (M05.32)

sarcoidosis (D86.87)

scleroderma (M34.82)

sicca syndrome [Sjögren] (M35.03)

systemic lupus erythematosus (M32.19)

CEREBRAL PALSY AND OTHER PARALYTIC SYNDROMES (G80-G83)

Definition: Cerebral palsy is a condition marked by impaired muscle coordination (spastic paralysis) and/or other disabilities, typically caused by damage to the brain before or at birth.

G80 **Cerebral palsy**

Excludes1: hereditary spastic paraplegia (G11.4)

G80.0 **Spastic quadriplegic cerebral palsy**

Congenital spastic paralysis (cerebral)

G80.1 **Spastic diplegic cerebral palsy**

Spastic cerebral palsy NOS

G80.2 **Spastic hemiplegic cerebral palsy**

G80.3 **Athetoid cerebral palsy**

Double athetosis (syndrome)

Dyskinetic cerebral palsy

Dystonic cerebral palsy

Vogt disease

G80.4 **Ataxic cerebral palsy**

G80.8 **Other cerebral palsy**

Mixed cerebral palsy syndromes

G80.9 **Cerebral palsy, unspecified**

Cerebral palsy NOS

G81 **Hemiplegia and hemiparesis**

Definition: Hemiplegia is defined as paralysis or loss of voluntary motion, on one side of the body; may include head and neck, trunk and/or limbs. Hemiparesis is weakness on one side of the body.

Note: This category is to be used only when hemiplegia (complete) (incomplete) is reported without further specification, or is stated to be old or longstanding but of unspecified cause. The category is also for use in multiple coding to identify these types of hemiplegia resulting from any cause.

Excludes1: congenital cerebral palsy (G80.-)

hemiplegia and hemiparesis due to sequela of cerebrovascular disease (I69.05-, I69.15-, I69.25-I69.35-, I69.85-, I69.95-)

G81.0 **Flaccid hemiplegia**

G81.00 **Flaccid hemiplegia affecting unspecified side**

G81.01 **Flaccid hemiplegia affecting right dominant side**

G81.02 **Flaccid hemiplegia affecting left dominant side**

G81.03 **Flaccid hemiplegia affecting right nondominant side**

G81.04 **Flaccid hemiplegia affecting left nondominant side**

G81.1 **Spastic hemiplegia**

G81.10 **Spastic hemiplegia affecting unspecified side**

G81.11 **Spastic hemiplegia affecting right dominant side**

G81.12 **Spastic hemiplegia affecting left dominant side**

G81.13 **Spastic hemiplegia affecting right nondominant side**

G81.14 **Spastic hemiplegia affecting left nondominant side**

G81.9 **Hemiplegia, unspecified**

G81.90 **Hemiplegia, unspecified affecting unspecified side**

G81.91 **Hemiplegia, unspecified affecting right dominant side**

G81.92 Hemiplegia, unspecified affecting left dominant side

G81.93 Hemiplegia, unspecified affecting right nondominant side

G81.94 Hemiplegia, unspecified affecting left nondominant side

G82 Paraplegia (paraparesis) and quadriplegia (quadriparesis)

Note: This category is to be used only when the listed conditions are reported without further specification, or are stated to be old or longstanding but of unspecified cause. The category is also for use in multiple coding to identify these conditions resulting from any cause

Excludes1: congenital cerebral palsy (G80.-)

functional quadriplegia (R53.2)

hysterical paralysis (F44.4)

G82.2 Paraplegia

Paralysis of both lower limbs NOS

Paraparesis (lower) NOS

Paraplegia (lower) NOS

G82.20 Paraplegia, unspecified

G82.21 Paraplegia, complete

G82.22 Paraplegia, incomplete

G82.5 Quadriplegia

G82.50 Quadriplegia, unspecified

G82.51 Quadriplegia, C1-C4 complete

G82.52 Quadriplegia, C1-C4 incomplete

G82.53 Quadriplegia, C5-C7 complete

G82.54 Quadriplegia, C5-C7 incomplete

G83 Other paralytic syndromes

Note: This category is to be used only when the listed conditions are reported without further specification, or are stated to be old or longstanding but of unspecified cause. The category is also for use in multiple coding to identify these conditions resulting from any cause.

Includes: paralysis (complete) (incomplete), except as in G80-G82

G83.0 Diplegia of upper limbs

Diplegia (upper)

Paralysis of both upper limbs

G83.1 Monoplegia of lower limb

Paralysis of lower limb

Excludes1: monoplegia of lower limbs due to sequela of cerebrovascular disease (I69.04-, I69.14-, I69.24-, I69.34-, I69.84-, I69.94-)

G83.10 Monoplegia of lower limb affecting unspecified side

G83.11 Monoplegia of lower limb affecting right dominant side

G83.12 Monoplegia of lower limb affecting left dominant side

G83.13 Monoplegia of lower limb affecting right nondominant side

G83.14 Monoplegia of lower limb affecting left nondominant side

G83.2 Monoplegia of upper limb

Paralysis of upper limb

Excludes1: monoplegia of upper limbs due to sequela of cerebrovascular disease (I69.03-, I69.13-, I69.23-, I69.33-, I69.83-, I69.93-)

G83.20 Monoplegia of upper limb affecting unspecified side

G83.21 Monoplegia of upper limb affecting right dominant side

G83.22 Monoplegia of upper limb affecting left dominant side

G83.23 Monoplegia of upper limb affecting right nondominant side

G83.24 Monoplegia of upper limb affecting left nondominant side

G83.3 Monoplegia, unspecified

G83.30 Monoplegia, unspecified affecting unspecified side

G83.31 Monoplegia, unspecified affecting right dominant side

G83.32 Monoplegia, unspecified affecting left dominant side

G83.33 Monoplegia, unspecified affecting right nondominant side

G83.34 Monoplegia, unspecified affecting left nondominant side

G83.4 Cauda equina syndrome

Neurogenic bladder due to cauda equina syndrome

Excludes1: cord bladder NOS (G95.89)

neurogenic bladder NOS (N31.9)

G83.5 Locked-in state

G83.8 Other specified paralytic syndromes

Excludes1: paralytic syndromes due to current spinal cord injury-code to spinal cord injury (S14, S24, S34)

G83.81 Brown-Séquard syndrome

G83.82 Anterior cord syndrome

G83.83 Posterior cord syndrome

G83.84 Todd's paralysis (postepileptic)

G83.89 Other specified paralytic syndromes

G83.9 Paralytic syndrome, unspecified

OTHER DISORDERS OF THE NERVOUS SYSTEM (G89-G99)

G89 Pain, not elsewhere classified

Code also related psychological factors associated with pain (F45.42)

Excludes1: generalized pain NOS (R52)

pain disorders exclusively related to psychological factors (F45.41)

pain NOS (R52)

Excludes2: atypical face pain (G50.1)

headache syndromes (G44.-)

localized pain, unspecified type - code to pain by site, such as: abdomen pain (R10.-)

back pain (M54.9)

breast pain (N64.4)

chest pain (R07.1-R07.9)

ear pain (H92.0-)

eye pain (H57.1)

headache (R51)

joint pain (M25.5-)

limb pain (M79.6-)

lumbar region pain (M54.5)

painful urination (R30.9)

pelvic and perineal pain (R10.2)

shoulder pain (M25.51-)

spine pain (M54.-)

throat pain (R07.0)

tongue pain (K14.6)

tooth pain (K08.8)

● New code ▲ Revised code **Excludes1:** Not coded here **Excludes2:** Not included here ⊗ Placeholder required ⑦ 7th digit required

renal colic (N23)

migraines (G43.-)

myalgia (M79.1)

pain from prosthetic devices, implants, and grafts (T82.84, T83.84, T84.84, T85.84-)

phantom limb syndrome with pain (G54.6)

vulvar vestibulitis (N94.810)

vulvodynia (N94.81-)

G89.0   Central pain syndrome

Déjérine-Roussy syndrome

Myelopathic pain syndrome

Thalamic pain syndrome (hyperesthetic)

G89.1   Acute pain, not elsewhere classified

G89.11   Acute pain due to trauma

G89.12   Acute post-thoracotomy pain

Post-thoracotomy pain NOS

G89.18   Other acute postprocedural pain

Postoperative pain NOS

Postprocedural pain NOS

G89.2   Chronic pain, not elsewhere classified

Excludes1: causalgia, lower limb (G57.7-)

causalgia, upper limb (G56.4-)

central pain syndrome (G89.0)

chronic pain syndrome (G89.4)

complex regional pain syndrome II, lower limb (G57.7-)

complex regional pain syndrome II, upper limb (G56.4-)

neoplasm related chronic pain (G89.3)

reflex sympathetic dystrophy (G90.5-)

G89.21   Chronic pain due to trauma

G89.22   Chronic post-thoracotomy pain

G89.28   Other chronic postprocedural pain

Other chronic postoperative pain

G89.29   Other chronic pain

G89.3   Neoplasm related pain (acute) (chronic)

Cancer associated pain

Pain due to malignancy (primary) (secondary)

Tumor associated pain

G89.4   Chronic pain syndrome

Chronic pain associated with significant psychosocial dysfunction

G90   Disorders of autonomic nervous system

Excludes1: dysfunction of the autonomic nervous system due to alcohol (G31.2)

G90.0   Idiopathic peripheral autonomic neuropathy

G90.01   Carotid sinus syncope

Carotid sinus syndrome

G90.09   Other idiopathic peripheral autonomic neuropathy

Idiopathic peripheral autonomic neuropathy NOS

G90.1   Familial dysautonomia [Riley-Day]

G90.2   Horner's syndrome

Bernard(-Horner) syndrome

Cervical sympathetic dystrophy or paralysis

G90.3   Multi-system degeneration of the autonomic nervous system

Neurogenic orthostatic hypotension [Shy-Drager]

Excludes1: orthostatic hypotension NOS (I95.1)

G90.4   Autonomic dysreflexia

Use additional code to identify the cause, such as:

fecal impaction (K56.41)

pressure ulcer (pressure area) (L89.-)

urinary tract infection (N39.0)

G90.5   Complex regional pain syndrome I (CRPS I)

Reflex sympathetic dystrophy

Excludes1: causalgia of lower limb (G57.7-)

causalgia of upper limb (G56.4-)

complex regional pain syndrome II of lower limb (G57.7-)

complex regional pain syndrome II of upper limb (G56.4-)

G90.50   Complex regional pain syndrome I, unspecified

G90.51   Complex regional pain syndrome I of upper limb

G90.511   Complex regional pain syndrome I of right upper limb

G90.512   Complex regional pain syndrome I of left upper limb

G90.513   Complex regional pain syndrome I of upper limb, bilateral

G90.519   Complex regional pain syndrome I of unspecified upper limb

G90.52   Complex regional pain syndrome I of lower limb

G90.521   Complex regional pain syndrome I of right lower limb

G90.522   Complex regional pain syndrome I of left lower limb

G90.523   Complex regional pain syndrome I of lower limb, bilateral

G90.529   Complex regional pain syndrome I of unspecified lower limb

G90.59   Complex regional pain syndrome I of other specified site

G90.8   Other disorders of autonomic nervous system

G90.9   Disorder of the autonomic nervous system, unspecified

G91   Hydrocephalus

Includes: acquired hydrocephalus

Excludes1: Arnold-Chiari syndrome with hydrocephalus (Q07.-)

congenital hydrocephalus (Q03.-)

spina bifida with hydrocephalus (Q05.-)

G91.0   Communicating hydrocephalus

Secondary normal pressure hydrocephalus

G91.1   Obstructive hydrocephalus

G91.2   (Idiopathic) normal pressure hydrocephalus

Normal pressure hydrocephalus NOS

G91.3   Post-traumatic hydrocephalus, unspecified

G91.4   Hydrocephalus in diseases classified elsewhere

Code first underlying condition, such as:

congenital syphilis (A50.4-)

neoplasm (C00-D49)

Excludes1: hydrocephalus due to congenital toxoplasmosis (P37.1)

G91.8   Other hydrocephalus

G91.9   Hydrocephalus, unspecified

G92   Toxic encephalopathy

Toxic encephalitis

Toxic metabolic encephalopathy

Code first, if applicable, drug induced (T36-T50)

Code first (T51-T65) to identify toxic agent

G93 **Other disorders of brain**

G93.0 **Cerebral cysts**

Arachnoid cyst

Porencephalic cyst, acquired

Excludes1: acquired periventricular cysts of newborn (P91.1)

congenital cerebral cysts (Q04.6)

G93.1 **Anoxic brain damage, not elsewhere classified**

Excludes1: cerebral anoxia due to anesthesia during labor and delivery (O74.3)

cerebral anoxia due to anesthesia during the puerperium (O89.2)

neonatal anoxia (P84)

G93.2 **Benign intracranial hypertension**

Excludes1: hypertensive encephalopathy (I67.4)

G93.3 **Postviral fatigue syndrome**

Benign myalgic encephalomyelitis

Excludes1: chronic fatigue syndrome NOS (R53.82)

G93.4 **Other and unspecified encephalopathy**

Excludes1: alcoholic encephalopathy (G31.2)

encephalopathy in diseases classified elsewhere (G94)

hypertensive encephalopathy (I67.4)

toxic (metabolic) encephalopathy (G92)

G93.40 **Encephalopathy, unspecified**

G93.41 **Metabolic encephalopathy**

Septic encephalopathy

G93.49 **Other encephalopathy**

Encephalopathy NEC

G93.5 **Compression of brain**

Arnold-Chiari type 1 compression of brain

Compression of brain (stem)

Herniation of brain (stem)

Excludes1: diffuse traumatic compression of brain (S06.2-)

focal traumatic compression of brain (S06.3-)

G93.6 **Cerebral edema**

Excludes1: cerebral edema due to birth injury (P11.0)

traumatic cerebral edema (S06.1-)

G93.7 **Reye's syndrome**

Code first poisoning due to salicylates, if applicable (T39.0-, with sixth character 1-4)

Use Additional code for adverse effect due to salicylates, if applicable (T39.0-, with sixth character 5)

G93.8 **Other specified disorders of brain**

G93.81 **Temporal sclerosis**

Hippocampal sclerosis

Mesial temporal sclerosis

G93.82 **Brain death**

G93.89 **Other specified disorders of brain**

Postradiation encephalopathy

G93.9 **Disorder of brain, unspecified**

G94 **Other disorders of brain in diseases classified elsewhere**

Code first underlying disease

Excludes1: encephalopathy in congenital syphilis (A50.49)

encephalopathy in influenza (J09.X9, J10.81, J11.81)

encephalopathy in syphilis (A52.19)

hydrocephalus in diseases classified elsewhere (G91.4)

G95 **Other and unspecified diseases of spinal cord**

Excludes2: myelitis (G04.-)

G95.0 **Syringomyelia and syringobulbia**

G95.1 **Vascular myelopathies**

Excludes2: intraspinal phlebitis and thrombophlebitis, except non-pyogenic (G08)

G95.11 **Acute infarction of spinal cord (embolic) (nonembolic)**

Anoxia of spinal cord

Arterial thrombosis of spinal cord

G95.19 **Other vascular myelopathies**

Edema of spinal cord

Hematomyelia

Nonpyogenic intraspinal phlebitis and thrombophlebitis

Subacute necrotic myelopathy

G95.2 **Other and unspecified cord compression**

G95.20 **Unspecified cord compression**

G95.29 **Other cord compression**

G95.8 **Other specified diseases of spinal cord**

Excludes1: neurogenic bladder NOS (N31.9)

neurogenic bladder due to cauda equina syndrome (G83.4)

neuromuscular dysfunction of bladder without spinal cord lesion (N31.-)

G95.81 **Conus medullaris syndrome**

G95.89 **Other specified diseases of spinal cord**

Cord bladder NOS

Drug-induced myelopathy

Radiation-induced myelopathy

Excludes1: myelopathy NOS (G95.9)

G95.9 **Disease of spinal cord, unspecified**

Myelopathy NOS

G96 **Other disorders of central nervous system**

G96.0 **Cerebrospinal fluid leak**

Excludes1: cerebrospinal fluid leak from spinal puncture (G97.0)

G96.1 **Disorders of meninges, not elsewhere classified**

G96.11 **Dural tear**

Excludes1: accidental puncture or laceration of dura during a procedure (G97.41)

G96.12 **Meningeal adhesions (cerebral) (spinal)**

G96.19 **Other disorders of meninges, not elsewhere classified**

G96.8 **Other specified disorders of central nervous system**

G96.9 **Disorder of central nervous system, unspecified**

G97 **Intraoperative and postprocedural complications and disorders of nervous system, not elsewhere classified**

Excludes2: intraoperative and postprocedural cerebrovascular infarction (I97.81-, I97.82-)

G97.0 **Cerebrospinal fluid leak from spinal puncture**

G97.1 **Other reaction to spinal and lumbar puncture**

Headache due to lumbar puncture

G97.2 **Intracranial hypotension following ventricular shunting**

G97.3 **Intraoperative hemorrhage and hematoma of a nervous system organ or structure complicating a procedure**

● New code ▲ Revised code **Excludes1:** Not coded here **Excludes2:** Not included here ⊗ Placeholder required ⑦ 7th digit required

Excludes1: intraoperative hemorrhage and hematoma of a nervous system organ or structure due to accidental puncture and laceration during a procedure (G97.4-)

G97.31 **Intraoperative hemorrhage and hematoma of a nervous system organ or structure complicating a nervous system procedure**

G97.32 **Intraoperative hemorrhage and hematoma of a nervous system organ or structure complicating other procedure**

G97.4 **Accidental puncture and laceration of a nervous system organ or structure during a procedure**

G97.41 **Accidental puncture or laceration of dura during a procedure** Incidental (inadvertent) durotomy

G97.48 **Accidental puncture and laceration of other nervous system organ or structure during a nervous system procedure**

G97.49 **Accidental puncture and laceration of other nervous system organ or structure during other procedure**

G97.5 **Postprocedural hemorrhage of a nervous system organ or structure following a procedure**

G97.51 **Postprocedural hemorrhage of a nervous system organ or structure following a nervous system procedure**

G97.52 **Postprocedural hemorrhage of a nervous system organ or structure following other procedure**

G97.6 **Postprocedural hematoma and seroma of a nervous system organ or structure following a procedure**

G97.61 **Postprocedural hematoma of a nervous system organ or structure following a nervous system procedure**

G97.62 **Postprocedural hematoma of a nervous system organ or structure following other procedure**

G97.63 **Postprocedural seroma of a nervous system organ or structure following a nervous system procedure**

G97.64 **Postprocedural seroma of a nervous system organ or structure following other procedure**

G97.8 **Other intraoperative and postprocedural complications and disorders of nervous system**

Use additional code to further specify disorder

G97.81 **Other intraoperative complications of nervous system**

G97.82 **Other postprocedural complications and disorders of nervous system**

G98 **Other disorders of nervous system not elsewhere classified**

Includes: nervous system disorder NOS

G98.0 **Neurogenic arthritis, not elsewhere classified**

Nonsyphilitic neurogenic arthropathy NEC Nonsyphilitic neurogenic spondylopathy NEC

Excludes1: spondylopathy (in):

syringomyelia and syringobulbia (G95.0)

tabes dorsalis (A52.11)

G98.8 **Other disorders of nervous system**

Nervous system disorder NOS

G99 **Other disorders of nervous system in diseases classified elsewhere**

G99.0 **Autonomic neuropathy in diseases classified elsewhere**

Code first underlying disease, such as:

amyloidosis (E85.-)

gout (M1A.-, M10.-)

hyperthyroidism (E05.-)

Excludes1: diabetic autonomic neuropathy (E08-E13 with .43)

G99.2 **Myelopathy in diseases classified elsewhere**

Code first underlying disease, such as:

neoplasm (C00-D49)

Excludes1: myelopathy in:

intervertebral disease (M50.0-, M51.0-)

spondylosis (M47.0-, M47.1-)

G99.8 **Other specified disorders of nervous system in diseases classified elsewhere**

Code first underlying disorder, such as:

amyloidosis (E85.-)

avitaminosis (E56.9)

Excludes1: nervous system involvement in:

cysticercosis (B69.0)

rubella (B06.0-)

syphilis (A52.1-)

● New code ▲ Revised code **Excludes1:** Not coded here **Excludes2:** Not included here ⊗ Placeholder required ⑦ 7th digit required

Chapter 7: Diseases Of The Eye And Adnexa (H00-H59)

DEFINITIONS

This chapter includes definitions of selected key words, terms and phrases and coding alerts for adding points to the clinical domain, and references to coding late effects where appropriate. An example from this chapter is as follows:

H16 **Keratitis**

Definition: Keratitis is an infection or inflammation of the cornea which can be caused by a variety of conditions, including infections, dry eyes, foreign objects, contact lenses, intense light, vitamin a deficiency or allergies.

MULTIPLE CODING FOR A SINGLE CONDITION

In addition to the etiology/manifestation convention that requires two codes to fully describe a single condition that affects multiple body systems, there are other single conditions that also require more than one code. "Use additional code" notes are found in the Tabular List at codes that are not part of an etiology/manifestation pair where a secondary code is useful to fully describe a condition. The sequencing rule is the same as the etiology/manifestation pair, "use additional code" indicates that a secondary code should be added.

For example, for bacterial infections that are not included in chapter 1, a secondary code from category B95, Streptococcus, Staphylococcus, and Enterococcus, as the cause of diseases classified elsewhere, or B96, Other bacterial agents as the cause of diseases classified elsewhere, may be required to identify the bacterial organism causing the infection. A "use additional code" note will normally be found at the infectious disease code, indicating a need for the organism code to be added as a secondary code.

"Code first" notes are also under certain codes that are not specifically manifestation codes but may be due to an underlying cause. When there is a "code first" note and an underlying condition is present, the underlying condition should be sequenced first.

"Code, if applicable, any causal condition first", notes indicate that this code may be assigned as a principal diagnosis when the causal condition is unknown or not applicable. If a causal condition is known, then the code for that condition should be sequenced as the principal or first-listed diagnosis.

Multiple codes may be needed for sequela, complication codes and obstetric codes to more fully describe a condition. See the specific guidelines for these conditions for further instruction.

COMBINATION CODE

A combination code is a single code used to classify: Two diagnoses, or a diagnosis with an associated secondary process (manifestation) A diagnosis with an associated complication

Combination codes are identified by referring to subterm entries in the Alphabetic Index and by reading the inclusion and exclusion notes in the Tabular List.

Assign only the combination code when that code fully identifies the diagnostic conditions involved or when the Alphabetic Index so directs. Multiple coding should not be used when the classification provides a combination code that clearly identifies all of the elements documented in the diagnosis. When the combination code lacks necessary specificity in describing the manifestation or complication, an additional code should be used as a secondary code.

SEQUELA (LATE EFFECTS)

A sequela is the residual effect (condition produced) after the acute phase of an illness or injury has terminated. There is no time limit on when a sequela code can be used. The residual may be apparent early, such as in cerebral infarction, or it may occur months or years later, such as that due to a previous injury. Coding of sequela generally requires two codes sequenced in the following order: The condition or nature of the sequela is sequenced first.

The sequela code is sequenced second.

An exception to the above guidelines are those instances where the code for the sequela is followed by a manifestation code identified in the Tabular List and title, or the sequela code has been expanded (at the fourth, fifth or sixth character levels) to include the manifestation(s). The code for the acute phase of an illness or injury that led to the sequela is never used with a code for the late effect.

GLAUCOMA

1) **Assigning Glaucoma Codes**

   Assign as many codes from category H40, Glaucoma, as needed to identify the type of glaucoma, the affected eye, and the glaucoma stage.

2) **Bilateral glaucoma with same type and stage**

   When a patient has bilateral glaucoma and both eyes are documented as being the same type and stage, and there is a code for bilateral glaucoma, report only the code for the type of glaucoma, bilateral, with the seventh character for the stage.

   When a patient has bilateral glaucoma and both eyes are documented as being the same type and stage, and the classification does not provide a code for bilateral glaucoma (i.e. subcategories H40.10, H40.11 and H40.20) report only one code for the type of glaucoma with the appropriate seventh character for the stage.

3) **Bilateral glaucoma stage with different types or stages**

When a patient has bilateral glaucoma and each eye is documented as having a different type or stage, and the classification distinguishes laterality, assign the appropriate code for each eye rather than the code for bilateral glaucoma.

When a patient has bilateral glaucoma and each eye is documented as having a different type, and the classification does not distinguish laterality (i.e. subcategories H40.10, H40.11 and H40.20), assign one code for each type of glaucoma with the appropriate seventh character for the stage.

When a patient has bilateral glaucoma and each eye is documented as having the same type, but different stage, and the classification does not distinguish laterality (i.e. subcategories H40.10, H40.11 and H40.20), assign a code for

the type of glaucoma for each eye with the seventh character for the specific glaucoma stage documented for each eye.

4) Patient admitted with glaucoma and stage evolves during the admission

If a patient is admitted with glaucoma and the stage progresses during the admission, assign the code for highest stage documented.

5) Indeterminate stage glaucoma

Assignment of the seventh character "4" for "indeterminate stage" should be based on the clinical documentation. The seventh character "4" is used for glaucomas whose stage cannot be clinically determined. This seventh character should not be confused with the seventh character "0", unspecified, which should be assigned when there is no documentation regarding the stage of the glaucoma.

● New code   ▲ Revised code   **Excludes1:** Not coded here   **Excludes2:** Not included here   ⊗ Placeholder required   ⑦7ᵗʰ digit required

Chapter 7

Diseases Of The Eye And Adnexa (H00-H59)

Note: Use an external cause code following the code for the eye condition, if applicable, to identify the cause of the eye condition

Excludes2: certain conditions originating in the perinatal period (P04-P96)

certain infectious and parasitic diseases (A00-B99)

complications of pregnancy, childbirth and the puerperium (O00-O9A)

congenital malformations, deformations, and chromosomal abnormalities (Q00-Q99)

diabetes mellitus related eye conditions (E09.3-, E10.3-, E11.3-, E13.3-)

endocrine, nutritional and metabolic diseases (E00-E88)

injury (trauma) of eye and orbit (S05.-)

injury, poisoning and certain other consequences of external causes (S00-T88)

neoplasms (C00-D49)

symptoms, signs and abnormal clinical and laboratory findings, not elsewhere classified (R00-R94)

syphilis related eye disorders (A50.01, A50.3-, A51.43, A52.71)

This chapter contains the following blocks:

H00-H05	Disorders of eyelid, lacrimal system and orbit
H10-H11	Disorders of conjunctiva
H15-H22	Disorders of sclera, cornea, iris and ciliary body
H25-H28	Disorders of lens
H30-H36	Disorders of choroid and retina
H40-H42	Glaucoma
H43-H44	Disorders of vitreous body and globe
H46-H47	Disorders of optic nerve and visual pathways
H49-H52	Disorders of ocular muscles, binocular movement, accommodation and refraction
H53-H54	Visual disturbances and blindness
H55-H57	Other disorders of eye and adnexa
H59	Intraoperative and postprocedural complications and disorders of eye and adnexa, not elsewhere classified

DISORDERS OF EYELID, LACRIMAL SYSTEM AND ORBIT (H00-H05)

Excludes2: open wound of eyelid (S01.1-)

superficial injury of eyelid (S00.1-, S00.2-)

H00   Hordeolum and chalazion

H00.0   Hordeolum (externum) (internum) of eyelid

H00.01   Hordeolum externum

Hordeolum NOS

Stye

H00.011   Hordeolum externum right upper eyelid

H00.012   Hordeolum externum right lower eyelid

H00.013   Hordeolum externum right eye, unspecified eyelid

H00.014   Hordeolum externum left upper eyelid

H00.015   Hordeolum externum left lower eyelid

H00.016   Hordeolum externum left eye, unspecified eyelid

H00.019   Hordeolum externum unspecified eye, unspecified eyelid

H00.02   Hordeolum internum

Infection of meibomian gland

H00.021   Hordeolum internum right upper eyelid

H00.022   Hordeolum internum right lower eyelid

H00.023   Hordeolum internum right eye, unspecified eyelid

H00.024   Hordeolum internum left upper eyelid

H00.025   Hordeolum internum left lower eyelid

H00.026   Hordeolum internum left eye, unspecified eyelid

H00.029   Hordeolum internum unspecified eye, unspecified eyelid

H00.03   Abscess of eyelid

Furuncle of eyelid

H00.031   Abscess of right upper eyelid

H00.032   Abscess of right lower eyelid

H00.033   Abscess of eyelid right eye, unspecified eyelid

H00.034   Abscess of left upper eyelid

H00.035   Abscess of left lower eyelid

H00.036   Abscess of eyelid left eye, unspecified eyelid

H00.039   Abscess of eyelid unspecified eye, unspecified eyelid

H00.1   Chalazion

Meibomian (gland) cyst

Excludes2: infected meibomian gland (H00.02-)

H00.11   Chalazion right upper eyelid

H00.12   Chalazion right lower eyelid

H00.13   Chalazion right eye, unspecified eyelid

H00.14   Chalazion left upper eyelid

H00.15   Chalazion left lower eyelid

H00.16   Chalazion left eye, unspecified eyelid

H00.19   Chalazion unspecified eye, unspecified eyelid

H01   Other inflammation of eyelid

H01.0   Blepharitis

Excludes1: blepharoconjunctivitis (H10.5-)

H01.00   Unspecified blepharitis

H01.001   Unspecified blepharitis right upper eyelid

H01.002   Unspecified blepharitis right lower eyelid

H01.003   Unspecified blepharitis right eye, unspecified eyelid

H01.004   Unspecified blepharitis left upper eyelid

H01.005   Unspecified blepharitis left lower eyelid

H01.006   Unspecified blepharitis left eye, unspecified eyelid

H01.009   Unspecified blepharitis unspecified eye, unspecified eyelid

H01.01   Ulcerative blepharitis

H01.011   Ulcerative blepharitis right upper eyelid

H01.012   Ulcerative blepharitis right lower eyelid

H01.013 Ulcerative blepharitis right eye, unspecified eyelid

H01.014 Ulcerative blepharitis left upper eyelid

H01.015 Ulcerative blepharitis left lower eyelid

H01.016 Ulcerative blepharitis left eye, unspecified eyelid

H01.019 Ulcerative blepharitis unspecified eye, unspecified eyelid

H01.02 **Squamous blepharitis**

H01.021 Squamous blepharitis right upper eyelid

H01.022 Squamous blepharitis right lower eyelid

H01.023 Squamous blepharitis right eye, unspecified eyelid

H01.024 Squamous blepharitis left upper eyelid

H01.025 Squamous blepharitis left lower eyelid

H01.026 Squamous blepharitis left eye, unspecified eyelid

H01.029 Squamous blepharitis unspecified eye, unspecified eyelid

H01.1 **Noninfectious dermatoses of eyelid**

H01.11 **Allergic dermatitis of eyelid**

Contact dermatitis of eyelid

H01.111 Allergic dermatitis of right upper eyelid

H01.112 Allergic dermatitis of right lower eyelid

H01.113 Allergic dermatitis of right eye, unspecified eyelid

H01.114 Allergic dermatitis of left upper eyelid

H01.115 Allergic dermatitis of left lower eyelid

H01.116 Allergic dermatitis of left eye, unspecified eyelid

H01.119 Allergic dermatitis of unspecified eye, unspecified eyelid

H01.12 **Discoid lupus erythematosus of eyelid**

H01.121 Discoid lupus erythematosus of right upper eyelid

H01.122 Discoid lupus erythematosus of right lower eyelid

H01.123 Discoid lupus erythematosus of right eye, unspecified eyelid

H01.124 Discoid lupus erythematosus of left upper eyelid

H01.125 Discoid lupus erythematosus of left lower eyelid

H01.126 Discoid lupus erythematosus of left eye, unspecified eyelid

H01.129 Discoid lupus erythematosus of unspecified eye, unspecified eyelid

H01.13 **Eczematous dermatitis of eyelid**

H01.131 Eczematous dermatitis of right upper eyelid

H01.132 Eczematous dermatitis of right lower eyelid

H01.133 Eczematous dermatitis of right eye, unspecified eyelid

H01.134 Eczematous dermatitis of left upper eyelid

H01.135 Eczematous dermatitis of left lower eyelid

H01.136 Eczematous dermatitis of left eye, unspecified eyelid

H01.139 Eczematous dermatitis of unspecified eye, unspecified eyelid

H01.14 **Xeroderma of eyelid**

H01.141 Xeroderma of right upper eyelid

H01.142 Xeroderma of right lower eyelid

H01.143 Xeroderma of right eye, unspecified eyelid

H01.144 Xeroderma of left upper eyelid

H01.145 Xeroderma of left lower eyelid

H01.146 Xeroderma of left eye, unspecified eyelid

H01.149 Xeroderma of unspecified eye, unspecified eyelid

H01.8 **Other specified inflammations of eyelid**

H01.9 **Unspecified inflammation of eyelid**

Inflammation of eyelid NOS

H02 Other disorders of eyelid

Excludes1: congenital malformations of eyelid (Q10.0-Q10.3)

H02.0 **Entropion and trichiasis of eyelid**

H02.00 **Unspecified entropion of eyelid**

H02.001 Unspecified entropion of right upper eyelid

H02.002 Unspecified entropion of right lower eyelid

H02.003 Unspecified entropion of right eye, unspecified eyelid

H02.004 Unspecified entropion of left upper eyelid

H02.005 Unspecified entropion of left lower eyelid

H02.006 Unspecified entropion of left eye, unspecified eyelid

H02.009 Unspecified entropion of unspecified eye, unspecified eyelid

H02.01 **Cicatricial entropion of eyelid**

H02.011 Cicatricial entropion of right upper eyelid

H02.012 Cicatricial entropion of right lower eyelid

H02.013 Cicatricial entropion of right eye, unspecified eyelid

H02.014 Cicatricial entropion of left upper eyelid

H02.015 Cicatricial entropion of left lower eyelid

H02.016 Cicatricial entropion of left eye, unspecified eyelid

H02.019 Cicatricial entropion of unspecified eye, unspecified eyelid

H02.02 **Mechanical entropion of eyelid**

H02.021 Mechanical entropion of right upper eyelid

H02.022 Mechanical entropion of right lower eyelid

H02.023 Mechanical entropion of right eye, unspecified eyelid

H02.024 Mechanical entropion of left upper eyelid

H02.025 Mechanical entropion of left lower eyelid

H02.026 Mechanical entropion of left eye, unspecified eyelid

H02.029 Mechanical entropion of unspecified eye, unspecified eyelid

H02.03 Senile entropion of eyelid

H02.031 Senile entropion of right upper eyelid

H02.032 Senile entropion of right lower eyelid

H02.033 Senile entropion of right eye, unspecified eyelid

H02.034 Senile entropion of left upper eyelid

H02.035 Senile entropion of left lower eyelid

H02.036 Senile entropion of left eye, unspecified eyelid

H02.039 Senile entropion of unspecified eye, unspecified eyelid

H02.04 Spastic entropion of eyelid

H02.041 Spastic entropion of right upper eyelid

H02.042 Spastic entropion of right lower eyelid

H02.043 Spastic entropion of right eye, unspecified eyelid

H02.044 Spastic entropion of left upper eyelid

H02.045 Spastic entropion of left lower eyelid

H02.046 Spastic entropion of left eye, unspecified eyelid

H02.049 Spastic entropion of unspecified eye, unspecified eyelid

▲H02.05 Trichiasis without entropion

▲H02.051 Trichiasis without entropion right upper eyelid

▲H02.052 Trichiasis without entropion right lower eyelid

▲H02.053 Trichiasis without entropion right eye, unspecified eyelid

▲H02.054 Trichiasis without entropion left upper eyelid

▲H02.055 Trichiasis without entropion left lower eyelid

▲H02.056 Trichiasis without entropion left eye, unspecified eyelid

▲H02.059 Trichiasis without entropion unspecified eye, unspecified eyelid

H02.1 Ectropion of eyelid

H02.10 Unspecified ectropion of eyelid

H02.101 Unspecified ectropion of right upper eyelid

H02.102 Unspecified ectropion of right lower eyelid

H02.103 Unspecified ectropion of right eye, unspecified eyelid

H02.104 Unspecified ectropion of left upper eyelid

H02.105 Unspecified ectropion of left lower eyelid

H02.106 Unspecified ectropion of left eye, unspecified eyelid

H02.109 Unspecified ectropion of unspecified eye, unspecified eyelid

H02.11 Cicatricial ectropion of eyelid

H02.111 Cicatricial ectropion of right upper eyelid

H02.112 Cicatricial ectropion of right lower eyelid

H02.113 Cicatricial ectropion of right eye, unspecified eyelid

H02.114 Cicatricial ectropion of left upper eyelid

H02.115 Cicatricial ectropion of left lower eyelid

H02.116 Cicatricial ectropion of left eye, unspecified eyelid

H02.119 Cicatricial ectropion of unspecified eye, unspecified eyelid

H02.12 Mechanical ectropion of eyelid

H02.121 Mechanical ectropion of right upper eyelid

H02.122 Mechanical ectropion of right lower eyelid

H02.123 Mechanical ectropion of right eye, unspecified eyelid

H02.124 Mechanical ectropion of left upper eyelid

H02.125 Mechanical ectropion of left lower eyelid

H02.126 Mechanical ectropion of left eye, unspecified eyelid

H02.129 Mechanical ectropion of unspecified eye, unspecified eyelid

H02.13 Senile ectropion of eyelid

H02.131 Senile ectropion of right upper eyelid

H02.132 Senile ectropion of right lower eyelid

H02.133 Senile ectropion of right eye, unspecified eyelid

H02.134 Senile ectropion of left upper eyelid

H02.135 Senile ectropion of left lower eyelid

H02.136 Senile ectropion of left eye, unspecified eyelid

H02.139 Senile ectropion of unspecified eye, unspecified eyelid

H02.14 Spastic ectropion of eyelid

H02.141 Spastic ectropion of right upper eyelid

H02.142 Spastic ectropion of right lower eyelid

H02.143 Spastic ectropion of right eye, unspecified eyelid

H02.144 Spastic ectropion of left upper eyelid

H02.145 Spastic ectropion of left lower eyelid

H02.146 Spastic ectropion of left eye, unspecified eyelid

H02.149 Spastic ectropion of unspecified eye, unspecified eyelid

H02.2 Lagophthalmos

H02.20 Unspecified lagophthalmos

H02.201 Unspecified lagophthalmos right upper eyelid

H02.202 Unspecified lagophthalmos right lower eyelid

H02.203 Unspecified lagophthalmos right eye, unspecified eyelid

H02.204 Unspecified lagophthalmos left upper eyelid

H02.205 Unspecified lagophthalmos left lower eyelid

H02.206 Unspecified lagophthalmos left eye, unspecified eyelid

H02.209 Unspecified lagophthalmos unspecified eye, unspecified eyelid

H02.21 Cicatricial lagophthalmos

H02.211 Cicatricial lagophthalmos right upper eyelid

H02.212 Cicatricial lagophthalmos right lower eyelid

H02.213 Cicatricial lagophthalmos right eye, unspecified eyelid

H02.214 Cicatricial lagophthalmos left upper eyelid

H02.215 Cicatricial lagophthalmos left lower eyelid

H02.216 Cicatricial lagophthalmos left eye, unspecified eyelid

H02.219 Cicatricial lagophthalmos unspecified eye, unspecified eyelid

H02.22 Mechanical lagophthalmos

H02.221 Mechanical lagophthalmos right upper eyelid

H02.222 Mechanical lagophthalmos right lower eyelid

H02.223 Mechanical lagophthalmos right eye, unspecified eyelid

H02.224 Mechanical lagophthalmos left upper eyelid

H02.225 Mechanical lagophthalmos left lower eyelid

H02.226 Mechanical lagophthalmos left eye, unspecified eyelid

H02.229 Mechanical lagophthalmos unspecified eye, unspecified eyelid

H02.23 Paralytic lagophthalmos

H02.231 Paralytic lagophthalmos right upper eyelid

H02.232 Paralytic lagophthalmos right lower eyelid

H02.233 Paralytic lagophthalmos right eye, unspecified eyelid

H02.234 Paralytic lagophthalmos left upper eyelid

H02.235 Paralytic lagophthalmos left lower eyelid

H02.236 Paralytic lagophthalmos left eye, unspecified eyelid

H02.239 Paralytic lagophthalmos unspecified eye, unspecified eyelid

H02.3 Blepharochalasis

Pseudoptosis

H02.30 Blepharochalasis unspecified eye, unspecified eyelid

H02.31 Blepharochalasis right upper eyelid

H02.32 Blepharochalasis right lower eyelid

H02.33 Blepharochalasis right eye, unspecified eyelid

H02.34 Blepharochalasis left upper eyelid

H02.35 Blepharochalasis left lower eyelid

H02.36 Blepharochalasis left eye, unspecified eyelid

H02.4 Ptosis of eyelid

H02.40 Unspecified ptosis of eyelid

H02.401 Unspecified ptosis of right eyelid

H02.402 Unspecified ptosis of left eyelid

H02.403 Unspecified ptosis of bilateral eyelids

H02.409 Unspecified ptosis of unspecified eyelid

H02.41 Mechanical ptosis of eyelid

H02.411 Mechanical ptosis of right eyelid

H02.412 Mechanical ptosis of left eyelid

H02.413 Mechanical ptosis of bilateral eyelids

H02.419 Mechanical ptosis of unspecified eyelid

H02.42 Myogenic ptosis of eyelid

H02.421 Myogenic ptosis of right eyelid

H02.422 Myogenic ptosis of left eyelid

H02.423 Myogenic ptosis of bilateral eyelids

H02.429 Myogenic ptosis of unspecified eyelid

H02.43 Paralytic ptosis of eyelid

Neurogenic ptosis of eyelid

H02.431 Paralytic ptosis of right eyelid

H02.432 Paralytic ptosis of left eyelid

H02.433 Paralytic ptosis of bilateral eyelids

H02.439 Paralytic ptosis unspecified eyelid

H02.5 Other disorders affecting eyelid function

Excludes2: blepharospasm (G24.5)

organic tic (G25.69)

psychogenic tic (F95.-)

H02.51 Abnormal innervation syndrome

H02.511 Abnormal innervation syndrome right upper eyelid

H02.512 Abnormal innervation syndrome right lower eyelid

H02.513 Abnormal innervation syndrome right eye, unspecified eyelid

H02.514 Abnormal innervation syndrome left upper eyelid

H02.515 Abnormal innervation syndrome left lower eyelid

H02.516 Abnormal innervation syndrome left eye, unspecified eyelid

H02.519 Abnormal innervation syndrome unspecified eye, unspecified eyelid

H02.52 Blepharophimosis

Ankyloblepharon

H02.521 Blepharophimosis right upper eyelid

H02.522 Blepharophimosis right lower eyelid

H02.523 Blepharophimosis right eye, unspecified eyelid

H02.524 Blepharophimosis left upper eyelid

H02.525 Blepharophimosis left lower eyelid

H02.526 Blepharophimosis left eye, unspecified eyelid

H02.529 Blepharophimosis unspecified eye, unspecified lid

H02.53 Eyelid retraction

Eyelid lag

H02.531 Eyelid retraction right upper eyelid

H02.532 Eyelid retraction right lower eyelid

● New code ▲ Revised code **Excludes1:** Not coded here **Excludes2:** Not included here ⊗ Placeholder required ⑦7th digit required

H02.533 Eyelid retraction right eye, unspecified eyelid

H02.534 Eyelid retraction left upper eyelid

H02.535 Eyelid retraction left lower eyelid

H02.536 Eyelid retraction left eye, unspecified eyelid

H02.539 Eyelid retraction unspecified eye, unspecified lid

H02.59 Other disorders affecting eyelid function

Deficient blink reflex

Sensory disorders

H02.6 Xanthelasma of eyelid

H02.60 Xanthelasma of unspecified eye, unspecified eyelid

H02.61 Xanthelasma of right upper eyelid

H02.62 Xanthelasma of right lower eyelid

H02.63 Xanthelasma of right eye, unspecified eyelid

H02.64 Xanthelasma of left upper eyelid

H02.65 Xanthelasma of left lower eyelid

H02.66 Xanthelasma of left eye, unspecified eyelid

H02.7 Other and unspecified degenerative disorders of eyelid and periocular area

H02.70 Unspecified degenerative disorders of eyelid and periocular area

H02.71 Chloasma of eyelid and periocular area

Dyspigmentation of eyelid

Hyperpigmentation of eyelid

H02.711 Chloasma of right upper eyelid and periocular area

H02.712 Chloasma of right lower eyelid and periocular area

H02.713 Chloasma of right eye, unspecified eyelid and periocular area

H02.714 Chloasma of left upper eyelid and periocular area

H02.715 Chloasma of left lower eyelid and periocular area

H02.716 Chloasma of left eye, unspecified eyelid and periocular area

H02.719 Chloasma of unspecified eye, unspecified eyelid and periocular area

H02.72 Madarosis of eyelid and periocular area

Hypotrichosis of eyelid

H02.721 Madarosis of right upper eyelid and periocular area

H02.722 Madarosis of right lower eyelid and periocular area

H02.723 Madarosis of right eye, unspecified eyelid and periocular area

H02.724 Madarosis of left upper eyelid and periocular area

H02.725 Madarosis of left lower eyelid and periocular area

H02.726 Madarosis of left eye, unspecified eyelid and periocular area

H02.729 Madarosis of unspecified eye, unspecified eyelid and periocular area

H02.73 Vitiligo of eyelid and periocular area

Hypopigmentation of eyelid

H02.731 Vitiligo of right upper eyelid and periocular area

H02.732 Vitiligo of right lower eyelid and periocular area

H02.733 Vitiligo of right eye, unspecified eyelid and periocular area

H02.734 Vitiligo of left upper eyelid and periocular area

H02.735 Vitiligo of left lower eyelid and periocular area

H02.736 Vitiligo of left eye, unspecified eyelid and periocular area

H02.739 Vitiligo of unspecified eye, unspecified eyelid and periocular area

H02.79 Other degenerative disorders of eyelid and periocular area

H02.8 Other specified disorders of eyelid

H02.81 Retained foreign body in eyelid

<u>Use additional code</u> to identify the type of retained foreign body (Z18.-)

Excludes1: laceration of eyelid with foreign body (S01.12-)

retained intraocular foreign body (H44.6-, H44.7-)

superficial foreign body of eyelid and periocular area (S00.25-)

H02.811 Retained foreign body in right upper eyelid

H02.812 Retained foreign body in right lower eyelid

H02.813 Retained foreign body in right eye, unspecified eyelid

H02.814 Retained foreign body in left upper eyelid

H02.815 Retained foreign body in left lower eyelid

H02.816 Retained foreign body in left eye, unspecified eyelid

H02.819 Retained foreign body in unspecified eye, unspecified eyelid

H02.82 Cysts of eyelid

Sebaceous cyst of eyelid

H02.821 Cysts of right upper eyelid

H02.822 Cysts of right lower eyelid

H02.823 Cysts of right eye, unspecified eyelid

H02.824 Cysts of left upper eyelid

H02.825 Cysts of left lower eyelid

H02.826 Cysts of left eye, unspecified eyelid

H02.829 Cysts of unspecified eye, unspecified eyelid

H02.83 Dermatochalasis of eyelid

H02.831 Dermatochalasis of right upper eyelid

H02.832 Dermatochalasis of right lower eyelid

H02.833 Dermatochalasis of right eye, unspecified eyelid

H02.834 Dermatochalasis of left upper eyelid

H02.835 Dermatochalasis of left lower eyelid

H02.836 Dermatochalasis of left eye, unspecified eyelid

H02.839 Dermatochalasis of unspecified eye, unspecified eyelid

H02.84 **Edema of eyelid**

Hyperemia of eyelid

H02.841 **Edema of right upper eyelid**

H02.842 **Edema of right lower eyelid**

H02.843 **Edema of right eye, unspecified eyelid**

H02.844 **Edema of left upper eyelid**

H02.845 **Edema of left lower eyelid**

H02.846 **Edema of left eye, unspecified eyelid**

H02.849 **Edema of unspecified eye, unspecified eyelid**

H02.85 **Elephantiasis of eyelid**

H02.851 **Elephantiasis of right upper eyelid**

H02.852 **Elephantiasis of right lower eyelid**

H02.853 **Elephantiasis of right eye, unspecified eyelid**

H02.854 **Elephantiasis of left upper eyelid**

H02.855 **Elephantiasis of left lower eyelid**

H02.856 **Elephantiasis of left eye, unspecified eyelid**

H02.859 **Elephantiasis of unspecified eye, unspecified eyelid**

H02.86 **Hypertrichosis of eyelid**

H02.861 **Hypertrichosis of right upper eyelid**

H02.862 **Hypertrichosis of right lower eyelid**

H02.863 **Hypertrichosis of right eye, unspecified eyelid**

H02.864 **Hypertrichosis of left upper eyelid**

H02.865 **Hypertrichosis of left lower eyelid**

H02.866 **Hypertrichosis of left eye, unspecified eyelid**

H02.869 **Hypertrichosis of unspecified eye, unspecified eyelid**

H02.87 **Vascular anomalies of eyelid**

H02.871 **Vascular anomalies of right upper eyelid**

H02.872 **Vascular anomalies of right lower eyelid**

H02.873 **Vascular anomalies of right eye, unspecified eyelid**

H02.874 **Vascular anomalies of left upper eyelid**

H02.875 **Vascular anomalies of left lower eyelid**

H02.876 **Vascular anomalies of left eye, unspecified eyelid**

H02.879 **Vascular anomalies of unspecified eye, unspecified eyelid**

H02.89 **Other specified disorders of eyelid**

Hemorrhage of eyelid

H02.9 **Unspecified disorder of eyelid**

Disorder of eyelid NOS

H04 **Disorders of lacrimal system**

Excludes1: congenital malformations of lacrimal system (Q10.4-Q10.6)

H04.0 **Dacryoadenitis**

H04.00 **Unspecified dacryoadenitis**

H04.001 **Unspecified dacryoadenitis, right lacrimal gland**

H04.002 **Unspecified dacryoadenitis, left lacrimal gland**

H04.003 **Unspecified dacryoadenitis, bilateral lacrimal glands**

H04.009 **Unspecified dacryoadenitis, unspecified lacrimal gland**

H04.01 **Acute dacryoadenitis**

H04.011 **Acute dacryoadenitis, right lacrimal gland**

H04.012 **Acute dacryoadenitis, left lacrimal gland**

H04.013 **Acute dacryoadenitis, bilateral lacrimal glands**

H04.019 **Acute dacryoadenitis, unspecified lacrimal gland**

H04.02 **Chronic dacryoadenitis**

H04.021 **Chronic dacryoadenitis, right lacrimal gland**

H04.022 **Chronic dacryoadenitis, left lacrimal gland**

H04.023 **Chronic dacryoadenitis, bilateral lacrimal glands**

H04.029 **Chronic dacryoadenitis, unspecified lacrimal gland**

H04.03 **Chronic enlargement of lacrimal gland**

H04.031 **Chronic enlargement of right lacrimal gland**

H04.032 **Chronic enlargement of left lacrimal gland**

H04.033 **Chronic enlargement of bilateral lacrimal glands**

H04.039 **Chronic enlargement of unspecified lacrimal gland**

H04.1 **Other disorders of lacrimal gland**

H04.11 **Dacryops**

H04.111 **Dacryops of right lacrimal gland**

H04.112 **Dacryops of left lacrimal gland**

H04.113 **Dacryops of bilateral lacrimal glands**

H04.119 **Dacryops of unspecified lacrimal gland**

H04.12 **Dry eye syndrome**

Tear film insufficiency, NOS

H04.121 **Dry eye syndrome of right lacrimal gland**

H04.122 **Dry eye syndrome of left lacrimal gland**

H04.123 **Dry eye syndrome of bilateral lacrimal glands**

H04.129 **Dry eye syndrome of unspecified lacrimal gland**

H04.13 **Lacrimal cyst**

Lacrimal cystic degeneration

H04.131 **Lacrimal cyst, right lacrimal gland**

H04.132 **Lacrimal cyst, left lacrimal gland**

H04.133 **Lacrimal cyst, bilateral lacrimal glands**

H04.139 **Lacrimal cyst, unspecified lacrimal gland**

H04.14 **Primary lacrimal gland atrophy**

H04.141 **Primary lacrimal gland atrophy, right lacrimal gland**

H04.142 **Primary lacrimal gland atrophy, left lacrimal gland**

H04.143 Primary lacrimal gland atrophy, bilateral lacrimal glands

H04.149 Primary lacrimal gland atrophy, unspecified lacrimal gland

H04.15 Secondary lacrimal gland atrophy

H04.151 Secondary lacrimal gland atrophy, right lacrimal gland

H04.152 Secondary lacrimal gland atrophy, left lacrimal gland

H04.153 Secondary lacrimal gland atrophy, bilateral lacrimal glands

H04.159 Secondary lacrimal gland atrophy, unspecified lacrimal gland

H04.16 Lacrimal gland dislocation

H04.161 Lacrimal gland dislocation, right lacrimal gland

H04.162 Lacrimal gland dislocation, left lacrimal gland

H04.163 Lacrimal gland dislocation, bilateral lacrimal glands

H04.169 Lacrimal gland dislocation, unspecified lacrimal gland

H04.19 Other specified disorders of lacrimal gland

H04.2 Epiphora

H04.20 Unspecified epiphora

H04.201 Unspecified epiphora, right lacrimal gland

H04.202 Unspecified epiphora, left lacrimal gland

H04.203 Unspecified epiphora, bilateral lacrimal glands

H04.209 Unspecified epiphora, unspecified lacrimal gland

H04.21 Epiphora due to excess lacrimation

H04.211 Epiphora due to excess lacrimation, right lacrimal gland

H04.212 Epiphora due to excess lacrimation, left lacrimal gland

H04.213 Epiphora due to excess lacrimation, bilateral lacrimal glands

H04.219 Epiphora due to excess lacrimation, unspecified lacrimal gland

H04.22 Epiphora due to insufficient drainage

H04.221 Epiphora due to insufficient drainage, right lacrimal gland

H04.222 Epiphora due to insufficient drainage, left lacrimal gland

H04.223 Epiphora due to insufficient drainage, bilateral lacrimal glands

H04.229 Epiphora due to insufficient drainage, unspecified lacrimal gland

H04.3 Acute and unspecified inflammation of lacrimal passages

Excludes1: neonatal dacryocystitis (P39.1)

H04.30 Unspecified dacryocystitis

H04.301 Unspecified dacryocystitis of right lacrimal passage

H04.302 Unspecified dacryocystitis of left lacrimal passage

H04.303 Unspecified dacryocystitis of bilateral lacrimal passages

H04.309 Unspecified dacryocystitis of unspecified lacrimal passage

H04.31 Phlegmonous dacryocystitis

H04.311 Phlegmonous dacryocystitis of right lacrimal passage

H04.312 Phlegmonous dacryocystitis of left lacrimal passage

H04.313 Phlegmonous dacryocystitis of bilateral lacrimal passages

H04.319 Phlegmonous dacryocystitis of unspecified lacrimal passage

H04.32 Acute dacryocystitis

Acute dacryopericystitis

H04.321 Acute dacryocystitis of right lacrimal passage

H04.322 Acute dacryocystitis of left lacrimal passage

H04.323 Acute dacryocystitis of bilateral lacrimal passages

H04.329 Acute dacryocystitis of unspecified lacrimal passage

H04.33 Acute lacrimal canaliculitis

H04.331 Acute lacrimal canaliculitis of right lacrimal passage

H04.332 Acute lacrimal canaliculitis of left lacrimal passage

H04.333 Acute lacrimal canaliculitis of bilateral lacrimal passages

H04.339 Acute lacrimal canaliculitis of unspecified lacrimal passage

H04.4 Chronic inflammation of lacrimal passages

H04.41 Chronic dacryocystitis

H04.411 Chronic dacryocystitis of right lacrimal passage

H04.412 Chronic dacryocystitis of left lacrimal passage

H04.413 Chronic dacryocystitis of bilateral lacrimal passages

H04.419 Chronic dacryocystitis of unspecified lacrimal passage

H04.42 Chronic lacrimal canaliculitis

H04.421 Chronic lacrimal canaliculitis of right lacrimal passage

H04.422 Chronic lacrimal canaliculitis of left lacrimal passage

H04.423 Chronic lacrimal canaliculitis of bilateral lacrimal passages

H04.429 Chronic lacrimal canaliculitis of unspecified lacrimal passage

H04.43 Chronic lacrimal mucocele

H04.431 Chronic lacrimal mucocele of right lacrimal passage

H04.432 Chronic lacrimal mucocele of left lacrimal passage

H04.433 Chronic lacrimal mucocele of bilateral lacrimal passages

H04.439 Chronic lacrimal mucocele of unspecified lacrimal passage

H04.5 Stenosis and insufficiency of lacrimal passages

H04.51 Dacryolith

H04.511 Dacryolith of right lacrimal passage

H04.512 Dacryolith of left lacrimal passage

H04.513 Dacryolith of bilateral lacrimal passages

H04.519 Dacryolith of unspecified lacrimal passage

| Add 4th-7th digits | Nonspecific code | Unspecified code | Manifestation code |

H04.52   Eversion of lacrimal punctum

    H04.521   Eversion of right lacrimal punctum

    H04.522   Eversion of left lacrimal punctum

    H04.523   Eversion of bilateral lacrimal punctum

    H04.529   Eversion of unspecified lacrimal punctum

H04.53   Neonatal obstruction of nasolacrimal duct

    Excludes1: congenital stenosis and stricture of lacrimal duct (Q10.5)

    H04.531   Neonatal obstruction of right nasolacrimal duct

    H04.532   Neonatal obstruction of left nasolacrimal duct

    H04.533   Neonatal obstruction of bilateral nasolacrimal duct

    H04.539   Neonatal obstruction of unspecified nasolacrimal duct

H04.54   Stenosis of lacrimal canaliculi

    H04.541   Stenosis of right lacrimal canaliculi

    H04.542   Stenosis of left lacrimal canaliculi

    H04.543   Stenosis of bilateral lacrimal canaliculi

    H04.549   Stenosis of unspecified lacrimal canaliculi

H04.55   Acquired stenosis of nasolacrimal duct

    H04.551   Acquired stenosis of right nasolacrimal duct

    H04.552   Acquired stenosis of left nasolacrimal duct

    H04.553   Acquired stenosis of bilateral nasolacrimal duct

    H04.559   Acquired stenosis of unspecified nasolacrimal duct

H04.56   Stenosis of lacrimal punctum

    H04.561   Stenosis of right lacrimal punctum

    H04.562   Stenosis of left lacrimal punctum

    H04.563   Stenosis of bilateral lacrimal punctum

    H04.569   Stenosis of unspecified lacrimal punctum

H04.57   Stenosis of lacrimal sac

    H04.571   Stenosis of right lacrimal sac

    H04.572   Stenosis of left lacrimal sac

    H04.573   Stenosis of bilateral lacrimal sac

    H04.579   Stenosis of unspecified lacrimal sac

H04.6   Other changes of lacrimal passages

  H04.61   Lacrimal fistula

    H04.611   Lacrimal fistula right lacrimal passage

    H04.612   Lacrimal fistula left lacrimal passage

    H04.613   Lacrimal fistula bilateral lacrimal passages

    H04.619   Lacrimal fistula unspecified lacrimal passage

  H04.69   Other changes of lacrimal passages

H04.8   Other disorders of lacrimal system

  H04.81   Granuloma of lacrimal passages

    H04.811   Granuloma of right lacrimal passage

    H04.812   Granuloma of left lacrimal passage

    H04.813   Granuloma of bilateral lacrimal passages

    H04.819   Granuloma of unspecified lacrimal passage

  H04.89   Other disorders of lacrimal system

H04.9   Disorder of lacrimal system, unspecified

H05   **Disorders of orbit**

  Excludes1: congenital malformation of orbit (Q10.7)

H05.0   Acute inflammation of orbit

  H05.00   Unspecified acute inflammation of orbit

  H05.01   Cellulitis of orbit

    Abscess of orbit

    H05.011   Cellulitis of right orbit

    H05.012   Cellulitis of left orbit

    H05.013   Cellulitis of bilateral orbits

    H05.019   Cellulitis of unspecified orbit

  H05.02   Osteomyelitis of orbit

    H05.021   Osteomyelitis of right orbit

    H05.022   Osteomyelitis of left orbit

    H05.023   Osteomyelitis of bilateral orbits

    H05.029   Osteomyelitis of unspecified orbit

  H05.03   Periostitis of orbit

    H05.031   Periostitis of right orbit

    H05.032   Periostitis of left orbit

    H05.033   Periostitis of bilateral orbits

    H05.039   Periostitis of unspecified orbit

  H05.04   Tenonitis of orbit

    H05.041   Tenonitis of right orbit

    H05.042   Tenonitis of left orbit

    H05.043   Tenonitis of bilateral orbits

    H05.049   Tenonitis of unspecified orbit

H05.1   Chronic inflammatory disorders of orbit

  H05.10   Unspecified chronic inflammatory disorders of orbit

  H05.11   Granuloma of orbit

    Pseudotumor (inflammatory) of orbit

    H05.111   Granuloma of right orbit

    H05.112   Granuloma of left orbit

    H05.113   Granuloma of bilateral orbits

    H05.119   Granuloma of unspecified orbit

  H05.12   Orbital myositis

    H05.121   Orbital myositis, right orbit

    H05.122   Orbital myositis, left orbit

    H05.123   Orbital myositis, bilateral

    H05.129   Orbital myositis, unspecified orbit

H05.2   Exophthalmic conditions

  H05.20   Unspecified exophthalmos

  H05.21   Displacement (lateral) of globe

    H05.211   Displacement (lateral) of globe, right eye

    H05.212   Displacement (lateral) of globe, left eye

    H05.213   Displacement (lateral) of globe, bilateral

    H05.219   Displacement (lateral) of globe, unspecified eye

  H05.22   Edema of orbit

    Orbital congestion

H05.221   Edema of right orbit

H05.222   Edema of left orbit

H05.223   Edema of bilateral orbit

H05.229   Edema of unspecified orbit

H05.23   Hemorrhage of orbit

H05.231   Hemorrhage of right orbit

H05.232   Hemorrhage of left orbit

H05.233   Hemorrhage of bilateral orbit

H05.239   Hemorrhage of unspecified orbit

H05.24   Constant exophthalmos

H05.241   Constant exophthalmos, right eye

H05.242   Constant exophthalmos, left eye

H05.243   Constant exophthalmos, bilateral

H05.249   Constant exophthalmos, unspecified eye

H05.25   Intermittent exophthalmos

H05.251   Intermittent exophthalmos, right eye

H05.252   Intermittent exophthalmos, left eye

H05.253   Intermittent exophthalmos, bilateral

H05.259   Intermittent exophthalmos, unspecified eye

H05.26   Pulsating exophthalmos

H05.261   Pulsating exophthalmos, right eye

H05.262   Pulsating exophthalmos, left eye

H05.263   Pulsating exophthalmos, bilateral

H05.269   Pulsating exophthalmos, unspecified eye

H05.3   **Deformity of orbit**

Excludes1: congenital deformity of orbit (Q10.7)

hypertelorism (Q75.2)

H05.30   Unspecified deformity of orbit

H05.31   Atrophy of orbit

H05.311   Atrophy of right orbit

H05.312   Atrophy of left orbit

H05.313   Atrophy of bilateral orbit

H05.319   Atrophy of unspecified orbit

H05.32   Deformity of orbit due to bone disease

Code also associated bone disease

H05.321   Deformity of right orbit due to bone disease

H05.322   Deformity of left orbit due to bone disease

H05.323   Deformity of bilateral orbits due to bone disease

H05.329   Deformity of unspecified orbit due to bone disease

H05.33   Deformity of orbit due to trauma or surgery

H05.331   Deformity of right orbit due to trauma or surgery

H05.332   Deformity of left orbit due to trauma or surgery

H05.333   Deformity of bilateral orbits due to trauma or surgery

H05.339   Deformity of unspecified orbit due to trauma or surgery

H05.34   Enlargement of orbit

H05.341   Enlargement of right orbit

H05.342   Enlargement of left orbit

H05.343   Enlargement of bilateral orbits

H05.349   Enlargement of unspecified orbit

H05.35   Exostosis of orbit

H05.351   Exostosis of right orbit

H05.352   Exostosis of left orbit

H05.353   Exostosis of bilateral orbits

H05.359   Exostosis of unspecified orbit

H05.4   **Enophthalmos**

H05.40   Unspecified enophthalmos

H05.401   Unspecified enophthalmos, right eye

H05.402   Unspecified enophthalmos, left eye

H05.403   Unspecified enophthalmos, bilateral

H05.409   Unspecified enophthalmos, unspecified eye

H05.41   Enophthalmos due to atrophy of orbital tissue

H05.411   Enophthalmos due to atrophy of orbital tissue, right eye

H05.412   Enophthalmos due to atrophy of orbital tissue, left eye

H05.413   Enophthalmos due to atrophy of orbital tissue, bilateral

H05.419   Enophthalmos due to atrophy of orbital tissue, unspecified eye

H05.42   Enophthalmos due to trauma or surgery

H05.421   Enophthalmos due to trauma or surgery, right eye

H05.422   Enophthalmos due to trauma or surgery, left eye

H05.423   Enophthalmos due to trauma or surgery, bilateral

H05.429   Enophthalmos due to trauma or surgery, unspecified eye

H05.5   **Retained (old) foreign body following penetrating wound of orbit**

Retrobulbar foreign body

Use additional code to identify the type of retained foreign body (Z18.-)

Excludes1: current penetrating wound of orbit (S05.4-)

Excludes2: retained foreign body of eyelid (H02.81-)

retained intraocular foreign body (H44.6-, H44.7-)

H05.50   Retained (old) foreign body following penetrating wound of unspecified orbit

H05.51   Retained (old) foreign body following penetrating wound of right orbit

H05.52   Retained (old) foreign body following penetrating wound of left orbit

H05.53   Retained (old) foreign body following penetrating wound of bilateral orbits

H05.8   **Other disorders of orbit**

H05.81   Cyst of orbit

Encephalocele of orbit

H05.811   Cyst of right orbit

H05.812   Cyst of left orbit

H05.813   Cyst of bilateral orbits

H05.819   Cyst of unspecified orbit

H05.82   Myopathy of extraocular muscles

H05.821   Myopathy of extraocular muscles, right orbit

H05.822   Myopathy of extraocular muscles, left orbit

H05.823 **Myopathy of extraocular muscles, bilateral**

H05.829 **Myopathy of extraocular muscles, unspecified orbit**

H05.89 **Other disorders of orbit**

H05.9 **Unspecified disorder of orbit**

DISORDERS OF CONJUNCTIVA (H10-H11)

Definition: Disorders of conjunctiva are disorders of the mucous membrane that lines the inner surface of the eyelid and the exposed surface of the eyeball.

H10 **Conjunctivitis**

Excludes1: keratoconjunctivitis (H16.2-)

H10.0 **Mucopurulent conjunctivitis**

H10.01 **Acute follicular conjunctivitis**

H10.011 **Acute follicular conjunctivitis, right eye**

H10.012 **Acute follicular conjunctivitis, left eye**

H10.013 **Acute follicular conjunctivitis, bilateral**

H10.019 **Acute follicular conjunctivitis, unspecified eye**

H10.02 **Other mucopurulent conjunctivitis**

H10.021 **Other mucopurulent conjunctivitis, right eye**

H10.022 **Other mucopurulent conjunctivitis, left eye**

H10.023 **Other mucopurulent conjunctivitis, bilateral**

H10.029 **Other mucopurulent conjunctivitis, unspecified eye**

H10.1 **Acute atopic conjunctivitis**

Acute papillary conjunctivitis

H10.10 **Acute atopic conjunctivitis, unspecified eye**

H10.11 **Acute atopic conjunctivitis, right eye**

H10.12 **Acute atopic conjunctivitis, left eye**

H10.13 **Acute atopic conjunctivitis, bilateral**

H10.2 **Other acute conjunctivitis**

H10.21 **Acute toxic conjunctivitis**

Acute chemical conjunctivitis

Code first (T51-T65) to identify chemical and intent

Excludes1: burn and corrosion of eye and adnexa (T26.-)

H10.211 **Acute toxic conjunctivitis, right eye**

H10.212 **Acute toxic conjunctivitis, left eye**

H10.213 **Acute toxic conjunctivitis, bilateral**

H10.219 **Acute toxic conjunctivitis, unspecified eye**

H10.22 **Pseudomembranous conjunctivitis**

H10.221 **Pseudomembranous conjunctivitis, right eye**

H10.222 **Pseudomembranous conjunctivitis, left eye**

H10.223 **Pseudomembranous conjunctivitis, bilateral**

H10.229 **Pseudomembranous conjunctivitis, unspecified eye**

H10.23 **Serous conjunctivitis, except viral**

Excludes1: viral conjunctivitis (B30.-)

H10.231 **Serous conjunctivitis, except viral, right eye**

H10.232 **Serous conjunctivitis, except viral, left eye**

H10.233 **Serous conjunctivitis, except viral, bilateral**

H10.239 **Serous conjunctivitis, except viral, unspecified eye**

H10.3 **Unspecified acute conjunctivitis**

Excludes1: ophthalmia neonatorum NOS (P39.1)

H10.30 **Unspecified acute conjunctivitis, unspecified eye**

H10.31 **Unspecified acute conjunctivitis, right eye**

H10.32 **Unspecified acute conjunctivitis, left eye**

H10.33 **Unspecified acute conjunctivitis, bilateral**

H10.4 **Chronic conjunctivitis**

H10.40 **Unspecified chronic conjunctivitis**

H10.401 **Unspecified chronic conjunctivitis, right eye**

H10.402 **Unspecified chronic conjunctivitis, left eye**

H10.403 **Unspecified chronic conjunctivitis, bilateral**

H10.409 **Unspecified chronic conjunctivitis, unspecified eye**

H10.41 **Chronic giant papillary conjunctivitis**

H10.411 **Chronic giant papillary conjunctivitis, right eye**

H10.412 **Chronic giant papillary conjunctivitis, left eye**

H10.413 **Chronic giant papillary conjunctivitis, bilateral**

H10.419 **Chronic giant papillary conjunctivitis, unspecified eye**

H10.42 **Simple chronic conjunctivitis**

H10.421 **Simple chronic conjunctivitis, right eye**

H10.422 **Simple chronic conjunctivitis, left eye**

H10.423 **Simple chronic conjunctivitis, bilateral**

H10.429 **Simple chronic conjunctivitis, unspecified eye**

H10.43 **Chronic follicular conjunctivitis**

H10.431 **Chronic follicular conjunctivitis, right eye**

H10.432 **Chronic follicular conjunctivitis, left eye**

H10.433 **Chronic follicular conjunctivitis, bilateral**

H10.439 **Chronic follicular conjunctivitis, unspecified eye**

H10.44 **Vernal conjunctivitis**

Excludes1: vernal keratoconjunctivitis with limbar and corneal involvement (H16.26-)

H10.45 **Other chronic allergic conjunctivitis**

H10.5 **Blepharoconjunctivitis**

H10.50 **Unspecified blepharoconjunctivitis**

H10.501 **Unspecified blepharoconjunctivitis, right eye**

H10.502 **Unspecified blepharoconjunctivitis, left eye**

● New code   ▲ Revised code   **Excludes1:** Not coded here   **Excludes2:** Not included here   ⊗ Placeholder required   ⑦7ᵗʰ digit required

H10.503 Unspecified blepharoconjunctivitis, bilateral

H10.509 Unspecified blepharoconjunctivitis, unspecified eye

H10.51 Ligneous conjunctivitis

H10.511 Ligneous conjunctivitis, right eye

H10.512 Ligneous conjunctivitis, left eye

H10.513 Ligneous conjunctivitis, bilateral

H10.519 Ligneous conjunctivitis, unspecified eye

H10.52 Angular blepharoconjunctivitis

H10.521 Angular blepharoconjunctivitis, right eye

H10.522 Angular blepharoconjunctivitis, left eye

H10.523 Angular blepharoconjunctivitis, bilateral

H10.529 Angular blepharoconjunctivitis, unspecified eye

H10.53 Contact blepharoconjunctivitis

H10.531 Contact blepharoconjunctivitis, right eye

H10.532 Contact blepharoconjunctivitis, left eye

H10.533 Contact blepharoconjunctivitis, bilateral

H10.539 Contact blepharoconjunctivitis, unspecified eye

H10.8 Other conjunctivitis

H10.81 Pingueculitis

Excludes1: pinguecula (H11.15-)

H10.811 Pingueculitis, right eye

H10.812 Pingueculitis, left eye

H10.813 Pingueculitis, bilateral

H10.819 Pingueculitis, unspecified eye

H10.89 Other conjunctivitis

H10.9 Unspecified conjunctivitis

H11 Other disorders of conjunctiva

Excludes1: keratoconjunctivitis (H16.2-)

H11.0 Pterygium of eye

Excludes1: pseudopterygium (H11.81-)

H11.00 Unspecified pterygium of eye

H11.001 Unspecified pterygium of right eye

H11.002 Unspecified pterygium of left eye

H11.003 Unspecified pterygium of eye, bilateral

H11.009 Unspecified pterygium of unspecified eye

H11.01 Amyloid pterygium

H11.011 Amyloid pterygium of right eye

H11.012 Amyloid pterygium of left eye

H11.013 Amyloid pterygium of eye, bilateral

H11.019 Amyloid pterygium of unspecified eye

H11.02 Central pterygium of eye

H11.021 Central pterygium of right eye

H11.022 Central pterygium of left eye

H11.023 Central pterygium of eye, bilateral

H11.029 Central pterygium of unspecified eye

H11.03 Double pterygium of eye

H11.031 Double pterygium of right eye

H11.032 Double pterygium of left eye

H11.033 Double pterygium of eye, bilateral

H11.039 Double pterygium of unspecified eye

H11.04 Peripheral pterygium of eye, stationary

H11.041 Peripheral pterygium, stationary, right eye

H11.042 Peripheral pterygium, stationary, left eye

H11.043 Peripheral pterygium, stationary, bilateral

H11.049 Peripheral pterygium, stationary, unspecified eye

H11.05 Peripheral pterygium of eye, progressive

H11.051 Peripheral pterygium, progressive, right eye

H11.052 Peripheral pterygium, progressive, left eye

H11.053 Peripheral pterygium, progressive, bilateral

H11.059 Peripheral pterygium, progressive, unspecified eye

H11.06 Recurrent pterygium of eye

H11.061 Recurrent pterygium of right eye

H11.062 Recurrent pterygium of left eye

H11.063 Recurrent pterygium of eye, bilateral

H11.069 Recurrent pterygium of unspecified eye

H11.1 Conjunctival degenerations and deposits

Excludes2: pseudopterygium (H11.81)

H11.10 Unspecified conjunctival degenerations

H11.11 Conjunctival deposits

H11.111 Conjunctival deposits, right eye

H11.112 Conjunctival deposits, left eye

H11.113 Conjunctival deposits, bilateral

H11.119 Conjunctival deposits, unspecified eye

H11.12 Conjunctival concretions

H11.121 Conjunctival concretions, right eye

H11.122 Conjunctival concretions, left eye

H11.123 Conjunctival concretions, bilateral

H11.129 Conjunctival concretions, unspecified eye

H11.13 Conjunctival pigmentations

Conjunctival argyrosis [argyria]

H11.131 Conjunctival pigmentations, right eye

H11.132 Conjunctival pigmentations, left eye

H11.133 Conjunctival pigmentations, bilateral

H11.139 Conjunctival pigmentations, unspecified eye

H11.14 Conjunctival xerosis, unspecified

Excludes1: xerosis of conjunctiva due to vitamin A deficiency (E50.0, E50.1)

H11.141 Conjunctival xerosis, unspecified, right eye

H11.142 Conjunctival xerosis, unspecified, left eye

H11.143 Conjunctival xerosis, unspecified, bilateral

Add 4th-7th digits   Nonspecific code   Unspecified code   Manifestation code

H11.149 Conjunctival xerosis, unspecified, unspecified eye

H11.15 Pinguecula

Excludes1: pingueculitis (H10.81-)

H11.151 Pinguecula, right eye

H11.152 Pinguecula, left eye

H11.153 Pinguecula, bilateral

H11.159 Pinguecula, unspecified eye

H11.2 Conjunctival scars

H11.21 Conjunctival adhesions and strands (localized)

H11.211 Conjunctival adhesions and strands (localized), right eye

H11.212 Conjunctival adhesions and strands (localized), left eye

H11.213 Conjunctival adhesions and strands (localized), bilateral

H11.219 Conjunctival adhesions and strands (localized), unspecified eye

H11.22 Conjunctival granuloma

H11.221 Conjunctival granuloma, right eye

H11.222 Conjunctival granuloma, left eye

H11.223 Conjunctival granuloma, bilateral

H11.229 Conjunctival granuloma, unspecified

H11.23 Symblepharon

H11.231 Symblepharon, right eye

H11.232 Symblepharon, left eye

H11.233 Symblepharon, bilateral

H11.239 Symblepharon, unspecified eye

H11.24 Scarring of conjunctiva

H11.241 Scarring of conjunctiva, right eye

H11.242 Scarring of conjunctiva, left eye

H11.243 Scarring of conjunctiva, bilateral

H11.249 Scarring of conjunctiva, unspecified eye

H11.3 Conjunctival hemorrhage

Subconjunctival hemorrhage

H11.30 Conjunctival hemorrhage, unspecified eye

H11.31 Conjunctival hemorrhage, right eye

H11.32 Conjunctival hemorrhage, left eye

H11.33 Conjunctival hemorrhage, bilateral

H11.4 Other conjunctival vascular disorders and cysts

H11.41 Vascular abnormalities of conjunctiva

Conjunctival aneurysm

H11.411 Vascular abnormalities of conjunctiva, right eye

H11.412 Vascular abnormalities of conjunctiva, left eye

H11.413 Vascular abnormalities of conjunctiva, bilateral

H11.419 Vascular abnormalities of conjunctiva, unspecified eye

H11.42 Conjunctival edema

H11.421 Conjunctival edema, right eye

H11.422 Conjunctival edema, left eye

H11.423 Conjunctival edema, bilateral

H11.429 Conjunctival edema, unspecified eye

H11.43 Conjunctival hyperemia

H11.431 Conjunctival hyperemia, right eye

H11.432 Conjunctival hyperemia, left eye

H11.433 Conjunctival hyperemia, bilateral

H11.439 Conjunctival hyperemia, unspecified eye

H11.44 Conjunctival cysts

H11.441 Conjunctival cysts, right eye

H11.442 Conjunctival cysts, left eye

H11.443 Conjunctival cysts, bilateral

H11.449 Conjunctival cysts, unspecified eye

H11.8 Other specified disorders of conjunctiva

H11.81 Pseudopterygium of conjunctiva

H11.811 Pseudopterygium of conjunctiva, right eye

H11.812 Pseudopterygium of conjunctiva, left eye

H11.813 Pseudopterygium of conjunctiva, bilateral

H11.819 Pseudopterygium of conjunctiva, unspecified eye

H11.82 Conjunctivochalasis

H11.821 Conjunctivochalasis, right eye

H11.822 Conjunctivochalasis, left eye

H11.823 Conjunctivochalasis, bilateral

H11.829 Conjunctivochalasis, unspecified eye

H11.89 Other specified disorders of conjunctiva

H11.9 Unspecified disorder of conjunctiva

DISORDERS OF SCLERA, CORNEA, IRIS AND CILIARY BODY (H15-H22)

H15 Disorders of sclera

H15.0 Scleritis

H15.00 Unspecified scleritis

H15.001 Unspecified scleritis, right eye

H15.002 Unspecified scleritis, left eye

H15.003 Unspecified scleritis, bilateral

H15.009 Unspecified scleritis, unspecified eye

H15.01 Anterior scleritis

H15.011 Anterior scleritis, right eye

H15.012 Anterior scleritis, left eye

H15.013 Anterior scleritis, bilateral

H15.019 Anterior scleritis, unspecified eye

H15.02 Brawny scleritis

H15.021 Brawny scleritis, right eye

H15.022 Brawny scleritis, left eye

H15.023 Brawny scleritis, bilateral

H15.029 Brawny scleritis, unspecified eye

H15.03 Posterior scleritis

Sclerotenonitis

H15.031 Posterior scleritis, right eye

H15.032 Posterior scleritis, left eye

H15.033 Posterior scleritis, bilateral

H15.039 Posterior scleritis, unspecified eye

H15.04 Scleritis with corneal involvement

H15.041 Scleritis with corneal involvement, right eye

H15.042 Scleritis with corneal involvement, left eye

H15.043 Scleritis with corneal involvement, bilateral

● New code   ▲ Revised code   Excludes1: Not coded here   Excludes2: Not included here   ⊗ Placeholder required   ⑦7th digit required

H15.049   Scleritis with corneal involvement, unspecified eye

H15.05   Scleromalacia perforans

     H15.051   Scleromalacia perforans, right eye

     H15.052   Scleromalacia perforans, left eye

     H15.053   Scleromalacia perforans, bilateral

     H15.059   Scleromalacia perforans, unspecified eye

H15.09   Other scleritis

     Scleral abscess

     H15.091   Other scleritis, right eye

     H15.092   Other scleritis, left eye

     H15.093   Other scleritis, bilateral

     H15.099   Other scleritis, unspecified eye

H15.1   **Episcleritis**

   H15.10   Unspecified episcleritis

     H15.101   Unspecified episcleritis, right eye

     H15.102   Unspecified episcleritis, left eye

     H15.103   Unspecified episcleritis, bilateral

     H15.109   Unspecified episcleritis, unspecified eye

   H15.11   Episcleritis periodica fugax

     H15.111   Episcleritis periodica fugax, right eye

     H15.112   Episcleritis periodica fugax, left eye

     H15.113   Episcleritis periodica fugax, bilateral

     H15.119   Episcleritis periodica fugax, unspecified eye

   H15.12   Nodular episcleritis

     H15.121   Nodular episcleritis, right eye

     H15.122   Nodular episcleritis, left eye

     H15.123   Nodular episcleritis, bilateral

     H15.129   Nodular episcleritis, unspecified eye

H15.8   **Other disorders of sclera**

   Excludes2: blue sclera (Q13.5)

     degenerative myopia (H44.2-)

   H15.81   Equatorial staphyloma

     H15.811   Equatorial staphyloma, right eye

     H15.812   Equatorial staphyloma, left eye

     H15.813   Equatorial staphyloma, bilateral

     H15.819   Equatorial staphyloma, unspecified eye

   H15.82   Localized anterior staphyloma

     H15.821   Localized anterior staphyloma, right eye

     H15.822   Localized anterior staphyloma, left eye

     H15.823   Localized anterior staphyloma, bilateral

     H15.829   Localized anterior staphyloma, unspecified eye

   H15.83   Staphyloma posticum

     H15.831   Staphyloma posticum, right eye

     H15.832   Staphyloma posticum, left eye

     H15.833   Staphyloma posticum, bilateral

     H15.839   Staphyloma posticum, unspecified eye

   H15.84   Scleral ectasia

     H15.841   Scleral ectasia, right eye

     H15.842   Scleral ectasia, left eye

     H15.843   Scleral ectasia, bilateral

     H15.849   Scleral ectasia, unspecified eye

   H15.85   Ring staphyloma

     H15.851   Ring staphyloma, right eye

     H15.852   Ring staphyloma, left eye

     H15.853   Ring staphyloma, bilateral

     H15.859   Ring staphyloma, unspecified eye

   H15.89   Other disorders of sclera

H15.9   **Unspecified disorder of sclera**

H16   **Keratitis**

   Definition: Keratitis is an infection or inflammation of the cornea which can be caused by a variety of conditions, including infections, dry eyes, foreign objects, contact lenses, intense light, vitamin a deficiency or allergies.

H16.0   **Corneal ulcer**

   H16.00   Unspecified corneal ulcer

     H16.001   Unspecified corneal ulcer, right eye

     H16.002   Unspecified corneal ulcer, left eye

     H16.003   Unspecified corneal ulcer, bilateral

     H16.009   Unspecified corneal ulcer, unspecified eye

   H16.01   Central corneal ulcer

     H16.011   Central corneal ulcer, right eye

     H16.012   Central corneal ulcer, left eye

     H16.013   Central corneal ulcer, bilateral

     H16.019   Central corneal ulcer, unspecified eye

   H16.02   Ring corneal ulcer

     H16.021   Ring corneal ulcer, right eye

     H16.022   Ring corneal ulcer, left eye

     H16.023   Ring corneal ulcer, bilateral

     H16.029   Ring corneal ulcer, unspecified eye

   H16.03   Corneal ulcer with hypopyon

     H16.031   Corneal ulcer with hypopyon, right eye

     H16.032   Corneal ulcer with hypopyon, left eye

     H16.033   Corneal ulcer with hypopyon, bilateral

     H16.039   Corneal ulcer with hypopyon, unspecified eye

   H16.04   Marginal corneal ulcer

     H16.041   Marginal corneal ulcer, right eye

     H16.042   Marginal corneal ulcer, left eye

     H16.043   Marginal corneal ulcer, bilateral

     H16.049   Marginal corneal ulcer, unspecified eye

   H16.05   Mooren's corneal ulcer

     H16.051   Mooren's corneal ulcer, right eye

     H16.052   Mooren's corneal ulcer, left eye

     H16.053   Mooren's corneal ulcer, bilateral

     H16.059   Mooren's corneal ulcer, unspecified eye

   H16.06   Mycotic corneal ulcer

     H16.061   Mycotic corneal ulcer, right eye

     H16.062   Mycotic corneal ulcer, left eye

     H16.063   Mycotic corneal ulcer, bilateral

     H16.069   Mycotic corneal ulcer, unspecified eye

Add 4th-7th digits   Nonspecific code   Unspecified code   Manifestation code

H16.07 **Perforated corneal ulcer**

    H16.071 **Perforated corneal ulcer, right eye**

    H16.072 **Perforated corneal ulcer, left eye**

    H16.073 **Perforated corneal ulcer, bilateral**

    H16.079 **Perforated corneal ulcer, unspecified eye**

H16.1 **Other and unspecified superficial keratitis without conjunctivitis**

    H16.10 **Unspecified superficial keratitis**

        H16.101 **Unspecified superficial keratitis, right eye**

        H16.102 **Unspecified superficial keratitis, left eye**

        H16.103 **Unspecified superficial keratitis, bilateral**

        H16.109 **Unspecified superficial keratitis, unspecified eye**

    H16.11 **Macular keratitis**

        Areolar keratitis

        Nummular keratitis \

        Stellate keratitis \

        Striate keratitis

        H16.111 **Macular keratitis, right eye**

        H16.112 **Macular keratitis, left eye**

        H16.113 **Macular keratitis, bilateral**

        H16.119 **Macular keratitis, unspecified eye**

    H16.12 **Filamentary keratitis**

        H16.121 **Filamentary keratitis, right eye**

        H16.122 **Filamentary keratitis, left eye**

        H16.123 **Filamentary keratitis, bilateral**

        H16.129 **Filamentary keratitis, unspecified eye**

    H16.13 **Photokeratitis**

        Snow blindness Welders keratitis

        H16.131 **Photokeratitis, right eye**

        H16.132 **Photokeratitis, left eye**

        H16.133 **Photokeratitis, bilateral**

        H16.139 **Photokeratitis, unspecified eye**

    H16.14 **Punctate keratitis**

        H16.141 **Punctate keratitis, right eye**

        H16.142 **Punctate keratitis, left eye**

        H16.143 **Punctate keratitis, bilateral**

        H16.149 **Punctate keratitis, unspecified eye**

H16.2 **Keratoconjunctivitis**

    H16.20 **Unspecified keratoconjunctivitis**

        Superficial keratitis with conjunctivitis NOS

        H16.201 **Unspecified keratoconjunctivitis, right eye**

        H16.202 **Unspecified keratoconjunctivitis, left eye**

        H16.203 **Unspecified keratoconjunctivitis, bilateral**

        H16.209 **Unspecified keratoconjunctivitis, unspecified eye**

    H16.21 **Exposure keratoconjunctivitis**

        H16.211 **Exposure keratoconjunctivitis, right eye**

        H16.212 **Exposure keratoconjunctivitis, left eye**

        H16.213 **Exposure keratoconjunctivitis, bilateral**

        H16.219 **Exposure keratoconjunctivitis, unspecified eye**

    H16.22 **Keratoconjunctivitis sicca, not specified as Sjögren's**

        Excludes1: Sjögren's syndrome (M35.01)

        H16.221 **Keratoconjunctivitis sicca, not specified as Sjögren's, right eye**

        H16.222 **Keratoconjunctivitis sicca, not specified as Sjögren's, left eye**

        H16.223 **Keratoconjunctivitis sicca, not specified as Sjögren's, bilateral**

        H16.229 **Keratoconjunctivitis sicca, not specified as Sjögren's, unspecified eye**

    H16.23 **Neurotrophic keratoconjunctivitis**

        H16.231 **Neurotrophic keratoconjunctivitis, right eye**

        H16.232 **Neurotrophic keratoconjunctivitis, left eye**

        H16.233 **Neurotrophic keratoconjunctivitis, bilateral**

        H16.239 **Neurotrophic keratoconjunctivitis, unspecified eye**

    H16.24 **Ophthalmia nodosa**

        H16.241 **Ophthalmia nodosa, right eye**

        H16.242 **Ophthalmia nodosa, left eye**

        H16.243 **Ophthalmia nodosa, bilateral**

        H16.249 **Ophthalmia nodosa, unspecified eye**

    H16.25 **Phlyctenular keratoconjunctivitis**

        H16.251 **Phlyctenular keratoconjunctivitis, right eye**

        H16.252 **Phlyctenular keratoconjunctivitis, left eye**

        H16.253 **Phlyctenular keratoconjunctivitis, bilateral**

        H16.259 **Phlyctenular keratoconjunctivitis, unspecified eye**

    H16.26 **Vernal keratoconjunctivitis, with limbar and corneal involvement**

        Excludes1: vernal conjunctivitis without limbar and corneal involvement (H10.44)

        H16.261 **Vernal keratoconjunctivitis, with limbar and corneal involvement, right eye**

        H16.262 **Vernal keratoconjunctivitis, with limbar and corneal involvement, left eye**

        H16.263 **Vernal keratoconjunctivitis, with limbar and corneal involvement, bilateral**

        H16.269 **Vernal keratoconjunctivitis, with limbar and corneal involvement, unspecified eye**

    H16.29 **Other keratoconjunctivitis**

        H16.291 **Other keratoconjunctivitis, right eye**

        H16.292 **Other keratoconjunctivitis, left eye**

        H16.293 **Other keratoconjunctivitis, bilateral**

        H16.299 **Other keratoconjunctivitis, unspecified eye**

H16.3 **Interstitial and deep keratitis**

● New code ▲ Revised code **Excludes1:** Not coded here **Excludes2:** Not included here ⊗ Placeholder required ⑦ 7ᵗʰ digit required

H16.30 Unspecified interstitial keratitis

    H16.301 Unspecified interstitial keratitis, right eye

    H16.302 Unspecified interstitial keratitis, left eye

    H16.303 Unspecified interstitial keratitis, bilateral

    H16.309 Unspecified interstitial keratitis, unspecified eye

H16.31 Corneal abscess

    H16.311 Corneal abscess, right eye

    H16.312 Corneal abscess, left eye

    H16.313 Corneal abscess, bilateral

    H16.319 Corneal abscess, unspecified eye

H16.32 Diffuse interstitial keratitis

    Cogan's syndrome

    H16.321 Diffuse interstitial keratitis, right eye

    H16.322 Diffuse interstitial keratitis, left eye

    H16.323 Diffuse interstitial keratitis, bilateral

    H16.329 Diffuse interstitial keratitis, unspecified eye

H16.33 Sclerosing keratitis

    H16.331 Sclerosing keratitis, right eye

    H16.332 Sclerosing keratitis, left eye

    H16.333 Sclerosing keratitis, bilateral

    H16.339 Sclerosing keratitis, unspecified eye

H16.39 Other interstitial and deep keratitis

    H16.391 Other interstitial and deep keratitis, right eye

    H16.392 Other interstitial and deep keratitis, left eye

    H16.393 Other interstitial and deep keratitis, bilateral

    H16.399 Other interstitial and deep keratitis, unspecified eye

H16.4 Corneal neovascularization

  H16.40 Unspecified corneal neovascularization

    H16.401 Unspecified corneal neovascularization, right eye

    H16.402 Unspecified corneal neovascularization, left eye

    H16.403 Unspecified corneal neovascularization, bilateral

    H16.409 Unspecified corneal neovascularization, unspecified eye

  H16.41 Ghost vessels (corneal)

    H16.411 Ghost vessels (corneal), right eye

    H16.412 Ghost vessels (corneal), left eye

    H16.413 Ghost vessels (corneal), bilateral

    H16.419 Ghost vessels (corneal), unspecified eye

  H16.42 Pannus (corneal)

    H16.421 Pannus (corneal), right eye

    H16.422 Pannus (corneal), left eye

    H16.423 Pannus (corneal), bilateral

    H16.429 Pannus (corneal), unspecified eye

  H16.43 Localized vascularization of cornea

    H16.431 Localized vascularization of cornea, right eye

    H16.432 Localized vascularization of cornea, left eye

    H16.433 Localized vascularization of cornea, bilateral

    H16.439 Localized vascularization of cornea, unspecified eye

  H16.44 Deep vascularization of cornea

    H16.441 Deep vascularization of cornea, right eye

    H16.442 Deep vascularization of cornea, left eye

    H16.443 Deep vascularization of cornea, bilateral

    H16.449 Deep vascularization of cornea, unspecified eye

H16.8 Other keratitis

H16.9 Unspecified keratitis

H17 Corneal scars and opacities

  H17.0 Adherent leukoma

    H17.00 Adherent leukoma, unspecified eye

    H17.01 Adherent leukoma, right eye

    H17.02 Adherent leukoma, left eye

    H17.03 Adherent leukoma, bilateral

  H17.1 Central corneal opacity

    Definition: Corneal opacity is a cloudy spot in the cornea, which is normally transparent. Causes include corneal scar tissue and infection.

    H17.10 Central corneal opacity, unspecified eye

    H17.11 Central corneal opacity, right eye

    H17.12 Central corneal opacity, left eye

    H17.13 Central corneal opacity, bilateral

  H17.8 Other corneal scars and opacities

    H17.81 Minor opacity of cornea

    Corneal nebula

    H17.811 Minor opacity of cornea, right eye

    H17.812 Minor opacity of cornea, left eye

    H17.813 Minor opacity of cornea, bilateral

    H17.819 Minor opacity of cornea, unspecified eye

    H17.82 Peripheral opacity of cornea

    H17.821 Peripheral opacity of cornea, right eye

    H17.822 Peripheral opacity of cornea, left eye

    H17.823 Peripheral opacity of cornea, bilateral

    H17.829 Peripheral opacity of cornea, unspecified eye

    H17.89 Other corneal scars and opacities

  H17.9 Unspecified corneal scar and opacity

H18 Other disorders of cornea

  H18.0 Corneal pigmentations and deposits

    H18.00 Unspecified corneal deposit

    H18.001 Unspecified corneal deposit, right eye

    H18.002 Unspecified corneal deposit, left eye

    H18.003 Unspecified corneal deposit, bilateral

    H18.009 Unspecified corneal deposit, unspecified eye

    H18.01 Anterior corneal pigmentations

    Staehlin's line

Add 4th-7th digits   Nonspecific code   Unspecified code   Manifestation code

H18.011 **Anterior corneal pigmentations, right eye**

H18.012 **Anterior corneal pigmentations, left eye**

H18.013 **Anterior corneal pigmentations, bilateral**

H18.019 **Anterior corneal pigmentations, unspecified eye**

H18.02 **Argentous corneal deposits**

H18.021 **Argentous corneal deposits, right eye**

H18.022 **Argentous corneal deposits, left eye**

H18.023 **Argentous corneal deposits, bilateral**

H18.029 **Argentous corneal deposits, unspecified eye**

H18.03 **Corneal deposits in metabolic disorders**

Code also associated metabolic disorder

H18.031 **Corneal deposits in metabolic disorders, right eye**

H18.032 **Corneal deposits in metabolic disorders, left eye**

H18.033 **Corneal deposits in metabolic disorders, bilateral**

H18.039 **Corneal deposits in metabolic disorders, unspecified eye**

H18.04 **Kayser-Fleischer ring**

Code also associated Wilson's disease (E83.01)

H18.041 **Kayser-Fleischer ring, right eye**

H18.042 **Kayser-Fleischer ring, left eye**

H18.043 **Kayser-Fleischer ring, bilateral**

H18.049 **Kayser-Fleischer ring, unspecified eye**

H18.05 **Posterior corneal pigmentations**

Krukenberg's spindle

H18.051 **Posterior corneal pigmentations, right eye**

H18.052 **Posterior corneal pigmentations, left eye**

H18.053 **Posterior corneal pigmentations, bilateral**

H18.059 **Posterior corneal pigmentations, unspecified eye**

H18.06 **Stromal corneal pigmentations**

Hematocornea

H18.061 **Stromal corneal pigmentations, right eye**

H18.062 **Stromal corneal pigmentations, left eye**

H18.063 **Stromal corneal pigmentations, bilateral**

H18.069 **Stromal corneal pigmentations, unspecified eye**

H18.1 **Bullous keratopathy**

H18.10 **Bullous keratopathy, unspecified eye**

H18.11 **Bullous keratopathy, right eye**

H18.12 **Bullous keratopathy, left eye**

H18.13 **Bullous keratopathy, bilateral**

H18.2 **Other and unspecified corneal edema**

H18.20 **Unspecified corneal edema**

H18.21 **Corneal edema secondary to contact lens**

Excludes2: Other corneal disorders due to contact lens (H18.82-)

H18.211 **Corneal edema secondary to contact lens, right eye**

H18.212 **Corneal edema secondary to contact lens, left eye**

H18.213 **Corneal edema secondary to contact lens, bilateral**

H18.219 **Corneal edema secondary to contact lens, unspecified eye**

H18.22 **Idiopathic corneal edema**

H18.221 **Idiopathic corneal edema, right eye**

H18.222 **Idiopathic corneal edema, left eye**

H18.223 **Idiopathic corneal edema, bilateral**

H18.229 **Idiopathic corneal edema, unspecified eye**

H18.23 **Secondary corneal edema**

H18.231 **Secondary corneal edema, right eye**

H18.232 **Secondary corneal edema, left eye**

H18.233 **Secondary corneal edema, bilateral**

H18.239 **Secondary corneal edema, unspecified eye**

H18.3 **Changes of corneal membranes**

H18.30 **Unspecified corneal membrane change**

H18.31 **Folds and rupture in Bowman's membrane**

H18.311 **Folds and rupture in Bowman's membrane, right eye**

H18.312 **Folds and rupture in Bowman's membrane, left eye**

H18.313 **Folds and rupture in Bowman's membrane, bilateral**

H18.319 **Folds and rupture in Bowman's membrane, unspecified eye**

H18.32 **Folds in Descemet's membrane**

H18.321 **Folds in Descemet's membrane, right eye**

H18.322 **Folds in Descemet's membrane, left eye**

H18.323 **Folds in Descemet's membrane, bilateral**

H18.329 **Folds in Descemet's membrane, unspecified eye**

H18.33 **Rupture in Descemet's membrane**

H18.331 **Rupture in Descemet's membrane, right eye**

H18.332 **Rupture in Descemet's membrane, left eye**

H18.333 **Rupture in Descemet's membrane, bilateral**

H18.339 **Rupture in Descemet's membrane, unspecified eye**

H18.4 **Corneal degeneration**

Excludes1: Mooren's ulcer (H16.0-)

recurrent erosion of cornea (H18.83-)

H18.40 **Unspecified corneal degeneration**

H18.41 **Arcus senilis**

Senile corneal changes

H18.411 **Arcus senilis, right eye**

H18.412 **Arcus senilis, left eye**

H18.413 **Arcus senilis, bilateral**

H18.419 **Arcus senilis, unspecified eye**

H18.42 **Band keratopathy**

H18.421 **Band keratopathy, right eye**

● New code ▲ Revised code **Excludes1:** Not coded here **Excludes2:** Not included here ⊗ Placeholder required ⑦7th digit required

H18.422   **Band keratopathy, left eye**

H18.423   **Band keratopathy, bilateral**

H18.429   **Band keratopathy, unspecified eye**

H18.43   **Other calcereous corneal degeneration**

H18.44   **Keratomalacia**

   Excludes1: keratomalacia due to vitamin A deficiency (E50.4)

H18.441   **Keratomalacia, right eye**

H18.442   **Keratomalacia, left eye**

H18.443   **Keratomalacia, bilateral**

H18.449   **Keratomalacia, unspecified eye**

H18.45   **Nodular corneal degeneration**

H18.451   **Nodular corneal degeneration, right eye**

H18.452   **Nodular corneal degeneration, left eye**

H18.453   **Nodular corneal degeneration, bilateral**

H18.459   **Nodular corneal degeneration, unspecified eye**

H18.46   **Peripheral corneal degeneration**

H18.461   **Peripheral corneal degeneration, right eye**

H18.462   **Peripheral corneal degeneration, left eye**

H18.463   **Peripheral corneal degeneration, bilateral**

H18.469   **Peripheral corneal degeneration, unspecified eye**

H18.49   **Other corneal degeneration**

H18.5   **Hereditary corneal dystrophies**

H18.50   **Unspecified hereditary corneal dystrophies**

H18.51   **Endothelial corneal dystrophy**

   Fuchs' dystrophy

H18.52   **Epithelial (juvenile) corneal dystrophy**

H18.53   **Granular corneal dystrophy**

H18.54   **Lattice corneal dystrophy**

H18.55   **Macular corneal dystrophy**

H18.59   **Other hereditary corneal dystrophies**

H18.6   **Keratoconus**

H18.60   **Keratoconus, unspecified**

H18.601   **Keratoconus, unspecified, right eye**

H18.602   **Keratoconus, unspecified, left eye**

H18.603   **Keratoconus, unspecified, bilateral**

H18.609   **Keratoconus, unspecified, unspecified eye**

H18.61   **Keratoconus, stable**

H18.611   **Keratoconus, stable, right eye**

H18.612   **Keratoconus, stable, left eye**

H18.613   **Keratoconus, stable, bilateral**

H18.619   **Keratoconus, stable, unspecified eye**

H18.62   **Keratoconus, unstable**

   Acute hydrops

H18.621   **Keratoconus, unstable, right eye**

H18.622   **Keratoconus, unstable, left eye**

H18.623   **Keratoconus, unstable, bilateral**

H18.629   **Keratoconus, unstable, unspecified eye**

H18.7   **Other and unspecified corneal deformities**

   Excludes1: congenital malformations of cornea (Q13.3-Q13.4)

H18.70   **Unspecified corneal deformity**

H18.71   **Corneal ectasia**

H18.711   **Corneal ectasia, right eye**

H18.712   **Corneal ectasia, left eye**

H18.713   **Corneal ectasia, bilateral**

H18.719   **Corneal ectasia, unspecified eye**

H18.72   **Corneal staphyloma**

H18.721   **Corneal staphyloma, right eye**

H18.722   **Corneal staphyloma, left eye**

H18.723   **Corneal staphyloma, bilateral**

H18.729   **Corneal staphyloma, unspecified eye**

H18.73   **Descemetocele**

H18.731   **Descemetocele, right eye**

H18.732   **Descemetocele, left eye**

H18.733   **Descemetocele, bilateral**

H18.739   **Descemetocele, unspecified eye**

H18.79   **Other corneal deformities**

H18.791   **Other corneal deformities, right eye**

H18.792   **Other corneal deformities, left eye**

H18.793   **Other corneal deformities, bilateral**

H18.799   **Other corneal deformities, unspecified eye**

H18.8   **Other specified disorders of cornea**

H18.81   **Anesthesia and hypoesthesia of cornea**

H18.811   **Anesthesia and hypoesthesia of cornea, right eye**

H18.812   **Anesthesia and hypoesthesia of cornea, left eye**

H18.813   **Anesthesia and hypoesthesia of cornea, bilateral**

H18.819   **Anesthesia and hypoesthesia of cornea, unspecified eye**

H18.82   **Corneal disorder due to contact lens**

   Excludes2: corneal edema due to contact lens (H18.21-)

H18.821   **Corneal disorder due to contact lens, right eye**

H18.822   **Corneal disorder due to contact lens, left eye**

H18.823   **Corneal disorder due to contact lens, bilateral**

H18.829   **Corneal disorder due to contact lens, unspecified eye**

H18.83   **Recurrent erosion of cornea**

H18.831   **Recurrent erosion of cornea, right eye**

H18.832   **Recurrent erosion of cornea, left eye**

H18.833   **Recurrent erosion of cornea, bilateral**

H18.839   **Recurrent erosion of cornea, unspecified eye**

H18.89   **Other specified disorders of cornea**

H18.891   **Other specified disorders of cornea, right eye**

H18.892   **Other specified disorders of cornea, left eye**

H18.893   **Other specified disorders of cornea, bilateral**

H18.899   **Other specified disorders of cornea, unspecified eye**

H18.9   **Unspecified disorder of cornea**

H20 **Iridocyclitis**

H20.0   **Acute and subacute iridocyclitis**

Acute anterior uveitis

Acute cyclitis

Acute iritis

Subacute anterior uveitis

Subacute cyclitis

Subacute iritis

Excludes1: iridocyclitis, iritis, uveitis (due to) (in) diabetes mellitus (E08-E13 with .39)

iridocyclitis, iritis, uveitis (due to) (in) diphtheria (A36.89)

iridocyclitis, iritis, uveitis (due to) (in) gonococcal (A54.32)

iridocyclitis, iritis, uveitis (due to) (in) herpes (simplex) (B00.51)

iridocyclitis, iritis, uveitis (due to) (in) herpes zoster (B02.32)

iridocyclitis, iritis, uveitis (due to) (in) late congenital syphilis (A50.39)

iridocyclitis, iritis, uveitis (due to) (in) late syphilis (A52.71)

iridocyclitis, iritis, uveitis (due to) (in) sarcoidosis (D86.83)

iridocyclitis, iritis, uveitis (due to) (in) syphilis (A51.43)

iridocyclitis, iritis, uveitis (due to) (in) toxoplasmosis (B58.09)

iridocyclitis, iritis, uveitis (due to) (in) tuberculosis (A18.54)

H20.00   **Unspecified acute and subacute iridocyclitis**

H20.01   **Primary iridocyclitis**

H20.011   **Primary iridocyclitis, right eye**

H20.012   **Primary iridocyclitis, left eye**

H20.013   **Primary iridocyclitis, bilateral**

H20.019   **Primary iridocyclitis, unspecified eye**

H20.02   **Recurrent acute iridocyclitis**

H20.021   **Recurrent acute iridocyclitis, right eye**

H20.022   **Recurrent acute iridocyclitis, left eye**

H20.023   **Recurrent acute iridocyclitis, bilateral**

H20.029   **Recurrent acute iridocyclitis, unspecified eye**

H20.03   **Secondary infectious iridocyclitis**

H20.031   **Secondary infectious iridocyclitis, right eye**

H20.032   **Secondary infectious iridocyclitis, left eye**

H20.033   **Secondary infectious iridocyclitis, bilateral**

H20.039   **Secondary infectious iridocyclitis, unspecified eye**

H20.04   **Secondary noninfectious iridocyclitis**

H20.041   **Secondary noninfectious iridocyclitis, right eye**

H20.042   **Secondary noninfectious iridocyclitis, left eye**

H20.043   **Secondary noninfectious iridocyclitis, bilateral**

H20.049   **Secondary noninfectious iridocyclitis, unspecified eye**

H20.05   **Hypopyon**

H20.051   **Hypopyon, right eye**

H20.052   **Hypopyon, left eye**

H20.053   **Hypopyon, bilateral**

H20.059   **Hypopyon, unspecified eye**

H20.1   **Chronic iridocyclitis**

Use additional code for any associated cataract (H26.21-)

Excludes2: posterior cyclitis (H30.2-)

H20.10   **Chronic iridocyclitis, unspecified eye**

H20.11   **Chronic iridocyclitis, right eye**

H20.12   **Chronic iridocyclitis, left eye**

H20.13   **Chronic iridocyclitis, bilateral**

H20.2   **Lens-induced iridocyclitis**

H20.20   **Lens-induced iridocyclitis, unspecified eye**

H20.21   **Lens-induced iridocyclitis, right eye**

H20.22   **Lens-induced iridocyclitis, left eye**

H20.23   **Lens-induced iridocyclitis, bilateral**

H20.8   **Other iridocyclitis**

Excludes2: glaucomatocyclitic crises (H40.4-)

posterior cyclitis (H30.2-) sympathetic uveitis (H44.13-)

H20.81   **Fuchs' heterochromic cyclitis**

H20.811   **Fuchs' heterochromic cyclitis, right eye**

H20.812   **Fuchs' heterochromic cyclitis, left eye**

H20.813   **Fuchs' heterochromic cyclitis, bilateral**

H20.819   **Fuchs' heterochromic cyclitis, unspecified eye**

H20.82   **Vogt-Koyanagi syndrome**

H20.821   **Vogt-Koyanagi syndrome, right eye**

H20.822   **Vogt-Koyanagi syndrome, left eye**

H20.823   **Vogt-Koyanagi syndrome, bilateral**

H20.829   **Vogt-Koyanagi syndrome, unspecified eye**

H20.9   **Unspecified iridocyclitis**

Uveitis NOS

H21 **Other disorders of iris and ciliary body**

Excludes2: sympathetic uveitis (H44.1-)

H21.0   **Hyphema**

Excludes1: traumatic hyphema (S05.1-)

H21.00   **Hyphema, unspecified eye**

H21.01   **Hyphema, right eye**

H21.02   **Hyphema, left eye**

H21.03   **Hyphema, bilateral**

H21.1   **Other vascular disorders of iris and ciliary body**

Neovascularization of iris or ciliary body

Rubeosis iridis

Rubeosis of iris

H21.1X   **Other vascular disorders of iris and ciliary body**

H21.1X1   **Other vascular disorders of iris and ciliary body, right eye**

  ● New code ▲ Revised code **Excludes1:** Not coded here **Excludes2:** Not included here ⊗ Placeholder required ⑦7th digit required

H21.1X2 Other vascular disorders of iris and ciliary body, left eye

H21.1X3 Other vascular disorders of iris and ciliary body, bilateral

H21.1X9 Other vascular disorders of iris and ciliary body, unspecified eye

H21.2 Degeneration of iris and ciliary body

H21.21 Degeneration of chamber angle

H21.211 Degeneration of chamber angle, right eye

H21.212 Degeneration of chamber angle, left eye

H21.213 Degeneration of chamber angle, bilateral

H21.219 Degeneration of chamber angle, unspecified eye

H21.22 Degeneration of ciliary body

H21.221 Degeneration of ciliary body, right eye

H21.222 Degeneration of ciliary body, left eye

H21.223 Degeneration of ciliary body, bilateral

H21.229 Degeneration of ciliary body, unspecified eye

H21.23 Degeneration of iris (pigmentary)

Translucency of iris

H21.231 Degeneration of iris (pigmentary), right eye

H21.232 Degeneration of iris (pigmentary), left eye

H21.233 Degeneration of iris (pigmentary), bilateral

H21.239 Degeneration of iris (pigmentary), unspecified eye

H21.24 Degeneration of pupillary margin

H21.241 Degeneration of pupillary margin, right eye

H21.242 Degeneration of pupillary margin, left eye

H21.243 Degeneration of pupillary margin, bilateral

H21.249 Degeneration of pupillary margin, unspecified eye

H21.25 Iridoschisis

H21.251 Iridoschisis, right eye

H21.252 Iridoschisis, left eye

H21.253 Iridoschisis, bilateral

H21.259 Iridoschisis, unspecified eye

H21.26 Iris atrophy (essential) (progressive)

H21.261 Iris atrophy (essential) (progressive), right eye

H21.262 Iris atrophy (essential) (progressive), left eye

H21.263 Iris atrophy (essential) (progressive), bilateral

H21.269 Iris atrophy (essential) (progressive), unspecified eye

H21.27 Miotic pupillary cyst

H21.271 Miotic pupillary cyst, right eye

H21.272 Miotic pupillary cyst, left eye

H21.273 Miotic pupillary cyst, bilateral

H21.279 Miotic pupillary cyst, unspecified eye

H21.29 Other iris atrophy

H21.3 Cyst of iris, ciliary body and anterior chamber

Excludes2: miotic pupillary cyst (H21.27-)

H21.30 Idiopathic cysts of iris, ciliary body or anterior chamber

Cyst of iris, ciliary body or anterior chamber NOS

H21.301 Idiopathic cysts of iris, ciliary body or anterior chamber, right eye

H21.302 Idiopathic cysts of iris, ciliary body or anterior chamber, left eye

H21.303 Idiopathic cysts of iris, ciliary body or anterior chamber, bilateral

H21.309 Idiopathic cysts of iris, ciliary body or anterior chamber, unspecified eye

H21.31 Exudative cysts of iris or anterior chamber

H21.311 Exudative cysts of iris or anterior chamber, right eye

H21.312 Exudative cysts of iris or anterior chamber, left eye

H21.313 Exudative cysts of iris or anterior chamber, bilateral

H21.319 Exudative cysts of iris or anterior chamber, unspecified eye

H21.32 Implantation cysts of iris, ciliary body or anterior chamber

H21.321 Implantation cysts of iris, ciliary body or anterior chamber, right eye

H21.322 Implantation cysts of iris, ciliary body or anterior chamber, left eye

H21.323 Implantation cysts of iris, ciliary body or anterior chamber, bilateral

H21.329 Implantation cysts of iris, ciliary body or anterior chamber, unspecified eye

H21.33 Parasitic cyst of iris, ciliary body or anterior chamber

H21.331 Parasitic cyst of iris, ciliary body or anterior chamber, right eye

H21.332 Parasitic cyst of iris, ciliary body or anterior chamber, left eye

H21.333 Parasitic cyst of iris, ciliary body or anterior chamber, bilateral

H21.339 Parasitic cyst of iris, ciliary body or anterior chamber, unspecified eye

H21.34 Primary cyst of pars plana

H21.341 Primary cyst of pars plana, right eye

H21.342 Primary cyst of pars plana, left eye

H21.343 Primary cyst of pars plana, bilateral

H21.349 Primary cyst of pars plana, unspecified eye

H21.35 Exudative cyst of pars plana

H21.351 Exudative cyst of pars plana, right eye

H21.352 Exudative cyst of pars plana, left eye

H21.353 Exudative cyst of pars plana, bilateral

H21.359 Exudative cyst of pars plana, unspecified eye

H21.4 Pupillary membranes

Iris bombé

Pupillary occlusion

Pupillary seclusion

| | Add 4th-7th digits | | Nonspecific code | | Unspecified code | | Manifestation code | 329 |

Excludes1: congenital pupillary membranes (Q13.8)

H21.40 **Pupillary membranes, unspecified eye**

H21.41 **Pupillary membranes, right eye**

H21.42 **Pupillary membranes, left eye**

H21.43 **Pupillary membranes, bilateral**

H21.5 **Other and unspecified adhesions and disruptions of iris and ciliary body**

Excludes1: corectopia (Q13.2)

H21.50 **Unspecified adhesions of iris**

Synechia (iris) NOS

H21.501 **Unspecified adhesions of iris, right eye**

H21.502 **Unspecified adhesions of iris, left eye**

H21.503 **Unspecified adhesions of iris, bilateral**

H21.509 **Unspecified adhesions of iris and ciliary body, unspecified eye**

H21.51 **Anterior synechiae (iris)**

H21.511 **Anterior synechiae (iris), right eye**

H21.512 **Anterior synechiae (iris), left eye**

H21.513 **Anterior synechiae (iris), bilateral**

H21.519 **Anterior synechiae (iris), unspecified eye**

H21.52 **Goniosynechiae**

H21.521 **Goniosynechiae, right eye**

H21.522 **Goniosynechiae, left eye**

H21.523 **Goniosynechiae, bilateral**

H21.529 **Goniosynechiae, unspecified eye**

H21.53 **Iridodialysis**

H21.531 **Iridodialysis, right eye**

H21.532 **Iridodialysis, left eye**

H21.533 **Iridodialysis, bilateral**

H21.539 **Iridodialysis, unspecified eye**

H21.54 **Posterior synechiae (iris)**

H21.541 **Posterior synechiae (iris), right eye**

H21.542 **Posterior synechiae (iris), left eye**

H21.543 **Posterior synechiae (iris), bilateral**

H21.549 **Posterior synechiae (iris), unspecified eye**

H21.55 **Recession of chamber angle**

H21.551 **Recession of chamber angle, right eye**

H21.552 **Recession of chamber angle, left eye**

H21.553 **Recession of chamber angle, bilateral**

H21.559 **Recession of chamber angle, unspecified eye**

H21.56 **Pupillary abnormalities**

Deformed pupil

Ectopic pupil

Rupture of sphincter, pupil

Excludes1: congenital deformity of pupil (Q13.2-)

H21.561 **Pupillary abnormality, right eye**

H21.562 **Pupillary abnormality, left eye**

H21.563 **Pupillary abnormality, bilateral**

H21.569 **Pupillary abnormality, unspecified eye**

H21.8 **Other specified disorders of iris and ciliary body**

H21.81 **Floppy iris syndrome**

Intraoperative floppy iris syndrome (IFIS)

Use additional code for adverse effect, if applicable, to identify drug (T36-T50 with fifth or sixth character 5)

H21.82 **Plateau iris syndrome (post-iridectomy) (postprocedural)**

H21.89 **Other specified disorders of iris and ciliary body**

H21.9 **Unspecified disorder of iris and ciliary body**

H22 **Disorders of iris and ciliary body in diseases classified elsewhere**

Code first underlying disease, such as:

gout (M1A.-, M10.-)

leprosy (A30.-)

parasitic disease (B89)

DISORDERS OF LENS (H25-H28)

H25 **Age-related cataract**

Definition: A cataract is a clouding that develops in the crystalline lens of the eye or in its envelope, varying in degree from slight to complete opacity and obstructing the passage of light.

Senile cataract

Excludes2: capsular glaucoma with pseudoexfoliation of lens (H40.1-)

H25.0 **Age-related incipient cataract**

H25.01 **Cortical age-related cataract**

H25.011 **Cortical age-related cataract, right eye**

H25.012 **Cortical age-related cataract, left eye**

H25.013 **Cortical age-related cataract, bilateral**

H25.019 **Cortical age-related cataract, unspecified eye**

H25.03 **Anterior subcapsular polar age-related cataract**

H25.031 **Anterior subcapsular polar age-related cataract, right eye**

H25.032 **Anterior subcapsular polar age-related cataract, left eye**

H25.033 **Anterior subcapsular polar age-related cataract, bilateral**

H25.039 **Anterior subcapsular polar age-related cataract, unspecified eye**

H25.04 **Posterior subcapsular polar age-related cataract**

H25.041 **Posterior subcapsular polar age-related cataract, right eye**

H25.042 **Posterior subcapsular polar age-related cataract, left eye**

H25.043 **Posterior subcapsular polar age-related cataract, bilateral**

H25.049 **Posterior subcapsular polar age-related cataract, unspecified eye**

H25.09 **Other age-related incipient cataract**

Coronary age-related cataract

Punctate age-related cataract

Water clefts

H25.091 **Other age-related incipient cataract, right eye**

H25.092 **Other age-related incipient cataract, left eye**

H25.093 **Other age-related incipient cataract, bilateral**

H25.099 **Other age-related incipient cataract, unspecified eye**

● New code ▲ Revised code **Excludes1:** Not coded here **Excludes2:** Not included here ⊗ Placeholder required ⑦7th digit required

H25.1   Age-related nuclear cataract

Cataracta brunescens Nuclear sclerosis cataract

   H25.10   Age-related nuclear cataract, unspecified eye

   H25.11   Age-related nuclear cataract, right eye

   H25.12   Age-related nuclear cataract, left eye

   H25.13   Age-related nuclear cataract, bilateral

H25.2   Age-related cataract, morgagnian type

Age-related hypermature cataract

   H25.20   Age-related cataract, morgagnian type, unspecified eye

   H25.21   Age-related cataract, morgagnian type, right eye

   H25.22   Age-related cataract, morgagnian type, left eye

   H25.23   Age-related cataract, morgagnian type, bilateral

H25.8   Other age-related cataract

   H25.81   Combined forms of age-related cataract

      H25.811   Combined forms of age-related cataract, right eye

      H25.812   Combined forms of age-related cataract, left eye

      H25.813   Combined forms of age-related cataract, bilateral

      H25.819   Combined forms of age-related cataract, unspecified eye

   H25.89   Other age-related cataract

H25.9   Unspecified age-related cataract

H26   Other cataract

Excludes1: congenital cataract (Q12.0)

H26.0   Infantile and juvenile cataract

   H26.00   Unspecified infantile and juvenile cataract

      H26.001   Unspecified infantile and juvenile cataract, right eye

      H26.002   Unspecified infantile and juvenile cataract, left eye

      H26.003   Unspecified infantile and juvenile cataract, bilateral

      H26.009   Unspecified infantile and juvenile cataract, unspecified eye

   H26.01   Infantile and juvenile cortical, lamellar, or zonular cataract

      H26.011   Infantile and juvenile cortical, lamellar, or zonular cataract, right eye

      H26.012   Infantile and juvenile cortical, lamellar, or zonular cataract, left eye

      H26.013   Infantile and juvenile cortical, lamellar, or zonular cataract, bilateral

      H26.019   Infantile and juvenile cortical, lamellar, or zonular cataract, unspecified eye

   H26.03   Infantile and juvenile nuclear cataract

      H26.031   Infantile and juvenile nuclear cataract, right eye

      H26.032   Infantile and juvenile nuclear cataract, left eye

      H26.033   Infantile and juvenile nuclear cataract, bilateral

      H26.039   Infantile and juvenile nuclear cataract, unspecified eye

H26.04   Anterior subcapsular polar infantile and juvenile cataract

      H26.041   Anterior subcapsular polar infantile and juvenile cataract, right eye

      H26.042   Anterior subcapsular polar infantile and juvenile cataract, left eye

      H26.043   Anterior subcapsular polar infantile and juvenile cataract, bilateral

      H26.049   Anterior subcapsular polar infantile and juvenile cataract, unspecified eye

H26.05   Posterior subcapsular polar infantile and juvenile cataract

      H26.051   Posterior subcapsular polar infantile and juvenile cataract, right eye

      H26.052   Posterior subcapsular polar infantile and juvenile cataract, left eye

      H26.053   Posterior subcapsular polar infantile and juvenile cataract, bilateral

      H26.059   Posterior subcapsular polar infantile and juvenile cataract, unspecified eye

H26.06   Combined forms of infantile and juvenile cataract

      H26.061   Combined forms of infantile and juvenile cataract, right eye

      H26.062   Combined forms of infantile and juvenile cataract, left eye

      H26.063   Combined forms of infantile and juvenile cataract, bilateral

      H26.069   Combined forms of infantile and juvenile cataract, unspecified eye

H26.09   Other infantile and juvenile cataract

H26.1   Traumatic cataract

Use additional code (Chapter 20) to identify external cause

   H26.10   Unspecified traumatic cataract

      H26.101   Unspecified traumatic cataract, right eye

      H26.102   Unspecified traumatic cataract, left eye

      H26.103   Unspecified traumatic cataract, bilateral

      H26.109   Unspecified traumatic cataract, unspecified eye

   H26.11   Localized traumatic opacities

      H26.111   Localized traumatic opacities, right eye

      H26.112   Localized traumatic opacities, left eye

      H26.113   Localized traumatic opacities, bilateral

      H26.119   Localized traumatic opacities, unspecified eye

   H26.12   Partially resolved traumatic cataract

      H26.121   Partially resolved traumatic cataract, right eye

      H26.122   Partially resolved traumatic cataract, left eye

      H26.123   Partially resolved traumatic cataract, bilateral

      H26.129   Partially resolved traumatic cataract, unspecified eye

   H26.13   Total traumatic cataract

      H26.131   Total traumatic cataract, right eye

      H26.132   Total traumatic cataract, left eye

H26.133　Total traumatic cataract, bilateral

H26.139　Total traumatic cataract, unspecified eye

H26.2　**Complicated cataract**

H26.20　Unspecified complicated cataract

Cataracta complicata NOS

H26.21　Cataract with neovascularization

Code also associated condition, such as:

chronic iridocyclitis (H20.1-)

H26.211　Cataract with neovascularization, right eye

H26.212　Cataract with neovascularization, left eye

H26.213　Cataract with neovascularization, bilateral

H26.219　Cataract with neovascularization, unspecified eye

H26.22　Cataract secondary to ocular disorders (degenerative) (inflammatory)

Code also associated ocular disorder

H26.221　Cataract secondary to ocular disorders (degenerative) (inflammatory), right eye

H26.222　Cataract secondary to ocular disorders (degenerative) (inflammatory), left eye

H26.223　Cataract secondary to ocular disorders (degenerative) (inflammatory), bilateral

H26.229　Cataract secondary to ocular disorders (degenerative) (inflammatory), unspecified eye

H26.23　Glaucomatous flecks (subcapsular)

Code first underlying glaucoma (H40-H42)

H26.231　Glaucomatous flecks (subcapsular), right eye

H26.232　Glaucomatous flecks (subcapsular), left eye

H26.233　Glaucomatous flecks (subcapsular), bilateral

H26.239　Glaucomatous flecks (subcapsular), unspecified eye

H26.3　**Drug-induced cataract**

Toxic cataract

Use additional code for adverse effect, if applicable, to identify drug (T36-T50 with fifth or sixth character 5)

H26.30　Drug-induced cataract, unspecified eye

H26.31　Drug-induced cataract, right eye

H26.32　Drug-induced cataract, left eye

H26.33　Drug-induced cataract, bilateral

H26.4　**Secondary cataract**

H26.40　Unspecified secondary cataract

H26.41　Soemmering's ring

H26.411　Soemmering's ring, right eye

H26.412　Soemmering's ring, left eye

H26.413　Soemmering's ring, bilateral

H26.419　Soemmering's ring, unspecified eye

H26.49　Other secondary cataract

H26.491　Other secondary cataract, right eye

H26.492　Other secondary cataract, left eye

H26.493　Other secondary cataract, bilateral

H26.499　Other secondary cataract, unspecified eye

H26.8　**Other specified cataract**

H26.9　**Unspecified cataract**

H27　**Other disorders of lens**

Excludes1: congenital lens malformations (Q12.-)

mechanical complications of intraocular lens implant (T85.2)

pseudophakia (Z96.1)

H27.0　**Aphakia**

Acquired absence of lens

Acquired aphakia

Aphakia due to trauma

Excludes1: cataract extraction status (Z98.4-)

congenital absence of lens (Q12.3)

congenital aphakia (Q12.3)

H27.00　Aphakia, unspecified eye

H27.01　Aphakia, right eye

H27.02　Aphakia, left eye

H27.03　Aphakia, bilateral

H27.1　**Dislocation of lens**

H27.10　Unspecified dislocation of lens

H27.11　Subluxation of lens

H27.111　Subluxation of lens, right eye

H27.112　Subluxation of lens, left eye

H27.113　Subluxation of lens, bilateral

H27.119　Subluxation of lens, unspecified eye

H27.12　Anterior dislocation of lens

H27.121　Anterior dislocation of lens, right eye

H27.122　Anterior dislocation of lens, left eye

H27.123　Anterior dislocation of lens, bilateral

H27.129　Anterior dislocation of lens, unspecified eye

H27.13　Posterior dislocation of lens

H27.131　Posterior dislocation of lens, right eye

H27.132　Posterior dislocation of lens, left eye

H27.133　Posterior dislocation of lens, bilateral

H27.139　Posterior dislocation of lens, unspecified eye

H27.8　**Other specified disorders of lens**

H27.9　**Unspecified disorder of lens**

H28　**Cataract in diseases classified elsewhere**

Code first underlying disease, such as:

hypoparathyroidism (E20.-)

myotonia (G71.1-)

myxedema (E03.-)

protein-calorie malnutrition (E40-E46)

Excludes1: cataract in diabetes mellitus (E08.36, E09.36, E10.36, E11.36, E13.36)

DISORDERS OF CHOROID AND RETINA (H30-H36)

H30　**Chorioretinal inflammation**

H30.0　**Focal chorioretinal inflammation**

Focal chorioretinitis

Focal choroiditis

Focal retinitis

Focal retinochoroiditis

H30.00 Unspecified focal chorioretinal inflammation

Focal chorioretinitis NOS

Focal choroiditis NOS

Focal retinitis NOS

Focal retinochoroiditis NOS

H30.001 Unspecified focal chorioretinal inflammation, right eye

H30.002 Unspecified focal chorioretinal inflammation, left eye

H30.003 Unspecified focal chorioretinal inflammation, bilateral

H30.009 Unspecified focal chorioretinal inflammation, unspecified eye

H30.01 Focal chorioretinal inflammation, juxtapapillary

H30.011 Focal chorioretinal inflammation, juxtapapillary, right eye

H30.012 Focal chorioretinal inflammation, juxtapapillary, left eye

H30.013 Focal chorioretinal inflammation, juxtapapillary, bilateral

H30.019 Focal chorioretinal inflammation, juxtapapillary, unspecified eye

H30.02 Focal chorioretinal inflammation of posterior pole

H30.021 Focal chorioretinal inflammation of posterior pole, right eye

H30.022 Focal chorioretinal inflammation of posterior pole, left eye

H30.023 Focal chorioretinal inflammation of posterior pole, bilateral

H30.029 Focal chorioretinal inflammation of posterior pole, unspecified eye

H30.03 Focal chorioretinal inflammation, peripheral

H30.031 Focal chorioretinal inflammation, peripheral, right eye

H30.032 Focal chorioretinal inflammation, peripheral, left eye

H30.033 Focal chorioretinal inflammation, peripheral, bilateral

H30.039 Focal chorioretinal inflammation, peripheral, unspecified eye

H30.04 Focal chorioretinal inflammation, macular or paramacular

H30.041 Focal chorioretinal inflammation, macular or paramacular, right eye

H30.042 Focal chorioretinal inflammation, macular or paramacular, left eye

H30.043 Focal chorioretinal inflammation, macular or paramacular, bilateral

H30.049 Focal chorioretinal inflammation, macular or paramacular, unspecified eye

H30.1 Disseminated chorioretinal inflammation

Disseminated chorioretinitis

Disseminated choroiditis

Disseminated retinitis

Disseminated retinochoroiditis

Excludes2: exudative retinopathy (H35.02-)

H30.10 Unspecified disseminated chorioretinal inflammation

Disseminated chorioretinitis NOS

Disseminated choroiditis NOS

Disseminated retinitis NOS

Disseminated retinochoroiditis NOS

H30.101 Unspecified disseminated chorioretinal inflammation, right eye

H30.102 Unspecified disseminated chorioretinal inflammation, left eye

H30.103 Unspecified disseminated chorioretinal inflammation, bilateral

H30.109 Unspecified disseminated chorioretinal inflammation, unspecified eye

H30.11 Disseminated chorioretinal inflammation of posterior pole

H30.111 Disseminated chorioretinal inflammation of posterior pole, right eye

H30.112 Disseminated chorioretinal inflammation of posterior pole, left eye

H30.113 Disseminated chorioretinal inflammation of posterior pole, bilateral

H30.119 Disseminated chorioretinal inflammation of posterior pole, unspecified eye

H30.12 Disseminated chorioretinal inflammation, peripheral

H30.121 Disseminated chorioretinal inflammation, peripheral right eye

H30.122 Disseminated chorioretinal inflammation, peripheral, left eye

H30.123 Disseminated chorioretinal inflammation, peripheral, bilateral

H30.129 Disseminated chorioretinal inflammation, peripheral, unspecified eye

H30.13 Disseminated chorioretinal inflammation, generalized

H30.131 Disseminated chorioretinal inflammation, generalized, right eye

H30.132 Disseminated chorioretinal inflammation, generalized, left eye

H30.133 Disseminated chorioretinal inflammation, generalized, bilateral

H30.139 Disseminated chorioretinal inflammation, generalized, unspecified eye

H30.14 Acute posterior multifocal placoid pigment epitheliopathy

H30.141 Acute posterior multifocal placoid pigment epitheliopathy, right eye

H30.142 Acute posterior multifocal placoid pigment epitheliopathy, left eye

H30.143 Acute posterior multifocal placoid pigment epitheliopathy, bilateral

H30.149 Acute posterior multifocal placoid pigment epitheliopathy, unspecified eye

H30.2 Posterior cyclitis

Pars planitis

H30.20 Posterior cyclitis, unspecified eye

H30.21 Posterior cyclitis, right eye

H30.22 Posterior cyclitis, left eye

H30.23 Posterior cyclitis, bilateral

H30.8 **Other chorioretinal inflammations**

    H30.81 **Harada's disease**

        H30.811 **Harada's disease, right eye**

        H30.812 **Harada's disease, left eye**

        H30.813 **Harada's disease, bilateral**

        H30.819 **Harada's disease, unspecified eye**

    H30.89 **Other chorioretinal inflammations**

        H30.891 **Other chorioretinal inflammations, right eye**

        H30.892 **Other chorioretinal inflammations, left eye**

        H30.893 **Other chorioretinal inflammations, bilateral**

        H30.899 **Other chorioretinal inflammations, unspecified eye**

H30.9 **Unspecified chorioretinal inflammation**

    Chorioretinitis NOS

    Choroiditis NOS Neuroretinitis NOS

    Retinitis NOS

    Retinochoroiditis NOS

    H30.90 **Unspecified chorioretinal inflammation, unspecified eye**

    H30.91 **Unspecified chorioretinal inflammation, right eye**

    H30.92 **Unspecified chorioretinal inflammation, left eye**

    H30.93 **Unspecified chorioretinal inflammation, bilateral**

H31 **Other disorders of choroid**

    H31.0 **Chorioretinal scars**

        Excludes2: postsurgical chorioretinal scars (H59.81-)

        H31.00 **Unspecified chorioretinal scars**

            H31.001 **Unspecified chorioretinal scars, right eye**

            H31.002 **Unspecified chorioretinal scars, left eye**

            H31.003 **Unspecified chorioretinal scars, bilateral**

            H31.009 **Unspecified chorioretinal scars, unspecified eye**

        H31.01 **Macula scars of posterior pole (postinflammatory) (post-traumatic)**

            Excludes1: postprocedural chorioretinal scar (H59.81-)

            H31.011 **Macula scars of posterior pole (postinflammatory) (post-traumatic), right eye**

            H31.012 **Macula scars of posterior pole (postinflammatory) (post-traumatic), left eye**

            H31.013 **Macula scars of posterior pole (postinflammatory) (post-traumatic), bilateral**

            H31.019 **Macula scars of posterior pole (postinflammatory) (post-traumatic), unspecified eye**

        H31.02 **Solar retinopathy**

            H31.021 **Solar retinopathy, right eye**

            H31.022 **Solar retinopathy, left eye**

            H31.023 **Solar retinopathy, bilateral**

            H31.029 **Solar retinopathy, unspecified eye**

        H31.09 **Other chorioretinal scars**

            H31.091 **Other chorioretinal scars, right eye**

            H31.092 **Other chorioretinal scars, left eye**

            H31.093 **Other chorioretinal scars, bilateral**

            H31.099 **Other chorioretinal scars, unspecified eye**

H31.1 **Choroidal degeneration**

    Excludes2: angioid streaks of macula (H35.33)

    H31.10 **Unspecified choroidal degeneration**

    Choroidal sclerosis NOS

        H31.101 **Choroidal degeneration, unspecified, right eye**

        H31.102 **Choroidal degeneration, unspecified, left eye**

        H31.103 **Choroidal degeneration, unspecified, bilateral**

        H31.109 **Choroidal degeneration, unspecified, unspecified eye**

    H31.11 **Age-related choroidal atrophy**

        H31.111 **Age-related choroidal atrophy, right eye**

        H31.112 **Age-related choroidal atrophy, left eye**

        H31.113 **Age-related choroidal atrophy, bilateral**

        H31.119 **Age-related choroidal atrophy, unspecified eye**

    H31.12 **Diffuse secondary atrophy of choroid**

        H31.121 **Diffuse secondary atrophy of choroid, right eye**

        H31.122 **Diffuse secondary atrophy of choroid, left eye**

        H31.123 **Diffuse secondary atrophy of choroid, bilateral**

        H31.129 **Diffuse secondary atrophy of choroid, unspecified eye**

H31.2 **Hereditary choroidal dystrophy**

    Excludes2: hyperornithinemia (E72.4)

        ornithinemia (E72.4)

    H31.20 **Hereditary choroidal dystrophy, unspecified**

    H31.21 **Choroideremia**

    H31.22 **Choroidal dystrophy (central areolar) (generalized) (peripapillary)**

    H31.23 **Gyrate atrophy, choroid**

    H31.29 **Other hereditary choroidal dystrophy**

H31.3 **Choroidal hemorrhage and rupture**

    H31.30 **Unspecified choroidal hemorrhage**

        H31.301 **Unspecified choroidal hemorrhage, right eye**

        H31.302 **Unspecified choroidal hemorrhage, left eye**

        H31.303 **Unspecified choroidal hemorrhage, bilateral**

        H31.309 **Unspecified choroidal hemorrhage, unspecified eye**

    H31.31 **Expulsive choroidal hemorrhage**

        H31.311 **Expulsive choroidal hemorrhage, right eye**

        H31.312 **Expulsive choroidal hemorrhage, left eye**

        H31.313 **Expulsive choroidal hemorrhage, bilateral**

        H31.319 **Expulsive choroidal hemorrhage, unspecified eye**

  ● New code ▲ Revised code **Excludes1:** Not coded here **Excludes2:** Not included here ⊗ Placeholder required ⑦ 7th digit required

H31.32 **Choroidal rupture**

H31.321 **Choroidal rupture, right eye**

H31.322 **Choroidal rupture, left eye**

H31.323 **Choroidal rupture, bilateral**

H31.329 **Choroidal rupture, unspecified eye**

H31.4 **Choroidal detachment**

H31.40 **Unspecified choroidal detachment**

H31.401 **Unspecified choroidal detachment, right eye**

H31.402 **Unspecified choroidal detachment, left eye**

H31.403 **Unspecified choroidal detachment, bilateral**

H31.409 **Unspecified choroidal detachment, unspecified eye**

H31.41 **Hemorrhagic choroidal detachment**

H31.411 **Hemorrhagic choroidal detachment, right eye**

H31.412 **Hemorrhagic choroidal detachment, left eye**

H31.413 **Hemorrhagic choroidal detachment, bilateral**

H31.419 **Hemorrhagic choroidal detachment, unspecified eye**

H31.42 **Serous choroidal detachment**

H31.421 **Serous choroidal detachment, right eye**

H31.422 **Serous choroidal detachment, left eye**

H31.423 **Serous choroidal detachment, bilateral**

H31.429 **Serous choroidal detachment, unspecified eye**

H31.8 **Other specified disorders of choroid**

H31.9 **Unspecified disorder of choroid**

H32 **Chorioretinal disorders in diseases classified elsewhere**

Code first underlying disease, such as:

congenital toxoplasmosis (P37.1)

histoplasmosis (B39.-)

leprosy (A30.-)

Excludes1: chorioretinitis (in):

toxoplasmosis (acquired) (B58.01)

tuberculosis (A18.53)

H33 **Retinal detachments and breaks**

Definition: Retinal detachment is a disorder of the eye in which the retina peels away from its underlying layer of support tissue.

Excludes1: detachment of retinal pigment epithelium (H35.72-, H35.73-)

H33.0 **Retinal detachment with retinal break**

Rhegmatogenous retinal detachment

Excludes1: serous retinal detachment (without retinal break) (H33.2-)

H33.00 **Unspecified retinal detachment with retinal break**

H33.001 **Unspecified retinal detachment with retinal break, right eye**

H33.002 **Unspecified retinal detachment with retinal break, left eye**

H33.003 **Unspecified retinal detachment with retinal break, bilateral**

H33.009 **Unspecified retinal detachment with retinal break, unspecified eye**

H33.01 **Retinal detachment with single break**

H33.011 **Retinal detachment with single break, right eye**

H33.012 **Retinal detachment with single break, left eye**

H33.013 **Retinal detachment with single break, bilateral**

H33.019 **Retinal detachment with single break, unspecified eye**

H33.02 **Retinal detachment with multiple breaks**

H33.021 **Retinal detachment with multiple breaks, right eye**

H33.022 **Retinal detachment with multiple breaks, left eye**

H33.023 **Retinal detachment with multiple breaks, bilateral**

H33.029 **Retinal detachment with multiple breaks, unspecified eye**

H33.03 **Retinal detachment with giant retinal tear**

H33.031 **Retinal detachment with giant retinal tear, right eye**

H33.032 **Retinal detachment with giant retinal tear, left eye**

H33.033 **Retinal detachment with giant retinal tear, bilateral**

H33.039 **Retinal detachment with giant retinal tear, unspecified eye**

H33.04 **Retinal detachment with retinal dialysis**

H33.041 **Retinal detachment with retinal dialysis, right eye**

H33.042 **Retinal detachment with retinal dialysis, left eye**

H33.043 **Retinal detachment with retinal dialysis, bilateral**

H33.049 **Retinal detachment with retinal dialysis, unspecified eye**

H33.05 **Total retinal detachment**

H33.051 **Total retinal detachment, right eye**

H33.052 **Total retinal detachment, left eye**

H33.053 **Total retinal detachment, bilateral**

H33.059 **Total retinal detachment, unspecified eye**

H33.1 **Retinoschisis and retinal cysts**

Excludes1: congenital retinoschisis (Q14.1)

microcystoid degeneration of retina (H35.42-)

H33.10 **Unspecified retinoschisis**

H33.101 **Unspecified retinoschisis, right eye**

H33.102 **Unspecified retinoschisis, left eye**

H33.103 **Unspecified retinoschisis, bilateral**

H33.109 **Unspecified retinoschisis, unspecified eye**

H33.11 **Cyst of ora serrata**

H33.111 **Cyst of ora serrata, right eye**

H33.112 **Cyst of ora serrata, left eye**

H33.113 **Cyst of ora serrata, bilateral**

H33.119 **Cyst of ora serrata, unspecified eye**

H33.12 **Parasitic cyst of retina**

H33.121 **Parasitic cyst of retina, right eye**

H33.122 **Parasitic cyst of retina, left eye**

H33.123 **Parasitic cyst of retina, bilateral**

H33.129 Parasitic cyst of retina, unspecified eye

H33.19 Other retinoschisis and retinal cysts

Pseudocyst of retina

H33.191 Other retinoschisis and retinal cysts, right eye

H33.192 Other retinoschisis and retinal cysts, left eye

H33.193 Other retinoschisis and retinal cysts, bilateral

H33.199 Other retinoschisis and retinal cysts, unspecified eye

H33.2 Serous retinal detachment

Retinal detachment NOS

Retinal detachment without retinal break

Excludes1: central serous chorioretinopathy (H35.71-)

H33.20 Serous retinal detachment, unspecified eye

H33.21 Serous retinal detachment, right eye

H33.22 Serous retinal detachment, left eye

H33.23 Serous retinal detachment, bilateral

H33.3 Retinal breaks without detachment

Excludes1: chorioretinal scars after surgery for detachment (H59.81-)

peripheral retinal degeneration without break (H35.4-)

H33.30 Unspecified retinal break

H33.301 Unspecified retinal break, right eye

H33.302 Unspecified retinal break, left eye

H33.303 Unspecified retinal break, bilateral

H33.309 Unspecified retinal break, unspecified eye

H33.31 Horseshoe tear of retina without detachment

Operculum of retina without detachment

H33.311 Horseshoe tear of retina without detachment, right eye

H33.312 Horseshoe tear of retina without detachment, left eye

H33.313 Horseshoe tear of retina without detachment, bilateral

H33.319 Horseshoe tear of retina without detachment, unspecified eye

H33.32 Round hole of retina without detachment

H33.321 Round hole, right eye

H33.322 Round hole, left eye

H33.323 Round hole, bilateral

H33.329 Round hole, unspecified eye

H33.33 Multiple defects of retina without detachment

H33.331 Multiple defects of retina without detachment, right eye

H33.332 Multiple defects of retina without detachment, left eye

H33.333 Multiple defects of retina without detachment, bilateral

H33.339 Multiple defects of retina without detachment, unspecified eye

H33.4 Traction detachment of retina

Proliferative vitreo-retinopathy with retinal detachment

H33.40 Traction detachment of retina, unspecified eye

H33.41 Traction detachment of retina, right eye

H33.42 Traction detachment of retina, left eye

H33.43 Traction detachment of retina, bilateral

H33.8 Other retinal detachments

H34 Retinal vascular occlusions

Excludes1: amaurosis fugax (G45.3)

H34.0 Transient retinal artery occlusion

H34.00 Transient retinal artery occlusion, unspecified eye

H34.01 Transient retinal artery occlusion, right eye

H34.02 Transient retinal artery occlusion, left eye

H34.03 Transient retinal artery occlusion, bilateral

H34.1 Central retinal artery occlusion

H34.10 Central retinal artery occlusion, unspecified eye

H34.11 Central retinal artery occlusion, right eye

H34.12 Central retinal artery occlusion, left eye

H34.13 Central retinal artery occlusion, bilateral

H34.2 Other retinal artery occlusions

H34.21 Partial retinal artery occlusion

Hollenhorst's plaque

Retinal microembolism

H34.211 Partial retinal artery occlusion, right eye

H34.212 Partial retinal artery occlusion, left eye

H34.213 Partial retinal artery occlusion, bilateral

H34.219 Partial retinal artery occlusion, unspecified eye

H34.23 Retinal artery branch occlusion

H34.231 Retinal artery branch occlusion, right eye

H34.232 Retinal artery branch occlusion, left eye

H34.233 Retinal artery branch occlusion, bilateral

H34.239 Retinal artery branch occlusion, unspecified eye

H34.8 Other retinal vascular occlusions

H34.81 Central retinal vein occlusion

One of the following 7th characters is to be assigned to codes in subcategory H34.81 to designate the severity of the occlusion:

0 - with macular edema

1 - with retinal neovascularization

2 – stable Old central retinal vein occlusion

⑦**H34.811** Central retinal vein occlusion, right eye

⑦**H34.812** Central retinal vein occlusion, left eye

⑦**H34.813** Central retinal vein occlusion, bilateral

⑦**H34.819** Central retinal vein occlusion, unspecified eye

H34.82 Venous engorgement

Incipient retinal vein occlusion

Partial retinal vein occlusion

H34.821 Venous engorgement, right eye

H34.822 Venous engorgement, left eye

H34.823 Venous engorgement, bilateral

H34.829 Venous engorgement, unspecified eye

H34.83 Tributary (branch) retinal vein occlusion

One of the following 7th characters is to be assigned to codes in subcategory H34.83 to designate the severity of the occlusion:

0 - with macular edema

1 - with retinal neovascularization

2 – stable Old tributary (branch) retinal vein occlusion

⑦H34.831　**Tributary (branch) retinal vein occlusion, right eye**

⑦H34.832　**Tributary (branch) retinal vein occlusion, left eye**

⑦H34.833　**Tributary (branch) retinal vein occlusion, bilateral**

⑦H34.839　**Tributary (branch) retinal vein occlusion, unspecified eye**

H34.9　**Unspecified retinal vascular occlusion**

H35　**Other retinal disorders**

Excludes2: diabetic retinal disorders (E08.311-E08.359, E09.311-E09.359, E10.311-E10.359, E11.311-E11.359, E13.311-E13.359)

H35.0　**Background retinopathy and retinal vascular changes**

Code also any associated hypertension (I10.-)

H35.00　**Unspecified background retinopathy**

H35.01　**Changes in retinal vascular appearance**

Retinal vascular sheathing

H35.011　**Changes in retinal vascular appearance, right eye**

H35.012　**Changes in retinal vascular appearance, left eye**

H35.013　**Changes in retinal vascular appearance, bilateral**

H35.019　**Changes in retinal vascular appearance, unspecified eye**

H35.02　**Exudative retinopathy**

Coats retinopathy

H35.021　**Exudative retinopathy, right eye**

H35.022　**Exudative retinopathy, left eye**

H35.023　**Exudative retinopathy, bilateral**

H35.029　**Exudative retinopathy, unspecified eye**

H35.03　**Hypertensive retinopathy**

H35.031　**Hypertensive retinopathy, right eye**

H35.032　**Hypertensive retinopathy, left eye**

H35.033　**Hypertensive retinopathy, bilateral**

H35.039　**Hypertensive retinopathy, unspecified eye**

H35.04　**Retinal micro-aneurysms, unspecified**

H35.041　**Retinal micro-aneurysms, unspecified, right eye**

H35.042　**Retinal micro-aneurysms, unspecified, left eye**

H35.043　**Retinal micro-aneurysms, unspecified, bilateral**

H35.049　**Retinal micro-aneurysms, unspecified, unspecified eye**

H35.05　**Retinal neovascularization, unspecified**

H35.051　**Retinal neovascularization, unspecified, right eye**

H35.052　**Retinal neovascularization, unspecified, left eye**

H35.053　**Retinal neovascularization, unspecified, bilateral**

H35.059　**Retinal neovascularization, unspecified, unspecified eye**

H35.06　**Retinal vasculitis**

Eales disease

Retinal perivasculitis

H35.061　**Retinal vasculitis, right eye**

H35.062　**Retinal vasculitis, left eye**

H35.063　**Retinal vasculitis, bilateral**

H35.069　**Retinal vasculitis, unspecified eye**

H35.07　**Retinal telangiectasis**

H35.071　**Retinal telangiectasis, right eye**

H35.072　**Retinal telangiectasis, left eye**

H35.073　**Retinal telangiectasis, bilateral**

H35.079　**Retinal telangiectasis, unspecified eye**

H35.09　**Other intraretinal microvascular abnormalities**

Retinal varices

H35.1　**Retinopathy of prematurity**

H35.10　**Retinopathy of prematurity, unspecified**

Retinopathy of prematurity NOS

H35.101　**Retinopathy of prematurity, unspecified, right eye**

H35.102　**Retinopathy of prematurity, unspecified, left eye**

H35.103　**Retinopathy of prematurity, unspecified, bilateral**

H35.109　**Retinopathy of prematurity, unspecified, unspecified eye**

H35.11　**Retinopathy of prematurity, stage 0**

H35.111　**Retinopathy of prematurity, stage 0, right eye**

H35.112　**Retinopathy of prematurity, stage 0, left eye**

H35.113　**Retinopathy of prematurity, stage 0, bilateral**

H35.119　**Retinopathy of prematurity, stage 0, unspecified eye**

H35.12　**Retinopathy of prematurity, stage 1**

H35.121　**Retinopathy of prematurity, stage 1, right eye**

H35.122　**Retinopathy of prematurity, stage 1, left eye**

H35.123　**Retinopathy of prematurity, stage 1, bilateral**

H35.129　**Retinopathy of prematurity, stage 1, unspecified eye**

H35.13　**Retinopathy of prematurity, stage 2**

H35.131　**Retinopathy of prematurity, stage 2, right eye**

H35.132　**Retinopathy of prematurity, stage 2, left eye**

H35.133　**Retinopathy of prematurity, stage 2, bilateral**

H35.139　**Retinopathy of prematurity, stage 2, unspecified eye**

H35.14　**Retinopathy of prematurity, stage 3**

H35.141　**Retinopathy of prematurity, stage 3, right eye**

H35.142　**Retinopathy of prematurity, stage 3, left eye**

H35.143　**Retinopathy of prematurity, stage 3, bilateral**

H35.149 Retinopathy of prematurity, stage 3, unspecified eye

H35.15 **Retinopathy of prematurity, stage 4**

H35.151 Retinopathy of prematurity, stage 4, right eye

H35.152 Retinopathy of prematurity, stage 4, left eye

H35.153 Retinopathy of prematurity, stage 4, bilateral

H35.159 Retinopathy of prematurity, stage 4, unspecified eye

H35.16 **Retinopathy of prematurity, stage 5**

H35.161 Retinopathy of prematurity, stage 5, right eye

H35.162 Retinopathy of prematurity, stage 5, left eye

H35.163 Retinopathy of prematurity, stage 5, bilateral

H35.169 Retinopathy of prematurity, stage 5, unspecified eye

H35.17 **Retrolental fibroplasia**

H35.171 Retrolental fibroplasia, right eye

H35.172 Retrolental fibroplasia, left eye

H35.173 Retrolental fibroplasia, bilateral

H35.179 Retrolental fibroplasia, unspecified eye

H35.2 **Other non-diabetic proliferative retinopathy**

Proliferative vitreo-retinopathy

Excludes1: proliferative vitreo-retinopathy with retinal detachment (H33.4-)

H35.20 **Other non-diabetic proliferative retinopathy, unspecified eye**

H35.21 **Other non-diabetic proliferative retinopathy, right eye**

H35.22 **Other non-diabetic proliferative retinopathy, left eye**

H35.23 **Other non-diabetic proliferative retinopathy, bilateral**

H35.3 **Degeneration of macula and posterior pole**

H35.30 **Unspecified macular degeneration**

Age-related macular degeneration

H35.31 **Nonexudative age-related macular degeneration**

Atrophic age-related macular degeneration

Dry age-related macular degeneration

One of the following 7th characters is to be assigned to codes in subcategory H35.31 to designate the stage of the disease:

0 - stage unspecified

1 - early dry stage

2 - intermediate dry stage

3 - advanced atrophic without subfoveal involvement advanced dry stage

4 - advanced atrophic with subfoveal involvement

⑦ H35.311 Nonexudative age-related macular degeneration, right eye

⑦ H35.312 Nonexudative age-related macular degeneration, left eye

⑦ H35.313 Nonexudative age-related macular degeneration, bilateral

⑦ H35.319 Nonexudative age-related macular degeneration, unspecified eye

H35.32 **Exudative age-related macular degeneration**

Wet age-related macular degeneration

One of the following 7th characters is to be assigned to codes in subcategory H35.32 to designate the stage of the disease:

0 - stage unspecified

1 - with active choroidal neovascularization

2 - with inactive choroidal neovascularization with involuted or regressed neovascularization

3 - with inactive scar

⑦ H35.321 Exudative age-related macular degeneration, right eye

⑦ H35.322 Exudative age-related macular degeneration, left eye

⑦ H35.323 Exudative age-related macular degeneration, bilateral

⑦ H35.329 Exudative age-related macular degeneration, unspecified eye

H35.33 **Angioid streaks of macula**

H35.34 **Macular cyst, hole, or pseudohole**

H35.341 Macular cyst, hole, or pseudohole, right eye

H35.342 Macular cyst, hole, or pseudohole, left eye

H35.343 Macular cyst, hole, or pseudohole, bilateral

H35.349 Macular cyst, hole, or pseudohole, unspecified eye

H35.35 **Cystoid macular degeneration**

Excludes1: cystoid macular edema following cataract surgery (H59.03-)

H35.351 Cystoid macular degeneration, right eye

H35.352 Cystoid macular degeneration, left eye

H35.353 Cystoid macular degeneration, bilateral

H35.359 Cystoid macular degeneration, unspecified eye

H35.36 **Drusen (degenerative) of macula**

H35.361 Drusen (degenerative) of macula, right eye

H35.362 Drusen (degenerative) of macula, left eye

H35.363 Drusen (degenerative) of macula, bilateral

H35.369 Drusen (degenerative) of macula, unspecified eye

H35.37 **Puckering of macula**

H35.371 Puckering of macula, right eye

H35.372 Puckering of macula, left eye

H35.373 Puckering of macula, bilateral

H35.379 Puckering of macula, unspecified eye

H35.38 **Toxic maculopathy**

Code first poisoning due to drug or toxin, if applicable (T36-T65 with fifth or sixth character 1-4 or 6)

Use additional code for adverse effect, if applicable, to identify drug (T36-T50 with fifth or sixth character 5)

H35.381 Toxic maculopathy, right eye

H35.382 Toxic maculopathy, left eye

● New code ▲ Revised code **Excludes1:** Not coded here **Excludes2:** Not included here ⊗ Placeholder required ⑦ 7th digit required

H35.383 **Toxic maculopathy, bilateral**

H35.389 **Toxic maculopathy, unspecified eye**

H35.4 **Peripheral retinal degeneration**

Excludes1: hereditary retinal degeneration (dystrophy) (H35.5-)

peripheral retinal degeneration with retinal break (H33.3-)

H35.40 **Unspecified peripheral retinal degeneration**

H35.41 **Lattice degeneration of retina**

Palisade degeneration of retina

H35.411 **Lattice degeneration of retina, right eye**

H35.412 **Lattice degeneration of retina, left eye**

H35.413 **Lattice degeneration of retina, bilateral**

H35.419 **Lattice degeneration of retina, unspecified eye**

H35.42 **Microcystoid degeneration of retina**

H35.421 **Microcystoid degeneration of retina, right eye**

H35.422 **Microcystoid degeneration of retina, left eye**

H35.423 **Microcystoid degeneration of retina, bilateral**

H35.429 **Microcystoid degeneration of retina, unspecified eye**

H35.43 **Paving stone degeneration of retina**

H35.431 **Paving stone degeneration of retina, right eye**

H35.432 **Paving stone degeneration of retina, left eye**

H35.433 **Paving stone degeneration of retina, bilateral**

H35.439 **Paving stone degeneration of retina, unspecified eye**

H35.44 **Age-related reticular degeneration of retina**

H35.441 **Age-related reticular degeneration of retina, right eye**

H35.442 **Age-related reticular degeneration of retina, left eye**

H35.443 **Age-related reticular degeneration of retina, bilateral**

H35.449 **Age-related reticular degeneration of retina, unspecified eye**

H35.45 **Secondary pigmentary degeneration**

H35.451 **Secondary pigmentary degeneration, right eye**

H35.452 **Secondary pigmentary degeneration, left eye**

H35.453 **Secondary pigmentary degeneration, bilateral**

H35.459 **Secondary pigmentary degeneration, unspecified eye**

H35.46 **Secondary vitreoretinal degeneration**

H35.461 **Secondary vitreoretinal degeneration, right eye**

H35.462 **Secondary vitreoretinal degeneration, left eye**

H35.463 **Secondary vitreoretinal degeneration, bilateral**

H35.469 **Secondary vitreoretinal degeneration, unspecified eye**

H35.5 **Hereditary retinal dystrophy**

Excludes1: dystrophies primarily involving Bruch's membrane (H31.1-)

H35.50 **Unspecified hereditary retinal dystrophy**

H35.51 **Vitreoretinal dystrophy**

H35.52 **Pigmentary retinal dystrophy**

Albipunctate retinal dystrophy

Retinitis pigmentosa

Tapetoretinal dystrophy

H35.53 **Other dystrophies primarily involving the sensory retina**

Stargardt's disease

H35.54 **Dystrophies primarily involving the retinal pigment epithelium**

Vitelliform retinal dystrophy

H35.6 **Retinal hemorrhage**

H35.60 **Retinal hemorrhage, unspecified eye**

H35.61 **Retinal hemorrhage, right eye**

H35.62 **Retinal hemorrhage, left eye**

H35.63 **Retinal hemorrhage, bilateral**

H35.7 **Separation of retinal layers**

Excludes1: retinal detachment (serous) (H33.2-)

rhegmatogenous retinal detachment (H33.0-)

H35.70 **Unspecified separation of retinal layers**

H35.71 **Central serous chorioretinopathy**

H35.711 **Central serous chorioretinopathy, right eye**

H35.712 **Central serous chorioretinopathy, left eye**

H35.713 **Central serous chorioretinopathy, bilateral**

H35.719 **Central serous chorioretinopathy, unspecified eye**

H35.72 **Serous detachment of retinal pigment epithelium**

H35.721 **Serous detachment of retinal pigment epithelium, right eye**

H35.722 **Serous detachment of retinal pigment epithelium, left eye**

H35.723 **Serous detachment of retinal pigment epithelium, bilateral**

H35.729 **Serous detachment of retinal pigment epithelium, unspecified eye**

H35.73 **Hemorrhagic detachment of retinal pigment epithelium**

H35.731 **Hemorrhagic detachment of retinal pigment epithelium, right eye**

H35.732 **Hemorrhagic detachment of retinal pigment epithelium, left eye**

H35.733 **Hemorrhagic detachment of retinal pigment epithelium, bilateral**

H35.739 **Hemorrhagic detachment of retinal pigment epithelium, unspecified eye**

H35.8 **Other specified retinal disorders**

Excludes2: retinal hemorrhage (H35.6-)

H35.81 **Retinal edema**

Retinal cotton wool spots

H35.82 **Retinal ischemia**

H35.89 **Other specified retinal disorders**

H35.9 **Unspecified retinal disorder**

H36 **Retinal disorders in diseases classified elsewhere**

Code first underlying disease, such as:

lipid storage disorders (E75.-)

sickle-cell disorders (D57.-)

Excludes1: arteriosclerotic retinopathy (H35.0-)

diabetic retinopathy (E08.3-, E09.3-, E10.3-, E11.3-, E13.3-)

GLAUCOMA (H40-H42)

Definition: Glaucoma is a group of eye diseases characterized by damage to the optic nerve usually due to excessively high intraocular pressure.

H40 Glaucoma

Excludes1: absolute glaucoma (H44.51-)

congenital glaucoma (Q15.0)

traumatic glaucoma due to birth injury (P15.3)

H40.0 Glaucoma suspect

H40.00 Preglaucoma, unspecified

H40.001 Preglaucoma, unspecified, right eye

H40.002 Preglaucoma, unspecified, left eye

H40.003 Preglaucoma, unspecified, bilateral

H40.009 Preglaucoma, unspecified, unspecified eye

H40.01 Open angle with borderline findings, low risk

Open angle, low risk

H40.011 Open angle with borderline findings, low risk, right eye

H40.012 Open angle with borderline findings, low risk, left eye

H40.013 Open angle with borderline findings, low risk, bilateral

H40.019 Open angle with borderline findings, low risk, unspecified eye

H40.02 Open angle with borderline findings, high risk

Open angle, high risk

H40.021 Open angle with borderline findings, high risk, right eye

H40.022 Open angle with borderline findings, high risk, left eye

H40.023 Open angle with borderline findings, high risk, bilateral

H40.029 Open angle with borderline findings, high risk, unspecified eye

H40.03 Anatomical narrow angle

Primary angle closure suspect

H40.031 Anatomical narrow angle, right eye

H40.032 Anatomical narrow angle, left eye

H40.033 Anatomical narrow angle, bilateral

H40.039 Anatomical narrow angle, unspecified eye

H40.04 Steroid responder

H40.041 Steroid responder, right eye

H40.042 Steroid responder, left eye

H40.043 Steroid responder, bilateral

H40.049 Steroid responder, unspecified eye

H40.05 Ocular hypertension

H40.051 Ocular hypertension, right eye

H40.052 Ocular hypertension, left eye

H40.053 Ocular hypertension, bilateral

H40.059 Ocular hypertension, unspecified eye

H40.06 Primary angle closure without glaucoma damage

H40.061 Primary angle closure without glaucoma damage, right eye

H40.062 Primary angle closure without glaucoma damage, left eye

H40.063 Primary angle closure without glaucoma damage, bilateral

H40.069 Primary angle closure without glaucoma damage, unspecified eye

H40.1 Open-angle glaucoma

⊗⑦**H40.10 Unspecified open-angle glaucoma**

One of the following 7th characters is to be assigned to code H40.10 to designate the stage of glaucoma

0 - stage unspecified

1 - mild stage

2 - moderate stage

3 - severe stage

4 - indeterminate stage

H40.11 Primary open-angle glaucoma

Chronic simple glaucoma

One of the following 7th characters is to be assigned to each code in subcategory H40.11 to designate the stage of glaucoma

0 - stage unspecified

1 - mild stage

2 - moderate stage

3 - severe stage

4 - indeterminate stage

⑦H40.111 Primary open-angle glaucoma, right eye

⑦H40.112 Primary open-angle glaucoma, left eye

⑦H40.113 Primary open-angle glaucoma, bilateral

⑦H40.119 Primary open-angle glaucoma, unspecified eye

H40.12 Low-tension glaucoma

One of the following 7th characters is to be assigned to each code in subcategory H40.12 to designate the stage of glaucoma

0 - stage unspecified

1 - mild stage

2 - moderate stage

3 - severe stage

4 - indeterminate stage

⑦H40.121 Low-tension glaucoma, right eye

⑦H40.122 Low-tension glaucoma, left eye

⑦H40.123 Low-tension glaucoma, bilateral

⑦H40.129 Low-tension glaucoma, unspecified eye

H40.13 Pigmentary glaucoma

One of the following 7th characters is to be assigned to each code in subcategory H40.13 to designate the stage of glaucoma

0 - stage unspecified

1 - mild stage

2 - moderate stage

3 - severe stage

4 - indeterminate stage

● New code ▲ Revised code Excludes1: Not coded here Excludes2: Not included here ⊗ Placeholder required ⑦ 7th digit required

⑦H40.131   **Pigmentary glaucoma, right eye**

⑦H40.132   **Pigmentary glaucoma, left eye**

⑦H40.133   **Pigmentary glaucoma, bilateral**

⑦H40.139   **Pigmentary glaucoma, unspecified eye**

H40.14   **Capsular glaucoma with pseudoexfoliation of lens**

One of the following 7th characters is to be assigned to each code in subcategory H40.14 to designate the stage of glaucoma

0 - stage unspecified

1 - mild stage

2 - moderate stage

3 - severe stage

4 - indeterminate stage

⑦H40.141   **Capsular glaucoma with pseudoexfoliation of lens, right eye**

⑦H40.142   **Capsular glaucoma with pseudoexfoliation of lens, left eye**

⑦H40.143   **Capsular glaucoma with pseudoexfoliation of lens, bilateral**

⑦H40.149   **Capsular glaucoma with pseudoexfoliation of lens, unspecified eye**

H40.15   **Residual stage of open-angle glaucoma**

H40.151   **Residual stage of open-angle glaucoma, right eye**

H40.152   **Residual stage of open-angle glaucoma, left eye**

H40.153   **Residual stage of open-angle glaucoma, bilateral**

H40.159   **Residual stage of open-angle glaucoma, unspecified eye**

H40.2   **Primary angle-closure glaucoma**

Excludes1: aqueous misdirection (H40.83-)

malignant glaucoma (H40.83-)

⊗⑦H40.20   **Unspecified primary angle-closure glaucoma**

One of the following 7th characters is to be assigned to code H40.20 to designate the stage of glaucoma

0 - stage unspecified

1 - mild stage

2 - moderate stage

3 - severe stage

4 - indeterminate stage

H40.21   **Acute angle-closure glaucoma**

Acute angle-closure glaucoma attack

Acute angle-closure glaucoma crisis

H40.211   **Acute angle-closure glaucoma, right eye**

H40.212   **Acute angle-closure glaucoma, left eye**

H40.213   **Acute angle-closure glaucoma, bilateral**

H40.219   **Acute angle-closure glaucoma, unspecified eye**

H40.22   **Chronic angle-closure glaucoma**

Chronic primary angle closure glaucoma

One of the following 7th characters is to be assigned to each code in subcategory H40.22 to designate the stage of glaucoma

0 - stage unspecified

1 - mild stage

2 - moderate stage

3 - severe stage

4 - indeterminate stage

⑦H40.221   **Chronic angle-closure glaucoma, right eye**

⑦H40.222   **Chronic angle-closure glaucoma, left eye**

⑦H40.223   **Chronic angle-closure glaucoma, bilateral**

⑦H40.229   **Chronic angle-closure glaucoma, unspecified eye**

H40.23   **Intermittent angle-closure glaucoma**

H40.231   **Intermittent angle-closure glaucoma, right eye**

H40.232   **Intermittent angle-closure glaucoma, left eye**

H40.233   **Intermittent angle-closure glaucoma, bilateral**

H40.239   **Intermittent angle-closure glaucoma, unspecified eye**

H40.24   **Residual stage of angle-closure glaucoma**

H40.241   **Residual stage of angle-closure glaucoma, right eye**

H40.242   **Residual stage of angle-closure glaucoma, left eye**

H40.243   **Residual stage of angle-closure glaucoma, bilateral**

H40.249   **Residual stage of angle-closure glaucoma, unspecified eye**

H40.3   **Glaucoma secondary to eye trauma**

Code also underlying condition

One of the following 7th characters is to be assigned to each code in subcategory H40.3 to designate the stage of glaucoma

0 - stage unspecified

1 - mild stage

2 - moderate stage

3 - severe stage

4 - indeterminate stage

⊗⑦H40.30   **Glaucoma secondary to eye trauma, unspecified eye**

⊗⑦H40.31   **Glaucoma secondary to eye trauma, right eye**

⊗⑦H40.32   **Glaucoma secondary to eye trauma, left eye**

⊗⑦H40.33   **Glaucoma secondary to eye trauma, bilateral**

H40.4   **Glaucoma secondary to eye inflammation**

Code also underlying condition

One of the following 7th characters is to be assigned to each code in subcategory H40.4 to designate the stage of glaucoma

0 - stage unspecified

1 - mild stage

2 - moderate stage

3 - severe stage

4 - indeterminate stage

⊗⑦H40.40   **Glaucoma secondary to eye inflammation, unspecified eye**

⊗⑦H40.41   **Glaucoma secondary to eye inflammation, right eye**

⊗⑦H40.42 Glaucoma secondary to eye inflammation, left eye

⊗⑦H40.43 Glaucoma secondary to eye inflammation, bilateral

H40.5 Glaucoma secondary to other eye disorders

Code also underlying eye disorder

One of the following 7th characters is to be assigned to each code in subcategory H40.5 to designate the stage of glaucoma

0 - stage unspecified

1 - mild stage

2 - moderate stage

3 - severe stage

4 - indeterminate stage

⊗⑦H40.50 Glaucoma secondary to other eye disorders, unspecified eye

⊗⑦H40.51 Glaucoma secondary to other eye disorders, right eye

⊗⑦H40.52 Glaucoma secondary to other eye disorders, left eye

⊗⑦H40.53 Glaucoma secondary to other eye disorders, bilateral

H40.6 Glaucoma secondary to drugs

Use additional code for adverse effect, if applicable, to identify drug (T36-T50 with fifth or sixth character 5)

One of the following 7th characters is to be assigned to each code in subcategory H40.6 to designate the stage of glaucoma

0 - stage unspecified

1 - mild stage

2 - moderate stage

3 - severe stage

4 - indeterminate stage

⊗⑦H40.60 Glaucoma secondary to drugs, unspecified eye

⊗⑦H40.61 Glaucoma secondary to drugs, right eye

⊗⑦H40.62 Glaucoma secondary to drugs, left eye

⊗⑦H40.63 Glaucoma secondary to drugs, bilateral

H40.8 Other glaucoma

H40.81 Glaucoma with increased episcleral venous pressure

H40.811 Glaucoma with increased episcleral venous pressure, right eye

H40.812 Glaucoma with increased episcleral venous pressure, left eye

H40.813 Glaucoma with increased episcleral venous pressure, bilateral

H40.819 Glaucoma with increased episcleral venous pressure, unspecified eye

H40.82 Hypersecretion glaucoma

H40.821 Hypersecretion glaucoma, right eye

H40.822 Hypersecretion glaucoma, left eye

H40.823 Hypersecretion glaucoma, bilateral

H40.829 Hypersecretion glaucoma, unspecified eye

H40.83 Aqueous misdirection

Malignant glaucoma

H40.831 Aqueous misdirection, right eye

H40.832 Aqueous misdirection, left eye

H40.833 Aqueous misdirection, bilateral

H40.839 Aqueous misdirection, unspecified eye

H40.89 Other specified glaucoma

H40.9 Unspecified glaucoma

H42 Glaucoma in diseases classified elsewhere

Code first underlying condition, such as:

amyloidosis (E85.-)

aniridia (Q13.1)

Lowe's syndrome (E72.03)

Rieger's anomaly (Q13.81)

specified metabolic disorder (E70-E88)

Excludes1: glaucoma (in) onchocerciasis (B73.02)

glaucoma (in) syphilis (A52.71)

glaucoma (in) tuberculous (A18.59)

DISORDERS OF VITREOUS BODY AND GLOBE (H43-H44)

H43 Disorders of vitreous body

H43.0 Vitreous prolapse

Excludes1: vitreous syndrome following cataract surgery (H59.0-)

traumatic vitreous prolapse (S05.2-)

H43.00 Vitreous prolapse, unspecified eye

H43.01 Vitreous prolapse, right eye

H43.02 Vitreous prolapse, left eye

H43.03 Vitreous prolapse, bilateral

H43.1 Vitreous hemorrhage

H43.10 Vitreous hemorrhage, unspecified eye

H43.11 Vitreous hemorrhage, right eye

H43.12 Vitreous hemorrhage, left eye

H43.13 Vitreous hemorrhage, bilateral

H43.2 Crystalline deposits in vitreous body

H43.20 Crystalline deposits in vitreous body, unspecified eye

H43.21 Crystalline deposits in vitreous body, right eye

H43.22 Crystalline deposits in vitreous body, left eye

H43.23 Crystalline deposits in vitreous body, bilateral

H43.3 Other vitreous opacities

H43.31 Vitreous membranes and strands

H43.311 Vitreous membranes and strands, right eye

H43.312 Vitreous membranes and strands, left eye

H43.313 Vitreous membranes and strands, bilateral

H43.319 Vitreous membranes and strands, unspecified eye

H43.39 Other vitreous opacities

Vitreous floaters

H43.391 Other vitreous opacities, right eye

H43.392 Other vitreous opacities, left eye

H43.393 Other vitreous opacities, bilateral

H43.399 Other vitreous opacities, unspecified eye

H43.8 Other disorders of vitreous body

Excludes1: proliferative vitreo-retinopathy with retinal detachment (H33.4-)

Excludes2: vitreous abscess (H44.02-)

H43.81 Vitreous degeneration

Vitreous detachment

H43.811 Vitreous degeneration, right eye

● New code ▲ Revised code **Excludes1:** Not coded here **Excludes2:** Not included here ⊗ Placeholder required ⑦ 7th digit required

H43.812   Vitreous degeneration, left eye

H43.813   Vitreous degeneration, bilateral

H43.819   Vitreous degeneration, unspecified eye

H43.82   **Vitreomacular adhesion**

Vitreomacular traction

H43.821   Vitreomacular adhesion, right eye

H43.822   Vitreomacular adhesion, left eye

H43.823   Vitreomacular adhesion, bilateral

H43.829   Vitreomacular adhesion, unspecified eye

H43.89   **Other disorders of vitreous body**

H43.9   **Unspecified disorder of vitreous body**

H44   **Disorders of globe**

Includes: disorders affecting multiple structures of eye

H44.0   **Purulent endophthalmitis**

Use additional code to identify organism

Excludes1: bleb associated endophthalmitis (H59.4-)

H44.00   **Unspecified purulent endophthalmitis**

H44.001   Unspecified purulent endophthalmitis, right eye

H44.002   Unspecified purulent endophthalmitis, left eye

H44.003   Unspecified purulent endophthalmitis, bilateral

H44.009   Unspecified purulent endophthalmitis, unspecified eye

H44.01   **Panophthalmitis (acute)**

H44.011   Panophthalmitis (acute), right eye

H44.012   Panophthalmitis (acute), left eye

H44.013   Panophthalmitis (acute), bilateral

H44.019   Panophthalmitis (acute), unspecified eye

H44.02   **Vitreous abscess (chronic)**

H44.021   Vitreous abscess (chronic), right eye

H44.022   Vitreous abscess (chronic), left eye

H44.023   Vitreous abscess (chronic), bilateral

H44.029   Vitreous abscess (chronic), unspecified eye

H44.1   **Other endophthalmitis**

Excludes1: bleb associated endophthalmitis (H59.4-)

Excludes2: ophthalmia nodosa (H16.2-)

H44.11   **Panuveitis**

H44.111   Panuveitis, right eye

H44.112   Panuveitis, left eye

H44.113   Panuveitis, bilateral

H44.119   Panuveitis, unspecified eye

H44.12   **Parasitic endophthalmitis, unspecified**

H44.121   Parasitic endophthalmitis, unspecified, right eye

H44.122   Parasitic endophthalmitis, unspecified, left eye

H44.123   Parasitic endophthalmitis, unspecified, bilateral

H44.129   Parasitic endophthalmitis, unspecified, unspecified eye

H44.13   **Sympathetic uveitis**

H44.131   Sympathetic uveitis, right eye

H44.132   Sympathetic uveitis, left eye

H44.133   Sympathetic uveitis, bilateral

H44.139   Sympathetic uveitis, unspecified eye

H44.19   **Other endophthalmitis**

H44.2   **Degenerative myopia**

Malignant myopia

H44.20   **Degenerative myopia, unspecified eye**

H44.21   **Degenerative myopia, right eye**

H44.22   **Degenerative myopia, left eye**

H44.23   **Degenerative myopia, bilateral**

•H44.2A   **Degenerative myopia with choroidal neovascularization**

Use Additional code for any associated choroid disorders (H31.-)

•H44.2A1   Degenerative myopia with choroidal neovascularization, right eye

•H44.2A2   Degenerative myopia with choroidal neovascularization, left eye

•H44.2A3   Degenerative myopia with choroidal neovascularization, bilateral eye

•H44.2A9   Degenerative myopia with choroidal neovascularization, unspecified eye

•H44.2B   **Degenerative myopia with macular hole**

•H44.2B1   Degenerative myopia with macular hole, right eye

•H44.2B2   Degenerative myopia with macular hole, left eye

•H44.2B3   Degenerative myopia with macular hole, bilateral eye

•H44.2B9   Degenerative myopia with macular hole, unspecified eye

•H44.2C   **Degenerative myopia with retinal detachment**

Use Additional code to identify the retinal detachment (H33.-)

•H44.2C1   Degenerative myopia with retinal detachment, right eye

•H44.2C2   Degenerative myopia with retinal detachment, left eye

•H44.2C3   Degenerative myopia with retinal detachment, bilateral eye

•H44.2C9   Degenerative myopia with retinal detachment, unspecified eye

•H44.2D   **Degenerative myopia with foveoschisis**

•H44.2D1   Degenerative myopia with foveoschisis, right eye

•H44.2D2   Degenerative myopia with foveoschisis, left eye

•H44.2D3   Degenerative myopia with foveoschisis, bilateral eye

•H44.2D9   Degenerative myopia with foveoschisis, unspecified eye

•H44.2E   **Degenerative myopia with other maculopathy**

•H44.2E1   Degenerative myopia with other maculopathy, right eye

•H44.2E2   Degenerative myopia with other maculopathy, left eye

•H44.2E3   Degenerative myopia with other maculopathy, bilateral eye

•H44.2E9   Degenerative myopia with other maculopathy, unspecified eye

H44.3 **Other and unspecified degenerative disorders of globe**

H44.30 Unspecified degenerative disorder of globe

H44.31 Chalcosis

H44.311 Chalcosis, right eye

H44.312 Chalcosis, left eye

H44.313 Chalcosis, bilateral

H44.319 Chalcosis, unspecified eye

H44.32 Siderosis of eye

H44.321 Siderosis of eye, right eye

H44.322 Siderosis of eye, left eye

H44.323 Siderosis of eye, bilateral

H44.329 Siderosis of eye, unspecified eye

H44.39 Other degenerative disorders of globe

H44.391 Other degenerative disorders of globe, right eye

H44.392 Other degenerative disorders of globe, left eye

H44.393 Other degenerative disorders of globe, bilateral

H44.399 Other degenerative disorders of globe, unspecified eye

H44.4 **Hypotony of eye**

H44.40 Unspecified hypotony of eye

H44.41 Flat anterior chamber hypotony of eye

H44.411 Flat anterior chamber hypotony of right eye

H44.412 Flat anterior chamber hypotony of left eye

H44.413 Flat anterior chamber hypotony of eye, bilateral

H44.419 Flat anterior chamber hypotony of unspecified eye

H44.42 Hypotony of eye due to ocular fistula

H44.421 Hypotony of right eye due to ocular fistula

H44.422 Hypotony of left eye due to ocular fistula

H44.423 Hypotony of eye due to ocular fistula, bilateral

H44.429 Hypotony of unspecified eye due to ocular fistula

H44.43 Hypotony of eye due to other ocular disorders

H44.431 Hypotony of eye due to other ocular disorders, right eye

H44.432 Hypotony of eye due to other ocular disorders, left eye

H44.433 Hypotony of eye due to other ocular disorders, bilateral

H44.439 Hypotony of eye due to other ocular disorders, unspecified eye

H44.44 Primary hypotony of eye

H44.441 Primary hypotony of right eye

H44.442 Primary hypotony of left eye

H44.443 Primary hypotony of eye, bilateral

H44.449 Primary hypotony of unspecified eye

H44.5 **Degenerated conditions of globe**

H44.50 Unspecified degenerated conditions of globe

H44.51 Absolute glaucoma

H44.511 Absolute glaucoma, right eye

H44.512 Absolute glaucoma, left eye

H44.513 Absolute glaucoma, bilateral

H44.519 Absolute glaucoma, unspecified eye

H44.52 Atrophy of globe

Phthisis bulbi

H44.521 Atrophy of globe, right eye

H44.522 Atrophy of globe, left eye

H44.523 Atrophy of globe, bilateral

H44.529 Atrophy of globe, unspecified eye

H44.53 Leucocoria

H44.531 Leucocoria, right eye

H44.532 Leucocoria, left eye

H44.533 Leucocoria, bilateral

H44.539 Leucocoria, unspecified eye

H44.6 **Retained (old) intraocular foreign body, magnetic**

Use additional code to identify magnetic foreign body (Z18.11)

Excludes1: current intraocular foreign body (S05.-)

Excludes2: retained foreign body in eyelid (H02.81-)

retained (old) foreign body following penetrating wound of orbit (H05.5-)

retained (old) intraocular foreign body, nonmagnetic (H44.7-)

H44.60 Unspecified retained (old) intraocular foreign body, magnetic

H44.601 Unspecified retained (old) intraocular foreign body, magnetic, right eye

H44.602 Unspecified retained (old) intraocular foreign body, magnetic, left eye

H44.603 Unspecified retained (old) intraocular foreign body, magnetic, bilateral

H44.609 Unspecified retained (old) intraocular foreign body, magnetic, unspecified eye

H44.61 Retained (old) magnetic foreign body in anterior chamber

H44.611 Retained (old) magnetic foreign body in anterior chamber, right eye

H44.612 Retained (old) magnetic foreign body in anterior chamber, left eye

H44.613 Retained (old) magnetic foreign body in anterior chamber, bilateral

H44.619 Retained (old) magnetic foreign body in anterior chamber, unspecified eye

H44.62 Retained (old) magnetic foreign body in iris or ciliary body

H44.621 Retained (old) magnetic foreign body in iris or ciliary body, right eye

H44.622 Retained (old) magnetic foreign body in iris or ciliary body, left eye

H44.623 Retained (old) magnetic foreign body in iris or ciliary body, bilateral

H44.629 Retained (old) magnetic foreign body in iris or ciliary body, unspecified eye

H44.63 Retained (old) magnetic foreign body in lens

H44.631 Retained (old) magnetic foreign body in lens, right eye

H44.632 Retained (old) magnetic foreign body in lens, left eye

H44.633 Retained (old) magnetic foreign body in lens, bilateral

H44.639 Retained (old) magnetic foreign body in lens, unspecified eye

H44.64 Retained (old) magnetic foreign body in posterior wall of globe

H44.641 Retained (old) magnetic foreign body in posterior wall of globe, right eye

H44.642 Retained (old) magnetic foreign body in posterior wall of globe, left eye

H44.643 Retained (old) magnetic foreign body in posterior wall of globe, bilateral

H44.649 Retained (old) magnetic foreign body in posterior wall of globe, unspecified eye

H44.65 Retained (old) magnetic foreign body in vitreous body

H44.651 Retained (old) magnetic foreign body in vitreous body, right eye

H44.652 Retained (old) magnetic foreign body in vitreous body, left eye

H44.653 Retained (old) magnetic foreign body in vitreous body, bilateral

H44.659 Retained (old) magnetic foreign body in vitreous body, unspecified eye

H44.69 Retained (old) intraocular foreign body, magnetic, in other or multiple sites

H44.691 Retained (old) intraocular foreign body, magnetic, in other or multiple sites, right eye

H44.692 Retained (old) intraocular foreign body, magnetic, in other or multiple sites, left eye

H44.693 Retained (old) intraocular foreign body, magnetic, in other or multiple sites, bilateral

H44.699 Retained (old) intraocular foreign body, magnetic, in other or multiple sites, unspecified eye

H44.7 Retained (old) intraocular foreign body, nonmagnetic

Use additional code to identify nonmagnetic foreign body (Z18.01-Z18.10, Z18.12, Z18.2-Z18.9)

Excludes1: current intraocular foreign body (S05.-)

Excludes2: retained foreign body in eyelid (H02.81-)

retained (old) foreign body following penetrating wound of orbit (H05.5-)

retained (old) intraocular foreign body, magnetic (H44.6-)

H44.70 Unspecified retained (old) intraocular foreign body, nonmagnetic

H44.701 Unspecified retained (old) intraocular foreign body, nonmagnetic, right eye

H44.702 Unspecified retained (old) intraocular foreign body, nonmagnetic, left eye

H44.703 Unspecified retained (old) intraocular foreign body, nonmagnetic, bilateral

H44.709 Unspecified retained (old) intraocular foreign body, nonmagnetic, unspecified eye

Retained (old) intraocular foreign body NOS

H44.71 Retained (nonmagnetic) (old) foreign body in anterior chamber

H44.711 Retained (nonmagnetic) (old) foreign body in anterior chamber, right eye

H44.712 Retained (nonmagnetic) (old) foreign body in anterior chamber, left eye

H44.713 Retained (nonmagnetic) (old) foreign body in anterior chamber, bilateral

H44.719 Retained (nonmagnetic) (old) foreign body in anterior chamber, unspecified eye

H44.72 Retained (nonmagnetic) (old) foreign body in iris or ciliary body

H44.721 Retained (nonmagnetic) (old) foreign body in iris or ciliary body, right eye

H44.722 Retained (nonmagnetic) (old) foreign body in iris or ciliary body, left eye

H44.723 Retained (nonmagnetic) (old) foreign body in iris or ciliary body, bilateral

H44.729 Retained (nonmagnetic) (old) foreign body in iris or ciliary body, unspecified eye

H44.73 Retained (nonmagnetic) (old) foreign body in lens

H44.731 Retained (nonmagnetic) (old) foreign body in lens, right eye

H44.732 Retained (nonmagnetic) (old) foreign body in lens, left eye

H44.733 Retained (nonmagnetic) (old) foreign body in lens, bilateral

H44.739 Retained (nonmagnetic) (old) foreign body in lens, unspecified eye

H44.74 Retained (nonmagnetic) (old) foreign body in posterior wall of globe

H44.741 Retained (nonmagnetic) (old) foreign body in posterior wall of globe, right eye

H44.742 Retained (nonmagnetic) (old) foreign body in posterior wall of globe, left eye

H44.743 Retained (nonmagnetic) (old) foreign body in posterior wall of globe, bilateral

H44.749 Retained (nonmagnetic) (old) foreign body in posterior wall of globe, unspecified eye

H44.75 Retained (nonmagnetic) (old) foreign body in vitreous body

H44.751 Retained (nonmagnetic) (old) foreign body in vitreous body, right eye

H44.752 Retained (nonmagnetic) (old) foreign body in vitreous body, left eye

H44.753 Retained (nonmagnetic) (old) foreign body in vitreous body, bilateral

H44.759 Retained (nonmagnetic) (old) foreign body in vitreous body, unspecified eye

H44.79 Retained (old) intraocular foreign body, nonmagnetic, in other or multiple sites

H44.791 Retained (old) intraocular foreign body, nonmagnetic, in other or multiple sites, right eye

H44.792 Retained (old) intraocular foreign body, nonmagnetic, in other or multiple sites, left eye

H44.793 Retained (old) intraocular foreign body, nonmagnetic, in other or multiple sites, bilateral

H44.799 Retained (old) intraocular foreign body, nonmagnetic, in other or multiple sites, unspecified eye

H44.8 **Other disorders of globe**

H44.81 **Hemophthalmos**

H44.811 Hemophthalmos, right eye

H44.812 Hemophthalmos, left eye

H44.813 Hemophthalmos, bilateral

H44.819 Hemophthalmos, unspecified eye

H44.82 **Luxation of globe**

H44.821 Luxation of globe, right eye

H44.822 Luxation of globe, left eye

H44.823 Luxation of globe, bilateral

H44.829 Luxation of globe, unspecified eye

H44.89 **Other disorders of globe**

H44.9 **Unspecified disorder of globe**

DISORDERS OF OPTIC NERVE AND VISUAL PATHWAYS (H46-H47)

H46 Optic neuritis

Excludes2: ischemic optic neuropathy (H47.01-)

neuromyelitis optica [Devic] (G36.0)

H46.0 **Optic papillitis**

H46.00 Optic papillitis, unspecified eye

H46.01 Optic papillitis, right eye

H46.02 Optic papillitis, left eye

H46.03 Optic papillitis, bilateral

H46.1 **Retrobulbar neuritis**

Retrobulbar neuritis NOS

Excludes1: syphilitic retrobulbar neuritis (A52.15)

H46.10 Retrobulbar neuritis, unspecified eye

H46.11 Retrobulbar neuritis, right eye

H46.12 Retrobulbar neuritis, left eye

H46.13 Retrobulbar neuritis, bilateral

H46.2 **Nutritional optic neuropathy**

H46.3 **Toxic optic neuropathy**

<u>Code first</u> (T51-T65) to identify cause

H46.8 **Other optic neuritis**

H46.9 **Unspecified optic neuritis**

H47 Other disorders of optic [2nd] nerve and visual pathways

H47.0 **Disorders of optic nerve, not elsewhere classified**

H47.01 **Ischemic optic neuropathy**

H47.011 Ischemic optic neuropathy, right eye

H47.012 Ischemic optic neuropathy, left eye

H47.013 Ischemic optic neuropathy, bilateral

H47.019 Ischemic optic neuropathy, unspecified eye

H47.02 **Hemorrhage in optic nerve sheath**

H47.021 Hemorrhage in optic nerve sheath, right eye

H47.022 Hemorrhage in optic nerve sheath, left eye

H47.023 Hemorrhage in optic nerve sheath, bilateral

H47.029 Hemorrhage in optic nerve sheath, unspecified eye

H47.03 **Optic nerve hypoplasia**

H47.031 Optic nerve hypoplasia, right eye

H47.032 Optic nerve hypoplasia, left eye

H47.033 Optic nerve hypoplasia, bilateral

H47.039 Optic nerve hypoplasia, unspecified eye

H47.09 **Other disorders of optic nerve, not elsewhere classified**

Compression of optic nerve

H47.091 Other disorders of optic nerve, not elsewhere classified, right eye

H47.092 Other disorders of optic nerve, not elsewhere classified, left eye

H47.093 Other disorders of optic nerve, not elsewhere classified, bilateral

H47.099 Other disorders of optic nerve, not elsewhere classified, unspecified eye

H47.1 **Papilledema**

H47.10 **Unspecified papilledema**

H47.11 **Papilledema associated with increased intracranial pressure**

H47.12 **Papilledema associated with decreased ocular pressure**

H47.13 **Papilledema associated with retinal disorder**

H47.14 **Foster-Kennedy syndrome**

H47.141 Foster-Kennedy syndrome, right eye

H47.142 Foster-Kennedy syndrome, left eye

H47.143 Foster-Kennedy syndrome, bilateral

H47.149 Foster-Kennedy syndrome, unspecified eye

H47.2 **Optic atrophy**

H47.20 **Unspecified optic atrophy**

H47.21 **Primary optic atrophy**

H47.211 Primary optic atrophy, right eye

H47.212 Primary optic atrophy, left eye

H47.213 Primary optic atrophy, bilateral

H47.219 Primary optic atrophy, unspecified eye

H47.22 **Hereditary optic atrophy**

Leber's optic atrophy

H47.23 **Glaucomatous optic atrophy**

H47.231 Glaucomatous optic atrophy, right eye

H47.232 Glaucomatous optic atrophy, left eye

H47.233 Glaucomatous optic atrophy, bilateral

H47.239 Glaucomatous optic atrophy, unspecified eye

H47.29 **Other optic atrophy**

Temporal pallor of optic disc

H47.291 Other optic atrophy, right eye

H47.292 Other optic atrophy, left eye

H47.293 Other optic atrophy, bilateral

H47.299 Other optic atrophy, unspecified eye

H47.3 **Other disorders of optic disc**

H47.31 **Coloboma of optic disc**

H47.311 Coloboma of optic disc, right eye

H47.312 Coloboma of optic disc, left eye

H47.313 Coloboma of optic disc, bilateral

H47.319 Coloboma of optic disc, unspecified eye

H47.32 **Drusen of optic disc**

● New code   ▲ Revised code   **Excludes1:** Not coded here   **Excludes2:** Not included here   ⊗ Placeholder required   ⑦7th digit required

H47.321   Drusen of optic disc, right eye

H47.322   Drusen of optic disc, left eye

H47.323   Drusen of optic disc, bilateral

H47.329   Drusen of optic disc, unspecified eye

H47.33   Pseudopapilledema of optic disc

H47.331   Pseudopapilledema of optic disc, right eye

H47.332   Pseudopapilledema of optic disc, left eye

H47.333   Pseudopapilledema of optic disc, bilateral

H47.339   Pseudopapilledema of optic disc, unspecified eye

H47.39   Other disorders of optic disc

H47.391   Other disorders of optic disc, right eye

H47.392   Other disorders of optic disc, left eye

H47.393   Other disorders of optic disc, bilateral

H47.399   Other disorders of optic disc, unspecified eye

H47.4   **Disorders of optic chiasm**

Code also underlying condition

H47.41   Disorders of optic chiasm in (due to) inflammatory disorders

H47.42   Disorders of optic chiasm in (due to) neoplasm

H47.43   Disorders of optic chiasm in (due to) vascular disorders

H47.49   Disorders of optic chiasm in (due to) other disorders

H47.5   **Disorders of other visual pathways**

Disorders of optic tracts, geniculate nuclei and optic radiations

Code also underlying condition

H47.51   Disorders of visual pathways in (due to) inflammatory disorders

H47.511   Disorders of visual pathways in (due to) inflammatory disorders, right side

H47.512   Disorders of visual pathways in (due to) inflammatory disorders, left side

H47.519   Disorders of visual pathways in (due to) inflammatory disorders, unspecified side

H47.52   Disorders of visual pathways in (due to) neoplasm

H47.521   Disorders of visual pathways in (due to) neoplasm, right side

H47.522   Disorders of visual pathways in (due to) neoplasm, left side

H47.529   Disorders of visual pathways in (due to) neoplasm, unspecified side

H47.53   Disorders of visual pathways in (due to) vascular disorders

H47.531   Disorders of visual pathways in (due to) vascular disorders, right side

H47.532   Disorders of visual pathways in (due to) vascular disorders, left side

H47.539   Disorders of visual pathways in (due to) vascular disorders, unspecified side

H47.6   **Disorders of visual cortex**

Code also underlying condition

Excludes1: injury to visual cortex S04.04

H47.61   Cortical blindness

H47.611   Cortical blindness, right side of brain

H47.612   Cortical blindness, left side of brain

H47.619   Cortical blindness, unspecified side of brain

H47.62   Disorders of visual cortex in (due to) inflammatory disorders

H47.621   Disorders of visual cortex in (due to) inflammatory disorders, right side of brain

H47.622   Disorders of visual cortex in (due to) inflammatory disorders, left side of brain

H47.629   Disorders of visual cortex in (due to) inflammatory disorders, unspecified side of brain

H47.63   Disorders of visual cortex in (due to) neoplasm

H47.631   Disorders of visual cortex in (due to) neoplasm, right side of brain

H47.632   Disorders of visual cortex in (due to) neoplasm, left side of brain

H47.639   Disorders of visual cortex in (due to) neoplasm, unspecified side of brain

H47.64   Disorders of visual cortex in (due to) vascular disorders

H47.641   Disorders of visual cortex in (due to) vascular disorders, right side of brain

H47.642   Disorders of visual cortex in (due to) vascular disorders, left side of brain

H47.649   Disorders of visual cortex in (due to) vascular disorders, unspecified side of brain

H47.9   **Unspecified disorder of visual pathways**

DISORDERS OF OCULAR MUSCLES, BINOCULAR MOVEMENT, ACCOMMODATION AND REFRACTION (H49-H52)

Definition: Refraction is the ability of the eye to bend light so that an image is focused on the retina. Accommodation is the automatic adjustment in focal length of the natural lens of the eye.

Excludes2: nystagmus and other irregular eye movements (H55)

H49   **Paralytic strabismus**

Definition: Strabismus, aka crossed eyes, is a visual defect in which the eyes are misaligned and point in different directions. Strabismus usually occurs in childhood but can occur later in life.

Excludes2: internal ophthalmoplegia (H52.51-)

internuclear ophthalmoplegia (H51.2-)

progressive supranuclear ophthalmoplegia (G23.1)

H49.0   **Third [oculomotor] nerve palsy**

H49.00   Third [oculomotor] nerve palsy, unspecified eye

H49.01   Third [oculomotor] nerve palsy, right eye

H49.02   Third [oculomotor] nerve palsy, left eye

H49.03   Third [oculomotor] nerve palsy, bilateral

H49.1   **Fourth [trochlear] nerve palsy**

H49.10   Fourth [trochlear] nerve palsy, unspecified eye

H49.11   Fourth [trochlear] nerve palsy, right eye

H49.12   Fourth [trochlear] nerve palsy, left eye

H49.13   Fourth [trochlear] nerve palsy, bilateral

H49.2   **Sixth [abducent] nerve palsy**

H49.20 Sixth [abducent] nerve palsy, unspecified eye
H49.21 Sixth [abducent] nerve palsy, right eye
H49.22 Sixth [abducent] nerve palsy, left eye
H49.23 Sixth [abducent] nerve palsy, bilateral
H49.3 Total (external) ophthalmoplegia
H49.30 Total (external) ophthalmoplegia, unspecified eye
H49.31 Total (external) ophthalmoplegia, right eye
H49.32 Total (external) ophthalmoplegia, left eye
H49.33 Total (external) ophthalmoplegia, bilateral
H49.4 Progressive external ophthalmoplegia
Excludes1: Kearns-Sayre syndrome (H49.81-)
H49.40 Progressive external ophthalmoplegia, unspecified eye
H49.41 Progressive external ophthalmoplegia, right eye
H49.42 Progressive external ophthalmoplegia, left eye
H49.43 Progressive external ophthalmoplegia, bilateral
H49.8 Other paralytic strabismus
H49.81 Kearns-Sayre syndrome
Progressive external ophthalmoplegia with pigmentary retinopathy
Use additional code for other manifestation, such as: heart block (I45.9)
H49.811 Kearns-Sayre syndrome, right eye
H49.812 Kearns-Sayre syndrome, left eye
H49.813 Kearns-Sayre syndrome, bilateral
H49.819 Kearns-Sayre syndrome, unspecified eye
H49.88 Other paralytic strabismus
External ophthalmoplegia NOS
H49.881 Other paralytic strabismus, right eye
H49.882 Other paralytic strabismus, left eye
H49.883 Other paralytic strabismus, bilateral
H49.889 Other paralytic strabismus, unspecified eye
H49.9 Unspecified paralytic strabismus
H50 Other strabismus
H50.0 Esotropia
Convergent concomitant strabismus
Excludes1: intermittent esotropia (H50.31-, H50.32)
H50.00 Unspecified esotropia
H50.01 Monocular esotropia
H50.011 Monocular esotropia, right eye
H50.012 Monocular esotropia, left eye
H50.02 Monocular esotropia with A pattern
H50.021 Monocular esotropia with A pattern, right eye
H50.022 Monocular esotropia with A pattern, left eye
H50.03 Monocular esotropia with V pattern
H50.031 Monocular esotropia with V pattern, right eye
H50.032 Monocular esotropia with V pattern, left eye
H50.04 Monocular esotropia with other noncomitancies
H50.041 Monocular esotropia with other noncomitancies, right eye
H50.042 Monocular esotropia with other noncomitancies, left eye

H50.05 Alternating esotropia
H50.06 Alternating esotropia with A pattern
H50.07 Alternating esotropia with V pattern
H50.08 Alternating esotropia with other noncomitancies
H50.1 Exotropia
Divergent concomitant strabismus
Excludes1: intermittent exotropia (H50.33-, H50.34)
H50.10 Unspecified exotropia
H50.11 Monocular exotropia
H50.111 Monocular exotropia, right eye
H50.112 Monocular exotropia, left eye
H50.12 Monocular exotropia with A pattern
H50.121 Monocular exotropia with A pattern, right eye
H50.122 Monocular exotropia with A pattern, left eye
H50.13 Monocular exotropia with V pattern
H50.131 Monocular exotropia with V pattern, right eye
H50.132 Monocular exotropia with V pattern, left eye
H50.14 Monocular exotropia with other noncomitancies
H50.141 Monocular exotropia with other noncomitancies, right eye
H50.142 Monocular exotropia with other noncomitancies, left eye
H50.15 Alternating exotropia
H50.16 Alternating exotropia with A pattern
H50.17 Alternating exotropia with V pattern
H50.18 Alternating exotropia with other noncomitancies
H50.2 Vertical strabismus
Hypertropia
H50.21 Vertical strabismus, right eye
H50.22 Vertical strabismus, left eye
H50.3 Intermittent heterotropia
H50.30 Unspecified intermittent heterotropia
H50.31 Intermittent monocular esotropia
H50.311 Intermittent monocular esotropia, right eye
H50.312 Intermittent monocular esotropia, left eye
H50.32 Intermittent alternating esotropia
H50.33 Intermittent monocular exotropia
H50.331 Intermittent monocular exotropia, right eye
H50.332 Intermittent monocular exotropia, left eye
H50.34 Intermittent alternating exotropia
H50.4 Other and unspecified heterotropia
H50.40 Unspecified heterotropia
H50.41 Cyclotropia
H50.411 Cyclotropia, right eye
H50.412 Cyclotropia, left eye
H50.42 Monofixation syndrome
H50.43 Accommodative component in esotropia
H50.5 Heterophoria
H50.50 Unspecified heterophoria

H50.51   Esophoria

H50.52   Exophoria

H50.53   Vertical heterophoria

H50.54   Cyclophoria

H50.55   Alternating heterophoria

H50.6   Mechanical strabismus

H50.60   Mechanical strabismus, unspecified

H50.61   Brown's sheath syndrome

H50.611   Brown's sheath syndrome, right eye

H50.612   Brown's sheath syndrome, left eye

H50.69   Other mechanical strabismus

Strabismus due to adhesions

Traumatic limitation of duction of eye muscle

H50.8   Other specified strabismus

H50.81   Duane's syndrome

H50.811   Duane's syndrome, right eye

H50.812   Duane's syndrome, left eye

H50.89   Other specified strabismus

H50.9   Unspecified strabismus

H51   Other disorders of binocular movement

H51.0   Palsy (spasm) of conjugate gaze

H51.1   Convergence insufficiency and excess

H51.11   Convergence insufficiency

H51.12   Convergence excess

H51.2   Internuclear ophthalmoplegia

H51.20   Internuclear ophthalmoplegia, unspecified eye

H51.21   Internuclear ophthalmoplegia, right eye

H51.22   Internuclear ophthalmoplegia, left eye

H51.23   Internuclear ophthalmoplegia, bilateral

H51.8   Other specified disorders of binocular movement

H51.9   Unspecified disorder of binocular movement

H52   Disorders of refraction and accommodation

H52.0   Hypermetropia

H52.00   Hypermetropia, unspecified eye

H52.01   Hypermetropia, right eye

H52.02   Hypermetropia, left eye

H52.03   Hypermetropia, bilateral

H52.1   Myopia

Excludes1: degenerative myopia (H44.2-)

H52.10   Myopia, unspecified eye

H52.11   Myopia, right eye

H52.12   Myopia, left eye

H52.13   Myopia, bilateral

H52.2   Astigmatism

H52.20   Unspecified astigmatism

H52.201   Unspecified astigmatism, right eye

H52.202   Unspecified astigmatism, left eye

H52.203   Unspecified astigmatism, bilateral

H52.209   Unspecified astigmatism, unspecified eye

H52.21   Irregular astigmatism

H52.211   Irregular astigmatism, right eye

H52.212   Irregular astigmatism, left eye

H52.213   Irregular astigmatism, bilateral

H52.219   Irregular astigmatism, unspecified eye

H52.22   Regular astigmatism

H52.221   Regular astigmatism, right eye

H52.222   Regular astigmatism, left eye

H52.223   Regular astigmatism, bilateral

H52.229   Regular astigmatism, unspecified eye

H52.3   Anisometropia and aniseikonia

H52.31   Anisometropia

H52.32   Aniseikonia

H52.4   Presbyopia

H52.5   Disorders of accommodation

H52.51   Internal ophthalmoplegia (complete) (total)

H52.511   Internal ophthalmoplegia (complete) (total), right eye

H52.512   Internal ophthalmoplegia (complete) (total), left eye

H52.513   Internal ophthalmoplegia (complete) (total), bilateral

H52.519   Internal ophthalmoplegia (complete) (total), unspecified eye

H52.52   Paresis of accommodation

H52.521   Paresis of accommodation, right eye

H52.522   Paresis of accommodation, left eye

H52.523   Paresis of accommodation, bilateral

H52.529   Paresis of accommodation, unspecified eye

H52.53   Spasm of accommodation

H52.531   Spasm of accommodation, right eye

H52.532   Spasm of accommodation, left eye

H52.533   Spasm of accommodation, bilateral

H52.539   Spasm of accommodation, unspecified eye

H52.6   Other disorders of refraction

H52.7   Unspecified disorder of refraction

VISUAL DISTURBANCES AND BLINDNESS (H53-H54)

H53   Visual disturbances

H53.0   Amblyopia ex anopsia

Excludes1: amblyopia due to vitamin A deficiency (E50.5)

H53.00   Unspecified amblyopia

H53.001   Unspecified amblyopia, right eye

H53.002   Unspecified amblyopia, left eye

H53.003   Unspecified amblyopia, bilateral

H53.009   Unspecified amblyopia, unspecified eye

H53.01   Deprivation amblyopia

H53.011   Deprivation amblyopia, right eye

H53.012   Deprivation amblyopia, left eye

H53.013   Deprivation amblyopia, bilateral

H53.019   Deprivation amblyopia, unspecified eye

H53.02   Refractive amblyopia

H53.021   Refractive amblyopia, right eye

H53.022   Refractive amblyopia, left eye

H53.023   Refractive amblyopia, bilateral

H53.029   Refractive amblyopia, unspecified eye

H53.03   Strabismic amblyopia

Excludes1: strabismus (H50.-)

H53.031   Strabismic amblyopia, right eye

H53.032   Strabismic amblyopia, left eye

Add 4th-7th digits   Nonspecific code   Unspecified code   Manifestation code

H53.033 Strabismic amblyopia, bilateral

H53.039 Strabismic amblyopia, unspecified eye

H53.04 Amblyopia suspect

H53.041 Amblyopia suspect, right eye

H53.042 Amblyopia suspect, left eye

H53.043 Amblyopia suspect, bilateral

H53.049 Amblyopia suspect, unspecified eye

H53.1 Subjective visual disturbances

subjective visual disturbances due to vitamin A deficiency (E50.5)

visual hallucinations (R44.1)

H53.10 Unspecified subjective visual disturbances

H53.11 Day blindness

Hemeralopia

H53.12 Transient visual loss

Scintillating scotoma amaurosis fugax (G45.3-)

transient retinal artery occlusion (H34.0-)

H53.121 Transient visual loss, right eye

H53.122 Transient visual loss, left eye

H53.123 Transient visual loss, bilateral

H53.129 Transient visual loss, unspecified eye

H53.13 Sudden visual loss

H53.131 Sudden visual loss, right eye

H53.132 Sudden visual loss, left eye

H53.133 Sudden visual loss, bilateral

H53.139 Sudden visual loss, unspecified eye

H53.14 Visual discomfort

Asthenopia

Photophobia

H53.141 Visual discomfort, right eye

H53.142 Visual discomfort, left eye

H53.143 Visual discomfort, bilateral

H53.149 Visual discomfort, unspecified

H53.15 Visual distortions of shape and size

Metamorphopsia

H53.16 Psychophysical visual disturbances

H53.19 Other subjective visual disturbances

Visual halos

H53.2 Diplopia

Double vision

H53.3 Other and unspecified disorders of binocular vision

H53.30 Unspecified disorder of binocular vision

H53.31 Abnormal retinal correspondence

H53.32 Fusion with defective stereopsis

H53.33 Simultaneous visual perception without fusion

H53.34 Suppression of binocular vision

H53.4 Visual field defects

H53.40 Unspecified visual field defects

H53.41 Scotoma involving central area

Central scotoma

H53.411 Scotoma involving central area, right eye

H53.412 Scotoma involving central area, left eye

H53.413 Scotoma involving central area, bilateral

H53.419 Scotoma involving central area, unspecified eye

H53.42 Scotoma of blind spot area

Enlarged blind spot

H53.421 Scotoma of blind spot area, right eye

H53.422 Scotoma of blind spot area, left eye

H53.423 Scotoma of blind spot area, bilateral

H53.429 Scotoma of blind spot area, unspecified eye

H53.43 Sector or arcuate defects

Arcuate scotoma

Bjerrum scotoma

H53.431 Sector or arcuate defects, right eye

H53.432 Sector or arcuate defects, left eye

H53.433 Sector or arcuate defects, bilateral

H53.439 Sector or arcuate defects, unspecified eye

H53.45 Other localized visual field defect

Peripheral visual field defect

Ring scotoma NOS

Scotoma NOS

H53.451 Other localized visual field defect, right eye

H53.452 Other localized visual field defect, left eye

H53.453 Other localized visual field defect, bilateral

H53.459 Other localized visual field defect, unspecified eye

H53.46 Homonymous bilateral field defects

Homonymous hemianopia

Homonymous hemianopsia

Quadrant anopia

Quadrant anopsia

H53.461 Homonymous bilateral field defects, right side

H53.462 Homonymous bilateral field defects, left side

H53.469 Homonymous bilateral field defects, unspecified side

Homonymous bilateral field defects NOS

H53.47 Heteronymous bilateral field defects

Heteronymous hemianop(s)ia

H53.48 Generalized contraction of visual field

H53.481 Generalized contraction of visual field, right eye

H53.482 Generalized contraction of visual field, left eye

H53.483 Generalized contraction of visual field, bilateral

H53.489 Generalized contraction of visual field, unspecified eye

H53.5 Color vision deficiencies

Color blindness

Excludes2: day blindness (H53.11)

H53.50 Unspecified color vision deficiencies

Color blindness NOS

H53.51 Achromatopsia

H53.52 Acquired color vision deficiency

H53.53 **Deuteranomaly**

Deuteranopia

H53.54 **Protanomaly**

Protanopia

H53.55 **Tritanomaly**

Tritanopia

H53.59 **Other color vision deficiencies**

H53.6 **Night blindness**

Excludes1: night blindness due to vitamin A deficiency (E50.5)

H53.60 **Unspecified night blindness**

H53.61 **Abnormal dark adaptation curve**

H53.62 **Acquired night blindness**

H53.63 **Congenital night blindness**

H53.69 **Other night blindness**

H53.7 **Vision sensitivity deficiencies**

H53.71 **Glare sensitivity**

H53.72 **Impaired contrast sensitivity**

H53.8 **Other visual disturbances**

H53.9 **Unspecified visual disturbance**

H54 Blindness and low vision

Note: For definition of visual impairment categories see table below

Code first any associated underlying cause of the blindness

Excludes1: amaurosis fugax (G45.3)

H54.0 **Blindness, both eyes**

Visual impairment categories 3, 4, 5 in both eyes.

• H54.0X **Blindness, both eyes, different category levels**

• H54.0X3 **Blindness right eye, category 3**

• H54.0X33 **Blindness right eye category 3, blindness left eye category 3**

• H54.0X34 **Blindness right eye category 3, blindness left eye category 4**

• H54.0X35 **Blindness right eye category 3, blindness left eye category 5**

• H54.0X4 **Blindness right eye, category 4**

• H54.0X43 **Blindness right eye category 4, blindness left eye category 3**

• H54.0X44 **Blindness right eye category 4, blindness left eye category 4**

• H54.0X45 **Blindness right eye category 4, blindness left eye category 5**

• H54.0X5 **Blindness right eye, category 5**

• H54.0X53 **Blindness right eye category 5, blindness left eye category 3**

• H54.0X54 **Blindness right eye category 5, blindness left eye category 4**

• H54.0X55 **Blindness right eye category 5, blindness left eye category 5**

H54.1 **Blindness, one eye, low vision other eye**

Visual impairment categories 3, 4, 5 in one eye, with categories 1 or 2 in the other eye.

H54.10 **Blindness, one eye, low vision other eye, unspecified eyes**

H54.11 **Blindness, right eye, low vision left eye**

• H54.113 **Blindness right eye category 3, low vision left eye**

• H54.1131 **Blindness right eye category 3, low vision left eye category 1**

• H54.1132 **Blindness right eye category 3, low vision left eye category 2**

• H54.114 **Blindness right eye category 4, low vision left eye**

• H54.1141 **Blindness right eye category 4, low vision left eye category 1**

• H54.1142 **Blindness right eye category 4, low vision left eye category 2**

• H54.115 **Blindness right eye category 5, low vision left eye**

• H54.1151 **Blindness right eye category 5, low vision left eye category 1**

• H54.1152 **Blindness right eye category 5, low vision left eye category 2**

H54.12 **Blindness, left eye, low vision right eye**

• H54.121 **Low vision right eye category 1, blindness left eye**

• H54.1213 **Low vision right eye category 1, blindness left eye category 3**

• H54.1214 **Low vision right eye category 1, blindness left eye category 4**

• H54.1215 **Low vision right eye category 1, blindness left eye category 5**

• H54.122 **Low vision right eye category 2, blindness left eye**

• H54.1223 **Low vision right eye category 2, blindness left eye category 3**

• H54.1224 **Low vision right eye category 2, blindness left eye category 4**

• H54.1225 **Low vision right eye category 2, blindness left eye category 5**

H54.2 **Low vision, both eyes**

Visual impairment categories 1 or 2 in both eyes.

• H54.2X **Low vision, both eyes, different category levels**

• H54.2X1 **Low vision, right eye, category 1**

• H54.2X11 **Low vision right eye category 1, low vision left eye category 1**

• H54.2X12 **Low vision right eye category 1, low vision left eye category 2**

• H54.2X2 **Low vision, right eye, category 2**

• H54.2X21 **Low vision right eye category 2, low vision left eye category 1**

• H54.2X22 **Low vision right eye category 2, low vision left eye category 2**

H54.3 Unqualified visual loss, both eyes

Visual impairment category 9 in both eyes.

H54.4 Blindness, one eye

Visual impairment categories 3, 4, 5 in one eye [normal vision in other eye]

H54.40 Blindness, one eye, unspecified eye

H54.41 Blindness, right eye, normal vision left eye

- **H54.413 Blindness, right eye, category 3**
  - **H54.413A Blindness right eye category 3, normal vision left eye**
- **H54.414 Blindness, right eye, category 4**
  - **H54.414A Blindness right eye category 4, normal vision left eye**
- **H54.415 Blindness, right eye, category 5**
  - **H54.415A Blindness right eye category 5, normal vision left eye**

H54.42 Blindness, left eye, normal vision right eye

- **H54.42A Blindness, left eye, category 3-5**
  - **H54.42A3 Blindness left eye category 3, normal vision right eye**
  - **H54.42A4 Blindness left eye category 4, normal vision right eye**
  - **H54.42A5 Blindness left eye category 5, normal vision right eye**

H54.5 Low vision, one eye

Visual impairment categories 1 or 2 in one eye [normal vision in other eye].

H54.50 Low vision, one eye, unspecified eye

H54.51 Low vision, right eye, normal vision left eye

- **H54.511 Low vision, right eye, category 1-2**
  - **H54.511A Low vision right eye category 1, normal vision left eye**
  - **H54.512A Low vision right eye category 2, normal vision left eye**

H54.52 Low vision, left eye, normal vision right eye

- **H54.52A Low vision, left eye, category 1-2**
  - **H54.52A1 Low vision left eye category 1, normal vision right eye**
  - **H54.52A2 Low vision left eye category 2, normal vision right eye**
- **H54.414 Blindness, right eye, category 4**
  - **H54.414A Blindness right eye category 4, normal vision left eye**
- **H54.415 Blindness, right eye, category 5**
  - **H54.415A Blindness right eye category 5, normal vision left eye**

H54.6 Unqualified visual loss, one eye

Visual impairment category 9 in one eye [normal vision in other eye].

H54.60 Unqualified visual loss, one eye, unspecified

H54.61 Unqualified visual loss, right eye, normal vision left eye

H54.62 Unqualified visual loss, left eye, normal vision right eye

H54.7 Unspecified visual loss

Visual impairment category 9 NOS

H54.8 Legal blindness, as defined in USA

Blindness NOS according to USA definition legal blindness with specification of impairment level (H54.0-H54.7)

Note: The table below gives a classification of severity of visual impairment recommended by a WHO Study Group on the Prevention of Blindness, Geneva, 6-10 November 1972.

The term 'low vision' in category H54 comprises categories 1 and 2 of the table, the term 'blindness' categories 3, 4 and 5, and the term 'unqualified visual loss' category 9.

If the extent of the visual field is taken into account, patients with a field no greater than 10 but greater than 5 around central fixation should be placed in category 3 and patients with a field no greater than 5 around central fixation should be placed in category 4, even if the central acuity is not impaired. (Document 508 compliance requires all cells in the following table to be filled.)

Category of visual impairment	Visual acuity with best possible correction	
	Maximum less than:	Minimum equal to or better than:
-	6/18	6/60
3/10(0.3)	1/10(0.1)	-
20/70	20/200	-
-	6/60	3/60
1/10(0.1)	1/20(0.05	-
20/200	20/400	-
-	3/60	1/60(finger counting at one meter)
1/200(0.05)	1/50(0.02)	-
20/400	5/300(20/1200)	-
-	1/60(finger counting at one meter)	Light perception
1/50(0.02)	-	-
5/300	-	-
-	No light perception	-
-	Undetermined or unspecified	-

OTHER DISORDERS OF EYE AND ADNEXA (H55-H57)

H55 Nystagmus and other irregular eye movements

H55.0 Nystagmus

H55.00 Unspecified nystagmus

H55.01 Congenital nystagmus

H55.02 Latent nystagmus

H55.03 Visual deprivation nystagmus

H55.04 Dissociated nystagmus

H55.09 Other forms of nystagmus

H55.8 Other irregular eye movements

H55.81 Saccadic eye movements

H55.89 Other irregular eye movements

H57 Other disorders of eye and adnexa

H57.0 Anomalies of pupillary function

H57.00 Unspecified anomaly of pupillary function

H57.01 Argyll Robertson pupil, atypical

Excludes1: syphilitic Argyll Robertson pupil (A52.19)

H57.02 Anisocoria

H57.03 Miosis

H57.04 Mydriasis

H57.05 Tonic pupil

● New code　▲ Revised code　**Excludes1:** Not coded here　**Excludes2:** Not included here　⊗ Placeholder required　⑦7th digit required

H57.051　Tonic pupil, right eye

H57.052　Tonic pupil, left eye

H57.053　Tonic pupil, bilateral

H57.059　Tonic pupil, unspecified eye

H57.09　Other anomalies of pupillary function

H57.1　Ocular pain

H57.10　Ocular pain, unspecified eye

H57.11　Ocular pain, right eye

H57.12　Ocular pain, left eye

H57.13　Ocular pain, bilateral

H57.8　Other specified disorders of eye and adnexa

H57.9　Unspecified disorder of eye and adnexa

INTRAOPERATIVE AND POSTPROCEDURAL COMPLICATIONS AND DISORDERS OF EYE AND ADNEXA, NOT ELSEWHERE CLASSIFIED (H59)

H59　Intraoperative and postprocedural complications and disorders of eye and adnexa, not elsewhere classified

Excludes1: mechanical complication of intraocular lens (T85.2)

mechanical complication of other ocular prosthetic devices, implants and grafts (T85.3)

pseudophakia (Z96.1)

secondary cataracts (H26.4-)

H59.0　Disorders of the eye following cataract surgery

H59.01　Keratopathy (bullous aphakic) following cataract surgery

Vitreal corneal syndrome

Vitreous (touch) syndrome

H59.011　Keratopathy (bullous aphakic) following cataract surgery, right eye

H59.012　Keratopathy (bullous aphakic) following cataract surgery, left eye

H59.013　Keratopathy (bullous aphakic) following cataract surgery, bilateral

H59.019　Keratopathy (bullous aphakic) following cataract surgery, unspecified eye

H59.02　Cataract (lens) fragments in eye following cataract surgery

H59.021　Cataract (lens) fragments in eye following cataract surgery, right eye

H59.022　Cataract (lens) fragments in eye following cataract surgery, left eye

H59.023　Cataract (lens) fragments in eye following cataract surgery, bilateral

H59.029　Cataract (lens) fragments in eye following cataract surgery, unspecified eye

H59.03　Cystoid macular edema following cataract surgery

H59.031　Cystoid macular edema following cataract surgery, right eye

H59.032　Cystoid macular edema following cataract surgery, left eye

H59.033　Cystoid macular edema following cataract surgery, bilateral

H59.039　Cystoid macular edema following cataract surgery, unspecified eye

H59.09　Other disorders of the eye following cataract surgery

H59.091　Other disorders of the right eye following cataract surgery

H59.092　Other disorders of the left eye following cataract surgery

H59.093　Other disorders of the eye following cataract surgery, bilateral

H59.099　Other disorders of unspecified eye following cataract surgery

H59.1　Intraoperative hemorrhage and hematoma of eye and adnexa complicating a procedure

Excludes1: intraoperative hemorrhage and hematoma of eye and adnexa due to accidental puncture or laceration during a procedure (H59.2-)

H59.11　Intraoperative hemorrhage and hematoma of eye and adnexa complicating an ophthalmic procedure

H59.111　Intraoperative hemorrhage and hematoma of right eye and adnexa complicating an ophthalmic procedure

H59.112　Intraoperative hemorrhage and hematoma of left eye and adnexa complicating an ophthalmic procedure

H59.113　Intraoperative hemorrhage and hematoma of eye and adnexa complicating an ophthalmic procedure, bilateral

H59.119　Intraoperative hemorrhage and hematoma of unspecified eye and adnexa complicating an ophthalmic procedure

H59.12　Intraoperative hemorrhage and hematoma of eye and adnexa complicating other procedure

H59.121　Intraoperative hemorrhage and hematoma of right eye and adnexa complicating other procedure

H59.122　Intraoperative hemorrhage and hematoma of left eye and adnexa complicating other procedure

H59.123　Intraoperative hemorrhage and hematoma of eye and adnexa complicating other procedure, bilateral

H59.129　Intraoperative hemorrhage and hematoma of unspecified eye and adnexa complicating other procedure

H59.2　Accidental puncture and laceration of eye and adnexa during a procedure

H59.21　Accidental puncture and laceration of eye and adnexa during an ophthalmic procedure

H59.211　Accidental puncture and laceration of right eye and adnexa during an ophthalmic procedure

H59.212　Accidental puncture and laceration of left eye and adnexa during an ophthalmic procedure

H59.213　Accidental puncture and laceration of eye and adnexa during an ophthalmic procedure, bilateral

H59.219　Accidental puncture and laceration of unspecified eye and adnexa during an ophthalmic procedure

H59.22　Accidental puncture and laceration of eye and adnexa during other procedure

H59.221　Accidental puncture and laceration of right eye and adnexa during other procedure

H59.222 Accidental puncture and laceration of left eye and adnexa during other procedure

H59.223 Accidental puncture and laceration of eye and adnexa during other procedure, bilateral

H59.229 Accidental puncture and laceration of unspecified eye and adnexa during other procedure

H59.3 **Postprocedural hemorrhage, hematoma, and seroma of eye and adnexa following a procedure**

  H59.31 Postprocedural hemorrhage of eye and adnexa following an ophthalmic procedure

    H59.311 Postprocedural hemorrhage of right eye and adnexa following an ophthalmic procedure

    H59.312 Postprocedural hemorrhage of left eye and adnexa following an ophthalmic procedure

    H59.313 Postprocedural hemorrhage of eye and adnexa following an ophthalmic procedure, bilateral

    H59.319 Postprocedural hemorrhage of unspecified eye and adnexa following an ophthalmic procedure

  H59.32 Postprocedural hemorrhage of eye and adnexa following other procedure

    H59.321 Postprocedural hemorrhage of right eye and adnexa following other procedure

    H59.322 Postprocedural hemorrhage of left eye and adnexa following other procedure

    H59.323 Postprocedural hemorrhage of eye and adnexa following other procedure, bilateral

    H59.329 Postprocedural hemorrhage of unspecified eye and adnexa following other procedure

  H59.33 Postprocedural hematoma of eye and adnexa following an ophthalmic procedure

    H59.331 Postprocedural hematoma of right eye and adnexa following an ophthalmic procedure

    H59.332 Postprocedural hematoma of left eye and adnexa following an ophthalmic procedure

    H59.333 Postprocedural hematoma of eye and adnexa following an ophthalmic procedure, bilateral

    H59.339 Postprocedural hematoma of unspecified eye and adnexa following an ophthalmic procedure

  H59.34 Postprocedural hematoma of eye and adnexa following other procedure

    H59.341 Postprocedural hematoma of right eye and adnexa following other procedure

    H59.342 Postprocedural hematoma of left eye and adnexa following other procedure

    H59.343 Postprocedural hematoma of eye and adnexa following other procedure, bilateral

    H59.349 Postprocedural hematoma of unspecified eye and adnexa following other procedure

  H59.35 Postprocedural seroma of eye and adnexa following an ophthalmic procedure

    H59.351 Postprocedural seroma of right eye and adnexa following an ophthalmic procedure

    H59.352 Postprocedural seroma of left eye and adnexa following an ophthalmic procedure

    H59.353 Postprocedural seroma of eye and adnexa following an ophthalmic procedure, bilateral

    H59.359 Postprocedural seroma of unspecified eye and adnexa following an ophthalmic procedure

  H59.36 Postprocedural seroma of eye and adnexa following other procedure

    H59.361 Postprocedural seroma of right eye and adnexa following other procedure

    H59.362 Postprocedural seroma of left eye and adnexa following other procedure

    H59.363 Postprocedural seroma of eye and adnexa following other procedure, bilateral

    H59.369 Postprocedural seroma of unspecified eye and adnexa following other procedure

H59.4 **Inflammation (infection) of postprocedural bleb**

Postprocedural blebitis

Excludes1: filtering (vitreous) bleb after glaucoma surgery status (Z98.83)

  H59.40 Inflammation (infection) of postprocedural bleb, unspecified

  H59.41 Inflammation (infection) of postprocedural bleb, stage 1

  H59.42 Inflammation (infection) of postprocedural bleb, stage 2

  H59.43 Inflammation (infection) of postprocedural bleb, stage 3

Bleb endophthalmitis

H59.8 **Other intraoperative and postprocedural complications and disorders of eye and adnexa, not elsewhere classified**

  H59.81 Chorioretinal scars after surgery for detachment

    H59.811 Chorioretinal scars after surgery for detachment, right eye

    H59.812 Chorioretinal scars after surgery for detachment, left eye

    H59.813 Chorioretinal scars after surgery for detachment, bilateral

    H59.819 Chorioretinal scars after surgery for detachment, unspecified eye

  H59.88 Other intraoperative complications of eye and adnexa, not elsewhere classified

  H59.89 Other postprocedural complications and disorders of eye and adnexa, not elsewhere classified

Chapter 8: Diseases Of The Ear And Mastoid Process (H60-H95)

DEFINITIONS

This chapter includes definitions of selected key words, terms and phrases and coding alerts for adding points to the clinical domain, and references to coding late effects where appropriate. An example from this chapter is as follows:

H65   Nonsuppurative otitis media

> **Definition:** Nonsuppurative otitis media and eustachian tube disorders, otitis media is an inflammation of the middle ear without the formation or discharge of pus.

MULTIPLE CODING FOR A SINGLE CONDITION

In addition to the etiology/manifestation convention that requires two codes to fully describe a single condition that affects multiple body systems, there are other single conditions that also require more than one code. "Use additional code" notes are found in the Tabular List at codes that are not part of an etiology/manifestation pair where a secondary code is useful to fully describe a condition. The sequencing rule is the same as the etiology/manifestation pair, "use additional code" indicates that a secondary code should be added.

For example, for bacterial infections that are not included in chapter 1, a secondary code from category B95, Streptococcus, Staphylococcus, and Enterococcus, as the cause of diseases classified elsewhere, or B96, Other bacterial agents as the cause of diseases classified elsewhere, may be required to identify the bacterial organism causing the infection. A "use additional code" note will normally be found at the infectious disease code, indicating a need for the organism code to be added as a secondary code.

"Code first" notes are also under certain codes that are not specifically manifestation codes but may be due to an underlying cause. When there is a "code first" note and an underlying condition is present, the underlying condition should be sequenced first.

"Code, if applicable, any causal condition first", notes indicate that this code may be assigned as a principal diagnosis when the causal condition is unknown or not applicable. If a causal condition is known, then the code for that condition should be sequenced as the principal or first-listed diagnosis.

Multiple codes may be needed for sequela, complication codes and obstetric codes to more fully describe a condition. See the specific guidelines for these conditions for further instruction.

COMBINATION CODE

A combination code is a single code used to classify: Two diagnoses, or a diagnosis with an associated secondary process (manifestation) A diagnosis with an associated complication

Combination codes are identified by referring to subterm entries in the Alphabetic Index and by reading the inclusion and exclusion notes in the Tabular List.

Assign only the combination code when that code fully identifies the diagnostic conditions involved or when the Alphabetic Index so directs. Multiple coding should not be used when the classification provides a combination code that clearly identifies all of the elements documented in the diagnosis. When the combination code lacks necessary specificity in describing the manifestation or complication, an additional code should be used as a secondary code.

SEQUELA (LATE EFFECTS)

A sequela is the residual effect (condition produced) after the acute phase of an illness or injury has terminated. There is no time limit on when a sequela code can be used. The residual may be apparent early, such as in cerebral infarction, or it may occur months or years later, such as that due to a previous injury. Coding of sequela generally requires two codes sequenced in the following order: The condition or nature of the sequela is sequenced first.

The sequela code is sequenced second.

An exception to the above guidelines are those instances where the code for the sequela is followed by a manifestation code identified in the Tabular List and title, or the sequela code has been expanded (at the fourth, fifth or sixth character levels) to include the manifestation(s). The code for the acute phase of an illness or injury that led to the sequela is never used with a code for the late effect.

Chapter 8

Diseases Of The Ear And Mastoid Process (H60-H95)

Note: Use an external cause code following the code for the ear condition, if applicable, to identify the cause of the ear condition

Excludes2: certain conditions originating in the perinatal period (P04-P96)

certain infectious and parasitic diseases (A00-B99)

complications of pregnancy, childbirth and the puerperium (O00-O9A)

congenital malformations, deformations and chromosomal abnormalities (Q00-Q99)

endocrine, nutritional and metabolic diseases (E00-E88)

injury, poisoning and certain other consequences of external causes (S00-T88)

neoplasms (C00-D49)

symptoms, signs and abnormal clinical and laboratory findings, not elsewhere classified (R00-R94)

This chapter contains the following blocks:

H60-H62	Diseases of external ear
H65-H75	Diseases of middle ear and mastoid
H80-H83	Diseases of inner ear
H90-H94	Other disorders of ear
H95	Intraoperative and postprocedural complications and disorders of ear and mastoid process, not elsewhere classified

DISEASES OF EXTERNAL EAR (H60-H62)

H60 Otitis externa

H60.0 Abscess of external ear

Boil of external ear

Carbuncle of auricle or external auditory canal

Furuncle of external ear

H60.00 Abscess of external ear, unspecified ear

H60.01 Abscess of right external ear

H60.02 Abscess of left external ear

H60.03 Abscess of external ear, bilateral

H60.1 Cellulitis of external ear

Cellulitis of auricle

Cellulitis of external auditory canal

H60.10 Cellulitis of external ear, unspecified ear

H60.11 Cellulitis of right external ear

H60.12 Cellulitis of left external ear

H60.13 Cellulitis of external ear, bilateral

H60.2 Malignant otitis externa

H60.20 Malignant otitis externa, unspecified ear

H60.21 Malignant otitis externa, right ear

H60.22 Malignant otitis externa, left ear

H60.23 Malignant otitis externa, bilateral

H60.3 Other infective otitis externa

H60.31 Diffuse otitis externa

H60.311 Diffuse otitis externa, right ear

H60.312 Diffuse otitis externa, left ear

H60.313 Diffuse otitis externa, bilateral

H60.319 Diffuse otitis externa, unspecified ear

H60.32 Hemorrhagic otitis externa

H60.321 Hemorrhagic otitis externa, right ear

H60.322 Hemorrhagic otitis externa, left ear

H60.323 Hemorrhagic otitis externa, bilateral

H60.329 Hemorrhagic otitis externa, unspecified ear

H60.33 Swimmer's ear

H60.331 Swimmer's ear, right ear

H60.332 Swimmer's ear, left ear

H60.333 Swimmer's ear, bilateral

H60.339 Swimmer's ear, unspecified ear

H60.39 Other infective otitis externa

H60.391 Other infective otitis externa, right ear

H60.392 Other infective otitis externa, left ear

H60.393 Other infective otitis externa, bilateral

H60.399 Other infective otitis externa, unspecified ear

H60.4 Cholesteatoma of external ear

Keratosis obturans of external ear (canal)

Excludes2: cholesteatoma of middle ear (H71.-)

recurrent cholesteatoma of postmastoidectomy cavity (H95.0-)

H60.40 Cholesteatoma of external ear, unspecified ear

H60.41 Cholesteatoma of right external ear

H60.42 Cholesteatoma of left external ear

H60.43 Cholesteatoma of external ear, bilateral

H60.5 Acute noninfective otitis externa

H60.50 Unspecified acute noninfective otitis externa

Acute otitis externa NOS

H60.501 Unspecified acute noninfective otitis externa, right ear

H60.502 Unspecified acute noninfective otitis externa, left ear

H60.503 Unspecified acute noninfective otitis externa, bilateral

H60.509 Unspecified acute noninfective otitis externa, unspecified ear

H60.51 Acute actinic otitis externa

H60.511 Acute actinic otitis externa, right ear

H60.512 Acute actinic otitis externa, left ear

H60.513 Acute actinic otitis externa, bilateral

H60.519 Acute actinic otitis externa, unspecified ear

H60.52 Acute chemical otitis externa

H60.521 Acute chemical otitis externa, right ear

H60.522 Acute chemical otitis externa, left ear

H60.523 Acute chemical otitis externa, bilateral

H60.529 Acute chemical otitis externa, unspecified ear

H60.53 Acute contact otitis externa

H60.531 Acute contact otitis externa, right ear

H60.532 Acute contact otitis externa, left ear

H60.533 Acute contact otitis externa, bilateral

H60.539 Acute contact otitis externa, unspecified ear

H60.54 Acute eczematoid otitis externa

H60.541 Acute eczematoid otitis externa, right ear

H60.542 Acute eczematoid otitis externa, left ear

H60.543 **Acute eczematoid otitis externa, bilateral**

H60.549 **Acute eczematoid otitis externa, unspecified ear**

H60.55 **Acute reactive otitis externa**

H60.551 **Acute reactive otitis externa, right ear**

H60.552 **Acute reactive otitis externa, left ear**

H60.553 **Acute reactive otitis externa, bilateral**

H60.559 **Acute reactive otitis externa, unspecified ear**

H60.59 **Other noninfective acute otitis externa**

H60.591 **Other noninfective acute otitis externa, right ear**

H60.592 **Other noninfective acute otitis externa, left ear**

H60.593 **Other noninfective acute otitis externa, bilateral**

H60.599 **Other noninfective acute otitis externa, unspecified ear**

H60.6 **Unspecified chronic otitis externa**

H60.60 **Unspecified chronic otitis externa, unspecified ear**

H60.61 **Unspecified chronic otitis externa, right ear**

H60.62 **Unspecified chronic otitis externa, left ear**

H60.63 **Unspecified chronic otitis externa, bilateral**

H60.8 **Other otitis externa**

H60.8X **Other otitis externa**

H60.8X1 **Other otitis externa, right ear**

H60.8X2 **Other otitis externa, left ear**

H60.8X3 **Other otitis externa, bilateral**

H60.8X9 **Other otitis externa, unspecified ear**

H60.9 **Unspecified otitis externa**

H60.90 **Unspecified otitis externa, unspecified ear**

H60.91 **Unspecified otitis externa, right ear**

H60.92 **Unspecified otitis externa, left ear**

H60.93 **Unspecified otitis externa, bilateral**

H61 **Other disorders of external ear**

H61.0 **Chondritis and perichondritis of external ear**

Chondrodermatitis nodularis chronica helicis

Perichondritis of auricle

Perichondritis of pinna

H61.00 **Unspecified perichondritis of external ear**

H61.001 **Unspecified perichondritis of right external ear**

H61.002 **Unspecified perichondritis of left external ear**

H61.003 **Unspecified perichondritis of external ear, bilateral**

H61.009 **Unspecified perichondritis of external ear, unspecified ear**

H61.01 **Acute perichondritis of external ear**

H61.011 **Acute perichondritis of right external ear**

H61.012 **Acute perichondritis of left external ear**

H61.013 **Acute perichondritis of external ear, bilateral**

H61.019 **Acute perichondritis of external ear, unspecified ear**

H61.02 **Chronic perichondritis of external ear**

H61.021 **Chronic perichondritis of right external ear**

H61.022 **Chronic perichondritis of left external ear**

H61.023 **Chronic perichondritis of external ear, bilateral**

H61.029 **Chronic perichondritis of external ear, unspecified ear**

H61.03 **Chondritis of external ear**

Chondritis of auricle

Chondritis of pinna

H61.031 **Chondritis of right external ear**

H61.032 **Chondritis of left external ear**

H61.033 **Chondritis of external ear, bilateral**

H61.039 **Chondritis of external ear, unspecified ear**

H61.1 **Noninfective disorders of pinna**

Excludes2: cauliflower ear (M95.1-)

gouty tophi of ear (M1A.-)

H61.10 **Unspecified noninfective disorders of pinna**

Disorder of pinna NOS

H61.101 **Unspecified noninfective disorders of pinna, right ear**

H61.102 **Unspecified noninfective disorders of pinna, left ear**

H61.103 **Unspecified noninfective disorders of pinna, bilateral**

H61.109 **Unspecified noninfective disorders of pinna, unspecified ear**

H61.11 **Acquired deformity of pinna**

Acquired deformity of auricle

Excludes2: cauliflower ear (M95.1-)

H61.111 **Acquired deformity of pinna, right ear**

H61.112 **Acquired deformity of pinna, left ear**

H61.113 **Acquired deformity of pinna, bilateral**

H61.119 **Acquired deformity of pinna, unspecified ear**

H61.12 **Hematoma of pinna**

Hematoma of auricle

H61.121 **Hematoma of pinna, right ear**

H61.122 **Hematoma of pinna, left ear**

H61.123 **Hematoma of pinna, bilateral**

H61.129 **Hematoma of pinna, unspecified ear**

H61.19 **Other noninfective disorders of pinna**

H61.191 **Noninfective disorders of pinna, right ear**

H61.192 **Noninfective disorders of pinna, left ear**

H61.193 **Noninfective disorders of pinna, bilateral**

H61.199 **Noninfective disorders of pinna, unspecified ear**

H61.2 **Impacted cerumen**

Wax in ear

H61.20 **Impacted cerumen, unspecified ear**

H61.21 **Impacted cerumen, right ear**

H61.22 **Impacted cerumen, left ear**

● New code   ▲ Revised code   **Excludes1:** Not coded here   **Excludes2:** Not included here   ⊗ Placeholder required   ⑦7th digit required

H61.23 **Impacted cerumen, bilateral**

H61.3 **Acquired stenosis of external ear canal**

Collapse of external ear canal

Excludes1: postprocedural stenosis of external ear canal (H95.81-)

H61.30 **Acquired stenosis of external ear canal, unspecified**

    H61.301 **Acquired stenosis of right external ear canal, unspecified**

    H61.302 **Acquired stenosis of left external ear canal, unspecified**

    H61.303 **Acquired stenosis of external ear canal, unspecified, bilateral**

    H61.309 **Acquired stenosis of external ear canal, unspecified, unspecified ear**

H61.31 **Acquired stenosis of external ear canal secondary to trauma**

    H61.311 **Acquired stenosis of right external ear canal secondary to trauma**

    H61.312 **Acquired stenosis of left external ear canal secondary to trauma**

    H61.313 **Acquired stenosis of external ear canal secondary to trauma, bilateral**

    H61.319 **Acquired stenosis of external ear canal secondary to trauma, unspecified ear**

H61.32 **Acquired stenosis of external ear canal secondary to inflammation and infection**

    H61.321 **Acquired stenosis of right external ear canal secondary to inflammation and infection**

    H61.322 **Acquired stenosis of left external ear canal secondary to inflammation and infection**

    H61.323 **Acquired stenosis of external ear canal secondary to inflammation and infection, bilateral**

    H61.329 **Acquired stenosis of external ear canal secondary to inflammation and infection, unspecified ear**

H61.39 **Other acquired stenosis of external ear canal**

    H61.391 **Other acquired stenosis of right external ear canal**

    H61.392 **Other acquired stenosis of left external ear canal**

    H61.393 **Other acquired stenosis of external ear canal, bilateral**

    H61.399 **Other acquired stenosis of external ear canal, unspecified ear**

H61.8 **Other specified disorders of external ear**

H61.81 **Exostosis of external canal**

    H61.811 **Exostosis of right external canal**

    H61.812 **Exostosis of left external canal**

    H61.813 **Exostosis of external canal, bilateral**

    H61.819 **Exostosis of external canal, unspecified ear**

H61.89 **Other specified disorders of external ear**

    H61.891 **Other specified disorders of right external ear**

    H61.892 **Other specified disorders of left external ear**

    H61.893 **Other specified disorders of external ear, bilateral**

    H61.899 **Other specified disorders of external ear, unspecified ear**

H61.9 **Disorder of external ear, unspecified**

H61.90 **Disorder of external ear, unspecified, unspecified ear**

H61.91 **Disorder of right external ear, unspecified**

H61.92 **Disorder of left external ear, unspecified**

H61.93 **Disorder of external ear, unspecified, bilateral**

H62 **Disorders of external ear in diseases classified elsewhere**

H62.4 **Otitis externa in other diseases classified elsewhere**

Code first underlying disease, such as:

erysipelas (A46)

impetigo (L01.0)

Excludes1: otitis externa (in):

candidiasis (B37.84)

herpes viral [herpes simplex] (B00.1)

herpes zoster (B02.8)

H62.40 **Otitis externa in other diseases classified elsewhere, unspecified ear**

H62.41 **Otitis externa in other diseases classified elsewhere, right ear**

H62.42 **Otitis externa in other diseases classified elsewhere, left ear**

H62.43 **Otitis externa in other diseases classified elsewhere, bilateral**

H62.8 **Other disorders of external ear in diseases classified elsewhere**

Code first underlying disease, such as:

gout (M1A.-, M10.-)

H62.8X **Other disorders of external ear in diseases classified elsewhere**

    H62.8X1 **Other disorders of right external ear in diseases classified elsewhere**

    H62.8X2 **Other disorders of left external ear in diseases classified elsewhere**

    H62.8X3 **Other disorders of external ear in diseases classified elsewhere, bilateral**

    H62.8X9 **Other disorders of external ear in diseases classified elsewhere, unspecified ear**

DISEASES OF MIDDLE EAR AND MASTOID (H65-H75)

H65 **Nonsuppurative otitis media**

Definition: Nonsuppurative otitis media and eustachian tube disorders, otitis media is an inflammation of the middle ear without the formation or discharge of pus.

Includes: nonsuppurative otitis media with myringitis

Use additional code for any associated perforated tympanic membrane (H72.-)

Use additional code to identify:

exposure to environmental tobacco smoke (Z77.22)

exposure to tobacco smoke in the perinatal period (P96.81)

history of tobacco dependence (Z87.891)

occupational exposure to environmental tobacco smoke (Z57.31)

tobacco dependence (F17.-)

tobacco use (Z72.0)

H65.0 **Acute serous otitis media**

Acute and subacute secretory otitis

H65.00 **Acute serous otitis media, unspecified ear**

H65.01 Acute serous otitis media, right ear

H65.02 Acute serous otitis media, left ear

H65.03 Acute serous otitis media, bilateral

H65.04 Acute serous otitis media, recurrent, right ear

H65.05 Acute serous otitis media, recurrent, left ear

H65.06 Acute serous otitis media, recurrent, bilateral

H65.07 Acute serous otitis media, recurrent, unspecified ear

H65.1 Other acute nonsuppurative otitis media

Excludes1: otitic barotrauma (T70.0)

otitis media (acute) NOS (H66.9)

H65.11 Acute and subacute allergic otitis media (mucoid) (sanguinous) (serous)

H65.111 Acute and subacute allergic otitis media (mucoid) (sanguinous) (serous), right ear

H65.112 Acute and subacute allergic otitis media (mucoid) (sanguinous) (serous), left ear

H65.113 Acute and subacute allergic otitis media (mucoid) (sanguinous) (serous), bilateral

H65.114 Acute and subacute allergic otitis media (mucoid) (sanguinous) (serous), recurrent, right ear

H65.115 Acute and subacute allergic otitis media (mucoid) (sanguinous) (serous), recurrent, left ear

H65.116 Acute and subacute allergic otitis media (mucoid) (sanguinous) (serous), recurrent, bilateral

H65.117 Acute and subacute allergic otitis media (mucoid) (sanguinous) (serous), recurrent, unspecified ear

H65.119 Acute and subacute allergic otitis media (mucoid) (sanguinous) (serous), unspecified ear

H65.19 Other acute nonsuppurative otitis media

Acute and subacute mucoid otitis media

Acute and subacute nonsuppurative otitis media NOS

Acute and subacute sanguinous otitis media

Acute and subacute seromucinous otitis media

H65.191 Other acute nonsuppurative otitis media, right ear

H65.192 Other acute nonsuppurative otitis media, left ear

H65.193 Other acute nonsuppurative otitis media, bilateral

H65.194 Other acute nonsuppurative otitis media, recurrent, right ear

H65.195 Other acute nonsuppurative otitis media, recurrent, left ear

H65.196 Other acute nonsuppurative otitis media, recurrent, bilateral

H65.197 Other acute nonsuppurative otitis media recurrent, unspecified ear

H65.199 Other acute nonsuppurative otitis media, unspecified ear

H65.2 Chronic serous otitis media

Chronic tubotympanal catarrh

H65.20 Chronic serous otitis media, unspecified ear

H65.21 Chronic serous otitis media, right ear

H65.22 Chronic serous otitis media, left ear

H65.23 Chronic serous otitis media, bilateral

H65.3 Chronic mucoid otitis media

Chronic mucinous otitis media

Chronic secretory otitis media

Chronic transudative otitis media Glue ear

Excludes1: adhesive middle ear disease (H74.1)

H65.30 Chronic mucoid otitis media, unspecified ear

H65.31 Chronic mucoid otitis media, right ear

H65.32 Chronic mucoid otitis media, left ear

H65.33 Chronic mucoid otitis media, bilateral

H65.4 Other chronic nonsuppurative otitis media

H65.41 Chronic allergic otitis media

H65.411 Chronic allergic otitis media, right ear

H65.412 Chronic allergic otitis media, left ear

H65.413 Chronic allergic otitis media, bilateral

H65.419 Chronic allergic otitis media, unspecified ear

H65.49 Other chronic nonsuppurative otitis media

Chronic exudative otitis media

Chronic nonsuppurative otitis media NOS

Chronic otitis media with effusion (nonpurulent)

Chronic seromucinous otitis media

H65.491 Other chronic nonsuppurative otitis media, right ear

H65.492 Other chronic nonsuppurative otitis media, left ear

H65.493 Other chronic nonsuppurative otitis media, bilateral

H65.499 Other chronic nonsuppurative otitis media, unspecified ear

H65.9 Unspecified nonsuppurative otitis media

Allergic otitis media NOS

Catarrhal otitis media NOS

Exudative otitis media NOS

Mucoid otitis media NOS

Otitis media with effusion (nonpurulent) NOS

Secretory otitis media NOS

Seromucinous otitis media NOS

Serous otitis media NOS

Transudative otitis media NOS

H65.90 Unspecified nonsuppurative otitis media, unspecified ear

H65.91 Unspecified nonsuppurative otitis media, right ear

H65.92 Unspecified nonsuppurative otitis media, left ear

H65.93 Unspecified nonsuppurative otitis media, bilateral

H66 Suppurative and unspecified otitis media

Definition: Suppurative and unspecified otitis media is an inflammation of the middle ear including the formation or discharge of pus.

Includes: suppurative and unspecified otitis media with myringitis

Use additional code to identify:

exposure to environmental tobacco smoke (Z77.22)

exposure to tobacco smoke in the perinatal period (P96.81)

history of tobacco dependence (Z87.891)

occupational exposure to environmental tobacco smoke (Z57.31)

tobacco dependence (F17.-)

tobacco use (Z72.0)

H66.0   Acute suppurative otitis media

 H66.00   Acute suppurative otitis media without spontaneous rupture of ear drum

  H66.001   Acute suppurative otitis media without spontaneous rupture of ear drum, right ear

  H66.002   Acute suppurative otitis media without spontaneous rupture of ear drum, left ear

  H66.003   Acute suppurative otitis media without spontaneous rupture of ear drum, bilateral

  H66.004   Acute suppurative otitis media without spontaneous rupture of ear drum, recurrent, right ear

  H66.005   Acute suppurative otitis media without spontaneous rupture of ear drum, recurrent, left ear

  H66.006   Acute suppurative otitis media without spontaneous rupture of ear drum, recurrent, bilateral

  H66.007   Acute suppurative otitis media without spontaneous rupture of ear drum, recurrent, unspecified ear

  H66.009   Acute suppurative otitis media without spontaneous rupture of ear drum, unspecified ear

 H66.01   Acute suppurative otitis media with spontaneous rupture of ear drum

  H66.011   Acute suppurative otitis media with spontaneous rupture of ear drum, right ear

  H66.012   Acute suppurative otitis media with spontaneous rupture of ear drum, left ear

  H66.013   Acute suppurative otitis media with spontaneous rupture of ear drum, bilateral

  H66.014   Acute suppurative otitis media with spontaneous rupture of ear drum, recurrent, right ear

  H66.015   Acute suppurative otitis media with spontaneous rupture of ear drum, recurrent, left ear

  H66.016   Acute suppurative otitis media with spontaneous rupture of ear drum, recurrent, bilateral

  H66.017   Acute suppurative otitis media with spontaneous rupture of ear drum, recurrent, unspecified ear

  H66.019   Acute suppurative otitis media with spontaneous rupture of ear drum, unspecified ear

H66.1   Chronic tubotympanic suppurative otitis media

Benign chronic suppurative otitis media

Chronic tubotympanic disease

Use additional code for any associated perforated tympanic membrane (H72.-)

 H66.10   Chronic tubotympanic suppurative otitis media, unspecified

 H66.11   Chronic tubotympanic suppurative otitis media, right ear

 H66.12   Chronic tubotympanic suppurative otitis media, left ear

 H66.13   Chronic tubotympanic suppurative otitis media, bilateral

H66.2   Chronic atticoantral suppurative otitis media

Chronic atticoantral disease

Use additional code for any associated perforated tympanic membrane (H72.-)

 H66.20   Chronic atticoantral suppurative otitis media, unspecified ear

 H66.21   Chronic atticoantral suppurative otitis media, right ear

 H66.22   Chronic atticoantral suppurative otitis media, left ear

 H66.23   Chronic atticoantral suppurative otitis media, bilateral

H66.3   Other chronic suppurative otitis media

Chronic suppurative otitis media NOS

Use additional code for any associated perforated tympanic membrane (H72.-)

Excludes1: tuberculous otitis media (A18.6)

 H66.3X   Other chronic suppurative otitis media

  H66.3X1   Other chronic suppurative otitis media, right ear

  H66.3X2   Other chronic suppurative otitis media, left ear

  H66.3X3   Other chronic suppurative otitis media, bilateral

  H66.3X9   Other chronic suppurative otitis media, unspecified ear

H66.4   Suppurative otitis media, unspecified

Purulent otitis media NOS

Use additional code for any associated perforated tympanic membrane (H72.-)

 H66.40   Suppurative otitis media, unspecified, unspecified ear

 H66.41   Suppurative otitis media, unspecified, right ear

 H66.42   Suppurative otitis media, unspecified, left ear

 H66.43   Suppurative otitis media, unspecified, bilateral

H66.9   Otitis media, unspecified

Otitis media NOS

Acute otitis media NOS

Chronic otitis media NOS

Use additional code for any associated perforated tympanic membrane (H72.-)

 H66.90   Otitis media, unspecified, unspecified ear

 H66.91   Otitis media, unspecified, right ear

 H66.92   Otitis media, unspecified, left ear

 H66.93   Otitis media, unspecified, bilateral

H67   Otitis media in diseases classified elsewhere

Code first underlying disease, such as:

viral disease NEC (B00-B34)

Use additional code for any associated perforated tympanic membrane (H72.-)

Excludes1: otitis media in:

influenza (J09.X9, J10.83, J11.83)

measles (B05.3)

scarlet fever (A38.0)

tuberculosis (A18.6)

H67.1   Otitis media in diseases classified elsewhere, right ear

H67.2   Otitis media in diseases classified elsewhere, left ear

H67.3   Otitis media in diseases classified elsewhere, bilateral

H67.9   Otitis media in diseases classified elsewhere, unspecified ear

H68   Eustachian salpingitis and obstruction

   H68.0   Eustachian salpingitis

     H68.00   Unspecified Eustachian salpingitis

       H68.001   Unspecified Eustachian salpingitis, right ear

       H68.002   Unspecified Eustachian salpingitis, left ear

       H68.003   Unspecified Eustachian salpingitis, bilateral

       H68.009   Unspecified Eustachian salpingitis, unspecified ear

     H68.01   Acute Eustachian salpingitis

       H68.011   Acute Eustachian salpingitis, right ear

       H68.012   Acute Eustachian salpingitis, left ear

       H68.013   Acute Eustachian salpingitis, bilateral

       H68.019   Acute Eustachian salpingitis, unspecified ear

     H68.02   Chronic Eustachian salpingitis

       H68.021   Chronic Eustachian salpingitis, right ear

       H68.022   Chronic Eustachian salpingitis, left ear

       H68.023   Chronic Eustachian salpingitis, bilateral

       H68.029   Chronic Eustachian salpingitis, unspecified ear

   H68.1   Obstruction of Eustachian tube

     Stenosis of Eustachian tube

     Stricture of Eustachian tube

     H68.10   Unspecified obstruction of Eustachian tube

       H68.101   Unspecified obstruction of Eustachian tube, right ear

       H68.102   Unspecified obstruction of Eustachian tube, left ear

       H68.103   Unspecified obstruction of Eustachian tube, bilateral

       H68.109   Unspecified obstruction of Eustachian tube, unspecified ear

     H68.11   Osseous obstruction of Eustachian tube

       H68.111   Osseous obstruction of Eustachian tube, right ear

       H68.112   Osseous obstruction of Eustachian tube, left ear

       H68.113   Osseous obstruction of Eustachian tube, bilateral

       H68.119   Osseous obstruction of Eustachian tube, unspecified ear

     H68.12   Intrinsic cartilaginous obstruction of Eustachian tube

       H68.121   Intrinsic cartilaginous obstruction of Eustachian tube, right ear

       H68.122   Intrinsic cartilaginous obstruction of Eustachian tube, left ear

       H68.123   Intrinsic cartilaginous obstruction of Eustachian tube, bilateral

       H68.129   Intrinsic cartilaginous obstruction of Eustachian tube, unspecified ear

     H68.13   Extrinsic cartilaginous obstruction of Eustachian tube

     Compression of Eustachian tube

       H68.131   Extrinsic cartilaginous obstruction of Eustachian tube, right ear

       H68.132   Extrinsic cartilaginous obstruction of Eustachian tube, left ear

       H68.133   Extrinsic cartilaginous obstruction of Eustachian tube, bilateral

       H68.139   Extrinsic cartilaginous obstruction of Eustachian tube, unspecified ear

H69   Other and unspecified disorders of Eustachian tube

   H69.0   Patulous Eustachian tube

     H69.00   Patulous Eustachian tube, unspecified ear

     H69.01   Patulous Eustachian tube, right ear

     H69.02   Patulous Eustachian tube, left ear

     H69.03   Patulous Eustachian tube, bilateral

   H69.8   Other specified disorders of Eustachian tube

     H69.80   Other specified disorders of Eustachian tube, unspecified ear

     H69.81   Other specified disorders of Eustachian tube, right ear

     H69.82   Other specified disorders of Eustachian tube, left ear

     H69.83   Other specified disorders of Eustachian tube, bilateral

   H69.9   Unspecified Eustachian tube disorder

     H69.90   Unspecified Eustachian tube disorder, unspecified ear

     H69.91   Unspecified Eustachian tube disorder, right ear

     H69.92   Unspecified Eustachian tube disorder, left ear

     H69.93   Unspecified Eustachian tube disorder, bilateral

H70   Mastoiditis and related conditions

   Definition: Mastoiditis is an infection of the spaces within the mastoid bone. It is almost always associated with otitis media, an infection of the middle ear. In the most serious cases, the bone itself becomes infected.

   H70.0   Acute mastoiditis

     Abscess of mastoid Empyema of mastoid

     H70.00   Acute mastoiditis without complications

       H70.001   Acute mastoiditis without complications, right ear

       H70.002   Acute mastoiditis without complications, left ear

       H70.003   Acute mastoiditis without complications, bilateral

       H70.009   Acute mastoiditis without complications, unspecified ear

     H70.01   Subperiosteal abscess of mastoid

       H70.011   Subperiosteal abscess of mastoid, right ear

       H70.012   Subperiosteal abscess of mastoid, left ear

       H70.013   Subperiosteal abscess of mastoid, bilateral

       H70.019   Subperiosteal abscess of mastoid, unspecified ear

     H70.09   Acute mastoiditis with other complications

H70.091 **Acute mastoiditis with other complications, right ear**

H70.092 **Acute mastoiditis with other complications, left ear**

H70.093 **Acute mastoiditis with other complications, bilateral**

H70.099 **Acute mastoiditis with other complications, unspecified ear**

H70.1 **Chronic mastoiditis**

Caries of mastoid

Fistula of mastoid

Excludes1: tuberculous mastoiditis (A18.03)

H70.10 **Chronic mastoiditis, unspecified ear**

H70.11 **Chronic mastoiditis, right ear**

H70.12 **Chronic mastoiditis, left ear**

H70.13 **Chronic mastoiditis, bilateral**

H70.2 **Petrositis**

Inflammation of petrous bone

H70.20 **Unspecified petrositis**

H70.201 **Unspecified petrositis, right ear**

H70.202 **Unspecified petrositis, left ear**

H70.203 **Unspecified petrositis, bilateral**

H70.209 **Unspecified petrositis, unspecified ear**

H70.21 **Acute petrositis**

H70.211 **Acute petrositis, right ear**

H70.212 **Acute petrositis, left ear**

H70.213 **Acute petrositis, bilateral**

H70.219 **Acute petrositis, unspecified ear**

H70.22 **Chronic petrositis**

H70.221 **Chronic petrositis, right ear**

H70.222 **Chronic petrositis, left ear**

H70.223 **Chronic petrositis, bilateral**

H70.229 **Chronic petrositis, unspecified ear**

H70.8 **Other mastoiditis and related conditions**

Excludes1: preauricular sinus and cyst (Q18.1)

sinus, fistula, and cyst of branchial cleft (Q18.0)

H70.81 **Postauricular fistula**

H70.811 **Postauricular fistula, right ear**

H70.812 **Postauricular fistula, left ear**

H70.813 **Postauricular fistula, bilateral**

H70.819 **Postauricular fistula, unspecified ear**

H70.89 **Other mastoiditis and related conditions**

H70.891 **Other mastoiditis and related conditions, right ear**

H70.892 **Other mastoiditis and related conditions, left ear**

H70.893 **Other mastoiditis and related conditions, bilateral**

H70.899 **Other mastoiditis and related conditions, unspecified ear**

H70.9 **Unspecified mastoiditis**

H70.90 **Unspecified mastoiditis, unspecified ear**

H70.91 **Unspecified mastoiditis, right ear**

H70.92 **Unspecified mastoiditis, left ear**

H70.93 **Unspecified mastoiditis, bilateral**

H71 **Cholesteatoma of middle ear**

Excludes2: cholesteatoma of external ear (H60.4-)

recurrent cholesteatoma of postmastoidectomy cavity (H95.0-)

H71.0 **Cholesteatoma of attic**

H71.00 **Cholesteatoma of attic, unspecified ear**

H71.01 **Cholesteatoma of attic, right ear**

H71.02 **Cholesteatoma of attic, left ear**

H71.03 **Cholesteatoma of attic, bilateral**

H71.1 **Cholesteatoma of tympanum**

H71.10 **Cholesteatoma of tympanum, unspecified ear**

H71.11 **Cholesteatoma of tympanum, right ear**

H71.12 **Cholesteatoma of tympanum, left ear**

H71.13 **Cholesteatoma of tympanum, bilateral**

H71.2 **Cholesteatoma of mastoid**

H71.20 **Cholesteatoma of mastoid, unspecified ear**

H71.21 **Cholesteatoma of mastoid, right ear**

H71.22 **Cholesteatoma of mastoid, left ear**

H71.23 **Cholesteatoma of mastoid, bilateral**

H71.3 **Diffuse cholesteatosis**

H71.30 **Diffuse cholesteatosis, unspecified ear**

H71.31 **Diffuse cholesteatosis, right ear**

H71.32 **Diffuse cholesteatosis, left ear**

H71.33 **Diffuse cholesteatosis, bilateral**

H71.9 **Unspecified cholesteatoma**

H71.90 **Unspecified cholesteatoma, unspecified ear**

H71.91 **Unspecified cholesteatoma, right ear**

H71.92 **Unspecified cholesteatoma, left ear**

H71.93 **Unspecified cholesteatoma, bilateral**

H72 **Perforation of tympanic membrane**

Includes: persistent post-traumatic perforation of ear drum

postinflammatory perforation of ear drum

Code first any associated otitis media (H65.-, H66.1-, H66.2-, H66.3-, H66.4-, H66.9-, H67.-)

Excludes1: acute suppurative otitis media with rupture of the tympanic membrane (H66.01-)

traumatic rupture of ear drum (S09.2-)

H72.0 **Central perforation of tympanic membrane**

H72.00 **Central perforation of tympanic membrane, unspecified ear**

H72.01 **Central perforation of tympanic membrane, right ear**

H72.02 **Central perforation of tympanic membrane, left ear**

H72.03 **Central perforation of tympanic membrane, bilateral**

H72.1 **Attic perforation of tympanic membrane**

Perforation of pars flaccida

H72.10 **Attic perforation of tympanic membrane, unspecified ear**

H72.11 **Attic perforation of tympanic membrane, right ear**

H72.12 **Attic perforation of tympanic membrane, left ear**

H72.13 **Attic perforation of tympanic membrane, bilateral**

H72.2 **Other marginal perforations of tympanic membrane**

H72.2X **Other marginal perforations of tympanic membrane**

H72.2X1 **Other marginal perforations of tympanic membrane, right ear**

H72.2X2 Other marginal perforations of tympanic membrane, left ear

H72.2X3 Other marginal perforations of tympanic membrane, bilateral

H72.2X9 Other marginal perforations of tympanic membrane, unspecified ear

H72.8 Other perforations of tympanic membrane

H72.81 Multiple perforations of tympanic membrane

H72.811 Multiple perforations of tympanic membrane, right ear

H72.812 Multiple perforations of tympanic membrane, left ear

H72.813 Multiple perforations of tympanic membrane, bilateral

H72.819 Multiple perforations of tympanic membrane, unspecified ear

H72.82 Total perforations of tympanic membrane

H72.821 Total perforations of tympanic membrane, right ear

H72.822 Total perforations of tympanic membrane, left ear

H72.823 Total perforations of tympanic membrane, bilateral

H72.829 Total perforations of tympanic membrane, unspecified ear

H72.9 Unspecified perforation of tympanic membrane

H72.90 Unspecified perforation of tympanic membrane, unspecified ear

H72.91 Unspecified perforation of tympanic membrane, right ear

H72.92 Unspecified perforation of tympanic membrane, left ear

H72.93 Unspecified perforation of tympanic membrane, bilateral

H73 Other disorders of tympanic membrane

H73.0 Acute myringitis

Excludes1: acute myringitis with otitis media (H65, H66)

H73.00 Unspecified acute myringitis

Acute tympanitis NOS

H73.001 Acute myringitis, right ear

H73.002 Acute myringitis, left ear

H73.003 Acute myringitis, bilateral

H73.009 Acute myringitis, unspecified ear

H73.01 Bullous myringitis

H73.011 Bullous myringitis, right ear

H73.012 Bullous myringitis, left ear

H73.013 Bullous myringitis, bilateral

H73.019 Bullous myringitis, unspecified ear

H73.09 Other acute myringitis

H73.091 Other acute myringitis, right ear

H73.092 Other acute myringitis, left ear

H73.093 Other acute myringitis, bilateral

H73.099 Other acute myringitis, unspecified ear

H73.1 Chronic myringitis

Chronic tympanitis

Excludes1: chronic myringitis with otitis media (H65, H66)

H73.10 Chronic myringitis, unspecified ear

H73.11 Chronic myringitis, right ear

H73.12 Chronic myringitis, left ear

H73.13 Chronic myringitis, bilateral

H73.2 Unspecified myringitis

H73.20 Unspecified myringitis, unspecified ear

H73.21 Unspecified myringitis, right ear

H73.22 Unspecified myringitis, left ear

H73.23 Unspecified myringitis, bilateral

H73.8 Other specified disorders of tympanic membrane

H73.81 Atrophic flaccid tympanic membrane

H73.811 Atrophic flaccid tympanic membrane, right ear

H73.812 Atrophic flaccid tympanic membrane, left ear

H73.813 Atrophic flaccid tympanic membrane, bilateral

H73.819 Atrophic flaccid tympanic membrane, unspecified ear

H73.82 Atrophic nonflaccid tympanic membrane

H73.821 Atrophic nonflaccid tympanic membrane, right ear

H73.822 Atrophic nonflaccid tympanic membrane, left ear

H73.823 Atrophic nonflaccid tympanic membrane, bilateral

H73.829 Atrophic nonflaccid tympanic membrane, unspecified ear

H73.89 Other specified disorders of tympanic membrane

H73.891 Other specified disorders of tympanic membrane, right ear

H73.892 Other specified disorders of tympanic membrane, left ear

H73.893 Other specified disorders of tympanic membrane, bilateral

H73.899 Other specified disorders of tympanic membrane, unspecified ear

H73.9 Unspecified disorder of tympanic membrane

H73.90 Unspecified disorder of tympanic membrane, unspecified ear

H73.91 Unspecified disorder of tympanic membrane, right ear

H73.92 Unspecified disorder of tympanic membrane, left ear

H73.93 Unspecified disorder of tympanic membrane, bilateral

H74 OTHER DISORDERS OF MIDDLE EAR MASTOID

Definition: The middle ear is the space between the eardrum and the inner ear that contains the three auditory ossicles, which convey vibrations through the oval window to the cochlea. The mastoid is the bone located directly behind the external ear.

Excludes2: mastoiditis (H70.-)

H74.0 Tympanosclerosis

H74.01 Tympanosclerosis, right ear

H74.02 Tympanosclerosis, left ear

H74.03 Tympanosclerosis, bilateral

H74.09 Tympanosclerosis, unspecified ear

H74.1 Adhesive middle ear disease

Adhesive otitis

Excludes1: glue ear (H65.3-)

H74.11 Adhesive right middle ear disease

H74.12 Adhesive left middle ear disease

● New code ▲ Revised code **Excludes1:** Not coded here **Excludes2:** Not included here ⊗ Placeholder required ⑦ 7th digit required

H74.13 Adhesive middle ear disease, bilateral

H74.19 Adhesive middle ear disease, unspecified ear

H74.2 Discontinuity and dislocation of ear ossicles

H74.20 Discontinuity and dislocation of ear ossicles, unspecified ear

H74.21 Discontinuity and dislocation of right ear ossicles

H74.22 Discontinuity and dislocation of left ear ossicles

H74.23 Discontinuity and dislocation of ear ossicles, bilateral

H74.3 Other acquired abnormalities of ear ossicles

H74.31 Ankylosis of ear ossicles

H74.311 Ankylosis of ear ossicles, right ear

H74.312 Ankylosis of ear ossicles, left ear

H74.313 Ankylosis of ear ossicles, bilateral

H74.319 Ankylosis of ear ossicles, unspecified ear

H74.32 Partial loss of ear ossicles

H74.321 Partial loss of ear ossicles, right ear

H74.322 Partial loss of ear ossicles, left ear

H74.323 Partial loss of ear ossicles, bilateral

H74.329 Partial loss of ear ossicles, unspecified ear

H74.39 Other acquired abnormalities of ear ossicles

H74.391 Other acquired abnormalities of right ear ossicles

H74.392 Other acquired abnormalities of left ear ossicles

H74.393 Other acquired abnormalities of ear ossicles, bilateral

H74.399 Other acquired abnormalities of ear ossicles, unspecified ear

H74.4 Polyp of middle ear

H74.40 Polyp of middle ear, unspecified ear

H74.41 Polyp of right middle ear

H74.42 Polyp of left middle ear

H74.43 Polyp of middle ear, bilateral

H74.8 Other specified disorders of middle ear and mastoid

H74.8X Other specified disorders of middle ear and mastoid

H74.8X1 Other specified disorders of right middle ear and mastoid

H74.8X2 Other specified disorders of left middle ear and mastoid

H74.8X3 Other specified disorders of middle ear and mastoid, bilateral

H74.8X9 Other specified disorders of middle ear and mastoid, unspecified ear

H74.9 Unspecified disorder of middle ear and mastoid

H74.90 Unspecified disorder of middle ear and mastoid, unspecified ear

H74.91 Unspecified disorder of right middle ear and mastoid

H74.92 Unspecified disorder of left middle ear and mastoid

H74.93 Unspecified disorder of middle ear and mastoid, bilateral

H75 OTHER DISORDERS OF MIDDLE EAR AND MASTOID IN DISEASES CLASSIFIED ELSEWHERE

Code first underlying disease

H75.0 Mastoiditis in infectious and parasitic diseases classified elsewhere

Excludes1: mastoiditis (in):

syphilis (A52.77)

tuberculosis (A18.03)

H75.00 Mastoiditis in infectious and parasitic diseases classified elsewhere, unspecified ear

H75.01 Mastoiditis in infectious and parasitic diseases classified elsewhere, right ear

H75.02 Mastoiditis in infectious and parasitic diseases classified elsewhere, left ear

H75.03 Mastoiditis in infectious and parasitic diseases classified elsewhere, bilateral

H75.8 Other specified disorders of middle ear and mastoid in diseases classified elsewhere

H75.80 Other specified disorders of middle ear and mastoid in diseases classified elsewhere, unspecified ear

H75.81 Other specified disorders of right middle ear and mastoid in diseases classified elsewhere

H75.82 Other specified disorders of left middle ear and mastoid in diseases classified elsewhere

H75.83 Other specified disorders of middle ear and mastoid in diseases classified elsewhere, bilateral

DISEASES OF INNER EAR (H80-H83)

H80 Otosclerosis

Includes: Otospongiosis

H80.0 Otosclerosis involving oval window, nonobliterative

H80.00 Otosclerosis involving oval window, nonobliterative, unspecified ear

H80.01 Otosclerosis involving oval window, nonobliterative, right ear

H80.02 Otosclerosis involving oval window, nonobliterative, left ear

H80.03 Otosclerosis involving oval window, nonobliterative, bilateral

H80.1 Otosclerosis involving oval window, obliterative

H80.10 Otosclerosis involving oval window, obliterative, unspecified ear

H80.11 Otosclerosis involving oval window, obliterative, right ear

H80.12 Otosclerosis involving oval window, obliterative, left ear

H80.13 Otosclerosis involving oval window, obliterative, bilateral

H80.2 Cochlear otosclerosis

Otosclerosis involving otic capsule

Otosclerosis involving round window

H80.20 Cochlear otosclerosis, unspecified ear

H80.21 Cochlear otosclerosis, right ear

H80.22 Cochlear otosclerosis, left ear

H80.23 Cochlear otosclerosis, bilateral

H80.8 Other otosclerosis

H80.80 Other otosclerosis, unspecified ear

H80.81 Other otosclerosis, right ear

H80.82 Other otosclerosis, left ear

H80.83 Other otosclerosis, bilateral

H80.9 Unspecified otosclerosis

H80.90 Unspecified otosclerosis, unspecified ear

Add 4th-7th digits   Nonspecific code   Unspecified code   Manifestation code

H80.91   Unspecified otosclerosis, right ear
H80.92   Unspecified otosclerosis, left ear
H80.93   Unspecified otosclerosis, bilateral

H81   **Disorders of vestibular function**

Excludes1: epidemic vertigo (A88.1)

vertigo NOS (R42)

H81.0   **Ménière's disease**

Labyrinthine hydrops

Ménière's syndrome or vertigo

H81.01   **Ménière's disease, right ear**
H81.02   **Ménière's disease, left ear**
H81.03   **Ménière's disease, bilateral**
H81.09   **Ménière's disease, unspecified ear**

H81.1   **Benign paroxysmal vertigo**

H81.10   **Benign paroxysmal vertigo, unspecified ear**
H81.11   **Benign paroxysmal vertigo, right ear**
H81.12   **Benign paroxysmal vertigo, left ear**
H81.13   **Benign paroxysmal vertigo, bilateral**

H81.2   **Vestibular neuronitis**

H81.20   **Vestibular neuronitis, unspecified ear**
H81.21   **Vestibular neuronitis, right ear**
H81.22   **Vestibular neuronitis, left ear**
H81.23   **Vestibular neuronitis, bilateral**

H81.3   **Other peripheral vertigo**

H81.31   **Aural vertigo**

H81.311   **Aural vertigo, right ear**
H81.312   **Aural vertigo, left ear**
H81.313   **Aural vertigo, bilateral**
H81.319   **Aural vertigo, unspecified ear**

H81.39   **Other peripheral vertigo**

Lermoyez' syndrome

Otogenic vertigo

Peripheral vertigo NOS

H81.391   **Other peripheral vertigo, right ear**
H81.392   **Other peripheral vertigo, left ear**
H81.393   **Other peripheral vertigo, bilateral**
H81.399   **Other peripheral vertigo, unspecified ear**

H81.4   **Vertigo of central origin**

Central positional nystagmus

H81.41   **Vertigo of central origin, right ear**
H81.42   **Vertigo of central origin, left ear**
H81.43   **Vertigo of central origin, bilateral**
H81.49   **Vertigo of central origin, unspecified ear**

H81.8   **Other disorders of vestibular function**

H81.8X   **Other disorders of vestibular function**

H81.8X1   **Other disorders of vestibular function, right ear**
H81.8X2   **Other disorders of vestibular function, left ear**
H81.8X3   **Other disorders of vestibular function, bilateral**
H81.8X9   **Other disorders of vestibular function, unspecified ear**

H81.9   **Unspecified disorder of vestibular function**

Vertiginous syndrome NOS

H81.90   **Unspecified disorder of vestibular function, unspecified ear**

H81.91   Unspecified disorder of vestibular function, right ear
H81.92   Unspecified disorder of vestibular function, left ear
H81.93   Unspecified disorder of vestibular function, bilateral

H82   **Vertiginous syndromes in diseases classified elsewhere**

Code first underlying disease

Excludes1: epidemic vertigo (A88.1)

H82.1   **Vertiginous syndromes in diseases classified elsewhere, right ear**
H82.2   **Vertiginous syndromes in diseases classified elsewhere, left ear**
H82.3   **Vertiginous syndromes in diseases classified elsewhere, bilateral**
H82.9   **Vertiginous syndromes in diseases classified elsewhere, unspecified ear**

H83   **Other diseases of inner ear**

H83.0   **Labyrinthitis**

H83.01   **Labyrinthitis, right ear**
H83.02   **Labyrinthitis, left ear**
H83.03   **Labyrinthitis, bilateral**
H83.09   **Labyrinthitis, unspecified ear**

H83.1   **Labyrinthine fistula**

H83.11   **Labyrinthine fistula, right ear**
H83.12   **Labyrinthine fistula, left ear**
H83.13   **Labyrinthine fistula, bilateral**
H83.19   **Labyrinthine fistula, unspecified ear**

H83.2   **Labyrinthine dysfunction**

Labyrinthine hypersensitivity

Labyrinthine hypofunction

Labyrinthine loss of function

H83.2X   **Labyrinthine dysfunction**

H83.2X1   **Labyrinthine dysfunction, right ear**
H83.2X2   **Labyrinthine dysfunction, left ear**
H83.2X3   **Labyrinthine dysfunction, bilateral**
H83.2X9   **Labyrinthine dysfunction, unspecified ear**

H83.3   **Noise effects on inner ear**

Acoustic trauma of inner ear

Noise-induced hearing loss of inner ear

H83.3X   **Noise effects on inner ear**

H83.3X1   **Noise effects on right inner ear**
H83.3X2   **Noise effects on left inner ear**
H83.3X3   **Noise effects on inner ear, bilateral**
H83.3X9   **Noise effects on inner ear, unspecified ear**

H83.8   **Other specified diseases of inner ear**

H83.8X   **Other specified diseases of inner ear**

H83.8X1   **Other specified diseases of right inner ear**
H83.8X2   **Other specified diseases of left inner ear**
H83.8X3   **Other specified diseases of inner ear, bilateral**
H83.8X9   **Other specified diseases of inner ear, unspecified ear**

H83.9   **Unspecified disease of inner ear**

H83.90   **Unspecified disease of inner ear, unspecified ear**
H83.91   **Unspecified disease of right inner ear**

● New code   ▲ Revised code   **Excludes1:** Not coded here   **Excludes2:** Not included here   ⊗ Placeholder required   ⑦7th digit required

H83.92 Unspecified disease of left inner ear

H83.93 Unspecified disease of inner ear, bilateral

OTHER DISORDERS OF EAR (H90-H94)

H90 **Conductive and sensorineural hearing loss**

Excludes1: deaf nonspeaking NEC (H91.3)

deafness NOS (H91.9-)

hearing loss NOS (H91.9-)

noise-induced hearing loss (H83.3-)

ototoxic hearing loss (H91.0-)

sudden (idiopathic) hearing loss (H91.2-)

H90.0 **Conductive hearing loss, bilateral**

H90.1 **Conductive hearing loss, unilateral with unrestricted hearing on the contralateral side**

H90.11 Conductive hearing loss, unilateral, right ear, with unrestricted hearing on the contralateral side

H90.12 Conductive hearing loss, unilateral, left ear, with unrestricted hearing on the contralateral side

H90.2 **Conductive hearing loss, unspecified**

Conductive deafness NOS

H90.3 **Sensorineural hearing loss, bilateral**

H90.4 **Sensorineural hearing loss, unilateral with unrestricted hearing on the contralateral side**

H90.41 Sensorineural hearing loss, unilateral, right ear, with unrestricted hearing on the contralateral side

H90.42 Sensorineural hearing loss, unilateral, left ear, with unrestricted hearing on the contralateral side

H90.5 **Unspecified sensorineural hearing loss**

Central hearing loss NOS

Congenital deafness NOS

Neural hearing loss NOS

Perceptive hearing loss NOS

Sensorineural deafness NOS

Sensory hearing loss NOS

Excludes1: abnormal auditory perception (H93.2-)

psychogenic deafness (F44.6)

H90.6 **Mixed conductive and sensorineural hearing loss, bilateral**

H90.7 **Mixed conductive and sensorineural hearing loss, unilateral with unrestricted hearing on the contralateral side**

H90.71 Mixed conductive and sensorineural hearing loss, unilateral, right ear, with unrestricted hearing on the contralateral side

H90.72 Mixed conductive and sensorineural hearing loss, unilateral, left ear, with unrestricted hearing on the contralateral side

H90.8 **Mixed conductive and sensorineural hearing loss, unspecified**

H90.A **Conductive and sensorineural hearing loss with restricted hearing on the contralateral side**

H90.A1 Conductive hearing loss, unilateral, with restricted hearing on the contralateral side

H90.A11 Conductive hearing loss, unilateral, right ear with restricted hearing on the contralateral side

H90.A12 Conductive hearing loss, unilateral, left ear with restricted hearing on the contralateral side

H90.A2 Sensorineural hearing loss, unilateral, with restricted hearing on the contralateral side

H90.A21 Sensorineural hearing loss, unilateral, right ear, with restricted hearing on the contralateral side

H90.A22 Sensorineural hearing loss, unilateral, left ear, with restricted hearing on the contralateral side

H90.A3 Mixed conductive and sensorineural hearing loss, unilateral with restricted hearing on the contralateral side

H90.A31 Mixed conductive and sensorineural hearing loss, unilateral, right ear with restricted hearing on the contralateral side

H90.A32 Mixed conductive and sensorineural hearing loss, unilateral, left ear with restricted hearing on the contralateral side

H91 **Other and unspecified hearing loss**

Excludes1: abnormal auditory perception (H93.2-)

hearing loss as classified in H90.-

impacted cerumen (H61.2-)

noise-induced hearing loss (H83.3-)

psychogenic deafness (F44.6)

transient ischemic deafness (H93.01-)

H91.0 **Ototoxic hearing loss**

Code first poisoning due to drug or toxin, if applicable (T36-T65 with fifth or sixth character 1-4 or 6)

Use additional code for adverse effect, if applicable, to identify drug (T36-T50 with fifth or sixth character 5)

H91.01 Ototoxic hearing loss, right ear

H91.02 Ototoxic hearing loss, left ear

H91.03 Ototoxic hearing loss, bilateral

H91.09 Ototoxic hearing loss, unspecified ear

H91.1 **Presbycusis**

Presbyacusia

H91.10 Presbycusis, unspecified ear

H91.11 Presbycusis, right ear

H91.12 Presbycusis, left ear

H91.13 Presbycusis, bilateral

H91.2 **Sudden idiopathic hearing loss**

Sudden hearing loss NOS

H91.20 Sudden idiopathic hearing loss, unspecified ear

H91.21 Sudden idiopathic hearing loss, right ear

H91.22 Sudden idiopathic hearing loss, left ear

H91.23 Sudden idiopathic hearing loss, bilateral

H91.3 **Deaf nonspeaking, not elsewhere classified**

H91.8 **Other specified hearing loss**

H91.8X Other specified hearing loss

H91.8X1 Other specified hearing loss, right ear

H91.8X2 Other specified hearing loss, left ear

H91.8X3 Other specified hearing loss, bilateral

H91.8X9 Other specified hearing loss, unspecified ear

H91.9 **Unspecified hearing loss**

Deafness NOS

Add 4th-7th digits	Nonspecific code	Unspecified code	Manifestation code

High frequency deafness

Low frequency deafness

H91.90 Unspecified hearing loss, unspecified ear

H91.91 Unspecified hearing loss, right ear

H91.92 Unspecified hearing loss, left ear

H91.93 Unspecified hearing loss, bilateral

H92 Otalgia and effusion of ear

H92.0 Otalgia

H92.01 Otalgia, right ear

H92.02 Otalgia, left ear

H92.03 Otalgia, bilateral

H92.09 Otalgia, unspecified ear

H92.1 Otorrhea

Excludes1: leakage of cerebrospinal fluid through ear (G96.0)

H92.10 Otorrhea, unspecified ear

H92.11 Otorrhea, right ear

H92.12 Otorrhea, left ear

H92.13 Otorrhea, bilateral

H92.2 Otorrhagia

Excludes1: traumatic otorrhagia - code to injury

H92.20 Otorrhagia, unspecified ear

H92.21 Otorrhagia, right ear

H92.22 Otorrhagia, left ear

H92.23 Otorrhagia, bilateral

H93 Other disorders of ear, not elsewhere classified

H93.0 Degenerative and vascular disorders of ear

Excludes1: presbycusis (H91.1)

H93.01 Transient ischemic deafness

H93.011 Transient ischemic deafness, right ear

H93.012 Transient ischemic deafness, left ear

H93.013 Transient ischemic deafness, bilateral

H93.019 Transient ischemic deafness, unspecified ear

H93.09 Unspecified degenerative and vascular disorders of ear

H93.091 Unspecified degenerative and vascular disorders of right ear

H93.092 Unspecified degenerative and vascular disorders of left ear

H93.093 Unspecified degenerative and vascular disorders of ear, bilateral

H93.099 Unspecified degenerative and vascular disorders of unspecified ear

H93.1 Tinnitus

H93.11 Tinnitus, right ear

H93.12 Tinnitus, left ear

H93.13 Tinnitus, bilateral

H93.19 Tinnitus, unspecified ear

H93.A Pulsatile tinnitus

H93.A1 Pulsatile tinnitus, right ear

H93.A2 Pulsatile tinnitus, left ear

H93.A3 Pulsatile tinnitus, bilateral

H93.A9 Pulsatile tinnitus, unspecified ear

H93.2 Other abnormal auditory perceptions

Excludes2: auditory hallucinations (R44.0)

H93.21 Auditory recruitment

H93.211 Auditory recruitment, right ear

H93.212 Auditory recruitment, left ear

H93.213 Auditory recruitment, bilateral

H93.219 Auditory recruitment, unspecified ear

H93.22 Diplacusis

H93.221 Diplacusis, right ear

H93.222 Diplacusis, left ear

H93.223 Diplacusis, bilateral

H93.229 Diplacusis, unspecified ear

H93.23 Hyperacusis

H93.231 Hyperacusis, right ear

H93.232 Hyperacusis, left ear

H93.233 Hyperacusis, bilateral

H93.239 Hyperacusis, unspecified ear

H93.24 Temporary auditory threshold shift

H93.241 Temporary auditory threshold shift, right ear

H93.242 Temporary auditory threshold shift, left ear

H93.243 Temporary auditory threshold shift, bilateral

H93.249 Temporary auditory threshold shift, unspecified ear

H93.25 Central auditory processing disorder

Congenital auditory imperception Word deafness

Excludes1: mixed receptive-expressive language disorder (F80.2)

H93.29 Other abnormal auditory perceptions

H93.291 Other abnormal auditory perceptions, right ear

H93.292 Other abnormal auditory perceptions, left ear

H93.293 Other abnormal auditory perceptions, bilateral

H93.299 Other abnormal auditory perceptions, unspecified ear

H93.3 Disorders of acoustic nerve

Disorder of 8th cranial nerve

Excludes1: acoustic neuroma (D33.3)

syphilitic acoustic neuritis (A52.15)

H93.3X Disorders of acoustic nerve

H93.3X1 Disorders of right acoustic nerve

H93.3X2 Disorders of left acoustic nerve

H93.3X3 Disorders of bilateral acoustic nerves

H93.3X9 Disorders of unspecified acoustic nerve

H93.8 Other specified disorders of ear

H93.8X Other specified disorders of ear

H93.8X1 Other specified disorders of right ear

H93.8X2 Other specified disorders of left ear

H93.8X3 Other specified disorders of ear, bilateral

H93.8X9 Other specified disorders of ear, unspecified ear

H93.9 Unspecified disorder of ear

H93.90 Unspecified disorder of ear, unspecified ear

H93.91 Unspecified disorder of right ear

H93.92 Unspecified disorder of left ear

H93.93 Unspecified disorder of ear, bilateral

● New code ▲ Revised code **Excludes1:** Not coded here **Excludes2:** Not included here ⊗ Placeholder required ⑦7th digit required

H94 **Other disorders of ear in diseases classified elsewhere**

H94.0 **Acoustic neuritis in infectious and parasitic diseases classified elsewhere**

<u>Code first</u> underlying disease, such as:

parasitic disease (B65-B89)

Excludes1: acoustic neuritis (in):

herpes zoster (B02.29)

syphilis (A52.15)

H94.00 **Acoustic neuritis in infectious and parasitic diseases classified elsewhere, unspecified ear**

H94.01 **Acoustic neuritis in infectious and parasitic diseases classified elsewhere, right ear**

H94.02 **Acoustic neuritis in infectious and parasitic diseases classified elsewhere, left ear**

H94.03 **Acoustic neuritis in infectious and parasitic diseases classified elsewhere, bilateral**

H94.8 **Other specified disorders of ear in diseases classified elsewhere**

<u>Code first</u> underlying disease, such as:

congenital syphilis (A50.0)

Excludes1: aural myiasis (B87.4)

syphilitic labyrinthitis (A52.79)

H94.80 **Other specified disorders of ear in diseases classified elsewhere, unspecified ear**

H94.81 **Other specified disorders of right ear in diseases classified elsewhere**

H94.82 **Other specified disorders of left ear in diseases classified elsewhere**

H94.83 **Other specified disorders of ear in diseases classified elsewhere, bilateral**

INTRAOPERATIVE AND POSTPROCEDURAL COMPLICATIONS AND DISORDERS OF EAR AND MASTOID PROCESS, NOT ELSEWHERE CLASSIFIED (H95)

H95 **Intraoperative and postprocedural complications and disorders of ear and mastoid process, not elsewhere classified**

H95.0 **Recurrent cholesteatoma of postmastoidectomy cavity**

H95.00 **Recurrent cholesteatoma of postmastoidectomy cavity, unspecified ear**

H95.01 **Recurrent cholesteatoma of postmastoidectomy cavity, right ear**

H95.02 **Recurrent cholesteatoma of postmastoidectomy cavity, left ear**

H95.03 **Recurrent cholesteatoma of postmastoidectomy cavity, bilateral ears**

H95.1 **Other disorders of ear and mastoid process following mastoidectomy**

H95.11 **Chronic inflammation of postmastoidectomy cavity**

H95.111 **Chronic inflammation of postmastoidectomy cavity, right ear**

H95.112 **Chronic inflammation of postmastoidectomy cavity, left ear**

H95.113 **Chronic inflammation of postmastoidectomy cavity, bilateral ears**

H95.119 **Chronic inflammation of postmastoidectomy cavity, unspecified ear**

H95.12 **Granulation of postmastoidectomy cavity**

H95.121 **Granulation of postmastoidectomy cavity, right ear**

H95.122 **Granulation of postmastoidectomy cavity, left ear**

H95.123 **Granulation of postmastoidectomy cavity, bilateral ears**

H95.129 **Granulation of postmastoidectomy cavity, unspecified ear**

H95.13 **Mucosal cyst of postmastoidectomy cavity**

H95.131 **Mucosal cyst of postmastoidectomy cavity, right ear**

H95.132 **Mucosal cyst of postmastoidectomy cavity, left ear**

H95.133 **Mucosal cyst of postmastoidectomy cavity, bilateral ears**

H95.139 **Mucosal cyst of postmastoidectomy cavity, unspecified ear**

H95.19 **Other disorders following mastoidectomy**

H95.191 **Other disorders following mastoidectomy, right ear**

H95.192 **Other disorders following mastoidectomy, left ear**

H95.193 **Other disorders following mastoidectomy, bilateral ears**

H95.199 **Other disorders following mastoidectomy, unspecified ear**

H95.2 **Intraoperative hemorrhage and hematoma of ear and mastoid process complicating a procedure**

Excludes1: intraoperative hemorrhage and hematoma of ear and mastoid process due to accidental puncture or laceration during a procedure (H95.3-)

H95.21 **Intraoperative hemorrhage and hematoma of ear and mastoid process complicating a procedure on the ear and mastoid process**

H95.22 **Intraoperative hemorrhage and hematoma of ear and mastoid process complicating other procedure**

H95.3 **Accidental puncture and laceration of ear and mastoid process during a procedure**

H95.31 **Accidental puncture and laceration of the ear and mastoid process during a procedure on the ear and mastoid process**

H95.32 **Accidental puncture and laceration of the ear and mastoid process during other procedure**

H95.4 **Postprocedural hemorrhage of ear and mastoid process following a procedure**

H95.41 **Postprocedural hemorrhage of ear and mastoid process following a procedure on the ear and mastoid process**

H95.42 **Postprocedural hemorrhage of ear and mastoid process following other procedure**

H95.5 **Postprocedural hematoma and seroma of ear and mastoid process following a procedure**

H95.51 **Postprocedural hematoma of ear and mastoid process following a procedure on the ear and mastoid process**

H95.52 **Postprocedural hematoma of ear and mastoid process following other procedure**

H95.53 **Postprocedural seroma of ear and mastoid process following a procedure on the ear and mastoid process**

H95.54 **Postprocedural seroma of ear and mastoid process following other procedure**

H95.8 **Other intraoperative and postprocedural complications and disorders of the ear and mastoid process, not elsewhere classified**

Excludes2: postprocedural complications and disorders following mastoidectomy (H95.0-, H95.1-)

H95.81 **Postprocedural stenosis of external ear canal**

    H95.811 **Postprocedural stenosis of right external ear canal**

    H95.812 **Postprocedural stenosis of left external ear canal**

    H95.813 **Postprocedural stenosis of external ear canal, bilateral**

    H95.819 **Postprocedural stenosis of unspecified external ear canal**

H95.88 **Other intraoperative complications and disorders of the ear and mastoid process, not elsewhere classified**

    <u>Use additional code</u> , if applicable, to further specify disorder

H95.89 **Other postprocedural complications and disorders of the ear and mastoid process, not elsewhere classified**

    <u>Use additional code</u>, if applicable, to further specify disorder

Chapter 9: Diseases Of The Circulatory System (I00-I99)

DEFINITIONS

This chapter includes definitions of selected key words, terms and phrases and coding alerts for adding points to the clinical domain, and references to coding late effects where appropriate. An example from this chapter is as follows:

I12   Hypertensive chronic kidney disease
Definition: Hypertensive chronic kidney disease, refers to diseases of the kidney caused by high blood pressure.

MULTIPLE CODING FOR A SINGLE CONDITION

In addition to the etiology/manifestation convention that requires two codes to fully describe a single condition that affects multiple body systems, there are other single conditions that also require more than one code. "Use additional code" notes are found in the Tabular List at codes that are not part of an etiology/manifestation pair where a secondary code is useful to fully describe a condition. The sequencing rule is the same as the etiology/manifestation pair, "use additional code" indicates that a secondary code should be added.

For example, for bacterial infections that are not included in chapter 1, a secondary code from category B95, Streptococcus, Staphylococcus, and Enterococcus, as the cause of diseases classified elsewhere, or B96, Other bacterial agents as the cause of diseases classified elsewhere, may be required to identify the bacterial organism causing the infection. A "use additional code" note will normally be found at the infectious disease code, indicating a need for the organism code to be added as a secondary code.

"Code first" notes are also under certain codes that are not specifically manifestation codes but may be due to an underlying cause. When there is a "code first" note and an underlying condition is present, the underlying condition should be sequenced first.

"Code, if applicable, any causal condition first", notes indicate that this code may be assigned as a principal diagnosis when the causal condition is unknown or not applicable. If a causal condition is known, then the code for that condition should be sequenced as the principal or first-listed diagnosis.

Multiple codes may be needed for sequela, complication codes and obstetric codes to more fully describe a condition. See the specific guidelines for these conditions for further instruction.

COMBINATION CODE

A combination code is a single code used to classify: Two diagnoses, or a diagnosis with an associated secondary process (manifestation) A diagnosis with an associated complication

Combination codes are identified by referring to subterm entries in the Alphabetic Index and by reading the inclusion and exclusion notes in the Tabular List.

Assign only the combination code when that code fully identifies the diagnostic conditions involved or when the Alphabetic Index so directs. Multiple coding should not be used when the classification provides a combination code that clearly identifies all of the elements documented in the diagnosis. When the combination code lacks necessary specificity in describing the manifestation or complication, an additional code should be used as a secondary code.

SEQUELA (LATE EFFECTS)

A sequela is the residual effect (condition produced) after the acute phase of an illness or injury has terminated. There is no time limit on when a sequela code can be used. The residual may be apparent early, such as in cerebral infarction, or it may occur months or years later, such as that due to a previous injury. Coding of sequela generally requires two codes sequenced in the following order: The condition or nature of the sequela is sequenced first.

The sequela code is sequenced second.

An exception to the above guidelines are those instances where the code for the sequela is followed by a manifestation code identified in the Tabular List and title, or the sequela code has been expanded (at the fourth, fifth or sixth character levels) to include the manifestation(s). The code for the acute phase of an illness or injury that led to the sequela is never used with a code for the late effect.

HYPERTENSION

The classification presumes a causal relationship between hypertension and heart involvement and between hypertension and kidney involvement, as the two conditions are linked by the term "with" in the Alphabetic Index. These conditions should be coded as related even in the absence of provider documentation explicitly linking them, unless the documentation clearly states the conditions are unrelated.

For hypertension and conditions not specifically linked by relational terms such as "with," "associated with" or "due to" in the classification, provider documentation must link the conditions in order to code them as related.

1)   **Hypertension with Heart Disease**

Hypertension with heart conditions classified to I50.- or I51.4-I51.9, are assigned to a code from category I11, Hypertensive heart disease. Use an additional code from category I50, Heart failure, to identify the type of heart failure in those patients with heart failure.

The same heart conditions (I50.-, I51.4-I51.9) with hypertension are coded separately if the provider has specifically documented a different cause. Sequence according to the circumstances of the admission/encounter.

2)   **Hypertensive Chronic Kidney Disease**

Assign codes from category I12, Hypertensive chronic kidney disease, when both hypertension and a condition classifiable to category N18, Chronic kidney disease (CKD), are present. CKD should not be coded as hypertensive if the physician has specifically documented a different cause.

The appropriate code from category N18 should be used as a secondary code with a code from category I12 to identify the stage of chronic kidney disease.

See Section I.C.14. Chronic kidney disease.

If a patient has hypertensive chronic kidney disease and acute renal failure, an additional code for the acute renal failure is required.

3) **Hypertensive Heart and Chronic Kidney Disease**

Assign codes from combination category I13, Hypertensive heart and chronic kidney disease, when there is hypertension with both heart and kidney involvement. If heart failure is present, assign an additional code from category I50 to identify the type of heart failure.

The appropriate code from category N18, Chronic kidney disease, should be used as a secondary code with a code from category I13 to identify the stage of chronic kidney disease.

See Section I.C.14. Chronic kidney disease.

The codes in category I13, Hypertensive heart and chronic kidney disease, are combination codes that include hypertension, heart disease and chronic kidney disease. The Includes note at I13 specifies that the conditions included at I11 and I12 are included together in I13. If a patient has hypertension, heart disease and chronic kidney disease, then a code from I13 should be used, not individual codes for hypertension, heart disease and chronic kidney disease, or codes from I11 or I12.

For patients with both acute renal failure and chronic kidney disease, an additional code for acute renal failure is required.

4) **Hypertensive Cerebrovascular Disease**

For hypertensive cerebrovascular disease, first assign the appropriate code from categories I60-I69, followed by the appropriate hypertension code.

5) **Hypertensive Retinopathy**

Subcategory H35.0, Background retinopathy and retinal vascular changes, should be used with a code from category I10 – I15, Hypertensive disease to include the systemic hypertension. The sequencing is based on the reason for the encounter.

6) **Hypertension, Secondary**

Secondary hypertension is due to an underlying condition. Two codes are required: one to identify the underlying etiology and one from category I15 to identify the hypertension. Sequencing of codes is determined by the reason for admission/encounter.

7) **Hypertension, Transient**

Assign code R03.0, Elevated blood pressure reading without diagnosis of hypertension, unless patient has an established diagnosis of hypertension. Assign code O13.-, Gestational [pregnancy-induced] hypertension without significant proteinuria, or O14.-, Pre-eclampsia, for transient hypertension of pregnancy.

8) **Hypertension, Controlled**

This diagnostic statement usually refers to an existing state of hypertension under control by therapy. Assign the appropriate code from categories I10-I15, Hypertensive diseases.

9) **Hypertension, Uncontrolled**

Uncontrolled hypertension may refer to untreated hypertension or hypertension not responding to current therapeutic regimen. In either case, assign the appropriate code from categories I10-I15, Hypertensive diseases.

10) **Hypertensive Crisis**

Assign a code from category I16, Hypertensive crisis, for documented hypertensive urgency, hypertensive emergency or unspecified hypertensive crisis. Code also any identified hypertensive disease (I10-I15). The sequencing is based on the reason for the encounter.

ATHEROSCLEROTIC CORONARY ARTERY DISEASE AND ANGINA

ICD-10-CM has combination codes for atherosclerotic heart disease with angina pectoris. The subcategories for these codes are I25.11, Atherosclerotic heart disease of native coronary artery with angina pectoris and I25.7, Atherosclerosis of coronary artery bypass graft(s) and coronary artery of transplanted heart with angina pectoris.

When using one of these combination codes it is not necessary to use an additional code for angina pectoris. A causal relationship can be assumed in a patient with both atherosclerosis and angina pectoris, unless the documentation indicates the angina is due to something other than the atherosclerosis.

If a patient with coronary artery disease is admitted due to an acute myocardial infarction (AMI), the AMI should be sequenced before the coronary artery disease.

See Section I.C.9. Acute myocardial infarction (AMI)

INTRAOPERATIVE AND POSTPROCEDURAL CEREBROVASCULAR ACCIDENT

● New code ▲ Revised code **Excludes1:** Not coded here **Excludes2:** Not included here ⊗ Placeholder required ⑦7th digit required

Medical record documentation should clearly specify the cause- and-effect relationship between the medical intervention and the cerebrovascular accident in order to assign a code for intraoperative or postprocedural cerebrovascular accident.

Proper code assignment depends on whether it was an infarction or hemorrhage and whether it occurred intraoperatively or postoperatively. If it was a cerebral hemorrhage, code assignment depends on the type of procedure performed.

SEQUELAE OF CEREBROVASCULAR DISEASE

1)   Category I69, Sequelae of Cerebrovascular disease

Category I69 is used to indicate conditions classifiable to categories I60-I67 as the causes of sequela (neurologic deficits), themselves classified elsewhere. These "late effects" include neurologic deficits that persist after initial onset of conditions classifiable to categories I60-I67. The neurologic deficits caused by cerebrovascular disease may be present from the onset or may arise at any time after the onset of the condition classifiable to categories I60-I67.

Codes from category I69, Sequelae of cerebrovascular disease, that specify hemiplegia, hemiparesis and monoplegia identify whether the dominant or nondominant side is affected. Should the affected side be documented, but not specified as dominant or nondominant, and the classification system does not indicate a default, code selection is as follows:

- For ambidextrous patients, the default should be dominant.

- If the left side is affected, the default is non-dominant.

- If the right side is affected, the default is dominant.

2)   Codes from category I69 with codes from I60-I67

Codes from category I69 may be assigned on a health care record with codes from I60-I67, if the patient has a current cerebrovascular disease and deficits from an old cerebrovascular disease.

3)   Codes from category I69 and Personal history of transient ischemic attack (TIA) and cerebral infarction (Z86.73)

Codes from category I69 should not be assigned if the patient does not have neurologic deficits.

See Section I.C.21. 4. History (of) for use of personal history codes

ACUTE MYOCARDIAL INFARCTION (AMI)

1)   ST elevation myocardial infarction (STEMI) and non ST elevation myocardial infarction (NSTEMI)

The ICD-10-CM codes for acute myocardial infarction (AMI) identify the site, such as anterolateral wall or true posterior wall. Subcategories I21.0-I21.2 and code I21.3 are used for ST elevation myocardial infarction (STEMI). Code I21.4, Non-ST elevation (NSTEMI) myocardial infarction, is used for non ST elevation myocardial infarction (NSTEMI) and nontransmural MIs.

If NSTEMI evolves to STEMI, assign the STEMI code. If STEMI converts to NSTEMI due to thrombolytic therapy, it is still coded as STEMI.

For encounters occurring while the myocardial infarction is equal to, or less than, four weeks old, including transfers to another acute setting or a postacute setting, and the myocardial infarction **meets** the definition for "other diagnoses" (see Section III, Reporting Additional Diagnoses), codes from category I21 may continue to be reported. For encounters after the 4 week time frame and the patient is still receiving care related to the myocardial infarction, the appropriate aftercare code should be assigned, rather than a code from category I21. For old or healed myocardial infarctions not requiring further care, code I25.2, Old myocardial infarction, may be assigned.

2)   Acute myocardial infarction, unspecified

Code I21.3, ST elevation (STEMI) myocardial infarction of unspecified site, is the default for unspecified acute myocardial infarction. If only STEMI or transmural MI without the site is documented, assign code I21.3.

3)   AMI documented as nontransmural or subendocardial but site provided

If an AMI is documented as nontransmural or subendocardial, but the site is provided, it is still coded as a subendocardial AMI.

See Section I.C.21.3 for information on coding status post administration of tPA in a different facility within the last 24 hours.

4)   Subsequent acute myocardial infarction

A code from category I22, Subsequent ST elevation (STEMI) and non ST elevation (NSTEMI) myocardial infarction, is to be used when a patient who has suffered an AMI has a new AMI within the 4 week time frame of the initial AMI. A code from category I22 must be used in conjunction with a code from category I21. The sequencing of the I22 and I21 codes depends on the circumstances of the encounter.

Chapter 9

Diseases Of The Circulatory System (I00-I99)

Excludes2: certain conditions originating in the perinatal period (P04-P96)

certain infectious and parasitic diseases (A00-B99)

complications of pregnancy, childbirth and the puerperium (O00-O9A)

congenital malformations, deformations, and chromosomal abnormalities (Q00-Q99)

endocrine, nutritional and metabolic diseases (E00-E88)

injury, poisoning and certain other consequences of external causes (S00-T88)

neoplasms (C00-D49)

symptoms, signs and abnormal clinical and laboratory findings, not elsewhere classified (R00-R94)

systemic connective tissue disorders (M30-M36)

transient cerebral ischemic attacks and related syndromes (G45.-)

This chapter contains the following blocks:

I00-I02   Acute rheumatic fever

I05-I09   Chronic rheumatic heart diseases

I10-I16   Hypertensive diseases

I20-I25   Ischemic heart diseases

I26-I28   Pulmonary heart disease and diseases of pulmonary circulation

I30-I52   Other forms of heart disease

I60-I69   Cerebrovascular diseases

I70-I79   Diseases of arteries, arterioles and capillaries

I80-I89   Diseases of veins, lymphatic vessels and lymph nodes, not elsewhere classified

I95-I99   Other and unspecified disorders of the circulatory system

ACUTE RHEUMATIC FEVER (I00-I02)

I00   Rheumatic fever without heart involvement

Includes: arthritis, rheumatic, acute or subacute

Excludes1: rheumatic fever with heart involvement (I01.0 -I01.9)

I01   Rheumatic fever with heart involvement

Excludes1: chronic diseases of rheumatic origin (I05-I09) unless rheumatic fever is also present or there is evidence of reactivation or activity of the rheumatic process.

I01.0   Acute rheumatic pericarditis

Any condition in I00 with pericarditis

Rheumatic pericarditis (acute)

Excludes1: acute pericarditis not specified as rheumatic (I30.-)

I01.1   Acute rheumatic endocarditis

Any condition in I00 with endocarditis or valvulitis

Acute rheumatic valvulitis

I01.2   Acute rheumatic myocarditis

Any condition in I00 with myocarditis

I01.8   Other acute rheumatic heart disease

Any condition in I00 **with other** or multiple types of heart involvement

Acute rheumatic pancarditis

I01.9   Acute rheumatic heart disease, unspecified

Any condition in I00 with unspecified type of heart involvement

Rheumatic carditis, acute

Rheumatic heart disease, active or acute

I02   Rheumatic chorea

Includes: Sydenham's chorea

Excludes1: chorea NOS (G25.5)

Huntington's chorea (G10)

I02.0   Rheumatic chorea with heart involvement

Chorea NOS with heart involvement

Rheumatic chorea with heart involvement of any type classifiable under I01.-

I02.9   Rheumatic chorea without heart involvement

Rheumatic chorea NOS

CHRONIC RHEUMATIC HEART DISEASES (I05-I09)

Definition: Rheumatic heart disease refers to a thickening and stenosis of one or more of the heart valves and often requires surgery to repair or replace the involved valve(s).

I05   Rheumatic mitral valve diseases

Includes: conditions classifiable to both I05.0 and I05.2-I05.9, whether specified as rheumatic or not

Excludes1: mitral valve disease specified as nonrheumatic (I34.-)

mitral valve disease with aortic and/or tricuspid valve involvement (I08.-)

I05.0   Rheumatic mitral stenosis

Mitral (valve) obstruction (rheumatic)

I05.1   Rheumatic mitral insufficiency

Rheumatic mitral incompetence

Rheumatic mitral regurgitation

Excludes1: mitral insufficiency not specified as rheumatic (I34.0)

I05.2   Rheumatic mitral stenosis with insufficiency

Rheumatic mitral stenosis with incompetence or regurgitation

I05.8   Other rheumatic mitral valve diseases

Rheumatic mitral (valve) failure

I05.9   Rheumatic mitral valve disease, unspecified

Rheumatic mitral (valve) disorder (chronic) NOS

I06   Rheumatic aortic valve diseases

Excludes1: aortic valve disease not specified as rheumatic (I35.-)

aortic valve disease with mitral and/or tricuspid valve involvement (I08.-)

I06.0   Rheumatic aortic stenosis

Rheumatic aortic (valve) obstruction

I06.1   Rheumatic aortic insufficiency

Rheumatic aortic incompetence

Rheumatic aortic regurgitation

I06.2   Rheumatic aortic stenosis with insufficiency

Rheumatic aortic stenosis with incompetence or regurgitation

I06.8   Other rheumatic aortic valve diseases

I06.9   Rheumatic aortic valve disease, unspecified

Rheumatic aortic (valve) disease NOS

I07   Rheumatic tricuspid valve diseases

Includes: rheumatic tricuspid valve diseases specified as rheumatic or unspecified

Excludes1: tricuspid valve disease specified as nonrheumatic (I36.-)

tricuspid valve disease with aortic and/or mitral valve involvement (I08.-)

I07.0   Rheumatic tricuspid stenosis

Tricuspid (valve) stenosis (rheumatic)

I07.1   Rheumatic tricuspid insufficiency

Tricuspid (valve) insufficiency (rheumatic)

I07.2 **Rheumatic tricuspid stenosis and insufficiency**

I07.8 **Other rheumatic tricuspid valve diseases**

I07.9 **Rheumatic tricuspid valve disease, unspecified**

Rheumatic tricuspid valve disorder NOS

I08 **Multiple valve diseases**

Includes: multiple valve diseases specified as rheumatic or unspecified

Excludes1: endocarditis, valve unspecified (I38)

multiple valve disease specified a nonrheumatic (I34.-, I35.-, I36.-, I37.-, I38.-, Q22.-, Q23.-, Q24.8-)

rheumatic valve disease NOS (I09.1)

I08.0 **Rheumatic disorders of both mitral and aortic valves**

Involvement of both mitral and aortic valves specified as rheumatic or unspecified

I08.1 **Rheumatic disorders of both mitral and tricuspid valves**

I08.2 **Rheumatic disorders of both aortic and tricuspid valves**

I08.3 **Combined rheumatic disorders of mitral, aortic and tricuspid valves**

I08.8 **Other rheumatic multiple valve diseases**

I08.9 **Rheumatic multiple valve disease, unspecified**

I09 **Other rheumatic heart diseases**

I09.0 **Rheumatic myocarditis**

Excludes1: myocarditis not specified as rheumatic (I51.4)

I09.1 **Rheumatic diseases of endocardium, valve unspecified**

Rheumatic endocarditis (chronic)

Rheumatic valvulitis (chronic)

Excludes1: endocarditis, valve unspecified (I38)

I09.2 **Chronic rheumatic pericarditis**

Adherent pericardium, rheumatic

Chronic rheumatic mediastinopericarditis

Chronic rheumatic myopericarditis

Excludes1: chronic pericarditis not specified as rheumatic (I31.-)

I09.8 **Other specified rheumatic heart diseases**

I09.81 **Rheumatic heart failure**

Use additional code to identify type of heart failure (I50.-)

I09.89 **Other specified rheumatic heart diseases**

Rheumatic disease of pulmonary valve

I09.9 **Rheumatic heart disease, unspecified**

Rheumatic carditis

Excludes1: rheumatoid carditis (M05.31)

HYPERTENSIVE DISEASES (I10-I16)

Definition: Hypertensive heart disease refers to heart disease caused by high blood pressure, especially localized high blood pressure.

Use additional code to identify:

exposure to environmental tobacco smoke (Z77.22)

history of tobacco dependence (Z87.891)

occupational exposure to environmental tobacco smoke (Z57.31)

tobacco dependence (F17.-)

tobacco use (Z72.0)

Excludes1: neonatal hypertension (P29.2)

primary pulmonary hypertension (I27.0)

Excludes2: hypertensive disease complicating pregnancy, childbirth and the puerperium (O10-O11, O13-O16)

I10 **Essential (primary) hypertension**

Includes: high blood pressure

hypertension (arterial) (benign) (essential) (malignant) (primary) (systemic)

Excludes1: hypertensive disease complicating pregnancy, childbirth and the puerperium (O10-O11, O13-O16)

Excludes2: essential (primary) hypertension involving vessels of brain (I60-I69)

essential (primary) hypertension involving vessels of eye (H35.0-)

I11 **Hypertensive heart disease**

Includes: any condition in I50.-, I51.4-I51.9 due to hypertension

I11.0 **Hypertensive heart disease with heart failure**

Hypertensive heart failure

Use additional code to identify type of heart failure (I50.-)

I11.9 **Hypertensive heart disease without heart failure**

Hypertensive heart disease NOS

I12 **Hypertensive chronic kidney disease**

Includes: any condition in N18 and N26 - due to hypertension

arteriosclerosis of kidney

arteriosclerotic nephritis (chronic) (interstitial) hypertensive nephropathy

nephrosclerosis

Excludes1: hypertension due to kidney disease (I15.0, I15.1)

renovascular hypertension (I15.0) secondary hypertension (I15.-)

Excludes2: acute kidney failure (N17.-)

I12.0 **Hypertensive chronic kidney disease with stage 5 chronic kidney disease or end stage renal disease**

Use additional code to identify the stage of chronic kidney disease (N18.5, N18.6)

I12.9 **Hypertensive chronic kidney disease with stage 1through stage 4 chronic kidney disease, or unspecified chronic kidney disease**

Hypertensive chronic kidney disease NOS Hypertensive renal disease NOS

Use additional code to identify the stage of chronic kidney disease (N18.1-N18.4, N18.9)

I13 **Hypertensive heart and chronic kidney disease**

Includes: any condition in I11.- with any condition in I12.-

cardiorenal disease cardiovascular renal disease

I13.0 **Hypertensive heart and chronic kidney disease with heart failure and stage 1through stage 4chronic kidney disease, or unspecified chronic kidney disease**

Use additional code to identify type of heart failure (I50.-)

Use additional code to identify stage of chronic kidney disease (N18.1-N18.4, N18.9)

I13.1 **Hypertensive heart and chronic kidney disease without heart failure**

I13.10 **Hypertensive heart and chronic kidney disease without heart failure, with stage 1through stage 4chronic kidney disease, or unspecified chronic kidney disease**

Hypertensive heart disease and hypertensive chronic kidney disease NOS

Use additional code to identify the stage of chronic kidney disease (N18.1-N18.4, N18.9)

I13.11 **Hypertensive heart and chronic kidney disease without heart failure, with stage 5 chronic kidney disease, or end stage renal disease**

Use additional code to identify the stage of chronic kidney disease (N18.5, N18.6)

I13.2 **Hypertensive heart and chronic kidney disease with heart failure and with stage 5 chronic kidney disease, or end stage renal disease**

Use additional code to identify type of heart failure (I50.-)

Use additional code to identify the stage of chronic kidney disease (N18.5, N18.6)

I15 **Secondary hypertension**

Definition: Secondary hypertension is a type of hypertension caused by an identifiable underlying secondary cause.

Code also underlying condition

Excludes1: postprocedural hypertension (I97.3)

Excludes2: secondary hypertension involving vessels of brain (I60-I69)

secondary hypertension involving vessels of eye (H35.0-)

I15.0 **Renovascular hypertension**

I15.1 **Hypertension secondary to other renal disorders**

I15.2 **Hypertension secondary to endocrine disorders**

I15.8 **Other secondary hypertension**

I15.9 **Secondary hypertension, unspecified**

I16 **Hypertensive crisis**

Code also any identified hypertensive disease (I10-I15)

I16.0 **Hypertensive urgency**

I16.1 **Hypertensive emergency**

I16.9 **Hypertensive crisis, unspecified**

ISCHEMIC HEART DISEASES (I20-I25)

Definition: Ischemic heart disease is a condition caused by a reduced amount of blood supplying the heart muscle. It can be caused by cholesterol and other lipids building up on the inner walls of arteries that supply the heart, forming a thick plaque that can reduce the amount of blood carrying nutrients and oxygen to heart tissue.

Use additional code to identify presence of hypertension (I10-I16)

I20 **Angina pectoris**

Use additional code to identify:

exposure to environmental tobacco smoke (Z77.22)

history of tobacco dependence (Z87.891)

occupational exposure to environmental tobacco smoke (Z57.31)

tobacco dependence (F17.-)

tobacco use (Z72.0)

Excludes1: angina pectoris with atherosclerotic heart disease of native coronary arteries (I25.1-)

atherosclerosis of coronary artery bypass graft(s) and coronary artery of transplanted heart with angina pectoris (I25.7-)

postinfarction angina (I23.7)

I20.0 **Unstable angina**

Accelerated angina

Crescendo angina

De novo effort angina

Intermediate coronary syndrome

Preinfarction syndrome

Worsening effort angina

I20.1 **Angina pectoris with documented spasm**

Angiospastic angina

Prinzmetal angina

Spasm-induced angina

Variant angina

I20.8 **Other forms of angina pectoris**

Angina equivalent

Angina of effort

Coronary slow flow syndrome

Stenocardia

Stable angina

Use additional code(s) for symptoms associated with angina equivalent

I20.9 **Angina pectoris, unspecified**

Angina NOS

Anginal syndrome

Cardiac angina

Ischemic chest pain

▲ **I21** **Acute myocardial infarction**

Definition: Myocardial infarction, commonly known as a heart attack, occurs when the blood supply to part of the heart is interrupted causing some heart cells to die.

Includes: cardiac infarction

coronary (artery) embolism

coronary (artery) occlusion

coronary (artery) rupture

coronary (artery) thrombosis

infarction of heart, myocardium, or ventricle

myocardial infarction specified as acute or with a stated duration of 4 weeks (28 days) or less from onset

Use additional code, if applicable, to identify:

exposure to environmental tobacco smoke (Z77.22)

history of tobacco dependence (Z87.891)

occupational exposure to environmental tobacco smoke (Z57.31)

status post administration of tPA (rtPA) in a different facility within the last 24 hours prior to admission to current facility (Z92.82)

tobacco dependence (F17.-)

tobacco use (Z72.0)

Excludes2: old myocardial infarction (I25.2)

postmyocardial infarction syndrome (I24.1)

subsequent type 1 myocardial infarction (I22.-)

I21.0 **ST elevation (STEMI) myocardial infarction of anterior wall**

Type 1 ST elevation myocardial infarction of anterior wall

I21.01 **ST elevation (STEMI) myocardial infarction involving left main coronary artery**

I21.02 **ST elevation (STEMI) myocardial infarction involving left anterior descending coronary artery**

ST elevation (STEMI) myocardial infarction involving diagonal coronary artery

I21.09 **ST elevation (STEMI) myocardial infarction involving other coronary artery of anterior wall**

Acute transmural myocardial infarction of anterior wall

Anteroapical transmural (Q wave) infarction (acute)

Anterolateral transmural (Q wave) infarction (acute)

Anteroseptal transmural (Q wave) infarction (acute)

Transmural (Q wave) infarction (acute) (of) anterior (wall) NOS

I21.1 **ST elevation (STEMI) myocardial infarction of inferior wall**

Type 1 ST elevation myocardial infarction of inferior wall

I21.11 **ST elevation (STEMI) myocardial infarction involving right coronary artery**

Inferoposterior transmural (Q wave) infarction (acute)

I21.19 **ST elevation (STEMI) myocardial infarction involving other coronary artery of inferior wall**

Acute transmural myocardial infarction of inferior wall

Inferolateral transmural (Q wave) infarction (acute)

Transmural (Q wave) infarction (acute) (of) diaphragmatic wall

Transmural (Q wave) infarction (acute) (of) inferior (wall) NOS

Excludes2: ST elevation (STEMI) myocardial infarction involving left circumflex coronary artery (I21.21)

I21.2 **ST elevation (STEMI) myocardial infarction of other sites**

Type 1 ST elevation myocardial infarction of other sites

I21.21 **ST elevation (STEMI) myocardial infarction involving left circumflex coronary artery**

ST elevation (STEMI) myocardial infarction involving oblique marginal coronary artery

I21.29 **ST elevation (STEMI) myocardial infarction involving other sites**

Acute transmural myocardial infarction **of other** sites

Apical-lateral transmural (Q wave) infarction (acute)

Basal-lateral transmural (Q wave) infarction (acute)

High lateral transmural (Q wave) infarction (acute)

Lateral (wall) NOS transmural (Q wave) infarction (acute)

Posterior (true) transmural (Q wave) infarction (acute)

Posterobasal transmural (Q wave) infarction (acute)

Posterolateral transmural (Q wave) infarction (acute)

Posteroseptal transmural (Q wave) infarction (acute)

Septal transmural (Q wave) infarction (acute) NOS

I21.3 **ST elevation (STEMI) myocardial infarction of unspecified site**

Acute transmural myocardial infarction of unspecified site

Type 1 ST elevation myocardial infarction of unspecified site

Transmural (Q wave) myocardial infarction NOS

I21.4 **Non-ST elevation (NSTEMI) myocardial infarction**

Acute subendocardial myocardial infarction

Non-Q wave myocardial infarction NOS

Nontransmural myocardial infarction NOS

Type 1 non-ST elevation myocardial infarction

●**I21.9** **Acute myocardial infarction, unspecified**

Myocardial infarction (acute) NOS

●**I21.A** **Other type of myocardial infarction**

●**I21.A1** **Myocardial infarction type 2**

Myocardial infarction due to demand ischemia

Myocardial infarction secondary to ischemic imbalance

Code also the underlying cause, if known and applicable, such as:

anemia (D50.0-D64.9)

chronic obstructive pulmonary disease (J44.-)

heart failure (I50.-)

paroxysmal tachycardia (I47.0-I47.9)

renal failure (N17.0-N19)

shock (R57.0-R57.9)

●**I21.A9** **Other myocardial infarction type**

Myocardial infarction associated with revascularization procedure

Myocardial infarction type 3

Myocardial infarction type 4a

Myocardial infarction type 4b

Myocardial infarction type 4c

Myocardial infarction type 5

Code first, if applicable, postprocedural myocardial infarction following cardiac surgery (I97.190), or postprocedural myocardial infarction during cardiac surgery (I97.790)

Code also complication, if known and applicable, such as:

(acute) stent occlusion (T82.897-)

(acute) stent stenosis (T82.857-)

(acute) stent thrombosis (T82.867-)

cardiac arrest due to underlying cardiac condition (I46.2)

complication of percutaneous coronary intervention (PCI) (I97.89)

occlusion of coronary artery bypass graft (T82.218-)

I22 **Subsequent ST elevation (STEMI) and non-ST elevation (NSTEMI) myocardial infarction**

Includes: acute myocardial infarction occurring within four weeks (28 days) of a previous acute myocardial infarction, regardless of site cardiac infarction

coronary (artery) embolism coronary (artery) occlusion

coronary (artery) rupture coronary (artery) thrombosis

infarction of heart, myocardium, or ventricle recurrent myocardial infarction

reinfarction of myocardium

rupture of heart, myocardium, or ventricle

subsequent type 1 myocardial infarction

Excludes1: subsequent myocardial infarction, type 2 (I21.A1)

subsequent myocardial infarction of other type (type 3) (type 4) (type 5) (I21.A9)

Use additional code, if applicable, to identify:

exposure to environmental tobacco smoke (Z77.22)

history of tobacco dependence (Z87.891)

occupational exposure to environmental tobacco smoke (Z57.31)

status post administration of tPA (rtPA) in a different facility within the last 24 hours prior to admission to current facility (Z92.82)

tobacco dependence (F17.-)

tobacco use (Z72.0)

I22.0 **Subsequent ST elevation (STEMI) myocardial infarction of anterior wall**

Subsequent acute transmural myocardial infarction of anterior wall

Subsequent transmural (Q wave) infarction (acute)(of) anterior (wall) NOS

● New code ▲ Revised code **Excludes1:** Not coded here **Excludes2:** Not included here ⊗ Placeholder required ⑦7th digit required

Subsequent anteroapical transmural (Q wave) infarction (acute)

Subsequent anterolateral transmural (Q wave) infarction (acute)

Subsequent anteroseptal transmural (Q wave) infarction (acute)

I22.1 **Subsequent ST elevation (STEMI) myocardial infarction of inferior wall**

Subsequent acute transmural myocardial infarction of inferior wall

Subsequent transmural (Q wave) infarction (acute)(of) diaphragmatic wall

Subsequent transmural (Q wave) infarction (acute)(of) inferior (wall) NOS

Subsequent inferolateral transmural (Q wave) infarction (acute)

Subsequent inferoposterior transmural (Q wave) infarction (acute)

I22.2 **Subsequent non-ST elevation (NSTEMI) myocardial infarction**

Subsequent acute subendocardial myocardial infarction

Subsequent non-Q wave myocardial infarction NOS

Subsequent nontransmural myocardial infarction NOS

I22.8 **Subsequent ST elevation (STEMI) myocardial infarction of other sites**

Subsequent acute transmural myocardial infarction **of other sites**

Subsequent apical-lateral transmural (Q wave) myocardial infarction (acute)

Subsequent basal-lateral transmural (Q wave) myocardial infarction (acute)

Subsequent high lateral transmural (Q wave) myocardial infarction (acute)

Subsequent transmural (Q wave) myocardial infarction (acute)(of) lateral (wall) NOS

Subsequent posterior (true)transmural (Q wave) myocardial infarction (acute)

Subsequent posterobasal transmural (Q wave) myocardial infarction (acute)

Subsequent posterolateral transmural (Q wave) myocardial infarction (acute)

Subsequent posteroseptal transmural (Q wave) myocardial infarction (acute)

Subsequent septal NOS transmural (Q wave) myocardial infarction (acute)

I22.9 **Subsequent ST elevation (STEMI) myocardial infarction of unspecified site**

Subsequent acute myocardial infarction of unspecified site

Subsequent myocardial infarction (acute) NOS

I23 **Certain current complications following ST elevation (STEMI) and non-ST elevation (NSTEMI) myocardial infarction (within the 28 day period)**

I23.0 **Hemopericardium as current complication following acute myocardial infarction**

Excludes1: hemopericardium not specified as current complication following acute myocardial infarction (I31.2)

I23.1 **Atrial septal defect as current complication following acute myocardial infarction**

Excludes1: acquired atrial septal defect not specified as current complication following acute myocardial infarction (I51.0)

I23.2 **Ventricular septal defect as current complication following acute myocardial infarction**

Excludes1: acquired ventricular septal defect not specified as current complication following acute myocardial infarction (I51.0)

I23.3 **Rupture of cardiac wall without hemopericardium as current complication following acute myocardial infarction**

I23.4 **Rupture of chordae tendineae as current complication following acute myocardial infarction**

Excludes1: rupture of chordae tendineae not specified as current complication following acute myocardial infarction (I51.1)

I23.5 **Rupture of papillary muscle as current complication following acute myocardial infarction**

Excludes1: rupture of papillary muscle not specified as current complication following acute myocardial infarction (I51.2)

I23.6 **Thrombosis of atrium, auricular appendage, and ventricle as current complications following acute myocardial infarction**

Excludes1: thrombosis of atrium, auricular appendage, and ventricle not specified as current complication following acute myocardial infarction (I51.3)

I23.7 **Postinfarction angina**

I23.8 **Other current complications following acute myocardial infarction**

I24 **Other acute ischemic heart diseases**

Excludes1: angina pectoris (I20.-)

transient myocardial ischemia in newborn (P29.4)

I24.0 **Acute coronary thrombosis not resulting in myocardial infarction**

Acute coronary (artery) (vein) embolism not resulting in myocardial infarction

Acute coronary (artery) (vein) occlusion not resulting in myocardial infarction

Acute coronary (artery) (vein) thromboembolism not resulting in myocardial infarction

Excludes1: atherosclerotic heart disease (I25.1-)

I24.1 **Dressler's syndrome**

Postmyocardial infarction syndrome

Excludes1: postinfarction angina (I23.7)

I24.8 **Other forms of acute ischemic heart disease**

Excludes1: myocardial infarction due to demand ischemia (I21.A1)

I24.9 **Acute ischemic heart disease, unspecified**

Excludes1: ischemic heart disease (chronic) NOS (I25.9)

I25 **Chronic ischemic heart disease**

Use additional code to identify:

chronic total occlusion of coronary artery (I25.82)

exposure to environmental tobacco smoke (Z77.22)

history of tobacco dependence (Z87.891)

occupational exposure to environmental tobacco smoke (Z57.31)

tobacco dependence (F17.-)

tobacco use (Z72.0)

I25.1 **Atherosclerotic heart disease of native coronary artery**

Atherosclerotic cardiovascular disease

Coronary (artery) atheroma

Coronary (artery) atherosclerosis

Coronary (artery) disease

Coronary (artery) sclerosis

Use additional code, if applicable, to identify:

coronary atherosclerosis due to calcified coronary lesion (I25.84)

| Add 4th-7th digits | Nonspecific code | Unspecified code | Manifestation code | 379 |

coronary atherosclerosis due to lipid rich plaque (I25.83)

Excludes2: atheroembolism (I75.-)

atherosclerosis of coronary artery bypass graft(s) and transplanted heart (I25.7-)

I25.10   Atherosclerotic heart disease of native coronary artery without angina pectoris

Atherosclerotic heart disease NOS

I25.11   Atherosclerotic heart disease of native coronary artery with angina pectoris

I25.110   Atherosclerotic heart disease of native coronary artery with unstable angina pectoris

Excludes1: unstable angina without atherosclerotic heart disease (I20.0)

I25.111   Atherosclerotic heart disease of native coronary artery with angina pectoris with documented spasm

Excludes1: angina pectoris with documented spasm without atherosclerotic heart disease (I20.1)

I25.118   Atherosclerotic heart disease of native coronary artery with other forms of angina pectoris

Excludes1: Other forms of angina pectoris without atherosclerotic heart disease (I20.8)

I25.119   Atherosclerotic heart disease of native coronary artery with unspecified angina pectoris

Atherosclerotic heart disease with angina NOS

Atherosclerotic heart disease with ischemic chest pain

Excludes1: unspecified angina pectoris without atherosclerotic heart disease (I20.9)

I25.2   Old myocardial infarction

Definition: Old myocardial infarction refers to an old occlusion or blockage of arteries supplying the muscles of the heart, resulting in injury or necrosis of the heart muscle.

Healed myocardial infarction

Past myocardial infarction diagnosed by ECG **or other** investigation, but currently presenting no symptoms

I25.3   Aneurysm of heart

Mural aneurysm

Ventricular aneurysm

I25.4   Coronary artery aneurysm and dissection

I25.41   Coronary artery aneurysm

Coronary arteriovenous fistula, acquired

Excludes1: congenital coronary (artery) aneurysm (Q24.5)

I25.42   Coronary artery dissection

I25.5   Ischemic cardiomyopathy

Excludes2: coronary atherosclerosis (I25.1-, I25.7-)

I25.6   Silent myocardial ischemia

I25.7   Atherosclerosis of coronary artery bypass graft(s) and coronary artery of transplanted heart with angina pectoris

Use additional code, if applicable, to identify:

coronary atherosclerosis due to calcified coronary lesion (I25.84)

coronary atherosclerosis due to lipid rich plaque (I25.83)

Excludes1: atherosclerosis of bypass graft(s) of transplanted heart without angina pectoris (I25.812)

atherosclerosis of coronary artery bypass graft(s) without angina pectoris (I25.810)

atherosclerosis of native coronary artery of transplanted heart without angina pectoris (I25.811)

I25.70   Atherosclerosis of coronary artery bypass graft(s), unspecified, with angina pectoris

I25.700   Atherosclerosis of coronary artery bypass graft(s), unspecified, with unstable angina pectoris

Excludes1: unstable angina pectoris without atherosclerosis of coronary artery bypass graft (I20.0)

I25.701   Atherosclerosis of coronary artery bypass graft(s), unspecified, with angina pectoris with documented spasm

Excludes1: angina pectoris with documented spasm without atherosclerosis of coronary artery bypass graft (I20.1)

I25.708   Atherosclerosis of coronary artery bypass graft(s), unspecified, with other forms of angina pectoris

Excludes1: Other forms of angina pectoris without atherosclerosis of coronary artery bypass graft (I20.8)

I25.709   Atherosclerosis of coronary artery bypass graft(s), unspecified, with unspecified angina pectoris

Excludes1: unspecified angina pectoris without atherosclerosis of coronary artery bypass graft (I20.9)

I25.71   Atherosclerosis of autologous vein coronary artery bypass graft(s) with angina pectoris

I25.710   Atherosclerosis of autologous vein coronary artery bypass graft(s) with unstable angina pectoris

Excludes1: unstable angina without atherosclerosis of autologous vein coronary artery bypass graft(s) (I20.0)

embolism or thrombus of coronary artery bypass graft(s) (T82.8-)

I25.711   Atherosclerosis of autologous vein coronary artery bypass graft(s) with angina pectoris with documented spasm

Excludes1: angina pectoris with documented spasm without atherosclerosis of autologous vein coronary artery bypass graft(s) (I20.1)

I25.718   Atherosclerosis of autologous vein coronary artery bypass graft(s) with other forms of angina pectoris

Excludes1: Other forms of angina

pectoris without atherosclerosis of autologous vein coronary artery bypass graft(s) (I20.8)

I25.719 **Atherosclerosis of autologous vein coronary artery bypass graft(s) with unspecified angina pectoris**

Excludes1: unspecified angina

pectoris without atherosclerosis of autologous vein coronary artery bypass graft(s) (I20.9)

I25.72 **Atherosclerosis of autologous artery coronary artery bypass graft(s) with angina pectoris**

Atherosclerosis of internal mammary artery graft with angina pectoris

I25.720 **Atherosclerosis of autologous artery coronary artery bypass graft(s) with unstable angina pectoris**

Excludes1: unstable angina without

atherosclerosis of autologous artery coronary artery bypass graft(s) (I20.0)

I25.721 **Atherosclerosis of autologous artery coronary artery bypass graft(s) with angina pectoris with documented spasm**

Excludes1: angina pectoris with

documented spasm without atherosclerosis of autologous artery coronary artery bypass graft(s) (I20.1)

I25.728 **Atherosclerosis of autologous artery coronary artery bypass graft(s) with other forms of angina pectoris**

Excludes1: Other forms of angina

pectoris without atherosclerosis of autologous artery coronary artery bypass graft(s) (I20.8)

I25.729 **Atherosclerosis of autologous artery coronary artery bypass graft(s) with unspecified angina pectoris**

Excludes1: unspecified angina

pectoris without atherosclerosis of autologous artery coronary artery bypass graft(s) (I20.9)

I25.73 **Atherosclerosis of nonautologous biological coronary artery bypass graft(s) with angina pectoris**

I25.730 **Atherosclerosis of nonautologous biological coronary artery bypass graft(s) with unstable angina pectoris**

Excludes1: unstable angina without

atherosclerosis of nonautologous biological coronary artery bypass graft(s) (I20.0)

I25.731 **Atherosclerosis of nonautologous biological coronary artery bypass graft(s) with angina pectoris with documented spasm**

Excludes1: angina pectoris with

documented spasm without atherosclerosis of nonautologous biological coronary artery bypass graft(s) (I20.1)

I25.738 **Atherosclerosis of nonautologous biological coronary artery bypass graft(s) with other forms of angina pectoris**

Excludes1: Other forms of angina

pectoris without atherosclerosis of nonautologous biological coronary artery bypass graft(s) (I20.8)

I25.739 **Atherosclerosis of nonautologous biological coronary artery bypass graft(s) with unspecified angina pectoris**

Excludes1: unspecified angina

pectoris without atherosclerosis of nonautologous biological coronary artery bypass graft(s) (I20.9)

I25.75 **Atherosclerosis of native coronary artery of transplanted heart with angina pectoris**

Excludes1: atherosclerosis of native coronary artery of transplanted heart without angina pectoris (I25.811)

I25.750 **Atherosclerosis of native coronary artery of transplanted heart with unstable angina**

I25.751 **Atherosclerosis of native coronary artery of transplanted heart with angina pectoris with documented spasm**

I25.758 **Atherosclerosis of native coronary artery of transplanted heart with other forms of angina pectoris**

I25.759 **Atherosclerosis of native coronary artery of transplanted heart with unspecified angina pectoris**

I25.76 **Atherosclerosis of bypass graft of coronary artery of transplanted heart with angina pectoris**

Excludes1: atherosclerosis of bypass graft of coronary artery of transplanted heart without angina pectoris (I25.812)

I25.760 **Atherosclerosis of bypass graft of coronary artery of transplanted heart with unstable angina**

I25.761 **Atherosclerosis of bypass graft of coronary artery of transplanted heart with angina pectoris with documented spasm**

I25.768 **Atherosclerosis of bypass graft of coronary artery of transplanted heart with other forms of angina pectoris**

I25.769 **Atherosclerosis of bypass graft of coronary artery of transplanted heart with unspecified angina pectoris**

I25.79 **Atherosclerosis of other coronary artery bypass graft(s) with angina pectoris**

Excludes1: angina pectoris with

I25.790 Atherosclerosis of other coronary artery bypass graft(s) with unstable angina pectoris

Excludes1: unstable angina without atherosclerosis of other coronary artery bypass graft(s) (I20.0)

I25.791 Atherosclerosis of other coronary artery bypass graft(s) with angina pectoris with documented spasm

Excludes1: angina pectoris with documented spasm without atherosclerosis of other coronary artery bypass graft(s) (I20.1)

I25.798 Atherosclerosis of other coronary artery bypass graft(s) with other forms of angina pectoris

Excludes1: Other forms of angina pectoris without atherosclerosis of other coronary artery bypass graft(s) (I20.8)

I25.799 Atherosclerosis of other coronary artery bypass graft(s) with unspecified angina pectoris

Excludes1: unspecified angina pectoris without atherosclerosis of other coronary artery bypass graft(s) (I20.9)

I25.8 Other forms of chronic ischemic heart disease

I25.81 Atherosclerosis of other coronary vessels without angina pectoris

<u>Use additional code</u>, if applicable, to identify:

coronary atherosclerosis due to calcified coronary lesion (I25.84)

coronary atherosclerosis due to lipid rich plaque (I25.83)

Excludes1: atherosclerotic heart disease of native coronary artery without angina pectoris (I25.10)

I25.810 Atherosclerosis of coronary artery bypass graft(s) without angina pectoris

Atherosclerosis of coronary artery bypass graft NOS

Excludes1: atherosclerosis of coronary bypass graft(s) with angina pectoris (I25.70-I25.73-, I25.79-)

I25.811 Atherosclerosis of native coronary artery of transplanted heart without angina pectoris

Atherosclerosis of native coronary artery of transplanted heart NOS

Excludes1: atherosclerosis of native coronary artery of transplanted heart with angina pectoris (I25.75-)

I25.812 Atherosclerosis of bypass graft of coronary artery of transplanted heart without angina pectoris

Atherosclerosis of bypass graft of transplanted heart NOS

Excludes1: atherosclerosis of bypass graft of transplanted heart with angina pectoris (I25.76)

I25.82 Chronic total occlusion of coronary artery

Complete occlusion of coronary artery

Total occlusion of coronary artery

<u>Code first</u> coronary atherosclerosis (I25.1-, I25.7-, I25.81-)

Excludes1: acute coronary occlusion with myocardial infarction (I21.0-I21.9, I22.-) acute coronary occlusion without myocardial infarction (I24.0)

I25.83 Coronary atherosclerosis due to lipid rich plaque

<u>Code first</u> coronary atherosclerosis (I25.1-, I25.7-, I25.81-)

I25.84 Coronary atherosclerosis due to calcified coronary lesion

Coronary atherosclerosis due to severely calcified coronary lesion

<u>Code first</u> coronary atherosclerosis (I25.1-, I25.7-, I25.81-)

I25.89 Other forms of chronic ischemic heart disease

I25.9 Chronic ischemic heart disease, unspecified

Ischemic heart disease (chronic) NOS

PULMONARY HEART DISEASE AND DISEASES OF PULMONARY CIRCULATION (I26-I28)

Definition: Pulmonary heart disease is the enlargement and eventual failure of the right ventricle of the heart due to disorders of the lungs or their blood vessels or chest wall abnormalities.

Definition: Pulmonary circulation is the circulation of blood through the lungs for the purpose of oxygenation and the release of carbon dioxide. Also known as lesser circulation.

I26 Pulmonary embolism

Includes: pulmonary (acute) (artery)(vein) infarction

pulmonary (acute) (artery)(vein) thromboembolism
pulmonary (acute) (artery)(vein) thrombosis

Excludes2: chronic pulmonary embolism (I27.82)

personal history of pulmonary embolism (Z86.711)

pulmonary embolism complicating abortion, ectopic or molar pregnancy (O00-O07, O08.2)

pulmonary embolism complicating pregnancy, childbirth and the puerperium (O88.-)

pulmonary embolism due to trauma (T79.0, T79.1)

pulmonary embolism due to complications of surgical and medical care (T80.0, T81.7-, T82.8-)

septic (non-pulmonary) arterial embolism (I76)

I26.0 Pulmonary embolism with acute cor pulmonale

I26.01 Septic pulmonary embolism with acute cor pulmonale

<u>Code first</u> underlying infection

I26.02 Saddle embolus of pulmonary artery with acute cor pulmonale

I26.09 Other pulmonary embolism with acute cor pulmonale

Acute cor pulmonale NOS

I26.9 Pulmonary embolism without acute cor pulmonale

I26.90 Septic pulmonary embolism without acute cor pulmonale

<u>Code first</u> underlying infection

I26.92   **Saddle embolus of pulmonary artery without acute cor pulmonale**

I26.99   **Other pulmonary embolism without acute cor pulmonale**

Acute pulmonary embolism NOS

Pulmonary embolism NOS

I27   **Other pulmonary heart diseases**

I27.0   **Primary pulmonary hypertension**

Heritable pulmonary arterial hypertension

Idiopathic pulmonary arterial hypertension

Primary group 1 pulmonary hypertension

Primary pulmonary arterial hypertension

Excludes1: persistent pulmonary hypertension of newborn (P29.30)

pulmonary hypertension NOS (I27.20)

secondary pulmonary arterial hypertension (I27.21)

secondary pulmonary hypertension (I27.29)

I27.1   **Kyphoscoliotic heart disease**

I27.2   **Other secondary pulmonary hypertension**

Code also associated underlying condition

Excludes1: Eisenmenger's syndrome (I27.83)

•I27.20   **Pulmonary hypertension, unspecified**

Pulmonary hypertension NOS

•I27.21   **Secondary pulmonary arterial hypertension**

(Associated) (drug-induced) (toxin-induced) pulmonary arterial hypertension NOS

(Associated) (drug-induced) (toxin-induced) (secondary) group 1 pulmonary hypertension

Code also associated conditions if applicable, or adverse effects of drugs or toxins, such as:

adverse effect of appetite depressants (T50.5X5)

congenital heart disease (Q20-Q28)

human immunodeficiency virus [HIV] disease (B20)

polymyositis (M33.2-)

portal hypertension (K76.6)

rheumatoid arthritis (M05.-)

schistosomiasis (B65.-)

Sjögren syndrome (M35.0-)

systemic sclerosis (M34.-)

•I27.22   **Pulmonary hypertension due to left heart disease**

Group 2 pulmonary hypertension

Code also associated left heart disease, if known, such as:

multiple valve disease (I08.-)

rheumatic mitral valve diseases (I05.-)

rheumatic aortic valve diseases (I06.-)

•I27.23   **Pulmonary hypertension due to lung diseases and hypoxia**

Group 3 pulmonary hypertension

Code also associated lung disease, if known, such as:

bronchiectasis (J47.-)

cystic fibrosis with pulmonary manifestations (E84.0)

interstitial lung disease (J84.-)

pleural effusion (J90)

sleep apnea (G47.3-)

•I27.24   **Chronic thromboembolic pulmonary hypertension**

Group 4 pulmonary hypertension

Code also associated pulmonary embolism, if applicable (I26.-, I27.82)

•I27.29   **Other secondary pulmonary hypertension**

Group 5 pulmonary hypertension

Pulmonary hypertension with unclear multifactorial mechanisms

Pulmonary hypertension due to hematologic disorders

Pulmonary hypertension due to metabolic disorders

Pulmonary hypertension due to other systemic disorders

Code also other associated disorders, if known, such as:

chronic myeloid leukemia (C92.10- C92.22)

essential thrombocythemia (D47.3)

Gaucher disease (E75.22)

hypertensive chronic kidney disease with end stage renal disease (I12.0, I12.11, I13.2)

hyperthyroidism (E05.-)

hypothyroidism (E00-E03)

polycythemia vera (D45)

sarcoidosis (D86.-)

I27.8   **Other specified pulmonary heart diseases**

I27.81   **Cor pulmonale (chronic)**

Cor pulmonale NOS

Excludes1: acute cor pulmonale (I26.0-)

I27.82   **Chronic pulmonary embolism**

Use additional code, if applicable, for associated long-term (current) use of anticoagulants (Z79.01)

Excludes1: personal history of pulmonary embolism (Z86.711)

•I27.83   **Eisenmenger's syndrome**

Eisenmenger's complex

(Irreversible) Eisenmenger's disease

Pulmonary hypertension with right to left shunt related to congenital heart disease

Code also underlying heart defect, if known, such as:

atrial septal defect (Q21.1)

Eisenmenger's defect (Q21.8)

patent ductus arteriosus (Q25.0)

ventricular septal defect (Q21.0)

I27.89   **Other specified pulmonary heart diseases**

I27.9   **Pulmonary heart disease, unspecified**

Chronic cardiopulmonary disease

I28   **Other diseases of pulmonary vessels**

I28.0   **Arteriovenous fistula of pulmonary vessels**

Excludes1: congenital arteriovenous fistula (Q25.72)

I28.1   **Aneurysm of pulmonary artery**

Excludes1: congenital aneurysm (Q25.79)

congenital arteriovenous aneurysm (Q25.72)

I28.8   **Other diseases of pulmonary vessels**

Pulmonary arteritis

Pulmonary endarteritis

Rupture of pulmonary vessels

Stenosis of pulmonary vessels

Stricture of pulmonary vessels

I28.9 **Disease of pulmonary vessels, unspecified**

OTHER FORMS OF HEART DISEASE (I30-I52)

I30 **Acute pericarditis**

Definition: Pericarditis is an inflammation of the two layers of the thin, sac-like membrane that surrounds the heart.

Includes: acute mediastinopericarditis

acute myopericarditis

acute pericardial effusion

acute pleuropericarditis

acute pneumopericarditis

Excludes1: Dressler's syndrome (I24.1)

rheumatic pericarditis (acute) (I01.0)

viral pericarditis due to Coxsackie virus (B33.23)

I30.0 **Acute nonspecific idiopathic pericarditis**

I30.1 **Infective pericarditis**

Pneumococcal pericarditis

Pneumopyopericardium

Purulent pericarditis

Pyopericarditis

Pyopericardium

Pyopneumopericardium

Staphylococcal pericarditis

Streptococcal pericarditis

Suppurative pericarditis

Viral pericarditis

Use additional code (B95-B97) to identify infectious agent

I30.8 **Other forms of acute pericarditis**

I30.9 **Acute pericarditis, unspecified**

I31 **Other diseases of pericardium**

Excludes1: diseases of pericardium specified as rheumatic (I09.2)

postcardiotomy syndrome (I97.0)

traumatic injury to pericardium (S26.-)

I31.0 **Chronic adhesive pericarditis**

Accretio cordis

Adherent pericardium

Adhesive mediastinopericarditis

I31.1 **Chronic constrictive pericarditis**

Concretio cordis

Pericardial calcification

I31.2 **Hemopericardium, not elsewhere classified**

Excludes1: hemopericardium as current complication following acute myocardial infarction (I23.0)

I31.3 **Pericardial effusion (noninflammatory)**

Chylopericardium

Excludes1: acute pericardial effusion (I30.9)

I31.4 **Cardiac tamponade**

Code first underlying cause

I31.8 **Other specified diseases of pericardium**

Epicardial plaques

Focal pericardial adhesions

I31.9 **Disease of pericardium, unspecified**

Pericarditis (chronic) NOS

I32 **Pericarditis in diseases classified elsewhere**

Code first underlying disease

Excludes1: pericarditis (in):

coxsackie (virus) (B33.23)

gonococcal (A54.83)

meningococcal (A39.53)

rheumatoid (arthritis) (M05.31)

syphilitic (A52.06)

systemic lupus erythematosus (M32.12)

tuberculosis (A18.84)

I33 **Acute and subacute endocarditis**

Definition: Endocarditis is an infection of the lining of the heart chambers and heart valves that is caused by bacteria, fungi, or other infectious substances.

Excludes1: acute rheumatic endocarditis (I01.1)

endocarditis NOS (I38)

I33.0 **Acute and subacute infective endocarditis**

Bacterial endocarditis (acute) (subacute)

Infective endocarditis (acute) (subacute) NOS

Endocarditis lenta (acute) (subacute)

Malignant endocarditis (acute) (subacute)

Purulent endocarditis (acute) (subacute)

Septic endocarditis (acute) (subacute)

Ulcerative endocarditis (acute) (subacute)

Vegetative endocarditis (acute) (subacute)

Use additional code (B95-B97) to identify infectious agent

I33.9 **Acute and subacute endocarditis, unspecified**

Acute endocarditis NOS

Acute myoendocarditis NOS

Acute Periendocarditis NOS

Subacute endocarditis NOS

Subacute myoendocarditis NOS

Subacute Periendocarditis NOS

I34 **Nonrheumatic mitral valve disorders**

Excludes1: mitral valve disease (I05.9)

mitral valve failure (I05.8)

mitral valve stenosis (I05.0)

mitral valve disorder of unspecified cause with diseases of aortic and/or tricuspid valve(s) (I08.-)

mitral valve disorder of unspecified cause with mitral stenosis or obstruction (I05.0)

mitral valve disorder specified as congenital (Q23.2, Q23.9)

mitral valve disorder specified as rheumatic (I05.-)

I34.0 **Nonrheumatic mitral (valve) insufficiency**

Nonrheumatic mitral (valve) incompetence NOS

Nonrheumatic mitral (valve) regurgitation NOS

I34.1 **Nonrheumatic mitral (valve) prolapse**

Floppy nonrheumatic mitral valve syndrome

Excludes1: Marfan's syndrome (Q87.4-)

I34.2 **Nonrheumatic mitral (valve) stenosis**

I34.8 **Other nonrheumatic mitral valve disorders**

I34.9 **Nonrheumatic mitral valve disorder, unspecified**

I35 **Nonrheumatic aortic valve disorders**

Excludes1: aortic valve disorder of unspecified cause but with diseases of mitral and/or tricuspid valve(s) (I08.-)

aortic valve disorder specified as congenital (Q23.0, Q23.1)

aortic valve disorder specified as rheumatic (I06.-)

hypertrophic subaortic stenosis (I42.1)

I35.0 **Nonrheumatic aortic (valve) stenosis**

I35.1 **Nonrheumatic aortic (valve) insufficiency**

Nonrheumatic aortic (valve) incompetence NOS

Nonrheumatic aortic (valve) regurgitation NOS

I35.2 **Nonrheumatic aortic (valve) stenosis with insufficiency**

I35.8 **Other nonrheumatic aortic valve disorders**

I35.9 **Nonrheumatic aortic valve disorder, unspecified**

I36 **Nonrheumatic tricuspid valve disorders**

Excludes1: tricuspid valve disorders of unspecified cause (I07.-)

tricuspid valve disorders specified as congenital (Q22.4, Q22.8, Q22.9)

tricuspid valve disorders specified as rheumatic (I07.-)

tricuspid valve disorders with aortic and/or mitral valve involvement (I08.-)

I36.0 **Nonrheumatic tricuspid (valve) stenosis**

I36.1 **Nonrheumatic tricuspid (valve) insufficiency**

Nonrheumatic tricuspid (valve) incompetence

Nonrheumatic tricuspid (valve) regurgitation

I36.2 **Nonrheumatic tricuspid (valve) stenosis with insufficiency**

I36.8 **Other nonrheumatic tricuspid valve disorders**

I36.9 **Nonrheumatic tricuspid valve disorder, unspecified**

I37 **Nonrheumatic pulmonary valve disorders**

Excludes1: pulmonary valve disorder specified as congenital (Q22.1, Q22.2, Q22.3)

pulmonary valve disorder specified as rheumatic (I09.89)

I37.0 **Nonrheumatic pulmonary valve stenosis**

I37.1 **Nonrheumatic pulmonary valve insufficiency**

Nonrheumatic pulmonary valve incompetence

Nonrheumatic pulmonary valve regurgitation

I37.2 **Nonrheumatic pulmonary valve stenosis with insufficiency**

I37.8 **Other nonrheumatic pulmonary valve disorders**

I37.9 **Nonrheumatic pulmonary valve disorder, unspecified**

I38 **Endocarditis, valve unspecified**

Includes: endocarditis (chronic) NOS

valvular incompetence NOS

valvular insufficiency NOS

valvular regurgitation NOS

valvular stenosis NOS

valvulitis (chronic) NOS

Excludes1: congenital insufficiency of cardiac valve NOS (Q24.8)

congenital stenosis of cardiac valve NOS (Q24.8)

endocardial fibroelastosis (I42.4)

endocarditis specified as rheumatic (I09.1)

I39 **Endocarditis and heart valve disorders in diseases classified elsewhere**

Code first underlying disease, such as:

Q fever (A78)

Excludes1: endocardial involvement in:

candidiasis (B37.6) gonococcal infection (A54.83)

Libman-Sacks disease (M32.11)

listerosis (A32.82)

meningococcal infection (A39.51)

rheumatoid arthritis (M05.31)

syphilis (A52.03)

tuberculosis (A18.84)

typhoid fever (A01.02)

I40 **Acute myocarditis**

Includes: subacute myocarditis

Excludes1: acute rheumatic myocarditis (I01.2)

I40.0 **Infective myocarditis**

Septic myocarditis

Use additional code (B95-B97) to identify infectious agent

I40.1 **Isolated myocarditis**

Fiedler's myocarditis

Giant cell myocarditis

Idiopathic myocarditis

I40.8 **Other acute myocarditis**

I40.9 **Acute myocarditis, unspecified**

I41 **Myocarditis in diseases classified elsewhere**

Code first underlying disease, such as:

typhus (A75.0-A75.9)

Excludes1: myocarditis (in):

Chagas' disease (chronic) (B57.2)

acute (B57.0)

coxsackie (virus) infection (B33.22)

diphtheritic (A36.81)

gonococcal (A54.83)

influenzal (J09.X9, J10.82, J11.82)

meningococcal (A39.52)

mumps (B26.82)

rheumatoid arthritis (M05.31)

sarcoid (D86.85)

syphilis (A52.06)

toxoplasmosis (B58.81)

tuberculous (A18.84)

I42 **Cardiomyopathy**

Definition: Cardiomyopathy is a weakening of the heart muscle or a change in heart muscle structure. It is often associated with inadequate heart pumping or other heart function problems.

Includes: myocardiopathy

Code first pre-existing cardiomyopathy complicating pregnancy and puerperium (O99.4)

Excludes2: ischemic cardiomyopathy (I25.5)

peripartum cardiomyopathy (O90.3)

ventricular hypertrophy (I51.7)

I42.0 **Dilated cardiomyopathy**

Congestive cardiomyopathy

I42.1 **Obstructive hypertrophic cardiomyopathy**

Hypertrophic subaortic stenosis (idiopathic)

I42.2 **Other hypertrophic cardiomyopathy**

Nonobstructive hypertrophic cardiomyopathy

I42.3 **Endomyocardial (eosinophilic) disease**

Endomyocardial (tropical) fibrosis

Löffler's endocarditis

I42.4 **Endocardial fibroelastosis**

Congenital cardiomyopathy

Elastomyofibrosis

I42.5 **Other restrictive cardiomyopathy**

Constrictive cardiomyopathy NOS

I42.6 **Alcoholic cardiomyopathy**

Code also presence of alcoholism (F10.-)

I42.7 **Cardiomyopathy due to drug and external agent**

Code first poisoning due to drug or toxin, if applicable (T36-T65 with fifth or sixth character 1-4 or 6)

Use additional code for adverse effect, if applicable, to identify drug (T36-T50 with fifth or sixth character 5)

I42.8 **Other cardiomyopathies**

I42.9 **Cardiomyopathy, unspecified**

Cardiomyopathy (primary) (secondary) NOS

I43 **Cardiomyopathy in diseases classified elsewhere**

Code first underlying disease, such as:

amyloidosis (E85.-)

glycogen storage disease (E74.0) gout (M10.0-)

thyrotoxicosis (E05.0-E05.9-)

Excludes1: cardiomyopathy (in):

coxsackie (virus) (B33.24)

diphtheria (A36.81)

sarcoidosis (D86.85)

tuberculosis (A18.84)

I44 **Atrioventricular and left bundle-branch block**

I44.0 **Atrioventricular block, first degree**

I44.1 **Atrioventricular block, second degree**

Atrioventricular block, type I and II

Mobitz block, type I and II

Second degree block, type I and II

Wenckebach's block

I44.2 **Atrioventricular block, complete**

Complete heart block NOS

Third degree block

I44.3 **Other and unspecified atrioventricular block**

Atrioventricular block NOS

I44.30 **Unspecified atrioventricular block**

I44.39 **Other atrioventricular block**

I44.4 **Left anterior fascicular block**

I44.5 **Left posterior fascicular block**

I44.6 **Other and unspecified fascicular block**

I44.60 **Unspecified fascicular block**

Left bundle-branch hemiblock NOS

I44.69 **Other fascicular block**

I44.7 **Left bundle-branch block, unspecified**

I45 **Other conduction disorders**

I45.0 **Right fascicular block**

I45.1 **Other and unspecified right bundle-branch block**

I45.10 **Unspecified right bundle-branch block**

Right bundle-branch block NOS

I45.19 **Other right bundle-branch block**

I45.2 **Bifascicular block**

I45.3 **Trifascicular block**

I45.4 **Nonspecific intraventricular block**

Bundle-branch block NOS

I45.5 **Other specified heart block**

Sinoatrial block

Sinoauricular block

Excludes1: heart block NOS (I45.9)

I45.6 **Pre-excitation syndrome**

Accelerated atrioventricular conduction

Accessory atrioventricular conduction

Anomalous atrioventricular excitation

Lown-Ganong-Levine syndrome

Pre-excitation atrioventricular conduction

Wolff-Parkinson-White syndrome

I45.8 **Other specified conduction disorders**

I45.81 **Long QT syndrome**

I45.89 **Other specified conduction disorders**

Atrioventricular [AV] dissociation

Interference dissociation

Isorhythmic dissociation

Nonparoxysmal AV nodal tachycardia

I45.9 **Conduction disorder, unspecified**

Heart block NOS

Stokes-Adams syndrome

I46 **Cardiac arrest**

Excludes1: cardiogenic shock (R57.0)

I46.2 **Cardiac arrest due to underlying cardiac condition**

Code first underlying cardiac condition

I46.8 **Cardiac arrest due to other underlying condition**

Code first underlying condition

I46.9 **Cardiac arrest, cause unspecified**

I47 **Paroxysmal tachycardia**

Code first tachycardia complicating:

abortion or ectopic or molar pregnancy (O00-O07, O08.8)

obstetric surgery and procedures (O75.4)

Excludes1: tachycardia NOS (R00.0)

sinoauricular tachycardia NOS (R00.0)

sinus [sinusal] tachycardia NOS (R00.0)

I47.0 **Re-entry ventricular arrhythmia**

I47.1 **Supraventricular tachycardia**

Atrial (paroxysmal) tachycardia

Atrioventricular [AV] (paroxysmal) tachycardia

Atrioventricular re-entrant (nodal) tachycardia [AVNRT] [AVRT]

Junctional (paroxysmal) tachycardia

Nodal (paroxysmal) tachycardia

I47.2 **Ventricular tachycardia**

I47.9 **Paroxysmal tachycardia, unspecified**

Bouveret (-Hoffman) syndrome

I48 **Atrial fibrillation and flutter**

I48.0 **Paroxysmal atrial fibrillation**

I48.1 **Persistent atrial fibrillation**

I48.2 **Chronic atrial fibrillation**

Permanent atrial fibrillation

I48.3 **Typical atrial flutter**

Type I atrial flutter

I48.4 **Atypical atrial flutter**

Type II atrial flutter

I48.9 **Unspecified atrial fibrillation and atrial flutter**

I48.91 **Unspecified atrial fibrillation**

I48.92 **Unspecified atrial flutter**

I49 **Other cardiac arrhythmias**

Code first cardiac arrhythmia complicating:

abortion or ectopic or molar pregnancy (O00-O07, O08.8)

obstetric surgery and procedures (O75.4)

Excludes1: neonatal dysrhythmia (P29.1-)

sinoatrial bradycardia (R00.1)

sinus bradycardia (R00.1)

vagal bradycardia (R00.1)

Excludes2: bradycardia NOS (R00.1)

I49.0 Ventricular fibrillation and flutter

    I49.01 Ventricular fibrillation

    I49.02 Ventricular flutter

I49.1 Atrial premature depolarization

    Atrial premature beats

I49.2 Junctional premature depolarization

I49.3 Ventricular premature depolarization

I49.4 Other and unspecified premature depolarization

    I49.40 Unspecified premature depolarization

        Premature beats NOS

    I49.49 Other premature depolarization

        Ectopic beats

        Extrasystoles

        Extrasystolic arrhythmias

        Premature contractions

I49.5 Sick sinus syndrome

    Tachycardia-bradycardia syndrome

I49.8 Other specified cardiac arrhythmias

    Brugada syndrome

    Coronary sinus rhythm disorder

    Ectopic rhythm disorder

    Nodal rhythm disorder

I49.9 Cardiac arrhythmia, unspecified

    Arrhythmia (cardiac) NOS

I50 Heart failure

Definition: Heart failure is a condition where there is ineffective pumping of the heart leading to an accumulation of fluid in the lungs. Typical symptoms include shortness of breath with exertion, difficulty breathing when lying flat and leg or ankle swelling.

Code first heart failure complicating abortion or ectopic or molar pregnancy (O00-O07, O08.8)

heart failure due to hypertension (I11.0)

heart failure due to hypertension with chronic kidney disease (I13.-)

heart failure following surgery (I97.13-)

obstetric surgery and procedures (O75.4)

rheumatic heart failure (I09.81)

Excludes1: neonatal cardiac failure (P29.0)

Excludes2: cardiac arrest (I46.-)

▲ I50.1 Left ventricular failure, unspecified

    Cardiac asthma

    Edema of lung with heart disease NOS

    Edema of lung with heart failure

    Left heart failure

    Pulmonary edema with heart disease NOS

    Pulmonary edema with heart failure

    Excludes1: edema of lung without heart disease or heart failure (J81.-)

        pulmonary edema without heart disease or failure (J81.-)

I50.2 Systolic (congestive) heart failure

    Heart failure with reduced ejection fraction [HFrEF]

    Systolic left ventricular heart failure

    Code also end stage heart failure, if applicable (I50.84)

    Excludes1: combined systolic (congestive) and diastolic (congestive) heart failure (I50.4-)

    I50.20 Unspecified systolic (congestive) heart failure

I50.21 Acute systolic (congestive) heart failure

I50.22 Chronic systolic (congestive) heart failure

I50.23 Acute on chronic systolic (congestive) heart failure

I50.3 Diastolic (congestive) heart failure

    Diastolic left ventricular heart failure

    Heart failure with normal ejection fraction

    Heart failure with preserved ejection fraction [HFpEF]

    Code also end stage heart failure, if applicable (I50.84)

    Excludes1: combined systolic (congestive) and diastolic (congestive) heart failure (I50.4-)

    I50.30 Unspecified diastolic (congestive) heart failure

    I50.31 Acute diastolic (congestive) heart failure

    I50.32 Chronic diastolic (congestive) heart failure

    I50.33 Acute on chronic diastolic (congestive) heart failure

I50.4 Combined systolic (congestive) and diastolic (congestive) heart failure

    Combined systolic and diastolic left ventricular heart failure

    Heart failure with reduced ejection fraction and diastolic dysfunction

    Code also end stage heart failure, if applicable (I50.84)

    I50.40 Unspecified combined systolic (congestive) and diastolic (congestive) heart failure

    I50.41 Acute combined systolic (congestive) and diastolic (congestive) heart failure

    I50.42 Chronic combined systolic (congestive) and diastolic (congestive) heart failure

    I50.43 Acute on chronic combined systolic (congestive) and diastolic (congestive) heart failure

●I50.8 Other heart failure

    ●I50.81 Right heart failure

        Right ventricular failure

        ●I50.810 Right heart failure, unspecified

            Right heart failure without mention of left heart failure

            Right ventricular failure NOS

        ●I50.811 Acute right heart failure

            Acute isolated right heart failure

            Acute (isolated) right ventricular failure

        ●I50.812 Chronic right heart failure

            Chronic isolated right heart failure

            Chronic (isolated) right ventricular failure

        ●I50.813 Acute on chronic right heart failure

            Acute on chronic isolated right heart failure

            Acute on chronic (isolated) right ventricular failure

            Acute decompensation of chronic (isolated) right ventricular failure

            Acute exacerbation of chronic (isolated) right ventricular failure

        ●I50.814 Right heart failure due to left heart failure

            Right ventricular failure secondary to left ventricular failure

            Code also the type of left ventricular failure, if known (I50.2-I50.43)

Excludes1: Right heart failure with but not due to left heart failure (I50.82)

- **I50.82 Biventricular heart failure**

  Code also the type of left ventricular failure as systolic, diastolic, or combined, if known (I50.2-I50.43)

- **I50.83 High output heart failure**

- **I50.84 End stage heart failure**

  Stage D heart failure

  Code also the type of heart failure as systolic, diastolic, or combined, if known (I50.2-I50.43)

- **I50.89 Other heart failure**

I50.9 Heart failure, unspecified

Cardiac, heart or myocardial failure NOS

Congestive heart disease

Congestive heart failure NOS

Excludes2: fluid overload (E87.70)

I51 Complications and ill-defined descriptions of heart disease

Excludes1: any condition in I51.4-I51.9 due to hypertension (I11.-)

any condition in I51.4-I51.9 due to hypertension and chronic kidney disease (I13.-)

heart disease specified as rheumatic (I00-I09)

I51.0 Cardiac septal defect, acquired

Acquired septal atrial defect (old)

Acquired septal auricular defect (old)

Acquired septal ventricular defect (old)

Excludes1: cardiac septal defect as current complication following acute myocardial infarction (I23.1, I23.2)

I51.1 Rupture of chordae tendineae, not elsewhere classified

Excludes1: rupture of chordae tendineae as current complication following acute myocardial infarction (I23.4)

I51.2 Rupture of papillary muscle, not elsewhere classified

Excludes1: rupture of papillary muscle as current complication following acute myocardial infarction (I23.5)

I51.3 Intracardiac thrombosis, not elsewhere classified

Apical thrombosis (old)

Atrial thrombosis (old)

Auricular thrombosis (old)

Mural thrombosis (old)

Ventricular thrombosis (old)

Excludes1: intracardiac thrombosis as current complication following acute myocardial infarction (I23.6)

I51.4 Myocarditis, unspecified

Chronic (interstitial) myocarditis

Myocardial fibrosis

Myocarditis NOS

Excludes1: acute or subacute myocarditis (I40.-)

I51.5 Myocardial degeneration

Fatty degeneration of heart or myocardium

Myocardial disease

Senile degeneration of heart or myocardium

I51.7 Cardiomegaly

Cardiac dilatation

Cardiac hypertrophy

Ventricular dilatation

I51.8 Other ill-defined heart diseases

I51.81 Takotsubo syndrome

Reversible left ventricular dysfunction following sudden emotional stress

Stress induced cardiomyopathy

Takotsubo cardiomyopathy

Transient left ventricular apical ballooning syndrome

I51.89 Other ill-defined heart diseases

Carditis (acute)(chronic)

Pancarditis (acute)(chronic)

I51.9 Heart disease, unspecified

I52 Other heart disorders in diseases classified elsewhere

Code first underlying disease, such as:

congenital syphilis (A50.5)

mucopolysaccharidosis (E76.3)

schistosomiasis (B65.0-B65.9)

Excludes1: heart disease (in):

gonococcal infection (A54.83)

meningococcal infection (A39.50)

rheumatoid arthritis (M05.31)

syphilis (A52.06)

CEREBROVASCULAR DISEASES (I60-I69)

Use additional code to identify presence of:

alcohol abuse and dependence (F10.-)

exposure to environmental tobacco smoke (Z77.22)

history of tobacco dependence (Z87.891) hypertension (I10-I15)

occupational exposure to environmental tobacco smoke (Z57.31)

tobacco dependence (F17.-)

tobacco use (Z72.0)

Excludes1: traumatic intracranial hemorrhage (S06.-)

I60 Nontraumatic subarachnoid hemorrhage

Definition: Subarachnoid hemorrhage refers to bleeding within the head into the space between two membranes that surround the brain.

Excludes1: syphilitic ruptured cerebral aneurysm (A52.05)

Excludes2: sequelae of subarachnoid hemorrhage (I69.0-)

I60.0 Nontraumatic subarachnoid hemorrhage from carotid siphon and bifurcation

I60.00 Nontraumatic subarachnoid hemorrhage from unspecified carotid siphon and bifurcation

I60.01 Nontraumatic subarachnoid hemorrhage from right carotid siphon and bifurcation

I60.02 Nontraumatic subarachnoid hemorrhage from left carotid siphon and bifurcation

I60.1 Nontraumatic subarachnoid hemorrhage from middle cerebral artery

I60.10 Nontraumatic subarachnoid hemorrhage from unspecified middle cerebral artery

I60.11 Nontraumatic subarachnoid hemorrhage from right middle cerebral artery

I60.12 Nontraumatic subarachnoid hemorrhage from left middle cerebral artery

I60.2 Nontraumatic subarachnoid hemorrhage from anterior communicating artery

I60.3 Nontraumatic subarachnoid hemorrhage from posterior communicating artery

I60.30 Nontraumatic subarachnoid hemorrhage from unspecified posterior communicating artery

● New code ▲ Revised code **Excludes1:** Not coded here **Excludes2:** Not included here ⊗ Placeholder required ⑦ 7th digit required

I60.31 **Nontraumatic subarachnoid hemorrhage from right posterior communicating artery**

I60.32 **Nontraumatic subarachnoid hemorrhage from left posterior communicating artery**

I60.4 **Nontraumatic subarachnoid hemorrhage from basilar artery**

I60.5 **Nontraumatic subarachnoid hemorrhage from vertebral artery**

I60.50 **Nontraumatic subarachnoid hemorrhage from unspecified vertebral artery**

I60.51 **Nontraumatic subarachnoid hemorrhage from right vertebral artery**

I60.52 **Nontraumatic subarachnoid hemorrhage from left vertebral artery**

I60.6 **Nontraumatic subarachnoid hemorrhage from other intracranial arteries**

I60.7 **Nontraumatic subarachnoid hemorrhage from unspecified intracranial artery**

Ruptured (congenital) berry aneurysm

Ruptured (congenital) cerebral aneurysm

Subarachnoid hemorrhage (nontraumatic) from cerebral artery NOS

Subarachnoid hemorrhage (nontraumatic) from communicating artery NOS

Excludes1: berry aneurysm, nonruptured (I67.1)

I60.8 **Other nontraumatic subarachnoid hemorrhage**

Meningeal hemorrhage

Rupture of cerebral arteriovenous malformation

I60.9 **Nontraumatic subarachnoid hemorrhage, unspecified**

I61 **Nontraumatic intracerebral hemorrhage**

Definition: Intracerebral hemorrhage is a medical condition indicated by the rupturing of a blood vessel in the brain and the subsequent bleeding into the tissues of the brain.

Excludes2: sequelae of intracerebral hemorrhage (I69.1-)

I61.0 **Nontraumatic intracerebral hemorrhage in hemisphere, subcortical**

Deep intracerebral hemorrhage (nontraumatic)

I61.1 **Nontraumatic intracerebral hemorrhage in hemisphere, cortical**

Cerebral lobe hemorrhage (nontraumatic)

Superficial intracerebral hemorrhage (nontraumatic)

I61.2 **Nontraumatic intracerebral hemorrhage in hemisphere, unspecified**

I61.3 **Nontraumatic intracerebral hemorrhage in brain stem**

I61.4 **Nontraumatic intracerebral hemorrhage in cerebellum**

I61.5 **Nontraumatic intracerebral hemorrhage, intraventricular**

I61.6 **Nontraumatic intracerebral hemorrhage, multiple localized**

I61.8 **Other nontraumatic intracerebral hemorrhage**

I61.9 **Nontraumatic intracerebral hemorrhage, unspecified**

I62 **Other and unspecified nontraumatic intracranial hemorrhage**

Definition: Intracranial hemorrhage is bleeding in the brain caused by the breaking (rupture) of a blood vessel in the head.

Excludes2: sequelae of intracranial hemorrhage (I69.2)

I62.0 **Nontraumatic subdural hemorrhage**

I62.00 **Nontraumatic subdural hemorrhage, unspecified**

I62.01 **Nontraumatic acute subdural hemorrhage**

I62.02 **Nontraumatic subacute subdural hemorrhage**

I62.03 **Nontraumatic chronic subdural hemorrhage**

I62.1 **Nontraumatic extradural hemorrhage**

Nontraumatic epidural hemorrhage

I62.9 **Nontraumatic intracranial hemorrhage, unspecified**

I63 **Cerebral infarction**

Includes: occlusion and stenosis of cerebral and precerebral arteries, resulting in cerebral infarction

Use additional code, if applicable, to identify status post administration of tPA (rtPA) in a different facility within the last 24 hours prior to admission to current facility (Z92.82)

Use additional code, if known, to indicate National Institutes of Health Stroke Scale (NIHSS) score (R29.7-)

Excludes2: sequelae of cerebral infarction (I69.3-)

I63.0 **Cerebral infarction due to thrombosis of precerebral arteries**

I63.00 **Cerebral infarction due to thrombosis of unspecified precerebral artery**

I63.01 **Cerebral infarction due to thrombosis of vertebral artery**

I63.011 **Cerebral infarction due to thrombosis of right vertebral artery**

I63.012 **Cerebral infarction due to thrombosis of left vertebral artery**

I63.013 **Cerebral infarction due to thrombosis of bilateral vertebral arteries**

I63.019 **Cerebral infarction due to thrombosis of unspecified vertebral artery**

I63.02 **Cerebral infarction due to thrombosis of basilar artery**

I63.03 **Cerebral infarction due to thrombosis of carotid artery**

I63.031 **Cerebral infarction due to thrombosis of right carotid artery**

I63.032 **Cerebral infarction due to thrombosis of left carotid artery**

I63.033 **Cerebral infarction due to thrombosis of bilateral carotid arteries**

I63.039 **Cerebral infarction due to thrombosis of unspecified carotid artery**

I63.09 **Cerebral infarction due to thrombosis of other precerebral artery**

I63.1 **Cerebral infarction due to embolism of precerebral arteries**

I63.10 **Cerebral infarction due to embolism of unspecified precerebral artery**

I63.11 **Cerebral infarction due to embolism of vertebral artery**

I63.111 **Cerebral infarction due to embolism of right vertebral artery**

I63.112 **Cerebral infarction due to embolism of left vertebral artery**

I63.113 **Cerebral infarction due to embolism of bilateral vertebral arteries**

I63.119 **Cerebral infarction due to embolism of unspecified vertebral artery**

I63.12 **Cerebral infarction due to embolism of basilar artery**

I63.13 **Cerebral infarction due to embolism of carotid artery**

I63.131 **Cerebral infarction due to embolism of right carotid artery**

I63.132 Cerebral infarction due to embolism of left carotid artery

I63.133 Cerebral infarction due to embolism of bilateral carotid arteries

I63.139 Cerebral infarction due to embolism of unspecified carotid artery

I63.19 Cerebral infarction due to embolism of other precerebral artery

I63.2 Cerebral infarction due to unspecified occlusion or stenosis of precerebral arteries

I63.20 Cerebral infarction due to unspecified occlusion or stenosis of unspecified precerebral arteries

I63.21 Cerebral infarction due to unspecified occlusion or stenosis of vertebral arteries

▲ **I63.211** Cerebral infarction due to unspecified occlusion or stenosis of right vertebral artery

▲ **I63.212** Cerebral infarction due to unspecified occlusion or stenosis of left vertebral arteries

I63.213 Cerebral infarction due to unspecified occlusion or stenosis of bilateral vertebral arteries

I63.219 Cerebral infarction due to unspecified occlusion or stenosis of unspecified vertebral arteries

▲ **I63.22** Cerebral infarction due to unspecified occlusion or stenosis of basilar artery

I63.23 Cerebral infarction due to unspecified occlusion or stenosis of carotid arteries

I63.231 Cerebral infarction due to unspecified occlusion or stenosis of right carotid arteries

I63.232 Cerebral infarction due to unspecified occlusion or stenosis of left carotid arteries

I63.233 Cerebral infarction due to unspecified occlusion or stenosis of bilateral carotid arteries

I63.239 Cerebral infarction due to unspecified occlusion or stenosis of unspecified carotid arteries

I63.29 Cerebral infarction due to unspecified occlusion or stenosis of other precerebral arteries

I63.3 Cerebral infarction due to thrombosis of cerebral arteries

I63.30 Cerebral infarction due to thrombosis of unspecified cerebral artery

I63.31 Cerebral infarction due to thrombosis of middle cerebral artery

I63.311 Cerebral infarction due to thrombosis of right middle cerebral artery

I63.312 Cerebral infarction due to thrombosis of left middle cerebral artery

I63.313 Cerebral infarction due to thrombosis of bilateral middle cerebral arteries

I63.319 Cerebral infarction due to thrombosis of unspecified middle cerebral artery

I63.32 Cerebral infarction due to thrombosis of anterior cerebral artery

I63.321 Cerebral infarction due to thrombosis of right anterior cerebral artery

I63.322 Cerebral infarction due to thrombosis of left anterior cerebral artery

▲ **I63.323** Cerebral infarction due to thrombosis of bilateral anterior cerebral arteries

I63.329 Cerebral infarction due to thrombosis of unspecified anterior cerebral artery

I63.33 Cerebral infarction due to thrombosis of posterior cerebral artery

I63.331 Cerebral infarction due to thrombosis of right posterior cerebral artery

I63.332 Cerebral infarction due to thrombosis of left posterior cerebral artery

▲ **I63.333** Cerebral infarction to thrombosis of bilateral posterior cerebral arteries

I63.339 Cerebral infarction due to thrombosis of unspecified posterior cerebral artery

I63.34 Cerebral infarction due to thrombosis of cerebellar artery

I63.341 Cerebral infarction due to thrombosis of right cerebellar artery

I63.342 Cerebral infarction due to thrombosis of left cerebellar artery

I63.343 Cerebral infarction to thrombosis of bilateral cerebellar arteries

I63.349 Cerebral infarction due to thrombosis of unspecified cerebellar artery

I63.39 Cerebral infarction due to thrombosis of other cerebral artery

I63.4 Cerebral infarction due to embolism of cerebral arteries

I63.40 Cerebral infarction due to embolism of unspecified cerebral artery

I63.41 Cerebral infarction due to embolism of middle cerebral artery

I63.411 Cerebral infarction due to embolism of right middle cerebral artery

I63.412 Cerebral infarction due to embolism of left middle cerebral artery

I63.413 Cerebral infarction due to embolism of bilateral middle cerebral arteries

I63.419 Cerebral infarction due to embolism of unspecified middle cerebral artery

I63.42 Cerebral infarction due to embolism of anterior cerebral artery

I63.421 Cerebral infarction due to embolism of right anterior cerebral artery

I63.422 Cerebral infarction due to embolism of left anterior cerebral artery

I63.423 Cerebral infarction due to embolism of bilateral anterior cerebral arteries

I63.429 Cerebral infarction due to embolism of unspecified anterior cerebral artery

I63.43 Cerebral infarction due to embolism of posterior cerebral artery

I63.431 Cerebral infarction due to embolism of right posterior cerebral artery

● New code   ▲ Revised code   **Excludes1:** Not coded here   **Excludes2:** Not included here   ⊗ Placeholder required   ⑦ 7th digit required

I63.432 Cerebral infarction due to embolism of left posterior cerebral artery

I63.433 Cerebral infarction due to embolism of bilateral posterior cerebral arteries

I63.439 Cerebral infarction due to embolism of unspecified posterior cerebral artery

I63.44 Cerebral infarction due to embolism of cerebellar artery

I63.441 Cerebral infarction due to embolism of right cerebellar artery

I63.442 Cerebral infarction due to embolism of left cerebellar artery

I63.443 Cerebral infarction due to embolism of bilateral cerebellar arteries

I63.449 Cerebral infarction due to embolism of unspecified cerebellar artery

I63.49 Cerebral infarction due to embolism of other cerebral artery

I63.5 Cerebral infarction due to unspecified occlusion or stenosis of cerebral arteries

I63.50 Cerebral infarction due to unspecified occlusion or stenosis of unspecified cerebral artery

I63.51 Cerebral infarction due to unspecified occlusion or stenosis of middle cerebral artery

I63.511 Cerebral infarction due to unspecified occlusion or stenosis of right middle cerebral artery

I63.512 Cerebral infarction due to unspecified occlusion or stenosis of left middle cerebral artery

▲ **I63.513** Cerebral infarction due to unspecified occlusion or stenosis of bilateral middle cerebral arteries

I63.519 Cerebral infarction due to unspecified occlusion or stenosis of unspecified middle cerebral artery

I63.52 Cerebral infarction due to unspecified occlusion or stenosis of anterior cerebral artery

I63.521 Cerebral infarction due to unspecified occlusion or stenosis of right anterior cerebral artery

I63.522 Cerebral infarction due to unspecified occlusion or stenosis of left anterior cerebral artery

▲ **I63.523** Cerebral infarction due to unspecified occlusion or stenosis of bilateral anterior cerebral arteries

I63.529 Cerebral infarction due to unspecified occlusion or stenosis of unspecified anterior cerebral artery

I63.53 Cerebral infarction due to unspecified occlusion or stenosis of posterior cerebral artery

I63.531 Cerebral infarction due to unspecified occlusion or stenosis of right posterior cerebral artery

I63.532 Cerebral infarction due to unspecified occlusion or stenosis of left posterior cerebral artery

▲ **I63.533** Cerebral infarction due to unspecified occlusion or stenosis of bilateral posterior cerebral arteries

I63.539 Cerebral infarction due to unspecified occlusion or stenosis of unspecified posterior cerebral artery

I63.54 Cerebral infarction due to unspecified occlusion or stenosis of cerebellar artery

I63.541 Cerebral infarction due to unspecified occlusion or stenosis of right cerebellar artery

I63.542 Cerebral infarction due to unspecified occlusion or stenosis of left cerebellar artery

I63.543 Cerebral infarction due to unspecified occlusion or stenosis of bilateral cerebellar arteries

I63.549 Cerebral infarction due to unspecified occlusion or stenosis of unspecified cerebellar artery

I63.59 Cerebral infarction due to unspecified occlusion or stenosis of other cerebral artery

I63.6 Cerebral infarction due to cerebral venous thrombosis, nonpyogenic

I63.8 Other cerebral infarction

I63.9 Cerebral infarction, unspecified

Stroke NOS

Excludes2: transient cerebral ischemic attacks and related syndromes (G45.-)

I65 **Occlusion and stenosis of precerebral arteries, not resulting in cerebral infarction**

Includes: embolism of precerebral artery

narrowing of precerebral artery

obstruction (complete) (partial) of precerebral artery

thrombosis of precerebral artery

Excludes1: insufficiency, NOS, of precerebral artery (G45.-)

insufficiency of precerebral arteries causing cerebral infarction (I63.0-I63.2)

I65.0 Occlusion and stenosis of vertebral artery

I65.01 Occlusion and stenosis of right vertebral artery

I65.02 Occlusion and stenosis of left vertebral artery

I65.03 Occlusion and stenosis of bilateral vertebral arteries

I65.09 Occlusion and stenosis of unspecified vertebral artery

I65.1 Occlusion and stenosis of basilar artery

I65.2 Occlusion and stenosis of carotid artery

I65.21 Occlusion and stenosis of right carotid artery

I65.22 Occlusion and stenosis of left carotid artery

I65.23 Occlusion and stenosis of bilateral carotid arteries

I65.29 Occlusion and stenosis of unspecified carotid artery

I65.8 Occlusion and stenosis of other precerebral arteries

I65.9 Occlusion and stenosis of unspecified precerebral artery

Occlusion and stenosis of precerebral artery NOS

I66 **Occlusion and stenosis of cerebral arteries, not resulting in cerebral infarction**

Includes: embolism of cerebral artery

narrowing of cerebral artery

obstruction (complete) (partial) of cerebral artery

thrombosis of cerebral artery

Excludes1: Occlusion and stenosis of cerebral artery causing cerebral infarction (I63.3-I63.5)

I66.0 Occlusion and stenosis of middle cerebral artery

I66.01 Occlusion and stenosis of right middle cerebral artery

I66.02 Occlusion and stenosis of left middle cerebral artery

I66.03 Occlusion and stenosis of bilateral middle cerebral arteries

I66.09 Occlusion and stenosis of unspecified middle cerebral artery

I66.1 Occlusion and stenosis of anterior cerebral artery

I66.11 Occlusion and stenosis of right anterior cerebral artery

I66.12 Occlusion and stenosis of left anterior cerebral artery

I66.13 Occlusion and stenosis of bilateral anterior cerebral arteries

I66.19 Occlusion and stenosis of unspecified anterior cerebral artery

I66.2 Occlusion and stenosis of posterior cerebral artery

I66.21 Occlusion and stenosis of right posterior cerebral artery

I66.22 Occlusion and stenosis of left posterior cerebral artery

I66.23 Occlusion and stenosis of bilateral posterior cerebral arteries

I66.29 Occlusion and stenosis of unspecified posterior cerebral artery

I66.3 Occlusion and stenosis of cerebellar arteries

I66.8 Occlusion and stenosis of other cerebral arteries

Occlusion and stenosis of perforating arteries

I66.9 Occlusion and stenosis of unspecified cerebral artery

I67 Other cerebrovascular diseases

Excludes2: sequelae of the listed conditions (I69.8)

I67.0 Dissection of cerebral arteries, nonruptured

Excludes1: ruptured cerebral arteries (I60.7)

I67.1 Cerebral aneurysm, nonruptured

Cerebral aneurysm NOS

Cerebral arteriovenous fistula, acquired

Internal carotid artery aneurysm, intracranial portion

Internal carotid artery aneurysm, NOS

Excludes1: congenital cerebral aneurysm, nonruptured (Q28.-)

ruptured cerebral aneurysm (I60.7)

I67.2 Cerebral atherosclerosis

Atheroma of cerebral and precerebral arteries

I67.3 Progressive vascular leukoencephalopathy

Binswanger's disease

I67.4 Hypertensive encephalopathy

Excludes2: insufficiency, NOS, of precerebral arteries (G45.2)

I67.5 Moyamoya disease

I67.6 Nonpyogenic thrombosis of intracranial venous system

Nonpyogenic thrombosis of cerebral vein

Nonpyogenic thrombosis of intracranial venous sinus

Excludes1: nonpyogenic thrombosis of intracranial venous system causing infarction (I63.6)

I67.7 Cerebral arteritis, not elsewhere classified

Granulomatous angiitis of the nervous system

Excludes1: allergic granulomatous angiitis (M30.1)

I67.8 Other specified cerebrovascular diseases

I67.81 Acute cerebrovascular insufficiency

Acute cerebrovascular insufficiency unspecified as to location or reversibility

I67.82 Cerebral ischemia

Chronic cerebral ischemia

I67.83 Posterior reversible encephalopathy syndrome

PRES

I67.84 Cerebral vasospasm and vasoconstriction

I67.841 Reversible cerebrovascular vasoconstriction syndrome

Call-Fleming syndrome

Code first underlying condition, if applicable, such as eclampsia (O15.00-O15.9)

I67.848 Other cerebrovascular vasospasm and vasoconstriction

I67.89 Other cerebrovascular disease

I67.9 Cerebrovascular disease, unspecified

I68 Cerebrovascular disorders in diseases classified elsewhere

I68.0 Cerebral amyloid angiopathy

Code first underlying amyloidosis (E85.-)

I68.2 Cerebral arteritis in other diseases classified elsewhere

Code first underlying disease

Excludes1: cerebral arteritis (in):

listerosis (A32.89)

systemic lupus erythematosus (M32.19)

syphilis (A52.04)

tuberculosis (A18.89)

I68.8 Other cerebrovascular disorders in diseases classified elsewhere

Code first underlying disease

Excludes1: syphilitic cerebral aneurysm (A52.05)

I69 Sequelae of cerebrovascular disease

Note: Category I69 is to be used to indicate conditions in I60-I67 as the cause of sequelae. The 'sequelae' include conditions specified as such or as residuals which may occur at any time after the onset of the causal condition

Excludes1: personal history of cerebral infarction without residual deficit (Z86.73)

personal history of prolonged reversible ischemic neurologic deficit (PRIND) (Z86.73)

personal history of reversible ischemic neurological deficit (RIND) (Z86.73)

sequelae of traumatic intracranial injury (S06.-)

I69.0 Sequelae of nontraumatic subarachnoid hemorrhage

I69.00 Unspecified sequelae of nontraumatic subarachnoid hemorrhage

I69.01 Cognitive deficits following nontraumatic subarachnoid hemorrhage

I69.010 Attention and concentration deficit following nontraumatic subarachnoid hemorrhage

I69.011 Memory deficit following nontraumatic subarachnoid hemorrhage

I69.012 Visuospatial deficit and spatial neglect following nontraumatic subarachnoid hemorrhage

I69.013 Psychomotor deficit following nontraumatic subarachnoid hemorrhage

I69.014 Frontal lobe and executive function deficit following nontraumatic subarachnoid hemorrhage

● New code ▲ Revised code **Excludes1:** Not coded here **Excludes2:** Not included here ⊗ Placeholder required ⑦ 7th digit required

I69.015　Cognitive social or emotional deficit following nontraumatic subarachnoid hemorrhage

I69.018　Other symptoms and signs involving cognitive functions following nontraumatic subarachnoid hemorrhage

I69.019　Unspecified symptoms and signs involving cognitive functions following nontraumatic subarachnoid hemorrhage

I69.02　Speech and language deficits following nontraumatic subarachnoid hemorrhage

I69.020　Aphasia following nontraumatic subarachnoid hemorrhage

I69.021　Dysphasia following nontraumatic subarachnoid hemorrhage

I69.022　Dysarthria following nontraumatic subarachnoid hemorrhage

I69.023　Fluency disorder following nontraumatic subarachnoid hemorrhage

Stuttering following nontraumatic subarachnoid hemorrhage

I69.028　Other speech and language deficits following nontraumatic subarachnoid hemorrhage

I69.03　Monoplegia of upper limb following nontraumatic subarachnoid hemorrhage

I69.031　Monoplegia of upper limb following nontraumatic subarachnoid hemorrhage affecting right dominant side

I69.032　Monoplegia of upper limb following nontraumatic subarachnoid hemorrhage affecting left dominant side

I69.033　Monoplegia of upper limb following nontraumatic subarachnoid hemorrhage affecting right non-dominant side

I69.034　Monoplegia of upper limb following nontraumatic subarachnoid hemorrhage affecting left non-dominant side

I69.039　Monoplegia of upper limb following nontraumatic subarachnoid hemorrhage affecting unspecified side

I69.04　Monoplegia of lower limb following nontraumatic subarachnoid hemorrhage

I69.041　Monoplegia of lower limb following nontraumatic subarachnoid hemorrhage affecting right dominant side

I69.042　Monoplegia of lower limb following nontraumatic subarachnoid hemorrhage affecting left dominant side

I69.043　Monoplegia of lower limb following nontraumatic subarachnoid hemorrhage affecting right non-dominant side

I69.044　Monoplegia of lower limb following nontraumatic subarachnoid hemorrhage affecting left non-dominant side

I69.049　Monoplegia of lower limb following nontraumatic subarachnoid

hemorrhage affecting unspecified side

I69.05　Hemiplegia and hemiparesis following nontraumatic subarachnoid hemorrhage

I69.051　Hemiplegia and hemiparesis following nontraumatic subarachnoid hemorrhage affecting right dominant side

I69.052　Hemiplegia and hemiparesis following nontraumatic subarachnoid hemorrhage affecting left dominant side

I69.053　Hemiplegia and hemiparesis following nontraumatic subarachnoid hemorrhage affecting right non-dominant side

I69.054　Hemiplegia and hemiparesis following nontraumatic subarachnoid hemorrhage affecting left non-dominant side

I69.059　Hemiplegia and hemiparesis following nontraumatic subarachnoid hemorrhage affecting unspecified side

I69.06　Other paralytic syndrome following nontraumatic subarachnoid hemorrhage

<u>Use additional code</u> to identify type of paralytic syndrome, such as:

locked-in state (G83.5)

quadriplegia (G82.5-)

Excludes1: hemiplegia/hemiparesis following nontraumatic subarachnoid hemorrhage (I69.05-)

monoplegia of lower limb following nontraumatic subarachnoid hemorrhage (I69.04-)

monoplegia of upper limb following nontraumatic subarachnoid hemorrhage (I69.03-)

I69.061　Other paralytic syndrome following nontraumatic subarachnoid hemorrhage affecting right dominant side

I69.062　Other paralytic syndrome following nontraumatic subarachnoid hemorrhage affecting left dominant side

I69.063　Other paralytic syndrome following nontraumatic subarachnoid hemorrhage affecting right non-dominant side

I69.064　Other paralytic syndrome following nontraumatic subarachnoid hemorrhage affecting left non-dominant side

I69.065　Other paralytic syndrome following nontraumatic subarachnoid hemorrhage, bilateral

I69.069　Other paralytic syndrome following nontraumatic subarachnoid hemorrhage affecting unspecified side

I69.09　Other sequelae of nontraumatic subarachnoid hemorrhage

I69.090　Apraxia following nontraumatic subarachnoid hemorrhage

I69.091 **Dysphagia following nontraumatic subarachnoid hemorrhage**

<u>Use additional code</u> to identify the type of dysphagia, if known (R13.1-)

I69.092 **Facial weakness following nontraumatic subarachnoid hemorrhage**

Facial droop following nontraumatic subarachnoid hemorrhage

I69.093 **Ataxia following nontraumatic subarachnoid hemorrhage**

I69.098 **Other sequelae following nontraumatic subarachnoid hemorrhage**

Alterations of sensation following nontraumatic subarachnoid hemorrhage

Disturbance of vision following nontraumatic subarachnoid hemorrhage

<u>Use additional code</u> to identify the sequelae

I69.1 **Sequelae of nontraumatic intracerebral hemorrhage**

I69.10 **Unspecified sequelae of nontraumatic intracerebral hemorrhage**

I69.11 **Cognitive deficits following nontraumatic intracerebral hemorrhage**

I69.110 **Attention and concentration deficit following nontraumatic intracerebral hemorrhage**

I69.111 **Memory deficit following nontraumatic intracerebral hemorrhage**

I69.112 **Visuospatial deficit and spatial neglect following nontraumatic intracerebral hemorrhage**

I69.113 **Psychomotor deficit following nontraumatic intracerebral hemorrhage**

I69.114 **Frontal lobe and executive function deficit following nontraumatic intracerebral hemorrhage**

I69.115 **Cognitive social or emotional deficit following nontraumatic intracerebral hemorrhage**

I69.118 **Other symptoms and signs involving cognitive functions following nontraumatic intracerebral hemorrhage**

I69.119 **Unspecified symptoms and signs involving cognitive functions following nontraumatic intracerebral hemorrhage**

I69.12 **Speech and language deficits following nontraumatic intracerebral hemorrhage**

I69.120 **Aphasia following nontraumatic intracerebral hemorrhage**

I69.121 **Dysphasia following nontraumatic intracerebral hemorrhage**

I69.122 **Dysarthria following nontraumatic intracerebral hemorrhage**

I69.123 **Fluency disorder following nontraumatic intracerebral hemorrhage**

Stuttering following nontraumatic intracerebral hemorrhage

I69.128 **Other speech and language deficits following nontraumatic intracerebral hemorrhage**

I69.13 **Monoplegia of upper limb following nontraumatic intracerebral hemorrhage**

I69.131 **Monoplegia of upper limb following nontraumatic intracerebral hemorrhage affecting right dominant side**

I69.132 **Monoplegia of upper limb following nontraumatic intracerebral hemorrhage affecting left dominant side**

I69.133 **Monoplegia of upper limb following nontraumatic intracerebral hemorrhage affecting right non-dominant side**

I69.134 **Monoplegia of upper limb following nontraumatic intracerebral hemorrhage affecting left non-dominant side**

I69.139 **Monoplegia of upper limb following nontraumatic intracerebral hemorrhage affecting unspecified side**

I69.14 **Monoplegia of lower limb following nontraumatic intracerebral hemorrhage**

I69.141 **Monoplegia of lower limb following nontraumatic intracerebral hemorrhage affecting right dominant side**

I69.142 **Monoplegia of lower limb following nontraumatic intracerebral hemorrhage affecting left dominant side**

I69.143 **Monoplegia of lower limb following nontraumatic intracerebral hemorrhage affecting right non-dominant side**

I69.144 **Monoplegia of lower limb following nontraumatic intracerebral hemorrhage affecting left non-dominant side**

I69.149 **Monoplegia of lower limb following nontraumatic intracerebral hemorrhage affecting unspecified side**

I69.15 **Hemiplegia and hemiparesis following nontraumatic intracerebral hemorrhage**

I69.151 **Hemiplegia and hemiparesis following nontraumatic intracerebral hemorrhage affecting right dominant side**

I69.152 **Hemiplegia and hemiparesis following nontraumatic intracerebral hemorrhage affecting left dominant side**

I69.153 **Hemiplegia and hemiparesis following nontraumatic intracerebral hemorrhage affecting right non-dominant side**

I69.154 **Hemiplegia and hemiparesis following nontraumatic intracerebral hemorrhage affecting left non-dominant side**

I69.159 **Hemiplegia and hemiparesis following nontraumatic intracerebral hemorrhage affecting unspecified side**

● New code ▲ Revised code **Excludes1:** Not coded here **Excludes2:** Not included here ⊗ Placeholder required ⑦ 7th digit required

I69.16 Other paralytic syndrome following nontraumatic intracerebral hemorrhage

Use additional code to identify type of paralytic syndrome, such as:

locked-in state (G83.5)

quadriplegia (G82.5-)

Excludes1: hemiplegia/hemiparesis following nontraumatic intracerebral hemorrhage (I69.15-)

monoplegia of lower limb following nontraumatic intracerebral hemorrhage (I69.14-)

monoplegia of upper limb following nontraumatic intracerebral hemorrhage (I69.13-)

I69.161 Other paralytic syndrome following nontraumatic intracerebral hemorrhage affecting right dominant side

I69.162 Other paralytic syndrome following nontraumatic intracerebral hemorrhage affecting left dominant side

I69.163 Other paralytic syndrome following nontraumatic intracerebral hemorrhage affecting right non-dominant side

I69.164 Other paralytic syndrome following nontraumatic intracerebral hemorrhage affecting left non-dominant side

I69.165 Other paralytic syndrome following nontraumatic intracerebral hemorrhage, bilateral

I69.169 Other paralytic syndrome following nontraumatic intracerebral hemorrhage affecting unspecified side

I69.19 Other sequelae of nontraumatic intracerebral hemorrhage

I69.190 Apraxia following nontraumatic intracerebral hemorrhage

I69.191 Dysphagia following nontraumatic intracerebral hemorrhage

Use additional code to identify the type of dysphagia, if known (R13.1-)

I69.192 Facial weakness following nontraumatic intracerebral hemorrhage

Facial droop following nontraumatic intracerebral hemorrhage

I69.193 Ataxia following nontraumatic intracerebral hemorrhage

I69.198 Other sequelae of nontraumatic intracerebral hemorrhage

Alteration of sensations following nontraumatic intracerebral hemorrhage

Disturbance of vision following nontraumatic intracerebral hemorrhage

Use additional code to identify the sequelae

I69.2 Sequelae of other nontraumatic intracranial hemorrhage

I69.20 Unspecified sequelae of other nontraumatic intracranial hemorrhage

I69.21 Cognitive deficits following other nontraumatic intracranial hemorrhage

I69.210 Attention and concentration deficit following other nontraumatic intracranial hemorrhage

I69.211 Memory deficit following other nontraumatic intracranial hemorrhage

I69.212 Visuospatial deficit and spatial neglect following other nontraumatic intracranial hemorrhage

I69.213 Psychomotor deficit following other nontraumatic intracranial hemorrhage

I69.214 Frontal lobe and executive function deficit following other nontraumatic intracranial hemorrhage

I69.215 Cognitive social or emotional deficit following other nontraumatic intracranial hemorrhage

I69.218 Other symptoms and signs involving cognitive functions following other nontraumatic intracranial hemorrhage

I69.219 Unspecified symptoms and signs involving cognitive functions following other nontraumatic intracranial hemorrhage

I69.22 Speech and language deficits following other nontraumatic intracranial hemorrhage

I69.220 Aphasia following other nontraumatic intracranial hemorrhage

I69.221 Dysphasia following other nontraumatic intracranial hemorrhage

I69.222 Dysarthria following other nontraumatic intracranial hemorrhage

I69.223 Fluency disorder following other nontraumatic intracranial hemorrhage

Stuttering following other nontraumatic intracranial hemorrhage

I69.228 Other speech and language deficits following other nontraumatic intracranial hemorrhage

I69.23 Monoplegia of upper limb following other nontraumatic intracranial hemorrhage

I69.231 Monoplegia of upper limb following other nontraumatic intracranial hemorrhage affecting right dominant side

I69.232 Monoplegia of upper limb following other nontraumatic intracranial hemorrhage affecting left dominant side

I69.233 Monoplegia of upper limb following other nontraumatic intracranial hemorrhage affecting right non-dominant side

I69.234 Monoplegia of upper limb following other nontraumatic intracranial hemorrhage affecting left non-dominant side

I69.239 Monoplegia of upper limb following other nontraumatic intracranial

▓ Add 4th-7th digits		Nonspecific code	Unspecified code	Manifestation code

hemorrhage affecting unspecified
side

I69.24 **Monoplegia of lower limb following other nontraumatic intracranial hemorrhage**

I69.241 **Monoplegia of lower limb following other nontraumatic intracranial hemorrhage affecting right dominant side**

I69.242 **Monoplegia of lower limb following other nontraumatic intracranial hemorrhage affecting left dominant side**

I69.243 **Monoplegia of lower limb following other nontraumatic intracranial hemorrhage affecting right non-dominant side**

I69.244 **Monoplegia of lower limb following other nontraumatic intracranial hemorrhage affecting left non-dominant side**

I69.249 **Monoplegia of lower limb following other nontraumatic intracranial hemorrhage affecting unspecified side**

I69.25 **Hemiplegia and hemiparesis following other nontraumatic intracranial hemorrhage**

I69.251 **Hemiplegia and hemiparesis following other nontraumatic intracranial hemorrhage affecting right dominant side**

I69.252 **Hemiplegia and hemiparesis following other nontraumatic intracranial hemorrhage affecting left dominant side**

I69.253 **Hemiplegia and hemiparesis following other nontraumatic intracranial hemorrhage affecting right non-dominant side**

I69.254 **Hemiplegia and hemiparesis following other nontraumatic intracranial hemorrhage affecting left non-dominant side**

I69.259 **Hemiplegia and hemiparesis following other nontraumatic intracranial hemorrhage affecting unspecified side**

I69.26 **Other paralytic syndrome following other nontraumatic intracranial hemorrhage**

Use additional code to identify type of paralytic syndrome, such as:

locked-in state (G83.5)

quadriplegia (G82.5-)

Excludes1: hemiplegia/hemiparesis following other nontraumatic intracranial hemorrhage (I69.25-)

monoplegia of lower limb following other nontraumatic intracranial hemorrhage (I69.24-)

monoplegia of upper limb following other nontraumatic intracranial hemorrhage (I69.23-)

I69.261 **Other paralytic syndrome following other nontraumatic intracranial hemorrhage affecting right dominant side**

I69.262 **Other paralytic syndrome following other nontraumatic intracranial**

hemorrhage affecting left dominant side

I69.263 **Other paralytic syndrome following other nontraumatic intracranial hemorrhage affecting right non-dominant side**

I69.264 **Other paralytic syndrome following other nontraumatic intracranial hemorrhage affecting left non-dominant side**

I69.265 **Other paralytic syndrome following other nontraumatic intracranial hemorrhage, bilateral**

I69.269 **Other paralytic syndrome following other nontraumatic intracranial hemorrhage affecting unspecified side**

I69.29 **Other sequelae of other nontraumatic intracranial hemorrhage**

I69.290 **Apraxia following other nontraumatic intracranial hemorrhage**

I69.291 **Dysphagia following other nontraumatic intracranial hemorrhage**

Use additional code to identify the type of dysphagia, if known (R13.1-)

I69.292 **Facial weakness following other nontraumatic intracranial hemorrhage**

Facial droop following other nontraumatic intracranial hemorrhage

I69.293 **Ataxia following other nontraumatic intracranial hemorrhage**

I69.298 **Other sequelae of other nontraumatic intracranial hemorrhage**

Alteration of sensation following other nontraumatic intracranial hemorrhage

Disturbance of vision following other nontraumatic intracranial hemorrhage

Use additional code to identify the sequelae

I69.3 **Sequelae of cerebral infarction**

Sequelae of stroke NOS

I69.30 **Unspecified sequelae of cerebral infarction**

I69.31 **Cognitive deficits following cerebral infarction**

I69.310 **Attention and concentration deficit following cerebral infarction**

I69.311 **Memory deficit following cerebral infarction**

I69.312 **Visuospatial deficit and spatial neglect following cerebral infarction**

I69.313 **Psychomotor deficit following cerebral infarction**

I69.314 **Frontal lobe and executive function deficit following cerebral infarction**

I69.315 **Cognitive social or emotional deficit following cerebral infarction**

I69.318 **Other symptoms and signs involving cognitive functions following cerebral infarction**

I69.319 **Unspecified symptoms and signs involving cognitive functions following cerebral infarction**

● New code ▲ Revised code **Excludes1:** Not coded here **Excludes2:** Not included here ⊗ Placeholder required ⑦ 7th digit required

I69.32 **Speech and language deficits following cerebral infarction**

    I69.320 **Aphasia following cerebral infarction**

    I69.321 **Dysphasia following cerebral infarction**

    I69.322 **Dysarthria following cerebral infarction**

        Excludes2: transient ischemic attack (TIA) (G45.9)

    I69.323 **Fluency disorder following cerebral infarction**

        Stuttering following cerebral infarction

    I69.328 **Other speech and language deficits following cerebral infarction**

I69.33 **Monoplegia of upper limb following cerebral infarction**

    I69.331 **Monoplegia of upper limb following cerebral infarction affecting right dominant side**

    I69.332 **Monoplegia of upper limb following cerebral infarction affecting left dominant side**

    I69.333 **Monoplegia of upper limb following cerebral infarction affecting right non-dominant side**

    I69.334 **Monoplegia of upper limb following cerebral infarction affecting left non-dominant side**

    I69.339 **Monoplegia of upper limb following cerebral infarction affecting unspecified side**

I69.34 **Monoplegia of lower limb following cerebral infarction**

    I69.341 **Monoplegia of lower limb following cerebral infarction affecting right dominant side**

    I69.342 **Monoplegia of lower limb following cerebral infarction affecting left dominant side**

    I69.343 **Monoplegia of lower limb following cerebral infarction affecting right non-dominant side**

    I69.344 **Monoplegia of lower limb following cerebral infarction affecting left non-dominant side**

    I69.349 **Monoplegia of lower limb following cerebral infarction affecting unspecified side**

I69.35 **Hemiplegia and hemiparesis following cerebral infarction**

    I69.351 **Hemiplegia and hemiparesis following cerebral infarction affecting right dominant side**

        Excludes2: precerebral artery, congential (nonruptured) (Q28.1)

    I69.352 **Hemiplegia and hemiparesis following cerebral infarction affecting left dominant side**

    I69.353 **Hemiplegia and hemiparesis following cerebral infarction affecting right non-dominant side**

    I69.354 **Hemiplegia and hemiparesis following cerebral infarction affecting left non-dominant side**

    I69.359 **Hemiplegia and hemiparesis following cerebral infarction affecting unspecified side**

I69.36 **Other paralytic syndrome following cerebral infarction**

    Use additional code to identify type of paralytic syndrome, such as:

    locked-in state (G83.5)

    quadriplegia (G82.5-)

    Excludes1: hemiplegia/hemiparesis following cerebral infarction (I69.35-)

        monoplegia of lower limb following cerebral infarction (I69.34-)

        monoplegia of upper limb following cerebral infarction (I69.33-)

    I69.361 **Other paralytic syndrome following cerebral infarction affecting right dominant side**

    I69.362 **Other paralytic syndrome following cerebral infarction affecting left dominant side**

    I69.363 **Other paralytic syndrome following cerebral infarction affecting right non-dominant side**

    I69.364 **Other paralytic syndrome following cerebral infarction affecting left non-dominant side**

    I69.365 **Other paralytic syndrome following cerebral infarction, bilateral**

    I69.369 **Other paralytic syndrome following cerebral infarction affecting unspecified side**

I69.39 **Other sequelae of cerebral infarction**

    I69.390 **Apraxia following cerebral infarction**

    I69.391 **Dysphagia following cerebral infarction**

        Use additional code to identify the type of dysphagia, if known (R13.1-)

    I69.392 **Facial weakness following cerebral infarction**

        Facial droop following cerebral infarction

    I69.393 **Ataxia following cerebral infarction**

    I69.398 **Other sequelae of cerebral infarction**

        Alteration of sensation following cerebral infarction

        Disturbance of vision following cerebral infarction

        Use additional code to identify the sequelae

I69.8 **Sequelae of other cerebrovascular diseases**

    Excludes1: sequelae of traumatic intracranial injury (S06.-)

I69.80 **Unspecified sequelae of other cerebrovascular disease**

I69.81 **Cognitive deficits following other cerebrovascular disease**

    I69.810 **Attention and concentration deficit following other cerebrovascular disease**

    I69.811 **Memory deficit following other cerebrovascular disease**

I69.812 Visuospatial deficit and spatial neglect following other cerebrovascular disease

I69.813 Psychomotor deficit following other cerebrovascular disease

I69.814 Frontal lobe and executive function deficit following other cerebrovascular disease

I69.815 Cognitive social or emotional deficit following other cerebrovascular disease

I69.818 Other symptoms and signs involving cognitive functions following other cerebrovascular disease

I69.819 Unspecified symptoms and signs involving cognitive functions following other cerebrovascular disease

I69.82 Speech and language deficits following other cerebrovascular disease

I69.820 Aphasia following other cerebrovascular disease

I69.821 Dysphasia following other cerebrovascular disease

I69.822 Dysarthria following other cerebrovascular disease

I69.823 Fluency disorder following other cerebrovascular disease

Stuttering following other cerebrovascular disease

I69.828 Other speech and language deficits following other cerebrovascular disease

I69.83 Monoplegia of upper limb following other cerebrovascular disease

I69.831 Monoplegia of upper limb following other cerebrovascular disease affecting right dominant side

I69.832 Monoplegia of upper limb following other cerebrovascular disease affecting left dominant side

I69.833 Monoplegia of upper limb following other cerebrovascular disease affecting right non-dominant side

I69.834 Monoplegia of upper limb following other cerebrovascular disease affecting left non-dominant side

I69.839 Monoplegia of upper limb following other cerebrovascular disease affecting unspecified side

I69.84 Monoplegia of lower limb following other cerebrovascular disease

I69.841 Monoplegia of lower limb following other cerebrovascular disease affecting right dominant side

I69.842 Monoplegia of lower limb following other cerebrovascular disease affecting left dominant side

I69.843 Monoplegia of lower limb following other cerebrovascular disease affecting right non-dominant side

I69.844 Monoplegia of lower limb following other cerebrovascular disease affecting left non-dominant side

I69.849 Monoplegia of lower limb following other cerebrovascular disease affecting unspecified side

I69.85 Hemiplegia and hemiparesis following other cerebrovascular disease

I69.851 Hemiplegia and hemiparesis following other cerebrovascular disease affecting right dominant side

I69.852 Hemiplegia and hemiparesis following other cerebrovascular disease affecting left dominant side

I69.853 Hemiplegia and hemiparesis following other cerebrovascular disease affecting right non-dominant side

I69.854 Hemiplegia and hemiparesis following other cerebrovascular disease affecting left non-dominant side

I69.859 Hemiplegia and hemiparesis following other cerebrovascular disease affecting unspecified side

I69.86 Other paralytic syndrome following other cerebrovascular disease

Use additional code to identify type of paralytic syndrome, such as:

locked-in state (G83.5)

quadriplegia (G82.5-)

Excludes1: hemiplegia/hemiparesis following other cerebrovascular disease (I69.85-)

monoplegia of lower limb following other cerebrovascular disease (I69.84-)

monoplegia of upper limb following other cerebrovascular disease (I69.83-)

I69.861 Other paralytic syndrome following other cerebrovascular disease affecting right dominant side

I69.862 Other paralytic syndrome following other cerebrovascular disease affecting left dominant side

I69.863 Other paralytic syndrome following other cerebrovascular disease affecting right non-dominant side

I69.864 Other paralytic syndrome following other cerebrovascular disease affecting left non-dominant side

I69.865 Other paralytic syndrome following other cerebrovascular disease, bilateral

I69.869 Other paralytic syndrome following other cerebrovascular disease affecting unspecified side

I69.89 Other sequelae of other cerebrovascular disease

I69.890 Apraxia following other cerebrovascular disease

I69.891 Dysphagia following other cerebrovascular disease

Use additional code to identify the type of dysphagia, if known (R13.1-)

I69.892 Facial weakness following other cerebrovascular disease

Facial droop following other cerebrovascular disease

I69.893 Ataxia following other cerebrovascular disease

● New code ▲ Revised code **Excludes1:** Not coded here **Excludes2:** Not included here ⊗ Placeholder required ⑦ 7th digit required

I69.898   **Other sequelae of other cerebrovascular disease**

Alteration of sensation following other cerebrovascular disease

Disturbance of vision following other cerebrovascular disease

<u>Use additional code</u> to identify the sequelae

I69.9   **Sequelae of unspecified cerebrovascular diseases**

Excludes1: sequelae of stroke (I69.3)

sequelae of traumatic intracranial injury (S06.-)

I69.90   **Unspecified sequelae of unspecified cerebrovascular disease**

I69.91   **Cognitive deficits following unspecified cerebrovascular disease**

I69.910   **Attention and concentration deficit following unspecified cerebrovascular disease**

I69.911   **Memory deficit following unspecified cerebrovascular disease**

I69.912   **Visuospatial deficit and spatial neglect following unspecified cerebrovascular disease**

I69.913   **Psychomotor deficit following unspecified cerebrovascular disease**

I69.914   **Frontal lobe and executive function deficit following unspecified cerebrovascular disease**

I69.915   **Cognitive social or emotional deficit following unspecified cerebrovascular disease**

I69.918   **Other symptoms and signs involving cognitive functions following unspecified cerebrovascular disease**

I69.919   **Unspecified symptoms and signs involving cognitive functions following unspecified cerebrovascular disease**

I69.92   **Speech and language deficits following unspecified cerebrovascular disease**

I69.920   **Aphasia following unspecified cerebrovascular disease**

I69.921   **Dysphasia following unspecified cerebrovascular disease**

I69.922   **Dysarthria following unspecified cerebrovascular disease**

I69.923   **Fluency disorder following unspecified cerebrovascular disease**

Stuttering following unspecified cerebrovascular disease

I69.928   **Other speech and language deficits following unspecified cerebrovascular disease**

I69.93   **Monoplegia of upper limb following unspecified cerebrovascular disease**

I69.931   **Monoplegia of upper limb following unspecified cerebrovascular disease affecting right dominant side**

I69.932   **Monoplegia of upper limb following unspecified cerebrovascular disease affecting left dominant side**

I69.933   **Monoplegia of upper limb following unspecified cerebrovascular disease affecting right non-dominant side**

I69.934   **Monoplegia of upper limb following unspecified cerebrovascular disease affecting left non-dominant side**

I69.939   **Monoplegia of upper limb following unspecified cerebrovascular disease affecting unspecified side**

I69.94   **Monoplegia of lower limb following unspecified cerebrovascular disease**

I69.941   **Monoplegia of lower limb following unspecified cerebrovascular disease affecting right dominant side**

I69.942   **Monoplegia of lower limb following unspecified cerebrovascular disease affecting left dominant side**

I69.943   **Monoplegia of lower limb following unspecified cerebrovascular disease affecting right non-dominant side**

I69.944   **Monoplegia of lower limb following unspecified cerebrovascular disease affecting left non-dominant side**

I69.949   **Monoplegia of lower limb following unspecified cerebrovascular disease affecting unspecified side**

I69.95   **Hemiplegia and hemiparesis following unspecified cerebrovascular disease**

I69.951   **Hemiplegia and hemiparesis following unspecified cerebrovascular disease affecting right dominant side**

I69.952   **Hemiplegia and hemiparesis following unspecified cerebrovascular disease affecting left dominant side**

I69.953   **Hemiplegia and hemiparesis following unspecified cerebrovascular disease affecting right non-dominant side**

I69.954   **Hemiplegia and hemiparesis following unspecified cerebrovascular disease affecting left non-dominant side**

I69.959   **Hemiplegia and hemiparesis following unspecified cerebrovascular disease affecting unspecified side**

I69.96   **Other paralytic syndrome following unspecified cerebrovascular disease**

<u>Use additional code</u> to identify type of paralytic syndrome, such as:

locked-in state (G83.5)

quadriplegia (G82.5-)

Excludes1: hemiplegia/hemiparesis following unspecified cerebrovascular disease (I69.95-)

monoplegia of lower limb following unspecified cerebrovascular disease (I69.94-)

monoplegia of upper limb following unspecified cerebrovascular disease (I69.93-)

I69.961   **Other paralytic syndrome following unspecified cerebrovascular disease affecting right dominant side**

I69.962   **Other paralytic syndrome following unspecified cerebrovascular disease affecting left dominant side**

I69.963   **Other paralytic syndrome following unspecified cerebrovascular disease affecting right non-dominant side**

I69.964   **Other paralytic syndrome following unspecified cerebrovascular disease affecting left non-dominant side**

I69.965   **Other paralytic syndrome following unspecified cerebrovascular disease, bilateral**

I69.969   **Other paralytic syndrome following unspecified cerebrovascular disease affecting unspecified side**

I69.99   **Other sequelae of unspecified cerebrovascular disease**

I69.990   **Apraxia following unspecified cerebrovascular disease**

I69.991   **Dysphagia following unspecified cerebrovascular disease**

Use additional code to identify the type of dysphagia, if known (R13.1-)

I69.992   **Facial weakness following unspecified cerebrovascular disease**

Facial droop following unspecified cerebrovascular disease

I69.993   **Ataxia following unspecified cerebrovascular disease**

I69.998   **Other sequelae following unspecified cerebrovascular disease**

Alteration in sensation following unspecified cerebrovascular disease

Disturbance of vision following unspecified cerebrovascular disease

Use additional code to identify the sequelae

DISEASES OF ARTERIES, ARTERIOLES AND CAPILLARIES (I70-I79)

I70   Atherosclerosis

Definition: Atherosclerosis is a condition in which an artery wall thickens as the result of a build up of fatty materials such as cholesterol. It is a syndrome affecting arterial blood vessels.

Includes: arteriolosclerosis

arterial degeneration arteriosclerosis

arteriosclerotic vascular disease

arteriovascular degeneration atheroma

endarteritis deformans or obliterans

senile arteritis

senile endarteritis vascular degeneration

Use additional code to identify:

exposure to environmental tobacco smoke (Z77.22) history of tobacco dependence (Z87.891)

occupational exposure to environmental tobacco smoke (Z57.31) tobacco dependence (F17.-)

tobacco use (Z72.0)

Excludes2: arteriosclerotic cardiovascular disease (I25.1-)

arteriosclerotic heart disease (I25.1-)

atheroembolism (I75.-)

cerebral atherosclerosis (I67.2)

coronary atherosclerosis (I25.1-)

mesenteric atherosclerosis (K55.1)

precerebral atherosclerosis (I67.2)

primary pulmonary atherosclerosis (I27.0)

I70.0   **Atherosclerosis of aorta**

I70.1   **Atherosclerosis of renal artery**

Goldblatt's kidney

Excludes2: atherosclerosis of renal arterioles (I12.-)

I70.2   **Atherosclerosis of native arteries of the extremities**

Mönckeberg's (medial) sclerosis

Use additional code, if applicable, to identify chronic total occlusion of artery of extremity (I70.92)

Excludes2: atherosclerosis of bypass graft of extremities (I70.30-I70.79)

I70.20   **Unspecified atherosclerosis of native arteries of extremities**

I70.201   **Unspecified atherosclerosis of native arteries of extremities, right leg**

I70.202   **Unspecified atherosclerosis of native arteries of extremities, left leg**

I70.203   **Unspecified atherosclerosis of native arteries of extremities, bilateral legs**

I70.208   **Unspecified atherosclerosis of native arteries of extremities, other extremity**

I70.209   **Unspecified atherosclerosis of native arteries of extremities, unspecified extremity**

I70.21   **Atherosclerosis of native arteries of extremities with intermittent claudication**

I70.211   **Atherosclerosis of native arteries of extremities with intermittent claudication, right leg**

I70.212   **Atherosclerosis of native arteries of extremities with intermittent claudication, left leg**

I70.213   **Atherosclerosis of native arteries of extremities with intermittent claudication, bilateral legs**

I70.218   **Atherosclerosis of native arteries of extremities with intermittent claudication, other extremity**

I70.219   **Atherosclerosis of native arteries of extremities with intermittent claudication, unspecified extremity**

I70.22   **Atherosclerosis of native arteries of extremities with rest pain**

Includes: any condition classifiable to I70.21-

I70.221   **Atherosclerosis of native arteries of extremities with rest pain, right leg**

I70.222   **Atherosclerosis of native arteries of extremities with rest pain, left leg**

I70.223   **Atherosclerosis of native arteries of extremities with rest pain, bilateral legs**

I70.228   **Atherosclerosis of native arteries of extremities with rest pain, other extremity**

I70.229   **Atherosclerosis of native arteries of extremities with rest pain, unspecified extremity**

I70.23   **Atherosclerosis of native arteries of right leg with ulceration**

Includes: any condition classifiable to I70.211 and I70.221

Use additional code to identify severity of ulcer (L97.-)

I70.231   Atherosclerosis of native arteries of right leg with ulceration of thigh

I70.232   Atherosclerosis of native arteries of right leg with ulceration of calf

I70.233   Atherosclerosis of native arteries of right leg with ulceration of ankle

I70.234   Atherosclerosis of native arteries of right leg with ulceration of heel and midfoot

Atherosclerosis of native arteries of right leg with ulceration of plantar surface of midfoot

I70.235   Atherosclerosis of native arteries of right leg with ulceration of other part of foot

Atherosclerosis of native arteries of right leg extremities with ulceration of toe

I70.238   Atherosclerosis of native arteries of right leg with ulceration of other part of lower right leg

I70.239   Atherosclerosis of native arteries of right leg with ulceration of unspecified site

I70.24   Atherosclerosis of native arteries of left leg with ulceration

Includes: any condition classifiable to I70.212 and I70.222

Use additional code to identify severity of ulcer (L97.-)

I70.241   Atherosclerosis of native arteries of left leg with ulceration of thigh

I70.242   Atherosclerosis of native arteries of left leg with ulceration of calf

I70.243   Atherosclerosis of native arteries of left leg with ulceration of ankle

I70.244   Atherosclerosis of native arteries of left leg with ulceration of heel and midfoot

Atherosclerosis of native arteries of left leg with ulceration of plantar surface of midfoot

I70.245   Atherosclerosis of native arteries of left leg with ulceration of other part of foot

Atherosclerosis of native arteries of left leg extremities with ulceration of toe

I70.248   Atherosclerosis of native arteries of left leg with ulceration of other part of lower left leg

I70.249   Atherosclerosis of native arteries of left leg with ulceration of unspecified site

I70.25   Atherosclerosis of native arteries of other extremities with ulceration

Includes: any condition classifiable to I70.218 and I70.228

Use additional code to identify the severity of the ulcer (L98.49-)

I70.26   Atherosclerosis of native arteries of extremities with gangrene

Includes: any condition classifiable to I70.21-, I70.22-, I70.23-, I70.24-, and I70.25-

Use additional code to identify the severity of any ulcer (L97.-, L98.49-), if applicable

I70.261   Atherosclerosis of native arteries of extremities with gangrene, right leg

I70.262   Atherosclerosis of native arteries of extremities with gangrene, left leg

I70.263   Atherosclerosis of native arteries of extremities with gangrene, bilateral legs

I70.268   Atherosclerosis of native arteries of extremities with gangrene, other extremity

I70.269   Atherosclerosis of native arteries of extremities with gangrene, unspecified extremity

I70.29   Other atherosclerosis of native arteries of extremities

I70.291   Other atherosclerosis of native arteries of extremities, right leg

I70.292   Other atherosclerosis of native arteries of extremities, left leg

I70.293   Other atherosclerosis of native arteries of extremities, bilateral legs

I70.298   Other atherosclerosis of native arteries of extremities, other extremity

I70.299   Other atherosclerosis of native arteries of extremities, unspecified extremity

I70.3   Atherosclerosis of unspecified type of bypass graft(s) of the extremities

Use additional code, if applicable, to identify chronic total occlusion of artery of extremity (I70.92)

Excludes1: embolism or thrombus of bypass graft(s) of extremities (T82.8-)

I70.30   Unspecified atherosclerosis of unspecified type of bypass graft(s) of the extremities

I70.301   Unspecified atherosclerosis of unspecified type of bypass graft(s) of the extremities, right leg

I70.302   Unspecified atherosclerosis of unspecified type of bypass graft(s) of the extremities, left leg

I70.303   Unspecified atherosclerosis of unspecified type of bypass graft(s) of the extremities, bilateral legs

I70.308   Unspecified atherosclerosis of unspecified type of bypass graft(s) of the extremities, other extremity

I70.309   Unspecified atherosclerosis of unspecified type of bypass graft(s) of the extremities, unspecified extremity

I70.31   Atherosclerosis of unspecified type of bypass graft(s) of the extremities with intermittent claudication

I70.311   Atherosclerosis of unspecified type of bypass graft(s) of the extremities with intermittent claudication, right leg

I70.312   Atherosclerosis of unspecified type of bypass graft(s) of the extremities with intermittent claudication, left leg

I70.313   Atherosclerosis of unspecified type of bypass graft(s) of the extremities with intermittent claudication, bilateral legs

I70.318 **Atherosclerosis of unspecified type of bypass graft(s) of the extremities with intermittent claudication, other extremity**

I70.319 **Atherosclerosis of unspecified type of bypass graft(s) of the extremities with intermittent claudication, unspecified extremity**

I70.32 **Atherosclerosis of unspecified type of bypass graft(s) of the extremities with rest pain**

Includes: any condition classifiable to I70.31-

I70.321 **Atherosclerosis of unspecified type of bypass graft(s) of the extremities with rest pain, right leg**

I70.322 **Atherosclerosis of unspecified type of bypass graft(s) of the extremities with rest pain, left leg**

I70.323 **Atherosclerosis of unspecified type of bypass graft(s) of the extremities with rest pain, bilateral legs**

I70.328 **Atherosclerosis of unspecified type of bypass graft(s) of the extremities with rest pain, other extremity**

I70.329 **Atherosclerosis of unspecified type of bypass graft(s) of the extremities with rest pain, unspecified extremity**

I70.33 **Atherosclerosis of unspecified type of bypass graft(s) of the right leg with ulceration**

Includes: any condition classifiable to I70.311 and I70.321

Use additional code to identify severity of ulcer (L97.-)

I70.331 **Atherosclerosis of unspecified type of bypass graft(s) of the right leg with ulceration of thigh**

I70.332 **Atherosclerosis of unspecified type of bypass graft(s) of the right leg with ulceration of calf**

I70.333 **Atherosclerosis of unspecified type of bypass graft(s) of the right leg with ulceration of ankle**

I70.334 **Atherosclerosis of unspecified type of bypass graft(s) of the right leg with ulceration of heel and midfoot**

Atherosclerosis of unspecified type of bypass graft(s) of right leg with ulceration of plantar surface of midfoot

I70.335 **Atherosclerosis of unspecified type of bypass graft(s) of the right leg with ulceration of other part of foot**

Atherosclerosis of unspecified type of bypass graft(s) of the right leg with ulceration of toe

I70.338 **Atherosclerosis of unspecified type of bypass graft(s) of the right leg with ulceration of other part of lower leg**

I70.339 **Atherosclerosis of unspecified type of bypass graft(s) of the right leg with ulceration of unspecified site**

I70.34 **Atherosclerosis of unspecified type of bypass graft(s) of the left leg with ulceration**

Includes: any condition classifiable to I70.312 and I70.322

Use additional code to identify severity of ulcer (L97.-)

I70.341 **Atherosclerosis of unspecified type of bypass graft(s) of the left leg with ulceration of thigh**

I70.342 **Atherosclerosis of unspecified type of bypass graft(s) of the left leg with ulceration of calf**

I70.343 **Atherosclerosis of unspecified type of bypass graft(s) of the left leg with ulceration of ankle**

I70.344 **Atherosclerosis of unspecified type of bypass graft(s) of the left leg with ulceration of heel and midfoot**

Atherosclerosis of unspecified type of bypass graft(s) of left leg with ulceration of plantar surface of midfoot

I70.345 **Atherosclerosis of unspecified type of bypass graft(s) of the left leg with ulceration of other part of foot**

Atherosclerosis of unspecified type of bypass graft(s) of the left leg with ulceration of toe

I70.348 **Atherosclerosis of unspecified type of bypass graft(s) of the left leg with ulceration of other part of lower leg**

I70.349 **Atherosclerosis of unspecified type of bypass graft(s) of the left leg with ulceration of unspecified site**

I70.35 **Atherosclerosis of unspecified type of bypass graft(s) of other extremity with ulceration**

Includes: any condition classifiable to I70.318 and I70.328

Use additional code to identify severity of ulcer (L98.49-)

I70.36 **Atherosclerosis of unspecified type of bypass graft(s) of the extremities with gangrene**

Includes: any condition classifiable to I70.31-, I70.32-, I70.33-, I70.34-, I70.35

Use additional code to identify the severity of any ulcer (L97.-, L98.49-), if applicable

I70.361 **Atherosclerosis of unspecified type of bypass graft(s) of the extremities with gangrene, right leg**

I70.362 **Atherosclerosis of unspecified type of bypass graft(s) of the extremities with gangrene, left leg**

I70.363 **Atherosclerosis of unspecified type of bypass graft(s) of the extremities with gangrene, bilateral legs**

I70.368 **Atherosclerosis of unspecified type of bypass graft(s) of the extremities with gangrene, other extremity**

I70.369 **Atherosclerosis of unspecified type of bypass graft(s) of the extremities with gangrene, unspecified extremity**

I70.39 **Other atherosclerosis of unspecified type of bypass graft(s) of the extremities**

I70.391 **Other atherosclerosis of unspecified type of bypass graft(s) of the extremities, right leg**

I70.392 **Other atherosclerosis of unspecified type of bypass graft(s) of the extremities, left leg**

I70.393 **Other atherosclerosis of unspecified type of bypass graft(s) of the extremities, bilateral legs**

● New code   ▲ Revised code   **Excludes1:** Not coded here   **Excludes2:** Not included here   ⊗ Placeholder required   ⑦ 7th digit required

I70.398 Other atherosclerosis of unspecified type of bypass graft(s) of the extremities, other extremity

I70.399 Other atherosclerosis of unspecified type of bypass graft(s) of the extremities, unspecified extremity

I70.4 Atherosclerosis of autologous vein bypass graft(s) of the extremities

Use additional code, if applicable, to identify chronic total occlusion of artery of extremity (I70.92)

I70.40 Unspecified atherosclerosis of autologous vein bypass graft(s) of the extremities

I70.401 Unspecified atherosclerosis of autologous vein bypass graft(s) of the extremities, right leg

I70.402 Unspecified atherosclerosis of autologous vein bypass graft(s) of the extremities, left leg

I70.403 Unspecified atherosclerosis of autologous vein bypass graft(s) of the extremities, bilateral legs

I70.408 Unspecified atherosclerosis of autologous vein bypass graft(s) of the extremities, other extremity

I70.409 Unspecified atherosclerosis of autologous vein bypass graft(s) of the extremities, unspecified extremity

I70.41 Atherosclerosis of autologous vein bypass graft(s) of the extremities with intermittent claudication

I70.411 Atherosclerosis of autologous vein bypass graft(s) of the extremities with intermittent claudication, right leg

I70.412 Atherosclerosis of autologous vein bypass graft(s) of the extremities with intermittent claudication, left leg

I70.413 Atherosclerosis of autologous vein bypass graft(s) of the extremities with intermittent claudication, bilateral legs

I70.418 Atherosclerosis of autologous vein bypass graft(s) of the extremities with intermittent claudication, other extremity

I70.419 Atherosclerosis of autologous vein bypass graft(s) of the extremities with intermittent claudication, unspecified extremity

I70.42 Atherosclerosis of autologous vein bypass graft(s) of the extremities with rest pain

Includes: any condition classifiable to I70.41-

I70.421 Atherosclerosis of autologous vein bypass graft(s) of the extremities with rest pain, right leg

I70.422 Atherosclerosis of autologous vein bypass graft(s) of the extremities with rest pain, left leg

I70.423 Atherosclerosis of autologous vein bypass graft(s) of the extremities with rest pain, bilateral legs

I70.428 Atherosclerosis of autologous vein bypass graft(s) of the extremities with rest pain, other extremity

I70.429 Atherosclerosis of autologous vein bypass graft(s) of the extremities with rest pain, unspecified extremity

I70.43 Atherosclerosis of autologous vein bypass graft(s) of the right leg with ulceration

Includes: any condition classifiable to I70.411 and I70.421

Use additional code to identify severity of ulcer (L97.-)

I70.431 Atherosclerosis of autologous vein bypass graft(s) of the right leg with ulceration of thigh

I70.432 Atherosclerosis of autologous vein bypass graft(s) of the right leg with ulceration of calf

I70.433 Atherosclerosis of autologous vein bypass graft(s) of the right leg with ulceration of ankle

I70.434 Atherosclerosis of autologous vein bypass graft(s) of the right leg with ulceration of heel and midfoot

Atherosclerosis of autologous vein bypass graft(s) of right leg with ulceration of plantar surface of midfoot

I70.435 Atherosclerosis of autologous vein bypass graft(s) of the right leg with ulceration of other part of foot

Atherosclerosis of autologous vein bypass graft(s) of right leg with ulceration of toe

I70.438 Atherosclerosis of autologous vein bypass graft(s) of the right leg with ulceration of other part of lower leg

I70.439 Atherosclerosis of autologous vein bypass graft(s) of the right leg with ulceration of unspecified site

I70.44 Atherosclerosis of autologous vein bypass graft(s) of the left leg with ulceration

Includes: any condition classifiable to I70.412 and I70.422

Use additional code to identify severity of ulcer (L97.-)

I70.441 Atherosclerosis of autologous vein bypass graft(s) of the left leg with ulceration of thigh

I70.442 Atherosclerosis of autologous vein bypass graft(s) of the left leg with ulceration of calf

I70.443 Atherosclerosis of autologous vein bypass graft(s) of the left leg with ulceration of ankle

I70.444 Atherosclerosis of autologous vein bypass graft(s) of the left leg with ulceration of heel and midfoot

Atherosclerosis of autologous vein bypass graft(s) of left leg with ulceration of plantar surface of midfoot

I70.445 Atherosclerosis of autologous vein bypass graft(s) of the left leg with ulceration of other part of foot

Atherosclerosis of autologous vein bypass graft(s) of left leg with ulceration of toe

I70.448 Atherosclerosis of autologous vein bypass graft(s) of the left leg with ulceration of other part of lower leg

Add 4th-7th digits   Nonspecific code   Unspecified code   Manifestation code

I70.449 Atherosclerosis of autologous vein bypass graft(s) of the left leg with ulceration of unspecified site

I70.45 Atherosclerosis of autologous vein bypass graft(s) of other extremity with ulceration

Includes: any condition classifiable to I70.418, I70.428, and I70.438

Use additional code to identify severity of ulcer (L98.49)

I70.46 Atherosclerosis of autologous vein bypass graft(s) of the extremities with gangrene

Includes: any condition classifiable to I70.41-, I70.42-, and I70.43-, I70.44-, I70.45

Use additional code to identify the severity of any ulcer (L97.-, L98.49-), if applicable

I70.461 Atherosclerosis of autologous vein bypass graft(s) of the extremities with gangrene, right leg

I70.462 Atherosclerosis of autologous vein bypass graft(s) of the extremities with gangrene, left leg

I70.463 Atherosclerosis of autologous vein bypass graft(s) of the extremities with gangrene, bilateral legs

I70.468 Atherosclerosis of autologous vein bypass graft(s) of the extremities with gangrene, other extremity

I70.469 Atherosclerosis of autologous vein bypass graft(s) of the extremities with gangrene, unspecified extremity

I70.49 Other atherosclerosis of autologous vein bypass graft(s) of the extremities

I70.491 Other atherosclerosis of autologous vein bypass graft(s) of the extremities, right leg

I70.492 Other atherosclerosis of autologous vein bypass graft(s) of the extremities, left leg

I70.493 Other atherosclerosis of autologous vein bypass graft(s) of the extremities, bilateral legs

I70.498 Other atherosclerosis of autologous vein bypass graft(s) of the extremities, other extremity

I70.499 Other atherosclerosis of autologous vein bypass graft(s) of the extremities, unspecified extremity

I70.5 Atherosclerosis of nonautologous biological bypass graft(s) of the extremities

Use additional code, if applicable, to identify chronic total occlusion of artery of extremity (I70.92)

I70.50 Unspecified atherosclerosis of nonautologous biological bypass graft(s) of the extremities

I70.501 Unspecified atherosclerosis of nonautologous biological bypass graft(s) of the extremities, right leg

I70.502 Unspecified atherosclerosis of nonautologous biological bypass graft(s) of the extremities, left leg

I70.503 Unspecified atherosclerosis of nonautologous biological bypass graft(s) of the extremities, bilateral legs

I70.508 Unspecified atherosclerosis of nonautologous biological bypass graft(s) of the extremities, other extremity

I70.509 Unspecified atherosclerosis of nonautologous biological bypass graft(s) of the extremities, unspecified extremity

I70.51 Atherosclerosis of nonautologous biological bypass graft(s) of the extremities intermittent claudication

I70.511 Atherosclerosis of nonautologous biological bypass graft(s) of the extremities with intermittent claudication, right leg

I70.512 Atherosclerosis of nonautologous biological bypass graft(s) of the extremities with intermittent claudication, left leg

I70.513 Atherosclerosis of nonautologous biological bypass graft(s) of the extremities with intermittent claudication, bilateral legs

I70.518 Atherosclerosis of nonautologous biological bypass graft(s) of the extremities with intermittent claudication, other extremity

I70.519 Atherosclerosis of nonautologous biological bypass graft(s) of the extremities with intermittent claudication, unspecified extremity

I70.52 Atherosclerosis of nonautologous biological bypass graft(s) of the extremities with rest pain

Includes: any condition classifiable to I70.51-

I70.521 Atherosclerosis of nonautologous biological bypass graft(s) of the extremities with rest pain, right leg

I70.522 Atherosclerosis of nonautologous biological bypass graft(s) of the extremities with rest pain, left leg

I70.523 Atherosclerosis of nonautologous biological bypass graft(s) of the extremities with rest pain, bilateral legs

I70.528 Atherosclerosis of nonautologous biological bypass graft(s) of the extremities with rest pain, other extremity

I70.529 Atherosclerosis of nonautologous biological bypass graft(s) of the extremities with rest pain, unspecified extremity

I70.53 Atherosclerosis of nonautologous biological bypass graft(s) of the right leg with ulceration

Includes: any condition classifiable to I70.511 and I70.521

Use additional code to identify severity of ulcer (L97.-)

I70.531 Atherosclerosis of nonautologous biological bypass graft(s) of the right leg with ulceration of thigh

I70.532 Atherosclerosis of nonautologous biological bypass graft(s) of the right leg with ulceration of calf

I70.533 Atherosclerosis of nonautologous biological bypass graft(s) of the right leg with ulceration of ankle

I70.534 Atherosclerosis of nonautologous biological bypass graft(s) of the right leg with ulceration of heel and midfoot

● New code ▲ Revised code **Excludes1:** Not coded here **Excludes2:** Not included here ⊗ Placeholder required ⑦ 7th digit required

Atherosclerosis of nonautologous biological bypass graft(s) of right leg with ulceration of plantar surface of midfoot

I70.535 **Atherosclerosis of nonautologous biological bypass graft(s) of the right leg with ulceration of other part of foot**

Atherosclerosis of nonautologous biological bypass graft(s) of the right leg with ulceration of toe

I70.538 **Atherosclerosis of nonautologous biological bypass graft(s) of the right leg with ulceration of other part of lower leg**

I70.539 **Atherosclerosis of nonautologous biological bypass graft(s) of the right leg with ulceration of unspecified site**

I70.54 **Atherosclerosis of nonautologous biological bypass graft(s) of the left leg with ulceration**

Includes: any condition classifiable to I70.512 and I70.522

Use additional code to identify severity of ulcer (L97.-)

I70.541 **Atherosclerosis of nonautologous biological bypass graft(s) of the left leg with ulceration of thigh**

I70.542 **Atherosclerosis of nonautologous biological bypass graft(s) of the left leg with ulceration of calf**

I70.543 **Atherosclerosis of nonautologous biological bypass graft(s) of the left leg with ulceration of ankle**

I70.544 **Atherosclerosis of nonautologous biological bypass graft(s) of the left leg with ulceration of heel and midfoot**

Atherosclerosis of nonautologous biological bypass graft(s) of left leg with ulceration of plantar surface of midfoot

I70.545 **Atherosclerosis of nonautologous biological bypass graft(s) of the left leg with ulceration of other part of foot**

Atherosclerosis of nonautologous biological bypass graft(s) of the left leg with ulceration of toe

I70.548 **Atherosclerosis of nonautologous biological bypass graft(s) of the left leg with ulceration of other part of lower leg**

I70.549 **Atherosclerosis of nonautologous biological bypass graft(s) of the left leg with ulceration of unspecified site**

I70.55 **Atherosclerosis of nonautologous biological bypass graft(s) of other extremity with ulceration**

Includes: any condition classifiable to I70.518, I70.528, and I70.538

Use additional code to identify severity of ulcer (L98.49)

I70.56 **Atherosclerosis of nonautologous biological bypass graft(s) of the extremities with gangrene**

Includes: any condition classifiable to I70.51-, I70.52-, and I70.53-, I70.54-, I70.55

Use additional code to identify the severity of any ulcer (L97.-, L98.49-), if applicable

I70.561 **Atherosclerosis of nonautologous biological bypass graft(s) of the extremities with gangrene, right leg**

I70.562 **Atherosclerosis of nonautologous biological bypass graft(s) of the extremities with gangrene, left leg**

I70.563 **Atherosclerosis of nonautologous biological bypass graft(s) of the extremities with gangrene, bilateral legs**

I70.568 **Atherosclerosis of nonautologous biological bypass graft(s) of the extremities with gangrene, other extremity**

I70.569 **Atherosclerosis of nonautologous biological bypass graft(s) of the extremities with gangrene, unspecified extremity**

I70.59 **Other atherosclerosis of nonautologous biological bypass graft(s) of the extremities**

I70.591 **Other atherosclerosis of nonautologous biological bypass graft(s) of the extremities, right leg**

I70.592 **Other atherosclerosis of nonautologous biological bypass graft(s) of the extremities, left leg**

I70.593 **Other atherosclerosis of nonautologous biological bypass graft(s) of the extremities, bilateral legs**

I70.598 **Other atherosclerosis of nonautologous biological bypass graft(s) of the extremities, other extremity**

I70.599 **Other atherosclerosis of nonautologous biological bypass graft(s) of the extremities, unspecified extremity**

I70.6 **Atherosclerosis of nonbiological bypass graft(s) of the extremities**

Use additional code, if applicable, to identify chronic total occlusion of artery of extremity (I70.92)

I70.60 **Unspecified atherosclerosis of nonbiological bypass graft(s) of the extremities**

I70.601 **Unspecified atherosclerosis of nonbiological bypass graft(s) of the extremities, right leg**

I70.602 **Unspecified atherosclerosis of nonbiological bypass graft(s) of the extremities, left leg**

I70.603 **Unspecified atherosclerosis of nonbiological bypass graft(s) of the extremities, bilateral legs**

I70.608 **Unspecified atherosclerosis of nonbiological bypass graft(s) of the extremities, other extremity**

I70.609 **Unspecified atherosclerosis of nonbiological bypass graft(s) of the extremities, unspecified extremity**

I70.61 **Atherosclerosis of nonbiological bypass graft(s) of the extremities with intermittent claudication**

I70.611 **Atherosclerosis of nonbiological bypass graft(s) of the extremities with intermittent claudication, right leg**

I70.612 Atherosclerosis of nonbiological bypass graft(s) of the extremities with intermittent claudication, left leg

I70.613 Atherosclerosis of nonbiological bypass graft(s) of the extremities with intermittent claudication, bilateral legs

I70.618 Atherosclerosis of nonbiological bypass graft(s) of the extremities with intermittent claudication, other extremity

I70.619 Atherosclerosis of nonbiological bypass graft(s) of the extremities with intermittent claudication, unspecified extremity

I70.62 Atherosclerosis of nonbiological bypass graft(s) of the extremities with rest pain

Includes: any condition classifiable to I70.61-

I70.621 Atherosclerosis of nonbiological bypass graft(s) of the extremities with rest pain, right leg

I70.622 Atherosclerosis of nonbiological bypass graft(s) of the extremities with rest pain, left leg

I70.623 Atherosclerosis of nonbiological bypass graft(s) of the extremities with rest pain, bilateral legs

I70.628 Atherosclerosis of nonbiological bypass graft(s) of the extremities with rest pain, other extremity

I70.629 Atherosclerosis of nonbiological bypass graft(s) of the extremities with rest pain, unspecified extremity

I70.63 Atherosclerosis of nonbiological bypass graft(s) of the right leg with ulceration

Includes: any condition classifiable to I70.611 and I70.621

Use additional code to identify severity of ulcer (L97.-)

I70.631 Atherosclerosis of nonbiological bypass graft(s) of the right leg with ulceration of thigh

I70.632 Atherosclerosis of nonbiological bypass graft(s) of the right leg with ulceration of calf

I70.633 Atherosclerosis of nonbiological bypass graft(s) of the right leg with ulceration of ankle

I70.634 Atherosclerosis of nonbiological bypass graft(s) of the right leg with ulceration of heel and midfoot

Atherosclerosis of nonbiological bypass graft(s) of right leg with ulceration of plantar surface of midfoot

I70.635 Atherosclerosis of nonbiological bypass graft(s) of the right leg with ulceration of other part of foot

Atherosclerosis of nonbiological bypass graft(s) of the right leg with ulceration of toe

I70.638 Atherosclerosis of nonbiological bypass graft(s) of the right leg with ulceration of other part of lower leg

I70.639 Atherosclerosis of nonbiological bypass graft(s) of the right leg with ulceration of unspecified site

I70.64 Atherosclerosis of nonbiological bypass graft(s) of the left leg with ulceration

Includes: any condition classifiable to I70.612 and I70.622

Use additional code to identify severity of ulcer (L97.-)

I70.641 Atherosclerosis of nonbiological bypass graft(s) of the left leg with ulceration of thigh

I70.642 Atherosclerosis of nonbiological bypass graft(s) of the left leg with ulceration of calf

I70.643 Atherosclerosis of nonbiological bypass graft(s) of the left leg with ulceration of ankle

I70.644 Atherosclerosis of nonbiological bypass graft(s) of the left leg with ulceration of heel and midfoot

Atherosclerosis of nonbiological bypass graft(s) of left leg with ulceration of plantar surface of midfoot

I70.645 Atherosclerosis of nonbiological bypass graft(s) of the left leg with ulceration of other part of foot

Atherosclerosis of nonbiological bypass graft(s) of the left leg with ulceration of toe

I70.648 Atherosclerosis of nonbiological bypass graft(s) of the left leg with ulceration of other part of lower leg

I70.649 Atherosclerosis of nonbiological bypass graft(s) of the left leg with ulceration of unspecified site

I70.65 Atherosclerosis of nonbiological bypass graft(s) of other extremity with ulceration

Includes: any condition classifiable to I70.618 and I70.628

Use additional code to identify severity of ulcer (L98.49)

I70.66 Atherosclerosis of nonbiological bypass graft(s) of the extremities with gangrene

Includes: any condition classifiable to I70.61-, I70.62-, I70.63-, I70.64-, I70.65

Use additional code to identify the severity of any ulcer (L97.-, L98.49-), if applicable

I70.661 Atherosclerosis of nonbiological bypass graft(s) of the extremities with gangrene, right leg

I70.662 Atherosclerosis of nonbiological bypass graft(s) of the extremities with gangrene, left leg

I70.663 Atherosclerosis of nonbiological bypass graft(s) of the extremities with gangrene, bilateral legs

I70.668 Atherosclerosis of nonbiological bypass graft(s) of the extremities with gangrene, other extremity

I70.669 Atherosclerosis of nonbiological bypass graft(s) of the extremities with gangrene, unspecified extremity

I70.69 Other atherosclerosis of nonbiological bypass graft(s) of the extremities

I70.691 Other atherosclerosis of nonbiological bypass graft(s) of the extremities, right leg

● New code ▲ Revised code **Excludes1:** Not coded here **Excludes2:** Not included here ⊗ Placeholder required ⑦7th digit required

I70.692   Other atherosclerosis of nonbiological bypass graft(s) of the extremities, left leg

I70.693   Other atherosclerosis of nonbiological bypass graft(s) of the extremities, bilateral legs

I70.698   Other atherosclerosis of nonbiological bypass graft(s) of the extremities, other extremity

I70.699   Other atherosclerosis of nonbiological bypass graft(s) of the extremities, unspecified extremity

I70.7   Atherosclerosis of other type of bypass graft(s) of the extremities

Use additional code, if applicable, to identify chronic total occlusion of artery of extremity (I70.92)

I70.70   Unspecified atherosclerosis of other type of bypass graft(s) of the extremities

I70.701   Unspecified atherosclerosis of other type of bypass graft(s) of the extremities, right leg

I70.702   Unspecified atherosclerosis of other type of bypass graft(s) of the extremities, left leg

I70.703   Unspecified atherosclerosis of other type of bypass graft(s) of the extremities, bilateral legs

I70.708   Unspecified atherosclerosis of other type of bypass graft(s) of the extremities, other extremity

I70.709   Unspecified atherosclerosis of other type of bypass graft(s) of the extremities, unspecified extremity

I70.71   Atherosclerosis of other type of bypass graft(s) of the extremities with intermittent claudication

I70.711   Atherosclerosis of other type of bypass graft(s) of the extremities with intermittent claudication, right leg

I70.712   Atherosclerosis of other type of bypass graft(s) of the extremities with intermittent claudication, left leg

I70.713   Atherosclerosis of other type of bypass graft(s) of the extremities with intermittent claudication, bilateral legs

I70.718   Atherosclerosis of other type of bypass graft(s) of the extremities with intermittent claudication, other extremity

I70.719   Atherosclerosis of other type of bypass graft(s) of the extremities with intermittent claudication, unspecified extremity

I70.72   Atherosclerosis of other type of bypass graft(s) of the extremities with rest pain

Includes: any condition classifiable to I70.71-

I70.721   Atherosclerosis of other type of bypass graft(s) of the extremities with rest pain, right leg

I70.722   Atherosclerosis of other type of bypass graft(s) of the extremities with rest pain, left leg

I70.723   Atherosclerosis of other type of bypass graft(s) of the extremities with rest pain, bilateral legs

I70.728   Atherosclerosis of other type of bypass graft(s) of the extremities with rest pain, other extremity

I70.729   Atherosclerosis of other type of bypass graft(s) of the extremities with rest pain, unspecified extremity

I70.73   Atherosclerosis of other type of bypass graft(s) of the right leg with ulceration

Includes: any condition classifiable to I70.711 and I70.721

Use additional code to identify severity of ulcer (L97.-)

I70.731   Atherosclerosis of other type of bypass graft(s) of the right leg with ulceration of thigh

I70.732   Atherosclerosis of other type of bypass graft(s) of the right leg with ulceration of calf

I70.733   Atherosclerosis of other type of bypass graft(s) of the right leg with ulceration of ankle

I70.734   Atherosclerosis of other type of bypass graft(s) of the right leg with ulceration of heel and midfoot

Atherosclerosis **of other** type of bypass graft(s) of right leg with ulceration of plantar surface of midfoot

I70.735   Atherosclerosis of other type of bypass graft(s) of the right leg with ulceration of other part of foot

Atherosclerosis **of other** type of bypass graft(s) of right leg with ulceration of toe

I70.738   Atherosclerosis of other type of bypass graft(s) of the right leg with ulceration of other part of lower leg

I70.739   Atherosclerosis of other type of bypass graft(s) of the right leg with ulceration of unspecified site

I70.74   Atherosclerosis of other type of bypass graft(s) of the left leg with ulceration

Includes: any condition classifiable to I70.712 and I70.722

Use additional code to identify severity of ulcer (L97.-)

I70.741   Atherosclerosis of other type of bypass graft(s) of the left leg with ulceration of thigh

I70.742   Atherosclerosis of other type of bypass graft(s) of the left leg with ulceration of calf

I70.743   Atherosclerosis of other type of bypass graft(s) of the left leg with ulceration of ankle

I70.744   Atherosclerosis of other type of bypass graft(s) of the left leg with ulceration of heel and midfoot

Atherosclerosis **of other** type of bypass graft(s) of left leg with ulceration of plantar surface of midfoot

I70.745   Atherosclerosis of other type of bypass graft(s) of the left leg with ulceration of other part of foot

Atherosclerosis **of other** type of bypass graft(s) of left leg with ulceration of toe

I70.748   **Atherosclerosis of other type of bypass graft(s) of the left leg with ulceration of other part of lower leg**

I70.749   **Atherosclerosis of other type of bypass graft(s) of the left leg with ulceration of unspecified site**

I70.75   **Atherosclerosis of other type of bypass graft(s) of other extremity with ulceration**

> **Includes:** any condition classifiable to I70.718 and I70.728

> **Use additional code** to identify severity of ulcer (L98.49)

I70.76   **Atherosclerosis of other type of bypass graft(s) of the extremities with gangrene**

> **Includes:** any condition classifiable to I70.71-, I70.72-, I70.73-, I70.74-, I70.75

> **Use additional code** to identify the severity of any ulcer (L97.-, L98.49-), if applicable

I70.761   **Atherosclerosis of other type of bypass graft(s) of the extremities with gangrene, right leg**

I70.762   **Atherosclerosis of other type of bypass graft(s) of the extremities with gangrene, left leg**

I70.763   **Atherosclerosis of other type of bypass graft(s) of the extremities with gangrene, bilateral legs**

I70.768   **Atherosclerosis of other type of bypass graft(s) of the extremities with gangrene, other extremity**

I70.769   **Atherosclerosis of other type of bypass graft(s) of the extremities with gangrene, unspecified extremity**

I70.79   **Other atherosclerosis of other type of bypass graft(s) of the extremities**

I70.791   **Other atherosclerosis of other type of bypass graft(s) of the extremities, right leg**

I70.792   **Other atherosclerosis of other type of bypass graft(s) of the extremities, left leg**

I70.793   **Other atherosclerosis of other type of bypass graft(s) of the extremities, bilateral legs**

I70.798   **Other atherosclerosis of other type of bypass graft(s) of the extremities, other extremity**

I70.799   **Other atherosclerosis of other type of bypass graft(s) of the extremities, unspecified extremity**

I70.8   **Atherosclerosis of other arteries**

I70.9   **Other and unspecified atherosclerosis**

I70.90   **Unspecified atherosclerosis**

I70.91   **Generalized atherosclerosis**

I70.92   **Chronic total occlusion of artery of the extremities**

> Complete occlusion of artery of the extremities

> Total occlusion of artery of the extremities

> **Code first** atherosclerosis of arteries of the extremities (I70.2-, I70.3-, I70.4-, I70.5-, I70.6-, I70.7-)

I71   **Aortic aneurysm and dissection**

> **Definition:** Aortic aneurysm and dissection is a localized, abnormal and persistent dilation of a section of the aorta. This usually results from a weakness in the vessel wall. If severe

enough, rupture of the aorta with severe hemorrhage is a potential hazard.

> **Excludes1:** aortic ectasia (I77.81-)
>> syphilitic aortic aneurysm (A52.01)
>> traumatic aortic aneurysm (S25.09, S35.09)

I71.0   **Dissection of aorta**

I71.00   **Dissection of unspecified site of aorta**

I71.01   **Dissection of thoracic aorta**

I71.02   **Dissection of abdominal aorta**

I71.03   **Dissection of thoracoabdominal aorta**

I71.1   **Thoracic aortic aneurysm, ruptured**

I71.2   **Thoracic aortic aneurysm, without rupture**

I71.3   **Abdominal aortic aneurysm, ruptured**

I71.4   **Abdominal aortic aneurysm, without rupture**

I71.5   **Thoracoabdominal aortic aneurysm, ruptured**

I71.6   **Thoracoabdominal aortic aneurysm, without rupture**

I71.8   **Aortic aneurysm of unspecified site, ruptured**

> Rupture of aorta NOS

I71.9   **Aortic aneurysm of unspecified site, without rupture**

> Aneurysm of aorta

> Dilatation of aorta

> Hyaline necrosis of aorta

I72   **Other aneurysm**

> **Includes:** aneurysm (cirsoid) (false) (ruptured)

> **Excludes2:** acquired aneurysm (I77.0)
>> aneurysm (of) aorta (I71.-)
>> aneurysm (of) arteriovenous NOS (Q27.3-)
>> carotid artery dissection (I77.71)
>> cerebral (nonruptured) aneurysm (I67.1)
>> coronary aneurysm (I25.4)
>> coronary artery dissection (I25.42)
>> dissection of artery NEC (I77.79)
>> dissection of precerebral artery, congenital (nonruptured) (Q28.1)
>> heart aneurysm (I25.3)
>> iliac artery dissection (I77.72)
>> pulmonary artery aneurysm (I28.1)
>> renal artery dissection (I77.73)
>> retinal aneurysm (H35.0)
>> ruptured cerebral aneurysm (I60.7)
>> varicose aneurysm (I77.0)
>> vertebral artery dissection (I77.74)

I72.0   **Aneurysm of carotid artery**

> Aneurysm of common carotid artery

> Aneurysm of external carotid artery

> Aneurysm of internal carotid artery, extracranial portion

> **Excludes1:** aneurysm of internal carotid artery, intracranial portion (I67.1)
>> aneurysm of internal carotid artery NOS (I67.1)

I72.1   **Aneurysm of artery of upper extremity**

I72.2   **Aneurysm of renal artery**

I72.3   **Aneurysm of iliac artery**

I72.4   **Aneurysm of artery of lower extremity**

I72.5   **Aneurysm of other precerebral arteries**

> Aneurysm of basilar artery (trunk)

> **Excludes2:** aneurysm of carotid artery (I72.0)
>> aneurysm of vertebral artery (I72.6)

dissection of carotid artery (I77.71)

dissection of other precerebral arteries (I77.75)

dissection of vertebral artery (I77.74)

I72.6 **Aneurysm of vertebral artery**

Excludes2: dissection of vertebral artery (I77.74)

I72.8 **Aneurysm of other specified arteries**

I72.9 **Aneurysm of unspecified site**

I73 **Other peripheral vascular diseases**

Excludes2: chilblains (T69.1)

frostbite (T33-T34)

immersion hand or foot (T69.0-)

spasm of cerebral artery (G45.9)

I73.0 **Raynaud's syndrome**

Raynaud's disease

Raynaud's phenomenon (secondary)

I73.00 **Raynaud's syndrome without gangrene**

I73.01 **Raynaud's syndrome with gangrene**

I73.1 **Thromboangiitis obliterans [Buerger's disease]**

I73.8 **Other specified peripheral vascular diseases**

Excludes1: diabetic (peripheral) angiopathy (E08-E13 with .51-.52)

I73.81 **Erythromelalgia**

I73.89 **Other specified peripheral vascular diseases**

Acrocyanosis

Erythrocyanosis

Simple acroparesthesia [Schultze's type]

Vasomotor acroparesthesia [Nothnagel's type]

I73.9 **Peripheral vascular disease, unspecified**

Intermittent claudication

Peripheral angiopathy NOS

Spasm of artery

Excludes1: atherosclerosis of the extremities (I70.2--I70.7-)

I74 **Arterial embolism and thrombosis**

Definition: An embolism is a sudden interruption in arterial blood flow to an organ or body extremity. The blockage is caused by a blood clot or foreign object. A Thrombosis is the formation or presence of a thrombus (a clot of coagulated blood) in a blood

Includes: embolic infarction

embolic occlusion thrombotic infarction thrombotic occlusion

Code first embolism and thrombosis complicating abortion or ectopic or molar pregnancy (O00-O07, O08.2)

embolism and thrombosis complicating pregnancy, childbirth and the puerperium (O88.-)

Excludes2: atheroembolism (I75.-)

basilar embolism and thrombosis (I63.0-I63.2, I65.1)

carotid embolism and thrombosis (I63.0-I63.2, I65.2)

cerebral embolism and thrombosis (I63.3-I63.5, I66.-)

coronary embolism and thrombosis (I21-I25)

mesenteric embolism and thrombosis (K55.0-)

ophthalmic embolism and thrombosis (H34.-)

precerebral embolism and thrombosis NOS (I63.0-I63.2, I65.9)

pulmonary embolism and thrombosis (I26.-)

renal embolism and thrombosis (N28.0)

retinal embolism and thrombosis (H34.-)

septic embolism and thrombosis (I76)

vertebral embolism and thrombosis (I63.0-I63.2, I65.0)

I74.0 **Embolism and thrombosis of abdominal aorta**

I74.01 **Saddle embolus of abdominal aorta**

I74.09 **Other arterial embolism and thrombosis of abdominal aorta**

Aortic bifurcation syndrome

Aortoiliac obstruction

Leriche's syndrome

I74.1 **Embolism and thrombosis of other and unspecified parts of aorta**

I74.10 **Embolism and thrombosis of unspecified parts of aorta**

I74.11 **Embolism and thrombosis of thoracic aorta**

I74.19 **Embolism and thrombosis of other parts of aorta**

I74.2 **Embolism and thrombosis of arteries of the upper extremities**

I74.3 **Embolism and thrombosis of arteries of the lower extremities**

I74.4 **Embolism and thrombosis of arteries of extremities, unspecified**

Peripheral arterial embolism NOS

I74.5 **Embolism and thrombosis of iliac artery**

I74.8 **Embolism and thrombosis of other arteries**

I74.9 **Embolism and thrombosis of unspecified artery**

I75 **Atheroembolism**

Includes: atherothrombotic microembolism

cholesterol embolism

I75.0 **Atheroembolism of extremities**

I75.01 **Atheroembolism of upper extremity**

I75.011 **Atheroembolism of right upper extremity**

I75.012 **Atheroembolism of left upper extremity**

I75.013 **Atheroembolism of bilateral upper extremities**

I75.019 **Atheroembolism of unspecified upper extremity**

I75.02 **Atheroembolism of lower extremity**

I75.021 **Atheroembolism of right lower extremity**

I75.022 **Atheroembolism of left lower extremity**

I75.023 **Atheroembolism of bilateral lower extremities**

I75.029 **Atheroembolism of unspecified lower extremity**

I75.8 **Atheroembolism of other sites**

I75.81 **Atheroembolism of kidney**

Use additional code for any associated acute kidney failure and chronic kidney disease (N17.-, N18.-)

I75.89 **Atheroembolism of other site**

I76 **Septic arterial embolism**

Code first underlying infection, such as:

infective endocarditis (I33.0)

lung abscess (J85.-)

Use additional code to identify the site of the embolism (I74.-)

Excludes2: septic pulmonary embolism (I26.01, I26.90)

I77 **Other disorders of arteries and arterioles**

Excludes2: collagen (vascular) diseases (M30-M36)

hypersensitivity angiitis (M31.0)

pulmonary artery (I28.-)

I77.0 **Arteriovenous fistula, acquired**

Aneurysmal varix

Arteriovenous aneurysm, acquired

Excludes1: arteriovenous aneurysm NOS (Q27.3-)

presence of arteriovenous shunt (fistula) for dialysis (Z99.2)

traumatic - see injury of blood vessel by body region

Excludes2: cerebral (I67.1)

coronary (I25.4)

I77.1 **Stricture of artery**

Narrowing of artery

I77.2 **Rupture of artery**

Erosion of artery

Fistula of artery

Ulcer of artery

Excludes1: traumatic rupture of artery - see injury of blood vessel by body region

I77.3 **Arterial fibromuscular dysplasia**

Fibromuscular hyperplasia (of) carotid artery

Fibromuscular hyperplasia (of) renal artery

I77.4 **Celiac artery compression syndrome**

I77.5 **Necrosis of artery**

I77.6 **Arteritis, unspecified**

Aortitis NOS

Endarteritis NOS

Excludes1: arteritis or endarteritis:

aortic arch (M31.4)

cerebral NEC (I67.7)

coronary (I25.89)

deformans (I70.-)

giant cell (M31.5., M31.6)

obliterans (I70.-)

senile (I70.-)

I77.7 **Other arterial dissection**

Excludes2: dissection of aorta (I71.0-)

dissection of coronary artery (I25.42)

I77.70 **Dissection of unspecified artery**

I77.71 **Dissection of carotid artery**

I77.72 **Dissection of iliac artery**

I77.73 **Dissection of renal artery**

I77.74 **Dissection of vertebral artery**

Excludes2: aneurysm of vertebral artery (I72.6)

I77.75 **Dissection of other precerebral arteries**

Dissection of basilar artery (trunk)

Excludes2: aneurysm of carotid artery (I72.0)

aneurysm **of other** precerebral arteries (I72.5)

aneurysm of vertebral artery (I72.6)

dissection of carotid artery (I77.71)

dissection of vertebral artery (I77.74)

I77.76 **Dissection of artery of upper extremity**

I77.77 **Dissection of artery of lower extremity**

I77.79 **Dissection of other specified artery**

I77.8 **Other specified disorders of arteries and arterioles**

I77.81 **Aortic ectasia**

Ectasis aorta

Excludes1: aortic aneurysm and dissection (I71.0-)

I77.810 **Thoracic aortic ectasia**

I77.811 **Abdominal aortic ectasia**

I77.812 **Thoracoabdominal aortic ectasia**

I77.819 **Aortic ectasia, unspecified site**

I77.89 **Other specified disorders of arteries and arterioles**

I77.9 **Disorder of arteries and arterioles, unspecified**

I78 **Diseases of capillaries**

I78.0 **Hereditary hemorrhagic telangiectasia**

Rendu-Osler-Weber disease

I78.1 **Nevus, non-neoplastic**

Araneus nevus

Senile nevus

Spider nevus

Stellar nevus

Excludes1: nevus NOS (D22.-)

vascular NOS (Q82.5)

Excludes2: blue nevus (D22.-)

flammeus nevus (Q82.5)

hairy nevus (D22.-)

melanocytic nevus (D22.-)

pigmented nevus (D22.-)

port-wine nevus (Q82.5)

sanguineous nevus (Q82.5)

strawberry nevus (Q82.5)

verrucous nevus (Q82.5)

I78.8 **Other diseases of capillaries**

I78.9 **Disease of capillaries, unspecified**

I79 **Disorders of arteries, arterioles and capillaries in diseases classified elsewhere**

I79.0 **Aneurysm of aorta in diseases classified elsewhere**

Code first underlying disease

Excludes1: syphilitic aneurysm (A52.01)

I79.1 **Aortitis in diseases classified elsewhere**

Code first underlying disease

Excludes1: syphilitic aortitis (A52.02)

I79.8 **Other disorders of arteries, arterioles and capillaries in diseases classified elsewhere**

Code first underlying disease, such as:

amyloidosis (E85.-)

Excludes1: diabetic (peripheral) angiopathy (E08-E13 with .51-.52)

syphilitic endarteritis (A52.09)

tuberculous endarteritis (A18.89)

DISEASES OF VEINS, LYMPHATIC VESSELS AND LYMPH NODES, NOT ELSEWHERE CLASSIFIED (I80-I89)

I80 **Phlebitis and thrombophlebitis**

Includes: endophlebitis

inflammation, vein periphlebitis suppurative phlebitis

Code first phlebitis and thrombophlebitis complicating abortion, ectopic or molar pregnancy (O00-O07, O08.7)

phlebitis and thrombophlebitis complicating pregnancy, childbirth and the puerperium (O22.-, O87.-)

● New code ▲ Revised code **Excludes1:** Not coded here **Excludes2:** Not included here ⊗ Placeholder required ⑦7th digit required

Excludes1: venous embolism and thrombosis of lower extremities (I82.4-, I82.5-, I82.81-)

I80.0 **Phlebitis and thrombophlebitis of superficial vessels of lower extremities**

Phlebitis and thrombophlebitis of femoropopliteal vein

I80.00 **Phlebitis and thrombophlebitis of superficial vessels of unspecified lower extremity**

I80.01 **Phlebitis and thrombophlebitis of superficial vessels of right lower extremity**

I80.02 **Phlebitis and thrombophlebitis of superficial vessels of left lower extremity**

I80.03 **Phlebitis and thrombophlebitis of superficial vessels of lower extremities, bilateral**

I80.1 **Phlebitis and thrombophlebitis of femoral vein**

I80.10 **Phlebitis and thrombophlebitis of unspecified femoral vein**

I80.11 **Phlebitis and thrombophlebitis of right femoral vein**

I80.12 **Phlebitis and thrombophlebitis of left femoral vein**

I80.13 **Phlebitis and thrombophlebitis of femoral vein, bilateral**

I80.2 **Phlebitis and thrombophlebitis of other and unspecified deep vessels of lower extremities**

I80.20 **Phlebitis and thrombophlebitis of unspecified deep vessels of lower extremities**

I80.201 **Phlebitis and thrombophlebitis of unspecified deep vessels of right lower extremity**

I80.202 **Phlebitis and thrombophlebitis of unspecified deep vessels of left lower extremity**

I80.203 **Phlebitis and thrombophlebitis of unspecified deep vessels of lower extremities, bilateral**

I80.209 **Phlebitis and thrombophlebitis of unspecified deep vessels of unspecified lower extremity**

I80.21 **Phlebitis and thrombophlebitis of iliac vein**

I80.211 **Phlebitis and thrombophlebitis of right iliac vein**

I80.212 **Phlebitis and thrombophlebitis of left iliac vein**

I80.213 **Phlebitis and thrombophlebitis of iliac vein, bilateral**

I80.219 **Phlebitis and thrombophlebitis of unspecified iliac vein**

I80.22 **Phlebitis and thrombophlebitis of popliteal vein**

I80.221 **Phlebitis and thrombophlebitis of right popliteal vein**

I80.222 **Phlebitis and thrombophlebitis of left popliteal vein**

I80.223 **Phlebitis and thrombophlebitis of popliteal vein, bilateral**

I80.229 **Phlebitis and thrombophlebitis of unspecified popliteal vein**

I80.23 **Phlebitis and thrombophlebitis of tibial vein**

I80.231 **Phlebitis and thrombophlebitis of right tibial vein**

I80.232 **Phlebitis and thrombophlebitis of left tibial vein**

I80.233 **Phlebitis and thrombophlebitis of tibial vein, bilateral**

I80.239 **Phlebitis and thrombophlebitis of unspecified tibial vein**

I80.29 **Phlebitis and thrombophlebitis of other deep vessels of lower extremities**

I80.291 **Phlebitis and thrombophlebitis of other deep vessels of right lower extremity**

I80.292 **Phlebitis and thrombophlebitis of other deep vessels of left lower extremity**

I80.293 **Phlebitis and thrombophlebitis of other deep vessels of lower extremity, bilateral**

I80.299 **Phlebitis and thrombophlebitis of other deep vessels of unspecified lower extremity**

I80.3 **Phlebitis and thrombophlebitis of lower extremities, unspecified**

I80.8 **Phlebitis and thrombophlebitis of other sites**

I80.9 **Phlebitis and thrombophlebitis of unspecified site**

I81 **Portal vein thrombosis**

Portal (vein) obstruction

Excludes2: hepatic vein thrombosis (I82.0)

phlebitis of portal vein (K75.1)

I82 **Other venous embolism and thrombosis**

Definition: Venous embolism and thrombosis is a mass of clotted blood or other material moved by the blood from one vein and forced into a smaller one.

Code first venous embolism and thrombosis complicating:

abortion, ectopic or molar pregnancy (O00-O07, O08.7)

pregnancy, childbirth and the puerperium (O22.-, O87.-)

Excludes2: venous embolism and thrombosis (of):

cerebral (I63.6, I67.6)

coronary (I21-I25)

intracranial and intraspinal, septic or NOS (G08)

intracranial, nonpyogenic (I67.6)

intraspinal, nonpyogenic (G95.1)

mesenteric (K55.0-)

portal (I81)

pulmonary (I26.-)

I82.0 **Budd-Chiari syndrome**

Hepatic vein thrombosis

I82.1 **Thrombophlebitis migrans**

I82.2 **Embolism and thrombosis of vena cava and other thoracic veins**

I82.21 **Embolism and thrombosis of superior vena cava**

I82.210 **Acute embolism and thrombosis of superior vena cava**

Embolism and thrombosis of superior vena cava NOS

I82.211 **Chronic embolism and thrombosis of superior vena cava**

I82.22 **Embolism and thrombosis of inferior vena cava**

I82.220 **Acute embolism and thrombosis of inferior vena cava**

Embolism and thrombosis of inferior vena cava NOS

I82.221 **Chronic embolism and thrombosis of inferior vena cava**

Add 4th-7th digits	Nonspecific code	Unspecified code	Manifestation code

I82.29 **Embolism and thrombosis of other thoracic veins**

Embolism and thrombosis of brachiocephalic (innominate) vein

I82.290 **Acute embolism and thrombosis of other thoracic veins**

I82.291 **Chronic embolism and thrombosis of other thoracic veins**

I82.3 **Embolism and thrombosis of renal vein**

I82.4 **Acute embolism and thrombosis of deep veins of lower extremity**

I82.40 **Acute embolism and thrombosis of unspecified deep veins of lower extremity**

Deep vein thrombosis NOS

DVT NOS

Excludes1: acute embolism and thrombosis of unspecified deep veins of distal lower extremity (I82.4Z-)

acute embolism and thrombosis of unspecified deep veins of proximal lower extremity (I82.4Y-)

I82.401 **Acute embolism and thrombosis of unspecified deep veins of right lower extremity**

I82.402 **Acute embolism and thrombosis of unspecified deep veins of left lower extremity**

I82.403 **Acute embolism and thrombosis of unspecified deep veins of lower extremity, bilateral**

I82.409 **Acute embolism and thrombosis of unspecified deep veins of unspecified lower extremity**

I82.41 **Acute embolism and thrombosis of femoral vein**

I82.411 **Acute embolism and thrombosis of right femoral vein**

I82.412 **Acute embolism and thrombosis of left femoral vein**

I82.413 **Acute embolism and thrombosis of femoral vein, bilateral**

I82.419 **Acute embolism and thrombosis of unspecified femoral vein**

I82.42 **Acute embolism and thrombosis of iliac vein**

I82.421 **Acute embolism and thrombosis of right iliac vein**

I82.422 **Acute embolism and thrombosis of left iliac vein**

I82.423 **Acute embolism and thrombosis of iliac vein, bilateral**

I82.429 **Acute embolism and thrombosis of unspecified iliac vein**

I82.43 **Acute embolism and thrombosis of popliteal vein**

I82.431 **Acute embolism and thrombosis of right popliteal vein**

I82.432 **Acute embolism and thrombosis of left popliteal vein**

I82.433 **Acute embolism and thrombosis of popliteal vein, bilateral**

I82.439 **Acute embolism and thrombosis of unspecified popliteal vein**

I82.44 **Acute embolism and thrombosis of tibial vein**

I82.441 **Acute embolism and thrombosis of right tibial vein**

I82.442 **Acute embolism and thrombosis of left tibial vein**

I82.443 **Acute embolism and thrombosis of tibial vein, bilateral**

I82.449 **Acute embolism and thrombosis of unspecified tibial vein**

I82.49 **Acute embolism and thrombosis of other specified deep vein of lower extremity**

I82.491 **Acute embolism and thrombosis of other specified deep vein of right lower extremity**

I82.492 **Acute embolism and thrombosis of other specified deep vein of left lower extremity**

I82.493 **Acute embolism and thrombosis of other specified deep vein of lower extremity, bilateral**

I82.499 **Acute embolism and thrombosis of other specified deep vein of unspecified lower extremity**

I82.4Y **Acute embolism and thrombosis of unspecified deep veins of proximal lower extremity**

Acute embolism and thrombosis of deep vein of thigh NOS

Acute embolism and thrombosis of deep vein of upper leg NOS

I82.4Y1 **Acute embolism and thrombosis of unspecified deep veins of right proximal lower extremity**

I82.4Y2 **Acute embolism and thrombosis of unspecified deep veins of left proximal lower extremity**

I82.4Y3 **Acute embolism and thrombosis of unspecified deep veins of proximal lower extremity, bilateral**

I82.4Y9 **Acute embolism and thrombosis of unspecified deep veins of unspecified proximal lower extremity**

I82.4Z **Acute embolism and thrombosis of unspecified deep veins of distal lower extremity**

Acute embolism and thrombosis of deep vein of calf NOS

Acute embolism and thrombosis of deep vein of lower leg NOS

I82.4Z1 **Acute embolism and thrombosis of unspecified deep veins of right distal lower extremity**

I82.4Z2 **Acute embolism and thrombosis of unspecified deep veins of left distal lower extremity**

I82.4Z3 **Acute embolism and thrombosis of unspecified deep veins of distal lower extremity, bilateral**

I82.4Z9 **Acute embolism and thrombosis of unspecified deep veins of unspecified distal lower extremity**

I82.5 **Chronic embolism and thrombosis of deep veins of lower extremity**

Use additional code, if applicable, for associated long-term (current) use of anticoagulants (Z79.01)

Excludes1: personal history of venous embolism and thrombosis (Z86.718)

I82.50 **Chronic embolism and thrombosis of unspecified deep veins of lower extremity**

● New code   ▲ Revised code   **Excludes1:** Not coded here   **Excludes2:** Not included here   ⊗ Placeholder required   ⑦ 7th digit required

Excludes1: chronic embolism and thrombosis of unspecified deep veins of distal lower extremity (I82.5Z-)

chronic embolism and thrombosis of unspecified deep veins of proximal lower extremity (I82.5Y-)

I82.501 Chronic embolism and thrombosis of unspecified deep veins of right lower extremity

I82.502 Chronic embolism and thrombosis of unspecified deep veins of left lower extremity

I82.503 Chronic embolism and thrombosis of unspecified deep veins of lower extremity, bilateral

I82.509 Chronic embolism and thrombosis of unspecified deep veins of unspecified lower extremity

I82.51 Chronic embolism and thrombosis of femoral vein

I82.511 Chronic embolism and thrombosis of right femoral vein

I82.512 Chronic embolism and thrombosis of left femoral vein

I82.513 Chronic embolism and thrombosis of femoral vein, bilateral

I82.519 Chronic embolism and thrombosis of unspecified femoral vein

I82.52 Chronic embolism and thrombosis of iliac vein

I82.521 Chronic embolism and thrombosis of right iliac vein

I82.522 Chronic embolism and thrombosis of left iliac vein

I82.523 Chronic embolism and thrombosis of iliac vein, bilateral

I82.529 Chronic embolism and thrombosis of unspecified iliac vein

I82.53 Chronic embolism and thrombosis of popliteal vein

I82.531 Chronic embolism and thrombosis of right popliteal vein

I82.532 Chronic embolism and thrombosis of left popliteal vein

I82.533 Chronic embolism and thrombosis of popliteal vein, bilateral

I82.539 Chronic embolism and thrombosis of unspecified popliteal vein

I82.54 Chronic embolism and thrombosis of tibial vein

I82.541 Chronic embolism and thrombosis of right tibial vein

I82.542 Chronic embolism and thrombosis of left tibial vein

I82.543 Chronic embolism and thrombosis of tibial vein, bilateral

I82.549 Chronic embolism and thrombosis of unspecified tibial vein

I82.59 Chronic embolism and thrombosis of other specified deep vein of lower extremity

I82.591 Chronic embolism and thrombosis of other specified deep vein of right lower extremity

I82.592 Chronic embolism and thrombosis of other specified deep vein of left lower extremity

I82.593 Chronic embolism and thrombosis of other specified deep vein of lower extremity, bilateral

I82.599 Chronic embolism and thrombosis of other specified deep vein of unspecified lower extremity

I82.5Y Chronic embolism and thrombosis of unspecified deep veins of proximal lower extremity

Chronic embolism and thrombosis of deep veins of thigh NOS

Chronic embolism and thrombosis of deep veins of upper leg NOS

I82.5Y1 Chronic embolism and thrombosis of unspecified deep veins of right proximal lower extremity

I82.5Y2 Chronic embolism and thrombosis of unspecified deep veins of left proximal lower extremity

I82.5Y3 Chronic embolism and thrombosis of unspecified deep veins of proximal lower extremity, bilateral

I82.5Y9 Chronic embolism and thrombosis of unspecified deep veins of unspecified proximal lower extremity

I82.5Z Chronic embolism and thrombosis of unspecified deep veins of distal lower extremity

Chronic embolism and thrombosis of deep veins of calf NOS

Chronic embolism and thrombosis of deep veins of lower leg NOS

I82.5Z1 Chronic embolism and thrombosis of unspecified deep veins of right distal lower extremity

I82.5Z2 Chronic embolism and thrombosis of unspecified deep veins of left distal lower extremity

I82.5Z3 Chronic embolism and thrombosis of unspecified deep veins of distal lower extremity, bilateral

I82.5Z9 Chronic embolism and thrombosis of unspecified deep veins of unspecified distal lower extremity

I82.6 Acute embolism and thrombosis of veins of upper extremity

I82.60 Acute embolism and thrombosis of unspecified veins of upper extremity

I82.601 Acute embolism and thrombosis of unspecified veins of right upper extremity

I82.602 Acute embolism and thrombosis of unspecified veins of left upper extremity

I82.603 Acute embolism and thrombosis of unspecified veins of upper extremity, bilateral

I82.609 Acute embolism and thrombosis of unspecified veins of unspecified upper extremity

I82.61 Acute embolism and thrombosis of superficial veins of upper extremity

Acute embolism and thrombosis of antecubital vein

Acute embolism and thrombosis of basilic vein

Acute embolism and thrombosis of cephalic vein

I82.611   **Acute embolism and thrombosis of superficial veins of right upper extremity**

I82.612   **Acute embolism and thrombosis of superficial veins of left upper extremity**

I82.613   **Acute embolism and thrombosis of superficial veins of upper extremity, bilateral**

I82.619   **Acute embolism and thrombosis of superficial veins of unspecified upper extremity**

I82.62   **Acute embolism and thrombosis of deep veins of upper extremity**

Acute embolism and thrombosis of brachial vein

Acute embolism and thrombosis of radial vein

Acute embolism and thrombosis of ulnar vein

I82.621   **Acute embolism and thrombosis of deep veins of right upper extremity**

I82.622   **Acute embolism and thrombosis of deep veins of left upper extremity**

I82.623   **Acute embolism and thrombosis of deep veins of upper extremity, bilateral**

I82.629   **Acute embolism and thrombosis of deep veins of unspecified upper extremity**

I82.7   **Chronic embolism and thrombosis of veins of upper extremity**

Use additional code, if applicable, for associated long-term (current) use of anticoagulants (Z79.01)

Excludes1: personal history of venous embolism and thrombosis (Z86.718)

I82.70   **Chronic embolism and thrombosis of unspecified veins of upper extremity**

I82.701   **Chronic embolism and thrombosis of unspecified veins of right upper extremity**

I82.702   **Chronic embolism and thrombosis of unspecified veins of left upper extremity**

I82.703   **Chronic embolism and thrombosis of unspecified veins of upper extremity, bilateral**

I82.709   **Chronic embolism and thrombosis of unspecified veins of unspecified upper extremity**

I82.71   **Chronic embolism and thrombosis of superficial veins of upper extremity**

Chronic embolism and thrombosis of antecubital vein

Chronic embolism and thrombosis of basilic vein

Chronic embolism and thrombosis of cephalic vein

I82.711   **Chronic embolism and thrombosis of superficial veins of right upper extremity**

I82.712   **Chronic embolism and thrombosis of superficial veins of left upper extremity**

I82.713   **Chronic embolism and thrombosis of superficial veins of upper extremity, bilateral**

I82.719   **Chronic embolism and thrombosis of superficial veins of unspecified upper extremity**

I82.72   **Chronic embolism and thrombosis of deep veins of upper extremity**

Chronic embolism and thrombosis of brachial vein

Chronic embolism and thrombosis of radial vein

Chronic embolism and thrombosis of ulnar vein

I82.721   **Chronic embolism and thrombosis of deep veins of right upper extremity**

I82.722   **Chronic embolism and thrombosis of deep veins of left upper extremity**

I82.723   **Chronic embolism and thrombosis of deep veins of upper extremity, bilateral**

I82.729   **Chronic embolism and thrombosis of deep veins of unspecified upper extremity**

I82.A   **Embolism and thrombosis of axillary vein**

I82.A1   **Acute embolism and thrombosis of axillary vein**

I82.A11   **Acute embolism and thrombosis of right axillary vein**

I82.A12   **Acute embolism and thrombosis of left axillary vein**

I82.A13   **Acute embolism and thrombosis of axillary vein, bilateral**

I82.A19   **Acute embolism and thrombosis of unspecified axillary vein**

I82.A2   **Chronic embolism and thrombosis of axillary vein**

I82.A21   **Chronic embolism and thrombosis of right axillary vein**

I82.A22   **Chronic embolism and thrombosis of left axillary vein**

I82.A23   **Chronic embolism and thrombosis of axillary vein, bilateral**

I82.A29   **Chronic embolism and thrombosis of unspecified axillary vein**

I82.B   **Embolism and thrombosis of subclavian vein**

I82.B1   **Acute embolism and thrombosis of subclavian vein**

I82.B11   **Acute embolism and thrombosis of right subclavian vein**

I82.B12   **Acute embolism and thrombosis of left subclavian vein**

I82.B13   **Acute embolism and thrombosis of subclavian vein, bilateral**

I82.B19   **Acute embolism and thrombosis of unspecified subclavian vein**

I82.B2   **Chronic embolism and thrombosis of subclavian vein**

I82.B21   **Chronic embolism and thrombosis of right subclavian vein**

I82.B22   **Chronic embolism and thrombosis of left subclavian vein**

I82.B23   **Chronic embolism and thrombosis of subclavian vein, bilateral**

I82.B29   **Chronic embolism and thrombosis of unspecified subclavian vein**

I82.C   **Embolism and thrombosis of internal jugular vein**

I82.C1   **Acute embolism and thrombosis of internal jugular vein**

I82.C11   **Acute embolism and thrombosis of right internal jugular vein**

I82.C12   **Acute embolism and thrombosis of left internal jugular vein**

  ● New code   ▲ Revised code   Excludes1: Not coded here   Excludes2: Not included here   ⊗ Placeholder required   ⑦ 7th digit required

I82.C13   **Acute embolism and thrombosis of internal jugular vein, bilateral**

I82.C19   **Acute embolism and thrombosis of unspecified internal jugular vein**

I82.C2   **Chronic embolism and thrombosis of internal jugular vein**

I82.C21   **Chronic embolism and thrombosis of right internal jugular vein**

I82.C22   **Chronic embolism and thrombosis of left internal jugular vein**

I82.C23   **Chronic embolism and thrombosis of internal jugular vein, bilateral**

I82.C29   **Chronic embolism and thrombosis of unspecified internal jugular vein**

I82.8   **Embolism and thrombosis of other specified veins**

Use additional code, if applicable, for associated long-term (current) use of anticoagulants (Z79.01)

I82.81   **Embolism and thrombosis of superficial veins of lower extremities**

Embolism and thrombosis of saphenous vein (greater) (lesser)

▲I82.811   **Embolism and thrombosis of superficial veins of right lower extremity**

▲I82.812   **Embolism and thrombosis of superficial veins of left lower extremity**

I82.813   **Embolism and thrombosis of superficial veins of lower extremity, bilateral**

▲I82.819   **Embolism and thrombosis of superficial veins of unspecified lower extremity**

I82.89   **Embolism and thrombosis of other specified veins**

I82.890   **Acute embolism and thrombosis of other specified veins**

I82.891   **Chronic embolism and thrombosis of other specified veins**

I82.9   **Embolism and thrombosis of unspecified vein**

I82.90   **Acute embolism and thrombosis of unspecified vein**

Embolism of vein NOS

Thrombosis (vein) NOS

I82.91   **Chronic embolism and thrombosis of unspecified vein**

I83   **Varicose veins of lower extremities**

Definition: Varicose veins are dilated (widened) tortuous (twisting) veins, usually involving a superficial vein in the leg, often associated with incompetency of the valves in the vein

Excludes1: varicose veins complicating pregnancy (O22.0-)
varicose veins complicating the puerperium (O87.4)

I83.0   **Varicose veins of lower extremities with ulcer**

Use additional code to identify severity of ulcer (L97.-)

I83.00   **Varicose veins of unspecified lower extremity with ulcer**

I83.001   **Varicose veins of unspecified lower extremity with ulcer of thigh**

I83.002   **Varicose veins of unspecified lower extremity with ulcer of calf**

I83.003   **Varicose veins of unspecified lower extremity with ulcer of ankle**

I83.004   **Varicose veins of unspecified lower extremity with ulcer of heel and midfoot**

Varicose veins of unspecified lower extremity with ulcer of plantar surface of midfoot

I83.005   **Varicose veins of unspecified lower extremity with ulcer other part of foot**

Varicose veins of unspecified lower extremity with ulcer of toe

I83.008   **Varicose veins of unspecified lower extremity with ulcer other part of lower leg**

I83.009   **Varicose veins of unspecified lower extremity with ulcer of unspecified site**

I83.01   **Varicose veins of right lower extremity with ulcer**

I83.011   **Varicose veins of right lower extremity with ulcer of thigh**

I83.012   **Varicose veins of right lower extremity with ulcer of calf**

I83.013   **Varicose veins of right lower extremity with ulcer of ankle**

I83.014   **Varicose veins of right lower extremity with ulcer of heel and midfoot**

Varicose veins of right lower extremity with ulcer of plantar surface of midfoot

I83.015   **Varicose veins of right lower extremity with ulcer other part of foot**

Varicose veins of right lower extremity with ulcer of toe

I83.018   **Varicose veins of right lower extremity with ulcer other part of lower leg**

I83.019   **Varicose veins of right lower extremity with ulcer of unspecified site**

I83.02   **Varicose veins of left lower extremity with ulcer**

I83.021   **Varicose veins of left lower extremity with ulcer of thigh**

I83.022   **Varicose veins of left lower extremity with ulcer of calf**

I83.023   **Varicose veins of left lower extremity with ulcer of ankle**

I83.024   **Varicose veins of left lower extremity with ulcer of heel and midfoot**

Varicose veins of left lower extremity with ulcer of plantar surface of midfoot

I83.025   **Varicose veins of left lower extremity with ulcer other part of foot**

Varicose veins of left lower extremity with ulcer of toe

I83.028   **Varicose veins of left lower extremity with ulcer other part of lower leg**

I83.029   **Varicose veins of left lower extremity with ulcer of unspecified site**

I83.1   **Varicose veins of lower extremities with inflammation**

I83.10   **Varicose veins of unspecified lower extremity with inflammation**

I83.11   **Varicose veins of right lower extremity with inflammation**

I83.12   Varicose veins of left lower extremity with inflammation

I83.2   Varicose veins of lower extremities with both ulcer and inflammation

Use additional code to identify severity of ulcer (L97.-)

I83.20   Varicose veins of unspecified lower extremity with both ulcer and inflammation

I83.201   Varicose veins of unspecified lower extremity with both ulcer of thigh and inflammation

I83.202   Varicose veins of unspecified lower extremity with both ulcer of calf and inflammation

I83.203   Varicose veins of unspecified lower extremity with both ulcer of ankle and inflammation

I83.204   Varicose veins of unspecified lower extremity with both ulcer of heel and midfoot and inflammation

Varicose veins of unspecified lower extremity with both ulcer of plantar surface of midfoot and inflammation

I83.205   Varicose veins of unspecified lower extremity with both ulcer other part of foot and inflammation

Varicose veins of unspecified lower extremity with both ulcer of toe and inflammation

I83.208   Varicose veins of unspecified lower extremity with both ulcer of other part of lower extremity and inflammation

I83.209   Varicose veins of unspecified lower extremity with both ulcer of unspecified site and inflammation

I83.21   Varicose veins of right lower extremity with both ulcer and inflammation

I83.211   Varicose veins of right lower extremity with both ulcer of thigh and inflammation

I83.212   Varicose veins of right lower extremity with both ulcer of calf and inflammation

I83.213   Varicose veins of right lower extremity with both ulcer of ankle and inflammation

I83.214   Varicose veins of right lower extremity with both ulcer of heel and midfoot and inflammation

Varicose veins of right lower extremity with both ulcer of plantar surface of midfoot and inflammation

I83.215   Varicose veins of right lower extremity with both ulcer other part of foot and inflammation

Varicose veins of right lower extremity with both ulcer of toe and inflammation

I83.218   Varicose veins of right lower extremity with both ulcer of other part of lower extremity and inflammation

I83.219   Varicose veins of right lower extremity with both ulcer of unspecified site and inflammation

I83.22   Varicose veins of left lower extremity with both ulcer and inflammation

I83.221   Varicose veins of left lower extremity with both ulcer of thigh and inflammation

I83.222   Varicose veins of left lower extremity with both ulcer of calf and inflammation

I83.223   Varicose veins of left lower extremity with both ulcer of ankle and inflammation

I83.224   Varicose veins of left lower extremity with both ulcer of heel and midfoot and inflammation

Varicose veins of left lower extremity with both ulcer of plantar surface of midfoot and inflammation

I83.225   Varicose veins of left lower extremity with both ulcer other part of foot and inflammation

Varicose veins of left lower extremity with both ulcer of toe and inflammation

I83.228   Varicose veins of left lower extremity with both ulcer of other part of lower extremity and inflammation

I83.229   Varicose veins of left lower extremity with both ulcer of unspecified site and inflammation

I83.8   Varicose veins of lower extremities with other complications

I83.81   Varicose veins of lower extremities with pain

▲**I83.811**   Varicose veins of right lower extremity with pain

▲**I83.812**   Varicose veins of left lower extremity with pain

I83.813   Varicose veins of bilateral lower extremity with pain

▲**I83.819**   Varicose veins of unspecified lower extremity with pain

I83.89   Varicose veins of lower extremities with other complications

Varicose veins of lower extremities with edema
Varicose veins of lower extremity with swelling

▲**I83.891**   Varicose veins of right lower extremity with other complications

▲**I83.892**   Varicose veins of left lower extremity with other complications

I83.893   Varicose veins of bilateral lower extremity with other complications

▲**I83.899**   Varicose veins of unspecified lower extremity with other complications

I83.9   Asymptomatic varicose veins of lower extremities

Phlebectasia of lower extremities

Varicose veins of lower extremities

Varix of lower extremities

I83.90   Asymptomatic varicose veins of unspecified lower extremity

Varicose veins NOS

I83.91   Asymptomatic varicose veins of right lower extremity

I83.92   Asymptomatic varicose veins of left lower extremity

I83.93   Asymptomatic varicose veins of bilateral lower extremities

I85   **Esophageal varices**

Use additional code to identify:

● New code   ▲ Revised code   **Excludes1:** Not coded here   **Excludes2:** Not included here   ⊗ Placeholder required   ⑦7th digit required

alcohol abuse and dependence (F10.-)

I85.0 **Esophageal varices**

Idiopathic esophageal varices

Primary esophageal varices

I85.00 **Esophageal varices without bleeding**

Esophageal varices NOS

I85.01 **Esophageal varices with bleeding**

I85.1 **Secondary esophageal varices**

Esophageal varices secondary to alcoholic liver disease

Esophageal varices secondary to cirrhosis of liver

Esophageal varices secondary to schistosomiasis

Esophageal varices secondary to toxic liver disease

<u>Code first</u> underlying disease

I85.10 **Secondary esophageal varices without bleeding**

I85.11 **Secondary esophageal varices with bleeding**

I86 **Varicose veins of other sites**

Excludes1: varicose veins of unspecified site (I83.9-)

Excludes2: retinal varices (H35.0-)

I86.0 **Sublingual varices**

I86.1 **Scrotal varices**

Varicocele

I86.2 **Pelvic varices**

I86.3 **Vulval varices**

Excludes1: vulval varices complicating childbirth and the puerperium (O87.8)

vulval varices complicating pregnancy (O22.1-)

I86.4 **Gastric varices**

I86.8 **Varicose veins of other specified sites**

Varicose ulcer of nasal septum

I87 **Other disorders of veins**

I87.0 **Postthrombotic syndrome**

Chronic venous hypertension due to deep vein thrombosis

Postphlebitic syndrome

Excludes1: chronic venous hypertension without deep vein thrombosis (I87.3-)

I87.00 **Postthrombotic syndrome without complications**

Asymptomatic Postthrombotic syndrome

I87.001 **Postthrombotic syndrome without complications of right lower extremity**

I87.002 **Postthrombotic syndrome without complications of left lower extremity**

I87.003 **Postthrombotic syndrome without complications of bilateral lower extremity**

I87.009 **Postthrombotic syndrome without complications of unspecified extremity**

Postthrombotic syndrome NOS

I87.01 **Postthrombotic syndrome with ulcer**

<u>Use additional code</u> to specify site and severity of ulcer (L97.-)

I87.011 **Postthrombotic syndrome with ulcer of right lower extremity**

I87.012 **Postthrombotic syndrome with ulcer of left lower extremity**

I87.013 **Postthrombotic syndrome with ulcer of bilateral lower extremity**

I87.019 **Postthrombotic syndrome with ulcer of unspecified lower extremity**

I87.02 **Postthrombotic syndrome with inflammation**

I87.021 **Postthrombotic syndrome with inflammation of right lower extremity**

I87.022 **Postthrombotic syndrome with inflammation of left lower extremity**

I87.023 **Postthrombotic syndrome with inflammation of bilateral lower extremity**

I87.029 **Postthrombotic syndrome with inflammation of unspecified lower extremity**

I87.03 **Postthrombotic syndrome with ulcer and inflammation**

<u>Use additional code</u> to specify site and severity of ulcer (L97.-)

I87.031 **Postthrombotic syndrome with ulcer and inflammation of right lower extremity**

I87.032 **Postthrombotic syndrome with ulcer and inflammation of left lower extremity**

I87.033 **Postthrombotic syndrome with ulcer and inflammation of bilateral lower extremity**

I87.039 **Postthrombotic syndrome with ulcer and inflammation of unspecified lower extremity**

I87.09 **Postthrombotic syndrome with other complications**

I87.091 **Postthrombotic syndrome with other complications of right lower extremity**

I87.092 **Postthrombotic syndrome with other complications of left lower extremity**

I87.093 **Postthrombotic syndrome with other complications of bilateral lower extremity**

I87.099 **Postthrombotic syndrome with other complications of unspecified lower extremity**

I87.1 **Compression of vein**

Stricture of vein

Vena cava syndrome (inferior) (superior)

Excludes2: compression of pulmonary vein (I28.8)

I87.2 **Venous insufficiency (chronic) (peripheral)**

Stasis dermatitis

Excludes1: stasis dermatitis with varicose veins of lower extremities (I83.1-, I83.2-)

I87.3 **Chronic venous hypertension (idiopathic)**

Stasis edema

Excludes1: chronic venous hypertension due to deep vein thrombosis (I87.0-)

varicose veins of lower extremities (I83.-)

I87.30 **Chronic venous hypertension (idiopathic) without complications**

Asymptomatic chronic venous hypertension (idiopathic)

I87.301 **Chronic venous hypertension (idiopathic) without complications of right lower extremity**

I87.302 **Chronic venous hypertension (idiopathic) without complications of left lower extremity**

I87.303 **Chronic venous hypertension (idiopathic) without complications of bilateral lower extremity**

I87.309 **Chronic venous hypertension (idiopathic) without complications of unspecified lower extremity**

Chronic venous hypertension NOS

I87.31 **Chronic venous hypertension (idiopathic) with ulcer**

Use additional code to specify site and severity of ulcer (L97.-)

I87.311 **Chronic venous hypertension (idiopathic) with ulcer of right lower extremity**

I87.312 **Chronic venous hypertension (idiopathic) with ulcer of left lower extremity**

I87.313 **Chronic venous hypertension (idiopathic) with ulcer of bilateral lower extremity**

I87.319 **Chronic venous hypertension (idiopathic) with ulcer of unspecified lower extremity**

I87.32 **Chronic venous hypertension (idiopathic) with inflammation**

I87.321 **Chronic venous hypertension (idiopathic) with inflammation of right lower extremity**

I87.322 **Chronic venous hypertension (idiopathic) with inflammation of left lower extremity**

I87.323 **Chronic venous hypertension (idiopathic) with inflammation of bilateral lower extremity**

I87.329 **Chronic venous hypertension (idiopathic) with inflammation of unspecified lower extremity**

I87.33 **Chronic venous hypertension (idiopathic) with ulcer and inflammation**

Use additional code to specify site and severity of ulcer (L97.-)

I87.331 **Chronic venous hypertension (idiopathic) with ulcer and inflammation of right lower extremity**

I87.332 **Chronic venous hypertension (idiopathic) with ulcer and inflammation of left lower extremity**

I87.333 **Chronic venous hypertension (idiopathic) with ulcer and inflammation of bilateral lower extremity**

I87.339 **Chronic venous hypertension (idiopathic) with ulcer and inflammation of unspecified lower extremity**

I87.39 **Chronic venous hypertension (idiopathic) with other complications**

I87.391 **Chronic venous hypertension (idiopathic) with other complications of right lower extremity**

I87.392 **Chronic venous hypertension (idiopathic) with other complications of left lower extremity**

I87.393 **Chronic venous hypertension (idiopathic) with other complications of bilateral lower extremity**

I87.399 **Chronic venous hypertension (idiopathic) with other complications of unspecified lower extremity**

I87.8 **Other specified disorders of veins**

Phlebosclerosis

Venofibrosis

I87.9 **Disorder of vein, unspecified**

I88 **Nonspecific lymphadenitis**

Excludes1: acute lymphadenitis, except mesenteric (L04.-)

enlarged lymph nodes NOS (R59.-)

human immunodeficiency virus [HIV] disease resulting in generalized lymphadenopathy (B20)

I88.0 **Nonspecific mesenteric lymphadenitis**

Mesenteric lymphadenitis (acute)(chronic)

I88.1 **Chronic lymphadenitis, except mesenteric**

Adenitis

Lymphadenitis

I88.8 **Other nonspecific lymphadenitis**

I88.9 **Nonspecific lymphadenitis, unspecified**

Lymphadenitis NOS

I89 **Other noninfective disorders of lymphatic vessels and lymph nodes**

Excludes1: chylocele, tunica vaginalis (nonfilarial) NOS (N50.89)

enlarged lymph nodes NOS (R59.-)

filarial chylocele (B74.-)

hereditary lymphedema (Q82.0)

I89.0 **Lymphedema, not elsewhere classified**

Elephantiasis (nonfilarial) NOS

Lymphangiectasis

Obliteration, lymphatic vessel

Praecox lymphedema

Secondary lymphedema

Excludes1: postmastectomy lymphedema (I97.2)

I89.1 **Lymphangitis**

Chronic lymphangitis

Lymphangitis NOS

Subacute lymphangitis

Excludes1: acute lymphangitis (L03.-)

I89.8 **Other specified noninfective disorders of lymphatic vessels and lymph nodes**

Chylocele (nonfilarial)

Chylous ascites

Chylous cyst

Lipomelanotic reticulosis

Lymph node or vessel fistula

Lymph node or vessel infarction

Lymph node or vessel rupture

I89.9 **Noninfective disorder of lymphatic vessels and lymph nodes, unspecified**

Disease of lymphatic vessels NOS

OTHER AND UNSPECIFIED DISORDERS OF THE CIRCULATORY SYSTEM (I95-I99)

I95 **Hypotension**

Excludes1: cardiovascular collapse (R57.9)

maternal hypotension syndrome (O26.5-)

nonspecific low blood pressure reading NOS (R03.1)

I95.0 Idiopathic hypotension

I95.1 Orthostatic hypotension

Hypotension, postural

Excludes1: neurogenic orthostatic hypotension [Shy-Drager] (G90.3)

orthostatic hypotension due to drugs (I95.2)

I95.2 Hypotension due to drugs

Orthostatic hypotension due to drugs

Use additional code for adverse effect, if applicable, to identify drug (T36-T50 with fifth or sixth character 5)

I95.3 Hypotension of hemodialysis

Intra-dialytic hypotension

I95.8 Other hypotension

I95.81 Postprocedural hypotension

I95.89 Other hypotension

Chronic hypotension

I95.9 Hypotension, unspecified

I96 Gangrene, not elsewhere classified

Gangrenous cellulitis

Excludes2: gangrene in atherosclerosis of native arteries of the extremities (I70.26)

gangrene in diabetes mellitus (E08-E13 with .52)

gangrene in hernia (K40.1, K40.4, K41.1, K41.4, K42.1, K43.1-, K44.1, K45.1, K46.1)

gangrene **in other** peripheral vascular diseases (I73.-)

gangrene of certain specified sites - see Alphabetical Index gas gangrene (A48.0)

pyoderma gangrenosum (L88)

I97 Intraoperative and postprocedural complications and disorders of circulatory system, not elsewhere classified

Excludes2: postprocedural shock (T81.1-)

I97.0 Postcardiotomy syndrome

I97.1 Other postprocedural cardiac functional disturbances

Excludes2: acute pulmonary insufficiency following thoracic surgery (J95.1)

intraoperative cardiac functional disturbances (I97.7-)

I97.11 Postprocedural cardiac insufficiency

I97.110 Postprocedural cardiac insufficiency following cardiac surgery

I97.111 Postprocedural cardiac insufficiency following other surgery

I97.12 Postprocedural cardiac arrest

I97.120 Postprocedural cardiac arrest following cardiac surgery

I97.121 Postprocedural cardiac arrest following other surgery

I97.13 Postprocedural heart failure

Use additional code to identify the heart failure (I50.-)

I97.130 Postprocedural heart failure following cardiac surgery

I97.131 Postprocedural heart failure following other surgery

I97.19 Other postprocedural cardiac functional disturbances

Use additional code, if applicable, to further specify disorder

I97.190 Other postprocedural cardiac functional disturbances following cardiac surgery

Use Additional code, if applicable, for type 4 or type 5 myocardial infarction, to further specify disorder

I97.191 Other postprocedural cardiac functional disturbances following other surgery

I97.2 Postmastectomy lymphedema syndrome

Elephantiasis due to mastectomy

Obliteration of lymphatic vessels

I97.3 Postprocedural hypertension

I97.4 Intraoperative hemorrhage and hematoma of a circulatory system organ or structure complicating a procedure

Excludes1: intraoperative hemorrhage and hematoma of a circulatory system organ or structure due to accidental puncture and laceration during a procedure (I97.5-)

Excludes2: intraoperative cerebrovascular hemorrhage complicating a procedure (G97.3-)

I97.41 Intraoperative hemorrhage and hematoma of a circulatory system organ or structure complicating a circulatory system procedure

I97.410 Intraoperative hemorrhage and hematoma of a circulatory system organ or structure complicating a cardiac catheterization

I97.411 Intraoperative hemorrhage and hematoma of a circulatory system organ or structure complicating a cardiac bypass

I97.418 Intraoperative hemorrhage and hematoma of a circulatory system organ or structure complicating other circulatory system procedure

I97.42 Intraoperative hemorrhage and hematoma of a circulatory system organ or structure complicating other procedure

I97.5 Accidental puncture and laceration of a circulatory system organ or structure during a procedure

Excludes2: accidental puncture and laceration of brain during a procedure (G97.4-)

I97.51 Accidental puncture and laceration of a circulatory system organ or structure during a circulatory system procedure

I97.52 Accidental puncture and laceration of a circulatory system organ or structure during other procedure

I97.6 Postprocedural hemorrhage, hematoma and seroma of a circulatory system organ or structure following a procedure

Excludes2: postprocedural cerebrovascular hemorrhage complicating a procedure (G97.5-)

I97.61 Postprocedural hemorrhage of a circulatory system organ or structure following a circulatory system procedure

I97.610 Postprocedural hemorrhage of a circulatory system organ or structure following a cardiac catheterization

I97.611 Postprocedural hemorrhage of a circulatory system organ or structure following cardiac bypass

I97.618 Postprocedural hemorrhage of a circulatory system organ or structure following other circulatory system procedure

I97.62 Postprocedural hemorrhage, hematoma and seroma of a circulatory system organ or structure following other procedure

I97.620 Postprocedural hemorrhage of a circulatory system organ or structure following other procedure

I97.621 Postprocedural hematoma of a circulatory system organ or structure following other procedure

I97.622 Postprocedural seroma of a circulatory system organ or structure following other procedure

I97.63 Postprocedural hematoma of a circulatory system organ or structure following a circulatory system procedure

I97.630 Postprocedural hematoma of a circulatory system organ or structure following a cardiac catheterization

I97.631 Postprocedural hematoma of a circulatory system organ or structure following cardiac bypass

I97.638 Postprocedural hematoma of a circulatory system organ or structure following other circulatory system procedure

I97.64 Postprocedural seroma of a circulatory system organ or structure following a circulatory system procedure

I97.640 Postprocedural seroma of a circulatory system organ or structure following a cardiac catheterization

I97.641 Postprocedural seroma of a circulatory system organ or structure following cardiac bypass

I97.648 Postprocedural seroma of a circulatory system organ or structure following other circulatory system procedure

I97.7 Intraoperative cardiac functional disturbances

Excludes2: acute pulmonary insufficiency following thoracic surgery (J95.1)

postprocedural cardiac functional disturbances (I97.1-)

I97.71 Intraoperative cardiac arrest

I97.710 Intraoperative cardiac arrest during cardiac surgery

I97.711 Intraoperative cardiac arrest during other surgery

I97.79 Other intraoperative cardiac functional disturbances

Use additional code, if applicable, to further specify disorder

I97.790 Other intraoperative cardiac functional disturbances during cardiac surgery

I97.791 Other intraoperative cardiac functional disturbances during other surgery

I97.8 Other intraoperative and postprocedural complications and disorders of the circulatory system, not elsewhere classified

Use additional code, if applicable, to further specify disorder

I97.81 Intraoperative cerebrovascular infarction

I97.810 Intraoperative cerebrovascular infarction during cardiac surgery

I97.811 Intraoperative cerebrovascular infarction during other surgery

I97.82 Postprocedural cerebrovascular infarction

I97.820 Postprocedural cerebrovascular infarction following cardiac surgery

I97.821 Postprocedural cerebrovascular infarction following other surgery

I97.88 Other intraoperative complications of the circulatory system, not elsewhere classified

I97.89 Other postprocedural complications and disorders of the circulatory system, not elsewhere classified

I99 Other and unspecified disorders of circulatory system

I99.8 Other disorder of circulatory system

I99.9 Unspecified disorder of circulatory system

● New code   ▲ Revised code   Excludes1: Not coded here   Excludes2: Not included here   ⊗ Placeholder required   ⑦ 7th digit required

Chapter 10: Diseases Of The Respiratory System (J00-J99)

DEFINITIONS

This chapter includes definitions of selected key words, terms and phrases and coding alerts for adding points to the clinical domain, and references to coding late effects where appropriate. An example from this chapter is as follows:

J01 Acute sinusitis

Definition: Sinusitis is an infection of the small, air-filled cavities inside the cheekbones and forehead.

MULTIPLE CODING FOR A SINGLE CONDITION

In addition to the etiology/manifestation convention that requires two codes to fully describe a single condition that affects multiple body systems, there are other single conditions that also require more than one code. "Use additional code" notes are found in the Tabular List at codes that are not part of an etiology/manifestation pair where a secondary code is useful to fully describe a condition. The sequencing rule is the same as the etiology/manifestation pair, "use additional code" indicates that a secondary code should be added.

For example, for bacterial infections that are not included in chapter 1, a secondary code from category B95, Streptococcus, Staphylococcus, and Enterococcus, as the cause of diseases classified elsewhere, or B96, Other bacterial agents as the cause of diseases classified elsewhere, may be required to identify the bacterial organism causing the infection. A "use additional code" note will normally be found at the infectious disease code, indicating a need for the organism code to be added as a secondary code.

"Code first" notes are also under certain codes that are not specifically manifestation codes but may be due to an underlying cause. When there is a "code first" note and an underlying condition is present, the underlying condition should be sequenced first.

"Code, if applicable, any causal condition first", notes indicate that this code may be assigned as a principal diagnosis when the causal condition is unknown or not applicable. If a causal condition is known, then the code for that condition should be sequenced as the principal or first-listed diagnosis.

Multiple codes may be needed for sequela, complication codes and obstetric codes to more fully describe a condition. See the specific guidelines for these conditions for further instruction.

COMBINATION CODE

A combination code is a single code used to classify: Two diagnoses, or a diagnosis with an associated secondary process (manifestation) A diagnosis with an associated complication

Combination codes are identified by referring to subterm entries in the Alphabetic Index and by reading the inclusion and exclusion notes in the Tabular List.

Assign only the combination code when that code fully identifies the diagnostic conditions involved or when the Alphabetic Index so directs. Multiple coding should not be used when the classification provides a combination code that clearly identifies all of the elements documented in the diagnosis. When the combination code lacks necessary specificity in describing the manifestation or complication, an additional code should be used as a secondary code.

SEQUELA (LATE EFFECTS)

A sequela is the residual effect (condition produced) after the acute phase of an illness or injury has terminated. There is no time limit on when a sequela code can be used. The residual may be apparent early, such as in cerebral infarction, or it may occur months or years later, such as that due to a previous injury. Coding of sequela generally requires two codes sequenced in the following order: The condition or nature of the sequela is sequenced first.

The sequela code is sequenced second.

An exception to the above guidelines are those instances where the code for the sequela is followed by a manifestation code identified in the Tabular List and title, or the sequela code has been expanded (at the fourth, fifth or sixth character levels) to include the manifestation(s). The code for the acute phase of an illness or injury that led to the sequela is never used with a code for the late effect.

CHRONIC OBSTRUCTIVE PULMONARY DISEASE [COPD] AND ASTHMA

1) **Acute exacerbation of chronic obstructive bronchitis and asthma**

   The codes in categories J44 and J45 distinguish between uncomplicated cases and those in acute exacerbation. An acute exacerbation is a worsening or a decompensation of a chronic condition. An acute exacerbation is not equivalent to an infection superimposed on a chronic condition, though an exacerbation may be triggered by an infection.

ACUTE RESPIRATORY FAILURE

1) **Acute respiratory failure as principal diagnosis**

   A code from subcategory J96.0, Acute respiratory failure, or subcategory J96.2, Acute and chronic respiratory failure, may be assigned as a principal diagnosis when it is the condition established after study to be chiefly responsible for occasioning the admission to the hospital, and the selection is supported by the Alphabetic Index and Tabular List. However, chapter-specific coding guidelines (such as obstetrics, poisoning, HIV, newborn) that provide sequencing direction take precedence.

2) **Acute respiratory failure as secondary diagnosis**

Add 4th-7th digits   Nonspecific code   Unspecified code   Manifestation code

Respiratory failure may be listed as a secondary diagnosis if it occurs after admission, or if it is present on admission, but does not meet the definition of principal diagnosis.

3) **Sequencing of acute respiratory failure and another acute condition**

When a patient is admitted with respiratory failure and another acute condition, (e.g., myocardial infarction, cerebrovascular accident, aspiration pneumonia), the principal diagnosis will not be the same in every situation. This applies whether the other acute condition is a respiratory or nonrespiratory condition. Selection of the principal diagnosis will be dependent on the circumstances of admission. If both the respiratory failure and the other acute condition are equally responsible for occasioning the admission to the hospital, and there are no chapter-specific sequencing rules, the guideline regarding two or more diagnoses that equally meet the definition for principal diagnosis *(Section II, C.)* may be applied in these situations.

If the documentation is not clear as to whether acute respiratory failure and another condition are equally responsible for occasioning the admission, query the provider for clarification.

INFLUENZA DUE TO CERTAIN IDENTIFIED INFLUENZA VIRUSES

Code only confirmed cases of influenza due to certain identified influenza viruses (category J09), and due to other identified influenza virus (category J10). This is an exception to the hospital inpatient guideline Section II, H. (Uncertain Diagnosis).

In this context, "confirmation" does not require documentation of positive laboratory testing specific for avian or other novel influenza A or other identified influenza virus. However, coding should be based on the provider's diagnostic statement that the patient has avian influenza, or other novel influenza A, for category J09, or has another particular identified strain of influenza, such as H1N1 or H3N2, but not identified as novel or variant, for category J10.

If the provider records "suspected" or "possible" or "probable" avian influenza, or novel influenza, or other identified influenza, then the appropriate influenza code from category J11, Influenza due to unidentified influenza virus, should be assigned. A code from category J09, Influenza due to certain identified influenza viruses, should not be assigned nor should a code from category J10, Influenza due to other identified influenza virus.

VENTILATOR ASSOCIATED PNEUMONIA

1) **Documentation of Ventilator associated Pneumonia**

As with all procedural or postprocedural complications, code assignment is based on the provider's documentation of the relationship between the condition and the procedure.

Code J95.851, Ventilator associated pneumonia, should be assigned only when the provider has documented ventilator associated pneumonia (VAP). An additional code to identify the organism (e.g., Pseudomonas aeruginosa, code B96.5) should also be assigned. Do not assign an additional code from categories J12-J18 to identify the type of pneumonia.

Code J95.851 should not be assigned for cases where the patient has pneumonia and is on a mechanical ventilator and the provider has not specifically stated that the pneumonia is ventilator-associated pneumonia. If the documentation is unclear as to whether the patient has a pneumonia that is a complication attributable to the mechanical ventilator, query the provider.

2) **Ventilator associated Pneumonia Develops after Admission**

A patient may be admitted with one type of pneumonia (e.g., code J13, Pneumonia due to Streptococcus pneumonia) and subsequently develop VAP. In this instance, the principal diagnosis would be the appropriate code from categories J12-

J18 for the pneumonia diagnosed at the time of admission. Code J95.851, Ventilator associated pneumonia, would be assigned as an additional diagnosis when the provider has also documented the presence of ventilator associated pneumonia.

Chapter 10
Diseases Of The Respiratory System (J00-J99)

Note: When a respiratory condition is described as occurring in more than one site and is not specifically indexed, it should be classified to the lower anatomic site (e.g. tracheobronchitis to bronchitis in J40).

<u>Use additional code</u>, where applicable, to identify:

exposure to environmental tobacco smoke (Z77.22)

exposure to tobacco smoke in the perinatal period (P96.81)

history of tobacco dependence (Z87.891)

occupational exposure to environmental tobacco smoke (Z57.31)

tobacco dependence (F17.-)

tobacco use (Z72.0)

Excludes2: certain conditions originating in the perinatal period (P04-P96)

certain infectious and parasitic diseases (A00-B99)

complications of pregnancy, childbirth and the puerperium (O00-O9A)

congenital malformations, deformations and chromosomal abnormalities (Q00-Q99)

endocrine, nutritional and metabolic diseases (E00-E88)

injury, poisoning and certain other consequences of external causes (S00-T88) neoplasms (C00-D49)

smoke inhalation (T59.81-)

symptoms, signs and abnormal clinical and laboratory findings, not elsewhere classified (R00-R94)

This chapter contains the following blocks:

J00-J06	Acute upper respiratory infections
J09-J18	Influenza and pneumonia
J20-J22	Other acute lower respiratory infections
J30-J39	Other diseases of upper respiratory tract
J40-J47	Chronic lower respiratory diseases
J60-J70	Lung diseases due to external agents
J80-J84	Other respiratory diseases principally affecting the interstitium
J85-J86	Suppurative and necrotic conditions of the lower respiratory tract
J90-J94	Other diseases of the pleura
J95	Intraoperative and postprocedural complications and disorders of respiratory system, not elsewhere classified
J96-J99	Other diseases of the respiratory system

ACUTE UPPER RESPIRATORY INFECTIONS (J00-J06)

Excludes1: chronic obstructive pulmonary disease with acute lower respiratory infection (J44.0)

influenza virus **with other** respiratory manifestations (J09.X2, J10.1, J11.1)

J00   Acute nasopharyngitis [common cold]

Acute rhinitis

Coryza (acute)

Infective nasopharyngitis NOS

Infective rhinitis

Nasal catarrh, acute Nasopharyngitis NOS

Excludes1: acute pharyngitis (J02.-)

acute sore throat NOS (J02.9)

pharyngitis NOS (J02.9)

rhinitis NOS (J31.0)

sore throat NOS (J02.9)

Excludes2: allergic rhinitis (J30.1-J30.9)

chronic pharyngitis (J31.2)

chronic rhinitis (J31.0)

chronic sore throat (J31.2)

nasopharyngitis, chronic (J31.1)

vasomotor rhinitis (J30.0)

J01   Acute sinusitis

Includes: acute abscess of sinus

acute empyema of sinus

acute infection of sinus

acute inflammation of sinus

acute suppuration of sinus

Use additional code (B95-B97) to identify infectious agent.

Excludes1: sinusitis NOS (J32.9)

Excludes2: chronic sinusitis (J32.0-J32.8)

J01.0   Acute maxillary sinusitis

Acute antritis

J01.00   Acute maxillary sinusitis, unspecified

J01.01   Acute recurrent maxillary sinusitis

J01.1   Acute frontal sinusitis

J01.10   Acute frontal sinusitis, unspecified

J01.11   Acute recurrent frontal sinusitis

J01.2   Acute ethmoidal sinusitis

J01.20   Acute ethmoidal sinusitis, unspecified

J01.21   Acute recurrent ethmoidal sinusitis

J01.3   Acute sphenoidal sinusitis

J01.30   Acute sphenoidal sinusitis, unspecified

J01.31   Acute recurrent sphenoidal sinusitis

J01.4   Acute pansinusitis

J01.40   Acute pansinusitis, unspecified

J01.41   Acute recurrent pansinusitis

J01.8   Other acute sinusitis

J01.80   Other acute sinusitis

Acute sinusitis involving more than one sinus but not pansinusitis

J01.81   Other acute recurrent sinusitis

Acute recurrent sinusitis involving more than one sinus but not pansinusitis

J01.9   Acute sinusitis, unspecified

J01.90   Acute sinusitis, unspecified

J01.91   Acute recurrent sinusitis, unspecified

J02   Acute pharyngitis

Includes: acute sore throat

Excludes1: acute laryngopharyngitis (J06.0)

peritonsillar abscess (J36)

pharyngeal abscess (J39.1)

retropharyngeal abscess (J39.0)

Excludes2: chronic pharyngitis (J31.2)

J02.0   Streptococcal pharyngitis

Septic pharyngitis

Streptococcal sore throat

Excludes2: scarlet fever (A38.-)

J02.8   Acute pharyngitis due to other specified organisms

Use additional code (B95-B97) to identify infectious agent

Excludes1: acute pharyngitis due to coxsackie virus (B08.5)

acute pharyngitis due to gonococcus (A54.5)

acute pharyngitis due to herpes [simplex] virus (B00.2)

acute pharyngitis due to infectious mononucleosis (B27.-)

enteroviral vesicular pharyngitis (B08.5)

J02.9 **Acute pharyngitis, unspecified**

Gangrenous pharyngitis (acute)

Infective pharyngitis (acute) NOS

Pharyngitis (acute) NOS

Sore throat (acute) NOS

Suppurative pharyngitis (acute)

Ulcerative pharyngitis (acute)

J03 **Acute tonsillitis**

Excludes1: acute sore throat (J02.-)

hypertrophy of tonsils (J35.1)

peritonsillar abscess (J36)

sore throat NOS (J02.9)

streptococcal sore throat (J02.0)

Excludes2: chronic tonsillitis (J35.0)

J03.0 **Streptococcal tonsillitis**

J03.00 **Acute streptococcal tonsillitis, unspecified**

J03.01 **Acute recurrent streptococcal tonsillitis**

J03.8 **Acute tonsillitis due to other specified organisms**

Use additional code (B95-B97) to identify infectious agent.

Excludes1: diphtheritic tonsillitis (A36.0)

herpesviral pharyngotonsillitis (B00.2)

streptococcal tonsillitis (J03.0)

tuberculous tonsillitis (A15.8)

Vincent's tonsillitis (A69.1)

J03.80 **Acute tonsillitis due to other specified organisms**

J03.81 **Acute recurrent tonsillitis due to other specified organisms**

J03.9 **Acute tonsillitis, unspecified**

Follicular tonsillitis (acute) Gangrenous tonsillitis (acute)

Infective tonsillitis (acute)

Tonsillitis (acute) NOS

Ulcerative tonsillitis (acute)

J03.90 **Acute tonsillitis, unspecified**

J03.91 **Acute recurrent tonsillitis, unspecified**

J04 **Acute laryngitis and tracheitis**

Use additional code (B95-B97) to identify infectious agent.

Excludes1: acute obstructive laryngitis [croup] and epiglottitis (J05.-)

Excludes2: laryngismus (stridulus) (J38.5)

J04.0 **Acute laryngitis**

Edematous laryngitis (acute)

Laryngitis (acute) NOS

Subglottic laryngitis (acute)

Suppurative laryngitis (acute)

Ulcerative laryngitis (acute)

Excludes1: acute obstructive laryngitis (J05.0)

Excludes2: chronic laryngitis (J37.0)

J04.1 **Acute tracheitis**

Acute viral tracheitis

Catarrhal tracheitis (acute)

Tracheitis (acute) NOS

Excludes2: chronic tracheitis (J42)

J04.10 **Acute tracheitis without obstruction**

J04.11 **Acute tracheitis with obstruction**

J04.2 **Acute laryngotracheitis**

Laryngotracheitis NOS

Tracheitis (acute) with laryngitis (acute)

Excludes1: acute obstructive laryngotracheitis (J05.0)

Excludes2: chronic laryngotracheitis (J37.1)

J04.3 **Supraglottitis, unspecified**

J04.30 **Supraglottitis, unspecified, without obstruction**

J04.31 **Supraglottitis, unspecified, with obstruction**

J05 **Acute obstructive laryngitis [croup] and epiglottitis**

Use additional code (B95-B97) to identify infectious agent.

J05.0 **Acute obstructive laryngitis [croup]**

Obstructive laryngitis (acute) NOS

Obstructive laryngotracheitis NOS

J05.1 **Acute epiglottitis**

Excludes2: epiglottitis, chronic (J37.0)

J05.10 **Acute epiglottitis without obstruction**

Epiglottitis NOS

J05.11 **Acute epiglottitis with obstruction**

J06 **Acute upper respiratory infections of multiple and unspecified sites**

Excludes1: acute respiratory infection NOS (J22)

streptococcal pharyngitis (J02.0)

J06.0 **Acute laryngopharyngitis**

J06.9 **Acute upper respiratory infection, unspecified**

Upper respiratory disease, acute

Upper respiratory infection NOS

INFLUENZA AND PNEUMONIA (J09-J18)

Excludes2: allergic or eosinophilic pneumonia (J82)

aspiration pneumonia NOS (J69.0)

meconium pneumonia (P24.01)

neonatal aspiration pneumonia (P24.-)

pneumonia due to solids and liquids (J69.-)

congenital pneumonia (P23.9)

lipid pneumonia (J69.1)

rheumatic pneumonia (I00)

ventilator associated pneumonia (J95.851)

J09 **Influenza due to certain identified influenza viruses**

Excludes1: influenza A/H1N1 (J10.-)

influenza due to other identified influenza virus (J10.-)

influenza due to unidentified influenza virus (J11.-)

seasonal influenza due **to other** identified influenza virus (J10.-)

seasonal influenza due to unidentified influenza virus (J11.-)

J09.X **Influenza due to identified novel influenza A virus**

Avian influenza

Bird influenza

Influenza A/H5N1

Influenza **of** other animal origin, not bird or swine

Swine influenza virus (viruses that normally cause infections in pigs)

J09.X1 **Influenza due to identified novel influenza A virus with pneumonia**

Code also, if applicable, associated:

lung abscess (J85.1)

Other specified type of pneumonia

J09.X2 **Influenza due to identified novel influenza A virus with other respiratory manifestations**

Influenza due to identified novel influenza A virus NOS

Influenza due to identified novel influenza A virus with laryngitis

Influenza due to identified novel influenza A virus with pharyngitis

Influenza due to identified novel influenza A virus with upper respiratory symptoms

Use additional code, if applicable, for associated:

pleural effusion (J91.8)

sinusitis (J01.-)

J09.X3 **Influenza due to identified novel influenza A virus with gastrointestinal manifestations**

Influenza due to identified novel influenza A virus gastroenteritis

Excludes1: 'intestinal flu' [viral gastroenteritis] (A08.-)

J09.X9 **Influenza due to identified novel influenza A virus with other manifestations**

Influenza due to identified novel influenza A virus with encephalopathy

Influenza due to identified novel influenza A virus with myocarditis

Influenza due to identified novel influenza A virus with otitis media

Use additional code to identify manifestation

J10 **Influenza due to other identified influenza virus**

Excludes1: influenza due to avian influenza virus (J09.X-)

influenza due to swine flu (J09.X-)

influenza due to unidentified influenza virus (J11.-)

J10.0 **Influenza due to other identified influenza virus with pneumonia**

Code also associated lung abscess, if applicable (J85.1)

J10.00 **Influenza due to other identified influenza virus with unspecified type of pneumonia**

J10.01 **Influenza due to other identified influenza virus with the same other identified influenza virus pneumonia**

J10.08 **Influenza due to other identified influenza virus with other specified pneumonia**

Code also other specified type of pneumonia

J10.1 **Influenza due to other identified influenza virus with other respiratory manifestations**

Influenza due to other identified influenza virus NOS

Influenza due to other identified influenza virus with laryngitis

Influenza due to other identified influenza virus with pharyngitis

Influenza due to other identified influenza virus with upper respiratory symptoms

Use additional code for associated pleural effusion, if applicable (J91.8)

Use additional code for associated sinusitis, if applicable (J01.-)

J10.2 **Influenza due to other identified influenza virus with gastrointestinal manifestations**

Influenza due to other identified influenza virus gastroenteritis

Excludes1: 'intestinal flu' [viral gastroenteritis] (A08.-)

J10.8 **Influenza due to other identified influenza virus with other manifestations**

J10.81 **Influenza due to other identified influenza virus with encephalopathy**

J10.82 **Influenza due to other identified influenza virus with myocarditis**

J10.83 **Influenza due to other identified influenza virus with otitis media**

Use additional code for any associated perforated tympanic membrane (H72.-)

J10.89 **Influenza due to other identified influenza virus with other manifestations**

Use additional codes to identify the manifestations

J11 **Influenza due to unidentified influenza virus**

J11.0 **Influenza due to unidentified influenza virus with pneumonia**

Code also associated lung abscess, if applicable (J85.1)

J11.00 **Influenza due to unidentified influenza virus with unspecified type of pneumonia**

Influenza with pneumonia NOS

J11.08 **Influenza due to unidentified influenza virus with specified pneumonia**

Code also other specified type of pneumonia

J11.1 **Influenza due to unidentified influenza virus with other respiratory manifestations**

Influenza NOS

Influenzal laryngitis NOS

Influenzal pharyngitis NOS

Influenza with upper respiratory symptoms NOS

Use additional code for associated pleural effusion, if applicable (J91.8)

Use additional code for associated sinusitis, if applicable (J01.-)

J11.2 **Influenza due to unidentified influenza virus with gastrointestinal manifestations**

Influenza gastroenteritis NOS

Excludes1: 'intestinal flu' [viral gastroenteritis] (A08.-)

J11.8 **Influenza due to unidentified influenza virus with other manifestations**

J11.81 **Influenza due to unidentified influenza virus with encephalopathy**

Influenzal encephalopathy NOS

J11.82 **Influenza due to unidentified influenza virus with myocarditis**

Influenzal myocarditis NOS

J11.83 **Influenza due to unidentified influenza virus with otitis media**

Influenzal otitis media NOS

Use additional code for any associated perforated tympanic membrane (H72.-)

J11.89 **Influenza due to unidentified influenza virus with other manifestations**

Use additional codes to identify the manifestations

J12 **Viral pneumonia, not elsewhere classified**

Includes: bronchopneumonia due to viruses other than influenza viruses

Code first associated influenza, if applicable (J09.X1, J10.0-, J11.0-)

Code also associated abscess, if applicable (J85.1)

Excludes1: aspiration pneumonia due to anesthesia during labor and delivery (O74.0)

aspiration pneumonia due to anesthesia during pregnancy (O29)

	Add 4th-7th digits		Nonspecific code		Unspecified code		Manifestation code

aspiration pneumonia due to anesthesia during puerperium (O89.0)

aspiration pneumonia due to solids and liquids (J69.-)

aspiration pneumonia NOS (J69.0)

congenital pneumonia (P23.0)

congenital rubella pneumonitis (P35.0)

interstitial pneumonia NOS (J84.9)

lipid pneumonia (J69.1)

neonatal aspiration pneumonia (P24.-)

J12.0 **Adenoviral pneumonia**

J12.1 **Respiratory syncytial virus pneumonia**

J12.2 **Parainfluenza virus pneumonia**

J12.3 **Human metapneumovirus pneumonia**

J12.8 **Other viral pneumonia**

    J12.81 **Pneumonia due to SARS-associated coronavirus**

        Severe acute respiratory syndrome NOS

    J12.89 **Other viral pneumonia**

J12.9 **Viral pneumonia, unspecified**

J13 **Pneumonia due to Streptococcus pneumoniae**

Bronchopneumonia due to S. pneumoniae

Code first associated influenza, if applicable (J09.X1, J10.0-, J11.0-)

Code also associated abscess, if applicable (J85.1)

Excludes1: congenital pneumonia due to S. pneumoniae (P23.6)

    lobar pneumonia, unspecified organism (J18.1)

    pneumonia due **to other** streptococci (J15.3-J15.4)

J14 **Pneumonia due to Hemophilus influenzae**

Bronchopneumonia due to H. influenzae

Code first associated influenza, if applicable (J09.X1, J10.0-, J11.0-)

Code also associated abscess, if applicable (J85.1)

Excludes1: congenital pneumonia due to H. influenzae (P23.6)

J15 **Bacterial pneumonia, not elsewhere classified**

Includes: bronchopneumonia due to bacteria other than S. pneumoniae and H. influenzae

Code first associated influenza, if applicable (J09.X1, J10.0-, J11.0-)

Code also associated abscess, if applicable (J85.1)

Excludes1: chlamydial pneumonia (J16.0)

    congenital pneumonia (P23.-)

    Legionnaires' disease (A48.1)

    spirochetal pneumonia (A69.8)

J15.0 **Pneumonia due to Klebsiella pneumoniae**

J15.1 **Pneumonia due to Pseudomonas**

J15.2 **Pneumonia due to staphylococcus**

    J15.20 **Pneumonia due to staphylococcus, unspecified**

    J15.21 **Pneumonia due to staphylococcus aureus**

        J15.211 **Pneumonia due to Methicillin susceptible Staphylococcus aureus**

            MSSA pneumonia

            Pneumonia due to Staphylococcus aureus NOS

        J15.212 **Pneumonia due to Methicillin resistant Staphylococcus aureus**

    J15.29 **Pneumonia due to other staphylococcus**

J15.3 **Pneumonia due to streptococcus, group B**

J15.4 **Pneumonia due to other streptococci**

    Excludes1: pneumonia due to streptococcus, group B (J15.3)

    pneumonia due to Streptococcus pneumoniae (J13)

J15.5 **Pneumonia due to Escherichia coli**

▲**J15.6** **Pneumonia due to other Gram-negative bacteria**

    Pneumonia due to Serratia marcescens

J15.7 **Pneumonia due to Mycoplasma pneumoniae**

J15.8 **Pneumonia due to other specified bacteria**

J15.9 **Unspecified bacterial pneumonia**

    Pneumonia due to gram-positive bacteria

J16 **Pneumonia due to other infectious organisms, not elsewhere classified**

Code first associated influenza, if applicable (J09.X1, J10.0-, J11.0-)

Code also associated abscess, if applicable (J85.1)

Excludes1: congenital pneumonia (P23.-)

    ornithosis (A70)

    pneumocystosis (B59)

    pneumonia NOS (J18.9)

J16.0 **Chlamydial pneumonia**

J16.8 **Pneumonia due to other specified infectious organisms**

J17 **Pneumonia in diseases classified elsewhere**

Code first underlying disease, such as:

Q fever (A78) rheumatic fever (I00)

schistosomiasis (B65.0-B65.9)

Excludes1: candidal pneumonia (B37.1)

    chlamydial pneumonia (J16.0)

    gonorrheal pneumonia (A54.84)

    histoplasmosis pneumonia (B39.0-B39.2)

    measles pneumonia (B05.2)

    nocardiosis pneumonia (A43.0)

    pneumocystosis (B59)

    pneumonia due to Pneumocystis carinii (B59)

    pneumonia due to Pneumocystis jiroveci (B59)

    pneumonia in actinomycosis (A42.0)

    pneumonia in anthrax (A22.1)

    pneumonia in ascariasis (B77.81)

    pneumonia in aspergillosis (B44.0-B44.1)

    pneumonia in coccidioidomycosis (B38.0-B38.2)

    pneumonia in cytomegalovirus disease (B25.0)

    pneumonia in toxoplasmosis (B58.3)

    rubella pneumonia (B06.81)

    salmonella pneumonia (A02.22)

    spirochetal infection NEC with pneumonia (A69.8)

    tularemia pneumonia (A21.2)

    typhoid fever with pneumonia (A01.03)

    varicella pneumonia (B01.2)

    whooping cough with pneumonia (A37 with fifth-character 1)

J18 **Pneumonia, unspecified organism**

Code first associated influenza, if applicable (J09.X1, J10.0-, J11.0-)

Excludes1: abscess of lung with pneumonia (J85.1)

    aspiration pneumonia due to anesthesia during labor and delivery (O74.0)

    aspiration pneumonia due to anesthesia during pregnancy (O29)

    aspiration pneumonia due to anesthesia during puerperium (O89.0)

    aspiration pneumonia due to solids and liquids (J69.-)

    aspiration pneumonia NOS (J69.0)

    congenital pneumonia (P23.0)

    drug-induced interstitial lung disorder (J70.2-J70.4)

interstitial pneumonia NOS (J84.9)

lipid pneumonia (J69.1)

neonatal aspiration pneumonia (P24.-)

pneumonitis due to external agents (J67-J70)

pneumonitis due to fumes and vapors (J68.0)

usual interstitial pneumonia (J84.17)

J18.0 Bronchopneumonia, unspecified organism

Definition: Bronchopneumonia is a pneumonia characterized by acute inflammation of the walls of the bronchioles

Excludes1: hypostatic bronchopneumonia (J18.2)

lipid pneumonia (J69.1)

Excludes2: acute bronchiolitis (J21.-)

chronic bronchiolitis (J44.9)

J18.1 Lobar pneumonia, unspecified organism

J18.2 Hypostatic pneumonia, unspecified organism

Hypostatic bronchopneumonia

Passive pneumonia

J18.8 Other pneumonia, unspecified organism

J18.9 Pneumonia, unspecified organism

OTHER ACUTE LOWER RESPIRATORY INFECTIONS (J20-J22)

Excludes2: chronic obstructive pulmonary disease with acute lower respiratory infection (J44.0)

J20 Acute bronchitis

Includes: acute and subacute bronchitis (with) bronchospasm

acute and subacute bronchitis (with) tracheitis

acute and subacute bronchitis (with) tracheobronchitis,

acute and subacute fibrinous bronchitis

acute and subacute membranous bronchitis acute and subacute purulent bronchitis acute and subacute septic bronchitis

Excludes1: bronchitis NOS (J40)

tracheobronchitis NOS (J40)

Excludes2: acute bronchitis with bronchiectasis (J47.0)

acute bronchitis with chronic obstructive asthma (J44.0)

acute bronchitis with chronic obstructive pulmonary disease (J44.0)

allergic bronchitis NOS (J45.909-)

bronchitis due to chemicals, fumes and vapors (J68.0)

chronic bronchitis NOS (J42)

chronic mucopurulent bronchitis (J41.1)

chronic obstructive bronchitis (J44.-)

chronic obstructive tracheobronchitis (J44.-)

chronic simple bronchitis (J41.0)

chronic tracheobronchitis (J42)

J20.0 Acute bronchitis due to Mycoplasma pneumoniae

J20.1 Acute bronchitis due to Hemophilus influenzae

J20.2 Acute bronchitis due to streptococcus

J20.3 Acute bronchitis due to coxsackievirus

J20.4 Acute bronchitis due to parainfluenza virus

J20.5 Acute bronchitis due to respiratory syncytial virus

J20.6 Acute bronchitis due to rhinovirus

J20.7 Acute bronchitis due to echovirus

J20.8 Acute bronchitis due to other specified organisms

J20.9 Acute bronchitis, unspecified

J21 Acute bronchiolitis

Includes: acute bronchiolitis with bronchospasm

Excludes2: respiratory bronchiolitis interstitial lung disease (J84.115)

J21.0 Acute bronchiolitis due to respiratory syncytial virus

J21.1 Acute bronchiolitis due to human metapneumovirus

J21.8 Acute bronchiolitis due to other specified organisms

J21.9 Acute bronchiolitis, unspecified

Bronchiolitis (acute)

Excludes1: chronic bronchiolitis (J44.-)

J22 Unspecified acute lower respiratory infection

Acute (lower) respiratory (tract) infection NOS

Excludes1: upper respiratory infection (acute) (J06.9)

OTHER DISEASES OF UPPER RESPIRATORY TRACT (J30-J39)

J30 Vasomotor and allergic rhinitis

Includes: spasmodic rhinorrhea

Excludes1: allergic rhinitis with asthma (bronchial) (J45.909)

rhinitis NOS (J31.0)

J30.0 Vasomotor rhinitis

J30.1 Allergic rhinitis due to pollen

Definition: Allergic rhinitis refers to a group of symptoms similar to those of a cold such as runny nose and sore throat, caused by an allergic reaction to an allergen such as dust, plant pollens or animal dander.

Allergy NOS due to pollen

Hay fever

Pollinosis

J30.2 Other seasonal allergic rhinitis

J30.5 Allergic rhinitis due to food

J30.8 Other allergic rhinitis

J30.81 Allergic rhinitis due to animal (cat) (dog) hair and dander

J30.89 Other allergic rhinitis

Perennial allergic rhinitis

J30.9 Allergic rhinitis, unspecified

J31 Chronic rhinitis, nasopharyngitis and pharyngitis

Use additional code to identify:

exposure to environmental tobacco smoke (Z77.22)

exposure to tobacco smoke in the perinatal period (P96.81)

history of tobacco dependence (Z87.891)

occupational exposure to environmental tobacco smoke (Z57.31)

tobacco dependence (F17.-)

tobacco use (Z72.0)

J31.0 Chronic rhinitis

Atrophic rhinitis (chronic)

Granulomatous rhinitis (chronic)

Hypertrophic rhinitis (chronic)

Obstructive rhinitis (chronic)

Ozena

Purulent rhinitis (chronic)

Rhinitis (chronic) NOS

Ulcerative rhinitis (chronic)

Excludes1: allergic rhinitis (J30.1-J30.9)

vasomotor rhinitis (J30.0)

J31.1 Chronic nasopharyngitis

Excludes2: acute nasopharyngitis (J00)

J31.2 Chronic pharyngitis

Chronic sore throat

Atrophic pharyngitis (chronic)

Granular pharyngitis (chronic)

Hypertrophic pharyngitis (chronic)

Excludes2: acute pharyngitis (J02.9)

J32   Chronic sinusitis

Includes: sinus abscess

sinus empyema

sinus infection

sinus suppuration

Use additional code to identify:

exposure to environmental tobacco smoke (Z77.22)

exposure to tobacco smoke in the perinatal period (P96.81)

history of tobacco dependence (Z87.891)

infectious agent (B95-B97)

occupational exposure to environmental tobacco smoke (Z57.31)

tobacco dependence (F17.-)

tobacco use (Z72.0)

Excludes2: acute sinusitis (J01.-)

J32.0   **Chronic maxillary sinusitis**

Antritis (chronic)

Maxillary sinusitis NOS

J32.1   **Chronic frontal sinusitis**

Frontal sinusitis NOS

J32.2   **Chronic ethmoidal sinusitis**

Ethmoidal sinusitis NOS

Excludes1: Woakes' ethmoiditis (J33.1)

J32.3   **Chronic sphenoidal sinusitis**

Sphenoidal sinusitis NOS

J32.4   **Chronic pansinusitis**

Pansinusitis NOS

J32.8   **Other chronic sinusitis**

Sinusitis (chronic) involving more than one sinus but not pansinusitis

J32.9   **Chronic sinusitis, unspecified**

Sinusitis (chronic) NOS

J33   Nasal polyp

Use additional code to identify:

exposure to environmental tobacco smoke (Z77.22)

exposure to tobacco smoke in the perinatal period (P96.81)

history of tobacco dependence (Z87.891)

occupational exposure to environmental tobacco smoke (Z57.31)

tobacco dependence (F17.-)

tobacco use (Z72.0)

Excludes1: adenomatous polyps (D14.0)

J33.0   **Polyp of nasal cavity**

Choanal polyp Nasopharyngeal polyp

J33.1   **Polypoid sinus degeneration**

Woakes' syndrome or ethmoiditis

J33.8   **Other polyp of sinus**

Accessory polyp of sinus

Ethmoidal polyp of sinus

Maxillary polyp of sinus \

Sphenoidal polyp of sinus

J33.9   **Nasal polyp, unspecified**

J34   Other and unspecified disorders of nose and nasal sinuses

Excludes2: varicose ulcer of nasal septum (I86.8)

J34.0   **Abscess, furuncle and carbuncle of nose**

Cellulitis of nose

Necrosis of nose

Ulceration of nose

J34.1   **Cyst and mucocele of nose and nasal sinus**

J34.2   **Deviated nasal septum**

Deflection or deviation of septum (nasal) (acquired)

Excludes1: congenital deviated nasal septum (Q67.4)

J34.3   **Hypertrophy of nasal turbinates**

J34.8   **Other specified disorders of nose and nasal sinuses**

J34.81   **Nasal mucositis (ulcerative)**

Code also type of associated therapy, such as:

antineoplastic and immunosuppressive drugs (T45.1X-)

radiological procedure and radiotherapy (Y84.2)

Excludes2: gastrointestinal mucositis (ulcerative) (K92.81)

mucositis (ulcerative) of vagina and vulva (N76.81)

oral mucositis (ulcerative) (K12.3-)

J34.89   **Other specified disorders of nose and nasal sinuses**

Perforation of nasal septum NOS

Rhinolith

J34.9   **Unspecified disorder of nose and nasal sinuses**

J35   Chronic diseases of tonsils and adenoids

Use additional code to identify:

exposure to environmental tobacco smoke (Z77.22)

exposure to tobacco smoke in the perinatal period (P96.81)

history of tobacco dependence (Z87.891)

occupational exposure to environmental tobacco smoke (Z57.31)

tobacco dependence (F17.-)

tobacco use (Z72.0)

J35.0   **Chronic tonsillitis and adenoiditis**

Excludes2: acute tonsillitis (J03.-)

J35.01   **Chronic tonsillitis**

J35.02   **Chronic adenoiditis**

J35.03   **Chronic tonsillitis and adenoiditis**

J35.1   **Hypertrophy of tonsils**

Enlargement of tonsils

Excludes1: hypertrophy of tonsils with tonsillitis (J35.0-)

J35.2   **Hypertrophy of adenoids**

Enlargement of adenoids

Excludes1: hypertrophy of adenoids with adenoiditis (J35.0-)

J35.3   **Hypertrophy of tonsils with hypertrophy of adenoids**

Excludes1: hypertrophy of tonsils and adenoids with tonsillitis and adenoiditis (J35.03)

J35.8   **Other chronic diseases of tonsils and adenoids**

Adenoid vegetations

Amygdalolith

Calculus, tonsil

Cicatrix of tonsil (and adenoid)

Tonsillar tag

Ulcer of tonsil

J35.9   **Chronic disease of tonsils and adenoids, unspecified**

Disease (chronic) of tonsils and adenoids NOS

J36   Peritonsillar abscess

Definition: A Peritonsillar abscess is an abscess forming in acute tonsillitis around one or both tonsils.

Includes: abscess of tonsil
> peritonsillar cellulitis quinsy

Use additional code (B95-B97) to identify infectious agent.

Excludes1: acute tonsillitis (J03.-)
> chronic tonsillitis (J35.0)
>
> retropharyngeal abscess (J39.0)
>
> tonsillitis NOS (J03.9-)

J37   Chronic laryngitis and laryngotracheitis

Use additional code to identify:

exposure to environmental tobacco smoke (Z77.22)

exposure to tobacco smoke in the perinatal period (P96.81)

history of tobacco dependence (Z87.891)

infectious agent (B95-B97)

occupational exposure to environmental tobacco smoke (Z57.31)

tobacco dependence (F17.-)

tobacco use (Z72.0)

J37.0   Chronic laryngitis

Catarrhal laryngitis

Hypertrophic laryngitis

Sicca laryngitis

Excludes2: acute laryngitis (J04.0)
> obstructive (acute) laryngitis (J05.0)

J37.1   Chronic laryngotracheitis

Laryngitis, chronic, with tracheitis (chronic)

Tracheitis, chronic, with laryngitis

Excludes1: chronic tracheitis (J42)

Excludes2: acute laryngotracheitis (J04.2)
> acute tracheitis (J04.1)

J38   Diseases of vocal cords and larynx, not elsewhere classified

Use additional code to identify:

exposure to environmental tobacco smoke (Z77.22)

exposure to tobacco smoke in the perinatal period (P96.81)

history of tobacco dependence (Z87.891)

occupational exposure to environmental tobacco smoke (Z57.31)

tobacco dependence (F17.-)

tobacco use (Z72.0)

Excludes1: congenital laryngeal stridor (P28.89)
> obstructive laryngitis (acute) (J05.0)
>
> postprocedural subglottic stenosis (J95.5)
>
> stridor (R06.1)
>
> ulcerative laryngitis (J04.0)

J38.0   Paralysis of vocal cords and larynx

Laryngoplegia

Paralysis of glottis

J38.00   Paralysis of vocal cords and larynx, unspecified

J38.01   Paralysis of vocal cords and larynx, unilateral

J38.02   Paralysis of vocal cords and larynx, bilateral

J38.1   Polyp of vocal cord and larynx

Excludes1: adenomatous polyps (D14.1)

J38.2   Nodules of vocal cords

Chorditis (fibrinous)(nodosa)(tuberosa)

Singer's nodes

Teacher's nodes

J38.3   Other diseases of vocal cords

Abscess of vocal cords

Cellulitis of vocal cords

Granuloma of vocal cords

Leukokeratosis of vocal cords

Leukoplakia of vocal cords

J38.4   Edema of larynx

Edema (of) glottis

Subglottic edema

Supraglottic edema

Excludes1: acute obstructive laryngitis [croup] (J05.0)
> edematous laryngitis (J04.0)

J38.5   Laryngeal spasm

Laryngismus (stridulus)

J38.6   Stenosis of larynx

J38.7   Other diseases of larynx

Abscess of larynx

Cellulitis of larynx

Disease of larynx NOS

Necrosis of larynx

Pachyderma of larynx

Perichondritis of larynx

Ulcer of larynx

J39   Other diseases of upper respiratory tract

Excludes1: acute respiratory infection NOS (J22)
> acute upper respiratory infection (J06.9)
>
> upper respiratory inflammation due to chemicals, gases, fumes or vapors (J68.2)

J39.0   Retropharyngeal and parapharyngeal abscess

Peripharyngeal abscess

Excludes1: peritonsillar abscess (J36)

J39.1   Other abscess of pharynx

Cellulitis of pharynx Nasopharyngeal abscess

J39.2   Other diseases of pharynx

Cyst of pharynx

Edema of pharynx

Excludes2: chronic pharyngitis (J31.2)
> ulcerative pharyngitis (J02.9)

J39.3   Upper respiratory tract hypersensitivity reaction, site unspecified

Excludes1: hypersensitivity reaction of upper respiratory tract, such as:
> extrinsic allergic alveolitis (J67.9)
>
> pneumoconiosis (J60-J67.9)

J39.8   Other specified diseases of upper respiratory tract

J39.9   Disease of upper respiratory tract, unspecified

CHRONIC LOWER RESPIRATORY DISEASES (J40-J47)

Excludes1: bronchitis due to chemicals, gases, fumes and vapors (J68.0)

Excludes2: cystic fibrosis (E84.-)

J40   Bronchitis, not specified as acute or chronic

Bronchitis NOS

Bronchitis with tracheitis NOS

Catarrhal bronchitis

Tracheobronchitis NOS

Use additional code to identify:

exposure to environmental tobacco smoke (Z77.22)

exposure to tobacco smoke in the perinatal period (P96.81)

history of tobacco dependence (Z87.891)

occupational exposure to environmental tobacco smoke (Z57.31) tobacco dependence (F17.-)

tobacco use (Z72.0)

Excludes1: acute bronchitis (J20.-)

allergic bronchitis NOS (J45.909-)

asthmatic bronchitis NOS (J45.9-)

bronchitis due to chemicals, gases, fumes and vapors (J68.0)

J41 **Simple and mucopurulent chronic bronchitis**

Use additional code to identify:

exposure to environmental tobacco smoke (Z77.22)

exposure to tobacco smoke in the perinatal period (P96.81)

history of tobacco dependence (Z87.891)

occupational exposure to environmental tobacco smoke (Z57.31)

tobacco dependence (F17.-)

tobacco use (Z72.0)

Excludes1: chronic bronchitis NOS (J42)

chronic obstructive bronchitis (J44.-)

J41.0 **Simple chronic bronchitis**

J41.1 **Mucopurulent chronic bronchitis**

J41.8 **Mixed simple and mucopurulent chronic bronchitis**

J42 **Unspecified chronic bronchitis**

Chronic bronchitis NOS

Chronic tracheitis

Chronic tracheobronchitis

Use additional code to identify:

exposure to environmental tobacco smoke (Z77.22)

exposure to tobacco smoke in the perinatal period (P96.81)

history of tobacco dependence (Z87.891)

occupational exposure to environmental tobacco smoke (Z57.31)

tobacco dependence (F17.-)

tobacco use (Z72.0)

Excludes1: chronic asthmatic bronchitis (J44.-)

chronic bronchitis with airways obstruction (J44.-)

chronic emphysematous bronchitis (J44.-)

chronic obstructive pulmonary disease NOS (J44.9)

simple and mucopurulent chronic bronchitis (J41.-)

J43 **Emphysema**

Definition: Emphysema is a chronic respiratory disease where there is over-inflation of the air sacs (alveoli) in the lungs, causing a decrease in lung function, and often, breathlessness.

Use additional code to identify:

exposure to environmental tobacco smoke (Z77.22)

history of tobacco dependence (Z87.891)

occupational exposure to environmental tobacco smoke (Z57.31)

tobacco dependence (F17.-)

tobacco use (Z72.0)

Excludes1: compensatory emphysema (J98.3)

emphysema due to inhalation of chemicals, gases, fumes or vapors (J68.4)

emphysema with chronic (obstructive)

bronchitis (J44.-)

emphysematous (obstructive) bronchitis (J44.-)

interstitial emphysema (J98.2)

mediastinal emphysema (J98.2)

neonatal interstitial emphysema (P25.0)

surgical (subcutaneous) emphysema (T81.82)

traumatic subcutaneous emphysema (T79.7)

J43.0 **Unilateral pulmonary emphysema [MacLeod's syndrome]**

Swyer-James syndrome

Unilateral emphysema

Unilateral hyperlucent lung

Unilateral pulmonary artery functional hypoplasia

Unilateral transparency of lung

J43.1 **Panlobular emphysema**

Panacinar emphysema

J43.2 **Centrilobular emphysema**

J43.8 **Other emphysema**

J43.9 **Emphysema, unspecified**

Bullous emphysema (lung)(pulmonary)

Emphysema (lung)(pulmonary) NOS

Emphysematous bleb

Vesicular emphysema (lung)(pulmonary)

J44 **Other chronic obstructive pulmonary disease**

Includes: asthma with chronic obstructive pulmonary disease

chronic asthmatic (obstructive) bronchitis

chronic bronchitis with airways obstruction

chronic bronchitis with emphysema

chronic emphysematous bronchitis

chronic obstructive asthma

chronic obstructive bronchitis

chronic obstructive tracheobronchitis

Code also type of asthma, if applicable (J45.-)

Use additional code to identify:

exposure to environmental tobacco smoke (Z77.22) history of tobacco dependence (Z87.891)

occupational exposure to environmental tobacco smoke (Z57.31) tobacco dependence (F17.-)

tobacco use (Z72.0)

Excludes1: bronchiectasis (J47.-)

chronic bronchitis NOS (J42)

chronic simple and mucopurulent bronchitis (J41.-)

chronic tracheitis (J42)

chronic tracheobronchitis (J42)

emphysema without chronic bronchitis (J43.-)

J44.0 **Chronic obstructive pulmonary disease with acute lower respiratory infection**

Code also to identify the infection

J44.1 **Chronic obstructive pulmonary disease with (acute) exacerbation**

Decompensated COPD

Decompensated COPD with (acute) exacerbation

Excludes2: chronic obstructive pulmonary disease [COPD] with acute bronchitis (J44.0)

lung diseases due to external agents (J60-J70)

J44.9 **Chronic obstructive pulmonary disease, unspecified**

Chronic obstructive airway disease NOS

Chronic obstructive lung disease NOS

Excludes2: lung diseases due to external agents (J60-J70)

J45 **Asthma**

Includes: allergic (predominantly) asthma

allergic bronchitis NOS

allergic rhinitis with asthma

atopic asthma

extrinsic allergic asthma

hay fever with asthma

idiosyncratic asthma

intrinsic nonallergic asthma

nonallergic asthma

Use additional code to identify:

exposure to environmental tobacco smoke (Z77.22)

exposure to tobacco smoke in the perinatal period (P96.81)

history of tobacco dependence (Z87.891)

occupational exposure to environmental tobacco smoke (Z57.31)

tobacco dependence (F17.-)

tobacco use (Z72.0)

Excludes1: detergent asthma (J69.8)

eosinophilic asthma (J82)

miner's asthma (J60)

wheezing NOS (R06.2)

wood asthma (J67.8)

Excludes2: asthma with chronic obstructive pulmonary disease (J44.9)

chronic asthmatic (obstructive) bronchitis (J44.9)

chronic obstructive asthma (J44.9)

J45.2   Mild intermittent asthma

    J45.20   Mild intermittent asthma, uncomplicated

        Mild intermittent asthma NOS

    J45.21   Mild intermittent asthma with (acute) exacerbation

    J45.22   Mild intermittent asthma with status asthmaticus

J45.3   Mild persistent asthma

    J45.30   Mild persistent asthma, uncomplicated

        Mild persistent asthma NOS

    J45.31   Mild persistent asthma with (acute) exacerbation

    J45.32   Mild persistent asthma with status asthmaticus

J45.4   Moderate persistent asthma

    J45.40   Moderate persistent asthma, uncomplicated

        Moderate persistent asthma NOS

    J45.41   Moderate persistent asthma with (acute) exacerbation

    J45.42   Moderate persistent asthma with status asthmaticus

J45.5   Severe persistent asthma

    J45.50   Severe persistent asthma, uncomplicated

        Severe persistent asthma NOS

    J45.51   Severe persistent asthma with (acute) exacerbation

    J45.52   Severe persistent asthma with status asthmaticus

J45.9   Other and unspecified asthma

    J45.90   Unspecified asthma

        Asthmatic bronchitis NOS

        Childhood asthma NOS

        Late onset asthma

    J45.901   Unspecified asthma with (acute) exacerbation

    J45.902   Unspecified asthma with status asthmaticus

    J45.909   Unspecified asthma, uncomplicated

        Asthma NOS

Excludes2: lung diseases due to external agents (J60-J70)

    J45.99   Other asthma

    J45.990   Exercise induced bronchospasm

    J45.991   Cough variant asthma

    J45.998   Other asthma

J47   Bronchiectasis

Definition: Bronchiectasis is a condition characterized by abnormal dilatation of the bronchi (airways) and excessive mucus production. The mucus accumulation may obstruct the bronchi. Is often associated with repeated bronchial infections.

Includes: bronchiolectasis

Use additional code to identify:

exposure to environmental tobacco smoke (Z77.22)

exposure to tobacco smoke in the perinatal period (P96.81)

history of tobacco dependence (Z87.891)

occupational exposure to environmental tobacco smoke (Z57.31)

tobacco dependence (F17.-)

tobacco use (Z72.0)

Excludes1: congenital bronchiectasis (Q33.4)

tuberculous bronchiectasis (current disease) (A15.0)

    J47.0   Bronchiectasis with acute lower respiratory infection

        Bronchiectasis with acute bronchitis

        Use additional code to identify the infection

    J47.1   Bronchiectasis with (acute) exacerbation

    J47.9   Bronchiectasis, uncomplicated

        Bronchiectasis NOS

LUNG DISEASES DUE TO EXTERNAL AGENTS (J60-J70)

Excludes2: asthma (J45.-)

malignant neoplasm of bronchus and lung (C34.-)

J60   Coalworker's pneumoconiosis

Anthracosilicosis

Anthracosis

Black lung disease

Coalworker's lung

Excludes1: coal worker pneumoconiosis with tuberculosis, any type in A15 (J65)

J61   Pneumoconiosis due to asbestos and other mineral fibers

Asbestosis

Excludes1: pleural plaque with asbestosis (J92.0)

pneumoconiosis with tuberculosis, any type in A15 (J65)

J62   Pneumoconiosis due to dust containing silica

Includes: silicotic fibrosis (massive) of lung

Excludes1: pneumoconiosis with tuberculosis, any type in A15 (J65)

    J62.0   Pneumoconiosis due to talc dust

    J62.8   Pneumoconiosis due to other dust containing silica

        Silicosis NOS

J63   Pneumoconiosis due to other inorganic dusts

Excludes1: pneumoconiosis with tuberculosis, any type in A15 (J65)

    J63.0   Aluminosis (of lung)

    J63.1   Bauxite fibrosis (of lung)

    J63.2   Berylliosis

    J63.3   Graphite fibrosis (of lung)

    J63.4   Siderosis

    J63.5   Stannosis

    J63.6   Pneumoconiosis due to other specified inorganic dusts

J64 **Unspecified pneumoconiosis**

Excludes1: pneumonoconiosis with tuberculosis, any type in A15 (J65)

J65 **Pneumoconiosis associated with tuberculosis**

Any condition in J60-J64 with tuberculosis, any type in A15

Silicotuberculosis

J66 **Airway disease due to specific organic dust**

Excludes2: allergic alveolitis (J67.-)

asbestosis (J61)

bagassosis (J67.1)

farmer's lung (J67.0)

hypersensitivity pneumonitis due to organic dust (J67.-)

reactive airways dysfunction syndrome (J68.3)

J66.0 **Byssinosis**

Airway disease due to cotton dust

J66.1 **Flax-dressers' disease**

J66.2 **Cannabinosis**

J66.8 **Airway disease due to other specific organic dusts**

J67 **Hypersensitivity pneumonitis due to organic dust**

Includes: allergic alveolitis and pneumonitis due to inhaled organic dust and particles of fungal, actinomycetic **or other** origin

Excludes1: pneumonitis due to inhalation of chemicals, gases, fumes or vapors (J68.0)

J67.0 **Farmer's lung**

Harvester's lung

Haymaker's lung

Moldy hay disease

J67.1 **Bagassosis**

Bagasse disease

Bagasse pneumonitis

J67.2 **Bird fancier's lung**

Budgerigar fancier's disease or lung

Pigeon fancier's disease or lung

J67.3 **Suberosis**

Cork handler's disease or lung

Cork worker's disease or lung

J67.4 **Maltworker's lung**

Alveolitis due to Aspergillus clavatus

J67.5 **Mushroom-worker's lung**

J67.6 **Maple-bark-stripper's lung**

Alveolitis due to

Cryptostroma corticale

Cryptostromosis

J67.7 **Air conditioner and humidifier lung**

Allergic alveolitis due to fungal, thermophilic actinomycetes **and other** organisms growing in ventilation [air conditioning] systems

J67.8 **Hypersensitivity pneumonitis due to other organic dusts**

Cheese-washer's lung

Coffee-worker's lung

Fish-meal worker's lung

Furrier's lung

Sequoiosis

J67.9 **Hypersensitivity pneumonitis due to unspecified organic dust**

Allergic alveolitis (extrinsic) NOS

Hypersensitivity pneumonitis NOS

J68 **Respiratory conditions due to inhalation of chemicals, gases, fumes and vapors**

Code first (T51-T65) to identify cause

Use additional code to identify associated respiratory conditions, such as:

acute respiratory failure (J96.0-)

J68.0 **Bronchitis and pneumonitis due to chemicals, gases, fumes and vapors**

Chemical bronchitis (acute)

J68.1 **Pulmonary edema due to chemicals, gases, fumes and vapors**

Chemical pulmonary edema (acute) (chronic)

Excludes1: pulmonary edema (acute) (chronic) NOS (J81.-)

J68.2 **Upper respiratory inflammation due to chemicals, gases, fumes and vapors, not elsewhere classified**

J68.3 **Other acute and subacute respiratory conditions due to chemicals, gases, fumes and vapors**

Reactive airways dysfunction syndrome

J68.4 **Chronic respiratory conditions due to chemicals, gases, fumes and vapors**

Emphysema (diffuse) (chronic) due to inhalation of chemicals, gases, fumes and vapors

Obliterative bronchiolitis (chronic) (subacute) due to inhalation of chemicals, gases, fumes and vapors

Pulmonary fibrosis (chronic) due to inhalation of chemicals, gases, fumes and vapors

Excludes1: chronic pulmonary edema due to chemicals, gases, fumes and vapors (J68.1)

J68.8 **Other respiratory conditions due to chemicals, gases, fumes and vapors**

J68.9 **Unspecified respiratory condition due to chemicals, gases, fumes and vapors**

J69 **Pneumonitis due to solids and liquids**

Excludes1: neonatal aspiration syndromes (P24.-)

postprocedural pneumonitis (J95.4)

J69.0 **Pneumonitis due to inhalation of food and vomit**

Aspiration pneumonia NOS

Aspiration pneumonia (due to) food (regurgitated)

Aspiration pneumonia (due to) gastric secretions

Aspiration pneumonia (due to) milk

Aspiration pneumonia (due to) vomit

Code also any associated foreign body in respiratory tract (T17.-)

Excludes1: chemical pneumonitis due to anesthesia (J95.4)

obstetric aspiration pneumonitis (O74.0)

J69.1 **Pneumonitis due to inhalation of oils and essences**

Exogenous lipoid pneumonia

Lipid pneumonia NOS

Code first (T51-T65) to identify substance

Excludes1: endogenous lipoid pneumonia (J84.89)

J69.8 **Pneumonitis due to inhalation of other solids and liquids**

Pneumonitis due to aspiration of blood

Pneumonitis due to aspiration of detergent

Code first (T51-T65) to identify substance

J70 **Respiratory conditions due to other external agents**

J70.0 **Acute pulmonary manifestations due to radiation**

Radiation pneumonitis

Use additional code (W88-W90, X39.0-) to identify the external cause

J70.1 **Chronic and other pulmonary manifestations due to radiation**

Fibrosis of lung following radiation

Use additional code (W88-W90, X39.0-) to identify the external cause

J70.2 **Acute drug-induced interstitial lung disorders**

Use additional code for adverse effect, if applicable, to identify drug (T36-T50 with fifth or sixth character 5)

Excludes1: interstitial pneumonia NOS (J84.9)

lymphoid interstitial pneumonia (J84.2)

J70.3 **Chronic drug-induced interstitial lung disorders**

Use additional code for adverse effect, if applicable, to identify drug (T36-T50 with fifth or sixth character 5)

Excludes1: interstitial pneumonia NOS (J84.9)

lymphoid interstitial pneumonia (J84.2)

J70.4 **Drug-induced interstitial lung disorders, unspecified**

Use additional code for adverse effect, if applicable, to identify drug (T36-T50 with fifth or sixth character 5)

Excludes1: interstitial pneumonia NOS (J84.9)

lymphoid interstitial pneumonia (J84.2)

J70.5 **Respiratory conditions due to smoke inhalation**

Smoke inhalation NOS

Excludes1: smoke inhalation due to chemicals, gases, fumes and vapors (J68.9)

J70.8 **Respiratory conditions due to other specified external agents**

Code first (T51-T65) to identify the external agent

J70.9 **Respiratory conditions due to unspecified external agent**

Code first (T51-T65) to identify the external agent

OTHER RESPIRATORY DISEASES PRINCIPALLY AFFECTING THE INTERSTITIUM (J80-J84)

J80 **Acute respiratory distress syndrome**

Acute respiratory distress syndrome in adult or child

Adult hyaline membrane disease

Excludes1: respiratory distress syndrome in newborn (perinatal) (P22.0)

J81 **Pulmonary edema**

Use additional code to identify:

exposure to environmental tobacco smoke (Z77.22)

history of tobacco dependence (Z87.891)

occupational exposure to environmental tobacco smoke (Z57.31)

tobacco dependence (F17.-)

tobacco use (Z72.0)

Excludes1: chemical (acute) pulmonary edema (J68.1)

hypostatic pneumonia (J18.2)

passive pneumonia (J18.2)

pulmonary edema due to external agents (J60-J70)

pulmonary edema with heart disease NOS (I50.1)

pulmonary edema with heart failure (I50.1)

J81.0 **Acute pulmonary edema**

Acute edema of lung

J81.1 **Chronic pulmonary edema**

Pulmonary congestion (chronic) (passive)

Pulmonary edema NOS

J82 **Pulmonary eosinophilia, not elsewhere classified**

Allergic pneumonia

Eosinophilic asthma

Eosinophilic pneumonia

Löffler's pneumonia

Tropical (pulmonary) eosinophilia NOS

Excludes1: pulmonary eosinophilia due to aspergillosis (B44.-)

pulmonary eosinophilia due to drugs (J70.2-J70.4)

pulmonary eosinophilia due to specified parasitic infection (B50-B83)

pulmonary eosinophilia due to systemic connective tissue disorders (M30-M36)

pulmonary infiltrate NOS (R91.8)

J84 **Other interstitial pulmonary diseases**

Excludes1: drug-induced interstitial lung disorders (J70.2-J70.4)

interstitial emphysema (J98.2)

Excludes2: lung diseases due to external agents (J60-J70)

J84.0 **Alveolar and parieto-alveolar conditions**

J84.01 **Alveolar proteinosis**

J84.02 **Pulmonary alveolar microlithiasis**

J84.03 **Idiopathic pulmonary hemosiderosis**

Essential brown induration of lung

Code first underlying disease, such as:

disorders of iron metabolism (E83.1-)

Excludes1: acute idiopathic pulmonary hemorrhage in infants [AIPHI] (R04.81)

J84.09 **Other alveolar and parieto-alveolar conditions**

J84.1 **Other interstitial pulmonary diseases with fibrosis**

Excludes1: pulmonary fibrosis (chronic) due to inhalation of chemicals, gases, fumes or vapors (J68.4)

pulmonary fibrosis (chronic) following radiation (J70.1)

J84.10 **Pulmonary fibrosis, unspecified**

Definition: Pulmonary fibrosis is a condition characterized by deposition of fibrous tissue in the lung. It decreases lung compliance and results in a restrictive ventilatory defect as seen in pulmonary function testing.

Capillary fibrosis of lung

Cirrhosis of lung (chronic) NOS

Fibrosis of lung (atrophic) (chronic) (confluent) (massive) (perialveolar) (peribronchial) NOS

Induration of lung (chronic) NOS

Postinflammatory pulmonary fibrosis

J84.11 **Idiopathic interstitial pneumonia**

Excludes1: lymphoid interstitial pneumonia (J84.2)

pneumocystis pneumonia (B59)

J84.111 **Idiopathic interstitial pneumonia, not otherwise specified**

J84.112 **Idiopathic pulmonary fibrosis**

Cryptogenic fibrosing alveolitis

Idiopathic fibrosing alveolitis

J84.113 **Idiopathic non-specific interstitial pneumonitis**

Excludes1: non-specific interstitial pneumonia NOS, or due to known underlying cause (J84.89)

J84.114 **Acute interstitial pneumonitis**

Hamman-Rich syndrome

Excludes1: pneumocystis pneumonia (B59)

J84.115 **Respiratory bronchiolitis interstitial lung disease**

J84.116 **Cryptogenic organizing pneumonia**

Excludes1: organizing pneumonia NOS, or due to known underlying cause (J84.89)

J84.117 **Desquamative interstitial pneumonia**

J84.17 **Other interstitial pulmonary diseases with fibrosis in diseases classified elsewhere**

Interstitial pneumonia (nonspecific) (usual) due to collagen vascular disease

Interstitial pneumonia (nonspecific) (usual) in diseases classified elsewhere

Organizing pneumonia due to collagen vascular disease

Organizing pneumonia in diseases classified elsewhere

Code first underlying disease, such as:

progressive systemic sclerosis (M34.0)

rheumatoid arthritis (M05.00-M06.9)

systemic lupus erythematosus (M32.0-M32.9)

J84.2 **Lymphoid interstitial pneumonia**

Lymphoid interstitial pneumonitis

J84.8 **Other specified interstitial pulmonary diseases**

Excludes1: exogenous lipoid pneumonia (J69.1)

unspecified lipoid pneumonia (J69.1)

J84.81 **Lymphangioleiomyomatosis**

Lymphangiomyomatosis

J84.82 **Adult pulmonary Langerhans cell histiocytosis**

Adult PLCH

J84.83 **Surfactant mutations of the lung**

J84.84 **Other interstitial lung diseases of childhood**

J84.841 **Neuroendocrine cell hyperplasia of infancy**

J84.842 **Pulmonary interstitial glycogenosis**

J84.843 **Alveolar capillary dysplasia with vein misalignment**

J84.848 **Other interstitial lung diseases of childhood**

J84.89 **Other specified interstitial pulmonary diseases**

Endogenous lipoid pneumonia

Interstitial pneumonitis

Non-specific interstitial pneumonitis NOS

Organizing pneumonia NOS

Code first, if applicable:

poisoning due to drug or toxin (T51-T65 with fifth or sixth character to indicate intent), for toxic pneumonopathy

underlying cause of pneumonopathy, if known

Use additional code, for adverse effect, to identify drug (T36-T50 with fifth or sixth character 5), if drug-induced

Excludes1: cryptogenic organizing pneumonia (J84.116)

idiopathic non-specific interstitial pneumonitis (J84.113)

lipoid pneumonia, exogenous or unspecified (J69.1)

lymphoid interstitial pneumonia (J84.2)

J84.9 **Interstitial pulmonary disease, unspecified**

Interstitial pneumonia NOS

SUPPURATIVE AND NECROTIC CONDITIONS OF THE LOWER RESPIRATORY TRACT (J85-J86)

J85 **Abscess of lung and mediastinum**

Use additional code (B95-B97) to identify infectious agent.

J85.0 **Gangrene and necrosis of lung**

J85.1 **Abscess of lung with pneumonia**

Code also the type of pneumonia

J85.2 **Abscess of lung without pneumonia**

Abscess of lung NOS

J85.3 **Abscess of mediastinum**

J86 **Pyothorax**

Use additional code (B95-B97) to identify infectious agent.

Excludes1: abscess of lung (J85.-)

pyothorax due to tuberculosis (A15.6)

J86.0 **Pyothorax with fistula**

Bronchocutaneous fistula

Bronchopleural fistula

Hepatopleural fistula

Mediastinal fistula

Pleural fistula

Thoracic fistula

Any condition classifiable to J86.9 with fistula

J86.9 **Pyothorax without fistula**

Abscess of pleura

Abscess of thorax

Empyema (chest) (lung) (pleura)

Fibrinopurulent pleurisy

Purulent pleurisy

Pyopneumothorax

Septic pleurisy

Seropurulent pleurisy

Suppurative pleurisy

OTHER DISEASES OF THE PLEURA (J90-J94)

J90 **Pleural effusion, not elsewhere classified**

Definition: Pleurisy is an inflammation of the membrane that surrounds and protects the lungs (the pleura). Inflammation occurs when an infection or damaging agent irritates the pleural surface.

Encysted pleurisy

Pleural effusion NOS

Pleurisy with effusion (exudative) (serous)

Excludes1: chylous (pleural) effusion (J94.0)

malignant pleural effusion (J91.0))

pleurisy NOS (R09.1)

tuberculous pleural effusion (A15.6)

J91 **Pleural effusion in conditions classified elsewhere**

Excludes2: pleural effusion in heart failure (I50.-)

pleural effusion in systemic lupus erythematosus (M32.13)

J91.0 **Malignant pleural effusion**

Code first underlying neoplasm

J91.8 **Pleural effusion in other conditions classified elsewhere**

Code first underlying disease, such as:

filariasis (B74.0-B74.9)

influenza (J09.X2, J10.1, J11.1)

J92 **Pleural plaque**

Includes: pleural thickening

● New code ▲ Revised code **Excludes1:** Not coded here **Excludes2:** Not included here ⊗ Placeholder required ⑦7th digit required

J92.0 **Pleural plaque with presence of asbestos**

J92.9 **Pleural plaque without asbestos**

Pleural plaque NOS

J93 **Pneumothorax and air leak**

Excludes1: congenital or perinatal pneumothorax (P25.1)

postprocedural air leak (J95.812)

postprocedural pneumothorax (J95.811)

traumatic pneumothorax (S27.0)

tuberculous (current disease)

pneumothorax (A15.-)

pyopneumothorax (J86.-)

J93.0 **Spontaneous tension pneumothorax**

J93.1 **Other spontaneous pneumothorax**

J93.11 **Primary spontaneous pneumothorax**

J93.12 **Secondary spontaneous pneumothorax**

Code first underlying condition, such as:

catamenial pneumothorax due to endometriosis (N80.8)

cystic fibrosis (E84.-)

eosinophilic pneumonia (J82)

lymphangioleiomyomatosis (J84.81)

malignant neoplasm of bronchus and lung (C34.-)

Marfan's syndrome (Q87.4)

pneumonia due to Pneumocystis carinii (B59)

secondary malignant neoplasm of lung (C78.0-)

spontaneous rupture of the esophagus (K22.3)

J93.8 **Other pneumothorax and air leak**

J93.81 **Chronic pneumothorax**

J93.82 **Other air leak**

Persistent air leak

J93.83 **Other pneumothorax**

Acute pneumothorax

Spontaneous pneumothorax NOS

J93.9 **Pneumothorax, unspecified**

Pneumothorax NOS

J94 **Other pleural conditions**

Excludes1: pleurisy NOS (R09.1)

traumatic hemopneumothorax (S27.2)

traumatic hemothorax (S27.1)

tuberculous pleural conditions (current disease) (A15.-)

J94.0 **Chylous effusion**

Chyliform effusion

J94.1 **Fibrothorax**

J94.2 **Hemothorax**

Hemopneumothorax

J94.8 **Other specified pleural conditions**

Hydropneumothorax

Hydrothorax

J94.9 **Pleural condition, unspecified**

INTRAOPERATIVE AND POSTPROCEDURAL COMPLICATIONS AND DISORDERS OF RESPIRATORY SYSTEM, NOT ELSEWHERE CLASSIFIED (J95)

J95 **Intraoperative and postprocedural complications and disorders of respiratory system, not elsewhere classified**

Excludes2: aspiration pneumonia (J69.-)

emphysema (subcutaneous) resulting from a procedure (T81.82)

hypostatic pneumonia (J18.2)

pulmonary manifestations due to radiation (J70.0-J70.1)

J95.0 **Tracheostomy complications**

J95.00 **Unspecified tracheostomy complication**

J95.01 **Hemorrhage from tracheostomy stoma**

J95.02 **Infection of tracheostomy stoma**

Use additional code to identify type of infection, such as:

cellulitis of neck (L03.221)

sepsis (A40, A41.-)

J95.03 **Malfunction of tracheostomy stoma**

Mechanical complication of tracheostomy stoma

Obstruction of tracheostomy airway

Tracheal stenosis due to tracheostomy

J95.04 **Tracheo-esophageal fistula following tracheostomy**

J95.09 **Other tracheostomy complication**

J95.1 **Acute pulmonary insufficiency following thoracic surgery**

Excludes2: Functional disturbances following cardiac surgery (I97.0, I97.1-)

J95.2 **Acute pulmonary insufficiency following nonthoracic surgery**

Excludes2: Functional disturbances following cardiac surgery (I97.0, I97.1-)

J95.3 **Chronic pulmonary insufficiency following surgery**

Excludes2: Functional disturbances following cardiac surgery (I97.0, I97.1-)

J95.4 **Chemical pneumonitis due to anesthesia**

Mendelson's syndrome

Postprocedural aspiration pneumonia

Use additional code for adverse effect, if applicable, to identify drug (T41.- with fifth or sixth character 5)

Excludes1: aspiration pneumonitis due to anesthesia complicating labor and delivery (O74.0)

aspiration pneumonitis due to anesthesia complicating pregnancy (O29)

aspiration pneumonitis due to anesthesia complicating the puerperium (O89.01)

J95.5 **Postprocedural subglottic stenosis**

J95.6 **Intraoperative hemorrhage and hematoma of a respiratory system organ or structure complicating a procedure**

Excludes1: intraoperative hemorrhage and hematoma of a respiratory system organ or structure due to accidental puncture and laceration during procedure (J95.7-)

J95.61 **Intraoperative hemorrhage and hematoma of a respiratory system organ or structure complicating a respiratory system procedure**

J95.62 **Intraoperative hemorrhage and hematoma of a respiratory system organ or structure complicating other procedure**

J95.7 **Accidental puncture and laceration of a respiratory system organ or structure during a procedure**

Excludes2: postprocedural pneumothorax (J95.811)

J95.71 **Accidental puncture and laceration of a respiratory system organ or structure during a respiratory system procedure**

J95.72 Accidental puncture and laceration of a respiratory system organ or structure during other procedure

J95.8 **Other intraoperative and postprocedural complications and disorders of respiratory system, not elsewhere classified**

    J95.81 Postprocedural pneumothorax and air leak

        J95.811 Postprocedural pneumothorax

        J95.812 Postprocedural air leak

    J95.82 Postprocedural respiratory failure

        Excludes1: Respiratory failure in other conditions (J96.-)

        J95.821 Acute postprocedural respiratory failure

            Postprocedural respiratory failure NOS

        J95.822 Acute and chronic postprocedural respiratory failure

    J95.83 Postprocedural hemorrhage of a respiratory system organ or structure following a procedure

        J95.830 Postprocedural hemorrhage of a respiratory system organ or structure following a respiratory system procedure

        J95.831 Postprocedural hemorrhage of a respiratory system organ or structure following other procedure

    J95.84 Transfusion-related acute lung injury (TRALI)

    J95.85 Complication of respirator [ventilator]

        J95.850 Mechanical complication of respirator

            Excludes1: encounter for respirator [ventilator] dependence during power failure (Z99.12)

        J95.851 Ventilator associated pneumonia

            Ventilator associated pneumonitis

            Use additional code to identify the organism, if known (B95.-, B96.-, B97.-)

            Excludes1: ventilator lung in newborn (P27.8)

        J95.859 Other complication of respirator [ventilator]

    J95.86 Postprocedural hematoma and seroma of a respiratory system organ or structure following a procedure

        J95.860 Postprocedural hematoma of a respiratory system organ or structure following a respiratory system procedure

        J95.861 Postprocedural hematoma of a respiratory system organ or structure following other procedure

        J95.862 Postprocedural seroma of a respiratory system organ or structure following a respiratory system procedure

        J95.863 Postprocedural seroma of a respiratory system organ or structure following other procedure

    J95.88 Other intraoperative complications of respiratory system, not elsewhere classified

J95.89 Other postprocedural complications and disorders of respiratory system, not elsewhere classified

    Use additional code to identify disorder, such as:

    aspiration pneumonia (J69.-)

    bacterial or viral pneumonia (J12-J18)

    Excludes2: acute pulmonary insufficiency following thoracic surgery (J95.1)

        postprocedural subglottic stenosis (J95.5)

OTHER DISEASES OF THE RESPIRATORY SYSTEM (J96-J99)

J96 **Respiratory failure, not elsewhere classified**

    Excludes1: acute respiratory distress syndrome (J80)

    cardiorespiratory failure (R09.2)

    newborn respiratory distress syndrome (P22.0)

    postprocedural respiratory failure (J95.82-)

    respiratory arrest (R09.2)

    respiratory arrest of newborn (P28.81)

    respiratory failure of newborn (P28.5)

    J96.0 Acute respiratory failure

        J96.00 Acute respiratory failure, unspecified whether with hypoxia or hypercapnia

        J96.01 Acute respiratory failure with hypoxia

        J96.02 Acute respiratory failure with hypercapnia

    J96.1 Chronic respiratory failure

        J96.10 Chronic respiratory failure, unspecified whether with hypoxia or hypercapnia

        J96.11 Chronic respiratory failure with hypoxia

        J96.12 Chronic respiratory failure with hypercapnia

    J96.2 Acute and chronic respiratory failure

        Acute on chronic respiratory failure

        J96.20 Acute and chronic respiratory failure, unspecified whether with hypoxia or hypercapnia

        J96.21 Acute and chronic respiratory failure with hypoxia

        J96.22 Acute and chronic respiratory failure with hypercapnia

    J96.9 Respiratory failure, unspecified

        J96.90 Respiratory failure, unspecified, unspecified whether with hypoxia or hypercapnia

        J96.91 Respiratory failure, unspecified with hypoxia

        J96.92 Respiratory failure, unspecified with hypercapnia

J98 **Other respiratory disorders**

    Use additional code to identify:

    exposure to environmental tobacco smoke (Z77.22)

    exposure to tobacco smoke in the perinatal period (P96.81)

    history of tobacco dependence (Z87.891)

    occupational exposure to environmental tobacco smoke (Z57.31)

    tobacco dependence (F17.-)

    tobacco use (Z72.0)

    Excludes1: newborn apnea (P28.4)

        newborn sleep apnea (P28.3)

    Excludes2: apnea NOS (R06.81)

        sleep apnea (G47.3-)

    J98.0 Diseases of bronchus, not elsewhere classified

        J98.01 Acute bronchospasm

● New code   ▲ Revised code   **Excludes1:** Not coded here   **Excludes2:** Not included here   ⊗ Placeholder required   ⑦ 7th digit required

Excludes1: acute bronchiolitis with bronchospasm (J21.-)

acute bronchitis with bronchospasm (J20.-)

asthma (J45.-)

exercise induced bronchospasm (J45.990)

J98.09 **Other diseases of bronchus, not elsewhere classified**

Broncholithiasis

Calcification of bronchus

Stenosis of bronchus

Tracheobronchial collapse

Tracheobronchial dyskinesia

Ulcer of bronchus

J98.1 **Pulmonary collapse**

Excludes1: therapeutic collapse of lung status (Z98.3)

J98.11 **Atelectasis**

Excludes1: newborn atelectasis

tuberculous atelectasis (current disease) (A15)

J98.19 **Other pulmonary collapse**

J98.2 **Interstitial emphysema**

Mediastinal emphysema

Excludes1: emphysema NOS (J43.9)

emphysema in newborn (P25.0)

surgical emphysema (subcutaneous) (T81.82)

traumatic subcutaneous emphysema (T79.7)

J98.3 **Compensatory emphysema**

J98.4 **Other disorders of lung**

Calcification of lung

Cystic lung disease (acquired)

Lung disease NOS

Pulmolithiasis

Excludes1: acute interstitial pneumonitis (J84.114)

pulmonary insufficiency following surgery (J95.1-J95.2)

J98.5 **Diseases of mediastinum, not elsewhere classified**

Excludes2: abscess of mediastinum (J85.3)

J98.51 **Mediastinitis**

Code first underlying condition, if applicable, such as postoperative mediastinitis (T81.-)

J98.59 **Other diseases of mediastinum, not elsewhere classified**

Fibrosis of mediastinum

Hernia of mediastinum

Retraction of mediastinum

J98.6 **Disorders of diaphragm**

Diaphragmatitis

Paralysis of diaphragm

Relaxation of diaphragm

Excludes1: congenital malformation of diaphragm NEC (Q79.1)

congenital diaphragmatic hernia (Q79.0)

Excludes2: diaphragmatic hernia (K44.-)

J98.8 **Other specified respiratory disorders**

J98.9 **Respiratory disorder, unspecified**

Respiratory disease (chronic) NOS

J99 **Respiratory disorders in diseases classified elsewhere**

Code first underlying disease, such as:

amyloidosis (E85.-)

ankylosing spondylitis (M45)

congenital syphilis (A50.5)

cryoglobulinemia (D89.1)

early congenital syphilis (A50.0)

schistosomiasis (B65.0-B65.9)

Excludes1: respiratory disorders in:

amebiasis (A06.5)

blastomycosis (B40.0-B40.2)

candidiasis (B37.1)

coccidioidomycosis (B38.0-B38.2)

cystic fibrosis with pulmonary manifestations (E84.0)

dermatomyositis (M33.01, M33.11)

histoplasmosis (B39.0-B39.2)

late syphilis (A52.72, A52.73)

polymyositis (M33.21)

sicca syndrome (M35.02)

systemic lupus erythematosus (M32.13)

systemic sclerosis (M34.81)

Wegener's granulomatosis (M31.30-M31.31)

Chapter 11: Diseases Of The Digestive System (K00-K95)

DEFINITIONS

This chapter includes definitions of selected key words, terms and phrases and coding alerts for adding points to the clinical domain, and references to coding late effects where appropriate. An example from this chapter is as follows:

K04 Diseases of pulp and periapical tissues
Definition: Pulp is the part in the center of a tooth made up of living soft tissue and cells called odontoblasts.

MULTIPLE CODING FOR A SINGLE CONDITION

In addition to the etiology/manifestation convention that requires two codes to fully describe a single condition that affects multiple body systems, there are other single conditions that also require more than one code. "Use additional code" notes are found in the Tabular List at codes that are not part of an etiology/manifestation pair where a secondary code is useful to fully describe a condition. The sequencing rule is the same as the etiology/manifestation pair, "use additional code" indicates that a secondary code should be added.

For example, for bacterial infections that are not included in chapter 1, a secondary code from category B95, Streptococcus, Staphylococcus, and Enterococcus, as the cause of diseases classified elsewhere, or B96, Other bacterial agents as the cause of diseases classified elsewhere, may be required to identify the bacterial organism causing the infection. A "use additional code" note will normally be found at the infectious disease code, indicating a need for the organism code to be added as a secondary code.

"Code first" notes are also under certain codes that are not specifically manifestation codes but may be due to an underlying cause. When there is a "code first" note and an underlying condition is present, the underlying condition should be sequenced first.

"Code, if applicable, any causal condition first", notes indicate that this code may be assigned as a principal diagnosis when the causal condition is unknown or not applicable. If a causal condition is known, then the code for that condition should be sequenced as the principal or first-listed diagnosis.

Multiple codes may be needed for sequela, complication codes and obstetric codes to more fully describe a condition. See the specific guidelines for these conditions for further instruction.

COMBINATION CODE

A combination code is a single code used to classify: Two diagnoses, or a diagnosis with an associated secondary process (manifestation) A diagnosis with an associated complication

Combination codes are identified by referring to subterm entries in the Alphabetic Index and by reading the inclusion and exclusion notes in the Tabular List.

Assign only the combination code when that code fully identifies the diagnostic conditions involved or when the Alphabetic Index so directs. Multiple coding should not be used when the classification provides a combination code that clearly identifies all of the elements documented in the diagnosis. When the combination code lacks necessary specificity in describing the manifestation or complication, an additional code should be used as a secondary code.

SEQUELA (LATE EFFECTS)

A sequela is the residual effect (condition produced) after the acute phase of an illness or injury has terminated. There is no time limit on when a sequela code can be used. The residual may be apparent early, such as in cerebral infarction, or it may occur months or years later, such as that due to a previous injury. Coding of sequela generally requires two codes sequenced in the following order: The condition or nature of the sequela is sequenced first.

The sequela code is sequenced second.

An exception to the above guidelines are those instances where the code for the sequela is followed by a manifestation code identified in the Tabular List and title, or the sequela code has been expanded (at the fourth, fifth or sixth character levels) to include the manifestation(s). The code for the acute phase of an illness or injury that led to the sequela is never used with a code for the late effect.

K00-K95

Chapter 11

Diseases Of The Digestive System (K00-K95)

Excludes2: certain conditions originating in the perinatal period (P04-P96)

certain infectious and parasitic diseases (A00-B99)

complications of pregnancy, childbirth and the puerperium (O00-O9A)

congenital malformations, deformations and chromosomal abnormalities (Q00-Q99)

endocrine, nutritional and metabolic diseases (E00-E88)

injury, poisoning and certain other consequences of external causes (S00-T88)

neoplasms (C00-D49)

symptoms, signs and abnormal clinical and laboratory findings, not elsewhere classified (R00-R94)

This chapter contains the following blocks:

K00-K14	Diseases of oral cavity and salivary glands
K20-K31	Diseases of esophagus, stomach and duodenum
K35-K38	Diseases of appendix
K40-K46	Hernia
K50-K52	Noninfective enteritis and colitis
K55-K64	Other diseases of intestines
K65-K68	Diseases of peritoneum and retroperitoneum
K70-K77	Diseases of liver
K80-K87	Disorders of gallbladder, biliary tract and pancreas
K90-K95	Other diseases of the digestive system

DISEASES OF ORAL CAVITY AND SALIVARY GLANDS (K00-K14)

K00 **Disorders of tooth development and eruption**

Excludes2: embedded and impacted teeth (K01.-)

K00.0 **Anodontia**

Hypodontia

Oligodontia

Excludes1: acquired absence of teeth (K08.1-)

K00.1 **Supernumerary teeth**

Distomolar Fourth molar

Mesiodens Paramolar

Supplementary teeth

Excludes2: supernumerary roots (K00.2)

K00.2 **Abnormalities of size and form of teeth**

Concrescence of teeth

Fusion of teeth

Gemination of teeth

Dens evaginatus

Dens in dente

Dens invaginatus

Enamel pearls

Macrodontia

Microdontia

Peg-shaped [conical] teeth

Supernumerary roots

Taurodontism

Tuberculum paramolare

Excludes1: abnormalities of teeth due to congenital syphilis (A50.5)

tuberculum Carabelli, which is regarded as a normal variation and should not be coded

K00.3 **Mottled teeth**

Dental fluorosis

Mottling of enamel

Nonfluoride enamel opacities

Excludes2: deposits [accretions] on teeth (K03.6)

K00.4 **Disturbances in tooth formation**

Aplasia and hypoplasia of cementum

Dilaceration of tooth

Enamel hypoplasia (neonatal) (postnatal) (prenatal)

Regional odontodysplasia

Turner's tooth

Excludes1: Hutchinson's teeth and mulberry molars in congenital syphilis (A50.5)

Excludes2: mottled teeth (K00.3)

K00.5 **Hereditary disturbances in tooth structure, not elsewhere classified**

Amelogenesis imperfecta

Dentinogenesis imperfecta

Odontogenesis imperfecta

Dentinal dysplasia

Shell teeth

K00.6 **Disturbances in tooth eruption**

Dentia praecox Natal tooth Neonatal tooth

Premature eruption of tooth

Premature shedding of primary [deciduous] tooth

Prenatal teeth

Retained [persistent] primary tooth

Excludes2: embedded and impacted teeth (K01.-)

K00.7 **Teething syndrome**

K00.8 **Other disorders of tooth development**

Color changes during tooth formation

Intrinsic staining of teeth NOS

Excludes2: posteruptive color changes (K03.7)

K00.9 **Disorder of tooth development, unspecified**

Disorder of odontogenesis NOS

K01 **Embedded and impacted teeth**

Excludes1: abnormal position of fully erupted teeth (M26.3-)

K01.0 **Embedded teeth**

K01.1 **Impacted teeth**

K02 **Dental caries**

Includes: caries of dentine

dental cavities

early childhood caries

pre-eruptive caries

recurrent caries (dentino enamel junction) (enamel) (to the pulp) tooth decay

K02.3 **Arrested dental caries**

Arrested coronal and root caries

K02.5 **Dental caries on pit and fissure surface**

Dental caries on chewing surface of tooth

K02.51 **Dental caries on pit and fissure surface limited to enamel**

White spot lesions [initial caries] on pit and fissure surface of tooth

---

K02.52 **Dental caries on pit and fissure surface penetrating into dentin**

Primary dental caries, cervical origin

K02.53 **Dental caries on pit and fissure surface penetrating into pulp**

K02.6 **Dental caries on smooth surface**

K02.61 **Dental caries on smooth surface limited to enamel**

White spot lesions [initial caries] on smooth surface of tooth

K02.62 **Dental caries on smooth surface penetrating into dentin**

K02.63 **Dental caries on smooth surface penetrating into pulp**

K02.7 **Dental root caries**

K02.9 **Dental caries, unspecified**

K03 **Other diseases of hard tissues of teeth**

Excludes2: bruxism (F45.8)

dental caries (K02.-)

teeth-grinding NOS (F45.8)

K03.0 **Excessive attrition of teeth**

Approximal wear of teeth

Occlusal wear of teeth

K03.1 **Abrasion of teeth**

Dentifrice abrasion of teeth

Habitual abrasion of teeth

Occupational abrasion of teeth

Ritual abrasion of teeth

Traditional abrasion of teeth Wedge defect NOS

K03.2 **Erosion of teeth**

Erosion of teeth due to diet

Erosion of teeth due to drugs and medicaments

Erosion of teeth due to persistent vomiting

Erosion of teeth NOS

Idiopathic erosion of teeth

Occupational erosion of teeth

K03.3 **Pathological resorption of teeth**

Internal granuloma of pulp

Resorption of teeth (external)

K03.4 **Hypercementosis**

Cementation hyperplasia

K03.5 **Ankylosis of teeth**

K03.6 **Deposits [accretions] on teeth**

Betel deposits [accretions] on teeth

Black deposits [accretions] on teeth

Extrinsic staining of teeth NOS

Green deposits [accretions] on teeth

Materia alba deposits [accretions] on teeth

Orange deposits [accretions] on teeth

Staining of teeth NOS

Subgingival dental calculus

Supragingival dental calculus

Tobacco deposits [accretions] on teeth

K03.7 **Posteruptive color changes of dental hard tissues**

Excludes2: deposits [accretions] on teeth (K03.6)

K03.8 **Other specified diseases of hard tissues of teeth**

K03.81 **Cracked tooth**

Excludes1: asymptomatic craze lines in enamel - omit code

broken or fractured tooth due to trauma (S02.5)

K03.89 **Other specified diseases of hard tissues of teeth**

K03.9 **Disease of hard tissues of teeth, unspecified**

K04 **Diseases of pulp and periapical tissues**

Definition: Pulp is the part in the center of a tooth made up of living soft tissue and cells called odontoblasts.

K04.0 **Pulpitis**

Acute pulpitis

Chronic (hyperplastic) (ulcerative) pulpitis

K04.01 **Reversible pulpitis**

K04.02 **Irreversible pulpitis**

K04.1 **Necrosis of pulp**

Pulpal gangrene

K04.2 **Pulp degeneration**

Denticles

Pulpal calcifications

Pulpal stones

K04.3 **Abnormal hard tissue formation in pulp**

Secondary or irregular dentine

K04.4 **Acute apical periodontitis of pulpal origin**

Acute apical periodontitis NOS

Excludes1: acute periodontitis (K05.2-)

K04.5 **Chronic apical periodontitis**

Apical or periapical granuloma

Apical periodontitis NOS

Excludes1: chronic periodontitis (K05.3-)

K04.6 **Periapical abscess with sinus**

Dental abscess with sinus

Dentoalveolar abscess with sinus

K04.7 **Periapical abscess without sinus**

Dental abscess without sinus

Dentoalveolar abscess without sinus

K04.8 **Radicular cyst**

Apical (periodontal) cyst

Periapical cyst

Residual radicular cyst

Excludes2: lateral periodontal cyst (K09.0)

K04.9 **Other and unspecified diseases of pulp and periapical tissues**

K04.90 **Unspecified diseases of pulp and periapical tissues**

K04.99 **Other diseases of pulp and periapical tissues**

K05 **Gingivitis and periodontal diseases**

Use additional code to identify:

alcohol abuse and dependence (F10.-)

exposure to environmental tobacco smoke (Z77.22)

exposure to tobacco smoke in the perinatal period (P96.81)

history of tobacco dependence (Z87.891)

occupational exposure to environmental tobacco smoke (Z57.31)

tobacco dependence (F17.-)

tobacco use (Z72.0)

K05.0 **Acute gingivitis**

Excludes1: acute necrotizing ulcerative gingivitis (A69.1)

herpesviral [herpes simplex] gingivostomatitis (B00.2)

K05.00   **Acute gingivitis, plaque induced**

Acute gingivitis NOS

Plaque induced gingival disease

K05.01   **Acute gingivitis, non-plaque induced**

K05.1   **Chronic gingivitis**

Desquamative gingivitis (chronic)

Gingivitis (chronic) NOS

Hyperplastic gingivitis (chronic)

Pregnancy associated gingivitis

Simple marginal gingivitis (chronic)

Ulcerative gingivitis (chronic)

Code first, if applicable, diseases of the digestive system complicating pregnancy (O99.61-)

K05.10   **Chronic gingivitis, plaque induced**

Chronic gingivitis NOS Gingivitis NOS

K05.11   **Chronic gingivitis, non-plaque induced**

K05.2   **Aggressive periodontitis**

Acute pericoronitis

Excludes1: acute apical periodontitis (K04.4)

periapical abscess (K04.7)

periapical abscess with sinus (K04.6)

K05.20   **Aggressive periodontitis, unspecified**

K05.21   **Aggressive periodontitis, localized**

Periodontal abscess

     K05.211   **Aggressive periodontitis, localized, slight**

     K05.212   **Aggressive periodontitis, localized, moderate**

     K05.213   **Aggressive periodontitis, localized, severe**

     K05.219   **Aggressive periodontitis, localized, unspecified severity**

K05.22   **Aggressive periodontitis, generalized**

     K05.221   **Aggressive periodontitis, generalized, slight**

     K05.222   **Aggressive periodontitis, generalized, moderate**

     K05.223   **Aggressive periodontitis, generalized, severe**

     K05.229   **Aggressive periodontitis, generalized, unspecified severity**

K05.3   **Chronic periodontitis**

Chronic pericoronitis

Complex periodontitis

Periodontitis NOS

Simplex periodontitis

Excludes1: chronic apical periodontitis (K04.5)

K05.30   **Chronic periodontitis, unspecified**

K05.31   **Chronic periodontitis, localized**

     K05.311   **Chronic periodontitis, localized, slight**

     K05.312   **Chronic periodontitis, localized, moderate**

     K05.313   **Chronic periodontitis, localized, severe**

     K05.319   **Chronic periodontitis, localized, unspecified severity**

K05.32   **Chronic periodontitis, generalized**

     K05.321   **Chronic periodontitis, generalized, slight**

     K05.322   **Chronic periodontitis, generalized, moderate**

     K05.323   **Chronic periodontitis, generalized, severe**

     K05.329   **Chronic periodontitis, generalized, unspecified severity**

K05.4   **Periodontosis**

Juvenile periodontosis

K05.5   **Other periodontal diseases**

Combined periodontic-endodontic lesion

Narrow gingival width (of periodontal soft tissue)

Excludes2: leukoplakia of gingiva (K13.21)

K05.6   **Periodontal disease, unspecified**

K06   **Other disorders of gingiva and edentulous alveolar ridge**

Excludes2: acute gingivitis (K05.0)

atrophy of edentulous alveolar ridge (K08.2)

chronic gingivitis (K05.1)

gingivitis NOS (K05.1)

K06.0   **Gingival recession**

Gingival recession (postinfective) (postprocedural)

•**K06.01**   **Gingival recession, localized**

     •**K06.010**   **Localized gingival recession, unspecified**

           Localized gingival recession, NOS

     •**K06.011**   **Localized gingival recession, minimal**

     •**K06.012**   **Localized gingival recession, moderate**

     •**K06.013**   **Localized gingival recession, severe**

•**K06.02**   **Gingival recession, generalized**

     •**K06.020**   **Generalized gingival recession, unspecified**

           Generalized gingival recession, NOS

     •**K06.021**   **Generalized gingival recession, minimal**

     •**K06.022**   **Generalized gingival recession, moderate**

     •**K06.023**   **Generalized gingival recession, severe**

K06.1   **Gingival enlargement**

Gingival fibromatosis

K06.2   **Gingival and edentulous alveolar ridge lesions associated with trauma**

Irritative hyperplasia of edentulous ridge [denture hyperplasia]

Use additional code (Chapter 20) to identify external cause or denture status (Z97.2)

K06.3   **Horizontal alveolar bone loss**

K06.8   **Other specified disorders of gingiva and edentulous alveolar ridge**

Fibrous epulis

Flabby alveolar ridge

Giant cell epulis

Peripheral giant cell granuloma of gingiva

Pyogenic granuloma of gingiva

Vertical ridge deficiency

Excludes2: gingival cyst (K09.0)

K06.9   **Disorder of gingiva and edentulous alveolar ridge, unspecified**

K08   **Other disorders of teeth and supporting structures**

Excludes2: dentofacial anomalies [including malocclusion] (M26.-)

disorders of jaw (M27.-)

K08.0 **Exfoliation of teeth due to systemic causes**

Code also underlying systemic condition

K08.1 **Complete loss of teeth**

Acquired loss of teeth, complete

Excludes1: congenital absence of teeth (K00.0)

exfoliation of teeth due to systemic causes (K08.0)

partial loss of teeth (K08.4-)

K08.10 **Complete loss of teeth, unspecified cause**

K08.101 **Complete loss of teeth, unspecified cause, class I**

K08.102 **Complete loss of teeth, unspecified cause, class II**

K08.103 **Complete loss of teeth, unspecified cause, class III**

K08.104 **Complete loss of teeth, unspecified cause, class IV**

K08.109 **Complete loss of teeth, unspecified cause, unspecified class**

Edentulism NOS

K08.11 **Complete loss of teeth due to trauma**

K08.111 **Complete loss of teeth due to trauma, class I**

K08.112 **Complete loss of teeth due to trauma, class II**

K08.113 **Complete loss of teeth due to trauma, class III**

K08.114 **Complete loss of teeth due to trauma, class IV**

K08.119 **Complete loss of teeth due to trauma, unspecified class**

K08.12 **Complete loss of teeth due to periodontal diseases**

K08.121 **Complete loss of teeth due to periodontal diseases, class I**

K08.122 **Complete loss of teeth due to periodontal diseases, class II**

K08.123 **Complete loss of teeth due to periodontal diseases, class III**

K08.124 **Complete loss of teeth due to periodontal diseases, class IV**

K08.129 **Complete loss of teeth due to periodontal diseases, unspecified class**

K08.13 **Complete loss of teeth due to caries**

K08.131 **Complete loss of teeth due to caries, class I**

K08.132 **Complete loss of teeth due to caries, class II**

K08.133 **Complete loss of teeth due to caries, class III**

K08.134 **Complete loss of teeth due to caries, class IV**

K08.139 **Complete loss of teeth due to caries, unspecified class**

K08.19 **Complete loss of teeth due to other specified cause**

K08.191 **Complete loss of teeth due to other specified cause, class I**

K08.192 **Complete loss of teeth due to other specified cause, class II**

K08.193 **Complete loss of teeth due to other specified cause, class III**

K08.194 **Complete loss of teeth due to other specified cause, class IV**

K08.199 **Complete loss of teeth due to other specified cause, unspecified class**

K08.2 **Atrophy of edentulous alveolar ridge**

K08.20 **Unspecified atrophy of edentulous alveolar ridge**

Atrophy of the mandible NOS

Atrophy of the maxilla NOS

K08.21 **Minimal atrophy of the mandible**

Minimal atrophy of the edentulous mandible

K08.22 **Moderate atrophy of the mandible**

Moderate atrophy of the edentulous mandible

K08.23 **Severe atrophy of the mandible**

Severe atrophy of the edentulous mandible

K08.24 **Minimal atrophy of maxilla**

Minimal atrophy of the edentulous maxilla

K08.25 **Moderate atrophy of the maxilla**

Moderate atrophy of the edentulous maxilla

K08.26 **Severe atrophy of the maxilla**

Severe atrophy of the edentulous maxilla

K08.3 **Retained dental root**

K08.4 **Partial loss of teeth**

Acquired loss of teeth, partial

Excludes1: complete loss of teeth (K08.1-)

congenital absence of teeth (K00.0)

Excludes2: exfoliation of teeth due to systemic causes (K08.0)

K08.40 **Partial loss of teeth, unspecified cause**

K08.401 **Partial loss of teeth, unspecified cause, class I**

K08.402 **Partial loss of teeth, unspecified cause, class II**

K08.403 **Partial loss of teeth, unspecified cause, class III**

K08.404 **Partial loss of teeth, unspecified cause, class IV**

K08.409 **Partial loss of teeth, unspecified cause, unspecified class**

Tooth extraction status NOS

K08.41 **Partial loss of teeth due to trauma**

K08.411 **Partial loss of teeth due to trauma, class I**

K08.412 **Partial loss of teeth due to trauma, class II**

K08.413 **Partial loss of teeth due to trauma, class III**

K08.414 **Partial loss of teeth due to trauma, class IV**

K08.419 **Partial loss of teeth due to trauma, unspecified class**

K08.42 **Partial loss of teeth due to periodontal diseases**

K08.421 **Partial loss of teeth due to periodontal diseases, class I**

K08.422 **Partial loss of teeth due to periodontal diseases, class II**

K08.423 **Partial loss of teeth due to periodontal diseases, class III**

K08.424   **Partial loss of teeth due to periodontal diseases, class IV**

K08.429   **Partial loss of teeth due to periodontal diseases, unspecified class**

K08.43   **Partial loss of teeth due to caries**

     K08.431   **Partial loss of teeth due to caries, class I**

     K08.432   **Partial loss of teeth due to caries, class II**

     K08.433   **Partial loss of teeth due to caries, class III**

     K08.434   **Partial loss of teeth due to caries, class IV**

     K08.439   **Partial loss of teeth due to caries, unspecified class**

K08.49   **Partial loss of teeth due to other specified cause**

     K08.491   **Partial loss of teeth due to other specified cause, class I**

     K08.492   **Partial loss of teeth due to other specified cause, class II**

     K08.493   **Partial loss of teeth due to other specified cause, class III**

     K08.494   **Partial loss of teeth due to other specified cause, class IV**

     K08.499   **Partial loss of teeth due to other specified cause, unspecified class**

K08.5   **Unsatisfactory restoration of tooth**

Defective bridge, crown, filling

Defective dental restoration

Excludes1: dental restoration status (Z98.811)

Excludes2: endosseous dental implant failure (M27.6-)

     unsatisfactory endodontic treatment (M27.5-)

   K08.50   **Unsatisfactory restoration of tooth, unspecified**

Defective dental restoration NOS

   K08.51   **Open restoration margins of tooth**

Dental restoration failure of marginal integrity

Open margin on tooth restoration

Poor gingival margin to tooth restoration

   K08.52   **Unrepairable overhanging of dental restorative materials**

Overhanging of tooth restoration

   K08.53   **Fractured dental restorative material**

Excludes1: cracked tooth (K03.81)

     traumatic fracture of tooth (S02.5)

     K08.530   **Fractured dental restorative material without loss of material**

     K08.531   **Fractured dental restorative material with loss of material**

     K08.539   **Fractured dental restorative material, unspecified**

   K08.54   **Contour of existing restoration of tooth biologically incompatible with oral health**

Dental restoration failure of periodontal anatomical integrity

Unacceptable contours of existing restoration of tooth

Unacceptable morphology of existing restoration of tooth

   K08.55   **Allergy to existing dental restorative material**

Use additional code to identify the specific type of allergy

   K08.56   **Poor aesthetic of existing restoration of tooth**

Dental restoration aesthetically inadequate or displeasing

   K08.59   **Other unsatisfactory restoration of tooth**

Other defective dental restoration

K08.8   **Other specified disorders of teeth and supporting structures**

   K08.81   **Primary occlusal trauma**

   K08.82   **Secondary occlusal trauma**

   K08.89   **Other specified disorders of teeth and supporting structures**

Enlargement of alveolar ridge NOS

Insufficient anatomic crown height

Insufficient clinical crown length

Irregular alveolar process

Toothache NOS

K08.9   **Disorder of teeth and supporting structures, unspecified**

K09   **Cysts of oral region, not elsewhere classified**

Includes: lesions showing histological features both of aneurysmal cyst and of another fibro-osseous lesion

Excludes2: cysts of jaw (M27.0-, M27.4-)

     radicular cyst (K04.8)

K09.0   **Developmental odontogenic cysts**

Dentigerous cyst

Eruption cyst

Follicular cyst

Gingival cyst

Lateral periodontal cyst

Primordial cyst

Excludes2: keratocysts (D16.4, D16.5)

     odontogenic keratocystic tumors (D16.4, D16.5)

K09.1   **Developmental (nonodontogenic) cysts of oral region**

Cyst (of) incisive canal

Cyst (of) palatine of papilla Globulomaxillary cyst

Median palatal cyst Nasoalveolar cyst Nasolabial cyst Nasopalatine duct cyst

K09.8   **Other cysts of oral region, not elsewhere classified**

Dermoid cyst

Epidermoid cyst

Lymphoepithelial cyst

Epstein's pearl

K09.9   **Cyst of oral region, unspecified**

K11   **Diseases of salivary glands**

Definition: The salivary gland is a gland that secretes saliva, especially any of three pairs of large glands, the parotid, submaxillary, and sublingual, whose secretions enter the mouth and mingle in saliva.

Use additional code to identify:

alcohol abuse and dependence (F10.-)

exposure to environmental tobacco smoke (Z77.22)

exposure to tobacco smoke in the perinatal period (P96.81)

history of tobacco dependence (Z87.891)

occupational exposure to environmental tobacco smoke (Z57.31)

tobacco dependence (F17.-)

tobacco use (Z72.0)

K11.0   **Atrophy of salivary gland**

K11.1   **Hypertrophy of salivary gland**

K11.2   **Sialoadenitis**

Parotitis

Excludes1: epidemic parotitis (B26.-)

mumps (B26.-)

uveoparotid fever [Heerfordt] (D86.89)

K11.20 Sialoadenitis, unspecified

K11.21 Acute sialoadenitis

Excludes1: acute recurrent sialoadenitis (K11.22)

K11.22 Acute recurrent sialoadenitis

K11.23 Chronic sialoadenitis

K11.3 Abscess of salivary gland

K11.4 Fistula of salivary gland

Excludes1: congenital fistula of salivary gland (Q38.4)

K11.5 Sialolithiasis

Calculus of salivary gland or duct

Stone of salivary gland or duct

K11.6 Mucocele of salivary gland

Mucous extravasation cyst of salivary gland

Mucous retention cyst of salivary gland

Ranula

K11.7 Disturbances of salivary secretion

Hypoptyalism

Ptyalism

Xerostomia

Excludes2: dry mouth NOS (R68.2)

K11.8 Other diseases of salivary glands

Benign lymphoepithelial lesion of salivary gland

Mikulicz' disease

Necrotizing sialometaplasia

Sialectasia

Stenosis of salivary duct

Stricture of salivary duct

Excludes1: sicca syndrome [Sjögren] (M35.0-)

K11.9 Disease of salivary gland, unspecified

Sialadenopathy NOS

K12 Stomatitis and related lesions

Use additional code to identify:

alcohol abuse and dependence (F10.-)

exposure to environmental tobacco smoke (Z77.22)

exposure to tobacco smoke in the perinatal period (P96.81)

history of tobacco dependence (Z87.891)

occupational exposure to environmental tobacco smoke (Z57.31)

tobacco dependence (F17.-)

tobacco use (Z72.0)

Excludes1: cancrum oris (A69.0)

cheilitis (K13.0)

gangrenous stomatitis (A69.0)

herpesviral [herpes simplex] gingivostomatitis (B00.2)

noma (A69.0)

K12.0 Recurrent oral aphthae

Aphthous stomatitis (major) (minor)

Bednar's aphthae

Periadenitis mucosa necrotica recurrens

Recurrent aphthous ulcer

Stomatitis herpetiformis

K12.1 Other forms of stomatitis

Stomatitis NOS

Denture stomatitis

Ulcerative stomatitis

Vesicular stomatitis

Excludes1: acute necrotizing ulcerative stomatitis (A69.1)

Vincent's stomatitis (A69.1)

K12.2 Cellulitis and abscess of mouth

Cellulitis of mouth (floor)

Submandibular abscess

Excludes2: abscess of salivary gland (K11.3)

abscess of tongue (K14.0)

periapical abscess (K04.6-K04.7)

periodontal abscess (K05.21)

peritonsillar abscess (J36)

K12.3 Oral mucositis (ulcerative)

Mucositis (oral) (oropharyngeal)

Excludes2: gastrointestinal mucositis (ulcerative) (K92.81)

mucositis (ulcerative) of vagina and vulva (N76.81)

nasal mucositis (ulcerative) (J34.81)

K12.30 Oral mucositis (ulcerative), unspecified

K12.31 Oral mucositis (ulcerative) due to antineoplastic therapy

Use additional code for adverse effect, if applicable, to identify antineoplastic and immunosuppressive drugs (T45.1X5)

Use additional code for other antineoplastic therapy, such as:

radiological procedure and radiotherapy (Y84.2)

K12.32 Oral mucositis (ulcerative) due to other drugs

Use additional code for adverse effect, if applicable, to identify drug (T36-T50 with fifth or sixth character 5)

K12.33 Oral mucositis (ulcerative) due to radiation

Use additional external cause code (W88-W90, X39.0-) to identify cause

K12.39 Other oral mucositis (ulcerative)

Viral oral mucositis (ulcerative)

K13 Other diseases of lip and oral mucosa

Includes: epithelial disturbances of tongue

Use additional code to identify:

alcohol abuse and dependence (F10.-)

exposure to environmental tobacco smoke (Z77.22)

exposure to tobacco smoke in the perinatal period (P96.81)

history of tobacco dependence (Z87.891)

occupational exposure to environmental tobacco smoke (Z57.31)

tobacco dependence (F17.-)

tobacco use (Z72.0)

Excludes2: certain disorders of gingiva and edentulous alveolar ridge (K05-K06)

cysts of oral region (K09.-)

diseases of tongue (K14.-)

stomatitis and related lesions (K12.-)

K13.0 Diseases of lips

Abscess of lips

Angular cheilitis

Cellulitis of lips

Cheilitis NOS

Cheilodynia

Cheilosis

Exfoliative cheilitis

Fistula of lips

Glandular cheilitis

Hypertrophy of lips

Perlèche NEC

> **Excludes1:** ariboflavinosis (E53.0)
>
> cheilitis due to radiation-related disorders (L55-L59)
>
> congenital fistula of lips (Q38.0)
>
> congenital hypertrophy of lips (Q18.6)
>
> Perlèche due to candidiasis (B37.83)
>
> Perlèche due to riboflavin deficiency (E53.0)

K13.1 **Cheek and lip biting**

K13.2 **Leukoplakia and other disturbances of oral epithelium, including tongue**

> **Excludes1:** carcinoma in situ of oral epithelium (D00.0-)
>
> hairy leukoplakia (K13.3)

K13.21 **Leukoplakia of oral mucosa, including tongue**

Leukokeratosis of oral mucosa

Leukoplakia of gingiva, lips, tongue

> **Excludes1:** hairy leukoplakia (K13.3)
>
> leukokeratosis nicotina palati (K13.24)

K13.22 **Minimal keratinized residual ridge mucosa**

Minimal keratinization of alveolar ridge mucosa

K13.23 **Excessive keratinized residual ridge mucosa**

Excessive keratinization of alveolar ridge mucosa

K13.24 **Leukokeratosis nicotina palati**

Smoker's palate

K13.29 **Other disturbances of oral epithelium, including tongue**

Erythroplakia of mouth or tongue

Focal epithelial hyperplasia of mouth or tongue

Leukoedema of mouth or tongue

Other oral epithelium disturbances

K13.3 **Hairy leukoplakia**

K13.4 **Granuloma and granuloma-like lesions of oral mucosa**

Eosinophilic granuloma pyogenicum

Verrucous xanthoma

K13.5 **Oral submucous fibrosis**

Submucous fibrosis of tongue

K13.6 **Irritative hyperplasia of oral mucosa**

> **Excludes2:** irritative hyperplasia of edentulous ridge [denture hyperplasia] (K06.2)

K13.7 **Other and unspecified lesions of oral mucosa**

K13.70 **Unspecified lesions of oral mucosa**

K13.79 **Other lesions of oral mucosa**

Focal oral mucinosis

K14 **Diseases of tongue**

Use additional code to identify:

alcohol abuse and dependence (F10.-)

exposure to environmental tobacco smoke (Z77.22)

history of tobacco dependence (Z87.891)

occupational exposure to environmental tobacco smoke (Z57.31)

tobacco dependence (F17.-)

tobacco use (Z72.0)

> **Excludes2:** erythroplakia (K13.29)
>
> focal epithelial hyperplasia (K13.29)

leukoedema of tongue (K13.29)

leukoplakia of tongue (K13.21)

hairy leukoplakia (K13.3)

macroglossia (congenital) (Q38.2)

submucous fibrosis of tongue (K13.5)

K14.0 **Glossitis**

Abscess of tongue

Ulceration (traumatic) of tongue

> **Excludes1:** atrophic glossitis (K14.4)

K14.1 **Geographic tongue**

Benign migratory glossitis

Glossitis areata exfoliativa

K14.2 **Median rhomboid glossitis**

K14.3 **Hypertrophy of tongue papillae**

Black hairy tongue

Coated tongue

Hypertrophy of foliate papillae

Lingua villosa nigra

K14.4 **Atrophy of tongue papillae**

Atrophic glossitis

K14.5 **Plicated tongue**

Fissured tongue

Furrowed tongue

Scrotal tongue

> **Excludes1:** fissured tongue, congenital (Q38.3)

K14.6 **Glossodynia**

Glossopyrosis

Painful tongue

K14.8 **Other diseases of tongue**

Atrophy of tongue

Crenated tongue

Enlargement of tongue

Glossocele

Glossoptosis

Hypertrophy of tongue

K14.9 **Disease of tongue, unspecified**

Glossopathy NOS

DISEASES OF ESOPHAGUS, STOMACH AND DUODENUM (K20-K31)

> **Excludes2:** hiatus hernia (K44.-)

K20 **Esophagitis**

Use additional code to identify:

alcohol abuse and dependence (F10.-)

> **Excludes1:** erosion of esophagus (K22.1-)
>
> esophagitis with gastro-esophageal reflux disease (K21.0)
>
> reflux esophagitis (K21.0)
>
> ulcerative esophagitis (K22.1-)

> **Excludes2:** eosinophilic gastritis or gastroenteritis (K52.81)

K20.0 **Eosinophilic esophagitis**

K20.8 **Other esophagitis**

Abscess of esophagus

K20.9 **Esophagitis, unspecified**

Esophagitis NOS

K21 **Gastro-esophageal reflux disease**

> **Excludes1:** newborn esophageal reflux (P78.83)

K21.0 **Gastro-esophageal reflux disease with esophagitis**

Reflux esophagitis

K21.9 **Gastro-esophageal reflux disease without esophagitis**

Esophageal reflux NOS

K22 **Other diseases of esophagus**

Excludes2: esophageal varices (I85.-)

K22.0 **Achalasia of cardia**

Achalasia NOS

Cardiospasm

Excludes1: congenital cardiospasm (Q39.5)

K22.1 **Ulcer of esophagus**

Barrett's ulcer

Erosion of esophagus

Fungal ulcer of esophagus

Peptic ulcer of esophagus

Ulcer of esophagus due to ingestion of chemicals

Ulcer of esophagus due to ingestion of drugs and medicaments

Ulcerative esophagitis

Code first poisoning due to drug or toxin, if applicable (T36-T65 with fifth or sixth character 1-4 or 6)

Use additional code for adverse effect, if applicable, to identify drug (T36-T50 with fifth or sixth character 5)

Excludes1: Barrett's esophagus (K22.7-)

K22.10 **Ulcer of esophagus without bleeding**

Ulcer of esophagus NOS

K22.11 **Ulcer of esophagus with bleeding**

Excludes2: bleeding esophageal varices (I85.01, I85.11)

K22.2 **Esophageal obstruction**

Compression of esophagus

Constriction of esophagus

Stenosis of esophagus

Stricture of esophagus

Excludes1: congenital stenosis or stricture of esophagus (Q39.3)

K22.3 **Perforation of esophagus**

Rupture of esophagus

Excludes1: traumatic perforation of (thoracic) esophagus (S27.8-)

K22.4 **Dyskinesia of esophagus**

Corkscrew esophagus

Diffuse esophageal spasm

Spasm of esophagus

Excludes1: cardiospasm (K22.0)

K22.5 **Diverticulum of esophagus, acquired**

Esophageal pouch, acquired

Excludes1: diverticulum of esophagus (congenital) (Q39.6)

K22.6 **Gastro-esophageal laceration-hemorrhage syndrome**

Mallory-Weiss syndrome

K22.7 **Barrett's esophagus**

Barrett's disease

Barrett's syndrome

Excludes1: Barrett's ulcer (K22.1)

malignant neoplasm of esophagus (C15.-)

K22.70 **Barrett's esophagus without dysplasia**

Barrett's esophagus NOS

K22.71 **Barrett's esophagus with dysplasia**

K22.710 **Barrett's esophagus with low grade dysplasia**

K22.711 **Barrett's esophagus with high grade dysplasia**

K22.719 **Barrett's esophagus with dysplasia, unspecified**

K22.8 **Other specified diseases of esophagus**

Hemorrhage of esophagus NOS

Excludes2: esophageal varices (I85.-)

Paterson-Kelly syndrome (D50.1)

K22.9 **Disease of esophagus, unspecified**

K23 **Disorders of esophagus in diseases classified elsewhere**

Code first underlying disease, such as:

congenital syphilis (A50.5)

Excludes1: late syphilis (A52.79)

megaesophagus due to Chagas' disease (B57.31)

tuberculosis (A18.83)

K25 **Gastric ulcer**

Definition: A Gastric ulcer is a hole in the lining of the stomach corroded by the acidic digestive juices which are secreted by the stomach cells.

Includes: erosion (acute) of stomach

pylorus ulcer (peptic) stomach ulcer (peptic)

Use additional code to identify:

alcohol abuse and dependence (F10.-)

Excludes1: acute gastritis (K29.0-)

peptic ulcer NOS (K27.-)

K25.0 **Acute gastric ulcer with hemorrhage**

K25.1 **Acute gastric ulcer with perforation**

K25.2 **Acute gastric ulcer with both hemorrhage and perforation**

K25.3 **Acute gastric ulcer without hemorrhage or perforation**

K25.4 **Chronic or unspecified gastric ulcer with hemorrhage**

K25.5 **Chronic or unspecified gastric ulcer with perforation**

K25.6 **Chronic or unspecified gastric ulcer with both hemorrhage and perforation**

K25.7 **Chronic gastric ulcer without hemorrhage or perforation**

K25.9 **Gastric ulcer, unspecified as acute or chronic, without hemorrhage or perforation**

K26 **Duodenal ulcer**

Definition: A Duodenal ulcer is a ulcer in the lining of the first part of the small intestine (duodenum).

Includes: erosion (acute) of duodenum

duodenum ulcer (peptic)

postpyloric ulcer (peptic)

Use additional code to identify:

alcohol abuse and dependence (F10.-)

Excludes1: peptic ulcer NOS (K27.-)

K26.0 **Acute duodenal ulcer with hemorrhage**

K26.1 **Acute duodenal ulcer with perforation**

K26.2 **Acute duodenal ulcer with both hemorrhage and perforation**

K26.3 **Acute duodenal ulcer without hemorrhage or perforation**

K26.4 **Chronic or unspecified duodenal ulcer with hemorrhage**

K26.5 **Chronic or unspecified duodenal ulcer with perforation**

K26.6 **Chronic or unspecified duodenal ulcer with both hemorrhage and perforation**

K26.7 Chronic duodenal ulcer without hemorrhage or perforation

K26.9 Duodenal ulcer, unspecified as acute or chronic, without hemorrhage or perforation

K27 Peptic ulcer, site unspecified

Definition: A Peptic ulcer is an ulcer of the mucous membrane lining of the alimentary tract

Includes: gastroduodenal ulcer NOS

peptic ulcer NOS

Use additional code to identify:

alcohol abuse and dependence (F10.-)

Excludes1: peptic ulcer of newborn (P78.82)

K27.0 Acute peptic ulcer, site unspecified, with hemorrhage

K27.1 Acute peptic ulcer, site unspecified, with perforation

K27.2 Acute peptic ulcer, site unspecified, with both hemorrhage and perforation

K27.3 Acute peptic ulcer, site unspecified, without hemorrhage or perforation

K27.4 Chronic or unspecified peptic ulcer, site unspecified, with hemorrhage

K27.5 Chronic or unspecified peptic ulcer, site unspecified, with perforation

K27.6 Chronic or unspecified peptic ulcer, site unspecified, with both hemorrhage and perforation

K27.7 Chronic peptic ulcer, site unspecified, without hemorrhage or perforation

K27.9 Peptic ulcer, site unspecified, unspecified as acute or chronic, without hemorrhage or perforation

K28 Gastrojejunal ulcer

Definition: A gastrojejunal ulcer is an ulcer that forms in the area between the stomach and the part of the small intestine known as the jejunum.

Includes: anastomotic ulcer (peptic) or erosion

gastrocolic ulcer (peptic) or erosion

gastrointestinal ulcer (peptic) or erosion

gastrojejunal ulcer (peptic) or erosion

jejunal ulcer (peptic) or erosion

marginal ulcer (peptic) or erosion

stomal ulcer (peptic) or erosion

Use additional code to identify:

alcohol abuse and dependence (F10.-)

Excludes1: primary ulcer of small intestine (K63.3)

K28.0 Acute gastrojejunal ulcer with hemorrhage

K28.1 Acute gastrojejunal ulcer with perforation

K28.2 Acute gastrojejunal ulcer with both hemorrhage and perforation

K28.3 Acute gastrojejunal ulcer without hemorrhage or perforation

K28.4 Chronic or unspecified gastrojejunal ulcer with hemorrhage

K28.5 Chronic or unspecified gastrojejunal ulcer with perforation

K28.6 Chronic or unspecified gastrojejunal ulcer with both hemorrhage and perforation

K28.7 Chronic gastrojejunal ulcer without hemorrhage or perforation

K28.9 Gastrojejunal ulcer, unspecified as acute or chronic, without hemorrhage or perforation

K29 Gastritis and duodenitis

Excludes1: eosinophilic gastritis or gastroenteritis (K52.81)

Zollinger-Ellison syndrome (E16.4)

K29.0 Acute gastritis

Use additional code to identify:

alcohol abuse and dependence (F10.-)

Excludes1: erosion (acute) of stomach (K25.-)

K29.00 Acute gastritis without bleeding

K29.01 Acute gastritis with bleeding

K29.2 Alcoholic gastritis

Use additional code to identify:

alcohol abuse and dependence (F10.-)

K29.20 Alcoholic gastritis without bleeding

K29.21 Alcoholic gastritis with bleeding

K29.3 Chronic superficial gastritis

K29.30 Chronic superficial gastritis without bleeding

K29.31 Chronic superficial gastritis with bleeding

K29.4 Chronic atrophic gastritis

Gastric atrophy

K29.40 Chronic atrophic gastritis without bleeding

K29.41 Chronic atrophic gastritis with bleeding

K29.5 Unspecified chronic gastritis

Chronic antral gastritis

Chronic fundal gastritis

K29.50 Unspecified chronic gastritis without bleeding

K29.51 Unspecified chronic gastritis with bleeding

K29.6 Other gastritis

Giant hypertrophic gastritis Granulomatous gastritis Ménétrier's disease

K29.60 Other gastritis without bleeding

K29.61 Other gastritis with bleeding

K29.7 Gastritis, unspecified

K29.70 Gastritis, unspecified, without bleeding

K29.71 Gastritis, unspecified, with bleeding

K29.8 Duodenitis

K29.80 Duodenitis without bleeding

K29.81 Duodenitis with bleeding

K29.9 Gastroduodenitis, unspecified

K29.90 Gastroduodenitis, unspecified, without bleeding

K29.91 Gastroduodenitis, unspecified, with bleeding

K30 Functional dyspepsia

Indigestion

Excludes1: dyspepsia NOS (R10.13)

heartburn (R12)

nervous dyspepsia (F45.8)

neurotic dyspepsia (F45.8)

psychogenic dyspepsia (F45.8)

K31 Other diseases of stomach and duodenum

Includes: functional disorders of stomach

Excludes2: diabetic gastroparesis (E08.43, E09.43, E10.43, E11.43, E13.43)

diverticulum of duodenum (K57.00-K57.13)

K31.0 Acute dilatation of stomach

Acute distention of stomach

K31.1 Adult hypertrophic pyloric stenosis

Pyloric stenosis NOS

Excludes1: congenital or infantile pyloric stenosis (Q40.0)

K31.2 Hourglass stricture and stenosis of stomach

Excludes1: congenital hourglass stomach (Q40.2)

hourglass contraction of stomach (K31.89)

K31.3 Pylorospasm, not elsewhere classified

> **Excludes1:** congenital or infantile pylorospasm (Q40.0)
>
> neurotic pylorospasm (F45.8)
>
> psychogenic pylorospasm (F45.8)

K31.4 Gastric diverticulum

> **Excludes1:** congenital diverticulum of stomach (Q40.2)

K31.5 Obstruction of duodenum

Constriction of duodenum

Duodenal ileus (chronic)

Stenosis of duodenum

Stricture of duodenum

Volvulus of duodenum

> **Excludes1:** congenital stenosis of duodenum (Q41.0)

K31.6 Fistula of stomach and duodenum

Gastrocolic fistula

Gastrojejunocolic fistula

K31.7 Polyp of stomach and duodenum

> **Excludes1:** adenomatous polyp of stomach (D13.1)

K31.8 Other specified diseases of stomach and duodenum

> **K31.81 Angiodysplasia of stomach and duodenum**
>
> > **K31.811 Angiodysplasia of stomach and duodenum with bleeding**
> >
> > **K31.819 Angiodysplasia of stomach and duodenum without bleeding**
> >
> > Angiodysplasia of stomach and duodenum NOS
>
> **K31.82 Dieulafoy lesion (hemorrhagic) of stomach and duodenum**
>
> > **Excludes2:** Dieulafoy lesion of intestine (K63.81)
>
> **K31.83 Achlorhydria**
>
> **K31.84 Gastroparesis**
>
> > Gastroparalysis
> >
> > **Code first** underlying disease, if known, such as:
> >
> > anorexia nervosa (F50.0-)
> >
> > diabetes mellitus (E08.43, E09.43, E10.43, E11.43, E13.43)
> >
> > scleroderma (M34.-)
>
> **K31.89 Other diseases of stomach and duodenum**

K31.9 Disease of stomach and duodenum, unspecified

DISEASES OF APPENDIX (K35-K38)

K35 Acute appendicitis

> **K35.2 Acute appendicitis with generalized peritonitis**
>
> Appendicitis (acute) with generalized (diffuse) peritonitis following rupture or perforation of appendix
>
> Perforated appendix NOS
>
> Ruptured appendix NOS
>
> **K35.3 Acute appendicitis with localized peritonitis**
>
> Acute appendicitis with or without perforation or rupture with peritonitis NOS
>
> Acute appendicitis with or without perforation or rupture with localized peritonitis
>
> Acute appendicitis with peritoneal abscess
>
> **K35.8 Other and unspecified acute appendicitis**
>
> > **K35.80 Unspecified acute appendicitis**
> >
> > Acute appendicitis NOS
> >
> > Acute appendicitis without (localized) (generalized) peritonitis

K35.89 Other acute appendicitis

K36 Other appendicitis

Chronic appendicitis

Recurrent appendicitis

K37 Unspecified appendicitis

> **Excludes1:** -unspecified appendicitis with peritonitis (K35.2-K35.3)

K38 Other diseases of appendix

> **K38.0 Hyperplasia of appendix**
>
> **K38.1 Appendicular concretions**
>
> Fecalith of appendix
>
> Stercolith of appendix
>
> **K38.2 Diverticulum of appendix**
>
> **K38.3 Fistula of appendix**
>
> **K38.8 Other specified diseases of appendix**
>
> Intussusception of appendix
>
> **K38.9 Disease of appendix, unspecified**

HERNIA (K40-K46)

Note: Hernia with both gangrene and obstruction is classified to hernia with gangrene.

Includes: acquired hernia

> congenital [except diaphragmatic or hiatus] hernia
>
> recurrent hernia

K40 Inguinal hernia

Includes: bubonocele

> direct inguinal hernia
>
> double inguinal hernia
>
> indirect inguinal hernia
>
> inguinal hernia NOS
>
> oblique inguinal hernia
>
> scrotal hernia

> **K40.0 Bilateral inguinal hernia, with obstruction, without gangrene**
>
> Inguinal hernia (bilateral) causing obstruction without gangrene
>
> Incarcerated inguinal hernia (bilateral) without gangrene
>
> Irreducible inguinal hernia (bilateral) without gangrene
>
> Strangulated inguinal hernia (bilateral) without gangrene
>
> > **K40.00 Bilateral inguinal hernia, with obstruction, without gangrene, not specified as recurrent**
> >
> > Bilateral inguinal hernia, with obstruction, without gangrene NOS
> >
> > **K40.01 Bilateral inguinal hernia, with obstruction, without gangrene, recurrent**
>
> **K40.1 Bilateral inguinal hernia, with gangrene**
>
> > **K40.10 Bilateral inguinal hernia, with gangrene, not specified as recurrent**
> >
> > Bilateral inguinal hernia, with gangrene NOS
> >
> > **K40.11 Bilateral inguinal hernia, with gangrene, recurrent**
>
> **K40.2 Bilateral inguinal hernia, without obstruction or gangrene**
>
> > **K40.20 Bilateral inguinal hernia, without obstruction or gangrene, not specified as recurrent**
> >
> > Bilateral inguinal hernia NOS
> >
> > **K40.21 Bilateral inguinal hernia, without obstruction or gangrene, recurrent**
>
> **K40.3 Unilateral inguinal hernia, with obstruction, without gangrene**

Inguinal hernia (unilateral) causing obstruction without gangrene

Incarcerated inguinal hernia (unilateral) without gangrene

Irreducible inguinal hernia (unilateral) without gangrene

Strangulated inguinal hernia (unilateral) without gangrene

K40.30 **Unilateral inguinal hernia, with obstruction, without gangrene, not specified as recurrent**

Inguinal hernia, with obstruction NOS

Unilateral inguinal hernia, with obstruction, without gangrene NOS

K40.31 **Unilateral inguinal hernia, with obstruction, without gangrene, recurrent**

K40.4 **Unilateral inguinal hernia, with gangrene**

K40.40 **Unilateral inguinal hernia, with gangrene, not specified as recurrent**

Inguinal hernia with gangrene NOS

Unilateral inguinal hernia with gangrene NOS

K40.41 **Unilateral inguinal hernia, with gangrene, recurrent**

K40.9 **Unilateral inguinal hernia, without obstruction or gangrene**

K40.90 **Unilateral inguinal hernia, without obstruction or gangrene, not specified as recurrent**

Inguinal hernia NOS

Unilateral inguinal hernia NOS

K40.91 **Unilateral inguinal hernia, without obstruction or gangrene, recurrent**

K41 **Femoral hernia**

K41.0 **Bilateral femoral hernia, with obstruction, without gangrene**

Femoral hernia (bilateral) causing obstruction, without gangrene

Incarcerated femoral hernia (bilateral), without gangrene

Irreducible femoral hernia (bilateral), without gangrene

Strangulated femoral hernia (bilateral), without gangrene

K41.00 **Bilateral femoral hernia, with obstruction, without gangrene, not specified as recurrent**

Bilateral femoral hernia, with obstruction, without gangrene NOS

K41.01 **Bilateral femoral hernia, with obstruction, without gangrene, recurrent**

K41.1 **Bilateral femoral hernia, with gangrene**

K41.10 **Bilateral femoral hernia, with gangrene, not specified as recurrent**

Bilateral femoral hernia, with gangrene NOS

K41.11 **Bilateral femoral hernia, with gangrene, recurrent**

K41.2 **Bilateral femoral hernia, without obstruction or gangrene**

K41.20 **Bilateral femoral hernia, without obstruction or gangrene, not specified as recurrent**

Bilateral femoral hernia NOS

K41.21 **Bilateral femoral hernia, without obstruction or gangrene, recurrent**

K41.3 **Unilateral femoral hernia, with obstruction, without gangrene**

Femoral hernia (unilateral) causing obstruction, without gangrene

Incarcerated femoral hernia (unilateral), without gangrene

Irreducible femoral hernia (unilateral), without gangrene

Strangulated femoral hernia (unilateral), without gangrene

K41.30 **Unilateral femoral hernia, with obstruction, without gangrene, not specified as recurrent**

Femoral hernia, with obstruction NOS

Unilateral femoral hernia, with obstruction NOS

K41.31 **Unilateral femoral hernia, with obstruction, without gangrene, recurrent**

K41.4 **Unilateral femoral hernia, with gangrene**

K41.40 **Unilateral femoral hernia, with gangrene, not specified as recurrent**

Femoral hernia, with gangrene NOS

Unilateral femoral hernia, with gangrene NOS

K41.41 **Unilateral femoral hernia, with gangrene, recurrent**

K41.9 **Unilateral femoral hernia, without obstruction or gangrene**

K41.90 **Unilateral femoral hernia, without obstruction or gangrene, not specified as recurrent**

Femoral hernia NOS

Unilateral femoral hernia NOS

K41.91 **Unilateral femoral hernia, without obstruction or gangrene, recurrent**

K42 **Umbilical hernia**

Includes: paraumbilical hernia

Excludes1: omphalocele (Q79.2)

K42.0 **Umbilical hernia with obstruction, without gangrene**

Umbilical hernia causing obstruction, without gangrene

Incarcerated umbilical hernia, without gangrene

Irreducible umbilical hernia, without gangrene

Strangulated umbilical hernia, without gangrene

K42.1 **Umbilical hernia with gangrene**

Gangrenous umbilical hernia

K42.9 **Umbilical hernia without obstruction or gangrene**

Umbilical hernia NOS

K43 **Ventral hernia**

K43.0 **Incisional hernia with obstruction, without gangrene**

Incisional hernia causing obstruction, without gangrene

Incarcerated incisional hernia, without gangrene

Irreducible incisional hernia, without gangrene

Strangulated incisional hernia, without gangrene

K43.1 **Incisional hernia with gangrene**

Gangrenous incisional hernia

K43.2 **Incisional hernia without obstruction or gangrene**

Incisional hernia NOS

K43.3 **Parastomal hernia with obstruction, without gangrene**

Incarcerated parastomal hernia, without gangrene

Irreducible parastomal hernia, without gangrene

Parastomal hernia causing obstruction, without gangrene

Strangulated parastomal hernia, without gangrene

K43.4 **Parastomal hernia with gangrene**

Gangrenous parastomal hernia

K43.5 **Parastomal hernia without obstruction or gangrene**

Parastomal hernia NOS

K43.6 **Other and unspecified ventral hernia with obstruction, without gangrene**

Epigastric hernia causing obstruction, without gangrene

Hypogastric hernia causing obstruction, without gangrene

Incarcerated epigastric hernia without gangrene

Incarcerated hypogastric hernia without gangrene

Incarcerated midline hernia without gangrene

Incarcerated spigelian hernia without gangrene

Incarcerated subxiphoid hernia without gangrene

Irreducible epigastric hernia without gangrene

Irreducible hypogastric hernia without gangrene

Irreducible midline hernia without gangrene

Irreducible spigelian hernia without gangrene

Irreducible subxiphoid hernia without gangrene

Midline hernia causing obstruction, without gangrene

Spigelian hernia causing obstruction, without gangrene

Strangulated epigastric hernia without gangrene

Strangulated hypogastric hernia without gangrene

Strangulated midline hernia without gangrene

Strangulated spigelian hernia without gangrene

Strangulated subxiphoid hernia without gangrene

Subxiphoid hernia causing obstruction, without gangrene

K43.7 **Other and unspecified ventral hernia with gangrene**

Any condition listed under K43.6 specified as gangrenous

K43.9 **Ventral hernia without obstruction or gangrene**

Epigastric hernia

Ventral hernia NOS

K44 **Diaphragmatic hernia**

Includes: hiatus hernia (esophageal) (sliding)

paraesophageal hernia

Excludes1: congenital diaphragmatic hernia (Q79.0)

congenital hiatus hernia (Q40.1)

K44.0 **Diaphragmatic hernia with obstruction, without gangrene**

Diaphragmatic hernia causing obstruction

Incarcerated diaphragmatic hernia

Irreducible diaphragmatic hernia

Strangulated diaphragmatic hernia

K44.1 **Diaphragmatic hernia with gangrene**

Gangrenous diaphragmatic hernia

K44.9 **Diaphragmatic hernia without obstruction or gangrene**

Diaphragmatic hernia NOS

K45 **Other abdominal hernia**

Includes: abdominal hernia, specified site NEC

lumbar hernia

obturator hernia

pudendal hernia

retroperitoneal hernia

sciatic hernia

K45.0 **Other specified abdominal hernia with obstruction, without gangrene**

Other specified abdominal hernia causing obstruction

Other specified incarcerated abdominal hernia

Other specified irreducible abdominal hernia

Other specified strangulated abdominal hernia

K45.1 **Other specified abdominal hernia with gangrene**

Any condition listed under K45 specified as gangrenous

K45.8 **Other specified abdominal hernia without obstruction or gangrene**

K46 **Unspecified abdominal hernia**

Includes: enterocele

epiplocele hernia NOS

interstitial hernia

intestinal hernia

intra-abdominal hernia

Excludes1: vaginal enterocele (N81.5)

K46.0 **Unspecified abdominal hernia with obstruction, without gangrene**

Unspecified abdominal hernia causing obstruction

Unspecified incarcerated abdominal hernia

Unspecified irreducible abdominal hernia

Unspecified strangulated abdominal hernia

K46.1 **Unspecified abdominal hernia with gangrene**

Any condition listed under K46 specified as gangrenous

K46.9 **Unspecified abdominal hernia without obstruction or gangrene**

Abdominal hernia NOS

NONINFECTIVE ENTERITIS AND COLITIS (K50-K52)

Includes: noninfective inflammatory bowel disease

Excludes1: irritable bowel syndrome (K58.-)

megacolon (K59.3-)

K50 **Crohn's disease [regional enteritis]**

Includes: granulomatous enteritis

Use additional code to identify manifestations, such as:

pyoderma gangrenosum (L88)

Excludes1: ulcerative colitis (K51.-)

K50.0 **Crohn's disease of small intestine**

Crohn's disease [regional enteritis] of duodenum

Crohn's disease [regional enteritis] of ileum

Crohn's disease [regional enteritis] of jejunum

Regional ileitis

Terminal ileitis

Excludes1: Crohn's disease of both small and large intestine (K50.8-)

K50.00 **Crohn's disease of small intestine without complications**

K50.01 **Crohn's disease of small intestine with complications**

K50.011 **Crohn's disease of small intestine with rectal bleeding**

K50.012 **Crohn's disease of small intestine with intestinal obstruction**

K50.013 **Crohn's disease of small intestine with fistula**

K50.014 **Crohn's disease of small intestine with abscess**

K50.018 **Crohn's disease of small intestine with other complication**

K50.019 **Crohn's disease of small intestine with unspecified complications**

K50.1 **Crohn's disease of large intestine**

Crohn's disease [regional enteritis] of colon

Crohn's disease [regional enteritis] of large bowel

Crohn's disease [regional enteritis] of rectum

Granulomatous colitis

Regional colitis

Excludes1: Crohn's disease of both small and large intestine (K50.8)

K50.10 **Crohn's disease of large intestine without complications**

K50.11 **Crohn's disease of large intestine with complications**

K50.111   Crohn's disease of large intestine with rectal bleeding

K50.112   Crohn's disease of large intestine with intestinal obstruction

K50.113   Crohn's disease of large intestine with fistula

K50.114   Crohn's disease of large intestine with abscess

K50.118   Crohn's disease of large intestine with other complication

K50.119   Crohn's disease of large intestine with unspecified complications

K50.8   Crohn's disease of both small and large intestine

K50.80   Crohn's disease of both small and large intestine without complications

K50.81   Crohn's disease of both small and large intestine with complications

K50.811   Crohn's disease of both small and large intestine with rectal bleeding

K50.812   Crohn's disease of both small and large intestine with intestinal obstruction

K50.813   Crohn's disease of both small and large intestine with fistula

K50.814   Crohn's disease of both small and large intestine with abscess

K50.818   Crohn's disease of both small and large intestine with other complication

K50.819   Crohn's disease of both small and large intestine with unspecified complications

K50.9   Crohn's disease, unspecified

K50.90   Crohn's disease, unspecified, without complications

Crohn's disease NOS

Regional enteritis NOS

K50.91   Crohn's disease, unspecified, with complications

K50.911   Crohn's disease, unspecified, with rectal bleeding

K50.912   Crohn's disease, unspecified, with intestinal obstruction

K50.913   Crohn's disease, unspecified, with fistula

K50.914   Crohn's disease, unspecified, with abscess

K50.918   Crohn's disease, unspecified, with other complication

K50.919   Crohn's disease, unspecified, with unspecified complications

K51   Ulcerative colitis

Definition: Ulcerative colitis ulcerative colitis is a form of inflammatory bowel disease (IBD). It causes swelling, ulcerations, and loss of function of the large intestine.

Use additional code to identify manifestations, such as: pyoderma gangrenosum (L88)

Excludes1: Crohn's disease [regional enteritis] (K50.-)

K51.0   Ulcerative (chronic) pancolitis

Backwash ileitis

K51.00   Ulcerative (chronic) pancolitis without complications

Ulcerative (chronic) pancolitis NOS

K51.01   Ulcerative (chronic) pancolitis with complications

K51.011   Ulcerative (chronic) pancolitis with rectal bleeding

K51.012   Ulcerative (chronic) pancolitis with intestinal obstruction

K51.013   Ulcerative (chronic) pancolitis with fistula

K51.014   Ulcerative (chronic) pancolitis with abscess

K51.018   Ulcerative (chronic) pancolitis with other complication

K51.019   Ulcerative (chronic) pancolitis with unspecified complications

K51.2   Ulcerative (chronic) proctitis

K51.20   Ulcerative (chronic) proctitis without complications

Ulcerative (chronic) proctitis NOS

K51.21   Ulcerative (chronic) proctitis with complications

K51.211   Ulcerative (chronic) proctitis with rectal bleeding

K51.212   Ulcerative (chronic) proctitis with intestinal obstruction

K51.213   Ulcerative (chronic) proctitis with fistula

K51.214   Ulcerative (chronic) proctitis with abscess

K51.218   Ulcerative (chronic) proctitis with other complication

K51.219   Ulcerative (chronic) proctitis with unspecified complications

K51.3   Ulcerative (chronic) rectosigmoiditis

K51.30   Ulcerative (chronic) rectosigmoiditis without complications

Ulcerative (chronic) rectosigmoiditis NOS

K51.31   Ulcerative (chronic) rectosigmoiditis with complications

K51.311   Ulcerative (chronic) rectosigmoiditis with rectal bleeding

K51.312   Ulcerative (chronic) rectosigmoiditis with intestinal obstruction

K51.313   Ulcerative (chronic) rectosigmoiditis with fistula

K51.314   Ulcerative (chronic) rectosigmoiditis with abscess

K51.318   Ulcerative (chronic) rectosigmoiditis with other complication

K51.319   Ulcerative (chronic) rectosigmoiditis with unspecified complications

K51.4   Inflammatory polyps of colon

Excludes1: adenomatous polyp of colon (D12.6)

polyposis of colon (D12.6) polyps of colon NOS (K63.5)

K51.40   Inflammatory polyps of colon without complications

Inflammatory polyps of colon NOS

K51.41   Inflammatory polyps of colon with complications

K51.411   Inflammatory polyps of colon with rectal bleeding

K51.412   Inflammatory polyps of colon with intestinal obstruction

K51.413 Inflammatory polyps of colon with fistula

K51.414 Inflammatory polyps of colon with abscess

K51.418 Inflammatory polyps of colon with other complication

K51.419 Inflammatory polyps of colon with unspecified complications

K51.5 **Left sided colitis**

Left Hemicolitis

K51.50 **Left sided colitis without complications**

Left sided colitis NOS

K51.51 **Left sided colitis with complications**

K51.511 Left sided colitis with rectal bleeding

K51.512 Left sided colitis with intestinal obstruction

K51.513 Left sided colitis with fistula

K51.514 Left sided colitis with abscess

K51.518 Left sided colitis with other complication

K51.519 Left sided colitis with unspecified complications

K51.8 **Other ulcerative colitis**

K51.80 **Other ulcerative colitis without complications**

K51.81 **Other ulcerative colitis with complications**

K51.811 Other ulcerative colitis with rectal bleeding

K51.812 Other ulcerative colitis with intestinal obstruction

K51.813 Other ulcerative colitis with fistula

K51.814 Other ulcerative colitis with abscess

K51.818 Other ulcerative colitis with other complication

K51.819 Other ulcerative colitis with unspecified complications

K51.9 **Ulcerative colitis, unspecified**

K51.90 **Ulcerative colitis, unspecified, without complications**

K51.91 **Ulcerative colitis, unspecified, with complications**

K51.911 Ulcerative colitis, unspecified with rectal bleeding

K51.912 Ulcerative colitis, unspecified with intestinal obstruction

K51.913 Ulcerative colitis, unspecified with fistula

K51.914 Ulcerative colitis, unspecified with abscess

K51.918 Ulcerative colitis, unspecified with other complication

K51.919 Ulcerative colitis, unspecified with unspecified complications

K52 **Other and unspecified noninfective gastroenteritis and colitis**

K52.0 **Gastroenteritis and colitis due to radiation**

K52.1 **Toxic gastroenteritis and colitis**

Drug-induced gastroenteritis and colitis

Code first (T51-T65) to identify toxic agent

Use additional code for adverse effect, if applicable, to identify drug (T36-T50 with fifth or sixth character 5)

K52.2 **Allergic and dietetic gastroenteritis and colitis**

Food hypersensitivity gastroenteritis or colitis

Use additional code to identify type of food allergy (Z91.01-, Z91.02-)

Excludes2: allergic eosinophilic colitis (K52.82)

allergic eosinophilic esophagitis (K20.0)

allergic eosinophilic gastritis (K52.81)

allergic eosinophilic gastroenteritis (K52.81)

food protein-induced proctocolitis (K52.82)

K52.21 **Food protein-induced enterocolitis syndrome**

Use additional code for hypovolemic shock, if present (R57.1)

K52.22 **Food protein-induced enteropathy**

K52.29 **Other allergic and dietetic gastroenteritis and colitis**

Food hypersensitivity gastroenteritis or colitis

Immediate gastrointestinal hypersensitivity

K52.3 **Indeterminate colitis**

Colonic inflammatory bowel disease unclassified (IBDU)

Excludes1: unspecified colitis (K52.9)

K52.8 **Other specified noninfective gastroenteritis and colitis**

K52.81 **Eosinophilic gastritis or gastroenteritis**

Eosinophilic enteritis

Excludes2: eosinophilic esophagitis (K20.0)

K52.82 **Eosinophilic colitis**

Allergic proctocolitis

Food-induced eosinophilic proctocolitis

Food protein-induced proctocolitis

Milk protein-induced proctocolitis

K52.83 **Microscopic colitis**

K52.831 Collagenous colitis

K52.832 Lymphocytic colitis

K52.838 Other microscopic colitis

K52.839 Microscopic colitis, unspecified

K52.89 **Other specified noninfective gastroenteritis and colitis**

K52.9 **Noninfective gastroenteritis and colitis, unspecified**

Colitis NOS

Enteritis NOS

Gastroenteritis NOS

Ileitis NOS

Jejunitis NOS

Sigmoiditis NOS

Excludes1: diarrhea NOS (R19.7)

functional diarrhea (K59.1)

infectious gastroenteritis and colitis NOS (A09)

neonatal diarrhea (noninfective) (P78.3)

psychogenic diarrhea (F45.8)

OTHER DISEASES OF INTESTINES (K55-K64)

K55 **Vascular disorders of intestine**

Excludes1: necrotizing enterocolitis of newborn (P77.-)

K55.0 **Acute vascular disorders of intestine**

Infarction of appendices epiploicae

Mesenteric (artery) (vein) embolism

Mesenteric (artery) (vein) infarction

Mesenteric (artery) (vein) thrombosis

K55.01 **Acute (reversible) ischemia of small intestine**

K55.011 Focal (segmental) acute (reversible) ischemia of small intestine

● New code   ▲ Revised code   **Excludes1:** Not coded here   **Excludes2:** Not included here   ⊗ Placeholder required   ⑦7th digit required

K55.012 Diffuse acute (reversible) ischemia of small intestine

K55.019 Acute (reversible) ischemia of small intestine, extent unspecified

K55.02 Acute infarction of small intestine

Gangrene of small intestine

Necrosis of small intestine

K55.021 Focal (segmental) acute infarction of small intestine

K55.022 Diffuse acute infarction of small intestine

K55.029 Acute infarction of small intestine, extent unspecified

K55.03 Acute (reversible) ischemia of large intestine

Acute fulminant ischemic colitis

Subacute ischemic colitis

K55.031 Focal (segmental) acute (reversible) ischemia of large intestine

K55.032 Diffuse acute (reversible) ischemia of large intestine

K55.039 Acute (reversible) ischemia of large intestine, extent unspecified

K55.04 Acute infarction of large intestine

Gangrene of large intestine

Necrosis of large intestine

K55.041 Focal (segmental) acute infarction of large intestine

K55.042 Diffuse acute infarction of large intestine

K55.049 Acute infarction of large intestine, extent unspecified

K55.05 Acute (reversible) ischemia of intestine, part unspecified

K55.051 Focal (segmental) acute (reversible) ischemia of intestine, part unspecified

K55.052 Diffuse acute (reversible) ischemia of intestine, part unspecified

K55.059 Acute (reversible) ischemia of intestine, part and extent unspecified

K55.06 Acute infarction of intestine, part unspecified

Acute intestinal infarction

Gangrene of intestine

Necrosis of intestine

K55.061 Focal (segmental) acute infarction of intestine, part unspecified

K55.062 Diffuse acute infarction of intestine, part unspecified

K55.069 Acute infarction of intestine, part and extent unspecified

K55.1 **Chronic vascular disorders of intestine**

Chronic ischemic colitis

Chronic ischemic enteritis

Chronic ischemic enterocolitis

Ischemic stricture of intestine

Mesenteric atherosclerosis

Mesenteric vascular insufficiency

K55.2 **Angiodysplasia of colon**

K55.20 Angiodysplasia of colon without hemorrhage

K55.21 Angiodysplasia of colon with hemorrhage

K55.3 **Necrotizing enterocolitis**

Excludes1: necrotizing enterocolitis of newborn (P77.-)

Excludes2: necrotizing enterocolitis due to Clostridium difficile (A04.7-)

K55.30 Necrotizing enterocolitis, unspecified

Necrotizing enterocolitis, NOS

K55.31 Stage 1 necrotizing enterocolitis

Necrotizing enterocolitis without pneumatosis, without perforation

K55.32 Stage 2 necrotizing enterocolitis

Necrotizing enterocolitis with pneumatosis, without perforation

K55.33 Stage 3 necrotizing enterocolitis

Necrotizing enterocolitis with perforation

Necrotizing enterocolitis with pneumatosis and perforation

K55.8 **Other vascular disorders of intestine**

K55.9 **Vascular disorder of intestine, unspecified**

Ischemic colitis Ischemic enteritis

Ischemic enterocolitis

K56 **Paralytic ileus and intestinal obstruction without hernia**

Excludes1: congenital stricture or stenosis of intestine (Q41-Q42)

cystic fibrosis with meconium ileus (E84.11)

ischemic stricture of intestine (K55.1)

meconium ileus NOS (P76.0)

neonatal intestinal obstructions classifiable to P76.-

obstruction of duodenum (K31.5)

postprocedural intestinal obstruction (K91.3-)

stenosis of anus or rectum (K62.4)

K56.0 **Paralytic ileus**

Paralysis of bowel

Paralysis of colon

Paralysis of intestine

Excludes1: gallstone ileus (K56.3)

ileus NOS (K56.7)

obstructive ileus NOS (K56.69-)

K56.1 **Intussusception**

Intussusception or invagination of bowel

Intussusception or invagination of colon

Intussusception or invagination of intestine

Intussusception or invagination of rectum

Excludes2: intussusception of appendix (K38.8)

K56.2 **Volvulus**

Strangulation of colon or intestine

Torsion of colon or intestine

Twist of colon or intestine

Excludes2: volvulus of duodenum (K31.5)

K56.3 **Gallstone ileus**

Obstruction of intestine by gallstone

K56.4 **Other impaction of intestine**

K56.41 Fecal impaction

Excludes1: constipation (K59.0-)

incomplete defecation (R15.0)

K56.49 Other impaction of intestine

▲**K56.5** **Intestinal adhesions [bands] with obstruction (postprocedural) (postinfection)**

Abdominal hernia due to adhesions with obstruction

Peritoneal adhesions [bands] with intestinal obstruction (postinfection)

● **K56.50** **Intestinal adhesions [bands], unspecified as to partial versus complete obstruction**

Intestinal adhesions with obstruction NOS

● **K56.51** **Intestinal adhesions [bands], with partial obstruction**

Intestinal adhesions with incomplete obstruction

● **K56.52** **Intestinal adhesions [bands] with complete obstruction**

K56.6 **Other and unspecified intestinal obstruction**

K56.60 **Unspecified intestinal obstruction**

Excludes1: intestinal obstruction due to specified condition-code to condition

● **K56.600** **Partial intestinal obstruction, unspecified as to cause**

Incomplete intestinal obstruction, NOS

● **K56.601** **Complete intestinal obstruction, unspecified as to cause**

● **K56.609** **Unspecified intestinal obstruction, unspecified as to partial versus complete obstruction**

Intestinal obstruction NOS

K56.69 **Other intestinal obstruction**

Enterostenosis NOS

Obstructive ileus NOS

Occlusion of colon or intestine NOS

Stenosis of colon or intestine NOS

Stricture of colon or intestine NOS

Excludes1: intestinal obstruction due to specified condition-code to condition

● **K56.690** **Other partial intestinal obstruction**

Other incomplete intestinal obstruction

● **K56.691** **Other complete intestinal obstruction**

● **K56.699** **Other intestinal obstruction unspecified as to partial versus complete obstruction**

Other intestinal obstruction, NEC

K56.7 **Ileus, unspecified**

Excludes1: obstructive ileus (K56.69-)

Excludes2: intestinal obstruction with hernia (K40-K46)

K57 **Diverticular disease of intestine**

Definition: Diverticulitis is a common digestive disease which involves the formation of pouches (diverticula) within the bowel wall. This process is known as diverticulosis, and typically occurs within the large intestine, or colon, although it can occasionally occur in the small intestine as well. Diverticulitis results when one of these diverticula becomes inflamed.

Excludes1: congenital diverticulum of intestine (Q43.8)

Meckel's diverticulum (Q43.0)

Excludes2: diverticulum of appendix (K38.2)

K57.0 **Diverticulitis of small intestine with perforation and abscess**

Diverticulitis of small intestine with peritonitis

Excludes1: diverticulitis of both small and large intestine with perforation and abscess (K57.4-)

K57.00 **Diverticulitis of small intestine with perforation and abscess without bleeding**

K57.01 **Diverticulitis of small intestine with perforation and abscess with bleeding**

K57.1 **Diverticular disease of small intestine without perforation or abscess**

Excludes1: diverticular disease of both small and large intestine without perforation or abscess (K57.5-)

K57.10 **Diverticulosis of small intestine without perforation or abscess without bleeding**

Diverticular disease of small intestine NOS

K57.11 **Diverticulosis of small intestine without perforation or abscess with bleeding**

K57.12 **Diverticulitis of small intestine without perforation or abscess without bleeding**

K57.13 **Diverticulitis of small intestine without perforation or abscess with bleeding**

K57.2 **Diverticulitis of large intestine with perforation and abscess**

Diverticulitis of colon with peritonitis

Excludes1: diverticulitis of both small and large intestine with perforation and abscess (K57.4-)

K57.20 **Diverticulitis of large intestine with perforation and abscess without bleeding**

K57.21 **Diverticulitis of large intestine with perforation and abscess with bleeding**

K57.3 **Diverticular disease of large intestine without perforation or abscess**

Excludes1: diverticular disease of both small and large intestine without perforation or abscess (K57.5-)

K57.30 **Diverticulosis of large intestine without perforation or abscess without bleeding**

Diverticular disease of colon NOS

K57.31 **Diverticulosis of large intestine without perforation or abscess with bleeding**

K57.32 **Diverticulitis of large intestine without perforation or abscess without bleeding**

K57.33 **Diverticulitis of large intestine without perforation or abscess with bleeding**

K57.4 **Diverticulitis of both small and large intestine with perforation and abscess**

Diverticulitis of both small and large intestine with peritonitis

K57.40 **Diverticulitis of both small and large intestine with perforation and abscess without bleeding**

K57.41 **Diverticulitis of both small and large intestine with perforation and abscess with bleeding**

K57.5 **Diverticular disease of both small and large intestine without perforation or abscess**

K57.50 **Diverticulosis of both small and large intestine without perforation or abscess without bleeding**

Diverticular disease of both small and large intestine NOS

K57.51 **Diverticulosis of both small and large intestine without perforation or abscess with bleeding**

K57.52 **Diverticulitis of both small and large intestine without perforation or abscess without bleeding**

K57.53 **Diverticulitis of both small and large intestine without perforation or abscess with bleeding**

K57.8 **Diverticulitis of intestine, part unspecified, with perforation and abscess**

Diverticulitis of intestine NOS with peritonitis

K57.80 **Diverticulitis of intestine, part unspecified, with perforation and abscess without bleeding**

K57.81 **Diverticulitis of intestine, part unspecified, with perforation and abscess with bleeding**

K57.9 **Diverticular disease of intestine, part unspecified, without perforation or abscess**

   K57.90 **Diverticulosis of intestine, part unspecified, without perforation or abscess without bleeding**

   Diverticular disease of intestine NOS

   K57.91 **Diverticulosis of intestine, part unspecified, without perforation or abscess with bleeding**

   K57.92 **Diverticulitis of intestine, part unspecified, without perforation or abscess without bleeding**

   K57.93 **Diverticulitis of intestine, part unspecified, without perforation or abscess with bleeding**

K58 **Irritable bowel syndrome**

Includes: irritable colon

   spastic colon

K58.0 **Irritable bowel syndrome with diarrhea**

K58.1 **Irritable bowel syndrome with constipation**

K58.2 **Mixed irritable bowel syndrome**

K58.8 **Other irritable bowel syndrome**

K58.9 **Irritable bowel syndrome without diarrhea**

   Irritable bowel syndrome NOS

K59 **Other functional intestinal disorders**

Excludes1: change in bowel habit NOS (R19.4)

   intestinal malabsorption (K90.-)

   psychogenic intestinal disorders (F45.8)

Excludes2: functional disorders of stomach (K31.-)

K59.0 **Constipation**

   Use additional code for adverse effect, if applicable, to identify drug (T36-T50 with fifth or sixth character 5)

   Excludes1: fecal impaction (K56.41)

     incomplete defecation (R15.0)

   K59.00 **Constipation, unspecified**

   K59.01 **Slow transit constipation**

   K59.02 **Outlet dysfunction constipation**

   K59.03 **Drug induced constipation**

     Use additional code for adverse effect, if applicable, to identify drug (T36-T50 with fifth or sixth character 5

   K59.04 **Chronic idiopathic constipation**

     Functional constipation

   K59.09 **Other constipation**

     Chronic constipation

K59.1 **Functional diarrhea**

   Excludes1: diarrhea NOS (R19.7)

     irritable bowel syndrome with diarrhea (K58.0)

K59.2 **Neurogenic bowel, not elsewhere classified**

K59.3 **Megacolon, not elsewhere classified**

   Dilatation of colon

   Code first, if applicable (T51-T65) to identify toxic agent

   Excludes1: congenital megacolon (aganglionic) (Q43.1)

     megacolon (due to) (in) Chagas' disease (B57.32)

     megacolon (due to) (in) Clostridium difficile (A04.7-)

     megacolon (due to) (in) Hirschsprung's disease (Q43.1)

   K59.31 **Toxic megacolon**

   K59.39 **Other megacolon**

     Megacolon NOS

K59.4 **Anal spasm**

   Proctalgia fugax

K59.8 **Other specified functional intestinal disorders**

   Atony of colon

   Pseudo-obstruction (acute) (chronic) of intestine

K59.9 **Functional intestinal disorder, unspecified**

K60 **Fissure and fistula of anal and rectal regions**

Excludes1: fissure and fistula of anal and rectal regions with abscess or cellulitis (K61.-)

Excludes2: anal sphincter tear (healed) (nontraumatic) (old) (K62.81)

K60.0 **Acute anal fissure**

K60.1 **Chronic anal fissure**

K60.2 **Anal fissure, unspecified**

K60.3 **Anal fistula**

K60.4 **Rectal fistula**

   Fistula of rectum to skin

   Excludes1: rectovaginal fistula (N82.3)

     vesicorectal fistula (N32.1)

K60.5 **Anorectal fistula**

K61 **Abscess of anal and rectal regions**

Includes: abscess of anal and rectal regions

   cellulitis of anal and rectal regions

K61.0 **Anal abscess**

   Perianal abscess

   Excludes1: intrasphincteric abscess (K61.4)

K61.1 **Rectal abscess**

   Perirectal abscess

   Excludes1: ischiorectal abscess (K61.3)

K61.2 **Anorectal abscess**

K61.3 **Ischiorectal abscess**

   Abscess of ischiorectal fossa

K61.4 **Intrasphincteric abscess**

K62 **Other diseases of anus and rectum**

Includes: anal canal

Excludes2: colostomy and enterostomy malfunction (K94.0-, K94.1-)

   fecal incontinence (R15.-)

   hemorrhoids (K64.-)

K62.0 **Anal polyp**

K62.1 **Rectal polyp**

   Excludes1: adenomatous polyp (D12.8)

K62.2 **Anal prolapse**

   Prolapse of anal canal

K62.3 **Rectal prolapse**

   Prolapse of rectal mucosa

K62.4 **Stenosis of anus and rectum**

   Stricture of anus (sphincter)

K62.5 **Hemorrhage of anus and rectum**

   Excludes1: gastrointestinal bleeding NOS (K92.2)

     melena (K92.1)

     neonatal rectal hemorrhage (P54.2)

K62.6 **Ulcer of anus and rectum**

   Solitary ulcer of anus and rectum

   Stercoral ulcer of anus and rectum

   Excludes1: fissure and fistula of anus and rectum (K60.-)

     ulcerative colitis (K51.-)

K62.7 **Radiation proctitis**

   Use additional code to identify the type of radiation (W90.-)

K62.8   **Other specified diseases of anus and rectum**

>   **Excludes2:** ulcerative proctitis (K51.2)

>   **K62.81**   **Anal sphincter tear (healed) (nontraumatic) (old)**
>
>   Tear of anus, nontraumatic
>
>   **Use additional code** for any associated fecal incontinence (R15.-)
>
>   >   **Excludes2:** anal fissure (K60.-)
>   >
>   >   anal sphincter tear (healed) (old) complicating delivery (O34.7-)
>   >
>   >   traumatic tear of anal sphincter (S31.831)

>   **K62.82**   **Dysplasia of anus**
>
>   Anal intraepithelial neoplasia I and II (AIN I and II) (histologically confirmed)
>
>   Dysplasia of anus NOS
>
>   Mild and moderate dysplasia of anus (histologically confirmed)
>
>   >   **Excludes1:** abnormal results from anal cytologic examination without histologic confirmation (R85.61-)
>   >
>   >   anal intraepithelial neoplasia III (D01.3)
>   >
>   >   carcinoma in situ of anus (D01.3)
>   >
>   >   HGSIL of anus (R85.613)
>   >
>   >   severe dysplasia of anus (D01.3)

>   **K62.89**   **Other specified diseases of anus and rectum**
>
>   Proctitis NOS
>
>   **Use additional code** for any associated fecal incontinence (R15.-)

K62.9   **Disease of anus and rectum, unspecified**

K63   **Other diseases of intestine**

K63.0   **Abscess of intestine**

>   **Excludes1:** abscess of intestine with Crohn's disease (K50.014, K50.114, K50.814, K50.914,)
>
>   abscess of intestine with diverticular disease (K57.0, K57.2, K57.4, K57.8)
>
>   abscess of intestine with ulcerative colitis (K51.014, K51.214, K51.314, K51.414, K51.514, K51.814, K51.914)
>
>   **Excludes2:** abscess of anal and rectal regions (K61.-)
>
>   abscess of appendix (K35.3)

K63.1   **Perforation of intestine (nontraumatic)**

>   Perforation (nontraumatic) of rectum
>
>   **Excludes1:** perforation (nontraumatic) of duodenum (K26.-)
>
>   perforation (nontraumatic) of intestine with diverticular disease (K57.0, K57.2, K57.4, K57.8)
>
>   **Excludes2:** perforation (nontraumatic) of appendix (K35.2, K35.3)

K63.2   **Fistula of intestine**

>   **Excludes1:** fistula of duodenum (K31.6)
>
>   fistula of intestine with Crohn's disease (K50.013, K50.113, K50.813, K50.913,)
>
>   fistula of intestine with ulcerative colitis (K51.013, K51.213, K51.313, K51.413, K51.513, K51.813, K51.913)
>
>   **Excludes2:** fistula of anal and rectal regions (K60.-)
>
>   fistula of appendix (K38.3)
>
>   intestinal-genital fistula, female (N82.2-N82.4)
>
>   vesicointestinal fistula (N32.1)

K63.3   **Ulcer of intestine**

Primary ulcer of small intestine

>   **Excludes1:** duodenal ulcer (K26.-)
>
>   gastrointestinal ulcer (K28.-)
>
>   gastrojejunal ulcer (K28.-)
>
>   jejunal ulcer (K28.-)
>
>   peptic ulcer, site unspecified (K27.-)
>
>   ulcer of intestine with perforation (K63.1)
>
>   ulcer of anus or rectum (K62.6)
>
>   ulcerative colitis (K51.-)

K63.4   **Enteroptosis**

K63.5   **Polyp of colon**

>   **Excludes1:** adenomatous polyp of colon (D12.6)
>
>   inflammatory polyp of colon (K51.4-)
>
>   polyposis of colon (D12.6)

K63.8   **Other specified diseases of intestine**

>   **K63.81**   **Dieulafoy lesion of intestine**
>
>   >   **Excludes2:** Dieulafoy lesion of stomach and duodenum (K31.82)

>   **K63.89**   **Other specified diseases of intestine**

K63.9   **Disease of intestine, unspecified**

K64   **Hemorrhoids and perianal venous thrombosis**

Includes: piles

Excludes1: hemorrhoids complicating childbirth and the puerperium (O87.2)

>   hemorrhoids complicating pregnancy (O22.4)

K64.0   **First degree hemorrhoids**

>   Grade/stage I hemorrhoids
>
>   Hemorrhoids (bleeding) without prolapse outside of anal canal

K64.1   **Second degree hemorrhoids**

>   Grade/stage II hemorrhoids
>
>   Hemorrhoids (bleeding) that prolapse with straining, but retract spontaneously

K64.2   **Third degree hemorrhoids**

>   Grade/stage III hemorrhoids
>
>   Hemorrhoids (bleeding) that prolapse with straining and require manual replacement back inside anal canal

K64.3   **Fourth degree hemorrhoids**

>   Grade/stage IV hemorrhoids
>
>   Hemorrhoids (bleeding) with prolapsed tissue that cannot be manually replaced

K64.4   **Residual hemorrhoidal skin tags**

>   External hemorrhoids, NOS
>
>   Skin tags of anus

K64.5   **Perianal venous thrombosis**

>   External hemorrhoids with thrombosis
>
>   Perianal hematoma
>
>   Thrombosed hemorrhoids NOS

K64.8   **Other hemorrhoids**

>   Internal hemorrhoids, without mention of degree
>
>   Prolapsed hemorrhoids, degree not specified

K64.9   **Unspecified hemorrhoids**

>   Hemorrhoids (bleeding) NOS
>
>   Hemorrhoids (bleeding) without mention of degree

DISEASES OF PERITONEUM AND RETROPERITONEUM (K65-K68)

K65   **Peritonitis**

Definition: Peritonitis is an inflammation of the membrane which

● New code   ▲ Revised code   **Excludes1:** Not coded here   **Excludes2:** Not included here   ⊗ Placeholder required   ⑦7th digit required

lines the inside of the abdomen and all of the internal organs.

Use additional code (B95-B97), to identify infectious agent

Excludes1: acute appendicitis with generalized peritonitis (K35.2)

    aseptic peritonitis (T81.6)

    benign paroxysmal peritonitis (E85.0)

    chemical peritonitis (T81.6)

    diverticulitis of both small and large intestine with peritonitis (K57.4-)

    diverticulitis of colon with peritonitis (K57.2-)

    diverticulitis of intestine, NOS, with peritonitis (K57.8-)

    diverticulitis of small intestine with peritonitis (K57.0-)

    gonococcal peritonitis (A54.85)

    neonatal peritonitis (P78.0-P78.1)

    pelvic peritonitis, female (N73.3-N73.5)

    periodic familial peritonitis (E85.0)

    peritonitis due to talc or other foreign substance (T81.6)

    peritonitis in chlamydia (A74.81)

    peritonitis in diphtheria (A36.89)

    peritonitis in syphilis (late) (A52.74)

    peritonitis in tuberculosis (A18.31)

    peritonitis with or following abortion or ectopic or molar pregnancy (O00-O07, O08.0)

    peritonitis with or following appendicitis (K35.-)

    peritonitis with or following diverticular disease of intestine (K57.-)

    puerperal peritonitis (O85)

    retroperitoneal infections (K68.-)

K65.0 **Generalized (acute) peritonitis**

    Pelvic peritonitis (acute), male

    Subphrenic peritonitis (acute)

    Suppurative peritonitis (acute)

K65.1 **Peritoneal abscess**

    Abdominopelvic abscess

    Abscess (of) omentum

    Abscess (of) peritoneum

    Mesenteric abscess

    Retrocecal abscess

    Subdiaphragmatic abscess

    Subhepatic abscess

    Subphrenic abscess

K65.2 **Spontaneous bacterial peritonitis**

    Excludes1: bacterial peritonitis NOS (K65.9)

K65.3 **Choleperitonitis**

    Peritonitis due to bile

K65.4 **Sclerosing mesenteritis**

    Fat necrosis of peritoneum (Idiopathic) sclerosing mesenteric fibrosis

    Mesenteric lipodystrophy

    Mesenteric panniculitis

    Retractile mesenteritis

K65.8 **Other peritonitis**

    Chronic proliferative peritonitis

    Peritonitis due to urine

K65.9 **Peritonitis, unspecified**

    Bacterial peritonitis NOS

K66 **Other disorders of peritoneum**

Excludes2: ascites (R18.-)

peritoneal effusion (chronic) (R18.8)

K66.0 **Peritoneal adhesions (postprocedural) (postinfection)**

    Adhesions (of) abdominal (wall)

    Adhesions (of) diaphragm

    Adhesions (of) intestine

    Adhesions (of) male pelvis

    Adhesions (of) omentum

    Adhesions (of) stomach

    Adhesive bands

    Mesenteric adhesions

    Excludes1: female pelvic adhesions [bands] (N73.6)

        peritoneal adhesions with intestinal obstruction (K56.5-)

K66.1 **Hemoperitoneum**

    Excludes1: traumatic hemoperitoneum (S36.8-)

K66.8 **Other specified disorders of peritoneum**

K66.9 **Disorder of peritoneum, unspecified**

K67 **Disorders of peritoneum in infectious diseases classified elsewhere**

Code first underlying disease, such as :

congenital syphilis (A50.0)

helminthiasis (B65.0 -B83.9)

Excludes1: peritonitis in chlamydia (A74.81)

    peritonitis in diphtheria (A36.89)

    peritonitis in gonococcal (A54.85)

    peritonitis in syphilis (late) (A52.74)

    peritonitis in tuberculosis (A18.31)

K68 **Disorders of retroperitoneum**

K68.1 **Retroperitoneal abscess**

    K68.11 **Postprocedural retroperitoneal abscess**

    K68.12 **Psoas muscle abscess**

    K68.19 **Other retroperitoneal abscess**

K68.9 **Other disorders of retroperitoneum**

DISEASES OF LIVER (K70-K77)

Excludes1: jaundice NOS (R17)

Excludes2: hemochromatosis (E83.11-)

Reye's syndrome (G93.7)

viral hepatitis (B15-B19)

Wilson's disease (E83.0)

K70 **Alcoholic liver disease**

Use additional code to identify:

    alcohol abuse and dependence (F10.-)

K70.0 **Alcoholic fatty liver**

K70.1 **Alcoholic hepatitis**

    K70.10 **Alcoholic hepatitis without ascites**

    K70.11 **Alcoholic hepatitis with ascites**

K70.2 **Alcoholic fibrosis and sclerosis of liver**

K70.3 **Alcoholic cirrhosis of liver**

    Alcoholic cirrhosis NOS

    K70.30 **Alcoholic cirrhosis of liver without ascites**

    K70.31 **Alcoholic cirrhosis of liver with ascites**

K70.4 **Alcoholic hepatic failure**

    Acute alcoholic hepatic failure

    Alcoholic hepatic failure NOS

    Chronic alcoholic hepatic failure

    Subacute alcoholic hepatic failure

K70.40　Alcoholic hepatic failure without coma

K70.41　Alcoholic hepatic failure with coma

K70.9　Alcoholic liver disease, unspecified

K71　Toxic liver disease

Includes: drug-induced idiosyncratic (unpredictable) liver disease

drug-induced toxic (predictable) liver disease

Code first poisoning due to drug or toxin, if applicable (T36-T65 with fifth or sixth character 1-4 or 6)

Use additional code for adverse effect, if applicable, to identify drug (T36-T50 with fifth or sixth character 5)

Excludes2: alcoholic liver disease (K70.-)

Budd-Chiari syndrome (I82.0)

K71.0　Toxic liver disease with cholestasis

Cholestasis with hepatocyte injury 'Pure' cholestasis

K71.1　Toxic liver disease with hepatic necrosis

Hepatic failure (acute) (chronic) due to drugs

K71.10　Toxic liver disease with hepatic necrosis, without coma

K71.11　Toxic liver disease with hepatic necrosis, with coma

K71.2　Toxic liver disease with acute hepatitis

K71.3　Toxic liver disease with chronic persistent hepatitis

K71.4　Toxic liver disease with chronic lobular hepatitis

K71.5　Toxic liver disease with chronic active hepatitis

Toxic liver disease with lupoid hepatitis

K71.50　Toxic liver disease with chronic active hepatitis without ascites

K71.51　Toxic liver disease with chronic active hepatitis with ascites

K71.6　Toxic liver disease with hepatitis, not elsewhere classified

K71.7　Toxic liver disease with fibrosis and cirrhosis of liver

K71.8　Toxic liver disease with other disorders of liver

Toxic liver disease with focal nodular hyperplasia

Toxic liver disease with hepatic granulomas

Toxic liver disease with peliosis hepatis

Toxic liver disease with veno-occlusive disease of liver

K71.9　Toxic liver disease, unspecified

K72　Hepatic failure, not elsewhere classified

Includes: fulminant hepatitis NEC, with hepatic failure

hepatic encephalopathy NOS

liver (cell) necrosis with hepatic failure

malignant hepatitis NEC, with hepatic failure yellow liver atrophy or dystrophy

Excludes1: alcoholic hepatic failure (K70.4)

hepatic failure with toxic liver disease (K71.1-)

icterus of newborn (P55-P59)

postprocedural hepatic failure (K91.82)

Excludes2: hepatic failure complicating abortion or ectopic or molar pregnancy (O00-O07, O08.8)

hepatic failure complicating pregnancy, childbirth and the puerperium (O26.6-)

viral hepatitis with hepatic coma (B15-B19)

K72.0　Acute and subacute hepatic failure

Acute non-viral hepatitis NOS

K72.00　Acute and subacute hepatic failure without coma

K72.01　Acute and subacute hepatic failure with coma

K72.1　Chronic hepatic failure

K72.10　Chronic hepatic failure without coma

K72.11　Chronic hepatic failure with coma

K72.9　Hepatic failure, unspecified

K72.90　Hepatic failure, unspecified without coma

K72.91　Hepatic failure, unspecified with coma

Hepatic coma NOS

K73　Chronic hepatitis, not elsewhere classified

Excludes1: alcoholic hepatitis (chronic) (K70.1-)

drug-induced hepatitis (chronic) (K71.-)

granulomatous hepatitis (chronic) NEC (K75.3)

reactive, nonspecific hepatitis (chronic) (K75.2)

viral hepatitis (chronic) (B15-B19)

K73.0　Chronic persistent hepatitis, not elsewhere classified

K73.1　Chronic lobular hepatitis, not elsewhere classified

K73.2　Chronic active hepatitis, not elsewhere classified

K73.8　Other chronic hepatitis, not elsewhere classified

K73.9　Chronic hepatitis, unspecified

K74　Fibrosis and cirrhosis of liver

Definition: Cirrhosis is the chronic scarring of the liver, leading to loss of normal liver function.

Code also, if applicable, viral hepatitis (acute) (chronic) (B15-B19)

Excludes1: alcoholic cirrhosis (of liver) (K70.3)

alcoholic fibrosis of liver (K70.2)

cardiac sclerosis of liver (K76.1)

cirrhosis (of liver) with toxic liver disease (K71.7)

congenital cirrhosis (of liver) (P78.81)

pigmentary cirrhosis (of liver) (E83.110)

K74.0　Hepatic fibrosis

K74.1　Hepatic sclerosis

K74.2　Hepatic fibrosis with hepatic sclerosis

K74.3　Primary biliary cirrhosis

Chronic nonsuppurative destructive cholangitis

K74.4　Secondary biliary cirrhosis

K74.5　Biliary cirrhosis, unspecified

K74.6　Other and unspecified cirrhosis of liver

K74.60　Unspecified cirrhosis of liver

Cirrhosis (of liver) NOS

K74.69　Other cirrhosis of liver

Cryptogenic cirrhosis (of liver)

Macronodular cirrhosis (of liver)

Micronodular cirrhosis (of liver)

Mixed type cirrhosis (of liver)

Portal cirrhosis (of liver)

Postnecrotic cirrhosis (of liver)

K75　Other inflammatory liver diseases

Excludes2: toxic liver disease (K71.-)

K75.0　Abscess of liver

Cholangitic hepatic abscess

Hematogenic hepatic abscess

Hepatic abscess NOS

Lymphogenic hepatic abscess

Pylephlebitic hepatic abscess

Excludes1: amebic liver abscess (A06.4)

cholangitis without liver abscess (K83.0)

pylephlebitis without liver abscess (K75.1)

Excludes2: acute or subacute hepatitis NOS (B17.9)

acute or subacute non-viral hepatitis (K72.0)

　●　New code　▲　Revised code　Excludes1: Not coded here　Excludes2: Not included here　⊗　Placeholder required　⑦ 7th digit required

chronic hepatitis NEC (K73.8)

K75.1 **Phlebitis of portal vein**

Pylephlebitis

Excludes1: pylephlebitic liver abscess (K75.0)

K75.2 **Nonspecific reactive hepatitis**

Excludes1: acute or subacute hepatitis (K72.0-)

chronic hepatitis NEC (K73.-)

viral hepatitis (B15-B19)

K75.3 **Granulomatous hepatitis, not elsewhere classified**

Excludes1: acute or subacute hepatitis (K72.0-)

chronic hepatitis NEC (K73.-)

viral hepatitis (B15-B19)

K75.4 **Autoimmune hepatitis**

Lupoid hepatitis NEC

K75.8 **Other specified inflammatory liver diseases**

K75.81 **Nonalcoholic steatohepatitis (NASH)**

K75.89 **Other specified inflammatory liver diseases**

K75.9 **Inflammatory liver disease, unspecified**

Hepatitis NOS

Excludes1: acute or subacute hepatitis (K72.0-)

chronic hepatitis NEC (K73.-)

viral hepatitis (B15-B19)

K76 **Other diseases of liver**

Excludes2: alcoholic liver disease (K70.-)

amyloid degeneration of liver (E85.-)

cystic disease of liver (congenital) (Q44.6)

hepatic vein thrombosis (I82.0)

hepatomegaly NOS (R16.0)

pigmentary cirrhosis (of liver) (E83.110)

portal vein thrombosis (I81)

toxic liver disease (K71.-)

K76.0 **Fatty (change of) liver, not elsewhere classified**

Nonalcoholic fatty liver disease (NAFLD)

Excludes1: nonalcoholic steatohepatitis (NASH) (K75.81)

K76.1 **Chronic passive congestion of liver**

Cardiac cirrhosis

Cardiac sclerosis

K76.2 **Central hemorrhagic necrosis of liver**

Excludes1: liver necrosis with hepatic failure (K72.-)

K76.3 **Infarction of liver**

K76.4 **Peliosis hepatis**

Hepatic angiomatosis

K76.5 **Hepatic veno-occlusive disease**

Excludes1: Budd-Chiari syndrome (I82.0)

K76.6 **Portal hypertension**

Use additional code for any associated complications, such as:

portal hypertensive gastropathy (K31.89)

K76.7 **Hepatorenal syndrome**

Excludes1: hepatorenal syndrome following labor and delivery (O90.4)

postprocedural hepatorenal syndrome (K91.83)

K76.8 **Other specified diseases of liver**

K76.81 **Hepatopulmonary syndrome**

Code first underlying liver disease, such as:

alcoholic cirrhosis of liver (K70.3-)

cirrhosis of liver without mention of alcohol (K74.6-)

K76.89 **Other specified diseases of liver**

Cyst (simple) of liver

Focal nodular hyperplasia of liver

Hepatoptosis

K76.9 **Liver disease, unspecified**

K77 **Liver disorders in diseases classified elsewhere**

Code first underlying disease, such as:

amyloidosis (E85.-)

congenital syphilis (A50.0, A50.5)

congenital toxoplasmosis (P37.1)

schistosomiasis (B65.0-B65.9)

Excludes1: alcoholic hepatitis (K70.1-)

alcoholic liver disease (K70.-)

cytomegaloviral hepatitis (B25.1)

herpesviral [herpes simplex] hepatitis (B00.81)

infectious mononucleosis with liver disease (B27.0-B27.9 with .9)

mumps hepatitis (B26.81)

sarcoidosis with liver disease (D86.89)

secondary syphilis with liver disease (A51.45)

syphilis (late) with liver disease (A52.74)

toxoplasmosis (acquired) hepatitis (B58.1)

tuberculosis with liver disease (A18.83)

DISORDERS OF GALLBLADDER, BILIARY TRACT AND PANCREAS (K80-K87)

K80 **Cholelithiasis**

Excludes1: retained cholelithiasis following cholecystectomy (K91.86)

K80.0 **Calculus of gallbladder with acute cholecystitis**

Any condition listed in K80.2 with acute cholecystitis

K80.00 **Calculus of gallbladder with acute cholecystitis without obstruction**

K80.01 **Calculus of gallbladder with acute cholecystitis with obstruction**

K80.1 **Calculus of gallbladder with other cholecystitis**

K80.10 **Calculus of gallbladder with chronic cholecystitis without obstruction**

Cholelithiasis with cholecystitis NOS

K80.11 **Calculus of gallbladder with chronic cholecystitis with obstruction**

K80.12 **Calculus of gallbladder with acute and chronic cholecystitis without obstruction**

K80.13 **Calculus of gallbladder with acute and chronic cholecystitis with obstruction**

K80.18 **Calculus of gallbladder with other cholecystitis without obstruction**

K80.19 **Calculus of gallbladder with other cholecystitis with obstruction**

K80.2 **Calculus of gallbladder without cholecystitis**

Cholecystolithiasis without cholecystitis

Cholelithiasis (without cholecystitis)

Colic (recurrent) of gallbladder (without cholecystitis)

Gallstone (impacted) of cystic duct (without cholecystitis)

Gallstone (impacted) of gallbladder (without cholecystitis)

K80.20 **Calculus of gallbladder without cholecystitis without obstruction**

K80.21 Calculus of gallbladder without cholecystitis with obstruction

K80.3 Calculus of bile duct with cholangitis

Any condition listed in K80.5 with cholangitis

K80.30 Calculus of bile duct with cholangitis, unspecified, without obstruction

K80.31 Calculus of bile duct with cholangitis, unspecified, with obstruction

K80.32 Calculus of bile duct with acute cholangitis without obstruction

K80.33 Calculus of bile duct with acute cholangitis with obstruction

K80.34 Calculus of bile duct with chronic cholangitis without obstruction

K80.35 Calculus of bile duct with chronic cholangitis with obstruction

K80.36 Calculus of bile duct with acute and chronic cholangitis without obstruction

K80.37 Calculus of bile duct with acute and chronic cholangitis with obstruction

K80.4 Calculus of bile duct with cholecystitis

Any condition listed in K80.5 with cholecystitis (with cholangitis)

K80.40 Calculus of bile duct with cholecystitis, unspecified, without obstruction

K80.41 Calculus of bile duct with cholecystitis, unspecified, with obstruction

K80.42 Calculus of bile duct with acute cholecystitis without obstruction

K80.43 Calculus of bile duct with acute cholecystitis with obstruction

K80.44 Calculus of bile duct with chronic cholecystitis without obstruction

K80.45 Calculus of bile duct with chronic cholecystitis with obstruction

K80.46 Calculus of bile duct with acute and chronic cholecystitis without obstruction

K80.47 Calculus of bile duct with acute and chronic cholecystitis with obstruction

K80.5 Calculus of bile duct without cholangitis or cholecystitis

Choledocholithiasis (without cholangitis or cholecystitis)

Gallstone (impacted) of bile duct NOS (without cholangitis or cholecystitis)

Gallstone (impacted) of common duct (without cholangitis or cholecystitis)

Gallstone (impacted) of hepatic duct (without cholangitis or cholecystitis)

Hepatic cholelithiasis (without cholangitis or cholecystitis)

Hepatic colic (recurrent) (without cholangitis or cholecystitis)

K80.50 Calculus of bile duct without cholangitis or cholecystitis without obstruction

K80.51 Calculus of bile duct without cholangitis or cholecystitis with obstruction

K80.6 Calculus of gallbladder and bile duct with cholecystitis

K80.60 Calculus of gallbladder and bile duct with cholecystitis, unspecified, without obstruction

K80.61 Calculus of gallbladder and bile duct with cholecystitis, unspecified, with obstruction

K80.62 Calculus of gallbladder and bile duct with acute cholecystitis without obstruction

K80.63 Calculus of gallbladder and bile duct with acute cholecystitis with obstruction

K80.64 Calculus of gallbladder and bile duct with chronic cholecystitis without obstruction

K80.65 Calculus of gallbladder and bile duct with chronic cholecystitis with obstruction

K80.66 Calculus of gallbladder and bile duct with acute and chronic cholecystitis without obstruction

K80.67 Calculus of gallbladder and bile duct with acute and chronic cholecystitis with obstruction

K80.7 Calculus of gallbladder and bile duct without cholecystitis

K80.70 Calculus of gallbladder and bile duct without cholecystitis without obstruction

K80.71 Calculus of gallbladder and bile duct without cholecystitis with obstruction

K80.8 Other cholelithiasis

K80.80 Other cholelithiasis without obstruction

K80.81 Other cholelithiasis with obstruction

K81 Cholecystitis

Excludes1: cholecystitis with cholelithiasis (K80.-)

K81.0 Acute cholecystitis

Abscess of gallbladder

Angiocholecystitis

Emphysematous (acute) cholecystitis

Empyema of gallbladder

Gangrene of gallbladder

Gangrenous cholecystitis

Suppurative cholecystitis

K81.1 Chronic cholecystitis

K81.2 Acute cholecystitis with chronic cholecystitis

K81.9 Cholecystitis, unspecified

K82 Other diseases of gallbladder

Excludes1: nonvisualization of gallbladder (R93.2)

postcholecystectomy syndrome (K91.5)

K82.0 Obstruction of gallbladder

Occlusion of cystic duct or gallbladder without cholelithiasis

Stenosis of cystic duct or gallbladder without cholelithiasis

Stricture of cystic duct or gallbladder without cholelithiasis

Excludes1: obstruction of gallbladder with cholelithiasis (K80.-)

K82.1 Hydrops of gallbladder

Mucocele of gallbladder

K82.2 Perforation of gallbladder

Rupture of cystic duct or gallbladder

K82.3 Fistula of gallbladder

Cholecystocolic fistula

Cholecystoduodenal fistula

K82.4 Cholesterolosis of gallbladder

Strawberry gallbladder

Excludes1: cholesterolosis of gallbladder with cholecystitis (K81.-)

cholesterolosis of gallbladder with cholelithiasis (K80.-)

K82.8 Other specified diseases of gallbladder

Adhesions of cystic duct or gallbladder

Atrophy of cystic duct or gallbladder

Cyst of cystic duct or gallbladder

Dyskinesia of cystic duct or gallbladder

Hypertrophy of cystic duct or gallbladder

● New code   ▲ Revised code   **Excludes1:** Not coded here   **Excludes2:** Not included here   ⊗ Placeholder required   ⑦7th digit required

Nonfunctioning of cystic duct or gallbladder

Ulcer of cystic duct or gallbladder

K82.9   **Disease of gallbladder, unspecified**

K83   **Other diseases of biliary tract**

Excludes1: postcholecystectomy syndrome (K91.5)

Excludes2: conditions involving the gallbladder (K81-K82)

conditions involving the cystic duct (K81-K82)

K83.0   **Cholangitis**

Ascending cholangitis

Cholangitis NOS

Primary cholangitis

Recurrent cholangitis

Sclerosing cholangitis

Secondary cholangitis

Stenosing cholangitis

Suppurative cholangitis

Excludes1: cholangitic liver abscess (K75.0)

cholangitis with choledocholithiasis (K80.3-, K80.4-)

chronic nonsuppurative destructive cholangitis (K74.3)

K83.1   **Obstruction of bile duct**

Occlusion of bile duct without cholelithiasis

Stenosis of bile duct without cholelithiasis

Stricture of bile duct without cholelithiasis

Excludes1: congenital obstruction of bile duct (Q44.3)

obstruction of bile duct with cholelithiasis (K80.-)

K83.2   **Perforation of bile duct**

Rupture of bile duct

K83.3   **Fistula of bile duct**

Choledochoduodenal fistula

K83.4   **Spasm of sphincter of Oddi**

K83.5   **Biliary cyst**

K83.8   **Other specified diseases of biliary tract**

Adhesions of biliary tract

Atrophy of biliary tract

Hypertrophy of biliary tract

Ulcer of biliary tract

K83.9   **Disease of biliary tract, unspecified**

K85   **Acute pancreatitis**

Includes: acute (recurrent) pancreatitis

subacute pancreatitis

K85.0   **Idiopathic acute pancreatitis**

K85.00   **Idiopathic acute pancreatitis without necrosis or infection**

K85.01   **Idiopathic acute pancreatitis with uninfected necrosis**

K85.02   **Idiopathic acute pancreatitis with infected necrosis**

K85.1   **Biliary acute pancreatitis**

Gallstone pancreatitis

K85.10   **Biliary acute pancreatitis without necrosis or infection**

K85.11   **Biliary acute pancreatitis with uninfected necrosis**

K85.12   **Biliary acute pancreatitis with infected necrosis**

K85.2   **Alcohol induced acute pancreatitis**

Excludes2: alcohol induced chronic pancreatitis (K86.0)

K85.20   **Alcohol induced acute pancreatitis without necrosis or infection**

K85.21   **Alcohol induced acute pancreatitis with uninfected necrosis**

K85.22   **Alcohol induced acute pancreatitis with infected necrosis**

K85.3   **Drug induced acute pancreatitis**

Use additional code for adverse effect, if applicable, to identify drug (T36-T50 with fifth or sixth character 5)

Use additional code to identify drug abuse and dependence (F11.-F17.-)

K85.30   **Drug induced acute pancreatitis without necrosis or infection**

K85.31   **Drug induced acute pancreatitis with uninfected necrosis**

K85.32   **Drug induced acute pancreatitis with infected necrosis**

K85.8   **Other acute pancreatitis**

K85.80   **Other acute pancreatitis without necrosis or infection**

K85.81   **Other acute pancreatitis with uninfected necrosis**

K85.82   **Other acute pancreatitis with infected necrosis**

K85.9   **Acute pancreatitis, unspecified**

Pancreatitis NOS

K85.90   **Acute pancreatitis without necrosis or infection, unspecified**

K85.91   **Acute pancreatitis with uninfected necrosis, unspecified**

K85.92   **Acute pancreatitis with infected necrosis, unspecified**

K86   **Other diseases of pancreas**

Excludes2: fibrocystic disease of pancreas (E84.-)

islet cell tumor (of pancreas) (D13.7)

pancreatic steatorrhea (K90.3)

K86.0   **Alcohol-induced chronic pancreatitis**

Use additional code to identify:

alcohol abuse and dependence (F10.-)

Code also exocrine pancreatic insufficiency (K86.81)

Excludes2: alcohol induced acute pancreatitis (K85.2-)

K86.1   **Other chronic pancreatitis**

Chronic pancreatitis NOS

Infectious chronic pancreatitis

Recurrent chronic pancreatitis

Relapsing chronic pancreatitis

Code also exocrine pancreatic insufficiency (K86.81)

K86.2   **Cyst of pancreas**

K86.3   **Pseudocyst of pancreas**

K86.8   **Other specified diseases of pancreas**

K86.81   **Exocrine pancreatic insufficiency**

K86.89   **Other specified diseases of pancreas**

Aseptic pancreatic necrosis, unrelated to acute pancreatitis

Atrophy of pancreas

Calculus of pancreas

Cirrhosis of pancreas

Fibrosis of pancreas

Pancreatic fat necrosis, unrelated to acute pancreatitis

Pancreatic infantilism

Pancreatic necrosis NOS, unrelated to acute pancreatitis

K86.9 Disease of pancreas, unspecified

K87 Disorders of gallbladder, biliary tract and pancreas in diseases classified elsewhere

Code first underlying disease

Excludes1: cytomegaloviral pancreatitis(B25.2)

mumps pancreatitis (B26.3)

syphilitic gallbladder (A52.74)

syphilitic pancreas (A52.74)

tuberculosis of gallbladder (A18.83)

tuberculosis of pancreas (A18.83)

OTHER DISEASES OF THE DIGESTIVE SYSTEM (K90-K95)

K90 Intestinal malabsorption

Definition: Intestinal malabsorption is a state arising from abnormality in digestion or absorption of food nutrients across the gastrointestinal(GI) tract.

Excludes1: intestinal malabsorption following gastrointestinal surgery (K91.2)

K90.0 Celiac disease

Celiac disease with steatorrhea

Celiac gluten-sensitive enteropathy Nontropical sprue

Use additional code for associated disorders including:

dermatitis herpetiformis (L13.0)

gluten ataxia (G32.81)

Code also exocrine pancreatic insufficiency (K86.81)

K90.1 Tropical sprue

Sprue NOS

Tropical steatorrhea

K90.2 Blind loop syndrome, not elsewhere classified

Blind loop syndrome NOS

Excludes1: congenital blind loop syndrome (Q43.8)

postsurgical blind loop syndrome (K91.2)

K90.3 Pancreatic steatorrhea

K90.4 Other malabsorption due to intolerance

Excludes2: celiac gluten-sensitive enteropathy (K90.0)

lactose intolerance (E73.-)

K90.41 Non-celiac gluten sensitivity

Gluten sensitivity NOS

Non-celiac gluten sensitive enteropathy

K90.49 Malabsorption due to intolerance, not elsewhere classified

Malabsorption due to intolerance to carbohydrate

Malabsorption due to intolerance to fat

Malabsorption due to intolerance to protein

Malabsorption due to intolerance to starch

K90.8 Other intestinal malabsorption

K90.81 Whipple's disease

K90.89 Other intestinal malabsorption

K90.9 Intestinal malabsorption, unspecified

K91 Intraoperative and postprocedural complications and disorders of digestive system, not elsewhere classified

Excludes2: complications of artificial opening of digestive system (K94.-)

complications of bariatric procedures (K95.-)

gastrojejunal ulcer (K28.-)

postprocedural (radiation) retroperitoneal abscess (K68.11)

radiation colitis (K52.0)

radiation gastroenteritis (K52.0)

radiation proctitis (K62.7)

K91.0 Vomiting following gastrointestinal surgery

K91.1 Postgastric surgery syndromes

Dumping syndrome

Postgastrectomy syndrome

Postvagotomy syndrome

K91.2 Postsurgical malabsorption, not elsewhere classified

Postsurgical blind loop syndrome

Excludes1: malabsorption osteomalacia in adults (M83.2)

malabsorption osteoporosis, postsurgical (M80.8-, M81.8)

K91.3 Postprocedural intestinal obstruction

●**K91.30 Postprocedural intestinal obstruction, unspecified as to partial versus complete**

Postprocedural intestinal obstruction NOS

●**K91.31 Postprocedural partial intestinal obstruction**

Postprocedural incomplete intestinal obstruction

●**K91.32 Postprocedural complete intestinal obstructionK91.5 Postcholecystectomy syndrome**

K91.6 Intraoperative hemorrhage and hematoma of a digestive system organ or structure complicating a procedure

Excludes1: intraoperative hemorrhage and hematoma of a digestive system organ or structure due to accidental puncture and laceration during a procedure (K91.7-)

K91.61 Intraoperative hemorrhage and hematoma of a digestive system organ or structure complicating a digestive system procedure

K91.62 Intraoperative hemorrhage and hematoma of a digestive system organ or structure complicating other procedure

K91.7 Accidental puncture and laceration of a digestive system organ or structure during a procedure

K91.71 Accidental puncture and laceration of a digestive system organ or structure during a digestive system procedure

K91.72 Accidental puncture and laceration of a digestive system organ or structure during other procedure

K91.8 Other intraoperative and postprocedural complications and disorders of digestive system

K91.81 Other intraoperative complications of digestive system

K91.82 Postprocedural hepatic failure

K91.83 Postprocedural hepatorenal syndrome

K91.84 Postprocedural hemorrhage of a digestive system organ or structure following a procedure

K91.840 Postprocedural hemorrhage of a digestive system organ or structure following a digestive system procedure

K91.841 Postprocedural hemorrhage of a digestive system organ or structure following other procedure

K91.85 Complications of intestinal pouch

K91.850 Pouchitis

Inflammation of internal ileoanal pouch

K91.858 Other complications of intestinal pouch

K91.86 Retained cholelithiasis following cholecystectomy

K91.87 Postprocedural hematoma and seroma of a digestive system organ or structure following a procedure

    K91.870 Postprocedural hematoma of a digestive system organ or structure following a digestive system procedure

    K91.871 Postprocedural hematoma of a digestive system organ or structure following other procedure

    K91.872 Postprocedural seroma of a digestive system organ or structure following a digestive system procedure

    K91.873 Postprocedural seroma of a digestive system organ or structure following other procedure

K91.89 Other postprocedural complications and disorders of digestive system

Use additional code, if applicable, to further specify disorder

Excludes2: postprocedural retroperitoneal abscess (K68.11)

K92 Other diseases of digestive system

Excludes1: neonatal gastrointestinal hemorrhage (P54.0-P54.3)

K92.0 Hematemesis

K92.1 Melena

Excludes1: occult blood in feces (R19.5)

K92.2 Gastrointestinal hemorrhage, unspecified

Gastric hemorrhage NOS

Intestinal hemorrhage NOS

Excludes1: acute hemorrhagic gastritis (K29.01)

hemorrhage of anus and rectum (K62.5)
angiodysplasia of stomach with hemorrhage (K31.811)
diverticular disease with hemorrhage (K57.-)
gastritis and duodenitis with hemorrhage (K29.-)
peptic ulcer with hemorrhage (K25-K28)

K92.8 Other specified diseases of the digestive system

    K92.81 Gastrointestinal mucositis (ulcerative)

Code also type of associated therapy, such as:

antineoplastic and immunosuppressive drugs (T45.1X-)

radiological procedure and radiotherapy (Y84.2)

Excludes2: mucositis (ulcerative) of vagina and vulva (N76.81)

nasal mucositis (ulcerative) (J34.81)

oral mucositis (ulcerative) (K12.3-)

    K92.89 Other specified diseases of the digestive system

K92.9 Disease of digestive system, unspecified

K94 Complications of artificial openings of the digestive system

K94.0 Colostomy complications

    K94.00 Colostomy complication, unspecified

    K94.01 Colostomy hemorrhage

    K94.02 Colostomy infection

Use additional code to specify type of infection, such as:

cellulitis of abdominal wall (L03.311) sepsis (A40.-, A41.-)

    K94.03 Colostomy malfunction

Mechanical complication of colostomy

    K94.09 Other complications of colostomy

K94.1 Enterostomy complications

    K94.10 Enterostomy complication, unspecified

    K94.11 Enterostomy hemorrhage

    K94.12 Enterostomy infection

Use additional code to specify type of infection, such as:

cellulitis of abdominal wall (L03.311) sepsis (A40.-, A41.-)

    K94.13 Enterostomy malfunction

Mechanical complication of enterostomy

    K94.19 Other complications of enterostomy

K94.2 Gastrostomy complications

    K94.20 Gastrostomy complication, unspecified

    K94.21 Gastrostomy hemorrhage

    K94.22 Gastrostomy infection

Use additional code to specify type of infection, such as:

cellulitis of abdominal wall (L03.311)

sepsis (A40.-, A41.-)

    K94.23 Gastrostomy malfunction

Mechanical complication of gastrostomy

    K94.29 Other complications of gastrostomy

K94.3 Esophagostomy complications

    K94.30 Esophagostomy complications, unspecified

    K94.31 Esophagostomy hemorrhage

    K94.32 Esophagostomy infection

Use additional code to identify the infection

    K94.33 Esophagostomy malfunction

Mechanical complication of esophagostomy

    K94.39 Other complications of esophagostomy

K95 Complications of bariatric procedures

K95.0 Complications of gastric band procedure

    K95.01 Infection due to gastric band procedure

Use additional code to specify type of infection or organism, such as:

bacterial and viral infectious agents (B95.-, B96.-)

cellulitis of abdominal wall (L03.311)

sepsis (A40.-, A41.-)

    K95.09 Other complications of gastric band procedure

Use additional code, if applicable, to further specify complication

K95.8 Complications of other bariatric procedure

Excludes1: complications of gastric band surgery (K95.0-)

    K95.81 Infection due to other bariatric procedure

Use additional code to specify type of infection or organism, such as:

bacterial and viral infectious agents (B95.-, B96.-)

cellulitis of abdominal wall (L03.311)

sepsis (A40.-, A41.-)

    K95.89 Other complications of other bariatric procedure

Use additional code, if applicable, to further specify complication

Chapter 12: Diseases Of The Skin And Subcutaneous Tissue (L00-L99)

DEFINITIONS

This chapter includes definitions of selected key words, terms and phrases and coding alerts for adding points to the clinical domain, and references to coding late effects where appropriate. An example from this chapter is as follows:

L49 Exfoliation due to erythematous conditions according to extent of body surface involved

> **Definition:** Erythematous conditions refers to conditions causing diffuse or patchy redness of skin.

MULTIPLE CODING FOR A SINGLE CONDITION

In addition to the etiology/manifestation convention that requires two codes to fully describe a single condition that affects multiple body systems, there are other single conditions that also require more than one code. "Use additional code" notes are found in the Tabular List at codes that are not part of an etiology/manifestation pair where a secondary code is useful to fully describe a condition. The sequencing rule is the same as the etiology/manifestation pair, "use additional code" indicates that a secondary code should be added.

For example, for bacterial infections that are not included in chapter 1, a secondary code from category B95, Streptococcus, Staphylococcus, and Enterococcus, as the cause of diseases classified elsewhere, or B96, Other bacterial agents as the cause of diseases classified elsewhere, may be required to identify the bacterial organism causing the infection. A "use additional code" note will normally be found at the infectious disease code, indicating a need for the organism code to be added as a secondary code.

"Code first" notes are also under certain codes that are not specifically manifestation codes but may be due to an underlying cause. When there is a "code first" note and an underlying condition is present, the underlying condition should be sequenced first.

"Code, if applicable, any causal condition first", notes indicate that this code may be assigned as a principal diagnosis when the causal condition is unknown or not applicable. If a causal condition is known, then the code for that condition should be sequenced as the principal or first-listed diagnosis.

Multiple codes may be needed for sequela, complication codes and obstetric codes to more fully describe a condition. See the specific guidelines for these conditions for further instruction.

COMBINATION CODE

A combination code is a single code used to classify: Two diagnoses, or a diagnosis with an associated secondary process (manifestation) A diagnosis with an associated complication

Combination codes are identified by referring to subterm entries in the Alphabetic Index and by reading the inclusion and exclusion notes in the Tabular List.

Assign only the combination code when that code fully identifies the diagnostic conditions involved or when the Alphabetic Index so directs. Multiple coding should not be used when the classification provides a combination code that clearly identifies all of the elements documented in the diagnosis. When the combination code lacks necessary specificity in describing the manifestation or complication, an additional code should be used as a secondary code.

SEQUELA (LATE EFFECTS)

A sequela is the residual effect (condition produced) after the acute phase of an illness or injury has terminated. There is no time limit on when a sequela code can be used. The residual may be apparent early, such as in cerebral infarction, or it may occur months or years later, such as that due to a previous injury. Coding of sequela generally requires two codes sequenced in the following order: The condition or nature of the sequela is sequenced first.

The sequela code is sequenced second.

An exception to the above guidelines are those instances where the code for the sequela is followed by a manifestation code identified in the Tabular List and title, or the sequela code has been expanded (at the fourth, fifth or sixth character levels) to include the manifestation(s). The code for the acute phase of an illness or injury that led to the sequela is never used with a code for the late effect.

PRESSURE ULCER STAGE CODES

1) Pressure ulcer stages

Codes from category L89, Pressure ulcer, identify the site of the pressure ulcer as well as the stage of the ulcer.
The ICD-10-CM classifies pressure ulcer stages based on severity, which is designated by stages 1-4, unspecified stage and unstageable.

Assign as many codes from category L89 as needed to identify all the pressure ulcers the patient has, if applicable.

2) Unstageable pressure ulcers

Assignment of the code for unstageable pressure ulcer (L89.--0) should be based on the clinical documentation. These codes are used for pressure ulcers whose stage cannot be clinically determined (e.g., the ulcer is covered by eschar or has been treated with a skin or muscle graft) and pressure ulcers that are documented as deep tissue injury but not documented as due to trauma. This code should not be confused with the codes for unspecified stage (L89.--9). When there is no documentation regarding the stage of the pressure ulcer, assign the appropriate code for unspecified stage (L89.--9).

L00-L99

| Add 4th-7th digits | Nonspecific code | Unspecified code | Manifestation code |

3) **Documented pressure ulcer stage**

Assignment of the pressure ulcer stage code should be guided by clinical documentation of the stage or documentation of the terms found in the Alphabetic Index. For clinical terms describing the stage that are not found in the Alphabetic Index, and there is no documentation of the stage, the provider should be queried.

4) **Patients admitted with pressure ulcers documented as healed**

No code is assigned if the documentation states that the pressure ulcer is completely healed.

5) **Patients admitted with pressure ulcers documented as healing**

Pressure ulcers described as healing should be assigned the appropriate pressure ulcer stage code based on the documentation in the medical record. If the documentation does not provide information about the stage of the healing pressure ulcer, assign the appropriate code for unspecified stage.

If the documentation is unclear as to whether the patient has a current (new) pressure ulcer or if the patient is being treated for a healing pressure ulcer, query the provider.

For ulcers that were present on admission but healed at the time of discharge, assign the code for the site and stage of the pressure ulcer at the time of admission.

6) **Patient admitted with pressure ulcer evolving into another stage during the admission**

If a patient is admitted with a pressure ulcer at one stage and it progresses to a higher stage, two separate codes should be assigned: one code for the site and stage of the ulcer on admission and a second code for the same ulcer site and the highest stage reported during the stay.

　● New code　▲ Revised code　Excludes1: Not coded here　Excludes2: Not included here　⊗ Placeholder required　⑦7th digit required

Chapter 12

Diseases Of The Skin And Subcutaneous Tissue (L00-L99)

Excludes2: certain conditions originating in the perinatal period (P04-P96)

certain infectious and parasitic diseases (A00-B99)

complications of pregnancy, childbirth and the puerperium (O00-O9A)

congenital malformations, deformations, and chromosomal abnormalities (Q00-Q99)

endocrine, nutritional and metabolic diseases (E00-E88)

lipomelanotic reticulosis (I89.8)

neoplasms (C00-D49)

symptoms, signs and abnormal clinical and laboratory findings, not elsewhere classified (R00-R94)

systemic connective tissue disorders (M30-M36)

viral warts (B07.-)

This chapter contains the following blocks:

L00-L08	Infections of the skin and subcutaneous tissue
L10-L14	Bullous disorders
L20-L30	Dermatitis and eczema
L40-L45	Papulosquamous disorders
L49-L54	Urticaria and erythema
L55-L59	Radiation-related disorders of the skin and subcutaneous tissue
L60-L75	Disorders of skin appendages
L76	Intraoperative and postprocedural complications of skin and subcutaneous tissue
L80-L99	Other disorders of the skin and subcutaneous tissue

INFECTIONS OF THE SKIN AND SUBCUTANEOUS TISSUE (L00-L08)

Use additional code (B95-B97) to identify infectious agent.

Excludes2: hordeolum (H00.0)

infective dermatitis (L30.3)

local infections of skin classified in Chapter 1

lupus panniculitis (L93.2)

panniculitis NOS (M79.3)

panniculitis of neck and back (M54.0-)

Perlèche NOS (K13.0)

Perlèche due to candidiasis (B37.0)

Perlèche due to riboflavin deficiency (E53.0)

pyogenic granuloma (L98.0)

relapsing panniculitis [Weber-Christian] (M35.6)

viral warts (B07.-)

zoster (B02.-)

L00   Staphylococcal scalded skin syndrome

Ritter's disease

Use additional code to identify percentage of skin exfoliation (L49.-)

Excludes1: bullous impetigo (L01.03)

pemphigus neonatorum (L01.03)

toxic epidermal necrolysis [Lyell] (L51.2)

L01   Impetigo

Excludes1: impetigo herpetiformis (L40.1)

L01.0   Impetigo

Impetigo contagiosa Impetigo vulgaris

L01.00   Impetigo, unspecified

Impetigo NOS

L01.01   Non-bullous impetigo

L01.02   Bockhart's impetigo

Impetigo follicularis

Perifolliculitis NOS

Superficial pustular perifolliculitis

L01.03   Bullous impetigo

Impetigo neonatorum

Pemphigus neonatorum

L01.09   Other impetigo

Ulcerative impetigo

L01.1   Impetiginization of other dermatoses

L02   Cutaneous abscess, furuncle and carbuncle

Definition: A carbuncle is an abscess larger than a boil, usually with one or more openings draining pus onto the skin. It is usually caused by bacterial infection, most commonly staphylococcus aureus. A furuncle is a skin disease caused by the infection of hair follicles, resulting in the localized accumulation of pus and dead tissue.

Use additional code to identify organism (B95-B96)

Excludes2: abscess of anus and rectal regions (K61.-)

abscess of female genital organs (external) (N76.4)

abscess of male genital organs (external) (N48.2, N49.-)

L02.0   Cutaneous abscess, furuncle and carbuncle of face

Excludes2: abscess of ear, external (H60.0)

abscess of eyelid (H00.0)

abscess of head [any part, except face] (L02.8)

abscess of lacrimal gland (H04.0)

abscess of lacrimal passages (H04.3)

abscess of mouth (K12.2)

abscess of nose (J34.0)

abscess of orbit (H05.0)

submandibular abscess (K12.2)

L02.01   Cutaneous abscess of face

L02.02   Furuncle of face

Boil of face

Folliculitis of face

L02.03   Carbuncle of face

L02.1   Cutaneous abscess, furuncle and carbuncle of neck

L02.11   Cutaneous abscess of neck

L02.12   Furuncle of neck

Boil of neck

Folliculitis of neck

L02.13   Carbuncle of neck

L02.2   Cutaneous abscess, furuncle and carbuncle of trunk

Excludes1: non-newborn omphalitis (L08.82)

omphalitis of newborn (P38.-)

Excludes2: abscess of breast (N61.1)

abscess of buttocks (L02.3)

abscess of female external genital organs (N76.4)

abscess of male external genital organs (N48.2, N49.-)

abscess of hip (L02.4)

L02.21   Cutaneous abscess of trunk

L02.211   Cutaneous abscess of abdominal wall

L02.212   Cutaneous abscess of back [any part, except buttock]

L02.213   Cutaneous abscess of chest wall

L02.214   Cutaneous abscess of groin

L02.215   Cutaneous abscess of perineum

L02.216   Cutaneous abscess of umbilicus

L02.219   Cutaneous abscess of trunk, unspecified

L02.22   **Furuncle of trunk**

Boil of trunk

Folliculitis of trunk

L02.221   Furuncle of abdominal wall

L02.222   Furuncle of back [any part, except buttock]

L02.223   Furuncle of chest wall

L02.224   Furuncle of groin

L02.225   Furuncle of perineum

L02.226   Furuncle of umbilicus

L02.229   Furuncle of trunk, unspecified

L02.23   **Carbuncle of trunk**

L02.231   Carbuncle of abdominal wall

L02.232   Carbuncle of back [any part, except buttock]

L02.233   Carbuncle of chest wall

L02.234   Carbuncle of groin

L02.235   Carbuncle of perineum

L02.236   Carbuncle of umbilicus

L02.239   Carbuncle of trunk, unspecified

L02.3   **Cutaneous abscess, furuncle and carbuncle of buttock**

Excludes1: pilonidal cyst with abscess (L05.01)

L02.31   **Cutaneous abscess of buttock**

Cutaneous abscess of gluteal region

L02.32   **Furuncle of buttock**

Boil of buttock

Folliculitis of buttock

Furuncle of gluteal region

L02.33   **Carbuncle of buttock**

Carbuncle of gluteal region

L02.4   **Cutaneous abscess, furuncle and carbuncle of limb**

Excludes2: Cutaneous abscess, furuncle and carbuncle of groin (L02.214, L02.224, L02.234)

Cutaneous abscess, furuncle and carbuncle of hand (L02.5-)

Cutaneous abscess, furuncle and carbuncle of foot (L02.6-)

L02.41   **Cutaneous abscess of limb**

L02.411   Cutaneous abscess of right axilla

L02.412   Cutaneous abscess of left axilla

L02.413   Cutaneous abscess of right upper limb

L02.414   Cutaneous abscess of left upper limb

L02.415   Cutaneous abscess of right lower limb

L02.416   Cutaneous abscess of left lower limb

L02.419   Cutaneous abscess of limb, unspecified

L02.42   **Furuncle of limb**

Boil of limb

Folliculitis of limb

L02.421   Furuncle of right axilla

L02.422   Furuncle of left axilla

L02.423   Furuncle of right upper limb

L02.424   Furuncle of left upper limb

L02.425   Furuncle of right lower limb

L02.426   Furuncle of left lower limb

L02.429   Furuncle of limb, unspecified

L02.43   **Carbuncle of limb**

L02.431   Carbuncle of right axilla

L02.432   Carbuncle of left axilla

L02.433   Carbuncle of right upper limb

L02.434   Carbuncle of left upper limb

L02.435   Carbuncle of right lower limb

L02.436   Carbuncle of left lower limb

L02.439   Carbuncle of limb, unspecified

L02.5   **Cutaneous abscess, furuncle and carbuncle of hand**

L02.51   **Cutaneous abscess of hand**

L02.511   Cutaneous abscess of right hand

L02.512   Cutaneous abscess of left hand

L02.519   Cutaneous abscess of unspecified hand

L02.52   **Furuncle hand**

Boil of hand

Folliculitis of hand

L02.521   Furuncle right hand

L02.522   Furuncle left hand

L02.529   Furuncle unspecified hand

L02.53   **Carbuncle of hand**

L02.531   Carbuncle of right hand

L02.532   Carbuncle of left hand

L02.539   Carbuncle of unspecified hand

L02.6   **Cutaneous abscess, furuncle and carbuncle of foot**

L02.61   **Cutaneous abscess of foot**

L02.611   Cutaneous abscess of right foot

L02.612   Cutaneous abscess of left foot

L02.619   Cutaneous abscess of unspecified foot

L02.62   **Furuncle of foot**

Boil of foot

Folliculitis of foot

L02.621   Furuncle of right foot

L02.622   Furuncle of left foot

L02.629   Furuncle of unspecified foot

L02.63   **Carbuncle of foot**

L02.631   Carbuncle of right foot

L02.632   Carbuncle of left foot

L02.639   Carbuncle of unspecified foot

L02.8   **Cutaneous abscess, furuncle and carbuncle of other sites**

L02.81   **Cutaneous abscess of other sites**

L02.811   Cutaneous abscess of head [any part, except face]

L02.818   Cutaneous abscess of other sites

L02.82   **Furuncle of other sites**

Boil of other sites

Folliculitis of other sites

● New code   ▲ Revised code   Excludes1: Not coded here   Excludes2: Not included here   ⊗ Placeholder required   ⑦7th digit required

L02.821   **Furuncle of head [any part, except face]**

L02.828   **Furuncle of other sites**

L02.83   **Carbuncle of other sites**

L02.831   **Carbuncle of head [any part, except face]**

L02.838   **Carbuncle of other sites**

L02.9   **Cutaneous abscess, furuncle and carbuncle, unspecified**

L02.91   **Cutaneous abscess, unspecified**

L02.92   **Furuncle, unspecified**

Boil NOS

Furunculosis NOS

L02.93   **Carbuncle, unspecified**

L03   **Cellulitis and acute lymphangitis**

Excludes2: cellulitis of anal and rectal region (K61.-)

cellulitis of external auditory canal (H60.1)

cellulitis of eyelid (H00.0)

cellulitis of female external genital organs (N76.4)

cellulitis of lacrimal apparatus (H04.3)

cellulitis of male external genital organs (N48.2, N49.-)

cellulitis of mouth (K12.2)

cellulitis of nose (J34.0)

eosinophilic cellulitis [Wells] (L98.3)

febrile neutrophilic dermatosis [Sweet] (L98.2)

lymphangitis (chronic) (subacute) (I89.1)

L03.0   **Cellulitis and acute lymphangitis of finger and toe**

Infection of nail

Onychia

Paronychia

Perionychia

L03.01   **Cellulitis of finger**

Felon Whitlow

Excludes1: herpetic whitlow (B00.89)

L03.011   **Cellulitis of right finger**

L03.012   **Cellulitis of left finger**

L03.019   **Cellulitis of unspecified finger**

L03.02   **Acute lymphangitis of finger**

Hangnail with lymphangitis of finger

L03.021   **Acute lymphangitis of right finger**

L03.022   **Acute lymphangitis of left finger**

L03.029   **Acute lymphangitis of unspecified finger**

L03.03   **Cellulitis of toe**

L03.031   **Cellulitis of right toe**

L03.032   **Cellulitis of left toe**

L03.039   **Cellulitis of unspecified toe**

L03.04   **Acute lymphangitis of toe**

Hangnail with lymphangitis of toe

L03.041   **Acute lymphangitis of right toe**

L03.042   **Acute lymphangitis of left toe**

L03.049   **Acute lymphangitis of unspecified toe**

L03.1   **Cellulitis and acute lymphangitis of other parts of limb**

L03.11   **Cellulitis of other parts of limb**

Excludes2: cellulitis of fingers (L03.01-)

cellulitis of toes (L03.03-)

groin (L03.314)

L03.111   **Cellulitis of right axilla**

L03.112   **Cellulitis of left axilla**

L03.113   **Cellulitis of right upper limb**

L03.114   **Cellulitis of left upper limb**

L03.115   **Cellulitis of right lower limb**

L03.116   **Cellulitis of left lower limb**

L03.119   **Cellulitis of unspecified part of limb**

L03.12   **Acute lymphangitis of other parts of limb**

Excludes2: acute lymphangitis of fingers (L03.2-)

acute lymphangitis of toes (L03.04-)

acute lymphangitis of groin (L03.324)

L03.121   **Acute lymphangitis of right axilla**

L03.122   **Acute lymphangitis of left axilla**

L03.123   **Acute lymphangitis of right upper limb**

L03.124   **Acute lymphangitis of left upper limb**

L03.125   **Acute lymphangitis of right lower limb**

L03.126   **Acute lymphangitis of left lower limb**

L03.129   **Acute lymphangitis of unspecified part of limb**

L03.2   **Cellulitis and acute lymphangitis of face and neck**

L03.21   **Cellulitis and acute lymphangitis of face**

L03.211   **Cellulitis of face**

Excludes2: abscess of orbit (H05.01-)

cellulitis of ear (H60.1-)

cellulitis of eyelid (H00.0-)

cellulitis of head (L03.81)

cellulitis of lacrimal apparatus (H04.3)

cellulitis of lip (K13.0)

cellulitis of mouth (K12.2)

cellulitis of nose (internal) (J34.0)

cellulitis of orbit (H05.01-)

cellulitis of scalp (L03.81)

L03.212   **Acute lymphangitis of face**

L03.213   **Periorbital cellulitis**

Preseptal cellulitis

L03.22   **Cellulitis and acute lymphangitis of neck**

L03.221   **Cellulitis of neck**

L03.222   **Acute lymphangitis of neck**

L03.3   **Cellulitis and acute lymphangitis of trunk**

L03.31   **Cellulitis of trunk**

Excludes2: cellulitis of anal and rectal regions (K61.-)

cellulitis of breast NOS (N61.0)

cellulitis of female external genital organs (N76.4)

cellulitis of male external genital organs (N48.2, N49.-)

omphalitis of newborn (P38.-)

puerperal cellulitis of breast (O91.2)

L03.311   **Cellulitis of abdominal wall**

Excludes2: cellulitis of umbilicus (L03.316)

cellulitis of groin (L03.314)

L03.312 **Cellulitis of back [any part except buttock]**

L03.313 **Cellulitis of chest wall**

L03.314 **Cellulitis of groin**

L03.315 **Cellulitis of perineum**

L03.316 **Cellulitis of umbilicus**

L03.317 **Cellulitis of buttock**

L03.319 **Cellulitis of trunk, unspecified**

L03.32 **Acute lymphangitis of trunk**

L03.321 **Acute lymphangitis of abdominal wall**

L03.322 **Acute lymphangitis of back [any part except buttock]**

L03.323 **Acute lymphangitis of chest wall**

L03.324 **Acute lymphangitis of groin**

L03.325 **Acute lymphangitis of perineum**

L03.326 **Acute lymphangitis of umbilicus**

L03.327 **Acute lymphangitis of buttock**

L03.329 **Acute lymphangitis of trunk, unspecified**

L03.8 **Cellulitis and acute lymphangitis of other sites**

L03.81 **Cellulitis of other sites**

L03.811 **Cellulitis of head [any part, except face]**

Cellulitis of scalp

Excludes2: cellulitis of face (L03.211)

L03.818 **Cellulitis of other sites**

L03.89 **Acute lymphangitis of other sites**

L03.891 **Acute lymphangitis of head [any part, except face]**

L03.898 **Acute lymphangitis of other sites**

L03.9 **Cellulitis and acute lymphangitis, unspecified**

L03.90 **Cellulitis, unspecified**

L03.91 **Acute lymphangitis, unspecified**

Excludes1: lymphangitis NOS (I89.1)

L04 **Acute lymphadenitis**

Definition: Lymphadenitis is an inflammation of a lymph node. It is often a complication of a bacterial infection of a wound, although it can also be caused by viruses or other disease agents.

Includes: abscess (acute) of lymph nodes, except mesenteric

acute lymphadenitis, except mesenteric

Excludes1: chronic or subacute lymphadenitis, except mesenteric (I88.1)

enlarged lymph nodes (R59.-)

human immunodeficiency virus [HIV] disease resulting in generalized lymphadenopathy (B20)

lymphadenitis NOS (I88.9)

nonspecific mesenteric lymphadenitis (I88.0)

L04.0 **Acute lymphadenitis of face, head and neck**

L04.1 **Acute lymphadenitis of trunk**

L04.2 **Acute lymphadenitis of upper limb**

Acute lymphadenitis of axilla

Acute lymphadenitis of shoulder

L04.3 **Acute lymphadenitis of lower limb**

Acute lymphadenitis of hip

Excludes2: acute lymphadenitis of groin (L04.1)

L04.8 **Acute lymphadenitis of other sites**

L04.9 **Acute lymphadenitis, unspecified**

L05 **Pilonidal cyst and sinus**

L05.0 **Pilonidal cyst and sinus with abscess**

L05.01 **Pilonidal cyst with abscess**

Pilonidal abscess

Pilonidal dimple with abscess

Postanal dimple with abscess

Excludes2: congenital sacral dimple (Q82.6)

parasacral dimple (Q82.6)

L05.02 **Pilonidal sinus with abscess**

Coccygeal fistula with abscess

Coccygeal sinus with abscess

Pilonidal fistula with abscess

L05.9 **Pilonidal cyst and sinus without abscess**

L05.91 **Pilonidal cyst without abscess**

Pilonidal dimple

Postanal dimple

Pilonidal cyst NOS

Excludes2: congenital sacral dimple (Q82.6)

parasacral dimple (Q82.6)

L05.92 **Pilonidal sinus without abscess**

Coccygeal fistula

Coccygeal sinus without abscess

Pilonidal fistula

L08 **Other local infections of skin and subcutaneous tissue**

L08.0 **Pyoderma**

Dermatitis gangrenosa

Purulent dermatitis

Septic dermatitis

Suppurative dermatitis

Excludes1: pyoderma gangrenosum (L88)

pyoderma vegetans (L08.81)

L08.1 **Erythrasma**

L08.8 **Other specified local infections of the skin and subcutaneous tissue**

L08.81 **Pyoderma vegetans**

Excludes1: pyoderma gangrenosum (L88)

pyoderma NOS (L08.0)

L08.82 **Omphalitis not of newborn**

Excludes1: omphalitis of newborn (P38.-)

L08.89 **Other specified local infections of the skin and subcutaneous tissue**

L08.9 **Local infection of the skin and subcutaneous tissue, unspecified**

BULLOUS DISORDERS (L10-L14)

Excludes1: benign familial pemphigus [Hailey-Hailey] (Q82.8)

staphylococcal scalded skin syndrome (L00)

toxic epidermal necrolysis [Lyell] (L51.2)

L10 **Pemphigus**

Excludes1: pemphigus neonatorum (L01.03)

L10.0 **Pemphigus vulgaris**

L10.1 **Pemphigus vegetans**

L10.2 **Pemphigus foliaceous**

L10.3 **Brazilian pemphigus [fogo selvagem]**

L10.4 **Pemphigus erythematosus**

Senear-Usher syndrome

L10.5 **Drug-induced pemphigus**

Use additional code for adverse effect, if applicable, to identify drug (T36-T50 with fifth or sixth character 5)

L10.8 **Other pemphigus**

L10.81 **Paraneoplastic pemphigus**

L10.89 **Other pemphigus**

L10.9 **Pemphigus, unspecified**

L11 **Other acantholytic disorders**

L11.0 **Acquired keratosis follicularis**

Excludes1: keratosis follicularis (congenital) [Darier-White] (Q82.8)

L11.1 **Transient acantholytic dermatosis [Grover]**

L11.8 **Other specified acantholytic disorders**

L11.9 **Acantholytic disorder, unspecified**

L12 **Pemphigoid**

Excludes1: herpes gestationis (O26.4-)

impetigo herpetiformis (L40.1)

L12.0 **Bullous pemphigoid**

L12.1 **Cicatricial pemphigoid**

Benign mucous membrane pemphigoid

L12.2 **Chronic bullous disease of childhood**

Juvenile dermatitis herpetiformis

L12.3 **Acquired epidermolysis bullosa**

Excludes1: epidermolysis bullosa (congenital) (Q81.-)

L12.30 **Acquired epidermolysis bullosa, unspecified**

L12.31 **Epidermolysis bullosa due to drug**

Use additional code for adverse effect, if applicable, to identify drug (T36-T50 with fifth or sixth character 5)

L12.35 **Other acquired epidermolysis bullosa**

L12.8 **Other pemphigoid**

L12.9 **Pemphigoid, unspecified**

L13 **Other bullous disorders**

L13.0 **Dermatitis herpetiformis**

Duhring's disease

Hydroa herpetiformis

Excludes1: juvenile dermatitis herpetiformis (L12.2)

senile dermatitis herpetiformis (L12.0)

L13.1 **Subcorneal pustular dermatitis**

Sneddon-Wilkinson disease

L13.8 **Other specified bullous disorders**

L13.9 **Bullous disorder, unspecified**

L14 **Bullous disorders in diseases classified elsewhere**

Code first underlying disease

DERMATITIS AND ECZEMA (L20-L30)

Note: In this block the terms dermatitis and eczema are used synonymously and interchangeably.

Excludes2: chronic (childhood) granulomatous disease (D71)

dermatitis gangrenosa (L08.0)

dermatitis herpetiformis (L13.0)

dry skin dermatitis (L85.3)

factitial dermatitis (L98.1)

perioral dermatitis (L71.0)

radiation-related disorders of the skin and subcutaneous tissue (L55-L59)

stasis dermatitis (I87.2)

L20 **Atopic dermatitis**

Definition: Atopic dermatitis and related conditions, aka eczema, is a chronic, recurring inflammatory skin disorder that usually first appears in babies or very young children and may last through adulthood. Eczema causes the skin to itch and develop a red, scaly, patchy rash.

L20.0 **Besnier's prurigo**

L20.8 **Other atopic dermatitis**

Excludes2: circumscribed neurodermatitis (L28.0)

L20.81 **Atopic neurodermatitis**

Diffuse neurodermatitis

L20.82 **Flexural eczema**

L20.83 **Infantile (acute) (chronic) eczema**

L20.84 **Intrinsic (allergic) eczema**

L20.89 **Other atopic dermatitis**

L20.9 **Atopic dermatitis, unspecified**

L21 **Seborrheic dermatitis**

Excludes2: infective dermatitis (L30.3)

seborrheic keratosis (L82.-)

L21.0 **Seborrhea capitis**

Cradle cap

L21.1 **Seborrheic infantile dermatitis**

L21.8 **Other seborrheic dermatitis**

L21.9 **Seborrheic dermatitis, unspecified**

Seborrhea NOS

L22 **Diaper dermatitis**

Diaper erythema

Diaper rash

Psoriasiform diaper rash

L23 **Allergic contact dermatitis**

Excludes1: allergy NOS (T78.40)

contact dermatitis NOS (L25.9)

dermatitis NOS (L30.9)

Excludes2: dermatitis due to substances taken internally (L27.-)

dermatitis of eyelid (H01.1-)

diaper dermatitis (L22)

eczema of external ear (H60.5-)

irritant contact dermatitis (L24.-)

perioral dermatitis (L71.0)

radiation-related disorders of the skin and subcutaneous tissue (L55-L59)

L23.0 **Allergic contact dermatitis due to metals**

Allergic contact dermatitis due to chromium

Allergic contact dermatitis due to nickel

L23.1 **Allergic contact dermatitis due to adhesives**

L23.2 **Allergic contact dermatitis due to cosmetics**

L23.3 **Allergic contact dermatitis due to drugs in contact with skin**

Use additional code for adverse effect, if applicable, to identify drug (T36-T50 with fifth or sixth character 5)

Excludes2: dermatitis due to ingested drugs and medicaments (L27.0-L27.1)

L23.4 **Allergic contact dermatitis due to dyes**

L23.5 **Allergic contact dermatitis due to other chemical products**

Allergic contact dermatitis due to cement

Allergic contact dermatitis due to insecticide

Allergic contact dermatitis due to plastic

Allergic contact dermatitis due to rubber

L23.6 **Allergic contact dermatitis due to food in contact with the skin**

Excludes2: dermatitis due to ingested food (L27.2)

L23.7 **Allergic contact dermatitis due to plants, except food**

Excludes2: allergy NOS due to pollen (J30.1)

L23.8 **Allergic contact dermatitis due to other agents**

L23.81 **Allergic contact dermatitis due to animal (cat) (dog) dander**

Allergic contact dermatitis due to animal (cat) (dog) hair

L23.89 **Allergic contact dermatitis due to other agents**

L23.9 **Allergic contact dermatitis, unspecified cause**

Allergic contact eczema NOS

L24 **Irritant contact dermatitis**

Excludes1: allergy NOS (T78.40)

contact dermatitis NOS (L25.9)

dermatitis NOS (L30.9)

Excludes2: allergic contact dermatitis (L23.-)

dermatitis due to substances taken internally (L27.-)

dermatitis of eyelid (H01.1-)

diaper dermatitis (L22)

eczema of external ear (H60.5-)

perioral dermatitis (L71.0)

radiation-related disorders of the skin and subcutaneous tissue (L55-L59)

L24.0 **Irritant contact dermatitis due to detergents**

L24.1 **Irritant contact dermatitis due to oils and greases**

L24.2 **Irritant contact dermatitis due to solvents**

Irritant contact dermatitis due to chlorocompound

Irritant contact dermatitis due to cyclohexane

Irritant contact dermatitis due to ester

Irritant contact dermatitis due to glycol

Irritant contact dermatitis due to hydrocarbon

Irritant contact dermatitis due to ketone

L24.3 **Irritant contact dermatitis due to cosmetics**

L24.4 **Irritant contact dermatitis due to drugs in contact with skin**

Use additional code for adverse effect, if applicable, to identify drug (T36-T50 with fifth or sixth character 5)

L24.5 **Irritant contact dermatitis due to other chemical products**

Irritant contact dermatitis due to cement

Irritant contact dermatitis due to insecticide

Irritant contact dermatitis due to plastic

Irritant contact dermatitis due to rubber

L24.6 **Irritant contact dermatitis due to food in contact with skin**

Excludes2: dermatitis due to ingested food (L27.2)

L24.7 **Irritant contact dermatitis due to plants, except food**

Excludes2: allergy NOS to pollen (J30.1)

L24.8 **Irritant contact dermatitis due to other agents**

L24.81 **Irritant contact dermatitis due to metals**

Irritant contact dermatitis due to chromium

Irritant contact dermatitis due to nickel

L24.89 **Irritant contact dermatitis due to other agents**

Irritant contact dermatitis due to dyes

L24.9 **Irritant contact dermatitis, unspecified cause**

Irritant contact eczema NOS

L25 **Unspecified contact dermatitis**

Excludes1: allergic contact dermatitis (L23.-)

allergy NOS (T78.40)

dermatitis NOS (L30.9)

irritant contact dermatitis (L24.-)

Excludes2: dermatitis due to ingested substances (L27.-)

dermatitis of eyelid (H01.1-)

eczema of external ear (H60.5-)

perioral dermatitis (L71.0)

radiation-related disorders of the skin and subcutaneous tissue (L55-L59)

L25.0 **Unspecified contact dermatitis due to cosmetics**

L25.1 **Unspecified contact dermatitis due to drugs in contact with skin**

Use additional code for adverse effect, if applicable, to identify drug (T36-T50 with fifth or sixth character 5)

Excludes2: dermatitis due to ingested drugs and medicaments (L27.0-L27.1)

L25.2 **Unspecified contact dermatitis due to dyes**

L25.3 **Unspecified contact dermatitis due to other chemical products**

Unspecified contact dermatitis due to cement

Unspecified contact dermatitis due to insecticide

L25.4 **Unspecified contact dermatitis due to food in contact with skin**

Excludes2: dermatitis due to ingested food (L27.2)

L25.5 **Unspecified contact dermatitis due to plants, except food**

Excludes1: nettle rash (L50.9)

Excludes2: allergy NOS due to pollen (J30.1)

L25.8 **Unspecified contact dermatitis due to other agents**

L25.9 **Unspecified contact dermatitis, unspecified cause**

Contact dermatitis (occupational) NOS

Contact eczema (occupational) NOS

L26 **Exfoliative dermatitis**

Hebra's pityriasis

Excludes1: Ritter's disease (L00)

L27 **Dermatitis due to substances taken internally**

Excludes1: allergy NOS (T78.40)

Excludes2: adverse food reaction, except dermatitis (T78.0-T78.1)

contact dermatitis (L23-L25)

drug photoallergic response (L56.1)

drug phototoxic response (L56.0)

urticaria (L50.-)

L27.0 **Generalized skin eruption due to drugs and medicaments taken internally**

Use additional code for adverse effect, if applicable, to identify drug (T36-T50 with fifth or sixth character 5)

L27.1 **Localized skin eruption due to drugs and medicaments taken internally**

Use additional code for adverse effect, if applicable, to identify drug (T36-T50 with fifth or sixth character 5)

L27.2 **Dermatitis due to ingested food**

Excludes2: dermatitis due to food in contact with skin (L23.6, L24.6, L25.4)

L27.8 **Dermatitis due to other substances taken internally**

L27.9 **Dermatitis due to unspecified substance taken internally**

L28 **Lichen simplex chronicus and prurigo**

● New code   ▲ Revised code   Excludes1: Not coded here   Excludes2: Not included here   ⊗ Placeholder required   ⑦7th digit required

L28.0 Lichen simplex chronicus

Circumscribed neurodermatitis

Lichen NOS

L28.1 Prurigo nodularis

L28.2 Other prurigo

Prurigo NOS

Prurigo Hebra

Prurigo mitis

Urticaria papulosa

L29 Pruritus

Excludes1: neurotic excoriation (L98.1)

psychogenic pruritus (F45.8)

L29.0 Pruritus ani

L29.1 Pruritus scroti

L29.2 Pruritus vulvae

L29.3 Anogenital pruritus, unspecified

L29.8 Other pruritus

L29.9 Pruritus, unspecified

Itch NOS

L30 Other and unspecified dermatitis

Excludes2: contact dermatitis (L23-L25)

dry skin dermatitis (L85.3)

small plaque parapsoriasis (L41.3)

stasis dermatitis (I87.2)

L30.0 Nummular dermatitis

L30.1 Dyshidrosis [pompholyx]

L30.2 Cutaneous autosensitization

Candidid [levurid]

Dermatophytid Eczematid

L30.3 Infective dermatitis

Infectious eczematoid dermatitis

L30.4 Erythema intertrigo

L30.5 Pityriasis alba

L30.8 Other specified dermatitis

L30.9 Dermatitis, unspecified

Eczema NOS

PAPULOSQUAMOUS DISORDERS (L40-L45)

L40 Psoriasis

L40.0 Psoriasis vulgaris

Nummular psoriasis

Plaque psoriasis

L40.1 Generalized pustular psoriasis

Impetigo herpetiformis

Von Zumbusch's disease

L40.2 Acrodermatitis continua

L40.3 Pustulosis palmaris et plantaris

L40.4 Guttate psoriasis

L40.5 Arthropathic psoriasis

L40.50 Arthropathic psoriasis, unspecified

L40.51 Distal interphalangeal psoriatic arthropathy

L40.52 Psoriatic arthritis mutilans

L40.53 Psoriatic spondylitis

L40.54 Psoriatic juvenile arthropathy

L40.59 Other psoriatic arthropathy

L40.8 Other psoriasis

Flexural psoriasis

L40.9 Psoriasis, unspecified

L41 Parapsoriasis

Excludes1: poikiloderma vasculare atrophicans (L94.5)

L41.0 Pityriasis lichenoides et varioliformis acuta

Mucha-Habermann disease

L41.1 Pityriasis lichenoides chronica

L41.3 Small plaque parapsoriasis

L41.4 Large plaque parapsoriasis

L41.5 Retiform parapsoriasis

L41.8 Other parapsoriasis

L41.9 Parapsoriasis, unspecified

L42 Pityriasis rosea

L43 Lichen planus

Excludes1: lichen planopilaris (L66.1)

L43.0 Hypertrophic lichen planus

L43.1 Bullous lichen planus

L43.2 Lichenoid drug reaction

Use additional code for adverse effect, if applicable, to identify drug (T36-T50 with fifth or sixth character 5)

L43.3 Subacute (active) lichen planus

Lichen planus tropicus

L43.8 Other lichen planus

L43.9 Lichen planus, unspecified

L44 Other papulosquamous disorders

L44.0 Pityriasis rubra pilaris

L44.1 Lichen nitidus

L44.2 Lichen striatus

L44.3 Lichen ruber moniliformis

L44.4 Infantile papular acrodermatitis [Gianotti-Crosti]

L44.8 Other specified papulosquamous disorders

L44.9 Papulosquamous disorder, unspecified

L45 Papulosquamous disorders in diseases classified elsewhere

Code first underlying disease.

URTICARIA AND ERYTHEMA (L49-L54)

Excludes1: Lyme disease (A69.2-)

rosacea (L71.-)

L49 Exfoliation due to erythematous conditions according to extent of body surface involved

Code first erythematous condition causing exfoliation, such as:

Ritter's disease (L00)

(Staphylococcal) scalded skin syndrome (L00)

Stevens-Johnson syndrome (L51.1)

Stevens-Johnson syndrome-toxic epidermal necrolysis overlap syndrome (L51.3)

Toxic epidermal necrolysis (L51.2)

L49.0 Exfoliation due to erythematous condition involving less than 10 percent of body surface

Exfoliation due to erythematous condition NOS

L49.1 Exfoliation due to erythematous condition involving 10-19 percent of body surface

L49.2 Exfoliation due to erythematous condition involving 20-29 percent of body surface

L49.3 Exfoliation due to erythematous condition involving 30-39 percent of body surface

L49.4 Exfoliation due to erythematous condition involving 40-49 percent of body surface

L49.5 Exfoliation due to erythematous condition involving 50-59 percent of body surface

L49.6 Exfoliation due to erythematous condition involving 60-69 percent of body surface

L49.7 Exfoliation due to erythematous condition involving 70-79 percent of body surface

L49.8 Exfoliation due to erythematous condition involving 80-89 percent of body surface

L49.9 Exfoliation due to erythematous condition involving 90 or more percent of body surface

L50 **Urticaria**

Excludes1: allergic contact dermatitis (L23.-)

angioneurotic edema (T78.3)

giant urticaria (T78.3)

hereditary angio-edema (D84.1)

Quincke's edema (T78.3)

serum urticaria (T80.6-)

solar urticaria (L56.3)

urticaria neonatorum (P83.8)

urticaria papulosa (L28.2)

urticaria pigmentosa (Q82.2)

L50.0 **Allergic urticaria**

L50.1 **Idiopathic urticaria**

L50.2 **Urticaria due to cold and heat**

Excludes2: familial cold urticaria (M04.2)

L50.3 **Dermatographic urticaria**

L50.4 **Vibratory urticaria**

L50.5 **Cholinergic urticaria**

L50.6 **Contact urticaria**

L50.8 **Other urticaria**

Chronic urticaria

Recurrent periodic urticaria

L50.9 **Urticaria, unspecified**

L51 **Erythema multiforme**

Use additional code for adverse effect, if applicable, to identify drug (T36-T50 with fifth or sixth character 5)

Use additional code to identify associated manifestations, such as:

arthropathy associated with dermatological disorders (M14.8-)

conjunctival edema (H11.42)

conjunctivitis (H10.22-)

corneal scars and opacities (H17.-)

corneal ulcer (H16.0-)

edema of eyelid (H02.84)

inflammation of eyelid (H01.8)

keratoconjunctivitis sicca (H16.22-)

mechanical lagophthalmos (H02.22-)

stomatitis (K12.-)

symblepharon (H11.23-)

Use additional code to identify percentage of skin exfoliation (L49.-)

Excludes1: staphylococcal scalded skin syndrome (L00)

Ritter's disease (L00)

L51.0 **Nonbullous erythema multiforme**

L51.1 **Stevens-Johnson syndrome**

L51.2 **Toxic epidermal necrolysis [Lyell]**

L51.3 **Stevens-Johnson syndrome-toxic epidermal necrolysis overlap syndrome**

SJS-TEN overlap syndrome

L51.8 **Other erythema multiforme**

L51.9 **Erythema multiforme, unspecified**

Erythema iris

Erythema multiforme major NOS

Erythema multiforme minor NOS

Herpes iris

L52 **Erythema nodosum**

Excludes1: tuberculous erythema nodosum (A18.4)

L53 **Other erythematous conditions**

Excludes1: erythema ab igne (L59.0)

erythema due to external agents in contact with skin (L23-L25)

erythema intertrigo (L30.4)

L53.0 **Toxic erythema**

Code first poisoning due to drug or toxin, if applicable (T36-T65 with fifth or sixth character 1-4 or 6)

Use additional code for adverse effect, if applicable, to identify drug (T36-T50 with fifth or sixth character 5)

Excludes1: neonatal erythema toxicum (P83.1)

L53.1 **Erythema annulare centrifugum**

L53.2 **Erythema marginatum**

L53.3 **Other chronic figurate erythema**

L53.8 **Other specified erythematous conditions**

L53.9 **Erythematous condition, unspecified**

Erythema NOS

Erythroderma NOS

L54 **Erythema in diseases classified elsewhere**

Code first underlying disease.

RADIATION-RELATED DISORDERS OF THE SKIN AND SUBCUTANEOUS TISSUE (L55-L59)

L55 **Sunburn**

L55.0 **Sunburn of first degree**

L55.1 **Sunburn of second degree**

L55.2 **Sunburn of third degree**

L55.9 **Sunburn, unspecified**

L56 **Other acute skin changes due to ultraviolet radiation**

Use additional code to identify the source of the ultraviolet radiation (W89, X32)

L56.0 **Drug phototoxic response**

Use additional code for adverse effect, if applicable, to identify drug (T36-T50 with fifth or sixth character 5)

L56.1 **Drug photoallergic response**

Use additional code for adverse effect, if applicable, to identify drug (T36-T50 with fifth or sixth character 5)

L56.2 **Photocontact dermatitis [berloque dermatitis]**

L56.3 **Solar urticaria**

L56.4 **Polymorphous light eruption**

L56.5 **Disseminated superficial actinic porokeratosis (DSAP)**

L56.8 **Other specified acute skin changes due to ultraviolet radiation**

L56.9 **Acute skin change due to ultraviolet radiation, unspecified**

L57 **Skin changes due to chronic exposure to nonionizing radiation**

Use additional code to identify the source of the ultraviolet radiation (W89)

L57.0 **Actinic keratosis**

Keratosis NOS

Senile keratosis

Solar keratosis

L57.1   Actinic reticuloid

L57.2   Cutis rhomboidalis nuchae

L57.3   Poikiloderma of Civatte

L57.4   Cutis laxa senilis

    Elastosis senilis

L57.5   Actinic granuloma

L57.8   Other skin changes due to chronic exposure to nonionizing radiation

    Farmer's skin

    Sailor's skin

    Solar dermatitis

L57.9   Skin changes due to chronic exposure to nonionizing radiation, unspecified

L58   Radiodermatitis

Use additional code to identify the source of the radiation (W88, W90)

L58.0   Acute radiodermatitis

L58.1   Chronic radiodermatitis

L58.9   Radiodermatitis, unspecified

L59   Other disorders of skin and subcutaneous tissue related to radiation

L59.0   Erythema ab igne [dermatitis ab igne]

L59.8   Other specified disorders of the skin and subcutaneous tissue related to radiation

L59.9   Disorder of the skin and subcutaneous tissue related to radiation, unspecified

DISORDERS OF SKIN APPENDAGES (L60-L75)

Excludes1: congenital malformations of integument (Q84.-)

L60   Nail disorders

Excludes2: clubbing of nails (R68.3)

    onychia and paronychia (L03.0-)

L60.0   Ingrowing nail

L60.1   Onycholysis

L60.2   Onychogryphosis

L60.3   Nail dystrophy

L60.4   Beau's lines

L60.5   Yellow nail syndrome

L60.8   Other nail disorders

L60.9   Nail disorder, unspecified

L62   Nail disorders in diseases classified elsewhere

Code first underlying disease, such as:

pachydermoperiostosis (M89.4-)

L63   Alopecia areata

L63.0   Alopecia (capitis) totalis

L63.1   Alopecia universalis

L63.2   Ophiasis

L63.8   Other alopecia areata

L63.9   Alopecia areata, unspecified

L64   Androgenic alopecia

Includes: male-pattern baldness

L64.0   Drug-induced androgenic alopecia

    Use additional code for adverse effect, if applicable, to identify drug (T36-T50 with fifth or sixth character 5)

L64.8   Other androgenic alopecia

L64.9   Androgenic alopecia, unspecified

L65   Other nonscarring hair loss

Use additional code for adverse effect, if applicable, to identify drug (T36-T50 with fifth or sixth character 5)

Excludes1: trichotillomania (F63.3)

L65.0   Telogen effluvium

L65.1   Anagen effluvium

L65.2   Alopecia mucinosa

L65.8   Other specified nonscarring hair loss

L65.9   Nonscarring hair loss, unspecified

    Alopecia NOS

L66   Cicatricial alopecia [scarring hair loss]

L66.0   Pseudopelade

L66.1   Lichen planopilaris

    Follicular lichen planus

L66.2   Folliculitis decalvans

L66.3   Perifolliculitis capitis abscedens

L66.4   Folliculitis ulerythematosa reticulata

L66.8   Other cicatricial alopecia

L66.9   Cicatricial alopecia, unspecified

L67   Hair color and hair shaft abnormalities

Excludes1: monilethrix (Q84.1)

    pili annulati (Q84.1)

    telogen effluvium (L65.0)

L67.0   Trichorrhexis nodosa

L67.1   Variations in hair color Canities

    Greyness, hair (premature)

    Heterochromia of hair

    Poliosis circumscripta, acquired

    Poliosis NOS

L67.8   Other hair color and hair shaft abnormalities

    Fragilitas crinium

L67.9   Hair color and hair shaft abnormality, unspecified

L68   Hypertrichosis

Includes: excess hair

Excludes1: congenital hypertrichosis (Q84.2)

    persistent lanugo (Q84.2)

L68.0   Hirsutism

L68.1   Acquired hypertrichosis lanuginosa

L68.2   Localized hypertrichosis

L68.3   Polytrichia

L68.8   Other hypertrichosis

L68.9   Hypertrichosis, unspecified

L70   Acne

Excludes2: acne keloid (L73.0)

L70.0   Acne vulgaris

L70.1   Acne conglobata

L70.2   Acne varioliformis

    Acne necrotica miliaris

L70.3   Acne tropica

L70.4   Infantile acne

L70.5   Acné excoriée

    Acné excoriée des jeunes filles

    Picker's acne

L70.8   Other acne

L70.9   Acne, unspecified

L71   Rosacea

Use additional code for adverse effect, if applicable, to identify drug (T36-T50 with fifth or sixth character 5)

L71.0   **Perioral dermatitis**

L71.1   **Rhinophyma**

L71.8   **Other rosacea**

L71.9   **Rosacea, unspecified**

L72   **Follicular cysts of skin and subcutaneous tissue**

    L72.0   **Epidermal cyst**

    L72.1   **Pilar and trichodermal cyst**

        L72.11   **Pilar cyst**

        L72.12   **Trichodermal cyst**

            Trichilemmal (proliferating) cyst

    L72.2   **Steatocystoma multiplex**

    L72.3   **Sebaceous cyst**

        Excludes2: pilar cyst (L72.11)

            trichilemmal (proliferating) cyst (L72.12)

    L72.8   **Other follicular cysts of the skin and subcutaneous tissue**

    L72.9   **Follicular cyst of the skin and subcutaneous tissue, unspecified**

L73   **Other follicular disorders**

    L73.0   **Acne keloid**

    L73.1   **Pseudofolliculitis barbae**

    L73.2   **Hidradenitis suppurativa**

    L73.8   **Other specified follicular disorders**

        Sycosis barbae

    L73.9   **Follicular disorder, unspecified**

L74   **Eccrine sweat disorders**

    Excludes2: generalized hyperhidrosis (R61)

    L74.0   **Miliaria rubra**

    L74.1   **Miliaria crystallina**

    L74.2   **Miliaria profunda**

        Miliaria tropicalis

    L74.3   **Miliaria, unspecified**

    L74.4   **Anhidrosis**

        Hypohidrosis

    L74.5   **Focal hyperhidrosis**

        L74.51   **Primary focal hyperhidrosis**

            L74.510   **Primary focal hyperhidrosis, axilla**

            L74.511   **Primary focal hyperhidrosis, face**

            L74.512   **Primary focal hyperhidrosis, palms**

            L74.513   **Primary focal hyperhidrosis, soles**

            L74.519   **Primary focal hyperhidrosis, unspecified**

        L74.52   **Secondary focal hyperhidrosis**

            Frey's syndrome

    L74.8   **Other eccrine sweat disorders**

    L74.9   **Eccrine sweat disorder, unspecified**

    Sweat gland disorder NOS

L75   **Apocrine sweat disorders**

    Excludes1: dyshidrosis (L30.1)

        hidradenitis suppurativa (L73.2)

    L75.0   **Bromhidrosis**

    L75.1   **Chromhidrosis**

    L75.2   **Apocrine miliaria**

        Fox-Fordyce disease

    L75.8   **Other apocrine sweat disorders**

    L75.9   **Apocrine sweat disorder, unspecified**

INTRAOPERATIVE AND POSTPROCEDURAL COMPLICATIONS OF SKIN AND SUBCUTANEOUS TISSUE (L76)

L76   **Intraoperative and postprocedural complications of skin and subcutaneous tissue**

    L76.0   **Intraoperative hemorrhage and hematoma of skin and subcutaneous tissue complicating a procedure**

        Excludes1: intraoperative hemorrhage and hematoma of skin and subcutaneous tissue due to accidental puncture and laceration during a procedure (L76.1-)

        L76.01   **Intraoperative hemorrhage and hematoma of skin and subcutaneous tissue complicating a dermatologic procedure**

        L76.02   **Intraoperative hemorrhage and hematoma of skin and subcutaneous tissue complicating other procedure**

    L76.1   **Accidental puncture and laceration of skin and subcutaneous tissue during a procedure**

        L76.11   **Accidental puncture and laceration of skin and subcutaneous tissue during a dermatologic procedure**

        L76.12   **Accidental puncture and laceration of skin and subcutaneous tissue during other procedure**

    L76.2   **Postprocedural hemorrhage of skin and subcutaneous tissue following a procedure**

        L76.21   **Postprocedural hemorrhage of skin and subcutaneous tissue following a dermatologic procedure**

        L76.22   **Postprocedural hemorrhage of skin and subcutaneous tissue following other procedure**

    L76.3   **Postprocedural hematoma and seroma of skin and subcutaneous tissue following a procedure**

        L76.31   **Postprocedural hematoma of skin and subcutaneous tissue following a dermatologic procedure**

        L76.32   **Postprocedural hematoma of skin and subcutaneous tissue following other procedure**

        L76.33   **Postprocedural seroma of skin and subcutaneous tissue following a dermatologic procedure**

        L76.34   **Postprocedural seroma of skin and subcutaneous tissue following other procedure**

    L76.8   **Other intraoperative and postprocedural complications of skin and subcutaneous tissue**

        Use additional code, if applicable, to further specify disorder

        L76.81   **Other intraoperative complications of skin and subcutaneous tissue**

        L76.82   **Other postprocedural complications of skin and subcutaneous tissue**

OTHER DISORDERS OF THE SKIN AND SUBCUTANEOUS TISSUE (L80-L99)

L80   **Vitiligo**

    Excludes2: vitiligo of eyelids (H02.73-)

        vitiligo of vulva (N90.89)

L81   **Other disorders of pigmentation**

    Excludes1: birthmark NOS (Q82.5)

        Peutz-Jeghers syndrome (Q85.8)

    Excludes2: nevus - see Alphabetical Index

    L81.0   **Postinflammatory hyperpigmentation**

    L81.1   **Chloasma**

    L81.2   **Freckles**

    L81.3   **Café au lait spots**

L81.4 **Other melanin hyperpigmentation**

Lentigo

L81.5 **Leukoderma, not elsewhere classified**

L81.6 **Other disorders of diminished melanin formation**

L81.7 **Pigmented purpuric dermatosis**

Angioma serpiginosum

L81.8 **Other specified disorders of pigmentation**

Iron pigmentation

Tattoo pigmentation

L81.9 **Disorder of pigmentation, unspecified**

L82 **Seborrheic keratosis**

Includes: basal cell papilloma

dermatosis papulosa nigra

Leser-Trélat disease

Excludes2: seborrheic dermatitis (L21.-)

L82.0 **Inflamed seborrheic keratosis**

L82.1 **Other seborrheic keratosis**

Seborrheic keratosis NOS

L83 **Acanthosis nigricans**

Confluent and reticulated papillomatosis

L84 **Corns and callosities**

Callus Clavus

L85 **Other epidermal thickening**

Excludes2: hypertrophic disorders of the skin (L91.-)

L85.0 **Acquired ichthyosis**

Excludes1: congenital ichthyosis (Q80.-)

L85.1 **Acquired keratosis [keratoderma] palmaris et plantaris**

Excludes1: inherited keratosis palmaris et plantaris (Q82.8)

L85.2 **Keratosis punctata (palmaris et plantaris)**

L85.3 **Xerosis cutis**

Dry skin dermatitis

L85.8 **Other specified epidermal thickening**

Cutaneous horn

L85.9 **Epidermal thickening, unspecified**

L86 **Keratoderma in diseases classified elsewhere**

Code first underlying disease, such as:

Reiter's disease (M02.3-)

Excludes1: gonococcal keratoderma (A54.89)

gonococcal keratosis (A54.89)

keratoderma due to vitamin A deficiency (E50.8)

keratosis due to vitamin A deficiency (E50.8)

xeroderma due to vitamin A deficiency (E50.8)

L87 **Transepidermal elimination disorders**

Excludes1: granuloma annulare (perforating) (L92.0)

L87.0 **Keratosis follicularis et parafollicularis in cutem penetrans**

Kyrle disease

Hyperkeratosis follicularis penetrans

L87.1 **Reactive perforating collagenosis**

L87.2 **Elastosis perforans serpiginosa**

L87.8 **Other transepidermal elimination disorders**

L87.9 **Transepidermal elimination disorder, unspecified**

L88 **Pyoderma gangrenosum**

Phagedenic pyoderma

Excludes1: dermatitis gangrenosa (L08.0)

L89 **Pressure ulcer**

Includes: bed sore

decubitus ulcer

plaster ulcer

pressure area

pressure sore

Code first any associated gangrene (I96)

Excludes2: decubitus (trophic) ulcer of cervix (uteri) (N86)

diabetic ulcers (E08.621, E08.622, E09.621, E09.622, E10.621, E10.622, E11.621, E11.622, E13.621, E13.622)

non-pressure chronic ulcer of skin (L97.-)

skin infections (L00-L08)

varicose ulcer (I83.0, I83.2)

L89.0 **Pressure ulcer of elbow**

L89.00 **Pressure ulcer of unspecified elbow**

L89.000 **Pressure ulcer of unspecified elbow, unstageable**

L89.001 **Pressure ulcer of unspecified elbow, stage 1**

Healing pressure ulcer of unspecified elbow, stage 1

Pressure pre-ulcer skin changes limited to persistent focal edema, unspecified elbow

L89.002 **Pressure ulcer of unspecified elbow, stage 2**

Healing pressure ulcer of unspecified elbow, stage 2

Pressure ulcer with abrasion, blister, partial thickness skin loss involving epidermis and/or dermis, unspecified elbow

L89.003 **Pressure ulcer of unspecified elbow, stage 3**

Healing pressure ulcer of unspecified elbow, stage 3

Pressure ulcer with full thickness skin loss involving damage or necrosis of subcutaneous tissue, unspecified elbow

L89.004 **Pressure ulcer of unspecified elbow, stage 4**

Healing pressure ulcer of unspecified elbow, stage 4

Pressure ulcer with necrosis of soft tissues through to underlying muscle, tendon, or bone, unspecified elbow

L89.009 **Pressure ulcer of unspecified elbow, unspecified stage**

Healing pressure ulcer of elbow NOS

Healing pressure ulcer of unspecified elbow, unspecified stage

L89.01 **Pressure ulcer of right elbow**

L89.010 **Pressure ulcer of right elbow, unstageable**

L89.011 **Pressure ulcer of right elbow, stage 1**

Healing pressure ulcer of right elbow, stage 1

Pressure pre-ulcer skin changes limited to persistent focal edema, right elbow

L89.012 **Pressure ulcer of right elbow, stage 2**

Healing pressure ulcer of right elbow, stage 2

Pressure ulcer with abrasion, blister, partial thickness skin loss involving epidermis and/or dermis, right elbow

---

Add 4th-7th digits   Nonspecific code   Unspecified code   Manifestation code

L89.013   Pressure ulcer of right elbow, stage 3

Healing pressure ulcer of right elbow, stage 3

Pressure ulcer with full thickness skin loss involving damage or necrosis of subcutaneous tissue, right elbow

L89.014   Pressure ulcer of right elbow, stage 4

Healing pressure ulcer of right elbow, stage 4

Pressure ulcer with necrosis of soft tissues through to underlying muscle, tendon, or bone, right elbow

L89.019   Pressure ulcer of right elbow, unspecified stage

Healing pressure right of elbow NOS

Healing pressure ulcer of right elbow, unspecified stage

L89.02   Pressure ulcer of left elbow

L89.020   Pressure ulcer of left elbow, unstageable

L89.021   Pressure ulcer of left elbow, stage 1

Healing pressure ulcer of left elbow, stage 1

Pressure pre-ulcer skin changes limited to persistent focal edema, left elbow

L89.022   Pressure ulcer of left elbow, stage 2

Healing pressure ulcer of left elbow, stage 2

Pressure ulcer with abrasion, blister, partial thickness skin loss involving epidermis and/or dermis, left elbow

L89.023   Pressure ulcer of left elbow, stage 3

Healing pressure ulcer of left elbow, stage 3

Pressure ulcer with full thickness skin loss involving damage or necrosis of subcutaneous tissue, left elbow

L89.024   Pressure ulcer of left elbow, stage 4

Healing pressure ulcer of left elbow, stage 4

Pressure ulcer with necrosis of soft tissues through to underlying muscle, tendon, or bone, left elbow

L89.029   Pressure ulcer of left elbow, unspecified stage

Healing pressure ulcer of left of elbow NOS

Healing pressure ulcer of left elbow, unspecified stage

L89.1   Pressure ulcer of back

L89.10   Pressure ulcer of unspecified part of back

L89.100   Pressure ulcer of unspecified part of back, unstageable

L89.101   Pressure ulcer of unspecified part of back, stage 1

Healing pressure ulcer of unspecified part of back, stage 1

Pressure pre-ulcer skin changes limited to persistent focal edema, unspecified part of back

L89.102   Pressure ulcer of unspecified part of back, stage 2

Healing pressure ulcer of unspecified part of back, stage 2

Pressure ulcer with abrasion, blister, partial thickness skin loss involving epidermis and/or dermis, unspecified part of back

L89.103   Pressure ulcer of unspecified part of back, stage 3

Healing pressure ulcer of unspecified part of back, stage 3

Pressure ulcer with full thickness skin loss involving damage or necrosis of subcutaneous tissue, unspecified part of back

L89.104   Pressure ulcer of unspecified part of back, stage 4

Healing pressure ulcer of unspecified part of back, stage 4

Pressure ulcer with necrosis of soft tissues through to underlying muscle, tendon, or bone, unspecified part of back

L89.109   Pressure ulcer of unspecified part of back, unspecified stage

Healing pressure ulcer of unspecified part of back NOS

Healing pressure ulcer of unspecified part of back, unspecified stage

L89.11   Pressure ulcer of right upper back

Pressure ulcer of right shoulder blade

L89.110   Pressure ulcer of right upper back, unstageable

L89.111   Pressure ulcer of right upper back, stage 1

Healing pressure ulcer of right upper back, stage 1

Pressure pre-ulcer skin changes limited to persistent focal edema, right upper back

L89.112   Pressure ulcer of right upper back, stage 2

Healing pressure ulcer of right upper back, stage 2

Pressure ulcer with abrasion, blister, partial thickness skin loss involving epidermis and/or dermis, right upper back

L89.113   Pressure ulcer of right upper back, stage 3

Healing pressure ulcer of right upper back, stage 3

Pressure ulcer with full thickness skin loss involving damage or necrosis of subcutaneous tissue, right upper back

L89.114   Pressure ulcer of right upper back, stage 4

Healing pressure ulcer of right upper back, stage 4

Pressure ulcer with necrosis of soft tissues through to underlying muscle, tendon, or bone, right upper back

L89.119   Pressure ulcer of right upper back, unspecified stage

Healing pressure ulcer of right upper back NOS

Healing pressure ulcer of right upper back, unspecified stage

● New code   ▲ Revised code   **Excludes1:** Not coded here   **Excludes2:** Not included here   ⊗ Placeholder required   ⑦ 7th digit required

L89.12 **Pressure ulcer of left upper back**

Pressure ulcer of left shoulder blade

L89.120 **Pressure ulcer of left upper back, unstageable**

L89.121 **Pressure ulcer of left upper back, stage 1**

Healing pressure ulcer of left upper back, stage 1

Pressure pre-ulcer skin changes limited to persistent focal edema, left upper back

L89.122 **Pressure ulcer of left upper back, stage 2**

Healing pressure ulcer of left upper back, stage 2

Pressure ulcer with abrasion, blister, partial thickness skin loss involving epidermis and/or dermis, left upper back

L89.123 **Pressure ulcer of left upper back, stage 3**

Healing pressure ulcer of left upper back, stage 3

Pressure ulcer with full thickness skin loss involving damage or necrosis of subcutaneous tissue, left upper back

L89.124 **Pressure ulcer of left upper back, stage 4**

Healing pressure ulcer of left upper back, stage 4

Pressure ulcer with necrosis of soft tissues through to underlying muscle, tendon, or bone, left upper back

L89.129 **Pressure ulcer of left upper back, unspecified stage**

Healing pressure ulcer of left upper back NOS

Healing pressure ulcer of left upper back, unspecified stage

L89.13 **Pressure ulcer of right lower back**

L89.130 **Pressure ulcer of right lower back, unstageable**

L89.131 **Pressure ulcer of right lower back, stage 1**

Healing pressure ulcer of right lower back, stage 1

Pressure pre-ulcer skin changes limited to persistent focal edema, right lower back

L89.132 **Pressure ulcer of right lower back, stage 2**

Healing pressure ulcer of right lower back, stage 2

Pressure ulcer with abrasion, blister, partial thickness skin loss involving epidermis and/or dermis, right lower back

L89.133 **Pressure ulcer of right lower back, stage 3**

Healing pressure ulcer of right lower back, stage 3

Pressure ulcer with full thickness skin loss involving damage or necrosis of subcutaneous tissue, right lower back

L89.134 **Pressure ulcer of right lower back, stage 4**

Healing pressure ulcer of right lower back, stage 4

Pressure ulcer with necrosis of soft tissues through to underlying muscle, tendon, or bone, right lower back

L89.139 **Pressure ulcer of right lower back, unspecified stage**

Healing pressure ulcer of right lower back NOS

Healing pressure ulcer of right lower back, unspecified stage

L89.14 **Pressure ulcer of left lower back**

L89.140 **Pressure ulcer of left lower back, unstageable**

L89.141 **Pressure ulcer of left lower back, stage 1**

Healing pressure ulcer of left lower back, stage 1

Pressure pre-ulcer skin changes limited to persistent focal edema, left lower back

L89.142 **Pressure ulcer of left lower back, stage 2**

Healing pressure ulcer of left lower back, stage 2

Pressure ulcer with abrasion, blister, partial thickness skin loss involving epidermis and/or dermis, left lower back

L89.143 **Pressure ulcer of left lower back, stage 3**

Healing pressure ulcer of left lower back, stage 3

Pressure ulcer with full thickness skin loss involving damage or necrosis of subcutaneous tissue, left lower back

L89.144 **Pressure ulcer of left lower back, stage 4**

Healing pressure ulcer of left lower back, stage 4

Pressure ulcer with necrosis of soft tissues through to underlying muscle, tendon, or bone, left lower back

L89.149 **Pressure ulcer of left lower back, unspecified stage**

Healing pressure ulcer of left lower back NOS

Healing pressure ulcer of left lower back, unspecified stage

L89.15 **Pressure ulcer of sacral region**

Pressure ulcer of coccyx

Pressure ulcer of tailbone

L89.150 **Pressure ulcer of sacral region, unstageable**

L89.151 **Pressure ulcer of sacral region, stage 1**

Healing pressure ulcer of sacral region, stage 1

Pressure pre-ulcer skin changes limited to persistent focal edema, sacral region

L89.152 **Pressure ulcer of sacral region, stage 2**

Healing pressure ulcer of sacral region, stage 2

Pressure ulcer with abrasion, blister, partial thickness skin loss involving epidermis and/or dermis, sacral region

L89.153 **Pressure ulcer of sacral region, stage 3**

Healing pressure ulcer of sacral region, stage 3

Pressure ulcer with full thickness skin loss involving damage or necrosis of subcutaneous tissue, sacral region

L89.154 **Pressure ulcer of sacral region, stage 4**

Healing pressure ulcer of sacral region, stage 4

Pressure ulcer with necrosis of soft tissues through to underlying muscle, tendon, or bone, sacral region

L89.159 **Pressure ulcer of sacral region, unspecified stage**

Healing pressure ulcer of sacral region NOS

Healing pressure ulcer of sacral region, unspecified stage

L89.2 **Pressure ulcer of hip**

L89.20 **Pressure ulcer of unspecified hip**

L89.200 **Pressure ulcer of unspecified hip, unstageable**

L89.201 **Pressure ulcer of unspecified hip, stage 1**

Healing pressure ulcer of unspecified hip back, stage 1

Pressure pre-ulcer skin changes limited to persistent focal edema, unspecified hip

L89.202 **Pressure ulcer of unspecified hip, stage 2**

Healing pressure ulcer of unspecified hip, stage 2

Pressure ulcer with abrasion, blister, partial thickness skin loss involving epidermis and/or dermis, unspecified hip

L89.203 **Pressure ulcer of unspecified hip, stage 3**

Healing pressure ulcer of unspecified hip, stage 3

Pressure ulcer with full thickness skin loss involving damage or necrosis of subcutaneous tissue, unspecified hip

L89.204 **Pressure ulcer of unspecified hip, stage 4**

Healing pressure ulcer of unspecified hip, stage 4

Pressure ulcer with necrosis of soft tissues through to underlying muscle, tendon, or bone, unspecified hip

L89.209 **Pressure ulcer of unspecified hip, unspecified stage**

Healing pressure ulcer of unspecified hip NOS

Healing pressure ulcer of unspecified hip, unspecified stage

L89.21 **Pressure ulcer of right hip**

L89.210 **Pressure ulcer of right hip, unstageable**

L89.211 **Pressure ulcer of right hip, stage 1**

Healing pressure ulcer of right hip back, stage 1

Pressure pre-ulcer skin changes limited to persistent focal edema, right hip

L89.212 **Pressure ulcer of right hip, stage 2**

Healing pressure ulcer of right hip, stage 2

Pressure ulcer with abrasion, blister, partial thickness skin loss involving epidermis and/or dermis, right hip

L89.213 **Pressure ulcer of right hip, stage 3**

Healing pressure ulcer of right hip, stage 3

Pressure ulcer with full thickness skin loss involving damage or necrosis of subcutaneous tissue, right hip

L89.214 **Pressure ulcer of right hip, stage 4**

Healing pressure ulcer of right hip, stage 4

Pressure ulcer with necrosis of soft tissues through to underlying muscle, tendon, or bone, right hip

L89.219 **Pressure ulcer of right hip, unspecified stage**

Healing pressure ulcer of right hip NOS

Healing pressure ulcer of right hip, unspecified stage

L89.22 **Pressure ulcer of left hip**

L89.220 **Pressure ulcer of left hip, unstageable**

L89.221 **Pressure ulcer of left hip, stage 1**

Healing pressure ulcer of left hip back, stage 1

Pressure pre-ulcer skin changes limited to persistent focal edema, left hip

L89.222 **Pressure ulcer of left hip, stage 2**

Healing pressure ulcer of left hip, stage 2

Pressure ulcer with abrasion, blister, partial thickness skin loss involving epidermis and/or dermis, left hip

L89.223 **Pressure ulcer of left hip, stage 3**

Healing pressure ulcer of left hip, stage 3

Pressure ulcer with full thickness skin loss involving damage or necrosis of subcutaneous tissue, left hip

L89.224 **Pressure ulcer of left hip, stage 4**

Healing pressure ulcer of left hip, stage 4

Pressure ulcer with necrosis of soft tissues through to underlying muscle, tendon, or bone, left hip

L89.229 **Pressure ulcer of left hip, unspecified stage**

Healing pressure ulcer of left hip NOS

Healing pressure ulcer of left hip, unspecified stage

L89.3 **Pressure ulcer of buttock**

L89.30 Pressure ulcer of unspecified buttock

    L89.300 **Pressure ulcer of unspecified buttock, unstageable**

    L89.301 **Pressure ulcer of unspecified buttock, stage 1**

        Healing pressure ulcer of unspecified buttock, stage 1

        Pressure pre-ulcer skin changes limited to persistent focal edema, unspecified buttock

    L89.302 **Pressure ulcer of unspecified buttock, stage 2**

        Healing pressure ulcer of unspecified buttock, stage 2

        Pressure ulcer with abrasion, blister, partial thickness skin loss involving epidermis and/or dermis, unspecified buttock

    L89.303 **Pressure ulcer of unspecified buttock, stage 3**

        Healing pressure ulcer of unspecified buttock, stage 3

        Pressure ulcer with full thickness skin loss involving damage or necrosis of subcutaneous tissue, unspecified buttock

    L89.304 **Pressure ulcer of unspecified buttock, stage 4**

        Healing pressure ulcer of unspecified buttock, stage 4

        Pressure ulcer with necrosis of soft tissues through to underlying muscle, tendon, or bone, unspecified buttock

    L89.309 **Pressure ulcer of unspecified buttock, unspecified stage**

        Healing pressure ulcer of unspecified buttock NOS

        Healing pressure ulcer of unspecified buttock, unspecified stage

L89.31 Pressure ulcer of right buttock

    L89.310 **Pressure ulcer of right buttock, unstageable**

    L89.311 **Pressure ulcer of right buttock, stage 1**

        Healing pressure ulcer of right buttock, stage 1

        Pressure pre-ulcer skin changes limited to persistent focal edema, right buttock

    L89.312 **Pressure ulcer of right buttock, stage 2**

        Healing pressure ulcer of right buttock, stage 2

        Pressure ulcer with abrasion, blister, partial thickness skin loss involving epidermis and/or dermis, right buttock

    L89.313 **Pressure ulcer of right buttock, stage 3**

        Healing pressure ulcer of right buttock, stage 3

        Pressure ulcer with full thickness skin loss involving damage or necrosis of subcutaneous tissue, right buttock

    L89.314 **Pressure ulcer of right buttock, stage 4**

        Healing pressure ulcer of right buttock, stage 4

        Pressure ulcer with necrosis of soft tissues through to underlying muscle, tendon, or bone, right buttock

    L89.319 **Pressure ulcer of right buttock, unspecified stage**

        Healing pressure ulcer of right buttock NOS

        Healing pressure ulcer of right buttock, unspecified stage

L89.32 Pressure ulcer of left buttock

    L89.320 **Pressure ulcer of left buttock, unstageable**

    L89.321 **Pressure ulcer of left buttock, stage 1**

        Healing pressure ulcer of left buttock, stage 1

        Pressure pre-ulcer skin changes limited to persistent focal edema, left buttock

    L89.322 **Pressure ulcer of left buttock, stage 2**

        Healing pressure ulcer of left buttock, stage 2

        Pressure ulcer with abrasion, blister, partial thickness skin loss involving epidermis and/or dermis, left buttock

    L89.323 **Pressure ulcer of left buttock, stage 3**

        Healing pressure ulcer of left buttock, stage 3

        Pressure ulcer with full thickness skin loss involving damage or necrosis of subcutaneous tissue, left buttock

    L89.324 **Pressure ulcer of left buttock, stage 4**

        Healing pressure ulcer of left buttock, stage 4

        Pressure ulcer with necrosis of soft tissues through to underlying muscle, tendon, or bone, left buttock

    L89.329 **Pressure ulcer of left buttock, unspecified stage**

        Healing pressure ulcer of left buttock NOS

        Healing pressure ulcer of left buttock, unspecified stage

L89.4 **Pressure ulcer of contiguous site of back, buttock and hip**

    L89.40 **Pressure ulcer of contiguous site of back, buttock and hip, unspecified stage**

        Healing pressure ulcer of contiguous site of back, buttock and hip NOS

        Healing pressure ulcer of contiguous site of back, buttock and hip, unspecified stage

    L89.41 **Pressure ulcer of contiguous site of back, buttock and hip, stage 1**

        Healing pressure ulcer of contiguous site of back, buttock and hip, stage 1

        Pressure pre-ulcer skin changes limited to persistent focal edema, contiguous site of back, buttock and hip

    L89.42 **Pressure ulcer of contiguous site of back, buttock and hip, stage 2**

        Healing pressure ulcer of contiguous site of back, buttock and hip, stage 2

Pressure ulcer with abrasion, blister, partial thickness skin loss involving epidermis and/or dermis, contiguous site of back, buttock and hip

L89.43 Pressure ulcer of contiguous site of back, buttock and hip, stage 3

Healing pressure ulcer of contiguous site of back, buttock and hip, stage 3

Pressure ulcer with full thickness skin loss involving damage or necrosis of subcutaneous tissue, contiguous site of back, buttock and hip

L89.44 Pressure ulcer of contiguous site of back, buttock and hip, stage 4

Healing pressure ulcer of contiguous site of back, buttock and hip, stage 4

Pressure ulcer with necrosis of soft tissues through to underlying muscle, tendon, or bone, contiguous site of back, buttock and hip

L89.45 Pressure ulcer of contiguous site of back, buttock and hip, unstageable

L89.5 Pressure ulcer of ankle

L89.50 Pressure ulcer of unspecified ankle

L89.500 Pressure ulcer of unspecified ankle, unstageable

L89.501 Pressure ulcer of unspecified ankle, stage 1

Healing pressure ulcer of unspecified ankle, stage 1

Pressure pre-ulcer skin changes limited to persistent focal edema, unspecified ankle

L89.502 Pressure ulcer of unspecified ankle, stage 2

Healing pressure ulcer of unspecified ankle, stage 2

Pressure ulcer with abrasion, blister, partial thickness skin loss involving epidermis and/or dermis, unspecified ankle

L89.503 Pressure ulcer of unspecified ankle, stage 3

Healing pressure ulcer of unspecified ankle, stage 3

Pressure ulcer with full thickness skin loss involving damage or necrosis of subcutaneous tissue, unspecified ankle

L89.504 Pressure ulcer of unspecified ankle, stage 4

Healing pressure ulcer of unspecified ankle, stage 4

Pressure ulcer with necrosis of soft tissues through to underlying muscle, tendon, or bone, unspecified ankle

L89.509 Pressure ulcer of unspecified ankle, unspecified stage

Healing pressure ulcer of unspecified ankle NOS

Healing pressure ulcer of unspecified ankle, unspecified stage

L89.51 Pressure ulcer of right ankle

L89.510 Pressure ulcer of right ankle, unstageable

L89.511 Pressure ulcer of right ankle, stage 1

Healing pressure ulcer of right ankle, stage 1

Pressure pre-ulcer skin changes limited to persistent focal edema, right ankle

L89.512 Pressure ulcer of right ankle, stage 2

Healing pressure ulcer of right ankle, stage 2

Pressure ulcer with abrasion, blister, partial thickness skin loss involving epidermis and/or dermis, right ankle

L89.513 Pressure ulcer of right ankle, stage 3

Healing pressure ulcer of right ankle, stage 3

Pressure ulcer with full thickness skin loss involving damage or necrosis of subcutaneous tissue, right ankle

L89.514 Pressure ulcer of right ankle, stage 4

Healing pressure ulcer of right ankle, stage 4

Pressure ulcer with necrosis of soft tissues through to underlying muscle, tendon, or bone, right ankle

L89.519 Pressure ulcer of right ankle, unspecified stage

Healing pressure ulcer of right ankle NOS

Healing pressure ulcer of right ankle, unspecified stage

L89.52 Pressure ulcer of left ankle

L89.520 Pressure ulcer of left ankle, unstageable

L89.521 Pressure ulcer of left ankle, stage 1

Healing pressure ulcer of left ankle, stage 1

Pressure pre-ulcer skin changes limited to persistent focal edema, left ankle

L89.522 Pressure ulcer of left ankle, stage 2

Healing pressure ulcer of left ankle, stage 2

Pressure ulcer with abrasion, blister, partial thickness skin loss involving epidermis and/or dermis, left ankle

L89.523 Pressure ulcer of left ankle, stage 3

Healing pressure ulcer of left ankle, stage 3

Pressure ulcer with full thickness skin loss involving damage or necrosis of subcutaneous tissue, left ankle

L89.524 Pressure ulcer of left ankle, stage 4

Healing pressure ulcer of left ankle, stage 4

Pressure ulcer with necrosis of soft tissues through to underlying muscle, tendon, or bone, left ankle

L89.529 Pressure ulcer of left ankle, unspecified stage

Healing pressure ulcer of left ankle NOS

Healing pressure ulcer of left ankle, unspecified stage

L89.6 Pressure ulcer of heel

L89.60 Pressure ulcer of unspecified heel

L89.600 Pressure ulcer of unspecified heel, unstageable

L89.601 Pressure ulcer of unspecified heel, stage 1

Healing pressure ulcer of unspecified heel, stage 1

Pressure pre-ulcer skin changes limited to persistent focal edema, unspecified heel

L89.602 **Pressure ulcer of unspecified heel, stage 2**

Healing pressure ulcer of unspecified heel, stage 2

Pressure ulcer with abrasion, blister, partial thickness skin loss involving epidermis and/or dermis, unspecified heel

L89.603 **Pressure ulcer of unspecified heel, stage 3**

Healing pressure ulcer of unspecified heel, stage 3

Pressure ulcer with full thickness skin loss involving damage or necrosis of subcutaneous tissue, unspecified heel

L89.604 **Pressure ulcer of unspecified heel, stage 4**

Healing pressure ulcer of unspecified heel, stage 4

Pressure ulcer with necrosis of soft tissues through to underlying muscle, tendon, or bone, unspecified heel

L89.609 **Pressure ulcer of unspecified heel, unspecified stage**

Healing pressure ulcer of unspecified heel NOS

Healing pressure ulcer of unspecified heel, unspecified stage

L89.61 **Pressure ulcer of right heel**

L89.610 **Pressure ulcer of right heel, unstageable**

L89.611 **Pressure ulcer of right heel, stage 1**

Healing pressure ulcer of right heel, stage 1

Pressure pre-ulcer skin changes limited to persistent focal edema, right heel

L89.612 **Pressure ulcer of right heel, stage 2**

Healing pressure ulcer of right heel, stage 2

Pressure ulcer with abrasion, blister, partial thickness skin loss involving epidermis and/or dermis, right heel

L89.613 **Pressure ulcer of right heel, stage 3**

Healing pressure ulcer of right heel, stage 3

Pressure ulcer with full thickness skin loss involving damage or necrosis of subcutaneous tissue, right heel

L89.614 **Pressure ulcer of right heel, stage 4**

Healing pressure ulcer of right heel, stage 4

Pressure ulcer with necrosis of soft tissues through to underlying muscle, tendon, or bone, right heel

L89.619 **Pressure ulcer of right heel, unspecified stage**

Healing pressure ulcer of right heel NOS

Healing pressure ulcer of right heel, unspecified stage

L89.62 **Pressure ulcer of left heel**

L89.620 **Pressure ulcer of left heel, unstageable**

L89.621 **Pressure ulcer of left heel, stage 1**

Healing pressure ulcer of left heel, stage 1

Pressure pre-ulcer skin changes limited to persistent focal edema, left heel

L89.622 **Pressure ulcer of left heel, stage 2**

Healing pressure ulcer of left heel, stage 2

Pressure ulcer with abrasion, blister, partial thickness skin loss involving epidermis and/or dermis, left heel

L89.623 **Pressure ulcer of left heel, stage 3**

Healing pressure ulcer of left heel, stage 3

Pressure ulcer with full thickness skin loss involving damage or necrosis of subcutaneous tissue, left heel

L89.624 **Pressure ulcer of left heel, stage 4**

Healing pressure ulcer of left heel, stage 4

Pressure ulcer with necrosis of soft tissues through to underlying muscle, tendon, or bone, left heel

L89.629 **Pressure ulcer of left heel, unspecified stage**

Healing pressure ulcer of left heel NOS

Healing pressure ulcer of left heel, unspecified stage

L89.8 **Pressure ulcer of other site**

L89.81 **Pressure ulcer of head**

Pressure ulcer of face

L89.810 **Pressure ulcer of head, unstageable**

L89.811 **Pressure ulcer of head, stage 1**

Healing pressure ulcer of head, stage 1

Pressure pre-ulcer skin changes limited to persistent focal edema, head

L89.812 **Pressure ulcer of head, stage 2**

Healing pressure ulcer of head, stage 2

Pressure ulcer with abrasion, blister, partial thickness skin loss involving epidermis and/or dermis, head

L89.813 **Pressure ulcer of head, stage 3**

Healing pressure ulcer of head, stage 3

Pressure ulcer with full thickness skin loss involving damage or necrosis of subcutaneous tissue, head

L89.814 **Pressure ulcer of head, stage 4**

Healing pressure ulcer of head, stage 4

Pressure ulcer with necrosis of soft tissues through to underlying muscle, tendon, or bone, head

L89.819 **Pressure ulcer of head, unspecified stage**

Healing pressure ulcer of head NOS

Healing pressure ulcer of head, unspecified stage

L89.89 **Pressure ulcer of other site**

L89.890 **Pressure ulcer of other site, unstageable**

| | Add 4th-7th digits | | Nonspecific code | | Unspecified code | | Manifestation code | 485 |

L89.891 **Pressure ulcer of other site, stage 1**

Healing pressure ulcer **of other** site, stage 1

Pressure pre-ulcer skin changes limited to persistent focal edema, **other** site

L89.892 **Pressure ulcer of other site, stage 2**

Healing pressure ulcer **of other** site, stage 2

Pressure ulcer with abrasion, blister, partial thickness skin loss involving epidermis and/or dermis, **other** site

L89.893 **Pressure ulcer of other site, stage 3**

Healing pressure ulcer **of other** site, stage 3

Pressure ulcer with full thickness skin loss involving damage or necrosis of subcutaneous tissue, **other** site

L89.894 **Pressure ulcer of other site, stage 4**

Healing pressure ulcer **of other** site, stage 4

Pressure ulcer with necrosis of soft tissues through to underlying muscle, tendon, or bone, **other** site

L89.899 **Pressure ulcer of other site, unspecified stage**

Healing pressure ulcer **of other** site NOS

Healing pressure ulcer **of other** site, unspecified stage

L89.9 **Pressure ulcer of unspecified site**

L89.90 **Pressure ulcer of unspecified site, unspecified stage**

Healing pressure ulcer of unspecified site NOS

Healing pressure ulcer of unspecified site, unspecified stage

L89.91 **Pressure ulcer of unspecified site, stage 1**

Healing pressure ulcer of unspecified site, stage 1

Pressure pre-ulcer skin changes limited to persistent focal edema, unspecified site

L89.92 **Pressure ulcer of unspecified site, stage 2**

Healing pressure ulcer of unspecified site, stage 2

Pressure ulcer with abrasion, blister, partial thickness skin loss involving epidermis and/or dermis, unspecified site

L89.93 **Pressure ulcer of unspecified site, stage 3**

Healing pressure ulcer of unspecified site, stage 3

Pressure ulcer with full thickness skin loss involving damage or necrosis of subcutaneous tissue, unspecified site

L89.94 **Pressure ulcer of unspecified site, stage 4**

Healing pressure ulcer of unspecified site, stage 4

Pressure ulcer with necrosis of soft tissues through to underlying muscle, tendon, or bone, unspecified site

L89.95 **Pressure ulcer of unspecified site, unstageable**

L90 **Atrophic disorders of skin**

L90.0 **Lichen sclerosus et atrophicus**

Excludes2: lichen sclerosus of external female genital organs (N90.4)

lichen sclerosus of external male genital organs (N48.0)

L90.1 **Anetoderma of Schweninger-Buzzi**

L90.2 **Anetoderma of Jadassohn-Pellizzari**

L90.3 **Atrophoderma of Pasini and Pierini**

L90.4 **Acrodermatitis chronica atrophicans**

L90.5 **Scar conditions and fibrosis of skin**

Adherent scar (skin)

Cicatrix

Disfigurement of skin due to scar

Fibrosis of skin NOS

Scar NOS

Excludes2: hypertrophic scar (L91.0)

keloid scar (L91.0)

L90.6 **Striae atrophicae**

L90.8 **Other atrophic disorders of skin**

L90.9 **Atrophic disorder of skin, unspecified**

L91 **Hypertrophic disorders of skin**

L91.0 **Hypertrophic scar**

Keloid

Keloid scar

Excludes2: acne keloid (L73.0)

scar NOS (L90.5)

L91.8 **Other hypertrophic disorders of the skin**

L91.9 **Hypertrophic disorder of the skin, unspecified**

L92 **Granulomatous disorders of skin and subcutaneous tissue**

Excludes2: actinic granuloma (L57.5)

L92.0 **Granuloma annulare**

Perforating granuloma annulare

L92.1 **Necrobiosis lipoidica, not elsewhere classified**

Excludes1: necrobiosis lipoidica associated with diabetes mellitus (E08-E13 with .620)

L92.2 **Granuloma faciale [eosinophilic granuloma of skin]**

L92.3 **Foreign body granuloma of the skin and subcutaneous tissue**

Use additional code to identify the type of retained foreign body (Z18.-)

L92.8 **Other granulomatous disorders of the skin and subcutaneous tissue**

L92.9 **Granulomatous disorder of the skin and subcutaneous tissue, unspecified**

Excludes2: umbilical granuloma (P83.81)

L93 **Lupus erythematosus**

Use additional code for adverse effect, if applicable, to identify drug (T36-T50 with fifth or sixth character 5)

Excludes1: lupus exedens (A18.4)

lupus vulgaris (A18.4)

scleroderma (M34.-)

systemic lupus erythematosus (M32.-)

L93.0 **Discoid lupus erythematosus**

Lupus erythematosus NOS

L93.1 **Subacute cutaneous lupus erythematosus**

L93.2 **Other local lupus erythematosus**

Lupus erythematosus profundus

Lupus panniculitis

L94 **Other localized connective tissue disorders**

Excludes1: systemic connective tissue disorders (M30-M36)

L94.0 **Localized scleroderma [morphea]**

Circumscribed scleroderma

L94.1 **Linear scleroderma**

En coup de sabre lesion

L94.2 **Calcinosis cutis**

● New code ▲ Revised code **Excludes1:** Not coded here **Excludes2:** Not included here ⊗ Placeholder required ⑦ 7th digit required

L94.3   Sclerodactyly

L94.4   Gottron's papules

L94.5   Poikiloderma vasculare atrophicans

L94.6   Ainhum

L94.8   Other specified localized connective tissue disorders

L94.9   Localized connective tissue disorder, unspecified

L95   Vasculitis limited to skin, not elsewhere classified

Excludes1: angioma serpiginosum (L81.7)

Henoch(-Schönlein) purpura (D69.0)

hypersensitivity angiitis (M31.0)

lupus panniculitis (L93.2)

panniculitis NOS (M79.3)

panniculitis of neck and back (M54.0-)

polyarteritis nodosa (M30.0)

relapsing panniculitis (M35.6)

rheumatoid vasculitis (M05.2)

serum sickness (T80.6-)

urticaria (L50.-)

Wegener's granulomatosis (M31.3-)

L95.0   Livedoid vasculitis

Atrophie blanche (en plaque)

L95.1   Erythema elevatum diutinum

L95.8   Other vasculitis limited to the skin

L95.9   Vasculitis limited to the skin, unspecified

L97   Non-pressure chronic ulcer of lower limb, not elsewhere classified

Includes: chronic ulcer of skin of lower limb NOS

non-healing ulcer of skin non-infected sinus of skin trophic ulcer NOS

tropical ulcer NOS

ulcer of skin of lower limb NOS

Code first any associated underlying condition, such as:

any associated gangrene (I96)

atherosclerosis of the lower extremities (I70.23-, I70.24-, I70.33-, I70.34-, I70.43-, I70.44-, I70.53-, I70.54-, I70.63-, I70.64-, I70.73-, I70.74-)

chronic venous hypertension (I87.31-, I87.33-)

diabetic ulcers (E08.621, E08.622, E09.621, E09.622, E10.621, E10.622, E11.621, E11.622, E13.621, E13.622)

postphlebitic syndrome (I87.01-, I87.03-)

postthrombotic syndrome (I87.01-, I87.03-)

varicose ulcer (I83.0-, I83.2-)

Excludes2: pressure ulcer (pressure area) (L89.-)

skin infections (L00-L08)

specific infections classified to A00-B99

L97.1   Non-pressure chronic ulcer of thigh

L97.10   Non-pressure chronic ulcer of unspecified thigh

L97.101   Non-pressure chronic ulcer of unspecified thigh limited to breakdown of skin

L97.102   Non-pressure chronic ulcer of unspecified thigh with fat layer exposed

L97.103   Non-pressure chronic ulcer of unspecified thigh with necrosis of muscle

L97.104   Non-pressure chronic ulcer of unspecified thigh with necrosis of bone

L97.105   Non-pressure chronic ulcer of unspecified thigh with muscle involvement without evidence of necrosis

L97.106   Non-pressure chronic ulcer of unspecified thigh with bone involvement without evidence of necrosis

L97.108   Non-pressure chronic ulcer of unspecified thigh with other specified severity

L97.109   Non-pressure chronic ulcer of unspecified thigh with unspecified severity

L97.11   Non-pressure chronic ulcer of right thigh

L97.111   Non-pressure chronic ulcer of right thigh limited to breakdown of skin

L97.112   Non-pressure chronic ulcer of right thigh with fat layer exposed

L97.113   Non-pressure chronic ulcer of right thigh with necrosis of muscle

L97.114   Non-pressure chronic ulcer of right thigh with necrosis of bone

L97.115   Non-pressure chronic ulcer of right thigh with muscle involvement without evidence of necrosis

L97.116   Non-pressure chronic ulcer of right thigh with bone involvement without evidence of necrosis

L97.118   Non-pressure chronic ulcer of right thigh with other specified severity

L97.119   Non-pressure chronic ulcer of right thigh with unspecified severity

L97.12   Non-pressure chronic ulcer of left thigh

L97.121   Non-pressure chronic ulcer of left thigh limited to breakdown of skin

L97.122   Non-pressure chronic ulcer of left thigh with fat layer exposed

L97.123   Non-pressure chronic ulcer of left thigh with necrosis of muscle

L97.124   Non-pressure chronic ulcer of left thigh with necrosis of bone

L97.125   Non-pressure chronic ulcer of left thigh with muscle involvement without evidence of necrosis

L97.126   Non-pressure chronic ulcer of left thigh with bone involvement without evidence of necrosis

L97.128   Non-pressure chronic ulcer of left thigh with other specified severity

L97.129   Non-pressure chronic ulcer of left thigh with unspecified severity

L97.2   Non-pressure chronic ulcer of calf

L97.20   Non-pressure chronic ulcer of unspecified calf

L97.201   Non-pressure chronic ulcer of unspecified calf limited to breakdown of skin

L97.202   Non-pressure chronic ulcer of unspecified calf with fat layer exposed

L97.203   Non-pressure chronic ulcer of unspecified calf with necrosis of muscle

L97.204   Non-pressure chronic ulcer of unspecified calf with necrosis of bone

●**L97.125** Non-pressure chronic ulcer of left thigh with muscle involvement without evidence of necrosis

●**L97.126** Non-pressure chronic ulcer of left thigh with bone involvement without evidence of necrosis

●**L97.128** Non-pressure chronic ulcer of left thigh with other specified severity

L97.209 Non-pressure chronic ulcer of unspecified calf with unspecified severity

L97.21 Non-pressure chronic ulcer of right calf

L97.211 Non-pressure chronic ulcer of right calf limited to breakdown of skin

L97.212 Non-pressure chronic ulcer of right calf with fat layer exposed

L97.213 Non-pressure chronic ulcer of right calf with necrosis of muscle

L97.214 Non-pressure chronic ulcer of right calf with necrosis of bone

●**L97.215** Non-pressure chronic ulcer of right calf with muscle involvement without evidence of necrosis

●**L97.216** Non-pressure chronic ulcer of right calf with bone involvement without evidence of necrosis

●**L97.218** Non-pressure chronic ulcer of right calf with other specified severity

L97.219 Non-pressure chronic ulcer of right calf with unspecified severity

L97.22 Non-pressure chronic ulcer of left calf

L97.221 Non-pressure chronic ulcer of left calf limited to breakdown of skin

L97.222 Non-pressure chronic ulcer of left calf with fat layer exposed

L97.223 Non-pressure chronic ulcer of left calf with necrosis of muscle

L97.224 Non-pressure chronic ulcer of left calf with necrosis of bone

●**L97.225** Non-pressure chronic ulcer of left calf with muscle involvement without evidence of necrosis

●**L97.226** Non-pressure chronic ulcer of left calf with bone involvement without evidence of necrosis

●**L97.228** Non-pressure chronic ulcer of left calf with other specified severity

L97.229 Non-pressure chronic ulcer of left calf with unspecified severity

L97.3 Non-pressure chronic ulcer of ankle

L97.30 Non-pressure chronic ulcer of unspecified ankle

L97.301 Non-pressure chronic ulcer of unspecified ankle limited to breakdown of skin

L97.302 Non-pressure chronic ulcer of unspecified ankle with fat layer exposed

L97.303 Non-pressure chronic ulcer of unspecified ankle with necrosis of muscle

L97.304 Non-pressure chronic ulcer of unspecified ankle with necrosis of bone

●**L97.305** Non-pressure chronic ulcer of unspecified ankle with muscle

involvement without evidence of necrosis

●**L97.306** Non-pressure chronic ulcer of unspecified ankle with bone involvement without evidence of necrosis

●**L97.308** Non-pressure chronic ulcer of unspecified ankle with other specified severity

L97.309 Non-pressure chronic ulcer of unspecified ankle with unspecified severity

L97.31 Non-pressure chronic ulcer of right ankle

L97.311 Non-pressure chronic ulcer of right ankle limited to breakdown of skin

L97.312 Non-pressure chronic ulcer of right ankle with fat layer exposed

L97.313 Non-pressure chronic ulcer of right ankle with necrosis of muscle

L97.314 Non-pressure chronic ulcer of right ankle with necrosis of bone

●**L97.315** Non-pressure chronic ulcer of right ankle with muscle involvement without evidence of necrosis

●**L97.316** Non-pressure chronic ulcer of right ankle with bone involvement without evidence of necrosis

●**L97.318** Non-pressure chronic ulcer of right ankle with other specified severity

L97.319 Non-pressure chronic ulcer of right ankle with unspecified severity

L97.32 Non-pressure chronic ulcer of left ankle

L97.321 Non-pressure chronic ulcer of left ankle limited to breakdown of skin

L97.322 Non-pressure chronic ulcer of left ankle with fat layer exposed

L97.323 Non-pressure chronic ulcer of left ankle with necrosis of muscle

L97.324 Non-pressure chronic ulcer of left ankle with necrosis of bone

●**L97.325** Non-pressure chronic ulcer of left ankle with muscle involvement without evidence of necrosis

●**L97.326** Non-pressure chronic ulcer of left ankle with bone involvement without evidence of necrosis

●**L97.328** Non-pressure chronic ulcer of left ankle with other specified severity

L97.329 Non-pressure chronic ulcer of left ankle with unspecified severity

L97.4 Non-pressure chronic ulcer of heel and midfoot

Non-pressure chronic ulcer of plantar surface of midfoot

L97.40 Non-pressure chronic ulcer of unspecified heel and midfoot

L97.401 Non-pressure chronic ulcer of unspecified heel and midfoot limited to breakdown of skin

L97.402 Non-pressure chronic ulcer of unspecified heel and midfoot with fat layer exposed

L97.403 Non-pressure chronic ulcer of unspecified heel and midfoot with necrosis of muscle

L97.404 Non-pressure chronic ulcer of unspecified heel and midfoot with necrosis of bone

- **L97.405** Non-pressure chronic ulcer of unspecified heel and midfoot with muscle involvement without evidence of necrosis

- **L97.406** Non-pressure chronic ulcer of unspecified heel and midfoot with bone involvement without evidence of necrosis

- **L97.408** Non-pressure chronic ulcer of unspecified heel and midfoot with other specified severity

L97.409 Non-pressure chronic ulcer of unspecified heel and midfoot with unspecified severity

L97.41 Non-pressure chronic ulcer of right heel and midfoot

L97.411 Non-pressure chronic ulcer of right heel and midfoot limited to breakdown of skin

L97.412 Non-pressure chronic ulcer of right heel and midfoot with fat layer exposed

L97.413 Non-pressure chronic ulcer of right heel and midfoot with necrosis of muscle

L97.414 Non-pressure chronic ulcer of right heel and midfoot with necrosis of bone

- **L97.415** Non-pressure chronic ulcer of right heel and midfoot with muscle involvement without evidence of necrosis

- **L97.416** Non-pressure chronic ulcer of right heel and midfoot with bone involvement without evidence of necrosis

- **L97.418** Non-pressure chronic ulcer of right heel and midfoot with other specified severity

L97.419 Non-pressure chronic ulcer of right heel and midfoot with unspecified severity

L97.42 Non-pressure chronic ulcer of left heel and midfoot

L97.421 Non-pressure chronic ulcer of left heel and midfoot limited to breakdown of skin

L97.422 Non-pressure chronic ulcer of left heel and midfoot with fat layer exposed

L97.423 Non-pressure chronic ulcer of left heel and midfoot with necrosis of muscle

L97.424 Non-pressure chronic ulcer of left heel and midfoot with necrosis of bone

- **L97.425** Non-pressure chronic ulcer of left heel and midfoot with muscle involvement without evidence of necrosis

- **L97.426** Non-pressure chronic ulcer of left heel and midfoot with bone involvement without evidence of necrosis

- **L97.428** Non-pressure chronic ulcer of left heel and midfoot with other specified severity

L97.429 Non-pressure chronic ulcer of left heel and midfoot with unspecified severity

L97.5 Non-pressure chronic ulcer of other part of foot

Non-pressure chronic ulcer of toe

L97.50 Non-pressure chronic ulcer of other part of unspecified foot

L97.501 Non-pressure chronic ulcer of other part of unspecified foot limited to breakdown of skin

L97.502 Non-pressure chronic ulcer of other part of unspecified foot with fat layer exposed

L97.503 Non-pressure chronic ulcer of other part of unspecified foot with necrosis of muscle

L97.504 Non-pressure chronic ulcer of other part of unspecified foot with necrosis of bone

- **L97.505** Non-pressure chronic ulcer of other part of unspecified foot with muscle involvement without evidence of necrosis

- **L97.506** Non-pressure chronic ulcer of other part of unspecified foot with bone involvement without evidence of necrosis

L97.508 Non-pressure chronic ulcer of other part of unspecified foot with other specified severity

L97.509 Non-pressure chronic ulcer of other part of unspecified foot with unspecified severity

L97.51 Non-pressure chronic ulcer of other part of right foot

L97.511 Non-pressure chronic ulcer of other part of right foot limited to breakdown of skin

L97.512 Non-pressure chronic ulcer of other part of right foot with fat layer exposed

L97.513 Non-pressure chronic ulcer of other part of right foot with necrosis of muscle

L97.514 Non-pressure chronic ulcer of other part of right foot with necrosis of bone

- **L97.515** Non-pressure chronic ulcer of other part of right foot with muscle involvement without evidence of necrosis

- **L97.516** Non-pressure chronic ulcer of other part of right foot with bone involvement without evidence of necrosis

- **L97.518** Non-pressure chronic ulcer of other part of right foot with other specified severity

L97.519 Non-pressure chronic ulcer of other part of right foot with unspecified severity

L97.52 Non-pressure chronic ulcer of other part of left foot

L97.521 Non-pressure chronic ulcer of other part of left foot limited to breakdown of skin

L97.522 Non-pressure chronic ulcer of other part of left foot with fat layer exposed

L97.523 Non-pressure chronic ulcer of other part of left foot with necrosis of muscle

L97.524 Non-pressure chronic ulcer of other part of left foot with necrosis of bone

● **L97.525** Non-pressure chronic ulcer of other part of left foot with muscle involvement without evidence of necrosis

● **L97.526** Non-pressure chronic ulcer of other part of left foot with bone involvement without evidence of necrosis

● **L97.528** Non-pressure chronic ulcer of other part of left foot with other specified severity

L97.529 Non-pressure chronic ulcer of other part of left foot with unspecified severity

L97.8 **Non-pressure chronic ulcer of other part of lower leg**

L97.80 **Non-pressure chronic ulcer of other part of unspecified lower leg**

L97.801 Non-pressure chronic ulcer of other part of unspecified lower leg limited to breakdown of skin

L97.802 Non-pressure chronic ulcer of other part of unspecified lower leg with fat layer exposed

L97.803 Non-pressure chronic ulcer of other part of unspecified lower leg with necrosis of muscle

L97.804 Non-pressure chronic ulcer of other part of unspecified lower leg with necrosis of bone

● **L97.805** Non-pressure chronic ulcer of other part of unspecified lower leg with muscle involvement without evidence of necrosis

● **L97.806** Non-pressure chronic ulcer of other part of unspecified lower leg with bone involvement without evidence of necrosis

● **L97.808** Non-pressure chronic ulcer of other part of unspecified lower leg with other specified severity

L97.809 Non-pressure chronic ulcer of other part of unspecified lower leg with unspecified severity

L97.81 **Non-pressure chronic ulcer of other part of right lower leg**

L97.811 Non-pressure chronic ulcer of other part of right lower leg limited to breakdown of skin

L97.812 Non-pressure chronic ulcer of other part of right lower leg with fat layer exposed

L97.813 Non-pressure chronic ulcer of other part of right lower leg with necrosis of muscle

L97.814 Non-pressure chronic ulcer of other part of right lower leg with necrosis of bone

● **L97.815** Non-pressure chronic ulcer of other part of right lower leg with muscle involvement without evidence of necrosis

● **L97.816** Non-pressure chronic ulcer of other part of right lower leg with bone involvement without evidence of necrosis

● **L97.818** Non-pressure chronic ulcer of other part of right lower leg with other specified severity

L97.819 Non-pressure chronic ulcer of other part of right lower leg with unspecified severity

L97.82 **Non-pressure chronic ulcer of other part of left lower leg**

L97.821 Non-pressure chronic ulcer of other part of left lower leg limited to breakdown of skin

L97.822 Non-pressure chronic ulcer of other part of left lower leg with fat layer exposed

L97.823 Non-pressure chronic ulcer of other part of left lower leg with necrosis of muscle

L97.824 Non-pressure chronic ulcer of other part of left lower leg with necrosis of bone

● **L97.825** Non-pressure chronic ulcer of other part of left lower leg with muscle involvement without evidence of necrosis

● **L97.826** Non-pressure chronic ulcer of other part of left lower leg with bone involvement without evidence of necrosis

● **L97.828** Non-pressure chronic ulcer of other part of left lower leg with other specified severity

L97.829 Non-pressure chronic ulcer of other part of left lower leg with unspecified severity

L97.9 **Non-pressure chronic ulcer of unspecified part of lower leg**

L97.90 **Non-pressure chronic ulcer of unspecified part of unspecified lower leg**

L97.901 Non-pressure chronic ulcer of unspecified part of unspecified lower leg limited to breakdown of skin

L97.902 Non-pressure chronic ulcer of unspecified part of unspecified lower leg with fat layer exposed

L97.903 Non-pressure chronic ulcer of unspecified part of unspecified lower leg with necrosis of muscle

L97.904 Non-pressure chronic ulcer of unspecified part of unspecified lower leg with necrosis of bone

● **L97.905** Non-pressure chronic ulcer of unspecified part of unspecified lower leg with muscle involvement without evidence of necrosis

● **L97.906** Non-pressure chronic ulcer of unspecified part of unspecified lower

● New code   ▲ Revised code   **Excludes1:** Not coded here   **Excludes2:** Not included here   ⊗ Placeholder required   ⑦ 7th digit required

leg with bone involvement without evidence of necrosis

• **L97.908** **Non-pressure chronic ulcer of unspecified part of unspecified lower leg with other specified severity**

L97.909 **Non-pressure chronic ulcer of unspecified part of unspecified lower leg with unspecified severity**

L97.91 **Non-pressure chronic ulcer of unspecified part of right lower leg**

L97.911 **Non-pressure chronic ulcer of unspecified part of right lower leg limited to breakdown of skin**

L97.912 **Non-pressure chronic ulcer of unspecified part of right lower leg with fat layer exposed**

L97.913 **Non-pressure chronic ulcer of unspecified part of right lower leg with necrosis of muscle**

L97.914 **Non-pressure chronic ulcer of unspecified part of right lower leg with necrosis of bone**

• **L97.915** **Non-pressure chronic ulcer of unspecified part of right lower leg with muscle involvement without evidence of necrosis**

• **L97.916** **Non-pressure chronic ulcer of unspecified part of right lower leg with bone involvement without evidence of necrosis**

• **L97.918** **Non-pressure chronic ulcer of unspecified part of right lower leg with other specified severity**

L97.919 **Non-pressure chronic ulcer of unspecified part of right lower leg with unspecified severity**

L97.92 **Non-pressure chronic ulcer of unspecified part of left lower leg**

L97.921 **Non-pressure chronic ulcer of unspecified part of left lower leg limited to breakdown of skin**

L97.922 **Non-pressure chronic ulcer of unspecified part of left lower leg with fat layer exposed**

L97.923 **Non-pressure chronic ulcer of unspecified part of left lower leg with necrosis of muscle**

L97.924 **Non-pressure chronic ulcer of unspecified part of left lower leg with necrosis of bone**

• **L97.925** **Non-pressure chronic ulcer of unspecified part of left lower leg with muscle involvement without evidence of necrosis**

• **L97.926** **Non-pressure chronic ulcer of unspecified part of left lower leg with bone involvement without evidence of necrosis**

• **L97.928** **Non-pressure chronic ulcer of unspecified part of left lower leg with other specified severity**

L97.929 **Non-pressure chronic ulcer of unspecified part of left lower leg with unspecified severity**

L98 **Other disorders of skin and subcutaneous tissue, not elsewhere classified**

L98.0 **Pyogenic granuloma**

Excludes2: pyogenic granuloma of gingiva (K06.8)

pyogenic granuloma of maxillary alveolar ridge (K04.5)

pyogenic granuloma of oral mucosa (K13.4)

L98.1 **Factitial dermatitis**

Neurotic excoriation

Excludes1: Excoriation (skin-picking) disorder (F42.4)

L98.2 **Febrile neutrophilic dermatosis [Sweet]**

L98.3 **Eosinophilic cellulitis [Wells]**

L98.4 **Non-pressure chronic ulcer of skin, not elsewhere classified**

Chronic ulcer of skin NOS

Tropical ulcer NOS

Ulcer of skin NOS

Excludes2: pressure ulcer (pressure area) (L89.-)

gangrene (I96)

skin infections (L00-L08)

specific infections classified to A00-B99

ulcer of lower limb NEC (L97.-)

varicose ulcer (I83.0-I82.2)

L98.41 **Non-pressure chronic ulcer of buttock**

L98.411 **Non-pressure chronic ulcer of buttock limited to breakdown of skin**

L98.412 **Non-pressure chronic ulcer of buttock with fat layer exposed**

L98.413 **Non-pressure chronic ulcer of buttock with necrosis of muscle**

L98.414 **Non-pressure chronic ulcer of buttock with necrosis of bone**

• **L98.415** **Non-pressure chronic ulcer of buttock with muscle involvement without evidence of necrosis**

• **L98.416** **Non-pressure chronic ulcer of buttock with bone involvement without evidence of necrosis**

• **L98.418** **Non-pressure chronic ulcer of buttock with other specified severity**

L98.419 **Non-pressure chronic ulcer of buttock with unspecified severity**

L98.42 **Non-pressure chronic ulcer of back**

L98.421 **Non-pressure chronic ulcer of back limited to breakdown of skin**

L98.422 **Non-pressure chronic ulcer of back with fat layer exposed**

L98.423 **Non-pressure chronic ulcer of back with necrosis of muscle**

L98.424 **Non-pressure chronic ulcer of back with necrosis of bone**

• **L98.425** **Non-pressure chronic ulcer of back with muscle involvement without evidence of necrosis**

• **L98.426** **Non-pressure chronic ulcer of back with bone involvement without evidence of necrosis**

• **L98.428** **Non-pressure chronic ulcer of back with other specified severity**

L98.429 **Non-pressure chronic ulcer of back with unspecified severity**

L98.49 **Non-pressure chronic ulcer of skin of other sites**

Non-pressure chronic ulcer of skin NOS

L98.491 **Non-pressure chronic ulcer of skin of other sites limited to breakdown of skin**

L98.492 Non-pressure chronic ulcer of skin of other sites with fat layer exposed

L98.493 Non-pressure chronic ulcer of skin of other sites with necrosis of muscle

L98.494 Non-pressure chronic ulcer of skin of other sites with necrosis of bone

● **L98.495** Non-pressure chronic ulcer of other sites with muscle involvement without evidence of necrosis

● **L98.496** Non-pressure chronic ulcer of other sites with bone involvement without evidence of necrosis

● **L98.498** Non-pressure chronic ulcer of other sites with other specified severity

L98.499 Non-pressure chronic ulcer of skin of other sites with unspecified severity

L98.5 Mucinosis of the skin

Focal mucinosis

Lichen myxedematosus

Reticular erythematous mucinosis

Excludes1: focal oral mucinosis (K13.79)

myxedema (E03.9)

L98.6 Other infiltrative disorders of the skin and subcutaneous tissue

Excludes1: hyalinosis cutis et mucosae (E78.89)

L98.7 Excessive and redundant skin and subcutaneous tissue

Loose or sagging skin following bariatric surgery weight loss

Loose or sagging skin following dietary weight loss

Loose or sagging skin, NOS

Excludes2: acquired excess or redundant skin of eyelid (H02.3-)

congenital excess or redundant skin of eyelid (Q10.3)

skin changes due to chronic exposure to nonionizing radiation (L57.-)

L98.8 Other specified disorders of the skin and subcutaneous tissue

L98.9 Disorder of the skin and subcutaneous tissue, unspecified

L99 Other disorders of skin and subcutaneous tissue in diseases classified elsewhere

Code first underlying disease, such as:

amyloidosis (E85.-)

Excludes1: skin disorders in diabetes (E08-E13 with .62)

skin disorders in gonorrhea (A54.89)

skin disorders in syphilis (A51.31, A52.79)

Chapter 13: Diseases Of The Musculoskeletal System And Connective Tissue (M00-M99)

DEFINITIONS

This chapter includes definitions of selected key words, terms and phrases and coding alerts for adding points to the clinical domain, and references to coding late effects where appropriate. An example from this chapter is as follows:

M05   Rheumatoid arthritis with rheumatoid factor

     Definition: Rheumatoid arthritis is a chronic, systemic inflammatory disorder that may affect many tissues and organs, but principally attacks the joints producing a inflammatory synovitis that often progresses to destruction of the articular cartilage and ankylosis of the joints.

MULTIPLE CODING FOR A SINGLE CONDITION

In addition to the etiology/manifestation convention that requires two codes to fully describe a single condition that affects multiple body systems, there are other single conditions that also require more than one code. "Use additional code" notes are found in the Tabular List at codes that are not part of an etiology/manifestation pair where a secondary code is useful to fully describe a condition. The sequencing rule is the same as the etiology/manifestation pair, "use additional code" indicates that a secondary code should be added.

For example, for bacterial infections that are not included in chapter 1, a secondary code from category B95, Streptococcus, Staphylococcus, and Enterococcus, as the cause of diseases classified elsewhere, or B96, Other bacterial agents as the cause of diseases classified elsewhere, may be required to identify the bacterial organism causing the infection. A "use additional code" note will normally be found at the infectious disease code, indicating a need for the organism code to be added as a secondary code.

"Code first" notes are also under certain codes that are not specifically manifestation codes but may be due to an underlying cause. When there is a "code first" note and an underlying condition is present, the underlying condition should be sequenced first.

"Code, if applicable, any causal condition first", notes indicate that this code may be assigned as a principal diagnosis when the causal condition is unknown or not applicable. If a causal condition is known, then the code for that condition should be sequenced as the principal or first-listed diagnosis.

Multiple codes may be needed for sequela, complication codes and obstetric codes to more fully describe a condition. See the specific guidelines for these conditions for further instruction.

COMBINATION CODE

A combination code is a single code used to classify: Two diagnoses, or a diagnosis with an associated secondary process (manifestation) A diagnosis with an associated complication

Combination codes are identified by referring to subterm entries in the Alphabetic Index and by reading the inclusion and exclusion notes in the Tabular List.

Assign only the combination code when that code fully identifies the diagnostic conditions involved or when the Alphabetic Index so directs. Multiple coding should not be used when the classification provides a combination code that clearly identifies all of the elements documented in the diagnosis. When the combination code lacks necessary specificity in describing the manifestation or complication, an additional code should be used as a secondary code.

SEQUELA (LATE EFFECTS)

A sequela is the residual effect (condition produced) after the acute phase of an illness or injury has terminated. There is no time limit on when a sequela code can be used. The residual may be apparent early, such as in cerebral infarction, or it may occur months or years later, such as that due to a previous injury. Coding of sequela generally requires two codes sequenced in the following order: The condition or nature of the sequela is sequenced first.

The sequela code is sequenced second.

An exception to the above guidelines are those instances where the code for the sequela is followed by a manifestation code identified in the Tabular List and title, or the sequela code has been expanded (at the fourth, fifth or sixth character levels) to include the manifestation(s). The code for the acute phase of an illness or injury that led to the sequela is never used with a code for the late effect.

SITE AND LATERALITY

Most of the codes within Chapter 13 have site and laterality designations. The site represents the bone, joint or the muscle involved. For some conditions where more than one bone, joint or muscle is usually involved, such as osteoarthritis, there is a "multiple sites" code available. For categories where no multiple site code is provided and more than one bone, joint or muscle is involved, multiple codes should be used to indicate the different sites involved.

1)   **Bone versus joint**

     For certain conditions, the bone may be affected at the upper or lower end, (e.g., avascular necrosis of bone, M87, Osteoporosis, M80, M81). Though the portion of the bone affected may be at the joint, the site designation will be the bone, not the joint.

ACUTE TRAUMATIC VERSUS CHRONIC OR RECURRENT MUSCULOSKELETAL CONDITIONS

Many musculoskeletal conditions are a result of previous injury or trauma to a site, or are recurrent conditions. Bone, joint or muscle conditions that are the result of a healed injury are usually found in chapter 13. Recurrent bone, joint or muscle conditions are also usually found in chapter 13. Any current, acute injury should be coded to the appropriate injury code from chapter 19. Chronic or recurrent conditions should generally be coded with a code from chapter 13. If it is difficult to determine from the documentation in the record which code is best to describe a condition, query the provider.

CODING OF PATHOLOGIC FRACTURES

7th character A is for use as long as the patient is receiving active treatment for the fracture. While the patient may be seen by a new or different provider over the course of treatment for a pathological fracture, assignment of the 7th character is based on whether the patient is undergoing active treatment and not whether the provider is seeing the patient for the first time.

7th character D is to be used for encounters after the patient has completed active treatment. The other 7th characters, listed under each subcategory in the Tabular List, are to be used for subsequent encounters for routine care of fractures during the healing and recovery phase as well as treatment of problems associated with the healing, such as malunions, nonunions, and sequelae.

Care for complications of surgical treatment for fracture repairs during the healing or recovery phase should be coded with the appropriate complication codes.

See Section I.C.19. Coding of traumatic fractures.

OSTEOPOROSIS

Osteoporosis is a systemic condition, meaning that all bones of the musculoskeletal system are affected. Therefore, site is not a component of the codes under category M81, Osteoporosis without current pathological fracture. The site codes under category M80, Osteoporosis with current pathological fracture, identify the site of the fracture, not the osteoporosis.

1) **Osteoporosis without pathological fracture**

   Category M81, Osteoporosis without current pathological fracture, is for use for patients with osteoporosis who do not currently have a pathologic fracture due to the osteoporosis, even if they have had a fracture in the past. For patients with a history of osteoporosis fractures, status code Z87.310, Personal history of (healed) osteoporosis fracture, should follow the code from M81.

2) **Osteoporosis with current pathological fracture**

   Category M80, Osteoporosis with current pathological fracture, is for patients who have a current pathologic fracture at the time of an encounter. The codes under M80 identify the site of the fracture. A code from category M80, not a traumatic fracture code, should be used for any patient with known osteoporosis who suffers a fracture, even if the patient had a minor fall or trauma, if that fall or trauma would not usually break a normal, healthy bone.

Chapter 13

Diseases Of The Musculoskeletal System And Connective Tissue (M00-M99)

Note: Use an external cause code following the code for the musculoskeletal condition, if applicable, to identify the cause of the musculoskeletal condition

Excludes2: arthropathic psoriasis (L40.5-)

certain conditions originating in the perinatal period (P04-P96)

certain infectious and parasitic diseases (A00-B99)

compartment syndrome (traumatic) (T79.A-)

complications of pregnancy, childbirth and the puerperium (O00-O9A)

congenital malformations, deformations, and chromosomal abnormalities (Q00-Q99)

endocrine, nutritional and metabolic diseases (E00-E88)

injury, poisoning and certain other consequences of external causes (S00-T88)

neoplasms (C00-D49)

symptoms, signs and abnormal clinical and laboratory findings, not elsewhere classified (R00-R94)

This chapter contains the following blocks:

M00-M02	Infectious arthropathies
M05-M14	Inflammatory polyarthropathies
M15-M19	Osteoarthritis
M20-M25	Other joint disorders
M26-M27	Dentofacial anomalies [including malocclusion] and other disorders of jaw
M30-M36	Systemic connective tissue disorders
M40-M43	Deforming dorsopathies
M45-M49	Spondylopathies
M50-M54	Other dorsopathies
M60-M63	Disorders of muscles
M65-M67	Disorders of synovium and tendon
M70-M79	Other soft tissue disorders
M80-M85	Disorders of bone density and structure
M86-M90	Other osteopathies
M91-M94	Chondropathies
M95	Other disorders of the musculoskeletal system and connective tissue
M96	Intraoperative and postprocedural complications and disorders of musculoskeletal system, not elsewhere classified
M99	Biomechanical lesions, not elsewhere classified

ARTHROPATHIES (M00-M25)

Includes: Disorders affecting predominantly peripheral (limb) joints

INFECTIOUS ARTHROPATHIES (M00-M02)

Note: This block comprises arthropathies due to microbiological agents. Distinction is made between the following types of etiological relationship:

a) direct infection of joint, where organisms invade synovial tissue and microbial antigen is present in the joint; b) indirect infection, which may be of two types: a reactive arthropathy, where microbial infection of the body is established but neither organisms nor antigens can be identified in the joint, and a postinfective arthropathy, where microbial antigen is present but recovery of an organism is inconstant and evidence of local multiplication is lacking.

M00 **Pyogenic arthritis**

   M00.0 **Staphylococcal arthritis and polyarthritis**

Use additional code (B95.61-B95.8) to identify bacterial agent

Excludes2: infection and inflammatory reaction due to internal joint prosthesis (T84.5-)

   M00.00 **Staphylococcal arthritis, unspecified joint**

   M00.01 **Staphylococcal arthritis, shoulder**

   M00.011 **Staphylococcal arthritis, right shoulder**

   M00.012 **Staphylococcal arthritis, left shoulder**

   M00.019 **Staphylococcal arthritis, unspecified shoulder**

   M00.02 **Staphylococcal arthritis, elbow**

   M00.021 **Staphylococcal arthritis, right elbow**

   M00.022 **Staphylococcal arthritis, left elbow**

   M00.029 **Staphylococcal arthritis, unspecified elbow**

   M00.03 **Staphylococcal arthritis, wrist**

   Staphylococcal arthritis of carpal bones

   M00.031 **Staphylococcal arthritis, right wrist**

   M00.032 **Staphylococcal arthritis, left wrist**

   M00.039 **Staphylococcal arthritis, unspecified wrist**

   M00.04 **Staphylococcal arthritis, hand**

   Staphylococcal arthritis of metacarpus and phalanges

   M00.041 **Staphylococcal arthritis, right hand**

   M00.042 **Staphylococcal arthritis, left hand**

   M00.049 **Staphylococcal arthritis, unspecified hand**

   M00.05 **Staphylococcal arthritis, hip**

   M00.051 **Staphylococcal arthritis, right hip**

   M00.052 **Staphylococcal arthritis, left hip**

   M00.059 **Staphylococcal arthritis, unspecified hip**

   M00.06 **Staphylococcal arthritis, knee**

   M00.061 **Staphylococcal arthritis, right knee**

   M00.062 **Staphylococcal arthritis, left knee**

   M00.069 **Staphylococcal arthritis, unspecified knee**

   M00.07 **Staphylococcal arthritis, ankle and foot**

   Staphylococcal arthritis, tarsus, metatarsus and phalanges

   M00.071 **Staphylococcal arthritis, right ankle and foot**

   M00.072 **Staphylococcal arthritis, left ankle and foot**

   M00.079 **Staphylococcal arthritis, unspecified ankle and foot**

   M00.08 **Staphylococcal arthritis, vertebrae**

   M00.09 **Staphylococcal polyarthritis**

M00.1 **Pneumococcal arthritis and polyarthritis**

   M00.10 **Pneumococcal arthritis, unspecified joint**

   M00.11 **Pneumococcal arthritis, shoulder**

   M00.111 **Pneumococcal arthritis, right shoulder**

   M00.112 **Pneumococcal arthritis, left shoulder**

   M00.119 **Pneumococcal arthritis, unspecified shoulder**

   M00.12 **Pneumococcal arthritis, elbow**

M00.121 Pneumococcal arthritis, right elbow

M00.122 Pneumococcal arthritis, left elbow

M00.129 Pneumococcal arthritis, unspecified elbow

M00.13 Pneumococcal arthritis, wrist

Pneumococcal arthritis of carpal bones

M00.131 Pneumococcal arthritis, right wrist

M00.132 Pneumococcal arthritis, left wrist

M00.139 Pneumococcal arthritis, unspecified wrist

M00.14 Pneumococcal arthritis, hand

Pneumococcal arthritis of metacarpus and phalanges

M00.141 Pneumococcal arthritis, right hand

M00.142 Pneumococcal arthritis, left hand

M00.149 Pneumococcal arthritis, unspecified hand

M00.15 Pneumococcal arthritis, hip

M00.151 Pneumococcal arthritis, right hip

M00.152 Pneumococcal arthritis, left hip

M00.159 Pneumococcal arthritis, unspecified hip

M00.16 Pneumococcal arthritis, knee

M00.161 Pneumococcal arthritis, right knee

M00.162 Pneumococcal arthritis, left knee

M00.169 Pneumococcal arthritis, unspecified knee

M00.17 Pneumococcal arthritis, ankle and foot

Pneumococcal arthritis, tarsus, metatarsus and phalanges

M00.171 Pneumococcal arthritis, right ankle and foot

M00.172 Pneumococcal arthritis, left ankle and foot

M00.179 Pneumococcal arthritis, unspecified ankle and foot

M00.18 Pneumococcal arthritis, vertebrae

M00.19 Pneumococcal polyarthritis

M00.2 Other streptococcal arthritis and polyarthritis

Use additional code (B95.0-B95.2, B95.4-B95.5) to identify bacterial agent

M00.20 Other streptococcal arthritis, unspecified joint

M00.21 Other streptococcal arthritis, shoulder

M00.211 Other streptococcal arthritis, right shoulder

M00.212 Other streptococcal arthritis, left shoulder

M00.219 Other streptococcal arthritis, unspecified shoulder

M00.22 Other streptococcal arthritis, elbow

M00.221 Other streptococcal arthritis, right elbow

M00.222 Other streptococcal arthritis, left elbow

M00.229 Other streptococcal arthritis, unspecified elbow

M00.23 Other streptococcal arthritis, wrist

Other streptococcal arthritis of carpal bones

M00.231 Other streptococcal arthritis, right wrist

M00.232 Other streptococcal arthritis, left wrist

M00.239 Other streptococcal arthritis, unspecified wrist

M00.24 Other streptococcal arthritis, hand

Other streptococcal arthritis metacarpus and phalanges

M00.241 Other streptococcal arthritis, right hand

M00.242 Other streptococcal arthritis, left hand

M00.249 Other streptococcal arthritis, unspecified hand

M00.25 Other streptococcal arthritis, hip

M00.251 Other streptococcal arthritis, right hip

M00.252 Other streptococcal arthritis, left hip

M00.259 Other streptococcal arthritis, unspecified hip

M00.26 Other streptococcal arthritis, knee

M00.261 Other streptococcal arthritis, right knee

M00.262 Other streptococcal arthritis, left knee

M00.269 Other streptococcal arthritis, unspecified knee

M00.27 Other streptococcal arthritis, ankle and foot

Other streptococcal arthritis, tarsus, metatarsus and phalanges

M00.271 Other streptococcal arthritis, right ankle and foot

M00.272 Other streptococcal arthritis, left ankle and foot

M00.279 Other streptococcal arthritis, unspecified ankle and foot

M00.28 Other streptococcal arthritis, vertebrae

M00.29 Other streptococcal polyarthritis

M00.8 Arthritis and polyarthritis due to other bacteria

Use additional code (B96) to identify bacteria

M00.80 Arthritis due to other bacteria, unspecified joint

M00.81 Arthritis due to other bacteria, shoulder

M00.811 Arthritis due to other bacteria, right shoulder

M00.812 Arthritis due to other bacteria, left shoulder

M00.819 Arthritis due to other bacteria, unspecified shoulder

M00.82 Arthritis due to other bacteria, elbow

M00.821 Arthritis due to other bacteria, right elbow

M00.822 Arthritis due to other bacteria, left elbow

M00.829 Arthritis due to other bacteria, unspecified elbow

M00.83 Arthritis due to other bacteria, wrist

Arthritis due to other bacteria, carpal bones

M00.831 Arthritis due to other bacteria, right wrist

M00.832 Arthritis due to other bacteria, left wrist

● New code ▲ Revised code **Excludes1:** Not coded here **Excludes2:** Not included here ⊗ Placeholder required ⑦ 7th digit required

M00.839   **Arthritis due to other bacteria, unspecified wrist**

M00.84   **Arthritis due to other bacteria, hand**

Arthritis due to other bacteria, metacarpus and phalanges

M00.841   **Arthritis due to other bacteria, right hand**

M00.842   **Arthritis due to other bacteria, left hand**

M00.849   **Arthritis due to other bacteria, unspecified hand**

M00.85   **Arthritis due to other bacteria, hip**

M00.851   **Arthritis due to other bacteria, right hip**

M00.852   **Arthritis due to other bacteria, left hip**

M00.859   **Arthritis due to other bacteria, unspecified hip**

M00.86   **Arthritis due to other bacteria, knee**

M00.861   **Arthritis due to other bacteria, right knee**

M00.862   **Arthritis due to other bacteria, left knee**

M00.869   **Arthritis due to other bacteria, unspecified knee**

M00.87   **Arthritis due to other bacteria, ankle and foot**

Arthritis due to other bacteria, tarsus, metatarsus, and phalanges

M00.871   **Arthritis due to other bacteria, right ankle and foot**

M00.872   **Arthritis due to other bacteria, left ankle and foot**

M00.879   **Arthritis due to other bacteria, unspecified ankle and foot**

M00.88   **Arthritis due to other bacteria, vertebrae**

M00.89   **Polyarthritis due to other bacteria**

M00.9   **Pyogenic arthritis, unspecified**

Infective arthritis NOS

M01   **Direct infections of joint in infectious and parasitic diseases classified elsewhere**

Code first underlying disease, such as:

leprosy [Hansen's disease] (A30.-)

mycoses (B35-B49)

O'nyong-nyong fever (A92.1)

paratyphoid fever (A01.1-A01.4)

Excludes1: arthropathy in Lyme disease (A69.23)

gonococcal arthritis (A54.42)

meningococcal arthritis (A39.83)

mumps arthritis (B26.85)

postinfective arthropathy (M02.-)

postmeningococcal arthritis (A39.84)

reactive arthritis (M02.3)

rubella arthritis (B06.82)

sarcoidosis arthritis (D86.86)

typhoid fever arthritis (A01.04)

tuberculosis arthritis (A18.01-A18.02)

M01.X   **Direct infection of joint in infectious and parasitic diseases classified elsewhere**

M01.X0   **Direct infection of unspecified joint in infectious and parasitic diseases classified elsewhere**

M01.X1   **Direct infection of shoulder joint in infectious and parasitic diseases classified elsewhere**

M01.X11   **Direct infection of right shoulder in infectious and parasitic diseases classified elsewhere**

M01.X12   **Direct infection of left shoulder in infectious and parasitic diseases classified elsewhere**

M01.X19   **Direct infection of unspecified shoulder in infectious and parasitic diseases classified elsewhere**

M01.X2   **Direct infection of elbow in infectious and parasitic diseases classified elsewhere**

M01.X21   **Direct infection of right elbow in infectious and parasitic diseases classified elsewhere**

M01.X22   **Direct infection of left elbow in infectious and parasitic diseases classified elsewhere**

M01.X29   **Direct infection of unspecified elbow in infectious and parasitic diseases classified elsewhere**

M01.X3   **Direct infection of wrist in infectious and parasitic diseases classified elsewhere**

Direct infection of carpal bones in infectious and parasitic diseases classified elsewhere

M01.X31   **Direct infection of right wrist in infectious and parasitic diseases classified elsewhere**

M01.X32   **Direct infection of left wrist in infectious and parasitic diseases classified elsewhere**

M01.X39   **Direct infection of unspecified wrist in infectious and parasitic diseases classified elsewhere**

M01.X4   **Direct infection of hand in infectious and parasitic diseases classified elsewhere**

Direct infection of metacarpus and phalanges in infectious and parasitic diseases classified elsewhere

M01.X41   **Direct infection of right hand in infectious and parasitic diseases classified elsewhere**

M01.X42   **Direct infection of left hand in infectious and parasitic diseases classified elsewhere**

M01.X49   **Direct infection of unspecified hand in infectious and parasitic diseases classified elsewhere**

M01.X5   **Direct infection of hip in infectious and parasitic diseases classified elsewhere**

M01.X51   **Direct infection of right hip in infectious and parasitic diseases classified elsewhere**

M01.X52   **Direct infection of left hip in infectious and parasitic diseases classified elsewhere**

M01.X59   **Direct infection of unspecified hip in infectious and parasitic diseases classified elsewhere**

M01.X6   **Direct infection of knee in infectious and parasitic diseases classified elsewhere**

M01.X61   **Direct infection of right knee in infectious and parasitic diseases classified elsewhere**

M01.X62 Direct infection of left knee in infectious and parasitic diseases classified elsewhere

M01.X69 Direct infection of unspecified knee in infectious and parasitic diseases classified elsewhere

M01.X7 Direct infection of ankle and foot in infectious and parasitic diseases classified elsewhere

Direct infection of tarsus, metatarsus and phalanges in infectious and parasitic diseases classified elsewhere

M01.X71 Direct infection of right ankle and foot in infectious and parasitic diseases classified elsewhere

M01.X72 Direct infection of left ankle and foot in infectious and parasitic diseases classified elsewhere

M01.X79 Direct infection of unspecified ankle and foot in infectious and parasitic diseases classified elsewhere

M01.X8 Direct infection of vertebrae in infectious and parasitic diseases classified elsewhere

M01.X9 Direct infection of multiple joints in infectious and parasitic diseases classified elsewhere

M02 **Postinfective and reactive arthropathies**

Code first underlying disease, such as:

congenital syphilis [Clutton's joints] (A50.5) enteritis due to Yersinia enterocolitica (A04.6)

infective endocarditis (I33.0)

viral hepatitis (B15-B19)

Excludes1: Behçet's disease (M35.2)

direct infections of joint in infectious and parasitic diseases classified elsewhere (M01.-)

postmeningococcal arthritis (A39.84)

mumps arthritis (B26.85)

rubella arthritis (B06.82)

syphilis arthritis (late) (A52.77)

rheumatic fever (I00)

tabetic arthropathy [Charcôt's] (A52.16)

M02.0 **Arthropathy following intestinal bypass**

M02.00 Arthropathy following intestinal bypass, unspecified site

M02.01 Arthropathy following intestinal bypass, shoulder

M02.011 Arthropathy following intestinal bypass, right shoulder

M02.012 Arthropathy following intestinal bypass, left shoulder

M02.019 Arthropathy following intestinal bypass, unspecified shoulder

M02.02 Arthropathy following intestinal bypass, elbow

M02.021 Arthropathy following intestinal bypass, right elbow

M02.022 Arthropathy following intestinal bypass, left elbow

M02.029 Arthropathy following intestinal bypass, unspecified elbow

M02.03 Arthropathy following intestinal bypass, wrist

Arthropathy following intestinal bypass, carpal bones

M02.031 Arthropathy following intestinal bypass, right wrist

M02.032 Arthropathy following intestinal bypass, left wrist

M02.039 Arthropathy following intestinal bypass, unspecified wrist

M02.04 Arthropathy following intestinal bypass, hand

Arthropathy following intestinal bypass, metacarpals and phalanges

M02.041 Arthropathy following intestinal bypass, right hand

M02.042 Arthropathy following intestinal bypass, left hand

M02.049 Arthropathy following intestinal bypass, unspecified hand

M02.05 Arthropathy following intestinal bypass, hip

M02.051 Arthropathy following intestinal bypass, right hip

M02.052 Arthropathy following intestinal bypass, left hip

M02.059 Arthropathy following intestinal bypass, unspecified hip

M02.06 Arthropathy following intestinal bypass, knee

M02.061 Arthropathy following intestinal bypass, right knee

M02.062 Arthropathy following intestinal bypass, left knee

M02.069 Arthropathy following intestinal bypass, unspecified knee

M02.07 Arthropathy following intestinal bypass, ankle and foot

Arthropathy following intestinal bypass, tarsus, metatarsus and phalanges

M02.071 Arthropathy following intestinal bypass, right ankle and foot

M02.072 Arthropathy following intestinal bypass, left ankle and foot

M02.079 Arthropathy following intestinal bypass, unspecified ankle and foot

M02.08 Arthropathy following intestinal bypass, vertebrae

M02.09 Arthropathy following intestinal bypass, multiple sites

M02.1 **Postdysenteric arthropathy**

M02.10 Postdysenteric arthropathy, unspecified site

M02.11 Postdysenteric arthropathy, shoulder

M02.111 Postdysenteric arthropathy, right shoulder

M02.112 Postdysenteric arthropathy, left shoulder

M02.119 Postdysenteric arthropathy, unspecified shoulder

M02.12 Postdysenteric arthropathy, elbow

M02.121 Postdysenteric arthropathy, right elbow

M02.122 Postdysenteric arthropathy, left elbow

M02.129 Postdysenteric arthropathy, unspecified elbow

M02.13 Postdysenteric arthropathy, wrist

Postdysenteric arthropathy, carpal bones

M02.131 Postdysenteric arthropathy, right wrist

M02.132 Postdysenteric arthropathy, left wrist

● New code   ▲ Revised code   **Excludes1:** Not coded here   **Excludes2:** Not included here   ⊗ Placeholder required   ⑦7ᵗʰ digit required

M02.139 Postdysenteric arthropathy, unspecified wrist

M02.14 Postdysenteric arthropathy, hand

Postdysenteric arthropathy, metacarpus and phalanges

    M02.141 Postdysenteric arthropathy, right hand

    M02.142 Postdysenteric arthropathy, left hand

    M02.149 Postdysenteric arthropathy, unspecified hand

M02.15 Postdysenteric arthropathy, hip

    M02.151 Postdysenteric arthropathy, right hip

    M02.152 Postdysenteric arthropathy, left hip

    M02.159 Postdysenteric arthropathy, unspecified hip

M02.16 Postdysenteric arthropathy, knee

    M02.161 Postdysenteric arthropathy, right knee

    M02.162 Postdysenteric arthropathy, left knee

    M02.169 Postdysenteric arthropathy, unspecified knee

M02.17 Postdysenteric arthropathy, ankle and foot

Postdysenteric arthropathy, tarsus, metatarsus and phalanges

    M02.171 Postdysenteric arthropathy, right ankle and foot

    M02.172 Postdysenteric arthropathy, left ankle and foot

    M02.179 Postdysenteric arthropathy, unspecified ankle and foot

M02.18 Postdysenteric arthropathy, vertebrae

M02.19 Postdysenteric arthropathy, multiple sites

M02.2 Postimmunization arthropathy

M02.20 Postimmunization arthropathy, unspecified site

M02.21 Postimmunization arthropathy, shoulder

    M02.211 Postimmunization arthropathy, right shoulder

    M02.212 Postimmunization arthropathy, left shoulder

    M02.219 Postimmunization arthropathy, unspecified shoulder

M02.22 Postimmunization arthropathy, elbow

    M02.221 Postimmunization arthropathy, right elbow

    M02.222 Postimmunization arthropathy, left elbow

    M02.229 Postimmunization arthropathy, unspecified elbow

M02.23 Postimmunization arthropathy, wrist

Postimmunization arthropathy, carpal bones

    M02.231 Postimmunization arthropathy, right wrist

    M02.232 Postimmunization arthropathy, left wrist

    M02.239 Postimmunization arthropathy, unspecified wrist

M02.24 Postimmunization arthropathy, hand

Postimmunization arthropathy, metacarpus and phalanges

    M02.241 Postimmunization arthropathy, right hand

    M02.242 Postimmunization arthropathy, left hand

    M02.249 Postimmunization arthropathy, unspecified hand

M02.25 Postimmunization arthropathy, hip

    M02.251 Postimmunization arthropathy, right hip

    M02.252 Postimmunization arthropathy, left hip

    M02.259 Postimmunization arthropathy, unspecified hip

M02.26 Postimmunization arthropathy, knee

    M02.261 Postimmunization arthropathy, right knee

    M02.262 Postimmunization arthropathy, left knee

    M02.269 Postimmunization arthropathy, unspecified knee

M02.27 Postimmunization arthropathy, ankle and foot

Postimmunization arthropathy, tarsus, metatarsus and phalanges

    M02.271 Postimmunization arthropathy, right ankle and foot

    M02.272 Postimmunization arthropathy, left ankle and foot

    M02.279 Postimmunization arthropathy, unspecified ankle and foot

M02.28 Postimmunization arthropathy, vertebrae

M02.29 Postimmunization arthropathy, multiple sites

M02.3 Reiter's disease

Reactive arthritis

M02.30 Reiter's disease, unspecified site

M02.31 Reiter's disease, shoulder

    M02.311 Reiter's disease, right shoulder

    M02.312 Reiter's disease, left shoulder

    M02.319 Reiter's disease, unspecified shoulder

M02.32 Reiter's disease, elbow

    M02.321 Reiter's disease, right elbow

    M02.322 Reiter's disease, left elbow

    M02.329 Reiter's disease, unspecified elbow

M02.33 Reiter's disease, wrist

Reiter's disease, carpal bones

    M02.331 Reiter's disease, right wrist

    M02.332 Reiter's disease, left wrist

    M02.339 Reiter's disease, unspecified wrist

M02.34 Reiter's disease, hand

Reiter's disease, metacarpus and phalanges

    M02.341 Reiter's disease, right hand

    M02.342 Reiter's disease, left hand

    M02.349 Reiter's disease, unspecified hand

M02.35 Reiter's disease, hip

    M02.351 Reiter's disease, right hip

    M02.352 Reiter's disease, left hip

    M02.359 Reiter's disease, unspecified hip

M02.36 Reiter's disease, knee

    M02.361 Reiter's disease, right knee

    M02.362 Reiter's disease, left knee

    M02.369 Reiter's disease, unspecified knee

M02.37 Reiter's disease, ankle and foot

Add 4th-7th digits   Nonspecific code   Unspecified code   Manifestation code

Reiter's disease, tarsus, metatarsus and phalanges

    M02.371 Reiter's disease, right ankle and foot

    M02.372 Reiter's disease, left ankle and foot

    M02.379 Reiter's disease, unspecified ankle and foot

  M02.38 Reiter's disease, vertebrae

  M02.39 Reiter's disease, multiple sites

M02.8 Other reactive arthropathies

  M02.80 Other reactive arthropathies, unspecified site

  M02.81 Other reactive arthropathies, shoulder

    M02.811 Other reactive arthropathies, right shoulder

    M02.812 Other reactive arthropathies, left shoulder

    M02.819 Other reactive arthropathies, unspecified shoulder

  M02.82 Other reactive arthropathies, elbow

    M02.821 Other reactive arthropathies, right elbow

    M02.822 Other reactive arthropathies, left elbow

    M02.829 Other reactive arthropathies, unspecified elbow

  M02.83 Other reactive arthropathies, wrist

Other reactive arthropathies, carpal bones

    M02.831 Other reactive arthropathies, right wrist

    M02.832 Other reactive arthropathies, left wrist

    M02.839 Other reactive arthropathies, unspecified wrist

  M02.84 Other reactive arthropathies, hand

Other reactive arthropathies, metacarpus and phalanges

    M02.841 Other reactive arthropathies, right hand

    M02.842 Other reactive arthropathies, left hand

    M02.849 Other reactive arthropathies, unspecified hand

  M02.85 Other reactive arthropathies, hip

    M02.851 Other reactive arthropathies, right hip

    M02.852 Other reactive arthropathies, left hip

    M02.859 Other reactive arthropathies, unspecified hip

  M02.86 Other reactive arthropathies, knee

    M02.861 Other reactive arthropathies, right knee

    M02.862 Other reactive arthropathies, left knee

    M02.869 Other reactive arthropathies, unspecified knee

  M02.87 Other reactive arthropathies, ankle and foot

Other reactive arthropathies, tarsus, metatarsus and phalanges

    M02.871 Other reactive arthropathies, right ankle and foot

    M02.872 Other reactive arthropathies, left ankle and foot

    M02.879 Other reactive arthropathies, unspecified ankle and foot

  M02.88 Other reactive arthropathies, vertebrae

  M02.89 Other reactive arthropathies, multiple sites

M02.9 Reactive arthropathy, unspecified

AUTOINFLAMMATORY SYNDROMES (M04)

M04 **Autoinflammatory syndromes**

  Excludes2: Crohn's disease (K50.-)

  M04.1 Periodic fever syndromes

Familial Mediterranean fever

Hyperimmunoglobin D syndrome

Mevalonate kinase deficiency

Tumor necrosis factor receptor associated periodic syndrome [TRAPS]

  M04.2 Cryopyrin-associated periodic syndromes

Chronic infantile neurological, cutaneous and articular syndrome [CINCA]

Familial cold autoinflammatory syndrome

Familial cold urticaria

Muckle-Wells syndrome

Neonatal onset multisystemic inflammatory disorder [NOMID]

  M04.8 Other autoinflammatory syndromes

Blau syndrome

Deficiency of interleukin 1 receptor antagonist [DIRA]

Majeed syndrome

Periodic fever, aphthous stomatitis, pharyngitis, and adenopathy syndrome [PFAPA]

Pyogenic arthritis, pyoderma gangrenosum, and acne syndrome [PAPA]

  M04.9 Autoinflammatory syndrome, unspecified

INFLAMMATORY POLYARTHROPATHIES (M05-M14)

M05 **Rheumatoid arthritis with rheumatoid factor**

  Definition: Rheumatoid arthritis is a chronic, systemic inflammatory disorder that may affect many tissues and organs, but principally attacks the joints producing a inflammatory synovitis that often progresses to destruction of the articular cartilage and ankylosis of the joints.

  Excludes1: rheumatic fever (I00)

juvenile rheumatoid arthritis (M08.-)

rheumatoid arthritis of spine (M45.-)

  M05.0 Felty's syndrome

Rheumatoid arthritis with splenoadenomegaly and leukopenia

  M05.00 Felty's syndrome, unspecified site

  M05.01 Felty's syndrome, shoulder

    M05.011 Felty's syndrome, right shoulder

    M05.012 Felty's syndrome, left shoulder

    M05.019 Felty's syndrome, unspecified shoulder

  M05.02 Felty's syndrome, elbow

    M05.021 Felty's syndrome, right elbow

    M05.022 Felty's syndrome, left elbow

    M05.029 Felty's syndrome, unspecified elbow

  M05.03 Felty's syndrome, wrist

Felty's syndrome, carpal bones

    M05.031 Felty's syndrome, right wrist

    M05.032 Felty's syndrome, left wrist

  ● New code ▲ Revised code **Excludes1:** Not coded here **Excludes2:** Not included here ⊗ Placeholder required ⑦7th digit required

M05.039   Felty's syndrome, unspecified wrist

M05.04   Felty's syndrome, hand

Felty's syndrome, metacarpus and phalanges

M05.041   Felty's syndrome, right hand

M05.042   Felty's syndrome, left hand

M05.049   Felty's syndrome, unspecified hand

M05.05   Felty's syndrome, hip

M05.051   Felty's syndrome, right hip

M05.052   Felty's syndrome, left hip

M05.059   Felty's syndrome, unspecified hip

M05.06   Felty's syndrome, knee

M05.061   Felty's syndrome, right knee

M05.062   Felty's syndrome, left knee

M05.069   Felty's syndrome, unspecified knee

M05.07   Felty's syndrome, ankle and foot

Felty's syndrome, tarsus, metatarsus and phalanges

M05.071   Felty's syndrome, right ankle and foot

M05.072   Felty's syndrome, left ankle and foot

M05.079   Felty's syndrome, unspecified ankle and foot

M05.09   Felty's syndrome, multiple sites

M05.1   Rheumatoid lung disease with rheumatoid arthritis

M05.10   Rheumatoid lung disease with rheumatoid arthritis of unspecified site

M05.11   Rheumatoid lung disease with rheumatoid arthritis of shoulder

M05.111   Rheumatoid lung disease with rheumatoid arthritis of right shoulder

M05.112   Rheumatoid lung disease with rheumatoid arthritis of left shoulder

M05.119   Rheumatoid lung disease with rheumatoid arthritis of unspecified shoulder

M05.12   Rheumatoid lung disease with rheumatoid arthritis of elbow

M05.121   Rheumatoid lung disease with rheumatoid arthritis of right elbow

M05.122   Rheumatoid lung disease with rheumatoid arthritis of left elbow

M05.129   Rheumatoid lung disease with rheumatoid arthritis of unspecified elbow

M05.13   Rheumatoid lung disease with rheumatoid arthritis of wrist

Rheumatoid lung disease with rheumatoid arthritis, carpal bones

M05.131   Rheumatoid lung disease with rheumatoid arthritis of right wrist

M05.132   Rheumatoid lung disease with rheumatoid arthritis of left wrist

M05.139   Rheumatoid lung disease with rheumatoid arthritis of unspecified wrist

M05.14   Rheumatoid lung disease with rheumatoid arthritis of hand

Rheumatoid lung disease with rheumatoid arthritis, metacarpus and phalanges

M05.141   Rheumatoid lung disease with rheumatoid arthritis of right hand

M05.142   Rheumatoid lung disease with rheumatoid arthritis of left hand

M05.149   Rheumatoid lung disease with rheumatoid arthritis of unspecified hand

M05.15   Rheumatoid lung disease with rheumatoid arthritis of hip

M05.151   Rheumatoid lung disease with rheumatoid arthritis of right hip

M05.152   Rheumatoid lung disease with rheumatoid arthritis of left hip

M05.159   Rheumatoid lung disease with rheumatoid arthritis of unspecified hip

M05.16   Rheumatoid lung disease with rheumatoid arthritis of knee

M05.161   Rheumatoid lung disease with rheumatoid arthritis of right knee

M05.162   Rheumatoid lung disease with rheumatoid arthritis of left knee

M05.169   Rheumatoid lung disease with rheumatoid arthritis of unspecified knee

M05.17   Rheumatoid lung disease with rheumatoid arthritis of ankle and foot

Rheumatoid lung disease with rheumatoid arthritis, tarsus, metatarsus and phalanges

M05.171   Rheumatoid lung disease with rheumatoid arthritis of right ankle and foot

M05.172   Rheumatoid lung disease with rheumatoid arthritis of left ankle and foot

M05.179   Rheumatoid lung disease with rheumatoid arthritis of unspecified ankle and foot

M05.19   Rheumatoid lung disease with rheumatoid arthritis of multiple sites

M05.2   Rheumatoid vasculitis with rheumatoid arthritis

M05.20   Rheumatoid vasculitis with rheumatoid arthritis of unspecified site

M05.21   Rheumatoid vasculitis with rheumatoid arthritis of shoulder

M05.211   Rheumatoid vasculitis with rheumatoid arthritis of right shoulder

M05.212   Rheumatoid vasculitis with rheumatoid arthritis of left shoulder

M05.219   Rheumatoid vasculitis with rheumatoid arthritis of unspecified shoulder

M05.22   Rheumatoid vasculitis with rheumatoid arthritis of elbow

M05.221   Rheumatoid vasculitis with rheumatoid arthritis of right elbow

M05.222   Rheumatoid vasculitis with rheumatoid arthritis of left elbow

M05.229   Rheumatoid vasculitis with rheumatoid arthritis of unspecified elbow

M05.23   Rheumatoid vasculitis with rheumatoid arthritis of wrist

Rheumatoid vasculitis with rheumatoid arthritis, carpal bones

M05.231   **Rheumatoid vasculitis with rheumatoid arthritis of right wrist**

M05.232   **Rheumatoid vasculitis with rheumatoid arthritis of left wrist**

M05.239   **Rheumatoid vasculitis with rheumatoid arthritis of unspecified wrist**

M05.24   **Rheumatoid vasculitis with rheumatoid arthritis of hand**

Rheumatoid vasculitis with rheumatoid arthritis, metacarpus and phalanges

M05.241   **Rheumatoid vasculitis with rheumatoid arthritis of right hand**

M05.242   **Rheumatoid vasculitis with rheumatoid arthritis of left hand**

M05.249   **Rheumatoid vasculitis with rheumatoid arthritis of unspecified hand**

M05.25   **Rheumatoid vasculitis with rheumatoid arthritis of hip**

M05.251   **Rheumatoid vasculitis with rheumatoid arthritis of right hip**

M05.252   **Rheumatoid vasculitis with rheumatoid arthritis of left hip**

M05.259   **Rheumatoid vasculitis with rheumatoid arthritis of unspecified hip**

M05.26   **Rheumatoid vasculitis with rheumatoid arthritis of knee**

M05.261   **Rheumatoid vasculitis with rheumatoid arthritis of right knee**

M05.262   **Rheumatoid vasculitis with rheumatoid arthritis of left knee**

M05.269   **Rheumatoid vasculitis with rheumatoid arthritis of unspecified knee**

M05.27   **Rheumatoid vasculitis with rheumatoid arthritis of ankle and foot**

Rheumatoid vasculitis with rheumatoid arthritis, tarsus, metatarsus and phalanges

M05.271   **Rheumatoid vasculitis with rheumatoid arthritis of right ankle and foot**

M05.272   **Rheumatoid vasculitis with rheumatoid arthritis of left ankle and foot**

M05.279   **Rheumatoid vasculitis with rheumatoid arthritis of unspecified ankle and foot**

M05.29   **Rheumatoid vasculitis with rheumatoid arthritis of multiple sites**

M05.3   **Rheumatoid heart disease with rheumatoid arthritis**

Rheumatoid carditis

Rheumatoid endocarditis

Rheumatoid myocarditis

Rheumatoid pericarditis

M05.30   **Rheumatoid heart disease with rheumatoid arthritis of unspecified site**

M05.31   **Rheumatoid heart disease with rheumatoid arthritis of shoulder**

M05.311   **Rheumatoid heart disease with rheumatoid arthritis of right shoulder**

M05.312   **Rheumatoid heart disease with rheumatoid arthritis of left shoulder**

M05.319   **Rheumatoid heart disease with rheumatoid arthritis of unspecified shoulder**

M05.32   **Rheumatoid heart disease with rheumatoid arthritis of elbow**

M05.321   **Rheumatoid heart disease with rheumatoid arthritis of right elbow**

M05.322   **Rheumatoid heart disease with rheumatoid arthritis of left elbow**

M05.329   **Rheumatoid heart disease with rheumatoid arthritis of unspecified elbow**

M05.33   **Rheumatoid heart disease with rheumatoid arthritis of wrist**

Rheumatoid heart disease with rheumatoid arthritis, carpal bones

M05.331   **Rheumatoid heart disease with rheumatoid arthritis of right wrist**

M05.332   **Rheumatoid heart disease with rheumatoid arthritis of left wrist**

M05.339   **Rheumatoid heart disease with rheumatoid arthritis of unspecified wrist**

M05.34   **Rheumatoid heart disease with rheumatoid arthritis of hand**

Rheumatoid heart disease with rheumatoid arthritis, metacarpus and phalanges

M05.341   **Rheumatoid heart disease with rheumatoid arthritis of right hand**

M05.342   **Rheumatoid heart disease with rheumatoid arthritis of left hand**

M05.349   **Rheumatoid heart disease with rheumatoid arthritis of unspecified hand**

M05.35   **Rheumatoid heart disease with rheumatoid arthritis of hip**

M05.351   **Rheumatoid heart disease with rheumatoid arthritis of right hip**

M05.352   **Rheumatoid heart disease with rheumatoid arthritis of left hip**

M05.359   **Rheumatoid heart disease with rheumatoid arthritis of unspecified hip**

M05.36   **Rheumatoid heart disease with rheumatoid arthritis of knee**

M05.361   **Rheumatoid heart disease with rheumatoid arthritis of right knee**

M05.362   **Rheumatoid heart disease with rheumatoid arthritis of left knee**

M05.369   **Rheumatoid heart disease with rheumatoid arthritis of unspecified knee**

M05.37   **Rheumatoid heart disease with rheumatoid arthritis of ankle and foot**

Rheumatoid heart disease with rheumatoid arthritis, tarsus, metatarsus and phalanges

M05.371   **Rheumatoid heart disease with rheumatoid arthritis of right ankle and foot**

M05.372   **Rheumatoid heart disease with rheumatoid arthritis of left ankle and foot**

M05.379   **Rheumatoid heart disease with rheumatoid arthritis of unspecified ankle and foot**

   ● New code   ▲ Revised code   **Excludes1:** Not coded here   **Excludes2:** Not included here   ⊗ Placeholder required   ⑦7th digit required

M05.39   Rheumatoid heart disease with rheumatoid
arthritis of multiple sites

M05.4   Rheumatoid myopathy with rheumatoid arthritis

M05.40   Rheumatoid myopathy with rheumatoid
arthritis of unspecified site

M05.41   Rheumatoid myopathy with rheumatoid
arthritis of shoulder

M05.411   Rheumatoid myopathy with
rheumatoid arthritis of right
shoulder

M05.412   Rheumatoid myopathy with
rheumatoid arthritis of left shoulder

M05.419   Rheumatoid myopathy with
rheumatoid arthritis of unspecified
shoulder

M05.42   Rheumatoid myopathy with rheumatoid
arthritis of elbow

M05.421   Rheumatoid myopathy with
rheumatoid arthritis of right elbow

M05.422   Rheumatoid myopathy with
rheumatoid arthritis of left elbow

M05.429   Rheumatoid myopathy with
rheumatoid arthritis of unspecified
elbow

M05.43   Rheumatoid myopathy with rheumatoid
arthritis of wrist

Rheumatoid myopathy with rheumatoid arthritis,
carpal bones

M05.431   Rheumatoid myopathy with
rheumatoid arthritis of right wrist

M05.432   Rheumatoid myopathy with
rheumatoid arthritis of left wrist

M05.439   Rheumatoid myopathy with
rheumatoid arthritis of unspecified
wrist

M05.44   Rheumatoid myopathy with rheumatoid
arthritis of hand

Rheumatoid myopathy with rheumatoid arthritis,
metacarpus and phalanges

M05.441   Rheumatoid myopathy with
rheumatoid arthritis of right hand

M05.442   Rheumatoid myopathy with
rheumatoid arthritis of left hand

M05.449   Rheumatoid myopathy with
rheumatoid arthritis of unspecified
hand

M05.45   Rheumatoid myopathy with rheumatoid
arthritis of hip

M05.451   Rheumatoid myopathy with
rheumatoid arthritis of right hip

M05.452   Rheumatoid myopathy with
rheumatoid arthritis of left hip

M05.459   Rheumatoid myopathy with
rheumatoid arthritis of unspecified
hip

M05.46   Rheumatoid myopathy with rheumatoid
arthritis of knee

M05.461   Rheumatoid myopathy with
rheumatoid arthritis of right knee

M05.462   Rheumatoid myopathy with
rheumatoid arthritis of left knee

M05.469   Rheumatoid myopathy with
rheumatoid arthritis of unspecified
knee

M05.47   Rheumatoid myopathy with rheumatoid
arthritis of ankle and foot

Rheumatoid myopathy with rheumatoid arthritis,
tarsus, metatarsus and phalanges

M05.471   Rheumatoid myopathy with
rheumatoid arthritis of right ankle
and foot

M05.472   Rheumatoid myopathy with
rheumatoid arthritis of left ankle and
foot

M05.479   Rheumatoid myopathy with
rheumatoid arthritis of unspecified
ankle and foot

M05.49   Rheumatoid myopathy with rheumatoid
arthritis of multiple sites

M05.5   Rheumatoid polyneuropathy with rheumatoid arthritis

M05.50   Rheumatoid polyneuropathy with rheumatoid
arthritis of unspecified site

M05.51   Rheumatoid polyneuropathy with rheumatoid
arthritis of shoulder

M05.511   Rheumatoid polyneuropathy with
rheumatoid arthritis of right
shoulder

M05.512   Rheumatoid polyneuropathy with
rheumatoid arthritis of left shoulder

M05.519   Rheumatoid polyneuropathy with
rheumatoid arthritis of unspecified
shoulder

M05.52   Rheumatoid polyneuropathy with rheumatoid
arthritis of elbow

M05.521   Rheumatoid polyneuropathy with
rheumatoid arthritis of right elbow

M05.522   Rheumatoid polyneuropathy with
rheumatoid arthritis of left elbow

M05.529   Rheumatoid polyneuropathy with
rheumatoid arthritis of unspecified
elbow

M05.53   Rheumatoid polyneuropathy with rheumatoid
arthritis of wrist

Rheumatoid polyneuropathy with rheumatoid
arthritis, carpal bones

M05.531   Rheumatoid polyneuropathy with
rheumatoid arthritis of right wrist

M05.532   Rheumatoid polyneuropathy with
rheumatoid arthritis of left wrist

M05.539   Rheumatoid polyneuropathy with
rheumatoid arthritis of unspecified
wrist

M05.54   Rheumatoid polyneuropathy with rheumatoid
arthritis of hand

Rheumatoid polyneuropathy with rheumatoid
arthritis, metacarpus and phalanges

M05.541   Rheumatoid polyneuropathy with
rheumatoid arthritis of right hand

M05.542   Rheumatoid polyneuropathy with
rheumatoid arthritis of left hand

M05.549   Rheumatoid polyneuropathy with
rheumatoid arthritis of unspecified
hand

M05.55   Rheumatoid polyneuropathy with rheumatoid
arthritis of hip

M05.551   Rheumatoid polyneuropathy with
rheumatoid arthritis of right hip

M05.552   Rheumatoid polyneuropathy with
rheumatoid arthritis of left hip

M05.559 Rheumatoid polyneuropathy with rheumatoid arthritis of unspecified hip

M05.56 Rheumatoid polyneuropathy with rheumatoid arthritis of knee

M05.561 Rheumatoid polyneuropathy with rheumatoid arthritis of right knee

M05.562 Rheumatoid polyneuropathy with rheumatoid arthritis of left knee

M05.569 Rheumatoid polyneuropathy with rheumatoid arthritis of unspecified knee

M05.57 Rheumatoid polyneuropathy with rheumatoid arthritis of ankle and foot

Rheumatoid polyneuropathy with rheumatoid arthritis, tarsus, metatarsus and phalanges

M05.571 Rheumatoid polyneuropathy with rheumatoid arthritis of right ankle and foot

M05.572 Rheumatoid polyneuropathy with rheumatoid arthritis of left ankle and foot

M05.579 Rheumatoid polyneuropathy with rheumatoid arthritis of unspecified ankle and foot

M05.59 Rheumatoid polyneuropathy with rheumatoid arthritis of multiple sites

M05.6 Rheumatoid arthritis with involvement of other organs and systems

M05.60 Rheumatoid arthritis of unspecified site with involvement of other organs and systems

M05.61 Rheumatoid arthritis of shoulder with involvement of other organs and systems

M05.611 Rheumatoid arthritis of right shoulder with involvement of other organs and systems

M05.612 Rheumatoid arthritis of left shoulder with involvement of other organs and systems

M05.619 Rheumatoid arthritis of unspecified shoulder with involvement of other organs and systems

M05.62 Rheumatoid arthritis of elbow with involvement of other organs and systems

M05.621 Rheumatoid arthritis of right elbow with involvement of other organs and systems

M05.622 Rheumatoid arthritis of left elbow with involvement of other organs and systems

M05.629 Rheumatoid arthritis of unspecified elbow with involvement of other organs and systems

M05.63 Rheumatoid arthritis of wrist with involvement of other organs and systems

Rheumatoid arthritis of carpal bones with involvement **of other** organs and systems

M05.631 Rheumatoid arthritis of right wrist with involvement of other organs and systems

M05.632 Rheumatoid arthritis of left wrist with involvement of other organs and systems

M05.639 Rheumatoid arthritis of unspecified wrist with involvement of other organs and systems

M05.64 Rheumatoid arthritis of hand with involvement of other organs and systems

Rheumatoid arthritis of metacarpus and phalanges with involvement **of other** organs and systems

M05.641 Rheumatoid arthritis of right hand with involvement of other organs and systems

M05.642 Rheumatoid arthritis of left hand with involvement of other organs and systems

M05.649 Rheumatoid arthritis of unspecified hand with involvement of other organs and systems

M05.65 Rheumatoid arthritis of hip with involvement of other organs and systems

M05.651 Rheumatoid arthritis of right hip with involvement of other organs and systems

M05.652 Rheumatoid arthritis of left hip with involvement of other organs and systems

M05.659 Rheumatoid arthritis of unspecified hip with involvement of other organs and systems

M05.66 Rheumatoid arthritis of knee with involvement of other organs and systems

M05.661 Rheumatoid arthritis of right knee with involvement of other organs and systems

M05.662 Rheumatoid arthritis of left knee with involvement of other organs and systems

M05.669 Rheumatoid arthritis of unspecified knee with involvement of other organs and systems

M05.67 Rheumatoid arthritis of ankle and foot with involvement of other organs and systems

Rheumatoid arthritis of tarsus, metatarsus and phalanges with involvement **of other** organs and systems

M05.671 Rheumatoid arthritis of right ankle and foot with involvement of other organs and systems

M05.672 Rheumatoid arthritis of left ankle and foot with involvement of other organs and systems

M05.679 Rheumatoid arthritis of unspecified ankle and foot with involvement of other organs and systems

M05.69 Rheumatoid arthritis of multiple sites with involvement of other organs and systems

M05.7 Rheumatoid arthritis with rheumatoid factor without organ or systems involvement

M05.70 Rheumatoid arthritis with rheumatoid factor of unspecified site without organ or systems involvement

M05.71 Rheumatoid arthritis with rheumatoid factor of shoulder without organ or systems involvement

M05.711 Rheumatoid arthritis with rheumatoid factor of right shoulder without organ or systems involvement

M05.712 Rheumatoid arthritis with rheumatoid factor of left shoulder without organ or systems involvement

M05.719 Rheumatoid arthritis with rheumatoid factor of unspecified shoulder without organ or systems involvement

M05.72 Rheumatoid arthritis with rheumatoid factor of elbow without organ or systems involvement

M05.721 Rheumatoid arthritis with rheumatoid factor of right elbow without organ or systems involvement

M05.722 Rheumatoid arthritis with rheumatoid factor of left elbow without organ or systems involvement

M05.729 Rheumatoid arthritis with rheumatoid factor of unspecified elbow without organ or systems involvement

M05.73 Rheumatoid arthritis with rheumatoid factor of wrist without organ or systems involvement

M05.731 Rheumatoid arthritis with rheumatoid factor of right wrist without organ or systems involvement

M05.732 Rheumatoid arthritis with rheumatoid factor of left wrist without organ or systems involvement

M05.739 Rheumatoid arthritis with rheumatoid factor of unspecified wrist without organ or systems involvement

M05.74 Rheumatoid arthritis with rheumatoid factor of hand without organ or systems involvement

M05.741 Rheumatoid arthritis with rheumatoid factor of right hand without organ or systems involvement

M05.742 Rheumatoid arthritis with rheumatoid factor of left hand without organ or systems involvement

M05.749 Rheumatoid arthritis with rheumatoid factor of unspecified hand without organ or systems involvement

M05.75 Rheumatoid arthritis with rheumatoid factor of hip without organ or systems involvement

M05.751 Rheumatoid arthritis with rheumatoid factor of right hip without organ or systems involvement

M05.752 Rheumatoid arthritis with rheumatoid factor of left hip without organ or systems involvement

M05.759 Rheumatoid arthritis with rheumatoid factor of unspecified hip without organ or systems involvement

M05.76 Rheumatoid arthritis with rheumatoid factor of knee without organ or systems involvement

M05.761 Rheumatoid arthritis with rheumatoid factor of right knee without organ or systems involvement

M05.762 Rheumatoid arthritis with rheumatoid factor of left knee

without organ or systems involvement

M05.769 Rheumatoid arthritis with rheumatoid factor of unspecified knee without organ or systems involvement

M05.77 Rheumatoid arthritis with rheumatoid factor of ankle and foot without organ or systems involvement

M05.771 Rheumatoid arthritis with rheumatoid factor of right ankle and foot without organ or systems involvement

M05.772 Rheumatoid arthritis with rheumatoid factor of left ankle and foot without organ or systems involvement

M05.779 Rheumatoid arthritis with rheumatoid factor of unspecified ankle and foot without organ or systems involvement

M05.79 Rheumatoid arthritis with rheumatoid factor of multiple sites without organ or systems involvement

M05.8 Other rheumatoid arthritis with rheumatoid factor

M05.80 Other rheumatoid arthritis with rheumatoid factor of unspecified site

M05.81 Other rheumatoid arthritis with rheumatoid factor of shoulder

M05.811 Other rheumatoid arthritis with rheumatoid factor of right shoulder

M05.812 Other rheumatoid arthritis with rheumatoid factor of left shoulder

M05.819 Other rheumatoid arthritis with rheumatoid factor of unspecified shoulder

M05.82 Other rheumatoid arthritis with rheumatoid factor of elbow

M05.821 Other rheumatoid arthritis with rheumatoid factor of right elbow

M05.822 Other rheumatoid arthritis with rheumatoid factor of left elbow

M05.829 Other rheumatoid arthritis with rheumatoid factor of unspecified elbow

M05.83 Other rheumatoid arthritis with rheumatoid factor of wrist

M05.831 Other rheumatoid arthritis with rheumatoid factor of right wrist

M05.832 Other rheumatoid arthritis with rheumatoid factor of left wrist

M05.839 Other rheumatoid arthritis with rheumatoid factor of unspecified wrist

M05.84 Other rheumatoid arthritis with rheumatoid factor of hand

M05.841 Other rheumatoid arthritis with rheumatoid factor of right hand

M05.842 Other rheumatoid arthritis with rheumatoid factor of left hand

M05.849 Other rheumatoid arthritis with rheumatoid factor of unspecified hand

M05.85 Other rheumatoid arthritis with rheumatoid factor of hip

M05.851 Other rheumatoid arthritis with rheumatoid factor of right hip

M05.852 Other rheumatoid arthritis with rheumatoid factor of left hip

M05.859 Other rheumatoid arthritis with rheumatoid factor of unspecified hip

M05.86 Other rheumatoid arthritis with rheumatoid factor of knee

M05.861 Other rheumatoid arthritis with rheumatoid factor of right knee

M05.862 Other rheumatoid arthritis with rheumatoid factor of left knee

M05.869 Other rheumatoid arthritis with rheumatoid factor of unspecified knee

M05.87 Other rheumatoid arthritis with rheumatoid factor of ankle and foot

M05.871 Other rheumatoid arthritis with rheumatoid factor of right ankle and foot

M05.872 Other rheumatoid arthritis with rheumatoid factor of left ankle and foot

M05.879 Other rheumatoid arthritis with rheumatoid factor of unspecified ankle and foot

M05.89 Other rheumatoid arthritis with rheumatoid factor of multiple sites

M05.9 Rheumatoid arthritis with rheumatoid factor, unspecified

M06 Other rheumatoid arthritis

M06.0 Rheumatoid arthritis without rheumatoid factor

M06.00 Rheumatoid arthritis without rheumatoid factor, unspecified site

M06.01 Rheumatoid arthritis without rheumatoid factor, shoulder

M06.011 Rheumatoid arthritis without rheumatoid factor, right shoulder

M06.012 Rheumatoid arthritis without rheumatoid factor, left shoulder

M06.019 Rheumatoid arthritis without rheumatoid factor, unspecified shoulder

M06.02 Rheumatoid arthritis without rheumatoid factor, elbow

M06.021 Rheumatoid arthritis without rheumatoid factor, right elbow

M06.022 Rheumatoid arthritis without rheumatoid factor, left elbow

M06.029 Rheumatoid arthritis without rheumatoid factor, unspecified elbow

M06.03 Rheumatoid arthritis without rheumatoid factor, wrist

M06.031 Rheumatoid arthritis without rheumatoid factor, right wrist

M06.032 Rheumatoid arthritis without rheumatoid factor, left wrist

M06.039 Rheumatoid arthritis without rheumatoid factor, unspecified wrist

M06.04 Rheumatoid arthritis without rheumatoid factor, hand

M06.041 Rheumatoid arthritis without rheumatoid factor, right hand

M06.042 Rheumatoid arthritis without rheumatoid factor, left hand

M06.049 Rheumatoid arthritis without rheumatoid factor, unspecified hand

M06.05 Rheumatoid arthritis without rheumatoid factor, hip

M06.051 Rheumatoid arthritis without rheumatoid factor, right hip

M06.052 Rheumatoid arthritis without rheumatoid factor, left hip

M06.059 Rheumatoid arthritis without rheumatoid factor, unspecified hip

M06.06 Rheumatoid arthritis without rheumatoid factor, knee

M06.061 Rheumatoid arthritis without rheumatoid factor, right knee

M06.062 Rheumatoid arthritis without rheumatoid factor, left knee

M06.069 Rheumatoid arthritis without rheumatoid factor, unspecified knee

M06.07 Rheumatoid arthritis without rheumatoid factor, ankle and foot

M06.071 Rheumatoid arthritis without rheumatoid factor, right ankle and foot

M06.072 Rheumatoid arthritis without rheumatoid factor, left ankle and foot

M06.079 Rheumatoid arthritis without rheumatoid factor, unspecified ankle and foot

M06.08 Rheumatoid arthritis without rheumatoid factor, vertebrae

M06.09 Rheumatoid arthritis without rheumatoid factor, multiple sites

M06.1 Adult-onset Still's disease

Excludes1: Still's disease NOS (M08.2-)

M06.2 Rheumatoid bursitis

M06.20 Rheumatoid bursitis, unspecified site

M06.21 Rheumatoid bursitis, shoulder

M06.211 Rheumatoid bursitis, right shoulder

M06.212 Rheumatoid bursitis, left shoulder

M06.219 Rheumatoid bursitis, unspecified shoulder

M06.22 Rheumatoid bursitis, elbow

M06.221 Rheumatoid bursitis, right elbow

M06.222 Rheumatoid bursitis, left elbow

M06.229 Rheumatoid bursitis, unspecified elbow

M06.23 Rheumatoid bursitis, wrist

M06.231 Rheumatoid bursitis, right wrist

M06.232 Rheumatoid bursitis, left wrist

M06.239 Rheumatoid bursitis, unspecified wrist

M06.24 Rheumatoid bursitis, hand

M06.241 Rheumatoid bursitis, right hand

M06.242 Rheumatoid bursitis, left hand

M06.249 Rheumatoid bursitis, unspecified hand

M06.25 Rheumatoid bursitis, hip

M06.251 Rheumatoid bursitis, right hip

M06.252 Rheumatoid bursitis, left hip

M06.259 Rheumatoid bursitis, unspecified hip

M06.26 Rheumatoid bursitis, knee

M06.261   Rheumatoid bursitis, right knee

M06.262   Rheumatoid bursitis, left knee

M06.269   Rheumatoid bursitis, unspecified knee

M06.27   Rheumatoid bursitis, ankle and foot

M06.271   Rheumatoid bursitis, right ankle and foot

M06.272   Rheumatoid bursitis, left ankle and foot

M06.279   Rheumatoid bursitis, unspecified ankle and foot

M06.28   Rheumatoid bursitis, vertebrae

M06.29   Rheumatoid bursitis, multiple sites

M06.3   Rheumatoid nodule

M06.30   Rheumatoid nodule, unspecified site

M06.31   Rheumatoid nodule, shoulder

M06.311   Rheumatoid nodule, right shoulder

M06.312   Rheumatoid nodule, left shoulder

M06.319   Rheumatoid nodule, unspecified shoulder

M06.32   Rheumatoid nodule, elbow

M06.321   Rheumatoid nodule, right elbow

M06.322   Rheumatoid nodule, left elbow

M06.329   Rheumatoid nodule, unspecified elbow

M06.33   Rheumatoid nodule, wrist

M06.331   Rheumatoid nodule, right wrist

M06.332   Rheumatoid nodule, left wrist

M06.339   Rheumatoid nodule, unspecified wrist

M06.34   Rheumatoid nodule, hand

M06.341   Rheumatoid nodule, right hand

M06.342   Rheumatoid nodule, left hand

M06.349   Rheumatoid nodule, unspecified hand

M06.35   Rheumatoid nodule, hip

M06.351   Rheumatoid nodule, right hip

M06.352   Rheumatoid nodule, left hip

M06.359   Rheumatoid nodule, unspecified hip

M06.36   Rheumatoid nodule, knee

M06.361   Rheumatoid nodule, right knee

M06.362   Rheumatoid nodule, left knee

M06.369   Rheumatoid nodule, unspecified knee

M06.37   Rheumatoid nodule, ankle and foot

M06.371   Rheumatoid nodule, right ankle and foot

M06.372   Rheumatoid nodule, left ankle and foot

M06.379   Rheumatoid nodule, unspecified ankle and foot

M06.38   Rheumatoid nodule, vertebrae

M06.39   Rheumatoid nodule, multiple sites

M06.4   Inflammatory polyarthropathy

Excludes1: polyarthritis NOS (M13.0)

M06.8   Other specified rheumatoid arthritis

M06.80   Other specified rheumatoid arthritis, unspecified site

M06.81   Other specified rheumatoid arthritis, shoulder

M06.811   Other specified rheumatoid arthritis, right shoulder

M06.812   Other specified rheumatoid arthritis, left shoulder

M06.819   Other specified rheumatoid arthritis, unspecified shoulder

M06.82   Other specified rheumatoid arthritis, elbow

M06.821   Other specified rheumatoid arthritis, right elbow

M06.822   Other specified rheumatoid arthritis, left elbow

M06.829   Other specified rheumatoid arthritis, unspecified elbow

M06.83   Other specified rheumatoid arthritis, wrist

M06.831   Other specified rheumatoid arthritis, right wrist

M06.832   Other specified rheumatoid arthritis, left wrist

M06.839   Other specified rheumatoid arthritis, unspecified wrist

M06.84   Other specified rheumatoid arthritis, hand

M06.841   Other specified rheumatoid arthritis, right hand

M06.842   Other specified rheumatoid arthritis, left hand

M06.849   Other specified rheumatoid arthritis, unspecified hand

M06.85   Other specified rheumatoid arthritis, hip

M06.851   Other specified rheumatoid arthritis, right hip

M06.852   Other specified rheumatoid arthritis, left hip

M06.859   Other specified rheumatoid arthritis, unspecified hip

M06.86   Other specified rheumatoid arthritis, knee

M06.861   Other specified rheumatoid arthritis, right knee

M06.862   Other specified rheumatoid arthritis, left knee

M06.869   Other specified rheumatoid arthritis, unspecified knee

M06.87   Other specified rheumatoid arthritis, ankle and foot

M06.871   Other specified rheumatoid arthritis, right ankle and foot

M06.872   Other specified rheumatoid arthritis, left ankle and foot

M06.879   Other specified rheumatoid arthritis, unspecified ankle and foot

M06.88   Other specified rheumatoid arthritis, vertebrae

M06.89   Other specified rheumatoid arthritis, multiple sites

M06.9   Rheumatoid arthritis, unspecified

M07   **Enteropathic arthropathies**

Code also associated enteropathy, such as:

regional enteritis [Crohn's disease] (K50.-)

ulcerative colitis (K51.-)

Excludes1: psoriatic arthropathies (L40.5-)

M07.6   Enteropathic arthropathies

M07.60   Enteropathic arthropathies, unspecified site

M07.61   Enteropathic arthropathies, shoulder

    Add 4th-7th digits   Nonspecific code   Unspecified code   Manifestation code   **507**

M07.611 Enteropathic arthropathies, right shoulder

M07.612 Enteropathic arthropathies, left shoulder

M07.619 Enteropathic arthropathies, unspecified shoulder

M07.62 Enteropathic arthropathies, elbow

M07.621 Enteropathic arthropathies, right elbow

M07.622 Enteropathic arthropathies, left elbow

M07.629 Enteropathic arthropathies, unspecified elbow

M07.63 Enteropathic arthropathies, wrist

M07.631 Enteropathic arthropathies, right wrist

M07.632 Enteropathic arthropathies, left wrist

M07.639 Enteropathic arthropathies, unspecified wrist

M07.64 Enteropathic arthropathies, hand

M07.641 Enteropathic arthropathies, right hand

M07.642 Enteropathic arthropathies, left hand

M07.649 Enteropathic arthropathies, unspecified hand

M07.65 Enteropathic arthropathies, hip

M07.651 Enteropathic arthropathies, right hip

M07.652 Enteropathic arthropathies, left hip

M07.659 Enteropathic arthropathies, unspecified hip

M07.66 Enteropathic arthropathies, knee

M07.661 Enteropathic arthropathies, right knee

M07.662 Enteropathic arthropathies, left knee

M07.669 Enteropathic arthropathies, unspecified knee

M07.67 Enteropathic arthropathies, ankle and foot

M07.671 Enteropathic arthropathies, right ankle and foot

M07.672 Enteropathic arthropathies, left ankle and foot

M07.679 Enteropathic arthropathies, unspecified ankle and foot

M07.68 Enteropathic arthropathies, vertebrae

M07.69 Enteropathic arthropathies, multiple sites

M08 **Juvenile arthritis**

Code also any associated underlying condition, such as:

regional enteritis [Crohn's disease] (K50.-)

ulcerative colitis (K51.-)

Excludes1: arthropathy in Whipple's disease (M14.8)

Felty's syndrome (M05.0)

juvenile dermatomyositis (M33.0-)

psoriatic juvenile arthropathy (L40.54)

M08.0 **Unspecified juvenile rheumatoid arthritis**

Juvenile rheumatoid arthritis with or without rheumatoid factor

M08.00 Unspecified juvenile rheumatoid arthritis of unspecified site

M08.01 Unspecified juvenile rheumatoid arthritis, shoulder

M08.011 Unspecified juvenile rheumatoid arthritis, right shoulder

M08.012 Unspecified juvenile rheumatoid arthritis, left shoulder

M08.019 Unspecified juvenile rheumatoid arthritis, unspecified shoulder

M08.02 Unspecified juvenile rheumatoid arthritis of elbow

M08.021 Unspecified juvenile rheumatoid arthritis, right elbow

M08.022 Unspecified juvenile rheumatoid arthritis, left elbow

M08.029 Unspecified juvenile rheumatoid arthritis, unspecified elbow

M08.03 Unspecified juvenile rheumatoid arthritis, wrist

M08.031 Unspecified juvenile rheumatoid arthritis, right wrist

M08.032 Unspecified juvenile rheumatoid arthritis, left wrist

M08.039 Unspecified juvenile rheumatoid arthritis, unspecified wrist

M08.04 Unspecified juvenile rheumatoid arthritis, hand

M08.041 Unspecified juvenile rheumatoid arthritis, right hand

M08.042 Unspecified juvenile rheumatoid arthritis, left hand

M08.049 Unspecified juvenile rheumatoid arthritis, unspecified hand

M08.05 Unspecified juvenile rheumatoid arthritis, hip

M08.051 Unspecified juvenile rheumatoid arthritis, right hip

M08.052 Unspecified juvenile rheumatoid arthritis, left hip

M08.059 Unspecified juvenile rheumatoid arthritis, unspecified hip

M08.06 Unspecified juvenile rheumatoid arthritis, knee

M08.061 Unspecified juvenile rheumatoid arthritis, right knee

M08.062 Unspecified juvenile rheumatoid arthritis, left knee

M08.069 Unspecified juvenile rheumatoid arthritis, unspecified knee

M08.07 Unspecified juvenile rheumatoid arthritis, ankle and foot

M08.071 Unspecified juvenile rheumatoid arthritis, right ankle and foot

M08.072 Unspecified juvenile rheumatoid arthritis, left ankle and foot

M08.079 Unspecified juvenile rheumatoid arthritis, unspecified ankle and foot

M08.08 Unspecified juvenile rheumatoid arthritis, vertebrae

M08.09 Unspecified juvenile rheumatoid arthritis, multiple sites

M08.1 **Juvenile ankylosing spondylitis**

Excludes1: ankylosing spondylitis in adults (M45.0-)

M08.2 **Juvenile rheumatoid arthritis with systemic onset**

Still's disease NOS

Excludes1: adult-onset Still's disease (M06.1-)

M08.20 Juvenile rheumatoid arthritis with systemic onset, unspecified site

● New code ▲ Revised code **Excludes1:** Not coded here **Excludes2:** Not included here ⊗ Placeholder required ⑦ 7th digit required

M08.21   Juvenile rheumatoid arthritis with systemic onset, shoulder

     M08.211   Juvenile rheumatoid arthritis with systemic onset, right shoulder

     M08.212   Juvenile rheumatoid arthritis with systemic onset, left shoulder

     M08.219   Juvenile rheumatoid arthritis with systemic onset, unspecified shoulder

M08.22   Juvenile rheumatoid arthritis with systemic onset, elbow

     M08.221   Juvenile rheumatoid arthritis with systemic onset, right elbow

     M08.222   Juvenile rheumatoid arthritis with systemic onset, left elbow

     M08.229   Juvenile rheumatoid arthritis with systemic onset, unspecified elbow

M08.23   Juvenile rheumatoid arthritis with systemic onset, wrist

     M08.231   Juvenile rheumatoid arthritis with systemic onset, right wrist

     M08.232   Juvenile rheumatoid arthritis with systemic onset, left wrist

     M08.239   Juvenile rheumatoid arthritis with systemic onset, unspecified wrist

M08.24   Juvenile rheumatoid arthritis with systemic onset, hand

     M08.241   Juvenile rheumatoid arthritis with systemic onset, right hand

     M08.242   Juvenile rheumatoid arthritis with systemic onset, left hand

     M08.249   Juvenile rheumatoid arthritis with systemic onset, unspecified hand

M08.25   Juvenile rheumatoid arthritis with systemic onset, hip

     M08.251   Juvenile rheumatoid arthritis with systemic onset, right hip

     M08.252   Juvenile rheumatoid arthritis with systemic onset, left hip

     M08.259   Juvenile rheumatoid arthritis with systemic onset, unspecified hip

M08.26   Juvenile rheumatoid arthritis with systemic onset, knee

     M08.261   Juvenile rheumatoid arthritis with systemic onset, right knee

     M08.262   Juvenile rheumatoid arthritis with systemic onset, left knee

     M08.269   Juvenile rheumatoid arthritis with systemic onset, unspecified knee

M08.27   Juvenile rheumatoid arthritis with systemic onset, ankle and foot

     M08.271   Juvenile rheumatoid arthritis with systemic onset, right ankle and foot

     M08.272   Juvenile rheumatoid arthritis with systemic onset, left ankle and foot

     M08.279   Juvenile rheumatoid arthritis with systemic onset, unspecified ankle and foot

M08.28   Juvenile rheumatoid arthritis with systemic onset, vertebrae

M08.29   Juvenile rheumatoid arthritis with systemic onset, multiple sites

M08.3   Juvenile rheumatoid polyarthritis (seronegative)

M08.4   Pauciarticular juvenile rheumatoid arthritis

M08.40   Pauciarticular juvenile rheumatoid arthritis, unspecified site

M08.41   Pauciarticular juvenile rheumatoid arthritis, shoulder

     M08.411   Pauciarticular juvenile rheumatoid arthritis, right shoulder

     M08.412   Pauciarticular juvenile rheumatoid arthritis, left shoulder

     M08.419   Pauciarticular juvenile rheumatoid arthritis, unspecified shoulder

M08.42   Pauciarticular juvenile rheumatoid arthritis, elbow

     M08.421   Pauciarticular juvenile rheumatoid arthritis, right elbow

     M08.422   Pauciarticular juvenile rheumatoid arthritis, left elbow

     M08.429   Pauciarticular juvenile rheumatoid arthritis, unspecified elbow

M08.43   Pauciarticular juvenile rheumatoid arthritis, wrist

     M08.431   Pauciarticular juvenile rheumatoid arthritis, right wrist

     M08.432   Pauciarticular juvenile rheumatoid arthritis, left wrist

     M08.439   Pauciarticular juvenile rheumatoid arthritis, unspecified wrist

M08.44   Pauciarticular juvenile rheumatoid arthritis, hand

     M08.441   Pauciarticular juvenile rheumatoid arthritis, right hand

     M08.442   Pauciarticular juvenile rheumatoid arthritis, left hand

     M08.449   Pauciarticular juvenile rheumatoid arthritis, unspecified hand

M08.45   Pauciarticular juvenile rheumatoid arthritis, hip

     M08.451   Pauciarticular juvenile rheumatoid arthritis, right hip

     M08.452   Pauciarticular juvenile rheumatoid arthritis, left hip

     M08.459   Pauciarticular juvenile rheumatoid arthritis, unspecified hip

M08.46   Pauciarticular juvenile rheumatoid arthritis, knee

     M08.461   Pauciarticular juvenile rheumatoid arthritis, right knee

     M08.462   Pauciarticular juvenile rheumatoid arthritis, left knee

     M08.469   Pauciarticular juvenile rheumatoid arthritis, unspecified knee

M08.47   Pauciarticular juvenile rheumatoid arthritis, ankle and foot

     M08.471   Pauciarticular juvenile rheumatoid arthritis, right ankle and foot

     M08.472   Pauciarticular juvenile rheumatoid arthritis, left ankle and foot

     M08.479   Pauciarticular juvenile rheumatoid arthritis, unspecified ankle and foot

M08.48   Pauciarticular juvenile rheumatoid arthritis, vertebrae

M08.8   Other juvenile arthritis

M08.80   Other juvenile arthritis, unspecified site

M08.81   Other juvenile arthritis, shoulder

M08.811 Other juvenile arthritis, right shoulder

M08.812 Other juvenile arthritis, left shoulder

M08.819 Other juvenile arthritis, unspecified shoulder

M08.82 Other juvenile arthritis, elbow

M08.821 Other juvenile arthritis, right elbow

M08.822 Other juvenile arthritis, left elbow

M08.829 Other juvenile arthritis, unspecified elbow

M08.83 Other juvenile arthritis, wrist

M08.831 Other juvenile arthritis, right wrist

M08.832 Other juvenile arthritis, left wrist

M08.839 Other juvenile arthritis, unspecified wrist

M08.84 Other juvenile arthritis, hand

M08.841 Other juvenile arthritis, right hand

M08.842 Other juvenile arthritis, left hand

M08.849 Other juvenile arthritis, unspecified hand

M08.85 Other juvenile arthritis, hip

M08.851 Other juvenile arthritis, right hip

M08.852 Other juvenile arthritis, left hip

M08.859 Other juvenile arthritis, unspecified hip

M08.86 Other juvenile arthritis, knee

M08.861 Other juvenile arthritis, right knee

M08.862 Other juvenile arthritis, left knee

M08.869 Other juvenile arthritis, unspecified knee

M08.87 Other juvenile arthritis, ankle and foot

M08.871 Other juvenile arthritis, right ankle and foot

M08.872 Other juvenile arthritis, left ankle and foot

M08.879 Other juvenile arthritis, unspecified ankle and foot

M08.88 Other juvenile arthritis, other specified site

Other juvenile arthritis, vertebrae

M08.89 Other juvenile arthritis, multiple sites

M08.9 Juvenile arthritis, unspecified

Excludes1: juvenile rheumatoid arthritis, unspecified (M08.0-)

M08.90 Juvenile arthritis, unspecified, unspecified site

M08.91 Juvenile arthritis, unspecified, shoulder

M08.911 Juvenile arthritis, unspecified, right shoulder

M08.912 Juvenile arthritis, unspecified, left shoulder

M08.919 Juvenile arthritis, unspecified, unspecified shoulder

M08.92 Juvenile arthritis, unspecified, elbow

M08.921 Juvenile arthritis, unspecified, right elbow

M08.922 Juvenile arthritis, unspecified, left elbow

M08.929 Juvenile arthritis, unspecified, unspecified elbow

M08.93 Juvenile arthritis, unspecified, wrist

M08.931 Juvenile arthritis, unspecified, right wrist

M08.932 Juvenile arthritis, unspecified, left wrist

M08.939 Juvenile arthritis, unspecified, unspecified wrist

M08.94 Juvenile arthritis, unspecified, hand

M08.941 Juvenile arthritis, unspecified, right hand

M08.942 Juvenile arthritis, unspecified, left hand

M08.949 Juvenile arthritis, unspecified, unspecified hand

M08.95 Juvenile arthritis, unspecified, hip

M08.951 Juvenile arthritis, unspecified, right hip

M08.952 Juvenile arthritis, unspecified, left hip

M08.959 Juvenile arthritis, unspecified, unspecified hip

M08.96 Juvenile arthritis, unspecified, knee

M08.961 Juvenile arthritis, unspecified, right knee

M08.962 Juvenile arthritis, unspecified, left knee

M08.969 Juvenile arthritis, unspecified, unspecified knee

M08.97 Juvenile arthritis, unspecified, ankle and foot

M08.971 Juvenile arthritis, unspecified, right ankle and foot

M08.972 Juvenile arthritis, unspecified, left ankle and foot

M08.979 Juvenile arthritis, unspecified, unspecified ankle and foot

M08.98 Juvenile arthritis, unspecified, vertebrae

M08.99 Juvenile arthritis, unspecified, multiple sites

M1A Chronic gout

Use additional code to identify:

Autonomic neuropathy in diseases classified elsewhere (G99.0)

Calculus of urinary tract in diseases classified elsewhere (N22)

Cardiomyopathy in diseases classified elsewhere (I43)

Disorders of external ear in diseases classified elsewhere (H61.1-, H62.8-)

Disorders of iris and ciliary body in diseases classified elsewhere (H22)

Glomerular disorders in diseases classified elsewhere (N08)

Excludes1: gout NOS (M10.-)

Excludes2: acute gout (M10.-)

The appropriate 7th character is to be added to each code from category M1A

0 - without tophus (tophi)

1 - with tophus (tophi)

M1A.0 Idiopathic chronic gout

Chronic gouty bursitis

Primary chronic gout

⊗⑦**M1A.00** Idiopathic chronic gout, unspecified site

M1A.01 Idiopathic chronic gout, shoulder

⑦**M1A.011** Idiopathic chronic gout, right shoulder

⑦**M1A.012** Idiopathic chronic gout, left shoulder

⑦**M1A.019** Idiopathic chronic gout, unspecified shoulder

M1A.02 Idiopathic chronic gout, elbow

⑦**M1A.021** Idiopathic chronic gout, right elbow

⑦**M1A.022** Idiopathic chronic gout, left elbow

⑦**M1A.029** Idiopathic chronic gout, unspecified elbow

M1A.03 Idiopathic chronic gout, wrist

⑦**M1A.031** Idiopathic chronic gout, right wrist

⑦**M1A.032** Idiopathic chronic gout, left wrist

⑦**M1A.039** Idiopathic chronic gout, unspecified wrist

M1A.04 Idiopathic chronic gout, hand

⑦**M1A.041** Idiopathic chronic gout, right hand

⑦**M1A.042** Idiopathic chronic gout, left hand

⑦**M1A.049** Idiopathic chronic gout, unspecified hand

M1A.05 Idiopathic chronic gout, hip

⑦**M1A.051** Idiopathic chronic gout, right hip

⑦**M1A.052** Idiopathic chronic gout, left hip

⑦**M1A.059** Idiopathic chronic gout, unspecified hip

M1A.06 Idiopathic chronic gout, knee

⑦**M1A.061** Idiopathic chronic gout, right knee

⑦**M1A.062** Idiopathic chronic gout, left knee

⑦**M1A.069** Idiopathic chronic gout, unspecified knee

M1A.07 Idiopathic chronic gout, ankle and foot

⑦**M1A.071** Idiopathic chronic gout, right ankle and foot

⑦**M1A.072** Idiopathic chronic gout, left ankle and foot

⑦**M1A.079** Idiopathic chronic gout, unspecified ankle and foot

⊗⑦**M1A.08** Idiopathic chronic gout, vertebrae

⊗⑦**M1A.09** Idiopathic chronic gout, multiple sites

M1A.1 Lead-induced chronic gout

Code first toxic effects of lead and its compounds (T56.0-)

⊗⑦**M1A.10** Lead-induced chronic gout, unspecified site

M1A.11 Lead-induced chronic gout, shoulder

⑦**M1A.111** Lead-induced chronic gout, right shoulder

⑦**M1A.112** Lead-induced chronic gout, left shoulder

⑦**M1A.119** Lead-induced chronic gout, unspecified shoulder

M1A.12 Lead-induced chronic gout, elbow

⑦**M1A.121** Lead-induced chronic gout, right elbow

⑦**M1A.122** Lead-induced chronic gout, left elbow

⑦**M1A.129** Lead-induced chronic gout, unspecified elbow

M1A.13 Lead-induced chronic gout, wrist

⑦**M1A.131** Lead-induced chronic gout, right wrist

⑦**M1A.132** Lead-induced chronic gout, left wrist

⑦**M1A.139** Lead-induced chronic gout, unspecified wrist

M1A.14 Lead-induced chronic gout, hand

⑦**M1A.141** Lead-induced chronic gout, right hand

⑦**M1A.142** Lead-induced chronic gout, left hand

⑦**M1A.149** Lead-induced chronic gout, unspecified hand

M1A.15 Lead-induced chronic gout, hip

⑦**M1A.151** Lead-induced chronic gout, right hip

⑦**M1A.152** Lead-induced chronic gout, left hip

⑦**M1A.159** Lead-induced chronic gout, unspecified hip

M1A.16 Lead-induced chronic gout, knee

⑦**M1A.161** Lead-induced chronic gout, right knee

⑦**M1A.162** Lead-induced chronic gout, left knee

⑦**M1A.169** Lead-induced chronic gout, unspecified knee

M1A.17 Lead-induced chronic gout, ankle and foot

⑦**M1A.171** Lead-induced chronic gout, right ankle and foot

⑦**M1A.172** Lead-induced chronic gout, left ankle and foot

⑦**M1A.179** Lead-induced chronic gout, unspecified ankle and foot

⊗⑦**M1A.18** Lead-induced chronic gout, vertebrae

⊗⑦**M1A.19** Lead-induced chronic gout, multiple sites

M1A.2 Drug-induced chronic gout

Use additional code for adverse effect, if applicable, to identify drug (T36-T50 with fifth or sixth character 5)

⊗⑦**M1A.20** Drug-induced chronic gout, unspecified site

M1A.21 Drug-induced chronic gout, shoulder

⑦**M1A.211** Drug-induced chronic gout, right shoulder

⑦**M1A.212** Drug-induced chronic gout, left shoulder

⑦**M1A.219** Drug-induced chronic gout, unspecified shoulder

M1A.22 Drug-induced chronic gout, elbow

⑦**M1A.221** Drug-induced chronic gout, right elbow

⑦**M1A.222** Drug-induced chronic gout, left elbow

⑦**M1A.229** Drug-induced chronic gout, unspecified elbow

M1A.23 Drug-induced chronic gout, wrist

⑦**M1A.231** Drug-induced chronic gout, right wrist

⑦**M1A.232** Drug-induced chronic gout, left wrist

⑦**M1A.239** Drug-induced chronic gout, unspecified wrist

M1A.24 Drug-induced chronic gout, hand

⑦**M1A.241** Drug-induced chronic gout, right hand

⑦**M1A.242** Drug-induced chronic gout, left hand

⑦**M1A.249** Drug-induced chronic gout, unspecified hand

M1A.25 Drug-induced chronic gout, hip

⑦**M1A.251** Drug-induced chronic gout, right hip

⑦**M1A.252** Drug-induced chronic gout, left hip

⑦**M1A.259** Drug-induced chronic gout, unspecified hip

M1A.26 Drug-induced chronic gout, knee

▓ Add 4th-7th digits	Nonspecific code	Unspecified code	Manifestation code

⑦M1A.261 Drug-induced chronic gout, right knee

⑦M1A.262 Drug-induced chronic gout, left knee

⑦M1A.269 Drug-induced chronic gout, unspecified knee

M1A.27 Drug-induced chronic gout, ankle and foot

⑦M1A.271 Drug-induced chronic gout, right ankle and foot

⑦M1A.272 Drug-induced chronic gout, left ankle and foot

⑦M1A.279 Drug-induced chronic gout, unspecified ankle and foot

⊗⑦M1A.28 Drug-induced chronic gout, vertebrae

⊗⑦M1A.29 Drug-induced chronic gout, multiple sites

M1A.3 Chronic gout due to renal impairment

Code first associated renal disease

⊗⑦M1A.30 Chronic gout due to renal impairment, unspecified site

M1A.31 Chronic gout due to renal impairment, shoulder

⑦M1A.311 Chronic gout due to renal impairment, right shoulder

⑦M1A.312 Chronic gout due to renal impairment, left shoulder

⑦M1A.319 Chronic gout due to renal impairment, unspecified shoulder

M1A.32 Chronic gout due to renal impairment, elbow

⑦M1A.321 Chronic gout due to renal impairment, right elbow

⑦M1A.322 Chronic gout due to renal impairment, left elbow

⑦M1A.329 Chronic gout due to renal impairment, unspecified elbow

M1A.33 Chronic gout due to renal impairment, wrist

⑦M1A.331 Chronic gout due to renal impairment, right wrist

⑦M1A.332 Chronic gout due to renal impairment, left wrist

⑦M1A.339 Chronic gout due to renal impairment, unspecified wrist

M1A.34 Chronic gout due to renal impairment, hand

⑦M1A.341 Chronic gout due to renal impairment, right hand

⑦M1A.342 Chronic gout due to renal impairment, left hand

⑦M1A.349 Chronic gout due to renal impairment, unspecified hand

M1A.35 Chronic gout due to renal impairment, hip

⑦M1A.351 Chronic gout due to renal impairment, right hip

⑦M1A.352 Chronic gout due to renal impairment, left hip

⑦M1A.359 Chronic gout due to renal impairment, unspecified hip

M1A.36 Chronic gout due to renal impairment, knee

⑦M1A.361 Chronic gout due to renal impairment, right knee

⑦M1A.362 Chronic gout due to renal impairment, left knee

⑦M1A.369 Chronic gout due to renal impairment, unspecified knee

M1A.37 Chronic gout due to renal impairment, ankle and foot

⑦M1A.371 Chronic gout due to renal impairment, right ankle and foot

⑦M1A.372 Chronic gout due to renal impairment, left ankle and foot

⑦M1A.379 Chronic gout due to renal impairment, unspecified ankle and foot

⊗⑦M1A.38 Chronic gout due to renal impairment, vertebrae

⊗⑦M1A.39 Chronic gout due to renal impairment, multiple sites

M1A.4 Other secondary chronic gout

Code first associated condition

⊗⑦M1A.40 Other secondary chronic gout, unspecified site

M1A.41 Other secondary chronic gout, shoulder

⑦M1A.411 Other secondary chronic gout, right shoulder

⑦M1A.412 Other secondary chronic gout, left shoulder

⑦M1A.419 Other secondary chronic gout, unspecified shoulder

M1A.42 Other secondary chronic gout, elbow

⑦M1A.421 Other secondary chronic gout, right elbow

⑦M1A.422 Other secondary chronic gout, left elbow

⑦M1A.429 Other secondary chronic gout, unspecified elbow

M1A.43 Other secondary chronic gout, wrist

⑦M1A.431 Other secondary chronic gout, right wrist

⑦M1A.432 Other secondary chronic gout, left wrist

⑦M1A.439 Other secondary chronic gout, unspecified wrist

M1A.44 Other secondary chronic gout, hand

⑦M1A.441 Other secondary chronic gout, right hand

⑦M1A.442 Other secondary chronic gout, left hand

⑦M1A.449 Other secondary chronic gout, unspecified hand

M1A.45 Other secondary chronic gout, hip

⑦M1A.451 Other secondary chronic gout, right hip

⑦M1A.452 Other secondary chronic gout, left hip

⑦M1A.459 Other secondary chronic gout, unspecified hip

M1A.46 Other secondary chronic gout, knee

⑦M1A.461 Other secondary chronic gout, right knee

⑦M1A.462 Other secondary chronic gout, left knee

⑦M1A.469 Other secondary chronic gout, unspecified knee

M1A.47 Other secondary chronic gout, ankle and foot

⑦M1A.471 Other secondary chronic gout, right ankle and foot

⑦M1A.472 Other secondary chronic gout, left ankle and foot

⑦M1A.479 Other secondary chronic gout, unspecified ankle and foot

● New code ▲ Revised code **Excludes1:** Not coded here **Excludes2:** Not included here ⊗ Placeholder required ⑦ 7th digit required

⊗⑦**M1A.48** Other secondary chronic gout, vertebrae
⊗⑦**M1A.49** Other secondary chronic gout, multiple sites
⊗⑦**M1A.9** Chronic gout, unspecified

M10 **Gout**
Acute gout
Gout attack
Gout flare
Podagra
Use additional code to identify:
Autonomic neuropathy in diseases classified elsewhere (G99.0)
Calculus of urinary tract in diseases classified elsewhere (N22)
Cardiomyopathy in diseases classified elsewhere (I43)
Disorders of external ear in diseases classified elsewhere (H61.1-, H62.8-)
Disorders of iris and ciliary body in diseases classified elsewhere (H22)
Glomerular disorders in diseases classified elsewhere (N08)
Excludes2: chronic gout (M1A.-)
M10.0 **Idiopathic gout**
Gouty bursitis
Primary gout
M10.00 Idiopathic gout, unspecified site
M10.01 Idiopathic gout, shoulder
M10.011 Idiopathic gout, right shoulder
M10.012 Idiopathic gout, left shoulder
M10.019 Idiopathic gout, unspecified shoulder
M10.02 Idiopathic gout, elbow
M10.021 Idiopathic gout, right elbow
M10.022 Idiopathic gout, left elbow
M10.029 Idiopathic gout, unspecified elbow
M10.03 Idiopathic gout, wrist
M10.031 Idiopathic gout, right wrist
M10.032 Idiopathic gout, left wrist
M10.039 Idiopathic gout, unspecified wrist
M10.04 Idiopathic gout, hand
M10.041 Idiopathic gout, right hand
M10.042 Idiopathic gout, left hand
M10.049 Idiopathic gout, unspecified hand
M10.05 Idiopathic gout, hip
M10.051 Idiopathic gout, right hip
M10.052 Idiopathic gout, left hip
M10.059 Idiopathic gout, unspecified hip
M10.06 Idiopathic gout, knee
M10.061 Idiopathic gout, right knee
M10.062 Idiopathic gout, left knee
M10.069 Idiopathic gout, unspecified knee
M10.07 Idiopathic gout, ankle and foot
M10.071 Idiopathic gout, right ankle and foot
M10.072 Idiopathic gout, left ankle and foot
M10.079 Idiopathic gout, unspecified ankle and foot
M10.08 Idiopathic gout, vertebrae
M10.09 Idiopathic gout, multiple sites
M10.1 **Lead-induced gout**
Code first toxic effects of lead and its compounds (T56.0-)
M10.10 Lead-induced gout, unspecified site

M10.11 Lead-induced gout, shoulder
M10.111 Lead-induced gout, right shoulder
M10.112 Lead-induced gout, left shoulder
M10.119 Lead-induced gout, unspecified shoulder
M10.12 Lead-induced gout, elbow
M10.121 Lead-induced gout, right elbow
M10.122 Lead-induced gout, left elbow
M10.129 Lead-induced gout, unspecified elbow
M10.13 Lead-induced gout, wrist
M10.131 Lead-induced gout, right wrist
M10.132 Lead-induced gout, left wrist
M10.139 Lead-induced gout, unspecified wrist
M10.14 Lead-induced gout, hand
M10.141 Lead-induced gout, right hand
M10.142 Lead-induced gout, left hand
M10.149 Lead-induced gout, unspecified hand
M10.15 Lead-induced gout, hip
M10.151 Lead-induced gout, right hip
M10.152 Lead-induced gout, left hip
M10.159 Lead-induced gout, unspecified hip
M10.16 Lead-induced gout, knee
M10.161 Lead-induced gout, right knee
M10.162 Lead-induced gout, left knee
M10.169 Lead-induced gout, unspecified knee
M10.17 Lead-induced gout, ankle and foot
M10.171 Lead-induced gout, right ankle and foot
M10.172 Lead-induced gout, left ankle and foot
M10.179 Lead-induced gout, unspecified ankle and foot
M10.18 Lead-induced gout, vertebrae
M10.19 Lead-induced gout, multiple sites
M10.2 **Drug-induced gout**
Use additional code for adverse effect, if applicable, to identify drug (T36-T50 with fifth or sixth character 5)
M10.20 Drug-induced gout, unspecified site
M10.21 Drug-induced gout, shoulder
M10.211 Drug-induced gout, right shoulder
M10.212 Drug-induced gout, left shoulder
M10.219 Drug-induced gout, unspecified shoulder
M10.22 Drug-induced gout, elbow
M10.221 Drug-induced gout, right elbow
M10.222 Drug-induced gout, left elbow
M10.229 Drug-induced gout, unspecified elbow
M10.23 Drug-induced gout, wrist
M10.231 Drug-induced gout, right wrist
M10.232 Drug-induced gout, left wrist
M10.239 Drug-induced gout, unspecified wrist
M10.24 Drug-induced gout, hand
M10.241 Drug-induced gout, right hand
M10.242 Drug-induced gout, left hand
M10.249 Drug-induced gout, unspecified hand
M10.25 Drug-induced gout, hip

Add 4th-7th digits   Nonspecific code   Unspecified code   Manifestation code   513

M10.251   Drug-induced gout, right hip

M10.252   Drug-induced gout, left hip

M10.259   Drug-induced gout, unspecified hip

M10.26   Drug-induced gout, knee

    M10.261   Drug-induced gout, right knee

    M10.262   Drug-induced gout, left knee

    M10.269   Drug-induced gout, unspecified knee

M10.27   Drug-induced gout, ankle and foot

    M10.271   Drug-induced gout, right ankle and foot

    M10.272   Drug-induced gout, left ankle and foot

    M10.279   Drug-induced gout, unspecified ankle and foot

M10.28   Drug-induced gout, vertebrae

M10.29   Drug-induced gout, multiple sites

M10.3   Gout due to renal impairment

    <u>Code first</u> associated renal disease

M10.30   Gout due to renal impairment, unspecified site

M10.31   Gout due to renal impairment, shoulder

    M10.311   Gout due to renal impairment, right shoulder

    M10.312   Gout due to renal impairment, left shoulder

    M10.319   Gout due to renal impairment, unspecified shoulder

M10.32   Gout due to renal impairment, elbow

    M10.321   Gout due to renal impairment, right elbow

    M10.322   Gout due to renal impairment, left elbow

    M10.329   Gout due to renal impairment, unspecified elbow

M10.33   Gout due to renal impairment, wrist

    M10.331   Gout due to renal impairment, right wrist

    M10.332   Gout due to renal impairment, left wrist

    M10.339   Gout due to renal impairment, unspecified wrist

M10.34   Gout due to renal impairment, hand

    M10.341   Gout due to renal impairment, right hand

    M10.342   Gout due to renal impairment, left hand

    M10.349   Gout due to renal impairment, unspecified hand

M10.35   Gout due to renal impairment, hip

    M10.351   Gout due to renal impairment, right hip

    M10.352   Gout due to renal impairment, left hip

    M10.359   Gout due to renal impairment, unspecified hip

M10.36   Gout due to renal impairment, knee

    M10.361   Gout due to renal impairment, right knee

    M10.362   Gout due to renal impairment, left knee

    M10.369   Gout due to renal impairment, unspecified knee

M10.37   Gout due to renal impairment, ankle and foot

    M10.371   Gout due to renal impairment, right ankle and foot

    M10.372   Gout due to renal impairment, left ankle and foot

    M10.379   Gout due to renal impairment, unspecified ankle and foot

M10.38   Gout due to renal impairment, vertebrae

M10.39   Gout due to renal impairment, multiple sites

M10.4   Other secondary gout

    <u>Code first</u> associated condition

M10.40   Other secondary gout, unspecified site

M10.41   Other secondary gout, shoulder

    M10.411   Other secondary gout, right shoulder

    M10.412   Other secondary gout, left shoulder

    M10.419   Other secondary gout, unspecified shoulder

M10.42   Other secondary gout, elbow

    M10.421   Other secondary gout, right elbow

    M10.422   Other secondary gout, left elbow

    M10.429   Other secondary gout, unspecified elbow

M10.43   Other secondary gout, wrist

    M10.431   Other secondary gout, right wrist

    M10.432   Other secondary gout, left wrist

    M10.439   Other secondary gout, unspecified wrist

M10.44   Other secondary gout, hand

    M10.441   Other secondary gout, right hand

    M10.442   Other secondary gout, left hand

    M10.449   Other secondary gout, unspecified hand

M10.45   Other secondary gout, hip

    M10.451   Other secondary gout, right hip

    M10.452   Other secondary gout, left hip

    M10.459   Other secondary gout, unspecified hip

M10.46   Other secondary gout, knee

    M10.461   Other secondary gout, right knee

    M10.462   Other secondary gout, left knee

    M10.469   Other secondary gout, unspecified knee

M10.47   Other secondary gout, ankle and foot

    M10.471   Other secondary gout, right ankle and foot

    M10.472   Other secondary gout, left ankle and foot

    M10.479   Other secondary gout, unspecified ankle and foot

M10.48   Other secondary gout, vertebrae

M10.49   Other secondary gout, multiple sites

M10.9   Gout, unspecified

    Gout NOS

M11   **Other crystal arthropathies**

    Definition: Crystal arthropathies refers to a type of arthropathy characterized by accumulation of crystals in joints.

M11.0   Hydroxyapatite deposition disease

    M11.00   Hydroxyapatite deposition disease, unspecified site

   ● New code   ▲ Revised code   **Excludes1:** Not coded here   **Excludes2:** Not included here   ⊗ Placeholder required   ⑦7th digit required

M11.01   Hydroxyapatite deposition disease, shoulder

     M11.011   Hydroxyapatite deposition disease, right shoulder

     M11.012   Hydroxyapatite deposition disease, left shoulder

     M11.019   Hydroxyapatite deposition disease, unspecified shoulder

M11.02   Hydroxyapatite deposition disease, elbow

     M11.021   Hydroxyapatite deposition disease, right elbow

     M11.022   Hydroxyapatite deposition disease, left elbow

     M11.029   Hydroxyapatite deposition disease, unspecified elbow

M11.03   Hydroxyapatite deposition disease, wrist

     M11.031   Hydroxyapatite deposition disease, right wrist

     M11.032   Hydroxyapatite deposition disease, left wrist

     M11.039   Hydroxyapatite deposition disease, unspecified wrist

M11.04   Hydroxyapatite deposition disease, hand

     M11.041   Hydroxyapatite deposition disease, right hand

     M11.042   Hydroxyapatite deposition disease, left hand

     M11.049   Hydroxyapatite deposition disease, unspecified hand

M11.05   Hydroxyapatite deposition disease, hip

     M11.051   Hydroxyapatite deposition disease, right hip

     M11.052   Hydroxyapatite deposition disease, left hip

     M11.059   Hydroxyapatite deposition disease, unspecified hip

M11.06   Hydroxyapatite deposition disease, knee

     M11.061   Hydroxyapatite deposition disease, right knee

     M11.062   Hydroxyapatite deposition disease, left knee

     M11.069   Hydroxyapatite deposition disease, unspecified knee

M11.07   Hydroxyapatite deposition disease, ankle and foot

     M11.071   Hydroxyapatite deposition disease, right ankle and foot

     M11.072   Hydroxyapatite deposition disease, left ankle and foot

     M11.079   Hydroxyapatite deposition disease, unspecified ankle and foot

M11.08   Hydroxyapatite deposition disease, vertebrae

M11.09   Hydroxyapatite deposition disease, multiple sites

M11.1   Familial chondrocalcinosis

   M11.10   Familial chondrocalcinosis, unspecified site

   M11.11   Familial chondrocalcinosis, shoulder

     M11.111   Familial chondrocalcinosis, right shoulder

     M11.112   Familial chondrocalcinosis, left shoulder

     M11.119   Familial chondrocalcinosis, unspecified shoulder

   M11.12   Familial chondrocalcinosis, elbow

     M11.121   Familial chondrocalcinosis, right elbow

     M11.122   Familial chondrocalcinosis, left elbow

     M11.129   Familial chondrocalcinosis, unspecified elbow

   M11.13   Familial chondrocalcinosis, wrist

     M11.131   Familial chondrocalcinosis, right wrist

     M11.132   Familial chondrocalcinosis, left wrist

     M11.139   Familial chondrocalcinosis, unspecified wrist

   M11.14   Familial chondrocalcinosis, hand

     M11.141   Familial chondrocalcinosis, right hand

     M11.142   Familial chondrocalcinosis, left hand

     M11.149   Familial chondrocalcinosis, unspecified hand

   M11.15   Familial chondrocalcinosis, hip

     M11.151   Familial chondrocalcinosis, right hip

     M11.152   Familial chondrocalcinosis, left hip

     M11.159   Familial chondrocalcinosis, unspecified hip

   M11.16   Familial chondrocalcinosis, knee

     M11.161   Familial chondrocalcinosis, right knee

     M11.162   Familial chondrocalcinosis, left knee

     M11.169   Familial chondrocalcinosis, unspecified knee

   M11.17   Familial chondrocalcinosis, ankle and foot

     M11.171   Familial chondrocalcinosis, right ankle and foot

     M11.172   Familial chondrocalcinosis, left ankle and foot

     M11.179   Familial chondrocalcinosis, unspecified ankle and foot

   M11.18   Familial chondrocalcinosis, vertebrae

   M11.19   Familial chondrocalcinosis, multiple sites

M11.2   Other chondrocalcinosis

Chondrocalcinosis NOS

   M11.20   Other chondrocalcinosis, unspecified site

   M11.21   Other chondrocalcinosis, shoulder

     M11.211   Other chondrocalcinosis, right shoulder

     M11.212   Other chondrocalcinosis, left shoulder

     M11.219   Other chondrocalcinosis, unspecified shoulder

   M11.22   Other chondrocalcinosis, elbow

     M11.221   Other chondrocalcinosis, right elbow

     M11.222   Other chondrocalcinosis, left elbow

     M11.229   Other chondrocalcinosis, unspecified elbow

   M11.23   Other chondrocalcinosis, wrist

     M11.231   Other chondrocalcinosis, right wrist

     M11.232   Other chondrocalcinosis, left wrist

     M11.239   Other chondrocalcinosis, unspecified wrist

   M11.24   Other chondrocalcinosis, hand

     M11.241   Other chondrocalcinosis, right hand

     M11.242   Other chondrocalcinosis, left hand

�as Add 4th-7th digits	Nonspecific code	Unspecified code	Manifestation code

M11.249 Other chondrocalcinosis, unspecified hand

M11.25 Other chondrocalcinosis, hip

M11.251 Other chondrocalcinosis, right hip

M11.252 Other chondrocalcinosis, left hip

M11.259 Other chondrocalcinosis, unspecified hip

M11.26 Other chondrocalcinosis, knee

M11.261 Other chondrocalcinosis, right knee

M11.262 Other chondrocalcinosis, left knee

M11.269 Other chondrocalcinosis, unspecified knee

M11.27 Other chondrocalcinosis, ankle and foot

M11.271 Other chondrocalcinosis, right ankle and foot

M11.272 Other chondrocalcinosis, left ankle and foot

M11.279 Other chondrocalcinosis, unspecified ankle and foot

M11.28 Other chondrocalcinosis, vertebrae

M11.29 Other chondrocalcinosis, multiple sites

M11.8 Other specified crystal arthropathies

M11.80 Other specified crystal arthropathies, unspecified site

M11.81 Other specified crystal arthropathies, shoulder

M11.811 Other specified crystal arthropathies, right shoulder

M11.812 Other specified crystal arthropathies, left shoulder

M11.819 Other specified crystal arthropathies, unspecified shoulder

M11.82 Other specified crystal arthropathies, elbow

M11.821 Other specified crystal arthropathies, right elbow

M11.822 Other specified crystal arthropathies, left elbow

M11.829 Other specified crystal arthropathies, unspecified elbow

M11.83 Other specified crystal arthropathies, wrist

M11.831 Other specified crystal arthropathies, right wrist

M11.832 Other specified crystal arthropathies, left wrist

M11.839 Other specified crystal arthropathies, unspecified wrist

M11.84 Other specified crystal arthropathies, hand

M11.841 Other specified crystal arthropathies, right hand

M11.842 Other specified crystal arthropathies, left hand

M11.849 Other specified crystal arthropathies, unspecified hand

M11.85 Other specified crystal arthropathies, hip

M11.851 Other specified crystal arthropathies, right hip

M11.852 Other specified crystal arthropathies, left hip

M11.859 Other specified crystal arthropathies, unspecified hip

M11.86 Other specified crystal arthropathies, knee

M11.861 Other specified crystal arthropathies, right knee

M11.862 Other specified crystal arthropathies, left knee

M11.869 Other specified crystal arthropathies, unspecified knee

M11.87 Other specified crystal arthropathies, ankle and foot

M11.871 Other specified crystal arthropathies, right ankle and foot

M11.872 Other specified crystal arthropathies, left ankle and foot

M11.879 Other specified crystal arthropathies, unspecified ankle and foot

M11.88 Other specified crystal arthropathies, vertebrae

M11.89 Other specified crystal arthropathies, multiple sites

M11.9 Crystal arthropathy, unspecified

M12 Other and unspecified arthropathy

Excludes1: arthrosis (M15-M19)

cricoarytenoid arthropathy (J38.7)

M12.0 Chronic postrheumatic arthropathy [Jaccoud]

M12.00 Chronic postrheumatic arthropathy [Jaccoud], unspecified site

M12.01 Chronic postrheumatic arthropathy [Jaccoud], shoulder

M12.011 Chronic postrheumatic arthropathy [Jaccoud], right shoulder

M12.012 Chronic postrheumatic arthropathy [Jaccoud], left shoulder

M12.019 Chronic postrheumatic arthropathy [Jaccoud], unspecified shoulder

M12.02 Chronic postrheumatic arthropathy [Jaccoud], elbow

M12.021 Chronic postrheumatic arthropathy [Jaccoud], right elbow

M12.022 Chronic postrheumatic arthropathy [Jaccoud], left elbow

M12.029 Chronic postrheumatic arthropathy [Jaccoud], unspecified elbow

M12.03 Chronic postrheumatic arthropathy [Jaccoud], wrist

M12.031 Chronic postrheumatic arthropathy [Jaccoud], right wrist

M12.032 Chronic postrheumatic arthropathy [Jaccoud], left wrist

M12.039 Chronic postrheumatic arthropathy [Jaccoud], unspecified wrist

M12.04 Chronic postrheumatic arthropathy [Jaccoud], hand

M12.041 Chronic postrheumatic arthropathy [Jaccoud], right hand

M12.042 Chronic postrheumatic arthropathy [Jaccoud], left hand

M12.049 Chronic postrheumatic arthropathy [Jaccoud], unspecified hand

M12.05 Chronic postrheumatic arthropathy [Jaccoud], hip

M12.051 Chronic postrheumatic arthropathy [Jaccoud], right hip

M12.052 Chronic postrheumatic arthropathy [Jaccoud], left hip

M12.059 Chronic postrheumatic arthropathy [Jaccoud], unspecified hip

M12.06 Chronic postrheumatic arthropathy [Jaccoud], knee

    M12.061 Chronic postrheumatic arthropathy [Jaccoud], right knee

    M12.062 Chronic postrheumatic arthropathy [Jaccoud], left knee

    M12.069 Chronic postrheumatic arthropathy [Jaccoud], unspecified knee

M12.07 Chronic postrheumatic arthropathy [Jaccoud], ankle and foot

    M12.071 Chronic postrheumatic arthropathy [Jaccoud], right ankle and foot

    M12.072 Chronic postrheumatic arthropathy [Jaccoud], left ankle and foot

    M12.079 Chronic postrheumatic arthropathy [Jaccoud], unspecified ankle and foot

M12.08 Chronic postrheumatic arthropathy [Jaccoud], other specified site

    Chronic postrheumatic arthropathy [Jaccoud], vertebrae

M12.09 Chronic postrheumatic arthropathy [Jaccoud], multiple sites

M12.1 Kaschin-Beck disease

    Osteochondroarthrosis deformans endemica

M12.10 Kaschin-Beck disease, unspecified site

M12.11 Kaschin-Beck disease, shoulder

    M12.111 Kaschin-Beck disease, right shoulder

    M12.112 Kaschin-Beck disease, left shoulder

    M12.119 Kaschin-Beck disease, unspecified shoulder

M12.12 Kaschin-Beck disease, elbow

    M12.121 Kaschin-Beck disease, right elbow

    M12.122 Kaschin-Beck disease, left elbow

    M12.129 Kaschin-Beck disease, unspecified elbow

M12.13 Kaschin-Beck disease, wrist

    M12.131 Kaschin-Beck disease, right wrist

    M12.132 Kaschin-Beck disease, left wrist

    M12.139 Kaschin-Beck disease, unspecified wrist

M12.14 Kaschin-Beck disease, hand

    M12.141 Kaschin-Beck disease, right hand

    M12.142 Kaschin-Beck disease, left hand

    M12.149 Kaschin-Beck disease, unspecified hand

M12.15 Kaschin-Beck disease, hip

    M12.151 Kaschin-Beck disease, right hip

    M12.152 Kaschin-Beck disease, left hip

    M12.159 Kaschin-Beck disease, unspecified hip

M12.16 Kaschin-Beck disease, knee

    M12.161 Kaschin-Beck disease, right knee

    M12.162 Kaschin-Beck disease, left knee

    M12.169 Kaschin-Beck disease, unspecified knee

M12.17 Kaschin-Beck disease, ankle and foot

    M12.171 Kaschin-Beck disease, right ankle and foot

    M12.172 Kaschin-Beck disease, left ankle and foot

    M12.179 Kaschin-Beck disease, unspecified ankle and foot

M12.18 Kaschin-Beck disease, vertebrae

M12.19 Kaschin-Beck disease, multiple sites

M12.2 Villonodular synovitis (pigmented)

M12.20 Villonodular synovitis (pigmented), unspecified site

M12.21 Villonodular synovitis (pigmented), shoulder

    M12.211 Villonodular synovitis (pigmented), right shoulder

    M12.212 Villonodular synovitis (pigmented), left shoulder

    M12.219 Villonodular synovitis (pigmented), unspecified shoulder

M12.22 Villonodular synovitis (pigmented), elbow

    M12.221 Villonodular synovitis (pigmented), right elbow

    M12.222 Villonodular synovitis (pigmented), left elbow

    M12.229 Villonodular synovitis (pigmented), unspecified elbow

M12.23 Villonodular synovitis (pigmented), wrist

    M12.231 Villonodular synovitis (pigmented), right wrist

    M12.232 Villonodular synovitis (pigmented), left wrist

    M12.239 Villonodular synovitis (pigmented), unspecified wrist

M12.24 Villonodular synovitis (pigmented), hand

    M12.241 Villonodular synovitis (pigmented), right hand

    M12.242 Villonodular synovitis (pigmented), left hand

    M12.249 Villonodular synovitis (pigmented), unspecified hand

M12.25 Villonodular synovitis (pigmented), hip

    M12.251 Villonodular synovitis (pigmented), right hip

    M12.252 Villonodular synovitis (pigmented), left hip

    M12.259 Villonodular synovitis (pigmented), unspecified hip

M12.26 Villonodular synovitis (pigmented), knee

    M12.261 Villonodular synovitis (pigmented), right knee

    M12.262 Villonodular synovitis (pigmented), left knee

    M12.269 Villonodular synovitis (pigmented), unspecified knee

M12.27 Villonodular synovitis (pigmented), ankle and foot

    M12.271 Villonodular synovitis (pigmented), right ankle and foot

    M12.272 Villonodular synovitis (pigmented), left ankle and foot

    M12.279 Villonodular synovitis (pigmented), unspecified ankle and foot

M12.28 Villonodular synovitis (pigmented), other specified site

    Villonodular synovitis (pigmented), vertebrae

M12.29 Villonodular synovitis (pigmented), multiple sites

M12.3 Palindromic rheumatism

    Add 4th-7th digits   Nonspecific code   Unspecified code   Manifestation code   517

M12.30 Palindromic rheumatism, unspecified site

M12.31 Palindromic rheumatism, shoulder

    M12.311 Palindromic rheumatism, right shoulder

    M12.312 Palindromic rheumatism, left shoulder

    M12.319 Palindromic rheumatism, unspecified shoulder

M12.32 Palindromic rheumatism, elbow

    M12.321 Palindromic rheumatism, right elbow

    M12.322 Palindromic rheumatism, left elbow

    M12.329 Palindromic rheumatism, unspecified elbow

M12.33 Palindromic rheumatism, wrist

    M12.331 Palindromic rheumatism, right wrist

    M12.332 Palindromic rheumatism, left wrist

    M12.339 Palindromic rheumatism, unspecified wrist

M12.34 Palindromic rheumatism, hand

    M12.341 Palindromic rheumatism, right hand

    M12.342 Palindromic rheumatism, left hand

    M12.349 Palindromic rheumatism, unspecified hand

M12.35 Palindromic rheumatism, hip

    M12.351 Palindromic rheumatism, right hip

    M12.352 Palindromic rheumatism, left hip

    M12.359 Palindromic rheumatism, unspecified hip

M12.36 Palindromic rheumatism, knee

    M12.361 Palindromic rheumatism, right knee

    M12.362 Palindromic rheumatism, left knee

    M12.369 Palindromic rheumatism, unspecified knee

M12.37 Palindromic rheumatism, ankle and foot

    M12.371 Palindromic rheumatism, right ankle and foot

    M12.372 Palindromic rheumatism, left ankle and foot

    M12.379 Palindromic rheumatism, unspecified ankle and foot

M12.38 Palindromic rheumatism, other specified site

    Palindromic rheumatism, vertebrae

M12.39 Palindromic rheumatism, multiple sites

M12.4 Intermittent hydrarthrosis

M12.40 Intermittent hydrarthrosis, unspecified site

M12.41 Intermittent hydrarthrosis, shoulder

    M12.411 Intermittent hydrarthrosis, right shoulder

    M12.412 Intermittent hydrarthrosis, left shoulder

    M12.419 Intermittent hydrarthrosis, unspecified shoulder

M12.42 Intermittent hydrarthrosis, elbow

    M12.421 Intermittent hydrarthrosis, right elbow

    M12.422 Intermittent hydrarthrosis, left elbow

    M12.429 Intermittent hydrarthrosis, unspecified elbow

M12.43 Intermittent hydrarthrosis, wrist

    M12.431 Intermittent hydrarthrosis, right wrist

    M12.432 Intermittent hydrarthrosis, left wrist

    M12.439 Intermittent hydrarthrosis, unspecified wrist

M12.44 Intermittent hydrarthrosis, hand

    M12.441 Intermittent hydrarthrosis, right hand

    M12.442 Intermittent hydrarthrosis, left hand

    M12.449 Intermittent hydrarthrosis, unspecified hand

M12.45 Intermittent hydrarthrosis, hip

    M12.451 Intermittent hydrarthrosis, right hip

    M12.452 Intermittent hydrarthrosis, left hip

    M12.459 Intermittent hydrarthrosis, unspecified hip

M12.46 Intermittent hydrarthrosis, knee

    M12.461 Intermittent hydrarthrosis, right knee

    M12.462 Intermittent hydrarthrosis, left knee

    M12.469 Intermittent hydrarthrosis, unspecified knee

M12.47 Intermittent hydrarthrosis, ankle and foot

    M12.471 Intermittent hydrarthrosis, right ankle and foot

    M12.472 Intermittent hydrarthrosis, left ankle and foot

    M12.479 Intermittent hydrarthrosis, unspecified ankle and foot

M12.48 Intermittent hydrarthrosis, other site

M12.49 Intermittent hydrarthrosis, multiple sites

M12.5 Traumatic arthropathy

    Excludes1: current injury-see Alphabetic Index

    post-traumatic osteoarthritis of first carpometacarpal joint (M18.2-M18.3)

    post-traumatic osteoarthritis of hip (M16.4-M16.5)

    post-traumatic osteoarthritis of knee (M17.2-M17.3)

    post-traumatic osteoarthritis NOS (M19.1-)

    post-traumatic osteoarthritis **of other** single joints (M19.1-)

M12.50 Traumatic arthropathy, unspecified site

M12.51 Traumatic arthropathy, shoulder

    M12.511 Traumatic arthropathy, right shoulder

    M12.512 Traumatic arthropathy, left shoulder

    M12.519 Traumatic arthropathy, unspecified shoulder

M12.52 Traumatic arthropathy, elbow

    M12.521 Traumatic arthropathy, right elbow

    M12.522 Traumatic arthropathy, left elbow

    M12.529 Traumatic arthropathy, unspecified elbow

M12.53 Traumatic arthropathy, wrist

    M12.531 Traumatic arthropathy, right wrist

    M12.532 Traumatic arthropathy, left wrist

    M12.539 Traumatic arthropathy, unspecified wrist

M12.54 Traumatic arthropathy, hand

    M12.541 Traumatic arthropathy, right hand

    M12.542 Traumatic arthropathy, left hand

M12.549 Traumatic arthropathy, unspecified hand

M12.55 Traumatic arthropathy, hip

M12.551 Traumatic arthropathy, right hip

M12.552 Traumatic arthropathy, left hip

M12.559 Traumatic arthropathy, unspecified hip

M12.56 Traumatic arthropathy, knee

M12.561 Traumatic arthropathy, right knee

M12.562 Traumatic arthropathy, left knee

M12.569 Traumatic arthropathy, unspecified knee

M12.57 Traumatic arthropathy, ankle and foot

M12.571 Traumatic arthropathy, right ankle and foot

M12.572 Traumatic arthropathy, left ankle and foot

M12.579 Traumatic arthropathy, unspecified ankle and foot

M12.58 Traumatic arthropathy, other specified site

Traumatic arthropathy, vertebrae

M12.59 Traumatic arthropathy, multiple sites

M12.8 Other specific arthropathies, not elsewhere classified

Transient arthropathy

M12.80 Other specific arthropathies, not elsewhere classified, unspecified site

M12.81 Other specific arthropathies, not elsewhere classified, shoulder

M12.811 Other specific arthropathies, not elsewhere classified, right shoulder

M12.812 Other specific arthropathies, not elsewhere classified, left shoulder

M12.819 Other specific arthropathies, not elsewhere classified, unspecified shoulder

M12.82 Other specific arthropathies, not elsewhere classified, elbow

M12.821 Other specific arthropathies, not elsewhere classified, right elbow

M12.822 Other specific arthropathies, not elsewhere classified, left elbow

M12.829 Other specific arthropathies, not elsewhere classified, unspecified elbow

M12.83 Other specific arthropathies, not elsewhere classified, wrist

M12.831 Other specific arthropathies, not elsewhere classified, right wrist

M12.832 Other specific arthropathies, not elsewhere classified, left wrist

M12.839 Other specific arthropathies, not elsewhere classified, unspecified wrist

M12.84 Other specific arthropathies, not elsewhere classified, hand

M12.841 Other specific arthropathies, not elsewhere classified, right hand

M12.842 Other specific arthropathies, not elsewhere classified, left hand

M12.849 Other specific arthropathies, not elsewhere classified, unspecified hand

M12.85 Other specific arthropathies, not elsewhere classified, hip

M12.851 Other specific arthropathies, not elsewhere classified, right hip

M12.852 Other specific arthropathies, not elsewhere classified, left hip

M12.859 Other specific arthropathies, not elsewhere classified, unspecified hip

M12.86 Other specific arthropathies, not elsewhere classified, knee

M12.861 Other specific arthropathies, not elsewhere classified, right knee

M12.862 Other specific arthropathies, not elsewhere classified, left knee

M12.869 Other specific arthropathies, not elsewhere classified, unspecified knee

M12.87 Other specific arthropathies, not elsewhere classified, ankle and foot

M12.871 Other specific arthropathies, not elsewhere classified, right ankle and foot

M12.872 Other specific arthropathies, not elsewhere classified, left ankle and foot

M12.879 Other specific arthropathies, not elsewhere classified, unspecified ankle and foot

M12.88 Other specific arthropathies, not elsewhere classified, other specified site

Other specific arthropathies, not elsewhere classified, vertebrae

M12.89 Other specific arthropathies, not elsewhere classified, multiple sites

M12.9 Arthropathy, unspecified

M13 Other arthritis

Excludes1: arthrosis (M15-M19)

osteoarthritis (M15-M19)

M13.0 Polyarthritis, unspecified

M13.1 Monoarthritis, not elsewhere classified

M13.10 Monoarthritis, not elsewhere classified, unspecified site

M13.11 Monoarthritis, not elsewhere classified, shoulder

M13.111 Monoarthritis, not elsewhere classified, right shoulder

M13.112 Monoarthritis, not elsewhere classified, left shoulder

M13.119 Monoarthritis, not elsewhere classified, unspecified shoulder

M13.12 Monoarthritis, not elsewhere classified, elbow

M13.121 Monoarthritis, not elsewhere classified, right elbow

M13.122 Monoarthritis, not elsewhere classified, left elbow

M13.129 Monoarthritis, not elsewhere classified, unspecified elbow

M13.13 Monoarthritis, not elsewhere classified, wrist

M13.131 Monoarthritis, not elsewhere classified, right wrist

M13.132 Monoarthritis, not elsewhere classified, left wrist

M13.139 Monoarthritis, not elsewhere classified, unspecified wrist

M13.14 Monoarthritis, not elsewhere classified, hand

M13.141 Monoarthritis, not elsewhere classified, right hand

M13.142 Monoarthritis, not elsewhere classified, left hand

M13.149 Monoarthritis, not elsewhere classified, unspecified hand

M13.15 Monoarthritis, not elsewhere classified, hip

M13.151 Monoarthritis, not elsewhere classified, right hip

M13.152 Monoarthritis, not elsewhere classified, left hip

M13.159 Monoarthritis, not elsewhere classified, unspecified hip

M13.16 Monoarthritis, not elsewhere classified, knee

M13.161 Monoarthritis, not elsewhere classified, right knee

M13.162 Monoarthritis, not elsewhere classified, left knee

M13.169 Monoarthritis, not elsewhere classified, unspecified knee

M13.17 Monoarthritis, not elsewhere classified, ankle and foot

M13.171 Monoarthritis, not elsewhere classified, right ankle and foot

M13.172 Monoarthritis, not elsewhere classified, left ankle and foot

M13.179 Monoarthritis, not elsewhere classified, unspecified ankle and foot

M13.8 **Other specified arthritis**

Allergic arthritis

Excludes1: osteoarthritis (M15-M19)

M13.80 Other specified arthritis, unspecified site

M13.81 Other specified arthritis, shoulder

M13.811 Other specified arthritis, right shoulder

M13.812 Other specified arthritis, left shoulder

M13.819 Other specified arthritis, unspecified shoulder

M13.82 Other specified arthritis, elbow

M13.821 Other specified arthritis, right elbow

M13.822 Other specified arthritis, left elbow

M13.829 Other specified arthritis, unspecified elbow

M13.83 Other specified arthritis, wrist

M13.831 Other specified arthritis, right wrist

M13.832 Other specified arthritis, left wrist

M13.839 Other specified arthritis, unspecified wrist

M13.84 Other specified arthritis, hand

M13.841 Other specified arthritis, right hand

M13.842 Other specified arthritis, left hand

M13.849 Other specified arthritis, unspecified hand

M13.85 Other specified arthritis, hip

M13.851 Other specified arthritis, right hip

M13.852 Other specified arthritis, left hip

M13.859 Other specified arthritis, unspecified hip

M13.86 Other specified arthritis, knee

M13.861 Other specified arthritis, right knee

M13.862 Other specified arthritis, left knee

M13.869 Other specified arthritis, unspecified knee

M13.87 Other specified arthritis, ankle and foot

M13.871 Other specified arthritis, right ankle and foot

M13.872 Other specified arthritis, left ankle and foot

M13.879 Other specified arthritis, unspecified ankle and foot

M13.88 Other specified arthritis, other site

M13.89 Other specified arthritis, multiple sites

M14 **Arthropathies in other diseases classified elsewhere**

Excludes1: arthropathy in:

diabetes mellitus (E08-E13 with .61-)

hematological disorders (M36.2-M36.3)

hypersensitivity reactions (M36.4)

neoplastic disease (M36.1)

neurosyphillis (A52.16)

sarcoidosis (D86.86)

enteropathic arthropathies (M07.-)

juvenile psoriatic arthropathy (L40.54)

lipoid dermatoarthritis (E78.81)

M14.6 **Charcôt's joint**

Neuropathic arthropathy

Excludes1: Charcôt's joint in diabetes mellitus (E08-E13 with .610)

Charcôt's joint in tabes dorsalis (A52.16)

M14.60 Charcôt's joint, unspecified site

M14.61 Charcôt's joint, shoulder

M14.611 Charcôt's joint, right shoulder

M14.612 Charcôt's joint, left shoulder

M14.619 Charcôt's joint, unspecified shoulder

M14.62 Charcôt's joint, elbow

M14.621 Charcôt's joint, right elbow

M14.622 Charcôt's joint, left elbow

M14.629 Charcôt's joint, unspecified elbow

M14.63 Charcôt's joint, wrist

M14.631 Charcôt's joint, right wrist

M14.632 Charcôt's joint, left wrist

M14.639 Charcôt's joint, unspecified wrist

M14.64 Charcôt's joint, hand

M14.641 Charcôt's joint, right hand

M14.642 Charcôt's joint, left hand

M14.649 Charcôt's joint, unspecified hand

M14.65 Charcôt's joint, hip

M14.651 Charcôt's joint, right hip

M14.652 Charcôt's joint, left hip

M14.659 Charcôt's joint, unspecified hip

M14.66 Charcôt's joint, knee

M14.661 Charcôt's joint, right knee

M14.662 Charcôt's joint, left knee

M14.669 Charcôt's joint, unspecified knee

M14.67 Charcôt's joint, ankle and foot

M14.671 Charcôt's joint, right ankle and foot

M14.672 Charcôt's joint, left ankle and foot

M14.679 Charcôt's joint, unspecified ankle and foot

● New code   ▲ Revised code   **Excludes1:** Not coded here   **Excludes2:** Not included here   ⊗ Placeholder required   ⑦ 7th digit required

M14.68 Charcôt's joint, vertebrae

M14.69 Charcôt's joint, multiple sites

M14.8 **Arthropathies in other specified diseases classified elsewhere**

Code first underlying disease, such as:

amyloidosis (E85.-)

erythema multiforme (L51.-)

erythema nodosum (L52)

hemochromatosis (E83.11-)

hyperparathyroidism (E21.-)

hypothyroidism (E00-E03)

sickle-cell disorders (D57.-)

thyrotoxicosis [hyperthyroidism] (E05.-)

Whipple's disease (K90.81)

M14.80 **Arthropathies in other specified diseases classified elsewhere, unspecified site**

M14.81 **Arthropathies in other specified diseases classified elsewhere, shoulder**

M14.811 **Arthropathies in other specified diseases classified elsewhere, right shoulder**

M14.812 **Arthropathies in other specified diseases classified elsewhere, left shoulder**

M14.819 **Arthropathies in other specified diseases classified elsewhere, unspecified shoulder**

M14.82 **Arthropathies in other specified diseases classified elsewhere, elbow**

M14.821 **Arthropathies in other specified diseases classified elsewhere, right elbow**

M14.822 **Arthropathies in other specified diseases classified elsewhere, left elbow**

M14.829 **Arthropathies in other specified diseases classified elsewhere, unspecified elbow**

M14.83 **Arthropathies in other specified diseases classified elsewhere, wrist**

M14.831 **Arthropathies in other specified diseases classified elsewhere, right wrist**

M14.832 **Arthropathies in other specified diseases classified elsewhere, left wrist**

M14.839 **Arthropathies in other specified diseases classified elsewhere, unspecified wrist**

M14.84 **Arthropathies in other specified diseases classified elsewhere, hand**

M14.841 **Arthropathies in other specified diseases classified elsewhere, right hand**

M14.842 **Arthropathies in other specified diseases classified elsewhere, left hand**

M14.849 **Arthropathies in other specified diseases classified elsewhere, unspecified hand**

M14.85 **Arthropathies in other specified diseases classified elsewhere, hip**

M14.851 **Arthropathies in other specified diseases classified elsewhere, right hip**

M14.852 **Arthropathies in other specified diseases classified elsewhere, left hip**

M14.859 **Arthropathies in other specified diseases classified elsewhere, unspecified hip**

M14.86 **Arthropathies in other specified diseases classified elsewhere, knee**

M14.861 **Arthropathies in other specified diseases classified elsewhere, right knee**

M14.862 **Arthropathies in other specified diseases classified elsewhere, left knee**

M14.869 **Arthropathies in other specified diseases classified elsewhere, unspecified knee**

M14.87 **Arthropathies in other specified diseases classified elsewhere, ankle and foot**

M14.871 **Arthropathies in other specified diseases classified elsewhere, right ankle and foot**

M14.872 **Arthropathies in other specified diseases classified elsewhere, left ankle and foot**

M14.879 **Arthropathies in other specified diseases classified elsewhere, unspecified ankle and foot**

M14.88 **Arthropathies in other specified diseases classified elsewhere, vertebrae**

M14.89 **Arthropathies in other specified diseases classified elsewhere, multiple sites**

OSTEOARTHRITIS (M15-M19)

Definition: Osteoarthritis (OA), which is also known as osteoarthrosis or degenerative joint disease (DJD), is a progressive disorder of the joints caused by gradual loss of cartilage and resulting in the development of bony spurs and cysts at the margins of the joints.

Excludes2: osteoarthritis of spine (M47.-)

M15 **Polyosteoarthritis**

Includes: arthritis of multiple sites

Excludes1: bilateral involvement of single joint (M16-M19)

M15.0 **Primary generalized (osteo)arthritis**

M15.1 **Heberden's nodes (with arthropathy)**

Interphalangeal distal osteoarthritis

M15.2 **Bouchard's nodes (with arthropathy)**

Juxtaphalangeal distal osteoarthritis

M15.3 **Secondary multiple arthritis**

Post-traumatic polyosteoarthritis

M15.4 **Erosive (osteo)arthritis**

M15.8 **Other polyosteoarthritis**

M15.9 **Polyosteoarthritis, unspecified**

Generalized osteoarthritis NOS

M16 **Osteoarthritis of hip**

M16.0 **Bilateral primary osteoarthritis of hip**

M16.1 **Unilateral primary osteoarthritis of hip**

Primary osteoarthritis of hip NOS

M16.10 **Unilateral primary osteoarthritis, unspecified hip**

M16.11 **Unilateral primary osteoarthritis, right hip**

M16.12 **Unilateral primary osteoarthritis, left hip**

M16.2   **Bilateral osteoarthritis resulting from hip dysplasia**

M16.3   **Unilateral osteoarthritis resulting from hip dysplasia**

Dysplastic osteoarthritis of hip NOS

     M16.30   **Unilateral osteoarthritis resulting from hip dysplasia, unspecified hip**

     M16.31   **Unilateral osteoarthritis resulting from hip dysplasia, right hip**

     M16.32   **Unilateral osteoarthritis resulting from hip dysplasia, left hip**

M16.4   **Bilateral post-traumatic osteoarthritis of hip**

M16.5   **Unilateral post-traumatic osteoarthritis of hip**

Post-traumatic osteoarthritis of hip NOS

     M16.50   **Unilateral post-traumatic osteoarthritis, unspecified hip**

     M16.51   **Unilateral post-traumatic osteoarthritis, right hip**

     M16.52   **Unilateral post-traumatic osteoarthritis, left hip**

M16.6   **Other bilateral secondary osteoarthritis of hip**

M16.7   **Other unilateral secondary osteoarthritis of hip**

Secondary osteoarthritis of hip NOS

M16.9   **Osteoarthritis of hip, unspecified**

M17   **Osteoarthritis of knee**

M17.0   **Bilateral primary osteoarthritis of knee**

M17.1   **Unilateral primary osteoarthritis of knee**

Primary osteoarthritis of knee NOS

     M17.10   **Unilateral primary osteoarthritis, unspecified knee**

     M17.11   **Unilateral primary osteoarthritis, right knee**

     M17.12   **Unilateral primary osteoarthritis, left knee**

M17.2   **Bilateral post-traumatic osteoarthritis of knee**

M17.3   **Unilateral post-traumatic osteoarthritis of knee**

Post-traumatic osteoarthritis of knee NOS

     M17.30   **Unilateral post-traumatic osteoarthritis, unspecified knee**

     M17.31   **Unilateral post-traumatic osteoarthritis, right knee**

     M17.32   **Unilateral post-traumatic osteoarthritis, left knee**

M17.4   **Other bilateral secondary osteoarthritis of knee**

M17.5   **Other unilateral secondary osteoarthritis of knee**

Secondary osteoarthritis of knee NOS

M17.9   **Osteoarthritis of knee, unspecified**

M18   **Osteoarthritis of first carpometacarpal joint**

M18.0   **Bilateral primary osteoarthritis of first carpometacarpal joints**

M18.1   **Unilateral primary osteoarthritis of first carpometacarpal joint**

Primary osteoarthritis of first carpometacarpal joint NOS

     M18.10   **Unilateral primary osteoarthritis of first carpometacarpal joint, unspecified hand**

     M18.11   **Unilateral primary osteoarthritis of first carpometacarpal joint, right hand**

     M18.12   **Unilateral primary osteoarthritis of first carpometacarpal joint, left hand**

M18.2   **Bilateral post-traumatic osteoarthritis of first carpometacarpal joints**

M18.3   **Unilateral post-traumatic osteoarthritis of first carpometacarpal joint**

Post-traumatic osteoarthritis of first carpometacarpal joint NOS

     M18.30   **Unilateral post-traumatic osteoarthritis of first carpometacarpal joint, unspecified hand**

     M18.31   **Unilateral post-traumatic osteoarthritis of first carpometacarpal joint, right hand**

     M18.32   **Unilateral post-traumatic osteoarthritis of first carpometacarpal joint, left hand**

M18.4   **Other bilateral secondary osteoarthritis of first carpometacarpal joints**

M18.5   **Other unilateral secondary osteoarthritis of first carpometacarpal joint**

Secondary osteoarthritis of first carpometacarpal joint NOS

     M18.50   **Other unilateral secondary osteoarthritis of first carpometacarpal joint, unspecified hand**

     M18.51   **Other unilateral secondary osteoarthritis of first carpometacarpal joint, right hand**

     M18.52   **Other unilateral secondary osteoarthritis of first carpometacarpal joint, left hand**

M18.9   **Osteoarthritis of first carpometacarpal joint, unspecified**

M19   **Other and unspecified osteoarthritis**

Excludes1: polyarthritis (M15.-)

Excludes2: arthrosis of spine (M47.-)

hallux rigidus (M20.2)

osteoarthritis of spine (M47.-)

M19.0   **Primary osteoarthritis of other joints**

     M19.01   **Primary osteoarthritis, shoulder**

         M19.011   **Primary osteoarthritis, right shoulder**

         M19.012   **Primary osteoarthritis, left shoulder**

         M19.019   **Primary osteoarthritis, unspecified shoulder**

     M19.02   **Primary osteoarthritis, elbow**

         M19.021   **Primary osteoarthritis, right elbow**

         M19.022   **Primary osteoarthritis, left elbow**

         M19.029   **Primary osteoarthritis, unspecified elbow**

     M19.03   **Primary osteoarthritis, wrist**

         M19.031   **Primary osteoarthritis, right wrist**

         M19.032   **Primary osteoarthritis, left wrist**

         M19.039   **Primary osteoarthritis, unspecified wrist**

     M19.04   **Primary osteoarthritis, hand**

Excludes2: primary osteoarthritis of first carpometacarpal joint (M18.0-, M18.1-)

         M19.041   **Primary osteoarthritis, right hand**

         M19.042   **Primary osteoarthritis, left hand**

         M19.049   **Primary osteoarthritis, unspecified hand**

     M19.07   **Primary osteoarthritis ankle and foot**

         M19.071   **Primary osteoarthritis, right ankle and foot**

         M19.072   **Primary osteoarthritis, left ankle and foot**

         M19.079   **Primary osteoarthritis, unspecified ankle and foot**

M19.1   **Post-traumatic osteoarthritis of other joints**

     M19.11   **Post-traumatic osteoarthritis, shoulder**

         M19.111   **Post-traumatic osteoarthritis, right shoulder**

         M19.112   **Post-traumatic osteoarthritis, left shoulder**

M19.119 Post-traumatic osteoarthritis, unspecified shoulder

M19.12 Post-traumatic osteoarthritis, elbow

M19.121 Post-traumatic osteoarthritis, right elbow

M19.122 Post-traumatic osteoarthritis, left elbow

M19.129 Post-traumatic osteoarthritis, unspecified elbow

M19.13 Post-traumatic osteoarthritis, wrist

M19.131 Post-traumatic osteoarthritis, right wrist

M19.132 Post-traumatic osteoarthritis, left wrist

M19.139 Post-traumatic osteoarthritis, unspecified wrist

M19.14 Post-traumatic osteoarthritis, hand

Excludes2: post-traumatic osteoarthritis of first carpometacarpal joint (M18.2-, M18.3-)

M19.141 Post-traumatic osteoarthritis, right hand

M19.142 Post-traumatic osteoarthritis, left hand

M19.149 Post-traumatic osteoarthritis, unspecified hand

M19.17 Post-traumatic osteoarthritis, ankle and foot

M19.171 Post-traumatic osteoarthritis, right ankle and foot

M19.172 Post-traumatic osteoarthritis, left ankle and foot

M19.179 Post-traumatic osteoarthritis, unspecified ankle and foot

M19.2 Secondary osteoarthritis of other joints

M19.21 Secondary osteoarthritis, shoulder

M19.211 Secondary osteoarthritis, right shoulder

M19.212 Secondary osteoarthritis, left shoulder

M19.219 Secondary osteoarthritis, unspecified shoulder

M19.22 Secondary osteoarthritis, elbow

M19.221 Secondary osteoarthritis, right elbow

M19.222 Secondary osteoarthritis, left elbow

M19.229 Secondary osteoarthritis, unspecified elbow

M19.23 Secondary osteoarthritis, wrist

M19.231 Secondary osteoarthritis, right wrist

M19.232 Secondary osteoarthritis, left wrist

M19.239 Secondary osteoarthritis, unspecified wrist

M19.24 Secondary osteoarthritis, hand

M19.241 Secondary osteoarthritis, right hand

M19.242 Secondary osteoarthritis, left hand

M19.249 Secondary osteoarthritis, unspecified hand

M19.27 Secondary osteoarthritis, ankle and foot

M19.271 Secondary osteoarthritis, right ankle and foot

M19.272 Secondary osteoarthritis, left ankle and foot

M19.279 Secondary osteoarthritis, unspecified ankle and foot

M19.9 Osteoarthritis, unspecified site

M19.90 Unspecified osteoarthritis, unspecified site

Arthrosis NOS

Arthritis NOS

Osteoarthritis NOS

M19.91 Primary osteoarthritis, unspecified site

Primary osteoarthritis NOS

M19.92 Post-traumatic osteoarthritis, unspecified site

Post-traumatic osteoarthritis NOS

M19.93 Secondary osteoarthritis, unspecified site

Secondary osteoarthritis NOS

OTHER JOINT DISORDERS (M20-M25)

Excludes2: joints of the spine (M40-M54)

M20 Acquired deformities of fingers and toes

Excludes1: acquired absence of fingers and toes (Z89.-)

congenital absence of fingers and toes (Q71.3-, Q72.3-)

congenital deformities and malformations of fingers and toes (Q66.-, Q68-Q70, Q74.-)

M20.0 Deformity of finger(s)

Excludes1: clubbing of fingers (R68.3)

palmar fascial fibromatosis [Dupuytren] (M72.0)

trigger finger (M65.3)

M20.00 Unspecified deformity of finger(s)

M20.001 Unspecified deformity of right finger(s)

M20.002 Unspecified deformity of left finger(s)

M20.009 Unspecified deformity of unspecified finger(s)

M20.01 Mallet finger

M20.011 Mallet finger of right finger(s)

M20.012 Mallet finger of left finger(s)

M20.019 Mallet finger of unspecified finger(s)

M20.02 Boutonnière deformity

M20.021 Boutonnière deformity of right finger(s)

M20.022 Boutonnière deformity of left finger(s)

M20.029 Boutonnière deformity of unspecified finger(s)

M20.03 Swan-neck deformity

M20.031 Swan-neck deformity of right finger(s)

M20.032 Swan-neck deformity of left finger(s)

M20.039 Swan-neck deformity of unspecified finger(s)

M20.09 Other deformity of finger(s)

M20.091 Other deformity of right finger(s)

M20.092 Other deformity of left finger(s)

M20.099 Other deformity of finger(s), unspecified finger(s)

M20.1 Hallux valgus (acquired)

Excludes2: bunion (M21.6-)

M20.10 Hallux valgus (acquired), unspecified foot

M20.11 Hallux valgus (acquired), right foot

M20.12 Hallux valgus (acquired), left foot

M20.2 Hallux rigidus

M20.20 Hallux rigidus, unspecified foot

▨ Add 4th-7th digits	▨ Nonspecific code	▨ Unspecified code	▨ Manifestation code

M20.21   Hallux rigidus, right foot

M20.22   Hallux rigidus, left foot

M20.3   Hallux varus (acquired)

M20.30   Hallux varus (acquired), unspecified foot

M20.31   Hallux varus (acquired), right foot

M20.32   Hallux varus (acquired), left foot

M20.4   Other hammer toe(s) (acquired)

M20.40   Other hammer toe(s) (acquired), unspecified foot

M20.41   Other hammer toe(s) (acquired), right foot

M20.42   Other hammer toe(s) (acquired), left foot

M20.5   Other deformities of toe(s) (acquired)

M20.5X   Other deformities of toe(s) (acquired)

M20.5X1   Other deformities of toe(s) (acquired), right foot

M20.5X2   Other deformities of toe(s) (acquired), left foot

M20.5X9   Other deformities of toe(s) (acquired), unspecified foot

M20.6   Acquired deformities of toe(s), unspecified

M20.60   Acquired deformities of toe(s), unspecified, unspecified foot

M20.61   Acquired deformities of toe(s), unspecified, right foot

M20.62   Acquired deformities of toe(s), unspecified, left foot

M21   **Other acquired deformities of limbs**

Excludes1: acquired absence of limb (Z89.-)

congenital absence of limbs (Q71-Q73)

congenital deformities and malformations of limbs (Q65-Q66, Q68-Q74)

Excludes2: acquired deformities of fingers or toes (M20.-)

coxa plana (M91.2)

M21.0   Valgus deformity, not elsewhere classified

Excludes1: metatarsus valgus (Q66.6)

talipes calcaneovalgus (Q66.4)

M21.00   Valgus deformity, not elsewhere classified, unspecified site

M21.02   Valgus deformity, not elsewhere classified, elbow

Cubitus valgus

M21.021   Valgus deformity, not elsewhere classified, right elbow

M21.022   Valgus deformity, not elsewhere classified, left elbow

M21.029   Valgus deformity, not elsewhere classified, unspecified elbow

M21.05   Valgus deformity, not elsewhere classified, hip

M21.051   Valgus deformity, not elsewhere classified, right hip

M21.052   Valgus deformity, not elsewhere classified, left hip

M21.059   Valgus deformity, not elsewhere classified, unspecified hip

M21.06   Valgus deformity, not elsewhere classified, knee

Genu valgum

Knock knee

M21.061   Valgus deformity, not elsewhere classified, right knee

M21.062   Valgus deformity, not elsewhere classified, left knee

M21.069   Valgus deformity, not elsewhere classified, unspecified knee

M21.07   Valgus deformity, not elsewhere classified, ankle

M21.071   Valgus deformity, not elsewhere classified, right ankle

M21.072   Valgus deformity, not elsewhere classified, left ankle

M21.079   Valgus deformity, not elsewhere classified, unspecified ankle

M21.1   Varus deformity, not elsewhere classified

Excludes1: metatarsus varus (Q66.22)

tibia vara (M92.5)

M21.10   Varus deformity, not elsewhere classified, unspecified site

M21.12   Varus deformity, not elsewhere classified, elbow

Cubitus varus, elbow

M21.121   Varus deformity, not elsewhere classified, right elbow

M21.122   Varus deformity, not elsewhere classified, left elbow

M21.129   Varus deformity, not elsewhere classified, unspecified elbow

M21.15   Varus deformity, not elsewhere classified, hip

M21.151   Varus deformity, not elsewhere classified, right hip

M21.152   Varus deformity, not elsewhere classified, left hip

M21.159   Varus deformity, not elsewhere classified, unspecified

M21.16   Varus deformity, not elsewhere classified, knee

Bow leg Genu varum

M21.161   Varus deformity, not elsewhere classified, right knee

M21.162   Varus deformity, not elsewhere classified, left knee

M21.169   Varus deformity, not elsewhere classified, unspecified knee

M21.17   Varus deformity, not elsewhere classified, ankle

M21.171   Varus deformity, not elsewhere classified, right ankle

M21.172   Varus deformity, not elsewhere classified, left ankle

M21.179   Varus deformity, not elsewhere classified, unspecified ankle

M21.2   Flexion deformity

M21.20   Flexion deformity, unspecified site

M21.21   Flexion deformity, shoulder

M21.211   Flexion deformity, right shoulder

M21.212   Flexion deformity, left shoulder

M21.219   Flexion deformity, unspecified shoulder

M21.22   Flexion deformity, elbow

M21.221   Flexion deformity, right elbow

M21.222   Flexion deformity, left elbow

M21.229   Flexion deformity, unspecified elbow

M21.23   Flexion deformity, wrist

M21.231   Flexion deformity, right wrist

M21.232   Flexion deformity, left wrist

M21.239   Flexion deformity, unspecified wrist

M21.24 Flexion deformity, finger joints

    M21.241 Flexion deformity, right finger joints

    M21.242 Flexion deformity, left finger joints

    M21.249 Flexion deformity, unspecified finger joints

M21.25 Flexion deformity, hip

    M21.251 Flexion deformity, right hip

    M21.252 Flexion deformity, left hip

    M21.259 Flexion deformity, unspecified hip

M21.26 Flexion deformity, knee

    M21.261 Flexion deformity, right knee

    M21.262 Flexion deformity, left knee

    M21.269 Flexion deformity, unspecified knee

M21.27 Flexion deformity, ankle and toes

    M21.271 Flexion deformity, right ankle and toes

    M21.272 Flexion deformity, left ankle and toes

    M21.279 Flexion deformity, unspecified ankle and toes

M21.3 Wrist or foot drop (acquired)

M21.33 Wrist drop (acquired)

    M21.331 Wrist drop, right wrist

    M21.332 Wrist drop, left wrist

    M21.339 Wrist drop, unspecified wrist

M21.37 Foot drop (acquired)

    M21.371 Foot drop, right foot

    M21.372 Foot drop, left foot

    M21.379 Foot drop, unspecified foot

M21.4 Flat foot [pes planus] (acquired)

    Excludes1: congenital pes planus (Q66.5-)

M21.40 Flat foot [pes planus] (acquired), unspecified foot

M21.41 Flat foot [pes planus] (acquired), right foot

M21.42 Flat foot [pes planus] (acquired), left foot

M21.5 Acquired clawhand, clubhand, clawfoot and clubfoot

    Excludes1: clubfoot, not specified as acquired (Q66.89)

M21.51 Acquired clawhand

    M21.511 Acquired clawhand, right hand

    M21.512 Acquired clawhand, left hand

    M21.519 Acquired clawhand, unspecified hand

M21.52 Acquired clubhand

    M21.521 Acquired clubhand, right hand

    M21.522 Acquired clubhand, left hand

    M21.529 Acquired clubhand, unspecified hand

M21.53 Acquired clawfoot

    M21.531 Acquired clawfoot, right foot

    M21.532 Acquired clawfoot, left foot

    M21.539 Acquired clawfoot, unspecified foot

M21.54 Acquired clubfoot

    M21.541 Acquired clubfoot, right foot

    M21.542 Acquired clubfoot, left foot

    M21.549 Acquired clubfoot, unspecified foot

M21.6 Other acquired deformities of foot

    Excludes2: deformities of toe (acquired) (M20.1-M20.6-)

M21.61 Bunion

    M21.611 Bunion of right foot

    M21.612 Bunion of left foot

    M21.619 Bunion of unspecified foot

M21.62 Bunionette

    M21.621 Bunionette of right foot

    M21.622 Bunionette of left foot

    M21.629 Bunionette of unspecified foot

M21.6X Other acquired deformities of foot

    M21.6X1 Other acquired deformities of right foot

    M21.6X2 Other acquired deformities of left foot

    M21.6X9 Other acquired deformities of unspecified foot

M21.7 Unequal limb length (acquired)

    Note: The site used should correspond to the shorter limb

M21.70 Unequal limb length (acquired), unspecified site

M21.72 Unequal limb length (acquired), humerus

    M21.721 Unequal limb length (acquired), right humerus

    M21.722 Unequal limb length (acquired), left humerus

    M21.729 Unequal limb length (acquired), unspecified humerus

M21.73 Unequal limb length (acquired), ulna and radius

    M21.731 Unequal limb length (acquired), right ulna

    M21.732 Unequal limb length (acquired), left ulna

    M21.733 Unequal limb length (acquired), right radius

    M21.734 Unequal limb length (acquired), left radius

    M21.739 Unequal limb length (acquired), unspecified ulna and radius

M21.75 Unequal limb length (acquired), femur

    M21.751 Unequal limb length (acquired), right femur

    M21.752 Unequal limb length (acquired), left femur

    M21.759 Unequal limb length (acquired), unspecified femur

M21.76 Unequal limb length (acquired), tibia and fibula

    M21.761 Unequal limb length (acquired), right tibia

    M21.762 Unequal limb length (acquired), left tibia

    M21.763 Unequal limb length (acquired), right fibula

    M21.764 Unequal limb length (acquired), left fibula

    M21.769 Unequal limb length (acquired), unspecified tibia and fibula

M21.8 Other specified acquired deformities of limbs

    Excludes2: coxa plana (M91.2)

M21.80 Other specified acquired deformities of unspecified limb

M21.82 Other specified acquired deformities of upper arm

    M21.821 Other specified acquired deformities of right upper arm

M21.822   Other specified acquired deformities of left upper arm

M21.829   Other specified acquired deformities of unspecified upper arm

M21.83   Other specified acquired deformities of forearm

M21.831   Other specified acquired deformities of right forearm

M21.832   Other specified acquired deformities of left forearm

M21.839   Other specified acquired deformities of unspecified forearm

M21.85   Other specified acquired deformities of thigh

M21.851   Other specified acquired deformities of right thigh

M21.852   Other specified acquired deformities of left thigh

M21.859   Other specified acquired deformities of unspecified thigh

M21.86   Other specified acquired deformities of lower leg

M21.861   Other specified acquired deformities of right lower leg

M21.862   Other specified acquired deformities of left lower leg

M21.869   Other specified acquired deformities of unspecified lower leg

M21.9   Unspecified acquired deformity of limb and hand

M21.90   Unspecified acquired deformity of unspecified limb

M21.92   Unspecified acquired deformity of upper arm

M21.921   Unspecified acquired deformity of right upper arm

M21.922   Unspecified acquired deformity of left upper arm

M21.929   Unspecified acquired deformity of unspecified upper arm

M21.93   Unspecified acquired deformity of forearm

M21.931   Unspecified acquired deformity of right forearm

M21.932   Unspecified acquired deformity of left forearm

M21.939   Unspecified acquired deformity of unspecified forearm

M21.94   Unspecified acquired deformity of hand

M21.941   Unspecified acquired deformity of hand, right hand

M21.942   Unspecified acquired deformity of hand, left hand

M21.949   Unspecified acquired deformity of hand, unspecified hand

M21.95   Unspecified acquired deformity of thigh

M21.951   Unspecified acquired deformity of right thigh

M21.952   Unspecified acquired deformity of left thigh

M21.959   Unspecified acquired deformity of unspecified thigh

M21.96   Unspecified acquired deformity of lower leg

M21.961   Unspecified acquired deformity of right lower leg

M21.962   Unspecified acquired deformity of left lower leg

M21.969   Unspecified acquired deformity of unspecified lower leg

M22   **Disorder of patella**

Excludes1: traumatic dislocation of patella (S83.0-)

M22.0   Recurrent dislocation of patella

M22.00   Recurrent dislocation of patella, unspecified knee

M22.01   Recurrent dislocation of patella, right knee

M22.02   Recurrent dislocation of patella, left knee

M22.1   Recurrent subluxation of patella

Incomplete dislocation of patella

M22.10   Recurrent subluxation of patella, unspecified knee

M22.11   Recurrent subluxation of patella, right knee

M22.12   Recurrent subluxation of patella, left knee

M22.2   Patellofemoral disorders

M22.2X   Patellofemoral disorders

M22.2X1   Patellofemoral disorders, right knee

M22.2X2   Patellofemoral disorders, left knee

M22.2X9   Patellofemoral disorders, unspecified knee

M22.3   Other derangements of patella

M22.3X   Other derangements of patella

M22.3X1   Other derangements of patella, right knee

M22.3X2   Other derangements of patella, left knee

M22.3X9   Other derangements of patella, unspecified knee

M22.4   Chondromalacia patellae

M22.40   Chondromalacia patellae, unspecified knee

M22.41   Chondromalacia patellae, right knee

M22.42   Chondromalacia patellae, left knee

M22.8   Other disorders of patella

M22.8X   Other disorders of patella

M22.8X1   Other disorders of patella, right knee

M22.8X2   Other disorders of patella, left knee

M22.8X9   Other disorders of patella, unspecified knee

M22.9   Unspecified disorder of patella

M22.90   Unspecified disorder of patella, unspecified knee

M22.91   Unspecified disorder of patella, right knee

M22.92   Unspecified disorder of patella, left knee

M23   **Internal derangement of knee**

Definition: Internal derangement of knee is a term that describes internal damage to the knee joint, generally caused by trauma. It is a nonspecific term that usually must be further refined by history, physical exam, x-rays, and frequently MRI studies.

Excludes1: ankylosis (M24.66)

current injury - see injury of knee and lower leg (S80-S89)

deformity of knee (M21.-)

osteochondritis dissecans (M93.2)

recurrent dislocation or subluxation of joints (M24.4)

recurrent dislocation or subluxation of patella (M22.0-M22.1)

M23.0   Cystic meniscus

M23.00   Cystic meniscus, unspecified meniscus

Cystic meniscus, unspecified lateral meniscus

Cystic meniscus, unspecified medial meniscus

M23.000   **Cystic meniscus, unspecified lateral meniscus, right knee**

M23.001   **Cystic meniscus, unspecified lateral meniscus, left knee**

M23.002   **Cystic meniscus, unspecified lateral meniscus, unspecified knee**

M23.003   **Cystic meniscus, unspecified medial meniscus, right knee**

M23.004   **Cystic meniscus, unspecified medial meniscus, left knee**

M23.005   **Cystic meniscus, unspecified medial meniscus, unspecified knee**

M23.006   **Cystic meniscus, unspecified meniscus, right knee**

M23.007   **Cystic meniscus, unspecified meniscus, left knee**

M23.009   **Cystic meniscus, unspecified meniscus, unspecified knee**

M23.01   **Cystic meniscus, anterior horn of medial meniscus**

M23.011   **Cystic meniscus, anterior horn of medial meniscus, right knee**

M23.012   **Cystic meniscus, anterior horn of medial meniscus, left knee**

M23.019   **Cystic meniscus, anterior horn of medial meniscus, unspecified knee**

M23.02   **Cystic meniscus, posterior horn of medial meniscus**

M23.021   **Cystic meniscus, posterior horn of medial meniscus, right knee**

M23.022   **Cystic meniscus, posterior horn of medial meniscus, left knee**

M23.029   **Cystic meniscus, posterior horn of medial meniscus, unspecified knee**

M23.03   **Cystic meniscus, other medial meniscus**

M23.031   **Cystic meniscus, other medial meniscus, right knee**

M23.032   **Cystic meniscus, other medial meniscus, left knee**

M23.039   **Cystic meniscus, other medial meniscus, unspecified knee**

M23.04   **Cystic meniscus, anterior horn of lateral meniscus**

M23.041   **Cystic meniscus, anterior horn of lateral meniscus, right knee**

M23.042   **Cystic meniscus, anterior horn of lateral meniscus, left knee**

M23.049   **Cystic meniscus, anterior horn of lateral meniscus, unspecified knee**

M23.05   **Cystic meniscus, posterior horn of lateral meniscus**

M23.051   **Cystic meniscus, posterior horn of lateral meniscus, right knee**

M23.052   **Cystic meniscus, posterior horn of lateral meniscus, left knee**

M23.059   **Cystic meniscus, posterior horn of lateral meniscus, unspecified knee**

M23.06   **Cystic meniscus, other lateral meniscus**

M23.061   **Cystic meniscus, other lateral meniscus, right knee**

M23.062   **Cystic meniscus, other lateral meniscus, left knee**

M23.069   **Cystic meniscus, other lateral meniscus, unspecified knee**

M23.2   **Derangement of meniscus due to old tear or injury**

Old bucket-handle tear

M23.20   **Derangement of unspecified meniscus due to old tear or injury**

Derangement of unspecified lateral meniscus due to old tear or injury

Derangement of unspecified medial meniscus due to old tear or injury

M23.200   **Derangement of unspecified lateral meniscus due to old tear or injury, right knee**

M23.201   **Derangement of unspecified lateral meniscus due to old tear or injury, left knee**

M23.202   **Derangement of unspecified lateral meniscus due to old tear or injury, unspecified knee**

M23.203   **Derangement of unspecified medial meniscus due to old tear or injury, right knee**

M23.204   **Derangement of unspecified medial meniscus due to old tear or injury, left knee**

M23.205   **Derangement of unspecified medial meniscus due to old tear or injury, unspecified knee**

M23.206   **Derangement of unspecified meniscus due to old tear or injury, right knee**

M23.207   **Derangement of unspecified meniscus due to old tear or injury, left knee**

M23.209   **Derangement of unspecified meniscus due to old tear or injury, unspecified knee**

M23.21   **Derangement of anterior horn of medial meniscus due to old tear or injury**

M23.211   **Derangement of anterior horn of medial meniscus due to old tear or injury, right knee**

M23.212   **Derangement of anterior horn of medial meniscus due to old tear or injury, left knee**

M23.219   **Derangement of anterior horn of medial meniscus due to old tear or injury, unspecified knee**

M23.22   **Derangement of posterior horn of medial meniscus due to old tear or injury**

M23.221   **Derangement of posterior horn of medial meniscus due to old tear or injury, right knee**

M23.222   **Derangement of posterior horn of medial meniscus due to old tear or injury, left knee**

M23.229   **Derangement of posterior horn of medial meniscus due to old tear or injury, unspecified knee**

M23.23   **Derangement of other medial meniscus due to old tear or injury**

M23.231   **Derangement of other medial meniscus due to old tear or injury, right knee**

M23.232   Derangement of other medial meniscus due to old tear or injury, left knee

M23.239   Derangement of other medial meniscus due to old tear or injury, unspecified knee

M23.24   Derangement of anterior horn of lateral meniscus due to old tear or injury

    M23.241   Derangement of anterior horn of lateral meniscus due to old tear or injury, right knee

    M23.242   Derangement of anterior horn of lateral meniscus due to old tear or injury, left knee

    M23.249   Derangement of anterior horn of lateral meniscus due to old tear or injury, unspecified knee

M23.25   Derangement of posterior horn of lateral meniscus due to old tear or injury

    M23.251   Derangement of posterior horn of lateral meniscus due to old tear or injury, right knee

    M23.252   Derangement of posterior horn of lateral meniscus due to old tear or injury, left knee

    M23.259   Derangement of posterior horn of lateral meniscus due to old tear or injury, unspecified knee

M23.26   Derangement of other lateral meniscus due to old tear or injury

    M23.261   Derangement of other lateral meniscus due to old tear or injury, right knee

    M23.262   Derangement of other lateral meniscus due to old tear or injury, left knee

    M23.269   Derangement of other lateral meniscus due to old tear or injury, unspecified knee

M23.3   **Other meniscus derangements**

   Degenerate meniscus

   Detached meniscus

   Retained meniscus

M23.30   Other meniscus derangements, unspecified meniscus

   Other meniscus derangements, unspecified lateral meniscus

   Other meniscus derangements, unspecified medial meniscus

    M23.300   Other meniscus derangements, unspecified lateral meniscus, right knee

    M23.301   Other meniscus derangements, unspecified lateral meniscus, left knee

    M23.302   Other meniscus derangements, unspecified lateral meniscus, unspecified knee

    M23.303   Other meniscus derangements, unspecified medial meniscus, right knee

    M23.304   Other meniscus derangements, unspecified medial meniscus, left knee

    M23.305   Other meniscus derangements, unspecified medial meniscus, unspecified knee

    M23.306   Other meniscus derangements, unspecified meniscus, right knee

    M23.307   Other meniscus derangements, unspecified meniscus, left knee

    M23.309   Other meniscus derangements, unspecified meniscus, unspecified knee

M23.31   Other meniscus derangements, anterior horn of medial meniscus

    M23.311   Other meniscus derangements, anterior horn of medial meniscus, right knee

    M23.312   Other meniscus derangements, anterior horn of medial meniscus, left knee

    M23.319   Other meniscus derangements, anterior horn of medial meniscus, unspecified knee

M23.32   Other meniscus derangements, posterior horn of medial meniscus

    M23.321   Other meniscus derangements, posterior horn of medial meniscus, right knee

    M23.322   Other meniscus derangements, posterior horn of medial meniscus, left knee

    M23.329   Other meniscus derangements, posterior horn of medial meniscus, unspecified knee

M23.33   Other meniscus derangements, other medial meniscus

    M23.331   Other meniscus derangements, other medial meniscus, right knee

    M23.332   Other meniscus derangements, other medial meniscus, left knee

    M23.339   Other meniscus derangements, other medial meniscus, unspecified knee

M23.34   Other meniscus derangements, anterior horn of lateral meniscus

    M23.341   Other meniscus derangements, anterior horn of lateral meniscus, right knee

    M23.342   Other meniscus derangements, anterior horn of lateral meniscus, left knee

    M23.349   Other meniscus derangements, anterior horn of lateral meniscus, unspecified knee

M23.35   Other meniscus derangements, posterior horn of lateral meniscus

    M23.351   Other meniscus derangements, posterior horn of lateral meniscus, right knee

    M23.352   Other meniscus derangements, posterior horn of lateral meniscus, left knee

    M23.359   Other meniscus derangements, posterior horn of lateral meniscus, unspecified knee

M23.36   Other meniscus derangements, other lateral meniscus

    M23.361   Other meniscus derangements, other lateral meniscus, right knee

M23.362   Other meniscus derangements, other lateral meniscus, left knee

M23.369   Other meniscus derangements, other lateral meniscus, unspecified knee

M23.4   **Loose body in knee**

M23.40   **Loose body in knee, unspecified knee**

M23.41   **Loose body in knee, right knee**

M23.42   **Loose body in knee, left knee**

M23.5   **Chronic instability of knee**

M23.50   **Chronic instability of knee, unspecified knee**

M23.51   **Chronic instability of knee, right knee**

M23.52   **Chronic instability of knee, left knee**

M23.6   **Other spontaneous disruption of ligament(s) of knee**

M23.60   **Other spontaneous disruption of unspecified ligament of knee**

M23.601   Other spontaneous disruption of unspecified ligament of right knee

M23.602   Other spontaneous disruption of unspecified ligament of left knee

M23.609   Other spontaneous disruption of unspecified ligament of unspecified knee

M23.61   **Other spontaneous disruption of anterior cruciate ligament of knee**

M23.611   Other spontaneous disruption of anterior cruciate ligament of right knee

M23.612   Other spontaneous disruption of anterior cruciate ligament of left knee

M23.619   Other spontaneous disruption of anterior cruciate ligament of unspecified knee

M23.62   **Other spontaneous disruption of posterior cruciate ligament of knee**

M23.621   Other spontaneous disruption of posterior cruciate ligament of right knee

M23.622   Other spontaneous disruption of posterior cruciate ligament of left knee

M23.629   Other spontaneous disruption of posterior cruciate ligament of unspecified knee

M23.63   **Other spontaneous disruption of medial collateral ligament of knee**

M23.631   Other spontaneous disruption of medial collateral ligament of right knee

M23.632   Other spontaneous disruption of medial collateral ligament of left knee

M23.639   Other spontaneous disruption of medial collateral ligament of unspecified knee

M23.64   **Other spontaneous disruption of lateral collateral ligament of knee**

M23.641   Other spontaneous disruption of lateral collateral ligament of right knee

M23.642   Other spontaneous disruption of lateral collateral ligament of left knee

M23.649   Other spontaneous disruption of lateral collateral ligament of unspecified knee

M23.67   **Other spontaneous disruption of capsular ligament of knee**

M23.671   Other spontaneous disruption of capsular ligament of right knee

M23.672   Other spontaneous disruption of capsular ligament of left knee

M23.679   Other spontaneous disruption of capsular ligament of unspecified knee

M23.8   **Other internal derangements of knee**

Laxity of ligament of knee

Snapping knee

M23.8X   **Other internal derangements of knee**

M23.8X1   Other internal derangements of right knee

M23.8X2   Other internal derangements of left knee

M23.8X9   Other internal derangements of unspecified knee

M23.9   **Unspecified internal derangement of knee**

M23.90   **Unspecified internal derangement of unspecified knee**

M23.91   **Unspecified internal derangement of right knee**

M23.92   **Unspecified internal derangement of left knee**

M24   **Other specific joint derangements**

Excludes1: current injury - see injury of joint by body region

Excludes2: ganglion (M67.4)

snapping knee (M23.8-)

temporomandibular joint disorders (M26.6-)

M24.0   **Loose body in joint**

Excludes2: loose body in knee (M23.4)

M24.00   **Loose body in unspecified joint**

M24.01   **Loose body in shoulder**

M24.011   Loose body in right shoulder

M24.012   Loose body in left shoulder

M24.019   Loose body in unspecified shoulder

M24.02   **Loose body in elbow**

M24.021   Loose body in right elbow

M24.022   Loose body in left elbow

M24.029   Loose body in unspecified elbow

M24.03   **Loose body in wrist**

M24.031   Loose body in right wrist

M24.032   Loose body in left wrist

M24.039   Loose body in unspecified wrist

M24.04   **Loose body in finger joints**

M24.041   Loose body in right finger joint(s)

M24.042   Loose body in left finger joint(s)

M24.049   Loose body in unspecified finger joint(s)

M24.05   **Loose body in hip**

M24.051   Loose body in right hip

M24.052   Loose body in left hip

M24.059   Loose body in unspecified hip

M24.07   **Loose body in ankle and toe joints**

M24.071   Loose body in right ankle

M24.072   Loose body in left ankle

M24.073   Loose body in unspecified ankle

M24.074   Loose body in right toe joint(s)

M24.075   Loose body in left toe joint(s)

M24.076   Loose body in unspecified toe joints

M24.08   Loose body, other site

M24.1   **Other articular cartilage disorders**

     Excludes2: chondrocalcinosis (M11.1, M11.2-)

           internal derangement of knee (M23.-)

           metastatic calcification (E83.5)

           ochronosis (E70.2)

M24.10   Other articular cartilage disorders, unspecified site

M24.11   Other articular cartilage disorders, shoulder

     M24.111   Other articular cartilage disorders, right shoulder

     M24.112   Other articular cartilage disorders, left shoulder

     M24.119   Other articular cartilage disorders, unspecified shoulder

M24.12   Other articular cartilage disorders, elbow

     M24.121   Other articular cartilage disorders, right elbow

     M24.122   Other articular cartilage disorders, left elbow

     M24.129   Other articular cartilage disorders, unspecified elbow

M24.13   Other articular cartilage disorders, wrist

     M24.131   Other articular cartilage disorders, right wrist

     M24.132   Other articular cartilage disorders, left wrist

     M24.139   Other articular cartilage disorders, unspecified wrist

M24.14   Other articular cartilage disorders, hand

     M24.141   Other articular cartilage disorders, right hand

     M24.142   Other articular cartilage disorders, left hand

     M24.149   Other articular cartilage disorders, unspecified hand

M24.15   Other articular cartilage disorders, hip

     M24.151   Other articular cartilage disorders, right hip

     M24.152   Other articular cartilage disorders, left hip

     M24.159   Other articular cartilage disorders, unspecified hip

M24.17   Other articular cartilage disorders, ankle and foot

     M24.171   Other articular cartilage disorders, right ankle

     M24.172   Other articular cartilage disorders, left ankle

     M24.173   Other articular cartilage disorders, unspecified ankle

     M24.174   Other articular cartilage disorders, right foot

     M24.175   Other articular cartilage disorders, left foot

     M24.176   Other articular cartilage disorders, unspecified foot

M24.2   **Disorder of ligament**

     Instability secondary to old ligament injury

     Ligamentous laxity NOS

     Excludes1: familial ligamentous laxity (M35.7)

Excludes2: internal derangement of knee (M23.5-M23.89)

M24.20   Disorder of ligament, unspecified site

M24.21   Disorder of ligament, shoulder

     M24.211   Disorder of ligament, right shoulder

     M24.212   Disorder of ligament, left shoulder

     M24.219   Disorder of ligament, unspecified shoulder

M24.22   Disorder of ligament, elbow

     M24.221   Disorder of ligament, right elbow

     M24.222   Disorder of ligament, left elbow

     M24.229   Disorder of ligament, unspecified elbow

M24.23   Disorder of ligament, wrist

     M24.231   Disorder of ligament, right wrist

     M24.232   Disorder of ligament, left wrist

     M24.239   Disorder of ligament, unspecified wrist

M24.24   Disorder of ligament, hand

     M24.241   Disorder of ligament, right hand

     M24.242   Disorder of ligament, left hand

     M24.249   Disorder of ligament, unspecified hand

M24.25   Disorder of ligament, hip

     M24.251   Disorder of ligament, right hip

     M24.252   Disorder of ligament, left hip

     M24.259   Disorder of ligament, unspecified hip

M24.27   Disorder of ligament, ankle and foot

     M24.271   Disorder of ligament, right ankle

     M24.272   Disorder of ligament, left ankle

     M24.273   Disorder of ligament, unspecified ankle

     M24.274   Disorder of ligament, right foot

     M24.275   Disorder of ligament, left foot

     M24.276   Disorder of ligament, unspecified foot

M24.28   Disorder of ligament, vertebrae

M24.3   **Pathological dislocation of joint, not elsewhere classified**

     Excludes1: congenital dislocation or displacement of joint-see congenital malformations and deformations of the musculoskeletal system (Q65-Q79)

           current injury - see injury of joints and ligaments by body region

           recurrent dislocation of joint (M24.4-)

M24.30   Pathological dislocation of unspecified joint, not elsewhere classified

M24.31   Pathological dislocation of shoulder, not elsewhere classified

     M24.311   Pathological dislocation of right shoulder, not elsewhere classified

     M24.312   Pathological dislocation of left shoulder, not elsewhere classified

     M24.319   Pathological dislocation of unspecified shoulder, not elsewhere classified

M24.32   Pathological dislocation of elbow, not elsewhere classified

     M24.321   Pathological dislocation of right elbow, not elsewhere classified

     M24.322   Pathological dislocation of left elbow, not elsewhere classified

M24.329　Pathological dislocation of unspecified elbow, not elsewhere classified

M24.33　Pathological dislocation of wrist, not elsewhere classified

M24.331　Pathological dislocation of right wrist, not elsewhere classified

M24.332　Pathological dislocation of left wrist, not elsewhere classified

M24.339　Pathological dislocation of unspecified wrist, not elsewhere classified

M24.34　Pathological dislocation of hand, not elsewhere classified

M24.341　Pathological dislocation of right hand, not elsewhere classified

M24.342　Pathological dislocation of left hand, not elsewhere classified

M24.349　Pathological dislocation of unspecified hand, not elsewhere classified

M24.35　Pathological dislocation of hip, not elsewhere classified

M24.351　Pathological dislocation of right hip, not elsewhere classified

M24.352　Pathological dislocation of left hip, not elsewhere classified

M24.359　Pathological dislocation of unspecified hip, not elsewhere classified

M24.36　Pathological dislocation of knee, not elsewhere classified

M24.361　Pathological dislocation of right knee, not elsewhere classified

M24.362　Pathological dislocation of left knee, not elsewhere classified

M24.369　Pathological dislocation of unspecified knee, not elsewhere classified

M24.37　Pathological dislocation of ankle and foot, not elsewhere classified

M24.371　Pathological dislocation of right ankle, not elsewhere classified

M24.372　Pathological dislocation of left ankle, not elsewhere classified

M24.373　Pathological dislocation of unspecified ankle, not elsewhere classified

M24.374　Pathological dislocation of right foot, not elsewhere classified

M24.375　Pathological dislocation of left foot, not elsewhere classified

M24.376　Pathological dislocation of unspecified foot, not elsewhere classified

M24.4　Recurrent dislocation of joint

Recurrent subluxation of joint

Excludes2: recurrent dislocation of patella (M22.0-M22.1)

recurrent vertebral dislocation (M43.3-, M43.4, M43.5-)

M24.40　Recurrent dislocation, unspecified joint

M24.41　Recurrent dislocation, shoulder

M24.411　Recurrent dislocation, right shoulder

M24.412　Recurrent dislocation, left shoulder

M24.419　Recurrent dislocation, unspecified shoulder

M24.42　Recurrent dislocation, elbow

M24.421　Recurrent dislocation, right elbow

M24.422　Recurrent dislocation, left elbow

M24.429　Recurrent dislocation, unspecified elbow

M24.43　Recurrent dislocation, wrist

M24.431　Recurrent dislocation, right wrist

M24.432　Recurrent dislocation, left wrist

M24.439　Recurrent dislocation, unspecified wrist

M24.44　Recurrent dislocation, hand and finger(s)

M24.441　Recurrent dislocation, right hand

M24.442　Recurrent dislocation, left hand

M24.443　Recurrent dislocation, unspecified hand

M24.444　Recurrent dislocation, right finger

M24.445　Recurrent dislocation, left finger

M24.446　Recurrent dislocation, unspecified finger

M24.45　Recurrent dislocation, hip

M24.451　Recurrent dislocation, right hip

M24.452　Recurrent dislocation, left hip

M24.459　Recurrent dislocation, unspecified hip

M24.46　Recurrent dislocation, knee

M24.461　Recurrent dislocation, right knee

M24.462　Recurrent dislocation, left knee

M24.469　Recurrent dislocation, unspecified knee

M24.47　Recurrent dislocation, ankle, foot and toes

M24.471　Recurrent dislocation, right ankle

M24.472　Recurrent dislocation, left ankle

M24.473　Recurrent dislocation, unspecified ankle

M24.474　Recurrent dislocation, right foot

M24.475　Recurrent dislocation, left foot

M24.476　Recurrent dislocation, unspecified foot

M24.477　Recurrent dislocation, right toe(s)

M24.478　Recurrent dislocation, left toe(s)

M24.479　Recurrent dislocation, unspecified toe(s)

M24.5　Contracture of joint

Excludes1: contracture of muscle without contracture of joint (M62.4-)

contracture of tendon (sheath) without contracture of joint (M62.4-)

Dupuytren's contracture (M72.0)

Excludes2: acquired deformities of limbs (M20-M21)

M24.50　Contracture, unspecified joint

M24.51　Contracture, shoulder

M24.511　Contracture, right shoulder

M24.512　Contracture, left shoulder

M24.519　Contracture, unspecified shoulder

M24.52　Contracture, elbow

M24.521　Contracture, right elbow

M24.522　Contracture, left elbow

M24.529　Contracture, unspecified elbow

M24.53　Contracture, wrist

　　M24.531　Contracture, right wrist

　　M24.532　Contracture, left wrist

　　M24.539　Contracture, unspecified wrist

M24.54　Contracture, hand

　　M24.541　Contracture, right hand

　　M24.542　Contracture, left hand

　　M24.549　Contracture, unspecified hand

M24.55　Contracture, hip

　　M24.551　Contracture, right hip

　　M24.552　Contracture, left hip

　　M24.559　Contracture, unspecified hip

M24.56　Contracture, knee

　　M24.561　Contracture, right knee

　　M24.562　Contracture, left knee

　　M24.569　Contracture, unspecified knee

M24.57　Contracture, ankle and foot

　　M24.571　Contracture, right ankle

　　M24.572　Contracture, left ankle

　　M24.573　Contracture, unspecified ankle

　　M24.574　Contracture, right foot

　　M24.575　Contracture, left foot

　　M24.576　Contracture, unspecified foot

M24.6　Ankylosis of joint

　Excludes1: stiffness of joint without ankylosis (M25.6-)

　Excludes2: spine (M43.2-)

M24.60　Ankylosis, unspecified joint

M24.61　Ankylosis, shoulder

　　M24.611　Ankylosis, right shoulder

　　M24.612　Ankylosis, left shoulder

　　M24.619　Ankylosis, unspecified shoulder

M24.62　Ankylosis, elbow

　　M24.621　Ankylosis, right elbow

　　M24.622　Ankylosis, left elbow

　　M24.629　Ankylosis, unspecified elbow

M24.63　Ankylosis, wrist

　　M24.631　Ankylosis, right wrist

　　M24.632　Ankylosis, left wrist

　　M24.639　Ankylosis, unspecified wrist

M24.64　Ankylosis, hand

　　M24.641　Ankylosis, right hand

　　M24.642　Ankylosis, left hand

　　M24.649　Ankylosis, unspecified hand

M24.65　Ankylosis, hip

　　M24.651　Ankylosis, right hip

　　M24.652　Ankylosis, left hip

　　M24.659　Ankylosis, unspecified hip

M24.66　Ankylosis, knee

　　M24.661　Ankylosis, right knee

　　M24.662　Ankylosis, left knee

　　M24.669　Ankylosis, unspecified knee

M24.67　Ankylosis, ankle and foot

　　M24.671　Ankylosis, right ankle

　　M24.672　Ankylosis, left ankle

　　M24.673　Ankylosis, unspecified ankle

　　M24.674　Ankylosis, right foot

　　M24.675　Ankylosis, left foot

　　M24.676　Ankylosis, unspecified foot

M24.7　Protrusio acetabuli

M24.8　Other specific joint derangements, not elsewhere classified

　Excludes2: iliotibial band syndrome (M76.3)

M24.80　Other specific joint derangements of unspecified joint, not elsewhere classified

M24.81　Other specific joint derangements of shoulder, not elsewhere classified

　　M24.811　Other specific joint derangements of right shoulder, not elsewhere classified

　　M24.812　Other specific joint derangements of left shoulder, not elsewhere classified

　　M24.819　Other specific joint derangements of unspecified shoulder, not elsewhere classified

M24.82　Other specific joint derangements of elbow, not elsewhere classified

　　M24.821　Other specific joint derangements of right elbow, not elsewhere classified

　　M24.822　Other specific joint derangements of left elbow, not elsewhere classified

　　M24.829　Other specific joint derangements of unspecified elbow, not elsewhere classified

M24.83　Other specific joint derangements of wrist, not elsewhere classified

　　M24.831　Other specific joint derangements of right wrist, not elsewhere classified

　　M24.832　Other specific joint derangements of left wrist, not elsewhere classified

　　M24.839　Other specific joint derangements of unspecified wrist, not elsewhere classified

M24.84　Other specific joint derangements of hand, not elsewhere classified

　　M24.841　Other specific joint derangements of right hand, not elsewhere classified

　　M24.842　Other specific joint derangements of left hand, not elsewhere classified

　　M24.849　Other specific joint derangements of unspecified hand, not elsewhere classified

M24.85　Other specific joint derangements of hip, not elsewhere classified

　　Irritable hip

　　M24.851　Other specific joint derangements of right hip, not elsewhere classified

　　M24.852　Other specific joint derangements of left hip, not elsewhere classified

　　M24.859　Other specific joint derangements of unspecified hip, not elsewhere classified

M24.87　Other specific joint derangements of ankle and foot, not elsewhere classified

　　M24.871　Other specific joint derangements of right ankle, not elsewhere classified

　　M24.872　Other specific joint derangements of left ankle, not elsewhere classified

M24.873   Other specific joint derangements of unspecified ankle, not elsewhere classified

M24.874   Other specific joint derangements of right foot, not elsewhere classified

M24.875   Other specific joint derangements left foot, not elsewhere classified

M24.876   Other specific joint derangements of unspecified foot, not elsewhere classified

M24.9   **Joint derangement, unspecified**

M25   **Other joint disorder, not elsewhere classified**

Excludes2: abnormality of gait and mobility (R26.-)

acquired deformities of limb (M20-M21)

calcification of bursa (M71.4-)

calcification of shoulder (joint) (M75.3)

calcification of tendon (M65.2-)

difficulty in walking (R26.2)

temporomandibular joint disorder (M26.6-)

M25.0   **Hemarthrosis**

Excludes1: current injury - see injury of joint by body region

hemophilic arthropathy (M36.2)

M25.00   Hemarthrosis, unspecified joint

M25.01   Hemarthrosis, shoulder

M25.011   Hemarthrosis, right shoulder

M25.012   Hemarthrosis, left shoulder

M25.019   Hemarthrosis, unspecified shoulder

M25.02   Hemarthrosis, elbow

M25.021   Hemarthrosis, right elbow

M25.022   Hemarthrosis, left elbow

M25.029   Hemarthrosis, unspecified elbow

M25.03   Hemarthrosis, wrist

M25.031   Hemarthrosis, right wrist

M25.032   Hemarthrosis, left wrist

M25.039   Hemarthrosis, unspecified wrist

M25.04   Hemarthrosis, hand

M25.041   Hemarthrosis, right hand

M25.042   Hemarthrosis, left hand

M25.049   Hemarthrosis, unspecified hand

M25.05   Hemarthrosis, hip

M25.051   Hemarthrosis, right hip

M25.052   Hemarthrosis, left hip

M25.059   Hemarthrosis, unspecified hip

M25.06   Hemarthrosis, knee

M25.061   Hemarthrosis, right knee

M25.062   Hemarthrosis, left knee

M25.069   Hemarthrosis, unspecified knee

M25.07   Hemarthrosis, ankle and foot

M25.071   Hemarthrosis, right ankle

M25.072   Hemarthrosis, left ankle

M25.073   Hemarthrosis, unspecified ankle

M25.074   Hemarthrosis, right foot

M25.075   Hemarthrosis, left foot

M25.076   Hemarthrosis, unspecified foot

M25.08   Hemarthrosis, other specified site

Hemarthrosis, vertebrae

M25.1   **Fistula of joint**

M25.10   Fistula, unspecified joint

M25.11   Fistula, shoulder

M25.111   Fistula, right shoulder

M25.112   Fistula, left shoulder

M25.119   Fistula, unspecified shoulder

M25.12   Fistula, elbow

M25.121   Fistula, right elbow

M25.122   Fistula, left elbow

M25.129   Fistula, unspecified elbow

M25.13   Fistula, wrist

M25.131   Fistula, right wrist

M25.132   Fistula, left wrist

M25.139   Fistula, unspecified wrist

M25.14   Fistula, hand

M25.141   Fistula, right hand

M25.142   Fistula, left hand

M25.149   Fistula, unspecified hand

M25.15   Fistula, hip

M25.151   Fistula, right hip

M25.152   Fistula, left hip

M25.159   Fistula, unspecified hip

M25.16   Fistula, knee

M25.161   Fistula, right knee

M25.162   Fistula, left knee

M25.169   Fistula, unspecified knee

M25.17   Fistula, ankle and foot

M25.171   Fistula, right ankle

M25.172   Fistula, left ankle

M25.173   Fistula, unspecified ankle

M25.174   Fistula, right foot

M25.175   Fistula, left foot

M25.176   Fistula, unspecified foot

M25.18   **Fistula, other specified site**

Fistula, vertebrae

M25.2   **Flail joint**

M25.20   Flail joint, unspecified joint

M25.21   Flail joint, shoulder

M25.211   Flail joint, right shoulder

M25.212   Flail joint, left shoulder

M25.219   Flail joint, unspecified shoulder

M25.22   Flail joint, elbow

M25.221   Flail joint, right elbow

M25.222   Flail joint, left elbow

M25.229   Flail joint, unspecified elbow

M25.23   Flail joint, wrist

M25.231   Flail joint, right wrist

M25.232   Flail joint, left wrist

M25.239   Flail joint, unspecified wrist

M25.24   Flail joint, hand

M25.241   Flail joint, right hand

M25.242   Flail joint, left hand

M25.249   Flail joint, unspecified hand

M25.25   Flail joint, hip

M25.251   Flail joint, right hip

M25.252   Flail joint, left hip

M25.259   Flail joint, unspecified hip

M25.26   Flail joint, knee
     M25.261   Flail joint, right knee
     M25.262   Flail joint, left knee
     M25.269   Flail joint, unspecified knee
M25.27   Flail joint, ankle and foot
     M25.271   Flail joint, right ankle and foot
     M25.272   Flail joint, left ankle and foot
     M25.279   Flail joint, unspecified ankle and foot
M25.28   Flail joint, other site

M25.3   **Other instability of joint**
   Excludes1: instability of joint secondary to old ligament injury (M24.2-)
     instability of joint secondary to removal of joint prosthesis (M96.8-)
   Excludes2: spinal instabilities (M53.2-)
M25.30   Other instability, unspecified joint
M25.31   Other instability, shoulder
     M25.311   Other instability, right shoulder
     M25.312   Other instability, left shoulder
     M25.319   Other instability, unspecified shoulder
M25.32   Other instability, elbow
     M25.321   Other instability, right elbow
     M25.322   Other instability, left elbow
     M25.329   Other instability, unspecified elbow
M25.33   Other instability, wrist
     M25.331   Other instability, right wrist
     M25.332   Other instability, left wrist
     M25.339   Other instability, unspecified wrist
M25.34   Other instability, hand
     M25.341   Other instability, right hand
     M25.342   Other instability, left hand
     M25.349   Other instability, unspecified hand
M25.35   Other instability, hip
     M25.351   Other instability, right hip
     M25.352   Other instability, left hip
     M25.359   Other instability, unspecified hip
M25.36   Other instability, knee
     M25.361   Other instability, right knee
     M25.362   Other instability, left knee
     M25.369   Other instability, unspecified knee
M25.37   Other instability, ankle and foot
     M25.371   Other instability, right ankle
     M25.372   Other instability, left ankle
     M25.373   Other instability, unspecified ankle
     M25.374   Other instability, right foot
     M25.375   Other instability, left foot
     M25.376   Other instability, unspecified foot

M25.4   **Effusion of joint**
   Excludes1: hydrarthrosis in yaws (A66.6)
     intermittent hydrarthrosis (M12.4-)
     Other infective (teno)synovitis (M65.1-)
M25.40   Effusion, unspecified joint
M25.41   Effusion, shoulder
     M25.411   Effusion, right shoulder
     M25.412   Effusion, left shoulder
     M25.419   Effusion, unspecified shoulder

M25.42   Effusion, elbow
     M25.421   Effusion, right elbow
     M25.422   Effusion, left elbow
     M25.429   Effusion, unspecified elbow
M25.43   Effusion, wrist
     M25.431   Effusion, right wrist
     M25.432   Effusion, left wrist
     M25.439   Effusion, unspecified wrist
M25.44   Effusion, hand
     M25.441   Effusion, right hand
     M25.442   Effusion, left hand
     M25.449   Effusion, unspecified hand
M25.45   Effusion, hip
     M25.451   Effusion, right hip
     M25.452   Effusion, left hip
     M25.459   Effusion, unspecified hip
M25.46   Effusion, knee
     M25.461   Effusion, right knee
     M25.462   Effusion, left knee
     M25.469   Effusion, unspecified knee
M25.47   Effusion, ankle and foot
     M25.471   Effusion, right ankle
     M25.472   Effusion, left ankle
     M25.473   Effusion, unspecified ankle
     M25.474   Effusion, right foot
     M25.475   Effusion, left foot
     M25.476   Effusion, unspecified foot
M25.48   Effusion, other site

M25.5   **Pain in joint**
   Excludes2: pain in hand (M79.64-)
     pain in fingers (M79.64-)
     pain in foot (M79.67-)
     pain in limb (M79.6-)
     pain in toes (M79.67-)
M25.50   Pain in unspecified joint
M25.51   Pain in shoulder
     M25.511   Pain in right shoulder
     M25.512   Pain in left shoulder
     M25.519   Pain in unspecified shoulder
M25.52   Pain in elbow
     M25.521   Pain in right elbow
     M25.522   Pain in left elbow
     M25.529   Pain in unspecified elbow
M25.53   Pain in wrist
     M25.531   Pain in right wrist
     M25.532   Pain in left wrist
     M25.539   Pain in unspecified wrist
M25.54   Pain in joints of hand
     M25.541   Pain in joints of right hand
     M25.542   Pain in joints of left hand
     M25.549   Pain in joints of unspecified hand
       Pain in joints of hand NOS
M25.55   Pain in hip
     M25.551   Pain in right hip
     M25.552   Pain in left hip
     M25.559   Pain in unspecified hip

   ● New code   ▲ Revised code   **Excludes1:** Not coded here   **Excludes2:** Not included here   ⊗ Placeholder required   ⑦ 7th digit required

M25.56 Pain in knee

    M25.561   Pain in right knee

    M25.562   Pain in left knee

    M25.569   Pain in unspecified knee

M25.57 Pain in ankle and joints of foot

    M25.571   Pain in right ankle and joints of right foot

    M25.572   Pain in left ankle and joints of left foot

    M25.579   Pain in unspecified ankle and joints of unspecified foot

M25.6 Stiffness of joint, not elsewhere classified

    Excludes1: ankylosis of joint (M24.6-)

             contracture of joint (M24.5-)

    M25.60   Stiffness of unspecified joint, not elsewhere classified

    M25.61   Stiffness of shoulder, not elsewhere classified

        M25.611   Stiffness of right shoulder, not elsewhere classified

        M25.612   Stiffness of left shoulder, not elsewhere classified

        M25.619   Stiffness of unspecified shoulder, not elsewhere classified

    M25.62   Stiffness of elbow, not elsewhere classified

        M25.621   Stiffness of right elbow, not elsewhere classified

        M25.622   Stiffness of left elbow, not elsewhere classified

        M25.629   Stiffness of unspecified elbow, not elsewhere classified

    M25.63   Stiffness of wrist, not elsewhere classified

        M25.631   Stiffness of right wrist, not elsewhere classified

        M25.632   Stiffness of left wrist, not elsewhere classified

        M25.639   Stiffness of unspecified wrist, not elsewhere classified

    M25.64   Stiffness of hand, not elsewhere classified

        M25.641   Stiffness of right hand, not elsewhere classified

        M25.642   Stiffness of left hand, not elsewhere classified

        M25.649   Stiffness of unspecified hand, not elsewhere classified

    M25.65   Stiffness of hip, not elsewhere classified

        M25.651   Stiffness of right hip, not elsewhere classified

        M25.652   Stiffness of left hip, not elsewhere classified

        M25.659   Stiffness of unspecified hip, not elsewhere classified

    M25.66   Stiffness of knee, not elsewhere classified

        M25.661   Stiffness of right knee, not elsewhere classified

        M25.662   Stiffness of left knee, not elsewhere classified

        M25.669   Stiffness of unspecified knee, not elsewhere classified

    M25.67   Stiffness of ankle and foot, not elsewhere classified

        M25.671   Stiffness of right ankle, not elsewhere classified

        M25.672   Stiffness of left ankle, not elsewhere classified

        M25.673   Stiffness of unspecified ankle, not elsewhere classified

        M25.674   Stiffness of right foot, not elsewhere classified

        M25.675   Stiffness of left foot, not elsewhere classified

        M25.676   Stiffness of unspecified foot, not elsewhere classified

M25.7 Osteophyte

    M25.70   Osteophyte, unspecified joint

    M25.71   Osteophyte, shoulder

        M25.711   Osteophyte, right shoulder

        M25.712   Osteophyte, left shoulder

        M25.719   Osteophyte, unspecified shoulder

    M25.72   Osteophyte, elbow

        M25.721   Osteophyte, right elbow

        M25.722   Osteophyte, left elbow

        M25.729   Osteophyte, unspecified elbow

    M25.73   Osteophyte, wrist

        M25.731   Osteophyte, right wrist

        M25.732   Osteophyte, left wrist

        M25.739   Osteophyte, unspecified wrist

    M25.74   Osteophyte, hand

        M25.741   Osteophyte, right hand

        M25.742   Osteophyte, left hand

        M25.749   Osteophyte, unspecified hand

    M25.75   Osteophyte, hip

        M25.751   Osteophyte, right hip

        M25.752   Osteophyte, left hip

        M25.759   Osteophyte, unspecified hip

    M25.76   Osteophyte, knee

        M25.761   Osteophyte, right knee

        M25.762   Osteophyte, left knee

        M25.769   Osteophyte, unspecified knee

    M25.77   Osteophyte, ankle and foot

        M25.771   Osteophyte, right ankle

        M25.772   Osteophyte, left ankle

        M25.773   Osteophyte, unspecified ankle

        M25.774   Osteophyte, right foot

        M25.775   Osteophyte, left foot

        M25.776   Osteophyte, unspecified foot

    M25.78   Osteophyte, vertebrae

M25.8 Other specified joint disorders

    M25.80   Other specified joint disorders, unspecified joint

    M25.81   Other specified joint disorders, shoulder

        M25.811   Other specified joint disorders, right shoulder

        M25.812   Other specified joint disorders, left shoulder

        M25.819   Other specified joint disorders, unspecified shoulder

    M25.82   Other specified joint disorders, elbow

        M25.821   Other specified joint disorders, right elbow

        M25.822   Other specified joint disorders, left elbow

M25.829 Other specified joint disorders, unspecified elbow

M25.83 Other specified joint disorders, wrist

M25.831 Other specified joint disorders, right wrist

M25.832 Other specified joint disorders, left wrist

M25.839 Other specified joint disorders, unspecified wrist

M25.84 Other specified joint disorders, hand

M25.841 Other specified joint disorders, right hand

M25.842 Other specified joint disorders, left hand

M25.849 Other specified joint disorders, unspecified hand

M25.85 Other specified joint disorders, hip

M25.851 Other specified joint disorders, right hip

M25.852 Other specified joint disorders, left hip

M25.859 Other specified joint disorders, unspecified hip

M25.86 Other specified joint disorders, knee

M25.861 Other specified joint disorders, right knee

M25.862 Other specified joint disorders, left knee

M25.869 Other specified joint disorders, unspecified knee

M25.87 Other specified joint disorders, ankle and foot

M25.871 Other specified joint disorders, right ankle and foot

M25.872 Other specified joint disorders, left ankle and foot

M25.879 Other specified joint disorders, unspecified ankle and foot

M25.9 Joint disorder, unspecified

DENTOFACIAL ANOMALIES [INCLUDING MALOCCLUSION] AND OTHER DISORDERS OF JAW (M26-M27)

Excludes1: hemifacial atrophy or hypertrophy (Q67.4)

unilateral condylar hyperplasia or hypoplasia (M27.8)

M26 Dentofacial anomalies [including malocclusion]

M26.0 Major anomalies of jaw size

Excludes1: acromegaly (E22.0)

Robin's syndrome (Q87.0)

M26.00 Unspecified anomaly of jaw size

M26.01 Maxillary hyperplasia

M26.02 Maxillary hypoplasia

M26.03 Mandibular hyperplasia

M26.04 Mandibular hypoplasia

M26.05 Macrogenia

M26.06 Microgenia

M26.07 Excessive tuberosity of jaw

Entire maxillary tuberosity

M26.09 Other specified anomalies of jaw size

M26.1 Anomalies of jaw-cranial base relationship

M26.10 Unspecified anomaly of jaw-cranial base relationship

M26.11 Maxillary asymmetry

M26.12 Other jaw asymmetry

M26.19 Other specified anomalies of jaw-cranial base relationship

M26.2 Anomalies of dental arch relationship

M26.20 Unspecified anomaly of dental arch relationship

M26.21 Malocclusion, Angle's class

M26.211 Malocclusion, Angle's class I

Neutro-occlusion

M26.212 Malocclusion, Angle's class II

Disto-occlusion Division I

Disto-occlusion Division II

M26.213 Malocclusion, Angle's class III

Mesio-occlusion

M26.219 Malocclusion, Angle's class, unspecified

M26.22 Open occlusal relationship

M26.220 Open anterior occlusal relationship

Anterior openbite

M26.221 Open posterior occlusal relationship

Posterior openbite

M26.23 Excessive horizontal overlap

Excessive horizontal overjet

M26.24 Reverse articulation

Crossbite (anterior) (posterior)

M26.25 Anomalies of interarch distance

M26.29 Other anomalies of dental arch relationship

Midline deviation of dental arch

Overbite (excessive) deep

Overbite (excessive) horizontal

Overbite (excessive) vertical

Posterior lingual occlusion of mandibular teeth

M26.3 Anomalies of tooth position of fully erupted tooth or teeth

Excludes2: embedded and impacted teeth (K01.-)

M26.30 Unspecified anomaly of tooth position of fully erupted tooth or teeth

Abnormal spacing of fully erupted tooth or teeth NOS

Displacement of fully erupted tooth or teeth NOS

Transposition of fully erupted tooth or teeth NOS

M26.31 Crowding of fully erupted teeth

M26.32 Excessive spacing of fully erupted teeth

Diastema of fully erupted tooth or teeth NOS

M26.33 Horizontal displacement of fully erupted tooth or teeth

Tipped tooth or teeth

Tipping of fully erupted tooth

M26.34 Vertical displacement of fully erupted tooth or teeth

Extruded tooth

Infraeruption of tooth or teeth

Supraeruption of tooth or teeth

M26.35 Rotation of fully erupted tooth or teeth

M26.36 Insufficient interocclusal distance of fully erupted teeth (ridge)

Lack of adequate intermaxillary vertical dimension of fully erupted teeth

M26.37 Excessive interocclusal distance of fully erupted teeth

Excessive intermaxillary vertical dimension of fully erupted teeth

Loss of occlusal vertical dimension of fully erupted teeth

M26.39 Other anomalies of tooth position of fully erupted tooth or teeth

M26.4 Malocclusion, unspecified

M26.5 Dentofacial functional abnormalities

> **Excludes1:** bruxism (F45.8)
>
> teeth-grinding NOS (F45.8)

M26.50 Dentofacial functional abnormalities, unspecified

M26.51 Abnormal jaw closure

M26.52 Limited mandibular range of motion

M26.53 Deviation in opening and closing of the mandible

M26.54 Insufficient anterior guidance

Insufficient anterior occlusal guidance

M26.55 Centric occlusion maximum intercuspation discrepancy

> **Excludes1:** centric occlusion NOS (M26.59)

M26.56 Non-working side interference

Balancing side interference

M26.57 Lack of posterior occlusal support

M26.59 Other dentofacial functional abnormalities

Centric occlusion (of teeth) NOS

Malocclusion due to abnormal swallowing

Malocclusion due to mouth breathing

Malocclusion due to tongue, lip or finger habits

M26.6 Temporomandibular joint disorders

> **Excludes2:** current temporomandibular joint dislocation (S03.0)
>
> current temporomandibular joint sprain (S03.4)

M26.60 Temporomandibular joint disorder, unspecified

M26.601 Right temporomandibular joint disorder, unspecified

M26.602 Left temporomandibular joint disorder, unspecified

M26.603 Bilateral temporomandibular joint disorder, unspecified

M26.609 Unspecified temporomandibular joint disorder, unspecified side

Temporomandibular joint disorder NOS

M26.61 Adhesions and ankylosis of temporomandibular joint

M26.611 Adhesions and ankylosis of right temporomandibular joint

M26.612 Adhesions and ankylosis of left temporomandibular joint

M26.613 Adhesions and ankylosis of bilateral temporomandibular joint

M26.619 Adhesions and ankylosis of temporomandibular joint, unspecified side

M26.62 Arthralgia of temporomandibular joint

M26.621 Arthralgia of right temporomandibular joint

M26.622 Arthralgia of left temporomandibular joint

M26.623 Arthralgia of bilateral temporomandibular joint

M26.629 Arthralgia of temporomandibular joint, unspecified side

M26.63 Articular disc disorder of temporomandibular joint

M26.631 Articular disc disorder of right temporomandibular joint

M26.632 Articular disc disorder of left temporomandibular joint

M26.633 Articular disc disorder of bilateral temporomandibular joint

M26.639 Articular disc disorder of temporomandibular joint, unspecified side

M26.69 Other specified disorders of temporomandibular joint

M26.7 Dental alveolar anomalies

M26.70 Unspecified alveolar anomaly

M26.71 Alveolar maxillary hyperplasia

M26.72 Alveolar mandibular hyperplasia

M26.73 Alveolar maxillary hypoplasia

M26.74 Alveolar mandibular hypoplasia

M26.79 Other specified alveolar anomalies

M26.8 Other dentofacial anomalies

M26.81 Anterior soft tissue impingement

Anterior soft tissue impingement on teeth

M26.82 Posterior soft tissue impingement

Posterior soft tissue impingement on teeth

M26.89 Other dentofacial anomalies

M26.9 Dentofacial anomaly, unspecified

M27 Other diseases of jaws

M27.0 Developmental disorders of jaws

Latent bone cyst of jaw

Stafne's cyst

Torus mandibularis

Torus palatinus

M27.1 Giant cell granuloma, central

Giant cell granuloma NOS

> **Excludes1:** peripheral giant cell granuloma (K06.8)

M27.2 Inflammatory conditions of jaws

Osteitis of jaw(s)

Osteomyelitis (neonatal) jaw(s)

Osteoradionecrosis jaw(s)

Periostitis jaw(s)

Sequestrum of jaw bone

> **Use additional code** (W88-W90, X39.0) to identify radiation, if radiation-induced
>
> **Excludes2:** osteonecrosis of jaw due to drug (M87.180)

M27.3 Alveolitis of jaws

Alveolar osteitis

Dry socket

M27.4 Other and unspecified cysts of jaw

> **Excludes1:** cysts of oral region (K09.-)
>
> latent bone cyst of jaw (M27.0)
>
> Stafne's cyst (M27.0)

M27.40 Unspecified cyst of jaw

Cyst of jaw NOS

M27.49 Other cysts of jaw

Aneurysmal cyst of jaw

Hemorrhagic cyst of jaw

Traumatic cyst of jaw

M27.5 **Periradicular pathology associated with previous endodontic treatment**

    M27.51 **Perforation of root canal space due to endodontic treatment**

    M27.52 **Endodontic overfill**

    M27.53 **Endodontic underfill**

    M27.59 **Other periradicular pathology associated with previous endodontic treatment**

M27.6 **Endosseous dental implant failure**

    M27.61 **Osseointegration failure of dental implant**

    Hemorrhagic complications of dental implant placement

    Iatrogenic osseointegration failure of dental implant

    Osseointegration failure of dental implant due to complications of systemic disease

    Osseointegration failure of dental implant due to poor bone quality

    Pre-integration failure of dental implant NOS

    Pre-osseointegration failure of dental implant

    M27.62 **Post-osseointegration biological failure of dental implant**

    Failure of dental implant due to lack of attached gingiva

    Failure of dental implant due to occlusal trauma (caused by poor prosthetic design)

    Failure of dental implant due to parafunctional habits

    Failure of dental implant due to periodontal infection (peri-implantitis)

    Failure of dental implant due to poor oral hygiene

    Iatrogenic post-osseointegration failure of dental implant

    Post-osseointegration failure of dental implant due to complications of systemic disease

    M27.63 **Post-osseointegration mechanical failure of dental implant**

    Failure of dental prosthesis causing loss of dental implant

    Fracture of dental implant

    Excludes2: cracked tooth (K03.81)

        fractured dental restorative material with loss of material (K08.531)

        fractured dental restorative material without loss of material (K08.530)

        fractured tooth (S02.5)

    M27.69 **Other endosseous dental implant failure**

    Dental implant failure NOS

M27.8 **Other specified diseases of jaws**

Cherubism

Exostosis

Fibrous dysplasia

Unilateral condylar hyperplasia

Unilateral condylar hypoplasia

Excludes1: jaw pain (R68.84)

M27.9 **Disease of jaws, unspecified**

SYSTEMIC CONNECTIVE TISSUE DISORDERS (M30-M36)

Includes: autoimmune disease NOS

collagen (vascular) disease NOS

systemic autoimmune disease systemic collagen (vascular) disease

Excludes1: autoimmune disease, single organ or single cell-type -code to relevant condition category

M30 **Polyarteritis nodosa and related conditions**

    Excludes1: microscopic polyarteritis (M31.7)

M30.0 **Polyarteritis nodosa**

M30.1 **Polyarteritis with lung involvement [Churg-Strauss]**

Allergic granulomatous angiitis

M30.2 **Juvenile polyarteritis**

M30.3 **Mucocutaneous lymph node syndrome [Kawasaki]**

M30.8 **Other conditions related to polyarteritis nodosa**

Polyangiitis overlap syndrome

M31 **Other necrotizing vasculopathies**

M31.0 **Hypersensitivity angiitis**

Goodpasture's syndrome

M31.1 **Thrombotic microangiopathy**

Thrombotic thrombocytopenic purpura

M31.2 **Lethal midline granuloma**

M31.3 **Wegener's granulomatosis**

Necrotizing respiratory granulomatosis

    M31.30 **Wegener's granulomatosis without renal involvement**

    Wegener's granulomatosis NOS

    M31.31 **Wegener's granulomatosis with renal involvement**

M31.4 **Aortic arch syndrome [Takayasu]**

M31.5 **Giant cell arteritis with polymyalgia rheumatica**

M31.6 **Other giant cell arteritis**

M31.7 **Microscopic polyangiitis**

Microscopic polyarteritis

    Excludes1: polyarteritis nodosa (M30.0)

M31.8 **Other specified necrotizing vasculopathies**

Hypocomplementemic vasculitis

Septic vasculitis

M31.9 **Necrotizing vasculopathy, unspecified**

M32 **Systemic lupus erythematosus (SLE)**

    Excludes1: lupus erythematosus (discoid) (NOS) (L93.0)

M32.0 **Drug-induced systemic lupus erythematosus**

    Use additional code for adverse effect, if applicable, to identify drug (T36-T50 with fifth or sixth character 5)

M32.1 **Systemic lupus erythematosus with organ or system involvement**

    M32.10 **Systemic lupus erythematosus, organ or system involvement unspecified**

    M32.11 **Endocarditis in systemic lupus erythematosus**

    Libman-Sacks disease

    M32.12 **Pericarditis in systemic lupus erythematosus**

    Lupus pericarditis

    M32.13 **Lung involvement in systemic lupus erythematosus**

    Pleural effusion due to systemic lupus erythematosus

    M32.14 **Glomerular disease in systemic lupus erythematosus**

    Lupus renal disease NOS

    M32.15 **Tubulo-interstitial nephropathy in systemic lupus erythematosus**

    M32.19 **Other organ or system involvement in systemic lupus erythematosus**

  ● New code ▲ Revised code **Excludes1:** Not coded here **Excludes2:** Not included here ⊗ Placeholder required ⑦7ᵗʰ digit required

M32.8   Other forms of systemic lupus erythematosus

M32.9   Systemic lupus erythematosus, unspecified

     SLE NOS

     Systemic lupus erythematosus NOS

     Systemic lupus erythematosus without organ involvement

M33   **Dermatopolymyositis**

▲**M33.0**   **Juvenile dermatomyositis**

     ▲**M33.00**   Juvenile dermatomyositis, organ involvement unspecified

     ▲**M33.01**   Juvenile dermatomyositis with respiratory involvement

     ▲**M33.02**   Juvenile dermatomyositis with myopathy

     ▲**M33.09**   Juvenile dermatomyositis with other organ involvement

M33.1   **Other dermatomyositis**

     ▲**M33.10**   Other dermatomyositis, organ involvement unspecified

     ▲**M33.11**   Other dermatomyositis with respiratory involvement

     ▲**M33.12**   Other dermatomyositis with myopathy

     ▲**M33.19**   Other dermatomyositis with other organ involvement

M33.2   **Polymyositis**

     M33.20   Polymyositis, organ involvement unspecified

     M33.21   Polymyositis with respiratory involvement

     M33.22   Polymyositis with myopathy

     M33.29   Polymyositis with other organ involvement

M33.9   **Dermatopolymyositis, unspecified**

     M33.90   Dermatopolymyositis, unspecified, organ involvement unspecified

     M33.91   Dermatopolymyositis, unspecified with respiratory involvement

     M33.92   Dermatopolymyositis, unspecified with myopathy

     ●**M33.93**   Dermatopolymyositis, unspecified without myopathy

     M33.99   Dermatopolymyositis, unspecified with other organ involvement

M34   **Systemic sclerosis [scleroderma]**

Excludes1: circumscribed scleroderma (L94.0)

     neonatal scleroderma (P83.8)

M34.0   **Progressive systemic sclerosis**

M34.1   **CR(E)ST syndrome**

     Combination of calcinosis, Raynaud's phenomenon, esophageal dysfunction, sclerodactyly, telangiectasia

M34.2   **Systemic sclerosis induced by drug and chemical**

     Code first poisoning due to drug or toxin, if applicable (T36-T65 with fifth or sixth character 1-4 or 6)

     Use additional code for adverse effect, if applicable, to identify drug (T36-T50 with fifth or sixth character 5)

M34.8   **Other forms of systemic sclerosis**

     M34.81   Systemic sclerosis with lung involvement

     M34.82   Systemic sclerosis with myopathy

     M34.83   Systemic sclerosis with polyneuropathy

     M34.89   Other systemic sclerosis

M34.9   **Systemic sclerosis, unspecified**

M35   **Other systemic involvement of connective tissue**

Excludes1: reactive perforating collagenosis (L87.1)

M35.0   **Sicca syndrome [Sjögren]**

     M35.00   Sicca syndrome, unspecified

     M35.01   Sicca syndrome with keratoconjunctivitis

     M35.02   Sicca syndrome with lung involvement

     M35.03   Sicca syndrome with myopathy

     M35.04   Sicca syndrome with tubulo-interstitial nephropathy

         Renal tubular acidosis in sicca syndrome

     M35.09   Sicca syndrome with other organ involvement

M35.1   **Other overlap syndromes**

     Mixed connective tissue disease

     Excludes1: polyangiitis overlap syndrome (M30.8)

M35.2   **Behçet's disease**

M35.3   **Polymyalgia rheumatica**

     Definition: Polymyalgia rheumatica is a rheumatic disorder that is associated with moderate to severe muscle pain and stiffness in the neck, shoulder and hip areas.

     Excludes1: polymyalgia rheumatica with giant cell arteritis (M31.5)

M35.4   **Diffuse (eosinophilic) fasciitis**

M35.5   **Multifocal fibrosclerosis**

M35.6   **Relapsing panniculitis [Weber-Christian]**

     Excludes1: lupus panniculitis (L93.2)

         panniculitis NOS (M79.3-)

M35.7   **Hypermobility syndrome**

     Familial ligamentous laxity

     Excludes1: Ehlers-Danlos syndrome (Q79.6)

         ligamentous laxity, NOS (M24.2-)

M35.8   **Other specified systemic involvement of connective tissue**

M35.9   **Systemic involvement of connective tissue, unspecified**

     Autoimmune disease (systemic) NOS

     Collagen (vascular) disease NOS

M36   **Systemic disorders of connective tissue in diseases classified elsewhere**

Excludes2: arthropathies in diseases classified elsewhere (M14.-)

M36.0   **Dermato(poly)myositis in neoplastic disease**

     Code first underlying neoplasm (C00-D49)

M36.1   **Arthropathy in neoplastic disease**

     Code first underlying neoplasm, such as:

         leukemia (C91-C95)

         malignant histiocytosis (C96.A)

         multiple myeloma (C90.0)

M36.2   **Hemophilic arthropathy**

     Hemarthrosis in hemophilic arthropathy

     Code first underlying disease, such as:

         factor VIII deficiency (D66)

         with vascular defect (D68.0)

         factor IX deficiency (D67)

         hemophilia (classical) (D66)

         hemophilia B (D67)

         hemophilia C (D68.1)

M36.3   **Arthropathy in other blood disorders**

M36.4   **Arthropathy in hypersensitivity reactions classified elsewhere**

     Code first underlying disease, such as:

         Henoch (-Schönlein) purpura (D69.0)

         serum sickness (T80.6-)

M36.8   **Systemic disorders of connective tissue in other diseases classified elsewhere**

Code first underlying disease, such as:

    alkaptonuria (E70.2)

    hypogammaglobulinemia (D80.-)

    ochronosis (E70.2)

DORSOPATHIES (M40-M54)
Deforming dorsopathies (M40-M43)

M40   **Kyphosis and lordosis**

    Excludes1: congenital kyphosis and lordosis (Q76.4)

        kyphoscoliosis (M41.-)

        postprocedural kyphosis and lordosis (M96.-)

    M40.0   **Postural kyphosis**

        Excludes1: osteochondrosis of spine (M42.-)

        M40.00   **Postural kyphosis, site unspecified**

        M40.03   **Postural kyphosis, cervicothoracic region**

        M40.04   **Postural kyphosis, thoracic region**

        M40.05   **Postural kyphosis, thoracolumbar region**

    M40.1   **Other secondary kyphosis**

        M40.10   **Other secondary kyphosis, site unspecified**

        M40.12   **Other secondary kyphosis, cervical region**

        M40.13   **Other secondary kyphosis, cervicothoracic region**

        M40.14   **Other secondary kyphosis, thoracic region**

        M40.15   **Other secondary kyphosis, thoracolumbar region**

    M40.2   **Other and unspecified kyphosis**

        M40.20   **Unspecified kyphosis**

            M40.202   **Unspecified kyphosis, cervical region**

            M40.203   **Unspecified kyphosis, cervicothoracic region**

            M40.204   **Unspecified kyphosis, thoracic region**

            M40.205   **Unspecified kyphosis, thoracolumbar region**

            M40.209   **Unspecified kyphosis, site unspecified**

        M40.29   **Other kyphosis**

            M40.292   **Other kyphosis, cervical region**

            M40.293   **Other kyphosis, cervicothoracic region**

            M40.294   **Other kyphosis, thoracic region**

            M40.295   **Other kyphosis, thoracolumbar region**

            M40.299   **Other kyphosis, site unspecified**

    M40.3   **Flatback syndrome**

        M40.30   **Flatback syndrome, site unspecified**

        M40.35   **Flatback syndrome, thoracolumbar region**

        M40.36   **Flatback syndrome, lumbar region**

        M40.37   **Flatback syndrome, lumbosacral region**

    M40.4   **Postural lordosis**

        Acquired lordosis

        M40.40   **Postural lordosis, site unspecified**

        M40.45   **Postural lordosis, thoracolumbar region**

        M40.46   **Postural lordosis, lumbar region**

        M40.47   **Postural lordosis, lumbosacral region**

    M40.5   **Lordosis, unspecified**

        M40.50   **Lordosis, unspecified, site unspecified**

        M40.55   **Lordosis, unspecified, thoracolumbar region**

        M40.56   **Lordosis, unspecified, lumbar region**

        M40.57   **Lordosis, unspecified, lumbosacral region**

M41   **Scoliosis**

    Includes: kyphoscoliosis

    Excludes1: congenital scoliosis NOS (Q67.5)

        congenital scoliosis due to bony malformation (Q76.3)

        postural congenital scoliosis (Q67.5)

        kyphoscoliotic heart disease (I27.1)

        postprocedural scoliosis (M96.-)

    M41.0   **Infantile idiopathic scoliosis**

        M41.00   **Infantile idiopathic scoliosis, site unspecified**

        M41.02   **Infantile idiopathic scoliosis, cervical region**

        M41.03   **Infantile idiopathic scoliosis, cervicothoracic region**

        M41.04   **Infantile idiopathic scoliosis, thoracic region**

        M41.05   **Infantile idiopathic scoliosis, thoracolumbar region**

        M41.06   **Infantile idiopathic scoliosis, lumbar region**

        M41.07   **Infantile idiopathic scoliosis, lumbosacral region**

        M41.08   **Infantile idiopathic scoliosis, sacral and sacrococcygeal region**

    M41.1   **Juvenile and adolescent idiopathic scoliosis**

        M41.11   **Juvenile idiopathic scoliosis**

            M41.112   **Juvenile idiopathic scoliosis, cervical region**

            M41.113   **Juvenile idiopathic scoliosis, cervicothoracic region**

            M41.114   **Juvenile idiopathic scoliosis, thoracic region**

            M41.115   **Juvenile idiopathic scoliosis, thoracolumbar region**

            M41.116   **Juvenile idiopathic scoliosis, lumbar region**

            M41.117   **Juvenile idiopathic scoliosis, lumbosacral region**

            M41.119   **Juvenile idiopathic scoliosis, site unspecified**

        M41.12   **Adolescent scoliosis**

            M41.122   **Adolescent idiopathic scoliosis, cervical region**

            M41.123   **Adolescent idiopathic scoliosis, cervicothoracic region**

            M41.124   **Adolescent idiopathic scoliosis, thoracic region**

            M41.125   **Adolescent idiopathic scoliosis, thoracolumbar region**

            M41.126   **Adolescent idiopathic scoliosis, lumbar region**

            M41.127   **Adolescent idiopathic scoliosis, lumbosacral region**

            M41.129   **Adolescent idiopathic scoliosis, site unspecified**

    M41.2   **Other idiopathic scoliosis**

        M41.20   **Other idiopathic scoliosis, site unspecified**

        M41.22   **Other idiopathic scoliosis, cervical region**

        M41.23   **Other idiopathic scoliosis, cervicothoracic region**

        M41.24   **Other idiopathic scoliosis, thoracic region**

        M41.25   **Other idiopathic scoliosis, thoracolumbar region**

        M41.26   **Other idiopathic scoliosis, lumbar region**

   ● New code   ▲ Revised code   **Excludes1:** Not coded here   **Excludes2:** Not included here   ⊗ Placeholder required   ⑦ 7th digit required

M41.27 **Other idiopathic scoliosis, lumbosacral region**

M41.3 Thoracogenic scoliosis

M41.30 **Thoracogenic scoliosis, site unspecified**

M41.34 **Thoracogenic scoliosis, thoracic region**

M41.35 **Thoracogenic scoliosis, thoracolumbar region**

M41.4 Neuromuscular scoliosis

Scoliosis secondary to cerebral palsy, Friedreich's ataxia, poliomyelitis **and other** neuromuscular disorders

<u>Code also</u> underlying condition

M41.40 **Neuromuscular scoliosis, site unspecified**

M41.41 **Neuromuscular scoliosis, occipito-atlanto-axial region**

M41.42 **Neuromuscular scoliosis, cervical region**

M41.43 **Neuromuscular scoliosis, cervicothoracic region**

M41.44 **Neuromuscular scoliosis, thoracic region**

M41.45 **Neuromuscular scoliosis, thoracolumbar region**

M41.46 **Neuromuscular scoliosis, lumbar region**

M41.47 **Neuromuscular scoliosis, lumbosacral region**

M41.5 Other secondary scoliosis

M41.50 **Other secondary scoliosis, site unspecified**

M41.52 **Other secondary scoliosis, cervical region**

M41.53 **Other secondary scoliosis, cervicothoracic region**

M41.54 **Other secondary scoliosis, thoracic region**

M41.55 **Other secondary scoliosis, thoracolumbar region**

M41.56 **Other secondary scoliosis, lumbar region**

M41.57 **Other secondary scoliosis, lumbosacral region**

M41.8 Other forms of scoliosis

M41.80 **Other forms of scoliosis, site unspecified**

M41.82 **Other forms of scoliosis, cervical region**

M41.83 **Other forms of scoliosis, cervicothoracic region**

M41.84 **Other forms of scoliosis, thoracic region**

M41.85 **Other forms of scoliosis, thoracolumbar region**

M41.86 **Other forms of scoliosis, lumbar region**

M41.87 **Other forms of scoliosis, lumbosacral region**

M41.9 Scoliosis, unspecified

M42 Spinal osteochondrosis

M42.0 Juvenile osteochondrosis of spine

Calvé's disease

Scheuermann's disease

Excludes1: postural kyphosis (M40.0)

M42.00 **Juvenile osteochondrosis of spine, site unspecified**

M42.01 **Juvenile osteochondrosis of spine, occipito-atlanto-axial region**

M42.02 **Juvenile osteochondrosis of spine, cervical region**

M42.03 **Juvenile osteochondrosis of spine, cervicothoracic region**

M42.04 **Juvenile osteochondrosis of spine, thoracic region**

M42.05 **Juvenile osteochondrosis of spine, thoracolumbar region**

M42.06 **Juvenile osteochondrosis of spine, lumbar region**

M42.07 **Juvenile osteochondrosis of spine, lumbosacral region**

M42.08 **Juvenile osteochondrosis of spine, sacral and sacrococcygeal region**

M42.09 **Juvenile osteochondrosis of spine, multiple sites in spine**

M42.1 Adult osteochondrosis of spine

M42.10 **Adult osteochondrosis of spine, site unspecified**

M42.11 **Adult osteochondrosis of spine, occipito-atlanto-axial region**

M42.12 **Adult osteochondrosis of spine, cervical region**

M42.13 **Adult osteochondrosis of spine, cervicothoracic region**

M42.14 **Adult osteochondrosis of spine, thoracic region**

M42.15 **Adult osteochondrosis of spine, thoracolumbar region**

M42.16 **Adult osteochondrosis of spine, lumbar region**

M42.17 **Adult osteochondrosis of spine, lumbosacral region**

M42.18 **Adult osteochondrosis of spine, sacral and sacrococcygeal region**

M42.19 **Adult osteochondrosis of spine, multiple sites in spine**

M42.9 Spinal osteochondrosis, unspecified

M43 Other deforming dorsopathies

Excludes1: congenital spondylolysis and spondylolisthesis (Q76.2)

hemivertebra (Q76.3-Q76.4)

Klippel-Feil syndrome (Q76.1)

lumbarization and sacralization (Q76.4)

platyspondylisis (Q76.4)

spina bifida occulta (Q76.0)

spinal curvature in osteoporosis (M80.-)

spinal curvature in

Paget's disease of bone [osteitis deformans] (M88.-)

M43.0 Spondylolysis

Excludes1: congenital spondylolysis (Q76.2)

spondylolisthesis (M43.1)

M43.00 **Spondylolysis, site unspecified**

M43.01 **Spondylolysis, occipito-atlanto-axial region**

M43.02 **Spondylolysis, cervical region**

M43.03 **Spondylolysis, cervicothoracic region**

M43.04 **Spondylolysis, thoracic region**

M43.05 **Spondylolysis, thoracolumbar region**

M43.06 **Spondylolysis, lumbar region**

M43.07 **Spondylolysis, lumbosacral region**

M43.08 **Spondylolysis, sacral and sacrococcygeal region**

M43.09 **Spondylolysis, multiple sites in spine**

M43.1 Spondylolisthesis

Excludes1: acute traumatic of lumbosacral region (S33.1)

acute traumatic of sites other than lumbosacral-code to Fracture, vertebra, by region congenital spondylolisthesis (Q76.2)

M43.10 **Spondylolisthesis, site unspecified**

M43.11 **Spondylolisthesis, occipito-atlanto-axial region**

M43.12 **Spondylolisthesis, cervical region**

M43.13 **Spondylolisthesis, cervicothoracic region**

M43.14 **Spondylolisthesis, thoracic region**

M43.15 **Spondylolisthesis, thoracolumbar region**

M43.16 **Spondylolisthesis, lumbar region**

M43.17 **Spondylolisthesis, lumbosacral region**

M43.18 **Spondylolisthesis, sacral and sacrococcygeal region**

M43.19 **Spondylolisthesis, multiple sites in spine**

M43.2 **Fusion of spine**

Ankylosis of spinal joint

Excludes1: ankylosing spondylitis (M45.0-)

congenital fusion of spine (Q76.4)

Excludes2: arthrodesis status (Z98.1)

pseudoarthrosis after fusion or arthrodesis (M96.0)

M43.20 **Fusion of spine, site unspecified**

M43.21 **Fusion of spine, occipito-atlanto-axial region**

M43.22 **Fusion of spine, cervical region**

M43.23 **Fusion of spine, cervicothoracic region**

M43.24 **Fusion of spine, thoracic region**

M43.25 **Fusion of spine, thoracolumbar region**

M43.26 **Fusion of spine, lumbar region**

M43.27 **Fusion of spine, lumbosacral region**

M43.28 **Fusion of spine, sacral and sacrococcygeal region**

M43.3 **Recurrent atlantoaxial dislocation with myelopathy**

M43.4 **Other recurrent atlantoaxial dislocation**

M43.5 **Other recurrent vertebral dislocation**

Excludes1: biomechanical lesions NEC (M99.-)

M43.5X **Other recurrent vertebral dislocation**

M43.5X2 **Other recurrent vertebral dislocation, cervical region**

M43.5X3 **Other recurrent vertebral dislocation, cervicothoracic region**

M43.5X4 **Other recurrent vertebral dislocation, thoracic region**

M43.5X5 **Other recurrent vertebral dislocation, thoracolumbar region**

M43.5X6 **Other recurrent vertebral dislocation, lumbar region**

M43.5X7 **Other recurrent vertebral dislocation, lumbosacral region**

M43.5X8 **Other recurrent vertebral dislocation, sacral and sacrococcygeal region**

M43.5X9 **Other recurrent vertebral dislocation, site unspecified**

M43.6 **Torticollis**

Excludes1: congenital (sternomastoid) torticollis (Q68.0)

current injury - see Injury, of spine, by body region ocular torticollis (R29.891)

psychogenic torticollis (F45.8)

spasmodic torticollis (G24.3)

torticollis due to birth injury (P15.2)

M43.8 **Other specified deforming dorsopathies**

Excludes2: kyphosis and lordosis (M40.-)

scoliosis (M41.-)

M43.8X **Other specified deforming dorsopathies**

M43.8X1 **Other specified deforming dorsopathies, occipito-atlanto-axial region**

M43.8X2 **Other specified deforming dorsopathies, cervical region**

M43.8X3 **Other specified deforming dorsopathies, cervicothoracic region**

M43.8X4 **Other specified deforming dorsopathies, thoracic region**

M43.8X5 **Other specified deforming dorsopathies, thoracolumbar region**

M43.8X6 **Other specified deforming dorsopathies, lumbar region**

M43.8X7 **Other specified deforming dorsopathies, lumbosacral region**

M43.8X8 **Other specified deforming dorsopathies, sacral and sacrococcygeal region**

M43.8X9 **Other specified deforming dorsopathies, site unspecified**

M43.9 **Deforming dorsopathy, unspecified**

Curvature of spine NOS

SPONDYLOPATHIES (M45-M49)

M45 **Ankylosing spondylitis**

Definition: Ankylosing spondylitis is a long-term disease that causes inflammation of the joints between the spinal bones and the joints between the spine and the pelvis. It eventually causes the affected spinal bones to join together.

Rheumatoid arthritis of spine

Excludes1: arthropathy in Reiter's disease (M02.3-)

juvenile (ankylosing) spondylitis (M08.1)

Excludes2: Behçet's disease (M35.2)

M45.0 **Ankylosing spondylitis of multiple sites in spine**

M45.1 **Ankylosing spondylitis of occipito-atlanto-axial region**

M45.2 **Ankylosing spondylitis of cervical region**

M45.3 **Ankylosing spondylitis of cervicothoracic region**

M45.4 **Ankylosing spondylitis of thoracic region**

M45.5 **Ankylosing spondylitis of thoracolumbar region**

M45.6 **Ankylosing spondylitis lumbar region**

M45.7 **Ankylosing spondylitis of lumbosacral region**

M45.8 **Ankylosing spondylitis sacral and sacrococcygeal region**

M45.9 **Ankylosing spondylitis of unspecified sites in spine**

M46 **Other inflammatory spondylopathies**

M46.0 **Spinal enthesopathy**

Definition: Enthesopathies are disorders of peripheral ligamentous or muscular attachments, abnormalities in the zones of attachment, for ligaments and tendons to bone.

Disorder of ligamentous or muscular attachments of spine

M46.00 **Spinal enthesopathy, site unspecified**

M46.01 **Spinal enthesopathy, occipito-atlanto-axial region**

M46.02 **Spinal enthesopathy, cervical region**

M46.03 **Spinal enthesopathy, cervicothoracic region**

M46.04 **Spinal enthesopathy, thoracic region**

M46.05 **Spinal enthesopathy, thoracolumbar region**

M46.06 **Spinal enthesopathy, lumbar region**

M46.07 **Spinal enthesopathy, lumbosacral region**

M46.08 **Spinal enthesopathy, sacral and sacrococcygeal region**

M46.09 **Spinal enthesopathy, multiple sites in spine**

M46.1 **Sacroiliitis, not elsewhere classified**

M46.2 **Osteomyelitis of vertebra**

Definition: Osteomyelitis is an inflammation of bone and bone marrow (usually caused by bacterial infection).

M46.20 **Osteomyelitis of vertebra, site unspecified**

M46.21 **Osteomyelitis of vertebra, occipito-atlanto-axial region**

M46.22 **Osteomyelitis of vertebra, cervical region**

M46.23 **Osteomyelitis of vertebra, cervicothoracic region**

M46.24 **Osteomyelitis of vertebra, thoracic region**

● New code   ▲ Revised code   **Excludes1:** Not coded here   **Excludes2:** Not included here   ⊗ Placeholder required   ⑦ 7th digit required

M46.25 Osteomyelitis of vertebra, thoracolumbar region

M46.26 Osteomyelitis of vertebra, lumbar region

M46.27 Osteomyelitis of vertebra, lumbosacral region

M46.28 Osteomyelitis of vertebra, sacral and sacrococcygeal region

M46.3 Infection of intervertebral disc (pyogenic)

Use additional code (B95-B97) to identify infectious agent.

M46.30 Infection of intervertebral disc (pyogenic), site unspecified

M46.31 Infection of intervertebral disc (pyogenic), occipito-atlanto-axial region

M46.32 Infection of intervertebral disc (pyogenic), cervical region

M46.33 Infection of intervertebral disc (pyogenic), cervicothoracic region

M46.34 Infection of intervertebral disc (pyogenic), thoracic region

M46.35 Infection of intervertebral disc (pyogenic), thoracolumbar region

M46.36 Infection of intervertebral disc (pyogenic), lumbar region

M46.37 Infection of intervertebral disc (pyogenic), lumbosacral region

M46.38 Infection of intervertebral disc (pyogenic), sacral and sacrococcygeal region

M46.39 Infection of intervertebral disc (pyogenic), multiple sites in spine

M46.4 Discitis, unspecified

M46.40 Discitis, unspecified, site unspecified

M46.41 Discitis, unspecified, occipito-atlanto-axial region

M46.42 Discitis, unspecified, cervical region

M46.43 Discitis, unspecified, cervicothoracic region

M46.44 Discitis, unspecified, thoracic region

M46.45 Discitis, unspecified, thoracolumbar region

M46.46 Discitis, unspecified, lumbar region

M46.47 Discitis, unspecified, lumbosacral region

M46.48 Discitis, unspecified, sacral and sacrococcygeal region

M46.49 Discitis, unspecified, multiple sites in spine

M46.5 Other infective spondylopathies

M46.50 Other infective spondylopathies, site unspecified

M46.51 Other infective spondylopathies, occipito-atlanto-axial region

M46.52 Other infective spondylopathies, cervical region

M46.53 Other infective spondylopathies, cervicothoracic region

M46.54 Other infective spondylopathies, thoracic region

M46.55 Other infective spondylopathies, thoracolumbar region

M46.56 Other infective spondylopathies, lumbar region

M46.57 Other infective spondylopathies, lumbosacral region

M46.58 Other infective spondylopathies, sacral and sacrococcygeal region

M46.59 Other infective spondylopathies, multiple sites in spine

M46.8 Other specified inflammatory spondylopathies

M46.80 Other specified inflammatory spondylopathies, site unspecified

M46.81 Other specified inflammatory spondylopathies, occipito-atlanto-axial region

M46.82 Other specified inflammatory spondylopathies, cervical region

M46.83 Other specified inflammatory spondylopathies, cervicothoracic region

M46.84 Other specified inflammatory spondylopathies, thoracic region

M46.85 Other specified inflammatory spondylopathies, thoracolumbar region

M46.86 Other specified inflammatory spondylopathies, lumbar region

M46.87 Other specified inflammatory spondylopathies, lumbosacral region

M46.88 Other specified inflammatory spondylopathies, sacral and sacrococcygeal region

M46.89 Other specified inflammatory spondylopathies, multiple sites in spine

M46.9 Unspecified inflammatory spondylopathy

M46.90 Unspecified inflammatory spondylopathy, site unspecified

M46.91 Unspecified inflammatory spondylopathy, occipito-atlanto-axial region

M46.92 Unspecified inflammatory spondylopathy, cervical region

M46.93 Unspecified inflammatory spondylopathy, cervicothoracic region

M46.94 Unspecified inflammatory spondylopathy, thoracic region

M46.95 Unspecified inflammatory spondylopathy, thoracolumbar region

M46.96 Unspecified inflammatory spondylopathy, lumbar region

M46.97 Unspecified inflammatory spondylopathy, lumbosacral region

M46.98 Unspecified inflammatory spondylopathy, sacral and sacrococcygeal region

M46.99 Unspecified inflammatory spondylopathy, multiple sites in spine

M47 Spondylosis

Definition: Spondylosis is degenerative arthritis (osteoarthritis) of the spinal vertebra and related tissue.

Includes: arthrosis or osteoarthritis of spine

degeneration of facet joints

M47.0 Anterior spinal and vertebral artery compression syndromes

M47.01 Anterior spinal artery compression syndromes

M47.011 Anterior spinal artery compression syndromes, occipito-atlanto-axial region

M47.012 Anterior spinal artery compression syndromes, cervical region

M47.013 Anterior spinal artery compression syndromes, cervicothoracic region

M47.014 Anterior spinal artery compression syndromes, thoracic region

M47.015 Anterior spinal artery compression syndromes, thoracolumbar region

M47.016 Anterior spinal artery compression syndromes, lumbar region

M47.019 Anterior spinal artery compression syndromes, site unspecified

---

Add 4th-7th digits	Nonspecific code	Unspecified code	Manifestation code	

M47.02 **Vertebral artery compression syndromes**

M47.021 **Vertebral artery compression syndromes, occipito-atlanto-axial region**

M47.022 **Vertebral artery compression syndromes, cervical region**

M47.029 **Vertebral artery compression syndromes, site unspecified**

M47.1 **Other spondylosis with myelopathy**

Spondylogenic compression of spinal cord

Excludes1: vertebral subluxation (M43.3-M43.59)

M47.10 **Other spondylosis with myelopathy, site unspecified**

M47.11 **Other spondylosis with myelopathy, occipito-atlanto-axial region**

M47.12 **Other spondylosis with myelopathy, cervical region**

M47.13 **Other spondylosis with myelopathy, cervicothoracic region**

M47.14 **Other spondylosis with myelopathy, thoracic region**

M47.15 **Other spondylosis with myelopathy, thoracolumbar region**

M47.16 **Other spondylosis with myelopathy, lumbar region**

M47.2 **Other spondylosis with radiculopathy**

M47.20 **Other spondylosis with radiculopathy, site unspecified**

M47.21 **Other spondylosis with radiculopathy, occipito-atlanto-axial region**

M47.22 **Other spondylosis with radiculopathy, cervical region**

M47.23 **Other spondylosis with radiculopathy, cervicothoracic region**

M47.24 **Other spondylosis with radiculopathy, thoracic region**

M47.25 **Other spondylosis with radiculopathy, thoracolumbar region**

M47.26 **Other spondylosis with radiculopathy, lumbar region**

M47.27 **Other spondylosis with radiculopathy, lumbosacral region**

M47.28 **Other spondylosis with radiculopathy, sacral and sacrococcygeal region**

M47.8 **Other spondylosis**

M47.81 **Spondylosis without myelopathy or radiculopathy**

M47.811 **Spondylosis without myelopathy or radiculopathy, occipito-atlanto-axial region**

M47.812 **Spondylosis without myelopathy or radiculopathy, cervical region**

M47.813 **Spondylosis without myelopathy or radiculopathy, cervicothoracic region**

M47.814 **Spondylosis without myelopathy or radiculopathy, thoracic region**

M47.815 **Spondylosis without myelopathy or radiculopathy, thoracolumbar region**

M47.816 **Spondylosis without myelopathy or radiculopathy, lumbar region**

M47.817 **Spondylosis without myelopathy or radiculopathy, lumbosacral region**

M47.818 **Spondylosis without myelopathy or radiculopathy, sacral and sacrococcygeal region**

M47.819 **Spondylosis without myelopathy or radiculopathy, site unspecified**

M47.89 **Other spondylosis**

M47.891 **Other spondylosis, occipito-atlanto-axial region**

M47.892 **Other spondylosis, cervical region**

M47.893 **Other spondylosis, cervicothoracic region**

M47.894 **Other spondylosis, thoracic region**

M47.895 **Other spondylosis, thoracolumbar region**

M47.896 **Other spondylosis, lumbar region**

M47.897 **Other spondylosis, lumbosacral region**

M47.898 **Other spondylosis, sacral and sacrococcygeal region**

M47.899 **Other spondylosis, site unspecified**

M47.9 **Spondylosis, unspecified**

M48 **Other spondylopathies**

M48.0 **Spinal stenosis**

Caudal stenosis

M48.00 **Spinal stenosis, site unspecified**

M48.01 **Spinal stenosis, occipito-atlanto-axial region**

M48.02 **Spinal stenosis, cervical region**

M48.03 **Spinal stenosis, cervicothoracic region**

M48.04 **Spinal stenosis, thoracic region**

M48.05 **Spinal stenosis, thoracolumbar region**

M48.06 **Spinal stenosis, lumbar region**

●M48.061 **Spinal stenosis, lumbar region without neurogenic claudication**

Spinal stenosis, lumbar region NOS

●M48.062 **Spinal stenosis, lumbar region with neurogenic claudication**

M48.07 **Spinal stenosis, lumbosacral region**

M48.08 **Spinal stenosis, sacral and sacrococcygeal region**

M48.1 **Ankylosing hyperostosis [Forestier]**

Diffuse idiopathic skeletal hyperostosis [DISH]

M48.10 **Ankylosing hyperostosis [Forestier], site unspecified**

M48.11 **Ankylosing hyperostosis [Forestier], occipito-atlanto-axial region**

M48.12 **Ankylosing hyperostosis [Forestier], cervical region**

M48.13 **Ankylosing hyperostosis [Forestier], cervicothoracic region**

M48.14 **Ankylosing hyperostosis [Forestier], thoracic region**

M48.15 **Ankylosing hyperostosis [Forestier], thoracolumbar region**

M48.16 **Ankylosing hyperostosis [Forestier], lumbar region**

M48.17 **Ankylosing hyperostosis [Forestier], lumbosacral region**

M48.18 **Ankylosing hyperostosis [Forestier], sacral and sacrococcygeal region**

M48.19 **Ankylosing hyperostosis [Forestier], multiple sites in spine**

M48.2 **Kissing spine**

M48.20 **Kissing spine, site unspecified**

● New code ▲ Revised code Excludes1: Not coded here Excludes2: Not included here ⊗ Placeholder required ⑦7th digit required

M48.21 Kissing spine, occipito-atlanto-axial region

M48.22 Kissing spine, cervical region

M48.23 Kissing spine, cervicothoracic region

M48.24 Kissing spine, thoracic region

M48.25 Kissing spine, thoracolumbar region

M48.26 Kissing spine, lumbar region

M48.27 Kissing spine, lumbosacral region

M48.3 Traumatic spondylopathy

M48.30 Traumatic spondylopathy, site unspecified

M48.31 Traumatic spondylopathy, occipito-atlanto-axial region

M48.32 Traumatic spondylopathy, cervical region

M48.33 Traumatic spondylopathy, cervicothoracic region

M48.34 Traumatic spondylopathy, thoracic region

M48.35 Traumatic spondylopathy, thoracolumbar region

M48.36 Traumatic spondylopathy, lumbar region

M48.37 Traumatic spondylopathy, lumbosacral region

M48.38 Traumatic spondylopathy, sacral and sacrococcygeal region

M48.4 Fatigue fracture of vertebra

Stress fracture of vertebra

Excludes1: pathological fracture NOS (M84.4-)

pathological fracture of vertebra due to neoplasm (M84.58)

pathological fracture of vertebra due to other diagnosis (M84.68)

pathological fracture of vertebra due to osteoporosis (M80.-)

traumatic fracture of vertebrae (S12.0-S12.3-, S22.0-, S32.0-)

The appropriate 7th character is to be added to each code from subcategory M48.4:

A - initial encounter for fracture

D - subsequent encounter for fracture with routine healing

G - subsequent encounter for fracture with delayed healing

S - sequela of fracture

⊗⑦M48.40 Fatigue fracture of vertebra, site unspecified

⊗⑦M48.41 Fatigue fracture of vertebra, occipito-atlanto-axial region

⊗⑦M48.42 Fatigue fracture of vertebra, cervical region

⊗⑦M48.43 Fatigue fracture of vertebra, cervicothoracic region

⊗⑦M48.44 Fatigue fracture of vertebra, thoracic region

⊗⑦M48.45 Fatigue fracture of vertebra, thoracolumbar region

⊗⑦M48.46 Fatigue fracture of vertebra, lumbar region

⊗⑦M48.47 Fatigue fracture of vertebra, lumbosacral region

⊗⑦M48.48 Fatigue fracture of vertebra, sacral and sacrococcygeal region

M48.5 Collapsed vertebra, not elsewhere classified

Collapsed vertebra NOS

Compression fracture of vertebra NOS

Wedging of vertebra NOS

Excludes1: current injury - see Injury of spine, by body region

fatigue fracture of vertebra (M48.4)

pathological fracture of vertebra due to neoplasm (M84.58)

pathological fracture of vertebra due to other diagnosis (M84.68)

pathological fracture of vertebra due to osteoporosis (M80.-)

pathological fracture NOS (M84.4-)

stress fracture of vertebra (M48.4-)

traumatic fracture of vertebra (S12.-, S22.-, S32.-)

The appropriate 7th character is to be added to each code from subcategory M48.5:

A - initial encounter for fracture

D - subsequent encounter for fracture with routine healing

G - subsequent encounter for fracture with delayed healing

S - sequela of fracture

⊗⑦M48.50 Collapsed vertebra, not elsewhere classified, site unspecified

⊗⑦M48.51 Collapsed vertebra, not elsewhere classified, occipito-atlanto-axial region

⊗⑦M48.52 Collapsed vertebra, not elsewhere classified, cervical region

⊗⑦M48.53 Collapsed vertebra, not elsewhere classified, cervicothoracic region

⊗⑦M48.54 Collapsed vertebra, not elsewhere classified, thoracic region

⊗⑦M48.55 Collapsed vertebra, not elsewhere classified, thoracolumbar region

⊗⑦M48.56 Collapsed vertebra, not elsewhere classified, lumbar region

⊗⑦M48.57 Collapsed vertebra, not elsewhere classified, lumbosacral region

⊗⑦M48.58 Collapsed vertebra, not elsewhere classified, sacral and sacrococcygeal region

M48.8 Other specified spondylopathies

Ossification of posterior longitudinal ligament

M48.8X Other specified spondylopathies

M48.8X1 Other specified spondylopathies, occipito-atlanto-axial region

M48.8X2 Other specified spondylopathies, cervical region

M48.8X3 Other specified spondylopathies, cervicothoracic region

M48.8X4 Other specified spondylopathies, thoracic region

M48.8X5 Other specified spondylopathies, thoracolumbar region

M48.8X6 Other specified spondylopathies, lumbar region

M48.8X7 Other specified spondylopathies, lumbosacral region

M48.8X8 Other specified spondylopathies, sacral and sacrococcygeal region

M48.8X9 Other specified spondylopathies, site unspecified

M48.9 Spondylopathy, unspecified

M49 Spondylopathies in diseases classified elsewhere

Includes: curvature of spine in diseases classified elsewhere

deformity of spine in diseases classified elsewhere

kyphosis in diseases classified elsewhere

scoliosis in diseases classified elsewhere

spondylopathy in diseases classified elsewhere

Add 4th-7th digits　　Nonspecific code　　Unspecified code　　Manifestation code

Code first underlying disease, such as:

brucellosis (A23.-)

Charcot-Marie-Tooth disease (G60.0)

enterobacterial infections (A01-A04)

osteitis fibrosa cystica (E21.0)

Excludes1: curvature of spine in tuberculosis [Pott's] (A18.01)

enteropathic arthropathies (M07.-)

gonococcal spondylitis (A54.41)

neuropathic [tabes dorsalis] spondylitis (A52.11)

neuropathic spondylopathy in syringomyelia (G95.0)

neuropathic spondylopathy in tabes dorsalis (A52.11)

nonsyphilitic neuropathic spondylopathy NEC (G98.0)

spondylitis in syphilis (acquired) (A52.77)

tuberculous spondylitis (A18.01)

typhoid fever spondylitis (A01.05)

M49.8 Spondylopathy in diseases classified elsewhere

M49.80 Spondylopathy in diseases classified elsewhere, site unspecified

M49.81 Spondylopathy in diseases classified elsewhere, occipito-atlanto-axial region

M49.82 Spondylopathy in diseases classified elsewhere, cervical region

M49.83 Spondylopathy in diseases classified elsewhere, cervicothoracic region

M49.84 Spondylopathy in diseases classified elsewhere, thoracic region

M49.85 Spondylopathy in diseases classified elsewhere, thoracolumbar region

M49.86 Spondylopathy in diseases classified elsewhere, lumbar region

M49.87 Spondylopathy in diseases classified elsewhere, lumbosacral region

M49.88 Spondylopathy in diseases classified elsewhere, sacral and sacrococcygeal region

M49.89 Spondylopathy in diseases classified elsewhere, multiple sites in spine

OTHER DORSOPATHIES (M50-M54)

Excludes1: current injury - see injury of spine by body region

discitis NOS (M46.4-)

M50 Cervical disc disorders

Note: code to the most superior level of disorder

Includes: cervicothoracic disc disorders with cervicalgia

cervicothoracic disc disorders

M50.0 Cervical disc disorder with myelopathy

M50.00 Cervical disc disorder with myelopathy, unspecified cervical region

M50.01 Cervical disc disorder with myelopathy, high cervical region

C2-C3 disc disorder with myelopathy

C3-C4 disc disorder with myelopathy

M50.02 Cervical disc disorder with myelopathy, mid-cervical region

M50.020 Cervical disc disorder with myelopathy, mid-cervical region, unspecified level

M50.021 Cervical disc disorder at C4-C5 level with myelopathy

C4-C5 disc disorder with myelopathy

M50.022 Cervical disc disorder at C5-C6 level with myelopathy

C5-C6 disc disorder with myelopathy

M50.023 Cervical disc disorder at C6-C7 level with myelopathy

C6-C7 disc disorder with myelopathy

M50.03 Cervical disc disorder with myelopathy, cervicothoracic region

C7-T1 disc disorder with myelopathy

M50.1 Cervical disc disorder with radiculopathy

Excludes2: brachial radiculitis NOS (M54.13)

M50.10 Cervical disc disorder with radiculopathy, unspecified cervical region

M50.11 Cervical disc disorder with radiculopathy, high cervical region

C2-C3 disc disorder with radiculopathy

C3 radiculopathy due to disc disorder

C3-C4 disc disorder with radiculopathy

C4 radiculopathy due to disc disorder

M50.12 Cervical disc disorder with radiculopathy, mid-cervical region

M50.120 Mid-cervical disc disorder, unspecified

M50.121 Cervical disc disorder at C4-C5 level with radiculopathy

C4-C5 disc disorder with radiculopathy

C5 radiculopathy due to disc disorder

M50.122 Cervical disc disorder at C5-C6 level with radiculopathy

C5-C6 disc disorder with radiculopathy

C6 radiculopathy due to disc disorder

M50.123 Cervical disc disorder at C6-C7 level with radiculopathy

C6-C7 disc disorder with radiculopathy

C7 radiculopathy due to disc disorder

M50.13 Cervical disc disorder with radiculopathy, cervicothoracic region

C7-T1 disc disorder with radiculopathy

C8 radiculopathy due to disc disorder

M50.2 Other cervical disc displacement

M50.20 Other cervical disc displacement, unspecified cervical region

M50.21 Other cervical disc displacement, high cervical region

Other C2-C3 cervical disc displacement

Other C3-C4 cervical disc displacement

M50.22 Other cervical disc displacement, mid-cervical region

M50.220 Other cervical disc displacement, mid-cervical region, unspecified level

M50.221 Other cervical disc displacement at C4-C5 level

Other C4-C5 cervical disc displacement

M50.222 Other cervical disc displacement at C5-C6 level

Other C5-C6 cervical disc displacement

M50.223 Other cervical disc displacement at C6-C7 level

● New code   ▲ Revised code   Excludes1: Not coded here   Excludes2: Not included here   ⊗ Placeholder required   ⑦7th digit required

Other C6-C7 cervical disc displacement

M50.23 Other cervical disc displacement, cervicothoracic region

Other C7-T1 cervical disc displacement

M50.3 Other cervical disc degeneration

M50.30 Other cervical disc degeneration, unspecified cervical region

M50.31 Other cervical disc degeneration, high cervical region

Other C2-C3 cervical disc degeneration

Other C3-C4 cervical disc degeneration

M50.32 Other cervical disc degeneration, mid-cervical region

M50.320 Other cervical disc degeneration, mid-cervical region, unspecified level

M50.321 Other cervical disc degeneration at C4-C5 level

Other C4-C5 cervical disc degeneration

M50.322 Other cervical disc degeneration at C5-C6 level

Other C5-C6 cervical disc degeneration

M50.323 Other cervical disc degeneration at C6-C7 level

Other C6-C7 cervical disc degeneration

M50.33 Other cervical disc degeneration, cervicothoracic region

Other C7-T1 cervical disc degeneration

M50.8 Other cervical disc disorders

M50.80 Other cervical disc disorders, unspecified cervical region

M50.81 Other cervical disc disorders, high cervical region

Other C2-C3 cervical disc disorders

Other C3-C4 cervical disc disorders

M50.82 Other cervical disc disorders, mid-cervical region

M50.820 Other cervical disc disorders, mid-cervical region, unspecified level

M50.821 Other cervical disc disorders at C4-C5 level

Other C4-C5 cervical disc disorders

M50.822 Other cervical disc disorders at C5-C6 level

Other C5-C6 cervical disc disorders

M50.823 Other cervical disc disorders at C6-C7 level

Other C6-C7 cervical disc disorders

M50.83 Other cervical disc disorders, cervicothoracic region

Other C7-T1 cervical disc disorders

M50.9 Cervical disc disorder, unspecified

M50.90 Cervical disc disorder, unspecified, unspecified cervical region

M50.91 Cervical disc disorder, unspecified, high cervical region

C2-C3 cervical disc disorder, unspecified

C3-C4 cervical disc disorder, unspecified

M50.92 Cervical disc disorder, unspecified, mid-cervical region

M50.920 Unspecified cervical disc disorder, mid-cervical region, unspecified level

M50.921 Unspecified cervical disc disorder at C4-C5 level

Unspecified C4-C5 cervical disc disorder

M50.922 Unspecified cervical disc disorder at C5-C6 level

Unspecified C5-C6 cervical disc disorder

M50.923 Unspecified cervical disc disorder at C6-C7 level

Unspecified C6-C7 cervical disc disorder

M50.93 Cervical disc disorder, unspecified, cervicothoracic region

C7-T1 cervical disc disorder, unspecified

M51 Thoracic, thoracolumbar, and lumbosacral intervertebral disc disorders

Definition: Intervertebral disc disorders result from a protrusion or herniation of one of the gel-like cushions (discs) that separate the vertebrae of the spine.

Excludes2: cervical and cervicothoracic disc disorders (M50.-)

sacral and sacrococcygeal disorders (M53.3)

M51.0 Thoracic, thoracolumbar and lumbosacral intervertebral disc disorders with myelopathy

M51.04 Intervertebral disc disorders with myelopathy, thoracic region

M51.05 Intervertebral disc disorders with myelopathy, thoracolumbar region

M51.06 Intervertebral disc disorders with myelopathy, lumbar region

M51.1 Thoracic, thoracolumbar and lumbosacral intervertebral disc disorders with radiculopathy

Sciatica due to intervertebral disc disorder

Excludes1: lumbar radiculitis NOS (M54.16)

sciatica NOS (M54.3)

M51.14 Intervertebral disc disorders with radiculopathy, thoracic region

M51.15 Intervertebral disc disorders with radiculopathy, thoracolumbar region

M51.16 Intervertebral disc disorders with radiculopathy, lumbar region

M51.17 Intervertebral disc disorders with radiculopathy, lumbosacral region

M51.2 Other thoracic, thoracolumbar and lumbosacral intervertebral disc displacement

Lumbago due to displacement of intervertebral disc

M51.24 Other intervertebral disc displacement, thoracic region

M51.25 Other intervertebral disc displacement, thoracolumbar region

M51.26 Other intervertebral disc displacement, lumbar region

M51.27 Other intervertebral disc displacement, lumbosacral region

M51.3 Other thoracic, thoracolumbar and lumbosacral intervertebral disc degeneration

M51.34 Other intervertebral disc degeneration, thoracic region

M51.35 Other intervertebral disc degeneration, thoracolumbar region

M51.36 Other intervertebral disc degeneration, lumbar region

Add 4th-7th digits　　　Nonspecific code　　　Unspecified code　　　Manifestation code

M51.37 Other intervertebral disc degeneration, lumbosacral region

M51.4 Schmorl's nodes

M51.44 Schmorl's nodes, thoracic region

M51.45 Schmorl's nodes, thoracolumbar region

M51.46 Schmorl's nodes, lumbar region

M51.47 Schmorl's nodes, lumbosacral region

M51.8 Other thoracic, thoracolumbar and lumbosacral intervertebral disc disorders

M51.84 Other intervertebral disc disorders, thoracic region

M51.85 Other intervertebral disc disorders, thoracolumbar region

M51.86 Other intervertebral disc disorders, lumbar region

M51.87 Other intervertebral disc disorders, lumbosacral region

M51.9 Unspecified thoracic, thoracolumbar and lumbosacral intervertebral disc disorder

M53 Other and unspecified dorsopathies, not elsewhere classified

M53.0 Cervicocranial syndrome

Posterior cervical sympathetic syndrome

M53.1 Cervicobrachial syndrome

Excludes2: cervical disc disorder (M50.-)

thoracic outlet syndrome (G54.0)

M53.2 Spinal instabilities

M53.2X Spinal instabilities

M53.2X1 Spinal instabilities, occipito-atlanto-axial region

M53.2X2 Spinal instabilities, cervical region

M53.2X3 Spinal instabilities, cervicothoracic region

M53.2X4 Spinal instabilities, thoracic region

M53.2X5 Spinal instabilities, thoracolumbar region

M53.2X6 Spinal instabilities, lumbar region

M53.2X7 Spinal instabilities, lumbosacral region

M53.2X8 Spinal instabilities, sacral and sacrococcygeal region

M53.2X9 Spinal instabilities, site unspecified

M53.3 Sacrococcygeal disorders, not elsewhere classified

Coccygodynia

M53.8 Other specified dorsopathies

M53.80 Other specified dorsopathies, site unspecified

M53.81 Other specified dorsopathies, occipito-atlanto-axial region

M53.82 Other specified dorsopathies, cervical region

M53.83 Other specified dorsopathies, cervicothoracic region

M53.84 Other specified dorsopathies, thoracic region

M53.85 Other specified dorsopathies, thoracolumbar region

M53.86 Other specified dorsopathies, lumbar region

M53.87 Other specified dorsopathies, lumbosacral region

M53.88 Other specified dorsopathies, sacral and sacrococcygeal region

M53.9 Dorsopathy, unspecified

M54 Dorsalgia

Excludes1: psychogenic dorsalgia (F45.41)

M54.0 Panniculitis affecting regions of neck and back

Excludes1: lupus panniculitis (L93.2)

panniculitis NOS (M79.3)

relapsing [Weber-Christian] panniculitis (M35.6)

M54.00 Panniculitis affecting regions of neck and back, site unspecified

M54.01 Panniculitis affecting regions of neck and back, occipito-atlanto-axial region

M54.02 Panniculitis affecting regions of neck and back, cervical region

M54.03 Panniculitis affecting regions of neck and back, cervicothoracic region

M54.04 Panniculitis affecting regions of neck and back, thoracic region

M54.05 Panniculitis affecting regions of neck and back, thoracolumbar region

M54.06 Panniculitis affecting regions of neck and back, lumbar region

M54.07 Panniculitis affecting regions of neck and back, lumbosacral region

M54.08 Panniculitis affecting regions of neck and back, sacral and sacrococcygeal region

M54.09 Panniculitis affecting regions, neck and back, multiple sites in spine

M54.1 Radiculopathy

Brachial neuritis or radiculitis NOS

Lumbar neuritis or radiculitis NOS

Lumbosacral neuritis or radiculitis NOS

Thoracic neuritis or radiculitis NOS

Radiculitis NOS

Excludes1: neuralgia and neuritis NOS (M79.2)

radiculopathy with cervical disc disorder (M50.1)

radiculopathy with lumbar **and other** intervertebral disc disorder (M51.1-)

radiculopathy with spondylosis (M47.2-)

M54.10 Radiculopathy, site unspecified

M54.11 Radiculopathy, occipito-atlanto-axial region

M54.12 Radiculopathy, cervical region

M54.13 Radiculopathy, cervicothoracic region

M54.14 Radiculopathy, thoracic region

M54.15 Radiculopathy, thoracolumbar region

M54.16 Radiculopathy, lumbar region

M54.17 Radiculopathy, lumbosacral region

M54.18 Radiculopathy, sacral and sacrococcygeal region

M54.2 Cervicalgia

Excludes1: cervicalgia due to intervertebral cervical disc disorder (M50.-)

M54.3 Sciatica

Excludes1: lesion of sciatic nerve (G57.0)

sciatica due to intervertebral disc disorder (M51.1-)

sciatica with lumbago (M54.4-)

M54.30 Sciatica, unspecified side

M54.31 Sciatica, right side

M54.32 Sciatica, left side

M54.4 Lumbago with sciatica

Excludes1: lumbago with sciatica due to intervertebral disc disorder (M51.1-)

● New code ▲ Revised code **Excludes1:** Not coded here **Excludes2:** Not included here ⊗ Placeholder required ⑦7th digit required

M54.40 Lumbago with sciatica, unspecified side

M54.41 Lumbago with sciatica, right side

M54.42 Lumbago with sciatica, left side

M54.5 Low back pain

Loin pain

Lumbago NOS

Excludes1: low back strain (S39.012)

lumbago due to intervertebral disc displacement (M51.2-)

lumbago with sciatica (M54.4-)

M54.6 Pain in thoracic spine

Excludes1: pain in thoracic spine due to intervertebral disc disorder (M51.-)

M54.8 Other dorsalgia

Excludes1: dorsalgia in thoracic region (M54.6)

low back pain (M54.5)

M54.81 Occipital neuralgia

M54.89 Other dorsalgia

M54.9 Dorsalgia, unspecified

Backache NOS

Back pain NOS

SOFT TISSUE DISORDERS (M60-M79)

DISORDERS OF MUSCLES (M60-M63)

Excludes1: dermatopolymyositis (M33.-)

muscular dystrophies and myopathies (G71-G72)

myopathy in amyloidosis (E85.-)

myopathy in polyarteritis nodosa (M30.0)

myopathy in rheumatoid arthritis (M05.32)

myopathy in scleroderma (M34.-)

myopathy in Sjögren's syndrome (M35.03)

myopathy in systemic lupus erythematosus (M32.-)

M60 Myositis

Excludes2: inclusion body myositis [IBM] (G72.41)

M60.0 Infective myositis

Tropical pyomyositis

Use additional code (B95-B97) to identify infectious agent

M60.00 Infective myositis, unspecified site

M60.000 Infective myositis, unspecified right arm

Infective myositis, right upper limb NOS

M60.001 Infective myositis, unspecified left arm

Infective myositis, left upper limb NOS

M60.002 Infective myositis, unspecified arm

Infective myositis, upper limb NOS

M60.003 Infective myositis, unspecified right leg

Infective myositis, right lower limb NOS

M60.004 Infective myositis, unspecified left leg

Infective myositis, left lower limb NOS

M60.005 Infective myositis, unspecified leg

Infective myositis, lower limb NOS

M60.009 Infective myositis, unspecified site

M60.01 Infective myositis, shoulder

M60.011 Infective myositis, right shoulder

M60.012 Infective myositis, left shoulder

M60.019 Infective myositis, unspecified shoulder

M60.02 Infective myositis, upper arm

M60.021 Infective myositis, right upper arm

M60.022 Infective myositis, left upper arm

M60.029 Infective myositis, unspecified upper arm

M60.03 Infective myositis, forearm

M60.031 Infective myositis, right forearm

M60.032 Infective myositis, left forearm

M60.039 Infective myositis, unspecified forearm

M60.04 Infective myositis, hand and fingers

M60.041 Infective myositis, right hand

M60.042 Infective myositis, left hand

M60.043 Infective myositis, unspecified hand

M60.044 Infective myositis, right finger(s)

M60.045 Infective myositis, left finger(s)

M60.046 Infective myositis, unspecified finger(s)

M60.05 Infective myositis, thigh

M60.051 Infective myositis, right thigh

M60.052 Infective myositis, left thigh

M60.059 Infective myositis, unspecified thigh

M60.06 Infective myositis, lower leg

M60.061 Infective myositis, right lower leg

M60.062 Infective myositis, left lower leg

M60.069 Infective myositis, unspecified lower leg

M60.07 Infective myositis, ankle, foot and toes

M60.070 Infective myositis, right ankle

M60.071 Infective myositis, left ankle

M60.072 Infective myositis, unspecified ankle

M60.073 Infective myositis, right foot

M60.074 Infective myositis, left foot

M60.075 Infective myositis, unspecified foot

M60.076 Infective myositis, right toe(s)

M60.077 Infective myositis, left toe(s)

M60.078 Infective myositis, unspecified toe(s)

M60.08 Infective myositis, other site

M60.09 Infective myositis, multiple sites

M60.1 Interstitial myositis

M60.10 Interstitial myositis of unspecified site

M60.11 Interstitial myositis, shoulder

M60.111 Interstitial myositis, right shoulder

M60.112 Interstitial myositis, left shoulder

M60.119 Interstitial myositis, unspecified shoulder

M60.12 Interstitial myositis, upper arm

M60.121 Interstitial myositis, right upper arm

M60.122 Interstitial myositis, left upper arm

M60.129 Interstitial myositis, unspecified upper arm

M60.13 Interstitial myositis, forearm

M60.131 Interstitial myositis, right forearm

M60.132 Interstitial myositis, left forearm

M60.139 Interstitial myositis, unspecified forearm

M60.14 Interstitial myositis, hand

M60.141 Interstitial myositis, right hand

M60.142 Interstitial myositis, left hand

M60.149 Interstitial myositis, unspecified hand

M60.15 Interstitial myositis, thigh

M60.151 Interstitial myositis, right thigh

M60.152 Interstitial myositis, left thigh

M60.159 Interstitial myositis, unspecified thigh

M60.16 Interstitial myositis, lower leg

M60.161 Interstitial myositis, right lower leg

M60.162 Interstitial myositis, left lower leg

M60.169 Interstitial myositis, unspecified lower leg

M60.17 Interstitial myositis, ankle and foot

M60.171 Interstitial myositis, right ankle and foot

M60.172 Interstitial myositis, left ankle and foot

M60.179 Interstitial myositis, unspecified ankle and foot

M60.18 Interstitial myositis, other site

M60.19 Interstitial myositis, multiple sites

M60.2 **Foreign body granuloma of soft tissue, not elsewhere classified**

Use additional code to identify the type of retained foreign body (Z18.-)

Excludes1: foreign body granuloma of skin and subcutaneous tissue (L92.3)

M60.20 Foreign body granuloma of soft tissue, not elsewhere classified, unspecified site

M60.21 Foreign body granuloma of soft tissue, not elsewhere classified, shoulder

M60.211 Foreign body granuloma of soft tissue, not elsewhere classified, right shoulder

M60.212 Foreign body granuloma of soft tissue, not elsewhere classified, left shoulder

M60.219 Foreign body granuloma of soft tissue, not elsewhere classified, unspecified shoulder

M60.22 Foreign body granuloma of soft tissue, not elsewhere classified, upper arm

M60.221 Foreign body granuloma of soft tissue, not elsewhere classified, right upper arm

M60.222 Foreign body granuloma of soft tissue, not elsewhere classified, left upper arm

M60.229 Foreign body granuloma of soft tissue, not elsewhere classified, unspecified upper arm

M60.23 Foreign body granuloma of soft tissue, not elsewhere classified, forearm

M60.231 Foreign body granuloma of soft tissue, not elsewhere classified, right forearm

M60.232 Foreign body granuloma of soft tissue, not elsewhere classified, left forearm

M60.239 Foreign body granuloma of soft tissue, not elsewhere classified, unspecified forearm

M60.24 Foreign body granuloma of soft tissue, not elsewhere classified, hand

M60.241 Foreign body granuloma of soft tissue, not elsewhere classified, right hand

M60.242 Foreign body granuloma of soft tissue, not elsewhere classified, left hand

M60.249 Foreign body granuloma of soft tissue, not elsewhere classified, unspecified hand

M60.25 Foreign body granuloma of soft tissue, not elsewhere classified, thigh

M60.251 Foreign body granuloma of soft tissue, not elsewhere classified, right thigh

M60.252 Foreign body granuloma of soft tissue, not elsewhere classified, left thigh

M60.259 Foreign body granuloma of soft tissue, not elsewhere classified, unspecified thigh

M60.26 Foreign body granuloma of soft tissue, not elsewhere classified, lower leg

M60.261 Foreign body granuloma of soft tissue, not elsewhere classified, right lower leg

M60.262 Foreign body granuloma of soft tissue, not elsewhere classified, left lower leg

M60.269 Foreign body granuloma of soft tissue, not elsewhere classified, unspecified lower leg

M60.27 Foreign body granuloma of soft tissue, not elsewhere classified, ankle and foot

M60.271 Foreign body granuloma of soft tissue, not elsewhere classified, right ankle and foot

M60.272 Foreign body granuloma of soft tissue, not elsewhere classified, left ankle and foot

M60.279 Foreign body granuloma of soft tissue, not elsewhere classified, unspecified ankle and foot

M60.28 Foreign body granuloma of soft tissue, not elsewhere classified, other site

M60.8 **Other myositis**

M60.80 Other myositis, unspecified site

M60.81 Other myositis shoulder

M60.811 Other myositis, right shoulder

M60.812 Other myositis, left shoulder

M60.819 Other myositis, unspecified shoulder

M60.82 Other myositis, upper arm

M60.821 Other myositis, right upper arm

M60.822 Other myositis, left upper arm

M60.829 Other myositis, unspecified upper arm

M60.83 Other myositis, forearm

M60.831 Other myositis, right forearm

M60.832   Other myositis, left forearm

M60.839   Other myositis, unspecified forearm

M60.84   Other myositis, hand

M60.841   Other myositis, right hand

M60.842   Other myositis, left hand

M60.849   Other myositis, unspecified hand

M60.85   Other myositis, thigh

M60.851   Other myositis, right thigh

M60.852   Other myositis, left thigh

M60.859   Other myositis, unspecified thigh

M60.86   Other myositis, lower leg

M60.861   Other myositis, right lower leg

M60.862   Other myositis, left lower leg

M60.869   Other myositis, unspecified lower leg

M60.87   Other myositis, ankle and foot

M60.871   Other myositis, right ankle and foot

M60.872   Other myositis, left ankle and foot

M60.879   Other myositis, unspecified ankle and foot

M60.88   Other myositis, other site

M60.89   Other myositis, multiple sites

M60.9   Myositis, unspecified

M61   Calcification and ossification of muscle

M61.0   Myositis ossificans traumatica

M61.00   Myositis ossificans traumatica, unspecified site

M61.01   Myositis ossificans traumatica, shoulder

M61.011   Myositis ossificans traumatica, right shoulder

M61.012   Myositis ossificans traumatica, left shoulder

M61.019   Myositis ossificans traumatica, unspecified shoulder

M61.02   Myositis ossificans traumatica, upper arm

M61.021   Myositis ossificans traumatica, right upper arm

M61.022   Myositis ossificans traumatica, left upper arm

M61.029   Myositis ossificans traumatica, unspecified upper arm

M61.03   Myositis ossificans traumatica, forearm

M61.031   Myositis ossificans traumatica, right forearm

M61.032   Myositis ossificans traumatica, left forearm

M61.039   Myositis ossificans traumatica, unspecified forearm

M61.04   Myositis ossificans traumatica, hand

M61.041   Myositis ossificans traumatica, right hand

M61.042   Myositis ossificans traumatica, left hand

M61.049   Myositis ossificans traumatica, unspecified hand

M61.05   Myositis ossificans traumatica, thigh

M61.051   Myositis ossificans traumatica, right thigh

M61.052   Myositis ossificans traumatica, left thigh

M61.059   Myositis ossificans traumatica, unspecified thigh

M61.06   Myositis ossificans traumatica, lower leg

M61.061   Myositis ossificans traumatica, right lower leg

M61.062   Myositis ossificans traumatica, left lower leg

M61.069   Myositis ossificans traumatica, unspecified lower leg

M61.07   Myositis ossificans traumatica, ankle and foot

M61.071   Myositis ossificans traumatica, right ankle and foot

M61.072   Myositis ossificans traumatica, left ankle and foot

M61.079   Myositis ossificans traumatica, unspecified ankle and foot

M61.08   Myositis ossificans traumatica, other site

M61.09   Myositis ossificans traumatica, multiple sites

M61.1   Myositis ossificans progressiva

Fibrodysplasia ossificans progressiva

M61.10   Myositis ossificans progressiva, unspecified site

M61.11   Myositis ossificans progressiva, shoulder

M61.111   Myositis ossificans progressiva, right shoulder

M61.112   Myositis ossificans progressiva, left shoulder

M61.119   Myositis ossificans progressiva, unspecified shoulder

M61.12   Myositis ossificans progressiva, upper arm

M61.121   Myositis ossificans progressiva, right upper arm

M61.122   Myositis ossificans progressiva, left upper arm

M61.129   Myositis ossificans progressiva, unspecified arm

M61.13   Myositis ossificans progressiva, forearm

M61.131   Myositis ossificans progressiva, right forearm

M61.132   Myositis ossificans progressiva, left forearm

M61.139   Myositis ossificans progressiva, unspecified forearm

M61.14   Myositis ossificans progressiva, hand and finger(s)

M61.141   Myositis ossificans progressiva, right hand

M61.142   Myositis ossificans progressiva, left hand

M61.143   Myositis ossificans progressiva, unspecified hand

M61.144   Myositis ossificans progressiva, right finger(s)

M61.145   Myositis ossificans progressiva, left finger(s)

M61.146   Myositis ossificans progressiva, unspecified finger(s)

M61.15   Myositis ossificans progressiva, thigh

M61.151   Myositis ossificans progressiva, right thigh

M61.152   Myositis ossificans progressiva, left thigh

M61.159   Myositis ossificans progressiva, unspecified thigh

M61.16   Myositis ossificans progressiva, lower leg

M61.161 Myositis ossificans progressiva, right lower leg

M61.162 Myositis ossificans progressiva, left lower leg

M61.169 Myositis ossificans progressiva, unspecified lower leg

M61.17 Myositis ossificans progressiva, ankle, foot and toe(s)

M61.171 Myositis ossificans progressiva, right ankle

M61.172 Myositis ossificans progressiva, left ankle

M61.173 Myositis ossificans progressiva, unspecified ankle

M61.174 Myositis ossificans progressiva, right foot

M61.175 Myositis ossificans progressiva, left foot

M61.176 Myositis ossificans progressiva, unspecified foot

M61.177 Myositis ossificans progressiva, right toe(s)

M61.178 Myositis ossificans progressiva, left toe(s)

M61.179 Myositis ossificans progressiva, unspecified toe(s)

M61.18 Myositis ossificans progressiva, other site

M61.19 Myositis ossificans progressiva, multiple sites

M61.2 Paralytic calcification and ossification of muscle

Myositis ossificans associated with quadriplegia or paraplegia

M61.20 Paralytic calcification and ossification of muscle, unspecified site

M61.21 Paralytic calcification and ossification of muscle, shoulder

M61.211 Paralytic calcification and ossification of muscle, right shoulder

M61.212 Paralytic calcification and ossification of muscle, left shoulder

M61.219 Paralytic calcification and ossification of muscle, unspecified shoulder

M61.22 Paralytic calcification and ossification of muscle, upper arm

M61.221 Paralytic calcification and ossification of muscle, right upper arm

M61.222 Paralytic calcification and ossification of muscle, left upper arm

M61.229 Paralytic calcification and ossification of muscle, unspecified upper arm

M61.23 Paralytic calcification and ossification of muscle, forearm

M61.231 Paralytic calcification and ossification of muscle, right forearm

M61.232 Paralytic calcification and ossification of muscle, left forearm

M61.239 Paralytic calcification and ossification of muscle, unspecified forearm

M61.24 Paralytic calcification and ossification of muscle, hand

M61.241 Paralytic calcification and ossification of muscle, right hand

M61.242 Paralytic calcification and ossification of muscle, left hand

M61.249 Paralytic calcification and ossification of muscle, unspecified hand

M61.25 Paralytic calcification and ossification of muscle, thigh

M61.251 Paralytic calcification and ossification of muscle, right thigh

M61.252 Paralytic calcification and ossification of muscle, left thigh

M61.259 Paralytic calcification and ossification of muscle, unspecified thigh

M61.26 Paralytic calcification and ossification of muscle, lower leg

M61.261 Paralytic calcification and ossification of muscle, right lower leg

M61.262 Paralytic calcification and ossification of muscle, left lower leg

M61.269 Paralytic calcification and ossification of muscle, unspecified lower leg

M61.27 Paralytic calcification and ossification of muscle, ankle and foot

M61.271 Paralytic calcification and ossification of muscle, right ankle and foot

M61.272 Paralytic calcification and ossification of muscle, left ankle and foot

M61.279 Paralytic calcification and ossification of muscle, unspecified ankle and foot

M61.28 Paralytic calcification and ossification of muscle, other site

M61.29 Paralytic calcification and ossification of muscle, multiple sites

M61.3 Calcification and ossification of muscles associated with burns

Myositis ossificans associated with burns

M61.30 Calcification and ossification of muscles associated with burns, unspecified site

M61.31 Calcification and ossification of muscles associated with burns, shoulder

M61.311 Calcification and ossification of muscles associated with burns, right shoulder

M61.312 Calcification and ossification of muscles associated with burns, left shoulder

M61.319 Calcification and ossification of muscles associated with burns, unspecified shoulder

M61.32 Calcification and ossification of muscles associated with burns, upper arm

M61.321 Calcification and ossification of muscles associated with burns, right upper arm

M61.322 Calcification and ossification of muscles associated with burns, left upper arm

● New code ▲ Revised code **Excludes1:** Not coded here **Excludes2:** Not included here ⊗ Placeholder required ⑦7th digit required

M61.329   Calcification and ossification of muscles associated with burns, unspecified upper arm

M61.33   Calcification and ossification of muscles associated with burns, forearm

M61.331   Calcification and ossification of muscles associated with burns, right forearm

M61.332   Calcification and ossification of muscles associated with burns, left forearm

M61.339   Calcification and ossification of muscles associated with burns, unspecified forearm

M61.34   Calcification and ossification of muscles associated with burns, hand

M61.341   Calcification and ossification of muscles associated with burns, right hand

M61.342   Calcification and ossification of muscles associated with burns, left hand

M61.349   Calcification and ossification of muscles associated with burns, unspecified hand

M61.35   Calcification and ossification of muscles associated with burns, thigh

M61.351   Calcification and ossification of muscles associated with burns, right thigh

M61.352   Calcification and ossification of muscles associated with burns, left thigh

M61.359   Calcification and ossification of muscles associated with burns, unspecified thigh

M61.36   Calcification and ossification of muscles associated with burns, lower leg

M61.361   Calcification and ossification of muscles associated with burns, right lower leg

M61.362   Calcification and ossification of muscles associated with burns, left lower leg

M61.369   Calcification and ossification of muscles associated with burns, unspecified lower leg

M61.37   Calcification and ossification of muscles associated with burns, ankle and foot

M61.371   Calcification and ossification of muscles associated with burns, right ankle and foot

M61.372   Calcification and ossification of muscles associated with burns, left ankle and foot

M61.379   Calcification and ossification of muscles associated with burns, unspecified ankle and foot

M61.38   Calcification and ossification of muscles associated with burns, other site

M61.39   Calcification and ossification of muscles associated with burns, multiple sites

M61.4   Other calcification of muscle

Excludes1: calcific tendinitis NOS (M65.2-)

calcific tendinitis of shoulder (M75.3)

M61.40   Other calcification of muscle, unspecified site

M61.41   Other calcification of muscle, shoulder

M61.411   Other calcification of muscle, right shoulder

M61.412   Other calcification of muscle, left shoulder

M61.419   Other calcification of muscle, unspecified shoulder

M61.42   Other calcification of muscle, upper arm

M61.421   Other calcification of muscle, right upper arm

M61.422   Other calcification of muscle, left upper arm

M61.429   Other calcification of muscle, unspecified upper arm

M61.43   Other calcification of muscle, forearm

M61.431   Other calcification of muscle, right forearm

M61.432   Other calcification of muscle, left forearm

M61.439   Other calcification of muscle, unspecified forearm

M61.44   Other calcification of muscle, hand

M61.441   Other calcification of muscle, right hand

M61.442   Other calcification of muscle, left hand

M61.449   Other calcification of muscle, unspecified hand

M61.45   Other calcification of muscle, thigh

M61.451   Other calcification of muscle, right thigh

M61.452   Other calcification of muscle, left thigh

M61.459   Other calcification of muscle, unspecified thigh

M61.46   Other calcification of muscle, lower leg

M61.461   Other calcification of muscle, right lower leg

M61.462   Other calcification of muscle, left lower leg

M61.469   Other calcification of muscle, unspecified lower leg

M61.47   Other calcification of muscle, ankle and foot

M61.471   Other calcification of muscle, right ankle and foot

M61.472   Other calcification of muscle, left ankle and foot

M61.479   Other calcification of muscle, unspecified ankle and foot

M61.48   Other calcification of muscle, other site

M61.49   Other calcification of muscle, multiple sites

M61.5   Other ossification of muscle

M61.50   Other ossification of muscle, unspecified site

M61.51   Other ossification of muscle, shoulder

M61.511   Other ossification of muscle, right shoulder

M61.512   Other ossification of muscle, left shoulder

M61.519   Other ossification of muscle, unspecified shoulder

M61.52   Other ossification of muscle, upper arm

M61.521   Other ossification of muscle, right upper arm

M61.522 Other ossification of muscle, left upper arm

M61.529 Other ossification of muscle, unspecified upper arm

M61.53 Other ossification of muscle, forearm

M61.531 Other ossification of muscle, right forearm

M61.532 Other ossification of muscle, left forearm

M61.539 Other ossification of muscle, unspecified forearm

M61.54 Other ossification of muscle, hand

M61.541 Other ossification of muscle, right hand

M61.542 Other ossification of muscle, left hand

M61.549 Other ossification of muscle, unspecified hand

M61.55 Other ossification of muscle, thigh

M61.551 Other ossification of muscle, right thigh

M61.552 Other ossification of muscle, left thigh

M61.559 Other ossification of muscle, unspecified thigh

M61.56 Other ossification of muscle, lower leg

M61.561 Other ossification of muscle, right lower leg

M61.562 Other ossification of muscle, left lower leg

M61.569 Other ossification of muscle, unspecified lower leg

M61.57 Other ossification of muscle, ankle and foot

M61.571 Other ossification of muscle, right ankle and foot

M61.572 Other ossification of muscle, left ankle and foot

M61.579 Other ossification of muscle, unspecified ankle and foot

M61.58 Other ossification of muscle, other site

M61.59 Other ossification of muscle, multiple sites

M61.9 Calcification and ossification of muscle, unspecified

M62 Other disorders of muscle

Excludes1: alcoholic myopathy (G72.1)

cramp and spasm (R25.2)

drug-induced myopathy (G72.0)

myalgia (M79.1)

stiff-man syndrome (G25.82)

Excludes2: nontraumatic hematoma of muscle (M79.81)

M62.0 Separation of muscle (nontraumatic)

Diastasis of muscle

Excludes1: diastasis recti complicating pregnancy, labor and delivery (O71.8)

traumatic separation of muscle- see strain of muscle by body region

M62.00 Separation of muscle (nontraumatic), unspecified site

M62.01 Separation of muscle (nontraumatic), shoulder

M62.011 Separation of muscle (nontraumatic), right shoulder

M62.012 Separation of muscle (nontraumatic), left shoulder

M62.019 Separation of muscle (nontraumatic), unspecified shoulder

M62.02 Separation of muscle (nontraumatic), upper arm

M62.021 Separation of muscle (nontraumatic), right upper arm

M62.022 Separation of muscle (nontraumatic), left upper arm

M62.029 Separation of muscle (nontraumatic), unspecified upper arm

M62.03 Separation of muscle (nontraumatic), forearm

M62.031 Separation of muscle (nontraumatic), right forearm

M62.032 Separation of muscle (nontraumatic), left forearm

M62.039 Separation of muscle (nontraumatic), unspecified forearm

M62.04 Separation of muscle (nontraumatic), hand

M62.041 Separation of muscle (nontraumatic), right hand

M62.042 Separation of muscle (nontraumatic), left hand

M62.049 Separation of muscle (nontraumatic), unspecified hand

M62.05 Separation of muscle (nontraumatic), thigh

M62.051 Separation of muscle (nontraumatic), right thigh

M62.052 Separation of muscle (nontraumatic), left thigh

M62.059 Separation of muscle (nontraumatic), unspecified thigh

M62.06 Separation of muscle (nontraumatic), lower leg

M62.061 Separation of muscle (nontraumatic), right lower leg

M62.062 Separation of muscle (nontraumatic), left lower leg

M62.069 Separation of muscle (nontraumatic), unspecified lower leg

M62.07 Separation of muscle (nontraumatic), ankle and foot

M62.071 Separation of muscle (nontraumatic), right ankle and foot

M62.072 Separation of muscle (nontraumatic), left ankle and foot

M62.079 Separation of muscle (nontraumatic), unspecified ankle and foot

M62.08 Separation of muscle (nontraumatic), other site

M62.1 Other rupture of muscle (nontraumatic)

Excludes1: traumatic rupture of muscle - see strain of muscle by body region

Excludes2: rupture of tendon (M66.-)

M62.10 Other rupture of muscle (nontraumatic), unspecified site

M62.11 Other rupture of muscle (nontraumatic), shoulder

M62.111 Other rupture of muscle (nontraumatic), right shoulder

M62.112 Other rupture of muscle (nontraumatic), left shoulder

M62.119 Other rupture of muscle (nontraumatic), unspecified shoulder

M62.12 Other rupture of muscle (nontraumatic), upper arm

M62.121   Other rupture of muscle (nontraumatic), right upper arm

M62.122   Other rupture of muscle (nontraumatic), left upper arm

M62.129   Other rupture of muscle (nontraumatic), unspecified upper arm

M62.13   Other rupture of muscle (nontraumatic), forearm

    M62.131   Other rupture of muscle (nontraumatic), right forearm

    M62.132   Other rupture of muscle (nontraumatic), left forearm

    M62.139   Other rupture of muscle (nontraumatic), unspecified forearm

M62.14   Other rupture of muscle (nontraumatic), hand

    M62.141   Other rupture of muscle (nontraumatic), right hand

    M62.142   Other rupture of muscle (nontraumatic), left hand

    M62.149   Other rupture of muscle (nontraumatic), unspecified hand

M62.15   Other rupture of muscle (nontraumatic), thigh

    M62.151   Other rupture of muscle (nontraumatic), right thigh

    M62.152   Other rupture of muscle (nontraumatic), left thigh

    M62.159   Other rupture of muscle (nontraumatic), unspecified thigh

M62.16   Other rupture of muscle (nontraumatic), lower leg

    M62.161   Other rupture of muscle (nontraumatic), right lower leg

    M62.162   Other rupture of muscle (nontraumatic), left lower leg

    M62.169   Other rupture of muscle (nontraumatic), unspecified lower leg

M62.17   Other rupture of muscle (nontraumatic), ankle and foot

    M62.171   Other rupture of muscle (nontraumatic), right ankle and foot

    M62.172   Other rupture of muscle (nontraumatic), left ankle and foot

    M62.179   Other rupture of muscle (nontraumatic), unspecified ankle and foot

M62.18   Other rupture of muscle (nontraumatic), other site

M62.2   **Nontraumatic ischemic infarction of muscle**

    Excludes1: compartment syndrome (traumatic) (T79.A-)

       nontraumatic compartment syndrome (M79.A-)

       traumatic ischemia of muscle (T79.6)

       rhabdomyolysis (M62.82)

       Volkmann's ischemic contracture (T79.6)

M62.20   Nontraumatic ischemic infarction of muscle, unspecified site

M62.21   Nontraumatic ischemic infarction of muscle, shoulder

    M62.211   Nontraumatic ischemic infarction of muscle, right shoulder

    M62.212   Nontraumatic ischemic infarction of muscle, left shoulder

    M62.219   Nontraumatic ischemic infarction of muscle, unspecified shoulder

M62.22   Nontraumatic ischemic infarction of muscle, upper arm

    M62.221   Nontraumatic ischemic infarction of muscle, right upper arm

    M62.222   Nontraumatic ischemic infarction of muscle, left upper arm

    M62.229   Nontraumatic ischemic infarction of muscle, unspecified upper arm

M62.23   Nontraumatic ischemic infarction of muscle, forearm

    M62.231   Nontraumatic ischemic infarction of muscle, right forearm

    M62.232   Nontraumatic ischemic infarction of muscle, left forearm

    M62.239   Nontraumatic ischemic infarction of muscle, unspecified forearm

M62.24   Nontraumatic ischemic infarction of muscle, hand

    M62.241   Nontraumatic ischemic infarction of muscle, right hand

    M62.242   Nontraumatic ischemic infarction of muscle, left hand

    M62.249   Nontraumatic ischemic infarction of muscle, unspecified hand

M62.25   Nontraumatic ischemic infarction of muscle, thigh

    M62.251   Nontraumatic ischemic infarction of muscle, right thigh

    M62.252   Nontraumatic ischemic infarction of muscle, left thigh

    M62.259   Nontraumatic ischemic infarction of muscle, unspecified thigh

M62.26   Nontraumatic ischemic infarction of muscle, lower leg

    M62.261   Nontraumatic ischemic infarction of muscle, right lower leg

    M62.262   Nontraumatic ischemic infarction of muscle, left lower leg

    M62.269   Nontraumatic ischemic infarction of muscle, unspecified lower leg

M62.27   Nontraumatic ischemic infarction of muscle, ankle and foot

    M62.271   Nontraumatic ischemic infarction of muscle, right ankle and foot

    M62.272   Nontraumatic ischemic infarction of muscle, left ankle and foot

    M62.279   Nontraumatic ischemic infarction of muscle, unspecified ankle and foot

M62.28   Nontraumatic ischemic infarction of muscle, other site

M62.3   **Immobility syndrome (paraplegic)**

M62.4   **Contracture of muscle**

    Contracture of tendon (sheath)

    Excludes1: contracture of joint (M24.5-)

M62.40   Contracture of muscle, unspecified site

M62.41   Contracture of muscle, shoulder

    M62.411   Contracture of muscle, right shoulder

    M62.412   Contracture of muscle, left shoulder

    M62.419   Contracture of muscle, unspecified shoulder

M62.42   Contracture of muscle, upper arm

M62.421 Contracture of muscle, right upper arm

M62.422 Contracture of muscle, left upper arm

M62.429 Contracture of muscle, unspecified upper arm

M62.43 Contracture of muscle, forearm

M62.431 Contracture of muscle, right forearm

M62.432 Contracture of muscle, left forearm

M62.439 Contracture of muscle, unspecified forearm

M62.44 Contracture of muscle, hand

M62.441 Contracture of muscle, right hand

M62.442 Contracture of muscle, left hand

M62.449 Contracture of muscle, unspecified hand

M62.45 Contracture of muscle, thigh

M62.451 Contracture of muscle, right thigh

M62.452 Contracture of muscle, left thigh

M62.459 Contracture of muscle, unspecified thigh

M62.46 Contracture of muscle, lower leg

M62.461 Contracture of muscle, right lower leg

M62.462 Contracture of muscle, left lower leg

M62.469 Contracture of muscle, unspecified lower leg

M62.47 Contracture of muscle, ankle and foot

M62.471 Contracture of muscle, right ankle and foot

M62.472 Contracture of muscle, left ankle and foot

M62.479 Contracture of muscle, unspecified ankle and foot

M62.48 Contracture of muscle, other site

M62.49 Contracture of muscle, multiple sites

M62.5 Muscle wasting and atrophy, not elsewhere classified

Disuse atrophy NEC

Excludes1: neuralgic amyotrophy (G54.5)

progressive muscular atrophy (G12.21)

sarcopenia (M62.84)

Excludes2: pelvic muscle wasting (N81.84)

M62.50 Muscle wasting and atrophy, not elsewhere classified, unspecified site

M62.51 Muscle wasting and atrophy, not elsewhere classified, shoulder

M62.511 Muscle wasting and atrophy, not elsewhere classified, right shoulder

M62.512 Muscle wasting and atrophy, not elsewhere classified, left shoulder

M62.519 Muscle wasting and atrophy, not elsewhere classified, unspecified shoulder

M62.52 Muscle wasting and atrophy, not elsewhere classified, upper arm

M62.521 Muscle wasting and atrophy, not elsewhere classified, right upper arm

M62.522 Muscle wasting and atrophy, not elsewhere classified, left upper arm

M62.529 Muscle wasting and atrophy, not elsewhere classified, unspecified upper arm

M62.53 Muscle wasting and atrophy, not elsewhere classified, forearm

M62.531 Muscle wasting and atrophy, not elsewhere classified, right forearm

M62.532 Muscle wasting and atrophy, not elsewhere classified, left forearm

M62.539 Muscle wasting and atrophy, not elsewhere classified, unspecified forearm

M62.54 Muscle wasting and atrophy, not elsewhere classified, hand

M62.541 Muscle wasting and atrophy, not elsewhere classified, right hand

M62.542 Muscle wasting and atrophy, not elsewhere classified, left hand

M62.549 Muscle wasting and atrophy, not elsewhere classified, unspecified hand

M62.55 Muscle wasting and atrophy, not elsewhere classified, thigh

M62.551 Muscle wasting and atrophy, not elsewhere classified, right thigh

M62.552 Muscle wasting and atrophy, not elsewhere classified, left thigh

M62.559 Muscle wasting and atrophy, not elsewhere classified, unspecified thigh

M62.56 Muscle wasting and atrophy, not elsewhere classified, lower leg

M62.561 Muscle wasting and atrophy, not elsewhere classified, right lower leg

M62.562 Muscle wasting and atrophy, not elsewhere classified, left lower leg

M62.569 Muscle wasting and atrophy, not elsewhere classified, unspecified lower leg

M62.57 Muscle wasting and atrophy, not elsewhere classified, ankle and foot

M62.571 Muscle wasting and atrophy, not elsewhere classified, right ankle and foot

M62.572 Muscle wasting and atrophy, not elsewhere classified, left ankle and foot

M62.579 Muscle wasting and atrophy, not elsewhere classified, unspecified ankle and foot

M62.58 Muscle wasting and atrophy, not elsewhere classified, other site

M62.59 Muscle wasting and atrophy, not elsewhere classified, multiple sites

M62.8 Other specified disorders of muscle

Excludes2: nontraumatic hematoma of muscle (M79.81)

M62.81 Muscle weakness (generalized)

Excludes1: muscle weakness in sarcopenia (M62.84)

M62.82 Rhabdomyolysis

Excludes1: traumatic rhabdomyolysis (T79.6)

M62.83 Muscle spasm

M62.830 Muscle spasm of back

M62.831 Muscle spasm of calf

Charley-horse

M62.838 Other muscle spasm

● New code ▲ Revised code **Excludes1:** Not coded here **Excludes2:** Not included here ⊗ Placeholder required ⑦ 7th digit required

M62.84 **Sarcopenia**

Age-related sarcopenia

Code first underlying disease, if applicable, such as:

disorders of myoneural junction and muscle disease in diseases classified elsewhere (G73.-)

Other and unspecified myopathies (G72.-)

primary disorders of muscles (G71.-)

M62.89 **Other specified disorders of muscle**

Muscle (sheath) hernia

M62.9 **Disorder of muscle, unspecified**

M63 **Disorders of muscle in diseases classified elsewhere**

Code first underlying disease, such as:

leprosy (A30.-)

neoplasm (C49.-, C79.89, D21.-, D48.1)

schistosomiasis (B65.-)

trichinellosis (B75)

Excludes1: myopathy in cysticercosis (B69.81)

myopathy in endocrine diseases (G73.7)

myopathy in metabolic diseases (G73.7)

myopathy in sarcoidosis (D86.87)

myopathy in secondary syphilis (A51.49)

myopathy in syphilis (late) (A52.78)

myopathy in toxoplasmosis (B58.82)

myopathy in tuberculosis (A18.09)

M63.8 **Disorders of muscle in diseases classified elsewhere**

M63.80 **Disorders of muscle in diseases classified elsewhere, unspecified site**

M63.81 **Disorders of muscle in diseases classified elsewhere, shoulder**

M63.811 **Disorders of muscle in diseases classified elsewhere, right shoulder**

M63.812 **Disorders of muscle in diseases classified elsewhere, left shoulder**

M63.819 **Disorders of muscle in diseases classified elsewhere, unspecified shoulder**

M63.82 **Disorders of muscle in diseases classified elsewhere, upper arm**

M63.821 **Disorders of muscle in diseases classified elsewhere, right upper arm**

M63.822 **Disorders of muscle in diseases classified elsewhere, left upper arm**

M63.829 **Disorders of muscle in diseases classified elsewhere, unspecified upper arm**

M63.83 **Disorders of muscle in diseases classified elsewhere, forearm**

M63.831 **Disorders of muscle in diseases classified elsewhere, right forearm**

M63.832 **Disorders of muscle in diseases classified elsewhere, left forearm**

M63.839 **Disorders of muscle in diseases classified elsewhere, unspecified forearm**

M63.84 **Disorders of muscle in diseases classified elsewhere, hand**

M63.841 **Disorders of muscle in diseases classified elsewhere, right hand**

M63.842 **Disorders of muscle in diseases classified elsewhere, left hand**

M63.849 **Disorders of muscle in diseases classified elsewhere, unspecified hand**

M63.85 **Disorders of muscle in diseases classified elsewhere, thigh**

M63.851 **Disorders of muscle in diseases classified elsewhere, right thigh**

M63.852 **Disorders of muscle in diseases classified elsewhere, left thigh**

M63.859 **Disorders of muscle in diseases classified elsewhere, unspecified thigh**

M63.86 **Disorders of muscle in diseases classified elsewhere, lower leg**

M63.861 **Disorders of muscle in diseases classified elsewhere, right lower leg**

M63.862 **Disorders of muscle in diseases classified elsewhere, left lower leg**

M63.869 **Disorders of muscle in diseases classified elsewhere, unspecified lower leg**

M63.87 **Disorders of muscle in diseases classified elsewhere, ankle and foot**

M63.871 **Disorders of muscle in diseases classified elsewhere, right ankle and foot**

M63.872 **Disorders of muscle in diseases classified elsewhere, left ankle and foot**

M63.879 **Disorders of muscle in diseases classified elsewhere, unspecified ankle and foot**

M63.88 **Disorders of muscle in diseases classified elsewhere, other site**

M63.89 **Disorders of muscle in diseases classified elsewhere, multiple sites**

DISORDERS OF SYNOVIUM AND TENDON (M65-M67)

M65 **Synovitis and tenosynovitis**

Excludes1: chronic crepitant synovitis of hand and wrist (M70.0-)

current injury - see injury of ligament or tendon by body region soft tissue disorders related to use, overuse and pressure (M70.-)

M65.0 **Abscess of tendon sheath**

Use additional code (B95-B96) to identify bacterial agent.

M65.00 **Abscess of tendon sheath, unspecified site**

M65.01 **Abscess of tendon sheath, shoulder**

M65.011 **Abscess of tendon sheath, right shoulder**

M65.012 **Abscess of tendon sheath, left shoulder**

M65.019 **Abscess of tendon sheath, unspecified shoulder**

M65.02 **Abscess of tendon sheath, upper arm**

M65.021 **Abscess of tendon sheath, right upper arm**

M65.022 **Abscess of tendon sheath, left upper arm**

M65.029 **Abscess of tendon sheath, unspecified upper arm**

M65.03 **Abscess of tendon sheath, forearm**

M65.031 **Abscess of tendon sheath, right forearm**

M65.032 Abscess of tendon sheath, left forearm

M65.039 Abscess of tendon sheath, unspecified forearm

M65.04 Abscess of tendon sheath, hand

M65.041 Abscess of tendon sheath, right hand

M65.042 Abscess of tendon sheath, left hand

M65.049 Abscess of tendon sheath, unspecified hand

M65.05 Abscess of tendon sheath, thigh

M65.051 Abscess of tendon sheath, right thigh

M65.052 Abscess of tendon sheath, left thigh

M65.059 Abscess of tendon sheath, unspecified thigh

M65.06 Abscess of tendon sheath, lower leg

M65.061 Abscess of tendon sheath, right lower leg

M65.062 Abscess of tendon sheath, left lower leg

M65.069 Abscess of tendon sheath, unspecified lower leg

M65.07 Abscess of tendon sheath, ankle and foot

M65.071 Abscess of tendon sheath, right ankle and foot

M65.072 Abscess of tendon sheath, left ankle and foot

M65.079 Abscess of tendon sheath, unspecified ankle and foot

M65.08 Abscess of tendon sheath, other site

M65.1 Other infective (teno)synovitis

M65.10 Other infective (teno)synovitis, unspecified site

M65.11 Other infective (teno)synovitis, shoulder

M65.111 Other infective (teno)synovitis, right shoulder

M65.112 Other infective (teno)synovitis, left shoulder

M65.119 Other infective (teno)synovitis, unspecified shoulder

M65.12 Other infective (teno)synovitis, elbow

M65.121 Other infective (teno)synovitis, right elbow

M65.122 Other infective (teno)synovitis, left elbow

M65.129 Other infective (teno)synovitis, unspecified elbow

M65.13 Other infective (teno)synovitis, wrist

M65.131 Other infective (teno)synovitis, right wrist

M65.132 Other infective (teno)synovitis, left wrist

M65.139 Other infective (teno)synovitis, unspecified wrist

M65.14 Other infective (teno)synovitis, hand

M65.141 Other infective (teno)synovitis, right hand

M65.142 Other infective (teno)synovitis, left hand

M65.149 Other infective (teno)synovitis, unspecified hand

M65.15 Other infective (teno)synovitis, hip

M65.151 Other infective (teno)synovitis, right hip

M65.152 Other infective (teno)synovitis, left hip

M65.159 Other infective (teno)synovitis, unspecified hip

M65.16 Other infective (teno)synovitis, knee

M65.161 Other infective (teno)synovitis, right knee

M65.162 Other infective (teno)synovitis, left knee

M65.169 Other infective (teno)synovitis, unspecified knee

M65.17 Other infective (teno)synovitis, ankle and foot

M65.171 Other infective (teno)synovitis, right ankle and foot

M65.172 Other infective (teno)synovitis, left ankle and foot

M65.179 Other infective (teno)synovitis, unspecified ankle and foot

M65.18 Other infective (teno)synovitis, other site

M65.19 Other infective (teno)synovitis, multiple sites

M65.2 Calcific tendinitis

Excludes1: tendinitis as classified in M75-M77

calcified tendinitis of shoulder (M75.3)

M65.20 Calcific tendinitis, unspecified site

M65.22 Calcific tendinitis, upper arm

M65.221 Calcific tendinitis, right upper arm

M65.222 Calcific tendinitis, left upper arm

M65.229 Calcific tendinitis, unspecified upper arm

M65.23 Calcific tendinitis, forearm

M65.231 Calcific tendinitis, right forearm

M65.232 Calcific tendinitis, left forearm

M65.239 Calcific tendinitis, unspecified forearm

M65.24 Calcific tendinitis, hand

M65.241 Calcific tendinitis, right hand

M65.242 Calcific tendinitis, left hand

M65.249 Calcific tendinitis, unspecified hand

M65.25 Calcific tendinitis, thigh

M65.251 Calcific tendinitis, right thigh

M65.252 Calcific tendinitis, left thigh

M65.259 Calcific tendinitis, unspecified thigh

M65.26 Calcific tendinitis, lower leg

M65.261 Calcific tendinitis, right lower leg

M65.262 Calcific tendinitis, left lower leg

M65.269 Calcific tendinitis, unspecified lower leg

M65.27 Calcific tendinitis, ankle and foot

M65.271 Calcific tendinitis, right ankle and foot

M65.272 Calcific tendinitis, left ankle and foot

M65.279 Calcific tendinitis, unspecified ankle and foot

M65.28 Calcific tendinitis, other site

M65.29 Calcific tendinitis, multiple sites

M65.3 Trigger finger

Nodular tendinous disease

M65.30 Trigger finger, unspecified finger

M65.31 Trigger thumb

M65.311 Trigger thumb, right thumb

M65.312 Trigger thumb, left thumb

M65.319 Trigger thumb, unspecified thumb

M65.32 **Trigger finger, index finger**

M65.321 Trigger finger, right index finger

M65.322 Trigger finger, left index finger

M65.329 Trigger finger, unspecified index finger

M65.33 **Trigger finger, middle finger**

M65.331 Trigger finger, right middle finger

M65.332 Trigger finger, left middle finger

M65.339 Trigger finger, unspecified middle finger

M65.34 **Trigger finger, ring finger**

M65.341 Trigger finger, right ring finger

M65.342 Trigger finger, left ring finger

M65.349 Trigger finger, unspecified ring finger

M65.35 **Trigger finger, little finger**

M65.351 Trigger finger, right little finger

M65.352 Trigger finger, left little finger

M65.359 Trigger finger, unspecified little finger

M65.4 **Radial styloid tenosynovitis [de Quervain]**

M65.8 **Other synovitis and tenosynovitis**

M65.80 **Other synovitis and tenosynovitis, unspecified site**

M65.81 **Other synovitis and tenosynovitis, shoulder**

M65.811 Other synovitis and tenosynovitis, right shoulder

M65.812 Other synovitis and tenosynovitis, left shoulder

M65.819 Other synovitis and tenosynovitis, unspecified shoulder

M65.82 **Other synovitis and tenosynovitis, upper arm**

M65.821 Other synovitis and tenosynovitis, right upper arm

M65.822 Other synovitis and tenosynovitis, left upper arm

M65.829 Other synovitis and tenosynovitis, unspecified upper arm

M65.83 **Other synovitis and tenosynovitis, forearm**

M65.831 Other synovitis and tenosynovitis, right forearm

M65.832 Other synovitis and tenosynovitis, left forearm

M65.839 Other synovitis and tenosynovitis, unspecified forearm

M65.84 **Other synovitis and tenosynovitis, hand**

M65.841 Other synovitis and tenosynovitis, right hand

M65.842 Other synovitis and tenosynovitis, left hand

M65.849 Other synovitis and tenosynovitis, unspecified hand

M65.85 **Other synovitis and tenosynovitis, thigh**

M65.851 Other synovitis and tenosynovitis, right thigh

M65.852 Other synovitis and tenosynovitis, left thigh

M65.859 Other synovitis and tenosynovitis, unspecified thigh

M65.86 **Other synovitis and tenosynovitis, lower leg**

M65.861 Other synovitis and tenosynovitis, right lower leg

M65.862 Other synovitis and tenosynovitis, left lower leg

M65.869 Other synovitis and tenosynovitis, unspecified lower leg

M65.87 **Other synovitis and tenosynovitis, ankle and foot**

M65.871 Other synovitis and tenosynovitis, right ankle and foot

M65.872 Other synovitis and tenosynovitis, left ankle and foot

M65.879 Other synovitis and tenosynovitis, unspecified ankle and foot

M65.88 **Other synovitis and tenosynovitis, other site**

M65.89 **Other synovitis and tenosynovitis, multiple sites**

M65.9 **Synovitis and tenosynovitis, unspecified**

M66 **Spontaneous rupture of synovium and tendon**

Includes: rupture that occurs when a normal force is applied to tissues that are inferred to have less than normal strength

Excludes2: rotator cuff syndrome (M75.1-)

rupture where an abnormal force is applied to normal tissue - see injury of tendon by body region

M66.0 **Rupture of popliteal cyst**

M66.1 **Rupture of synovium**

Rupture of synovial cyst

Excludes2: rupture of popliteal cyst (M66.0)

M66.10 **Rupture of synovium, unspecified joint**

M66.11 **Rupture of synovium, shoulder**

M66.111 Rupture of synovium, right shoulder

M66.112 Rupture of synovium, left shoulder

M66.119 Rupture of synovium, unspecified shoulder

M66.12 **Rupture of synovium, elbow**

M66.121 Rupture of synovium, right elbow

M66.122 Rupture of synovium, left elbow

M66.129 Rupture of synovium, unspecified elbow

M66.13 **Rupture of synovium, wrist**

M66.131 Rupture of synovium, right wrist

M66.132 Rupture of synovium, left wrist

M66.139 Rupture of synovium, unspecified wrist

M66.14 **Rupture of synovium, hand and fingers**

M66.141 Rupture of synovium, right hand

M66.142 Rupture of synovium, left hand

M66.143 Rupture of synovium, unspecified hand

M66.144 Rupture of synovium, right finger(s)

M66.145 Rupture of synovium, left finger(s)

M66.146 Rupture of synovium, unspecified finger(s)

M66.15 **Rupture of synovium, hip**

M66.151 Rupture of synovium, right hip

M66.152 Rupture of synovium, left hip

M66.159 Rupture of synovium, unspecified hip

M66.17 Rupture of synovium, ankle, foot and toes

    M66.171 Rupture of synovium, right ankle

    M66.172 Rupture of synovium, left ankle

    M66.173 Rupture of synovium, unspecified ankle

    M66.174 Rupture of synovium, right foot

    M66.175 Rupture of synovium, left foot

    M66.176 Rupture of synovium, unspecified foot

    M66.177 Rupture of synovium, right toe(s)

    M66.178 Rupture of synovium, left toe(s)

    M66.179 Rupture of synovium, unspecified toe(s)

M66.18 Rupture of synovium, other site

M66.2 Spontaneous rupture of extensor tendons

   M66.20 Spontaneous rupture of extensor tendons, unspecified site

   M66.21 Spontaneous rupture of extensor tendons, shoulder

    M66.211 Spontaneous rupture of extensor tendons, right shoulder

    M66.212 Spontaneous rupture of extensor tendons, left shoulder

    M66.219 Spontaneous rupture of extensor tendons, unspecified shoulder

   M66.22 Spontaneous rupture of extensor tendons, upper arm

    M66.221 Spontaneous rupture of extensor tendons, right upper arm

    M66.222 Spontaneous rupture of extensor tendons, left upper arm

    M66.229 Spontaneous rupture of extensor tendons, unspecified upper arm

   M66.23 Spontaneous rupture of extensor tendons, forearm

    M66.231 Spontaneous rupture of extensor tendons, right forearm

    M66.232 Spontaneous rupture of extensor tendons, left forearm

    M66.239 Spontaneous rupture of extensor tendons, unspecified forearm

   M66.24 Spontaneous rupture of extensor tendons, hand

    M66.241 Spontaneous rupture of extensor tendons, right hand

    M66.242 Spontaneous rupture of extensor tendons, left hand

    M66.249 Spontaneous rupture of extensor tendons, unspecified hand

   M66.25 Spontaneous rupture of extensor tendons, thigh

    M66.251 Spontaneous rupture of extensor tendons, right thigh

    M66.252 Spontaneous rupture of extensor tendons, left thigh

    M66.259 Spontaneous rupture of extensor tendons, unspecified thigh

   M66.26 Spontaneous rupture of extensor tendons, lower leg

    M66.261 Spontaneous rupture of extensor tendons, right lower leg

    M66.262 Spontaneous rupture of extensor tendons, left lower leg

    M66.269 Spontaneous rupture of extensor tendons, unspecified lower leg

   M66.27 Spontaneous rupture of extensor tendons, ankle and foot

    M66.271 Spontaneous rupture of extensor tendons, right ankle and foot

    M66.272 Spontaneous rupture of extensor tendons, left ankle and foot

    M66.279 Spontaneous rupture of extensor tendons, unspecified ankle and foot

   M66.28 Spontaneous rupture of extensor tendons, other site

   M66.29 Spontaneous rupture of extensor tendons, multiple sites

M66.3 Spontaneous rupture of flexor tendons

   M66.30 Spontaneous rupture of flexor tendons, unspecified site

   M66.31 Spontaneous rupture of flexor tendons, shoulder

    M66.311 Spontaneous rupture of flexor tendons, right shoulder

    M66.312 Spontaneous rupture of flexor tendons, left shoulder

    M66.319 Spontaneous rupture of flexor tendons, unspecified shoulder

   M66.32 Spontaneous rupture of flexor tendons, upper arm

    M66.321 Spontaneous rupture of flexor tendons, right upper arm

    M66.322 Spontaneous rupture of flexor tendons, left upper arm

    M66.329 Spontaneous rupture of flexor tendons, unspecified upper arm

   M66.33 Spontaneous rupture of flexor tendons, forearm

    M66.331 Spontaneous rupture of flexor tendons, right forearm

    M66.332 Spontaneous rupture of flexor tendons, left forearm

    M66.339 Spontaneous rupture of flexor tendons, unspecified forearm

   M66.34 Spontaneous rupture of flexor tendons, hand

    M66.341 Spontaneous rupture of flexor tendons, right hand

    M66.342 Spontaneous rupture of flexor tendons, left hand

    M66.349 Spontaneous rupture of flexor tendons, unspecified hand

   M66.35 Spontaneous rupture of flexor tendons, thigh

    M66.351 Spontaneous rupture of flexor tendons, right thigh

    M66.352 Spontaneous rupture of flexor tendons, left thigh

    M66.359 Spontaneous rupture of flexor tendons, unspecified thigh

   M66.36 Spontaneous rupture of flexor tendons, lower leg

    M66.361 Spontaneous rupture of flexor tendons, right lower leg

    M66.362 Spontaneous rupture of flexor tendons, left lower leg

    M66.369 Spontaneous rupture of flexor tendons, unspecified lower leg

   M66.37 Spontaneous rupture of flexor tendons, ankle and foot

    M66.371 Spontaneous rupture of flexor tendons, right ankle and foot

● New code   ▲ Revised code   **Excludes1:** Not coded here   **Excludes2:** Not included here   ⊗ Placeholder required   ⑦7th digit required

M66.372 Spontaneous rupture of flexor tendons, left ankle and foot

M66.379 Spontaneous rupture of flexor tendons, unspecified ankle and foot

M66.38 Spontaneous rupture of flexor tendons, other site

M66.39 Spontaneous rupture of flexor tendons, multiple sites

M66.8 Spontaneous rupture of other tendons

M66.80 Spontaneous rupture of other tendons, unspecified site

M66.81 Spontaneous rupture of other tendons, shoulder

M66.811 Spontaneous rupture of other tendons, right shoulder

M66.812 Spontaneous rupture of other tendons, left shoulder

M66.819 Spontaneous rupture of other tendons, unspecified shoulder

M66.82 Spontaneous rupture of other tendons, upper arm

M66.821 Spontaneous rupture of other tendons, right upper arm

M66.822 Spontaneous rupture of other tendons, left upper arm

M66.829 Spontaneous rupture of other tendons, unspecified upper arm

M66.83 Spontaneous rupture of other tendons, forearm

M66.831 Spontaneous rupture of other tendons, right forearm

M66.832 Spontaneous rupture of other tendons, left forearm

M66.839 Spontaneous rupture of other tendons, unspecified forearm

M66.84 Spontaneous rupture of other tendons, hand

M66.841 Spontaneous rupture of other tendons, right hand

M66.842 Spontaneous rupture of other tendons, left hand

M66.849 Spontaneous rupture of other tendons, unspecified hand

M66.85 Spontaneous rupture of other tendons, thigh

M66.851 Spontaneous rupture of other tendons, right thigh

M66.852 Spontaneous rupture of other tendons, left thigh

M66.859 Spontaneous rupture of other tendons, unspecified thigh

M66.86 Spontaneous rupture of other tendons, lower leg

M66.861 Spontaneous rupture of other tendons, right lower leg

M66.862 Spontaneous rupture of other tendons, left lower leg

M66.869 Spontaneous rupture of other tendons, unspecified lower leg

M66.87 Spontaneous rupture of other tendons, ankle and foot

M66.871 Spontaneous rupture of other tendons, right ankle and foot

M66.872 Spontaneous rupture of other tendons, left ankle and foot

M66.879 Spontaneous rupture of other tendons, unspecified ankle and foot

M66.88 Spontaneous rupture of other tendons, other

M66.89 Spontaneous rupture of other tendons, multiple sites

M66.9 Spontaneous rupture of unspecified tendon

Rupture at musculotendinous junction, nontraumatic

M67 Other disorders of synovium and tendon

Excludes1: palmar fascial fibromatosis [Dupuytren] (M72.0)

tendinitis NOS (M77.9-)

xanthomatosis localized to tendons (E78.2)

M67.0 Short Achilles tendon (acquired)

M67.00 Short Achilles tendon (acquired), unspecified ankle

M67.01 Short Achilles tendon (acquired), right ankle

M67.02 Short Achilles tendon (acquired), left ankle

M67.2 Synovial hypertrophy, not elsewhere classified

Excludes1: villonodular synovitis (pigmented) (M12.2-)

M67.20 Synovial hypertrophy, not elsewhere classified, unspecified site

M67.21 Synovial hypertrophy, not elsewhere classified, shoulder

M67.211 Synovial hypertrophy, not elsewhere classified, right shoulder

M67.212 Synovial hypertrophy, not elsewhere classified, left shoulder

M67.219 Synovial hypertrophy, not elsewhere classified, unspecified shoulder

M67.22 Synovial hypertrophy, not elsewhere classified, upper arm

M67.221 Synovial hypertrophy, not elsewhere classified, right upper arm

M67.222 Synovial hypertrophy, not elsewhere classified, left upper arm

M67.229 Synovial hypertrophy, not elsewhere classified, unspecified upper arm

M67.23 Synovial hypertrophy, not elsewhere classified, forearm

M67.231 Synovial hypertrophy, not elsewhere classified, right forearm

M67.232 Synovial hypertrophy, not elsewhere classified, left forearm

M67.239 Synovial hypertrophy, not elsewhere classified, unspecified forearm

M67.24 Synovial hypertrophy, not elsewhere classified, hand

M67.241 Synovial hypertrophy, not elsewhere classified, right hand

M67.242 Synovial hypertrophy, not elsewhere classified, left hand

M67.249 Synovial hypertrophy, not elsewhere classified, unspecified hand

M67.25 Synovial hypertrophy, not elsewhere classified, thigh

M67.251 Synovial hypertrophy, not elsewhere classified, right thigh

M67.252 Synovial hypertrophy, not elsewhere classified, left thigh

M67.259 Synovial hypertrophy, not elsewhere classified, unspecified thigh

M67.26 Synovial hypertrophy, not elsewhere classified, lower leg

M67.261 Synovial hypertrophy, not elsewhere classified, right lower leg

M67.262 Synovial hypertrophy, not elsewhere classified, left lower leg

M67.269 Synovial hypertrophy, not elsewhere classified, unspecified lower leg

M67.27 Synovial hypertrophy, not elsewhere classified, ankle and foot

    M67.271 Synovial hypertrophy, not elsewhere classified, right ankle and foot

    M67.272 Synovial hypertrophy, not elsewhere classified, left ankle and foot

    M67.279 Synovial hypertrophy, not elsewhere classified, unspecified ankle and foot

M67.28 Synovial hypertrophy, not elsewhere classified, other site

M67.29 Synovial hypertrophy, not elsewhere classified, multiple sites

M67.3 **Transient synovitis**

Toxic synovitis

Excludes1: palindromic rheumatism (M12.3-)

M67.30 Transient synovitis, unspecified site

M67.31 Transient synovitis, shoulder

    M67.311 Transient synovitis, right shoulder

    M67.312 Transient synovitis, left shoulder

    M67.319 Transient synovitis, unspecified shoulder

M67.32 Transient synovitis, elbow

    M67.321 Transient synovitis, right elbow

    M67.322 Transient synovitis, left elbow

    M67.329 Transient synovitis, unspecified elbow

M67.33 Transient synovitis, wrist

    M67.331 Transient synovitis, right wrist

    M67.332 Transient synovitis, left wrist

    M67.339 Transient synovitis, unspecified wrist

M67.34 Transient synovitis, hand

    M67.341 Transient synovitis, right hand

    M67.342 Transient synovitis, left hand

    M67.349 Transient synovitis, unspecified hand

M67.35 Transient synovitis, hip

    M67.351 Transient synovitis, right hip

    M67.352 Transient synovitis, left hip

    M67.359 Transient synovitis, unspecified hip

M67.36 Transient synovitis, knee

    M67.361 Transient synovitis, right knee

    M67.362 Transient synovitis, left knee

    M67.369 Transient synovitis, unspecified knee

M67.37 Transient synovitis, ankle and foot

    M67.371 Transient synovitis, right ankle and foot

    M67.372 Transient synovitis, left ankle and foot

    M67.379 Transient synovitis, unspecified ankle and foot

M67.38 Transient synovitis, other site

M67.39 Transient synovitis, multiple sites

M67.4 **Ganglion**

Ganglion of joint or tendon (sheath)

Excludes1: ganglion in yaws (A66.6)

Excludes2: cyst of bursa (M71.2-M71.3)

cyst of synovium (M71.2-M71.3)

M67.40 Ganglion, unspecified site

M67.41 Ganglion, shoulder

    M67.411 Ganglion, right shoulder

    M67.412 Ganglion, left shoulder

    M67.419 Ganglion, unspecified shoulder

M67.42 Ganglion, elbow

    M67.421 Ganglion, right elbow

    M67.422 Ganglion, left elbow

    M67.429 Ganglion, unspecified elbow

M67.43 Ganglion, wrist

    M67.431 Ganglion, right wrist

    M67.432 Ganglion, left wrist

    M67.439 Ganglion, unspecified wrist

M67.44 Ganglion, hand

    M67.441 Ganglion, right hand

    M67.442 Ganglion, left hand

    M67.449 Ganglion, unspecified hand

M67.45 Ganglion, hip

    M67.451 Ganglion, right hip

    M67.452 Ganglion, left hip

    M67.459 Ganglion, unspecified hip

M67.46 Ganglion, knee

    M67.461 Ganglion, right knee

    M67.462 Ganglion, left knee

    M67.469 Ganglion, unspecified knee

M67.47 Ganglion, ankle and foot

    M67.471 Ganglion, right ankle and foot

    M67.472 Ganglion, left ankle and foot

    M67.479 Ganglion, unspecified ankle and foot

M67.48 Ganglion, other site

M67.49 Ganglion, multiple sites

M67.5 **Plica syndrome**

Plica knee

M67.50 Plica syndrome, unspecified knee

M67.51 Plica syndrome, right knee

M67.52 Plica syndrome, left knee

M67.8 **Other specified disorders of synovium and tendon**

M67.80 Other specified disorders of synovium and tendon, unspecified site

M67.81 Other specified disorders of synovium and tendon, shoulder

    M67.811 Other specified disorders of synovium, right shoulder

    M67.812 Other specified disorders of synovium, left shoulder

    M67.813 Other specified disorders of tendon, right shoulder

    M67.814 Other specified disorders of tendon, left shoulder

    M67.819 Other specified disorders of synovium and tendon, unspecified shoulder

M67.82 Other specified disorders of synovium and tendon, elbow

    M67.821 Other specified disorders of synovium, right elbow

    M67.822 Other specified disorders of synovium, left elbow

    M67.823 Other specified disorders of tendon, right elbow

M67.824 Other specified disorders of tendon, left elbow

M67.829 Other specified disorders of synovium and tendon, unspecified elbow

M67.83 Other specified disorders of synovium and tendon, wrist

M67.831 Other specified disorders of synovium, right wrist

M67.832 Other specified disorders of synovium, left wrist

M67.833 Other specified disorders of tendon, right wrist

M67.834 Other specified disorders of tendon, left wrist

M67.839 Other specified disorders of synovium and tendon, unspecified forearm

M67.84 Other specified disorders of synovium and tendon, hand

M67.841 Other specified disorders of synovium, right hand

M67.842 Other specified disorders of synovium, left hand

M67.843 Other specified disorders of tendon, right hand

M67.844 Other specified disorders of tendon, left hand

M67.849 Other specified disorders of synovium and tendon, unspecified hand

M67.85 Other specified disorders of synovium and tendon, hip

M67.851 Other specified disorders of synovium, right hip

M67.852 Other specified disorders of synovium, left hip

M67.853 Other specified disorders of tendon, right hip

M67.854 Other specified disorders of tendon, left hip

M67.859 Other specified disorders of synovium and tendon, unspecified hip

M67.86 Other specified disorders of synovium and tendon, knee

M67.861 Other specified disorders of synovium, right knee

M67.862 Other specified disorders of synovium, left knee

M67.863 Other specified disorders of tendon, right knee

M67.864 Other specified disorders of tendon, left knee

M67.869 Other specified disorders of synovium and tendon, unspecified knee

M67.87 Other specified disorders of synovium and tendon, ankle and foot

M67.871 Other specified disorders of synovium, right ankle and foot

M67.872 Other specified disorders of synovium, left ankle and foot

M67.873 Other specified disorders of tendon, right ankle and foot

M67.874 Other specified disorders of tendon, left ankle and foot

M67.879 Other specified disorders of synovium and tendon, unspecified ankle and foot

M67.88 Other specified disorders of synovium and tendon, other site

M67.89 Other specified disorders of synovium and tendon, multiple sites

M67.9 Unspecified disorder of synovium and tendon

M67.90 Unspecified disorder of synovium and tendon, unspecified site

M67.91 Unspecified disorder of synovium and tendon, shoulder

M67.911 Unspecified disorder of synovium and tendon, right shoulder

M67.912 Unspecified disorder of synovium and tendon, left shoulder

M67.919 Unspecified disorder of synovium and tendon, unspecified shoulder

M67.92 Unspecified disorder of synovium and tendon, upper arm

M67.921 Unspecified disorder of synovium and tendon, right upper arm

M67.922 Unspecified disorder of synovium and tendon, left upper arm

M67.929 Unspecified disorder of synovium and tendon, unspecified upper arm

M67.93 Unspecified disorder of synovium and tendon, forearm

M67.931 Unspecified disorder of synovium and tendon, right forearm

M67.932 Unspecified disorder of synovium and tendon, left forearm

M67.939 Unspecified disorder of synovium and tendon, unspecified forearm

M67.94 Unspecified disorder of synovium and tendon, hand

M67.941 Unspecified disorder of synovium and tendon, right hand

M67.942 Unspecified disorder of synovium and tendon, left hand

M67.949 Unspecified disorder of synovium and tendon, unspecified hand

M67.95 Unspecified disorder of synovium and tendon, thigh

M67.951 Unspecified disorder of synovium and tendon, right thigh

M67.952 Unspecified disorder of synovium and tendon, left thigh

M67.959 Unspecified disorder of synovium and tendon, unspecified thigh

M67.96 Unspecified disorder of synovium and tendon, lower leg

M67.961 Unspecified disorder of synovium and tendon, right lower leg

M67.962 Unspecified disorder of synovium and tendon, left lower leg

M67.969 Unspecified disorder of synovium and tendon, unspecified lower leg

M67.97 Unspecified disorder of synovium and tendon, ankle and foot

M67.971 Unspecified disorder of synovium and tendon, right ankle and foot

M67.972   **Unspecified disorder of synovium and tendon, left ankle and foot**

M67.979   **Unspecified disorder of synovium and tendon, unspecified ankle and foot**

M67.98   **Unspecified disorder of synovium and tendon, other site**

M67.99   **Unspecified disorder of synovium and tendon, multiple sites**

OTHER SOFT TISSUE DISORDERS (M70-M79)

M70   **Soft tissue disorders related to use, overuse and pressure**

Includes: soft tissue disorders of occupational origin

Use additional external cause code to identify activity causing disorder (Y93.-)

Excludes1: bursitis NOS (M71.9-)

Excludes2: bursitis of shoulder (M75.5)

enthesopathies (M76-M77)

pressure ulcer (pressure area) (L89.-)

M70.0   **Crepitant synovitis (acute) (chronic) of hand and wrist**

M70.03   **Crepitant synovitis (acute) (chronic), wrist**

M70.031   **Crepitant synovitis (acute) (chronic), right wrist**

M70.032   **Crepitant synovitis (acute) (chronic), left wrist**

M70.039   **Crepitant synovitis (acute) (chronic), unspecified wrist**

M70.04   **Crepitant synovitis (acute) (chronic), hand**

M70.041   **Crepitant synovitis (acute) (chronic), right hand**

M70.042   **Crepitant synovitis (acute) (chronic), left hand**

M70.049   **Crepitant synovitis (acute) (chronic), unspecified hand**

M70.1   **Bursitis of hand**

M70.10   **Bursitis, unspecified hand**

M70.11   **Bursitis, right hand**

M70.12   **Bursitis, left hand**

M70.2   **Olecranon bursitis**

M70.20   **Olecranon bursitis, unspecified elbow**

M70.21   **Olecranon bursitis, right elbow**

M70.22   **Olecranon bursitis, left elbow**

M70.3   **Other bursitis of elbow**

M70.30   **Other bursitis of elbow, unspecified elbow**

M70.31   **Other bursitis of elbow, right elbow**

M70.32   **Other bursitis of elbow, left elbow**

M70.4   **Prepatellar bursitis**

M70.40   **Prepatellar bursitis, unspecified knee**

M70.41   **Prepatellar bursitis, right knee**

M70.42   **Prepatellar bursitis, left knee**

M70.5   **Other bursitis of knee**

M70.50   **Other bursitis of knee, unspecified knee**

M70.51   **Other bursitis of knee, right knee**

M70.52   **Other bursitis of knee, left knee**

M70.6   **Trochanteric bursitis**

Trochanteric tendinitis

M70.60   **Trochanteric bursitis, unspecified hip**

M70.61   **Trochanteric bursitis, right hip**

M70.62   **Trochanteric bursitis, left hip**

M70.7   **Other bursitis of hip**

Ischial bursitis

M70.70   **Other bursitis of hip, unspecified hip**

M70.71   **Other bursitis of hip, right hip**

M70.72   **Other bursitis of hip, left hip**

M70.8   **Other soft tissue disorders related to use, overuse and pressure**

M70.80   **Other soft tissue disorders related to use, overuse and pressure of unspecified site**

M70.81   **Other soft tissue disorders related to use, overuse and pressure of shoulder**

M70.811   **Other soft tissue disorders related to use, overuse and pressure, right shoulder**

M70.812   **Other soft tissue disorders related to use, overuse and pressure, left shoulder**

M70.819   **Other soft tissue disorders related to use, overuse and pressure, unspecified shoulder**

M70.82   **Other soft tissue disorders related to use, overuse and pressure of upper arm**

M70.821   **Other soft tissue disorders related to use, overuse and pressure, right upper arm**

M70.822   **Other soft tissue disorders related to use, overuse and pressure, left upper arm**

M70.829   **Other soft tissue disorders related to use, overuse and pressure, unspecified upper arms**

M70.83   **Other soft tissue disorders related to use, overuse and pressure of forearm**

M70.831   **Other soft tissue disorders related to use, overuse and pressure, right forearm**

M70.832   **Other soft tissue disorders related to use, overuse and pressure, left forearm**

M70.839   **Other soft tissue disorders related to use, overuse and pressure, unspecified forearm**

M70.84   **Other soft tissue disorders related to use, overuse and pressure of hand**

M70.841   **Other soft tissue disorders related to use, overuse and pressure, right hand**

M70.842   **Other soft tissue disorders related to use, overuse and pressure, left hand**

M70.849   **Other soft tissue disorders related to use, overuse and pressure, unspecified hand**

M70.85   **Other soft tissue disorders related to use, overuse and pressure of thigh**

M70.851   **Other soft tissue disorders related to use, overuse and pressure, right thigh**

M70.852   **Other soft tissue disorders related to use, overuse and pressure, left thigh**

M70.859   **Other soft tissue disorders related to use, overuse and pressure, unspecified thigh**

M70.86   **Other soft tissue disorders related to use, overuse and pressure lower leg**

M70.861 Other soft tissue disorders related to use, overuse and pressure, right lower leg

M70.862 Other soft tissue disorders related to use, overuse and pressure, left lower leg

M70.869 Other soft tissue disorders related to use, overuse and pressure, unspecified leg

M70.87 Other soft tissue disorders related to use, overuse and pressure of ankle and foot

M70.871 Other soft tissue disorders related to use, overuse and pressure, right ankle and foot

M70.872 Other soft tissue disorders related to use, overuse and pressure, left ankle and foot

M70.879 Other soft tissue disorders related to use, overuse and pressure, unspecified ankle and foot

M70.88 Other soft tissue disorders related to use, overuse and pressure other site

M70.89 Other soft tissue disorders related to use, overuse and pressure multiple sites

M70.9 Unspecified soft tissue disorder related to use, overuse and pressure

M70.90 Unspecified soft tissue disorder related to use, overuse and pressure of unspecified site

M70.91 Unspecified soft tissue disorder related to use, overuse and pressure of shoulder

M70.911 Unspecified soft tissue disorder related to use, overuse and pressure, right shoulder

M70.912 Unspecified soft tissue disorder related to use, overuse and pressure, left shoulder

M70.919 Unspecified soft tissue disorder related to use, overuse and pressure, unspecified shoulder

M70.92 Unspecified soft tissue disorder related to use, overuse and pressure of upper arm

M70.921 Unspecified soft tissue disorder related to use, overuse and pressure, right upper arm

M70.922 Unspecified soft tissue disorder related to use, overuse and pressure, left upper arm

M70.929 Unspecified soft tissue disorder related to use, overuse and pressure, unspecified upper arm

M70.93 Unspecified soft tissue disorder related to use, overuse and pressure of forearm

M70.931 Unspecified soft tissue disorder related to use, overuse and pressure, right forearm

M70.932 Unspecified soft tissue disorder related to use, overuse and pressure, left forearm

M70.939 Unspecified soft tissue disorder related to use, overuse and pressure, unspecified forearm

M70.94 Unspecified soft tissue disorder related to use, overuse and pressure of hand

M70.941 Unspecified soft tissue disorder related to use, overuse and pressure, right hand

M70.942 Unspecified soft tissue disorder related to use, overuse and pressure, left hand

M70.949 Unspecified soft tissue disorder related to use, overuse and pressure, unspecified hand

M70.95 Unspecified soft tissue disorder related to use, overuse and pressure of thigh

M70.951 Unspecified soft tissue disorder related to use, overuse and pressure, right thigh

M70.952 Unspecified soft tissue disorder related to use, overuse and pressure, left thigh

M70.959 Unspecified soft tissue disorder related to use, overuse and pressure, unspecified thigh

M70.96 Unspecified soft tissue disorder related to use, overuse and pressure lower leg

M70.961 Unspecified soft tissue disorder related to use, overuse and pressure, right lower leg

M70.962 Unspecified soft tissue disorder related to use, overuse and pressure, left lower leg

M70.969 Unspecified soft tissue disorder related to use, overuse and pressure, unspecified lower leg

M70.97 Unspecified soft tissue disorder related to use, overuse and pressure of ankle and foot

M70.971 Unspecified soft tissue disorder related to use, overuse and pressure, right ankle and foot

M70.972 Unspecified soft tissue disorder related to use, overuse and pressure, left ankle and foot

M70.979 Unspecified soft tissue disorder related to use, overuse and pressure, unspecified ankle and foot

M70.98 Unspecified soft tissue disorder related to use, overuse and pressure other

M70.99 Unspecified soft tissue disorder related to use, overuse and pressure multiple sites

M71 **Other bursopathies**

Excludes1: bunion (M20.1)

bursitis related to use, overuse or pressure (M70.-)

enthesopathies (M76-M77)

M71.0 **Abscess of bursa**

Use additional code (B95.-, B96.-) to identify causative organism

M71.00 Abscess of bursa, unspecified site

M71.01 Abscess of bursa, shoulder

M71.011 Abscess of bursa, right shoulder

M71.012 Abscess of bursa, left shoulder

M71.019 Abscess of bursa, unspecified shoulder

M71.02 Abscess of bursa, elbow

M71.021 Abscess of bursa, right elbow

M71.022 Abscess of bursa, left elbow

M71.029 Abscess of bursa, unspecified elbow

M71.03 Abscess of bursa, wrist

M71.031 Abscess of bursa, right wrist

M71.032 Abscess of bursa, left wrist

M71.039 Abscess of bursa, unspecified wrist

M71.04 Abscess of bursa, hand
  M71.041 Abscess of bursa, right hand
  M71.042 Abscess of bursa, left hand
  M71.049 Abscess of bursa, unspecified hand

M71.05 Abscess of bursa, hip
  M71.051 Abscess of bursa, right hip
  M71.052 Abscess of bursa, left hip
  M71.059 Abscess of bursa, unspecified hip

M71.06 Abscess of bursa, knee
  M71.061 Abscess of bursa, right knee
  M71.062 Abscess of bursa, left knee
  M71.069 Abscess of bursa, unspecified knee

M71.07 Abscess of bursa, ankle and foot
  M71.071 Abscess of bursa, right ankle and foot
  M71.072 Abscess of bursa, left ankle and foot
  M71.079 Abscess of bursa, unspecified ankle and foot

M71.08 Abscess of bursa, other site

M71.09 Abscess of bursa, multiple sites

M71.1 Other infective bursitis
  Use additional code (B95.-, B96.-) to identify causative organism

M71.10 Other infective bursitis, unspecified site

M71.11 Other infective bursitis, shoulder
  M71.111 Other infective bursitis, right shoulder
  M71.112 Other infective bursitis, left shoulder
  M71.119 Other infective bursitis, unspecified shoulder

M71.12 Other infective bursitis, elbow
  M71.121 Other infective bursitis, right elbow
  M71.122 Other infective bursitis, left elbow
  M71.129 Other infective bursitis, unspecified elbow

M71.13 Other infective bursitis, wrist
  M71.131 Other infective bursitis, right wrist
  M71.132 Other infective bursitis, left wrist
  M71.139 Other infective bursitis, unspecified wrist

M71.14 Other infective bursitis, hand
  M71.141 Other infective bursitis, right hand
  M71.142 Other infective bursitis, left hand
  M71.149 Other infective bursitis, unspecified hand

M71.15 Other infective bursitis, hip
  M71.151 Other infective bursitis, right hip
  M71.152 Other infective bursitis, left hip
  M71.159 Other infective bursitis, unspecified hip

M71.16 Other infective bursitis, knee
  M71.161 Other infective bursitis, right knee
  M71.162 Other infective bursitis, left knee
  M71.169 Other infective bursitis, unspecified knee

M71.17 Other infective bursitis, ankle and foot
  M71.171 Other infective bursitis, right ankle and foot
  M71.172 Other infective bursitis, left ankle and foot
  M71.179 Other infective bursitis, unspecified ankle and foot

M71.18 Other infective bursitis, other site

M71.19 Other infective bursitis, multiple sites

M71.2 Synovial cyst of popliteal space [Baker]
  Excludes1: synovial cyst of popliteal space with rupture (M66.0)

M71.20 Synovial cyst of popliteal space [Baker], unspecified knee

M71.21 Synovial cyst of popliteal space [Baker], right knee

M71.22 Synovial cyst of popliteal space [Baker], left knee

M71.3 Other bursal cyst
  Synovial cyst NOS
  Excludes1: synovial cyst with rupture (M66.1-)

M71.30 Other bursal cyst, unspecified site

M71.31 Other bursal cyst, shoulder
  M71.311 Other bursal cyst, right shoulder
  M71.312 Other bursal cyst, left shoulder
  M71.319 Other bursal cyst, unspecified shoulder

M71.32 Other bursal cyst, elbow
  M71.321 Other bursal cyst, right elbow
  M71.322 Other bursal cyst, left elbow
  M71.329 Other bursal cyst, unspecified elbow

M71.33 Other bursal cyst, wrist
  M71.331 Other bursal cyst, right wrist
  M71.332 Other bursal cyst, left wrist
  M71.339 Other bursal cyst, unspecified wrist

M71.34 Other bursal cyst, hand
  M71.341 Other bursal cyst, right hand
  M71.342 Other bursal cyst, left hand
  M71.349 Other bursal cyst, unspecified hand

M71.35 Other bursal cyst, hip
  M71.351 Other bursal cyst, right hip
  M71.352 Other bursal cyst, left hip
  M71.359 Other bursal cyst, unspecified hip

M71.37 Other bursal cyst, ankle and foot
  M71.371 Other bursal cyst, right ankle and foot
  M71.372 Other bursal cyst, left ankle and foot
  M71.379 Other bursal cyst, unspecified ankle and foot

M71.38 Other bursal cyst, other site

M71.39 Other bursal cyst, multiple sites

M71.4 Calcium deposit in bursa
  Excludes2: calcium deposit in bursa of shoulder (M75.3)

M71.40 Calcium deposit in bursa, unspecified site

M71.42 Calcium deposit in bursa, elbow
  M71.421 Calcium deposit in bursa, right elbow
  M71.422 Calcium deposit in bursa, left elbow
  M71.429 Calcium deposit in bursa, unspecified elbow

M71.43 Calcium deposit in bursa, wrist
  M71.431 Calcium deposit in bursa, right wrist

M71.432 Calcium deposit in bursa, left wrist

M71.439 Calcium deposit in bursa, unspecified wrist

M71.44 Calcium deposit in bursa, hand

M71.441 Calcium deposit in bursa, right hand

M71.442 Calcium deposit in bursa, left hand

M71.449 Calcium deposit in bursa, unspecified hand

M71.45 Calcium deposit in bursa, hip

M71.451 Calcium deposit in bursa, right hip

M71.452 Calcium deposit in bursa, left hip

M71.459 Calcium deposit in bursa, unspecified hip

M71.46 Calcium deposit in bursa, knee

M71.461 Calcium deposit in bursa, right knee

M71.462 Calcium deposit in bursa, left knee

M71.469 Calcium deposit in bursa, unspecified knee

M71.47 Calcium deposit in bursa, ankle and foot

M71.471 Calcium deposit in bursa, right ankle and foot

M71.472 Calcium deposit in bursa, left ankle and foot

M71.479 Calcium deposit in bursa, unspecified ankle and foot

M71.48 Calcium deposit in bursa, other site

M71.49 Calcium deposit in bursa, multiple sites

M71.5 Other bursitis, not elsewhere classified

Excludes1: bursitis NOS (M71.9-)

Excludes2: bursitis of shoulder (M75.5)

bursitis of tibial collateral [Pellegrini-Stieda] (M76.4-)

M71.50 Other bursitis, not elsewhere classified, unspecified site

M71.52 Other bursitis, not elsewhere classified, elbow

M71.521 Other bursitis, not elsewhere classified, right elbow

M71.522 Other bursitis, not elsewhere classified, left elbow

M71.529 Other bursitis, not elsewhere classified, unspecified elbow

M71.53 Other bursitis, not elsewhere classified, wrist

M71.531 Other bursitis, not elsewhere classified, right wrist

M71.532 Other bursitis, not elsewhere classified, left wrist

M71.539 Other bursitis, not elsewhere classified, unspecified wrist

M71.54 Other bursitis, not elsewhere classified, hand

M71.541 Other bursitis, not elsewhere classified, right hand

M71.542 Other bursitis, not elsewhere classified, left hand

M71.549 Other bursitis, not elsewhere classified, unspecified hand

M71.55 Other bursitis, not elsewhere classified, hip

M71.551 Other bursitis, not elsewhere classified, right hip

M71.552 Other bursitis, not elsewhere classified, left hip

M71.559 Other bursitis, not elsewhere classified, unspecified hip

M71.56 Other bursitis, not elsewhere classified, knee

M71.561 Other bursitis, not elsewhere classified, right knee

M71.562 Other bursitis, not elsewhere classified, left knee

M71.569 Other bursitis, not elsewhere classified, unspecified knee

M71.57 Other bursitis, not elsewhere classified, ankle and foot

M71.571 Other bursitis, not elsewhere classified, right ankle and foot

M71.572 Other bursitis, not elsewhere classified, left ankle and foot

M71.579 Other bursitis, not elsewhere classified, unspecified ankle and foot

M71.58 Other bursitis, not elsewhere classified, other site

M71.8 Other specified bursopathies

M71.80 Other specified bursopathies, unspecified site

M71.81 Other specified bursopathies, shoulder

M71.811 Other specified bursopathies, right shoulder

M71.812 Other specified bursopathies, left shoulder

M71.819 Other specified bursopathies, unspecified shoulder

M71.82 Other specified bursopathies, elbow

M71.821 Other specified bursopathies, right elbow

M71.822 Other specified bursopathies, left elbow

M71.829 Other specified bursopathies, unspecified elbow

M71.83 Other specified bursopathies, wrist

M71.831 Other specified bursopathies, right wrist

M71.832 Other specified bursopathies, left wrist

M71.839 Other specified bursopathies, unspecified wrist

M71.84 Other specified bursopathies, hand

M71.841 Other specified bursopathies, right hand

M71.842 Other specified bursopathies, left hand

M71.849 Other specified bursopathies, unspecified hand

M71.85 Other specified bursopathies, hip

M71.851 Other specified bursopathies, right hip

M71.852 Other specified bursopathies, left hip

M71.859 Other specified bursopathies, unspecified hip

M71.86 Other specified bursopathies, knee

M71.861 Other specified bursopathies, right knee

M71.862 Other specified bursopathies, left knee

M71.869 Other specified bursopathies, unspecified knee

M71.87 Other specified bursopathies, ankle and foot

M71.871 Other specified bursopathies, right ankle and foot

M71.872 Other specified bursopathies, left ankle and foot

M71.879 Other specified bursopathies, unspecified ankle and foot

M71.88 Other specified bursopathies, other site

M71.89 Other specified bursopathies, multiple sites

M71.9 Bursopathy, unspecified

Bursitis NOS

M72 Fibroblastic disorders

Excludes2: retroperitoneal fibromatosis (D48.3)

M72.0 Palmar fascial fibromatosis [Dupuytren]

M72.1 Knuckle pads

M72.2 Plantar fascial fibromatosis

Plantar fasciitis

M72.4 Pseudosarcomatous fibromatosis

Nodular fasciitis

M72.6 Necrotizing fasciitis

Use additional code (B95.-, B96.-) to identify causative organism

M72.8 Other fibroblastic disorders

Abscess of fascia

Fasciitis NEC

Other infective fasciitis

Use additional code to (B95.-, B96.-) identify causative organism

Excludes1: diffuse (eosinophilic) fasciitis (M35.4)

necrotizing fasciitis (M72.6)

nodular fasciitis (M72.4)

perirenal fasciitis NOS (N13.5)

perirenal fasciitis with infection (N13.6)

plantar fasciitis (M72.2)

M72.9 Fibroblastic disorder, unspecified

Fasciitis NOS

Fibromatosis NOS

M75 Shoulder lesions

Excludes2: shoulder-hand syndrome (M89.0-)

M75.0 Adhesive capsulitis of shoulder

Frozen shoulder

Periarthritis of shoulder

M75.00 Adhesive capsulitis of unspecified shoulder

M75.01 Adhesive capsulitis of right shoulder

M75.02 Adhesive capsulitis of left shoulder

M75.1 Rotator cuff tear or rupture, not specified as traumatic

Rotator cuff syndrome

Supraspinatus tear or rupture, not specified as traumatic

Supraspinatus syndrome

Excludes1: tear of rotator cuff, traumatic (S46.01-)

M75.10 Unspecified rotator cuff tear or rupture, not specified as traumatic

M75.100 Unspecified rotator cuff tear or rupture of unspecified shoulder, not specified as traumatic

M75.101 Unspecified rotator cuff tear or rupture of right shoulder, not specified as traumatic

M75.102 Unspecified rotator cuff tear or rupture of left shoulder, not specified as traumatic

M75.11 Incomplete rotator cuff tear or rupture not specified as traumatic

M75.110 Incomplete rotator cuff tear or rupture of unspecified shoulder, not specified as traumatic

M75.111 Incomplete rotator cuff tear or rupture of right shoulder, not specified as traumatic

M75.112 Incomplete rotator cuff tear or rupture of left shoulder, not specified as traumatic

M75.12 Complete rotator cuff tear or rupture not specified as traumatic

M75.120 Complete rotator cuff tear or rupture of unspecified shoulder, not specified as traumatic

M75.121 Complete rotator cuff tear or rupture of right shoulder, not specified as traumatic

M75.122 Complete rotator cuff tear or rupture of left shoulder, not specified as traumatic

M75.2 Bicipital tendinitis

M75.20 Bicipital tendinitis, unspecified shoulder

M75.21 Bicipital tendinitis, right shoulder

M75.22 Bicipital tendinitis, left shoulder

M75.3 Calcific tendinitis of shoulder

Calcified bursa of shoulder

M75.30 Calcific tendinitis of unspecified shoulder

M75.31 Calcific tendinitis of right shoulder

M75.32 Calcific tendinitis of left shoulder

M75.4 Impingement syndrome of shoulder

M75.40 Impingement syndrome of unspecified shoulder

M75.41 Impingement syndrome of right shoulder

M75.42 Impingement syndrome of left shoulder

M75.5 Bursitis of shoulder

M75.50 Bursitis of unspecified shoulder

M75.51 Bursitis of right shoulder

M75.52 Bursitis of left shoulder

M75.8 Other shoulder lesions

M75.80 Other shoulder lesions, unspecified shoulder

M75.81 Other shoulder lesions, right shoulder

M75.82 Other shoulder lesions, left shoulder

M75.9 Shoulder lesion, unspecified

M75.90 Shoulder lesion, unspecified, unspecified shoulder

M75.91 Shoulder lesion, unspecified, right shoulder

M75.92 Shoulder lesion, unspecified, left shoulder

M76 Enthesopathies, lower limb, excluding foot

Excludes2: bursitis due to use, overuse and pressure (M70.-)

enthesopathies of ankle and foot (M77.5-)

M76.0 Gluteal tendinitis

M76.00 Gluteal tendinitis, unspecified hip

M76.01 Gluteal tendinitis, right hip

M76.02 Gluteal tendinitis, left hip

M76.1 Psoas tendinitis

M76.10 Psoas tendinitis, unspecified hip

M76.11 Psoas tendinitis, right hip

M76.12 Psoas tendinitis, left hip

M76.2 Iliac crest spur

● New code ▲ Revised code **Excludes1:** Not coded here **Excludes2:** Not included here ⊗ Placeholder required ⑦7th digit required

M76.20   Iliac crest spur, unspecified hip

M76.21   Iliac crest spur, right hip

M76.22   Iliac crest spur, left hip

M76.3   Iliotibial band syndrome

M76.30   Iliotibial band syndrome, unspecified leg

M76.31   Iliotibial band syndrome, right leg

M76.32   Iliotibial band syndrome, left leg

M76.4   Tibial collateral bursitis [Pellegrini-Stieda]

M76.40   Tibial collateral bursitis [Pellegrini-Stieda], unspecified leg

M76.41   Tibial collateral bursitis [Pellegrini-Stieda], right leg

M76.42   Tibial collateral bursitis [Pellegrini-Stieda], left leg

M76.5   Patellar tendinitis

M76.50   Patellar tendinitis, unspecified knee

M76.51   Patellar tendinitis, right knee

M76.52   Patellar tendinitis, left knee

M76.6   Achilles tendinitis

Achilles bursitis

M76.60   Achilles tendinitis, unspecified leg

M76.61   Achilles tendinitis, right leg

M76.62   Achilles tendinitis, left leg

M76.7   Peroneal tendinitis

M76.70   Peroneal tendinitis, unspecified leg

M76.71   Peroneal tendinitis, right leg

M76.72   Peroneal tendinitis, left leg

M76.8   Other specified enthesopathies of lower limb, excluding foot

M76.81   Anterior tibial syndrome

M76.811   Anterior tibial syndrome, right leg

M76.812   Anterior tibial syndrome, left leg

M76.819   Anterior tibial syndrome, unspecified leg

M76.82   Posterior tibial tendinitis

M76.821   Posterior tibial tendinitis, right leg

M76.822   Posterior tibial tendinitis, left leg

M76.829   Posterior tibial tendinitis, unspecified leg

M76.89   Other specified enthesopathies of lower limb, excluding foot

M76.891   Other specified enthesopathies of right lower limb, excluding foot

M76.892   Other specified enthesopathies of left lower limb, excluding foot

M76.899   Other specified enthesopathies of unspecified lower limb, excluding foot

M76.9   Unspecified enthesopathy, lower limb, excluding foot

M77   **Other enthesopathies**

Excludes1: bursitis NOS (M71.9-)

Excludes2: bursitis due to use, overuse and pressure (M70.-)

osteophyte (M25.7)

spinal enthesopathy (M46.0-)

M77.0   Medial epicondylitis

M77.00   Medial epicondylitis, unspecified elbow

M77.01   Medial epicondylitis, right elbow

M77.02   Medial epicondylitis, left elbow

M77.1   Lateral epicondylitis

Tennis elbow

M77.10   Lateral epicondylitis, unspecified elbow

M77.11   Lateral epicondylitis, right elbow

M77.12   Lateral epicondylitis, left elbow

M77.2   Periarthritis of wrist

M77.20   Periarthritis, unspecified wrist

M77.21   Periarthritis, right wrist

M77.22   Periarthritis, left wrist

M77.3   Calcaneal spur

M77.30   Calcaneal spur, unspecified foot

M77.31   Calcaneal spur, right foot

M77.32   Calcaneal spur, left foot

M77.4   Metatarsalgia

Excludes1: Morton's metatarsalgia (G57.6)

M77.40   Metatarsalgia, unspecified foot

M77.41   Metatarsalgia, right foot

M77.42   Metatarsalgia, left foot

M77.5   Other enthesopathy of foot

M77.50   Other enthesopathy of unspecified foot

M77.51   Other enthesopathy of right foot

M77.52   Other enthesopathy of left foot

M77.8   Other enthesopathies, not elsewhere classified

M77.9   Enthesopathy, unspecified

Bone spur NOS

Capsulitis NOS

Periarthritis NOS

Tendinitis NOS

M79   **Other and unspecified soft tissue disorders, not elsewhere classified**

Excludes1: psychogenic rheumatism (F45.8)

soft tissue pain, psychogenic (F45.41)

M79.0   Rheumatism, unspecified

Definition: Rheumatism refers to 1) any painful disorder of the joints or muscles or connective tissues or 2) a chronic autoimmune disease with inflammation of the joints and marked deformities.

Excludes1: fibromyalgia (M79.7)

palindromic rheumatism (M12.3-)

M79.1   Myalgia

Myofascial pain syndrome

Excludes1: fibromyalgia (M79.7)

myositis (M60.-)

M79.2   Neuralgia and neuritis, unspecified

Excludes1: brachial radiculitis NOS (M54.1)

lumbosacral radiculitis NOS (M54.1)

mononeuropathies (G56-G58)

radiculitis NOS (M54.1)

sciatica (M54.3-M54.4)

M79.3   Panniculitis, unspecified

Excludes1: lupus panniculitis (L93.2)

neck and back panniculitis (M54.0-)

relapsing [Weber-Christian] panniculitis (M35.6)

M79.4   Hypertrophy of (infrapatellar) fat pad

M79.5   Residual foreign body in soft tissue

Excludes1: foreign body granuloma of skin and subcutaneous tissue (L92.3)

foreign body granuloma of soft tissue (M60.2-)

M79.6   Pain in limb, hand, foot, fingers and toes

Excludes2: pain in joint (M25.5-)

M79.60 Pain in limb, unspecified

    M79.601 Pain in right arm
        Pain in right upper limb NOS

    M79.602 Pain in left arm
        Pain in left upper limb NOS

    M79.603 Pain in arm, unspecified
        Pain in upper limb NOS

    M79.604 Pain in right leg
        Pain in right lower limb NOS

    M79.605 Pain in left leg
        Pain in left lower limb NOS

    M79.606 Pain in leg, unspecified
        Pain in lower limb NOS

    M79.609 Pain in unspecified limb
        Pain in limb NOS

M79.62 Pain in upper arm
    Pain in axillary region

    M79.621 Pain in right upper arm

    M79.622 Pain in left upper arm

    M79.629 Pain in unspecified upper arm

M79.63 Pain in forearm

    M79.631 Pain in right forearm

    M79.632 Pain in left forearm

    M79.639 Pain in unspecified forearm

M79.64 Pain in hand and fingers

    M79.641 Pain in right hand

    M79.642 Pain in left hand

    M79.643 Pain in unspecified hand

    M79.644 Pain in right finger(s)

    M79.645 Pain in left finger(s)

    M79.646 Pain in unspecified finger(s)

M79.65 Pain in thigh

    M79.651 Pain in right thigh

    M79.652 Pain in left thigh

    M79.659 Pain in unspecified thigh

M79.66 Pain in lower leg

    M79.661 Pain in right lower leg

    M79.662 Pain in left lower leg

    M79.669 Pain in unspecified lower leg

M79.67 Pain in foot and toes

    M79.671 Pain in right foot

    M79.672 Pain in left foot

    M79.673 Pain in unspecified foot

    M79.674 Pain in right toe(s)

    M79.675 Pain in left toe(s)

    M79.676 Pain in unspecified toe(s)

M79.7 Fibromyalgia
    Fibromyositis
    Fibrositis
    Myofibrositis

M79.A Nontraumatic compartment syndrome
    Code first, if applicable, associated postprocedural complication
    Excludes1: compartment syndrome NOS (T79.A-)
        fibromyalgia (M79.7)

        nontraumatic ischemic infarction of muscle (M62.2-)
        traumatic compartment syndrome (T79.A-)

    M79.A1 Nontraumatic compartment syndrome of upper extremity
        Nontraumatic compartment syndrome of shoulder, arm, forearm, wrist, hand, and fingers

        M79.A11 Nontraumatic compartment syndrome of right upper extremity

        M79.A12 Nontraumatic compartment syndrome of left upper extremity

        M79.A19 Nontraumatic compartment syndrome of unspecified upper extremity

    M79.A2 Nontraumatic compartment syndrome of lower extremity
        Nontraumatic compartment syndrome of hip, buttock, thigh, leg, foot, and toes

        M79.A21 Nontraumatic compartment syndrome of right lower extremity

        M79.A22 Nontraumatic compartment syndrome of left lower extremity

        M79.A29 Nontraumatic compartment syndrome of unspecified lower extremity

    M79.A3 Nontraumatic compartment syndrome of abdomen

    M79.A9 Nontraumatic compartment syndrome of other sites

M79.8 Other specified soft tissue disorders

    M79.81 Nontraumatic hematoma of soft tissue
        Nontraumatic hematoma of muscle
        Nontraumatic seroma of muscle and soft tissue

    M79.89 Other specified soft tissue disorders
        Polyalgia

M79.9 Soft tissue disorder, unspecified

OSTEOPATHIES AND CHONDROPATHIES (M80-M94)

DISORDERS OF BONE DENSITY AND STRUCTURE (M80-M85)

M80 Osteoporosis with current pathological fracture

    Includes: osteoporosis with current fragility fracture

    Use additional code to identify major osseous defect, if applicable (M89.7-)

    Excludes1: collapsed vertebra NOS (M48.5)
        pathological fracture NOS (M84.4)
        wedging of vertebra NOS (M48.5)

    Excludes2: personal history of (healed) osteoporosis fracture (Z87.310)

    The appropriate 7th character is to be added to each code from category M80:

    A - initial encounter for fracture

    D - subsequent encounter for fracture with routine healing

    G - subsequent encounter for fracture with delayed healing

    K - subsequent encounter for fracture with nonunion

    P - subsequent encounter for fracture with malunion

    S - sequela

    M80.0 Age-related osteoporosis with current pathological fracture
        Involutional osteoporosis with current pathological fracture
        Osteoporosis NOS with current pathological fracture

Postmenopausal osteoporosis with current pathological fracture

Senile osteoporosis with current pathological fracture

⊗⑦**M80.00** **Age-related osteoporosis with current pathological fracture, unspecified site**

M80.01 **Age-related osteoporosis with current pathological fracture, shoulder**

⑦**M80.011** **Age-related osteoporosis with current pathological fracture, right shoulder**

⑦**M80.012** **Age-related osteoporosis with current pathological fracture, left shoulder**

⑦**M80.019** **Age-related osteoporosis with current pathological fracture, unspecified shoulder**

M80.02 **Age-related osteoporosis with current pathological fracture, humerus**

⑦**M80.021** **Age-related osteoporosis with current pathological fracture, right humerus**

⑦**M80.022** **Age-related osteoporosis with current pathological fracture, left humerus**

⑦**M80.029** **Age-related osteoporosis with current pathological fracture, unspecified humerus**

M80.03 **Age-related osteoporosis with current pathological fracture, forearm**

Age-related osteoporosis with current pathological fracture of wrist

⑦**M80.031** **Age-related osteoporosis with current pathological fracture, right forearm**

⑦**M80.032** **Age-related osteoporosis with current pathological fracture, left forearm**

⑦**M80.039** **Age-related osteoporosis with current pathological fracture, unspecified forearm**

M80.04 **Age-related osteoporosis with current pathological fracture, hand**

⑦**M80.041** **Age-related osteoporosis with current pathological fracture, right hand**

⑦**M80.042** **Age-related osteoporosis with current pathological fracture, left hand**

⑦**M80.049** **Age-related osteoporosis with current pathological fracture, unspecified hand**

M80.05 **Age-related osteoporosis with current pathological fracture, femur**

Age-related osteoporosis with current pathological fracture of hip

⑦**M80.051** **Age-related osteoporosis with current pathological fracture, right femur**

⑦**M80.052** **Age-related osteoporosis with current pathological fracture, left femur**

⑦**M80.059** **Age-related osteoporosis with current pathological fracture, unspecified femur**

M80.06 **Age-related osteoporosis with current pathological fracture, lower leg**

⑦**M80.061** **Age-related osteoporosis with current pathological fracture, right lower leg**

⑦**M80.062** **Age-related osteoporosis with current pathological fracture, left lower leg**

⑦**M80.069** **Age-related osteoporosis with current pathological fracture, unspecified lower leg**

M80.07 **Age-related osteoporosis with current pathological fracture, ankle and foot**

⑦**M80.071** **Age-related osteoporosis with current pathological fracture, right ankle and foot**

⑦**M80.072** **Age-related osteoporosis with current pathological fracture, left ankle and foot**

⑦**M80.079** **Age-related osteoporosis with current pathological fracture, unspecified ankle and foot**

⊗⑦**M80.08** **Age-related osteoporosis with current pathological fracture, vertebra(e)**

M80.8 **Other osteoporosis with current pathological fracture**

Drug-induced osteoporosis with current pathological fracture

Idiopathic osteoporosis with current pathological fracture

Osteoporosis of disuse with current pathological fracture

Postoophorectomy osteoporosis with current pathological fracture

Postsurgical malabsorption osteoporosis with current pathological fracture

Post-traumatic osteoporosis with current pathological fracture

Use additional code for adverse effect, if applicable, to identify drug (T36-T50 with fifth or sixth character 5)

⊗⑦**M80.80** **Other osteoporosis with current pathological fracture, unspecified site**

M80.81 **Other osteoporosis with pathological fracture, shoulder**

⑦**M80.811** **Other osteoporosis with current pathological fracture, right shoulder**

⑦**M80.812** **Other osteoporosis with current pathological fracture, left shoulder**

⑦**M80.819** **Other osteoporosis with current pathological fracture, unspecified shoulder**

M80.82 **Other osteoporosis with current pathological fracture, humerus**

⑦**M80.821** **Other osteoporosis with current pathological fracture, right humerus**

⑦**M80.822** **Other osteoporosis with current pathological fracture, left humerus**

⑦**M80.829** **Other osteoporosis with current pathological fracture, unspecified humerus**

M80.83 **Other osteoporosis with current pathological fracture, forearm**

Other osteoporosis with current pathological fracture of wrist

⑦**M80.831** **Other osteoporosis with current pathological fracture, right forearm**

⑦**M80.832** **Other osteoporosis with current pathological fracture, left forearm**

⑦ **M80.839** Other osteoporosis with current pathological fracture, unspecified forearm

M80.84 Other osteoporosis with current pathological fracture, hand

⑦ **M80.841** Other osteoporosis with current pathological fracture, right hand

⑦ **M80.842** Other osteoporosis with current pathological fracture, left hand

⑦ **M80.849** Other osteoporosis with current pathological fracture, unspecified hand

M80.85 Other osteoporosis with current pathological fracture, femur

Other osteoporosis with current pathological fracture of hip

⑦ **M80.851** Other osteoporosis with current pathological fracture, right femur

⑦ **M80.852** Other osteoporosis with current pathological fracture, left femur

⑦ **M80.859** Other osteoporosis with current pathological fracture, unspecified femur

M80.86 Other osteoporosis with current pathological fracture, lower leg

⑦ **M80.861** Other osteoporosis with current pathological fracture, right lower leg

⑦ **M80.862** Other osteoporosis with current pathological fracture, left lower leg

⑦ **M80.869** Other osteoporosis with current pathological fracture, unspecified lower leg

M80.87 Other osteoporosis with current pathological fracture, ankle and foot

⑦ **M80.871** Other osteoporosis with current pathological fracture, right ankle and foot

⑦ **M80.872** Other osteoporosis with current pathological fracture, left ankle and foot

⑦ **M80.879** Other osteoporosis with current pathological fracture, unspecified ankle and foot

⊗⑦ **M80.88** Other osteoporosis with current pathological fracture, vertebra(e)

M81 Osteoporosis without current pathological fracture

Use additional code to identify:

major osseous defect, if applicable (M89.7-)

personal history of (healed) osteoporosis fracture, if applicable (Z87.310)

Excludes1: osteoporosis with current pathological fracture (M80.-)

Sudeck's atrophy (M89.0)

M81.0 Age-related osteoporosis without current pathological fracture

Involutional osteoporosis without current pathological fracture

Osteoporosis NOS

Postmenopausal osteoporosis without current pathological fracture

Senile osteoporosis without current pathological fracture

M81.6 Localized osteoporosis [Lequesne]

Excludes1: Sudeck's atrophy (M89.0)

M81.8 Other osteoporosis without current pathological fracture

Drug-induced osteoporosis without current pathological fracture

Idiopathic osteoporosis without current pathological fracture

Osteoporosis of disuse without current pathological fracture

Postoophorectomy osteoporosis without current pathological fracture

Postsurgical malabsorption osteoporosis without current pathological fracture

Post-traumatic osteoporosis without current pathological fracture

Use additional code for adverse effect, if applicable, to identify drug (T36-T50 with fifth or sixth character 5)

M83 Adult osteomalacia

Excludes1: infantile and juvenile osteomalacia (E55.0)

renal osteodystrophy (N25.0)

rickets (active) (E55.0)

rickets (active) sequelae (E64.3)

vitamin D-resistant osteomalacia (E83.3)

vitamin D-resistant rickets (active) (E83.3)

M83.0 Puerperal osteomalacia

M83.1 Senile osteomalacia

M83.2 Adult osteomalacia due to malabsorption

Postsurgical malabsorption osteomalacia in adults

M83.3 Adult osteomalacia due to malnutrition

M83.4 Aluminum bone disease

M83.5 Other drug-induced osteomalacia in adults

Use additional code for adverse effect, if applicable, to identify drug (T36-T50 with fifth or sixth character 5)

M83.8 Other adult osteomalacia

M83.9 Adult osteomalacia, unspecified

M84 Disorder of continuity of bone

Excludes2: traumatic fracture of bone-see fracture, by site

M84.3 Stress fracture

Fatigue fracture

March fracture

Stress fracture NOS

Stress reaction

Use additional external cause code(s) to identify the cause of the stress fracture

Excludes1: pathological fracture NOS (M84.4.-)

pathological fracture due to osteoporosis (M80.-)

traumatic fracture (S12.-, S22.-, S32.-, S42.-, S52.-, S62.-, S72.-, S82.-, S92.-)

Excludes2: personal history of (healed) stress (fatigue) fracture (Z87.312)

stress fracture of vertebra (M48.4-)

The appropriate 7th character is to be added to each code from subcategory M84.3:

A - initial encounter for fracture

D - subsequent encounter for fracture with routine healing

G - subsequent encounter for fracture with delayed healing

K - subsequent encounter for fracture with nonunion

P - subsequent encounter for fracture with malunion S - sequela

⊗⑦ **M84.30** Stress fracture, unspecified site

M84.31 Stress fracture, shoulder

⑦ **M84.311** Stress fracture, right shoulder

⑦ **M84.312** Stress fracture, left shoulder

⑦ **M84.319** Stress fracture, unspecified shoulder

● New code ▲ Revised code **Excludes1:** Not coded here **Excludes2:** Not included here ⊗ Placeholder required ⑦ 7th digit required

M84.32 Stress fracture, humerus
- ⑦M84.321   Stress fracture, right humerus
- ⑦M84.322   Stress fracture, left humerus
- ⑦M84.329   Stress fracture, unspecified humerus

M84.33 Stress fracture, ulna and radius
- ⑦M84.331   Stress fracture, right ulna
- ⑦M84.332   Stress fracture, left ulna
- ⑦M84.333   Stress fracture, right radius
- ⑦M84.334   Stress fracture, left radius
- ⑦M84.339   Stress fracture, unspecified ulna and radius

M84.34 Stress fracture, hand and fingers
- ⑦M84.341   Stress fracture, right hand
- ⑦M84.342   Stress fracture, left hand
- ⑦M84.343   Stress fracture, unspecified hand
- ⑦M84.344   Stress fracture, right finger(s)
- ⑦M84.345   Stress fracture, left finger(s)
- ⑦M84.346   Stress fracture, unspecified finger(s)

M84.35 Stress fracture, pelvis and femur
Stress fracture, hip
- ⑦M84.350   Stress fracture, pelvis
- ⑦M84.351   Stress fracture, right femur
- ⑦M84.352   Stress fracture, left femur
- ⑦M84.353   Stress fracture, unspecified femur
- ⑦M84.359   Stress fracture, hip, unspecified

M84.36 Stress fracture, tibia and fibula
- ⑦M84.361   Stress fracture, right tibia
- ⑦M84.362   Stress fracture, left tibia
- ⑦M84.363   Stress fracture, right fibula
- ⑦M84.364   Stress fracture, left fibula
- ⑦M84.369   Stress fracture, unspecified tibia and fibula

M84.37 Stress fracture, ankle, foot and toes
- ⑦M84.371   Stress fracture, right ankle
- ⑦M84.372   Stress fracture, left ankle
- ⑦M84.373   Stress fracture, unspecified ankle
- ⑦M84.374   Stress fracture, right foot
- ⑦M84.375   Stress fracture, left foot
- ⑦M84.376   Stress fracture, unspecified foot
- ⑦M84.377   Stress fracture, right toe(s)
- ⑦M84.378   Stress fracture, left toe(s)
- ⑦M84.379   Stress fracture, unspecified toe(s)

⊗⑦M84.38 Stress fracture, other site
> Excludes2: stress fracture of vertebra (M48.4-)

M84.4 Pathological fracture, not elsewhere classified
Chronic fracture
Pathological fracture NOS
> Excludes1: collapsed vertebra NEC (M48.5)
> pathological fracture in neoplastic disease (M84.5-)
> pathological fracture in osteoporosis (M80.-)
> pathological fracture in other disease (M84.6-)
> stress fracture (M84.3-)
> traumatic fracture (S12.-, S22.-, S32.-, S42.-, S52.-, S62.-, S72.-, S82.-, S92.-)

> Excludes2: personal history of (healed) pathological fracture (Z87.311)

The appropriate 7th character is to be added to each code from subcategory M84.4:
A - initial encounter for fracture
D - subsequent encounter for fracture with routine healing
G - subsequent encounter for fracture with delayed healing
K - subsequent encounter for fracture with nonunion
P - subsequent encounter for fracture with malunion
S - sequela

⊗⑦M84.40 Pathological fracture, unspecified site

M84.41 Pathological fracture, shoulder
- ⑦M84.411   Pathological fracture, right shoulder
- ⑦M84.412   Pathological fracture, left shoulder
- ⑦M84.419   Pathological fracture, unspecified shoulder

M84.42 Pathological fracture, humerus
- ⑦M84.421   Pathological fracture, right humerus
- ⑦M84.422   Pathological fracture, left humerus
- ⑦M84.429   Pathological fracture, unspecified humerus

M84.43 Pathological fracture, ulna and radius
- ⑦M84.431   Pathological fracture, right ulna
- ⑦M84.432   Pathological fracture, left ulna
- ⑦M84.433   Pathological fracture, right radius
- ⑦M84.434   Pathological fracture, left radius
- ⑦M84.439   Pathological fracture, unspecified ulna and radius

M84.44 Pathological fracture, hand and fingers
- ⑦M84.441   Pathological fracture, right hand
- ⑦M84.442   Pathological fracture, left hand
- ⑦M84.443   Pathological fracture, unspecified hand
- ⑦M84.444   Pathological fracture, right finger(s)
- ⑦M84.445   Pathological fracture, left finger(s)
- ⑦M84.446   Pathological fracture, unspecified finger(s)

M84.45 Pathological fracture, femur and pelvis
- ⑦M84.451   Pathological fracture, right femur
- ⑦M84.452   Pathological fracture, left femur
- ⑦M84.453   Pathological fracture, unspecified femur
- ⑦M84.454   Pathological fracture, pelvis
- ⑦M84.459   Pathological fracture, hip, unspecified

M84.46 Pathological fracture, tibia and fibula
- ⑦M84.461   Pathological fracture, right tibia
- ⑦M84.462   Pathological fracture, left tibia
- ⑦M84.463   Pathological fracture, right fibula
- ⑦M84.464   Pathological fracture, left fibula
- ⑦M84.469   Pathological fracture, unspecified tibia and fibula

M84.47 Pathological fracture, ankle, foot and toes
- ⑦M84.471   Pathological fracture, right ankle
- ⑦M84.472   Pathological fracture, left ankle
- ⑦M84.473   Pathological fracture, unspecified ankle
- ⑦M84.474   Pathological fracture, right foot
- ⑦M84.475   Pathological fracture, left foot
- ⑦M84.476   Pathological fracture, unspecified foot

⑦ **M84.477** Pathological fracture, right toe(s)

⑦ **M84.478** Pathological fracture, left toe(s)

⑦ **M84.479** Pathological fracture, unspecified toe(s)

⊗⑦ **M84.48** Pathological fracture, other site

M84.5 Pathological fracture in neoplastic disease

<u>Code also</u> underlying neoplasm

The appropriate 7th character is to be added to each code from subcategory M84.5:

A - initial encounter for fracture

D - subsequent encounter for fracture with routine healing

G - subsequent encounter for fracture with delayed healing

K - subsequent encounter for fracture with nonunion

P - subsequent encounter for fracture with malunion

S - sequela

⊗⑦ **M84.50** Pathological fracture in neoplastic disease, unspecified site

M84.51 Pathological fracture in neoplastic disease, shoulder

⑦ **M84.511** Pathological fracture in neoplastic disease, right shoulder

⑦ **M84.512** Pathological fracture in neoplastic disease, left shoulder

⑦ **M84.519** Pathological fracture in neoplastic disease, unspecified shoulder

M84.52 Pathological fracture in neoplastic disease, humerus

⑦ **M84.521** Pathological fracture in neoplastic disease, right humerus

⑦ **M84.522** Pathological fracture in neoplastic disease, left humerus

⑦ **M84.529** Pathological fracture in neoplastic disease, unspecified humerus

M84.53 Pathological fracture in neoplastic disease, ulna and radius

⑦ **M84.531** Pathological fracture in neoplastic disease, right ulna

⑦ **M84.532** Pathological fracture in neoplastic disease, left ulna

⑦ **M84.533** Pathological fracture in neoplastic disease, right radius

⑦ **M84.534** Pathological fracture in neoplastic disease, left radius

⑦ **M84.539** Pathological fracture in neoplastic disease, unspecified ulna and radius

M84.54 Pathological fracture in neoplastic disease, hand

⑦ **M84.541** Pathological fracture in neoplastic disease, right hand

⑦ **M84.542** Pathological fracture in neoplastic disease, left hand

⑦ **M84.549** Pathological fracture in neoplastic disease, unspecified hand

M84.55 Pathological fracture in neoplastic disease, pelvis and femur

⑦ **M84.550** Pathological fracture in neoplastic disease, pelvis

⑦ **M84.551** Pathological fracture in neoplastic disease, right femur

⑦ **M84.552** Pathological fracture in neoplastic disease, left femur

⑦ **M84.553** Pathological fracture in neoplastic disease, unspecified femur

⑦ **M84.559** Pathological fracture in neoplastic disease, hip, unspecified

M84.56 Pathological fracture in neoplastic disease, tibia and fibula

⑦ **M84.561** Pathological fracture in neoplastic disease, right tibia

⑦ **M84.562** Pathological fracture in neoplastic disease, left tibia

⑦ **M84.563** Pathological fracture in neoplastic disease, right fibula

⑦ **M84.564** Pathological fracture in neoplastic disease, left fibula

⑦ **M84.569** Pathological fracture in neoplastic disease, unspecified tibia and fibula

M84.57 Pathological fracture in neoplastic disease, ankle and foot

⑦ **M84.571** Pathological fracture in neoplastic disease, right ankle

⑦ **M84.572** Pathological fracture in neoplastic disease, left ankle

⑦ **M84.573** Pathological fracture in neoplastic disease, unspecified ankle

⑦ **M84.574** Pathological fracture in neoplastic disease, right foot

⑦ **M84.575** Pathological fracture in neoplastic disease, left foot

⑦ **M84.576** Pathological fracture in neoplastic disease, unspecified foot

⊗⑦ **M84.58** Pathological fracture in neoplastic disease, other specified site

Pathological fracture in neoplastic disease, vertebrae

M84.6 Pathological fracture in other disease

<u>Code also</u> underlying condition

Excludes1: pathological fracture in osteoporosis (M80.-)

The appropriate 7th character is to be added to each code from subcategory M84.6:

A - initial encounter for fracture

D - subsequent encounter for fracture with routine healing

G - subsequent encounter for fracture with delayed healing

K - subsequent encounter for fracture with nonunion

P - subsequent encounter for fracture with malunion

S - sequela

⊗⑦ **M84.60** Pathological fracture in other disease, unspecified site

M84.61 Pathological fracture in other disease, shoulder

⑦ **M84.611** Pathological fracture in other disease, right shoulder

⑦ **M84.612** Pathological fracture in other disease, left shoulder

⑦ **M84.619** Pathological fracture in other disease, unspecified shoulder

M84.62 Pathological fracture in other disease, humerus

⑦ **M84.621** Pathological fracture in other disease, right humerus

⑦ **M84.622** Pathological fracture in other disease, left humerus

⑦ **M84.629** Pathological fracture in other disease, unspecified humerus

M84.63 Pathological fracture in other disease, ulna and radius

⑦ **M84.631** Pathological fracture in other disease, right ulna

⑦M84.632   **Pathological fracture in other disease, left ulna**

⑦M84.633   **Pathological fracture in other disease, right radius**

⑦M84.634   **Pathological fracture in other disease, left radius**

⑦M84.639   **Pathological fracture in other disease, unspecified ulna and radius**

M84.64   **Pathological fracture in other disease, hand**

⑦M84.641   **Pathological fracture in other disease, right hand**

⑦M84.642   **Pathological fracture in other disease, left hand**

⑦M84.649   **Pathological fracture in other disease, unspecified hand**

M84.65   **Pathological fracture in other disease, pelvis and femur**

⑦M84.650   **Pathological fracture in other disease, pelvis**

⑦M84.651   **Pathological fracture in other disease, right femur**

⑦M84.652   **Pathological fracture in other disease, left femur**

⑦M84.653   **Pathological fracture in other disease, unspecified femur**

⑦M84.659   **Pathological fracture in other disease, hip, unspecified**

M84.66   **Pathological fracture in other disease, tibia and fibula**

⑦M84.661   **Pathological fracture in other disease, right tibia**

⑦M84.662   **Pathological fracture in other disease, left tibia**

⑦M84.663   **Pathological fracture in other disease, right fibula**

⑦M84.664   **Pathological fracture in other disease, left fibula**

⑦M84.669   **Pathological fracture in other disease, unspecified tibia and fibula**

M84.67   **Pathological fracture in other disease, ankle and foot**

⑦M84.671   **Pathological fracture in other disease, right ankle**

⑦M84.672   **Pathological fracture in other disease, left ankle**

⑦M84.673   **Pathological fracture in other disease, unspecified ankle**

⑦M84.674   **Pathological fracture in other disease, right foot**

⑦M84.675   **Pathological fracture in other disease, left foot**

⑦M84.676   **Pathological fracture in other disease, unspecified foot**

⊗⑦M84.68   **Pathological fracture in other disease, other site**

M84.7   **Nontraumatic fracture, not elsewhere classified**

M84.75   **Atypical femoral fracture**

The appropriate 7th character is to be added to each code from M84.75:

A - initial encounter for fracture

D - subsequent encounter for fracture with routine healing

G - subsequent encounter for fracture with delayed healing

K - subsequent encounter for fracture with nonunion

P - subsequent encounter for fracture with malunion

S - sequela

⑦M84.750   **Atypical femoral fracture, unspecified**

⑦M84.751   **Incomplete atypical femoral fracture, right leg**

⑦M84.752   **Incomplete atypical femoral fracture, left leg**

⑦M84.753   **Incomplete atypical femoral fracture, unspecified leg**

⑦M84.754   **Complete transverse atypical femoral fracture, right leg**

⑦M84.755   **Complete transverse atypical femoral fracture, left leg**

⑦M84.756   **Complete transverse atypical femoral fracture, unspecified leg**

⑦M84.757   **Complete oblique atypical femoral fracture, right leg**

⑦M84.758   **Complete oblique atypical femoral fracture, left leg**

⑦M84.759   **Complete oblique atypical femoral fracture, unspecified leg**

M84.8   **Other disorders of continuity of bone**

⊗⑦M84.80   **Other disorders of continuity of bone, unspecified site**

M84.81   **Other disorders of continuity of bone, shoulder**

⑦M84.811   **Other disorders of continuity of bone, right shoulder**

⑦M84.812   **Other disorders of continuity of bone, left shoulder**

⑦M84.819   **Other disorders of continuity of bone, unspecified shoulder**

M84.82   **Other disorders of continuity of bone, humerus**

⑦M84.821   **Other disorders of continuity of bone, right humerus**

⑦M84.822   **Other disorders of continuity of bone, left humerus**

⑦M84.829   **Other disorders of continuity of bone, unspecified humerus**

M84.83   **Other disorders of continuity of bone, ulna and radius**

⑦M84.831   **Other disorders of continuity of bone, right ulna**

⑦M84.832   **Other disorders of continuity of bone, left ulna**

⑦M84.833   **Other disorders of continuity of bone, right radius**

⑦M84.834   **Other disorders of continuity of bone, left radius**

⑦M84.839   **Other disorders of continuity of bone, unspecified ulna and radius**

M84.84   **Other disorders of continuity of bone, hand**

⑦M84.841   **Other disorders of continuity of bone, right hand**

⑦M84.842   **Other disorders of continuity of bone, left hand**

⑦M84.849   **Other disorders of continuity of bone, unspecified hand**

M84.85   **Other disorders of continuity of bone, pelvic region and thigh**

---

⑦ **M84.851**   Other disorders of continuity of bone, right pelvic region and thigh

⑦ **M84.852**   Other disorders of continuity of bone, left pelvic region and thigh

⑦ **M84.859**   Other disorders of continuity of bone, unspecified pelvic region and thigh

M84.86   Other disorders of continuity of bone, tibia and fibula

⑦ **M84.861**   Other disorders of continuity of bone, right tibia

⑦ **M84.862**   Other disorders of continuity of bone, left tibia

⑦ **M84.863**   Other disorders of continuity of bone, right fibula

⑦ **M84.864**   Other disorders of continuity of bone, left fibula

⑦ **M84.869**   Other disorders of continuity of bone, unspecified tibia and fibula

M84.87   Other disorders of continuity of bone, ankle and foot

⑦ **M84.871**   Other disorders of continuity of bone, right ankle and foot

⑦ **M84.872**   Other disorders of continuity of bone, left ankle and foot

⑦ **M84.879**   Other disorders of continuity of bone, unspecified ankle and foot

⊗⑦ **M84.88**   Other disorders of continuity of bone, other site

⊗⑦ **M84.9**   Disorder of continuity of bone, unspecified

M85   **Other disorders of bone density and structure**

Excludes1: osteogenesis imperfecta (Q78.0)

osteopetrosis (Q78.2)

osteopoikilosis (Q78.8)

polyostotic fibrous dysplasia (Q78.1)

M85.0   **Fibrous dysplasia (monostotic)**

Excludes2: fibrous dysplasia of jaw (M27.8)

M85.00   Fibrous dysplasia (monostotic), unspecified site

M85.01   Fibrous dysplasia (monostotic), shoulder

M85.011   Fibrous dysplasia (monostotic), right shoulder

M85.012   Fibrous dysplasia (monostotic), left shoulder

M85.019   Fibrous dysplasia (monostotic), unspecified shoulder

M85.02   Fibrous dysplasia (monostotic), upper arm

M85.021   Fibrous dysplasia (monostotic), right upper arm

M85.022   Fibrous dysplasia (monostotic), left upper arm

M85.029   Fibrous dysplasia (monostotic), unspecified upper arm

M85.03   Fibrous dysplasia (monostotic), forearm

M85.031   Fibrous dysplasia (monostotic), right forearm

M85.032   Fibrous dysplasia (monostotic), left forearm

M85.039   Fibrous dysplasia (monostotic), unspecified forearm

M85.04   Fibrous dysplasia (monostotic), hand

M85.041   Fibrous dysplasia (monostotic), right hand

M85.042   Fibrous dysplasia (monostotic), left hand

M85.049   Fibrous dysplasia (monostotic), unspecified hand

M85.05   Fibrous dysplasia (monostotic), thigh

M85.051   Fibrous dysplasia (monostotic), right thigh

M85.052   Fibrous dysplasia (monostotic), left thigh

M85.059   Fibrous dysplasia (monostotic), unspecified thigh

M85.06   Fibrous dysplasia (monostotic), lower leg

M85.061   Fibrous dysplasia (monostotic), right lower leg

M85.062   Fibrous dysplasia (monostotic), left lower leg

M85.069   Fibrous dysplasia (monostotic), unspecified lower leg

M85.07   Fibrous dysplasia (monostotic), ankle and foot

M85.071   Fibrous dysplasia (monostotic), right ankle and foot

M85.072   Fibrous dysplasia (monostotic), left ankle and foot

M85.079   Fibrous dysplasia (monostotic), unspecified ankle and foot

M85.08   Fibrous dysplasia (monostotic), other site

M85.09   Fibrous dysplasia (monostotic), multiple sites

M85.1   **Skeletal fluorosis**

M85.10   Skeletal fluorosis, unspecified site

M85.11   Skeletal fluorosis, shoulder

M85.111   Skeletal fluorosis, right shoulder

M85.112   Skeletal fluorosis, left shoulder

M85.119   Skeletal fluorosis, unspecified shoulder

M85.12   Skeletal fluorosis, upper arm

M85.121   Skeletal fluorosis, right upper arm

M85.122   Skeletal fluorosis, left upper arm

M85.129   Skeletal fluorosis, unspecified upper arm

M85.13   Skeletal fluorosis, forearm

M85.131   Skeletal fluorosis, right forearm

M85.132   Skeletal fluorosis, left forearm

M85.139   Skeletal fluorosis, unspecified forearm

M85.14   Skeletal fluorosis, hand

M85.141   Skeletal fluorosis, right hand

M85.142   Skeletal fluorosis, left hand

M85.149   Skeletal fluorosis, unspecified hand

M85.15   Skeletal fluorosis, thigh

M85.151   Skeletal fluorosis, right thigh

M85.152   Skeletal fluorosis, left thigh

M85.159   Skeletal fluorosis, unspecified thigh

M85.16   Skeletal fluorosis, lower leg

M85.161   Skeletal fluorosis, right lower leg

M85.162   Skeletal fluorosis, left lower leg

M85.169   Skeletal fluorosis, unspecified lower leg

M85.17   Skeletal fluorosis, ankle and foot

M85.171   Skeletal fluorosis, right ankle and foot

M85.172   Skeletal fluorosis, left ankle and foot

M85.179   Skeletal fluorosis, unspecified ankle and foot

M85.18   Skeletal fluorosis, other site

M85.19   Skeletal fluorosis, multiple sites

M85.2   Hyperostosis of skull

M85.3   Osteitis condensans

M85.30   Osteitis condensans, unspecified site

M85.31   Osteitis condensans, shoulder

M85.311   Osteitis condensans, right shoulder

M85.312   Osteitis condensans, left shoulder

M85.319   Osteitis condensans, unspecified shoulder

M85.32   Osteitis condensans, upper arm

M85.321   Osteitis condensans, right upper arm

M85.322   Osteitis condensans, left upper arm

M85.329   Osteitis condensans, unspecified upper arm

M85.33   Osteitis condensans, forearm

M85.331   Osteitis condensans, right forearm

M85.332   Osteitis condensans, left forearm

M85.339   Osteitis condensans, unspecified forearm

M85.34   Osteitis condensans, hand

M85.341   Osteitis condensans, right hand

M85.342   Osteitis condensans, left hand

M85.349   Osteitis condensans, unspecified hand

M85.35   Osteitis condensans, thigh

M85.351   Osteitis condensans, right thigh

M85.352   Osteitis condensans, left thigh

M85.359   Osteitis condensans, unspecified thigh

M85.36   Osteitis condensans, lower leg

M85.361   Osteitis condensans, right lower leg

M85.362   Osteitis condensans, left lower leg

M85.369   Osteitis condensans, unspecified lower leg

M85.37   Osteitis condensans, ankle and foot

M85.371   Osteitis condensans, right ankle and foot

M85.372   Osteitis condensans, left ankle and foot

M85.379   Osteitis condensans, unspecified ankle and foot

M85.38   Osteitis condensans, other site

M85.39   Osteitis condensans, multiple sites

M85.4   Solitary bone cyst

Excludes2: solitary cyst of jaw (M27.4)

M85.40   Solitary bone cyst, unspecified site

M85.41   Solitary bone cyst, shoulder

M85.411   Solitary bone cyst, right shoulder

M85.412   Solitary bone cyst, left shoulder

M85.419   Solitary bone cyst, unspecified shoulder

M85.42   Solitary bone cyst, humerus

M85.421   Solitary bone cyst, right humerus

M85.422   Solitary bone cyst, left humerus

M85.429   Solitary bone cyst, unspecified humerus

M85.43   Solitary bone cyst, ulna and radius

M85.431   Solitary bone cyst, right ulna and radius

M85.432   Solitary bone cyst, left ulna and radius

M85.439   Solitary bone cyst, unspecified ulna and radius

M85.44   Solitary bone cyst, hand

M85.441   Solitary bone cyst, right hand

M85.442   Solitary bone cyst, left hand

M85.449   Solitary bone cyst, unspecified hand

M85.45   Solitary bone cyst, pelvis

M85.451   Solitary bone cyst, right pelvis

M85.452   Solitary bone cyst, left pelvis

M85.459   Solitary bone cyst, unspecified pelvis

M85.46   Solitary bone cyst, tibia and fibula

M85.461   Solitary bone cyst, right tibia and fibula

M85.462   Solitary bone cyst, left tibia and fibula

M85.469   Solitary bone cyst, unspecified tibia and fibula

M85.47   Solitary bone cyst, ankle and foot

M85.471   Solitary bone cyst, right ankle and foot

M85.472   Solitary bone cyst, left ankle and foot

M85.479   Solitary bone cyst, unspecified ankle and foot

M85.48   Solitary bone cyst, other site

M85.5   Aneurysmal bone cyst

Excludes2: aneurysmal cyst of jaw (M27.4)

M85.50   Aneurysmal bone cyst, unspecified site

M85.51   Aneurysmal bone cyst, shoulder

M85.511   Aneurysmal bone cyst, right shoulder

M85.512   Aneurysmal bone cyst, left shoulder

M85.519   Aneurysmal bone cyst, unspecified shoulder

M85.52   Aneurysmal bone cyst, upper arm

M85.521   Aneurysmal bone cyst, right upper arm

M85.522   Aneurysmal bone cyst, left upper arm

M85.529   Aneurysmal bone cyst, unspecified upper arm

M85.53   Aneurysmal bone cyst, forearm

M85.531   Aneurysmal bone cyst, right forearm

M85.532   Aneurysmal bone cyst, left forearm

M85.539   Aneurysmal bone cyst, unspecified forearm

M85.54   Aneurysmal bone cyst, hand

M85.541   Aneurysmal bone cyst, right hand

M85.542   Aneurysmal bone cyst, left hand

M85.549   Aneurysmal bone cyst, unspecified hand

M85.55   Aneurysmal bone cyst, thigh

M85.551   Aneurysmal bone cyst, right thigh

M85.552   Aneurysmal bone cyst, left thigh

M85.559 Aneurysmal bone cyst, unspecified thigh

M85.56 Aneurysmal bone cyst, lower leg

M85.561 Aneurysmal bone cyst, right lower leg

M85.562 Aneurysmal bone cyst, left lower leg

M85.569 Aneurysmal bone cyst, unspecified lower leg

M85.57 Aneurysmal bone cyst, ankle and foot

M85.571 Aneurysmal bone cyst, right ankle and foot

M85.572 Aneurysmal bone cyst, left ankle and foot

M85.579 Aneurysmal bone cyst, unspecified ankle and foot

M85.58 Aneurysmal bone cyst, other site

M85.59 Aneurysmal bone cyst, multiple sites

M85.6 Other cyst of bone

Excludes1: cyst of jaw NEC (M27.4)

osteitis fibrosa cystica generalisata [von

Recklinghausen's disease of bone] (E21.0)

M85.60 Other cyst of bone, unspecified site

M85.61 Other cyst of bone, shoulder

M85.611 Other cyst of bone, right shoulder

M85.612 Other cyst of bone, left shoulder

M85.619 Other cyst of bone, unspecified shoulder

M85.62 Other cyst of bone, upper arm

M85.621 Other cyst of bone, right upper arm

M85.622 Other cyst of bone, left upper arm

M85.629 Other cyst of bone, unspecified upper arm

M85.63 Other cyst of bone, forearm

M85.631 Other cyst of bone, right forearm

M85.632 Other cyst of bone, left forearm

M85.639 Other cyst of bone, unspecified forearm

M85.64 Other cyst of bone, hand

M85.641 Other cyst of bone, right hand

M85.642 Other cyst of bone, left hand

M85.649 Other cyst of bone, unspecified hand

M85.65 Other cyst of bone, thigh

M85.651 Other cyst of bone, right thigh

M85.652 Other cyst of bone, left thigh

M85.659 Other cyst of bone, unspecified thigh

M85.66 Other cyst of bone, lower leg

M85.661 Other cyst of bone, right lower leg

M85.662 Other cyst of bone, left lower leg

M85.669 Other cyst of bone, unspecified lower leg

M85.67 Other cyst of bone, ankle and foot

M85.671 Other cyst of bone, right ankle and foot

M85.672 Other cyst of bone, left ankle and foot

M85.679 Other cyst of bone, unspecified ankle and foot

M85.68 Other cyst of bone, other site

M85.69 Other cyst of bone, multiple sites

M85.8 Other specified disorders of bone density and structure

Hyperostosis of bones, except skull

Osteosclerosis, acquired

Excludes1: diffuse idiopathic skeletal hyperostosis [DISH] (M48.1)

osteosclerosis congenita (Q77.4)

osteosclerosis fragilitas (generalisata) (Q78.2)

osteosclerosis myelofibrosis (D75.81)

M85.80 Other specified disorders of bone density and structure, unspecified site

M85.81 Other specified disorders of bone density and structure, shoulder

M85.811 Other specified disorders of bone density and structure, right shoulder

M85.812 Other specified disorders of bone density and structure, left shoulder

M85.819 Other specified disorders of bone density and structure, unspecified shoulder

M85.82 Other specified disorders of bone density and structure, upper arm

M85.821 Other specified disorders of bone density and structure, right upper arm

M85.822 Other specified disorders of bone density and structure, left upper arm

M85.829 Other specified disorders of bone density and structure, unspecified upper arm

M85.83 Other specified disorders of bone density and structure, forearm

M85.831 Other specified disorders of bone density and structure, right forearm

M85.832 Other specified disorders of bone density and structure, left forearm

M85.839 Other specified disorders of bone density and structure, unspecified forearm

M85.84 Other specified disorders of bone density and structure, hand

M85.841 Other specified disorders of bone density and structure, right hand

M85.842 Other specified disorders of bone density and structure, left hand

M85.849 Other specified disorders of bone density and structure, unspecified hand

M85.85 Other specified disorders of bone density and structure, thigh

M85.851 Other specified disorders of bone density and structure, right thigh

M85.852 Other specified disorders of bone density and structure, left thigh

M85.859 Other specified disorders of bone density and structure, unspecified thigh

M85.86 Other specified disorders of bone density and structure, lower leg

M85.861 Other specified disorders of bone density and structure, right lower leg

M85.862 Other specified disorders of bone density and structure, left lower leg

● New code　　▲ Revised code　　**Excludes1:** Not coded here　　**Excludes2:** Not included here　　⊗ Placeholder required　　⑦7th digit required

M85.869 Other specified disorders of bone density and structure, unspecified lower leg

M85.87 Other specified disorders of bone density and structure, ankle and foot

M85.871 Other specified disorders of bone density and structure, right ankle and foot

M85.872 Other specified disorders of bone density and structure, left ankle and foot

M85.879 Other specified disorders of bone density and structure, unspecified ankle and foot

M85.88 Other specified disorders of bone density and structure, other site

M85.89 Other specified disorders of bone density and structure, multiple sites

M85.9 Disorder of bone density and structure, unspecified

OTHER OSTEOPATHIES (M86-M90)

Excludes1: postprocedural osteopathies (M96.-)

M86 **Osteomyelitis**

Use additional code (B95-B97) to identify infectious agent

Use additional code to identify major osseous defect, if applicable (M89.7-)

Excludes1: osteomyelitis due to:

echinococcus (B67.2)

gonococcus (A54.43)

salmonella (A02.24)

Excludes2: osteomyelitis of:

orbit (H05.0-)

petrous bone (H70.2-)

vertebra (M46.2-)

M86.0 Acute hematogenous osteomyelitis

M86.00 Acute hematogenous osteomyelitis, unspecified site

M86.01 Acute hematogenous osteomyelitis, shoulder

M86.011 Acute hematogenous osteomyelitis, right shoulder

M86.012 Acute hematogenous osteomyelitis, left shoulder

M86.019 Acute hematogenous osteomyelitis, unspecified shoulder

M86.02 Acute hematogenous osteomyelitis, humerus

M86.021 Acute hematogenous osteomyelitis, right humerus

M86.022 Acute hematogenous osteomyelitis, left humerus

M86.029 Acute hematogenous osteomyelitis, unspecified humerus

M86.03 Acute hematogenous osteomyelitis, radius and ulna

M86.031 Acute hematogenous osteomyelitis, right radius and ulna

M86.032 Acute hematogenous osteomyelitis, left radius and ulna

M86.039 Acute hematogenous osteomyelitis, unspecified radius and ulna

M86.04 Acute hematogenous osteomyelitis, hand

M86.041 Acute hematogenous osteomyelitis, right hand

M86.042 Acute hematogenous osteomyelitis, left hand

M86.049 Acute hematogenous osteomyelitis, unspecified hand

M86.05 Acute hematogenous osteomyelitis, femur

M86.051 Acute hematogenous osteomyelitis, right femur

M86.052 Acute hematogenous osteomyelitis, left femur

M86.059 Acute hematogenous osteomyelitis, unspecified femur

M86.06 Acute hematogenous osteomyelitis, tibia and fibula

M86.061 Acute hematogenous osteomyelitis, right tibia and fibula

M86.062 Acute hematogenous osteomyelitis, left tibia and fibula

M86.069 Acute hematogenous osteomyelitis, unspecified tibia and fibula

M86.07 Acute hematogenous osteomyelitis, ankle and foot

M86.071 Acute hematogenous osteomyelitis, right ankle and foot

M86.072 Acute hematogenous osteomyelitis, left ankle and foot

M86.079 Acute hematogenous osteomyelitis, unspecified ankle and foot

M86.08 Acute hematogenous osteomyelitis, other sites

M86.09 Acute hematogenous osteomyelitis, multiple sites

M86.1 Other acute osteomyelitis

M86.10 Other acute osteomyelitis, unspecified site

M86.11 Other acute osteomyelitis, shoulder

M86.111 Other acute osteomyelitis, right shoulder

M86.112 Other acute osteomyelitis, left shoulder

M86.119 Other acute osteomyelitis, unspecified shoulder

M86.12 Other acute osteomyelitis, humerus

M86.121 Other acute osteomyelitis, right humerus

M86.122 Other acute osteomyelitis, left humerus

M86.129 Other acute osteomyelitis, unspecified humerus

M86.13 Other acute osteomyelitis, radius and ulna

M86.131 Other acute osteomyelitis, right radius and ulna

M86.132 Other acute osteomyelitis, left radius and ulna

M86.139 Other acute osteomyelitis, unspecified radius and ulna

M86.14 Other acute osteomyelitis, hand

M86.141 Other acute osteomyelitis, right hand

M86.142 Other acute osteomyelitis, left hand

M86.149 Other acute osteomyelitis, unspecified hand

M86.15 Other acute osteomyelitis, femur

M86.151 Other acute osteomyelitis, right femur

M86.152 Other acute osteomyelitis, left femur

Add 4th-7th digits   Nonspecific code   Unspecified code   Manifestation code

M86.159   Other acute osteomyelitis, unspecified femur

M86.16   Other acute osteomyelitis, tibia and fibula

     M86.161   Other acute osteomyelitis, right tibia and fibula

     M86.162   Other acute osteomyelitis, left tibia and fibula

     M86.169   Other acute osteomyelitis, unspecified tibia and fibula

M86.17   Other acute osteomyelitis, ankle and foot

     M86.171   Other acute osteomyelitis, right ankle and foot

     M86.172   Other acute osteomyelitis, left ankle and foot

     M86.179   Other acute osteomyelitis, unspecified ankle and foot

M86.18   Other acute osteomyelitis, other site

M86.19   Other acute osteomyelitis, multiple sites

M86.2   Subacute osteomyelitis

   M86.20   Subacute osteomyelitis, unspecified site

   M86.21   Subacute osteomyelitis, shoulder

     M86.211   Subacute osteomyelitis, right shoulder

     M86.212   Subacute osteomyelitis, left shoulder

     M86.219   Subacute osteomyelitis, unspecified shoulder

   M86.22   Subacute osteomyelitis, humerus

     M86.221   Subacute osteomyelitis, right humerus

     M86.222   Subacute osteomyelitis, left humerus

     M86.229   Subacute osteomyelitis, unspecified humerus

   M86.23   Subacute osteomyelitis, radius and ulna

     M86.231   Subacute osteomyelitis, right radius and ulna

     M86.232   Subacute osteomyelitis, left radius and ulna

     M86.239   Subacute osteomyelitis, unspecified radius and ulna

   M86.24   Subacute osteomyelitis, hand

     M86.241   Subacute osteomyelitis, right hand

     M86.242   Subacute osteomyelitis, left hand

     M86.249   Subacute osteomyelitis, unspecified hand

   M86.25   Subacute osteomyelitis, femur

     M86.251   Subacute osteomyelitis, right femur

     M86.252   Subacute osteomyelitis, left femur

     M86.259   Subacute osteomyelitis, unspecified femur

   M86.26   Subacute osteomyelitis, tibia and fibula

     M86.261   Subacute osteomyelitis, right tibia and fibula

     M86.262   Subacute osteomyelitis, left tibia and fibula

     M86.269   Subacute osteomyelitis, unspecified tibia and fibula

   M86.27   Subacute osteomyelitis, ankle and foot

     M86.271   Subacute osteomyelitis, right ankle and foot

     M86.272   Subacute osteomyelitis, left ankle and foot

     M86.279   Subacute osteomyelitis, unspecified ankle and foot

   M86.28   Subacute osteomyelitis, other site

   M86.29   Subacute osteomyelitis, multiple sites

M86.3   Chronic multifocal osteomyelitis

   M86.30   Chronic multifocal osteomyelitis, unspecified site

   M86.31   Chronic multifocal osteomyelitis, shoulder

     M86.311   Chronic multifocal osteomyelitis, right shoulder

     M86.312   Chronic multifocal osteomyelitis, left shoulder

     M86.319   Chronic multifocal osteomyelitis, unspecified shoulder

   M86.32   Chronic multifocal osteomyelitis, humerus

     M86.321   Chronic multifocal osteomyelitis, right humerus

     M86.322   Chronic multifocal osteomyelitis, left humerus

     M86.329   Chronic multifocal osteomyelitis, unspecified humerus

   M86.33   Chronic multifocal osteomyelitis, radius and ulna

     M86.331   Chronic multifocal osteomyelitis, right radius and ulna

     M86.332   Chronic multifocal osteomyelitis, left radius and ulna

     M86.339   Chronic multifocal osteomyelitis, unspecified radius and ulna

   M86.34   Chronic multifocal osteomyelitis, hand

     M86.341   Chronic multifocal osteomyelitis, right hand

     M86.342   Chronic multifocal osteomyelitis, left hand

     M86.349   Chronic multifocal osteomyelitis, unspecified hand

   M86.35   Chronic multifocal osteomyelitis, femur

     M86.351   Chronic multifocal osteomyelitis, right femur

     M86.352   Chronic multifocal osteomyelitis, left femur

     M86.359   Chronic multifocal osteomyelitis, unspecified femur

   M86.36   Chronic multifocal osteomyelitis, tibia and fibula

     M86.361   Chronic multifocal osteomyelitis, right tibia and fibula

     M86.362   Chronic multifocal osteomyelitis, left tibia and fibula

     M86.369   Chronic multifocal osteomyelitis, unspecified tibia and fibula

   M86.37   Chronic multifocal osteomyelitis, ankle and foot

     M86.371   Chronic multifocal osteomyelitis, right ankle and foot

     M86.372   Chronic multifocal osteomyelitis, left ankle and foot

     M86.379   Chronic multifocal osteomyelitis, unspecified ankle and foot

   M86.38   Chronic multifocal osteomyelitis, other site

   M86.39   Chronic multifocal osteomyelitis, multiple sites

M86.4   Chronic osteomyelitis with draining sinus

   M86.40   Chronic osteomyelitis with draining sinus, unspecified site

● New code   ▲ Revised code   **Excludes1:** Not coded here   **Excludes2:** Not included here   ⊗ Placeholder required   ⑦ 7th digit required

M86.41   **Chronic osteomyelitis with draining sinus, shoulder**

     M86.411   **Chronic osteomyelitis with draining sinus, right shoulder**

     M86.412   **Chronic osteomyelitis with draining sinus, left shoulder**

     M86.419   **Chronic osteomyelitis with draining sinus, unspecified shoulder**

M86.42   **Chronic osteomyelitis with draining sinus, humerus**

     M86.421   **Chronic osteomyelitis with draining sinus, right humerus**

     M86.422   **Chronic osteomyelitis with draining sinus, left humerus**

     M86.429   **Chronic osteomyelitis with draining sinus, unspecified humerus**

M86.43   **Chronic osteomyelitis with draining sinus, radius and ulna**

     M86.431   **Chronic osteomyelitis with draining sinus, right radius and ulna**

     M86.432   **Chronic osteomyelitis with draining sinus, left radius and ulna**

     M86.439   **Chronic osteomyelitis with draining sinus, unspecified radius and ulna**

M86.44   **Chronic osteomyelitis with draining sinus, hand**

     M86.441   **Chronic osteomyelitis with draining sinus, right hand**

     M86.442   **Chronic osteomyelitis with draining sinus, left hand**

     M86.449   **Chronic osteomyelitis with draining sinus, unspecified hand**

M86.45   **Chronic osteomyelitis with draining sinus, femur**

     M86.451   **Chronic osteomyelitis with draining sinus, right femur**

     M86.452   **Chronic osteomyelitis with draining sinus, left femur**

     M86.459   **Chronic osteomyelitis with draining sinus, unspecified femur**

M86.46   **Chronic osteomyelitis with draining sinus, tibia and fibula**

     M86.461   **Chronic osteomyelitis with draining sinus, right tibia and fibula**

     M86.462   **Chronic osteomyelitis with draining sinus, left tibia and fibula**

     M86.469   **Chronic osteomyelitis with draining sinus, unspecified tibia and fibula**

M86.47   **Chronic osteomyelitis with draining sinus, ankle and foot**

     M86.471   **Chronic osteomyelitis with draining sinus, right ankle and foot**

     M86.472   **Chronic osteomyelitis with draining sinus, left ankle and foot**

     M86.479   **Chronic osteomyelitis with draining sinus, unspecified ankle and foot**

M86.48   **Chronic osteomyelitis with draining sinus, other site**

M86.49   **Chronic osteomyelitis with draining sinus, multiple sites**

M86.5   **Other chronic hematogenous osteomyelitis**

   M86.50   **Other chronic hematogenous osteomyelitis, unspecified site**

   M86.51   **Other chronic hematogenous osteomyelitis, shoulder**

     M86.511   **Other chronic hematogenous osteomyelitis, right shoulder**

     M86.512   **Other chronic hematogenous osteomyelitis, left shoulder**

     M86.519   **Other chronic hematogenous osteomyelitis, unspecified shoulder**

   M86.52   **Other chronic hematogenous osteomyelitis, humerus**

     M86.521   **Other chronic hematogenous osteomyelitis, right humerus**

     M86.522   **Other chronic hematogenous osteomyelitis, left humerus**

     M86.529   **Other chronic hematogenous osteomyelitis, unspecified humerus**

   M86.53   **Other chronic hematogenous osteomyelitis, radius and ulna**

     M86.531   **Other chronic hematogenous osteomyelitis, right radius and ulna**

     M86.532   **Other chronic hematogenous osteomyelitis, left radius and ulna**

     M86.539   **Other chronic hematogenous osteomyelitis, unspecified radius and ulna**

   M86.54   **Other chronic hematogenous osteomyelitis, hand**

     M86.541   **Other chronic hematogenous osteomyelitis, right hand**

     M86.542   **Other chronic hematogenous osteomyelitis, left hand**

     M86.549   **Other chronic hematogenous osteomyelitis, unspecified hand**

   M86.55   **Other chronic hematogenous osteomyelitis, femur**

     M86.551   **Other chronic hematogenous osteomyelitis, right femur**

     M86.552   **Other chronic hematogenous osteomyelitis, left femur**

     M86.559   **Other chronic hematogenous osteomyelitis, unspecified femur**

   M86.56   **Other chronic hematogenous osteomyelitis, tibia and fibula**

     M86.561   **Other chronic hematogenous osteomyelitis, right tibia and fibula**

     M86.562   **Other chronic hematogenous osteomyelitis, left tibia and fibula**

     M86.569   **Other chronic hematogenous osteomyelitis, unspecified tibia and fibula**

   M86.57   **Other chronic hematogenous osteomyelitis, ankle and foot**

     M86.571   **Other chronic hematogenous osteomyelitis, right ankle and foot**

     M86.572   **Other chronic hematogenous osteomyelitis, left ankle and foot**

     M86.579   **Other chronic hematogenous osteomyelitis, unspecified ankle and foot**

   M86.58   **Other chronic hematogenous osteomyelitis, other site**

   M86.59   **Other chronic hematogenous osteomyelitis, multiple sites**

M86.6   **Other chronic osteomyelitis**

   M86.60   **Other chronic osteomyelitis, unspecified site**

   M86.61   **Other chronic osteomyelitis, shoulder**

	Add 4th-7th digits		Nonspecific code		Unspecified code		Manifestation code

M86.611 Other chronic osteomyelitis, right shoulder

M86.612 Other chronic osteomyelitis, left shoulder

M86.619 Other chronic osteomyelitis, unspecified shoulder

M86.62 Other chronic osteomyelitis, humerus

M86.621 Other chronic osteomyelitis, right humerus

M86.622 Other chronic osteomyelitis, left humerus

M86.629 Other chronic osteomyelitis, unspecified humerus

M86.63 Other chronic osteomyelitis, radius and ulna

M86.631 Other chronic osteomyelitis, right radius and ulna

M86.632 Other chronic osteomyelitis, left radius and ulna

M86.639 Other chronic osteomyelitis, unspecified radius and ulna

M86.64 Other chronic osteomyelitis, hand

M86.641 Other chronic osteomyelitis, right hand

M86.642 Other chronic osteomyelitis, left hand

M86.649 Other chronic osteomyelitis, unspecified hand

M86.65 Other chronic osteomyelitis, thigh

M86.651 Other chronic osteomyelitis, right thigh

M86.652 Other chronic osteomyelitis, left thigh

M86.659 Other chronic osteomyelitis, unspecified thigh

M86.66 Other chronic osteomyelitis, tibia and fibula

M86.661 Other chronic osteomyelitis, right tibia and fibula

M86.662 Other chronic osteomyelitis, left tibia and fibula

M86.669 Other chronic osteomyelitis, unspecified tibia and fibula

M86.67 Other chronic osteomyelitis, ankle and foot

M86.671 Other chronic osteomyelitis, right ankle and foot

M86.672 Other chronic osteomyelitis, left ankle and foot

M86.679 Other chronic osteomyelitis, unspecified ankle and foot

M86.68 Other chronic osteomyelitis, other site

M86.69 Other chronic osteomyelitis, multiple sites

M86.8 Other osteomyelitis

Brodie's abscess

M86.8X Other osteomyelitis

M86.8X0 Other osteomyelitis, multiple sites

M86.8X1 Other osteomyelitis, shoulder

M86.8X2 Other osteomyelitis, upper arm

M86.8X3 Other osteomyelitis, forearm

M86.8X4 Other osteomyelitis, hand

M86.8X5 Other osteomyelitis, thigh

M86.8X6 Other osteomyelitis, lower leg

M86.8X7 Other osteomyelitis, ankle and foot

M86.8X8 Other osteomyelitis, other site

M86.8X9 Other osteomyelitis, unspecified sites

M86.9 Osteomyelitis, unspecified

Infection of bone NOS

Periostitis without osteomyelitis

M87 **Osteonecrosis**

Includes: avascular necrosis of bone

Use additional code to identify major osseous defect, if applicable (M89.7-)

Excludes1: juvenile osteonecrosis (M91-M92)

osteochondropathies (M90-M93)

M87.0 Idiopathic aseptic necrosis of bone

M87.00 Idiopathic aseptic necrosis of unspecified bone

M87.01 Idiopathic aseptic necrosis of shoulder

Idiopathic aseptic necrosis of clavicle and scapula

M87.011 Idiopathic aseptic necrosis of right shoulder

M87.012 Idiopathic aseptic necrosis of left shoulder

M87.019 Idiopathic aseptic necrosis of unspecified shoulder

M87.02 Idiopathic aseptic necrosis of humerus

M87.021 Idiopathic aseptic necrosis of right humerus

M87.022 Idiopathic aseptic necrosis of left humerus

M87.029 Idiopathic aseptic necrosis of unspecified humerus

M87.03 Idiopathic aseptic necrosis of radius, ulna and carpus

M87.031 Idiopathic aseptic necrosis of right radius

M87.032 Idiopathic aseptic necrosis of left radius

M87.033 Idiopathic aseptic necrosis of unspecified radius

M87.034 Idiopathic aseptic necrosis of right ulna

M87.035 Idiopathic aseptic necrosis of left ulna

M87.036 Idiopathic aseptic necrosis of unspecified ulna

M87.037 Idiopathic aseptic necrosis of right carpus

M87.038 Idiopathic aseptic necrosis of left carpus

M87.039 Idiopathic aseptic necrosis of unspecified carpus

M87.04 Idiopathic aseptic necrosis of hand and fingers

Idiopathic aseptic necrosis of metacarpals and phalanges of hands

M87.041 Idiopathic aseptic necrosis of right hand

M87.042 Idiopathic aseptic necrosis of left hand

M87.043 Idiopathic aseptic necrosis of unspecified hand

M87.044 Idiopathic aseptic necrosis of right finger(s)

M87.045 Idiopathic aseptic necrosis of left finger(s)

● New code   ▲ Revised code   Excludes1: Not coded here   Excludes2: Not included here   ⊗ Placeholder required   ⑦ 7th digit required

M87.046　Idiopathic aseptic necrosis of unspecified finger(s)

M87.05　Idiopathic aseptic necrosis of pelvis and femur

M87.050　Idiopathic aseptic necrosis of pelvis

M87.051　Idiopathic aseptic necrosis of right femur

M87.052　Idiopathic aseptic necrosis of left femur

M87.059　Idiopathic aseptic necrosis of unspecified femur

Idiopathic aseptic necrosis of hip NOS

M87.06　Idiopathic aseptic necrosis of tibia and fibula

M87.061　Idiopathic aseptic necrosis of right tibia

M87.062　Idiopathic aseptic necrosis of left tibia

M87.063　Idiopathic aseptic necrosis of unspecified tibia

M87.064　Idiopathic aseptic necrosis of right fibula

M87.065　Idiopathic aseptic necrosis of left fibula

M87.066　Idiopathic aseptic necrosis of unspecified fibula

M87.07　Idiopathic aseptic necrosis of ankle, foot and toes

Idiopathic aseptic necrosis of metatarsus, tarsus, and phalanges of toes

M87.071　Idiopathic aseptic necrosis of right ankle

M87.072　Idiopathic aseptic necrosis of left ankle

M87.073　Idiopathic aseptic necrosis of unspecified ankle

M87.074　Idiopathic aseptic necrosis of right foot

M87.075　Idiopathic aseptic necrosis of left foot

M87.076　Idiopathic aseptic necrosis of unspecified foot

M87.077　Idiopathic aseptic necrosis of right toe(s)

M87.078　Idiopathic aseptic necrosis of left toe(s)

M87.079　Idiopathic aseptic necrosis of unspecified toe(s)

M87.08　Idiopathic aseptic necrosis of bone, other site

M87.09　Idiopathic aseptic necrosis of bone, multiple sites

M87.1　Osteonecrosis due to drugs

Use additional code for adverse effect, if applicable, to identify drug (T36-T50 with fifth or sixth character 5)

M87.10　Osteonecrosis due to drugs, unspecified bone

M87.11　Osteonecrosis due to drugs, shoulder

M87.111　Osteonecrosis due to drugs, right shoulder

M87.112　Osteonecrosis due to drugs, left shoulder

M87.119　Osteonecrosis due to drugs, unspecified shoulder

M87.12　Osteonecrosis due to drugs, humerus

M87.121　Osteonecrosis due to drugs, right humerus

M87.122　Osteonecrosis due to drugs, left humerus

M87.129　Osteonecrosis due to drugs, unspecified humerus

M87.13　Osteonecrosis due to drugs of radius, ulna and carpus

M87.131　Osteonecrosis due to drugs of right radius

M87.132　Osteonecrosis due to drugs of left radius

M87.133　Osteonecrosis due to drugs of unspecified radius

M87.134　Osteonecrosis due to drugs of right ulna

M87.135　Osteonecrosis due to drugs of left ulna

M87.136　Osteonecrosis due to drugs of unspecified ulna

M87.137　Osteonecrosis due to drugs of right carpus

M87.138　Osteonecrosis due to drugs of left carpus

M87.139　Osteonecrosis due to drugs of unspecified carpus

M87.14　Osteonecrosis due to drugs, hand and fingers

M87.141　Osteonecrosis due to drugs, right hand

M87.142　Osteonecrosis due to drugs, left hand

M87.143　Osteonecrosis due to drugs, unspecified hand

M87.144　Osteonecrosis due to drugs, right finger(s)

M87.145　Osteonecrosis due to drugs, left finger(s)

M87.146　Osteonecrosis due to drugs, unspecified finger(s)

M87.15　Osteonecrosis due to drugs, pelvis and femur

M87.150　Osteonecrosis due to drugs, pelvis

M87.151　Osteonecrosis due to drugs, right femur

M87.152　Osteonecrosis due to drugs, left femur

M87.159　Osteonecrosis due to drugs, unspecified femur

M87.16　Osteonecrosis due to drugs, tibia and fibula

M87.161　Osteonecrosis due to drugs, right tibia

M87.162　Osteonecrosis due to drugs, left tibia

M87.163　Osteonecrosis due to drugs, unspecified tibia

M87.164　Osteonecrosis due to drugs, right fibula

M87.165　Osteonecrosis due to drugs, left fibula

M87.166　Osteonecrosis due to drugs, unspecified fibula

M87.17　Osteonecrosis due to drugs, ankle, foot and toes

M87.171　Osteonecrosis due to drugs, right ankle

M87.172　Osteonecrosis due to drugs, left ankle

M87.173　Osteonecrosis due to drugs, unspecified ankle

M87.174 Osteonecrosis due to drugs, right foot

M87.175 Osteonecrosis due to drugs, left foot

M87.176 Osteonecrosis due to drugs, unspecified foot

M87.177 Osteonecrosis due to drugs, right toe(s)

M87.178 Osteonecrosis due to drugs, left toe(s)

M87.179 Osteonecrosis due to drugs, unspecified toe(s)

M87.18 Osteonecrosis due to drugs, other site

M87.180 Osteonecrosis due to drugs, jaw

M87.188 Osteonecrosis due to drugs, other site

M87.19 Osteonecrosis due to drugs, multiple sites

M87.2 Osteonecrosis due to previous trauma

M87.20 Osteonecrosis due to previous trauma, unspecified bone

M87.21 Osteonecrosis due to previous trauma, shoulder

M87.211 Osteonecrosis due to previous trauma, right shoulder

M87.212 Osteonecrosis due to previous trauma, left shoulder

M87.219 Osteonecrosis due to previous trauma, unspecified shoulder

M87.22 Osteonecrosis due to previous trauma, humerus

M87.221 Osteonecrosis due to previous trauma, right humerus

M87.222 Osteonecrosis due to previous trauma, left humerus

M87.229 Osteonecrosis due to previous trauma, unspecified humerus

M87.23 Osteonecrosis due to previous trauma of radius, ulna and carpus

M87.231 Osteonecrosis due to previous trauma of right radius

M87.232 Osteonecrosis due to previous trauma of left radius

M87.233 Osteonecrosis due to previous trauma of unspecified radius

M87.234 Osteonecrosis due to previous trauma of right ulna

M87.235 Osteonecrosis due to previous trauma of left ulna

M87.236 Osteonecrosis due to previous trauma of unspecified ulna

M87.237 Osteonecrosis due to previous trauma of right carpus

M87.238 Osteonecrosis due to previous trauma of left carpus

M87.239 Osteonecrosis due to previous trauma of unspecified carpus

M87.24 Osteonecrosis due to previous trauma, hand and fingers

M87.241 Osteonecrosis due to previous trauma, right hand

M87.242 Osteonecrosis due to previous trauma, left hand

M87.243 Osteonecrosis due to previous trauma, unspecified hand

M87.244 Osteonecrosis due to previous trauma, right finger(s)

M87.245 Osteonecrosis due to previous trauma, left finger(s)

M87.246 Osteonecrosis due to previous trauma, unspecified finger(s)

M87.25 Osteonecrosis due to previous trauma, pelvis and femur

M87.250 Osteonecrosis due to previous trauma, pelvis

M87.251 Osteonecrosis due to previous trauma, right femur

M87.252 Osteonecrosis due to previous trauma, left femur

M87.256 Osteonecrosis due to previous trauma, unspecified femur

M87.26 Osteonecrosis due to previous trauma, tibia and fibula

M87.261 Osteonecrosis due to previous trauma, right tibia

M87.262 Osteonecrosis due to previous trauma, left tibia

M87.263 Osteonecrosis due to previous trauma, unspecified tibia

M87.264 Osteonecrosis due to previous trauma, right fibula

M87.265 Osteonecrosis due to previous trauma, left fibula

M87.266 Osteonecrosis due to previous trauma, unspecified fibula

M87.27 Osteonecrosis due to previous trauma, ankle, foot and toes

M87.271 Osteonecrosis due to previous trauma, right ankle

M87.272 Osteonecrosis due to previous trauma, left ankle

M87.273 Osteonecrosis due to previous trauma, unspecified ankle

M87.274 Osteonecrosis due to previous trauma, right foot

M87.275 Osteonecrosis due to previous trauma, left foot

M87.276 Osteonecrosis due to previous trauma, unspecified foot

M87.277 Osteonecrosis due to previous trauma, right toe(s)

M87.278 Osteonecrosis due to previous trauma, left toe(s)

M87.279 Osteonecrosis due to previous trauma, unspecified toe(s)

M87.28 Osteonecrosis due to previous trauma, other site

M87.29 Osteonecrosis due to previous trauma, multiple sites

M87.3 Other secondary osteonecrosis

M87.30 Other secondary osteonecrosis, unspecified bone

M87.31 Other secondary osteonecrosis, shoulder

M87.311 Other secondary osteonecrosis, right shoulder

M87.312 Other secondary osteonecrosis, left shoulder

M87.319 Other secondary osteonecrosis, unspecified shoulder

M87.32 Other secondary osteonecrosis, humerus

M87.321 Other secondary osteonecrosis, right humerus

● New code   ▲ Revised code   Excludes1: Not coded here   Excludes2: Not included here   ⊗ Placeholder required   ⑦ 7th digit required

M87.322   Other secondary osteonecrosis, left humerus

M87.329   Other secondary osteonecrosis, unspecified humerus

M87.33   Other secondary osteonecrosis of radius, ulna and carpus

M87.331   Other secondary osteonecrosis of right radius

M87.332   Other secondary osteonecrosis of left radius

M87.333   Other secondary osteonecrosis of unspecified radius

M87.334   Other secondary osteonecrosis of right ulna

M87.335   Other secondary osteonecrosis of left ulna

M87.336   Other secondary osteonecrosis of unspecified ulna

M87.337   Other secondary osteonecrosis of right carpus

M87.338   Other secondary osteonecrosis of left carpus

M87.339   Other secondary osteonecrosis of unspecified carpus

M87.34   Other secondary osteonecrosis, hand and fingers

M87.341   Other secondary osteonecrosis, right hand

M87.342   Other secondary osteonecrosis, left hand

M87.343   Other secondary osteonecrosis, unspecified hand

M87.344   Other secondary osteonecrosis, right finger(s)

M87.345   Other secondary osteonecrosis, left finger(s)

M87.346   Other secondary osteonecrosis, unspecified finger(s)

M87.35   Other secondary osteonecrosis, pelvis and femur

M87.350   Other secondary osteonecrosis, pelvis

M87.351   Other secondary osteonecrosis, right femur

M87.352   Other secondary osteonecrosis, left femur

M87.353   Other secondary osteonecrosis, unspecified femur

M87.36   Other secondary osteonecrosis, tibia and fibula

M87.361   Other secondary osteonecrosis, right tibia

M87.362   Other secondary osteonecrosis, left tibia

M87.363   Other secondary osteonecrosis, unspecified tibia

M87.364   Other secondary osteonecrosis, right fibula

M87.365   Other secondary osteonecrosis, left fibula

M87.366   Other secondary osteonecrosis, unspecified fibula

M87.37   Other secondary osteonecrosis, ankle and foot

M87.371   Other secondary osteonecrosis, right ankle

M87.372   Other secondary osteonecrosis, left ankle

M87.373   Other secondary osteonecrosis, unspecified ankle

M87.374   Other secondary osteonecrosis, right foot

M87.375   Other secondary osteonecrosis, left foot

M87.376   Other secondary osteonecrosis, unspecified foot

M87.377   Other secondary osteonecrosis, right toe(s)

M87.378   Other secondary osteonecrosis, left toe(s)

M87.379   Other secondary osteonecrosis, unspecified toe(s)

M87.38   Other secondary osteonecrosis, other site

M87.39   Other secondary osteonecrosis, multiple sites

M87.8   Other osteonecrosis

M87.80   Other osteonecrosis, unspecified bone

M87.81   Other osteonecrosis, shoulder

M87.811   Other osteonecrosis, right shoulder

M87.812   Other osteonecrosis, left shoulder

M87.819   Other osteonecrosis, unspecified shoulder

M87.82   Other osteonecrosis, humerus

M87.821   Other osteonecrosis, right humerus

M87.822   Other osteonecrosis, left humerus

M87.829   Other osteonecrosis, unspecified humerus

M87.83   Other osteonecrosis of radius, ulna and carpus

M87.831   Other osteonecrosis of right radius

M87.832   Other osteonecrosis of left radius

M87.833   Other osteonecrosis of unspecified radius

M87.834   Other osteonecrosis of right ulna

M87.835   Other osteonecrosis of left ulna

M87.836   Other osteonecrosis of unspecified ulna

M87.837   Other osteonecrosis of right carpus

M87.838   Other osteonecrosis of left carpus

M87.839   Other osteonecrosis of unspecified carpus

M87.84   Other osteonecrosis, hand and fingers

M87.841   Other osteonecrosis, right hand

M87.842   Other osteonecrosis, left hand

M87.843   Other osteonecrosis, unspecified hand

M87.844   Other osteonecrosis, right finger(s)

M87.845   Other osteonecrosis, left finger(s)

M87.849   Other osteonecrosis, unspecified finger(s)

M87.85   Other osteonecrosis, pelvis and femur

M87.850   Other osteonecrosis, pelvis

M87.851   Other osteonecrosis, right femur

M87.852   Other osteonecrosis, left femur

M87.859   Other osteonecrosis, unspecified femur

M87.86   Other osteonecrosis, tibia and fibula

M87.861   Other osteonecrosis, right tibia

M87.862 Other osteonecrosis, left tibia

M87.863 Other osteonecrosis, unspecified tibia

M87.864 Other osteonecrosis, right fibula

M87.865 Other osteonecrosis, left fibula

M87.869 Other osteonecrosis, unspecified fibula

M87.87 Other osteonecrosis, ankle, foot and toes

M87.871 Other osteonecrosis, right ankle

M87.872 Other osteonecrosis, left ankle

M87.873 Other osteonecrosis, unspecified ankle

M87.874 Other osteonecrosis, right foot

M87.875 Other osteonecrosis, left foot

M87.876 Other osteonecrosis, unspecified foot

M87.877 Other osteonecrosis, right toe(s)

M87.878 Other osteonecrosis, left toe(s)

M87.879 Other osteonecrosis, unspecified toe(s)

M87.88 Other osteonecrosis, other site

M87.89 Other osteonecrosis, multiple sites

M87.9 Osteonecrosis, unspecified

Necrosis of bone NOS

M88 Osteitis deformans [Paget's disease of bone]

Definition: Osteitis deformans, aka Paget's disease, is a disease of bone occurring in the middle aged and elderly; excessive bone destruction sometimes leading to bone pain and fractures and skeletal deformities.

Excludes1: osteitis deformans in neoplastic disease (M90.6)

M88.0 Osteitis deformans of skull

M88.1 Osteitis deformans of vertebrae

M88.8 Osteitis deformans of other bones

M88.81 Osteitis deformans of shoulder

M88.811 Osteitis deformans of right shoulder

M88.812 Osteitis deformans of left shoulder

M88.819 Osteitis deformans of unspecified shoulder

M88.82 Osteitis deformans of upper arm

M88.821 Osteitis deformans of right upper arm

M88.822 Osteitis deformans of left upper arm

M88.829 Osteitis deformans of unspecified upper arm

M88.83 Osteitis deformans of forearm

M88.831 Osteitis deformans of right forearm

M88.832 Osteitis deformans of left forearm

M88.839 Osteitis deformans of unspecified forearm

M88.84 Osteitis deformans of hand

M88.841 Osteitis deformans of right hand

M88.842 Osteitis deformans of left hand

M88.849 Osteitis deformans of unspecified hand

M88.85 Osteitis deformans of thigh

M88.851 Osteitis deformans of right thigh

M88.852 Osteitis deformans of left thigh

M88.859 Osteitis deformans of unspecified thigh

M88.86 Osteitis deformans of lower leg

M88.861 Osteitis deformans of right lower leg

M88.862 Osteitis deformans of left lower leg

M88.869 Osteitis deformans of unspecified lower leg

M88.87 Osteitis deformans of ankle and foot

M88.871 Osteitis deformans of right ankle and foot

M88.872 Osteitis deformans of left ankle and foot

M88.879 Osteitis deformans of unspecified ankle and foot

M88.88 Osteitis deformans of other bones

Excludes2: osteitis deformans of skull (M88.0)

osteitis deformans of vertebrae (M88.1)

M88.89 Osteitis deformans of multiple sites

M88.9 Osteitis deformans of unspecified bone

M89 Other disorders of bone

M89.0 Algoneurodystrophy

Shoulder-hand syndrome

Sudeck's atrophy

Excludes1: causalgia, lower limb (G57.7-)

causalgia, upper limb (G56.4-)

complex regional pain syndrome II, lower limb (G57.7-)

complex regional pain syndrome II, upper limb (G56.4-)

reflex sympathetic dystrophy (G90.5-)

M89.00 Algoneurodystrophy, unspecified site

M89.01 Algoneurodystrophy, shoulder

M89.011 Algoneurodystrophy, right shoulder

M89.012 Algoneurodystrophy, left shoulder

M89.019 Algoneurodystrophy, unspecified shoulder

M89.02 Algoneurodystrophy, upper arm

M89.021 Algoneurodystrophy, right upper arm

M89.022 Algoneurodystrophy, left upper arm

M89.029 Algoneurodystrophy, unspecified upper arm

M89.03 Algoneurodystrophy, forearm

M89.031 Algoneurodystrophy, right forearm

M89.032 Algoneurodystrophy, left forearm

M89.039 Algoneurodystrophy, unspecified forearm

M89.04 Algoneurodystrophy, hand

M89.041 Algoneurodystrophy, right hand

M89.042 Algoneurodystrophy, left hand

M89.049 Algoneurodystrophy, unspecified hand

M89.05 Algoneurodystrophy, thigh

M89.051 Algoneurodystrophy, right thigh

M89.052 Algoneurodystrophy, left thigh

M89.059 Algoneurodystrophy, unspecified thigh

M89.06 Algoneurodystrophy, lower leg

M89.061 Algoneurodystrophy, right lower leg

M89.062 Algoneurodystrophy, left lower leg

M89.069 Algoneurodystrophy, unspecified lower leg

● New code   ▲ Revised code   Excludes1: Not coded here   Excludes2: Not included here   ⊗ Placeholder required   ⑦ 7th digit required

M89.07   Algoneurodystrophy, ankle and foot

     M89.071   Algoneurodystrophy, right ankle and foot

     M89.072   Algoneurodystrophy, left ankle and foot

     M89.079   Algoneurodystrophy, unspecified ankle and foot

M89.08   Algoneurodystrophy, other site

M89.09   Algoneurodystrophy, multiple sites

M89.1   Physeal arrest

Arrest of growth plate

Epiphyseal arrest

Growth plate arrest

M89.12   Physeal arrest, humerus

     M89.121   Complete physeal arrest, right proximal humerus

     M89.122   Complete physeal arrest, left proximal humerus

     M89.123   Partial physeal arrest, right proximal humerus

     M89.124   Partial physeal arrest, left proximal humerus

     M89.125   Complete physeal arrest, right distal humerus

     M89.126   Complete physeal arrest, left distal humerus

     M89.127   Partial physeal arrest, right distal humerus

     M89.128   Partial physeal arrest, left distal humerus

     M89.129   Physeal arrest, humerus, unspecified

M89.13   Physeal arrest, forearm

     M89.131   Complete physeal arrest, right distal radius

     M89.132   Complete physeal arrest, left distal radius

     M89.133   Partial physeal arrest, right distal radius

     M89.134   Partial physeal arrest, left distal radius

     M89.138   Other physeal arrest of forearm

     M89.139   Physeal arrest, forearm, unspecified

M89.15   Physeal arrest, femur

     M89.151   Complete physeal arrest, right proximal femur

     M89.152   Complete physeal arrest, left proximal femur

     M89.153   Partial physeal arrest, right proximal femur

     M89.154   Partial physeal arrest, left proximal femur

     M89.155   Complete physeal arrest, right distal femur

     M89.156   Complete physeal arrest, left distal femur

     M89.157   Partial physeal arrest, right distal femur

     M89.158   Partial physeal arrest, left distal femur

     M89.159   Physeal arrest, femur, unspecified

M89.16   Physeal arrest, lower leg

     M89.160   Complete physeal arrest, right proximal tibia

     M89.161   Complete physeal arrest, left proximal tibia

     M89.162   Partial physeal arrest, right proximal tibia

     M89.163   Partial physeal arrest, left proximal tibia

     M89.164   Complete physeal arrest, right distal tibia

     M89.165   Complete physeal arrest, left distal tibia

     M89.166   Partial physeal arrest, right distal tibia

     M89.167   Partial physeal arrest, left distal tibia

     M89.168   Other physeal arrest of lower leg

     M89.169   Physeal arrest, lower leg, unspecified

M89.18   Physeal arrest, other site

M89.2   Other disorders of bone development and growth

M89.20   Other disorders of bone development and growth, unspecified site

M89.21   Other disorders of bone development and growth, shoulder

     M89.211   Other disorders of bone development and growth, right shoulder

     M89.212   Other disorders of bone development and growth, left shoulder

     M89.219   Other disorders of bone development and growth, unspecified shoulder

M89.22   Other disorders of bone development and growth, humerus

     M89.221   Other disorders of bone development and growth, right humerus

     M89.222   Other disorders of bone development and growth, left humerus

     M89.229   Other disorders of bone development and growth, unspecified humerus

M89.23   Other disorders of bone development and growth, ulna and radius

     M89.231   Other disorders of bone development and growth, right ulna

     M89.232   Other disorders of bone development and growth, left ulna

     M89.233   Other disorders of bone development and growth, right radius

     M89.234   Other disorders of bone development and growth, left radius

     M89.239   Other disorders of bone development and growth, unspecified ulna and radius

M89.24   Other disorders of bone development and growth, hand

     M89.241   Other disorders of bone development and growth, right hand

     M89.242   Other disorders of bone development and growth, left hand

     M89.249   Other disorders of bone development and growth, unspecified hand

M89.25   Other disorders of bone development and growth, femur

     M89.251   Other disorders of bone development and growth, right femur

     M89.252   Other disorders of bone development and growth, left femur

Add 4th-7th digits	Nonspecific code	Unspecified code	Manifestation code

M89.259 Other disorders of bone development and growth, unspecified femur

M89.26 Other disorders of bone development and growth, tibia and fibula

M89.261 Other disorders of bone development and growth, right tibia

M89.262 Other disorders of bone development and growth, left tibia

M89.263 Other disorders of bone development and growth, right fibula

M89.264 Other disorders of bone development and growth, left fibula

M89.269 Other disorders of bone development and growth, unspecified lower leg

M89.27 Other disorders of bone development and growth, ankle and foot

M89.271 Other disorders of bone development and growth, right ankle and foot

M89.272 Other disorders of bone development and growth, left ankle and foot

M89.279 Other disorders of bone development and growth, unspecified ankle and foot

M89.28 Other disorders of bone development and growth, other site

M89.29 Other disorders of bone development and growth, multiple sites

M89.3 Hypertrophy of bone

M89.30 Hypertrophy of bone, unspecified site

M89.31 Hypertrophy of bone, shoulder

M89.311 Hypertrophy of bone, right shoulder

M89.312 Hypertrophy of bone, left shoulder

M89.319 Hypertrophy of bone, unspecified shoulder

M89.32 Hypertrophy of bone, humerus

M89.321 Hypertrophy of bone, right humerus

M89.322 Hypertrophy of bone, left humerus

M89.329 Hypertrophy of bone, unspecified humerus

M89.33 Hypertrophy of bone, ulna and radius

M89.331 Hypertrophy of bone, right ulna

M89.332 Hypertrophy of bone, left ulna

M89.333 Hypertrophy of bone, right radius

M89.334 Hypertrophy of bone, left radius

M89.339 Hypertrophy of bone, unspecified ulna and radius

M89.34 Hypertrophy of bone, hand

M89.341 Hypertrophy of bone, right hand

M89.342 Hypertrophy of bone, left hand

M89.349 Hypertrophy of bone, unspecified hand

M89.35 Hypertrophy of bone, femur

M89.351 Hypertrophy of bone, right femur

M89.352 Hypertrophy of bone, left femur

M89.359 Hypertrophy of bone, unspecified femur

M89.36 Hypertrophy of bone, tibia and fibula

M89.361 Hypertrophy of bone, right tibia

M89.362 Hypertrophy of bone, left tibia

M89.363 Hypertrophy of bone, right fibula

M89.364 Hypertrophy of bone, left fibula

M89.369 Hypertrophy of bone, unspecified tibia and fibula

M89.37 Hypertrophy of bone, ankle and foot

M89.371 Hypertrophy of bone, right ankle and foot

M89.372 Hypertrophy of bone, left ankle and foot

M89.379 Hypertrophy of bone, unspecified ankle and foot

M89.38 Hypertrophy of bone, other site

M89.39 Hypertrophy of bone, multiple sites

M89.4 Other hypertrophic osteoarthropathy

Marie-Bamberger disease

Pachydermoperiostosis

M89.40 Other hypertrophic osteoarthropathy, unspecified site

M89.41 Other hypertrophic osteoarthropathy, shoulder

M89.411 Other hypertrophic osteoarthropathy, right shoulder

M89.412 Other hypertrophic osteoarthropathy, left shoulder

M89.419 Other hypertrophic osteoarthropathy, unspecified shoulder

M89.42 Other hypertrophic osteoarthropathy, upper arm

M89.421 Other hypertrophic osteoarthropathy, right upper arm

M89.422 Other hypertrophic osteoarthropathy, left upper arm

M89.429 Other hypertrophic osteoarthropathy, unspecified upper arm

M89.43 Other hypertrophic osteoarthropathy, forearm

M89.431 Other hypertrophic osteoarthropathy, right forearm

M89.432 Other hypertrophic osteoarthropathy, left forearm

M89.439 Other hypertrophic osteoarthropathy, unspecified forearm

M89.44 Other hypertrophic osteoarthropathy, hand

M89.441 Other hypertrophic osteoarthropathy, right hand

M89.442 Other hypertrophic osteoarthropathy, left hand

M89.449 Other hypertrophic osteoarthropathy, unspecified hand

M89.45 Other hypertrophic osteoarthropathy, thigh

M89.451 Other hypertrophic osteoarthropathy, right thigh

M89.452 Other hypertrophic osteoarthropathy, left thigh

M89.459 Other hypertrophic osteoarthropathy, unspecified thigh

M89.46 Other hypertrophic osteoarthropathy, lower leg

M89.461 Other hypertrophic osteoarthropathy, right lower leg

M89.462 Other hypertrophic osteoarthropathy, left lower leg

M89.469 Other hypertrophic osteoarthropathy, unspecified lower leg

M89.47 **Other hypertrophic osteoarthropathy, ankle and foot**

M89.471 **Other hypertrophic osteoarthropathy, right ankle and foot**

M89.472 **Other hypertrophic osteoarthropathy, left ankle and foot**

M89.479 **Other hypertrophic osteoarthropathy, unspecified ankle and foot**

M89.48 **Other hypertrophic osteoarthropathy, other site**

M89.49 **Other hypertrophic osteoarthropathy, multiple sites**

M89.5 **Osteolysis**

Use additional code to identify major osseous defect, if applicable (M89.7-)

Excludes2: periprosthetic osteolysis of internal prosthetic joint (T84.05-)

M89.50 **Osteolysis, unspecified site**

M89.51 **Osteolysis, shoulder**

M89.511 **Osteolysis, right shoulder**

M89.512 **Osteolysis, left shoulder**

M89.519 **Osteolysis, unspecified shoulder**

M89.52 **Osteolysis, upper arm**

M89.521 **Osteolysis, right upper arm**

M89.522 **Osteolysis, left upper arm**

M89.529 **Osteolysis, unspecified upper arm**

M89.53 **Osteolysis, forearm**

M89.531 **Osteolysis, right forearm**

M89.532 **Osteolysis, left forearm**

M89.539 **Osteolysis, unspecified forearm**

M89.54 **Osteolysis, hand**

M89.541 **Osteolysis, right hand**

M89.542 **Osteolysis, left hand**

M89.549 **Osteolysis, unspecified hand**

M89.55 **Osteolysis, thigh**

M89.551 **Osteolysis, right thigh**

M89.552 **Osteolysis, left thigh**

M89.559 **Osteolysis, unspecified thigh**

M89.56 **Osteolysis, lower leg**

M89.561 **Osteolysis, right lower leg**

M89.562 **Osteolysis, left lower leg**

M89.569 **Osteolysis, unspecified lower leg**

M89.57 **Osteolysis, ankle and foot**

M89.571 **Osteolysis, right ankle and foot**

M89.572 **Osteolysis, left ankle and foot**

M89.579 **Osteolysis, unspecified ankle and foot**

M89.58 **Osteolysis, other site**

M89.59 **Osteolysis, multiple sites**

M89.6 **Osteopathy after poliomyelitis**

Use additional code (B91) to identify previous poliomyelitis

Excludes1: postpolio syndrome (G14)

M89.60 **Osteopathy after poliomyelitis, unspecified site**

M89.61 **Osteopathy after poliomyelitis, shoulder**

M89.611 **Osteopathy after poliomyelitis, right shoulder**

M89.612 **Osteopathy after poliomyelitis, left shoulder**

M89.619 **Osteopathy after poliomyelitis, unspecified shoulder**

M89.62 **Osteopathy after poliomyelitis, upper arm**

M89.621 **Osteopathy after poliomyelitis, right upper arm**

M89.622 **Osteopathy after poliomyelitis, left upper arm**

M89.629 **Osteopathy after poliomyelitis, unspecified upper arm**

M89.63 **Osteopathy after poliomyelitis, forearm**

M89.631 **Osteopathy after poliomyelitis, right forearm**

M89.632 **Osteopathy after poliomyelitis, left forearm**

M89.639 **Osteopathy after poliomyelitis, unspecified forearm**

M89.64 **Osteopathy after poliomyelitis, hand**

M89.641 **Osteopathy after poliomyelitis, right hand**

M89.642 **Osteopathy after poliomyelitis, left hand**

M89.649 **Osteopathy after poliomyelitis, unspecified hand**

M89.65 **Osteopathy after poliomyelitis, thigh**

M89.651 **Osteopathy after poliomyelitis, right thigh**

M89.652 **Osteopathy after poliomyelitis, left thigh**

M89.659 **Osteopathy after poliomyelitis, unspecified thigh**

M89.66 **Osteopathy after poliomyelitis, lower leg**

M89.661 **Osteopathy after poliomyelitis, right lower leg**

M89.662 **Osteopathy after poliomyelitis, left lower leg**

M89.669 **Osteopathy after poliomyelitis, unspecified lower leg**

M89.67 **Osteopathy after poliomyelitis, ankle and foot**

M89.671 **Osteopathy after poliomyelitis, right ankle and foot**

M89.672 **Osteopathy after poliomyelitis, left ankle and foot**

M89.679 **Osteopathy after poliomyelitis, unspecified ankle and foot**

M89.68 **Osteopathy after poliomyelitis, other site**

M89.69 **Osteopathy after poliomyelitis, multiple sites**

M89.7 **Major osseous defect**

Code first underlying disease, if known, such as:

aseptic necrosis of bone (M87.-)

malignant neoplasm of bone (C40.-)

osteolysis (M89.5)

osteomyelitis (M86.-)

osteonecrosis (M87.-)

osteoporosis (M80.-, M81.-)

periprosthetic osteolysis (T84.05-)

M89.70 **Major osseous defect, unspecified site**

M89.71 **Major osseous defect, shoulder region**

Major osseous defect clavicle or scapula

M89.711 **Major osseous defect, right shoulder region**

M89.712 **Major osseous defect, left shoulder region**

M89.719 Major osseous defect, unspecified shoulder region

M89.72 Major osseous defect, humerus

M89.721 Major osseous defect, right humerus

M89.722 Major osseous defect, left humerus

M89.729 Major osseous defect, unspecified humerus

M89.73 Major osseous defect, forearm

Major osseous defect of radius and ulna

M89.731 Major osseous defect, right forearm

M89.732 Major osseous defect, left forearm

M89.739 Major osseous defect, unspecified forearm

M89.74 Major osseous defect, hand

Major osseous defect of carpus, fingers, metacarpus

M89.741 Major osseous defect, right hand

M89.742 Major osseous defect, left hand

M89.749 Major osseous defect, unspecified hand

M89.75 Major osseous defect, pelvic region and thigh

Major osseous defect of femur and pelvis

M89.751 Major osseous defect, right pelvic region and thigh

M89.752 Major osseous defect, left pelvic region and thigh

M89.759 Major osseous defect, unspecified pelvic region and thigh

M89.76 Major osseous defect, lower leg

Major osseous defect of fibula and tibia

M89.761 Major osseous defect, right lower leg

M89.762 Major osseous defect, left lower leg

M89.769 Major osseous defect, unspecified lower leg

M89.77 Major osseous defect, ankle and foot

Major osseous defect of metatarsus, tarsus, toes

M89.771 Major osseous defect, right ankle and foot

M89.772 Major osseous defect, left ankle and foot

M89.779 Major osseous defect, unspecified ankle and foot

M89.78 Major osseous defect, other site

M89.79 Major osseous defect, multiple sites

M89.8 Other specified disorders of bone

Infantile cortical hyperostoses

Post-traumatic subperiosteal ossification

M89.8X Other specified disorders of bone

M89.8X0 Other specified disorders of bone, multiple sites

M89.8X1 Other specified disorders of bone, shoulder

M89.8X2 Other specified disorders of bone, upper arm

M89.8X3 Other specified disorders of bone, forearm

M89.8X4 Other specified disorders of bone, hand

M89.8X5 Other specified disorders of bone, thigh

M89.8X6 Other specified disorders of bone, lower leg

M89.8X7 Other specified disorders of bone, ankle and foot

M89.8X8 Other specified disorders of bone, other site

M89.8X9 Other specified disorders of bone, unspecified site

M89.9 Disorder of bone, unspecified

M90 Osteopathies in diseases classified elsewhere

Excludes1: osteochondritis, osteomyelitis, and osteopathy (in):

cryptococcosis (B45.3)

diabetes mellitus (E08-E13 with .69-)

gonococcal (A54.43)

neurogenic syphilis (A52.11)

renal osteodystrophy (N25.0)

salmonellosis (A02.24)

secondary syphilis (A51.46)

syphilis (late) (A52.77)

M90.5 Osteonecrosis in diseases classified elsewhere

Code first underlying disease, such as:

caisson disease (T70.3)

hemoglobinopathy (D50-D64)

M90.50 Osteonecrosis in diseases classified elsewhere, unspecified site

M90.51 Osteonecrosis in diseases classified elsewhere, shoulder

M90.511 Osteonecrosis in diseases classified elsewhere, right shoulder

M90.512 Osteonecrosis in diseases classified elsewhere, left shoulder

M90.519 Osteonecrosis in diseases classified elsewhere, unspecified shoulder

M90.52 Osteonecrosis in diseases classified elsewhere, upper arm

M90.521 Osteonecrosis in diseases classified elsewhere, right upper arm

M90.522 Osteonecrosis in diseases classified elsewhere, left upper arm

M90.529 Osteonecrosis in diseases classified elsewhere, unspecified upper arm

M90.53 Osteonecrosis in diseases classified elsewhere, forearm

M90.531 Osteonecrosis in diseases classified elsewhere, right forearm

M90.532 Osteonecrosis in diseases classified elsewhere, left forearm

M90.539 Osteonecrosis in diseases classified elsewhere, unspecified forearm

M90.54 Osteonecrosis in diseases classified elsewhere, hand

M90.541 Osteonecrosis in diseases classified elsewhere, right hand

M90.542 Osteonecrosis in diseases classified elsewhere, left hand

M90.549 Osteonecrosis in diseases classified elsewhere, unspecified hand

M90.55 Osteonecrosis in diseases classified elsewhere, thigh

M90.551 Osteonecrosis in diseases classified elsewhere, right thigh

● New code   ▲ Revised code   **Excludes1:** Not coded here   **Excludes2:** Not included here   ⊗ Placeholder required   ⑦ 7th digit required

M90.552   Osteonecrosis in diseases classified elsewhere, left thigh

M90.559   Osteonecrosis in diseases classified elsewhere, unspecified thigh

M90.56   Osteonecrosis in diseases classified elsewhere, lower leg

M90.561   Osteonecrosis in diseases classified elsewhere, right lower leg

M90.562   Osteonecrosis in diseases classified elsewhere, left lower leg

M90.569   Osteonecrosis in diseases classified elsewhere, unspecified lower leg

M90.57   Osteonecrosis in diseases classified elsewhere, ankle and foot

M90.571   Osteonecrosis in diseases classified elsewhere, right ankle and foot

M90.572   Osteonecrosis in diseases classified elsewhere, left ankle and foot

M90.579   Osteonecrosis in diseases classified elsewhere, unspecified ankle and foot

M90.58   Osteonecrosis in diseases classified elsewhere, other site

M90.59   Osteonecrosis in diseases classified elsewhere, multiple sites

M90.6   **Osteitis deformans in neoplastic diseases**

Osteitis deformans in malignant neoplasm of bone

Code first the neoplasm (C40.-, C41.-)

Excludes1: osteitis deformans [Paget's disease of bone] (M88.-)

M90.60   Osteitis deformans in neoplastic diseases, unspecified site

M90.61   Osteitis deformans in neoplastic diseases, shoulder

M90.611   Osteitis deformans in neoplastic diseases, right shoulder

M90.612   Osteitis deformans in neoplastic diseases, left shoulder

M90.619   Osteitis deformans in neoplastic diseases, unspecified shoulder

M90.62   Osteitis deformans in neoplastic diseases, upper arm

M90.621   Osteitis deformans in neoplastic diseases, right upper arm

M90.622   Osteitis deformans in neoplastic diseases, left upper arm

M90.629   Osteitis deformans in neoplastic diseases, unspecified upper arm

M90.63   Osteitis deformans in neoplastic diseases, forearm

M90.631   Osteitis deformans in neoplastic diseases, right forearm

M90.632   Osteitis deformans in neoplastic diseases, left forearm

M90.639   Osteitis deformans in neoplastic diseases, unspecified forearm

M90.64   Osteitis deformans in neoplastic diseases, hand

M90.641   Osteitis deformans in neoplastic diseases, right hand

M90.642   Osteitis deformans in neoplastic diseases, left hand

M90.649   Osteitis deformans in neoplastic diseases, unspecified hand

M90.65   Osteitis deformans in neoplastic diseases, thigh

M90.651   Osteitis deformans in neoplastic diseases, right thigh

M90.652   Osteitis deformans in neoplastic diseases, left thigh

M90.659   Osteitis deformans in neoplastic diseases, unspecified thigh

M90.66   Osteitis deformans in neoplastic diseases, lower leg

M90.661   Osteitis deformans in neoplastic diseases, right lower leg

M90.662   Osteitis deformans in neoplastic diseases, left lower leg

M90.669   Osteitis deformans in neoplastic diseases, unspecified lower leg

M90.67   Osteitis deformans in neoplastic diseases, ankle and foot

M90.671   Osteitis deformans in neoplastic diseases, right ankle and foot

M90.672   Osteitis deformans in neoplastic diseases, left ankle and foot

M90.679   Osteitis deformans in neoplastic diseases, unspecified ankle and foot

M90.68   Osteitis deformans in neoplastic diseases, other site

M90.69   Osteitis deformans in neoplastic diseases, multiple sites

M90.8   **Osteopathy in diseases classified elsewhere**

Code first underlying disease, such as:

rickets (E55.0)

vitamin-D-resistant rickets (E83.3)

M90.80   Osteopathy in diseases classified elsewhere, unspecified site

M90.81   Osteopathy in diseases classified elsewhere, shoulder

M90.811   Osteopathy in diseases classified elsewhere, right shoulder

M90.812   Osteopathy in diseases classified elsewhere, left shoulder

M90.819   Osteopathy in diseases classified elsewhere, unspecified shoulder

M90.82   Osteopathy in diseases classified elsewhere, upper arm

M90.821   Osteopathy in diseases classified elsewhere, right upper arm

M90.822   Osteopathy in diseases classified elsewhere, left upper arm

M90.829   Osteopathy in diseases classified elsewhere, unspecified upper arm

M90.83   Osteopathy in diseases classified elsewhere, forearm

M90.831   Osteopathy in diseases classified elsewhere, right forearm

M90.832   Osteopathy in diseases classified elsewhere, left forearm

M90.839   Osteopathy in diseases classified elsewhere, unspecified forearm

M90.84   Osteopathy in diseases classified elsewhere, hand

M90.841   Osteopathy in diseases classified elsewhere, right hand

M90.842   Osteopathy in diseases classified elsewhere, left hand

M90.849   Osteopathy in diseases classified elsewhere, unspecified hand

| Add 4th-7th digits | Nonspecific code | Unspecified code | Manifestation code | 591 |

M90.85 **Osteopathy in diseases classified elsewhere, thigh**

    M90.851 **Osteopathy in diseases classified elsewhere, right thigh**

    M90.852 **Osteopathy in diseases classified elsewhere, left thigh**

    M90.859 **Osteopathy in diseases classified elsewhere, unspecified thigh**

M90.86 **Osteopathy in diseases classified elsewhere, lower leg**

    M90.861 **Osteopathy in diseases classified elsewhere, right lower leg**

    M90.862 **Osteopathy in diseases classified elsewhere, left lower leg**

    M90.869 **Osteopathy in diseases classified elsewhere, unspecified lower leg**

M90.87 **Osteopathy in diseases classified elsewhere, ankle and foot**

    M90.871 **Osteopathy in diseases classified elsewhere, right ankle and foot**

    M90.872 **Osteopathy in diseases classified elsewhere, left ankle and foot**

    M90.879 **Osteopathy in diseases classified elsewhere, unspecified ankle and foot**

M90.88 **Osteopathy in diseases classified elsewhere, other site**

M90.89 **Osteopathy in diseases classified elsewhere, multiple sites**

CHONDROPATHIES (M91-M94)

Excludes1: postprocedural chondropathies (M96.-)

M91 Juvenile osteochondrosis of hip and pelvis

    Excludes1: slipped upper femoral epiphysis (nontraumatic) (M93.0)

M91.0 **Juvenile osteochondrosis of pelvis**

    Osteochondrosis (juvenile) of acetabulum

    Osteochondrosis (juvenile) of iliac crest [Buchanan]

    Osteochondrosis (juvenile) of ischiopubic synchondrosis [van Neck]

    Osteochondrosis (juvenile) of symphysis pubis [Pierson]

M91.1 **Juvenile osteochondrosis of head of femur [Legg-Calvé-Perthes]**

    M91.10 **Juvenile osteochondrosis of head of femur [Legg-Calvé-Perthes], unspecified leg**

    M91.11 **Juvenile osteochondrosis of head of femur [Legg-Calvé-Perthes], right leg**

    M91.12 **Juvenile osteochondrosis of head of femur [Legg-Calvé-Perthes], left leg**

M91.2 **Coxa plana**

    Hip deformity due to previous juvenile osteochondrosis

    M91.20 **Coxa plana, unspecified hip**

    M91.21 **Coxa plana, right hip**

    M91.22 **Coxa plana, left hip**

M91.3 **Pseudocoxalgia**

    M91.30 **Pseudocoxalgia, unspecified hip**

    M91.31 **Pseudocoxalgia, right hip**

    M91.32 **Pseudocoxalgia, left hip**

M91.4 **Coxa magna**

    M91.40 **Coxa magna, unspecified hip**

    M91.41 **Coxa magna, right hip**

    M91.42 **Coxa magna, left hip**

M91.8 **Other juvenile osteochondrosis of hip and pelvis**

    Juvenile osteochondrosis after reduction of congenital dislocation of hip

    M91.80 **Other juvenile osteochondrosis of hip and pelvis, unspecified leg**

    M91.81 **Other juvenile osteochondrosis of hip and pelvis, right leg**

    M91.82 **Other juvenile osteochondrosis of hip and pelvis, left leg**

M91.9 **Juvenile osteochondrosis of hip and pelvis, unspecified**

    M91.90 **Juvenile osteochondrosis of hip and pelvis, unspecified, unspecified leg**

    M91.91 **Juvenile osteochondrosis of hip and pelvis, unspecified, right leg**

    M91.92 **Juvenile osteochondrosis of hip and pelvis, unspecified, left leg**

M92 Other juvenile osteochondrosis

M92.0 **Juvenile osteochondrosis of humerus**

    Osteochondrosis (juvenile) of capitulum of humerus [Panner]

    Osteochondrosis (juvenile) of head of humerus [Haas]

    M92.00 **Juvenile osteochondrosis of humerus, unspecified arm**

    M92.01 **Juvenile osteochondrosis of humerus, right arm**

    M92.02 **Juvenile osteochondrosis of humerus, left arm**

M92.1 **Juvenile osteochondrosis of radius and ulna**

    Osteochondrosis (juvenile) of lower ulna [Burns]

    Osteochondrosis (juvenile) of radial head [Brailsford]

    M92.10 **Juvenile osteochondrosis of radius and ulna, unspecified arm**

    M92.11 **Juvenile osteochondrosis of radius and ulna, right arm**

    M92.12 **Juvenile osteochondrosis of radius and ulna, left arm**

M92.2 **Juvenile osteochondrosis, hand**

    M92.20 **Unspecified juvenile osteochondrosis, hand**

        M92.201 **Unspecified juvenile osteochondrosis, right hand**

        M92.202 **Unspecified juvenile osteochondrosis, left hand**

        M92.209 **Unspecified juvenile osteochondrosis, unspecified hand**

    M92.21 **Osteochondrosis (juvenile) of carpal lunate [Kienböck]**

        M92.211 **Osteochondrosis (juvenile) of carpal lunate [Kienböck], right hand**

        M92.212 **Osteochondrosis (juvenile) of carpal lunate [Kienböck], left hand**

        M92.219 **Osteochondrosis (juvenile) of carpal lunate [Kienböck], unspecified hand**

    M92.22 **Osteochondrosis (juvenile) of metacarpal heads [Mauclaire]**

        M92.221 **Osteochondrosis (juvenile) of metacarpal heads [Mauclaire], right hand**

        M92.222 **Osteochondrosis (juvenile) of metacarpal heads [Mauclaire], left hand**

        M92.229 **Osteochondrosis (juvenile) of metacarpal heads [Mauclaire], unspecified hand**

    M92.29 **Other juvenile osteochondrosis, hand**

        M92.291 **Other juvenile osteochondrosis, right hand**

M92.292 Other juvenile osteochondrosis, left hand

M92.299 Other juvenile osteochondrosis, unspecified hand

M92.3 Other juvenile osteochondrosis, upper limb

M92.30 Other juvenile osteochondrosis, unspecified upper limb

M92.31 Other juvenile osteochondrosis, right upper limb

M92.32 Other juvenile osteochondrosis, left upper limb

M92.4 Juvenile osteochondrosis of patella

Osteochondrosis (juvenile) of primary patellar center [Köhler]

Osteochondrosis (juvenile) of secondary patellar centre [Sinding Larsen]

M92.40 Juvenile osteochondrosis of patella, unspecified knee

M92.41 Juvenile osteochondrosis of patella, right knee

M92.42 Juvenile osteochondrosis of patella, left knee

M92.5 Juvenile osteochondrosis of tibia and fibula

Osteochondrosis (juvenile) of proximal tibia [Blount]

Osteochondrosis (juvenile) of tibial tubercle [Osgood-Schlatter]

Tibia vara

M92.50 Juvenile osteochondrosis of tibia and fibula, unspecified leg

M92.51 Juvenile osteochondrosis of tibia and fibula, right leg

M92.52 Juvenile osteochondrosis of tibia and fibula, left leg

M92.6 Juvenile osteochondrosis of tarsus

Osteochondrosis (juvenile) of calcaneum [Sever]

Osteochondrosis (juvenile) of os tibiale externum [Haglund]

Osteochondrosis (juvenile) of talus [Diaz]

Osteochondrosis (juvenile) of tarsal navicular [Köhler]

M92.60 Juvenile osteochondrosis of tarsus, unspecified ankle

M92.61 Juvenile osteochondrosis of tarsus, right ankle

M92.62 Juvenile osteochondrosis of tarsus, left ankle

M92.7 Juvenile osteochondrosis of metatarsus

Osteochondrosis (juvenile) of fifth metatarsus [Iselin]

Osteochondrosis (juvenile) of second metatarsus [Freiberg]

M92.70 Juvenile osteochondrosis of metatarsus, unspecified foot

M92.71 Juvenile osteochondrosis of metatarsus, right foot

M92.72 Juvenile osteochondrosis of metatarsus, left foot

M92.8 Other specified juvenile osteochondrosis

Calcaneal apophysitis

M92.9 Juvenile osteochondrosis, unspecified

Juvenile apophysitis NOS

Juvenile epiphysitis NOS

Juvenile osteochondritis NOS

Juvenile osteochondrosis NOS

M93 Other osteochondropathies

Excludes2: osteochondrosis of spine (M42.-)

M93.0 Slipped upper femoral epiphysis (nontraumatic)

Use additional code for associated chondrolysis (M94.3)

M93.00 Unspecified slipped upper femoral epiphysis (nontraumatic)

M93.001 Unspecified slipped upper femoral epiphysis (nontraumatic), right hip

M93.002 Unspecified slipped upper femoral epiphysis (nontraumatic), left hip

M93.003 Unspecified slipped upper femoral epiphysis (nontraumatic), unspecified hip

M93.01 Acute slipped upper femoral epiphysis (nontraumatic)

M93.011 Acute slipped upper femoral epiphysis (nontraumatic), right hip

M93.012 Acute slipped upper femoral epiphysis (nontraumatic), left hip

M93.013 Acute slipped upper femoral epiphysis (nontraumatic), unspecified hip

M93.02 Chronic slipped upper femoral epiphysis (nontraumatic)

M93.021 Chronic slipped upper femoral epiphysis (nontraumatic), right hip

M93.022 Chronic slipped upper femoral epiphysis (nontraumatic), left hip

M93.023 Chronic slipped upper femoral epiphysis (nontraumatic), unspecified hip

M93.03 Acute on chronic slipped upper femoral epiphysis (nontraumatic)

M93.031 Acute on chronic slipped upper femoral epiphysis (nontraumatic), right hip

M93.032 Acute on chronic slipped upper femoral epiphysis (nontraumatic), left hip

M93.033 Acute on chronic slipped upper femoral epiphysis (nontraumatic), unspecified hip

M93.1 Kienböck's disease of adults

Adult osteochondrosis of carpal lunates

M93.2 Osteochondritis dissecans

M93.20 Osteochondritis dissecans of unspecified site

M93.21 Osteochondritis dissecans of shoulder

M93.211 Osteochondritis dissecans, right shoulder

M93.212 Osteochondritis dissecans, left shoulder

M93.219 Osteochondritis dissecans, unspecified shoulder

M93.22 Osteochondritis dissecans of elbow

M93.221 Osteochondritis dissecans, right elbow

M93.222 Osteochondritis dissecans, left elbow

M93.229 Osteochondritis dissecans, unspecified elbow

M93.23 Osteochondritis dissecans of wrist

M93.231 Osteochondritis dissecans, right wrist

M93.232 Osteochondritis dissecans, left wrist

M93.239 Osteochondritis dissecans, unspecified wrist

M93.24 Osteochondritis dissecans of joints of hand

M93.241 Osteochondritis dissecans, joints of right hand

M93.242 Osteochondritis dissecans, joints of left hand

M93.249 Osteochondritis dissecans, joints of unspecified hand

M93.25 Osteochondritis dissecans of hip

M93.251 Osteochondritis dissecans, right hip

M93.252 Osteochondritis dissecans, left hip

M93.259 Osteochondritis dissecans, unspecified hip

M93.26 Osteochondritis dissecans knee

M93.261 Osteochondritis dissecans, right knee

M93.262 Osteochondritis dissecans, left knee

M93.269 Osteochondritis dissecans, unspecified knee

M93.27 Osteochondritis dissecans of ankle and joints of foot

M93.271 Osteochondritis dissecans, right ankle and joints of right foot

M93.272 Osteochondritis dissecans, left ankle and joints of left foot

M93.279 Osteochondritis dissecans, unspecified ankle and joints of foot

M93.28 Osteochondritis dissecans other site

M93.29 Osteochondritis dissecans multiple sites

M93.8 Other specified osteochondropathies

M93.80 Other specified osteochondropathies of unspecified site

M93.81 Other specified osteochondropathies of shoulder

M93.811 Other specified osteochondropathies, right shoulder

M93.812 Other specified osteochondropathies, left shoulder

M93.819 Other specified osteochondropathies, unspecified shoulder

M93.82 Other specified osteochondropathies of upper arm

M93.821 Other specified osteochondropathies, right upper arm

M93.822 Other specified osteochondropathies, left upper arm

M93.829 Other specified osteochondropathies, unspecified upper arm

M93.83 Other specified osteochondropathies of forearm

M93.831 Other specified osteochondropathies, right forearm

M93.832 Other specified osteochondropathies, left forearm

M93.839 Other specified osteochondropathies, unspecified forearm

M93.84 Other specified osteochondropathies of hand

M93.841 Other specified osteochondropathies, right hand

M93.842 Other specified osteochondropathies, left hand

M93.849 Other specified osteochondropathies, unspecified hand

M93.85 Other specified osteochondropathies of thigh

M93.851 Other specified osteochondropathies, right thigh

M93.852 Other specified osteochondropathies, left thigh

M93.859 Other specified osteochondropathies, unspecified thigh

M93.86 Other specified osteochondropathies lower leg

M93.861 Other specified osteochondropathies, right lower leg

M93.862 Other specified osteochondropathies, left lower leg

M93.869 Other specified osteochondropathies, unspecified lower leg

M93.87 Other specified osteochondropathies of ankle and foot

M93.871 Other specified osteochondropathies, right ankle and foot

M93.872 Other specified osteochondropathies, left ankle and foot

M93.879 Other specified osteochondropathies, unspecified ankle and foot

M93.88 Other specified osteochondropathies other

M93.89 Other specified osteochondropathies multiple sites

M93.9 Osteochondropathy, unspecified

Apophysitis NOS

Epiphysitis NOS

Osteochondritis NOS

Osteochondrosis NOS

M93.90 Osteochondropathy, unspecified of unspecified site

M93.91 Osteochondropathy, unspecified of shoulder

M93.911 Osteochondropathy, unspecified, right shoulder

M93.912 Osteochondropathy, unspecified, left shoulder

M93.919 Osteochondropathy, unspecified, unspecified shoulder

M93.92 Osteochondropathy, unspecified of upper arm

M93.921 Osteochondropathy, unspecified, right upper arm

M93.922 Osteochondropathy, unspecified, left upper arm

M93.929 Osteochondropathy, unspecified, unspecified upper arm

M93.93 Osteochondropathy, unspecified of forearm

M93.931 Osteochondropathy, unspecified, right forearm

M93.932 Osteochondropathy, unspecified, left forearm

M93.939 Osteochondropathy, unspecified, unspecified forearm

M93.94 Osteochondropathy, unspecified of hand

M93.941 Osteochondropathy, unspecified, right hand

M93.942 Osteochondropathy, unspecified, left hand

M93.949 Osteochondropathy, unspecified, unspecified hand

M93.95 Osteochondropathy, unspecified of thigh

M93.951 Osteochondropathy, unspecified, right thigh

M93.952 Osteochondropathy, unspecified, left thigh

M93.959 Osteochondropathy, unspecified, unspecified thigh

M93.96 Osteochondropathy, unspecified lower leg

● New code ▲ Revised code **Excludes1:** Not coded here **Excludes2:** Not included here ⊗ Placeholder required ⑦7th digit required

M93.961 Osteochondropathy, unspecified, right lower leg

M93.962 Osteochondropathy, unspecified, left lower leg

M93.969 Osteochondropathy, unspecified, unspecified lower leg

M93.97 Osteochondropathy, unspecified of ankle and foot

M93.971 Osteochondropathy, unspecified, right ankle and foot

M93.972 Osteochondropathy, unspecified, left ankle and foot

M93.979 Osteochondropathy, unspecified, unspecified ankle and foot

M93.98 Osteochondropathy, unspecified other

M93.99 Osteochondropathy, unspecified multiple sites

M94 **Other disorders of cartilage**

M94.0 **Chondrocostal junction syndrome [Tietze]**
Costochondritis

M94.1 **Relapsing polychondritis**

M94.2 **Chondromalacia**

Excludes1: chondromalacia patellae (M22.4)

M94.20 Chondromalacia, unspecified site

M94.21 Chondromalacia, shoulder

M94.211 Chondromalacia, right shoulder

M94.212 Chondromalacia, left shoulder

M94.219 Chondromalacia, unspecified shoulder

M94.22 Chondromalacia, elbow

M94.221 Chondromalacia, right elbow

M94.222 Chondromalacia, left elbow

M94.229 Chondromalacia, unspecified elbow

M94.23 Chondromalacia, wrist

M94.231 Chondromalacia, right wrist

M94.232 Chondromalacia, left wrist

M94.239 Chondromalacia, unspecified wrist

M94.24 Chondromalacia, joints of hand

M94.241 Chondromalacia, joints of right hand

M94.242 Chondromalacia, joints of left hand

M94.249 Chondromalacia, joints of unspecified hand

M94.25 Chondromalacia, hip

M94.251 Chondromalacia, right hip

M94.252 Chondromalacia, left hip

M94.259 Chondromalacia, unspecified hip

M94.26 Chondromalacia, knee

M94.261 Chondromalacia, right knee

M94.262 Chondromalacia, left knee

M94.269 Chondromalacia, unspecified knee

M94.27 Chondromalacia, ankle and joints of foot

M94.271 Chondromalacia, right ankle and joints of right foot

M94.272 Chondromalacia, left ankle and joints of left foot

M94.279 Chondromalacia, unspecified ankle and joints of foot

M94.28 Chondromalacia, other site

M94.29 Chondromalacia, multiple sites

M94.3 **Chondrolysis**

Code first any associated slipped upper femoral epiphysis (nontraumatic) (M93.0-)

M94.35 Chondrolysis, hip

M94.351 Chondrolysis, right hip

M94.352 Chondrolysis, left hip

M94.359 Chondrolysis, unspecified hip

M94.8 **Other specified disorders of cartilage**

M94.8X Other specified disorders of cartilage

M94.8X0 Other specified disorders of cartilage, multiple sites

M94.8X1 Other specified disorders of cartilage, shoulder

M94.8X2 Other specified disorders of cartilage, upper arm

M94.8X3 Other specified disorders of cartilage, forearm

M94.8X4 Other specified disorders of cartilage, hand

M94.8X5 Other specified disorders of cartilage, thigh

M94.8X6 Other specified disorders of cartilage, lower leg

M94.8X7 Other specified disorders of cartilage, ankle and foot

M94.8X8 Other specified disorders of cartilage, other site

M94.8X9 Other specified disorders of cartilage, unspecified sites

M94.9 **Disorder of cartilage, unspecified**

OTHER DISORDERS OF THE MUSCULOSKELETAL SYSTEM AND CONNECTIVE TISSUE (M95)

M95 **Other acquired deformities of musculoskeletal system and connective tissue**

Excludes2: acquired absence of limbs and organs (Z89-Z90)

acquired deformities of limbs (M20-M21)

congenital malformations and deformations of the musculoskeletal system (Q65-Q79)

deforming dorsopathies (M40-M43)

dentofacial anomalies [including malocclusion] (M26.-)

postprocedural musculoskeletal disorders (M96.-)

M95.0 **Acquired deformity of nose**

Excludes2: deviated nasal septum (J34.2)

M95.1 **Cauliflower ear**

Excludes2: Other acquired deformities of ear (H61.1)

M95.10 Cauliflower ear, unspecified ear

M95.11 Cauliflower ear, right ear

M95.12 Cauliflower ear, left ear

M95.2 **Other acquired deformity of head**

M95.3 **Acquired deformity of neck**

M95.4 **Acquired deformity of chest and rib**

M95.5 **Acquired deformity of pelvis**

Excludes1: maternal care for known or suspected disproportion (O33.-)

M95.8 **Other specified acquired deformities of musculoskeletal system**

M95.9 **Acquired deformity of musculoskeletal system, unspecified**

INTRAOPERATIVE AND POSTPROCEDURAL COMPLICATIONS AND DISORDERS OF MUSCULOSKELETAL SYSTEM, NOT ELSEWHERE CLASSIFIED (M96)

M96 **Intraoperative and postprocedural complications and disorders of musculoskeletal system, not elsewhere classified**

> **Excludes2:** arthropathy following intestinal bypass (M02.0-)
>
> complications of internal orthopedic prosthetic devices, implants and grafts (T84.-)
>
> disorders associated with osteoporosis (M80)
>
> periprosthetic fracture around internal prosthetic joint (M97.-)
>
> presence of functional implants **and other** devices (Z96-Z97)

M96.0 **Pseudarthrosis after fusion or arthrodesis**

M96.1 **Postlaminectomy syndrome, not elsewhere classified**

M96.2 **Postradiation kyphosis**

M96.3 **Postlaminectomy kyphosis**

M96.4 **Postsurgical lordosis**

M96.5 **Postradiation scoliosis**

M96.6 **Fracture of bone following insertion of orthopedic implant, joint prosthesis, or bone plate**

> Intraoperative fracture of bone during insertion of orthopedic implant, joint prosthesis, or bone plate
>
> **Excludes2:** complication of internal orthopedic devices, implants or grafts (T84.-)

M96.62 **Fracture of humerus following insertion of orthopedic implant, joint prosthesis, or bone plate**

M96.621 **Fracture of humerus following insertion of orthopedic implant, joint prosthesis, or bone plate, right arm**

M96.622 **Fracture of humerus following insertion of orthopedic implant, joint prosthesis, or bone plate, left arm**

M96.629 **Fracture of humerus following insertion of orthopedic implant, joint prosthesis, or bone plate, unspecified arm**

M96.63 **Fracture of radius or ulna following insertion of orthopedic implant, joint prosthesis, or bone plate**

M96.631 **Fracture of radius or ulna following insertion of orthopedic implant, joint prosthesis, or bone plate, right arm**

M96.632 **Fracture of radius or ulna following insertion of orthopedic implant, joint prosthesis, or bone plate, left arm**

M96.639 **Fracture of radius or ulna following insertion of orthopedic implant, joint prosthesis, or bone plate, unspecified arm**

M96.65 **Fracture of pelvis following insertion of orthopedic implant, joint prosthesis, or bone plate**

M96.66 **Fracture of femur following insertion of orthopedic implant, joint prosthesis, or bone plate**

M96.661 **Fracture of femur following insertion of orthopedic implant, joint prosthesis, or bone plate, right leg**

M96.662 **Fracture of femur following insertion of orthopedic implant, joint prosthesis, or bone plate, left leg**

M96.669 **Fracture of femur following insertion of orthopedic implant, joint prosthesis, or bone plate, unspecified leg**

M96.67 **Fracture of tibia or fibula following insertion of orthopedic implant, joint prosthesis, or bone plate**

M96.671 **Fracture of tibia or fibula following insertion of orthopedic implant, joint prosthesis, or bone plate, right leg**

M96.672 **Fracture of tibia or fibula following insertion of orthopedic implant, joint prosthesis, or bone plate, left leg**

M96.679 **Fracture of tibia or fibula following insertion of orthopedic implant, joint prosthesis, or bone plate, unspecified leg**

M96.69 **Fracture of other bone following insertion of orthopedic implant, joint prosthesis, or bone plate**

M96.8 **Other intraoperative and postprocedural complications and disorders of musculoskeletal system, not elsewhere classified**

M96.81 **Intraoperative hemorrhage and hematoma of a musculoskeletal structure complicating a procedure**

> **Excludes1:** intraoperative hemorrhage and hematoma of a musculoskeletal structure due to accidental puncture and laceration during a procedure (M96.82-)

M96.810 **Intraoperative hemorrhage and hematoma of a musculoskeletal structure complicating a musculoskeletal system procedure**

M96.811 **Intraoperative hemorrhage and hematoma of a musculoskeletal structure complicating other procedure**

M96.82 **Accidental puncture and laceration of a musculoskeletal structure during a procedure**

M96.820 **Accidental puncture and laceration of a musculoskeletal structure during a musculoskeletal system procedure**

M96.821 **Accidental puncture and laceration of a musculoskeletal structure during other procedure**

M96.83 **Postprocedural hemorrhage of a musculoskeletal structure following a procedure**

M96.830 **Postprocedural hemorrhage of a musculoskeletal structure following a musculoskeletal system procedure**

M96.831 **Postprocedural hemorrhage of a musculoskeletal structure following other procedure**

M96.84 **Postprocedural hematoma and seroma of a musculoskeletal structure following a procedure**

M96.840 **Postprocedural hematoma of a musculoskeletal structure following a musculoskeletal system procedure**

M96.841 **Postprocedural hematoma of a musculoskeletal structure following other procedure**

M96.842 **Postprocedural seroma of a musculoskeletal structure following a musculoskeletal system procedure**

M96.843 **Postprocedural seroma of a musculoskeletal structure following other procedure**

● New code   ▲ Revised code   **Excludes1:** Not coded here   **Excludes2:** Not included here   ⊗ Placeholder required   ⑦ 7th digit required

M96.89 **Other intraoperative and postprocedural complications and disorders of the musculoskeletal system**

Instability of joint secondary to removal of joint prosthesis

Use additional code, if applicable, to further specify disorder

PERIPROSTHETIC FRACTURE AROUND INTERNAL PROSTHETIC JOINT (M97)

M97 **Periprosthetic fracture around internal prosthetic joint**

Excludes2: fracture of bone following insertion of orthopedic implant, joint prosthesis or bone plate (M96.6-)

breakage (fracture) of prosthetic joint (T84.01-)

The appropriate 7th character is to be added to each code from category M97

A - initial encounter

D - subsequent encounter

S - sequela

M97.0 **Periprosthetic fracture around internal prosthetic hip joint**

⊗⑦**M97.01** **Periprosthetic fracture around internal prosthetic right hip joint**

⊗⑦**M97.02** **Periprosthetic fracture around internal prosthetic left hip joint**

M97.1 **Periprosthetic fracture around internal prosthetic knee joint**

⊗⑦**M97.11** **Periprosthetic fracture around internal prosthetic right knee joint**

⊗⑦**M97.12** **Periprosthetic fracture around internal prosthetic left knee joint**

M97.2 **Periprosthetic fracture around internal prosthetic ankle joint**

⊗⑦**M97.21** **Periprosthetic fracture around internal prosthetic right ankle joint**

⊗⑦**M97.22** **Periprosthetic fracture around internal prosthetic left ankle joint**

M97.3 **Periprosthetic fracture around internal prosthetic shoulder joint**

⊗⑦**M97.31** **Periprosthetic fracture around internal prosthetic right shoulder joint**

⊗⑦**M97.32** **Periprosthetic fracture around internal prosthetic left shoulder joint**

M97.4 **Periprosthetic fracture around internal prosthetic elbow joint**

⊗⑦**M97.41** **Periprosthetic fracture around internal prosthetic right elbow joint**

⊗⑦**M97.42** **Periprosthetic fracture around internal prosthetic left elbow joint**

⊗⑦**M97.8** **Periprosthetic fracture around other internal prosthetic joint**

Periprosthetic fracture around internal prosthetic finger joint

Periprosthetic fracture around internal prosthetic spinal joint

Periprosthetic fracture around internal prosthetic toe joint

Periprosthetic fracture around internal prosthetic wrist joint

Use additional code to identify the joint (Z96.6-)

⊗⑦**M97.9** **Periprosthetic fracture around unspecified internal prosthetic joint**

BIOMECHANICAL LESIONS, NOT ELSEWHERE CLASSIFIED (M99)

M99 **Biomechanical lesions, not elsewhere classified**

Note: This category should not be used if the condition can be classified elsewhere.

M99.0 **Segmental and somatic dysfunction**

M99.00 **Segmental and somatic dysfunction of head region**

M99.01 **Segmental and somatic dysfunction of cervical region**

M99.02 **Segmental and somatic dysfunction of thoracic region**

M99.03 **Segmental and somatic dysfunction of lumbar region**

M99.04 **Segmental and somatic dysfunction of sacral region**

M99.05 **Segmental and somatic dysfunction of pelvic region**

M99.06 **Segmental and somatic dysfunction of lower extremity**

M99.07 **Segmental and somatic dysfunction of upper extremity**

M99.08 **Segmental and somatic dysfunction of rib cage**

M99.09 **Segmental and somatic dysfunction of abdomen and other regions**

M99.1 **Subluxation complex (vertebral)**

M99.10 **Subluxation complex (vertebral) of head region**

M99.11 **Subluxation complex (vertebral) of cervical region**

M99.12 **Subluxation complex (vertebral) of thoracic region**

M99.13 **Subluxation complex (vertebral) of lumbar region**

M99.14 **Subluxation complex (vertebral) of sacral region**

M99.15 **Subluxation complex (vertebral) of pelvic region**

M99.16 **Subluxation complex (vertebral) of lower extremity**

M99.17 **Subluxation complex (vertebral) of upper extremity**

M99.18 **Subluxation complex (vertebral) of rib cage**

M99.19 **Subluxation complex (vertebral) of abdomen and other regions**

M99.2 **Subluxation stenosis of neural canal**

M99.20 **Subluxation stenosis of neural canal of head region**

M99.21 **Subluxation stenosis of neural canal of cervical region**

M99.22 **Subluxation stenosis of neural canal of thoracic region**

M99.23 **Subluxation stenosis of neural canal of lumbar region**

M99.24 **Subluxation stenosis of neural canal of sacral region**

M99.25 **Subluxation stenosis of neural canal of pelvic region**

M99.26 **Subluxation stenosis of neural canal of lower extremity**

M99.27 **Subluxation stenosis of neural canal of upper extremity**

M99.28 **Subluxation stenosis of neural canal of rib cage**

M99.29 **Subluxation stenosis of neural canal of abdomen and other regions**

M99.3 **Osseous stenosis of neural canal**

M99.30 **Osseous stenosis of neural canal of head region**

M99.31 **Osseous stenosis of neural canal of cervical region**

M99.32   Osseous stenosis of neural canal of thoracic region

M99.33   Osseous stenosis of neural canal of lumbar region

M99.34   Osseous stenosis of neural canal of sacral region

M99.35   Osseous stenosis of neural canal of pelvic region

M99.36   Osseous stenosis of neural canal of lower extremity

M99.37   Osseous stenosis of neural canal of upper extremity

M99.38   Osseous stenosis of neural canal of rib cage

M99.39   Osseous stenosis of neural canal of abdomen and other regions

M99.4   Connective tissue stenosis of neural canal

M99.40   Connective tissue stenosis of neural canal of head region

M99.41   Connective tissue stenosis of neural canal of cervical region

M99.42   Connective tissue stenosis of neural canal of thoracic region

M99.43   Connective tissue stenosis of neural canal of lumbar region

M99.44   Connective tissue stenosis of neural canal of sacral region

M99.45   Connective tissue stenosis of neural canal of pelvic region

M99.46   Connective tissue stenosis of neural canal of lower extremity

M99.47   Connective tissue stenosis of neural canal of upper extremity

M99.48   Connective tissue stenosis of neural canal of rib cage

M99.49   Connective tissue stenosis of neural canal of abdomen and other regions

M99.5   Intervertebral disc stenosis of neural canal

M99.50   Intervertebral disc stenosis of neural canal of head region

M99.51   Intervertebral disc stenosis of neural canal of cervical region

M99.52   Intervertebral disc stenosis of neural canal of thoracic region

M99.53   Intervertebral disc stenosis of neural canal of lumbar region

M99.54   Intervertebral disc stenosis of neural canal of sacral region

M99.55   Intervertebral disc stenosis of neural canal of pelvic region

M99.56   Intervertebral disc stenosis of neural canal of lower extremity

M99.57   Intervertebral disc stenosis of neural canal of upper extremity

M99.58   Intervertebral disc stenosis of neural canal of rib cage

M99.59   Intervertebral disc stenosis of neural canal of abdomen and other regions

M99.6   Osseous and subluxation stenosis of intervertebral foramina

M99.60   Osseous and subluxation stenosis of intervertebral foramina of head region

M99.61   Osseous and subluxation stenosis of intervertebral foramina of cervical region

M99.62   Osseous and subluxation stenosis of intervertebral foramina of thoracic region

M99.63   Osseous and subluxation stenosis of intervertebral foramina of lumbar region

M99.64   Osseous and subluxation stenosis of intervertebral foramina of sacral region

M99.65   Osseous and subluxation stenosis of intervertebral foramina of pelvic region

M99.66   Osseous and subluxation stenosis of intervertebral foramina of lower extremity

M99.67   Osseous and subluxation stenosis of intervertebral foramina of upper extremity

M99.68   Osseous and subluxation stenosis of intervertebral foramina of rib cage

M99.69   Osseous and subluxation stenosis of intervertebral foramina of abdomen and other regions

M99.7   Connective tissue and disc stenosis of intervertebral foramina

M99.70   Connective tissue and disc stenosis of intervertebral foramina of head region

M99.71   Connective tissue and disc stenosis of intervertebral foramina of cervical region

M99.72   Connective tissue and disc stenosis of intervertebral foramina of thoracic region

M99.73   Connective tissue and disc stenosis of intervertebral foramina of lumbar region

M99.74   Connective tissue and disc stenosis of intervertebral foramina of sacral region

M99.75   Connective tissue and disc stenosis of intervertebral foramina of pelvic region

M99.76   Connective tissue and disc stenosis of intervertebral foramina of lower extremity

M99.77   Connective tissue and disc stenosis of intervertebral foramina of upper extremity

M99.78   Connective tissue and disc stenosis of intervertebral foramina of rib cage

M99.79   Connective tissue and disc stenosis of intervertebral foramina of abdomen and other regions

M99.8   Other biomechanical lesions

M99.80   Other biomechanical lesions of head region

M99.81   Other biomechanical lesions of cervical region

M99.82   Other biomechanical lesions of thoracic region

M99.83   Other biomechanical lesions of lumbar region

M99.84   Other biomechanical lesions of sacral region

M99.85   Other biomechanical lesions of pelvic region

M99.86   Other biomechanical lesions of lower extremity

M99.87   Other biomechanical lesions of upper extremity

M99.88   Other biomechanical lesions of rib cage

M99.89   Other biomechanical lesions of abdomen and other regions

M99.9   Biomechanical lesion, unspecified

Chapter 14: Diseases Of The Genitourinary System (N00-N99)

DEFINITIONS

This chapter includes definitions of selected key words, terms and phrases and coding alerts for adding points to the clinical domain, and references to coding late effects where appropriate. An example from this chapter is as follows:

N03   Chronic nephritic syndrome
    Definition: Nephritic syndrome is a collection of signs associated with disorders affecting the kidneys, more specifically glomerular disorders.

MULTIPLE CODING FOR A SINGLE CONDITION

In addition to the etiology/manifestation convention that requires two codes to fully describe a single condition that affects multiple body systems, there are other single conditions that also require more than one code. "Use additional code" notes are found in the Tabular List at codes that are not part of an etiology/manifestation pair where a secondary code is useful to fully describe a condition. The sequencing rule is the same as the etiology/manifestation pair, "use additional code" indicates that a secondary code should be added.

For example, for bacterial infections that are not included in chapter 1, a secondary code from category B95, Streptococcus, Staphylococcus, and Enterococcus, as the cause of diseases classified elsewhere, or B96, Other bacterial agents as the cause of diseases classified elsewhere, may be required to identify the bacterial organism causing the infection. A "use additional code" note will normally be found at the infectious disease code, indicating a need for the organism code to be added as a secondary code.

"Code first" notes are also under certain codes that are not specifically manifestation codes but may be due to an underlying cause. When there is a "code first" note and an underlying condition is present, the underlying condition should be sequenced first.

"Code, if applicable, any causal condition first", notes indicate that this code may be assigned as a principal diagnosis when the causal condition is unknown or not applicable. If a causal condition is known, then the code for that condition should be sequenced as the principal or first-listed diagnosis.

Multiple codes may be needed for sequela, complication codes and obstetric codes to more fully describe a condition. See the specific guidelines for these conditions for further instruction.

COMBINATION CODE

A combination code is a single code used to classify: Two diagnoses, or a diagnosis with an associated secondary process (manifestation) A diagnosis with an associated complication

Combination codes are identified by referring to subterm entries in the Alphabetic Index and by reading the inclusion and exclusion notes in the Tabular List.

Assign only the combination code when that code fully identifies the diagnostic conditions involved or when the Alphabetic Index so directs. Multiple coding should not be used when the classification provides a combination code that clearly identifies all of the elements documented in the diagnosis. When the combination code lacks necessary specificity in describing the manifestation or complication, an additional code should be used as a secondary code.

SEQUELA (LATE EFFECTS)

A sequela is the residual effect (condition produced) after the acute phase of an illness or injury has terminated. There is no time limit on when a sequela code can be used. The residual may be apparent early, such as in cerebral infarction, or it may occur months or years later, such as that due to a previous injury. Coding of sequela generally requires two codes sequenced in the following order: The condition or nature of the sequela is sequenced first.

The sequela code is sequenced second.

An exception to the above guidelines are those instances where the code for the sequela is followed by a manifestation code identified in the Tabular List and title, or the sequela code has been expanded (at the fourth, fifth or sixth character levels) to include the manifestation(s). The code for the acute phase of an illness or injury that led to the sequela is never used with a code for the late effect.

CHRONIC KIDNEY DISEASE

1)   **Stages of chronic kidney disease (CKD)**

The ICD-10-CM classifies CKD based on severity. The severity of CKD is designated by stages 1-5. Stage 2, code N18.2, equates to mild CKD; stage 3, code N18.3, equates to moderate CKD; and stage 4, code N18.4, equates to severe CKD. Code N18.6, End stage renal disease (ESRD), is assigned when the provider has documented end-stage-renal disease (ESRD).

If both a stage of CKD and ESRD are documented, assign code N18.6 only.

2)   **Chronic kidney disease and kidney transplant status**

Patients who have undergone kidney transplant may still have some form of chronic kidney disease (CKD) because the kidney transplant may not fully restore kidney function. Therefore, the presence of CKD alone does not constitute a transplant complication. Assign the appropriate N18 code for the patient's stage of CKD and code Z94.0, Kidney transplant status. If a transplant complication such as failure or rejection or other transplant complication is documented, see section I.C.19.g for information on coding complications of a kidney transplant. If the documentation is unclear as to whether the patient has a complication of the transplant, query the provider.

3)   **Chronic kidney disease with other conditions**

Patients with CKD may also suffer from other serious conditions, most commonly diabetes mellitus and hypertension. The sequencing of the CKD code in relationship to codes for other contributing conditions is based on the conventions in the Tabular List.

See I.C.9. Hypertensive chronic kidney disease.
See I.C.19. Chronic kidney disease and kidney transplant complications.

● New code   ▲ Revised code   **Excludes1:** Not coded here   **Excludes2:** Not included here   ⊗ Placeholder required   ⑦7ᵗʰ digit required

Chapter 14
Diseases Of The Genitourinary System
(N00-N99)

Excludes2: certain conditions originating in the perinatal period (P04-P96)

certain infectious and parasitic diseases (A00-B99)

complications of pregnancy, childbirth and the puerperium (O00-O9A)

congenital malformations, deformations and chromosomal abnormalities (Q00-Q99)

endocrine, nutritional and metabolic diseases (E00-E88)

injury, poisoning and certain other consequences of external causes (S00-T88)

neoplasms (C00-D49)

symptoms, signs and abnormal clinical and laboratory findings, not elsewhere classified (R00-R94)

This chapter contains the following blocks: N00-N08 Glomerular diseases

N10-N16	Renal tubulo-interstitial diseases
N17-N19	Acute kidney failure and chronic kidney disease
N20-N23	Urolithiasis
N25-N29	Other disorders of kidney and ureter
N30-N39	Other diseases of the urinary system
N40-N53	Diseases of male genital organs
N60-N65	Disorders of breast
N70-N77	Inflammatory diseases of female pelvic organs
N80-N98	Noninflammatory disorders of female genital tract
N99	Intraoperative and postprocedural complications and disorders of genitourinary system, not elsewhere classified

GLOMERULAR DISEASES (N00-N08)

Definition: Glomerulonephritis is a form of nephritis with inflammation of the capillary loops in the renal glomeruli. The acute form is characterized by proteinuria, edema, hematuria, renal failure, and hypertension, sometimes preceded by tonsillitis or febrile pharyngitis.

Code also any associated kidney failure (N17-N19).

Excludes1: hypertensive chronic kidney disease (I12.-)

N00   Acute nephritic syndrome

Includes: acute glomerular disease

acute glomerulonephritis acute nephritis

Excludes1: acute tubulo-interstitial nephritis (N10)

nephritic syndrome NOS (N05.-)

N00.0   Acute nephritic syndrome with minor glomerular abnormality

Acute nephritic syndrome with minimal change lesion

N00.1   Acute nephritic syndrome with focal and segmental glomerular lesions

Acute nephritic syndrome with focal and segmental hyalinosis

Acute nephritic syndrome with focal and segmental sclerosis

Acute nephritic syndrome with focal glomerulonephritis

N00.2   Acute nephritic syndrome with diffuse membranous glomerulonephritis

N00.3   Acute nephritic syndrome with diffuse mesangial proliferative glomerulonephritis

N00.4   Acute nephritic syndrome with diffuse endocapillary proliferative glomerulonephritis

N00.5   Acute nephritic syndrome with diffuse mesangiocapillary glomerulonephritis

Acute nephritic syndrome with membranoproliferative glomerulonephritis, types 1 and 3, or NOS

N00.6   Acute nephritic syndrome with dense deposit disease

Acute nephritic syndrome with membranoproliferative glomerulonephritis, type 2

N00.7   Acute nephritic syndrome with diffuse crescentic glomerulonephritis

Acute nephritic syndrome with extracapillary glomerulonephritis

N00.8   Acute nephritic syndrome with other morphologic changes

Acute nephritic syndrome with proliferative glomerulonephritis NOS

N00.9   Acute nephritic syndrome with unspecified morphologic changes

N01   Rapidly progressive nephritic syndrome

Includes: rapidly progressive glomerular disease

rapidly progressive glomerulonephritis rapidly progressive nephritis

Excludes1: nephritic syndrome NOS (N05.-)

N01.0   Rapidly progressive nephritic syndrome with minor glomerular abnormality

Rapidly progressive nephritic syndrome with minimal change lesion

N01.1   Rapidly progressive nephritic syndrome with focal and segmental glomerular lesions

Rapidly progressive nephritic syndrome with focal and segmental hyalinosis

Rapidly progressive nephritic syndrome with focal and segmental sclerosis

Rapidly progressive nephritic syndrome with focal glomerulonephritis

N01.2   Rapidly progressive nephritic syndrome with diffuse membranous glomerulonephritis

N01.3   Rapidly progressive nephritic syndrome with diffuse mesangial proliferative glomerulonephritis

N01.4   Rapidly progressive nephritic syndrome with diffuse endocapillary proliferative glomerulonephritis

N01.5   Rapidly progressive nephritic syndrome with diffuse mesangiocapillary glomerulonephritis

Rapidly progressive nephritic syndrome with membranoproliferative glomerulonephritis, types 1 and 3, or NOS

N01.6   Rapidly progressive nephritic syndrome with dense deposit disease

Rapidly progressive nephritic syndrome with membranoproliferative glomerulonephritis, type 2

N01.7   Rapidly progressive nephritic syndrome with diffuse crescentic glomerulonephritis

Rapidly progressive nephritic syndrome with extracapillary glomerulonephritis

N01.8   Rapidly progressive nephritic syndrome with other morphologic changes

Rapidly progressive nephritic syndrome with proliferative glomerulonephritis NOS

N01.9   Rapidly progressive nephritic syndrome with unspecified morphologic changes

N02   Recurrent and persistent hematuria

Excludes1: acute cystitis with hematuria (N30.01)

hematuria NOS (R31.9)

hematuria not associated with specified morphologic lesions (R31.-)

	Add 4th-7th digits		Nonspecific code		Unspecified code		Manifestation code	

N02.0 **Recurrent and persistent hematuria with minor glomerular abnormality**

Recurrent and persistent hematuria with minimal change lesion

N02.1 **Recurrent and persistent hematuria with focal and segmental glomerular lesions**

Recurrent and persistent hematuria with focal and segmental hyalinosis

Recurrent and persistent hematuria with focal and segmental sclerosis

Recurrent and persistent hematuria with focal glomerulonephritis

N02.2 **Recurrent and persistent hematuria with diffuse membranous glomerulonephritis**

N02.3 **Recurrent and persistent hematuria with diffuse mesangial proliferative glomerulonephritis**

N02.4 **Recurrent and persistent hematuria with diffuse endocapillary proliferative glomerulonephritis**

N02.5 **Recurrent and persistent hematuria with diffuse mesangiocapillary glomerulonephritis**

Recurrent and persistent hematuria with membranoproliferative glomerulonephritis, types 1 and 3, or NOS

N02.6 **Recurrent and persistent hematuria with dense deposit disease**

Recurrent and persistent hematuria with membranoproliferative glomerulonephritis, type 2

N02.7 **Recurrent and persistent hematuria with diffuse crescentic glomerulonephritis**

Recurrent and persistent hematuria with extracapillary glomerulonephritis

N02.8 **Recurrent and persistent hematuria with other morphologic changes**

Recurrent and persistent hematuria with proliferative glomerulonephritis NOS

N02.9 **Recurrent and persistent hematuria with unspecified morphologic changes**

N03 **Chronic nephritic syndrome**

Definition: Nephritic syndrome is a collection of signs associated with disorders affecting the kidneys, more specifically glomerular disorders.

Includes: chronic glomerular disease

chronic glomerulonephritis chronic nephritis

Excludes1: chronic tubulo-interstitial nephritis (N11.-)

diffuse sclerosing glomerulonephritis (N05.8-)

nephritic syndrome NOS (N05.-)

N03.0 **Chronic nephritic syndrome with minor glomerular abnormality**

Chronic nephritic syndrome with minimal change lesion

N03.1 **Chronic nephritic syndrome with focal and segmental glomerular lesions**

Chronic nephritic syndrome with focal and segmental hyalinosis

Chronic nephritic syndrome with focal and segmental sclerosis

Chronic nephritic syndrome with focal glomerulonephritis

N03.2 **Chronic nephritic syndrome with diffuse membranous glomerulonephritis**

N03.3 **Chronic nephritic syndrome with diffuse mesangial proliferative glomerulonephritis**

N03.4 **Chronic nephritic syndrome with diffuse endocapillary proliferative glomerulonephritis**

N03.5 **Chronic nephritic syndrome with diffuse mesangiocapillary glomerulonephritis**

Chronic nephritic syndrome with membranoproliferative glomerulonephritis, types 1 and 3, or NOS

N03.6 **Chronic nephritic syndrome with dense deposit disease**

Chronic nephritic syndrome with membranoproliferative glomerulonephritis, type 2

N03.7 **Chronic nephritic syndrome with diffuse crescentic glomerulonephritis**

Chronic nephritic syndrome with extracapillary glomerulonephritis

N03.8 **Chronic nephritic syndrome with other morphologic changes**

Chronic nephritic syndrome with proliferative glomerulonephritis NOS

N03.9 **Chronic nephritic syndrome with unspecified morphologic changes**

N04 **Nephrotic syndrome**

Definition: Nephrotic syndrome is a collection of symptoms which occur because the glomeruli (tiny blood vessels) in the kidney become leaky. This allows protein, normally never passed out in the urine, to leave the body in large amounts.

Includes: congenital nephrotic syndrome

lipoid nephrosis

N04.0 **Nephrotic syndrome with minor glomerular abnormality**

Nephrotic syndrome with minimal change lesion

N04.1 **Nephrotic syndrome with focal and segmental glomerular lesions**

Nephrotic syndrome with focal and segmental hyalinosis

Nephrotic syndrome with focal and segmental sclerosis

Nephrotic syndrome with focal glomerulonephritis

N04.2 **Nephrotic syndrome with diffuse membranous glomerulonephritis**

N04.3 **Nephrotic syndrome with diffuse mesangial proliferative glomerulonephritis**

N04.4 **Nephrotic syndrome with diffuse endocapillary proliferative glomerulonephritis**

N04.5 **Nephrotic syndrome with diffuse mesangiocapillary glomerulonephritis**

Nephrotic syndrome with membranoproliferative glomerulonephritis, types 1 and 3, or NOS

N04.6 **Nephrotic syndrome with dense deposit disease**

Nephrotic syndrome with membranoproliferative glomerulonephritis, type 2

N04.7 **Nephrotic syndrome with diffuse crescentic glomerulonephritis**

Nephrotic syndrome with extracapillary glomerulonephritis

N04.8 **Nephrotic syndrome with other morphologic changes**

Nephrotic syndrome with proliferative glomerulonephritis NOS

N04.9 **Nephrotic syndrome with unspecified morphologic changes**

N05 **Unspecified nephritic syndrome**

Includes: glomerular disease NOS

glomerulonephritis NOS nephritis NOS

nephropathy NOS and renal disease NOS with morphological lesion specified in .0-.8

Excludes1: nephropathy NOS with no stated morphological lesion (N28.9)

renal disease NOS with no stated morphological lesion (N28.9)

tubulo-interstitial nephritis NOS (N12)

N05.0   **Unspecified nephritic syndrome with minor glomerular abnormality**

Unspecified nephritic syndrome with minimal change lesion

N05.1   **Unspecified nephritic syndrome with focal and segmental glomerular lesions**

Unspecified nephritic syndrome with focal and segmental hyalinosis

Unspecified nephritic syndrome with focal and segmental sclerosis

Unspecified nephritic syndrome with focal glomerulonephritis

N05.2   **Unspecified nephritic syndrome with diffuse membranous glomerulonephritis**

N05.3   **Unspecified nephritic syndrome with diffuse mesangial proliferative glomerulonephritis**

N05.4   **Unspecified nephritic syndrome with diffuse endocapillary proliferative glomerulonephritis**

N05.5   **Unspecified nephritic syndrome with diffuse mesangiocapillary glomerulonephritis**

Unspecified nephritic syndrome with membranoproliferative glomerulonephritis, types 1 and 3, or NOS

N05.6   **Unspecified nephritic syndrome with dense deposit disease**

Unspecified nephritic syndrome with membranoproliferative glomerulonephritis, type 2

N05.7   **Unspecified nephritic syndrome with diffuse crescentic glomerulonephritis**

Unspecified nephritic syndrome with extracapillary glomerulonephritis

N05.8   **Unspecified nephritic syndrome with other morphologic changes**

Unspecified nephritic syndrome with proliferative glomerulonephritis NOS

N05.9   **Unspecified nephritic syndrome with unspecified morphologic changes**

N06   **Isolated proteinuria with specified morphological lesion**

Excludes1: Proteinuria not associated with specific morphologic lesions (R80.0)

N06.0   **Isolated proteinuria with minor glomerular abnormality**

Isolated proteinuria with minimal change lesion

N06.1   **Isolated proteinuria with focal and segmental glomerular lesions**

Isolated proteinuria with focal and segmental hyalinosis

Isolated proteinuria with focal and segmental sclerosis

Isolated proteinuria with focal glomerulonephritis

N06.2   **Isolated proteinuria with diffuse membranous glomerulonephritis**

N06.3   **Isolated proteinuria with diffuse mesangial proliferative glomerulonephritis**

N06.4   **Isolated proteinuria with diffuse endocapillary proliferative glomerulonephritis**

N06.5   **Isolated proteinuria with diffuse mesangiocapillary glomerulonephritis**

Isolated proteinuria with membranoproliferative glomerulonephritis, types 1 and 3, or NOS

N06.6   **Isolated proteinuria with dense deposit disease**

Isolated proteinuria with membranoproliferative glomerulonephritis, type 2

N06.7   **Isolated proteinuria with diffuse crescentic glomerulonephritis**

Isolated proteinuria with extracapillary glomerulonephritis

N06.8   **Isolated proteinuria with other morphologic lesion**

Isolated proteinuria with proliferative glomerulonephritis NOS

N06.9   **Isolated proteinuria with unspecified morphologic lesion**

N07   **Hereditary nephropathy, not elsewhere classified**

Excludes2: Alport's syndrome (Q87.81-)

hereditary amyloid nephropathy (E85.-)

nail patella syndrome (Q87.2)

non-neuropathic heredofamilial amyloidosis (E85.-)

N07.0   **Hereditary nephropathy, not elsewhere classified with minor glomerular abnormality**

Hereditary nephropathy, not elsewhere classified with minimal change lesion

N07.1   **Hereditary nephropathy, not elsewhere classified with focal and segmental glomerular lesions**

Hereditary nephropathy, not elsewhere classified with focal and segmental hyalinosis

Hereditary nephropathy, not elsewhere classified with focal and segmental sclerosis

Hereditary nephropathy, not elsewhere classified with focal glomerulonephritis

N07.2   **Hereditary nephropathy, not elsewhere classified with diffuse membranous glomerulonephritis**

N07.3   **Hereditary nephropathy, not elsewhere classified with diffuse mesangial proliferative glomerulonephritis**

N07.4   **Hereditary nephropathy, not elsewhere classified with diffuse endocapillary proliferative glomerulonephritis**

N07.5   **Hereditary nephropathy, not elsewhere classified with diffuse mesangiocapillary glomerulonephritis**

Hereditary nephropathy, not elsewhere classified with membranoproliferative glomerulonephritis, types 1 and 3, or NOS

N07.6   **Hereditary nephropathy, not elsewhere classified with dense deposit disease**

Hereditary nephropathy, not elsewhere classified with membranoproliferative glomerulonephritis, type 2

N07.7   **Hereditary nephropathy, not elsewhere classified with diffuse crescentic glomerulonephritis**

Hereditary nephropathy, not elsewhere classified with extracapillary glomerulonephritis

N07.8   **Hereditary nephropathy, not elsewhere classified with other morphologic lesions**

Hereditary nephropathy, not elsewhere classified with proliferative glomerulonephritis NOS

N07.9   **Hereditary nephropathy, not elsewhere classified with unspecified morphologic lesions**

N08   **Glomerular disorders in diseases classified elsewhere**

Glomerulonephritis Nephritis Nephropathy

Code first underlying disease, such as:

amyloidosis (E85.-)

congenital syphilis (A50.5)

cryoglobulinemia (D89.1)

disseminated intravascular coagulation (D65)

gout (M1A.-, M10.-)

microscopic polyangiitis (M31.7)

multiple myeloma (C90.0-)

sepsis (A40.0-A41.9)

sickle-cell disease (D57.0-D57.8)

Excludes1: glomerulonephritis, nephritis and nephropathy (in):

antiglomerular basement membrane disease (M31.0)

diabetes (E08-E13 with .21)

gonococcal (A54.21)

Goodpasture's syndrome (M31.0)

hemolytic-uremic syndrome (D59.3)

lupus (M32.14)

mumps (B26.83)

syphilis (A52.75)

systemic lupus erythematosus (M32.14)

Wegener's granulomatosis (M31.31)

pyelonephritis in diseases classified elsewhere (N16)

renal tubulo-interstitial disorders classified elsewhere (N16)

RENAL TUBULO-INTERSTITIAL DISEASES (N10-N16)

Includes: pyelonephritis

Excludes1: pyeloureteritis cystica (N28.85)

N10   Acute pyelonephritis

Acute infectious interstitial nephritis

Acute pyelitis

Acute tubulo-interstitial nephritis

Hemoglobin nephrosis

Myoglobin nephrosis

Use additional code (B95-B97), to identify infectious agent.

N11   Chronic tubulo-interstitial nephritis

Includes: chronic infectious interstitial nephritis

chronic pyelitis chronic pyelonephritis

Use additional code (B95-B97), to identify infectious agent.

N11.0   Nonobstructive reflux-associated chronic pyelonephritis

Pyelonephritis (chronic) associated with (vesicoureteral) reflux

Excludes1: vesicoureteral reflux NOS (N13.70)

N11.1   Chronic obstructive pyelonephritis

Pyelonephritis (chronic) associated with anomaly of pelviureteric junction

Pyelonephritis (chronic) associated with anomaly of pyeloureteric junction

Pyelonephritis (chronic) associated with crossing of vessel

Pyelonephritis (chronic) associated with kinking of ureter

Pyelonephritis (chronic) associated with obstruction of ureter

Pyelonephritis (chronic) associated with stricture of pelviureteric junction

Pyelonephritis (chronic) associated with stricture of ureter

Excludes1: calculus pyelonephritis (N20.9)

obstructive uropathy (N13.-)

N11.8   Other chronic tubulo-interstitial nephritis

Nonobstructive chronic pyelonephritis NOS

N11.9   Chronic tubulo-interstitial nephritis, unspecified

Chronic interstitial nephritis NOS

Chronic pyelitis NOS

Chronic pyelonephritis NOS

N12   Tubulo-interstitial nephritis, not specified as acute or chronic

Interstitial nephritis NOS

Pyelitis NOS

Pyelonephritis NOS

Excludes1: calculous pyelonephritis (N20.9)

N13   Obstructive and reflux uropathy

Excludes2: calculus of kidney and ureter without hydronephrosis (N20.-)

congenital obstructive defects of renal pelvis and ureter (Q62.0-Q62.3)

hydronephrosis with ureteropelvic junction obstruction (Q62.11)

obstructive pyelonephritis (N11.1)

N13.0   Hydronephrosis with ureteropelvic junction obstruction

Definition: Hydronephrosis is a condition that occurs as a result of urine accumulation in the upper urinary tract. This usually occurs from a blockage somewhere along the urinary tract.

Hydronephrosis due to acquired occlusion of ureteropelvic junction

Excludes2: Hydronephrosis with ureteropelvic junction obstruction due to calculus (N13.2)

N13.1   Hydronephrosis with ureteral stricture, not elsewhere classified

Excludes1: Hydronephrosis with ureteral stricture with infection (N13.6)

N13.2   Hydronephrosis with renal and ureteral calculous obstruction

Excludes1: Hydronephrosis with renal and ureteral calculous obstruction with infection (N13.6)

N13.3   Other and unspecified hydronephrosis

Excludes1: hydronephrosis with infection (N13.6)

N13.30   Unspecified hydronephrosis

N13.39   Other hydronephrosis

N13.4   Hydroureter

Excludes1: congenital hydroureter (Q62.3-)

hydroureter with infection (N13.6)

vesicoureteral-reflux with hydroureter (N13.73-)

N13.5   Crossing vessel and stricture of ureter without hydronephrosis

Kinking and stricture of ureter without hydronephrosis

Excludes1: Crossing vessel and stricture of ureter without hydronephrosis with infection (N13.6)

N13.6   Pyonephrosis

Conditions in N13.0-N13.5 with infection

Obstructive uropathy with infection

Use additional code (B95-B97), to identify infectious agent.

N13.7   Vesicoureteral-reflux

Excludes1: reflux-associated pyelonephritis (N11.0)

N13.70   Vesicoureteral-reflux, unspecified

Vesicoureteral-reflux NOS

N13.71   Vesicoureteral-reflux without reflux nephropathy

N13.72   Vesicoureteral-reflux with reflux nephropathy without hydroureter

N13.721   Vesicoureteral-reflux with reflux nephropathy without hydroureter, unilateral

N13.722   Vesicoureteral-reflux with reflux nephropathy without hydroureter, bilateral

N13.729   Vesicoureteral-reflux with reflux nephropathy without hydroureter, unspecified

N13.731   Vesicoureteral-reflux with reflux nephropathy with hydroureter, unilateral

N13.732   Vesicoureteral-reflux with reflux nephropathy with hydroureter, bilateral

N13.739   **Vesicoureteral-reflux with reflux nephropathy with hydroureter, unspecified**

N13.8   **Other obstructive and reflux uropathy**

Urinary tract obstruction due to specified cause

Code first, if applicable, any causal condition, such as:

enlarged prostate (N40.1)

N13.9   **Obstructive and reflux uropathy, unspecified**

Urinary tract obstruction NOS

N14   **Drug- and heavy-metal-induced tubulo-interstitial and tubular conditions**

Code first poisoning due to drug or toxin, if applicable (T36-T65 with fifth or sixth character 1-4 or 6)

Use additional code for adverse effect, if applicable, to identify drug (T36-T50 with fifth or sixth character 5)

N14.0   **Analgesic nephropathy**

N14.1   **Nephropathy induced by other drugs, medicaments and biological substances**

N14.2   **Nephropathy induced by unspecified drug, medicament or biological substance**

N14.3   **Nephropathy induced by heavy metals**

N14.4   **Toxic nephropathy, not elsewhere classified**

N15   **Other renal tubulo-interstitial diseases**

N15.0   **Balkan nephropathy**

Balkan endemic nephropathy

N15.1   **Renal and perinephric abscess**

N15.8   **Other specified renal tubulo-interstitial diseases**

N15.9   **Renal tubulo-interstitial disease, unspecified**

Infection of kidney NOS

Excludes1: urinary tract infection NOS (N39.0)

N16   **Renal tubulo-interstitial disorders in diseases classified elsewhere**

Pyelonephritis

Tubulo-interstitial nephritis

Code first underlying disease, such as:

brucellosis (A23.0-A23.9)

cryoglobulinemia (D89.1)

glycogen storage disease (E74.0)

leukemia (C91-C95)

lymphoma (C81.0-C85.9, C96.0-C96.9)

multiple myeloma (C90.0-)

sepsis (A40.0-A41.9)

Wilson's disease (E83.0)

Excludes1: diphtheritic pyelonephritis and tubulo-interstitial nephritis (A36.84)

pyelonephritis and tubulo-interstitial nephritis in candidiasis (B37.49)

pyelonephritis and tubulo-interstitial nephritis in cystinosis (E72.04)

pyelonephritis and tubulo-interstitial nephritis in salmonella infection (A02.25)

pyelonephritis and tubulo-interstitial nephritis in sarcoidosis (D86.84)

pyelonephritis and tubulo-interstitial nephritis in sicca syndrome [Sjogren's] (M35.04)

pyelonephritis and tubulo-interstitial nephritis in systemic lupus erythematosus (M32.15)

pyelonephritis and tubulo-interstitial nephritis in toxoplasmosis (B58.83)

renal tubular degeneration in diabetes (E08-E13 with .29)

syphilitic pyelonephritis and tubulo-interstitial nephritis (A52.75)

ACUTE KIDNEY FAILURE AND CHRONIC KIDNEY DISEASE (N17-N19)

Excludes2: congenital renal failure (P96.0)

drug- and heavy-metal-induced tubulo-interstitial and tubular conditions (N14.-)

extrarenal uremia (R39.2)

hemolytic-uremic syndrome (D59.3)

hepatorenal syndrome (K76.7)

postpartum hepatorenal syndrome (O90.4)

posttraumatic renal failure (T79.5)

prerenal uremia (R39.2)

renal failure complicating abortion or ectopic or molar pregnancy (O00-O07, O08.4)

renal failure following labor and delivery (O90.4)

renal failure postprocedural (N99.0)

N17   **Acute kidney failure**

Code also associated underlying condition

Excludes1: posttraumatic renal failure (T79.5)

N17.0   **Acute kidney failure with tubular necrosis**

Acute tubular necrosis

Renal tubular necrosis

Tubular necrosis NOS

N17.1   **Acute kidney failure with acute cortical necrosis**

Acute cortical necrosis

Cortical necrosis NOS

Renal cortical necrosis

N17.2   **Acute kidney failure with medullary necrosis**

Medullary [papillary] necrosis NOS

Acute medullary [papillary] necrosis

Renal medullary [papillary] necrosis

N17.8   **Other acute kidney failure**

N17.9   **Acute kidney failure, unspecified**

Acute kidney injury (nontraumatic)

Excludes2: traumatic kidney injury (S37.0-)

N18   **Chronic kidney disease (CKD)**

Definition: Chronic kidney disease (CKD), aka chronic renal disease, is a progressive loss of renal function over a period of months or years.

Code first any associated:

diabetic chronic kidney disease (E08.22, E09.22, E10.22, E11.22, E13.22)

hypertensive chronic kidney disease (I12.-, I13.-)

Use additional code to identify kidney transplant status, if applicable, (Z94.0)

N18.1   **Chronic kidney disease, stage 1**

N18.2   **Chronic kidney disease, stage 2 (mild)**

N18.3   **Chronic kidney disease, stage 3 (moderate)**

N18.4   **Chronic kidney disease, stage 4 (severe)**

N18.5   **Chronic kidney disease, stage 5**

Excludes1: chronic kidney disease, stage 5 requiring chronic dialysis (N18.6)

N18.6   **End stage renal disease**

Chronic kidney disease requiring chronic dialysis

Use additional code to identify dialysis status (Z99.2)

N18.9   **Chronic kidney disease, unspecified**

Chronic renal disease

Chronic renal failure NOS

Chronic renal insufficiency

Chronic uremia NOS

Diffuse sclerosing glomerulonephritis NOS

N19   Unspecified kidney failure

Uremia NOS

Excludes1: acute kidney failure (N17.-)

chronic kidney disease (N18.-)

chronic uremia (N18.9)

extrarenal uremia (R39.2)

prerenal uremia (R39.2)

renal insufficiency (acute) (N28.9)

uremia of newborn (P96.0)

UROLITHIASIS (N20-N23)

N20   Calculus of kidney and ureter

Calculous pyelonephritis

Excludes1: nephrocalcinosis (E83.5)

that with hydronephrosis (N13.2)

N20.0   Calculus of kidney

Nephrolithiasis NOS

Renal calculus

Renal stone

Staghorn calculus

Stone in kidney

N20.1   Calculus of ureter

Ureteric stone

N20.2   Calculus of kidney with calculus of ureter

N20.9   Urinary calculus, unspecified

N21   Calculus of lower urinary tract

Includes: calculus of lower urinary tract with cystitis and urethritis

N21.0   Calculus in bladder

Calculus in diverticulum of bladder

Urinary bladder stone

Excludes2: staghorn calculus (N20.0)

N21.1   Calculus in urethra

Excludes2: calculus of prostate (N42.0)

N21.8   Other lower urinary tract calculus

N21.9   Calculus of lower urinary tract, unspecified

Excludes1: calculus of urinary tract NOS (N20.9)

N22   Calculus of urinary tract in diseases classified elsewhere

Code first underlying disease, such as:

gout (M1A.-, M10.-)

schistosomiasis (B65.0-B65.9)

N23   Unspecified renal colic

OTHER DISORDERS OF KIDNEY AND URETER (N25-N29)

Excludes2: disorders of kidney and ureter with urolithiasis (N20-N23)

N25   Disorders resulting from impaired renal tubular function

N25.0   Renal osteodystrophy

Azotemic osteodystrophy

Phosphate-losing tubular disorders

Renal rickets

Renal short stature

Excludes2: metabolic disorders classifiable to E70-E88

N25.1   Nephrogenic diabetes insipidus

Excludes1: diabetes insipidus NOS (E23.2)

N25.8   Other disorders resulting from impaired renal tubular function

N25.81   Secondary hyperparathyroidism of renal origin

Excludes1: secondary hyperparathyroidism, non-renal (E21.1)

Excludes2: metabolic disorders classifiable to E70-E88

N25.89   Other disorders resulting from impaired renal tubular function

Hypokalemic nephropathy

Lightwood-Albright syndrome

Renal tubular acidosis NOS

N25.9   Disorder resulting from impaired renal tubular function, unspecified

N26   Unspecified contracted kidney

Excludes1: contracted kidney due to hypertension (I12.-)

diffuse sclerosing glomerulonephritis (N05.8.-)

hypertensive nephrosclerosis (arteriolar) (arteriosclerotic) (I12.-)

small kidney of unknown cause (N27.-)

N26.1   Atrophy of kidney (terminal)

N26.2   Page kidney

N26.9   Renal sclerosis, unspecified

N27   Small kidney of unknown cause

Includes: oligonephronia

N27.0   Small kidney, unilateral

N27.1   Small kidney, bilateral

N27.9   Small kidney, unspecified

N28   Other disorders of kidney and ureter, not elsewhere classified

N28.0   Ischemia and infarction of kidney

Renal artery embolism

Renal artery obstruction

Renal artery occlusion

Renal artery thrombosis

Renal infarct

Excludes1: atherosclerosis of renal artery (extrarenal part) (I70.1)

congenital stenosis of renal artery (Q27.1)

Goldblatt's kidney (I70.1)

N28.1   Cyst of kidney, acquired

Cyst (multiple) (solitary) of kidney, acquired

Excludes1: cystic kidney disease (congenital) (Q61.-)

N28.8   Other specified disorders of kidney and ureter

Excludes1: hydroureter (N13.4)

ureteric stricture with hydronephrosis (N13.1)

ureteric stricture without hydronephrosis (N13.5)

N28.81   Hypertrophy of kidney

N28.82   Megaloureter

N28.83   Nephroptosis

N28.84   Pyelitis cystica

N28.85   Pyeloureteritis cystica

N28.86   Ureteritis cystica

N28.89   Other specified disorders of kidney and ureter

N28.9   Disorder of kidney and ureter, unspecified

Nephropathy NOS

Renal disease (acute) NOS

Renal insufficiency (acute)

Excludes1: chronic renal insufficiency (N18.9)

unspecified nephritic syndrome (N05.-)

N29 Other disorders of kidney and ureter in diseases classified elsewhere

Code first underlying disease, such as:

amyloidosis (E85.-)

nephrocalcinosis (E83.5)

schistosomiasis (B65.0-B65.9)

Excludes1: disorders of kidney and ureter in:

cystinosis (E72.0)

gonorrhea (A54.21)

syphilis (A52.75)

tuberculosis (A18.11)

OTHER DISEASES OF THE URINARY SYSTEM (N30-N39)

Excludes1: urinary infection (complicating):

abortion or ectopic or molar pregnancy (O00-O07, O08.8)

pregnancy, childbirth and the puerperium (O23.-, O75.3, O86.2-)

N30 Cystitis

Use additional code to identify infectious agent (B95-B97)

Excludes1: prostatocystitis (N41.3)

N30.0 Acute cystitis

Excludes1: irradiation cystitis (N30.4-)

trigonitis (N30.3-)

N30.00 Acute cystitis without hematuria

N30.01 Acute cystitis with hematuria

N30.1 Interstitial cystitis (chronic)

N30.10 Interstitial cystitis (chronic) without hematuria

N30.11 Interstitial cystitis (chronic) with hematuria

N30.2 Other chronic cystitis

N30.20 Other chronic cystitis without hematuria

N30.21 Other chronic cystitis with hematuria

N30.3 Trigonitis

Urethrotrigonitis

N30.30 Trigonitis without hematuria

N30.31 Trigonitis with hematuria

N30.4 Irradiation cystitis

N30.40 Irradiation cystitis without hematuria

N30.41 Irradiation cystitis with hematuria

N30.8 Other cystitis

Abscess of bladder

N30.80 Other cystitis without hematuria

N30.81 Other cystitis with hematuria

N30.9 Cystitis, unspecified

N30.90 Cystitis, unspecified without hematuria

N30.91 Cystitis, unspecified with hematuria

N31 Neuromuscular dysfunction of bladder, not elsewhere classified

Use additional code to identify any associated urinary incontinence (N39.3-N39.4-)

Excludes1: cord bladder NOS (G95.89)

neurogenic bladder due to cauda equina syndrome (G83.4)

neuromuscular dysfunction due to spinal cord lesion (G95.89)

N31.0 Uninhibited neuropathic bladder, not elsewhere classified

N31.1 Reflex neuropathic bladder, not elsewhere classified

N31.2 Flaccid neuropathic bladder, not elsewhere classified

Atonic (motor) (sensory) neuropathic bladder

Autonomous neuropathic bladder

Nonreflex neuropathic bladder

N31.8 Other neuromuscular dysfunction of bladder

N31.9 Neuromuscular dysfunction of bladder, unspecified

Neurogenic bladder dysfunction NOS

N32 Other disorders of bladder

Excludes2: calculus of bladder (N21.0)

cystocele (N81.1-)

hernia or prolapse of bladder, female (N81.1-)

N32.0 Bladder-neck obstruction

Bladder-neck stenosis (acquired)

Excludes1: congenital bladder-neck obstruction (Q64.3-)

N32.1 Vesicointestinal fistula

Vesicorectal fistula

N32.2 Vesical fistula, not elsewhere classified

Excludes1: fistula between bladder and female genital tract (N82.0-N82.1)

N32.3 Diverticulum of bladder

Excludes1: congenital diverticulum of bladder (Q64.6)

diverticulitis of bladder (N30.8-)

N32.8 Other specified disorders of bladder

N32.81 Overactive bladder

Detrusor muscle hyperactivity

Excludes1: frequent urination due to specified bladder condition- code to condition

N32.89 Other specified disorders of bladder

Bladder hemorrhage

Bladder hypertrophy

Calcified bladder

Contracted bladder

N32.9 Bladder disorder, unspecified

N33 Bladder disorders in diseases classified elsewhere

Code first underlying disease, such as:

schistosomiasis (B65.0-B65.9)

Excludes1: bladder disorder in syphilis (A52.76)

bladder disorder in tuberculosis (A18.12)

candidal cystitis (B37.41)

chlamydial cystitis (A56.01)

cystitis in gonorrhea (A54.01)

cystitis in neurogenic bladder (N31.-)

diphtheritic cystitis (A36.85)

syphilitic cystitis (A52.76)

trichomonal cystitis (A59.03)

N34 Urethritis and urethral syndrome

Use additional code (B95-B97), to identify infectious agent.

Excludes2: Reiter's disease (M02.3-)

urethritis in diseases with a predominantly sexual mode of transmission (A50-A64)

urethrotrigonitis (N30.3-)

N34.0 Urethral abscess

Abscess (of) Cowper's gland

Abscess (of) Littre's gland

Abscess (of) urethral (gland)

Periurethral abscess

Excludes1: urethral caruncle (N36.2)

N34.1 **Nonspecific urethritis**

Nongonococcal urethritis Nonvenereal urethritis

N34.2 **Other urethritis**

Meatitis, urethral

Postmenopausal urethritis

Ulcer of urethra (meatus)

Urethritis NOS

N34.3 **Urethral syndrome, unspecified**

N35 **Urethral stricture**

Excludes1: congenital urethral stricture (Q64.3-)

postprocedural urethral stricture (N99.1-)

N35.0 **Post-traumatic urethral stricture**

Urethral stricture due to injury

Excludes1: postprocedural urethral stricture (N99.1-)

N35.01 **Post-traumatic urethral stricture, male**

N35.010 **Post-traumatic urethral stricture, male, meatal**

N35.011 **Post-traumatic bulbous urethral stricture**

N35.012 **Post-traumatic membranous urethral stricture**

N35.013 **Post-traumatic anterior urethral stricture**

N35.014 **Post-traumatic urethral stricture, male, unspecified**

N35.02 **Post-traumatic urethral stricture, female**

N35.021 **Urethral stricture due to childbirth**

N35.028 **Other post-traumatic urethral stricture, female**

N35.1 **Postinfective urethral stricture, not elsewhere classified**

Excludes1: urethral stricture associated with schistosomiasis (B65.-, N29)

gonococcal urethral stricture (A54.01)

syphilitic urethral stricture (A52.76)

N35.11 **Postinfective urethral stricture, not elsewhere classified, male**

N35.111 **Postinfective urethral stricture, not elsewhere classified, male, meatal**

▲**N35.112** **Postinfective bulbous urethral stricture, not elsewhere classified, male**

▲**N35.113** **Postinfective membranous urethral stricture, not elsewhere classified, male**

▲**N35.114** **Postinfective anterior urethral stricture, not elsewhere classified, male**

N35.119 **Postinfective urethral stricture, not elsewhere classified, male, unspecified**

N35.12 **Postinfective urethral stricture, not elsewhere classified, female**

N35.8 **Other urethral stricture**

Excludes1: postprocedural urethral stricture (N99.1-)

N35.9 **Urethral stricture, unspecified**

N36 **Other disorders of urethra**

N36.0 **Urethral fistula**

Urethroperineal fistula

Urethrorectal fistula

Urinary fistula NOS

Excludes1: urethroscrotal fistula (N50.89)

urethrovaginal fistula (N82.1)

urethrovesicovaginal fistula (N82.1)

N36.1 **Urethral diverticulum**

N36.2 **Urethral caruncle**

N36.4 **Urethral functional and muscular disorders**

Use additional code to identify associated urinary stress incontinence (N39.3)

N36.41 **Hypermobility of urethra**

N36.42 **Intrinsic sphincter deficiency (ISD)**

N36.43 **Combined hypermobility of urethra and intrinsic sphincter deficiency**

N36.44 **Muscular disorders of urethra**

Bladder sphincter dyssynergy

N36.5 **Urethral false passage**

N36.8 **Other specified disorders of urethra**

Excludes1: congenital urethrocele (Q64.7)

female urethrocele (N81.0)

N36.9 **Urethral disorder, unspecified**

N37 **Urethral disorders in diseases classified elsewhere**

Code first underlying disease

Excludes1: urethritis (in):

candidal infection (B37.41)

chlamydial (A56.01)

gonorrhea (A54.01)

syphilis (A52.76)

trichomonal infection (A59.03)

tuberculosis (A18.13)

N39 **Other disorders of urinary system**

Excludes2: hematuria NOS (R31.-)

recurrent or persistent hematuria (N02.-)

recurrent or persistent hematuria with specified morphological lesion (N02.-)

proteinuria NOS (R80.-)

N39.0 **Urinary tract infection, site not specified**

Use additional code (B95-B97), to identify infectious agent.

Excludes1: candidiasis of urinary tract (B37.4-)

neonatal urinary tract infection (P39.3)

urinary tract infection of specified site, such as: cystitis (N30.-)

urethritis (N34.-)

N39.3 **Stress incontinence (female) (male)**

Code also any associated overactive bladder (N32.81)

Excludes1: mixed incontinence (N39.46)

N39.4 **Other specified urinary incontinence**

Code also any associated overactive bladder (N32.81)

Excludes1: enuresis NOS (R32)

functional urinary incontinence (R39.81)

urinary incontinence associated with cognitive impairment (R39.81)

urinary incontinence NOS (R32)

urinary incontinence of nonorganic origin (F98.0)

N39.41 **Urge incontinence**

Excludes1: mixed incontinence (N39.46)

N39.42 **Incontinence without sensory awareness**

Insensible (urinary) incontinence

N39.43 **Post-void dribbling**

N39.44 **Nocturnal enuresis**

● New code   ▲ Revised code   **Excludes1:** Not coded here   **Excludes2:** Not included here   ⊗ Placeholder required   ⑦ 7th digit required

N39.45 **Continuous leakage**

N39.46 **Mixed incontinence**

Urge and stress incontinence

N39.49 **Other specified urinary incontinence**

N39.490 **Overflow incontinence**

N39.491 **Coital incontinence**

N39.492 **Postural (urinary) incontinence**

N39.498 **Other specified urinary incontinence**

Reflex incontinence

Total incontinence

N39.8 **Other specified disorders of urinary system**

N39.9 **Disorder of urinary system, unspecified**

DISEASES OF MALE GENITAL ORGANS (N40-N53)

NOTE: ALL DIAGNOSIS CODES IN THIS SECTION APPLY TO MALE PATIENTS ONLY

N40 **Benign prostatic hyperplasia**

Includes: adenofibromatous hypertrophy of prostate

benign hypertrophy of the prostate

benign prostatic hypertrophy

BPH

enlarged prostate nodular prostate

polyp of prostate

Excludes1: benign neoplasms of prostate (adenoma, benign) (fibroadenoma) (fibroma) (myoma) (D29.1)

Excludes2: malignant neoplasm of prostate (C61)

N40.0 **Benign prostatic hyperplasia without lower urinary tract symptoms**

Enlarged prostate without LUTS

Enlarged prostate NOS

N40.1 **Benign prostatic hyperplasia with lower urinary tract symptoms**

Enlarged prostate with LUTS

Use additional code for associated symptoms, when specified:

incomplete bladder emptying (R39.14)

nocturia (R35.1)

straining on urination (R39.16)

urinary frequency (R35.0)

urinary hesitancy (R39.11)

urinary incontinence (N39.4-)

urinary obstruction (N13.8)

urinary retention (R33.8)

urinary urgency (R39.15)

weak urinary stream (R39.12)

N40.2 **Nodular prostate without lower urinary tract symptoms**

Nodular prostate without LUTS

N40.3 **Nodular prostate with lower urinary tract symptoms**

Use additional code for associated symptoms, when specified:

incomplete bladder emptying (R39.14)

nocturia (R35.1)

straining on urination (R39.16)

urinary frequency (R35.0)

urinary hesitancy (R39.11)

urinary incontinence (N39.4-)

urinary obstruction (N13.8)

urinary retention (R33.8)

urinary urgency (R39.15)

weak urinary stream (R39.12)

N41 **Inflammatory diseases of prostate**

Use additional code (B95-B97), to identify infectious agent.

N41.0 **Acute prostatitis**

N41.1 **Chronic prostatitis**

N41.2 **Abscess of prostate**

N41.3 **Prostatocystitis**

N41.4 **Granulomatous prostatitis**

N41.8 **Other inflammatory diseases of prostate**

N41.9 **Inflammatory disease of prostate, unspecified**

Prostatitis NOS

N42 **Other and unspecified disorders of prostate**

N42.0 **Calculus of prostate**

Prostatic stone

N42.1 **Congestion and hemorrhage of prostate**

Excludes1: enlarged prostate (N40.-)

hematuria (R31.-)

hyperplasia of prostate (N40.-)

inflammatory diseases of prostate (N41.-)

N42.3 **Dysplasia of prostate**

N42.30 **Unspecified dysplasia of prostate**

N42.31 **Prostatic intraepithelial neoplasia**

PIN

Prostatic intraepithelial neoplasia I (PIN I)

Prostatic intraepithelial neoplasia II (PIN II)

Excludes1: prostatic intraepithelial neoplasia III (PIN III) (D07.5)

N42.32 **Atypical small acinar proliferation of prostate**

N42.39 **Other dysplasia of prostate**

N42.8 **Other specified disorders of prostate**

N42.81 **Prostatodynia syndrome**

Painful prostate syndrome

N42.82 **Prostatosis syndrome**

N42.83 **Cyst of prostate**

N42.89 **Other specified disorders of prostate**

N42.9 **Disorder of prostate, unspecified**

N43 **Hydrocele and spermatocele**

Definition: A Hydrocele is a painless swelling of the scrotum, caused by a collection of fluid around the testicle; commonly occurs in middle-aged men.

Includes: hydrocele of spermatic cord, testis or tunica vaginalis

Excludes1: congenital hydrocele (P83.5)

N43.0 **Encysted hydrocele**

N43.1 **Infected hydrocele**

Use additional code (B95-B97), to identify infectious agent

N43.2 **Other hydrocele**

N43.3 **Hydrocele, unspecified**

N43.4 **Spermatocele of epididymis**

Spermatic cyst

N43.40 **Spermatocele of epididymis, unspecified**

N43.41 **Spermatocele of epididymis, single**

N43.42 **Spermatocele of epididymis, multiple**

N44 **Noninflammatory disorders of testis**

N44.0 **Torsion of testis**

N44.00   Torsion of testis, unspecified

N44.01   Extravaginal torsion of spermatic cord

N44.02   Intravaginal torsion of spermatic cord

      Torsion of spermatic cord NOS

N44.03   Torsion of appendix testis

N44.04   Torsion of appendix epididymis

N44.1   Cyst of tunica albuginea testis

N44.2   Benign cyst of testis

N44.8   Other noninflammatory disorders of the testis

N45   **Orchitis and epididymitis**

Definition: Orchitis is the inflammation and swelling of the testes as a result of infection or physical injury. Epididymitis is an inflammation of the epididymis which is located along the posterior aspect of the testicle.

Use additional code (B95-B97), to identify infectious agent.

N45.1   Epididymitis

N45.2   Orchitis

N45.3   Epididymo-orchitis

N45.4   Abscess of epididymis or testis

N46   **Male infertility**

Excludes1: vasectomy status (Z98.52)

N46.0   Azoospermia

      Absolute male infertility

      Male infertility due to germinal (cell) aplasia

      Male infertility due to spermatogenic arrest (complete)

N46.01   Organic azoospermia

      Azoospermia NOS

N46.02   Azoospermia due to extratesticular causes

      Code also associated cause

      N46.021   Azoospermia due to drug therapy

      N46.022   Azoospermia due to infection

      N46.023   Azoospermia due to obstruction of efferent ducts

      N46.024   Azoospermia due to radiation

      N46.025   Azoospermia due to systemic disease

      N46.029   Azoospermia due to other extratesticular causes

N46.1   Oligospermia

      Male infertility due to germinal cell desquamation

      Male infertility due to hypospermatogenesis

      Male infertility due to incomplete spermatogenic arrest

N46.11   Organic oligospermia

      Oligospermia NOS

N46.12   Oligospermia due to extratesticular causes

      Code also associated cause

      N46.121   Oligospermia due to drug therapy

      N46.122   Oligospermia due to infection

      N46.123   Oligospermia due to obstruction of efferent ducts

      N46.124   Oligospermia due to radiation

      N46.125   Oligospermia due to systemic disease

      N46.129   Oligospermia due to other extratesticular causes

N46.8   Other male infertility

N46.9   Male infertility, unspecified

N47   **Disorders of prepuce**

N47.0   Adherent prepuce, newborn

N47.1   Phimosis

N47.2   Paraphimosis

N47.3   Deficient foreskin

N47.4   Benign cyst of prepuce

N47.5   Adhesions of prepuce and glans penis

N47.6   Balanoposthitis

      Use additional code (B95-B97), to identify infectious agent.

      Excludes1: balanitis (N48.1)

N47.7   Other inflammatory diseases of prepuce

      Use additional code (B95-B97), to identify infectious agent.

N47.8   Other disorders of prepuce

N48   **Other disorders of penis**

N48.0   Leukoplakia of penis

      Balanitis xerotica obliterans

      Kraurosis of penis

      Lichen sclerosus of external male genital organs

      Excludes1: carcinoma in situ of penis (D07.4)

N48.1   Balanitis

      Use additional code (B95-B97), to identify infectious agent

      Excludes1: amebic balanitis (A06.8)

            balanitis xerotica obliterans (N48.0)

            candidal balanitis (B37.42)

            gonococcal balanitis (A54.23)

            herpesviral [herpes simplex] balanitis (A60.01)

N48.2   Other inflammatory disorders of penis

      Use additional code (B95-B97), to identify infectious agent.

      Excludes1: balanitis (N48.1)

            balanitis xerotica obliterans (N48.0)

            balanoposthitis (N47.6)

      N48.21   Abscess of corpus cavernosum and penis

      N48.22   Cellulitis of corpus cavernosum and penis

      N48.29   Other inflammatory disorders of penis

N48.3   Priapism

      Painful erection

      Code first underlying cause

      N48.30   Priapism, unspecified

      N48.31   Priapism due to trauma

      N48.32   Priapism due to disease classified elsewhere

      N48.33   Priapism, drug-induced

      N48.39   Other priapism

N48.5   Ulcer of penis

N48.6   Induration penis plastica

      Peyronie's disease

      Plastic induration of penis

N48.8   Other specified disorders of penis

      N48.81   Thrombosis of superficial vein of penis

      N48.82   Acquired torsion of penis

            Acquired torsion of penis NOS

            Excludes1: congenital torsion of penis (Q55.63)

      N48.83   Acquired buried penis

            Excludes1: congenital hidden penis (Q55.64)

      N48.89   Other specified disorders of penis

N48.9   Disorder of penis, unspecified

N49   **Inflammatory disorders of male genital organs, not elsewhere classified**

   ● New code   ▲ Revised code   **Excludes1:** Not coded here   **Excludes2:** Not included here   ⊗ Placeholder required   ⑦7th digit required

Use additional code (B95-B97), to identify infectious agent

Excludes1: inflammation of penis (N48.1, N48.2-)

orchitis and epididymitis (N45.-)

N49.0 **Inflammatory disorders of seminal vesicle**

Vesiculitis NOS

N49.1 **Inflammatory disorders of spermatic cord, tunica vaginalis and vas deferens**

Vasitis

N49.2 **Inflammatory disorders of scrotum**

N49.3 **Fournier gangrene**

N49.8 **Inflammatory disorders of other specified male genital organs**

Inflammation of multiple sites in male genital organs

N49.9 **Inflammatory disorder of unspecified male genital organ**

Abscess of unspecified male genital organ

Boil of unspecified male genital organ

Carbuncle of unspecified male genital organ

Cellulitis of unspecified male genital organ

N50 **Other and unspecified disorders of male genital organs**

Excludes2: torsion of testis (N44.0-)

N50.0 **Atrophy of testis**

N50.1 **Vascular disorders of male genital organs**

Hematocele, NOS, of male genital organs

Hemorrhage of male genital organs

Thrombosis of male genital organs

N50.3 **Cyst of epididymis**

N50.8 **Other specified disorders of male genital organs**

N50.81 **Testicular pain**

N50.811 **Right testicular pain**

N50.812 **Left testicular pain**

N50.819 **Testicular pain, unspecified**

N50.82 **Scrotal pain**

N50.89 **Other specified disorders of the male genital organs**

Atrophy of scrotum, seminal vesicle, spermatic cord, tunica vaginalis and vas deferens

Chylocele, tunica vaginalis (nonfilarial) NOS

Edema of scrotum, seminal vesicle, spermatic cord, tunica vaginalis and vas deferens

Hypertrophy of scrotum, seminal vesicle, spermatic cord, tunica vaginalis and vas deferens

Stricture of spermatic cord, tunica vaginalis, and vas deferens

Ulcer of scrotum, seminal vesicle, spermatic cord, testis, tunica vaginalis and vas deferens

Urethroscrotal fistula

N50.9 **Disorder of male genital organs, unspecified**

N51 **Disorders of male genital organs in diseases classified elsewhere**

Code first underlying disease, such as:

filariasis (B74.0-B74.9)

Excludes1: amebic balanitis (A06.8)

candidal balanitis (B37.42)

gonococcal balanitis (A54.23)

gonococcal prostatitis (A54.22)

herpesviral [herpes simplex] balanitis (A60.01)

trichomonal prostatitis (A59.02)

tuberculous prostatitis (A18.14)

N52 **Male erectile dysfunction**

Excludes1: psychogenic impotence (F52.21)

N52.0 **Vasculogenic erectile dysfunction**

N52.01 **Erectile dysfunction due to arterial insufficiency**

N52.02 **Corporo-venous occlusive erectile dysfunction**

N52.03 **Combined arterial insufficiency and corporo-venous occlusive erectile dysfunction**

N52.1 **Erectile dysfunction due to diseases classified elsewhere**

Code first underlying disease

N52.2 **Drug-induced erectile dysfunction**

N52.3 **Postprocedural erectile dysfunction**

N52.31 **Erectile dysfunction following radical prostatectomy**

N52.32 **Erectile dysfunction following radical cystectomy**

N52.33 **Erectile dysfunction following urethral surgery**

N52.34 **Erectile dysfunction following simple prostatectomy**

N52.35 **Erectile dysfunction following radiation therapy**

N52.36 **Erectile dysfunction following interstitial seed therapy**

N52.37 **Erectile dysfunction following prostate ablative therapy**

Erectile dysfunction following cryotherapy

Erectile dysfunction following other prostate ablative therapies

Erectile dysfunction following ultrasound ablative therapies

N52.39 **Other and unspecified postprocedural erectile dysfunction**

N52.8 **Other male erectile dysfunction**

N52.9 **Male erectile dysfunction, unspecified**

Impotence NOS

N53 **Other male sexual dysfunction**

Excludes1: psychogenic sexual dysfunction (F52.-)

N53.1 **Ejaculatory dysfunction**

Excludes1: premature ejaculation (F52.4)

N53.11 **Retarded ejaculation**

N53.12 **Painful ejaculation**

N53.13 **Anejaculatory orgasm**

N53.14 **Retrograde ejaculation**

N53.19 **Other ejaculatory dysfunction**

Ejaculatory dysfunction NOS

N53.8 **Other male sexual dysfunction**

N53.9 **Unspecified male sexual dysfunction**

DISORDERS OF BREAST (N60-N65)

Excludes1: disorders of breast associated with childbirth (O91-O92)

N60 **Benign mammary dysplasia**

Definition: Mammary dysplasia is a common condition marked by benign (noncancerous) changes in breast tissue. These changes may include irregular lumps or cysts, breast discomfort, sensitive nipples, and itching.

Includes: fibrocystic mastopathy

N60.0 **Solitary cyst of breast**

Cyst of breast

N60.01 **Solitary cyst of right breast**

N60.02 **Solitary cyst of left breast**

Add 4th-7th digits	Nonspecific code	Unspecified code	Manifestation code

N60.09 Solitary cyst of unspecified breast

N60.1 **Diffuse cystic mastopathy**

Cystic breast

Fibrocystic disease of breast

Excludes1: diffuse cystic mastopathy with epithelial proliferation (N60.3-)

N60.11 Diffuse cystic mastopathy of right breast

N60.12 Diffuse cystic mastopathy of left breast

N60.19 Diffuse cystic mastopathy of unspecified breast

N60.2 **Fibroadenosis of breast**

Adenofibrosis of breast

Excludes2: fibroadenoma of breast (D24.-)

N60.21 Fibroadenosis of right breast

N60.22 Fibroadenosis of left breast ●

N60.29 Fibroadenosis of unspecified breast

N60.3 **Fibrosclerosis of breast**

Cystic mastopathy with epithelial proliferation

N60.31 Fibrosclerosis of right breast

N60.32 Fibrosclerosis of left breast

N60.39 Fibrosclerosis of unspecified breast

N60.4 **Mammary duct ectasia**

N60.41 Mammary duct ectasia of right breast

N60.42 Mammary duct ectasia of left breast

N60.49 Mammary duct ectasia of unspecified breast

N60.8 **Other benign mammary dysplasias**

N60.81 Other benign mammary dysplasias of right breast

N60.82 Other benign mammary dysplasias of left breast

N60.89 Other benign mammary dysplasias of unspecified breast

N60.9 **Unspecified benign mammary dysplasia**

N60.91 Unspecified benign mammary dysplasia of right breast

N60.92 Unspecified benign mammary dysplasia of left breast

N60.99 Unspecified benign mammary dysplasia of unspecified breast

N61 **Inflammatory disorders of breast**

Excludes1: inflammatory carcinoma of breast (C50.9)

inflammatory disorder of breast associated with childbirth (O91.-)

neonatal infective mastitis (P39.0)

thrombophlebitis of breast [Mondor's disease] (I80.8)

N61.0 **Mastitis without abscess**

Infective mastitis (acute) (nonpuerperal) (subacute)

Mastitis (acute) (nonpuerperal) (subacute) NOS

Cellulitis (acute) (nonpuerperal) (subacute) of breast NOS

Cellulitis (acute) (nonpuerperal) (subacute) of nipple NOS

N61.1 **Abscess of the breast and nipple**

Abscess (acute) (chronic) (nonpuerperal) of areola

Abscess (acute) (chronic) (nonpuerperal) of breast

Carbuncle of breast

Mastitis with abscess

N62 **Hypertrophy of breast**

Gynecomastia

Hypertrophy of breast NOS

Massive pubertal hypertrophy of breast

Excludes1: breast engorgement of newborn (P83.4)

disproportion of reconstructed breast (N65.1)

N63 **Unspecified lump in breast**

Nodule(s) NOS in breast

●**N63.0** Unspecified lump in unspecified breast

●**N63.1** Unspecified lump in the right breast

●**N63.10** Unspecified lump in the right breast, unspecified quadrant

●**N63.11** Unspecified lump in the right breast, upper outer quadrant

●**N63.12** Unspecified lump in the right breast, upper inner quadrant

●**N63.13** Unspecified lump in the right breast, lower outer quadrant

●**N63.14** Unspecified lump in the right breast, lower inner quadrant

●**N63.2** Unspecified lump in the left breast

●**N63.20** Unspecified lump in the left breast, unspecified quadrant

●**N63.21** Unspecified lump in the left breast, upper outer quadrant

●**N63.22** Unspecified lump in the left breast, upper inner quadrant

●**N63.23** Unspecified lump in the left breast, lower outer quadrant

●**N63.24** Unspecified lump in the left breast, lower inner quadrant

●**N63.3** Unspecified lump in axillary tail

●**N63.31** Unspecified lump in axillary tail of the right breast

●**N63.32** Unspecified lump in axillary tail of the left breast

●**N63.4** Unspecified lump in breast, subareolar

●**N63.41** Unspecified lump in right breast, subareolar

●**N63.42** Unspecified lump in left breast, subareolar

N64 **Other disorders of breast**

Excludes2: mechanical complication of breast prosthesis and implant (T85.4-)

N64.0 **Fissure and fistula of nipple**

N64.1 **Fat necrosis of breast**

Fat necrosis (segmental) of breast

Code first breast necrosis due to breast graft (T85.898)

N64.2 **Atrophy of breast**

N64.3 **Galactorrhea not associated with childbirth**

N64.4 **Mastodynia**

N64.5 **Other signs and symptoms in breast**

Excludes2: abnormal findings on diagnostic imaging of breast (R92.-)

N64.51 Induration of breast

N64.52 Nipple discharge

Excludes1: abnormal findings in nipple discharge (R89.-)

N64.53 Retraction of nipple

N64.59 Other signs and symptoms in breast

N64.8 **Other specified disorders of breast**

N64.81 Ptosis of breast

Excludes1: ptosis of native breast in relation to reconstructed breast (N65.1)

N64.82 Hypoplasia of breast

Micromastia

● New code ▲ Revised code **Excludes1:** Not coded here **Excludes2:** Not included here ⊗ Placeholder required ⑦ 7th digit required

Excludes1: congenital absence of breast (Q83.0)

hypoplasia of native breast in relation to reconstructed breast (N65.1)

N64.89   Other specified disorders of breast

Galactocele

Subinvolution of breast (postlactational)

N64.9   Disorder of breast, unspecified

N65   Deformity and disproportion of reconstructed breast

N65.0   Deformity of reconstructed breast

Contour irregularity in reconstructed breast

Excess tissue in reconstructed breast

Misshapen reconstructed breast

N65.1   Disproportion of reconstructed breast

Breast asymmetry between native breast and reconstructed breast

Disproportion between native breast and reconstructed breast

INFLAMMATORY DISEASES OF FEMALE PELVIC ORGANS (N70-N77)

NOTE: ALL DIAGNOSIS CODES IN THIS SECTION APPLY TO FEMALE PATIENTS ONLY

Excludes1: inflammatory diseases of female pelvic organs complicating:

abortion or ectopic or molar pregnancy (O00-O07, O08.0)

pregnancy, childbirth and the puerperium (O23.-, O75.3, O85, O86.-)

N70   Salpingitis and oophoritis

Includes: abscess (of) fallopian tube

abscess (of) ovary pyosalpinx salpingo-oophoritis

tubo-ovarian abscess

tubo-ovarian inflammatory disease

Use additional code (B95-B97), to identify infectious agent

Excludes1: gonococcal infection (A54.24)

tuberculous infection (A18.17)

N70.0   Acute salpingitis and oophoritis

N70.01   Acute salpingitis

N70.02   Acute oophoritis

N70.03   Acute salpingitis and oophoritis

N70.1   Chronic salpingitis and oophoritis

Hydrosalpinx

N70.11   Chronic salpingitis

N70.12   Chronic oophoritis

N70.13   Chronic salpingitis and oophoritis

N70.9   Salpingitis and oophoritis, unspecified

N70.91   Salpingitis, unspecified

N70.92   Oophoritis, unspecified

N70.93   Salpingitis and oophoritis, unspecified

N71   Inflammatory disease of uterus, except cervix

Includes: endo (myo) metritis

metritis myometritis pyometra uterine abscess

Use additional code (B95-B97), to identify infectious agent

Excludes1: hyperplastic endometritis (N85.0-)

infection of uterus following delivery (O85, O86.-)

N71.0   Acute inflammatory disease of uterus

N71.1   Chronic inflammatory disease of uterus

N71.9   Inflammatory disease of uterus, unspecified

N72   Inflammatory disease of cervix uteri

Includes: cervicitis (with or without erosion or ectropion)

endocervicitis (with or without erosion or ectropion)

exocervicitis (with or without erosion or ectropion)

Use additional code (B95-B97), to identify infectious agent

Excludes1: erosion and ectropion of cervix without cervicitis (N86)

N73   Other female pelvic inflammatory diseases

Use additional code (B95-B97), to identify infectious agent.

N73.0   Acute parametritis and pelvic cellulitis

Abscess of broad ligament

Abscess of parametrium

Pelvic cellulitis, female

N73.1   Chronic parametritis and pelvic cellulitis

Any condition in N73.0 specified as chronic

Excludes1: tuberculous parametritis and pelvic cellulitis (A18.17)

N73.2   Unspecified parametritis and pelvic cellulitis

Any condition in N73.0 unspecified whether acute or chronic

N73.3   Female acute pelvic peritonitis

N73.4   Female chronic pelvic peritonitis

Excludes1: tuberculous pelvic (female) peritonitis (A18.17)

N73.5   Female pelvic peritonitis, unspecified

N73.6   Female pelvic peritoneal adhesions (postinfective)

Excludes2: postprocedural pelvic peritoneal adhesions (N99.4)

N73.8   Other specified female pelvic inflammatory diseases

N73.9   Female pelvic inflammatory disease, unspecified

Female pelvic infection or inflammation NOS

N74   Female pelvic inflammatory disorders in diseases classified elsewhere

Code first underlying disease

Excludes1: chlamydial cervicitis (A56.02)

chlamydial pelvic inflammatory disease (A56.11)

gonococcal cervicitis (A54.03)

gonococcal pelvic inflammatory disease (A54.24)

herpesviral [herpes simplex] cervicitis (A60.03)

herpesviral [herpes simplex] pelvic inflammatory disease (A60.09)

syphilitic cervicitis (A52.76)

syphilitic pelvic inflammatory disease (A52.76)

trichomonal cervicitis (A59.09)

tuberculous cervicitis (A18.16)

tuberculous pelvic inflammatory disease (A18.17)

N75   Diseases of Bartholin's gland

N75.0   Cyst of Bartholin's gland

N75.1   Abscess of Bartholin's gland

N75.8   Other diseases of Bartholin's gland

Bartholinitis

N75.9   Disease of Bartholin's gland, unspecified

N76   Other inflammation of vagina and vulva

Use additional code (B95-B97), to identify infectious agent

Excludes2: senile (atrophic) vaginitis (N95.2)

vulvar vestibulitis (N94.810)

N76.0   Acute vaginitis

Acute vulvovaginitis

Vaginitis NOS

Vulvovaginitis NOS

N76.1 **Subacute and chronic vaginitis**

Chronic vulvovaginitis

Subacute vulvovaginitis

N76.2 **Acute vulvitis**

Vulvitis NOS

N76.3 **Subacute and chronic vulvitis**

N76.4 **Abscess of vulva**

Furuncle of vulva

N76.5 **Ulceration of vagina**

N76.6 **Ulceration of vulva**

N76.8 **Other specified inflammation of vagina and vulva**

N76.81 **Mucositis (ulcerative) of vagina and vulva**

Code also type of associated therapy, such as:

antineoplastic and immunosuppressive drugs (T45.1X-)

radiological procedure and radiotherapy (Y84.2)

Excludes2: gastrointestinal mucositis (ulcerative) (K92.81)

nasal mucositis (ulcerative) (J34.81)

oral mucositis (ulcerative) (K12.3-)

N76.89 **Other specified inflammation of vagina and vulva**

N77 **Vulvovaginal ulceration and inflammation in diseases classified elsewhere**

N77.0 **Ulceration of vulva in diseases classified elsewhere**

Code first underlying disease, such as:

Behçet's disease (M35.2)

Excludes1: ulceration of vulva in gonococcal infection (A54.02)

ulceration of vulva in herpesviral [herpes simplex] infection (A60.04)

ulceration of vulva in syphilis (A51.0)

ulceration of vulva in tuberculosis (A18.18)

N77.1 **Vaginitis, vulvitis and vulvovaginitis in diseases classified elsewhere**

Code first underlying disease, such as:

pinworm (B80)

Excludes1: candidal vulvovaginitis (B37.3)

chlamydial vulvovaginitis (A56.02)

gonococcal vulvovaginitis (A54.02)

herpesviral [herpes simplex] vulvovaginitis (A60.04)

trichomonal vulvovaginitis (A59.01)

tuberculous vulvovaginitis (A18.18)

vulvovaginitis in early syphilis (A51.0)

vulvovaginitis in late syphilis (A52.76)

NONINFLAMMATORY DISORDERS OF FEMALE GENITAL TRACT (N80-N98)

N80 **Endometriosis**

Definition: Endometriosis is a condition where tissue that normally lines the uterus grows in other areas of the body. This can cause pain, irregular menstrual bleeding, and infertility for some women.

N80.0 **Endometriosis of uterus**

Adenomyosis

Excludes1: stromal endometriosis (D39.0)

N80.1 **Endometriosis of ovary**

N80.2 **Endometriosis of fallopian tube**

N80.3 **Endometriosis of pelvic peritoneum**

N80.4 **Endometriosis of rectovaginal septum and vagina**

N80.5 **Endometriosis of intestine**

N80.6 **Endometriosis in cutaneous scar**

N80.8 **Other endometriosis**

Endometriosis of thorax

N80.9 **Endometriosis, unspecified**

N81 **Female genital prolapse**

Definition: Genital prolapse is a condition in which the vaginal wall or uterus descend below their normal positions; part of the bladder or rectum may protrude from the vagina.

Excludes1: genital prolapse complicating pregnancy, labor or delivery (O34.5-)

prolapse and hernia of ovary and fallopian tube (N83.4-)

prolapse of vaginal vault after hysterectomy (N99.3)

N81.0 **Urethrocele**

Excludes1: urethrocele with cystocele (N81.1-)

urethrocele with prolapse of uterus (N81.2-N81.4)

N81.1 **Cystocele**

Cystocele with urethrocele

Cystourethrocele

Excludes1: cystocele with prolapse of uterus (N81.2-N81.4)

N81.10 **Cystocele, unspecified**

Prolapse of (anterior) vaginal wall NOS

N81.11 **Cystocele, midline**

N81.12 **Cystocele, lateral**

Paravaginal cystocele

N81.2 **Incomplete uterovaginal prolapse**

First degree uterine prolapse

Prolapse of cervix NOS

Second degree uterine prolapse

Excludes1: cervical stump prolapse (N81.85)

N81.3 **Complete uterovaginal prolapse**

Procidentia (uteri) NOS

Third degree uterine prolapse

N81.4 **Uterovaginal prolapse, unspecified**

Prolapse of uterus NOS

N81.5 **Vaginal enterocele**

Excludes1: enterocele with prolapse of uterus (N81.2-N81.4)

N81.6 **Rectocele**

Prolapse of posterior vaginal wall

Use additional code for any associated fecal incontinence, if applicable (R15.-)

Excludes2: perineocele (N81.81)

rectal prolapse (K62.3)

rectocele with prolapse of uterus (N81.2-N81.4)

N81.8 **Other female genital prolapse**

N81.81 **Perineocele**

N81.82 **Incompetence or weakening of pubocervical tissue**

N81.83 **Incompetence or weakening of rectovaginal tissue**

N81.84 **Pelvic muscle wasting**

Disuse atrophy of pelvic muscles and anal sphincter

N81.85 **Cervical stump prolapse**

● New code ▲ Revised code **Excludes1:** Not coded here **Excludes2:** Not included here ⊗ Placeholder required ⑦7th digit required

N81.89 Other female genital prolapse

Deficient perineum

Old laceration of muscles of pelvic floor

N81.9 Female genital prolapse, unspecified

N82 **Fistulae involving female genital tract**

Definition: A fistula involving female genital tract is a fistula that has formed in the wall of the vagina. A vaginal fistula may open into the urinary tract, the rectum, the colon, or the small bowel.

Excludes1: vesicointestinal fistulae (N32.1)

N82.0 Vesicovaginal fistula

N82.1 Other female urinary-genital tract fistulae

Cervicovesical fistula

Ureterovaginal fistula

Urethrovaginal fistula

Uteroureteric fistula

Uterovesical fistula

N82.2 Fistula of vagina to small intestine

N82.3 Fistula of vagina to large intestine

Rectovaginal fistula

N82.4 Other female intestinal-genital tract fistulae

Intestinouterine fistula

N82.5 Female genital tract-skin fistulae

Uterus to abdominal wall fistula

Vaginoperineal fistula

N82.8 Other female genital tract fistulae

N82.9 Female genital tract fistula, unspecified

N83 **Noninflammatory disorders of ovary, fallopian tube and broad ligament**

Excludes2: hydrosalpinx (N70.1-)

N83.0 Follicular cyst of ovary

Cyst of graafian follicle

Hemorrhagic follicular cyst (of ovary)

N83.00 Follicular cyst of ovary, unspecified side

N83.01 Follicular cyst of right ovary

N83.02 Follicular cyst of left ovary

N83.1 Corpus luteum cyst

Hemorrhagic corpus luteum cyst

N83.10 Corpus luteum cyst of ovary, unspecified side

N83.11 Corpus luteum cyst of right ovary

N83.12 Corpus luteum cyst of left ovary

N83.2 Other and unspecified ovarian cysts

Excludes1: developmental ovarian cyst (Q50.1)

neoplastic ovarian cyst (D27.-)

polycystic ovarian syndrome (E28.2)

Stein-Leventhal syndrome (E28.2)

N83.20 Unspecified ovarian cysts

N83.201 Unspecified ovarian cyst, right side

N83.202 Unspecified ovarian cyst, left side

N83.209 Unspecified ovarian cyst, unspecified side

Ovarian cyst, NOS

N83.29 Other ovarian cysts

Retention cyst of ovary

Simple cyst of ovary

N83.291 Other ovarian cyst, right side

N83.292 Other ovarian cyst, left side

N83.299 Other ovarian cyst, unspecified side

N83.3 Acquired atrophy of ovary and fallopian tube

N83.31 Acquired atrophy of ovary

N83.311 Acquired atrophy of right ovary

N83.312 Acquired atrophy of left ovary

N83.319 Acquired atrophy of ovary, unspecified side

Acquired atrophy of ovary, NOS

N83.32 Acquired atrophy of fallopian tube

N83.321 Acquired atrophy of right fallopian tube

N83.322 Acquired atrophy of left fallopian tube

N83.329 Acquired atrophy of fallopian tube, unspecified side

Acquired atrophy of fallopian tube, NOS

N83.33 Acquired atrophy of ovary and fallopian tube

N83.331 Acquired atrophy of right ovary and fallopian tube

N83.332 Acquired atrophy of left ovary and fallopian tube

N83.339 Acquired atrophy of ovary and fallopian tube, unspecified side

Acquired atrophy of ovary and fallopian tube, NOS

N83.4 Prolapse and hernia of ovary and fallopian tube

N83.40 Prolapse and hernia of ovary and fallopian tube, unspecified side

Prolapse and hernia of ovary and fallopian tube, NOS

N83.41 Prolapse and hernia of right ovary and fallopian tube

N83.42 Prolapse and hernia of left ovary and fallopian tube

N83.5 Torsion of ovary, ovarian pedicle and fallopian tube

Torsion of accessory tube

N83.51 Torsion of ovary and ovarian pedicle

N83.511 Torsion of right ovary and ovarian pedicle

N83.512 Torsion of left ovary and ovarian pedicle

N83.519 Torsion of ovary and ovarian pedicle, unspecified side

Torsion of ovary and ovarian pedicle, NOS

N83.52 Torsion of fallopian tube

Torsion of hydatid of Morgagni

N83.521 Torsion of right fallopian tube

N83.522 Torsion of left fallopian tube

N83.529 Torsion of fallopian tube, unspecified side

Torsion of fallopian tube, NOS

N83.53 Torsion of ovary, ovarian pedicle and fallopian tube

N83.6 Hematosalpinx

Excludes1: hematosalpinx (with) (in):

hematocolpos (N89.7)

hematometra (N85.7)

tubal pregnancy (O00.1-)

N83.7 Hematoma of broad ligament

N83.8 **Other noninflammatory disorders of ovary, fallopian tube and broad ligament**

Broad ligament laceration syndrome [Allen-Masters]

N83.9 **Noninflammatory disorder of ovary, fallopian tube and broad ligament, unspecified**

N84 **Polyp of female genital tract**

Excludes1: adenomatous polyp (D28.-)

placental polyp (O90.89)

N84.0 **Polyp of corpus uteri**

Polyp of endometrium

Polyp of uterus NOS

Excludes1: polypoid endometrial hyperplasia (N85.0-)

N84.1 **Polyp of cervix uteri**

Mucous polyp of cervix

N84.2 **Polyp of vagina**

N84.3 **Polyp of vulva**

Polyp of labia

N84.8 **Polyp of other parts of female genital tract**

N84.9 **Polyp of female genital tract, unspecified**

N85 **Other noninflammatory disorders of uterus, except cervix**

Excludes1: endometriosis (N80.-)

inflammatory diseases of uterus (N71.-)

noninflammatory disorders of cervix, except malposition (N86-N88)

polyp of corpus uteri (N84.0)

uterine prolapse (N81.-)

N85.0 **Endometrial hyperplasia**

N85.00 **Endometrial hyperplasia, unspecified**

Hyperplasia (adenomatous) (cystic) (glandular) of endometrium

Hyperplastic endometritis

N85.01 **Benign endometrial hyperplasia**

Endometrial hyperplasia (complex) (simple) without atypia

N85.02 **Endometrial intraepithelial neoplasia [EIN]**

Endometrial hyperplasia with atypia

Excludes1: malignant neoplasm of endometrium (with endometrial intraepithelial neoplasia [EIN]) (C54.1)

N85.2 **Hypertrophy of uterus**

Bulky or enlarged uterus

Excludes1: puerperal hypertrophy of uterus (O90.89)

N85.3 **Subinvolution of uterus**

Excludes1: puerperal subinvolution of uterus (O90.89)

N85.4 **Malposition of uterus**

Anteversion of uterus

Retroflexion of uterus

Retroversion of uterus

Excludes1: malposition of uterus complicating pregnancy, labor or delivery (O34.5-, O65.5)

N85.5 **Inversion of uterus**

Excludes1: current obstetric trauma (O71.2)

postpartum inversion of uterus (O71.2)

N85.6 **Intrauterine synechiae**

N85.7 **Hematometra**

Hematosalpinx with hematometra

Excludes1: hematometra with hematocolpos (N89.7)

N85.8 **Other specified noninflammatory disorders of uterus**

Atrophy of uterus, acquired

Fibrosis of uterus NOS

N85.9 **Noninflammatory disorder of uterus, unspecified**

Disorder of uterus NOS

N86 **Erosion and ectropion of cervix uteri**

Decubitus (trophic) ulcer of cervix

Eversion of cervix

Excludes1: erosion and ectropion of cervix with cervicitis (N72)

N87 **Dysplasia of cervix uteri**

Excludes1: abnormal results from cervical cytologic examination without histologic confirmation (R87.61-)

carcinoma in situ of cervix uteri (D06.-)

cervical intraepithelial neoplasia III [CIN III] (D06.-)

HGSIL of cervix (R87.613)

severe dysplasia of cervix uteri (D06.-)

N87.0 **Mild cervical dysplasia**

Cervical intraepithelial neoplasia I [CIN I]

N87.1 **Moderate cervical dysplasia**

Cervical intraepithelial neoplasia II [CIN II]

N87.9 **Dysplasia of cervix uteri, unspecified**

Anaplasia of cervix

Cervical atypism

Cervical dysplasia NOS

N88 **Other noninflammatory disorders of cervix uteri**

Excludes2: inflammatory disease of cervix (N72)

polyp of cervix (N84.1)

N88.0 **Leukoplakia of cervix uteri**

N88.1 **Old laceration of cervix uteri**

Adhesions of cervix

Excludes1: current obstetric trauma (O71.3)

N88.2 **Stricture and stenosis of cervix uteri**

Excludes1: stricture and stenosis of cervix uteri complicating labor (O65.5)

N88.3 **Incompetence of cervix uteri**

Investigation and management of (suspected) cervical incompetence in a nonpregnant woman

Excludes1: cervical incompetence complicating pregnancy (O34.3-)

N88.4 **Hypertrophic elongation of cervix uteri**

N88.8 **Other specified noninflammatory disorders of cervix uteri**

Excludes1: current obstetric trauma (O71.3)

N88.9 **Noninflammatory disorder of cervix uteri, unspecified**

N89 **Other noninflammatory disorders of vagina**

Excludes1: abnormal results from vaginal cytologic examination without histologic confirmation (R87.62-)

carcinoma in situ of vagina (D07.2)

HGSIL of vagina (R87.623)

inflammation of vagina (N76.-)

senile (atrophic) vaginitis (N95.2)

severe dysplasia of vagina (D07.2)

trichomonal leukorrhea (A59.00)

vaginal intraepithelial neoplasia [VAIN], grade III (D07.2)

N89.0 **Mild vaginal dysplasia**

Vaginal intraepithelial neoplasia [VAIN], grade I

N89.1 **Moderate vaginal dysplasia**

Vaginal intraepithelial neoplasia [VAIN], grade II

● New code ▲ Revised code **Excludes1:** Not coded here **Excludes2:** Not included here ⊗ Placeholder required ⑦7th digit required

N89.3 **Dysplasia of vagina, unspecified**

N89.4 **Leukoplakia of vagina**

N89.5 **Stricture and atresia of vagina**

Vaginal adhesions

Vaginal stenosis

Excludes1: congenital atresia or stricture (Q52.4)

postprocedural adhesions of vagina (N99.2)

N89.6 **Tight hymenal ring**

Rigid hymen

Tight introitus

Excludes1: imperforate hymen (Q52.3)

N89.7 **Hematocolpos**

Hematocolpos with hematometra or hematosalpinx

N89.8 **Other specified noninflammatory disorders of vagina**

Leukorrhea NOS

Old vaginal laceration

Pessary ulcer of vagina

Excludes1: current obstetric trauma (O70.-, O71.4, O71.7-O71.8)

old laceration involving muscles of pelvic floor (N81.8)

N89.9 **Noninflammatory disorder of vagina, unspecified**

N90 **Other noninflammatory disorders of vulva and perineum**

Excludes1: anogenital (venereal) warts (A63.0)

carcinoma in situ of vulva (D07.1)

condyloma acuminatum (A63.0)

current obstetric trauma (O70.-, O71.7-O71.8)

inflammation of vulva (N76.-)

severe dysplasia of vulva (D07.1)

vulvar intraepithelial neoplasm III [VIN III] (D07.1)

N90.0 **Mild vulvar dysplasia**

Vulvar intraepithelial neoplasia [VIN], grade I

N90.1 **Moderate vulvar dysplasia**

Vulvar intraepithelial neoplasia [VIN], grade II

N90.3 **Dysplasia of vulva, unspecified**

N90.4 **Leukoplakia of vulva**

Dystrophy of vulva

Kraurosis of vulva

Lichen sclerosus of external female genital organs

N90.5 **Atrophy of vulva**

Stenosis of vulva

N90.6 **Hypertrophy of vulva**

N90.60 **Unspecified hypertrophy of vulva**

Unspecified hypertrophy of labia

N90.61 **Childhood asymmetric labium majus enlargement**

CALME

N90.69 **Other specified hypertrophy of vulva**

Other specified hypertrophy of labia

N90.7 **Vulvar cyst**

N90.8 **Other specified noninflammatory disorders of vulva and perineum**

N90.81 **Female genital mutilation status**

Female genital cutting status

N90.810 **Female genital mutilation status, unspecified**

Female genital cutting status, unspecified

Female genital mutilation status NOS

N90.811 **Female genital mutilation Type I status**

Clitorectomy status

Female genital cutting Type I status

N90.812 **Female genital mutilation Type II status**

Clitorectomy with excision of labia minora status

Female genital cutting Type II status

N90.813 **Female genital mutilation Type III status**

Female genital cutting Type III status

Infibulation status

N90.818 **Other female genital mutilation status**

Female genital cutting Type IV status

Female genital mutilation Type IV status

Other female genital cutting status

N90.89 **Other specified noninflammatory disorders of vulva and perineum**

Adhesions of vulva

Hypertrophy of clitoris

N90.9 **Noninflammatory disorder of vulva and perineum, unspecified**

N91 **Absent, scanty and rare menstruation**

Excludes1: ovarian dysfunction (E28.-)

N91.0 **Primary amenorrhea**

N91.1 **Secondary amenorrhea**

N91.2 **Amenorrhea, unspecified**

N91.3 **Primary oligomenorrhea**

N91.4 **Secondary oligomenorrhea**

N91.5 **Oligomenorrhea, unspecified**

Hypomenorrhea NOS

N92 **Excessive, frequent and irregular menstruation**

Excludes1: postmenopausal bleeding (N95.0)

precocious puberty (menstruation) (E30.1)

N92.0 **Excessive and frequent menstruation with regular cycle**

Heavy periods NOS

Menorrhagia NOS

Polymenorrhea

N92.1 **Excessive and frequent menstruation with irregular cycle**

Irregular intermenstrual bleeding

Irregular, shortened intervals between menstrual bleeding

Menometrorrhagia

Metrorrhagia

N92.2 **Excessive menstruation at puberty**

Excessive bleeding associated with onset of menstrual periods

Pubertal menorrhagia

Puberty bleeding

N92.3 **Ovulation bleeding**

Regular intermenstrual bleeding

N92.4 **Excessive bleeding in the premenopausal period**

Climacteric menorrhagia or metrorrhagia

Menopausal menorrhagia or metrorrhagia

Preclimacteric menorrhagia or metrorrhagia

Premenopausal menorrhagia or metrorrhagia

N92.5 Other specified irregular menstruation

N92.6 Irregular menstruation, unspecified

Irregular bleeding NOS

Irregular periods NOS

> **Excludes1:** irregular menstruation with:
>
> > lengthened intervals or scanty bleeding (N91.3-N91.5)
> >
> > shortened intervals or excessive bleeding (N92.1)

N93 Other abnormal uterine and vaginal bleeding

> **Excludes1:** neonatal vaginal hemorrhage (P54.6)
>
> precocious puberty (menstruation) (E30.1)
>
> pseudomenses (P54.6)

N93.0 Postcoital and contact bleeding

N93.1 Pre-pubertal vaginal bleeding

N93.8 Other specified abnormal uterine and vaginal bleeding

Dysfunctional or functional uterine or vaginal bleeding NOS

N93.9 Abnormal uterine and vaginal bleeding, unspecified

N94 Pain and other conditions associated with female genital organs and menstrual cycle

N94.0 Mittelschmerz

N94.1 Dyspareunia

> **Excludes1:** psychogenic dyspareunia (F52.6)

N94.10 Unspecified dyspareunia

N94.11 Superficial (introital) dyspareunia

N94.12 Deep dyspareunia

N94.19 Other specified dyspareunia

N94.2 Vaginismus

> **Excludes1:** psychogenic vaginismus (F52.5)

N94.3 Premenstrual tension syndrome

> **Code also** associated menstrual migraine (G43.82-, G43.83-)
>
> **Excludes1:** Premenstrual dysphoric disorder (F32.81)

N94.4 Primary dysmenorrhea

N94.5 Secondary dysmenorrhea

N94.6 Dysmenorrhea, unspecified

> **Excludes1:** psychogenic dysmenorrhea (F45.8)

N94.8 Other specified conditions associated with female genital organs and menstrual cycle

N94.81 Vulvodynia

N94.810 Vulvar vestibulitis

N94.818 Other vulvodynia

N94.819 Vulvodynia, unspecified

Vulvodynia NOS

N94.89 Other specified conditions associated with female genital organs and menstrual cycle

N94.9 Unspecified condition associated with female genital organs and menstrual cycle

N95 Menopausal and other perimenopausal disorders

Menopausal **and other** perimenopausal disorders due to naturally occurring (age-related) menopause and perimenopause

> **Excludes1:** excessive bleeding in the premenopausal period (N92.4)
>
> menopausal and perimenopausal disorders due to artificial or premature menopause (E89.4-, E28.31-)
>
> premature menopause (E28.31-)
>
> **Excludes2:** postmenopausal osteoporosis (M81.0-)

postmenopausal osteoporosis with current pathological fracture (M80.0-)

postmenopausal urethritis (N34.2)

N95.0 Postmenopausal bleeding

N95.1 Menopausal and female climacteric states

Symptoms such as flushing, sleeplessness, headache, lack of concentration, associated with natural (age-related) menopause

> **Use additional code** for associated symptoms
>
> **Excludes1:** asymptomatic menopausal state (Z78.0)
>
> > symptoms associated with artificial menopause (E89.41)
> >
> > symptoms associated with premature menopause (E28.310)

N95.2 Postmenopausal atrophic vaginitis

Senile (atrophic) vaginitis

N95.8 Other specified menopausal and perimenopausal disorders

N95.9 Unspecified menopausal and perimenopausal disorder

N96 Recurrent pregnancy loss

Investigation or care in a nonpregnant woman with history of recurrent pregnancy loss

> **Excludes1:** recurrent pregnancy loss with current pregnancy (O26.2-)

N97 Female infertility

> **Includes:** inability to achieve a pregnancy
>
> sterility, female NOS
>
> **Excludes1:** female infertility associated with:
>
> hypopituitarism (E23.0)
>
> Stein-Leventhal syndrome (E28.2)
>
> **Excludes2:** incompetence of cervix uteri (N88.3)

N97.0 Female infertility associated with anovulation

N97.1 Female infertility of tubal origin

Female infertility associated with congenital anomaly of tube female infertility due to tubal block

Female infertility due to tubal occlusion female infertility due to tubal stenosis

N97.2 Female infertility of uterine origin

Female infertility associated with congenital anomaly of uterus female infertility due to nonimplantation of ovum

N97.8 Female infertility of other origin

N97.9 Female infertility, unspecified

N98 Complications associated with artificial fertilization

N98.0 Infection associated with artificial insemination

N98.1 Hyperstimulation of ovaries

Hyperstimulation of ovaries NOS

Hyperstimulation of ovaries associated with induced ovulation

N98.2 Complications of attempted introduction of fertilized ovum following in vitro fertilization

N98.3 Complications of attempted introduction of embryo in embryo transfer

N98.8 Other complications associated with artificial fertilization

N98.9 Complication associated with artificial fertilization, unspecified

INTRAOPERATIVE AND POSTPROCEDURAL COMPLICATIONS AND DISORDERS OF GENITOURINARY SYSTEM, NOT ELSEWHERE CLASSIFIED (N99)

N99 **Intraoperative and postprocedural complications and disorders of genitourinary system, not elsewhere classified**

Excludes2: irradiation cystitis (N30.4-)

postoophorectomy osteoporosis with current pathological fracture (M80.8-)

postoophorectomy osteoporosis without current pathological fracture (M81.8)

N99.0 **Postprocedural (acute) (chronic) kidney failure**

<u>Use additional code</u> to type of kidney disease

N99.1 **Postprocedural urethral stricture**

Postcatheterization urethral stricture

N99.11 **Postprocedural urethral stricture, male**

N99.110 **Postprocedural urethral stricture, male, meatal**

▲**N99.111** **Postprocedural bulbous urethral stricture, male**

▲**N99.112** **Postprocedural membranous urethral stricture, male**

▲**N99.113** **Postprocedural anterior bulbous urethral stricture, male**

N99.114 **Postprocedural urethral stricture, male, unspecified**

N99.115 **Postprocedural fossa navicularis urethral stricture**

N99.12 **Postprocedural urethral stricture, female**

N99.2 **Postprocedural adhesions of vagina**

N99.3 **Prolapse of vaginal vault after hysterectomy**

N99.4 **Postprocedural pelvic peritoneal adhesions**

Excludes2: pelvic peritoneal adhesions NOS (N73.6)

postinfective pelvic peritoneal adhesions (N73.6)

N99.5 **Complications of stoma of urinary tract**

Excludes2: mechanical complication of urinary catheter (T83.0-)

N99.51 **Complication of cystostomy**

N99.510 **Cystostomy hemorrhage**

N99.511 **Cystostomy infection**

N99.512 **Cystostomy malfunction**

N99.518 **Other cystostomy complication**

N99.52 **Complication of incontinent external stoma of urinary tract**

N99.520 **Hemorrhage of incontinent external stoma of urinary tract**

N99.521 **Infection of incontinent external stoma of urinary tract**

N99.522 **Malfunction of incontinent external stoma of urinary tract**

N99.523 **Herniation of incontinent stoma of urinary tract**

N99.524 **Stenosis of incontinent stoma of urinary tract**

N99.528 **Other complication of incontinent external stoma of urinary tract**

N99.53 **Complication of continent stoma of urinary tract**

N99.530 **Hemorrhage of continent stoma of urinary tract**

N99.531 **Infection of continent stoma of urinary tract**

N99.532 **Malfunction of continent stoma of urinary tract**

N99.533 **Herniation of continent stoma of urinary tract**

N99.534 **Stenosis of continent stoma of urinary tract**

N99.538 **Other complication of continent stoma of urinary tract**

N99.6 **Intraoperative hemorrhage and hematoma of a genitourinary system organ or structure complicating a procedure**

Excludes1: intraoperative hemorrhage and hematoma of a genitourinary system organ or structure due to accidental puncture or laceration during a procedure (N99.7-)

N99.61 **Intraoperative hemorrhage and hematoma of a genitourinary system organ or structure complicating a genitourinary system procedure**

N99.62 **Intraoperative hemorrhage and hematoma of a genitourinary system organ or structure complicating other procedure**

N99.7 **Accidental puncture and laceration of a genitourinary system organ or structure during a procedure**

N99.71 **Accidental puncture and laceration of a genitourinary system organ or structure during a genitourinary system procedure**

N99.72 **Accidental puncture and laceration of a genitourinary system organ or structure during other procedure**

N99.8 **Other intraoperative and postprocedural complications and disorders of genitourinary system**

N99.81 **Other intraoperative complications of genitourinary system**

N99.82 **Postprocedural hemorrhage of a genitourinary system organ or structure following a procedure**

N99.820 **Postprocedural hemorrhage of a genitourinary system organ or structure following a genitourinary system procedure**

N99.821 **Postprocedural hemorrhage of a genitourinary system organ or structure following other procedure**

N99.83 **Residual ovary syndrome**

N99.84 **Postprocedural hematoma and seroma of a genitourinary system organ or structure following a procedure**

N99.840 **Postprocedural hematoma of a genitourinary system organ or structure following a genitourinary system procedure**

N99.841 **Postprocedural hematoma of a genitourinary system organ or structure following other procedure**

N99.842 **Postprocedural seroma of a genitourinary system organ or structure following a genitourinary system procedure**

N99.843 **Postprocedural seroma of a genitourinary system organ or structure following other procedure**

N99.89 **Other postprocedural complications and disorders of genitourinary system**

Chapter 15: Pregnancy, Childbirth And The Puerperium (O00-O9A)

DEFINITIONS

This chapter includes definitions of selected key words, terms and phrases and coding alerts for adding points to the clinical domain, and references to coding late effects where appropriate. An example from this chapter is as follows:

O03   Spontaneous abortion

> **Definition:** *Spontaneous abortion* refers to the loss of pregnancy before 20 weeks of gestation without outside intervention.

MULTIPLE CODING FOR A SINGLE CONDITION

In addition to the etiology/manifestation convention that requires two codes to fully describe a single condition that affects multiple body systems, there are other single conditions that also require more than one code. "Use additional code" notes are found in the Tabular List at codes that are not part of an etiology/manifestation pair where a secondary code is useful to fully describe a condition. The sequencing rule is the same as the etiology/manifestation pair, "use additional code" indicates that a secondary code should be added.

For example, for bacterial infections that are not included in chapter 1, a secondary code from category B95, Streptococcus, Staphylococcus, and Enterococcus, as the cause of diseases classified elsewhere, or B96, Other bacterial agents as the cause of diseases classified elsewhere, may be required to identify the bacterial organism causing the infection. A "use additional code" note will normally be found at the infectious disease code, indicating a need for the organism code to be added as a secondary code.

"Code first" notes are also under certain codes that are not specifically manifestation codes but may be due to an underlying cause. When there is a "code first" note and an underlying condition is present, the underlying condition should be sequenced first.

"Code, if applicable, any causal condition first", notes indicate that this code may be assigned as a principal diagnosis when the causal condition is unknown or not applicable. If a causal condition is known, then the code for that condition should be sequenced as the principal or first-listed diagnosis.

Multiple codes may be needed for sequela, complication codes and obstetric codes to more fully describe a condition. See the specific guidelines for these conditions for further instruction.

COMBINATION CODE

A combination code is a single code used to classify: Two diagnoses, or a diagnosis with an associated secondary process (manifestation) A diagnosis with an associated complication

Combination codes are identified by referring to subterm entries in the Alphabetic Index and by reading the inclusion and exclusion notes in the Tabular List.

Assign only the combination code when that code fully identifies the diagnostic conditions involved or when the Alphabetic Index so directs. Multiple coding should not be used when the classification provides a combination code that clearly identifies all of the elements documented in the diagnosis. When the combination code lacks necessary specificity in describing the manifestation or complication, an additional code should be used as a secondary code.

SEQUELA (LATE EFFECTS)

A sequela is the residual effect (condition produced) after the acute phase of an illness or injury has terminated. There is no time limit on when a sequela code can be used. The residual may be apparent early, such as in cerebral infarction, or it may occur months or years later, such as that due to a previous injury. Coding of sequela generally requires two codes sequenced in the following order: The condition or nature of the sequela is sequenced first.

The sequela code is sequenced second.

An exception to the above guidelines are those instances where the code for the sequela is followed by a manifestation code identified in the Tabular List and title, or the sequela code has been expanded (at the fourth, fifth or sixth character levels) to include the manifestation(s). The code for the acute phase of an illness or injury that led to the sequela is never used with a code for the late effect.

GENERAL RULES FOR OBSTETRIC CASES

1)   Codes from chapter 15 and sequencing priority

Obstetric cases require codes from chapter 15, codes in the range O00-O9A, Pregnancy, Childbirth, and the Puerperium. Chapter 15 codes have sequencing priority over codes from other chapters. Additional codes from other chapters may be used in conjunction with chapter 15 codes to further specify conditions. Should the provider document that the pregnancy is incidental to the encounter, then code Z33.1, Pregnant state, incidental, should be used in place of any chapter 15 codes. It is the provider's responsibility to state that the condition being treated is not affecting the pregnancy.

2)   Chapter 15 codes used only on the maternal record

Chapter 15 codes are to be used only on the maternal record, never on the record of the newborn.

3)   Final character for trimester

The majority of codes in Chapter 15 have a final character indicating the trimester of pregnancy. The timeframes for the trimesters are indicated at the beginning of the chapter. If trimester is not a component of a code, it is because the condition always occurs in a specific trimester, or the concept of trimester of pregnancy is not applicable. Certain codes have characters for only certain trimesters because the condition does not occur in all trimesters, but it may occur in more than just one.

Assignment of the final character for trimester should be based on the provider's documentation of the trimester (or number of weeks) for the current admission/encounter. This applies to the assignment of trimester for pre-existing conditions as well as those that develop during or are due to the pregnancy. The provider's documentation of the number of weeks may be used to assign the appropriate code identifying the trimester.

Whenever delivery occurs during the current admission, and there is an "in childbirth" option for the obstetric complication being coded, the "in childbirth" code should be assigned.

4) Selection of trimester for inpatient admissions that encompass more than one trimester

In instances when a patient is admitted to a hospital for complications of pregnancy during one trimester and remains in the hospital into a subsequent trimester, the trimester character for the antepartum complication code should be assigned on the basis of the trimester when the complication developed, not the trimester of the discharge. If the condition developed prior to the current admission/encounter or represents a pre-existing condition, the trimester character for the trimester at the time of the admission/encounter should be assigned.

5) Unspecified trimester

Each category that includes codes for trimester has a code for "unspecified trimester." The "unspecified trimester" code should rarely be used, such as when the documentation in the record is insufficient to determine the trimester and it is not possible to obtain clarification.

6) 7th character for Fetus Identification

Where applicable, a 7th character is to be assigned for certain categories (O31, O32, O33.3 - O33.6, O35, O36, O40, O41, O60.1, O60.2, O64, and O69) to identify the fetus for which the complication code applies.

Assign 7th character "0":

- For single gestations

- When the documentation in the record is insufficient to determine the fetus affected and it is not possible to obtain clarification.

- When it is not possible to clinically determine which fetus is affected.

SELECTION OF OB PRINCIPAL OR FIRST-LISTED DIAGNOSIS

1) Routine outpatient prenatal visits

For routine outpatient prenatal visits when no complications are present, a code from category Z34, Encounter for supervision of normal pregnancy, should be used as the first-listed diagnosis. These codes should not be used in conjunction with chapter 15 codes.

2) Supervision of High-Risk Pregnancy

Codes from category O09, Supervision of high-risk pregnancy, are intended for use only during the prenatal period. For complications during the labor or delivery episode as a result of a high-risk pregnancy, assign the applicable complication codes from Chapter 15. If there are no complications during the labor or delivery episode, assign code O80, Encounter for full-term uncomplicated delivery.

For routine prenatal outpatient visits for patients with high-risk pregnancies, a code from category O09, Supervision of high-risk pregnancy, should be used as the first-listed diagnosis. Secondary chapter 15 codes may be used in conjunction with these codes if appropriate.

3) Episodes when no delivery occurs

In episodes when no delivery occurs, the principal diagnosis should correspond to the principal complication of the pregnancy which necessitated the encounter. Should more than one complication exist, all of which are treated or monitored, any of the complications codes may be sequenced first.

4) When a delivery occurs

When an obstetric patient is admitted and delivers during that admission, the condition that prompted the admission should be sequenced as the principal diagnosis. If multiple conditions prompted the admission, sequence the one most related to the delivery as the principal diagnosis. A code for any complication of the delivery should be assigned as an additional diagnosis. In cases of cesarean delivery, if the patient was admitted with a condition that resulted in the performance of a cesarean procedure, that condition should be selected as the principal diagnosis. If the reason for the admission was unrelated to the condition resulting in the cesarean delivery, the condition related to the reason for the admission should be selected as the principal diagnosis.

5) Outcome of delivery

A code from category Z37, Outcome of delivery, should be included on every maternal record when a delivery has occurred. These codes are not to be used on subsequent records or on the newborn record.

PRE-EXISTING CONDITIONS VERSUS CONDITIONS DUE TO THE PREGNANCY

Certain categories in Chapter 15 distinguish between conditions of the mother that existed prior to pregnancy (pre-existing) and those that are a direct result of pregnancy. When assigning codes from Chapter 15, it is important to assess if a condition was pre-existing prior to pregnancy or developed during or due to the pregnancy in order to assign the correct code.

Categories that do not distinguish between pre-existing and pregnancy-related conditions may be used for either. It is acceptable to use codes specifically for the puerperium with codes complicating pregnancy and childbirth if a condition arises postpartum during the delivery encounter.

PRE-EXISTING HYPERTENSION IN PREGNANCY

Category O10, Pre-existing hypertension complicating pregnancy, childbirth and the puerperium, includes codes for hypertensive heart and hypertensive chronic kidney disease. When assigning one of the O10 codes that includes hypertensive heart disease or hypertensive chronic kidney disease, it is necessary to add a secondary code from the appropriate hypertension category to specify the type of heart failure or chronic kidney disease.

See Section I.C.9. Hypertension.

FETAL CONDITIONS AFFECTING THE MANAGEMENT OF THE MOTHER

1) **Codes from categories O35 and O36**

   Codes from categories O35, Maternal care for known or suspected fetal abnormality and damage, and O36, Maternal care for other fetal problems, are assigned only when the fetal condition is actually responsible for modifying the management of the mother, i.e., by requiring diagnostic studies, additional observation, special care, or termination of pregnancy. The fact that the fetal condition exists does not justify assigning a code from this series to the mother's record.

2) **In utero surgery**

   In cases when surgery is performed on the fetus, a diagnosis code from category O35, Maternal care for known or suspected fetal abnormality and damage, should be assigned identifying the fetal condition. Assign the appropriate procedure code for the procedure performed.

   No code from Chapter 16, the perinatal codes, should be used on the mother's record to identify fetal conditions. Surgery performed in utero on a fetus is still to be coded as an obstetric encounter.

HIV INFECTION IN PREGNANCY, CHILDBIRTH AND THE PUERPERIUM

During pregnancy, childbirth or the puerperium, a patient admitted because of an HIV-related illness should receive a principal diagnosis from subcategory O98.7-, Human immunodeficiency [HIV] disease complicating pregnancy, childbirth and the puerperium, followed by the code(s) for the HIV-related illness(es).

Patients with asymptomatic HIV infection status admitted during pregnancy, childbirth, or the puerperium should receive codes of O98.7- and Z21, Asymptomatic human immunodeficiency virus [HIV] infection status.

DIABETES MELLITUS IN PREGNANCY

Diabetes mellitus is a significant complicating factor in pregnancy. Pregnant women who are diabetic should be assigned a code from category O24, Diabetes mellitus in pregnancy, childbirth, and the puerperium, first, followed by the appropriate diabetes code(s) (E08-E13) from Chapter 4.

LONG TERM USE OF INSULIN AND ORAL HYPOGLYCEMICS

Code Z79.4, Long-term (current) use of insulin, or code Z79.84, Long-term (current) use of oral hypoglycemic drugs, should also be assigned if the diabetes mellitus is being treated with insulin or oral medications. If the patient is treated with both oral medications and insulin, only the code for insulin-controlled should be assigned.

GESTATIONAL (PREGNANCY INDUCED) DIABETES

Gestational (pregnancy induced) diabetes can occur during the second and third trimester of pregnancy in women who were not diabetic prior to pregnancy. Gestational diabetes can cause complications in the pregnancy similar to those of pre-existing diabetes mellitus. It also puts the woman at greater risk of developing diabetes after the pregnancy. Codes for gestational diabetes are in subcategory O24.4, Gestational diabetes mellitus. No other code from category O24, Diabetes mellitus in pregnancy, childbirth, and the puerperium, should be used with a code from O24.4.

The codes under subcategory O24.4 include diet controlled, insulin controlled, and controlled by oral hypoglycemic drugs. If a patient with gestational diabetes is treated with both diet and insulin, only the code for insulin-controlled is required. If a patient with gestational diabetes is treated with both diet and oral hypoglycemic medications, only the code for "controlled by oral hypoglycemic drugs" is required. Code Z79.4, Long-term (current) use of insulin or code Z79.84, Long-term (current) use of oral hypoglycemic drugs, should not be assigned with codes from subcategory O24.4. An abnormal glucose tolerance in pregnancy is assigned a code from subcategory O99.81, Abnormal glucose complicating pregnancy, childbirth, and the puerperium.

SEPSIS AND SEPTIC SHOCK COMPLICATING ABORTION, PREGNANCY, CHILDBIRTH AND THE PUERPERIUM

When assigning a chapter 15 code for sepsis complicating abortion, pregnancy, childbirth, and the puerperium, a code for the specific type of infection should be assigned as an additional diagnosis. If severe sepsis is present, a code from subcategory R65.2, Severe sepsis, and code(s) for associated organ dysfunction(s) should also be assigned as additional diagnoses.

PUERPERAL SEPSIS

Code O85, Puerperal sepsis, should be assigned with a secondary code to identify the causal organism (e.g., for a bacterial infection, assign a code from category B95-B96, Bacterial infections in conditions classified elsewhere). A code from category A40, Streptococcal sepsis, or A41, Other sepsis, should not be used for puerperal sepsis. If applicable, use additional codes to identify severe sepsis (R65.2-) and any associated acute organ dysfunction.

ALCOHOL AND TOBACCO USE DURING PREGNANCY, CHILDBIRTH AND THE PUERPERIUM

1) Alcohol use during pregnancy, childbirth and the puerperium

Codes under subcategory O99.31, Alcohol use complicating pregnancy, childbirth, and the puerperium, should be assigned for any pregnancy case when a mother uses alcohol during the pregnancy or postpartum. A secondary code from category F10, Alcohol related disorders, should also be assigned to identify manifestations of the alcohol use.

2) Tobacco use during pregnancy, childbirth and the puerperium

Codes under subcategory O99.33, Smoking (tobacco) complicating pregnancy, childbirth, and the puerperium, should be assigned for any pregnancy case when a mother uses any type of tobacco product during the pregnancy or postpartum. A secondary code from category F17, Nicotine dependence, should also be assigned to identify the type of nicotine dependence.

POISONING, TOXIC EFFECTS, ADVERSE EFFECTS AND UNDERDOSING IN A PREGNANT PATIENT

A code from subcategory O9A.2, Injury, poisoning and certain other consequences of external causes complicating pregnancy, childbirth, and the puerperium, should be sequenced first, followed by the appropriate injury, poisoning, toxic effect, adverse effect or underdosing code, and then the additional code(s) that specifies the condition caused by the poisoning, toxic effect, adverse effect or underdosing.

See Section I.C.19. Adverse effects, poisoning, underdosing and toxic effects.

NORMAL DELIVERY, CODE O80

1) Encounter for full term uncomplicated delivery

Code O80 should be assigned when a woman is admitted for a full-term normal delivery and delivers a single, healthy infant without any complications antepartum, during the delivery, or postpartum during the delivery episode. Code O80 is always a principal diagnosis. It is not to be used if any other code from chapter 15 is needed to describe a current complication of the antenatal, delivery, or perinatal period. Additional codes from other chapters may be used with code O80 if they are not related to or are in any way complicating the pregnancy.

2) Uncomplicated delivery with resolved antepartum complication

Code O80 may be used if the patient had a complication at some point during the pregnancy, but the complication is not present at the time of the admission for delivery.

3) Outcome of delivery for O80

Z37.0, Single live birth, is the only outcome of delivery code appropriate for use with O80.

THE PERIPARTUM AND POSTPARTUM PERIODS

1) Peripartum and Postpartum periods

The postpartum period begins immediately after delivery and continues for six weeks following delivery. The peripartum period is defined as the last month of pregnancy to five months postpartum.

2) Peripartum and postpartum complication

A postpartum complication is any complication occurring within the six-week period.

3) Pregnancy-related complications after 6 week period

Chapter 15 codes may also be used to describe pregnancy-related complications after the peripartum or postpartum period if the provider documents that a condition is pregnancy related.

4) Admission for routine postpartum care following delivery outside hospital

When the mother delivers outside the hospital prior to admission and is admitted for routine postpartum care and no complications are noted, code Z39.0, Encounter for care and examination of mother immediately after delivery, should be assigned as the principal diagnosis.

5) Pregnancy associated cardiomyopathy

Pregnancy associated cardiomyopathy, code O90.3, is unique in that it may be diagnosed in the third trimester of pregnancy but may continue to progress months after delivery. For this reason, it is referred to as peripartum cardiomyopathy. Code O90.3 is only for use when the cardiomyopathy develops as a result of pregnancy in a woman who did not have pre-existing heart disease.

CODE O94, SEQUELAE OF COMPLICATION OF PREGNANCY, CHILDBIRTH, AND THE PUERPERIUM

1) Code O94

Code O94, Sequelae of complication of pregnancy, childbirth, and the puerperium, is for use in those cases when an initial complication of a pregnancy develops a sequelae requiring care or treatment at a future date.

2) After the initial postpartum period

This code may be used at any time after the initial postpartum period.

3) Sequencing of Code O94

This code, like all sequela codes, is to be sequenced following the code describing the sequelae of the complication.

TERMINATION OF PREGNANCY AND SPONTANEOUS ABORTIONS

1) Abortion with Liveborn Fetus

When an attempted termination of pregnancy results in a liveborn fetus, assign code Z33.2, Encounter for elective termination of pregnancy and a code from category Z37, Outcome of Delivery.

2) Retained Products of Conception following an abortion

Subsequent encounters for retained products of conception following a spontaneous abortion or elective termination of pregnancy are assigned the appropriate code from category O03, Spontaneous abortion, or codes O07.4, Failed attempted termination of pregnancy without complication and Z33.2, Encounter for elective termination of pregnancy. This advice is appropriate even when the patient was discharged previously with a discharge diagnosis of complete abortion.

3) Complications leading to abortion

Codes from Chapter 15 may be used as additional codes to identify any documented complications of the pregnancy in conjunction with codes in categories in O07 and O08.

ABUSE IN A PREGNANT PATIENT

For suspected or confirmed cases of abuse of a pregnant patient, a code(s) from subcategories O9A.3, Physical abuse complicating pregnancy, childbirth, and the puerperium, O9A.4, Sexual abuse complicating pregnancy, childbirth, and the puerperium, and O9A.5, Psychological abuse complicating pregnancy, childbirth, and the puerperium, should be sequenced first, followed by the appropriate codes (if applicable) to identify any associated current injury due to physical abuse, sexual abuse, and the perpetrator of abuse.

See Section I.C.19. Adult and child abuse, neglect and other maltreatment.

Chapter 15

Pregnancy, Childbirth And The Puerperium (O00-O9A)

NOTE: ALL DIAGNOSIS CODES IN THIS CHAPTER APPLY TO FEMALE PATIENTS ONLY

NOTE: CODES FROM THIS CHAPTER ARE FOR USE ONLY ON MATERNAL RECORDS, NEVER ON NEWBORN RECORDS

Codes from this chapter are for use for conditions related to or aggravated by the pregnancy, childbirth, or by the puerperium (maternal causes or obstetric causes) trimesters are counted from the first day of the last menstrual period. They are defined as follows:

1st trimester- less than 14 weeks 0 days

2nd trimester- 14 weeks 0 days to less than 28 weeks 0 days

3rd trimester- 28 weeks 0 days until delivery

Use additional code from category Z3A, Weeks of gestation, to identify the specific week of the pregnancy, if known.

Excludes1: supervision of normal pregnancy (Z34.-)

Excludes2: mental and behavioral disorders associated with the puerperium (F53)

obstetrical tetanus (A34)

postpartum necrosis of pituitary gland (E23.0)

puerperal osteomalacia (M83.0)

This chapter contains the following blocks:

O00-O08	Pregnancy with abortive outcome
O09	Supervision of high risk pregnancy
O10-O16	Edema, proteinuria and hypertensive disorders in pregnancy, childbirth and the puerperium
O20-O29	Other maternal disorders predominantly related to pregnancy
O30-O48	Maternal care related to the fetus and amniotic cavity and possible delivery problems
O60-O77	Complications of labor and delivery
O80-O82	Encounter for delivery
O85-O92	Complications predominantly related to the puerperium
O94-O9A	Other obstetric conditions, not elsewhere classified

PREGNANCY WITH ABORTIVE OUTCOME (O00-O08)

Excludes1: continuing pregnancy in multiple gestation after abortion of one fetus or more (O31.1-, O31.3-)

O00   Ectopic pregnancy

Includes: ruptured ectopic pregnancy

Use additional code from category O08 to identify any associated complication

O00.0   Abdominal pregnancy

Excludes1: maternal care for viable fetus in abdominal pregnancy (O36.7-)

O00.00   Abdominal pregnancy without intrauterine pregnancy

Abdominal pregnancy NOS

O00.01   Abdominal pregnancy with intrauterine pregnancy

O00.1   Tubal pregnancy

Fallopian pregnancy

Rupture of (fallopian) tube due to pregnancy

Tubal abortion

O00.10   Tubal pregnancy without intrauterine pregnancy

Tubal pregnancy NOS

- **O00.101   Right tubal pregnancy without intrauterine pregnancy**
- **O00.102   Left tubal pregnancy without intrauterine pregnancy**
- **O00.109   Unspecified tubal pregnancy without intrauterine pregnancy**

O00.11   Tubal pregnancy with intrauterine pregnancy

- **O00.111   Right tubal pregnancy with intrauterine pregnancy**
- **O00.112   Left tubal pregnancy with intrauterine pregnancy**
- **O00.119   Unspecified tubal pregnancy with intrauterine pregnancy**

O00.2   Ovarian pregnancy

O00.20   Ovarian pregnancy without intrauterine pregnancy

Ovarian pregnancy NOS

- **O00.201   Right ovarian pregnancy without intrauterine pregnancy**
- **O00.202   Left ovarian pregnancy without intrauterine pregnancy**
- **O00.209   Unspecified ovarian pregnancy without intrauterine pregnancy**

O00.21   Ovarian pregnancy with intrauterine pregnancy

- **O00.211   Right ovarian pregnancy with intrauterine pregnancy**
- **O00.212   Left ovarian pregnancy with intrauterine pregnancy**
- **O00.219   Unspecified ovarian pregnancy with intrauterine pregnancy**

O00.8   Other ectopic pregnancy

Definition: Ectopic pregnancy occurs with the implantation and subsequent development of a fertilized ovum outside the uterus, as in a fallopian tube.

Cervical pregnancy

Cornual pregnancy

Intraligamentous pregnancy

Mural pregnancy

O00.80   Other ectopic pregnancy without intrauterine pregnancy

Other ectopic pregnancy NOS

O00.81   Other ectopic pregnancy with intrauterine pregnancy

O00.9   Ectopic pregnancy, unspecified

O00.90   Unspecified ectopic pregnancy without intrauterine pregnancy

Ectopic pregnancy NOS

O00.91   Unspecified ectopic pregnancy with intrauterine pregnancy

O01   Hydatidiform mole

Definition: A Hydatidiform mole is a rare mass or growth that forms inside the uterus at the beginning of a pregnancy. It is a type of gestational trophoblastic disease (GTD).

Use additional code from category O08 to identify any associated complication.

Excludes1: chorioadenoma (destruens) (D39.2)

malignant hydatidiform mole (D39.2)

O01.0   Classical hydatidiform mole

Complete hydatidiform mole

O01.1   Incomplete and partial hydatidiform mole

O01.9 **Hydatidiform mole, unspecified**

Trophoblastic disease NOS

Vesicular mole NOS

O02 **Other abnormal products of conception**

Use additional code from category O08 to identify any associated complication.

Excludes1: papyraceous fetus (O31.0-)

O02.0 **Blighted ovum and nonhydatidiform mole**

Carneous mole

Fleshy mole

Intrauterine mole NOS

Molar pregnancy NEC

Pathological ovum

O02.1 **Missed abortion**

Definition: A missed abortion is an abortion in which the fetus dies but is retained within the uterus for two months or longer.

Early fetal death, before completion of 20 weeks of gestation, with retention of dead fetus

Excludes1: failed induced abortion (O07.-)

fetal death (intrauterine) (late) (O36.4)

missed abortion with blighted ovum (O02.0)

missed abortion with hydatidiform mole (O01.-)

missed abortion with nonhydatidiform (O02.0)

missed abortion with other abnormal products of conception (O02.8-)

missed delivery (O36.4)

stillbirth (P95)

O02.8 **Other specified abnormal products of conception**

Excludes1: abnormal products of conception with blighted ovum (O02.0)

abnormal products of conception with hydatidiform mole (O01.-)

abnormal products of conception with nonhydatidiform mole (O02.0)

O02.81 **Inappropriate change in quantitative human chorionic gonadotropin (hCG) in early pregnancy**

Biochemical pregnancy

Chemical pregnancy

Inappropriate level of quantitative human chorionic gonadotropin (hCG) for gestational age in early pregnancy

O02.89 **Other abnormal products of conception**

O02.9 **Abnormal product of conception, unspecified**

O03 **Spontaneous abortion**

Definition: Spontaneous abortion refers to the loss of pregnancy before 20 weeks of gestation without outside intervention.

Note: Incomplete abortion includes retained products of conception following spontaneous abortion

Includes: miscarriage

O03.0 **Genital tract and pelvic infection following incomplete spontaneous abortion**

Endometritis following incomplete spontaneous abortion

Oophoritis following incomplete spontaneous abortion

Parametritis following incomplete spontaneous abortion

Pelvic peritonitis following incomplete spontaneous abortion

Salpingitis following incomplete spontaneous abortion

Salpingo-oophoritis following incomplete spontaneous abortion

Excludes1: sepsis following incomplete spontaneous abortion (O03.37)

urinary tract infection following incomplete spontaneous abortion (O03.38)

O03.1 **Delayed or excessive hemorrhage following incomplete spontaneous abortion**

Afibrinogenemia following incomplete spontaneous abortion

Defibrination syndrome following incomplete spontaneous abortion

Hemolysis following incomplete spontaneous abortion

Intravascular coagulation following incomplete spontaneous abortion

O03.2 **Embolism following incomplete spontaneous abortion**

Air embolism following incomplete spontaneous abortion

Amniotic fluid embolism following incomplete spontaneous abortion

Blood-clot embolism following incomplete spontaneous abortion

Embolism NOS following incomplete spontaneous abortion

Fat embolism following incomplete spontaneous abortion

Pulmonary embolism following incomplete spontaneous abortion

Pyemic embolism following incomplete spontaneous abortion

Septic or septicopyemic embolism following incomplete spontaneous abortion

Soap embolism following incomplete spontaneous abortion

O03.3 **Other and unspecified complications following incomplete spontaneous abortion**

O03.30 **Unspecified complication following incomplete spontaneous abortion**

O03.31 **Shock following incomplete spontaneous abortion**

Circulatory collapse following incomplete spontaneous abortion

Shock (postprocedural) following incomplete spontaneous abortion

Excludes1: shock due to infection following incomplete spontaneous abortion (O03.37)

O03.32 **Renal failure following incomplete spontaneous abortion**

Kidney failure (acute) following incomplete spontaneous abortion

Oliguria following incomplete spontaneous abortion

Renal shutdown following incomplete spontaneous abortion

Renal tubular necrosis following incomplete spontaneous abortion

Uremia following incomplete spontaneous abortion

O03.33 **Metabolic disorder following incomplete spontaneous abortion**

O03.34 **Damage to pelvic organs following incomplete spontaneous abortion**

Laceration, perforation, tear or chemical damage of bladder following incomplete spontaneous abortion

Laceration, perforation, tear or chemical damage of bowel following incomplete spontaneous abortion

Laceration, perforation, tear or chemical damage of broad ligament following incomplete spontaneous abortion

Laceration, perforation, tear or chemical damage of cervix following incomplete spontaneous abortion

Laceration, perforation, tear or chemical damage of periurethral tissue following incomplete spontaneous abortion

Laceration, perforation, tear or chemical damage of uterus following incomplete spontaneous abortion

Laceration, perforation, tear or chemical damage of vagina following incomplete spontaneous abortion

O03.35   Other venous complications following incomplete spontaneous abortion

O03.36   Cardiac arrest following incomplete spontaneous abortion

O03.37   Sepsis following incomplete spontaneous abortion

Use additional code to identify infectious agent (B95-B97)

Use additional code to identify severe sepsis, if applicable (R65.2-)

Excludes1: septic or septicopyemic embolism following incomplete spontaneous abortion (O03.2)

O03.38   Urinary tract infection following incomplete spontaneous abortion

Cystitis following incomplete spontaneous abortion

O03.39   Incomplete spontaneous abortion with other complications

O03.4   Incomplete spontaneous abortion without complication

O03.5   Genital tract and pelvic infection following complete or unspecified spontaneous abortion

Endometritis following complete or unspecified spontaneous abortion

Oophoritis following complete or unspecified spontaneous abortion

Parametritis following complete or unspecified spontaneous abortion

Pelvic peritonitis following complete or unspecified spontaneous abortion

Salpingitis following complete or unspecified spontaneous abortion

Salpingo-oophoritis following complete or unspecified spontaneous abortion

Excludes1: sepsis following complete or unspecified spontaneous abortion (O03.87)

urinary tract infection following complete or unspecified spontaneous abortion (O03.88)

O03.6   Delayed or excessive hemorrhage following complete or unspecified spontaneous abortion

Afibrinogenemia following complete or unspecified spontaneous abortion

Defibrination syndrome following complete or unspecified spontaneous abortion

Hemolysis following complete or unspecified spontaneous abortion

Intravascular coagulation following complete or unspecified spontaneous abortion

O03.7   Embolism following complete or unspecified spontaneous abortion

Air embolism following complete or unspecified spontaneous abortion

Amniotic fluid embolism following complete or unspecified spontaneous abortion

Blood-clot embolism following complete or unspecified spontaneous abortion

Embolism NOS following complete or unspecified spontaneous abortion

Fat embolism following complete or unspecified spontaneous abortion

Pulmonary embolism following complete or unspecified spontaneous abortion

Pyemic embolism following complete or unspecified spontaneous abortion

Septic or septicopyemic embolism following complete or unspecified spontaneous abortion

Soap embolism following complete or unspecified spontaneous abortion

O03.8   Other and unspecified complications following complete or unspecified spontaneous abortion

O03.80   Unspecified complication following complete or unspecified spontaneous abortion

O03.81   Shock following complete or unspecified spontaneous abortion

Circulatory collapse following complete or unspecified spontaneous abortion

Shock (postprocedural) following complete or unspecified spontaneous abortion

Excludes1: shock due to infection following complete or unspecified spontaneous abortion (O03.87)

O03.82   Renal failure following complete or unspecified spontaneous abortion

Kidney failure (acute) following complete or unspecified spontaneous abortion

Oliguria following complete or unspecified spontaneous abortion

Renal shutdown following complete or unspecified spontaneous abortion

Renal tubular necrosis following complete or unspecified spontaneous abortion

Uremia following complete or unspecified spontaneous abortion

O03.83   Metabolic disorder following complete or unspecified spontaneous abortion

O03.84   Damage to pelvic organs following complete or unspecified spontaneous abortion

Laceration, perforation, tear or chemical damage of bladder following complete or unspecified spontaneous abortion

Laceration, perforation, tear or chemical damage of bowel following complete or unspecified spontaneous abortion

Laceration, perforation, tear or chemical damage of broad ligament following complete or unspecified spontaneous abortion

Laceration, perforation, tear or chemical damage of cervix following complete or unspecified spontaneous abortion

Laceration, perforation, tear or chemical damage of periurethral tissue following complete or unspecified spontaneous abortion

Laceration, perforation, tear or chemical damage of uterus following complete or unspecified spontaneous abortion

Laceration, perforation, tear or chemical damage of vagina following complete or unspecified spontaneous abortion

O03.85 **Other venous complications following complete or unspecified spontaneous abortion**

O03.86 **Cardiac arrest following complete or unspecified spontaneous abortion**

O03.87 **Sepsis following complete or unspecified spontaneous abortion**

Use additional code to identify infectious agent (B95-B97)

Use additional code to identify severe sepsis, if applicable (R65.2-)

Excludes1: septic or septicopyemic embolism following complete or unspecified spontaneous abortion (O03.7)

O03.88 **Urinary tract infection following complete or unspecified spontaneous abortion**

Cystitis following complete or unspecified spontaneous abortion

O03.89 **Complete or unspecified spontaneous abortion with other complications**

O03.9 **Complete or unspecified spontaneous abortion without complication**

Miscarriage NOS

Spontaneous abortion NOS

O04 **Complications following (induced) termination of pregnancy**

Includes: complications following (induced) termination of pregnancy

Excludes1: encounter for elective termination of pregnancy, uncomplicated (Z33.2)

failed attempted termination of pregnancy (O07.-)

O04.5 **Genital tract and pelvic infection following (induced) termination of pregnancy**

Endometritis following (induced) termination of pregnancy

Oophoritis following (induced) termination of pregnancy

Parametritis following (induced) termination of pregnancy

Pelvic peritonitis following (induced) termination of pregnancy

Salpingitis following (induced) termination of pregnancy

Salpingo-oophoritis following (induced) termination of pregnancy

Excludes1: sepsis following (induced) termination of pregnancy (O04.87)

urinary tract infection following (induced) termination of pregnancy (O04.88)

O04.6 **Delayed or excessive hemorrhage following (induced) termination of pregnancy**

Afibrinogenemia following (induced) termination of pregnancy

Defibrination syndrome following (induced) termination of pregnancy

Hemolysis following (induced) termination of pregnancy

Intravascular coagulation following (induced) termination of pregnancy

O04.7 **Embolism following (induced) termination of pregnancy**

Air embolism following (induced) termination of pregnancy

Amniotic fluid embolism following (induced) termination of pregnancy

Blood-clot embolism following (induced) termination of pregnancy

Embolism NOS following (induced) termination of pregnancy

Fat embolism following (induced) termination of pregnancy

Pulmonary embolism following (induced) termination of pregnancy

Pyemic embolism following (induced) termination of pregnancy

Septic or septicopyemic embolism following (induced) termination of pregnancy

Soap embolism following (induced) termination of pregnancy

O04.8 **(Induced) termination of pregnancy with other and unspecified complications**

O04.80 **(Induced) termination of pregnancy with unspecified complications**

O04.81 **Shock following (induced) termination of pregnancy**

Circulatory collapse following (induced) termination of pregnancy

Shock (postprocedural) following (induced) termination of pregnancy

Excludes1: shock due to infection following (induced) termination of pregnancy (O04.87)

O04.82 **Renal failure following (induced) termination of pregnancy**

Kidney failure (acute) following (induced) termination of pregnancy

Oliguria following (induced) termination of pregnancy

Renal shutdown following (induced) termination of pregnancy

Renal tubular necrosis following (induced) termination of pregnancy

Uremia following (induced) termination of pregnancy

O04.83 **Metabolic disorder following (induced) termination of pregnancy**

O04.84 **Damage to pelvic organs following (induced) termination of pregnancy**

Laceration, perforation, tear or chemical damage of bladder following (induced) termination of pregnancy

Laceration, perforation, tear or chemical damage of bowel following (induced) termination of pregnancy

Laceration, perforation, tear or chemical damage of broad ligament following (induced) termination of pregnancy

Laceration, perforation, tear or chemical damage of cervix following (induced) termination of pregnancy

Laceration, perforation, tear or chemical damage of periurethral tissue following (induced) termination of pregnancy

Laceration, perforation, tear or chemical damage of uterus following (induced) termination of pregnancy

Laceration, perforation, tear or chemical damage of vagina following (induced) termination of pregnancy

O04.85 **Other venous complications following (induced) termination of pregnancy**

O04.86 **Cardiac arrest following (induced) termination of pregnancy**

O04.87 **Sepsis following (induced) termination of pregnancy**

Use additional code to identify infectious agent (B95-B97)

Use additional code to identify severe sepsis, if applicable (R65.2-)

Excludes1: septic or septicopyemic embolism following (induced) termination of pregnancy (O04.7)

O04.88 **Urinary tract infection following (induced) termination of pregnancy**

Cystitis following (induced) termination of pregnancy

O04.89 **(Induced) termination of pregnancy with other complications**

O07 **Failed attempted termination of pregnancy**

Includes: failure of attempted induction of termination of pregnancy

incomplete elective abortion

Excludes1: incomplete spontaneous abortion (O03.0-)

O07.0 **Genital tract and pelvic infection following failed attempted termination of pregnancy**

Endometritis following failed attempted termination of pregnancy

Oophoritis following failed attempted termination of pregnancy

Parametritis following failed attempted termination of pregnancy

Pelvic peritonitis following failed attempted termination of pregnancy

Salpingitis following failed attempted termination of pregnancy

Salpingo-oophoritis following failed attempted termination of pregnancy

Excludes1: sepsis following failed attempted termination of pregnancy (O07.37)

urinary tract infection following failed attempted termination of pregnancy (O07.38)

O07.1 **Delayed or excessive hemorrhage following failed attempted termination of pregnancy**

Afibrinogenemia following failed attempted termination of pregnancy

Defibrination syndrome following failed attempted termination of pregnancy

Hemolysis following failed attempted termination of pregnancy

Intravascular coagulation following failed attempted termination of pregnancy

O07.2 **Embolism following failed attempted termination of pregnancy**

Air embolism following failed attempted termination of pregnancy

Amniotic fluid embolism following failed attempted termination of pregnancy

Blood-clot embolism following failed attempted termination of pregnancy

Embolism NOS following failed attempted termination of pregnancy

Fat embolism following failed attempted termination of pregnancy

Pulmonary embolism following failed attempted termination of pregnancy

Pyemic embolism following failed attempted termination of pregnancy

Septic or septicopyemic embolism following failed attempted termination of pregnancy

Soap embolism following failed attempted termination of pregnancy

O07.3 **Failed attempted termination of pregnancy with other and unspecified complications**

O07.30 **Failed attempted termination of pregnancy with unspecified complications**

O07.31 **Shock following failed attempted termination of pregnancy**

Circulatory collapse following failed attempted termination of pregnancy

Shock (postprocedural) following failed attempted termination of pregnancy

Excludes1: shock due to infection following failed attempted termination of pregnancy (O07.37)

O07.32 **Renal failure following failed attempted termination of pregnancy**

Kidney failure (acute) following failed attempted termination of pregnancy

Oliguria following failed attempted termination of pregnancy

Renal shutdown following failed attempted termination of pregnancy

Renal tubular necrosis following failed attempted termination of pregnancy

Uremia following failed attempted termination of pregnancy

O07.33 **Metabolic disorder following failed attempted termination of pregnancy**

O07.34 **Damage to pelvic organs following failed attempted termination of pregnancy**

Laceration, perforation, tear or chemical damage of bladder following failed attempted termination of pregnancy

Laceration, perforation, tear or chemical damage of bowel following failed attempted termination of pregnancy

Laceration, perforation, tear or chemical damage of broad ligament following failed attempted termination of pregnancy

Laceration, perforation, tear or chemical damage of cervix following failed attempted termination of pregnancy

Laceration, perforation, tear or chemical damage of periurethral tissue following failed attempted termination of pregnancy

Laceration, perforation, tear or chemical damage of uterus following failed attempted termination of pregnancy

Laceration, perforation, tear or chemical damage of vagina following failed attempted termination of pregnancy

O07.35 **Other venous complications following failed attempted termination of pregnancy**

O07.36 **Cardiac arrest following failed attempted termination of pregnancy**

Add 4th-7th digits   Nonspecific code   Unspecified code   Manifestation code

O07.37 Sepsis following failed attempted termination of pregnancy

Use additional code (B95-B97), to identify infectious agent

Use additional code (R65.2-) to identify severe sepsis, if applicable

Excludes1: septic or septicopyemic embolism following failed attempted termination of pregnancy (O07.2)

O07.38 Urinary tract infection following failed attempted termination of pregnancy

Cystitis following failed attempted termination of pregnancy

O07.39 Failed attempted termination of pregnancy with other complications

O07.4 Failed attempted termination of pregnancy without complication

O08 Complications following ectopic and molar pregnancy

This category is for use with categories O00-O02 to identify any associated complications

O08.0 Genital tract and pelvic infection following ectopic and molar pregnancy

Endometritis following ectopic and molar pregnancy

Oophoritis following ectopic and molar pregnancy

Parametritis following ectopic and molar pregnancy

Pelvic peritonitis following ectopic and molar pregnancy

Salpingitis following ectopic and molar pregnancy

Salpingo-oophoritis following ectopic and molar pregnancy

Excludes1: sepsis following ectopic and molar pregnancy (O08.82)

urinary tract infection (O08.83)

O08.1 Delayed or excessive hemorrhage following ectopic and molar pregnancy

Afibrinogenemia following ectopic and molar pregnancy

Defibrination syndrome following ectopic and molar pregnancy

Hemolysis following ectopic and molar pregnancy

Intravascular coagulation following ectopic and molar pregnancy

Excludes1: delayed or excessive hemorrhage due to incomplete abortion (O03.1)

O08.2 Embolism following ectopic and molar pregnancy

Air embolism following ectopic and molar pregnancy

Amniotic fluid embolism following ectopic and molar pregnancy

Blood-clot embolism following ectopic and molar pregnancy

Embolism NOS following ectopic and molar pregnancy

Fat embolism following ectopic and molar pregnancy

Pulmonary embolism following ectopic and molar pregnancy

Pyemic embolism following ectopic and molar pregnancy

Septic or septicopyemic embolism following ectopic and molar pregnancy

Soap embolism following ectopic and molar pregnancy

O08.3 Shock following ectopic and molar pregnancy

Circulatory collapse following ectopic and molar pregnancy

Shock (postprocedural) following ectopic and molar pregnancy

Excludes1: shock due to infection following ectopic and molar pregnancy (O08.82)

O08.4 Renal failure following ectopic and molar pregnancy

Kidney failure (acute) following ectopic and molar pregnancy

Oliguria following ectopic and molar pregnancy

Renal shutdown following ectopic and molar pregnancy

Renal tubular necrosis following ectopic and molar pregnancy

Uremia following ectopic and molar pregnancy

O08.5 Metabolic disorders following an ectopic and molar pregnancy

O08.6 Damage to pelvic organs and tissues following an ectopic and molar pregnancy

Laceration, perforation, tear or chemical damage of bladder following an ectopic and molar pregnancy

Laceration, perforation, tear or chemical damage of bowel following an ectopic and molar pregnancy

Laceration, perforation, tear or chemical damage of broad ligament following an ectopic and molar pregnancy

Laceration, perforation, tear or chemical damage of cervix following an ectopic and molar pregnancy

Laceration, perforation, tear or chemical damage of periurethral tissue following an ectopic and molar pregnancy

Laceration, perforation, tear or chemical damage of uterus following an ectopic and molar pregnancy

Laceration, perforation, tear or chemical damage of vagina following an ectopic and molar pregnancy

O08.7 Other venous complications following an ectopic and molar pregnancy

O08.8 Other complications following an ectopic and molar pregnancy

O08.81 Cardiac arrest following an ectopic and molar pregnancy

O08.82 Sepsis following ectopic and molar pregnancy

Use additional code (B95-B97), to identify infectious agent

Use additional code (R65.2-) to identify severe sepsis, if applicable

Excludes1: septic or septicopyemic embolism following ectopic and molar pregnancy (O08.2)

O08.83 Urinary tract infection following an ectopic and molar pregnancy

Cystitis following an ectopic and molar pregnancy

O08.89 Other complications following an ectopic and molar pregnancy

O08.9 Unspecified complication following an ectopic and molar pregnancy

SUPERVISION OF HIGH RISK PREGNANCY (O09)

O09 Supervision of high risk pregnancy

O09.0 Supervision of pregnancy with history of infertility

O09.00 Supervision of pregnancy with history of infertility, unspecified trimester

O09.01 Supervision of pregnancy with history of infertility, first trimester

O09.02 Supervision of pregnancy with history of infertility, second trimester

O09.03 Supervision of pregnancy with history of infertility, third trimester

O09.1 Supervision of pregnancy with history of ectopic pregnancy

O09.10   Supervision of pregnancy with history of ectopic pregnancy, unspecified trimester

O09.11   Supervision of pregnancy with history of ectopic pregnancy, first trimester

O09.12   Supervision of pregnancy with history of ectopic pregnancy, second trimester

O09.13   Supervision of pregnancy with history of ectopic pregnancy, third trimester

O09.A   **Supervision of pregnancy with history of molar pregnancy**

O09.A0   Supervision of pregnancy with history of molar pregnancy, unspecified trimester

O09.A1   Supervision of pregnancy with history of molar pregnancy, first trimester

O09.A2   Supervision of pregnancy with history of molar pregnancy, second trimester

O09.A3   Supervision of pregnancy with history of molar pregnancy, third trimester

O09.2   **Supervision of pregnancy with other poor reproductive or obstetric history**

> **Excludes2:** pregnancy care for patient with history of recurrent pregnancy loss (O26.2-)

O09.21   Supervision of pregnancy with history of pre-term labor

O09.211   Supervision of pregnancy with history of pre-term labor, first trimester

O09.212   Supervision of pregnancy with history of pre-term labor, second trimester

O09.213   Supervision of pregnancy with history of pre-term labor, third trimester

O09.219   Supervision of pregnancy with history of pre-term labor, unspecified trimester

O09.29   Supervision of pregnancy with other poor reproductive or obstetric history

Supervision of pregnancy with history of neonatal death

Supervision of pregnancy with history of stillbirth

O09.291   Supervision of pregnancy with other poor reproductive or obstetric history, first trimester

O09.292   Supervision of pregnancy with other poor reproductive or obstetric history, second trimester

O09.293   Supervision of pregnancy with other poor reproductive or obstetric history, third trimester

O09.299   Supervision of pregnancy with other poor reproductive or obstetric history, unspecified trimester

O09.3   **Supervision of pregnancy with insufficient antenatal care**

Supervision of concealed pregnancy

Supervision of hidden pregnancy

O09.30   Supervision of pregnancy with insufficient antenatal care, unspecified trimester

O09.31   Supervision of pregnancy with insufficient antenatal care, first trimester

O09.32   Supervision of pregnancy with insufficient antenatal care, second trimester

O09.33   Supervision of pregnancy with insufficient antenatal care, third trimester

O09.4   **Supervision of pregnancy with grand multiparity**

O09.40   Supervision of pregnancy with grand multiparity, unspecified trimester

O09.41   Supervision of pregnancy with grand multiparity, first trimester

O09.42   Supervision of pregnancy with grand multiparity, second trimester

O09.43   Supervision of pregnancy with grand multiparity, third trimester

O09.5   **Supervision of elderly primigravida and multigravida**

Pregnancy for a female 35 years and older at expected date of delivery

O09.51   Supervision of elderly primigravida

O09.511   Supervision of elderly primigravida, first trimester

O09.512   Supervision of elderly primigravida, second trimester

O09.513   Supervision of elderly primigravida, third trimester

O09.519   Supervision of elderly primigravida, unspecified trimester

O09.52   Supervision of elderly multigravida

O09.521   Supervision of elderly multigravida, first trimester

O09.522   Supervision of elderly multigravida, second trimester

O09.523   Supervision of elderly multigravida, third trimester

O09.529   Supervision of elderly multigravida, unspecified trimester

O09.6   **Supervision of young primigravida and multigravida**

Supervision of pregnancy for a female less than 16 years old at expected date of delivery

O09.61   Supervision of young primigravida

O09.611   Supervision of young primigravida, first trimester

O09.612   Supervision of young primigravida, second trimester

O09.613   Supervision of young primigravida, third trimester

O09.619   Supervision of young primigravida, unspecified trimester

O09.62   Supervision of young multigravida

O09.621   Supervision of young multigravida, first trimester

O09.622   Supervision of young multigravida, second trimester

O09.623   Supervision of young multigravida, third trimester

O09.629   Supervision of young multigravida, unspecified trimester

O09.7   **Supervision of high risk pregnancy due to social problems**

O09.70   Supervision of high risk pregnancy due to social problems, unspecified trimester

O09.71   Supervision of high risk pregnancy due to social problems, first trimester

O09.72   Supervision of high risk pregnancy due to social problems, second trimester

O09.73   Supervision of high risk pregnancy due to social problems, third trimester

O09.8   **Supervision of other high risk pregnancies**

O09.81   Supervision of pregnancy resulting from assisted reproductive technology

Supervision of pregnancy resulting from in-vitro fertilization

Excludes2: gestational carrier status (Z33.3)

O09.811   Supervision of pregnancy resulting from assisted reproductive technology, first trimester

O09.812   Supervision of pregnancy resulting from assisted reproductive technology, second trimester

O09.813   Supervision of pregnancy resulting from assisted reproductive technology, third trimester

O09.819   Supervision of pregnancy resulting from assisted reproductive technology, unspecified trimester

O09.82   Supervision of pregnancy with history of in utero procedure during previous pregnancy

O09.821   Supervision of pregnancy with history of in utero procedure during previous pregnancy, first trimester

O09.822   Supervision of pregnancy with history of in utero procedure during previous pregnancy, second trimester

O09.823   Supervision of pregnancy with history of in utero procedure during previous pregnancy, third trimester

O09.829   Supervision of pregnancy with history of in utero procedure during previous pregnancy, unspecified trimester

Excludes1: supervision of pregnancy affected by in utero procedure during current pregnancy (O35.7)

O09.89   Supervision of other high risk pregnancies

O09.891   Supervision of other high risk pregnancies, first trimester

O09.892   Supervision of other high risk pregnancies, second trimester

O09.893   Supervision of other high risk pregnancies, third trimester

O09.899   Supervision of other high risk pregnancies, unspecified trimester

O09.9   Supervision of high risk pregnancy, unspecified

O09.90   Supervision of high risk pregnancy, unspecified, unspecified trimester

O09.91   Supervision of high risk pregnancy, unspecified, first trimester

O09.92   Supervision of high risk pregnancy, unspecified, second trimester

O09.93   Supervision of high risk pregnancy, unspecified, third trimester

EDEMA, PROTEINURIA AND HYPERTENSIVE DISORDERS IN PREGNANCY, CHILDBIRTH AND THE PUERPERIUM (O10-O16)

O10   Pre-existing hypertension complicating pregnancy, childbirth and the puerperium

Includes: pre-existing hypertension with pre-existing proteinuria complicating pregnancy, childbirth and the puerperium

Excludes2: pre-existing hypertension with superimposed pre-eclampsia complicating pregnancy, childbirth and the puerperium (O11.-)

O10.0   Pre-existing essential hypertension complicating pregnancy, childbirth and the puerperium

Any condition in I10 specified as a reason for obstetric care during pregnancy, childbirth or the puerperium

O10.01   Pre-existing essential hypertension complicating pregnancy

O10.011   Pre-existing essential hypertension complicating pregnancy, first trimester

O10.012   Pre-existing essential hypertension complicating pregnancy, second trimester

O10.013   Pre-existing essential hypertension complicating pregnancy, third trimester

O10.019   Pre-existing essential hypertension complicating pregnancy, unspecified trimester

O10.02   Pre-existing essential hypertension complicating childbirth

O10.03   Pre-existing essential hypertension complicating the puerperium

O10.1   Pre-existing hypertensive heart disease complicating pregnancy, childbirth and the puerperium

Any condition in I11 specified as a reason for obstetric care during pregnancy, childbirth or the puerperium

Use additional code from I11 to identify the type of hypertensive heart disease

O10.11   Pre-existing hypertensive heart disease complicating pregnancy

O10.111   Pre-existing hypertensive heart disease complicating pregnancy, first trimester

O10.112   Pre-existing hypertensive heart disease complicating pregnancy, second trimester

O10.113   Pre-existing hypertensive heart disease complicating pregnancy, third trimester

O10.119   Pre-existing hypertensive heart disease complicating pregnancy, unspecified trimester

O10.12   Pre-existing hypertensive heart disease complicating childbirth

O10.13   Pre-existing hypertensive heart disease complicating the puerperium

O10.2   Pre-existing hypertensive chronic kidney disease complicating pregnancy, childbirth and the puerperium

Any condition in I12 specified as a reason for obstetric care during pregnancy, childbirth or the puerperium

Use additional code from I12 to identify the type of hypertensive chronic kidney disease

O10.21   Pre-existing hypertensive chronic kidney disease complicating pregnancy

O10.211   Pre-existing hypertensive chronic kidney disease complicating pregnancy, first trimester

O10.212   Pre-existing hypertensive chronic kidney disease complicating pregnancy, second trimester

O10.213   Pre-existing hypertensive chronic kidney disease complicating pregnancy, third trimester

O10.219   Pre-existing hypertensive chronic kidney disease complicating pregnancy, unspecified trimester

O10.22 Pre-existing hypertensive chronic kidney disease complicating childbirth

O10.23 Pre-existing hypertensive chronic kidney disease complicating the puerperium

O10.3 Pre-existing hypertensive heart and chronic kidney disease complicating pregnancy, childbirth and the puerperium

Any condition in I13 specified as a reason for obstetric care during pregnancy, childbirth or the puerperium

Use additional code from I13 to identify the type of hypertensive heart and chronic kidney disease

O10.31 Pre-existing hypertensive heart and chronic kidney disease complicating pregnancy

O10.311 Pre-existing hypertensive heart and chronic kidney disease complicating pregnancy, first trimester

O10.312 Pre-existing hypertensive heart and chronic kidney disease complicating pregnancy, second trimester

O10.313 Pre-existing hypertensive heart and chronic kidney disease complicating pregnancy, third trimester

O10.319 Pre-existing hypertensive heart and chronic kidney disease complicating pregnancy, unspecified trimester

O10.32 Pre-existing hypertensive heart and chronic kidney disease complicating childbirth

O10.33 Pre-existing hypertensive heart and chronic kidney disease complicating the puerperium

O10.4 Pre-existing secondary hypertension complicating pregnancy, childbirth and the puerperium

Any condition in I15 specified as a reason for obstetric care during pregnancy, childbirth or the puerperium

Use additional code from I15 to identify the type of secondary hypertension

O10.41 Pre-existing secondary hypertension complicating pregnancy

O10.411 Pre-existing secondary hypertension complicating pregnancy, first trimester

O10.412 Pre-existing secondary hypertension complicating pregnancy, second trimester

O10.413 Pre-existing secondary hypertension complicating pregnancy, third trimester

O10.419 Pre-existing secondary hypertension complicating pregnancy, unspecified trimester

O10.42 Pre-existing secondary hypertension complicating childbirth

O10.43 Pre-existing secondary hypertension complicating the puerperium

O10.9 Unspecified pre-existing hypertension complicating pregnancy, childbirth and the puerperium

O10.91 Unspecified pre-existing hypertension complicating pregnancy

O10.911 Unspecified pre-existing hypertension complicating pregnancy, first trimester

O10.912 Unspecified pre-existing hypertension complicating pregnancy, second trimester

O10.913 Unspecified pre-existing hypertension complicating pregnancy, third trimester

O10.919 Unspecified pre-existing hypertension complicating pregnancy, unspecified trimester

O10.92 Unspecified pre-existing hypertension complicating childbirth

O10.93 Unspecified pre-existing hypertension complicating the puerperium

O11 Pre-existing hypertension with pre-eclampsia

Includes: conditions in O10 complicated by pre-eclampsia

pre-eclampsia superimposed pre-existing hypertension

Use additional code from O10 to identify the type of hypertension

O11.1 Pre-existing hypertension with pre-eclampsia, first trimester

O11.2 Pre-existing hypertension with pre-eclampsia, second trimester

O11.3 Pre-existing hypertension with pre-eclampsia, third trimester

O11.4 Pre-existing hypertension with pre-eclampsia, complicating childbirth

O11.5 Pre-existing hypertension with pre-eclampsia, complicating the puerperium

O11.9 Pre-existing hypertension with pre-eclampsia, unspecified trimester

O12 Gestational [pregnancy-induced] edema and proteinuria without hypertension

O12.0 Gestational edema

O12.00 Gestational edema, unspecified trimester

O12.01 Gestational edema, first trimester

O12.02 Gestational edema, second trimester

O12.03 Gestational edema, third trimester

O12.04 Gestational edema, complicating childbirth

O12.05 Gestational edema, complicating the puerperium

O12.1 Gestational proteinuria

O12.10 Gestational proteinuria, unspecified trimester

O12.11 Gestational proteinuria, first trimester

O12.12 Gestational proteinuria, second trimester

O12.13 Gestational proteinuria, third trimester

O12.14 Gestational proteinuria, complicating childbirth

O12.15 Gestational proteinuria, complicating the puerperium

O12.2 Gestational edema with proteinuria

O12.20 Gestational edema with proteinuria, unspecified trimester

O12.21 Gestational edema with proteinuria, first trimester

O12.22 Gestational edema with proteinuria, second trimester

O12.23 Gestational edema with proteinuria, third trimester

O12.24 Gestational edema with proteinuria, complicating childbirth

O12.25 Gestational edema with proteinuria, complicating the puerperium

O13 Gestational [pregnancy-induced] hypertension without significant proteinuria

Includes: gestational hypertension NOS

transient hypertension of pregnancy

O13.1 Gestational [pregnancy-induced] hypertension without significant proteinuria, first trimester

O13.2 Gestational [pregnancy-induced] hypertension without significant proteinuria, second trimester

O13.3 Gestational [pregnancy-induced] hypertension without significant proteinuria, third trimester

O13.4 Gestational [pregnancy-induced] hypertension without significant proteinuria, complicating childbirth

O13.5 Gestational [pregnancy-induced] hypertension without significant proteinuria, complicating the puerperium

O13.9 Gestational [pregnancy-induced] hypertension without significant proteinuria, unspecified trimester

O14 Pre-eclampsia

Excludes1: pre-existing hypertension with pre-eclampsia (O11)

O14.0 Mild to moderate pre-eclampsia

    O14.00 Mild to moderate pre-eclampsia, unspecified trimester

    O14.02 Mild to moderate pre-eclampsia, second trimester

    O14.03 Mild to moderate pre-eclampsia, third trimester

    O14.04 Mild to moderate pre-eclampsia, complicating childbirth

    O14.05 Mild to moderate pre-eclampsia, complicating the puerperium

O14.1 Severe pre-eclampsia

    Excludes1: HELLP syndrome (O14.2-)

    O14.10 Severe pre-eclampsia, unspecified trimester

    O14.12 Severe pre-eclampsia, second trimester

    O14.13 Severe pre-eclampsia, third trimester

    O14.14 Severe pre-eclampsia complicating childbirth

    O14.15 Severe pre-eclampsia, complicating the puerperium

O14.2 HELLP syndrome

    Severe pre-eclampsia with hemolysis, elevated liver enzymes and low platelet count (HELLP)

    O14.20 HELLP syndrome (HELLP), unspecified trimester

    O14.22 HELLP syndrome (HELLP), second trimester

    O14.23 HELLP syndrome (HELLP), third trimester

    O14.24 HELLP syndrome, complicating childbirth

    O14.25 HELLP syndrome, complicating the puerperium

O14.9 Unspecified pre-eclampsia

    O14.90 Unspecified pre-eclampsia, unspecified trimester

    O14.92 Unspecified pre-eclampsia, second trimester

    O14.93 Unspecified pre-eclampsia, third trimester

    O14.94 Unspecified pre-eclampsia, complicating childbirth

    O14.95 Unspecified pre-eclampsia, complicating the puerperium

O15 Eclampsia

Includes: convulsions following conditions in O10-O14 and O16

O15.0 Eclampsia complicating pregnancy

    O15.00 Eclampsia complicating pregnancy, unspecified trimester

    O15.02 Eclampsia complicating pregnancy, second trimester

    O15.03 Eclampsia complicating pregnancy, third trimester

O15.1 Eclampsia complicating labor

O15.2 Eclampsia complicating the puerperium

O15.9 Eclampsia, unspecified as to time period

    Eclampsia NOS

O16 Unspecified maternal hypertension

O16.1 Unspecified maternal hypertension, first trimester

O16.2 Unspecified maternal hypertension, second trimester

O16.3 Unspecified maternal hypertension, third trimester

O16.4 Unspecified maternal hypertension, complicating childbirth

O16.5 Unspecified maternal hypertension, complicating the puerperium

O16.9 Unspecified maternal hypertension, unspecified trimester

OTHER MATERNAL DISORDERS PREDOMINANTLY RELATED TO PREGNANCY (O20-O29)

Excludes2: maternal care related to the fetus and amniotic cavity and possible delivery problems (O30-O48)

maternal diseases classifiable elsewhere but complicating pregnancy, labor and delivery, and the puerperium (O98-O99)

O20 Hemorrhage in early pregnancy

Includes: hemorrhage before completion of 20 weeks gestation

Excludes1: pregnancy with abortive outcome (O00-O08)

O20.0 Threatened abortion

    Hemorrhage specified as due to threatened abortion

O20.8 Other hemorrhage in early pregnancy

O20.9 Hemorrhage in early pregnancy, unspecified

O21 Excessive vomiting in pregnancy

O21.0 Mild hyperemesis gravidarum

    Hyperemesis gravidarum, mild or unspecified, starting before the end of the 20th week of gestation

O21.1 Hyperemesis gravidarum with metabolic disturbance

    Hyperemesis gravidarum, starting before the end of the 20th week of gestation, with metabolic disturbance such as carbohydrate depletion

    Hyperemesis gravidarum, starting before the end of the 20th week of gestation, with metabolic disturbance such as dehydration

    Hyperemesis gravidarum, starting before the end of the 20th week of gestation, with metabolic disturbance such as electrolyte imbalance

O21.2 Late vomiting of pregnancy

    Excessive vomiting starting after 20 completed weeks of gestation

O21.8 Other vomiting complicating pregnancy

    Vomiting due to diseases classified elsewhere, complicating pregnancy

    Use additional code, to identify cause.

O21.9 Vomiting of pregnancy, unspecified

O22 Venous complications and hemorrhoids in pregnancy

Excludes1: venous complications of:

    abortion NOS (O03.9)

    ectopic or molar pregnancy (O08.7)

    failed attempted abortion (O07.35)

    induced abortion (O04.85)

    spontaneous abortion (O03.89)

Excludes2: obstetric pulmonary embolism (O88.-)

    venous complications and hemorrhoids of childbirth and the puerperium (O87.-)

O22.0 Varicose veins of lower extremity in pregnancy

    Varicose veins NOS in pregnancy

O22.00   Varicose veins of lower extremity in pregnancy, unspecified trimester

O22.01   Varicose veins of lower extremity in pregnancy, first trimester

O22.02   Varicose veins of lower extremity in pregnancy, second trimester

O22.03   Varicose veins of lower extremity in pregnancy, third trimester

O22.1   **Genital varices in pregnancy**

Perineal varices in pregnancy

Vaginal varices in pregnancy

Vulval varices in pregnancy

O22.10   Genital varices in pregnancy, unspecified trimester

O22.11   Genital varices in pregnancy, first trimester

O22.12   Genital varices in pregnancy, second trimester

O22.13   Genital varices in pregnancy, third trimester

O22.2   **Superficial thrombophlebitis in pregnancy**

Phlebitis in pregnancy NOS

Thrombophlebitis of legs in pregnancy

Thrombosis in pregnancy NOS

<u>Use additional code</u> to identify the superficial thrombophlebitis (I80.0-)

O22.20   Superficial thrombophlebitis in pregnancy, unspecified trimester

O22.21   Superficial thrombophlebitis in pregnancy, first trimester

O22.22   Superficial thrombophlebitis in pregnancy, second trimester

O22.23   Superficial thrombophlebitis in pregnancy, third trimester

O22.3   **Deep phlebothrombosis in pregnancy**

Deep vein thrombosis, antepartum

<u>Use additional code</u> to identify the deep vein thrombosis (I82.4-, I82.5-, I82.62-. I82.72-)

<u>Use additional code</u>, if applicable, for associated long-term (current) use of anticoagulants (Z79.01)

O22.30   Deep phlebothrombosis in pregnancy, unspecified trimester

O22.31   Deep phlebothrombosis in pregnancy, first trimester

O22.32   Deep phlebothrombosis in pregnancy, second trimester

O22.33   Deep phlebothrombosis in pregnancy, third trimester

O22.4   **Hemorrhoids in pregnancy**

O22.40   Hemorrhoids in pregnancy, unspecified trimester

O22.41   Hemorrhoids in pregnancy, first trimester

O22.42   Hemorrhoids in pregnancy, second trimester

O22.43   Hemorrhoids in pregnancy, third trimester

O22.5   **Cerebral venous thrombosis in pregnancy**

Cerebrovenous sinus thrombosis in pregnancy

O22.50   Cerebral venous thrombosis in pregnancy, unspecified trimester

O22.51   Cerebral venous thrombosis in pregnancy, first trimester

O22.52   Cerebral venous thrombosis in pregnancy, second trimester

O22.53   Cerebral venous thrombosis in pregnancy, third trimester

O22.8   **Other venous complications in pregnancy**

O22.8X   Other venous complications in pregnancy

O22.8X1   Other venous complications in pregnancy, first trimester

O22.8X2   Other venous complications in pregnancy, second trimester

O22.8X3   Other venous complications in pregnancy, third trimester

O22.8X9   Other venous complications in pregnancy, unspecified trimester

O22.9   **Venous complication in pregnancy, unspecified**

Gestational phlebitis NOS

Gestational phlebopathy NOS

Gestational thrombosis NOS

O22.90   Venous complication in pregnancy, unspecified, unspecified trimester

O22.91   Venous complication in pregnancy, unspecified, first trimester

O22.92   Venous complication in pregnancy, unspecified, second trimester

O22.93   Venous complication in pregnancy, unspecified, third trimester

O23   **Infections of genitourinary tract in pregnancy**

<u>Use additional code</u> to identify organism (B95.-, B96.-)

Excludes2: gonococcal infections complicating pregnancy, childbirth and the puerperium (O98.2)

infections with a predominantly sexual mode of transmission NOS complicating pregnancy, childbirth and the puerperium (O98.3)

syphilis complicating pregnancy, childbirth and the puerperium (O98.1)

tuberculosis of genitourinary system complicating pregnancy, childbirth and the puerperium (O98.0)

venereal disease NOS complicating pregnancy, childbirth and the puerperium (O98.3)

O23.0   **Infections of kidney in pregnancy**

Pyelonephritis in pregnancy

O23.00   Infections of kidney in pregnancy, unspecified trimester

O23.01   Infections of kidney in pregnancy, first trimester

O23.02   Infections of kidney in pregnancy, second trimester

O23.03   Infections of kidney in pregnancy, third trimester

O23.1   **Infections of bladder in pregnancy**

O23.10   Infections of bladder in pregnancy, unspecified trimester

O23.11   Infections of bladder in pregnancy, first trimester

O23.12   Infections of bladder in pregnancy, second trimester

O23.13   Infections of bladder in pregnancy, third trimester

O23.2   **Infections of urethra in pregnancy**

O23.20   Infections of urethra in pregnancy, unspecified trimester

O23.21   Infections of urethra in pregnancy, first trimester

O23.22   Infections of urethra in pregnancy, second trimester

O23.23   Infections of urethra in pregnancy, third trimester

O23.3   **Infections of other parts of urinary tract in pregnancy**

O23.30 Infections of other parts of urinary tract in pregnancy, unspecified trimester

O23.31 Infections of other parts of urinary tract in pregnancy, first trimester

O23.32 Infections of other parts of urinary tract in pregnancy, second trimester

O23.33 Infections of other parts of urinary tract in pregnancy, third trimester

O23.4 Unspecified infection of urinary tract in pregnancy

O23.40 Unspecified infection of urinary tract in pregnancy, unspecified trimester

O23.41 Unspecified infection of urinary tract in pregnancy, first trimester

O23.42 Unspecified infection of urinary tract in pregnancy, second trimester

O23.43 Unspecified infection of urinary tract in pregnancy, third trimester

O23.5 Infections of the genital tract in pregnancy

O23.51 Infection of cervix in pregnancy

O23.511 Infections of cervix in pregnancy, first trimester

O23.512 Infections of cervix in pregnancy, second trimester

O23.513 Infections of cervix in pregnancy, third trimester

O23.519 Infections of cervix in pregnancy, unspecified trimester

O23.52 Salpingo-oophoritis in pregnancy

Oophoritis in pregnancy

Salpingitis in pregnancy

O23.521 Salpingo-oophoritis in pregnancy, first trimester

O23.522 Salpingo-oophoritis in pregnancy, second trimester

O23.523 Salpingo-oophoritis in pregnancy, third trimester

O23.529 Salpingo-oophoritis in pregnancy, unspecified trimester

O23.59 Infection of other part of genital tract in pregnancy

O23.591 Infection of other part of genital tract in pregnancy, first trimester

O23.592 Infection of other part of genital tract in pregnancy, second trimester

O23.593 Infection of other part of genital tract in pregnancy, third trimester

O23.599 Infection of other part of genital tract in pregnancy, unspecified trimester

O23.9 Unspecified genitourinary tract infection in pregnancy

Genitourinary tract infection in pregnancy NOS

O23.90 Unspecified genitourinary tract infection in pregnancy, unspecified trimester

O23.91 Unspecified genitourinary tract infection in pregnancy, first trimester

O23.92 Unspecified genitourinary tract infection in pregnancy, second trimester

O23.93 Unspecified genitourinary tract infection in pregnancy, third trimester

O24 Diabetes mellitus in pregnancy, childbirth, and the puerperium

O24.0 Pre-existing type 1 diabetes mellitus, in pregnancy, childbirth and the puerperium

Juvenile onset diabetes mellitus, in pregnancy, childbirth and the puerperium

Ketosis-prone diabetes mellitus in pregnancy, childbirth and the puerperium

Use additional code from category E10 to further identify any manifestations

O24.01 Pre-existing type 1 Diabetes mellitus, in pregnancy

O24.011 Pre-existing type 1 diabetes mellitus, in pregnancy, first trimester

O24.012 Pre-existing type 1 diabetes mellitus, in pregnancy, second trimester

O24.013 Pre-existing type 1 diabetes mellitus, in pregnancy, third trimester

O24.019 Pre-existing type 1 diabetes mellitus, in pregnancy, unspecified trimester

O24.02 Pre-existing type 1 diabetes mellitus, in childbirth

O24.03 Pre-existing type 1 diabetes mellitus, in the puerperium

O24.1 Pre-existing type 2 diabetes mellitus, in pregnancy, childbirth and the puerperium

Insulin-resistant diabetes mellitus in pregnancy, childbirth and the puerperium

Use additional code (for):

from category E11 to further identify any manifestations

long-term (current) use of insulin (Z79.4)

O24.11 Pre-existing type 2 diabetes mellitus, in pregnancy

O24.111 Pre-existing type 2 diabetes mellitus, in pregnancy, first trimester

O24.112 Pre-existing type 2 diabetes mellitus, in pregnancy, second trimester

O24.113 Pre-existing type 2 diabetes mellitus, in pregnancy, third trimester

O24.119 Pre-existing type 2 diabetes mellitus, in pregnancy, unspecified trimester

O24.12 Pre-existing type 2 diabetes mellitus, in childbirth

O24.13 Pre-existing type 2 diabetes mellitus, in the puerperium

O24.3 Unspecified pre-existing diabetes mellitus in pregnancy, childbirth and the puerperium

Use additional code (for):

from category E11 to further identify any manifestation

long-term (current) use of insulin (Z79.4)

O24.31 Unspecified pre-existing diabetes mellitus in pregnancy

O24.311 Unspecified pre-existing diabetes mellitus in pregnancy, first trimester

O24.312 Unspecified pre-existing diabetes mellitus in pregnancy, second trimester

O24.313 Unspecified pre-existing diabetes mellitus in pregnancy, third trimester

O24.319 Unspecified pre-existing diabetes mellitus in pregnancy, unspecified trimester

O24.32 Unspecified pre-existing diabetes mellitus in childbirth

O24.33 Unspecified pre-existing diabetes mellitus in the puerperium

O24.4 Gestational diabetes mellitus

● New code   ▲ Revised code   **Excludes1:** Not coded here   **Excludes2:** Not included here   ⊗ Placeholder required   ⑦ 7th digit required

Diabetes mellitus arising in pregnancy

Gestational diabetes mellitus NOS

O24.41 Gestational diabetes mellitus in pregnancy

- **O24.410 Gestational diabetes mellitus in pregnancy, diet controlled**
- **O24.414 Gestational diabetes mellitus in pregnancy, insulin controlled**
- **O24.415 Gestational diabetes mellitus in pregnancy, controlled by oral hypoglycemic drugs**

  Gestational diabetes mellitus in pregnancy, controlled by oral antidiabetic drugs

- **O24.419 Gestational diabetes mellitus in pregnancy, unspecified control**

O24.42 Gestational diabetes mellitus in childbirth

- **O24.420 Gestational diabetes mellitus in childbirth, diet controlled**
- **O24.424 Gestational diabetes mellitus in childbirth, insulin controlled**
- **O24.425 Gestational diabetes mellitus in childbirth, controlled by oral hypoglycemic drugs**

  Gestational diabetes mellitus in childbirth, controlled by oral antidiabetic drugs

- **O24.429 Gestational diabetes mellitus in childbirth, unspecified control**

O24.43 Gestational diabetes mellitus in the puerperium

- **O24.430 Gestational diabetes mellitus in the puerperium, diet controlled**
- **O24.434 Gestational diabetes mellitus in the puerperium, insulin controlled**
- **O24.435 Gestational diabetes mellitus in puerperium, controlled by oral hypoglycemic drugs**

  Gestational diabetes mellitus in puerperium, controlled by oral antidiabetic drugs

- **O24.439 Gestational diabetes mellitus in the puerperium, unspecified control**

O24.8 Other pre-existing diabetes mellitus in pregnancy, childbirth, and the puerperium

Use additional code (for):

from categories E08, E09 and E13 to further identify any manifestation long-term (current) use of insulin (Z79.4)

O24.81 Other pre-existing diabetes mellitus in pregnancy

- **O24.811 Other pre-existing diabetes mellitus in pregnancy, first trimester**
- **O24.812 Other pre-existing diabetes mellitus in pregnancy, second trimester**
- **O24.813 Other pre-existing diabetes mellitus in pregnancy, third trimester**
- **O24.819 Other pre-existing diabetes mellitus in pregnancy, unspecified trimester**

O24.82 Other pre-existing diabetes mellitus in childbirth

O24.83 Other pre-existing diabetes mellitus in the puerperium

O24.9 Unspecified diabetes mellitus in pregnancy, childbirth and the puerperium

Use additional code for long-term (current) use of insulin (Z79.4)

O24.91 Unspecified diabetes mellitus in pregnancy

- **O24.911 Unspecified diabetes mellitus in pregnancy, first trimester**
- **O24.912 Unspecified diabetes mellitus in pregnancy, second trimester**
- **O24.913 Unspecified diabetes mellitus in pregnancy, third trimester**
- **O24.919 Unspecified diabetes mellitus in pregnancy, unspecified trimester**

O24.92 Unspecified diabetes mellitus in childbirth

O24.93 Unspecified diabetes mellitus in the puerperium

O25 Malnutrition in pregnancy, childbirth and the puerperium

O25.1 Malnutrition in pregnancy

- **O25.10 Malnutrition in pregnancy, unspecified trimester**
- **O25.11 Malnutrition in pregnancy, first trimester**
- **O25.12 Malnutrition in pregnancy, second trimester**
- **O25.13 Malnutrition in pregnancy, third trimester**

O25.2 Malnutrition in childbirth

O25.3 Malnutrition in the puerperium

O26 Maternal care for other conditions predominantly related to pregnancy

O26.0 Excessive weight gain in pregnancy

Excludes2: gestational edema (O12.0, O12.2)

- **O26.00 Excessive weight gain in pregnancy, unspecified trimester**
- **O26.01 Excessive weight gain in pregnancy, first trimester**
- **O26.02 Excessive weight gain in pregnancy, second trimester**
- **O26.03 Excessive weight gain in pregnancy, third trimester**

O26.1 Low weight gain in pregnancy

- **O26.10 Low weight gain in pregnancy, unspecified trimester**
- **O26.11 Low weight gain in pregnancy, first trimester**
- **O26.12 Low weight gain in pregnancy, second trimester**
- **O26.13 Low weight gain in pregnancy, third trimester**

O26.2 Pregnancy care for patient with recurrent pregnancy loss

- **O26.20 Pregnancy care for patient with recurrent pregnancy loss, unspecified trimester**
- **O26.21 Pregnancy care for patient with recurrent pregnancy loss, first trimester**
- **O26.22 Pregnancy care for patient with recurrent pregnancy loss, second trimester**
- **O26.23 Pregnancy care for patient with recurrent pregnancy loss, third trimester**

O26.3 Retained intrauterine contraceptive device in pregnancy

- **O26.30 Retained intrauterine contraceptive device in pregnancy, unspecified trimester**
- **O26.31 Retained intrauterine contraceptive device in pregnancy, first trimester**
- **O26.32 Retained intrauterine contraceptive device in pregnancy, second trimester**
- **O26.33 Retained intrauterine contraceptive device in pregnancy, third trimester**

O26.4 Herpes gestationis

- **O26.40 Herpes gestationis, unspecified trimester**
- **O26.41 Herpes gestationis, first trimester**
- **O26.42 Herpes gestationis, second trimester**

	Add 4th-7th digits		Nonspecific code		Unspecified code		Manifestation code

O26.43   Herpes gestationis, third trimester

O26.5   **Maternal hypotension syndrome**

Supine hypotensive syndrome

   O26.50   **Maternal hypotension syndrome, unspecified trimester**

   O26.51   **Maternal hypotension syndrome, first trimester**

   O26.52   **Maternal hypotension syndrome, second trimester**

   O26.53   **Maternal hypotension syndrome, third trimester**

O26.6   **Liver and biliary tract disorders in pregnancy, childbirth and the puerperium**

   Use additional code to identify the specific disorder

   Excludes2: hepatorenal syndrome following labor and delivery (O90.4)

   O26.61   **Liver and biliary tract disorders in pregnancy**

     O26.611   **Liver and biliary tract disorders in pregnancy, first trimester**

     O26.612   **Liver and biliary tract disorders in pregnancy, second trimester**

     O26.613   **Liver and biliary tract disorders in pregnancy, third trimester**

     O26.619   **Liver and biliary tract disorders in pregnancy, unspecified trimester**

   O26.62   **Liver and biliary tract disorders in childbirth**

   O26.63   **Liver and biliary tract disorders in the puerperium**

O26.7   **Subluxation of symphysis (pubis) in pregnancy, childbirth and the puerperium**

   Excludes1: traumatic separation of symphysis (pubis) during childbirth (O71.6)

   O26.71   **Subluxation of symphysis (pubis) in pregnancy**

     O26.711   **Subluxation of symphysis (pubis) in pregnancy, first trimester**

     O26.712   **Subluxation of symphysis (pubis) in pregnancy, second trimester**

     O26.713   **Subluxation of symphysis (pubis) in pregnancy, third trimester**

     O26.719   **Subluxation of symphysis (pubis) in pregnancy, unspecified trimester**

   O26.72   **Subluxation of symphysis (pubis) in childbirth**

   O26.73   **Subluxation of symphysis (pubis) in the puerperium**

O26.8   **Other specified pregnancy related conditions**

   O26.81   **Pregnancy related exhaustion and fatigue**

     O26.811   **Pregnancy related exhaustion and fatigue, first trimester**

     O26.812   **Pregnancy related exhaustion and fatigue, second trimester**

     O26.813   **Pregnancy related exhaustion and fatigue, third trimester**

     O26.819   **Pregnancy related exhaustion and fatigue, unspecified trimester**

   O26.82   **Pregnancy related peripheral neuritis**

     O26.821   **Pregnancy related peripheral neuritis, first trimester**

     O26.822   **Pregnancy related peripheral neuritis, second trimester**

     O26.823   **Pregnancy related peripheral neuritis, third trimester**

     O26.829   **Pregnancy related peripheral neuritis, unspecified trimester**

O26.83   **Pregnancy related renal disease**

   Use additional code to identify the specific disorder

     O26.831   **Pregnancy related renal disease, first trimester**

     O26.832   **Pregnancy related renal disease, second trimester**

     O26.833   **Pregnancy related renal disease, third trimester**

     O26.839   **Pregnancy related renal disease, unspecified trimester**

O26.84   **Uterine size-date discrepancy complicating pregnancy**

   Excludes1: encounter for suspected problem with fetal growth ruled out (Z03.74)

     O26.841   **Uterine size-date discrepancy, first trimester**

     O26.842   **Uterine size-date discrepancy, second trimester**

     O26.843   **Uterine size-date discrepancy, third trimester**

     O26.849   **Uterine size-date discrepancy, unspecified trimester**

O26.85   **Spotting complicating pregnancy**

     O26.851   **Spotting complicating pregnancy, first trimester**

     O26.852   **Spotting complicating pregnancy, second trimester**

     O26.853   **Spotting complicating pregnancy, third trimester**

     O26.859   **Spotting complicating pregnancy, unspecified trimester**

O26.86   **Pruritic urticarial papules and plaques of pregnancy (PUPPP)**

Polymorphic eruption of pregnancy

O26.87   **Cervical shortening**

   Excludes1: encounter for suspected cervical shortening ruled out (Z03.75)

     O26.872   **Cervical shortening, second trimester**

     O26.873   **Cervical shortening, third trimester**

     O26.879   **Cervical shortening, unspecified trimester**

O26.89   **Other specified pregnancy related conditions**

     O26.891   **Other specified pregnancy related conditions, first trimester**

     O26.892   **Other specified pregnancy related conditions, second trimester**

     O26.893   **Other specified pregnancy related conditions, third trimester**

     O26.899   **Other specified pregnancy related conditions, unspecified trimester**

O26.9   **Pregnancy related conditions, unspecified**

   O26.90   **Pregnancy related conditions, unspecified, unspecified trimester**

   O26.91   **Pregnancy related conditions, unspecified, first trimester**

   O26.92   **Pregnancy related conditions, unspecified, second trimester**

   O26.93   **Pregnancy related conditions, unspecified, third trimester**

O28   **Abnormal findings on antenatal screening of mother**

   Excludes1: diagnostic findings classified elsewhere - see

Alphabetical Index

O28.0   **Abnormal hematological finding on antenatal screening of mother**

O28.1   **Abnormal biochemical finding on antenatal screening of mother**

O28.2   **Abnormal cytological finding on antenatal screening of mother**

O28.3   **Abnormal ultrasonic finding on antenatal screening of mother**

O28.4   **Abnormal radiological finding on antenatal screening of mother**

O28.5   **Abnormal chromosomal and genetic finding on antenatal screening of mother**

O28.8   **Other abnormal findings on antenatal screening of mother**

O28.9   **Unspecified abnormal findings on antenatal screening of mother**

O29   **Complications of anesthesia during pregnancy**

Includes: maternal complications arising from the administration of a general, regional or local anesthetic, analgesic **or other** sedation during pregnancy

Use additional code, if necessary, to identify the complication

Excludes2: complications of anesthesia during labor and delivery (O74.-)

complications of anesthesia during the puerperium (O89.-)

O29.0   **Pulmonary complications of anesthesia during pregnancy**

     O29.01   **Aspiration pneumonitis due to anesthesia during pregnancy**

       Inhalation of stomach contents or secretions NOS due to anesthesia during pregnancy

       Mendelson's syndrome due to anesthesia during pregnancy

       O29.011   **Aspiration pneumonitis due to anesthesia during pregnancy, first trimester**

       O29.012   **Aspiration pneumonitis due to anesthesia during pregnancy, second trimester**

       O29.013   **Aspiration pneumonitis due to anesthesia during pregnancy, third trimester**

       O29.019   **Aspiration pneumonitis due to anesthesia during pregnancy, unspecified trimester**

     O29.02   **Pressure collapse of lung due to anesthesia during pregnancy**

       O29.021   **Pressure collapse of lung due to anesthesia during pregnancy, first trimester**

       O29.022   **Pressure collapse of lung due to anesthesia during pregnancy, second trimester**

       O29.023   **Pressure collapse of lung due to anesthesia during pregnancy, third trimester**

       O29.029   **Pressure collapse of lung due to anesthesia during pregnancy, unspecified trimester**

     O29.09   **Other pulmonary complications of anesthesia during pregnancy**

       O29.091   **Other pulmonary complications of anesthesia during pregnancy, first trimester**

       O29.092   **Other pulmonary complications of anesthesia during pregnancy, second trimester**

       O29.093   **Other pulmonary complications of anesthesia during pregnancy, third trimester**

       O29.099   **Other pulmonary complications of anesthesia during pregnancy, unspecified trimester**

O29.1   **Cardiac complications of anesthesia during pregnancy**

     O29.11   **Cardiac arrest due to anesthesia during pregnancy**

       O29.111   **Cardiac arrest due to anesthesia during pregnancy, first trimester**

       O29.112   **Cardiac arrest due to anesthesia during pregnancy, second trimester**

       O29.113   **Cardiac arrest due to anesthesia during pregnancy, third trimester**

       O29.119   **Cardiac arrest due to anesthesia during pregnancy, unspecified trimester**

     O29.12   **Cardiac failure due to anesthesia during pregnancy**

       O29.121   **Cardiac failure due to anesthesia during pregnancy, first trimester**

       O29.122   **Cardiac failure due to anesthesia during pregnancy, second trimester**

       O29.123   **Cardiac failure due to anesthesia during pregnancy, third trimester**

       O29.129   **Cardiac failure due to anesthesia during pregnancy, unspecified trimester**

     O29.19   **Other cardiac complications of anesthesia during pregnancy**

       O29.191   **Other cardiac complications of anesthesia during pregnancy, first trimester**

       O29.192   **Other cardiac complications of anesthesia during pregnancy, second trimester**

       O29.193   **Other cardiac complications of anesthesia during pregnancy, third trimester**

       O29.199   **Other cardiac complications of anesthesia during pregnancy, unspecified trimester**

O29.2   **Central nervous system complications of anesthesia during pregnancy**

     O29.21   **Cerebral anoxia due to anesthesia during pregnancy**

       O29.211   **Cerebral anoxia due to anesthesia during pregnancy, first trimester**

       O29.212   **Cerebral anoxia due to anesthesia during pregnancy, second trimester**

       O29.213   **Cerebral anoxia due to anesthesia during pregnancy, third trimester**

       O29.219   **Cerebral anoxia due to anesthesia during pregnancy, unspecified trimester**

     O29.29   **Other central nervous system complications of anesthesia during pregnancy**

       O29.291   **Other central nervous system complications of anesthesia during pregnancy, first trimester**

O29.292 Other central nervous system complications of anesthesia during pregnancy, second trimester

O29.293 Other central nervous system complications of anesthesia during pregnancy, third trimester

O29.299 Other central nervous system complications of anesthesia during pregnancy, unspecified trimester

O29.3 Toxic reaction to local anesthesia during pregnancy

O29.3X Toxic reaction to local anesthesia during pregnancy

O29.3X1 Toxic reaction to local anesthesia during pregnancy, first trimester

O29.3X2 Toxic reaction to local anesthesia during pregnancy, second trimester

O29.3X3 Toxic reaction to local anesthesia during pregnancy, third trimester

O29.3X9 Toxic reaction to local anesthesia during pregnancy, unspecified trimester

O29.4 Spinal and epidural anesthesia induced headache during pregnancy

O29.40 Spinal and epidural anesthesia induced headache during pregnancy, unspecified trimester

O29.41 Spinal and epidural anesthesia induced headache during pregnancy, first trimester

O29.42 Spinal and epidural anesthesia induced headache during pregnancy, second trimester

O29.43 Spinal and epidural anesthesia induced headache during pregnancy, third trimester

O29.5 Other complications of spinal and epidural anesthesia during pregnancy

O29.5X Other complications of spinal and epidural anesthesia during pregnancy

O29.5X1 Other complications of spinal and epidural anesthesia during pregnancy, first trimester

O29.5X2 Other complications of spinal and epidural anesthesia during pregnancy, second trimester

O29.5X3 Other complications of spinal and epidural anesthesia during pregnancy, third trimester

O29.5X9 Other complications of spinal and epidural anesthesia during pregnancy, unspecified trimester

O29.6 Failed or difficult intubation for anesthesia during pregnancy

O29.60 Failed or difficult intubation for anesthesia during pregnancy, unspecified trimester

O29.61 Failed or difficult intubation for anesthesia during pregnancy, first trimester

O29.62 Failed or difficult intubation for anesthesia during pregnancy, second trimester

O29.63 Failed or difficult intubation for anesthesia during pregnancy, third trimester

O29.8 Other complications of anesthesia during pregnancy

O29.8X Other complications of anesthesia during pregnancy

O29.8X1 Other complications of anesthesia during pregnancy, first trimester

O29.8X2 Other complications of anesthesia during pregnancy, second trimester

O29.8X3 Other complications of anesthesia during pregnancy, third trimester

O29.8X9 Other complications of anesthesia during pregnancy, unspecified trimester

O29.9 Unspecified complication of anesthesia during pregnancy

O29.90 Unspecified complication of anesthesia during pregnancy, unspecified trimester

O29.91 Unspecified complication of anesthesia during pregnancy, first trimester

O29.92 Unspecified complication of anesthesia during pregnancy, second trimester

O29.93 Unspecified complication of anesthesia during pregnancy, third trimester

MATERNAL CARE RELATED TO THE FETUS AND AMNIOTIC CAVITY AND POSSIBLE DELIVERY PROBLEMS (O30-O48)

O30 Multiple gestation

Code also any complications specific to multiple gestation

O30.0 Twin pregnancy

O30.00 Twin pregnancy, unspecified number of placenta and unspecified number of amniotic sacs

O30.001 Twin pregnancy, unspecified number of placenta and unspecified number of amniotic sacs, first trimester

O30.002 Twin pregnancy, unspecified number of placenta and unspecified number of amniotic sacs, second trimester

O30.003 Twin pregnancy, unspecified number of placenta and unspecified number of amniotic sacs, third trimester

O30.009 Twin pregnancy, unspecified number of placenta and unspecified number of amniotic sacs, unspecified trimester

O30.01 Twin pregnancy, monochorionic/ monoamniotic

Twin pregnancy, one placenta, one amniotic sac

Excludes1: conjoined twins (O30.02-)

O30.011 Twin pregnancy, monochorionic/monoamniotic, first trimester

O30.012 Twin pregnancy, monochorionic/monoamniotic, second trimester

O30.013 Twin pregnancy, monochorionic/monoamniotic, third trimester

O30.019 Twin pregnancy, monochorionic/monoamniotic, unspecified trimester

O30.02 Conjoined twin pregnancy

O30.021 Conjoined twin pregnancy, first trimester

O30.022 Conjoined twin pregnancy, second trimester

O30.023 Conjoined twin pregnancy, third trimester

O30.029 Conjoined twin pregnancy, unspecified trimester

O30.03 Twin pregnancy, monochorionic/ diamniotic
Twin pregnancy, one placenta, two amniotic sacs

O30.031 Twin pregnancy, monochorionic/ diamniotic, first trimester

● New code ▲ Revised code **Excludes1:** Not coded here **Excludes2:** Not included here ⊗ Placeholder required ⑦7th digit required

O30.032   Twin pregnancy, monochorionic/
diamniotic, second trimester

O30.033   Twin pregnancy, monochorionic/
diamniotic, third trimester

O30.039   Twin pregnancy, monochorionic/
diamniotic, unspecified trimester

O30.04   Twin pregnancy, dichorionic/diamniotic Twin
pregnancy, two placentae, two amniotic sacs

O30.041   Twin pregnancy, dichorionic/
diamniotic, first trimester

O30.042   Twin pregnancy, dichorionic/
diamniotic, second trimester

O30.043   Twin pregnancy, dichorionic/
diamniotic, third trimester

O30.049   Twin pregnancy, dichorionic/
diamniotic, unspecified trimester

O30.09   Twin pregnancy, unable to determine number
of placenta and number of amniotic sacs

O30.091   Twin pregnancy, unable to
determine number of placenta and
number of amniotic sacs, first
trimester

O30.092   Twin pregnancy, unable to
determine number of placenta and
number of amniotic sacs, second
trimester

O30.093   Twin pregnancy, unable to
determine number of placenta and
number of amniotic sacs, third
trimester

O30.099   Twin pregnancy, unable to
determine number of placenta and
number of amniotic sacs, unspecified
trimester

O30.1   Triplet pregnancy

O30.10   Triplet pregnancy, unspecified number of
placenta and unspecified number of amniotic
sacs

O30.101   Triplet pregnancy, unspecified
number of placenta and unspecified
number of amniotic sacs, first
trimester

O30.102   Triplet pregnancy, unspecified
number of placenta and unspecified
number of amniotic sacs, second
trimester

O30.103   Triplet pregnancy, unspecified
number of placenta and unspecified
number of amniotic sacs, third
trimester

O30.109   Triplet pregnancy, unspecified
number of placenta and unspecified
number of amniotic sacs, unspecified
trimester

O30.11   Triplet pregnancy with two or more
monochorionic fetuses

O30.111   Triplet pregnancy with two or more
monochorionic fetuses, first
trimester

O30.112   Triplet pregnancy with two or more
monochorionic fetuses, second
trimester

O30.113   Triplet pregnancy with two or more
monochorionic fetuses, third
trimester

O30.119   Triplet pregnancy with two or more
monochorionic fetuses, unspecified
trimester

O30.12   Triplet pregnancy with two or more
monoamniotic fetuses

O30.121   Triplet pregnancy with two or more
monoamniotic fetuses, first trimester

O30.122   Triplet pregnancy with two or more
monoamniotic fetuses, second
trimester

O30.123   Triplet pregnancy with two or more
monoamniotic fetuses, third
trimester

O30.129   Triplet pregnancy with two or more
monoamniotic fetuses, unspecified
trimester

O30.19   Triplet pregnancy, unable to determine number
of placenta and number of amniotic sacs

O30.191   Triplet pregnancy, unable to
determine number of placenta and
number of amniotic sacs, first
trimester

O30.192   Triplet pregnancy, unable to
determine number of placenta and
number of amniotic sacs, second
trimester

O30.193   Triplet pregnancy, unable to
determine number of placenta and
number of amniotic sacs, third
trimester

O30.199   Triplet pregnancy, unable to
determine number of placenta and
number of amniotic sacs, unspecified
trimester

O30.2   Quadruplet pregnancy

O30.20   Quadruplet pregnancy, unspecified number of
placenta and unspecified number of amniotic
sacs

O30.201   Quadruplet pregnancy, unspecified
number of placenta and unspecified
number of amniotic sacs, first
trimester

O30.202   Quadruplet pregnancy, unspecified
number of placenta and unspecified
number of amniotic sacs, second
trimester

O30.203   Quadruplet pregnancy, unspecified
number of placenta and unspecified
number of amniotic sacs, third
trimester

O30.209   Quadruplet pregnancy, unspecified
number of placenta and unspecified
number of amniotic sacs, unspecified
trimester

O30.21   Quadruplet pregnancy with two or more
monochorionic fetuses

O30.211   Quadruplet pregnancy with two or
more monochorionic fetuses, first
trimester

O30.212   Quadruplet pregnancy with two or
more monochorionic fetuses, second
trimester

O30.213   Quadruplet pregnancy with two or
more monochorionic fetuses, third
trimester

O30.219   Quadruplet pregnancy with two or
more monochorionic fetuses,
unspecified trimester

Add 4th-7th digits	Nonspecific code	Unspecified code	Manifestation code

O30.22 **Quadruplet pregnancy with two or more monoamniotic fetuses**

    O30.221 Quadruplet pregnancy with two or more monoamniotic fetuses, first trimester

    O30.222 Quadruplet pregnancy with two or more monoamniotic fetuses, second trimester

    O30.223 Quadruplet pregnancy with two or more monoamniotic fetuses, third trimester

    O30.229 Quadruplet pregnancy with two or more monoamniotic fetuses, unspecified trimester

O30.29 **Quadruplet pregnancy, unable to determine number of placenta and number of amniotic sacs**

    O30.291 Quadruplet pregnancy, unable to determine number of placenta and number of amniotic sacs, first trimester

    O30.292 Quadruplet pregnancy, unable to determine number of placenta and number of amniotic sacs, second trimester

    O30.293 Quadruplet pregnancy, unable to determine number of placenta and number of amniotic sacs, third trimester

    O30.299 Quadruplet pregnancy, unable to determine number of placenta and number of amniotic sacs, unspecified trimester

O30.8 **Other specified multiple gestation**

    Multiple gestation pregnancy greater then quadruplets

O30.80 **Other specified multiple gestation, unspecified number of placenta and unspecified number of amniotic sacs**

    O30.801 Other specified multiple gestation, unspecified number of placenta and unspecified number of amniotic sacs, first trimester

    O30.802 Other specified multiple gestation, unspecified number of placenta and unspecified number of amniotic sacs, second trimester

    O30.803 Other specified multiple gestation, unspecified number of placenta and unspecified number of amniotic sacs, third trimester

    O30.809 Other specified multiple gestation, unspecified number of placenta and unspecified number of amniotic sacs, unspecified trimester

O30.81 **Other specified multiple gestation with two or more monochorionic fetuses**

    O30.811 Other specified multiple gestation with two or more monochorionic fetuses, first trimester

    O30.812 Other specified multiple gestation with two or more monochorionic fetuses, second trimester

    O30.813 Other specified multiple gestation with two or more monochorionic fetuses, third trimester

    O30.819 Other specified multiple gestation with two or more monochorionic fetuses, unspecified trimester

O30.82 **Other specified multiple gestation with two or more monoamniotic fetuses**

    O30.821 Other specified multiple gestation with two or more monoamniotic fetuses, first trimester

    O30.822 Other specified multiple gestation with two or more monoamniotic fetuses, second trimester

    O30.823 Other specified multiple gestation with two or more monoamniotic fetuses, third trimester

    O30.829 Other specified multiple gestation with two or more monoamniotic fetuses, unspecified trimester

O30.89 **Other specified multiple gestation, unable to determine number of placenta and number of amniotic sacs**

    O30.891 Other specified multiple gestation, unable to determine number of placenta and number of amniotic sacs, first trimester

    O30.892 Other specified multiple gestation, unable to determine number of placenta and number of amniotic sacs, second trimester

    O30.893 Other specified multiple gestation, unable to determine number of placenta and number of amniotic sacs, third trimester

    O30.899 Other specified multiple gestation, unable to determine number of placenta and number of amniotic sacs, unspecified trimester

O30.9 **Multiple gestation, unspecified**

    Multiple pregnancy NOS

    O30.90 Multiple gestation, unspecified, unspecified trimester

    O30.91 Multiple gestation, unspecified, first trimester

    O30.92 Multiple gestation, unspecified, second trimester

    O30.93 Multiple gestation, unspecified, third trimester

O31 **Complications specific to multiple gestation**

Excludes2: delayed delivery of second twin, triplet, etc. (O63.2)

    malpresentation of one fetus or more (O32.9)

    placental transfusion syndromes (O43.0-)

One of the following 7th characters is to be assigned to each code under category O31. 7th character 0 is for single gestations and multiple gestations where the fetus is unspecified. 7th characters 1 through 9 are for cases of multiple gestations to identify the fetus for which the code applies. The appropriate code from category O30, Multiple gestation, must also be assigned when assigning a code from category O31 that has a 7th character of 1 through 9.

0 - not applicable or unspecified

1 - fetus 1

2 - fetus 2

3 - fetus 3

4 - fetus 4

5 - fetus 5

9 - Other fetus

O31.0 **Papyraceous fetus**

    Fetus compressus

    ⊗⑦O31.00 Papyraceous fetus, unspecified trimester

    ⊗⑦O31.01 Papyraceous fetus, first trimester

    ⊗⑦O31.02 Papyraceous fetus, second trimester

● New code   ▲ Revised code   **Excludes1:** Not coded here   **Excludes2:** Not included here   ⊗ Placeholder required   ⑦ 7th digit required

⊗⑦**O31.03** **Papyraceous fetus, third trimester**

O31.1 **Continuing pregnancy after spontaneous abortion of one fetus or more**

⊗⑦**O31.10** Continuing pregnancy after spontaneous abortion of one fetus or more, unspecified trimester

⊗⑦**O31.11** Continuing pregnancy after spontaneous abortion of one fetus or more, first trimester

⊗⑦**O31.12** Continuing pregnancy after spontaneous abortion of one fetus or more, second trimester

⊗⑦**O31.13** Continuing pregnancy after spontaneous abortion of one fetus or more, third trimester

O31.2 **Continuing pregnancy after intrauterine death of one fetus or more**

⊗⑦**O31.20** Continuing pregnancy after intrauterine death of one fetus or more, unspecified trimester

⊗⑦**O31.21** Continuing pregnancy after intrauterine death of one fetus or more, first trimester

⊗⑦**O31.22** Continuing pregnancy after intrauterine death of one fetus or more, second trimester

⊗⑦**O31.23** Continuing pregnancy after intrauterine death of one fetus or more, third trimester

O31.3 **Continuing pregnancy after elective fetal reduction of one fetus or more**

Continuing pregnancy after selective termination of one fetus or more

⊗⑦**O31.30** Continuing pregnancy after elective fetal reduction of one fetus or more, unspecified trimester

⊗⑦**O31.31** Continuing pregnancy after elective fetal reduction of one fetus or more, first trimester

⊗⑦**O31.32** Continuing pregnancy after elective fetal reduction of one fetus or more, second trimester

⊗⑦**O31.33** Continuing pregnancy after elective fetal reduction of one fetus or more, third trimester

O31.8 **Other complications specific to multiple gestation**

O31.8X **Other complications specific to multiple gestation**

⑦**O31.8X1** Other complications specific to multiple gestation, first trimester

⑦**O31.8X2** Other complications specific to multiple gestation, second trimester

⑦**O31.8X3** Other complications specific to multiple gestation, third trimester

⑦**O31.8X9** Other complications specific to multiple gestation, unspecified trimester

O32 **Maternal care for malpresentation of fetus**

Includes: the listed conditions as a reason for observation, hospitalization or other obstetric care of the mother, or for cesarean delivery before onset of labor

Excludes1: malpresentation of fetus with obstructed labor (O64.-)

One of the following 7th characters is to be assigned to each code under category O32. 7th character 0 is for single gestations and multiple gestations where the fetus is unspecified. 7th characters 1 through 9 are for cases of multiple gestations to identify the fetus for which the code applies. The appropriate code from category O30, Multiple gestation, must also be assigned when assigning a code from category O32 that has a 7th character of 1 through 9.

0 - not applicable or unspecified

1 - fetus 1

2 - fetus 2

3 - fetus 3

4 - fetus 4

5 - fetus 5

9 - Other fetus

⊗⑦**O32.0** **Maternal care for unstable lie**

⊗⑦**O32.1** **Maternal care for breech presentation**

Maternal care for buttocks presentation

Maternal care for complete breech

Maternal care for frank breech

Excludes1: footling presentation (O32.8)

incomplete breech (O32.8)

⊗⑦**O32.2** **Maternal care for transverse and oblique lie**

Maternal care for oblique presentation

Maternal care for transverse presentation

⊗⑦**O32.3** **Maternal care for face, brow and chin presentation**

⊗⑦**O32.4** **Maternal care for high head at term**

Maternal care for failure of head to enter pelvic brim

⊗⑦**O32.6** **Maternal care for compound presentation**

⊗⑦**O32.8** **Maternal care for other malpresentation of fetus**

Maternal care for footling presentation

Maternal care for incomplete breech

⊗⑦**O32.9** **Maternal care for malpresentation of fetus, unspecified**

O33 **Maternal care for disproportion**

Includes: the listed conditions as a reason for observation, hospitalization **or other** obstetric care of the mother, or for cesarean delivery before onset of labor

Excludes1: disproportion with obstructed labor (O65-O66)

O33.0 **Maternal care for disproportion due to deformity of maternal pelvic bones**

Maternal care for disproportion due to pelvic deformity causing disproportion NOS

O33.1 **Maternal care for disproportion due to generally contracted pelvis**

Maternal care for disproportion due to contracted pelvis NOS causing disproportion

O33.2 **Maternal care for disproportion due to inlet contraction of pelvis**

Maternal care for disproportion due to inlet contraction (pelvis) causing disproportion

⊗⑦**O33.3** **Maternal care for disproportion due to outlet contraction of pelvis**

Maternal care for disproportion due to mid-cavity contraction (pelvis)

Maternal care for disproportion due to outlet contraction (pelvis)

One of the following 7th characters is to be assigned to code O33.3. 7th character 0 is for single gestations and multiple gestations where the fetus is unspecified. 7th characters 1 through 9 are for cases of multiple gestations to identify the fetus for which the code applies. The appropriate code from category O30, Multiple gestation, must also be assigned when assigning code O33.3 with a 7th character of 1 through 9.

0 - not applicable or unspecified

1 - fetus 1

2 - fetus 2

3 - fetus 3

4 - fetus 4

5 - fetus 5

9 - Other fetus

⊗⑦**O33.4** **Maternal care for disproportion of mixed maternal and fetal origin**

One of the following 7th characters is to be assigned to code O33.4. 7th character 0 is for single gestations and multiple gestations where the fetus is unspecified. 7th characters 1 through 9 are for cases of multiple gestations to identify the fetus for which the code applies. The appropriate code from category O30,

Multiple gestation, must also be assigned when assigning code O33.4 with a 7th character of 1 through 9.

0 - not applicable or unspecified

1 - fetus 1

2 - fetus 2

3 - fetus 3

4 - fetus 4

5 - fetus 5

9 - Other fetus

⊗⑦**O33.5** **Maternal care for disproportion due to unusually large fetus**

Maternal care for disproportion due to disproportion of fetal origin with normally formed fetus

Maternal care for disproportion due to fetal disproportion NOS

One of the following 7th characters is to be assigned to code O33.5. 7th character 0 is for single gestations and multiple gestations where the fetus is unspecified. 7th characters 1 through 9 are for cases of multiple gestations to identify the fetus for which the code applies. The appropriate code from category O30,

Multiple gestation, must also be assigned when assigning code O33.5 with a 7th character of 1 through 9.

0 - not applicable or unspecified

1 - fetus 1

2 - fetus 2

3 - fetus 3

4 - fetus 4

5 - fetus 5

9 - Other fetus

⊗⑦**O33.6** **Maternal care for disproportion due to hydrocephalic fetus**

One of the following 7th characters is to be assigned to code O33.6. 7th character 0 is for single gestations and multiple gestations where the fetus is unspecified. 7th characters 1 through 9 are for cases of multiple gestations to identify the fetus for which the code applies. The appropriate code from category O30,

Multiple gestation, must also be assigned when assigning code O33.6 with a 7th character of 1 through 9.

0 - not applicable or unspecified

1 - fetus 1

2 - fetus 2

3 - fetus 3

4 - fetus 4

5 - fetus 5

9 - Other fetus

⊗⑦**O33.7** **Maternal care for disproportion due to other fetal deformities**

Maternal care for disproportion due to fetal ascites

Maternal care for disproportion due to fetal hydrops

Maternal care for disproportion due to fetal meningomyelocele

Maternal care for disproportion due to fetal sacral teratoma

Maternal care for disproportion due to fetal tumor

One of the following 7th characters is to be assigned to code O33.7. 7th character 0 is for single gestations and multiple gestations where the fetus is unspecified. 7th characters 1 through 9 are for cases of multiple gestations to identify the fetus for which the code applies. The appropriate code from category O30,

Multiple gestation, must also be assigned when assigning code O33.7 with a 7th character of 1 through 9.

0 - not applicable or unspecified

1 - fetus 1

2 - fetus 2

3 - fetus 3

4 - fetus 4

5 - fetus 5

9 - Other fetus

Excludes1: obstructed labor due to other fetal deformities (O66.3)

O33.8 **Maternal care for disproportion of other origin**

O33.9 **Maternal care for disproportion, unspecified**

Maternal care for disproportion due to cephalopelvic disproportion NOS

Maternal care for disproportion due to fetopelvic disproportion NOS

O34 **Maternal care for abnormality of pelvic organs**

Includes: the listed conditions as a reason for hospitalization or **other** obstetric care of the mother, or for cesarean

delivery before onset of labor

Code first any associated obstructed labor (O65.5)

Use additional code for specific condition

O34.0 **Maternal care for congenital malformation of uterus**

Maternal care for double uterus

Maternal care for uterus bicornis

O34.00 **Maternal care for unspecified congenital malformation of uterus, unspecified trimester**

O34.01 **Maternal care for unspecified congenital malformation of uterus, first trimester**

O34.02 **Maternal care for unspecified congenital malformation of uterus, second trimester**

O34.03 **Maternal care for unspecified congenital malformation of uterus, third trimester**

O34.1 **Maternal care for benign tumor of corpus uteri**

Excludes2: maternal care for benign tumor of cervix (O34.4-)

maternal care for malignant neoplasm of uterus (O9A.1-)

O34.10 **Maternal care for benign tumor of corpus uteri, unspecified trimester**

O34.11 **Maternal care for benign tumor of corpus uteri, first trimester**

O34.12 **Maternal care for benign tumor of corpus uteri, second trimester**

O34.13 **Maternal care for benign tumor of corpus uteri, third trimester**

O34.2 **Maternal care due to uterine scar from previous surgery**

O34.21 **Maternal care for scar from previous cesarean delivery**

O34.211 **Maternal care for low transverse scar from previous cesarean delivery**

O34.212 **Maternal care for vertical scar from previous cesarean delivery**

Maternal care for classical scar from previous cesarean delivery

O34.219 **Maternal care for unspecified type scar from previous cesarean delivery**

O34.29 **Maternal care due to uterine scar from other previous surgery**

Maternal care due to uterine scar **from other** transmural uterine incision

O34.3 **Maternal care for cervical incompetence**

Maternal care for cerclage with or without cervical incompetence

Maternal care for Shirodkar suture with or without cervical incompetence

O34.30 **Maternal care for cervical incompetence, unspecified trimester**

O34.31 **Maternal care for cervical incompetence, first trimester**

O34.32 **Maternal care for cervical incompetence, second trimester**

O34.33 **Maternal care for cervical incompetence, third trimester**

O34.4 **Maternal care for other abnormalities of cervix**

O34.40 **Maternal care for other abnormalities of cervix, unspecified trimester**

O34.41 **Maternal care for other abnormalities of cervix, first trimester**

O34.42 **Maternal care for other abnormalities of cervix, second trimester**

O34.43 **Maternal care for other abnormalities of cervix, third trimester**

O34.5 **Maternal care for other abnormalities of gravid uterus**

O34.51 **Maternal care for incarceration of gravid uterus**

O34.511 **Maternal care for incarceration of gravid uterus, first trimester**

O34.512 **Maternal care for incarceration of gravid uterus, second trimester**

O34.513 **Maternal care for incarceration of gravid uterus, third trimester**

O34.519 **Maternal care for incarceration of gravid uterus, unspecified trimester**

O34.52 **Maternal care for prolapse of gravid uterus**

O34.521 **Maternal care for prolapse of gravid uterus, first trimester**

O34.522 **Maternal care for prolapse of gravid uterus, second trimester**

O34.523 **Maternal care for prolapse of gravid uterus, third trimester**

O34.529 **Maternal care for prolapse of gravid uterus, unspecified trimester**

O34.53 **Maternal care for retroversion of gravid uterus**

O34.531 **Maternal care for retroversion of gravid uterus, first trimester**

O34.532 **Maternal care for retroversion of gravid uterus, second trimester**

O34.533 **Maternal care for retroversion of gravid uterus, third trimester**

O34.539 **Maternal care for retroversion of gravid uterus, unspecified trimester**

O34.59 **Maternal care for other abnormalities of gravid uterus**

O34.591 **Maternal care for other abnormalities of gravid uterus, first trimester**

O34.592 **Maternal care for other abnormalities of gravid uterus, second trimester**

O34.593 **Maternal care for other abnormalities of gravid uterus, third trimester**

O34.599 **Maternal care for other abnormalities of gravid uterus, unspecified trimester**

O34.6 **Maternal care for abnormality of vagina**

Excludes2: maternal care for vaginal varices in pregnancy (O22.1-)

O34.60 **Maternal care for abnormality of vagina, unspecified trimester**

O34.61 **Maternal care for abnormality of vagina, first trimester**

O34.62 **Maternal care for abnormality of vagina, second trimester**

O34.63 **Maternal care for abnormality of vagina, third trimester**

O34.7 **Maternal care for abnormality of vulva and perineum**

Excludes2: maternal care for perineal and vulval varices in pregnancy (O22.1-)

O34.70 **Maternal care for abnormality of vulva and perineum, unspecified trimester**

O34.71 **Maternal care for abnormality of vulva and perineum, first trimester**

O34.72 **Maternal care for abnormality of vulva and perineum, second trimester**

O34.73 **Maternal care for abnormality of vulva and perineum, third trimester**

O34.8 **Maternal care for other abnormalities of pelvic organs**

O34.80 **Maternal care for other abnormalities of pelvic organs, unspecified trimester**

O34.81 **Maternal care for other abnormalities of pelvic organs, first trimester**

O34.82 **Maternal care for other abnormalities of pelvic organs, second trimester**

O34.83 **Maternal care for other abnormalities of pelvic organs, third trimester**

O34.9 **Maternal care for abnormality of pelvic organ, unspecified**

O34.90 **Maternal care for abnormality of pelvic organ, unspecified, unspecified trimester**

O34.91 **Maternal care for abnormality of pelvic organ, unspecified, first trimester**

O34.92 **Maternal care for abnormality of pelvic organ, unspecified, second trimester**

O34.93 **Maternal care for abnormality of pelvic organ, unspecified, third trimester**

O35 **Maternal care for known or suspected fetal abnormality and damage**

Includes: the listed conditions in the fetus as a reason for hospitalization **or other** obstetric care to the mother, or for termination of pregnancy

Code also any associated maternal condition

Excludes1: encounter for suspected maternal and fetal conditions ruled out (Z03.7-)

One of the following 7th characters is to be assigned to each code under category O35. 7th character 0 is for single gestations and multiple gestations where the fetus is unspecified. 7th characters 1 through 9 are for cases of multiple gestations to identify the fetus for which the code applies. The appropriate code from category O30,

Multiple gestation, must also be assigned when assigning a code from category O35 that has a 7th character of 1 through 9.

0 - not applicable or unspecified
1 - fetus 1
2 - fetus 2
3 - fetus 3
4 - fetus 4
5 - fetus 5
9 - Other fetus

⊗⑦**O35.0** **Maternal care for (suspected) central nervous system malformation in fetus**

Maternal care for fetal anencephaly

Maternal care for fetal hydrocephalus

Maternal care for fetal spina bifida

Excludes2: chromosomal abnormality in fetus (O35.1)

⊗⑦**O35.1** **Maternal care for (suspected) chromosomal abnormality in fetus**

⊗⑦**O35.2** **Maternal care for (suspected) hereditary disease in fetus**

Excludes2: chromosomal abnormality in fetus (O35.1)

⊗⑦**O35.3** **Maternal care for (suspected) damage to fetus from viral disease in mother**

Maternal care for damage to fetus from maternal cytomegalovirus infection

Maternal care for damage to fetus from maternal rubella

⊗⑦**O35.4** **Maternal care for (suspected) damage to fetus from alcohol**

⊗⑦**O35.5** **Maternal care for (suspected) damage to fetus by drugs**

Maternal care for damage to fetus from drug addiction

⊗⑦**O35.6** **Maternal care for (suspected) damage to fetus by radiation**

⊗⑦**O35.7** **Maternal care for (suspected) damage to fetus by other medical procedures**

Maternal care for damage to fetus by amniocentesis

Maternal care for damage to fetus by biopsy procedures

Maternal care for damage to fetus by hematological investigation

Maternal care for damage to fetus by intrauterine contraceptive device

Maternal care for damage to fetus by intrauterine surgery

⊗⑦**O35.8** **Maternal care for other (suspected) fetal abnormality and damage**

Maternal care for damage to fetus from maternal listeriosis

Maternal care for damage to fetus from maternal toxoplasmosis

⊗⑦**O35.9** **Maternal care for (suspected) fetal abnormality and damage, unspecified**

O36 **Maternal care for other fetal problems**

Includes: the listed conditions in the fetus as a reason for hospitalization or other obstetric care of the mother, or for termination of pregnancy

Excludes1: encounter for suspected maternal and fetal conditions ruled out (Z03.7-)

placental transfusion syndromes (O43.0-)

Excludes2: labor and delivery complicated by fetal stress (O77.-)

One of the following 7th characters is to be assigned to each code under category O36. 7th character 0 is for single gestations and multiple gestations where the fetus is unspecified. 7th characters 1 through 9 are for cases of multiple gestations to identify the fetus for which the code applies. The appropriate code from category O30, Multiple gestation, must also be assigned when assigning a code from category O36 that has a 7th character of 1 through 9.

0 - not applicable or unspecified
1 - fetus 1
2 - fetus 2
3 - fetus 3
4 - fetus 4
5 - fetus 5
9 - Other fetus

O36.0 **Maternal care for rhesus isoimmunization**

Maternal care for Rh incompatibility (with hydrops fetalis)

O36.01 **Maternal care for anti-D [Rh] antibodies**

⑦**O36.011** **Maternal care for anti-D [Rh] antibodies, first trimester**

⑦**O36.012** **Maternal care for anti-D [Rh] antibodies, second trimester**

⑦**O36.013** **Maternal care for anti-D [Rh] antibodies, third trimester**

⑦**O36.019** **Maternal care for anti-D [Rh] antibodies, unspecified trimester**

O36.09 **Maternal care for other rhesus isoimmunization**

⑦**O36.091** **Maternal care for other rhesus isoimmunization, first trimester**

⑦**O36.092** **Maternal care for other rhesus isoimmunization, second trimester**

⑦**O36.093** **Maternal care for other rhesus isoimmunization, third trimester**

⑦**O36.099** **Maternal care for other rhesus isoimmunization, unspecified trimester**

O36.1 **Maternal care for other isoimmunization**

Maternal care for ABO isoimmunization

O36.11 **Maternal care for Anti-A sensitization**

Maternal care for isoimmunization NOS (with hydrops fetalis)

⑦**O36.111** **Maternal care for Anti-A sensitization, first trimester**

⑦**O36.112** **Maternal care for Anti-A sensitization, second trimester**

⑦**O36.113** **Maternal care for Anti-A sensitization, third trimester**

⑦**O36.119** **Maternal care for Anti-A sensitization, unspecified trimester**

O36.19 **Maternal care for other isoimmunization**

Maternal care for Anti-B sensitization

⑦**O36.191** **Maternal care for other isoimmunization, first trimester**

⑦**O36.192** **Maternal care for other isoimmunization, second trimester**

⑦**O36.193** **Maternal care for other isoimmunization, third trimester**

⑦**O36.199** **Maternal care for other isoimmunization, unspecified trimester**

O36.2 **Maternal care for hydrops fetalis**

Maternal care for hydrops fetalis NOS

Maternal care for hydrops fetalis not associated with isoimmunization

Excludes1: hydrops fetalis associated with ABO isoimmunization (O36.1-)

hydrops fetalis associated with rhesus isoimmunization (O36.0-)

● New code ▲ Revised code Excludes1: Not coded here Excludes2: Not included here ⊗ Placeholder required ⑦7th digit required

⊗⑦O36.20 **Maternal care for hydrops fetalis, unspecified trimester**

⊗⑦O36.21 **Maternal care for hydrops fetalis, first trimester**

⊗⑦O36.22 **Maternal care for hydrops fetalis, second trimester**

⊗⑦O36.23 **Maternal care for hydrops fetalis, third trimester**

⊗⑦O36.4 **Maternal care for intrauterine death**

Maternal care for intrauterine fetal death NOS

Maternal care for intrauterine fetal death after completion of 20 weeks of gestation

Maternal care for late fetal death

Maternal care for missed delivery

Excludes1: missed abortion (O02.1)

stillbirth (P95)

O36.5 **Maternal care for known or suspected poor fetal growth**

O36.51 **Maternal care for known or suspected placental insufficiency**

⑦O36.511 **Maternal care for known or suspected placental insufficiency, first trimester**

⑦O36.512 **Maternal care for known or suspected placental insufficiency, second trimester**

⑦O36.513 **Maternal care for known or suspected placental insufficiency, third trimester**

⑦O36.519 **Maternal care for known or suspected placental insufficiency, unspecified trimester**

O36.59 **Maternal care for other known or suspected poor fetal growth**

Maternal care for known or suspected light-for-dates NOS

Maternal care for known or suspected small-for-dates NOS

⑦O36.591 **Maternal care for other known or suspected poor fetal growth, first trimester**

⑦O36.592 **Maternal care for other known or suspected poor fetal growth, second trimester**

⑦O36.593 **Maternal care for other known or suspected poor fetal growth, third trimester**

⑦O36.599 **Maternal care for other known or suspected poor fetal growth, unspecified trimester**

O36.6 **Maternal care for excessive fetal growth**

Maternal care for known or suspected large-for-dates

⊗⑦O36.60 **Maternal care for excessive fetal growth, unspecified trimester**

⊗⑦O36.61 **Maternal care for excessive fetal growth, first trimester**

⊗⑦O36.62 **Maternal care for excessive fetal growth, second trimester**

⊗⑦O36.63 **Maternal care for excessive fetal growth, third trimester**

O36.7 **Maternal care for viable fetus in abdominal pregnancy**

⊗⑦O36.70 **Maternal care for viable fetus in abdominal pregnancy, unspecified trimester**

⊗⑦O36.71 **Maternal care for viable fetus in abdominal pregnancy, first trimester**

⊗⑦O36.72 **Maternal care for viable fetus in abdominal pregnancy, second trimester**

⊗⑦O36.73 **Maternal care for viable fetus in abdominal pregnancy, third trimester**

O36.8 **Maternal care for other specified fetal problems**

⊗⑦O36.80 **Pregnancy with inconclusive fetal viability**

Encounter to determine fetal viability of pregnancy

O36.81 **Decreased fetal movements**

⑦O36.812 **Decreased fetal movements, second trimester**

⑦O36.813 **Decreased fetal movements, third trimester**

⑦O36.819 **Decreased fetal movements, unspecified trimester**

•O36.83 **Maternal care for abnormalities of the fetal heart rate or rhythm**

•⑦O36.831 **Maternal care for abnormalities of the fetal heart rate or rhythm, first trimester**

•⑦O36.832 **Maternal care for abnormalities of the fetal heart rate or rhythm, second trimester**

•⑦O36.833 **Maternal care for abnormalities of the fetal heart rate or rhythm, third trimester**

•⑦O36.839 **Maternal care for abnormalities of the fetal heart rate or rhythm, unspecified trimester**

O36.82 **Fetal anemia and thrombocytopenia**

⑦O36.821 **Fetal anemia and thrombocytopenia, first trimester**

⑦O36.822 **Fetal anemia and thrombocytopenia, second trimester**

⑦O36.823 **Fetal anemia and thrombocytopenia, third trimester**

⑦O36.829 **Fetal anemia and thrombocytopenia, unspecified trimester**

O36.89 **Maternal care for other specified fetal problems**

⑦O36.891 **Maternal care for other specified fetal problems, first trimester**

⑦O36.892 **Maternal care for other specified fetal problems, second trimester**

⑦O36.893 **Maternal care for other specified fetal problems, third trimester**

⑦O36.899 **Maternal care for other specified fetal problems, unspecified trimester**

O36.9 **Maternal care for fetal problem, unspecified**

⊗⑦O36.90 **Maternal care for fetal problem, unspecified, unspecified trimester**

⊗⑦O36.91 **Maternal care for fetal problem, unspecified, first trimester**

⊗⑦O36.92 **Maternal care for fetal problem, unspecified, second trimester**

⊗⑦O36.93 **Maternal care for fetal problem, unspecified, third trimester**

O40 **Polyhydramnios**

Definition: Polyhydramnios is a condition that exists when there is too much amniotic fluid in the uterus.

Includes: hydramnios

Excludes1: encounter for suspected maternal and fetal conditions ruled out (Z03.7-)

| Add 4th-7th digits | | Nonspecific code | Unspecified code | Manifestation code | 649 |

One of the following 7th characters is to be assigned to each code under category O40. 7th character 0 is for single gestations and multiple gestations where the fetus is unspecified. 7th characters 1 through 9 are for cases of multiple gestations to identify the fetus for which the code applies. The appropriate code from category O30,

Multiple gestation, must also be assigned when assigning a code from category O40 that has a 7th character of 1 through 9.

0 - not applicable or unspecified

1 - fetus 1

2 - fetus 2

3 - fetus 3

4 - fetus 4

5 - fetus 5

9 - Other fetus

⊗⑦**O40.1** **Polyhydramnios, first trimester**

⊗⑦**O40.2** **Polyhydramnios, second trimester**

⊗⑦**O40.3** **Polyhydramnios, third trimester**

⊗⑦**O40.9** **Polyhydramnios, unspecified trimester**

O41 **Other disorders of amniotic fluid and membranes**

Excludes1: encounter for suspected maternal and fetal conditions ruled out (Z03.7-)

One of the following 7th characters is to be assigned to each code under category O41. 7th character 0 is for single gestations and multiple gestations where the fetus is unspecified. 7th characters 1 through 9 are for cases of multiple gestations to identify the fetus for which the code applies. The appropriate code from category O30,

Multiple gestation, must also be assigned when assigning a code from category O41 that has a 7th character of 1 through 9.

0 - not applicable or unspecified

1 - fetus 1

2 - fetus 2

3 - fetus 3

4 - fetus 4

5 - fetus 5

9 - Other fetus

O41.0 **Oligohydramnios**

Oligohydramnios without rupture of membranes

⊗⑦**O41.00** **Oligohydramnios, unspecified trimester**

⊗⑦**O41.01** **Oligohydramnios, first trimester**

⊗⑦**O41.02** **Oligohydramnios, second trimester**

⊗⑦**O41.03** **Oligohydramnios, third trimester**

O41.1 **Infection of amniotic sac and membranes**

O41.10 **Infection of amniotic sac and membranes, unspecified**

⑦**O41.101** **Infection of amniotic sac and membranes, unspecified, first trimester**

⑦**O41.102** **Infection of amniotic sac and membranes, unspecified, second trimester**

⑦**O41.103** **Infection of amniotic sac and membranes, unspecified, third trimester**

⑦**O41.109** **Infection of amniotic sac and membranes, unspecified, unspecified trimester**

O41.12 **Chorioamnionitis**

⑦**O41.121** **Chorioamnionitis, first trimester**

⑦**O41.122** **Chorioamnionitis, second trimester**

⑦**O41.123** **Chorioamnionitis, third trimester**

⑦**O41.129** **Chorioamnionitis, unspecified trimester**

O41.14 **Placentitis**

⑦**O41.141** **Placentitis, first trimester**

⑦**O41.142** **Placentitis, second trimester**

⑦**O41.143** **Placentitis, third trimester**

⑦**O41.149** **Placentitis, unspecified trimester**

O41.8 **Other specified disorders of amniotic fluid and membranes**

O41.8X **Other specified disorders of amniotic fluid and membranes**

⑦**O41.8X1** **Other specified disorders of amniotic fluid and membranes, first trimester**

⑦**O41.8X2** **Other specified disorders of amniotic fluid and membranes, second trimester**

⑦**O41.8X3** **Other specified disorders of amniotic fluid and membranes, third trimester**

⑦**O41.8X9** **Other specified disorders of amniotic fluid and membranes, unspecified trimester**

O41.9 **Disorder of amniotic fluid and membranes, unspecified**

⊗⑦**O41.90** **Disorder of amniotic fluid and membranes, unspecified, unspecified trimester**

⊗⑦**O41.91** **Disorder of amniotic fluid and membranes, unspecified, first trimester**

⊗⑦**O41.92** **Disorder of amniotic fluid and membranes, unspecified, second trimester**

⊗⑦**O41.93** **Disorder of amniotic fluid and membranes, unspecified, third trimester**

O42 **Premature rupture of membranes**

O42.0 **Premature rupture of membranes, onset of labor within 24 hours of rupture**

O42.00 **Premature rupture of membranes, onset of labor within 24 hours of rupture, unspecified weeks of gestation**

O42.01 **Preterm premature rupture of membranes, onset of labor within 24 hours of rupture**

Premature rupture of membranes before 37 completed weeks of gestation

O42.011 **Preterm premature rupture of membranes, onset of labor within 24 hours of rupture, first trimester**

O42.012 **Preterm premature rupture of membranes, onset of labor within 24 hours of rupture, second trimester**

O42.013 **Preterm premature rupture of membranes, onset of labor within 24 hours of rupture, third trimester**

O42.019 **Preterm premature rupture of membranes, onset of labor within 24 hours of rupture, unspecified trimester**

O42.02 **Full-term premature rupture of membranes, onset of labor within 24 hours of rupture**

Premature rupture of membranes at or after 37 completed weeks of gestation, onset of labor within 24 hours of rupture

O42.1 **Premature rupture of membranes, onset of labor more than 24 hours following rupture**

O42.10 **Premature rupture of membranes, onset of labor more than 24 hours following rupture, unspecified weeks of gestation**

● New code　▲ Revised code　**Excludes1:** Not coded here　**Excludes2:** Not included here　⊗ Placeholder required　⑦ 7th digit required

O42.11 **Preterm premature rupture of membranes, onset of labor more than 24 hours following rupture**

Premature rupture of membranes before 37 completed weeks of gestation

O42.111 **Preterm premature rupture of membranes, onset of labor more than 24 hours following rupture, first trimester**

O42.112 **Preterm premature rupture of membranes, onset of labor more than 24 hours following rupture, second trimester**

O42.113 **Preterm premature rupture of membranes, onset of labor more than 24 hours following rupture, third trimester**

O42.119 **Preterm premature rupture of membranes, onset of labor more than 24 hours following rupture, unspecified trimester**

O42.12 **Full-term premature rupture of membranes, onset of labor more than 24 hours following rupture**

Premature rupture of membranes at or after 37 completed weeks of gestation, onset of labor more than 24 hours following rupture

O42.9 **Premature rupture of membranes, unspecified as to length of time between rupture and onset of labor**

O42.90 **Premature rupture of membranes, unspecified as to length of time between rupture and onset of labor, unspecified weeks of gestation**

O42.91 **Preterm premature rupture of membranes, unspecified as to length of time between rupture and onset of labor**

Premature rupture of membranes before 37 completed weeks of gestation

O42.911 **Preterm premature rupture of membranes, unspecified as to length of time between rupture and onset of labor, first trimester**

O42.912 **Preterm premature rupture of membranes, unspecified as to length of time between rupture and onset of labor, second trimester**

O42.913 **Preterm premature rupture of membranes, unspecified as to length of time between rupture and onset of labor, third trimester**

O42.919 **Preterm premature rupture of membranes, unspecified as to length of time between rupture and onset of labor, unspecified trimester**

O42.92 **Full-term premature rupture of membranes, unspecified as to length of time between rupture and onset of labor**

Premature rupture of membranes at or after 37 completed weeks of gestation, unspecified as to length of time between rupture and onset of labor

O43 **Placental disorders**

Excludes2: maternal care for poor fetal growth due to placental insufficiency (O36.5-)

placenta previa (O44.-)

placental polyp (O90.89)

placentitis (O41.14-)

premature separation of placenta [abruptio placentae] (O45.-)

O43.0 **Placental transfusion syndromes**

O43.01 **Fetomaternal placental transfusion syndrome**

Maternofetal placental transfusion syndrome

O43.011 **Fetomaternal placental transfusion syndrome, first trimester**

O43.012 **Fetomaternal placental transfusion syndrome, second trimester**

O43.013 **Fetomaternal placental transfusion syndrome, third trimester**

O43.019 **Fetomaternal placental transfusion syndrome, unspecified trimester**

O43.02 **Fetus-to-fetus placental transfusion syndrome**

O43.021 **Fetus-to-fetus placental transfusion syndrome, first trimester**

O43.022 **Fetus-to-fetus placental transfusion syndrome, second trimester**

O43.023 **Fetus-to-fetus placental transfusion syndrome, third trimester**

O43.029 **Fetus-to-fetus placental transfusion syndrome, unspecified trimester**

O43.1 **Malformation of placenta**

O43.10 **Malformation of placenta, unspecified**

Abnormal placenta NOS

O43.101 **Malformation of placenta, unspecified, first trimester**

O43.102 **Malformation of placenta, unspecified, second trimester**

O43.103 **Malformation of placenta, unspecified, third trimester**

O43.109 **Malformation of placenta, unspecified, unspecified trimester**

O43.11 **Circumvallate placenta**

O43.111 **Circumvallate placenta, first trimester**

O43.112 **Circumvallate placenta, second trimester**

O43.113 **Circumvallate placenta, third trimester**

O43.119 **Circumvallate placenta, unspecified trimester**

O43.12 **Velamentous insertion of umbilical cord**

O43.121 **Velamentous insertion of umbilical cord, first trimester**

O43.122 **Velamentous insertion of umbilical cord, second trimester**

O43.123 **Velamentous insertion of umbilical cord, third trimester**

O43.129 **Velamentous insertion of umbilical cord, unspecified trimester**

O43.19 **Other malformation of placenta**

O43.191 **Other malformation of placenta, first trimester**

O43.192 **Other malformation of placenta, second trimester**

O43.193 **Other malformation of placenta, third trimester**

O43.199 **Other malformation of placenta, unspecified trimester**

O43.2 **Morbidly adherent placenta**

Code also associated third stage postpartum hemorrhage, if applicable (O72.0)

Excludes1: retained placenta (O73.-)

O43.21 **Placenta accreta**

| Add 4th-7th digits | Nonspecific code | Unspecified code | Manifestation code | 651 |

O43.211 Placenta accreta, first trimester

O43.212 Placenta accreta, second trimester

O43.213 Placenta accreta, third trimester

O43.219 Placenta accreta, unspecified trimester

O43.22 Placenta increta

O43.221 Placenta increta, first trimester

O43.222 Placenta increta, second trimester

O43.223 Placenta increta, third trimester

O43.229 Placenta increta, unspecified trimester

O43.23 Placenta percreta

O43.231 Placenta percreta, first trimester

O43.232 Placenta percreta, second trimester

O43.233 Placenta percreta, third trimester

O43.239 Placenta percreta, unspecified trimester

O43.8 Other placental disorders

O43.81 Placental infarction

O43.811 Placental infarction, first trimester

O43.812 Placental infarction, second trimester

O43.813 Placental infarction, third trimester

O43.819 Placental infarction, unspecified trimester

O43.89 Other placental disorders

Placental dysfunction

O43.891 Other placental disorders, first trimester

O43.892 Other placental disorders, second trimester

O43.893 Other placental disorders, third trimester

O43.899 Other placental disorders, unspecified trimester

O43.9 Unspecified placental disorder

O43.90 Unspecified placental disorder, unspecified trimester

O43.91 Unspecified placental disorder, first trimester

O43.92 Unspecified placental disorder, second trimester

O43.93 Unspecified placental disorder, third trimester

O44 Placenta previa

O44.0 Complete placenta previa NOS or without hemorrhage

Placenta previa NOS

O44.00 Complete placenta previa NOS or without hemorrhage, unspecified trimester

O44.01 Complete placenta previa NOS or without hemorrhage, first trimester

O44.02 Complete placenta previa NOS or without hemorrhage, second trimester

O44.03 Complete placenta previa NOS or without hemorrhage, third trimester

O44.1 Complete placenta previa with hemorrhage

Excludes1: labor and delivery complicated by hemorrhage from vasa previa (O69.4)

O44.10 Complete placenta previa with hemorrhage, unspecified trimester

O44.11 Complete placenta previa with hemorrhage, first trimester

O44.12 Complete placenta previa with hemorrhage, second trimester

O44.13 Complete placenta previa with hemorrhage, third trimester

O44.2 Partial placenta previa without hemorrhage

Marginal placenta previa, NOS or without hemorrhage

O44.20 Partial placenta previa NOS or without hemorrhage, unspecified trimester

O44.21 Partial placenta previa NOS or without hemorrhage, first trimester

O44.22 Partial placenta previa NOS or without hemorrhage, second trimester

O44.23 Partial placenta previa NOS or without hemorrhage, third trimester

O44.3 Partial placenta previa with hemorrhage

Marginal placenta previa with hemorrhage

O44.30 Partial placenta previa with hemorrhage, unspecified trimester

O44.31 Partial placenta previa with hemorrhage, first trimester

O44.32 Partial placenta previa with hemorrhage, second trimester

O44.33 Partial placenta previa with hemorrhage, third trimester

O44.4 Low lying placenta NOS or without hemorrhage

Low implantation of placenta NOS or without hemorrhage

O44.40 Low lying placenta NOS or without hemorrhage, unspecified trimester

O44.41 Low lying placenta NOS or without hemorrhage, first trimester

O44.42 Low lying placenta NOS or without hemorrhage, second trimester

O44.43 Low lying placenta NOS or without hemorrhage, third trimester

O44.5 Low lying placenta with hemorrhage

Low implantation of placenta with hemorrhage

O44.50 Low lying placenta with hemorrhage, unspecified trimester

O44.51 Low lying placenta with hemorrhage, first trimester

O44.52 Low lying placenta with hemorrhage, second trimester

O44.53 Low lying placenta with hemorrhage, third trimester

O45 Premature separation of placenta [abruptio placentae]

O45.0 Premature separation of placenta with coagulation defect

O45.00 Premature separation of placenta with coagulation defect, unspecified

O45.001 Premature separation of placenta with coagulation defect, unspecified, first trimester

O45.002 Premature separation of placenta with coagulation defect, unspecified, second trimester

O45.003 Premature separation of placenta with coagulation defect, unspecified, third trimester

O45.009 Premature separation of placenta with coagulation defect, unspecified, unspecified trimester

O45.01 Premature separation of placenta with afibrinogenemia

Premature separation of placenta with hypofibrinogenemia

O45.011 **Premature separation of placenta with afibrinogenemia, first trimester**

O45.012 **Premature separation of placenta with afibrinogenemia, second trimester**

O45.013 **Premature separation of placenta with afibrinogenemia, third trimester**

O45.019 **Premature separation of placenta with afibrinogenemia, unspecified trimester**

O45.02 **Premature separation of placenta with disseminated intravascular coagulation**

O45.021 **Premature separation of placenta with disseminated intravascular coagulation, first trimester**

O45.022 **Premature separation of placenta with disseminated intravascular coagulation, second trimester**

O45.023 **Premature separation of placenta with disseminated intravascular coagulation, third trimester**

O45.029 **Premature separation of placenta with disseminated intravascular coagulation, unspecified trimester**

O45.09 **Premature separation of placenta with other coagulation defect**

O45.091 **Premature separation of placenta with other coagulation defect, first trimester**

O45.092 **Premature separation of placenta with other coagulation defect, second trimester**

O45.093 **Premature separation of placenta with other coagulation defect, third trimester**

O45.099 **Premature separation of placenta with other coagulation defect, unspecified trimester**

O45.8 **Other premature separation of placenta**

O45.8X **Other premature separation of placenta**

O45.8X1 **Other premature separation of placenta, first trimester**

O45.8X2 **Other premature separation of placenta, second trimester**

O45.8X3 **Other premature separation of placenta, third trimester**

O45.8X9 **Other premature separation of placenta, unspecified trimester**

O45.9 **Premature separation of placenta, unspecified**

Abruptio placentae NOS

O45.90 **Premature separation of placenta, unspecified, unspecified trimester**

O45.91 **Premature separation of placenta, unspecified, first trimester**

O45.92 **Premature separation of placenta, unspecified, second trimester**

O45.93 **Premature separation of placenta, unspecified, third trimester**

O46 **Antepartum hemorrhage, not elsewhere classified**

Excludes1: hemorrhage in early pregnancy (O20.-)

intrapartum hemorrhage NEC (O67.-)

placenta previa (O44.-)

premature separation of placenta [abruptio placentae] (O45.-)

O46.0 **Antepartum hemorrhage with coagulation defect**

O46.00 **Antepartum hemorrhage with coagulation defect, unspecified**

O46.001 **Antepartum hemorrhage with coagulation defect, unspecified, first trimester**

O46.002 **Antepartum hemorrhage with coagulation defect, unspecified, second trimester**

O46.003 **Antepartum hemorrhage with coagulation defect, unspecified, third trimester**

O46.009 **Antepartum hemorrhage with coagulation defect, unspecified, unspecified trimester**

O46.01 **Antepartum hemorrhage with afibrinogenemia**

Antepartum hemorrhage with hypofibrinogenemia

O46.011 **Antepartum hemorrhage with afibrinogenemia, first trimester**

O46.012 **Antepartum hemorrhage with afibrinogenemia, second trimester**

O46.013 **Antepartum hemorrhage with afibrinogenemia, third trimester**

O46.019 **Antepartum hemorrhage with afibrinogenemia, unspecified trimester**

O46.02 **Antepartum hemorrhage with disseminated intravascular coagulation**

O46.021 **Antepartum hemorrhage with disseminated intravascular coagulation, first trimester**

O46.022 **Antepartum hemorrhage with disseminated intravascular coagulation, second trimester**

O46.023 **Antepartum hemorrhage with disseminated intravascular coagulation, third trimester**

O46.029 **Antepartum hemorrhage with disseminated intravascular coagulation, unspecified trimester**

O46.09 **Antepartum hemorrhage with other coagulation defect**

O46.091 **Antepartum hemorrhage with other coagulation defect, first trimester**

O46.092 **Antepartum hemorrhage with other coagulation defect, second trimester**

O46.093 **Antepartum hemorrhage with other coagulation defect, third trimester**

O46.099 **Antepartum hemorrhage with other coagulation defect, unspecified trimester**

O46.8 **Other antepartum hemorrhage**

O46.8X **Other antepartum hemorrhage**

O46.8X1 **Other antepartum hemorrhage, first trimester**

O46.8X2 **Other antepartum hemorrhage, second trimester**

O46.8X3 **Other antepartum hemorrhage, third trimester**

O46.8X9 **Other antepartum hemorrhage, unspecified trimester**

O46.9 **Antepartum hemorrhage, unspecified**

O46.90 **Antepartum hemorrhage, unspecified, unspecified trimester**

O46.91 Antepartum hemorrhage, unspecified, first trimester

O46.92 Antepartum hemorrhage, unspecified, second trimester

O46.93 Antepartum hemorrhage, unspecified, third trimester

O47 **False labor**

Includes: Braxton Hicks contractions

threatened labor

Excludes1: preterm labor (O60.-)

O47.0 **False labor before 37completed weeks of gestation**

O47.00 False labor before 37 completed weeks of gestation, unspecified trimester

O47.02 False labor before 37 completed weeks of gestation, second trimester

O47.03 False labor before 37 completed weeks of gestation, third trimester

O47.1 **False labor at or after 37completed weeks of gestation**

O47.9 **False labor, unspecified**

O48 **Late pregnancy**

O48.0 **Post-term pregnancy**

Pregnancy over 40 completed weeks to 42 completed weeks gestation

O48.1 **Prolonged pregnancy**

Pregnancy which has advanced beyond 42 completed weeks gestation

COMPLICATIONS OF LABOR AND DELIVERY (O60-O77)

O60 **Preterm labor**

Includes: onset (spontaneous) of labor before 37 completed weeks of gestation

Excludes1: false labor (O47.0-)

threatened labor NOS (O47.0-)

O60.0 **Preterm labor without delivery**

O60.00 Preterm labor without delivery, unspecified trimester

O60.02 Preterm labor without delivery, second trimester

O60.03 Preterm labor without delivery, third trimester

O60.1 **Preterm labor with preterm delivery**

One of the following 7th characters is to be assigned to each code under subcategory O60.1. 7th character 0 is for single gestations and multiple gestations where the fetus is unspecified. 7th characters 1 through 9 are for cases of multiple gestations to identify the fetus for which the code applies. The appropriate code from category O30, Multiple gestation, must also be assigned when assigning a code from subcategory O60.1 that has a 7th character of 1 through 9.

0 - not applicable or unspecified

1 - fetus 1

2 - fetus 2

3 - fetus 3

4 - fetus 4

5 - fetus 5

9 - Other fetus

⊗⑦**O60.10** Preterm labor with preterm delivery, unspecified trimester

Preterm labor with delivery NOS

⊗⑦**O60.12** Preterm labor second trimester with preterm delivery second trimester

⊗⑦**O60.13** Preterm labor second trimester with preterm delivery third trimester

⊗⑦**O60.14** Preterm labor third trimester with preterm delivery third trimester

O60.2 **Term delivery with preterm labor**

One of the following 7th characters is to be assigned to each code under subcategory O60.2. 7th character 0 is for single gestations and multiple gestations where the fetus is unspecified. 7th characters 1 through 9 are for cases of multiple gestations to identify the fetus for which the code applies. The appropriate code from category O30, Multiple gestation, must also be assigned when assigning a code from subcategory O60.2 that has a 7th character of 1 through 9.

0 - not applicable or unspecified

1 - fetus 1

2 - fetus 2

3 - fetus 3

4 - fetus 4

5 - fetus 5

9 - Other fetus

⊗⑦**O60.20** Term delivery with preterm labor, unspecified trimester

⊗⑦**O60.22** Term delivery with preterm labor, second trimester

⊗⑦**O60.23** Term delivery with preterm labor, third trimester

O61 **Failed induction of labor**

O61.0 **Failed medical induction of labor**

Failed induction (of labor) by oxytocin

Failed induction (of labor) by prostaglandins

O61.1 **Failed instrumental induction of labor**

Failed mechanical induction (of labor)

Failed surgical induction (of labor)

O61.8 **Other failed induction of labor**

O61.9 **Failed induction of labor, unspecified**

O62 **Abnormalities of forces of labor**

O62.0 **Primary inadequate contractions**

Failure of cervical dilatation

Primary hypotonic uterine dysfunction

Uterine inertia during latent phase of labor

O62.1 **Secondary uterine inertia**

Arrested active phase of labor

Secondary hypotonic uterine dysfunction

O62.2 **Other uterine inertia**

Atony of uterus without hemorrhage

Atony of uterus NOS

Desultory labor

Hypotonic uterine dysfunction NOS

Irregular labor

Poor contractions

Slow slope active phase of labor

Uterine inertia NOS

Excludes1: atony of uterus with hemorrhage (postpartum) (O72.1)

postpartum atony of uterus without hemorrhage (O75.89)

O62.3 **Precipitate labor**

O62.4 **Hypertonic, incoordinate, and prolonged uterine contractions**

Cervical spasm

● New code ▲ Revised code **Excludes1:** Not coded here **Excludes2:** Not included here ⊗ Placeholder required ⑦7th digit required

Contraction ring dystocia

Dyscoordinate labor hour-glass contraction of uterus

Hypertonic uterine dysfunction

Incoordinate uterine action

Tetanic contractions

Uterine dystocia NOS

Uterine spasm

Excludes1: dystocia (fetal) (maternal) NOS (O66.9)

O62.8 **Other abnormalities of forces of labor**

O62.9 **Abnormality of forces of labor, unspecified**

O63 **Long labor**

O63.0 **Prolonged first stage (of labor)**

O63.1 **Prolonged second stage (of labor)**

O63.2 **Delayed delivery of second twin, triplet, etc.**

O63.9 **Long labor, unspecified**

Prolonged labor NOS

O64 **Obstructed labor due to malposition and malpresentation of fetus**

Definition: Malposition and malpresentation of fetus refers to presentation of the fetal parts in inappropriate positions for the easiest passage through the cervix, e.g. Retention of the head, breech presentation.

One of the following 7th characters is to be assigned to each code under category O64. 7th character 0 is for single gestations and multiple gestations where the fetus is unspecified. 7th characters 1 through 9 are for cases of multiple gestations to identify the fetus for which the code applies. The appropriate code from category O30, Multiple gestation, must also be assigned when assigning a code from category O64 that has a 7th character of 1 through 9.

0 - not applicable or unspecified

1 - fetus 1

2 - fetus 2

3 - fetus 3

4 - fetus 4

5 - fetus 5

9 - Other fetus

⊗⑦**O64.0** **Obstructed labor due to incomplete rotation of fetal head**

Deep transverse arrest

Obstructed labor due to persistent occipitoiliac (position)

Obstructed labor due to persistent occipitoposterior (position)

Obstructed labor due to persistent occipitosacral (position)

Obstructed labor due to persistent occipitotransverse (position)

⊗⑦**O64.1** **Obstructed labor due to breech presentation**

Obstructed labor due to buttocks presentation

Obstructed labor due to complete breech presentation

Obstructed labor due to frank breech presentation

⊗⑦**O64.2** **Obstructed labor due to face presentation**

Obstructed labor due to chin presentation

⊗⑦**O64.3** **Obstructed labor due to brow presentation**

⊗⑦**O64.4** **Obstructed labor due to shoulder presentation**

Prolapsed arm

Excludes1: impacted shoulders (O66.0)

shoulder dystocia (O66.0)

⊗⑦**O64.5** **Obstructed labor due to compound presentation**

⊗⑦**O64.8** **Obstructed labor due to other malposition and malpresentation**

Obstructed labor due to footling presentation

Obstructed labor due to incomplete breech presentation

⊗⑦**O64.9** **Obstructed labor due to malposition and malpresentation, unspecified**

O65 **Obstructed labor due to maternal pelvic abnormality**

O65.0 **Obstructed labor due to deformed pelvis**

O65.1 **Obstructed labor due to generally contracted pelvis**

O65.2 **Obstructed labor due to pelvic inlet contraction**

O65.3 **Obstructed labor due to pelvic outlet and mid-cavity contraction**

O65.4 **Obstructed labor due to fetopelvic disproportion, unspecified**

Excludes1: dystocia due to abnormality of fetus (O66.2-O66.3)

O65.5 **Obstructed labor due to abnormality of maternal pelvic organs**

Obstructed labor due to conditions listed in O34.-

Use additional code to identify abnormality of pelvic organs O34.-

O65.8 **Obstructed labor due to other maternal pelvic abnormalities**

O65.9 **Obstructed labor due to maternal pelvic abnormality, unspecified**

O66 **Other obstructed labor**

O66.0 **Obstructed labor due to shoulder dystocia**

Impacted shoulders

O66.1 **Obstructed labor due to locked twins**

O66.2 **Obstructed labor due to unusually large fetus**

O66.3 **Obstructed labor due to other abnormalities of fetus**

Dystocia due to fetal ascites

Dystocia due to fetal hydrops

Dystocia due to fetal meningomyelocele

Dystocia due to fetal sacral teratoma

Dystocia due to fetal tumor

Dystocia due to hydrocephalic fetus

Use additional code to identify cause of obstruction

O66.4 **Failed trial of labor O66.40 Failed trial of labor, unspecified**

O66.40 **Failed trial of labor, unspecified**

O66.41 **Failed attempted vaginal birth after previous cesarean delivery**

Code first rupture of uterus, if applicable (O71.0-O71.1)

O66.5 **Attempted application of vacuum extractor and forceps**

Attempted application of vacuum or forceps, with subsequent delivery by forceps or cesarean delivery

O66.6 **Obstructed labor due to other multiple fetuses**

O66.8 **Other specified obstructed labor**

Use additional code to identify cause of obstruction

O66.9 **Obstructed labor, unspecified**

Dystocia NOS

Fetal dystocia NOS

Maternal dystocia NOS

O67 **Labor and delivery complicated by intrapartum hemorrhage, not elsewhere classified**

Excludes1: antepartum hemorrhage NEC (O46.-)

placenta previa (O44.-)

premature separation of placenta [abruptio placentae] (O45.-)

Excludes2: postpartum hemorrhage (O72.-)

O67.0 **Intrapartum hemorrhage with coagulation defect**

Intrapartum hemorrhage (excessive) associated with afibrinogenemia

Add 4th-7th digits   Nonspecific code   Unspecified code   Manifestation code

Intrapartum hemorrhage (excessive) associated with disseminated intravascular coagulation

Intrapartum hemorrhage (excessive) associated with hyperfibrinolysis

Intrapartum hemorrhage (excessive) associated with hypofibrinogenemia

O67.8   Other intrapartum hemorrhage

Excessive intrapartum hemorrhage

O67.9   Intrapartum hemorrhage, unspecified

O68   Labor and delivery complicated by abnormality of fetal acid-base balance

Fetal acidemia complicating labor and delivery

Fetal acidosis complicating labor and delivery

Fetal alkalosis complicating labor and delivery

Fetal metabolic acidemia complicating labor and delivery

Excludes1: fetal stress NOS (O77.9)

labor and delivery complicated by electrocardiographic evidence of fetal stress (O77.8)

labor and delivery complicated by ultrasonic evidence of fetal stress (O77.8)

Excludes2: abnormality in fetal heart rate or rhythm (O76)

labor and delivery complicated by meconium in amniotic fluid (O77.0)

O69   Labor and delivery complicated by umbilical cord complications

One of the following 7th characters is to be assigned to each code under category O69. 7th character 0 is for single gestations and multiple gestations where the fetus is unspecified. 7th characters 1 through 9 are for cases of multiple gestations to identify the fetus for which the code applies. The appropriate code from category O30, Multiple gestation, must also be assigned when assigning a code from category O69 that has a 7th character of 1 through 9.

0 - not applicable or unspecified

1 - fetus 1

2 - fetus 2

3 - fetus 3

4 - fetus 4

5 - fetus 5

9 - Other fetus

⊗⑦**O69.0   Labor and delivery complicated by prolapse of cord**

⊗⑦**O69.1   Labor and delivery complicated by cord around neck, with compression**

Excludes1: labor and delivery complicated by cord around neck, without compression (O69.81)

⊗⑦**O69.2   Labor and delivery complicated by other cord entanglement, with compression**

Labor and delivery complicated by compression of cord NOS

Labor and delivery complicated by entanglement of cords of twins in monoamniotic sac

Labor and delivery complicated by knot in cord

Excludes1: labor and delivery complicated by other cord entanglement, without compression (O69.82)

⊗⑦**O69.3   Labor and delivery complicated by short cord**

⊗⑦**O69.4   Labor and delivery complicated by vasa previa**

Labor and delivery complicated by hemorrhage from vasa previa

⊗⑦**O69.5   Labor and delivery complicated by vascular lesion of cord**

Labor and delivery complicated by cord bruising

Labor and delivery complicated by cord hematoma

Labor and delivery complicated by thrombosis of umbilical vessels

O69.8   Labor and delivery complicated by other cord complications

⊗⑦**O69.81   Labor and delivery complicated by cord around neck, without compression**

⊗⑦**O69.82   Labor and delivery complicated by other cord entanglement, without compression**

⊗⑦**O69.89   Labor and delivery complicated by other cord complications**

⊗⑦**O69.9   Labor and delivery complicated by cord complication, unspecified**

O70   Perineal laceration during delivery

Includes: episiotomy extended by laceration

Excludes1: obstetric high vaginal laceration alone (O71.4)

O70.0   First degree perineal laceration during delivery

Perineal laceration, rupture or tear involving fourchette during delivery

Perineal laceration, rupture or tear involving labia during delivery

Perineal laceration, rupture or tear involving skin during delivery

Perineal laceration, rupture or tear involving vagina during delivery

Perineal laceration, rupture or tear involving vulva during delivery

Slight perineal laceration, rupture or tear during delivery

O70.1   Second degree perineal laceration during delivery

Perineal laceration, rupture or tear during delivery as in O70.0, also involving pelvic floor

Perineal laceration, rupture or tear during delivery as in O70.0, also involving perineal muscles

Perineal laceration, rupture or tear during delivery as in O70.0, also involving vaginal muscles

Excludes1: perineal laceration involving anal sphincter (O70.2)

O70.2   Third degree perineal laceration during delivery

Perineal laceration, rupture or tear during delivery as in O70.1, also involving anal sphincter

Perineal laceration, rupture or tear during delivery as in O70.1, also involving rectovaginal septum

Perineal laceration, rupture or tear during delivery as in O70.1, also involving sphincter NOS

Excludes1: anal sphincter tear during delivery without third degree perineal laceration (O70.4)

perineal laceration involving anal or rectal mucosa (O70.3)

O70.20   Third degree perineal laceration during delivery, unspecified

O70.21   Third degree perineal laceration during delivery, IIIa

Third degree perineal laceration during delivery with less than 50% of external anal sphincter (EAS) thickness torn

O70.22   Third degree perineal laceration during delivery, IIIb

Third degree perineal laceration during delivery with more than 50% external anal sphincter (EAS) thickness torn

O70.23   Third degree perineal laceration during delivery, IIIC

Third degree perineal laceration during delivery with both external anal sphincter (EAS) and internal anal sphincter (IAS) torn

O70.3   Fourth degree perineal laceration during delivery

Perineal laceration, rupture or tear during delivery as in O70.2, also involving anal mucosa

Perineal laceration, rupture or tear during delivery as in O70.2, also involving rectal mucosa

O70.4 **Anal sphincter tear complicating delivery, not associated with third degree laceration**

> **Excludes1:** anal sphincter tear with third degree perineal laceration (O70.2)

O70.9 **Perineal laceration during delivery, unspecified**

O71 **Other obstetric trauma**

Includes: obstetric damage from instruments

O71.0 **Rupture of uterus (spontaneous) before onset of labor**

> **Excludes1:** disruption of (current) cesarean delivery wound (O90.0)
>
> laceration of uterus, NEC (O71.81)

O71.00 **Rupture of uterus before onset of labor, unspecified trimester**

O71.02 **Rupture of uterus before onset of labor, second trimester**

O71.03 **Rupture of uterus before onset of labor, third trimester**

O71.1 **Rupture of uterus during labor**

Rupture of uterus not stated as occurring before onset of labor

> **Excludes1:** disruption of cesarean delivery wound (O90.0)
>
> laceration of uterus, NEC (O71.81)

O71.2 **Postpartum inversion of uterus**

O71.3 **Obstetric laceration of cervix**

Annular detachment of cervix

O71.4 **Obstetric high vaginal laceration alone**

Laceration of vaginal wall without perineal laceration

> **Excludes1:** obstetric high vaginal laceration with perineal laceration (O70.-)

O71.5 **Other obstetric injury to pelvic organs**

Obstetric injury to bladder

Obstetric injury to urethra

> **Excludes2:** obstetric periurethral trauma (O71.82)

O71.6 **Obstetric damage to pelvic joints and ligaments**

Obstetric avulsion of inner symphyseal cartilage

Obstetric damage to coccyx

Obstetric traumatic separation of symphysis (pubis)

O71.7 **Obstetric hematoma of pelvis**

Obstetric hematoma of perineum

Obstetric hematoma of vagina

Obstetric hematoma of vulva

O71.8 **Other specified obstetric trauma**

O71.81 **Laceration of uterus, not elsewhere classified**

O71.82 **Other specified trauma to perineum and vulva**

Obstetric periurethral trauma

O71.89 **Other specified obstetric trauma**

O71.9 **Obstetric trauma, unspecified**

O72 **Postpartum hemorrhage**

Includes: hemorrhage after delivery of fetus or infant

O72.0 **Third-stage hemorrhage**

Hemorrhage associated with retained, trapped or adherent placenta

Retained placenta NOS

Code also type of adherent placenta (O43.2-)

O72.1 **Other immediate postpartum hemorrhage**

Hemorrhage following delivery of placenta

Postpartum hemorrhage (atonic) NOS

Uterine atony with hemorrhage

> **Excludes1:** uterine atony NOS (O62.2)
>
> uterine atony without hemorrhage (O62.2)
>
> postpartum atony of uterus without hemorrhage (O75.89)

O72.2 **Delayed and secondary postpartum hemorrhage**

Hemorrhage associated with retained portions of placenta or membranes after the first 24 hours following delivery of placenta

Retained products of conception NOS, following delivery

O72.3 **Postpartum coagulation defects**

Postpartum afibrinogenemia

Postpartum fibrinolysis

O73 **Retained placenta and membranes, without hemorrhage**

Excludes1: placenta accreta (O43.21-)

> placenta increta (O43.22-)
>
> placenta percreta (O43.23-)

O73.0 **Retained placenta without hemorrhage**

Adherent placenta, without hemorrhage

Trapped placenta without hemorrhage

O73.1 **Retained portions of placenta and membranes, without hemorrhage**

Retained products of conception following delivery, without hemorrhage

O74 **Complications of anesthesia during labor and delivery**

Includes: maternal complications arising from the administration of a general, regional or local anesthetic, analgesic or other sedation during labor and delivery

Use additional code, if applicable, to identify specific complication

O74.0 **Aspiration pneumonitis due to anesthesia during labor and delivery**

Inhalation of stomach contents or secretions NOS due to anesthesia during labor and delivery

Mendelson's syndrome due to anesthesia during labor and delivery

O74.1 **Other pulmonary complications of anesthesia during labor and delivery**

O74.2 **Cardiac complications of anesthesia during labor and delivery**

O74.3 **Central nervous system complications of anesthesia during labor and delivery**

O74.4 **Toxic reaction to local anesthesia during labor and delivery**

O74.5 **Spinal and epidural anesthesia-induced headache during labor and delivery**

O74.6 **Other complications of spinal and epidural anesthesia during labor and delivery**

O74.7 **Failed or difficult intubation for anesthesia during labor and delivery**

O74.8 **Other complications of anesthesia during labor and delivery**

O74.9 **Complication of anesthesia during labor and delivery, unspecified**

O75 **Other complications of labor and delivery, not elsewhere classified**

Excludes2: puerperal (postpartum) infection (O86.-)

> puerperal (postpartum) sepsis (O85)

O75.0 **Maternal distress during labor and delivery**

O75.1 **Shock during or following labor and delivery**

Obstetric shock following labor and delivery

O75.2 Pyrexia during labor, not elsewhere classified

O75.3 Other infection during labor Sepsis during labor **Use additional code** (B95-B97), to identify infectious agent

O75.4 Other complications of obstetric surgery and procedures

Cardiac arrest following obstetric surgery or procedures

Cardiac failure following obstetric surgery or procedures

Cerebral anoxia following obstetric surgery or procedures

Pulmonary edema following obstetric surgery or procedures

Use additional code to identify specific complication

Excludes2: complications of anesthesia during labor and delivery (O74.-)

disruption of obstetrical (surgical) wound (O90.0-O90.1)

hematoma of obstetrical (surgical) wound (O90.2)

infection of obstetrical (surgical) wound (O86.0)

O75.5 Delayed delivery after artificial rupture of membranes

O75.8 Other specified complications of labor and delivery

O75.81 Maternal exhaustion complicating labor and delivery

O75.82 Onset (spontaneous) of labor after 37 completed weeks of gestation but before 39 completed weeks gestation, with delivery by (planned) cesarean section

Delivery by (planned) cesarean section occurring after 37 completed weeks of gestation but before 39 completed weeks gestation due to (spontaneous) onset of labor

Code first to specify reason for planned cesarean section such as:

cephalopelvic disproportion (normally formed fetus) (O33.9)

previous cesarean delivery (O34.21)

O75.89 Other specified complications of labor and delivery

O75.9 Complication of labor and delivery, unspecified

O76 Abnormality in fetal heart rate and rhythm complicating labor and delivery

Depressed fetal heart rate tones complicating labor and delivery

Fetal bradycardia complicating labor and delivery

Fetal heart rate decelerations complicating labor and delivery

Fetal heart rate irregularity complicating labor and delivery

Fetal heart rate abnormal variability complicating labor and delivery

Fetal tachycardia complicating labor and delivery

Non-reassuring fetal heart rate or rhythm complicating labor and delivery

Excludes1: fetal stress NOS (O77.9)

labor and delivery complicated by electrocardiographic evidence of fetal stress (O77.8)

labor and delivery complicated by ultrasonic evidence of fetal stress (O77.8)

Excludes2: fetal metabolic acidemia (O68)

Other fetal stress (O77.0-O77.1)

O77 Other fetal stress complicating labor and delivery

O77.0 Labor and delivery complicated by meconium in amniotic fluid

O77.1 Fetal stress in labor or delivery due to drug administration

O77.8 Labor and delivery complicated by other evidence of fetal stress

Labor and delivery complicated by electrocardiographic evidence of fetal stress

Labor and delivery complicated by ultrasonic evidence of fetal stress

Excludes1: abnormality of fetal acid-base balance (O68)

abnormality in fetal heart rate or rhythm (O76)

fetal metabolic acidemia (O68)

O77.9 Labor and delivery complicated by fetal stress, unspecified

Excludes1: abnormality of fetal acid-base balance (O68)

abnormality in fetal heart rate or rhythm (O76)

fetal metabolic acidemia (O68)

ENCOUNTER FOR DELIVERY (O80-O82)

O80 Encounter for full-term uncomplicated delivery

Delivery requiring minimal or no assistance, with or without episiotomy, without fetal manipulation [e.g., rotation version] or instrumentation [forceps] of a spontaneous, cephalic, vaginal, full-term, single, live-born infant. This code is for use as a single diagnosis code and is not to be used with any other code from chapter 15.

Use additional code to indicate outcome of delivery (Z37.0)

O82 Encounter for cesarean delivery without indication

Use additional code to indicate outcome of delivery (Z37.0)

COMPLICATIONS PREDOMINANTLY RELATED TO THE PUERPERIUM (O85-O92)

Excludes2: mental and behavioral disorders associated with the puerperium (F53)

obstetrical tetanus (A34)

puerperal osteomalacia (M83.0)

O85 Puerperal sepsis

Postpartum sepsis

Puerperal peritonitis

Puerperal pyemia

Use additional code (B95-B97), to identify infectious agent

Use additional code (R65.2-) to identify severe sepsis, if applicable

Excludes1: fever of unknown origin following delivery (O86.4)

genital tract infection following delivery (O86.1-)

obstetric pyemic and septic embolism (O88.3-)

puerperal septic thrombophlebitis (O86.81)

urinary tract infection following delivery (O86.2-)

Excludes2: sepsis during labor (O75.3)

O86 Other puerperal infections

Use additional code (B95-B97), to identify infectious agent

Excludes2: infection during labor (O75.3)

obstetrical tetanus (A34)

O86.0 Infection of obstetric surgical wound

Infected cesarean delivery wound following delivery

Infected perineal repair following delivery

O86.1 Other infection of genital tract following delivery

O86.11 Cervicitis following delivery

O86.12 Endometritis following delivery

O86.13 Vaginitis following delivery

O86.19 Other infection of genital tract following delivery

O86.2 Urinary tract infection following delivery

O86.20 Urinary tract infection following delivery, unspecified

Puerperal urinary tract infection NOS

O86.21 **Infection of kidney following delivery**

O86.22 **Infection of bladder following delivery**

Infection of urethra following delivery

O86.29 **Other urinary tract infection following delivery**

O86.4 **Pyrexia of unknown origin following delivery**

Puerperal infection NOS following delivery

Puerperal pyrexia NOS following delivery

Excludes2: pyrexia during labor (O75.2)

O86.8 **Other specified puerperal infections**

O86.81 **Puerperal septic thrombophlebitis**

O86.89 **Other specified puerperal infections**

O87 **Venous complications and hemorrhoids in the puerperium**

Includes: venous complications in labor, delivery and the puerperium

Excludes2: obstetric embolism (O88.-)

puerperal septic thrombophlebitis (O86.81)

venous complications in pregnancy (O22.-)

O87.0 **Superficial thrombophlebitis in the puerperium**

Puerperal phlebitis NOS

Puerperal thrombosis NOS

O87.1 **Deep phlebothrombosis in the puerperium**

Deep vein thrombosis, postpartum

Pelvic thrombophlebitis, postpartum

Use additional code to identify the deep vein thrombosis (I82.4-, I82.5-, I82.62-. I82.72-)

Use additional code, if applicable, for associated long-term (current) use of anticoagulants (Z79.01)

O87.2 **Hemorrhoids in the puerperium**

O87.3 **Cerebral venous thrombosis in the puerperium**

Cerebrovenous sinus thrombosis in the puerperium

O87.4 **Varicose veins of lower extremity in the puerperium**

O87.8 **Other venous complications in the puerperium**

Genital varices in the puerperium

O87.9 **Venous complication in the puerperium, unspecified**

Puerperal phlebopathy NOS

O88 **Obstetric embolism**

Excludes1: embolism complicating abortion NOS (O03.2)

embolism complicating ectopic or molar pregnancy (O08.2)

embolism complicating failed attempted abortion (O07.2)

embolism complicating induced abortion (O04.7)

embolism complicating spontaneous abortion (O03.2, O03.7)

O88.0 **Obstetric air embolism**

O88.01 **Obstetric air embolism in pregnancy**

O88.011 **Air embolism in pregnancy, first trimester**

O88.012 **Air embolism in pregnancy, second trimester**

O88.013 **Air embolism in pregnancy, third trimester**

O88.019 **Air embolism in pregnancy, unspecified trimester**

O88.02 **Air embolism in childbirth**

O88.03 **Air embolism in the puerperium**

O88.1 **Amniotic fluid embolism**

Anaphylactoid syndrome in pregnancy

O88.11 **Amniotic fluid embolism in pregnancy**

O88.111 **Amniotic fluid embolism in pregnancy, first trimester**

O88.112 **Amniotic fluid embolism in pregnancy, second trimester**

O88.113 **Amniotic fluid embolism in pregnancy, third trimester**

O88.119 **Amniotic fluid embolism in pregnancy, unspecified trimester**

O88.12 **Amniotic fluid embolism in childbirth**

O88.13 **Amniotic fluid embolism in the puerperium**

O88.2 **Obstetric thromboembolism**

O88.21 **Thromboembolism in pregnancy**

Obstetric (pulmonary) embolism NOS

O88.211 **Thromboembolism in pregnancy, first trimester**

O88.212 **Thromboembolism in pregnancy, second trimester**

O88.213 **Thromboembolism in pregnancy, third trimester**

O88.219 **Thromboembolism in pregnancy, unspecified trimester**

O88.22 **Thromboembolism in childbirth**

O88.23 **Thromboembolism in the puerperium**

Puerperal (pulmonary) embolism NOS

O88.3 **Obstetric pyemic and septic embolism**

O88.31 **Pyemic and septic embolism in pregnancy**

O88.311 **Pyemic and septic embolism in pregnancy, first trimester**

O88.312 **Pyemic and septic embolism in pregnancy, second trimester**

O88.313 **Pyemic and septic embolism in pregnancy, third trimester**

O88.319 **Pyemic and septic embolism in pregnancy, unspecified trimester**

O88.32 **Pyemic and septic embolism in childbirth**

O88.33 **Pyemic and septic embolism in the puerperium**

O88.8 **Other obstetric embolism**

Obstetric fat embolism

O88.81 **Other embolism in pregnancy**

O88.811 **Other embolism in pregnancy, first trimester**

O88.812 **Other embolism in pregnancy, second trimester**

O88.813 **Other embolism in pregnancy, third trimester**

O88.819 **Other embolism in pregnancy, unspecified trimester**

O88.82 **Other embolism in childbirth**

O88.83 **Other embolism in the puerperium**

O89 **Complications of anesthesia during the puerperium**

Includes: maternal complications arising from the administration of a general, regional or local anesthetic, analgesic **or other** sedation during the puerperium

Use additional code, if applicable, to identify specific complication

O89.0 **Pulmonary complications of anesthesia during the puerperium**

O89.01 **Aspiration pneumonitis due to anesthesia during the puerperium**

Inhalation of stomach contents or secretions NOS due to anesthesia during the puerperium

Mendelson's syndrome due to anesthesia during the puerperium

O89.09 Other pulmonary complications of anesthesia during the puerperium

O89.1 Cardiac complications of anesthesia during the puerperium

O89.2 Central nervous system complications of anesthesia during the puerperium

O89.3 Toxic reaction to local anesthesia during the puerperium

O89.4 Spinal and epidural anesthesia-induced headache during the puerperium

O89.5 Other complications of spinal and epidural anesthesia during the puerperium

O89.6 Failed or difficult intubation for anesthesia during the puerperium

O89.8 Other complications of anesthesia during the puerperium

O89.9 Complication of anesthesia during the puerperium, unspecified

O90 **Complications of the puerperium, not elsewhere classified**

O90.0 Disruption of cesarean delivery wound

Dehiscence of cesarean delivery wound

Excludes1: rupture of uterus (spontaneous) before onset of labor (O71.0-)

rupture of uterus during labor (O71.1)

O90.1 Disruption of perineal obstetric wound

Disruption of wound of episiotomy

Disruption of wound of perineal laceration

Secondary perineal tear

O90.2 Hematoma of obstetric wound

O90.3 Peripartum cardiomyopathy

Conditions in I42.- arising during pregnancy and the puerperium

Excludes1: pre-existing heart disease complicating pregnancy and the puerperium (O99.4-)

O90.4 Postpartum acute kidney failure

Hepatorenal syndrome following labor and delivery

O90.5 Postpartum thyroiditis

O90.6 Postpartum mood disturbance

Postpartum blues

Postpartum dysphoria

Postpartum sadness

Excludes1: postpartum depression (F53)

puerperal psychosis (F53)

O90.8 Other complications of the puerperium, not elsewhere classified

O90.81 Anemia of the puerperium

Postpartum anemia NOS

Excludes1: pre-existing anemia complicating the puerperium (O99.03)

O90.89 Other complications of the puerperium, not elsewhere classified

Placental polyp

O90.9 Complication of the puerperium, unspecified

O91 **Infections of breast associated with pregnancy, the puerperium and lactation**

Use additional code to identify infection

O91.0 Infection of nipple associated with pregnancy, the puerperium and lactation

O91.01 Infection of nipple associated with pregnancy

Gestational abscess of nipple

O91.011 Infection of nipple associated with pregnancy, first trimester

O91.012 Infection of nipple associated with pregnancy, second trimester

O91.013 Infection of nipple associated with pregnancy, third trimester

O91.019 Infection of nipple associated with pregnancy, unspecified trimester

O91.02 Infection of nipple associated with the puerperium

Puerperal abscess of nipple

O91.03 Infection of nipple associated with lactation

Abscess of nipple associated with lactation

O91.1 Abscess of breast associated with pregnancy, the puerperium and lactation

O91.11 Abscess of breast associated with pregnancy

Gestational mammary abscess

Gestational purulent mastitis

Gestational subareolar abscess

O91.111 Abscess of breast associated with pregnancy, first trimester

O91.112 Abscess of breast associated with pregnancy, second trimester

O91.113 Abscess of breast associated with pregnancy, third trimester

O91.119 Abscess of breast associated with pregnancy, unspecified trimester

O91.12 Abscess of breast associated with the puerperium

Puerperal mammary abscess

Puerperal purulent mastitis

Puerperal subareolar abscess

O91.13 Abscess of breast associated with lactation

Mammary abscess associated with lactation

Purulent mastitis associated with lactation

Subareolar abscess associated with lactation

O91.2 Nonpurulent mastitis associated with pregnancy, the puerperium and lactation

O91.21 Nonpurulent mastitis associated with pregnancy

Gestational interstitial mastitis

Gestational lymphangitis of breast

Gestational mastitis NOS

Gestational parenchymatous mastitis

O91.211 Nonpurulent mastitis associated with pregnancy, first trimester

O91.212 Nonpurulent mastitis associated with pregnancy, second trimester

O91.213 Nonpurulent mastitis associated with pregnancy, third trimester

O91.219 Nonpurulent mastitis associated with pregnancy, unspecified trimester

O91.22 Nonpurulent mastitis associated with the puerperium

Puerperal interstitial mastitis

Puerperal lymphangitis of breast

Puerperal mastitis NOS

Puerperal parenchymatous mastitis

O91.23 Nonpurulent mastitis associated with lactation

Interstitial mastitis associated with lactation

Lymphangitis of breast associated with lactation

● New code   ▲ Revised code   **Excludes1:** Not coded here   **Excludes2:** Not included here   ⊗ Placeholder required   ⑦ 7ᵗʰ digit required

Mastitis NOS associated with lactation

Parenchymatous mastitis associated with lactation

O92 **Other disorders of breast and disorders of lactation associated with pregnancy and the puerperium**

O92.0 **Retracted nipple associated with pregnancy, the puerperium, and lactation**

    O92.01 **Retracted nipple associated with pregnancy**

      O92.011 **Retracted nipple associated with pregnancy, first trimester**

      O92.012 **Retracted nipple associated with pregnancy, second trimester**

      O92.013 **Retracted nipple associated with pregnancy, third trimester**

      O92.019 **Retracted nipple associated with pregnancy, unspecified trimester**

    O92.02 **Retracted nipple associated with the puerperium**

    O92.03 **Retracted nipple associated with lactation**

O92.1 **Cracked nipple associated with pregnancy, the puerperium, and lactation**

Fissure of nipple, gestational or puerperal

    O92.11 **Cracked nipple associated with pregnancy**

      O92.111 **Cracked nipple associated with pregnancy, first trimester**

      O92.112 **Cracked nipple associated with pregnancy, second trimester**

      O92.113 **Cracked nipple associated with pregnancy, third trimester**

      O92.119 **Cracked nipple associated with pregnancy, unspecified trimester**

    O92.12 **Cracked nipple associated with the puerperium**

    O92.13 **Cracked nipple associated with lactation**

O92.2 **Other and unspecified disorders of breast associated with pregnancy and the puerperium**

    O92.20 **Unspecified disorder of breast associated with pregnancy and the puerperium**

    O92.29 **Other disorders of breast associated with pregnancy and the puerperium**

O92.3 **Agalactia**

Primary agalactia

Excludes1: Elective agalactia (O92.5)

    Secondary agalactia (O92.5)

    Therapeutic agalactia (O92.5)

O92.4 **Hypogalactia**

O92.5 **Suppressed lactation**

Elective agalactia

Secondary agalactia

Therapeutic agalactia

Excludes1: primary agalactia (O92.3)

O92.6 **Galactorrhea**

O92.7 **Other and unspecified disorders of lactation**

    O92.70 **Unspecified disorders of lactation**

    O92.79 **Other disorders of lactation**

Puerperal galactocele

OTHER OBSTETRIC CONDITIONS, NOT ELSEWHERE CLASSIFIED (O94-O9A)

O94 **Sequelae of complication of pregnancy, childbirth, and the puerperium**

Note: This category is to be used to indicate conditions in O00-O77.-, O85-O94 and O98-O9A.- as the cause of late effects. The sequelae

include conditions specified as such, or as late effects, which may occur at any time after the puerperium

Code first condition resulting from (sequela) of complication of pregnancy, childbirth, and the puerperium

O98 **Maternal infectious and parasitic diseases classifiable elsewhere but complicating pregnancy, childbirth and the puerperium**

Includes: the listed conditions when complicating the pregnant state, when aggravated by the pregnancy, or as a reason for obstetric care

Use additional code (Chapter 1), to identify specific infectious or parasitic disease

Excludes2: herpes gestationis (O26.4-)

    infectious carrier state (O99.82-, O99.83-)

    obstetrical tetanus (A34)

    puerperal infection (O86.-)

    puerperal sepsis (O85)

    when the reason for maternal care is that the disease is known or suspected to have affected the fetus (O35-O36)

O98.0 **Tuberculosis complicating pregnancy, childbirth and the puerperium**

Conditions in A15-A19

    O98.01 **Tuberculosis complicating pregnancy**

      O98.011 **Tuberculosis complicating pregnancy, first trimester**

      O98.012 **Tuberculosis complicating pregnancy, second trimester**

      O98.013 **Tuberculosis complicating pregnancy, third trimester**

      O98.019 **Tuberculosis complicating pregnancy, unspecified trimester**

    O98.02 **Tuberculosis complicating childbirth**

    O98.03 **Tuberculosis complicating the puerperium**

O98.1 **Syphilis complicating pregnancy, childbirth and the puerperium**

Conditions in A50-A53

    O98.11 **Syphilis complicating pregnancy**

      O98.111 **Syphilis complicating pregnancy, first trimester**

      O98.112 **Syphilis complicating pregnancy, second trimester**

      O98.113 **Syphilis complicating pregnancy, third trimester**

      O98.119 **Syphilis complicating pregnancy, unspecified trimester**

    O98.12 **Syphilis complicating childbirth**

    O98.13 **Syphilis complicating the puerperium**

O98.2 **Gonorrhea complicating pregnancy, childbirth and the puerperium**

Conditions in A54.-

    O98.21 **Gonorrhea complicating pregnancy**

      O98.211 **Gonorrhea complicating pregnancy, first trimester**

      O98.212 **Gonorrhea complicating pregnancy, second trimester**

      O98.213 **Gonorrhea complicating pregnancy, third trimester**

      O98.219 **Gonorrhea complicating pregnancy, unspecified trimester**

    O98.22 **Gonorrhea complicating childbirth**

    O98.23 **Gonorrhea complicating the puerperium**

O98.3 **Other infections with a predominantly sexual mode of transmission complicating pregnancy, childbirth and the puerperium** Conditions in A55-A64

O98.31 Other infections with a predominantly sexual mode of transmission complicating pregnancy

    O98.311 Other infections with a predominantly sexual mode of transmission complicating pregnancy, first trimester

    O98.312 Other infections with a predominantly sexual mode of transmission complicating pregnancy, second trimester

    O98.313 Other infections with a predominantly sexual mode of transmission complicating pregnancy, third trimester

    O98.319 Other infections with a predominantly sexual mode of transmission complicating pregnancy, unspecified trimester

O98.32 Other infections with a predominantly sexual mode of transmission complicating childbirth

O98.33 Other infections with a predominantly sexual mode of transmission complicating the puerperium

O98.4 Viral hepatitis complicating pregnancy, childbirth and the puerperium

Conditions in B15-B19

O98.41 Viral hepatitis complicating pregnancy

    O98.411 Viral hepatitis complicating pregnancy, first trimester

    O98.412 Viral hepatitis complicating pregnancy, second trimester

    O98.413 Viral hepatitis complicating pregnancy, third trimester

    O98.419 Viral hepatitis complicating pregnancy, unspecified trimester

O98.42 Viral hepatitis complicating childbirth

O98.43 Viral hepatitis complicating the puerperium

O98.5 Other viral diseases complicating pregnancy, childbirth and the puerperium

Conditions in A80-B09, B25-B34, R87.81-, R87.82-

Excludes1: human immunodeficiency virus [HIV] disease complicating pregnancy, childbirth and the puerperium (O98.7-)

O98.51 Other viral diseases complicating pregnancy

    O98.511 Other viral diseases complicating pregnancy, first trimester

    O98.512 Other viral diseases complicating pregnancy, second trimester

    O98.513 Other viral diseases complicating pregnancy, third trimester

    O98.519 Other viral diseases complicating pregnancy, unspecified trimester

O98.52 Other viral diseases complicating childbirth

O98.53 Other viral diseases complicating the puerperium

O98.6 Protozoal diseases complicating pregnancy, childbirth and the puerperium

Conditions in B50-B64

O98.61 Protozoal diseases complicating pregnancy

    O98.611 Protozoal diseases complicating pregnancy, first trimester

    O98.612 Protozoal diseases complicating pregnancy, second trimester

    O98.613 Protozoal diseases complicating pregnancy, third trimester

    O98.619 Protozoal diseases complicating pregnancy, unspecified trimester

O98.62 Protozoal diseases complicating childbirth

O98.63 Protozoal diseases complicating the puerperium

O98.7 Human immunodeficiency virus [HIV] disease complicating pregnancy, childbirth and the puerperium

Use additional code to identify the type of HIV disease:

Acquired immune deficiency syndrome (AIDS) (B20)

Asymptomatic HIV status (Z21)

HIV positive NOS (Z21)

Symptomatic HIV disease (B20)

O98.71 Human immunodeficiency virus [HIV] disease complicating pregnancy

    O98.711 Human immunodeficiency virus [HIV] disease complicating pregnancy, first trimester

    O98.712 Human immunodeficiency virus [HIV] disease complicating pregnancy, second trimester

    O98.713 Human immunodeficiency virus [HIV] disease complicating pregnancy, third trimester

    O98.719 Human immunodeficiency virus [HIV] disease complicating pregnancy, unspecified trimester

O98.72 Human immunodeficiency virus [HIV] disease complicating childbirth

O98.73 Human immunodeficiency virus [HIV] disease complicating the puerperium

O98.8 Other maternal infectious and parasitic diseases complicating pregnancy, childbirth and the puerperium

O98.81 Other maternal infectious and parasitic diseases complicating pregnancy

    O98.811 Other maternal infectious and parasitic diseases complicating pregnancy, first trimester

    O98.812 Other maternal infectious and parasitic diseases complicating pregnancy, second trimester

    O98.813 Other maternal infectious and parasitic diseases complicating pregnancy, third trimester

    O98.819 Other maternal infectious and parasitic diseases complicating pregnancy, unspecified trimester

O98.82 Other maternal infectious and parasitic diseases complicating childbirth

O98.83 Other maternal infectious and parasitic diseases complicating the puerperium

O98.9 Unspecified maternal infectious and parasitic disease complicating pregnancy, childbirth and the puerperium

O98.91 Unspecified maternal infectious and parasitic disease complicating pregnancy

    O98.911 Unspecified maternal infectious and parasitic disease complicating pregnancy, first trimester

    O98.912 Unspecified maternal infectious and parasitic disease complicating pregnancy, second trimester

    O98.913 Unspecified maternal infectious and parasitic disease complicating pregnancy, third trimester

O98.919   Unspecified maternal infectious and parasitic disease complicating pregnancy, unspecified trimester

O98.92   Unspecified maternal infectious and parasitic disease complicating childbirth

O98.93   Unspecified maternal infectious and parasitic disease complicating the puerperium

O99   Other maternal diseases classifiable elsewhere but complicating pregnancy, childbirth and the puerperium

Includes: conditions which complicate the pregnant state, are aggravated by the pregnancy or are a main reason for obstetric care

Use additional code to identify specific condition

Excludes2: when the reason for maternal care is that the condition is known or suspected to have affected the fetus (O35-O36)

O99.0   Anemia complicating pregnancy, childbirth and the puerperium

Conditions in D50-D64

Excludes1: anemia arising in the puerperium (O90.81)

postpartum anemia NOS (O90.81)

O99.01   Anemia complicating pregnancy

O99.011   Anemia complicating pregnancy, first trimester

O99.012   Anemia complicating pregnancy, second trimester

O99.013   Anemia complicating pregnancy, third trimester

O99.019   Anemia complicating pregnancy, unspecified trimester

O99.02   Anemia complicating childbirth

O99.03   Anemia complicating the puerperium

Excludes1: postpartum anemia not pre-existing prior to delivery (O90.81)

O99.1   Other diseases of the blood and blood-forming organs and certain disorders involving the immune mechanism complicating pregnancy, childbirth and the puerperium

Conditions in D65-D89

Excludes1: hemorrhage with coagulation defects (O45.-, O46.0-, O67.0, O72.3)

O99.11   Other diseases of the blood and blood-forming organs and certain disorders involving the immune mechanism complicating pregnancy

O99.111   Other diseases of the blood and blood-forming organs and certain disorders involving the immune mechanism complicating pregnancy, first trimester

O99.112   Other diseases of the blood and blood-forming organs and certain disorders involving the immune mechanism complicating pregnancy, second trimester

O99.113   Other diseases of the blood and blood-forming organs and certain disorders involving the immune mechanism complicating pregnancy, third trimester

O99.119   Other diseases of the blood and blood-forming organs and certain disorders involving the immune mechanism complicating pregnancy, unspecified trimester

O99.12   Other diseases of the blood and blood-forming organs and certain disorders involving the immune mechanism complicating childbirth

O99.13   Other diseases of the blood and blood-forming organs and certain disorders involving the immune mechanism complicating the puerperium

O99.2   Endocrine, nutritional and metabolic diseases complicating pregnancy, childbirth and the puerperium

Conditions in E00-E88

Excludes2: diabetes mellitus (O24.-)

malnutrition (O25.-)

postpartum thyroiditis (O90.5)

O99.21   Obesity complicating pregnancy, childbirth, and the puerperium

Use additional code to identify the type of obesity (E66.-)

O99.210   Obesity complicating pregnancy, unspecified trimester

O99.211   Obesity complicating pregnancy, first trimester

O99.212   Obesity complicating pregnancy, second trimester

O99.213   Obesity complicating pregnancy, third trimester

O99.214   Obesity complicating childbirth

O99.215   Obesity complicating the puerperium

O99.28   Other endocrine, nutritional and metabolic diseases complicating pregnancy, childbirth and the puerperium

O99.280   Endocrine, nutritional and metabolic diseases complicating pregnancy, unspecified trimester

O99.281   Endocrine, nutritional and metabolic diseases complicating pregnancy, first trimester

O99.282   Endocrine, nutritional and metabolic diseases complicating pregnancy, second trimester

O99.283   Endocrine, nutritional and metabolic diseases complicating pregnancy, third trimester

O99.284   Endocrine, nutritional and metabolic diseases complicating childbirth

O99.285   Endocrine, nutritional and metabolic diseases complicating the puerperium

O99.3   Mental disorders and diseases of the nervous system complicating pregnancy, childbirth and the puerperium

O99.31   Alcohol use complicating pregnancy, childbirth, and the puerperium

Use additional code(s) from F10 to identify manifestations of the alcohol use

O99.310   Alcohol use complicating pregnancy, unspecified trimester

O99.311   Alcohol use complicating pregnancy, first trimester

O99.312   Alcohol use complicating pregnancy, second trimester

O99.313   Alcohol use complicating pregnancy, third trimester

O99.314   Alcohol use complicating childbirth

O99.315   Alcohol use complicating the puerperium

O99.32   Drug use complicating pregnancy, childbirth, and the puerperium

Use additional code(s) from F11-F16 and F18-F19 to identify manifestations of the drug use

O99.320 **Drug use complicating pregnancy, unspecified trimester**

O99.321 **Drug use complicating pregnancy, first trimester**

O99.322 **Drug use complicating pregnancy, second trimester**

O99.323 **Drug use complicating pregnancy, third trimester**

O99.324 **Drug use complicating childbirth**

O99.325 **Drug use complicating the puerperium**

O99.33 **Tobacco use disorder complicating pregnancy, childbirth, and the puerperium**

Smoking complicating pregnancy, childbirth, and the puerperium

Use additional code from category F17 to identify type of tobacco nicotine dependence

O99.330 **Smoking (tobacco) complicating pregnancy, unspecified trimester**

O99.331 **Smoking (tobacco) complicating pregnancy, first trimester**

O99.332 **Smoking (tobacco) complicating pregnancy, second trimester**

O99.333 **Smoking (tobacco) complicating pregnancy, third trimester**

O99.334 **Smoking (tobacco) complicating childbirth**

O99.335 **Smoking (tobacco) complicating the puerperium**

O99.34 **Other mental disorders complicating pregnancy, childbirth, and the puerperium**

Conditions in F01-F09 and F20-F99

Excludes2: postpartum mood disturbance (O90.6)

postnatal psychosis (F53)

puerperal psychosis (F53)

O99.340 **Other mental disorders complicating pregnancy, unspecified trimester**

O99.341 **Other mental disorders complicating pregnancy, first trimester**

O99.342 **Other mental disorders complicating pregnancy, second trimester**

O99.343 **Other mental disorders complicating pregnancy, third trimester**

O99.344 **Other mental disorders complicating childbirth**

O99.345 **Other mental disorders complicating the puerperium**

O99.35 **Diseases of the nervous system complicating pregnancy, childbirth, and the puerperium**

Conditions in G00-G99

Excludes2: pregnancy related peripheral neuritis (O26.8-)

O99.350 **Diseases of the nervous system complicating pregnancy, unspecified trimester**

O99.351 **Diseases of the nervous system complicating pregnancy, first trimester**

O99.352 **Diseases of the nervous system complicating pregnancy, second trimester**

O99.353 **Diseases of the nervous system complicating pregnancy, third trimester**

O99.354 **Diseases of the nervous system complicating childbirth**

O99.355 **Diseases of the nervous system complicating the puerperium**

O99.4 **Diseases of the circulatory system complicating pregnancy, childbirth and the puerperium**

Conditions in I00-I99

Excludes1: peripartum cardiomyopathy (O90.3)

Excludes2: hypertensive disorders (O10-O16)

obstetric embolism (O88.-)

venous complications and cerebrovenous sinus thrombosis in labor, childbirth and the puerperium (O87.-)

venous complications and cerebrovenous sinus thrombosis in pregnancy (O22.-)

O99.41 **Diseases of the circulatory system complicating pregnancy**

O99.411 **Diseases of the circulatory system complicating pregnancy, first trimester**

O99.412 **Diseases of the circulatory system complicating pregnancy, second trimester**

O99.413 **Diseases of the circulatory system complicating pregnancy, third trimester**

O99.419 **Diseases of the circulatory system complicating pregnancy, unspecified trimester**

O99.42 **Diseases of the circulatory system complicating childbirth**

O99.43 **Diseases of the circulatory system complicating the puerperium**

O99.5 **Diseases of the respiratory system complicating pregnancy, childbirth and the puerperium**

Conditions in J00-J99

O99.51 **Diseases of the respiratory system complicating pregnancy**

O99.511 **Diseases of the respiratory system complicating pregnancy, first trimester**

O99.512 **Diseases of the respiratory system complicating pregnancy, second trimester**

O99.513 **Diseases of the respiratory system complicating pregnancy, third trimester**

O99.519 **Diseases of the respiratory system complicating pregnancy, unspecified trimester**

O99.52 **Diseases of the respiratory system complicating childbirth**

O99.53 **Diseases of the respiratory system complicating the puerperium**

O99.6 **Diseases of the digestive system complicating pregnancy, childbirth and the puerperium**

Conditions in K00-K93

Excludes2: hemorrhoids in pregnancy (O22.4-)

liver and biliary tract disorders in pregnancy, childbirth and the puerperium (O26.6-)

O99.61 **Diseases of the digestive system complicating pregnancy**

● New code   ▲ Revised code   **Excludes1:** Not coded here   **Excludes2:** Not included here   ⊗ Placeholder required   ⑦ 7th digit required

O99.611 Diseases of the digestive system complicating pregnancy, first trimester

O99.612 Diseases of the digestive system complicating pregnancy, second trimester

O99.613 Diseases of the digestive system complicating pregnancy, third trimester

O99.619 Diseases of the digestive system complicating pregnancy, unspecified trimester

O99.62 Diseases of the digestive system complicating childbirth

O99.63 Diseases of the digestive system complicating the puerperium

O99.7 Diseases of the skin and subcutaneous tissue complicating pregnancy, childbirth and the puerperium

Conditions in L00-L99

Excludes2: herpes gestationis (O26.4)

pruritic urticarial papules and plaques of pregnancy (PUPPP) (O26.86)

O99.71 Diseases of the skin and subcutaneous tissue complicating pregnancy

O99.711 Diseases of the skin and subcutaneous tissue complicating pregnancy, first trimester

O99.712 Diseases of the skin and subcutaneous tissue complicating pregnancy, second trimester

O99.713 Diseases of the skin and subcutaneous tissue complicating pregnancy, third trimester

O99.719 Diseases of the skin and subcutaneous tissue complicating pregnancy, unspecified trimester

O99.72 Diseases of the skin and subcutaneous tissue complicating childbirth

O99.73 Diseases of the skin and subcutaneous tissue complicating the puerperium

O99.8 Other specified diseases and conditions complicating pregnancy, childbirth and the puerperium

Conditions in D00-D48, H00-H95, M00-N99, and Q00-Q99

Use additional code to identify condition

Excludes2: genitourinary infections in pregnancy (O23.-)

infection of genitourinary tract following delivery (O86.1-O86.3)

malignant neoplasm complicating pregnancy, childbirth and the puerperium (O9A.1-)

maternal care for known or suspected abnormality of maternal pelvic organs (O34.-)

postpartum acute kidney failure (O90.4)

traumatic injuries in pregnancy (O9A.2-)

O99.81 Abnormal glucose complicating pregnancy, childbirth and the puerperium

Excludes1: gestational diabetes (O24.4-)

O99.810 Abnormal glucose complicating pregnancy

O99.814 Abnormal glucose complicating childbirth

O99.815 Abnormal glucose complicating the puerperium

O99.82 Streptococcus B carrier state complicating pregnancy, childbirth and the puerperium

Excludes1: Carrier of streptococcus group B (GBS) in a nonpregnant woman (Z22.330)

O99.820 Streptococcus B carrier state complicating pregnancy

O99.824 Streptococcus B carrier state complicating childbirth

O99.825 Streptococcus B carrier state complicating the puerperium

O99.83 Other infection carrier state complicating pregnancy, childbirth and the puerperium

Use additional code to identify the carrier state (Z22.-)

O99.830 Other infection carrier state complicating pregnancy

O99.834 Other infection carrier state complicating childbirth

O99.835 Other infection carrier state complicating the puerperium

O99.84 Bariatric surgery status complicating pregnancy, childbirth and the puerperium

Gastric banding status complicating pregnancy, childbirth and the puerperium

Gastric bypass status for obesity complicating pregnancy, childbirth and the puerperium

Obesity surgery status complicating pregnancy, childbirth and the puerperium

O99.840 Bariatric surgery status complicating pregnancy, unspecified trimester

O99.841 Bariatric surgery status complicating pregnancy, first trimester

O99.842 Bariatric surgery status complicating pregnancy, second trimester

O99.843 Bariatric surgery status complicating pregnancy, third trimester

O99.844 Bariatric surgery status complicating childbirth

O99.845 Bariatric surgery status complicating the puerperium

O99.89 Other specified diseases and conditions complicating pregnancy, childbirth and the puerperium

O9A Maternal malignant neoplasms, traumatic injuries and abuse classifiable elsewhere but complicating pregnancy, childbirth and the puerperium

O9A.1 Malignant neoplasm complicating pregnancy, childbirth and the puerperium

Conditions in C00-C96

Use additional code to identify neoplasm

Excludes2: maternal care for benign tumor of corpus uteri (O34.1-)

maternal care for benign tumor of cervix (O34.4-)

O9A.11 Malignant neoplasm complicating pregnancy

O9A.111 Malignant neoplasm complicating pregnancy, first trimester

O9A.112 Malignant neoplasm complicating pregnancy, second trimester

O9A.113 Malignant neoplasm complicating pregnancy, third trimester

O9A.119 Malignant neoplasm complicating pregnancy, unspecified trimester

O9A.12 Malignant neoplasm complicating childbirth

O9A.13 **Malignant neoplasm complicating the puerperium**

O9A.2 **Injury, poisoning and certain other consequences of external causes complicating pregnancy, childbirth and the puerperium**

Conditions in S00-T88, except T74 and T76

Use additional code(s) to identify the injury or poisoning

Excludes2: physical, sexual and psychological abuse complicating pregnancy, childbirth and the puerperium (O9A.3-, O9A.4-, O9A.5-)

O9A.21 **Injury, poisoning and certain other consequences of external causes complicating pregnancy**

O9A.211 **Injury, poisoning and certain other consequences of external causes complicating pregnancy, first trimester**

O9A.212 **Injury, poisoning and certain other consequences of external causes complicating pregnancy, second trimester**

O9A.213 **Injury, poisoning and certain other consequences of external causes complicating pregnancy, third trimester**

O9A.219 **Injury, poisoning and certain other consequences of external causes complicating pregnancy, unspecified trimester**

O9A.22 **Injury, poisoning and certain other consequences of external causes complicating childbirth**

O9A.23 **Injury, poisoning and certain other consequences of external causes complicating the puerperium**

O9A.3 **Physical abuse complicating pregnancy, childbirth and the puerperium**

Conditions in T74.11 or T76.11

Use additional code (if applicable):

to identify any associated current injury due to physical abuse to identify the perpetrator of abuse (Y07.-)

Excludes2: sexual abuse complicating pregnancy, childbirth and the puerperium (O9A.4)

O9A.31 **Physical abuse complicating pregnancy**

O9A.311 **Physical abuse complicating pregnancy, first trimester**

O9A.312 **Physical abuse complicating pregnancy, second trimester**

O9A.313 **Physical abuse complicating pregnancy, third trimester**

O9A.319 **Physical abuse complicating pregnancy, unspecified trimester**

O9A.32 **Physical abuse complicating childbirth**

O9A.33 **Physical abuse complicating the puerperium**

O9A.4 **Sexual abuse complicating pregnancy, childbirth and the puerperium**

Conditions in T74.21 or T76.21

Use additional code (if applicable):

to identify any associated current injury due to sexual abuse to identify the perpetrator of abuse (Y07.-)

O9A.41 **Sexual abuse complicating pregnancy**

O9A.411 **Sexual abuse complicating pregnancy, first trimester**

O9A.412 **Sexual abuse complicating pregnancy, second trimester**

O9A.413 **Sexual abuse complicating pregnancy, third trimester**

O9A.419 **Sexual abuse complicating pregnancy, unspecified trimester**

O9A.42 **Sexual abuse complicating childbirth**

O9A.43 **Sexual abuse complicating the puerperium**

O9A.5 **Psychological abuse complicating pregnancy, childbirth and the puerperium**

Conditions in T74.31 or T76.31

Use additional code to identify the perpetrator of abuse (Y07.-)

O9A.51 **Psychological abuse complicating pregnancy**

O9A.511 **Psychological abuse complicating pregnancy, first trimester**

O9A.512 **Psychological abuse complicating pregnancy, second trimester**

O9A.513 **Psychological abuse complicating pregnancy, third trimester**

O9A.519 **Psychological abuse complicating pregnancy, unspecified trimester**

O9A.52 **Psychological abuse complicating childbirth**

O9A.53 **Psychological abuse complicating the puerperium**

● New code ▲ Revised code Excludes1: Not coded here Excludes2: Not included here ⊗ Placeholder required ⑦7th digit required

Chapter 16: Certain Conditions Originating In The Perinatal Period (P00-P96)

DEFINITIONS

This chapter includes definitions of selected key words, terms and phrases and coding alerts for adding points to the clinical domain, and references to coding late effects where appropriate. An example from this chapter is as follows:

P36   Bacterial sepsis of newborn

         Definition: Neonatal sepsis is a blood infection that occurs in an infant younger than 90 days old. Early-onset sepsis is seen in the first week of life.

MULTIPLE CODING FOR A SINGLE CONDITION

In addition to the etiology/manifestation convention that requires two codes to fully describe a single condition that affects multiple body systems, there are other single conditions that also require more than one code. "Use additional code" notes are found in the Tabular List at codes that are not part of an etiology/manifestation pair where a secondary code is useful to fully describe a condition. The sequencing rule is the same as the etiology/manifestation pair, "use additional code" indicates that a secondary code should be added.

For example, for bacterial infections that are not included in chapter 1, a secondary code from category B95, Streptococcus, Staphylococcus, and Enterococcus, as the cause of diseases classified elsewhere, or B96, Other bacterial agents as the cause of diseases classified elsewhere, may be required to identify the bacterial organism causing the infection. A "use additional code" note will normally be found at the infectious disease code, indicating a need for the organism code to be added as a secondary code.

"**Code first**" notes are also under certain codes that are not specifically manifestation codes but may be due to an underlying cause. When there is a "**Code first**" note and an underlying condition is present, the underlying condition should be sequenced first.

"Code, if applicable, any causal condition first", notes indicate that this code may be assigned as a principal diagnosis when the causal condition is unknown or not applicable. If a causal condition is known, then the code for that condition should be sequenced as the principal or first-listed diagnosis.

Multiple codes may be needed for sequela, complication codes and obstetric codes to more fully describe a condition. See the specific guidelines for these conditions for further instruction.

COMBINATION CODE

A combination code is a single code used to classify: Two diagnoses, or a diagnosis with an associated secondary process (manifestation) A diagnosis with an associated complication

Combination codes are identified by referring to subterm entries in the Alphabetic Index and by reading the inclusion and exclusion notes in the Tabular List.

Assign only the combination code when that code fully identifies the diagnostic conditions involved or when the Alphabetic Index so directs. Multiple coding should not be used when the classification provides a combination code that clearly identifies all of the elements documented in the diagnosis. When the combination code lacks necessary specificity in describing the manifestation or complication, an additional code should be used as a secondary code.

SEQUELA (LATE EFFECTS)

A sequela is the residual effect (condition produced) after the acute phase of an illness or injury has terminated. There is no time limit on when a sequela code can be used. The residual may be apparent early, such as in cerebral infarction, or it may occur months or years later, such as that due to a previous injury. Coding of sequela generally requires two codes sequenced in the following order: The condition or nature of the sequela is sequenced first.

The sequela code is sequenced second.

An exception to the above guidelines are those instances where the code for the sequela is followed by a manifestation code identified in the Tabular List and title, or the sequela code has been expanded (at the fourth, fifth or sixth character levels) to include the manifestation(s). The code for the acute phase of an illness or injury that led to the sequela is never used with a code for the late effect.

GENERAL PERINATAL RULES

1) Use of Chapter 16 Codes

Codes in this chapter are <u>never</u> for use on the maternal record. Codes from Chapter 15, the obstetric chapter, are never permitted on the newborn record. Chapter 16 codes may be used throughout the life of the patient if the condition is still present.

2) Principal Diagnosis for Birth Record

When coding the birth episode in a newborn record, assign a code from category Z38, Liveborn infants according to place of birth and type of delivery, as the principal diagnosis. A code from category Z38 is assigned only once, to a newborn at the time of birth. If a newborn is transferred to another institution, a code from category Z38 should not be used at the receiving hospital.

A code from category Z38 is used only on the newborn record, not on the mother's record.

3) Use of Codes from other Chapters with Codes from Chapter 16

Codes from other chapters may be used with codes from chapter 16 if the codes from the other chapters provide more specific detail. Codes for signs and symptoms may be assigned when a definitive diagnosis has not been established. If the reason for the encounter is a perinatal condition, the code from chapter 16 should be sequenced first.

Add 4th-7th digits	Nonspecific code	Unspecified code	Manifestation code

4) **Use of Chapter 16 Codes after the Perinatal Period**

Should a condition originate in the perinatal period, and continue throughout the life of the patient, the perinatal code should continue to be used regardless of the patient's age.

5) **Birth process or community acquired conditions**

If a newborn has a condition that may be either due to the birth process or community acquired and the documentation does not indicate which it is, the default is due to the birth process and the code from Chapter 16 should be used. If the condition is community-acquired, a code from Chapter 16 should not be assigned.

6) **Code all clinically significant conditions**

All clinically significant conditions noted on routine newborn examination should be coded. A condition is clinically significant if it requires:

§ clinical evaluation; or

§ therapeutic treatment; or

§ diagnostic procedures; or

§ extended length of hospital stay; or

§ increased nursing care and/or monitoring; or

§ has implications for future health care needs

Note: The perinatal guidelines listed above are the same as the general coding guidelines for "additional diagnoses", except for the final point regarding implications for future health care needs. Codes should be assigned for conditions that have been specified by the provider as having implications for future health care needs.

OBSERVATION AND EVALUATION OF NEWBORNS FOR SUSPECTED CONDITIONS NOT FOUND

1) Assign a code from category Z05, Observation and evaluation of newborns and infants for suspected conditions ruled out, to identify those instances when a healthy newborn is evaluated for a suspected condition that is determined after study not to be present. Do not use a code from category Z05 when the patient has identified signs or symptoms of a suspected problem; in such cases code the sign or symptom.

2) A code from category Z05 may also be assigned as a principal or first-listed code for readmissions or encounters when the code from category Z38 code no longer applies. Codes from category Z05 are for use only for healthy newborns and infants for which no condition after study is found to be present.

3) Z05 on a birth record

A code from category Z05 is to be used as a secondary code after the code from category Z38, liveborn infants according to place of birth and type of delivery.

CODING ADDITIONAL PERINATAL DIAGNOSES

1) **Assigning codes for conditions that require treatment**

Assign codes for conditions that require treatment or further investigation, prolong the length of stay, or require resource utilization.

2) **Codes for conditions specified as having implications for future health care needs**

Assign codes for conditions that have been specified by the provider as having implications for future health care needs.

Note: This guideline should not be used for adult patients.

PREMATURITY AND FETAL GROWTH RETARDATION

Providers utilize different criteria in determining prematurity. A code for prematurity should not be assigned unless it is documented. Assignment of codes in categories P05, Disorders of newborn related to slow fetal growth and fetal malnutrition, and P07, Disorders of newborn related to short gestation and low birth weight, not elsewhere classified, should be based on the recorded birth weight and estimated gestational age. Codes from category P05 should not be assigned with codes from category P07.

When both birth weight and gestational age are available, two codes from category P07 should be assigned, with the code for birth weight sequenced before the code for gestational age.

LOW BIRTH WEIGHT AND IMMATURITY STATUS

Codes from category P07, Disorders of newborn related to short gestation and low birth weight, not elsewhere classified, are for use for a child or adult who was premature or had a low birth weight as a newborn and this is affecting the patient's current health status.

See Section I.C.21. Factors influencing health status and contact with health services, Status.

BACTERIAL SEPSIS OF NEWBORN

Category P36, Bacterial sepsis of newborn, includes congenital sepsis. If a perinate is documented as having sepsis without documentation of congenital or community acquired, the default is congenital and a code from category P36 should be assigned. If the P36 code includes the causal organism, an additional code from category B95, Streptococcus, Staphylococcus, and Enterococcus as the cause of diseases classified elsewhere, or B96, Other bacterial agents as the cause of diseases classified elsewhere, should not be assigned. If the P36 code does not include the causal organism, assign an additional code from category B96. If applicable, use additional codes to identify severe sepsis (R65.2-) and any associated acute organ dysfunction.

STILLBIRTH

Code P95, Stillbirth, is only for use in institutions that maintain separate records for stillbirths. No other code should be used with P95. Code P95 should not be used on the mother's record.

● New code ▲ Revised code **Excludes1:** Not coded here **Excludes2:** Not included here ⊗ Placeholder required ⑦ 7th digit required

Chapter 16

Certain Conditions Originating In The Perinatal Period (P00-P96)

NOTE: CODES FROM THIS CHAPTER ARE FOR USE ON NEWBORN RECORDS ONLY, NEVER ON MATERNAL RECORDS

Includes: conditions that have their origin in the fetal or perinatal period (before birth through the first 28 days after birth) even if morbidity occurs later

Excludes2: congenital malformations, deformations and chromosomal

abnormalities (Q00-Q99)

endocrine, nutritional and metabolic diseases (E00-E88)

injury, poisoning and certain other consequences of external causes (S00-T88)

neoplasms (C00-D49)

tetanus neonatorum (A33)

This chapter contains the following blocks:

P00-P04	Newborn affected by maternal factors and by complications of pregnancy, labor, and delivery
P05-P08	Disorders of newborn related to length of gestation and fetal growth
P09	Abnormal findings on neonatal screening
P10-P15	Birth trauma
P19-P29	Respiratory and cardiovascular disorders specific to the perinatal period
P35-P39	Infections specific to the perinatal period
P50-P61	Hemorrhagic and hematological disorders of newborn
P70-P74	Transitory endocrine and metabolic disorders specific to newborn
P76-P78	Digestive system disorders of newborn
P80-P83	Conditions involving the integument and temperature regulation of newborn
P84	Other problems with newborn
P90-P96	Other disorders originating in the perinatal period

NEWBORN AFFECTED BY MATERNAL FACTORS AND BY COMPLICATIONS OF PREGNANCY, LABOR, AND DELIVERY (P00-P04)

Note: These codes are for use when the listed maternal conditions are specified as the cause of confirmed morbidity or potential morbidity which have their origin in the perinatal period (before birth through the first 28 days after birth).

P00 Newborn affected by maternal conditions that may be unrelated to present pregnancy

Code first any current condition in newborn

Excludes2: encounter for observation of newborn for suspected

diseases and conditions ruled out (Z05.-)

newborn affected by maternal complications of pregnancy (P01.-)

newborn affected by maternal endocrine and metabolic disorders (P70-P74)

newborn affected by noxious substances transmitted via placenta or breast milk (P04.-)

P00.0 **Newborn affected by maternal hypertensive disorders**

Newborn affected by maternal conditions classifiable to O10-O11, O13-O16

P00.1 **Newborn affected by maternal renal and urinary tract diseases**

Newborn affected by maternal conditions classifiable to N00-N39

P00.2 **Newborn affected by maternal infectious and parasitic diseases**

Newborn affected by maternal infectious disease classifiable to A00-B99, J09 and J10

Excludes2: infections specific to the perinatal period (P35-P39)

maternal genital tract or other localized infections (P00.8)

P00.3 **Newborn affected by other maternal circulatory and respiratory diseases**

Newborn affected by maternal conditions classifiable to I00-I99, J00-J99, Q20-Q34 and not included in P00.0, P00.2

P00.4 **Newborn affected by maternal nutritional disorders**

Newborn affected by maternal disorders classifiable to E40-E64

Maternal malnutrition NOS

P00.5 **Newborn affected by maternal injury**

Newborn affected by maternal conditions classifiable to O9A.2-

P00.6 **Newborn affected by surgical procedure on mother**

Newborn affected by amniocentesis

Excludes1: Cesarean delivery for present delivery (P03.4)

damage to placenta from amniocentesis, Cesarean delivery or surgical induction (P02.1)

previous surgery to uterus or pelvic organs (P03.89)

Excludes2: newborn affected by complication of (fetal) intrauterine procedure (P96.5)

P00.7 **Newborn affected by other medical procedures on mother, not elsewhere classified**

Newborn affected by radiation to mother

Excludes1: damage to placenta from amniocentesis, cesarean delivery or surgical induction (P02.1)

newborn affected by other complications of labor and delivery (P03.-)

P00.8 **Newborn affected by other maternal conditions**

P00.81 **Newborn affected by periodontal disease in mother**

P00.89 **Newborn affected by other maternal conditions**

Newborn affected by conditions classifiable to T80-T88

Newborn affected by maternal genital tract or other localized infections

Newborn affected by maternal systemic lupus erythematosus

P00.9 **Newborn affected by unspecified maternal condition**

P01 **Newborn affected by maternal complications of pregnancy**

Code first any current condition in newborn

Excludes2: encounter for observation of newborn for suspected

diseases and conditions ruled out (Z05.-)

P01.0 **Newborn affected by incompetent cervix**

P01.1 **Newborn affected by premature rupture of membranes**

P01.2 **Newborn affected by oligohydramnios**

Excludes1: oligohydramnios due to premature rupture of membranes (P01.1)

P01.3 **Newborn affected by polyhydramnios**

Newborn affected by hydramnios

P01.4 **Newborn affected by ectopic pregnancy**

Newborn affected by abdominal pregnancy

P01.5 **Newborn affected by multiple pregnancy**

Newborn affected by triplet (pregnancy)

Newborn affected by twin (pregnancy)

P01.6 **Newborn affected by maternal death**

P01.7 **Newborn affected by malpresentation before labor**
Newborn affected by breech presentation before labor
Newborn affected by external version before labor
Newborn affected by face presentation before labor
Newborn affected by transverse lie before labor
Newborn affected by unstable lie before labor

P01.8 **Newborn affected by other maternal complications of pregnancy**

P01.9 **Newborn affected by maternal complication of pregnancy, unspecified**

P02 **Newborn affected by complications of placenta, cord and membranes**
Code first any current condition in newborn
Excludes2: encounter for observation of newborn for suspected diseases and conditions ruled out (Z05.-)

P02.0 **Newborn affected by placenta previa**

P02.1 **Newborn affected by other forms of placental separation and hemorrhage**
Newborn affected by abruptio placenta
Newborn affected by accidental hemorrhage
Newborn affected by antepartum hemorrhage
Newborn affected by damage to placenta from amniocentesis, cesarean delivery or surgical induction
Newborn affected by maternal blood loss
Newborn affected by premature separation of placenta

P02.2 **Newborn affected by other and unspecified morphological and functional abnormalities of placenta**

P02.20 **Newborn affected by unspecified morphological and functional abnormalities of placenta**

P02.29 **Newborn affected by other morphological and functional abnormalities of placenta**
Newborn affected by placental dysfunction
Newborn affected by placental infarction
Newborn affected by placental insufficiency

P02.3 **Newborn affected by placental transfusion syndromes**
Newborn affected by placental and cord abnormalities resulting in twin-to-twin or other transplacental transfusion

P02.4 **Newborn affected by prolapsed cord**

P02.5 **Newborn affected by other compression of umbilical cord**
Newborn affected by umbilical cord (tightly) around neck
Newborn affected by entanglement of umbilical cord
Newborn affected by knot in umbilical cord

P02.6 **Newborn affected by other and unspecified conditions of umbilical cord**

P02.60 **Newborn affected by unspecified conditions of umbilical cord**

P02.69 **Newborn affected by other conditions of umbilical cord**
Newborn affected by short umbilical cord
Newborn affected by vasa previa
Excludes1: newborn affected by single umbilical artery (Q27.0)

P02.7 **Newborn affected by chorioamnionitis**
Newborn affected by amnionitis
Newborn affected by membranitis
Newborn affected by placentitis

P02.8 **Newborn affected by other abnormalities of membranes**

P02.9 **Newborn affected by abnormality of membranes, unspecified**

P03 **Newborn affected by other complications of labor and delivery**
Code first any current condition in newborn
Excludes2: encounter for observation of newborn for suspected diseases and conditions ruled out (Z05.-)

P03.0 **Newborn affected by breech delivery and extraction**

P03.1 **Newborn affected by other malpresentation, malposition and disproportion during labor and delivery**
Newborn affected by contracted pelvis
Newborn affected by conditions classifiable to O64-O66
Newborn affected by persistent occipitoposterior
Newborn affected by transverse lie

P03.2 **Newborn affected by forceps delivery**

P03.3 **Newborn affected by delivery by vacuum extractor [ventouse]**

P03.4 **Newborn affected by Cesarean delivery**

P03.5 **Newborn affected by precipitate delivery**
Newborn affected by rapid second stage

P03.6 **Newborn affected by abnormal uterine contractions**
Newborn affected by conditions classifiable to O62.-, except O62.3
Newborn affected by hypertonic labor
Newborn affected by uterine inertia

P03.8 **Newborn affected by other specified complications of labor and delivery**

P03.81 **Newborn affected by abnormality in fetal (intrauterine) heart rate or rhythm**
Excludes1: neonatal cardiac dysrhythmia (P29.1-)

P03.810 **Newborn affected by abnormality in fetal (intrauterine) heart rate or rhythm before the onset of labor**

P03.811 **Newborn affected by abnormality in fetal (intrauterine) heart rate or rhythm during labor**

P03.819 **Newborn affected by abnormality in fetal (intrauterine) heart rate or rhythm, unspecified as to time of onset**

P03.82 **Meconium passage during delivery**
Excludes1: meconium aspiration (P24.00, P24.01)
meconium staining (P96.83)

P03.89 **Newborn affected by other specified complications of labor and delivery**
Newborn affected by abnormality of maternal soft tissues
Newborn affected by conditions classifiable to O60-O75 and by procedures used in labor and delivery not included in P02.- and P03.0-P03.6
Newborn affected by induction of labor

P03.9 **Newborn affected by complication of labor and delivery, unspecified**

P04 **Newborn affected by noxious substances transmitted via placenta or breast milk**
Includes: nonteratogenic effects of substances transmitted via placenta
Excludes2: congenital malformations (Q00-Q99)
encounter for observation of newborn for suspected diseases and conditions ruled out (Z05.-)
neonatal jaundice from excessive hemolysis due to drugs or toxins transmitted from mother (P58.4)

● New code ▲ Revised code Excludes1: Not coded here Excludes2: Not included here ⊗ Placeholder required ⑦ 7th digit required

newborn in contact with and (suspected) exposures hazardous to health not transmitted via placenta or breast milk (Z77.-)

P04.0 **Newborn affected by maternal anesthesia and analgesia in pregnancy, labor and delivery**

Newborn affected by reactions and intoxications from maternal opiates and tranquilizers administered during labor and delivery

P04.1 **Newborn affected by other maternal medication**

Newborn affected by cancer chemotherapy

Newborn affected by cytotoxic drugs

Excludes1: dysmorphism due to warfarin (Q86.2)

fetal hydantoin syndrome (Q86.1)

maternal use of drugs of addiction (P04.4-)

P04.2 **Newborn affected by maternal use of tobacco**

Newborn affected by exposure in utero to tobacco smoke

Excludes2: newborn exposure to environmental tobacco smoke (P96.81)

P04.3 **Newborn affected by maternal use of alcohol**

Excludes1: fetal alcohol syndrome (Q86.0)

P04.4 **Newborn affected by maternal use of drugs of addiction**

P04.41 **Newborn affected by maternal use of cocaine**

'Crack baby'

P04.49 **Newborn affected by maternal use of other drugs of addiction**

Excludes2: newborn affected by maternal anesthesia and analgesia (P04.0)

withdrawal symptoms from maternal use of drugs of addiction (P96.1)

P04.5 **Newborn affected by maternal use of nutritional chemical substances**

P04.6 **Newborn affected by maternal exposure to environmental chemical substances**

P04.8 **Newborn affected by other maternal noxious substances**

P04.9 **Newborn affected by maternal noxious substance, unspecified**

DISORDERS OF NEWBORN RELATED TO LENGTH OF GESTATION AND FETAL GROWTH (P05-P08)

P05 **Disorders of newborn related to slow fetal growth and fetal malnutrition**

P05.0 **Newborn light for gestational age**

Newborn light-for-dates

Weight below but length above 10th percentile for gestational age

P05.00 **Newborn light for gestational age, unspecified weight**

P05.01 **Newborn light for gestational age, less than 500 grams**

P05.02 **Newborn light for gestational age, 500-749 grams**

P05.03 **Newborn light for gestational age, 750-999 grams**

P05.04 **Newborn light for gestational age, 1000-1249 grams**

P05.05 **Newborn light for gestational age, 1250-1499 grams**

P05.06 **Newborn light for gestational age, 1500-1749 grams**

P05.07 **Newborn light for gestational age, 1750-1999 grams**

P05.08 **Newborn light for gestational age, 2000-2499 grams**

P05.09 **Newborn light for gestational age, 2500 grams and over**

Newborn light for gestational age, other

P05.1 **Newborn small for gestational age**

Newborn small-and-light-for-dates

Newborn small-for-dates

Weight and length below 10th percentile for gestational age

P05.10 **Newborn small for gestational age, unspecified weight**

P05.11 **Newborn small for gestational age, less than 500 grams**

P05.12 **Newborn small for gestational age, 500-749 grams**

P05.13 **Newborn small for gestational age, 750-999 grams**

P05.14 **Newborn small for gestational age, 1000-1249 grams**

P05.15 **Newborn small for gestational age, 1250-1499 grams**

P05.16 **Newborn small for gestational age, 1500-1749 grams**

P05.17 **Newborn small for gestational age, 1750-1999 grams**

P05.18 **Newborn small for gestational age, 2000-2499 grams**

P05.19 **Newborn small for gestational age, other**

Newborn small for gestational age, 2500 grams and over

P05.2 **Newborn affected by fetal (intrauterine) malnutrition not light or small for gestational age**

Infant, not light or small for gestational age, showing signs of fetal malnutrition, such as dry, peeling skin and loss of subcutaneous tissue

Excludes1: newborn affected by fetal malnutrition with light for gestational age (P05.0-)

newborn affected by fetal malnutrition with small for gestational age (P05.1-)

P05.9 **Newborn affected by slow intrauterine growth, unspecified**

Newborn affected by fetal growth retardation NOS

P07 **Disorders of newborn related to short gestation and low birth weight, not elsewhere classified**

Note: When both birth weight and gestational age of the newborn are available, both should be coded with birth weight sequenced before gestational age

Includes: the listed conditions, without further specification, as the cause of morbidity or additional care, in newborn

P07.0 **Extremely low birth weight newborn**

Newborn birth weight 999 g. or less

Excludes1: low birth weight due to slow fetal growth and fetal malnutrition (P05.-)

P07.00 **Extremely low birth weight newborn, unspecified weight**

P07.01 **Extremely low birth weight newborn, less than 500 grams**

P07.02 **Extremely low birth weight newborn, 500-749 grams**

P07.03 **Extremely low birth weight newborn, 750-999 grams**

P07.1 **Other low birth weight newborn**

Newborn birth weight 1000-2499 g.

Excludes1: low birth weight due to slow fetal growth and fetal malnutrition (P05.-)

P07.10 **Other low birth weight newborn, unspecified weight**

P07.14 **Other low birth weight newborn, 1000-1249 grams**

P07.15 **Other low birth weight newborn, 1250-1499 grams**

P07.16 **Other low birth weight newborn, 1500-1749 grams**

P07.17 **Other low birth weight newborn, 1750-1999 grams**

P07.18 **Other low birth weight newborn, 2000-2499 grams**

P07.2 **Extreme immaturity of newborn**

Less than 28 completed weeks (less than 196 completed days) of gestation.

P07.20 **Extreme immaturity of newborn, unspecified weeks of gestation**

Gestational age less than 28 completed weeks NOS

P07.21 **Extreme immaturity of newborn, gestational age less than 23 completed weeks**

Extreme immaturity of newborn, gestational age less than 23 weeks, 0 days

P07.22 **Extreme immaturity of newborn, gestational age 23 completed weeks**

Extreme immaturity of newborn, gestational age 23 weeks, 0 days through 23 weeks, 6 days

P07.23 **Extreme immaturity of newborn, gestational age 24 completed weeks**

Extreme immaturity of newborn, gestational age 24 weeks, 0 days through 24 weeks, 6 days

P07.24 **Extreme immaturity of newborn, gestational age 25 completed weeks**

Extreme immaturity of newborn, gestational age 25 weeks, 0 days through 25 weeks, 6 days

P07.25 **Extreme immaturity of newborn, gestational age 26 completed weeks**

Extreme immaturity of newborn, gestational age 26 weeks, 0 days through 26 weeks, 6 days

P07.26 **Extreme immaturity of newborn, gestational age 27 completed weeks**

Extreme immaturity of newborn, gestational age 27 weeks, 0 days through 27 weeks, 6 days

P07.3 **Preterm [premature] newborn [Other]**

28 completed weeks or more but less than 37 completed weeks (196 completed days but less than 259 completed days) of gestation.

Prematurity NOS

P07.30 **Preterm newborn, unspecified weeks of gestation**

P07.31 **Preterm newborn, gestational age 28 completed weeks**

Preterm newborn, gestational age 28 weeks, 0 days through 28 weeks, 6 days

P07.32 **Preterm newborn, gestational age 29 completed weeks**

Preterm newborn, gestational age 29 weeks, 0 days through 29 weeks, 6 days

P07.33 **Preterm newborn, gestational age 30 completed weeks**

Preterm newborn, gestational age 30 weeks, 0 days through 30 weeks, 6 days

P07.34 **Preterm newborn, gestational age 31 completed weeks**

Preterm newborn, gestational age 31 weeks, 0 days through 31 weeks, 6 days

P07.35 **Preterm newborn, gestational age 32 completed weeks**

Preterm newborn, gestational age 32 weeks, 0 days through 32 weeks, 6 days

P07.36 **Preterm newborn, gestational age 33 completed weeks**

Preterm newborn, gestational age 33 weeks, 0 days through 33 weeks, 6 days

P07.37 **Preterm newborn, gestational age 34 completed weeks**

Preterm newborn, gestational age 34 weeks, 0 days through 34 weeks, 6 days

P07.38 **Preterm newborn, gestational age 35 completed weeks**

Preterm newborn, gestational age 35 weeks, 0 days through 35 weeks, 6 days

P07.39 **Preterm newborn, gestational age 36 completed weeks**

Preterm newborn, gestational age 36 weeks, 0 days through 36 weeks, 6 days

P08 **Disorders of newborn related to long gestation and high birth weight**

Note: When both birth weight and gestational age of the newborn are available, priority of assignment should be given to birth weight

Includes: the listed conditions, without further specification, as causes of morbidity or additional care, in newborn

P08.0 **Exceptionally large newborn baby**

Usually implies a birth weight of 4500 g. or more

Excludes1: syndrome of infant of diabetic mother (P70.1)

syndrome of infant of mother with gestational diabetes (P70.0)

P08.1 **Other heavy for gestational age newborn**

Other newborn heavy- or large-for-dates regardless of period of gestation Usually implies a birth weight of 4000 g. to 4499 g.

Excludes1: newborn with a birth weight of 4500 or more (P08.0)

syndrome of infant of diabetic mother (P70.1)

syndrome of infant of mother with gestational diabetes (P70.0).

P08.2 **Late newborn, not heavy for gestational age**

P08.21 **Post-term newborn**

Newborn with gestation period over 40 completed weeks to 42 completed weeks

P08.22 **Prolonged gestation of newborn**

Newborn with gestation period over 42 completed weeks (294 days or more), not heavy- or large-for-dates.

Postmaturity NOS

ABNORMAL FINDINGS ON NEONATAL SCREENING (P09)

P09 **Abnormal findings on neonatal screening**

Use additional code to identify signs, symptoms and conditions associated with the screening

Excludes2: nonspecific serologic evidence of human immunodeficiency virus [HIV] (R75)

BIRTH TRAUMA (P10-P15)

Definition: Birth trauma refers to: 1) a physical injury sustained by an infant during birth; or 2) the psychological shock said to be experienced by an infant during birth.

P10 **Intracranial laceration and hemorrhage due to birth injury**

> **Excludes1:** intracranial hemorrhage of newborn NOS (P52.9)
>
> intracranial hemorrhage of newborn due to anoxia or hypoxia (P52.-)
>
> nontraumatic intracranial hemorrhage of newborn (P52.-)

P10.0 **Subdural hemorrhage due to birth injury**

Subdural hematoma (localized) due to birth injury

> **Excludes1:** subdural hemorrhage accompanying tentorial tear (P10.4)

P10.1 **Cerebral hemorrhage due to birth injury**

P10.2 **Intraventricular hemorrhage due to birth injury**

P10.3 **Subarachnoid hemorrhage due to birth injury**

P10.4 **Tentorial tear due to birth injury**

P10.8 **Other intracranial lacerations and hemorrhages due to birth injury**

P10.9 **Unspecified intracranial laceration and hemorrhage due to birth injury**

P11 **Other birth injuries to central nervous system**

P11.0 **Cerebral edema due to birth injury**

P11.1 **Other specified brain damage due to birth injury**

P11.2 **Unspecified brain damage due to birth injury**

P11.3 **Birth injury to facial nerve**

Facial palsy due to birth injury

P11.4 **Birth injury to other cranial nerves**

P11.5 **Birth injury to spine and spinal cord**

Fracture of spine due to birth injury

P11.9 **Birth injury to central nervous system, unspecified**

P12 **Birth injury to scalp**

P12.0 **Cephalhematoma due to birth injury**

P12.1 **Chignon (from vacuum extraction) due to birth injury**

P12.2 **Epicranial subaponeurotic hemorrhage due to birth injury**

Subgaleal hemorrhage

P12.3 **Bruising of scalp due to birth injury**

P12.4 **Injury of scalp of newborn due to monitoring equipment**

Sampling incision of scalp of newborn

Scalp clip (electrode) injury of newborn

P12.8 **Other birth injuries to scalp**

P12.81 **Caput succedaneum**

P12.89 **Other birth injuries to scalp**

P12.9 **Birth injury to scalp, unspecified**

P13 **Birth injury to skeleton**

> **Excludes2:** birth injury to spine (P11.5)

P13.0 **Fracture of skull due to birth injury**

P13.1 **Other birth injuries to skull**

> **Excludes1:** cephalhematoma (P12.0)

P13.2 **Birth injury to femur**

P13.3 **Birth injury to other long bones**

P13.4 **Fracture of clavicle due to birth injury**

P13.8 **Birth injuries to other parts of skeleton**

P13.9 **Birth injury to skeleton, unspecified**

P14 **Birth injury to peripheral nervous system**

P14.0 **Erb's paralysis due to birth injury**

P14.1 **Klumpke's paralysis due to birth injury**

P14.2 **Phrenic nerve paralysis due to birth injury**

P14.3 **Other brachial plexus birth injuries**

P14.8 **Birth injuries to other parts of peripheral nervous system**

P14.9 **Birth injury to peripheral nervous system, unspecified**

P15 **Other birth injuries**

P15.0 **Birth injury to liver**

Rupture of liver due to birth injury

P15.1 **Birth injury to spleen**

Rupture of spleen due to birth injury

P15.2 **Sternomastoid injury due to birth injury**

P15.3 **Birth injury to eye**

Subconjunctival hemorrhage due to birth injury

Traumatic glaucoma due to birth injury

P15.4 **Birth injury to face**

Facial congestion due to birth injury

P15.5 **Birth injury to external genitalia**

P15.6 **Subcutaneous fat necrosis due to birth injury**

P15.8 **Other specified birth injuries**

P15.9 **Birth injury, unspecified**

RESPIRATORY AND CARDIOVASCULAR DISORDERS SPECIFIC TO THE PERINATAL PERIOD (P19-P29)

P19 **Metabolic acidemia in newborn**

> **Includes:** metabolic acidemia in newborn

P19.0 **Metabolic acidemia in newborn first noted before onset of labor**

P19.1 **Metabolic acidemia in newborn first noted during labor**

P19.2 **Metabolic acidemia noted at birth**

P19.9 **Metabolic acidemia, unspecified**

P22 **Respiratory distress of newborn**

> **Excludes1:** respiratory arrest of newborn (P28.81)
>
> respiratory failure of newborn NOS (P28.5)

P22.0 **Respiratory distress syndrome of newborn**

> **Definition:** Respiratory distress syndrome (RDS), formerly known as hyaline membrane disease, is a syndrome of respiratory difficulty in newborn infants caused by a deficiency of a molecule called surfactant.

Cardiorespiratory distress syndrome of newborn

Hyaline membrane disease

Idiopathic respiratory distress syndrome [IRDS or RDS] of newborn

Pulmonary hypoperfusion syndrome

Respiratory distress syndrome, type I

P22.1 **Transient tachypnea of newborn**

Idiopathic tachypnea of newborn

Respiratory distress syndrome, type II

Wet lung syndrome

P22.8 **Other respiratory distress of newborn**

P22.9 **Respiratory distress of newborn, unspecified**

P23 **Congenital pneumonia**

> **Includes:** infective pneumonia acquired in utero or during birth
>
> **Excludes1:** neonatal pneumonia resulting from aspiration (P24.-)

P23.0 **Congenital pneumonia due to viral agent**

> **Use additional code** (B97) to identify organism
>
> **Excludes1:** congenital rubella pneumonitis (P35.0)

P23.1 **Congenital pneumonia due to Chlamydia**

P23.2 **Congenital pneumonia due to staphylococcus**

P23.3 **Congenital pneumonia due to streptococcus, group B**

P23.4   Congenital pneumonia due to Escherichia coli

P23.5   Congenital pneumonia due to Pseudomonas

P23.6   Congenital pneumonia due to other bacterial agents

Congenital pneumonia due to Hemophilus influenzae

Congenital pneumonia due to Klebsiella pneumoniae

Congenital pneumonia due to Mycoplasma

Congenital pneumonia due to Streptococcus, except group B

<u>Use additional code</u> (B95-B96) to identify organism

P23.8   Congenital pneumonia due to other organisms

P23.9   Congenital pneumonia, unspecified

P24   Neonatal aspiration

Includes: aspiration in utero and during delivery

P24.0   Meconium aspiration

Excludes1: meconium passage (without aspiration) during delivery (P03.82)

meconium staining (P96.83)

P24.00   Meconium aspiration without respiratory symptoms

Meconium aspiration NOS

P24.01   Meconium aspiration with respiratory symptoms

Meconium aspiration pneumonia

Meconium aspiration pneumonitis

Meconium aspiration syndrome NOS

<u>Use additional code</u> to identify any secondary pulmonary hypertension, if applicable (I27.2-)

P24.1   Neonatal aspiration of (clear) amniotic fluid and mucus

Neonatal aspiration of liquor (amnii)

P24.10   Neonatal aspiration of (clear) amniotic fluid and mucus without respiratory symptoms

Neonatal aspiration of amniotic fluid and mucus NOS

P24.11   Neonatal aspiration of (clear) amniotic fluid and mucus with respiratory symptoms

Neonatal aspiration of amniotic fluid and mucus with pneumonia

Neonatal aspiration of amniotic fluid and mucus with pneumonitis

<u>Use additional code</u> to identify any secondary pulmonary hypertension, if applicable (I27.2-)

P24.2   Neonatal aspiration of blood

P24.20   Neonatal aspiration of blood without respiratory symptoms

Neonatal aspiration of blood NOS

P24.21   Neonatal aspiration of blood with respiratory symptoms

Neonatal aspiration of blood with pneumonia

Neonatal aspiration of blood with pneumonitis

<u>Use additional code</u> to identify any secondary pulmonary hypertension, if applicable (I27.2-)

P24.3   Neonatal aspiration of milk and regurgitated food

Neonatal aspiration of stomach contents

P24.30   Neonatal aspiration of milk and regurgitated food without respiratory symptoms

Neonatal aspiration of milk and regurgitated food NOS

P24.31   Neonatal aspiration of milk and regurgitated food with respiratory symptoms

Neonatal aspiration of milk and regurgitated food with pneumonia

Neonatal aspiration of milk and regurgitated food with pneumonitis

<u>Use additional code</u> to identify any secondary pulmonary hypertension, if applicable (I27.2-)

P24.8   Other neonatal aspiration

P24.80   Other neonatal aspiration without respiratory symptoms

Neonatal aspiration NEC

P24.81   Other neonatal aspiration with respiratory symptoms

Neonatal aspiration pneumonia NEC

Neonatal aspiration with pneumonitis NEC

Neonatal aspiration with pneumonia NOS

Neonatal aspiration with pneumonitis NOS

<u>Use additional code</u> to identify any secondary pulmonary hypertension, if applicable (I27.2-)

P24.9   Neonatal aspiration, unspecified

P25   Interstitial emphysema and related conditions originating in the perinatal period

P25.0   Interstitial emphysema originating in the perinatal period

P25.1   Pneumothorax originating in the perinatal period

P25.2   Pneumomediastinum originating in the perinatal period

P25.3   Pneumopericardium originating in the perinatal period

P25.8   Other conditions related to interstitial emphysema originating in the perinatal period

P26   Pulmonary hemorrhage originating in the perinatal period

Excludes1: acute idiopathic hemorrhage in infants over 28 days old (R04.81)

P26.0   Tracheobronchial hemorrhage originating in the perinatal period

P26.1   Massive pulmonary hemorrhage originating in the perinatal period

P26.8   Other pulmonary hemorrhages originating in the perinatal period

P26.9   Unspecified pulmonary hemorrhage originating in the perinatal period

P27   Chronic respiratory disease originating in the perinatal period

Excludes2: respiratory distress of newborn (P22.0-P22.9)

P27.0   Wilson-Mikity syndrome

Pulmonary dysmaturity

P27.1   Bronchopulmonary dysplasia originating in the perinatal period

P27.8   Other chronic respiratory diseases originating in the perinatal period

Congenital pulmonary fibrosis

Ventilator lung in newborn

P27.9   Unspecified chronic respiratory disease originating in the perinatal period

P28   Other respiratory conditions originating in the perinatal period

Excludes1: congenital malformations of the respiratory system (Q30-Q34)

P28.0   Primary atelectasis of newborn

Primary failure to expand terminal respiratory units

Pulmonary hypoplasia associated with short gestation

Pulmonary immaturity NOS

P28.1   Other and unspecified atelectasis of newborn

P28.10   Unspecified atelectasis of newborn

Atelectasis of newborn NOS

P28.11 **Resorption atelectasis without respiratory distress syndrome**
Excludes1: resorption atelectasis with respiratory distress syndrome (P22.0)

P28.19 **Other atelectasis of newborn**
Partial atelectasis of newborn
Secondary atelectasis of newborn

P28.2 **Cyanotic attacks of newborn**
Excludes1: apnea of newborn (P28.3-P28.4)

P28.3 **Primary sleep apnea of newborn**
Central sleep apnea of newborn
Obstructive sleep apnea of newborn
Sleep apnea of newborn NOS

P28.4 **Other apnea of newborn**
Apnea of prematurity
Obstructive apnea of newborn
Excludes1: obstructive sleep apnea of newborn (P28.3)

P28.5 **Respiratory failure of newborn**
Excludes1: respiratory arrest of newborn (P28.81)
respiratory distress of newborn (P22.0-)

P28.8 **Other specified respiratory conditions of newborn**

P28.81 **Respiratory arrest of newborn**

P28.89 **Other specified respiratory conditions of newborn**
Congenital laryngeal stridor
Sniffles in newborn
Snuffles in newborn
Excludes1: early congenital syphilitic rhinitis A50.05)

P28.9 **Respiratory condition of newborn, unspecified**
Respiratory depression in newborn

P29 **Cardiovascular disorders originating in the perinatal period**
Excludes1: congenital malformations of the circulatory system (Q20-Q28)

P29.0 **Neonatal cardiac failure**

P29.1 **Neonatal cardiac dysrhythmia**

P29.11 **Neonatal tachycardia**

P29.12 **Neonatal bradycardia**

P29.2 **Neonatal hypertension**

P29.3 **Persistent fetal circulation**

•**P29.30** **Pulmonary hypertension of newborn**
Persistent pulmonary hypertension of newborn

•**P29.38** **Other persistent fetal circulation**
Delayed closure of ductus arteriosus

P29.4 **Transient myocardial ischemia in newborn**

P29.8 **Other cardiovascular disorders originating in the perinatal period**

P29.81 **Cardiac arrest of newborn**

P29.89 **Other cardiovascular disorders originating in the perinatal period**

P29.9 **Cardiovascular disorder originating in the perinatal period, unspecified**

INFECTIONS SPECIFIC TO THE PERINATAL PERIOD (P35-P39)

Infections acquired in utero, during birth via the umbilicus, or during the first 28 days after birth

Excludes2: asymptomatic human immunodeficiency virus [HIV] infection status (Z21)
congenital gonococcal infection (A54.-)
congenital pneumonia (P23.-)
congenital syphilis (A50.-)
human immunodeficiency virus [HIV] disease (B20)
infant botulism (A48.51)
infectious diseases not specific to the perinatal period (A00-B99, J09, J10.-)
intestinal infectious disease (A00-A09)
laboratory evidence of human immunodeficiency virus [HIV] (R75)
tetanus neonatorum (A33)

P35 **Congenital viral diseases**
Includes: infections acquired in utero or during birth

P35.0 **Congenital rubella syndrome**
Congenital rubella pneumonitis

P35.1 **Congenital cytomegalovirus infection**

P35.2 **Congenital herpesviral [herpes simplex] infection**

P35.3 **Congenital viral hepatitis**

P35.8 **Other congenital viral diseases**
Congenital varicella [chickenpox]

P35.9 **Congenital viral disease, unspecified**

P36 **Bacterial sepsis of newborn**
Definition: Neonatal sepsis is a blood infection that occurs in an infant younger than 90 days old. Early-onset sepsis is seen in the first week of life. Late-onset sepsis occurs between days 8 and 89.
Includes: congenital sepsis
Use additional code(s), if applicable, to identify severe sepsis (R652-) and associated acute organ dysfunction(s)

P36.0 **Sepsis of newborn due to streptococcus, group B**

P36.1 **Sepsis of newborn due to other and unspecified streptococci**

P36.10 **Sepsis of newborn due to unspecified streptococci**

P36.19 **Sepsis of newborn due to other streptococci**

P36.2 **Sepsis of newborn due to Staphylococcus aureus**

P36.3 **Sepsis of newborn due to other and unspecified staphylococci**

P36.30 **Sepsis of newborn due to unspecified staphylococci**

P36.39 **Sepsis of newborn due to other staphylococci**

P36.4 **Sepsis of newborn due to Escherichia coli**

P36.5 **Sepsis of newborn due to anaerobes**

P36.8 **Other bacterial sepsis of newborn**
Use additional code from category B96 to identify organism

P36.9 **Bacterial sepsis of newborn, unspecified**

P37 **Other congenital infectious and parasitic diseases**
Excludes2: congenital syphilis (A50.-)
infectious neonatal diarrhea (A00-A09)
necrotizing enterocolitis in newborn (P77.-)
noninfectious neonatal diarrhea (P78.3)
ophthalmia neonatorum due to gonococcus (A54.31)
tetanus neonatorum (A33)

P37.0 **Congenital tuberculosis**

P37.1 **Congenital toxoplasmosis**
Hydrocephalus due to congenital toxoplasmosis

P37.2 **Neonatal (disseminated) listeriosis**

Add 4th-7th digits   Nonspecific code   Unspecified code   Manifestation code

P37.3   **Congenital falciparum malaria**

P37.4   **Other congenital malaria**

P37.5   **Neonatal candidiasis**

P37.8   **Other specified congenital infectious and parasitic diseases**

P37.9   **Congenital infectious or parasitic disease, unspecified**

P38   **Omphalitis of newborn**

Definition: Omphalitis is the medical term for inflammation of the umbilical cord stump in the neonatal newborn period, most commonly attributed to a bacterial infection.

Excludes1: omphalitis not of newborn (L08.82)

    tetanus omphalitis (A33)

    umbilical hemorrhage of newborn (P51.-)

P38.1   **Omphalitis with mild hemorrhage**

P38.9   **Omphalitis without hemorrhage**

    Omphalitis of newborn NOS

P39   **Other infections specific to the perinatal period**

Use additional code to identify organism or specific infection

P39.0   **Neonatal infective mastitis**

    Excludes1: breast engorgement of newborn (P83.4)

        noninfective mastitis of newborn (P83.4)

P39.1   **Neonatal conjunctivitis and dacryocystitis**

    Neonatal chlamydial conjunctivitis

    Ophthalmia neonatorum NOS

    Excludes1: gonococcal conjunctivitis (A54.31)

P39.2   **Intra-amniotic infection affecting newborn, not elsewhere classified**

P39.3   **Neonatal urinary tract infection**

P39.4   **Neonatal skin infection**

    Neonatal pyoderma

    Excludes1: pemphigus neonatorum (L00)

        staphylococcal scalded skin syndrome (L00)

P39.8   **Other specified infections specific to the perinatal period**

P39.9   **Infection specific to the perinatal period, unspecified**

HEMORRHAGIC AND HEMATOLOGICAL DISORDERS OF NEWBORN (P50-P61)

Excludes1: congenital stenosis and stricture of bile ducts (Q44.3)

    Crigler-Najjar syndrome (E80.5)

    Dubin-Johnson syndrome (E80.6)

    Gilbert syndrome (E80.4)

    hereditary hemolytic anemias (D55-D58)

P50   **Newborn affected by intrauterine (fetal) blood loss**

    Excludes1: congenital anemia from intrauterine (fetal) blood loss (P61.3)

P50.0   **Newborn affected by intrauterine (fetal) blood loss from vasa previa**

P50.1   **Newborn affected by intrauterine (fetal) blood loss from ruptured cord**

P50.2   **Newborn affected by intrauterine (fetal) blood loss from placenta**

P50.3   **Newborn affected by hemorrhage into co-twin**

P50.4   **Newborn affected by hemorrhage into maternal circulation**

P50.5   **Newborn affected by intrauterine (fetal) blood loss from cut end of co-twin's cord**

P50.8   **Newborn affected by other intrauterine (fetal) blood loss**

P50.9   **Newborn affected by intrauterine (fetal) blood loss, unspecified**

Newborn affected by fetal hemorrhage NOS

P51   **Umbilical hemorrhage of newborn**

    Excludes1: omphalitis with mild hemorrhage (P38.1)

    umbilical hemorrhage from cut end of co-twins cord (P50.5)

P51.0   **Massive umbilical hemorrhage of newborn**

P51.8   **Other umbilical hemorrhages of newborn**

    Slipped umbilical ligature NOS

P51.9   **Umbilical hemorrhage of newborn, unspecified**

P52   **Intracranial nontraumatic hemorrhage of newborn**

Includes: intracranial hemorrhage due to anoxia or hypoxia

Excludes1: intracranial hemorrhage due to birth injury (P10.-)

    intracranial hemorrhage due to other injury (S06.-)

P52.0   **Intraventricular (nontraumatic) hemorrhage, grade 1, of newborn**

    Subependymal hemorrhage (without intraventricular extension)

    Bleeding into germinal matrix

P52.1   **Intraventricular (nontraumatic) hemorrhage, grade 2, of newborn**

    Subependymal hemorrhage with intraventricular extension

    Bleeding into ventricle

P52.2   **Intraventricular (nontraumatic) hemorrhage, grade 3and grade 4, of newborn**

    P52.21   **Intraventricular (nontraumatic) hemorrhage, grade 3, of newborn**

        Subependymal hemorrhage with intraventricular extension with enlargement of ventricle

    P52.22   **Intraventricular (nontraumatic) hemorrhage, grade 4, of newborn**

        Bleeding into cerebral cortex

        Subependymal hemorrhage with intracerebral extension

P52.3   **Unspecified intraventricular (nontraumatic) hemorrhage of newborn**

P52.4   **Intracerebral (nontraumatic) hemorrhage of newborn**

P52.5   **Subarachnoid (nontraumatic) hemorrhage of newborn**

P52.6   **Cerebellar (nontraumatic) and posterior fossa hemorrhage of newborn**

P52.8   **Other intracranial (nontraumatic) hemorrhages of newborn**

P52.9   **Intracranial (nontraumatic) hemorrhage of newborn, unspecified**

P53   **Hemorrhagic disease of newborn**

    Vitamin K deficiency of newborn

P54   **Other neonatal hemorrhages**

    Excludes1: newborn affected by (intrauterine) blood loss (P50.-)

    pulmonary hemorrhage originating in the perinatal period (P26.-)

P54.0   **Neonatal hematemesis**

    Excludes1: neonatal hematemesis due to swallowed maternal blood (P78.2)

P54.1   **Neonatal melena**

    Excludes1: neonatal melena due to swallowed maternal blood (P78.2)

P54.2   **Neonatal rectal hemorrhage**

P54.3   **Other neonatal gastrointestinal hemorrhage**

P54.4   **Neonatal adrenal hemorrhage**

P54.5   **Neonatal cutaneous hemorrhage**

    Neonatal bruising

Neonatal ecchymoses

Neonatal petechiae

Neonatal superficial hematomata

Excludes2: bruising of scalp due to birth injury (P12.3)

cephalhematoma due to birth injury (P12.0)

P54.6 Neonatal vaginal hemorrhage

Neonatal pseudomenses

P54.8 Other specified neonatal hemorrhages

P54.9 Neonatal hemorrhage, unspecified

P55 Hemolytic disease of newborn

P55.0 Rh isoimmunization of newborn

P55.1 ABO isoimmunization of newborn

P55.8 Other hemolytic diseases of newborn

P55.9 Hemolytic disease of newborn, unspecified

P56 Hydrops fetalis due to hemolytic disease

Excludes1: hydrops fetalis NOS (P83.2)

P56.0 Hydrops fetalis due to isoimmunization

P56.9 Hydrops fetalis due to other and unspecified hemolytic disease

P56.90 Hydrops fetalis due to unspecified hemolytic disease

P56.99 Hydrops fetalis due to other hemolytic disease

P57 Kernicterus

Definition: Kernicterus is a disorder that is due to severe jaundice in the newborn, with deposition of the pigment bilirubin in the brain that causes damage to the brain, potentially leading to athetoid cerebral palsy, hearing loss, vision problems, or mental retardation.

P57.0 Kernicterus due to isoimmunization

P57.8 Other specified kernicterus

Excludes1: Crigler-Najjar syndrome (E80.5)

P57.9 Kernicterus, unspecified

P58 Neonatal jaundice due to other excessive hemolysis

Excludes1: jaundice due to isoimmunization (P55-P57)

P58.0 Neonatal jaundice due to bruising

P58.1 Neonatal jaundice due to bleeding

P58.2 Neonatal jaundice due to infection

P58.3 Neonatal jaundice due to polycythemia

P58.4 Neonatal jaundice due to drugs or toxins transmitted from mother or given to newborn

Code first poisoning due to drug or toxin, if applicable (T36-T65 with fifth or sixth character 1-4 or 6)

Use additional code for adverse effect, if applicable, to identify drug (T36-T50 with fifth or sixth character 5)

P58.41 Neonatal jaundice due to drugs or toxins transmitted from mother

P58.42 Neonatal jaundice due to drugs or toxins given to newborn

P58.5 Neonatal jaundice due to swallowed maternal blood

P58.8 Neonatal jaundice due to other specified excessive hemolysis

P58.9 Neonatal jaundice due to excessive hemolysis, unspecified

P59 Neonatal jaundice from other and unspecified causes

Excludes1: jaundice due to inborn errors of metabolism (E70-E88)

kernicterus (P57.-)

P59.0 Neonatal jaundice associated with preterm delivery

Hyperbilirubinemia of prematurity

Jaundice due to delayed conjugation associated with preterm delivery

P59.1 Inspissated bile syndrome

P59.2 Neonatal jaundice from other and unspecified hepatocellular damage

Excludes1: congenital viral hepatitis (P35.3)

P59.20 Neonatal jaundice from unspecified hepatocellular damage

P59.29 Neonatal jaundice from other hepatocellular damage

Neonatal giant cell hepatitis

Neonatal (idiopathic) hepatitis

P59.3 Neonatal jaundice from breast milk inhibitor

P59.8 Neonatal jaundice from other specified causes

P59.9 Neonatal jaundice, unspecified

Neonatal physiological jaundice (intense)(prolonged) NOS

P60 Disseminated intravascular coagulation of newborn

Defibrination syndrome of newborn

P61 Other perinatal hematological disorders

Excludes1: transient hypogammaglobulinemia of infancy (D80.7)

P61.0 Transient neonatal thrombocytopenia

Neonatal thrombocytopenia due to exchange transfusion

Neonatal thrombocytopenia due to idiopathic maternal thrombocytopenia

Neonatal thrombocytopenia due to isoimmunization

P61.1 Polycythemia neonatorum

P61.2 Anemia of prematurity

P61.3 Congenital anemia from fetal blood loss

P61.4 Other congenital anemias, not elsewhere classified

Congenital anemia NOS

P61.5 Transient neonatal neutropenia

Excludes1: congenital neutropenia (non transient) (D70.0)

P61.6 Other transient neonatal disorders of coagulation

P61.8 Other specified perinatal hematological disorders

P61.9 Perinatal hematological disorder, unspecified

TRANSITORY ENDOCRINE AND METABOLIC DISORDERS SPECIFIC TO NEWBORN (P70-P74)

Includes: transitory endocrine and metabolic disturbances caused by the infant's response to maternal endocrine and metabolic factors, or its adjustment to extrauterine environment

P70 Transitory disorders of carbohydrate metabolism specific to newborn

P70.0 Syndrome of infant of mother with gestational diabetes

Newborn (with hypoglycemia) affected by maternal gestational diabetes

Excludes1: newborn (with hypoglycemia) affected by maternal (pre-existing) diabetes mellitus (P70.1)

syndrome of infant of a diabetic mother (P70.1)

P70.1 Syndrome of infant of a diabetic mother

Newborn (with hypoglycemia) affected by maternal (pre-existing) diabetes mellitus

Excludes1: newborn (with hypoglycemia) affected by maternal gestational diabetes (P70.0)

syndrome of infant of mother with gestational diabetes (P70.0)

P70.2 Neonatal diabetes mellitus

P70.3 Iatrogenic neonatal hypoglycemia

P70.4 Other neonatal hypoglycemia

Transitory neonatal hypoglycemia

P70.8 **Other transitory disorders of carbohydrate metabolism of newborn**

P70.9 **Transitory disorder of carbohydrate metabolism of newborn, unspecified**

P71 **Transitory neonatal disorders of calcium and magnesium metabolism**

P71.0 **Cow's milk hypocalcemia in newborn**

P71.1 **Other neonatal hypocalcemia**

Excludes1: neonatal hypoparathyroidism (P71.4)

P71.2 **Neonatal hypomagnesemia**

P71.3 **Neonatal tetany without calcium or magnesium deficiency**

Neonatal tetany NOS

P71.4 **Transitory neonatal hypoparathyroidism**

P71.8 **Other transitory neonatal disorders of calcium and magnesium metabolism**

P71.9 **Transitory neonatal disorder of calcium and magnesium metabolism, unspecified**

P72 **Other transitory neonatal endocrine disorders**

Excludes1: congenital hypothyroidism with or without goiter (E03.0-E03.1)

Dyshormogenetic goiter (E07.1)

Pendred's syndrome (E07.1)

P72.0 **Neonatal goiter, not elsewhere classified**

Transitory congenital goiter with normal functioning

P72.1 **Transitory neonatal hyperthyroidism**

Neonatal thyrotoxicosis

P72.2 **Other transitory neonatal disorders of thyroid function, not elsewhere classified**

Transitory neonatal hypothyroidism

P72.8 **Other specified transitory neonatal endocrine disorders**

P72.9 **Transitory neonatal endocrine disorder, unspecified**

P74 **Other transitory neonatal electrolyte and metabolic disturbances**

P74.0 **Late metabolic acidosis of newborn**

Excludes1: (fetal) metabolic acidosis of newborn (P19)

P74.1 **Dehydration of newborn**

P74.2 **Disturbances of sodium balance of newborn**

P74.3 **Disturbances of potassium balance of newborn**

P74.4 **Other transitory electrolyte disturbances of newborn**

P74.5 **Transitory tyrosinemia of newborn**

P74.6 **Transitory hyperammonemia of newborn**

P74.8 **Other transitory metabolic disturbances of newborn**

Amino-acid metabolic disorders described as transitory

P74.9 **Transitory metabolic disturbance of newborn, unspecified**

DIGESTIVE SYSTEM DISORDERS OF NEWBORN (P76-P78)

P76 **Other intestinal obstruction of newborn**

P76.0 **Meconium plug syndrome**

Meconium ileus NOS

Excludes1: meconium ileus in cystic fibrosis (E84.11)

P76.1 **Transitory ileus of newborn**

Excludes1: Hirschsprung's disease (Q43.1)

P76.2 **Intestinal obstruction due to inspissated milk**

P76.8 **Other specified intestinal obstruction of newborn**

Excludes1: intestinal obstruction classifiable to K56.-

P76.9 **Intestinal obstruction of newborn, unspecified**

P77 **Necrotizing enterocolitis of newborn**

P77.1 **Stage 1 necrotizing enterocolitis in newborn**

Necrotizing enterocolitis without pneumatosis, without perforation

P77.2 **Stage 2 necrotizing enterocolitis in newborn**

Necrotizing enterocolitis with pneumatosis, without perforation

P77.3 **Stage 3 necrotizing enterocolitis in newborn**

Necrotizing enterocolitis with perforation

Necrotizing enterocolitis with pneumatosis and perforation

P77.9 **Necrotizing enterocolitis in newborn, unspecified**

Necrotizing enterocolitis in newborn, NOS

P78 **Other perinatal digestive system disorders**

Excludes1: cystic fibrosis (E84.0-E84.9)

neonatal gastrointestinal hemorrhages (P54.0-P54.3)

P78.0 **Perinatal intestinal perforation**

Meconium peritonitis

P78.1 **Other neonatal peritonitis**

Neonatal peritonitis NOS

P78.2 **Neonatal hematemesis and melena due to swallowed maternal blood**

P78.3 **Noninfective neonatal diarrhea**

Neonatal diarrhea NOS

P78.8 **Other specified perinatal digestive system disorders**

P78.81 **Congenital cirrhosis (of liver)**

P78.82 **Peptic ulcer of newborn**

P78.83 **Newborn esophageal reflux**

Neonatal esophageal reflux

• **P78.84** **Gestational alloimmune liver disease**

GALD

Neonatal hemochromatosis

Excludes 1: hemochromatosis (E83.11-)

P78.89 **Other specified perinatal digestive system disorders**

P78.9 **Perinatal digestive system disorder, unspecified**

CONDITIONS INVOLVING THE INTEGUMENT AND TEMPERATURE REGULATION OF NEWBORN (P80-P83)

P80 **Hypothermia of newborn**

P80.0 **Cold injury syndrome**

Severe and usually chronic hypothermia associated with a pink flushed appearance, edema and neurological and biochemical abnormalities.

Excludes1: mild hypothermia of newborn (P80.8)

P80.8 **Other hypothermia of newborn**

Mild hypothermia of newborn

P80.9 **Hypothermia of newborn, unspecified**

P81 **Other disturbances of temperature regulation of newborn**

P81.0 **Environmental hyperthermia of newborn**

P81.8 **Other specified disturbances of temperature regulation of newborn**

P81.9 **Disturbance of temperature regulation of newborn, unspecified**

Fever of newborn NOS

P83 **Other conditions of integument specific to newborn**

Excludes1: congenital malformations of skin and integument (Q80-Q84)

hydrops fetalis due to hemolytic disease (P56.-)

neonatal skin infection (P39.4)

● New code   ▲ Revised code   Excludes1: Not coded here   Excludes2: Not included here   ⊗ Placeholder required   ⑦ 7th digit required

staphylococcal scalded skin syndrome (L00)

Excludes2: cradle cap (L21.0)

diaper [napkin] dermatitis (L22)

P83.0 **Sclerema neonatorum**

P83.1 **Neonatal erythema toxicum**

P83.2 **Hydrops fetalis not due to hemolytic disease**

Hydrops fetalis NOS

P83.3 **Other and unspecified edema specific to newborn**

P83.30 **Unspecified edema specific to newborn**

P83.39 **Other edema specific to newborn**

P83.4 **Breast engorgement of newborn**

Noninfective mastitis of newborn

P83.5 **Congenital hydrocele**

P83.6 **Umbilical polyp of newborn**

P83.8 **Other specified conditions of integument specific to newborn**

•P83.81 **Umbilical granuloma**

Excludes2: Granulomatous disorder of the skin and subcutaneous tissue, unspecified (L92.9)

•P83.88 **Other specified conditions of integument specific to newborn**

Bronze baby syndrome

Neonatal scleroderma

Urticaria neonatorum

P83.9 **Condition of the integument specific to newborn, unspecified**

OTHER PROBLEMS WITH NEWBORN (P84)

P84 **Other problems with newborn**

Acidemia of newborn

Acidosis of newborn

Anoxia of newborn NOS

Asphyxia of newborn NOS

Hypercapnia of newborn

Hypoxemia of newborn

Hypoxia of newborn NOS

Mixed metabolic and respiratory acidosis of newborn

Excludes1: intracranial hemorrhage due to anoxia or hypoxia (P52.-)

hypoxic ischemic encephalopathy [HIE] (P91.6-)

late metabolic acidosis of newborn (P74.0)

OTHER DISORDERS ORIGINATING IN THE PERINATAL PERIOD (P90-P96)

P90 **Convulsions of newborn**

Excludes1: benign myoclonic epilepsy in infancy (G40.3-)

benign neonatal convulsions (familial) (G40.3-)

P91 **Other disturbances of cerebral status of newborn**

P91.0 **Neonatal cerebral ischemia**

P91.1 **Acquired periventricular cysts of newborn**

P91.2 **Neonatal cerebral leukomalacia**

Periventricular leukomalacia

P91.3 **Neonatal cerebral irritability**

P91.4 **Neonatal cerebral depression**

P91.5 **Neonatal coma**

P91.6 **Hypoxic ischemic encephalopathy [HIE]**

Excludes1: Neonatal cerebral depression (P91.4)

Neonatal cerebral irritability (P91.3)

Neonatal coma (P91.5)

P91.60 **Hypoxic ischemic encephalopathy [HIE], unspecified**

P91.61 **Mild hypoxic ischemic encephalopathy [HIE]**

P91.62 **Moderate hypoxic ischemic encephalopathy [HIE]**

P91.63 **Severe hypoxic ischemic encephalopathy [HIE]**

P91.8 **Other specified disturbances of cerebral status of newborn**

•P91.81 **Neonatal encephalopathy**

•P91.811 **Neonatal encephalopathy in diseases classified elsewhere**

Code first underlying condition, if known, such as:

congenital cirrhosis (of liver) (P78.71)

intracranial nontraumatic hemorrhage of newborn (P52.-)

kernicterus (P57.-)

•P91.819 **Neonatal encephalopathy, unspecified**

•P91.88 **Other specified disturbances of cerebral status of newborn**

P91.9 **Disturbance of cerebral status of newborn, unspecified**

P92 **Feeding problems of newborn**

Excludes1: eating disorders (F50.-)

Feeding problems in child over 28 days old (R63.3)

P92.0 **Vomiting of newborn**

Excludes1: vomiting of child over 28 days old (R11.-)

P92.01 **Bilious vomiting of newborn**

Excludes1: bilious vomiting in child over 28 days old (R11.14)

P92.09 **Other vomiting of newborn**

Excludes1: regurgitation of food in newborn (P92.1)

P92.1 **Regurgitation and rumination of newborn**

P92.2 **Slow feeding of newborn**

P92.3 **Underfeeding of newborn**

P92.4 **Overfeeding of newborn**

P92.5 **Neonatal difficulty in feeding at breast**

P92.6 **Failure to thrive in newborn**

Excludes1: failure to thrive in child over 28 days old (R62.51)

P92.8 **Other feeding problems of newborn**

P92.9 **Feeding problem of newborn, unspecified**

P93 **Reactions and intoxications due to drugs administered to newborn**

Includes: reactions and intoxications due to drugs administered to fetus affecting newborn

Excludes1: jaundice due to drugs or toxins transmitted from mother or given to newborn (P58.4-)

reactions and intoxications from maternal opiates, tranquilizers **and other** medication (P04.0-P04.1, P04.4)

withdrawal symptoms from maternal use of drugs of addiction (P96.1)

withdrawal symptoms from therapeutic use of drugs in newborn (P96.2)

P93.0 **Grey baby syndrome**

Grey syndrome from chloramphenicol administration in newborn

P93.8 **Other reactions and intoxications due to drugs administered to newborn**

<u>Use additional code</u> for adverse effect, if applicable, to identify drug (T36-T50 with fifth or sixth character 5)

P94 **Disorders of muscle tone of newborn**

P94.0 **Transient neonatal myasthenia gravis**

Excludes1: myasthenia gravis (G70.0)

P94.1 **Congenital hypertonia**

P94.2 **Congenital hypotonia**

Floppy baby syndrome, unspecified

P94.8 **Other disorders of muscle tone of newborn**

P94.9 **Disorder of muscle tone of newborn, unspecified**

P95 **Stillbirth**

Dead born fetus NOS

Fetal death of unspecified cause

Stillbirth NOS

Excludes1: maternal care for intrauterine death (O36.4)

missed abortion (O02.1)

outcome of delivery, stillbirth (Z37.1, Z37.3, Z37.4, Z37.7)

P96 **Other conditions originating in the perinatal period**

P96.0 **Congenital renal failure**

Uremia of newborn

P96.1 **Neonatal withdrawal symptoms from maternal use of drugs of addiction**

Drug withdrawal syndrome in infant of dependent mother

Neonatal abstinence syndrome

Excludes1: reactions and intoxications from maternal opiates and tranquilizers administered during labor and delivery (P04.0)

P96.2 **Withdrawal symptoms from therapeutic use of drugs in newborn**

P96.3 **Wide cranial sutures of newborn**

Neonatal craniotabes

P96.5 **Complication to newborn due to (fetal) intrauterine procedure**

Excludes2: newborn affected by amniocentesis (P00.6)

P96.8 **Other specified conditions originating in the perinatal period**

P96.81 **Exposure to (parental) (environmental) tobacco smoke in the perinatal period**

Excludes2: newborn affected by in utero exposure to tobacco (P04.2)

exposure to environmental tobacco smoke after the perinatal period (Z77.22)

P96.82 **Delayed separation of umbilical cord**

P96.83 **Meconium staining**

Excludes1: meconium aspiration (P24.00, P24.01)

meconium passage during delivery (P03.82)

P96.89 **Other specified conditions originating in the perinatal period**

<u>Use additional code</u> to specify condition

P96.9 **Condition originating in the perinatal period, unspecified**

Congenital debility NOS

● New code   ▲ Revised code   Excludes1: Not coded here   Excludes2: Not included here   ⊗ Placeholder required   ⑦7th digit required

Chapter 17: Congenital Malformations, Deformations And Chromosomal Abnormalities (Q00-Q99)

DEFINITIONS

This chapter includes definitions of selected key words, terms and phrases and coding alerts for adding points to the clinical domain, and references to coding late effects where appropriate. An example from this chapter is as follows:

Q11   Anophthalmos, microphthalmos and macrophthalmos
    Definition: Anophthalmos is the absence of one or both eyes. Both the globe and the ocular tissue are missing from the orbit.

MULTIPLE CODING FOR A SINGLE CONDITION

In addition to the etiology/manifestation convention that requires two codes to fully describe a single condition that affects multiple body systems, there are other single conditions that also require more than one code. "Use additional code" notes are found in the Tabular List at codes that are not part of an etiology/manifestation pair where a secondary code is useful to fully describe a condition. The sequencing rule is the same as the etiology/manifestation pair, "use additional code" indicates that a secondary code should be added.

For example, for bacterial infections that are not included in chapter 1, a secondary code from category B95, Streptococcus, Staphylococcus, and Enterococcus, as the cause of diseases classified elsewhere, or B96, Other bacterial agents as the cause of diseases classified elsewhere, may be required to identify the bacterial organism causing the infection. A "use additional code" note will normally be found at the infectious disease code, indicating a need for the organism code to be added as a secondary code.

"Code first" notes are also under certain codes that are not specifically manifestation codes but may be due to an underlying cause. When there is a "code first" note and an underlying condition is present, the underlying condition should be sequenced first.

"Code, if applicable, any causal condition first", notes indicate that this code may be assigned as a principal diagnosis when the causal condition is unknown or not applicable. If a causal condition is known, then the code for that condition should be sequenced as the principal or first-listed diagnosis.

Multiple codes may be needed for sequela, complication codes and obstetric codes to more fully describe a condition. See the specific guidelines for these conditions for further instruction.

COMBINATION CODE

A combination code is a single code used to classify: Two diagnoses, or a diagnosis with an associated secondary process (manifestation) A diagnosis with an associated complication

Combination codes are identified by referring to subterm entries in the Alphabetic Index and by reading the inclusion and exclusion notes in the Tabular List.

Assign only the combination code when that code fully identifies the diagnostic conditions involved or when the Alphabetic Index so directs. Multiple coding should not be used when the classification provides a combination code that clearly identifies all of the elements documented in the diagnosis. When the combination code lacks necessary specificity in describing the manifestation or complication, an additional code should be used as a secondary code.

SEQUELA (LATE EFFECTS)

A sequela is the residual effect (condition produced) after the acute phase of an illness or injury has terminated. There is no time limit on when a sequela code can be used. The residual may be apparent early, such as in cerebral infarction, or it may occur months or years later, such as that due to a previous injury. Coding of sequela generally requires two codes sequenced in the following order: The condition or nature of the sequela is sequenced first.

The sequela code is sequenced second.

An exception to the above guidelines are those instances where the code for the sequela is followed by a manifestation code identified in the Tabular List and title, or the sequela code has been expanded (at the fourth, fifth or sixth character levels) to include the manifestation(s). The code for the acute phase of an illness or injury that led to the sequela is never used with a code for the late effect.

Assign an appropriate code(s) from categories Q00-Q99, Congenital malformations, deformations, and chromosomal abnormalities when a malformation/deformation or chromosomal abnormality is documented. A malformation/deformation/or chromosomal abnormality may be the principal/first-listed diagnosis on a record or a secondary diagnosis.

When a malformation/deformation or chromosomal abnormality does not have a unique code assignment, assign additional code(s) for any manifestations that may be present.

When the code assignment specifically identifies the malformation/deformation or chromosomal abnormality, manifestations that are an inherent component of the anomaly should not be coded separately. Additional codes should be assigned for manifestations that are not an inherent component.

Codes from Chapter 17 may be used throughout the life of the patient. If a congenital malformation or deformity has been corrected, a personal history code should be used to identify the history of the malformation or deformity. Although present at birth, malformation/deformation/or chromosomal abnormality may not be identified until later in life. Whenever the condition is diagnosed by the physician, it is appropriate to assign a code from codes Q00-Q99.For the birth admission, the appropriate code from category Z38, Liveborn infants, according to place of birth and type of delivery, should be sequenced as the principal diagnosis, followed by any congenital anomaly codes, Q00-Q99.

Q00-Q99

• New code ▲ Revised code **Excludes1:** Not coded here **Excludes2:** Not included here ⊗ Placeholder required ⑦ 7th digit required

Chapter 17

Congenital Malformations, Deformations And Chromosomal Abnormalities (Q00-Q99)

Note: Codes from this chapter are not for use on maternal or fetal records

Excludes2: inborn errors of metabolism (E70-E88)

This chapter contains the following blocks:

Q00-Q07	Congenital malformations of the nervous system
Q10-Q18	Congenital malformations of eye, ear, face and neck
Q20-Q28	Congenital malformations of the circulatory system
Q30-Q34	Congenital malformations of the respiratory system
Q35-Q37	Cleft lip and cleft palate
Q38-Q45	Other congenital malformations of the digestive system
Q50-Q56	Congenital malformations of genital organs
Q60-Q64	Congenital malformations of the urinary system
Q65-Q79	Congenital malformations and deformations of the musculoskeletal system
Q80-Q89	Other congenital malformations
Q90-Q99	Chromosomal abnormalities, not elsewhere classified

CONGENITAL MALFORMATIONS OF THE NERVOUS SYSTEM (Q00-Q07)

Q00 Anencephaly and similar malformations

Definition: Anencephaly is the absence of a major portion of the brain, skull, and scalp that occurs during embryonic development.

Q00.0 Anencephaly

Acephaly

Acrania

Amyelencephaly

Hemianencephaly

Hemicephaly

Q00.1 Craniorachischisis

Q00.2 Iniencephaly

Q01 Encephalocele

Includes: Arnold-Chiari syndrome, type III

encephalocystocele

encephalomyelocele

hydroencephalocele

hydromeningocele, cranial meningocele, cerebral meningoencephalocele

Excludes1: Meckel-Gruber syndrome (Q61.9)

Q01.0 Frontal encephalocele

Q01.1 Nasofrontal encephalocele

Q01.2 Occipital encephalocele

Q01.8 Encephalocele of other sites

Q01.9 Encephalocele, unspecified

Q02 Microcephaly

Includes: hydromicrocephaly

micrencephalon

Excludes1: Meckel-Gruber syndrome (Q61.9)

Q03 Congenital hydrocephalus

Includes: hydrocephalus in newborn

Excludes1: Arnold-Chiari syndrome, type II (Q07.0-)

acquired hydrocephalus (G91.-)

hydrocephalus due to congenital toxoplasmosis (P37.1)

hydrocephalus with spina bifida (Q05.0-Q05.4)

Q03.0 Malformations of aqueduct of Sylvius

Anomaly of aqueduct of Sylvius

Obstruction of aqueduct of Sylvius, congenital

Stenosis of aqueduct of Sylvius

Q03.1 Atresia of foramina of Magendie and Luschka

Dandy-Walker syndrome

Q03.8 Other congenital hydrocephalus

Q03.9 Congenital hydrocephalus, unspecified

Q04 Other congenital malformations of brain

Excludes1: cyclopia (Q87.0)

macrocephaly (Q75.3)

Q04.0 Congenital malformations of corpus callosum

Agenesis of corpus callosum

Q04.1 Arhinencephaly

Q04.2 Holoprosencephaly

Q04.3 Other reduction deformities of brain

Absence of part of brain

Agenesis of part of brain

Agyria

Aplasia of part of brain

Hydranencephaly

Hypoplasia of part of brain

Lissencephaly

Microgyria

Pachygyria

Excludes1: congenital malformations of corpus callosum (Q04.0)

Q04.4 Septo-optic dysplasia of brain

Q04.5 Megalencephaly

Q04.6 Congenital cerebral cysts

Porencephaly

Schizencephaly

Excludes1: acquired porencephalic cyst (G93.0)

Q04.8 Other specified congenital malformations of brain

Arnold-Chiari syndrome, type IV

Macrogyria

Q04.9 Congenital malformation of brain, unspecified

Congenital anomaly NOS of brain

Congenital deformity NOS of brain

Congenital disease or lesion NOS of brain

Multiple anomalies NOS of brain, congenital

Q05 Spina bifida

Definition: Spina bifida is a serious birth abnormality in which the spinal cord is malformed and lacks its usual protective skeletal and soft tissue coverings.

Includes: hydromeningocele (spinal)

meningocele (spinal)

meningomyelocele

myelocele

myelomeningocele

rachischisis

spina bifida (aperta)(cystica)

syringomyelocele

Use additional code for any associated paraplegia (paraparesis) (G82.2-)

Add 4th-7th digits	Nonspecific code	Unspecified code	Manifestation code

Excludes1: Arnold-Chiari syndrome, type II (Q07.0-)

　　　 spina bifida occulta (Q76.0)

Q05.0　**Cervical spina bifida with hydrocephalus**

Q05.1　**Thoracic spina bifida with hydrocephalus**

　　　 Dorsal spina bifida with hydrocephalus

　　　 Thoracolumbar spina bifida with hydrocephalus

Q05.2　**Lumbar spina bifida with hydrocephalus**

　　　 Lumbosacral spina bifida with hydrocephalus

Q05.3　**Sacral spina bifida with hydrocephalus**

Q05.4　**Unspecified spina bifida with hydrocephalus**

Q05.5　**Cervical spina bifida without hydrocephalus**

Q05.6　**Thoracic spina bifida without hydrocephalus**

　　　 Dorsal spina bifida NOS

　　　 Thoracolumbar spina bifida NOS

Q05.7　**Lumbar spina bifida without hydrocephalus**

　　　 Lumbosacral spina bifida NOS

Q05.8　**Sacral spina bifida without hydrocephalus**

Q05.9　**Spina bifida, unspecified**

Q06　**Other congenital malformations of spinal cord**

Q06.0　**Amyelia**

Q06.1　**Hypoplasia and dysplasia of spinal cord**

　　　 Atelomyelia

　　　 Myelatelia

　　　 Myelodysplasia of spinal cord

Q06.2　**Diastematomyelia**

Q06.3　**Other congenital cauda equina malformations**

Q06.4　**Hydromyelia**

　　　 Hydrorachis

Q06.8　**Other specified congenital malformations of spinal cord**

Q06.9　**Congenital malformation of spinal cord, unspecified**

　　　 Congenital anomaly NOS of spinal cord

　　　 Congenital deformity NOS of spinal cord

　　　 Congenital disease or lesion NOS of spinal cord

Q07　**Other congenital malformations of nervous system**

　　　Excludes2: congenital central alveolar hypoventilation syndrome (G47.35)

　　　 familial dysautonomia [Riley-Day] (G90.1)

　　　 neurofibromatosis (nonmalignant) (Q85.0-)

Q07.0　**Arnold-Chiari syndrome**

　　　 Arnold-Chiari syndrome, type II

　　　Excludes1: Arnold-Chiari syndrome, type III (Q01.-)

　　　　　 Arnold-Chiari syndrome, type IV (Q04.8)

　　Q07.00　**Arnold-Chiari syndrome without spina bifida or hydrocephalus**

　　Q07.01　**Arnold-Chiari syndrome with spina bifida**

　　Q07.02　**Arnold-Chiari syndrome with hydrocephalus**

　　Q07.03　**Arnold-Chiari syndrome with spina bifida and hydrocephalus**

Q07.8　**Other specified congenital malformations of nervous system**

　　　 Agenesis of nerve

　　　 Displacement of brachial plexus Jaw-winking syndrome

　　　 Marcus Gunn's syndrome

Q07.9　**Congenital malformation of nervous system, unspecified**

　　　 Congenital anomaly NOS of nervous system

　　　 Congenital deformity NOS of nervous system

Congenital disease or lesion NOS of nervous system

CONGENITAL MALFORMATIONS OF EYE, EAR, FACE AND NECK (Q10-Q18)

Excludes2: cleft lip and cleft palate (Q35-Q37)

　　　 congenital malformation of cervical spine (Q05.0, Q05.5, Q67.5, Q76.0-Q76.4)

　　　 congenital malformation of larynx (Q31.-)

　　　 congenital malformation of lip NEC (Q38.0)

　　　 congenital malformation of nose (Q30.-)

　　　 congenital malformation of parathyroid gland (Q89.2)

　　　 congenital malformation of thyroid gland (Q89.2)

Q10　**Congenital malformations of eyelid, lacrimal apparatus and orbit**

　　　Excludes1: cryptophthalmos NOS (Q11.2)

　　　　　 cryptophthalmos syndrome (Q87.0)

Q10.0　**Congenital ptosis**

Q10.1　**Congenital ectropion**

Q10.2　**Congenital entropion**

Q10.3　**Other congenital malformations of eyelid**

　　　 Ablepharon

　　　 Blepharophimosis, congenital

　　　 Coloboma of eyelid

　　　 Congenital absence or agenesis of cilia

　　　 Congenital absence or agenesis of eyelid

　　　 Congenital accessory eyelid

　　　 Congenital accessory eye muscle

　　　 Congenital malformation of eyelid NOS

Q10.4　**Absence and agenesis of lacrimal apparatus**

　　　 Congenital absence of punctum lacrimale

Q10.5　**Congenital stenosis and stricture of lacrimal duct**

Q10.6　**Other congenital malformations of lacrimal apparatus**

　　　 Congenital malformation of lacrimal apparatus NOS

Q10.7　**Congenital malformation of orbit**

Q11　**Anophthalmos, microphthalmos and macrophthalmos**

Q11.0　**Cystic eyeball**

Q11.1　**Other anophthalmos**

　　　 Anophthalmos NOS

　　　 Agenesis of eye

　　　 Aplasia of eye

Q11.2　**Microphthalmos**

　　　 Cryptophthalmos NOS

　　　 Dysplasia of eye

　　　 Hypoplasia of eye

　　　 Rudimentary eye

　　　Excludes1: cryptophthalmos syndrome (Q87.0)

Q11.3　**Macrophthalmos**

　　　Excludes1: macrophthalmos in congenital glaucoma (Q15.0)

Q12　**Congenital lens malformations**

Q12.0　**Congenital cataract**

Q12.1　**Congenital displaced lens**

Q12.2　**Coloboma of lens**

Q12.3　**Congenital aphakia**

Q12.4　**Spherophakia**

Q12.8　**Other congenital lens malformations**

　　　 Microphakia

Q12.9 **Congenital lens malformation, unspecified**

Q13 **Congenital malformations of anterior segment of eye**

Q13.0 **Coloboma of iris**

Coloboma NOS

Q13.1 **Absence of iris**

Aniridia

<u>Use additional code</u> for associated glaucoma (H42)

Q13.2 **Other congenital malformations of iris**

Anisocoria, congenital

Atresia of pupil

Congenital malformation of iris NOS

Corectopia

Q13.3 **Congenital corneal opacity**

Q13.4 **Other congenital corneal malformations**

Congenital malformation of cornea NOS

Microcornea

Peter's anomaly

Q13.5 **Blue sclera**

Q13.8 **Other congenital malformations of anterior segment of eye**

Q13.81 **Rieger's anomaly**

<u>Use additional code</u> for associated glaucoma (H42)

Q13.89 **Other congenital malformations of anterior segment of eye**

Q13.9 **Congenital malformation of anterior segment of eye, unspecified**

Q14 **Congenital malformations of posterior segment of eye**

Excludes2: optic nerve hypoplasia (H47.03-)

Q14.0 **Congenital malformation of vitreous humor**

Congenital vitreous opacity

Q14.1 **Congenital malformation of retina**

Congenital retinal aneurysm

Q14.2 **Congenital malformation of optic disc**

Coloboma of optic disc

Q14.3 **Congenital malformation of choroid**

Q14.8 **Other congenital malformations of posterior segment of eye**

Coloboma of the fundus

Q14.9 **Congenital malformation of posterior segment of eye, unspecified**

Q15 **Other congenital malformations of eye**

Excludes1: congenital nystagmus (H55.01)

ocular albinism (E70.31-)

optic nerve hypoplasia (H47.03-)

retinitis pigmentosa (H35.52)

Q15.0 **Congenital glaucoma**

Axenfeld's anomaly

Buphthalmos Glaucoma of childhood Glaucoma of newborn Hydrophthalmos

Keratoglobus, congenital, with glaucoma

Macrocornea with glaucoma

Macrophthalmos in congenital glaucoma

Megalocornea with glaucoma

Q15.8 **Other specified congenital malformations of eye**

Q15.9 **Congenital malformation of eye, unspecified**

Congenital anomaly of eye

Congenital deformity of eye

Q16 **Congenital malformations of ear causing impairment of hearing**

Excludes1: congenital deafness (H90.-)

Q16.0 **Congenital absence of (ear) auricle**

Q16.1 **Congenital absence, atresia and stricture of auditory canal (external)**

Congenital atresia or stricture of osseous meatus

Q16.2 **Absence of eustachian tube**

Q16.3 **Congenital malformation of ear ossicles**

Congenital fusion of ear ossicles

Q16.4 **Other congenital malformations of middle ear**

Congenital malformation of middle ear NOS

Q16.5 **Congenital malformation of inner ear**

Congenital anomaly of membranous labyrinth

Congenital anomaly of organ of Corti

Q16.9 **Congenital malformation of ear causing impairment of hearing, unspecified**

Congenital absence of ear NOS

Q17 **Other congenital malformations of ear**

Excludes1: congenital malformations of ear with impairment of hearing (Q16.0-Q16.9)

preauricular sinus (Q18.1)

Q17.0 **Accessory auricle**

Accessory tragus

Polyotia

Preauricular appendage or tag

Supernumerary ear

Supernumerary lobule

Q17.1 **Macrotia**

Q17.2 **Microtia**

Q17.3 **Other misshapen ear**

Pointed ear

Q17.4 **Misplaced ear**

Low-set ears

Excludes1: cervical auricle (Q18.2)

Q17.5 **Prominent ear**

Bat ear

Q17.8 **Other specified congenital malformations of ear**

Congenital absence of lobe of ear

Q17.9 **Congenital malformation of ear, unspecified**

Congenital anomaly of ear NOS

Q18 **Other congenital malformations of face and neck**

Excludes1: cleft lip and cleft palate (Q35-Q37)

conditions classified to Q67.0-Q67.4

congenital malformations of skull and face bones (Q75.-)

cyclopia (Q87.0)

dentofacial anomalies [including malocclusion] (M26.-)

malformation syndromes affecting facial appearance (Q87.0)

persistent thyroglossal duct (Q89.2)

Q18.0 **Sinus, fistula and cyst of branchial cleft** Branchial vestige

Q18.1 **Preauricular sinus and cyst**

Fistula of auricle, congenital

Cervicoaural fistula

Q18.2 **Other branchial cleft malformations**

Branchial cleft malformation NOS

Cervical auricle

Otocephaly

Q18.3 **Webbing of neck**

Pterygium colli

Q18.4 **Macrostomia**

Q18.5 **Microstomia**

Q18.6 **Macrocheilia**

Hypertrophy of lip, congenital

Q18.7 **Microcheilia**

Q18.8 **Other specified congenital malformations of face and neck**

Medial cyst of face and neck

Medial fistula of face and neck

Medial sinus of face and neck

Q18.9 **Congenital malformation of face and neck, unspecified**

Congenital anomaly NOS of face and neck

CONGENITAL MALFORMATIONS OF THE CIRCULATORY SYSTEM (Q20-Q28)

Q20 **Congenital malformations of cardiac chambers and connections**

Excludes1: dextrocardia with situs inversus (Q89.3)

mirror-image atrial arrangement with situs inversus (Q89.3)

Q20.0 **Common arterial trunk**

Persistent truncus arteriosus

Excludes1: aortic septal defect (Q21.4)

Q20.1 **Double outlet right ventricle**

Taussig-Bing syndrome

Q20.2 **Double outlet left ventricle**

Q20.3 **Discordant ventriculoarterial connection**

Dextrotransposition of aorta

Transposition of great vessels (complete)

Q20.4 **Double inlet ventricle**

Common ventricle

Cor triloculare biatriatum

Single ventricle

Q20.5 **Discordant atrioventricular connection**

Corrected transposition

Levotransposition

Ventricular inversion

Q20.6 **Isomerism of atrial appendages**

Isomerism of atrial appendages with asplenia or polysplenia

Q20.8 **Other congenital malformations of cardiac chambers and connections**

Cor binoculare

Q20.9 **Congenital malformation of cardiac chambers and connections, unspecified**

Q21 **Congenital malformations of cardiac septa**

Excludes1: acquired cardiac septal defect (I51.0)

Q21.0 **Ventricular septal defect**

Roger's disease

Q21.1 **Atrial septal defect**

Coronary sinus defect

Patent or persistent foramen ovale

Patent or persistent ostium secundum defect (type II)

Patent or persistent sinus venosus defect

Q21.2 **Atrioventricular septal defect**

Common atrioventricular canal

Endocardial cushion defect

Ostium primum atrial septal defect (type I)

Q21.3 **Tetralogy of Fallot**

Definition: Tetralogy of Fallot, which is one of the most common congenital heart disorders, comprises right ventricular (RV) outflow tract obstruction (RVOTO) (infundibular stenosis), ventricular septal defect (VSD), aorta dextroposition, and RV hypertrophy.

Ventricular septal defect with pulmonary stenosis or atresia, dextroposition of aorta and hypertrophy of right ventricle.

Q21.4 **Aortopulmonary septal defect**

Aortic septal defect

Aortopulmonary window

Q21.8 **Other congenital malformations of cardiac septa**

Eisenmenger's defect

Pentalogy of Fallot

Code also if applicable:

Eisenmenger's complex (I27.83)

Eisenmenger's syndrome (I27.83)

Q21.9 **Congenital malformation of cardiac septum, unspecified**

Septal (heart) defect NOS

Q22 **Congenital malformations of pulmonary and tricuspid valves**

Q22.0 **Pulmonary valve atresia**

Q22.1 **Congenital pulmonary valve stenosis**

Q22.2 **Congenital pulmonary valve insufficiency**

Congenital pulmonary valve regurgitation

Q22.3 **Other congenital malformations of pulmonary valve**

Congenital malformation of pulmonary valve NOS

Supernumerary cusps of pulmonary valve

Q22.4 **Congenital tricuspid stenosis**

Congenital tricuspid atresia

Q22.5 **Ebstein's anomaly**

Q22.6 **Hypoplastic right heart syndrome**

Q22.8 **Other congenital malformations of tricuspid valve**

Q22.9 **Congenital malformation of tricuspid valve, unspecified**

Q23 **Congenital malformations of aortic and mitral valves**

Q23.0 **Congenital stenosis of aortic valve**

Congenital aortic atresia

Congenital aortic stenosis NOS

Excludes1: congenital stenosis of aortic valve in hypoplastic left heart syndrome (Q23.4)

congenital subaortic stenosis (Q24.4)

supravalvular aortic stenosis (congenital) (Q25.3)

Q23.1 **Congenital insufficiency of aortic valve**

Bicuspid aortic valve

Congenital aortic insufficiency

Q23.2 **Congenital mitral stenosis**

Congenital mitral atresia

Q23.3 **Congenital mitral insufficiency**

Q23.4 **Hypoplastic left heart syndrome**

Q23.8 **Other congenital malformations of aortic and mitral valves**

Q23.9 **Congenital malformation of aortic and mitral valves, unspecified**

● New code ▲ Revised code **Excludes1:** Not coded here **Excludes2:** Not included here ⊗ Placeholder required ⑦7th digit required

Q24 **Other congenital malformations of heart**

Excludes1: endocardial fibroelastosis (I42.4)

Q24.0 **Dextrocardia**

Excludes1: dextrocardia with situs inversus (Q89.3)

isomerism of atrial appendages (with asplenia or polysplenia) (Q20.6)

mirror-image atrial arrangement with situs inversus (Q89.3)

Q24.1 **Levocardia**

Q24.2 **Cor triatriatum**

Q24.3 **Pulmonary infundibular stenosis**

Subvalvular pulmonic stenosis

Q24.4 **Congenital subaortic stenosis**

Q24.5 **Malformation of coronary vessels**

Congenital coronary (artery) aneurysm

Q24.6 **Congenital heart block**

Q24.8 **Other specified congenital malformations of heart**

Congenital diverticulum of left ventricle

Congenital malformation of myocardium

Congenital malformation of pericardium

Malposition of heart

Uhl's disease

Q24.9 **Congenital malformation of heart, unspecified**

Congenital anomaly of heart

Congenital disease of heart

Q25 **Congenital malformations of great arteries**

Q25.0 **Patent ductus arteriosus**

Patent ductus

Botallo

Persistent ductus arteriosus

Q25.1 **Coarctation of aorta**

Coarctation of aorta (preductal) (postductal)

Stenosis of aorta

Q25.2 **Atresia of aorta**

Q25.21 **Interruption of aortic arch**

Atresia of aortic arch

Q25.29 **Other atresia of aorta**

Atresia of aorta

Q25.3 **Supravalvular aortic stenosis**

Excludes1: congenital aortic stenosis NOS (Q23.0)

congenital stenosis of aortic valve (Q23.0)

Q25.4 **Other congenital malformations of aorta**

Excludes1: hypoplasia of aorta in hypoplastic left heart syndrome (Q23.4)

Q25.40 **Congenital malformation of aorta unspecified**

Q25.41 **Absence and aplasia of aorta**

Q25.42 **Hypoplasia of aorta**

Q25.43 **Congenital aneurysm of aorta**

Congenital aneurysm of aortic root

Congenital aneurysm of aortic sinus

Q25.44 **Congenital dilation of aorta**

Q25.45 **Double aortic arch**

Vascular ring of aorta

Q25.46 **Tortuous aortic arch**

Persistent convolutions of aortic arch

Q25.47 **Right aortic arch**

Persistent right aortic arch

Q25.48 **Anomalous origin of subclavian artery**

Q25.49 **Other congenital malformations of aorta**

Aortic arch

Bovine arch

Q25.5 **Atresia of pulmonary artery**

Q25.6 **Stenosis of pulmonary artery**

Supravalvular pulmonary stenosis

Q25.7 **Other congenital malformations of pulmonary artery**

Q25.71 **Coarctation of pulmonary artery**

Q25.72 **Congenital pulmonary arteriovenous malformation**

Congenital pulmonary arteriovenous aneurysm

Q25.79 **Other congenital malformations of pulmonary artery**

Aberrant pulmonary artery

Agenesis of pulmonary artery

Congenital aneurysm of pulmonary artery

Congenital anomaly of pulmonary artery

Hypoplasia of pulmonary artery

Q25.8 **Other congenital malformations of other great arteries**

Q25.9 **Congenital malformation of great arteries, unspecified**

Q26 **Congenital malformations of great veins**

Q26.0 **Congenital stenosis of vena cava**

Congenital stenosis of vena cava (inferior)(superior)

Q26.1 **Persistent left superior vena cava**

Q26.2 **Total anomalous pulmonary venous connection**

Total anomalous pulmonary venous return [TAPVR], subdiaphragmatic

Total anomalous pulmonary venous return [TAPVR], supradiaphragmatic

Q26.3 **Partial anomalous pulmonary venous connection**

Partial anomalous pulmonary venous return

Q26.4 **Anomalous pulmonary venous connection, unspecified**

Q26.5 **Anomalous portal venous connection**

Q26.6 **Portal vein-hepatic artery fistula**

Q26.8 **Other congenital malformations of great veins**

Absence of vena cava (inferior) (superior)

Azygos continuation of inferior vena cava

Persistent left posterior cardinal vein

Scimitar syndrome

Q26.9 **Congenital malformation of great vein, unspecified**

Congenital anomaly of vena cava (inferior) (superior) NOS

Q27 **Other congenital malformations of peripheral vascular system**

Excludes2: anomalies of cerebral and precerebral vessels (Q28.0-Q28.3)

anomalies of coronary vessels (Q24.5)

anomalies of pulmonary artery (Q25.5-Q25.7)

congenital retinal aneurysm (Q14.1)

hemangioma and lymphangioma (D18.-)

Q27.0 **Congenital absence and hypoplasia of umbilical artery**

Single umbilical artery

Q27.1 **Congenital renal artery stenosis**

Q27.2 **Other congenital malformations of renal artery**

Congenital malformation of renal artery NOS

Multiple renal arteries

Q27.3 **Arteriovenous malformation (peripheral)**

Arteriovenous aneurysm

Excludes1: acquired arteriovenous aneurysm (I77.0)

Excludes2: arteriovenous malformation of cerebral vessels (Q28.2)

arteriovenous malformation of precerebral vessels (Q28.0)

Q27.30 **Arteriovenous malformation, site unspecified**

Q27.31 **Arteriovenous malformation of vessel of upper limb**

Q27.32 **Arteriovenous malformation of vessel of lower limb**

Q27.33 **Arteriovenous malformation of digestive system vessel**

Q27.34 **Arteriovenous malformation of renal vessel**

Q27.39 **Arteriovenous malformation, other site**

Q27.4 **Congenital phlebectasia**

Q27.8 **Other specified congenital malformations of peripheral vascular system**

Absence of peripheral vascular system

Atresia of peripheral vascular system

Congenital aneurysm (peripheral)

Congenital stricture, artery

Congenital varix

Excludes1: arteriovenous malformation (Q27.3-)

Q27.9 **Congenital malformation of peripheral vascular system, unspecified**

Anomaly of artery or vein NOS

Q28 **Other congenital malformations of circulatory system**

Excludes1: congenital aneurysm NOS (Q27.8)

congenital coronary aneurysm (Q24.5)

ruptured cerebral arteriovenous malformation (I60.8)

ruptured malformation of precerebral vessels (I72.0)

Excludes2: congenital peripheral aneurysm (Q27.8)

congenital pulmonary aneurysm (Q25.79)

congenital retinal aneurysm (Q14.1)

Q28.0 **Arteriovenous malformation of precerebral vessels**

Congenital arteriovenous precerebral aneurysm (nonruptured)

Q28.1 **Other malformations of precerebral vessels**

Congenital malformation of precerebral vessels NOS

Congenital precerebral aneurysm (nonruptured)

Q28.2 **Arteriovenous malformation of cerebral vessels**

Arteriovenous malformation of brain NOS

Congenital arteriovenous cerebral aneurysm (nonruptured)

Q28.3 **Other malformations of cerebral vessels**

Congenital cerebral aneurysm (nonruptured)

Congenital malformation of cerebral vessels NOS

Developmental venous anomaly

Q28.8 **Other specified congenital malformations of circulatory system**

Congenital aneurysm, specified site NEC

Spinal vessel anomaly

Q28.9 **Congenital malformation of circulatory system, unspecified**

CONGENITAL MALFORMATIONS OF THE RESPIRATORY SYSTEM (Q30-Q34)

Q30 **Congenital malformations of nose**

Excludes1: congenital deviation of nasal septum (Q67.4)

Q30.0 **Choanal atresia**

Atresia of nares (anterior) (posterior)

Congenital stenosis of nares (anterior) (posterior)

Q30.1 **Agenesis and underdevelopment of nose**

Congenital absent of nose

Q30.2 **Fissured, notched and cleft nose**

Q30.3 **Congenital perforated nasal septum**

Q30.8 **Other congenital malformations of nose**

Accessory nose

Congenital anomaly of nasal sinus wall

Q30.9 **Congenital malformation of nose, unspecified**

Q31 **Congenital malformations of larynx**

Excludes1: congenital laryngeal stridor NOS (P28.89)

Q31.0 **Web of larynx**

Glottic web of larynx

Subglottic web of larynx

Web of larynx NOS

Q31.1 **Congenital subglottic stenosis**

Q31.2 **Laryngeal hypoplasia**

Q31.3 **Laryngocele**

Q31.5 **Congenital laryngomalacia**

Q31.8 **Other congenital malformations of larynx**

Absence of larynx

Agenesis of larynx

Atresia of larynx

Congenital cleft thyroid cartilage

Congenital fissure of epiglottis

Congenital stenosis of larynx NEC

Posterior cleft of cricoid cartilage

Q31.9 **Congenital malformation of larynx, unspecified**

Q32 **Congenital malformations of trachea and bronchus**

Excludes1: congenital bronchiectasis (Q33.4)

Q32.0 **Congenital tracheomalacia**

Q32.1 **Other congenital malformations of trachea**

Atresia of trachea

Congenital anomaly of tracheal cartilage

Congenital dilatation of trachea

Congenital malformation of trachea

Congenital stenosis of trachea

Congenital tracheocele

Q32.2 **Congenital bronchomalacia**

Q32.3 **Congenital stenosis of bronchus**

Q32.4 **Other congenital malformations of bronchus**

Absence of bronchus

Agenesis of bronchus

Atresia of bronchus

Congenital diverticulum of bronchus

Congenital malformation of bronchus NOS

Q33 **Congenital malformations of lung**

Q33.0 **Congenital cystic lung**

Congenital cystic lung disease

Congenital honeycomb lung

Congenital polycystic lung disease

Excludes1: cystic fibrosis (E84.0)

cystic lung disease, acquired or unspecified (J98.4)

Q33.1 **Accessory lobe of lung**

● New code ▲ Revised code **Excludes1:** Not coded here **Excludes2:** Not included here ⊗ Placeholder required ⑦7th digit required

Azygos lobe (fissured), lung

Q33.2 **Sequestration of lung**

Q33.3 **Agenesis of lung**

Congenital absence of lung (lobe)

Q33.4 **Congenital bronchiectasis**

Q33.5 **Ectopic tissue in lung**

Q33.6 **Congenital hypoplasia and dysplasia of lung**

Excludes1: pulmonary hypoplasia associated with short gestation (P28.0)

Q33.8 **Other congenital malformations of lung**

Q33.9 **Congenital malformation of lung, unspecified**

Q34 **Other congenital malformations of respiratory system**

Excludes2: congenital central alveolar hypoventilation syndrome (G47.35)

Q34.0 **Anomaly of pleura**

Q34.1 **Congenital cyst of mediastinum**

Q34.8 **Other specified congenital malformations of respiratory system**

Atresia of nasopharynx

Q34.9 **Congenital malformation of respiratory system, unspecified**

Congenital absence of respiratory system

Congenital anomaly of respiratory system NOS

CLEFT LIP AND CLEFT PALATE (Q35-Q37)

Definition: Cleft lip is a congenital deformity characterized by a vertical cleft or pair of clefts in the upper lip, with or without involvement of the palate. Cleft palate is a congenital fissure in the roof of the mouth, resulting from incomplete fusion of the palate during embryonic development.

Use additional code to identify associated malformation of the nose (Q30.2)

Excludes1: Robin's syndrome (Q87.0)

Q35 **Cleft palate**

Includes: fissure of palate

palatoschisis

Excludes1: cleft palate with cleft lip (Q37.-)

Q35.1 **Cleft hard palate**

Q35.3 **Cleft soft palate**

Q35.5 **Cleft hard palate with cleft soft palate**

Q35.7 **Cleft uvula**

Q35.9 **Cleft palate, unspecified**

Cleft palate NOS

Q36 **Cleft lip**

Includes: cheiloschisis

congenital fissure of lip harelip

labium leporinum

Excludes1: cleft lip with cleft palate (Q37.-)

Q36.0 **Cleft lip, bilateral**

Q36.1 **Cleft lip, median**

Q36.9 **Cleft lip, unilateral**

Cleft lip NOS

Q37 **Cleft palate with cleft lip**

Includes: cheilopalatoschisis

Q37.0 **Cleft hard palate with bilateral cleft lip**

Q37.1 **Cleft hard palate with unilateral cleft lip**

Cleft hard palate with cleft lip NOS

Q37.2 **Cleft soft palate with bilateral cleft lip**

Q37.3 **Cleft soft palate with unilateral cleft lip**

Cleft soft palate with cleft lip NOS

Q37.4 **Cleft hard and soft palate with bilateral cleft lip**

Q37.5 **Cleft hard and soft palate with unilateral cleft lip**

Cleft hard and soft palate with cleft lip NOS

Q37.8 **Unspecified cleft palate with bilateral cleft lip**

Q37.9 **Unspecified cleft palate with unilateral cleft lip**

Cleft palate with cleft lip NOS

OTHER CONGENITAL MALFORMATIONS OF THE DIGESTIVE SYSTEM (Q38-Q45)

Q38 **Other congenital malformations of tongue, mouth and pharynx**

Excludes1: dentofacial anomalies (M26.-)

macrostomia (Q18.4) microstomia (Q18.5)

Q38.0 **Congenital malformations of lips, not elsewhere classified**

Congenital fistula of lip

Congenital malformation of lip NOS

Van der Woude's syndrome

Excludes1: cleft lip (Q36.-)

cleft lip with cleft palate (Q37.-)

macrocheilia (Q18.6)

microcheilia (Q18.7)

Q38.1 **Ankyloglossia**

Tongue tie

Q38.2 **Macroglossia**

Congenital hypertrophy of tongue

Q38.3 **Other congenital malformations of tongue**

Aglossia

Bifid tongue

Congenital adhesion of tongue

Congenital fissure of tongue

Congenital malformation of tongue NOS

Double tongue

Hypoglossia

Hypoplasia of tongue

Microglossia

Q38.4 **Congenital malformations of salivary glands and ducts**

Atresia of salivary glands and ducts

Congenital absence of salivary glands and ducts

Congenital accessory salivary glands and ducts

Congenital fistula of salivary gland

Q38.5 **Congenital malformations of palate, not elsewhere classified**

Congenital absence of uvula

Congenital malformation of palate NOS

Congenital high arched palate

Excludes1: cleft palate (Q35.-)

cleft palate with cleft lip (Q37.-)

Q38.6 **Other congenital malformations of mouth**

Congenital malformation of mouth NOS

Q38.7 **Congenital pharyngeal pouch**

Congenital diverticulum of pharynx

Excludes1: pharyngeal pouch syndrome (D82.1)

Q38.8 **Other congenital malformations of pharynx**

Congenital malformation of pharynx NOS

Imperforate pharynx

Q39 **Congenital malformations of esophagus**

Q39.0 **Atresia of esophagus without fistula**

Atresia of esophagus NOS

Q39.1 **Atresia of esophagus with tracheo-esophageal fistula**

Atresia of esophagus with broncho-esophageal fistula

Q39.2 **Congenital tracheo-esophageal fistula without atresia**

Congenital tracheo-esophageal fistula NOS

Q39.3 **Congenital stenosis and stricture of esophagus**

Q39.4 **Esophageal web**

Q39.5 **Congenital dilatation of esophagus**

Congenital cardiospasm

Q39.6 **Congenital diverticulum of esophagus**

Congenital esophageal pouch

Q39.8 **Other congenital malformations of esophagus**

Congenital absence of esophagus

Congenital displacement of esophagus

Congenital duplication of esophagus

Q39.9 **Congenital malformation of esophagus, unspecified**

Q40 **Other congenital malformations of upper alimentary tract**

Q40.0 **Congenital hypertrophic pyloric stenosis**

Congenital or infantile constriction

Congenital or infantile hypertrophy

Congenital or infantile spasm

Congenital or infantile stenosis

Congenital or infantile stricture

Q40.1 **Congenital hiatus hernia**

Congenital displacement of cardia through esophageal hiatus

Excludes1: congenital diaphragmatic hernia (Q79.0)

Q40.2 **Other specified congenital malformations of stomach**

Congenital displacement of stomach

Congenital diverticulum of stomach

Congenital hourglass stomach

Congenital duplication of stomach

Megalogastria

Microgastria

Q40.3 **Congenital malformation of stomach, unspecified**

Q40.8 **Other specified congenital malformations of upper alimentary tract**

Q40.9 **Congenital malformation of upper alimentary tract, unspecified**

Congenital anomaly of upper alimentary tract

Congenital deformity of upper alimentary tract

Q41 **Congenital absence, atresia and stenosis of small intestine**

Includes: congenital obstruction, occlusion or stricture of small intestine or intestine NOS

Excludes1: cystic fibrosis with intestinal manifestation (E84.11)

meconium ileus NOS (without cystic fibrosis) (P76.0)

Q41.0 **Congenital absence, atresia and stenosis of duodenum**

Q41.1 **Congenital absence, atresia and stenosis of jejunum**

Apple peel syndrome

Imperforate jejunum

Q41.2 **Congenital absence, atresia and stenosis of ileum**

Q41.8 **Congenital absence, atresia and stenosis of other specified parts of small intestine**

Q41.9 **Congenital absence, atresia and stenosis of small intestine, part unspecified**

Congenital absence, atresia and stenosis of intestine NOS

Q42 **Congenital absence, atresia and stenosis of large intestine**

Includes: congenital obstruction, occlusion and stricture of large intestine

Q42.0 **Congenital absence, atresia and stenosis of rectum with fistula**

Q42.1 **Congenital absence, atresia and stenosis of rectum without fistula**

Imperforate rectum

Q42.2 **Congenital absence, atresia and stenosis of anus with fistula**

Q42.3 **Congenital absence, atresia and stenosis of anus without fistula**

Imperforate anus

Q42.8 **Congenital absence, atresia and stenosis of other parts of large intestine**

Q42.9 **Congenital absence, atresia and stenosis of large intestine, part unspecified**

Q43 **Other congenital malformations of intestine**

Q43.0 **Meckel's diverticulum (displaced) (hypertrophic)**

Persistent omphalomesenteric duct

Persistent vitelline duct

Q43.1 **Hirschsprung's disease**

Aganglionosis

Congenital (aganglionic) megacolon

Q43.2 **Other congenital functional disorders of colon**

Congenital dilatation of colon

Q43.3 **Congenital malformations of intestinal fixation**

Congenital omental, anomalous adhesions [bands]

Congenital peritoneal adhesions [bands]

Incomplete rotation of cecum and colon

Insufficient rotation of cecum and colon

Jackson's membrane

Malrotation of colon

Rotation failure of cecum and colon

Universal mesentery

Q43.4 **Duplication of intestine**

Q43.5 **Ectopic anus**

Q43.6 **Congenital fistula of rectum and anus**

Excludes1: congenital fistula of anus with absence, atresia and stenosis (Q42.2)

congenital fistula of rectum with absence, atresia and stenosis (Q42.0)

congenital rectovaginal fistula (Q52.2)

congenital urethrorectal fistula (Q64.73)

pilonidal fistula or sinus (L05.-)

Q43.7 **Persistent cloaca**

Cloaca NOS

Q43.8 **Other specified congenital malformations of intestine**

Congenital blind loop syndrome

Congenital diverticulitis, colon

Congenital diverticulum, intestine

Dolichocolon

Megaloappendix

Megaloduodenum

Microcolon

Transposition of appendix

Transposition of colon

Transposition of intestine

● New code ▲ Revised code **Excludes1:** Not coded here **Excludes2:** Not included here ⊗ Placeholder required ⑦7th digit required

Q43.9 Congenital malformation of intestine, unspecified

Q44 Congenital malformations of gallbladder, bile ducts and liver

Q44.0 Agenesis, aplasia and hypoplasia of gallbladder

Congenital absence of gallbladder

Q44.1 Other congenital malformations of gallbladder

Congenital malformation of gallbladder NOS

Intrahepatic gallbladder

Q44.2 Atresia of bile ducts

Q44.3 Congenital stenosis and stricture of bile ducts

Q44.4 Choledochal cyst

Q44.5 Other congenital malformations of bile ducts

Accessory hepatic duct

Biliary duct duplication

Congenital malformation of bile duct NOS

Cystic duct duplication

Q44.6 Cystic disease of liver

Fibrocystic disease of liver

Q44.7 Other congenital malformations of liver

Accessory liver

Alagille's syndrome

Congenital absence of liver

Congenital hepatomegaly

Congenital malformation of liver NOS

Q45 Other congenital malformations of digestive system

Excludes2: congenital diaphragmatic hernia (Q79.0)

congenital hiatus hernia (Q40.1)

Q45.0 Agenesis, aplasia and hypoplasia of pancreas

Congenital absence of pancreas

Q45.1 Annular pancreas

Q45.2 Congenital pancreatic cyst

Q45.3 Other congenital malformations of pancreas and pancreatic duct

Accessory pancreas

Congenital malformation of pancreas or pancreatic duct NOS

Excludes1: congenital diabetes mellitus (E10.-)

cystic fibrosis (E84.0-E84.9)

fibrocystic disease of pancreas (E84.-)

neonatal diabetes mellitus (P70.2)

Q45.8 Other specified congenital malformations of digestive system

Absence (complete) (partial) of alimentary tract NOS

Duplication of digestive system

Malposition, congenital of digestive system

Q45.9 Congenital malformation of digestive system, unspecified

Congenital anomaly of digestive system

Congenital deformity of digestive system

CONGENITAL MALFORMATIONS OF GENITAL ORGANS (Q50-Q56)

Excludes1: androgen insensitivity syndrome (E34.5-)

syndromes associated with anomalies in the number and form of chromosomes (Q90-Q99)

Q50 Congenital malformations of ovaries, fallopian tubes and broad ligaments

Q50.0 Congenital absence of ovary

Excludes1: Turner's syndrome (Q96.-)

Q50.01 Congenital absence of ovary, unilateral

Q50.02 Congenital absence of ovary, bilateral

Q50.1 Developmental ovarian cyst

Q50.2 Congenital torsion of ovary

Q50.3 Other congenital malformations of ovary

Q50.31 Accessory ovary

Q50.32 Ovarian streak

46, XX with streak gonads

Q50.39 Other congenital malformation of ovary

Congenital malformation of ovary NOS

Q50.4 Embryonic cyst of fallopian tube

Fimbrial cyst

Q50.5 Embryonic cyst of broad ligament

Epoophoron cyst

Parovarian cyst

Q50.6 Other congenital malformations of fallopian tube and broad ligament

Absence of fallopian tube and broad ligament

Accessory fallopian tube and broad ligament

Atresia of fallopian tube and broad ligament

Congenital malformation of fallopian tube or broad ligament NOS

Q51 Congenital malformations of uterus and cervix

Q51.0 Agenesis and aplasia of uterus

Congenital absence of uterus

Q51.1 Doubling of uterus with doubling of cervix and vagina

Q51.10 Doubling of uterus with doubling of cervix and vagina without obstruction

Doubling of uterus with doubling of cervix and vagina NOS

Q51.11 Doubling of uterus with doubling of cervix and vagina with obstruction

Q51.2 Other doubling of uterus

Doubling of uterus NOS

Septate uterus, complete or partial

Q51.3 Bicornate uterus

Bicornate uterus, complete or partial

Q51.4 Unicornate uterus

Unicornate uterus with or without a separate uterine horn

Uterus with only one functioning horn

Q51.5 Agenesis and aplasia of cervix

Congenital absence of cervix

Q51.6 Embryonic cyst of cervix

Q51.7 Congenital fistulae between uterus and digestive and urinary tracts

Q51.8 Other congenital malformations of uterus and cervix

Q51.81 Other congenital malformations of uterus

Q51.810 Arcuate uterus

Arcuatus uterus

Q51.811 Hypoplasia of uterus

Q51.818 Other congenital malformations of uterus

Müllerian anomaly of uterus NEC

Q51.82 Other congenital malformations of cervix

Q51.820 Cervical duplication

Q51.821 Hypoplasia of cervix

Q51.828 Other congenital malformations of cervix

Q51.9 **Congenital malformation of uterus and cervix, unspecified**

Q52 **Other congenital malformations of female genitalia**

Q52.0 **Congenital absence of vagina**

Vaginal agenesis, total or partial

Q52.1 **Doubling of vagina**

Excludes1: doubling of vagina with doubling of uterus and cervix (Q51.1-)

Q52.10 **Doubling of vagina, unspecified**

Septate vagina NOS

Q52.11 **Transverse vaginal septum**

Q52.12 **Longitudinal vaginal septum**

Q52.120 **Longitudinal vaginal septum, nonobstructing**

Q52.121 **Longitudinal vaginal septum, obstructing, right side**

Q52.122 **Longitudinal vaginal septum, obstructing, left side**

Q52.123 **Longitudinal vaginal septum, microperforate, right side**

Q52.124 **Longitudinal vaginal septum, microperforate, left side**

Q52.129 **Other and unspecified longitudinal vaginal septum**

Q52.2 **Congenital rectovaginal fistula**

Excludes1: cloaca (Q43.7)

Q52.3 **Imperforate hymen**

Q52.4 **Other congenital malformations of vagina**

Canal of Nuck cyst, congenital

Congenital malformation of vagina NOS

Embryonic vaginal cyst

Gartner's duct cyst

Q52.5 **Fusion of labia**

Q52.6 **Congenital malformation of clitoris**

Q52.7 **Other and unspecified congenital malformations of vulva**

Q52.70 **Unspecified congenital malformations of vulva**

Congenital malformation of vulva NOS

Q52.71 **Congenital absence of vulva**

Q52.79 **Other congenital malformations of vulva**

Congenital cyst of vulva

Q52.8 **Other specified congenital malformations of female genitalia**

Q52.9 **Congenital malformation of female genitalia, unspecified**

Q53 **Undescended and ectopic testicle**

Q53.0 **Ectopic testis**

Q53.00 **Ectopic testis, unspecified**

Q53.01 **Ectopic testis, unilateral**

Q53.02 **Ectopic testes, bilateral**

Q53.1 **Undescended testicle, unilateral**

Q53.10 **Unspecified undescended testicle, unilateral**

Q53.11 **Abdominal testis, unilateral**

●Q53.111 **Unilateral intraabdominal testis**

●Q53.112 **Unilateral inguinal testis**

Q53.12 **Ectopic perineal testis, unilateral**

●Q53.13 **Unilateral high scrotal testis**

Q53.2 **Undescended testicle, bilateral**

Q53.20 **Undescended testicle, unspecified, bilateral**

Q53.21 **Abdominal testis, bilateral**

●Q53.211 **Bilateral intraabdominal testes**

●Q53.212 **Bilateral inguinal testes**

Q53.22 **Ectopic perineal testis, bilateral**

●Q53.23 **Bilateral high scrotal testes**

Q53.9 **Undescended testicle, unspecified**

Cryptorchism NOS

Q54 **Hypospadias**

Excludes1: epispadias (Q64.0)

Q54.0 **Hypospadias, balanic**

Hypospadias, coronal

Hypospadias, glandular

Q54.1 **Hypospadias, penile**

Q54.2 **Hypospadias, penoscrotal**

Q54.3 **Hypospadias, perineal**

Q54.4 **Congenital chordee**

Chordee without hypospadias

Q54.8 **Other hypospadias**

Hypospadias with intersex state

Q54.9 **Hypospadias, unspecified**

Q55 **Other congenital malformations of male genital organs**

Excludes1: congenital hydrocele (P83.5)

hypospadias (Q54.-)

Q55.0 **Absence and aplasia of testis**

Monorchism

Q55.1 **Hypoplasia of testis and scrotum**

Fusion of testes

Q55.2 **Other and unspecified congenital malformations of testis and scrotum**

Q55.20 **Unspecified congenital malformations of testis and scrotum**

Congenital malformation of testis or scrotum NOS

Q55.21 **Polyorchism**

Q55.22 **Retractile testis**

Q55.23 **Scrotal transposition**

Q55.29 **Other congenital malformations of testis and scrotum**

Q55.3 **Atresia of vas deferens**

Code first any associated cystic fibrosis (E84.-)

Q55.4 **Other congenital malformations of vas deferens, epididymis, seminal vesicles and prostate**

Absence or aplasia of prostate

Absence or aplasia of spermatic cord

Congenital malformation of vas deferens, epididymis, seminal vesicles or prostate NOS

Q55.5 **Congenital absence and aplasia of penis**

Q55.6 **Other congenital malformations of penis**

Q55.61 **Curvature of penis (lateral)**

Q55.62 **Hypoplasia of penis**

Micropenis

Q55.63 **Congenital torsion of penis**

Excludes1: acquired torsion of penis (N48.82)

Q55.64 **Hidden penis**

Buried penis

Concealed penis

Excludes1: acquired buried penis (N48.83)

● New code ▲ Revised code **Excludes1:** Not coded here **Excludes2:** Not included here ⊗ Placeholder required ⑦7th digit required

Q55.69 Other congenital malformation of penis

Congenital malformation of penis NOS

Q55.7 Congenital vasocutaneous fistula

Q55.8 Other specified congenital malformations of male genital organs

Q55.9 Congenital malformation of male genital organ, unspecified

Congenital anomaly of male genital organ

Congenital deformity of male genital organ

Q56 Indeterminate sex and pseudohermaphroditism

Excludes1: 46,XX true hermaphrodite (Q99.1)

androgen insensitivity syndrome (E34.5-)

chimera 46,XX/46,XY true hermaphrodite (Q99.0)

female pseudohermaphroditism with adrenocortical disorder (E25.-)

pseudohermaphroditism with specified chromosomal anomaly (Q96-Q99)

pure gonadal dysgenesis (Q99.1)

Q56.0 Hermaphroditism, not elsewhere classified

Ovotestis

Q56.1 Male pseudohermaphroditism, not elsewhere classified

46, XY with streak gonads

Male pseudohermaphroditism NOS

Q56.2 Female pseudohermaphroditism, not elsewhere classified

Female pseudohermaphroditism NOS

Q56.3 Pseudohermaphroditism, unspecified

Q56.4 Indeterminate sex, unspecified

Ambiguous genitalia

CONGENITAL MALFORMATIONS OF THE URINARY SYSTEM (Q60-Q64)

Q60 Renal agenesis and other reduction defects of kidney

Includes: congenital absence of kidney

congenital atrophy of kidney infantile atrophy of kidney

Q60.0 Renal agenesis, unilateral

Q60.1 Renal agenesis, bilateral

Q60.2 Renal agenesis, unspecified

Q60.3 Renal hypoplasia, unilateral

Q60.4 Renal hypoplasia, bilateral

Q60.5 Renal hypoplasia, unspecified

Q60.6 Potter's syndrome

Q61 Cystic kidney disease

Excludes1: acquired cyst of kidney (N28.1)

Potter's syndrome (Q60.6)

Q61.0 Congenital renal cyst

Q61.00 Congenital renal cyst, unspecified

Cyst of kidney NOS (congenital)

Q61.01 Congenital single renal cyst

Q61.02 Congenital multiple renal cysts

Q61.1 Polycystic kidney, infantile type

Polycystic kidney, autosomal recessive

Q61.11 Cystic dilatation of collecting ducts

Q61.19 Other polycystic kidney, infantile type

Q61.2 Polycystic kidney, adult type

Polycystic kidney, autosomal dominant

Q61.3 Polycystic kidney, unspecified

Q61.4 Renal dysplasia

Multicystic dysplastic kidney

Multicystic kidney (development)

Multicystic kidney disease

Multicystic renal dysplasia

Excludes1: polycystic kidney disease (Q61.11-Q61.3)

Q61.5 Medullary cystic kidney

Nephronophthisis

Sponge kidney NOS

Q61.8 Other cystic kidney diseases

Fibrocystic kidney

Fibrocystic renal degeneration or disease

Q61.9 Cystic kidney disease, unspecified

Meckel-Gruber syndrome

Q62 Congenital obstructive defects of renal pelvis and congenital malformations of ureter

Q62.0 Congenital hydronephrosis

Q62.1 Congenital occlusion of ureter

Atresia and stenosis of ureter

Q62.10 Congenital occlusion of ureter, unspecified

Q62.11 Congenital occlusion of ureteropelvic junction

Q62.12 Congenital occlusion of ureterovesical orifice

Q62.2 Congenital megaureter

Congenital dilatation of ureter

Q62.3 Other obstructive defects of renal pelvis and ureter

Q62.31 Congenital ureterocele, orthotopic

Q62.32 Cecoureterocele

Ectopic ureterocele

Q62.39 Other obstructive defects of renal pelvis and ureter

Ureteropelvic junction obstruction NOS

Q62.4 Agenesis of ureter

Congenital absence ureter

Q62.5 Duplication of ureter

Accessory ureter

Double ureter

Q62.6 Malposition of ureter

Q62.60 Malposition of ureter, unspecified

Q62.61 Deviation of ureter

Q62.62 Displacement of ureter

Q62.63 Anomalous implantation of ureter

Ectopia of ureter

Ectopic ureter

Q62.69 Other malposition of ureter

Q62.7 Congenital vesico-uretero-renal reflux

Q62.8 Other congenital malformations of ureter

Anomaly of ureter NOS

Q63 Other congenital malformations of kidney

Excludes1: congenital nephrotic syndrome (N04.-)

Q63.0 Accessory kidney

Q63.1 Lobulated, fused and horseshoe kidney

Q63.2 Ectopic kidney

Congenital displaced kidney

Malrotation of kidney

Q63.3 Hyperplastic and giant kidney

Compensatory hypertrophy of kidney

Q63.8 Other specified congenital malformations of kidney

Congenital renal calculi

	Add 4th-7th digits		Nonspecific code		Unspecified code		Manifestation code

Q63.9 Congenital malformation of kidney, unspecified

Q64 **Other congenital malformations of urinary system**

Q64.0 **Epispadias**

Excludes1: hypospadias (Q54.-)

Q64.1 **Exstrophy of urinary bladder**

Q64.10 **Exstrophy of urinary bladder, unspecified**

Ectopia vesicae

Q64.11 **Supravesical fissure of urinary bladder**

▲Q64.12 **Cloacal exstrophy of urinary bladder**

Q64.19 **Other exstrophy of urinary bladder**

Extroversion of bladder

Q64.2 **Congenital posterior urethral valves**

Q64.3 **Other atresia and stenosis of urethra and bladder neck**

Q64.31 **Congenital bladder neck obstruction**

Congenital obstruction of vesicourethral orifice

Q64.32 **Congenital stricture of urethra**

Q64.33 **Congenital stricture of urinary meatus**

Q64.39 **Other atresia and stenosis of urethra and bladder neck**

Atresia and stenosis of urethra and bladder neck NOS

Q64.4 **Malformation of urachus**

Cyst of urachus

Patent urachus

Prolapse of urachus

Q64.5 **Congenital absence of bladder and urethra**

Q64.6 **Congenital diverticulum of bladder**

Q64.7 **Other and unspecified congenital malformations of bladder and urethra**

Excludes1: congenital prolapse of bladder (mucosa) (Q79.4)

Q64.70 **Unspecified congenital malformation of bladder and urethra**

Malformation of bladder or urethra NOS

Q64.71 **Congenital prolapse of urethra**

Q64.72 **Congenital prolapse of urinary meatus**

Q64.73 **Congenital urethrorectal fistula**

Q64.74 **Double urethra**

Q64.75 **Double urinary meatus**

Q64.79 **Other congenital malformations of bladder and urethra**

Q64.8 **Other specified congenital malformations of urinary system**

Q64.9 **Congenital malformation of urinary system, unspecified**

Congenital anomaly NOS of urinary system

Congenital deformity NOS of urinary system

CONGENITAL MALFORMATIONS AND DEFORMATIONS OF THE MUSCULOSKELETAL SYSTEM (Q65-Q79)

Q65 **Congenital deformities of hip**

Excludes1: clicking hip (R29.4)

Q65.0 **Congenital dislocation of hip, unilateral**

Q65.00 **Congenital dislocation of unspecified hip, unilateral**

Q65.01 **Congenital dislocation of right hip, unilateral**

Q65.02 **Congenital dislocation of left hip, unilateral**

Q65.1 **Congenital dislocation of hip, bilateral**

Q65.2 **Congenital dislocation of hip, unspecified**

Q65.3 **Congenital partial dislocation of hip, unilateral**

Q65.30 **Congenital partial dislocation of unspecified hip, unilateral**

Q65.31 **Congenital partial dislocation of right hip, unilateral**

Q65.32 **Congenital partial dislocation of left hip, unilateral**

Q65.4 **Congenital partial dislocation of hip, bilateral**

Q65.5 **Congenital partial dislocation of hip, unspecified**

Q65.6 **Congenital unstable hip**

Congenital dislocatable hip

Q65.8 **Other congenital deformities of hip**

Q65.81 **Congenital coxa valga**

Q65.82 **Congenital coxa vara**

Q65.89 **Other specified congenital deformities of hip**

Anteversion of femoral neck

Congenital acetabular dysplasia

Q65.9 **Congenital deformity of hip, unspecified**

Q66 **Congenital deformities of feet**

Excludes1: reduction defects of feet (Q72.-)

valgus deformities (acquired) (M21.0-)

varus deformities (acquired) (M21.1-)

Q66.0 **Congenital talipes equinovarus**

Q66.1 **Congenital talipes calcaneovarus**

Q66.2 **Congenital metatarsus (primus) varus**

Q66.21 **Congenital metatarsus primus varus**

Q66.22 **Congenital metatarsus adductus**

Congenital metatarsus varus

Q66.3 **Other congenital varus deformities of feet**

Hallux varus, congenital

Q66.4 **Congenital talipes calcaneovalgus**

Q66.5 **Congenital pes planus**

Congenital flat foot

Congenital rigid flat foot

Congenital spastic (everted) flat foot

Excludes1: pes planus, acquired (M21.4)

Q66.50 **Congenital pes planus, unspecified foot**

Q66.51 **Congenital pes planus, right foot**

Q66.52 **Congenital pes planus, left foot**

Q66.6 **Other congenital valgus deformities of feet**

Congenital metatarsus valgus

Q66.7 **Congenital pes cavus**

Q66.8 **Other congenital deformities of feet**

Q66.80 **Congenital vertical talus deformity, unspecified foot**

Q66.81 **Congenital vertical talus deformity, right foot**

Q66.82 **Congenital vertical talus deformity, left foot**

Q66.89 **Other specified congenital deformities of feet**

Congenital asymmetric talipes

Congenital clubfoot NOS

Congenital talipes NOS

Congenital tarsal coalition

Hammer toe, congenital

Q66.9 **Congenital deformity of feet, unspecified**

Q67 **Congenital musculoskeletal deformities of head, face, spine and chest**

Excludes1: congenital malformation syndromes classified to Q87.-

Potter's syndrome (Q60.6)

● New code ▲ Revised code **Excludes1:** Not coded here **Excludes2:** Not included here ⊗ Placeholder required ⑦ 7th digit required

Q67.0   **Congenital facial asymmetry**

Q67.1   **Congenital compression facies**

Q67.2   **Dolichocephaly**

Q67.3   **Plagiocephaly**

Q67.4   **Other congenital deformities of skull, face and jaw**

     Congenital depressions in skull

     Congenital hemifacial atrophy or hypertrophy

     Deviation of nasal septum, congenital

     Squashed or bent nose, congenital

     Excludes1: dentofacial anomalies [including malocclusion] (M26.-)

         syphilitic saddle nose (A50.5)

Q67.5   **Congenital deformity of spine**

     Congenital postural scoliosis

     Congenital scoliosis NOS

     Excludes1: infantile idiopathic scoliosis (M41.0)

         scoliosis due to congenital bony malformation (Q76.3)

Q67.6   **Pectus excavatum**

     Congenital funnel chest

Q67.7   **Pectus carinatum**

     Congenital pigeon chest

Q67.8   **Other congenital deformities of chest**

     Congenital deformity of chest wall NOS

Q68   **Other congenital musculoskeletal deformities**

     Excludes1: reduction defects of limb(s) (Q71-Q73)

     Excludes2: congenital myotonic chondrodystrophy (G71.13)

Q68.0   **Congenital deformity of sternocleidomastoid muscle**

     Congenital contracture of sternocleidomastoid (muscle)

     Congenital (sternomastoid) torticollis

     Sternomastoid tumor (congenital)

Q68.1   **Congenital deformity of finger(s) and hand**

     Congenital club finger

     Spade-like hand (congenital)

Q68.2   **Congenital deformity of knee**

     Congenital dislocation of knee

     Congenital genu recurvatum

Q68.3   **Congenital bowing of femur**

     Excludes1: anteversion of femur (neck) (Q65.89)

Q68.4   **Congenital bowing of tibia and fibula**

Q68.5   **Congenital bowing of long bones of leg, unspecified**

Q68.6   **Discoid meniscus**

Q68.8   **Other specified congenital musculoskeletal deformities**

     Congenital deformity of clavicle

     Congenital deformity of elbow

     Congenital deformity of forearm

     Congenital deformity of scapula

     Congenital deformity of wrist

     Congenital dislocation of elbow

     Congenital dislocation of shoulder

     Congenital dislocation of wrist

Q69   **Polydactyly**

Q69.0   **Accessory finger(s)**

Q69.1   **Accessory thumb(s)**

Q69.2   **Accessory toe(s)**

     Accessory hallux

Q69.9   **Polydactyly, unspecified**

     Supernumerary digit(s) NOS

Q70   **Syndactyly**

Q70.0   **Fused fingers**

     Complex syndactyly of fingers with synostosis

     Q70.00   **Fused fingers, unspecified hand**

     Q70.01   **Fused fingers, right hand**

     Q70.02   **Fused fingers, left hand**

     Q70.03   **Fused fingers, bilateral**

Q70.1   **Webbed fingers**

     Simple syndactyly of fingers without synostosis

     Q70.10   **Webbed fingers, unspecified hand**

     Q70.11   **Webbed fingers, right hand**

     Q70.12   **Webbed fingers, left hand**

     Q70.13   **Webbed fingers, bilateral**

Q70.2   **Fused toes**

     Complex syndactyly of toes with synostosis

     Q70.20   **Fused toes, unspecified foot**

     Q70.21   **Fused toes, right foot**

     Q70.22   **Fused toes, left foot**

     Q70.23   **Fused toes, bilateral**

Q70.3   **Webbed toes**

     Simple syndactyly of toes without synostosis

     Q70.30   **Webbed toes, unspecified foot**

     Q70.31   **Webbed toes, right foot**

     Q70.32   **Webbed toes, left foot**

     Q70.33   **Webbed toes, bilateral**

Q70.4   **Polysyndactyly, unspecified**

     Excludes1: specified syndactyly of hand and feet - code to specified conditions (Q70.0- -Q70.3-)

Q70.9   **Syndactyly, unspecified**

     Symphalangy NOS

Q71   **Reduction defects of upper limb**

Q71.0   **Congenital complete absence of upper limb**

     Q71.00   **Congenital complete absence of unspecified upper limb**

     Q71.01   **Congenital complete absence of right upper limb**

     Q71.02   **Congenital complete absence of left upper limb**

     Q71.03   **Congenital complete absence of upper limb, bilateral**

Q71.1   **Congenital absence of upper arm and forearm with hand present**

     Q71.10   **Congenital absence of unspecified upper arm and forearm with hand present**

     Q71.11   **Congenital absence of right upper arm and forearm with hand present**

     Q71.12   **Congenital absence of left upper arm and forearm with hand present**

     Q71.13   **Congenital absence of upper arm and forearm with hand present, bilateral**

Q71.2   **Congenital absence of both forearm and hand**

     Q71.20   **Congenital absence of both forearm and hand, unspecified upper limb**

     Q71.21   **Congenital absence of both forearm and hand, right upper limb**

     Q71.22   **Congenital absence of both forearm and hand, left upper limb**

     Q71.23   **Congenital absence of both forearm and hand, bilateral**

Q71.3 **Congenital absence of hand and finger**

   Q71.30   Congenital absence of unspecified hand and finger

   Q71.31   Congenital absence of right hand and finger

   Q71.32   Congenital absence of left hand and finger

   Q71.33   Congenital absence of hand and finger, bilateral

Q71.4 **Longitudinal reduction defect of radius**

   Clubhand (congenital)

   Radial clubhand

   Q71.40   Longitudinal reduction defect of unspecified radius

   Q71.41   Longitudinal reduction defect of right radius

   Q71.42   Longitudinal reduction defect of left radius

   Q71.43   Longitudinal reduction defect of radius, bilateral

Q71.5 **Longitudinal reduction defect of ulna**

   Q71.50   Longitudinal reduction defect of unspecified ulna

   Q71.51   Longitudinal reduction defect of right ulna

   Q71.52   Longitudinal reduction defect of left ulna

   Q71.53   Longitudinal reduction defect of ulna, bilateral

Q71.6 **Lobster-claw hand**

   Q71.60   Lobster-claw hand, unspecified hand

   Q71.61   Lobster-claw right hand

   Q71.62   Lobster-claw left hand

   Q71.63   Lobster-claw hand, bilateral

Q71.8 **Other reduction defects of upper limb**

   Q71.81   Congenital shortening of upper limb

      Q71.811   Congenital shortening of right upper limb

      Q71.812   Congenital shortening of left upper limb

      Q71.813   Congenital shortening of upper limb, bilateral

      Q71.819   Congenital shortening of unspecified upper limb

   Q71.89   Other reduction defects of upper limb

      Q71.891   Other reduction defects of right upper limb

      Q71.892   Other reduction defects of left upper limb

      Q71.893   Other reduction defects of upper limb, bilateral

      Q71.899   Other reduction defects of unspecified upper limb

Q71.9 **Unspecified reduction defect of upper limb**

   Q71.90   Unspecified reduction defect of unspecified upper limb

   Q71.91   Unspecified reduction defect of right upper limb

   Q71.92   Unspecified reduction defect of left upper limb

   Q71.93   Unspecified reduction defect of upper limb, bilateral

Q72 **Reduction defects of lower limb**

Q72.0 **Congenital complete absence of lower limb**

   Q72.00   Congenital complete absence of unspecified lower limb

   Q72.01   Congenital complete absence of right lower limb

   Q72.02   Congenital complete absence of left lower limb

   Q72.03   Congenital complete absence of lower limb, bilateral

Q72.1 **Congenital absence of thigh and lower leg with foot present**

   Q72.10   Congenital absence of unspecified thigh and lower leg with foot present

   Q72.11   Congenital absence of right thigh and lower leg with foot present

   Q72.12   Congenital absence of left thigh and lower leg with foot present

   Q72.13   Congenital absence of thigh and lower leg with foot present, bilateral

Q72.2 **Congenital absence of both lower leg and foot**

   Q72.20   Congenital absence of both lower leg and foot, unspecified lower limb

   Q72.21   Congenital absence of both lower leg and foot, right lower limb

   Q72.22   Congenital absence of both lower leg and foot, left lower limb

   Q72.23   Congenital absence of both lower leg and foot, bilateral

Q72.3 **Congenital absence of foot and toe(s)**

   Q72.30   Congenital absence of unspecified foot and toe(s)

   Q72.31   Congenital absence of right foot and toe(s)

   Q72.32   Congenital absence of left foot and toe(s)

   Q72.33   Congenital absence of foot and toe(s), bilateral

Q72.4 **Longitudinal reduction defect of femur**

   Proximal femoral focal deficiency

   Q72.40   Longitudinal reduction defect of unspecified femur

   Q72.41   Longitudinal reduction defect of right femur

   Q72.42   Longitudinal reduction defect of left femur

   Q72.43   Longitudinal reduction defect of femur, bilateral

Q72.5 **Longitudinal reduction defect of tibia**

   Q72.50   Longitudinal reduction defect of unspecified tibia

   Q72.51   Longitudinal reduction defect of right tibia

   Q72.52   Longitudinal reduction defect of left tibia

   Q72.53   Longitudinal reduction defect of tibia, bilateral

Q72.6 **Longitudinal reduction defect of fibula**

   Q72.60   Longitudinal reduction defect of unspecified fibula

   Q72.61   Longitudinal reduction defect of right fibula

   Q72.62   Longitudinal reduction defect of left fibula

   Q72.63   Longitudinal reduction defect of fibula, bilateral

Q72.7 **Split foot**

   Q72.70   Split foot, unspecified lower limb

   Q72.71   Split foot, right lower limb

   Q72.72   Split foot, left lower limb

   Q72.73   Split foot, bilateral

Q72.8 **Other reduction defects of lower limb**

   Q72.81   Congenital shortening of lower limb

   ● New code   ▲ Revised code   **Excludes1:** Not coded here   **Excludes2:** Not included here   ⊗ Placeholder required   ⑦7th digit required

Q72.811 **Congenital shortening of right lower limb**

Q72.812 **Congenital shortening of left lower limb**

Q72.813 **Congenital shortening of lower limb, bilateral**

Q72.819 **Congenital shortening of unspecified lower limb**

Q72.89 **Other reduction defects of lower limb**

Q72.891 **Other reduction defects of right lower limb**

Q72.892 **Other reduction defects of left lower limb**

Q72.893 **Other reduction defects of lower limb, bilateral**

Q72.899 **Other reduction defects of unspecified lower limb**

Q72.9 **Unspecified reduction defect of lower limb**

Q72.90 **Unspecified reduction defect of unspecified lower limb**

Q72.91 **Unspecified reduction defect of right lower limb**

Q72.92 **Unspecified reduction defect of left lower limb**

Q72.93 **Unspecified reduction defect of lower limb, bilateral**

Q73 **Reduction defects of unspecified limb**

Q73.0 **Congenital absence of unspecified limb(s)**

Amelia NOS

Q73.1 **Phocomelia, unspecified limb(s)**

Phocomelia NOS

Q73.8 **Other reduction defects of unspecified limb(s)**

Longitudinal reduction deformity of unspecified limb(s)

Ectromelia of limb NOS

Hemimelia of limb NOS

Reduction defect of limb NOS

Q74 **Other congenital malformations of limb(s)**

Excludes1: polydactyly (Q69.-)

reduction defect of limb (Q71-Q73)

syndactyly (Q70.-)

Q74.0 **Other congenital malformations of upper limb(s), including shoulder girdle**

Accessory carpal bones

Cleidocranial dysostosis

Congenital pseudarthrosis of clavicle

Macrodactylia (fingers)

Madelung's deformity

Radioulnar synostosis

Sprengel's deformity

Triphalangeal thumb

Q74.1 **Congenital malformation of knee**

Congenital absence of patella

Congenital dislocation of patella

Congenital genu valgum

Congenital genu varum

Rudimentary patella

Excludes1: congenital dislocation of knee (Q68.2)

congenital genu recurvatum (Q68.2)

nail patella syndrome (Q87.2)

Q74.2 **Other congenital malformations of lower limb(s), including pelvic girdle**

Congenital fusion of sacroiliac joint

Congenital malformation of ankle joint

Congenital malformation of sacroiliac joint

Excludes1: anteversion of femur (neck) (Q65.89)

Q74.3 **Arthrogryposis multiplex congenita**

Q74.8 **Other specified congenital malformations of limb(s)**

Q74.9 **Unspecified congenital malformation of limb(s)**

Congenital anomaly of limb(s) NOS

Q75 **Other congenital malformations of skull and face bones**

Excludes1: congenital malformation of face NOS (Q18.-)

congenital malformation syndromes classified to Q87.-

dentofacial anomalies [including malocclusion] (M26.-)

musculoskeletal deformities of head and face (Q67.0-Q67.4)

skull defects associated with congenital anomalies of brain such as: anencephaly (Q00.0)

encephalocele (Q01.-)

hydrocephalus (Q03.-)

microcephaly (Q02)

Q75.0 **Craniosynostosis**

Acrocephaly

Imperfect fusion of skull

Oxycephaly

Trigonocephaly

Q75.1 **Craniofacial dysostosis**

Crouzon's disease

Q75.2 **Hypertelorism**

Q75.3 **Macrocephaly**

Q75.4 **Mandibulofacial dysostosis**

Franceschetti syndrome

Treacher Collins syndrome

Q75.5 **Oculomandibular dysostosis**

Q75.8 **Other specified congenital malformations of skull and face bones**

Absence of skull bone, congenital

Congenital deformity of forehead

Platybasia

Q75.9 **Congenital malformation of skull and face bones, unspecified**

Congenital anomaly of face bones NOS

Congenital anomaly of skull NOS

Q76 **Congenital malformations of spine and bony thorax**

Excludes1: congenital musculoskeletal deformities of spine and chest (Q67.5-Q67.8)

Q76.0 **Spina bifida occulta**

Excludes1: meningocele (spinal) (Q05.-)

spina bifida (aperta) (cystica) (Q05.-)

Q76.1 **Klippel-Feil syndrome**

Cervical fusion syndrome

Q76.2 **Congenital spondylolisthesis**

Congenital spondylolysis

Excludes1: spondylolisthesis (acquired) (M43.1-)

spondylolysis (acquired) (M43.0-)

Q76.3 **Congenital scoliosis due to congenital bony malformation**

Hemivertebra fusion or failure of segmentation with scoliosis

Q76.4 Other congenital malformations of spine, not associated with scoliosis

Q76.41 Congenital kyphosis

Q76.411 Congenital kyphosis, occipito-atlanto-axial region

Q76.412 Congenital kyphosis, cervical region

Q76.413 Congenital kyphosis, cervicothoracic region

Q76.414 Congenital kyphosis, thoracic region

Q76.415 Congenital kyphosis, thoracolumbar region

Q76.419 Congenital kyphosis, unspecified region

Q76.42 Congenital lordosis

Q76.425 Congenital lordosis, thoracolumbar region

Q76.426 Congenital lordosis, lumbar region

Q76.427 Congenital lordosis, lumbosacral region

Q76.428 Congenital lordosis, sacral and sacrococcygeal region

Q76.429 Congenital lordosis, unspecified region

Q76.49 Other congenital malformations of spine, not associated with scoliosis

Congenital absence of vertebra NOS

Congenital fusion of spine NOS

Congenital malformation of lumbosacral (joint) (region) NOS

Congenital malformation of spine NOS

Hemivertebra NOS

Malformation of spine NOS

Platyspondylisis NOS

Supernumerary vertebra NOS

Q76.5 Cervical rib

Supernumerary rib in cervical region

Q76.6 Other congenital malformations of ribs

Accessory rib

Congenital absence of rib

Congenital fusion of ribs

Congenital malformation of ribs NOS

Excludes1: short rib syndrome (Q77.2)

Q76.7 Congenital malformation of sternum

Congenital absence of sternum

Sternum bifidum

Q76.8 Other congenital malformations of bony thorax

Q76.9 Congenital malformation of bony thorax, unspecified

Q77 Osteochondrodysplasia with defects of growth of tubular bones and spine

Excludes1: mucopolysaccharidosis (E76.0-E76.3)

Excludes2: congenital myotonic chondrodystrophy (G71.13)

Q77.0 Achondrogenesis

Hypochondrogenesis

Q77.1 Thanatophoric short stature

Q77.2 Short rib syndrome

Asphyxiating thoracic dysplasia [Jeune]

Q77.3 Chondrodysplasia punctata

Excludes1: Rhizomelic chondrodysplasia punctata (E71.43)

Q77.4 Achondroplasia

Hypochondroplasia

Osteosclerosis congenita

Q77.5 Diastrophic dysplasia

Q77.6 Chondroectodermal dysplasia

Ellis-van Creveld syndrome

Q77.7 Spondyloepiphyseal dysplasia

Q77.8 Other osteochondrodysplasia with defects of growth of tubular bones and spine

Q77.9 Osteochondrodysplasia with defects of growth of tubular bones and spine, unspecified

Q78 Other osteochondrodysplasias

Excludes2: congenital myotonic chondrodystrophy (G71.13)

Q78.0 Osteogenesis imperfecta

Fragilitas ossium

Osteopsathyrosis

Q78.1 Polyostotic fibrous dysplasia

Albright(-McCune)(-Sternberg) syndrome

Q78.2 Osteopetrosis

Albers-Schönberg syndrome

Osteosclerosis NOS

Q78.3 Progressive diaphyseal dysplasia

Camurati-Engelmann syndrome

Q78.4 Enchondromatosis

Maffucci's syndrome

Ollier's disease

Q78.5 Metaphyseal dysplasia

Pyle's syndrome

Q78.6 Multiple congenital exostoses

Diaphyseal aclasis

Q78.8 Other specified osteochondrodysplasias

Osteopoikilosis

Q78.9 Osteochondrodysplasia, unspecified

Chondrodystrophy NOS

Osteodystrophy NOS

Q79 Congenital malformations of musculoskeletal system, not elsewhere classified

Excludes2: congenital (sternomastoid) torticollis (Q68.0)

Q79.0 Congenital diaphragmatic hernia

Excludes1: congenital hiatus hernia (Q40.1)

Q79.1 Other congenital malformations of diaphragm

Absence of diaphragm

Congenital malformation of diaphragm NOS

Eventration of diaphragm

Q79.2 Exomphalos

Omphalocele

Excludes1: umbilical hernia (K42.-)

Q79.3 Gastroschisis

Q79.4 Prune belly syndrome

Congenital prolapse of bladder mucosa

Eagle-Barrett syndrome

Q79.5 Other congenital malformations of abdominal wall

Excludes1: umbilical hernia (K42.-)

Q79.51 Congenital hernia of bladder

● New code ▲ Revised code **Excludes1:** Not coded here **Excludes2:** Not included here ⊗ Placeholder required ⑦ 7th digit required

Q79.59 **Other congenital malformations of abdominal wall**

Q79.6 **Ehlers-Danlos syndrome**

Q79.8 **Other congenital malformations of musculoskeletal system**

Absence of muscle

Absence of tendon

Accessory muscle

Amyotrophia congenita

Congenital constricting bands

Congenital shortening of tendon

Poland syndrome

Q79.9 **Congenital malformation of musculoskeletal system, unspecified**

Congenital anomaly of musculoskeletal system NOS

Congenital deformity of musculoskeletal system NOS

OTHER CONGENITAL MALFORMATIONS (Q80-Q89)

Q80 **Congenital ichthyosis**

Excludes1: Refsum's disease (G60.1)

Q80.0 **Ichthyosis vulgaris**

Q80.1 **X-linked ichthyosis**

Q80.2 **Lamellar ichthyosis**

Collodion baby

Q80.3 **Congenital bullous ichthyosiform erythroderma**

Q80.4 **Harlequin fetus**

Q80.8 **Other congenital ichthyosis**

Q80.9 **Congenital ichthyosis, unspecified**

Q81 **Epidermolysis bullosa**

Q81.0 **Epidermolysis bullosa simplex**

Excludes1: Cockayne's syndrome (Q87.1)

Q81.1 **Epidermolysis bullosa letalis**

Herlitz' syndrome

Q81.2 **Epidermolysis bullosa dystrophica**

Q81.8 **Other epidermolysis bullosa**

Q81.9 **Epidermolysis bullosa, unspecified**

Q82 **Other congenital malformations of skin**

Excludes1: acrodermatitis enteropathica (E83.2)

congenital erythropoietic porphyria (E80.0)

pilonidal cyst or sinus (L05.-)

Sturge-Weber (-Dimitri) syndrome (Q85.8)

Q82.0 **Hereditary lymphedema**

Q82.1 **Xeroderma pigmentosum**

▲Q82.2 **Congenital cutaneous mastocytosis**

Congenital diffuse cutaneous mastocytosis

Congenital maculopapular cutaneous mastocytosis

Congenital urticaria pigmentosa

Excludes1:

cutaneous mastocytosis NOS (D47.01)

diffuse cutaneous mastocytosis (with onset after newborn period) (D47.01)

malignant mastocytosis (C96.2-)

systemic mastocytosis (D47.02)

urticaria pigmentosa (non-congenital) (with onset after newborn period) (D47.01)

Q82.3 **Incontinentia pigmenti**

Q82.4 **Ectodermal dysplasia (anhidrotic)**

Excludes1: Ellis-van Creveld syndrome (Q77.6)

Q82.5 **Congenital non-neoplastic nevus**

Birthmark NOS

Flammeus Nevus

Port-wine Nevus

Sanguineous Nevus

Strawberry Nevus

Vascular Nevus NOS

Verrucous Nevus

Excludes2: Café au lait spots (L81.3)

lentigo (L81.4)

araneus nevus (I78.1)

melanocytic nevus (D22.-)

nevus NOS (D22.-)

pigmented nevus (D22.-)

spider nevus (I78.1)

stellar nevus (I78.1)

Q82.6 **Congenital sacral dimple**

Parasacral dimple

Excludes2: pilonidal cyst with abscess (L05.01)

pilonidal cyst without abscess (L05.91)

Q82.8 **Other specified congenital malformations of skin**

Abnormal palmar creases

Accessory skin tags

Benign familial pemphigus [Hailey-Hailey]

Congenital poikiloderma

Cutis laxa (hyperelastica)

Dermatoglyphic anomalies

Inherited keratosis palmaris et plantaris

Keratosis follicularis [Darier-White]

Excludes1: Ehlers-Danlos syndrome (Q79.6)

Q82.9 **Congenital malformation of skin, unspecified**

Q83 **Congenital malformations of breast**

Excludes2: absence of pectoral muscle (Q79.8)

hypoplasia of breast (N64.82)

micromastia (N64.82)

Q83.0 **Congenital absence of breast with absent nipple**

Q83.1 **Accessory breast**

Supernumerary breast

Q83.2 **Absent nipple**

Q83.3 **Accessory nipple**

Supernumerary nipple

Q83.8 **Other congenital malformations of breast**

Q83.9 **Congenital malformation of breast, unspecified**

Q84 **Other congenital malformations of integument**

Q84.0 **Congenital alopecia**

Congenital atrichosis

Q84.1 **Congenital morphological disturbances of hair, not elsewhere classified**

Beaded hair

Monilethrix

Pili annulati

Excludes1: Menkes' kinky hair syndrome (E83.0)

Q84.2 **Other congenital malformations of hair**

Congenital hypertrichosis

Congenital malformation of hair NOS

Persistent lanugo

Q84.3 **Anonychia**

Excludes1: nail patella syndrome (Q87.2)

Q84.4 **Congenital leukonychia**

Q84.5 **Enlarged and hypertrophic nails**

Congenital onychauxis

Pachyonychia

Q84.6 **Other congenital malformations of nails**

Congenital club nail

Congenital koilonychia

Congenital malformation of nail NOS

Q84.8 **Other specified congenital malformations of integument**

Aplasia cutis congenita

Q84.9 **Congenital malformation of integument, unspecified**

Congenital anomaly of integument NOS

Congenital deformity of integument NOS

Q85 **Phakomatoses, not elsewhere classified**

Excludes1: ataxia telangiectasia [Louis-Bar] (G11.3)

familial dysautonomia [Riley-Day] (G90.1)

Q85.0 **Neurofibromatosis (nonmalignant)**

Q85.00 **Neurofibromatosis, unspecified**

Q85.01 **Neurofibromatosis, type 1**

Von Recklinghausen disease

Q85.02 **Neurofibromatosis, type 2**

Acoustic neurofibromatosis

Q85.03 **Schwannomatosis**

Q85.09 **Other neurofibromatosis**

Q85.1 **Tuberous sclerosis**

Bourneville's disease

Epiloia

Q85.8 **Other phakomatoses, not elsewhere classified**

Peutz-Jeghers Syndrome

Sturge-Weber(-Dimitri) syndrome von Hippel-Lindau syndrome

Excludes1: Meckel-Gruber syndrome (Q61.9)

Q85.9 **Phakomatosis, unspecified**

Hamartoses NOS

Q86 **Congenital malformation syndromes due to known exogenous causes, not elsewhere classified**

Excludes2: iodine-deficiency-related hypothyroidism (E00-E02)

nonteratogenic effects of substances transmitted via placenta or breast milk (P04.-)

Q86.0 **Fetal alcohol syndrome (dysmorphic)**

Q86.1 **Fetal hydantoin syndrome**

Meadow's syndrome

Q86.2 **Dysmorphism due to warfarin**

Q86.8 **Other congenital malformation syndromes due to known exogenous causes**

Q87 **Other specified congenital malformation syndromes affecting multiple systems**

Use additional code(s) to identify all associated manifestations

Q87.0 **Congenital malformation syndromes predominantly affecting facial appearance**

Acrocephalopolysyndactyly

Acrocephalosyndactyly [Apert]

Cryptophthalmos syndrome

Cyclopia

Goldenhar syndrome

Moebius syndrome

Oro-facial-digital syndrome

Robin syndrome

Whistling face

Q87.1 **Congenital malformation syndromes predominantly associated with short stature**

Aarskog syndrome

Cockayne syndrome

De Lange syndrome

Dubowitz syndrome Noonan syndrome

Prader-Willi syndrome

Robinow-Silverman-Smith syndrome

Russell-Silver syndrome

Seckel syndrome

Excludes1: Ellis-van Creveld syndrome (Q77.6)

Smith-Lemli-Opitz syndrome (E78.72)

Q87.2 **Congenital malformation syndromes predominantly involving limbs**

Holt-Oram syndrome

Klippel-Trenaunay-Weber syndrome Nail patella syndrome

Rubinstein-Taybi syndrome

Sirenomelia syndrome

Thrombocytopenia with absent radius [TAR] syndrome

VATER syndrome

Q87.3 **Congenital malformation syndromes involving early overgrowth**

Beckwith-Wiedemann syndrome

Sotos syndrome

Weaver syndrome

Q87.4 **Marfan's syndrome**

Q87.40 **Marfan's syndrome, unspecified**

Q87.41 **Marfan's syndrome with cardiovascular manifestations**

Q87.410 **Marfan's syndrome with aortic dilation**

Q87.418 **Marfan's syndrome with other cardiovascular manifestations**

Q87.42 **Marfan's syndrome with ocular manifestations**

Q87.43 **Marfan's syndrome with skeletal manifestation**

Q87.5 **Other congenital malformation syndromes with other skeletal changes**

Q87.8 **Other specified congenital malformation syndromes, not elsewhere classified**

Excludes1: Zellweger syndrome (E71.510)

Q87.81 **Alport syndrome**

Use additional code to identify stage of chronic kidney disease (N18.1-N18.6)

Q87.82 **Arterial tortuosity syndrome**

Q87.89 **Other specified congenital malformation syndromes, not elsewhere classified**

Laurence-Moon (-Bardet)-Biedl syndrome

Q89 **Other congenital malformations, not elsewhere classified**

Q89.0 **Congenital absence and malformations of spleen**

Excludes1: isomerism of atrial appendages (with asplenia or polysplenia) (Q20.6)

Q89.01 **Asplenia (congenital)**

Q89.09 **Congenital malformations of spleen**

Congenital splenomegaly

Q89.1 Congenital malformations of adrenal gland

> **Excludes1:** adrenogenital disorders (E25.-)
>
> congenital adrenal hyperplasia (E25.0)

Q89.2 Congenital malformations of other endocrine glands

Congenital malformation of parathyroid or thyroid gland

Persistent thyroglossal duct

Thyroglossal cyst

> **Excludes1:** congenital goiter (E03.0)
>
> congenital hypothyroidism (E03.1)

Q89.3 Situs inversus

Dextrocardia with situs inversus

Mirror-image atrial arrangement with situs inversus

Situs inversus or transversus abdominalis

Situs inversus or transversus thoracis

Transposition of abdominal viscera

Transposition of thoracic viscera

> **Excludes1:** dextrocardia NOS (Q24.0)

Q89.4 Conjoined twins

Craniopagus

Dicephaly

Pygopagus

Thoracopagus

Q89.7 Multiple congenital malformations, not elsewhere classified

Multiple congenital anomalies NOS

Multiple congenital deformities NOS

> **Excludes1:** congenital malformation syndromes affecting multiple systems (Q87.-)

Q89.8 Other specified congenital malformations

> **Use additional code**(s) to identify all associated manifestations

Q89.9 Congenital malformation, unspecified

Congenital anomaly NOS

Congenital deformity NOS

CHROMOSOMAL ABNORMALITIES, NOT ELSEWHERE CLASSIFIED (Q90-Q99)

Excludes2: mitochondrial metabolic disorders (E88.4-)

Q90 Down syndrome

> **Use additional code**(s) to identify any associated physical conditions and degree of intellectual disabilities (F70-F79)

Q90.0 Trisomy 21, nonmosaicism (meiotic nondisjunction)

Q90.1 Trisomy 21, mosaicism (mitotic nondisjunction)

Q90.2 Trisomy 21, translocation

Q90.9 Down syndrome, unspecified

Trisomy 21 NOS

Q91 Trisomy 18 and Trisomy 13

Q91.0 Trisomy 18, nonmosaicism (meiotic nondisjunction)

Q91.1 Trisomy 18, mosaicism (mitotic nondisjunction)

Q91.2 Trisomy 18, translocation

Q91.3 Trisomy 18, unspecified

Q91.4 Trisomy 13, nonmosaicism (meiotic nondisjunction)

Q91.5 Trisomy 13, mosaicism (mitotic nondisjunction)

Q91.6 Trisomy 13, translocation

Q91.7 Trisomy 13, unspecified

Q92 Other trisomies and partial trisomies of the autosomes, not elsewhere classified

Includes: unbalanced translocations and insertions

Excludes1: trisomies of chromosomes 13, 18, 21 (Q90-Q91)

Q92.0 Whole chromosome trisomy, nonmosaicism (meiotic nondisjunction)

Q92.1 Whole chromosome trisomy, mosaicism (mitotic nondisjunction)

Q92.2 Partial trisomy

Less than whole arm duplicated Whole arm or more duplicated

> **Excludes1:** partial trisomy due to unbalanced translocation (Q92.5)

Q92.5 Duplications with other complex rearrangements

Partial trisomy due to unbalanced translocations

> **Code also** any associated deletions due to unbalanced translocations, inversions and insertions (Q93.7)

Q92.6 Marker chromosomes

Trisomies due to dicentrics

Trisomies due to extra rings

Trisomies due to isochromosomes

Individual with marker heterochromatin

> **Q92.61 Marker chromosomes in normal individual**
>
> **Q92.62 Marker chromosomes in abnormal individual**

Q92.7 Triploidy and polyploidy

Q92.8 Other specified trisomies and partial trisomies of autosomes

Duplications identified by fluorescence in situ hybridization (FISH)

Duplications identified by in situ hybridization (ISH)

Duplications seen only at prometaphase

Q92.9 Trisomy and partial trisomy of autosomes, unspecified

Q93 Monosomies and deletions from the autosomes, not elsewhere classified

Q93.0 Whole chromosome monosomy, nonmosaicism (meiotic nondisjunction)

Q93.1 Whole chromosome monosomy, mosaicism (mitotic nondisjunction)

Q93.2 Chromosome replaced with ring, dicentric or isochromosome

Q93.3 Deletion of short arm of chromosome 4

Wolff-Hirschorn syndrome

Q93.4 Deletion of short arm of chromosome 5

Cri-du-chat syndrome

Q93.5 Other deletions of part of a chromosome

Angelman syndrome

Q93.7 Deletions with other complex rearrangements

Deletions due to unbalanced translocations, inversions and insertions

> **Code also** any associated duplications due to unbalanced translocations, inversions and insertions (Q92.5)

Q93.8 Other deletions from the autosomes

> **Q93.81 Velo-cardio-facial syndrome**
>
> Deletion 22q11.2

> **Q93.88 Other microdeletions**
>
> Miller-Dieker syndrome
>
> Smith-Magenis syndrome

> **Q93.89 Other deletions from the autosomes**
>
> Deletions identified by fluorescence in situ hybridization (FISH)
>
> Deletions identified by in situ hybridization (ISH)

Deletions seen only at prometaphase

Q93.9   Deletion from autosomes, unspecified

Q95   **Balanced rearrangements and structural markers, not elsewhere classified**

Includes: Robertsonian and balanced reciprocal translocations and insertions

Q95.0   Balanced translocation and insertion in normal individual

Q95.1   Chromosome inversion in normal individual

Q95.2   Balanced autosomal rearrangement in abnormal individual

Q95.3   Balanced sex/autosomal rearrangement in abnormal individual

Q95.5   Individual with autosomal fragile site

Q95.8   Other balanced rearrangements and structural markers

Q95.9   Balanced rearrangement and structural marker, unspecified

Q96   **Turner's syndrome**

Excludes1: Noonan syndrome (Q87.1)

Q96.0   Karyotype 45, X

Q96.1   Karyotype 46, X iso (Xq)

Karyotype 46, isochromosome Xq

Q96.2   Karyotype 46, X with abnormal sex chromosome, except iso (Xq)

Karyotype 46, X with abnormal sex chromosome, except isochromosome Xq

Q96.3   Mosaicism, 45, X/46, XX or XY

Q96.4   Mosaicism, 45, X/Other cell line(s) with abnormal sex chromosome

Q96.8   Other variants of Turner's syndrome

Q96.9   Turner's syndrome, unspecified

Q97   **Other sex chromosome abnormalities, female phenotype, not elsewhere classified**

Excludes1: Turner's syndrome (Q96.-)

Q97.0   Karyotype 47, XXX

Q97.1   Female with more than three X chromosomes

Q97.2   Mosaicism, lines with various numbers of X chromosomes

Q97.3   Female with 46, XY karyotype

Q97.8   Other specified sex chromosome abnormalities, female phenotype

Q97.9   Sex chromosome abnormality, female phenotype, unspecified

Q98   **Other sex chromosome abnormalities, male phenotype, not elsewhere classified**

Q98.0   Klinefelter syndrome karyotype 47, XXY

Q98.1   Klinefelter syndrome, male with more than two X chromosomes

Q98.3   Other male with 46, XX karyotype

Q98.4   Klinefelter syndrome, unspecified

Q98.5   Karyotype 47, XYY

Q98.6   Male with structurally abnormal sex chromosome

Q98.7   Male with sex chromosome mosaicism

Q98.8   Other specified sex chromosome abnormalities, male phenotype

Q98.9   Sex chromosome abnormality, male phenotype, unspecified

Q99   **Other chromosome abnormalities, not elsewhere classified**

Q99.0   Chimera 46, XX/46, XY

Chimera 46, XX/46, XY true hermaphrodite

Q99.1   **46, XX true hermaphrodite**

46, XX with streak gonads

46, XY with streak gonads

Pure gonadal dysgenesis

Q99.2   **Fragile X chromosome**

Fragile X syndrome

Q99.8   **Other specified chromosome abnormalities**

Q99.9   **Chromosomal abnormality, unspecified**

● New code   ▲ Revised code   **Excludes1:** Not coded here   **Excludes2:** Not included here   ⊗ Placeholder required   ⑦7th digit required

Chapter 18: Symptoms, Signs And Abnormal Clinical And Laboratory Findings, Not Elsewhere Classified (R00-R99)

DEFINITIONS

This chapter includes definitions of selected key words, terms and phrases and coding alerts for adding points to the clinical domain, and references to coding late effects where appropriate. An example from this chapter is as follows:

R16 Hepatomegaly and splenomegaly, not elsewhere classified
Definition: Hepatomegaly refers to abnormal enlargement of the liver. Splenomegaly refers to abnormal enlargement of the spleen.

MULTIPLE CODING FOR A SINGLE CONDITION

In addition to the etiology/manifestation convention that requires two codes to fully describe a single condition that affects multiple body systems, there are other single conditions that also require more than one code. "Use additional code" notes are found in the Tabular List at codes that are not part of an etiology/manifestation pair where a secondary code is useful to fully describe a condition. The sequencing rule is the same as the etiology/manifestation pair, "use additional code" indicates that a secondary code should be added.

For example, for bacterial infections that are not included in chapter 1, a secondary code from category B95, Streptococcus, Staphylococcus, and Enterococcus, as the cause of diseases classified elsewhere, or B96, Other bacterial agents as the cause of diseases classified elsewhere, may be required to identify the bacterial organism causing the infection. A "use additional code" note will normally be found at the infectious disease code, indicating a need for the organism code to be added as a secondary code.

"Code first" notes are also under certain codes that are not specifically manifestation codes but may be due to an underlying cause. When there is a "code first" note and an underlying condition is present, the underlying condition should be sequenced first.

"Code, if applicable, any causal condition first", notes indicate that this code may be assigned as a principal diagnosis when the causal condition is unknown or not applicable. If a causal condition is known, then the code for that condition should be sequenced as the principal or first-listed diagnosis.

Multiple codes may be needed for sequela, complication codes and obstetric codes to more fully describe a condition. See the specific guidelines for these conditions for further instruction.

COMBINATION CODE

A combination code is a single code used to classify: Two diagnoses, or a diagnosis with an associated secondary process (manifestation) A diagnosis with an associated complication

Combination codes are identified by referring to subterm entries in the Alphabetic Index and by reading the inclusion and exclusion notes in the Tabular List.

Assign only the combination code when that code fully identifies the diagnostic conditions involved or when the Alphabetic Index so directs. Multiple coding should not be used when the classification provides a combination code that clearly identifies all of the elements documented in the diagnosis. When the combination code lacks necessary specificity in describing the manifestation or complication, an additional code should be used as a secondary code.

SEQUELA (LATE EFFECTS)

A sequela is the residual effect (condition produced) after the acute phase of an illness or injury has terminated. There is no time limit on when a sequela code can be used. The residual may be apparent early, such as in cerebral infarction, or it may occur months or years later, such as that due to a previous injury. Coding of sequela generally requires two codes sequenced in the following order: The condition or nature of the sequela is sequenced first.

The sequela code is sequenced second.

An exception to the above guidelines are those instances where the code for the sequela is followed by a manifestation code identified in the Tabular List and title, or the sequela code has been expanded (at the fourth, fifth or sixth character levels) to include the manifestation(s). The code for the acute phase of an illness or injury that led to the sequela is never used with a code for the late effect.

Chapter 18 includes symptoms, signs, abnormal results of clinical or other investigative procedures, and ill-defined conditions regarding which no diagnosis classifiable elsewhere is recorded. Signs and symptoms that point to a specific diagnosis have been assigned to a category in other chapters of the classification.

USE OF SYMPTOM CODES

Codes that describe symptoms and signs are acceptable for reporting purposes when a related definitive diagnosis has not been established (confirmed) by the provider.

USE OF A SYMPTOM CODE WITH A DEFINITIVE DIAGNOSIS CODE

Codes for signs and symptoms may be reported in addition to a related definitive diagnosis when the sign or symptom is not routinely associated with that diagnosis, such as the various signs and symptoms associated with complex syndromes. The definitive diagnosis code should be sequenced before the symptom code.

Signs or symptoms that are associated routinely with a disease process should not be assigned as additional codes, unless otherwise instructed by the classification.

COMBINATION CODES THAT INCLUDE SYMPTOMS

ICD-10-CM contains a number of combination codes that identify both the definitive diagnosis and common symptoms of that diagnosis. When using one of these combination codes, an additional code should not be assigned for the symptom.

REPEATED FALLS

Code R29.6, Repeated falls, is for use for encounters when a patient has recently fallen and the reason for the fall is being investigated.

Code Z91.81, History of falling, is for use when a patient has fallen in the past and is at risk for future falls. When appropriate, both codes R29.6 and Z91.81 may be assigned together.

COMA SCALE

The coma scale codes (R40.2-) can be used in conjunction with traumatic brain injury codes, acute cerebrovascular disease or sequelae of cerebrovascular disease codes. These codes are primarily for use by trauma registries, but they may be used in any setting where this information is collected. The coma scale may also be used to assess the status of the central nervous system for other non-trauma conditions, such as monitoring patients in the intensive care unit regardless of medical condition. The coma scale codes should be sequenced after the diagnosis code(s).

These codes, one from each subcategory, are needed to complete the scale. The 7th character indicates when the scale was recorded. The 7th character should match for all three codes.

At a minimum, report the initial score documented on presentation at your facility. This may be a score from the emergency medicine technician (EMT) or in the emergency department. If desired, a facility may choose to capture multiple coma scale scores.

Assign code R40.24, Glasgow coma scale, total score, when only the total score is documented in the medical record and not the individual score(s).

FUNCTIONAL QUADRIPLEGIA

Functional quadriplegia (code R53.2) is the lack of ability to use one's limbs or to ambulate due to extreme debility. It is not associated with neurologic deficit or injury, and code R53.2 should not be used for cases of neurologic quadriplegia. It should only be assigned if functional quadriplegia is specifically documented in the medical record.

SIRS DUE TO NON-INFECTIOUS PROCESS

The systemic inflammatory response syndrome (SIRS) can develop as a result of certain non-infectious disease processes, such as trauma, malignant neoplasm, or pancreatitis. When SIRS is documented with a noninfectious condition, and no subsequent infection is documented, the code for the underlying condition, such as an injury, should be assigned, followed by code R65.10, Systemic inflammatory response syndrome (SIRS) of non-infectious origin without acute organ dysfunction, or code R65.11, Systemic inflammatory response syndrome (SIRS) of non-infectious origin with acute organ dysfunction. If an associated acute organ dysfunction is documented, the appropriate code(s) for the specific type of organ dysfunction(s) should be assigned in addition to code R65.11. If acute organ dysfunction is documented, but it cannot be determined if the acute organ dysfunction is associated with SIRS or due to another condition (e.g., directly due to the trauma), the provider should be queried.

DEATH NOS

Code R99, Ill-defined and unknown cause of mortality, is only for use in the very limited circumstance when a patient who has already died is brought into an emergency department or other healthcare facility and is pronounced dead upon arrival. It does not represent the discharge disposition of death.

NIHSS STROKE SCALE

The NIH stroke scale (NIHSS) codes (R29.7- -) can be used in conjunction with acute stroke codes (I63) to identify the patient's neurological status and the severity of the stroke. The stroke scale codes should be sequenced after the acute stroke diagnosis code(s).

At a minimum, report the initial score documented. If desired, a facility may choose to capture multiple stroke scale scores.

See Section I.B.14.for information concerning the medical record documentation that may be used for assignment of the NIHSS codes.

Chapter 18
Symptoms, Signs And Abnormal Clinical And Laboratory Findings, Not Elsewhere Classified (R00-R99)

Note: This chapter includes symptoms, signs, abnormal results of clinical or other investigative procedures, and ill-defined conditions regarding which no diagnosis classifiable elsewhere is recorded.

Signs and symptoms that point rather definitely to a given diagnosis have been assigned to a category in other chapters of the classification. In general, categories in this chapter include the less well-defined conditions and symptoms that, without the necessary study of the case to establish a final diagnosis, point perhaps equally to two or more diseases or to two or more systems of the body. Practically all categories in the chapter could be designated 'not otherwise specified', 'unknown etiology' or 'transient'. The Alphabetical Index should be consulted to determine which symptoms and signs are to be allocated here and which to other chapters. The residual subcategories, numbered .8, are generally provided for other relevant symptoms that cannot be allocated elsewhere in the classification.

The conditions and signs or symptoms included in categories R00-R94 consist of: (a) cases for which no more specific diagnosis can be made even after all the facts bearing on the case have been investigated; (b) signs or symptoms existing at the time of initial encounter that proved to be transient and whose causes could not be determined; (c) provisional diagnosis in a patient who failed to return for further investigation or care; (d) cases referred elsewhere for investigation or treatment before the diagnosis was made; (e) cases in which a more precise diagnosis was not available for any other reason; (f) certain symptoms, for which supplementary information is provided, that represent important problems in medical care in their own right.

Excludes2: abnormal findings on antenatal screening of mother (O28.-)
certain conditions originating in the perinatal period (P04-P96)
signs and symptoms classified in the body system chapters signs and symptoms of breast (N63, N64.5)

This chapter contains the following blocks:

R00-R09	Symptoms and signs involving the circulatory and respiratory systems
R10-R19	Symptoms and signs involving the digestive system and abdomen
R20-R23	Symptoms and signs involving the skin and subcutaneous tissue
R25-R29	Symptoms and signs involving the nervous and musculoskeletal systems
R30-R39	Symptoms and signs involving the genitourinary system
R40-R46	Symptoms and signs involving cognition, perception, emotional state and behavior
R47-R49	Symptoms and signs involving speech and voice
R50-R69	General symptoms and signs
R70-R79	Abnormal findings on examination of blood, without diagnosis
R80-R82	Abnormal findings on examination of urine, without diagnosis
R83-R89	Abnormal findings on examination of other body fluids, substances and tissues, without diagnosis
R90-R94	Abnormal findings on diagnostic imaging and in function studies, without diagnosis
R97	Abnormal tumor markers
R99	Ill-defined and unknown cause of mortality

SYMPTOMS AND SIGNS INVOLVING THE CIRCULATORY AND RESPIRATORY SYSTEMS (R00-R09)

R00   **Abnormalities of heart beat**

Excludes1: abnormalities originating in the perinatal period (P29.1-)

Excludes2: specified arrhythmias (I47-I49)

R00.0   Tachycardia, unspecified

Rapid heart beat

Sinoauricular tachycardia NOS

Sinus [sinusal] tachycardia NOS

Excludes1: neonatal tachycardia (P29.11)

paroxysmal tachycardia (I47.-)

R00.1   Bradycardia, unspecified

Sinoatrial bradycardia

Sinus bradycardia

Slow heart beat

Vagal bradycardia

Use additional code for adverse effect, if applicable, to identify drug (T36-T50 with fifth or sixth character 5)

Excludes1: neonatal bradycardia (P29.12)

R00.2   Palpitations

Awareness of heart beat

R00.8   Other abnormalities of heart beat

R00.9   Unspecified abnormalities of heart beat

R01   **Cardiac murmurs and other cardiac sounds**

Excludes1: cardiac murmurs and sounds originating in the perinatal period (P29.8)

R01.0   Benign and innocent cardiac murmurs

Functional cardiac murmur

R01.1   Cardiac murmur, unspecified

Cardiac bruit NOS

Heart murmur NOS

Systolic murmur NOS

R01.2   Other cardiac sounds

Cardiac dullness, increased or decreased

Precordial friction

R03   **Abnormal blood-pressure reading, without diagnosis**

R03.0   Elevated blood-pressure reading, without diagnosis of hypertension

Note: This category is to be used to record an episode of elevated blood pressure in a patient in whom no formal diagnosis of hypertension has been made, or as an isolated incidental finding.

R03.1   Nonspecific low blood-pressure reading

Excludes1: hypotension (I95.-)

maternal hypotension syndrome (O26.5-)

neurogenic orthostatic hypotension (G90.3)

R04   **Hemorrhage from respiratory passages**

R04.0   Epistaxis

Hemorrhage from nose Nosebleed

R04.1   Hemorrhage from throat

Excludes2: hemoptysis (R04.2)

R04.2   Hemoptysis

Blood-stained sputum

Cough with hemorrhage

R04.8   Hemorrhage from other sites in respiratory passages

R04.81   Acute idiopathic pulmonary hemorrhage in infants

AIPHI

Acute idiopathic hemorrhage in infants over 28 days old

> **Excludes1:** perinatal pulmonary hemorrhage (P26.-)
>
> von Willebrand's disease (D68.0)

R04.89 **Hemorrhage from other sites in respiratory passages**

Pulmonary hemorrhage NOS

R04.9 **Hemorrhage from respiratory passages, unspecified**

R05 **Cough**

> **Excludes1:** cough with hemorrhage (R04.2)
>
> smoker's cough (J41.0)

R06 **Abnormalities of breathing**

> **Excludes1:** acute respiratory distress syndrome (J80)
>
> respiratory arrest (R09.2)
>
> respiratory arrest of newborn (P28.81)
>
> respiratory distress syndrome of newborn (P22.-)
>
> respiratory failure (J96.-)
>
> respiratory failure of newborn (P28.5)

R06.0 **Dyspnea**

> **Excludes1:** tachypnea NOS (R06.82)
>
> transient tachypnea of newborn (P22.1)

R06.00 **Dyspnea, unspecified**

R06.01 **Orthopnea**

R06.02 **Shortness of breath**

● **R06.03** **Acute respiratory distress**

R06.09 **Other forms of dyspnea**

R06.1 **Stridor**

> **Excludes1:** congenital laryngeal stridor (P28.89)
>
> laryngismus (stridulus) (J38.5)

R06.2 **Wheezing**

> **Excludes1:** Asthma (J45.-)

R06.3 **Periodic breathing**

Cheyne-Stokes breathing

R06.4 **Hyperventilation**

> **Excludes1:** psychogenic hyperventilation (F45.8)

R06.5 **Mouth breathing**

> **Excludes2:** dry mouth NOS (R68.2)

R06.6 **Hiccough**

> **Excludes1:** psychogenic hiccough (F45.8)

R06.7 **Sneezing**

R06.8 **Other abnormalities of breathing**

R06.81 **Apnea, not elsewhere classified**

Apnea NOS

> **Excludes1:** apnea (of) newborn (P28.4)
>
> sleep apnea (G47.3-)
>
> sleep apnea of newborn (primary) (P28.3)

R06.82 **Tachypnea, not elsewhere classified**

Tachypnea NOS

> **Excludes1:** transitory tachypnea of newborn (P22.1)

R06.83 **Snoring**

R06.89 **Other abnormalities of breathing**

Breath-holding (spells)

Sighing

R06.9 **Unspecified abnormalities of breathing**

R07 **Pain in throat and chest**

> **Excludes1:** epidemic myalgia (B33.0)
>
> **Excludes2:** jaw pain R68.84
>
> pain in breast (N64.4)

R07.0 **Pain in throat**

> **Excludes1:** chronic sore throat (J31.2)
>
> sore throat (acute) NOS (J02.9)
>
> **Excludes2:** dysphagia (R13.1-)
>
> pain in neck (M54.2)

R07.1 **Chest pain on breathing**

Painful respiration

R07.2 **Precordial pain**

R07.8 **Other chest pain**

R07.81 **Pleurodynia**

Pleurodynia NOS

> **Excludes1:** epidemic pleurodynia (B33.0)

R07.82 **Intercostal pain**

R07.89 **Other chest pain**

Anterior chest-wall pain NOS

R07.9 **Chest pain, unspecified**

R09 **Other symptoms and signs involving the circulatory and respiratory system**

> **Excludes1:** acute respiratory distress syndrome (J80)
>
> respiratory arrest of newborn (P28.81)
>
> respiratory distress syndrome of newborn (P22.0)
>
> respiratory failure (J96.-)
>
> respiratory failure of newborn (P28.5)

R09.0 **Asphyxia and hypoxemia**

> **Excludes1:** asphyxia due to carbon monoxide (T58.-)
>
> asphyxia due to foreign body in respiratory tract (T17.-)
>
> birth (intrauterine) asphyxia (P84)
>
> hyperventilation (R06.4) traumatic asphyxia (T71.-)
>
> **Excludes2:** hypercapnia (R06.89)

R09.01 **Asphyxia**

R09.02 **Hypoxemia**

R09.1 **Pleurisy**

> **Excludes1:** pleurisy with effusion (J90)

R09.2 **Respiratory arrest**

Cardiorespiratory failure

> **Excludes1:** cardiac arrest (I46.-)
>
> respiratory arrest of newborn (P28.81)
>
> respiratory distress of newborn (P22.0)
>
> respiratory failure (J96.-)
>
> respiratory failure of newborn (P28.5)
>
> respiratory insufficiency (R06.89)
>
> respiratory insufficiency of newborn (P28.5)

R09.3 **Abnormal sputum**

Abnormal amount of sputum

Abnormal color of sputum

Abnormal odor of sputum

Excessive sputum

> **Excludes1:** blood-stained sputum (R04.2)

R09.8 **Other specified symptoms and signs involving the circulatory and respiratory systems**

R09.81 **Nasal congestion**

R09.82 **Postnasal drip**

R09.89 **Other specified symptoms and signs involving the circulatory and respiratory systems**

Bruit (arterial)

Abnormal chest percussion

Feeling of foreign body in throat

Friction sounds in chest

Chest tympany Choking sensation

Rales

Weak pulse

> **Excludes2:** foreign body in throat (T17.2-)
>
> wheezing (R06.2)

SYMPTOMS AND SIGNS INVOLVING THE DIGESTIVE SYSTEM AND ABDOMEN (R10-R19)

Excludes2: congenital or infantile pylorospasm (Q40.0)

gastrointestinal hemorrhage (K92.0-K92.2)

intestinal obstruction (K56.-)

newborn gastrointestinal hemorrhage (P54.0-P54.3)

newborn intestinal obstruction (P76.-)

pylorospasm (K31.3)

signs and symptoms involving the urinary system (R30-R39)

symptoms referable to female genital organs (N94.-)

symptoms referable to male genital organs (N48-N50)

R10   Abdominal and pelvic pain

> **Excludes1:** renal colic (N23)
>
> **Excludes2:** dorsalgia (M54.-)
>
> flatulence and related conditions (R14.-)

R10.0   Acute abdomen

Severe abdominal pain (generalized) (with abdominal rigidity)

> **Excludes1:** abdominal rigidity NOS (R19.3)
>
> generalized abdominal pain NOS (R10.84)
>
> localized abdominal pain (R10.1-R10.3-)

R10.1   Pain localized to upper abdomen

R10.10   Upper abdominal pain, unspecified

R10.11   Right upper quadrant pain

R10.12   Left upper quadrant pain

R10.13   Epigastric pain

Dyspepsia

> **Excludes1:** functional dyspepsia (K30)

R10.2   Pelvic and perineal pain

> **Excludes1:** vulvodynia (N94.81)

R10.3   Pain localized to other parts of lower abdomen

R10.30   Lower abdominal pain, unspecified

R10.31   Right lower quadrant pain

R10.32   Left lower quadrant pain

R10.33   Periumbilical pain

R10.8   Other abdominal pain

R10.81   Abdominal tenderness

Abdominal tenderness NOS

R10.811   Right upper quadrant abdominal tenderness

R10.812   Left upper quadrant abdominal tenderness

R10.813   Right lower quadrant abdominal tenderness

R10.814   Left lower quadrant abdominal tenderness

R10.815   Periumbilic abdominal tenderness

R10.816   Epigastric abdominal tenderness

R10.817   Generalized abdominal tenderness

R10.819   Abdominal tenderness, unspecified site

R10.82   Rebound abdominal tenderness

R10.821   Right upper quadrant rebound abdominal tenderness

R10.822   Left upper quadrant rebound abdominal tenderness

R10.823   Right lower quadrant rebound abdominal tenderness

R10.824   Left lower quadrant rebound abdominal tenderness

R10.825   Periumbilic rebound abdominal tenderness

R10.826   Epigastric rebound abdominal tenderness

R10.827   Generalized rebound abdominal tenderness

R10.829   Rebound abdominal tenderness, unspecified site

R10.83   Colic

Colic NOS

Infantile colic

> **Excludes1:** colic in adult and child over 12 months old (R10.84)

R10.84   Generalized abdominal pain

> **Excludes1:** generalized abdominal pain associated with acute abdomen (R10.0)

R10.9   Unspecified abdominal pain

R11   Nausea and vomiting

> **Excludes1:** cyclical vomiting associated with migraine (G43.A-)
>
> excessive vomiting in pregnancy (O21.-)
>
> hematemesis (K92.0)
>
> neonatal hematemesis (P54.0)
>
> newborn vomiting (P92.0-)
>
> psychogenic vomiting (F50.89)
>
> vomiting associated with bulimia nervosa (F50.2)
>
> vomiting following gastrointestinal surgery (K91.0)

R11.0   Nausea

Nausea NOS

Nausea without vomiting

R11.1   Vomiting

R11.10   Vomiting, unspecified

Vomiting NOS

R11.11   Vomiting without nausea

R11.12   Projectile vomiting

R11.13   Vomiting of fecal matter

R11.14   Bilious vomiting

Bilious emesis

R11.2   Nausea with vomiting, unspecified

Persistent nausea with vomiting NOS

R12   Heartburn

> **Excludes1:** dyspepsia NOS (R10.13)
>
> functional dyspepsia (K30)

R13   Aphagia and dysphagia

R13.0   Aphagia

Inability to swallow

> **Excludes1:** psychogenic aphagia (F50.9)

R13.1   Dysphagia

Code first, if applicable, dysphagia following cerebrovascular disease (I69. with final characters -91)

Excludes1: psychogenic dysphagia (F45.8)

R13.10 Dysphagia, unspecified

Difficulty in swallowing NOS

R13.11 Dysphagia, oral phase

R13.12 Dysphagia, oropharyngeal phase

R13.13 Dysphagia, pharyngeal phase

R13.14 Dysphagia, pharyngoesophageal phase

R13.19 Other dysphagia

Cervical dysphagia Neurogenic dysphagia

R14 Flatulence and related conditions

Excludes1: psychogenic aerophagy (F45.8)

R14.0 Abdominal distension (gaseous)

Bloating

Tympanites (abdominal) (intestinal)

R14.1 Gas pain

R14.2 Eructation

R14.3 Flatulence

R15 Fecal incontinence

Includes: encopresis NOS

Excludes1: fecal incontinence of nonorganic origin (F98.1)

R15.0 Incomplete defecation

Excludes1: constipation (K59.0-)

fecal impaction (K56.41)

R15.1 Fecal smearing

Fecal soiling

R15.2 Fecal urgency

R15.9 Full incontinence of feces

Fecal incontinence NOS

R16 Hepatomegaly and splenomegaly, not elsewhere classified

Definition: Cleft lip is a congenital deformity characterized by a vertical cleft or pair of clefts in the upper lip, with or without involvement of the palate. Cleft palate is a congenital fissure in the roof of the mouth, resulting from incomplete fusion of the palate during embryonic development.

R16.0 Hepatomegaly, not elsewhere classified

Hepatomegaly NOS

R16.1 Splenomegaly, not elsewhere classified

Splenomegaly NOS

R16.2 Hepatomegaly with splenomegaly, not elsewhere classified

Hepatosplenomegaly NOS

R17 Unspecified jaundice

Excludes1: neonatal jaundice (P55, P57-P59)

R18 Ascites

Includes: fluid in peritoneal cavity

Excludes1: ascites in alcoholic cirrhosis (K70.31)

ascites in alcoholic hepatitis (K70.11)

ascites in toxic liver disease with chronic active hepatitis (K71.51)

R18.0 Malignant ascites

Code first malignancy, such as:

malignant neoplasm of ovary (C56.-)

secondary malignant neoplasm of retroperitoneum and peritoneum (C78.6)

R18.8 Other ascites

Ascites NOS

Peritoneal effusion (chronic)

R19 Other symptoms and signs involving the digestive system and abdomen

Excludes1: acute abdomen (R10.0)

R19.0 Intra-abdominal and pelvic swelling, mass and lump

Excludes1: abdominal distension (gaseous) (R14.-)

ascites (R18.-)

R19.00 Intra-abdominal and pelvic swelling, mass and lump, unspecified site

R19.01 Right upper quadrant abdominal swelling, mass and lump

R19.02 Left upper quadrant abdominal swelling, mass and lump

R19.03 Right lower quadrant abdominal swelling, mass and lump

R19.04 Left lower quadrant abdominal swelling, mass and lump

R19.05 Periumbilic swelling, mass or lump

Diffuse or generalized umbilical swelling or mass

R19.06 Epigastric swelling, mass or lump

R19.07 Generalized intra-abdominal and pelvic swelling, mass and lump

Diffuse or generalized intra-abdominal swelling or mass NOS

Diffuse or generalized pelvic swelling or mass NOS

R19.09 Other intra-abdominal and pelvic swelling, mass and lump

R19.1 Abnormal bowel sounds

R19.11 Absent bowel sounds

R19.12 Hyperactive bowel sounds

R19.15 Other abnormal bowel sounds

Abnormal bowel sounds NOS

R19.2 Visible peristalsis

Definition: Peristalsis is the involuntary constriction and relaxation of the muscles of the intestine or another canal, creating wavelike movements that push the contents of the canal forward.

Hyperperistalsis

R19.3 Abdominal rigidity

Excludes1: abdominal rigidity with severe abdominal pain (R10.0)

R19.30 Abdominal rigidity, unspecified site

R19.31 Right upper quadrant abdominal rigidity

R19.32 Left upper quadrant abdominal rigidity

R19.33 Right lower quadrant abdominal rigidity

R19.34 Left lower quadrant abdominal rigidity

R19.35 Periumbilic abdominal rigidity

R19.36 Epigastric abdominal rigidity

R19.37 Generalized abdominal rigidity

R19.4 Change in bowel habit

Excludes1: constipation (K59.0-)

functional diarrhea (K59.1)

R19.5 Other fecal abnormalities

Abnormal stool color

Bulky stools

Mucus in stools

Occult blood in feces

Occult blood in stools

Excludes1: melena (K92.1)

    neonatal melena (P54.1)

R19.6   **Halitosis**

R19.7   **Diarrhea, unspecified**

  Diarrhea NOS

  Excludes1: functional diarrhea (K59.1)

    neonatal diarrhea (P78.3)

    psychogenic diarrhea (F45.8)

R19.8   **Other specified symptoms and signs involving the digestive system and abdomen**

SYMPTOMS AND SIGNS INVOLVING THE SKIN AND SUBCUTANEOUS TISSUE (R20-R23)

Excludes2: symptoms relating to breast (N64.4-N64.5)

R20   **Disturbances of skin sensation**

  Excludes1: dissociative anesthesia and sensory loss (F44.6)

    psychogenic disturbances (F45.8)

R20.0   **Anesthesia of skin**

R20.1   **Hypoesthesia of skin**

R20.2   **Paresthesia of skin**

  Formication

  Pins and needles

  Tingling skin

  Excludes1: acroparesthesia (I73.8)

R20.3   **Hyperesthesia**

R20.8   **Other disturbances of skin sensation**

R20.9   **Unspecified disturbances of skin sensation**

R21   **Rash and other nonspecific skin eruption**

  Includes: rash NOS

  Excludes1: specified type of rash- code to condition

    vesicular eruption (R23.8)

R22   **Localized swelling, mass and lump of skin and subcutaneous tissue**

  Includes: subcutaneous nodules (localized)(superficial)

  Excludes1: abnormal findings on diagnostic imaging (R90-R93)

    edema (R60.-)

    enlarged lymph nodes (R59.-) \

    localized adiposity (E65)

    swelling of joint (M25.4-)

R22.0   **Localized swelling, mass and lump, head**

R22.1   **Localized swelling, mass and lump, neck**

R22.2   **Localized swelling, mass and lump, trunk**

  Excludes1: intra-abdominal or pelvic mass and lump (R19.0-)

    intra-abdominal or pelvic swelling (R19.0-)

  Excludes2: breast mass and lump (N63)

R22.3   **Localized swelling, mass and lump, upper limb**

  R22.30   **Localized swelling, mass and lump, unspecified upper limb**

  R22.31   **Localized swelling, mass and lump, right upper limb**

  R22.32   **Localized swelling, mass and lump, left upper limb**

  R22.33   **Localized swelling, mass and lump, upper limb, bilateral**

R22.4   **Localized swelling, mass and lump, lower limb**

  R22.40   **Localized swelling, mass and lump, unspecified lower limb**

  R22.41   **Localized swelling, mass and lump, right lower limb**

  R22.42   **Localized swelling, mass and lump, left lower limb**

  R22.43   **Localized swelling, mass and lump, lower limb, bilateral**

R22.9   **Localized swelling, mass and lump, unspecified**

R23   **Other skin changes**

R23.0   **Cyanosis**

  Excludes1: acrocyanosis (I73.8)

    cyanotic attacks of newborn (P28.2)

R23.1   **Pallor** Clammy skin

R23.2   **Flushing**

  Excessive blushing

  Code first, if applicable, menopausal and female climacteric states (N95.1)

R23.3   **Spontaneous ecchymoses**

  Petechiae

  Excludes1: ecchymoses of newborn (P54.5)

    purpura (D69.-)

R23.4   **Changes in skin texture**

  Desquamation of skin

  Induration of skin

  Scaling of skin

  Excludes1: epidermal thickening NOS (L85.9)

R23.8   **Other skin changes**

R23.9   **Unspecified skin changes**

SYMPTOMS AND SIGNS INVOLVING THE NERVOUS AND MUSCULOSKELETAL SYSTEMS (R25-R29)

R25   **Abnormal involuntary movements**

  Excludes1: specific movement disorders (G20-G26)

    stereotyped movement disorders (F98.4)

    tic disorders (F95.-)

R25.0   **Abnormal head movements**

R25.1   **Tremor, unspecified**

  Excludes1: chorea NOS (G25.5)

    essential tremor (G25.0)

    hysterical tremor (F44.4)

    intention tremor (G25.2)

R25.2   **Cramp and spasm**

  Excludes2: carpopedal spasm (R29.0)

    charley-horse (M62.831)

    infantile spasms (G40.4-)

    muscle spasm of back (M62.830)

    muscle spasm of calf (M62.831)

R25.3   **Fasciculation**

  Twitching NOS

R25.8   **Other abnormal involuntary movements**

R25.9   **Unspecified abnormal involuntary movements**

R26   **Abnormalities of gait and mobility**

  Excludes1: ataxia NOS (R27.0)

    hereditary ataxia (G11.-)

    locomotor (syphilitic) ataxia (A52.11)

    immobility syndrome (paraplegic) (M62.3)

R26.0   **Ataxic gait**

  Staggering gait

R26.1   **Paralytic gait**

Spastic gait

R26.2 **Difficulty in walking, not elsewhere classified**

Excludes1: falling (R29.6)

unsteadiness on feet (R26.81)

R26.8 **Other abnormalities of gait and mobility**

R26.81 **Unsteadiness on feet**

R26.89 **Other abnormalities of gait and mobility**

R26.9 **Unspecified abnormalities of gait and mobility**

R27 **Other lack of coordination**

Excludes1: ataxic gait (R26.0)

hereditary ataxia (G11.-)

vertigo NOS (R42)

R27.0 **Ataxia, unspecified**

Excludes1: ataxia following cerebrovascular disease (I69. with final characters -93)

R27.8 **Other lack of coordination**

R27.9 **Unspecified lack of coordination**

R29 **Other symptoms and signs involving the nervous and musculoskeletal systems**

R29.0 **Tetany** Carpopedal spasm

Excludes1: hysterical tetany (F44.5)

neonatal tetany (P71.3)

parathyroid tetany (E20.9)

post-thyroidectomy tetany (E89.2)

R29.1 **Meningismus**

R29.2 **Abnormal reflex**

Excludes2: abnormal pupillary reflex (H57.0)

hyperactive gag reflex (J39.2)

vasovagal reaction or syncope (R55)

R29.3 **Abnormal posture**

R29.4 **Clicking hip**

Excludes1: congenital deformities of hip (Q65.-)

R29.5 **Transient paralysis**

Code first any associated spinal cord injury (S14.0, S14.1-, S24.0, S24.1-, S34.0-, S34.1-)

Excludes1: transient ischemic attack (G45.9)

R29.6 **Repeated falls**

Falling

Tendency to fall

Excludes2: at risk for falling (Z91.81)

history of falling (Z91.81)

R29.7 **National Institutes of Health Stroke Scale (NIHSS) score**

Code first the type of cerebral infarction (I63-)

R29.70 **NIHSS score 0-9**

R29.700 **NIHSS score 0**

R29.701 **NIHSS score 1**

R29.702 **NIHSS score 2**

R29.703 **NIHSS score 3**

R29.704 **NIHSS score 4**

R29.705 **NIHSS score 5**

R29.706 **NIHSS score 6**

R29.707 **NIHSS score 7**

R29.708 **NIHSS score 8**

R29.709 **NIHSS score 9**

R29.71 **NIHSS score 10-19**

R29.710 **NIHSS score 10**

R29.711 **NIHSS score 11**

R29.712 **NIHSS score 12**

R29.713 **NIHSS score 13**

R29.714 **NIHSS score 14**

R29.715 **NIHSS score 15**

R29.716 **NIHSS score 16**

R29.717 **NIHSS score 17**

R29.718 **NIHSS score 18**

R29.719 **NIHSS score 19**

R29.72 **NIHSS score 20-29**

R29.720 **NIHSS score 20**

R29.721 **NIHSS score 21**

R29.722 **NIHSS score 22**

R29.723 **NIHSS score 23**

R29.724 **NIHSS score 24**

R29.725 **NIHSS score 25**

R29.726 **NIHSS score 26**

R29.727 **NIHSS score 27**

R29.728 **NIHSS score 28**

R29.729 **NIHSS score 29**

R29.73 **NIHSS score 30-39**

R29.730 **NIHSS score 30**

R29.731 **NIHSS score 31**

R29.732 **NIHSS score 32**

R29.733 **NIHSS score 33**

R29.734 **NIHSS score 34**

R29.735 **NIHSS score 35**

R29.736 **NIHSS score 36**

R29.737 **NIHSS score 37**

R29.738 **NIHSS score 38**

R29.739 **NIHSS score 39**

R29.74 **NIHSS score 40-42**

R29.740 **NIHSS score 40**

R29.741 **NIHSS score 41**

R29.742 **NIHSS score 42**

R29.8 **Other symptoms and signs involving the nervous and musculoskeletal systems**

R29.81 **Other symptoms and signs involving the nervous system**

R29.810 **Facial weakness**

Facial droop

Excludes1: Bell's palsy (G51.0)

facial weakness following cerebrovascular disease (I69. with final characters -92)

R29.818 **Other symptoms and signs involving the nervous system**

R29.89 **Other symptoms and signs involving the musculoskeletal system**

Excludes2: pain in limb (M79.6-)

R29.890 **Loss of height**

Excludes1: osteoporosis (M80-M81)

R29.891 **Ocular torticollis**

Excludes1: congenital (sternomastoid) torticollis Q68.0

psychogenic torticollis (F45.8)

spasmodic torticollis (G24.3)

torticollis due to birth injury

(P15.8)

torticollis NOS M43.6

R29.898 **Other symptoms and signs involving the musculoskeletal system**

R29.9 **Unspecified symptoms and signs involving the nervous and musculoskeletal systems**

R29.90 **Unspecified symptoms and signs involving the nervous system**

R29.91 **Unspecified symptoms and signs involving the musculoskeletal system**

SYMPTOMS AND SIGNS INVOLVING THE GENITOURINARY SYSTEM (R30-R39)

R30 **Pain associated with micturition**

Excludes1: psychogenic pain associated with micturition (F45.8)

R30.0 **Dysuria**

Strangury

R30.1 **Vesical tenesmus**

R30.9 **Painful micturition, unspecified**

Painful urination NOS

R31 **Hematuria**

Excludes1: hematuria included with underlying conditions, such as:

acute cystitis with hematuria (N30.01)

recurrent and persistent hematuria in glomerular diseases (N02.-)

R31.0 **Gross hematuria**

R31.1 **Benign essential microscopic hematuria**

R31.2 **Other microscopic hematuria**

R31.21 **Asymptomatic microscopic hematuria**

AMH

R31.29 **Other microscopic hematuria**

R31.9 **Hematuria, unspecified**

R32 **Unspecified urinary incontinence**

Enuresis NOS

Excludes1: functional urinary incontinence (R39.81)

nonorganic enuresis (F98.0)

stress incontinence and other specified urinary incontinence (N39.3-N39.4-)

urinary incontinence associated with cognitive impairment (R39.81)

R33 **Retention of urine**

Excludes1: psychogenic retention of urine (F45.8)

R33.0 **Drug induced retention of urine**

Use additional code for adverse effect, if applicable, to identify drug (T36-T50 with fifth or sixth character 5)

R33.8 **Other retention of urine**

Code first, if applicable, any causal condition, such as:

enlarged prostate (N40.1)

R33.9 **Retention of urine, unspecified**

R34 **Anuria and oliguria**

Excludes1: anuria and oliguria complicating abortion or ectopic or molar pregnancy (O00-O07, O08.4)

anuria and oliguria complicating pregnancy (O26.83-)

anuria and oliguria complicating the puerperium (O90.4)

R35 **Polyuria**

Code first, if applicable, any causal condition, such as:

enlarged prostate (N40.1)

Excludes1: psychogenic polyuria (F45.8)

R35.0 **Frequency of micturition**

R35.1 **Nocturia**

R35.8 **Other polyuria**

Polyuria NOS

R36 **Urethral discharge**

R36.0 **Urethral discharge without blood**

R36.1 **Hematospermia**

R36.9 **Urethral discharge, unspecified**

Penile discharge NOS

Urethrorrhea

R37 **Sexual dysfunction, unspecified**

R39 **Other and unspecified symptoms and signs involving the genitourinary system**

R39.0 **Extravasation of urine**

R39.1 **Other difficulties with micturition**

Code first, if applicable, any causal condition, such as:

enlarged prostate (N40.1)

R39.11 **Hesitancy of micturition**

R39.12 **Poor urinary stream**

Weak urinary steam

R39.13 **Splitting of urinary stream**

R39.14 **Feeling of incomplete bladder emptying**

R39.15 **Urgency of urination**

Excludes1: urge incontinence (N39.41, N39.46)

R39.16 **Straining to void**

R39.19 **Other difficulties with micturition**

R39.191 **Need to immediately re-void**

R39.192 **Position dependent micturition**

R39.198 **Other difficulties with micturition**

R39.2 **Extrarenal uremia**

Prerenal uremia

Excludes1: uremia NOS (N19)

R39.8 **Other symptoms and signs involving the genitourinary system**

R39.81 **Functional urinary incontinence**

Urinary incontinence due to cognitive impairment, or severe physical disability or immobility

Excludes1: stress incontinence and other specified urinary incontinence (N39.3-N39.4-)

urinary incontinence NOS (R32)

R39.82 **Chronic bladder pain**

• R39.83 **Unilateral non-palpable testicle**

• R39.84 **Bilateral non-palpable testicles**

R39.89 **Other symptoms and signs involving the genitourinary system**

R39.9 **Unspecified symptoms and signs involving the genitourinary system**

SYMPTOMS AND SIGNS INVOLVING COGNITION, PERCEPTION, EMOTIONAL STATE AND BEHAVIOR (R40-R46)

Excludes2: symptoms and signs constituting part of a pattern of mental disorder (F01-F99)

R40 **Somnolence, stupor and coma**

Definition: Somnolence (or "drowsiness") is a state of near-sleep, a strong desire for sleep, or sleeping for unusually long periods (cf. hypersomnia).

Excludes1: neonatal coma (P91.5)

somnolence, stupor and coma in diabetes (E08-E13)

somnolence, stupor and coma in hepatic failure (K72.-)

somnolence, stupor and coma in hypoglycemia (nondiabetic) (E15)

R40.0 **Somnolence**

Drowsiness

Excludes1: coma (R40.2-)

R40.1 **Stupor** Catatonic stupor

Semicoma

Excludes1: catatonic schizophrenia (F20.2)

coma (R40.2-)

depressive stupor (F31-F33)

dissociative stupor (F44.2)

manic stupor (F30.2)

R40.2 **Coma**

Code first any associated:

fracture of skull (S02.-)

intracranial injury (S06.-)

Note: One code from each subcategory, R40.21-R40.23, is required to complete the coma scale

R40.20 **Unspecified coma**

Coma NOS

Unconsciousness NOS

R40.21 **Coma scale, eyes open**

The following appropriate 7th character is to be added to subcategory R40.21-:

0 - unspecified time

1 - in the field [EMT or ambulance]

2 - at arrival to emergency department

3 - at hospital admission

4 - 24 hours or more after hospital admission

⑦**R40.211** **Coma scale, eyes open, never**

⑦**R40.212** **Coma scale, eyes open, to pain**

⑦**R40.213** **Coma scale, eyes open, to sound**

⑦**R40.214** **Coma scale, eyes open, spontaneous**

R40.22 **Coma scale, best verbal response**

The following appropriate 7th character is to be added to subcategory R40.22-:

0 - unspecified time

1 - in the field [EMT or ambulance]

2 - at arrival to emergency department

3 - at hospital admission

4 - 24 hours or more after hospital admission

⑦**R40.221** **Coma scale, best verbal response, none**

⑦**R40.222** **Coma scale, best verbal response, incomprehensible words**

Incomprehensible sounds (2-5 years of age)

Moans/grunts to pain; restless (<2 years old)

⑦**R40.223** **Coma scale, best verbal response, inappropriate words**

Inappropriate crying or screaming (< 2 years of age)

Screaming (2-5 years of age)

⑦**R40.224** **Coma scale, best verbal response, confused conversation**

Inappropriate words (2-5 years of age)

Irritable cries (< 2 years of age)

⑦**R40.225** **Coma scale, best verbal response, oriented**

Cooing or babbling or crying appropriately (< 2 years of age)

Uses appropriate words (2- 5 years of age)

R40.23 **Coma scale, best motor response**

The following appropriate 7th character is to be added to subcategory R40.23-:

0 - unspecified time

1 - in the field [EMT or ambulance]

2 - at arrival to emergency department

3 - at hospital admission

4 - 24 hours or more after hospital admission

⑦**R40.231** **Coma scale, best motor response, none**

⑦**R40.232** **Coma scale, best motor response, extension**

Abnormal extensor posturing to pain or noxious stimuli (< 2 years of age)

Extensor posturing to pain or noxious stimuli (2-5 years of age)

⑦**R40.233** **Coma scale, best motor response, abnormal**

Abnormal flexure posturing to pain or noxious stimuli (0-5 years of age)

Flexion/decorticate posturing (< 2 years of age)

⑦**R40.234** **Coma scale, best motor response, flexion withdrawal**

Withdraws from pain or noxious stimuli (0-5 years of age)

⑦**R40.235** **Coma scale, best motor response, localizes pain**

Localizes pain (2-5 years of age)

Withdraws to touch (< 2 years of age)

⑦**R40.236** **Coma scale, best motor response, obeys commands**

Normal or spontaneous movement (< 2 years of age)

Obeys commands (2-5 years of age)

R40.24 **Glasgow coma scale, total score**

Note: Assign a code from subcategory R40.24, when only the total coma score is documented

The following appropriate 7th character is to be added to subcategory R40.24-:

0 - unspecified time

1 - in the field [EMT or ambulance]

2 - at arrival to emergency department

3 - at hospital admission

4 - 24 hours or more after hospital admission

⑦**R40.241** **Glasgow coma scale score 13-15**

⑦**R40.242** **Glasgow coma scale score 9-12**

⑦**R40.243** **Glasgow coma scale score 3-8**

⑦**R40.244** **Other coma, without documented Glasgow coma scale score, or with partial score reported**

R40.3 **Persistent vegetative state**

R40.4 **Transient alteration of awareness**

R41 **Other symptoms and signs involving cognitive functions and awareness**

Excludes1: dissociative [conversion] disorders (F44.-)

mild cognitive impairment, so stated (G31.84)

R41.0 **Disorientation, unspecified**

Confusion NOS

Delirium NOS

R41.1 **Anterograde amnesia**

R41.2 **Retrograde amnesia**

R41.3 **Other amnesia**

Amnesia NOS

Memory loss NOS

Excludes1: amnestic disorder due to known physiologic condition (F04)

amnestic syndrome due to psychoactive substance use (F10-F19 with 5th character .6)

mild memory disturbance due to known physiological condition (F06.8)

transient global amnesia (G45.4)

R41.4 **Neurologic neglect syndrome**

Asomatognosia

Hemi-akinesia

Hemi-inattention

Hemispatial neglect

Left-sided neglect

Sensory neglect

Visuospatial neglect

Excludes1: visuospatial deficit (R41.842)

R41.8 **Other symptoms and signs involving cognitive functions and awareness**

R41.81 **Age-related cognitive decline**

Senility NOS

R41.82 **Altered mental status, unspecified**

Change in mental status NOS

Excludes1: altered level of consciousness (R40.-)

altered mental status due to known condition - code to condition delirium NOS (R41.0)

R41.83 **Borderline intellectual functioning**

IQ level 71 to 84

Excludes1: intellectual disabilities (F70-F79)

R41.84 **Other specified cognitive deficit**

Excludes1: cognitive deficits as sequelae of cerebrovascular disease (I69.01-, I69.11-, I69.21-, I69.31-, I69.81-, I69.91-)

R41.840 **Attention and concentration deficit**

Excludes1: attention-deficit hyperactivity disorders (F90.-)

R41.841 **Cognitive communication deficit**

R41.842 **Visuospatial deficit**

R41.843 **Psychomotor deficit**

R41.844 **Frontal lobe and executive function deficit**

R41.89 **Other symptoms and signs involving cognitive functions and awareness**

Anosognosia

R41.9 **Unspecified symptoms and signs involving cognitive functions and awareness**

Unspecified neurocognitive disorder

R42 **Dizziness and giddiness**

Light-headedness

Vertigo NOS

Excludes1: vertiginous syndromes (H81.-)

vertigo from infrasound (T75.23)

R43 **Disturbances of smell and taste**

R43.0 **Anosmia**

R43.1 **Parosmia**

R43.2 **Parageusia**

R43.8 **Other disturbances of smell and taste**

Mixed disturbance of smell and taste

R43.9 **Unspecified disturbances of smell and taste**

R44 **Other symptoms and signs involving general sensations and perceptions**

Excludes1: alcoholic hallucinations (F1.5)

hallucinations in drug psychosis (F11-F19 with .5)

hallucinations in mood disorders with psychotic symptoms (F30.2, F31.5, F32.3, F33.3)

hallucinations in schizophrenia, schizotypal and delusional disorders (F20-F29)

Excludes2: disturbances of skin sensation (R20.-)

R44.0 **Auditory hallucinations**

R44.1 **Visual hallucinations**

R44.2 **Other hallucinations**

R44.3 **Hallucinations, unspecified**

R44.8 **Other symptoms and signs involving general sensations and perceptions**

R44.9 **Unspecified symptoms and signs involving general sensations and perceptions**

R45 **Symptoms and signs involving emotional state**

R45.0 **Nervousness**

Nervous tension

R45.1 **Restlessness and agitation**

R45.2 **Unhappiness**

R45.3 **Demoralization and apathy**

Excludes1: anhedonia (R45.84)

R45.4 **Irritability and anger**

R45.5 **Hostility**

R45.6 **Violent behavior**

R45.7 **State of emotional shock and stress, unspecified**

R45.8 **Other symptoms and signs involving emotional state**

R45.81 **Low self-esteem**

R45.82 **Worries**

R45.83 **Excessive crying of child, adolescent or adult**

Excludes1: excessive crying of infant (baby) R68.11

R45.84 **Anhedonia**

R45.85 **Homicidal and suicidal ideations**

Excludes1: suicide attempt (T14.91)

R45.850 **Homicidal ideations**

R45.851 **Suicidal ideations**

R45.86 **Emotional lability**

R45.87 **Impulsiveness**

R45.89 **Other symptoms and signs involving emotional state**

R46 **Symptoms and signs involving appearance and behavior**

Excludes1: appearance and behavior in schizophrenia, schizotypal and delusional disorders (F20-F29)

mental and behavioral disorders (F01-F99)

R46.0   Very low level of personal hygiene

R46.1   Bizarre personal appearance

R46.2   Strange and inexplicable behavior

R46.3   Overactivity

R46.4   Slowness and poor responsiveness

    Excludes1: stupor (R40.1)

R46.5   Suspiciousness and marked evasiveness

R46.6   Undue concern and preoccupation with stressful events

R46.7   Verbosity and circumstantial detail obscuring reason for contact

R46.8   Other symptoms and signs involving appearance and behavior

    R46.81   Obsessive-compulsive behavior

        Excludes1: obsessive-compulsive disorder (F42-)

    R46.89   Other symptoms and signs involving appearance and behavior

SYMPTOMS AND SIGNS INVOLVING SPEECH AND VOICE (R47-R49)

R47   Speech disturbances, not elsewhere classified

    Excludes1: autism (F84.0)

        cluttering (F80.81)

        specific developmental disorders of speech and language (F80.-)

        stuttering (F80.81)

R47.0   Dysphasia and aphasia

    R47.01   Aphasia

        Excludes1: aphasia following cerebrovascular disease (I69. with final characters -20)

            progressive isolated aphasia (G31.01)

    R47.02   Dysphasia

        Excludes1: dysphasia following cerebrovascular disease (I69. with final characters -21)

R47.1   Dysarthria and anarthria

    Excludes1: dysarthria following cerebrovascular disease (I69. with final characters -22)

R47.8   Other speech disturbances

    Excludes1: dysarthria following cerebrovascular disease (I69. with final characters -28)

    R47.81   Slurred speech

    R47.82   Fluency disorder in conditions classified elsewhere

        Stuttering in conditions classified elsewhere

        Code first underlying disease or condition, such as:

        Parkinson's disease (G20)

        Excludes1: adult onset fluency disorder (F98.5)

            childhood onset fluency disorder (F80.81)

            fluency disorder (stuttering) following cerebrovascular disease (I69. with final characters -23)

    R47.89   Other speech disturbances

R47.9   Unspecified speech disturbances

R48   Dyslexia and other symbolic dysfunctions, not elsewhere classified

    Definition: Dyslexia is a general term for disorders that involve difficulty in learning to read or interpret words, letters, and other symbols, but that do not affect general intelligence.

    Excludes1: specific developmental disorders of scholastic skills (F81.-)

R48.0   Dyslexia and alexia

R48.1   Agnosia

    Astereognosia (astereognosis)

    Autotopagnosia

    Excludes1: visual object agnosia (R48.3)

R48.2   Apraxia

    Excludes1: apraxia following cerebrovascular disease (I69. with final characters -90)

R48.3   Visual agnosia

    Prosopagnosia

    Simultanagnosia (asimultagnosia)

R48.8   Other symbolic dysfunctions

    Acalculia

    Agraphia

R48.9   Unspecified symbolic dysfunctions

R49   Voice and resonance disorders

    Excludes1: psychogenic voice and resonance disorders (F44.4)

R49.0   Dysphonia

    Hoarseness

R49.1   Aphonia

    Loss of voice

R49.2   Hypernasality and hyponasality

    R49.21   Hypernasality

    R49.22   Hyponasality

R49.8   Other voice and resonance disorders

R49.9   Unspecified voice and resonance disorder

    Change in voice NOS Resonance disorder NOS

GENERAL SYMPTOMS AND SIGNS (R50-R69)

R50   Fever of other and unknown origin

    Excludes1: chills without fever (R68.83)

        febrile convulsions (R56.0-)

        fever of unknown origin during labor (O75.2)

        fever of unknown origin in newborn (P81.9)

        hypothermia due to illness (R68.0)

        malignant hyperthermia due to anesthesia (T88.3)

        puerperal pyrexia NOS (O86.4)

R50.2   Drug induced fever

    Use additional code for adverse effect, if applicable, to identify drug (T36-T50 with fifth or sixth character 5)

    Excludes1: postvaccination (postimmunization) fever (R50.83)

R50.8   Other specified fever

    R50.81   Fever presenting with conditions classified elsewhere

        Code first underlying condition when associated fever is present, such as with:

        leukemia (C91-C95)

        neutropenia (D70.-)

        sickle-cell disease (D57.-)

    R50.82   Postprocedural fever

        Excludes1: postprocedural infection (T81.4-)

            posttransfusion fever (R50.84)

            postvaccination (postimmunization) fever (R50.83)

    R50.83   Postvaccination fever

Postimmunization fever

R50.84   Febrile nonhemolytic transfusion reaction

FNHTR Posttransfusion fever

R50.9   Fever, unspecified

Fever NOS

Fever of unknown origin [FUO]

Fever with chills

Fever with rigors

Hyperpyrexia NOS

Persistent fever

Pyrexia NOS

R51   Headache

Facial pain NOS

Excludes1: atypical face pain (G50.1)

migraine **and other** headache syndromes (G43-G44)

trigeminal neuralgia (G50.0)

R52   Pain, unspecified

Acute pain NOS

Generalized pain NOS

Pain NOS

Excludes1: acute and chronic pain, not elsewhere classified (G89.-)

localized pain, unspecified type - code to pain by site, such as: abdomen pain (R10.-)

back pain (M54.9)

breast pain (N64.4)

chest pain (R07.1-R07.9)

ear pain (H92.0-)

eye pain (H57.1)

headache (R51)

joint pain (M25.5-)

limb pain (M79.6-)

lumbar region pain (M54.5)

pelvic and perineal pain (R10.2)

shoulder pain (M25.51-)

spine pain (M54.-)

throat pain (R07.0)

tongue pain (K14.6)

tooth pain (K08.8)

renal colic (N23)

pain disorders exclusively related to psychological factors (F45.41)

R53   Malaise and fatigue

R53.0   Neoplastic (malignant) related fatigue

Code first associated neoplasm

R53.1   Weakness

Asthenia NOS

Excludes1: age-related weakness (R54)

muscle weakness (M62.8-)

sarcopenia (M62.84)

senile asthenia (R54)

R53.2   Functional quadriplegia

Complete immobility due to severe physical disability or frailty

Excludes1: frailty NOS (R54)

hysterical paralysis (F44.4)

immobility syndrome (M62.3)

neurologic quadriplegia (G82.5-)

quadriplegia (G82.50)

R53.8   Other malaise and fatigue

Excludes1: combat exhaustion and fatigue (F43.0)

congenital debility (P96.9)

exhaustion and fatigue due to excessive exertion (T73.3)

exhaustion and fatigue due to exposure (T73.2)

exhaustion and fatigue due to heat (T67.-)

exhaustion and fatigue due to pregnancy (O26.8-)

exhaustion and fatigue due to recurrent depressive episode (F33)

exhaustion and fatigue due to depressive episode (F32.-)

R53.81   Other malaise

Chronic debility

Debility NOS

General physical deterioration

Malaise NOS

Nervous debility

Excludes1: age-related physical debility (R54)

R53.82   Chronic fatigue, unspecified

Chronic fatigue syndrome NOS

Excludes1: postviral fatigue syndrome (G93.3)

R53.83   Other fatigue

Excludes2: exhaustion and fatigue due to depressive episode (F32.-)

Fatigue NOS

Lack of energy

Lethargy

Tiredness

R54   Age-related physical debility

Frailty

Old age

Senescence

Senile asthenia

Senile debility

Excludes1: age-related cognitive decline (R41.81)

sarcopenia (M62.84)

senile psychosis (F03)

senility NOS (R41.81)

R55   Syncope and collapse

Blackout

Fainting

Vasovagal attack

Excludes1: cardiogenic shock (R57.0)

carotid sinus syncope (G90.01) heat syncope (T67.1)

neurocirculatory asthenia (F45.8)

neurogenic orthostatic hypotension (G90.3)

orthostatic hypotension (I95.1)

postprocedural shock (T81.1-)

psychogenic syncope (F48.8)

shock NOS (R57.9)

shock complicating or following abortion or ectopic or molar pregnancy (O00-O07, O08.3)

shock complicating or following labor and delivery (O75.1)

Stokes-Adams attack (I45.9)

unconsciousness NOS (R40.2-)

R56 Convulsions, not elsewhere classified

Excludes1: dissociative convulsions and seizures (F44.5)

epileptic convulsions and seizures (G40.-)

newborn convulsions and seizures (P90)

R56.0 Febrile convulsions

R56.00 Simple febrile convulsions

Febrile convulsion NOS

Febrile seizure NOS

R56.01 Complex febrile convulsions

Atypical febrile seizure

Complex febrile seizure

Complicated febrile seizure

Excludes1: status epilepticus (G40.901)

R56.1 Post traumatic seizures

Excludes1: post traumatic epilepsy (G40.-)

R56.9 Unspecified convulsions

Convulsion disorder

Fit NOS

Recurrent convulsions

Seizure(s) (convulsive) NOS

R57 Shock, not elsewhere classified

Excludes1: anaphylactic shock NOS (T78.2)

anaphylactic reaction or shock due to adverse food reaction (T78.0-)

anaphylactic shock due to adverse effect of correct drug or medicament properly administered (T88.6)

anaphylactic shock due to serum (T80.5-)

anesthetic shock (T88.3)

electric shock (T75.4)

obstetric shock (O75.1)

postprocedural shock (T81.1-)

psychic shock (F43.0)

shock complicating or following ectopic or molar pregnancy (O00-O07, O08.3)

shock due to lightning (T75.01)

traumatic shock (T79.4)

toxic shock syndrome (A48.3)

R57.0 Cardiogenic shock

Excludes2: septic shock (R65.21)

R57.1 Hypovolemic shock

R57.8 Other shock

R57.9 Shock, unspecified

Failure of peripheral circulation NOS

R58 Hemorrhage, not elsewhere classified

Hemorrhage NOS

Excludes1: hemorrhage included with underlying conditions, such as:

acute duodenal ulcer with hemorrhage (K26.0)

acute gastritis with bleeding (K29.01)

ulcerative enterocolitis with rectal bleeding (K51.01)

R59 Enlarged lymph nodes

Includes: swollen glands

Excludes1: lymphadenitis NOS (I88.9)

acute lymphadenitis (L04.-)

chronic lymphadenitis (I88.1)

mesenteric (acute) (chronic) lymphadenitis (I88.0)

R59.0 Localized enlarged lymph nodes

R59.1 Generalized enlarged lymph nodes

Lymphadenopathy NOS

R59.9 Enlarged lymph nodes, unspecified

R60 Edema, not elsewhere classified

Excludes1: angioneurotic edema (T78.3)

ascites (R18.-)

cerebral edema (G93.6)

cerebral edema due to birth injury (P11.0)

edema of larynx (J38.4)

edema of nasopharynx (J39.2)

edema of pharynx (J39.2)

gestational edema (O12.0-)

hereditary edema (Q82.0)

hydrops fetalis NOS (P83.2)

hydrothorax (J94.8)

hydrops fetalis NOS (P83.2)

newborn edema (P83.3)

pulmonary edema (J81.-)

R60.0 Localized edema

R60.1 Generalized edema

Excludes2: nutritional edema (E40-E46)

R60.9 Edema, unspecified

Fluid retention NOS

R61 Generalized hyperhidrosis

Excessive sweating Night sweats

Secondary hyperhidrosis

Code first, if applicable, menopausal and female climacteric states (N95.1)

Excludes1: focal (primary) (secondary) hyperhidrosis (L74.5-)

Frey's syndrome (L74.52)

localized (primary) (secondary) hyperhidrosis (L74.5-)

R62 Lack of expected normal physiological development in childhood and adults

Excludes1: delayed puberty (E30.0)

gonadal dysgenesis (Q99.1)

hypopituitarism (E23.0)

R62.0 Delayed milestone in childhood

Delayed attainment of expected physiological developmental stage

Late talker

Late walker

R62.5 Other and unspecified lack of expected normal physiological development in childhood

Excludes1: HIV disease resulting in failure to thrive (B20)

physical retardation due to malnutrition (E45)

R62.50 Unspecified lack of expected normal physiological development in childhood

Infantilism NOS

R62.51 Failure to thrive (child)

Failure to gain weight

Excludes1: failure to thrive in child under 28 days old (P92.6)

R62.52 Short stature (child)

Lack of growth

Physical retardation

Short stature NOS

> Excludes1: short stature due to endocrine disorder (E34.3)

R62.59 **Other lack of expected normal physiological development in childhood**

R62.7 **Adult failure to thrive**

R63 **Symptoms and signs concerning food and fluid intake**

> Excludes1: bulimia NOS (F50.2)
>
> eating disorders of nonorganic origin (F50.-)
>
> malnutrition (E40-E46)

R63.0 **Anorexia**

Loss of appetite

> Excludes1: anorexia nervosa (F50.0-)
>
> loss of appetite of nonorganic origin (F50.89)

R63.1 **Polydipsia**

Excessive thirst

R63.2 **Polyphagia**

Excessive eating

Hyperalimentation NOS

R63.3 **Feeding difficulties**

Feeding problem (elderly) (infant) NOS

Picky eater

> Excludes1: eating disorders (F50.-):
>
> feeding problems of newborn (P92.-)
>
> infant feeding disorder of nonorganic origin (F98.2-)

R63.4 **Abnormal weight loss**

R63.5 **Abnormal weight gain**

> Excludes1: excessive weight gain in pregnancy (O26.0-)
>
> obesity (E66.-)

R63.6 **Underweight**

Use additional code to identify body mass index (BMI), if known (Z68.-)

> Excludes1: abnormal weight loss (R63.4)
>
> anorexia nervosa (F50.0-)
>
> malnutrition (E40-E46)

R63.8 **Other symptoms and signs concerning food and fluid intake**

R64 **Cachexia**

Wasting syndrome

Code first underlying condition, if known

> Excludes1: abnormal weight loss (R63.4)
>
> nutritional marasmus (E41)

R65 **Symptoms and signs specifically associated with systemic inflammation and infection**

R65.1 **Systemic inflammatory response syndrome (SIRS) of non-infectious origin**

Code first underlying condition, such as:

heatstroke (T67.0)

injury and trauma (S00-T88)

> Excludes1: sepsis- code to infection
>
> severe sepsis (R65.2)

R65.10 **Systemic inflammatory response syndrome (SIRS) of non-infectious origin without acute organ dysfunction**

Systemic inflammatory response syndrome (SIRS) NOS

R65.11 **Systemic inflammatory response syndrome (SIRS) of non-infectious origin with acute organ dysfunction**

Use additional code to identify specific acute organ dysfunction, such as:

acute kidney failure (N17.-)

acute respiratory failure (J96.0-)

critical illness myopathy (G72.81)

critical illness polyneuropathy (G62.81)

disseminated intravascular coagulopathy [DIC] (D65)

encephalopathy (metabolic) (septic) (G93.41)

hepatic failure (K72.0-)

R65.2 **Severe sepsis**

Infection with associated acute organ dysfunction

Sepsis with acute organ dysfunction

Sepsis with multiple organ dysfunction

Systemic inflammatory response syndrome due to infectious process with acute organ dysfunction

Code first underlying infection, such as:

infection following a procedure (T81.4-)

infections following infusion, transfusion and therapeutic injection (T80.2-)

puerperal sepsis (O85)

sepsis following complete or unspecified spontaneous abortion (O03.87)

sepsis following ectopic and molar pregnancy (O08.82)

sepsis following incomplete spontaneous abortion (O03.37)

sepsis following (induced) termination of pregnancy (O04.87)

sepsis NOS (A41.9)

Use additional code to identify specific acute organ dysfunction, such as:

acute kidney failure (N17.-)

acute respiratory failure (J96.0-)

critical illness myopathy (G72.81)

critical illness polyneuropathy (G62.81)

disseminated intravascular coagulopathy [DIC] (D65)

encephalopathy (metabolic) (septic) (G93.41)

hepatic failure (K72.0-)

R65.20 **Severe sepsis without septic shock**

Severe sepsis NOS

R65.21 **Severe sepsis with septic shock**

R68 **Other general symptoms and signs**

R68.0 **Hypothermia, not associated with low environmental temperature**

> Excludes1: hypothermia NOS (accidental) (T68)
>
> hypothermia due to anesthesia (T88.51)
>
> hypothermia due to low environmental temperature (T68)
>
> newborn hypothermia (P80.-)

R68.1 **Nonspecific symptoms peculiar to infancy**

> Excludes1: colic, infantile (R10.83)
>
> neonatal cerebral irritability (P91.3)
>
> teething syndrome (K00.7)

R68.11 **Excessive crying of infant (baby)**

> Excludes1: excessive crying of child, adolescent, or adult (R45.83)

R68.12 **Fussy infant (baby)**

Irritable infant

R68.13 **Apparent life threatening event in infant (ALTE)**

Apparent life threatening event in newborn

Code first confirmed diagnosis, if known

Use additional code(s) for associated signs and symptoms if no confirmed diagnosis established, or if signs and symptoms are not associated routinely with confirmed diagnosis, or provide additional information for cause of ALTE

R68.19 **Other nonspecific symptoms peculiar to infancy**

R68.2 **Dry mouth, unspecified**

Excludes1: dry mouth due to dehydration (E86.0)

dry mouth due to sicca syndrome [Sjögren] (M35.0-)

salivary gland hyposecretion (K11.7)

R68.3 **Clubbing of fingers**

Clubbing of nails

Excludes1: congenital club finger (Q68.1)

R68.8 **Other general symptoms and signs**

R68.81 **Early satiety**

R68.82 **Decreased libido**

Decreased sexual desire

R68.83 **Chills (without fever)**

Chills NOS

Excludes1: chills with fever (R50.9)

R68.84 **Jaw pain**

Mandibular pain

Maxilla pain

Excludes1: temporomandibular joint arthralgia (M26.62-)

R68.89 **Other general symptoms and signs**

R69 **Illness, unspecified**

Unknown and unspecified cases of morbidity

ABNORMAL FINDINGS ON EXAMINATION OF BLOOD, WITHOUT DIAGNOSIS (R70-R79)

Excludes2: abnormal findings on antenatal screening of mother (O28.-)

abnormalities of lipids (E78.-)

abnormalities of platelets and thrombocytes (D69.-)

abnormalities of white blood cells classified elsewhere (D70-D72)

coagulation hemorrhagic disorders (D65-D68)

diagnostic abnormal findings classified elsewhere - see Alphabetical Index hemorrhagic and hematological disorders of newborn (P50-P61)

R70 **Elevated erythrocyte sedimentation rate and abnormality of plasma viscosity**

R70.0 **Elevated erythrocyte sedimentation rate**

R70.1 **Abnormal plasma viscosity**

R71 **Abnormality of red blood cells**

Excludes1: anemias (D50-D64)

anemia of premature infant (P61.2)

benign (familial) polycythemia (D75.0)

congenital anemias (P61.2-P61.4)

newborn anemia due to isoimmunization (P55.-)

polycythemia neonatorum (P61.1)

polycythemia NOS (D75.1)

polycythemia vera (D45) secondary polycythemia (D75.1)

R71.0 **Precipitous drop in hematocrit**

Drop (precipitous) in hemoglobin

Drop in hematocrit

R71.8 **Other abnormality of red blood cells**

Abnormal red-cell morphology NOS

Abnormal red-cell volume NOS

Anisocytosis

Poikilocytosis

R73 **Elevated blood glucose level**

Excludes1: diabetes mellitus (E08-E13)

diabetes mellitus in pregnancy, childbirth and the puerperium (O24.-)

neonatal disorders (P70.0-P70.2)

postsurgical hypoinsulinemia (E89.1)

R73.0 **Abnormal glucose**

Excludes1: abnormal glucose in pregnancy (O99.81-)

diabetes mellitus (E08-E13)

dysmetabolic syndrome X (E88.81)

gestational diabetes (O24.4-)

glycosuria (R81)

hypoglycemia (E16.2)

R73.01 **Impaired fasting glucose**

Elevated fasting glucose

R73.02 **Impaired glucose tolerance (oral)**

Elevated glucose tolerance

R73.03 **Prediabetes**

Latent diabetes

R73.09 **Other abnormal glucose**

Abnormal glucose NOS

Abnormal non-fasting glucose tolerance

R73.9 **Hyperglycemia, unspecified**

R74 **Abnormal serum enzyme levels**

R74.0 **Nonspecific elevation of levels of transaminase and lactic acid dehydrogenase [LDH]**

R74.8 **Abnormal levels of other serum enzymes**

Abnormal level of acid phosphatase

Abnormal level of alkaline phosphatase

Abnormal level of amylase

Abnormal level of lipase [triacylglycerol lipase]

R74.9 **Abnormal serum enzyme level, unspecified**

R75 **Inconclusive laboratory evidence of human immunodeficiency virus [HIV]**

Nonconclusive HIV-test finding in infants

Excludes1: asymptomatic human immunodeficiency virus [HIV] infection status (Z21)

human immunodeficiency virus [HIV] disease (B20)

R76 **Other abnormal immunological findings in serum**

R76.0 **Raised antibody titer**

Excludes1: isoimmunization in pregnancy (O36.0-O36.1)

isoimmunization affecting newborn (P55.-)

R76.1 **Nonspecific reaction to test for tuberculosis**

R76.11 **Nonspecific reaction to tuberculin skin test without active tuberculosis**

Abnormal result of Mantoux test

PPD positive

Tuberculin (skin test) positive

Tuberculin (skin test) reactor

Excludes1: nonspecific reaction to cell mediated immunity measurement of gamma

● New code ▲ Revised code **Excludes1:** Not coded here **Excludes2:** Not included here ⊗ Placeholder required ⑦ 7th digit required

interferon antigen response without active tuberculosis (R76.12)

R76.12 **Nonspecific reaction to cell mediated immunity measurement of gamma interferon antigen response without active tuberculosis**

Nonspecific reaction to QuantiFERON-TB test (QFT) without active tuberculosis

Excludes1: nonspecific reaction to tuberculin skin test without active tuberculosis (R76.11)

positive tuberculin skin test (R76.11)

R76.8 **Other specified abnormal immunological findings in serum**

Raised level of immunoglobulins NOS

R76.9 **Abnormal immunological finding in serum, unspecified**

R77 **Other abnormalities of plasma proteins**

Excludes1: disorders of plasma-protein metabolism (E88.0)

R77.0 **Abnormality of albumin**

R77.1 **Abnormality of globulin**

Hyperglobulinemia NOS

R77.2 **Abnormality of alphafetoprotein**

R77.8 **Other specified abnormalities of plasma proteins**

R77.9 **Abnormality of plasma protein, unspecified**

R78 **Findings of drugs and other substances, not normally found in blood**

Use additional code to identify the any retained foreign body, if applicable (Z18.-)

Excludes1: mental or behavioral disorders due to psychoactive substance use (F10-F19)

R78.0 **Finding of alcohol in blood**

Use additional external cause code (Y90.-), for detail regarding alcohol level.

R78.1 **Finding of opiate drug in blood**

R78.2 **Finding of cocaine in blood**

R78.3 **Finding of hallucinogen in blood**

R78.4 **Finding of other drugs of addictive potential in blood**

R78.5 **Finding of other psychotropic drug in blood**

R78.6 **Finding of steroid agent in blood**

R78.7 **Finding of abnormal level of heavy metals in blood**

R78.71 **Abnormal lead level in blood**

Excludes1: lead poisoning (T56.0-)

R78.79 **Finding of abnormal level of heavy metals in blood**

R78.8 **Finding of other specified substances, not normally found in blood**

R78.81 **Bacteremia**

Excludes1: sepsis-code to specified infection

R78.89 **Finding of other specified substances, not normally found in blood**

Finding of abnormal level of lithium in blood

R78.9 **Finding of unspecified substance, not normally found in blood**

R79 **Other abnormal findings of blood chemistry**

Use additional code to identify any retained foreign body, if applicable (Z18.-)

Excludes1: asymptomatic hyperuricemia (E79.0)

hyperglycemia NOS (R73.9) hypoglycemia NOS (E16.2)

neonatal hypoglycemia (P70.3-P70.4)

specific findings indicating disorder of amino-acid metabolism (E70-E72)

specific findings indicating disorder of carbohydrate metabolism (E73-E74)

specific findings indicating disorder of lipid metabolism (E75.-)

R79.0 **Abnormal level of blood mineral**

Abnormal blood level of cobalt

Abnormal blood level of copper

Abnormal blood level of iron

Abnormal blood level of magnesium

Abnormal blood level of mineral NEC

Abnormal blood level of zinc

Excludes1: abnormal level of lithium (R78.89)

disorders of mineral metabolism (E83.-)

neonatal hypomagnesemia (P71.2)

nutritional mineral deficiency (E58-E61)

R79.1 **Abnormal coagulation profile**

Abnormal or prolonged bleeding time

Abnormal or prolonged coagulation time

Abnormal or prolonged partial thromboplastin time [PTT]

Abnormal or prolonged prothrombin time [PT]

Excludes1: coagulation defects (D68.-)

Excludes2: abnormality of fluid, electrolyte or acid-base balance (E86-E87)

R79.8 **Other specified abnormal findings of blood chemistry**

R79.81 **Abnormal blood-gas level**

R79.82 **Elevated C-reactive protein (CRP)**

R79.89 **Other specified abnormal findings of blood chemistry**

R79.9 **Abnormal finding of blood chemistry, unspecified**

ABNORMAL FINDINGS ON EXAMINATION OF URINE, WITHOUT DIAGNOSIS (R80-R82)

Excludes1: abnormal findings on antenatal screening of mother (O28.-)

diagnostic abnormal findings classified elsewhere - see Alphabetical Index

specific findings indicating disorder of amino-acid metabolism (E70-E72)

specific findings indicating disorder of carbohydrate metabolism (E73-E74)

R80 **Proteinuria**

Excludes1: gestational proteinuria (O12.1-)

R80.0 **Isolated proteinuria**

Idiopathic proteinuria

Excludes1: isolated proteinuria with specific morphological lesion (N06.-)

R80.1 **Persistent proteinuria, unspecified**

R80.2 **Orthostatic proteinuria, unspecified**

Postural proteinuria

R80.3 **Bence Jones proteinuria**

R80.8 **Other proteinuria**

R80.9 **Proteinuria, unspecified**

Albuminuria NOS

R81 **Glycosuria**

Excludes1: renal glycosuria (E74.8)

R82 **Other and unspecified abnormal findings in urine**

Includes: chromoabnormalities in urine

Use additional code to identify any retained foreign body, if applicable (Z18.-)

Excludes2: hematuria (R31.-)

R82.0 **Chyluria**

Excludes1: filarial chyluria (B74.-)

R82.1 **Myoglobinuria**

R82.2 **Biliuria**

R82.3 **Hemoglobinuria**

Excludes1: hemoglobinuria due to hemolysis from external causes NEC (D59.6)

hemoglobinuria due to paroxysmal nocturnal [Marchiafava-Micheli] (D59.5)

R82.4 **Acetonuria**

Ketonuria

R82.5 **Elevated urine levels of drugs, medicaments and biological substances**

Elevated urine levels of catecholamines

Elevated urine levels of indoleacetic acid

Elevated urine levels of 17-ketosteroids

Elevated urine levels of steroids

R82.6 **Abnormal urine levels of substances chiefly nonmedicinal as to source**

Abnormal urine level of heavy metals

R82.7 **Abnormal findings on microbiological examination of urine**

Excludes1: colonization status (Z22.-)

R82.71 **Bacteriuria**

R82.79 **Other abnormal findings on microbiological examination of urine**

Positive culture findings of urine

R82.8 **Abnormal findings on cytological and histological examination of urine**

R82.9 **Other and unspecified abnormal findings in urine**

R82.90 **Unspecified abnormal findings in urine**

R82.91 **Other chromoabnormalities of urine**

Chromoconversion (dipstick)

Idiopathic dipstick converts positive for blood with no cellular forms in sediment

Excludes1: hemoglobinuria (R82.3)

myoglobinuria (R82.1)

R82.99 **Other abnormal findings in urine**

Cells and casts in urine

Crystalluria

Melanuria

ABNORMAL FINDINGS ON EXAMINATION OF OTHER BODY FLUIDS, SUBSTANCES AND TISSUES, WITHOUT DIAGNOSIS (R83-R89)

Excludes1: abnormal findings on antenatal screening of mother (O28.-)

diagnostic abnormal findings classified elsewhere - see Alphabetical Index

Excludes2: abnormal findings on examination of blood, without diagnosis (R70-R79)

abnormal findings on examination of urine, without diagnosis (R80-R82)

abnormal tumor markers (R97.-)

R83 **Abnormal findings in cerebrospinal fluid**

R83.0 **Abnormal level of enzymes in cerebrospinal fluid**

R83.1 **Abnormal level of hormones in cerebrospinal fluid**

R83.2 **Abnormal level of other drugs, medicaments and biological substances in cerebrospinal fluid**

R83.3 **Abnormal level of substances chiefly nonmedicinal as to source in cerebrospinal fluid**

R83.4 **Abnormal immunological findings in cerebrospinal fluid**

R83.5 **Abnormal microbiological findings in cerebrospinal fluid**

Positive culture findings in cerebrospinal fluid

Excludes1: colonization status (Z22.-)

R83.6 **Abnormal cytological findings in cerebrospinal fluid**

R83.8 **Other abnormal findings in cerebrospinal fluid**

Abnormal chromosomal findings in cerebrospinal fluid

R83.9 **Unspecified abnormal finding in cerebrospinal fluid**

R84 **Abnormal findings in specimens from respiratory organs and thorax**

Includes: abnormal findings in bronchial washings

abnormal findings in nasal secretions

abnormal findings in pleural fluid

abnormal findings in sputum

abnormal findings in throat scrapings

Excludes1: blood-stained sputum (R04.2)

R84.0 **Abnormal level of enzymes in specimens from respiratory organs and thorax**

R84.1 **Abnormal level of hormones in specimens from respiratory organs and thorax**

R84.2 **Abnormal level of other drugs, medicaments and biological substances in specimens from respiratory organs and thorax**

R84.3 **Abnormal level of substances chiefly nonmedicinal as to source in specimens from respiratory organs and thorax**

R84.4 **Abnormal immunological findings in specimens from respiratory organs and thorax**

R84.5 **Abnormal microbiological findings in specimens from respiratory organs and thorax**

Positive culture findings in specimens from respiratory organs and thorax

Excludes1: colonization status (Z22.-)

R84.6 **Abnormal cytological findings in specimens from respiratory organs and thorax**

R84.7 **Abnormal histological findings in specimens from respiratory organs and thorax**

R84.8 **Other abnormal findings in specimens from respiratory organs and thorax**

Abnormal chromosomal findings in specimens from respiratory organs and thorax

R84.9 **Unspecified abnormal finding in specimens from respiratory organs and thorax**

R85 **Abnormal findings in specimens from digestive organs and abdominal cavity**

Includes: abnormal findings in peritoneal fluid

abnormal findings in saliva

Excludes1: cloudy peritoneal dialysis effluent (R88.0)

fecal abnormalities (R19.5)

R85.0 **Abnormal level of enzymes in specimens from digestive organs and abdominal cavity**

R85.1 **Abnormal level of hormones in specimens from digestive organs and abdominal cavity**

R85.2 **Abnormal level of other drugs, medicaments and biological substances in specimens from digestive organs and abdominal cavity**

R85.3 **Abnormal level of substances chiefly nonmedicinal as to source in specimens from digestive organs and abdominal cavity**

R85.4 **Abnormal immunological findings in specimens from digestive organs and abdominal cavity**

R85.5 **Abnormal microbiological findings in specimens from digestive organs and abdominal cavity**

● New code ▲ Revised code **Excludes1:** Not coded here **Excludes2:** Not included here ⊗ Placeholder required ⑦ 7th digit required

Positive culture findings in specimens from digestive organs and abdominal cavity

> **Excludes1:** colonization status (Z22.-)

R85.6 **Abnormal cytological findings in specimens from digestive organs and abdominal cavity**

R85.61 **Abnormal cytologic smear of anus**

> **Excludes1:** abnormal cytological findings in specimens from other digestive organs and abdominal cavity (R85.69)
>
> carcinoma in situ of anus (histologically confirmed) (D01.3)
>
> anal intraepithelial neoplasia I [AIN I] (K62.82)
>
> anal intraepithelial neoplasia II [AIN II] (K62.82)
>
> anal intraepithelial neoplasia III [AIN III] (D01.3)
>
> dysplasia (mild) (moderate) of anus (histologically confirmed) (K62.82)
>
> severe dysplasia of anus (histologically confirmed) (D01.3)

> **Excludes2:** anal high risk human papillomavirus (HPV) DNA test positive (R85.81)
>
> anal low risk human papillomavirus (HPV) DNA test positive (R85.82)

R85.610 **Atypical squamous cells of undetermined significance on cytologic smear of anus (ASC-US)**

R85.611 **Atypical squamous cells cannot exclude high grade squamous intraepithelial lesion on cytologic smear of anus (ASC-H)**

R85.612 **Low grade squamous intraepithelial lesion on cytologic smear of anus (LGSIL)**

R85.613 **High grade squamous intraepithelial lesion on cytologic smear of anus (HGSIL)**

R85.614 **Cytologic evidence of malignancy on smear of anus**

R85.615 **Unsatisfactory cytologic smear of anus**

Inadequate sample of cytologic smear of anus

R85.616 **Satisfactory anal smear but lacking transformation zone**

R85.618 **Other abnormal cytological findings on specimens from anus**

R85.619 **Unspecified abnormal cytological findings in specimens from anus**

Abnormal anal cytology NOS

Atypical glandular cells of anus NOS

R85.69 **Abnormal cytological findings in specimens from other digestive organs and abdominal cavity**

R85.7 **Abnormal histological findings in specimens from digestive organs and abdominal cavity**

R85.8 **Other abnormal findings in specimens from digestive organs and abdominal cavity**

R85.81 **Anal high risk human papillomavirus (HPV) DNA test positive**

> **Excludes1:** anogenital warts due to human papillomavirus (HPV) (A63.0)
>
> condyloma acuminatum (A63.0)

R85.82 **Anal low risk human papillomavirus (HPV) DNA test positive**

> **Use additional code** for associated human papillomavirus (B97.7)

R85.89 **Other abnormal findings in specimens from digestive organs and abdominal cavity**

Abnormal chromosomal findings in specimens from digestive organs and abdominal cavity

R85.9 **Unspecified abnormal finding in specimens from digestive organs and abdominal cavity**

R86 **Abnormal findings in specimens from male genital organs**

> **Includes:** abnormal findings in prostatic secretions
>
> abnormal findings in semen, seminal fluid
>
> abnormal spermatozoa

> **Excludes1:** azoospermia (N46.0-)
>
> oligospermia (N46.1-)

R86.0 **Abnormal level of enzymes in specimens from male genital organs**

R86.1 **Abnormal level of hormones in specimens from male genital organs**

R86.2 **Abnormal level of other drugs, medicaments and biological substances in specimens from male genital organs**

R86.3 **Abnormal level of substances chiefly nonmedicinal as to source in specimens from male genital organs**

R86.4 **Abnormal immunological findings in specimens from male genital organs**

R86.5 **Abnormal microbiological findings in specimens from male genital organs**

Positive culture findings in specimens from male genital organs

> **Excludes1:** colonization status (Z22.-)

R86.6 **Abnormal cytological findings in specimens from male genital organs**

R86.7 **Abnormal histological findings in specimens from male genital organs**

R86.8 **Other abnormal findings in specimens from male genital organs**

Abnormal chromosomal findings in specimens from male genital organs

R86.9 **Unspecified abnormal finding in specimens from male genital organs**

R87 **Abnormal findings in specimens from female genital organs**

> **Includes:** abnormal findings in secretion and smears from cervix uteri
>
> abnormal findings in secretion and smears from vagina
>
> abnormal findings in secretion and smears from vulva

R87.0 **Abnormal level of enzymes in specimens from female genital organs**

R87.1 **Abnormal level of hormones in specimens from female genital organs**

R87.2 **Abnormal level of other drugs, medicaments and biological substances in specimens from female genital organs**

R87.3 **Abnormal level of substances chiefly nonmedicinal as to source in specimens from female genital organs**

R87.4 **Abnormal immunological findings in specimens from female genital organs**

R87.5 **Abnormal microbiological findings in specimens from female genital organs**

Positive culture findings in specimens from female genital organs

> **Excludes1:** colonization status (Z22.-)

R87.6 **Abnormal cytological findings in specimens from female genital organs**

R87.61 Abnormal cytological findings in specimens from cervix uteri

Excludes1: abnormal cytological findings in specimens from other female genital organs (R87.69)

abnormal cytological findings in specimens from vagina (R87.62-)

carcinoma in situ of cervix uteri (histologically confirmed) (D06.-)

cervical intraepithelial neoplasia I [CIN I] (N87.0)

cervical intraepithelial neoplasia II [CIN II] (N87.1)

cervical intraepithelial neoplasia III [CIN III] (D06.-)

dysplasia (mild) (moderate) of cervix uteri (histologically confirmed) (N87.-)

severe dysplasia of cervix uteri (histologically confirmed) (D06.-)

Excludes2: cervical high risk human papillomavirus (HPV) DNA test positive (R87.810)

cervical low risk human papillomavirus (HPV) DNA test positive (R87.820)

R87.610 Atypical squamous cells of undetermined significance on cytologic smear of cervix (ASC-US)

R87.611 Atypical squamous cells cannot exclude high grade squamous intraepithelial lesion on cytologic smear of cervix (ASC-H)

R87.612 Low grade squamous intraepithelial lesion on cytologic smear of cervix (LGSIL)

R87.613 High grade squamous intraepithelial lesion on cytologic smear of cervix (HGSIL)

R87.614 Cytologic evidence of malignancy on smear of cervix

R87.615 Unsatisfactory cytologic smear of cervix

Inadequate sample of cytologic smear of cervix

R87.616 Satisfactory cervical smear but lacking transformation zone

R87.618 Other abnormal cytological findings on specimens from cervix uteri

R87.619 Unspecified abnormal cytological findings in specimens from cervix uteri

Abnormal cervical cytology NOS

Abnormal Papanicolaou smear of cervix NOS

Abnormal thin preparation smear of cervix NOS

Atypical endocervical cells of cervix NOS

Atypical endometrial cells of cervix NOS

Atypical glandular cells of cervix NOS

R87.62 Abnormal cytological findings in specimens from vagina

Use additional code to identify acquired absence of uterus and cervix, if applicable (Z90.71-)

Excludes1: abnormal cytological findings in specimens from cervix uteri (R87.61-)

abnormal cytological findings in specimens from other female genital organs (R87.69)

carcinoma in situ of vagina (histologically confirmed) (D07.2)

vaginal intraepithelial neoplasia I [VAIN I] (N89.0)

vaginal intraepithelial neoplasia II [VAIN II] (N89.1)

vaginal intraepithelial neoplasia III [VAIN III] (D07.2)

dysplasia (mild) (moderate) of vagina (histologically confirmed) (N89.-)

severe dysplasia of vagina (histologically confirmed) (D07.2)

Excludes2: vaginal high risk human papillomavirus (HPV) DNA test positive (R87.811)

vaginal low risk human papillomavirus (HPV) DNA test positive (R87.821)

R87.620 Atypical squamous cells of undetermined significance on cytologic smear of vagina (ASC-US)

R87.621 Atypical squamous cells cannot exclude high grade squamous intraepithelial lesion on cytologic smear of vagina (ASC-H)

R87.622 Low grade squamous intraepithelial lesion on cytologic smear of vagina (LGSIL)

R87.623 High grade squamous intraepithelial lesion on cytologic smear of vagina (HGSIL)

R87.624 Cytologic evidence of malignancy on smear of vagina

R87.625 Unsatisfactory cytologic smear of vagina

Inadequate sample of cytologic smear of vagina

R87.628 Other abnormal cytological findings on specimens from vagina

R87.629 Unspecified abnormal cytological findings in specimens from vagina

Abnormal Papanicolaou smear of vagina NOS

Abnormal thin preparation smear of vagina NOS

Abnormal vaginal cytology NOS

Atypical endocervical cells of vagina NOS

Atypical endometrial cells of vagina NOS

Atypical glandular cells of vagina NOS

R87.69 Abnormal cytological findings in specimens from other female genital organs

Abnormal cytological findings in specimens from female genital organs NOS

Excludes1: dysplasia of vulva (histologically confirmed) (N90.0-N90.3)

R87.7 Abnormal histological findings in specimens from female genital organs

● New code ▲ Revised code **Excludes1:** Not coded here **Excludes2:** Not included here ⊗ Placeholder required ⑦ 7th digit required

Excludes1: carcinoma in situ (histologically confirmed) of female genital organs (D06-D07.3)

cervical intraepithelial neoplasia I [CIN I] (N87.0)

cervical intraepithelial neoplasia II [CIN II] (N87.1)

cervical intraepithelial neoplasia III [CIN III] (D06.-)

dysplasia (mild) (moderate) of cervix uteri (histologically confirmed) (N87.-)

dysplasia (mild) (moderate) of vagina (histologically confirmed) (N89.-)

vaginal intraepithelial neoplasia I [VAIN I] (N89.0)

vaginal intraepithelial neoplasia II [VAIN II] (N89.1)

vaginal intraepithelial neoplasia III [VAIN III] (D07.2)

severe dysplasia of cervix uteri (histologically confirmed) (D06.-)

severe dysplasia of vagina (histologically confirmed) (D07.2)

R87.8 **Other abnormal findings in specimens from female genital organs**

R87.81 **High risk human papillomavirus (HPV) DNA test positive from female genital organs**

Excludes1: anogenital warts due to human papillomavirus (HPV) (A63.0)

condyloma acuminatum (A63.0)

R87.810 **Cervical high risk human papillomavirus (HPV) DNA test positive**

R87.811 **Vaginal high risk human papillomavirus (HPV) DNA test positive**

R87.82 **Low risk human papillomavirus (HPV) DNA test positive from female genital organs**

Use additional code for associated human papillomavirus (B97.7)

R87.820 **Cervical low risk human papillomavirus (HPV) DNA test positive**

R87.821 **Vaginal low risk human papillomavirus (HPV) DNA test positive**

R87.89 **Other abnormal findings in specimens from female genital organs**

Abnormal chromosomal findings in specimens from female genital organs

R87.9 **Unspecified abnormal finding in specimens from female genital organs**

R88 **Abnormal findings in other body fluids and substances**

R88.0 **Cloudy (hemodialysis) (peritoneal) dialysis effluent**

R88.8 **Abnormal findings in other body fluids and substances**

R89 **Abnormal findings in specimens from other organs, systems and tissues**

Includes: abnormal findings in nipple discharge

abnormal findings in synovial fluid abnormal findings in wound secretions

R89.0 **Abnormal level of enzymes in specimens from other organs, systems and tissues**

R89.1 **Abnormal level of hormones in specimens from other organs, systems and tissues**

R89.2 **Abnormal level of other drugs, medicaments and biological substances in specimens from other organs, systems and tissues**

R89.3 **Abnormal level of substances chiefly nonmedicinal as to source in specimens from other organs, systems and tissues**

R89.4 **Abnormal immunological findings in specimens from other organs, systems and tissues**

R89.5 **Abnormal microbiological findings in specimens from other organs, systems and tissues**

Positive culture findings in specimens **from other** organs, systems and tissues

Excludes1: colonization status (Z22.-)

R89.6 **Abnormal cytological findings in specimens from other organs, systems and tissues**

R89.7 **Abnormal histological findings in specimens from other organs, systems and tissues**

R89.8 **Other abnormal findings in specimens from other organs, systems and tissues**

Abnormal chromosomal findings in specimens **from other** organs, systems and tissues

R89.9 **Unspecified abnormal finding in specimens from other organs, systems and tissues**

ABNORMAL FINDINGS ON DIAGNOSTIC IMAGING AND IN FUNCTION STUDIES, WITHOUT DIAGNOSIS (R90-R94)

Includes: nonspecific abnormal findings on diagnostic imaging by computerized axial tomography [CAT scan]

nonspecific abnormal findings on diagnostic imaging by magnetic resonance imaging [MRI][NMR]

nonspecific abnormal findings on diagnostic imaging by positron emission tomography [PET scan]

nonspecific abnormal findings on diagnostic imaging by thermography

nonspecific abnormal findings on diagnostic imaging by ultrasound [echogram]

nonspecific abnormal findings on diagnostic imaging by X-ray examination

Excludes1: abnormal findings on antenatal screening of mother (O28.-)

diagnostic abnormal findings classified elsewhere - see Alphabetical Index

R90 **Abnormal findings on diagnostic imaging of central nervous system**

R90.0 **Intracranial space-occupying lesion found on diagnostic imaging of central nervous system**

R90.8 **Other abnormal findings on diagnostic imaging of central nervous system**

R90.81 **Abnormal echoencephalogram**

R90.82 **White matter disease, unspecified**

R90.89 **Other abnormal findings on diagnostic imaging of central nervous system**

Other cerebrovascular abnormality found on diagnostic imaging of central nervous system

R91 **Abnormal findings on diagnostic imaging of lung**

R91.1 **Solitary pulmonary nodule**

Coin lesion lung

Solitary pulmonary nodule, subsegmental branch of the bronchial tree

R91.8 **Other nonspecific abnormal finding of lung field**

Lung mass NOS found on diagnostic imaging of lung

Pulmonary infiltrate NOS

Shadow, lung

R92 **Abnormal and inconclusive findings on diagnostic imaging of breast**

R92.0 **Mammographic microcalcification found on diagnostic imaging of breast**

> **Excludes2:** mammographic calcification (calculus) found on diagnostic imaging of breast (R92.1)

R92.1 **Mammographic calcification found on diagnostic imaging of breast**

Mammographic calculus found on diagnostic imaging of breast

R92.2 **Inconclusive mammogram**

Dense breasts NOS

Inconclusive mammogram NEC

Inconclusive mammography due to dense breasts

Inconclusive mammography NEC

R92.8 **Other abnormal and inconclusive findings on diagnostic imaging of breast**

R93 **Abnormal findings on diagnostic imaging of other body structures**

R93.0 **Abnormal findings on diagnostic imaging of skull and head, not elsewhere classified**

> **Excludes1:** intracranial space-occupying lesion found on diagnostic imaging (R90.0)

R93.1 **Abnormal findings on diagnostic imaging of heart and coronary circulation**

Abnormal echocardiogram NOS

Abnormal heart shadow

R93.2 **Abnormal findings on diagnostic imaging of liver and biliary tract**

Nonvisualization of gallbladder

R93.3 **Abnormal findings on diagnostic imaging of other parts of digestive tract**

R93.4 **Abnormal findings on diagnostic imaging of urinary organs**

> **Excludes2:** hypertrophy of kidney (N28.81)

R93.41 **Abnormal radiologic findings on diagnostic imaging of renal pelvis, ureter, or bladder**

Filling defect of bladder found on diagnostic imaging

Filling defect of renal pelvis found on diagnostic imaging

Filling defect of ureter found on diagnostic imaging

R93.42 **Abnormal radiologic findings on diagnostic imaging of kidney**

R93.421 **Abnormal radiologic findings on diagnostic imaging of right kidney**

R93.422 **Abnormal radiologic findings on diagnostic imaging of left kidney**

R93.429 **Abnormal radiologic findings on diagnostic imaging of unspecified kidney**

R93.49 **Abnormal radiologic findings on diagnostic imaging of other urinary organs**

R93.5 **Abnormal findings on diagnostic imaging of other abdominal regions, including retroperitoneum**

R93.6 **Abnormal findings on diagnostic imaging of limbs**

> **Excludes2:** abnormal finding in skin and subcutaneous tissue (R93.8)

R93.7 **Abnormal findings on diagnostic imaging of other parts of musculoskeletal system**

> **Excludes2:** abnormal findings on diagnostic imaging of skull (R93.0)

R93.8 **Abnormal findings on diagnostic imaging of other specified body structures**

Abnormal finding by radioisotope localization of placenta

Abnormal radiological finding in skin and subcutaneous tissue

Mediastinal shift

R93.9 **Diagnostic imaging inconclusive due to excess body fat of patient**

R94 **Abnormal results of function studies**

> **Includes:** abnormal results of radionuclide [radioisotope] uptake studies
>
> abnormal results of scintigraphy

R94.0 **Abnormal results of function studies of central nervous system**

R94.01 **Abnormal electroencephalogram [EEG]**

R94.02 **Abnormal brain scan**

R94.09 **Abnormal results of other function studies of central nervous system**

R94.1 **Abnormal results of function studies of peripheral nervous system and special senses**

R94.11 **Abnormal results of function studies of eye**

R94.110 **Abnormal electro-oculogram [EOG]**

R94.111 **Abnormal electroretinogram [ERG]**

Abnormal retinal function study

R94.112 **Abnormal visually evoked potential [VEP]**

R94.113 **Abnormal oculomotor study**

R94.118 **Abnormal results of other function studies of eye**

R94.12 **Abnormal results of function studies of ear and other special senses**

R94.120 **Abnormal auditory function study**

R94.121 **Abnormal vestibular function study**

R94.128 **Abnormal results of other function studies of ear and other special senses**

R94.13 **Abnormal results of function studies of peripheral nervous system**

R94.130 **Abnormal response to nerve stimulation, unspecified**

R94.131 **Abnormal electromyogram [EMG]**

> **Excludes1:** electromyogram of eye (R94.113)

R94.138 **Abnormal results of other function studies of peripheral nervous system**

R94.2 **Abnormal results of pulmonary function studies**

Reduced ventilatory capacity Reduced vital capacity

R94.3 **Abnormal results of cardiovascular function studies**

R94.30 **Abnormal result of cardiovascular function study, unspecified**

R94.31 **Abnormal electrocardiogram [ECG] [EKG]**

> **Excludes1:** long QT syndrome (I45.81)

R94.39 **Abnormal result of other cardiovascular function study**

Abnormal electrophysiological intracardiac studies

Abnormal phonocardiogram

Abnormal vectorcardiogram

R94.4 **Abnormal results of kidney function studies**

Abnormal renal function test

R94.5 **Abnormal results of liver function studies**

R94.6 **Abnormal results of thyroid function studies**

R94.7 **Abnormal results of other endocrine function studies**

● New code ▲ Revised code **Excludes1:** Not coded here **Excludes2:** Not included here ⊗ Placeholder required ⑦ 7th digit required

Excludes2: abnormal glucose (R73.0-)

R94.8 **Abnormal results of function studies of other organs and systems**

Abnormal basal metabolic rate [BMR]

Abnormal bladder function test

Abnormal splenic function test

ABNORMAL TUMOR MARKERS (R97)

Definition: A tumor marker is a biomarker found in the blood, urine, or body tissues that can be elevated in cancer, among other tissue types. There are many different **tumor** markers, each indicative of a particular disease process, and they are used in oncology to help detect the presence of cancer.

R97 **Abnormal tumor markers**

Elevated tumor associated antigens [TAA]

Elevated tumor specific antigens [TSA]

R97.0 **Elevated carcinoembryonic antigen [CEA]**

R97.1 **Elevated cancer antigen 125 [CA 125]**

R97.2 **Elevated prostate specific antigen [PSA]**

R97.20 **Elevated prostate specific antigen [PSA]**

R97.21 **Rising PSA following treatment for malignant neoplasm of prostate**

R97.8 **Other abnormal tumor markers**

ILL-DEFINED AND UNKNOWN CAUSE OF MORTALITY (R99)

R99 **Ill-defined and unknown cause of mortality**

Death (unexplained) NOS

Unspecified cause of mortality

● New code   ▲ Revised code   **Excludes1:** Not coded here   **Excludes2:** Not included here   ⊗ Placeholder required   ⑦ 7th digit required

Chapter 19: Injury, Poisoning And Certain Other Consequences Of External Causes (S00-T88)

DEFINITIONS

This chapter includes definitions of selected key words, terms and phrases and coding alerts for adding points to the clinical domain, and references to coding late effects where appropriate. An example from this chapter is as follows:

S05.7   Avulsion of eye

Traumatic enucleation

Definition: An avulsion is an injury in which a body structure is forcibly detached from its normal point of insertion by either trauma or surgery (from the Latin *avellere*, meaning "to tear off"). The term most commonly refers to a surface trauma where all layers of the skin have been torn away, exposing the underlying structures (i.e., subcutaneous tissue, muscle, tendons, or bone).

MULTIPLE CODING FOR A SINGLE CONDITION

In addition to the etiology/manifestation convention that requires two codes to fully describe a single condition that affects multiple body systems, there are other single conditions that also require more than one code. "Use additional code" notes are found in the Tabular List at codes that are not part of an etiology/manifestation pair where a secondary code is useful to fully describe a condition. The sequencing rule is the same as the etiology/manifestation pair, "use additional code" indicates that a secondary code should be added.

For example, for bacterial infections that are not included in chapter 1, a secondary code from category B95, Streptococcus, Staphylococcus, and Enterococcus, as the cause of diseases classified elsewhere, or B96, Other bacterial agents as the cause of diseases classified elsewhere, may be required to identify the bacterial organism causing the infection. A "use additional code" note will normally be found at the infectious disease code, indicating a need for the organism code to be added as a secondary code.

"**Code first**" notes are also under certain codes that are not specifically manifestation codes but may be due to an underlying cause. When there is a "**Code first**" note and an underlying condition is present, the underlying condition should be sequenced first.

"Code, if applicable, any causal condition first", notes indicate that this code may be assigned as a principal diagnosis when the causal condition is unknown or not applicable. If a causal condition is known, then the code for that condition should be sequenced as the principal or first-listed diagnosis.

Multiple codes may be needed for sequela, complication codes and obstetric codes to more fully describe a condition. See the specific guidelines for these conditions for further instruction.

COMBINATION CODE

A combination code is a single code used to classify: Two diagnoses, or a diagnosis with an associated secondary process (manifestation) A diagnosis with an associated complication

Combination codes are identified by referring to subterm entries in the Alphabetic Index and by reading the inclusion and exclusion notes in the Tabular List.

Assign only the combination code when that code fully identifies the diagnostic conditions involved or when the Alphabetic Index so directs. Multiple coding should not be used when the classification provides a combination code that clearly identifies all of the elements documented in the diagnosis. When the combination code lacks necessary specificity in describing the manifestation or complication, an additional code should be used as a secondary code.

SEQUELA (LATE EFFECTS)

A sequela is the residual effect (condition produced) after the acute phase of an illness or injury has terminated. There is no time limit on when a sequela code can be used. The residual may be apparent early, such as in cerebral infarction, or it may occur months or years later, such as that due to a previous injury. Coding of sequela generally requires two codes sequenced in the following order: The condition or nature of the sequela is sequenced first.

The sequela code is sequenced second.

An exception to the above guidelines are those instances where the code for the sequela is followed by a manifestation code identified in the Tabular List and title, or the sequela code has been expanded (at the fourth, fifth or sixth character levels) to include the manifestation(s). The code for the acute phase of an illness or injury that led to the sequela is never used with a code for the late effect.

APPLICATION OF 7TH CHARACTERS IN CHAPTER 19

Most categories in chapter 19 have a 7th character requirement for each applicable code. Most categories in this chapter have three 7th character values (with the exception of fractures): A, initial encounter, D, subsequent encounter and S, sequela. Categories for traumatic fractures have additional 7th character values. While the patient may be seen by a new or different provider over the course of treatment for an injury, assignment of the 7th character is based on whether the patient is undergoing active treatment and not whether the provider is seeing the patient for the first time.

For complication codes, active treatment refers to treatment for the condition described by the code, even though it may be related to an earlier precipitating problem. For example, code T84.50XA, Infection and inflammatory reaction due to unspecified internal joint prosthesis, initial encounter, is used when active treatment is provided for the infection, even though the condition relates to the prosthetic device, implant or graft that was placed at a previous encounter.

7th character "A", initial encounter is used for each encounter where the patient is receiving active treatment for the condition.

S00-T88

7th character "D" subsequent encounter is used for encounters after the patient has completed active treatment of the condition and is receiving routine care for the condition during the healing or recovery phase.

The aftercare Z codes should not be used for aftercare for conditions such as injuries or poisonings, where 7th characters are provided to identify subsequent care. For example, for aftercare of an injury, assign the acute injury code with the 7th character "D" (subsequent encounter).

7th character "S", sequela, is for use for complications or conditions that arise as a direct result of a condition, such as scar formation after a burn. The scars are sequelae of the burn. When using 7th character "S", it is necessary to use both the injury code that precipitated the sequela and the code for the sequela itself. The "S" is added only to the injury code, not the sequela code. The 7th character "S" identifies the injury responsible for the sequela. The specific type of sequela (e.g. scar) is sequenced first, followed by the injury code.

See Section I.B.10 Sequelae, (Late Effects)

CODING OF INJURIES

When coding injuries, assign separate codes for each injury unless a combination code is provided, in which case the combination code is assigned. Code T07, Unspecified multiple injuries should not be assigned in the inpatient setting unless information for a more specific code is not available. Traumatic injury codes (S00-T14.9) are not to be used for normal, healing surgical wounds or to identify complications of surgical wounds.

The code for the most serious injury, as determined by the provider and the focus of treatment, is sequenced first.

1) **Superficial injuries**

Superficial injuries such as abrasions or contusions are not coded when associated with more severe injuries of the same site.

2) **Primary injury with damage to nerves/blood vessels**

When a primary injury results in minor damage to peripheral nerves or blood vessels, the primary injury is sequenced first with additional code(s) for injuries to nerves and spinal cord (such as category S04), and/or injury to blood vessels (such as category S15). When the primary injury is to the blood vessels or nerves, that injury should be sequenced first.

CODING OF TRAUMATIC FRACTURES

The principles of multiple coding of injuries should be followed in coding fractures. Fractures of specified sites are coded individually by site in accordance with both the provisions within categories S02, S12, S22, S32, S42, S49, S52, S59, S62, S72, S79, S82, S89, S92 and the level of detail furnished by medical record content.

A fracture not indicated as open or closed should be coded to closed. A fracture not indicated whether displaced or not displaced should be coded to displaced.

More specific guidelines are as follows:

1) **Initial vs. Subsequent Encounter for Fractures**

Traumatic fractures are coded using the appropriate 7th character for initial encounter (A, B, C) for each encounter where the patient is receiving active treatment for the fracture. The appropriate 7th character for initial encounter should also be assigned for a patient who delayed seeking treatment for the fracture or nonunion.

Fractures are coded using the appropriate 7th character for subsequent care for encounters after the patient has completed active treatment of the fracture and is receiving routine care for the fracture during the healing or recovery phase.

Care for complications of surgical treatment for fracture repairs during the healing or recovery phase should be coded with the appropriate complication codes.

Care of complications of fractures, such as malunion and nonunion, should be reported with the appropriate 7th character for subsequent care with nonunion (K, M, N,) or subsequent care with malunion (P, Q, R).

Malunion/nonunion: The appropriate 7th character for initial encounter should also be assigned for a patient who delayed seeking treatment for the fracture or nonunion.

The open fracture designations in the assignment of the 7th character for fractures of the forearm, femur and lower leg, including ankle are based on the Gustilo open fracture classification. When the Gustilo classification type is not specified for an open fracture, the 7th character for open fracture type I or II should be assigned (B, E, H, M, Q).

A code from category M80, not a traumatic fracture code, should be used for any patient with known osteoporosis who suffers a fracture, even if the patient had a minor fall or trauma, if that fall or trauma would not usually break a normal, healthy bone.

See Section I.C.13. Osteoporosis.

The aftercare Z codes should not be used for aftercare for traumatic fractures. For aftercare of a traumatic fracture, assign the acute fracture code with the appropriate 7th character.

2) **Multiple fractures sequencing**

Multiple fractures are sequenced in accordance with the severity of the fracture.

CODING OF BURNS AND CORROSIONS

The ICD-10-CM makes a distinction between burns and corrosions. The burn codes are for thermal burns, except sunburns, that come from a heat source, such as a fire or hot appliance. The burn codes are also for burns resulting from electricity and radiation. Corrosions are burns due to chemicals. The guidelines are the same for burns and corrosions.

Current burns (T20-T25) are classified by depth, extent and by agent (X code). Burns are classified by depth as first degree (erythema), second degree (blistering), and third degree (full-thickness involvement). Burns of the eye and internal organs (T26-T28) are classified by site, but not by degree.

1) **Sequencing of burn and related condition codes**

> Sequence first the code that reflects the highest degree of burn when more than one burn is present.

> a. When the reason for the admission or encounter is for treatment of external multiple burns, sequence first the code that reflects the burn of the highest degree.

> b. When a patient has both internal and external burns, the circumstances of admission govern the selection of the principal diagnosis or first-listed diagnosis.

> c. When a patient is admitted for burn injuries and other related conditions such as smoke inhalation and/or respiratory failure, the circumstances of admission govern the selection of the principal or first-listed diagnosis.

2) **Burns of the same local site**

> Classify burns of the same local site (three-character category level, T20-T28) but of different degrees to the subcategory identifying the highest degree recorded in the diagnosis.

3) **Non-healing burns**

> Non-healing burns are coded as acute burns.

> Necrosis of burned skin should be coded as a non-healed burn.

4) **Infected Burn**

> For any documented infected burn site, use an additional code for the infection.

5) **Assign separate codes for each burn site**

> When coding burns, assign separate codes for each burn site. Category T30, Burn and corrosion, body region unspecified is extremely vague and should rarely be used.

6) **Burns and Corrosions Classified According to Extent of Body Surface Involved**

> Assign codes from category T31, Burns classified according to extent of body surface involved, or T32, Corrosions classified according to extent of body surface involved, when the site of the burn is not specified or when there is a need for additional data. It is advisable to use category T31 as additional coding when needed to provide data for evaluating burn mortality, such as that needed by burn units. It is also advisable to use category T31 as an additional code for reporting purposes when there is mention of a third-degree burn involving 20 percent or more of the body surface.

> Categories T31 and T32 are based on the classic "rule of nines" in estimating body surface involved: head and neck are assigned nine percent, each arm nine percent, each leg 18 percent, the anterior trunk 18 percent, posterior trunk 18 percent, and genitalia one percent. Providers may change these percentage assignments where necessary to accommodate infants and children who have proportionately larger heads than adults, and patients who have large buttocks, thighs, or abdomen that involve burns.

7) **Encounters for treatment of sequela of burns**

> Encounters for the treatment of the late effects of burns or corrosions (i.e., scars or joint contractures) should be coded with a burn or corrosion code with the 7th character "S" for sequela.

8) **Sequelae with a late effect code and current burn**

> When appropriate, both a code for a current burn or corrosion with 7th character "A" or "D" and a burn or corrosion code with 7th character "S" may be assigned on the same record (when both a current burn and sequelae of an old burn exist). Burns and corrosions do not heal at the same rate and a current healing wound may still exist with sequela of a healed burn or corrosion.

> *See Section I.B.10 Sequela (Late Effects)*

9) **Use of an external cause code with burns and corrosions**

> An external cause code should be used with burns and corrosions to identify the source and intent of the burn, as well as the place where it occurred.

ADVERSE EFFECTS, POISONING, UNDERDOSING AND TOXIC EFFECTS

Codes in categories T36-T65 are combination codes that include the substance that was taken as well as the intent. No additional external cause code is required for poisonings, toxic effects, adverse effects and underdosing codes.

1) **Do not code directly from the Table of Drugs**

   Do not code directly from the Table of Drugs and Chemicals. Always refer back to the Tabular List.

2) **Use as many codes as necessary to describe**

   Use as many codes as necessary to describe completely all drugs, medicinal or biological substances.

3) **If the same code would describe the causative agent**

   If the same code would describe the causative agent for more than one adverse reaction, poisoning, toxic effect or underdosing, assign the code only once.

4) **If two or more drugs, medicinal or biological substances**

   If two or more drugs, medicinal or biological substances are reported, code each individually unless a combination code is listed in the Table of Drugs and Chemicals.

5) **The occurrence of drug toxicity is classified in ICD-10-CM as follows:**

   (a) **Adverse Effect**

   When coding an adverse effect of a drug that has been correctly prescribed and properly administered, assign the appropriate code for the nature of the adverse effect followed by the appropriate code for the adverse effect of the drug (T36-T50). The code for the drug should have a 5th or 6th character "5" (for example T36.0X5-) Examples of the nature of an adverse effect are tachycardia, delirium, gastrointestinal hemorrhaging, vomiting, hypokalemia, hepatitis, renal failure, or respiratory failure.

   (b) **Poisoning**

   When coding a poisoning or reaction to the improper use of a medication (e.g., overdose, wrong substance given or taken in error, wrong route of administration), first assign the appropriate code from categories T36-T50. The poisoning codes have an associated intent as their 5th or 6th character (accidental, intentional self-harm, assault and undetermined. If the intent of the poisoning is unknown or unspecified, code the intent as accidental intent. The undetermined intent is only for use if the documentation in the record specifies that the intent cannot be determined. Use additional code(s) for all manifestations of poisonings.

   If there is also a diagnosis of abuse or dependence of the substance, the abuse or dependence is assigned as an additional code.

   Examples of poisoning include:

   (i) Error was made in drug prescription Errors made in drug prescription or in the administration of the drug by provider, nurse, patient, or other person.

   (ii) Overdose of a drug intentionally taken

   If an overdose of a drug was intentionally taken or administered and resulted in drug toxicity, it would be coded as a poisoning.

   (iii) Nonprescribed drug taken with correctly prescribed and properly administered drug

   If a nonprescribed drug or medicinal agent was taken in combination with a correctly prescribed and properly administered drug, any drug toxicity or other reaction resulting from the interaction of the two drugs would be classified as a poisoning.

   (iv) Interaction of drug(s) and alcohol

   When a reaction results from the interaction of a drug(s) and alcohol, this would be classified as poisoning.

   See Section I.C.4. if poisoning is the result of insulin pump malfunctions.

   (c) **Underdosing**

   Underdosing refers to taking less of a medication than is prescribed by a provider or a manufacturer's instruction. For underdosing, assign the code from categories T36-T50 (fifth or sixth character "6").

   Codes for underdosing should never be assigned as principal or first-listed codes. If a patient has a relapse or exacerbation of the medical condition for which the drug is prescribed because of the reduction in dose, then the medical condition itself should be coded.

   Noncompliance (Z91.12-, Z91.13-) or complication of care (Y63.6-Y63.9) codes are to be used with an underdosing code to indicate intent, if known.

   (d) **Toxic Effects**

● New code   ▲ Revised code   **Excludes1:** Not coded here   **Excludes2:** Not included here   ⊗ Placeholder required   ⑦ 7th digit required

When a harmful substance is ingested or comes in contact with a person, this is classified as a toxic effect. The toxic effect codes are in categories T51-T65.

Toxic effect codes have an associated intent: accidental, intentional self-harm, assault and undetermined.

ADULT AND CHILD ABUSE, NEGLECT AND OTHER MALTREATMENT

Sequence first the appropriate code from categories T74.- (Adult and child abuse, neglect and other maltreatment, confirmed) or T76.-(Adult and child abuse, neglect and other maltreatment, suspected) for abuse, neglect and other maltreatment, followed by any accompanying mental health or injury code(s).

If the documentation in the medical record states abuse or neglect it is coded as confirmed (T74.-). It is coded as suspected if it is documented as suspected (T76.-).

For cases of confirmed abuse or neglect an external cause code from the assault section (X92-**Y09**) should be added to identify the cause of any physical injuries. A perpetrator code (Y07) should be added when the perpetrator of the abuse is known. For suspected cases of abuse or neglect, do not report external cause or perpetrator code.

If a suspected case of abuse, neglect or mistreatment is ruled out during an encounter code Z04.71, Encounter for examination and observation following alleged physical adult abuse, ruled out, or code Z04.72, Encounter for examination and observation following alleged child physical abuse, ruled out, should be used, not a code from T76.

If a suspected case of alleged rape or sexual abuse is ruled out during an encounter code Z04.41, Encounter for examination and observation following alleged adult rape or code Z04.42, Encounter for examination and observation following alleged **child** rape, should be used, not a code from T76.

See Section I.C.15. Abuse in a pregnant patient.

COMPLICATIONS OF CARE

1) **General guidelines for complications of care**

    (a) **Documentation of complications of care**

        See Section I.B.16. for information on documentation of complications of care.

2) **Pain due to medical devices**

    Pain associated with devices, implants or grafts left in a surgical site (for example painful hip prosthesis) is assigned to the appropriate code(s) found in Chapter 19, Injury, poisoning, and certain other consequences of external causes. Specific codes for pain due to medical devices are found in the T code section of the ICD-10-CM. Use additional code(s) from category G89 to identify acute or chronic pain due to presence of the device, implant or graft (G89.18 or G89.28).

3) **Transplant complications**

    (a) **Transplant complications other than kidney**

        Codes under category T86, Complications of transplanted organs and tissues, are for use for both complications and rejection of transplanted organs. A transplant complication code is only assigned if the complication affects the function of the transplanted organ. Two codes are required to fully describe a transplant complication: the appropriate code from category T86 and a secondary code that identifies the complication.

        Pre-existing conditions or conditions that develop after the transplant are not coded as complications unless they affect the function of the transplanted organs.

        See I.C.21. for transplant organ removal status See I.C.2. for malignant neoplasm associated with transplanted organ.

    (b) **Kidney transplant complications**

        Patients who have undergone kidney transplant may still have some form of chronic kidney disease (CKD) because the kidney transplant may not fully restore kidney function. Code T86.1- should be assigned for documented complications of a kidney transplant, such as transplant failure or rejection or other transplant complication. Code T86.1- should not be assigned for post kidney transplant patients who have chronic kidney (CKD) unless a transplant complication such as transplant failure or rejection is documented. If the documentation is unclear as to whether the patient has a complication of the transplant, query the provider.

        Conditions that affect the function of the transplanted kidney, other than CKD, should be assigned a code from subcategory T86.1, Complications of transplanted organ, Kidney, and a secondary code that identifies the complication.

        For patients with CKD following a kidney transplant, but who do not have a complication such as failure or rejection, *see section I.C.14. Chronic kidney disease and kidney transplant status.*

4) **Complication codes that include the external cause**

    As with certain other T codes, some of the complications of care codes have the external cause included in the code. The code includes the nature of the complication as well as the type of procedure that caused the complication. No external cause code indicating the type of procedure is necessary for these codes.

5) **Complications of care codes within the body system chapters**

| | Add 4th-7th digits | Nonspecific code | Unspecified code | Manifestation code | 733 |

Intraoperative and postprocedural complication codes are found within the body system chapters with codes specific to the organs and structures of that body system. These codes should be sequenced first, followed by a code(s) for the specific complication, if applicable.

● New code   ▲ Revised code   **Excludes1:** Not coded here   **Excludes2:** Not included here   ⊗ Placeholder required   ⑦ 7th digit required

Chapter 19

Injury, Poisoning And Certain Other Consequences Of External Causes (S00-T88)

Note: Use secondary code(s) from Chapter 20, External causes of morbidity, to indicate cause of injury. Codes within the T section that include the external cause do not require an additional external cause code

Use additional code to identify any retained foreign body, if applicable (Z18.-)

Excludes1: birth trauma (P10-P15)

> obstetric trauma (O70-O71)

This chapter contains the following blocks:

S00-S09	Injuries to the head
S10-S19	Injuries to the neck
S20-S29	Injuries to the thorax
S30-S39	Injuries to the abdomen, lower back, lumbar spine, pelvis and external genitals
S40-S49	Injuries to the shoulder and upper arm
S50-S59	Injuries to the elbow and forearm
S60-S69	Injuries to the wrist, hand and fingers
S70-S79	Injuries to the hip and thigh
S80-S89	Injuries to the knee and lower leg
S90-S99	Injuries to the ankle and foot
T07	Injuries involving multiple body regions
T14	Injury of unspecified body region
T15-T19	Effects of foreign body entering through natural orifice
T20-T32	Burns and corrosions
T20-T25	Burns and corrosions of external body surface, specified by site
T26-T28	Burns and corrosions confined to eye and internal organs
T30-T32	Burns and corrosions of multiple and unspecified body regions
T33-T34	Frostbite
T36-T50	Poisoning by, adverse effect of and underdosing of drugs, medicaments and biological substances
T51-T65	Toxic effects of substances chiefly nonmedicinal as to source
T66-T78	Other and unspecified effects of external causes
T79	Certain early complications of trauma
T80-T88	Complications of surgical and medical care, not elsewhere classified

Note: The chapter uses the S-section for coding different types of injuries related to single body regions and the T-section to cover injuries to unspecified body regions as well as poisoning and certain other consequences of external causes.

INJURIES TO THE HEAD (S00-S09)

Includes: injuries of ear

injuries of eye

injuries of face [any part] injuries of gum

injuries of jaw injuries of oral cavity injuries of palate

injuries of periocular area injuries of scalp

injuries of temporomandibular joint area injuries of tongue

injuries of tooth

Code also for any associated infection

Excludes2: burns and corrosions (T20-T32)

> effects of foreign body in ear (T16)
>
> effects of foreign body in larynx (T17.3)
>
> effects of foreign body in mouth NOS (T18.0)
>
> effects of foreign body in nose (T17.0-T17.1)

effects of foreign body in pharynx (T17.2)

effects of foreign body on external eye (T15.-)

frostbite (T33-T34)

insect bite or sting, venomous (T63.4)

S00 Superficial injury of head

Excludes1: diffuse cerebral contusion (S06.2-)

> focal cerebral contusion (S06.3-)
>
> injury of eye and orbit (S05.-)
>
> open wound of head (S01.-)

The appropriate 7th character is to be added to each code from category S00

A - initial encounter

D - subsequent encounter

S - sequela

S00.0 Superficial injury of scalp

  ⊗⑦**S00.00 Unspecified superficial injury of scalp**

  ⊗⑦**S00.01 Abrasion of scalp**

  ⊗⑦**S00.02 Blister (nonthermal) of scalp**

  ⊗⑦**S00.03 Contusion of scalp**

      Bruise of scalp

      Hematoma of scalp

  ⊗⑦**S00.04 External constriction of part of scalp**

  ⊗⑦**S00.05 Superficial foreign body of scalp**

      Splinter in the scalp

  ⊗⑦**S00.06 Insect bite (nonvenomous) of scalp**

  ⊗⑦**S00.07 Other superficial bite of scalp**

    Excludes1: open bite of scalp (S01.05)

S00.1 Contusion of eyelid and periocular area

  Black eye

  Excludes2: contusion of eyeball and orbital tissues (S05.1)

  ⊗⑦**S00.10 Contusion of unspecified eyelid and periocular area**

  ⊗⑦**S00.11 Contusion of right eyelid and periocular area**

  ⊗⑦**S00.12 Contusion of left eyelid and periocular area**

S00.2 Other and unspecified superficial injuries of eyelid and periocular area

  Excludes2: superficial injury of conjunctiva and cornea (S05.0-)

  S00.20 Unspecified superficial injury of eyelid and periocular area

    ⑦**S00.201 Unspecified superficial injury of right eyelid and periocular area**

    ⑦**S00.202 Unspecified superficial injury of left eyelid and periocular area**

    ⑦**S00.209 Unspecified superficial injury of unspecified eyelid and periocular area**

  S00.21 Abrasion of eyelid and periocular area

    ⑦**S00.211 Abrasion of right eyelid and periocular area**

    ⑦**S00.212 Abrasion of left eyelid and periocular area**

    ⑦**S00.219 Abrasion of unspecified eyelid and periocular area**

  S00.22 Blister (nonthermal) of eyelid and periocular area

    ⑦**S00.221 Blister (nonthermal) of right eyelid and periocular area**

⑦S00.222 **Blister (nonthermal) of left eyelid and periocular area**

⑦S00.229 **Blister (nonthermal) of unspecified eyelid and periocular area**

S00.24 **External constriction of eyelid and periocular area**

⑦S00.241 **External constriction of right eyelid and periocular area**

⑦S00.242 **External constriction of left eyelid and periocular area**

⑦S00.249 **External constriction of unspecified eyelid and periocular area**

S00.25 **Superficial foreign body of eyelid and periocular area**

Splinter of eyelid and periocular area

Excludes2: retained foreign body in eyelid (H02.81-)

⑦S00.251 **Superficial foreign body of right eyelid and periocular area**

⑦S00.252 **Superficial foreign body of left eyelid and periocular area**

⑦S00.259 **Superficial foreign body of unspecified eyelid and periocular area**

S00.26 **Insect bite (nonvenomous) of eyelid and periocular area**

⑦S00.261 **Insect bite (nonvenomous) of right eyelid and periocular area**

⑦S00.262 **Insect bite (nonvenomous) of left eyelid and periocular area**

⑦S00.269 **Insect bite (nonvenomous) of unspecified eyelid and periocular area**

S00.27 **Other superficial bite of eyelid and periocular area**

Excludes1: open bite of eyelid and periocular area (S01.15)

⑦S00.271 **Other superficial bite of right eyelid and periocular area**

⑦S00.272 **Other superficial bite of left eyelid and periocular area**

⑦S00.279 **Other superficial bite of unspecified eyelid and periocular area**

S00.3 **Superficial injury of nose**

⊗⑦S00.30 **Unspecified superficial injury of nose**

⊗⑦S00.31 **Abrasion of nose**

⊗⑦S00.32 **Blister (nonthermal) of nose**

⊗⑦S00.33 **Contusion of nose**

Bruise of nose

Hematoma of nose

⊗⑦S00.34 **External constriction of nose**

⊗⑦S00.35 **Superficial foreign body of nose**

Splinter in the nose

⊗⑦S00.36 **Insect bite (nonvenomous) of nose**

⊗⑦S00.37 **Other superficial bite of nose**

Excludes1: open bite of nose (S01.25)

S00.4 **Superficial injury of ear**

S00.40 **Unspecified superficial injury of ear**

⑦S00.401 **Unspecified superficial injury of right ear**

⑦S00.402 **Unspecified superficial injury of left ear**

⑦S00.409 **Unspecified superficial injury of unspecified ear**

S00.41 **Abrasion of ear**

⑦S00.411 **Abrasion of right ear**

⑦S00.412 **Abrasion of left ear**

⑦S00.419 **Abrasion of unspecified ear**

S00.42 **Blister (nonthermal) of ear**

⑦S00.421 **Blister (nonthermal) of right ear**

⑦S00.422 **Blister (nonthermal) of left ear**

⑦S00.429 **Blister (nonthermal) of unspecified ear**

S00.43 **Contusion of ear**

Bruise of ear

Hematoma of ear

⑦S00.431 **Contusion of right ear**

⑦S00.432 **Contusion of left ear**

⑦S00.439 **Contusion of unspecified ear**

S00.44 **External constriction of ear**

⑦S00.441 **External constriction of right ear**

⑦S00.442 **External constriction of left ear**

⑦S00.449 **External constriction of unspecified ear**

S00.45 **Superficial foreign body of ear**

Splinter in the ear

⑦S00.451 **Superficial foreign body of right ear**

⑦S00.452 **Superficial foreign body of left ear**

⑦S00.459 **Superficial foreign body of unspecified ear**

S00.46 **Insect bite (nonvenomous) of ear**

⑦S00.461 **Insect bite (nonvenomous) of right ear**

⑦S00.462 **Insect bite (nonvenomous) of left ear**

⑦S00.469 **Insect bite (nonvenomous) of unspecified ear**

S00.47 **Other superficial bite of ear**

Excludes1: open bite of ear (S01.35)

⑦S00.471 **Other superficial bite of right ear**

⑦S00.472 **Other superficial bite of left ear**

⑦S00.479 **Other superficial bite of unspecified ear**

S00.5 **Superficial injury of lip and oral cavity**

S00.50 **Unspecified superficial injury of lip and oral cavity**

⑦S00.501 **Unspecified superficial injury of lip**

⑦S00.502 **Unspecified superficial injury of oral cavity**

S00.51 **Abrasion of lip and oral cavity**

⑦S00.511 **Abrasion of lip**

⑦S00.512 **Abrasion of oral cavity**

S00.52 **Blister (nonthermal) of lip and oral cavity**

⑦S00.521 **Blister (nonthermal) of lip**

⑦S00.522 **Blister (nonthermal) of oral cavity**

S00.53 **Contusion of lip and oral cavity**

⑦S00.531 **Contusion of lip**

Bruise of lip

Hematoma of lip

⑦S00.532 **Contusion of oral cavity**

Bruise of oral cavity

● New code   ▲ Revised code   **Excludes1:** Not coded here   **Excludes2:** Not included here   ⊗ Placeholder required   ⑦7th digit required

Hematoma of oral cavity

S00.54   **External constriction of lip and oral cavity**

⑦S00.541   **External constriction of lip**

⑦S00.542   **External constriction of oral cavity**

S00.55   **Superficial foreign body of lip and oral cavity**

⑦S00.551   **Superficial foreign body of lip**

Splinter of lip and oral cavity

⑦S00.552   **Superficial foreign body of oral cavity**

Splinter of lip and oral cavity

S00.56   **Insect bite (nonvenomous) of lip and oral cavity**

⑦S00.561   **Insect bite (nonvenomous) of lip**

⑦S00.562   **Insect bite (nonvenomous) of oral cavity**

S00.57   **Other superficial bite of lip and oral cavity**

⑦S00.571   **Other superficial bite of lip**

Excludes1: open bite of lip (S01.551)

⑦S00.572   **Other superficial bite of oral cavity**

Excludes1: open bite of oral cavity (S01.552)

S00.8   **Superficial injury of other parts of head**

Superficial injuries of face [any part]

⊗⑦S00.80   **Unspecified superficial injury of other part of head**

⊗⑦S00.81   **Abrasion of other part of head**

⊗⑦S00.82   **Blister (nonthermal) of other part of head**

⊗⑦S00.83   **Contusion of other part of head**

Bruise of other part of head

Hematoma of other part of head

⊗⑦S00.84   **External constriction of other part of head**

⊗⑦S00.85   **Superficial foreign body of other part of head**

Splinter in other part of head

⊗⑦S00.86   **Insect bite (nonvenomous) of other part of head**

⊗⑦S00.87   **Other superficial bite of other part of head**

Excludes1: open bite of other part of head (S01.85)

S00.9   **Superficial injury of unspecified part of head**

⊗⑦S00.90   **Unspecified superficial injury of unspecified part of head**

⊗⑦S00.91   **Abrasion of unspecified part of head**

⊗⑦S00.92   **Blister (nonthermal) of unspecified part of head**

⊗⑦S00.93   **Contusion of unspecified part of head**

Bruise of head

Hematoma of head

⊗⑦S00.94   **External constriction of unspecified part of head**

⊗⑦S00.95   **Superficial foreign body of unspecified part of head**

Splinter of head

⊗⑦S00.96   **Insect bite (nonvenomous) of unspecified part of head**

⊗⑦S00.97   **Other superficial bite of unspecified part of head**

Excludes1: open bite of head (S01.95)

S01   Open wound of head

Code also any associated:

injury of cranial nerve (S04.-)

injury of muscle and tendon of head (S09.1-)

intracranial injury (S06.-)

wound infection

Excludes1: open skull fracture (S02.- with 7th character B)

Excludes2: injury of eye and orbit (S05.-)

traumatic amputation of part of head (S08.-)

The appropriate 7th character is to be added to each code from category S01

A - initial encounter

D - subsequent encounter

S - sequela

S01.0   **Open wound of scalp**

Excludes1: avulsion of scalp (S08.0)

⊗⑦S01.00   **Unspecified open wound of scalp**

⊗⑦S01.01   **Laceration without foreign body of scalp**

⊗⑦S01.02   **Laceration with foreign body of scalp**

⊗⑦S01.03   **Puncture wound without foreign body of scalp**

⊗⑦S01.04   **Puncture wound with foreign body of scalp**

⊗⑦S01.05   **Open bite of scalp**

Bite of scalp NOS

Excludes1: superficial bite of scalp (S00.06, S00.07-)

S01.1   **Open wound of eyelid and periocular area**

Open wound of eyelid and periocular area with or without involvement of lacrimal passages

S01.10   **Unspecified open wound of eyelid and periocular area**

⑦S01.101   **Unspecified open wound of right eyelid and periocular area**

⑦S01.102   **Unspecified open wound of left eyelid and periocular area**

⑦S01.109   **Unspecified open wound of unspecified eyelid and periocular area**

S01.11   **Laceration without foreign body of eyelid and periocular area**

⑦S01.111   **Laceration without foreign body of right eyelid and periocular area**

⑦S01.112   **Laceration without foreign body of left eyelid and periocular area**

⑦S01.119   **Laceration without foreign body of unspecified eyelid and periocular area**

S01.12   **Laceration with foreign body of eyelid and periocular area**

⑦S01.121   **Laceration with foreign body of right eyelid and periocular area**

⑦S01.122   **Laceration with foreign body of left eyelid and periocular area**

⑦S01.129   **Laceration with foreign body of unspecified eyelid and periocular area**

S01.13   **Puncture wound without foreign body of eyelid and periocular area**

⑦S01.131   **Puncture wound without foreign body of right eyelid and periocular area**

⑦S01.132   **Puncture wound without foreign body of left eyelid and periocular area**

⑦S01.139   **Puncture wound without foreign body of unspecified eyelid and periocular area**

S01.14   **Puncture wound with foreign body of eyelid and periocular area**

⑦S01.141   **Puncture wound with foreign body of right eyelid and periocular area**

⑦S01.142   **Puncture wound with foreign body of left eyelid and periocular area**

⑦S01.149   **Puncture wound with foreign body of unspecified eyelid and periocular area**

S01.15   **Open bite of eyelid and periocular area**

Bite of eyelid and periocular area NOS

Excludes1: superficial bite of eyelid and periocular area (S00.26, S00.27)

⑦S01.151   **Open bite of right eyelid and periocular area**

⑦S01.152   **Open bite of left eyelid and periocular area**

⑦S01.159   **Open bite of unspecified eyelid and periocular area**

S01.2   **Open wound of nose**

⊗⑦S01.20   **Unspecified open wound of nose**

⊗⑦S01.21   **Laceration without foreign body of nose**

⊗⑦S01.22   **Laceration with foreign body of nose**

⊗⑦S01.23   **Puncture wound without foreign body of nose**

⊗⑦S01.24   **Puncture wound with foreign body of nose**

⊗⑦S01.25   **Open bite of nose**

Bite of nose NOS

Excludes1: superficial bite of nose (S00.36, S00.37)

S01.3   **Open wound of ear**

S01.30   **Unspecified open wound of ear**

⑦S01.301   **Unspecified open wound of right ear**

⑦S01.302   **Unspecified open wound of left ear**

⑦S01.309   **Unspecified open wound of unspecified ear**

S01.31   **Laceration without foreign body of ear**

⑦S01.311   **Laceration without foreign body of right ear**

⑦S01.312   **Laceration without foreign body of left ear**

⑦S01.319   **Laceration without foreign body of unspecified ear**

S01.32   **Laceration with foreign body of ear**

⑦S01.321   **Laceration with foreign body of right ear**

⑦S01.322   **Laceration with foreign body of left ear**

⑦S01.329   **Laceration with foreign body of unspecified ear**

S01.33   **Puncture wound without foreign body of ear**

⑦S01.331   **Puncture wound without foreign body of right ear**

⑦S01.332   **Puncture wound without foreign body of left ear**

⑦S01.339   **Puncture wound without foreign body of unspecified ear**

S01.34   **Puncture wound with foreign body of ear**

⑦S01.341   **Puncture wound with foreign body of right ear**

⑦S01.342   **Puncture wound with foreign body of left ear**

⑦S01.349   **Puncture wound with foreign body of unspecified ear**

S01.35   **Open bite of ear**

Bite of ear NOS

Excludes1: superficial bite of ear (S00.46, S00.47)

⑦S01.351   **Open bite of right ear**

⑦S01.352   **Open bite of left ear**

⑦S01.359   **Open bite of unspecified ear**

S01.4   **Open wound of cheek and temporomandibular area**

S01.40   **Unspecified open wound of cheek and temporomandibular area**

⑦S01.401   **Unspecified open wound of right cheek and temporomandibular area**

⑦S01.402   **Unspecified open wound of left cheek and temporomandibular area**

⑦S01.409   **Unspecified open wound of unspecified cheek and temporomandibular area**

S01.41   **Laceration without foreign body of cheek and temporomandibular area**

⑦S01.411   **Laceration without foreign body of right cheek and temporomandibular area**

⑦S01.412   **Laceration without foreign body of left cheek and temporomandibular area**

⑦S01.419   **Laceration without foreign body of unspecified cheek and temporomandibular area**

S01.42   **Laceration with foreign body of cheek and temporomandibular area**

⑦S01.421   **Laceration with foreign body of right cheek and temporomandibular area**

⑦S01.422   **Laceration with foreign body of left cheek and temporomandibular area**

⑦S01.429   **Laceration with foreign body of unspecified cheek and temporomandibular area**

S01.43   **Puncture wound without foreign body of cheek and temporomandibular area**

⑦S01.431   **Puncture wound without foreign body of right cheek and temporomandibular area**

⑦S01.432   **Puncture wound without foreign body of left cheek and temporomandibular area**

⑦S01.439   **Puncture wound without foreign body of unspecified cheek and temporomandibular area**

S01.44   **Puncture wound with foreign body of cheek and temporomandibular area**

⑦S01.441   **Puncture wound with foreign body of right cheek and temporomandibular area**

⑦S01.442   **Puncture wound with foreign body of left cheek and temporomandibular area**

⑦S01.449   **Puncture wound with foreign body of unspecified cheek and temporomandibular area**

S01.45   **Open bite of cheek and temporomandibular area**

Bite of cheek and temporomandibular area NOS

Excludes2: superficial bite of cheek and temporomandibular area (S00.86, S00.87)

⑦**S01.451**   **Open bite of right cheek and temporomandibular area**

⑦**S01.452**   **Open bite of left cheek and temporomandibular area**

⑦**S01.459**   **Open bite of unspecified cheek and temporomandibular area**

S01.5   **Open wound of lip and oral cavity**

Excludes2: tooth dislocation (S03.2)

tooth fracture (S02.5)

S01.50   **Unspecified open wound of lip and oral cavity**

⑦**S01.501**   **Unspecified open wound of lip**

⑦**S01.502**   **Unspecified open wound of oral cavity**

S01.51   **Laceration of lip and oral cavity without foreign body**

⑦**S01.511**   **Laceration without foreign body of lip**

⑦**S01.512**   **Laceration without foreign body of oral cavity**

S01.52   **Laceration of lip and oral cavity with foreign body**

⑦**S01.521**   **Laceration with foreign body of lip**

⑦**S01.522**   **Laceration with foreign body of oral cavity**

S01.53   **Puncture wound of lip and oral cavity without foreign body**

⑦**S01.531**   **Puncture wound without foreign body of lip**

⑦**S01.532**   **Puncture wound without foreign body of oral cavity**

S01.54   **Puncture wound of lip and oral cavity with foreign body**

⑦**S01.541**   **Puncture wound with foreign body of lip**

⑦**S01.542**   **Puncture wound with foreign body of oral cavity**

S01.55   **Open bite of lip and oral cavity**

⑦**S01.551**   **Open bite of lip**

Bite of lip NOS

Excludes1: superficial bite of lip (S00.571)

⑦**S01.552**   **Open bite of oral cavity**

Bite of oral cavity NOS

Excludes1: superficial bite of oral cavity (S00.572)

S01.8   **Open wound of other parts of head**

⊗⑦**S01.80**   **Unspecified open wound of other part of head**

⊗⑦**S01.81**   **Laceration without foreign body of other part of head**

⊗⑦**S01.82**   **Laceration with foreign body of other part of head**

⊗⑦**S01.83**   **Puncture wound without foreign body of other part of head**

⊗⑦**S01.84**   **Puncture wound with foreign body of other part of head**

⊗⑦**S01.85**   **Open bite of other part of head**

Bite **of other** part of head NOS

Excludes1: superficial bite **of other** part of head (S00.87)

S01.9   **Open wound of unspecified part of head**

⊗⑦**S01.90**   **Unspecified open wound of unspecified part of head**

⊗⑦**S01.91**   **Laceration without foreign body of unspecified part of head**

⊗⑦**S01.92**   **Laceration with foreign body of unspecified part of head**

⊗⑦**S01.93**   **Puncture wound without foreign body of unspecified part of head**

⊗⑦**S01.94**   **Puncture wound with foreign body of unspecified part of head**

⊗⑦**S01.95**   **Open bite of unspecified part of head**

Bite of head NOS

Excludes1: superficial bite of head NOS (S00.97)

S02   **Fracture of skull and facial bones**

Note: A fracture not indicated as open or closed should be coded to closed

Code also any associated intracranial injury (S06.-)

The appropriate 7th character is to be added to each code from category S02

A - initial encounter for closed fracture

B - initial encounter for open fracture

D - subsequent encounter for fracture with routine healing

G - subsequent encounter for fracture with delayed healing

K - subsequent encounter for fracture with nonunion

S - sequela

⊗⑦**S02.0**   **Fracture of vault of skull**

Fracture of frontal bone

Fracture of parietal bone

S02.1   **Fracture of base of skull**

Excludes1: orbit NOS (S02.8)

Excludes2: orbital floor (S02.3-)

S02.10   **Unspecified fracture of base of skull**

⑦**S02.101**   **Fracture of base of skull, right side**

⑦**S02.102**   **Fracture of base of skull, left side**

⑦**S02.109**   **Fracture of base of skull, unspecified side**

S02.11   **Fracture of occiput**

⑦**S02.110**   **Type I occipital condyle fracture, unspecified side**

⑦**S02.111**   **Type II occipital condyle fracture, unspecified side**

⑦**S02.112**   **Type III occipital condyle fracture, unspecified side**

⑦**S02.113**   **Unspecified occipital condyle fracture**

⑦**S02.118**   **Other fracture of occiput, unspecified side**

⑦**S02.119**   **Unspecified fracture of occiput**

⑦**S02.11A**   **Type I occipital condyle fracture, right side**

⑦**S02.11B**   **Type I occipital condyle fracture, left side**

⑦**S02.11C**   **Type II occipital condyle fracture, right side**

⑦**S02.11D**   **Type II occipital condyle fracture, left side**

⑦**S02.11E**   **Type III occipital condyle fracture, right side**

⑦**S02.11F**   **Type III occipital condyle fracture, left side**

⑦**S02.11G**   **Other fracture of occiput, right side**

▨   Add 4th-7th digits   Nonspecific code   Unspecified code   Manifestation code   **739**

⊘⑦**S02.11H**   **Other fracture of occiput, left side**

⊗⑦S02.19   **Other fracture of base of skull**

Fracture of anterior fossa of base of skull

Fracture of ethmoid sinus

Fracture of frontal sinus

Fracture of middle fossa of base of skull

Fracture of orbital roof

Fracture of posterior fossa of base of skull

Fracture of sphenoid

Fracture of temporal bone

⊗⑦S02.2   **Fracture of nasal bones**

S02.3   **Fracture of orbital floor**

Excludes1: orbit NOS (S02.8)

Excludes2: orbital roof (S02.1-)

⊗⑦S02.30   **Fracture of orbital floor, unspecified side**

⊗⑦S02.31   **Fracture of orbital floor, right side**

⊗⑦S02.32   **Fracture of orbital floor, left side**

S02.4   **Fracture of malar, maxillary and zygoma bones**

Fracture of superior maxilla

Fracture of upper jaw (bone)

Fracture of zygomatic process of temporal bone

S02.40   **Fracture of malar, maxillary and zygoma bones, unspecified**

⑦S02.400   **Malar fracture, unspecified side**

⑦S02.401   **Maxillary fracture, unspecified side**

⑦S02.402   **Zygomatic fracture, unspecified side**

⑦S02.40A   **Malar fracture, right side**

⑦S02.40B   **Malar fracture, left side**

⑦S02.40C   **Maxillary fracture, right side**

⑦S02.40D   **Maxillary fracture, left side**

⑦S02.40E   **Zygomatic fracture, right side**

⑦S02.40F   **Zygomatic fracture, left side**

S02.41   **LeFort fracture**

⑦S02.411   **LeFort I fracture**

⑦S02.412   **LeFort II fracture**

⑦S02.413   **LeFort III fracture**

⊗⑦S02.42   **Fracture of alveolus of maxilla**

⊗⑦S02.5   **Fracture of tooth (traumatic)**

Broken tooth

Excludes1: cracked tooth (nontraumatic) (K03.81)

S02.6   **Fracture of mandible**

Fracture of lower jaw (bone)

S02.60   **Fracture of mandible, unspecified**

⑦S02.600   **Fracture of unspecified part of body of mandible, unspecified side**

⑦S02.601   **Fracture of unspecified part of body of right mandible**

⑦S02.602   **Fracture of unspecified part of body of left mandible**

⑦S02.609   **Fracture of mandible, unspecified**

S02.61   **Fracture of condylar process of mandible**

⑦S02.610   **Fracture of condylar process of mandible, unspecified side**

⑦S02.611   **Fracture of condylar process of right mandible**

⑦S02.612   **Fracture of condylar process of left mandible**

S02.62   **Fracture of subcondylar process of mandible**

⑦S02.620   **Fracture of subcondylar process of mandible, unspecified side**

⑦S02.621   **Fracture of subcondylar process of right mandible**

⑦S02.622   **Fracture of subcondylar process of left mandible**

S02.63   **Fracture of coronoid process of mandible**

⑦S02.630   **Fracture of coronoid process of mandible, unspecified side**

⑦S02.631   **Fracture of coronoid process of right mandible**

⑦S02.632   **Fracture of coronoid process of left mandible**

S02.64   **Fracture of ramus of mandible**

⑦S02.640   **Fracture of ramus of mandible, unspecified side**

⑦S02.641   **Fracture of ramus of right mandible**

⑦S02.642   **Fracture of ramus of left mandible**

S02.65   **Fracture of angle of mandible**

⑦S02.650   **Fracture of angle of mandible, unspecified side**

⑦S02.651   **Fracture of angle of right mandible**

⑦S02.652   **Fracture of angle of left mandible**

⊗⑦S02.66   **Fracture of symphysis of mandible**

S02.67   **Fracture of alveolus of mandible**

⑦S02.670   **Fracture of alveolus of mandible, unspecified side**

⑦S02.671   **Fracture of alveolus of right mandible**

⑦S02.672   **Fracture of alveolus of left mandible**

⊗⑦S02.69   **Fracture of mandible of other specified site**

S02.8   **Fractures of other specified skull and facial bones**

Fracture of orbit NOS

Fracture of palate

Excludes1: fracture of orbital floor (S02.3-)

fracture of orbital roof (S02.1-)

⊗⑦S02.80   **Fracture of other specified skull and facial bones, unspecified side**

⊗⑦S02.81   **Fracture of other specified skull and facial bones, right side**

⊗⑦S02.82   **Fracture of other specified skull and facial bones, left side**

S02.9   **Fracture of unspecified skull and facial bones**

⊗⑦S02.91   **Unspecified fracture of skull**

⊗⑦S02.92   **Unspecified fracture of facial bones**

S03   **Dislocation and sprain of joints and ligaments of head**

Includes: avulsion of joint (capsule) or ligament of head

laceration of cartilage, joint (capsule) or ligament of head sprain of cartilage, joint (capsule) or ligament of head

traumatic hemarthrosis of joint or ligament of head

traumatic rupture of joint or ligament of head

traumatic subluxation of joint or ligament of head

traumatic tear of joint or ligament of head

Code also any associated open wound

Excludes2: Strain of muscle or tendon of head (S09.1)

The appropriate 7th character is to be added to each code from category S03

A - initial encounter

D - subsequent encounter

S - sequela

S03.0   **Dislocation of jaw**

Dislocation of jaw (cartilage) (meniscus)

Dislocation of mandible

Dislocation of temporomandibular (joint)

⊗⑦**S03.00**   **Dislocation of jaw, unspecified side**

⊗⑦**S03.01**   **Dislocation of jaw, right side**

⊗⑦**S03.02**   **Dislocation of jaw, left side**

⊗⑦**S03.03**   **Dislocation of jaw, bilateral**

⊗⑦**S03.1**   **Dislocation of septal cartilage of nose**

⊗⑦**S03.2**   **Dislocation of tooth**

S03.4   **Sprain of jaw**

Sprain of temporomandibular (joint) (ligament)

⊗⑦**S03.40**   **Sprain of jaw, unspecified side**

⊗⑦**S03.41**   **Sprain of jaw, right side**

⊗⑦**S03.42**   **Sprain of jaw, left side**

⊗⑦**S03.43**   **Sprain of jaw, bilateral**

⊗⑦**S03.8**   **Sprain of joints and ligaments of other parts of head**

⊗⑦**S03.9**   **Sprain of joints and ligaments of unspecified parts of head**

S04   **Injury of cranial nerve**

The selection of side should be based on the side of the body being affected

Code first any associated intracranial injury (S06.-)

Code also any associated:

open wound of head (S01.-)

skull fracture (S02.-)

The appropriate 7th character is to be added to each code from category S04

A - initial encounter

D - subsequent encounter

S - sequela

S04.0   **Injury of optic nerve and pathways**

Use additional code to identify any visual field defect or blindness (H53.4-, H54-)

S04.01   **Injury of optic nerve**

Injury of 2nd cranial nerve

⑦**S04.011**   **Injury of optic nerve, right eye**

⑦**S04.012**   **Injury of optic nerve, left eye**

⑦**S04.019**   **Injury of optic nerve, unspecified eye**

Injury of optic nerve NOS

⊗⑦**S04.02**   **Injury of optic chiasm**

S04.03   **Injury of optic tract and pathways**

Injury of optic radiation

▲⑦**S04.031**   **Injury of optic tract and pathways, right side**

▲⑦**S04.032**   **Injury of optic tract and pathways, left side**

▲⑦**S04.039**   **Injury of optic tract and pathways, unspecified side**

Injury of optic tract and pathways NOS

S04.04   **Injury of visual cortex**

▲⑦**S04.041**   **Injury of visual cortex, right side**

▲⑦**S04.042**   **Injury of visual cortex, left side**

▲⑦**S04.049**   **Injury of visual cortex, unspecified side**

Injury of visual cortex NOS

S04.1   **Injury of oculomotor nerve**

Injury of 3rd cranial nerve

⊗⑦**S04.10**   **Injury of oculomotor nerve, unspecified side**

⊗⑦**S04.11**   **Injury of oculomotor nerve, right side**

⊗⑦**S04.12**   **Injury of oculomotor nerve, left side**

S04.2   **Injury of trochlear nerve**

Injury of 4th cranial nerve

⊗⑦**S04.20**   **Injury of trochlear nerve, unspecified side**

⊗⑦**S04.21**   **Injury of trochlear nerve, right side**

⊗⑦**S04.22**   **Injury of trochlear nerve, left side**

S04.3   **Injury of trigeminal nerve**

Injury of 5th cranial nerve

⊗⑦**S04.30**   **Injury of trigeminal nerve, unspecified side**

⊗⑦**S04.31**   **Injury of trigeminal nerve, right side**

⊗⑦**S04.32**   **Injury of trigeminal nerve, left side**

S04.4   **Injury of abducent nerve**

Injury of 6th cranial nerve

⊗⑦**S04.40**   **Injury of abducent nerve, unspecified side**

⊗⑦**S04.41**   **Injury of abducent nerve, right side**

⊗⑦**S04.42**   **Injury of abducent nerve, left side**

S04.5   **Injury of facial nerve**

Injury of 7th cranial nerve

⊗⑦**S04.50**   **Injury of facial nerve, unspecified side**

⊗⑦**S04.51**   **Injury of facial nerve, right side**

⊗⑦**S04.52**   **Injury of facial nerve, left side**

S04.6   **Injury of acoustic nerve**

Injury of auditory nerve Injury of 8th cranial nerve

⊗⑦**S04.60**   **Injury of acoustic nerve, unspecified side**

⊗⑦**S04.61**   **Injury of acoustic nerve, right side**

⊗⑦**S04.62**   **Injury of acoustic nerve, left side**

S04.7   **Injury of accessory nerve**

Injury of 11th cranial nerve

⊗⑦**S04.70**   **Injury of accessory nerve, unspecified side**

⊗⑦**S04.71**   **Injury of accessory nerve, right side**

⊗⑦**S04.72**   **Injury of accessory nerve, left side**

S04.8   **Injury of other cranial nerves**

S04.81   **Injury of olfactory [1st] nerve**

⑦**S04.811**   **Injury of olfactory [1st] nerve, right side**

⑦**S04.812**   **Injury of olfactory [1st] nerve, left side**

⑦**S04.819**   **Injury of olfactory [1st] nerve, unspecified side**

S04.89   **Injury of other cranial nerves**

Injury of vagus [10th] nerve

⑦**S04.891**   **Injury of other cranial nerves, right side**

⑦**S04.892**   **Injury of other cranial nerves, left side**

⑦**S04.899**   **Injury of other cranial nerves, unspecified side**

⊗⑦**S04.9**   **Injury of unspecified cranial nerve**

S05   **Injury of eye and orbit**

Includes: open wound of eye and orbit

Excludes2: 2nd cranial [optic] nerve injury (S04.0-)

3rd cranial [oculomotor] nerve injury (S04.1-)

open wound of eyelid and periocular area (S01.1-)

orbital bone fracture (S02.1-, S02.3-, S02.8-)

superficial injury of eyelid (S00.1-S00.2)

The appropriate 7th character is to be added to each code from category S05

A - initial encounter

D - subsequent encounter

S - sequela

S05.0   Injury of conjunctiva and corneal abrasion without foreign body

> **Excludes1:** foreign body in conjunctival sac (T15.1)
>
> foreign body in cornea (T15.0)

⊗⑦**S05.00   Injury of conjunctiva and corneal abrasion without foreign body, unspecified eye**

⊗⑦**S05.01   Injury of conjunctiva and corneal abrasion without foreign body, right eye**

⊗⑦**S05.02   Injury of conjunctiva and corneal abrasion without foreign body, left eye**

S05.1   Contusion of eyeball and orbital tissues

Traumatic hyphema

> **Excludes2:** black eye NOS (S00.1)
>
> contusion of eyelid and periocular area (S00.1)

⊗⑦**S05.10   Contusion of eyeball and orbital tissues, unspecified eye**

⊗⑦**S05.11   Contusion of eyeball and orbital tissues, right eye**

⊗⑦**S05.12   Contusion of eyeball and orbital tissues, left eye**

S05.2   Ocular laceration and rupture with prolapse or loss of intraocular tissue

⊗⑦**S05.20   Ocular laceration and rupture with prolapse or loss of intraocular tissue, unspecified eye**

⊗⑦**S05.21   Ocular laceration and rupture with prolapse or loss of intraocular tissue, right eye**

⊗⑦**S05.22   Ocular laceration and rupture with prolapse or loss of intraocular tissue, left eye**

S05.3   Ocular laceration without prolapse or loss of intraocular tissue

Laceration of eye NOS

⊗⑦**S05.30   Ocular laceration without prolapse or loss of intraocular tissue, unspecified eye**

⊗⑦**S05.31   Ocular laceration without prolapse or loss of intraocular tissue, right eye**

⊗⑦**S05.32   Ocular laceration without prolapse or loss of intraocular tissue, left eye**

S05.4   Penetrating wound of orbit with or without foreign body

> **Excludes2:** retained (old) foreign body following penetrating wound in orbit (H05.5-)

⊗⑦**S05.40   Penetrating wound of orbit with or without foreign body, unspecified eye**

⊗⑦**S05.41   Penetrating wound of orbit with or without foreign body, right eye**

⊗⑦**S05.42   Penetrating wound of orbit with or without foreign body, left eye**

S05.5   Penetrating wound with foreign body of eyeball

> **Excludes2:** retained (old) intraocular foreign body (H44.6-, H44.7)

⊗⑦**S05.50   Penetrating wound with foreign body of unspecified eyeball**

⊗⑦**S05.51   Penetrating wound with foreign body of right eyeball**

⊗⑦**S05.52   Penetrating wound with foreign body of left eyeball**

S05.6   Penetrating wound without foreign body of eyeball

Ocular penetration NOS

⊗⑦**S05.60   Penetrating wound without foreign body of unspecified eyeball**

⊗⑦**S05.61   Penetrating wound without foreign body of right eyeball**

⊗⑦**S05.62   Penetrating wound without foreign body of left eyeball**

S05.7   Avulsion of eye

> **Definition:** An avulsion is an injury in which a body structure is forcibly detached from its normal point of insertion by either trauma or surgery.

Traumatic enucleation

⊗⑦**S05.70   Avulsion of unspecified eye**

⊗⑦**S05.71   Avulsion of right eye**

⊗⑦**S05.72   Avulsion of left eye**

S05.8   Other injuries of eye and orbit

Lacrimal duct injury

S05.8X   Other injuries of eye and orbit

⑦**S05.8X1   Other injuries of right eye and orbit**

⑦**S05.8X2   Other injuries of left eye and orbit**

⑦**S05.8X9   Other injuries of unspecified eye and orbit**

S05.9   Unspecified injury of eye and orbit

Injury of eye NOS

⊗⑦**S05.90   Unspecified injury of unspecified eye and orbit**

⊗⑦**S05.91   Unspecified injury of right eye and orbit**

⊗⑦**S05.92   Unspecified injury of left eye and orbit**

S06   Intracranial injury

Includes: traumatic brain injury

Code also any associated:

open wound of head (S01.-)

skull fracture (S02.-)

Excludes1: head injury NOS (S09.90)

The appropriate 7th character is to be added to each code from category S06

A - initial encounter

D - subsequent encounter

S – sequela

Note: 7th characters D and S do not apply to codes in category S06 with 6th character 7 - death due to brain injury prior to regaining consciousness, or 8 - death due to other cause prior to regaining consciousness.

S06.0   Concussion

Commotio cerebri

> **Excludes1:** concussion with other intracranial injuries classified in subcategories S06.1- to S06.6- , S06.81- and S06.82- code to specified intracranial injury

S06.0X   Concussion

⑦**S06.0X0   Concussion without loss of consciousness**

⑦**S06.0X1   Concussion with loss of consciousness of 30 minutes or less**

⑦**S06.0X9   Concussion with loss of consciousness of unspecified duration**

Concussion NOS

S06.1   Traumatic cerebral edema

Diffuse traumatic cerebral edema

Focal traumatic cerebral edema

S06.1X   Traumatic cerebral edema

⑦S06.1X0   **Traumatic cerebral edema without loss of consciousness**

⑦S06.1X1   **Traumatic cerebral edema with loss of consciousness of 30 minutes or less**

⑦S06.1X2   **Traumatic cerebral edema with loss of consciousness of 31 minutes to 59 minutes**

⑦S06.1X3   **Traumatic cerebral edema with loss of consciousness of 1hour to 5 hours 59 minutes**

⑦S06.1X4   **Traumatic cerebral edema with loss of consciousness of 6 hours to 24 hours**

⑦S06.1X5   **Traumatic cerebral edema with loss of consciousness greater than 24 hours with return to pre-existing conscious level**

⑦S06.1X6   **Traumatic cerebral edema with loss of consciousness greater than 24 hours without return to pre-existing conscious level with patient surviving**

⑦S06.1X7   **Traumatic cerebral edema with loss of consciousness of any duration with death due to brain injury prior to regaining consciousness**

⑦S06.1X8   **Traumatic cerebral edema with loss of consciousness of any duration with death due to other cause prior to regaining consciousness**

⑦S06.1X9   **Traumatic cerebral edema with loss of consciousness of unspecified duration**

Traumatic cerebral edema NOS

S06.2   Diffuse traumatic brain injury

Diffuse axonal brain injury

Excludes1: traumatic diffuse cerebral edema (S06.1X-)

S06.2X   Diffuse traumatic brain injury

⑦S06.2X0   **Diffuse traumatic brain injury without loss of consciousness**

⑦S06.2X1   **Diffuse traumatic brain injury with loss of consciousness of 30 minutes or less**

⑦S06.2X2   **Diffuse traumatic brain injury with loss of consciousness of 31 minutes to 59 minutes**

⑦S06.2X3   **Diffuse traumatic brain injury with loss of consciousness of 1 hour to 5 hours 59 minutes**

⑦S06.2X4   **Diffuse traumatic brain injury with loss of consciousness of 6 hours to 24 hours**

⑦S06.2X5   **Diffuse traumatic brain injury with loss of consciousness greater than 24 hours with return to pre-existing conscious levels**

⑦S06.2X6   **Diffuse traumatic brain injury with loss of consciousness greater than 24 hours without return to pre-existing conscious level with patient surviving**

⑦S06.2X7   **Diffuse traumatic brain injury with loss of consciousness of any duration with death due to brain injury prior to regaining consciousness**

⑦S06.2X8   **Diffuse traumatic brain injury with loss of consciousness of any duration with death due to other cause prior to regaining consciousness**

⑦S06.2X9   **Diffuse traumatic brain injury with loss of consciousness of unspecified duration**

Diffuse traumatic brain injury NOS

S06.3   Focal traumatic brain injury

Excludes1: any condition classifiable to S06.4-S06.6

focal cerebral edema (S06.1)

S06.30   Unspecified focal traumatic brain injury

⑦S06.300   **Unspecified focal traumatic brain injury without loss of consciousness**

⑦S06.301   **Unspecified focal traumatic brain injury with loss of consciousness of 30 minutes or less**

⑦S06.302   **Unspecified focal traumatic brain injury with loss of consciousness of 31 minutes to 59 minutes**

⑦S06.303   **Unspecified focal traumatic brain injury with loss of consciousness of 1 hour to 5 hours 59 minutes**

⑦S06.304   **Unspecified focal traumatic brain injury with loss of consciousness of 6 hours to 24 hours**

⑦S06.305   **Unspecified focal traumatic brain injury with loss of consciousness greater than 24 hours with return to pre-existing conscious level**

⑦S06.306   **Unspecified focal traumatic brain injury with loss of consciousness greater than 24 hours without return to pre-existing conscious level with patient surviving**

⑦S06.307   **Unspecified focal traumatic brain injury with loss of consciousness of any duration with death due to brain injury prior to regaining consciousness**

⑦S06.308   **Unspecified focal traumatic brain injury with loss of consciousness of any duration with death due to other cause prior to regaining consciousness**

⑦S06.309   **Unspecified focal traumatic brain injury with loss of consciousness of unspecified duration**

Unspecified focal traumatic brain injury NOS

S06.31   Contusion and laceration of right cerebrum

⑦S06.310   **Contusion and laceration of right cerebrum without loss of consciousness**

⑦S06.311   **Contusion and laceration of right cerebrum with loss of consciousness of 30 minutes or less**

⑦S06.312   **Contusion and laceration of right cerebrum with loss of consciousness of 31 minutes to 59 minutes**

⑦S06.313   **Contusion and laceration of right cerebrum with loss of consciousness of 1 hour to 5 hours 59 minutes**

⑦S06.314   **Contusion and laceration of right cerebrum with loss of consciousness of 6 hours to 24 hours**

⑦S06.315   **Contusion and laceration of right cerebrum with loss of consciousness greater than 24 hours with return to pre-existing conscious level**

---

⑦S06.316   Contusion and laceration of right cerebrum with loss of consciousness greater than 24 hours without return to pre-existing conscious level with patient surviving

⑦S06.317   Contusion and laceration of right cerebrum with loss of consciousness of any duration with death due to brain injury prior to regaining consciousness

⑦S06.318   Contusion and laceration of right cerebrum with loss of consciousness of any duration with death due to other cause prior to regaining consciousness

⑦S06.319   Contusion and laceration of right cerebrum with loss of consciousness of unspecified duration

Contusion and laceration of right cerebrum NOS

S06.32   **Contusion and laceration of left cerebrum**

⑦S06.320   Contusion and laceration of left cerebrum without loss of consciousness

⑦S06.321   Contusion and laceration of left cerebrum with loss of consciousness of 30 minutes or less

⑦S06.322   Contusion and laceration of left cerebrum with loss of consciousness of 31 minutes to59 minutes

⑦S06.323   Contusion and laceration of left cerebrum with loss of consciousness of 1 hour to 5 hours 59 minutes

⑦S06.324   Contusion and laceration of left cerebrum with loss of consciousness of 6 hours to 24 hours

⑦S06.325   Contusion and laceration of left cerebrum with loss of consciousness greater than 24 hours with return to pre-existing conscious level

⑦S06.326   Contusion and laceration of left cerebrum with loss of consciousness greater than 24 hours without return to pre-existing conscious level with patient surviving

⑦S06.327   Contusion and laceration of left cerebrum with loss of consciousness of any duration with death due to brain injury prior to regaining consciousness

⑦S06.328   Contusion and laceration of left cerebrum with loss of consciousness of any duration with death due to other cause prior to regaining consciousness

⑦S06.329   Contusion and laceration of left cerebrum with loss of consciousness of unspecified duration

Contusion and laceration of left cerebrum NOS

S06.33   **Contusion and laceration of cerebrum, unspecified**

⑦S06.330   Contusion and laceration of cerebrum, unspecified, without loss of consciousness

⑦S06.331   Contusion and laceration of cerebrum, unspecified, with loss of consciousness of 30 minutes or less

⑦S06.332   Contusion and laceration of cerebrum, unspecified, with loss of consciousness of 31 minutes to 59 minutes

⑦S06.333   Contusion and laceration of cerebrum, unspecified, with loss of consciousness of 1 hour to 5 hours 59 minutes

⑦S06.334   Contusion and laceration of cerebrum, unspecified, with loss of consciousness of 6 hours to 24 hours

⑦S06.335   Contusion and laceration of cerebrum, unspecified, with loss of consciousness greater than 24 hours with return to pre-existing conscious level

⑦S06.336   Contusion and laceration of cerebrum, unspecified, with loss of consciousness greater than 24 hours without return to pre-existing conscious level with patient surviving

⑦S06.337   Contusion and laceration of cerebrum, unspecified, with loss of consciousness of any duration with death due to brain injury prior to regaining consciousness

⑦S06.338   Contusion and laceration of cerebrum, unspecified, with loss of consciousness of any duration with death due to other cause prior to regaining consciousness

⑦S06.339   Contusion and laceration of cerebrum, unspecified, with loss of consciousness of unspecified duration

Contusion and laceration of cerebrum NOS

S06.34   **Traumatic hemorrhage of right cerebrum**

Traumatic intracerebral hemorrhage and hematoma of right cerebrum

⑦S06.340   Traumatic hemorrhage of right cerebrum without loss of consciousness

⑦S06.341   Traumatic hemorrhage of right cerebrum with loss of consciousness of 30 minutes or less

⑦S06.342   Traumatic hemorrhage of right cerebrum with loss of consciousness of 31 minutes to 59 minutes

⑦S06.343   Traumatic hemorrhage of right cerebrum with loss of consciousness of 1 hours to 5 hours 59 minutes

⑦S06.344   Traumatic hemorrhage of right cerebrum with loss of consciousness of 6 hours to 24 hours

⑦S06.345   Traumatic hemorrhage of right cerebrum with loss of consciousness greater than 24 hours with return to pre-existing conscious level

⑦S06.346   Traumatic hemorrhage of right cerebrum with loss of consciousness greater than 24 hours without return to pre-existing conscious level with patient surviving

⑦S06.347   Traumatic hemorrhage of right cerebrum with loss of consciousness of any duration with death due to brain injury prior to regaining consciousness

  ● New code   ▲ Revised code   **Excludes1:** Not coded here   **Excludes2:** Not included here   ⊗ Placeholder required   ⑦7ᵗʰ digit required

⑦**S06.348** **Traumatic hemorrhage of right cerebrum with loss of consciousness of any duration with death due to other cause prior to regaining consciousness**

⑦**S06.349** **Traumatic hemorrhage of right cerebrum with loss of consciousness of unspecified duration**

Traumatic hemorrhage of right cerebrum NOS

S06.35 **Traumatic hemorrhage of left cerebrum**

Traumatic intracerebral hemorrhage and hematoma of left cerebrum

⑦**S06.350** **Traumatic hemorrhage of left cerebrum without loss of consciousness**

⑦**S06.351** **Traumatic hemorrhage of left cerebrum with loss of consciousness of 30 minutes or less**

⑦**S06.352** **Traumatic hemorrhage of left cerebrum with loss of consciousness of 31 minutes to 59 minutes**

⑦**S06.353** **Traumatic hemorrhage of left cerebrum with loss of consciousness of 1 hours to 5 hours 59 minutes**

⑦**S06.354** **Traumatic hemorrhage of left cerebrum with loss of consciousness of 6 hours to 24 hours**

⑦**S06.355** **Traumatic hemorrhage of left cerebrum with loss of consciousness greater than 24 hours with return to pre-existing conscious level**

⑦**S06.356** **Traumatic hemorrhage of left cerebrum with loss of consciousness greater than 24 hours without return to pre-existing conscious level with patient surviving**

⑦**S06.357** **Traumatic hemorrhage of left cerebrum with loss of consciousness of any duration with death due to brain injury prior to regaining consciousness**

⑦**S06.358** **Traumatic hemorrhage of left cerebrum with loss of consciousness of any duration with death due to other cause prior to regaining consciousness**

⑦**S06.359** **Traumatic hemorrhage of left cerebrum with loss of consciousness of unspecified duration**

Traumatic hemorrhage of left cerebrum NOS

S06.36 **Traumatic hemorrhage of cerebrum, unspecified**

Traumatic intracerebral hemorrhage and hematoma, unspecified

⑦**S06.360** **Traumatic hemorrhage of cerebrum, unspecified, without loss of consciousness**

⑦**S06.361** **Traumatic hemorrhage of cerebrum, unspecified, with loss of consciousness of 30 minutes or less**

⑦**S06.362** **Traumatic hemorrhage of cerebrum, unspecified, with loss of consciousness of 31 minutes to 59 minutes**

⑦**S06.363** **Traumatic hemorrhage of cerebrum, unspecified, with loss of**

consciousness of 1 hours to 5 hours 59 minutes

⑦**S06.364** **Traumatic hemorrhage of cerebrum, unspecified, with loss of consciousness of 6 hours to 24 hours**

⑦**S06.365** **Traumatic hemorrhage of cerebrum, unspecified, with loss of consciousness greater than 24 hours with return to pre-existing conscious level**

⑦**S06.366** **Traumatic hemorrhage of cerebrum, unspecified, with loss of consciousness greater than 24 hours without return to pre-existing conscious level with patient surviving**

⑦**S06.367** **Traumatic hemorrhage of cerebrum, unspecified, with loss of consciousness of any duration with death due to brain injury prior to regaining consciousness**

⑦**S06.368** **Traumatic hemorrhage of cerebrum, unspecified, with loss of consciousness of any duration with death due to other cause prior to regaining consciousness**

⑦**S06.369** **Traumatic hemorrhage of cerebrum, unspecified, with loss of consciousness of unspecified duration**

Traumatic hemorrhage of cerebrum NOS

S06.37 **Contusion, laceration, and hemorrhage of cerebellum**

⑦**S06.370** **Contusion, laceration, and hemorrhage of cerebellum without loss of consciousness**

⑦**S06.371** **Contusion, laceration, and hemorrhage of cerebellum with loss of consciousness of 30 minutes or less**

⑦**S06.372** **Contusion, laceration, and hemorrhage of cerebellum with loss of consciousness of 31 minutes to 59 minutes**

⑦**S06.373** **Contusion, laceration, and hemorrhage of cerebellum with loss of consciousness of 1 hour to 5 hours 59 minutes**

⑦**S06.374** **Contusion, laceration, and hemorrhage of cerebellum with loss of consciousness of 6 hours to 24 hours**

⑦**S06.375** **Contusion, laceration, and hemorrhage of cerebellum with loss of consciousness greater than 24 hours with return to pre-existing conscious level**

⑦**S06.376** **Contusion, laceration, and hemorrhage of cerebellum with loss of consciousness greater than 24 hours without return to pre-existing conscious level with patient surviving**

⑦**S06.377** **Contusion, laceration, and hemorrhage of cerebellum with loss of consciousness of any duration with death due to brain injury prior to regaining consciousness**

⑦**S06.378** **Contusion, laceration, and hemorrhage of cerebellum with loss of consciousness of any duration with death due to other cause prior to regaining consciousness**

⑦S06.379 Contusion, laceration, and hemorrhage of cerebellum with loss of consciousness of unspecified duration

Contusion, laceration, and hemorrhage of cerebellum NOS

S06.38 Contusion, laceration, and hemorrhage of brainstem

⑦S06.380 Contusion, laceration, and hemorrhage of brainstem without loss of consciousness

⑦S06.381 Contusion, laceration, and hemorrhage of brainstem with loss of consciousness of 30 minutes or less

⑦S06.382 Contusion, laceration, and hemorrhage of brainstem with loss of consciousness of 31 minutes to 59 minutes

⑦S06.383 Contusion, laceration, and hemorrhage of brainstem with loss of consciousness of 1 hour to 5 hours 59 minutes

⑦S06.384 Contusion, laceration, and hemorrhage of brainstem with loss of consciousness of 6 hours to 24 hours

⑦S06.385 Contusion, laceration, and hemorrhage of brainstem with loss of consciousness greater than 24 hours with return to pre-existing conscious level

⑦S06.386 Contusion, laceration, and hemorrhage of brainstem with loss of consciousness greater than 24 hours without return to pre-existing conscious level with patient surviving

⑦S06.387 Contusion, laceration, and hemorrhage of brainstem with loss of consciousness of any duration with death due to brain injury prior to regaining consciousness

⑦S06.388 Contusion, laceration, and hemorrhage of brainstem with loss of consciousness of any duration with death due to other cause prior to regaining consciousness

⑦S06.389 Contusion, laceration, and hemorrhage of brainstem with loss of consciousness of unspecified duration

Contusion, laceration, and hemorrhage of brainstem NOS

S06.4 Epidural hemorrhage

Extradural hemorrhage NOS

Extradural hemorrhage (traumatic)

S06.4X Epidural hemorrhage

⑦S06.4X0 Epidural hemorrhage without loss of consciousness

⑦S06.4X1 Epidural hemorrhage with loss of consciousness of 30 minutes or less

⑦S06.4X2 Epidural hemorrhage with loss of consciousness of 31 minutes to 59 minutes

⑦S06.4X3 Epidural hemorrhage with loss of consciousness of 1 hour to 5 hours 59 minutes

⑦S06.4X4 Epidural hemorrhage with loss of consciousness of 6 hours to 24 hours

⑦S06.4X5 Epidural hemorrhage with loss of consciousness greater than 24 hours with return to pre-existing conscious level

⑦S06.4X6 Epidural hemorrhage with loss of consciousness greater than 24 hours without return to pre-existing conscious level with patient surviving

⑦S06.4X7 Epidural hemorrhage with loss of consciousness of any duration with death due to brain injury prior to regaining consciousness

⑦S06.4X8 Epidural hemorrhage with loss of consciousness of any duration with death due to other causes prior to regaining consciousness

⑦S06.4X9 Epidural hemorrhage with loss of consciousness of unspecified duration

Epidural hemorrhage NOS

S06.5 Traumatic subdural hemorrhage

S06.5X Traumatic subdural hemorrhage

⑦S06.5X0 Traumatic subdural hemorrhage without loss of consciousness

⑦S06.5X1 Traumatic subdural hemorrhage with loss of consciousness of 30 minutes or less

⑦S06.5X2 Traumatic subdural hemorrhage with loss of consciousness of 31 minutes to 59 minutes

⑦S06.5X3 Traumatic subdural hemorrhage with loss of consciousness of 1 hour to 5 hours 59 minutes

⑦S06.5X4 Traumatic subdural hemorrhage with loss of consciousness of 6 hours to 24 hours

⑦S06.5X5 Traumatic subdural hemorrhage with loss of consciousness greater than 24 hours with return to pre-existing conscious level

⑦S06.5X6 Traumatic subdural hemorrhage with loss of consciousness greater than 24 hours without return to pre-existing conscious level with patient surviving

⑦S06.5X7 Traumatic subdural hemorrhage with loss of consciousness of any duration with death due to brain injury before regaining consciousness

⑦S06.5X8 Traumatic subdural hemorrhage with loss of consciousness of any duration with death due to other cause before regaining consciousness

⑦S06.5X9 Traumatic subdural hemorrhage with loss of consciousness of unspecified duration

Traumatic subdural hemorrhage NOS

S06.6 Traumatic subarachnoid hemorrhage

S06.6X Traumatic subarachnoid hemorrhage

⑦S06.6X0 Traumatic subarachnoid hemorrhage without loss of consciousness

⑦S06.6X1 Traumatic subarachnoid hemorrhage with loss of consciousness of 30 minutes or less

⑦S06.6X2 Traumatic subarachnoid hemorrhage with loss of

consciousness of 31 minutes to 59 minutes

⑦S06.6X3   **Traumatic subarachnoid hemorrhage with loss of consciousness of 1 hour to 5 hours 59 minutes**

⑦S06.6X4   **Traumatic subarachnoid hemorrhage with loss of consciousness of 6 hours to 24 hours**

⑦S06.6X5   **Traumatic subarachnoid hemorrhage with loss of consciousness greater than 24 hours with return to pre-existing conscious level**

⑦S06.6X6   **Traumatic subarachnoid hemorrhage with loss of consciousness greater than 24 hours without return to pre-existing conscious level with patient**

⑦S06.6X7   **Traumatic subarachnoid hemorrhage with loss of consciousness of any duration with death due to brain injury prior to regaining consciousness**

⑦S06.6X8   **Traumatic subarachnoid hemorrhage with loss of consciousness of any duration with death due to other cause prior to regaining consciousness**

⑦S06.6X9   **Traumatic subarachnoid hemorrhage with loss of consciousness of unspecified duration**

Traumatic subarachnoid hemorrhage NOS

S06.8   **Other specified intracranial injuries**

S06.81   **Injury of right internal carotid artery, intracranial portion, not elsewhere classified**

⑦S06.810   **Injury of right internal carotid artery, intracranial portion, not elsewhere classified without loss of consciousness**

⑦S06.811   **Injury of right internal carotid artery, intracranial portion, not elsewhere classified with loss of consciousness of 30 minutes or less**

⑦S06.812   **Injury of right internal carotid artery, intracranial portion, not elsewhere classified with loss of consciousness of 31 minutes to 59 minutes**

⑦S06.813   **Injury of right internal carotid artery, intracranial portion, not elsewhere classified with loss of consciousness of 1 hour to 5 hours 59 minutes**

⑦S06.814   **Injury of right internal carotid artery, intracranial portion, not elsewhere classified with loss of consciousness of 6 hours to 24 hours**

⑦S06.815   **Injury of right internal carotid artery, intracranial portion, not elsewhere classified with loss of consciousness greater than 24 hours with return to pre-existing conscious level**

⑦S06.816   **Injury of right internal carotid artery, intracranial portion, not elsewhere classified with loss of consciousness greater than 24 hours**

without return to pre-existing conscious level with patient surviving

⑦S06.817   **Injury of right internal carotid artery, intracranial portion, not elsewhere classified with loss of consciousness of any duration with death due to brain injury prior to regaining consciousness**

⑦S06.818   **Injury of right internal carotid artery, intracranial portion, not elsewhere classified with loss of consciousness of any duration with death due to other cause prior to regaining consciousness**

⑦S06.819   **Injury of right internal carotid artery, intracranial portion, not elsewhere classified with loss of consciousness of unspecified duration**

Injury of right internal carotid artery, intracranial portion, not elsewhere classified NOS

S06.82   **Injury of left internal carotid artery, intracranial portion, not elsewhere classified**

⑦S06.820   **Injury of left internal carotid artery, intracranial portion, not elsewhere classified without loss of consciousness**

⑦S06.821   **Injury of left internal carotid artery, intracranial portion, not elsewhere classified with loss of consciousness of 30 minutes or less**

⑦S06.822   **Injury of left internal carotid artery, intracranial portion, not elsewhere classified with loss of consciousness of 31 minutes to 59 minutes**

⑦S06.823   **Injury of left internal carotid artery, intracranial portion, not elsewhere classified with loss of consciousness of 1 hour to 5 hours 59 minutes**

⑦S06.824   **Injury of left internal carotid artery, intracranial portion, not elsewhere classified with loss of consciousness of 6 hours to 24 hours**

⑦S06.825   **Injury of left internal carotid artery, intracranial portion, not elsewhere classified with loss of consciousness greater than 24 hours with return to pre-existing conscious level**

⑦S06.826   **Injury of left internal carotid artery, intracranial portion, not elsewhere classified with loss of consciousness greater than 24 hours without return to pre-existing conscious level with patient surviving**

⑦S06.827   **Injury of left internal carotid artery, intracranial portion, not elsewhere classified with loss of consciousness of any duration with death due to brain injury prior to regaining consciousness**

⑦S06.828   **Injury of left internal carotid artery, intracranial portion, not elsewhere classified with loss of consciousness of any duration with death due to other cause prior to regaining consciousness**

⑦S06.829   **Injury of left internal carotid artery, intracranial portion, not elsewhere classified with loss of consciousness of unspecified duration**

Injury of left internal carotid artery, intracranial portion, not elsewhere classified NOS

S06.89   Other specified intracranial injury

Excludes1: concussion (S06.0X-)

⑦**S06.890   Other specified intracranial injury without loss of consciousness**

⑦**S06.891   Other specified intracranial injury with loss of consciousness of 30 minutes or less**

⑦**S06.892   Other specified intracranial injury with loss of consciousness of 31 minutes to 59 minutes**

⑦**S06.893   Other specified intracranial injury with loss of consciousness of 1 hour to 5 hours 59 minutes**

⑦**S06.894   Other specified intracranial injury with loss of consciousness of 6 hours to 24 hours**

⑦**S06.895   Other specified intracranial injury with loss of consciousness greater than 24 hours with return to pre-existing conscious level**

⑦**S06.896   Other specified intracranial injury with loss of consciousness greater than 24 hours without return to pre-existing conscious level with patient surviving**

⑦**S06.897   Other specified intracranial injury with loss of consciousness of any duration with death due to brain injury prior to regaining consciousness**

⑦**S06.898   Other specified intracranial injury with loss of consciousness of any duration with death due to other cause prior to regaining consciousness**

⑦**S06.899   Other specified intracranial injury with loss of consciousness of unspecified duration**

S06.9   Unspecified intracranial injury

Brain injury NOS

Head injury NOS with loss of consciousness

Traumatic brain injury NOS

Excludes1: conditions classifiable to S06.0- to S06.8-code to specified intracranial injury

head injury NOS (S09.90)

S06.9X   Unspecified intracranial injury

⑦**S06.9X0   Unspecified intracranial injury without loss of consciousness**

⑦**S06.9X1   Unspecified intracranial injury with loss of consciousness of 30 minutes or less**

⑦**S06.9X2   Unspecified intracranial injury with loss of consciousness of 31 minutes to 59 minutes**

⑦**S06.9X3   Unspecified intracranial injury with loss of consciousness of 1 hour to 5 hours 59 minutes**

⑦**S06.9X4   Unspecified intracranial injury with loss of consciousness of 6 hours to 24 hours**

⑦**S06.9X5   Unspecified intracranial injury with loss of consciousness greater than 24**

hours with return to pre-existing conscious level

⑦**S06.9X6   Unspecified intracranial injury with loss of consciousness greater than 24 hours without return to pre-existing conscious level with patient surviving**

⑦**S06.9X7   Unspecified intracranial injury with loss of consciousness of any duration with death due to brain injury prior to regaining consciousness**

⑦**S06.9X8   Unspecified intracranial injury with loss of consciousness of any duration with death due to other cause prior to regaining consciousness**

⑦**S06.9X9   Unspecified intracranial injury with loss of consciousness of unspecified duration**

S07   Crushing injury of head

Use additional code for all associated injuries, such as:

intracranial injuries (S06.-)

skull fractures (S02.-)

The appropriate 7th character is to be added to each code from category S07

A - initial encounter

D - subsequent encounter

S - sequela

⊗⑦**S07.0   Crushing injury of face**

⊗⑦**S07.1   Crushing injury of skull**

⊗⑦**S07.8   Crushing injury of other parts of head**

⊗⑦**S07.9   Crushing injury of head, part unspecified**

S08   Avulsion and traumatic amputation of part of head

An amputation not identified as partial or complete should be coded to complete

The appropriate 7th character is to be added to each code from category S08

A - initial encounter

D - subsequent encounter

S - sequela

⊗⑦**S08.0   Avulsion of scalp**

S08.1   Traumatic amputation of ear

S08.11   Complete traumatic amputation of ear

⑦**S08.111   Complete traumatic amputation of right ear**

⑦**S08.112   Complete traumatic amputation of left ear**

⑦**S08.119   Complete traumatic amputation of unspecified ear**

S08.12   Partial traumatic amputation of ear

⑦**S08.121   Partial traumatic amputation of right ear**

⑦**S08.122   Partial traumatic amputation of left ear**

⑦**S08.129   Partial traumatic amputation of unspecified ear**

S08.8   Traumatic amputation of other parts of head

S08.81   Traumatic amputation of nose

⑦**S08.811   Complete traumatic amputation of nose**

⑦**S08.812   Partial traumatic amputation of nose**

⊗⑦**S08.89   Traumatic amputation of other parts of head**

S09   Other and unspecified injuries of head

The appropriate 7th character is to be added to each code from category S09

A - initial encounter

D - subsequent encounter

S - sequela

⊗⑦**S09.0** **Injury of blood vessels of head, not elsewhere classified**

    Excludes1: injury of cerebral blood vessels (S06.-)

        injury of precerebral blood vessels (S15.-)

S09.1 **Injury of muscle and tendon of head**

    Code also any associated open wound (S01.-)

    Excludes2: sprain to joints and ligament of head (S03.9)

  ⊗⑦**S09.10** **Unspecified injury of muscle and tendon of head**

    Injury of muscle and tendon of head NOS

  ⊗⑦**S09.11** **Strain of muscle and tendon of head**

  ⊗⑦**S09.12** **Laceration of muscle and tendon of head**

  ⊗⑦**S09.19** **Other specified injury of muscle and tendon of head**

S09.2 **Traumatic rupture of ear drum**

    Excludes1: traumatic rupture of ear drum due to blast injury (S09.31-)

  ⊗⑦**S09.20** **Traumatic rupture of unspecified ear drum**

  ⊗⑦**S09.21** **Traumatic rupture of right ear drum**

  ⊗⑦**S09.22** **Traumatic rupture of left ear drum**

S09.3 **Other specified and unspecified injury of middle and inner ear**

    Excludes1: injury to ear NOS (S09.91-)

    Excludes2: injury to external ear (S00.4-, S01.3-, S08.1-)

  S09.30 **Unspecified injury of middle and inner ear**

    ⑦**S09.301** **Unspecified injury of right middle and inner ear**

    ⑦**S09.302** **Unspecified injury of left middle and inner ear**

    ⑦**S09.309** **Unspecified injury of unspecified middle and inner ear**

  S09.31 **Primary blast injury of ear**

    Blast injury of ear NOS

    ⑦**S09.311** **Primary blast injury of right ear**

    ⑦**S09.312** **Primary blast injury of left ear**

    ⑦**S09.313** **Primary blast injury of ear, bilateral**

    ⑦**S09.319** **Primary blast injury of unspecified ear**

  S09.39 **Other specified injury of middle and inner ear**

    Secondary blast injury to ear

    ⑦**S09.391** **Other specified injury of right middle and inner ear**

    ⑦**S09.392** **Other specified injury of left middle and inner ear**

    ⑦**S09.399** **Other specified injury of unspecified middle and inner ear**

⊗⑦**S09.8** **Other specified injuries of head**

S09.9 **Unspecified injury of face and head**

  ⊗⑦**S09.90** **Unspecified injury of head**

    Head injury NOS

    Excludes1: brain injury NOS (S06.9-)

        head injury NOS with loss of consciousness (S06.9-)

        intracranial injury NOS (S06.9-)

  ⊗⑦**S09.91** **Unspecified injury of ear**

    Injury of ear NOS

  ⊗⑦**S09.92** **Unspecified injury of nose**

    Injury of nose NOS

  ⊗⑦**S09.93** **Unspecified injury of face**

    Injury of face NOS

INJURIES TO THE NECK (S10-S19)

Includes: injuries of nape

injuries of supraclavicular region injuries of throat

Excludes2: burns and corrosions (T20-T32)

    effects of foreign body in esophagus (T18.1)

    effects of foreign body in larynx (T17.3)

    effects of foreign body in pharynx (T17.2)

    effects of foreign body in trachea (T17.4)

    frostbite (T33-T34)

    insect bite or sting, venomous (T63.4)

S10 **Superficial injury of neck**

The appropriate 7th character is to be added to each code from category S10

A - initial encounter

D - subsequent encounter

S - sequela

⊗⑦**S10.0** **Contusion of throat**

    Contusion of cervical esophagus

    Contusion of larynx

    Contusion of pharynx

    Contusion of trachea

S10.1 **Other and unspecified superficial injuries of throat**

  ⊗⑦**S10.10** **Unspecified superficial injuries of throat**

  ⊗⑦**S10.11** **Abrasion of throat**

  ⊗⑦**S10.12** **Blister (nonthermal) of throat**

  ⊗⑦**S10.14** **External constriction of part of throat**

  ⊗⑦**S10.15** **Superficial foreign body of throat**

    Splinter in the throat

  ⊗⑦**S10.16** **Insect bite (nonvenomous) of throat**

  ⊗⑦**S10.17** **Other superficial bite of throat**

    Excludes1: open bite of throat (S11.85)

S10.8 **Superficial injury of other specified parts of neck**

  ⊗⑦**S10.80** **Unspecified superficial injury of other specified part of neck**

  ⊗⑦**S10.81** **Abrasion of other specified part of neck**

  ⊗⑦**S10.82** **Blister (nonthermal) of other specified part of neck**

  ⊗⑦**S10.83** **Contusion of other specified part of neck**

  ⊗⑦**S10.84** **External constriction of other specified part of neck**

  ⊗⑦**S10.85** **Superficial foreign body of other specified part of neck**

    Splinter in other specified part of neck

  ⊗⑦**S10.86** **Insect bite of other specified part of neck**

  ⊗⑦**S10.87** **Other superficial bite of other specified part of neck**

    Excludes1: open bite of other specified parts of neck (S11.85)

S10.9 **Superficial injury of unspecified part of neck**

  ⊗⑦**S10.90** **Unspecified superficial injury of unspecified part of neck**

  ⊗⑦**S10.91** **Abrasion of unspecified part of neck**

⊗⑦S10.92   Blister (nonthermal) of unspecified part of neck

⊗⑦S10.93   Contusion of unspecified part of neck

⊗⑦S10.94   External constriction of unspecified part of neck

⊗⑦S10.95   Superficial foreign body of unspecified part of neck

⊗⑦S10.96   Insect bite of unspecified part of neck

⊗⑦S10.97   Other superficial bite of unspecified part of neck

S11   Open wound of neck

Code also any associated:

spinal cord injury (S14.0, S14.1-)

wound infection

Excludes2: open fracture of vertebra (S12.- with 7th character B)

The appropriate 7th character is to be added to each code from category S11

A - initial encounter

D - subsequent encounter

S - sequela

S11.0   Open wound of larynx and trachea

S11.01   Open wound of larynx

Excludes2: open wound of vocal cord (S11.03)

⑦S11.011   Laceration without foreign body of larynx

⑦S11.012   Laceration with foreign body of larynx

⑦S11.013   Puncture wound without foreign body of larynx

⑦S11.014   Puncture wound with foreign body of larynx

⑦S11.015   Open bite of larynx

Bite of larynx NOS

⑦S11.019   Unspecified open wound of larynx

S11.02   Open wound of trachea

Open wound of cervical trachea

Open wound of trachea NOS

Excludes2: open wound of thoracic trachea (S27.5-)

⑦S11.021   Laceration without foreign body of trachea

⑦S11.022   Laceration with foreign body of trachea

⑦S11.023   Puncture wound without foreign body of trachea

⑦S11.024   Puncture wound with foreign body of trachea

⑦S11.025   Open bite of trachea

Bite of trachea NOS

⑦S11.029   Unspecified open wound of trachea

S11.03   Open wound of vocal cord

⑦S11.031   Laceration without foreign body of vocal cord

⑦S11.032   Laceration with foreign body of vocal cord

⑦S11.033   Puncture wound without foreign body of vocal cord

⑦S11.034   Puncture wound with foreign body of vocal cord

⑦S11.035   Open bite of vocal cord

Bite of vocal cord NOS

⑦S11.039   Unspecified open wound of vocal cord

S11.1   Open wound of thyroid gland

⊗⑦S11.10   Unspecified open wound of thyroid gland

⊗⑦S11.11   Laceration without foreign body of thyroid gland

⊗⑦S11.12   Laceration with foreign body of thyroid gland

⊗⑦S11.13   Puncture wound without foreign body of thyroid gland

⊗⑦S11.14   Puncture wound with foreign body of thyroid gland

⊗⑦S11.15   Open bite of thyroid gland

Bite of thyroid gland NOS

S11.2   Open wound of pharynx and cervical esophagus

Excludes1: open wound of esophagus NOS (S27.8-)

⊗⑦S11.20   Unspecified open wound of pharynx and cervical esophagus

⊗⑦S11.21   Laceration without foreign body of pharynx and cervical esophagus

⊗⑦S11.22   Laceration with foreign body of pharynx and cervical esophagus

⊗⑦S11.23   Puncture wound without foreign body of pharynx and cervical esophagus

⊗⑦S11.24   Puncture wound with foreign body of pharynx and cervical esophagus

⊗⑦S11.25   Open bite of pharynx and cervical esophagus

Bite of pharynx and cervical esophagus NOS

S11.8   Open wound of other specified parts of neck

⊗⑦S11.80   Unspecified open wound of other specified part of neck

⊗⑦S11.81   Laceration without foreign body of other specified part of neck

⊗⑦S11.82   Laceration with foreign body of other specified part of neck

⊗⑦S11.83   Puncture wound without foreign body of other specified part of neck

⊗⑦S11.84   Puncture wound with foreign body of other specified part of neck

⊗⑦S11.85   Open bite of other specified part of neck

Bite of other specified part of neck NOS

Excludes1: superficial bite of other specified part of neck (S10.87)

⊗⑦S11.89   Other open wound of other specified part of neck

S11.9   Open wound of unspecified part of neck

⊗⑦S11.90   Unspecified open wound of unspecified part of neck

⊗⑦S11.91   Laceration without foreign body of unspecified part of neck

⊗⑦S11.92   Laceration with foreign body of unspecified part of neck

⊗⑦S11.93   Puncture wound without foreign body of unspecified part of neck

⊗⑦S11.94   Puncture wound with foreign body of unspecified part of neck

⊗⑦S11.95   Open bite of unspecified part of neck

Bite of neck NOS

Excludes1: superficial bite of neck (S10.97)

S12   Fracture of cervical vertebra and other parts of neck

Note: A fracture not indicated as displaced or nondisplaced should be coded to displaced

A fracture not indicated as open or closed should be coded to closed

Includes: fracture of cervical neural arch

fracture of cervical spine

fracture of cervical spinous process

fracture of cervical transverse process

fracture of cervical vertebral arch fracture of neck

<u>Code first</u> any associated cervical spinal cord injury (S14.0, S14.1-)

The appropriate 7th character is to be added to all codes from subcategories S12.0-S12.6

A - initial encounter for closed fracture

B - initial encounter for open fracture

D - subsequent encounter for fracture with routine healing

G - subsequent encounter for fracture with delayed healing

K - subsequent encounter for fracture with nonunion

S - sequela

S12.0   **Fracture of first cervical vertebra**

Atlas

    S12.00   **Unspecified fracture of first cervical vertebra**

       ⑦**S12.000**   **Unspecified displaced fracture of first cervical vertebra**

       ⑦**S12.001**   **Unspecified nondisplaced fracture of first cervical vertebra**

   ⊗⑦**S12.01**   **Stable burst fracture of first cervical vertebra**

   ⊗⑦**S12.02**   **Unstable burst fracture of first cervical vertebra**

    S12.03   **Posterior arch fracture of first cervical vertebra**

       ⑦**S12.030**   **Displaced posterior arch fracture of first cervical vertebra**

       ⑦**S12.031**   **Nondisplaced posterior arch fracture of first cervical vertebra**

    S12.04   **Lateral mass fracture of first cervical vertebra**

       ⑦**S12.040**   **Displaced lateral mass fracture of first cervical vertebra**

       ⑦**S12.041**   **Nondisplaced lateral mass fracture of first cervical vertebra**

    S12.09   **Other fracture of first cervical vertebra**

       ⑦**S12.090**   **Other displaced fracture of first cervical vertebra**

       ⑦**S12.091**   **Other nondisplaced fracture of first cervical vertebra**

S12.1   **Fracture of second cervical vertebra**

Axis

    S12.10   **Unspecified fracture of second cervical vertebra**

       ⑦**S12.100**   **Unspecified displaced fracture of second cervical vertebra**

       ⑦**S12.101**   **Unspecified nondisplaced fracture of second cervical vertebra**

    S12.11   **Type II dens fracture**

       ⑦**S12.110**   **Anterior displaced Type II dens fracture**

       ⑦**S12.111**   **Posterior displaced Type II dens fracture**

       ⑦**S12.112 Nondisplaced Type II dens fracture**

    S12.12   **Other dens fracture**

       ⑦**S12.120**   **Other displaced dens fracture**

       ⑦**S12.121**   **Other nondisplaced dens fracture**

    S12.13   **Unspecified traumatic spondylolisthesis of second cervical vertebra**

       ⑦**S12.130**   **Unspecified traumatic displaced spondylolisthesis of second cervical vertebra**

       ⑦**S12.131**   **Unspecified traumatic nondisplaced spondylolisthesis of second cervical vertebra**

   ⊗⑦**S12.14**   **Type III traumatic spondylolisthesis of second cervical vertebra**

    S12.15   **Other traumatic spondylolisthesis of second cervical vertebra**

       ⑦**S12.150**   **Other traumatic displaced spondylolisthesis of second cervical vertebra**

       ⑦**S12.151**   **Other traumatic nondisplaced spondylolisthesis of second cervical vertebra**

    S12.19   **Other fracture of second cervical vertebra**

       ⑦**S12.190**   **Other displaced fracture of second cervical vertebra**

       ⑦**S12.191**   **Other nondisplaced fracture of second cervical vertebra**

S12.2   **Fracture of third cervical vertebra**

    S12.20   **Unspecified fracture of third cervical vertebra**

       ⑦**S12.200**   **Unspecified displaced fracture of third cervical vertebra**

       ⑦**S12.201**   **Unspecified nondisplaced fracture of third cervical vertebra**

    S12.23   **Unspecified traumatic spondylolisthesis of third cervical vertebra**

       ⑦**S12.230**   **Unspecified traumatic displaced spondylolisthesis of third cervical vertebra**

       ⑦**S12.231**   **Unspecified traumatic nondisplaced spondylolisthesis of third cervical vertebra**

   ⊗⑦**S12.24**   **Type III traumatic spondylolisthesis of third cervical vertebra**

    S12.25   **Other traumatic spondylolisthesis of third cervical vertebra**

       ⑦**S12.250**   **Other traumatic displaced spondylolisthesis of third cervical vertebra**

       ⑦**S12.251**   **Other traumatic nondisplaced spondylolisthesis of third cervical vertebra**

    S12.29   **Other fracture of third cervical vertebra**

       ⑦**S12.290 Other displaced fracture of third cervical vertebra**

       ⑦**S12.291 Other nondisplaced fracture of third cervical vertebra**

S12.3   **Fracture of fourth cervical vertebra**

    S12.30   **Unspecified fracture of fourth cervical vertebra**

       ⑦**S12.300**   **Unspecified displaced fracture of fourth cervical vertebra**

       ⑦**S12.301**   **Unspecified nondisplaced fracture of fourth cervical vertebra**

    S12.33   **Unspecified traumatic spondylolisthesis of fourth cervical vertebra**

       ⑦**S12.330**   **Unspecified traumatic displaced spondylolisthesis of fourth cervical vertebra**

       ⑦**S12.331**   **Unspecified traumatic nondisplaced spondylolisthesis of fourth cervical vertebra**

⊗⑦**S12.34** Type III traumatic spondylolisthesis of fourth cervical vertebra

S12.35 Other traumatic spondylolisthesis of fourth cervical vertebra

⑦**S12.350** Other traumatic displaced spondylolisthesis of fourth cervical vertebra

⑦**S12.351** Other traumatic nondisplaced spondylolisthesis of fourth cervical vertebra

S12.39 Other fracture of fourth cervical vertebra

⑦**S12.390** Other displaced fracture of fourth cervical vertebra

⑦**S12.391** Other nondisplaced fracture of fourth cervical vertebra

S12.4 Fracture of fifth cervical vertebra

S12.40 Unspecified fracture of fifth cervical vertebra

⑦**S12.400** Unspecified displaced fracture of fifth cervical vertebra

⑦**S12.401** Unspecified nondisplaced fracture of fifth cervical vertebra

S12.43 Unspecified traumatic spondylolisthesis of fifth cervical vertebra

⑦**S12.430** Unspecified traumatic displaced spondylolisthesis of fifth cervical vertebra

⑦**S12.431** Unspecified traumatic nondisplaced spondylolisthesis of fifth cervical vertebra

⊗⑦**S12.44** Type III traumatic spondylolisthesis of fifth cervical vertebra

S12.45 Other traumatic spondylolisthesis of fifth cervical vertebra

⑦**S12.450** Other traumatic displaced spondylolisthesis of fifth cervical vertebra

⑦**S12.451** Other traumatic nondisplaced spondylolisthesis of fifth cervical vertebra

S12.49 Other fracture of fifth cervical vertebra

⑦**S12.490** Other displaced fracture of fifth cervical vertebra

⑦**S12.491** Other nondisplaced fracture of fifth cervical vertebra

S12.5 Fracture of sixth cervical vertebra

S12.50 Unspecified fracture of sixth cervical vertebra

⑦**S12.500** Unspecified displaced fracture of sixth cervical vertebra

⑦**S12.501** Unspecified nondisplaced fracture of sixth cervical vertebra

S12.53 Unspecified traumatic spondylolisthesis of sixth cervical vertebra

⑦**S12.530** Unspecified traumatic displaced spondylolisthesis of sixth cervical vertebra

⑦**S12.531** Unspecified traumatic nondisplaced spondylolisthesis of sixth cervical vertebra

⊗⑦**S12.54** Type III traumatic spondylolisthesis of sixth cervical vertebra

S12.55 Other traumatic spondylolisthesis of sixth cervical vertebra

⑦**S12.550** Other traumatic displaced spondylolisthesis of sixth cervical vertebra

⑦**S12.551** Other traumatic nondisplaced spondylolisthesis of sixth cervical vertebra

S12.59 Other fracture of sixth cervical vertebra

⑦**S12.590** Other displaced fracture of sixth cervical vertebra

⑦**S12.591** Other nondisplaced fracture of sixth cervical vertebra

S12.6 Fracture of seventh cervical vertebra

S12.60 Unspecified fracture of seventh cervical vertebra

⑦**S12.600** Unspecified displaced fracture of seventh cervical vertebra

⑦**S12.601** Unspecified nondisplaced fracture of seventh cervical vertebra

S12.63 Unspecified traumatic spondylolisthesis of seventh cervical vertebra

⑦**S12.630** Unspecified traumatic displaced spondylolisthesis of seventh cervical vertebra

⑦**S12.631** Unspecified traumatic nondisplaced spondylolisthesis of seventh cervical vertebra

⑦**S12.64** Type III traumatic spondylolisthesis of seventh cervical vertebra

S12.65 Other traumatic spondylolisthesis of seventh cervical vertebra

⑦**S12.650** Other traumatic displaced spondylolisthesis of seventh cervical vertebra

⑦**S12.651** Other traumatic nondisplaced spondylolisthesis of seventh cervical vertebra

S12.69 Other fracture of seventh cervical vertebra

⑦**S12.690** Other displaced fracture of seventh cervical vertebra

⑦**S12.691** Other nondisplaced fracture of seventh cervical vertebra

⊗⑦**S12.8** Fracture of other parts of neck

Hyoid bone

Larynx

Thyroid cartilage

Trachea

The appropriate 7th character is to be added to code S12.8

A - initial encounter

D - subsequent encounter

S - sequela

⊗⑦**S12.9** Fracture of neck, unspecified

Fracture of neck NOS

Fracture of cervical spine NOS

Fracture of cervical vertebra NOS

The appropriate 7th character is to be added to code S12.9

A - initial encounter

D - subsequent encounter

S - sequela

S13 Dislocation and sprain of joints and ligaments at neck level

Includes: avulsion of joint or ligament at neck level

laceration of cartilage, joint or ligament at neck level

sprain of cartilage, joint or ligament at neck level

traumatic hemarthrosis of joint or ligament at neck level

traumatic rupture of joint or ligament at neck level

● New code ▲ Revised code **Excludes1:** Not coded here **Excludes2:** Not included here ⊗ Placeholder required ⑦7th digit required

traumatic subluxation of joint or ligament at neck level

traumatic tear of joint or ligament at neck level

Code also any associated open wound

Excludes2: strain of muscle or tendon at neck level (S16.1)

The appropriate 7th character is to be added to each code from category S13

A - initial encounter

D - subsequent encounter

S - sequela

⊗⑦**S13.0** **Traumatic rupture of cervical intervertebral disc**

    Excludes1: rupture or displacement (nontraumatic) of cervical intervertebral disc NOS (M50.-)

S13.1 **Subluxation and dislocation of cervical vertebrae**

    Definition: Subluxation is a condition that occurs when a joint begins to dislocate. Instead of the joint surfaces completely losing contact, a subluxation can be considered a "partial dislocation." A subluxation can be the result of a trauma or acute injury. In these cases, the injury can be quite painful. Subluxations can also occur as a result of loose joints.

    Code also any associated:

    open wound of neck (S11.-)

    spinal cord injury (S14.1-)

    Excludes2: fracture of cervical vertebrae (S12.0-S12.3-)

S13.10 **Subluxation and dislocation of unspecified cervical vertebrae**

    ⑦**S13.100** **Subluxation of unspecified cervical vertebrae**

    ⑦**S13.101** **Dislocation of unspecified cervical vertebrae**

S13.11 **Subluxation and dislocation of C0/C1 cervical vertebrae**

    Subluxation and dislocation of atlantooccipital joint

    Subluxation and dislocation of atloido-occipital joint

    Subluxation and dislocation of occipitoatloid joint

    ⑦**S13.110** **Subluxation of C0/C1 cervical vertebrae**

    ⑦**S13.111** **Dislocation of C0/C1 cervical vertebrae**

S13.12 **Subluxation and dislocation of C1/C2 cervical vertebrae**

    Subluxation and dislocation of atlantoaxial joint

    ⑦**S13.120** **Subluxation of C1/C2 cervical vertebrae**

    ⑦**S13.121** **Dislocation of C1/C2 cervical vertebrae**

S13.13 **Subluxation and dislocation of C2/C3 cervical vertebrae**

    ⑦**S13.130** **Subluxation of C2/C3 cervical vertebrae**

    ⑦**S13.131** **Dislocation of C2/C3 cervical vertebrae**

S13.14 **Subluxation and dislocation of C3/C4 cervical vertebrae**

    ⑦**S13.140** **Subluxation of C3/C4 cervical vertebrae**

    ⑦**S13.141** **Dislocation of C3/C4 cervical vertebrae**

S13.15 **Subluxation and dislocation of C4/C5 cervical vertebrae**

⑦**S13.150** **Subluxation of C4/C5 cervical vertebrae**

⑦**S13.151** **Dislocation of C4/C5 cervical vertebrae**

S13.16 **Subluxation and dislocation of C5/C6 cervical vertebrae**

    ⑦**S13.160** **Subluxation of C5/C6 cervical vertebrae**

    ⑦**S13.161** **Dislocation of C5/C6 cervical vertebrae**

S13.17 **Subluxation and dislocation of C6/C7 cervical vertebrae**

    ⑦**S13.170** **Subluxation of C6/C7 cervical vertebrae**

    ⑦**S13.171** **Dislocation of C6/C7 cervical vertebrae**

S13.18 **Subluxation and dislocation of C7/T1 cervical vertebrae**

    ⑦**S13.180** **Subluxation of C7/T1 cervical vertebrae**

    ⑦**S13.181** **Dislocation of C7/T1 cervical vertebrae**

S13.2 **Dislocation of other and unspecified parts of neck**

    ⊗⑦**S13.20** **Dislocation of unspecified parts of neck**

    ⊗⑦**S13.29** **Dislocation of other parts of neck**

⊗⑦**S13.4** **Sprain of ligaments of cervical spine**

    Sprain of anterior longitudinal (ligament), cervical

    Sprain of atlanto-axial (joints)

    Sprain of atlanto-occipital (joints)

    Whiplash injury of cervical spine

⊗⑦**S13.5** **Sprain of thyroid region**

    Sprain of cricoarytenoid (joint) (ligament)

    Sprain of cricothyroid (joint) (ligament)

    Sprain of thyroid cartilage

⊗⑦**S13.8** **Sprain of joints and ligaments of other parts of neck**

⊗⑦**S13.9** **Sprain of joints and ligaments of unspecified parts of neck**

S14 **Injury of nerves and spinal cord at neck level**

    Note: Code to highest level of cervical cord injury

    Code also any associated:

    fracture of cervical vertebra (S12.0--S12.6.-)

    open wound of neck (S11.-)

    transient paralysis (R29.5)

The appropriate 7th character is to be added to each code from category S14

A - initial encounter

D - subsequent encounter

S - sequela

⊗⑦**S14.0** **Concussion and edema of cervical spinal cord**

S14.1 **Other and unspecified injuries of cervical spinal cord**

    S14.10 **Unspecified injury of cervical spinal cord**

        ⑦**S14.101** **Unspecified injury at C1 level of cervical spinal cord**

        ⑦**S14.102** **Unspecified injury at C2 level of cervical spinal cord**

        ⑦**S14.103** **Unspecified injury at C3 level of cervical spinal cord**

        ⑦**S14.104** **Unspecified injury at C4 level of cervical spinal cord**

        ⑦**S14.105** **Unspecified injury at C5 level of cervical spinal cord**

⑦S14.106   **Unspecified injury at C6 level of cervical spinal cord**

⑦S14.107   **Unspecified injury at C7 level of cervical spinal cord**

⑦S14.108   **Unspecified injury at C8 level of cervical spinal cord**

⑦S14.109   **Unspecified injury at unspecified level of cervical spinal cord**

      Injury of cervical spinal cord NOS

S14.11   **Complete lesion of cervical spinal cord**

⑦S14.111   **Complete lesion at C1 level of cervical spinal cord**

⑦S14.112   **Complete lesion at C2 level of cervical spinal cord**

⑦S14.113   **Complete lesion at C3 level of cervical spinal cord**

⑦S14.114   **Complete lesion at C4 level of cervical spinal cord**

⑦S14.115   **Complete lesion at C5 level of cervical spinal cord**

⑦S14.116   **Complete lesion at C6 level of cervical spinal cord**

⑦S14.117   **Complete lesion at C7 level of cervical spinal cord**

⑦S14.118   **Complete lesion at C8 level of cervical spinal cord**

⑦S14.119   **Complete lesion at unspecified level of cervical spinal cord**

S14.12   **Central cord syndrome of cervical spinal cord**

⑦S14.121   **Central cord syndrome at C1 level of cervical spinal cord**

⑦S14.122   **Central cord syndrome at C2 level of cervical spinal cord**

⑦S14.123   **Central cord syndrome at C3 level of cervical spinal cord**

⑦S14.124   **Central cord syndrome at C4 level of cervical spinal cord**

⑦S14.125   **Central cord syndrome at C5 level of cervical spinal cord**

⑦S14.126   **Central cord syndrome at C6 level of cervical spinal cord**

⑦S14.127   **Central cord syndrome at C7 level of cervical spinal cord**

⑦S14.128   **Central cord syndrome at C8 level of cervical spinal cord**

⑦S14.129   **Central cord syndrome at unspecified level of cervical spinal cord**

S14.13   **Anterior cord syndrome of cervical spinal cord**

⑦S14.131   **Anterior cord syndrome at C1 level of cervical spinal cord**

⑦S14.132   **Anterior cord syndrome at C2 level of cervical spinal cord**

⑦S14.133   **Anterior cord syndrome at C3 level of cervical spinal cord**

⑦S14.134   **Anterior cord syndrome at C4 level of cervical spinal cord**

⑦S14.135   **Anterior cord syndrome at C5 level of cervical spinal cord**

⑦S14.136   **Anterior cord syndrome at C6 level of cervical spinal cord**

⑦S14.137   **Anterior cord syndrome at C7 level of cervical spinal cord**

⑦S14.138   **Anterior cord syndrome at C8 level of cervical spinal cord**

⑦S14.139   **Anterior cord syndrome at unspecified level of cervical spinal cord**

S14.14   **Brown-Séquard syndrome of cervical spinal cord**

⑦S14.141   **Brown-Séquard syndrome at C1 level of cervical spinal cord**

⑦S14.142   **Brown-Séquard syndrome at C2 level of cervical spinal cord**

⑦S14.143   **Brown-Séquard syndrome at C3 level of cervical spinal cord**

⑦S14.144   **Brown-Séquard syndrome at C4 level of cervical spinal cord**

⑦S14.145   **Brown-Séquard syndrome at C5 level of cervical spinal cord**

⑦S14.146   **Brown-Séquard syndrome at C6 level of cervical spinal cord**

⑦S14.147   **Brown-Séquard syndrome at C7 level of cervical spinal cord**

⑦S14.148   **Brown-Séquard syndrome at C8 level of cervical spinal cord**

⑦S14.149   **Brown-Séquard syndrome at unspecified level of cervical spinal cord**

S14.15   **Other incomplete lesions of cervical spinal cord**

      Incomplete lesion of cervical spinal cord NOS

      Posterior cord syndrome of cervical spinal cord

⑦S14.151   **Other incomplete lesion at C1 level of cervical spinal cord**

⑦S14.152   **Other incomplete lesion at C2 level of cervical spinal cord**

⑦S14.153   **Other incomplete lesion at C3 level of cervical spinal cord**

⑦S14.154   **Other incomplete lesion at C4 level of cervical spinal cord**

⑦S14.155   **Other incomplete lesion at C5 level of cervical spinal cord**

⑦S14.156   **Other incomplete lesion at C6 level of cervical spinal cord**

⑦S14.157   **Other incomplete lesion at C7 level of cervical spinal cord**

⑦S14.158   **Other incomplete lesion at C8 level of cervical spinal cord**

⑦S14.159   **Other incomplete lesion at unspecified level of cervical spinal cord**

⊗⑦S14.2   **Injury of nerve root of cervical spine**

⊗⑦S14.3   **Injury of brachial plexus**

⊗⑦S14.4   **Injury of peripheral nerves of neck**

⊗⑦S14.5   **Injury of cervical sympathetic nerves**

⊗⑦S14.8   **Injury of other specified nerves of neck**

⊗⑦S14.9   **Injury of unspecified nerves of neck**

S15   **Injury of blood vessels at neck level**

    Code also any associated open wound (S11.-)

    The appropriate 7th character is to be added to each code from category S15

    A - initial encounter

    D - subsequent encounter

    S - sequela

S15.0   **Injury of carotid artery of neck**

Injury of carotid artery (common) (external) (internal, extracranial portion)

Injury of carotid artery NOS

Excludes1: injury of internal carotid artery, intracranial portion (S06.8)

S15.00   Unspecified injury of carotid artery

⑦ **S15.001   Unspecified injury of right carotid artery**

⑦ **S15.002   Unspecified injury of left carotid artery**

⑦ **S15.009   Unspecified injury of unspecified carotid artery**

S15.01   Minor laceration of carotid artery

Incomplete transection of carotid artery

Laceration of carotid artery NOS

Superficial laceration of carotid artery

⑦ **S15.011   Minor laceration of right carotid artery**

⑦ **S15.012   Minor laceration of left carotid artery**

⑦ **S15.019   Minor laceration of unspecified carotid artery**

S15.02   Major laceration of carotid artery

Complete transection of carotid artery

Traumatic rupture of carotid artery

⑦ **S15.021   Major laceration of right carotid artery**

⑦ **S15.022   Major laceration of left carotid artery**

⑦ **S15.029   Major laceration of unspecified carotid artery**

S15.09   Other specified injury of carotid artery

⑦ **S15.091   Other specified injury of right carotid artery**

⑦ **S15.092   Other specified injury of left carotid artery**

⑦ **S15.099   Other specified injury of unspecified carotid artery**

S15.1   Injury of vertebral artery

S15.10   Unspecified injury of vertebral artery

⑦ **S15.101   Unspecified injury of right vertebral artery**

⑦ **S15.102   Unspecified injury of left vertebral artery**

⑦ **S15.109   Unspecified injury of unspecified vertebral artery**

S15.11   Minor laceration of vertebral artery

Incomplete transection of vertebral artery

Laceration of vertebral artery NOS

Superficial laceration of vertebral artery

⑦ **S15.111 Minor laceration of right vertebral artery**

⑦ **S15.112 Minor laceration of left vertebral artery**

⑦ **S15.119 Minor laceration of unspecified vertebral artery**

S15.12   Major laceration of vertebral artery

Complete transection of vertebral artery

Traumatic rupture of vertebral artery

⑦ **S15.121   Major laceration of right vertebral artery**

⑦ **S15.122   Major laceration of left vertebral artery**

⑦ **S15.129   Major laceration of unspecified vertebral artery**

S15.19   Other specified injury of vertebral artery

⑦ **S15.191   Other specified injury of right vertebral artery**

⑦ **S15.192   Other specified injury of left vertebral artery**

⑦ **S15.199   Other specified injury of unspecified vertebral artery**

S15.2   Injury of external jugular vein

S15.20   Unspecified injury of external jugular vein

⑦ **S15.201   Unspecified injury of right external jugular vein**

⑦ **S15.202   Unspecified injury of left external jugular vein**

⑦ **S15.209   Unspecified injury of unspecified external jugular vein**

S15.21   Minor laceration of external jugular vein

Incomplete transection of external jugular vein

Laceration of external jugular vein NOS

Superficial laceration of external jugular vein

⑦ **S15.211   Minor laceration of right external jugular vein**

⑦ **S15.212   Minor laceration of left external jugular vein**

⑦ **S15.219   Minor laceration of unspecified external jugular vein**

S15.22   Major laceration of external jugular vein

Complete transection of external jugular vein

Traumatic rupture of external jugular vein

⑦ **S15.221   Major laceration of right external jugular vein**

⑦ **S15.222   Major laceration of left external jugular vein**

⑦ **S15.229   Major laceration of unspecified external jugular vein**

S15.29   Other specified injury of external jugular vein

⑦ **S15.291   Other specified injury of right external jugular vein**

⑦ **S15.292   Other specified injury of left external jugular vein**

⑦ **S15.299   Other specified injury of unspecified external jugular vein**

S15.3   Injury of internal jugular vein

S15.30   Unspecified injury of internal jugular vein

⑦ **S15.301   Unspecified injury of right internal jugular vein**

⑦ **S15.302   Unspecified injury of left internal jugular vein**

⑦ **S15.309   Unspecified injury of unspecified internal jugular vein**

S15.31   Minor laceration of internal jugular vein

Incomplete transection of internal jugular vein

Laceration of internal jugular vein NOS

Superficial laceration of internal jugular vein

⑦ **S15.311   Minor laceration of right internal jugular vein**

⑦ **S15.312   Minor laceration of left internal jugular vein**

⑦**S15.319** **Minor laceration of unspecified internal jugular vein**

⑦**S15.32** **Major laceration of internal jugular vein**

Complete transection of internal jugular vein

Traumatic rupture of internal jugular vein

⑦**S15.321** **Major laceration of right internal jugular vein**

⑦**S15.322** **Major laceration of left internal jugular vein**

⑦**S15.329** **Major laceration of unspecified internal jugular vein**

⑦**S15.39** **Other specified injury of internal jugular vein**

⑦**S15.391** **Other specified injury of right internal jugular vein**

⑦**S15.392** **Other specified injury of left internal jugular vein**

⑦**S15.399** **Other specified injury of unspecified internal jugular vein**

⊗⑦**S15.8** **Injury of other specified blood vessels at neck level**

⊗⑦**S15.9** **Injury of unspecified blood vessel at neck level**

S16 **Injury of muscle, fascia and tendon at neck level**

Code also any associated open wound (S11.-)

Excludes2: sprain of joint or ligament at neck level (S13.9)

The appropriate 7th character is to be added to each code from category S16

A - initial encounter

D - subsequent encounter

S - sequela

⊗⑦**S16.1** **Strain of muscle, fascia and tendon at neck level**

⊗⑦**S16.2** **Laceration of muscle, fascia and tendon at neck level**

⊗⑦**S16.8** **Other specified injury of muscle, fascia and tendon at neck level**

⊗⑦**S16.9** **Unspecified injury of muscle, fascia and tendon at neck level**

S17 **Crushing injury of neck**

Use additional code for all associated injuries, such as:

injury of blood vessels (S15.-)

open wound of neck (S11.-)

spinal cord injury (S14.0, S14.1-)

vertebral fracture (S12.0--S12.3-)

The appropriate 7th character is to be added to each code from category S17

A - initial encounter

D - subsequent encounter

S - sequela

⊗⑦**S17.0** **Crushing injury of larynx and trachea**

⊗⑦**S17.8** **Crushing injury of other specified parts of neck**

⊗⑦**S17.9** **Crushing injury of neck, part unspecified**

S19 **Other specified and unspecified injuries of neck**

The appropriate 7th character is to be added to each code from category S19

A - initial encounter

D - subsequent encounter

S - sequela

S19.8 **Other specified injuries of neck**

⊗⑦**S19.80** **Other specified injuries of unspecified part of neck**

⊗⑦**S19.81** **Other specified injuries of larynx**

⊗⑦**S19.82** **Other specified injuries of cervical trachea**

Excludes2: Other specified injury of thoracic trachea (S27.5-)

⊗⑦**S19.83** **Other specified injuries of vocal cord**

⊗⑦**S19.84** **Other specified injuries of thyroid gland**

⊗⑦**S19.85** **Other specified injuries of pharynx and cervical esophagus**

⊗⑦**S19.89** **Other specified injuries of other specified part of neck**

⊗⑦**S19.9** **Unspecified injury of neck**

INJURIES TO THE THORAX (S20-S29)

Includes: injuries of breast

injuries of chest (wall)

injuries of interscapular area

Excludes2: burns and corrosions (T20-T32)

effects of foreign body in bronchus (T17.5)

effects of foreign body in esophagus (T18.1)

effects of foreign body in lung (T17.8)

effects of foreign body in trachea (T17.4)

frostbite (T33-T34)

injuries of axilla injuries of clavicle

injuries of scapular region injuries of shoulder insect bite or sting, venomous (T63.4)

S20 **Superficial injury of thorax**

The appropriate 7th character is to be added to each code from category S20

A - initial encounter

D - subsequent encounter

S - sequela

S20.0 **Contusion of breast**

⊗⑦**S20.00** **Contusion of breast, unspecified breast**

⊗⑦**S20.01** **Contusion of right breast**

⊗⑦**S20.02** **Contusion of left breast**

S20.1 **Other and unspecified superficial injuries of breast**

S20.10 **Unspecified superficial injuries of breast**

⑦**S20.101** **Unspecified superficial injuries of breast, right breast**

⑦**S20.102** **Unspecified superficial injuries of breast, left breast**

⑦**S20.109** **Unspecified superficial injuries of breast, unspecified breast**

S20.11 **Abrasion of breast**

⑦**S20.111** **Abrasion of breast, right breast**

⑦**S20.112** **Abrasion of breast, left breast**

⑦**S20.119** **Abrasion of breast, unspecified breast**

S20.12 **Blister (nonthermal) of breast**

⑦**S20.121** **Blister (nonthermal) of breast, right breast**

⑦**S20.122** **Blister (nonthermal) of breast, left breast**

⑦**S20.129** **Blister (nonthermal) of breast, unspecified breast**

S20.14 **External constriction of part of breast**

⑦**S20.141** **External constriction of part of breast, right breast**

⑦**S20.142** **External constriction of part of breast, left breast**

⑦**S20.149** **External constriction of part of breast, unspecified breast**

● New code   ▲ Revised code   **Excludes1:** Not coded here   **Excludes2:** Not included here   ⊗ Placeholder required   ⑦ 7th digit required

S20.15 ⑦**Superficial foreign body of breast**

Splinter in the breast

  ⑦**S20.151** **Superficial foreign body of breast, right breast**

  ⑦**S20.152** **Superficial foreign body of breast, left breast**

  ⑦**S20.159** **Superficial foreign body of breast, unspecified breast**

S20.16 **Insect bite (nonvenomous) of breast**

  ⑦**S20.161** **Insect bite (nonvenomous) of breast, right breast**

  ⑦**S20.162** **Insect bite (nonvenomous) of breast, left breast**

  ⑦**S20.169** **Insect bite (nonvenomous) of breast, unspecified breast**

S20.17 **Other superficial bite of breast**

  Excludes1: open bite of breast (S21.05-)

  ⑦**S20.171** **Other superficial bite of breast, right breast**

  ⑦**S20.172** **Other superficial bite of breast, left breast**

  ⑦**S20.179** **Other superficial bite of breast, unspecified breast**

S20.2 **Contusion of thorax**

⊗⑦**S20.20** **Contusion of thorax, unspecified**

S20.21 **Contusion of front wall of thorax**

  ⑦**S20.211** **Contusion of right front wall of thorax**

  ⑦**S20.212** **Contusion of left front wall of thorax**

  ⑦**S20.219** **Contusion of unspecified front wall of thorax**

S20.22 **Contusion of back wall of thorax**

  ⑦**S20.221** **Contusion of right back wall of thorax**

  ⑦**S20.222** **Contusion of left back wall of thorax**

  ⑦**S20.229** **Contusion of unspecified back wall of thorax**

S20.3 **Other and unspecified superficial injuries of front wall of thorax**

S20.30 **Unspecified superficial injuries of front wall of thorax**

  ⑦**S20.301** **Unspecified superficial injuries of right front wall of thorax**

  ⑦**S20.302** **Unspecified superficial injuries of left front wall of thorax**

  ⑦**S20.309** **Unspecified superficial injuries of unspecified front wall of thorax**

S20.31 **Abrasion of front wall of thorax**

  ⑦**S20.311** **Abrasion of right front wall of thorax**

  ⑦**S20.312** **Abrasion of left front wall of thorax**

  ⑦**S20.319** **Abrasion of unspecified front wall of thorax**

S20.32 **Blister (nonthermal) of front wall of thorax**

  ⑦**S20.321** **Blister (nonthermal) of right front wall of thorax**

  ⑦**S20.322** **Blister (nonthermal) of left front wall of thorax**

  ⑦**S20.329** **Blister (nonthermal) of unspecified front wall of thorax**

S20.34 **External constriction of front wall of thorax**

  ⑦**S20.341** **External constriction of right front wall of thorax**

  ⑦**S20.342** **External constriction of left front wall of thorax**

  ⑦**S20.349** **External constriction of unspecified front wall of thorax**

S20.35 **Superficial foreign body of front wall of thorax**

Splinter in front wall of thorax

  ⑦**S20.351** ⑦**Superficial foreign body of right front wall of thorax**

  ⑦**S20.352** ⑦**Superficial foreign body of left front wall of thorax**

  ⑦**S20.359** ⑦**Superficial foreign body of unspecified front wall of thorax**

S20.36 **Insect bite (nonvenomous) of front wall of thorax**

  ⑦**S20.361** **Insect bite (nonvenomous) of right front wall of thorax**

  ⑦**S20.362** **Insect bite (nonvenomous) of left front wall of thorax**

  ⑦**S20.369** **Insect bite (nonvenomous) of unspecified front wall of thorax**

S20.37 **Other superficial bite of front wall of thorax**

  Excludes1: open bite of front wall of thorax (S21.14)

  ⑦**S20.371** **Other superficial bite of right front wall of thorax**

  ⑦**S20.372** **Other superficial bite of left front wall of thorax**

  ⑦**S20.379** **Other superficial bite of unspecified front wall of thorax**

S20.4 **Other and unspecified superficial injuries of back wall of thorax**

S20.40 **Unspecified superficial injuries of back wall of thorax**

  ⑦**S20.401** **Unspecified superficial injuries of right back wall of thorax**

  ⑦**S20.402** **Unspecified superficial injuries of left back wall of thorax**

  ⑦**S20.409** **Unspecified superficial injuries of unspecified back wall of thorax**

S20.41 **Abrasion of back wall of thorax**

  ⑦**S20.411** **Abrasion of right back wall of thorax**

  ⑦**S20.412** **Abrasion of left back wall of thorax**

  ⑦**S20.419** **Abrasion of unspecified back wall of thorax**

S20.42 **Blister (nonthermal) of back wall of thorax**

  ⑦**S20.421** **Blister (nonthermal) of right back wall of thorax**

  ⑦**S20.422** **Blister (nonthermal) of left back wall of thorax**

  ⑦**S20.429** **Blister (nonthermal) of unspecified back wall of thorax**

S20.44 **External constriction of back wall of thorax**

  ⑦**S20.441** **External constriction of right back wall of thorax**

  ⑦**S20.442** **External constriction of left back wall of thorax**

  ⑦**S20.449** **External constriction of unspecified back wall of thorax**

S20.45 **Superficial foreign body of back wall of thorax**

Splinter of back wall of thorax

⑦S20.451 **Superficial foreign body of right back wall of thorax**

⑦S20.452 **Superficial foreign body of left back wall of thorax**

⑦S20.459 **Superficial foreign body of unspecified back wall of thorax**

S20.46 **Insect bite (nonvenomous) of back wall of thorax**

⑦S20.461 **Insect bite (nonvenomous) of right back wall of thorax**

⑦S20.462 **Insect bite (nonvenomous) of left back wall of thorax**

⑦S20.469 **Insect bite (nonvenomous) of unspecified back wall of thorax**

S20.47 **Other superficial bite of back wall of thorax**

> Excludes1: open bite of back wall of thorax (S21.24)

⑦S20.471 **Other superficial bite of right back wall of thorax**

⑦S20.472 **Other superficial bite of left back wall of thorax**

⑦S20.479 **Other superficial bite of unspecified back wall of thorax**

S20.9 **Superficial injury of unspecified parts of thorax**

> Excludes1: contusion of thorax NOS (S20.20)

⊗⑦S20.90 **Unspecified superficial injury of unspecified parts of thorax**

Superficial injury of thoracic wall NOS

⊗⑦S20.91 **Abrasion of unspecified parts of thorax**

⊗⑦S20.92 **Blister (nonthermal) of unspecified parts of thorax**

⊗⑦S20.94 **External constriction of unspecified parts of thorax**

⊗⑦S20.95 **Superficial foreign body of unspecified parts of thorax**

Splinter in thorax NOS

⊗⑦S20.96 **Insect bite (nonvenomous) of unspecified parts of thorax**

⊗⑦S20.97 **Other superficial bite of unspecified parts of thorax**

> Excludes1: open bite of thorax NOS (S21.95)

S21 **Open wound of thorax**

Code also any associated injury, such as:

injury of heart (S26.-)

injury of intrathoracic organs (S27.-)

rib fracture (S22.3-, S22.4-)

spinal cord injury (S24.0-, S24.1-)

traumatic hemopneumothorax (S27.3)

traumatic hemothorax (S27.1)

traumatic pneumothorax (S27.0) wound infection

> Excludes1: traumatic amputation (partial) of thorax (S28.1)

The appropriate 7th character is to be added to each code from category S21

A - initial encounter

D - subsequent encounter

S - sequela

S21.0 **Open wound of breast**

S21.00 **Unspecified open wound of breast**

⑦S21.001 **Unspecified open wound of right breast**

⑦S21.002 **Unspecified open wound of left breast**

⑦S21.009 **Unspecified open wound of unspecified breast**

S21.01 **Laceration without foreign body of breast**

⑦S21.011 **Laceration without foreign body of right breast**

⑦S21.012 **Laceration without foreign body of left breast**

⑦S21.019 **Laceration without foreign body of unspecified breast**

S21.02 **Laceration with foreign body of breast**

⑦S21.021 **Laceration with foreign body of right breast**

⑦S21.022 **Laceration with foreign body of left breast**

⑦S21.029 **Laceration with foreign body of unspecified breast**

S21.03 **Puncture wound without foreign body of breast**

⑦S21.031 **Puncture wound without foreign body of right breast**

⑦S21.032 **Puncture wound without foreign body of left breast**

⑦S21.039 **Puncture wound without foreign body of unspecified breast**

S21.04 **Puncture wound with foreign body of breast**

⑦S21.041 **Puncture wound with foreign body of right breast**

⑦S21.042 **Puncture wound with foreign body of left breast**

⑦S21.049 **Puncture wound with foreign body of unspecified breast**

S21.05 **Open bite of breast**

Bite of breast NOS

> Excludes1: superficial bite of breast (S20.17)

⑦S21.051 **Open bite of right breast**

⑦S21.052 **Open bite of left breast**

⑦S21.059 **Open bite of unspecified breast**

S21.1 **Open wound of front wall of thorax without penetration into thoracic cavity**

Open wound of chest without penetration into thoracic cavity

S21.10 **Unspecified open wound of front wall of thorax without penetration into thoracic cavity**

⑦S21.101 **Unspecified open wound of right front wall of thorax without penetration into thoracic cavity**

⑦S21.102 **Unspecified open wound of left front wall of thorax without penetration into thoracic cavity**

⑦S21.109 **Unspecified open wound of unspecified front wall of thorax without penetration into thoracic cavity**

S21.11 **Laceration without foreign body of front wall of thorax without penetration into thoracic cavity**

⑦S21.111 **Laceration without foreign body of right front wall of thorax without penetration into thoracic cavity**

⑦S21.112 **Laceration without foreign body of left front wall of thorax without penetration into thoracic cavity**

⑦S21.119 **Laceration without foreign body of unspecified front wall of thorax**

● New code   ▲ Revised code   Excludes1: Not coded here   Excludes2: Not included here   ⊗ Placeholder required   ⑦ 7th digit required

without penetration into thoracic cavity

S21.12 Laceration with foreign body of front wall of thorax without penetration into thoracic cavity

⑦**S21.121** Laceration with foreign body of right front wall of thorax without penetration into thoracic cavity

⑦**S21.122** Laceration with foreign body of left front wall of thorax without penetration into thoracic cavity

⑦**S21.129** Laceration with foreign body of unspecified front wall of thorax without penetration into thoracic cavity

S21.13 Puncture wound without foreign body of front wall of thorax without penetration into thoracic cavity

⑦**S21.131** Puncture wound without foreign body of right front wall of thorax without penetration into thoracic cavity

⑦**S21.132** Puncture wound without foreign body of left front wall of thorax without penetration into thoracic cavity

⑦**S21.139** Puncture wound without foreign body of unspecified front wall of thorax without penetration into thoracic cavity

S21.14 Puncture wound with foreign body of front wall of thorax without penetration into thoracic cavity

⑦**S21.141** Puncture wound with foreign body of right front wall of thorax without penetration into thoracic cavity

⑦**S21.142** Puncture wound with foreign body of left front wall of thorax without penetration into thoracic cavity

⑦**S21.149** Puncture wound with foreign body of unspecified front wall of thorax without penetration into thoracic cavity

S21.15 Open bite of front wall of thorax without penetration into thoracic cavity

Bite of front wall of thorax NOS

Excludes1: superficial bite of front wall of thorax (S20.37)

⑦**S21.151** Open bite of right front wall of thorax without penetration into thoracic cavity

⑦**S21.152** Open bite of left front wall of thorax without penetration into thoracic cavity

⑦**S21.159** Open bite of unspecified front wall of thorax without penetration into thoracic cavity

S21.2 Open wound of back wall of thorax without penetration into thoracic cavity

S21.20 Unspecified open wound of back wall of thorax without penetration into thoracic cavity

⑦**S21.201** Unspecified open wound of right back wall of thorax without penetration into thoracic cavity

⑦**S21.202** Unspecified open wound of left back wall of thorax without penetration into thoracic cavity

⑦**S21.209** Unspecified open wound of unspecified back wall of thorax without penetration into thoracic cavity

S21.21 Laceration without foreign body of back wall of thorax without penetration into thoracic cavity

⑦**S21.211** Laceration without foreign body of right back wall of thorax without penetration into thoracic cavity

⑦**S21.212** Laceration without foreign body of left back wall of thorax without penetration into thoracic cavity

⑦**S21.219** Laceration without foreign body of unspecified back wall of thorax without penetration into thoracic cavity

S21.22 Laceration with foreign body of back wall of thorax without penetration into thoracic cavity

⑦**S21.221** Laceration with foreign body of right back wall of thorax without penetration into thoracic cavity

⑦**S21.222** Laceration with foreign body of left back wall of thorax without penetration into thoracic cavity

⑦**S21.229** Laceration with foreign body of unspecified back wall of thorax without penetration into thoracic cavity

S21.23 Puncture wound without foreign body of back wall of thorax without penetration into thoracic cavity

⑦**S21.231** Puncture wound without foreign body of right back wall of thorax without penetration into thoracic cavity

⑦**S21.232** Puncture wound without foreign body of left back wall of thorax without penetration into thoracic cavity

⑦**S21.239** Puncture wound without foreign body of unspecified back wall of thorax without penetration into thoracic cavity

S21.24 Puncture wound with foreign body of back wall of thorax without penetration into thoracic cavity

⑦**S21.241** Puncture wound with foreign body of right back wall of thorax without penetration into thoracic cavity

⑦**S21.242** Puncture wound with foreign body of left back wall of thorax without penetration into thoracic cavity

⑦**S21.249** Puncture wound with foreign body of unspecified back wall of thorax without penetration into thoracic cavity

S21.25 Open bite of back wall of thorax without penetration into thoracic cavity

Bite of back wall of thorax NOS

Excludes1: superficial bite of back wall of thorax (S20.47)

⑦**S21.251** Open bite of right back wall of thorax without penetration into thoracic cavity

⑦**S21.252** Open bite of left back wall of thorax without penetration into thoracic cavity

Add 4th-7th digits   Nonspecific code   Unspecified code   Manifestation code

⑦**S21.259** Open bite of unspecified back wall of thorax without penetration into thoracic cavity

S21.3 Open wound of front wall of thorax with penetration into thoracic cavity

Open wound of chest with penetration into thoracic cavity

S21.30 Unspecified open wound of front wall of thorax with penetration into thoracic cavity

⑦**S21.301** Unspecified open wound of right front wall of thorax with penetration into thoracic cavity

⑦**S21.302** Unspecified open wound of left front wall of thorax with penetration into thoracic cavity

⑦**S21.309** Unspecified open wound of unspecified front wall of thorax with penetration into thoracic cavity

S21.31 Laceration without foreign body of front wall of thorax with penetration into thoracic cavity

⑦**S21.311** Laceration without foreign body of right front wall of thorax with penetration into thoracic cavity

⑦**S21.312** Laceration without foreign body of left front wall of thorax with penetration into thoracic cavity

⑦**S21.319** Laceration without foreign body of unspecified front wall of thorax with penetration into thoracic cavity

S21.32 Laceration with foreign body of front wall of thorax with penetration into thoracic cavity

⑦**S21.321** Laceration with foreign body of right front wall of thorax with penetration into thoracic cavity

⑦**S21.322** Laceration with foreign body of left front wall of thorax with penetration into thoracic cavity

⑦**S21.329** Laceration with foreign body of unspecified front wall of thorax with penetration into thoracic cavity

S21.33 Puncture wound without foreign body of front wall of thorax with penetration into thoracic cavity

⑦**S21.331** Puncture wound without foreign body of right front wall of thorax with penetration into thoracic cavity

⑦**S21.332** Puncture wound without foreign body of left front wall of thorax with penetration into thoracic cavity

⑦**S21.339** Puncture wound without foreign body of unspecified front wall of thorax with penetration into thoracic cavity

S21.34 Puncture wound with foreign body of front wall of thorax with penetration into thoracic cavity

⑦**S21.341** Puncture wound with foreign body of right front wall of thorax with penetration into thoracic cavity

⑦**S21.342** Puncture wound with foreign body of left front wall of thorax with penetration into thoracic cavity

⑦**S21.349** Puncture wound with foreign body of unspecified front wall of thorax with penetration into thoracic cavity

S21.35 Open bite of front wall of thorax with penetration into thoracic cavity

Excludes1: superficial bite of front wall of thorax

(S20.37)

⑦**S21.351** Open bite of right front wall of thorax with penetration into thoracic cavity

⑦**S21.352** Open bite of left front wall of thorax with penetration into thoracic cavity

⑦**S21.359** Open bite of unspecified front wall of thorax with penetration into thoracic cavity

S21.4 Open wound of back wall of thorax with penetration into thoracic cavity

S21.40 Unspecified open wound of back wall of thorax with penetration into thoracic cavity

⑦**S21.401** Unspecified open wound of right back wall of thorax with penetration into thoracic cavity

⑦**S21.402** Unspecified open wound of left back wall of thorax with penetration into thoracic cavity

⑦**S21.409** Unspecified open wound of unspecified back wall of thorax with penetration into thoracic cavity

S21.41 Laceration without foreign body of back wall of thorax with penetration into thoracic cavity

⑦**S21.411** Laceration without foreign body of right back wall of thorax with penetration into thoracic cavity

⑦**S21.412** Laceration without foreign body of left back wall of thorax with penetration into thoracic cavity

⑦**S21.419** Laceration without foreign body of unspecified back wall of thorax with penetration into thoracic cavity

S21.42 Laceration with foreign body of back wall of thorax with penetration into thoracic cavity

⑦**S21.421** Laceration with foreign body of right back wall of thorax with penetration into thoracic cavity

⑦**S21.422** Laceration with foreign body of left back wall of thorax with penetration into thoracic cavity

⑦**S21.429** Laceration with foreign body of unspecified back wall of thorax with penetration into thoracic cavity

S21.43 Puncture wound without foreign body of back wall of thorax with penetration into thoracic cavity

⑦**S21.431** Puncture wound without foreign body of right back wall of thorax with penetration into thoracic cavity

⑦**S21.432** Puncture wound without foreign body of left back wall of thorax with penetration into thoracic cavity

⑦**S21.439** Puncture wound without foreign body of unspecified back wall of thorax with penetration into thoracic cavity

S21.44 Puncture wound with foreign body of back wall of thorax with penetration into thoracic cavity

⑦**S21.441** Puncture wound with foreign body of right back wall of thorax with penetration into thoracic cavity

⑦**S21.442** Puncture wound with foreign body of left back wall of thorax with penetration into thoracic cavity

⑦S21.449 **Puncture wound with foreign body of unspecified back wall of thorax with penetration into thoracic cavity**

S21.45 **Open bite of back wall of thorax with penetration into thoracic cavity**

Bite of back wall of thorax NOS

Excludes1: superficial bite of back wall of thorax (S20.47)

⑦S21.451 **Open bite of right back wall of thorax with penetration into thoracic cavity**

⑦S21.452 **Open bite of left back wall of thorax with penetration into thoracic cavity**

⑦S21.459 **Open bite of unspecified back wall of thorax with penetration into thoracic cavity**

S21.9 **Open wound of unspecified part of thorax**

Open wound of thoracic wall NOS

⊗⑦S21.90 **Unspecified open wound of unspecified part of thorax**

⊗⑦S21.91 **Laceration without foreign body of unspecified part of thorax**

⊗⑦S21.92 **Laceration with foreign body of unspecified part of thorax**

⊗⑦S21.93 **Puncture wound without foreign body of unspecified part of thorax**

⊗⑦S21.94 **Puncture wound with foreign body of unspecified part of thorax**

⊗⑦S21.95 **Open bite of unspecified part of thorax**

Excludes1: superficial bite of thorax (S20.97)

S22 **Fracture of rib(s), sternum and thoracic spine**

Note: A fracture not indicated as displaced or nondisplaced should be coded to displaced

A fracture not indicated as open or closed should be coded to closed

Includes: fracture of thoracic neural arch

fracture of thoracic spinous process

fracture of thoracic transverse process

fracture of thoracic vertebra

fracture of thoracic vertebral arch

Code first any associated:

injury of intrathoracic organ (S27.-)

spinal cord injury (S24.0-, S24.1-)

Excludes1: transection of thorax (S28.1)

Excludes2: fracture of clavicle (S42.0-)

fracture of scapula (S42.1-)

The appropriate 7th character is to be added to each code from category S22

A - initial encounter for closed fracture

B - initial encounter for open fracture

D - subsequent encounter for fracture with routine healing

G - subsequent encounter for fracture with delayed healing

K - subsequent encounter for fracture with nonunion

S - sequela

S22.0 **Fracture of thoracic vertebra**

S22.00 **Fracture of unspecified thoracic vertebra**

⑦S22.000 **Wedge compression fracture of unspecified thoracic vertebra**

⑦S22.001 **Stable burst fracture of unspecified thoracic vertebra**

⑦S22.002 **Unstable burst fracture of unspecified thoracic vertebra**

⑦S22.008 **Other fracture of unspecified thoracic vertebra**

⑦S22.009 **Unspecified fracture of unspecified thoracic vertebra**

S22.01 **Fracture of first thoracic vertebra**

⑦S22.010 **Wedge compression fracture of first thoracic vertebra**

⑦S22.011 **Stable burst fracture of first thoracic vertebra**

⑦S22.012 **Unstable burst fracture of first thoracic vertebra**

⑦S22.018 **Other fracture of first thoracic vertebra**

⑦S22.019 **Unspecified fracture of first thoracic vertebra**

S22.02 **Fracture of second thoracic vertebra**

⑦S22.020 **Wedge compression fracture of second thoracic vertebra**

⑦S22.021 **Stable burst fracture of second thoracic vertebra**

⑦S22.022 **Unstable burst fracture of second thoracic vertebra**

⑦S22.028 **Other fracture of second thoracic vertebra**

⑦S22.029 **Unspecified fracture of second thoracic vertebra**

S22.03 **Fracture of third thoracic vertebra**

⑦S22.030 **Wedge compression fracture of third thoracic vertebra**

⑦S22.031 **Stable burst fracture of third thoracic vertebra**

⑦S22.032 **Unstable burst fracture of third thoracic vertebra**

⑦S22.038 **Other fracture of third thoracic vertebra**

⑦S22.039 **Unspecified fracture of third thoracic vertebra**

S22.04 **Fracture of fourth thoracic vertebra**

⑦S22.040 **Wedge compression fracture of fourth thoracic vertebra**

⑦S22.041 **Stable burst fracture of fourth thoracic vertebra**

⑦S22.042 **Unstable burst fracture of fourth thoracic vertebra**

⑦S22.048 **Other fracture of fourth thoracic vertebra**

⑦S22.049 **Unspecified fracture of fourth thoracic vertebra**

S22.05 **Fracture of T5-T6 vertebra**

⑦S22.050 **Wedge compression fracture of T5-T6 vertebra**

⑦S22.051 **Stable burst fracture of T5-T6 vertebra**

⑦S22.052 **Unstable burst fracture of T5-T6 vertebra**

⑦S22.058 **Other fracture of T5-T6 vertebra**

⑦S22.059 **Unspecified fracture of T5-T6 vertebra**

S22.06 **Fracture of T7-T8 vertebra**

⑦S22.060 **Wedge compression fracture of T7-T8 vertebra**

⑦S22.061 **Stable burst fracture of T7-T8 vertebra**

⑦**S22.062** Unstable burst fracture of T7-T8 vertebra

⑦**S22.068** Other fracture of T7-T8 thoracic vertebra

⑦**S22.069** Unspecified fracture of T7-T8 vertebra

S22.07 Fracture of T9-T10 vertebra

⑦**S22.070** Wedge compression fracture of T9-T10 vertebra

⑦**S22.071** Stable burst fracture of T9-T10 vertebra

⑦**S22.072** Unstable burst fracture of T9-T10 vertebra

⑦**S22.078** Other fracture of T9-T10 vertebra

⑦**S22.079** Unspecified fracture of T9-T10 vertebra

S22.08 Fracture of T11-T12 vertebra

⑦**S22.080** Wedge compression fracture of T11-T12 vertebra

⑦**S22.081** Stable burst fracture of T11-T12 vertebra

⑦**S22.082** Unstable burst fracture of T11-T12 vertebra

⑦**S22.088** Other fracture of T11-T12 vertebra

⑦**S22.089** Unspecified fracture of T11-T12 vertebra

S22.2 **Fracture of sternum**

⊗⑦**S22.20** Unspecified fracture of sternum

⊗⑦**S22.21** Fracture of manubrium

⊗⑦**S22.22** Fracture of body of sternum

⊗⑦**S22.23** Sternal manubrial dissociation

⊗⑦**S22.24** Fracture of xiphoid process

S22.3 **Fracture of one rib**

⊗⑦**S22.31** Fracture of one rib, right side

⊗⑦**S22.32** Fracture of one rib, left side

⊗⑦**S22.39** Fracture of one rib, unspecified side

S22.4 **Multiple fractures of ribs**

Fractures of two or more ribs

Excludes1: flail chest (S22.5-)

⊗⑦**S22.41** Multiple fractures of ribs, right side

⊗⑦**S22.42** Multiple fractures of ribs, left side

⊗⑦**S22.43** Multiple fractures of ribs, bilateral

⊗⑦**S22.49** Multiple fractures of ribs, unspecified side

⊗⑦**S22.5** **Flail chest**

⊗⑦**S22.9** **Fracture of bony thorax, part unspecified**

S23 **Dislocation and sprain of joints and ligaments of thorax**

Includes: avulsion of joint or ligament of thorax

laceration of cartilage, joint or ligament of thorax

sprain of cartilage, joint or ligament of thorax

traumatic hemarthrosis of joint or ligament of thorax

traumatic rupture of joint or ligament of thorax

traumatic subluxation of joint or ligament of thorax

traumatic tear of joint or ligament of thorax

Code also any associated open wound

Excludes2: dislocation, sprain of sternoclavicular joint (S43.2, S43.6)

strain of muscle or tendon of thorax (S29.01-)

The appropriate 7th character is to be added to each code from category S23

A - initial encounter

D - subsequent encounter

S - sequela

⊗⑦**S23.0** **Traumatic rupture of thoracic intervertebral disc**

Excludes1: rupture or displacement (nontraumatic) of thoracic intervertebral disc NOS (M51.- with fifth character 4)

S23.1 **Subluxation and dislocation of thoracic vertebra**

Code also any associated

open wound of thorax (S21.-)

spinal cord injury (S24.0-, S24.1-)

Excludes2: fracture of thoracic vertebrae (S22.0-)

S23.10 Subluxation and dislocation of unspecified thoracic vertebra

⑦**S23.100** Subluxation of unspecified thoracic vertebra

⑦**S23.101** Dislocation of unspecified thoracic vertebra

S23.11 Subluxation and dislocation of T1/T2 thoracic vertebra

⑦**S23.110** Subluxation of T1/T2 thoracic vertebra

⑦**S23.111** Dislocation of T1/T2 thoracic vertebra

S23.12 Subluxation and dislocation of T2/T3-T3/T4 thoracic vertebra

⑦**S23.120** Subluxation of T2/T3 thoracic vertebra

⑦**S23.121** Dislocation of T2/T3 thoracic vertebra

⑦**S23.122** Subluxation of T3/T4 thoracic vertebra

⑦**S23.123** Dislocation of T3/T4 thoracic vertebra

S23.13 Subluxation and dislocation of T4/T5-T5/T6 thoracic vertebra

⑦**S23.130** Subluxation of T4/T5 thoracic vertebra

⑦**S23.131** Dislocation of T4/T5 thoracic vertebra

⑦**S23.132** Subluxation of T5/T6 thoracic vertebra

⑦**S23.133** Dislocation of T5/T6 thoracic vertebra

S23.14 Subluxation and dislocation of T6/T7-T7/T8 thoracic vertebra

⑦**S23.140** Subluxation of T6/T7 thoracic vertebra

⑦**S23.141** Dislocation of T6/T7 thoracic vertebra

⑦**S23.142** Subluxation of T7/T8 thoracic vertebra

⑦**S23.143** Dislocation of T7/T8thoracic vertebra

S23.15 Subluxation and dislocation of T8/T9-T9/T10 thoracic vertebra

⑦**S23.150** Subluxation of T8/T9thoracic vertebra

⑦**S23.151** Dislocation of T8/T9thoracic vertebra

⑦**S23.152** Subluxation of T9/T10thoracic vertebra

● New code ▲ Revised code **Excludes1:** Not coded here **Excludes2:** Not included here ⊗ Placeholder required ⑦7th digit required

⑦S23.153   **Dislocation of T9/T10thoracic vertebra**

S23.16   **Subluxation and dislocation of T10/T11-T11/T12 thoracic vertebra**

⑦S23.160   **Subluxation of T10/T11thoracic vertebra**

⑦S23.161   **Dislocation of T10/T11thoracic vertebra**

⑦S23.162   **Subluxation of T11/T12thoracic vertebra**

⑦S23.163   **Dislocation of T11/T12thoracic vertebra**

S23.17   **Subluxation and dislocation of T12/L1 thoracic vertebra**

⑦S23.170   **Subluxation of T12/L1 thoracic vertebra**

⑦S23.171   **Dislocation of T12/L1 thoracic vertebra**

S23.2   **Dislocation of other and unspecified parts of thorax**

⊗⑦S23.20   **Dislocation of unspecified part of thorax**

⊗⑦S23.29   **Dislocation of other parts of thorax**

⊗⑦S23.3   **Sprain of ligaments of thoracic spine**

S23.4   **Sprain of ribs and sternum**

⊗⑦S23.41   **Sprain of ribs**

S23.42   **Sprain of sternum**

⑦S23.420   **Sprain of sternoclavicular (joint) (ligament)**

⑦S23.421   **Sprain of chondrosternal joint**

⑦S23.428   **Other sprain of sternum**

⑦S23.429   **Unspecified sprain of sternum**

⊗⑦S23.8   **Sprain of other specified parts of thorax**

⊗⑦S23.9   **Sprain of unspecified parts of thorax**

S24   **Injury of nerves and spinal cord at thorax level**

Note: Code to highest level of thoracic spinal cord injury

Injuries to the spinal cord (S24.0 and S24.1) refer to the cord level and not bone level injury, and can affect nerve roots at and below the level given.

Code also any associated:

fracture of thoracic vertebra (S22.0-)

open wound of thorax (S21.-)

transient paralysis (R29.5)

Excludes2: injury of brachial plexus (S14.3)

The appropriate 7th character is to be added to each code from category S24

A - initial encounter

D - subsequent encounter

S - sequela

⊗⑦S24.0   **Concussion and edema of thoracic spinal cord**

S24.1   **Other and unspecified injuries of thoracic spinal cord**

S24.10   **Unspecified injury of thoracic spinal cord**

⑦S24.101   **Unspecified injury at T1 level of thoracic spinal cord**

⑦S24.102   **Unspecified injury at T2-T6 level of thoracic spinal cord**

⑦S24.103   **Unspecified injury at T7-T10 level of thoracic spinal cord**

⑦S24.104   **Unspecified injury at T11-T12 level of thoracic spinal cord**

⑦S24.109   **Unspecified injury at unspecified level of thoracic spinal cord**

Injury of thoracic spinal cord NOS

S24.11   **Complete lesion of thoracic spinal cord**

⑦S24.111   **Complete lesion at T1 level of thoracic spinal cord**

⑦S24.112   **Complete lesion at T2-T6 level of thoracic spinal cord**

⑦S24.113   **Complete lesion at T7-T10 level of thoracic spinal cord**

⑦S24.114   **Complete lesion at T11-T12 level of thoracic spinal cord**

⑦S24.119   **Complete lesion at unspecified level of thoracic spinal cord**

S24.13   **Anterior cord syndrome of thoracic spinal cord**

⑦S24.131   **Anterior cord syndrome at T1 level of thoracic spinal cord**

⑦S24.132   **Anterior cord syndrome at T2-T6 level of thoracic spinal cord**

⑦S24.133   **Anterior cord syndrome at T7-T10 level of thoracic spinal cord**

⑦S24.134   **Anterior cord syndrome at T11-T12 level of thoracic spinal cord**

⑦S24.139   **Anterior cord syndrome at unspecified level of thoracic spinal cord**

S24.14   **Brown-Séquard syndrome of thoracic spinal cord**

⑦S24.141   **Brown-Séquard syndrome at T1 level of thoracic spinal cord**

⑦S24.142   **Brown-Séquard syndrome at T2-T6 level of thoracic spinal cord**

⑦S24.143   **Brown-Séquard syndrome at T7-T10 level of thoracic spinal cord**

⑦S24.144   **Brown-Séquard syndrome at T11-T12 level of thoracic spinal cord**

⑦S24.149   **Brown-Séquard syndrome at unspecified level of thoracic spinal cord**

⑦S24.15   **Other incomplete lesions of thoracic spinal cord**

Incomplete lesion of thoracic spinal cord NOS

Posterior cord syndrome of thoracic spinal cord

⑦S24.151   **Other incomplete lesion at T1 level of thoracic spinal cord**

⑦S24.152   **Other incomplete lesion at T2-T6 level of thoracic spinal cord**

⑦S24.153   **Other incomplete lesion at T7-T10 level of thoracic spinal cord**

⑦S24.154   **Other incomplete lesion at T11-T12 level of thoracic spinal cord**

⑦S24.159   **Other incomplete lesion at unspecified level of thoracic spinal cord**

⊗⑦S24.2   **Injury of nerve root of thoracic spine**

⊗⑦S24.3   **Injury of peripheral nerves of thorax**

⊗⑦S24.4   **Injury of thoracic sympathetic nervous system**

Injury of cardiac plexus

Injury of esophageal plexus

Injury of pulmonary plexus

Injury of stellate ganglion

Injury of thoracic sympathetic ganglion

⊗⑦S24.8   **Injury of other specified nerves of thorax**

⊗⑦S24.9   **Injury of unspecified nerve of thorax**

S25   **Injury of blood vessels of thorax**

Code also any associated open wound (S21.-)

Add 4th-7th digits	Nonspecific code	Unspecified code	Manifestation code

The appropriate 7th character is to be added to each code from category S25

A - initial encounter

D - subsequent encounter

S - sequela

S25.0   Injury of thoracic aorta

Injury of aorta NOS

⊗⑦**S25.00   Unspecified injury of thoracic aorta**

⊗⑦**S25.01   Minor laceration of thoracic aorta**

Incomplete transection of thoracic aorta

Laceration of thoracic aorta NOS

Superficial laceration of thoracic aorta

⊗⑦**S25.02   Major laceration of thoracic aorta**

Complete transection of thoracic aorta

Traumatic rupture of thoracic aorta

⊗⑦**S25.09   Other specified injury of thoracic aorta**

S25.1   Injury of innominate or subclavian artery

S25.10   Unspecified injury of innominate or subclavian artery

⑦**S25.101   Unspecified injury of right innominate or subclavian artery**

injury of left innominate or subclavian artery

⑦**S25.109   Unspecified injury of unspecified innominate or subclavian artery**

S25.11   Minor laceration of innominate or subclavian artery

Incomplete transection of innominate or subclavian artery

Laceration of innominate or subclavian artery NOS

Superficial laceration of innominate or subclavian artery

⑦**S25.111   Minor laceration of right innominate or subclavian artery**

⑦**S25.112   Minor laceration of left innominate or subclavian artery**

⑦**S25.119   Minor laceration of unspecified innominate or subclavian artery**

S25.12   Major laceration of innominate or subclavian artery

Complete transection of innominate or subclavian artery

Traumatic rupture of innominate or subclavian artery

⑦**S25.121   Major laceration of right innominate or subclavian artery**

⑦**S25.122   Major laceration of left innominate or subclavian artery**

⑦**S25.129   Major laceration of unspecified innominate or subclavian artery**

S25.19   Other specified injury of innominate or subclavian artery

⑦**S25.191   Other specified injury of right innominate or subclavian artery**

⑦**S25.192   Other specified injury of left innominate or subclavian artery**

⑦**S25.199   Other specified injury of unspecified innominate or subclavian artery**

S25.2   Injury of superior vena cava

Injury of vena cava NOS

⊗⑦**S25.20   Unspecified injury of superior vena cava**

⊗⑦**S25.21   Minor laceration of superior vena cava**

Incomplete transection of superior vena cava

Laceration of superior vena cava NOS

Superficial laceration of superior vena cava

⊗⑦**S25.22   Major laceration of superior vena cava**

Complete transection of superior vena cava

Traumatic rupture of superior vena cava

⊗⑦**S25.29   Other specified injury of superior vena cava**

S25.3   Injury of innominate or subclavian vein

S25.30   Unspecified injury of innominate or subclavian vein

⑦**S25.301   Unspecified injury of right innominate or subclavian vein**

⑦**S25.302   Unspecified injury of left innominate or subclavian vein**

⑦**S25.309   Unspecified injury of unspecified innominate or subclavian vein**

S25.31   Minor laceration of innominate or subclavian vein

Incomplete transection of innominate or subclavian vein

Laceration of innominate or subclavian vein NOS

Superficial laceration of innominate or subclavian vein

⑦**S25.311   Minor laceration of right innominate or subclavian vein**

⑦**S25.312   Minor laceration of left innominate or subclavian vein**

⑦**S25.319   Minor laceration of unspecified innominate or subclavian vein**

S25.32   Major laceration of innominate or subclavian vein

Complete transection of innominate or subclavian vein

Traumatic rupture of innominate or subclavian vein

⑦**S25.321   Major laceration of right innominate or subclavian vein**

⑦**S25.322   Major laceration of left innominate or subclavian vein**

⑦**S25.329   Major laceration of unspecified innominate or subclavian vein**

S25.39   Other specified injury of innominate or subclavian vein

⑦**S25.391   Other specified injury of right innominate or subclavian vein**

⑦**S25.392   Other specified injury of left innominate or subclavian vein**

⑦**S25.399   Other specified injury of unspecified innominate or subclavian vein**

S25.4   Injury of pulmonary blood vessels

S25.40   Unspecified injury of pulmonary blood vessels

⑦**S25.401   Unspecified injury of right pulmonary blood vessels**

⑦**S25.402   Unspecified injury of left pulmonary blood vessels**

⑦**S25.409   Unspecified injury of unspecified pulmonary blood vessels**

S25.41   Minor laceration of pulmonary blood vessels

Incomplete transection of pulmonary blood vessels

Laceration of pulmonary blood vessels NOS

Superficial laceration of pulmonary blood vessels

⑦S25.411 **Minor laceration of right pulmonary blood vessels**

⑦S25.412 **Minor laceration of left pulmonary blood vessels**

⑦S25.419 **Minor laceration of unspecified pulmonary blood vessels**

S25.42 **Major laceration of pulmonary blood vessels**

Complete transection of pulmonary blood vessels

Traumatic rupture of pulmonary blood vessels

⑦S25.421 **Major laceration of right pulmonary blood vessels**

⑦S25.422 **Major laceration of left pulmonary blood vessels**

⑦S25.429 **Major laceration of unspecified pulmonary blood vessels**

S25.49 **Other specified injury of pulmonary blood vessels**

⑦S25.491 **Other specified injury of right pulmonary blood vessels**

⑦S25.492 **Other specified injury of left pulmonary blood vessels**

⑦S25.499 **Other specified injury of unspecified pulmonary blood vessels**

S25.5 **Injury of intercostal blood vessels**

S25.50 **Unspecified injury of intercostal blood vessels**

⑦S25.501 **Unspecified injury of intercostal blood vessels, right side**

⑦S25.502 **Unspecified injury of intercostal blood vessels, left side**

⑦S25.509 **Unspecified injury of intercostal blood vessels, unspecified side**

S25.51 **Laceration of intercostal blood vessels**

⑦S25.511 **Laceration of intercostal blood vessels, right side**

⑦S25.512 **Laceration of intercostal blood vessels, left side**

⑦S25.519 **Laceration of intercostal blood vessels, unspecified side**

S25.59 **Other specified injury of intercostal blood vessels**

⑦S25.591 **Other specified injury of intercostal blood vessels, right side**

⑦S25.592 **Other specified injury of intercostal blood vessels, left side**

⑦S25.599 **Other specified injury of intercostal blood vessels, unspecified side**

S25.8 **Injury of other blood vessels of thorax**

Injury of azygos vein

Injury of mammary artery or vein

S25.80 **Unspecified injury of other blood vessels of thorax**

⑦S25.801 **Unspecified injury of other blood vessels of thorax, right side**

⑦S25.802 **Unspecified injury of other blood vessels of thorax, left side**

⑦S25.809 **Unspecified injury of other blood vessels of thorax, unspecified side**

S25.81 **Laceration of other blood vessels of thorax**

⑦S25.811 **Laceration of other blood vessels of thorax, right side**

⑦S25.812 **Laceration of other blood vessels of thorax, left side**

⑦S25.819 **Laceration of other blood vessels of thorax, unspecified side**

S25.89 **Other specified injury of other blood vessels of thorax**

⑦S25.891 **Other specified injury of other blood vessels of thorax, right side**

⑦S25.892 **Other specified injury of other blood vessels of thorax, left side**

⑦S25.899 **Other specified injury of other blood vessels of thorax, unspecified side**

S25.9 **Injury of unspecified blood vessel of thorax**

⑦S25.90 **Unspecified injury of unspecified blood vessel of thorax**

⑦S25.91 **Laceration of unspecified blood vessel of thorax**

⑦S25.99 **Other specified injury of unspecified blood vessel of thorax**

S26 **Injury of heart**

Code also any associated:

open wound of thorax (S21.-)

traumatic hemopneumothorax (S27.2)

traumatic hemothorax (S27.1)

traumatic pneumothorax (S27.0)

The appropriate 7th character is to be added to each code from category S26

A - initial encounter

D - subsequent encounter

S - sequela

S26.0 **Injury of heart with hemopericardium**

⊗⑦S26.00 **Unspecified injury of heart with hemopericardium**

⊗⑦S26.01 **Contusion of heart with hemopericardium**

S26.02 **Laceration of heart with hemopericardium**

⑦S26.020 **Mild laceration of heart with hemopericardium**

Laceration of heart without penetration of heart chamber

⑦S26.021 **Moderate laceration of heart with hemopericardium**

Laceration of heart with penetration of heart chamber

⑦S26.022 **Major laceration of heart with hemopericardium**

Laceration of heart with penetration of multiple heart chambers

⊗⑦S26.09 **Other injury of heart with hemopericardium**

S26.1 **Injury of heart without hemopericardium**

⊗⑦S26.10 **Unspecified injury of heart without hemopericardium**

⊗⑦S26.11 **Contusion of heart without hemopericardium**

⊗⑦S26.12 **Laceration of heart without hemopericardium**

⊗⑦S26.19 **Other injury of heart without hemopericardium**

S26.9 **Injury of heart, unspecified with or without hemopericardium**

⊗⑦S26.90 **Unspecified injury of heart, unspecified with or without hemopericardium**

⊗⑦S26.91 **Contusion of heart, unspecified with or without hemopericardium**

⊗⑦S26.92 **Laceration of heart, unspecified with or without hemopericardium**

Laceration of heart NOS

⊗⑦S26.99 **Other injury of heart, unspecified with or without hemopericardium**

S27 **Injury of other and unspecified intrathoracic organs**

Code also any associated open wound of thorax (S21.-)

Excludes2: injury of cervical esophagus (S10-S19)

injury of trachea (cervical) (S10-S19)

The appropriate 7th character is to be added to each code from category S27

A - initial encounter

D - subsequent encounter

S - sequela

⊗⑦S27.0 **Traumatic pneumothorax**

Excludes1: spontaneous pneumothorax (J93.-)

⊗⑦S27.1 **Traumatic hemothorax**

⊗⑦S27.2 **Traumatic hemopneumothorax**

⊗⑦S27.3 **Other and unspecified injuries of lung**

S27.30 **Unspecified injury of lung**

⑦S27.301 **Unspecified injury of lung, unilateral**

⑦S27.302 **Unspecified injury of lung, bilateral**

⑦S27.309 **Unspecified injury of lung, unspecified**

S27.31 **Primary blast injury of lung**

Blast injury of lung NOS

⑦S27.311 **Primary blast injury of lung, unilateral**

⑦S27.312 **Primary blast injury of lung, bilateral**

⑦S27.319 **Primary blast injury of lung, unspecified**

S27.32 **Contusion of lung**

⑦S27.321 **Contusion of lung, unilateral**

⑦S27.322 **Contusion of lung, bilateral**

⑦S27.329 **Contusion of lung, unspecified**

S27.33 **Laceration of lung**

⑦S27.331 **Laceration of lung, unilateral**

⑦S27.332 **Laceration of lung, bilateral**

⑦S27.339 **Laceration of lung, unspecified**

S27.39 **Other injuries of lung**

Secondary blast injury of lung

⑦S27.391 **Other injuries of lung, unilateral**

⑦S27.392 **Other injuries of lung, bilateral**

⑦S27.399 **Other injuries of lung, unspecified**

S27.4 **Injury of bronchus**

S27.40 **Unspecified injury of bronchus**

⑦S27.401 **Unspecified injury of bronchus, unilateral**

⑦S27.402 **Unspecified injury of bronchus, bilateral**

⑦S27.409 **Unspecified injury of bronchus, unspecified**

S27.41 **Primary blast injury of bronchus**

Blast injury of bronchus NOS

⑦S27.411 **Primary blast injury of bronchus, unilateral**

⑦S27.412 **Primary blast injury of bronchus, bilateral**

⑦S27.419 **Primary blast injury of bronchus, unspecified**

S27.42 **Contusion of bronchus**

⑦S27.421 **Contusion of bronchus, unilateral**

⑦S27.422 **Contusion of bronchus, bilateral**

⑦S27.429 **Contusion of bronchus, unspecified**

S27.43 **Laceration of bronchus**

⑦S27.431 **Laceration of bronchus, unilateral**

⑦S27.432 **Laceration of bronchus, bilateral**

⑦S27.439 **Laceration of bronchus, unspecified**

S27.49 **Other injury of bronchus**

Secondary blast injury of bronchus

⑦S27.491 **Other injury of bronchus, unilateral**

⑦S27.492 **Other injury of bronchus, bilateral**

⑦S27.499 **Other injury of bronchus, unspecified**

S27.5 **Injury of thoracic trachea**

⊗⑦S27.50 **Unspecified injury of thoracic trachea**

⊗⑦S27.51 **Primary blast injury of thoracic trachea**

Blast injury of thoracic trachea NOS

⊗⑦S27.52 **Contusion of thoracic trachea**

⊗⑦S27.53 **Laceration of thoracic trachea**

⊗⑦S27.59 **Other injury of thoracic trachea**

Secondary blast injury of thoracic trachea

S27.6 **Injury of pleura**

⊗⑦S27.60 **Unspecified injury of pleura**

⊗⑦S27.63 **Laceration of pleura**

⊗⑦S27.69 **Other injury of pleura**

S27.8 **Injury of other specified intrathoracic organs**

S27.80 **Injury of diaphragm**

⑦S27.802 **Contusion of diaphragm**

⑦S27.803 **Laceration of diaphragm**

⑦S27.808 **Other injury of diaphragm**

⑦S27.809 **Unspecified injury of diaphragm**

S27.81 **Injury of esophagus (thoracic part)**

⑦S27.812 **Contusion of esophagus (thoracic part)**

⑦S27.813 **Laceration of esophagus (thoracic part)**

⑦S27.818 **Other injury of esophagus (thoracic part)**

⑦S27.819 **Unspecified injury of esophagus (thoracic part)**

S27.89 **Injury of other specified intrathoracic organs**

Injury of lymphatic thoracic duct

Injury of thymus gland

⑦S27.892 **Contusion of other specified intrathoracic organs**

⑦S27.893 **Laceration of other specified intrathoracic organs**

⑦S27.898 **Other injury of other specified intrathoracic organs**

⑦S27.899 **Unspecified injury of other specified intrathoracic organs**

⊗⑦S27.9 **Injury of unspecified intrathoracic organ**

S28 **Crushing injury of thorax, and traumatic amputation of part of thorax**

The appropriate 7th character is to be added to each code from category S28

A - initial encounter

D - subsequent encounter

S - sequela

● New code ▲ Revised code **Excludes1:** Not coded here **Excludes2:** Not included here ⊗ Placeholder required ⑦ 7th digit required

⊗⑦**S28.0**   **Crushed chest**

Use additional code for all associated injuries

Excludes1: flail chest (S22.5)

⊗⑦**S28.1**   **Traumatic amputation (partial) of part of thorax, except breast**

S28.2   **Traumatic amputation of breast**

  S28.21   **Complete traumatic amputation of breast**

    Traumatic amputation of breast NOS

    ⑦**S28.211**   **Complete traumatic amputation of right breast**

    ⑦**S28.212**   **Complete traumatic amputation of left breast**

    ⑦**S28.219**   **Complete traumatic amputation of unspecified breast**

  S28.22   **Partial traumatic amputation of breast**

    ⑦**S28.221**   **Partial traumatic amputation of right breast**

    ⑦**S28.222**   **Partial traumatic amputation of left breast**

    ⑦**S28.229**   **Partial traumatic amputation of unspecified breast**

S29   **Other and unspecified injuries of thorax**

Code also any associated open wound (S21.-)

The appropriate 7th character is to be added to each code from category S29

A - initial encounter

D - subsequent encounter

S - sequela

S29.0   **Injury of muscle and tendon at thorax level**

  S29.00   **Unspecified injury of muscle and tendon of thorax**

    ⑦**S29.001**   **Unspecified injury of muscle and tendon of front wall of thorax**

    ⑦**S29.002**   **Unspecified injury of muscle and tendon of back wall of thorax**

    ⑦**S29.009**   **Unspecified injury of muscle and tendon of unspecified wall of thorax**

  S29.01   **Strain of muscle and tendon of thorax**

    ⑦**S29.011**   **Strain of muscle and tendon of front wall of thorax**

    ⑦**S29.012**   **Strain of muscle and tendon of back wall of thorax**

    ⑦**S29.019**   **Strain of muscle and tendon of unspecified wall of thorax**

  S29.02   **Laceration of muscle and tendon of thorax**

    ⑦**S29.021**   **Laceration of muscle and tendon of front wall of thorax**

    ⑦**S29.022**   **Laceration of muscle and tendon of back wall of thorax**

    ⑦**S29.029**   **Laceration of muscle and tendon of unspecified wall of thorax**

  S29.09   **Other injury of muscle and tendon of thorax**

    ⑦**S29.091**   **Other injury of muscle and tendon of front wall of thorax**

    ⑦**S29.092**   **Other injury of muscle and tendon of back wall of thorax**

    ⑦**S29.099**   **Other injury of muscle and tendon of unspecified wall of thorax**

⊗⑦**S29.8**   **Other specified injuries of thorax**

⊗⑦**S29.9**   **Unspecified injury of thorax**

INJURIES TO THE ABDOMEN, LOWER BACK, LUMBAR SPINE, PELVIS AND EXTERNAL GENITALS (S30-S39)

Includes: injuries to the abdominal wall

  injuries to the anus injuries to the buttock

  injuries to the external genitalia injuries to the flank

  injuries to the groin

Excludes2: burns and corrosions (T20-T32)

  effects of foreign body in anus and rectum (T18.5)

  effects of foreign body in genitourinary tract (T19.-)

  effects of foreign body in stomach, small intestine and colon (T18.2-T18.4)

  frostbite (T33-T34)

  insect bite or sting, venomous (T63.4)

S30   **Superficial injury of abdomen, lower back, pelvis and external genitals**

Excludes2: superficial injury of hip (S70.-)

The appropriate 7th character is to be added to each code from category S30

A - initial encounter

D - subsequent encounter

S - sequela

⊗⑦**S30.0**   **Contusion of lower back and pelvis**

  Contusion of buttock

⊗⑦**S30.1**   **Contusion of abdominal wall**

  Contusion of flank

  Contusion of groin

S30.2   **Contusion of external genital organs**

  S30.20   **Contusion of unspecified external genital organ**

    ⑦**S30.201**   **Contusion of unspecified external genital organ, male**

    ⑦**S30.202**   **Contusion of unspecified external genital organ, female**

  ⊗⑦**S30.21**   **Contusion of penis**

  ⊗⑦**S30.22**   **Contusion of scrotum and testes**

  ⊗⑦**S30.23**   **Contusion of vagina and vulva**

S30.3   **Contusion of anus**

S30.8   **Other superficial injuries of abdomen, lower back, pelvis and external genitals**

  S30.81   **Abrasion of abdomen, lower back, pelvis and external genitals**

    ⑦**S30.810**   **Abrasion of lower back and pelvis**

    ⑦**S30.811**   **Abrasion of abdominal wall**

    ⑦**S30.812**   **Abrasion of penis**

    ⑦**S30.813**   **Abrasion of scrotum and testes**

    ⑦**S30.814**   **Abrasion of vagina and vulva**

    ⑦**S30.815**   **Abrasion of unspecified external genital organs, male**

    ⑦**S30.816**   **Abrasion of unspecified external genital organs, female**

    ⑦**S30.817**   **Abrasion of anus**

  S30.82   **Blister (nonthermal) of abdomen, lower back, pelvis and external genitals**

    ⑦**S30.820**   **Blister (nonthermal) of lower back and pelvis**

    ⑦**S30.821**   **Blister (nonthermal) of abdominal wall**

    ⑦**S30.822**   **Blister (nonthermal) of penis**

    ⑦**S30.823**   **Blister (nonthermal) of scrotum and testes**

| | Add 4th-7th digits | | Nonspecific code | | Unspecified code | | Manifestation code | 767 |

⑦S30.824 **Blister (nonthermal) of vagina and vulva**

⑦S30.825 **Blister (nonthermal) of unspecified external genital organs, male**

⑦S30.826 **Blister (nonthermal) of unspecified external genital organs, female**

⑦S30.827 **Blister (nonthermal) of anus**

S30.84 **External constriction of abdomen, lower back, pelvis and external genitals**

⑦S30.840 **External constriction of lower back and pelvis**

⑦S30.841 **External constriction of abdominal wall**

⑦S30.842 **External constriction of penis**

Hair tourniquet syndrome of penis

Use additional cause code to identify the constricting item (W49.0-)

⑦S30.843 **External constriction of scrotum and testes**

⑦S30.844 **External constriction of vagina and vulva**

⑦S30.845 **External constriction of unspecified external genital organs, male**

⑦S30.846 **External constriction of unspecified external genital organs, female**

S30.85 **Superficial foreign body of abdomen, lower back, pelvis and external genitals**

Splinter in the abdomen, lower back, pelvis and external genitals

⑦S30.850 **Superficial foreign body of lower back and pelvis**

⑦S30.851 **Superficial foreign body of abdominal wall**

⑦S30.852 **Superficial foreign body of penis**

⑦S30.853 **Superficial foreign body of scrotum and testes**

⑦S30.854 **Superficial foreign body of vagina and vulva**

⑦S30.855 **Superficial foreign body of unspecified external genital organs, male**

⑦S30.856 **Superficial foreign body of unspecified external genital organs, female**

⑦S30.857 **Superficial foreign body of anus**

S30.86 **Insect bite (nonvenomous) of abdomen, lower back, pelvis and external genitals**

⑦S30.860 **Insect bite (nonvenomous) of lower back and pelvis**

⑦S30.861 **Insect bite (nonvenomous) of abdominal wall**

⑦S30.862 **Insect bite (nonvenomous) of penis**

⑦S30.863 **Insect bite (nonvenomous) of scrotum and testes**

⑦S30.864 **Insect bite (nonvenomous) of vagina and vulva**

⑦S30.865 **Insect bite (nonvenomous) of unspecified external genital organs, male**

⑦S30.866 **Insect bite (nonvenomous) of unspecified external genital organs, female**

⑦S30.867 **Insect bite (nonvenomous) of anus**

S30.87 **Other superficial bite of abdomen, lower back, pelvis and external genitals**

Excludes1: open bite of abdomen, lower back, pelvis and external genitals (S31.05, S31.15, S31.25, S31.35, S31.45, S31.55)

⑦S30.870 **Other superficial bite of lower back and pelvis**

⑦S30.871 **Other superficial bite of abdominal wall**

⑦S30.872 **Other superficial bite of penis**

⑦S30.873 **Other superficial bite of scrotum and testes**

⑦S30.874 **Other superficial bite of vagina and vulva**

⑦S30.875 **Other superficial bite of unspecified external genital organs, male**

⑦S30.876 **Other superficial bite of unspecified external genital organs, female**

⑦S30.877 **Other superficial bite of anus**

S30.9 **Unspecified superficial injury of abdomen, lower back, pelvis and external genitals**

⊗⑦S30.91 **Unspecified superficial injury of lower back and pelvis**

⊗⑦S30.92 **Unspecified superficial injury of abdominal wall**

⊗⑦S30.93 **Unspecified superficial injury of penis**

⊗⑦S30.94 **Unspecified superficial injury of scrotum and testes**

⊗⑦S30.95 **Unspecified superficial injury of vagina and vulva**

⊗⑦S30.96 **Unspecified superficial injury of unspecified external genital organs, male**

⊗⑦S30.97 **Unspecified superficial injury of unspecified external genital organs, female**

⊗⑦S30.98 **Unspecified superficial injury of anus**

S31 **Open wound of abdomen, lower back, pelvis and external genitals**

Code also any associated:

spinal cord injury (S24.0, S24.1-, S34.0-, S34.1-)

wound infection

Excludes1: traumatic amputation of part of abdomen, lower back and pelvis (S38.2-, S38.3)

Excludes2: open wound of hip (S71.00-S71.02)

open fracture of pelvis (S32.1--S32.9 with 7th character B)

The appropriate 7th character is to be added to each code from category S31

A - initial encounter

D - subsequent encounter

S - sequela

S31.0 **Open wound of lower back and pelvis**

S31.00 **Unspecified open wound of lower back and pelvis**

⑦S31.000 **Unspecified open wound of lower back and pelvis without penetration into retroperitoneum**

Unspecified open wound of lower back and pelvis NOS

⑦S31.001 **Unspecified open wound of lower back and pelvis with penetration into retroperitoneum**

S31.01 **Laceration without foreign body of lower back and pelvis**

● New code   ▲ Revised code   **Excludes1:** Not coded here   **Excludes2:** Not included here   ⊗ Placeholder required   ⑦7th digit required

⑦S31.010 **Laceration without foreign body of lower back and pelvis without penetration into retroperitoneum**

Laceration without foreign body of lower back and pelvis NOS

⑦S31.011 **Laceration without foreign body of lower back and pelvis with penetration into retroperitoneum**

S31.02 **Laceration with foreign body of lower back and pelvis**

⑦S31.020 **Laceration with foreign body of lower back and pelvis without penetration into retroperitoneum**

Laceration with foreign body of lower back and pelvis NOS

⑦S31.021 **Laceration with foreign body of lower back and pelvis with penetration into retroperitoneum**

S31.03 **Puncture wound without foreign body of lower back and pelvis**

⑦S31.030 **Puncture wound without foreign body of lower back and pelvis without penetration into retroperitoneum**

Puncture wound without foreign body of lower back and pelvis NOS

⑦S31.031 **Puncture wound without foreign body of lower back and pelvis with penetration into retroperitoneum**

S31.04 **Puncture wound with foreign body of lower back and pelvis**

⑦S31.040 **Puncture wound with foreign body of lower back and pelvis without penetration into retroperitoneum**

Puncture wound with foreign body of lower back and pelvis NOS

⑦S31.041 **Puncture wound with foreign body of lower back and pelvis with penetration into retroperitoneum**

S31.05 **Open bite of lower back and pelvis**

Bite of lower back and pelvis NOS

Excludes1: superficial bite of lower back and pelvis (S30.860, S30.870)

⑦S31.050 **Open bite of lower back and pelvis without penetration into retroperitoneum**

Open bite of lower back and pelvis NOS

⑦S31.051 **Open bite of lower back and pelvis with penetration into retroperitoneum**

S31.1 **Open wound of abdominal wall without penetration into peritoneal cavity**

Open wound of abdominal wall NOS

Excludes2: open wound of abdominal wall with penetration into peritoneal cavity (S31.6-)

S31.10 **Unspecified open wound of abdominal wall without penetration into peritoneal cavity**

⑦S31.100 **Unspecified open wound of abdominal wall, right upper quadrant without penetration into peritoneal cavity**

⑦S31.101 **Unspecified open wound of abdominal wall, left upper quadrant without penetration into peritoneal cavity**

⑦S31.102 **Unspecified open wound of abdominal wall, epigastric region without penetration into peritoneal cavity**

⑦S31.103 **Unspecified open wound of abdominal wall, right lower quadrant without penetration into peritoneal cavity**

⑦S31.104 **Unspecified open wound of abdominal wall, left lower quadrant without penetration into peritoneal cavity**

⑦S31.105 **Unspecified open wound of abdominal wall, periumbilic region without penetration into peritoneal cavity**

⑦S31.109 **Unspecified open wound of abdominal wall, unspecified quadrant without penetration into peritoneal cavity**

Unspecified open wound of abdominal wall NOS

⑦S31.11 **Laceration without foreign body of abdominal wall without penetration into peritoneal cavity**

⑦S31.110 **Laceration without foreign body of abdominal wall, right upper quadrant without penetration into peritoneal cavity**

⑦S31.111 **Laceration without foreign body of abdominal wall, left upper quadrant without penetration into peritoneal cavity**

⑦S31.112 **Laceration without foreign body of abdominal wall, epigastric region without penetration into peritoneal cavity**

⑦S31.113 **Laceration without foreign body of abdominal wall, right lower quadrant without penetration into peritoneal cavity**

⑦S31.114 **Laceration without foreign body of abdominal wall, left lower quadrant without penetration into peritoneal cavity**

⑦S31.115 **Laceration without foreign body of abdominal wall, periumbilic region without penetration into peritoneal cavity**

⑦S31.119 **Laceration without foreign body of abdominal wall, unspecified quadrant without penetration into peritoneal cavity**

S31.12 **Laceration with foreign body of abdominal wall without penetration into peritoneal cavity**

⑦S31.120 **Laceration of abdominal wall with foreign body, right upper quadrant without penetration into peritoneal cavity**

⑦S31.121 **Laceration of abdominal wall with foreign body, left upper quadrant without penetration into peritoneal cavity**

⑦S31.122 **Laceration of abdominal wall with foreign body, epigastric region without penetration into peritoneal cavity**

⑦S31.123 **Laceration of abdominal wall with foreign body, right lower quadrant** without penetration into peritoneal cavity

⑦S31.124   **Laceration of abdominal wall with foreign body, left lower quadrant without penetration into peritoneal cavity**

⑦S31.125   **Laceration of abdominal wall with foreign body, periumbilic region without penetration into peritoneal cavity**

⑦S31.129   **Laceration of abdominal wall with foreign body, unspecified quadrant without penetration into peritoneal cavity**

S31.13   **Puncture wound of abdominal wall without foreign body without penetration into peritoneal cavity**

⑦S31.130   **Puncture wound of abdominal wall without foreign body, right upper quadrant without penetration into peritoneal cavity**

⑦S31.131   **Puncture wound of abdominal wall without foreign body, left upper quadrant without penetration into peritoneal cavity**

⑦S31.132   **Puncture wound of abdominal wall without foreign body, epigastric region without penetration into peritoneal cavity**

⑦S31.133   **Puncture wound of abdominal wall without foreign body, right lower quadrant without penetration into peritoneal cavity**

⑦S31.134   **Puncture wound of abdominal wall without foreign body, left lower quadrant without penetration into peritoneal cavity**

⑦S31.135   **Puncture wound of abdominal wall without foreign body, periumbilic region without penetration into peritoneal cavity**

⑦S31.139   **Puncture wound of abdominal wall without foreign body, unspecified quadrant without penetration into peritoneal cavity**

S31.14   **Puncture wound of abdominal wall with foreign body without penetration into peritoneal cavity**

⑦S31.140   **Puncture wound of abdominal wall with foreign body, right upper quadrant without penetration into peritoneal cavity**

⑦S31.141   **Puncture wound of abdominal wall with foreign body, left upper quadrant without penetration into peritoneal cavity**

⑦S31.142   **Puncture wound of abdominal wall with foreign body, epigastric region without penetration into peritoneal cavity**

⑦S31.143   **Puncture wound of abdominal wall with foreign body, right lower quadrant without penetration into peritoneal cavity**

⑦S31.144   **Puncture wound of abdominal wall with foreign body, left lower quadrant without penetration into peritoneal cavity**

⑦S31.145   **Puncture wound of abdominal wall with foreign body, periumbilic region**

without penetration into peritoneal cavity

⑦S31.149   **Puncture wound of abdominal wall with foreign body, unspecified quadrant without penetration into peritoneal cavity**

S31.15   **Open bite of abdominal wall without penetration into peritoneal cavity**

Bite of abdominal wall NOS

Excludes1: superficial bite of abdominal wall (S30.871)

⑦S31.150   **Open bite of abdominal wall, right upper quadrant without penetration into peritoneal cavity**

⑦S31.151   **Open bite of abdominal wall, left upper quadrant without penetration into peritoneal cavity**

⑦S31.152   **Open bite of abdominal wall, epigastric region without penetration into peritoneal cavity**

⑦S31.153   **Open bite of abdominal wall, right lower quadrant without penetration into peritoneal cavity**

⑦S31.154   **Open bite of abdominal wall, left lower quadrant without penetration into peritoneal cavity**

⑦S31.155   **Open bite of abdominal wall, periumbilic region without penetration into peritoneal cavity**

⑦S31.159   **Open bite of abdominal wall, unspecified quadrant without penetration into peritoneal cavity**

S31.2   **Open wound of penis**

⊗⑦S31.20   **Unspecified open wound of penis**

⊗⑦S31.21   **Laceration without foreign body of penis**

⊗⑦S31.22   **Laceration with foreign body of penis**

⊗⑦S31.23   **Puncture wound without foreign body of penis**

⊗⑦S31.24   **Puncture wound with foreign body of penis**

⊗⑦S31.25   **Open bite of penis**

Bite of penis NOS

Excludes1: superficial bite of penis (S30.862, S30.872)

S31.3   **Open wound of scrotum and testes**

⊗⑦S31.30   **Unspecified open wound of scrotum and testes**

⊗⑦S31.31   **Laceration without foreign body of scrotum and testes**

⊗⑦S31.32   **Laceration with foreign body of scrotum and testes**

⊗⑦S31.33   **Puncture wound without foreign body of scrotum and testes**

⊗⑦S31.34   **Puncture wound with foreign body of scrotum and testes**

⊗⑦S31.35   **Open bite of scrotum and testes**

Bite of scrotum and testes NOS

Excludes1: superficial bite of scrotum and testes (S30.863, S30.873)

S31.4   **Open wound of vagina and vulva**

Excludes1: injury to vagina and vulva during delivery (O70.-, O71.4)

⊗⑦S31.40   **Unspecified open wound of vagina and vulva**

⊗⑦S31.41   **Laceration without foreign body of vagina and vulva**

  ● New code   ▲ Revised code   **Excludes1:** Not coded here   **Excludes2:** Not included here   ⊗ Placeholder required   ⑦ 7th digit required

⊗⑦**S31.42** **Laceration with foreign body of vagina and vulva**

⊗⑦**S31.43** **Puncture wound without foreign body of vagina and vulva**

⊗⑦**S31.44** **Puncture wound with foreign body of vagina and vulva**

⊗⑦**S31.45** **Open bite of vagina and vulva**

Bite of vagina and vulva NOS

Excludes1: superficial bite of vagina and vulva (S30.864, S30.874)

S31.5 **Open wound of unspecified external genital organs**

Excludes1: traumatic amputation of external genital organs (S38.21, S38.22)

S31.50 **Unspecified open wound of unspecified external genital organs**

⑦**S31.501** **Unspecified open wound of unspecified external genital organs, male**

⑦**S31.502** **Unspecified open wound of unspecified external genital organs, female**

S31.51 **Laceration without foreign body of unspecified external genital organs**

⑦**S31.511** **Laceration without foreign body of unspecified external genital organs, male**

⑦**S31.512** **Laceration without foreign body of unspecified external genital organs, female**

S31.52 **Laceration with foreign body of unspecified external genital organs**

⑦**S31.521** **Laceration with foreign body of unspecified external genital organs, male**

⑦**S31.522** **Laceration with foreign body of unspecified external genital organs, female**

S31.53 **Puncture wound without foreign body of unspecified external genital organs**

⑦**S31.531** **Puncture wound without foreign body of unspecified external genital organs, male**

⑦**S31.532** **Puncture wound without foreign body of unspecified external genital organs, female**

S31.54 **Puncture wound with foreign body of unspecified external genital organs**

⑦**S31.541** **Puncture wound with foreign body of unspecified external genital organs, male**

⑦**S31.542** **Puncture wound with foreign body of unspecified external genital organs, female**

S31.55 **Open bite of unspecified external genital organs**

Bite of unspecified external genital organs NOS

Excludes1: superficial bite of unspecified external genital organs (S30.865, S30.866, S30.875, S30.876)

⑦**S31.551** **Open bite of unspecified external genital organs, male**

⑦**S31.552** **Open bite of unspecified external genital organs, female**

S31.6 **Open wound of abdominal wall with penetration into peritoneal cavity**

S31.60 **Unspecified open wound of abdominal wall with penetration into peritoneal cavity**

⑦**S31.600** **Unspecified open wound of abdominal wall, right upper quadrant with penetration into peritoneal cavity**

⑦**S31.601** **Unspecified open wound of abdominal wall, left upper quadrant with penetration into peritoneal cavity**

⑦**S31.602** **Unspecified open wound of abdominal wall, epigastric region with penetration into peritoneal cavity**

⑦**S31.603** **Unspecified open wound of abdominal wall, right lower quadrant with penetration into peritoneal cavity**

⑦**S31.604** **Unspecified open wound of abdominal wall, left lower quadrant with penetration into peritoneal cavity**

⑦**S31.605** **Unspecified open wound of abdominal wall, periumbilic region with penetration into peritoneal cavity**

⑦**S31.609** **Unspecified open wound of abdominal wall, unspecified quadrant with penetration into peritoneal cavity**

S31.61 **Laceration without foreign body of abdominal wall with penetration into peritoneal cavity**

⑦**S31.610** **Laceration without foreign body of abdominal wall, right upper quadrant with penetration into peritoneal cavity**

⑦**S31.611** **Laceration without foreign body of abdominal wall, left upper quadrant with penetration into peritoneal cavity**

⑦**S31.612** **Laceration without foreign body of abdominal wall, epigastric region with penetration into peritoneal cavity**

⑦**S31.613** **Laceration without foreign body of abdominal wall, right lower quadrant with penetration into peritoneal cavity**

⑦**S31.614** **Laceration without foreign body of abdominal wall, left lower quadrant with penetration into peritoneal cavity**

⑦**S31.615** **Laceration without foreign body of abdominal wall, periumbilic region with penetration into peritoneal cavity**

⑦**S31.619** **Laceration without foreign body of abdominal wall, unspecified quadrant with penetration into peritoneal cavity**

S31.62 **Laceration with foreign body of abdominal wall with penetration into peritoneal cavity**

⑦**S31.620** **Laceration with foreign body of abdominal wall, right upper quadrant with penetration into peritoneal cavity**

⑦**S31.621** **Laceration with foreign body of abdominal wall, left upper quadrant** with penetration into peritoneal cavity

⑦ **S31.622** **Laceration with foreign body of abdominal wall, epigastric region with penetration into peritoneal cavity**

⑦ **S31.623** **Laceration with foreign body of abdominal wall, right lower quadrant with penetration into peritoneal cavity**

⑦ **S31.624** **Laceration with foreign body of abdominal wall, left lower quadrant with penetration into peritoneal cavity**

⑦ **S31.625** **Laceration with foreign body of abdominal wall, periumbilic region with penetration into peritoneal cavity**

⑦ **S31.629** **Laceration with foreign body of abdominal wall, unspecified quadrant with penetration into peritoneal cavity**

S31.63 **Puncture wound without foreign body of abdominal wall with penetration into peritoneal cavity**

⑦ **S31.630** **Puncture wound without foreign body of abdominal wall, right upper quadrant with penetration into peritoneal cavity**

⑦ **S31.631** **Puncture wound without foreign body of abdominal wall, left upper quadrant with penetration into peritoneal cavity**

⑦ **S31.632** **Puncture wound without foreign body of abdominal wall, epigastric region with penetration into peritoneal cavity**

⑦ **S31.633** **Puncture wound without foreign body of abdominal wall, right lower quadrant with penetration into peritoneal cavity**

⑦ **S31.634** **Puncture wound without foreign body of abdominal wall, left lower quadrant with penetration into peritoneal cavity**

⑦ **S31.635** **Puncture wound without foreign body of abdominal wall, periumbilic region with penetration into peritoneal cavity**

⑦ **S31.639** **Puncture wound without foreign body of abdominal wall, unspecified quadrant with penetration into peritoneal cavity**

S31.64 **Puncture wound with foreign body of abdominal wall with penetration into peritoneal cavity**

⑦ **S31.640** **Puncture wound with foreign body of abdominal wall, right upper quadrant with penetration into peritoneal cavity**

⑦ **S31.641** **Puncture wound with foreign body of abdominal wall, left upper quadrant with penetration into peritoneal cavity**

⑦ **S31.642** **Puncture wound with foreign body of abdominal wall, epigastric region with penetration into peritoneal cavity**

⑦ **S31.643** **Puncture wound with foreign body of abdominal wall, right lower quadrant with penetration into peritoneal cavity**

⑦ **S31.644** **Puncture wound with foreign body of abdominal wall, left lower quadrant with penetration into peritoneal cavity**

⑦ **S31.645** **Puncture wound with foreign body of abdominal wall, periumbilic region with penetration into peritoneal cavity**

⑦ **S31.649** **Puncture wound with foreign body of abdominal wall, unspecified quadrant with penetration into peritoneal cavity**

S31.65 **Open bite of abdominal wall with penetration into peritoneal cavity**

Excludes1: superficial bite of abdominal wall (S30.861, S30.871)

⑦ **S31.650** **Open bite of abdominal wall, right upper quadrant with penetration into peritoneal cavity**

⑦ **S31.651** **Open bite of abdominal wall, left upper quadrant with penetration into peritoneal cavity**

⑦ **S31.652** **Open bite of abdominal wall, epigastric region with penetration into peritoneal cavity**

⑦ **S31.653** **Open bite of abdominal wall, right lower quadrant with penetration into peritoneal cavity**

⑦ **S31.654** **Open bite of abdominal wall, left lower quadrant with penetration into peritoneal cavity**

⑦ **S31.655** **Open bite of abdominal wall, periumbilic region with penetration into peritoneal cavity**

⑦ **S31.659** **Open bite of abdominal wall, unspecified quadrant with penetration into peritoneal cavity**

S31.8 **Open wound of other parts of abdomen, lower back and pelvis**

S31.80 **Open wound of unspecified buttock**

⑦ **S31.801** **Laceration without foreign body of unspecified buttock**

⑦ **S31.802** **Laceration with foreign body of unspecified buttock**

⑦ **S31.803** **Puncture wound without foreign body of unspecified buttock**

⑦ **S31.804** **Puncture wound with foreign body of unspecified buttock**

⑦ **S31.805** **Open bite of unspecified buttock**

Bite of buttock NOS

Excludes1: superficial bite of buttock (S30.870)

⑦ **S31.809** **Unspecified open wound of unspecified buttock**

S31.81 **Open wound of right buttock**

⑦ **S31.811** **Laceration without foreign body of right buttock**

⑦ **S31.812** **Laceration with foreign body of right buttock**

⑦ **S31.813** **Puncture wound without foreign body of right buttock**

● New code ▲ Revised code **Excludes1:** Not coded here **Excludes2:** Not included here ⊗ Placeholder required ⑦ 7ᵗʰ digit required

⑦S31.814 **Puncture wound with foreign body of right buttock**

⑦S31.815 **Open bite of right buttock**

Bite of right buttock NOS

Excludes1: superficial bite of buttock (S30.870)

⑦S31.819 **Unspecified open wound of right buttock**

S31.82 **Open wound of left buttock**

⑦S31.821 **Laceration without foreign body of left buttock**

⑦S31.822 **Laceration with foreign body of left buttock**

⑦S31.823 **Puncture wound without foreign body of left buttock**

⑦S31.824 **Puncture wound with foreign body of left buttock**

⑦S31.825 **Open bite of left buttock**

Bite of left buttock NOS

Excludes1: superficial bite of buttock (S30.870)

⑦S31.829 **Unspecified open wound of left buttock**

⑦S31.83 **Open wound of anus**

⑦S31.831 **Laceration without foreign body of anus**

⑦S31.832 **Laceration with foreign body of anus**

⑦S31.833 **Puncture wound without foreign body of anus**

⑦S31.834 **Puncture wound with foreign body of anus**

⑦S31.835 **Open bite of anus**

Bite of anus NOS

Excludes1: superficial bite of anus (S30.877)

⑦S31.839 **Unspecified open wound of anus**

S32 **Fracture of lumbar spine and pelvis**

Note: A fracture not indicated as displaced or nondisplaced should be coded to displaced

A fracture not indicated as opened or closed should be coded to closed

Includes: fracture of lumbosacral neural arch

fracture of lumbosacral spinous process

fracture of lumbosacral transverse process

fracture of lumbosacral vertebra

fracture of lumbosacral vertebral arch

Code first any associated spinal cord and spinal nerve injury (S34.-)

Excludes1: transection of abdomen (S38.3)

Excludes2: fracture of hip NOS (S72.0-)

The appropriate 7th character is to be added to each code from category S32

A - initial encounter for closed fracture

B - initial encounter for open fracture

D - subsequent encounter for fracture with routine healing

G - subsequent encounter for fracture with delayed healing

K - subsequent encounter for fracture with nonunion

S - sequela

S32.0 **Fracture of lumbar vertebra**

Fracture of lumbar spine NOS

S32.00 **Fracture of unspecified lumbar vertebra**

⑦S32.000 **Wedge compression fracture of unspecified lumbar vertebra**

⑦S32.001 **Stable burst fracture of unspecified lumbar vertebra**

⑦S32.002 **Unstable burst fracture of unspecified lumbar vertebra**

⑦S32.008 **Other fracture of unspecified lumbar vertebra**

⑦S32.009 **Unspecified fracture of unspecified lumbar vertebra**

S32.01 **Fracture of first lumbar vertebra**

⑦S32.010 **Wedge compression fracture of first lumbar vertebra**

⑦S32.011 **Stable burst fracture of first lumbar vertebra**

⑦S32.012 **Unstable burst fracture of first lumbar vertebra**

⑦S32.018 **Other fracture of first lumbar vertebra**

⑦S32.019 **Unspecified fracture of first lumbar vertebra**

S32.02 **Fracture of second lumbar vertebra**

⑦S32.020 **Wedge compression fracture of second lumbar vertebra**

⑦S32.021 **Stable burst fracture of second lumbar vertebra**

⑦S32.022 **Unstable burst fracture of second lumbar vertebra**

⑦S32.028 **Other fracture of second lumbar vertebra**

⑦S32.029 **Unspecified fracture of second lumbar vertebra**

S32.03 **Fracture of third lumbar vertebra**

⑦S32.030 **Wedge compression fracture of third lumbar vertebra**

⑦S32.031 **Stable burst fracture of third lumbar vertebra**

⑦S32.032 **Unstable burst fracture of third lumbar vertebra**

⑦S32.038 **Other fracture of third lumbar vertebra**

⑦S32.039 **Unspecified fracture of third lumbar vertebra**

S32.04 **Fracture of fourth lumbar vertebra**

⑦S32.040 **Wedge compression fracture of fourth lumbar vertebra**

⑦S32.041 **Stable burst fracture of fourth lumbar vertebra**

⑦S32.042 **Unstable burst fracture of fourth lumbar vertebra**

⑦S32.048 **Other fracture of fourth lumbar vertebra**

⑦S32.049 **Unspecified fracture of fourth lumbar vertebra**

S32.05 **Fracture of fifth lumbar vertebra**

⑦S32.050 **Wedge compression fracture of fifth lumbar vertebra**

⑦S32.051 **Stable burst fracture of fifth lumbar vertebra**

⑦S32.052 **Unstable burst fracture of fifth lumbar vertebra**

⑦S32.058 **Other fracture of fifth lumbar vertebra**

⑦ S32.059   **Unspecified fracture of fifth lumbar vertebra**

S32.1   **Fracture of sacrum**

For vertical fractures, code to most medial fracture extension

Use two codes if both a vertical and transverse fracture are present

<u>Code also</u> any associated fracture of pelvic ring (S32.8-)

⊗⑦ S32.10   **Unspecified fracture of sacrum**

S32.11   **Zone I fracture of sacrum**

Vertical sacral ala fracture of sacrum

⑦ S32.110   **Nondisplaced Zone I fracture of sacrum**

⑦ S32.111   **Minimally displaced Zone I fracture of sacrum**

⑦ S32.112   **Severely displaced Zone I fracture of sacrum**

⑦ S32.119   **Unspecified Zone I fracture of sacrum**

S32.12   **Zone II fracture of sacrum**

Vertical foraminal region fracture of sacrum

⑦ S32.120   **Nondisplaced Zone II fracture of sacrum**

⑦ S32.121   **Minimally displaced Zone II fracture of sacrum**

⑦ S32.122   **Severely displaced Zone II fracture of sacrum**

⑦ S32.129   **Unspecified Zone II fracture of sacrum**

S32.13   **Zone III fracture of sacrum**

Vertical fracture into spinal canal region of sacrum

⑦ S32.130   **Nondisplaced Zone III fracture of sacrum**

⑦ S32.131   **Minimally displaced Zone III fracture of sacrum**

⑦ S32.132   **Severely displaced Zone III fracture of sacrum**

⑦ S32.139   **Unspecified Zone III fracture of sacrum**

S32.14   **Type 1   fracture of sacrum**

Transverse flexion fracture of sacrum without displacement

⊗⑦ S32.15   **Type 2 fracture of sacrum**

Transverse flexion fracture of sacrum with posterior displacement

⊗⑦ S32.16   **Type 3 fracture of sacrum**

Transverse extension fracture of sacrum with anterior displacement

⊗⑦ S32.17   **Type 4 fracture of sacrum**

Transverse segmental comminution of upper sacrum

⊗⑦ S32.19   **Other fracture of sacrum**

⊗⑦ S32.2   **Fracture of coccyx**

S32.3   **Fracture of ilium**

Excludes1: fracture of ilium with associated disruption of pelvic ring (S32.8-)

S32.30   **Unspecified fracture of ilium**

⑦ S32.301   **Unspecified fracture of right ilium**

⑦ S32.302   **Unspecified fracture of left ilium**

⑦ S32.309   **Unspecified fracture of unspecified ilium**

S32.31   **Avulsion fracture of ilium**

⑦ S32.311   **Displaced avulsion fracture of right ilium**

⑦ S32.312   **Displaced avulsion fracture of left ilium**

⑦ S32.313   **Displaced avulsion fracture of unspecified ilium**

⑦ S32.314   **Nondisplaced avulsion fracture of right ilium**

⑦ S32.315   **Nondisplaced avulsion fracture of left ilium**

⑦ S32.316   **Nondisplaced avulsion fracture of unspecified ilium**

S32.39   **Other fracture of ilium**

⑦ S32.391   **Other fracture of right ilium**

⑦ S32.392   **Other fracture of left ilium**

⑦ S32.399   **Other fracture of unspecified ilium**

S32.4   **Fracture of acetabulum**

<u>Code also</u> any associated fracture of pelvic ring (S32.8-)

S32.40   **Unspecified fracture of acetabulum**

⑦ S32.401   **Unspecified fracture of right acetabulum**

⑦ S32.402   **Unspecified fracture of left acetabulum**

⑦ S32.409   **Unspecified fracture of unspecified acetabulum**

S32.41   **Fracture of anterior wall of acetabulum**

⑦ S32.411   **Displaced fracture of anterior wall of right acetabulum**

⑦ S32.412   **Displaced fracture of anterior wall of left acetabulum**

⑦ S32.413   **Displaced fracture of anterior wall of unspecified acetabulum**

⑦ S32.414   **Nondisplaced fracture of anterior wall of right acetabulum**

⑦ S32.415   **Nondisplaced fracture of anterior wall of left acetabulum**

⑦ S32.416   **Nondisplaced fracture of anterior wall of unspecified acetabulum**

S32.42   **Fracture of posterior wall of acetabulum**

⑦ S32.421   **Displaced fracture of posterior wall of right acetabulum**

⑦ S32.422   **Displaced fracture of posterior wall of left acetabulum**

⑦ S32.423   **Displaced fracture of posterior wall of unspecified acetabulum**

⑦ S32.424   **Nondisplaced fracture of posterior wall of right acetabulum**

⑦ S32.425   **Nondisplaced fracture of posterior wall of left acetabulum**

⑦ S32.426   **Nondisplaced fracture of posterior wall of unspecified acetabulum**

S32.43   **Fracture of anterior column [iliopubic] of acetabulum**

⑦ S32.431   **Displaced fracture of anterior column [iliopubic] of right acetabulum**

⑦ S32.432   **Displaced fracture of anterior column [iliopubic] of left acetabulum**

⑦ S32.433   **Displaced fracture of anterior column [iliopubic] of unspecified acetabulum**

⑦S32.434   Nondisplaced fracture of anterior column [iliopubic] of right acetabulum

⑦S32.435   Nondisplaced fracture of anterior column [iliopubic] of left acetabulum

⑦S32.436   Nondisplaced fracture of anterior column [iliopubic] of unspecified acetabulum

S32.44   Fracture of posterior column [ilioischial] of acetabulum

⑦S32.441   Displaced fracture of posterior column [ilioischial] of right acetabulum

⑦S32.442   Displaced fracture of posterior column [ilioischial] of left acetabulum

⑦S32.443   Displaced fracture of posterior column [ilioischial] of unspecified acetabulum

⑦S32.444   Nondisplaced fracture of posterior column [ilioischial] of right acetabulum

⑦S32.445   Nondisplaced fracture of posterior column [ilioischial] of left acetabulum

⑦S32.446   Nondisplaced fracture of posterior column [ilioischial] of unspecified acetabulum

S32.45   Transverse fracture of acetabulum

⑦S32.451   Displaced transverse fracture of right acetabulum

⑦S32.452   Displaced transverse fracture of left acetabulum

⑦S32.453   Displaced transverse fracture of unspecified acetabulum

⑦S32.454   Nondisplaced transverse fracture of right acetabulum

⑦S32.455   Nondisplaced transverse fracture of left acetabulum

⑦S32.456   Nondisplaced transverse fracture of unspecified acetabulum

S32.46   Associated transverse-posterior fracture of acetabulum

⑦S32.461   Displaced associated transverse-posterior fracture of right acetabulum

⑦S32.462   Displaced associated transverse-posterior fracture of left acetabulum

⑦S32.463   Displaced associated transverse-posterior fracture of unspecified acetabulum

⑦S32.464   Nondisplaced associated transverse-posterior fracture of right acetabulum

⑦S32.465   Nondisplaced associated transverse-posterior fracture of left acetabulum

⑦S32.466   Nondisplaced associated transverse-posterior fracture of unspecified acetabulum

S32.47   Fracture of medial wall of acetabulum

⑦S32.471   Displaced fracture of medial wall of right acetabulum

⑦S32.472   Displaced fracture of medial wall of left acetabulum

⑦S32.473   Displaced fracture of medial wall of unspecified acetabulum

⑦S32.474   Nondisplaced fracture of medial wall of right acetabulum

⑦S32.475   Nondisplaced fracture of medial wall of left acetabulum

⑦S32.476   Nondisplaced fracture of medial wall of unspecified acetabulum

S32.48   Dome fracture of acetabulum

⑦S32.481   Displaced dome fracture of right acetabulum

⑦S32.482   Displaced dome fracture of left acetabulum

⑦S32.483   Displaced dome fracture of unspecified acetabulum

⑦S32.484   Nondisplaced dome fracture of right acetabulum

⑦S32.485   Nondisplaced dome fracture of left acetabulum

⑦S32.486   Nondisplaced dome fracture of unspecified acetabulum

S32.49   Other specified fracture of acetabulum

⑦S32.491   Other specified fracture of right acetabulum

⑦S32.492   Other specified fracture of left acetabulum

⑦S32.499   Other specified fracture of unspecified acetabulum

S32.5   Fracture of pubis

Excludes1: fracture of pubis with associated disruption of pelvic ring (S32.8-)

S32.50   Unspecified fracture of pubis

⑦S32.501   Unspecified fracture of right pubis

⑦S32.502   Unspecified fracture of left pubis

⑦S32.509   Unspecified fracture of unspecified pubis

S32.51   Fracture of superior rim of pubis

⑦S32.511   Fracture of superior rim of right pubis

⑦S32.512   Fracture of superior rim of left pubis

⑦S32.519   Fracture of superior rim of unspecified pubis

S32.59   Other specified fracture of pubis

⑦S32.591   Other specified fracture of right pubis

⑦S32.592   Other specified fracture of left pubis

⑦S32.599   Other specified fracture of unspecified pubis

S32.6   Fracture of ischium

Excludes1: fracture of ischium with associated disruption of pelvic ring (S32.8-)

S32.60   Unspecified fracture of ischium

⑦S32.601   Unspecified fracture of right ischium

⑦S32.602   Unspecified fracture of left ischium

⑦S32.609   Unspecified fracture of unspecified ischium

S32.61   Avulsion fracture of ischium

⑦S32.611   Displaced avulsion fracture of right ischium

⑦S32.612   Displaced avulsion fracture of left ischium

⑦S32.613   Displaced avulsion fracture of unspecified ischium

⑦S32.614 **Nondisplaced avulsion fracture of right ischium**

⑦S32.615 **Nondisplaced avulsion fracture of left ischium**

⑦S32.616 **Nondisplaced avulsion fracture of unspecified ischium**

S32.69 **Other specified fracture of ischium**

⑦S32.691 **Other specified fracture of right ischium**

⑦S32.692 **Other specified fracture of left ischium**

⑦S32.699 **Other specified fracture of unspecified ischium**

S32.8 **Fracture of other parts of pelvis**

Code also any associated:

fracture of acetabulum (S32.4-)

sacral fracture (S32.1-)

S32.81 **Multiple fractures of pelvis with disruption of pelvic ring**

Multiple pelvic fractures with disruption of pelvic circle

⑦S32.810 **Multiple fractures of pelvis with stable disruption of pelvic ring**

⑦S32.811 **Multiple fractures of pelvis with unstable disruption of pelvic ring**

⊗⑦S32.82 **Multiple fractures of pelvis without disruption of pelvic ring**

Multiple pelvic fractures without disruption of pelvic circle

⊗⑦S32.89 **Fracture of other parts of pelvis**

S32.9 **Fracture of unspecified parts of lumbosacral spine and pelvis**

Fracture of lumbosacral spine NOS

Fracture of pelvis NOS

S33 **Dislocation and sprain of joints and ligaments of lumbar spine and pelvis**

Includes: avulsion of joint or ligament of lumbar spine and pelvis

laceration of cartilage, joint or ligament of lumbar spine and pelvis

sprain of cartilage, joint or ligament of lumbar spine and pelvis

traumatic hemarthrosis of joint or ligament of lumbar spine and pelvis

traumatic rupture of joint or ligament of lumbar spine and pelvis

traumatic subluxation of joint or ligament of lumbar spine and pelvis

traumatic tear of joint or ligament of lumbar spine and pelvis

Code also any associated open wound

Excludes1: nontraumatic rupture or displacement of lumbar intervertebral disc NOS (M51.-)

obstetric damage to pelvic joints and ligaments (O71.6)

Excludes2: dislocation and sprain of joints and ligaments of hip (S73.-)

strain of muscle of lower back and pelvis (S39.01-)

The appropriate 7th character is to be added to each code from category S33

A - initial encounter

D - subsequent encounter

S - sequela

⊗⑦S33.0 **Traumatic rupture of lumbar intervertebral disc**

Excludes1: rupture or displacement (nontraumatic) of lumbar intervertebral disc NOS (M51.- with fifth character 6)

S33.1 **Subluxation and dislocation of lumbar vertebra**

Code also any associated:

open wound of abdomen, lower back and pelvis (S31)

spinal cord injury (S24.0, S24.1-, S34.0-, S34.1-)

Excludes2: fracture of lumbar vertebrae (S32.0-)

S33.10 **Subluxation and dislocation of unspecified lumbar vertebra**

⑦S33.100 **Subluxation of unspecified lumbar vertebra**

⑦S33.101 **Dislocation of unspecified lumbar vertebra**

S33.11 **Subluxation and dislocation of L1/L2 lumbar vertebra**

⑦S33.110 **Subluxation of L1/L2 lumbar vertebra**

⑦S33.111 **Dislocation of L1/L2 lumbar vertebra**

S33.12 **Subluxation and dislocation of L2/L3 lumbar vertebra**

⑦S33.120 **Subluxation of L2/L3 lumbar vertebra**

⑦S33.121 **Dislocation of L2/L3 lumbar vertebra**

S33.13 **Subluxation and dislocation of L3/L4 lumbar vertebra**

⑦S33.130 **Subluxation of L3/L4 lumbar vertebra**

⑦S33.131 **Dislocation of L3/L4 lumbar vertebra**

⑦S33.14 **Subluxation and dislocation of L4/L5 lumbar vertebra**

⑦S33.140 **Subluxation of L4/L5 lumbar vertebra**

⑦S33.141 **Dislocation of L4/L5 lumbar vertebra**

⊗⑦S33.2 **Dislocation of sacroiliac and sacrococcygeal joint**

S33.3 **Dislocation of other and unspecified parts of lumbar spine and pelvis**

⊗⑦S33.30 **Dislocation of unspecified parts of lumbar spine and pelvis**

⊗⑦S33.39 **Dislocation of other parts of lumbar spine and pelvis**

⊗⑦S33.4 **Traumatic rupture of symphysis pubis**

⊗⑦S33.5 **Sprain of ligaments of lumbar spine**

⊗⑦S33.6 **Sprain of sacroiliac joint**

⊗⑦S33.8 **Sprain of other parts of lumbar spine and pelvis**

⊗⑦S33.9 **Sprain of unspecified parts of lumbar spine and pelvis**

S34 **Injury of lumbar and sacral spinal cord and nerves at abdomen, lower back and pelvis level**

Note: Code to highest level of lumbar cord injury

Injuries to the spinal cord (S34.0 and S34.1) refer to the cord level and not bone level injury, and can affect nerve roots at and below the level given.

Code also any associated:

fracture of vertebra (S22.0-, S32.0-)

open wound of abdomen, lower back and pelvis (S31.-)

transient paralysis (R29.5)

The appropriate 7th character is to be added to each code from category S34

A - initial encounter

D - subsequent encounter

S - sequela

S34.0 **Concussion and edema of lumbar and sacral spinal cord**

● New code   ▲ Revised code   Excludes1: Not coded here   Excludes2: Not included here   ⊗ Placeholder required   ⑦ 7th digit required

⊗⑦S34.01   **Concussion and edema of lumbar spinal cord**

⊗⑦S34.02   **Concussion and edema of sacral spinal cord**

   Concussion and edema of conus medullaris

S34.1   **Other and unspecified injury of lumbar and sacral spinal cord**

  S34.10 **Unspecified injury to lumbar spinal cord**

    ⑦**S34.101**   **Unspecified injury to L1 level of lumbar spinal cord**

       Unspecified injury to lumbar spinal cord level 1

    ⑦**S34.102**   **Unspecified injury to L2 level of lumbar spinal cord**

       Unspecified injury to lumbar spinal cord level 2

    ⑦**S34.103**   **Unspecified injury to L3 level of lumbar spinal cord**

       Unspecified injury to lumbar spinal cord level 3

    ⑦**S34.104**   **Unspecified injury to L4 level of lumbar spinal cord**

       Unspecified injury to lumbar spinal cord level 4

    ⑦**S34.105**   **Unspecified injury to L5 level of lumbar spinal cord**

       Unspecified injury to lumbar spinal cord level 5

    ⑦**S34.109**   **Unspecified injury to unspecified level of lumbar spinal cord**

  S34.11 **Complete lesion of lumbar spinal cord**

    ⑦S34.111   **Complete lesion of L1 level of lumbar spinal cord**

       Complete lesion of lumbar spinal cord level 1

    ⑦S34.112   **Complete lesion of L2 level of lumbar spinal cord**

       Complete lesion of lumbar spinal cord level 2

    ⑦S34.113   **Complete lesion of L3 level of lumbar spinal cord**

       Complete lesion of lumbar spinal cord level 3

    ⑦S34.114   **Complete lesion of L4 level of lumbar spinal cord**

       Complete lesion of lumbar spinal cord level 4

    ⑦S34.115   **Complete lesion of L5 level of lumbar spinal cord**

       Complete lesion of lumbar spinal cord level 5

    ⑦**S34.119**   **Complete lesion of unspecified level of lumbar spinal cord**

  S34.12 **Incomplete lesion of lumbar spinal cord**

    ⑦S34.121   **Incomplete lesion of L1 level of lumbar spinal cord**

       Incomplete lesion of lumbar spinal cord level 1

    ⑦S34.122   **Incomplete lesion of L2 level of lumbar spinal cord**

       Incomplete lesion of lumbar spinal cord level 2

    ⑦S34.123   **Incomplete lesion of L3 level of lumbar spinal cord**

       Incomplete lesion of lumbar spinal cord level 3

    ⑦S34.124   **Incomplete lesion of L4 level of lumbar spinal cord**

       Incomplete lesion of lumbar spinal cord level 4

    ⑦S34.125   **Incomplete lesion of L5 level of lumbar spinal cord**

       Incomplete lesion of lumbar spinal cord level 5

    ⑦**S34.129**   **Incomplete lesion of unspecified level of lumbar spinal cord**

  S34.13 **Other and unspecified injury to sacral spinal cord**

    Other injury to conus medullaris

    ⑦S34.131   **Complete lesion of sacral spinal cord**

       Complete lesion of conus medullaris

    ⑦S34.132   **Incomplete lesion of sacral spinal cord**

       Incomplete lesion of conus medullaris

    ⑦S34.139   **Unspecified injury to sacral spinal cord**

       Unspecified injury of conus medullaris

S34.2   **Injury of nerve root of lumbar and sacral spine**

  ⊗⑦S34.21 **Injury of nerve root of lumbar spine**

  ⊗⑦S34.22 **Injury of nerve root of sacral spine**

⊗⑦S34.3   **Injury of cauda equina**

⊗⑦S34.4   **Injury of lumbosacral plexus**

⊗⑦S34.5   **Injury of lumbar, sacral and pelvic sympathetic nerves**

   Injury of celiac ganglion or plexus

   Injury of hypogastric plexus

   Injury of mesenteric plexus (inferior) (superior)

   Injury of splanchnic nerve

⊗⑦S34.6   **Injury of peripheral nerve(s) at abdomen, lower back and pelvis level**

⊗⑦S34.8   **Injury of other nerves at abdomen, lower back and pelvis level**

⊗⑦S34.9   **Injury of unspecified nerves at abdomen, lower back and pelvis level**

S35   **Injury of blood vessels at abdomen, lower back and pelvis level**

  Code also any associated open wound (S31.-)

  The appropriate 7th character is to be added to each code from category S35

  A - initial encounter

  D - subsequent encounter

  S - sequela

  S35.0   **Injury of abdominal aorta**

    Excludes1: injury of aorta NOS (S25.0)

    ⊗⑦S35.00   **Unspecified injury of abdominal aorta**

    ⊗⑦S35.01   **Minor laceration of abdominal aorta**

       Incomplete transection of abdominal aorta

       Laceration of abdominal aorta NOS

       Superficial laceration of abdominal aorta

    ⊗⑦S35.02   **Major laceration of abdominal aorta**

       Complete transection of abdominal aorta

       Traumatic rupture of abdominal aorta

    ⊗⑦S35.09   **Other injury of abdominal aorta**

  S35.1   **Injury of inferior vena cava**

    Injury of hepatic vein

    Excludes1: injury of vena cava NOS (S25.2)

    ⊗⑦S35.10   **Unspecified injury of inferior vena cava**

⊗⑦S35.11 **Minor laceration of inferior vena cava**

Incomplete transection of inferior vena cava

Laceration of inferior vena cava NOS

Superficial laceration of inferior vena cava

⊗⑦S35.12 **Major laceration of inferior vena cava**

Complete transection of inferior vena cava

Traumatic rupture of inferior vena cava

⊗⑦**S35.19** **Other injury of inferior vena cava**

S35.2 **Injury of celiac or mesenteric artery and branches**

S35.21 **Injury of celiac artery**

⑦S35.211 **Minor laceration of celiac artery**

Incomplete transection of celiac artery

Laceration of celiac artery NOS

Superficial laceration of celiac artery

⑦S35.212 **Major laceration of celiac artery**

Complete transection of celiac artery

Traumatic rupture of celiac artery

⑦**S35.218** **Other injury of celiac artery**

⑦S35.219 **Unspecified injury of celiac artery**

S35.22 **Injury of superior mesenteric artery**

⑦S35.221 **Minor laceration of superior mesenteric artery**

Incomplete transection of superior mesenteric artery

Laceration of superior mesenteric artery NOS

Superficial laceration of superior mesenteric artery

⑦S35.222 **Major laceration of superior mesenteric artery**

Complete transection of superior mesenteric artery

Traumatic rupture of superior mesenteric artery

⑦**S35.228** **Other injury of superior mesenteric artery**

⑦S35.229 **Unspecified injury of superior mesenteric artery**

S35.23 **Injury of inferior mesenteric artery**

⑦S35.231 **Minor laceration of inferior mesenteric artery**

Incomplete transection of inferior mesenteric artery

Laceration of inferior mesenteric artery NOS

Superficial laceration of inferior mesenteric artery

⑦S35.232 **Major laceration of inferior mesenteric artery**

Complete transection of inferior mesenteric artery

Traumatic rupture of inferior mesenteric artery

⑦**S35.238** **Other injury of inferior mesenteric artery**

⑦S35.239 **Unspecified injury of inferior mesenteric artery**

S35.29 **Injury of branches of celiac and mesenteric artery**

Injury of gastric artery

Injury of gastroduodenal artery

Injury of hepatic artery

Injury of splenic artery

⑦S35.291 **Minor laceration of branches of celiac and mesenteric artery**

Incomplete transection of branches of celiac and mesenteric artery

Laceration of branches of celiac and mesenteric artery NOS

Superficial laceration of branches of celiac and mesenteric artery

⑦S35.292 **Major laceration of branches of celiac and mesenteric artery**

Complete transection of branches of celiac and mesenteric artery

Traumatic rupture of branches of celiac and mesenteric artery

⑦**S35.298** **Other injury of branches of celiac and mesenteric artery**

⑦S35.299 **Unspecified injury of branches of celiac and mesenteric artery**

S35.3 **Injury of portal or splenic vein and branches**

S35.31 **Injury of portal vein**

⑦S35.311 **Laceration of portal vein**

⑦S35.318 **Other specified injury of portal vein**

⑦S35.319 **Unspecified injury of portal vein**

S35.32 **Injury of splenic vein**

⑦S35.321 **Laceration of splenic vein**

⑦S35.328 **Other specified injury of splenic vein**

⑦S35.329 **Unspecified injury of splenic vein**

S35.33 **Injury of superior mesenteric vein**

⑦S35.331 **Laceration of superior mesenteric vein**

⑦S35.338 **Other specified injury of superior mesenteric vein**

⑦**S35.339** **Unspecified injury of superior mesenteric vein**

S35.34 **Injury of inferior mesenteric vein**

⑦S35.341 **Laceration of inferior mesenteric vein**

⑦S35.348 **Other specified injury of inferior mesenteric vein**

⑦S35.349 **Unspecified injury of inferior mesenteric vein**

S35.4 **Injury of renal blood vessels**

S35.40 **Unspecified injury of renal blood vessel**

⑦S35.401 **Unspecified injury of right renal artery**

⑦S35.402 **Unspecified injury of left renal artery**

⑦S35.403 **Unspecified injury of unspecified renal artery**

⑦S35.404 **Unspecified injury of right renal vein**

⑦S35.405 **Unspecified injury of left renal vein**

⑦S35.406 **Unspecified injury of unspecified renal vein**

S35.41 **Laceration of renal blood vessel**

⑦S35.411 **Laceration of right renal artery**

⑦S35.412 **Laceration of left renal artery**

⑦S35.413 **Laceration of unspecified renal artery**

⑦S35.414 **Laceration of right renal vein**

● New code ▲ Revised code **Excludes1:** Not coded here **Excludes2:** Not included here ⊗ Placeholder required ⑦7ᵗʰ digit required

⑦S35.415　**Laceration of left renal vein**

⑦S35.416　**Laceration of unspecified renal vein**

S35.49　**Other specified injury of renal blood vessel**

⑦S35.491　**Other specified injury of right renal artery**

⑦S35.492　**Other specified injury of left renal artery**

⑦S35.493　**Other specified injury of unspecified renal artery**

⑦S35.494　**Other specified injury of right renal vein**

⑦S35.495　**Other specified injury of left renal vein**

⑦S35.496　**Other specified injury of unspecified renal vein**

S35.5　**Injury of iliac blood vessels**

⊗⑦S35.50　**Injury of unspecified iliac blood vessel(s)**

S35.51　**Injury of iliac artery or vein**

Injury of hypogastric artery or vein

⑦S35.511　**Injury of right iliac artery**

⑦S35.512　**Injury of left iliac artery**

⑦S35.513　**Injury of unspecified iliac artery**

⑦S35.514　**Injury of right iliac vein**

⑦S35.515　**Injury of left iliac vein**

⑦S35.516　**Injury of unspecified iliac vein**

S35.53　**Injury of uterine artery or vein**

⑦S35.531　**Injury of right uterine artery**

⑦S35.532　**Injury of left uterine artery**

⑦S35.533　**Injury of unspecified uterine artery**

⑦S35.534　**Injury of right uterine vein**

⑦S35.535　**Injury of left uterine vein**

⑦S35.536　**Injury of unspecified uterine vein**

⊗⑦S35.59　**Injury of other iliac blood vessels**

S35.8　**Injury of other blood vessels at abdomen, lower back and pelvis level**

Injury of ovarian artery or vein

S35.8X　**Injury of other blood vessels at abdomen, lower back and pelvis level**

⑦S35.8X1　**Laceration of other blood vessels at abdomen, lower back and pelvis level**

⑦S35.8X8　**Other specified injury of other blood vessels at abdomen, lower back and pelvis level**

⑦S35.8X9　**Unspecified injury of other blood vessels at abdomen, lower back and pelvis level**

S35.9　**Injury of unspecified blood vessel at abdomen, lower back and pelvis level**

⊗⑦S35.90　**Unspecified injury of unspecified blood vessel at abdomen, lower back and pelvis level**

⊗⑦S35.91　**Laceration of unspecified blood vessel at abdomen, lower back and pelvis level**

⊗⑦S35.99　**Other specified injury of unspecified blood vessel at abdomen, lower back and pelvis level**

S36　**Injury of intra-abdominal organs**

Code also any associated open wound (S31.-)

The appropriate 7th character is to be added to each code from category S36

A - initial encounter

D - subsequent encounter

S - sequela

S36.0　**Injury of spleen**

⊗⑦S36.00　**Unspecified injury of spleen**

S36.02　**Contusion of spleen**

⑦S36.020　**Minor contusion of spleen**

Contusion of spleen less than 2 cm

⑦S36.021　**Major contusion of spleen**

Contusion of spleen greater than 2 cm

⑦S36.029　**Unspecified contusion of spleen**

S36.03　**Laceration of spleen**

⑦S36.030　**Superficial (capsular) laceration of spleen**

Laceration of spleen less than 1 cm

Minor laceration of spleen

⑦S36.031　**Moderate laceration of spleen**

Laceration of spleen 1 to 3 cm

⑦S36.032　**Major laceration of spleen**

Avulsion of spleen

Laceration of spleen greater than 3 cm

Massive laceration of spleen

Multiple moderate lacerations of spleen
Stellate laceration of spleen

⑦S36.039　**Unspecified laceration of spleen**

S36.09　**Other injury of spleen**

S36.1　**Injury of liver and gallbladder and bile duct**

S36.11　**Injury of liver**

⑦S36.112　**Contusion of liver**

⑦S36.113　**Laceration of liver, unspecified degree**

⑦S36.114　**Minor laceration of liver**

Laceration involving capsule only, or, without significant involvement of hepatic parenchyma [i.e., less than 1 cm deep]

⑦S36.115　**Moderate laceration of liver**

Laceration involving parenchyma but without major disruption of parenchyma [i.e., less than 10 cm long and less than 3 cm deep]

⑦S36.116　**Major laceration of liver**

Laceration with significant disruption of hepatic parenchyma [i.e., greater than 10 cm long and 3 cm deep]

Multiple moderate lacerations, with or without hematoma

Stellate laceration of liver

⑦S36.118　**Other injury of liver**

⑦S36.119　**Unspecified injury of liver**

S36.12　**Injury of gallbladder**

⑦S36.122　**Contusion of gallbladder**

⑦S36.123　**Laceration of gallbladder**

⑦S36.128　**Other injury of gallbladder**

⑦S36.129　**Unspecified injury of gallbladder**

⊗⑦S36.13　**Injury of bile duct**

S36.2　**Injury of pancreas**

S36.20　**Unspecified injury of pancreas**

⑦S36.200　**Unspecified injury of head of pancreas**

⑦S36.201　**Unspecified injury of body of pancreas**

⑦S36.202　**Unspecified injury of tail of pancreas**

⑦ S36.209 Unspecified injury of unspecified part of pancreas

S36.22 **Contusion of pancreas**
⑦ S36.220 Contusion of head of pancreas
⑦ S36.221 Contusion of body of pancreas
⑦ S36.222 Contusion of tail of pancreas
⑦ S36.229 Contusion of unspecified part of pancreas

S36.23 **Laceration of pancreas, unspecified degree**
⑦ S36.230 Laceration of head of pancreas, unspecified degree
⑦ S36.231 Laceration of body of pancreas, unspecified degree
⑦ S36.232 Laceration of tail of pancreas, unspecified degree
⑦ S36.239 Laceration of unspecified part of pancreas, unspecified degree

S36.24 **Minor laceration of pancreas**
⑦ S36.240 Minor laceration of head of pancreas
⑦ S36.241 Minor laceration of body of pancreas
⑦ S36.242 Minor laceration of tail of pancreas
⑦ S36.249 Minor laceration of unspecified part of pancreas

S36.25 **Moderate laceration of pancreas**
⑦ S36.250 Moderate laceration of head of pancreas
⑦ S36.251 Moderate laceration of body of pancreas
⑦ S36.252 Moderate laceration of tail of pancreas
⑦ S36.259 Moderate laceration of unspecified part of pancreas

S36.26 **Major laceration of pancreas**
⑦ S36.260 Major laceration of head of pancreas
⑦ S36.261 Major laceration of body of pancreas
⑦ S36.262 Major laceration of tail of pancreas
⑦ S36.269 Major laceration of unspecified part of pancreas

S36.29 **Other injury of pancreas**
⑦ S36.290 Other injury of head of pancreas
⑦ S36.291 Other injury of body of pancreas
⑦ S36.292 Other injury of tail of pancreas
⑦ S36.299 Other injury of unspecified part of pancreas

S36.3 **Injury of stomach**
⊗⑦ S36.30 Unspecified injury of stomach
⊗⑦ S36.32 Contusion of stomach
⊗⑦ S36.33 Laceration of stomach
⊗⑦ S36.39 Other injury of stomach

S36.4 **Injury of small intestine**
S36.40 **Unspecified injury of small intestine**
⑦ S36.400 Unspecified injury of duodenum
⑦ S36.408 Unspecified injury of other part of small intestine
⑦ S36.409 Unspecified injury of unspecified part of small intestine

S36.41 **Primary blast injury of small intestine**
Blast injury of small intestine NOS
⑦ S36.410 Primary blast injury of duodenum

⑦ S36.418 Primary blast injury of other part of small intestine
⑦ S36.419 Primary blast injury of unspecified part of small intestine

S36.42 **Contusion of small intestine**
⑦ S36.420 Contusion of duodenum
⑦ S36.428 Contusion of other part of small intestine
⑦ S36.429 Contusion of unspecified part of small intestine

S36.43 **Laceration of small intestine**
⑦ S36.430 Laceration of duodenum
⑦ S36.438 Laceration of other part of small intestine
⑦ S36.439 Laceration of unspecified part of small intestine

S36.49 **Other injury of small intestine**
⑦ S36.490 Other injury of duodenum
⑦ S36.498 Other injury of other part of small intestine
⑦ S36.499 Other injury of unspecified part of small intestine

S36.5 **Injury of colon**
Excludes2: injury of rectum (S36.6-)
S36.50 **Unspecified injury of colon**
⑦ S36.500 Unspecified injury of ascending [right] colon
⑦ S36.501 Unspecified injury of transverse colon
⑦ S36.502 Unspecified injury of descending [left] colon
⑦ S36.503 Unspecified injury of sigmoid colon
⑦ S36.508 Unspecified injury of other part of colon
⑦ S36.509 Unspecified injury of unspecified part of colon

S36.51 **Primary blast injury of colon**
Blast injury of colon NOS
⑦ S36.510 Primary blast injury of ascending [right] colon
⑦ S36.511 Primary blast injury of transverse colon
⑦ S36.512 Primary blast injury of descending [left] colon
⑦ S36.513 Primary blast injury of sigmoid colon
⑦ S36.518 Primary blast injury of other part of colon
⑦ S36.519 Primary blast injury of unspecified part of colon

S36.52 **Contusion of colon**
⑦ S36.520 Contusion of ascending [right] colon
⑦ S36.521 Contusion of transverse colon
⑦ S36.522 Contusion of descending [left] colon
⑦ S36.523 Contusion of sigmoid colon
⑦ S36.528 Contusion of other part of colon
⑦ S36.529 Contusion of unspecified part of colon

S36.53 **Laceration of colon**
⑦ S36.530 Laceration of ascending [right] colon
⑦ S36.531 Laceration of transverse colon

⑦S36.532   **Laceration of descending [left] colon**

⑦S36.533   **Laceration of sigmoid colon**

⑦S36.538   **Laceration of other part of colon**

⑦S36.539   **Laceration of unspecified part of colon**

S36.59   **Other injury of colon**

Secondary blast injury of colon

⑦S36.590   **Other injury of ascending [right] colon**

⑦S36.591   **Other injury of transverse colon**

⑦S36.592   **Other injury of descending [left] colon**

⑦S36.593   **Other injury of sigmoid colon**

⑦S36.598   **Other injury of other part of colon**

⑦S36.599   **Other injury of unspecified part of colon**

S36.6   **Injury of rectum**

⊗⑦S36.60   **Unspecified injury of rectum**

⊗⑦S36.61   **Primary blast injury of rectum**

Blast injury of rectum NOS

⊗⑦S36.62   **Contusion of rectum**

⊗⑦S36.63   **Laceration of rectum**

⊗⑦S36.69   **Other injury of rectum**

Secondary blast injury of rectum

S36.8   **Injury of other intra-abdominal organs**

⊗⑦S36.81   **Injury of peritoneum**

S36.89   **Injury of other intra-abdominal organs**

Injury of retroperitoneum

⑦S36.892   **Contusion of other intra-abdominal organs**

⑦S36.893   **Laceration of other intra-abdominal organs**

⑦S36.898   **Other injury of other intra-abdominal organs**

⑦S36.899   **Unspecified injury of other intra-abdominal organs**

S36.9   **Injury of unspecified intra-abdominal organ**

⊗⑦S36.90   **Unspecified injury of unspecified intra-abdominal organ**

⊗⑦S36.92   **Contusion of unspecified intra-abdominal organ**

⊗⑦S36.93   **Laceration of unspecified intra-abdominal organ**

⊗⑦S36.99   **Other injury of unspecified intra-abdominal organ**

S37   **Injury of urinary and pelvic organs**

Code also any associated open wound (S31.-)

Excludes1: obstetric trauma to pelvic organs (O71.-)

Excludes2: injury of peritoneum (S36.81)

injury of retroperitoneum (S36.89-)

The appropriate 7th character is to be added to each code from category S37

A - initial encounter

D - subsequent encounter

S - sequela

S37.0   **Injury of kidney**

Excludes2: acute kidney injury (nontraumatic) (N17.9)

S37.00   **Unspecified injury of kidney**

⑦S37.001   **Unspecified injury of right kidney**

⑦S37.002   **Unspecified injury of left kidney**

⑦S37.009   **Unspecified injury of unspecified kidney**

S37.01   **Minor contusion of kidney**

Contusion of kidney less than 2 cm

Contusion of kidney NOS

⑦S37.011   **Minor contusion of right kidney**

⑦S37.012   **Minor contusion of left kidney**

⑦S37.019   **Minor contusion of unspecified kidney**

S37.02   **Major contusion of kidney**

Contusion of kidney greater than 2 cm

⑦S37.021   **Major contusion of right kidney**

⑦S37.022   **Major contusion of left kidney**

⑦S37.029   **Major contusion of unspecified kidney**

S37.03   **Laceration of kidney, unspecified degree**

⑦S37.031   **Laceration of right kidney, unspecified degree**

⑦S37.032   **Laceration of left kidney, unspecified degree**

⑦S37.039   **Laceration of unspecified kidney, unspecified degree**

S37.04   **Minor laceration of kidney**

Laceration of kidney less than 1 cm

⑦S37.041   **Minor laceration of right kidney**

⑦S37.042   **Minor laceration of left kidney**

⑦S37.049   **Minor laceration of unspecified kidney**

S37.05   **Moderate laceration of kidney**

Laceration of kidney 1 to 3 cm

⑦S37.051   **Moderate laceration of right kidney**

⑦S37.052   **Moderate laceration of left kidney**

⑦S37.059   **Moderate laceration of unspecified kidney**

S37.06   **Major laceration of kidney**

Avulsion of kidney

Laceration of kidney greater than 3 cm

Massive laceration of kidney

Multiple moderate lacerations of kidney

Stellate laceration of kidney

⑦S37.061   **Major laceration of right kidney**

⑦S37.062   **Major laceration of left kidney**

⑦S37.069   **Major laceration of unspecified kidney**

S37.09   **Other injury of kidney**

⑦S37.091   **Other injury of right kidney**

⑦S37.092   **Other injury of left kidney**

⑦S37.099   **Other injury of unspecified kidney**

S37.1   **Injury of ureter**

⊗⑦S37.10   **Unspecified injury of ureter**

⊗⑦S37.12   **Contusion of ureter**

⊗⑦S37.13   **Laceration of ureter**

⊗⑦S37.19   **Other injury of ureter**

S37.2   **Injury of bladder**

⊗⑦S37.20   **Unspecified injury of bladder**

⊗⑦S37.22   **Contusion of bladder**

⊗⑦S37.23   **Laceration of bladder**

⊗⑦S37.29   **Other injury of bladder**

S37.3   **Injury of urethra**

| ▆ | Add 4th-7th digits | ▆ | Nonspecific code | ▆ | Unspecified code | ▆ | Manifestation code | **781** |

⊗⑦S37.30   Unspecified injury of urethra

⊗⑦S37.32   Contusion of urethra

⊗⑦S37.33   Laceration of urethra

⊗⑦S37.39   Other injury of urethra

S37.4   Injury of ovary

   S37.40   Unspecified injury of ovary

     ⑦ S37.401   Unspecified injury of ovary, unilateral

     ⑦ S37.402   Unspecified injury of ovary, bilateral

     ⑦ S37.409   Unspecified injury of ovary, unspecified

   S37.42   Contusion of ovary

     ⑦ S37.421   Contusion of ovary, unilateral

     ⑦ S37.422   Contusion of ovary, bilateral

     ⑦ S37.429   Contusion of ovary, unspecified

   S37.43   Laceration of ovary

     ⑦ S37.431   Laceration of ovary, unilateral

     ⑦ S37.432   Laceration of ovary, bilateral

     ⑦ S37.439   Laceration of ovary, unspecified

   S37.49   Other injury of ovary

     ⑦ S37.491   Other injury of ovary, unilateral

     ⑦ S37.492   Other injury of ovary, bilateral

     ⑦ S37.499   Other injury of ovary, unspecified

S37.5   Injury of fallopian tube

   S37.50   Unspecified injury of fallopian tube

     ⑦ S37.501   Unspecified injury of fallopian tube, unilateral

     ⑦ S37.502   Unspecified injury of fallopian tube, bilateral

     ⑦ S37.509   Unspecified injury of fallopian tube, unspecified

   S37.51   Primary blast injury of fallopian tube

     Blast injury of fallopian tube NOS

     ⑦ S37.511   Primary blast injury of fallopian tube, unilateral

     ⑦ S37.512   Primary blast injury of fallopian tube, bilateral

     ⑦ S37.519   Primary blast injury of fallopian tube, unspecified

   S37.52   Contusion of fallopian tube

     ⑦ S37.521   Contusion of fallopian tube, unilateral

     ⑦ S37.522   Contusion of fallopian tube, bilateral

     ⑦ S37.529   Contusion of fallopian tube, unspecified

   S37.53   Laceration of fallopian tube

     ⑦ S37.531   Laceration of fallopian tube, unilateral

     ⑦ S37.532   Laceration of fallopian tube, bilateral

     ⑦ S37.539   Laceration of fallopian tube, unspecified

   S37.59   Other injury of fallopian tube

     Secondary blast injury of fallopian tube

     ⑦ S37.591   Other injury of fallopian tube, unilateral

     ⑦ S37.592   Other injury of fallopian tube, bilateral

     ⑦ S37.599   Other injury of fallopian tube, unspecified

S37.6   Injury of uterus

     Excludes1: injury to gravid uterus (O9A.2-)

         injury to uterus during delivery (O71.-)

   ⊗⑦S37.60   Unspecified injury of uterus

   ⊗⑦S37.62   Contusion of uterus

   ⊗⑦S37.63   Laceration of uterus

   ⊗⑦S37.69   Other injury of uterus

S37.8   Injury of other urinary and pelvic organs

   S37.81   Injury of adrenal gland

     ⑦ S37.812   Contusion of adrenal gland

     ⑦ S37.813   Laceration of adrenal gland

     ⑦ S37.818   Other injury of adrenal gland

     ⑦ S37.819   Unspecified injury of adrenal gland

   S37.82   Injury of prostate

     ⑦ S37.822   Contusion of prostate

     ⑦ S37.823   Laceration of prostate

     ⑦ S37.828   Other injury of prostate

     ⑦ S37.829   Unspecified injury of prostate

   S37.89   Injury of other urinary and pelvic organ

     ⑦ S37.892   Contusion of other urinary and pelvic organ

     ⑦ S37.893   Laceration of other urinary and pelvic organ

     ⑦ S37.898   Other injury of other urinary and pelvic organ

     ⑦ S37.899   Unspecified injury of other urinary and pelvic organ

S37.9   Injury of unspecified urinary and pelvic organ

   ⊗⑦S37.90   Unspecified injury of unspecified urinary and pelvic organ

   ⊗⑦S37.92   Contusion of unspecified urinary and pelvic organ

   ⊗⑦S37.93   Laceration of unspecified urinary and pelvic organ

   ⊗⑦S37.99   Other injury of unspecified urinary and pelvic organ

S38   **Crushing injury and traumatic amputation of abdomen, lower back, pelvis and external genitals**

An amputation not identified as partial or complete should be coded to complete

The appropriate 7th character is to be added to each code from category S38

A - initial encounter

D - subsequent encounter

S - sequela

   S38.0   Crushing injury of external genital organs

     <u>Use additional code</u> for any associated injuries

     S38.00   Crushing injury of unspecified external genital organs

       ⑦ S38.001   Crushing injury of unspecified external genital organs, male

       ⑦ S38.002   Crushing injury of unspecified external genital organs, female

     ⊗⑦S38.01   Crushing injury of penis

     ⊗⑦S38.02   Crushing injury of scrotum and testis

     ⊗⑦S38.03   Crushing injury of vulva

   S38.1   Crushing injury of abdomen, lower back, and pelvis

     <u>Use additional code</u> for all associated injuries, such as:

     fracture of thoracic or lumbar spine and pelvis (S22.0-, S32.-)

     injury to intra-abdominal organs (S36.-)

injury to urinary and pelvic organs (S37.-)

open wound of abdominal wall (S31.-)

spinal cord injury (S34.0, S34.1-)

Excludes2: crushing injury of external genital organs (S38.0-)

S38.2 **Traumatic amputation of external genital organs**

   S38.21 **Traumatic amputation of female external genital organs**

      Traumatic amputation of clitoris

      Traumatic amputation of labium (majus) (minus)

      Traumatic amputation of vulva

      ⑦S38.211 **Complete traumatic amputation of female external genital organs**

      ⑦S38.212 **Partial traumatic amputation of female external genital organs**

   S38.22 **Traumatic amputation of penis**

      ⑦S38.221 **Complete traumatic amputation of penis**

      ⑦S38.222 **Partial traumatic amputation of penis**

   S38.23 **Traumatic amputation of scrotum and testis**

      ⑦S38.231 **Complete traumatic amputation of scrotum and testis**

      ⑦S38.232 **Partial traumatic amputation of scrotum and testis**

⊗⑦S38.3 **Transection (partial) of abdomen**

S39 **Other and unspecified injuries of abdomen, lower back, pelvis and external genitals**

Code also any associated open wound (S31.-)

Excludes2: sprain of joints and ligaments of lumbar spine and pelvis (S33.-)

The appropriate 7th character is to be added to each code from category S39

A - initial encounter

D - subsequent encounter

S - sequela

S39.0 **Injury of muscle, fascia and tendon of abdomen, lower back and pelvis**

   S39.00 **Unspecified injury of muscle, fascia and tendon of abdomen, lower back and pelvis**

      ⑦S39.001 **Unspecified injury of muscle, fascia and tendon of abdomen**

      ⑦S39.002 **Unspecified injury of muscle, fascia and tendon of lower back**

      ⑦S39.003 **Unspecified injury of muscle, fascia and tendon of pelvis**

   S39.01 **Strain of muscle, fascia and tendon of abdomen, lower back and pelvis**

      ⑦S39.011 **Strain of muscle, fascia and tendon of abdomen**

      ⑦S39.012 **Strain of muscle, fascia and tendon of lower back**

      ⑦S39.013 **Strain of muscle, fascia and tendon of pelvis**

   S39.02 **Laceration of muscle, fascia and tendon of abdomen, lower back and pelvis**

      ⑦S39.021 **Laceration of muscle, fascia and tendon of abdomen**

      ⑦S39.022 **Laceration of muscle, fascia and tendon of lower back**

      ⑦S39.023 **Laceration of muscle, fascia and tendon of pelvis**

   S39.09 **Other injury of muscle, fascia and tendon of abdomen, lower back and pelvis**

      ⑦S39.091 **Other injury of muscle, fascia and tendon of abdomen**

      ⑦S39.092 **Other injury of muscle, fascia and tendon of lower back**

      ⑦S39.093 **Other injury of muscle, fascia and tendon of pelvis**

S39.8 **Other specified injuries of abdomen, lower back, pelvis and external genitals**

   ⊗⑦S39.81 **Other specified injuries of abdomen**

   ⊗⑦S39.82 **Other specified injuries of lower back**

   ⊗⑦S39.83 **Other specified injuries of pelvis**

   S39.84 **Other specified injuries of external genitals**

      ⑦S39.840 **Fracture of corpus cavernosum penis**

      ⑦S39.848 **Other specified injuries of external genitals**

S39.9 **Unspecified injury of abdomen, lower back, pelvis and external genitals**

   ⊗⑦S39.91 **Unspecified injury of abdomen**

   ⊗⑦S39.92 **Unspecified injury of lower back**

   ⊗⑦S39.93 **Unspecified injury of pelvis**

   ⊗⑦S39.94 **Unspecified injury of external genitals**

INJURIES TO THE SHOULDER AND UPPER ARM (S40-S49)

Includes: injuries of axilla

injuries of scapular region

Excludes2: burns and corrosions (T20-T32)

frostbite (T33-T34)

injuries of elbow (S50-S59)

insect bite or sting, venomous (T63.4)

S40 **Superficial injury of shoulder and upper arm**

The appropriate 7th character is to be added to each code from category S40

A - initial encounter

D - subsequent encounter

S - sequela

S40.0 **Contusion of shoulder and upper arm**

   S40.01 **Contusion of shoulder**

      ⑦S40.011 **Contusion of right shoulder**

      ⑦S40.012 **Contusion of left shoulder**

      ⑦S40.019 **Contusion of unspecified shoulder**

   S40.02 **Contusion of upper arm**

      ⑦S40.021 **Contusion of right upper arm**

      ⑦S40.022 **Contusion of left upper arm**

      ⑦S40.029 **Contusion of unspecified upper arm**

S40.2 **Other superficial injuries of shoulder**

   S40.21 **Abrasion of shoulder**

      ⑦S40.211 **Abrasion of right shoulder**

      ⑦S40.212 **Abrasion of left shoulder**

      ⑦S40.219 **Abrasion of unspecified shoulder**

   S40.22 **Blister (nonthermal) of shoulder**

      ⑦S40.221 **Blister (nonthermal) of right shoulder**

      ⑦S40.222 **Blister (nonthermal) of left shoulder**

      ⑦S40.229 **Blister (nonthermal) of unspecified shoulder**

   S40.24 **External constriction of shoulder**

⑦S40.241 **External constriction of right shoulder**

⑦S40.242 **External constriction of left shoulder**

⑦S40.249 **External constriction of unspecified shoulder**

S40.25 **Superficial foreign body of shoulder**

Splinter in the shoulder

⑦S40.251 **Superficial foreign body of right shoulder**

⑦S40.252 **Superficial foreign body of left shoulder**

⑦S40.259 **Superficial foreign body of unspecified shoulder**

S40.26 **Insect bite (nonvenomous) of shoulder**

⑦S40.261 **Insect bite (nonvenomous) of right shoulder**

⑦S40.262 **Insect bite (nonvenomous) of left shoulder**

⑦S40.269 **Insect bite (nonvenomous) of unspecified shoulder**

S40.27 **Other superficial bite of shoulder**

Excludes1: open bite of shoulder (S41.05)

⑦S40.271 **Other superficial bite of right shoulder**

⑦S40.272 **Other superficial bite of left shoulder**

⑦S40.279 **Other superficial bite of unspecified shoulder**

S40.8 **Other superficial injuries of upper arm**

S40.81 **Abrasion of upper arm**

⑦S40.811 **Abrasion of right upper arm**

⑦S40.812 **Abrasion of left upper arm**

⑦S40.819 **Abrasion of unspecified upper arm**

S40.82 **Blister (nonthermal) of upper arm**

⑦S40.821 **Blister (nonthermal) of right upper arm**

⑦S40.822 **Blister (nonthermal) of left upper arm**

⑦S40.829 **Blister (nonthermal) of unspecified upper arm**

S40.84 **External constriction of upper arm**

⑦S40.841 **External constriction of right upper arm**

⑦S40.842 **External constriction of left upper arm**

⑦S40.849 **External constriction of unspecified upper arm**

S40.85 **Superficial foreign body of upper arm**

Splinter in the upper arm

⑦S40.851 **Superficial foreign body of right upper arm**

⑦S40.852 **Superficial foreign body of left upper arm**

⑦S40.859 **Superficial foreign body of unspecified upper arm**

S40.86 **Insect bite (nonvenomous) of upper arm**

⑦S40.861 **Insect bite (nonvenomous) of right upper arm**

⑦S40.862 **Insect bite (nonvenomous) of left upper arm**

⑦S40.869 **Insect bite (nonvenomous) of unspecified upper arm**

S40.87 **Other superficial bite of upper arm**

Excludes1: open bite of upper arm (S41.14)

Excludes2: Other superficial bite of shoulder (S40.27-)

⑦S40.871 **Other superficial bite of right upper arm**

⑦S40.872 **Other superficial bite of left upper arm**

⑦S40.879 **Other superficial bite of unspecified upper arm**

S40.9 **Unspecified superficial injury of shoulder and upper arm**

S40.91 **Unspecified superficial injury of shoulder**

⑦S40.911 **Unspecified superficial injury of right shoulder**

⑦S40.912 **Unspecified superficial injury of left shoulder**

⑦S40.919 **Unspecified superficial injury of unspecified shoulder**

S40.92 **Unspecified superficial injury of upper arm**

⑦S40.921 **Unspecified superficial injury of right upper arm**

⑦S40.922 **Unspecified superficial injury of left upper arm**

⑦S40.929 **Unspecified superficial injury of unspecified upper arm**

S41 **Open wound of shoulder and upper arm**

Code also any associated wound infection

Excludes1: traumatic amputation of shoulder and upper arm (S48.-)

Excludes2: open fracture of shoulder and upper arm (S42.- with 7th character B or C)

The appropriate 7th character is to be added to each code from category S41

A - initial encounter

D - subsequent encounter

S - sequela

S41.0 **Open wound of shoulder**

S41.00 **Unspecified open wound of shoulder**

⑦S41.001 **Unspecified open wound of right shoulder**

⑦S41.002 **Unspecified open wound of left shoulder**

⑦S41.009 **Unspecified open wound of unspecified shoulder**

S41.01 **Laceration without foreign body of shoulder**

⑦S41.011 **Laceration without foreign body of right shoulder**

⑦S41.012 **Laceration without foreign body of left shoulder**

⑦S41.019 **Laceration without foreign body of unspecified shoulder**

S41.02 **Laceration with foreign body of shoulder**

⑦S41.021 **Laceration with foreign body of right shoulder**

⑦S41.022 **Laceration with foreign body of left shoulder**

⑦S41.029 **Laceration with foreign body of unspecified shoulder**

S41.03 **Puncture wound without foreign body of shoulder**

⑦S41.031 **Puncture wound without foreign body of right shoulder**

⑦S41.032 **Puncture wound without foreign body of left shoulder**

● New code ▲ Revised code **Excludes1:** Not coded here **Excludes2:** Not included here ⊗ Placeholder required ⑦7th digit required

⑦S41.039   **Puncture wound without foreign body of unspecified shoulder**

S41.04   **Puncture wound with foreign body of shoulder**

⑦S41.041   **Puncture wound with foreign body of right shoulder**

⑦S41.042   **Puncture wound with foreign body of left shoulder**

⑦S41.049   **Puncture wound with foreign body of unspecified shoulder**

S41.05   **Open bite of shoulder**

Bite of shoulder NOS

Excludes1: superficial bite of shoulder (S40.27)

⑦S41.051   **Open bite of right shoulder**

⑦S41.052   **Open bite of left shoulder**

⑦S41.059   **Open bite of unspecified shoulder**

S41.1   **Open wound of upper arm**

S41.10   **Unspecified open wound of upper arm**

⑦S41.101   **Unspecified open wound of right upper arm**

⑦S41.102   **Unspecified open wound of left upper arm**

⑦S41.109   **Unspecified open wound of unspecified upper arm**

S41.11   **Laceration without foreign body of upper arm**

⑦S41.111   **Laceration without foreign body of right upper arm**

⑦S41.112   **Laceration without foreign body of left upper arm**

⑦S41.119   **Laceration without foreign body of unspecified upper arm**

S41.12   **Laceration with foreign body of upper arm**

⑦S41.121   **Laceration with foreign body of right upper arm**

⑦S41.122   **Laceration with foreign body of left upper arm**

⑦S41.129   **Laceration with foreign body of unspecified upper arm**

S41.13   **Puncture wound without foreign body of upper arm**

⑦S41.131   **Puncture wound without foreign body of right upper arm**

⑦S41.132   **Puncture wound without foreign body of left upper arm**

⑦S41.139   **Puncture wound without foreign body of unspecified upper arm**

S41.14   **Puncture wound with foreign body of upper arm**

⑦S41.141   **Puncture wound with foreign body of right upper arm**

⑦S41.142   **Puncture wound with foreign body of left upper arm**

⑦S41.149   **Puncture wound with foreign body of unspecified upper arm**

S41.15   **Open bite of upper arm**

Bite of upper arm NOS

Excludes1: superficial bite of upper arm (S40.87)

⑦S41.151   **Open bite of right upper arm**

⑦S41.152   **Open bite of left upper arm**

⑦S41.159   **Open bite of unspecified upper arm**

S42   **Fracture of shoulder and upper arm**

Note: A fracture not indicated as displaced or nondisplaced should be coded to displaced

A fracture not indicated as open or closed should be coded to closed

Excludes1: traumatic amputation of shoulder and upper arm (S48.-)

The appropriate 7th character is to be added to all codes from category S42

A - initial encounter for closed fracture

B - initial encounter for open fracture

D - subsequent encounter for fracture with routine healing

G - subsequent encounter for fracture with delayed healing

K - subsequent encounter for fracture with nonunion

P - subsequent encounter for fracture with malunion

S - sequela

S42.0   **Fracture of clavicle**

S42.00   **Fracture of unspecified part of clavicle**

⑦S42.001   **Fracture of unspecified part of right clavicle**

⑦S42.002   **Fracture of unspecified part of left clavicle**

⑦S42.009   **Fracture of unspecified part of unspecified clavicle**

S42.01   **Fracture of sternal end of clavicle**

⑦S42.011   **Anterior displaced fracture of sternal end of right clavicle**

⑦S42.012   **Anterior displaced fracture of sternal end of left clavicle**

⑦S42.013   **Anterior displaced fracture of sternal end of unspecified clavicle**

Displaced fracture of sternal end of clavicle NOS

⑦S42.014   **Posterior displaced fracture of sternal end of right clavicle**

⑦S42.015   **Posterior displaced fracture of sternal end of left clavicle**

⑦S42.016   **Posterior displaced fracture of sternal end of unspecified clavicle**

⑦S42.017   **Nondisplaced fracture of sternal end of right clavicle**

⑦S42.018   **Nondisplaced fracture of sternal end of left clavicle**

⑦S42.019   **Nondisplaced fracture of sternal end of unspecified clavicle**

S42.02   **Fracture of shaft of clavicle**

⑦S42.021   **Displaced fracture of shaft of right clavicle**

⑦S42.022   **Displaced fracture of shaft of left clavicle**

⑦S42.023   **Displaced fracture of shaft of unspecified clavicle**

⑦S42.024   **Nondisplaced fracture of shaft of right clavicle**

⑦S42.025   **Nondisplaced fracture of shaft of left clavicle**

⑦S42.026   **Nondisplaced fracture of shaft of unspecified clavicle**

S42.03   **Fracture of lateral end of clavicle**

Fracture of acromial end of clavicle

⑦S42.031   **Displaced fracture of lateral end of right clavicle**

⑦S42.032   **Displaced fracture of lateral end of left clavicle**

⑦S42.033   **Displaced fracture of lateral end of unspecified clavicle**

⑦S42.034   **Nondisplaced fracture of lateral end of right clavicle**

⑦S42.035   **Nondisplaced fracture of lateral end of left clavicle**

⑦S42.036   **Nondisplaced fracture of lateral end of unspecified clavicle**

S42.1   **Fracture of scapula**

   S42.10   **Fracture of unspecified part of scapula**

     ⑦S42.101   **Fracture of unspecified part of scapula, right shoulder**

     ⑦S42.102   **Fracture of unspecified part of scapula, left shoulder**

     ⑦S42.109   **Fracture of unspecified part of scapula, unspecified shoulder**

   S42.11   **Fracture of body of scapula**

     ⑦S42.111   **Displaced fracture of body of scapula, right shoulder**

     ⑦S42.112   **Displaced fracture of body of scapula, left shoulder**

     ⑦S42.113   **Displaced fracture of body of scapula, unspecified shoulder**

     ⑦S42.114   **Nondisplaced fracture of body of scapula, right shoulder**

     ⑦S42.115   **Nondisplaced fracture of body of scapula, left shoulder**

     ⑦S42.116   **Nondisplaced fracture of body of scapula, unspecified shoulder**

   S42.12   **Fracture of acromial process**

     ⑦S42.121   **Displaced fracture of acromial process, right shoulder**

     ⑦S42.122   **Displaced fracture of acromial process, left shoulder**

     ⑦S42.123   **Displaced fracture of acromial process, unspecified shoulder**

     ⑦S42.124   **Nondisplaced fracture of acromial process, right shoulder**

     ⑦S42.125   **Nondisplaced fracture of acromial process, left shoulder**

     ⑦S42.126   **Nondisplaced fracture of acromial process, unspecified shoulder**

   S42.13   **Fracture of coracoid process**

     ⑦S42.131   **Displaced fracture of coracoid process, right shoulder**

     ⑦S42.132   **Displaced fracture of coracoid process, left shoulder**

     ⑦S42.133   **Displaced fracture of coracoid process, unspecified shoulder**

     ⑦S42.134   **Nondisplaced fracture of coracoid process, right shoulder**

     ⑦S42.135   **Nondisplaced fracture of coracoid process, left shoulder**

     ⑦S42.136   **Nondisplaced fracture of coracoid process, unspecified shoulder**

   S42.14   **Fracture of glenoid cavity of scapula**

     ⑦S42.141   **Displaced fracture of glenoid cavity of scapula, right shoulder**

     ⑦S42.142   **Displaced fracture of glenoid cavity of scapula, left shoulder**

     ⑦S42.143   **Displaced fracture of glenoid cavity of scapula, unspecified shoulder**

     ⑦S42.144   **Nondisplaced fracture of glenoid cavity of scapula, right shoulder**

     ⑦S42.145   **Nondisplaced fracture of glenoid cavity of scapula, left shoulder**

     ⑦S42.146   **Nondisplaced fracture of glenoid cavity of scapula, unspecified shoulder**

   S42.15   **Fracture of neck of scapula**

     ⑦S42.151   **Displaced fracture of neck of scapula, right shoulder**

     ⑦S42.152   **Displaced fracture of neck of scapula, left shoulder**

     ⑦S42.153   **Displaced fracture of neck of scapula, unspecified shoulder**

     ⑦S42.154   **Nondisplaced fracture of neck of scapula, right shoulder**

     ⑦S42.155   **Nondisplaced fracture of neck of scapula, left shoulder**

     ⑦S42.156   **Nondisplaced fracture of neck of scapula, unspecified shoulder**

   S42.19   **Fracture of other part of scapula**

     ⑦S42.191   **Fracture of other part of scapula, right shoulder**

     ⑦S42.192   **Fracture of other part of scapula, left shoulder**

     ⑦S42.199   **Fracture of other part of scapula, unspecified shoulder**

S42.2   **Fracture of upper end of humerus**

   Fracture of proximal end of humerus

   Excludes2: fracture of shaft of humerus (S42.3-)

     physeal fracture of upper end of humerus (S49.0-)

   S42.20   **Unspecified fracture of upper end of humerus**

     ⑦S42.201   **Unspecified fracture of upper end of right humerus**

     ⑦S42.202   **Unspecified fracture of upper end of left humerus**

     ⑦S42.209   **Unspecified fracture of upper end of unspecified humerus**

   S42.21   **Unspecified fracture of surgical neck of humerus**

     Fracture of neck of humerus NOS

     ⑦S42.211   **Unspecified displaced fracture of surgical neck of right humerus**

     ⑦S42.212   **Unspecified displaced fracture of surgical neck of left humerus**

     ⑦S42.213   **Unspecified displaced fracture of surgical neck of unspecified humerus**

     ⑦S42.214   **Unspecified nondisplaced fracture of surgical neck of right humerus**

     ⑦S42.215   **Unspecified nondisplaced fracture of surgical neck of left humerus**

     ⑦S42.216   **Unspecified nondisplaced fracture of surgical neck of unspecified humerus**

   S42.22   **2-part fracture of surgical neck of humerus**

     ⑦S42.221   **2-part displaced fracture of surgical neck of right humerus**

     ⑦S42.222   **2-part displaced fracture of surgical neck of left humerus**

     ⑦S42.223   **2-part displaced fracture of surgical neck of unspecified humerus**

     ⑦S42.224   **2-part nondisplaced fracture of surgical neck of right humerus**

     ⑦S42.225   **2-part nondisplaced fracture of surgical neck of left humerus**

     ⑦S42.226   **2-part nondisplaced fracture of surgical neck of unspecified humerus**

   ● New code   ▲ Revised code   **Excludes1:** Not coded here   **Excludes2:** Not included here   ⊗ Placeholder required   ⑦7th digit required

S42.23   **3-part fracture of surgical neck of humerus**

⑦S42.231   3-part fracture of surgical neck of right humerus

⑦S42.232   3-part fracture of surgical neck of left humerus

⑦S42.239   3-part fracture of surgical neck of unspecified humerus

S42.24   **4-part fracture of surgical neck of humerus**

⑦S42.241   4-part fracture of surgical neck of right humerus

⑦S42.242   4-part fracture of surgical neck of left humerus

⑦S42.249   4-part fracture of surgical neck of unspecified humerus

S42.25   **Fracture of greater tuberosity of humerus**

⑦S42.251   Displaced fracture of greater tuberosity of right humerus

⑦S42.252   Displaced fracture of greater tuberosity of left humerus

⑦S42.253   Displaced fracture of greater tuberosity of unspecified humerus

⑦S42.254   Nondisplaced fracture of greater tuberosity of right humerus

⑦S42.255   Nondisplaced fracture of greater tuberosity of left humerus

⑦S42.256   Nondisplaced fracture of greater tuberosity of unspecified humerus

S42.26   **Fracture of lesser tuberosity of humerus**

⑦S42.261   Displaced fracture of lesser tuberosity of right humerus

⑦S42.262   Displaced fracture of lesser tuberosity of left humerus

⑦S42.263   Displaced fracture of lesser tuberosity of unspecified humerus

⑦S42.264   Nondisplaced fracture of lesser tuberosity of right humerus

⑦S42.265   Nondisplaced fracture of lesser tuberosity of left humerus

⑦S42.266   Nondisplaced fracture of lesser tuberosity of unspecified humerus

S42.27   **Torus fracture of upper end of humerus**

The appropriate 7th character is to be added to all codes in subcategory S42.27

A - initial encounter for closed fracture

D - subsequent encounter for fracture with routine healing

G - subsequent encounter for fracture with delayed healing

K - subsequent encounter for fracture with nonunion

P - subsequent encounter for fracture with malunion S - sequela

⑦S42.271   **Torus fracture of upper end of right humerus**

⑦S42.272   **Torus fracture of upper end of left humerus**

⑦S42.279   **Torus fracture of upper end of unspecified humerus**

S42.29   **Other fracture of upper end of humerus**

Fracture of anatomical neck of humerus

Fracture of articular head of humerus

⑦S42.291   **Other displaced fracture of upper end of right humerus**

⑦S42.292   **Other displaced fracture of upper end of left humerus**

⑦S42.293   **Other displaced fracture of upper end of unspecified humerus**

⑦S42.294   **Other nondisplaced fracture of upper end of right humerus**

⑦S42.295   **Other nondisplaced fracture of upper end of left humerus**

⑦S42.296   **Other nondisplaced fracture of upper end of unspecified humerus**

S42.3   **Fracture of shaft of humerus**

Fracture of humerus NOS

Fracture of upper arm NOS

Excludes2: physeal fractures of upper end of humerus (S49.0-)

physeal fractures of lower end of humerus (S49.1-)

S42.30   **Unspecified fracture of shaft of humerus**

⑦S42.301   Unspecified fracture of shaft of humerus, right arm

⑦S42.302   Unspecified fracture of shaft of humerus, left arm

⑦S42.309   Unspecified fracture of shaft of humerus, unspecified arm

S42.31   **Greenstick fracture of shaft of humerus**

The appropriate 7th character is to be added to all codes in subcategory S42.31

A - initial encounter for closed fracture

D - subsequent encounter for fracture with routine healing

G - subsequent encounter for fracture with delayed healing

K - subsequent encounter for fracture with nonunion

P - subsequent encounter for fracture with malunion S - sequela

⑦S42.311   **Greenstick fracture of shaft of humerus, right arm**

⑦S42.312   **Greenstick fracture of shaft of humerus, left arm**

⑦S42.319   **Greenstick fracture of shaft of humerus, unspecified arm**

S42.32   **Transverse fracture of shaft of humerus**

⑦S42.321   Displaced transverse fracture of shaft of humerus, right arm

⑦S42.322   Displaced transverse fracture of shaft of humerus, left arm

⑦S42.323   Displaced transverse fracture of shaft of humerus, unspecified arm

⑦S42.324   Nondisplaced transverse fracture of shaft of humerus, right arm

⑦S42.325   Nondisplaced transverse fracture of shaft of humerus, left arm

⑦S42.326   Nondisplaced transverse fracture of shaft of humerus, unspecified arm

S42.33   **Oblique fracture of shaft of humerus**

⑦S42.331   Displaced oblique fracture of shaft of humerus, right arm

⑦S42.332   Displaced oblique fracture of shaft of humerus, left arm

⑦S42.333   Displaced oblique fracture of shaft of humerus, unspecified arm

⑦S42.334   Nondisplaced oblique fracture of shaft of humerus, right arm

---

| � | Add 4th-7th digits | Nonspecific code | Unspecified code | Manifestation code | 787 |

⑦S42.335 Nondisplaced oblique fracture of shaft of humerus, left arm

⑦S42.336 Nondisplaced oblique fracture of shaft of humerus, unspecified arm

S42.34 ⑦Spiral fracture of shaft of humerus

⑦S42.341 Displaced spiral fracture of shaft of humerus, right arm

⑦S42.342 Displaced spiral fracture of shaft of humerus, left arm

⑦S42.343 Displaced spiral fracture of shaft of humerus, unspecified arm

⑦S42.344 Nondisplaced spiral fracture of shaft of humerus, right arm

⑦S42.345 Nondisplaced spiral fracture of shaft of humerus, left arm

⑦S42.346 Nondisplaced spiral fracture of shaft of humerus, unspecified arm

S42.35 Comminuted fracture of shaft of humerus

⑦S42.351 Displaced comminuted fracture of shaft of humerus, right arm

⑦S42.352 Displaced comminuted fracture of shaft of humerus, left arm

⑦S42.353 Displaced comminuted fracture of shaft of humerus, unspecified arm

⑦S42.354 Nondisplaced comminuted fracture of shaft of humerus, right arm

⑦S42.355 Nondisplaced comminuted fracture of shaft of humerus, left arm

⑦S42.356 Nondisplaced comminuted fracture of shaft of humerus, unspecified arm

S42.36 Segmental fracture of shaft of humerus

⑦S42.361 Displaced segmental fracture of shaft of humerus, right arm

⑦S42.362 Displaced segmental fracture of shaft of humerus, left arm

⑦S42.363 Displaced segmental fracture of shaft of humerus, unspecified arm

⑦S42.364 Nondisplaced segmental fracture of shaft of humerus, right arm

⑦S42.365 Nondisplaced segmental fracture of shaft of humerus, left arm

⑦S42.366 Nondisplaced segmental fracture of shaft of humerus, unspecified arm

S42.39 Other fracture of shaft of humerus

⑦S42.391 Other fracture of shaft of right humerus

⑦S42.392 Other fracture of shaft of left humerus

⑦S42.399 Other fracture of shaft of unspecified humerus

S42.4 Fracture of lower end of humerus

Fracture of distal end of humerus

Excludes2: fracture of shaft of humerus (S42.3-)

physeal fracture of lower end of humerus (S49.1-)

S42.40 Unspecified fracture of lower end of humerus

Fracture of elbow NOS

⑦S42.401 Unspecified fracture of lower end of right humerus

⑦S42.402 Unspecified fracture of lower end of left humerus

⑦S42.409 Unspecified fracture of lower end of unspecified humerus

S42.41 Simple supracondylar fracture without intercondylar fracture of humerus

⑦S42.411 Displaced simple supracondylar fracture without intercondylar fracture of right humerus

⑦S42.412 Displaced simple supracondylar fracture without intercondylar fracture of left humerus

⑦S42.413 Displaced simple supracondylar fracture without intercondylar fracture of unspecified humerus

⑦S42.414 Nondisplaced simple supracondylar fracture without intercondylar fracture of right humerus

⑦S42.415 Nondisplaced simple supracondylar fracture without intercondylar fracture of left humerus

⑦S42.416 Nondisplaced simple supracondylar fracture without intercondylar fracture of unspecified humerus

S42.42 Comminuted supracondylar fracture without intercondylar fracture of humerus

⑦S42.421 Displaced comminuted supracondylar fracture without intercondylar fracture of right humerus

⑦S42.422 Displaced comminuted supracondylar fracture without intercondylar fracture of left humerus

⑦S42.423 Displaced comminuted supracondylar fracture without intercondylar fracture of unspecified humerus

⑦S42.424 Nondisplaced comminuted supracondylar fracture without intercondylar fracture of right humerus

⑦S42.425 Nondisplaced comminuted supracondylar fracture without intercondylar fracture of left humerus

⑦S42.426 Nondisplaced comminuted supracondylar fracture without intercondylar fracture of unspecified humerus

S42.43 Fracture (avulsion) of lateral epicondyle of humerus

⑦S42.431 Displaced fracture (avulsion) of lateral epicondyle of right humerus

⑦S42.432 Displaced fracture (avulsion) of lateral epicondyle of left humerus

⑦S42.433 Displaced fracture (avulsion) of lateral epicondyle of unspecified humerus

⑦S42.434 Nondisplaced fracture (avulsion) of lateral epicondyle of right humerus

⑦S42.435 Nondisplaced fracture (avulsion) of lateral epicondyle of left humerus

⑦S42.436 Nondisplaced fracture (avulsion) of lateral epicondyle of unspecified humerus

S42.44 Fracture (avulsion) of medial epicondyle of humerus

⑦S42.441 Displaced fracture (avulsion) of medial epicondyle of right humerus

⑦S42.442   **Displaced fracture (avulsion) of medial epicondyle of left humerus**

⑦S42.443   **Displaced fracture (avulsion) of medial epicondyle of unspecified humerus**

⑦S42.444   **Nondisplaced fracture (avulsion) of medial epicondyle of right humerus**

⑦S42.445   **Nondisplaced fracture (avulsion) of medial epicondyle of left humerus**

⑦S42.446   **Nondisplaced fracture (avulsion) of medial epicondyle of unspecified humerus**

⑦S42.447   **Incarcerated fracture (avulsion) of medial epicondyle of right humerus**

⑦S42.448   **Incarcerated fracture (avulsion) of medial epicondyle of left humerus**

⑦S42.449   **Incarcerated fracture (avulsion) of medial epicondyle of unspecified humerus**

S42.45   **Fracture of lateral condyle of humerus**

Fracture of capitellum of humerus

⑦S42.451   **Displaced fracture of lateral condyle of right humerus**

⑦S42.452   **Displaced fracture of lateral condyle of left humerus**

⑦S42.453   **Displaced fracture of lateral condyle of unspecified humerus**

⑦S42.454   **Nondisplaced fracture of lateral condyle of right humerus**

⑦S42.455   **Nondisplaced fracture of lateral condyle of left humerus**

⑦S42.456   **Nondisplaced fracture of lateral condyle of unspecified humerus**

S42.46   **Fracture of medial condyle of humerus**

Trochlea fracture of humerus

⑦S42.461   **Displaced fracture of medial condyle of right humerus**

⑦S42.462   **Displaced fracture of medial condyle of left humerus**

⑦S42.463   **Displaced fracture of medial condyle of unspecified humerus**

⑦S42.464   **Nondisplaced fracture of medial condyle of right humerus**

⑦S42.465   **Nondisplaced fracture of medial condyle of left humerus**

⑦S42.466   **Nondisplaced fracture of medial condyle of unspecified humerus**

S42.47   **Transcondylar fracture of humerus**

⑦S42.471   **Displaced transcondylar fracture of right humerus**

⑦S42.472   **Displaced transcondylar fracture of left humerus**

⑦S42.473   **Displaced transcondylar fracture of unspecified humerus**

⑦S42.474   **Nondisplaced transcondylar fracture of right humerus**

⑦S42.475   **Nondisplaced transcondylar fracture of left humerus**

⑦S42.476   **Nondisplaced transcondylar fracture of unspecified humerus**

S42.48   **Torus fracture of lower end of humerus**

The appropriate 7th character is to be added to all codes in subcategory S42.48

A - initial encounter for closed fracture

D - subsequent encounter for fracture with routine healing

G - subsequent encounter for fracture with delayed healing

K - subsequent encounter for fracture with nonunion

P - subsequent encounter for fracture with malunion

S - sequela

⑦S42.481   **Torus fracture of lower end of right humerus**

⑦S42.482   **Torus fracture of lower end of left humerus**

⑦S42.489   **Torus fracture of lower end of unspecified humerus**

S42.49   **Other fracture of lower end of humerus**

⑦S42.491   **Other displaced fracture of lower end of right humerus**

⑦S42.492   **Other displaced fracture of lower end of left humerus**

⑦S42.493   **Other displaced fracture of lower end of unspecified humerus**

⑦S42.494   **Other nondisplaced fracture of lower end of right humerus**

⑦S42.495   **Other nondisplaced fracture of lower end of left humerus**

⑦S42.496   **Other nondisplaced fracture of lower end of unspecified humerus**

S42.9   **Fracture of shoulder girdle, part unspecified**

Fracture of shoulder NOS

⊗⑦S42.90   **Fracture of unspecified shoulder girdle, part unspecified**

⊗⑦S42.91   **Fracture of right shoulder girdle, part unspecified**

⊗⑦S42.92   **Fracture of left shoulder girdle, part unspecified**

S43   **Dislocation and sprain of joints and ligaments of shoulder girdle**

Includes: avulsion of joint or ligament of shoulder girdle

laceration of cartilage, joint or ligament of shoulder girdle

sprain of cartilage, joint or ligament of shoulder girdle

traumatic hemarthrosis of joint or ligament of shoulder girdle

traumatic rupture of joint or ligament of shoulder girdle

traumatic subluxation of joint or ligament of shoulder girdle

traumatic tear of joint or ligament of shoulder girdle

Code also any associated open wound

Excludes2: strain of muscle, fascia and tendon of shoulder and upper arm (S46.-)

The appropriate 7th character is to be added to each code from category S43

A - initial encounter

D - subsequent encounter

S - sequela

S43.0   **Subluxation and dislocation of shoulder joint**

Dislocation of glenohumeral joint

Subluxation of glenohumeral joint

S43.00   **Unspecified subluxation and dislocation of shoulder joint**

Dislocation of humerus NOS

Subluxation of humerus NOS

⑦S43.001   **Unspecified subluxation of right shoulder joint**

---

⑦S43.002   Unspecified subluxation of left shoulder joint

⑦S43.003   Unspecified subluxation of unspecified shoulder joint

⑦S43.004   Unspecified dislocation of right shoulder joint

⑦S43.005   Unspecified dislocation of left shoulder joint

⑦S43.006   Unspecified dislocation of unspecified shoulder joint

S43.01   **Anterior subluxation and dislocation of humerus**

⑦S43.011   Anterior subluxation of right humerus

⑦S43.012   Anterior subluxation of left humerus

⑦S43.013   Anterior subluxation of unspecified humerus

⑦S43.014   Anterior dislocation of right humerus

⑦S43.015   Anterior dislocation of left humerus

⑦S43.016   Anterior dislocation of unspecified humerus

S43.02   **Posterior subluxation and dislocation of humerus**

⑦S43.021   Posterior subluxation of right humerus

⑦S43.022   Posterior subluxation of left humerus

⑦S43.023   Posterior subluxation of unspecified humerus

⑦S43.024   Posterior dislocation of right humerus

⑦S43.025   Posterior dislocation of left humerus

⑦S43.026   Posterior dislocation of unspecified humerus

S43.03   **Inferior subluxation and dislocation of humerus**

⑦S43.031   Inferior subluxation of right humerus

⑦S43.032   Inferior subluxation of left humerus

⑦S43.033   Inferior subluxation of unspecified humerus

⑦S43.034   Inferior dislocation of right humerus

⑦S43.035   Inferior dislocation of left humerus

⑦S43.036   Inferior dislocation of unspecified humerus

S43.08   **Other subluxation and dislocation of shoulder joint**

⑦S43.081   Other subluxation of right shoulder joint

⑦S43.082   Other subluxation of left shoulder joint

⑦S43.083   Other subluxation of unspecified shoulder joint

⑦S43.084   Other dislocation of right shoulder joint

⑦S43.085   Other dislocation of left shoulder joint

⑦S43.086   Other dislocation of unspecified shoulder joint

S43.1   **Subluxation and dislocation of acromioclavicular joint**

S43.10   **Unspecified dislocation of acromioclavicular joint**

⑦S43.101   Unspecified dislocation of right acromioclavicular joint

⑦S43.102   Unspecified dislocation of left acromioclavicular joint

⑦S43.109   Unspecified dislocation of unspecified acromioclavicular joint

S43.11   **Subluxation of acromioclavicular joint**

⑦S43.111   Subluxation of right acromioclavicular joint

⑦S43.112   Subluxation of left acromioclavicular joint

⑦S43.119   Subluxation of unspecified acromioclavicular joint

S43.12   **Dislocation of acromioclavicular joint, 100%-200% displacement**

⑦S43.121   Dislocation of right acromioclavicular joint, 100%-200% displacement

⑦S43.122   Dislocation of left acromioclavicular joint, 100%-200% displacement

⑦S43.129   Dislocation of unspecified acromioclavicular joint, 100%-200% displacement

S43.13   **Dislocation of acromioclavicular joint, greater than 200% displacement**

⑦S43.131   Dislocation of right acromioclavicular joint, greater than 200% displacement

⑦S43.132   Dislocation of left acromioclavicular joint, greater than 200% displacement

⑦S43.139   Dislocation of unspecified acromioclavicular joint, greater than 200% displacement

S43.14   **Inferior dislocation of acromioclavicular joint**

⑦S43.141   Inferior dislocation of right acromioclavicular joint

⑦S43.142   Inferior dislocation of left acromioclavicular joint

⑦S43.149   Inferior dislocation of unspecified acromioclavicular joint

S43.15   **Posterior dislocation of acromioclavicular joint**

⑦S43.151   Posterior dislocation of right acromioclavicular joint

⑦S43.152   Posterior dislocation of left acromioclavicular joint

⑦S43.159   Posterior dislocation of unspecified acromioclavicular joint

S43.2   **Subluxation and dislocation of sternoclavicular joint**

S43.20   **Unspecified subluxation and dislocation of sternoclavicular joint**

⑦S43.201   Unspecified subluxation of right sternoclavicular joint

⑦S43.202   Unspecified subluxation of left sternoclavicular joint

⑦S43.203   Unspecified subluxation of unspecified sternoclavicular joint

⑦S43.204   Unspecified dislocation of right sternoclavicular joint

⑦S43.205   Unspecified dislocation of left sternoclavicular joint

⑦S43.206   Unspecified dislocation of unspecified sternoclavicular joint

   ● New code   ▲ Revised code   **Excludes1:** Not coded here   **Excludes2:** Not included here   ⊗ Placeholder required   ⑦7th digit required

S43.21 Anterior subluxation and dislocation of sternoclavicular joint

⑦ **S43.211** Anterior subluxation of right sternoclavicular joint

⑦ **S43.212** Anterior subluxation of left sternoclavicular joint

⑦ **S43.213** Anterior subluxation of unspecified sternoclavicular joint

⑦ **S43.214** Anterior dislocation of right sternoclavicular joint

⑦ **S43.215** Anterior dislocation of left sternoclavicular joint

⑦ **S43.216** Anterior dislocation of unspecified sternoclavicular joint

S43.22 Posterior subluxation and dislocation of sternoclavicular joint

⑦ **S43.221** Posterior subluxation of right sternoclavicular joint

⑦ **S43.222** Posterior subluxation of left sternoclavicular joint

⑦ **S43.223** Posterior subluxation of unspecified sternoclavicular joint

⑦ **S43.224** Posterior dislocation of right sternoclavicular joint

⑦ **S43.225** Posterior dislocation of left sternoclavicular joint

⑦ **S43.226** Posterior dislocation of unspecified sternoclavicular joint

S43.3 Subluxation and dislocation of other and unspecified parts of shoulder girdle

S43.30 Subluxation and dislocation of unspecified parts of shoulder girdle

Dislocation of shoulder girdle NOS

Subluxation of shoulder girdle NOS

⑦ **S43.301** Subluxation of unspecified parts of right shoulder girdle

⑦ **S43.302** Subluxation of unspecified parts of left shoulder girdle

⑦ **S43.303** Subluxation of unspecified parts of unspecified shoulder girdle

⑦ **S43.304** Dislocation of unspecified parts of right shoulder girdle

⑦ **S43.305** Dislocation of unspecified parts of left shoulder girdle

⑦ **S43.306** Dislocation of unspecified parts of unspecified shoulder girdle

S43.31 Subluxation and dislocation of scapula

⑦ **S43.311** Subluxation of right scapula

⑦ **S43.312** Subluxation of left scapula

⑦ **S43.313** Subluxation of unspecified scapula

⑦ **S43.314** Dislocation of right scapula

⑦ **S43.315** Dislocation of left scapula

⑦ **S43.316** Dislocation of unspecified scapula

S43.39 Subluxation and dislocation of other parts of shoulder girdle

⑦ **S43.391** Subluxation of other parts of right shoulder girdle

⑦ **S43.392** Subluxation of other parts of left shoulder girdle

⑦ **S43.393** Subluxation of other parts of unspecified shoulder girdle

⑦ **S43.394** Dislocation of other parts of right shoulder girdle

⑦ **S43.395** Dislocation of other parts of left shoulder girdle

⑦ **S43.396** Dislocation of other parts of unspecified shoulder girdle

S43.4 Sprain of shoulder joint

S43.40 Unspecified sprain of shoulder joint

⑦ **S43.401** Unspecified sprain of right shoulder joint

⑦ **S43.402** Unspecified sprain of left shoulder joint

⑦ **S43.409** Unspecified sprain of unspecified shoulder joint

S43.41 Sprain of coracohumeral (ligament)

⑦ **S43.411** Sprain of right coracohumeral (ligament)

⑦ **S43.412** Sprain of left coracohumeral (ligament)

⑦ **S43.419** Sprain of unspecified coracohumeral (ligament)

S43.42 Sprain of rotator cuff capsule

Excludes1: rotator cuff syndrome (complete)(incomplete), not specified as traumatic (M75.1-)

Excludes2: injury of tendon of rotator cuff (S46.0-)

⑦ **S43.421** Sprain of right rotator cuff capsule

⑦ **S43.422** Sprain of left rotator cuff capsule

⑦ **S43.429** Sprain of unspecified rotator cuff capsule

S43.43 Superior glenoid labrum lesion

SLAP lesion

⑦ **S43.431** Superior glenoid labrum lesion of right shoulder

⑦ **S43.432** Superior glenoid labrum lesion of left shoulder

⑦ **S43.439** Superior glenoid labrum lesion of unspecified shoulder

S43.49 Other sprain of shoulder joint

⑦ **S43.491** Other sprain of right shoulder joint

⑦ **S43.492** Other sprain of left shoulder joint

⑦ **S43.499** Other sprain of unspecified shoulder joint

S43.5 Sprain of acromioclavicular joint

Sprain of acromioclavicular ligament

⊗⑦ **S43.50** Sprain of unspecified acromioclavicular joint

⊗⑦ **S43.51** Sprain of right acromioclavicular joint

⊗⑦ **S43.52** Sprain of left acromioclavicular joint

S43.6 Sprain of sternoclavicular joint

⊗⑦ **S43.60** Sprain of unspecified sternoclavicular joint

⊗⑦ **S43.61** Sprain of right sternoclavicular joint

⊗⑦ **S43.62** Sprain of left sternoclavicular joint

S43.8 Sprain of other specified parts of shoulder girdle

⊗⑦ **S43.80** Sprain of other specified parts of unspecified shoulder girdle

⊗⑦ **S43.81** Sprain of other specified parts of right shoulder girdle

⊗⑦ **S43.82** Sprain of other specified parts of left shoulder girdle

S43.9 Sprain of unspecified parts of shoulder girdle

⊗⑦ **S43.90** Sprain of unspecified parts of unspecified shoulder girdle

Sprain of shoulder girdle NOS

⊗⑦**S43.91**   **Sprain of unspecified parts of right shoulder girdle**

⊗⑦**S43.92**   **Sprain of unspecified parts of left shoulder girdle**

S44   **Injury of nerves at shoulder and upper arm level**

Code also any associated open wound (S41.-)

Excludes2: injury of brachial plexus (S14.3-)

The appropriate 7th character is to be added to each code from category S44

A - initial encounter

D - subsequent encounter

S - sequela

S44.0   **Injury of ulnar nerve at upper arm level**

Excludes1: ulnar nerve NOS (S54.0)

⊗⑦**S44.00**   **Injury of ulnar nerve at upper arm level, unspecified arm**

⊗⑦**S44.01**   **Injury of ulnar nerve at upper arm level, right arm**

⊗⑦**S44.02**   **Injury of ulnar nerve at upper arm level, left arm**

S44.1   **Injury of median nerve at upper arm level**

Excludes1: median nerve NOS (S54.1)

⊗⑦**S44.10**   **Injury of median nerve at upper arm level, unspecified arm**

⊗⑦**S44.11**   **Injury of median nerve at upper arm level, right arm**

⊗⑦**S44.12**   **Injury of median nerve at upper arm level, left arm**

S44.2   **Injury of radial nerve at upper arm level**

Excludes1: radial nerve NOS (S54.2)

⊗⑦**S44.20**   **Injury of radial nerve at upper arm level, unspecified arm**

⊗⑦**S44.21**   **Injury of radial nerve at upper arm level, right arm**

⊗⑦**S44.22**   **Injury of radial nerve at upper arm level, left arm**

S44.3   **Injury of axillary nerve**

⊗⑦**S44.30**   **Injury of axillary nerve, unspecified arm**

⊗⑦**S44.31**   **Injury of axillary nerve, right arm**

⊗⑦**S44.32**   **Injury of axillary nerve, left arm**

S44.4   **Injury of musculocutaneous nerve**

⊗⑦**S44.40**   **Injury of musculocutaneous nerve, unspecified arm**

⊗⑦**S44.41**   **Injury of musculocutaneous nerve, right arm**

⊗⑦**S44.42**   **Injury of musculocutaneous nerve, left arm**

S44.5   **Injury of cutaneous sensory nerve at shoulder and upper arm level**

⊗⑦**S44.50**   **Injury of cutaneous sensory nerve at shoulder and upper arm level, unspecified arm**

⊗⑦**S44.51**   **Injury of cutaneous sensory nerve at shoulder and upper arm level, right arm**

⊗⑦**S44.52**   **Injury of cutaneous sensory nerve at shoulder and upper arm level, left arm**

S44.8   **Injury of other nerves at shoulder and upper arm level**

S44.8X   **Injury of other nerves at shoulder and upper arm level**

⑦**S44.8X1**   **Injury of other nerves at shoulder and upper arm level, right arm**

⑦**S44.8X2**   **Injury of other nerves at shoulder and upper arm level, left arm**

⑦**S44.8X9**   **Injury of other nerves at shoulder and upper arm level, unspecified arm**

S44.9   **Injury of unspecified nerve at shoulder and upper arm level**

⊗⑦**S44.90**   **Injury of unspecified nerve at shoulder and upper arm level, unspecified arm**

⊗⑦**S44.91**   **Injury of unspecified nerve at shoulder and upper arm level, right arm**

⊗⑦**S44.92**   **Injury of unspecified nerve at shoulder and upper arm level, left arm**

S45   **Injury of blood vessels at shoulder and upper arm level**

Code also any associated open wound (S41.-)

Excludes2: injury of subclavian artery (S25.1)

injury of subclavian vein (S25.3)

The appropriate 7th character is to be added to each code from category S45

A - initial encounter

D - subsequent encounter

S - sequela

S45.0   **Injury of axillary artery**

S45.00   **Unspecified injury of axillary artery**

⑦**S45.001**   **Unspecified injury of axillary artery, right side**

⑦**S45.002**   **Unspecified injury of axillary artery, left side**

⑦**S45.009**   **Unspecified injury of axillary artery, unspecified side**

S45.01   **Laceration of axillary artery**

⑦**S45.011**   **Laceration of axillary artery, right side**

⑦**S45.012**   **Laceration of axillary artery, left side**

⑦**S45.019**   **Laceration of axillary artery, unspecified side**

S45.09   **Other specified injury of axillary artery**

⑦**S45.091**   **Other specified injury of axillary artery, right side**

⑦**S45.092**   **Other specified injury of axillary artery, left side**

⑦**S45.099**   **Other specified injury of axillary artery, unspecified side**

S45.1   **Injury of brachial artery**

S45.10   **Unspecified injury of brachial artery**

⑦**S45.101**   **Unspecified injury of brachial artery, right side**

⑦**S45.102**   **Unspecified injury of brachial artery, left side**

⑦**S45.109**   **Unspecified injury of brachial artery, unspecified side**

S45.11   **Laceration of brachial artery**

⑦**S45.111 Laceration of brachial artery, right side**

⑦**S45.112 Laceration of brachial artery, left side**

⑦**S45.119 Laceration of brachial artery, unspecified side**

S45.19   **Other specified injury of brachial artery**

⑦**S45.191**   **Other specified injury of brachial artery, right side**

⑦**S45.192**   **Other specified injury of brachial artery, left side**

⑦S45.199 Other specified injury of brachial artery, unspecified side

S45.2 Injury of axillary or brachial vein

S45.20 Unspecified injury of axillary or brachial vein

⑦S45.201 Unspecified injury of axillary or brachial vein, right side

⑦S45.202 Unspecified injury of axillary or brachial vein, left side

⑦S45.209 Unspecified injury of axillary or brachial vein, unspecified side

S45.21 Laceration of axillary or brachial vein

⑦S45.211 Laceration of axillary or brachial vein, right side

⑦S45.212 Laceration of axillary or brachial vein, left side

⑦S45.219 Laceration of axillary or brachial vein, unspecified side

S45.29 Other specified injury of axillary or brachial vein

⑦S45.291 Other specified injury of axillary or brachial vein, right side

⑦S45.292 Other specified injury of axillary or brachial vein, left side

⑦S45.299 Other specified injury of axillary or brachial vein, unspecified side

S45.3 Injury of superficial vein at shoulder and upper arm level

S45.30 Unspecified injury of superficial vein at shoulder and upper arm level

⑦S45.301 Unspecified injury of superficial vein at shoulder and upper arm level, right arm

⑦S45.302 Unspecified injury of superficial vein at shoulder and upper arm level, left arm

⑦S45.309 Unspecified injury of superficial vein at shoulder and upper arm level, unspecified arm

S45.31 Laceration of superficial vein at shoulder and upper arm level

⑦S45.311 Laceration of superficial vein at shoulder and upper arm level, right arm

⑦S45.312 Laceration of superficial vein at shoulder and upper arm level, left arm

⑦S45.319 Laceration of superficial vein at shoulder and upper arm level, unspecified arm

S45.39 Other specified injury of superficial vein at shoulder and upper arm level

⑦S45.391 Other specified injury of superficial vein at shoulder and upper arm level, right arm

⑦S45.392 Other specified injury of superficial vein at shoulder and upper arm level, left arm

⑦S45.399 Other specified injury of superficial vein at shoulder and upper arm level, unspecified arm

S45.8 Injury of other specified blood vessels at shoulder and upper arm level

S45.80 Unspecified injury of other specified blood vessels at shoulder and upper arm level

⑦S45.801 Unspecified injury of other specified blood vessels at shoulder and upper arm level, right arm

⑦S45.802 Unspecified injury of other specified blood vessels at shoulder and upper arm level, left arm

⑦S45.809 Unspecified injury of other specified blood vessels at shoulder and upper arm level, unspecified arm

S45.81 Laceration of other specified blood vessels at shoulder and upper arm level

⑦S45.811 Laceration of other specified blood vessels at shoulder and upper arm level, right arm

⑦S45.812 Laceration of other specified blood vessels at shoulder and upper arm level, left arm

⑦S45.819 Laceration of other specified blood vessels at shoulder and upper arm level, unspecified arm

S45.89 Other specified injury of other specified blood vessels at shoulder and upper arm level

⑦S45.891 Other specified injury of other specified blood vessels at shoulder and upper arm level, right arm

⑦S45.892 Other specified injury of other specified blood vessels at shoulder and upper arm level, left arm

⑦S45.899 Other specified injury of other specified blood vessels at shoulder and upper arm level, unspecified arm

S45.9 Injury of unspecified blood vessel at shoulder and upper arm level

S45.90 Unspecified injury of unspecified blood vessel at shoulder and upper arm level

⑦S45.901 Unspecified injury of unspecified blood vessel at shoulder and upper arm level, right arm

⑦S45.902 Unspecified injury of unspecified blood vessel at shoulder and upper arm level, left arm

⑦S45.909 Unspecified injury of unspecified blood vessel at shoulder and upper arm level, unspecified arm

S45.91 Laceration of unspecified blood vessel at shoulder and upper arm level

⑦S45.911 Laceration of unspecified blood vessel at shoulder and upper arm level, right arm

⑦S45.912 Laceration of unspecified blood vessel at shoulder and upper arm level, left arm

⑦S45.919 Laceration of unspecified blood vessel at shoulder and upper arm level, unspecified arm

S45.99 Other specified injury of unspecified blood vessel at shoulder and upper arm level

⑦S45.991 Other specified injury of unspecified blood vessel at shoulder and upper arm level, right arm

⑦S45.992 Other specified injury of unspecified blood vessel at shoulder and upper arm level, left arm

⑦S45.999 Other specified injury of unspecified blood vessel at shoulder and upper arm level, unspecified arm

S46 **Injury of muscle, fascia and tendon at shoulder and upper arm level**

Code also any associated open wound (S41.-)

Excludes2: injury of muscle, fascia and tendon at elbow (S56.-)

sprain of joints and ligaments of shoulder girdle (S43.9)

The appropriate 7th character is to be added to each code from category S46

A - initial encounter

D - subsequent encounter

S - sequela

S46.0 **Injury of muscle(s) and tendon(s) of the rotator cuff of shoulder**

  S46.00 **Unspecified injury of muscle(s) and tendon(s) of the rotator cuff of shoulder**

    ⑦ **S46.001** Unspecified injury of muscle(s) and tendon(s) of the rotator cuff of right shoulder

    ⑦ **S46.002** Unspecified injury of muscle(s) and tendon(s) of the rotator cuff of left shoulder

    ⑦ **S46.009** Unspecified injury of muscle(s) and tendon(s) of the rotator cuff of unspecified shoulder

  S46.01 **Strain of muscle(s) and tendon(s) of the rotator cuff of shoulder**

    ⑦ **S46.011** Strain of muscle(s) and tendon(s) of the rotator cuff of right shoulder

    ⑦ **S46.012** Strain of muscle(s) and tendon(s) of the rotator cuff of left shoulder

    ⑦ **S46.019** Strain of muscle(s) and tendon(s) of the rotator cuff of unspecified shoulder

  S46.02 **Laceration of muscle(s) and tendon(s) of the rotator cuff of shoulder**

    ⑦ **S46.021** Laceration of muscle(s) and tendon(s) of the rotator cuff of right shoulder

    ⑦ **S46.022** Laceration of muscle(s) and tendon(s) of the rotator cuff of left shoulder

    ⑦ **S46.029** Laceration of muscle(s) and tendon(s) of the rotator cuff of unspecified shoulder

  S46.09 **Other injury of muscle(s) and tendon(s) of the rotator cuff of shoulder**

    ⑦ **S46.091** Other injury of muscle(s) and tendon(s) of the rotator cuff of right shoulder

    ⑦ **S46.092** Other injury of muscle(s) and tendon(s) of the rotator cuff of left shoulder

    ⑦ **S46.099** Other injury of muscle(s) and tendon(s) of the rotator cuff of unspecified shoulder

S46.1 **Injury of muscle, fascia and tendon of long head of biceps**

  S46.10 **Unspecified injury of muscle, fascia and tendon of long head of biceps**

    ⑦ **S46.101** Unspecified injury of muscle, fascia and tendon of long head of biceps, right arm

    ⑦ **S46.102** Unspecified injury of muscle, fascia and tendon of long head of biceps, left arm

    ⑦ **S46.109** Unspecified injury of muscle, fascia and tendon of long head of biceps, unspecified arm

  S46.11 **Strain of muscle, fascia and tendon of long head of biceps**

    ⑦ **S46.111** Strain of muscle, fascia and tendon of long head of biceps, right arm

    ⑦ **S46.112** Strain of muscle, fascia and tendon of long head of biceps, left arm

    ⑦ **S46.119** Strain of muscle, fascia and tendon of long head of biceps, unspecified arm

  S46.12 **Laceration of muscle, fascia and tendon of long head of biceps**

    ⑦ **S46.121** Laceration of muscle, fascia and tendon of long head of biceps, right arm

    ⑦ **S46.122** Laceration of muscle, fascia and tendon of long head of biceps, left arm

    ⑦ **S46.129** Laceration of muscle, fascia and tendon of long head of biceps, unspecified arm

  S46.19 **Other injury of muscle, fascia and tendon of long head of biceps**

    ⑦ **S46.191** Other injury of muscle, fascia and tendon of long head of biceps, right arm

    ⑦ **S46.192** Other injury of muscle, fascia and tendon of long head of biceps, left arm

    ⑦ **S46.199** Other injury of muscle, fascia and tendon of long head of biceps, unspecified arm

S46.2 **Injury of muscle, fascia and tendon of other parts of biceps**

  S46.20 **Unspecified injury of muscle, fascia and tendon of other parts of biceps**

    ⑦ **S46.201** Unspecified injury of muscle, fascia and tendon of other parts of biceps, right arm

    ⑦ **S46.202** Unspecified injury of muscle, fascia and tendon of other parts of biceps, left arm

    ⑦ **S46.209** Unspecified injury of muscle, fascia and tendon of other parts of biceps, unspecified arm

  S46.21 **Strain of muscle, fascia and tendon of other parts of biceps**

    ⑦ **S46.211** Strain of muscle, fascia and tendon of other parts of biceps, right arm

    ⑦ **S46.212** Strain of muscle, fascia and tendon of other parts of biceps, left arm

    ⑦ **S46.219** Strain of muscle, fascia and tendon of other parts of biceps, unspecified arm

  S46.22 **Laceration of muscle, fascia and tendon of other parts of biceps**

    ⑦ **S46.221** Laceration of muscle, fascia and tendon of other parts of biceps, right arm

    ⑦ **S46.222** Laceration of muscle, fascia and tendon of other parts of biceps, left arm

● New code   ▲ Revised code   **Excludes1:** Not coded here   **Excludes2:** Not included here   ⊗ Placeholder required   ⑦ 7th digit required

⑦S46.229 Laceration of muscle, fascia and tendon of other parts of biceps, unspecified arm

S46.29 Other injury of muscle, fascia and tendon of other parts of biceps

⑦S46.291 Other injury of muscle, fascia and tendon of other parts of biceps, right arm

⑦S46.292 Other injury of muscle, fascia and tendon of other parts of biceps, left arm

⑦S46.299 Other injury of muscle, fascia and tendon of other parts of biceps, unspecified arm

S46.3 Injury of muscle, fascia and tendon of triceps

S46.30 Unspecified injury of muscle, fascia and tendon of triceps

⑦S46.301 Unspecified injury of muscle, fascia and tendon of triceps, right arm

⑦S46.302 Unspecified injury of muscle, fascia and tendon of triceps, left arm

⑦S46.309 Unspecified injury of muscle, fascia and tendon of triceps, unspecified arm

S46.31 Strain of muscle, fascia and tendon of triceps

⑦S46.311 Strain of muscle, fascia and tendon of triceps, right arm

⑦S46.312 Strain of muscle, fascia and tendon of triceps, left arm

⑦S46.319 Strain of muscle, fascia and tendon of triceps, unspecified arm

S46.32 Laceration of muscle, fascia and tendon of triceps

⑦S46.321 Laceration of muscle, fascia and tendon of triceps, right arm

⑦S46.322 Laceration of muscle, fascia and tendon of triceps, left arm

⑦S46.329 Laceration of muscle, fascia and tendon of triceps, unspecified arm

S46.39 Other injury of muscle, fascia and tendon of triceps

⑦S46.391 Other injury of muscle, fascia and tendon of triceps, right arm

⑦S46.392 Other injury of muscle, fascia and tendon of triceps, left arm

⑦S46.399 Other injury of muscle, fascia and tendon of triceps, unspecified arm

S46.8 Injury of other muscles, fascia and tendons at shoulder and upper arm level

S46.80 Unspecified injury of other muscles, fascia and tendons at shoulder and upper arm level

⑦S46.801 Unspecified injury of other muscles, fascia and tendons at shoulder and upper arm level, right arm

⑦S46.802 Unspecified injury of other muscles, fascia and tendons at shoulder and upper arm level, left arm

⑦S46.809 Unspecified injury of other muscles, fascia and tendons at shoulder and upper arm level, unspecified arm

S46.81 Strain of other muscles, fascia and tendons at shoulder and upper arm level

⑦S46.811 Strain of other muscles, fascia and tendons at shoulder and upper arm level, right arm

⑦S46.812 Strain of other muscles, fascia and tendons at shoulder and upper arm level, left arm

⑦S46.819 Strain of other muscles, fascia and tendons at shoulder and upper arm level, unspecified arm

S46.82 Laceration of other muscles, fascia and tendons at shoulder and upper arm level

⑦S46.821 Laceration of other muscles, fascia and tendons at shoulder and upper arm level, right arm

⑦S46.822 Laceration of other muscles, fascia and tendons at shoulder and upper arm level, left arm

⑦S46.829 Laceration of other muscles, fascia and tendons at shoulder and upper arm level, unspecified arm

S46.89 Other injury of other muscles, fascia and tendons at shoulder and upper arm level

⑦S46.891 Other injury of other muscles, fascia and tendons at shoulder and upper arm level, right arm

⑦S46.892 Other injury of other muscles, fascia and tendons at shoulder and upper arm level, left arm

⑦S46.899 Other injury of other muscles, fascia and tendons at shoulder and upper arm level, unspecified arm

S46.9 Injury of unspecified muscle, fascia and tendon at shoulder and upper arm level

S46.90 Unspecified injury of unspecified muscle, fascia and tendon at shoulder and upper arm level

⑦S46.901 Unspecified injury of unspecified muscle, fascia and tendon at shoulder and upper arm level, right arm

⑦S46.902 Unspecified injury of unspecified muscle, fascia and tendon at shoulder and upper arm level, left arm

⑦S46.909 Unspecified injury of unspecified muscle, fascia and tendon at shoulder and upper arm level, unspecified arm

S46.91 Strain of unspecified muscle, fascia and tendon at shoulder and upper arm level

⑦S46.911 Strain of unspecified muscle, fascia and tendon at shoulder and upper arm level, right arm

⑦S46.912 Strain of unspecified muscle, fascia and tendon at shoulder and upper arm level, left arm

⑦S46.919 Strain of unspecified muscle, fascia and tendon at shoulder and upper arm level, unspecified arm

S46.92 Laceration of unspecified muscle, fascia and tendon at shoulder and upper arm level

⑦S46.921 Laceration of unspecified muscle, fascia and tendon at shoulder and upper arm level, right arm

⑦S46.922 Laceration of unspecified muscle, fascia and tendon at shoulder and upper arm level, left arm

⑦S46.929 Laceration of unspecified muscle, fascia and tendon at shoulder and upper arm level, unspecified arm

S46.99   **Other injury of unspecified muscle, fascia and tendon at shoulder and upper arm level**

⑦**S46.991**   Other injury of unspecified muscle, fascia and tendon at shoulder and upper arm level, right arm

⑦**S46.992**   Other injury of unspecified muscle, fascia and tendon at shoulder and upper arm level, left arm

⑦**S46.999**   Other injury of unspecified muscle, fascia and tendon at shoulder and upper arm level, unspecified arm

S47   **Crushing injury of shoulder and upper arm**

<u>Use additional code</u> for all associated injuries

Excludes2: crushing injury of elbow (S57.0-)

The appropriate 7th character is to be added to each code from category S47

A - initial encounter

D - subsequent encounter

S - sequela

⊗⑦**S47.1**   **Crushing injury of right shoulder and upper arm**

⊗⑦**S47.2**   **Crushing injury of left shoulder and upper arm**

⊗⑦**S47.9**   **Crushing injury of shoulder and upper arm, unspecified arm**

S48   **Traumatic amputation of shoulder and upper arm**

An amputation not identified as partial or complete should be coded to complete

Excludes1: traumatic amputation at elbow level (S58.0)

The appropriate 7th character is to be added to each code from category S48

A - initial encounter

D - subsequent encounter

S - sequela

S48.0   **Traumatic amputation at shoulder joint**

S48.01   **Complete traumatic amputation at shoulder joint**

⑦**S48.011**   Complete traumatic amputation at right shoulder joint

⑦**S48.012**   Complete traumatic amputation at left shoulder joint

⑦**S48.019**   Complete traumatic amputation at unspecified shoulder joint

S48.02   **Partial traumatic amputation at shoulder joint**

⑦**S48.021**   Partial traumatic amputation at right shoulder joint

⑦**S48.022**   Partial traumatic amputation at left shoulder joint

⑦**S48.029**   Partial traumatic amputation at unspecified shoulder joint

S48.1   **Traumatic amputation at level between shoulder and elbow**

S48.11   **Complete traumatic amputation at level between shoulder and elbow**

⑦**S48.111**   Complete traumatic amputation at level between right shoulder and elbow

⑦**S48.112**   Complete traumatic amputation at level between left shoulder and elbow

⑦**S48.119**   Complete traumatic amputation at level between unspecified shoulder and elbow

S48.12   **Partial traumatic amputation at level between shoulder and elbow**

⑦**S48.121**   Partial traumatic amputation at level between right shoulder and elbow

⑦**S48.122**   Partial traumatic amputation at level between left shoulder and elbow

⑦**S48.129**   Partial traumatic amputation at level between unspecified shoulder and elbow

S48.9   **Traumatic amputation of shoulder and upper arm, level unspecified**

S48.91   **Complete traumatic amputation of shoulder and upper arm, level unspecified**

⑦**S48.911**   Complete traumatic amputation of right shoulder and upper arm, level unspecified

⑦**S48.912**   Complete traumatic amputation of left shoulder and upper arm, level unspecified

⑦**S48.919**   Complete traumatic amputation of unspecified shoulder and upper arm, level unspecified

S48.92   **Partial traumatic amputation of shoulder and upper arm, level unspecified**

⑦**S48.921**   Partial traumatic amputation of right shoulder and upper arm, level unspecified

⑦**S48.922**   Partial traumatic amputation of left shoulder and upper arm, level unspecified

⑦**S48.929**   Partial traumatic amputation of unspecified shoulder and upper arm, level unspecified

S49   **Other and unspecified injuries of shoulder and upper arm**

The appropriate 7th character is to be added to each code from subcategories S49.0 and S49.1

A - initial encounter for closed fracture

D - subsequent encounter for fracture with routine healing

G - subsequent encounter for fracture with delayed healing

K - subsequent encounter for fracture with nonunion

P - subsequent encounter for fracture with malunion

S - sequela

S49.0   **Physeal fracture of upper end of humerus**

S49.00   **Unspecified physeal fracture of upper end of humerus**

⑦**S49.001**   Unspecified physeal fracture of upper end of humerus, right arm

⑦**S49.002**   Unspecified physeal fracture of upper end of humerus, left arm

⑦**S49.009**   Unspecified physeal fracture of upper end of humerus, unspecified arm

S49.01   **Salter-Harris Type I physeal fracture of upper end of humerus**

⑦**S49.011**   Salter-Harris Type I physeal fracture of upper end of humerus, right arm

⑦**S49.012**   Salter-Harris Type I physeal fracture of upper end of humerus, left arm

⑦**S49.019**   Salter-Harris Type I physeal fracture of upper end of humerus, unspecified arm

S49.02   **Salter-Harris Type II physeal fracture of upper end of humerus**

   ● New code   ▲ Revised code   **Excludes1:** Not coded here   **Excludes2:** Not included here   ⊗ Placeholder required   ⑦ 7th digit required

⑦S49.021 Salter-Harris Type II physeal fracture of upper end of humerus, right arm

⑦S49.022 Salter-Harris Type II physeal fracture of upper end of humerus, left arm

⑦S49.029 Salter-Harris Type II physeal fracture of upper end of humerus, unspecified arm

S49.03 Salter-Harris Type III physeal fracture of upper end of humerus

⑦S49.031 Salter-Harris Type III physeal fracture of upper end of humerus, right arm

⑦S49.032 Salter-Harris Type III physeal fracture of upper end of humerus, left arm

⑦S49.039 Salter-Harris Type III physeal fracture of upper end of humerus, unspecified arm

S49.04 Salter-Harris Type IV physeal fracture of upper end of humerus

⑦S49.041 Salter-Harris Type IV physeal fracture of upper end of humerus, right arm

⑦S49.042 Salter-Harris Type IV physeal fracture of upper end of humerus, left arm

⑦S49.049 Salter-Harris Type IV physeal fracture of upper end of humerus, unspecified arm

S49.09 Other physeal fracture of upper end of humerus

⑦S49.091 Other physeal fracture of upper end of humerus, right arm

⑦S49.092 Other physeal fracture of upper end of humerus, left arm

⑦S49.099 Other physeal fracture of upper end of humerus, unspecified arm

S49.1 Physeal fracture of lower end of humerus

S49.10 Unspecified physeal fracture of lower end of humerus

⑦S49.101 Unspecified physeal fracture of lower end of humerus, right arm

⑦S49.102 Unspecified physeal fracture of lower end of humerus, left arm

⑦S49.109 Unspecified physeal fracture of lower end of humerus, unspecified arm

S49.11 Salter-Harris Type I physeal fracture of lower end of humerus

⑦S49.111 Salter-Harris Type I physeal fracture of lower end of humerus, right arm

⑦S49.112 Salter-Harris Type I physeal fracture of lower end of humerus, left arm

⑦S49.119 Salter-Harris Type I physeal fracture of lower end of humerus, unspecified arm

S49.12 Salter-Harris Type II physeal fracture of lower end of humerus

⑦S49.121 Salter-Harris Type II physeal fracture of lower end of humerus, right arm

⑦S49.122 Salter-Harris Type II physeal fracture of lower end of humerus, left arm

⑦S49.129 Salter-Harris Type II physeal fracture of lower end of humerus, unspecified arm

S49.13 Salter-Harris Type III physeal fracture of lower end of humerus

⑦S49.131 Salter-Harris Type III physeal fracture of lower end of humerus, right arm

⑦S49.132 Salter-Harris Type III physeal fracture of lower end of humerus, left arm

⑦S49.139 Salter-Harris Type III physeal fracture of lower end of humerus, unspecified arm

S49.14 Salter-Harris Type IV physeal fracture of lower end of humerus

⑦S49.141 Salter-Harris Type IV physeal fracture of lower end of humerus, right arm

⑦S49.142 Salter-Harris Type IV physeal fracture of lower end of humerus, left arm

⑦S49.149 Salter-Harris Type IV physeal fracture of lower end of humerus, unspecified arm

S49.19 Other physeal fracture of lower end of humerus

⑦S49.191 Other physeal fracture of lower end of humerus, right arm

⑦S49.192 Other physeal fracture of lower end of humerus, left arm

⑦S49.199 Other physeal fracture of lower end of humerus, unspecified arm

S49.8 Other specified injuries of shoulder and upper arm

The appropriate 7th character is to be added to each code in subcategory S49.8

A - initial encounter

D - subsequent encounter

S - sequela

⊗⑦S49.80 Other specified injuries of shoulder and upper arm, unspecified arm

⊗⑦S49.81 Other specified injuries of right shoulder and upper arm

⊗⑦S49.82 Other specified injuries of left shoulder and upper arm

S49.9 Unspecified injury of shoulder and upper arm

The appropriate 7th character is to be added to each code in subcategory S49.9

A - initial encounter

D - subsequent encounter

S - sequela

⊗⑦S49.90 Unspecified injury of shoulder and upper arm, unspecified arm

⊗⑦S49.91 Unspecified injury of right shoulder and upper arm

⊗⑦S49.92 Unspecified injury of left shoulder and upper arm

INJURIES TO THE ELBOW AND FOREARM (S50-S59)

Excludes2: burns and corrosions (T20-T32)

frostbite (T33-T34)

injuries of wrist and hand (S60-S69)

insect bite or sting, venomous (T63.4)

S50 Superficial injury of elbow and forearm

Excludes2: superficial injury of wrist and hand (S60.-)

The appropriate 7th character is to be added to each code from category S50

A - initial encounter

D - subsequent encounter

S - sequela

S50.0 Contusion of elbow

⊗⑦**S50.00** Contusion of unspecified elbow

⊗⑦**S50.01** Contusion of right elbow

⊗⑦**S50.02** Contusion of left elbow

S50.1 Contusion of forearm

⊗⑦**S50.10** Contusion of unspecified forearm

⊗⑦**S50.11** Contusion of right forearm

⊗⑦**S50.12** Contusion of left forearm

S50.3 Other superficial injuries of elbow

S50.31 Abrasion of elbow

⑦**S50.311** Abrasion of right elbow

⑦**S50.312** Abrasion of left elbow

⑦**S50.319** Abrasion of unspecified elbow

S50.32 Blister (nonthermal) of elbow

⑦**S50.321** Blister (nonthermal) of right elbow

⑦**S50.322** Blister (nonthermal) of left elbow

⑦**S50.329** Blister (nonthermal) of unspecified elbow

S50.34 External constriction of elbow

⑦**S50.341** External constriction of right elbow

⑦**S50.342** External constriction of left elbow

⑦**S50.349** External constriction of unspecified elbow

S50.35 Superficial foreign body of elbow

Splinter in the elbow

⑦**S50.351** Superficial foreign body of right elbow

⑦**S50.352** Superficial foreign body of left elbow

⑦**S50.359** Superficial foreign body of unspecified elbow

S50.36 Insect bite (nonvenomous) of elbow

⑦**S50.361** Insect bite (nonvenomous) of right elbow

⑦**S50.362** Insect bite (nonvenomous) of left elbow

⑦**S50.369** Insect bite (nonvenomous) of unspecified elbow

S50.37 Other superficial bite of elbow

Excludes1: open bite of elbow (S51.04)

⑦**S50.371** Other superficial bite of right elbow

⑦**S50.372** Other superficial bite of left elbow

⑦**S50.379** Other superficial bite of unspecified elbow

S50.8 Other superficial injuries of forearm

S50.81 Abrasion of forearm

⑦**S50.811** Abrasion of right forearm

⑦**S50.812** Abrasion of left forearm

⑦**S50.819** Abrasion of unspecified forearm

S50.82 Blister (nonthermal) of forearm

⑦**S50.821** Blister (nonthermal) of right forearm

⑦**S50.822** Blister (nonthermal) of left forearm

⑦**S50.829** Blister (nonthermal) of unspecified forearm

S50.84 External constriction of forearm

⑦**S50.841** External constriction of right forearm

⑦**S50.842** External constriction of left forearm

⑦**S50.849** External constriction of unspecified forearm

S50.85 Superficial foreign body of forearm

Splinter in the forearm

⑦**S50.851** Superficial foreign body of right forearm

⑦**S50.852** Superficial foreign body of left forearm

⑦**S50.859** Superficial foreign body of unspecified forearm

S50.86 Insect bite (nonvenomous) of forearm

⑦**S50.861** Insect bite (nonvenomous) of right forearm

⑦**S50.862** Insect bite (nonvenomous) of left forearm

⑦**S50.869** Insect bite (nonvenomous) of unspecified forearm

S50.87 Other superficial bite of forearm

Excludes1: open bite of forearm (S51.84)

⑦**S50.871** Other superficial bite of right forearm

⑦**S50.872** Other superficial bite of left forearm

⑦**S50.879** Other superficial bite of unspecified forearm

S50.9 Unspecified superficial injury of elbow and forearm

S50.90 Unspecified superficial injury of elbow

⑦**S50.901** Unspecified superficial injury of right elbow

⑦**S50.902** Unspecified superficial injury of left elbow

⑦**S50.909** Unspecified superficial injury of unspecified elbow

S50.91 Unspecified superficial injury of forearm

⑦**S50.911** Unspecified superficial injury of right forearm

⑦**S50.912** Unspecified superficial injury of left forearm

⑦**S50.919** Unspecified superficial injury of unspecified forearm

S51 Open wound of elbow and forearm

Code also any associated wound infection

Excludes1: open fracture of elbow and forearm (S52.- with open fracture 7th character)

traumatic amputation of elbow and forearm (S58.-)

Excludes2: open wound of wrist and hand (S61.-)

The appropriate 7th character is to be added to each code from category S51

A - initial encounter

D - subsequent encounter

S - sequela

S51.0 Open wound of elbow

S51.00 Unspecified open wound of elbow

⑦**S51.001** Unspecified open wound of right elbow

● New code   ▲ Revised code   **Excludes1:** Not coded here   **Excludes2:** Not included here   ⊗ Placeholder required   ⑦7th digit required

⑦ S51.002 Unspecified open wound of left elbow

⑦ S51.009 Unspecified open wound of unspecified elbow

Open wound of elbow NOS

S51.01 Laceration without foreign body of elbow

⑦ S51.011 Laceration without foreign body of right elbow

⑦ S51.012 Laceration without foreign body of left elbow

⑦ S51.019 Laceration without foreign body of unspecified elbow

S51.02 Laceration with foreign body of elbow

⑦ S51.021 Laceration with foreign body of right elbow

⑦ S51.022 Laceration with foreign body of left elbow

⑦ S51.029 Laceration with foreign body of unspecified elbow

S51.03 Puncture wound without foreign body of elbow

⑦ S51.031 Puncture wound without foreign body of right elbow

⑦ S51.032 Puncture wound without foreign body of left elbow

⑦ S51.039 Puncture wound without foreign body of unspecified elbow

S51.04 Puncture wound with foreign body of elbow

⑦ S51.041 Puncture wound with foreign body of right elbow

⑦ S51.042 Puncture wound with foreign body of left elbow

⑦ S51.049 Puncture wound with foreign body of unspecified elbow

S51.05 Open bite of elbow

Bite of elbow NOS

Excludes1: superficial bite of elbow (S50.36, S50.37)

⑦ S51.051 Open bite, right elbow

⑦ S51.052 Open bite, left elbow

⑦ S51.059 Open bite, unspecified elbow

S51.8 Open wound of forearm

Excludes2: open wound of elbow (S51.0-)

S51.80 Unspecified open wound of forearm

⑦ S51.801 Unspecified open wound of right forearm

⑦ S51.802 Unspecified open wound of left forearm

⑦ S51.809 Unspecified open wound of unspecified forearm

Open wound of forearm NOS

S51.81 Laceration without foreign body of forearm

⑦ S51.811 Laceration without foreign body of right forearm

⑦ S51.812 Laceration without foreign body of left forearm

⑦ S51.819 Laceration without foreign body of unspecified forearm

S51.82 Laceration with foreign body of forearm

⑦ S51.821 Laceration with foreign body of right forearm

⑦ S51.822 Laceration with foreign body of left forearm

⑦ S51.829 Laceration with foreign body of unspecified forearm

S51.83 Puncture wound without foreign body of forearm

⑦ S51.831 Puncture wound without foreign body of right forearm

⑦ S51.832 Puncture wound without foreign body of left forearm

⑦ S51.839 Puncture wound without foreign body of unspecified forearm

S51.84 Puncture wound with foreign body of forearm

⑦ S51.841 Puncture wound with foreign body of right forearm

⑦ S51.842 Puncture wound with foreign body of left forearm

⑦ S51.849 Puncture wound with foreign body of unspecified forearm

S51.85 Open bite of forearm

Bite of forearm NOS

Excludes1: superficial bite of forearm (S50.86, S50.87)

⑦ S51.851 Open bite of right forearm

⑦ S51.852 Open bite of left forearm

⑦ S51.859 Open bite of unspecified forearm

S52 Fracture of forearm

Note: A fracture not indicated as displaced or nondisplaced should be coded to displaced

A fracture not indicated as open or closed should be coded to closed

The open fracture designations are based on the Gustilo open fracture classification

Excludes1: traumatic amputation of forearm (S58.-)

Excludes2: fracture at wrist and hand level (S62.-)

The appropriate 7th character is to be added to all codes from category S52

A - initial encounter for closed fracture

B - initial encounter for open fracture type I or II initial encounter for open fracture NOS

C - initial encounter for open fracture type IIIA, IIIB, or IIIC

D - subsequent encounter for closed fracture with routine healing

E - subsequent encounter for open fracture type I or II with routine healing

F - subsequent encounter for open fracture type IIIA, IIIB, or IIIC with routine healing

G - subsequent encounter for closed fracture with delayed healing

H - subsequent encounter for open fracture type I or II with delayed healing

J - subsequent encounter for open fracture type IIIA, IIIB, or IIIC with delayed healing

K - subsequent encounter for closed fracture with nonunion

M - subsequent encounter for open fracture type I or II with nonunion

N - subsequent encounter for open fracture type IIIA, IIIB, or IIIC with nonunion P - subsequent encounter for closed fracture with malunion

Q - subsequent encounter for open fracture type I or II with malunion

R - subsequent encounter for open fracture type IIIA, IIIB, or IIIC with malunion

S - sequela

S52.0 Fracture of upper end of ulna

Fracture of proximal end of ulna

Excludes2: fracture of elbow NOS (S42.40-)

| | Add 4th-7th digits | | Nonspecific code | | Unspecified code | | Manifestation code | 799 |

fractures of shaft of ulna (S52.2-)

S52.00 Unspecified fracture of upper end of ulna

⑦**S52.001** Unspecified fracture of upper end of right ulna

⑦**S52.002** Unspecified fracture of upper end of left ulna

⑦**S52.009** Unspecified fracture of upper end of unspecified ulna

S52.01 Torus fracture of upper end of ulna

The appropriate 7th character is to be added to all codes in subcategory S52.01

A - initial encounter for closed fracture

D - subsequent encounter for fracture with routine healing

G - subsequent encounter for fracture with delayed healing

K - subsequent encounter for fracture with nonunion

P - subsequent encounter for fracture with malunion S - sequela

⑦**S52.011** Torus fracture of upper end of right ulna

⑦**S52.012** Torus fracture of upper end of left ulna

⑦**S52.019** Torus fracture of upper end of unspecified ulna

S52.02 Fracture of olecranon process without intraarticular extension of ulna

⑦**S52.021** Displaced fracture of olecranon process without intraarticular extension of right ulna

⑦**S52.022** Displaced fracture of olecranon process without intraarticular extension of left ulna

⑦**S52.023** Displaced fracture of olecranon process without intraarticular extension of unspecified ulna

⑦**S52.024** Nondisplaced fracture of olecranon process without intraarticular extension of right ulna

⑦**S52.025** Nondisplaced fracture of olecranon process without intraarticular extension of left ulna

⑦**S52.026** Nondisplaced fracture of olecranon process without intraarticular extension of unspecified ulna

S52.03 Fracture of olecranon process with intraarticular extension of ulna

⑦**S52.031** Displaced fracture of olecranon process with intraarticular extension of right ulna

⑦**S52.032** Displaced fracture of olecranon process with intraarticular extension of left ulna

⑦**S52.033** Displaced fracture of olecranon process with intraarticular extension of unspecified ulna

⑦**S52.034** Nondisplaced fracture of olecranon process with intraarticular extension of right ulna

⑦**S52.035** Nondisplaced fracture of olecranon process with intraarticular extension of left ulna

⑦**S52.036** Nondisplaced fracture of olecranon process with intraarticular extension of unspecified ulna

S52.04 Fracture of coronoid process of ulna

⑦**S52.041** Displaced fracture of coronoid process of right ulna

⑦**S52.042** Displaced fracture of coronoid process of left ulna

⑦**S52.043** Displaced fracture of coronoid process of unspecified ulna

⑦**S52.044** Nondisplaced fracture of coronoid process of right ulna

⑦**S52.045** Nondisplaced fracture of coronoid process of left ulna

⑦**S52.046** Nondisplaced fracture of coronoid process of unspecified ulna

S52.09 Other fracture of upper end of ulna

⑦**S52.091** Other fracture of upper end of right ulna

⑦**S52.092** Other fracture of upper end of left ulna

⑦**S52.099** Other fracture of upper end of unspecified ulna

S52.1 Fracture of upper end of radius

Fracture of proximal end of radius

Excludes2: physeal fractures of upper end of radius (S59.2-)

fracture of shaft of radius (S52.3-)

S52.10 Unspecified fracture of upper end of radius

⑦**S52.101** Unspecified fracture of upper end of right radius

⑦**S52.102** Unspecified fracture of upper end of left radius

⑦**S52.109** Unspecified fracture of upper end of unspecified radius

S52.11 Torus fracture of upper end of radius

The appropriate 7th character is to be added to all codes in subcategory S52.11

A - initial encounter for closed fracture

D - subsequent encounter for fracture with routine healing

G - subsequent encounter for fracture with delayed healing

K - subsequent encounter for fracture with nonunion

P - subsequent encounter for fracture with malunion S - sequela

⑦**S52.111** Torus fracture of upper end of right radius

⑦**S52.112** Torus fracture of upper end of left radius

⑦**S52.119** Torus fracture of upper end of unspecified radius

S52.12 Fracture of head of radius

⑦**S52.121** Displaced fracture of head of right radius

⑦**S52.122** Displaced fracture of head of left radius

⑦**S52.123** Displaced fracture of head of unspecified radius

⑦**S52.124** Nondisplaced fracture of head of right radius

⑦**S52.125** Nondisplaced fracture of head of left radius

● New code   ▲ Revised code   **Excludes1:** Not coded here   **Excludes2:** Not included here   ⊗ Placeholder required   ⑦7th digit required

⑦**S52.126**   **Nondisplaced fracture of head of unspecified radius**

S52.13   **Fracture of neck of radius**

⑦**S52.131**   **Displaced fracture of neck of right radius**

⑦**S52.132**   **Displaced fracture of neck of left radius**

⑦**S52.133**   **Displaced fracture of neck of unspecified radius**

⑦**S52.134**   **Nondisplaced fracture of neck of right radius**

⑦**S52.135**   **Nondisplaced fracture of neck of left radius**

⑦**S52.136**   **Nondisplaced fracture of neck of unspecified radius**

S52.18   **Other fracture of upper end of radius**

⑦**S52.181**   **Other fracture of upper end of right radius**

⑦**S52.182**   **Other fracture of upper end of left radius**

⑦**S52.189**   **Other fracture of upper end of unspecified radius**

S52.2   **Fracture of shaft of ulna**

S52.20   **Unspecified fracture of shaft of ulna**
Fracture of ulna NOS

⑦**S52.201**   **Unspecified fracture of shaft of right ulna**

⑦**S52.202**   **Unspecified fracture of shaft of left ulna**

⑦**S52.209**   **Unspecified fracture of shaft of unspecified ulna**

S52.21   **Greenstick fracture of shaft of ulna**

The appropriate 7th character is to be added to all codes in subcategory S52.21

A - initial encounter for closed fracture

D - subsequent encounter for fracture with routine healing

G - subsequent encounter for fracture with delayed healing

K - subsequent encounter for fracture with nonunion

P - subsequent encounter for fracture with malunion

S - sequela

⑦**S52.211**   **Greenstick fracture of shaft of right ulna**

⑦**S52.212**   **Greenstick fracture of shaft of left ulna**

⑦**S52.219**   **Greenstick fracture of shaft of unspecified ulna**

S52.22   **Transverse fracture of shaft of ulna**

⑦**S52.221**   **Displaced transverse fracture of shaft of right ulna**

⑦**S52.222**   **Displaced transverse fracture of shaft of left ulna**

⑦**S52.223**   **Displaced transverse fracture of shaft of unspecified ulna**

⑦**S52.224**   **Nondisplaced transverse fracture of shaft of right ulna**

⑦**S52.225**   **Nondisplaced transverse fracture of shaft of left ulna**

⑦**S52.226**   **Nondisplaced transverse fracture of shaft of unspecified ulna**

S52.23   **Oblique fracture of shaft of ulna**

⑦**S52.231**   **Displaced oblique fracture of shaft of right ulna**

⑦**S52.232**   **Displaced oblique fracture of shaft of left ulna**

⑦**S52.233**   **Displaced oblique fracture of shaft of unspecified ulna**

⑦**S52.234**   **Nondisplaced oblique fracture of shaft of right ulna**

⑦**S52.235**   **Nondisplaced oblique fracture of shaft of left ulna**

⑦**S52.236**   **Nondisplaced oblique fracture of shaft of unspecified ulna**

S52.24   **Spiral fracture of shaft of ulna**

⑦**S52.241**   **Displaced spiral fracture of shaft of ulna, right arm**

⑦**S52.242**   **Displaced spiral fracture of shaft of ulna, left arm**

⑦**S52.243**   **Displaced spiral fracture of shaft of ulna, unspecified arm**

⑦**S52.244**   **Nondisplaced spiral fracture of shaft of ulna, right arm**

⑦**S52.245**   **Nondisplaced spiral fracture of shaft of ulna, left arm**

⑦**S52.246**   **Nondisplaced spiral fracture of shaft of ulna, unspecified arm**

S52.25   **Comminuted fracture of shaft of ulna**

⑦**S52.251**   **Displaced comminuted fracture of shaft of ulna, right arm**

⑦**S52.252**   **Displaced comminuted fracture of shaft of ulna, left arm**

⑦**S52.253**   **Displaced comminuted fracture of shaft of ulna, unspecified arm**

⑦**S52.254**   **Nondisplaced comminuted fracture of shaft of ulna, right arm**

⑦**S52.255**   **Nondisplaced comminuted fracture of shaft of ulna, left arm**

⑦**S52.256**   **Nondisplaced comminuted fracture of shaft of ulna, unspecified arm**

S52.26   **Segmental fracture of shaft of ulna**

⑦**S52.261**   **Displaced segmental fracture of shaft of ulna, right arm**

⑦**S52.262**   **Displaced segmental fracture of shaft of ulna, left arm**

⑦**S52.263**   **Displaced segmental fracture of shaft of ulna, unspecified arm**

⑦**S52.264**   **Nondisplaced segmental fracture of shaft of ulna, right arm**

⑦**S52.265**   **Nondisplaced segmental fracture of shaft of ulna, left arm**

⑦**S52.266**   **Nondisplaced segmental fracture of shaft of ulna, unspecified arm**

S52.27   **Monteggia's fracture of ulna**
Fracture of upper shaft of ulna with dislocation of radial head

⑦**S52.271**   **Monteggia's fracture of right ulna**

⑦**S52.272**   **Monteggia's fracture of left ulna**

⑦**S52.279**   **Monteggia's fracture of unspecified ulna**

S52.28   **Bent bone of ulna**

⑦**S52.281**   **Bent bone of right ulna**

⑦**S52.282**   **Bent bone of left ulna**

⑦**S52.283**   **Bent bone of unspecified ulna**

Add 4th-7th digits   Nonspecific code   Unspecified code   Manifestation code

S52.29   Other fracture of shaft of ulna

⑦ S52.291   Other fracture of shaft of right ulna

⑦ S52.292   Other fracture of shaft of left ulna

⑦ S52.299   Other fracture of shaft of unspecified ulna

S52.3   Fracture of shaft of radius

S52.30   Unspecified fracture of shaft of radius

⑦ S52.301   Unspecified fracture of shaft of right radius

⑦ S52.302   Unspecified fracture of shaft of left radius

⑦ S52.309   Unspecified fracture of shaft of unspecified radius

S52.31   Greenstick fracture of shaft of radius

The appropriate 7th character is to be added to all codes in subcategory S52.31

A - initial encounter for closed fracture

D - subsequent encounter for fracture with routine healing

G - subsequent encounter for fracture with delayed healing

K - subsequent encounter for fracture with nonunion

P - subsequent encounter for fracture with malunion S - sequela

⑦ S52.311   Greenstick fracture of shaft of radius, right arm

⑦ S52.312   Greenstick fracture of shaft of radius, left arm

⑦ S52.319   Greenstick fracture of shaft of radius, unspecified arm

S52.32   Transverse fracture of shaft of radius

⑦ S52.321   Displaced transverse fracture of shaft of right radius

⑦ S52.322   Displaced transverse fracture of shaft of left radius

⑦ S52.323   Displaced transverse fracture of shaft of unspecified radius

⑦ S52.324   Nondisplaced transverse fracture of shaft of right radius

⑦ S52.325   Nondisplaced transverse fracture of shaft of left radius

⑦ S52.326   Nondisplaced transverse fracture of shaft of unspecified radius

S52.33   Oblique fracture of shaft of radius

⑦ S52.331   Displaced oblique fracture of shaft of right radius

⑦ S52.332   Displaced oblique fracture of shaft of left radius

⑦ S52.333   Displaced oblique fracture of shaft of unspecified radius

⑦ S52.334   Nondisplaced oblique fracture of shaft of right radius

⑦ S52.335   Nondisplaced oblique fracture of shaft of left radius

⑦ S52.336   Nondisplaced oblique fracture of shaft of unspecified radius

S52.34   Spiral fracture of shaft of radius

⑦ S52.341   Displaced spiral fracture of shaft of radius, right arm

⑦ S52.342   Displaced spiral fracture of shaft of radius, left arm

⑦ S52.343   Displaced spiral fracture of shaft of radius, unspecified arm

⑦ S52.344   Nondisplaced spiral fracture of shaft of radius, right arm

⑦ S52.345   Nondisplaced spiral fracture of shaft of radius, left arm

⑦ S52.346   Nondisplaced spiral fracture of shaft of radius, unspecified arm

S52.35   Comminuted fracture of shaft of radius

⑦ S52.351   Displaced comminuted fracture of shaft of radius, right arm

⑦ S52.352   Displaced comminuted fracture of shaft of radius, left arm

⑦ S52.353   Displaced comminuted fracture of shaft of radius, unspecified arm

⑦ S52.354   Nondisplaced comminuted fracture of shaft of radius, right arm

⑦ S52.355   Nondisplaced comminuted fracture of shaft of radius, left arm

⑦ S52.356   Nondisplaced comminuted fracture of shaft of radius, unspecified arm

S52.36   Segmental fracture of shaft of radius

⑦ S52.361   Displaced segmental fracture of shaft of radius, right arm

⑦ S52.362   Displaced segmental fracture of shaft of radius, left arm

⑦ S52.363   Displaced segmental fracture of shaft of radius, unspecified arm

⑦ S52.364   Nondisplaced segmental fracture of shaft of radius, right arm

⑦ S52.365   Nondisplaced segmental fracture of shaft of radius, left arm

⑦ S52.366   Nondisplaced segmental fracture of shaft of radius, unspecified arm

S52.37   Galeazzi's fracture

Fracture of lower shaft of radius with radioulnar joint dislocation

⑦ S52.371   Galeazzi's fracture of right radius

⑦ S52.372   Galeazzi's fracture of left radius

⑦ S52.379   Galeazzi's fracture of unspecified radius

S52.38   Bent bone of radius

⑦ S52.381   Bent bone of right radius

⑦ S52.382   Bent bone of left radius

⑦ S52.389   Bent bone of unspecified radius

S52.39   Other fracture of shaft of radius

⑦ S52.391   Other fracture of shaft of radius, right arm

⑦ S52.392   Other fracture of shaft of radius, left arm

⑦ S52.399   Other fracture of shaft of radius, unspecified arm

S52.5   Fracture of lower end of radius

Fracture of distal end of radius

Excludes2: physeal fractures of lower end of radius (S59.2-)

S52.50   Unspecified fracture of the lower end of radius

⑦ S52.501   Unspecified fracture of the lower end of right radius

⑦ S52.502   Unspecified fracture of the lower end of left radius

⑦ S52.509   Unspecified fracture of the lower end of unspecified radius

S52.51   **Fracture of radial styloid process**

⑦S52.511   **Displaced fracture of right radial styloid process**

⑦S52.512   **Displaced fracture of left radial styloid process**

⑦S52.513   **Displaced fracture of unspecified radial styloid process**

⑦S52.514   **Nondisplaced fracture of right radial styloid process**

⑦S52.515   **Nondisplaced fracture of left radial styloid process**

⑦S52.516   **Nondisplaced fracture of unspecified radial styloid process**

S52.52   **Torus fracture of lower end of radius**

The appropriate 7th character is to be added to all codes in subcategory S52.52

A - initial encounter for closed fracture

D - subsequent encounter for fracture with routine healing

G - subsequent encounter for fracture with delayed healing

K - subsequent encounter for fracture with nonunion

P - subsequent encounter for fracture with malunion

S - sequela

⑦S52.521   **Torus fracture of lower end of right radius**

⑦S52.522   **Torus fracture of lower end of left radius**

⑦S52.529   **Torus fracture of lower end of unspecified radius**

S52.53   **Colles' fracture**

⑦S52.531   **Colles' fracture of right radius**

⑦S52.532   **Colles' fracture of left radius**

⑦S52.539   **Colles' fracture of unspecified radius**

S52.54   **Smith's fracture**

⑦S52.541   **Smith's fracture of right radius**

⑦S52.542   **Smith's fracture of left radius**

⑦S52.549   **Smith's fracture of unspecified radius**

S52.55   **Other extraarticular fracture of lower end of radius**

⑦S52.551   **Other extraarticular fracture of lower end of right radius**

⑦S52.552   **Other extraarticular fracture of lower end of left radius**

⑦S52.559   **Other extraarticular fracture of lower end of unspecified radius**

S52.56   **Barton's fracture**

⑦S52.561   **Barton's fracture of right radius**

⑦S52.562   **Barton's fracture of left radius**

⑦S52.569   **Barton's fracture of unspecified radius**

S52.57   **Other intraarticular fracture of lower end of radius**

⑦S52.571   **Other intraarticular fracture of lower end of right radius**

⑦S52.572   **Other intraarticular fracture of lower end of left radius**

⑦S52.579   **Other intraarticular fracture of lower end of unspecified radius**

S52.59   **Other fractures of lower end of radius**

⑦S52.591   **Other fractures of lower end of right radius**

⑦S52.592   **Other fractures of lower end of left radius**

⑦S52.599   **Other fractures of lower end of unspecified radius**

S52.6   **Fracture of lower end of ulna**

S52.60   **Unspecified fracture of lower end of ulna**

⑦S52.601   **Unspecified fracture of lower end of right ulna**

⑦S52.602   **Unspecified fracture of lower end of left ulna**

⑦S52.609   **Unspecified fracture of lower end of unspecified ulna**

S52.61   **Fracture of ulna styloid process**

⑦S52.611   **Displaced fracture of right ulna styloid process**

⑦S52.612   **Displaced fracture of left ulna styloid process**

⑦S52.613   **Displaced fracture of unspecified ulna styloid process**

⑦S52.614   **Nondisplaced fracture of right ulna styloid process**

⑦S52.615   **Nondisplaced fracture of left ulna styloid process**

⑦S52.616   **Nondisplaced fracture of unspecified ulna styloid process**

S52.62   **Torus fracture of lower end of ulna**

The appropriate 7th character is to be added to all codes in subcategory S52.62

A - initial encounter for closed fracture

D - subsequent encounter for fracture with routine healing

G - subsequent encounter for fracture with delayed healing

K - subsequent encounter for fracture with nonunion

P - subsequent encounter for fracture with malunion

S - sequela

⑦S52.621   **Torus fracture of lower end of right ulna**

⑦S52.622   **Torus fracture of lower end of left ulna**

⑦S52.629   **Torus fracture of lower end of unspecified ulna**

S52.69   **Other fracture of lower end of ulna**

⑦S52.691   **Other fracture of lower end of right ulna**

⑦S52.692   **Other fracture of lower end of left ulna**

⑦S52.699   **Other fracture of lower end of unspecified ulna**

S52.9   **Unspecified fracture of forearm**

⊗⑦S52.90   **Unspecified fracture of unspecified forearm**

⊗⑦S52.91   **Unspecified fracture of right forearm**

⊗⑦S52.92   **Unspecified fracture of left forearm**

S53   **Dislocation and sprain of joints and ligaments of elbow**

Includes: avulsion of joint or ligament of elbow

laceration of cartilage, joint or ligament of elbow sprain of cartilage, joint or ligament of elbow

---

traumatic hemarthrosis of joint or ligament of elbow

traumatic rupture of joint or ligament of elbow

traumatic subluxation of joint or ligament of elbow

traumatic tear of joint or ligament of elbow

Code also any associated open wound

Excludes2: strain of muscle, fascia and tendon at forearm level (S56.-)

The appropriate 7th character is to be added to each code from category S53

A - initial encounter

D - subsequent encounter

S - sequela

S53.0   Subluxation and dislocation of radial head

Dislocation of radiohumeral joint

Subluxation of radiohumeral joint

Excludes1: Monteggia's fracture-dislocation (S52.27-)

S53.00   Unspecified subluxation and dislocation of radial head

⑦S53.001   **Unspecified subluxation of right radial head**

⑦S53.002   **Unspecified subluxation of left radial head**

⑦S53.003   **Unspecified subluxation of unspecified radial head**

⑦S53.004   **Unspecified dislocation of right radial head**

⑦S53.005   **Unspecified dislocation of left radial head**

⑦S53.006   **Unspecified dislocation of unspecified radial head**

S53.01   Anterior subluxation and dislocation of radial head

Anteromedial subluxation and dislocation of radial head

⑦S53.011   **Anterior subluxation of right radial head**

⑦S53.012   **Anterior subluxation of left radial head**

⑦S53.013   **Anterior subluxation of unspecified radial head**

⑦S53.014   **Anterior dislocation of right radial head**

⑦S53.015   **Anterior dislocation of left radial head**

⑦S53.016   **Anterior dislocation of unspecified radial head**

S53.02   Posterior subluxation and dislocation of radial head

Posterolateral subluxation and dislocation of radial head

⑦S53.021   **Posterior subluxation of right radial head**

⑦S53.022   **Posterior subluxation of left radial head**

⑦S53.023   **Posterior subluxation of unspecified radial head**

⑦S53.024   **Posterior dislocation of right radial head**

⑦S53.025   **Posterior dislocation of left radial head**

⑦S53.026   **Posterior dislocation of unspecified radial head**

S53.03   Nursemaid's elbow

⑦S53.031   **Nursemaid's elbow, right elbow**

⑦S53.032   **Nursemaid's elbow, left elbow**

⑦S53.033   **Nursemaid's elbow, unspecified elbow**

S53.09   Other subluxation and dislocation of radial head

⑦S53.091   **Other subluxation of right radial head**

⑦S53.092   **Other subluxation of left radial head**

⑦S53.093   **Other subluxation of unspecified radial head**

⑦S53.094   **Other dislocation of right radial head**

⑦S53.095   **Other dislocation of left radial head**

⑦S53.096   **Other dislocation of unspecified radial head**

S53.1   Subluxation and dislocation of ulnohumeral joint

Subluxation and dislocation of elbow NOS

Excludes1: dislocation of radial head alone (S53.0-)

S53.10   Unspecified subluxation and dislocation of ulnohumeral joint

⑦S53.101   **Unspecified subluxation of right ulnohumeral joint**

⑦S53.102   **Unspecified subluxation of left ulnohumeral joint**

⑦S53.103   **Unspecified subluxation of unspecified ulnohumeral joint**

⑦S53.104   **Unspecified dislocation of right ulnohumeral joint**

⑦S53.105   **Unspecified dislocation of left ulnohumeral joint**

⑦S53.106   **Unspecified dislocation of unspecified ulnohumeral joint**

S53.11   Anterior subluxation and dislocation of ulnohumeral joint

⑦S53.111   **Anterior subluxation of right ulnohumeral joint**

⑦S53.112   **Anterior subluxation of left ulnohumeral joint**

⑦S53.113   **Anterior subluxation of unspecified ulnohumeral joint**

⑦S53.114   **Anterior dislocation of right ulnohumeral joint**

⑦S53.115   **Anterior dislocation of left ulnohumeral joint**

⑦S53.116   **Anterior dislocation of unspecified ulnohumeral joint**

S53.12   Posterior subluxation and dislocation of ulnohumeral joint

⑦S53.121   **Posterior subluxation of right ulnohumeral joint**

⑦S53.122   **Posterior subluxation of left ulnohumeral joint**

⑦S53.123   **Posterior subluxation of unspecified ulnohumeral joint**

⑦S53.124   **Posterior dislocation of right ulnohumeral joint**

⑦S53.125   **Posterior dislocation of left ulnohumeral joint**

⑦S53.126   **Posterior dislocation of unspecified ulnohumeral joint**

S53.13   Medial subluxation and dislocation of ulnohumeral joint

● New code   ▲ Revised code   **Excludes1:** Not coded here   **Excludes2:** Not included here   ⊗ Placeholder required   ⑦7th digit required

⑦S53.131 **Medial subluxation of right ulnohumeral joint**

⑦S53.132 **Medial subluxation of left ulnohumeral joint**

⑦S53.133 **Medial subluxation of unspecified ulnohumeral joint**

⑦S53.134 **Medial dislocation of right ulnohumeral joint**

⑦S53.135 **Medial dislocation of left ulnohumeral joint**

⑦S53.136 **Medial dislocation of unspecified ulnohumeral joint**

S53.14 **Lateral subluxation and dislocation of ulnohumeral joint**

⑦S53.141 **Lateral subluxation of right ulnohumeral joint**

⑦S53.142 **Lateral subluxation of left ulnohumeral joint**

⑦S53.143 **Lateral subluxation of unspecified ulnohumeral joint**

⑦S53.144 **Lateral dislocation of right ulnohumeral joint**

⑦S53.145 **Lateral dislocation of left ulnohumeral joint**

⑦S53.146 **Lateral dislocation of unspecified ulnohumeral joint**

S53.19 **Other subluxation and dislocation of ulnohumeral joint**

⑦S53.191 **Other subluxation of right ulnohumeral joint**

⑦S53.192 **Other subluxation of left ulnohumeral joint**

⑦S53.193 **Other subluxation of unspecified ulnohumeral joint**

⑦S53.194 **Other dislocation of right ulnohumeral joint**

⑦S53.195 **Other dislocation of left ulnohumeral joint**

⑦S53.196 **Other dislocation of unspecified ulnohumeral joint**

S53.2 **Traumatic rupture of radial collateral ligament**

Excludes1: sprain of radial collateral ligament NOS (S53.43-)

⊗⑦S53.20 **Traumatic rupture of unspecified radial collateral ligament**

⊗⑦S53.21 **Traumatic rupture of right radial collateral ligament**

⊗⑦S53.22 **Traumatic rupture of left radial collateral ligament**

S53.3 **Traumatic rupture of ulnar collateral ligament**

Excludes1: sprain of ulnar collateral ligament (S53.44-)

⊗⑦S53.30 **Traumatic rupture of unspecified ulnar collateral ligament**

⊗⑦S53.31 **Traumatic rupture of right ulnar collateral ligament**

⊗⑦S53.32 **Traumatic rupture of left ulnar collateral ligament**

S53.4 **Sprain of elbow**

Excludes2: traumatic rupture of radial collateral ligament (S53.2-)

traumatic rupture of ulnar collateral ligament (S53.3-)

S53.40 **Unspecified sprain of elbow**

⑦S53.401 **Unspecified sprain of right elbow**

⑦S53.402 **Unspecified sprain of left elbow**

⑦S53.409 **Unspecified sprain of unspecified elbow**

Sprain of elbow NOS

S53.41 **Radiohumeral (joint) sprain**

⑦S53.411 **Radiohumeral (joint) sprain of right elbow**

⑦S53.412 **Radiohumeral (joint) sprain of left elbow**

⑦S53.419 **Radiohumeral (joint) sprain of unspecified elbow**

S53.42 **Ulnohumeral (joint) sprain**

⑦S53.421 **Ulnohumeral (joint) sprain of right elbow**

⑦S53.422 **Ulnohumeral (joint) sprain of left elbow**

⑦S53.429 **Ulnohumeral (joint) sprain of unspecified elbow**

S53.43 **Radial collateral ligament sprain**

⑦S53.431 **Radial collateral ligament sprain of right elbow**

⑦S53.432 **Radial collateral ligament sprain of left elbow**

⑦S53.439 **Radial collateral ligament sprain of unspecified elbow**

S53.44 **Ulnar collateral ligament sprain**

⑦S53.441 **Ulnar collateral ligament sprain of right elbow**

⑦S53.442 **Ulnar collateral ligament sprain of left elbow**

⑦S53.449 **Ulnar collateral ligament sprain of unspecified elbow**

S53.49 **Other sprain of elbow**

⑦S53.491 **Other sprain of right elbow**

⑦S53.492 **Other sprain of left elbow**

⑦S53.499 **Other sprain of unspecified elbow**

S54 **Injury of nerves at forearm level**

Code also any associated open wound (S51.-)

Excludes2: injury of nerves at wrist and hand level (S64.-)

The appropriate 7th character is to be added to each code from category S54

A - initial encounter

D - subsequent encounter

S - sequela

S54.0 **Injury of ulnar nerve at forearm level**

Injury of ulnar nerve NOS

⊗⑦S54.00 **Injury of ulnar nerve at forearm level, unspecified arm**

⊗⑦S54.01 **Injury of ulnar nerve at forearm level, right arm**

⊗⑦S54.02 **Injury of ulnar nerve at forearm level, left arm**

S54.1 **Injury of median nerve at forearm level**

Injury of median nerve NOS

⊗⑦S54.10 **Injury of median nerve at forearm level, unspecified arm**

⊗⑦S54.11 **Injury of median nerve at forearm level, right arm**

⊗⑦S54.12 **Injury of median nerve at forearm level, left arm**

S54.2 **Injury of radial nerve at forearm level**

Injury of radial nerve NOS

⊗⑦**S54.20** **Injury of radial nerve at forearm level, unspecified arm**

⊗⑦**S54.21** **Injury of radial nerve at forearm level, right arm**

⊗⑦**S54.22** **Injury of radial nerve at forearm level, left arm**

S54.3 **Injury of cutaneous sensory nerve at forearm level**

⊗⑦**S54.30** **Injury of cutaneous sensory nerve at forearm level, unspecified arm**

⊗⑦**S54.31** **Injury of cutaneous sensory nerve at forearm level, right arm**

⊗⑦**S54.32** **Injury of cutaneous sensory nerve at forearm level, left arm**

S54.8 **Injury of other nerves at forearm level**

S54.8X **Injury of other nerves at forearm level**

⑦**S54.8X1** **Injury of other nerves at forearm level, right arm**

⑦**S54.8X2** **Injury of other nerves at forearm level, left arm**

⑦**S54.8X9** **Injury of other nerves at forearm level, unspecified arm**

S54.9 **Injury of unspecified nerve at forearm level**

⊗⑦**S54.90** **Injury of unspecified nerve at forearm level, unspecified arm**

⊗⑦**S54.91** **Injury of unspecified nerve at forearm level, right arm**

⊗⑦**S54.92** **Injury of unspecified nerve at forearm level, left arm**

S55 **Injury of blood vessels at forearm level**

Code also any associated open wound (S51.-)

Excludes2: injury of blood vessels at wrist and hand level (S65.-)

injury of brachial vessels (S45.1-S45.2)

The appropriate 7th character is to be added to each code from category S55

A - initial encounter

D - subsequent encounter

S - sequela

S55.0 **Injury of ulnar artery at forearm level**

S55.00 **Unspecified injury of ulnar artery at forearm level**

⑦**S55.001** **Unspecified injury of ulnar artery at forearm level, right arm**

⑦**S55.002** **Unspecified injury of ulnar artery at forearm level, left arm**

⑦**S55.009** **Unspecified injury of ulnar artery at forearm level, unspecified arm**

S55.01 **Laceration of ulnar artery at forearm level**

⑦**S55.011** **Laceration of ulnar artery at forearm level, right arm**

⑦**S55.012** **Laceration of ulnar artery at forearm level, left arm**

⑦**S55.019** **Laceration of ulnar artery at forearm level, unspecified arm**

S55.09 **Other specified injury of ulnar artery at forearm level**

⑦**S55.091** **Other specified injury of ulnar artery at forearm level, right arm**

⑦**S55.092** **Other specified injury of ulnar artery at forearm level, left arm**

⑦**S55.099** **Other specified injury of ulnar artery at forearm level, unspecified arm**

S55.1 **Injury of radial artery at forearm level**

S55.10 **Unspecified injury of radial artery at forearm level**

⑦**S55.101** **Unspecified injury of radial artery at forearm level, right arm**

⑦**S55.102** **Unspecified injury of radial artery at forearm level, left arm**

⑦**S55.109** **Unspecified injury of radial artery at forearm level, unspecified arm**

S55.11 **Laceration of radial artery at forearm level**

⑦**S55.111** **Laceration of radial artery at forearm level, right arm**

⑦**S55.112** **Laceration of radial artery at forearm level, left arm**

⑦**S55.119** **Laceration of radial artery at forearm level, unspecified arm**

S55.19 **Other specified injury of radial artery at forearm level**

⑦**S55.191** **Other specified injury of radial artery at forearm level, right arm**

⑦**S55.192** **Other specified injury of radial artery at forearm level, left arm**

⑦**S55.199** **Other specified injury of radial artery at forearm level, unspecified arm**

S55.2 **Injury of vein at forearm level**

S55.20 **Unspecified injury of vein at forearm level**

⑦**S55.201** **Unspecified injury of vein at forearm level, right arm**

⑦**S55.202** **Unspecified injury of vein at forearm level, left arm**

⑦**S55.209** **Unspecified injury of vein at forearm level, unspecified arm**

S55.21 **Laceration of vein at forearm level**

⑦**S55.211** **Laceration of vein at forearm level, right arm**

⑦**S55.212** **Laceration of vein at forearm level, left arm**

⑦**S55.219** **Laceration of vein at forearm level, unspecified arm**

S55.29 **Other specified injury of vein at forearm level**

⑦**S55.291** **Other specified injury of vein at forearm level, right arm**

⑦**S55.292** **Other specified injury of vein at forearm level, left arm**

⑦**S55.299** **Other specified injury of vein at forearm level, unspecified arm**

S55.8 **Injury of other blood vessels at forearm level**

S55.80 **Unspecified injury of other blood vessels at forearm level**

⑦**S55.801** **Unspecified injury of other blood vessels at forearm level, right arm**

⑦**S55.802** **Unspecified injury of other blood vessels at forearm level, left arm**

⑦**S55.809** **Unspecified injury of other blood vessels at forearm level, unspecified arm**

S55.81 **Laceration of other blood vessels at forearm level**

⑦**S55.811** **Laceration of other blood vessels at forearm level, right arm**

⑦**S55.812** **Laceration of other blood vessels at forearm level, left arm**

● New code ▲ Revised code **Excludes1:** Not coded here **Excludes2:** Not included here ⊗ Placeholder required ⑦7th digit required

⑦**S55.819**   Laceration of other blood vessels at forearm level, unspecified arm

S55.89   Other specified injury of other blood vessels at forearm level

⑦**S55.891**   Other specified injury of other blood vessels at forearm level, right arm

⑦**S55.892**   Other specified injury of other blood vessels at forearm level, left arm

⑦**S55.899**   Other specified injury of other blood vessels at forearm level, unspecified arm

S55.9   Injury of unspecified blood vessel at forearm level

S55.90   Unspecified injury of unspecified blood vessel at forearm level

⑦**S55.901**   Unspecified injury of unspecified blood vessel at forearm level, right arm

⑦**S55.902**   Unspecified injury of unspecified blood vessel at forearm level, left arm

⑦**S55.909**   Unspecified injury of unspecified blood vessel at forearm level, unspecified arm

S55.91   Laceration of unspecified blood vessel at forearm level

⑦**S55.911**   Laceration of unspecified blood vessel at forearm level, right arm

⑦**S55.912**   Laceration of unspecified blood vessel at forearm level, left arm

⑦**S55.919**   Laceration of unspecified blood vessel at forearm level, unspecified arm

S55.99   Other specified injury of unspecified blood vessel at forearm level

⑦**S55.991**   Other specified injury of unspecified blood vessel at forearm level, right arm

⑦**S55.992**   Other specified injury of unspecified blood vessel at forearm level, left arm

⑦**S55.999**   Other specified injury of unspecified blood vessel at forearm level, unspecified arm

S56   Injury of muscle, fascia and tendon at forearm level

Code also any associated open wound (S51.-)

Excludes2: injury of muscle, fascia and tendon at or below wrist (S66.-)

sprain of joints and ligaments of elbow (S53.4-)

The appropriate 7th character is to be added to each code from category S56

A - initial encounter

D - subsequent encounter

S - sequela

S56.0   Injury of flexor muscle, fascia and tendon of thumb at forearm level

S56.00   Unspecified injury of flexor muscle, fascia and tendon of thumb at forearm level

⑦**S56.001**   Unspecified injury of flexor muscle, fascia and tendon of right thumb at forearm level

⑦**S56.002**   Unspecified injury of flexor muscle, fascia and tendon of left thumb at forearm level

⑦**S56.009**   Unspecified injury of flexor muscle, fascia and tendon of unspecified thumb at forearm level

S56.01   Strain of flexor muscle, fascia and tendon of thumb at forearm level

⑦**S56.011**   Strain of flexor muscle, fascia and tendon of right thumb at forearm level

⑦**S56.012**   Strain of flexor muscle, fascia and tendon of left thumb at forearm level

⑦**S56.019**   Strain of flexor muscle, fascia and tendon of unspecified thumb at forearm level

S56.02   Laceration of flexor muscle, fascia and tendon of thumb at forearm level

⑦**S56.021**   Laceration of flexor muscle, fascia and tendon of right thumb at forearm level

⑦**S56.022**   Laceration of flexor muscle, fascia and tendon of left thumb at forearm level

⑦**S56.029**   Laceration of flexor muscle, fascia and tendon of unspecified thumb at forearm level

S56.09   Other injury of flexor muscle, fascia and tendon of thumb at forearm level

⑦**S56.091**   Other injury of flexor muscle, fascia and tendon of right thumb at forearm level

⑦**S56.092**   Other injury of flexor muscle, fascia and tendon of left thumb at forearm level

⑦**S56.099**   Other injury of flexor muscle, fascia and tendon of unspecified thumb at forearm level

S56.1   Injury of flexor muscle, fascia and tendon of other and unspecified finger at forearm level

S56.10   Unspecified injury of flexor muscle, fascia and tendon of other and unspecified finger at forearm level

⑦**S56.101**   Unspecified injury of flexor muscle, fascia and tendon of right index finger at forearm level

⑦**S56.102**   Unspecified injury of flexor muscle, fascia and tendon of left index finger at forearm level

⑦**S56.103**   Unspecified injury of flexor muscle, fascia and tendon of right middle finger at forearm level

⑦**S56.104**   Unspecified injury of flexor muscle, fascia and tendon of left middle finger at forearm level

⑦**S56.105**   Unspecified injury of flexor muscle, fascia and tendon of right ring finger at forearm level

⑦**S56.106**   Unspecified injury of flexor muscle, fascia and tendon of left ring finger at forearm level

⑦**S56.107**   Unspecified injury of flexor muscle, fascia and tendon of right little finger at forearm level

⑦**S56.108**   Unspecified injury of flexor muscle, fascia and tendon of left little finger at forearm level

⑦**S56.109**   Unspecified injury of flexor muscle, fascia and tendon of unspecified finger at forearm level

S56.11 Strain of flexor muscle, fascia and tendon of other and unspecified finger at forearm level

⑦S56.111 Strain of flexor muscle, fascia and tendon of right index finger at forearm level

⑦S56.112 Strain of flexor muscle, fascia and tendon of left index finger at forearm level

⑦S56.113 Strain of flexor muscle, fascia and tendon of right middle finger at forearm level

⑦S56.114 Strain of flexor muscle, fascia and tendon of left middle finger at forearm level

⑦S56.115 Strain of flexor muscle, fascia and tendon of right ring finger at forearm level

⑦S56.116 Strain of flexor muscle, fascia and tendon of left ring finger at forearm level

⑦S56.117 Strain of flexor muscle, fascia and tendon of right little finger at forearm level

⑦S56.118 Strain of flexor muscle, fascia and tendon of left little finger at forearm level

⑦S56.119 Strain of flexor muscle, fascia and tendon of finger of unspecified finger at forearm level

S56.12 Laceration of flexor muscle, fascia and tendon of other and unspecified finger at forearm level

⑦S56.121 Laceration of flexor muscle, fascia and tendon of right index finger at forearm level

⑦S56.122 Laceration of flexor muscle, fascia and tendon of left index finger at forearm level

⑦S56.123 Laceration of flexor muscle, fascia and tendon of right middle finger at forearm level

⑦S56.124 Laceration of flexor muscle, fascia and tendon of left middle finger at forearm level

⑦S56.125 Laceration of flexor muscle, fascia and tendon of right ring finger at forearm level

⑦S56.126 Laceration of flexor muscle, fascia and tendon of left ring finger at forearm level

⑦S56.127 Laceration of flexor muscle, fascia and tendon of right little finger at forearm level

⑦S56.128 Laceration of flexor muscle, fascia and tendon of left little finger at forearm level

⑦S56.129 Laceration of flexor muscle, fascia and tendon of unspecified finger at forearm level

S56.19 Other injury of flexor muscle, fascia and tendon of other and unspecified finger at forearm level

⑦S56.191 Other injury of flexor muscle, fascia and tendon of right index finger at forearm level

⑦S56.192 Other injury of flexor muscle, fascia and tendon of left index finger at forearm level

⑦S56.193 Other injury of flexor muscle, fascia and tendon of right middle finger at forearm level

⑦S56.194 Other injury of flexor muscle, fascia and tendon of left middle finger at forearm level

⑦S56.195 Other injury of flexor muscle, fascia and tendon of right ring finger at forearm level

⑦S56.196 Other injury of flexor muscle, fascia and tendon of left ring finger at forearm level

⑦S56.197 Other injury of flexor muscle, fascia and tendon of right little finger at forearm level

⑦S56.198 Other injury of flexor muscle, fascia and tendon of left little finger at forearm level

⑦S56.199 Other injury of flexor muscle, fascia and tendon of unspecified finger at forearm level

S56.2 Injury of other flexor muscle, fascia and tendon at forearm level

S56.20 Unspecified injury of other flexor muscle, fascia and tendon at forearm level

⑦S56.201 Unspecified injury of other flexor muscle, fascia and tendon at forearm level, right arm

⑦S56.202 Unspecified injury of other flexor muscle, fascia and tendon at forearm level, left arm

⑦S56.209 Unspecified injury of other flexor muscle, fascia and tendon at forearm level, unspecified arm

S56.21 Strain of other flexor muscle, fascia and tendon at forearm level

⑦S56.211 Strain of other flexor muscle, fascia and tendon at forearm level, right arm

⑦S56.212 Strain of other flexor muscle, fascia and tendon at forearm level, left arm

⑦S56.219 Strain of other flexor muscle, fascia and tendon at forearm level, unspecified arm

S56.22 Laceration of other flexor muscle, fascia and tendon at forearm level

⑦S56.221 Laceration of other flexor muscle, fascia and tendon at forearm level, right arm

⑦S56.222 Laceration of other flexor muscle, fascia and tendon at forearm level, left arm

⑦S56.229 Laceration of other flexor muscle, fascia and tendon at forearm level, unspecified arm

S56.29 Other injury of other flexor muscle, fascia and tendon at forearm level

⑦S56.291 Other injury of other flexor muscle, fascia and tendon at forearm level, right arm

⑦S56.292 Other injury of other flexor muscle, fascia and tendon at forearm level, left arm

⑦S56.299 Other injury of other flexor muscle, fascia and tendon at forearm level, unspecified arm

● New code   ▲ Revised code   **Excludes1:** Not coded here   **Excludes2:** Not included here   ⊗ Placeholder required   ⑦ 7th digit required

S56.3 Injury of extensor or abductor muscles, fascia and tendons of thumb at forearm level

S56.30 Unspecified injury of extensor or abductor muscles, fascia and tendons of thumb at forearm level

⑦S56.301 Unspecified injury of extensor or abductor muscles, fascia and tendons of right thumb at forearm level

⑦S56.302 Unspecified injury of extensor or abductor muscles, fascia and tendons of left thumb at forearm level

⑦S56.309 Unspecified injury of extensor or abductor muscles, fascia and tendons of unspecified thumb at forearm level

S56.31 Strain of extensor or abductor muscles, fascia and tendons of thumb at forearm level

⑦S56.311 Strain of extensor or abductor muscles, fascia and tendons of right thumb at forearm level

⑦S56.312 Strain of extensor or abductor muscles, fascia and tendons of left thumb at forearm level

⑦S56.319 Strain of extensor or abductor muscles, fascia and tendons of unspecified thumb at forearm level

S56.32 Laceration of extensor or abductor muscles, fascia and tendons of thumb at forearm level

⑦S56.321 Laceration of extensor or abductor muscles, fascia and tendons of right thumb at forearm level

⑦S56.322 Laceration of extensor or abductor muscles, fascia and tendons of left thumb at forearm level

⑦S56.329 Laceration of extensor or abductor muscles, fascia and tendons of unspecified thumb at forearm level

S56.39 Other injury of extensor or abductor muscles, fascia and tendons of thumb at forearm level

⑦S56.391 Other injury of extensor or abductor muscles, fascia and tendons of right thumb at forearm level

⑦S56.392 Other injury of extensor or abductor muscles, fascia and tendons of left thumb at forearm level

⑦S56.399 Other injury of extensor or abductor muscles, fascia and tendons of unspecified thumb at forearm level

S56.4 Injury of extensor muscle, fascia and tendon of other and unspecified finger at forearm level

S56.40 Unspecified injury of extensor muscle, fascia and tendon of other and unspecified finger at forearm level

⑦S56.401 Unspecified injury of extensor muscle, fascia and tendon of right index finger at forearm level

⑦S56.402 Unspecified injury of extensor muscle, fascia and tendon of left index finger at forearm level

⑦S56.403 Unspecified injury of extensor muscle, fascia and tendon of right middle finger at forearm level

⑦S56.404 Unspecified injury of extensor muscle, fascia and tendon of left middle finger at forearm level

⑦S56.405 Unspecified injury of extensor muscle, fascia and tendon of right ring finger at forearm level

⑦S56.406 Unspecified injury of extensor muscle, fascia and tendon of left ring finger at forearm level

⑦S56.407 Unspecified injury of extensor muscle, fascia and tendon of right little finger at forearm level

⑦S56.408 Unspecified injury of extensor muscle, fascia and tendon of left little finger at forearm level

⑦S56.409 Unspecified injury of extensor muscle, fascia and tendon of unspecified finger at forearm level

S56.41 Strain of extensor muscle, fascia and tendon of other and unspecified finger at forearm level

⑦S56.411 Strain of extensor muscle, fascia and tendon of right index finger at forearm level

⑦S56.412 Strain of extensor muscle, fascia and tendon of left index finger at forearm level

⑦S56.413 Strain of extensor muscle, fascia and tendon of right middle finger at forearm level

⑦S56.414 Strain of extensor muscle, fascia and tendon of left middle finger at forearm level

⑦S56.415 Strain of extensor muscle, fascia and tendon of right ring finger at forearm level

⑦S56.416 Strain of extensor muscle, fascia and tendon of left ring finger at forearm level

⑦S56.417 Strain of extensor muscle, fascia and tendon of right little finger at forearm level

⑦S56.418 Strain of extensor muscle, fascia and tendon of left little finger at forearm level

⑦S56.419 Strain of extensor muscle, fascia and tendon of finger, unspecified finger at forearm level

S56.42 Laceration of extensor muscle, fascia and tendon of other and unspecified finger at forearm level

⑦S56.421 Laceration of extensor muscle, fascia and tendon of right index finger at forearm level

⑦S56.422 Laceration of extensor muscle, fascia and tendon of left index finger at forearm level

⑦S56.423 Laceration of extensor muscle, fascia and tendon of right middle finger at forearm level

⑦S56.424 Laceration of extensor muscle, fascia and tendon of left middle finger at forearm level

⑦S56.425 Laceration of extensor muscle, fascia and tendon of right ring finger at forearm level

⑦S56.426 Laceration of extensor muscle, fascia and tendon of left ring finger at forearm level

⑦ S56.427 Laceration of extensor muscle, fascia and tendon of right little finger at forearm level

⑦ S56.428 Laceration of extensor muscle, fascia and tendon of left little finger at forearm level

⑦ S56.429 Laceration of extensor muscle, fascia and tendon of unspecified finger at forearm level

S56.49 **Other injury of extensor muscle, fascia and tendon of other and unspecified finger at forearm level**

⑦ S56.491 Other injury of extensor muscle, fascia and tendon of right index finger at forearm level

⑦ S56.492 Other injury of extensor muscle, fascia and tendon of left index finger at forearm level

⑦ S56.493 Other injury of extensor muscle, fascia and tendon of right middle finger at forearm level

⑦ S56.494 Other injury of extensor muscle, fascia and tendon of left middle finger at forearm level

⑦ S56.495 Other injury of extensor muscle, fascia and tendon of right ring finger at forearm level

⑦ S56.496 Other injury of extensor muscle, fascia and tendon of left ring finger at forearm level

⑦ S56.497 Other injury of extensor muscle, fascia and tendon of right little finger at forearm level

⑦ S56.498 Other injury of extensor muscle, fascia and tendon of left little finger at forearm level

⑦ S56.499 Other injury of extensor muscle, fascia and tendon of unspecified finger at forearm level

S56.5 **Injury of other extensor muscle, fascia and tendon at forearm level**

S56.50 **Unspecified injury of other extensor muscle, fascia and tendon at forearm level**

⑦ S56.501 Unspecified injury of other extensor muscle, fascia and tendon at forearm level, right arm

⑦ S56.502 Unspecified injury of other extensor muscle, fascia and tendon at forearm level, left arm

⑦ S56.509 Unspecified injury of other extensor muscle, fascia and tendon at forearm level, unspecified arm

S56.51 **Strain of other extensor muscle, fascia and tendon at forearm level**

⑦ S56.511 Strain of other extensor muscle, fascia and tendon at forearm level, right arm

⑦ S56.512 Strain of other extensor muscle, fascia and tendon at forearm level, left arm

⑦ S56.519 Strain of other extensor muscle, fascia and tendon at forearm level, unspecified arm

S56.52 **Laceration of other extensor muscle, fascia and tendon at forearm level**

⑦ S56.521 Laceration of other extensor muscle, fascia and tendon at forearm level, right arm

⑦ S56.522 Laceration of other extensor muscle, fascia and tendon at forearm level, left arm

⑦ S56.529 Laceration of other extensor muscle, fascia and tendon at forearm level, unspecified arm

S56.59 **Other injury of other extensor muscle, fascia and tendon at forearm level**

⑦ S56.591 Other injury of other extensor muscle, fascia and tendon at forearm level, right arm

⑦ S56.592 Other injury of other extensor muscle, fascia and tendon at forearm level, left arm

⑦ S56.599 Other injury of other extensor muscle, fascia and tendon at forearm level, unspecified arm

S56.8 **Injury of other muscles, fascia and tendons at forearm level**

S56.80 **Unspecified injury of other muscles, fascia and tendons at forearm level**

⑦ S56.801 Unspecified injury of other muscles, fascia and tendons at forearm level, right arm

⑦ S56.802 Unspecified injury of other muscles, fascia and tendons at forearm level, left arm

⑦ S56.809 Unspecified injury of other muscles, fascia and tendons at forearm level, unspecified arm

S56.81 **Strain of other muscles, fascia and tendons at forearm level**

⑦ S56.811 Strain of other muscles, fascia and tendons at forearm level, right arm

⑦ S56.812 Strain of other muscles, fascia and tendons at forearm level, left arm

⑦ S56.819 Strain of other muscles, fascia and tendons at forearm level, unspecified arm

S56.82 **Laceration of other muscles, fascia and tendons at forearm level**

⑦ S56.821 Laceration of other muscles, fascia and tendons at forearm level, right arm

⑦ S56.822 Laceration of other muscles, fascia and tendons at forearm level, left arm

⑦ S56.829 Laceration of other muscles, fascia and tendons at forearm level, unspecified arm

S56.89 **Other injury of other muscles, fascia and tendons at forearm level**

⑦ S56.891 Other injury of other muscles, fascia and tendons at forearm level, right arm

⑦ S56.892 Other injury of other muscles, fascia and tendons at forearm level, left arm

⑦ S56.899 Other injury of other muscles, fascia and tendons at forearm level, unspecified arm

S56.9 **Injury of unspecified muscles, fascia and tendons at forearm level**

● New code ▲ Revised code **Excludes1:** Not coded here **Excludes2:** Not included here ⊗ Placeholder required ⑦ 7ᵗʰ digit required

S56.90   Unspecified injury of unspecified muscles, fascia and tendons at forearm level

⑦S56.901   Unspecified injury of unspecified muscles, fascia and tendons at forearm level, right arm

⑦S56.902   Unspecified injury of unspecified muscles, fascia and tendons at forearm level, left arm

⑦S56.909   Unspecified injury of unspecified muscles, fascia and tendons at forearm level, unspecified arm

S56.91   Strain of unspecified muscles, fascia and tendons at forearm level

⑦S56.911   Strain of unspecified muscles, fascia and tendons at forearm level, right arm

⑦S56.912   Strain of unspecified muscles, fascia and tendons at forearm level, left arm

⑦S56.919   Strain of unspecified muscles, fascia and tendons at forearm level, unspecified arm

S56.92   Laceration of unspecified muscles, fascia and tendons at forearm level

⑦S56.921   Laceration of unspecified muscles, fascia and tendons at forearm level, right arm

⑦S56.922   Laceration of unspecified muscles, fascia and tendons at forearm level, left arm

⑦S56.929   Laceration of unspecified muscles, fascia and tendons at forearm level, unspecified arm

S56.99   Other injury of unspecified muscles, fascia and tendons at forearm level

⑦S56.991   Other injury of unspecified muscles, fascia and tendons at forearm level, right arm

⑦S56.992   Other injury of unspecified muscles, fascia and tendons at forearm level, left arm

⑦S56.999   Other injury of unspecified muscles, fascia and tendons at forearm level, unspecified arm

S57   Crushing injury of elbow and forearm

Use additional code(s) for all associated injuries

Excludes2: crushing injury of wrist and hand (S67.-)

The appropriate 7th character is to be added to each code from category S57

A - initial encounter

D - subsequent encounter

S - sequela

S57.0   Crushing injury of elbow

⊗⑦S57.00   Crushing injury of unspecified elbow

⊗⑦S57.01   Crushing injury of right elbow

⊗⑦S57.02   Crushing injury of left elbow

S57.8   Crushing injury of forearm

⊗⑦S57.80   Crushing injury of unspecified forearm

⊗⑦S57.81   Crushing injury of right forearm

⊗⑦S57.82   Crushing injury of left forearm

S58   Traumatic amputation of elbow and forearm

An amputation not identified as partial or complete should be coded to complete

Excludes1: traumatic amputation of wrist and hand (S68.-)

The appropriate 7th character is to be added to each code from category S58

A - initial encounter

D - subsequent encounter

S - sequela

S58.0   Traumatic amputation at elbow level

S58.01   Complete traumatic amputation at elbow level

⑦S58.011   Complete traumatic amputation at elbow level, right arm

⑦S58.012   Complete traumatic amputation at elbow level, left arm

⑦S58.019   Complete traumatic amputation at elbow level, unspecified arm

S58.02   Partial traumatic amputation at elbow level

⑦S58.021   Partial traumatic amputation at elbow level, right arm

⑦S58.022   Partial traumatic amputation at elbow level, left arm

⑦S58.029   Partial traumatic amputation at elbow level, unspecified arm

S58.1   Traumatic amputation at level between elbow and wrist

S58.11   Complete traumatic amputation at level between elbow and wrist

⑦S58.111   Complete traumatic amputation at level between elbow and wrist, right arm

⑦S58.112   Complete traumatic amputation at level between elbow and wrist, left arm

⑦S58.119   Complete traumatic amputation at level between elbow and wrist, unspecified arm

S58.12   Partial traumatic amputation at level between elbow and wrist

⑦S58.121   Partial traumatic amputation at level between elbow and wrist, right arm

⑦S58.122   Partial traumatic amputation at level between elbow and wrist, left arm

⑦S58.129   Partial traumatic amputation at level between elbow and wrist, unspecified arm

S58.9   Traumatic amputation of forearm, level unspecified

Excludes1: traumatic amputation of wrist (S68.-)

S58.91   Complete traumatic amputation of forearm, level unspecified

⑦S58.911   Complete traumatic amputation of right forearm, level unspecified

⑦S58.912   Complete traumatic amputation of left forearm, level unspecified

⑦S58.919   Complete traumatic amputation of unspecified forearm, level unspecified

S58.92   Partial traumatic amputation of forearm, level unspecified

⑦S58.921   Partial traumatic amputation of right forearm, level unspecified

⑦S58.922   Partial traumatic amputation of left forearm, level unspecified

⑦S58.929   Partial traumatic amputation of unspecified forearm, level unspecified

S59   Other and unspecified injuries of elbow and forearm

Excludes2: Other and unspecified injuries of wrist and hand (S69.-)

    Add 4th-7th digits   Nonspecific code   Unspecified code   Manifestation code

The appropriate 7th character is to be added to each code from subcategories S59.0, S59.1, and S59.2

A - initial encounter for closed fracture

D - subsequent encounter for fracture with routine healing

G - subsequent encounter for fracture with delayed healing

K - subsequent encounter for fracture with nonunion

P - subsequent encounter for fracture with malunion

S - sequela

S59.0　Physeal fracture of lower end of ulna

　　S59.00　Unspecified physeal fracture of lower end of ulna

　　　⑦ S59.001　Unspecified physeal fracture of lower end of ulna, right arm

　　　⑦ S59.002　Unspecified physeal fracture of lower end of ulna, left arm

　　　⑦ S59.009　Unspecified physeal fracture of lower end of ulna, unspecified arm

　　S59.01　Salter-Harris Type I physeal fracture of lower end of ulna

　　　⑦ S59.011　Salter-Harris Type I physeal fracture of lower end of ulna, right arm

　　　⑦ S59.012　Salter-Harris Type I physeal fracture of lower end of ulna, left arm

　　　⑦ S59.019　Salter-Harris Type I physeal fracture of lower end of ulna, unspecified arm

　　S59.02　Salter-Harris Type II physeal fracture of lower end of ulna

　　　⑦ S59.021　Salter-Harris Type II physeal fracture of lower end of ulna, right arm

　　　⑦ S59.022　Salter-Harris Type II physeal fracture of lower end of ulna, left arm

　　　⑦ S59.029　Salter-Harris Type II physeal fracture of lower end of ulna, unspecified arm

　　S59.03　Salter-Harris Type III physeal fracture of lower end of ulna

　　　⑦ S59.031　Salter-Harris Type III physeal fracture of lower end of ulna, right arm

　　　⑦ S59.032　Salter-Harris Type III physeal fracture of lower end of ulna, left arm

　　　⑦ S59.039　Salter-Harris Type III physeal fracture of lower end of ulna, unspecified arm

　　S59.04　Salter-Harris Type IV physeal fracture of lower end of ulna

　　　⑦ S59.041　Salter-Harris Type IV physeal fracture of lower end of ulna, right arm

　　　⑦ S59.042　Salter-Harris Type IV physeal fracture of lower end of ulna, left arm

　　　⑦ S59.049　Salter-Harris Type IV physeal fracture of lower end of ulna, unspecified arm

　　S59.09　Other physeal fracture of lower end of ulna

　　　⑦ S59.091　Other physeal fracture of lower end of ulna, right arm

　　　⑦ S59.092　Other physeal fracture of lower end of ulna, left arm

　　　⑦ S59.099　Other physeal fracture of lower end of ulna, unspecified arm

S59.1　Physeal fracture of upper end of radius

　　S59.10　Unspecified physeal fracture of upper end of radius

　　　⑦ S59.101　Unspecified physeal fracture of upper end of radius, right arm

　　　⑦ S59.102　Unspecified physeal fracture of upper end of radius, left arm

　　　⑦ S59.109　Unspecified physeal fracture of upper end of radius, unspecified arm

　　S59.11　Salter-Harris Type I physeal fracture of upper end of radius

　　　⑦ S59.111　Salter-Harris Type I physeal fracture of upper end of radius, right arm

　　　⑦ S59.112　Salter-Harris Type I physeal fracture of upper end of radius, left arm

　　　⑦ S59.119　Salter-Harris Type I physeal fracture of upper end of radius, unspecified arm

　　S59.12　Salter-Harris Type II physeal fracture of upper end of radius

　　　⑦ S59.121　Salter-Harris Type II physeal fracture of upper end of radius, right arm

　　　⑦ S59.122　Salter-Harris Type II physeal fracture of upper end of radius, left arm

　　　⑦ S59.129　Salter-Harris Type II physeal fracture of upper end of radius, unspecified arm

　　S59.13　Salter-Harris Type III physeal fracture of upper end of radius

　　　⑦ S59.131　Salter-Harris Type III physeal fracture of upper end of radius, right arm

　　　⑦ S59.132　Salter-Harris Type III physeal fracture of upper end of radius, left arm

　　　⑦ S59.139　Salter-Harris Type III physeal fracture of upper end of radius, unspecified arm

　　S59.14　Salter-Harris Type IV physeal fracture of upper end of radius

　　　⑦ S59.141　Salter-Harris Type IV physeal fracture of upper end of radius, right arm

　　　⑦ S59.142　Salter-Harris Type IV physeal fracture of upper end of radius, left arm

　　　⑦ S59.149　Salter-Harris Type IV physeal fracture of upper end of radius, unspecified arm

　　S59.19　Other physeal fracture of upper end of radius

　　　S59.191　Other physeal fracture of upper end of radius, right arm

　　　⑦ S59.192　Other physeal fracture of upper end of radius, left arm

　　　⑦ S59.199　Other physeal fracture of upper end of radius, unspecified arm

S59.2　Physeal fracture of lower end of radius

　● New code　▲ Revised code　Excludes1: Not coded here　Excludes2: Not included here　⊗ Placeholder required　⑦ 7th digit required

S59.20 Unspecified physeal fracture of lower end of radius

⑦**S59.201** Unspecified physeal fracture of lower end of radius, right arm

⑦**S59.202** Unspecified physeal fracture of lower end of radius, left arm

⑦**S59.209** Unspecified physeal fracture of lower end of radius, unspecified arm

S59.21 Salter-Harris Type I physeal fracture of lower end of radius

⑦**S59.211** Salter-Harris Type I physeal fracture of lower end of radius, right arm

⑦**S59.212** Salter-Harris Type I physeal fracture of lower end of radius, left arm

⑦**S59.219** Salter-Harris Type I physeal fracture of lower end of radius, unspecified arm

S59.22 Salter-Harris Type II physeal fracture of lower end of radius

⑦**S59.221** Salter-Harris Type II physeal fracture of lower end of radius, right arm

⑦**S59.222** Salter-Harris Type II physeal fracture of lower end of radius, left arm

⑦**S59.229** Salter-Harris Type II physeal fracture of lower end of radius, unspecified arm

S59.23 Salter-Harris Type III physeal fracture of lower end of radius

⑦**S59.231** Salter-Harris Type III physeal fracture of lower end of radius, right arm

⑦**S59.232** Salter-Harris Type III physeal fracture of lower end of radius, left arm

⑦**S59.239** Salter-Harris Type III physeal fracture of lower end of radius, unspecified arm

S59.24 Salter-Harris Type IV physeal fracture of lower end of radius

⑦**S59.241** Salter-Harris Type IV physeal fracture of lower end of radius, right arm

⑦**S59.242** Salter-Harris Type IV physeal fracture of lower end of radius, left arm

⑦**S59.249** Salter-Harris Type IV physeal fracture of lower end of radius, unspecified arm

S59.29 Other physeal fracture of lower end of radius

⑦**S59.291** Other physeal fracture of lower end of radius, right arm

⑦**S59.292** Other physeal fracture of lower end of radius, left arm

⑦**S59.299** Other physeal fracture of lower end of radius, unspecified arm

S59.8 Other specified injuries of elbow and forearm

The appropriate 7th character is to be added to each code in subcategory S59.8

A - initial encounter

D - subsequent encounter

S - sequela

S59.80 Other specified injuries of elbow

⑦**S59.801** Other specified injuries of right elbow

⑦**S59.802** Other specified injuries of left elbow

⑦**S59.809** Other specified injuries of unspecified elbow

S59.81 Other specified injuries of forearm

⑦**S59.811** Other specified injuries right forearm

⑦**S59.812** Other specified injuries left forearm

⑦**S59.819** Other specified injuries unspecified forearm

S59.9 Unspecified injury of elbow and forearm

The appropriate 7th character is to be added to each code in subcategory S59.9

A - initial encounter

D - subsequent encounter

S - sequela

S59.90 Unspecified injury of elbow

⑦**S59.901** Unspecified injury of right elbow

⑦**S59.902** Unspecified injury of left elbow

⑦**S59.909** Unspecified injury of unspecified elbow

S59.91 Unspecified injury of forearm

⑦**S59.911** Unspecified injury of right forearm

⑦**S59.912** Unspecified injury of left forearm

⑦**S59.919** Unspecified injury of unspecified forearm

INJURIES TO THE WRIST, HAND AND FINGERS (S60-S69)

Excludes2: burns and corrosions (T20-T32)

frostbite (T33-T34)

insect bite or sting, venomous (T63.4)

S60 **Superficial injury of wrist, hand and fingers**

The appropriate 7th character is to be added to each code from category S60

A - initial encounter

D - subsequent encounter

S - sequela

S60.0 Contusion of finger without damage to nail

Excludes1: contusion involving nail (matrix) (S60.1)

⊗⑦**S60.00** Contusion of unspecified finger without damage to nail

Contusion of finger(s) NOS

S60.01 Contusion of thumb without damage to nail

⑦**S60.011** Contusion of right thumb without damage to nail

⑦**S60.012** Contusion of left thumb without damage to nail

⑦**S60.019** Contusion of unspecified thumb without damage to nail

S60.02 Contusion of index finger without damage to nail

⑦**S60.021** Contusion of right index finger without damage to nail

⑦**S60.022** Contusion of left index finger without damage to nail

⑦**S60.029** Contusion of unspecified index finger without damage to nail

S60.03 Contusion of middle finger without damage to nail

⑦ S60.031   Contusion of right middle finger without damage to nail

⑦ S60.032   Contusion of left middle finger without damage to nail

⑦ S60.039   Contusion of unspecified middle finger without damage to nail

S60.04   Contusion of ring finger without damage to nail

⑦ S60.041   Contusion of right ring finger without damage to nail

⑦ S60.042   Contusion of left ring finger without damage to nail

⑦ S60.049   Contusion of unspecified ring finger without damage to nail

S60.05   Contusion of little finger without damage to nail

⑦ S60.051   Contusion of right little finger without damage to nail

⑦ S60.052   Contusion of left little finger without damage to nail

⑦ S60.059   Contusion of unspecified little finger without damage to nail

S60.1   Contusion of finger with damage to nail

⊗⑦ S60.10   Contusion of unspecified finger with damage to nail

S60.11   Contusion of thumb with damage to nail

⑦ S60.111   Contusion of right thumb with damage to nail

⑦ S60.112   Contusion of left thumb with damage to nail

⑦ S60.119   Contusion of unspecified thumb with damage to nail

S60.12   Contusion of index finger with damage to nail

⑦ S60.121   Contusion of right index finger with damage to nail

⑦ S60.122   Contusion of left index finger with damage to nail

⑦ S60.129   Contusion of unspecified index finger with damage to nail

S60.13   Contusion of middle finger with damage to nail

⑦ S60.131   Contusion of right middle finger with damage to nail

⑦ S60.132   Contusion of left middle finger with damage to nail

⑦ S60.139   Contusion of unspecified middle finger with damage to nail

S60.14   Contusion of ring finger with damage to nail

⑦ S60.141   Contusion of right ring finger with damage to nail

⑦ S60.142   Contusion of left ring finger with damage to nail

⑦ S60.149   Contusion of unspecified ring finger with damage to nail

S60.15   Contusion of little finger with damage to nail

⑦ S60.151   Contusion of right little finger with damage to nail

⑦ S60.152   Contusion of left little finger with damage to nail

⑦ S60.159   Contusion of unspecified little finger with damage to nail

S60.2   Contusion of wrist and hand

Excludes2: contusion of fingers (S60.0-, S60.1-)

S60.21   Contusion of wrist

⑦ S60.211   Contusion of right wrist

⑦ S60.212   Contusion of left wrist

⑦ S60.219   Contusion of unspecified wrist

S60.22   Contusion of hand

⑦ S60.221   Contusion of right hand

⑦ S60.222   Contusion of left hand

⑦ S60.229   Contusion of unspecified hand

S60.3   Other superficial injuries of thumb

S60.31   Abrasion of thumb

⑦ S60.311   Abrasion of right thumb

⑦ S60.312   Abrasion of left thumb

⑦ S60.319   Abrasion of unspecified thumb

S60.32   Blister (nonthermal) of thumb

⑦ S60.321   Blister (nonthermal) of right thumb

⑦ S60.322   Blister (nonthermal) of left thumb

⑦ S60.329   Blister (nonthermal) of unspecified thumb

S60.34   External constriction of thumb

Hair tourniquet syndrome of thumb

Use additional cause code to identify the constricting item (W49.0-)

⑦ S60.341   External constriction of right thumb

⑦ S60.342   External constriction of left thumb

⑦ S60.349   External constriction of unspecified thumb

S60.35   Superficial foreign body of thumb

Splinter in the thumb

⑦ S60.351   Superficial foreign body of right thumb

⑦ S60.352   Superficial foreign body of left thumb

⑦ S60.359   Superficial foreign body of unspecified thumb

S60.36   Insect bite (nonvenomous) of thumb

⑦ S60.361   Insect bite (nonvenomous) of right thumb

⑦ S60.362   Insect bite (nonvenomous) of left thumb

⑦ S60.369   Insect bite (nonvenomous) of unspecified thumb

S60.37   Other superficial bite of thumb

Excludes1: open bite of thumb (S61.05-, S61.15-)

⑦ S60.371   Other superficial bite of right thumb

⑦ S60.372   Other superficial bite of left thumb

⑦ S60.379   Other superficial bite of unspecified thumb

S60.39   Other superficial injuries of thumb

⑦ S60.391   Other superficial injuries of right thumb

⑦ S60.392   Other superficial injuries of left thumb

⑦ S60.399   Other superficial injuries of unspecified thumb

S60.4   Other superficial injuries of other fingers

S60.41   Abrasion of fingers

⑦ S60.410   Abrasion of right index finger

⑦ S60.411   Abrasion of left index finger

⑦ S60.412   Abrasion of right middle finger

⑦ S60.413   Abrasion of left middle finger

   ● New code   ▲ Revised code   **Excludes1:** Not coded here   **Excludes2:** Not included here   ⊗ Placeholder required   ⑦ 7ᵗʰ digit required

⑦S60.414   **Abrasion of right ring finger**

⑦S60.415   **Abrasion of left ring finger**

⑦S60.416   **Abrasion of right little finger**

⑦S60.417   **Abrasion of left little finger**

⑦S60.418   **Abrasion of other finger**

     Abrasion of specified finger with unspecified laterality

⑦S60.419   **Abrasion of unspecified finger**

S60.42   **Blister (nonthermal) of fingers**

⑦S60.420   **Blister (nonthermal) of right index finger**

⑦S60.421   **Blister (nonthermal) of left index finger**

⑦S60.422   **Blister (nonthermal) of right middle finger**

⑦S60.423   **Blister (nonthermal) of left middle finger**

⑦S60.424   **Blister (nonthermal) of right ring finger**

⑦S60.425   **Blister (nonthermal) of left ring finger**

⑦S60.426   **Blister (nonthermal) of right little finger**

⑦S60.427   **Blister (nonthermal) of left little finger**

⑦S60.428   **Blister (nonthermal) of other finger**

     Blister (nonthermal) of specified finger with unspecified laterality

⑦S60.429   **Blister (nonthermal) of unspecified finger**

S60.44   **External constriction of fingers**

     Hair tourniquet syndrome of finger

     Use additional cause code to identify the constricting item (W49.0-)

⑦S60.440   **External constriction of right index finger**

⑦S60.441   **External constriction of left index finger**

⑦S60.442   **External constriction of right middle finger**

⑦S60.443   **External constriction of left middle finger**

⑦S60.444   **External constriction of right ring finger**

⑦S60.445   **External constriction of left ring finger**

⑦S60.446   **External constriction of right little finger**

⑦S60.447   **External constriction of left little finger**

⑦S60.448   **External constriction of other finger**

     External constriction of specified finger with unspecified laterality

⑦S60.449   **External constriction of unspecified finger**

S60.45   **Superficial foreign body of fingers**

     Splinter in the finger(s)

⑦S60.450   **Superficial foreign body of right index finger**

⑦S60.451   **Superficial foreign body of left index finger**

⑦S60.452   **Superficial foreign body of right middle finger**

⑦S60.453   **Superficial foreign body of left middle finger**

⑦S60.454   **Superficial foreign body of right ring finger**

⑦S60.455   **Superficial foreign body of left ring finger**

⑦S60.456   **Superficial foreign body of right little finger**

⑦S60.457   **Superficial foreign body of left little finger**

⑦S60.458   **Superficial foreign body of other finger**

     Superficial foreign body of specified finger with unspecified laterality

⑦S60.459   **Superficial foreign body of unspecified finger**

S60.46   **Insect bite (nonvenomous) of fingers**

⑦S60.460   **Insect bite (nonvenomous) of right index finger**

⑦S60.461   **Insect bite (nonvenomous) of left index finger**

⑦S60.462   **Insect bite (nonvenomous) of right middle finger**

⑦S60.463   **Insect bite (nonvenomous) of left middle finger**

⑦S60.464   **Insect bite (nonvenomous) of right ring finger**

⑦S60.465   **Insect bite (nonvenomous) of left ring finger**

⑦S60.466   **Insect bite (nonvenomous) of right little finger**

⑦S60.467   **Insect bite (nonvenomous) of left little finger**

⑦S60.468   **Insect bite (nonvenomous) of other finger**

     Insect bite (nonvenomous) of specified finger with unspecified laterality

⑦S60.469   **Insect bite (nonvenomous) of unspecified finger**

S60.47   **Other superficial bite of fingers**

     Excludes1: open bite of fingers (S61.25-, S61.35-)

⑦S60.470   **Other superficial bite of right index finger**

⑦S60.471   **Other superficial bite of left index finger**

⑦S60.472   **Other superficial bite of right middle finger**

⑦S60.473   **Other superficial bite of left middle finger**

⑦S60.474   **Other superficial bite of right ring finger**

⑦S60.475   **Other superficial bite of left ring finger**

⑦S60.476   **Other superficial bite of right little finger**

⑦S60.477   **Other superficial bite of left little finger**

⑦S60.478   **Other superficial bite of other finger**

     Other superficial bite of specified finger with unspecified laterality

⑦S60.479   **Other superficial bite of unspecified finger**

S60.5   **Other superficial injuries of hand**

     Excludes2: superficial injuries of fingers (S60.3-, S60.4-)

S60.51　**Abrasion of hand**

⑦S60.511　**Abrasion of right hand**

⑦S60.512　**Abrasion of left hand**

⑦S60.519　**Abrasion of unspecified hand**

S60.52　**Blister (nonthermal) of hand**

⑦S60.521　**Blister (nonthermal) of right hand**

⑦S60.522　**Blister (nonthermal) of left hand**

⑦S60.529　**Blister (nonthermal) of unspecified hand**

S60.54　**External constriction of hand**

⑦S60.541　**External constriction of right hand**

⑦S60.542　**External constriction of left hand**

⑦S60.549　**External constriction of unspecified hand**

S60.55　**Superficial foreign body of hand**

Splinter in the hand

⑦S60.551　**Superficial foreign body of right hand**

⑦S60.552　**Superficial foreign body of left hand**

⑦S60.559　**Superficial foreign body of unspecified hand**

S60.56　**Insect bite (nonvenomous) of hand**

⑦S60.561　**Insect bite (nonvenomous) of right hand**

⑦S60.562　**Insect bite (nonvenomous) of left hand**

⑦S60.569　**Insect bite (nonvenomous) of unspecified hand**

S60.57　**Other superficial bite of hand**

Excludes1: open bite of hand (S61.45-)

⑦S60.571　**Other superficial bite of hand of right hand**

⑦S60.572　**Other superficial bite of hand of left hand**

⑦S60.579　**Other superficial bite of hand of unspecified hand**

S60.8　**Other superficial injuries of wrist**

S60.81　**Abrasion of wrist**

⑦S60.811　**Abrasion of right wrist**

⑦S60.812　**Abrasion of left wrist**

⑦S60.819　**Abrasion of unspecified wrist**

S60.82　**Blister (nonthermal) of wrist**

⑦S60.821　**Blister (nonthermal) of right wrist**

⑦S60.822　**Blister (nonthermal) of left wrist**

⑦S60.829　**Blister (nonthermal) of unspecified wrist**

S60.84　**External constriction of wrist**

⑦S60.841　**External constriction of right wrist**

⑦S60.842　**External constriction of left wrist**

⑦S60.849　**External constriction of unspecified wrist**

S60.85　**Superficial foreign body of wrist**

Splinter in the wrist

⑦S60.851　**Superficial foreign body of right wrist**

⑦S60.852　**Superficial foreign body of left wrist**

⑦S60.859　**Superficial foreign body of unspecified wrist**

S60.86　**Insect bite (nonvenomous) of wrist**

⑦S60.861　**Insect bite (nonvenomous) of right wrist**

⑦S60.862　**Insect bite (nonvenomous) of left wrist**

⑦S60.869　**Insect bite (nonvenomous) of unspecified wrist**

S60.87　**Other superficial bite of wrist**

Excludes1: open bite of wrist (S61.55)

⑦S60.871　**Other superficial bite of right wrist**

⑦S60.872　**Other superficial bite of left wrist**

⑦S60.879　**Other superficial bite of unspecified wrist**

S60.9　**Unspecified superficial injury of wrist, hand and fingers**

S60.91　**Unspecified superficial injury of wrist**

⑦S60.911　**Unspecified superficial injury of right wrist**

⑦S60.912　**Unspecified superficial injury of left wrist**

⑦S60.919　**Unspecified superficial injury of unspecified wrist**

S60.92　**Unspecified superficial injury of hand**

⑦S60.921　**Unspecified superficial injury of right hand**

⑦S60.922　**Unspecified superficial injury of left hand**

⑦S60.929　**Unspecified superficial injury of unspecified hand**

S60.93　**Unspecified superficial injury of thumb**

⑦S60.931　**Unspecified superficial injury of right thumb**

⑦S60.932　**Unspecified superficial injury of left thumb**

⑦S60.939　**Unspecified superficial injury of unspecified thumb**

S60.94　**Unspecified superficial injury of other fingers**

⑦S60.940　**Unspecified superficial injury of right index finger**

⑦S60.941　**Unspecified superficial injury of left index finger**

⑦S60.942　**Unspecified superficial injury of right middle finger**

⑦S60.943　**Unspecified superficial injury of left middle finger**

⑦S60.944　**Unspecified superficial injury of right ring finger**

⑦S60.945　**Unspecified superficial injury of left ring finger**

⑦S60.946　**Unspecified superficial injury of right little finger**

⑦S60.947　**Unspecified superficial injury of left little finger**

⑦S60.948　**Unspecified superficial injury of other finger**

Unspecified superficial injury of specified finger with unspecified laterality

⑦S60.949　**Unspecified superficial injury of unspecified finger**

S61　**Open wound of wrist, hand and fingers**

Code also any associated wound infection

Excludes1: open fracture of wrist, hand and finger (S62.- with 7th character B)

　● New code　▲ Revised code　**Excludes1:** Not coded here　**Excludes2:** Not included here　⊗ Placeholder required　⑦7ᵗʰ digit required

traumatic amputation of wrist and hand (S68.-)

The appropriate 7th character is to be added to each code from category S61

A - initial encounter

D - subsequent encounter

S - sequela

S61.0   Open wound of thumb without damage to nail

> Excludes1: open wound of thumb with damage to nail (S61.1-)

S61.00   Unspecified open wound of thumb without damage to nail

⑦**S61.001   Unspecified open wound of right thumb without damage to nail**

⑦**S61.002   Unspecified open wound of left thumb without damage to nail**

⑦**S61.009   Unspecified open wound of unspecified thumb without damage to nail**

⑦**S61.01 Laceration without foreign body of thumb without damage to nail**

⑦**S61.011   Laceration without foreign body of right thumb without damage to nail**

⑦**S61.012   Laceration without foreign body of left thumb without damage to nail**

⑦**S61.019   Laceration without foreign body of unspecified thumb without damage to nail**

S61.02   Laceration with foreign body of thumb without damage to nail

⑦**S61.021   Laceration with foreign body of right thumb without damage to nail**

⑦**S61.022   Laceration with foreign body of left thumb without damage to nail**

⑦**S61.029   Laceration with foreign body of unspecified thumb without damage to nail**

S61.03   Puncture wound without foreign body of thumb without damage to nail

⑦**S61.031   Puncture wound without foreign body of right thumb without damage to nail**

⑦**S61.032   Puncture wound without foreign body of left thumb without damage to nail**

⑦**S61.039   Puncture wound without foreign body of unspecified thumb without damage to nail**

S61.04   Puncture wound with foreign body of thumb without damage to nail

⑦**S61.041   Puncture wound with foreign body of right thumb without damage to nail**

⑦**S61.042   Puncture wound with foreign body of left thumb without damage to nail**

⑦**S61.049   Puncture wound with foreign body of unspecified thumb without damage to nail**

S61.05   Open bite of thumb without damage to nail

Bite of thumb NOS

> Excludes1: superficial bite of thumb (S60.36-, S60.37-)

⑦**S61.051   Open bite of right thumb without damage to nail**

⑦**S61.052   Open bite of left thumb without damage to nail**

⑦**S61.059   Open bite of unspecified thumb without damage to nail**

S61.1   Open wound of thumb with damage to nail

S61.10   Unspecified open wound of thumb with damage to nail

⑦**S61.101   Unspecified open wound of right thumb with damage to nail**

⑦**S61.102   Unspecified open wound of left thumb with damage to nail**

⑦**S61.109   Unspecified open wound of unspecified thumb with damage to nail**

S61.11   Laceration without foreign body of thumb with damage to nail

⑦**S61.111   Laceration without foreign body of right thumb with damage to nail**

⑦**S61.112   Laceration without foreign body of left thumb with damage to nail**

⑦**S61.119   Laceration without foreign body of unspecified thumb with damage to nail**

S61.12   Laceration with foreign body of thumb with damage to nail

⑦**S61.121   Laceration with foreign body of right thumb with damage to nail**

⑦**S61.122   Laceration with foreign body of left thumb with damage to nail**

⑦**S61.129   Laceration with foreign body of unspecified thumb with damage to nail**

S61.13   Puncture wound without foreign body of thumb with damage to nail

⑦**S61.131   Puncture wound without foreign body of right thumb with damage to nail**

⑦**S61.132   Puncture wound without foreign body of left thumb with damage to nail**

⑦**S61.139   Puncture wound without foreign body of unspecified thumb with damage to nail**

S61.14   Puncture wound with foreign body of thumb with damage to nail

⑦**S61.141   Puncture wound with foreign body of right thumb with damage to nail**

⑦**S61.142   Puncture wound with foreign body of left thumb with damage to nail**

⑦**S61.149   Puncture wound with foreign body of unspecified thumb with damage to nail**

S61.15   Open bite of thumb with damage to nail

Bite of thumb with damage to nail NOS

> Excludes1: superficial bite of thumb (S60.36-, S60.37-)

⑦**S61.151   Open bite of right thumb with damage to nail**

⑦**S61.152   Open bite of left thumb with damage to nail**

⑦**S61.159   Open bite of unspecified thumb with damage to nail**

S61.2   Open wound of other finger without damage to nail

> Excludes1: open wound of finger involving nail (matrix) (S61.3-)

> Excludes2: open wound of thumb without damage to nail (S61.0-)

S61.20 Unspecified open wound of other finger without damage to nail

⑦ **S61.200 Unspecified open wound of right index finger without damage to nail**

⑦ **S61.201 Unspecified open wound of left index finger without damage to nail**

⑦ **S61.202 Unspecified open wound of right middle finger without damage to nail**

⑦ **S61.203 Unspecified open wound of left middle finger without damage to nail**

⑦ **S61.204 Unspecified open wound of right ring finger without damage to nail**

⑦ **S61.205 Unspecified open wound of left ring finger without damage to nail**

⑦ **S61.206 Unspecified open wound of right little finger without damage to nail**

⑦ **S61.207 Unspecified open wound of left little finger without damage to nail**

⑦ **S61.208 Unspecified open wound of other finger without damage to nail**

Unspecified open wound of specified finger with unspecified laterality without damage to nail

⑦ **S61.209 Unspecified open wound of unspecified finger without damage to nail**

S61.21 Laceration without foreign body of finger without damage to nail

⑦ **S61.210 Laceration without foreign body of right index finger without damage to nail**

⑦ **S61.211 Laceration without foreign body of left index finger without damage to nail**

⑦ **S61.212 Laceration without foreign body of right middle finger without damage to nail**

⑦ **S61.213 Laceration without foreign body of left middle finger without damage to nail**

⑦ **S61.214 Laceration without foreign body of right ring finger without damage to nail**

⑦ **S61.215 Laceration without foreign body of left ring finger without damage to nail**

⑦ **S61.216 Laceration without foreign body of right little finger without damage to nail**

⑦ **S61.217 Laceration without foreign body of left little finger without damage to nail**

⑦ **S61.218 Laceration without foreign body of other finger without damage to nail**

Laceration without foreign body of specified finger with unspecified laterality without damage to nail

⑦ **S61.219 Laceration without foreign body of unspecified finger without damage to nail**

S61.22 Laceration with foreign body of finger without damage to nail

⑦ **S61.220 Laceration with foreign body of right index finger without damage to nail**

⑦ **S61.221 Laceration with foreign body of left index finger without damage to nail**

⑦ **S61.222 Laceration with foreign body of right middle finger without damage to nail**

⑦ **S61.223 Laceration with foreign body of left middle finger without damage to nail**

⑦ **S61.224 Laceration with foreign body of right ring finger without damage to nail**

⑦ **S61.225 Laceration with foreign body of left ring finger without damage to nail**

⑦ **S61.226 Laceration with foreign body of right little finger without damage to nail**

⑦ **S61.227 Laceration with foreign body of left little finger without damage to nail**

⑦ **S61.228 Laceration with foreign body of other finger without damage to nail**

Laceration with foreign body of specified finger with unspecified laterality without damage to nail

⑦ **S61.229 Laceration with foreign body of unspecified finger without damage to nail**

S61.23 Puncture wound without foreign body of finger without damage to nail

⑦ **S61.230 Puncture wound without foreign body of right index finger without damage to nail**

⑦ **S61.231 Puncture wound without foreign body of left index finger without damage to nail**

⑦ **S61.232 Puncture wound without foreign body of right middle finger without damage to nail**

⑦ **S61.233 Puncture wound without foreign body of left middle finger without damage to nail**

⑦ **S61.234 Puncture wound without foreign body of right ring finger without damage to nail**

⑦ **S61.235 Puncture wound without foreign body of left ring finger without damage to nail**

⑦ **S61.236 Puncture wound without foreign body of right little finger without damage to nail**

⑦ **S61.237 Puncture wound without foreign body of left little finger without damage to nail**

⑦ **S61.238 Puncture wound without foreign body of other finger without damage to nail**

Puncture wound without foreign body of specified finger with unspecified laterality without damage to nail

⑦ **S61.239 Puncture wound without foreign body of unspecified finger without damage to nail**

S61.24 Puncture wound with foreign body of finger without damage to nail

⑦ **S61.240 Puncture wound with foreign body of right index finger without damage to nail**

⑦ **S61.241 Puncture wound with foreign body of left index finger without damage to nail**

⑦ **S61.242 Puncture wound with foreign body of right middle finger without damage to nail**

● New code   ▲ Revised code   **Excludes1:** Not coded here   **Excludes2:** Not included here   ⊗ Placeholder required   ⑦ 7th digit required

⑦S61.243　Puncture wound with foreign body of left middle finger without damage to nail

⑦S61.244　Puncture wound with foreign body of right ring finger without damage to nail

⑦S61.245　Puncture wound with foreign body of left ring finger without damage to nail

⑦S61.246　Puncture wound with foreign body of right little finger without damage to nail

⑦S61.247　Puncture wound with foreign body of left little finger without damage to nail

⑦S61.248　Puncture wound with foreign body of other finger without damage to nail

Puncture wound with foreign body of specified finger with unspecified laterality without damage to nail

⑦S61.249　Puncture wound with foreign body of unspecified finger without damage to nail

S61.25　Open bite of finger without damage to nail

Bite of finger without damage to nail NOS

Excludes1: superficial bite of finger (S60.46-, S60.47-)

⑦S61.250　Open bite of right index finger without damage to nail

⑦S61.251　Open bite of left index finger without damage to nail

⑦S61.252　Open bite of right middle finger without damage to nail

⑦S61.253　Open bite of left middle finger without damage to nail

⑦S61.254　Open bite of right ring finger without damage to nail

⑦S61.255　Open bite of left ring finger without damage to nail

⑦S61.256　Open bite of right little finger without damage to nail

⑦S61.257　Open bite of left little finger without damage to nail

⑦S61.258　Open bite of other finger without damage to nail

Open bite of specified finger with unspecified laterality without damage to nail

⑦S61.259　Open bite of unspecified finger without damage to nail

S61.3　Open wound of other finger with damage to nail

S61.30　Unspecified open wound of finger with damage to nail

⑦S61.300　Unspecified open wound of right index finger with damage to nail

⑦S61.301　Unspecified open wound of left index finger with damage to nail

⑦S61.302　Unspecified open wound of right middle finger with damage to nail

⑦S61.303　Unspecified open wound of left middle finger with damage to nail

⑦S61.304　Unspecified open wound of right ring finger with damage to nail

⑦S61.305　Unspecified open wound of left ring finger with damage to nail

⑦S61.306　Unspecified open wound of right little finger with damage to nail

⑦S61.307　Unspecified open wound of left little finger with damage to nail

⑦S61.308　Unspecified open wound of other finger with damage to nail

Unspecified open wound of specified finger with unspecified laterality with damage to nail

⑦S61.309　Unspecified open wound of unspecified finger with damage to nail

S61.31　Laceration without foreign body of finger with damage to nail

⑦S61.310　Laceration without foreign body of right index finger with damage to nail

⑦S61.311　Laceration without foreign body of left index finger with damage to nail

⑦S61.312　Laceration without foreign body of right middle finger with damage to nail

⑦S61.313　Laceration without foreign body of left middle finger with damage to nail

⑦S61.314　Laceration without foreign body of right ring finger with damage to nail

⑦S61.315　Laceration without foreign body of left ring finger with damage to nail

⑦S61.316　Laceration without foreign body of right little finger with damage to nail

⑦S61.317　Laceration without foreign body of left little finger with damage to nail

⑦S61.318　Laceration without foreign body of other finger with damage to nail

Laceration without foreign body of specified finger with unspecified laterality with damage to nail

⑦S61.319　Laceration without foreign body of unspecified finger with damage to nail

S61.32　Laceration with foreign body of finger with damage to nail

⑦S61.320　Laceration with foreign body of right index finger with damage to nail

⑦S61.321　Laceration with foreign body of left index finger with damage to nail

⑦S61.322　Laceration with foreign body of right middle finger with damage to nail

⑦S61.323　Laceration with foreign body of left middle finger with damage to nail

⑦S61.324　Laceration with foreign body of right ring finger with damage to nail

⑦S61.325　Laceration with foreign body of left ring finger with damage to nail

⑦S61.326　Laceration with foreign body of right little finger with damage to nail

⑦S61.327　Laceration with foreign body of left little finger with damage to nail

⑦S61.328　Laceration with foreign body of other finger with damage to nail

Laceration with foreign body of specified finger with unspecified laterality with damage to nail

| ▓ Add 4th-7th digits | Nonspecific code | Unspecified code | Manifestation code | 819 |

⑦ **S61.329** Laceration with foreign body of unspecified finger with damage to nail

S61.33 **Puncture wound without foreign body of finger with damage to nail**

⑦ **S61.330** Puncture wound without foreign body of right index finger with damage to nail

⑦ **S61.331** Puncture wound without foreign body of left index finger with damage to nail

⑦ **S61.332** Puncture wound without foreign body of right middle finger with damage to nail

⑦ **S61.333** Puncture wound without foreign body of left middle finger with damage to nail

⑦ **S61.334** Puncture wound without foreign body of right ring finger with damage to nail

⑦ **S61.335** Puncture wound without foreign body of left ring finger with damage to nail

⑦ **S61.336** Puncture wound without foreign body of right little finger with damage to nail

⑦ **S61.337** Puncture wound without foreign body of left little finger with damage to nail

⑦ **S61.338** Puncture wound without foreign body of other finger with damage to nail

Puncture wound without foreign body of specified finger with unspecified laterality with damage to nail

⑦ **S61.339** Puncture wound without foreign body of unspecified finger with damage to nail

S61.34 **Puncture wound with foreign body of finger with damage to nail**

⑦ **S61.340** Puncture wound with foreign body of right index finger with damage to nail

⑦ **S61.341** Puncture wound with foreign body of left index finger with damage to nail

⑦ **S61.342** Puncture wound with foreign body of right middle finger with damage to nail

⑦ **S61.343** Puncture wound with foreign body of left middle finger with damage to nail

⑦ **S61.344** Puncture wound with foreign body of right ring finger with damage to nail

⑦ **S61.345** Puncture wound with foreign body of left ring finger with damage to nail

⑦ **S61.346** Puncture wound with foreign body of right little finger with damage to nail

⑦ **S61.347** Puncture wound with foreign body of left little finger with damage to nail

⑦ **S61.348** Puncture wound with foreign body of other finger with damage to nail

Puncture wound with foreign body of specified finger with unspecified laterality with damage to nail

⑦ **S61.349** Puncture wound with foreign body of unspecified finger with damage to nail

S61.35 **Open bite of finger with damage to nail**

Bite of finger with damage to nail NOS

Excludes1: superficial bite of finger (S60.46-, S60.47-)

⑦ **S61.350** Open bite of right index finger with damage to nail

⑦ **S61.351** Open bite of left index finger with damage to nail

⑦ **S61.352** Open bite of right middle finger with damage to nail

⑦ **S61.353** Open bite of left middle finger with damage to nail

⑦ **S61.354** Open bite of right ring finger with damage to nail

⑦ **S61.355** Open bite of left ring finger with damage to nail

⑦ **S61.356** Open bite of right little finger with damage to nail

⑦ **S61.357** Open bite of left little finger with damage to nail

⑦ **S61.358** Open bite of other finger with damage to nail

Open bite of specified finger with unspecified laterality with damage to nail

⑦ **S61.359** Open bite of unspecified finger with damage to nail

S61.4 **Open wound of hand**

S61.40 **Unspecified open wound of hand**

⑦ **S61.401** Unspecified open wound of right hand

⑦ **S61.402** Unspecified open wound of left hand

⑦ **S61.409** Unspecified open wound of unspecified hand

S61.41 **Laceration without foreign body of hand**

⑦ **S61.411** Laceration without foreign body of right hand

⑦ **S61.412** Laceration without foreign body of left hand

⑦ **S61.419** Laceration without foreign body of unspecified hand

S61.42 **Laceration with foreign body of hand**

⑦ **S61.421** Laceration with foreign body of right hand

⑦ **S61.422** Laceration with foreign body of left hand

⑦ **S61.429** Laceration with foreign body of unspecified hand

S61.43 **Puncture wound without foreign body of hand**

⑦ **S61.431** Puncture wound without foreign body of right hand

⑦ **S61.432** Puncture wound without foreign body of left hand

⑦ **S61.439** Puncture wound without foreign body of unspecified hand

S61.44 **Puncture wound with foreign body of hand**

⑦ **S61.441** Puncture wound with foreign body of right hand

⑦ **S61.442** Puncture wound with foreign body of left hand

S61.449 Puncture wound with foreign body of unspecified hand

S61.45 **Open bite of hand**

● New code ▲ Revised code **Excludes1:** Not coded here **Excludes2:** Not included here ⊗ Placeholder required ⑦ 7th digit required

Bite of hand NOS

Excludes1: superficial bite of hand (S60.56-, S60.57-)

⑦S61.451   **Open bite of right hand**

⑦S61.452   **Open bite of left hand**

⑦S61.459   **Open bite of unspecified hand**

S61.5   Open wound of wrist

S61.50   Unspecified open wound of wrist

⑦S61.501   **Unspecified open wound of right wrist**

⑦S61.502   **Unspecified open wound of left wrist**

⑦S61.509   **Unspecified open wound of unspecified wrist**

S61.51   Laceration without foreign body of wrist

⑦S61.511   **Laceration without foreign body of right wrist**

⑦S61.512   **Laceration without foreign body of left wrist**

⑦S61.519   **Laceration without foreign body of unspecified wrist**

S61.52   Laceration with foreign body of wrist

⑦S61.521   **Laceration with foreign body of right wrist**

⑦S61.522   **Laceration with foreign body of left wrist**

⑦S61.529   **Laceration with foreign body of unspecified wrist**

S61.53   Puncture wound without foreign body of wrist

⑦S61.531   **Puncture wound without foreign body of right wrist**

⑦S61.532   **Puncture wound without foreign body of left wrist**

⑦S61.539   **Puncture wound without foreign body of unspecified wrist**

S61.54   Puncture wound with foreign body of wrist

⑦S61.541   **Puncture wound with foreign body of right wrist**

⑦S61.542   **Puncture wound with foreign body of left wrist**

⑦S61.549   **Puncture wound with foreign body of unspecified wrist**

S61.55   Open bite of wrist

Bite of wrist NOS

Excludes1: superficial bite of wrist (S60.86-, S60.87-)

⑦S61.551   **Open bite of right wrist**

⑦S61.552   **Open bite of left wrist**

⑦S61.559   **Open bite of unspecified wrist**

S62   Fracture at wrist and hand level

Note: A fracture not indicated as displaced or nondisplaced should be coded to displaced

A fracture not indicated as open or closed should be coded to closed

Excludes1: traumatic amputation of wrist and hand (S68.-)

Excludes2: fracture of distal parts of ulna and radius (S52.-)

The appropriate 7th character is to be added to each code from category S62

A - initial encounter for closed fracture

B - initial encounter for open fracture

D - subsequent encounter for fracture with routine healing

G - subsequent encounter for fracture with delayed healing

K - subsequent encounter for fracture with nonunion

P - subsequent encounter for fracture with malunion

S - sequela

S62.0   Fracture of navicular [scaphoid] bone of wrist

S62.00   Unspecified fracture of navicular [scaphoid] bone of wrist

⑦S62.001   **Unspecified fracture of navicular [scaphoid] bone of right wrist**

⑦S62.002   **Unspecified fracture of navicular [scaphoid] bone of left wrist**

⑦S62.009   **Unspecified fracture of navicular [scaphoid] bone of unspecified wrist**

S62.01   Fracture of distal pole of navicular [scaphoid] bone of wrist

Fracture of volar tuberosity of navicular [scaphoid] bone of wrist

⑦S62.011   **Displaced fracture of distal pole of navicular [scaphoid] bone of right wrist**

⑦S62.012   **Displaced fracture of distal pole of navicular [scaphoid] bone of left wrist**

⑦S62.013   **Displaced fracture of distal pole of navicular [scaphoid] bone of unspecified wrist**

⑦S62.014   **Nondisplaced fracture of distal pole of navicular [scaphoid] bone of right wrist**

⑦S62.015   **Nondisplaced fracture of distal pole of navicular [scaphoid] bone of left wrist**

⑦S62.016   **Nondisplaced fracture of distal pole of navicular [scaphoid] bone of unspecified wrist**

S62.02   Fracture of middle third of navicular [scaphoid] bone of wrist

⑦S62.021   **Displaced fracture of middle third of navicular [scaphoid] bone of right wrist**

⑦S62.022   **Displaced fracture of middle third of navicular [scaphoid] bone of left wrist**

⑦S62.023   **Displaced fracture of middle third of navicular [scaphoid] bone of unspecified wrist**

⑦S62.024   **Nondisplaced fracture of middle third of navicular [scaphoid] bone of right wrist**

⑦S62.025   **Nondisplaced fracture of middle third of navicular [scaphoid] bone of left wrist**

⑦S62.026   **Nondisplaced fracture of middle third of navicular [scaphoid] bone of unspecified wrist**

S62.03   Fracture of proximal third of navicular [scaphoid] bone of wrist

⑦S62.031   **Displaced fracture of proximal third of navicular [scaphoid] bone of right wrist**

⑦S62.032   **Displaced fracture of proximal third of navicular [scaphoid] bone of left wrist**

⑦S62.033   **Displaced fracture of proximal third of navicular [scaphoid] bone of unspecified wrist**

⑦ S62.034 Nondisplaced fracture of proximal third of navicular [scaphoid] bone of right wrist

⑦ S62.035 Nondisplaced fracture of proximal third of navicular [scaphoid] bone of left wrist

⑦ S62.036 Nondisplaced fracture of proximal third of navicular [scaphoid] bone of unspecified wrist

S62.1 **Fracture of other and unspecified carpal bone(s)**

Excludes2: fracture of scaphoid of wrist (S62.0-)

S62.10 **Fracture of unspecified carpal bone**

Fracture of wrist NOS

⑦ S62.101 Fracture of unspecified carpal bone, right wrist

⑦ S62.102 Fracture of unspecified carpal bone, left wrist

⑦ S62.109 Fracture of unspecified carpal bone, unspecified wrist

S62.11 **Fracture of triquetrum [cuneiform] bone of wrist**

⑦ S62.111 Displaced fracture of triquetrum [cuneiform] bone, right wrist

⑦ S62.112 Displaced fracture of triquetrum [cuneiform] bone, left wrist

⑦ S62.113 Displaced fracture of triquetrum [cuneiform] bone, unspecified wrist

⑦ S62.114 Nondisplaced fracture of triquetrum [cuneiform] bone, right wrist

⑦ S62.115 Nondisplaced fracture of triquetrum [cuneiform] bone, left wrist

⑦ S62.116 Nondisplaced fracture of triquetrum [cuneiform] bone, unspecified wrist

S62.12 **Fracture of lunate [semilunar]**

⑦ S62.121 Displaced fracture of lunate [semilunar], right wrist

⑦ S62.122 Displaced fracture of lunate [semilunar], left wrist

⑦ S62.123 Displaced fracture of lunate [semilunar], unspecified wrist

⑦ S62.124 Nondisplaced fracture of lunate [semilunar], right wrist

⑦ S62.125 Nondisplaced fracture of lunate [semilunar], left wrist

⑦ S62.126 Nondisplaced fracture of lunate [semilunar], unspecified wrist

S62.13 **Fracture of capitate [os magnum] bone**

⑦ S62.131 Displaced fracture of capitate [os magnum] bone, right wrist

⑦ S62.132 Displaced fracture of capitate [os magnum] bone, left wrist

⑦ S62.133 Displaced fracture of capitate [os magnum] bone, unspecified wrist

⑦ S62.134 Nondisplaced fracture of capitate [os magnum] bone, right wrist

⑦ S62.135 Nondisplaced fracture of capitate [os magnum] bone, left wrist

⑦ S62.136 Nondisplaced fracture of capitate [os magnum] bone, unspecified wrist

S62.14 **Fracture of body of hamate [unciform] bone**

Fracture of hamate [unciform] bone NOS

⑦ S62.141 Displaced fracture of body of hamate [unciform] bone, right wrist

⑦ S62.142 Displaced fracture of body of hamate [unciform] bone, left wrist

⑦ S62.143 Displaced fracture of body of hamate [unciform] bone, unspecified wrist

⑦ S62.144 Nondisplaced fracture of body of hamate [unciform] bone, right wrist

⑦ S62.145 Nondisplaced fracture of body of hamate [unciform] bone, left wrist

⑦ S62.146 Nondisplaced fracture of body of hamate [unciform] bone, unspecified wrist

S62.15 **Fracture of hook process of hamate [unciform] bone**

Fracture of unciform process of hamate [unciform] bone

⑦ S62.151 Displaced fracture of hook process of hamate [unciform] bone, right wrist

⑦ S62.152 Displaced fracture of hook process of hamate [unciform] bone, left wrist

⑦ S62.153 Displaced fracture of hook process of hamate [unciform] bone, unspecified wrist

⑦ S62.154 Nondisplaced fracture of hook process of hamate [unciform] bone, right wrist

⑦ S62.155 Nondisplaced fracture of hook process of hamate [unciform] bone, left wrist

⑦ S62.156 Nondisplaced fracture of hook process of hamate [unciform] bone, unspecified wrist

S62.16 **Fracture of pisiform**

⑦ S62.161 Displaced fracture of pisiform, right wrist

⑦ S62.162 Displaced fracture of pisiform, left wrist

⑦ S62.163 Displaced fracture of pisiform, unspecified wrist

⑦ S62.164 Nondisplaced fracture of pisiform, right wrist

⑦ S62.165 Nondisplaced fracture of pisiform, left wrist

⑦ S62.166 Nondisplaced fracture of pisiform, unspecified wrist

S62.17 **Fracture of trapezium [larger multangular]**

⑦ S62.171 Displaced fracture of trapezium [larger multangular], right wrist

⑦ S62.172 Displaced fracture of trapezium [larger multangular], left wrist

⑦ S62.173 Displaced fracture of trapezium [larger multangular], unspecified wrist

⑦ S62.174 Nondisplaced fracture of trapezium [larger multangular], right wrist

⑦ S62.175 Nondisplaced fracture of trapezium [larger multangular], left wrist

⑦ S62.176 Nondisplaced fracture of trapezium [larger multangular], unspecified wrist

S62.18 **Fracture of trapezoid [smaller multangular]**

⑦ S62.181 Displaced fracture of trapezoid [smaller multangular], right wrist

⑦ S62.182 Displaced fracture of trapezoid [smaller multangular], left wrist

⑦S62.183   Displaced fracture of trapezoid [smaller multangular], unspecified wrist

⑦S62.184   Nondisplaced fracture of trapezoid [smaller multangular], right wrist

⑦S62.185   Nondisplaced fracture of trapezoid [smaller multangular], left wrist

⑦S62.186   Nondisplaced fracture of trapezoid [smaller multangular], unspecified wrist

S62.2   Fracture of first metacarpal bone

    S62.20   Unspecified fracture of first metacarpal bone

        ⑦S62.201   Unspecified fracture of first metacarpal bone, right hand

        ⑦S62.202   Unspecified fracture of first metacarpal bone, left hand

        ⑦S62.209   Unspecified fracture of first metacarpal bone, unspecified hand

    S62.21   Bennett's fracture

        ⑦S62.211   Bennett's fracture, right hand

        ⑦S62.212   Bennett's fracture, left hand

        ⑦S62.213   Bennett's fracture, unspecified hand

    S62.22   Rolando's fracture

        ⑦S62.221   Displaced Rolando's fracture, right hand

        ⑦S62.222   Displaced Rolando's fracture, left hand

        ⑦S62.223   Displaced Rolando's fracture, unspecified hand

        ⑦S62.224   Nondisplaced Rolando's fracture, right hand

        ⑦S62.225   Nondisplaced Rolando's fracture, left hand

        ⑦S62.226   Nondisplaced Rolando's fracture, unspecified hand

    S62.23   Other fracture of base of first metacarpal bone

        ⑦S62.231   Other displaced fracture of base of first metacarpal bone, right hand

        ⑦S62.232   Other displaced fracture of base of first metacarpal bone, left hand

        ⑦S62.233   Other displaced fracture of base of first metacarpal bone, unspecified hand

        ⑦S62.234   Other nondisplaced fracture of base of first metacarpal bone, right hand

        ⑦S62.235   Other nondisplaced fracture of base of first metacarpal bone, left hand

        ⑦S62.236   Other nondisplaced fracture of base of first metacarpal bone, unspecified hand

    S62.24   Fracture of shaft of first metacarpal bone

        ⑦S62.241   Displaced fracture of shaft of first metacarpal bone, right hand

        ⑦S62.242   Displaced fracture of shaft of first metacarpal bone, left hand

        ⑦S62.243   Displaced fracture of shaft of first metacarpal bone, unspecified hand

        ⑦S62.244   Nondisplaced fracture of shaft of first metacarpal bone, right hand

        ⑦S62.245   Nondisplaced fracture of shaft of first metacarpal bone, left hand

        ⑦S62.246   Nondisplaced fracture of shaft of first metacarpal bone, unspecified hand

    S62.25   Fracture of neck of first metacarpal bone

        ⑦S62.251   Displaced fracture of neck of first metacarpal bone, right hand

        ⑦S62.252   Displaced fracture of neck of first metacarpal bone, left hand

        ⑦S62.253   Displaced fracture of neck of first metacarpal bone, unspecified hand

        ⑦S62.254   Nondisplaced fracture of neck of first metacarpal bone, right hand

        ⑦S62.255   Nondisplaced fracture of neck of first metacarpal bone, left hand

        ⑦S62.256   Nondisplaced fracture of neck of first metacarpal bone, unspecified hand

    S62.29   Other fracture of first metacarpal bone

        ⑦S62.291   Other fracture of first metacarpal bone, right hand

        ⑦S62.292   Other fracture of first metacarpal bone, left hand

        ⑦S62.299   Other fracture of first metacarpal bone, unspecified hand

S62.3   Fracture of other and unspecified metacarpal bone

    Excludes2: fracture of first metacarpal bone (S62.2-)

    S62.30   Unspecified fracture of other metacarpal bone

        ⑦S62.300   Unspecified fracture of second metacarpal bone, right hand

        ⑦S62.301   Unspecified fracture of second metacarpal bone, left hand

        ⑦S62.302   Unspecified fracture of third metacarpal bone, right hand

        ⑦S62.303   Unspecified fracture of third metacarpal bone, left hand

        ⑦S62.304   Unspecified fracture of fourth metacarpal bone, right hand

        ⑦S62.305   Unspecified fracture of fourth metacarpal bone, left hand

        ⑦S62.306   Unspecified fracture of fifth metacarpal bone, right hand

        ⑦S62.307   Unspecified fracture of fifth metacarpal bone, left hand

        ⑦S62.308   Unspecified fracture of other metacarpal bone

                Unspecified fracture of specified metacarpal bone with unspecified laterality

        ⑦S62.309   Unspecified fracture of unspecified metacarpal bone

    S62.31   Displaced fracture of base of other metacarpal bone

        ⑦S62.310   Displaced fracture of base of second metacarpal bone, right hand

        ▲⑦S62.311   Displaced fracture of base of second metacarpal bone, left hand

        ⑦S62.312   Displaced fracture of base of third metacarpal bone, right hand

        ⑦S62.313   Displaced fracture of base of third metacarpal bone, left hand

        ⑦S62.314   Displaced fracture of base of fourth metacarpal bone, right hand

        ⑦S62.315   Displaced fracture of base of fourth metacarpal bone, left hand

        ⑦S62.316   Displaced fracture of base of fifth metacarpal bone, right hand

        ▲⑦S62.317   Displaced fracture of base of fifth metacarpal bone. left hand

---

⑦**S62.318** Displaced fracture of base of other metacarpal bone

Displaced fracture of base of specified metacarpal bone with unspecified laterality

⑦**S62.319** Displaced fracture of base of unspecified metacarpal bone

S62.32 Displaced fracture of shaft of other metacarpal bone

⑦**S62.320** Displaced fracture of shaft of second metacarpal bone, right hand

⑦**S62.321** Displaced fracture of shaft of second metacarpal bone, left hand

⑦**S62.322** Displaced fracture of shaft of third metacarpal bone, right hand

⑦**S62.323** Displaced fracture of shaft of third metacarpal bone, left hand

⑦**S62.324** Displaced fracture of shaft of fourth metacarpal bone, right hand

⑦**S62.325** Displaced fracture of shaft of fourth metacarpal bone, left hand

⑦**S62.326** Displaced fracture of shaft of fifth metacarpal bone, right hand

⑦**S62.327** Displaced fracture of shaft of fifth metacarpal bone, left hand

⑦**S62.328** Displaced fracture of shaft of other metacarpal bone

Displaced fracture of shaft of specified metacarpal bone with unspecified laterality

⑦**S62.329** Displaced fracture of shaft of unspecified metacarpal bone

S62.33 Displaced fracture of neck of other metacarpal bone

⑦**S62.330** Displaced fracture of neck of second metacarpal bone, right hand

⑦**S62.331** Displaced fracture of neck of second metacarpal bone, left hand

⑦**S62.332** Displaced fracture of neck of third metacarpal bone, right hand

⑦**S62.333** Displaced fracture of neck of third metacarpal bone, left hand

⑦**S62.334** Displaced fracture of neck of fourth metacarpal bone, right hand

⑦**S62.335** Displaced fracture of neck of fourth metacarpal bone, left hand

⑦**S62.336** Displaced fracture of neck of fifth metacarpal bone, right hand

⑦**S62.337** Displaced fracture of neck of fifth metacarpal bone, left hand

⑦**S62.338** Displaced fracture of neck of other metacarpal bone

Displaced fracture of neck of specified metacarpal bone with unspecified laterality

⑦**S62.339** Displaced fracture of neck of unspecified metacarpal bone

S62.34 Nondisplaced fracture of base of other metacarpal bone

⑦**S62.340** Nondisplaced fracture of base of second metacarpal bone, right hand

▲⑦**S62.341** Nondisplaced fracture of base of second metacarpal bone, left hand

⑦**S62.342** Nondisplaced fracture of base of third metacarpal bone, right hand

⑦**S62.343** Nondisplaced fracture of base of third metacarpal bone, left hand

⑦**S62.344** Nondisplaced fracture of base of fourth metacarpal bone, right hand

⑦**S62.345** Nondisplaced fracture of base of fourth metacarpal bone, left hand

⑦**S62.346** Nondisplaced fracture of base of fifth metacarpal bone, right hand

▲⑦**S62.347** Nondisplaced fracture of base of fifth metacarpal bone, left hand

⑦**S62.348** Nondisplaced fracture of base of other metacarpal bone

Nondisplaced fracture of base of specified metacarpal bone with unspecified laterality

⑦**S62.349** Nondisplaced fracture of base of unspecified metacarpal bone

S62.35 Nondisplaced fracture of shaft of other metacarpal bone

⑦**S62.350** Nondisplaced fracture of shaft of second metacarpal bone, right hand

⑦**S62.351** Nondisplaced fracture of shaft of second metacarpal bone, left hand

⑦**S62.352** Nondisplaced fracture of shaft of third metacarpal bone, right hand

⑦**S62.353** Nondisplaced fracture of shaft of third metacarpal bone, left hand

⑦**S62.354** Nondisplaced fracture of shaft of fourth metacarpal bone, right hand

⑦**S62.355** Nondisplaced fracture of shaft of fourth metacarpal bone, left hand

⑦**S62.356** Nondisplaced fracture of shaft of fifth metacarpal bone, right hand

⑦**S62.357** Nondisplaced fracture of shaft of fifth metacarpal bone, left hand

⑦**S62.358** Nondisplaced fracture of shaft of other metacarpal bone

Nondisplaced fracture of shaft of specified metacarpal bone with unspecified laterality

⑦**S62.359** Nondisplaced fracture of shaft of unspecified metacarpal bone

S62.36 Nondisplaced fracture of neck of other metacarpal bone

⑦**S62.360** Nondisplaced fracture of neck of second metacarpal bone, right hand

⑦**S62.361** Nondisplaced fracture of neck of second metacarpal bone, left hand

⑦**S62.362** Nondisplaced fracture of neck of third metacarpal bone, right hand

⑦**S62.363** Nondisplaced fracture of neck of third metacarpal bone, left hand

⑦**S62.364** Nondisplaced fracture of neck of fourth metacarpal bone, right hand

⑦**S62.365** Nondisplaced fracture of neck of fourth metacarpal bone, left hand

⑦**S62.366** Nondisplaced fracture of neck of fifth metacarpal bone, right hand

⑦**S62.367** Nondisplaced fracture of neck of fifth metacarpal bone, left hand

⑦**S62.368** Nondisplaced fracture of neck of other metacarpal bone

Nondisplaced fracture of neck of specified metacarpal bone with unspecified laterality

● New code   ▲ Revised code   **Excludes1:** Not coded here   **Excludes2:** Not included here   ⊗ Placeholder required   ⑦7th digit required

⑦S62.369 Nondisplaced fracture of neck of unspecified metacarpal bone

S62.39 Other fracture of other metacarpal bone

⑦S62.390 Other fracture of second metacarpal bone, right hand

⑦S62.391 Other fracture of second metacarpal bone, left hand

⑦S62.392 Other fracture of third metacarpal bone, right hand

⑦S62.393 Other fracture of third metacarpal bone, left hand

⑦S62.394 Other fracture of fourth metacarpal bone, right hand

⑦S62.395 Other fracture of fourth metacarpal bone, left hand

⑦S62.396 Other fracture of fifth metacarpal bone, right hand

⑦S62.397 Other fracture of fifth metacarpal bone, left hand

⑦S62.398 Other fracture of other metacarpal bone

Other fracture of specified metacarpal bone with unspecified laterality

⑦S62.399 Other fracture of unspecified metacarpal bone

S62.5 Fracture of thumb

S62.50 Fracture of unspecified phalanx of thumb

⑦S62.501 Fracture of unspecified phalanx of right thumb

⑦S62.502 Fracture of unspecified phalanx of left thumb

⑦S62.509 Fracture of unspecified phalanx of unspecified thumb

S62.51 Fracture of proximal phalanx of thumb

⑦S62.511 Displaced fracture of proximal phalanx of right thumb

⑦S62.512 Displaced fracture of proximal phalanx of left thumb

⑦S62.513 Displaced fracture of proximal phalanx of unspecified thumb

⑦S62.514 Nondisplaced fracture of proximal phalanx of right thumb

⑦S62.515 Nondisplaced fracture of proximal phalanx of left thumb

⑦S62.516 Nondisplaced fracture of proximal phalanx of unspecified thumb

S62.52 Fracture of distal phalanx of thumb

⑦S62.521 Displaced fracture of distal phalanx of right thumb

⑦S62.522 Displaced fracture of distal phalanx of left thumb

⑦S62.523 Displaced fracture of distal phalanx of unspecified thumb

⑦S62.524 Nondisplaced fracture of distal phalanx of right thumb

⑦S62.525 Nondisplaced fracture of distal phalanx of left thumb

⑦S62.526 Nondisplaced fracture of distal phalanx of unspecified thumb

S62.6 Fracture of other and unspecified finger(s)

Excludes2: fracture of thumb (S62.5-)

S62.60 Fracture of unspecified phalanx of finger

⑦S62.600 Fracture of unspecified phalanx of right index finger

⑦S62.601 Fracture of unspecified phalanx of left index finger

⑦S62.602 Fracture of unspecified phalanx of right middle finger

⑦S62.603 Fracture of unspecified phalanx of left middle finger

⑦S62.604 Fracture of unspecified phalanx of right ring finger

⑦S62.605 Fracture of unspecified phalanx of left ring finger

⑦S62.606 Fracture of unspecified phalanx of right little finger

⑦S62.607 Fracture of unspecified phalanx of left little finger

⑦S62.608 Fracture of unspecified phalanx of other finger

Fracture of unspecified phalanx of specified finger with unspecified laterality

⑦S62.609 Fracture of unspecified phalanx of unspecified finger

S62.61 Displaced fracture of proximal phalanx of finger

⑦S62.610 Displaced fracture of proximal phalanx of right index finger

⑦S62.611 Displaced fracture of proximal phalanx of left index finger

⑦S62.612 Displaced fracture of proximal phalanx of right middle finger

⑦S62.613 Displaced fracture of proximal phalanx of left middle finger

⑦S62.614 Displaced fracture of proximal phalanx of right ring finger

⑦S62.615 Displaced fracture of proximal phalanx of left ring finger

⑦S62.616 Displaced fracture of proximal phalanx of right little finger

⑦S62.617 Displaced fracture of proximal phalanx of left little finger

⑦S62.618 Displaced fracture of proximal phalanx of other finger

Displaced fracture of proximal phalanx of specified finger with unspecified laterality

⑦S62.619 Displaced fracture of proximal phalanx of unspecified finger

▲S62.62 Displaced fracture of middle phalanx of finger

▲⑦S62.620 Displaced fracture of middle phalanx of right index finger

▲⑦S62.621 Displaced fracture of middle phalanx of left index finger

▲⑦S62.622 Displaced fracture of middle phalanx of right middle finger

▲⑦S62.623 Displaced fracture of middle phalanx of left middle finger

▲⑦S62.624 Displaced fracture of middle phalanx of right ring finger

▲⑦S62.625 Displaced fracture of middle phalanx of left ring finger

⑦S62.626 Displaced fracture of middle phalanx of right little finger

▨ Add 4th-7th digits		Nonspecific code	Unspecified code	Manifestation code

⑦S62.627 Displaced fracture of middle phalanx of left little finger

⑦**S62.628** Displaced fracture of middle phalanx of other finger

Displaced fracture of middle phalanx of specified finger with unspecified laterality

⑦S62.629 Displaced fracture of middle phalanx of unspecified finger

S62.63 Displaced fracture of distal phalanx of finger

⑦S62.630 Displaced fracture of distal phalanx of right index finger

⑦S62.631 Displaced fracture of distal phalanx of left index finger

⑦S62.632 Displaced fracture of distal phalanx of right middle finger

⑦S62.633 Displaced fracture of distal phalanx of left middle finger

⑦S62.634 Displaced fracture of distal phalanx of right ring finger

⑦S62.635 Displaced fracture of distal phalanx of left ring finger

⑦S62.636 Displaced fracture of distal phalanx of right little finger

⑦S62.637 Displaced fracture of distal phalanx of left little finger

⑦**S62.638** Displaced fracture of distal phalanx of other finger

Displaced fracture of distal phalanx of specified finger with unspecified laterality

⑦**S62.639** Displaced fracture of distal phalanx of unspecified finger

S62.64 Nondisplaced fracture of proximal phalanx of finger

⑦S62.640 Nondisplaced fracture of proximal phalanx of right index finger

⑦S62.641 Nondisplaced fracture of proximal phalanx of left index finger

⑦S62.642 Nondisplaced fracture of proximal phalanx of right middle finger

⑦S62.643 Nondisplaced fracture of proximal phalanx of left middle finger

⑦S62.644 Nondisplaced fracture of proximal phalanx of right ring finger

⑦S62.645 Nondisplaced fracture of proximal phalanx of left ring finger

⑦S62.646 Nondisplaced fracture of proximal phalanx of right little finger

⑦S62.647 Nondisplaced fracture of proximal phalanx of left little finger

⑦**S62.648** Nondisplaced fracture of proximal phalanx of other finger

Nondisplaced fracture of proximal phalanx of specified finger with unspecified laterality

⑦S62.649 Nondisplaced fracture of proximal phalanx of unspecified finger

▲S62.65 Nondisplaced fracture of middle phalanx of finger

▲⑦S62.650 Nondisplaced fracture of middle phalanx of right index finger

▲⑦S62.651 Nondisplaced fracture of middle phalanx of left index finger

▲⑦S62.652 Nondisplaced fracture of middle phalanx of right middle finger

▲⑦S62.653 Nondisplaced fracture of middle phalanx of left middle finger

⑦S62.654 Nondisplaced fracture of middle phalanx of right ring finger

⑦S62.655 Nondisplaced fracture of middle phalanx of left ring finger

⑦S62.656 Nondisplaced fracture of middle phalanx of right little finger

⑦S62.657 Nondisplaced fracture of middle phalanx of left little finger

⑦**S62.658** Nondisplaced fracture of middle phalanx of other finger

Nondisplaced fracture of medial phalanx of specified finger with unspecified laterality

⑦**S62.659** Nondisplaced fracture of middle phalanx of unspecified finger

S62.66 Nondisplaced fracture of distal phalanx of finger

⑦S62.660 Nondisplaced fracture of distal phalanx of right index finger

⑦S62.661 Nondisplaced fracture of distal phalanx of left index finger

⑦S62.662 Nondisplaced fracture of distal phalanx of right middle finger

⑦S62.663 Nondisplaced fracture of distal phalanx of left middle finger

⑦S62.664 Nondisplaced fracture of distal phalanx of right ring finger

⑦S62.665 Nondisplaced fracture of distal phalanx of left ring finger

⑦S62.666 Nondisplaced fracture of distal phalanx of right little finger

⑦S62.667 Nondisplaced fracture of distal phalanx of left little finger

⑦**S62.668** Nondisplaced fracture of distal phalanx of other finger

Nondisplaced fracture of distal phalanx of specified finger with unspecified laterality

⑦S62.669 Nondisplaced fracture of distal phalanx of unspecified finger

S62.9 Unspecified fracture of wrist and hand

⊗⑦**S62.90** Unspecified fracture of unspecified wrist and hand

⊗⑦**S62.91** Unspecified fracture of right wrist and hand

⊗⑦**S62.92** Unspecified fracture of left wrist and hand

S63 Dislocation and sprain of joints and ligaments at wrist and hand level

Includes: avulsion of joint or ligament at wrist and hand level

laceration of cartilage, joint or ligament at wrist and hand level

sprain of cartilage, joint or ligament at wrist and hand level

traumatic hemarthrosis of joint or ligament at wrist and hand level

traumatic rupture of joint or ligament at wrist and hand level

traumatic subluxation of joint or ligament at wrist and hand level

traumatic tear of joint or ligament at wrist and hand level

Code also any associated open wound

● New code   ▲ Revised code   **Excludes1:** Not coded here   **Excludes2:** Not included here   ⊗ Placeholder required   ⑦ 7th digit required

Excludes2: strain of muscle, fascia and tendon of wrist and hand (S66.-)

The appropriate 7th character is to be added to each code from category S63

A - initial encounter

D - subsequent encounter

S - sequela

S63.0 **Subluxation and dislocation of wrist and hand joints**

    S63.00 **Unspecified subluxation and dislocation of wrist and hand**

        Dislocation of carpal bone NOS

        Dislocation of distal end of radius NOS

        Subluxation of carpal bone NOS

        Subluxation of distal end of radius NOS

      ⑦S63.001 **Unspecified subluxation of right wrist and hand**

      ⑦S63.002 **Unspecified subluxation of left wrist and hand**

      ⑦S63.003 **Unspecified subluxation of unspecified wrist and hand**

      ⑦S63.004 **Unspecified dislocation of right wrist and hand**

      ⑦S63.005 **Unspecified dislocation of left wrist and hand**

      ⑦S63.006 **Unspecified dislocation of unspecified wrist and hand**

    S63.01 **Subluxation and dislocation of distal radioulnar joint**

      ⑦S63.011 **Subluxation of distal radioulnar joint of right wrist**

      ⑦S63.012 **Subluxation of distal radioulnar joint of left wrist**

      ⑦S63.013 **Subluxation of distal radioulnar joint of unspecified wrist**

      ⑦S63.014 **Dislocation of distal radioulnar joint of right wrist**

      ⑦S63.015 **Dislocation of distal radioulnar joint of left wrist**

      ⑦S63.016 **Dislocation of distal radioulnar joint of unspecified wrist**

    S63.02 **Subluxation and dislocation of radiocarpal joint**

      ⑦S63.021 **Subluxation of radiocarpal joint of right wrist**

      ⑦S63.022 **Subluxation of radiocarpal joint of left wrist**

      ⑦S63.023 **Subluxation of radiocarpal joint of unspecified wrist**

      ⑦S63.024 **Dislocation of radiocarpal joint of right wrist**

      ⑦S63.025 **Dislocation of radiocarpal joint of left wrist**

      ⑦S63.026 **Dislocation of radiocarpal joint of unspecified wrist**

    S63.03 **Subluxation and dislocation of midcarpal joint**

      ⑦S63.031 **Subluxation of midcarpal joint of right wrist**

      ⑦S63.032 **Subluxation of midcarpal joint of left wrist**

      ⑦S63.033 **Subluxation of midcarpal joint of unspecified wrist**

      ⑦S63.034 **Dislocation of midcarpal joint of right wrist**

      ⑦S63.035 **Dislocation of midcarpal joint of left wrist**

      ⑦S63.036 **Dislocation of midcarpal joint of unspecified wrist**

    S63.04 **Subluxation and dislocation of carpometacarpal joint of thumb**

      Excludes2: interphalangeal subluxation and dislocation of thumb (S63.1-)

      ⑦S63.041 **Subluxation of carpometacarpal joint of right thumb**

      ⑦S63.042 **Subluxation of carpometacarpal joint of left thumb**

      ⑦S63.043 **Subluxation of carpometacarpal joint of unspecified thumb**

      ⑦S63.044 **Dislocation of carpometacarpal joint of right thumb**

      ⑦S63.045 **Dislocation of carpometacarpal joint of left thumb**

      ⑦S63.046 **Dislocation of carpometacarpal joint of unspecified thumb**

    S63.05 **Subluxation and dislocation of other carpometacarpal joint**

      Excludes2: subluxation and dislocation of carpometacarpal joint of thumb (S63.04-)

      ⑦S63.051 **Subluxation of other carpometacarpal joint of right hand**

      ⑦S63.052 **Subluxation of other carpometacarpal joint of left hand**

      ⑦S63.053 **Subluxation of other carpometacarpal joint of unspecified hand**

      ⑦S63.054 **Dislocation of other carpometacarpal joint of right hand**

      ⑦S63.055 **Dislocation of other carpometacarpal joint of left hand**

      ⑦S63.056 **Dislocation of other carpometacarpal joint of unspecified hand**

    S63.06 **Subluxation and dislocation of metacarpal (bone), proximal end**

      ⑦S63.061 **Subluxation of metacarpal (bone), proximal end of right hand**

      ⑦S63.062 **Subluxation of metacarpal (bone), proximal end of left hand**

      ⑦S63.063 **Subluxation of metacarpal (bone), proximal end of unspecified hand**

      ⑦S63.064 **Dislocation of metacarpal (bone), proximal end of right hand**

      ⑦S63.065 **Dislocation of metacarpal (bone), proximal end of left hand**

      ⑦S63.066 **Dislocation of metacarpal (bone), proximal end of unspecified hand**

    S63.07 **Subluxation and dislocation of distal end of ulna**

      ⑦S63.071 **Subluxation of distal end of right ulna**

      ⑦S63.072 **Subluxation of distal end of left ulna**

      ⑦S63.073 **Subluxation of distal end of unspecified ulna**

      ⑦S63.074 **Dislocation of distal end of right ulna**

      ⑦S63.075 **Dislocation of distal end of left ulna**

      ⑦S63.076 **Dislocation of distal end of unspecified ulna**

S63.09 **Other subluxation and dislocation of wrist and hand**

⑦ **S63.091** Other subluxation of right wrist and hand

⑦ **S63.092** Other subluxation of left wrist and hand

⑦ **S63.093** Other subluxation of unspecified wrist and hand

⑦ **S63.094** Other dislocation of right wrist and hand

⑦ **S63.095** Other dislocation of left wrist and hand

⑦ **S63.096** Other dislocation of unspecified wrist and hand

S63.1 **Subluxation and dislocation of thumb**

S63.10 **Unspecified subluxation and dislocation of thumb**

⑦ **S63.101** Unspecified subluxation of right thumb

⑦ **S63.102** Unspecified subluxation of left thumb

⑦ **S63.103** Unspecified subluxation of unspecified thumb

⑦ **S63.104** Unspecified dislocation of right thumb

⑦ **S63.105** Unspecified dislocation of left thumb

⑦ **S63.106** Unspecified dislocation of unspecified thumb

S63.11 **Subluxation and dislocation of metacarpophalangeal joint of thumb**

⑦ **S63.111** Subluxation of metacarpophalangeal joint of right thumb

⑦ **S63.112** Subluxation of metacarpophalangeal joint of left thumb

⑦ **S63.113** Subluxation of metacarpophalangeal joint of unspecified thumb

⑦ **S63.114** Dislocation of metacarpophalangeal joint of right thumb

⑦ **S63.115** Dislocation of metacarpophalangeal joint of left thumb

⑦ **S63.116** Dislocation of metacarpophalangeal joint of unspecified thumb

▲ **S63.12** **Subluxation and dislocation of interphalangeal joint of thumb**

▲⑦ **S63.121** Subluxation of interphalangeal joint of right thumb

▲⑦ **S63.122** Subluxation of interphalangeal joint of left thumb

▲⑦ **S63.123** Subluxation of interphalangeal joint of unspecified thumb

▲⑦ **S63.124** Dislocation of interphalangeal joint of right thumb

▲⑦ **S63.125** Dislocation of interphalangeal joint of left thumb

▲⑦ **S63.126** Dislocation of interphalangeal joint of unspecified thumb

S63.2 **Subluxation and dislocation of other finger(s)**

Excludes2: subluxation and dislocation of thumb (S63.1-)

S63.20 **Unspecified subluxation of other finger**

⑦ **S63.200** Unspecified subluxation of right index finger

⑦ **S63.201** Unspecified subluxation of left index finger

⑦ **S63.202** Unspecified subluxation of right middle finger

⑦ **S63.203** Unspecified subluxation of left middle finger

⑦ **S63.204** Unspecified subluxation of right ring finger

⑦ **S63.205** Unspecified subluxation of left ring finger

⑦ **S63.206** Unspecified subluxation of right little finger

⑦ **S63.207** Unspecified subluxation of left little finger

⑦ **S63.208** Unspecified subluxation of other finger

Unspecified subluxation of specified finger with unspecified laterality

⑦ **S63.209** Unspecified subluxation of unspecified finger

S63.21 **Subluxation of metacarpophalangeal joint of finger**

⑦ **S63.210** Subluxation of metacarpophalangeal joint of right index finger

⑦ **S63.211** Subluxation of metacarpophalangeal joint of left index finger

⑦ **S63.212** Subluxation of metacarpophalangeal joint of right middle finger

⑦ **S63.213** Subluxation of metacarpophalangeal joint of left middle finger

⑦ **S63.214** Subluxation of metacarpophalangeal joint of right ring finger

⑦ **S63.215** Subluxation of metacarpophalangeal joint of left ring finger

⑦ **S63.216** Subluxation of metacarpophalangeal joint of right little finger

⑦ **S63.217** Subluxation of metacarpophalangeal joint of left little finger

⑦ **S63.218** Subluxation of metacarpophalangeal joint of other finger

Subluxation of metacarpophalangeal joint of specified finger with unspecified laterality

⑦ **S63.219** Subluxation of metacarpophalangeal joint of unspecified finger

S63.22 **Subluxation of unspecified interphalangeal joint of finger**

⑦ **S63.220** Subluxation of unspecified interphalangeal joint of right index finger

⑦ **S63.221** Subluxation of unspecified interphalangeal joint of left index finger

⑦ **S63.222** Subluxation of unspecified interphalangeal joint of right middle finger

⑦ **S63.223** Subluxation of unspecified interphalangeal joint of left middle finger

⑦ **S63.224** Subluxation of unspecified interphalangeal joint of right ring finger

⑦ **S63.225** Subluxation of unspecified interphalangeal joint of left ring finger

● New code   ▲ Revised code   **Excludes1:** Not coded here   **Excludes2:** Not included here   ⊗ Placeholder required   ⑦ 7th digit required

⑦S63.226 **Subluxation of unspecified interphalangeal joint of right little finger**

⑦S63.227 **Subluxation of unspecified interphalangeal joint of left little finger**

⑦S63.228 **Subluxation of unspecified interphalangeal joint of other finger**

Subluxation of unspecified interphalangeal joint of specified finger with unspecified laterality

⑦S63.229 **Subluxation of unspecified interphalangeal joint of unspecified finger**

S63.23 **Subluxation of proximal interphalangeal joint of finger**

⑦S63.230 **Subluxation of proximal interphalangeal joint of right index finger**

⑦S63.231 **Subluxation of proximal interphalangeal joint of left index finger**

⑦S63.232 **Subluxation of proximal interphalangeal joint of right middle finger**

⑦S63.233 **Subluxation of proximal interphalangeal joint of left middle finger**

⑦S63.234 **Subluxation of proximal interphalangeal joint of right ring finger**

⑦S63.235 **Subluxation of proximal interphalangeal joint of left ring finger**

⑦S63.236 **Subluxation of proximal interphalangeal joint of right little finger**

⑦S63.237 **Subluxation of proximal interphalangeal joint of left little finger**

⑦S63.238 **Subluxation of proximal interphalangeal joint of other finger**

Subluxation of proximal interphalangeal joint of specified finger with unspecified laterality

⑦S63.239 **Subluxation of proximal interphalangeal joint of unspecified finger**

S63.24 **Subluxation of distal interphalangeal joint of finger**

⑦S63.240 **Subluxation of distal interphalangeal joint of right index finger**

⑦S63.241 **Subluxation of distal interphalangeal joint of left index finger**

⑦S63.242 **Subluxation of distal interphalangeal joint of right middle finger**

⑦S63.243 **Subluxation of distal interphalangeal joint of left middle finger**

⑦S63.244 **Subluxation of distal interphalangeal joint of right ring finger**

⑦S63.245 **Subluxation of distal interphalangeal joint of left ring finger**

⑦S63.246 **Subluxation of distal interphalangeal joint of right little finger**

⑦S63.247 **Subluxation of distal interphalangeal joint of left little finger**

⑦S63.248 **Subluxation of distal interphalangeal joint of other finger**

Subluxation of distal interphalangeal joint of specified finger with unspecified laterality

⑦S63.249 **Subluxation of distal interphalangeal joint of unspecified finger**

S63.25 **Unspecified dislocation of other finger**

⑦S63.250 **Unspecified dislocation of right index finger**

⑦S63.251 **Unspecified dislocation of left index finger**

⑦S63.252 **Unspecified dislocation of right middle finger**

⑦S63.253 **Unspecified dislocation of left middle finger**

⑦S63.254 **Unspecified dislocation of right ring finger**

⑦S63.255 **Unspecified dislocation of left ring finger**

⑦S63.256 **Unspecified dislocation of right little finger**

⑦S63.257 **Unspecified dislocation of left little finger**

⑦S63.258 **Unspecified dislocation of other finger**

Unspecified dislocation of specified finger with unspecified laterality

⑦S63.259 **Unspecified dislocation of unspecified finger**

Unspecified dislocation of unspecified finger with unspecified laterality

S63.26 **Dislocation of metacarpophalangeal joint of finger**

⑦S63.260 **Dislocation of metacarpophalangeal joint of right index finger**

⑦S63.261 **Dislocation of metacarpophalangeal joint of left index finger**

⑦S63.262 **Dislocation of metacarpophalangeal joint of right middle finger**

⑦S63.263 **Dislocation of metacarpophalangeal joint of left middle finger**

⑦S63.264 **Dislocation of metacarpophalangeal joint of right ring finger**

⑦S63.265 **Dislocation of metacarpophalangeal joint of left ring finger**

⑦S63.266 **Dislocation of metacarpophalangeal joint of right little finger**

⑦S63.267 **Dislocation of metacarpophalangeal joint of left little finger**

⑦S63.268 **Dislocation of metacarpophalangeal joint of other finger**

Dislocation of metacarpophalangeal joint of specified finger with unspecified laterality

⑦S63.269 **Dislocation of metacarpophalangeal joint of unspecified finger**

S63.27 **Dislocation of unspecified interphalangeal joint of finger**

⑦S63.270 **Dislocation of unspecified interphalangeal joint of right index finger**

⑦S63.271 **Dislocation of unspecified interphalangeal joint of left index finger**

⑦S63.272 **Dislocation of unspecified interphalangeal joint of right middle finger**

⑦S63.273 **Dislocation of unspecified interphalangeal joint of left middle finger**

⑦S63.274 **Dislocation of unspecified interphalangeal joint of right ring finger**

⑦S63.275 **Dislocation of unspecified interphalangeal joint of left ring finger**

⑦S63.276 **Dislocation of unspecified interphalangeal joint of right little finger**

⑦S63.277 **Dislocation of unspecified interphalangeal joint of left little finger**

⑦S63.278 **Dislocation of unspecified interphalangeal joint of other finger**

Dislocation of unspecified interphalangeal joint of specified finger with unspecified laterality

⑦S63.279 **Dislocation of unspecified interphalangeal joint of unspecified finger**

Dislocation of unspecified interphalangeal joint of unspecified finger without specified laterality

S63.28 **Dislocation of proximal interphalangeal joint of finger**

⑦S63.280 **Dislocation of proximal interphalangeal joint of right index finger**

⑦S63.281 **Dislocation of proximal interphalangeal joint of left index finger**

⑦S63.282 **Dislocation of proximal interphalangeal joint of right middle finger**

⑦S63.283 **Dislocation of proximal interphalangeal joint of left middle finger**

⑦S63.284 **Dislocation of proximal interphalangeal joint of right ring finger**

⑦S63.285 **Dislocation of proximal interphalangeal joint of left ring finger**

⑦S63.286 **Dislocation of proximal interphalangeal joint of right little finger**

⑦S63.287 **Dislocation of proximal interphalangeal joint of left little finger**

⑦S63.288 **Dislocation of proximal interphalangeal joint of other finger**

Dislocation of proximal interphalangeal joint of specified finger with unspecified laterality

⑦S63.289 **Dislocation of proximal interphalangeal joint of unspecified finger**

S63.29 **Dislocation of distal interphalangeal joint of finger**

⑦S63.290 **Dislocation of distal interphalangeal joint of right index finger**

⑦S63.291 **Dislocation of distal interphalangeal joint of left index finger**

⑦S63.292 **Dislocation of distal interphalangeal joint of right middle finger**

⑦S63.293 **Dislocation of distal interphalangeal joint of left middle finger**

⑦S63.294 **Dislocation of distal interphalangeal joint of right ring finger**

⑦S63.295 **Dislocation of distal interphalangeal joint of left ring finger**

⑦S63.296 **Dislocation of distal interphalangeal joint of right little finger**

⑦S63.297 **Dislocation of distal interphalangeal joint of left little finger**

⑦S63.298 **Dislocation of distal interphalangeal joint of other finger**

Dislocation of distal interphalangeal joint of specified finger with unspecified laterality

⑦S63.299 **Dislocation of distal interphalangeal joint of unspecified finger**

S63.3 **Traumatic rupture of ligament of wrist**

S63.30 **Traumatic rupture of unspecified ligament of wrist**

⑦S63.301 **Traumatic rupture of unspecified ligament of right wrist**

⑦S63.302 **Traumatic rupture of unspecified ligament of left wrist**

⑦S63.309 **Traumatic rupture of unspecified ligament of unspecified wrist**

S63.31 **Traumatic rupture of collateral ligament of wrist**

⑦S63.311 **Traumatic rupture of collateral ligament of right wrist**

⑦S63.312 **Traumatic rupture of collateral ligament of left wrist**

⑦S63.319 **Traumatic rupture of collateral ligament of unspecified wrist**

S63.32 **Traumatic rupture of radiocarpal ligament**

⑦S63.321 **Traumatic rupture of right radiocarpal ligament**

⑦S63.322 **Traumatic rupture of left radiocarpal ligament**

⑦S63.329 **Traumatic rupture of unspecified radiocarpal ligament**

S63.33 **Traumatic rupture of ulnocarpal (palmar) ligament**

⑦S63.331 **Traumatic rupture of right ulnocarpal (palmar) ligament**

⑦S63.332 **Traumatic rupture of left ulnocarpal (palmar) ligament**

⑦S63.339 **Traumatic rupture of unspecified ulnocarpal (palmar) ligament**

S63.39 **Traumatic rupture of other ligament of wrist**

⑦S63.391 **Traumatic rupture of other ligament of right wrist**

⑦S63.392 **Traumatic rupture of other ligament of left wrist**

⑦S63.399 **Traumatic rupture of other ligament of unspecified wrist**

S63.4 **Traumatic rupture of ligament of finger at metacarpophalangeal and interphalangeal joint(s)**

● New code ▲ Revised code **Excludes1:** Not coded here **Excludes2:** Not included here ⊗ Placeholder required ⑦ 7th digit required

S63.40　Traumatic rupture of unspecified ligament of finger at metacarpophalangeal and interphalangeal joint

⑦S63.400　Traumatic rupture of unspecified ligament of right index finger at metacarpophalangeal and interphalangeal joint

⑦S63.401　Traumatic rupture of unspecified ligament of left index finger at metacarpophalangeal and interphalangeal joint

⑦S63.402　Traumatic rupture of unspecified ligament of right middle finger at metacarpophalangeal and interphalangeal joint

⑦S63.403　Traumatic rupture of unspecified ligament of left middle finger at metacarpophalangeal and interphalangeal joint

⑦S63.404　Traumatic rupture of unspecified ligament of right ring finger at metacarpophalangeal and interphalangeal joint

⑦S63.405　Traumatic rupture of unspecified ligament of left ring finger at metacarpophalangeal and interphalangeal joint

⑦S63.406　Traumatic rupture of unspecified ligament of right little finger at metacarpophalangeal and interphalangeal joint

⑦S63.407　Traumatic rupture of unspecified ligament of left little finger at metacarpophalangeal and interphalangeal joint

⑦S63.408　Traumatic rupture of unspecified ligament of other finger at metacarpophalangeal and interphalangeal joint

Traumatic rupture of unspecified ligament of specified finger with unspecified laterality at metacarpophalangeal and interphalangeal joint

⑦S63.409　Traumatic rupture of unspecified ligament of unspecified finger at metacarpophalangeal and interphalangeal joint

S63.41　Traumatic rupture of collateral ligament of finger at metacarpophalangeal and interphalangeal joint

⑦S63.410　Traumatic rupture of collateral ligament of right index finger at metacarpophalangeal and interphalangeal joint

⑦S63.411　Traumatic rupture of collateral ligament of left index finger at metacarpophalangeal and interphalangeal joint

⑦S63.412　Traumatic rupture of collateral ligament of right middle finger at metacarpophalangeal and interphalangeal joint

⑦S63.413　Traumatic rupture of collateral ligament of left middle finger at metacarpophalangeal and interphalangeal joint

⑦S63.414　Traumatic rupture of collateral ligament of right ring finger at

metacarpophalangeal and interphalangeal joint

⑦S63.415　Traumatic rupture of collateral ligament of left ring finger at metacarpophalangeal and interphalangeal joint

⑦S63.416　Traumatic rupture of collateral ligament of right little finger at metacarpophalangeal and interphalangeal joint

⑦S63.417　Traumatic rupture of collateral ligament of left little finger at metacarpophalangeal and interphalangeal joint

⑦S63.418　Traumatic rupture of collateral ligament of other finger at metacarpophalangeal and interphalangeal joint

Traumatic rupture of collateral ligament of specified finger with unspecified laterality at metacarpophalangeal and interphalangeal joint

⑦S63.419　Traumatic rupture of collateral ligament of unspecified finger at metacarpophalangeal and interphalangeal joint

S63.42　Traumatic rupture of palmar ligament of finger at metacarpophalangeal and interphalangeal joint

⑦S63.420　Traumatic rupture of palmar ligament of right index finger at metacarpophalangeal and interphalangeal joint

⑦S63.421　Traumatic rupture of palmar ligament of left index finger at metacarpophalangeal and interphalangeal joint

⑦S63.422　Traumatic rupture of palmar ligament of right middle finger at metacarpophalangeal and interphalangeal joint

⑦S63.423　Traumatic rupture of palmar ligament of left middle finger at metacarpophalangeal and interphalangeal joint

⑦S63.424　Traumatic rupture of palmar ligament of right ring finger at metacarpophalangeal and interphalangeal joint

⑦S63.425　Traumatic rupture of palmar ligament of left ring finger at metacarpophalangeal and interphalangeal joint

⑦S63.426　Traumatic rupture of palmar ligament of right little finger at metacarpophalangeal and interphalangeal joint

⑦S63.427　Traumatic rupture of palmar ligament of left little finger at metacarpophalangeal and interphalangeal joint

⑦S63.428　Traumatic rupture of palmar ligament of other finger at metacarpophalangeal and interphalangeal joint

Traumatic rupture of palmar ligament of specified finger with unspecified laterality at metacarpophalangeal and interphalangeal joint

⑦**S63.429** **Traumatic rupture of palmar ligament of unspecified finger at metacarpophalangeal and interphalangeal joint**

S63.43 **Traumatic rupture of volar plate of finger at metacarpophalangeal and interphalangeal joint**

⑦**S63.430** **Traumatic rupture of volar plate of right index finger at metacarpophalangeal and interphalangeal joint**

⑦**S63.431** **Traumatic rupture of volar plate of left index finger at metacarpophalangeal and interphalangeal joint**

⑦**S63.432** **Traumatic rupture of volar plate of right middle finger at metacarpophalangeal and interphalangeal joint**

⑦**S63.433** **Traumatic rupture of volar plate of left middle finger at metacarpophalangeal and interphalangeal joint**

⑦**S63.434** **Traumatic rupture of volar plate of right ring finger at metacarpophalangeal and interphalangeal joint**

⑦**S63.435** **Traumatic rupture of volar plate of left ring finger at metacarpophalangeal and interphalangeal joint**

⑦**S63.436** **Traumatic rupture of volar plate of right little finger at metacarpophalangeal and interphalangeal joint**

⑦**S63.437** **Traumatic rupture of volar plate of left little finger at metacarpophalangeal and interphalangeal joint**

⑦**S63.438** **Traumatic rupture of volar plate of other finger at metacarpophalangeal and interphalangeal joint**

Traumatic rupture of volar plate of specified finger with unspecified laterality at metacarpophalangeal and interphalangeal joint

⑦**S63.439** **Traumatic rupture of volar plate of unspecified finger at metacarpophalangeal and interphalangeal joint**

S63.49 **Traumatic rupture of other ligament of finger at metacarpophalangeal and interphalangeal joint**

⑦**S63.490** **Traumatic rupture of other ligament of right index finger at metacarpophalangeal and interphalangeal joint**

⑦**S63.491** **Traumatic rupture of other ligament of left index finger at metacarpophalangeal and interphalangeal joint**

⑦**S63.492** **Traumatic rupture of other ligament of right middle finger at metacarpophalangeal and interphalangeal joint**

⑦**S63.493** **Traumatic rupture of other ligament of left middle finger at**

metacarpophalangeal and interphalangeal joint

⑦**S63.494** **Traumatic rupture of other ligament of right ring finger at metacarpophalangeal and interphalangeal joint**

⑦**S63.495** **Traumatic rupture of other ligament of left ring finger at metacarpophalangeal and interphalangeal joint**

⑦**S63.496** **Traumatic rupture of other ligament of right little finger at metacarpophalangeal and interphalangeal joint**

⑦**S63.497** **Traumatic rupture of other ligament of left little finger at metacarpophalangeal and interphalangeal joint**

⑦**S63.498** **Traumatic rupture of other ligament of other finger at metacarpophalangeal and interphalangeal joint**

Traumatic rupture of ligament of specified finger with unspecified laterality at metacarpophalangeal and interphalangeal joint

⑦**S63.499** **Traumatic rupture of other ligament of unspecified finger at metacarpophalangeal and interphalangeal joint**

S63.5 **Other and unspecified sprain of wrist**

S63.50 **Unspecified sprain of wrist**

⑦**S63.501** **Unspecified sprain of right wrist**

⑦**S63.502** **Unspecified sprain of left wrist**

⑦**S63.509** **Unspecified sprain of unspecified wrist**

S63.51 **Sprain of carpal (joint)**

⑦**S63.511** **Sprain of carpal joint of right wrist**

⑦**S63.512** **Sprain of carpal joint of left wrist**

⑦**S63.519** **Sprain of carpal joint of unspecified wrist**

S63.52 **Sprain of radiocarpal joint**

Excludes1: traumatic rupture of radiocarpal ligament (S63.32-)

⑦**S63.521** **Sprain of radiocarpal joint of right wrist**

⑦**S63.522** **Sprain of radiocarpal joint of left wrist**

⑦**S63.529** **Sprain of radiocarpal joint of unspecified wrist**

S63.59 **Other specified sprain of wrist**

⑦**S63.591** **Other specified sprain of right wrist**

⑦**S63.592** **Other specified sprain of left wrist**

⑦**S63.599** **Other specified sprain of unspecified wrist**

S63.6 **Other and unspecified sprain of finger(s)**

Excludes1: traumatic rupture of ligament of finger at metacarpophalangeal and interphalangeal joint(s) (S63.4-)

S63.60 **Unspecified sprain of thumb**

⑦**S63.601** **Unspecified sprain of right thumb**

⑦**S63.602** **Unspecified sprain of left thumb**

⑦**S63.609** **Unspecified sprain of unspecified thumb**

S63.61 Unspecified sprain of other and unspecified finger(s)

⑦**S63.610** Unspecified sprain of right index finger

⑦**S63.611** Unspecified sprain of left index finger

⑦**S63.612** Unspecified sprain of right middle finger

⑦**S63.613** Unspecified sprain of left middle finger

⑦**S63.614** Unspecified sprain of right ring finger

⑦**S63.615** Unspecified sprain of left ring finger

⑦**S63.616** Unspecified sprain of right little finger

⑦**S63.617** Unspecified sprain of left little finger

⑦**S63.618** Unspecified sprain of other finger

Unspecified sprain of specified finger with unspecified laterality

⑦**S63.619** Unspecified sprain of unspecified finger

S63.62 Sprain of interphalangeal joint of thumb

⑦**S63.621** Sprain of interphalangeal joint of right thumb

⑦**S63.622** Sprain of interphalangeal joint of left thumb

⑦**S63.629** Sprain of interphalangeal joint of unspecified thumb

S63.63 Sprain of interphalangeal joint of other and unspecified finger(s)

⑦**S63.630** Sprain of interphalangeal joint of right index finger

⑦**S63.631** Sprain of interphalangeal joint of left index finger

⑦**S63.632** Sprain of interphalangeal joint of right middle finger

⑦**S63.633** Sprain of interphalangeal joint of left middle finger

⑦**S63.634** Sprain of interphalangeal joint of right ring finger

⑦**S63.635** Sprain of interphalangeal joint of left ring finger

⑦**S63.636** Sprain of interphalangeal joint of right little finger

⑦**S63.637** Sprain of interphalangeal joint of left little finger

⑦**S63.638** Sprain of interphalangeal joint of other finger

⑦**S63.639** Sprain of interphalangeal joint of unspecified finger

S63.64 Sprain of metacarpophalangeal joint of thumb

⑦**S63.641** Sprain of metacarpophalangeal joint of right thumb

⑦**S63.642** Sprain of metacarpophalangeal joint of left thumb

S63.649 Sprain of metacarpophalangeal joint of unspecified thumb

S63.65 Sprain of metacarpophalangeal joint of other and unspecified finger(s)

⑦**S63.650** Sprain of metacarpophalangeal joint of right index finger

⑦**S63.651** Sprain of metacarpophalangeal joint of left index finger

⑦**S63.652** Sprain of metacarpophalangeal joint of right middle finger

⑦**S63.653** Sprain of metacarpophalangeal joint of left middle finger

⑦**S63.654** Sprain of metacarpophalangeal joint of right ring finger

⑦**S63.655** Sprain of metacarpophalangeal joint of left ring finger

⑦**S63.656** Sprain of metacarpophalangeal joint of right little finger

⑦**S63.657** Sprain of metacarpophalangeal joint of left little finger

⑦**S63.658** Sprain of metacarpophalangeal joint of other finger

Sprain of metacarpophalangeal joint of specified finger with unspecified laterality

⑦**S63.659** Sprain of metacarpophalangeal joint of unspecified finger

S63.68 Other sprain of thumb

⑦**S63.681** Other sprain of right thumb

⑦**S63.682** Other sprain of left thumb

⑦**S63.689** Other sprain of unspecified thumb

S63.69 Other sprain of other and unspecified finger(s)

⑦**S63.690** Other sprain of right index finger

⑦**S63.691** Other sprain of left index finger

⑦**S63.692** Other sprain of right middle finger

⑦**S63.693** Other sprain of left middle finger

⑦**S63.694** Other sprain of right ring finger

⑦**S63.695** Other sprain of left ring finger

⑦**S63.696** Other sprain of right little finger

⑦**S63.697** Other sprain of left little finger

⑦**S63.698** Other sprain of other finger

Other sprain of specified finger with unspecified laterality

⑦**S63.699** Other sprain of unspecified finger

S63.8 Sprain of other part of wrist and hand

S63.8X Sprain of other part of wrist and hand

⑦**S63.8X1** Sprain of other part of right wrist and hand

⑦**S63.8X2** Sprain of other part of left wrist and hand

⑦**S63.8X9** Sprain of other part of unspecified wrist and hand

S63.9 Sprain of unspecified part of wrist and hand

⊗⑦**S63.90** Sprain of unspecified part of unspecified wrist and hand

⊗⑦**S63.91** Sprain of unspecified part of right wrist and hand

⊗⑦**S63.92** Sprain of unspecified part of left wrist and hand

S64 **Injury of nerves at wrist and hand level**

<u>Code also</u> any associated open wound (S61.-)

The appropriate 7th character is to be added to each code from category S64

A - initial encounter

D - subsequent encounter

S - sequela

S64.0 Injury of ulnar nerve at wrist and hand level

⊗⑦**S64.00** Injury of ulnar nerve at wrist and hand level of unspecified arm

⊗⑦**S64.01** Injury of ulnar nerve at wrist and hand level of right arm

⊗⑦**S64.02** Injury of ulnar nerve at wrist and hand level of left arm

S64.1 Injury of median nerve at wrist and hand level

⊗⑦**S64.10** Injury of median nerve at wrist and hand level of unspecified arm

⊗⑦**S64.11** Injury of median nerve at wrist and hand level of right arm

⊗⑦**S64.12** Injury of median nerve at wrist and hand level of left arm

S64.2 Injury of radial nerve at wrist and hand level

⊗⑦**S64.20** Injury of radial nerve at wrist and hand level of unspecified arm

⊗⑦**S64.21** Injury of radial nerve at wrist and hand level of right arm

⊗⑦**S64.22** Injury of radial nerve at wrist and hand level of left arm

S64.3 Injury of digital nerve of thumb

⊗⑦**S64.30** Injury of digital nerve of unspecified thumb

⊗⑦**S64.31** Injury of digital nerve of right thumb

⊗⑦**S64.32** Injury of digital nerve of left thumb

S64.4 Injury of digital nerve of other and unspecified finger

⊗⑦**S64.40** Injury of digital nerve of unspecified finger

S64.49 Injury of digital nerve of other finger

⑦**S64.490** Injury of digital nerve of right index finger

⑦**S64.491** Injury of digital nerve of left index finger

⑦**S64.492** Injury of digital nerve of right middle finger

⑦**S64.493** Injury of digital nerve of left middle finger

⑦**S64.494** Injury of digital nerve of right ring finger

⑦**S64.495** Injury of digital nerve of left ring finger

⑦**S64.496** Injury of digital nerve of right little finger

⑦**S64.497** Injury of digital nerve of left little finger

⑦**S64.498** Injury of digital nerve of other finger

Injury of digital nerve of specified finger with unspecified laterality

S64.8 Injury of other nerves at wrist and hand level

S64.8X Injury of other nerves at wrist and hand level

⑦**S64.8X1** Injury of other nerves at wrist and hand level of right arm

⑦**S64.8X2** Injury of other nerves at wrist and hand level of left arm

⑦**S64.8X9** Injury of other nerves at wrist and hand level of unspecified arm

S64.9 Injury of unspecified nerve at wrist and hand level

⊗⑦**S64.90** Injury of unspecified nerve at wrist and hand level of unspecified arm

⊗⑦**S64.91** Injury of unspecified nerve at wrist and hand level of right arm

⊗⑦**S64.92** Injury of unspecified nerve at wrist and hand level of left arm

S65 Injury of blood vessels at wrist and hand level

Code also any associated open wound (S61.-)

The appropriate 7th character is to be added to each code from category S65

A - initial encounter

D - subsequent encounter

S - sequela

S65.0 Injury of ulnar artery at wrist and hand level

S65.00 Unspecified injury of ulnar artery at wrist and hand level

⑦**S65.001** Unspecified injury of ulnar artery at wrist and hand level of right arm

⑦**S65.002** Unspecified injury of ulnar artery at wrist and hand level of left arm

⑦**S65.009** Unspecified injury of ulnar artery at wrist and hand level of unspecified arm

S65.01 Laceration of ulnar artery at wrist and hand level

⑦**S65.011** Laceration of ulnar artery at wrist and hand level of right arm

⑦**S65.012** Laceration of ulnar artery at wrist and hand level of left arm

⑦**S65.019** Laceration of ulnar artery at wrist and hand level of unspecified arm

S65.09 Other specified injury of ulnar artery at wrist and hand level

⑦**S65.091** Other specified injury of ulnar artery at wrist and hand level of right arm

⑦**S65.092** Other specified injury of ulnar artery at wrist and hand level of left arm

⑦**S65.099** Other specified injury of ulnar artery at wrist and hand level of unspecified arm

S65.1 Injury of radial artery at wrist and hand level

S65.10 Unspecified injury of radial artery at wrist and hand level

⑦**S65.101** Unspecified injury of radial artery at wrist and hand level of right arm

⑦**S65.102** Unspecified injury of radial artery at wrist and hand level of left arm

⑦**S65.109** Unspecified injury of radial artery at wrist and hand level of unspecified arm

S65.11 Laceration of radial artery at wrist and hand level

⑦**S65.111** Laceration of radial artery at wrist and hand level of right arm

⑦**S65.112** Laceration of radial artery at wrist and hand level of left arm

⑦**S65.119** Laceration of radial artery at wrist and hand level of unspecified arm

S65.19 Other specified injury of radial artery at wrist and hand level

⑦**S65.191** Other specified injury of radial artery at wrist and hand level of right arm

⑦**S65.192** Other specified injury of radial artery at wrist and hand level of left arm

⑦**S65.199** Other specified injury of radial artery at wrist and hand level of unspecified arm

S65.2 Injury of superficial palmar arch

● New code ▲ Revised code **Excludes1:** Not coded here **Excludes2:** Not included here ⊗ Placeholder required ⑦ 7th digit required

S65.20 Unspecified injury of superficial palmar arch

⑦ **S65.201** Unspecified injury of superficial palmar arch of right hand

⑦ **S65.202** Unspecified injury of superficial palmar arch of left hand

⑦ **S65.209** Unspecified injury of superficial palmar arch of unspecified hand

S65.21 Laceration of superficial palmar arch

⑦ **S65.211** Laceration of superficial palmar arch of right hand

⑦ **S65.212** Laceration of superficial palmar arch of left hand

⑦ **S65.219** Laceration of superficial palmar arch of unspecified hand

S65.29 Other specified injury of superficial palmar arch

⑦ **S65.291** Other specified injury of superficial palmar arch of right hand

⑦ **S65.292** Other specified injury of superficial palmar arch of left hand

⑦ **S65.299** Other specified injury of superficial palmar arch of unspecified hand

S65.3 Injury of deep palmar arch

S65.30 Unspecified injury of deep palmar arch

⑦ **S65.301** Unspecified injury of deep palmar arch of right hand

⑦ **S65.302** Unspecified injury of deep palmar arch of left hand

⑦ **S65.309** Unspecified injury of deep palmar arch of unspecified hand

S65.31 Laceration of deep palmar arch

⑦ **S65.311** Laceration of deep palmar arch of right hand

⑦ **S65.312** Laceration of deep palmar arch of left hand

⑦ **S65.319** Laceration of deep palmar arch of unspecified hand

S65.39 Other specified injury of deep palmar arch

⑦ **S65.391** Other specified injury of deep palmar arch of right hand

⑦ **S65.392** Other specified injury of deep palmar arch of left hand

⑦ **S65.399** Other specified injury of deep palmar arch of unspecified hand

S65.4 Injury of blood vessel of thumb

S65.40 Unspecified injury of blood vessel of thumb

⑦ **S65.401** Unspecified injury of blood vessel of right thumb

⑦ **S65.402** Unspecified injury of blood vessel of left thumb

⑦ **S65.409** Unspecified injury of blood vessel of unspecified thumb

S65.41 Laceration of blood vessel of thumb

⑦ **S65.411** Laceration of blood vessel of right thumb

⑦ **S65.412** Laceration of blood vessel of left thumb

⑦ **S65.419** Laceration of blood vessel of unspecified thumb

S65.49 Other specified injury of blood vessel of thumb

⑦ **S65.491** Other specified injury of blood vessel of right thumb

⑦ **S65.492** Other specified injury of blood vessel of left thumb

⑦ **S65.499** Other specified injury of blood vessel of unspecified thumb

S65.5 Injury of blood vessel of other and unspecified finger

S65.50 Unspecified injury of blood vessel of other and unspecified finger

⑦ **S65.500** Unspecified injury of blood vessel of right index finger

⑦ **S65.501** Unspecified injury of blood vessel of left index finger

⑦ **S65.502** Unspecified injury of blood vessel of right middle finger

⑦ **S65.503** Unspecified injury of blood vessel of left middle finger

⑦ **S65.504** Unspecified injury of blood vessel of right ring finger

⑦ **S65.505** Unspecified injury of blood vessel of left ring finger

⑦ **S65.506** Unspecified injury of blood vessel of right little finger

⑦ **S65.507** Unspecified injury of blood vessel of left little finger

⑦ **S65.508** Unspecified injury of blood vessel of other finger

Unspecified injury of blood vessel of specified finger with unspecified laterality

⑦ **S65.509** Unspecified injury of blood vessel of unspecified finger

S65.51 Laceration of blood vessel of other and unspecified finger

⑦ **S65.510** Laceration of blood vessel of right index finger

⑦ **S65.511** Laceration of blood vessel of left index finger

⑦ **S65.512** Laceration of blood vessel of right middle finger

⑦ **S65.513** Laceration of blood vessel of left middle finger

⑦ **S65.514** Laceration of blood vessel of right ring finger

⑦ **S65.515** Laceration of blood vessel of left ring finger

⑦ **S65.516** Laceration of blood vessel of right little finger

⑦ **S65.517** Laceration of blood vessel of left little finger

⑦ **S65.518** Laceration of blood vessel of other finger

Laceration of blood vessel of specified finger with unspecified laterality

⑦ **S65.519** Laceration of blood vessel of unspecified finger

S65.59 Other specified injury of blood vessel of other and unspecified finger

⑦ **S65.590** Other specified injury of blood vessel of right index finger

⑦ **S65.591** Other specified injury of blood vessel of left index finger

⑦ **S65.592** Other specified injury of blood vessel of right middle finger

⑦ **S65.593** Other specified injury of blood vessel of left middle finger

⑦**S65.594** Other specified injury of blood vessel of right ring finger

⑦**S65.595** Other specified injury of blood vessel of left ring finger

⑦**S65.596** Other specified injury of blood vessel of right little finger

⑦**S65.597** Other specified injury of blood vessel of left little finger

⑦**S65.598** Other specified injury of blood vessel of other finger

Other specified injury of blood vessel of specified finger with unspecified laterality

⑦**S65.599** Other specified injury of blood vessel of unspecified finger

S65.8 Injury of other blood vessels at wrist and hand level

S65.80 Unspecified injury of other blood vessels at wrist and hand level

⑦**S65.801** Unspecified injury of other blood vessels at wrist and hand level of right arm

⑦**S65.802** Unspecified injury of other blood vessels at wrist and hand level of left arm

⑦**S65.809** Unspecified injury of other blood vessels at wrist and hand level of unspecified arm

S65.81 Laceration of other blood vessels at wrist and hand level

⑦**S65.811** Laceration of other blood vessels at wrist and hand level of right arm

⑦**S65.812** Laceration of other blood vessels at wrist and hand level of left arm

⑦**S65.819** Laceration of other blood vessels at wrist and hand level of unspecified arm

S65.89 Other specified injury of other blood vessels at wrist and hand level

⑦**S65.891** Other specified injury of other blood vessels at wrist and hand level of right arm

⑦**S65.892** Other specified injury of other blood vessels at wrist and hand level of left arm

⑦**S65.899** Other specified injury of other blood vessels at wrist and hand level of unspecified arm

S65.9 Injury of unspecified blood vessel at wrist and hand level

S65.90 Unspecified injury of unspecified blood vessel at wrist and hand level

⑦**S65.901** Unspecified injury of unspecified blood vessel at wrist and hand level of right arm

⑦**S65.902** Unspecified injury of unspecified blood vessel at wrist and hand level of left arm

⑦**S65.909** Unspecified injury of unspecified blood vessel at wrist and hand level of unspecified arm

S65.91 Laceration of unspecified blood vessel at wrist and hand level

⑦**S65.911** Laceration of unspecified blood vessel at wrist and hand level of right arm

⑦**S65.912** Laceration of unspecified blood vessel at wrist and hand level of left arm

⑦**S65.919** Laceration of unspecified blood vessel at wrist and hand level of unspecified arm

S65.99 Other specified injury of unspecified blood vessel at wrist and hand level

⑦**S65.991** Other specified injury of unspecified blood vessel at wrist and hand of right arm

⑦**S65.992** Other specified injury of unspecified blood vessel at wrist and hand of left arm

⑦**S65.999** Other specified injury of unspecified blood vessel at wrist and hand of unspecified arm

S66 Injury of muscle, fascia and tendon at wrist and hand level

Code also any associated open wound (S61.-)

Excludes2: sprain of joints and ligaments of wrist and hand (S63.-)

The appropriate 7th character is to be added to each code from category S66

A - initial encounter

D - subsequent encounter

S - sequela

S66.0 Injury of long flexor muscle, fascia and tendon of thumb at wrist and hand level

S66.00 Unspecified injury of long flexor muscle, fascia and tendon of thumb at wrist and hand level

⑦**S66.001** Unspecified injury of long flexor muscle, fascia and tendon of right thumb at wrist and hand level

⑦**S66.002** Unspecified injury of long flexor muscle, fascia and tendon of left thumb at wrist and hand level

⑦**S66.009** Unspecified injury of long flexor muscle, fascia and tendon of unspecified thumb at wrist and hand level

S66.01 Strain of long flexor muscle, fascia and tendon of thumb at wrist and hand level

⑦**S66.011** Strain of long flexor muscle, fascia and tendon of right thumb at wrist and hand level

⑦**S66.012** Strain of long flexor muscle, fascia and tendon of left thumb at wrist and hand level

⑦**S66.019** Strain of long flexor muscle, fascia and tendon of unspecified thumb at wrist and hand level

S66.02 Laceration of long flexor muscle, fascia and tendon of thumb at wrist and hand level

⑦**S66.021** Laceration of long flexor muscle, fascia and tendon of right thumb at wrist and hand level

⑦**S66.022** Laceration of long flexor muscle, fascia and tendon of left thumb at wrist and hand level

⑦**S66.029** Laceration of long flexor muscle, fascia and tendon of unspecified thumb at wrist and hand level

S66.09 Other specified injury of long flexor muscle, fascia and tendon of thumb at wrist and hand level

● New code ▲ Revised code **Excludes1:** Not coded here **Excludes2:** Not included here ⊗ Placeholder required ⑦7ᵗʰ digit required

⑦S66.091   **Other specified injury of long flexor muscle, fascia and tendon of right thumb at wrist and hand level**

⑦S66.092   **Other specified injury of long flexor muscle, fascia and tendon of left thumb at wrist and hand level**

⑦S66.099   **Other specified injury of long flexor muscle, fascia and tendon of unspecified thumb at wrist and hand level**

S66.1   **Injury of flexor muscle, fascia and tendon of other and unspecified finger at wrist and hand level**

Excludes2: Injury of long flexor muscle, fascia and tendon of thumb at wrist and hand level (S66.0-)

S66.10   **Unspecified injury of flexor muscle, fascia and tendon of other and unspecified finger at wrist and hand level**

⑦S66.100   **Unspecified injury of flexor muscle, fascia and tendon of right index finger at wrist and hand level**

⑦S66.101   **Unspecified injury of flexor muscle, fascia and tendon of left index finger at wrist and hand level**

⑦S66.102   **Unspecified injury of flexor muscle, fascia and tendon of right middle finger at wrist and hand level**

⑦S66.103   **Unspecified injury of flexor muscle, fascia and tendon of left middle finger at wrist and hand level**

⑦S66.104   **Unspecified injury of flexor muscle, fascia and tendon of right ring finger at wrist and hand level**

⑦S66.105   **Unspecified injury of flexor muscle, fascia and tendon of left ring finger at wrist and hand level**

⑦S66.106   **Unspecified injury of flexor muscle, fascia and tendon of right little finger at wrist and hand level**

⑦S66.107   **Unspecified injury of flexor muscle, fascia and tendon of left little finger at wrist and hand level**

⑦S66.108   **Unspecified injury of flexor muscle, fascia and tendon of other finger at wrist and hand level**

Unspecified injury of flexor muscle, fascia and tendon of specified finger with unspecified laterality at wrist and hand level

⑦S66.109   **Unspecified injury of flexor muscle, fascia and tendon of unspecified finger at wrist and hand level**

S66.11   **Strain of flexor muscle, fascia and tendon of other and unspecified finger at wrist and hand level**

⑦S66.110   **Strain of flexor muscle, fascia and tendon of right index finger at wrist and hand level**

⑦S66.111   **Strain of flexor muscle, fascia and tendon of left index finger at wrist and hand level**

⑦S66.112   **Strain of flexor muscle, fascia and tendon of right middle finger at wrist and hand level**

⑦S66.113   **Strain of flexor muscle, fascia and tendon of left middle finger at wrist and hand level**

⑦S66.114   **Strain of flexor muscle, fascia and tendon of right ring finger at wrist and hand level**

⑦S66.115   **Strain of flexor muscle, fascia and tendon of left ring finger at wrist and hand level**

⑦S66.116   **Strain of flexor muscle, fascia and tendon of right little finger at wrist and hand level**

⑦S66.117   **Strain of flexor muscle, fascia and tendon of left little finger at wrist and hand level**

⑦S66.118   **Strain of flexor muscle, fascia and tendon of other finger at wrist and hand level**

Strain of flexor muscle, fascia and tendon of specified finger with unspecified laterality at wrist and hand level

⑦S66.119   **Strain of flexor muscle, fascia and tendon of unspecified finger at wrist and hand level**

S66.12   **Laceration of flexor muscle, fascia and tendon of other and unspecified finger at wrist and hand level**

⑦S66.120   **Laceration of flexor muscle, fascia and tendon of right index finger at wrist and hand level**

⑦S66.121   **Laceration of flexor muscle, fascia and tendon of left index finger at wrist and hand level**

⑦S66.122   **Laceration of flexor muscle, fascia and tendon of right middle finger at wrist and hand level**

⑦S66.123   **Laceration of flexor muscle, fascia and tendon of left middle finger at wrist and hand level**

⑦S66.124   **Laceration of flexor muscle, fascia and tendon of right ring finger at wrist and hand level**

⑦S66.125   **Laceration of flexor muscle, fascia and tendon of left ring finger at wrist and hand level**

⑦S66.126   **Laceration of flexor muscle, fascia and tendon of right little finger at wrist and hand level**

⑦S66.127   **Laceration of flexor muscle, fascia and tendon of left little finger at wrist and hand level**

⑦S66.128   **Laceration of flexor muscle, fascia and tendon of other finger at wrist and hand level**

Laceration of flexor muscle, fascia and tendon of specified finger with unspecified laterality at wrist and hand level

⑦S66.129   **Laceration of flexor muscle, fascia and tendon of unspecified finger at wrist and hand level**

S66.19   **Other injury of flexor muscle, fascia and tendon of other and unspecified finger at wrist and hand level**

⑦S66.190   **Other injury of flexor muscle, fascia and tendon of right index finger at wrist and hand level**

⑦S66.191   **Other injury of flexor muscle, fascia and tendon of left index finger at wrist and hand level**

⑦ S66.192 Other injury of flexor muscle, fascia and tendon of right middle finger at wrist and hand level

⑦ S66.193 Other injury of flexor muscle, fascia and tendon of left middle finger at wrist and hand level

⑦ S66.194 Other injury of flexor muscle, fascia and tendon of right ring finger at wrist and hand level

⑦ S66.195 Other injury of flexor muscle, fascia and tendon of left ring finger at wrist and hand level

⑦ S66.196 Other injury of flexor muscle, fascia and tendon of right little finger at wrist and hand level

⑦ S66.197 Other injury of flexor muscle, fascia and tendon of left little finger at wrist and hand level

⑦ S66.198 Other injury of flexor muscle, fascia and tendon of other finger at wrist and hand level

Other injury of flexor muscle, fascia and tendon of specified finger with unspecified laterality at wrist and hand level

⑦ S66.199 Other injury of flexor muscle, fascia and tendon of unspecified finger at wrist and hand level

S66.2 **Injury of extensor muscle, fascia and tendon of thumb at wrist and hand level**

S66.20 Unspecified injury of extensor muscle, fascia and tendon of thumb at wrist and hand level

⑦ S66.201 Unspecified injury of extensor muscle, fascia and tendon of right thumb at wrist and hand level

⑦ S66.202 Unspecified injury of extensor muscle, fascia and tendon of left thumb at wrist and hand level

⑦ S66.209 Unspecified injury of extensor muscle, fascia and tendon of unspecified thumb at wrist and hand level

S66.21 Strain of extensor muscle, fascia and tendon of thumb at wrist and hand level

⑦ S66.211 Strain of extensor muscle, fascia and tendon of right thumb at wrist and hand level

⑦ S66.212 Strain of extensor muscle, fascia and tendon of left thumb at wrist and hand level

⑦ S66.219 Strain of extensor muscle, fascia and tendon of unspecified thumb at wrist and hand level

S66.22 Laceration of extensor muscle, fascia and tendon of thumb at wrist and hand level

⑦ S66.221 Laceration of extensor muscle, fascia and tendon of right thumb at wrist and hand level

⑦ S66.222 Laceration of extensor muscle, fascia and tendon of left thumb at wrist and hand level

⑦ S66.229 Laceration of extensor muscle, fascia and tendon of unspecified thumb at wrist and hand level

S66.29 Other specified injury of extensor muscle, fascia and tendon of thumb at wrist and hand level

⑦ S66.291 Other specified injury of extensor muscle, fascia and tendon of right thumb at wrist and hand level

⑦ S66.292 Other specified injury of extensor muscle, fascia and tendon of left thumb at wrist and hand level

⑦ S66.299 Other specified injury of extensor muscle, fascia and tendon of unspecified thumb at wrist and hand level

S66.3 **Injury of extensor muscle, fascia and tendon of other and unspecified finger at wrist and hand level**

Excludes2: Injury of extensor muscle, fascia and tendon of thumb at wrist and hand level (S66.2-)

S66.30 Unspecified injury of extensor muscle, fascia and tendon of other and unspecified finger at wrist and hand level

⑦ S66.300 Unspecified injury of extensor muscle, fascia and tendon of right index finger at wrist and hand level

⑦ S66.301 Unspecified injury of extensor muscle, fascia and tendon of left index finger at wrist and hand level

⑦ S66.302 Unspecified injury of extensor muscle, fascia and tendon of right middle finger at wrist and hand level

⑦ S66.303 Unspecified injury of extensor muscle, fascia and tendon of left middle finger at wrist and hand level

⑦ S66.304 Unspecified injury of extensor muscle, fascia and tendon of right ring finger at wrist and hand level

⑦ S66.305 Unspecified injury of extensor muscle, fascia and tendon of left ring finger at wrist and hand level

⑦ S66.306 Unspecified injury of extensor muscle, fascia and tendon of right little finger at wrist and hand level

⑦ S66.307 Unspecified injury of extensor muscle, fascia and tendon of left little finger at wrist and hand level

⑦ S66.308 Unspecified injury of extensor muscle, fascia and tendon of other finger at wrist and hand level

Unspecified injury of extensor muscle, fascia and tendon of specified finger with unspecified laterality at wrist and hand level

⑦ S66.309 Unspecified injury of extensor muscle, fascia and tendon of unspecified finger at wrist and hand level

S66.31 Strain of extensor muscle, fascia and tendon of other and unspecified finger at wrist and hand level

⑦ S66.310 Strain of extensor muscle, fascia and tendon of right index finger at wrist and hand level

⑦ S66.311 Strain of extensor muscle, fascia and tendon of left index finger at wrist and hand level

⑦ S66.312 Strain of extensor muscle, fascia and tendon of right middle finger at wrist and hand level

⑦ S66.313 Strain of extensor muscle, fascia and tendon of left middle finger at wrist and hand level

● New code ▲ Revised code **Excludes1:** Not coded here **Excludes2:** Not included here ⊗ Placeholder required ⑦ 7th digit required

⑦**S66.314** Strain of extensor muscle, fascia and tendon of right ring finger at wrist and hand level

⑦**S66.315** Strain of extensor muscle, fascia and tendon of left ring finger at wrist and hand level

⑦**S66.316** Strain of extensor muscle, fascia and tendon of right little finger at wrist and hand level

⑦**S66.317** Strain of extensor muscle, fascia and tendon of left little finger at wrist and hand level

⑦**S66.318** Strain of extensor muscle, fascia and tendon of other finger at wrist and hand level

Strain of extensor muscle, fascia and tendon of specified finger with unspecified laterality at wrist and hand level

⑦**S66.319** Strain of extensor muscle, fascia and tendon of unspecified finger at wrist and hand level

S66.32 Laceration of extensor muscle, fascia and tendon of other and unspecified finger at wrist and hand level

⑦**S66.320** Laceration of extensor muscle, fascia and tendon of right index finger at wrist and hand level

⑦**S66.321** Laceration of extensor muscle, fascia and tendon of left index finger at wrist and hand level

⑦**S66.322** Laceration of extensor muscle, fascia and tendon of right middle finger at wrist and hand level

⑦**S66.323** Laceration of extensor muscle, fascia and tendon of left middle finger at wrist and hand level

⑦**S66.324** Laceration of extensor muscle, fascia and tendon of right ring finger at wrist and hand level

⑦**S66.325** Laceration of extensor muscle, fascia and tendon of left ring finger at wrist and hand level

⑦**S66.326** Laceration of extensor muscle, fascia and tendon of right little finger at wrist and hand level

⑦**S66.327** Laceration of extensor muscle, fascia and tendon of left little finger at wrist and hand level

⑦**S66.328** Laceration of extensor muscle, fascia and tendon of other finger at wrist and hand level

Laceration of extensor muscle, fascia and tendon of specified finger with unspecified laterality at wrist and hand level

⑦**S66.329** Laceration of extensor muscle, fascia and tendon of unspecified finger at wrist and hand level

S66.39 Other injury of extensor muscle, fascia and tendon of other and unspecified finger at wrist and hand level

⑦**S66.390** Other injury of extensor muscle, fascia and tendon of right index finger at wrist and hand level

⑦**S66.391** Other injury of extensor muscle, fascia and tendon of left index finger at wrist and hand level

⑦**S66.392** Other injury of extensor muscle, fascia and tendon of right middle finger at wrist and hand level

⑦**S66.393** Other injury of extensor muscle, fascia and tendon of left middle finger at wrist and hand level

⑦**S66.394** Other injury of extensor muscle, fascia and tendon of right ring finger at wrist and hand level

⑦**S66.395** Other injury of extensor muscle, fascia and tendon of left ring finger at wrist and hand level

⑦**S66.396** Other injury of extensor muscle, fascia and tendon of right little finger at wrist and hand level

⑦**S66.397** Other injury of extensor muscle, fascia and tendon of left little finger at wrist and hand level

⑦**S66.398** Other injury of extensor muscle, fascia and tendon of other finger at wrist and hand level

Other injury of extensor muscle, fascia and tendon of specified finger with unspecified laterality at wrist and hand level

⑦**S66.399** Other injury of extensor muscle, fascia and tendon of unspecified finger at wrist and hand level

S66.4 Injury of intrinsic muscle, fascia and tendon of thumb at wrist and hand level

S66.40 Unspecified injury of intrinsic muscle, fascia and tendon of thumb at wrist and hand level

⑦**S66.401** Unspecified injury of intrinsic muscle, fascia and tendon of right thumb at wrist and hand level

⑦**S66.402** Unspecified injury of intrinsic muscle, fascia and tendon of left thumb at wrist and hand level

⑦**S66.409** Unspecified injury of intrinsic muscle, fascia and tendon of unspecified thumb at wrist and hand level

S66.41 Strain of intrinsic muscle, fascia and tendon of thumb at wrist and hand level

⑦**S66.411** Strain of intrinsic muscle, fascia and tendon of right thumb at wrist and hand level

⑦**S66.412** Strain of intrinsic muscle, fascia and tendon of left thumb at wrist and hand level

⑦**S66.419** Strain of intrinsic muscle, fascia and tendon of unspecified thumb at wrist and hand level

S66.42 Laceration of intrinsic muscle, fascia and tendon of thumb at wrist and hand level

⑦**S66.421** Laceration of intrinsic muscle, fascia and tendon of right thumb at wrist and hand level

⑦**S66.422** Laceration of intrinsic muscle, fascia and tendon of left thumb at wrist and hand level

⑦**S66.429** Laceration of intrinsic muscle, fascia and tendon of unspecified thumb at wrist and hand level

S66.49 Other specified injury of intrinsic muscle, fascia and tendon of thumb at wrist and hand level

---

Add 4th-7th digits   Nonspecific code   Unspecified code   Manifestation code

⑦**S66.491** Other specified injury of intrinsic muscle, fascia and tendon of right thumb at wrist and hand level

⑦**S66.492** Other specified injury of intrinsic muscle, fascia and tendon of left thumb at wrist and hand level

⑦**S66.499** Other specified injury of intrinsic muscle, fascia and tendon of unspecified thumb at wrist and hand level

S66.5 **Injury of intrinsic muscle, fascia and tendon of other and unspecified finger at wrist and hand level**

Excludes2: injury of intrinsic muscle, fascia and tendon of thumb at wrist and hand level (S66.4-)

S66.50 Unspecified injury of intrinsic muscle, fascia and tendon of other and unspecified finger at wrist and hand level

⑦**S66.500** Unspecified injury of intrinsic muscle, fascia and tendon of right index finger at wrist and hand level

⑦**S66.501** Unspecified injury of intrinsic muscle, fascia and tendon of left index finger at wrist and hand level

⑦**S66.502** Unspecified injury of intrinsic muscle, fascia and tendon of right middle finger at wrist and hand level

⑦**S66.503** Unspecified injury of intrinsic muscle, fascia and tendon of left middle finger at wrist and hand level

⑦**S66.504** Unspecified injury of intrinsic muscle, fascia and tendon of right ring finger at wrist and hand level

⑦**S66.505** Unspecified injury of intrinsic muscle, fascia and tendon of left ring finger at wrist and hand level

⑦**S66.506** Unspecified injury of intrinsic muscle, fascia and tendon of right little finger at wrist and hand level

⑦**S66.507** Unspecified injury of intrinsic muscle, fascia and tendon of left little finger at wrist and hand level

⑦**S66.508** Unspecified injury of intrinsic muscle, fascia and tendon of other finger at wrist and hand level

Unspecified injury of intrinsic muscle, fascia and tendon of specified finger with unspecified laterality at wrist and hand level

⑦**S66.509** Unspecified injury of intrinsic muscle, fascia and tendon of unspecified finger at wrist and hand level

S66.51 Strain of intrinsic muscle, fascia and tendon of other and unspecified finger at wrist and hand level

⑦**S66.510** Strain of intrinsic muscle, fascia and tendon of right index finger at wrist and hand level

⑦**S66.511** Strain of intrinsic muscle, fascia and tendon of left index finger at wrist and hand level

⑦**S66.512** Strain of intrinsic muscle, fascia and tendon of right middle finger at wrist and hand level

⑦**S66.513** Strain of intrinsic muscle, fascia and tendon of left middle finger at wrist and hand level

⑦**S66.514** Strain of intrinsic muscle, fascia and tendon of right ring finger at wrist and hand level

⑦**S66.515** Strain of intrinsic muscle, fascia and tendon of left ring finger at wrist and hand level

⑦**S66.516** Strain of intrinsic muscle, fascia and tendon of right little finger at wrist and hand level

⑦**S66.517** Strain of intrinsic muscle, fascia and tendon of left little finger at wrist and hand level

⑦**S66.518** Strain of intrinsic muscle, fascia and tendon of other finger at wrist and hand level

Strain of intrinsic muscle, fascia and tendon of specified finger with unspecified laterality at wrist and hand level

⑦**S66.519** Strain of intrinsic muscle, fascia and tendon of unspecified finger at wrist and hand level

S66.52 Laceration of intrinsic muscle, fascia and tendon of other and unspecified finger at wrist and hand level

⑦**S66.520** Laceration of intrinsic muscle, fascia and tendon of right index finger at wrist and hand level

⑦**S66.521** Laceration of intrinsic muscle, fascia and tendon of left index finger at wrist and hand level

⑦**S66.522** Laceration of intrinsic muscle, fascia and tendon of right middle finger at wrist and hand level

⑦**S66.523** Laceration of intrinsic muscle, fascia and tendon of left middle finger at wrist and hand level

⑦**S66.524** Laceration of intrinsic muscle, fascia and tendon of right ring finger at wrist and hand level

⑦**S66.525** Laceration of intrinsic muscle, fascia and tendon of left ring finger at wrist and hand level

⑦**S66.526** Laceration of intrinsic muscle, fascia and tendon of right little finger at wrist and hand level

⑦**S66.527** Laceration of intrinsic muscle, fascia and tendon of left little finger at wrist and hand level

⑦**S66.528** Laceration of intrinsic muscle, fascia and tendon of other finger at wrist and hand level

Laceration of intrinsic muscle, fascia and tendon of specified finger with unspecified laterality at wrist and hand level

⑦**S66.529** Laceration of intrinsic muscle, fascia and tendon of unspecified finger at wrist and hand level

S66.59 Other injury of intrinsic muscle, fascia and tendon of other and unspecified finger at wrist and hand level

⑦**S66.590** Other injury of intrinsic muscle, fascia and tendon of right index finger at wrist and hand level

⑦**S66.591** Other injury of intrinsic muscle, fascia and tendon of left index finger at wrist and hand level

● New code ▲ Revised code **Excludes1:** Not coded here **Excludes2:** Not included here ⊗ Placeholder required ⑦7th digit required

⑦S66.592　Other injury of intrinsic muscle, fascia and tendon of right middle finger at wrist and hand level

⑦S66.593　Other injury of intrinsic muscle, fascia and tendon of left middle finger at wrist and hand level

⑦S66.594　Other injury of intrinsic muscle, fascia and tendon of right ring finger at wrist and hand level

⑦S66.595　Other injury of intrinsic muscle, fascia and tendon of left ring finger at wrist and hand level

⑦S66.596　Other injury of intrinsic muscle, fascia and tendon of right little finger at wrist and hand level

⑦S66.597　Other injury of intrinsic muscle, fascia and tendon of left little finger at wrist and hand level

⑦S66.598　Other injury of intrinsic muscle, fascia and tendon of other finger at wrist and hand level

Other injury of intrinsic muscle, fascia and tendon of specified finger with unspecified laterality at wrist and hand level

⑦S66.599　Other injury of intrinsic muscle, fascia and tendon of unspecified finger at wrist and hand level

S66.8　Injury of other specified muscles, fascia and tendons at wrist and hand level

S66.80　Unspecified injury of other specified muscles, fascia and tendons at wrist and hand level

⑦S66.801　Unspecified injury of other specified muscles, fascia and tendons at wrist and hand level, right hand

⑦S66.802　Unspecified injury of other specified muscles, fascia and tendons at wrist and hand level, left hand

⑦S66.809　Unspecified injury of other specified muscles, fascia and tendons at wrist and hand level, unspecified hand

S66.81　Strain of other specified muscles, fascia and tendons at wrist and hand level

⑦S66.811　Strain of other specified muscles, fascia and tendons at wrist and hand level, right hand

⑦S66.812　Strain of other specified muscles, fascia and tendons at wrist and hand level, left hand

⑦S66.819　Strain of other specified muscles, fascia and tendons at wrist and hand level, unspecified hand

S66.82　Laceration of other specified muscles, fascia and tendons at wrist and hand level

⑦S66.821　Laceration of other specified muscles, fascia and tendons at wrist and hand level, right hand

⑦S66.822　Laceration of other specified muscles, fascia and tendons at wrist and hand level, left hand

⑦S66.829　Laceration of other specified muscles, fascia and tendons at wrist and hand level, unspecified hand

S66.89　Other injury of other specified muscles, fascia and tendons at wrist and hand level

⑦S66.891　Other injury of other specified muscles, fascia and tendons at wrist and hand level, right hand

⑦S66.892　Other injury of other specified muscles, fascia and tendons at wrist and hand level, left hand

⑦S66.899　Other injury of other specified muscles, fascia and tendons at wrist and hand level, unspecified hand

S66.9　Injury of unspecified muscle, fascia and tendon at wrist and hand level

S66.90　Unspecified injury of unspecified muscle, fascia and tendon at wrist and hand level

⑦S66.901　Unspecified injury of unspecified muscle, fascia and tendon at wrist and hand level, right hand

⑦S66.902　Unspecified injury of unspecified muscle, fascia and tendon at wrist and hand level, left hand

⑦S66.909　Unspecified injury of unspecified muscle, fascia and tendon at wrist and hand level, unspecified hand

S66.91　Strain of unspecified muscle, fascia and tendon at wrist and hand level

⑦S66.911　Strain of unspecified muscle, fascia and tendon at wrist and hand level, right hand

⑦S66.912　Strain of unspecified muscle, fascia and tendon at wrist and hand level, left hand

⑦S66.919　Strain of unspecified muscle, fascia and tendon at wrist and hand level, unspecified hand

S66.92　Laceration of unspecified muscle, fascia and tendon at wrist and hand level

⑦S66.921　Laceration of unspecified muscle, fascia and tendon at wrist and hand level, right hand

⑦S66.922　Laceration of unspecified muscle, fascia and tendon at wrist and hand level, left hand

⑦S66.929　Laceration of unspecified muscle, fascia and tendon at wrist and hand level, unspecified hand

S66.99　Other injury of unspecified muscle, fascia and tendon at wrist and hand level

⑦S66.991　Other injury of unspecified muscle, fascia and tendon at wrist and hand level, right hand

⑦S66.992　Other injury of unspecified muscle, fascia and tendon at wrist and hand level, left hand

⑦S66.999　Other injury of unspecified muscle, fascia and tendon at wrist and hand level, unspecified hand

S67　**Crushing injury of wrist, hand and fingers**

Use additional code for all associated injuries, such as:

fracture of wrist and hand (S62.-) open wound of wrist and hand (S61.-)

The appropriate 7th character is to be added to each code from category S67

A - initial encounter

D - subsequent encounter

S - sequela

S67.0　Crushing injury of thumb

⊗⑦**S67.00**   **Crushing injury of unspecified thumb**

⊗⑦**S67.01**   **Crushing injury of right thumb**

⊗⑦**S67.02**   **Crushing injury of left thumb**

S67.1   **Crushing injury of other and unspecified finger(s)**

    Excludes2: crushing injury of thumb (S67.0-)

⊗⑦**S67.10**   **Crushing injury of unspecified finger(s)**

S67.19   **Crushing injury of other finger(s)**

    ⑦**S67.190**   **Crushing injury of right index finger**

    ⑦**S67.191**   **Crushing injury of left index finger**

    ⑦**S67.192**   **Crushing injury of right middle finger**

    ⑦**S67.193**   **Crushing injury of left middle finger**

    ⑦**S67.194**   **Crushing injury of right ring finger**

    ⑦**S67.195**   **Crushing injury of left ring finger**

    ⑦**S67.196**   **Crushing injury of right little finger**

    ⑦**S67.197**   **Crushing injury of left little finger**

    ⑦**S67.198**   **Crushing injury of other finger**

      Crushing injury of specified finger with unspecified laterality

S67.2   **Crushing injury of hand**

    Excludes2: crushing injury of fingers (S67.1-)

           crushing injury of thumb (S67.0-)

⊗⑦**S67.20**   **Crushing injury of unspecified hand**

⊗⑦**S67.21**   **Crushing injury of right hand**

⊗⑦**S67.22**   **Crushing injury of left hand**

S67.3   **Crushing injury of wrist**

⊗⑦**S67.30**   **Crushing injury of unspecified wrist**

⊗⑦**S67.31**   **Crushing injury of right wrist**

⊗⑦**S67.32**   **Crushing injury of left wrist**

S67.4   **Crushing injury of wrist and hand**

    Excludes1: crushing injury of hand alone (S67.2-)

           crushing injury of wrist alone (S67.3-)

    Excludes2: crushing injury of fingers (S67.1-)

           crushing injury of thumb (S67.0-)

⊗⑦**S67.40**   **Crushing injury of unspecified wrist and hand**

⊗⑦**S67.41**   **Crushing injury of right wrist and hand**

⊗⑦**S67.42**   **Crushing injury of left wrist and hand**

S67.9   **Crushing injury of unspecified part(s) of wrist, hand and fingers**

⊗⑦**S67.90**   **Crushing injury of unspecified part(s) of unspecified wrist, hand and fingers**

⊗⑦**S67.91**   **Crushing injury of unspecified part(s) of right wrist, hand and fingers**

⊗⑦**S67.92**   **Crushing injury of unspecified part(s) of left wrist, hand and fingers**

S68   **Traumatic amputation of wrist, hand and fingers**

An amputation not identified as partial or complete should be coded to complete

The appropriate 7th character is to be added to each code from category S68

A - initial encounter

D - subsequent encounter

S - sequela

S68.0   **Traumatic metacarpophalangeal amputation of thumb**

    Traumatic amputation of thumb NOS

S68.01   **Complete traumatic metacarpophalangeal amputation of thumb**

⑦**S68.011**   **Complete traumatic metacarpophalangeal amputation of right thumb**

⑦**S68.012**   **Complete traumatic metacarpophalangeal amputation of left thumb**

⑦**S68.019**   **Complete traumatic metacarpophalangeal amputation of unspecified thumb**

S68.02   **Partial traumatic metacarpophalangeal amputation of thumb**

⑦**S68.021**   **Partial traumatic metacarpophalangeal amputation of right thumb**

⑦**S68.022**   **Partial traumatic metacarpophalangeal amputation of left thumb**

⑦**S68.029**   **Partial traumatic metacarpophalangeal amputation of unspecified thumb**

S68.1   **Traumatic metacarpophalangeal amputation of other and unspecified finger**

    Traumatic amputation of finger NOS

    Excludes2: traumatic metacarpophalangeal amputation of thumb (S68.0-)

S68.11   **Complete traumatic metacarpophalangeal amputation of other and unspecified finger**

⑦**S68.110**   **Complete traumatic metacarpophalangeal amputation of right index finger**

⑦**S68.111**   **Complete traumatic metacarpophalangeal amputation of left index finger**

⑦**S68.112**   **Complete traumatic metacarpophalangeal amputation of right middle finger**

⑦**S68.113**   **Complete traumatic metacarpophalangeal amputation of left middle finger**

⑦**S68.114**   **Complete traumatic metacarpophalangeal amputation of right ring finger**

⑦**S68.115**   **Complete traumatic metacarpophalangeal amputation of left ring finger**

⑦**S68.116**   **Complete traumatic metacarpophalangeal amputation of right little finger**

⑦**S68.117**   **Complete traumatic metacarpophalangeal amputation of left little finger**

⑦**S68.118**   **Complete traumatic metacarpophalangeal amputation of other finger**

      Complete traumatic metacarpophalangeal amputation of specified finger with unspecified laterality

⑦**S68.119**   **Complete traumatic metacarpophalangeal amputation of unspecified finger**

S68.12   **Partial traumatic metacarpophalangeal amputation of other and unspecified finger**

⑦**S68.120**   **Partial traumatic metacarpophalangeal amputation of right index finger**

⑦S68.121　Partial traumatic metacarpophalangeal amputation of left index finger

⑦S68.122　Partial traumatic metacarpophalangeal amputation of right middle finger

⑦S68.123　Partial traumatic metacarpophalangeal amputation of left middle finger

⑦S68.124　Partial traumatic metacarpophalangeal amputation of right ring finger

⑦S68.125　Partial traumatic metacarpophalangeal amputation of left ring finger

⑦S68.126　Partial traumatic metacarpophalangeal amputation of right little finger

⑦S68.127　Partial traumatic metacarpophalangeal amputation of left little finger

⑦S68.128　Partial traumatic metacarpophalangeal amputation of other finger

　　　　Partial traumatic metacarpophalangeal amputation of specified finger with unspecified laterality

⑦S68.129　Partial traumatic metacarpophalangeal amputation of unspecified finger

S68.4　**Traumatic amputation of hand at wrist level**

Traumatic amputation of hand NOS

Traumatic amputation of wrist

S68.41　**Complete traumatic amputation of hand at wrist level**

⑦S68.411　Complete traumatic amputation of right hand at wrist level

⑦S68.412　Complete traumatic amputation of left hand at wrist level

⑦S68.419　Complete traumatic amputation of unspecified hand at wrist level

S68.42　**Partial traumatic amputation of hand at wrist level**

⑦S68.421　Partial traumatic amputation of right hand at wrist level

⑦S68.422　Partial traumatic amputation of left hand at wrist level

⑦S68.429　Partial traumatic amputation of unspecified hand at wrist level

S68.5　**Traumatic transphalangeal amputation of thumb**

Traumatic interphalangeal joint amputation of thumb

S68.51　**Complete traumatic transphalangeal amputation of thumb**

⑦S68.511　Complete traumatic transphalangeal amputation of right thumb

⑦S68.512　Complete traumatic transphalangeal amputation of left thumb

⑦S68.519　Complete traumatic transphalangeal amputation of unspecified thumb

S68.52　**Partial traumatic transphalangeal amputation of thumb**

⑦S68.521　Partial traumatic transphalangeal amputation of right thumb

⑦S68.522　Partial traumatic transphalangeal amputation of left thumb

⑦S68.529　Partial traumatic transphalangeal amputation of unspecified thumb

S68.6　**Traumatic transphalangeal amputation of other and unspecified finger**

S68.61　**Complete traumatic transphalangeal amputation of other and unspecified finger(s)**

⑦S68.610　Complete traumatic transphalangeal amputation of right index finger

⑦S68.611　Complete traumatic transphalangeal amputation of left index finger

⑦S68.612　Complete traumatic transphalangeal amputation of right middle finger

⑦S68.613　Complete traumatic transphalangeal amputation of left middle finger

⑦S68.614　Complete traumatic transphalangeal amputation of right ring finger

⑦S68.615　Complete traumatic transphalangeal amputation of left ring finger

⑦S68.616　Complete traumatic transphalangeal amputation of right little finger

⑦S68.617　Complete traumatic transphalangeal amputation of left little finger

⑦S68.618　Complete traumatic transphalangeal amputation of other finger

　　　　Complete traumatic transphalangeal amputation of specified finger with unspecified laterality

⑦S68.619　Complete traumatic transphalangeal amputation of unspecified finger

S68.62　**Partial traumatic transphalangeal amputation of other and unspecified finger**

⑦S68.620　Partial traumatic transphalangeal amputation of right index finger

⑦S68.621　Partial traumatic transphalangeal amputation of left index finger

⑦S68.622　Partial traumatic transphalangeal amputation of right middle finger

⑦S68.623　Partial traumatic transphalangeal amputation of left middle finger

⑦S68.624　Partial traumatic transphalangeal amputation of right ring finger

⑦S68.625　Partial traumatic transphalangeal amputation of left ring finger

⑦S68.626　Partial traumatic transphalangeal amputation of right little finger

⑦S68.627　Partial traumatic transphalangeal amputation of left little finger

⑦S68.628　Partial traumatic transphalangeal amputation of other finger

　　　　Partial traumatic transphalangeal amputation of specified finger with unspecified laterality

⑦S68.629　Partial traumatic transphalangeal amputation of unspecified finger

S68.7　**Traumatic transmetacarpal amputation of hand**

S68.71　**Complete traumatic transmetacarpal amputation of hand**

⑦S68.711　Complete traumatic transmetacarpal amputation of right hand

⑦S68.712　Complete traumatic transmetacarpal amputation of left hand

⑦S68.719　Complete traumatic transmetacarpal amputation of unspecified hand

---

S68.72 **Partial traumatic transmetacarpal amputation of hand**

⑦S68.721 **Partial traumatic transmetacarpal amputation of right hand**

⑦S68.722 **Partial traumatic transmetacarpal amputation of left hand**

⑦S68.729 **Partial traumatic transmetacarpal amputation of unspecified hand**

S69 **Other and unspecified injuries of wrist, hand and finger(s)**

The appropriate 7th character is to be added to each code from category S69

A - initial encounter

D - subsequent encounter

S - sequela

S69.8 **Other specified injuries of wrist, hand and finger(s)**

⊗⑦**S69.80** **Other specified injuries of unspecified wrist, hand and finger(s)**

⊗⑦**S69.81** **Other specified injuries of right wrist, hand and finger(s)**

⊗⑦**S69.82** **Other specified injuries of left wrist, hand and finger(s)**

S69.9 **Unspecified injury of wrist, hand and finger(s)**

⊗⑦**S69.90** **Unspecified injury of unspecified wrist, hand and finger(s)**

⊗⑦**S69.91** **Unspecified injury of right wrist, hand and finger(s)**

⊗⑦**S69.92** **Unspecified injury of left wrist, hand and finger(s)**

INJURIES TO THE HIP AND THIGH (S70-S79)

Excludes2: burns and corrosions (T20-T32)

frostbite (T33-T34) snake bite (T63.0-)

venomous insect bite or sting (T63.4-)

S70 **Superficial injury of hip and thigh**

The appropriate 7th character is to be added to each code from category S70

A - initial encounter

D - subsequent encounter

S - sequela

S70.0 **Contusion of hip**

⊗⑦**S70.00** **Contusion of unspecified hip**

⊗⑦**S70.01** **Contusion of right hip**

⊗⑦**S70.02** **Contusion of left hip**

S70.1 **Contusion of thigh**

⊗⑦**S70.10** **Contusion of unspecified thigh**

⊗⑦**S70.11** **Contusion of right thigh**

⊗⑦**S70.12** **Contusion of left thigh**

S70.2 **Other superficial injuries of hip**

S70.21 **Abrasion of hip**

⑦S70.211 **Abrasion, right hip**

⑦S70.212 **Abrasion, left hip**

⑦S70.219 **Abrasion, unspecified hip**

S70.22 **Blister (nonthermal) of hip**

⑦S70.221 **Blister (nonthermal), right hip**

⑦S70.222 **Blister (nonthermal), left hip**

⑦S70.229 **Blister (nonthermal), unspecified hip**

S70.24 **External constriction of hip**

⑦S70.241 **External constriction, right hip**

⑦S70.242 **External constriction, left hip**

⑦S70.249 **External constriction, unspecified hip**

S70.25 **Superficial foreign body of hip**

Splinter in the hip

⑦S70.251 **Superficial foreign body, right hip**

⑦S70.252 **Superficial foreign body, left hip**

⑦S70.259 **Superficial foreign body, unspecified hip**

S70.26 **Insect bite (nonvenomous) of hip**

⑦S70.261 **Insect bite (nonvenomous), right hip**

⑦S70.262 **Insect bite (nonvenomous), left hip**

⑦S70.269 **Insect bite (nonvenomous), unspecified hip**

S70.27 **Other superficial bite of hip**

Excludes1: open bite of hip (S71.05-)

⑦**S70.271** **Other superficial bite of hip, right hip**

⑦**S70.272** **Other superficial bite of hip, left hip**

⑦**S70.279** **Other superficial bite of hip, unspecified hip**

S70.3 **Other superficial injuries of thigh**

S70.31 **Abrasion of thigh**

⑦S70.311 **Abrasion, right thigh**

⑦S70.312 **Abrasion, left thigh**

⑦S70.319 **Abrasion, unspecified thigh**

S70.32 **Blister (nonthermal) of thigh**

⑦S70.321 **Blister (nonthermal), right thigh**

⑦S70.322 **Blister (nonthermal), left thigh**

⑦S70.329 **Blister (nonthermal), unspecified thigh**

S70.34 **External constriction of thigh**

⑦S70.341 **External constriction, right thigh**

⑦S70.342 **External constriction, left thigh**

⑦S70.349 **External constriction, unspecified thigh**

S70.35 **Superficial foreign body of thigh**

Splinter in the thigh

⑦S70.351 **Superficial foreign body, right thigh**

⑦S70.352 **Superficial foreign body, left thigh**

⑦S70.359 **Superficial foreign body, unspecified thigh**

S70.36 **Insect bite (nonvenomous) of thigh**

⑦S70.361 **Insect bite (nonvenomous), right thigh**

⑦S70.362 **Insect bite (nonvenomous), left thigh**

⑦S70.369 **Insect bite (nonvenomous), unspecified thigh**

S70.37 **Other superficial bite of thigh**

Excludes1: open bite of thigh (S71.15)

⑦**S70.371** **Other superficial bite of right thigh**

⑦**S70.372** **Other superficial bite of left thigh**

⑦**S70.379** **Other superficial bite of unspecified thigh**

S70.9 **Unspecified superficial injury of hip and thigh**

S70.91 **Unspecified superficial injury of hip**

⑦S70.911 **Unspecified superficial injury of right hip**

⑦S70.912 **Unspecified superficial injury of left hip**

⑦**S70.919** Unspecified superficial injury of unspecified hip

S70.92 Unspecified superficial injury of thigh

⑦**S70.921** Unspecified superficial injury of right thigh

⑦**S70.922** Unspecified superficial injury of left thigh

⑦**S70.929** Unspecified superficial injury of unspecified thigh

S71 Open wound of hip and thigh

Code also any associated wound infection

Excludes1: open fracture of hip and thigh (S72.-)

traumatic amputation of hip and thigh (S78.-)

Excludes2: bite of venomous animal (T63.-)

open wound of ankle, foot and toes (S91.-)

open wound of knee and lower leg (S81.-)

The appropriate 7th character is to be added to each code from category S71

A - initial encounter

D - subsequent encounter

S - sequela

S71.0 Open wound of hip

S71.00 Unspecified open wound of hip

⑦**S71.001** Unspecified open wound, right hip

⑦**S71.002** Unspecified open wound, left hip

⑦**S71.009** Unspecified open wound, unspecified hip

S71.01 Laceration without foreign body of hip

⑦**S71.011** Laceration without foreign body, right hip

⑦**S71.012** Laceration without foreign body, left hip

⑦**S71.019** Laceration without foreign body, unspecified hip

S71.02 Laceration with foreign body of hip

⑦**S71.021** Laceration with foreign body, right hip

⑦**S71.022** Laceration with foreign body, left hip

⑦**S71.029** Laceration with foreign body, unspecified hip

S71.03 Puncture wound without foreign body of hip

⑦**S71.031** Puncture wound without foreign body, right hip

⑦**S71.032** Puncture wound without foreign body, left hip

⑦**S71.039** Puncture wound without foreign body, unspecified hip

S71.04 Puncture wound with foreign body of hip

⑦**S71.041** Puncture wound with foreign body, right hip

⑦**S71.042** Puncture wound with foreign body, left hip

⑦**S71.049** Puncture wound with foreign body, unspecified hip

S71.05 Open bite of hip

Bite of hip NOS

Excludes1: superficial bite of hip (S70.26, S70.27)

⑦**S71.051** Open bite, right hip

⑦**S71.052** Open bite, left hip

⑦**S71.059** Open bite, unspecified hip

S71.1 Open wound of thigh

S71.10 Unspecified open wound of thigh

⑦**S71.101** Unspecified open wound, right thigh

⑦**S71.102** Unspecified open wound, left thigh

⑦**S71.109** Unspecified open wound, unspecified thigh

S71.11 Laceration without foreign body of thigh

⑦**S71.111** Laceration without foreign body, right thigh

⑦**S71.112** Laceration without foreign body, left thigh

⑦**S71.119** Laceration without foreign body, unspecified thigh

S71.12 Laceration with foreign body of thigh

⑦**S71.121** Laceration with foreign body, right thigh

⑦**S71.122** Laceration with foreign body, left thigh

⑦**S71.129** Laceration with foreign body, unspecified thigh

S71.13 Puncture wound without foreign body of thigh

⑦**S71.131** Puncture wound without foreign body, right thigh

⑦**S71.132** Puncture wound without foreign body, left thigh

⑦**S71.139** Puncture wound without foreign body, unspecified thigh

S71.14 Puncture wound with foreign body of thigh

⑦**S71.141** Puncture wound with foreign body, right thigh

⑦**S71.142** Puncture wound with foreign body, left thigh

⑦**S71.149** Puncture wound with foreign body, unspecified thigh

S71.15 Open bite of thigh

Bite of thigh NOS

Excludes1: superficial bite of thigh (S70.37-)

⑦**S71.151** Open bite, right thigh

⑦**S71.152** Open bite, left thigh

⑦**S71.159** Open bite, unspecified thigh

S72 Fracture of femur

Note: A fracture not indicated as displaced or nondisplaced should be coded to displaced

A fracture not indicated as open or closed should be coded to closed

The open fracture designations are based on the Gustilo open fracture classification

Excludes1: traumatic amputation of hip and thigh (S78.-)

Excludes2: fracture of lower leg and ankle (S82.-)

fracture of foot (S92.-)

periprosthetic fracture of prosthetic implant of hip (M97.0-)

The appropriate 7th character is to be added to all codes from category S72

A - initial encounter for closed fracture

B - initial encounter for open fracture type I or II initial encounter for open fracture NOS

C - initial encounter for open fracture type IIIA, IIIB, or IIIC

D - subsequent encounter for closed fracture with routine healing

E - subsequent encounter for open fracture type I or II with routine healing

F - subsequent encounter for open fracture type IIIA, IIIB, or IIIC with routine healing

G - subsequent encounter for closed fracture with delayed healing

H - subsequent encounter for open fracture type I or II with delayed healing

J - subsequent encounter for open fracture type IIIA, IIIB, or IIIC with delayed healing

K - subsequent encounter for closed fracture with nonunion

M - subsequent encounter for open fracture type I or II with nonunion

N - subsequent encounter for open fracture type IIIA, IIIB, or IIIC with nonunion

P - subsequent encounter for closed fracture with malunion

Q - subsequent encounter for open fracture type I or II with malunion

R - subsequent encounter for open fracture type IIIA, IIIB, or IIIC with malunion

S - sequela

S72.0   Fracture of head and neck of femur

> **Excludes2:** physeal fracture of upper end of femur (S79.0-)

> **S72.00   Fracture of unspecified part of neck of femur**
>
> > Fracture of hip NOS
> >
> > Fracture of neck of femur NOS
> >
> > ⑦**S72.001   Fracture of unspecified part of neck of right femur**
> >
> > ⑦**S72.002   Fracture of unspecified part of neck of left femur**
> >
> > ⑦**S72.009   Fracture of unspecified part of neck of unspecified femur**

> **S72.01   Unspecified intracapsular fracture of femur**
>
> > Subcapital fracture of femur
> >
> > ⑦**S72.011   Unspecified intracapsular fracture of right femur**
> >
> > ⑦**S72.012   Unspecified intracapsular fracture of left femur**
> >
> > ⑦**S72.019   Unspecified intracapsular fracture of unspecified femur**

> **S72.02   Fracture of epiphysis (separation) (upper) of femur**
>
> > Transepiphyseal fracture of femur
> >
> > **Excludes1:** capital femoral epiphyseal fracture (pediatric) of femur (S79.01-)
> >
> > Salter-Harris Type I physeal fracture of upper end of femur (S79.01-)
> >
> > ⑦**S72.021   Displaced fracture of epiphysis (separation) (upper) of right femur**
> >
> > ⑦**S72.022   Displaced fracture of epiphysis (separation) (upper) of left femur**
> >
> > ⑦**S72.023   Displaced fracture of epiphysis (separation) (upper) of unspecified femur**
> >
> > ⑦**S72.024   Nondisplaced fracture of epiphysis (separation) (upper) of right femur**
> >
> > ⑦**S72.025   Nondisplaced fracture of epiphysis (separation) (upper) of left femur**
> >
> > ⑦**S72.026   Nondisplaced fracture of epiphysis (separation) (upper) of unspecified femur**

> **S72.03   Midcervical fracture of femur**
>
> > Transcervical fracture of femur NOS
> >
> > ⑦**S72.031   Displaced midcervical fracture of right femur**

> > ⑦**S72.032   Displaced midcervical fracture of left femur**
> >
> > ⑦**S72.033   Displaced midcervical fracture of unspecified femur**
> >
> > ⑦**S72.034   Nondisplaced midcervical fracture of right femur**
> >
> > ⑦**S72.035   Nondisplaced midcervical fracture of left femur**
> >
> > ⑦**S72.036   Nondisplaced midcervical fracture of unspecified femur**

> **S72.04   Fracture of base of neck of femur**
>
> > Cervicotrochanteric fracture of femur
> >
> > ⑦**S72.041   Displaced fracture of base of neck of right femur**
> >
> > ⑦**S72.042   Displaced fracture of base of neck of left femur**
> >
> > ⑦**S72.043   Displaced fracture of base of neck of unspecified femur**
> >
> > ⑦**S72.044   Nondisplaced fracture of base of neck of right femur**
> >
> > ⑦**S72.045   Nondisplaced fracture of base of neck of left femur**
> >
> > ⑦**S72.046   Nondisplaced fracture of base of neck of unspecified femur**

> **S72.05   Unspecified fracture of head of femur**
>
> > Fracture of head of femur NOS
> >
> > ⑦**S72.051   Unspecified fracture of head of right femur**
> >
> > ⑦**S72.052   Unspecified fracture of head of left femur**
> >
> > ⑦**S72.059   Unspecified fracture of head of unspecified femur**

> **S72.06   Articular fracture of head of femur**
>
> > ⑦**S72.061   Displaced articular fracture of head of right femur**
> >
> > ⑦**S72.062   Displaced articular fracture of head of left femur**
> >
> > ⑦**S72.063   Displaced articular fracture of head of unspecified femur**
> >
> > ⑦**S72.064   Nondisplaced articular fracture of head of right femur**
> >
> > ⑦**S72.065   Nondisplaced articular fracture of head of left femur**
> >
> > ⑦**S72.066   Nondisplaced articular fracture of head of unspecified femur**

> **S72.09   Other fracture of head and neck of femur**
>
> > ⑦**S72.091   Other fracture of head and neck of right femur**
> >
> > ⑦**S72.092   Other fracture of head and neck of left femur**
> >
> > ⑦**S72.099   Other fracture of head and neck of unspecified femur**

S72.1   Pertrochanteric fracture

> **S72.10   Unspecified trochanteric fracture of femur**
>
> > Fracture of trochanter NOS
> >
> > ⑦**S72.101   Unspecified trochanteric fracture of right femur**
> >
> > ⑦**S72.102   Unspecified trochanteric fracture of left femur**
> >
> > ⑦**S72.109   Unspecified trochanteric fracture of unspecified femur**

> **S72.11   Fracture of greater trochanter of femur**

⑦S72.111   **Displaced fracture of greater trochanter of right femur**

⑦S72.112   **Displaced fracture of greater trochanter of left femur**

⑦S72.113   **Displaced fracture of greater trochanter of unspecified femur**

⑦S72.114   **Nondisplaced fracture of greater trochanter of right femur**

⑦S72.115   **Nondisplaced fracture of greater trochanter of left femur**

⑦S72.116   **Nondisplaced fracture of greater trochanter of unspecified femur**

S72.12   **Fracture of lesser trochanter of femur**

⑦S72.121   **Displaced fracture of lesser trochanter of right femur**

⑦S72.122   **Displaced fracture of lesser trochanter of left femur**

⑦S72.123   **Displaced fracture of lesser trochanter of unspecified femur**

⑦S72.124   **Nondisplaced fracture of lesser trochanter of right femur**

⑦S72.125   **Nondisplaced fracture of lesser trochanter of left femur**

⑦S72.126   **Nondisplaced fracture of lesser trochanter of unspecified femur**

S72.13   **Apophyseal fracture of femur**

Excludes1: chronic (nontraumatic) slipped upper femoral epiphysis (M93.0-)

⑦S72.131   **Displaced apophyseal fracture of right femur**

⑦S72.132   **Displaced apophyseal fracture of left femur**

⑦S72.133   **Displaced apophyseal fracture of unspecified femur**

⑦S72.134   **Nondisplaced apophyseal fracture of right femur**

⑦S72.135   **Nondisplaced apophyseal fracture of left femur**

⑦S72.136   **Nondisplaced apophyseal fracture of unspecified femur**

S72.14   **Intertrochanteric fracture of femur**

⑦S72.141   **Displaced intertrochanteric fracture of right femur**

⑦S72.142   **Displaced intertrochanteric fracture of left femur**

⑦S72.143   **Displaced intertrochanteric fracture of unspecified femur**

⑦S72.144   **Nondisplaced intertrochanteric fracture of right femur**

⑦S72.145   **Nondisplaced intertrochanteric fracture of left femur**

⑦S72.146   **Nondisplaced intertrochanteric fracture of unspecified femur**

S72.2   **Subtrochanteric fracture of femur**

⊗⑦S72.21   **Displaced subtrochanteric fracture of right femur**

⊗⑦S72.22   **Displaced subtrochanteric fracture of left femur**

⊗⑦S72.23   **Displaced subtrochanteric fracture of unspecified femur**

⊗⑦S72.24   **Nondisplaced subtrochanteric fracture of right femur**

⊗⑦S72.25   **Nondisplaced subtrochanteric fracture of left femur**

⊗⑦S72.26   **Nondisplaced subtrochanteric fracture of unspecified femur**

S72.3   **Fracture of shaft of femur**

S72.30   **Unspecified fracture of shaft of femur**

⑦S72.301   **Unspecified fracture of shaft of right femur**

⑦S72.302   **Unspecified fracture of shaft of left femur**

⑦S72.309   **Unspecified fracture of shaft of unspecified femur**

S72.32   **Transverse fracture of shaft of femur**

⑦S72.321   **Displaced transverse fracture of shaft of right femur**

⑦S72.322   **Displaced transverse fracture of shaft of left femur**

⑦S72.323   **Displaced transverse fracture of shaft of unspecified femur**

⑦S72.324   **Nondisplaced transverse fracture of shaft of right femur**

⑦S72.325   **Nondisplaced transverse fracture of shaft of left femur**

⑦S72.326   **Nondisplaced transverse fracture of shaft of unspecified femur**

S72.33   **Oblique fracture of shaft of femur**

⑦S72.331   **Displaced oblique fracture of shaft of right femur**

⑦S72.332   **Displaced oblique fracture of shaft of left femur**

⑦S72.333   **Displaced oblique fracture of shaft of unspecified femur**

⑦S72.334   **Nondisplaced oblique fracture of shaft of right femur**

⑦S72.335   **Nondisplaced oblique fracture of shaft of left femur**

⑦S72.336   **Nondisplaced oblique fracture of shaft of unspecified femur**

S72.34   **Spiral fracture of shaft of femur**

⑦S72.341   **Displaced spiral fracture of shaft of right femur**

⑦S72.342   **Displaced spiral fracture of shaft of left femur**

⑦S72.343   **Displaced spiral fracture of shaft of unspecified femur**

⑦S72.344   **Nondisplaced spiral fracture of shaft of right femur**

⑦S72.345   **Nondisplaced spiral fracture of shaft of left femur**

⑦S72.346   **Nondisplaced spiral fracture of shaft of unspecified femur**

S72.35   **Comminuted fracture of shaft of femur**

⑦S72.351   **Displaced comminuted fracture of shaft of right femur**

⑦S72.352   **Displaced comminuted fracture of shaft of left femur**

⑦S72.353   **Displaced comminuted fracture of shaft of unspecified femur**

⑦S72.354   **Nondisplaced comminuted fracture of shaft of right femur**

⑦S72.355   **Nondisplaced comminuted fracture of shaft of left femur**

⑦S72.356   **Nondisplaced comminuted fracture of shaft of unspecified femur**

S72.36   **Segmental fracture of shaft of femur**

⑦S72.361　Displaced segmental fracture of shaft of right femur

⑦S72.362　Displaced segmental fracture of shaft of left femur

⑦S72.363　Displaced segmental fracture of shaft of unspecified femur

⑦S72.364　Nondisplaced segmental fracture of shaft of right femur

⑦S72.365　Nondisplaced segmental fracture of shaft of left femur

⑦S72.366　Nondisplaced segmental fracture of shaft of unspecified femur

S72.39　Other fracture of shaft of femur

⑦S72.391　Other fracture of shaft of right femur

⑦S72.392　Other fracture of shaft of left femur

⑦S72.399　Other fracture of shaft of unspecified femur

S72.4　Fracture of lower end of femur

Fracture of distal end of femur

Excludes2: fracture of shaft of femur (S72.3-)

physeal fracture of lower end of femur (S79.1-)

S72.40　Unspecified fracture of lower end of femur

⑦S72.401　Unspecified fracture of lower end of right femur

⑦S72.402　Unspecified fracture of lower end of left femur

⑦S72.409　Unspecified fracture of lower end of unspecified femur

S72.41　Unspecified condyle fracture of lower end of femur

Condyle fracture of femur NOS

⑦S72.411　Displaced unspecified condyle fracture of lower end of right femur

⑦S72.412　Displaced unspecified condyle fracture of lower end of left femur

⑦S72.413　Displaced unspecified condyle fracture of lower end of unspecified femur

⑦S72.414　Nondisplaced unspecified condyle fracture of lower end of right femur

⑦S72.415　Nondisplaced unspecified condyle fracture of lower end of left femur

⑦S72.416　Nondisplaced unspecified condyle fracture of lower end of unspecified femur

S72.42　Fracture of lateral condyle of femur

⑦S72.421　Displaced fracture of lateral condyle of right femur

⑦S72.422　Displaced fracture of lateral condyle of left femur

⑦S72.423　Displaced fracture of lateral condyle of unspecified femur

⑦S72.424　Nondisplaced fracture of lateral condyle of right femur

⑦S72.425　Nondisplaced fracture of lateral condyle of left femur

⑦S72.426　Nondisplaced fracture of lateral condyle of unspecified femur

S72.43　Fracture of medial condyle of femur

⑦S72.431　Displaced fracture of medial condyle of right femur

⑦S72.432　Displaced fracture of medial condyle of left femur

⑦S72.433　Displaced fracture of medial condyle of unspecified femur

⑦S72.434　Nondisplaced fracture of medial condyle of right femur

⑦S72.435　Nondisplaced fracture of medial condyle of left femur

⑦S72.436　Nondisplaced fracture of medial condyle of unspecified femur

S72.44　Fracture of lower epiphysis (separation) of femur

Excludes1: Salter-Harris Type I physeal fracture of lower end of femur (S79.11-)

⑦S72.441　Displaced fracture of lower epiphysis (separation) of right femur

⑦S72.442　Displaced fracture of lower epiphysis (separation) of left femur

⑦S72.443　Displaced fracture of lower epiphysis (separation) of unspecified femur

⑦S72.444　Nondisplaced fracture of lower epiphysis (separation) of right femur

⑦S72.445　Nondisplaced fracture of lower epiphysis (separation) of left femur

⑦S72.446　Nondisplaced fracture of lower epiphysis (separation) of unspecified femur

S72.45　Supracondylar fracture without intracondylar extension of lower end of femur

Supracondylar fracture of lower end of femur NOS

Excludes1: supracondylar fracture with intracondylar extension of lower end of femur (S72.46-)

⑦S72.451　Displaced supracondylar fracture without intracondylar extension of lower end of right femur

⑦S72.452　Displaced supracondylar fracture without intracondylar extension of lower end of left femur

⑦S72.453　Displaced supracondylar fracture without intracondylar extension of lower end of unspecified femur

⑦S72.454　Nondisplaced supracondylar fracture without intracondylar extension of lower end of right femur

⑦S72.455　Nondisplaced supracondylar fracture without intracondylar extension of lower end of left femur

⑦S72.456　Nondisplaced supracondylar fracture without intracondylar extension of lower end of unspecified femur

S72.46　Supracondylar fracture with intracondylar extension of lower end of femur

Excludes1: supracondylar fracture without intracondylar extension of lower end of femur (S72.45-)

⑦S72.461　Displaced supracondylar fracture with intracondylar extension of lower end of right femur

⑦S72.462　Displaced supracondylar fracture with intracondylar extension of lower end of left femur

⑦S72.463　Displaced supracondylar fracture with intracondylar extension of lower end of unspecified femur

　● New code　▲ Revised code　Excludes1: Not coded here　Excludes2: Not included here　⊗ Placeholder required　⑦ 7th digit required

⑦S72.464   **Nondisplaced supracondylar fracture with intracondylar extension of lower end of right femur**

⑦S72.465   **Nondisplaced supracondylar fracture with intracondylar extension of lower end of left femur**

⑦S72.466   **Nondisplaced supracondylar fracture with intracondylar extension of lower end of unspecified femur**

S72.47   **Torus fracture of lower end of femur**

The appropriate 7th character is to be added to all codes in subcategory S72.47

A - initial encounter for closed fracture

D - subsequent encounter for fracture with routine healing

G - subsequent encounter for fracture with delayed healing

K - subsequent encounter for fracture with nonunion

P - subsequent encounter for fracture with malunion

S - sequela

⑦S72.471   **Torus fracture of lower end of right femur**

⑦S72.472   **Torus fracture of lower end of left femur**

⑦S72.479   **Torus fracture of lower end of unspecified femur**

S72.49   **Other fracture of lower end of femur**

⑦S72.491   **Other fracture of lower end of right femur**

⑦S72.492   **Other fracture of lower end of left femur**

⑦S72.499   **Other fracture of lower end of unspecified femur**

S72.8   **Other fracture of femur**

S72.8X   **Other fracture of femur**

⑦S72.8X1   **Other fracture of right femur**

⑦S72.8X2   **Other fracture of left femur**

⑦S72.8X9   **Other fracture of unspecified femur**

S72.9   **Unspecified fracture of femur**

Fracture of thigh NOS

Fracture of upper leg NOS

Excludes1: fracture of hip NOS (S72.00-, S72.01-)

⊗⑦S72.90   **Unspecified fracture of unspecified femur**

⊗⑦S72.91   **Unspecified fracture of right femur**

⊗⑦S72.92   **Unspecified fracture of left femur**

S73   **Dislocation and sprain of joint and ligaments of hip**

Includes: avulsion of joint or ligament of hip

laceration of cartilage, joint or ligament of hip sprain of cartilage, joint or ligament of hip

traumatic hemarthrosis of joint or ligament of hip

traumatic rupture of joint or ligament of hip

traumatic subluxation of joint or ligament of hip

traumatic tear of joint or ligament of hip

Code also any associated open wound

Excludes2: strain of muscle, fascia and tendon of hip and thigh (S76.-)

The appropriate 7th character is to be added to each code from category S73

A - initial encounter

D - subsequent encounter

S - sequela

S73.0   **Subluxation and dislocation of hip**

Excludes2: dislocation and subluxation of hip prosthesis (T84.020, T84.021)

S73.00   **Unspecified subluxation and dislocation of hip**

Dislocation of hip NOS Subluxation of hip NOS

⑦S73.001   **Unspecified subluxation of right hip**

⑦S73.002   **Unspecified subluxation of left hip**

⑦S73.003   **Unspecified subluxation of unspecified hip**

⑦S73.004   **Unspecified dislocation of right hip**

⑦S73.005   **Unspecified dislocation of left hip**

⑦S73.006   **Unspecified dislocation of unspecified hip**

S73.01   **Posterior subluxation and dislocation of hip**

⑦S73.011   **Posterior subluxation of right hip**

⑦S73.012   **Posterior subluxation of left hip**

⑦S73.013   **Posterior subluxation of unspecified hip**

⑦S73.014   **Posterior dislocation of right hip**

⑦S73.015   **Posterior dislocation of left hip**

⑦S73.016   **Posterior dislocation of unspecified hip**

S73.02   **Obturator subluxation and dislocation of hip**

⑦S73.021   **Obturator subluxation of right hip**

⑦S73.022   **Obturator subluxation of left hip**

⑦S73.023   **Obturator subluxation of unspecified hip**

⑦S73.024   **Obturator dislocation of right hip**

⑦S73.025   **Obturator dislocation of left hip**

⑦S73.026   **Obturator dislocation of unspecified hip**

▲S73.03   **Other anterior subluxation and dislocation of hip**

⑦S73.031   **Other anterior subluxation of right hip**

⑦S73.032   **Other anterior subluxation of left hip**

⑦S73.033   **Other anterior subluxation of unspecified hip**

⑦S73.034   **Other anterior dislocation of right hip**

⑦S73.035   **Other anterior dislocation of left hip**

⑦S73.036   **Other anterior dislocation of unspecified hip**

▲S73.04   **Central subluxation and dislocation of hip**

⑦S73.041   **Central subluxation of right hip**

⑦S73.042   **Central subluxation of left hip**

⑦S73.043   **Central subluxation of unspecified hip**

⑦S73.044   **Central dislocation of right hip**

⑦S73.045   **Central dislocation of left hip**

⑦S73.046   **Central dislocation of unspecified hip**

S73.1   **Sprain of hip**

S73.10   **Unspecified sprain of hip**

⑦S73.101   **Unspecified sprain of right hip**

⑦S73.102   **Unspecified sprain of left hip**

⑦S73.109   **Unspecified sprain of unspecified hip**

S73.11   **Iliofemoral ligament sprain of hip**

Add 4th-7th digits   Nonspecific code   Unspecified code   Manifestation code

⑦**S73.111** **Iliofemoral ligament sprain of right hip**

⑦**S73.112** **Iliofemoral ligament sprain of left hip**

⑦**S73.119** **Iliofemoral ligament sprain of unspecified hip**

S73.12 **Ischiocapsular (ligament) sprain of hip**

⑦**S73.121** **Ischiocapsular ligament sprain of right hip**

⑦**S73.122** **Ischiocapsular ligament sprain of left hip**

⑦**S73.129** **Ischiocapsular ligament sprain of unspecified hip**

S73.19 **Other sprain of hip**

⑦**S73.191** **Other sprain of right hip**

⑦**S73.192** **Other sprain of left hip**

⑦**S73.199** **Other sprain of unspecified hip**

S74 **Injury of nerves at hip and thigh level**

Code also any associated open wound (S71.-)

Excludes2: injury of nerves at ankle and foot level (S94.-)

injury of nerves at lower leg level (S84.-)

The appropriate 7th character is to be added to each code from category S74

A - initial encounter

D - subsequent encounter

S - sequela

S74.0 **Injury of sciatic nerve at hip and thigh level**

⊗⑦**S74.00** **Injury of sciatic nerve at hip and thigh level, unspecified leg**

⊗⑦**S74.01** **Injury of sciatic nerve at hip and thigh level, right leg**

⊗⑦**S74.02** **Injury of sciatic nerve at hip and thigh level, left leg**

S74.1 **Injury of femoral nerve at hip and thigh level**

⊗⑦**S74.10** **Injury of femoral nerve at hip and thigh level, unspecified leg**

⊗⑦**S74.11** **Injury of femoral nerve at hip and thigh level, right leg**

⊗⑦**S74.12** **Injury of femoral nerve at hip and thigh level, left leg**

S74.2 **Injury of cutaneous sensory nerve at hip and thigh level**

⊗⑦**S74.20** **Injury of cutaneous sensory nerve at hip and thigh level, unspecified leg**

⊗⑦**S74.21** **Injury of cutaneous sensory nerve at hip and high level, right leg**

⊗⑦**S74.22** **Injury of cutaneous sensory nerve at hip and thigh level, left leg**

S74.8 **Injury of other nerves at hip and thigh level**

S74.8X **Injury of other nerves at hip and thigh level**

⑦**S74.8X1** **Injury of other nerves at hip and thigh level, right leg**

⑦**S74.8X2** **Injury of other nerves at hip and thigh level, left leg**

⑦**S74.8X9** **Injury of other nerves at hip and thigh level, unspecified leg**

S74.9 **Injury of unspecified nerve at hip and thigh level**

⊗⑦**S74.90** **Injury of unspecified nerve at hip and thigh level, unspecified leg**

⊗⑦**S74.91** **Injury of unspecified nerve at hip and thigh level, right leg**

⊗⑦**S74.92** **Injury of unspecified nerve at hip and thigh level, left leg**

S75 **Injury of blood vessels at hip and thigh level**

Code also any associated open wound (S71.-)

Excludes2: injury of blood vessels at lower leg level (S85.-)

injury of popliteal artery (S85.0)

The appropriate 7th character is to be added to each code from category S75

A - initial encounter

D - subsequent encounter

S - sequela

S75.0 **Injury of femoral artery**

S75.00 **Unspecified injury of femoral artery**

⑦**S75.001** **Unspecified injury of femoral artery, right leg**

⑦**S75.002** **Unspecified injury of femoral artery, left leg**

⑦**S75.009** **Unspecified injury of femoral artery, unspecified leg**

S75.01 **Minor laceration of femoral artery**

Incomplete transection of femoral artery

Laceration of femoral artery NOS

Superficial laceration of femoral artery

⑦**S75.011** **Minor laceration of femoral artery, right leg**

⑦**S75.012** **Minor laceration of femoral artery, left leg**

⑦**S75.019** **Minor laceration of femoral artery, unspecified leg**

S75.02 **Major laceration of femoral artery**

Complete transection of femoral artery

Traumatic rupture of femoral artery

⑦**S75.021** **Major laceration of femoral artery, right leg**

⑦**S75.022** **Major laceration of femoral artery, left leg**

⑦**S75.029** **Major laceration of femoral artery, unspecified leg**

S75.09 **Other specified injury of femoral artery**

⑦**S75.091** **Other specified injury of femoral artery, right leg**

⑦**S75.092** **Other specified injury of femoral artery, left leg**

⑦**S75.099** **Other specified injury of femoral artery, unspecified leg**

S75.1 **Injury of femoral vein at hip and thigh level**

S75.10 **Unspecified injury of femoral vein at hip and thigh level**

⑦**S75.101** **Unspecified injury of femoral vein at hip and thigh level, right leg**

⑦**S75.102** **Unspecified injury of femoral vein at hip and thigh level, left leg**

⑦**S75.109** **Unspecified injury of femoral vein at hip and thigh level, unspecified leg**

S75.11 **Minor laceration of femoral vein at hip and thigh level**

Incomplete transection of femoral vein at hip and thigh level

Laceration of femoral vein at hip and thigh level NOS

Superficial laceration of femoral vein at hip and thigh level

⑦**S75.111** **Minor laceration of femoral vein at hip and thigh level, right leg**

⑦S75.112   Minor laceration of femoral vein at hip and thigh level, left leg

⑦S75.119   Minor laceration of femoral vein at hip and thigh level, unspecified leg

S75.12   Major laceration of femoral vein at hip and thigh level

Complete transection of femoral vein at hip and thigh level

Traumatic rupture of femoral vein at hip and thigh level

⑦S75.121   Major laceration of femoral vein at hip and thigh level, right leg

⑦S75.122   Major laceration of femoral vein at hip and thigh level, left leg

⑦S75.129   Major laceration of femoral vein at hip and thigh level, unspecified leg

S75.19   Other specified injury of femoral vein at hip and thigh level

⑦S75.191   Other specified injury of femoral vein at hip and thigh level, right leg

⑦S75.192   Other specified injury of femoral vein at hip and thigh level, left leg

⑦S75.199   Other specified injury of femoral vein at hip and thigh level, unspecified leg

S75.2   Injury of greater saphenous vein at hip and thigh level

Excludes1: greater saphenous vein NOS (S85.3)

S75.20   Unspecified injury of greater saphenous vein at hip and thigh level

⑦S75.201   Unspecified injury of greater saphenous vein at hip and thigh level, right leg

⑦S75.202   Unspecified injury of greater saphenous vein at hip and thigh level, left leg

⑦S75.209   Unspecified injury of greater saphenous vein at hip and thigh level, unspecified leg

S75.21   Minor laceration of greater saphenous vein at hip and thigh level

Incomplete transection of greater saphenous vein at hip and thigh level

Laceration of greater saphenous vein at hip and thigh level NOS

Superficial laceration of greater saphenous vein at hip and thigh level

⑦S75.211   Minor laceration of greater saphenous vein at hip and thigh level, right leg

⑦S75.212   Minor laceration of greater saphenous vein at hip and thigh level, left leg

⑦S75.219   Minor laceration of greater saphenous vein at hip and thigh level, unspecified leg

S75.22   Major laceration of greater saphenous vein at hip and thigh level

Complete transection of greater saphenous vein at hip and thigh level

Traumatic rupture of greater saphenous vein at hip and thigh level

⑦S75.221   Major laceration of greater saphenous vein at hip and thigh level, right leg

⑦S75.222   Major laceration of greater saphenous vein at hip and thigh level, left leg

⑦S75.229   Major laceration of greater saphenous vein at hip and thigh level, unspecified leg

S75.29   Other specified injury of greater saphenous vein at hip and thigh level

⑦S75.291   Other specified injury of greater saphenous vein at hip and thigh level, right leg

⑦S75.292   Other specified injury of greater saphenous vein at hip and thigh level, left leg

⑦S75.299   Other specified injury of greater saphenous vein at hip and thigh level, unspecified leg

S75.8   Injury of other blood vessels at hip and thigh level

S75.80   Unspecified injury of other blood vessels at hip and thigh level

⑦S75.801   Unspecified injury of other blood vessels at hip and thigh level, right leg

⑦S75.802   Unspecified injury of other blood vessels at hip and thigh level, left leg

⑦S75.809   Unspecified injury of other blood vessels at hip and thigh level, unspecified leg

S75.81   Laceration of other blood vessels at hip and thigh level

⑦S75.811   Laceration of other blood vessels at hip and thigh level, right leg

⑦S75.812   Laceration of other blood vessels at hip and thigh level, left leg

⑦S75.819   Laceration of other blood vessels at hip and thigh level, unspecified leg

S75.89   Other specified injury of other blood vessels at hip and thigh level

⑦S75.891   Other specified injury of other blood vessels at hip and thigh level, right leg

⑦S75.892   Other specified injury of other blood vessels at hip and thigh level, left leg

⑦S75.899   Other specified injury of other blood vessels at hip and thigh level, unspecified leg

S75.9   Injury of unspecified blood vessel at hip and thigh level

S75.90   Unspecified injury of unspecified blood vessel at hip and thigh level

⑦S75.901   Unspecified injury of unspecified blood vessel at hip and thigh level, right leg

⑦S75.902   Unspecified injury of unspecified blood vessel at hip and thigh level, left leg

⑦S75.909   Unspecified injury of unspecified blood vessel at hip and thigh level, unspecified leg

S75.91   Laceration of unspecified blood vessel at hip and thigh level

⑦S75.911   Laceration of unspecified blood vessel at hip and thigh level, right leg

⑦S75.912   Laceration of unspecified blood vessel at hip and thigh level, left leg

⑦S75.919 Laceration of unspecified blood vessel at hip and thigh level, unspecified leg

S75.99 Other specified injury of unspecified blood vessel at hip and thigh level

⑦S75.991 Other specified injury of unspecified blood vessel at hip and thigh level, right leg

⑦S75.992 Other specified injury of unspecified blood vessel at hip and thigh level, left leg

⑦S75.999 Other specified injury of unspecified blood vessel at hip and thigh level, unspecified leg

S76 Injury of muscle, fascia and tendon at hip and thigh level

Code also any associated open wound (S71.-)

Excludes2: injury of muscle, fascia and tendon at lower leg level (S86)

sprain of joint and ligament of hip (S73.1)

The appropriate 7th character is to be added to each code from category S76

A - initial encounter

D - subsequent encounter

S - sequela

S76.0 Injury of muscle, fascia and tendon of hip

S76.00 Unspecified injury of muscle, fascia and tendon of hip

⑦S76.001 Unspecified injury of muscle, fascia and tendon of right hip

⑦S76.002 Unspecified injury of muscle, fascia and tendon of left hip

⑦S76.009 Unspecified injury of muscle, fascia and tendon of unspecified hip

S76.01 Strain of muscle, fascia and tendon of hip

⑦S76.011 Strain of muscle, fascia and tendon of right hip

⑦S76.012 Strain of muscle, fascia and tendon of left hip

⑦S76.019 Strain of muscle, fascia and tendon of unspecified hip

S76.02 Laceration of muscle, fascia and tendon of hip

⑦S76.021 Laceration of muscle, fascia and tendon of right hip

⑦S76.022 Laceration of muscle, fascia and tendon of left hip

⑦S76.029 Laceration of muscle, fascia and tendon of unspecified hip

S76.09 Other specified injury of muscle, fascia and tendon of hip

⑦S76.091 Other specified injury of muscle, fascia and tendon of right hip

⑦S76.092 Other specified injury of muscle, fascia and tendon of left hip

⑦S76.099 Other specified injury of muscle, fascia and tendon of unspecified hip

S76.1 Injury of quadriceps muscle, fascia and tendon

Injury of patellar ligament (tendon)

S76.10 Unspecified injury of quadriceps muscle, fascia and tendon

⑦S76.101 Unspecified injury of right quadriceps muscle, fascia and tendon

⑦S76.102 Unspecified injury of left quadriceps muscle, fascia and tendon

⑦S76.109 Unspecified injury of unspecified quadriceps muscle, fascia and tendon

S76.11 Strain of quadriceps muscle, fascia and tendon

⑦S76.111 Strain of right quadriceps muscle, fascia and tendon

⑦S76.112 Strain of left quadriceps muscle, fascia and tendon

⑦S76.119 Strain of unspecified quadriceps muscle, fascia and tendon

S76.12 Laceration of quadriceps muscle, fascia and tendon

⑦S76.121 Laceration of right quadriceps muscle, fascia and tendon

⑦S76.122 Laceration of left quadriceps muscle, fascia and tendon

⑦S76.129 Laceration of unspecified quadriceps muscle, fascia and tendon

S76.19 Other specified injury of quadriceps muscle, fascia and tendon

⑦S76.191 Other specified injury of right quadriceps muscle, fascia and tendon

⑦S76.192 Other specified injury of left quadriceps muscle, fascia and tendon

⑦S76.199 Other specified injury of unspecified quadriceps muscle, fascia and tendon

S76.2 Injury of adductor muscle, fascia and tendon of thigh

S76.20 Unspecified injury of adductor muscle, fascia and tendon of thigh

⑦S76.201 Unspecified injury of adductor muscle, fascia and tendon of right thigh

⑦S76.202 Unspecified injury of adductor muscle, fascia and tendon of left thigh

⑦S76.209 Unspecified injury of adductor muscle, fascia and tendon of unspecified thigh

S76.21 Strain of adductor muscle, fascia and tendon of thigh

⑦S76.211 Strain of adductor muscle, fascia and tendon of right thigh

⑦S76.212 Strain of adductor muscle, fascia and tendon of left thigh

⑦S76.219 Strain of adductor muscle, fascia and tendon of unspecified thigh

S76.22 Laceration of adductor muscle, fascia and tendon of thigh

⑦S76.221 Laceration of adductor muscle, fascia and tendon of right thigh

⑦S76.222 Laceration of adductor muscle, fascia and tendon of left thigh

⑦S76.229 Laceration of adductor muscle, fascia and tendon of unspecified thigh

S76.29 Other injury of adductor muscle, fascia and tendon of thigh

⑦S76.291 Other injury of adductor muscle, fascia and tendon of right thigh

⑦S76.292 Other injury of adductor muscle, fascia and tendon of left thigh

⑦S76.299 Other injury of adductor muscle, fascia and tendon of unspecified thigh

S76.3 Injury of muscle, fascia and tendon of the posterior muscle group at thigh level

● New code ▲ Revised code **Excludes1:** Not coded here **Excludes2:** Not included here ⊗ Placeholder required ⑦7th digit required

S76.30   **Unspecified injury of muscle, fascia and tendon of the posterior muscle group at thigh level**

    ⑦S76.301   **Unspecified injury of muscle, fascia and tendon of the posterior muscle group at thigh level, right thigh**

    ⑦S76.302   **Unspecified injury of muscle, fascia and tendon of the posterior muscle group at thigh level, left thigh**

    ⑦S76.309   **Unspecified injury of muscle, fascia and tendon of the posterior muscle group at thigh level, unspecified thigh**

S76.31   **Strain of muscle, fascia and tendon of the posterior muscle group at thigh level**

    ⑦S76.311   **Strain of muscle, fascia and tendon of the posterior muscle group at thigh level, right thigh**

    ⑦S76.312   **Strain of muscle, fascia and tendon of the posterior muscle group at thigh level, left thigh**

    ⑦S76.319   **Strain of muscle, fascia and tendon of the posterior muscle group at thigh level, unspecified thigh**

S76.32   **Laceration of muscle, fascia and tendon of the posterior muscle group at thigh level**

    ⑦S76.321   **Laceration of muscle, fascia and tendon of the posterior muscle group at thigh level, right thigh**

    ⑦S76.322   **Laceration of muscle, fascia and tendon of the posterior muscle group at thigh level, left thigh**

    ⑦S76.329   **Laceration of muscle, fascia and tendon of the posterior muscle group at thigh level, unspecified thigh**

S76.39   **Other specified injury of muscle, fascia and tendon of the posterior muscle group at thigh level**

    ⑦S76.391   **Other specified injury of muscle, fascia and tendon of the posterior muscle group at thigh level, right thigh**

    ⑦S76.392   **Other specified injury of muscle, fascia and tendon of the posterior muscle group at thigh level, left thigh**

    ⑦S76.399   **Other specified injury of muscle, fascia and tendon of the posterior muscle group at thigh level, unspecified thigh**

S76.8   **Injury of other specified muscles, fascia and tendons at thigh level**

S76.80   **Unspecified injury of other specified muscles, fascia and tendons at thigh level**

    ⑦S76.801   **Unspecified injury of other specified muscles, fascia and tendons at thigh level, right thigh**

    ⑦S76.802   **Unspecified injury of other specified muscles, fascia and tendons at thigh level, left thigh**

    ⑦S76.809   **Unspecified injury of other specified muscles, fascia and tendons at thigh level, unspecified thigh**

S76.81   **Strain of other specified muscles, fascia and tendons at thigh level**

    ⑦S76.811   **Strain of other specified muscles, fascia and tendons at thigh level, right thigh**

    ⑦S76.812   **Strain of other specified muscles, fascia and tendons at thigh level, left thigh**

    ⑦S76.819   **Strain of other specified muscles, fascia and tendons at thigh level, unspecified thigh**

S76.82   **Laceration of other specified muscles, fascia and tendons at thigh level**

    ⑦S76.821   **Laceration of other specified muscles, fascia and tendons at thigh level, right thigh**

    ⑦S76.822   **Laceration of other specified muscles, fascia and tendons at thigh level, left thigh**

    ⑦S76.829   **Laceration of other specified muscles, fascia and tendons at thigh level, unspecified thigh**

S76.89   **Other injury of other specified muscles, fascia and tendons at thigh level**

    ⑦S76.891   **Other injury of other specified muscles, fascia and tendons at thigh level, right thigh**

    ⑦S76.892   **Other injury of other specified muscles, fascia and tendons at thigh level, left thigh**

    ⑦S76.899   **Other injury of other specified muscles, fascia and tendons at thigh level, unspecified thigh**

S76.9   **Injury of unspecified muscles, fascia and tendons at thigh level**

S76.90   **Unspecified injury of unspecified muscles, fascia and tendons at thigh level**

    ⑦S76.901   **Unspecified injury of unspecified muscles, fascia and tendons at thigh level, right thigh**

    ⑦S76.902   **Unspecified injury of unspecified muscles, fascia and tendons at thigh level, left thigh**

    ⑦S76.909   **Unspecified injury of unspecified muscles, fascia and tendons at thigh level, unspecified thigh**

S76.91   **Strain of unspecified muscles, fascia and tendons at thigh level**

    ⑦S76.911   **Strain of unspecified muscles, fascia and tendons at thigh level, right thigh**

    ⑦S76.912   **Strain of unspecified muscles, fascia and tendons at thigh level, left thigh**

    ⑦S76.919   **Strain of unspecified muscles, fascia and tendons at thigh level, unspecified thigh**

S76.92   **Laceration of unspecified muscles, fascia and tendons at thigh level**

    ⑦S76.921   **Laceration of unspecified muscles, fascia and tendons at thigh level, right thigh**

    ⑦S76.922   **Laceration of unspecified muscles, fascia and tendons at thigh level, left thigh**

    ⑦S76.929   **Laceration of unspecified muscles, fascia and tendons at thigh level, unspecified thigh**

S76.99   **Other specified injury of unspecified muscles, fascia and tendons at thigh level**

    ⑦S76.991   **Other specified injury of unspecified muscles, fascia and tendons at thigh level, right thigh**

⑦**S76.992** Other specified injury of unspecified muscles, fascia and tendons at thigh level, left thigh

⑦**S76.999** Other specified injury of unspecified muscles, fascia and tendons at thigh level, unspecified thigh

S77 Crushing injury of hip and thigh

Use additional code(s) for all associated injuries

Excludes2: crushing injury of ankle and foot (S97.-)

crushing injury of lower leg (S87.-)

The appropriate 7th character is to be added to each code from category S77

A - initial encounter

D - subsequent encounter

S - sequela

S77.0 Crushing injury of hip

⊗⑦**S77.00** Crushing injury of unspecified hip

⊗⑦**S77.01** Crushing injury of right hip

⊗⑦**S77.02** Crushing injury of left hip

S77.1 Crushing injury of thigh

⊗⑦**S77.10** Crushing injury of unspecified thigh

⊗⑦**S77.11** Crushing injury of right thigh

⊗⑦**S77.12** Crushing injury of left thigh

S77.2 Crushing injury of hip with thigh

⊗⑦**S77.20** Crushing injury of unspecified hip with thigh

⊗⑦**S77.21** Crushing injury of right hip with thigh

⊗⑦**S77.22** Crushing injury of left hip with thigh

S78 Traumatic amputation of hip and thigh

An amputation not identified as partial or complete should be coded to complete

Excludes1: traumatic amputation of knee (S88.0-)

The appropriate 7th character is to be added to each code from category S78

A - initial encounter

D - subsequent encounter

S - sequela

S78.0 Traumatic amputation at hip joint

S78.01 Complete traumatic amputation at hip joint

⑦**S78.011** Complete traumatic amputation at right hip joint

⑦**S78.012** Complete traumatic amputation at left hip joint

⑦**S78.019** Complete traumatic amputation at unspecified hip joint

S78.02 Partial traumatic amputation at hip joint

⑦**S78.021** Partial traumatic amputation at right hip joint

⑦**S78.022** Partial traumatic amputation at left hip joint

⑦**S78.029** Partial traumatic amputation at unspecified hip joint

S78.1 Traumatic amputation at level between hip and knee

Excludes1: traumatic amputation of knee (S88.0-)

S78.11 Complete traumatic amputation at level between hip and knee

⑦**S78.111** Complete traumatic amputation at level between right hip and knee

⑦**S78.112** Complete traumatic amputation at level between left hip and knee

⑦**S78.119** Complete traumatic amputation at level between unspecified hip and knee

S78.12 Partial traumatic amputation at level between hip and knee

⑦**S78.121** Partial traumatic amputation at level between right hip and knee

⑦**S78.122** Partial traumatic amputation at level between left hip and knee

⑦**S78.129** Partial traumatic amputation at level between unspecified hip and knee

S78.9 Traumatic amputation of hip and thigh, level unspecified

S78.91 Complete traumatic amputation of hip and thigh, level unspecified

⑦**S78.911** Complete traumatic amputation of right hip and thigh, level unspecified

⑦**S78.912** Complete traumatic amputation of left hip and thigh, level unspecified

⑦**S78.919** Complete traumatic amputation of unspecified hip and thigh, level unspecified

S78.92 Partial traumatic amputation of hip and thigh, level unspecified

⑦**S78.921** Partial traumatic amputation of right hip and thigh, level unspecified

⑦**S78.922** Partial traumatic amputation of left hip and thigh, level unspecified

⑦**S78.929** Partial traumatic amputation of unspecified hip and thigh, level unspecified

S79 Other and unspecified injuries of hip and thigh

Note: A fracture not indicated as open or closed should be coded to closed

The appropriate 7th character is to be added to each code from subcategories S79.0 and S79.1

A - initial encounter for closed fracture

D - subsequent encounter for fracture with routine healing

G - subsequent encounter for fracture with delayed healing

K - subsequent encounter for fracture with nonunion

P - subsequent encounter for fracture with malunion

S - sequela

S79.0 Physeal fracture of upper end of femur

Excludes1: apophyseal fracture of upper end of femur (S72.13-)

nontraumatic slipped upper femoral epiphysis (M93.0-)

S79.00 Unspecified physeal fracture of upper end of femur

⑦**S79.001** Unspecified physeal fracture of upper end of right femur

⑦**S79.002** Unspecified physeal fracture of upper end of left femur

⑦**S79.009** Unspecified physeal fracture of upper end of unspecified femur

S79.01 Salter-Harris Type I physeal fracture of upper end of femur

Acute on chronic slipped capital femoral epiphysis (traumatic)

Acute slipped capital femoral epiphysis (traumatic)

Capital femoral epiphyseal fracture

Excludes1: chronic slipped upper femoral

epiphysis (nontraumatic) (M93.02-)

⑦S79.011   Salter-Harris Type I physeal fracture of upper end of right femur

⑦S79.012   Salter-Harris Type I physeal fracture of upper end of left femur

⑦S79.019   Salter-Harris Type I physeal fracture of upper end of unspecified femur

S79.09   Other physeal fracture of upper end of femur

⑦S79.091   Other physeal fracture of upper end of right femur

⑦S79.092   Other physeal fracture of upper end of left femur

⑦S79.099   Other physeal fracture of upper end of unspecified femur

S79.1   Physeal fracture of lower end of femur

S79.10   Unspecified physeal fracture of lower end of femur

⑦S79.101   Unspecified physeal fracture of lower end of right femur

⑦S79.102   Unspecified physeal fracture of lower end of left femur

⑦S79.109   Unspecified physeal fracture of lower end of unspecified femur

S79.11   Salter-Harris Type I physeal fracture of lower end of femur

⑦S79.111   Salter-Harris Type I physeal fracture of lower end of right femur

⑦S79.112   Salter-Harris Type I physeal fracture of lower end of left femur

⑦S79.119   Salter-Harris Type I physeal fracture of lower end of unspecified femur

S79.12   Salter-Harris Type II physeal fracture of lower end of femur

⑦S79.121   Salter-Harris Type II physeal fracture of lower end of right femur

⑦S79.122   Salter-Harris Type II physeal fracture of lower end of left femur

⑦S79.129   Salter-Harris Type II physeal fracture of lower end of unspecified femur

S79.13   Salter-Harris Type III physeal fracture of lower end of femur

⑦S79.131   Salter-Harris Type III physeal fracture of lower end of right femur

⑦S79.132   Salter-Harris Type III physeal fracture of lower end of left femur

⑦S79.139   Salter-Harris Type III physeal fracture of lower end of unspecified femur

S79.14   Salter-Harris Type IV physeal fracture of lower end of femur

⑦S79.141   Salter-Harris Type IV physeal fracture of lower end of right femur

⑦S79.142   Salter-Harris Type IV physeal fracture of lower end of left femur

⑦S79.149   Salter-Harris Type IV physeal fracture of lower end of unspecified femur

S79.19   Other physeal fracture of lower end of femur

⑦S79.191   Other physeal fracture of lower end of right femur

⑦S79.192   Other physeal fracture of lower end of left femur

⑦S79.199   Other physeal fracture of lower end of unspecified femur

S79.8   Other specified injuries of hip and thigh

The appropriate 7th character is to be added to each code in subcategory S79.8

A - initial encounter

D - subsequent encounter

S - sequela

S79.81   Other specified injuries of hip

⑦S79.811   Other specified injuries of right hip

⑦S79.812   Other specified injuries of left hip

⑦S79.819   Other specified injuries of unspecified hip

S79.82   Other specified injuries of thigh

⑦S79.821   Other specified injuries of right thigh

⑦S79.822   Other specified injuries of left thigh

⑦S79.829   Other specified injuries of unspecified thigh

S79.9   Unspecified injury of hip and thigh

The appropriate 7th character is to be added to each code in subcategory S79.9

A - initial encounter

D - subsequent encounter

S - sequela

S79.91   Unspecified injury of hip

⑦S79.911   Unspecified injury of right hip

⑦S79.912   Unspecified injury of left hip

⑦S79.919   Unspecified injury of unspecified hip

S79.92   Unspecified injury of thigh

⑦S79.921   Unspecified injury of right thigh

⑦S79.922   Unspecified injury of left thigh

⑦S79.929   Unspecified injury of unspecified thigh

INJURIES TO THE KNEE AND LOWER LEG (S80-S89)

Excludes2: burns and corrosions (T20-T32)

frostbite (T33-T34)

injuries of ankle and foot, except fracture of ankle and malleolus (S90-S99)

insect bite or sting, venomous (T63.4)

S80   Superficial injury of knee and lower leg

Excludes2: superficial injury of ankle and foot (S90.-)

The appropriate 7th character is to be added to each code from category S80

A - initial encounter

D - subsequent encounter

S - sequela

S80.0   Contusion of knee

⊗⑦S80.00   Contusion of unspecified knee

⊗⑦S80.01   Contusion of right knee

⊗⑦S80.02   Contusion of left knee

S80.1   Contusion of lower leg

⊗⑦S80.10   Contusion of unspecified lower leg

⊗⑦S80.11   Contusion of right lower leg

⊗⑦S80.12   Contusion of left lower leg

S80.2   Other superficial injuries of knee

S80.21   Abrasion of knee

⑦S80.211   Abrasion, right knee

⑦S80.212   Abrasion, left knee

⑦S80.219   Abrasion, unspecified knee

S80.22   Blister (nonthermal) of knee

⑦S80.221   Blister (nonthermal), right knee

⑦S80.222   Blister (nonthermal), left knee

⑦S80.229   Blister (nonthermal), unspecified knee

S80.24   External constriction of knee

⑦S80.241   External constriction, right knee

⑦S80.242   External constriction, left knee

⑦S80.249   External constriction, unspecified knee

S80.25   Superficial foreign body of knee

Splinter in the knee

⑦S80.251   Superficial foreign body, right knee

⑦S80.252   Superficial foreign body, left knee

⑦S80.259   Superficial foreign body, unspecified knee

S80.26   Insect bite (nonvenomous) of knee

⑦S80.261   Insect bite (nonvenomous), right knee

⑦S80.262   Insect bite (nonvenomous), left knee

⑦S80.269   Insect bite (nonvenomous), unspecified knee

S80.27   Other superficial bite of knee

Excludes1: open bite of knee (S81.05-)

⑦S80.271   Other superficial bite of right knee

⑦S80.272   Other superficial bite of left knee

⑦S80.279   Other superficial bite of unspecified knee

S80.8   Other superficial injuries of lower leg

S80.81   Abrasion of lower leg

⑦S80.811   Abrasion, right lower leg

⑦S80.812   Abrasion, left lower leg

⑦S80.819   Abrasion, unspecified lower leg

S80.82   Blister (nonthermal) of lower leg

⑦S80.821   Blister (nonthermal), right lower leg

⑦S80.822   Blister (nonthermal), left lower leg

⑦S80.829   Blister (nonthermal), unspecified lower leg

S80.84   External constriction of lower leg

⑦S80.841   External constriction, right lower leg

⑦S80.842   External constriction, left lower leg

⑦S80.849   External constriction, unspecified lower leg

S80.85   Superficial foreign body of lower leg

Splinter in the lower leg

⑦S80.851   Superficial foreign body, right lower leg

⑦S80.852   Superficial foreign body, left lower leg

⑦S80.859   Superficial foreign body, unspecified lower leg

S80.86   Insect bite (nonvenomous) of lower leg

⑦S80.861   Insect bite (nonvenomous), right lower leg

⑦S80.862   Insect bite (nonvenomous), left lower leg

⑦S80.869   Insect bite (nonvenomous), unspecified lower leg

S80.87   Other superficial bite of lower leg

Excludes1: open bite of lower leg (S81.85-)

⑦S80.871   Other superficial bite, right lower leg

⑦S80.872   Other superficial bite, left lower leg

⑦S80.879   Other superficial bite, unspecified lower leg

S80.9   Unspecified superficial injury of knee and lower leg

S80.91   Unspecified superficial injury of knee

⑦S80.911   Unspecified superficial injury of right knee

⑦S80.912   Unspecified superficial injury of left knee

⑦S80.919   Unspecified superficial injury of unspecified knee

S80.92   Unspecified superficial injury of lower leg

⑦S80.921   Unspecified superficial injury of right lower leg

⑦S80.922   Unspecified superficial injury of left lower leg

⑦S80.929   Unspecified superficial injury of unspecified lower leg

S81   **Open wound of knee and lower leg**

<u>Code also</u> any associated wound infection

Excludes1: open fracture of knee and lower leg (S82.-)

traumatic amputation of lower leg (S88.-)

Excludes2: open wound of ankle and foot (S91.-)

The appropriate 7th character is to be added to each code from category S81

A - initial encounter

D - subsequent encounter

S - sequela

S81.0   Open wound of knee

S81.00   Unspecified open wound of knee

⑦S81.001   Unspecified open wound, right knee

⑦S81.002   Unspecified open wound, left knee

⑦S81.009   Unspecified open wound, unspecified knee

S81.01   Laceration without foreign body of knee

⑦S81.011   Laceration without foreign body, right knee

⑦S81.012   Laceration without foreign body, left knee

⑦S81.019   Laceration without foreign body, unspecified knee

S81.02   Laceration with foreign body of knee

⑦S81.021   Laceration with foreign body, right knee

⑦S81.022   Laceration with foreign body, left knee

⑦S81.029   Laceration with foreign body, unspecified knee

S81.03   Puncture wound without foreign body of knee

⑦S81.031   Puncture wound without foreign body, right knee

⑦S81.032   Puncture wound without foreign body, left knee

⑦S81.039   Puncture wound without foreign body, unspecified knee

S81.04   Puncture wound with foreign body of knee

⑦S81.041 **Puncture wound with foreign body, right knee**

⑦S81.042 **Puncture wound with foreign body, left knee**

⑦S81.049 **Puncture wound with foreign body, unspecified knee**

S81.05 **Open bite of knee**

Bite of knee NOS

Excludes1: superficial bite of knee (S80.27-)

⑦S81.051 **Open bite, right knee**

⑦S81.052 **Open bite, left knee**

⑦S81.059 **Open bite, unspecified knee**

S81.8 **Open wound of lower leg**

S81.80 **Unspecified open wound of lower leg**

⑦S81.801 **Unspecified open wound, right lower leg**

⑦S81.802 **Unspecified open wound, left lower leg**

⑦S81.809 **Unspecified open wound, unspecified lower leg**

S81.81 **Laceration without foreign body of lower leg**

⑦S81.811 **Laceration without foreign body, right lower leg**

⑦S81.812 **Laceration without foreign body, left lower leg**

⑦S81.819 **Laceration without foreign body, unspecified lower leg**

S81.82 **Laceration with foreign body of lower leg**

⑦S81.821 **Laceration with foreign body, right lower leg**

⑦S81.822 **Laceration with foreign body, left lower leg**

⑦S81.829 **Laceration with foreign body, unspecified lower leg**

S81.83 **Puncture wound without foreign body of lower leg**

⑦S81.831 **Puncture wound without foreign body, right lower leg**

⑦S81.832 **Puncture wound without foreign body, left lower leg**

⑦S81.839 **Puncture wound without foreign body, unspecified lower leg**

S81.84 **Puncture wound with foreign body of lower leg**

⑦S81.841 **Puncture wound with foreign body, right lower leg**

⑦S81.842 **Puncture wound with foreign body, left lower leg**

⑦S81.849 **Puncture wound with foreign body, unspecified lower leg**

S81.85 **Open bite of lower leg**

Bite of lower leg NOS

Excludes1: superficial bite of lower leg (S80.86-S80.87-)

⑦S81.851 **Open bite, right lower leg**

⑦S81.852 **Open bite, left lower leg**

⑦S81.859 **Open bite, unspecified lower leg**

S82 **Fracture of lower leg, including ankle**

Note: A fracture not indicated as displaced or nondisplaced should be coded to displaced

A fracture not indicated as open or closed should be coded to closed

The open fracture designations are based on the Gustilo open fracture classification

Includes: fracture of malleolus

Excludes1: traumatic amputation of lower leg (S88.-)

Excludes2: fracture of foot, except ankle (S92.-)

periprosthetic fracture of prosthetic implant of knee (M97.0-)

The appropriate 7th character is to be added to all codes from category S82

A - initial encounter for closed fracture

B - initial encounter for open fracture type I or II initial encounter for open fracture NOS

C - initial encounter for open fracture type IIIA, IIIB, or IIIC

D - subsequent encounter for closed fracture with routine healing

E - subsequent encounter for open fracture type I or II with routine healing

F - subsequent encounter for open fracture type IIIA, IIIB, or IIIC with routine healing

G - subsequent encounter for closed fracture with delayed healing

H - subsequent encounter for open fracture type I or II with delayed healing

J - subsequent encounter for open fracture type IIIA, IIIB, or IIIC with delayed healing

K - subsequent encounter for closed fracture with nonunion

M - subsequent encounter for open fracture type I or II with nonunion

N - subsequent encounter for open fracture type IIIA, IIIB, or IIIC with nonunion

P - subsequent encounter for closed fracture with malunion

Q - subsequent encounter for open fracture type I or II with malunion

R - subsequent encounter for open fracture type IIIA, IIIB, or IIIC with malunion

S - sequela

S82.0 **Fracture of patella**

Knee cap

S82.00 **Unspecified fracture of patella**

⑦S82.001 **Unspecified fracture of right patella**

⑦S82.002 **Unspecified fracture of left patella**

⑦S82.009 **Unspecified fracture of unspecified patella**

S82.01 **Osteochondral fracture of patella**

⑦S82.011 **Displaced osteochondral fracture of right patella**

⑦S82.012 **Displaced osteochondral fracture of left patella**

⑦S82.013 **Displaced osteochondral fracture of unspecified patella**

⑦S82.014 **Nondisplaced osteochondral fracture of right patella**

⑦S82.015 **Nondisplaced osteochondral fracture of left patella**

⑦S82.016 **Nondisplaced osteochondral fracture of unspecified patella**

S82.02 **Longitudinal fracture of patella**

⑦S82.021 **Displaced longitudinal fracture of right patella**

⑦S82.022 **Displaced longitudinal fracture of left patella**

⑦S82.023 **Displaced longitudinal fracture of unspecified patella**

⑦S82.024 **Nondisplaced longitudinal fracture of right patella**

⑦S82.025 **Nondisplaced longitudinal fracture of left patella**

⑦S82.026   Nondisplaced longitudinal fracture of unspecified patella

S82.03   Transverse fracture of patella

⑦S82.031   Displaced transverse fracture of right patella

⑦S82.032   Displaced transverse fracture of left patella

⑦S82.033   Displaced transverse fracture of unspecified patella

⑦S82.034   Nondisplaced transverse fracture of right patella

⑦S82.035   Nondisplaced transverse fracture of left patella

⑦S82.036   Nondisplaced transverse fracture of unspecified patella

S82.04   Comminuted fracture of patella

⑦S82.041   Displaced comminuted fracture of right patella

⑦S82.042   Displaced comminuted fracture of left patella

⑦S82.043   Displaced comminuted fracture of unspecified patella

⑦S82.044   Nondisplaced comminuted fracture of right patella

⑦S82.045   Nondisplaced comminuted fracture of left patella

⑦S82.046   Nondisplaced comminuted fracture of unspecified patella

S82.09   Other fracture of patella

⑦S82.091   Other fracture of right patella

⑦S82.092   Other fracture of left patella

⑦S82.099   Other fracture of unspecified patella

S82.1   Fracture of upper end of tibia

Fracture of proximal end of tibia

Excludes2: fracture of shaft of tibia (S82.2-)

physeal fracture of upper end of tibia (S89.0-)

S82.10   Unspecified fracture of upper end of tibia

⑦S82.101   Unspecified fracture of upper end of right tibia

⑦S82.102   Unspecified fracture of upper end of left tibia

⑦S82.109   Unspecified fracture of upper end of unspecified tibia

S82.11   Fracture of tibial spine

⑦S82.111   Displaced fracture of right tibial spine

⑦S82.112   Displaced fracture of left tibial spine

⑦S82.113   Displaced fracture of unspecified tibial spine

⑦S82.114   Nondisplaced fracture of right tibial spine

⑦S82.115   Nondisplaced fracture of left tibial spine

⑦S82.116   Nondisplaced fracture of unspecified tibial spine

S82.12   Fracture of lateral condyle of tibia

⑦S82.121   Displaced fracture of lateral condyle of right tibia

⑦S82.122   Displaced fracture of lateral condyle of left tibia

⑦S82.123   Displaced fracture of lateral condyle of unspecified tibia

⑦S82.124   Nondisplaced fracture of lateral condyle of right tibia

⑦S82.125   Nondisplaced fracture of lateral condyle of left tibia

⑦S82.126   Nondisplaced fracture of lateral condyle of unspecified tibia

S82.13   Fracture of medial condyle of tibia

⑦S82.131   Displaced fracture of medial condyle of right tibia

⑦S82.132   Displaced fracture of medial condyle of left tibia

⑦S82.133   Displaced fracture of medial condyle of unspecified tibia

⑦S82.134   Nondisplaced fracture of medial condyle of right tibia

⑦S82.135   Nondisplaced fracture of medial condyle of left tibia

⑦S82.136   Nondisplaced fracture of medial condyle of unspecified tibia

S82.14   Bicondylar fracture of tibia

Fracture of tibial plateau NOS

⑦S82.141   Displaced bicondylar fracture of right tibia

⑦S82.142   Displaced bicondylar fracture of left tibia

⑦S82.143   Displaced bicondylar fracture of unspecified tibia

⑦S82.144   Nondisplaced bicondylar fracture of right tibia

⑦S82.145   Nondisplaced bicondylar fracture of left tibia

⑦S82.146   Nondisplaced bicondylar fracture of unspecified tibia

S82.15   Fracture of tibial tuberosity

⑦S82.151   Displaced fracture of right tibial tuberosity

⑦82.152   Displaced fracture of left tibial tuberosity

⑦S82.153   Displaced fracture of unspecified tibial tuberosity

⑦S82.154   Nondisplaced fracture of right tibial tuberosity

⑦S82.155   Nondisplaced fracture of left tibial tuberosity

⑦S82.156   Nondisplaced fracture of unspecified tibial tuberosity

S82.16   Torus fracture of upper end of tibia

The appropriate 7th character is to be added to all codes in subcategory S82.16

A - initial encounter for closed fracture

D - subsequent encounter for fracture with routine healing

G - subsequent encounter for fracture with delayed healing

K - subsequent encounter for fracture with nonunion

P - subsequent encounter for fracture with malunion

S - sequela

⑦S82.161   Torus fracture of upper end of right tibia

⑦S82.162   Torus fracture of upper end of left tibia

⑦S82.169 Torus fracture of upper end of unspecified tibia

S82.19 Other fracture of upper end of tibia

⑦S82.191 Other fracture of upper end of right tibia

⑦S82.192 Other fracture of upper end of left tibia

⑦S82.199 Other fracture of upper end of unspecified tibia

S82.2 Fracture of shaft of tibia

S82.20 Unspecified fracture of shaft of tibia

Fracture of tibia NOS

⑦S82.201 Unspecified fracture of shaft of right tibia

⑦S82.202 Unspecified fracture of shaft of left tibia

⑦S82.209 Unspecified fracture of shaft of unspecified tibia

S82.22 Transverse fracture of shaft of tibia

⑦S82.221 Displaced transverse fracture of shaft of right tibia

⑦S82.222 Displaced transverse fracture of shaft of left tibia

⑦S82.223 Displaced transverse fracture of shaft of unspecified tibia

⑦S82.224 Nondisplaced transverse fracture of shaft of right tibia

⑦S82.225 Nondisplaced transverse fracture of shaft of left tibia

⑦S82.226 Nondisplaced transverse fracture of shaft of unspecified tibia

S82.23 Oblique fracture of shaft of tibia

⑦S82.231 Displaced oblique fracture of shaft of right tibia

⑦S82.232 Displaced oblique fracture of shaft of left tibia

⑦S82.233 Displaced oblique fracture of shaft of unspecified tibia

⑦S82.234 Nondisplaced oblique fracture of shaft of right tibia

⑦S82.235 Nondisplaced oblique fracture of shaft of left tibia

⑦S82.236 Nondisplaced oblique fracture of shaft of unspecified tibia

S82.24 Spiral fracture of shaft of tibia

Toddler fracture

⑦S82.241 Displaced spiral fracture of shaft of right tibia

⑦S82.242 Displaced spiral fracture of shaft of left tibia

⑦S82.243 Displaced spiral fracture of shaft of unspecified tibia

⑦S82.244 Nondisplaced spiral fracture of shaft of right tibia

⑦S82.245 Nondisplaced spiral fracture of shaft of left tibia

⑦S82.246 Nondisplaced spiral fracture of shaft of unspecified tibia

S82.25 Comminuted fracture of shaft of tibia

⑦S82.251 Displaced comminuted fracture of shaft of right tibia

⑦S82.252 Displaced comminuted fracture of shaft of left tibia

⑦S82.253 Displaced comminuted fracture of shaft of unspecified tibia

⑦S82.254 Nondisplaced comminuted fracture of shaft of right tibia

⑦S82.255 Nondisplaced comminuted fracture of shaft of left tibia

⑦S82.256 Nondisplaced comminuted fracture of shaft of unspecified tibia

S82.26 Segmental fracture of shaft of tibia

⑦S82.261 Displaced segmental fracture of shaft of right tibia

⑦S82.262 Displaced segmental fracture of shaft of left tibia

⑦S82.263 Displaced segmental fracture of shaft of unspecified tibia

⑦S82.264 Nondisplaced segmental fracture of shaft of right tibia

⑦S82.265 Nondisplaced segmental fracture of shaft of left tibia

⑦S82.266 Nondisplaced segmental fracture of shaft of unspecified tibia

S82.29 Other fracture of shaft of tibia

⑦S82.291 Other fracture of shaft of right tibia

⑦S82.292 Other fracture of shaft of left tibia

⑦S82.299 Other fracture of shaft of unspecified tibia

S82.3 Fracture of lower end of tibia

Excludes1: bimalleolar fracture of lower leg (S82.84-)
fracture of medial malleolus alone (S82.5-)
Maisonneuve's fracture (S82.86-)
pilon fracture of distal tibia (S82.87-)
trimalleolar fractures of lower leg (S82.85-)

S82.30 Unspecified fracture of lower end of tibia

⑦S82.301 Unspecified fracture of lower end of right tibia

⑦S82.302 Unspecified fracture of lower end of left tibia

⑦S82.309 Unspecified fracture of lower end of unspecified tibia

S82.31 Torus fracture of lower end of tibia

The appropriate 7th character is to be added to all codes in subcategory S82.31

A - initial encounter for closed fracture

D - subsequent encounter for fracture with routine healing

G - subsequent encounter for fracture with delayed healing

K - subsequent encounter for fracture with nonunion

P - subsequent encounter for fracture with malunion

S - sequela

⑦S82.311 Torus fracture of lower end of right tibia

⑦S82.312 Torus fracture of lower end of left tibia

⑦S82.319 Torus fracture of lower end of unspecified tibia

S82.39 Other fracture of lower end of tibia

⑦S82.391 Other fracture of lower end of right tibia

⑦ **S82.392** Other fracture of lower end of left tibia

⑦ **S82.399** Other fracture of lower end of unspecified tibia

S82.4 Fracture of shaft of fibula

Excludes2: fracture of lateral malleolus alone (S82.6-)

S82.40 Unspecified fracture of shaft of fibula

⑦ **S82.401** Unspecified fracture of shaft of right fibula

⑦ **S82.402** Unspecified fracture of shaft of left fibula

⑦ **S82.409** Unspecified fracture of shaft of unspecified fibula

S82.42 Transverse fracture of shaft of fibula

⑦ **S82.421** Displaced transverse fracture of shaft of right fibula

⑦ **S82.422** Displaced transverse fracture of shaft of left fibula

⑦ **S82.423** Displaced transverse fracture of shaft of unspecified fibula

⑦ **S82.424** Nondisplaced transverse fracture of shaft of right fibula

⑦ **S82.425** Nondisplaced transverse fracture of shaft of left fibula

⑦ **S82.426** Nondisplaced transverse fracture of shaft of unspecified fibula

S82.43 Oblique fracture of shaft of fibula

⑦ **S82.431** Displaced oblique fracture of shaft of right fibula

⑦ **S82.432** Displaced oblique fracture of shaft of left fibula

⑦ **S82.433** Displaced oblique fracture of shaft of unspecified fibula

⑦ **S82.434** Nondisplaced oblique fracture of shaft of right fibula

⑦ **S82.435** Nondisplaced oblique fracture of shaft of left fibula

⑦ **S82.436** Nondisplaced oblique fracture of shaft of unspecified fibula

S82.44 Spiral fracture of shaft of fibula

⑦ **S82.441** Displaced spiral fracture of shaft of right fibula

⑦ **S82.442** Displaced spiral fracture of shaft of left fibula

⑦ **S82.443** Displaced spiral fracture of shaft of unspecified fibula

⑦ **S82.444** Nondisplaced spiral fracture of shaft of right fibula

⑦ **S82.445** Nondisplaced spiral fracture of shaft of left fibula

⑦ **S82.446** Nondisplaced spiral fracture of shaft of unspecified fibula

S82.45 Comminuted fracture of shaft of fibula

⑦ **S82.451** Displaced comminuted fracture of shaft of right fibula

⑦ **S82.452** Displaced comminuted fracture of shaft of left fibula

⑦ **S82.453** Displaced comminuted fracture of shaft of unspecified fibula

⑦ **S82.454** Nondisplaced comminuted fracture of shaft of right fibula

⑦ **S82.455** Nondisplaced comminuted fracture of shaft of left fibula

⑦ **S82.456** Nondisplaced comminuted fracture of shaft of unspecified fibula

S82.46 Segmental fracture of shaft of fibula

⑦ **S82.461** Displaced segmental fracture of shaft of right fibula

⑦ **S82.462** Displaced segmental fracture of shaft of left fibula

⑦ **S82.463** Displaced segmental fracture of shaft of unspecified fibula

⑦ **S82.464** Nondisplaced segmental fracture of shaft of right fibula

⑦ **S82.465** Nondisplaced segmental fracture of shaft of left fibula

⑦ **S82.466** Nondisplaced segmental fracture of shaft of unspecified fibula

S82.49 Other fracture of shaft of fibula

⑦ **S82.491** Other fracture of shaft of right fibula

⑦ **S82.492** Other fracture of shaft of left fibula

⑦ **S82.499** Other fracture of shaft of unspecified fibula

S82.5 Fracture of medial malleolus

Excludes1: pilon fracture of distal tibia (S82.87-)

Salter-Harris type III of lower end of tibia (S89.13-)

Salter-Harris type IV of lower end of tibia (S89.14-)

⊗⑦ **S82.51** Displaced fracture of medial malleolus of right tibia

⊗⑦ **S82.52** Displaced fracture of medial malleolus of left tibia

⊗⑦ **S82.53** Displaced fracture of medial malleolus of unspecified tibia

⊗⑦ **S82.54** Nondisplaced fracture of medial malleolus of right tibia

⊗⑦ **S82.55** Nondisplaced fracture of medial malleolus of left tibia

⊗⑦ **S82.56** Nondisplaced fracture of medial malleolus of unspecified tibia

S82.6 Fracture of lateral malleolus

Excludes1: pilon fracture of distal tibia (S82.87-)

⊗⑦ **S82.61** Displaced fracture of lateral malleolus of right fibula

⊗⑦ **S82.62** Displaced fracture of lateral malleolus of left fibula

⊗⑦ **S82.63** Displaced fracture of lateral malleolus of unspecified fibula

⊗⑦ **S82.64** Nondisplaced fracture of lateral malleolus of right fibula

⊗⑦ **S82.65** Nondisplaced fracture of lateral malleolus of left fibula

⊗⑦ **S82.66** Nondisplaced fracture of lateral malleolus of unspecified fibula

S82.8 Other fractures of lower leg

S82.81 Torus fracture of upper end of fibula

The appropriate 7th character is to be added to all codes in subcategory S82.81

A - initial encounter for closed fracture

D - subsequent encounter for fracture with routine healing

G - subsequent encounter for fracture with delayed healing

K - subsequent encounter for fracture with nonunion

● New code ▲ Revised code **Excludes1:** Not coded here **Excludes2:** Not included here ⊗ Placeholder required ⑦ 7th digit required

P - subsequent encounter for fracture with malunion

S - sequela

⑦S82.811   **Torus fracture of upper end of right fibula**

⑦S82.812   **Torus fracture of upper end of left fibula**

⑦S82.819   **Torus fracture of upper end of unspecified fibula**

S82.82   **Torus fracture of lower end of fibula**

The appropriate 7th character is to be added to all codes in subcategory S82.82

A - initial encounter for closed fracture

D - subsequent encounter for fracture with routine healing

G - subsequent encounter for fracture with delayed healing

K - subsequent encounter for fracture with nonunion

P - subsequent encounter for fracture with malunion

S - sequela

⑦S82.821   **Torus fracture of lower end of right fibula**

⑦S82.822   **Torus fracture of lower end of left fibula**

⑦S82.829   **Torus fracture of lower end of unspecified fibula**

S82.83   **Other fracture of upper and lower end of fibula**

⑦S82.831   **Other fracture of upper and lower end of right fibula**

⑦S82.832   **Other fracture of upper and lower end of left fibula**

⑦S82.839   **Other fracture of upper and lower end of unspecified fibula**

S82.84   **Bimalleolar fracture of lower leg**

⑦S82.841   Displaced bimalleolar fracture of right lower leg

⑦S82.842   Displaced bimalleolar fracture of left lower leg

⑦S82.843   Displaced bimalleolar fracture of unspecified lower leg

⑦S82.844   Nondisplaced bimalleolar fracture of right lower leg

⑦S82.845   Nondisplaced bimalleolar fracture of left lower leg

⑦S82.846   Nondisplaced bimalleolar fracture of unspecified lower leg

S82.85   **Trimalleolar fracture of lower leg**

⑦S82.851   Displaced trimalleolar fracture of right lower leg

⑦S82.852   Displaced trimalleolar fracture of left lower leg

⑦S82.853   Displaced trimalleolar fracture of unspecified lower leg

⑦S82.854   Nondisplaced trimalleolar fracture of right lower leg

⑦S82.855   Nondisplaced trimalleolar fracture of left lower leg

⑦S82.856   Nondisplaced trimalleolar fracture of unspecified lower leg

S82.86   **Maisonneuve's fracture**

⑦S82.861   **Displaced Maisonneuve's fracture of right leg**

⑦S82.862   **Displaced Maisonneuve's fracture of left leg**

⑦S82.863   **Displaced Maisonneuve's fracture of unspecified leg**

⑦S82.864   **Nondisplaced Maisonneuve's fracture of right leg**

⑦S82.865   **Nondisplaced Maisonneuve's fracture of left leg**

⑦S82.866   **Nondisplaced Maisonneuve's fracture of unspecified leg**

S82.87   **Pilon fracture of tibia**

⑦S82.871   **Displaced pilon fracture of right tibia**

⑦S82.872   **Displaced pilon fracture of left tibia**

⑦S82.873   **Displaced pilon fracture of unspecified tibia**

⑦S82.874   **Nondisplaced pilon fracture of right tibia**

⑦S82.875   **Nondisplaced pilon fracture of left tibia**

⑦S82.876   **Nondisplaced pilon fracture of unspecified tibia**

S82.89   **Other fractures of lower leg**

Fracture of ankle NOS

⑦S82.891   **Other fracture of right lower leg**

⑦S82.892   **Other fracture of left lower leg**

⑦ S82.899   **Other fracture of unspecified lower leg**

S82.9   **Unspecified fracture of lower leg**

⊗⑦S82.90   **Unspecified fracture of unspecified lower leg**

⊗⑦S82.91   **Unspecified fracture of right lower leg**

⊗⑦S82.92   **Unspecified fracture of left lower leg**

S83   **Dislocation and sprain of joints and ligaments of knee**

Includes: avulsion of joint or ligament of knee

laceration of cartilage, joint or ligament of knee

sprain of cartilage, joint or ligament of knee

traumatic hemarthrosis of joint or ligament of knee

traumatic rupture of joint or ligament of knee

traumatic subluxation of joint or ligament of knee

traumatic tear of joint or ligament of knee

Code also any associated open wound

Excludes1: derangement of patella (M22.0-M22.3)

injury of patellar ligament (tendon) (S76.1-)

internal derangement of knee (M23.-)

old dislocation of knee (M24.36)

pathological dislocation of knee (M24.36)

recurrent dislocation of knee (M22.0)

Excludes2: strain of muscle, fascia and tendon of lower leg (S86.-)

The appropriate 7th character is to be added to each code from category S83

A - initial encounter

D - subsequent encounter

S - sequela

S83.0   **Subluxation and dislocation of patella**

S83.00   **Unspecified subluxation and dislocation of patella**

⑦S83.001   **Unspecified subluxation of right patella**

⑦ S83.002　Unspecified subluxation of left patella

⑦ S83.003　Unspecified subluxation of unspecified patella

⑦ S83.004　Unspecified dislocation of right patella

⑦ S83.005　Unspecified dislocation of left patella

⑦ S83.006　Unspecified dislocation of unspecified patella

S83.01　Lateral subluxation and dislocation of patella

⑦ S83.011　Lateral subluxation of right patella

⑦ S83.012　Lateral subluxation of left patella

⑦ S83.013　Lateral subluxation of unspecified patella

⑦ S83.014　Lateral dislocation of right patella

⑦ S83.015　Lateral dislocation of left patella

⑦ S83.016　Lateral dislocation of unspecified patella

S83.09　Other subluxation and dislocation of patella

⑦ S83.091　Other subluxation of right patella

⑦ S83.092　Other subluxation of left patella

⑦ S83.093　Other subluxation of unspecified patella

⑦ S83.094　Other dislocation of right patella

⑦ S83.095　Other dislocation of left patella

⑦ S83.096　Other dislocation of unspecified patella

S83.1　Subluxation and dislocation of knee

Excludes2: instability of knee prosthesis (T84.022, T84.023)

S83.10　Unspecified subluxation and dislocation of knee

⑦ S83.101　Unspecified subluxation of right knee

⑦ S83.102　Unspecified subluxation of left knee

⑦ S83.103　Unspecified subluxation of unspecified knee

⑦ S83.104　Unspecified dislocation of right knee

⑦ S83.105　Unspecified dislocation of left knee

⑦ S83.106　Unspecified dislocation of unspecified knee

S83.11　Anterior subluxation and dislocation of proximal end of tibia

Posterior subluxation and dislocation of distal end of femur

⑦ S83.111　Anterior subluxation of proximal end of tibia, right knee

⑦ S83.112　Anterior subluxation of proximal end of tibia, left knee

⑦ S83.113　Anterior subluxation of proximal end of tibia, unspecified knee

⑦ S83.114　Anterior dislocation of proximal end of tibia, right knee

⑦ S83.115　Anterior dislocation of proximal end of tibia, left knee

⑦ S83.116　Anterior dislocation of proximal end of tibia, unspecified knee

S83.12　Posterior subluxation and dislocation of proximal end of tibia

Anterior dislocation of distal end of femur

⑦ S83.121　Posterior subluxation of proximal end of tibia, right knee

⑦ S83.122　Posterior subluxation of proximal end of tibia, left knee

⑦ S83.123　Posterior subluxation of proximal end of tibia, unspecified knee

⑦ S83.124　Posterior dislocation of proximal end of tibia, right knee

⑦ S83.125　Posterior dislocation of proximal end of tibia, left knee

⑦ S83.126　Posterior dislocation of proximal end of tibia, unspecified knee

S83.13　Medial subluxation and dislocation of proximal end of tibia

⑦ S83.131　Medial subluxation of proximal end of tibia, right knee

⑦ S83.132　Medial subluxation of proximal end of tibia, left knee

⑦ S83.133　Medial subluxation of proximal end of tibia, unspecified knee

⑦ S83.134　Medial dislocation of proximal end of tibia, right knee

⑦ S83.135　Medial dislocation of proximal end of tibia, left knee

⑦ S83.136　Medial dislocation of proximal end of tibia, unspecified knee

S83.14　Lateral subluxation and dislocation of proximal end of tibia

⑦ S83.141　Lateral subluxation of proximal end of tibia, right knee

⑦ S83.142　Lateral subluxation of proximal end of tibia, left knee

⑦ S83.143　Lateral subluxation of proximal end of tibia, unspecified knee

⑦ S83.144　Lateral dislocation of proximal end of tibia, right knee

⑦ S83.145　Lateral dislocation of proximal end of tibia, left knee

⑦ S83.146　Lateral dislocation of proximal end of tibia, unspecified knee

S83.19　Other subluxation and dislocation of knee

⑦ S83.191　Other subluxation of right knee

⑦ S83.192　Other subluxation of left knee

⑦ S83.193　Other subluxation of unspecified knee

⑦ S83.194　Other dislocation of right knee

⑦ S83.195　Other dislocation of left knee

⑦ S83.196　Other dislocation of unspecified knee

S83.2　Tear of meniscus, current injury

Excludes1: old bucket-handle tear (M23.2)

S83.20　Tear of unspecified meniscus, current injury

Tear of meniscus of knee NOS

⑦ S83.200　Bucket-handle tear of unspecified meniscus, current injury, right knee

⑦ S83.201　Bucket-handle tear of unspecified meniscus, current injury, left knee

⑦ S83.202　Bucket-handle tear of unspecified meniscus, current injury, unspecified knee

⑦ S83.203　Other tear of unspecified meniscus, current injury, right knee

⑦ S83.204　Other tear of unspecified meniscus, current injury, left knee

⑦ S83.205　Other tear of unspecified meniscus, current injury, unspecified knee

⑦S83.206　Unspecified tear of unspecified meniscus, current injury, right knee

⑦S83.207　Unspecified tear of unspecified meniscus, current injury, left knee

⑦S83.209　Unspecified tear of unspecified meniscus, current injury, unspecified knee

S83.21　Bucket-handle tear of medial meniscus, current injury

　　⑦S83.211　Bucket-handle tear of medial meniscus, current injury, right knee

　　⑦S83.212　Bucket-handle tear of medial meniscus, current injury, left knee

　　⑦S83.219　Bucket-handle tear of medial meniscus, current injury, unspecified knee

S83.22　Peripheral tear of medial meniscus, current injury

　　⑦S83.221　Peripheral tear of medial meniscus, current injury, right knee

　　⑦S83.222　Peripheral tear of medial meniscus, current injury, left knee

　　⑦S83.229　Peripheral tear of medial meniscus, current injury, unspecified knee

S83.23　Complex tear of medial meniscus, current injury

　　⑦S83.231　Complex tear of medial meniscus, current injury, right knee

　　⑦S83.232　Complex tear of medial meniscus, current injury, left knee

　　⑦S83.239　Complex tear of medial meniscus, current injury, unspecified knee

S83.24　Other tear of medial meniscus, current injury

　　⑦S83.241　Other tear of medial meniscus, current injury, right knee

　　⑦S83.242　Other tear of medial meniscus, current injury, left knee

　　⑦S83.249　Other tear of medial meniscus, current injury, unspecified knee

S83.25　Bucket-handle tear of lateral meniscus, current injury

　　⑦S83.251　Bucket-handle tear of lateral meniscus, current injury, right knee

　　⑦S83.252　Bucket-handle tear of lateral meniscus, current injury, left knee

　　⑦S83.259　Bucket-handle tear of lateral meniscus, current injury, unspecified knee

S83.26　Peripheral tear of lateral meniscus, current injury

　　⑦S83.261　Peripheral tear of lateral meniscus, current injury, right knee

　　⑦S83.262　Peripheral tear of lateral meniscus, current injury, left knee

　　⑦S83.269　Peripheral tear of lateral meniscus, current injury, unspecified knee

S83.27　Complex tear of lateral meniscus, current injury

　　⑦S83.271　Complex tear of lateral meniscus, current injury, right knee

　　⑦S83.272　Complex tear of lateral meniscus, current injury, left knee

　　⑦S83.279　Complex tear of lateral meniscus, current injury, unspecified knee

S83.28　Other tear of lateral meniscus, current injury

　　⑦S83.281　Other tear of lateral meniscus, current injury, right knee

　　⑦S83.282　Other tear of lateral meniscus, current injury, left knee

　　⑦S83.289　Other tear of lateral meniscus, current injury, unspecified knee

S83.3　Tear of articular cartilage of knee, current

　　⊗⑦S83.30　Tear of articular cartilage of unspecified knee, current

　　⊗⑦S83.31　Tear of articular cartilage of right knee, current

　　⊗⑦S83.32　Tear of articular cartilage of left knee, current

S83.4　Sprain of collateral ligament of knee

　　S83.40　Sprain of unspecified collateral ligament of knee

　　　　⑦S83.401　Sprain of unspecified collateral ligament of right knee

　　　　⑦S83.402　Sprain of unspecified collateral ligament of left knee

　　　　⑦S83.409　Sprain of unspecified collateral ligament of unspecified knee

　　S83.41　Sprain of medial collateral ligament of knee
　　　　Sprain of tibial collateral ligament

　　　　⑦S83.411　Sprain of medial collateral ligament of right knee

　　　　⑦S83.412　Sprain of medial collateral ligament of left knee

　　　　⑦S83.419　Sprain of medial collateral ligament of unspecified knee

　　S83.42　Sprain of lateral collateral ligament of knee
　　　　Sprain of fibular collateral ligament

　　　　⑦S83.421　Sprain of lateral collateral ligament of right knee

　　　　⑦S83.422　Sprain of lateral collateral ligament of left knee

　　　　⑦S83.429　Sprain of lateral collateral ligament of unspecified knee

S83.5　Sprain of cruciate ligament of knee

　　S83.50　Sprain of unspecified cruciate ligament of knee

　　　　⑦S83.501　Sprain of unspecified cruciate ligament of right knee

　　　　⑦S83.502　Sprain of unspecified cruciate ligament of left knee

　　　　⑦S83.509　Sprain of unspecified cruciate ligament of unspecified knee

　　S83.51　Sprain of anterior cruciate ligament of knee

　　　　⑦S83.511　Sprain of anterior cruciate ligament of right knee

　　　　⑦S83.512　Sprain of anterior cruciate ligament of left knee

　　　　⑦S83.519　Sprain of anterior cruciate ligament of unspecified knee

　　S83.52　Sprain of posterior cruciate ligament of knee

　　　　⑦S83.521　Sprain of posterior cruciate ligament of right knee

　　　　⑦S83.522　Sprain of posterior cruciate ligament of left knee

　　　　⑦S83.529　Sprain of posterior cruciate ligament of unspecified knee

S83.6　Sprain of the superior tibiofibular joint and ligament

　　⊗⑦S83.60　Sprain of the superior tibiofibular joint and ligament, unspecified knee

⊗⑦S83.61 **Sprain of the superior tibiofibular joint and ligament, right knee**

⊗⑦S83.62 **Sprain of the superior tibiofibular joint and ligament, left knee**

S83.8 **Sprain of other specified parts of knee**

S83.8X **Sprain of other specified parts of knee**

⑦ S83.8X1 **Sprain of other specified parts of right knee**

⑦ S83.8X2 **Sprain of other specified parts of left knee**

⑦ S83.8X9 **Sprain of other specified parts of unspecified knee**

S83.9 **Sprain of unspecified site of knee**

⊗⑦S83.90 **Sprain of unspecified site of unspecified knee**

⊗⑦S83.91 **Sprain of unspecified site of right knee**

⊗⑦S83.92 **Sprain of unspecified site of left knee**

S84 **Injury of nerves at lower leg level**

Code also any associated open wound (S81.-)

Excludes2: injury of nerves at ankle and foot level (S94.-)

The appropriate 7th character is to be added to each code from category S84

A - initial encounter

D - subsequent encounter

S - sequela

S84.0 **Injury of tibial nerve at lower leg level**

⊗⑦S84.00 **Injury of tibial nerve at lower leg level, unspecified leg**

⊗⑦S84.01 **Injury of tibial nerve at lower leg level, right leg**

⊗⑦S84.02 **Injury of tibial nerve at lower leg level, left leg**

S84.1 **Injury of peroneal nerve at lower leg level**

⊗⑦S84.10 **Injury of peroneal nerve at lower leg level, unspecified leg**

⊗⑦S84.11 **Injury of peroneal nerve at lower leg level, right leg**

⊗⑦S84.12 **Injury of peroneal nerve at lower leg level, left leg**

S84.2 **Injury of cutaneous sensory nerve at lower leg level**

⊗⑦S84.20 **Injury of cutaneous sensory nerve at lower leg level, unspecified leg**

⊗⑦S84.21 **Injury of cutaneous sensory nerve at lower leg level, right leg**

⊗⑦S84.22 **Injury of cutaneous sensory nerve at lower leg level, left leg**

S84.8 **Injury of other nerves at lower leg level**

S84.80 **Injury of other nerves at lower leg level**

⑦ S84.801 **Injury of other nerves at lower leg level, right leg**

⑦ S84.802 **Injury of other nerves at lower leg level, left leg**

⑦ S84.809 **Injury of other nerves at lower leg level, unspecified leg**

S84.9 **Injury of unspecified nerve at lower leg level**

⊗⑦S84.90 **Injury of unspecified nerve at lower leg level, unspecified leg**

⊗⑦S84.91 **Injury of unspecified nerve at lower leg level, right leg**

⊗⑦S84.92 **Injury of unspecified nerve at lower leg level, left leg**

S85 **Injury of blood vessels at lower leg level**

Code also any associated open wound (S81.-)

Excludes2: injury of blood vessels at ankle and foot level (S95.-)

The appropriate 7th character is to be added to each code from category S85

A - initial encounter

D - subsequent encounter

S - sequela

S85.0 **Injury of popliteal artery**

S85.00 **Unspecified injury of popliteal artery**

⑦ S85.001 **Unspecified injury of popliteal artery, right leg**

⑦ S85.002 **Unspecified injury of popliteal artery, left leg**

⑦ S85.009 **Unspecified injury of popliteal artery, unspecified leg**

S85.01 **Laceration of popliteal artery**

⑦ S85.011 **Laceration of popliteal artery, right leg**

⑦ S85.012 **Laceration of popliteal artery, left leg**

⑦ S85.019 **Laceration of popliteal artery, unspecified leg**

S85.09 **Other specified injury of popliteal artery**

⑦ S85.091 **Other specified injury of popliteal artery, right leg**

⑦ S85.092 **Other specified injury of popliteal artery, left leg**

⑦ S85.099 **Other specified injury of popliteal artery, unspecified leg**

S85.1 **Injury of tibial artery**

S85.10 **Unspecified injury of unspecified tibial artery**

Injury of tibial artery NOS

⑦ S85.101 **Unspecified injury of unspecified tibial artery, right leg**

⑦ S85.102 **Unspecified injury of unspecified tibial artery, left leg**

⑦ S85.109 **Unspecified injury of unspecified tibial artery, unspecified leg**

S85.11 **Laceration of unspecified tibial artery**

⑦ S85.111 **Laceration of unspecified tibial artery, right leg**

⑦ S85.112 **Laceration of unspecified tibial artery, left leg**

⑦ S85.119 **Laceration of unspecified tibial artery, unspecified leg**

S85.12 **Other specified injury of unspecified tibial artery**

⑦ S85.121 **Other specified injury of unspecified tibial artery, right leg**

⑦ S85.122 **Other specified injury of unspecified tibial artery, left leg**

⑦ S85.129 **Other specified injury of unspecified tibial artery, unspecified leg**

S85.13 **Unspecified injury of anterior tibial artery**

⑦ S85.131 **Unspecified injury of anterior tibial artery, right leg**

⑦ S85.132 **Unspecified injury of anterior tibial artery, left leg**

⑦ S85.139 **Unspecified injury of anterior tibial artery, unspecified leg**

S85.14 **Laceration of anterior tibial artery**

⑦ S85.141 **Laceration of anterior tibial artery, right leg**

● New code ▲ Revised code **Excludes1:** Not coded here **Excludes2:** Not included here ⊗ Placeholder required ⑦7th digit required

⑦S85.142   **Laceration of anterior tibial artery, left leg**

⑦S85.149   **Laceration of anterior tibial artery, unspecified leg**

S85.15   **Other specified injury of anterior tibial artery**

⑦S85.151   **Other specified injury of anterior tibial artery, right leg**

⑦S85.152   **Other specified injury of anterior tibial artery, left leg**

⑦S85.159   **Other specified injury of anterior tibial artery, unspecified leg**

S85.16   **Unspecified injury of posterior tibial artery**

⑦S85.161   **Unspecified injury of posterior tibial artery, right leg**

⑦S85.162   **Unspecified injury of posterior tibial artery, left leg**

⑦S85.169   **Unspecified injury of posterior tibial artery, unspecified leg**

S85.17   **Laceration of posterior tibial artery**

⑦S85.171   **Laceration of posterior tibial artery, right leg**

⑦S85.172   **Laceration of posterior tibial artery, left leg**

⑦S85.179   **Laceration of posterior tibial artery, unspecified leg**

S85.18   **Other specified injury of posterior tibial artery**

⑦S85.181   **Other specified injury of posterior tibial artery, right leg**

⑦S85.182   **Other specified injury of posterior tibial artery, left leg**

⑦S85.189   **Other specified injury of posterior tibial artery, unspecified leg**

S85.2   **Injury of peroneal artery**

S85.20   **Unspecified injury of peroneal artery**

⑦S85.201   **Unspecified injury of peroneal artery, right leg**

⑦S85.202   **Unspecified injury of peroneal artery, left leg**

⑦S85.209   **Unspecified injury of peroneal artery, unspecified leg**

S85.21   **Laceration of peroneal artery**

⑦S85.211   **Laceration of peroneal artery, right leg**

⑦S85.212   **Laceration of peroneal artery, left leg**

⑦S85.219   **Laceration of peroneal artery, unspecified leg**

S85.29   **Other specified injury of peroneal artery**

⑦S85.291   **Other specified injury of peroneal artery, right leg**

⑦S85.292   **Other specified injury of peroneal artery, left leg**

⑦S85.299   **Other specified injury of peroneal artery, unspecified leg**

S85.3   **Injury of greater saphenous vein at lower leg level**

Injury of greater saphenous vein NOS

Injury of saphenous vein NOS

S85.30   **Unspecified injury of greater saphenous vein at lower leg level**

⑦S85.301   **Unspecified injury of greater saphenous vein at lower leg level, right leg**

⑦S85.302   **Unspecified injury of greater saphenous vein at lower leg level, left leg**

⑦S85.309   **Unspecified injury of greater saphenous vein at lower leg level, unspecified leg**

S85.31   **Laceration of greater saphenous vein at lower leg level**

⑦S85.311   **Laceration of greater saphenous vein at lower leg level, right leg**

⑦S85.312   **Laceration of greater saphenous vein at lower leg level, left leg**

⑦S85.319   **Laceration of greater saphenous vein at lower leg level, unspecified leg**

S85.39   **Other specified injury of greater saphenous vein at lower leg level**

⑦S85.391   **Other specified injury of greater saphenous vein at lower leg level, right leg**

⑦S85.392   **Other specified injury of greater saphenous vein at lower leg level, left leg**

⑦S85.399   **Other specified injury of greater saphenous vein at lower leg level, unspecified leg**

S85.4   **Injury of lesser saphenous vein at lower leg level**

S85.40   **Unspecified injury of lesser saphenous vein at lower leg level**

⑦S85.401   **Unspecified injury of lesser saphenous vein at lower leg level, right leg**

⑦S85.402   **Unspecified injury of lesser saphenous vein at lower leg level, left leg**

⑦S85.409   **Unspecified injury of lesser saphenous vein at lower leg level, unspecified leg**

S85.41   **Laceration of lesser saphenous vein at lower leg level**

⑦S85.411   **Laceration of lesser saphenous vein at lower leg level, right leg**

⑦S85.412   **Laceration of lesser saphenous vein at lower leg level, left leg**

⑦S85.419   **Laceration of lesser saphenous vein at lower leg level, unspecified leg**

S85.49   **Other specified injury of lesser saphenous vein at lower leg level**

⑦S85.491   **Other specified injury of lesser saphenous vein at lower leg level, right leg**

⑦S85.492   **Other specified injury of lesser saphenous vein at lower leg level, left leg**

⑦S85.499   **Other specified injury of lesser saphenous vein at lower leg level, unspecified leg**

S85.5   **Injury of popliteal vein**

S85.50   **Unspecified injury of popliteal vein**

⑦S85.501   **Unspecified injury of popliteal vein, right leg**

⑦S85.502   **Unspecified injury of popliteal vein, left leg**

⑦S85.509   **Unspecified injury of popliteal vein, unspecified leg**

S85.51   **Laceration of popliteal vein**

---

⑦ S85.511   **Laceration of popliteal vein, right leg**

⑦ S85.512   **Laceration of popliteal vein, left leg**

⑦ S85.519   **Laceration of popliteal vein, unspecified leg**

    S85.59   **Other specified injury of popliteal vein**

⑦ S85.591   **Other specified injury of popliteal vein, right leg**

⑦ S85.592   **Other specified injury of popliteal vein, left leg**

⑦ S85.599   **Other specified injury of popliteal vein, unspecified leg**

  S85.8   **Injury of other blood vessels at lower leg level**

    S85.80   **Unspecified injury of other blood vessels at lower leg level**

⑦ S85.801   **Unspecified injury of other blood vessels at lower leg level, right leg**

⑦ S85.802   **Unspecified injury of other blood vessels at lower leg level, left leg**

⑦ S85.809   **Unspecified injury of other blood vessels at lower leg level, unspecified leg**

    S85.81   **Laceration of other blood vessels at lower leg level**

⑦ S85.811   **Laceration of other blood vessels at lower leg level, right leg**

⑦ S85.812   **Laceration of other blood vessels at lower leg level, left leg**

⑦ S85.819   **Laceration of other blood vessels at lower leg level, unspecified leg**

    S85.89   **Other specified injury of other blood vessels at lower leg level**

⑦ S85.891   **Other specified injury of other blood vessels at lower leg level, right leg**

⑦ S85.892   **Other specified injury of other blood vessels at lower leg level, left leg**

⑦ S85.899   **Other specified injury of other blood vessels at lower leg level, unspecified leg**

  S85.9   **Injury of unspecified blood vessel at lower leg level**

    S85.90   **Unspecified injury of unspecified blood vessel at lower leg level**

⑦ S85.901   **Unspecified injury of unspecified blood vessel at lower leg level, right leg**

⑦ S85.902   **Unspecified injury of unspecified blood vessel at lower leg level, left leg**

⑦ S85.909   **Unspecified injury of unspecified blood vessel at lower leg level, unspecified leg**

    S85.91   **Laceration of unspecified blood vessel at lower leg level**

⑦ S85.911   **Laceration of unspecified blood vessel at lower leg level, right leg**

⑦ S85.912   **Laceration of unspecified blood vessel at lower leg level, left leg**

⑦ S85.919   **Laceration of unspecified blood vessel at lower leg level, unspecified leg**

    S85.99   **Other specified injury of unspecified blood vessel at lower leg level**

⑦ S85.991   **Other specified injury of unspecified blood vessel at lower leg level, right leg**

⑦ S85.992   **Other specified injury of unspecified blood vessel at lower leg level, left leg**

⑦ S85.999   **Other specified injury of unspecified blood vessel at lower leg level, unspecified leg**

S86   **Injury of muscle, fascia and tendon at lower leg level**

  <u>**Code also**</u> any associated open wound (S81.-)

  Excludes2: injury of muscle, fascia and tendon at ankle (S96.-)

    injury of patellar ligament (tendon) (S76.1-)

    sprain of joints and ligaments of knee (S83.-)

The appropriate 7th character is to be added to each code from category S86

A - initial encounter

D - subsequent encounter

S - sequela

  S86.0   **Injury of Achilles tendon**

    S86.00   **Unspecified injury of Achilles tendon**

⑦ S86.001   **Unspecified injury of right Achilles tendon**

⑦ S86.002   **Unspecified injury of left Achilles tendon**

⑦ S86.009   **Unspecified injury of unspecified Achilles tendon**

    S86.01   **Strain of Achilles tendon**

⑦ S86.011   **Strain of right Achilles tendon**

⑦ S86.012   **Strain of left Achilles tendon**

⑦ S86.019   **Strain of unspecified Achilles tendon**

    S86.02   **Laceration of Achilles tendon**

⑦ S86.021   **Laceration of right Achilles tendon**

⑦ S86.022   **Laceration of left Achilles tendon**

⑦ S86.029   **Laceration of unspecified Achilles tendon**

    S86.09   **Other specified injury of Achilles tendon**

⑦ S86.091   **Other specified injury of right Achilles tendon**

⑦ S86.092   **Other specified injury of left Achilles tendon**

⑦ S86.099   **Other specified injury of unspecified Achilles tendon**

  S86.1   **Injury of other muscle(s) and tendon(s) of posterior muscle group at lower leg level**

    S86.10   **Unspecified injury of other muscle(s) and tendon(s) of posterior muscle group at lower leg level**

⑦ S86.101   **Unspecified injury of other muscle(s) and tendon(s) of posterior muscle group at lower leg level, right leg**

⑦ S86.102   **Unspecified injury of other muscle(s) and tendon(s) of posterior muscle group at lower leg level, left leg**

⑦ S86.109   **Unspecified injury of other muscle(s) and tendon(s) of posterior muscle group at lower leg level, unspecified leg**

    S86.11   **Strain of other muscle(s) and tendon(s) of posterior muscle group at lower leg level**

⑦ S86.111   **Strain of other muscle(s) and tendon(s) of posterior muscle group at lower leg level, right leg**

⑦ S86.112   **Strain of other muscle(s) and tendon(s) of posterior muscle group at lower leg level, left leg**

⑦**S86.119** Strain of other muscle(s) and tendon(s) of posterior muscle group at lower leg level, unspecified leg

S86.12 Laceration of other muscle(s) and tendon(s) of posterior muscle group at lower leg level

⑦**S86.121** Laceration of other muscle(s) and tendon(s) of posterior muscle group at lower leg level, right leg

⑦**S86.122** Laceration of other muscle(s) and tendon(s) of posterior muscle group at lower leg level, left leg

⑦**S86.129** Laceration of other muscle(s) and tendon(s) of posterior muscle group at lower leg level, unspecified leg

S86.19 Other injury of other muscle(s) and tendon(s) of posterior muscle group at lower leg level

⑦**S86.191** Other injury of other muscle(s) and tendon(s) of posterior muscle group at lower leg level, right leg

⑦**S86.192** Other injury of other muscle(s) and tendon(s) of posterior muscle group at lower leg level, left leg

⑦**S86.199** Other injury of other muscle(s) and tendon(s) of posterior muscle group at lower leg level, unspecified leg

S86.2 Injury of muscle(s) and tendon(s) of anterior muscle group at lower leg level

S86.20 Unspecified injury of muscle(s) and tendon(s) of anterior muscle group at lower leg level

⑦**S86.201** Unspecified injury of muscle(s) and tendon(s) of anterior muscle group at lower leg level, right leg

⑦**S86.202** Unspecified injury of muscle(s) and tendon(s) of anterior muscle group at lower leg level, left leg

⑦**S86.209** Unspecified injury of muscle(s) and tendon(s) of anterior muscle group at lower leg level, unspecified leg

S86.21 Strain of muscle(s) and tendon(s) of anterior muscle group at lower leg level

⑦**S86.211** Strain of muscle(s) and tendon(s) of anterior muscle group at lower leg level, right leg

⑦**S86.212** Strain of muscle(s) and tendon(s) of anterior muscle group at lower leg level, left leg

⑦**S86.219** Strain of muscle(s) and tendon(s) of anterior muscle group at lower leg level, unspecified leg

S86.22 Laceration of muscle(s) and tendon(s) of anterior muscle group at lower leg level

⑦**S86.221** Laceration of muscle(s) and tendon(s) of anterior muscle group at lower leg level, right leg

⑦**S86.222** Laceration of muscle(s) and tendon(s) of anterior muscle group at lower leg level, left leg

⑦**S86.229** Laceration of muscle(s) and tendon(s) of anterior muscle group at lower leg level, unspecified leg

S86.29 Other injury of muscle(s) and tendon(s) of anterior muscle group at lower leg level

⑦**S86.291** Other injury of muscle(s) and tendon(s) of anterior muscle group at lower leg level, right leg

⑦**S86.292** Other injury of muscle(s) and tendon(s) of anterior muscle group at lower leg level, left leg

⑦**S86.299** Other injury of muscle(s) and tendon(s) of anterior muscle group at lower leg level, unspecified leg

S86.3 Injury of muscle(s) and tendon(s) of peroneal muscle group at lower leg level

S86.30 Unspecified injury of muscle(s) and tendon(s) of peroneal muscle group at lower leg level

⑦**S86.301** Unspecified injury of muscle(s) and tendon(s) of peroneal muscle group at lower leg level, right leg

⑦**S86.302** Unspecified injury of muscle(s) and tendon(s) of peroneal muscle group at lower leg level, left leg

⑦**S86.309** Unspecified injury of muscle(s) and tendon(s) of peroneal muscle group at lower leg level, unspecified leg

S86.31 Strain of muscle(s) and tendon(s) of peroneal muscle group at lower leg level

⑦**S86.311** Strain of muscle(s) and tendon(s) of peroneal muscle group at lower leg level, right leg

⑦**S86.312** Strain of muscle(s) and tendon(s) of peroneal muscle group at lower leg level, left leg

⑦**S86.319** Strain of muscle(s) and tendon(s) of peroneal muscle group at lower leg level, unspecified leg

S86.32 Laceration of muscle(s) and tendon(s) of peroneal muscle group at lower leg level

⑦**S86.321** Laceration of muscle(s) and tendon(s) of peroneal muscle group at lower leg level, right leg

⑦**S86.322** Laceration of muscle(s) and tendon(s) of peroneal muscle group at lower leg level, left leg

⑦**S86.329** Laceration of muscle(s) and tendon(s) of peroneal muscle group at lower leg level, unspecified leg

S86.39 Other injury of muscle(s) and tendon(s) of peroneal muscle group at lower leg level

⑦**S86.391** Other injury of muscle(s) and tendon(s) of peroneal muscle group at lower leg level, right leg

⑦**S86.392** Other injury of muscle(s) and tendon(s) of peroneal muscle group at lower leg level, left leg

⑦**S86.399** Other injury of muscle(s) and tendon(s) of peroneal muscle group at lower leg level, unspecified leg

S86.8 Injury of other muscles and tendons at lower leg level

S86.80 Unspecified injury of other muscles and tendons at lower leg level

⑦**S86.801** Unspecified injury of other muscle(s) and tendon(s) at lower leg level, right leg

⑦**S86.802** Unspecified injury of other muscle(s) and tendon(s) at lower leg level, left leg

⑦**S86.809** Unspecified injury of other muscle(s) and tendon(s) at lower leg level, unspecified leg

S86.81 Strain of other muscles and tendons at lower leg level

---

Add 4th-7th digits   Nonspecific code   Unspecified code   Manifestation code   867

⑦ **S86.811** Strain of other muscle(s) and tendon(s) at lower leg level, right leg

⑦ **S86.812** Strain of other muscle(s) and tendon(s) at lower leg level, left leg

⑦ **S86.819** Strain of other muscle(s) and tendon(s) at lower leg level, unspecified leg

S86.82 Laceration of other muscles and tendons at lower leg level

⑦ **S86.821** Laceration of other muscle(s) and tendon(s) at lower leg level, right leg

⑦ **S86.822** Laceration of other muscle(s) and tendon(s) at lower leg level, left leg

⑦ **S86.829** Laceration of other muscle(s) and tendon(s) at lower leg level, unspecified leg

S86.89 Other injury of other muscles and tendons at lower leg level

⑦ **S86.891** Other injury of other muscle(s) and tendon(s) at lower leg level, right leg

⑦ **S86.892** Other injury of other muscle(s) and tendon(s) at lower leg level, left leg

⑦ **S86.899** Other injury of other muscle(s) and tendon(s) at lower leg level, unspecified leg

S86.9 Injury of unspecified muscle and tendon at lower leg level

S86.90 Unspecified injury of unspecified muscle and tendon at lower leg level

⑦ **S86.901** Unspecified injury of unspecified muscle(s) and tendon(s) at lower leg level, right leg

⑦ **S86.902** Unspecified injury of unspecified muscle(s) and tendon(s) at lower leg level, left leg

⑦ **S86.909** Unspecified injury of unspecified muscle(s) and tendon(s) at lower leg level, unspecified leg

S86.91 Strain of unspecified muscle and tendon at lower leg level

⑦ **S86.911** Strain of unspecified muscle(s) and tendon(s) at lower leg level, right leg

⑦ **S86.912** Strain of unspecified muscle(s) and tendon(s) at lower leg level, left leg

⑦ **S86.919** Strain of unspecified muscle(s) and tendon(s) at lower leg level, unspecified leg

S86.92 Laceration of unspecified muscle and tendon at lower leg level

⑦ **S86.921** Laceration of unspecified muscle(s) and tendon(s) at lower leg level, right leg

⑦ **S86.922** Laceration of unspecified muscle(s) and tendon(s) at lower leg level, left leg

⑦ **S86.929** Laceration of unspecified muscle(s) and tendon(s) at lower leg level, unspecified leg

S86.99 Other injury of unspecified muscle and tendon at lower leg level

⑦ **S86.991** Other injury of unspecified muscle(s) and tendon(s) at lower leg level, right leg

⑦ **S86.992** Other injury of unspecified muscle(s) and tendon(s) at lower leg level, left leg

⑦ **S86.999** Other injury of unspecified muscle(s) and tendon(s) at lower leg level, unspecified leg

S87 **Crushing injury of lower leg**

Use additional code(s) for all associated injuries

Excludes2: crushing injury of ankle and foot (S97.-)

The appropriate 7th character is to be added to each code from category S87

A - initial encounter

D - subsequent encounter

S - sequela

S87.0 **Crushing injury of knee**

⊗⑦**S87.00** Crushing injury of unspecified knee

⊗⑦**S87.01** Crushing injury of right knee

⊗⑦**S87.02** Crushing injury of left knee

S87.8 **Crushing injury of lower leg**

⊗⑦**S87.80** Crushing injury of unspecified lower leg

⊗⑦**S87.81** Crushing injury of right lower leg

⊗⑦**S87.82** Crushing injury of left lower leg

S88 **Traumatic amputation of lower leg**

An amputation not identified as partial or complete should be coded to complete

Excludes1: traumatic amputation of ankle and foot (S98.-)

The appropriate 7th character is to be added to each code from category S88

A - initial encounter

D - subsequent encounter

S - sequela

S88.0 **Traumatic amputation at knee level**

S88.01 Complete traumatic amputation at knee level

⑦ **S88.011** Complete traumatic amputation at knee level, right lower leg

⑦ **S88.012** Complete traumatic amputation at knee level, left lower leg

⑦ **S88.019** Complete traumatic amputation at knee level, unspecified lower leg

S88.02 Partial traumatic amputation at knee level

⑦ **S88.021** Partial traumatic amputation at knee level, right lower leg

⑦ **S88.022** Partial traumatic amputation at knee level, left lower leg

⑦ **S88.029** Partial traumatic amputation at knee level, unspecified lower leg

S88.1 **Traumatic amputation at level between knee and ankle**

S88.11 Complete traumatic amputation at level between knee and ankle

⑦ **S88.111** Complete traumatic amputation at level between knee and ankle, right lower leg

⑦ **S88.112** Complete traumatic amputation at level between knee and ankle, left lower leg

⑦ **S88.119** Complete traumatic amputation at level between knee and ankle, unspecified lower leg

S88.12 Partial traumatic amputation at level between knee and ankle

⑦ **S88.121** Partial traumatic amputation at level between knee and ankle, right lower leg

● New code ▲ Revised code **Excludes1:** Not coded here **Excludes2:** Not included here ⊗ Placeholder required ⑦ 7th digit required

⑦S88.122 **Partial traumatic amputation at level between knee and ankle, left lower leg**

⑦S88.129 **Partial traumatic amputation at level between knee and ankle, unspecified lower leg**

S88.9 **Traumatic amputation of lower leg, level unspecified**

S88.91 **Complete traumatic amputation of lower leg, level unspecified**

⑦S88.911 **Complete traumatic amputation of right lower leg, level unspecified**

⑦S88.912 **Complete traumatic amputation of left lower leg, level unspecified**

⑦S88.919 **Complete traumatic amputation of unspecified lower leg, level unspecified**

S88.92 **Partial traumatic amputation of lower leg, level unspecified**

⑦S88.921 **Partial traumatic amputation of right lower leg, level unspecified**

⑦S88.922 **Partial traumatic amputation of left lower leg, level unspecified**

⑦S88.929 **Partial traumatic amputation of unspecified lower leg, level unspecified**

S89 **Other and unspecified injuries of lower leg**

Note: A fracture not indicated as open or closed should be coded to closed

Excludes2: Other and unspecified injuries of ankle and foot (S99.-)

The appropriate 7th character is to be added to each code from subcategories S89.0, S89.1, S89.2, and S89.3

A - initial encounter for closed fracture

D - subsequent encounter for fracture with routine healing

G - subsequent encounter for fracture with delayed healing

K - subsequent encounter for fracture with nonunion

P - subsequent encounter for fracture with malunion

S - sequela

S89.0 **Physeal fracture of upper end of tibia**

S89.00 **Unspecified physeal fracture of upper end of tibia**

⑦S89.001 **Unspecified physeal fracture of upper end of right tibia**

⑦S89.002 **Unspecified physeal fracture of upper end of left tibia**

⑦S89.009 **Unspecified physeal fracture of upper end of unspecified tibia**

S89.01 **Salter-Harris Type I physeal fracture of upper end of tibia**

⑦S89.011 **Salter-Harris Type I physeal fracture of upper end of right tibia**

⑦S89.012 **Salter-Harris Type I physeal fracture of upper end of left tibia**

⑦S89.019 **Salter-Harris Type I physeal fracture of upper end of unspecified tibia**

S89.02 **Salter-Harris Type II physeal fracture of upper end of tibia**

⑦S89.021 **Salter-Harris Type II physeal fracture of upper end of right tibia**

⑦S89.022 **Salter-Harris Type II physeal fracture of upper end of left tibia**

⑦S89.029 **Salter-Harris Type II physeal fracture of upper end of unspecified tibia**

S89.03 **Salter-Harris Type III physeal fracture of upper end of tibia**

⑦S89.031 **Salter-Harris Type III physeal fracture of upper end of right tibia**

⑦S89.032 **Salter-Harris Type III physeal fracture of upper end of left tibia**

⑦S89.039 **Salter-Harris Type III physeal fracture of upper end of unspecified tibia**

S89.04 **Salter-Harris Type IV physeal fracture of upper end of tibia**

⑦S89.041 **Salter-Harris Type IV physeal fracture of upper end of right tibia**

⑦S89.042 **Salter-Harris Type IV physeal fracture of upper end of left tibia**

⑦S89.049 **Salter-Harris Type IV physeal fracture of upper end of unspecified tibia**

S89.09 **Other physeal fracture of upper end of tibia**

⑦S89.091 **Other physeal fracture of upper end of right tibia**

⑦S89.092 **Other physeal fracture of upper end of left tibia**

⑦S89.099 **Other physeal fracture of upper end of unspecified tibia**

S89.1 **Physeal fracture of lower end of tibia**

S89.10 **Unspecified physeal fracture of lower end of tibia**

⑦S89.101 **Unspecified physeal fracture of lower end of right tibia**

⑦S89.102 **Unspecified physeal fracture of lower end of left tibia**

⑦S89.109 **Unspecified physeal fracture of lower end of unspecified tibia**

S89.11 **Salter-Harris Type I physeal fracture of lower end of tibia**

⑦S89.111 **Salter-Harris Type I physeal fracture of lower end of right tibia**

⑦S89.112 **Salter-Harris Type I physeal fracture of lower end of left tibia**

⑦S89.119 **Salter-Harris Type I physeal fracture of lower end of unspecified tibia**

S89.12 **Salter-Harris Type II physeal fracture of lower end of tibia**

⑦S89.121 **Salter-Harris Type II physeal fracture of lower end of right tibia**

⑦S89.122 **Salter-Harris Type II physeal fracture of lower end of left tibia**

⑦S89.129 **Salter-Harris Type II physeal fracture of lower end of unspecified tibia**

S89.13 **Salter-Harris Type III physeal fracture of lower end of tibia**

Excludes1: fracture of medial malleolus (adult) (S82.5-)

⑦S89.131 **Salter-Harris Type III physeal fracture of lower end of right tibia**

⑦S89.132 **Salter-Harris Type III physeal fracture of lower end of left tibia**

⑦ **S89.139** Salter-Harris Type III physeal fracture of lower end of unspecified tibia

S89.14 Salter-Harris Type IV physeal fracture of lower end of tibia

Excludes1: fracture of medial malleolus (adult) (S82.5-)

⑦ **S89.141** Salter-Harris Type IV physeal fracture of lower end of right tibia

⑦ **S89.142** Salter-Harris Type IV physeal fracture of lower end of left tibia

⑦ **S89.149** Salter-Harris Type IV physeal fracture of lower end of unspecified tibia

S89.19 Other physeal fracture of lower end of tibia

⑦ **S89.191** Other physeal fracture of lower end of right tibia

⑦ **S89.192** Other physeal fracture of lower end of left tibia

⑦ **S89.199** Other physeal fracture of lower end of unspecified tibia

S89.2 Physeal fracture of upper end of fibula

S89.20 Unspecified physeal fracture of upper end of fibula

⑦ **S89.201** Unspecified physeal fracture of upper end of right fibula

⑦ **S89.202** Unspecified physeal fracture of upper end of left fibula

⑦ **S89.209** Unspecified physeal fracture of upper end of unspecified fibula

S89.21 Salter-Harris Type I physeal fracture of upper end of fibula

⑦ **S89.211** Salter-Harris Type I physeal fracture of upper end of right fibula

⑦ **S89.212** Salter-Harris Type I physeal fracture of upper end of left fibula

⑦ **S89.219** Salter-Harris Type I physeal fracture of upper end of unspecified fibula

S89.22 Salter-Harris Type II physeal fracture of upper end of fibula

⑦ **S89.221** Salter-Harris Type II physeal fracture of upper end of right fibula

⑦ **S89.222** Salter-Harris Type II physeal fracture of upper end of left fibula

⑦ **S89.229** Salter-Harris Type II physeal fracture of upper end of unspecified fibula

S89.29 Other physeal fracture of upper end of fibula

⑦ **S89.291** Other physeal fracture of upper end of right fibula

⑦ **S89.292** Other physeal fracture of upper end of left fibula

⑦ **S89.299** Other physeal fracture of upper end of unspecified fibula

S89.3 Physeal fracture of lower end of fibula

S89.30 Unspecified physeal fracture of lower end of fibula

⑦ **S89.301** Unspecified physeal fracture of lower end of right fibula

⑦ **S89.302** Unspecified physeal fracture of lower end of left fibula

⑦ **S89.309** Unspecified physeal fracture of lower end of unspecified fibula

S89.31 Salter-Harris Type I physeal fracture of lower end of fibula

⑦ **S89.311** Salter-Harris Type I physeal fracture of lower end of right fibula

⑦ **S89.312** Salter-Harris Type I physeal fracture of lower end of left fibula

⑦ **S89.319** Salter-Harris Type I physeal fracture of lower end of unspecified fibula

S89.32 Salter-Harris Type II physeal fracture of lower end of fibula

⑦ **S89.321** Salter-Harris Type II physeal fracture of lower end of right fibula

⑦ **S89.322** Salter-Harris Type II physeal fracture of lower end of left fibula

⑦ **S89.329** Salter-Harris Type II physeal fracture of lower end of unspecified fibula

S89.39 Other physeal fracture of lower end of fibula

⑦ **S89.391** Other physeal fracture of lower end of right fibula

⑦ **S89.392** Other physeal fracture of lower end of left fibula

⑦ **S89.399** Other physeal fracture of lower end of unspecified fibula

S89.8 Other specified injuries of lower leg

The appropriate 7th character is to be added to each code in subcategory S89.8

A - initial encounter

D - subsequent encounter

S - sequela

⊗⑦ **S89.80** Other specified injuries of unspecified lower leg

⊗⑦ **S89.81** Other specified injuries of right lower leg

⊗⑦ **S89.82** Other specified injuries of left lower leg

S89.9 Unspecified injury of lower leg

The appropriate 7th character is to be added to each code in subcategory S89.9

A - initial encounter

D - subsequent encounter

S - sequela

⊗⑦ **S89.90** Unspecified injury of unspecified lower leg

⊗⑦ **S89.91** Unspecified injury of right lower leg

⊗⑦ **S89.92** Unspecified injury of left lower leg

INJURIES TO THE ANKLE AND FOOT (S90-S99)

Excludes2: burns and corrosions (T20-T32)

fracture of ankle and malleolus (S82.-)

frostbite (T33-T34)

insect bite or sting, venomous (T63.4)

S90 Superficial injury of ankle, foot and toes

The appropriate 7th character is to be added to each code from category S90

A - initial encounter

D - subsequent encounter

S - sequela

S90.0 Contusion of ankle

⊗⑦ **S90.00** Contusion of unspecified ankle

⊗⑦ **S90.01** Contusion of right ankle

⊗⑦ **S90.02** Contusion of left ankle

S90.1 Contusion of toe without damage to nail

● New code ▲ Revised code **Excludes1:** Not coded here **Excludes2:** Not included here ⊗ Placeholder required ⑦ 7th digit required

S90.11　Contusion of great toe without damage to nail

⑦S90.111　Contusion of right great toe without damage to nail

⑦S90.112　Contusion of left great toe without damage to nail

⑦S90.119　Contusion of unspecified great toe without damage to nail

S90.12　Contusion of lesser toe without damage to nail

⑦S90.121　Contusion of right lesser toe(s) without damage to nail

⑦S90.122　Contusion of left lesser toe(s) without damage to nail

⑦S90.129　Contusion of unspecified lesser toe(s) without damage to nail

Contusion of toe NOS

S90.2　Contusion of toe with damage to nail

S90.21　Contusion of great toe with damage to nail

⑦S90.211　Contusion of right great toe with damage to nail

⑦S90.212　Contusion of left great toe with damage to nail

⑦S90.219　Contusion of unspecified great toe with damage to nail

S90.22　Contusion of lesser toe with damage to nail

⑦S90.221　Contusion of right lesser toe(s) with damage to nail

⑦S90.222　Contusion of left lesser toe(s) with damage to nail

⑦S90.229　Contusion of unspecified lesser toe(s) with damage to nail

S90.3　Contusion of foot

Excludes2: contusion of toes (S90.1-, S90.2-)

⊗⑦S90.30　Contusion of unspecified foot

Contusion of foot NOS

⊗⑦S90.31　Contusion of right foot

⊗⑦S90.32　Contusion of left foot

S90.4　Other superficial injuries of toe

S90.41　Abrasion of toe

⑦S90.411　Abrasion, right great toe

⑦S90.412　Abrasion, left great toe

⑦S90.413　Abrasion, unspecified great toe

⑦S90.414　Abrasion, right lesser toe(s)

⑦S90.415　Abrasion, left lesser toe(s)

⑦S90.416　Abrasion, unspecified lesser toe(s)

S90.42　Blister (nonthermal) of toe

⑦S90.421　Blister (nonthermal), right great toe

⑦S90.422　Blister (nonthermal), left great toe

⑦S90.423　Blister (nonthermal), unspecified great toe

⑦S90.424　Blister (nonthermal), right lesser toe(s)

⑦S90.425　Blister (nonthermal), left lesser toe(s)

⑦S90.426　Blister (nonthermal), unspecified lesser toe(s)

S90.44　External constriction of toe

Hair tourniquet syndrome of toe

⑦S90.441　External constriction, right great toe

⑦S90.442　External constriction, left great toe

⑦S90.443　External constriction, unspecified great toe

⑦S90.444　External constriction, right lesser toe(s)

⑦S90.445　External constriction, left lesser toe(s)

⑦S90.446　External constriction, unspecified lesser toe(s)

S90.45　Superficial foreign body of toe

Splinter in the toe

⑦S90.451　Superficial foreign body, right great toe

⑦S90.452　Superficial foreign body, left great toe

⑦S90.453　Superficial foreign body, unspecified great toe

⑦S90.454　Superficial foreign body, right lesser toe(s)

⑦S90.455　Superficial foreign body, left lesser toe(s)

⑦S90.456　Superficial foreign body, unspecified lesser toe(s)

S90.46　Insect bite (nonvenomous) of toe

⑦S90.461　Insect bite (nonvenomous), right great toe

⑦S90.462　Insect bite (nonvenomous), left great toe

⑦S90.463　Insect bite (nonvenomous), unspecified great toe

⑦S90.464　Insect bite (nonvenomous), right lesser toe(s)

⑦S90.465　Insect bite (nonvenomous), left lesser toe(s)

⑦S90.466　Insect bite (nonvenomous), unspecified lesser toe(s)

S90.47　Other superficial bite of toe

Excludes1: open bite of toe (S91.15-, S91.25-)

⑦S90.471　Other superficial bite of right great toe

⑦S90.472　Other superficial bite of left great toe

⑦S90.473　Other superficial bite of unspecified great toe

⑦S90.474　Other superficial bite of right lesser toe(s)

⑦S90.475　Other superficial bite of left lesser toe(s)

⑦S90.476　Other superficial bite of unspecified lesser toe(s)

S90.5　Other superficial injuries of ankle

S90.51　Abrasion of ankle

⑦S90.511　Abrasion, right ankle

⑦S90.512　Abrasion, left ankle

⑦S90.519　Abrasion, unspecified ankle

S90.52　Blister (nonthermal) of ankle

⑦S90.521　Blister (nonthermal), right ankle

⑦S90.522　Blister (nonthermal), left ankle

⑦S90.529　Blister (nonthermal), unspecified ankle

S90.54　External constriction of ankle

⑦S90.541　External constriction, right ankle

⑦S90.542　External constriction, left ankle

⑦S90.549　External constriction, unspecified ankle

S90.55　Superficial foreign body of ankle

Splinter in the ankle

⑦ S90.551 Superficial foreign body, right ankle

⑦ S90.552 Superficial foreign body, left ankle

⑦ S90.559 Superficial foreign body, unspecified ankle

S90.56 Insect bite (nonvenomous) of ankle

⑦ S90.561 Insect bite (nonvenomous), right ankle

⑦ S90.562 Insect bite (nonvenomous), left ankle

⑦ S90.569 Insect bite (nonvenomous), unspecified ankle

S90.57 Other superficial bite of ankle

Excludes1: open bite of ankle (S91.05-)

⑦ S90.571 Other superficial bite of ankle, right ankle

⑦ S90.572 Other superficial bite of ankle, left ankle

⑦ S90.579 Other superficial bite of ankle, unspecified ankle

S90.8 Other superficial injuries of foot

S90.81 Abrasion of foot

⑦ S90.811 Abrasion, right foot

⑦ S90.812 Abrasion, left foot

⑦ S90.819 Abrasion, unspecified foot

S90.82 Blister (nonthermal) of foot

⑦ S90.821 Blister (nonthermal), right foot

⑦ S90.822 Blister (nonthermal), left foot

⑦ S90.829 Blister (nonthermal), unspecified foot

S90.84 External constriction of foot

⑦ S90.841 External constriction, right foot

⑦ S90.842 External constriction, left foot

⑦ S90.849 External constriction, unspecified foot

S90.85 Superficial foreign body of foot

Splinter in the foot

⑦ S90.851 Superficial foreign body, right foot

⑦ S90.852 Superficial foreign body, left foot

⑦ S90.859 Superficial foreign body, unspecified foot

S90.86 Insect bite (nonvenomous) of foot

⑦ S90.861 Insect bite (nonvenomous), right foot

⑦ S90.862 Insect bite (nonvenomous), left foot

⑦ S90.869 Insect bite (nonvenomous), unspecified foot

S90.87 Other superficial bite of foot

Excludes1: open bite of foot (S91.35-)

⑦ S90.871 Other superficial bite of right foot

⑦ S90.872 Other superficial bite of left foot

⑦ S90.879 Other superficial bite of unspecified foot

S90.9 Unspecified superficial injury of ankle, foot and toe

S90.91 Unspecified superficial injury of ankle

⑦ S90.911 Unspecified superficial injury of right ankle

⑦ S90.912 Unspecified superficial injury of left ankle

⑦ S90.919 Unspecified superficial injury of unspecified ankle

S90.92 Unspecified superficial injury of foot

⑦ S90.921 Unspecified superficial injury of right foot

⑦ S90.922 Unspecified superficial injury of left foot

⑦ S90.929 Unspecified superficial injury of unspecified foot

S90.93 Unspecified superficial injury of toes

⑦ S90.931 Unspecified superficial injury of right great toe

⑦ S90.932 Unspecified superficial injury of left great toe

⑦ S90.933 Unspecified superficial injury of unspecified great toe

⑦ S90.934 Unspecified superficial injury of right lesser toe(s)

⑦ S90.935 Unspecified superficial injury of left lesser toe(s)

⑦ S90.936 Unspecified superficial injury of unspecified lesser toe(s)

S91 Open wound of ankle, foot and toes

Code also any associated wound infection

Excludes1: open fracture of ankle, foot and toes (S92.-with 7th character B)

traumatic amputation of ankle and foot (S98.-)

The appropriate 7th character is to be added to each code from category S91

A - initial encounter

D - subsequent encounter

S - sequela

S91.0 Open wound of ankle

S91.00 Unspecified open wound of ankle

⑦ S91.001 Unspecified open wound, right ankle

⑦ S91.002 Unspecified open wound, left ankle

⑦ S91.009 Unspecified open wound, unspecified ankle

S91.01 Laceration without foreign body of ankle

⑦ S91.011 Laceration without foreign body, right ankle

⑦ S91.012 Laceration without foreign body, left ankle

⑦ S91.019 Laceration without foreign body, unspecified ankle

S91.02 Laceration with foreign body of ankle

⑦ S91.021 Laceration with foreign body, right ankle

⑦ S91.022 Laceration with foreign body, left ankle

⑦ S91.029 Laceration with foreign body, unspecified ankle

S91.03 Puncture wound without foreign body of ankle

⑦ S91.031 Puncture wound without foreign body, right ankle

⑦ S91.032 Puncture wound without foreign body, left ankle

⑦ S91.039 Puncture wound without foreign body, unspecified ankle

S91.04 Puncture wound with foreign body of ankle

⑦ S91.041 Puncture wound with foreign body, right ankle

⑦ S91.042 Puncture wound with foreign body, left ankle

● New code ▲ Revised code **Excludes1:** Not coded here **Excludes2:** Not included here ⊗ Placeholder required ⑦ 7th digit required

⑦S91.049   **Puncture wound with foreign body, unspecified ankle**

S91.05   **Open bite of ankle**

Excludes1: superficial bite of ankle (S90.56-, S90.57-)

⑦S91.051   **Open bite, right ankle**

⑦S91.052   **Open bite, left ankle**

⑦S91.059   **Open bite, unspecified ankle**

S91.1   **Open wound of toe without damage to nail**

S91.10   **Unspecified open wound of toe without damage to nail**

⑦S91.101   **Unspecified open wound of right great toe without damage to nail**

⑦S91.102   **Unspecified open wound of left great toe without damage to nail**

⑦S91.103   **Unspecified open wound of unspecified great toe without damage to nail**

⑦S91.104   **Unspecified open wound of right lesser toe(s) without damage to nail**

⑦S91.105   **Unspecified open wound of left lesser toe(s) without damage to nail**

⑦S91.106   **Unspecified open wound of unspecified lesser toe(s) without damage to nail**

⑦S91.109   **Unspecified open wound of unspecified toe(s) without damage to nail**

S91.11   **Laceration without foreign body of toe without damage to nail**

⑦S91.111   **Laceration without foreign body of right great toe without damage to nail**

⑦S91.112   **Laceration without foreign body of left great toe without damage to nail**

⑦S91.113   **Laceration without foreign body of unspecified great toe without damage to nail**

⑦S91.114   **Laceration without foreign body of right lesser toe(s) without damage to nail**

⑦S91.115   **Laceration without foreign body of left lesser toe(s) without damage to nail**

⑦S91.116   **Laceration without foreign body of unspecified lesser toe(s) without damage to nail**

⑦S91.119   **Laceration without foreign body of unspecified toe without damage to nail**

S91.12   **Laceration with foreign body of toe without damage to nail**

⑦S91.121   **Laceration with foreign body of right great toe without damage to nail**

⑦S91.122   **Laceration with foreign body of left great toe without damage to nail**

⑦S91.123   **Laceration with foreign body of unspecified great toe without damage to nail**

⑦S91.124   **Laceration with foreign body of right lesser toe(s) without damage to nail**

⑦S91.125   **Laceration with foreign body of left lesser toe(s) without damage to nail**

⑦S91.126   **Laceration with foreign body of unspecified lesser toe(s) without damage to nail**

⑦S91.129   **Laceration with foreign body of unspecified toe(s) without damage to nail**

S91.13   **Puncture wound without foreign body of toe without damage to nail**

⑦S91.131   **Puncture wound without foreign body of right great toe without damage to nail**

⑦S91.132   **Puncture wound without foreign body of left great toe without damage to nail**

⑦S91.133   **Puncture wound without foreign body of unspecified great toe without damage to nail**

⑦S91.134   **Puncture wound without foreign body of right lesser toe(s) without damage to nail**

⑦S91.135   **Puncture wound without foreign body of left lesser toe(s) without damage to nail**

⑦S91.136   **Puncture wound without foreign body of unspecified lesser toe(s) without damage to nail**

⑦S91.139   **Puncture wound without foreign body of unspecified toe(s) without damage to nail**

S91.14   **Puncture wound with foreign body of toe without damage to nail**

⑦S91.141   **Puncture wound with foreign body of right great toe without damage to nail**

⑦S91.142   **Puncture wound with foreign body of left great toe without damage to nail**

⑦S91.143   **Puncture wound with foreign body of unspecified great toe without damage to nail**

⑦S91.144   **Puncture wound with foreign body of right lesser toe(s) without damage to nail**

⑦S91.145   **Puncture wound with foreign body of left lesser toe(s) without damage to nail**

⑦S91.146   **Puncture wound with foreign body of unspecified lesser toe(s) without damage to nail**

⑦S91.149   **Puncture wound with foreign body of unspecified toe(s) without damage to nail**

S91.15   **Open bite of toe without damage to nail**

Bite of toe NOS

Excludes1: superficial bite of toe (S90.46-, S90.47-)

⑦S91.151   **Open bite of right great toe without damage to nail**

⑦S91.152   **Open bite of left great toe without damage to nail**

⑦S91.153   **Open bite of unspecified great toe without damage to nail**

⑦S91.154   **Open bite of right lesser toe(s) without damage to nail**

⑦S91.155   **Open bite of left lesser toe(s) without damage to nail**

⑦S91.156 Open bite of unspecified lesser toe(s) without damage to nail

⑦S91.159 Open bite of unspecified toe(s) without damage to nail

S91.2 **Open wound of toe with damage to nail**

S91.20 Unspecified open wound of toe with damage to nail

⑦S91.201 Unspecified open wound of right great toe with damage to nail

⑦S91.202 Unspecified open wound of left great toe with damage to nail

⑦S91.203 Unspecified open wound of unspecified great toe with damage to nail

⑦S91.204 Unspecified open wound of right lesser toe(s) with damage to nail

⑦S91.205 Unspecified open wound of left lesser toe(s) with damage to nail

⑦S91.206 Unspecified open wound of unspecified lesser toe(s) with damage to nail

⑦S91.209 Unspecified open wound of unspecified toe(s) with damage to nail

S91.21 Laceration without foreign body of toe with damage to nail

⑦S91.211 Laceration without foreign body of right great toe with damage to nail

⑦S91.212 Laceration without foreign body of left great toe with damage to nail

⑦S91.213 Laceration without foreign body of unspecified great toe with damage to nail

⑦S91.214 Laceration without foreign body of right lesser toe(s) with damage to nail

⑦S91.215 Laceration without foreign body of left lesser toe(s) with damage to nail

⑦S91.216 Laceration without foreign body of unspecified lesser toe(s) with damage to nail

⑦S91.219 Laceration without foreign body of unspecified toe(s) with damage to nail

S91.22 Laceration with foreign body of toe with damage to nail

⑦S91.221 Laceration with foreign body of right great toe with damage to nail

⑦S91.222 Laceration with foreign body of left great toe with damage to nail

⑦S91.223 Laceration with foreign body of unspecified great toe with damage to nail

⑦S91.224 Laceration with foreign body of right lesser toe(s) with damage to nail

⑦S91.225 Laceration with foreign body of left lesser toe(s) with damage to nail

⑦S91.226 Laceration with foreign body of unspecified lesser toe(s) with damage to nail

⑦S91.229 Laceration with foreign body of unspecified toe(s) with damage to nail

S91.23 Puncture wound without foreign body of toe with damage to nail

⑦S91.231 Puncture wound without foreign body of right great toe with damage to nail

⑦S91.232 Puncture wound without foreign body of left great toe with damage to nail

⑦S91.233 Puncture wound without foreign body of unspecified great toe with damage to nail

⑦S91.234 Puncture wound without foreign body of right lesser toe(s) with damage to nail

⑦S91.235 Puncture wound without foreign body of left lesser toe(s) with damage to nail

⑦S91.236 Puncture wound without foreign body of unspecified lesser toe(s) with damage to nail

⑦S91.239 Puncture wound without foreign body of unspecified toe(s) with damage to nail

S91.24 Puncture wound with foreign body of toe with damage to nail

⑦S91.241 Puncture wound with foreign body of right great toe with damage to nail

⑦S91.242 Puncture wound with foreign body of left great toe with damage to nail

⑦S91.243 Puncture wound with foreign body of unspecified great toe with damage to nail

⑦S91.244 Puncture wound with foreign body of right lesser toe(s) with damage to nail

⑦S91.245 Puncture wound with foreign body of left lesser toe(s) with damage to nail

⑦S91.246 Puncture wound with foreign body of unspecified lesser toe(s) with damage to nail

⑦S91.249 Puncture wound with foreign body of unspecified toe(s) with damage to nail

S91.25 Open bite of toe with damage to nail

Bite of toe with damage to nail NOS

Excludes1: superficial bite of toe (S90.46-, S90.47-)

⑦S91.251 Open bite of right great toe with damage to nail

⑦S91.252 Open bite of left great toe with damage to nail

⑦S91.253 Open bite of unspecified great toe with damage to nail

⑦S91.254 Open bite of right lesser toe(s) with damage to nail

⑦S91.255 Open bite of left lesser toe(s) with damage to nail

⑦S91.256 Open bite of unspecified lesser toe(s) with damage to nail

⑦S91.259 Open bite of unspecified toe(s) with damage to nail

S91.3 **Open wound of foot**

S91.30 Unspecified open wound of foot

⑦S91.301 Unspecified open wound, right foot

⑦S91.302 Unspecified open wound, left foot

⑦S91.309 Unspecified open wound, unspecified foot

● New code ▲ Revised code **Excludes1:** Not coded here **Excludes2:** Not included here ⊗ Placeholder required ⑦7th digit required

S91.31   Laceration without foreign body of foot

⑦S91.311   Laceration without foreign body, right foot

⑦S91.312   Laceration without foreign body, left foot

⑦S91.319   Laceration without foreign body, unspecified foot

S91.32   Laceration with foreign body of foot

⑦S91.321   Laceration with foreign body, right foot

⑦S91.322   Laceration with foreign body, left foot

⑦S91.329   Laceration with foreign body, unspecified foot

S91.33   Puncture wound without foreign body of foot

⑦S91.331   Puncture wound without foreign body, right foot

⑦S91.332   Puncture wound without foreign body, left foot

⑦S91.339   Puncture wound without foreign body, unspecified foot

S91.34   Puncture wound with foreign body of foot

⑦S91.341   Puncture wound with foreign body, right foot

⑦S91.342   Puncture wound with foreign body, left foot

⑦S91.349   Puncture wound with foreign body, unspecified foot

S91.35   Open bite of foot

Excludes1: superficial bite of foot (S90.86-, S90.87-)

⑦S91.351   Open bite, right foot

⑦S91.352   Open bite, left foot

⑦S91.359   Open bite, unspecified foot

S92   Fracture of foot and toe, except ankle

Note: A fracture not indicated as displaced or nondisplaced should be coded to displaced

A fracture not indicated as open or closed should be coded to closed

Excludes1: traumatic amputation of ankle and foot (S98.-)

Excludes2: fracture of ankle (S82.-)

fracture of malleolus (S82.-)

The appropriate 7th character is to be added to each code from category S92

A - initial encounter for closed fracture

B - initial encounter for open fracture

D - subsequent encounter for fracture with routine healing

G - subsequent encounter for fracture with delayed healing

K - subsequent encounter for fracture with nonunion

P - subsequent encounter for fracture with malunion

S - sequela

S92.0   Fracture of calcaneus

Heel bone Os calcis

Excludes2: Physeal fracture of calcaneus (S99.0-)

S92.00   Unspecified fracture of calcaneus

⑦S92.001   Unspecified fracture of right calcaneus

⑦S92.002   Unspecified fracture of left calcaneus

⑦S92.009   Unspecified fracture of unspecified calcaneus

S92.01   Fracture of body of calcaneus

⑦S92.011   Displaced fracture of body of right calcaneus

⑦S92.012   Displaced fracture of body of left calcaneus

⑦S92.013   Displaced fracture of body of unspecified calcaneus

⑦S92.014   Nondisplaced fracture of body of right calcaneus

⑦S92.015   Nondisplaced fracture of body of left calcaneus

⑦S92.016   Nondisplaced fracture of body of unspecified calcaneus

S92.02   Fracture of anterior process of calcaneus

⑦S92.021   Displaced fracture of anterior process of right calcaneus

⑦S92.022   Displaced fracture of anterior process of left calcaneus

⑦S92.023   Displaced fracture of anterior process of unspecified calcaneus

⑦S92.024   Nondisplaced fracture of anterior process of right calcaneus

⑦S92.025   Nondisplaced fracture of anterior process of left calcaneus

⑦S92.026   Nondisplaced fracture of anterior process of unspecified calcaneus

S92.03   Avulsion fracture of tuberosity of calcaneus

⑦S92.031   Displaced avulsion fracture of tuberosity of right calcaneus

⑦S92.032   Displaced avulsion fracture of tuberosity of left calcaneus

⑦S92.033   Displaced avulsion fracture of tuberosity of unspecified calcaneus

⑦S92.034   Nondisplaced avulsion fracture of tuberosity of right calcaneus

⑦S92.035   Nondisplaced avulsion fracture of tuberosity of left calcaneus

⑦S92.036   Nondisplaced avulsion fracture of tuberosity of unspecified calcaneus

S92.04   Other fracture of tuberosity of calcaneus

⑦S92.041   Displaced other fracture of tuberosity of right calcaneus

⑦S92.042   Displaced other fracture of tuberosity of left calcaneus

⑦S92.043   Displaced other fracture of tuberosity of unspecified calcaneus

⑦S92.044   Nondisplaced other fracture of tuberosity of right calcaneus

⑦S92.045   Nondisplaced other fracture of tuberosity of left calcaneus

⑦S92.046   Nondisplaced other fracture of tuberosity of unspecified calcaneus

S92.05   Other extraarticular fracture of calcaneus

⑦S92.051   Displaced other extraarticular fracture of right calcaneus

⑦S92.052   Displaced other extraarticular fracture of left calcaneus

⑦S92.053   Displaced other extraarticular fracture of unspecified calcaneus

⑦S92.054   Nondisplaced other extraarticular fracture of right calcaneus

⑦S92.055   Nondisplaced other extraarticular fracture of left calcaneus

⑦S92.056   Nondisplaced other extraarticular fracture of unspecified calcaneus

S92.06 Intraarticular fracture of calcaneus

⑦ S92.061 Displaced intraarticular fracture of right calcaneus

⑦ S92.062 Displaced intraarticular fracture of left calcaneus

⑦ S92.063 Displaced intraarticular fracture of unspecified calcaneus

⑦ S92.064 Nondisplaced intraarticular fracture of right calcaneus

⑦ S92.065 Nondisplaced intraarticular fracture of left calcaneus

⑦ S92.066 Nondisplaced intraarticular fracture of unspecified calcaneus

S92.1 Fracture of talus

Astragalus

S92.10 Unspecified fracture of talus

⑦ S92.101 Unspecified fracture of right talus

⑦ S92.102 Unspecified fracture of left talus

⑦ S92.109 Unspecified fracture of unspecified talus

S92.11 Fracture of neck of talus

⑦ S92.111 Displaced fracture of neck of right talus

⑦ S92.112 Displaced fracture of neck of left talus

⑦ S92.113 Displaced fracture of neck of unspecified talus

⑦ S92.114 Nondisplaced fracture of neck of right talus

⑦ S92.115 Nondisplaced fracture of neck of left talus

⑦ S92.116 Nondisplaced fracture of neck of unspecified talus

S92.12 Fracture of body of talus

⑦ S92.121 Displaced fracture of body of right talus

⑦ S92.122 Displaced fracture of body of left talus

⑦ S92.123 Displaced fracture of body of unspecified talus

⑦ S92.124 Nondisplaced fracture of body of right talus

⑦ S92.125 Nondisplaced fracture of body of left talus

⑦ S92.126 Nondisplaced fracture of body of unspecified talus

S92.13 Fracture of posterior process of talus

⑦ S92.131 Displaced fracture of posterior process of right talus

⑦ S92.132 Displaced fracture of posterior process of left talus

⑦ S92.133 Displaced fracture of posterior process of unspecified talus

⑦ S92.134 Nondisplaced fracture of posterior process of right talus

⑦ S92.135 Nondisplaced fracture of posterior process of left talus

⑦ S92.136 Nondisplaced fracture of posterior process of unspecified talus

S92.14 Dome fracture of talus

Excludes1: osteochondritis dissecans (M93.2)

⑦ S92.141 Displaced dome fracture of right talus

⑦ S92.142 Displaced dome fracture of left talus

⑦ S92.143 Displaced dome fracture of unspecified talus

⑦ S92.144 Nondisplaced dome fracture of right talus

⑦ S92.145 Nondisplaced dome fracture of left talus

⑦ S92.146 Nondisplaced dome fracture of unspecified talus

S92.15 Avulsion fracture (chip fracture) of talus

⑦ S92.151 Displaced avulsion fracture (chip fracture) of right talus

⑦ S92.152 Displaced avulsion fracture (chip fracture) of left talus

⑦ S92.153 Displaced avulsion fracture (chip fracture) of unspecified talus

⑦ S92.154 Nondisplaced avulsion fracture (chip fracture) of right talus

⑦ S92.155 Nondisplaced avulsion fracture (chip fracture) of left talus

⑦ S92.156 Nondisplaced avulsion fracture (chip fracture) of unspecified talus

S92.19 Other fracture of talus

⑦ S92.191 Other fracture of right talus

⑦ S92.192 Other fracture of left talus

⑦ S92.199 Other fracture of unspecified talus

S92.2 Fracture of other and unspecified tarsal bone(s)

S92.20 Fracture of unspecified tarsal bone(s)

⑦ S92.201 Fracture of unspecified tarsal bone(s) of right foot

⑦ S92.202 Fracture of unspecified tarsal bone(s) of left foot

⑦ S92.209 Fracture of unspecified tarsal bone(s) of unspecified foot

S92.21 Fracture of cuboid bone

⑦ S92.211 Displaced fracture of cuboid bone of right foot

⑦ S92.212 Displaced fracture of cuboid bone of left foot

⑦ S92.213 Displaced fracture of cuboid bone of unspecified foot

⑦ S92.214 Nondisplaced fracture of cuboid bone of right foot

⑦ S92.215 Nondisplaced fracture of cuboid bone of left foot

⑦ S92.216 Nondisplaced fracture of cuboid bone of unspecified foot

S92.22 Fracture of lateral cuneiform

⑦ S92.221 Displaced fracture of lateral cuneiform of right foot

⑦ S92.222 Displaced fracture of lateral cuneiform of left foot

⑦ S92.223 Displaced fracture of lateral cuneiform of unspecified foot

⑦ S92.224 Nondisplaced fracture of lateral cuneiform of right foot

⑦ S92.225 Nondisplaced fracture of lateral cuneiform of left foot

⑦ S92.226 Nondisplaced fracture of lateral cuneiform of unspecified foot

S92.23 Fracture of intermediate cuneiform

⑦ S92.231 Displaced fracture of intermediate cuneiform of right foot

● New code ▲ Revised code **Excludes1:** Not coded here **Excludes2:** Not included here ⊗ Placeholder required ⑦ 7th digit required

⑦S92.232   Displaced fracture of intermediate cuneiform of left foot

⑦S92.233   Displaced fracture of intermediate cuneiform of unspecified foot

⑦S92.234   Nondisplaced fracture of intermediate cuneiform of right foot

⑦S92.235   Nondisplaced fracture of intermediate cuneiform of left foot

⑦S92.236   Nondisplaced fracture of intermediate cuneiform of unspecified foot

S92.24   **Fracture of medial cuneiform**

⑦S92.241   Displaced fracture of medial cuneiform of right foot

⑦S92.242   Displaced fracture of medial cuneiform of left foot

⑦S92.243   Displaced fracture of medial cuneiform of unspecified foot

⑦S92.244   Nondisplaced fracture of medial cuneiform of right foot

⑦S92.245   Nondisplaced fracture of medial cuneiform of left foot

⑦S92.246   Nondisplaced fracture of medial cuneiform of unspecified foot

S92.25   **Fracture of navicular [scaphoid] of foot**

⑦S92.251   Displaced fracture of navicular [scaphoid] of right foot

⑦S92.252   Displaced fracture of navicular [scaphoid] of left foot

⑦S92.253   Displaced fracture of navicular [scaphoid] of unspecified foot

⑦S92.254   Nondisplaced fracture of navicular [scaphoid] of right foot

⑦S92.255   Nondisplaced fracture of navicular [scaphoid] of left foot

⑦S92.256   Nondisplaced fracture of navicular [scaphoid] of unspecified foot

S92.3   **Fracture of metatarsal bone(s)**

Excludes2: Physeal fracture of metatarsal (S99.1-)

S92.30   **Fracture of unspecified metatarsal bone(s)**

⑦S92.301   Fracture of unspecified metatarsal bone(s), right foot

⑦S92.302   Fracture of unspecified metatarsal bone(s), left foot

⑦S92.309   Fracture of unspecified metatarsal bone(s), unspecified foot

S92.31   **Fracture of first metatarsal bone**

⑦S92.311   Displaced fracture of first metatarsal bone, right foot

⑦S92.312   Displaced fracture of first metatarsal bone, left foot

⑦S92.313   Displaced fracture of first metatarsal bone, unspecified foot

⑦S92.314   Nondisplaced fracture of first metatarsal bone, right foot

⑦S92.315   Nondisplaced fracture of first metatarsal bone, left foot

⑦S92.316   Nondisplaced fracture of first metatarsal bone, unspecified foot

S92.32   **Fracture of second metatarsal bone**

⑦S92.321   Displaced fracture of second metatarsal bone, right foot

⑦S92.322   Displaced fracture of second metatarsal bone, left foot

⑦S92.323   Displaced fracture of second metatarsal bone, unspecified foot

⑦S92.324   Nondisplaced fracture of second metatarsal bone, right foot

⑦S92.325   Nondisplaced fracture of second metatarsal bone, left foot

⑦S92.326   Nondisplaced fracture of second metatarsal bone, unspecified foot

S92.33   **Fracture of third metatarsal bone**

⑦S92.331   Displaced fracture of third metatarsal bone, right foot

⑦S92.332   Displaced fracture of third metatarsal bone, left foot

⑦S92.333   Displaced fracture of third metatarsal bone, unspecified foot

⑦S92.334   Nondisplaced fracture of third metatarsal bone, right foot

⑦S92.335   Nondisplaced fracture of third metatarsal bone, left foot

⑦S92.336   Nondisplaced fracture of third metatarsal bone, unspecified foot

S92.34   **Fracture of fourth metatarsal bone**

⑦S92.341   Displaced fracture of fourth metatarsal bone, right foot

⑦S92.342   Displaced fracture of fourth metatarsal bone, left foot

⑦S92.343   Displaced fracture of fourth metatarsal bone, unspecified foot

⑦S92.344   Nondisplaced fracture of fourth metatarsal bone, right foot

⑦S92.345   Nondisplaced fracture of fourth metatarsal bone, left foot

⑦S92.346   Nondisplaced fracture of fourth metatarsal bone, unspecified foot

S92.35   **Fracture of fifth metatarsal bone**

⑦S92.351   Displaced fracture of fifth metatarsal bone, right foot

⑦S92.352   Displaced fracture of fifth metatarsal bone, left foot

⑦S92.353   Displaced fracture of fifth metatarsal bone, unspecified foot

⑦S92.354   Nondisplaced fracture of fifth metatarsal bone, right foot

⑦S92.355   Nondisplaced fracture of fifth metatarsal bone, left foot

⑦S92.356   Nondisplaced fracture of fifth metatarsal bone, unspecified foot

S92.4   **Fracture of great toe**

Excludes2: Physeal fracture of phalanx of toe (S99.2-)

S92.40   **Unspecified fracture of great toe**

⑦S92.401   Displaced unspecified fracture of right great toe

⑦S92.402   Displaced unspecified fracture of left great toe

⑦S92.403   Displaced unspecified fracture of unspecified great toe

⑦S92.404   Nondisplaced unspecified fracture of right great toe

⑦S92.405   Nondisplaced unspecified fracture of left great toe

⑦S92.406   Nondisplaced unspecified fracture of unspecified great toe

S92.41   **Fracture of proximal phalanx of great toe**

⑦ S92.411 Displaced fracture of proximal phalanx of right great toe

⑦ S92.412 Displaced fracture of proximal phalanx of left great toe

⑦ S92.413 Displaced fracture of proximal phalanx of unspecified great toe

⑦ S92.414 Nondisplaced fracture of proximal phalanx of right great toe

⑦ S92.415 Nondisplaced fracture of proximal phalanx of left great toe

⑦ S92.416 Nondisplaced fracture of proximal phalanx of unspecified great toe

S92.42 Fracture of distal phalanx of great toe

⑦ S92.421 Displaced fracture of distal phalanx of right great toe

⑦ S92.422 Displaced fracture of distal phalanx of left great toe

⑦ S92.423 Displaced fracture of distal phalanx of unspecified great toe

⑦ S92.424 Nondisplaced fracture of distal phalanx of right great toe

⑦ S92.425 Nondisplaced fracture of distal phalanx of left great toe

⑦ S92.426 Nondisplaced fracture of distal phalanx of unspecified great toe

S92.49 Other fracture of great toe

⑦ S92.491 Other fracture of right great toe

⑦ S92.492 Other fracture of left great toe

⑦ S92.499 Other fracture of unspecified great toe

S92.5 Fracture of lesser toe(s)

Excludes2: Physeal fracture of phalanx of toe (S99.2-)

S92.50 Unspecified fracture of lesser toe(s)

⑦ S92.501 Displaced unspecified fracture of right lesser toe(s)

⑦ S92.502 Displaced unspecified fracture of left lesser toe(s)

⑦ S92.503 Displaced unspecified fracture of unspecified lesser toe(s)

⑦ S92.504 Nondisplaced unspecified fracture of right lesser toe(s)

⑦ S92.505 Nondisplaced unspecified fracture of left lesser toe(s)

⑦ S92.506 Nondisplaced unspecified fracture of unspecified lesser toe(s)

S92.51 Fracture of proximal phalanx of lesser toe(s)

⑦ S92.511 Displaced fracture of proximal phalanx of right lesser toe(s)

⑦ S92.512 Displaced fracture of proximal phalanx of left lesser toe(s)

⑦ S92.513 Displaced fracture of proximal phalanx of unspecified lesser toe(s)

⑦ S92.514 Nondisplaced fracture of proximal phalanx of right lesser toe(s)

⑦ S92.515 Nondisplaced fracture of proximal phalanx of left lesser toe(s)

⑦ S92.516 Nondisplaced fracture of proximal phalanx of unspecified lesser toe(s)

▲S92.52 Fracture of middle phalanx of lesser toe(s)

▲⑦ S92.521 Displaced fracture of middle phalanx of right lesser toe(s)

▲⑦ S92.522 Displaced fracture of middle phalanx of left lesser toe(s)

▲⑦ S92.523 Displaced fracture of middle phalanx of unspecified lesser toe(s)

▲⑦ S92.524 Nondisplaced fracture of middle phalanx of right lesser toe(s)

▲⑦ S92.525 Nondisplaced fracture of middle phalanx of left lesser toe(s)

▲⑦ S92.526 Nondisplaced fracture of middle phalanx of unspecified lesser toe(s)

S92.53 Fracture of distal phalanx of lesser toe(s)

⑦ S92.531 Displaced fracture of distal phalanx of right lesser toe(s)

⑦ S92.532 Displaced fracture of distal phalanx of left lesser toe(s)

⑦ S92.533 Displaced fracture of distal phalanx of unspecified lesser toe(s)

⑦ S92.534 Nondisplaced fracture of distal phalanx of right lesser toe(s)

⑦ S92.535 Nondisplaced fracture of distal phalanx of left lesser toe(s)

⑦ S92.536 Nondisplaced fracture of distal phalanx of unspecified lesser toe(s)

S92.59 Other fracture of lesser toe(s)

⑦ S92.591 Other fracture of right lesser toe(s)

⑦ S92.592 Other fracture of left lesser toe(s)

⑦ S92.599 Other fracture of unspecified lesser toe(s)

S92.8 Other fracture of foot, except ankle

S92.81 Other fracture of foot

Sesamoid fracture of foot

⑦ S92.811 Other fracture of right foot

⑦ S92.812 Other fracture of left foot

⑦ S92.819 Other fracture of unspecified foot

S92.9 Unspecified fracture of foot and toe

S92.90 Unspecified fracture of foot

⑦ S92.901 Unspecified fracture of right foot

⑦ S92.902 Unspecified fracture of left foot

⑦ S92.909 Unspecified fracture of unspecified foot

S92.91 Unspecified fracture of toe

⑦ S92.911 Unspecified fracture of right toe(s)

⑦ S92.912 Unspecified fracture of left toe(s)

⑦ S92.919 Unspecified fracture of unspecified toe(s)

S93 Dislocation and sprain of joints and ligaments at ankle, foot and toe level

Includes: avulsion of joint or ligament of ankle, foot and toe

laceration of cartilage, joint or ligament of ankle, foot and toe

sprain of cartilage, joint or ligament of ankle, foot and toe

traumatic hemarthrosis of joint or ligament of ankle, foot and toe

traumatic rupture of joint or ligament of ankle, foot and toe

traumatic subluxation of joint or ligament of ankle, foot and toe

traumatic tear of joint or ligament of ankle, foot and toe

Code also any associated open wound

Excludes2: strain of muscle and tendon of ankle and foot (S96.-)

The appropriate 7th character is to be added to each code from category S93

A - initial encounter

D - subsequent encounter

S - sequela

S93.0 Subluxation and dislocation of ankle joint

● New code ▲ Revised code **Excludes1:** Not coded here **Excludes2:** Not included here ⊗ Placeholder required ⑦ 7th digit required

Subluxation and dislocation of astragalus Subluxation and dislocation of fibula, lower end Subluxation and dislocation of talus Subluxation and dislocation of tibia, lower end

⊗⑦**S93.01**　**Subluxation of right ankle joint**

⊗⑦**S93.02**　**Subluxation of left ankle joint**

⊗⑦**S93.03**　**Subluxation of unspecified ankle joint**

⊗⑦**S93.04**　**Dislocation of right ankle joint**

⊗⑦**S93.05**　**Dislocation of left ankle joint**

⊗⑦**S93.06**　**Dislocation of unspecified ankle joint**

S93.1　**Subluxation and dislocation of toe**

　　S93.10　**Unspecified subluxation and dislocation of toe**

　　　Dislocation of toe NOS Subluxation of toe NOS

　　　⑦**S93.101**　**Unspecified subluxation of right toe(s)**

　　　⑦**S93.102**　**Unspecified subluxation of left toe(s)**

　　　⑦**S93.103**　**Unspecified subluxation of unspecified toe(s)**

　　　⑦**S93.104**　**Unspecified dislocation of right toe(s)**

　　　⑦**S93.105**　**Unspecified dislocation of left toe(s)**

　　　⑦**S93.106**　**Unspecified dislocation of unspecified toe(s)**

　　S93.11　**Dislocation of interphalangeal joint**

　　　⑦**S93.111**　**Dislocation of interphalangeal joint of right great toe**

　　　⑦**S93.112**　**Dislocation of interphalangeal joint of left great toe**

　　　⑦**S93.113**　**Dislocation of interphalangeal joint of unspecified great toe**

　　　⑦**S93.114**　**Dislocation of interphalangeal joint of right lesser toe(s)**

　　　⑦**S93.115**　**Dislocation of interphalangeal joint of left lesser toe(s)**

　　　⑦**S93.116**　**Dislocation of interphalangeal joint of unspecified lesser toe(s)**

　　　⑦**S93.119**　**Dislocation of interphalangeal joint of unspecified toe(s)**

　　⑦**S93.12 Dislocation of metatarsophalangeal joint**

　　　⑦**S93.121**　**Dislocation of metatarsophalangeal joint of right great toe**

　　　⑦**S93.122**　**Dislocation of metatarsophalangeal joint of left great toe**

　　　⑦**S93.123**　**Dislocation of metatarsophalangeal joint of unspecified great toe**

　　　⑦**S93.124**　**Dislocation of metatarsophalangeal joint of right lesser toe(s)**

　　　⑦**S93.125**　**Dislocation of metatarsophalangeal joint of left lesser toe(s)**

　　　⑦**S93.126**　**Dislocation of metatarsophalangeal joint of unspecified lesser toe(s)**

　　　⑦**S93.129**　**Dislocation of metatarsophalangeal joint of unspecified toe(s)**

　　S93.13　**Subluxation of interphalangeal joint**

　　　⑦**S93.131**　**Subluxation of interphalangeal joint of right great toe**

　　　⑦**S93.132**　**Subluxation of interphalangeal joint of left great toe**

　　　⑦**S93.133**　**Subluxation of interphalangeal joint of unspecified great toe**

　　　⑦**S93.134**　**Subluxation of interphalangeal joint of right lesser toe(s)**

　　　⑦**S93.135**　**Subluxation of interphalangeal joint of left lesser toe(s)**

　　　⑦**S93.136**　**Subluxation of interphalangeal joint of unspecified lesser toe(s)**

　　　⑦**S93.139**　**Subluxation of interphalangeal joint of unspecified toe(s)**

　　S93.14　**Subluxation of metatarsophalangeal joint**

　　　⑦**S93.141**　**Subluxation of metatarsophalangeal joint of right great toe**

　　　⑦**S93.142**　**Subluxation of metatarsophalangeal joint of left great toe**

　　　⑦**S93.143**　**Subluxation of metatarsophalangeal joint of unspecified great toe**

　　　⑦**S93.144**　**Subluxation of metatarsophalangeal joint of right lesser toe(s)**

　　　⑦**S93.145**　**Subluxation of metatarsophalangeal joint of left lesser toe(s)**

　　　⑦**S93.146**　**Subluxation of metatarsophalangeal joint of unspecified lesser toe(s)**

　　　⑦**S93.149**　**Subluxation of metatarsophalangeal joint of unspecified toe(s)**

S93.3　**Subluxation and dislocation of foot**

　　Excludes2: dislocation of toe (S93.1-)

　　S93.30　**Unspecified subluxation and dislocation of foot**

　　　Dislocation of foot NOS

　　　Subluxation of foot NOS

　　　⑦**S93.301**　**Unspecified subluxation of right foot**

　　　⑦**S93.302**　**Unspecified subluxation of left foot**

　　　⑦**S93.303**　**Unspecified subluxation of unspecified foot**

　　　⑦**S93.304**　**Unspecified dislocation of right foot**

　　　⑦**S93.305**　**Unspecified dislocation of left foot**

　　　⑦**S93.306**　**Unspecified dislocation of unspecified foot**

　　S93.31　**Subluxation and dislocation of tarsal joint**

　　　⑦**S93.311**　**Subluxation of tarsal joint of right foot**

　　　⑦**S93.312**　**Subluxation of tarsal joint of left foot**

　　　⑦**S93.313**　**Subluxation of tarsal joint of unspecified foot**

　　　⑦**S93.314**　**Dislocation of tarsal joint of right foot**

　　　⑦**S93.315**　**Dislocation of tarsal joint of left foot**

　　　⑦**S93.316**　**Dislocation of tarsal joint of unspecified foot**

　　S93.32　**Subluxation and dislocation of tarsometatarsal joint**

　　　⑦**S93.321**　**Subluxation of tarsometatarsal joint of right foot**

　　　⑦**S93.322**　**Subluxation of tarsometatarsal joint of left foot**

　　　⑦**S93.323**　**Subluxation of tarsometatarsal joint of unspecified foot**

　　　⑦**S93.324**　**Dislocation of tarsometatarsal joint of right foot**

　　　⑦**S93.325**　**Dislocation of tarsometatarsal joint of left foot**

　　　⑦**S93.326**　**Dislocation of tarsometatarsal joint of unspecified foot**

　　S93.33　**Other subluxation and dislocation of foot**

　　　⑦**S93.331**　**Other subluxation of right foot**

　　　⑦**S93.332**　**Other subluxation of left foot**

　　　⑦**S93.333**　**Other subluxation of unspecified foot**

　　　⑦**S93.334**　**Other dislocation of right foot**

| ▨ | Add 4th-7th digits | ▨ | Nonspecific code | ▨ | Unspecified code | ▨ | Manifestation code |

⑦ **S93.335**   **Other dislocation of left foot**

⑦ **S93.336**   **Other dislocation of unspecified foot**

S93.4   **Sprain of ankle**

   Excludes2: injury of Achilles tendon (S86.0-)

   S93.40   **Sprain of unspecified ligament of ankle**

     Sprain of ankle NOS

     Sprained ankle NOS

     ⑦ **S93.401**   **Sprain of unspecified ligament of right ankle**

     ⑦ **S93.402**   **Sprain of unspecified ligament of left ankle**

     ⑦ **S93.409**   **Sprain of unspecified ligament of unspecified ankle**

   S93.41   **Sprain of calcaneofibular ligament**

     ⑦ **S93.411**   **Sprain of calcaneofibular ligament of right ankle**

     ⑦ **S93.412**   **Sprain of calcaneofibular ligament of left ankle**

     ⑦ **S93.419**   **Sprain of calcaneofibular ligament of unspecified ankle**

   S93.42   **Sprain of deltoid ligament**

     ⑦ **S93.421**   **Sprain of deltoid ligament of right ankle**

     ⑦ **S93.422**   **Sprain of deltoid ligament of left ankle**

     ⑦ **S93.429**   **Sprain of deltoid ligament of unspecified ankle**

   S93.43   **Sprain of tibiofibular ligament**

     ⑦ **S93.431**   **Sprain of tibiofibular ligament of right ankle**

     ⑦ **S93.432**   **Sprain of tibiofibular ligament of left ankle**

     ⑦ **S93.439**   **Sprain of tibiofibular ligament of unspecified ankle**

   S93.49   **Sprain of other ligament of ankle**

     Sprain of internal collateral ligament

     Sprain of talofibular ligament

     ⑦ **S93.491**   **Sprain of other ligament of right ankle**

     ⑦ **S93.492**   **Sprain of other ligament of left ankle**

     ⑦ **S93.499**   **Sprain of other ligament of unspecified ankle**

S93.5   **Sprain of toe**

   S93.50   **Unspecified sprain of toe**

     ⑦ **S93.501**   **Unspecified sprain of right great toe**

     ⑦ **S93.502**   **Unspecified sprain of left great toe**

     ⑦ **S93.503**   **Unspecified sprain of unspecified great toe**

     ⑦ **S93.504**   **Unspecified sprain of right lesser toe(s)**

     ⑦ **S93.505**   **Unspecified sprain of left lesser toe(s)**

     ⑦ **S93.506**   **Unspecified sprain of unspecified lesser toe(s)**

     ⑦ **S93.509**   **Unspecified sprain of unspecified toe(s)**

   S93.51   **Sprain of interphalangeal joint of toe**

     ⑦ **S93.511**   **Sprain of interphalangeal joint of right great toe**

     ⑦ **S93.512**   **Sprain of interphalangeal joint of left great toe**

⑦ **S93.513**   **Sprain of interphalangeal joint of unspecified great toe**

⑦ **S93.514**   **Sprain of interphalangeal joint of right lesser toe(s)**

⑦ **S93.515**   **Sprain of interphalangeal joint of left lesser toe(s)**

⑦ **S93.516**   **Sprain of interphalangeal joint of unspecified lesser toe(s)**

⑦ **S93.519**   **Sprain of interphalangeal joint of unspecified toe(s)**

   S93.52   **Sprain of metatarsophalangeal joint of toe**

     ⑦ **S93.521**   **Sprain of metatarsophalangeal joint of right great toe**

     ⑦ **S93.522**   **Sprain of metatarsophalangeal joint of left great toe**

     ⑦ **S93.523**   **Sprain of metatarsophalangeal joint of unspecified great toe**

     ⑦ **S93.524**   **Sprain of metatarsophalangeal joint of right lesser toe(s)**

     ⑦ **S93.525**   **Sprain of metatarsophalangeal joint of left lesser toe(s)**

     ⑦ **S93.526**   **Sprain of metatarsophalangeal joint of unspecified lesser toe(s)**

     ⑦ **S93.529**   **Sprain of metatarsophalangeal joint of unspecified toe(s)**

S93.6   **Sprain of foot**

   Excludes2: sprain of metatarsophalangeal joint of toe (S93.52-)

     sprain of toe (S93.5-)

   S93.60   **Unspecified sprain of foot**

     ⑦ **S93.601**   **Unspecified sprain of right foot**

     ⑦ **S93.602**   **Unspecified sprain of left foot**

     ⑦ **S93.609**   **Unspecified sprain of unspecified foot**

   S93.61   **Sprain of tarsal ligament of foot**

     ⑦ **S93.611**   **Sprain of tarsal ligament of right foot**

     ⑦ **S93.612**   **Sprain of tarsal ligament of left foot**

     ⑦ **S93.619**   **Sprain of tarsal ligament of unspecified foot**

   S93.62   **Sprain of tarsometatarsal ligament of foot**

     ⑦ **S93.621**   **Sprain of tarsometatarsal ligament of right foot**

     ⑦ **S93.622**   **Sprain of tarsometatarsal ligament of left foot**

     ⑦ **S93.629**   **Sprain of tarsometatarsal ligament of unspecified foot**

   S93.69   **Other sprain of foot**

     ⑦ **S93.691**   **Other sprain of right foot**

     ⑦ **S93.692**   **Other sprain of left foot**

     ⑦ **S93.699**   **Other sprain of unspecified foot**

S94   **Injury of nerves at ankle and foot level**

   Code also any associated open wound (S91.-)

   The appropriate 7th character is to be added to each code from category S94

   A - initial encounter

   D - subsequent encounter

   S - sequela

   S94.0   **Injury of lateral plantar nerve**

     ⊗⑦ **S94.00**   **Injury of lateral plantar nerve, unspecified leg**

     ⊗⑦ **S94.01**   **Injury of lateral plantar nerve, right leg**

  ● New code   ▲ Revised code   **Excludes1:** Not coded here   **Excludes2:** Not included here   ⊗ Placeholder required   ⑦ 7ᵗʰ digit required

⊗⑦**S94.02**   **Injury of lateral plantar nerve, left leg**

S94.1   **Injury of medial plantar nerve**

⊗⑦**S94.10**   **Injury of medial plantar nerve, unspecified leg**

⊗⑦**S94.11**   **Injury of medial plantar nerve, right leg**

⊗⑦**S94.12**   **Injury of medial plantar nerve, left leg**

S94.2   **Injury of deep peroneal nerve at ankle and foot level**

Injury of terminal, lateral branch of deep peroneal nerve

⊗⑦**S94.20**   **Injury of deep peroneal nerve at ankle and foot level, unspecified leg**

⊗⑦**S94.21**   **Injury of deep peroneal nerve at ankle and foot level, right leg**

⊗⑦**S94.22**   **Injury of deep peroneal nerve at ankle and foot level, left leg**

S94.3   **Injury of cutaneous sensory nerve at ankle and foot level**

⊗⑦**S94.30**   **Injury of cutaneous sensory nerve at ankle and foot level, unspecified leg**

⊗⑦**S94.31**   **Injury of cutaneous sensory nerve at ankle and foot level, right leg**

⊗⑦**S94.32**   **Injury of cutaneous sensory nerve at ankle and foot level, left leg**

S94.8   **Injury of other nerves at ankle and foot level**

S94.8X   **Injury of other nerves at ankle and foot level**

⑦**S94.8X1**   **Injury of other nerves at ankle and foot level, right leg**

⑦**S94.8X2**   **Injury of other nerves at ankle and foot level, left leg**

⑦**S94.8X9**   **Injury of other nerves at ankle and foot level, unspecified leg**

S94.9   **Injury of unspecified nerve at ankle and foot level**

⊗⑦**S94.90**   **Injury of unspecified nerve at ankle and foot level, unspecified leg**

⊗⑦**S94.91**   **Injury of unspecified nerve at ankle and foot level, right leg**

⊗⑦**S94.92**   **Injury of unspecified nerve at ankle and foot level, left leg**

S95   **Injury of blood vessels at ankle and foot level**

Code also any associated open wound (S91.-)

Excludes2: injury of posterior tibial artery and vein (S85.1-, S85.8-)

The appropriate 7th character is to be added to each code from category S95

A - initial encounter

D - subsequent encounter

S - sequela

S95.0   **Injury of dorsal artery of foot**

S95.00   **Unspecified injury of dorsal artery of foot**

⑦**S95.001**   **Unspecified injury of dorsal artery of right foot**

⑦**S95.002**   **Unspecified injury of dorsal artery of left foot**

⑦**S95.009**   **Unspecified injury of dorsal artery of unspecified foot**

S95.01   **Laceration of dorsal artery of foot**

⑦**S95.011**   **Laceration of dorsal artery of right foot**

⑦**S95.012**   **Laceration of dorsal artery of left foot**

⑦**S95.019**   **Laceration of dorsal artery of unspecified foot**

S95.09   **Other specified injury of dorsal artery of foot**

⑦**S95.091**   **Other specified injury of dorsal artery of right foot**

⑦**S95.092**   **Other specified injury of dorsal artery of left foot**

⑦**S95.099**   **Other specified injury of dorsal artery of unspecified foot**

S95.1   **Injury of plantar artery of foot**

S95.10   **Unspecified injury of plantar artery of foot**

⑦**S95.101**   **Unspecified injury of plantar artery of right foot**

⑦**S95.102**   **Unspecified injury of plantar artery of left foot**

⑦**S95.109**   **Unspecified injury of plantar artery of unspecified foot**

S95.11   **Laceration of plantar artery of foot**

⊗⑦**S95.111**   **Laceration of plantar artery of right foot**

⑦**S95.112**   **Laceration of plantar artery of left foot**

⑦**S95.119**   **Laceration of plantar artery of unspecified foot**

S95.19   **Other specified injury of plantar artery of foot**

⑦**S95.191**   **Other specified injury of plantar artery of right foot**

⑦**S95.192**   **Other specified injury of plantar artery of left foot**

⑦**S95.199**   **Other specified injury of plantar artery of unspecified foot**

S95.2   **Injury of dorsal vein of foot**

S95.20   **Unspecified injury of dorsal vein of foot**

⑦**S95.201**   **Unspecified injury of dorsal vein of right foot**

⑦**S95.202**   **Unspecified injury of dorsal vein of left foot**

⑦**S95.209**   **Unspecified injury of dorsal vein of unspecified foot**

S95.21   **Laceration of dorsal vein of foot**

⑦**S95.211**   **Laceration of dorsal vein of right foot**

⑦**S95.212**   **Laceration of dorsal vein of left foot**

⑦**S95.219**   **Laceration of dorsal vein of unspecified foot**

S95.29   **Other specified injury of dorsal vein of foot**

⑦**S95.291**   **Other specified injury of dorsal vein of right foot**

⑦**S95.292**   **Other specified injury of dorsal vein of left foot**

⑦**S95.299**   **Other specified injury of dorsal vein of unspecified foot**

S95.8   **Injury of other blood vessels at ankle and foot level**

S95.80   **Unspecified injury of other blood vessels at ankle and foot level**

⑦**S95.801**   **Unspecified injury of other blood vessels at ankle and foot level, right leg**

⑦**S95.802**   **Unspecified injury of other blood vessels at ankle and foot level, left leg**

⑦**S95.809**   **Unspecified injury of other blood vessels at ankle and foot level, unspecified leg**

S95.81   **Laceration of other blood vessels at ankle and foot level**

⑦ **S95.811** Laceration of other blood vessels at ankle and foot level, right leg

⑦ **S95.812** Laceration of other blood vessels at ankle and foot level, left leg

⑦ **S95.819** Laceration of other blood vessels at ankle and foot level, unspecified leg

S95.89 Other specified injury of other blood vessels at ankle and foot level

⑦ **S95.891** Other specified injury of other blood vessels at ankle and foot level, right leg

⑦ **S95.892** Other specified injury of other blood vessels at ankle and foot level, left leg

⑦ **S95.899** Other specified injury of other blood vessels at ankle and foot level, unspecified leg

S95.9 Injury of unspecified blood vessel at ankle and foot level

S95.90 Unspecified injury of unspecified blood vessel at ankle and foot level

⑦ **S95.901** Unspecified injury of unspecified blood vessel at ankle and foot level, right leg

⑦ **S95.902** Unspecified injury of unspecified blood vessel at ankle and foot level, left leg

⑦ **S95.909** Unspecified injury of unspecified blood vessel at ankle and foot level, unspecified leg

S95.91 Laceration of unspecified blood vessel at ankle and foot level

⑦ **S95.911** Laceration of unspecified blood vessel at ankle and foot level, right leg

⑦ **S95.912** Laceration of unspecified blood vessel at ankle and foot level, left leg

⑦ **S95.919** Laceration of unspecified blood vessel at ankle and foot level, unspecified leg

S95.99 Other specified injury of unspecified blood vessel at ankle and foot level

⑦ **S95.991** Other specified injury of unspecified blood vessel at ankle and foot level, right leg

⑦ **S95.992** Other specified injury of unspecified blood vessel at ankle and foot level, left leg

⑦ **S95.999** Other specified injury of unspecified blood vessel at ankle and foot level, unspecified leg

S96 Injury of muscle and tendon at ankle and foot level

Code also any associated open wound (S91.-)

Excludes2: injury of Achilles tendon (S86.0-)

sprain of joints and ligaments of ankle and foot (S93.-)

The appropriate 7th character is to be added to each code from category S96

A - initial encounter

D - subsequent encounter

S - sequela

S96.0 Injury of muscle and tendon of long flexor muscle of toe at ankle and foot level

S96.00 Unspecified injury of muscle and tendon of long flexor muscle of toe at ankle and foot level

⑦ **S96.001** Unspecified injury of muscle and tendon of long flexor muscle of toe at ankle and foot level, right foot

⑦ **S96.002** Unspecified injury of muscle and tendon of long flexor muscle of toe at ankle and foot level, left foot

⑦ **S96.009** Unspecified injury of muscle and tendon of long flexor muscle of toe at ankle and foot level, unspecified foot

S96.01 Strain of muscle and tendon of long flexor muscle of toe at ankle and foot level

⑦ **S96.011** Strain of muscle and tendon of long flexor muscle of toe at ankle and foot level, right foot

⑦ **S96.012** Strain of muscle and tendon of long flexor muscle of toe at ankle and foot level, left foot

⑦ **S96.019** Strain of muscle and tendon of long flexor muscle of toe at ankle and foot level, unspecified foot

S96.02 Laceration of muscle and tendon of long flexor muscle of toe at ankle and foot level

⑦ **S96.021** Laceration of muscle and tendon of long flexor muscle of toe at ankle and foot level, right foot

⑦ **S96.022** Laceration of muscle and tendon of long flexor muscle of toe at ankle and foot level, left foot

⑦ **S96.029** Laceration of muscle and tendon of long flexor muscle of toe at ankle and foot level, unspecified foot

S96.09 Other injury of muscle and tendon of long flexor muscle of toe at ankle and foot level

⑦ **S96.091** Other injury of muscle and tendon of long flexor muscle of toe at ankle and foot level, right foot

⑦ **S96.092** Other injury of muscle and tendon of long flexor muscle of toe at ankle and foot level, left foot

⑦ **S96.099** Other injury of muscle and tendon of long flexor muscle of toe at ankle and foot level, unspecified foot

S96.1 Injury of muscle and tendon of long extensor muscle of toe at ankle and foot level

S96.10 Unspecified injury of muscle and tendon of long extensor muscle of toe at ankle and foot level

⑦ **S96.101** Unspecified injury of muscle and tendon of long extensor muscle of toe at ankle and foot level, right foot

⑦ **S96.102** Unspecified injury of muscle and tendon of long extensor muscle of toe at ankle and foot level, left foot

⑦ **S96.109** Unspecified injury of muscle and tendon of long extensor muscle of toe at ankle and foot level, unspecified foot

S96.11 Strain of muscle and tendon of long extensor muscle of toe at ankle and foot level

⑦ **S96.111** Strain of muscle and tendon of long extensor muscle of toe at ankle and foot level, right foot

⑦ **S96.112** Strain of muscle and tendon of long extensor muscle of toe at ankle and foot level, left foot

⑦ **S96.119** Strain of muscle and tendon of long extensor muscle of toe at ankle and foot level, unspecified foot

S96.12 Laceration of muscle and tendon of long extensor muscle of toe at ankle and foot level

• New code ▲ Revised code **Excludes1:** Not coded here **Excludes2:** Not included here ⊗ Placeholder required ⑦7th digit required

⑦S96.121　Laceration of muscle and tendon of long extensor muscle of toe at ankle and foot level, right foot

⑦S96.122　Laceration of muscle and tendon of long extensor muscle of toe at ankle and foot level, left foot

⑦S96.129　Laceration of muscle and tendon of long extensor muscle of toe at ankle and foot level, unspecified foot

S96.19　Other specified injury of muscle and tendon of long extensor muscle of toe at ankle and foot level

⑦S96.191　Other specified injury of muscle and tendon of long extensor muscle of toe at ankle and foot level, right foot

⑦S96.192　Other specified injury of muscle and tendon of long extensor muscle of toe at ankle and foot level, left foot

⑦S96.199　Other specified injury of muscle and tendon of long extensor muscle of toe at ankle and foot level, unspecified foot

S96.2　Injury of intrinsic muscle and tendon at ankle and foot level

S96.20　Unspecified injury of intrinsic muscle and tendon at ankle and foot level

⑦S96.201　Unspecified injury of intrinsic muscle and tendon at ankle and foot level, right foot

⑦S96.202　Unspecified injury of intrinsic muscle and tendon at ankle and foot level, left foot

⑦S96.209　Unspecified injury of intrinsic muscle and tendon at ankle and foot level, unspecified foot

S96.21　Strain of intrinsic muscle and tendon at ankle and foot level

⑦S96.211　Strain of intrinsic muscle and tendon at ankle and foot level, right foot

⑦S96.212　Strain of intrinsic muscle and tendon at ankle and foot level, left foot

⑦S96.219　Strain of intrinsic muscle and tendon at ankle and foot level, unspecified foot

S96.22　Laceration of intrinsic muscle and tendon at ankle and foot level

⑦S96.221　Laceration of intrinsic muscle and tendon at ankle and foot level, right foot

⑦S96.222　Laceration of intrinsic muscle and tendon at ankle and foot level, left foot

⑦S96.229　Laceration of intrinsic muscle and tendon at ankle and foot level, unspecified foot

S96.29　Other specified injury of intrinsic muscle and tendon at ankle and foot level

⑦S96.291　Other specified injury of intrinsic muscle and tendon at ankle and foot level, right foot

⑦S96.292　Other specified injury of intrinsic muscle and tendon at ankle and foot level, left foot

⑦S96.299　Other specified injury of intrinsic muscle and tendon at ankle and foot level, unspecified foot

S96.8　Injury of other specified muscles and tendons at ankle and foot level

S96.80　Unspecified injury of other specified muscles and tendons at ankle and foot level

⑦S96.801　Unspecified injury of other specified muscles and tendons at ankle and foot level, right foot

⑦S96.802　Unspecified injury of other specified muscles and tendons at ankle and foot level, left foot

⑦S96.809　Unspecified injury of other specified muscles and tendons at ankle and foot level, unspecified foot

S96.81　Strain of other specified muscles and tendons at ankle and foot level

⑦S96.811　Strain of other specified muscles and tendons at ankle and foot level, right foot

⑦S96.812　Strain of other specified muscles and tendons at ankle and foot level, left foot

⑦S96.819　Strain of other specified muscles and tendons at ankle and foot level, unspecified foot

S96.82　Laceration of other specified muscles and tendons at ankle and foot level

⑦S96.821　Laceration of other specified muscles and tendons at ankle and foot level, right foot

⑦S96.822　Laceration of other specified muscles and tendons at ankle and foot level, left foot

⑦S96.829　Laceration of other specified muscles and tendons at ankle and foot level, unspecified foot

S96.89　Other specified injury of other specified muscles and tendons at ankle and foot level

⑦S96.891　Other specified injury of other specified muscles and tendons at ankle and foot level, right foot

⑦S96.892　Other specified injury of other specified muscles and tendons at ankle and foot level, left foot

⑦S96.899　Other specified injury of other specified muscles and tendons at ankle and foot level, unspecified foot

S96.9　Injury of unspecified muscle and tendon at ankle and foot level

S96.90　Unspecified injury of unspecified muscle and tendon at ankle and foot level

⑦S96.901　Unspecified injury of unspecified muscle and tendon at ankle and foot level, right foot

⑦S96.902　Unspecified injury of unspecified muscle and tendon at ankle and foot level, left foot

⑦S96.909　Unspecified injury of unspecified muscle and tendon at ankle and foot level, unspecified foot

S96.91　Strain of unspecified muscle and tendon at ankle and foot level

⑦S96.911　Strain of unspecified muscle and tendon at ankle and foot level, right foot

⑦S96.912　Strain of unspecified muscle and tendon at ankle and foot level, left foot

⑦**S96.919** Strain of unspecified muscle and tendon at ankle and foot level, unspecified foot

S96.92 Laceration of unspecified muscle and tendon at ankle and foot level

⑦**S96.921** Laceration of unspecified muscle and tendon at ankle and foot level, right foot

⑦**S96.922** Laceration of unspecified muscle and tendon at ankle and foot level, left foot

⑦**S96.929** Laceration of unspecified muscle and tendon at ankle and foot level, unspecified foot

S96.99 Other specified injury of unspecified muscle and tendon at ankle and foot level

⑦**S96.991** Other specified injury of unspecified muscle and tendon at ankle and foot level, right foot

⑦**S96.992** Other specified injury of unspecified muscle and tendon at ankle and foot level, left foot

⑦**S96.999** Other specified injury of unspecified muscle and tendon at ankle and foot level, unspecified foot

S97 **Crushing injury of ankle and foot**

<u>Use additional code</u>(s) for all associated injuries

The appropriate 7th character is to be added to each code from category S97

A - initial encounter

D - subsequent encounter

S - sequela

S97.0 **Crushing injury of ankle**

⊗⑦**S97.00** Crushing injury of unspecified ankle

⊗⑦**S97.01** Crushing injury of right ankle

⊗⑦**S97.02** Crushing injury of left ankle

S97.1 **Crushing injury of toe**

S97.10 Crushing injury of unspecified toe(s)

⑦**S97.101** Crushing injury of unspecified right toe(s)

⑦**S97.102** Crushing injury of unspecified left toe(s)

⑦**S97.109** Crushing injury of unspecified toe(s)

Crushing injury of toe NOS

S97.11 Crushing injury of great toe

⑦**S97.111** Crushing injury of right great toe

⑦**S97.112** Crushing injury of left great toe

⑦**S97.119** Crushing injury of unspecified great toe

S97.12 Crushing injury of lesser toe(s)

⑦**S97.121** Crushing injury of right lesser toe(s)

⑦**S97.122** Crushing injury of left lesser toe(s)

⑦**S97.129** Crushing injury of unspecified lesser toe(s)

S97.8 **Crushing injury of foot**

⊗⑦**S97.80** Crushing injury of unspecified foot

Crushing injury of foot NOS

⊗⑦**S97.81** Crushing injury of right foot

⊗⑦**S97.82** Crushing injury of left foot

S98 **Traumatic amputation of ankle and foot**

An amputation not identified as partial or complete should be coded to complete

The appropriate 7th character is to be added to each code from category S98

A - initial encounter

D - subsequent encounter

S - sequela

S98.0 **Traumatic amputation of foot at ankle level**

S98.01 Complete traumatic amputation of foot at ankle level

⑦**S98.011** Complete traumatic amputation of right foot at ankle level

⑦**S98.012** Complete traumatic amputation of left foot at ankle level

⑦**S98.019** Complete traumatic amputation of unspecified foot at ankle level

S98.02 Partial traumatic amputation of foot at ankle level

⑦**S98.021** Partial traumatic amputation of right foot at ankle level

⑦**S98.022** Partial traumatic amputation of left foot at ankle level

⑦**S98.029** Partial traumatic amputation of unspecified foot at ankle level

S98.1 **Traumatic amputation of one toe**

S98.11 Complete traumatic amputation of great toe

⑦**S98.111** Complete traumatic amputation of right great toe

⑦**S98.112** Complete traumatic amputation of left great toe

⑦**S98.119** Complete traumatic amputation of unspecified great toe

S98.12 Partial traumatic amputation of great toe

⑦**S98.121** Partial traumatic amputation of right great toe

⑦**S98.122** Partial traumatic amputation of left great toe

⑦**S98.129** Partial traumatic amputation of unspecified great toe

S98.13 Complete traumatic amputation of one lesser toe

Traumatic amputation of toe NOS

⑦**S98.131** Complete traumatic amputation of one right lesser toe

⑦**S98.132** Complete traumatic amputation of one left lesser toe

⑦**S98.139** Complete traumatic amputation of one unspecified lesser toe

S98.14 Partial traumatic amputation of one lesser toe

⑦**S98.141** Partial traumatic amputation of one right lesser toe

⑦**S98.142** Partial traumatic amputation of one left lesser toe

⑦**S98.149** Partial traumatic amputation of one unspecified lesser toe

S98.2 **Traumatic amputation of two or more lesser toes**

S98.21 Complete traumatic amputation of two or more lesser toes

⑦**S98.211** Complete traumatic amputation of two or more right lesser toes

⑦**S98.212** Complete traumatic amputation of two or more left lesser toes

⑦**S98.219** Complete traumatic amputation of two or more unspecified lesser toes

S98.22   **Partial traumatic amputation of two or more lesser toes**

⑦S98.221   **Partial traumatic amputation of two or more right lesser toes**

⑦S98.222   **Partial traumatic amputation of two or more left lesser toes**

⑦S98.229   **Partial traumatic amputation of two or more unspecified lesser toes**

S98.3   **Traumatic amputation of midfoot**

S98.31   **Complete traumatic amputation of midfoot**

⑦S98.311   **Complete traumatic amputation of right midfoot**

⑦S98.312   **Complete traumatic amputation of left midfoot**

⑦S98.319   **Complete traumatic amputation of unspecified midfoot**

S98.32   **Partial traumatic amputation of midfoot**

⑦S98.321   **Partial traumatic amputation of right midfoot**

⑦S98.322   **Partial traumatic amputation of left midfoot**

⑦S98.329   **Partial traumatic amputation of unspecified midfoot**

S98.9   **Traumatic amputation of foot, level unspecified**

S98.91   **Complete traumatic amputation of foot, level unspecified**

⑦S98.911   **Complete traumatic amputation of right foot, level unspecified**

⑦S98.912   **Complete traumatic amputation of left foot, level unspecified**

⑦S98.919   **Complete traumatic amputation of unspecified foot, level unspecified**

S98.92   **Partial traumatic amputation of foot, level unspecified**

⑦S98.921   **Partial traumatic amputation of right foot, level unspecified**

⑦S98.922   **Partial traumatic amputation of left foot, level unspecified**

⑦S98.929   **Partial traumatic amputation of unspecified foot, level unspecified**

S99   **Other and unspecified injuries of ankle and foot**

S99.0   **Physeal fracture of calcaneus**

The appropriate 7th character is to be added to each code from subcategories S99.0

A - initial encounter for closed fracture

B - initial encounter for open fracture

D - subsequent encounter for fracture with routine healing

G - subsequent encounter for fracture with delayed healing

K - subsequent encounter for fracture with nonunion

P - subsequent encounter for fracture with malunion

S - sequela

S99.00   **Unspecified physeal fracture of calcaneus**

⑦S99.001   **Unspecified physeal fracture of right calcaneus**

⑦S99.002   **Unspecified physeal fracture of left calcaneus**

⑦S99.009   **Unspecified physeal fracture of unspecified calcaneus**

S99.01   **Salter-Harris Type I physeal fracture of calcaneus**

⑦S99.011   **Salter-Harris Type I physeal fracture of right calcaneus**

⑦S99.012   **Salter-Harris Type I physeal fracture of left calcaneus**

⑦S99.019   **Salter-Harris Type I physeal fracture of unspecified calcaneus**

S99.02   **Salter-Harris Type II physeal fracture of calcaneus**

⑦S99.021   **Salter-Harris Type II physeal fracture of right calcaneus**

⑦S99.022   **Salter-Harris Type II physeal fracture of left calcaneus**

⑦S99.029   **Salter-Harris Type II physeal fracture of unspecified calcaneus**

S99.03   **Salter-Harris Type III physeal fracture of calcaneus**

⑦S99.031   **Salter-Harris Type III physeal fracture of right calcaneus**

⑦S99.032   **Salter-Harris Type III physeal fracture of left calcaneus**

⑦S99.039   **Salter-Harris Type III physeal fracture of unspecified calcaneus**

S99.04   **Salter-Harris Type IV physeal fracture of calcaneus**

⑦S99.041   **Salter-Harris Type IV physeal fracture of right calcaneus**

⑦S99.042   **Salter-Harris Type IV physeal fracture of left calcaneus**

⑦S99.049   **Salter-Harris Type IV physeal fracture of unspecified calcaneus**

S99.09   **Other physeal fracture of calcaneus**

⑦S99.091   **Other physeal fracture of right calcaneus**

⑦S99.092   **Other physeal fracture of left calcaneus**

⑦S99.099   **Other physeal fracture of unspecified calcaneus**

S99.1   **Physeal fracture of metatarsal**

The appropriate 7th character is to be added to each code from subcategories S99.1

A - initial encounter for closed fracture

B - initial encounter for open fracture

D - subsequent encounter for fracture with routine healing

G - subsequent encounter for fracture with delayed healing

K - subsequent encounter for fracture with nonunion

P - subsequent encounter for fracture with malunion

S - sequela

S99.10   **Unspecified physeal fracture of metatarsal**

⑦S99.101   **Unspecified physeal fracture of right metatarsal**

⑦S99.102   **Unspecified physeal fracture of left metatarsal**

⑦S99.109   **Unspecified physeal fracture of unspecified metatarsal**

S99.11   **Salter-Harris Type I physeal fracture of metatarsal**

⑦S99.111   **Salter-Harris Type I physeal fracture of right metatarsal**

⑦S99.112   **Salter-Harris Type I physeal fracture of left metatarsal**

⑦S99.119   **Salter-Harris Type I physeal fracture of unspecified metatarsal**

S99.12   **Salter-Harris Type II physeal fracture of metatarsal**

⑦S99.121   Salter-Harris Type II physeal fracture of right metatarsal

⑦S99.122   Salter-Harris Type II physeal fracture of left metatarsal

⑦S99.129   Salter-Harris Type II physeal fracture of unspecified metatarsal

S99.13   Salter-Harris Type III physeal fracture of metatarsal

⑦S99.131   Salter-Harris Type III physeal fracture of right metatarsal

⑦S99.132   Salter-Harris Type III physeal fracture of left metatarsal

⑦S99.139   Salter-Harris Type III physeal fracture of unspecified metatarsal

S99.14   Salter-Harris Type IV physeal fracture of metatarsal

⑦S99.141   Salter-Harris Type IV physeal fracture of right metatarsal

⑦S99.142   Salter-Harris Type IV physeal fracture of left metatarsal

⑦S99.149   Salter-Harris Type IV physeal fracture of unspecified metatarsal

S99.19   Other physeal fracture of metatarsal

⑦S99.191   Other physeal fracture of right metatarsal

⑦S99.192   Other physeal fracture of left metatarsal

⑦S99.199   Other physeal fracture of unspecified metatarsal

S99.2   **Physeal fracture of phalanx of toe**

The appropriate 7th character is to be added to each code from subcategories S99.2

A - initial encounter for closed fracture

B - initial encounter for open fracture

D - subsequent encounter for fracture with routine healing

G - subsequent encounter for fracture with delayed healing

K - subsequent encounter for fracture with nonunion

P - subsequent encounter for fracture with malunion

S - sequela

S99.20   Unspecified physeal fracture of phalanx of toe

⑦S99.201   Unspecified physeal fracture of phalanx of right toe

⑦S99.202   Unspecified physeal fracture of phalanx of left toe

⑦S99.209   Unspecified physeal fracture of phalanx of unspecified toe

S99.21   Salter-Harris Type I physeal fracture of phalanx of toe

⑦S99.211   Salter-Harris Type I physeal fracture of phalanx of right toe

⑦S99.212   Salter-Harris Type I physeal fracture of phalanx of left toe

⑦S99.219   Salter-Harris Type I physeal fracture of phalanx of unspecified toe

S99.22   Salter-Harris Type II physeal fracture of phalanx of toe

⑦S99.221   Salter-Harris Type II physeal fracture of phalanx of right toe

⑦S99.222   Salter-Harris Type II physeal fracture of phalanx of left toe

⑦S99.229   Salter-Harris Type II physeal fracture of phalanx of unspecified toe

S99.23   Salter-Harris Type III physeal fracture of phalanx of toe

⑦S99.231   Salter-Harris Type III physeal fracture of phalanx of right toe

⑦S99.232   Salter-Harris Type III physeal fracture of phalanx of left toe

⑦S99.239   Salter-Harris Type III physeal fracture of phalanx of unspecified toe

S99.24   Salter-Harris Type IV physeal fracture of phalanx of toe

⑦S99.241   Salter-Harris Type IV physeal fracture of phalanx of right toe

⑦S99.242   Salter-Harris Type IV physeal fracture of phalanx of left toe

⑦S99.249   Salter-Harris Type IV physeal fracture of phalanx of unspecified toe

S99.29   Other physeal fracture of phalanx of toe

⑦S99.291   Other physeal fracture of phalanx of right toe

⑦S99.292   Other physeal fracture of phalanx of left toe

⑦S99.299   Other physeal fracture of phalanx of unspecified toe

S99.8   **Other specified injuries of ankle and foot**

The appropriate 7th character is to be added to each code from subcategory S99.8

A - initial encounter

D - subsequent encounter

S - sequela

S99.81   Other specified injuries of ankle

⑦S99.811   Other specified injuries of right ankle

⑦S99.812   Other specified injuries of left ankle

⑦S99.819   Other specified injuries of unspecified ankle

S99.82   Other specified injuries of foot

⑦S99.821   Other specified injuries of right foot

⑦S99.822   Other specified injuries of left foot

⑦S99.829   Other specified injuries of unspecified foot

S99.9   **Unspecified injury of ankle and foot**

The appropriate 7th character is to be added to each code from subcategory S99.9

A - initial encounter

D - subsequent encounter

S - sequela

S99.91   Unspecified injury of ankle

⑦S99.911   Unspecified injury of right ankle

⑦S99.912   Unspecified injury of left ankle

⑦S99.919   Unspecified injury of unspecified ankle

S99.92   Unspecified injury of foot

⑦S99.921   Unspecified injury of right foot

⑦S99.922   Unspecified injury of left foot

⑦S99.929   Unspecified injury of unspecified foot

INJURY, POISONING AND CERTAIN OTHER CONSEQUENCES OF EXTERNAL CAUSES (T07-T88)

INJURIES INVOLVING MULTIPLE BODY REGIONS (T07)

   ● New code   ▲ Revised code   **Excludes1:** Not coded here   **Excludes2:** Not included here   ⊗ Placeholder required   ⑦7th digit required

Excludes1: burns and corrosions (T20-T32)

frostbite (T33-T34)

insect bite or sting, venomous (T63.4)

sunburn (L55.-)

⊗⑦**T07** **Unspecified multiple injuries**

Excludes1: injury NOS (T14.90)

The appropriate 7th character is to be added to code T07

A initial encounter

D subsequent encounter

S sequela

INJURY OF UNSPECIFIED BODY REGION (T14)

T14 **Injury of unspecified body region**

The appropriate 7th character is to be added to each code from category T14

A initial encounter

D subsequent encounter

S sequela

Excludes1: multiple unspecified injuries (T07)

⊗⑦**T14.8** **Other injury of unspecified body region**

Abrasion NOS

Contusion NOS

Crush injury NOS

Fracture NOS

Skin injury NOS

Vascular injury NOS

Wound NOS

T14.9 **Unspecified injury**

⊗⑦**T14.90** **Injury, unspecified**

Injury NOS

⊗⑦**T14.91** **Suicide attempt**

Attempted suicide NOS

EFFECTS OF FOREIGN BODY ENTERING THROUGH NATURAL ORIFICE (T15-T19)

Excludes2: foreign body accidentally left in operation wound (T81.5-)

foreign body in penetrating wound - See open wound by body region residual foreign body in soft tissue (M79.5)

splinter, without open wound - See superficial injury by body region

T15 **Foreign body on external eye**

Excludes2: foreign body in penetrating wound of orbit and eye ball (S05.4-, S05.5-)

open wound of eyelid and periocular area (S01.1-)

retained foreign body in eyelid (H02.8-)

retained (old) foreign body in penetrating wound of orbit and eye ball (H05.5-, H44.6-, H44.7-)

superficial foreign body of eyelid and periocular area (S00.25-)

The appropriate 7th character is to be added to each code from category T15

A - initial encounter

D - subsequent encounter

S - sequela

T15.0 **Foreign body in cornea**

⊗⑦**T15.00** **Foreign body in cornea, unspecified eye**

⊗⑦**T15.01** **Foreign body in cornea, right eye**

⊗⑦**T15.02** **Foreign body in cornea, left eye**

T15.1 **Foreign body in conjunctival sac**

⊗⑦**T15.10** **Foreign body in conjunctival sac, unspecified eye**

⊗⑦**T15.11** **Foreign body in conjunctival sac, right eye**

⊗⑦**T15.12** **Foreign body in conjunctival sac, left eye**

T15.8 **Foreign body in other and multiple parts of external eye**

Foreign body in lacrimal punctum

⊗⑦**T15.80** **Foreign body in other and multiple parts of external eye, unspecified eye**

⊗⑦**T15.81** **Foreign body in other and multiple parts of external eye, right eye**

⊗⑦**T15.82** **Foreign body in other and multiple parts of external eye, left eye**

T15.9 **Foreign body on external eye, part unspecified**

⊗⑦**T15.90** **Foreign body on external eye, part unspecified, unspecified eye**

⊗⑦**T15.91** **Foreign body on external eye, part unspecified, right eye**

⊗⑦**T15.92** **Foreign body on external eye, part unspecified, left eye**

T16 **Foreign body in ear**

Includes: foreign body in auditory canal

The appropriate 7th character is to be added to each code from category T16

A - initial encounter

D - subsequent encounter

S - sequela

⊗⑦**T16.1** **Foreign body in right ear**

⊗⑦**T16.2** **Foreign body in left ear**

⊗⑦**T16.9** **Foreign body in ear, unspecified ear**

T17 **Foreign body in respiratory tract**

The appropriate 7th character is to be added to each code from category T17

A - initial encounter

D - subsequent encounter

S - sequela

⊗⑦**T17.0** **Foreign body in nasal sinus**

⊗⑦**T17.1** **Foreign body in nostril**

Foreign body in nose NOS

T17.2 **Foreign body in pharynx**

Foreign body in nasopharynx

Foreign body in throat NOS

T17.20 **Unspecified foreign body in pharynx**

⑦**T17.200** **Unspecified foreign body in pharynx causing asphyxiation**

⑦**T17.208** **Unspecified foreign body in pharynx causing other injury**

T17.21 **Gastric contents in pharynx**

Aspiration of gastric contents into pharynx

Vomitus in pharynx

⑦**T17.210** **Gastric contents in pharynx causing asphyxiation**

⑦**T17.218** **Gastric contents in pharynx causing other injury**

T17.22 **Food in pharynx**

Bones in pharynx

Seeds in pharynx

⑦**T17.220** **Food in pharynx causing asphyxiation**

⑦**T17.228** **Food in pharynx causing other injury**

T17.29　Other foreign object in pharynx

⑦T17.290　Other foreign object in pharynx causing asphyxiation

⑦T17.298　Other foreign object in pharynx causing other injury

T17.3　Foreign body in larynx

T17.30　Unspecified foreign body in larynx

⑦T17.300　Unspecified foreign body in larynx causing asphyxiation

⑦T17.308　Unspecified foreign body in larynx causing other injury

T17.31　Gastric contents in larynx

Aspiration of gastric contents into larynx

Vomitus in larynx

⑦T17.310　Gastric contents in larynx causing asphyxiation

⑦T17.318　Gastric contents in larynx causing other injury

T17.32　Food in larynx

Bones in larynx

Seeds in larynx

⑦T17.320　Food in larynx causing asphyxiation

⑦T17.328　Food in larynx causing other injury

T17.39　Other foreign object in larynx

⑦T17.390　Other foreign object in larynx causing asphyxiation

⑦T17.398　Other foreign object in larynx causing other injury

T17.4　Foreign body in trachea

T17.40　Unspecified foreign body in trachea

⑦T17.400　Unspecified foreign body in trachea causing asphyxiation

⑦T17.408　Unspecified foreign body in trachea causing other injury

T17.41　Gastric contents in trachea

Aspiration of gastric contents into trachea

Vomitus in trachea

⑦T17.410　Gastric contents in trachea causing asphyxiation

⑦T17.418　Gastric contents in trachea causing other injury

T17.42　Food in trachea

Bones in trachea

Seeds in trachea

⑦T17.420　Food in trachea causing asphyxiation

⑦T17.428　Food in trachea causing other injury

T17.49　Other foreign object in trachea

⑦T17.490　Other foreign object in trachea causing asphyxiation

⑦T17.498　Other foreign object in trachea causing other injury

T17.5　Foreign body in bronchus

T17.50　Unspecified foreign body in bronchus

⑦T17.500　Unspecified foreign body in bronchus causing asphyxiation

⑦T17.508　Unspecified foreign body in bronchus causing other injury

T17.51　Gastric contents in bronchus

Aspiration of gastric contents into bronchus

Vomitus in bronchus

⑦T17.510　Gastric contents in bronchus causing asphyxiation

⑦T17.518　Gastric contents in bronchus causing other injury

T17.52　Food in bronchus

Bones in bronchus

Seeds in bronchus

⑦T17.520　Food in bronchus causing asphyxiation

⑦T17.528　Food in bronchus causing other injury

T17.59　Other foreign object in bronchus

⑦T17.590　Other foreign object in bronchus causing asphyxiation

⑦T17.598　Other foreign object in bronchus causing other injury

T17.8　Foreign body in other parts of respiratory tract

Foreign body in bronchioles

Foreign body in lung

T17.80　Unspecified foreign body in other parts of respiratory tract

⑦T17.800　Unspecified foreign body in other parts of respiratory tract causing asphyxiation

⑦T17.808　Unspecified foreign body in other parts of respiratory tract causing other injury

T17.81　Gastric contents in other parts of respiratory tract

Aspiration of gastric contents into other parts of respiratory tract

Vomitus in other parts of respiratory tract

⑦T17.810　Gastric contents in other parts of respiratory tract causing asphyxiation

⑦T17.818　Gastric contents in other parts of respiratory tract causing other injury

T17.82　Food in other parts of respiratory tract

Bones in other parts of respiratory tract

Seeds in other parts of respiratory tract

⑦T17.820　Food in other parts of respiratory tract causing asphyxiation

⑦T17.828　Food in other parts of respiratory tract causing other injury

T17.89　Other foreign object in other parts of respiratory tract

⑦T17.890　Other foreign object in other parts of respiratory tract causing asphyxiation

⑦T17.898　Other foreign object in other parts of respiratory tract causing other injury

T17.9　Foreign body in respiratory tract, part unspecified

T17.90　Unspecified foreign body in respiratory tract, part unspecified

⑦T17.900　Unspecified foreign body in respiratory tract, part unspecified causing asphyxiation

⑦T17.908　Unspecified foreign body in respiratory tract, part unspecified causing other injury

T17.91　Gastric contents in respiratory tract, part unspecified

● New code　▲ Revised code　**Excludes1:** Not coded here　**Excludes2:** Not included here　⊗ Placeholder required　⑦7th digit required

Aspiration of gastric contents into respiratory tract, part unspecified

Vomitus in trachea respiratory tract, part unspecified

⑦ **T17.910** **Gastric contents in respiratory tract, part unspecified causing asphyxiation**

⑦ **T17.918** **Gastric contents in respiratory tract, part unspecified causing other injury**

T17.92 **Food in respiratory tract, part unspecified**

Bones in respiratory tract, part unspecified

Seeds in respiratory tract, part unspecified

⑦ **T17.920** **Food in respiratory tract, part unspecified causing asphyxiation**

⑦ **T17.928** **Food in respiratory tract, part unspecified causing other injury**

T17.99 **Other foreign object in respiratory tract, part unspecified**

⑦ **T17.990** **Other foreign object in respiratory tract, part unspecified in causing asphyxiation**

⑦ **T17.998** **Other foreign object in respiratory tract, part unspecified causing other injury**

T18 **Foreign body in alimentary tract**

Excludes2: foreign body in pharynx (T17.2-)

The appropriate 7th character is to be added to each code from category T18

A - initial encounter

D - subsequent encounter

S - sequela

⊗⑦**T18.0** **Foreign body in mouth**

T18.1 **Foreign body in esophagus**

Excludes2: foreign body in respiratory tract (T17.-)

T18.10 **Unspecified foreign body in esophagus**

⑦ **T18.100** **Unspecified foreign body in esophagus causing compression of trachea**

Unspecified foreign body in esophagus causing obstruction of respiration

⑦ **T18.108** **Unspecified foreign body in esophagus causing other injury**

T18.11 **Gastric contents in esophagus**

Vomitus in esophagus

⑦ **T18.110** **Gastric contents in esophagus causing compression of trachea**

Gastric contents in esophagus causing obstruction of respiration

⑦ **T18.118** **Gastric contents in esophagus causing other injury**

T18.12 **Food in esophagus**

Bones in esophagus

Seeds in esophagus

⑦ **T18.120** **Food in esophagus causing compression of trachea**

Food in esophagus causing obstruction of respiration

⑦ **T18.128** **Food in esophagus causing other injury**

T18.19 **Other foreign object in esophagus**

⑦ **T18.190** **Other foreign object in esophagus causing compression of trachea**

Other foreign body in esophagus causing obstruction of respiration

⑦ **T18.198** **Other foreign object in esophagus causing other injury**

⊗⑦**T18.2** **Foreign body in stomach**

⊗⑦**T18.3** **Foreign body in small intestine**

⊗⑦**T18.4** **Foreign body in colon**

⊗⑦**T18.5** **Foreign body in anus and rectum**

Foreign body in rectosigmoid (junction)

⊗⑦**T18.8** **Foreign body in other parts of alimentary tract**

⊗⑦**T18.9** **Foreign body of alimentary tract, part unspecified**

Foreign body in digestive system NOS

Swallowed foreign body NOS

T19 **Foreign body in genitourinary tract**

Excludes2: complications due to implanted mesh (T83.7-)

mechanical complications of contraceptive device (intrauterine) (vaginal) (T83.3-)

presence of contraceptive device (intrauterine) (vaginal) (Z97.5)

The appropriate 7th character is to be added to each code from category T19

A - initial encounter

D - subsequent encounter

S - sequela

⊗⑦**T19.0** **Foreign body in urethra**

⊗⑦**T19.1** **Foreign body in bladder**

⊗⑦**T19.2** **Foreign body in vulva and vagina**

⊗⑦**T19.3** **Foreign body in uterus**

⊗⑦**T19.4** **Foreign body in penis**

⊗⑦**T19.8** **Foreign body in other parts of genitourinary tract**

⊗⑦**T19.9** **Foreign body in genitourinary tract, part unspecified**

BURNS AND CORROSIONS (T20-T32)

Includes: burns (thermal) from electrical heating appliances

burns (thermal) from electricity

burns (thermal) from flame

burns (thermal) from friction

burns (thermal) from hot air and hot gases

burns (thermal) from hot objects

burns (thermal) from lightning

burns (thermal) from radiation

chemical burn [corrosion] (external) (internal) scalds

Excludes2: erythema [dermatitis] ab igne (L59.0)

radiation-related disorders of the skin and subcutaneous tissue (L55-L59)

sunburn (L55.-)

BURNS AND CORROSIONS OF EXTERNAL BODY SURFACE, SPECIFIED BY SITE (T20-T25)

Includes: burns and corrosions of first degree [erythema]

burns and corrosions of second degree [blisters][epidermal loss]

burns and corrosions of third degree [deep necrosis of underlying tissue] [full- thickness skin loss]

Use additional code from category T31 or T32 to identify extent of body surface involved

T20 **Burn and corrosion of head, face, and neck**

Excludes2: burn and corrosion of ear drum (T28.41, T28.91)

burn and corrosion of eye and adnexa (T26.-)

burn and corrosion of mouth and pharynx (T28.0)

| | Add 4th-7th digits | Nonspecific code | Unspecified code | Manifestation code |

The appropriate 7th character is to be added to each code from category T20

A - initial encounter

D - subsequent encounter

S - sequela

T20.0   Burn of unspecified degree of head, face, and neck

Use additional external cause code to identify the source, place and intent of the burn (X00-X19, X75-X77, X96-X98, Y92)

⊗⑦**T20.00**   **Burn of unspecified degree of head, face, and neck, unspecified site**

T20.01   **Burn of unspecified degree of ear [any part, except ear drum]**

Excludes2: burn of ear drum (T28.41-)

⑦**T20.011**   **Burn of unspecified degree of right ear [any part, except ear drum]**

⑦**T20.012**   **Burn of unspecified degree of left ear [any part, except ear drum]**

⑦**T20.019**   **Burn of unspecified degree of unspecified ear [any part, except ear drum]**

⊗⑦**T20.02**   **Burn of unspecified degree of lip(s)**

⊗⑦**T20.03**   **Burn of unspecified degree of chin**

⊗⑦**T20.04**   **Burn of unspecified degree of nose (septum)**

⊗⑦**T20.05**   **Burn of unspecified degree of scalp [any part]**

⊗⑦**T20.06**   **Burn of unspecified degree of forehead and cheek**

⊗⑦**T20.07**   **Burn of unspecified degree of neck**

⊗⑦**T20.09**   **Burn of unspecified degree of multiple sites of head, face, and neck**

T20.1   Burn of first degree of head, face, and neck

Use additional external cause code to identify the source, place and intent of the burn (X00-X19, X75-X77, X96-X98, Y92)

⊗⑦**T20.10**   **Burn of first degree of head, face, and neck, unspecified site**

T20.11   **Burn of first degree of ear [any part, except ear drum]**

Excludes2: burn of ear drum (T28.41-)

⑦**T20.111**   **Burn of first degree of right ear [any part, except ear drum]**

⑦**T20.112**   **Burn of first degree of left ear [any part, except ear drum]**

⑦**T20.119**   **Burn of first degree of unspecified ear [any part, except ear drum]**

⊗⑦**T20.12**   **Burn of first degree of lip(s)**

⊗⑦**T20.13**   **Burn of first degree of chin**

⊗⑦**T20.14**   **Burn of first degree of nose (septum)**

⊗⑦**T20.15**   **Burn of first degree of scalp [any part]**

⊗⑦**T20.16**   **Burn of first degree of forehead and cheek**

⊗⑦**T20.17**   **Burn of first degree of neck**

⊗⑦**T20.19**   **Burn of first degree of multiple sites of head, face, and neck**

T20.2   Burn of second degree of head, face, and neck

Use additional external cause code to identify the source, place and intent of the burn (X00-X19, X75-X77, X96-X98, Y92)

⊗⑦**T20.20**   **Burn of second degree of head, face, and neck, unspecified site**

T20.21   **Burn of second degree of ear [any part, except ear drum]**

Excludes2: burn of ear drum (T28.41-)

⑦**T20.211**   **Burn of second degree of right ear [any part, except ear drum]**

⑦**T20.212**   **Burn of second degree of left ear [any part, except ear drum]**

⑦**T20.219**   **Burn of second degree of unspecified ear [any part, except ear drum]**

⊗⑦**T20.22**   **Burn of second degree of lip(s)**

⊗⑦**T20.23**   **Burn of second degree of chin**

⊗⑦**T20.24**   **Burn of second degree of nose (septum)**

⊗⑦**T20.25**   **Burn of second degree of scalp [any part]**

⊗⑦**T20.26**   **Burn of second degree of forehead and cheek**

⊗⑦**T20.27**   **Burn of second degree of neck**

⊗⑦**T20.29**   **Burn of second degree of multiple sites of head, face, and neck**

T20.3   Burn of third degree of head, face, and neck

Use additional external cause code to identify the source, place and intent of the burn (X00-X19, X75-X77, X96-X98, Y92)

⊗⑦**T20.30**   **Burn of third degree of head, face, and neck, unspecified site**

T20.31   **Burn of third degree of ear [any part, except ear drum]**

Excludes2: burn of ear drum (T28.41-)

⑦**T20.311**   **Burn of third degree of right ear [any part, except ear drum]**

⑦**T20.312**   **Burn of third degree of left ear [any part, except ear drum]**

⑦**T20.319**   **Burn of third degree of unspecified ear [any part, except ear drum]**

⊗⑦**T20.32**   **Burn of third degree of lip(s)**

⊗⑦**T20.33**   **Burn of third degree of chin**

⊗⑦**T20.34**   **Burn of third degree of nose (septum)**

⊗⑦**T20.35**   **Burn of third degree of scalp [any part]**

⊗⑦**T20.36**   **Burn of third degree of forehead and cheek**

⊗⑦**T20.37**   **Burn of third degree of neck**

⊗⑦**T20.39**   **Burn of third degree of multiple sites of head, face, and neck**

T20.4   Corrosion of unspecified degree of head, face, and neck

Code first (T51-T65) to identify chemical and intent

Use additional external cause code to identify place (Y92)

⊗⑦**T20.40**   **Corrosion of unspecified degree of head, face, and neck, unspecified site**

T20.41   **Corrosion of unspecified degree of ear [any part, except ear drum]**

Excludes2: corrosion of ear drum (T28.91-)

⑦**T20.411**   **Corrosion of unspecified degree of right ear [any part, except ear drum]**

⑦**T20.412**   **Corrosion of unspecified degree of left ear [any part, except ear drum]**

⑦**T20.419**   **Corrosion of unspecified degree of unspecified ear [any part, except ear drum]**

⊗⑦**T20.42**   **Corrosion of unspecified degree of lip(s)**

⊗⑦**T20.43**   **Corrosion of unspecified degree of chin**

⊗⑦**T20.44**   **Corrosion of unspecified degree of nose (septum)**

⊗⑦**T20.45**   **Corrosion of unspecified degree of scalp [any part]**

⊗⑦**T20.46**   **Corrosion of unspecified degree of forehead and cheek**

⊗⑦**T20.47**   **Corrosion of unspecified degree of neck**

● New code   ▲ Revised code   **Excludes1:** Not coded here   **Excludes2:** Not included here   ⊗ Placeholder required   ⑦7th digit required

⊗7**T20.49** Corrosion of unspecified degree of multiple sites of head, face, and neck

T20.5 Corrosion of first degree of head, face, and neck

Code first (T51-T65) to identify chemical and intent

Use additional external cause code to identify place (Y92)

⊗7**T20.50** Corrosion of first degree of head, face, and neck, unspecified site

T20.51 Corrosion of first degree of ear [any part, except ear drum]

Excludes2: corrosion of ear drum (T28.91-)

7**T20.511** Corrosion of first degree of right ear [any part, except ear drum]

7**T20.512** Corrosion of first degree of left ear [any part, except ear drum]

7**T20.519** Corrosion of first degree of unspecified ear [any part, except ear drum]

⊗7**T20.52** Corrosion of first degree of lip(s)

⊗7**T20.53** Corrosion of first degree of chin

⊗7**T20.54** Corrosion of first degree of nose (septum)

⊗7**T20.55** Corrosion of first degree of scalp [any part]

⊗7**T20.56** Corrosion of first degree of forehead and cheek

⊗7**T20.57** Corrosion of first degree of neck

⊗7**T20.59** Corrosion of first degree of multiple sites of head, face, and neck

T20.6 Corrosion of second degree of head, face, and neck

Code first (T51-T65) to identify chemical and intent

Use additional external cause code to identify place (Y92)

⊗7**T20.60** Corrosion of second degree of head, face, and neck, unspecified site

T20.61 Corrosion of second degree of ear [any part, except ear drum]

Excludes2: corrosion of ear drum (T28.91-)

7**T20.611** Corrosion of second degree of right ear [any part, except ear drum]

7**T20.612** Corrosion of second degree of left ear [any part, except ear drum]

7**T20.619** Corrosion of second degree of unspecified ear [any part, except ear drum]

⊗7**T20.62** Corrosion of second degree of lip(s)

⊗7**T20.63** Corrosion of second degree of chin

⊗7**T20.64** Corrosion of second degree of nose (septum)

⊗7**T20.65** Corrosion of second degree of scalp [any part]

⊗7**T20.66** Corrosion of second degree of forehead and cheek

⊗7**T20.67** Corrosion of second degree of neck

⊗7**T20.69** Corrosion of second degree of multiple sites of head, face, and neck

T20.7 Corrosion of third degree of head, face, and neck

Code first (T51-T65) to identify chemical and intent

Use additional external cause code to identify place (Y92)

⊗7**T20.70** Corrosion of third degree of head, face, and neck, unspecified site

T20.71 Corrosion of third degree of ear [any part, except ear drum]

Excludes2: corrosion of ear drum (T28.91-)

7**T20.711** Corrosion of third degree of right ear [any part, except ear drum]

7**T20.712** Corrosion of third degree of left ear [any part, except ear drum]

7**T20.719** Corrosion of third degree of unspecified ear [any part, except ear drum]

⊗7**T20.72** Corrosion of third degree of lip(s)

⊗7**T20.73** Corrosion of third degree of chin

⊗7**T20.74** Corrosion of third degree of nose (septum)

⊗7**T20.75** Corrosion of third degree of scalp [any part]

⊗7**T20.76** Corrosion of third degree of forehead and cheek

⊗7**T20.77** Corrosion of third degree of neck

⊗7**T20.79** Corrosion of third degree of multiple sites of head, face, and neck

T21 **Burn and corrosion of trunk**

Includes: burns and corrosion of hip region

Excludes2: burns and corrosion of axilla (T22.- with fifth character 4)

burns and corrosion of scapular region (T22.- with fifth character 6)

burns and corrosion of shoulder (T22.- with fifth character 5)

The appropriate 7th character is to be added to each code from category T21

A - initial encounter

D - subsequent encounter

S - sequela

T21.0 Burn of unspecified degree of trunk

Use additional external cause code to identify the source, place and intent of the burn (X00-X19, X75-X77, X96-X98, Y92)

⊗7**T21.00** Burn of unspecified degree of trunk, unspecified site

⊗7**T21.01** Burn of unspecified degree of chest wall

urn of unspecified degree of breast

⊗7**T21.02** Burn of unspecified degree of abdominal wall

Burn of unspecified degree of flank

Burn of unspecified degree of groin

⊗7**T21.03** Burn of unspecified degree of upper back

urn of unspecified degree of interscapular region

⊗7**T21.04** Burn of unspecified degree of lower back

⊗7**T21.05** Burn of unspecified degree of buttock

urn of unspecified degree of anus

⊗7**T21.06** Burn of unspecified degree of male genital region

urn of unspecified degree of penis

urn of unspecified degree of scrotum

urn of unspecified degree of testis

⊗7**T21.07** Burn of unspecified degree of female genital region

urn of unspecified degree of labium (majus) (minus)

urn of unspecified degree of perineum

urn of unspecified degree of vulva

Excludes2: burn of vagina (T28.3)

⊗7**T21.09** Burn of unspecified degree of other site of trunk

T21.1 Burn of first degree of trunk

Use additional external cause code to identify the source, place and intent of the burn (X00-X19, X75-X77, X96-X98, Y92)

⊗7**T21.10** Burn of first degree of trunk, unspecified site

⊗7**T21.11** Burn of first degree of chest wall

Burn of first degree of breast

⊗⑦**T21.12** **Burn of first degree of abdominal wall**

Burn of first degree of flank

Burn of first degree of groin

⊗⑦**T21.13** **Burn of first degree of upper back**

Burn of first degree of interscapular region

⊗⑦**T21.14** **Burn of first degree of lower back**

⊗⑦**T21.15** **Burn of first degree of buttock**

Burn of first degree of anus

⊗⑦**T21.16** **Burn of first degree of male genital region**

Burn of first degree of penis

Burn of first degree of scrotum

Burn of first degree of testis

⊗⑦**T21.17** **Burn of first degree of female genital region**

Burn of first degree of labium (majus) (minus)

Burn of first degree of perineum

Burn of first degree of vulva

Excludes2: burn of vagina (T28.3)

⊗⑦**T21.19** **Burn of first degree of other site of trunk**

T21.2 **Burn of second degree of trunk**

Use additional external cause code to identify the source, place and intent of the burn (X00-X19, X75-X77, X96-X98, Y92)

⊗⑦**T21.20** **Burn of second degree of trunk, unspecified site**

⊗⑦**T21.21** **Burn of second degree of chest wall**

Burn of second degree of breast

⊗⑦**T21.22** **Burn of second degree of abdominal wall**

Burn of second degree of flank

Burn of second degree of groin

T21.23 **Burn of second degree of upper back**

Burn of second degree of interscapular region

⊗⑦**T21.24** **Burn of second degree of lower back**

⊗⑦**T21.25** **Burn of second degree of buttock**

Burn of second degree of anus

⊗⑦**T21.26** **Burn of second degree of male genital region**

Burn of second degree of penis

Burn of second degree of scrotum

Burn of second degree of testis

⊗⑦**T21.27** **Burn of second degree of female genital region**

Burn of second degree of labium (majus) (minus)

Burn of second degree of perineum

Burn of second degree of vulva

Excludes2: burn of vagina (T28.3)

⊗⑦**T21.29** **Burn of second degree of other site of trunk**

T21.3 **Burn of third degree of trunk**

Use additional external cause code to identify the source, place and intent of the burn (X00-X19, X75-X77, X96-X98, Y92)

⊗⑦**T21.30** **Burn of third degree of trunk, unspecified site**

⊗⑦**T21.31** **Burn of third degree of chest wall**

Burn of third degree of breast

⊗⑦**T21.32** **Burn of third degree of abdominal wall**

Burn of third degree of flank

Burn of third degree of groin

⊗⑦**T21.33** **Burn of third degree of upper back**

Burn of third degree of interscapular region

⊗⑦**T21.34** **Burn of third degree of lower back**

⊗⑦**T21.35** **Burn of third degree of buttock**

Burn of third degree of anus

⊗⑦**T21.36** **Burn of third degree of male genital region**

Burn of third degree of penis

Burn of third degree of scrotum

Burn of third degree of testis

⊗⑦**T21.37** **Burn of third degree of female genital region**

Burn of third degree of labium (majus) (minus)

Burn of third degree of perineum

Burn of third degree of vulva

Excludes2: burn of vagina (T28.3)

⊗⑦**T21.39** **Burn of third degree of other site of trunk**

T21.4 **Corrosion of unspecified degree of trunk**

Code first (T51-T65) to identify chemical and intent

Use additional external cause code to identify place (Y92)

⊗⑦**T21.40** **Corrosion of unspecified degree of trunk, unspecified site**

⊗⑦**T21.41** **Corrosion of unspecified degree of chest wall**

Corrosion of unspecified degree of breast

⊗⑦**T21.42** **Corrosion of unspecified degree of abdominal wall**

Corrosion of unspecified degree of flank

Corrosion of unspecified degree of groin

⊗⑦**T21.43** **Corrosion of unspecified degree of upper back**

Corrosion of unspecified degree of interscapular region

⊗⑦**T21.44** **Corrosion of unspecified degree of lower back**

⊗⑦**T21.45** **Corrosion of unspecified degree of buttock**

Corrosion of unspecified degree of anus

⊗⑦**T21.46** **Corrosion of unspecified degree of male genital region**

Corrosion of unspecified degree of penis

Corrosion of unspecified degree of scrotum

Corrosion of unspecified degree of testis

⊗⑦**T21.47** **Corrosion of unspecified degree of female genital region**

Corrosion of unspecified degree of labium (majus) (minus)

Corrosion of unspecified degree of perineum

Corrosion of unspecified degree of vulva

Excludes2: corrosion of vagina (T28.8)

⊗⑦**T21.49** **Corrosion of unspecified degree of other site of trunk**

T21.5 **Corrosion of first degree of trunk**

Code first (T51-T65) to identify chemical and intent

Use additional external cause code to identify place (Y92)

⊗⑦**T21.50** **Corrosion of first degree of trunk, unspecified site**

⊗⑦**T21.51** **Corrosion of first degree of chest wall**

Corrosion of first degree of breast

⊗⑦**T21.52** **Corrosion of first degree of abdominal wall**

Corrosion of first degree of flank

Corrosion of first degree of groin

⊗⑦**T21.53** **Corrosion of first degree of upper back**

Corrosion of first degree of interscapular region

⊗⑦**T21.54** **Corrosion of first degree of lower back**

⊗⑦**T21.55** **Corrosion of first degree of buttock**

Corrosion of first degree of anus

● New code   ▲ Revised code   **Excludes1:** Not coded here   **Excludes2:** Not included here   ⊗ Placeholder required   ⑦ 7th digit required

⊗⑦**T21.56** **Corrosion of first degree of male genital region**

Corrosion of first degree of penis

Corrosion of first degree of scrotum

Corrosion of first degree of testis

⊗⑦**T21.57** **Corrosion of first degree of female genital region**

Corrosion of first degree of labium (majus) (minus)

Corrosion of first degree of perineum

Corrosion of first degree of vulva

Excludes2: corrosion of vagina (T28.8)

⊗⑦**T21.59** **Corrosion of first degree of other site of trunk**

T21.6 **Corrosion of second degree of trunk**

Code first (T51-T65) to identify chemical and intent

Use additional external cause code to identify place (Y92)

⊗⑦**T21.60** **Corrosion of second degree of trunk, unspecified site**

⊗⑦**T21.61** **Corrosion of second degree of chest wall**

Corrosion of second degree of breast

⊗⑦**T21.62** **Corrosion of second degree of abdominal wall**

Corrosion of second degree of flank

Corrosion of second degree of groin

⊗⑦**T21.63** **Corrosion of second degree of upper back**

Corrosion of second degree of interscapular region

⊗⑦**T21.64** **Corrosion of second degree of lower back**

⊗⑦**T21.65** **Corrosion of second degree of buttock**

Corrosion of second degree of anus

⊗⑦**T21.66** **Corrosion of second degree of male genital region**

Corrosion of second degree of penis

Corrosion of second degree of scrotum

Corrosion of second degree of testis

⊗⑦**T21.67** **Corrosion of second degree of female genital region**

Corrosion of second degree of labium (majus) (minus)

Corrosion of second degree of perineum

Corrosion of second degree of vulva

Excludes2: corrosion of vagina (T28.8)

⊗⑦**T21.69** **Corrosion of second degree of other site of trunk**

T21.7 **Corrosion of third degree of trunk**

Code first (T51-T65) to identify chemical and intent

Use additional external cause code to identify place (Y92)

⊗⑦**T21.70** **Corrosion of third degree of trunk, unspecified site**

⊗⑦**T21.71** **Corrosion of third degree of chest wall**

Corrosion of third degree of breast

⊗⑦**T21.72** **Corrosion of third degree of abdominal wall**

Corrosion of third degree of flank

Corrosion of third degree of groin

⊗⑦**T21.73** **Corrosion of third degree of upper back**

Corrosion of third degree of interscapular region

⊗⑦**T21.74** **Corrosion of third degree of lower back**

⊗⑦**T21.75** **Corrosion of third degree of buttock**

Corrosion of third degree of anus

⊗⑦**T21.76** **Corrosion of third degree of male genital region**

Corrosion of third degree of penis

Corrosion of third degree of scrotum

Corrosion of third degree of testis

⊗⑦**T21.77** **Corrosion of third degree of female genital region**

Corrosion of third degree of labium (majus) (minus)

Corrosion of third degree of perineum

Corrosion of third degree of vulva

Excludes2: corrosion of vagina (T28.8)

⊗⑦**T21.79** **Corrosion of third degree of other site of trunk**

T22 **Burn and corrosion of shoulder and upper limb, except wrist and hand**

Excludes2: burn and corrosion of interscapular region (T21.-)

burn and corrosion of wrist and hand (T23.-)

The appropriate 7th character is to be added to each code from category T22

A - initial encounter

D - subsequent encounter

S - sequela

T22.0 **Burn of unspecified degree of shoulder and upper limb, except wrist and hand**

Use additional external cause code to identify the source, place and intent of the burn (X00-X19, X75-X77, X96-X98, Y92)

⊗⑦**T22.00** **Burn of unspecified degree of shoulder and upper limb, except wrist and hand, unspecified site**

T22.01 **Burn of unspecified degree of forearm**

⑦**T22.011** **Burn of unspecified degree of right forearm**

⑦**T22.012** **Burn of unspecified degree of left forearm**

⑦**T22.019** **Burn of unspecified degree of unspecified forearm**

T22.02 **Burn of unspecified degree of elbow**

⑦**T22.021** **Burn of unspecified degree of right elbow**

⑦**T22.022** **Burn of unspecified degree of left elbow**

⑦**T22.029** **Burn of unspecified degree of unspecified elbow**

T22.03 **Burn of unspecified degree of upper arm**

⑦**T22.031** **Burn of unspecified degree of right upper arm**

⑦**T22.032** **Burn of unspecified degree of left upper arm**

⑦**T22.039** **Burn of unspecified degree of unspecified upper arm**

T22.04 **Burn of unspecified degree of axilla**

⑦**T22.041** **Burn of unspecified degree of right axilla**

⑦**T22.042** **Burn of unspecified degree of left axilla**

⑦**T22.049** **Burn of unspecified degree of unspecified axilla**

T22.05 **Burn of unspecified degree of shoulder**

⑦**T22.051** **Burn of unspecified degree of right shoulder**

⑦**T22.052** **Burn of unspecified degree of left shoulder**

⑦**T22.059** **Burn of unspecified degree of unspecified shoulder**

T22.06   **Burn of unspecified degree of scapular region**

⑦T22.061   **Burn of unspecified degree of right scapular region**

⑦T22.062   **Burn of unspecified degree of left scapular region**

⑦T22.069   **Burn of unspecified degree of unspecified scapular region**

T22.09   **Burn of unspecified degree of multiple sites of shoulder and upper limb, except wrist and hand**

⑦T22.091   **Burn of unspecified degree of multiple sites of right shoulder and upper limb, except wrist and hand**

⑦T22.092   **Burn of unspecified degree of multiple sites of left shoulder and upper limb, except wrist and hand**

⑦T22.099   **Burn of unspecified degree of multiple sites of unspecified shoulder and upper limb, except wrist and hand**

T22.1   **Burn of first degree of shoulder and upper limb, except wrist and hand**

Use **additional** external cause code to identify the source, place and intent of the burn (X00-X19, X75-X77, X96-X98, Y92)

⊗⑦T22.10   **Burn of first degree of shoulder and upper limb, except wrist and hand, unspecified site**

T22.11   **Burn of first degree of forearm**

⑦T22.111   **Burn of first degree of right forearm**

⑦T22.112   **Burn of first degree of left forearm**

⑦T22.119   **Burn of first degree of unspecified forearm**

T22.12   **Burn of first degree of elbow**

⑦T22.121   **Burn of first degree of right elbow**

⑦T22.122   **Burn of first degree of left elbow**

⑦T22.129   **Burn of first degree of unspecified elbow**

T22.13   **Burn of first degree of upper arm**

⑦T22.131   **Burn of first degree of right upper arm**

⑦T22.132   **Burn of first degree of left upper arm**

⑦T22.139   **Burn of first degree of unspecified upper arm**

T22.14   **Burn of first degree of axilla**

⑦T22.141   **Burn of first degree of right axilla**

⑦T22.142   **Burn of first degree of left axilla**

⑦T22.149   **Burn of first degree of unspecified axilla**

T22.15   **Burn of first degree of shoulder**

⑦T22.151   **Burn of first degree of right shoulder**

⑦T22.152   **Burn of first degree of left shoulder**

⑦T22.159   **Burn of first degree of unspecified shoulder**

T22.16   **Burn of first degree of scapular region**

⑦T22.161   **Burn of first degree of right scapular region**

⑦T22.162   **Burn of first degree of left scapular region**

⑦T22.169   **Burn of first degree of unspecified scapular region**

T22.19   **Burn of first degree of multiple sites of shoulder and upper limb, except wrist and hand**

⑦T22.191   **Burn of first degree of multiple sites of right shoulder and upper limb, except wrist and hand**

⑦T22.192   **Burn of first degree of multiple sites of left shoulder and upper limb, except wrist and hand**

⑦T22.199   **Burn of first degree of multiple sites of unspecified shoulder and upper limb, except wrist and hand**

T22.2   **Burn of second degree of shoulder and upper limb, except wrist and hand**

Use **additional** external cause code to identify the source, place and intent of the burn (X00-X19, X75-X77, X96-X98, Y92)

⊗⑦T22.20   **Burn of second degree of shoulder and upper limb, except wrist and hand, unspecified site**

T22.21   **Burn of second degree of forearm**

⑦T22.211   **Burn of second degree of right forearm**

⑦T22.212   **Burn of second degree of left forearm**

⑦T22.219   **Burn of second degree of unspecified forearm**

T22.22   **Burn of second degree of elbow**

⑦T22.221   **Burn of second degree of right elbow**

⑦T22.222   **Burn of second degree of left elbow**

⑦T22.229   **Burn of second degree of unspecified elbow**

T22.23   **Burn of second degree of upper arm**

⑦T22.231   **Burn of second degree of right upper arm**

⑦T22.232   **Burn of second degree of left upper arm**

⑦T22.239   **Burn of second degree of unspecified upper arm**

T22.24   **Burn of second degree of axilla**

⑦T22.241   **Burn of second degree of right axilla**

⑦T22.242   **Burn of second degree of left axilla**

⑦T22.249   **Burn of second degree of unspecified axilla**

T22.25   **Burn of second degree of shoulder**

⑦T22.251   **Burn of second degree of right shoulder**

⑦T22.252   **Burn of second degree of left shoulder**

⑦T22.259   **Burn of second degree of unspecified shoulder**

T22.26   **Burn of second degree of scapular region**

⑦T22.261   **Burn of second degree of right scapular region**

⑦T22.262   **Burn of second degree of left scapular region**

⑦T22.269   **Burn of second degree of unspecified scapular region**

T22.29   **Burn of second degree of multiple sites of shoulder and upper limb, except wrist and hand**

⑦T22.291   **Burn of second degree of multiple sites of right shoulder and upper limb, except wrist and hand**

⑦T22.292   **Burn of second degree of multiple sites of left shoulder and upper limb, except wrist and hand**

● New code   ▲ Revised code   **Excludes1:** Not coded here   **Excludes2:** Not included here   ⊗ Placeholder required   ⑦7th digit required

⑦ **T22.299** Burn of second degree of multiple sites of unspecified shoulder and upper limb, except wrist and hand

T22.3 **Burn of third degree of shoulder and upper limb, except wrist and hand**

Use additional external cause code to identify the source, place and intent of the burn (X00-X19, X75-X77, X96-X98, Y92)

⊗⑦ **T22.30** Burn of third degree of shoulder and upper limb, except wrist and hand, unspecified site

T22.31 Burn of third degree of forearm

⑦ **T22.311** Burn of third degree of right forearm

⑦ **T22.312** Burn of third degree of left forearm

⑦ **T22.319** Burn of third degree of unspecified forearm

T22.32 Burn of third degree of elbow

⑦ **T22.321** Burn of third degree of right elbow

⑦ **T22.322** Burn of third degree of left elbow

⑦ **T22.329** Burn of third degree of unspecified elbow

T22.33 Burn of third degree of upper arm

⑦ **T22.331** Burn of third degree of right upper arm

⑦ **T22.332** Burn of third degree of left upper arm

⑦ **T22.339** Burn of third degree of unspecified upper arm

T22.34 Burn of third degree of axilla

⑦ **T22.341** Burn of third degree of right axilla

⑦ **T22.342** Burn of third degree of left axilla

⑦ **T22.349** Burn of third degree of unspecified axilla

T22.35 Burn of third degree of shoulder

⑦ **T22.351** Burn of third degree of right shoulder

⑦ **T22.352** Burn of third degree of left shoulder

⑦ **T22.359** Burn of third degree of unspecified shoulder

T22.36 Burn of third degree of scapular region

⑦ **T22.361** Burn of third degree of right scapular region

⑦ **T22.362** Burn of third degree of left scapular region

⑦ **T22.369** Burn of third degree of unspecified scapular region

T22.39 Burn of third degree of multiple sites of shoulder and upper limb, except wrist and hand

⑦ **T22.391** Burn of third degree of multiple sites of right shoulder and upper limb, except wrist and hand

⑦ **T22.392** Burn of third degree of multiple sites of left shoulder and upper limb, except wrist and hand

⑦ **T22.399** Burn of third degree of multiple sites of unspecified shoulder and upper limb, except wrist and hand

T22.4 **Corrosion of unspecified degree of shoulder and upper limb, except wrist and hand**

Code first (T51-T65) to identify chemical and intent

Use additional external cause code to identify place (Y92)

⊗⑦ **T22.40** Corrosion of unspecified degree of shoulder and upper limb, except wrist and hand, unspecified site

T22.41 Corrosion of unspecified degree of forearm

⑦ **T22.411** Corrosion of unspecified degree of right forearm

⑦ **T22.412** Corrosion of unspecified degree of left forearm

⑦ **T22.419** Corrosion of unspecified degree of unspecified forearm

T22.42 Corrosion of unspecified degree of elbow

⑦ **T22.421** Corrosion of unspecified degree of right elbow

⑦ **T22.422** Corrosion of unspecified degree of left elbow

⑦ **T22.429** Corrosion of unspecified degree of unspecified elbow

T22.43 Corrosion of unspecified degree of upper arm

⑦ **T22.431** Corrosion of unspecified degree of right upper arm

⑦ **T22.432** Corrosion of unspecified degree of left upper arm

⑦ **T22.439** Corrosion of unspecified degree of unspecified upper arm

T22.44 Corrosion of unspecified degree of axilla

⑦ **T22.441** Corrosion of unspecified degree of right axilla

⑦ **T22.442** Corrosion of unspecified degree of left axilla

⑦ **T22.449** Corrosion of unspecified degree of unspecified axilla

T22.45 Corrosion of unspecified degree of shoulder

⑦ **T22.451** Corrosion of unspecified degree of right shoulder

⑦ **T22.452** Corrosion of unspecified degree of left shoulder

⑦ **T22.459** Corrosion of unspecified degree of unspecified shoulder

T22.46 Corrosion of unspecified degree of scapular region

⑦ **T22.461** Corrosion of unspecified degree of right scapular region

⑦ **T22.462** Corrosion of unspecified degree of left scapular region

⑦ **T22.469** Corrosion of unspecified degree of unspecified scapular region

T22.49 Corrosion of unspecified degree of multiple sites of shoulder and upper limb, except wrist and hand

⑦ **T22.491** Corrosion of unspecified degree of multiple sites of right shoulder and upper limb, except wrist and hand

⑦ **T22.492** Corrosion of unspecified degree of multiple sites of left shoulder and upper limb, except wrist and hand

⑦ **T22.499** Corrosion of unspecified degree of multiple sites of unspecified shoulder and upper limb, except wrist and hand

T22.5 **Corrosion of first degree of shoulder and upper limb, except wrist and hand**

Code first (T51-T65) to identify chemical and intent

Use additional external cause code to identify place (Y92)

Add 4th-7th digits   Nonspecific code   Unspecified code   Manifestation code

⊗⑦**T22.50** Corrosion of first degree of shoulder and upper limb, except wrist and hand unspecified site

T22.51 Corrosion of first degree of forearm

⑦**T22.511** Corrosion of first degree of right forearm

⑦**T22.512** Corrosion of first degree of left forearm

⑦**T22.519** Corrosion of first degree of unspecified forearm

T22.52 Corrosion of first degree of elbow

⑦**T22.521** Corrosion of first degree of right elbow

⑦**T22.522** Corrosion of first degree of left elbow

⑦**T22.529** Corrosion of first degree of unspecified elbow

T22.53 Corrosion of first degree of upper arm

⑦**T22.531** Corrosion of first degree of right upper arm

⑦**T22.532** Corrosion of first degree of left upper arm

⑦**T22.539** Corrosion of first degree of unspecified upper arm

T22.54 Corrosion of first degree of axilla

⑦**T22.541** Corrosion of first degree of right axilla

⑦**T22.542** Corrosion of first degree of left axilla

⑦**T22.549** Corrosion of first degree of unspecified axilla

T22.55 Corrosion of first degree of shoulder

⑦**T22.551** Corrosion of first degree of right shoulder

⑦**T22.552** Corrosion of first degree of left shoulder

⑦**T22.559** Corrosion of first degree of unspecified shoulder

T22.56 Corrosion of first degree of scapular region

⑦**T22.561** Corrosion of first degree of right scapular region

⑦**T22.562** Corrosion of first degree of left scapular region

⑦**T22.569** Corrosion of first degree of unspecified scapular region

T22.59 Corrosion of first degree of multiple sites of shoulder and upper limb, except wrist and hand

⑦**T22.591** Corrosion of first degree of multiple sites of right shoulder and upper limb, except wrist and hand

⑦**T22.592** Corrosion of first degree of multiple sites of left shoulder and upper limb, except wrist and hand

⑦**T22.599** Corrosion of first degree of multiple sites of unspecified shoulder and upper limb, except wrist and hand

T22.6 Corrosion of second degree of shoulder and upper limb, except wrist and hand

Code first (T51-T65) to identify chemical and intent

Use additional external cause code to identify place (Y92)

⊗⑦**T22.60** Corrosion of second degree of shoulder and upper limb, except wrist and hand, unspecified site

T22.61 Corrosion of second degree of forearm

⑦**T22.611** Corrosion of second degree of right forearm

⑦**T22.612** Corrosion of second degree of left forearm

⑦**T22.619** Corrosion of second degree of unspecified forearm

T22.62 Corrosion of second degree of elbow

⑦**T22.621** Corrosion of second degree of right elbow

⑦**T22.622** Corrosion of second degree of left elbow

⑦**T22.629** Corrosion of second degree of unspecified elbow

T22.63 Corrosion of second degree of upper arm

⑦**T22.631** Corrosion of second degree of right upper arm

⑦**T22.632** Corrosion of second degree of left upper arm

⑦**T22.639** Corrosion of second degree of unspecified upper arm

T22.64 Corrosion of second degree of axilla

⑦**T22.641** Corrosion of second degree of right axilla

⑦**T22.642** Corrosion of second degree of left axilla

⑦**T22.649** Corrosion of second degree of unspecified axilla

T22.65 Corrosion of second degree of shoulder

⑦**T22.651** Corrosion of second degree of right shoulder

⑦**T22.652** Corrosion of second degree of left shoulder

⑦**T22.659** Corrosion of second degree of unspecified shoulder

T22.66 Corrosion of second degree of scapular region

⑦**T22.661** Corrosion of second degree of right scapular region

⑦**T22.662** Corrosion of second degree of left scapular region

⑦**T22.669** Corrosion of second degree of unspecified scapular region

T22.69 Corrosion of second degree of multiple sites of shoulder and upper limb, except wrist and hand

⑦**T22.691** Corrosion of second degree of multiple sites of right shoulder and upper limb, except wrist and hand

⑦**T22.692** Corrosion of second degree of multiple sites of left shoulder and upper limb, except wrist and hand

⑦**T22.699** Corrosion of second degree of multiple sites of unspecified shoulder and upper limb, except wrist and hand

T22.7 Corrosion of third degree of shoulder and upper limb, except wrist and hand

Code first (T51-T65) to identify chemical and intent

Use additional external cause code to identify place (Y92)

⊗⑦**T22.70** Corrosion of third degree of shoulder and upper limb, except wrist and hand, unspecified site

T22.71 Corrosion of third degree of forearm

⑦**T22.711** Corrosion of third degree of right forearm

● New code ▲ Revised code **Excludes1:** Not coded here **Excludes2:** Not included here ⊗ Placeholder required ⑦ 7th digit required

⑦T22.712   Corrosion of third degree of left forearm

⑦T22.719   Corrosion of third degree of unspecified forearm

T22.72   Corrosion of third degree of elbow

⑦T22.721   Corrosion of third degree of right elbow

⑦T22.722   Corrosion of third degree of left elbow

⑦T22.729   Corrosion of third degree of unspecified elbow

T22.73   Corrosion of third degree of upper arm

⑦T22.731   Corrosion of third degree of right upper arm

⑦T22.732   Corrosion of third degree of left upper arm

⑦T22.739   Corrosion of third degree of unspecified upper arm

T22.74   Corrosion of third degree of axilla

⑦T22.741   Corrosion of third degree of right axilla

⑦T22.742   Corrosion of third degree of left axilla

⑦T22.749   Corrosion of third degree of unspecified axilla

T22.75   Corrosion of third degree of shoulder

⑦T22.751   Corrosion of third degree of right shoulder

⑦T22.752   Corrosion of third degree of left shoulder

⑦T22.759   Corrosion of third degree of unspecified shoulder

T22.76   Corrosion of third degree of scapular region

⑦T22.761   Corrosion of third degree of right scapular region

⑦T22.762   Corrosion of third degree of left scapular region

⑦T22.769   Corrosion of third degree of unspecified scapular region

T22.79   Corrosion of third degree of multiple sites of shoulder and upper limb, except wrist and hand

⑦T22.791   Corrosion of third degree of multiple sites of right shoulder and upper limb, except wrist and hand

⑦T22.792   Corrosion of third degree of multiple sites of left shoulder and upper limb, except wrist and hand

⑦T22.799   Corrosion of third degree of multiple sites of unspecified shoulder and upper limb, except wrist and hand

T23   Burn and corrosion of wrist and hand

The appropriate 7th character is to be added to each code from category T23

A - initial encounter

D - subsequent encounter

S - sequela

T23.0   Burn of unspecified degree of wrist and hand

Use additional external cause code to identify the source, place and intent of the burn (X00-X19, X75-X77, X96-X98, Y92)

T23.00   Burn of unspecified degree of hand, unspecified site

⑦T23.001   Burn of unspecified degree of right hand, unspecified site

⑦T23.002   Burn of unspecified degree of left hand, unspecified site

⑦T23.009   Burn of unspecified degree of unspecified hand, unspecified site

T23.01   Burn of unspecified degree of thumb (nail)

⑦T23.011   Burn of unspecified degree of right thumb (nail)

⑦T23.012   Burn of unspecified degree of left thumb (nail)

⑦T23.019   Burn of unspecified degree of unspecified thumb (nail)

T23.02   Burn of unspecified degree of single finger (nail) except thumb

⑦T23.021   Burn of unspecified degree of single right finger (nail) except thumb

⑦T23.022   Burn of unspecified degree of single left finger (nail) except thumb

⑦T23.029   Burn of unspecified degree of unspecified single finger (nail) except thumb

T23.03   Burn of unspecified degree of multiple fingers (nail), not including thumb

⑦T23.031   Burn of unspecified degree of multiple right fingers (nail), not including thumb

⑦T23.032   Burn of unspecified degree of multiple left fingers (nail), not including thumb

⑦T23.039   Burn of unspecified degree of unspecified multiple fingers (nail), not including thumb

T23.04   Burn of unspecified degree of multiple fingers (nail), including thumb

⑦T23.041   Burn of unspecified degree of multiple right fingers (nail), including thumb

⑦T23.042   Burn of unspecified degree of multiple left fingers (nail), including thumb

⑦T23.049   Burn of unspecified degree of unspecified multiple fingers (nail), including thumb

T23.05   Burn of unspecified degree of palm

⑦T23.051   Burn of unspecified degree of right palm

⑦T23.052   Burn of unspecified degree of left palm

⑦T23.059   Burn of unspecified degree of unspecified palm

T23.06   Burn of unspecified degree of back of hand

⑦T23.061   Burn of unspecified degree of back of right hand

⑦T23.062   Burn of unspecified degree of back of left hand

⑦T23.069   Burn of unspecified degree of back of unspecified hand

T23.07   Burn of unspecified degree of wrist

⑦T23.071   Burn of unspecified degree of right wrist

⑦T23.072   Burn of unspecified degree of left wrist

⑦T23.079   Burn of unspecified degree of unspecified wrist

▓ Add 4th-7th digits	Nonspecific code	Unspecified code	Manifestation code	

T23.09 **Burn of unspecified degree of multiple sites of wrist and hand**

⑦T23.091 **Burn of unspecified degree of multiple sites of right wrist and hand**

⑦T23.092 **Burn of unspecified degree of multiple sites of left wrist and hand**

⑦T23.099 **Burn of unspecified degree of multiple sites of unspecified wrist and hand**

T23.1 **Burn of first degree of wrist and hand**

Use additional external cause code to identify the source, place and intent of the burn (X00-X19, X75-X77, X96-X98, Y92)

T23.10 **Burn of first degree of hand, unspecified site**

⑦T23.101 **Burn of first degree of right hand, unspecified site**

⑦T23.102 **Burn of first degree of left hand, unspecified site**

⑦T23.109 **Burn of first degree of unspecified hand, unspecified site**

T23.11 **Burn of first degree of thumb (nail)**

⑦T23.111 **Burn of first degree of right thumb (nail)**

⑦T23.112 **Burn of first degree of left thumb (nail)**

⑦T23.119 **Burn of first degree of unspecified thumb (nail)**

T23.12 **Burn of first degree of single finger (nail) except thumb**

⑦T23.121 **Burn of first degree of single right finger (nail) except thumb**

⑦T23.122 **Burn of first degree of single left finger (nail) except thumb**

⑦T23.129 **Burn of first degree of unspecified single finger (nail) except thumb**

T23.13 **Burn of first degree of multiple fingers (nail), not including thumb**

⑦T23.131 **Burn of first degree of multiple right fingers (nail), not including thumb**

⑦T23.132 **Burn of first degree of multiple left fingers (nail), not including thumb**

⑦T23.139 **Burn of first degree of unspecified multiple fingers (nail), not including thumb**

T23.14 **Burn of first degree of multiple fingers (nail), including thumb**

⑦T23.141 **Burn of first degree of multiple right fingers (nail), including thumb**

⑦T23.142 **Burn of first degree of multiple left fingers (nail), including thumb**

⑦T23.149 **Burn of first degree of unspecified multiple fingers (nail), including thumb**

T23.15 **Burn of first degree of palm**

⑦T23.151 **Burn of first degree of right palm**

⑦T23.152 **Burn of first degree of left palm**

⑦T23.159 **Burn of first degree of unspecified palm**

T23.16 **Burn of first degree of back of hand**

⑦T23.161 **Burn of first degree of back of right hand**

⑦T23.162 **Burn of first degree of back of left hand**

⑦T23.169 **Burn of first degree of back of unspecified hand**

⑦T23.17 **Burn of first degree of wrist**

⑦T23.171 **Burn of first degree of right wrist**

⑦T23.172 **Burn of first degree of left wrist**

T23.179 **Burn of first degree of unspecified wrist**

⑦T23.19 **Burn of first degree of multiple sites of wrist and hand**

⑦T23.191 **Burn of first degree of multiple sites of right wrist and hand**

⑦T23.192 **Burn of first degree of multiple sites of left wrist and hand**

⑦T23.199 **Burn of first degree of multiple sites of unspecified wrist and hand**

T23.2 **Burn of second degree of wrist and hand**

Use additional external cause code to identify the source, place and intent of the burn (X00-X19, X75-X77, X96-X98, Y92)

T23.20 **Burn of second degree of hand, unspecified site**

⑦T23.201 **Burn of second degree of right hand, unspecified site**

⑦T23.202 **Burn of second degree of left hand, unspecified site**

⑦T23.209 **Burn of second degree of unspecified hand, unspecified site**

T23.21 **Burn of second degree of thumb (nail)**

⑦T23.211 **Burn of second degree of right thumb (nail)**

⑦T23.212 **Burn of second degree of left thumb (nail)**

⑦T23.219 **Burn of second degree of unspecified thumb (nail)**

T23.22 **Burn of second degree of single finger (nail) except thumb**

⑦T23.221 **Burn of second degree of single right finger (nail) except thumb**

⑦T23.222 **Burn of second degree of single left finger (nail) except thumb**

⑦T23.229 **Burn of second degree of unspecified single finger (nail) except thumb**

T23.23 **Burn of second degree of multiple fingers (nail), not including thumb**

⑦T23.231 **Burn of second degree of multiple right fingers (nail), not including thumb**

⑦T23.232 **Burn of second degree of multiple left fingers (nail), not including thumb**

⑦T23.239 **Burn of second degree of unspecified multiple fingers (nail), not including thumb**

T23.24 **Burn of second degree of multiple fingers (nail), including thumb**

⑦T23.241 **Burn of second degree of multiple right fingers (nail), including thumb**

⑦T23.242 **Burn of second degree of multiple left fingers (nail), including thumb**

⑦T23.249 **Burn of second degree of unspecified multiple fingers (nail), including thumb**

T23.25 **Burn of second degree of palm**

⑦T23.251 **Burn of second degree of right palm**

⑦T23.252 **Burn of second degree of left palm**

● New code ▲ Revised code **Excludes1:** Not coded here **Excludes2:** Not included here ⊗ Placeholder required ⑦7ᵗʰ digit required

⑦**T23.259** Burn of second degree of unspecified palm

T23.26 Burn of second degree of back of hand

⑦**T23.261** Burn of second degree of back of right hand

⑦**T23.262** Burn of second degree of back of left hand

⑦**T23.269** Burn of second degree of back of unspecified hand

T23.27 Burn of second degree of wrist

⑦**T23.271** Burn of second degree of right wrist

⑦**T23.272** Burn of second degree of left wrist

⑦**T23.279** Burn of second degree of unspecified wrist

T23.29 Burn of second degree of multiple sites of wrist and hand

⑦**T23.291** Burn of second degree of multiple sites of right wrist and hand

⑦**T23.292** Burn of second degree of multiple sites of left wrist and hand

⑦**T23.299** Burn of second degree of multiple sites of unspecified wrist and hand

T23.3 **Burn of third degree of wrist and hand**

Use additional external cause code to identify the source, place and intent of the burn (X00-X19, X75-X77, X96-X98, Y92)

T23.30 Burn of third degree of hand, unspecified site

⑦**T23.301** Burn of third degree of right hand, unspecified site

⑦**T23.302** Burn of third degree of left hand, unspecified site

⑦**T23.309** Burn of third degree of unspecified hand, unspecified site

T23.31 Burn of third degree of thumb (nail)

⑦**T23.311** Burn of third degree of right thumb (nail)

⑦**T23.312** Burn of third degree of left thumb (nail)

⑦**T23.319** Burn of third degree of unspecified thumb (nail)

T23.32 Burn of third degree of single finger (nail) except thumb

⑦**T23.321** Burn of third degree of single right finger (nail) except thumb

⑦**T23.322** Burn of third degree of single left finger (nail) except thumb

⑦**T23.329** Burn of third degree of unspecified single finger (nail) except thumb

T23.33 Burn of third degree of multiple fingers (nail), not including thumb

⑦**T23.331** Burn of third degree of multiple right fingers (nail), not including thumb

⑦**T23.332** Burn of third degree of multiple left fingers (nail), not including thumb

⑦**T23.339** Burn of third degree of unspecified multiple fingers (nail), not including thumb

T23.34 Burn of third degree of multiple fingers (nail), including thumb

⑦**T23.341** Burn of third degree of multiple right fingers (nail), including thumb

⑦**T23.342** Burn of third degree of multiple left fingers (nail), including thumb

⑦**T23.349** Burn of third degree of unspecified multiple fingers (nail), including thumb

T23.35 Burn of third degree of palm

⑦**T23.351** Burn of third degree of right palm

⑦**T23.352** Burn of third degree of left palm

⑦**T23.359** Burn of third degree of unspecified palm

T23.36 Burn of third degree of back of hand

⑦**T23.361** Burn of third degree of back of right hand

⑦**T23.362** Burn of third degree of back of left hand

⑦**T23.369** Burn of third degree of back of unspecified hand

T23.37 Burn of third degree of wrist

⑦**T23.371** Burn of third degree of right wrist

⑦**T23.372** Burn of third degree of left wrist

⑦**T23.379** Burn of third degree of unspecified wrist

T23.39 Burn of third degree of multiple sites of wrist and hand

⑦**T23.391** Burn of third degree of multiple sites of right wrist and hand

⑦**T23.392** Burn of third degree of multiple sites of left wrist and hand

⑦**T23.399** Burn of third degree of multiple sites of unspecified wrist and hand

T23.4 **Corrosion of unspecified degree of wrist and hand**

Code first (T51-T65) to identify chemical and intent

Use additional external cause code to identify place (Y92)

T23.40 Corrosion of unspecified degree of hand, unspecified site

⑦**T23.401** Corrosion of unspecified degree of right hand, unspecified site

⑦**T23.402** Corrosion of unspecified degree of left hand, unspecified site

⑦**T23.409** Corrosion of unspecified degree of unspecified hand, unspecified site

T23.41 Corrosion of unspecified degree of thumb (nail)

⑦**T23.411** Corrosion of unspecified degree of right thumb (nail)

⑦**T23.412** Corrosion of unspecified degree of left thumb (nail)

⑦**T23.419** Corrosion of unspecified degree of unspecified thumb (nail)

T23.42 Corrosion of unspecified degree of single finger (nail) except thumb

⑦**T23.421** Corrosion of unspecified degree of single right finger (nail) except thumb

⑦**T23.422** Corrosion of unspecified degree of single left finger (nail) except thumb

⑦**T23.429** Corrosion of unspecified degree of unspecified single finger (nail) except thumb

T23.43 Corrosion of unspecified degree of multiple fingers (nail), not including thumb

⑦**T23.431** Corrosion of unspecified degree of multiple right fingers (nail), not including thumb

⑦**T23.432** Corrosion of unspecified degree of multiple left fingers (nail), not including thumb

⑦T23.439 Corrosion of unspecified degree of unspecified multiple fingers (nail), not including thumb

T23.44 Corrosion of unspecified degree of multiple fingers (nail), including thumb

⑦T23.441 Corrosion of unspecified degree of multiple right fingers (nail), including thumb

⑦T23.442 Corrosion of unspecified degree of multiple left fingers (nail), including thumb

⑦T23.449 Corrosion of unspecified degree of unspecified multiple fingers (nail), including thumb

T23.45 Corrosion of unspecified degree of palm

⑦T23.451 Corrosion of unspecified degree of right palm

⑦T23.452 Corrosion of unspecified degree of left palm

⑦T23.459 Corrosion of unspecified degree of unspecified palm

T23.46 Corrosion of unspecified degree of back of hand

⑦T23.461 Corrosion of unspecified degree of back of right hand

⑦T23.462 Corrosion of unspecified degree of back of left hand

⑦T23.469 Corrosion of unspecified degree of back of unspecified hand

T23.47 Corrosion of unspecified degree of wrist

⑦T23.471 Corrosion of unspecified degree of right wrist

⑦T23.472 Corrosion of unspecified degree of left wrist

⑦T23.479 Corrosion of unspecified degree of unspecified wrist

T23.49 Corrosion of unspecified degree of multiple sites of wrist and hand

⑦T23.491 Corrosion of unspecified degree of multiple sites of right wrist and hand

⑦T23.492 Corrosion of unspecified degree of multiple sites of left wrist and hand

⑦T23.499 Corrosion of unspecified degree of multiple sites of unspecified wrist and hand

T23.5 **Corrosion of first degree of wrist and hand**

Code first (T51-T65) to identify chemical and intent

Use additional external cause code to identify place (Y92)

T23.50 Corrosion of first degree of hand, unspecified site

⑦T23.501 Corrosion of first degree of right hand, unspecified site

⑦T23.502 Corrosion of first degree of left hand, unspecified site

⑦T23.509 Corrosion of first degree of unspecified hand, unspecified site

T23.51 Corrosion of first degree of thumb (nail)

⑦T23.511 Corrosion of first degree of right thumb (nail)

⑦T23.512 Corrosion of first degree of left thumb (nail)

⑦T23.519 Corrosion of first degree of unspecified thumb (nail)

T23.52 Corrosion of first degree of single finger (nail) except thumb

⑦T23.521 Corrosion of first degree of single right finger (nail) except thumb

⑦T23.522 Corrosion of first degree of single left finger (nail) except thumb

⑦T23.529 Corrosion of first degree of unspecified single finger (nail) except thumb

T23.53 Corrosion of first degree of multiple fingers (nail), not including thumb

⑦T23.531 Corrosion of first degree of multiple right fingers (nail), not including thumb

⑦T23.532 Corrosion of first degree of multiple left fingers (nail), not including thumb

⑦T23.539 Corrosion of first degree of unspecified multiple fingers (nail), not including thumb

T23.54 Corrosion of first degree of multiple fingers (nail), including thumb

⑦T23.541 Corrosion of first degree of multiple right fingers (nail), including thumb

⑦T23.542 Corrosion of first degree of multiple left fingers (nail), including thumb

⑦T23.549 Corrosion of first degree of unspecified multiple fingers (nail), including thumb

T23.55 Corrosion of first degree of palm

⑦T23.551 Corrosion of first degree of right palm

⑦T23.552 Corrosion of first degree of left palm

⑦T23.559 Corrosion of first degree of unspecified palm

T23.56 Corrosion of first degree of back of hand

⑦T23.561 Corrosion of first degree of back of right hand

⑦T23.562 Corrosion of first degree of back of left hand

⑦T23.569 Corrosion of first degree of back of unspecified hand

T23.57 Corrosion of first degree of wrist

⑦T23.571 Corrosion of first degree of right wrist

⑦T23.572 Corrosion of first degree of left wrist

⑦T23.579 Corrosion of first degree of unspecified wrist

T23.59 Corrosion of first degree of multiple sites of wrist and hand

⑦T23.591 Corrosion of first degree of multiple sites of right wrist and hand

⑦T23.592 Corrosion of first degree of multiple sites of left wrist and hand

⑦T23.599 Corrosion of first degree of multiple sites of unspecified wrist and hand

T23.6 **Corrosion of second degree of wrist and hand**

Code first (T51-T65) to identify chemical and intent

Use additional external cause code to identify place (Y92)

T23.60 Corrosion of second degree of hand, unspecified site

⑦T23.601 Corrosion of second degree of right hand, unspecified site

⑦T23.602 Corrosion of second degree of left hand, unspecified site

● New code   ▲ Revised code   **Excludes1:** Not coded here   **Excludes2:** Not included here   ⊗ Placeholder required   ⑦7ᵗʰ digit required

⑦T23.609 Corrosion of second degree of unspecified hand, unspecified site

T23.61 Corrosion of second degree of thumb (nail)

⑦T23.611 Corrosion of second degree of right thumb (nail)

⑦T23.612 Corrosion of second degree of left thumb (nail)

⑦T23.619 Corrosion of second degree of unspecified thumb (nail)

T23.62 Corrosion of second degree of single finger (nail) except thumb

⑦T23.621 Corrosion of second degree of single right finger (nail) except thumb

⑦T23.622 Corrosion of second degree of single left finger (nail) except thumb

⑦T23.629 Corrosion of second degree of unspecified single finger (nail) except thumb

T23.63 Corrosion of second degree of multiple fingers (nail), not including thumb

⑦T23.631 Corrosion of second degree of multiple right fingers (nail), not including thumb

⑦T23.632 Corrosion of second degree of multiple left fingers (nail), not including thumb

⑦T23.639 Corrosion of second degree of unspecified multiple fingers (nail), not including thumb

T23.64 Corrosion of second degree of multiple fingers (nail), including thumb

⑦T23.641 Corrosion of second degree of multiple right fingers (nail), including thumb

⑦T23.642 Corrosion of second degree of multiple left fingers (nail), including thumb

⑦T23.649 Corrosion of second degree of unspecified multiple fingers (nail), including thumb

T23.65 Corrosion of second degree of palm

⑦T23.651 Corrosion of second degree of right palm

⑦T23.652 Corrosion of second degree of left palm

⑦T23.659 Corrosion of second degree of unspecified palm

T23.66 Corrosion of second degree of back of hand

⑦T23.661 Corrosion of second degree back of right hand

⑦T23.662 Corrosion of second degree back of left hand

⑦T23.669 Corrosion of second degree back of unspecified hand

T23.67 Corrosion of second degree of wrist

⑦T23.671 Corrosion of second degree of right wrist

⑦T23.672 Corrosion of second degree of left wrist

⑦T23.679 Corrosion of second degree of unspecified wrist

T23.69 Corrosion of second degree of multiple sites of wrist and hand

⑦T23.691 Corrosion of second degree of multiple sites of right wrist and hand

⑦T23.692 Corrosion of second degree of multiple sites of left wrist and hand

⑦T23.699 Corrosion of second degree of multiple sites of unspecified wrist and hand

T23.7 Corrosion of third degree of wrist and hand

Code first (T51-T65) to identify chemical and intent

Use additional external cause code to identify place (Y92)

T23.70 Corrosion of third degree of hand, unspecified site

⑦T23.701 Corrosion of third degree of right hand, unspecified site

⑦T23.702 Corrosion of third degree of left hand, unspecified site

⑦T23.709 Corrosion of third degree of unspecified hand, unspecified site

T23.71 Corrosion of third degree of thumb (nail)

⑦T23.711 Corrosion of third degree of right thumb (nail)

⑦T23.712 Corrosion of third degree of left thumb (nail)

⑦T23.719 Corrosion of third degree of unspecified thumb (nail)

T23.72 Corrosion of third degree of single finger (nail) except thumb

⑦T23.721 Corrosion of third degree of single right finger (nail) except thumb

⑦T23.722 Corrosion of third degree of single left finger (nail) except thumb

⑦T23.729 Corrosion of third degree of unspecified single finger (nail) except thumb

T23.73 Corrosion of third degree of multiple fingers (nail), not including thumb

⑦T23.731 Corrosion of third degree of multiple right fingers (nail), not including thumb

⑦T23.732 Corrosion of third degree of multiple left fingers (nail), not including thumb

⑦T23.739 Corrosion of third degree of unspecified multiple fingers (nail), not including thumb

T23.74 Corrosion of third degree of multiple fingers (nail), including thumb

⑦T23.741 Corrosion of third degree of multiple right fingers (nail), including thumb

⑦T23.742 Corrosion of third degree of multiple left fingers (nail), including thumb

⑦T23.749 Corrosion of third degree of unspecified multiple fingers (nail), including thumb

T23.75 Corrosion of third degree of palm

⑦T23.751 Corrosion of third degree of right palm

⑦T23.752 Corrosion of third degree of left palm

⑦T23.759 Corrosion of third degree of unspecified palm

T23.76 Corrosion of third degree of back of hand

⑦T23.761 Corrosion of third degree of back of right hand

⑦T23.762 Corrosion of third degree of back of left hand

⑦ **T23.769** Corrosion of third degree back of unspecified hand

T23.77 Corrosion of third degree of wrist

⑦ **T23.771** Corrosion of third degree of right wrist

⑦ **T23.772** Corrosion of third degree of left wrist

⑦ **T23.779** Corrosion of third degree of unspecified wrist

T23.79 Corrosion of third degree of multiple sites of wrist and hand

⑦ **T23.791** Corrosion of third degree of multiple sites of right wrist and hand

⑦ **T23.792** Corrosion of third degree of multiple sites of left wrist and hand

⑦ **T23.799** Corrosion of third degree of multiple sites of unspecified wrist and hand

T24 **Burn and corrosion of lower limb, except ankle and foot**

Excludes2: burn and corrosion of ankle and foot (T25.-)

burn and corrosion of hip region (T21.-)

The appropriate 7th character is to be added to each code from category T24

A - initial encounter

D - subsequent encounter

S - sequela

T24.0 **Burn of unspecified degree of lower limb, except ankle and foot**

Use additional external cause code to identify the source, place and intent of the burn (X00-X19, X75-X77, X96-X98, Y92)

T24.00 Burn of unspecified degree of unspecified site of lower limb, except ankle and foot

⑦ **T24.001** Burn of unspecified degree of unspecified site of right lower limb, except ankle and foot

⑦ **T24.002** Burn of unspecified degree of unspecified site of left lower limb, except ankle and foot

⑦ **T24.009** Burn of unspecified degree of unspecified site of unspecified lower limb, except ankle and foot

T24.01 Burn of unspecified degree of thigh

⑦ **T24.011** Burn of unspecified degree of right thigh

⑦ **T24.012** Burn of unspecified degree of left thigh

⑦ **T24.019** Burn of unspecified degree of unspecified thigh

T24.02 Burn of unspecified degree of knee

⑦ **T24.021** Burn of unspecified degree of right knee

⑦ **T24.022** Burn of unspecified degree of left knee

⑦ **T24.029** Burn of unspecified degree of unspecified knee

T24.03 Burn of unspecified degree of lower leg

⑦ **T24.031** Burn of unspecified degree of right lower leg

⑦ **T24.032** Burn of unspecified degree of left lower leg

⑦ **T24.039** Burn of unspecified degree of unspecified lower leg

T24.09 **Burn of unspecified degree of multiple sites of lower limb, except ankle and foot**

⑦ **T24.091** Burn of unspecified degree of multiple sites of right lower limb, except ankle and foot

⑦ **T24.092** Burn of unspecified degree of multiple sites of left lower limb, except ankle and foot

⑦ **T24.099** Burn of unspecified degree of multiple sites of unspecified lower limb, except ankle and foot

T24.1 **Burn of first degree of lower limb, except ankle and foot**

Use additional external cause code to identify the source, place and intent of the burn (X00-X19, X75-X77, X96-X98, Y92)

T24.10 **Burn of first degree of unspecified site of lower limb, except ankle and foot**

⑦ **T24.101** Burn of first degree of unspecified site of right lower limb, except ankle and foot

⑦ **T24.102** Burn of first degree of unspecified site of left lower limb, except ankle and foot

⑦ **T24.109** Burn of first degree of unspecified site of unspecified lower limb, except ankle and foot

T24.11 Burn of first degree of thigh

⑦ **T24.111** Burn of first degree of right thigh

⑦ **T24.112** Burn of first degree of left thigh

⑦ **T24.119** Burn of first degree of unspecified thigh

T24.12 Burn of first degree of knee

⑦ **T24.121** Burn of first degree of right knee

⑦ **T24.122** Burn of first degree of left knee

⑦ **T24.129** Burn of first degree of unspecified knee

T24.13 Burn of first degree of lower leg

⑦ **T24.131** Burn of first degree of right lower leg

⑦ **T24.132** Burn of first degree of left lower leg

⑦ **T24.139** Burn of first degree of unspecified lower leg

T24.19 **Burn of first degree of multiple sites of lower limb, except ankle and foot**

⑦ **T24.191** Burn of first degree of multiple sites of right lower limb, except ankle and foot

⑦ **T24.192** Burn of first degree of multiple sites of left lower limb, except ankle and foot

⑦ **T24.199** Burn of first degree of multiple sites of unspecified lower limb, except ankle and foot

T24.2 **Burn of second degree of lower limb, except ankle and foot**

Use additional external cause code to identify the source, place and intent of the burn (X00-X19, X75-X77, X96-X98, Y92)

T24.20 **Burn of second degree of unspecified site of lower limb, except ankle and foot**

⑦ **T24.201** Burn of second degree of unspecified site of right lower limb, except ankle and foot

⑦ **T24.202** Burn of second degree of unspecified site of left lower limb, except ankle and foot

⑦ **T24.209**   Burn of second degree of unspecified site of unspecified lower limb, except ankle and foot

T24.21   Burn of second degree of thigh

⑦ **T24.211**   Burn of second degree of right thigh

⑦ **T24.212**   Burn of second degree of left thigh

⑦ **T24.219**   Burn of second degree of unspecified thigh

T24.22   Burn of second degree of knee

⑦ **T24.221**   Burn of second degree of right knee

⑦ **T24.222**   Burn of second degree of left knee

⑦ **T24.229**   Burn of second degree of unspecified knee

T24.23   Burn of second degree of lower leg

⑦ **T24.231**   Burn of second degree of right lower leg

⑦ **T24.232**   Burn of second degree of left lower leg

⑦ **T24.239**   Burn of second degree of unspecified lower leg

T24.29   Burn of second degree of multiple sites of lower limb, except ankle and foot

⑦ **T24.291**   Burn of second degree of multiple sites of right lower limb, except ankle and foot

⑦ **T24.292**   Burn of second degree of multiple sites of left lower limb, except ankle and foot

⑦ **T24.299**   Burn of second degree of multiple sites of unspecified lower limb, except ankle and foot

T24.3   Burn of third degree of lower limb, except ankle and foot

Use additional external cause code to identify the source, place and intent of the burn (X00-X19, X75-X77, X96-X98, Y92)

T24.30   Burn of third degree of unspecified site of lower limb, except ankle and foot

⑦ **T24.301**   Burn of third degree of unspecified site of right lower limb, except ankle and foot

⑦ **T24.302**   Burn of third degree of unspecified site of left lower limb, except ankle and foot

⑦ **T24.309**   Burn of third degree of unspecified site of unspecified lower limb, except ankle and foot

T24.31   Burn of third degree of thigh

⑦ **T24.311**   Burn of third degree of right thigh

⑦ **T24.312**   Burn of third degree of left thigh

⑦ **T24.319**   Burn of third degree of unspecified thigh

T24.32   Burn of third degree of knee

⑦ **T24.321**   Burn of third degree of right knee

⑦ **T24.322**   Burn of third degree of left knee

⑦ **T24.329**   Burn of third degree of unspecified knee

T24.33   Burn of third degree of lower leg

⑦ **T24.331**   Burn of third degree of right lower leg

⑦ **T24.332**   Burn of third degree of left lower leg

⑦ **T24.339**   Burn of third degree of unspecified lower leg

T24.39   Burn of third degree of multiple sites of lower limb, except ankle and foot

⑦ **T24.391**   Burn of third degree of multiple sites of right lower limb, except ankle and foot

⑦ **T24.392**   Burn of third degree of multiple sites of left lower limb, except ankle and foot

⑦ **T24.399**   Burn of third degree of multiple sites of unspecified lower limb, except ankle and foot

T24.4   Corrosion of unspecified degree of lower limb, except ankle and foot

Code first (T51-T65) to identify chemical and intent

Use additional external cause code to identify place (Y92)

T24.40   Corrosion of unspecified degree of unspecified site of lower limb, except ankle and foot

⑦ **T24.401**   Corrosion of unspecified degree of unspecified site of right lower limb, except ankle and foot

⑦ **T24.402**   Corrosion of unspecified degree of unspecified site of left lower limb, except ankle and foot

⑦ **T24.409**   Corrosion of unspecified degree of unspecified site of unspecified lower limb, except ankle and foot

T24.41   Corrosion of unspecified degree of thigh

⑦ **T24.411**   Corrosion of unspecified degree of right thigh

⑦ **T24.412**   Corrosion of unspecified degree of left thigh

⑦ **T24.419**   Corrosion of unspecified degree of unspecified thigh

T24.42   Corrosion of unspecified degree of knee

⑦ **T24.421**   Corrosion of unspecified degree of right knee

⑦ **T24.422**   Corrosion of unspecified degree of left knee

⑦ **T24.429**   Corrosion of unspecified degree of unspecified knee

T24.43   Corrosion of unspecified degree of lower leg

⑦ **T24.431**   Corrosion of unspecified degree of right lower leg

⑦ **T24.432**   Corrosion of unspecified degree of left lower leg

⑦ **T24.439**   Corrosion of unspecified degree of unspecified lower leg

T24.49   Corrosion of unspecified degree of multiple sites of lower limb, except ankle and foot

⑦ **T24.491**   Corrosion of unspecified degree of multiple sites of right lower limb, except ankle and foot

⑦ **T24.492**   Corrosion of unspecified degree of multiple sites of left lower limb, except ankle and foot

⑦ **T24.499**   Corrosion of unspecified degree of multiple sites of unspecified lower limb, except ankle and foot

T24.5   Corrosion of first degree of lower limb, except ankle and foot

Code first (T51-T65) to identify chemical and intent

Use additional external cause code to identify place (Y92)

T24.50   Corrosion of first degree of unspecified site of lower limb, except ankle and foot

---

| | Add 4th-7th digits | Nonspecific code | Unspecified code | Manifestation code | 903 |

⑦**T24.501** Corrosion of first degree of unspecified site of right lower limb, except ankle and foot

⑦**T24.502** Corrosion of first degree of unspecified site of left lower limb, except ankle and foot

⑦**T24.509** Corrosion of first degree of unspecified site of unspecified lower limb, except ankle and foot

T24.51 Corrosion of first degree of thigh

⑦**T24.511** Corrosion of first degree of right thigh

⑦**T24.512** Corrosion of first degree of left thigh

⑦**T24.519** Corrosion of first degree of unspecified thigh

T24.52 Corrosion of first degree of knee

⑦**T24.521** Corrosion of first degree of right knee

⑦**T24.522** Corrosion of first degree of left knee

⑦**T24.529** Corrosion of first degree of unspecified knee

T24.53 Corrosion of first degree of lower leg

⑦**T24.531** Corrosion of first degree of right lower leg

⑦**T24.532** Corrosion of first degree of left lower leg

⑦**T24.539** Corrosion of first degree of unspecified lower leg

T24.59 Corrosion of first degree of multiple sites of lower limb, except ankle and foot

⑦**T24.591** Corrosion of first degree of multiple sites of right lower limb, except ankle and foot

⑦**T24.592** Corrosion of first degree of multiple sites of left lower limb, except ankle and foot

⑦**T24.599** Corrosion of first degree of multiple sites of unspecified lower limb, except ankle and foot

T24.6 Corrosion of second degree of lower limb, except ankle and foot

Code first (T51-T65) to identify chemical and intent

Use additional external cause code to identify place (Y92)

T24.60 Corrosion of second degree of unspecified site of lower limb, except ankle and foot

⑦**T24.601** Corrosion of second degree of unspecified site of right lower limb, except ankle and foot

⑦**T24.602** Corrosion of second degree of unspecified site of left lower limb, except ankle and foot

⑦**T24.609** Corrosion of second degree of unspecified site of unspecified lower limb, except ankle and foot

T24.61 Corrosion of second degree of thigh

⑦**T24.611** Corrosion of second degree of right thigh

⑦**T24.612** Corrosion of second degree of left thigh

⑦**T24.619** Corrosion of second degree of unspecified thigh

T24.62 Corrosion of second degree of knee

⑦**T24.621** Corrosion of second degree of right knee

⑦**T24.622** Corrosion of second degree of left knee

⑦**T24.629** Corrosion of second degree of unspecified knee

T24.63 Corrosion of second degree of lower leg

⑦**T24.631** Corrosion of second degree of right lower leg

⑦**T24.632** Corrosion of second degree of left lower leg

⑦**T24.639** Corrosion of second degree of unspecified lower leg

T24.69 Corrosion of second degree of multiple sites of lower limb, except ankle and foot

⑦**T24.691** Corrosion of second degree of multiple sites of right lower limb, except ankle and foot

⑦**T24.692** Corrosion of second degree of multiple sites of left lower limb, except ankle and foot

⑦**T24.699** Corrosion of second degree of multiple sites of unspecified lower limb, except ankle and foot

T24.7 Corrosion of third degree of lower limb, except ankle and foot

Code first (T51-T65) to identify chemical and intent

Use additional external cause code to identify place (Y92)

T24.70 Corrosion of third degree of unspecified site of lower limb, except ankle and foot

⑦**T24.701** Corrosion of third degree of unspecified site of right lower limb, except ankle and foot

⑦**T24.702** Corrosion of third degree of unspecified site of left lower limb, except ankle and foot

⑦**T24.709** Corrosion of third degree of unspecified site of unspecified lower limb, except ankle and foot

T24.71 Corrosion of third degree of thigh

⑦**T24.711** Corrosion of third degree of right thigh

⑦**T24.712** Corrosion of third degree of left thigh

⑦**T24.719** Corrosion of third degree of unspecified thigh

T24.72 Corrosion of third degree of knee

⑦**T24.721** Corrosion of third degree of right knee

⑦**T24.722** Corrosion of third degree of left knee

⑦**T24.729** Corrosion of third degree of unspecified knee

T24.73 Corrosion of third degree of lower leg

⑦**T24.731** Corrosion of third degree of right lower leg

⑦**T24.732** Corrosion of third degree of left lower leg

⑦**T24.739** Corrosion of third degree of unspecified lower leg

T24.79 Corrosion of third degree of multiple sites of lower limb, except ankle and foot

⑦**T24.791** Corrosion of third degree of multiple sites of right lower limb, except ankle and foot

● New code ▲ Revised code **Excludes1:** Not coded here **Excludes2:** Not included here ⊗ Placeholder required ⑦7ᵗʰ digit required

⑦**T24.792** **Corrosion of third degree of multiple sites of left lower limb, except ankle and foot**

⑦**T24.799** **Corrosion of third degree of multiple sites of unspecified lower limb, except ankle and foot**

T25 **Burn and corrosion of ankle and foot**

The appropriate 7th character is to be added to each code from category T25

A - initial encounter

D - subsequent encounter

S - sequela

T25.0 **Burn of unspecified degree of ankle and foot**

Use additional external cause code to identify the source, place and intent of the burn (X00-X19, X75-X77, X96-X98, Y92)

T25.01 **Burn of unspecified degree of ankle**

⑦**T25.011** **Burn of unspecified degree of right ankle**

⑦**T25.012** **Burn of unspecified degree of left ankle**

⑦**T25.019** **Burn of unspecified degree of unspecified ankle**

T25.02 **Burn of unspecified degree of foot**

Excludes2: burn of unspecified degree of toe(s) (nail) (T25.03-)

⑦**T25.021** **Burn of unspecified degree of right foot**

⑦**T25.022** **Burn of unspecified degree of left foot**

⑦**T25.029** **Burn of unspecified degree of unspecified foot**

T25.03 **Burn of unspecified degree of toe(s) (nail)**

⑦**T25.031** **Burn of unspecified degree of right toe(s) (nail)**

⑦**T25.032** **Burn of unspecified degree of left toe(s) (nail)**

⑦**T25.039** **Burn of unspecified degree of unspecified toe(s) (nail)**

T25.09 **Burn of unspecified degree of multiple sites of ankle and foot**

⑦**T25.091** **Burn of unspecified degree of multiple sites of right ankle and foot**

⑦**T25.092** **Burn of unspecified degree of multiple sites of left ankle and foot**

⑦**T25.099** **Burn of unspecified degree of multiple sites of unspecified ankle and foot**

T25.1 **Burn of first degree of ankle and foot**

Use additional external cause code to identify the source, place and intent of the burn (X00-X19, X75-X77, X96-X98, Y92)

T25.11 **Burn of first degree of ankle**

⑦**T25.111** **Burn of first degree of right ankle**

⑦**T25.112** **Burn of first degree of left ankle**

⑦**T25.119** **Burn of first degree of unspecified ankle**

T25.12 **Burn of first degree of foot**

Excludes2: burn of first degree of toe(s) (nail) (T25.13-)

⑦**T25.121** **Burn of first degree of right foot**

⑦**T25.122** **Burn of first degree of left foot**

⑦**T25.129** **Burn of first degree of unspecified foot**

T25.13 **Burn of first degree of toe(s) (nail)**

⑦**T25.131** **Burn of first degree of right toe(s) (nail)**

⑦**T25.132** **Burn of first degree of left toe(s) (nail)**

⑦**T25.139** **Burn of first degree of unspecified toe(s) (nail)**

T25.19 **Burn of first degree of multiple sites of ankle and foot**

⑦**T25.191** **Burn of first degree of multiple sites of right ankle and foot**

⑦**T25.192** **Burn of first degree of multiple sites of left ankle and foot**

⑦**T25.199** **Burn of first degree of multiple sites of unspecified ankle and foot**

T25.2 **Burn of second degree of ankle and foot**

Use additional external cause code to identify the source, place and intent of the burn (X00-X19, X75-X77, X96-X98, Y92)

T25.21 **Burn of second degree of ankle**

⑦**T25.211** **Burn of second degree of right ankle**

⑦**T25.212** **Burn of second degree of left ankle**

⑦**T25.219** **Burn of second degree of unspecified ankle**

T25.22 **Burn of second degree of foot**

Excludes2: burn of second degree of toe(s) (nail) (T25.23-)

⑦**T25.221** **Burn of second degree of right foot**

⑦**T25.222** **Burn of second degree of left foot**

⑦**T25.229** **Burn of second degree of unspecified foot**

T25.23 **Burn of second degree of toe(s) (nail)**

⑦**T25.231** **Burn of second degree of right toe(s) (nail)**

⑦**T25.232** **Burn of second degree of left toe(s) (nail)**

⑦**T25.239** **Burn of second degree of unspecified toe(s) (nail)**

T25.29 **Burn of second degree of multiple sites of ankle and foot**

⑦**T25.291** **Burn of second degree of multiple sites of right ankle and foot**

⑦**T25.292** **Burn of second degree of multiple sites of left ankle and foot**

⑦**T25.299** **Burn of second degree of multiple sites of unspecified ankle and foot**

T25.3 **Burn of third degree of ankle and foot**

Use additional external cause code to identify the source, place and intent of the burn (X00-X19, X75-X77, X96-X98, Y92)

T25.31 **Burn of third degree of ankle**

⑦**T25.311** **Burn of third degree of right ankle**

⑦**T25.312** **Burn of third degree of left ankle**

⑦**T25.319** **Burn of third degree of unspecified ankle**

T25.32 **Burn of third degree of foot**

Excludes2: burn of third degree of toe(s) (nail) (T25.33-)

⑦**T25.321** **Burn of third degree of right foot**

⑦**T25.322** **Burn of third degree of left foot**

⑦**T25.329** **Burn of third degree of unspecified foot**

T25.33 **Burn of third degree of toe(s) (nail)**

⑦**T25.331** **Burn of third degree of right toe(s) (nail)**

⑦**T25.332** **Burn of third degree of left toe(s) (nail)**

⑦**T25.339** **Burn of third degree of unspecified toe(s) (nail)**

T25.39 **Burn of third degree of multiple sites of ankle and foot**

⑦**T25.391** **Burn of third degree of multiple sites of right ankle and foot**

⑦**T25.392** **Burn of third degree of multiple sites of left ankle and foot**

⑦**T25.399** **Burn of third degree of multiple sites of unspecified ankle and foot**

T25.4 **Corrosion of unspecified degree of ankle and foot**

Code first (T51-T65) to identify chemical and intent

Use additional external cause code to identify place (Y92)

T25.41 **Corrosion of unspecified degree of ankle**

⑦**T25.411** **Corrosion of unspecified degree of right ankle**

⑦**T25.412** **Corrosion of unspecified degree of left ankle**

⑦**T25.419** **Corrosion of unspecified degree of unspecified ankle**

T25.42 **Corrosion of unspecified degree of foot**

Excludes2: corrosion of unspecified degree of toe(s) (nail) (T25.43-)

⑦**T25.421** **Corrosion of unspecified degree of right foot**

⑦**T25.422** **Corrosion of unspecified degree of left foot**

⑦**T25.429** **Corrosion of unspecified degree of unspecified foot**

T25.43 **Corrosion of unspecified degree of toe(s) (nail)**

⑦**T25.431** **Corrosion of unspecified degree of right toe(s) (nail)**

⑦**T25.432** **Corrosion of unspecified degree of left toe(s) (nail)**

⑦**T25.439** **Corrosion of unspecified degree of unspecified toe(s) (nail)**

T25.49 **Corrosion of unspecified degree of multiple sites of ankle and foot**

⑦**T25.491** **Corrosion of unspecified degree of multiple sites of right ankle and foot**

⑦**T25.492** **Corrosion of unspecified degree of multiple sites of left ankle and foot**

⑦**T25.499** **Corrosion of unspecified degree of multiple sites of unspecified ankle and foot**

T25.5 **Corrosion of first degree of ankle and foot**

Code first (T51-T65) to identify chemical and intent

Use additional external cause code to identify place (Y92)

T25.51 **Corrosion of first degree of ankle**

⑦**T25.511** **Corrosion of first degree of right ankle**

⑦**T25.512** **Corrosion of first degree of left ankle**

⑦**T25.519** **Corrosion of first degree of unspecified ankle**

T25.52 **Corrosion of first degree of foot**

Excludes2: corrosion of first degree of toe(s) (nail) (T25.53-)

⑦**T25.521** **Corrosion of first degree of right foot**

⑦**T25.522** **Corrosion of first degree of left foot**

⑦**T25.529** **Corrosion of first degree of unspecified foot**

T25.53 **Corrosion of first degree of toe(s) (nail)**

⑦**T25.531** **Corrosion of first degree of right toe(s) (nail)**

⑦**T25.532** **Corrosion of first degree of left toe(s) (nail)**

⑦**T25.539** **Corrosion of first degree of unspecified toe(s) (nail)**

T25.59 **Corrosion of first degree of multiple sites of ankle and foot**

⑦**T25.591** **Corrosion of first degree of multiple sites of right ankle and foot**

⑦**T25.592** **Corrosion of first degree of multiple sites of left ankle and foot**

⑦**T25.599** **Corrosion of first degree of multiple sites of unspecified ankle and foot**

T25.6 **Corrosion of second degree of ankle and foot**

Code first (T51-T65) to identify chemical and intent

Use additional external cause code to identify place (Y92)

T25.61 **Corrosion of second degree of ankle**

⑦**T25.611** **Corrosion of second degree of right ankle**

⑦**T25.612** **Corrosion of second degree of left ankle**

⑦**T25.619** **Corrosion of second degree of unspecified ankle**

T25.62 **Corrosion of second degree of foot**

Excludes2: corrosion of second degree of toe(s) (nail) (T25.63-)

⑦**T25.621** **Corrosion of second degree of right foot**

⑦**T25.622** **Corrosion of second degree of left foot**

⑦**T25.629** **Corrosion of second degree of unspecified foot**

T25.63 **Corrosion of second degree of toe(s) (nail)**

⑦**T25.631** **Corrosion of second degree of right toe(s) (nail)**

⑦**T25.632** **Corrosion of second degree of left toe(s) (nail)**

⑦**T25.639** **Corrosion of second degree of unspecified toe(s) (nail)**

⑦**T25.69** **Corrosion of second degree of multiple sites of ankle and foot**

⑦**T25.691** **Corrosion of second degree of right ankle and foot**

⑦**T25.692** **Corrosion of second degree of left ankle and foot**

⑦**T25.699** **Corrosion of second degree of unspecified ankle and foot**

T25.7 **Corrosion of third degree of ankle and foot**

Code first (T51-T65) to identify chemical and intent

Use additional external cause code to identify place (Y92)

T25.71 **Corrosion of third degree of ankle**

⑦**T25.711** **Corrosion of third degree of right ankle**

● New code   ▲ Revised code   **Excludes1:** Not coded here   **Excludes2:** Not included here   ⊗ Placeholder required   ⑦7th digit required

⑦T25.712   **Corrosion of third degree of left ankle**

⑦T25.719   **Corrosion of third degree of unspecified ankle**

T25.72   **Corrosion of third degree of foot**

> **Excludes2:** corrosion of third degree of toe(s) (nail) (T25.73-)

⑦T25.721   **Corrosion of third degree of right foot**

⑦T25.722   **Corrosion of third degree of left foot**

⑦T25.729   **Corrosion of third degree of unspecified foot**

⑦T25.73   **Corrosion of third degree of toe(s) (nail)**

⑦T25.731   **Corrosion of third degree of right toe(s) (nail)**

⑦T25.732   **Corrosion of third degree of left toe(s) (nail)**

⑦T25.739   **Corrosion of third degree of unspecified toe(s) (nail)**

T25.79   **Corrosion of third degree of multiple sites of ankle and foot**

⑦T25.791   **Corrosion of third degree of multiple sites of right ankle and foot**

⑦T25.792   **Corrosion of third degree of multiple sites of left ankle and foot**

⑦T25.799   **Corrosion of third degree of multiple sites of unspecified ankle and foot**

BURNS AND CORROSIONS CONFINED TO EYE AND INTERNAL ORGANS (T26-T28)

T26   **Burn and corrosion confined to eye and adnexa**

The appropriate 7th character is to be added to each code from category T26

A - initial encounter

D - subsequent encounter

S - sequela

T26.0   **Burn of eyelid and periocular area**

> **Use additional** external cause code to identify the source, place and intent of the burn (X00-X19, X75-X77, X96-X98, Y92)

⊗⑦T26.00   **Burn of unspecified eyelid and periocular area**

⊗⑦T26.01   **Burn of right eyelid and periocular area**

⊗⑦T26.02   **Burn of left eyelid and periocular area**

T26.1   **Burn of cornea and conjunctival sac**

> **Use additional** external cause code to identify the source, place and intent of the burn (X00-X19, X75-X77, X96-X98, Y92)

⊗⑦T26.10   **Burn of cornea and conjunctival sac, unspecified eye**

⊗⑦T26.11   **Burn of cornea and conjunctival sac, right eye**

⊗⑦T26.12   **Burn of cornea and conjunctival sac, left eye**

T26.2   **Burn with resulting rupture and destruction of eyeball**

> **Use additional** external cause code to identify the source, place and intent of the burn (X00-X19, X75-X77, X96-X98, Y92)

⊗⑦T26.20   **Burn with resulting rupture and destruction of unspecified eyeball**

⊗⑦T26.21   **Burn with resulting rupture and destruction of right eyeball**

⊗⑦T26.22   **Burn with resulting rupture and destruction of left eyeball**

T26.3   **Burns of other specified parts of eye and adnexa**

> **Use additional** external cause code to identify the source, place and intent of the burn (X00-X19, X75-X77, X96-X98, Y92)

⊗⑦T26.30   **Burns of other specified parts of unspecified eye and adnexa**

⊗⑦T26.31   **Burns of other specified parts of right eye and adnexa**

⊗⑦T26.32   **Burns of other specified parts of left eye and adnexa**

T26.4   **Burn of eye and adnexa, part unspecified**

> **Use additional** external cause code to identify the source, place and intent of the burn (X00-X19, X75-X77, X96-X98, Y92)

⊗⑦T26.40   **Burn of unspecified eye and adnexa, part unspecified**

⊗⑦T26.41   **Burn of right eye and adnexa, part unspecified**

⊗⑦T26.42   **Burn of left eye and adnexa, part unspecified**

T26.5   **Corrosion of eyelid and periocular area**

> **Code first** (T51-T65) to identify chemical and intent
>
> **Use additional** external cause code to identify place (Y92)

⊗⑦T26.50   **Corrosion of unspecified eyelid and periocular area**

⊗⑦T26.51   **Corrosion of right eyelid and periocular area**

⊗⑦T26.52   **Corrosion of left eyelid and periocular area**

T26.6   **Corrosion of cornea and conjunctival sac**

> **Code first** (T51-T65) to identify chemical and intent
>
> **Use additional** external cause code to identify place (Y92)

⊗⑦T26.60   **Corrosion of cornea and conjunctival sac, unspecified eye**

⊗⑦T26.61   **Corrosion of cornea and conjunctival sac, right eye**

⊗⑦T26.62   **Corrosion of cornea and conjunctival sac, left eye**

T26.7   **Corrosion with resulting rupture and destruction of eyeball**

> **Code first** (T51-T65) to identify chemical and intent
>
> **Use additional** external cause code to identify place (Y92)

⊗⑦T26.70   **Corrosion with resulting rupture and destruction of unspecified eyeball**

⊗⑦T26.71   **Corrosion with resulting rupture and destruction of right eyeball**

⊗⑦T26.72   **Corrosion with resulting rupture and destruction of left eyeball**

T26.8   **Corrosions of other specified parts of eye and adnexa**

> **Code first** (T51-T65) to identify chemical and intent
>
> **Use additional** external cause code to identify place (Y92)

⊗⑦T26.80   **Corrosions of other specified parts of unspecified eye and adnexa**

⊗⑦T26.81   **Corrosions of other specified parts of right eye and adnexa**

⊗⑦T26.82   **Corrosions of other specified parts of left eye and adnexa**

⑦T26.9   **Corrosion of eye and adnexa, part unspecified**

> **Code first** (T51-T65) to identify chemical and intent
>
> **Use additional** external cause code to identify place (Y92)

⊗⑦T26.90   **Corrosion of unspecified eye and adnexa, part unspecified**

⊗⑦T26.91   **Corrosion of right eye and adnexa, part unspecified**

⊗⑦T26.92   **Corrosion of left eye and adnexa, part unspecified**

T27   **Burn and corrosion of respiratory tract**

| Add 4th-7th digits | Nonspecific code | Unspecified code | Manifestation code |

Use additional external cause code to identify the source and intent of the burn (X00-X19, X75-X77, X96-X98)

Use additional external cause code to identify place (Y92)

The appropriate 7th character is to be added to each code from category T27

A - initial encounter

D - subsequent encounter

S - sequela

⊗⑦ **T27.0** **Burn of larynx and trachea**

⊗⑦ **T27.1** **Burn involving larynx and trachea with lung**

⊗⑦ **T27.2** **Burn of other parts of respiratory tract**

Burn of thoracic cavity

⊗⑦ **T27.3** **Burn of respiratory tract, part unspecified**

⊗⑦ **T27.4** **Corrosion of larynx and trachea**

Code first (T51-T65) to identify chemical and intent

⊗⑦ **T27.5** **Corrosion involving larynx and trachea with lung**

⊗⑦ **T27.6** **Corrosion of other parts of respiratory tract**

Code first (T51-T65) to identify chemical and intent

⊗⑦ **T27.7** **Corrosion of respiratory tract, part unspecified**

Code first (T51-T65) to identify chemical and intent

T28 **Burn and corrosion of other internal organs**

Use additional external cause code to identify the source and intent of the burn (X00-X19, X75-X77, X96-X98)

Use additional external cause code to identify place (Y92)

The appropriate 7th character is to be added to each code from category T28

A - initial encounter

D - subsequent encounter

S - sequela

⊗⑦ **T28.0** **Burn of mouth and pharynx**

⊗⑦ **T28.1** **Burn of esophagus**

⊗⑦ **T28.2** **Burn of other parts of alimentary tract**

⊗⑦ **T28.3** **Burn of internal genitourinary organs**

T28.4 **Burns of other and unspecified internal organs**

Code first (T51-T65) to identify chemical and intent

⊗⑦ **T28.40** **Burn of unspecified internal organ**

T28.41 **Burn of ear drum**

⑦ **T28.411** **Burn of right ear drum**

⑦ **T28.412** **Burn of left ear drum**

⑦ **T28.419** **Burn of unspecified ear drum**

⊗⑦ **T28.49** **Burn of other internal organ**

⊗⑦ **T28.5** **Corrosion of mouth and pharynx**

Code first (T51-T65) to identify chemical and intent

⊗⑦ **T28.6** **Corrosion of esophagus**

Code first (T51-T65) to identify chemical and intent

⊗⑦ **T28.7** **Corrosion of other parts of alimentary tract**

Code first (T51-T65) to identify chemical and intent

⊗⑦ **T28.8** **Corrosion of internal genitourinary organs**

Code first (T51-T65) to identify chemical and intent

T28.9 **Corrosions of other and unspecified internal organs**

Code first (T51-T65) to identify chemical and intent

⊗⑦ **T28.90** **Corrosions of unspecified internal organs**

T28.91 **Corrosions of ear drum**

⑦ **T28.911** **Corrosions of right ear drum**

⑦ **T28.912** **Corrosions of left ear drum**

⑦ **T28.919** **Corrosions of unspecified ear drum**

⊗⑦ **T28.99** **Corrosions of other internal organs**

BURNS AND CORROSIONS OF MULTIPLE AND UNSPECIFIED BODY REGIONS (T30-T32)

T30 **Burn and corrosion, body region unspecified**

T30.0 **Burn of unspecified body region, unspecified degree**

This code is not for inpatient use. Code to specified site and degree of burns

Burn NOS

Multiple burns NOS

T30.4 **Corrosion of unspecified body region, unspecified degree**

This code is not for inpatient use. Code to specified site and degree of corrosion

Corrosion NOS

Multiple corrosion NOS

T31 **Burns classified according to extent of body surface involved**

Note: This category is to be used as the primary code only when the site of the burn is unspecified. It should be used as a supplementary code with categories T20-T25 when the site is specified.

T31.0 **Burns involving less than 10% of body surface**

T31.1 **Burns involving 10-19% of body surface**

T31.10 **Burns involving 10-19% of body surface with 0% to 9% third degree burns**

Burns involving 10-19% of body surface NOS

T31.11 **Burns involving 10-19% of body surface with 10-19% third degree burns**

T31.2 **Burns involving 20-29% of body surface**

T31.20 **Burns involving 20-29% of body surface with 0% to 9% third degree burns**

Burns involving 20-29% of body surface NOS

T31.21 **Burns involving 20-29% of body surface with 10-19% third degree burns**

T31.22 **Burns involving 20-29% of body surface with 20-29% third degree burns**

T31.3 **Burns involving 30-39% of body surface**

T31.30 **Burns involving 30-39% of body surface with 0% to 9% third degree burns**

Burns involving 30-39% of body surface NOS

T31.31 **Burns involving 30-39% of body surface with 10-19% third degree burns**

T31.32 **Burns involving 30-39% of body surface with 20-29% third degree burns**

T31.33 **Burns involving 30-39% of body surface with 30-39% third degree burns**

T31.4 **Burns involving 40-49% of body surface**

T31.40 **Burns involving 40-49% of body surface with 0% to 9% third degree burns**

Burns involving 40-49% of body surface NOS

T31.41 **Burns involving 40-49% of body surface with 10-19% third degree burns**

T31.42 **Burns involving 40-49% of body surface with 20-29% third degree burns**

T31.43 **Burns involving 40-49% of body surface with 30-39% third degree burns**

T31.44 **Burns involving 40-49% of body surface with 40-49% third degree burns**

T31.5 **Burns involving 50-59% of body surface**

T31.50 **Burns involving 50-59% of body surface with 0% to 9% third degree burns**

Burns involving 50-59% of body surface NOS

T31.51 **Burns involving 50-59% of body surface with 10-19% third degree burns**

● New code ▲ Revised code **Excludes1:** Not coded here **Excludes2:** Not included here ⊗ Placeholder required ⑦ 7th digit required

T31.52 Burns involving 50-59% of body surface with 20-29% third degree burns

T31.53 Burns involving 50-59% of body surface with 30-39% third degree burns

T31.54 Burns involving 50-59% of body surface with 40-49% third degree burns

T31.55 Burns involving 50-59% of body surface with 50-59% third degree burns

T31.6 Burns involving 60-69% of body surface

T31.60 Burns involving 60-69% of body surface with 0% to 9% third degree burns

Burns involving 60-69% of body surface NOS

T31.61 Burns involving 60-69% of body surface with 10-19% third degree burns

T31.62 Burns involving 60-69% of body surface with 20-29% third degree burns

T31.63 Burns involving 60-69% of body surface with 30-39% third degree burns

T31.64 Burns involving 60-69% of body surface with 40-49% third degree burns

T31.65 Burns involving 60-69% of body surface with 50-59% third degree burns

T31.66 Burns involving 60-69% of body surface with 60-69% third degree burns

T31.7 Burns involving 70-79% of body surface

T31.70 Burns involving 70-79% of body surface with 0% to 9% third degree burns

Burns involving 70-79% of body surface NOS

T31.71 Burns involving 70-79% of body surface with 10-19% third degree burns

T31.72 Burns involving 70-79% of body surface with 20-29% third degree burns

T31.73 Burns involving 70-79% of body surface with 30-39% third degree burns

T31.74 Burns involving 70-79% of body surface with 40-49% third degree burns

T31.75 Burns involving 70-79% of body surface with 50-59% third degree burns

T31.76 Burns involving 70-79% of body surface with 60-69% third degree burns

T31.77 Burns involving 70-79% of body surface with 70-79% third degree burns

T31.8 Burns involving 80-89% of body surface

T31.80 Burns involving 80-89% of body surface with 0% to 9% third degree burns

Burns involving 80-89% of body surface NOS

T31.81 Burns involving 80-89% of body surface with 10-19% third degree burns

T31.82 Burns involving 80-89% of body surface with 20-29% third degree burns

T31.83 Burns involving 80-89% of body surface with 30-39% third degree burns

T31.84 Burns involving 80-89% of body surface with 40-49% third degree burns

T31.85 Burns involving 80-89% of body surface with 50-59% third degree burns

T31.86 Burns involving 80-89% of body surface with 60-69% third degree burns

T31.87 Burns involving 80-89% of body surface with 70-79% third degree burns

T31.88 Burns involving 80-89% of body surface with 80-89% third degree burns

T31.9 Burns involving 90% or more of body surface

T31.90 Burns involving 90% or more of body surface with 0% to 9% third degree burns

Burns involving 90% or more of body surface NOS

T31.91 Burns involving 90% or more of body surface with 10-19% third degree burns

T31.92 Burns involving 90% or more of body surface with 20-29% third degree burns

T31.93 Burns involving 90% or more of body surface with 30-39% third degree burns

T31.94 Burns involving 90% or more of body surface with 40-49% third degree burns

T31.95 Burns involving 90% or more of body surface with 50-59% third degree burns

T31.96 Burns involving 90% or more of body surface with 60-69% third degree burns

T31.97 Burns involving 90% or more of body surface with 70-79% third degree burns

T31.98 Burns involving 90% or more of body surface with 80-89% third degree burns

T31.99 Burns involving 90% or more of body surface with 90% or more third degree burns

T32 Corrosions classified according to extent of body surface involved

Note: This category is to be used as the primary code only when the site of the corrosion is unspecified. It may be used as a supplementary code with categories T20-T25 when the site is specified.

T32.0 Corrosions involving less than 10% of body surface

T32.1 Corrosions involving 10-19% of body surface

T32.10 Corrosions involving 10-19% of body surface with 0% to 9% third degree corrosion

Corrosions involving 10-19% of body surface NOS

T32.11 Corrosions involving 10-19% of body surface with 10-19% third degree corrosion

T32.2 Corrosions involving 20-29% of body surface

T32.20 Corrosions involving 20-29% of body surface with 0% to 9% third degree corrosion

T32.21 Corrosions involving 20-29% of body surface with 10-19% third degree corrosion

T32.22 Corrosions involving 20-29% of body surface with 20-29% third degree corrosion

T32.3 Corrosions involving 30-39% of body surface

T32.30 Corrosions involving 30-39% of body surface with 0% to 9% third degree corrosion

T32.31 Corrosions involving 30-39% of body surface with 10-19% third degree corrosion

T32.32 Corrosions involving 30-39% of body surface with 20-29% third degree corrosion

T32.33 Corrosions involving 30-39% of body surface with 30-39% third degree corrosion

T32.4 Corrosions involving 40-49% of body surface

T32.40 Corrosions involving 40-49% of body surface with 0% to 9% third degree corrosion

T32.41 Corrosions involving 40-49% of body surface with 10-19% third degree corrosion

T32.42 Corrosions involving 40-49% of body surface with 20-29% third degree corrosion

T32.43 Corrosions involving 40-49% of body surface with 30-39% third degree corrosion

T32.44 Corrosions involving 40-49% of body surface with 40-49% third degree corrosion

T32.5 Corrosions involving 50-59% of body surface

T32.50 Corrosions involving 50-59% of body surface with 0% to 9% third degree corrosion

T32.51 Corrosions involving 50-59% of body surface with 10-19% third degree corrosion

T32.52 Corrosions involving 50-59% of body surface with 20-29% third degree corrosion

T32.53 Corrosions involving 50-59% of body surface with 30-39% third degree corrosion

T32.54 Corrosions involving 50-59% of body surface with 40-49% third degree corrosion

T32.55 Corrosions involving 50-59% of body surface with 50-59% third degree corrosion

T32.6 Corrosions involving 60-69% of body surface

T32.60 Corrosions involving 60-69% of body surface with 0% to 9% third degree corrosion

T32.61 Corrosions involving 60-69% of body surface with 10-19% third degree corrosion

T32.62 Corrosions involving 60-69% of body surface with 20-29% third degree corrosion

T32.63 Corrosions involving 60-69% of body surface with 30-39% third degree corrosion

T32.64 Corrosions involving 60-69% of body surface with 40-49% third degree corrosion

T32.65 Corrosions involving 60-69% of body surface with 50-59% third degree corrosion

T32.66 Corrosions involving 60-69% of body surface with 60-69% third degree corrosion

T32.7 Corrosions involving 70-79% of body surface

T32.70 Corrosions involving 70-79% of body surface with 0% to 9% third degree corrosion

T32.71 Corrosions involving 70-79% of body surface with 10-19% third degree corrosion

T32.72 Corrosions involving 70-79% of body surface with 20-29% third degree corrosion

T32.73 Corrosions involving 70-79% of body surface with 30-39% third degree corrosion

T32.74 Corrosions involving 70-79% of body surface with 40-49% third degree corrosion

T32.75 Corrosions involving 70-79% of body surface with 50-59% third degree corrosion

T32.76 Corrosions involving 70-79% of body surface with 60-69% third degree corrosion

T32.77 Corrosions involving 70-79% of body surface with 70-79% third degree corrosion

T32.8 Corrosions involving 80-89% of body surface

T32.80 Corrosions involving 80-89% of body surface with 0% to 9% third degree corrosion

T32.81 Corrosions involving 80-89% of body surface with 10-19% third degree corrosion

T32.82 Corrosions involving 80-89% of body surface with 20-29% third degree corrosion

T32.83 Corrosions involving 80-89% of body surface with 30-39% third degree corrosion

T32.84 Corrosions involving 80-89% of body surface with 40-49% third degree corrosion

T32.85 Corrosions involving 80-89% of body surface with 50-59% third degree corrosion

T32.86 Corrosions involving 80-89% of body surface with 60-69% third degree corrosion

T32.87 Corrosions involving 80-89% of body surface with 70-79% third degree corrosion

T32.88 Corrosions involving 80-89% of body surface with 80-89% third degree corrosion

T32.9 Corrosions involving 90% or more of body surface

T32.90 Corrosions involving 90% or more of body surface with 0% to 9% third degree corrosion

T32.91 Corrosions involving 90% or more of body surface with 10-19% third degree corrosion

T32.92 Corrosions involving 90% or more of body surface with 20-29% third degree corrosion

T32.93 Corrosions involving 90% or more of body surface with 30-39% third degree corrosion

T32.94 Corrosions involving 90% or more of body surface with 40-49% third degree corrosion

T32.95 Corrosions involving 90% or more of body surface with 50-59% third degree corrosion

T32.96 Corrosions involving 90% or more of body surface with 60-69% third degree corrosion

T32.97 Corrosions involving 90% or more of body surface with 70-79% third degree corrosion

T32.98 Corrosions involving 90% or more of body surface with 80-89% third degree corrosion

T32.99 Corrosions involving 90% or more of body surface with 90% or more third degree corrosion

FROSTBITE (T33-T34)

Excludes2: hypothermia **and other** effects of reduced temperature (T68, T69.-)

T33 Superficial frostbite

Includes: frostbite with partial thickness skin loss

The appropriate 7th character is to be added to each code from category T33

A - initial encounter

D - subsequent encounter

S - sequela

T33.0 Superficial frostbite of head

    T33.01 Superficial frostbite of ear

        ⑦T33.011 Superficial frostbite of right ear

        ⑦T33.012 Superficial frostbite of left ear

        ⑦T33.019 Superficial frostbite of unspecified ear

⊗⑦T33.02 Superficial frostbite of nose

⊗⑦T33.09 Superficial frostbite of other part of head

⊗⑦T33.1 Superficial frostbite of neck

⊗⑦T33.2 Superficial frostbite of thorax

⊗⑦T33.3 Superficial frostbite of abdominal wall, lower back and pelvis

T33.4 Superficial frostbite of arm

    Excludes2: superficial frostbite of wrist and hand (T33.5-)

⊗⑦T33.40 Superficial frostbite of unspecified arm

⊗⑦T33.41 Superficial frostbite of right arm

⊗⑦T33.42 Superficial frostbite of left arm

T33.5 Superficial frostbite of wrist, hand, and fingers

    T33.51 Superficial frostbite of wrist

        ⑦T33.511 Superficial frostbite of right wrist

        ⑦T33.512 Superficial frostbite of left wrist

        ⑦T33.519 Superficial frostbite of unspecified wrist

    T33.52 Superficial frostbite of hand

    Excludes2: superficial frostbite of fingers (T33.53-)

        ⑦T33.521 Superficial frostbite of right hand

        ⑦T33.522 Superficial frostbite of left hand

● New code ▲ Revised code **Excludes1:** Not coded here **Excludes2:** Not included here ⊗ Placeholder required ⑦ 7th digit required

⑦T33.529　**Superficial frostbite of unspecified hand**

T33.53　**Superficial frostbite of finger(s)**

⑦T33.531　**Superficial frostbite of right finger(s)**

⑦T33.532　**Superficial frostbite of left finger(s)**

⑦T33.539　**Superficial frostbite of unspecified finger(s)**

T33.6　**Superficial frostbite of hip and thigh**

⊗⑦T33.60　**Superficial frostbite of unspecified hip and thigh**

⊗⑦T33.61　**Superficial frostbite of right hip and thigh**

⊗⑦T33.62　**Superficial frostbite of left hip and thigh**

T33.7　**Superficial frostbite of knee and lower leg**

Excludes2: superficial frostbite of ankle and foot (T33.8-)

⊗⑦T33.70　**Superficial frostbite of unspecified knee and lower leg**

⊗⑦T33.71　**Superficial frostbite of right knee and lower leg**

⊗⑦T33.72　**Superficial frostbite of left knee and lower leg**

T33.8　**Superficial frostbite of ankle, foot, and toe(s)**

T33.81　**Superficial frostbite of ankle**

⑦T33.811　**Superficial frostbite of right ankle**

⑦T33.812　**Superficial frostbite of left ankle**

⑦T33.819　**Superficial frostbite of unspecified ankle**

T33.82　**Superficial frostbite of foot**

⑦T33.821　**Superficial frostbite of right foot**

⑦T33.822　**Superficial frostbite of left foot**

⑦T33.829　**Superficial frostbite of unspecified foot**

T33.83　**Superficial frostbite of toe(s)**

⑦T33.831　**Superficial frostbite of right toe(s)**

⑦T33.832　**Superficial frostbite of left toe(s)**

⑦T33.839　**Superficial frostbite of unspecified toe(s)**

T33.9　**Superficial frostbite of other and unspecified sites**

⊗⑦T33.90　**Superficial frostbite of unspecified sites**

Superficial frostbite NOS

⊗⑦T33.99　**Superficial frostbite of other sites**

Superficial frostbite of leg NOS

Superficial frostbite of trunk NOS

T34　**Frostbite with tissue necrosis**

The appropriate 7th character is to be added to each code from category T34

A - initial encounter

D - subsequent encounter

S - sequela

T34.0　**Frostbite with tissue necrosis of head**

T34.01　**Frostbite with tissue necrosis of ear**

⑦T34.011　**Frostbite with tissue necrosis of right ear**

⑦T34.012　**Frostbite with tissue necrosis of left ear**

⑦T34.019　**Frostbite with tissue necrosis of unspecified ear**

⊗⑦T34.02　**Frostbite with tissue necrosis of nose**

⊗⑦T34.09　**Frostbite with tissue necrosis of other part of head**

⊗⑦T34.1　**Frostbite with tissue necrosis of neck**

⊗⑦T34.2　**Frostbite with tissue necrosis of thorax**

⊗⑦T34.3　**Frostbite with tissue necrosis of abdominal wall, lower back and pelvis**

T34.4　**Frostbite with tissue necrosis of arm**

Excludes2: frostbite with tissue necrosis of wrist and hand (T34.5-)

⊗⑦T34.40　**Frostbite with tissue necrosis of unspecified arm**

⊗⑦T34.41　**Frostbite with tissue necrosis of right arm**

⊗⑦T34.42　**Frostbite with tissue necrosis of left arm**

T34.5　**Frostbite with tissue necrosis of wrist, hand, and finger(s)**

T34.51　**Frostbite with tissue necrosis of wrist**

⑦T34.511　**Frostbite with tissue necrosis of right wrist**

⑦T34.512　**Frostbite with tissue necrosis of left wrist**

⑦T34.519　**Frostbite with tissue necrosis of unspecified wrist**

T34.52　**Frostbite with tissue necrosis of hand**

Excludes2: frostbite with tissue necrosis of finger(s) (T34.53-)

⑦T34.521　**Frostbite with tissue necrosis of right hand**

⑦T34.522　**Frostbite with tissue necrosis of left hand**

⑦T34.529　**Frostbite with tissue necrosis of unspecified hand**

T34.53　**Frostbite with tissue necrosis of finger(s)**

⑦T34.531　**Frostbite with tissue necrosis of right finger(s)**

⑦T34.532　**Frostbite with tissue necrosis of left finger(s)**

⑦T34.539　**Frostbite with tissue necrosis of unspecified finger(s)**

T34.6　**Frostbite with tissue necrosis of hip and thigh**

⊗⑦T34.60　**Frostbite with tissue necrosis of unspecified hip and thigh**

⊗⑦T34.61　**Frostbite with tissue necrosis of right hip and thigh**

⊗⑦T34.62　**Frostbite with tissue necrosis of left hip and thigh**

T34.7　**Frostbite with tissue necrosis of knee and lower leg**

Excludes2: frostbite with tissue necrosis of ankle and foot (T34.8-)

⊗⑦T34.70　**Frostbite with tissue necrosis of unspecified knee and lower leg**

⊗⑦T34.71　**Frostbite with tissue necrosis of right knee and lower leg**

⊗⑦T34.72　**Frostbite with tissue necrosis of left knee and lower leg**

T34.8　**Frostbite with tissue necrosis of ankle, foot, and toe(s)**

T34.81　**Frostbite with tissue necrosis of ankle**

⑦T34.811　**Frostbite with tissue necrosis of right ankle**

⑦T34.812　**Frostbite with tissue necrosis of left ankle**

⑦T34.819　**Frostbite with tissue necrosis of unspecified ankle**

T34.82　**Frostbite with tissue necrosis of foot**

⑦T34.821　**Frostbite with tissue necrosis of right foot**

⑦T34.822　**Frostbite with tissue necrosis of left foot**

⑦**T34.829** **Frostbite with tissue necrosis of unspecified foot**

T34.83 **Frostbite with tissue necrosis of toe(s)**

⑦**T34.831** **Frostbite with tissue necrosis of right toe(s)**

⑦**T34.832** **Frostbite with tissue necrosis of left toe(s)**

⑦**T34.839** **Frostbite with tissue necrosis of unspecified toe(s)**

T34.9 **Frostbite with tissue necrosis of other and unspecified sites**

⊗⑦**T34.90** **Frostbite with tissue necrosis of unspecified sites**

Frostbite with tissue necrosis NOS

⊗⑦**T34.99** **Frostbite with tissue necrosis of other sites**

Frostbite with tissue necrosis of leg NOS

Frostbite with tissue necrosis of trunk NOS

POISONING BY, ADVERSE EFFECTS OF AND UNDERDOSING OF DRUGS, MEDICAMENTS AND BIOLOGICAL SUBSTANCES (T36-T50)

Includes: adverse effect of correct substance properly administered

poisoning by overdose of substance

poisoning by wrong substance given or taken in error underdosing by (inadvertently) (deliberately) taking less substance than prescribed or instructed

Code first, for adverse effects, the nature of the adverse effect, such as:

adverse effect NOS (T88.7)

aspirin gastritis (K29.-)

blood disorders (D56-D76)

contact dermatitis (L23-L25)

dermatitis due to substances taken internally (L27.-)

nephropathy (N14.0-N14.2)

Note: The drug giving rise to the adverse effect should be identified by use of codes from categories T36-T50 with fifth or sixth character 5.

Use additional code(s) to specify:

manifestations of poisoning

underdosing or failure in dosage during medical and surgical care (Y63.6, Y63.8-Y63.9)

underdosing of medication regimen (Z91.12-, Z91.13-)

Excludes1: toxic reaction to local anesthesia in pregnancy (O29.3-)

Excludes2: abuse and dependence of psychoactive substances (F10-F19)

abuse of non-dependence-producing substances (F55.-)

drug reaction and poisoning affecting newborn (P00-P96)

pathological drug intoxication (inebriation) (F10-F19)

T36 **Poisoning by, adverse effect of and underdosing of systemic antibiotics**

Excludes1: antineoplastic antibiotics (T45.1-)

locally applied antibiotic NEC (T49.0)

topically used antibiotic for ear, nose and throat (T49.6)

topically used antibiotic for eye (T49.5)

The appropriate 7th character is to be added to each code from category T36

A - initial encounter

D - subsequent encounter

S - sequela

T36.0 **Poisoning by, adverse effect of and underdosing of penicillins**

T36.0X **Poisoning by, adverse effect of and underdosing of penicillins**

⑦**T36.0X1** **Poisoning by penicillins, accidental (unintentional)**

Poisoning by penicillins NOS

⑦**T36.0X2** **Poisoning by penicillins, intentional self-harm**

⑦**T36.0X3** **Poisoning by penicillins, assault**

⑦**T36.0X4** **Poisoning by penicillins, undetermined**

⑦**T36.0X5** **Adverse effect of penicillins**

⑦**T36.0X6** **Underdosing of penicillins**

T36.1 **Poisoning by, adverse effect of and underdosing of cephalosporins and other beta-lactam antibiotics**

T36.1X **Poisoning by, adverse effect of and underdosing of cephalosporins and other beta-lactam antibiotics**

⑦**T36.1X1** **Poisoning by cephalosporins and other beta-lactam antibiotics, accidental (unintentional)**

Poisoning by cephalosporins **and other** beta-lactam antibiotics NOS

⑦**T36.1X2** **Poisoning by cephalosporins and other beta-lactam antibiotics, intentional self-harm**

⑦**T36.1X3** **Poisoning by cephalosporins and other beta-lactam antibiotics, assault**

⑦**T36.1X4** **Poisoning by cephalosporins and other beta-lactam antibiotics, undetermined**

⑦**T36.1X5** **Adverse effect of cephalosporins and other beta-lactam antibiotics**

⑦**T36.1X6** **Underdosing of cephalosporins and other beta-lactam antibiotics**

T36.2 **Poisoning by, adverse effect of and underdosing of chloramphenicol group**

T36.2X **Poisoning by, adverse effect of and underdosing of chloramphenicol group**

⑦**T36.2X1** **Poisoning by chloramphenicol group, accidental (unintentional)**

Poisoning by chloramphenicol group NOS

⑦**T36.2X2** **Poisoning by chloramphenicol group, intentional self-harm**

⑦**T36.2X3** **Poisoning by chloramphenicol group, assault**

⑦**T36.2X4** **Poisoning by chloramphenicol group, undetermined**

⑦**T36.2X5** **Adverse effect of chloramphenicol group**

⑦**T36.2X6** **Underdosing of chloramphenicol group**

T36.3 **Poisoning by, adverse effect of and underdosing of macrolides**

T36.3X **Poisoning by, adverse effect of and underdosing of macrolides**

⑦**T36.3X1** **Poisoning by macrolides, accidental (unintentional)**

Poisoning by macrolides NOS

⑦**T36.3X2** **Poisoning by macrolides, intentional self-harm**

⑦**T36.3X3** **Poisoning by macrolides, assault**

⑦**T36.3X4** **Poisoning by macrolides, undetermined**

⑦**T36.3X5**   **Adverse effect of macrolides**

⑦**T36.3X6**   **Underdosing of macrolides**

T36.4   **Poisoning by, adverse effect of and underdosing of tetracyclines**

T36.4X   **Poisoning by, adverse effect of and underdosing of tetracyclines**

⑦**T36.4X1**   **Poisoning by tetracyclines, accidental (unintentional)**

Poisoning by tetracyclines NOS

⑦**T36.4X2**   **Poisoning by tetracyclines, intentional self-harm**

⑦**T36.4X3**   **Poisoning by tetracyclines, assault**

⑦**T36.4X4**   **Poisoning by tetracyclines, undetermined**

⑦**T36.4X5**   **Adverse effect of tetracyclines**

⑦**T36.4X6**   **Underdosing of tetracyclines**

T36.5   **Poisoning by, adverse effect of and underdosing of aminoglycosides**

Poisoning by, adverse effect of and underdosing of streptomycin

T36.5X   **Poisoning by, adverse effect of and underdosing of aminoglycosides**

⑦**T36.5X1**   **Poisoning by aminoglycosides, accidental (unintentional)**

Poisoning by aminoglycosides NOS

⑦**T36.5X2**   **Poisoning by aminoglycosides, intentional self-harm**

⑦**T36.5X3**   **Poisoning by aminoglycosides, assault**

⑦**T36.5X4**   **Poisoning by aminoglycosides, undetermined**

⑦**T36.5X5**   **Adverse effect of aminoglycosides**

⑦**T36.5X6**   **Underdosing of aminoglycosides**

T36.6   **Poisoning by, adverse effect of and underdosing of rifampicins**

T36.6X   **Poisoning by, adverse effect of and underdosing of rifampicins**

⑦**T36.6X1**   **Poisoning by rifampicins, accidental (unintentional)**

Poisoning by rifampicins NOS

⑦**T36.6X2**   **Poisoning by rifampicins, intentional self-harm**

⑦**T36.6X3**   **Poisoning by rifampicins, assault**

⑦**T36.6X4**   **Poisoning by rifampicins, undetermined**

⑦**T36.6X5**   **Adverse effect of rifampicins**

⑦**T36.6X6**   **Underdosing of rifampicins**

T36.7   **Poisoning by, adverse effect of and underdosing of antifungal antibiotics, systemically used**

T36.7X   **Poisoning by, adverse effect of and underdosing of antifungal antibiotics, systemically used**

⑦**T36.7X1**   **Poisoning by antifungal antibiotics, systemically used, accidental (unintentional)**

Poisoning by antifungal antibiotics, systemically used NOS

⑦**T36.7X2**   **Poisoning by antifungal antibiotics, systemically used, intentional self-harm**

⑦**T36.7X3**   **Poisoning by antifungal antibiotics, systemically used, assault**

⑦**T36.7X4**   **Poisoning by antifungal antibiotics, systemically used, undetermined**

⑦**T36.7X5**   **Adverse effect of antifungal antibiotics, systemically used**

⑦**T36.7X6**   **Underdosing of antifungal antibiotics, systemically used**

T36.8   **Poisoning by, adverse effect of and underdosing of other systemic antibiotics**

T36.8X   **Poisoning by, adverse effect of and underdosing of other systemic antibiotics**

⑦**T36.8X1**   **Poisoning by other systemic antibiotics, accidental (unintentional)**

Poisoning by other systemic antibiotics NOS

⑦**T36.8X2**   **Poisoning by other systemic antibiotics, intentional self-harm**

⑦**T36.8X3**   **Poisoning by other systemic antibiotics, assault**

⑦**T36.8X4**   **Poisoning by other systemic antibiotics, undetermined**

⑦**T36.8X5**   **Adverse effect of other systemic antibiotics**

⑦**T36.8X6**   **Underdosing of other systemic antibiotics**

T36.9   **Poisoning by, adverse effect of and underdosing of unspecified systemic antibiotic**

⊗⑦**T36.91**   **Poisoning by unspecified systemic antibiotic, accidental (unintentional)**

Poisoning by systemic antibiotic NOS

⊗⑦**T36.92**   **Poisoning by unspecified systemic antibiotic, intentional self-harm**

⊗⑦**T36.93**   **Poisoning by unspecified systemic antibiotic, assault**

⊗⑦**T36.94**   **Poisoning by unspecified systemic antibiotic, undetermined**

⊗⑦**T36.95**   **Adverse effect of unspecified systemic antibiotic**

⊗⑦**T36.96**   **Underdosing of unspecified systemic antibiotic**

T37   **Poisoning by, adverse effect of and underdosing of other systemic anti- infectives and antiparasitics**

Excludes1: anti-infectives topically used for ear, nose and throat (T49.6-)

anti-infectives topically used for eye (T49.5-)

locally applied anti-infectives NEC (T49.0-)

The appropriate 7th character is to be added to each code from category T37

A - initial encounter

D - subsequent encounter

S - sequela

T37.0   **Poisoning by, adverse effect of and underdosing of sulfonamides**

T37.0X   **Poisoning by, adverse effect of and underdosing of sulfonamides**

⑦**T37.0X1**   **Poisoning by sulfonamides, accidental (unintentional)**

Poisoning by sulfonamides NOS

⑦**T37.0X2**   **Poisoning by sulfonamides, intentional self-harm**

⑦**T37.0X3**   **Poisoning by sulfonamides, assault**

⑦**T37.0X4**   **Poisoning by sulfonamides, undetermined**

⑦**T37.0X5**   **Adverse effect of sulfonamides**

⑦**T37.0X6**   **Underdosing of sulfonamides**

T37.1   **Poisoning by, adverse effect of and underdosing of antimycobacterial drugs**

Excludes1: rifampicins (T36.6-)

---

streptomycin (T36.5-)

T37.1X Poisoning by, adverse effect of and underdosing of antimycobacterial drugs

⑦ **T37.1X1 Poisoning by antimycobacterial drugs, accidental (unintentional)**

Poisoning by antimycobacterial drugs NOS

⑦ **T37.1X2 Poisoning by antimycobacterial drugs, intentional self-harm**

⑦ **T37.1X3 Poisoning by antimycobacterial drugs, assault**

⑦ **T37.1X4 Poisoning by antimycobacterial drugs, undetermined**

⑦ **T37.1X5 Adverse effect of antimycobacterial drugs**

⑦ **T37.1X6 Underdosing of antimycobacterial drugs**

T37.2 Poisoning by, adverse effect of and underdosing of antimalarials and drugs acting on other blood protozoa

Excludes1: hydroxyquinoline derivatives (T37.8-)

T37.2X Poisoning by, adverse effect of and underdosing of antimalarials and drugs acting on other blood protozoa

⑦ **T37.2X1 Poisoning by antimalarials and drugs acting on other blood protozoa, accidental (unintentional)**

Poisoning by antimalarials and drugs acting on other blood protozoa NOS

⑦ **T37.2X2 Poisoning by antimalarials and drugs acting on other blood protozoa, intentional self-harm**

⑦ **T37.2X3 Poisoning by antimalarials and drugs acting on other blood protozoa, assault**

⑦ **T37.2X4 Poisoning by antimalarials and drugs acting on other blood protozoa, undetermined**

⑦ **T37.2X5 Adverse effect of antimalarials and drugs acting on other blood protozoa**

⑦ **T37.2X6 Underdosing of antimalarials and drugs acting on other blood protozoa**

T37.3 Poisoning by, adverse effect of and underdosing of other antiprotozoal drugs

T37.3X Poisoning by, adverse effect of and underdosing of other antiprotozoal drugs

⑦ **T37.3X1 Poisoning by other antiprotozoal drugs, accidental (unintentional)**

Poisoning by other antiprotozoal drugs NOS

⑦ **T37.3X2 Poisoning by other antiprotozoal drugs, intentional self-harm**

⑦ **T37.3X3 Poisoning by other antiprotozoal drugs, assault**

⑦ **T37.3X4 Poisoning by other antiprotozoal drugs, undetermined**

⑦ **T37.3X5 Adverse effect of other antiprotozoal drugs**

⑦ **T37.3X6 Underdosing of other antiprotozoal drugs**

T37.4 Poisoning by, adverse effect of and underdosing of anthelminthics

T37.4X Poisoning by, adverse effect of and underdosing of anthelminthics

⑦ **T37.4X1 Poisoning by anthelminthics, accidental (unintentional)**

Poisoning by anthelminthics NOS

⑦ **T37.4X2 Poisoning by anthelminthics, intentional self-harm**

⑦ **T37.4X3 Poisoning by anthelminthics, assault**

⑦ **T37.4X4 Poisoning by anthelminthics, undetermined**

⑦ **T37.4X5 Adverse effect of anthelminthics**

⑦ **T37.4X6 Underdosing of anthelminthics**

T37.5 Poisoning by, adverse effect of and underdosing of antiviral drugs

Excludes1: amantadine (T42.8-)

cytarabine (T45.1-)

T37.5X Poisoning by, adverse effect of and underdosing of antiviral drugs

⑦ **T37.5X1 Poisoning by antiviral drugs, accidental (unintentional)**

Poisoning by antiviral drugs NOS

⑦ **T37.5X2 Poisoning by antiviral drugs, intentional self-harm**

⑦ **T37.5X3 Poisoning by antiviral drugs, assault**

⑦ **T37.5X4 Poisoning by antiviral drugs, undetermined**

⑦ **T37.5X5 Adverse effect of antiviral drugs**

⑦ **T37.5X6 Underdosing of antiviral drugs**

T37.8 Poisoning by, adverse effect of and underdosing of other specified systemic anti-infectives and antiparasitics

Poisoning by, adverse effect of and underdosing of hydroxyquinoline derivatives

Excludes1: antimalarial drugs (T37.2-)

T37.8X Poisoning by, adverse effect of and underdosing of other specified systemic anti-infectives and antiparasitics

⑦ **T37.8X1 Poisoning by other specified systemic anti-infectives and antiparasitics, accidental (unintentional)**

Poisoning by other specified systemic anti-infectives and antiparasitics NOS

⑦ **T37.8X2 Poisoning by other specified systemic anti-infectives and antiparasitics, intentional self-harm**

⑦ **T37.8X3 Poisoning by other specified systemic anti-infectives and antiparasitics, assault**

⑦ **T37.8X4 Poisoning by other specified systemic anti-infectives and antiparasitics, undetermined**

⑦ **T37.8X5 Adverse effect of other specified systemic anti-infectives and antiparasitics**

⑦ **T37.8X6 Underdosing of other specified systemic anti-infectives and antiparasitics**

⑦ **T37.9 Poisoning by, adverse effect of and underdosing of unspecified systemic anti-infective and antiparasitics**

⊗⑦ **T37.91 Poisoning by unspecified systemic anti-infective and antiparasitics, accidental (unintentional)**

Poisoning by, adverse effect of and underdosing of systemic anti-infective and antiparasitics NOS

⊗⑦ **T37.92 Poisoning by unspecified systemic anti-infective and antiparasitics, intentional self-harm**

⊗⑦ **T37.93 Poisoning by unspecified systemic anti-infective and antiparasitics, assault**

⊗⑦ **T37.94 Poisoning by unspecified systemic anti-infective and antiparasitics, undetermined**

⊗⑦**T37.95** **Adverse effect of unspecified systemic anti-infective and antiparasitic**

⊗⑦**T37.96** **Underdosing of unspecified systemic anti-infectives and antiparasitics**

T38 **Poisoning by, adverse effect of and underdosing of hormones and their synthetic substitutes and antagonists, not elsewhere classified**

Excludes1: mineralocorticoids and their antagonists (T50.0-)

oxytocic hormones (T48.0-)

parathyroid hormones and derivatives (T50.9-)

The appropriate 7th character is to be added to each code from category T38

A - initial encounter

D - subsequent encounter

S - sequela

T38.0 **Poisoning by, adverse effect of and underdosing of glucocorticoids and synthetic analogues**

Excludes1: glucocorticoids, topically used (T49.-)

T38.0X **Poisoning by, adverse effect of and underdosing of glucocorticoids and synthetic analogues**

⑦**T38.0X1** **Poisoning by glucocorticoids and synthetic analogues, accidental (unintentional)**

Poisoning by glucocorticoids and synthetic analogues NOS

⑦**T38.0X2** **Poisoning by glucocorticoids and synthetic analogues, intentional self-harm**

⑦**T38.0X3** **Poisoning by glucocorticoids and synthetic analogues, assault**

⑦**T38.0X4** **Poisoning by glucocorticoids and synthetic analogues, undetermined**

⑦**T38.0X5** **Adverse effect of glucocorticoids and synthetic analogues**

⑦**T38.0X6** **Underdosing of glucocorticoids and synthetic analogues**

T38.1 **Poisoning by, adverse effect of and underdosing of thyroid hormones and substitutes**

T38.1X **Poisoning by, adverse effect of and underdosing of thyroid hormones and substitutes**

⑦**T38.1X1** **Poisoning by thyroid hormones and substitutes, accidental (unintentional)**

Poisoning by thyroid hormones and substitutes NOS

⑦**T38.1X2** **Poisoning by thyroid hormones and substitutes, intentional self-harm**

⑦**T38.1X3** **Poisoning by thyroid hormones and substitutes, assault**

⑦**T38.1X4** **Poisoning by thyroid hormones and substitutes, undetermined**

⑦**T38.1X5** **Adverse effect of thyroid hormones and substitutes**

⑦**T38.1X6** **Underdosing of thyroid hormones and substitutes**

T38.2 **Poisoning by, adverse effect of and underdosing of antithyroid drugs**

T38.2X **Poisoning by, adverse effect of and underdosing of antithyroid drugs**

⑦**T38.2X1** **Poisoning by antithyroid drugs, accidental (unintentional)**

Poisoning by antithyroid drugs NOS

⑦**T38.2X2** **Poisoning by antithyroid drugs, intentional self-harm**

⑦**T38.2X3** **Poisoning by antithyroid drugs, assault**

⑦**T38.2X4** **Poisoning by antithyroid drugs, undetermined**

⑦**T38.2X5** **Adverse effect of antithyroid drugs**

⑦**T38.2X6** **Underdosing of antithyroid drugs**

T38.3 **Poisoning by, adverse effect of and underdosing of insulin and oral hypoglycemic [antidiabetic] drugs**

T38.3X **Poisoning by, adverse effect of and underdosing of insulin and oral hypoglycemic [antidiabetic] drugs**

⑦**T38.3X1** **Poisoning by insulin and oral hypoglycemic [antidiabetic] drugs, accidental (unintentional)**

Poisoning by insulin and oral hypoglycemic [antidiabetic] drugs NOS

⑦**T38.3X2** **Poisoning by insulin and oral hypoglycemic [antidiabetic] drugs, intentional self-harm**

⑦**T38.3X3** **Poisoning by insulin and oral hypoglycemic [antidiabetic] drugs, assault**

⑦**T38.3X4** **Poisoning by insulin and oral hypoglycemic [antidiabetic] drugs, undetermined**

⑦**T38.3X5** **Adverse effect of insulin and oral hypoglycemic [antidiabetic] drugs**

⑦**T38.3X6** **Underdosing of insulin and oral hypoglycemic [antidiabetic] drugs**

T38.4 **Poisoning by, adverse effect of and underdosing of oral contraceptives**

Poisoning by, adverse effect of and underdosing of multiple- and single-ingredient oral contraceptive preparations

T38.4X **Poisoning by, adverse effect of and underdosing of oral contraceptives**

⑦**T38.4X1** **Poisoning by oral contraceptives, accidental (unintentional)**

Poisoning by oral contraceptives NOS

⑦**T38.4X2** **Poisoning by oral contraceptives, intentional self-harm**

⑦**T38.4X3** **Poisoning by oral contraceptives, assault**

⑦**T38.4X4** **Poisoning by oral contraceptives, undetermined**

⑦**T38.4X5** **Adverse effect of oral contraceptives**

⑦**T38.4X6** **Underdosing of oral contraceptives**

T38.5 **Poisoning by, adverse effect of and underdosing of other estrogens and progestogens**

Poisoning by, adverse effect of and underdosing of estrogens and progestogens mixtures and substitutes

T38.5X **Poisoning by, adverse effect of and underdosing of other estrogens and progestogens**

⑦**T38.5X1** **Poisoning by other estrogens and progestogens, accidental (unintentional)**

Poisoning by other estrogens and progestogens NOS

⑦**T38.5X2** **Poisoning by other estrogens and progestogens, intentional self-harm**

⑦**T38.5X3** **Poisoning by other estrogens and progestogens, assault**

⑦**T38.5X4** **Poisoning by other estrogens and progestogens, undetermined**

⑦ **T38.5X5**   Adverse effect of other estrogens and progestogens

⑦ **T38.5X6**   Underdosing of other estrogens and progestogens

T38.6   Poisoning by, adverse effect of and underdosing of antigonadotrophins, antiestrogens, antiandrogens, not elsewhere classified

Poisoning by, adverse effect of and underdosing of tamoxifen

T38.6X   Poisoning by, adverse effect of and underdosing of antigonadotrophins, antiestrogens, antiandrogens, not elsewhere classified

⑦ **T38.6X1**   Poisoning by antigonadotrophins, antiestrogens, antiandrogens, not elsewhere classified, accidental (unintentional)

Poisoning by antigonadotrophins, antiestrogens, antiandrogens, not elsewhere classified NOS

⑦ **T38.6X2**   Poisoning by antigonadotrophins, antiestrogens, antiandrogens, not elsewhere classified, intentional self-harm

⑦ **T38.6X3**   Poisoning by antigonadotrophins, antiestrogens, antiandrogens, not elsewhere classified, assault

⑦ **T38.6X4**   Poisoning by antigonadotrophins, antiestrogens, antiandrogens, not elsewhere classified, undetermined

⑦ **T38.6X5**   Adverse effect of antigonadotrophins, antiestrogens, antiandrogens, not elsewhere classified

⑦ **T38.6X6**   Underdosing of antigonadotrophins, antiestrogens, antiandrogens, not elsewhere classified

T38.7   Poisoning by, adverse effect of and underdosing of androgens and anabolic congeners

T38.7X   Poisoning by, adverse effect of and underdosing of androgens and anabolic congeners

⑦ **T38.7X1**   Poisoning by androgens and anabolic congeners, accidental (unintentional)

Poisoning by androgens and anabolic congeners NOS

⑦ **T38.7X2**   Poisoning by androgens and anabolic congeners, intentional self-harm

⑦ **T38.7X3**   Poisoning by androgens and anabolic congeners, assault

⑦ **T38.7X4**   Poisoning by androgens and anabolic congeners, undetermined

⑦ **T38.7X5**   Adverse effect of androgens and anabolic congeners

⑦ **T38.7X6**   Underdosing of androgens and anabolic congeners

T38.8   Poisoning by, adverse effect of and underdosing of other and unspecified hormones and synthetic substitutes

⑦ **T38.80** Poisoning by, adverse effect of and underdosing of unspecified hormones and synthetic substitutes

⑦ **T38.801**   Poisoning by unspecified hormones and synthetic substitutes, accidental (unintentional)

Poisoning by unspecified hormones and synthetic substitutes NOS

⑦ **T38.802**   Poisoning by unspecified hormones and synthetic substitutes, intentional self-harm

⑦ **T38.803**   Poisoning by unspecified hormones and synthetic substitutes, assault

⑦ **T38.804**   Poisoning by unspecified hormones and synthetic substitutes, undetermined

⑦ **T38.805**   Adverse effect of unspecified hormones and synthetic substitutes

⑦ **T38.806**   Underdosing of unspecified hormones and synthetic substitutes

T38.81   Poisoning by, adverse effect of and underdosing of anterior pituitary [adenohypophyseal] hormones

⑦ **T38.811**   Poisoning by anterior pituitary [adenohypophyseal] hormones, accidental (unintentional)

Poisoning by anterior pituitary [adenohypophyseal] hormones NOS

⑦ **T38.812**   Poisoning by anterior pituitary [adenohypophyseal] hormones, intentional self-harm

⑦ **T38.813**   Poisoning by anterior pituitary [adenohypophyseal] hormones, assault

⑦ **T38.814**   Poisoning by anterior pituitary [adenohypophyseal] hormones, undetermined

⑦ **T38.815**   Adverse effect of anterior pituitary [adenohypophyseal] hormones

⑦ **T38.816**   Underdosing of anterior pituitary [adenohypophyseal] hormones

T38.89   Poisoning by, adverse effect of and underdosing of other hormones and synthetic substitutes

⑦ **T38.891**   Poisoning by other hormones and synthetic substitutes, accidental (unintentional)

Poisoning by other hormones and synthetic substitutes NOS

⑦ **T38.892**   Poisoning by other hormones and synthetic substitutes, intentional self-harm

⑦ **T38.893**   Poisoning by other hormones and synthetic substitutes, assault

⑦ **T38.894**   Poisoning by other hormones and synthetic substitutes, undetermined

⑦ **T38.895**   Adverse effect of other hormones and synthetic substitutes

⑦ **T38.896**   Underdosing of other hormones and synthetic substitutes

T38.9   Poisoning by, adverse effect of and underdosing of other and unspecified hormone antagonists

T38.90   Poisoning by, adverse effect of and underdosing of unspecified hormone antagonists

⑦ **T38.901**   Poisoning by unspecified hormone antagonists, accidental (unintentional)

Poisoning by unspecified hormone antagonists NOS

⑦ **T38.902**   Poisoning by unspecified hormone antagonists, intentional self-harm

⑦ **T38.903**   Poisoning by unspecified hormone antagonists, assault

⑦ **T38.904**   Poisoning by unspecified hormone antagonists, undetermined

● New code   ▲ Revised code   **Excludes1:** Not coded here   **Excludes2:** Not included here   ⊗ Placeholder required   ⑦ 7ᵗʰ digit required

⑦**T38.905** **Adverse effect of unspecified hormone antagonists**

⑦**T38.906** **Underdosing of unspecified hormone antagonists**

T38.99 **Poisoning by, adverse effect of and underdosing of other hormone antagonists**

⑦**T38.991** **Poisoning by other hormone antagonists, accidental (unintentional)**

Poisoning by other hormone antagonists NOS

⑦**T38.992** **Poisoning by other hormone antagonists, intentional self-harm**

⑦**T38.993** **Poisoning by other hormone antagonists, assault**

⑦**T38.994** **Poisoning by other hormone antagonists, undetermined**

⑦**T38.995** **Adverse effect of other hormone antagonists**

⑦**T38.996** **Underdosing of other hormone antagonists**

T39 **Poisoning by, adverse effect of and underdosing of nonopioid analgesics, antipyretics and antirheumatics**

The appropriate 7th character is to be added to each code from category T39

A - initial encounter

D - subsequent encounter

S - sequela

T39.0 **Poisoning by, adverse effect of and underdosing of salicylates**

T39.01 **Poisoning by, adverse effect of and underdosing of aspirin**

Poisoning by, adverse effect of and underdosing of acetylsalicylic acid

⑦**T39.011** **Poisoning by aspirin, accidental (unintentional)**

⑦**T39.012** **Poisoning by aspirin, intentional self-harm**

⑦**T39.013** **Poisoning by aspirin, assault**

⑦**T39.014** **Poisoning by aspirin, undetermined**

⑦**T39.015** **Adverse effect of aspirin**

⑦**T39.016** **Underdosing of aspirin**

T39.09 **Poisoning by, adverse effect of and underdosing of other salicylates**

⑦**T39.091** **Poisoning by salicylates, accidental (unintentional)**

Poisoning by salicylates NOS

⑦**T39.092** **Poisoning by salicylates, intentional self-harm**

⑦**T39.093** **Poisoning by salicylates, assault**

⑦**T39.094** **Poisoning by salicylates, undetermined**

⑦**T39.095** **Adverse effect of salicylates**

⑦**T39.096** **Underdosing of salicylates**

T39.1 **Poisoning by, adverse effect of and underdosing of 4-Aminophenol derivatives**

T39.1X **Poisoning by, adverse effect of and underdosing of 4-Aminophenol derivatives**

⑦**T39.1X1** **Poisoning by 4-Aminophenol derivatives, accidental (unintentional)**

Poisoning by 4-Aminophenol derivatives NOS

⑦**T39.1X2** **Poisoning by 4-Aminophenol derivatives, intentional self-harm**

⑦**T39.1X3** **Poisoning by 4-Aminophenol derivatives, assault**

⑦**T39.1X4** **Poisoning by 4-Aminophenol derivatives, undetermined**

⑦**T39.1X5** **Adverse effect of 4-Aminophenol derivatives**

⑦**T39.1X6** **Underdosing of 4-Aminophenol derivatives**

T39.2 **Poisoning by, adverse effect of and underdosing of pyrazolone derivatives**

T39.2X **Poisoning by, adverse effect of and underdosing of pyrazolone derivatives**

⑦**T39.2X1** **Poisoning by pyrazolone derivatives, accidental (unintentional)**

Poisoning by pyrazolone derivatives NOS

⑦**T39.2X2** **Poisoning by pyrazolone derivatives, intentional self-harm**

⑦**T39.2X3** **Poisoning by pyrazolone derivatives, assault**

⑦**T39.2X4** **Poisoning by pyrazolone derivatives, undetermined**

⑦**T39.2X5** **Adverse effect of pyrazolone derivatives**

⑦**T39.2X6** **Underdosing of pyrazolone derivatives**

T39.3 **Poisoning by, adverse effect of and underdosing of other nonsteroidal anti-inflammatory drugs [NSAID]**

T39.31 **Poisoning by, adverse effect of and underdosing of propionic acid derivatives**

Poisoning by, adverse effect of and underdosing of fenoprofen

Poisoning by, adverse effect of and underdosing of flurbiprofen

Poisoning by, adverse effect of and underdosing of ibuprofen

Poisoning by, adverse effect of and underdosing of ketoprofen

Poisoning by, adverse effect of and underdosing of naproxen

Poisoning by, adverse effect of and underdosing of oxaprozin

⑦**T39.311** **Poisoning by propionic acid derivatives, accidental (unintentional)**

⑦**T39.312** **Poisoning by propionic acid derivatives, intentional self-harm**

⑦**T39.313** **Poisoning by propionic acid derivatives, assault**

⑦**T39.314** **Poisoning by propionic acid derivatives, undetermined**

⑦**T39.315** **Adverse effect of propionic acid derivatives**

⑦**T39.316** **Underdosing of propionic acid derivatives**

T39.39 **Poisoning by, adverse effect of and underdosing of other nonsteroidal anti-inflammatory drugs [NSAID]**

⑦**T39.391** **Poisoning by other nonsteroidal anti-inflammatory drugs [NSAID], accidental (unintentional)**

Poisoning by other nonsteroidal anti-inflammatory drugs NOS

⑦ **T39.392** **Poisoning by other nonsteroidal anti-inflammatory drugs [NSAID], intentional self-harm**

⑦ **T39.393** **Poisoning by other nonsteroidal anti-inflammatory drugs [NSAID], assault**

⑦ **T39.394** **Poisoning by other nonsteroidal anti-inflammatory drugs [NSAID], undetermined**

⑦ **T39.395** **Adverse effect of other nonsteroidal anti-inflammatory drugs [NSAID]**

⑦ **T39.396** **Underdosing of other nonsteroidal anti-inflammatory drugs [NSAID]**

T39.4 **Poisoning by, adverse effect of and underdosing of antirheumatics, not elsewhere classified**

Excludes1: poisoning by, adverse effect of and underdosing of glucocorticoids (T38.0-)

poisoning by, adverse effect of and underdosing of salicylates (T39.0-)

T39.4X **Poisoning by, adverse effect of and underdosing of antirheumatics, not elsewhere classified**

⑦ **T39.4X1** **Poisoning by antirheumatics, not elsewhere classified, accidental (unintentional)**

Poisoning by antirheumatics, not elsewhere classified NOS

⑦ **T39.4X2** **Poisoning by antirheumatics, not elsewhere classified, intentional self-harm**

⑦ **T39.4X3** **Poisoning by antirheumatics, not elsewhere classified, assault**

⑦ **T39.4X4** **Poisoning by antirheumatics, not elsewhere classified, undetermined**

⑦ **T39.4X5** **Adverse effect of antirheumatics, not elsewhere classified**

⑦ **T39.4X6** **Underdosing of antirheumatics, not elsewhere classified**

T39.8 **Poisoning by, adverse effect of and underdosing of other nonopioid analgesics and antipyretics, not elsewhere classified**

T39.8X **Poisoning by, adverse effect of and underdosing of other nonopioid analgesics and antipyretics, not elsewhere classified**

⑦ **T39.8X1** **Poisoning by other nonopioid analgesics and antipyretics, not elsewhere classified, accidental (unintentional)**

Poisoning by other nonopioid analgesics and antipyretics, not elsewhere classified NOS

⑦ **T39.8X2** **Poisoning by other nonopioid analgesics and antipyretics, not elsewhere classified, intentional self-harm**

⑦ **T39.8X3** **Poisoning by other nonopioid analgesics and antipyretics, not elsewhere classified, assault**

⑦ **T39.8X4** **Poisoning by other nonopioid analgesics and antipyretics, not elsewhere classified, undetermined**

⑦ **T39.8X5** **Adverse effect of other nonopioid analgesics and antipyretics, not elsewhere classified**

⑦ **T39.8X6** **Underdosing of other nonopioid analgesics and antipyretics, not elsewhere classified**

T39.9 **Poisoning by, adverse effect of and underdosing of unspecified nonopioid analgesic, antipyretic and antirheumatic**

⊗⑦ **T39.91** **Poisoning by unspecified nonopioid analgesic, antipyretic and antirheumatic, accidental (unintentional)**

Poisoning by nonopioid analgesic, antipyretic and antirheumatic NOS

⊗⑦ **T39.92** **Poisoning by unspecified nonopioid analgesic, antipyretic and antirheumatic, intentional self-harm**

⊗⑦ **T39.93** **Poisoning by unspecified nonopioid analgesic, antipyretic and antirheumatic, assault**

⊗⑦ **T39.94** **Poisoning by unspecified nonopioid analgesic, antipyretic and antirheumatic, undetermined**

⊗⑦ **T39.95** **Adverse effect of unspecified nonopioid analgesic, antipyretic and antirheumatic**

⊗⑦ **T39.96** **Underdosing of unspecified nonopioid analgesic, antipyretic and antirheumatic**

T40 **Poisoning by, adverse effect of and underdosing of narcotics and psychodysleptics [hallucinogens]**

Excludes2: drug dependence and related mental and behavioral disorders due to psychoactive substance use (F10.-F19.-)

The appropriate 7th character is to be added to each code from category T40

A - initial encounter

D - subsequent encounter

S - sequela

T40.0 **Poisoning by, adverse effect of and underdosing of opium**

T40.0X **Poisoning by, adverse effect of and underdosing of opium**

⑦ **T40.0X1** **Poisoning by opium, accidental (unintentional)**

Poisoning by opium NOS

⑦ **T40.0X2** **Poisoning by opium, intentional self-harm**

⑦ **T40.0X3** **Poisoning by opium, assault**

⑦ **T40.0X4** **Poisoning by opium, undetermined**

⑦ **T40.0X5** **Adverse effect of opium**

⑦ **T40.0X6** **Underdosing of opium**

T40.1 **Poisoning by and adverse effect of heroin**

T40.1X **Poisoning by and adverse effect of heroin**

⑦ **T40.1X1** **Poisoning by heroin, accidental (unintentional)**

Poisoning by heroin NOS

⑦ **T40.1X2** **Poisoning by heroin, intentional self-harm**

⑦ **T40.1X3** **Poisoning by heroin, assault**

⑦ **T40.1X4** **Poisoning by heroin, undetermined**

T40.2 **Poisoning by, adverse effect of and underdosing of other opioids**

T40.2X **Poisoning by, adverse effect of and underdosing of other opioids**

⑦ **T40.2X1** **Poisoning by other opioids, accidental (unintentional)**

Poisoning by other opioids NOS

⑦ **T40.2X2** **Poisoning by other opioids, intentional self-harm**

⑦ **T40.2X3** **Poisoning by other opioids, assault**

⑦ **T40.2X4** **Poisoning by other opioids, undetermined**

● New code ▲ Revised code **Excludes1:** Not coded here **Excludes2:** Not included here ⊗ Placeholder required ⑦ 7th digit required

⑦T40.2X5   Adverse effect of other opioids

⑦T40.2X6   Underdosing of other opioids

T40.3   Poisoning by, adverse effect of and underdosing of methadone

    T40.3X   Poisoning by, adverse effect of and underdosing of methadone

      ⑦T40.3X1   Poisoning by methadone, accidental (unintentional)

        Poisoning by methadone NOS

      ⑦T40.3X2   Poisoning by methadone, intentional self-harm

      ⑦T40.3X3   Poisoning by methadone, assault

      ⑦T40.3X4   Poisoning by methadone, undetermined

      ⑦T40.3X5   Adverse effect of methadone

      ⑦T40.3X6   Underdosing of methadone

T40.4   Poisoning by, adverse effect of and underdosing of other synthetic narcotics

    T40.4X   Poisoning by, adverse effect of and underdosing of other synthetic narcotics

      ⑦T40.4X1   Poisoning by other synthetic narcotics, accidental (unintentional)

        Poisoning by other synthetic narcotics NOS

      ⑦T40.4X2   Poisoning by other synthetic narcotics, intentional self-harm

      ⑦T40.4X3   Poisoning by other synthetic narcotics, assault

      ⑦T40.4X4   Poisoning by other synthetic narcotics, undetermined

      ⑦T40.4X5   Adverse effect of other synthetic narcotics

      ⑦T40.4X6   Underdosing of other synthetic narcotics

T40.5   Poisoning by, adverse effect of and underdosing of cocaine

    T40.5X   Poisoning by, adverse effect of and underdosing of cocaine

      ⑦T40.5X1   Poisoning by cocaine, accidental (unintentional)

        Poisoning by cocaine NOS

      ⑦T40.5X2   Poisoning by cocaine, intentional self-harm

      ⑦T40.5X3   Poisoning by cocaine, assault

      ⑦T40.5X4   Poisoning by cocaine, undetermined

      ⑦T40.5X5   Adverse effect of cocaine

      ⑦T40.5X6   Underdosing of cocaine

T40.6   Poisoning by, adverse effect of and underdosing of other and unspecified narcotics

    T40.60   Poisoning by, adverse effect of and underdosing of unspecified narcotics

      ⑦T40.601   Poisoning by unspecified narcotics, accidental (unintentional)

        Poisoning by narcotics NOS

      ⑦T40.602   Poisoning by unspecified narcotics, intentional self-harm

      ⑦T40.603   Poisoning by unspecified narcotics, assault

      ⑦T40.604   Poisoning by unspecified narcotics, undetermined

      ⑦T40.605   Adverse effect of unspecified narcotics

      ⑦T40.606   Underdosing of unspecified narcotics

T40.69   Poisoning by, adverse effect of and underdosing of other narcotics

      ⑦T40.691   Poisoning by other narcotics, accidental (unintentional)

        Poisoning by other narcotics NOS

      ⑦T40.692   Poisoning by other narcotics, intentional self-harm

      ⑦T40.693   Poisoning by other narcotics, assault

      ⑦T40.694   Poisoning by other narcotics, undetermined

      ⑦T40.695   Adverse effect of other narcotics

      ⑦T40.696   Underdosing of other narcotics

T40.7   Poisoning by, adverse effect of and underdosing of cannabis (derivatives)

    T40.7X   Poisoning by, adverse effect of and underdosing of cannabis (derivatives)

      ⑦T40.7X1   Poisoning by cannabis (derivatives), accidental (unintentional)

        Poisoning by cannabis NOS

      ⑦T40.7X2   Poisoning by cannabis (derivatives), intentional self-harm

      ⑦T40.7X3   Poisoning by cannabis (derivatives), assault

      ⑦T40.7X4   Poisoning by cannabis (derivatives), undetermined

      ⑦T40.7X5   Adverse effect of cannabis (derivatives)

      ⑦T40.7X6   Underdosing of cannabis (derivatives)

T40.8   Poisoning by and adverse effect of lysergide [LSD]

    T40.8X   Poisoning by and adverse effect of lysergide [LSD]

      ⑦T40.8X1   Poisoning by lysergide [LSD], accidental (unintentional)

        Poisoning by lysergide [LSD]NOS

      ⑦T40.8X2   Poisoning by lysergide [LSD], intentional self-harm

      ⑦T40.8X3   Poisoning by lysergide [LSD], assault

      ⑦T40.8X4   Poisoning by lysergide [LSD], undetermined

T40.9   Poisoning by, adverse effect of and underdosing of other and unspecified psychodysleptics [hallucinogens]

    T40.90   Poisoning by, adverse effect of and underdosing of unspecified psychodysleptics [hallucinogens]

      ⑦T40.901   Poisoning by unspecified psychodysleptics [hallucinogens], accidental (unintentional)

      ⑦T40.902   Poisoning by unspecified psychodysleptics [hallucinogens], intentional self-harm

      ⑦T40.903   Poisoning by unspecified psychodysleptics [hallucinogens], assault

      ⑦T40.904   Poisoning by unspecified psychodysleptics [hallucinogens], undetermined

      ⑦T40.905   Adverse effect of unspecified psychodysleptics [hallucinogens]

      ⑦T40.906   Underdosing of unspecified psychodysleptics

    T40.99   Poisoning by, adverse effect of and underdosing of other psychodysleptics [hallucinogens]

■ Add 4th-7th digits   Nonspecific code   Unspecified code   Manifestation code

⑦**T40.991** **Poisoning by other psychodysleptics [hallucinogens], accidental (unintentional)**

Poisoning by other psychodysleptics [hallucinogens] NOS

⑦**T40.992** **Poisoning by other psychodysleptics [hallucinogens], intentional self-harm**

⑦**T40.993** **Poisoning by other psychodysleptics [hallucinogens], assault**

⑦**T40.994** **Poisoning by other psychodysleptics [hallucinogens], undetermined**

⑦**T40.995** **Adverse effect of other psychodysleptics [hallucinogens]**

⑦**T40.996** **Underdosing of other psychodysleptics**

T41 **Poisoning by, adverse effect of and underdosing of anesthetics and therapeutic gases**

Excludes1: benzodiazepines (T42.4-)

cocaine (T40.5-)

complications of anesthesia during pregnancy (O29.-)

complications of anesthesia during labor and delivery (O74.-)

complications of anesthesia during the puerperium (O89.-)

opioids (T40.0-T40.2-)

The appropriate 7th character is to be added to each code from category T41

A - initial encounter

D - subsequent encounter

S - sequela

T41.0 **Poisoning by, adverse effect of and underdosing of inhaled anesthetics**

Excludes1: oxygen (T41.5-)

T41.0X **Poisoning by, adverse effect of and underdosing of inhaled anesthetics**

⑦**T41.0X1** **Poisoning by inhaled anesthetics, accidental (unintentional)**

Poisoning by inhaled anesthetics NOS

⑦**T41.0X2** **Poisoning by inhaled anesthetics, intentional self-harm**

⑦**T41.0X3** **Poisoning by inhaled anesthetics, assault**

⑦**T41.0X4** **Poisoning by inhaled anesthetics, undetermined**

⑦**T41.0X5** **Adverse effect of inhaled anesthetics**

⑦**T41.0X6** **Underdosing of inhaled anesthetics**

T41.1 **Poisoning by, adverse effect of and underdosing of intravenous anesthetics**

Poisoning by, adverse effect of and underdosing of thiobarbiturates

T41.1X **Poisoning by, adverse effect of and underdosing of intravenous anesthetics**

⑦**T41.1X1** **Poisoning by intravenous anesthetics, accidental (unintentional)**

Poisoning by intravenous anesthetics NOS

⑦**T41.1X2** **Poisoning by intravenous anesthetics, intentional self-harm**

⑦**T41.1X3** **Poisoning by intravenous anesthetics, assault**

⑦**T41.1X4** **Poisoning by intravenous anesthetics, undetermined**

⑦**T41.1X5** **Adverse effect of intravenous anesthetics**

⑦**T41.1X6** **Underdosing of intravenous anesthetics**

T41.2 **Poisoning by, adverse effect of and underdosing of other and unspecified general anesthetics**

T41.20 **Poisoning by, adverse effect of and underdosing of unspecified general anesthetics**

⑦**T41.201** **Poisoning by unspecified general anesthetics, accidental (unintentional)**

Poisoning by general anesthetics NOS

⑦**T41.202** **Poisoning by unspecified general anesthetics, intentional self-harm**

⑦**T41.203** **Poisoning by unspecified general anesthetics, assault**

⑦**T41.204** **Poisoning by unspecified general anesthetics, undetermined**

⑦**T41.205** **Adverse effect of unspecified general anesthetics**

⑦**T41.206** **Underdosing of unspecified general anesthetics**

T41.29 **Poisoning by, adverse effect of and underdosing of other general anesthetics**

⑦**T41.291** **Poisoning by other general anesthetics, accidental (unintentional)**

Poisoning by other general anesthetics NOS

⑦**T41.292** **Poisoning by other general anesthetics, intentional self-harm**

⑦**T41.293** **Poisoning by other general anesthetics, assault**

⑦**T41.294** **Poisoning by other general anesthetics, undetermined**

⑦**T41.295** **Adverse effect of other general anesthetics**

⑦**T41.296** **Underdosing of other general anesthetics**

T41.3 **Poisoning by, adverse effect of and underdosing of local anesthetics**

Cocaine (topical)

Excludes2: poisoning by cocaine used as a central nervous system stimulant (T40.5X1-T40.5X4)

T41.3X **Poisoning by, adverse effect of and underdosing of local anesthetics**

⑦**T41.3X1** **Poisoning by local anesthetics, accidental (unintentional)**

Poisoning by local anesthetics NOS

⑦**T41.3X2** **Poisoning by local anesthetics, intentional self-harm**

⑦**T41.3X3** **Poisoning by local anesthetics, assault**

⑦**T41.3X4** **Poisoning by local anesthetics, undetermined**

⑦**T41.3X5** **Adverse effect of local anesthetics**

⑦**T41.3X6** **Underdosing of local anesthetics**

T41.4 **Poisoning by, adverse effect of and underdosing of unspecified anesthetic**

⊗⑦**T41.41** **Poisoning by unspecified anesthetic, accidental (unintentional)**

Poisoning by anesthetic NOS

⊗⑦**T41.42** **Poisoning by unspecified anesthetic, intentional self-harm**

⊗⑦**T41.43** **Poisoning by unspecified anesthetic, assault**

⊗⑦**T41.44** **Poisoning by unspecified anesthetic, undetermined**

⊗⑦**T41.45** **Adverse effect of unspecified anesthetic**

⊗⑦**T41.46** **Underdosing of unspecified anesthetics**

T41.5 **Poisoning by, adverse effect of and underdosing of therapeutic gases**

T41.5X **Poisoning by, adverse effect of and underdosing of therapeutic gases**

⑦**T41.5X1** **Poisoning by therapeutic gases, accidental (unintentional)**

Poisoning by therapeutic gases NOS

⑦**T41.5X2** **Poisoning by therapeutic gases, intentional self-harm**

⑦**T41.5X3** **Poisoning by therapeutic gases, assault**

⑦**T41.5X4** **Poisoning by therapeutic gases, undetermined**

⑦**T41.5X5** **Adverse effect of therapeutic gases**

⑦**T41.5X6** **Underdosing of therapeutic gases**

T42 **Poisoning by, adverse effect of and underdosing of antiepileptic, sedative- hypnotic and antiparkinsonism drugs**

Excludes2: drug dependence and related mental and behavioral disorders due to psychoactive substance use (F10.--F19.-)

The appropriate 7th character is to be added to each code from category T42

A - initial encounter

D - subsequent encounter

S - sequela

T42.0 **Poisoning by, adverse effect of and underdosing of hydantoin derivatives**

T42.0X **Poisoning by, adverse effect of and underdosing of hydantoin derivatives**

⑦**T42.0X1** **Poisoning by hydantoin derivatives, accidental (unintentional)**

Poisoning by hydantoin derivatives NOS

⑦**T42.0X2** **Poisoning by hydantoin derivatives, intentional self-harm**

⑦**T42.0X3** **Poisoning by hydantoin derivatives, assault**

⑦**T42.0X4** **Poisoning by hydantoin derivatives, undetermined**

⑦**T42.0X5** **Adverse effect of hydantoin derivatives**

⑦**T42.0X6** **Underdosing of hydantoin derivatives**

T42.1 **Poisoning by, adverse effect of and underdosing of iminostilbenes**

Poisoning by, adverse effect of and underdosing of carbamazepine

T42.1X **Poisoning by, adverse effect of and underdosing of iminostilbenes**

⑦**T42.1X1** **Poisoning by iminostilbenes, accidental (unintentional)**

Poisoning by iminostilbenes NOS

⑦**T42.1X2** **Poisoning by iminostilbenes, intentional self-harm**

⑦**T42.1X3** **Poisoning by iminostilbenes, assault**

⑦**T42.1X4** **Poisoning by iminostilbenes, undetermined**

⑦**T42.1X5** **Adverse effect of iminostilbenes**

⑦**T42.1X6** **Underdosing of iminostilbenes**

T42.2 **Poisoning by, adverse effect of and underdosing of succinimides and oxazolidinediones**

T42.2X **Poisoning by, adverse effect of and underdosing of succinimides and oxazolidinediones**

⑦**T42.2X1** **Poisoning by succinimides and oxazolidinediones, accidental (unintentional)**

Poisoning by succinimides and oxazolidinediones NOS

⑦**T42.2X2** **Poisoning by succinimides and oxazolidinediones, intentional self-harm**

⑦**T42.2X3** **Poisoning by succinimides and oxazolidinediones, assault**

⑦**T42.2X4** **Poisoning by succinimides and oxazolidinediones, undetermined**

⑦**T42.2X5** **Adverse effect of succinimides and oxazolidinediones**

⑦**T42.2X6** **Underdosing of succinimides and oxazolidinediones**

T42.3 **Poisoning by, adverse effect of and underdosing of barbiturates**

Excludes1: poisoning by, adverse effect of and underdosing of thiobarbiturates (T41.1-)

T42.3X **Poisoning by, adverse effect of and underdosing of barbiturates**

⑦**T42.3X1** **Poisoning by barbiturates, accidental (unintentional)**

Poisoning by barbiturates NOS

⑦**T42.3X2** **Poisoning by barbiturates, intentional self-harm**

⑦**T42.3X3** **Poisoning by barbiturates, assault**

⑦**T42.3X4** **Poisoning by barbiturates, undetermined**

⑦**T42.3X5** **Adverse effect of barbiturates**

⑦**T42.3X6** **Underdosing of barbiturates**

T42.4 **Poisoning by, adverse effect of and underdosing of benzodiazepines**

T42.4X **Poisoning by, adverse effect of and underdosing of benzodiazepines**

⑦**T42.4X1** **Poisoning by benzodiazepines, accidental (unintentional)**

Poisoning by benzodiazepines NOS

⑦**T42.4X2** **Poisoning by benzodiazepines, intentional self-harm**

⑦**T42.4X3** **Poisoning by benzodiazepines, assault**

⑦**T42.4X4** **Poisoning by benzodiazepines, undetermined**

⑦**T42.4X5** **Adverse effect of benzodiazepines**

⑦**T42.4X6** **Underdosing of benzodiazepines**

T42.5 **Poisoning by, adverse effect of and underdosing of mixed antiepileptics**

T42.5X **Poisoning by, adverse effect of and underdosing of antiepileptics**

⑦**T42.5X1** **Poisoning by mixed antiepileptics, accidental (unintentional)**

Poisoning by mixed antiepileptics NOS

⑦**T42.5X2** **Poisoning by mixed antiepileptics, intentional self-harm**

⑦**T42.5X3** **Poisoning by mixed antiepileptics, assault**

⑦ **T42.5X4** **Poisoning by mixed antiepileptics, undetermined**

⑦ **T42.5X5** **Adverse effect of mixed antiepileptics**

⑦ **T42.5X6** **Underdosing of mixed antiepileptics**

T42.6 **Poisoning by, adverse effect of and underdosing of other antiepileptic and sedative-hypnotic drugs**

Poisoning by, adverse effect of and underdosing of methaqualone

Poisoning by, adverse effect of and underdosing of valproic acid

Excludes1: poisoning by, adverse effect of and underdosing of carbamazepine (T42.1-)

T42.6X **Poisoning by, adverse effect of and underdosing of other antiepileptic and sedative-hypnotic drugs**

⑦ **T42.6X1** **Poisoning by other antiepileptic and sedative-hypnotic drugs, accidental (unintentional)**

Poisoning by other antiepileptic and sedative-hypnotic drugs NOS

⑦ **T42.6X2** **Poisoning by other antiepileptic and sedative-hypnotic drugs, intentional self-harm**

⑦ **T42.6X3** **Poisoning by other antiepileptic and sedative-hypnotic drugs, assault**

⑦ **T42.6X4** **Poisoning by other antiepileptic and sedative-hypnotic drugs, undetermined**

⑦ **T42.6X5** **Adverse effect of other antiepileptic and sedative-hypnotic drugs**

⑦ **T42.6X6** **Underdosing of other antiepileptic and sedative-hypnotic drugs**

T42.7 **Poisoning by, adverse effect of and underdosing of unspecified antiepileptic and sedative-hypnotic drugs**

⊗⑦ **T42.71** **Poisoning by unspecified antiepileptic and sedative-hypnotic drugs, accidental (unintentional)**

Poisoning by antiepileptic and sedative-hypnotic drugs NOS

⊗⑦ **T42.72** **Poisoning by unspecified antiepileptic and sedative-hypnotic drugs, intentional self-harm**

⊗⑦ **T42.73** **Poisoning by unspecified antiepileptic and sedative-hypnotic drugs, assault**

⊗⑦ **T42.74** **Poisoning by unspecified antiepileptic and sedative-hypnotic drugs, undetermined**

⊗⑦ **T42.75** **Adverse effect of unspecified antiepileptic and sedative-hypnotic drugs**

⊗⑦ **T42.76** **Underdosing of unspecified antiepileptic and sedative-hypnotic drugs**

T42.8 **Poisoning by, adverse effect of and underdosing of antiparkinsonism drugs and other central muscle-tone depressants**

Poisoning by, adverse effect of and underdosing of amantadine

T42.8X **Poisoning by, adverse effect of and underdosing of antiparkinsonism drugs and other central muscle-tone depressants**

⑦ **T42.8X1** **Poisoning by antiparkinsonism drugs and other central muscle-tone depressants, accidental (unintentional)**

Poisoning by antiparkinsonism drugs and other central muscle-tone depressants NOS

⑦ **T42.8X2** **Poisoning by antiparkinsonism drugs and other central muscle-tone depressants, intentional self-harm**

⑦ **T42.8X3** **Poisoning by antiparkinsonism drugs and other central muscle-tone depressants, assault**

⑦ **T42.8X4** **Poisoning by antiparkinsonism drugs and other central muscle-tone depressants, undetermined**

⑦ **T42.8X5** **Adverse effect of antiparkinsonism drugs and other central muscle-tone depressants**

⑦ **T42.8X6** **Underdosing of antiparkinsonism drugs and other central muscle-tone depressants**

T43 **Poisoning by, adverse effect of and underdosing of psychotropic drugs, not elsewhere classified**

Excludes1: appetite depressants (T50.5-)

barbiturates (T42.3-)

benzodiazepines (T42.4-)

methaqualone (T42.6-)

psychodysleptics [hallucinogens] (T40.7-T40.9-)

Excludes2: drug dependence and related mental and behavioral disorders due to psychoactive substance use (F10.--F19.-)

The appropriate 7th character is to be added to each code from category T43

A - initial encounter

D - subsequent encounter

S - sequela

T43.0 **Poisoning by, adverse effect of and underdosing of tricyclic and tetracyclic antidepressants**

T43.01 **Poisoning by, adverse effect of and underdosing of tricyclic antidepressants**

⑦ **T43.011** **Poisoning by tricyclic antidepressants, accidental (unintentional)**

Poisoning by tricyclic antidepressants NOS

⑦ **T43.012** **Poisoning by tricyclic antidepressants, intentional self-harm**

⑦ **T43.013** **Poisoning by tricyclic antidepressants, assault**

⑦ **T43.014** **Poisoning by tricyclic antidepressants, undetermined**

⑦ **T43.015** **Adverse effect of tricyclic antidepressants**

⑦ **T43.016** **Underdosing of tricyclic antidepressants**

T43.02 **Poisoning by, adverse effect of and underdosing of tetracyclic antidepressants**

⑦ **T43.021** **Poisoning by tetracyclic antidepressants, accidental (unintentional)**

Poisoning by tetracyclic antidepressants NOS

⑦ **T43.022** **Poisoning by tetracyclic antidepressants, intentional self-harm**

⑦ **T43.023** **Poisoning by tetracyclic antidepressants, assault**

⑦ **T43.024** **Poisoning by tetracyclic antidepressants, undetermined**

⑦T43.025 **Adverse effect of tetracyclic antidepressants**

⑦T43.026 **Underdosing of tetracyclic antidepressants**

T43.1 **Poisoning by, adverse effect of and underdosing of monoamine-oxidase-inhibitor antidepressants**

    T43.1X **Poisoning by, adverse effect of and underdosing of monoamine-oxidase-inhibitor antidepressants**

        ⑦T43.1X1 **Poisoning by monoamine-oxidase-inhibitor antidepressants, accidental (unintentional)**

            Poisoning by monoamine-oxidase-inhibitor antidepressants NOS

        ⑦T43.1X2 **Poisoning by monoamine-oxidase-inhibitor antidepressants, intentional self-harm**

        ⑦T43.1X3 **Poisoning by monoamine-oxidase-inhibitor antidepressants, assault**

        ⑦T43.1X4 **Poisoning by monoamine-oxidase-inhibitor antidepressants, undetermined**

        ⑦T43.1X5 **Adverse effect of monoamine-oxidase-inhibitor antidepressants**

        ⑦T43.1X6 **Underdosing of monoamine-oxidase-inhibitor antidepressants**

T43.2 **Poisoning by, adverse effect of and underdosing of other and unspecified antidepressants**

    T43.20 **Poisoning by, adverse effect of and underdosing of unspecified antidepressants**

        ⑦T43.201 **Poisoning by unspecified antidepressants, accidental (unintentional)**

            Poisoning by antidepressants NOS

        ⑦T43.202 **Poisoning by unspecified antidepressants, intentional self-harm**

        ⑦T43.203 **Poisoning by unspecified antidepressants, assault**

        ⑦T43.204 **Poisoning by unspecified antidepressants, undetermined**

        ⑦T43.205 **Adverse effect of unspecified antidepressants**

            Antidepressant discontinuation syndrome

        ⑦T43.206 **Underdosing of unspecified antidepressants**

    T43.21 **Poisoning by, adverse effect of and underdosing of selective serotonin and norepinephrine reuptake inhibitors**

        Poisoning by, adverse effect of and underdosing of SSNRI antidepressants

        ⑦T43.211 **Poisoning by selective serotonin and norepinephrine reuptake inhibitors, accidental (unintentional)**

        ⑦T43.212 **Poisoning by selective serotonin and norepinephrine reuptake inhibitors, intentional self-harm**

        ⑦T43.213 **Poisoning by selective serotonin and norepinephrine reuptake inhibitors, assault**

        ⑦T43.214 **Poisoning by selective serotonin and norepinephrine reuptake inhibitors, undetermined**

⑦T43.215 **Adverse effect of selective serotonin and norepinephrine reuptake inhibitors**

⑦T43.216 **Underdosing of selective serotonin and norepinephrine reuptake inhibitors**

    T43.22 **Poisoning by, adverse effect of and underdosing of selective serotonin reuptake inhibitors**

        Poisoning by, adverse effect of and underdosing of SSRI antidepressants

        ⑦T43.221 **Poisoning by selective serotonin reuptake inhibitors, accidental (unintentional)**

        ⑦T43.222 **Poisoning by selective serotonin reuptake inhibitors, intentional self-harm**

        ⑦T43.223 **Poisoning by selective serotonin reuptake inhibitors, assault**

        ⑦T43.224 **Poisoning by selective serotonin reuptake inhibitors, undetermined**

        ⑦T43.225 **Adverse effect of selective serotonin reuptake inhibitors**

        ⑦T43.226 **Underdosing of selective serotonin reuptake inhibitors**

    T43.29 **Poisoning by, adverse effect of and underdosing of other antidepressants**

        ⑦T43.291 **Poisoning by other antidepressants, accidental (unintentional)**

            Poisoning by other antidepressants NOS

        ⑦T43.292 **Poisoning by other antidepressants, intentional self-harm**

        ⑦T43.293 **Poisoning by other antidepressants, assault**

        ⑦T43.294 **Poisoning by other antidepressants, undetermined**

        ⑦T43.295 **Adverse effect of other antidepressants**

        ⑦T43.296 **Underdosing of other antidepressants**

T43.3 **Poisoning by, adverse effect of and underdosing of phenothiazine antipsychotics and neuroleptics**

    T43.3X **Poisoning by, adverse effect of and underdosing of phenothiazine antipsychotics and neuroleptics**

        ⑦T43.3X1 **Poisoning by phenothiazine antipsychotics and neuroleptics, accidental (unintentional)**

            Poisoning by phenothiazine antipsychotics and neuroleptics NOS

        ⑦T43.3X2 **Poisoning by phenothiazine antipsychotics and neuroleptics, intentional self-harm**

        ⑦T43.3X3 **Poisoning by phenothiazine antipsychotics and neuroleptics, assault**

        ⑦T43.3X4 **Poisoning by phenothiazine antipsychotics and neuroleptics, undetermined**

        ⑦T43.3X5 **Adverse effect of phenothiazine antipsychotics and neuroleptics**

        ⑦T43.3X6 **Underdosing of phenothiazine antipsychotics and neuroleptics**

T43.4 **Poisoning by, adverse effect of and underdosing of butyrophenone and thiothixene neuroleptics**

▓ Add 4th-7th digits	Nonspecific code	Unspecified code	Manifestation code

T43.4X **Poisoning by, adverse effect of and underdosing of butyrophenone and thiothixene neuroleptics**

⑦ **T43.4X1** **Poisoning by butyrophenone and thiothixene neuroleptics, accidental (unintentional)**

Poisoning by butyrophenone and thiothixene neuroleptics NOS

⑦ **T43.4X2** **Poisoning by butyrophenone and thiothixene neuroleptics, intentional self-harm**

⑦ **T43.4X3** **Poisoning by butyrophenone and thiothixene neuroleptics, assault**

⑦ **T43.4X4** **Poisoning by butyrophenone and thiothixene neuroleptics, undetermined**

⑦ **T43.4X5** **Adverse effect of butyrophenone and thiothixene neuroleptics**

⑦ **T43.4X6** **Underdosing of butyrophenone and thiothixene neuroleptics**

T43.5 **Poisoning by, adverse effect of and underdosing of other and unspecified antipsychotics and neuroleptics**

Excludes1: poisoning by, adverse effect of and underdosing of rauwolfia (T46.5-)

T43.50 **Poisoning by, adverse effect of and underdosing of unspecified antipsychotics and neuroleptics**

⑦ **T43.501** **Poisoning by unspecified antipsychotics and neuroleptics, accidental (unintentional)**

Poisoning by antipsychotics and neuroleptics NOS

⑦ **T43.502** **Poisoning by unspecified antipsychotics and neuroleptics, intentional self-harm**

⑦ **T43.503** **Poisoning by unspecified antipsychotics and neuroleptics, assault**

⑦ **T43.504** **Poisoning by unspecified antipsychotics and neuroleptics, undetermined**

⑦ **T43.505** **Adverse effect of unspecified antipsychotics and neuroleptics**

⑦ **T43.506** **Underdosing of unspecified antipsychotics and neuroleptics**

T43.59 **Poisoning by, adverse effect of and underdosing of other antipsychotics and neuroleptics**

⑦ **T43.591** **Poisoning by other antipsychotics and neuroleptics, accidental (unintentional)**

Poisoning by other antipsychotics and neuroleptics NOS

⑦ **T43.592** **Poisoning by other antipsychotics and neuroleptics, intentional self-harm**

⑦ **T43.593** **Poisoning by other antipsychotics and neuroleptics, assault**

⑦ **T43.594** **Poisoning by other antipsychotics and neuroleptics, undetermined**

⑦ **T43.595** **Adverse effect of other antipsychotics and neuroleptics**

⑦ **T43.596** **Underdosing of other antipsychotics and neuroleptics**

T43.6 **Poisoning by, adverse effect of and underdosing of psychostimulants**

Excludes1: poisoning by, adverse effect of and underdosing of cocaine (T40.5-)

T43.60 **Poisoning by, adverse effect of and underdosing of unspecified psychostimulant**

⑦ **T43.601** **Poisoning by unspecified psychostimulants, accidental (unintentional)**

Poisoning by psychostimulants NOS

⑦ **T43.602** **Poisoning by unspecified psychostimulants, intentional self-harm**

⑦ **T43.603** **Poisoning by unspecified psychostimulants, assault**

⑦ **T43.604** **Poisoning by unspecified psychostimulants, undetermined**

⑦ **T43.605** **Adverse effect of unspecified psychostimulants**

⑦ **T43.606** **Underdosing of unspecified psychostimulants**

T43.61 **Poisoning by, adverse effect of and underdosing of caffeine**

⑦ **T43.611** **Poisoning by caffeine, accidental (unintentional)**

Poisoning by caffeine NOS

⑦ **T43.612** **Poisoning by caffeine, intentional self-harm**

⑦ **T43.613** **Poisoning by caffeine, assault**

⑦ **T43.614** **Poisoning by caffeine, undetermined**

⑦ **T43.615** **Adverse effect of caffeine**

⑦ **T43.616** **Underdosing of caffeine**

T43.62 **Poisoning by, adverse effect of and underdosing of amphetamines**

Poisoning by, adverse effect of and underdosing of methamphetamines

⑦ **T43.621** **Poisoning by amphetamines, accidental (unintentional)**

Poisoning by amphetamines NOS

⑦ **T43.622** **Poisoning by amphetamines, intentional self-harm**

⑦ **T43.623** **Poisoning by amphetamines, assault**

⑦ **T43.624** **Poisoning by amphetamines, undetermined**

⑦ **T43.625** **Adverse effect of amphetamines**

⑦ **T43.626** **Underdosing of amphetamines**

T43.63 **Poisoning by, adverse effect of and underdosing of methylphenidate**

⑦ **T43.631** **Poisoning by methylphenidate, accidental (unintentional)**

Poisoning by methylphenidate NOS

⑦ **T43.632** **Poisoning by methylphenidate, intentional self-harm**

⑦ **T43.633** **Poisoning by methylphenidate, assault**

⑦ **T43.634** **Poisoning by methylphenidate, undetermined**

⑦ **T43.635** **Adverse effect of methylphenidate**

⑦ **T43.636** **Underdosing of methylphenidate**

T43.69 **Poisoning by, adverse effect of and underdosing of other psychostimulants**

⑦ **T43.691** **Poisoning by other psychostimulants, accidental (unintentional)**

Poisoning by other psychostimulants NOS

⑦ **T43.692** **Poisoning by other psychostimulants, intentional self-harm**

● New code ▲ Revised code Excludes1: Not coded here Excludes2: Not included here ⊗ Placeholder required ⑦ 7th digit required

⑦T43.693 **Poisoning by other psychostimulants, assault**

⑦T43.694 **Poisoning by other psychostimulants, undetermined**

⑦T43.695 **Adverse effect of other psychostimulants**

⑦T43.696 **Underdosing of other psychostimulants**

T43.8 **Poisoning by, adverse effect of and underdosing of other psychotropic drugs**

T43.8X **Poisoning by, adverse effect of and underdosing of other psychotropic drugs**

⑦T43.8X1 **Poisoning by other psychotropic drugs, accidental (unintentional)**

Poisoning by other psychotropic drugs NOS

⑦T43.8X2 **Poisoning by other psychotropic drugs, intentional self-harm**

⑦T43.8X3 **Poisoning by other psychotropic drugs, assault**

⑦T43.8X4 **Poisoning by other psychotropic drugs, undetermined**

⑦T43.8X5 **Adverse effect of other psychotropic drugs**

⑦T43.8X6 **Underdosing of other psychotropic drugs**

T43.9 **Poisoning by, adverse effect of and underdosing of unspecified psychotropic drug**

⊗⑦T43.91 **Poisoning by unspecified psychotropic drug, accidental (unintentional)**

Poisoning by psychotropic drug NOS

⊗⑦T43.92 **Poisoning by unspecified psychotropic drug, intentional self-harm**

⊗⑦T43.93 **Poisoning by unspecified psychotropic drug, assault**

⊗⑦T43.94 **Poisoning by unspecified psychotropic drug, undetermined**

⊗⑦T43.95 **Adverse effect of unspecified psychotropic drug**

⊗⑦T43.96 **Underdosing of unspecified psychotropic drug**

T44 **Poisoning by, adverse effect of and underdosing of drugs primarily affecting the autonomic nervous system**

The appropriate 7th character is to be added to each code from category T44

A - initial encounter

D - subsequent encounter

S - sequela

T44.0 **Poisoning by, adverse effect of and underdosing of anticholinesterase agents**

T44.0X **Poisoning by, adverse effect of and underdosing of anticholinesterase agents**

⑦T44.0X1 **Poisoning by anticholinesterase agents, accidental (unintentional)**

poisoning by anticholinesterase agents NOS

⑦T44.0X2 **Poisoning by anticholinesterase agents, intentional self-harm**

⑦T44.0X3 **Poisoning by anticholinesterase agents, assault**

⑦T44.0X4 **Poisoning by anticholinesterase agents, undetermined**

⑦T44.0X5 **Adverse effect of anticholinesterase agents**

⑦T44.0X6 **Underdosing of anticholinesterase agents**

T44.1 **Poisoning by, adverse effect of and underdosing of other parasympathomimetics [cholinergics]**

T44.1X **Poisoning by, adverse effect of and underdosing of other parasympathomimetics [cholinergics]**

⑦T44.1X1 **Poisoning by other parasympathomimetics [cholinergics], accidental (unintentional)**

Poisoning by other parasympathomimetics [cholinergics] NOS

⑦T44.1X2 **Poisoning by other parasympathomimetics [cholinergics], intentional self-harm**

⑦T44.1X3 **Poisoning by other parasympathomimetics [cholinergics], assault**

⑦T44.1X4 **Poisoning by other parasympathomimetics [cholinergics], undetermined**

⑦T44.1X5 **Adverse effect of other parasympathomimetics [cholinergics]**

⑦T44.1X6 **Underdosing of other parasympathomimetics**

T44.2 **Poisoning by, adverse effect of and underdosing of ganglionic blocking drugs**

T44.2X **Poisoning by, adverse effect of and underdosing of ganglionic blocking drugs**

⑦T44.2X1 **Poisoning by ganglionic blocking drugs, accidental (unintentional)**

Poisoning by ganglionic blocking drugs NOS

⑦T44.2X2 **Poisoning by ganglionic blocking drugs, intentional self-harm**

⑦T44.2X3 **Poisoning by ganglionic blocking drugs, assault**

⑦T44.2X4 **Poisoning by ganglionic blocking drugs, undetermined**

⑦T44.2X5 **Adverse effect of ganglionic blocking drugs**

⑦T44.2X6 **Underdosing of ganglionic blocking drugs**

T44.3 **Poisoning by, adverse effect of and underdosing of other parasympatholytics [anticholinergics and antimuscarinics] and spasmolytics**

Poisoning by, adverse effect of and underdosing of papaverine

T44.3X **Poisoning by, adverse effect of and underdosing of other parasympatholytics [anticholinergics and antimuscarinics] and spasmolytics**

⑦T44.3X1 **Poisoning by other parasympatholytics [anticholinergics and antimuscarinics] and spasmolytics, accidental (unintentional)**

Poisoning by other parasympatholytics [anticholinergics and antimuscarinics] and spasmolytics NOS

⑦T44.3X2 **Poisoning by other parasympatholytics [anticholinergics and antimuscarinics] and spasmolytics, intentional self-harm**

⑦T44.3X3 **Poisoning by other parasympatholytics [anticholinergics and antimuscarinics] and spasmolytics, assault**

⑦ **T44.3X4** **Poisoning by other parasympatholytics [anticholinergics and antimuscarinics] and spasmolytics, undetermined**

⑦ **T44.3X5** **Adverse effect of other parasympatholytics [anticholinergics and antimuscarinics] and spasmolytics**

⑦ **T44.3X6** **Underdosing of other parasympatholytics [anticholinergics and antimuscarinics] and spasmolytics**

T44.4 **Poisoning by, adverse effect of and underdosing of predominantly alpha-adrenoreceptor agonists**

Poisoning by, adverse effect of and underdosing of metaraminol

T44.4X **Poisoning by, adverse effect of and underdosing of predominantly alpha-adrenoreceptor agonists**

⑦ **T44.4X1** **Poisoning by predominantly alpha-adrenoreceptor agonists, accidental (unintentional)**

Poisoning by predominantly alpha-adrenoreceptor agonists NOS

⑦ **T44.4X2** **Poisoning by predominantly alpha-adrenoreceptor agonists, intentional self-harm**

⑦ **T44.4X3** **Poisoning by predominantly alpha-adrenoreceptor agonists, assault**

⑦ **T44.4X4** **Poisoning by predominantly alpha-adrenoreceptor agonists, undetermined**

⑦ **T44.4X5** **Adverse effect of predominantly alpha-adrenoreceptor agonists**

⑦ **T44.4X6** **Underdosing of predominantly alpha-adrenoreceptor agonists**

T44.5 **Poisoning by, adverse effect of and underdosing of predominantly beta-adrenoreceptor agonists**

Excludes1: poisoning by, adverse effect of and underdosing of beta-adrenoreceptor agonists used in asthma therapy (T48.6-)

T44.5X **Poisoning by, adverse effect of and underdosing of predominantly beta-adrenoreceptor agonists**

⑦ **T44.5X1** **Poisoning by predominantly beta-adrenoreceptor agonists, accidental (unintentional)**

Poisoning by predominantly beta-adrenoreceptor agonists NOS

⑦ **T44.5X2** **Poisoning by predominantly beta-adrenoreceptor agonists, intentional self-harm**

⑦ **T44.5X3** **Poisoning by predominantly beta-adrenoreceptor agonists, assault**

⑦ **T44.5X4** **Poisoning by predominantly beta-adrenoreceptor agonists, undetermined**

⑦ **T44.5X5** **Adverse effect of predominantly beta-adrenoreceptor agonists**

⑦ **T44.5X6** **Underdosing of predominantly beta-adrenoreceptor agonists**

T44.6 **Poisoning by, adverse effect of and underdosing of alpha-adrenoreceptor antagonists**

Excludes1: poisoning by, adverse effect of and underdosing of ergot alkaloids (T48.0)

T44.6X **Poisoning by, adverse effect of and underdosing of alpha-adrenoreceptor antagonists**

⑦ **T44.6X1** **Poisoning by alpha-adrenoreceptor antagonists, accidental (unintentional)**

Poisoning by alpha-adrenoreceptor antagonists NOS

⑦ **T44.6X2** **Poisoning by alpha-adrenoreceptor antagonists, intentional self-harm**

⑦ **T44.6X3** **Poisoning by alpha-adrenoreceptor antagonists, assault**

⑦ **T44.6X4** **Poisoning by alpha-adrenoreceptor antagonists, undetermined**

⑦ **T44.6X5** **Adverse effect of alpha-adrenoreceptor antagonists**

⑦ **T44.6X6** **Underdosing of alpha-adrenoreceptor antagonists**

T44.7 **Poisoning by, adverse effect of and underdosing of beta-adrenoreceptor antagonists**

T44.7X **Poisoning by, adverse effect of and underdosing of beta-adrenoreceptor antagonists**

⑦ **T44.7X1** **Poisoning by beta-adrenoreceptor antagonists, accidental (unintentional)**

Poisoning by beta-adrenoreceptor antagonists NOS

⑦ **T44.7X2** **Poisoning by beta-adrenoreceptor antagonists, intentional self-harm**

⑦ **T44.7X3** **Poisoning by beta-adrenoreceptor antagonists, assault**

⑦ **T44.7X4** **Poisoning by beta-adrenoreceptor antagonists, undetermined**

⑦ **T44.7X5** **Adverse effect of beta-adrenoreceptor antagonists**

⑦ **T44.7X6** **Underdosing of beta-adrenoreceptor antagonists**

T44.8 **Poisoning by, adverse effect of and underdosing of centrally-acting and adrenergic-neuron- blocking agents**

Excludes1: poisoning by, adverse effect of and underdosing of clonidine (T46.5)

poisoning by, adverse effect of and underdosing of guanethidine (T46.5)

T44.8X **Poisoning by, adverse effect of and underdosing of centrally-acting and adrenergic- neuron- blocking agents**

⑦ **T44.8X1** **Poisoning by centrally-acting and adrenergic-neuron-blocking agents, accidental (unintentional)**

Poisoning by centrally-acting and adrenergic-neuron-blocking agents NOS

⑦ **T44.8X2** **Poisoning by centrally-acting and adrenergic-neuron-blocking agents, intentional self-harm**

⑦ **T44.8X3** **Poisoning by centrally-acting and adrenergic-neuron-blocking agents, assault**

⑦ **T44.8X4** **Poisoning by centrally-acting and adrenergic-neuron-blocking agents, undetermined**

⑦ **T44.8X5** **Adverse effect of centrally-acting and adrenergic-neuron-blocking agents**

⑦ **T44.8X6** **Underdosing of centrally-acting and adrenergic-neuron-blocking agents**

● New code ▲ Revised code **Excludes1:** Not coded here **Excludes2:** Not included here ⊗ Placeholder required ⑦ 7th digit required

T44.9 **Poisoning by, adverse effect of and underdosing of other and unspecified drugs primarily affecting the autonomic nervous system**

Poisoning by, adverse effect of and underdosing of drug stimulating both alpha and beta-adrenoreceptors

T44.90 **Poisoning by, adverse effect of and underdosing of unspecified drugs primarily affecting the autonomic nervous system**

⑦**T44.901** **Poisoning by unspecified drugs primarily affecting the autonomic nervous system, accidental (unintentional)**

Poisoning by unspecified drugs primarily affecting the autonomic nervous system NOS

⑦**T44.902** **Poisoning by unspecified drugs primarily affecting the autonomic nervous system, intentional self-harm**

⑦**T44.903** **Poisoning by unspecified drugs primarily affecting the autonomic nervous system, assault**

⑦**T44.904** **Poisoning by unspecified drugs primarily affecting the autonomic nervous system, undetermined**

⑦**T44.905** **Adverse effect of unspecified drugs primarily affecting the autonomic nervous system**

⑦**T44.906** **Underdosing of unspecified drugs primarily affecting the autonomic nervous system**

T44.99 **Poisoning by, adverse effect of and underdosing of other drugs primarily affecting the autonomic nervous system**

⑦**T44.991** **Poisoning by other drug primarily affecting the autonomic nervous system, accidental (unintentional)**

Poisoning by other drugs primarily affecting the autonomic nervous system NOS

⑦**T44.992** **Poisoning by other drug primarily affecting the autonomic nervous system, intentional self-harm**

⑦**T44.993** **Poisoning by other drug primarily affecting the autonomic nervous system, assault**

⑦**T44.994** **Poisoning by other drug primarily affecting the autonomic nervous system, undetermined**

⑦**T44.995** **Adverse effect of other drug primarily affecting the autonomic nervous system**

⑦**T44.996** **Underdosing of other drug primarily affecting the autonomic nervous system**

T45 **Poisoning by, adverse effect of and underdosing of primarily systemic and hematological agents, not elsewhere classified**

The appropriate 7th character is to be added to each code from category T45

A - initial encounter

D - subsequent encounter

S - sequela

T45.0 **Poisoning by, adverse effect of and underdosing of antiallergic and antiemetic drugs**

Excludes1: poisoning by, adverse effect of and underdosing of phenothiazine-based neuroleptics (T43.3)

T45.0X **Poisoning by, adverse effect of and underdosing of antiallergic and antiemetic drugs**

⑦**T45.0X1** **Poisoning by antiallergic and antiemetic drugs, accidental (unintentional)**

Poisoning by antiallergic and antiemetic drugs NOS

⑦**T45.0X2** **Poisoning by antiallergic and antiemetic drugs, intentional self-harm**

⑦**T45.0X3** **Poisoning by antiallergic and antiemetic drugs, assault**

⑦**T45.0X4** **Poisoning by antiallergic and antiemetic drugs, undetermined**

⑦**T45.0X5** **Adverse effect of antiallergic and antiemetic drugs**

⑦**T45.0X6** **Underdosing of antiallergic and antiemetic drugs**

T45.1 **Poisoning by, adverse effect of and underdosing of antineoplastic and immunosuppressive drugs**

Excludes1: poisoning by, adverse effect of and underdosing of tamoxifen (T38.6)

T45.1X **Poisoning by, adverse effect of and underdosing of antineoplastic and immunosuppressive drugs**

⑦**T45.1X1** **Poisoning by antineoplastic and immunosuppressive drugs, accidental (unintentional)**

Poisoning by antineoplastic and immunosuppressive drugs NOS

⑦**T45.1X2** **Poisoning by antineoplastic and immunosuppressive drugs, intentional self-harm**

⑦**T45.1X3** **Poisoning by antineoplastic and immunosuppressive drugs, assault**

⑦**T45.1X4** **Poisoning by antineoplastic and immunosuppressive drugs, undetermined**

⑦**T45.1X5** **Adverse effect of antineoplastic and immunosuppressive drugs**

⑦**T45.1X6** **Underdosing of antineoplastic and immunosuppressive drugs**

T45.2 **Poisoning by, adverse effect of and underdosing of vitamins**

Excludes2: poisoning by, adverse effect of and underdosing of nicotinic acid (derivatives) (T46.7)

poisoning by, adverse effect of and underdosing of iron (T45.4)

poisoning by, adverse effect of and underdosing of vitamin K (T45.7)

T45.2X **Poisoning by, adverse effect of and underdosing of vitamins**

⑦**T45.2X1** **Poisoning by vitamins, accidental (unintentional)**

Poisoning by vitamins NOS

⑦**T45.2X2** **Poisoning by vitamins, intentional self-harm**

⑦**T45.2X3** **Poisoning by vitamins, assault**

⑦**T45.2X4** **Poisoning by vitamins, undetermined**

⑦**T45.2X5** **Adverse effect of vitamins**

⑦**T45.2X6** **Underdosing of vitamins**

Excludes1: vitamin deficiencies (E50-E56)

T45.3 **Poisoning by, adverse effect of and underdosing of enzymes**

T45.3X   **Poisoning by, adverse effect of and underdosing of enzymes**

⑦T45.3X1   **Poisoning by enzymes, accidental (unintentional)**

Poisoning by enzymes NOS

⑦T45.3X2   **Poisoning by enzymes, intentional self-harm**

⑦T45.3X3   **Poisoning by enzymes, assault**

⑦T45.3X4   **Poisoning by enzymes, undetermined**

⑦T45.3X5   **Adverse effect of enzymes**

⑦T45.3X6   **Underdosing of enzymes**

T45.4   **Poisoning by, adverse effect of and underdosing of iron and its compounds**

T45.4X   **Poisoning by, adverse effect of and underdosing of iron and its compounds**

⑦T45.4X1   **Poisoning by iron and its compounds, accidental (unintentional)**

Poisoning by iron and its compounds NOS

⑦T45.4X2   **Poisoning by iron and its compounds, intentional self-harm**

⑦T45.4X3   **Poisoning by iron and its compounds, assault**

⑦T45.4X4   **Poisoning by iron and its compounds, undetermined**

⑦T45.4X5   **Adverse effect of iron and its compounds**

⑦T45.4X6   **Underdosing of iron and its compounds**
Excludes1: iron deficiency (E61.1)

T45.5   **Poisoning by, adverse effect of and underdosing of anticoagulants and antithrombotic drugs**

T45.51   **Poisoning by, adverse effect of and underdosing of anticoagulants**

⑦T45.511   **Poisoning by anticoagulants, accidental (unintentional)**

Poisoning by anticoagulants NOS

⑦T45.512   **Poisoning by anticoagulants, intentional self-harm**

⑦T45.513   **Poisoning by anticoagulants, assault**

⑦T45.514   **Poisoning by anticoagulants, undetermined**

⑦T45.515   **Adverse effect of anticoagulants**

⑦T45.516   **Underdosing of anticoagulants**

T45.52   **Poisoning by, adverse effect of and underdosing of antithrombotic drugs**

Poisoning by, adverse effect of and underdosing of antiplatelet drugs

Excludes2: poisoning by, adverse effect of and underdosing of aspirin (T39.01-)

poisoning by, adverse effect of and underdosing of acetylsalicylic acid (T39.01-)

⑦T45.521   **Poisoning by antithrombotic drugs, accidental (unintentional)**

Poisoning by antithrombotic drug NOS

⑦T45.522   **Poisoning by antithrombotic drugs, intentional self-harm**

⑦T45.523   **Poisoning by antithrombotic drugs, assault**

⑦T45.524   **Poisoning by antithrombotic drugs, undetermined**

⑦T45.525   **Adverse effect of antithrombotic drugs**

⑦T45.526   **Underdosing of antithrombotic drugs**

T45.6   **Poisoning by, adverse effect of and underdosing of fibrinolysis-affecting drugs**

T45.60   **Poisoning by, adverse effect of and underdosing of unspecified fibrinolysis-affecting drugs**

⑦T45.601   **Poisoning by unspecified fibrinolysis-affecting drugs, accidental (unintentional)**

Poisoning by fibrinolysis-affecting drug NOS

⑦T45.602   **Poisoning by unspecified fibrinolysis-affecting drugs, intentional self-harm**

⑦T45.603   **Poisoning by unspecified fibrinolysis-affecting drugs, assault**

⑦T45.604   **Poisoning by unspecified fibrinolysis-affecting drugs, undetermined**

⑦T45.605   **Adverse effect of unspecified fibrinolysis-affecting drugs**

⑦T45.606   **Underdosing of unspecified fibrinolysis-affecting drugs**

T45.61   **Poisoning by, adverse effect of and underdosing of thrombolytic drugs**

⑦T45.611   **Poisoning by thrombolytic drug, accidental (unintentional)**

Poisoning by thrombolytic drug NOS

⑦T45.612   **Poisoning by thrombolytic drug, intentional self-harm**

⑦T45.613   **Poisoning by thrombolytic drug, assault**

⑦T45.614   **Poisoning by thrombolytic drug, undetermined**

⑦T45.615   **Adverse effect of thrombolytic drugs**

⑦T45.616   **Underdosing of thrombolytic drugs**

T45.62   **Poisoning by, adverse effect of and underdosing of hemostatic drugs**

⑦T45.621   **Poisoning by hemostatic drug, accidental (unintentional)**

Poisoning by hemostatic drug NOS

⑦T45.622   **Poisoning by hemostatic drug, intentional self-harm**

⑦T45.623   **Poisoning by hemostatic drug, assault**

⑦T45.624   **Poisoning by hemostatic drug, undetermined**

⑦T45.625   **Adverse effect of hemostatic drug**

⑦T45.626   **Underdosing of hemostatic drugs**

T45.69   **Poisoning by, adverse effect of and underdosing of other fibrinolysis-affecting drugs**

⑦T45.691   **Poisoning by other fibrinolysis-affecting drugs, accidental (unintentional)**

Poisoning by other fibrinolysis-affecting drug NOS

⑦T45.692   **Poisoning by other fibrinolysis-affecting drugs, intentional self-harm**

⑦T45.693   **Poisoning by other fibrinolysis-affecting drugs, assault**

⑦T45.694   **Poisoning by other fibrinolysis-affecting drugs, undetermined**

⑦T45.695   **Adverse effect of other fibrinolysis-affecting drugs**

⑦**T45.696** **Underdosing of other fibrinolysis-affecting drugs**

T45.7 **Poisoning by, adverse effect of and underdosing of anticoagulant antagonists, vitamin K and other coagulants**

T45.7X **Poisoning by, adverse effect of and underdosing of anticoagulant antagonists, vitamin K and other coagulants**

⑦**T45.7X1** **Poisoning by anticoagulant antagonists, vitamin K and other coagulants, accidental (unintentional)**

Poisoning by anticoagulant antagonists, vitamin K and other coagulants NOS

⑦**T45.7X2** **Poisoning by anticoagulant antagonists, vitamin K and other coagulants, intentional self-harm**

⑦**T45.7X3** **Poisoning by anticoagulant antagonists, vitamin K and other coagulants, assault**

⑦**T45.7X4** **Poisoning by anticoagulant antagonists, vitamin K and other coagulants, undetermined**

⑦**T45.7X5** **Adverse effect of anticoagulant antagonists, vitamin K and other coagulants**

⑦**T45.7X6** **Underdosing of anticoagulant antagonist, vitamin K and other coagulants**

Excludes1: vitamin K deficiency (E56.1)

T45.8 **Poisoning by, adverse effect of and underdosing of other primarily systemic and hematological agents**

Poisoning by, adverse effect of and underdosing of liver preparations **and other** antianemic agents

Poisoning by, adverse effect of and underdosing of natural blood and blood products

Poisoning by, adverse effect of and underdosing of plasma substitute

Excludes2: poisoning by, adverse effect of and underdosing of immunoglobulin (T50.Z1)

poisoning by, adverse effect of and underdosing of iron (T45.4) transfusion reactions (T80.-)

T45.8X **Poisoning by, adverse effect of and underdosing of other primarily systemic and hematological agents**

⑦**T45.8X1** **Poisoning by other primarily systemic and hematological agents, accidental (unintentional)**

Poisoning by other primarily systemic and hematological agents NOS

⑦**T45.8X2** **Poisoning by other primarily systemic and hematological agents, intentional self-harm**

⑦**T45.8X3** **Poisoning by other primarily systemic and hematological agents, assault**

⑦**T45.8X4** **Poisoning by other primarily systemic and hematological agents, undetermined**

⑦**T45.8X5** **Adverse effect of other primarily systemic and hematological agents**

⑦**T45.8X6** **Underdosing of other primarily systemic and hematological agents**

T45.9 **Poisoning by, adverse effect of and underdosing of unspecified primarily systemic and hematological agent**

T45.91 **Poisoning by unspecified primarily systemic and hematological agent, accidental (unintentional)**

Poisoning by primarily systemic and hematological agent NOS

T45.92 **Poisoning by unspecified primarily systemic and hematological agent, intentional self-harm**

T45.93 **Poisoning by unspecified primarily systemic and hematological agent, assault**

T45.94 **Poisoning by unspecified primarily systemic and hematological agent, undetermined**

T45.95 **Adverse effect of unspecified primarily systemic and hematological agent**

T45.96 **Underdosing of unspecified primarily systemic and hematological agent**

T46 **Poisoning by, adverse effect of and underdosing of agents primarily affecting the cardiovascular system**

Excludes1: poisoning by, adverse effect of and underdosing of metaraminol (T44.4)

The appropriate 7th character is to be added to each code from category T46

A - initial encounter

D - subsequent encounter

S - sequela

T46.0 **Poisoning by, adverse effect of and underdosing of cardiac-stimulant glycosides and drugs of similar action**

T46.0X **Poisoning by, adverse effect of and underdosing of cardiac-stimulant glycosides and drugs of similar action**

⑦**T46.0X1** **Poisoning by cardiac-stimulant glycosides and drugs of similar action, accidental (unintentional)**

Poisoning by cardiac-stimulant glycosides and drugs of similar action NOS

⑦**T46.0X2** **Poisoning by cardiac-stimulant glycosides and drugs of similar action, intentional self-harm**

⑦**T46.0X3** **Poisoning by cardiac-stimulant glycosides and drugs of similar action, assault**

⑦**T46.0X4** **Poisoning by cardiac-stimulant glycosides and drugs of similar action, undetermined**

⑦**T46.0X5** **Adverse effect of cardiac-stimulant glycosides and drugs of similar action**

⑦**T46.0X6** **Underdosing of cardiac-stimulant glycosides and drugs of similar action**

T46.1 **Poisoning by, adverse effect of and underdosing of calcium-channel blockers**

T46.1X **Poisoning by, adverse effect of and underdosing of calcium-channel blockers**

⑦**T46.1X1** **Poisoning by calcium-channel blockers, accidental (unintentional)**

Poisoning by calcium-channel blockers NOS

⑦**T46.1X2** **Poisoning by calcium-channel blockers, intentional self-harm**

⑦**T46.1X3** **Poisoning by calcium-channel blockers, assault**

⑦**T46.1X4** **Poisoning by calcium-channel blockers, undetermined**

⑦ **T46.1X5** Adverse effect of calcium-channel blockers

⑦ **T46.1X6** Underdosing of calcium-channel blockers

T46.2 Poisoning by, adverse effect of and underdosing of other antidysrhythmic drugs, not elsewhere classified

Excludes1: poisoning by, adverse effect of and underdosing of beta-adrenoreceptor antagonists (T44.7-)

T46.2X Poisoning by, adverse effect of and underdosing of other antidysrhythmic drugs

⑦ **T46.2X1** Poisoning by other antidysrhythmic drugs, accidental (unintentional)

Poisoning by other antidysrhythmic drugs NOS

⑦ **T46.2X2** Poisoning by other antidysrhythmic drugs, intentional self-harm

⑦ **T46.2X3** Poisoning by other antidysrhythmic drugs, assault

⑦ **T46.2X4** Poisoning by other antidysrhythmic drugs, undetermined

⑦ **T46.2X5** Adverse effect of other antidysrhythmic drugs

⑦ **T46.2X6** Underdosing of other antidysrhythmic drugs

T46.3 Poisoning by, adverse effect of and underdosing of coronary vasodilators

Poisoning by, adverse effect of and underdosing of dipyridamole

Excludes1: poisoning by, adverse effect of and underdosing of calcium-channel blockers (T46.1)

T46.3X Poisoning by, adverse effect of and underdosing of coronary vasodilators

⑦ **T46.3X1** Poisoning by coronary vasodilators, accidental (unintentional)

Poisoning by coronary vasodilators NOS

⑦ **T46.3X2** Poisoning by coronary vasodilators, intentional self-harm

⑦ **T46.3X3** Poisoning by coronary vasodilators, assault

⑦ **T46.3X4** Poisoning by coronary vasodilators, undetermined

⑦ **T46.3X5** Adverse effect of coronary vasodilators

⑦ **T46.3X6** Underdosing of coronary vasodilators

T46.4 Poisoning by, adverse effect of and underdosing of angiotensin-converting-enzyme inhibitors

T46.4X Poisoning by, adverse effect of and underdosing of angiotensin-converting-enzyme inhibitors

⑦ **T46.4X1** Poisoning by angiotensin-converting-enzyme inhibitors, accidental (unintentional)

Poisoning by angiotensin-converting-enzyme inhibitors NOS

⑦ **T46.4X2** Poisoning by angiotensin-converting-enzyme inhibitors, intentional self-harm

⑦ **T46.4X3** Poisoning by angiotensin-converting-enzyme inhibitors, assault

⑦ **T46.4X4** Poisoning by angiotensin-converting-enzyme inhibitors, undetermined

⑦ **T46.4X5** Adverse effect of angiotensin-converting-enzyme inhibitors

⑦ **T46.4X6** Underdosing of angiotensin-converting-enzyme inhibitors

T46.5 Poisoning by, adverse effect of and underdosing of other antihypertensive drugs

Excludes2: poisoning by, adverse effect of and underdosing of beta-adrenoreceptor antagonists (T44.7)

poisoning by, adverse effect of and underdosing of calcium-channel blockers (T46.1) \

poisoning by, adverse effect of and underdosing of diuretics (T50.0-T50.2)

T46.5X Poisoning by, adverse effect of and underdosing of other antihypertensive drugs

⑦ **T46.5X1** Poisoning by other antihypertensive drugs, accidental (unintentional)

Poisoning by other antihypertensive drugs NOS

⑦ **T46.5X2** Poisoning by other antihypertensive drugs, intentional self-harm

⑦ **T46.5X3** Poisoning by other antihypertensive drugs, assault

⑦ **T46.5X4** Poisoning by other antihypertensive drugs, undetermined

⑦ **T46.5X5** Adverse effect of other antihypertensive drugs

⑦ **T46.5X6** Underdosing of other antihypertensive drugs

T46.6 Poisoning by, adverse effect of and underdosing of antihyperlipidemic and antiarteriosclerotic drugs

T46.6X Poisoning by, adverse effect of and underdosing of antihyperlipidemic and antiarteriosclerotic drugs

⑦ **T46.6X1** Poisoning by antihyperlipidemic and antiarteriosclerotic drugs, accidental (unintentional)

Poisoning by antihyperlipidemic and antiarteriosclerotic drugs NOS

⑦ **T46.6X2** Poisoning by antihyperlipidemic and antiarteriosclerotic drugs, intentional self-harm

⑦ **T46.6X3** Poisoning by antihyperlipidemic and antiarteriosclerotic drugs, assault

⑦ **T46.6X4** Poisoning by antihyperlipidemic and antiarteriosclerotic drugs, undetermined

⑦ **T46.6X5** Adverse effect of antihyperlipidemic and antiarteriosclerotic drugs

⑦ **T46.6X6** Underdosing of antihyperlipidemic and antiarteriosclerotic drugs

T46.7 Poisoning by, adverse effect of and underdosing of peripheral vasodilators

Poisoning by, adverse effect of and underdosing of nicotinic acid (derivatives)

Excludes1: poisoning by, adverse effect of and underdosing of papaverine (T44.3)

T46.7X Poisoning by, adverse effect of and underdosing of peripheral vasodilators

⑦ **T46.7X1** Poisoning by peripheral vasodilators, accidental (unintentional)

Poisoning by peripheral vasodilators NOS

⑦ **T46.7X2** Poisoning by peripheral vasodilators, intentional self-harm

⑦ **T46.7X3** Poisoning by peripheral vasodilators, assault

● New code ▲ Revised code **Excludes1:** Not coded here **Excludes2:** Not included here ⊗ Placeholder required ⑦ 7th digit required

⑦T46.7X4 **Poisoning by peripheral vasodilators, undetermined**

⑦T46.7X5 **Adverse effect of peripheral vasodilators**

⑦T46.7X6 **Underdosing of peripheral vasodilators**

T46.8 **Poisoning by, adverse effect of and underdosing of antivaricose drugs, including sclerosing agents**

T46.8X **Poisoning by, adverse effect of and underdosing of antivaricose drugs, including sclerosing agents**

⑦T46.8X1 **Poisoning by antivaricose drugs, including sclerosing agents, accidental (unintentional)**

Poisoning by antivaricose drugs, including sclerosing agents NOS

⑦T46.8X2 **Poisoning by antivaricose drugs, including sclerosing agents, intentional self-harm**

⑦T46.8X3 **Poisoning by antivaricose drugs, including sclerosing agents, assault**

⑦T46.8X4 **Poisoning by antivaricose drugs, including sclerosing agents, undetermined**

⑦T46.8X5 **Adverse effect of antivaricose drugs, including sclerosing agents**

⑦T46.8X6 **Underdosing of antivaricose drugs, including sclerosing agents**

T46.9 **Poisoning by, adverse effect of and underdosing of other and unspecified agents primarily affecting the cardiovascular system**

T46.90 **Poisoning by, adverse effect of and underdosing of unspecified agents primarily affecting the cardiovascular system**

⑦T46.901 **Poisoning by unspecified agents primarily affecting the cardiovascular system, accidental (unintentional)**

⑦T46.902 **Poisoning by unspecified agents primarily affecting the cardiovascular system, intentional self-harm**

⑦T46.903 **Poisoning by unspecified agents primarily affecting the cardiovascular system, assault**

⑦T46.904 **Poisoning by unspecified agents primarily affecting the cardiovascular system, undetermined**

⑦T46.905 **Adverse effect of unspecified agents primarily affecting the cardiovascular system**

⑦T46.906 **Underdosing of unspecified agents primarily affecting the cardiovascular system**

T46.99 **Poisoning by, adverse effect of and underdosing of other agents primarily affecting the cardiovascular system**

⑦T46.991 **Poisoning by other agents primarily affecting the cardiovascular system, accidental (unintentional)**

⑦T46.992 **Poisoning by other agents primarily affecting the cardiovascular system, intentional self-harm**

⑦T46.993 **Poisoning by other agents primarily affecting the cardiovascular system, assault**

⑦T46.994 **Poisoning by other agents primarily affecting the cardiovascular system, undetermined**

⑦T46.995 **Adverse effect of other agents primarily affecting the cardiovascular system**

⑦T46.996 **Underdosing of other agents primarily affecting the cardiovascular system**

T47 **Poisoning by, adverse effect of and underdosing of agents primarily affecting the gastrointestinal system**

The appropriate 7th character is to be added to each code from category T47

A - initial encounter

D - subsequent encounter

S - sequela

T47.0 **Poisoning by, adverse effect of and underdosing of histamine H2-receptor blockers**

T47.0X **Poisoning by, adverse effect of and underdosing of histamine H2-receptor blockers**

⑦T47.0X1 **Poisoning by histamine H2-receptor blockers, accidental (unintentional)**

Poisoning by histamine H2-receptor blockers NOS

⑦T47.0X2 **Poisoning by histamine H2-receptor blockers, intentional self-harm**

⑦T47.0X3 **Poisoning by histamine H2-receptor blockers, assault**

⑦T47.0X4 **Poisoning by histamine H2-receptor blockers, undetermined**

⑦T47.0X5 **Adverse effect of histamine H2-receptor blockers**

⑦T47.0X6 **Underdosing of histamine H2-receptor blockers**

T47.1 **Poisoning by, adverse effect of and underdosing of other antacids and anti-gastric-secretion drugs**

T47.1X **Poisoning by, adverse effect of and underdosing of other antacids and anti-gastric-secretion drugs**

⑦T47.1X1 **Poisoning by other antacids and anti-gastric-secretion drugs, accidental (unintentional)**

Poisoning by other antacids and anti-gastric-secretion drugs NOS

⑦T47.1X2 **Poisoning by other antacids and anti-gastric-secretion drugs, intentional self-harm**

⑦T47.1X3 **Poisoning by other antacids and anti-gastric-secretion drugs, assault**

⑦T47.1X4 **Poisoning by other antacids and anti-gastric-secretion drugs, undetermined**

⑦T47.1X5 **Adverse effect of other antacids and anti-gastric-secretion drugs**

⑦T47.1X6 **Underdosing of other antacids and anti-gastric-secretion drugs**

T47.2 **Poisoning by, adverse effect of and underdosing of stimulant laxatives**

T47.2X **Poisoning by, adverse effect of and underdosing of stimulant laxatives**

⑦T47.2X1 **Poisoning by stimulant laxatives, accidental (unintentional)**

Poisoning by stimulant laxatives NOS

⑦T47.2X2 **Poisoning by stimulant laxatives, intentional self-harm**

⑦T47.2X3 **Poisoning by stimulant laxatives, assault**

⑦T47.2X4 **Poisoning by stimulant laxatives, undetermined**

⑦T47.2X5 **Adverse effect of stimulant laxatives**

⑦T47.2X6 **Underdosing of stimulant laxatives**

T47.3 **Poisoning by, adverse effect of and underdosing of saline and osmotic laxatives**

T47.3X **Poisoning by and adverse effect of saline and osmotic laxatives**

⑦T47.3X1 **Poisoning by saline and osmotic laxatives, accidental (unintentional)**

Poisoning by saline and osmotic laxatives NOS

⑦T47.3X2 **Poisoning by saline and osmotic laxatives, intentional self-harm**

⑦T47.3X3 **Poisoning by saline and osmotic laxatives, assault**

⑦T47.3X4 **Poisoning by saline and osmotic laxatives, undetermined**

⑦T47.3X5 **Adverse effect of saline and osmotic laxatives**

⑦T47.3X6 **Underdosing of saline and osmotic laxatives**

T47.4 **Poisoning by, adverse effect of and underdosing of other laxatives**

T47.4X **Poisoning by, adverse effect of and underdosing of other laxatives**

⑦T47.4X1 **Poisoning by other laxatives, accidental (unintentional)**

Poisoning by other laxatives NOS

⑦T47.4X2 **Poisoning by other laxatives, intentional self-harm**

⑦T47.4X3 **Poisoning by other laxatives, assault**

⑦T47.4X4 **Poisoning by other laxatives, undetermined**

⑦T47.4X5 **Adverse effect of other laxatives**

⑦T47.4X6 **Underdosing of other laxatives**

T47.5 **Poisoning by, adverse effect of and underdosing of digestants**

T47.5X **Poisoning by, adverse effect of and underdosing of digestants**

⑦T47.5X1 **Poisoning by digestants, accidental (unintentional)**

Poisoning by digestants NOS

⑦T47.5X2 **Poisoning by digestants, intentional self-harm**

⑦T47.5X3 **Poisoning by digestants, assault**

⑦T47.5X4 **Poisoning by digestants, undetermined**

⑦T47.5X5 **Adverse effect of digestants**

⑦T47.5X6 **Underdosing of digestants**

T47.6 **Poisoning by, adverse effect of and underdosing of antidiarrheal drugs**

Excludes2: poisoning by, adverse effect of and underdosing of systemic antibiotics and other anti-infectives (T36-T37)

T47.6X **Poisoning by, adverse effect of and underdosing of antidiarrheal drugs**

⑦T47.6X1 **Poisoning by antidiarrheal drugs, accidental (unintentional)**

Poisoning by antidiarrheal drugs NOS

⑦T47.6X2 **Poisoning by antidiarrheal drugs, intentional self-harm**

⑦T47.6X3 **Poisoning by antidiarrheal drugs, assault**

⑦T47.6X4 **Poisoning by antidiarrheal drugs, undetermined**

⑦T47.6X5 **Adverse effect of antidiarrheal drugs**

⑦T47.6X6 **Underdosing of antidiarrheal drugs**

T47.7 **Poisoning by, adverse effect of and underdosing of emetics**

T47.7X **Poisoning by, adverse effect of and underdosing of emetics**

⑦T47.7X1 **Poisoning by emetics, accidental (unintentional)**

Poisoning by emetics NOS

⑦T47.7X2 **Poisoning by emetics, intentional self-harm**

⑦T47.7X3 **Poisoning by emetics, assault**

⑦T47.7X4 **Poisoning by emetics, undetermined**

⑦T47.7X5 **Adverse effect of emetics**

⑦T47.7X6 **Underdosing of emetics**

T47.8 **Poisoning by, adverse effect of and underdosing of other agents primarily affecting gastrointestinal system**

T47.8X **Poisoning by, adverse effect of and underdosing of other agents primarily affecting gastrointestinal system**

⑦T47.8X1 **Poisoning by other agents primarily affecting gastrointestinal system, accidental (unintentional)**

Poisoning by other agents primarily affecting gastrointestinal system NOS

⑦T47.8X2 **Poisoning by other agents primarily affecting gastrointestinal system, intentional self-harm**

⑦T47.8X3 **Poisoning by other agents primarily affecting gastrointestinal system, assault**

⑦T47.8X4 **Poisoning by other agents primarily affecting gastrointestinal system, undetermined**

⑦T47.8X5 **Adverse effect of other agents primarily affecting gastrointestinal system**

⑦T47.8X6 **Underdosing of other agents primarily affecting gastrointestinal system**

T47.9 **Poisoning by, adverse effect of and underdosing of unspecified agents primarily affecting the gastrointestinal system**

⊗⑦T47.91 **Poisoning by unspecified agents primarily affecting the gastrointestinal system, accidental (unintentional)**

Poisoning by agents primarily affecting the gastrointestinal system NOS

⊗⑦T47.92 **Poisoning by unspecified agents primarily affecting the gastrointestinal system, intentional self-harm**

⊗⑦T47.93 **Poisoning by unspecified agents primarily affecting the gastrointestinal system, assault**

⊗⑦T47.94 **Poisoning by unspecified agents primarily affecting the gastrointestinal system, undetermined**

⊗⑦T47.95 **Adverse effect of unspecified agents primarily affecting the gastrointestinal system**

● New code ▲ Revised code **Excludes1:** Not coded here **Excludes2:** Not included here ⊗ Placeholder required ⑦ 7th digit required

⊗⑦**T47.96**   **Underdosing of unspecified agents primarily affecting the gastrointestinal system**

T48   **Poisoning by, adverse effect of and underdosing of agents primarily acting on smooth and skeletal muscles and the respiratory system**

The appropriate 7th character is to be added to each code from category T48

A - initial encounter

D - subsequent encounter

S - sequela

T48.0   **Poisoning by, adverse effect of and underdosing of oxytocic drugs**

     Excludes1: poisoning by, adverse effect of and underdosing of estrogens, progestogens and antagonists (T38.4-T38.6)

     T48.0X   **Poisoning by, adverse effect of and underdosing of oxytocic drugs**

       ⑦**T48.0X1**   **Poisoning by oxytocic drugs, accidental (unintentional)**

           Poisoning by oxytocic drugs NOS

       ⑦**T48.0X2**   **Poisoning by oxytocic drugs, intentional self-harm**

       ⑦**T48.0X3**   **Poisoning by oxytocic drugs, assault**

       ⑦**T48.0X4**   **Poisoning by oxytocic drugs, undetermined**

       ⑦**T48.0X5**   **Adverse effect of oxytocic drugs**

       ⑦**T48.0X6**   **Underdosing of oxytocic drugs**

T48.1   **Poisoning by, adverse effect of and underdosing of skeletal muscle relaxants [neuromuscular blocking agents]**

     T48.1X   **Poisoning by, adverse effect of and underdosing of skeletal muscle relaxants [neuromuscular blocking agents]**

       ⑦**T48.1X1**   **Poisoning by skeletal muscle relaxants [neuromuscular blocking agents], accidental (unintentional)**

           Poisoning by skeletal muscle relaxants [neuromuscular blocking agents] NOS

       ⑦**T48.1X2**   **Poisoning by skeletal muscle relaxants [neuromuscular blocking agents], intentional self-harm**

       ⑦**T48.1X3**   **Poisoning by skeletal muscle relaxants [neuromuscular blocking agents], assault**

       ⑦**T48.1X4**   **Poisoning by skeletal muscle relaxants [neuromuscular blocking agents], undetermined**

       ⑦**T48.1X5**   **Adverse effect of skeletal muscle relaxants [neuromuscular blocking agents]**

       ⑦**T48.1X6**   **Underdosing of skeletal muscle relaxants [neuromuscular blocking agents]**

T48.2   **Poisoning by, adverse effect of and underdosing of other and unspecified drugs acting on muscles**

     T48.20   **Poisoning by, adverse effect of and underdosing of unspecified drugs acting on muscles**

       ⑦**T48.201**   **Poisoning by unspecified drugs acting on muscles, accidental (unintentional)**

           Poisoning by unspecified drugs acting on muscles NOS

       ⑦**T48.202**   **Poisoning by unspecified drugs acting on muscles, intentional self-harm**

⑦**T48.203**   **Poisoning by unspecified drugs acting on muscles, assault**

⑦**T48.204**   **Poisoning by unspecified drugs acting on muscles, undetermined**

⑦**T48.205**   **Adverse effect of unspecified drugs acting on muscles**

⑦**T48.206**   **Underdosing of unspecified drugs acting on muscles**

     T48.29   **Poisoning by, adverse effect of and underdosing of other drugs acting on muscles**

       ⑦**T48.291**   **Poisoning by other drugs acting on muscles, accidental (unintentional)**

           Poisoning by other drugs acting on muscles NOS

       ⑦**T48.292**   **Poisoning by other drugs acting on muscles, intentional self-harm**

       ⑦**T48.293**   **Poisoning by other drugs acting on muscles, assault**

       ⑦**T48.294**   **Poisoning by other drugs acting on muscles, undetermined**

       ⑦**T48.295**   **Adverse effect of other drugs acting on muscles**

       ⑦**T48.296**   **Underdosing of other drugs acting on muscles**

T48.3   **Poisoning by, adverse effect of and underdosing of antitussives**

     T48.3X   **Poisoning by, adverse effect of and underdosing of antitussives**

       ⑦**T48.3X1**   **Poisoning by antitussives, accidental (unintentional)**

           Poisoning by antitussives NOS

       ⑦**T48.3X2**   **Poisoning by antitussives, intentional self-harm**

       ⑦**T48.3X3**   **Poisoning by antitussives, assault**

       ⑦**T48.3X4**   **Poisoning by antitussives, undetermined**

       ⑦**T48.3X5**   **Adverse effect of antitussives**

       ⑦**T48.3X6**   **Underdosing of antitussives**

T48.4   **Poisoning by, adverse effect of and underdosing of expectorants**

     T48.4X   **Poisoning by, adverse effect of and underdosing of expectorants**

       ⑦**T48.4X1**   **Poisoning by expectorants, accidental (unintentional)**

           Poisoning by expectorants NOS

       ⑦**T48.4X2**   **Poisoning by expectorants, intentional self-harm**

       ⑦**T48.4X3**   **Poisoning by expectorants, assault**

       ⑦**T48.4X4**   **Poisoning by expectorants, undetermined**

       ⑦**T48.4X5**   **Adverse effect of expectorants**

       ⑦**T48.4X6**   **Underdosing of expectorants**

T48.5   **Poisoning by, adverse effect of and underdosing of other anti-common-cold drugs**

     Poisoning by, adverse effect of and underdosing of decongestants

     Excludes2: poisoning by, adverse effect of and underdosing of antipyretics, NEC (T39.9-)

       poisoning by, adverse effect of and underdosing of non-steroidal antiinflammatory drugs (T39.3-)

       poisoning by, adverse effect of and underdosing of salicylates (T39.0-)

T48.5X Poisoning by, adverse effect of and underdosing of other anti-common-cold drugs

⑦ **T48.5X1** Poisoning by other anti-common-cold drugs, accidental (unintentional)

Poisoning by other anti-common-cold drugs NOS

⑦ **T48.5X2** Poisoning by other anti-common-cold drugs, intentional self-harm

⑦ **T48.5X3** Poisoning by other anti-common-cold drugs, assault

⑦ **T48.5X4** Poisoning by other anti-common-cold drugs, undetermined

⑦ **T48.5X5** Adverse effect of other anti-common-cold drugs

⑦ **T48.5X6** Underdosing of other anti-common-cold drugs

T48.6 Poisoning by, adverse effect of and underdosing of antiasthmatics, not elsewhere classified

Poisoning by, adverse effect of and underdosing of beta-adrenoreceptor agonists used in asthma therapy

Excludes1: poisoning by, adverse effect of and underdosing of beta-adrenoreceptor agonists not used in asthma therapy (T44.5)

poisoning by, adverse effect of and underdosing of anterior pituitary [adenohypophyseal] hormones (T38.8)

T48.6X Poisoning by, adverse effect of and underdosing of antiasthmatics

⑦ **T48.6X1** Poisoning by antiasthmatics, accidental (unintentional)

Poisoning by antiasthmatics NOS

⑦ **T48.6X2** Poisoning by antiasthmatics, intentional self-harm

⑦ **T48.6X3** Poisoning by antiasthmatics, assault

⑦ **T48.6X4** Poisoning by antiasthmatics, undetermined

⑦ **T48.6X5** Adverse effect of antiasthmatics

⑦ **T48.6X6** Underdosing of antiasthmatics

T48.9 Poisoning by, adverse effect of and underdosing of other and unspecified agents primarily acting on the respiratory system

T48.90 Poisoning by, adverse effect of and underdosing of unspecified agents primarily acting on the respiratory system

⑦ **T48.901** Poisoning by unspecified agents primarily acting on the respiratory system, accidental (unintentional)

⑦ **T48.902** Poisoning by unspecified agents primarily acting on the respiratory system, intentional self-harm

⑦ **T48.903** Poisoning by unspecified agents primarily acting on the respiratory system, assault

⑦ **T48.904** Poisoning by unspecified agents primarily acting on the respiratory system, undetermined

⑦ **T48.905** Adverse effect of unspecified agents primarily acting on the respiratory system

⑦ **T48.906** Underdosing of unspecified agents primarily acting on the respiratory system

T48.99 Poisoning by, adverse effect of and underdosing of other agents primarily acting on the respiratory system

⑦ **T48.991** Poisoning by other agents primarily acting on the respiratory system, accidental (unintentional)

⑦ **T48.992** Poisoning by other agents primarily acting on the respiratory system, intentional self-harm

⑦ **T48.993** Poisoning by other agents primarily acting on the respiratory system, assault

⑦ **T48.994** Poisoning by other agents primarily acting on the respiratory system, undetermined

⑦ **T48.995** Adverse effect of other agents primarily acting on the respiratory system

⑦ **T48.996** Underdosing of other agents primarily acting on the respiratory system

T49 Poisoning by, adverse effect of and underdosing of topical agents primarily affecting skin and mucous membrane and by ophthalmological, otorhinolaryngological and dental drugs

Includes: poisoning by, adverse effect of and underdosing of glucocorticoids, topically used

The appropriate 7th character is to be added to each code from category T49

A - initial encounter

D - subsequent encounter \

S - sequela

T49.0 Poisoning by, adverse effect of and underdosing of local antifungal, anti-infective and anti-inflammatory drugs

T49.0X Poisoning by, adverse effect of and underdosing of local antifungal, anti-infective and anti-inflammatory drugs

⑦ **T49.0X1** Poisoning by local antifungal, anti-infective and anti-inflammatory drugs, accidental (unintentional)

Poisoning by local antifungal, anti-infective and anti-inflammatory drugs NOS

⑦ **T49.0X2** Poisoning by local antifungal, anti-infective and anti-inflammatory drugs, intentional self-harm

⑦ **T49.0X3** Poisoning by local antifungal, anti-infective and anti-inflammatory drugs, assault

⑦ **T49.0X4** Poisoning by local antifungal, anti-infective and anti-inflammatory drugs, undetermined

⑦ **T49.0X5** Adverse effect of local antifungal, anti-infective and anti-inflammatory drugs

⑦ **T49.0X6** Underdosing of local antifungal, anti-infective and anti-inflammatory drugs

T49.1 Poisoning by, adverse effect of and underdosing of antipruritics

T49.1X Poisoning by, adverse effect of and underdosing of antipruritics

⑦ **T49.1X1** Poisoning by antipruritics, accidental (unintentional)

Poisoning by antipruritics NOS

⑦ **T49.1X2** Poisoning by antipruritics, intentional self-harm

⑦ **T49.1X3** Poisoning by antipruritics, assault

⑦ **T49.1X4** Poisoning by antipruritics, undetermined

● New code ▲ Revised code **Excludes1:** Not coded here **Excludes2:** Not included here ⊗ Placeholder required ⑦7th digit required

⑦T49.1X5   Adverse effect of antipruritics

⑦T49.1X6   Underdosing of antipruritics

T49.2   Poisoning by, adverse effect of and underdosing of local astringents and local detergents

    T49.2X   Poisoning by, adverse effect of and underdosing of local astringents and local detergents

      ⑦T49.2X1   Poisoning by local astringents and local detergents, accidental (unintentional)

            Poisoning by local astringents and local detergents NOS

      ⑦T49.2X2   Poisoning by local astringents and local detergents, intentional self-harm

      ⑦T49.2X3   Poisoning by local astringents and local detergents, assault

      ⑦T49.2X4   Poisoning by local astringents and local detergents, undetermined

      ⑦T49.2X5   Adverse effect of local astringents and local detergents

      ⑦T49.2X6   Underdosing of local astringents and local detergents

T49.3   Poisoning by, adverse effect of and underdosing of emollients, demulcents and protectants

    T49.3X   Poisoning by, adverse effect of and underdosing of emollients, demulcents and protectants

      ⑦T49.3X1   Poisoning by emollients, demulcents and protectants, accidental (unintentional)

            Poisoning by emollients, demulcents and protectants NOS

      ⑦T49.3X2   Poisoning by emollients, demulcents and protectants, intentional self-harm

      ⑦T49.3X3   Poisoning by emollients, demulcents and protectants, assault

      ⑦T49.3X4   Poisoning by emollients, demulcents and protectants, undetermined

      ⑦T49.3X5   Adverse effect of emollients, demulcents and protectants

      ⑦T49.3X6   Underdosing of emollients, demulcents and protectants

T49.4   Poisoning by, adverse effect of and underdosing of keratolytics, keratoplastics, and other hair treatment drugs and preparations

    T49.4X   Poisoning by, adverse effect of and underdosing of keratolytics, keratoplastics, and other hair treatment drugs and preparations

      ⑦T49.4X1   Poisoning by keratolytics, keratoplastics, and other hair treatment drugs and preparations, accidental (unintentional)

            Poisoning by keratolytics, keratoplastics, **and other** hair treatment drugs and preparations NOS

      ⑦T49.4X2   Poisoning by keratolytics, keratoplastics, and other hair treatment drugs and preparations, intentional self-harm

      ⑦T49.4X3   Poisoning by keratolytics, keratoplastics, and other hair treatment drugs and preparations, assault

      ⑦T49.4X4   Poisoning by keratolytics, keratoplastics, and other hair

            treatment drugs and preparations, undetermined

      ⑦T49.4X5   Adverse effect of keratolytics, keratoplastics, and other hair treatment drugs and preparations

      ⑦T49.4X6   Underdosing of keratolytics, keratoplastics, and other hair treatment drugs and preparations

T49.5   Poisoning by, adverse effect of and underdosing of ophthalmological drugs and preparations

    T49.5X   Poisoning by, adverse effect of and underdosing of ophthalmological drugs and preparations

      ⑦T49.5X1   Poisoning by ophthalmological drugs and preparations, accidental (unintentional)

            Poisoning by ophthalmological drugs and preparations NOS

      ⑦T49.5X2   Poisoning by ophthalmological drugs and preparations, intentional self-harm

      ⑦T49.5X3   Poisoning by ophthalmological drugs and preparations, assault

      ⑦T49.5X4   Poisoning by ophthalmological drugs and preparations, undetermined

      ⑦T49.5X5   Adverse effect of ophthalmological drugs and preparations

      ⑦T49.5X6   Underdosing of ophthalmological drugs and preparations

T49.6   Poisoning by, adverse effect of and underdosing of otorhinolaryngological drugs and preparations

    T49.6X   Poisoning by, adverse effect of and underdosing of otorhinolaryngological drugs and preparations

      ⑦T49.6X1   Poisoning by otorhinolaryngological drugs and preparations, accidental (unintentional)

            Poisoning by otorhinolaryngological drugs and preparations NOS

      ⑦T49.6X2   Poisoning by otorhinolaryngological drugs and preparations, intentional self-harm

      ⑦T49.6X3   Poisoning by otorhinolaryngological drugs and preparations, assault

      ⑦T49.6X4   Poisoning by otorhinolaryngological drugs and preparations, undetermined

      ⑦T49.6X5   Adverse effect of otorhinolaryngological drugs and preparations

      ⑦T49.6X6   Underdosing of otorhinolaryngological drugs and preparations

T49.7   Poisoning by, adverse effect of and underdosing of dental drugs, topically applied

    T49.7X   Poisoning by, adverse effect of and underdosing of dental drugs, topically applied

      ⑦T49.7X1   Poisoning by dental drugs, topically applied, accidental (unintentional)

            Poisoning by dental drugs, topically applied NOS

      ⑦T49.7X2   Poisoning by dental drugs, topically applied, intentional self-harm

      ⑦T49.7X3   Poisoning by dental drugs, topically applied, assault

      ⑦T49.7X4   Poisoning by dental drugs, topically applied, undetermined

---

▓ Add 4th-7th digits   Nonspecific code   ▓ Unspecified code   ▓ Manifestation code

⑦T49.7X5   **Adverse effect of dental drugs, topically applied**

⑦T49.7X6   **Underdosing of dental drugs, topically applied**

T49.8   **Poisoning by, adverse effect of and underdosing of other topical agents**

Poisoning by, adverse effect of and underdosing of spermicides

T49.8X   **Poisoning by, adverse effect of and underdosing of other topical agents**

⑦T49.8X1   **Poisoning by other topical agents, accidental (unintentional)**

Poisoning by other topical agents NOS

⑦T49.8X2   **Poisoning by other topical agents, intentional self-harm**

⑦T49.8X3   **Poisoning by other topical agents, assault**

⑦T49.8X4   **Poisoning by other topical agents, undetermined**

⑦T49.8X5   **Adverse effect of other topical agents**

⑦T49.8X6   **Underdosing of other topical agents**

T49.9   **Poisoning by, adverse effect of and underdosing of unspecified topical agent**

⊗⑦T49.91   **Poisoning by unspecified topical agent, accidental (unintentional)**

⊗⑦T49.92   **Poisoning by unspecified topical agent, intentional self-harm**

⊗⑦T49.93   **Poisoning by unspecified topical agent, assault**

⊗⑦T49.94   **Poisoning by unspecified topical agent, undetermined**

⊗⑦T49.95   **Adverse effect of unspecified topical agent**

⊗⑦T49.96   **Underdosing of unspecified topical agent**

T50   **Poisoning by, adverse effect of and underdosing of diuretics and other and unspecified drugs, medicaments and biological substances**

The appropriate 7th character is to be added to each code from category T50

A - initial encounter

D - subsequent encounter

S - sequela

T50.0   **Poisoning by, adverse effect of and underdosing of mineralocorticoids and their antagonists**

T50.0X   **Poisoning by, adverse effect of and underdosing of mineralocorticoids and their antagonists**

⑦T50.0X1   **Poisoning by mineralocorticoids and their antagonists, accidental (unintentional)**

Poisoning by mineralocorticoids and their antagonists NOS

⑦T50.0X2   **Poisoning by mineralocorticoids and their antagonists, intentional self-harm**

⑦T50.0X3   **Poisoning by mineralocorticoids and their antagonists, assault**

⑦T50.0X4   **Poisoning by mineralocorticoids and their antagonists, undetermined**

⑦T50.0X5   **Adverse effect of mineralocorticoids and their antagonists**

⑦T50.0X6   **Underdosing of mineralocorticoids and their antagonists**

T50.1   **Poisoning by, adverse effect of and underdosing of loop [high-ceiling] diuretics**

T50.1X   **Poisoning by, adverse effect of and underdosing of loop [high-ceiling] diuretics**

⑦T50.1X1   **Poisoning by loop [high-ceiling] diuretics, accidental (unintentional)**

Poisoning by loop [high-ceiling] diuretics NOS

⑦T50.1X2   **Poisoning by loop [high-ceiling] diuretics, intentional self-harm**

⑦T50.1X3   **Poisoning by loop [high-ceiling] diuretics, assault**

⑦T50.1X4   **Poisoning by loop [high-ceiling] diuretics, undetermined**

⑦T50.1X5   **Adverse effect of loop [high-ceiling] diuretics**

⑦T50.1X6   **Underdosing of loop [high-ceiling] diuretics**

T50.2   **Poisoning by, adverse effect of and underdosing of carbonic-anhydrase inhibitors, benzothiadiazides and other diuretics**

Poisoning by, adverse effect of and underdosing of acetazolamide

T50.2X   **Poisoning by, adverse effect of and underdosing of carbonic-anhydrase inhibitors, benzothiadiazides and other diuretics**

⑦T50.2X1   **Poisoning by carbonic-anhydrase inhibitors, benzothiadiazides and other diuretics, accidental (unintentional)**

Poisoning by carbonic-anhydrase inhibitors, benzothiadiazides **and other** diuretics NOS

⑦T50.2X2   **Poisoning by carbonic-anhydrase inhibitors, benzothiadiazides and other diuretics, intentional self-harm**

⑦T50.2X3   **Poisoning by carbonic-anhydrase inhibitors, benzothiadiazides and other diuretics, assault**

⑦T50.2X4   **Poisoning by carbonic-anhydrase inhibitors, benzothiadiazides and other diuretics, undetermined**

⑦T50.2X5   **Adverse effect of carbonic-anhydrase inhibitors, benzothiadiazides and other diuretics**

⑦T50.2X6   **Underdosing of carbonic-anhydrase inhibitors, benzothiadiazides and other diuretics**

T50.3   **Poisoning by, adverse effect of and underdosing of electrolytic, caloric and water-balance agents**

Poisoning by, adverse effect of and underdosing of oral rehydration salts

T50.3X   **Poisoning by, adverse effect of and underdosing of electrolytic, caloric and water-balance agents**

⑦T50.3X1   **Poisoning by electrolytic, caloric and water-balance agents, accidental (unintentional)**

Poisoning by electrolytic, caloric and water-balance agents NOS

⑦T50.3X2   **Poisoning by electrolytic, caloric and water-balance agents, intentional self-harm**

⑦T50.3X3   **Poisoning by electrolytic, caloric and water-balance agents, assault**

⑦T50.3X4   **Poisoning by electrolytic, caloric and water-balance agents, undetermined**

⑦T50.3X5   **Adverse effect of electrolytic, caloric and water-balance agents**

● New code   ▲ Revised code   **Excludes1:** Not coded here   **Excludes2:** Not included here   ⊗ Placeholder required   ⑦7th digit required

⑦T50.3X6 **Underdosing of electrolytic, caloric and water-balance agents**

T50.4 **Poisoning by, adverse effect of and underdosing of drugs affecting uric acid metabolism**

　T50.4X **Poisoning by, adverse effect of and underdosing of drugs affecting uric acid metabolism**

　　⑦T50.4X1 **Poisoning by drugs affecting uric acid metabolism, accidental (unintentional)**

　　　Poisoning by drugs affecting uric acid metabolism NOS

　　⑦T50.4X2 **Poisoning by drugs affecting uric acid metabolism, intentional self-harm**

　　⑦T50.4X3 **Poisoning by drugs affecting uric acid metabolism, assault**

　　⑦T50.4X4 **Poisoning by drugs affecting uric acid metabolism, undetermined**

　　⑦T50.4X5 **Adverse effect of drugs affecting uric acid metabolism**

　　⑦T50.4X6 **Underdosing of drugs affecting uric acid metabolism**

T50.5 **Poisoning by, adverse effect of and underdosing of appetite depressants**

　T50.5X **Poisoning by, adverse effect of and underdosing of appetite depressants**

　　⑦T50.5X1 **Poisoning by appetite depressants, accidental (unintentional)**

　　　Poisoning by appetite depressants NOS

　　⑦T50.5X2 **Poisoning by appetite depressants, intentional self-harm**

　　⑦T50.5X3 **Poisoning by appetite depressants, assault**

　　⑦T50.5X4 **Poisoning by appetite depressants, undetermined**

　　⑦T50.5X5 **Adverse effect of appetite depressants**

　　⑦T50.5X6 **Underdosing of appetite depressants**

T50.6 **Poisoning by, adverse effect of and underdosing of antidotes and chelating agents**

　Poisoning by, adverse effect of and underdosing of alcohol deterrents

　T50.6X **Poisoning by, adverse effect of and underdosing of antidotes and chelating agents**

　　⑦T50.6X1 **Poisoning by antidotes and chelating agents, accidental (unintentional)**

　　　Poisoning by antidotes and chelating agents NOS

　　⑦T50.6X2 **Poisoning by antidotes and chelating agents, intentional self-harm**

　　⑦T50.6X3 **Poisoning by antidotes and chelating agents, assault**

　　⑦T50.6X4 **Poisoning by antidotes and chelating agents, undetermined**

　　⑦T50.6X5 **Adverse effect of antidotes and chelating agents**

　　⑦T50.6X6 **Underdosing of antidotes and chelating agents**

T50.7 **Poisoning by, adverse effect of and underdosing of analeptics and opioid receptor antagonists**

　T50.7X **Poisoning by, adverse effect of and underdosing of analeptics and opioid receptor antagonists**

　　⑦T50.7X1 **Poisoning by analeptics and opioid receptor antagonists, accidental (unintentional)**

　　　Poisoning by analeptics and opioid receptor antagonists NOS

　　⑦T50.7X2 **Poisoning by analeptics and opioid receptor antagonists, intentional self-harm**

　　⑦T50.7X3 **Poisoning by analeptics and opioid receptor antagonists, assault**

　　⑦T50.7X4 **Poisoning by analeptics and opioid receptor antagonists, undetermined**

　　⑦T50.7X5 **Adverse effect of analeptics and opioid receptor antagonists**

　　⑦T50.7X6 **Underdosing of analeptics and opioid receptor antagonists**

T50.8 **Poisoning by, adverse effect of and underdosing of diagnostic agents**

　T50.8X **Poisoning by, adverse effect of and underdosing of diagnostic agents**

　　⑦T50.8X1 **Poisoning by diagnostic agents, accidental (unintentional)**

　　　Poisoning by diagnostic agents NOS

　　⑦T50.8X2 **Poisoning by diagnostic agents, intentional self-harm**

　　⑦T50.8X3 **Poisoning by diagnostic agents, assault**

　　⑦T50.8X4 **Poisoning by diagnostic agents, undetermined**

　　⑦T50.8X5 **Adverse effect of diagnostic agents**

　　⑦T50.8X6 **Underdosing of diagnostic agents**

T50.A **Poisoning by, adverse effect of and underdosing of bacterial vaccines**

　T50.A1 **Poisoning by, adverse effect of and underdosing of pertussis vaccine, including combinations with a pertussis component**

　　⑦T50.A11 **Poisoning by pertussis vaccine, including combinations with a pertussis component, accidental (unintentional)**

　　⑦T50.A12 **Poisoning by pertussis vaccine, including combinations with a pertussis component, intentional self-harm**

　　⑦T50.A13 **Poisoning by pertussis vaccine, including combinations with a pertussis component, assault**

　　⑦T50.A14 **Poisoning by pertussis vaccine, including combinations with a pertussis component, undetermined**

　　⑦T50.A15 **Adverse effect of pertussis vaccine, including combinations with a pertussis component**

　　⑦T50.A16 **Underdosing of pertussis vaccine, including combinations with a pertussis component**

　T50.A2 **Poisoning by, adverse effect of and underdosing of mixed bacterial vaccines without a pertussis component**

　　⑦T50.A21 **Poisoning by mixed bacterial vaccines without a pertussis component, accidental (unintentional)**

　　⑦T50.A22 **Poisoning by mixed bacterial vaccines without a pertussis component, intentional self-harm**

⑦T50.A23 Poisoning by mixed bacterial vaccines without a pertussis component, assault

⑦T50.A24 Poisoning by mixed bacterial vaccines without a pertussis component, undetermined

⑦T50.A25 Adverse effect of mixed bacterial vaccines without a pertussis component

⑦T50.A26 Underdosing of mixed bacterial vaccines without a pertussis component

T50.A9 Poisoning by, adverse effect of and underdosing of other bacterial vaccines

⑦T50.A91 Poisoning by other bacterial vaccines, accidental (unintentional)

⑦T50.A92 Poisoning by other bacterial vaccines, intentional self-harm

⑦T50.A93 Poisoning by other bacterial vaccines, assault

⑦T50.A94 Poisoning by other bacterial vaccines, undetermined

⑦T50.A95 Adverse effect of other bacterial vaccines

⑦T50.A96 Underdosing of other bacterial vaccines

T50.B Poisoning by, adverse effect of and underdosing of viral vaccines

T50.B1 Poisoning by, adverse effect of and underdosing of smallpox vaccines

⑦T50.B11 Poisoning by smallpox vaccines, accidental (unintentional)

⑦T50.B12 Poisoning by smallpox vaccines, intentional self-harm

⑦T50.B13 Poisoning by smallpox vaccines, assault

⑦T50.B14 Poisoning by smallpox vaccines, undetermined

⑦T50.B15 Adverse effect of smallpox vaccines

⑦T50.B16 Underdosing of smallpox vaccines

T50.B9 Poisoning by, adverse effect of and underdosing of other viral vaccines

⑦T50.B91 Poisoning by other viral vaccines, accidental (unintentional)

⑦T50.B92 Poisoning by other viral vaccines, intentional self-harm

⑦T50.B93 Poisoning by other viral vaccines, assault

⑦T50.B94 Poisoning by other viral vaccines, undetermined

⑦T50.B95 Adverse effect of other viral vaccines

⑦T50.B96 Underdosing of other viral vaccines

T50.Z Poisoning by, adverse effect of and underdosing of other vaccines and biological substances

T50.Z1 Poisoning by, adverse effect of and underdosing of immunoglobulin

⑦T50.Z11 Poisoning by immunoglobulin, accidental (unintentional)

⑦T50.Z12 Poisoning by immunoglobulin, intentional self-harm

⑦T50.Z13 Poisoning by immunoglobulin, assault

⑦T50.Z14 Poisoning by immunoglobulin, undetermined

⑦T50.Z15 Adverse effect of immunoglobulin

⑦T50.Z16 Underdosing of immunoglobulin

T50.Z9 Poisoning by, adverse effect of and underdosing of other vaccines and biological substances

⑦T50.Z91 Poisoning by other vaccines and biological substances, accidental (unintentional)

⑦T50.Z92 Poisoning by other vaccines and biological substances, intentional self-harm

⑦T50.Z93 Poisoning by other vaccines and biological substances, assault

⑦T50.Z94 Poisoning by other vaccines and biological substances, undetermined

⑦T50.Z95 Adverse effect of other vaccines and biological substances

⑦T50.Z96 Underdosing of other vaccines and biological substances

T50.9 Poisoning by, adverse effect of and underdosing of other and unspecified drugs, medicaments and biological substances

T50.90 Poisoning by, adverse effect of and underdosing of unspecified drugs, medicaments and biological substances

⑦T50.901 Poisoning by unspecified drugs, medicaments and biological substances, accidental (unintentional)

⑦T50.902 Poisoning by unspecified drugs, medicaments and biological substances, intentional self-harm

⑦T50.903 Poisoning by unspecified drugs, medicaments and biological substances, assault

⑦T50.904 Poisoning by unspecified drugs, medicaments and biological substances, undetermined

⑦T50.905 Adverse effect of unspecified drugs, medicaments and biological substances

⑦T50.906 Underdosing of unspecified drugs, medicaments and biological substances

T50.99 Poisoning by, adverse effect of and underdosing of other drugs, medicaments and biological substances

⑦T50.991 Poisoning by other drugs, medicaments and biological substances, accidental (unintentional)

⑦T50.992 Poisoning by other drugs, medicaments and biological substances, intentional self-harm

⑦T50.993 Poisoning by other drugs, medicaments and biological substances, assault

⑦T50.994 Poisoning by other drugs, medicaments and biological substances, undetermined

⑦T50.995 Adverse effect of other drugs, medicaments and biological substances

⑦T50.996 Underdosing of other drugs, medicaments and biological substances

TOXIC EFFECTS OF SUBSTANCES CHIEFLY NONMEDICINAL AS TO SOURCE (T51-T65)

Note: When no intent is indicated code to accidental. Undetermined intent is only for use when there is specific documentation in the record that the intent of the toxic effect cannot be determined.

<u>Use additional code</u>(s):

for all associated manifestations of toxic effect, such as: respiratory conditions due to external agents (J60-J70)

personal history of foreign body fully removed (Z87.821)

to identify any retained foreign body, if applicable (Z18.-)

Excludes1: contact with and (suspected) exposure to toxic substances (Z77.-)

T51   Toxic effect of alcohol

The appropriate 7th character is to be added to each code from category T51

A - initial encounter

D - subsequent encounter

S - sequela

T51.0   Toxic effect of ethanol

Toxic effect of ethyl alcohol

Excludes2: acute alcohol intoxication or 'hangover' effects (F10.129, F10.229, F10.929)

drunkenness (F10.129, F10.229, F10.929)

pathological alcohol intoxication (F10.129, F10.229, F10.929)

T51.0X   Toxic effect of ethanol

⑦**T51.0X1   Toxic effect of ethanol, accidental (unintentional)**

Toxic effect of ethanol NOS

⑦**T51.0X2   Toxic effect of ethanol, intentional self-harm**

⑦**T51.0X3   Toxic effect of ethanol, assault**

⑦**T51.0X4   Toxic effect of ethanol, undetermined**

T51.1   Toxic effect of methanol

Toxic effect of methyl alcohol

T51.1X   Toxic effect of methanol

⑦**T51.1X1   Toxic effect of methanol, accidental (unintentional)**

Toxic effect of methanol NOS

⑦**T51.1X2   Toxic effect of methanol, intentional self-harm**

⑦**T51.1X3   Toxic effect of methanol, assault**

⑦**T51.1X4   Toxic effect of methanol, undetermined**

T51.2   Toxic effect of 2-Propanol

Toxic effect of isopropyl alcohol

T51.2X   Toxic effect of 2-Propanol

⑦**T51.2X1   Toxic effect of 2-Propanol, accidental (unintentional)**

Toxic effect of 2-Propanol NOS

⑦**T51.2X2   Toxic effect of 2-Propanol, intentional self-harm**

⑦**T51.2X3   Toxic effect of 2-Propanol, assault**

⑦**T51.2X4   Toxic effect of 2-Propanol, undetermined**

T51.3   Toxic effect of fusel oil

Toxic effect of amyl alcohol

Toxic effect of butyl [1-butanol] alcohol

Toxic effect of propyl [1-propanol] alcohol

T51.3X   Toxic effect of fusel oil

⑦**T51.3X1   Toxic effect of fusel oil, accidental (unintentional)**

Toxic effect of fusel oil NOS

⑦**T51.3X2   Toxic effect of fusel oil, intentional self-harm**

⑦**T51.3X3   Toxic effect of fusel oil, assault**

⑦**T51.3X4   Toxic effect of fusel oil, undetermined**

T51.8   Toxic effect of other alcohols

T51.8X   Toxic effect of other alcohols

⑦**T51.8X1   Toxic effect of other alcohols, accidental (unintentional)**

Toxic effect of other alcohols NOS

⑦**T51.8X2   Toxic effect of other alcohols, intentional self-harm**

⑦**T51.8X3   Toxic effect of other alcohols, assault**

⑦**T51.8X4   Toxic effect of other alcohols, undetermined**

T51.9   Toxic effect of unspecified alcohol

⊗⑦**T51.91   Toxic effect of unspecified alcohol, accidental (unintentional)**

⊗⑦**T51.92   Toxic effect of unspecified alcohol, intentional self-harm**

⊗⑦**T51.93   Toxic effect of unspecified alcohol, assault**

⊗⑦**T51.94   Toxic effect of unspecified alcohol, undetermined**

T52   Toxic effect of organic solvents

Excludes1: halogen derivatives of aliphatic and aromatic hydrocarbons (T53.-)

The appropriate 7th character is to be added to each code from category T52

A - initial encounter

D - subsequent encounter

S - sequela

⑦**T52.0 Toxic effects of petroleum products**

Toxic effects of gasoline [petrol]

Toxic effects of kerosene [paraffin oil]

Toxic effects of paraffin wax

Toxic effects of ether petroleum

Toxic effects of naphtha petroleum

Toxic effects of spirit petroleum

T52.0X   Toxic effects of petroleum products

⑦**T52.0X1   Toxic effect of petroleum products, accidental (unintentional)**

Toxic effects of petroleum products NOS

⑦**T52.0X2   Toxic effect of petroleum products, intentional self-harm**

⑦**T52.0X3   Toxic effect of petroleum products, assault**

⑦**T52.0X4   Toxic effect of petroleum products, undetermined**

T52.1   Toxic effects of benzene

Excludes1: homologues of benzene (T52.2)

nitroderivatives and aminoderivatives of benzene and its homologues (T65.3)

T52.1X   Toxic effects of benzene

⑦**T52.1X1   Toxic effect of benzene, accidental (unintentional)**

Toxic effects of benzene NOS

⑦**T52.1X2 Toxic effect of benzene, intentional self-harm**

⑦**T52.1X3 Toxic effect of benzene, assault**

⑦**T52.1X4 Toxic effect of benzene, undetermined**

T52.2 Toxic effects of homologues of benzene

Toxic effects of toluene [methylbenzene]

Toxic effects of xylene [dimethylbenzene]

T52.2X Toxic effects of homologues of benzene

⑦**T52.2X1 Toxic effect of homologues of benzene, accidental (unintentional)**

Toxic effects of homologues of benzene NOS

⑦**T52.2X2 Toxic effect of homologues of benzene, intentional self-harm**

⑦**T52.2X3 Toxic effect of homologues of benzene, assault**

⑦**T52.2X4 Toxic effect of homologues of benzene, undetermined**

T52.3 Toxic effects of glycols

T52.3X Toxic effects of glycols

⑦**T52.3X1 Toxic effect of glycols, accidental (unintentional)**

Toxic effects of glycols NOS

⑦**T52.3X2 Toxic effect of glycols, intentional self-harm**

⑦**T52.3X3 Toxic effect of glycols, assault**

⑦**T52.3X4 Toxic effect of glycols, undetermined**

T52.4 Toxic effects of ketones

T52.4X Toxic effects of ketones

⑦**T52.4X1 Toxic effect of ketones, accidental (unintentional)**

Toxic effects of ketones NOS

⑦**T52.4X2 Toxic effect of ketones, intentional self-harm**

⑦**T52.4X3 Toxic effect of ketones, assault**

⑦**T52.4X4 Toxic effect of ketones, undetermined**

T52.8 Toxic effects of other organic solvents

T52.8X Toxic effects of other organic solvents

⑦**T52.8X1 Toxic effect of other organic solvents, accidental (unintentional)**

Toxic effects **of other** organic solvents NOS

⑦**T52.8X2 Toxic effect of other organic solvents, intentional self-harm**

⑦**T52.8X3 Toxic effect of other organic solvents, assault**

⑦**T52.8X4 Toxic effect of other organic solvents, undetermined**

T52.9 Toxic effects of unspecified organic solvent

⊗⑦**T52.91 Toxic effect of unspecified organic solvent, accidental (unintentional)**

⊗⑦**T52.92 Toxic effect of unspecified organic solvent, intentional self-harm**

⊗⑦**T52.93 Toxic effect of unspecified organic solvent, assault**

⊗⑦**T52.94 Toxic effect of unspecified organic solvent, undetermined**

T53 Toxic effect of halogen derivatives of aliphatic and aromatic hydrocarbons

The appropriate 7th character is to be added to each code from category T53

A - initial encounter

D - subsequent encounter

S - sequela

T53.0 Toxic effects of carbon tetrachloride

Toxic effects of tetrachloromethane

T53.0X Toxic effects of carbon tetrachloride

⑦**T53.0X1 Toxic effect of carbon tetrachloride, accidental (unintentional)**

Toxic effects of carbon tetrachloride NOS

⑦**T53.0X2 Toxic effect of carbon tetrachloride, intentional self-harm**

⑦**T53.0X3 Toxic effect of carbon tetrachloride, assault**

⑦**T53.0X4 Toxic effect of carbon tetrachloride, undetermined**

T53.1 Toxic effects of chloroform

Toxic effects of trichloromethane

T53.1X Toxic effects of chloroform

⑦**T53.1X1 Toxic effect of chloroform, accidental (unintentional)**

Toxic effects of chloroform NOS

⑦**T53.1X2 Toxic effect of chloroform, intentional self-harm**

⑦**T53.1X3 Toxic effect of chloroform, assault**

⑦**T53.1X4 Toxic effect of chloroform, undetermined**

T53.2 Toxic effects of trichloroethylene

Toxic effects of trichloroethene

T53.2X Toxic effects of trichloroethylene

⑦**T53.2X1 Toxic effect of trichloroethylene, accidental (unintentional)**

Toxic effects of trichloroethylene NOS

⑦**T53.2X2 Toxic effect of trichloroethylene, intentional self-harm**

⑦**T53.2X3 Toxic effect of trichloroethylene, assault**

⑦**T53.2X4 Toxic effect of trichloroethylene, undetermined**

T53.3 Toxic effects of tetrachloroethylene

Toxic effects of perchloroethylene

Toxic effect of tetrachloroethane

T53.3X Toxic effects of tetrachloroethylene

⑦**T53.3X1 Toxic effect of tetrachloroethylene, accidental (unintentional)**

toxic effects of tetrachloroethylene NOS

⑦**T53.3X2 Toxic effect of tetrachloroethylene, intentional self-harm**

⑦**T53.3X3 Toxic effect of tetrachloroethylene, assault**

⑦**T53.3X4 Toxic effect of tetrachloroethylene, undetermined**

T53.4 Toxic effects of dichloromethane

Toxic effects of methylene chloride

T53.4X Toxic effects of dichloromethane

⑦**T53.4X1 Toxic effect of dichloromethane, accidental (unintentional)**

Toxic effects of dichloromethane NOS

⑦T53.4X2 Toxic effect of dichloromethane, intentional self-harm

⑦T53.4X3 Toxic effect of dichloromethane, assault

⑦T53.4X4 Toxic effect of dichloromethane, undetermined

T53.5 Toxic effects of chlorofluorocarbons

　　T53.5X Toxic effects of chlorofluorocarbons

　　　　⑦T53.5X1 Toxic effect of chlorofluorocarbons, accidental (unintentional)

　　　　　　Toxic effects of chlorofluorocarbons NOS

　　　　⑦T53.5X2 Toxic effect of chlorofluorocarbons, intentional self-harm

　　　　⑦T53.5X3 Toxic effect of chlorofluorocarbons, assault

　　　　⑦T53.5X4 Toxic effect of chlorofluorocarbons, undetermined

T53.6 Toxic effects of other halogen derivatives of aliphatic hydrocarbons

　　T53.6X Toxic effects of other halogen derivatives of aliphatic hydrocarbons

　　　　⑦T53.6X1 Toxic effect of other halogen derivatives of aliphatic hydrocarbons, accidental (unintentional)

　　　　　　Toxic effects of other halogen derivatives of aliphatic hydrocarbons NOS

　　　　⑦T53.6X2 Toxic effect of other halogen derivatives of aliphatic hydrocarbons, intentional self-harm

　　　　⑦T53.6X3 Toxic effect of other halogen derivatives of aliphatic hydrocarbons, assault

　　　　⑦T53.6X4 Toxic effect of other halogen derivatives of aliphatic hydrocarbons, undetermined

T53.7 Toxic effects of other halogen derivatives of aromatic hydrocarbons

　　T53.7X Toxic effects of other halogen derivatives of aromatic hydrocarbons

　　　　⑦T53.7X1 Toxic effect of other halogen derivatives of aromatic hydrocarbons, accidental (unintentional)

　　　　　　Toxic effects of other halogen derivatives of aromatic hydrocarbons NOS

　　　　⑦T53.7X2 Toxic effect of other halogen derivatives of aromatic hydrocarbons, intentional self-harm

　　　　⑦T53.7X3 Toxic effect of other halogen derivatives of aromatic hydrocarbons, assault

　　　　⑦T53.7X4 Toxic effect of other halogen derivatives of aromatic hydrocarbons, undetermined

T53.9 Toxic effects of unspecified halogen derivatives of aliphatic and aromatic hydrocarbons

　　⊗⑦T53.91 Toxic effect of unspecified halogen derivatives of aliphatic and aromatic hydrocarbons, accidental (unintentional)

　　⊗⑦T53.92 Toxic effect of unspecified halogen derivatives of aliphatic and aromatic hydrocarbons, intentional self-harm

⊗⑦T53.93 Toxic effect of unspecified halogen derivatives of aliphatic and aromatic hydrocarbons, assault

⊗⑦T53.94 Toxic effect of unspecified halogen derivatives of aliphatic and aromatic hydrocarbons, undetermined

T54 Toxic effect of corrosive substances

The appropriate 7th character is to be added to each code from category T54

A - initial encounter

D - subsequent encounter

S - sequela

T54.0 Toxic effects of phenol and phenol homologues

　　T54.0X Toxic effects of phenol and phenol homologues

　　　　⑦T54.0X1 Toxic effect of phenol and phenol homologues, accidental (unintentional)

　　　　　　Toxic effects of phenol and phenol homologues NOS

　　　　⑦T54.0X2 Toxic effect of phenol and phenol homologues, intentional self-harm

　　　　⑦T54.0X3 Toxic effect of phenol and phenol homologues, assault

　　　　⑦T54.0X4 Toxic effect of phenol and phenol homologues, undetermined

T54.1 Toxic effects of other corrosive organic compounds

　　T54.1X Toxic effects of other corrosive organic compounds

　　　　⑦T54.1X1 Toxic effect of other corrosive organic compounds, accidental (unintentional)

　　　　　　Toxic effects of other corrosive organic compounds NOS

　　　　⑦T54.1X2 Toxic effect of other corrosive organic compounds, intentional self-harm

　　　　⑦T54.1X3 Toxic effect of other corrosive organic compounds, assault

　　　　⑦T54.1X4 Toxic effect of other corrosive organic compounds, undetermined

T54.2 Toxic effects of corrosive acids and acid-like substances

Toxic effects of hydrochloric acid

Toxic effects of sulfuric acid

　　T54.2X Toxic effects of corrosive acids and acid-like substances

　　　　⑦T54.2X1 Toxic effect of corrosive acids and acid-like substances, accidental (unintentional)

　　　　　　Toxic effects of corrosive acids and acid-like substances NOS

　　　　⑦T54.2X2 Toxic effect of corrosive acids and acid-like substances, intentional self-harm

　　　　⑦T54.2X3 Toxic effect of corrosive acids and acid-like substances, assault

　　　　⑦T54.2X4 Toxic effect of corrosive acids and acid-like substances, undetermined

T54.3 Toxic effects of corrosive alkalis and alkali-like substances

Toxic effects of potassium hydroxide

Toxic effects of sodium hydroxide

　　T54.3X Toxic effects of corrosive alkalis and alkali-like substances

⑦**T54.3X1** Toxic effect of corrosive alkalis and alkali-like substances, accidental (unintentional)

Toxic effects of corrosive alkalis and alkali-like substances NOS

⑦**T54.3X2** Toxic effect of corrosive alkalis and alkali-like substances, intentional self-harm

⑦**T54.3X3** Toxic effect of corrosive alkalis and alkali-like substances, assault

⑦**T54.3X4** Toxic effect of corrosive alkalis and alkali-like substances, undetermined

T54.9 Toxic effects of unspecified corrosive substance

⊗⑦**T54.91** Toxic effect of unspecified corrosive substance, accidental (unintentional)

⊗⑦**T54.92** Toxic effect of unspecified corrosive substance, intentional self-harm

⊗⑦**T54.93** Toxic effect of unspecified corrosive substance, assault

⊗⑦**T54.94** Toxic effect of unspecified corrosive substance, undetermined

T55 **Toxic effect of soaps and detergents**

The appropriate 7th character is to be added to each code from category T55

A - initial encounter

D - subsequent encounter

S - sequela

T55.0 **Toxic effect of soaps**

T55.0X **Toxic effect of soaps**

⑦**T55.0X1** Toxic effect of soaps, accidental (unintentional)

Toxic effect of soaps NOS

⑦**T55.0X2** Toxic effect of soaps, intentional self-harm

⑦**T55.0X3** Toxic effect of soaps, assault

⑦**T55.0X4** Toxic effect of soaps, undetermined

T55.1 **Toxic effect of detergents**

T55.1X **Toxic effect of detergents**

⑦**T55.1X1** Toxic effect of detergents, accidental (unintentional)

Toxic effect of detergents NOS

⑦**T55.1X2** Toxic effect of detergents, intentional self-harm

⑦**T55.1X3** Toxic effect of detergents, assault

⑦**T55.1X4** Toxic effect of detergents, undetermined

T56 **Toxic effect of metals**

Includes: toxic effects of fumes and vapors of metals

toxic effects of metals from all sources, except medicinal substances

Use additional code to identify any retained metal foreign body, if applicable (Z18.0-, T18.1-)

Excludes1: arsenic and its compounds (T57.0)

manganese and its compounds (T57.2)

The appropriate 7th character is to be added to each code from category T56

A - initial encounter

D - subsequent encounter

S - sequela

T56.0 **Toxic effects of lead and its compounds**

T56.0X **Toxic effects of lead and its compounds**

⑦**T56.0X1** Toxic effect of lead and its compounds, accidental (unintentional)

Toxic effects of lead and its compounds NOS

⑦**T56.0X2** Toxic effect of lead and its compounds, intentional self-harm

⑦**T56.0X3** Toxic effect of lead and its compounds, assault

⑦**T56.0X4** Toxic effect of lead and its compounds, undetermined

T56.1 **Toxic effects of mercury and its compounds**

⑦**T56.1X** Toxic effects of mercury and its compounds

⑦**T56.1X1** Toxic effect of mercury and its compounds, accidental (unintentional)

Toxic effects of mercury and its compounds NOS

⑦**T56.1X2** Toxic effect of mercury and its compounds, intentional self-harm

⑦**T56.1X3** Toxic effect of mercury and its compounds, assault

⑦**T56.1X4** Toxic effect of mercury and its compounds, undetermined

T56.2 **Toxic effects of chromium and its compounds**

T56.2X **Toxic effects of chromium and its compounds**

⑦**T56.2X1** Toxic effect of chromium and its compounds, accidental (unintentional)

Toxic effects of chromium and its compounds NOS

⑦**T56.2X2** Toxic effect of chromium and its compounds, intentional self-harm

⑦**T56.2X3** Toxic effect of chromium and its compounds, assault

⑦**T56.2X4** Toxic effect of chromium and its compounds, undetermined

T56.3 **Toxic effects of cadmium and its compounds**

T56.3X **Toxic effects of cadmium and its compounds**

⑦**T56.3X1** Toxic effect of cadmium and its compounds, accidental (unintentional)

Toxic effects of cadmium and its compounds NOS

⑦**T56.3X2** Toxic effect of cadmium and its compounds, intentional self-harm

⑦**T56.3X3** Toxic effect of cadmium and its compounds, assault

⑦**T56.3X4** Toxic effect of cadmium and its compounds, undetermined

T56.4 **Toxic effects of copper and its compounds**

T56.4X **Toxic effects of copper and its compounds**

⑦**T56.4X1** Toxic effect of copper and its compounds, accidental (unintentional)

Toxic effects of copper and its compounds NOS

⑦**T56.4X2** Toxic effect of copper and its compounds, intentional self-harm

⑦**T56.4X3** Toxic effect of copper and its compounds, assault

⑦**T56.4X4** Toxic effect of copper and its compounds, undetermined

● New code ▲ Revised code **Excludes1:** Not coded here **Excludes2:** Not included here ⊗ Placeholder required ⑦ 7ᵗʰ digit required

T56.5 **Toxic effects of zinc and its compounds**

    T56.5X **Toxic effects of zinc and its compounds**

       ⑦**T56.5X1** **Toxic effect of zinc and its compounds, accidental (unintentional)**

          Toxic effects of zinc and its compounds NOS

       ⑦**T56.5X2** **Toxic effect of zinc and its compounds, intentional self-harm**

       ⑦**T56.5X3** **Toxic effect of zinc and its compounds, assault**

       ⑦**T56.5X4** **Toxic effect of zinc and its compounds, undetermined**

T56.6 **Toxic effects of tin and its compounds**

    T56.6X **Toxic effects of tin and its compounds**

       ⑦**T56.6X1** **Toxic effect of tin and its compounds, accidental (unintentional)**

          Toxic effects of tin and its compounds NOS

       ⑦**T56.6X2** **Toxic effect of tin and its compounds, intentional self-harm**

       ⑦**T56.6X3** **Toxic effect of tin and its compounds, assault**

       ⑦**T56.6X4** **Toxic effect of tin and its compounds, undetermined**

T56.7 **Toxic effects of beryllium and its compounds**

    T56.7X **Toxic effects of beryllium and its compounds**

       ⑦**T56.7X1** **Toxic effect of beryllium and its compounds, accidental (unintentional)**

          Toxic effects of beryllium and its compounds NOS

       ⑦**T56.7X2** **Toxic effect of beryllium and its compounds, intentional self-harm**

       ⑦**T56.7X3** **Toxic effect of beryllium and its compounds, assault**

       ⑦**T56.7X4** **Toxic effect of beryllium and its compounds, undetermined**

T56.8 **Toxic effects of other metals**

    T56.81 **Toxic effect of thallium**

       ⑦**T56.811** **Toxic effect of thallium, accidental (unintentional)**

          Toxic effect of thallium NOS

       ⑦**T56.812** **Toxic effect of thallium, intentional self-harm**

       ⑦**T56.813** **Toxic effect of thallium, assault**

       ⑦**T56.814** **Toxic effect of thallium, undetermined**

    T56.89 **Toxic effects of other metals**

       ⑦**T56.891** **Toxic effect of other metals, accidental (unintentional)**

          Toxic effects of other metals NOS

       ⑦**T56.892** **Toxic effect of other metals, intentional self-harm**

       ⑦**T56.893** **Toxic effect of other metals, assault**

       ⑦**T56.894** **Toxic effect of other metals, undetermined**

T56.9 **Toxic effects of unspecified metal**

    ⊗⑦**T56.91** **Toxic effect of unspecified metal, accidental (unintentional)**

    ⊗⑦**T56.92** **Toxic effect of unspecified metal, intentional self-harm**

    ⊗⑦**T56.93** **Toxic effect of unspecified metal, assault**

    ⊗⑦**T56.94** **Toxic effect of unspecified metal, undetermined**

T57 **Toxic effect of other inorganic substances**

The appropriate 7th character is to be added to each code from category T57

A - initial encounter

D - subsequent encounter

S - sequela

T57.0 **Toxic effect of arsenic and its compounds**

    T57.0X **Toxic effect of arsenic and its compounds**

       ⑦**T57.0X1** **Toxic effect of arsenic and its compounds, accidental (unintentional)**

          Toxic effect of arsenic and its compounds NOS

       ⑦**T57.0X2** **Toxic effect of arsenic and its compounds, intentional self-harm**

       ⑦**T57.0X3** **Toxic effect of arsenic and its compounds, assault**

       ⑦**T57.0X4** **Toxic effect of arsenic and its compounds, undetermined**

T57.1 **Toxic effect of phosphorus and its compounds**

    Excludes1: organophosphate insecticides (T60.0)

    T57.1X **Toxic effect of phosphorus and its compounds**

       ⑦**T57.1X1** **Toxic effect of phosphorus and its compounds, accidental (unintentional)**

          Toxic effect of phosphorus and its compounds NOS

       ⑦**T57.1X2** **Toxic effect of phosphorus and its compounds, intentional self-harm**

       ⑦**T57.1X3** **Toxic effect of phosphorus and its compounds, assault**

       ⑦**T57.1X4** **Toxic effect of phosphorus and its compounds, undetermined**

T57.2 **Toxic effect of manganese and its compounds**

    T57.2X **Toxic effect of manganese and its compounds**

       ⑦**T57.2X1** **Toxic effect of manganese and its compounds, accidental (unintentional)**

          Toxic effect of manganese and its compounds NOS

       ⑦**T57.2X2** **Toxic effect of manganese and its compounds, intentional self-harm**

       ⑦**T57.2X3** **Toxic effect of manganese and its compounds, assault**

       ⑦**T57.2X4** **Toxic effect of manganese and its compounds, undetermined**

T57.3 **Toxic effect of hydrogen cyanide**

    T57.3X **Toxic effect of hydrogen cyanide**

       ⑦**T57.3X1** **Toxic effect of hydrogen cyanide, accidental (unintentional)**

          Toxic effect of hydrogen cyanide NOS

       ⑦**T57.3X2** **Toxic effect of hydrogen cyanide, intentional self-harm**

       ⑦**T57.3X3** **Toxic effect of hydrogen cyanide, assault**

       ⑦**T57.3X4** **Toxic effect of hydrogen cyanide, undetermined**

T57.8 **Toxic effect of other specified inorganic substances**

    T57.8X **Toxic effect of other specified inorganic substances**

⑦**T57.8X1** Toxic effect of other specified inorganic substances, accidental (unintentional)

Toxic effect of other specified inorganic substances NOS

⑦**T57.8X2** Toxic effect of other specified inorganic substances, intentional self-harm

⑦**T57.8X3** Toxic effect of other specified inorganic substances, assault

⑦**T57.8X4** Toxic effect of other specified inorganic substances, undetermined

T57.9 **Toxic effect of unspecified inorganic substance**

⊗⑦**T57.91** Toxic effect of unspecified inorganic substance, accidental (unintentional)

⊗⑦**T57.92** Toxic effect of unspecified inorganic substance, intentional self-harm

⊗⑦**T57.93** Toxic effect of unspecified inorganic substance, assault

⊗⑦**T57.94** Toxic effect of unspecified inorganic substance, undetermined

T58 **Toxic effect of carbon monoxide**

Includes: asphyxiation from carbon monoxide

toxic effect of carbon monoxide from all sources

The appropriate 7th character is to be added to each code from category T58

A - initial encounter

D - subsequent encounter

S - sequela

T58.0 **Toxic effect of carbon monoxide from motor vehicle exhaust**

Toxic effect of exhaust gas from gas engine

Toxic effect of exhaust gas from motor pump

⊗⑦**T58.01** Toxic effect of carbon monoxide from motor vehicle exhaust, accidental (unintentional)

⊗⑦**T58.02** Toxic effect of carbon monoxide from motor vehicle exhaust, intentional self-harm

⊗⑦**T58.03** Toxic effect of carbon monoxide from motor vehicle exhaust, assault

⊗⑦**T58.04** Toxic effect of carbon monoxide from motor vehicle exhaust, undetermined

T58.1 **Toxic effect of carbon monoxide from utility gas**

Toxic effect of acetylene

Toxic effect of gas NOS used for lighting, heating, cooking

Toxic effect of water gas

⊗⑦**T58.11** Toxic effect of carbon monoxide from utility gas, accidental (unintentional)

⊗⑦**T58.12** Toxic effect of carbon monoxide from utility gas, intentional self-harm

⊗⑦**T58.13** Toxic effect of carbon monoxide from utility gas, assault

⊗⑦**T58.14** Toxic effect of carbon monoxide from utility gas, undetermined

T58.2 **Toxic effect of carbon monoxide from incomplete combustion of other domestic fuels**

Toxic effect of carbon monoxide from incomplete combustion of coal, coke, kerosene, wood

T58.2X **Toxic effect of carbon monoxide from incomplete combustion of other domestic fuels**

⑦**T58.2X1** Toxic effect of carbon monoxide from incomplete combustion of other domestic fuels, accidental (unintentional)

⑦**T58.2X2** Toxic effect of carbon monoxide from incomplete combustion of other domestic fuels, intentional self-harm

⑦**T58.2X3** Toxic effect of carbon monoxide from incomplete combustion of other domestic fuels, assault

⑦**T58.2X4** Toxic effect of carbon monoxide from incomplete combustion of other domestic fuels, undetermined

T58.8 **Toxic effect of carbon monoxide from other source**

Toxic effect of carbon monoxide from blast furnace gas

Toxic effect of carbon monoxide from fuels in industrial use

Toxic effect of carbon monoxide from kiln vapor

T58.8X **Toxic effect of carbon monoxide from other source**

⑦**T58.8X1** Toxic effect of carbon monoxide from other source, accidental (unintentional)

⑦**T58.8X2** Toxic effect of carbon monoxide from other source, intentional self-harm

⑦**T58.8X3** Toxic effect of carbon monoxide from other source, assault

⑦**T58.8X4** Toxic effect of carbon monoxide from other source, undetermined

T58.9 **Toxic effect of carbon monoxide from unspecified source**

⊗⑦**T58.91** Toxic effect of carbon monoxide from unspecified source, accidental (unintentional)

⊗⑦**T58.92** Toxic effect of carbon monoxide from unspecified source, intentional self-harm

⊗⑦**T58.93** Toxic effect of carbon monoxide from unspecified source, assault

⊗⑦**T58.94** Toxic effect of carbon monoxide from unspecified source, undetermined

T59 **Toxic effect of other gases, fumes and vapors**

Includes: aerosol propellants

Excludes1: chlorofluorocarbons (T53.5)

The appropriate 7th character is to be added to each code from category T59

A - initial encounter

D - subsequent encounter

S - sequela

T59.0 **Toxic effect of nitrogen oxides**

T59.0X **Toxic effect of nitrogen oxides**

⑦**T59.0X1** Toxic effect of nitrogen oxides, accidental (unintentional)

Toxic effect of nitrogen oxides NOS

⑦**T59.0X2** Toxic effect of nitrogen oxides, intentional self-harm

⑦**T59.0X3** Toxic effect of nitrogen oxides, assault

⑦**T59.0X4** Toxic effect of nitrogen oxides, undetermined

T59.1 **Toxic effect of sulfur dioxide**

T59.1X **Toxic effect of sulfur dioxide**

⑦**T59.1X1** Toxic effect of sulfur dioxide, accidental (unintentional)

Toxic effect of sulfur dioxide NOS

⑦**T59.1X2** Toxic effect of sulfur dioxide, intentional self-harm

⑦**T59.1X3** Toxic effect of sulfur dioxide, assault

⑦T59.1X4 Toxic effect of sulfur dioxide, undetermined

T59.2 **Toxic effect of formaldehyde**

T59.2X **Toxic effect of formaldehyde**

⑦T59.2X1 Toxic effect of formaldehyde, accidental (unintentional)

Toxic effect of formaldehyde NOS

⑦T59.2X2 Toxic effect of formaldehyde, intentional self-harm

⑦T59.2X3 Toxic effect of formaldehyde, assault

⑦T59.2X4 Toxic effect of formaldehyde, undetermined

T59.3 **Toxic effect of lacrimogenic gas**

Toxic effect of tear gas

T59.3X **Toxic effect of lacrimogenic gas**

⑦T59.3X1 Toxic effect of lacrimogenic gas, accidental (unintentional)

Toxic effect of lacrimogenic gas NOS

⑦T59.3X2 Toxic effect of lacrimogenic gas, intentional self-harm

⑦T59.3X3 Toxic effect of lacrimogenic gas, assault

⑦T59.3X4 Toxic effect of lacrimogenic gas, undetermined

T59.4 **Toxic effect of chlorine gas**

T59.4X **Toxic effect of chlorine gas**

⑦T59.4X1 Toxic effect of chlorine gas, accidental (unintentional)

Toxic effect of chlorine gas NOS

⑦T59.4X2 Toxic effect of chlorine gas, intentional self-harm

⑦T59.4X3 Toxic effect of chlorine gas, assault

⑦T59.4X4 Toxic effect of chlorine gas, undetermined

T59.5 **Toxic effect of fluorine gas and hydrogen fluoride**

T59.5X **Toxic effect of fluorine gas and hydrogen fluoride**

⑦T59.5X1 Toxic effect of fluorine gas and hydrogen fluoride, accidental (unintentional)

Toxic effect of fluorine gas and hydrogen fluoride NOS

⑦T59.5X2 Toxic effect of fluorine gas and hydrogen fluoride, intentional self-harm

⑦T59.5X3 Toxic effect of fluorine gas and hydrogen fluoride, assault

⑦T59.5X4 Toxic effect of fluorine gas and hydrogen fluoride, undetermined

T59.6 **Toxic effect of hydrogen sulfide**

T59.6X **Toxic effect of hydrogen sulfide**

⑦T59.6X1 Toxic effect of hydrogen sulfide, accidental (unintentional)

Toxic effect of hydrogen sulfide NOS

⑦T59.6X2 Toxic effect of hydrogen sulfide, intentional self-harm

⑦T59.6X3 Toxic effect of hydrogen sulfide, assault

⑦T59.6X4 Toxic effect of hydrogen sulfide, undetermined

T59.7 **Toxic effect of carbon dioxide**

T59.7X **Toxic effect of carbon dioxide**

⑦T59.7X1 Toxic effect of carbon dioxide, accidental (unintentional)

Toxic effect of carbon dioxide NOS

⑦T59.7X2 Toxic effect of carbon dioxide, intentional self-harm

⑦T59.7X3 Toxic effect of carbon dioxide, assault

⑦T59.7X4 Toxic effect of carbon dioxide, undetermined

T59.8 **Toxic effect of other specified gases, fumes and vapors**

T59.81 **Toxic effect of smoke**

Smoke inhalation

Excludes2: toxic effect of cigarette (tobacco) smoke (T65.22-)

⑦T59.811 Toxic effect of smoke, accidental (unintentional)

Toxic effect of smoke NOS

⑦T59.812 Toxic effect of smoke, intentional self-harm

⑦T59.813 Toxic effect of smoke, assault

⑦T59.814 Toxic effect of smoke, undetermined

T59.89 **Toxic effect of other specified gases, fumes and vapors**

⑦T59.891 Toxic effect of other specified gases, fumes and vapors, accidental (unintentional)

⑦T59.892 Toxic effect of other specified gases, fumes and vapors, intentional self-harm

⑦T59.893 Toxic effect of other specified gases, fumes and vapors, assault

⑦T59.894 Toxic effect of other specified gases, fumes and vapors, undetermined

T59.9 **Toxic effect of unspecified gases, fumes and vapors**

⊗⑦T59.91 Toxic effect of unspecified gases, fumes and vapors, accidental (unintentional)

⊗⑦T59.92 Toxic effect of unspecified gases, fumes and vapors, intentional self-harm

⊗⑦T59.93 Toxic effect of unspecified gases, fumes and vapors, assault

⊗⑦T59.94 Toxic effect of unspecified gases, fumes and vapors, undetermined

T60 **Toxic effect of pesticides**

Includes: toxic effect of wood preservatives

The appropriate 7th character is to be added to each code from category T60

A - initial encounter

D - subsequent encounter

S - sequela

T60.0 **Toxic effect of organophosphate and carbamate insecticides**

T60.0X **Toxic effect of organophosphate and carbamate insecticides**

⑦T60.0X1 Toxic effect of organophosphate and carbamate insecticides, accidental (unintentional)

Toxic effect of organophosphate and carbamate insecticides NOS

⑦T60.0X2 Toxic effect of organophosphate and carbamate insecticides, intentional self-harm

⑦T60.0X3 Toxic effect of organophosphate and carbamate insecticides, assault

⑦ **T60.0X4** **Toxic effect of organophosphate and carbamate insecticides, undetermined**

T60.1 **Toxic effect of halogenated insecticides**

> **Excludes1:** chlorinated hydrocarbon (T53.-)

T60.1X **Toxic effect of halogenated insecticides**

⑦ **T60.1X1** **Toxic effect of halogenated insecticides, accidental (unintentional)**

Toxic effect of halogenated insecticides NOS

⑦ **T60.1X2** **Toxic effect of halogenated insecticides, intentional self-harm**

⑦ **T60.1X3** **Toxic effect of halogenated insecticides, assault**

⑦ **T60.1X4** **Toxic effect of halogenated insecticides, undetermined**

T60.2 **Toxic effect of other insecticides**

T60.2X **Toxic effect of other insecticides**

⑦ **T60.2X1** **Toxic effect of other insecticides, accidental (unintentional)**

Toxic effect of other insecticides NOS

⑦ **T60.2X2** **Toxic effect of other insecticides, intentional self-harm**

⑦ **T60.2X3** **Toxic effect of other insecticides, assault**

⑦ **T60.2X4** **Toxic effect of other insecticides, undetermined**

T60.3 **Toxic effect of herbicides and fungicides**

T60.3X **Toxic effect of herbicides and fungicides**

⑦ **T60.3X1** **Toxic effect of herbicides and fungicides, accidental (unintentional)**

Toxic effect of herbicides and fungicides NOS

⑦ **T60.3X2** **Toxic effect of herbicides and fungicides, intentional self-harm**

⑦ **T60.3X3** **Toxic effect of herbicides and fungicides, assault**

⑦ **T60.3X4** **Toxic effect of herbicides and fungicides, undetermined**

T60.4 **Toxic effect of rodenticides**

> **Excludes1:** strychnine and its salts (T65.1)
>
> thallium (T56.81-)

T60.4X **Toxic effect of rodenticides**

⑦ **T60.4X1** **Toxic effect of rodenticides, accidental (unintentional)**

Toxic effect of rodenticides NOS

⑦ **T60.4X2** **Toxic effect of rodenticides, intentional self-harm**

⑦ **T60.4X3** **Toxic effect of rodenticides, assault**

⑦ **T60.4X4** **Toxic effect of rodenticides, undetermined**

T60.8 **Toxic effect of other pesticides**

T60.8X **Toxic effect of other pesticides**

⑦ **T60.8X1** **Toxic effect of other pesticides, accidental (unintentional)**

Toxic effect of other pesticides NOS

⑦ **T60.8X2** **Toxic effect of other pesticides, intentional self-harm**

⑦ **T60.8X3** **Toxic effect of other pesticides, assault**

⑦ **T60.8X4** **Toxic effect of other pesticides, undetermined**

T60.9 **Toxic effect of unspecified pesticide**

⊗⑦ **T60.91** **Toxic effect of unspecified pesticide, accidental (unintentional)**

⊗⑦ **T60.92** **Toxic effect of unspecified pesticide, intentional self-harm**

⊗⑦ **T60.93** **Toxic effect of unspecified pesticide, assault**

⊗⑦ **T60.94** **Toxic effect of unspecified pesticide, undetermined**

T61 **Toxic effect of noxious substances eaten as seafood**

> **Excludes1:** allergic reaction to food, such as:
>
> anaphylactic reaction or shock due to adverse food reaction (T78.0-)
>
> bacterial foodborne intoxications (A05.-)
>
> dermatitis (L23.6, L25.4, L27.2)
>
> food protein-induced enterocolitis syndrome (K52.21)
>
> food protein-induced enteropathy (K52.22)
>
> gastroenteritis (noninfective) (K52.29)
>
> toxic effect of aflatoxin **and other** mycotoxins (T64)
>
> toxic effect of cyanides (T65.0-)
>
> toxic effect of harmful algae bloom (T65.82-)
>
> toxic effect of hydrogen cyanide (T57.3-)
>
> toxic effect of mercury (T56.1-)
>
> toxic effect of red tide (T65.82-)

The appropriate 7th character is to be added to each code from category T61

A - initial encounter

D - subsequent encounter

S - sequela

T61.0 **Ciguatera fish poisoning**

⊗⑦ **T61.01** **Ciguatera fish poisoning, accidental (unintentional)**

⊗⑦ **T61.02** **Ciguatera fish poisoning, intentional self-harm**

⊗⑦ **T61.03** **Ciguatera fish poisoning, assault**

⊗⑦ **T61.04** **Ciguatera fish poisoning, undetermined**

T61.1 **Scombroid fish poisoning**

Histamine-like syndrome

⊗⑦ **T61.11** **Scombroid fish poisoning, accidental (unintentional)**

⊗⑦ **T61.12** **Scombroid fish poisoning, intentional self-harm**

⊗⑦ **T61.13** **Scombroid fish poisoning, assault**

⊗⑦ **T61.14** **Scombroid fish poisoning, undetermined**

T61.7 **Other fish and shellfish poisoning**

T61.77 **Other fish poisoning**

⑦ **T61.771** **Other fish poisoning, accidental (unintentional)**

⑦ **T61.772** **Other fish poisoning, intentional self-harm**

⑦ **T61.773** **Other fish poisoning, assault**

⑦ **T61.774** **Other fish poisoning, undetermined**

T61.78 **Other shellfish poisoning**

⑦ **T61.781** **Other shellfish poisoning, accidental (unintentional)**

⑦ **T61.782** **Other shellfish poisoning, intentional self-harm**

⑦ **T61.783** **Other shellfish poisoning, assault**

⑦ **T61.784** **Other shellfish poisoning, undetermined**

T61.8 **Toxic effect of other seafood**

T61.8X **Toxic effect of other seafood**

⑦ **T61.8X1** Toxic effect of other seafood, accidental (unintentional)

⑦ **T61.8X2** Toxic effect of other seafood, intentional self-harm

⑦ **T61.8X3** Toxic effect of other seafood, assault

⑦ **T61.8X4** Toxic effect of other seafood, undetermined

T61.9 Toxic effect of unspecified seafood

⊗⑦ **T61.91** Toxic effect of unspecified seafood, accidental (unintentional)

⊗⑦ **T61.92** Toxic effect of unspecified seafood, intentional self-harm

⊗⑦ **T61.93** Toxic effect of unspecified seafood, assault

⊗⑦ **T61.94** Toxic effect of unspecified seafood, undetermined

T62 **Toxic effect of other noxious substances eaten as food**

Excludes1: allergic reaction to food, such as:

anaphylactic shock (reaction) due to adverse food reaction (T78.0-)

bacterial food borne intoxications (A05.-)

dermatitis (L23.6, L25.4, L27.2)

food protein-induced enterocolitis syndrome (K52.21)

food protein-induced enteropathy (K52.22)

gastroenteritis (noninfective) (K52.29)

toxic effect of aflatoxin **and other** mycotoxins (T64)

toxic effect of cyanides (T65.0-)

toxic effect of hydrogen cyanide (T57.3-)

toxic effect of mercury (T56.1-)

The appropriate 7th character is to be added to each code from category T62

A - initial encounter

D - subsequent encounter

S - sequela

T62.0 **Toxic effect of ingested mushrooms**

T62.0X **Toxic effect of ingested mushrooms**

⑦ **T62.0X1** Toxic effect of ingested mushrooms, accidental (unintentional)

Toxic effect of ingested mushrooms NOS

⑦ **T62.0X2** Toxic effect of ingested mushrooms, intentional self-harm

⑦ **T62.0X3** Toxic effect of ingested mushrooms, assault

⑦ **T62.0X4** Toxic effect of ingested mushrooms, undetermined

T62.1 **Toxic effect of ingested berries**

T62.1X **Toxic effect of ingested berries**

⑦ **T62.1X1** Toxic effect of ingested berries, accidental (unintentional)

Toxic effect of ingested berries NOS

⑦ **T62.1X2** Toxic effect of ingested berries, intentional self-harm

⑦ **T62.1X3** Toxic effect of ingested berries, assault

⑦ **T62.1X4** Toxic effect of ingested berries, undetermined

T62.2 **Toxic effect of other ingested (parts of) plant(s)**

T62.2X **Toxic effect of other ingested (parts of) plant(s)**

⑦ **T62.2X1** Toxic effect of other ingested (parts of) plant(s), accidental (unintentional)

Toxic effect **of other** ingested (parts of) plant(s) NOS

⑦ **T62.2X2** Toxic effect of other ingested (parts of) plant(s), intentional self-harm

⑦ **T62.2X3** Toxic effect of other ingested (parts of) plant(s), assault

⑦ **T62.2X4** Toxic effect of other ingested (parts of) plant(s), undetermined

T62.8 **Toxic effect of other specified noxious substances eaten as food**

T62.8X **Toxic effect of other specified noxious substances eaten as food**

⑦ **T62.8X1** Toxic effect of other specified noxious substances eaten as food, accidental (unintentional)

Toxic effect **of other** specified noxious substances eaten as food NOS

⑦ **T62.8X2** Toxic effect of other specified noxious substances eaten as food, intentional self-harm

⑦ **T62.8X3** Toxic effect of other specified noxious substances eaten as food, assault

⑦ **T62.8X4** Toxic effect of other specified noxious substances eaten as food, undetermined

T62.9 **Toxic effect of unspecified noxious substance eaten as food**

⊗⑦ **T62.91** Toxic effect of unspecified noxious substance eaten as food, accidental (unintentional)

Toxic effect of unspecified noxious substance eaten as food NOS

⊗⑦ **T62.92** Toxic effect of unspecified noxious substance eaten as food, intentional self-harm

⊗⑦ **T62.93** Toxic effect of unspecified noxious substance eaten as food, assault

⊗⑦ **T62.94** Toxic effect of unspecified noxious substance eaten as food, undetermined

T63 **Toxic effect of contact with venomous animals and plants**

Includes: bite or touch of venomous animal

pricked or stuck by thorn or leaf

Excludes2: ingestion of toxic animal or plant (T61.-, T62.-)

The appropriate 7th character is to be added to each code from category T63

A - initial encounter

D - subsequent encounter

S - sequela

T63.0 **Toxic effect of snake venom**

T63.00 **Toxic effect of unspecified snake venom**

⑦ **T63.001** Toxic effect of unspecified snake venom, accidental (unintentional)

Toxic effect of unspecified snake venom NOS

T63.002 Toxic effect of unspecified snake venom, intentional self-harm

⑦ **T63.003** Toxic effect of unspecified snake venom, assault

⑦ **T63.004** Toxic effect of unspecified snake venom, undetermined

T63.01 **Toxic effect of rattlesnake venom**

⑦ **T63.011** Toxic effect of rattlesnake venom, accidental (unintentional)

Toxic effect of rattlesnake venom NOS

⑦ **T63.012** **Toxic effect of rattlesnake venom, intentional self-harm**

⑦ **T63.013** **Toxic effect of rattlesnake venom, assault**

⑦ **T63.014** **Toxic effect of rattlesnake venom, undetermined**

T63.02 **Toxic effect of coral snake venom**

⑦ **T63.021** **Toxic effect of coral snake venom, accidental (unintentional)**

Toxic effect of coral snake venom NOS

⑦ **T63.022** **Toxic effect of coral snake venom, intentional self-harm**

⑦ **T63.023** **Toxic effect of coral snake venom, assault**

⑦ **T63.024** **Toxic effect of coral snake venom, undetermined**

T63.03 **Toxic effect of taipan venom**

⑦ **T63.031** **Toxic effect of taipan venom, accidental (unintentional)**

Toxic effect of taipan venom NOS

⑦ **T63.032** **Toxic effect of taipan venom, intentional self-harm**

⑦ **T63.033** **Toxic effect of taipan venom, assault**

⑦ **T63.034** **Toxic effect of taipan venom, undetermined**

T63.04 **Toxic effect of cobra venom**

⑦ **T63.041** **Toxic effect of cobra venom, accidental (unintentional)**

Toxic effect of cobra venom NOS

⑦ **T63.042** **Toxic effect of cobra venom, intentional self-harm**

⑦ **T63.043** **Toxic effect of cobra venom, assault**

⑦ **T63.044** **Toxic effect of cobra venom, undetermined**

T63.06 **Toxic effect of venom of other North and South American snake**

⑦ **T63.061** **Toxic effect of venom of other North and South American snake, accidental (unintentional)**

Toxic effect of venom of other North and South American snake NOS

⑦ **T63.062** **Toxic effect of venom of other North and South American snake, intentional self-harm**

⑦ **T63.063** **Toxic effect of venom of other North and South American snake, assault**

⑦ **T63.064** **Toxic effect of venom of other North and South American snake, undetermined**

T63.07 **Toxic effect of venom of other Australian snake**

⑦ **T63.071** **Toxic effect of venom of other Australian snake, accidental (unintentional)**

Toxic effect of venom of other Australian snake NOS

⑦ **T63.072** **Toxic effect of venom of other Australian snake, intentional self-harm**

⑦ **T63.073** **Toxic effect of venom of other Australian snake, assault**

⑦ **T63.074** **Toxic effect of venom of other Australian snake, undetermined**

T63.08 **Toxic effect of venom of other African and Asian snake**

⑦ **T63.081** **Toxic effect of venom of other African and Asian snake, accidental (unintentional)**

Toxic effect of venom of other African and Asian snake NOS

⑦ **T63.082** **Toxic effect of venom of other African and Asian snake, intentional self-harm**

⑦ **T63.083** **Toxic effect of venom of other African and Asian snake, assault**

⑦ **T63.084** **Toxic effect of venom of other African and Asian snake, undetermined**

T63.09 **Toxic effect of venom of other snake**

⑦ **T63.091** **Toxic effect of venom of other snake, accidental (unintentional)**

Toxic effect of venom of other snake NOS

⑦ **T63.092** **Toxic effect of venom of other snake, intentional self-harm**

⑦ **T63.093** **Toxic effect of venom of other snake, assault**

⑦ **T63.094** **Toxic effect of venom of other snake, undetermined**

T63.1 **Toxic effect of venom of other reptiles**

T63.11 **Toxic effect of venom of gila monster**

⑦ **T63.111** **Toxic effect of venom of gila monster, accidental (unintentional)**

Toxic effect of venom of gila monster NOS

⑦ **T63.112** **Toxic effect of venom of gila monster, intentional self-harm**

⑦ **T63.113** **Toxic effect of venom of gila monster, assault**

⑦ **T63.114** **Toxic effect of venom of gila monster, undetermined**

T63.12 **Toxic effect of venom of other venomous lizard**

⑦ **T63.121** **Toxic effect of venom of other venomous lizard, accidental (unintentional)**

Toxic effect of venom of other venomous lizard NOS

⑦ **T63.122** **Toxic effect of venom of other venomous lizard, intentional self-harm**

⑦ **T63.123** **Toxic effect of venom of other venomous lizard, assault**

⑦ **T63.124** **Toxic effect of venom of other venomous lizard, undetermined**

T63.19 **Toxic effect of venom of other reptiles**

⑦ **T63.191** **Toxic effect of venom of other reptiles, accidental (unintentional)**

Toxic effect of venom of other reptiles NOS

⑦ **T63.192** **Toxic effect of venom of other reptiles, intentional self-harm**

⑦ **T63.193** **Toxic effect of venom of other reptiles, assault**

⑦ **T63.194** **Toxic effect of venom of other reptiles, undetermined**

T63.2 **Toxic effect of venom of scorpion**

T63.2X **Toxic effect of venom of scorpion**

⑦ **T63.2X1** **Toxic effect of venom of scorpion, accidental (unintentional)**

Toxic effect of venom of scorpion NOS

⑦T63.2X2 **Toxic effect of venom of scorpion, intentional self-harm**

⑦T63.2X3 **Toxic effect of venom of scorpion, assault**

⑦T63.2X4 **Toxic effect of venom of scorpion, undetermined**

T63.3 **Toxic effect of venom of spider**

  T63.30 **Toxic effect of unspecified spider venom**

    ⑦T63.301 **Toxic effect of unspecified spider venom, accidental (unintentional)**

    ⑦T63.302 **Toxic effect of unspecified spider venom, intentional self-harm**

    ⑦T63.303 **Toxic effect of unspecified spider venom, assault**

    ⑦T63.304 **Toxic effect of unspecified spider venom, undetermined**

  T63.31 **Toxic effect of venom of black widow spider**

    ⑦T63.311 **Toxic effect of venom of black widow spider, accidental (unintentional)**

    ⑦T63.312 **Toxic effect of venom of black widow spider, intentional self-harm**

    ⑦T63.313 **Toxic effect of venom of black widow spider, assault**

    ⑦T63.314 **Toxic effect of venom of black widow spider, undetermined**

  T63.32 **Toxic effect of venom of tarantula**

    ⑦T63.321 **Toxic effect of venom of tarantula, accidental (unintentional)**

    ⑦T63.322 **Toxic effect of venom of tarantula, intentional self-harm**

    ⑦T63.323 **Toxic effect of venom of tarantula, assault**

    ⑦T63.324 **Toxic effect of venom of tarantula, undetermined**

  T63.33 **Toxic effect of venom of brown recluse spider**

    ⑦T63.331 **Toxic effect of venom of brown recluse spider, accidental (unintentional)**

    ⑦T63.332 **Toxic effect of venom of brown recluse spider, intentional self-harm**

    ⑦T63.333 **Toxic effect of venom of brown recluse spider, assault**

    ⑦T63.334 **Toxic effect of venom of brown recluse spider, undetermined**

  T63.39 **Toxic effect of venom of other spider**

    ⑦T63.391 **Toxic effect of venom of other spider, accidental (unintentional)**

    ⑦T63.392 **Toxic effect of venom of other spider, intentional self-harm**

    ⑦T63.393 **Toxic effect of venom of other spider, assault**

    ⑦T63.394 **Toxic effect of venom of other spider, undetermined**

T63.4 **Toxic effect of venom of other arthropods**

  T63.41 **Toxic effect of venom of centipedes and venomous millipedes**

    ⑦T63.411 **Toxic effect of venom of centipedes and venomous millipedes, accidental (unintentional)**

    ⑦T63.412 **Toxic effect of venom of centipedes and venomous millipedes, intentional self-harm**

⑦T63.413 **Toxic effect of venom of centipedes and venomous millipedes, assault**

⑦T63.414 **Toxic effect of venom of centipedes and venomous millipedes, undetermined**

  T63.42 **Toxic effect of venom of ants**

    ⑦T63.421 **Toxic effect of venom of ants, accidental (unintentional)**

    ⑦T63.422 **Toxic effect of venom of ants, intentional self-harm**

    ⑦T63.423 **Toxic effect of venom of ants, assault**

    ⑦T63.424 **Toxic effect of venom of ants, undetermined**

  T63.43 **Toxic effect of venom of caterpillars**

    ⑦T63.431 **Toxic effect of venom of caterpillars, accidental (unintentional)**

    ⑦T63.432 **Toxic effect of venom of caterpillars, intentional self-harm**

    ⑦T63.433 **Toxic effect of venom of caterpillars, assault**

    ⑦T63.434 **Toxic effect of venom of caterpillars, undetermined**

  T63.44 **Toxic effect of venom of bees**

    ⑦T63.441 **Toxic effect of venom of bees, accidental (unintentional)**

    ⑦T63.442 **Toxic effect of venom of bees, intentional self-harm**

    ⑦T63.443 **Toxic effect of venom of bees, assault**

    ⑦T63.444 **Toxic effect of venom of bees, undetermined**

  T63.45 **Toxic effect of venom of hornets**

    ⑦T63.451 **Toxic effect of venom of hornets, accidental (unintentional)**

    ⑦T63.452 **Toxic effect of venom of hornets, intentional self-harm**

    ⑦T63.453 **Toxic effect of venom of hornets, assault**

    ⑦T63.454 **Toxic effect of venom of hornets, undetermined**

  T63.46 **Toxic effect of venom of wasps**

Toxic effect of yellow jacket

    ⑦T63.461 **Toxic effect of venom of wasps, accidental (unintentional)**

    ⑦T63.462 **Toxic effect of venom of wasps, intentional self-harm**

    ⑦T63.463 **Toxic effect of venom of wasps, assault**

    ⑦T63.464 **Toxic effect of venom of wasps, undetermined**

  T63.48 **Toxic effect of venom of other arthropod**

    ⑦T63.481 **Toxic effect of venom of other arthropod, accidental (unintentional)**

    ⑦T63.482 **Toxic effect of venom of other arthropod, intentional self-harm**

    ⑦T63.483 **Toxic effect of venom of other arthropod, assault**

    ⑦T63.484 **Toxic effect of venom of other arthropod, undetermined**

T63.5 **Toxic effect of contact with venomous fish**

Excludes2: poisoning by ingestion of fish (T61.-)

  T63.51 **Toxic effect of contact with stingray**

    ⑦T63.511 **Toxic effect of contact with stingray, accidental (unintentional)**

⑦T63.512 Toxic effect of contact with stingray, intentional self-harm

⑦T63.513 Toxic effect of contact with stingray, assault

⑦T63.514 Toxic effect of contact with stingray, undetermined

T63.59 Toxic effect of contact with other venomous fish

⑦**T63.591** Toxic effect of contact with other venomous fish, accidental (unintentional)

⑦**T63.592** Toxic effect of contact with other venomous fish, intentional self-harm

⑦**T63.593** Toxic effect of contact with other venomous fish, assault

⑦**T63.594** Toxic effect of contact with other venomous fish, undetermined

T63.6 Toxic effect of contact with other venomous marine animals

Excludes1: sea-snake venom (T63.09)

Excludes2: poisoning by ingestion of shellfish (T61.78-)

T63.61 Toxic effect of contact with Portuguese Man-o-war

Toxic effect of contact with bluebottle

⑦T63.611 Toxic effect of contact with Portuguese Man-o-war, accidental (unintentional)

⑦T63.612 Toxic effect of contact with Portuguese Man-o-war, intentional self-harm

⑦T63.613 Toxic effect of contact with Portuguese Man-o-war, assault

⑦T63.614 Toxic effect of contact with Portuguese Man-o-war, undetermined

T63.62 Toxic effect of contact with other jellyfish

⑦**T63.621** Toxic effect of contact with other jellyfish, accidental (unintentional)

⑦**T63.622** Toxic effect of contact with other jellyfish, intentional self-harm

⑦**T63.623** Toxic effect of contact with other jellyfish, assault

⑦**T63.624** Toxic effect of contact with other jellyfish, undetermined

T63.63 Toxic effect of contact with sea anemone

⑦T63.631 Toxic effect of contact with sea anemone, accidental (unintentional)

⑦T63.632 Toxic effect of contact with sea anemone, intentional self-harm

⑦T63.633 Toxic effect of contact with sea anemone, assault

⑦T63.634 Toxic effect of contact with sea anemone, undetermined

T63.69 Toxic effect of contact with other venomous marine animals

⑦**T63.691** Toxic effect of contact with other venomous marine animals, accidental (unintentional)

⑦**T63.692** Toxic effect of contact with other venomous marine animals, intentional self-harm

⑦**T63.693** Toxic effect of contact with other venomous marine animals, assault

⑦**T63.694** Toxic effect of contact with other venomous marine animals, undetermined

T63.7 Toxic effect of contact with venomous plant

T63.71 Toxic effect of contact with venomous marine plant

⑦T63.711 Toxic effect of contact with venomous marine plant, accidental (unintentional)

⑦T63.712 Toxic effect of contact with venomous marine plant, intentional self-harm

⑦T63.713 Toxic effect of contact with venomous marine plant, assault

⑦T63.714 Toxic effect of contact with venomous marine plant, undetermined

T63.79 Toxic effect of contact with other venomous plant

⑦**T63.791** Toxic effect of contact with other venomous plant, accidental (unintentional)

⑦**T63.792** Toxic effect of contact with other venomous plant, intentional self-harm

⑦T63.793 Toxic effect of contact with other venomous plant, assault

⑦T63.794 Toxic effect of contact with other venomous plant, undetermined

T63.8 Toxic effect of contact with other venomous animals

T63.81 Toxic effect of contact with venomous frog

Excludes1: contact with nonvenomous frog (W62.0)

⑦T63.811 Toxic effect of contact with venomous frog, accidental (unintentional)

⑦T63.812 Toxic effect of contact with venomous frog, intentional self-harm

⑦T63.813 Toxic effect of contact with venomous frog, assault

⑦T63.814 Toxic effect of contact with venomous frog, undetermined

T63.82 Toxic effect of contact with venomous toad

Excludes1: contact with nonvenomous toad (W62.1)

⑦T63.821 Toxic effect of contact with venomous toad, accidental (unintentional)

⑦T63.822 Toxic effect of contact with venomous toad, intentional self-harm

⑦T63.823 Toxic effect of contact with venomous toad, assault

⑦T63.824 Toxic effect of contact with venomous toad, undetermined

T63.83 Toxic effect of contact with other venomous amphibian

Excludes1: contact with nonvenomous amphibian (W62.9)

⑦**T63.831** Toxic effect of contact with other venomous amphibian, accidental (unintentional)

⑦**T63.832** Toxic effect of contact with other venomous amphibian, intentional self-harm

● New code ▲ Revised code **Excludes1:** Not coded here **Excludes2:** Not included here ⊗ Placeholder required ⑦7th digit required

⑦ **T63.833** Toxic effect of contact with other venomous amphibian, assault

⑦ **T63.834** Toxic effect of contact with other venomous amphibian, undetermined

T63.89 Toxic effect of contact with other venomous animals

⑦ **T63.891** Toxic effect of contact with other venomous animals, accidental (unintentional)

⑦ **T63.892** Toxic effect of contact with other venomous animals, intentional self-harm

⑦ **T63.893** Toxic effect of contact with other venomous animals, assault

⑦ **T63.894** Toxic effect of contact with other venomous animals, undetermined

T63.9 Toxic effect of contact with unspecified venomous animal

⊗⑦ **T63.91** Toxic effect of contact with unspecified venomous animal, accidental (unintentional)

⊗⑦ **T63.92** Toxic effect of contact with unspecified venomous animal, intentional self-harm

⊗⑦ **T63.93** Toxic effect of contact with unspecified venomous animal, assault

⊗⑦ **T63.94** Toxic effect of contact with unspecified venomous animal, undetermined

T64 Toxic effect of aflatoxin and other mycotoxin food contaminants

The appropriate 7th character is to be added to each code from category T64

A - initial encounter

D - subsequent encounter

S - sequela

T64.0 Toxic effect of aflatoxin

⊗⑦ **T64.01** Toxic effect of aflatoxin, accidental (unintentional)

⊗⑦ **T64.02** Toxic effect of aflatoxin, intentional self-harm

⊗⑦ **T64.03** Toxic effect of aflatoxin, assault

⊗⑦ **T64.04** Toxic effect of aflatoxin, undetermined

T64.8 Toxic effect of other mycotoxin food contaminants

⊗⑦ **T64.81** Toxic effect of other mycotoxin food contaminants, accidental (unintentional)

⊗⑦ **T64.82** Toxic effect of other mycotoxin food contaminants, intentional self-harm

⊗⑦ **T64.83** Toxic effect of other mycotoxin food contaminants, assault

⊗⑦ **T64.84** Toxic effect of other mycotoxin food contaminants, undetermined

T65 Toxic effect of other and unspecified substances

The appropriate 7th character is to be added to each code from category T65

A - initial encounter

D - subsequent encounter

S - sequela

T65.0 Toxic effect of cyanides

Excludes1: hydrogen cyanide (T57.3-)

T65.0X Toxic effect of cyanides

⑦ **T65.0X1** Toxic effect of cyanides, accidental (unintentional)

Toxic effect of cyanides NOS

⑦ **T65.0X2** Toxic effect of cyanides, intentional self-harm

⑦ **T65.0X3** Toxic effect of cyanides, assault

⑦ **T65.0X4** Toxic effect of cyanides, undetermined

T65.1 Toxic effect of strychnine and its salts

T65.1X Toxic effect of strychnine and its salts

⑦ **T65.1X1** Toxic effect of strychnine and its salts, accidental (unintentional)

Toxic effect of strychnine and its salts NOS

⑦ **T65.1X2** Toxic effect of strychnine and its salts, intentional self-harm

⑦ **T65.1X3** Toxic effect of strychnine and its salts, assault

⑦ **T65.1X4** Toxic effect of strychnine and its salts, undetermined

T65.2 Toxic effect of tobacco and nicotine

Excludes2: nicotine dependence (F17.-)

T65.21 Toxic effect of chewing tobacco

⑦ **T65.211** Toxic effect of chewing tobacco, accidental (unintentional)

Toxic effect of chewing tobacco NOS

⑦ **T65.212** Toxic effect of chewing tobacco, intentional self-harm

⑦ **T65.213** Toxic effect of chewing tobacco, assault

⑦ **T65.214** Toxic effect of chewing tobacco, undetermined

T65.22 Toxic effect of tobacco cigarettes

Toxic effect of tobacco smoke

Use additional code for exposure to second hand tobacco smoke (Z57.31, Z77.22)

⑦ **T65.221** Toxic effect of tobacco cigarettes, accidental (unintentional)

Toxic effect of tobacco cigarettes NOS

⑦ **T65.222** Toxic effect of tobacco cigarettes, intentional self-harm

⑦ **T65.223** Toxic effect of tobacco cigarettes, assault

⑦ **T65.224** Toxic effect of tobacco cigarettes, undetermined

T65.29 Toxic effect of other tobacco and nicotine

⑦ **T65.291** Toxic effect of other tobacco and nicotine, accidental (unintentional)

Toxic effect of other tobacco and nicotine NOS

⑦ **T65.292** Toxic effect of other tobacco and nicotine, intentional self-harm

⑦ **T65.293** Toxic effect of other tobacco and nicotine, assault

⑦ **T65.294** Toxic effect of other tobacco and nicotine, undetermined

T65.3 Toxic effect of nitroderivatives and aminoderivatives of benzene and its homologues

Toxic effect of anilin [benzeneamine]

Toxic effect of nitrobenzene

Toxic effect of trinitrotoluene

T65.3X Toxic effect of nitroderivatives and aminoderivatives of benzene and its homologues

⑦ **T65.3X1** Toxic effect of nitroderivatives and aminoderivatives of benzene and its homologues, accidental (unintentional)

	Add 4th-7th digits		Nonspecific code		Unspecified code		Manifestation code

Toxic effect of nitroderivatives and aminoderivatives of benzene and its homologues NOS

⑦T65.3X2 **Toxic effect of nitroderivatives and aminoderivatives of benzene and its homologues, intentional self-harm**

⑦T65.3X3 **Toxic effect of nitroderivatives and aminoderivatives of benzene and its homologues, assault**

⑦T65.3X4 **Toxic effect of nitroderivatives and aminoderivatives of benzene and its homologues, undetermined**

T65.4 **Toxic effect of carbon disulfide**

T65.4X **Toxic effect of carbon disulfide**

⑦T65.4X1 **Toxic effect of carbon disulfide, accidental (unintentional)**

Toxic effect of carbon disulfide NOS

⑦T65.4X2 **Toxic effect of carbon disulfide, intentional self-harm**

⑦T65.4X3 **Toxic effect of carbon disulfide, assault**

⑦T65.4X4 **Toxic effect of carbon disulfide, undetermined**

T65.5 **Toxic effect of nitroglycerin and other nitric acids and esters**

Toxic effect of 1,2,3-Propanetriol trinitrate

T65.5X **Toxic effect of nitroglycerin and other nitric acids and esters**

⑦T65.5X1 **Toxic effect of nitroglycerin and other nitric acids and esters, accidental (unintentional)**

Toxic effect of nitroglycerin **and other** nitric acids and esters NOS

⑦T65.5X2 **Toxic effect of nitroglycerin and other nitric acids and esters, intentional self-harm**

⑦T65.5X3 **Toxic effect of nitroglycerin and other nitric acids and esters, assault**

⑦T65.5X4 **Toxic effect of nitroglycerin and other nitric acids and esters, undetermined**

T65.6 **Toxic effect of paints and dyes, not elsewhere classified**

T65.6X **Toxic effect of paints and dyes, not elsewhere classified**

⑦T65.6X1 **Toxic effect of paints and dyes, not elsewhere classified, accidental (unintentional)**

Toxic effect of paints and dyes NOS

⑦T65.6X2 **Toxic effect of paints and dyes, not elsewhere classified, intentional self-harm**

⑦T65.6X3 **Toxic effect of paints and dyes, not elsewhere classified, assault**

⑦T65.6X4 **Toxic effect of paints and dyes, not elsewhere classified, undetermined**

T65.8 **Toxic effect of other specified substances**

T65.81 **Toxic effect of latex**

⑦T65.811 **Toxic effect of latex, accidental (unintentional)**

Toxic effect of latex NOS

⑦T65.812 **Toxic effect of latex, intentional self-harm**

⑦T65.813 **Toxic effect of latex, assault**

⑦T65.814 **Toxic effect of latex, undetermined**

T65.82 **Toxic effect of harmful algae and algae toxins**

Toxic effect of (harmful) algae bloom NOS

Toxic effect of blue-green algae bloom

Toxic effect of brown tide

Toxic effect of cyanobacteria bloom

Toxic effect of Florida red tide

Toxic effect of pfiesteria piscicida

Toxic effect of red tide

⑦T65.821 **Toxic effect of harmful algae and algae toxins, accidental (unintentional)**

Toxic effect of harmful algae and algae toxins NOS

⑦T65.822 **Toxic effect of harmful algae and algae toxins, intentional self-harm**

⑦T65.823 **Toxic effect of harmful algae and algae toxins, assault**

⑦T65.824 **Toxic effect of harmful algae and algae toxins, undetermined**

T65.83 **Toxic effect of fiberglass**

⑦T65.831 **Toxic effect of fiberglass, accidental (unintentional)**

Toxic effect of fiberglass NOS

⑦T65.832 **Toxic effect of fiberglass, intentional self-harm**

⑦T65.833 **Toxic effect of fiberglass, assault**

⑦T65.834 **Toxic effect of fiberglass, undetermined**

T65.89 **Toxic effect of other specified substances**

⑦T65.891 **Toxic effect of other specified substances, accidental (unintentional)**

Toxic effect of other specified substances NOS

⑦T65.892 **Toxic effect of other specified substances, intentional self-harm**

⑦T65.893 **Toxic effect of other specified substances, assault**

⑦T65.894 **Toxic effect of other specified substances, undetermined**

T65.9 **Toxic effect of unspecified substance**

⊗⑦T65.91 **Toxic effect of unspecified substance, accidental (unintentional)**

Poisoning NOS

⊗⑦T65.92 **Toxic effect of unspecified substance, intentional self-harm**

⊗⑦T65.93 **Toxic effect of unspecified substance, assault**

⊗⑦T65.94 **Toxic effect of unspecified substance, undetermined**

OTHER AND UNSPECIFIED EFFECTS OF EXTERNAL CAUSES (T66-T78)

⊗⑦**T66** **Radiation sickness, unspecified**

Excludes1: specified adverse effects of radiation, such as:

burns (T20-T31)

leukemia (C91-C95)

radiation gastroenteritis and colitis (K52.0)

radiation pneumonitis (J70.0)

radiation related disorders of the skin and subcutaneous tissue (L55-L59)

sunburn (L55.-)

The appropriate 7th character is to be added to code T66

A - initial encounter

D - subsequent encounter

S - sequela

T67   Effects of heat and light

Excludes1: erythema [dermatitis] ab igne (L59.0)

malignant hyperpyrexia due to anesthesia (T88.3)

radiation-related disorders of the skin and subcutaneous tissue (L55-L59)

Excludes2: burns (T20-T31)

sunburn (L55.-)

sweat disorder due to heat (L74-L75)

The appropriate 7th character is to be added to each code from category T67

A - initial encounter

D - subsequent encounter

S - sequela

⊗⑦**T67.0   Heatstroke and sunstroke**

Heat apoplexy

Heat pyrexia

Siriasis

Thermoplegia

Use additional code(s) to identify any associated complications of heatstroke, such as:

coma and stupor (R40.-)

systemic inflammatory response syndrome (R65.1-)

⊗⑦**T67.1   Heat syncope**

Heat collapse

⊗⑦**T67.2   Heat cramp**

⊗⑦**T67.3   Heat exhaustion, anhydrotic**

Heat prostration due to water depletion

Excludes1: heat exhaustion due to salt depletion (T67.4)

⊗⑦**T67.4   Heat exhaustion due to salt depletion**

Heat prostration due to salt (and water) depletion

⊗⑦**T67.5   Heat exhaustion, unspecified**

Heat prostration NOS

⊗⑦**T67.6   Heat fatigue, transient**

⊗⑦**T67.7   Heat edema**

⊗⑦**T67.8   Other effects of heat and light**

⊗⑦**T67.9   Effect of heat and light, unspecified**

⊗⑦**T68   Hypothermia**

Accidental hypothermia

Hypothermia NOS

Use additional code to identify source of exposure:

Exposure to excessive cold of man-made origin (W93)

Exposure to excessive cold of natural origin (X31)

Excludes1: hypothermia following anesthesia (T88.51)

hypothermia not associated with low environmental temperature (R68.0)

hypothermia of newborn (P80.-)

Excludes2: frostbite (T33-T34)

The appropriate 7th character is to be added to code T68

A - initial encounter

D - subsequent encounter

S - sequela

T69   Other effects of reduced temperature

Use additional code to identify source of exposure:

Exposure to excessive cold of man-made origin (W93)

Exposure to excessive cold of natural origin (X31)

Excludes2: frostbite (T33-T34)

The appropriate 7th character is to be added to each code from category T69

A - initial encounter

D - subsequent encounter

S - sequela

T69.0   Immersion hand and foot

T69.01   Immersion hand

⑦**T69.011   Immersion hand, right hand**

⑦**T69.012   Immersion hand, left hand**

⑦**T69.019   Immersion hand, unspecified hand**

T69.02   Immersion foot

Trench foot

⑦**T69.021   Immersion foot, right foot**

⑦**T69.022   Immersion foot, left foot**

⑦**T69.029   Immersion foot, unspecified foot**

⊗⑦**T69.1   Chilblains**

⊗⑦**T69.8   Other specified effects of reduced temperature**

⊗⑦**T69.9   Effect of reduced temperature, unspecified**

T70   Effects of air pressure and water pressure

The appropriate 7th character is to be added to each code from category T70

A - initial encounter

D - subsequent encounter

S - sequela

⊗⑦**T70.0   Otitic barotrauma**

Aero-otitis media

Effects of change in ambient atmospheric pressure or water pressure on ears

⊗⑦**T70.1   Sinus barotrauma**

Aerosinusitis

Effects of change in ambient atmospheric pressure on sinuses

T70.2   Other and unspecified effects of high altitude

Excludes2: polycythemia due to high altitude (D75.1)

⊗⑦**T70.20   Unspecified effects of high altitude**

⊗⑦**T70.29   Other effects of high altitude**

Alpine sickness

Anoxia due to high altitude

Barotrauma NOS

Hypobaropathy

Mountain sickness

⊗⑦**T70.3   Caisson disease [decompression sickness]**

Compressed-air disease

Diver's palsy or paralysis

⊗⑦**T70.4   Effects of high-pressure fluids**

Hydraulic jet injection (industrial)

Pneumatic jet injection (industrial)

Traumatic jet injection (industrial)

⊗⑦**T70.8   Other effects of air pressure and water pressure**

⊗⑦**T70.9   Effect of air pressure and water pressure, unspecified**

T71   Asphyxiation

Mechanical suffocation

Traumatic suffocation

Excludes1: acute respiratory distress (syndrome) (J80)

anoxia due to high altitude (T70.2) asphyxia NOS (R09.01)

asphyxia from carbon monoxide (T58.-)

asphyxia from inhalation of food or foreign body (T17.-)

asphyxia from other gases, fumes and vapors (T59.-)

respiratory distress (syndrome) in newborn (P22.-)

The appropriate 7th character is to be added to each code from category T71

A - initial encounter

D - subsequent encounter

S - sequela

T71.1   Asphyxiation due to mechanical threat to breathing

Suffocation due to mechanical threat to breathing

T71.11   Asphyxiation due to smothering under pillow

⑦**T71.111   Asphyxiation due to smothering under pillow, accidental**

Asphyxiation due to smothering under pillow NOS

⑦**T71.112   Asphyxiation due to smothering under pillow, intentional self-harm**

⑦**T71.113   Asphyxiation due to smothering under pillow, assault**

⑦**T71.114   Asphyxiation due to smothering under pillow, undetermined**

T71.12   Asphyxiation due to plastic bag

⑦**T71.121   Asphyxiation due to plastic bag, accidental**

Asphyxiation due to plastic bag NOS

⑦**T71.122   Asphyxiation due to plastic bag, intentional self-harm**

⑦**T71.123   Asphyxiation due to plastic bag, assault**

⑦**T71.124   Asphyxiation due to plastic bag, undetermined**

T71.13   Asphyxiation due to being trapped in bed linens

⑦**T71.131   Asphyxiation due to being trapped in bed linens, accidental**

Asphyxiation due to being trapped in bed linens NOS

⑦**T71.132   Asphyxiation due to being trapped in bed linens, intentional self-harm**

⑦**T71.133   Asphyxiation due to being trapped in bed linens, assault**

⑦**T71.134   Asphyxiation due to being trapped in bed linens, undetermined**

T71.14   Asphyxiation due to smothering under another person's body (in bed)

⑦**T71.141   Asphyxiation due to smothering under another person's body (in bed), accidental**

Asphyxiation due to smothering under another person's body (in bed) NOS

⑦**T71.143   Asphyxiation due to smothering under another person's body (in bed), assault**

⑦**T71.144   Asphyxiation due to smothering under another person's body (in bed), undetermined**

T71.15   Asphyxiation due to smothering in furniture

⑦**T71.151   Asphyxiation due to smothering in furniture, accidental**

Asphyxiation due to smothering in furniture NOS

⑦**T71.152   Asphyxiation due to smothering in furniture, intentional self-harm**

⑦**T71.153   Asphyxiation due to smothering in furniture, assault**

⑦**T71.154   Asphyxiation due to smothering in furniture, undetermined**

T71.16   Asphyxiation due to hanging

Hanging by window shade cord

Use additional code for any associated injuries, such as:

crushing injury of neck (S17.-)

fracture of cervical vertebrae (S12.0-S12.2-)

open wound of neck (S11.-)

⑦**T71.161   Asphyxiation due to hanging, accidental**

Asphyxiation due to hanging NOS

Hanging NOS

⑦**T71.162   Asphyxiation due to hanging, intentional self-harm**

⑦**T71.163   Asphyxiation due to hanging, assault**

⑦**T71.164   Asphyxiation due to hanging, undetermined**

T71.19   Asphyxiation due to mechanical threat to breathing due to other causes

⑦**T71.191   Asphyxiation due to mechanical threat to breathing due to other causes, accidental**

Asphyxiation due **to other** causes NOS

⑦**T71.192   Asphyxiation due to mechanical threat to breathing due to other causes, intentional self-harm**

⑦**T71.193   Asphyxiation due to mechanical threat to breathing due to other causes, assault**

⑦**T71.194   Asphyxiation due to mechanical threat to breathing due to other causes, undetermined**

T71.2   Asphyxiation due to systemic oxygen deficiency due to low oxygen content in ambient air

Suffocation due to systemic oxygen deficiency due to low oxygen content in ambient air

⊗⑦**T71.20   Asphyxiation due to systemic oxygen deficiency due to low oxygen content in ambient air due to unspecified cause**

⊗⑦**T71.21   Asphyxiation due to cave-in or falling earth**

Use additional code for any associated cataclysm (X34-X38)

T71.22   Asphyxiation due to being trapped in a car trunk

⑦**T71.221   Asphyxiation due to being trapped in a car trunk, accidental**

⑦**T71.222   Asphyxiation due to being trapped in a car trunk, intentional self-harm**

⑦**T71.223   Asphyxiation due to being trapped in a car trunk, assault**

⑦**T71.224   Asphyxiation due to being trapped in a car trunk, undetermined**

T71.23   Asphyxiation due to being trapped in a (discarded) refrigerator

⑦**T71.231   Asphyxiation due to being trapped in a (discarded) refrigerator, accidental**

⑦T71.232   **Asphyxiation due to being trapped in a (discarded) refrigerator, intentional self-harm**

⑦T71.233   **Asphyxiation due to being trapped in a (discarded) refrigerator, assault**

⑦T71.234   **Asphyxiation due to being trapped in a (discarded) refrigerator, undetermined**

⊗⑦**T71.29**   **Asphyxiation due to being trapped in other low oxygen environment**

⊗⑦**T71.9**   **Asphyxiation due to unspecified cause**

Suffocation (by strangulation) due to unspecified cause

Suffocation NOS

Systemic oxygen deficiency due to low oxygen content in ambient air due to unspecified cause

Systemic oxygen deficiency due to mechanical threat to breathing due to unspecified cause

Traumatic asphyxia NOS

T73   **Effects of other deprivation**

The appropriate 7th character is to be added to each code from category T73

A - initial encounter

D - subsequent encounter

S - sequela

⊗⑦**T73.0**   **Starvation**

Deprivation of food

⊗⑦**T73.1**   **Deprivation of water**

⊗⑦**T73.2**   **Exhaustion due to exposure**

⊗⑦**T73.3**   **Exhaustion due to excessive exertion**

Exhaustion due to overexertion

⊗⑦**T73.8**   **Other effects of deprivation**

⊗⑦**T73.9**   **Effect of deprivation, unspecified**

T74   **Adult and child abuse, neglect and other maltreatment, confirmed**

Use additional code, if applicable, to identify any associated current injury

Use additional external cause code to identify perpetrator, if known (Y07.-)

Excludes1: abuse and maltreatment in pregnancy (O9A.3-, O9A.4-, O9A.5-)

adult and child maltreatment, suspected (T76.-)

The appropriate 7th character is to be added to each code from category T74

A - initial encounter

D - subsequent encounter

S - sequela

T74.0   **Neglect or abandonment, confirmed**

⊗⑦**T74.01**   **Adult neglect or abandonment, confirmed**

⊗⑦**T74.02**   **Child neglect or abandonment, confirmed**

T74.1   **Physical abuse, confirmed**

Excludes2: sexual abuse (T74.2-)

⊗⑦**T74.11**   **Adult physical abuse, confirmed**

⊗⑦**T74.12**   **Child physical abuse, confirmed**

Excludes2: shaken infant syndrome (T74.4)

T74.2   **Sexual abuse, confirmed**

Rape, confirmed

Sexual assault, confirmed

⊗⑦**T74.21**   **Adult sexual abuse, confirmed**

⊗⑦**T74.22**   **Child sexual abuse, confirmed**

T74.3   **Psychological abuse, confirmed**

⊗⑦**T74.31**   **Adult psychological abuse, confirmed**

⊗⑦**T74.32**   **Child psychological abuse, confirmed**

T74.4   **Shaken infant syndrome**

T74.9   **Unspecified maltreatment, confirmed**

⊗⑦**T74.91**   **Unspecified adult maltreatment, confirmed**

⊗⑦**T74.92**   **Unspecified child maltreatment, confirmed**

T75   **Other and unspecified effects of other external causes**

Excludes1: adverse effects NEC (T78.-)

Excludes2: burns (electric) (T20-T31)

The appropriate 7th character is to be added to each code from category T75

A - initial encounter

D - subsequent encounter

S - sequela

T75.0   **Effects of lightning**

Struck by lightning

⊗⑦**T75.00**   **Unspecified effects of lightning**

Struck by lightning NOS

⊗⑦**T75.01**   **Shock due to being struck by lightning**

⊗⑦**T75.09**   **Other effects of lightning**

Use additional code for other effects of lightning

⊗⑦**T75.1**   **Unspecified effects of drowning and nonfatal submersion**

Immersion

Excludes1: specified effects of drowning- code to effects

T75.2   **Effects of vibration**

⊗⑦**T75.20**   **Unspecified effects of vibration**

⊗⑦**T75.21**   **Pneumatic hammer syndrome**

⊗⑦**T75.22**   **Traumatic vasospastic syndrome**

⊗⑦**T75.23**   **Vertigo from infrasound**

Excludes1: vertigo NOS (R42)

⊗⑦**T75.29**   **Other effects of vibration**

⊗⑦**T75.3**   **Motion sickness**

Airsickness

Seasickness

Travel sickness

Use additional external cause code to identify vehicle or type of motion (Y92.81-, Y93.5-)

⊗⑦**T75.4**   **Electrocution**

Shock from electric current

Shock from electroshock gun (taser)

T75.8   **Other specified effects of external causes**

⊗⑦**T75.81**   **Effects of abnormal gravitation [G] forces**

⊗⑦**T75.82**   **Effects of weightlessness**

⊗⑦**T75.89**   **Other specified effects of external causes**

T76   **Adult and child abuse, neglect and other maltreatment, suspected**

Use additional code, if applicable, to identify any associated current injury

Excludes1: adult and child maltreatment, confirmed (T74.-)

suspected abuse and maltreatment in pregnancy (O9A.3-, O9A.4-, O9A.5-)

suspected adult physical abuse, ruled out (Z04.71)

suspected adult sexual abuse, ruled out (Z04.41)

suspected child physical abuse, ruled out (Z04.72)

suspected child sexual abuse, ruled out (Z04.42)

The appropriate 7th character is to be added to each code from category T76

A - initial encounter

| | Add 4th-7th digits | | Nonspecific code | | Unspecified code | | Manifestation code | 955 |

D - subsequent encounter

S - sequela

T76.0 Neglect or abandonment, suspected

⊗⑦**T76.01 Adult neglect or abandonment, suspected**

⊗⑦**T76.02 Child neglect or abandonment, suspected**

T76.1 Physical abuse, suspected

⊗⑦**T76.11 Adult physical abuse, suspected**

⊗⑦**T76.12 Child physical abuse, suspected**

T76.2 Sexual abuse, suspected

Rape, suspected

Excludes1: alleged abuse, ruled out (Z04.7)

⊗⑦**T76.21 Adult sexual abuse, suspected**

⊗⑦**T76.22 Child sexual abuse, suspected**

T76.3 Psychological abuse, suspected

⊗⑦**T76.31 Adult psychological abuse, suspected**

⊗⑦**T76.32 Child psychological abuse, suspected**

T76.9 Unspecified maltreatment, suspected

⊗⑦**T76.91 Unspecified adult maltreatment, suspected**

⊗⑦**T76.92 Unspecified child maltreatment, suspected**

T78 Adverse effects, not elsewhere classified

Excludes2: complications of surgical and medical care NEC (T80-T88)

The appropriate 7th character is to be added to each code from category T78

A - initial encounter

D - subsequent encounter

S - sequela

T78.0 Anaphylactic reaction due to food

Anaphylactic reaction due to adverse food reaction

Anaphylactic shock or reaction due to nonpoisonous foods

Anaphylactoid reaction due to food

⊗⑦**T78.00 Anaphylactic reaction due to unspecified food**

⊗⑦**T78.01 Anaphylactic reaction due to peanuts**

⊗⑦**T78.02 Anaphylactic reaction due to shellfish (crustaceans)**

⊗⑦**T78.03 Anaphylactic reaction due to other fish**

⊗⑦**T78.04 Anaphylactic reaction due to fruits and vegetables**

⊗⑦**T78.05 Anaphylactic reaction due to tree nuts and seeds**

Excludes2: anaphylactic reaction due to peanuts (T78.01)

⊗⑦**T78.06 Anaphylactic reaction due to food additives**

⊗⑦**T78.07 Anaphylactic reaction due to milk and dairy products**

⊗⑦**T78.08 Anaphylactic reaction due to eggs**

⊗⑦**T78.09 Anaphylactic reaction due to other food products**

⊗⑦**T78.1 Other adverse food reactions, not elsewhere classified**

Use additional code to identify the type of reaction, if applicable

Excludes1: anaphylactic reaction or shock due to adverse food reaction (T78.0-)

anaphylactic reaction due to food (T78.0-)

bacterial food borne intoxications (A05.-)

Excludes2: allergic and dietetic gastroenteritis and colitis (K52.29)

allergic rhinitis due to food (J30.5)

dermatitis due to food in contact with skin (L23.6, L24.6, L25.4)

dermatitis due to ingested food (L27.2)

food protein-induced enterocolitis syndrome (K52.21)

food protein-induced enteropathy (K52.22)

⊗⑦**T78.2 Anaphylactic shock, unspecified**

Allergic shock

Anaphylactic reaction

Anaphylaxis

Excludes1: anaphylactic reaction or shock due to adverse effect of correct medicinal substance properly administered (T88.6)

anaphylactic reaction or shock due to adverse food reaction (T78.0-)

anaphylactic reaction or shock due to serum (T80.5-)

⊗⑦**T78.3 Angioneurotic edema**

Allergic angioedema Giant urticaria Quincke's edema

Excludes1: serum urticaria (T80.6-)

urticaria (L50.-)

T78.4 Other and unspecified allergy

Excludes1: specified types of allergic reaction such as:

allergic diarrhea (K52.29)

allergic gastroenteritis and colitis (K52.29)

dermatitis (L23-L25, L27.-)

food protein-induced enterocolitis syndrome (K52.21)

food protein-induced enteropathy (K52.22)

hay fever (J30.1)

⊗⑦**T78.40 Allergy, unspecified**

Allergic reaction NOS

Hypersensitivity NOS

⊗⑦**T78.41 Arthus phenomenon**

Arthus reaction

⊗⑦**T78.49 Other allergy**

⊗⑦**T78.8 Other adverse effects, not elsewhere classified**

CERTAIN EARLY COMPLICATIONS OF TRAUMA (T79)

T79 Certain early complications of trauma, not elsewhere classified

Excludes2: acute respiratory distress syndrome (J80)

complications occurring during or following medical procedures (T80-T88)

complications of surgical and medical care NEC (T80-T88)

newborn respiratory distress syndrome (P22.0)

The appropriate 7th character is to be added to each code from category T79

A - initial encounter

D - subsequent encounter

S - sequela

⊗⑦**T79.0 Air embolism (traumatic)**

Excludes1: air embolism complicating abortion or ectopic or molar pregnancy (O00-O07, O08.2)

air embolism complicating pregnancy, childbirth and the puerperium (O88.0)

air embolism following infusion, transfusion, and therapeutic injection (T80.0)

air embolism following procedure NEC (T81.7-)

⊗⑦**T79.1 Fat embolism (traumatic)**

Excludes1: fat embolism complicating:

abortion or ectopic or molar pregnancy (O00-O07, O08.2)

pregnancy, childbirth and the puerperium (O88.8)

⊗⑦**T79.2** **Traumatic secondary and recurrent hemorrhage and seroma**

⊗⑦**T79.4** **Traumatic shock**

Shock (immediate) (delayed) following injury

Excludes1: anaphylactic shock due to adverse food reaction (T78.0-)

anaphylactic shock due to correct medicinal substance properly administered (T88.6)

anaphylactic shock due to serum (T80.5-)

anaphylactic shock NOS (T78.2)

anesthetic shock (T88.2)

electric shock (T75.4)

nontraumatic shock NEC (R57.-)

obstetric shock (O75.1)

postprocedural shock (T81.1-)

septic shock (R65.21)

shock complicating abortion or ectopic or molar pregnancy (O00-O07, O08.3)

shock due to lightning (T75.01)

shock NOS (R57.9)

⊗⑦**T79.5** **Traumatic anuria**

Crush syndrome

Renal failure following crushing

⊗⑦**T79.6** **Traumatic ischemia of muscle**

Traumatic rhabdomyolysis

Volkmann's ischemic contracture

Excludes2: anterior tibial syndrome (M76.8)

compartment syndrome (traumatic) (T79.A-)

nontraumatic ischemia of muscle (M62.2-)

⊗⑦**T79.7** **Traumatic subcutaneous emphysema**

Excludes1: emphysema NOS (J43)

emphysema (subcutaneous) resulting from a procedure (T81.82)

T79.A **Traumatic compartment syndrome**

Excludes1: fibromyalgia (M79.7)

nontraumatic compartment syndrome (M79.A-)

traumatic ischemic infarction of muscle (T79.6)

⊗⑦**T79.A0** **Compartment syndrome, unspecified**

Compartment syndrome NOS

T79.A1 **Traumatic compartment syndrome of upper extremity**

Traumatic compartment syndrome of shoulder, arm, forearm, wrist, hand, and fingers

⑦**T79.A11** **Traumatic compartment syndrome of right upper extremity**

⑦**T79.A12** **Traumatic compartment syndrome of left upper extremity**

⑦**T79.A19** **Traumatic compartment syndrome of unspecified upper extremity**

T79.A2 **Traumatic compartment syndrome of lower extremity**

Traumatic compartment syndrome of hip, buttock, thigh, leg, foot, and toes

⑦**T79.A21** **Traumatic compartment syndrome of right lower extremity**

⑦**T79.A22** **Traumatic compartment syndrome of left lower extremity**

⑦**T79.A29** **Traumatic compartment syndrome of unspecified lower extremity**

⊗⑦**T79.A3** **Traumatic compartment syndrome of abdomen**

⊗⑦**T79.A9** **Traumatic compartment syndrome of other sites**

⊗⑦**T79.8** **Other early complications of trauma**

⊗⑦**T79.9** **Unspecified early complication of trauma**

COMPLICATIONS OF SURGICAL AND MEDICAL CARE, NOT ELSEWHERE CLASSIFIED (T80-T88)

Use additional code for adverse effect, if applicable, to identify drug (T36-T50 with fifth or sixth character 5)

Use additional code(s) to identify the specified condition resulting from the complication

Use additional code to identify devices involved and details of circumstances (Y62-Y82)

Excludes2: any encounters with medical care for postprocedural conditions in which no complications are present, such as:

artificial opening status (Z93.-) closure of external stoma (Z43.-)

fitting and adjustment of external prosthetic device (Z44.-)

burns and corrosions from local applications and irradiation (T20-T32)

complications of surgical procedures during pregnancy, childbirth and the puerperium (O00-O9A)

mechanical complication of respirator [ventilator] (J95.850)

poisoning and toxic effects of drugs and chemicals (T36-T65 with fifth or sixth character 1-4 or 6)

postprocedural fever (R50.82)

specified complications classified elsewhere, such as: cerebrospinal fluid leak from spinal puncture (G97.0)

colostomy malfunction (K94.0-)

disorders of fluid and electrolyte imbalance (E86-E87) f

functional disturbances following cardiac surgery (I97.0-I97.1)

intraoperative and postprocedural complications of specified body systems (D78.-, E36.-, E89.-, G97.3-, G97.4, H59.3-, H59.-, H95.2-, H95.3, I97.4-, I97.5, J95.6-, J95.7, K91.6-, L76.-, M96.-, N99.-)

ostomy complications (J95.0-, K94.-, N99.5-)

postgastric surgery syndromes (K91.1)

postlaminectomy syndrome NEC (M96.1)

postmastectomy lymphedema syndrome (I97.2)

postsurgical blind-loop syndrome (K91.2)

ventilator associated pneumonia (J95.851)

T80 **Complications following infusion, transfusion and therapeutic injection**

Includes: complications following perfusion

Excludes2: bone marrow transplant rejection (T86.01)

febrile nonhemolytic transfusion reaction (R50.84)

fluid overload due to transfusion (E87.71)

posttransfusion purpura (D69.51)

transfusion associated circulatory overload (TACO) (E87.71)

transfusion (red blood cell) associated hemochromatosis (E83.111)

transfusion related acute lung injury (TRALI) (J95.84)

The appropriate 7th character is to be added to each code from category T80

A - initial encounter

D - subsequent encounter

S - sequela

⊗⑦**T80.0** **Air embolism following infusion, transfusion and therapeutic injection**

⊗⑦**T80.1** **Vascular complications following infusion, transfusion and therapeutic injection**

Use additional code to identify the vascular complication

Excludes2: extravasation of vesicant agent (T80.81-)

infiltration of vesicant agent (T80.81-)

vascular complications specified as due to prosthetic devices, implants and grafts (T82.8-, T83.8-,T84.8-, T85.8-)

postprocedural vascular complications (T81.7-)

T80.2 **Infections following infusion, transfusion and therapeutic injection**

Use additional code to identify the specific infection, such as:

sepsis (A41.9)

Use additional code (R65.2-) to identify severe sepsis, if applicable

Excludes2: infections specified as due to prosthetic devices, implants and grafts (T82.6-T82.7, T83.5-T83.6, T84.5-T84.7, T85.7)

postprocedural infections (T81.4-)

T80.21 **Infection due to central venous catheter**

Infection due to pulmonary artery catheter (Swan-Ganz catheter)

⑦ **T80.211** **Bloodstream infection due to central venous catheter**

Catheter-related bloodstream infection (CRBSI) NOS

Central line-associated bloodstream infection (CLABSI)

Bloodstream infection due to Hickman catheter

Bloodstream infection due to peripherally inserted central catheter (PICC)

Bloodstream infection due to portacath (port-a-cath)

Bloodstream infection due to pulmonary artery catheter

Bloodstream infection due to triple lumen catheter

Bloodstream infection due to umbilical venous catheter

⑦ **T80.212** **Local infection due to central venous catheter**

Exit or insertion site infection

Local infection due to Hickman catheter

Local infection due to peripherally inserted central catheter (PICC)

Local infection due to portacath (port-a-cath)

Local infection due to pulmonary artery catheter

Local infection due to triple lumen catheter

Local infection due to umbilical venous catheter

Port or reservoir infection

Tunnel infection

⑦ **T80.218** **Other infection due to central venous catheter**

Other central line-associated infection

Other infection due to Hickman catheter

Other infection due to peripherally inserted central catheter (PICC)

Other infection due to portacath (port-a-cath)

Other infection due to pulmonary artery catheter

Other infection due to triple lumen catheter

Other infection due to umbilical venous catheter

⑦ **T80.219** **Unspecified infection due to central venous catheter**

Central line-associated infection NOS

Unspecified infection due to Hickman catheter

Unspecified infection due to peripherally inserted central catheter (PICC)

Unspecified infection due to portacath (port-a-cath)

Unspecified infection due to pulmonary artery catheter

Unspecified infection due to triple lumen catheter

Unspecified infection due to umbilical venous catheter

⊗⑦**T80.22** **Acute infection following transfusion, infusion, or injection of blood and blood products**

⊗⑦**T80.29** **Infection following other infusion, transfusion and therapeutic injection**

T80.3 **ABO incompatibility reaction due to transfusion of blood or blood products**

Excludes1: minor blood group antigens reactions (Duffy) (E) (K(ell)) (Kidd) (Lewis) (M) (N) (P) (S) (T80.A)

⊗⑦**T80.30** **ABO incompatibility reaction due to transfusion of blood or blood products, unspecified**

ABO incompatibility blood transfusion NOS

Reaction to ABO incompatibility from transfusion NOS

T80.31 **ABO incompatibility with hemolytic transfusion reaction**

⑦ **T80.310** **ABO incompatibility with acute hemolytic transfusion reaction**

ABO incompatibility with hemolytic transfusion reaction less than 24 hours after transfusion

Acute hemolytic transfusion reaction (AHTR) due to ABO incompatibility

⑦ **T80.311** **ABO incompatibility with delayed hemolytic transfusion reaction**

ABO incompatibility with hemolytic transfusion reaction 24 hours or more after transfusion

Delayed hemolytic transfusion reaction (DHTR) due to ABO incompatibility

⑦ **T80.319** **ABO incompatibility with hemolytic transfusion reaction, unspecified**

ABO incompatibility with hemolytic transfusion reaction at unspecified time after transfusion

● New code ▲ Revised code **Excludes1:** Not coded here **Excludes2:** Not included here ⊗ Placeholder required ⑦ 7th digit required

Hemolytic transfusion reaction (HTR) due to ABO incompatibility NOS

⑦**T80.39** **Other ABO incompatibility reaction due to transfusion of blood or blood products**

Delayed serologic transfusion reaction (DSTR) from ABO incompatibility

Other ABO incompatible blood transfusion

Other reaction to ABO incompatible blood transfusion

T80.4 **Rh incompatibility reaction due to transfusion of blood or blood products**

Reaction due to incompatibility of Rh antigens (C) (c) (D) (E) (e)

⊗⑦**T80.40** **Rh incompatibility reaction due to transfusion of blood or blood products, unspecified**

Reaction due to Rh factor in transfusion NOS

Rh incompatible blood transfusion NOS

T80.41 **Rh incompatibility with hemolytic transfusion reaction**

⑦**T80.410** **Rh incompatibility with acute hemolytic transfusion reaction**

Acute hemolytic transfusion reaction (AHTR) due to Rh incompatibility

Rh incompatibility with hemolytic transfusion reaction less than 24 hours after transfusion

⑦**T80.411** **Rh incompatibility with delayed hemolytic transfusion reaction**

Delayed hemolytic transfusion reaction (DHTR) due to Rh incompatibility

Rh incompatibility with hemolytic transfusion reaction 24 hours or more after transfusion

⑦**T80.419** **Rh incompatibility with hemolytic transfusion reaction, unspecified**

Rh incompatibility with hemolytic transfusion reaction at unspecified time after transfusion

Hemolytic transfusion reaction (HTR) due to Rh incompatibility NOS

⊗⑦**T80.49** **Other Rh incompatibility reaction due to transfusion of blood or blood products**

Delayed serologic transfusion reaction (DSTR) from Rh incompatibility

Other reaction to Rh incompatible blood transfusion

T80.A **Non-ABO incompatibility reaction due to transfusion of blood or blood products**

Reaction due to incompatibility of minor antigens (Duffy) (Kell) (Kidd) (Lewis) (M) (N) (P) (S)

⊗⑦**T80.A0** **Non-ABO incompatibility reaction due to transfusion of blood or blood products, unspecified**

Non-ABO antigen incompatibility reaction from transfusion NOS

T80.A1 **Non-ABO incompatibility with hemolytic transfusion reaction**

⑦**T80.A10** **Non-ABO incompatibility with acute hemolytic transfusion reaction**

Acute hemolytic transfusion reaction (AHTR) due to non-ABO incompatibility

Non-ABO incompatibility with hemolytic transfusion reaction less than 24 hours after transfusion

⑦**T80.A11** **Non-ABO incompatibility with delayed hemolytic transfusion reaction**

Delayed hemolytic transfusion reaction (DHTR) due to non-ABO incompatibility

Non-ABO incompatibility with hemolytic transfusion reaction 24 or more hours after transfusion

⑦**T80.A19** **Non-ABO incompatibility with hemolytic transfusion reaction, unspecified**

Hemolytic transfusion reaction (HTR) due to non-ABO incompatibility NOS

Non-ABO incompatibility with hemolytic transfusion reaction at unspecified time after transfusion

⊗⑦**T80.A9** **Other non-ABO incompatibility reaction due to transfusion of blood or blood products**

Delayed serologic transfusion reaction (DSTR) from non-ABO incompatibility

Other reaction to non-ABO incompatible blood transfusion

T80.5 **Anaphylactic reaction due to serum**

Allergic shock due to serum

Anaphylactic shock due to serum

Anaphylactoid reaction due to serum

Anaphylaxis due to serum

Excludes1: ABO incompatibility reaction due to transfusion of blood or blood products (T80.3-)

allergic reaction or shock NOS (T78.2) anaphylactic reaction or shock NOS (T78.2)

anaphylactic reaction or shock due to adverse effect of correct medicinal substance properly administered (T88.6) **Other** serum reaction (T80.6-)

⊗⑦**T80.51** **Anaphylactic reaction due to administration of blood and blood products**

⊗⑦**T80.52** **Anaphylactic reaction due to vaccination**

⊗⑦**T80.59** **Anaphylactic reaction due to other serum**

T80.6 **Other serum reactions into** xication by serum

Protein sickness

Serum rash

Serum sickness

Serum urticaria

Excludes2: serum hepatitis (B16-B19)

⊗⑦**T80.61** **Other serum reaction due to administration of blood and blood products**

⊗⑦**T80.62** **Other serum reaction due to vaccination**

⊗⑦**T80.69** **Other serum reaction due to other serum**

Code also, if applicable, arthropathy in hypersensitivity reactions classified elsewhere (M36.4)

T80.8 **Other complications following infusion, transfusion and therapeutic injection**

T80.81 **Extravasation of vesicant agent**

Infiltration of vesicant agent

⑦**T80.810** **Extravasation of vesicant antineoplastic chemotherapy**

Infiltration of vesicant antineoplastic chemotherapy

⑦**T80.818** **Extravasation of other vesicant agent**

Infiltration **of other** vesicant agent

Add 4th-7th digits	Nonspecific code	Unspecified code	Manifestation code

⊗⑦**T80.89** **Other complications following infusion, transfusion and therapeutic injection**

Delayed serologic transfusion reaction (DSTR), unspecified incompatibility

Use additional code to identify graft-versus-host reaction, if applicable, (D89.81-)

T80.9 **Unspecified complication following infusion, transfusion and therapeutic injection**

⊗⑦**T80.90** **Unspecified complication following infusion and therapeutic injection**

T80.91 **Hemolytic transfusion reaction, unspecified incompatibility**

Excludes1: ABO incompatibility with hemolytic transfusion reaction (T80.31-)

Non-ABO incompatibility with hemolytic transfusion reaction (T80.A1-)

Rh incompatibility with hemolytic transfusion reaction (T80.41-)

⑦ **T80.910** **Acute hemolytic transfusion reaction, unspecified incompatibility**

⑦ **T80.911** **Delayed hemolytic transfusion reaction, unspecified incompatibility**

⑦ **T80.919** **Hemolytic transfusion reaction, unspecified incompatibility, unspecified as acute or delayed**

Hemolytic transfusion reaction NOS

⊗⑦**T80.92** **Unspecified transfusion reaction**

Transfusion reaction NOS

T81 **Complications of procedures, not elsewhere classified**

Use additional code for adverse effect, if applicable, to identify drug (T36-T50 with fifth or sixth character 5)

Excludes2: complications following immunization (T88.0-T88.1)

complications following infusion, transfusion and therapeutic injection (T80.-)

complications of transplanted organs and tissue (T86.-)

specified complications classified elsewhere, such as: complication of prosthetic devices, implants and grafts (T82-T85)

dermatitis due to drugs and medicaments (L23.3, L24.4, L25.1, L27.0-L27.1)

endosseous dental implant failure (M27.6-)

floppy iris syndrome (IFIS) (intraoperative) H21.81

intraoperative and postprocedural complications of specific body system (D78.-, E36.-, E89.-, G97.3-, G97.4, H59.3-, H59.-, H95.2-, H95.3, I97.4-, I97.5, J95, K91.-, L76.-, M96.-, N99.-)

ostomy complications (J95.0-, K94.-, N99.5-)

plateau iris syndrome (post-iridectomy) (postprocedural) H21.82

poisoning and toxic effects of drugs and chemicals (T36-T65 with fifth or sixth character 1-4 or 6)

The appropriate 7th character is to be added to each code from category T81

A - initial encounter

D - subsequent encounter

S - sequela

T81.1 **Postprocedural shock**

Shock during or resulting from a procedure, not elsewhere classified

Excludes1: anaphylactic shock NOS (T78.2)

anaphylactic shock due to correct substance properly administered (T88.6)

anaphylactic shock due to serum (T80.5-)

anesthetic shock (T88.2)

electric shock (T75.4)

obstetric shock (O75.1)

septic shock (R65.21)

shock following abortion or ectopic or molar pregnancy (O00-O07, O08.3)

traumatic shock (T79.4)

⊗⊗⑦**T81.10** **Postprocedural shock unspecified**

Collapse NOS during or resulting from a procedure, not elsewhere classified

Postprocedural failure of peripheral circulation

Postprocedural shock NOS

⊗⑦**T81.11** **Postprocedural cardiogenic shock**

⊗⑦**T81.12** **Postprocedural septic shock**

Postprocedural endotoxic shock resulting from a procedure, not elsewhere classified

Postprocedural gram-negative shock resulting from a procedure, not elsewhere classified

Code first underlying infection

Use additional code, to identify any associated acute organ dysfunction, if applicable

⊗⑦**T81.19** **Other postprocedural shock**

Postprocedural hypovolemic shock

T81.3 **Disruption of wound, not elsewhere classified**

Disruption of any suture materials or other closure methods

Excludes1: breakdown (mechanical) of permanent sutures (T85.612)

displacement of permanent sutures (T85.622)

disruption of cesarean delivery wound (O90.0)

disruption of perineal obstetric wound (O90.1)

mechanical complication of permanent sutures NEC (T85.692)

⊗⑦**T81.30** **Disruption of wound, unspecified**

Disruption of wound NOS

⊗⑦**T81.31** **Disruption of external operation (surgical) wound, not elsewhere classified**

Dehiscence of operation wound NOS

Disruption of operation wound NOS

Disruption or dehiscence of closure of cornea

Disruption or dehiscence of closure of mucosa

Disruption or dehiscence of closure of skin and subcutaneous tissue

Full-thickness skin disruption or dehiscence

Superficial disruption or dehiscence of operation wound

Excludes1: dehiscence of amputation stump (T87.81)

⊗⑦**T81.32** **Disruption of internal operation (surgical) wound, not elsewhere classified**

Deep disruption or dehiscence of operation wound NOS

Disruption or dehiscence of closure of internal organ or other internal tissue

Disruption or dehiscence of closure of muscle or muscle flap

Disruption or dehiscence of closure of ribs or rib cage

Disruption or dehiscence of closure of skull or craniotomy

● New code   ▲ Revised code   **Excludes1:** Not coded here   **Excludes2:** Not included here   ⊗ Placeholder required   ⑦ 7th digit required

Disruption or dehiscence of closure of sternum or sternotomy

Disruption or dehiscence of closure of tendon or ligament

Disruption or dehiscence of closure of superficial or muscular fascia

⊗⑦**T81.33**   **Disruption of traumatic injury wound repair**

Disruption or dehiscence of closure of traumatic laceration (external) (internal)

⊗⑦**T81.4**   **Infection following a procedure**

Intra-abdominal abscess following a procedure

Postprocedural infection, not elsewhere classified

Sepsis following a procedure

Stitch abscess following a procedure

Subphrenic abscess following a procedure

Wound abscess following a procedure

<u>Use additional code</u> to identify infection

<u>Use additional code</u> (R65.2-) to identify severe sepsis, if applicable

Excludes1: obstetric surgical wound infection (O86.0)

postprocedural fever NOS (R50.82)

postprocedural retroperitoneal abscess (K68.11)

Excludes2: bleb associated endophthalmitis (H59.4-)

infection due to infusion, transfusion and therapeutic injection (T80.2-)

infection due to prosthetic devices, implants and grafts (T82.6-T82.7, T83.5-T83.6, T84.5-T84.7, T85.7)

T81.5   **Complications of foreign body accidentally left in body following procedure**

T81.50   **Unspecified complication of foreign body accidentally left in body following procedure**

⑦**T81.500**   **Unspecified complication of foreign body accidentally left in body following surgical operation**

⑦**T81.501**   **Unspecified complication of foreign body accidentally left in body following infusion or transfusion**

⑦**T81.502**   **Unspecified complication of foreign body accidentally left in body following kidney dialysis**

⑦**T81.503**   **Unspecified complication of foreign body accidentally left in body following injection or immunization**

⑦**T81.504**   **Unspecified complication of foreign body accidentally left in body following endoscopic examination**

⑦**T81.505**   **Unspecified complication of foreign body accidentally left in body following heart catheterization**

⑦**T81.506**   **Unspecified complication of foreign body accidentally left in body following aspiration, puncture or other catheterization**

⑦**T81.507**   **Unspecified complication of foreign body accidentally left in body following removal of catheter or packing**

⑦**T81.508**   **Unspecified complication of foreign body accidentally left in body following other procedure**

⑦**T81.509**   **Unspecified complication of foreign body accidentally left in body following unspecified procedure**

T81.51   **Adhesions due to foreign body accidentally left in body following procedure**

⑦**T81.510**   **Adhesions due to foreign body accidentally left in body following surgical operation**

⑦**T81.511**   **Adhesions due to foreign body accidentally left in body following infusion or transfusion**

⑦**T81.512**   **Adhesions due to foreign body accidentally left in body following kidney dialysis**

⑦**T81.513**   **Adhesions due to foreign body accidentally left in body following injection or immunization**

⑦**T81.514**   **Adhesions due to foreign body accidentally left in body following endoscopic examination**

⑦**T81.515**   **Adhesions due to foreign body accidentally left in body following heart catheterization**

⑦**T81.516**   **Adhesions due to foreign body accidentally left in body following aspiration, puncture or other catheterization**

⑦**T81.517**   **Adhesions due to foreign body accidentally left in body following removal of catheter or packing**

⑦**T81.518**   **Adhesions due to foreign body accidentally left in body following other procedure**

⑦**T81.519**   **Adhesions due to foreign body accidentally left in body following unspecified procedure**

T81.52   **Obstruction due to foreign body accidentally left in body following procedure**

⑦**T81.520**   **Obstruction due to foreign body accidentally left in body following surgical operation**

⑦**T81.521**   **Obstruction due to foreign body accidentally left in body following infusion or transfusion**

⑦**T81.522**   **Obstruction due to foreign body accidentally left in body following kidney dialysis**

⑦**T81.523**   **Obstruction due to foreign body accidentally left in body following injection or immunization**

⑦**T81.524**   **Obstruction due to foreign body accidentally left in body following endoscopic examination**

⑦**T81.525**   **Obstruction due to foreign body accidentally left in body following heart catheterization**

⑦**T81.526**   **Obstruction due to foreign body accidentally left in body following aspiration, puncture or other catheterization**

⑦**T81.527**   **Obstruction due to foreign body accidentally left in body following removal of catheter or packing**

⑦**T81.528**   **Obstruction due to foreign body accidentally left in body following other procedure**

⑦**T81.529**   **Obstruction due to foreign body accidentally left in body following unspecified procedure**

T81.53 Perforation due to foreign body accidentally left in body following procedure

⑦ **T81.530** Perforation due to foreign body accidentally left in body following surgical operation

⑦ **T81.531** Perforation due to foreign body accidentally left in body following infusion or transfusion

⑦ **T81.532** Perforation due to foreign body accidentally left in body following kidney dialysis

⑦ **T81.533** Perforation due to foreign body accidentally left in body following injection or immunization

⑦ **T81.534** Perforation due to foreign body accidentally left in body following endoscopic examination

⑦ **T81.535** Perforation due to foreign body accidentally left in body following heart catheterization

⑦ **T81.536** Perforation due to foreign body accidentally left in body following aspiration, puncture or other catheterization

⑦ **T81.537** Perforation due to foreign body accidentally left in body following removal of catheter or packing

⑦ **T81.538** Perforation due to foreign body accidentally left in body following other procedure

⑦ **T81.539** Perforation due to foreign body accidentally left in body following unspecified procedure

T81.59 Other complications of foreign body accidentally left in body following procedure

Excludes2: obstruction or perforation due to prosthetic devices and implants intentionally left in body (T82.0-T82.5, T83.0-T83.4, T83.7, T84.0-T84.4, T85.0-T85.6)

⑦ **T81.590** Other complications of foreign body accidentally left in body following surgical operation

⑦ **T81.591** Other complications of foreign body accidentally left in body following infusion or transfusion

⑦ **T81.592** Other complications of foreign body accidentally left in body following kidney dialysis

⑦ **T81.593** Other complications of foreign body accidentally left in body following injection or immunization

⑦ **T81.594** Other complications of foreign body accidentally left in body following endoscopic examination

⑦ **T81.595** Other complications of foreign body accidentally left in body following heart catheterization

⑦ **T81.596** Other complications of foreign body accidentally left in body following aspiration, puncture or other catheterization

⑦ **T81.597** Other complications of foreign body accidentally left in body following removal of catheter or packing

⑦ **T81.598** Other complications of foreign body accidentally left in body following other procedure

⑦ **T81.599** Other complications of foreign body accidentally left in body following unspecified procedure

T81.6 Acute reaction to foreign substance accidentally left during a procedure

Excludes2: complications of foreign body accidentally left in body cavity or operation wound following procedure (T81.5-)

⊗⑦**T81.60** Unspecified acute reaction to foreign substance accidentally left during a procedure

⊗⑦**T81.61** Aseptic peritonitis due to foreign substance accidentally left during a procedure

Chemical peritonitis

⊗⑦**T81.69** Other acute reaction to foreign substance accidentally left during a procedure

T81.7 Vascular complications following a procedure, not elsewhere classified

Air embolism following procedure NEC

Phlebitis or thrombophlebitis resulting from a procedure

Excludes1: embolism complicating abortion or ectopic or molar pregnancy (O00-O07, O08.2)

embolism complicating pregnancy, childbirth and the puerperium (O88.-)

traumatic embolism (T79.0)

Excludes2: embolism due to prosthetic devices, implants and grafts (T82.8-, T83.81, T84.8-, T85.81-)

embolism following infusion, transfusion and therapeutic injection (T80.0)

T81.71 Complication of artery following a procedure, not elsewhere classified

⑦ **T81.710** Complication of mesenteric artery following a procedure, not elsewhere classified

⑦ **T81.711** Complication of renal artery following a procedure, not elsewhere classified

⑦ **T81.718** Complication of other artery following a procedure, not elsewhere classified

⑦ **T81.719** Complication of unspecified artery following a procedure, not elsewhere classified

⊗⑦**T81.72** Complication of vein following a procedure, not elsewhere classified

T81.8 Other complications of procedures, not elsewhere classified

Excludes2: hypothermia following anesthesia (T88.51)

malignant hyperpyrexia due to anesthesia (T88.3)

⊗⑦**T81.81** Complication of inhalation therapy

⊗⑦**T81.82** Emphysema (subcutaneous) resulting from a procedure

⊗⑦**T81.83** Persistent postprocedural fistula

⊗⑦**T81.89** Other complications of procedures, not elsewhere classified

Use additional code to specify complication, such as:

postprocedural delirium (F05)

⊗⑦**T81.9** Unspecified complication of procedure

T82 Complications of cardiac and vascular prosthetic devices, implants and grafts

Excludes2: failure and rejection of transplanted organs and tissue (T86.-)

● New code   ▲ Revised code   **Excludes1:** Not coded here   **Excludes2:** Not included here   ⊗ Placeholder required   ⑦7th digit required

The appropriate 7th character is to be added to each code from category T82

A - initial encounter

D - subsequent encounter

S - sequela

T82.0   Mechanical complication of heart valve prosthesis

Mechanical complication of artificial heart valve

Excludes1: mechanical complication of biological heart valve graft (T82.22-)

⊗⑦**T82.01   Breakdown (mechanical) of heart valve prosthesis**

⊗⑦**T82.02   Displacement of heart valve prosthesis**

Malposition of heart valve prosthesis

⊗⑦**T82.03   Leakage of heart valve prosthesis**

⊗⑦**T82.09   Other mechanical complication of heart valve prosthesis**

Obstruction (mechanical) of heart valve prosthesis

Perforation of heart valve prosthesis

Protrusion of heart valve prosthesis

T82.1   Mechanical complication of cardiac electronic device

T82.11   Breakdown (mechanical) of cardiac electronic device

⑦**T82.110   Breakdown (mechanical) of cardiac electrode**

⑦**T82.111   Breakdown (mechanical) of cardiac pulse generator (battery)**

⑦**T82.118   Breakdown (mechanical) of other cardiac electronic device**

⑦**T82.119   Breakdown (mechanical) of unspecified cardiac electronic device**

T82.12   Displacement of cardiac electronic device

Malposition of cardiac electronic device

⑦**T82.120   Displacement of cardiac electrode**

⑦**T82.121   Displacement of cardiac pulse generator (battery)**

⑦**T82.128   Displacement of other cardiac electronic device**

⑦**T82.129   Displacement of unspecified cardiac electronic device**

T82.19   Other mechanical complication of cardiac electronic device

Leakage of cardiac electronic device

Obstruction of cardiac electronic device

Perforation of cardiac electronic device

Protrusion of cardiac electronic device

⑦**T82.190   Other mechanical complication of cardiac electrode**

⑦**T82.191   Other mechanical complication of cardiac pulse generator (battery)**

⑦**T82.198   Other mechanical complication of other cardiac electronic device**

⑦**T82.199   Other mechanical complication of unspecified cardiac device**

T82.2   Mechanical complication of coronary artery bypass graft and biological heart valve graft

Excludes1: mechanical complication of artificial heart valve prosthesis (T82.0-)

T82.21   Mechanical complication of coronary artery bypass graft

⑦**T82.211   Breakdown (mechanical) of coronary artery bypass graft**

⑦**T82.212   Displacement of coronary artery bypass graft**

Malposition of coronary artery bypass graft

⑦**T82.213   Leakage of coronary artery bypass graft**

⑦**T82.218   Other mechanical complication of coronary artery bypass graft**

Obstruction, mechanical of coronary artery bypass graft

Perforation of coronary artery bypass graft

Protrusion of coronary artery bypass graft

T82.22   Mechanical complication of biological heart valve graft

⑦**T82.221   Breakdown (mechanical) of biological heart valve graft**

⑦**T82.222   Displacement of biological heart valve graft**

Malposition of biological heart valve graft

⑦**T82.223   Leakage of biological heart valve graft**

⑦**T82.228   Other mechanical complication of biological heart valve graft**

Obstruction of biological heart valve graft

Perforation of biological heart valve graft

Protrusion of biological heart valve graft

T82.3   Mechanical complication of other vascular grafts

T82.31   Breakdown (mechanical) of other vascular grafts

⑦**T82.310   Breakdown (mechanical) of aortic (bifurcation) graft (replacement)**

⑦**T82.311   Breakdown (mechanical) of carotid arterial graft (bypass)**

⑦**T82.312   Breakdown (mechanical) of femoral arterial graft (bypass)**

⑦**T82.318   Breakdown (mechanical) of other vascular grafts**

⑦**T82.319   Breakdown (mechanical) of unspecified vascular grafts**

T82.32   Displacement of other vascular grafts

Malposition **of other** vascular grafts

⑦**T82.320   Displacement of aortic (bifurcation) graft (replacement)**

⑦**T82.321   Displacement of carotid arterial graft (bypass)**

⑦**T82.322   Displacement of femoral arterial graft (bypass)**

⑦**T82.328   Displacement of other vascular grafts**

⑦**T82.329   Displacement of unspecified vascular grafts**

T82.33   Leakage of other vascular grafts

⑦**T82.330   Leakage of aortic (bifurcation) graft (replacement)**

⑦**T82.331   Leakage of carotid arterial graft (bypass)**

⑦**T82.332   Leakage of femoral arterial graft (bypass)**

▨ Add 4th-7th digits   ▨ Nonspecific code   ▨ Unspecified code   ▨ Manifestation code

⑦ **T82.338** **Leakage of other vascular grafts**

⑦ **T82.339** **Leakage of unspecified vascular graft**

T82.39 **Other mechanical complication of other vascular grafts**

Obstruction (mechanical) of other vascular grafts

Perforation of other vascular grafts

Protrusion of other vascular grafts

⑦ **T82.390** **Other mechanical complication of aortic (bifurcation) graft (replacement)**

⑦ **T82.391** **Other mechanical complication of carotid arterial graft (bypass)**

⑦ **T82.392** **Other mechanical complication of femoral arterial graft (bypass)**

⑦ **T82.398** **Other mechanical complication of other vascular grafts**

⑦ **T82.399** **Other mechanical complication of unspecified vascular grafts**

T82.4 **Mechanical complication of vascular dialysis catheter**

Mechanical complication of hemodialysis catheter

Excludes1: mechanical complication of intraperitoneal dialysis catheter (T85.62)

⊗⑦ **T82.41** **Breakdown (mechanical) of vascular dialysis catheter**

⊗⑦ **T82.42** **Displacement of vascular dialysis catheter**

Malposition of vascular dialysis catheter

⊗⑦ **T82.43** **Leakage of vascular dialysis catheter**

⊗⑦ **T82.49** **Other complication of vascular dialysis catheter**

Obstruction (mechanical) of vascular dialysis catheter

Perforation of vascular dialysis catheter

Protrusion of vascular dialysis catheter

T82.5 **Mechanical complication of other cardiac and vascular devices and implants**

Excludes2: mechanical complication of epidural and subdural infusion catheter (T85.61)

T82.51 **Breakdown (mechanical) of other cardiac and vascular devices and implants**

⑦ **T82.510** **Breakdown (mechanical) of surgically created arteriovenous fistula**

⑦ **T82.511** **Breakdown (mechanical) of surgically created arteriovenous shunt**

⑦ **T82.512** **Breakdown (mechanical) of artificial heart**

⑦ **T82.513** **Breakdown (mechanical) of balloon (counterpulsation) device**

⑦ **T82.514** **Breakdown (mechanical) of infusion catheter**

⑦ **T82.515** **Breakdown (mechanical) of umbrella device**

⑦ **T82.518** **Breakdown (mechanical) of other cardiac and vascular devices and implants**

⑦ **T82.519** **Breakdown (mechanical) of unspecified cardiac and vascular devices and implants**

T82.52 **Displacement of other cardiac and vascular devices and implants**

Malposition **of other** cardiac and vascular devices and implants

⑦ **T82.520** **Displacement of surgically created arteriovenous fistula**

⑦ **T82.521** **Displacement of surgically created arteriovenous shunt**

⑦ **T82.522** **Displacement of artificial heart**

⑦ **T82.523** **Displacement of balloon (counterpulsation) device**

⑦ **T82.524** **Displacement of infusion catheter**

⑦ **T82.525** **Displacement of umbrella device**

⑦ **T82.528** **Displacement of other cardiac and vascular devices and implants**

⑦ **T82.529** **Displacement of unspecified cardiac and vascular devices and implants**

T82.53 **Leakage of other cardiac and vascular devices and implants**

⑦ **T82.530** **Leakage of surgically created arteriovenous fistula**

⑦ **T82.531** **Leakage of surgically created arteriovenous shunt**

⑦ **T82.532** **Leakage of artificial heart**

⑦ **T82.533** **Leakage of balloon (counterpulsation) device**

⑦ **T82.534** **Leakage of infusion catheter**

⑦ **T82.535** **Leakage of umbrella device**

⑦ **T82.538** **Leakage of other cardiac and vascular devices and implants**

⑦ **T82.539** **Leakage of unspecified cardiac and vascular devices and implants**

T82.59 **Other mechanical complication of other cardiac and vascular devices and implants**

Obstruction (mechanical) **of other** cardiac and vascular devices and implants

Perforation **of other** cardiac and vascular devices and implants

Protrusion **of other** cardiac and vascular devices and implants

⑦ **T82.590** **Other mechanical complication of surgically created arteriovenous fistula**

⑦ **T82.591** **Other mechanical complication of surgically created arteriovenous shunt**

⑦ **T82.592** **Other mechanical complication of artificial heart**

⑦ **T82.593** **Other mechanical complication of balloon (counterpulsation) device**

⑦ **T82.594** **Other mechanical complication of infusion catheter**

⑦ **T82.595** **Other mechanical complication of umbrella device**

⑦ **T82.598** **Other mechanical complication of other cardiac and vascular devices and implants**

⑦ **T82.599** **Other mechanical complication of unspecified cardiac and vascular devices and implants**

⊗⑦ **T82.6** **Infection and inflammatory reaction due to cardiac valve prosthesis**

Use additional code to identify infection

⊗⑦ **T82.7** **Infection and inflammatory reaction due to other cardiac and vascular devices, implants and grafts**

Use additional code to identify infection

T82.8 **Other specified complications of cardiac and vascular prosthetic devices, implants and grafts**

● New code   ▲ Revised code   **Excludes1:** Not coded here   **Excludes2:** Not included here   ⊗ Placeholder required   ⑦ 7ᵗʰ digit required

T82.81 Embolism due to cardiac and vascular prosthetic devices, implants and grafts

⑦**T82.817** Embolism due to cardiac prosthetic devices, implants and grafts

⑦**T82.818** Embolism due to vascular prosthetic devices, implants and grafts

T82.82 Fibrosis due to cardiac and vascular prosthetic devices, implants and grafts

⑦**T82.827** Fibrosis due to cardiac prosthetic devices, implants and grafts

⑦**T82.828** Fibrosis due to vascular prosthetic devices, implants and grafts

T82.83 Hemorrhage due to cardiac and vascular prosthetic devices, implants and grafts

⑦**T82.837** Hemorrhage due to cardiac prosthetic devices, implants and grafts

⑦**T82.838** Hemorrhage due to vascular prosthetic devices, implants and grafts

T82.84 Pain due to cardiac and vascular prosthetic devices, implants and grafts

⑦**T82.847** Pain due to cardiac prosthetic devices, implants and grafts

⑦**T82.848** Pain due to vascular prosthetic devices, implants and grafts

T82.85 Stenosis due to cardiac and vascular prosthetic devices, implants and grafts

⑦**T82.855** Stenosis of coronary artery stent

In-stent stenosis (restenosis) of coronary artery stent

Restenosis of coronary artery stent

⑦**T82.856** Stenosis of peripheral vascular stent

In-stent stenosis (restenosis) of peripheral vascular stent

Restenosis of peripheral vascular stent

⑦**T82.857** Stenosis of other cardiac prosthetic devices, implants and grafts

⑦**T82.858** Stenosis of other vascular prosthetic devices, implants and grafts

T82.86 Thrombosis of cardiac and vascular prosthetic devices, implants and grafts

⑦**T82.867** Thrombosis due to cardiac prosthetic devices, implants and grafts

⑦**T82.868** Thrombosis due to vascular prosthetic devices, implants and grafts

T82.89 Other specified complication of cardiac and vascular prosthetic devices, implants and grafts

⑦**T82.897** Other specified complication of cardiac prosthetic devices, implants and grafts

⑦**T82.898** Other specified complication of vascular prosthetic devices, implants and grafts

⊗⑦**T82.9** Unspecified complication of cardiac and vascular prosthetic device, implant and graft

T83 **Complications of genitourinary prosthetic devices, implants and grafts**

Excludes2: failure and rejection of transplanted organs and tissue (T86.-)

The appropriate 7th character is to be added to each code from category T83

A - initial encounter

D - subsequent encounter

S - sequela

T83.0 **Mechanical complication of urinary catheter**

Excludes2: complications of stoma of urinary tract N99.5-)

T83.01 Breakdown (mechanical) of urinary catheter

⑦**T83.010** Breakdown (mechanical) of cystostomy catheter

⑦**T83.011** Breakdown (mechanical) of indwelling urethral catheter

⑦**T83.012** Breakdown (mechanical) of nephrostomy catheter

⑦**T83.018** Breakdown (mechanical) of other urinary catheter

Breakdown (mechanical) of Hopkins catheter

Breakdown (mechanical) of ileostomy catheter

Breakdown (mechanical) urostomy catheter

⑦**T83.02** Displacement of urinary catheter

Malposition of urinary catheter

⑦**T83.020** Displacement of cystostomy catheter

⑦**T83.021** Displacement of indwelling urethral catheter

⑦**T83.022** Displacement of nephrostomy catheter

⑦**T83.028** Displacement of other urinary catheter

Displacement of Hopkins catheter

Displacement of ileostomy catheter

Displacement of urostomy catheter

T83.03 Leakage of urinary catheter

⑦**T83.030** Leakage of cystostomy catheter

⑦**T83.031** Leakage of indwelling urethral catheter

⑦**T83.032** Leakage of nephrostomy catheter

⑦**T83.038** Leakage of other urinary catheter

Leakage of Hopkins catheter

Leakage of ileostomy catheter

Leakage of urostomy catheter

T83.09 Other mechanical complication of urinary catheter

Obstruction (mechanical) of urinary catheter

Perforation of urinary catheter

Protrusion of urinary catheter

⑦**T83.090** Other mechanical complication of cystostomy catheter

⑦**T83.091** Other mechanical complication of indwelling urethral catheter

⑦**T83.092** Other mechanical complication of nephrostomy catheter

⑦**T83.098** Other mechanical complication of other urinary catheter

Other mechanical complication of Hopkins catheter

Other mechanical complication of ileostomy catheter

Other mechanical complication of urostomy catheter

T83.1 **Mechanical complication of other urinary devices and implants**

T83.11 **Breakdown (mechanical) of other urinary devices and implants**

⑦ **T83.110** **Breakdown (mechanical) of urinary electronic stimulator device**

Excludes2: Breakdown (mechanical) of electrode (lead) for sacral nerve neurostimulator (T85.111)

Breakdown mechanical) of implanted electronic sacral neurostimulator, pulse generator or receiver (T85.113)

⑦ **T83.111** **Breakdown (mechanical) of implanted urinary sphincter**

⑦ **T83.112** **Breakdown (mechanical) of indwelling ureteral stent**

⑦ **T83.113** **Breakdown (mechanical) of other urinary stents**

Breakdown (mechanical) of ileal conduit stent

Breakdown (mechanical) of nephroureteral stent

⑦ **T83.118** **Breakdown (mechanical) of other urinary devices and implants**

T83.12 **Displacement of other urinary devices and implants**

Malposition of other urinary devices and implants

⑦ **T83.120** **Displacement of urinary electronic stimulator device**

Excludes2: Displacement of electrode (lead) for sacral nerve neurostimulator (T85.121)

Displacement of implanted electronic sacral neurostimulator, pulse generator or receiver (T85.123)

⑦ **T83.121** **Displacement of implanted urinary sphincter**

⑦ **T83.122** **Displacement of indwelling ureteral stent**

⑦ **T83.123** **Displacement of other urinary stents**

Displacement of ileal conduit stent

Displacement of nephroureteral stent

⑦ **T83.128** **Displacement of other urinary devices and implants**

⑦ **T83.19** **Other mechanical complication of other urinary devices and implants**

Leakage of other urinary devices and implants

Obstruction (mechanical) of other urinary devices and implants

Perforation of other urinary devices and implants

Protrusion of other urinary devices and implants

⑦ **T83.190** **Other mechanical complication of urinary electronic stimulator device**

Excludes2: Other mechanical complication of electrode (lead) for sacral nerve neurostimulator (T85.191)

Other mechanical complication of implanted electronic sacral

neurostimulator, pulse generator or receiver (T85.193)

⑦ **T83.191** **Other mechanical complication of implanted urinary sphincter**

⑦ **T83.192** **Other mechanical complication of indwelling ureteral stent**

⑦ **T83.193** **Other mechanical complication of other urinary stent**

Other mechanical complication of ileal conduit stent

Other mechanical complication of nephroureteral stent

⑦ **T83.198** **Other mechanical complication of other urinary devices and implants**

T83.2 **Mechanical complication of graft of urinary organ**

⊗⑦**T83.21** **Breakdown (mechanical) of graft of urinary organ**

⊗⑦**T83.22** **Displacement of graft of urinary organ**

Malposition of graft of urinary organ

⊗⑦**T83.23** **Leakage of graft of urinary organ**

⊗⑦**T83.24** **Erosion of graft of urinary organ**

⊗⑦**T83.25** **Exposure of graft of urinary organ**

⊗⑦**T83.29** **Other mechanical complication of graft of urinary organ**

Obstruction (mechanical) of graft of urinary organ

Perforation of graft of urinary organ

Protrusion of graft of urinary organ

T83.3 **Mechanical complication of intrauterine contraceptive device**

⊗⑦**T83.31** **Breakdown (mechanical) of intrauterine contraceptive device**

⊗⑦**T83.32** **Displacement of intrauterine contraceptive device**

Malposition of intrauterine contraceptive device

Missing string of intrauterine contraceptive device

⊗⑦**T83.39** **Other mechanical complication of intrauterine contraceptive device**

Leakage of intrauterine contraceptive device

Obstruction (mechanical) of intrauterine contraceptive device

Perforation of intrauterine contraceptive device

Protrusion of intrauterine contraceptive device

T83.4 **Mechanical complication of other prosthetic devices, implants and grafts of genital tract**

T83.41 **Breakdown (mechanical) of other prosthetic devices, implants and grafts of genital tract**

⑦ **T83.410** **Breakdown (mechanical) of implanted penile prosthesis**

Breakdown (mechanical) of penile prosthesis cylinder

Breakdown (mechanical) of penile prosthesis pump

Breakdown (mechanical) of penile prosthesis reservoir

⑦ **T83.411** **Breakdown (mechanical) of implanted testicular prosthesis**

⑦ **T83.418** **Breakdown (mechanical) of other prosthetic devices, implants and grafts of genital tract**

T83.42 **Displacement of other prosthetic devices, implants and grafts of genital tract**

● New code ▲ Revised code Excludes1: Not coded here Excludes2: Not included here ⊗ Placeholder required ⑦ 7th digit required

Malposition **of other** prosthetic devices, implants and grafts of genital tract

⑦**T83.420** **Displacement of implanted penile prosthesis**

Displacement of penile prosthesis cylinder

Displacement of penile prosthesis pump

Displacement of penile prosthesis reservoir

⑦**T83.421** **Displacement of implanted testicular prosthesis**

⑦**T83.428** **Displacement of other prosthetic devices, implants and grafts of genital tract**

T83.49 **Other mechanical complication of other prosthetic devices, implants and grafts of genital tract**

Leakage **of** other prosthetic devices, implants and grafts of genital tract

Obstruction, mechanical of other prosthetic devices, implants and grafts of genital tract

Perforation of other prosthetic devices, implants and grafts of genital tract

Protrusion **of other** prosthetic devices, implants and grafts of genital tract

⑦**T83.490** **Other mechanical complication of implanted penile prosthesis**

Other mechanical complication of penile prosthesis cylinder

Other mechanical complication of penile prosthesis pump

Other mechanical complication of penile prosthesis reservoir

⑦**T83.491** **Other mechanical complication of implanted testicular prosthesis**

⑦**T83.498** **Other mechanical complication of other prosthetic devices, implants and grafts of genital tract**

T83.5 **Infection and inflammatory reaction due to prosthetic device, implant and graft in urinary system**

Use additional code to identify infection

T83.51 **Infection and inflammatory reaction due to urinary catheter**

Excludes2: complications of stoma of urinary tract (N99.5-)

⑦**T83.510** **Infection and inflammatory reaction due to cystostomy catheter**

⑦**T83.511** **Infection and inflammatory reaction due to indwelling urethral catheter**

⑦**T83.512** **Infection and inflammatory reaction due to nephrostomy catheter**

⑦**T83.518** **Infection and inflammatory reaction due to other urinary catheter**

Infection and inflammatory reaction due to Hopkins catheter

Infection and inflammatory reaction due to ileostomy catheter

Infection and inflammatory reaction due to urostomy catheter

T83.59 **Infection and inflammatory reaction due to prosthetic device, implant and graft in urinary system**

⑦**T83.590** **Infection and inflammatory reaction due to implanted urinary neurostimulation device**

Excludes2: Infection and inflammatory reaction due to electrode lead of sacral nerve neurostimulator (T85.732)

Infection and inflammatory reaction due to pulse generator or receiver of sacral nerve neurostimulator (T85.734)

⑦**T83.591** **Infection and inflammatory reaction due to implanted urinary sphincter**

⑦**T83.592** **Infection and inflammatory reaction due to indwelling ureteral stent**

⑦**T83.593** **Infection and inflammatory reaction due to other urinary stents**

Infection and inflammatory reaction due to ileal conduit stents

Infection and inflammatory reaction due to nephroureteral stent

⑦**T83.598** **Infection and inflammatory reaction due to other prosthetic device, implant and graft in urinary system**

T83.6 **Infection and inflammatory reaction due to prosthetic device, implant and graft in genital tract**

Use additional code to identify infection

⊗⑦**T83.61** **Infection and inflammatory reaction due to implanted penile prosthesis**

Infection and inflammatory reaction due to penile prosthesis cylinder

Infection and inflammatory reaction due to penile prosthesis pump

Infection and inflammatory reaction due to penile prosthesis reservoir

⊗⑦**T83.62** **Infection and inflammatory reaction due to implanted testicular prosthesis**

⊗⑦**T83.69** **Infection and inflammatory reaction due to other prosthetic device, implant and graft in genital tract**

T83.7 **Complications due to implanted mesh and other prosthetic materials**

T83.71 **Erosion of implanted mesh and other prosthetic materials to surrounding organ or tissue**

⑦**T83.711** **Erosion of implanted vaginal mesh to surrounding organ or tissue**

Erosion of implanted vaginal mesh into pelvic floor muscles

⑦**T83.712** **Erosion of implanted urethral mesh to surrounding organ or tissue**

Erosion of implanted female urethral sling

Erosion of implanted male urethral sling

Erosion of implanted urethral mesh into pelvic floor muscles

⑦**T83.713** **Erosion of implanted urethral bulking agent to surrounding organ or tissue**

⑦**T83.714** **Erosion of implanted ureteral bulking agent to surrounding organ or tissue**

⑦**T83.718** **Erosion of other implanted mesh to organ or tissue**

⑦ **T83.719**   **Erosion of other prosthetic materials to surrounding organ or tissue**

T83.72   **Exposure of implanted mesh and other prosthetic materials into surrounding organ or tissue**

Extrusion of implanted mesh

⑦ **T83.721**   **Exposure of implanted vaginal mesh into vagina**

Exposure of implanted vaginal mesh through vaginal wall

⑦ **T83.722**   **Exposure of implanted urethral mesh into urethra**

Exposure of implanted female urethral sling

Exposure of implanted male urethral sling

Exposure of implanted urethral mesh through urethral wall

⑦ **T83.723**   **Exposure of implanted urethral bulking agent into urethra**

⑦ **T83.724**   **Exposure of implanted ureteral bulking agent into ureter**

⑦ **T83.728**   **Exposure of other implanted mesh into organ or tissue**

⑦ **T83.729**   **Exposure of other prosthetic materials into organ or tissue**

⊗⑦ **T83.79**   **Other specified complications due to other genitourinary prosthetic materials**

T83.8   **Other specified complications of genitourinary prosthetic devices, implants and grafts**

⊗⑦ **T83.81**   **Embolism due to genitourinary prosthetic devices, implants and grafts**

⊗⑦ **T83.82**   **Fibrosis due to genitourinary prosthetic devices, implants and grafts**

⊗⑦ **T83.83**   **Hemorrhage due to genitourinary prosthetic devices, implants and grafts**

⊗⑦ **T83.84**   **Pain due to genitourinary prosthetic devices, implants and grafts**

⊗⑦ **T83.85**   **Stenosis due to genitourinary prosthetic devices, implants and grafts**

⊗⑦ **T83.86**   **Thrombosis due to genitourinary prosthetic devices, implants and grafts**

⊗⑦ **T83.89**   **Other specified complication of genitourinary prosthetic devices, implants and grafts**

⑦ **T83.9**   **Unspecified complication of genitourinary prosthetic device, implant and graft**

T84   **Complications of internal orthopedic prosthetic devices, implants and grafts**

> **Excludes2:** failure and rejection of transplanted organs and tissues (T86.-)

fracture of bone following insertion of orthopedic implant, joint prosthesis or bone plate (M96.6)

The appropriate 7th character is to be added to each code from category T84

A - initial encounter

D - subsequent encounter

S - sequela

T84.0   **Mechanical complication of internal joint prosthesis**

T84.01   **Broken internal joint prosthesis**

Breakage (fracture) of prosthetic joint

Broken prosthetic joint implant

> **Excludes1:** periprosthetic joint implant fracture (M97-)

⑦ **T84.010**   **Broken internal right hip prosthesis**

⑦ **T84.011**   **Broken internal left hip prosthesis**

⑦ **T84.012**   **Broken internal right knee prosthesis**

⑦ **T84.013**   **Broken internal left knee prosthesis**

⑦ **T84.018**   **Broken internal joint prosthesis, other site**

> **Use additional code** to identify the joint (Z96.6-)

⑦ **T84.019**   **Broken internal joint prosthesis, unspecified site**

T84.02   **Dislocation of internal joint prosthesis**

Instability of internal joint prosthesis

Subluxation of internal joint prosthesis

⑦ **T84.020**   **Dislocation of internal right hip prosthesis**

⑦ **T84.021**   **Dislocation of internal left hip prosthesis**

⑦ **T84.022**   **Instability of internal right knee prosthesis**

⑦ **T84.023**   **Instability of internal left knee prosthesis**

⑦ **T84.028**   **Dislocation of other internal joint prosthesis**

> **Use additional code** to identify the joint (Z96.6-)

⑦ **T84.029**   **Dislocation of unspecified internal joint prosthesis**

T84.03   **Mechanical loosening of internal prosthetic joint**

Aseptic loosening of prosthetic joint

⑦ **T84.030**   **Mechanical loosening of internal right hip prosthetic joint**

⑦ **T84.031**   **Mechanical loosening of internal left hip prosthetic joint**

⑦ **T84.032**   **Mechanical loosening of internal right knee prosthetic joint**

⑦ **T84.033**   **Mechanical loosening of internal left knee prosthetic joint**

⑦ **T84.038**   **Mechanical loosening of other internal prosthetic joint**

> **Use additional code** to identify the joint (Z96.6-)

⑦ **T84.039**   **Mechanical loosening of unspecified internal prosthetic joint**

T84.05   **Periprosthetic osteolysis of internal prosthetic joint**

> **Use additional code** to identify major osseous defect, if applicable (M89.7-)

⑦ **T84.050**   **Periprosthetic osteolysis of internal prosthetic right hip joint**

⑦ **T84.051**   **Periprosthetic osteolysis of internal prosthetic left hip joint**

⑦ **T84.052**   **Periprosthetic osteolysis of internal prosthetic right knee joint**

⑦ **T84.053**   **Periprosthetic osteolysis of internal prosthetic left knee joint**

⑦ **T84.058**   **Periprosthetic osteolysis of other internal prosthetic joint**

> **Use additional code** to identify the joint (Z96.6-)

⑦ **T84.059**   **Periprosthetic osteolysis of unspecified internal prosthetic joint**

T84.06   **Wear of articular bearing surface of internal prosthetic joint**

⑦T84.060   **Wear of articular bearing surface of internal prosthetic right hip joint**

⑦T84.061   **Wear of articular bearing surface of internal prosthetic left hip joint**

⑦T84.062   **Wear of articular bearing surface of internal prosthetic right knee joint**

⑦T84.063   **Wear of articular bearing surface of internal prosthetic left knee joint**

⑦T84.068   **Wear of articular bearing surface of other internal prosthetic joint**

Use additional code to identify the joint (Z96.6-)

⑦T84.069   **Wear of articular bearing surface of unspecified internal prosthetic joint**

T84.09   **Other mechanical complication of internal joint prosthesis**

Prosthetic joint implant failure NOS

⑦T84.090   **Other mechanical complication of internal right hip prosthesis**

⑦T84.091   **Other mechanical complication of internal left hip prosthesis**

⑦T84.092   **Other mechanical complication of internal right knee prosthesis**

⑦T84.093   **Other mechanical complication of internal left knee prosthesis**

⑦T84.098   **Other mechanical complication of other internal joint prosthesis**

Use additional code to identify the joint (Z96.6-)

⑦T84.099   **Other mechanical complication of unspecified internal joint prosthesis**

T84.1   **Mechanical complication of internal fixation device of bones of limb**

Excludes2: mechanical complication of internal fixation device of bones of feet (T84.2-)

mechanical complication of internal fixation device of bones of fingers (T84.2-)

mechanical complication of internal fixation device of bones of hands (T84.2-)

mechanical complication of internal fixation device of bones of toes (T84.2-)

T84.11   **Breakdown (mechanical) of internal fixation device of bones of limb**

⑦T84.110   **Breakdown (mechanical) of internal fixation device of right humerus**

⑦T84.111   **Breakdown (mechanical) of internal fixation device of left humerus**

⑦T84.112   **Breakdown (mechanical) of internal fixation device of bone of right forearm**

⑦T84.113   **Breakdown (mechanical) of internal fixation device of bone of left forearm**

⑦T84.114   **Breakdown (mechanical) of internal fixation device of right femur**

⑦T84.115   **Breakdown (mechanical) of internal fixation device of left femur**

⑦T84.116   **Breakdown (mechanical) of internal fixation device of bone of right lower leg**

⑦T84.117   **Breakdown (mechanical) of internal fixation device of bone of left lower leg**

⑦T84.119   **Breakdown (mechanical) of internal fixation device of unspecified bone of limb**

T84.12   **Displacement of internal fixation device of bones of limb**

Malposition of internal fixation device of bones of limb

⑦T84.120   **Displacement of internal fixation device of right humerus**

⑦T84.121   **Displacement of internal fixation device of left humerus**

⑦T84.122   **Displacement of internal fixation device of bone of right forearm**

⑦T84.123   **Displacement of internal fixation device of bone of left forearm**

⑦T84.124   **Displacement of internal fixation device of right femur**

⑦T84.125   **Displacement of internal fixation device of left femur**

⑦T84.126   **Displacement of internal fixation device of bone of right lower leg**

⑦T84.127   **Displacement of internal fixation device of bone of left lower leg**

⑦T84.129   **Displacement of internal fixation device of unspecified bone of limb**

T84.19   **Other mechanical complication of internal fixation device of bones of limb**

Obstruction (mechanical) of internal fixation device of bones of limb

Perforation of internal fixation device of bones of limb

Protrusion of internal fixation device of bones of limb

⑦T84.190   **Other mechanical complication of internal fixation device of right humerus**

⑦T84.191   **Other mechanical complication of internal fixation device of left humerus**

⑦T84.192   **Other mechanical complication of internal fixation device of bone of right forearm**

⑦T84.193   **Other mechanical complication of internal fixation device of bone of left forearm**

⑦T84.194   **Other mechanical complication of internal fixation device of right femur**

⑦T84.195   **Other mechanical complication of internal fixation device of left femur**

⑦T84.196   **Other mechanical complication of internal fixation device of bone of right lower leg**

⑦T84.197   **Other mechanical complication of internal fixation device of bone of left lower leg**

⑦T84.199   **Other mechanical complication of internal fixation device of unspecified bone of limb**

T84.2   **Mechanical complication of internal fixation device of other bones**

T84.21   **Breakdown (mechanical) of internal fixation device of other bones**

⑦T84.210   **Breakdown (mechanical) of internal fixation device of bones of hand and fingers**

⑦ T84.213   Breakdown (mechanical) of internal fixation device of bones of foot and toes

⑦ T84.216   Breakdown (mechanical) of internal fixation device of vertebrae

⑦ T84.218   Breakdown (mechanical) of internal fixation device of other bones

T84.22   Displacement of internal fixation device of other bones

Malposition of internal fixation device of other bones

⑦ T84.220   Displacement of internal fixation device of bones of hand and fingers

⑦ T84.223   Displacement of internal fixation device of bones of foot and toes

⑦ T84.226   Displacement of internal fixation device of vertebrae

⑦ T84.228   Displacement of internal fixation device of other bones

T84.29   Other mechanical complication of internal fixation device of other bones

Obstruction (mechanical) of internal fixation device of other bones

Perforation of internal fixation device of other bones

Protrusion of internal fixation device of other bones

⑦ T84.290   Other mechanical complication of internal fixation device of bones of hand and fingers

⑦ T84.293   Other mechanical complication of internal fixation device of bones of foot and toes

⑦ T84.296   Other mechanical complication of internal fixation device of vertebrae

⑦ T84.298   Other mechanical complication of internal fixation device of other bones

T84.3   Mechanical complication of other bone devices, implants and grafts

Excludes2: Other complications of bone graft (T86.83-)

T84.31   Breakdown (mechanical) of other bone devices, implants and grafts

⑦ T84.310   Breakdown (mechanical) of electronic bone stimulator

⑦ T84.318   Breakdown (mechanical) of other bone devices, implants and grafts

T84.32   Displacement of other bone devices, implants and grafts

Malposition of other bone devices, implants and grafts

⑦ T84.320   Displacement of electronic bone stimulator

⑦ T84.328   Displacement of other bone devices, implants and grafts

T84.39   Other mechanical complication of other bone devices, implants and grafts

Obstruction (mechanical) of other bone devices, implants and grafts

Perforation of other bone devices, implants and grafts

Protrusion of other bone devices, implants and grafts

⑦ T84.390   Other mechanical complication of electronic bone stimulator

⑦ T84.398   Other mechanical complication of other bone devices, implants and grafts

T84.4   Mechanical complication of other internal orthopedic devices, implants and grafts

T84.41   Breakdown (mechanical) of other internal orthopedic devices, implants and grafts

⑦ T84.410   Breakdown (mechanical) of muscle and tendon graft

⑦ T84.418   Breakdown (mechanical) of other internal orthopedic devices, implants and grafts

T84.42   Displacement of other internal orthopedic devices, implants and grafts

Malposition of other internal orthopedic devices, implants and grafts

⑦ T84.420   Displacement of muscle and tendon graft

⑦ T84.428   Displacement of other internal orthopedic devices, implants and grafts

T84.49   Other mechanical complication of other internal orthopedic devices, implants and grafts

Mechanical complication of other internal orthopedic devices, implants and grafts NOS

Obstruction (mechanical) of other internal orthopedic devices, implants and grafts

Perforation of other internal orthopedic devices, implants and grafts

Protrusion of other internal orthopedic devices, implants and grafts

⑦ T84.490   Other mechanical complication of muscle and tendon graft

⑦ T84.498   Other mechanical complication of other internal orthopedic devices, implants and grafts

T84.5   Infection and inflammatory reaction due to internal joint prosthesis

<u>Use additional code</u> to identify infection

⊗⑦ T84.50   Infection and inflammatory reaction due to unspecified internal joint prosthesis

⊗⑦ T84.51   Infection and inflammatory reaction due to internal right hip prosthesis

⊗⑦ T84.52   Infection and inflammatory reaction due to internal left hip prosthesis

⊗⑦ T84.53   Infection and inflammatory reaction due to internal right knee prosthesis

⊗⑦ T84.54   Infection and inflammatory reaction due to internal left knee prosthesis

⊗⑦ T84.59   Infection and inflammatory reaction due to other internal joint prosthesis

T84.6   Infection and inflammatory reaction due to internal fixation device

<u>Use additional code</u> to identify infection

⊗⑦ T84.60   Infection and inflammatory reaction due to internal fixation device of unspecified site

T84.61   Infection and inflammatory reaction due to internal fixation device of arm

⑦ T84.610   Infection and inflammatory reaction due to internal fixation device of right humerus

⑦ T84.611   Infection and inflammatory reaction due to internal fixation device of left humerus

⑦T84.612   **Infection and inflammatory reaction due to internal fixation device of right radius**

⑦T84.613   **Infection and inflammatory reaction due to internal fixation device of left radius**

⑦T84.614   **Infection and inflammatory reaction due to internal fixation device of right ulna**

⑦T84.615   **Infection and inflammatory reaction due to internal fixation device of left ulna**

⑦T84.619   **Infection and inflammatory reaction due to internal fixation device of unspecified bone of arm**

T84.62   **Infection and inflammatory reaction due to internal fixation device of leg**

⑦T84.620   **Infection and inflammatory reaction due to internal fixation device of right femur**

⑦T84.621   **Infection and inflammatory reaction due to internal fixation device of left femur**

⑦T84.622   **Infection and inflammatory reaction due to internal fixation device of right tibia**

⑦T84.623   **Infection and inflammatory reaction due to internal fixation device of left tibia**

⑦T84.624   **Infection and inflammatory reaction due to internal fixation device of right fibula**

⑦T84.625   **Infection and inflammatory reaction due to internal fixation device of left fibula**

⑦T84.629   **Infection and inflammatory reaction due to internal fixation device of unspecified bone of leg**

⊗⑦T84.63   **Infection and inflammatory reaction due to internal fixation device of spine**

⊗⑦T84.69   **Infection and inflammatory reaction due to internal fixation device of other site**

⊗⑦T84.7   **Infection and inflammatory reaction due to other internal orthopedic prosthetic devices, implants and grafts**

<u>Use additional code</u> to identify infection

T84.8   **Other specified complications of internal orthopedic prosthetic devices, implants and grafts**

⊗⑦T84.81   **Embolism due to internal orthopedic prosthetic devices, implants and grafts**

⊗⑦T84.82   **Fibrosis due to internal orthopedic prosthetic devices, implants and grafts**

⊗⑦T84.83   **Hemorrhage due to internal orthopedic prosthetic devices, implants and grafts**

⊗⑦T84.84   **Pain due to internal orthopedic prosthetic devices, implants and grafts**

⊗⑦T84.85   **Stenosis due to internal orthopedic prosthetic devices, implants and grafts**

⊗⑦T84.86   **Thrombosis due to internal orthopedic prosthetic devices, implants and grafts**

⊗⑦T84.89   **Other specified complication of internal orthopedic prosthetic devices, implants and grafts**

⊗⑦T84.9   **Unspecified complication of internal orthopedic prosthetic device, implant and graft**

T85   **Complications of other internal prosthetic devices, implants and grafts**

Excludes2: failure and rejection of transplanted organs and tissue (T86.-)

The appropriate 7th character is to be added to each code from category T85

A - initial encounter

D - subsequent encounter

S - sequela

T85.0   **Mechanical complication of ventricular intracranial (communicating) shunt**

⊗⑦T85.01   **Breakdown (mechanical) of ventricular intracranial (communicating) shunt**

⊗⑦T85.02   **Displacement of ventricular intracranial (communicating) shunt**

Malposition of ventricular intracranial (communicating) shunt

⊗⑦T85.03   **Leakage of ventricular intracranial (communicating) shunt**

⊗⑦T85.09   **Other mechanical complication of ventricular intracranial (communicating) shunt**

Obstruction (mechanical) of ventricular intracranial (communicating) shunt

Perforation of ventricular intracranial (communicating) shunt

Protrusion of ventricular intracranial (communicating) shunt

T85.1   **Mechanical complication of implanted electronic stimulator of nervous system**

T85.11   **Breakdown (mechanical) of implanted electronic stimulator of nervous system**

⑦T85.110   **Breakdown (mechanical) of implanted electronic neurostimulator of brain electrode (lead)**

⑦T85.111   **Breakdown (mechanical) of implanted electronic neurostimulator of peripheral nerve electrode (lead)**

Breakdown of electrode (lead) for cranial nerve neurostimulators

Breakdown of electrode (lead) for gastric neurostimulator

Breakdown of electrode (lead) for sacral nerve neurostimulator

Breakdown of electrode (lead) for vagal nerve neurostimulators

⑦T85.112   **Breakdown (mechanical) of implanted electronic neurostimulator of spinal cord electrode (lead)**

⑦T85.113   **Breakdown (mechanical) of implanted electronic neurostimulator, generator**

Breakdown (mechanical) of implanted electronic neurostimulator generator, brain, peripheral, gastric, spinal

Breakdown (mechanical) of implanted electronic sacral neurostimulator, pulse generator or receiver

⑦T85.118   **Breakdown (mechanical) of other implanted electronic stimulator of nervous system**

T85.12   **Displacement of implanted electronic stimulator of nervous system**

Malposition of implanted electronic stimulator of nervous system

---

| | Add 4th-7th digits | | Nonspecific code | | Unspecified code | | Manifestation code |

⑦ **T85.120** **Displacement of implanted electronic neurostimulator of brain electrode (lead)**

⑦ **T85.121** **Displacement of implanted electronic neurostimulator of peripheral nerve electrode (lead)**

Displacement of electrode (lead) for cranial nerve neurostimulators

Displacement of electrode (lead) for gastric neurostimulator

Displacement of electrode (lead) for sacral nerve neurostimulator

Displacement of electrode (lead) for vagal nerve neurostimulators

⑦ **T85.122** **Displacement of implanted electronic neurostimulator of spinal cord electrode (lead)**

⑦ **T85.123** **Displacement of implanted electronic neurostimulator, generator**

Displacement of implanted electronic neurostimulator generator, brain, peripheral, gastric, spinal

Displacement of implanted electronic sacral neurostimulator, pulse generator or receiver

⑦ **T85.128** **Displacement of other implanted electronic stimulator of nervous system**

T85.19 **Other mechanical complication of implanted electronic stimulator of nervous system**

Leakage of implanted electronic stimulator of nervous system

Obstruction (mechanical) of implanted electronic stimulator of nervous system

Perforation of implanted electronic stimulator of nervous system

Protrusion of implanted electronic stimulator of nervous system

⑦ **T85.190** **Other mechanical complication of implanted electronic neurostimulator of brain electrode (lead)**

⑦ **T85.191** **Other mechanical complication of implanted electronic neurostimulator of peripheral nerve electrode (lead)**

Other mechanical complication of electrode (lead) for cranial nerve neurostimulators

Other mechanical complication of electrode (lead) for gastric neurostimulator

Other mechanical complication of electrode (lead) for sacral nerve neurostimulator

Other mechanical complication of electrode (lead) for vagal nerve neurostimulators

⑦ **T85.192** **Other mechanical complication of implanted electronic neurostimulator of spinal cord electrode (lead)**

⑦ **T85.193** **Other mechanical complication of implanted electronic neurostimulator, generator**

Other mechanical complication of implanted electronic neurostimulator generator, brain, peripheral, gastric, spinal

Other mechanical complication of implanted electronic sacral neurostimulator, pulse generator or receiver

⑦ **T85.199** **Other mechanical complication of other implanted electronic stimulator of nervous system**

T85.2 **Mechanical complication of intraocular lens**

⊗⑦ **T85.21** **Breakdown (mechanical) of intraocular lens**

⊗⑦ **T85.22** **Displacement of intraocular lens**

Malposition of intraocular lens

⊗⑦ **T85.29** **Other mechanical complication of intraocular lens**

Obstruction (mechanical) of intraocular lens

Perforation of intraocular lens

Protrusion of intraocular lens

T85.3 **Mechanical complication of other ocular prosthetic devices, implants and grafts**

Excludes2: Other complications of corneal graft (T86.84-)

T85.31 **Breakdown (mechanical) of other ocular prosthetic devices, implants and grafts**

⑦ **T85.310** **Breakdown (mechanical) of prosthetic orbit of right eye**

⑦ **T85.311** **Breakdown (mechanical) of prosthetic orbit of left eye**

⑦ **T85.318** **Breakdown (mechanical) of other ocular prosthetic devices, implants and grafts**

T85.32 **Displacement of other ocular prosthetic devices, implants and grafts**

Malposition of other ocular prosthetic devices, implants and grafts

⑦ **T85.320** **Displacement of prosthetic orbit of right eye**

⑦ **T85.321** **Displacement of prosthetic orbit of left eye**

⑦ **T85.328** **Displacement of other ocular prosthetic devices, implants and grafts**

T85.39 **Other mechanical complication of other ocular prosthetic devices, implants and grafts**

Obstruction (mechanical) of other ocular prosthetic devices, implants and grafts

Perforation of other ocular prosthetic devices, implants and grafts

Protrusion of other ocular prosthetic devices, implants and grafts

⑦ **T85.390** **Other mechanical complication of prosthetic orbit of right eye**

⑦ **T85.391** **Other mechanical complication of prosthetic orbit of left eye**

⑦ **T85.398** **Other mechanical complication of other ocular prosthetic devices, implants and grafts**

T85.4 **Mechanical complication of breast prosthesis and implant**

⊗⑦ **T85.41** **Breakdown (mechanical) of breast prosthesis and implant**

⊗⑦ **T85.42** **Displacement of breast prosthesis and implant**

Malposition of breast prosthesis and implant

⊗⑦ **T85.43** **Leakage of breast prosthesis and implant**

⊗⑦ **T85.44** **Capsular contracture of breast implant**

● New code ▲ Revised code **Excludes1:** Not coded here **Excludes2:** Not included here ⊗ Placeholder required ⑦ 7ᵗʰ digit required

⊗⑦**T85.49** **Other mechanical complication of breast prosthesis and implant**

Obstruction (mechanical) of breast prosthesis and implant

Perforation of breast prosthesis and implant

Protrusion of breast prosthesis and implant

T85.5 **Mechanical complication of gastrointestinal prosthetic devices, implants and grafts**

T85.51 **Breakdown (mechanical) of gastrointestinal prosthetic devices, implants and grafts**

⑦**T85.510** **Breakdown (mechanical) of bile duct prosthesis**

⑦**T85.511** **Breakdown (mechanical) of esophageal anti-reflux device**

⑦**T85.518** **Breakdown (mechanical) of other gastrointestinal prosthetic devices, implants and grafts**

T85.52 **Displacement of gastrointestinal prosthetic devices, implants and grafts**

Malposition of gastrointestinal prosthetic devices, implants and grafts

⑦**T85.520** **Displacement of bile duct prosthesis**

⑦**T85.521** **Displacement of esophageal anti-reflux device**

⑦**T85.528** **Displacement of other gastrointestinal prosthetic devices, implants and grafts**

T85.59 **Other mechanical complication of gastrointestinal prosthetic devices, implants and**

Obstruction, mechanical of gastrointestinal prosthetic devices, implants and grafts

Perforation of gastrointestinal prosthetic devices, implants and grafts

Protrusion of gastrointestinal prosthetic devices, implants and grafts

⑦**T85.590** **Other mechanical complication of bile duct prosthesis**

⑦**T85.591** **Other mechanical complication of esophageal anti-reflux device**

⑦**T85.598** **Other mechanical complication of other gastrointestinal prosthetic devices, implants and grafts**

T85.6 **Mechanical complication of other specified internal and external prosthetic devices, implants and grafts**

T85.61 **Breakdown (mechanical) of other specified internal prosthetic devices, implants and grafts**

⑦**T85.610** **Breakdown (mechanical) of cranial or spinal infusion catheter**

Breakdown (mechanical) of epidural infusion catheter

Breakdown (mechanical) of intrathecal infusion catheter

Breakdown (mechanical) of subarachnoid infusion catheter

Breakdown (mechanical) of subdural infusion catheter

⑦**T85.611** **Breakdown (mechanical) of intraperitoneal dialysis catheter**

Excludes1: mechanical complication of vascular dialysis catheter (T82.4-)

⑦**T85.612** **Breakdown (mechanical) of permanent sutures**

Excludes1: mechanical complication of permanent (wire) suture used in bone repair (T84.1-T84.2)

⑦**T85.613** **Breakdown (mechanical) of artificial skin graft and decellularized allodermis**

Failure of artificial skin graft and decellularized allodermis

Non-adherence of artificial skin graft and decellularized allodermis

Poor incorporation of artificial skin graft and decellularized allodermis

Shearing of artificial skin graft and decellularized allodermis

⑦**T85.614** **Breakdown (mechanical) of insulin pump**

⑦**T85.615** **Breakdown (mechanical) of other nervous system device, implant or graft**

Breakdown (mechanical) of intrathecal infusion pump

⑦**T85.618** **Breakdown (mechanical) of other specified internal prosthetic devices, implants and grafts**

T85.62 **Displacement of other specified internal prosthetic devices, implants and grafts**

Malposition of other specified internal prosthetic devices, implants and grafts

⑦**T85.620** **Displacement of cranial or spinal infusion catheter**

Displacement of epidural infusion catheter

Displacement of intrathecal infusion catheter

Displacement of subarachnoid infusion catheter

Displacement of subdural infusion catheter

⑦**T85.621** **Displacement of intraperitoneal dialysis catheter**

Excludes1: mechanical complication of vascular dialysis catheter (T82.4-)

⑦**T85.622** **Displacement of permanent sutures**

Excludes1: mechanical complication of permanent (wire) suture used in bone repair (T84.1-T84.2)

⑦**T85.623** **Displacement of artificial skin graft and decellularized allodermis**

Dislodgement of artificial skin graft and decellularized allodermis

⑦**T85.624** **Displacement of insulin pump**

⑦**T85.625** **Displacement of other nervous system device, implant or graft**

Displacement of intrathecal infusion pump

⑦**T85.628** **Displacement of other specified internal prosthetic devices, implants and grafts**

T85.63 **Leakage of other specified internal prosthetic devices, implants and grafts**

⑦**T85.630** **Leakage of cranial or spinal infusion catheter**

Leakage of epidural infusion catheter

Leakage of intrathecal infusion catheter infusion catheter

Leakage of subdural infusion catheter

Leakage of subarachnoid infusion catheter

⑦ **T85.631 Leakage of intraperitoneal dialysis catheter**

Excludes1: mechanical complication of vascular dialysis catheter (T82.4)

⑦ **T85.633 Leakage of insulin pump**

⑦ **T85.635 Leakage of other nervous system device, implant or graft**

Leakage of intrathecal infusion pump

⑦ **T85.638 Leakage of other specified internal prosthetic devices, implants and grafts**

T85.69 Other mechanical complication of other specified internal prosthetic devices, implants and grafts

Obstruction, mechanical of other specified internal prosthetic devices, implants and grafts

Perforation of other specified internal prosthetic devices, implants and grafts

Protrusion of other specified internal prosthetic devices, implants and grafts

⑦ **T85.690 Other mechanical complication of cranial or spinal infusion catheter**

Other mechanical complication of epidural infusion catheter

Other mechanical complication of intrathecal infusion catheter

Other mechanical complication of subarachnoid infusion catheter

Other mechanical complication of subdural infusion catheter

⑦ **T85.691 Other mechanical complication of intraperitoneal dialysis catheter**

Excludes1: mechanical complication of vascular dialysis catheter (T82.4)

⑦ **T85.692 Other mechanical complication of permanent sutures**

Excludes1: mechanical complication of permanent (wire) suture used in bone repair (T84.1-T84.2)

⑦ **T85.693 Other mechanical complication of artificial skin graft and decellularized allodermis**

⑦ **T85.694 Other mechanical complication of insulin pump**

⑦ **T85.695 Other mechanical complication of other nervous system device, implant or graft**

Other mechanical complication of intrathecal infusion pump

⑦ **T85.698 Other mechanical complication of other specified internal prosthetic devices, implants and grafts**

Mechanical complication of nonabsorbable surgical material NOS

T85.7 Infection and inflammatory reaction due to other internal prosthetic devices, implants and grafts

Use additional code to identify infection

⊗⑦ **T85.71 Infection and inflammatory reaction due to peritoneal dialysis catheter**

⊗⑦ **T85.72 Infection and inflammatory reaction due to insulin pump**

T85.73 Infection and inflammatory reaction due to nervous system devices, implants and graft

⑦ **T85.730 Infection and inflammatory reaction due to ventricular intracranial (communicating) shunt**

⑦ **T85.731 Infection and inflammatory reaction due to implanted electronic neurostimulator of brain, electrode (lead)**

⑦ **T85.732 Infection and inflammatory reaction due to implanted electronic neurostimulator of peripheral nerve, electrode (lead)**

Infection and inflammatory reaction due to electrode (lead) for cranial nerve neurostimulators

Infection and inflammatory reaction due to electrode (lead) for gastric neurostimulator

Infection and inflammatory reaction due to electrode (lead) for sacral nerve neurostimulator

Infection and inflammatory reaction due to electrode (lead) for vagal nerve neurostimulators

⑦ **T85.733 Infection and inflammatory reaction due to implanted electronic neurostimulator of spinal cord, electrode (lead)**

⑦ **T85.734 Infection and inflammatory reaction due to implanted electronic neurostimulator, generator** pocket infection

⑦ **T85.735 Infection and inflammatory reaction due to cranial or spinal infusion catheter**

Infection and inflammatory reaction due to epidural catheter

Infection and inflammatory reaction due to intrathecal infusion catheter

Infection and inflammatory reaction due to subarachnoid catheter

Infection and inflammatory reaction due to subdural catheter

⑦ **T85.738 Infection and inflammatory reaction due to other nervous system device, implant or graft**

Infection and inflammatory reaction due to intrathecal infusion pump

⊗⑦ **T85.79 Infection and inflammatory reaction due to other internal prosthetic devices, implants and grafts**

T85.8 Other specified complications of internal prosthetic devices, implants and grafts, not elsewhere classified

T85.81 Embolism due to internal prosthetic devices, implants and grafts, not elsewhere classified

⑦ **T85.810 Embolism due to nervous system prosthetic devices, implants and grafts**

⑦ **T85.818 Embolism due to other internal prosthetic devices, implants and grafts**

● New code   ▲ Revised code   **Excludes1:** Not coded here   **Excludes2:** Not included here   ⊗ Placeholder required   ⑦ 7th digit required

T85.82 **Fibrosis due to internal prosthetic devices, implants and grafts, not elsewhere classified**

⑦T85.820 **Fibrosis due to nervous system prosthetic devices, implants and grafts**

⑦T85.828 **Fibrosis due to other internal prosthetic devices, implants and grafts**

T85.83 **Hemorrhage due to internal prosthetic devices, implants and grafts, not elsewhere classified**

⑦T85.830 **Hemorrhage due to nervous system prosthetic devices, implants and grafts**

⑦T85.838 **Hemorrhage due to other internal prosthetic devices, implants and grafts**

T85.84 **Pain due to internal prosthetic devices, implants and grafts, not elsewhere classified**

⑦T85.840 **Pain due to nervous system prosthetic devices, implants and grafts**

⑦T85.848 **Pain due to other internal prosthetic devices, implants and grafts**

T85.85 **Stenosis due to internal prosthetic devices, implants and grafts, not elsewhere classified**

⑦T85.850 **Stenosis due to nervous system prosthetic devices, implants and grafts**

⑦T85.858 **Stenosis due to other internal prosthetic devices, implants and grafts**

T85.86 **Thrombosis due to internal prosthetic devices, implants and grafts, not elsewhere classified**

⑦T85.860 **Thrombosis due to nervous system prosthetic devices, implants and grafts**

⑦T85.868 **Thrombosis due to other internal prosthetic devices, implants and grafts**

T85.89 **Other specified complication of internal prosthetic devices, implants and grafts, not elsewhere classified**

Erosion or breakdown of subcutaneous device pocket

⑦T85.890 **Other specified complication of nervous system prosthetic devices, implants and grafts**

⑦T85.898 **Other specified complication of other internal prosthetic devices, implants and grafts**

⑦T85.9 **Unspecified complication of internal prosthetic device, implant and graft**

Complication of internal prosthetic device, implant and graft NOS

T86 **Complications of transplanted organs and tissue**

Use additional code to identify **Other** transplant complications, such as:

graft-versus-host disease (D89.81-)

malignancy associated with organ transplant (C80.2)

post-transplant lymphoproliferative disorders (PTLD) (D47.Z1)

T86.0 **Complications of bone marrow transplant**

T86.00 **Unspecified complication of bone marrow transplant**

T86.01 **Bone marrow transplant rejection**

T86.02 **Bone marrow transplant failure**

T86.03 **Bone marrow transplant infection**

T86.09 **Other complications of bone marrow transplant**

T86.1 **Complications of kidney transplant**

T86.10 **Unspecified complication of kidney transplant**

T86.11 **Kidney transplant rejection**

T86.12 **Kidney transplant failure**

T86.13 **Kidney transplant infection**

Use additional code to specify infection

T86.19 **Other complication of kidney transplant**

T86.2 **Complications of heart transplant**

Excludes1: complication of: artificial heart device (T82.5)

heart-lung transplant (T86.3)

T86.20 **Unspecified complication of heart transplant**

T86.21 **Heart transplant rejection**

T86.22 **Heart transplant failure**

T86.23 **Heart transplant infection**

Use additional code to specify infection

T86.29 **Other complications of heart transplant**

T86.290 **Cardiac allograft vasculopathy**

Excludes1: atherosclerosis of coronary arteries (I25.75-, I25.76-, I25.81-)

T86.298 **Other complications of heart transplant**

T86.3 **Complications of heart-lung transplant**

T86.30 **Unspecified complication of heart-lung transplant**

T86.31 **Heart-lung transplant rejection**

T86.32 **Heart-lung transplant failure**

T86.33 **Heart-lung transplant infection**

Use additional code to specify infection

T86.39 **Other complications of heart-lung transplant**

T86.4 **Complications of liver transplant**

T86.40 **Unspecified complication of liver transplant**

T86.41 **Liver transplant rejection**

T86.42 **Liver transplant failure**

T86.43 **Liver transplant infection**

Use additional code to identify infection, such as:

Cytomegalovirus (CMV) infection (B25.-)

T86.49 **Other complications of liver transplant**

T86.5 **Complications of stem cell transplant**

Complications from stem cells from peripheral blood

Complications from stem cells from umbilical cord

T86.8 **Complications of other transplanted organs and tissues**

T86.81 **Complications of lung transplant**

Excludes1: complication of heart-lung transplant (T86.3-)

T86.810 **Lung transplant rejection**

T86.811 **Lung transplant failure**

T86.812 **Lung transplant infection**

Use additional code to specify infection

T86.818 **Other complications of lung transplant**

T86.819 **Unspecified complication of lung transplant**

T86.82 **Complications of skin graft (allograft) (autograft)**

Excludes2: complication of artificial skin graft (T85.693)

T86.820   Skin graft (allograft) rejection

T86.821   Skin graft (allograft) (autograft) failure

T86.822   Skin graft (allograft) (autograft) infection

Use additional code to specify infection

T86.828   Other complications of skin graft (allograft) (autograft)

T86.829   Unspecified complication of skin graft (allograft) (autograft)

T86.83   Complications of bone graft

Excludes2: mechanical complications of bone graft (T84.3-)

T86.830   Bone graft rejection

T86.831   Bone graft failure

T86.832   Bone graft infection

Use additional code to specify infection

T86.838   Other complications of bone graft

T86.839   Unspecified complication of bone graft

T86.84   Complications of corneal transplant

Excludes2: mechanical complications of corneal graft (T85.3-)

T86.840   Corneal transplant rejection

T86.841   Corneal transplant failure

T86.842   Corneal transplant infection

Use additional code to specify infection

T86.848   Other complications of corneal transplant

T86.849   Unspecified complication of corneal transplant

T86.85   Complication of intestine transplant

T86.850   Intestine transplant rejection

T86.851   Intestine transplant failure

T86.852   Intestine transplant infection

Use additional code to specify infection

T86.858   Other complications of intestine transplant

T86.859   Unspecified complication of intestine transplant

T86.89   Complications of other transplanted tissue

Transplant failure or rejection of pancreas

T86.890   Other transplanted tissue rejection

T86.891   Other transplanted tissue failure

T86.892   Other transplanted tissue infection

Use additional code to specify infection

T86.898   Other complications of other transplanted tissue

T86.899   Unspecified complication of other transplanted tissue

T86.9   Complication of unspecified transplanted organ and tissue

T86.90   Unspecified complication of unspecified transplanted organ and tissue

T86.91   Unspecified transplanted organ and tissue rejection

T86.92   Unspecified transplanted organ and tissue failure

T86.93   Unspecified transplanted organ and tissue infection

Use additional code to specify infection

T86.99   Other complications of unspecified transplanted organ and tissue

T87   **Complications peculiar to reattachment and amputation**

T87.0   Complications of reattached (part of) upper extremity

T87.0X   Complications of reattached (part of) upper extremity

T87.0X1   Complications of reattached (part of) right upper extremity

T87.0X2   Complications of reattached (part of) left upper extremity

T87.0X9   Complications of reattached (part of) unspecified upper extremity

T87.1   Complications of reattached (part of) lower extremity

T87.1X   Complications of reattached (part of) lower extremity

T87.1X1   Complications of reattached (part of) right lower extremity

T87.1X2   Complications of reattached (part of) left lower extremity

T87.1X9   Complications of reattached (part of) unspecified lower extremity

T87.2   Complications of other reattached body part

T87.3   Neuroma of amputation stump

T87.30   Neuroma of amputation stump, unspecified extremity

T87.31   Neuroma of amputation stump, right upper extremity

T87.32   Neuroma of amputation stump, left upper extremity

T87.33   Neuroma of amputation stump, right lower extremity

T87.34   Neuroma of amputation stump, left lower extremity

T87.4   Infection of amputation stump

T87.40   Infection of amputation stump, unspecified extremity

T87.41   Infection of amputation stump, right upper extremity

T87.42   Infection of amputation stump, left upper extremity

T87.43   Infection of amputation stump, right lower extremity

T87.44   Infection of amputation stump, left lower extremity

T87.5   Necrosis of amputation stump

T87.50   Necrosis of amputation stump, unspecified extremity

T87.51   Necrosis of amputation stump, right upper extremity

T87.52   Necrosis of amputation stump, left upper extremity

T87.53   Necrosis of amputation stump, right lower extremity

T87.54   Necrosis of amputation stump, left lower extremity

T87.8   Other complications of amputation stump

● New code   ▲ Revised code   Excludes1: Not coded here   Excludes2: Not included here   ⊗ Placeholder required   ⑦7th digit required

T87.81 **Dehiscence of amputation stump**

T87.89 **Other complications of amputation stump**

Amputation stump contracture

Amputation stump contracture of next proximal joint

Amputation stump flexion

Amputation stump edema

Amputation stump hematoma

Excludes2: phantom limb syndrome (G54.6-G54.7)

T87.9 **Unspecified complications of amputation stump**

T88 **Other complications of surgical and medical care, not elsewhere classified**

Excludes2: complication following infusion, transfusion and therapeutic injection (T80.-)

complication following procedure NEC (T81.-)

complications of anesthesia in labor and delivery (O74.-)

complications of anesthesia in pregnancy (O29.-)

complications of anesthesia in puerperium (O89.-)

complications of devices, implants and grafts (T82-T85)

complications of obstetric surgery and procedure (O75.4)

dermatitis due to drugs and medicaments (L23.3, L24.4, L25.1, L27.0-L27.1)

poisoning and toxic effects of drugs and chemicals (T36-T65 with fifth or sixth character 1-4 or 6) specified complications classified elsewhere

The appropriate 7th character is to be added to each code from category T88

A - initial encounter

D - subsequent encounter

S - sequela

⊗⑦**T88.0** **Infection following immunization**

Sepsis following immunization

⊗⑦**T88.1** **Other complications following immunization, not elsewhere classified**

Generalized vaccinia

Rash following immunization

Excludes1: vaccinia not from vaccine (B08.011)

Excludes2: anaphylactic shock due to serum (T80.5-)

Other serum reactions (T80.6-)

postimmunization arthropathy (M02.2)

postimmunization encephalitis (G04.02)

postimmunization fever (R50.83)

⊗⑦**T88.2** **Shock due to anesthesia**

Use additional code for adverse effect, if applicable, to identify drug (T41.- with fifth or sixth character 5)

Excludes1: complications of anesthesia (in):

labor and delivery (O74.-)

pregnancy (O29.-)

puerperium (O89.-)

postprocedural shock NOS (T81.1-)

⊗⑦**T88.3** **Malignant hyperthermia due to anesthesia**

Use additional code for adverse effect, if applicable, to identify drug (T41.- with fifth or sixth character 5)

⊗⑦**T88.4** **Failed or difficult intubation**

T88.5 **Other complications of anesthesia**

Use additional code for adverse effect, if applicable, to identify drug (T41.- with fifth or sixth character 5)

⊗⑦**T88.51** **Hypothermia following anesthesia**

⊗⑦**T88.52** **Failed moderate sedation during procedure**

Failed conscious sedation during procedure

Excludes2: personal history of failed moderate sedation (Z92.83)

⊗⑦**T88.53** **Unintended awareness under general anesthesia during procedure**

Excludes2: personal history of unintended awareness under general anesthesia (Z92.84)

⊗⑦**T88.59** **Other complications of anesthesia**

⊗⑦**T88.6** **Anaphylactic reaction due to adverse effect of correct drug or medicament properly administered**

Anaphylactic shock due to adverse effect of correct drug or medicament properly administered

Anaphylactoid reaction NOS

Use additional code for adverse effect, if applicable, to identify drug (T36-T50 with fifth or sixth character 5)

Excludes1: anaphylactic reaction due to serum (T80.5-)

anaphylactic shock or reaction due to adverse food reaction (T78.0-)

⊗⑦**T88.7** **Unspecified adverse effect of drug or medicament**

Drug hypersensitivity NOS

Drug reaction NOS

Use additional code for adverse effect, if applicable, to identify drug (T36-T50 with fifth or sixth character 5)

Excludes1: specified adverse effects of drugs and medicaments (A00-R94 and T80-T88.6, T88.8)

⊗⑦**T88.8** **Other specified complications of surgical and medical care, not elsewhere classified**

Use additional code to identify the complication

⊗⑦**T88.9** **Complication of surgical and medical care, unspecified**

Chapter 20: External Causes Of Morbidity (V00-Y99)

MULTIPLE CODING FOR A SINGLE CONDITION

In addition to the etiology/manifestation convention that requires two codes to fully describe a single condition that affects multiple body systems, there are other single conditions that also require more than one code. "Use additional code" notes are found in the Tabular List at codes that are not part of an etiology/manifestation pair where a secondary code is useful to fully describe a condition. The sequencing rule is the same as the etiology/manifestation pair, "use additional code" indicates that a secondary code should be added.

For example, for bacterial infections that are not included in chapter 1, a secondary code from category B95, Streptococcus, Staphylococcus, and Enterococcus, as the cause of diseases classified elsewhere, or B96, Other bacterial agents as the cause of diseases classified elsewhere, may be required to identify the bacterial organism causing the infection. A "use additional code" note will normally be found at the infectious disease code, indicating a need for the organism code to be added as a secondary code.

 "Code first" notes are also under certain codes that are not specifically manifestation codes but may be due to an underlying cause. When there is a "code first" note and an underlying condition is present, the underlying condition should be sequenced first.

"Code, if applicable, any causal condition first", notes indicate that this code may be assigned as a principal diagnosis when the causal condition is unknown or not applicable. If a causal condition is known, then the code for that condition should be sequenced as the principal or first-listed diagnosis.

Multiple codes may be needed for sequela, complication codes and obstetric codes to more fully describe a condition. See the specific guidelines for these conditions for further instruction.

COMBINATION CODE

A combination code is a single code used to classify: Two diagnoses, or a diagnosis with an associated secondary process (manifestation) A diagnosis with an associated complication

Combination codes are identified by referring to subterm entries in the Alphabetic Index and by reading the inclusion and exclusion notes in the Tabular List.

Assign only the combination code when that code fully identifies the diagnostic conditions involved or when the Alphabetic Index so directs. Multiple coding should not be used when the classification provides a combination code that clearly identifies all of the elements documented in the diagnosis. When the combination code lacks necessary specificity in describing the manifestation or complication, an additional code should be used as a secondary code.

SEQUELA (LATE EFFECTS)

A sequela is the residual effect (condition produced) after the acute phase of an illness or injury has terminated. There is no time limit on when a sequela code can be used. The residual may be apparent early, such as in cerebral infarction, or it may occur months or years later, such as that due to a previous injury. Coding of sequela generally requires two codes sequenced in the following order: The condition or nature of the sequela is sequenced first.

The sequela code is sequenced second.

An exception to the above guidelines are those instances where the code for the sequela is followed by a manifestation code identified in the Tabular List and title, or the sequela code has been expanded (at the fourth, fifth or sixth character levels) to include the manifestation(s). The code for the acute phase of an illness or injury that led to the sequela is never used with a code for the late effect.

GENERAL

The external causes of morbidity codes should never be sequenced as the first-listed or principal diagnosis.

External cause codes are intended to provide data for injury research and evaluation of injury prevention strategies. These codes capture how the injury or health condition happened (cause), the intent (unintentional or accidental; or intentional, such as suicide or assault), the place where the event occurred the activity of the patient at the time of the event, and the person's status (e.g., civilian, military).

There is no national requirement for mandatory ICD-10-CM external cause code reporting. Unless a provider is subject to a state-based external cause code reporting mandate or these codes are required by a particular payer, reporting of ICD-10-CM codes in Chapter 20, External Causes of Morbidity, is not required. In the absence of a mandatory reporting requirement, providers are encouraged to voluntarily report external cause codes, as they provide valuable data for injury research and evaluation of injury prevention strategies.

The external causes of morbidity codes should never be sequenced as the first-listed or principal diagnosis.

External cause codes are intended to provide data for injury research and evaluation of injury prevention strategies. These codes capture how the injury or health condition happened (cause), the intent (unintentional or accidental; or intentional, such as suicide or assault), the place where the event occurred the activity of the patient at the time of the event, and the person's status (e.g., civilian, military).

There is no national requirement for mandatory ICD-10-CM external cause code reporting. Unless a provider is subject to a state-based external cause code reporting mandate or these codes are required by a particular payer, reporting of ICD-10-CM codes in Chapter 20, External Causes of Morbidity, is not required. In the absence of a mandatory reporting requirement, providers are encouraged to voluntarily report external cause codes, as they provide valuable data for injury research and evaluation of injury prevention strategies.

GENERAL EXTERNAL CAUSE CODING GUIDELINES

1)   Used with any code in the range of A00.0-T88.9, Z00-Z99

| Add 4th-7th digits | Nonspecific code | Unspecified code | Manifestation code | 979 |

An external cause code may be used with any code in the range of A00.0-T88.9, Z00-Z99, classification that is a health condition due to an external cause. Though they are most applicable to injuries, they are also valid for use with such things as infections or diseases due to an external source, and other health conditions, such as a heart attack that occurs during strenuous physical activity.

2) External cause code used for length of treatment

Assign the external cause code, with the appropriate 7th character (initial encounter, subsequent encounter or sequela) for each encounter for which the injury or condition is being treated.

Most categories in chapter 20 have a 7th character requirement for each applicable code. Most categories in this chapter have three 7th character values: A, initial encounter, D, subsequent encounter and S, sequela. While the patient may be seen by a new or different provider over the course of treatment for an injury or condition, assignment of the 7th character for external cause should match the 7th character of the code assigned for the associated injury or condition for the encounter.

3) Use the full range of external cause codes

Use the full range of external cause codes to completely describe the cause, the intent, the place of occurrence, and if applicable, the activity of the patient at the time of the event, and the patient's status, for all injuries, and other health conditions due to an external cause.

4) Assign as many external cause codes as necessary

Assign as many external cause codes as necessary to fully explain each cause. If only one external code can be recorded, assign the code most related to the principal diagnosis.

5) The selection of the appropriate external cause code

The selection of the appropriate external cause code is guided by the Alphabetic Index of External Causes and by Inclusion and Exclusion notes in the Tabular List.

6) External cause code can never be a principal diagnosis

An external cause code can never be a principal (first-listed) diagnosis.

7) Combination external cause codes

Certain of the external cause codes are combination codes that identify sequential events that result in an injury, such as a fall which results in striking against an object. The injury may be due to either event or both. The combination external cause code used should correspond to the sequence of events regardless of which caused the most serious injury.

8) No external cause code needed in certain circumstances

No external cause code from Chapter 20 is needed if the external cause and intent are included in a code from another chapter (e.g. T36.0X1- Poisoning by penicillins, accidental (unintentional)).

PLACE OF OCCURRENCE GUIDELINE

Codes from category Y92, Place of occurrence of the external cause, are secondary codes for use after other external cause codes to identify the location of the patient at the time of injury or other condition.

Generally, a place of occurrence code is assigned only once, at the initial encounter for treatment. However, in the rare instance that a new injury occurs during hospitalization, an additional place of occurrence code may be assigned. No 7th characters are used for Y92.

Do not use place of occurrence code Y92.9 if the place is not stated or is not applicable.

ACTIVITY CODE

Assign a code from category Y93, Activity code, to describe the activity of the patient at the time the injury or other health condition occurred.

An activity code is used only once, at the initial encounter for treatment. Only one code from Y93 should be recorded on a medical record.

The activity codes are not applicable to poisonings, adverse effects, misadventures or sequela.

Do not assign Y93.9, Unspecified activity, if the activity is not stated.

A code from category Y93 is appropriate for use with external cause and intent codes if identifying the activity provides additional information about the event.

PLACE OF OCCURRENCE, ACTIVITY, AND STATUS CODES USED WITH OTHER EXTERNAL CAUSE CODE

When applicable, place of occurrence, activity, and external cause status codes are sequenced after the main external cause code(s). Regardless of the number of external cause codes assigned, generally there should be only one place of occurrence code, one activity code, and one external cause status code assigned to an encounter. However, in the rare instance that a new injury occurs during hospitalization, an additional place of occurrence code may be assigned.

IF THE REPORTING FORMAT LIMITS THE NUMBER OF EXTERNAL CAUSE CODES

If the reporting format limits the number of external cause codes that can be used in reporting clinical data, report the code for the cause/intent most related to the principal diagnosis. If the format permits capture of additional external cause codes, the cause/intent, including medical misadventures, of the additional events should be reported rather than the codes for place, activity, or external status.

MULTIPLE EXTERNAL CAUSE CODING GUIDELINES

More than one external cause code is required to fully describe the external cause of an illness or injury. The assignment of external cause codes should be sequenced in the following priority:

If two or more events cause separate injuries, an external cause code should be assigned for each cause. The first-listed external cause code will be selected in the following order:

External codes for child and adult abuse take priority over all other external cause codes.

See Section I.C.19., Child and Adult abuse guidelines.

External cause codes for terrorism events take priority over all other external cause codes except child and adult abuse.

External cause codes for cataclysmic events take priority over all other external cause codes except child and adult abuse and terrorism.

External cause codes for transport accidents take priority over all other external cause codes except cataclysmic events, child and adult abuse and terrorism.

Activity and external cause status codes are assigned following all causal (intent) external cause codes.

The first-listed external cause code should correspond to the cause of the most serious diagnosis due to an assault, accident, or self-harm, following the order of hierarchy listed above.

CHILD AND ADULT ABUSE GUIDELINE

Adult and child abuse, neglect and maltreatment are classified as assault. Any of the assault codes may be used to indicate the external cause of any injury resulting from the confirmed abuse.

For confirmed cases of abuse, neglect and maltreatment, when the perpetrator is known, a code from Y07, Perpetrator of maltreatment and neglect, should accompany any other assault codes.

See Section I.C.19. Adult and child abuse, neglect and other maltreatment

UNKNOWN OR UNDETERMINED INTENT GUIDELINE

If the intent (accident, self-harm, assault) of the cause of an injury or other condition is unknown or unspecified, code the intent as accidental intent. All transport accident categories assume accidental intent.

1) **Use of undetermined intent**

   External cause codes for events of undetermined intent are only for use if the documentation in the record specifies that the intent cannot be determined.

SEQUELAE (LATE EFFECTS) OF EXTERNAL CAUSE GUIDELINES

1) **Sequelae external cause codes**

   Sequela are reported using the external cause code with the 7th character "S" for sequela. These codes should be used with any report of a late effect or sequela resulting from a previous injury.

   See Section I.B.10 Sequela (Late Effects)

2) **Sequela external cause code with a related current injury**

   A sequela external cause code should never be used with a related current nature of injury code.

3) **Use of sequela external cause codes for subsequent visits**

   Use a late effect external cause code for subsequent visits when a late effect of the initial injury is being treated. Do not use a late effect external cause code for subsequent visits for follow-up care (e.g., to assess healing, to receive rehabilitative therapy) of the injury when no late effect of the injury has been documented.

TERRORISM GUIDELINES

1) **Cause of injury identified by the Federal Government (FBI) as terrorism**

   When the cause of an injury is identified by the Federal Government (FBI) as terrorism, the first-listed external cause code should be a code from category Y38, Terrorism. The definition of terrorism employed by the FBI is found at the inclusion note at the beginning of category Y38. Use additional code for place of occurrence (Y92.-). More than one Y38 code may be assigned if the injury is the result of more than one mechanism of terrorism.

2) **Cause of an injury is suspected to be the result of terrorism**

| | Add 4th-7th digits | | Nonspecific code | | Unspecified code | | Manifestation code | 981 |

When the cause of an injury is suspected to be the result of terrorism a code from category Y38 should not be assigned. Suspected cases should be classified as assault.

3) Code Y38.9, Terrorism, secondary effects

Assign code Y38.9, Terrorism, secondary effects, for conditions occurring subsequent to the terrorist event. This code should not be assigned for conditions that are due to the initial terrorist act.

It is acceptable to assign code Y38.9 with another code from Y38 if there is an injury due to the initial terrorist event and an injury that is a subsequent result of the terrorist event.

EXTERNAL CAUSE STATUS

A code from category Y99, External cause status, should be assigned whenever any other external cause code is assigned for an encounter, including an Activity code, except for the events noted below. Assign a code from category Y99, External cause status, to indicate the work status of the person at the time the event occurred. The status code indicates whether the event occurred during military activity, whether a non-military person was at work, whether an individual including a student or volunteer was involved in a non-work activity at the time of the causal event.

A code from Y99, External cause status, should be assigned, when applicable, with other external cause codes, such as transport accidents and falls. The external cause status codes are not applicable to poisonings, adverse effects, misadventures or late effects.

Do not assign a code from category Y99 if no other external cause codes (cause, activity) are applicable for the encounter.

An external cause status code is used only once, at the initial encounter for treatment. Only one code from Y99 should be recorded on a medical record.

Do not assign code Y99.9, Unspecified external cause status, if the status is not stated.

Chapter 20

External Causes Of Morbidity (V00-Y99)

Note: This chapter permits the classification of environmental events and circumstances as the cause of injury, and other adverse effects. Where a code from this section is applicable, it is intended that it shall be used secondary to a code from another chapter of the Classification indicating the nature of the condition.

Most often, the condition will be classifiable to Chapter 19, Injury, poisoning and certain other consequences of external causes (S00-T88). Other conditions that may be stated to be due to external causes are classified in Chapters I to XVIII. For these conditions, codes from Chapter 20 should be used to provide additional information as to the cause of the condition.

This chapter contains the following blocks: V00-X58 Accidents

V00-V99	Transport accidents
V00-V09	Pedestrian injured in transport accident
V10-V19	Pedal cycle rider injured in transport accident
V20-V29	Motorcycle rider injured in transport accident
V30-V39	Occupant of three-wheeled motor vehicle injured in transport accident
V40-V49	Car occupant injured in transport accident
V50-V59	Occupant of pick-up truck or van injured in transport accident
V60-V69	Occupant of heavy transport vehicle injured in transport accident
V70-V79	Bus occupant injured in transport accident
V80-V89	Other land transport accidents
V90-V94	Water transport accidents
V95-V97	Air and space transport accidents
V98-V99	Other and unspecified transport accidents
W00-X58	Other external causes of accidental injury
W00-W19	Slipping, tripping, stumbling and falls
W20-W49	Exposure to inanimate mechanical forces
W50-W64	Exposure to animate mechanical forces
W65-W74	Accidental non-transport drowning and submersion
W85-W99	Exposure to electric current, radiation and extreme ambient air temperature and pressure
X00-X08	Exposure to smoke, fire and flames
X10-X19	Contact with heat and hot substances
X30-X39	Exposure to forces of nature
X52-X58	Accidental exposure **to other** specified factors
X71-X83	Intentional self-harm
X92-Y09	Assault
Y21-Y33	Event of undetermined intent
Y35-Y38	Legal intervention, operations of war, military operations, and terrorism
Y62-Y84	Complications of medical and surgical care
Y62-Y69	Misadventures to patients during surgical and medical care
Y70-Y82	Medical devices associated with adverse incidents in diagnostic and therapeutic use
Y83-Y84	Surgical and other medical procedures as the cause of abnormal reaction of the patient, or of later complication, without mention of misadventure at the time of the procedure
Y90-Y99	Supplementary factors related to causes of morbidity classified elsewhere

ACCIDENTS (V00-X58)

TRANSPORT ACCIDENTS (V00-V99)

Note: This section is structured in 12 groups. Those relating to land transport accidents (V00-V89) reflect the victim's mode of transport and are subdivided to identify the victim's 'counterpart' or the type of event. The vehicle of which the injured person is an occupant is identified in the first two characters since it is seen as the most important factor to identify for prevention purposes. A transport accident is one in which the vehicle involved must be moving or running or in use for transport purposes at the time of the accident.

Use additional code to identify:

Airbag injury (W22.1)

Type of street or road (Y92.4-)

Use of cellular telephone and other electronic equipment at the time of the transport accident (Y93.C-)

Excludes1: agricultural vehicles in stationary use or maintenance (W31.-)

assault by crashing of motor vehicle (Y03.-)

automobile or motor cycle in stationary use or maintenance- code to type of accident crashing of motor vehicle, undetermined intent (Y32)

intentional self-harm by crashing of motor vehicle (X82)

Excludes2: transport accidents due to cataclysm (X34-X38)

Note: Definitions related to transport accidents:

a) A transport accident (V00-V99) is any accident involving a device designed primarily for, or used at the time primarily for, conveying persons or good from one place to another.

b) A public highway [traffic way] or street is the entire width between property lines (or other boundary lines) of land open to the public as a matter of right or custom for purposes of moving persons or property from one place to another. A roadway is that part of the public highway designed, improved and customarily used for vehicular traffic.

c) A traffic accident is any vehicle accident occurring on the public highway [i.e. originating on, terminating on, or involving a vehicle partially on the highway]. A vehicle accident is assumed to have occurred on the public highway unless another place is specified, except in the case of accidents involving only off-road motor vehicles, which are classified as nontraffic accidents unless the contrary is stated.

d) A nontraffic accident is any vehicle accident that occurs entirely in any place other than a public highway.

e) A pedestrian is any person involved in an accident who was not at the time of the accident riding in or on a motor vehicle, railway train, streetcar or animal-drawn or other vehicle, or on a pedal cycle or animal. This includes, a person changing a tire, working on a parked car, or a person on foot. It also includes the user of a pedestrian conveyance such as a babystroller, ice-skates, skis, sled, roller skates, a skateboard, nonmotorized or motorized wheelchair, motorized mobility scooter, or nonmotorized scooter.

f) A driver is an occupant of a transport vehicle who is operating or intending to operate it.

g) A passenger is any occupant of a transport vehicle other than the driver, except a person traveling on the outside of the vehicle.

h) A person on the outside of a vehicle is any person being transported by a vehicle but not occupying the space normally reserved for the driver or passengers, or the space intended for the transport of property. This includes a person travelling on the bodywork, bumper, fender, roof, running board or step of a vehicle, as well as, hanging on the outside of the vehicle.

i) A pedal cycle is any land transport vehicle operated solely by nonmotorized pedals including a bicycle or tricycle.

j) A pedal cyclist is any person riding a pedal cycle or in a sidecar or trailer attached to a pedal cycle.

k) A motorcycle is a two-wheeled motor vehicle with one or two riding saddles and sometimes with a third wheel for the support of a sidecar. The sidecar is considered part of the motorcycle. This includes a moped, motor scooter, or motorized bicycle.

l) A motorcycle rider is any person riding a motorcycle or in a sidecar or trailer attached to the motorcycle.

m) A three-wheeled motor vehicle is a motorized tricycle designed primarily for on-road use. This includes a motor-driven tricycle, a motorized rickshaw, or a three-wheeled motor car.

n) A car [automobile] is a four-wheeled motor vehicle designed primarily for carrying up to 7 persons. A trailer being towed by the car is considered part of the car. It does not include a van or minivan - see definition

o) A pick-up truck or van is a four or six-wheeled motor vehicle designed for carrying passengers as well as property or cargo weighing less than the local limit for classification as a heavy goods vehicle, and not requiring a special driver's license. This includes a minivan and a sport-utility vehicle (SUV).

p) A heavy transport vehicle is a motor vehicle designed primarily for carrying property, meeting local criteria for classification as a heavy goods vehicle in terms of weight and requiring a special driver's license.

q) A bus (coach) is a motor vehicle designed or adapted primarily for carrying more than 10 passengers, and requiring a special driver's license.

r) A railway train or railway vehicle is any device, with or without freight or passenger cars couple to it, designed for traffic on a railway track. This includes subterranean (subways) or elevated trains.

s) A streetcar, is a device designed and used primarily for transporting passengers within a municipality, running on rails, usually subject to normal traffic control signals, and operated principally on a right-of-way that forms part of the roadway. This includes a tram or trolley that runs on rails. A trailer being towed by a streetcar is considered part of the streetcar.

t) A special vehicle mainly used on industrial premises is a motor vehicle designed primarily for use within the buildings and premises of industrial or commercial establishments. This includes battery-powered airport passenger vehicles or baggage/mail trucks, forklifts, coal-cars in a coal mine, logging cars and trucks used in mines or quarries.

u) A special vehicle mainly used in agriculture is a motor vehicle designed specifically for use in farming and agriculture (horticulture), to work the land, tend and harvest crops and transport materials on the farm. This includes harvesters, farm machinery and tractor and trailers.

v) A special construction vehicle is a motor vehicle designed specifically for use on construction and demolition sites. This includes bulldozers, diggers, earth levellers, dump trucks. backhoes, front-end loaders, pavers, and mechanical shovels.

w) A special all-terrain vehicle is a motor vehicle of special design to enable it to negotiate over rough or soft terrain , snow or sand. Examples of special design are high construction, special wheels and tires, tracks, and support on a cushion of air. This includes snow mobiles, All-terrain vehicles (ATV), and dune buggies. It does not include passenger vehicle designated as Sport Utility Vehicles. (SUV)

x) A watercraft is any device designed for transporting passengers or goods on water. This includes motor or sail boats, ships, and hovercraft.

y) An aircraft is any device for transporting passengers or goods in the air. This includes hot-air balloons, gliders, helicopters and airplanes. (z) A military vehicle is any motorized vehicle operating on a public roadway owned by the military and being operated by a member of the military.

PEDESTRIAN INJURED IN TRANSPORT ACCIDENT (V00-V09)

Includes: person changing tire on transport vehicle

person examining engine of vehicle broken down in (on side of) road

Excludes1: fall due to non-transport collision with other person (W03)

pedestrian on foot falling (slipping) on ice and snow (W00.-)

struck or bumped by another person (W51)

V00 Pedestrian conveyance accident

Use additional place of occurrence and activity external cause codes, if known (Y92.-, Y93.-)

Excludes1: collision with another person without fall (W51)

fall due to person on foot colliding with another person on foot (W03)

fall from non-moving wheelchair, nonmotorized scooter and motorized mobility scooter without collision (W05.-)

pedestrian (conveyance) collision with other land transport vehicle (V01-V09)

pedestrian on foot falling (slipping) on ice and snow (W00.-)

The appropriate 7th character is to be added to each code from category V00

A - initial encounter

D - subsequent encounter

S - sequela

V00.0 Pedestrian on foot injured in collision with pedestrian conveyance

⊗⑦**V00.01 Pedestrian on foot injured in collision with roller-skater**

⊗⑦**V00.02 Pedestrian on foot injured in collision with skateboarder**

⊗⑦**V00.09 Pedestrian on foot injured in collision with other pedestrian conveyance**

V00.1 Rolling-type pedestrian conveyance accident

Excludes1: accident with babystroller (V00.82-)

accident with wheelchair (powered) (V00.81-)

accident with motorized mobility scooter (V00.83-)

V00.11 In-line roller-skate accident

⑦**V00.111 Fall from in-line roller-skates**

⑦**V00.112 In-line roller-skater colliding with stationary object**

⑦**V00.118 Other in-line roller-skate accident**

Excludes1: roller-skater collision with other land transport vehicle (V01-V09 with 5th character 1)

V00.12 Non-in- line roller-skate accident

⑦**V00.121 Fall from non-in-line roller-skates**

⑦**V00.122 Non-in-line roller-skater colliding with stationary object**

⑦**V00.128 Other non-in-line roller-skating accident**

Excludes1: roller-skater collision with other land transport vehicle (V01-V09 with 5th character 1)

V00.13 Skateboard accident

⑦**V00.131 Fall from skateboard**

⑦**V00.132 Skateboarder colliding with stationary object**

⑦**V00.138 Other skateboard accident**

Excludes1: skateboarder collision with other land transport vehicle (V01-V09 with 5th character 2)

V00.14 Scooter (nonmotorized) accident

Excludes1: motor scooter accident (V20-V29)

⑦**V00.141 Fall from scooter (nonmotorized)**

● New code   ▲ Revised code   **Excludes1:** Not coded here   **Excludes2:** Not included here   ⊗ Placeholder required   ⑦7th digit required

⑦**V00.142** **Scooter (nonmotorized) colliding with stationary object**

⑦**V00.148** **Other scooter (nonmotorized) accident**

Excludes1: scooter (nonmotorized) collision with other land transport vehicle (V01-V09 with fifth character 9)

V00.15 **Heelies accident**

Rolling shoe Wheeled shoe Wheelies accident

⑦**V00.151** **Fall from heelies**

⑦**V00.152** **Heelies colliding with stationary object**

⑦**V00.158** **Other heelies accident**

V00.18 **Accident on other rolling-type pedestrian conveyance**

⑦**V00.181** **Fall from other rolling-type pedestrian conveyance**

⑦**V00.182** **Pedestrian on other rolling-type pedestrian conveyance colliding with stationary object**

⑦**V00.188** **Other accident on other rolling-type pedestrian conveyance**

V00.2 **Gliding-type pedestrian conveyance accident**

V00.21 **Ice-skates accident**

⑦**V00.211** **Fall from ice-skates**

⑦**V00.212** **Ice-skater colliding with stationary object**

⑦**V00.218** **Other ice-skates accident**

Excludes1: ice-skater collision with other land transport vehicle (V01-V09 with 5th digit 9)

V00.22 **Sled accident**

⑦**V00.221** **Fall from sled**

⑦**V00.222** **Sledder colliding with stationary object**

⑦**V00.228** **Other sled accident**

Excludes1: sled collision with other land transport vehicle (V01-V09 with 5th digit 9)

V00.28 **Other gliding-type pedestrian conveyance accident**

⑦**V00.281** **Fall from other gliding-type pedestrian conveyance**

⑦**V00.282** **Pedestrian on other gliding-type pedestrian conveyance colliding with stationary object**

⑦**V00.288** **Other accident on other gliding-type pedestrian conveyance**

Excludes1: gliding-type pedestrian conveyance collision with other land transport vehicle (V01-V09 with 5th digit 9)

V00.3 **Flat-bottomed pedestrian conveyance accident**

V00.31 **Snowboard accident**

⑦**V00.311** **Fall from snowboard**

⑦**V00.312** **Snowboarder colliding with stationary object**

⑦**V00.318** **Other snowboard accident**

Excludes1: snowboarder collision with other land transport vehicle (V01-V09 with 5th digit 9)

V00.32 **Snow-ski accident**

⑦**V00.321** **Fall from snow-skis**

⑦**V00.322** **Snow-skier colliding with stationary object**

⑦**V00.328** **Other snow-ski accident**

Excludes1: snow-skier collision with other land transport vehicle (V01-V09 with 5th digit 9)

V00.38 **Other flat-bottomed pedestrian conveyance accident**

⑦**V00.381** **Fall from other flat-bottomed pedestrian conveyance**

⑦**V00.382** **Pedestrian on other flat-bottomed pedestrian conveyance colliding with stationary object**

⑦**V00.388** **Other accident on other flat-bottomed pedestrian conveyance**

V00.8 **Accident on other pedestrian conveyance**

V00.81 **Accident with wheelchair (powered)**

⑦**V00.811** **Fall from moving wheelchair (powered)**

Excludes1: fall from non-moving wheelchair (W05.0)

⑦**V00.812** **Wheelchair (powered) colliding with stationary object**

⑦**V00.818** **Other accident with wheelchair (powered)**

V00.82 **Accident with babystroller**

⑦**V00.821** **Fall from babystroller**

⑦**V00.822** **Babystroller colliding with stationary object**

⑦**V00.828** **Other accident with babystroller**

V00.83 **Accident with motorized mobility scooter**

⑦**V00.831** **Fall from motorized mobility scooter**

Excludes1: fall from non-moving motorized mobility scooter (W05.2)

⑦**V00.832** **Motorized mobility scooter colliding with stationary object**

⑦**V00.838** **Other accident with motorized mobility scooter**

V00.89 **Accident on other pedestrian conveyance**

⑦**V00.891** **Fall from other pedestrian conveyance**

⑦**V00.892** **Pedestrian on other pedestrian conveyance colliding with stationary object**

⑦**V00.898** **Other accident on other pedestrian conveyance**

Excludes1: Other pedestrian (conveyance) collision with other land transport vehicle (V01-V09 with 5th digit 9)

V01 **Pedestrian injured in collision with pedal cycle**

The appropriate 7th character is to be added to each code from category V01

A - initial encounter

D - subsequent encounter

S - sequela

V01.0 **Pedestrian injured in collision with pedal cycle in nontraffic accident**

⊗⑦**V01.00** **Pedestrian on foot injured in collision with pedal cycle in nontraffic accident**

Add 4th-7th digits   Nonspecific code   Unspecified code   Manifestation code

Pedestrian NOS injured in collision with pedal cycle in nontraffic accident

⊗⑦**V01.01** **Pedestrian on roller-skates injured in collision with pedal cycle in nontraffic accident**

⊗⑦**V01.02** **Pedestrian on skateboard injured in collision with pedal cycle in nontraffic accident**

⊗⑦**V01.09** **Pedestrian with other conveyance injured in collision with pedal cycle in nontraffic accident**

Pedestrian with babystroller injured in collision with pedal cycle in nontraffic accident

Pedestrian on ice-skates injured in collision with pedal cycle in nontraffic accident

Pedestrian on nonmotorized scooter injured in collision with pedal cycle in nontraffic accident

Pedestrian on sled injured in collision with pedal cycle in nontraffic accident

Pedestrian on snowboard injured in collision with pedal cycle in nontraffic accident

Pedestrian on snow-skis injured in collision with pedal cycle in nontraffic accident

Pedestrian in wheelchair (powered) injured in collision with pedal cycle in nontraffic accident

Pedestrian in motorized mobility scooter injured in collision with pedal cycle in nontraffic accident

V01.1 **Pedestrian injured in collision with pedal cycle in traffic accident**

⊗⑦**V01.10** **Pedestrian on foot injured in collision with pedal cycle in traffic accident**

Pedestrian NOS injured in collision with pedal cycle in traffic accident

⊗⑦**V01.11** **Pedestrian on roller-skates injured in collision with pedal cycle in traffic accident**

⊗⑦**V01.12** **Pedestrian on skateboard injured in collision with pedal cycle in traffic accident**

⊗⑦**V01.19** **Pedestrian with other conveyance injured in collision with pedal cycle in traffic accident**

Pedestrian with babystroller injured in collision with pedal cycle in traffic accident

Pedestrian on ice-skates injured in collision with pedal cycle in traffic accident

Pedestrian on nonmotorized scooter injured in collision with pedal cycle in traffic accident

Pedestrian on sled injured in collision with pedal cycle in traffic accident

Pedestrian on snowboard injured in collision with pedal cycle in traffic accident

Pedestrian on snow-skis injured in collision with pedal cycle in traffic accident

Pedestrian in wheelchair (powered) injured in collision with pedal cycle in traffic accident

Pedestrian in motorized mobility scooter injured in collision with pedal cycle in traffic accident

V01.9 **Pedestrian injured in collision with pedal cycle, unspecified whether traffic or nontraffic accident**

⊗⑦**V01.90** **Pedestrian on foot injured in collision with pedal cycle, unspecified whether traffic or nontraffic accident**

Pedestrian NOS injured in collision with pedal cycle, unspecified whether traffic or nontraffic accident

⊗⑦**V01.91** **Pedestrian on roller-skates injured in collision with pedal cycle, unspecified whether traffic or nontraffic accident**

⊗⑦**V01.92** **Pedestrian on skateboard injured in collision with pedal cycle, unspecified whether traffic or nontraffic accident**

⊗⑦**V01.99** **Pedestrian with other conveyance injured in collision with pedal cycle, unspecified whether traffic or nontraffic accident**

Pedestrian with babystroller injured in collision with pedal cycle, unspecified whether traffic or nontraffic accident

Pedestrian on ice-skates injured in collision with pedal cycle unspecified, whether traffic or nontraffic accident

Pedestrian on nonmotorized scooter injured in collision with pedal cycle, unspecified whether traffic or nontraffic accident

Pedestrian on sled injured in collision with pedal cycle unspecified, whether traffic or nontraffic accident

Pedestrian on snowboard injured in collision with pedal cycle, unspecified whether traffic or nontraffic accident

Pedestrian on snow-skis injured in collision with pedal cycle, unspecified whether traffic or nontraffic accident

Pedestrian in wheelchair (powered) injured in collision with pedal cycle, unspecified whether traffic or nontraffic accident

Pedestrian in motorized mobility scooter injured in collision with pedal cycle, unspecified whether traffic or nontraffic accident

V02 **Pedestrian injured in collision with two- or three-wheeled motor vehicle**

The appropriate 7th character is to be added to each code from category V02

A - initial encounter

D - subsequent encounter

S - sequela

V02.0 **Pedestrian injured in collision with two- or three-wheeled motor vehicle in nontraffic accident**

⊗⑦**V02.00** **Pedestrian on foot injured in collision with two- or three-wheeled motor vehicle in nontraffic accident**

Pedestrian NOS injured in collision with two- or three-wheeled motor vehicle in nontraffic accident

⊗⑦**V02.01** **Pedestrian on roller-skates injured in collision with two- or three-wheeled motor vehicle in nontraffic accident**

⊗⑦**V02.02** **Pedestrian on skateboard injured in collision with two- or three-wheeled motor vehicle in nontraffic accident**

⊗⑦**V02.09** **Pedestrian with other conveyance injured in collision with two- or three-wheeled motor vehicle in nontraffic accident**

Pedestrian with babystroller injured in collision with two- or three-wheeled motor vehicle in nontraffic accident

Pedestrian on ice-skates injured in collision with two- or three-wheeled motor vehicle in nontraffic accident

Pedestrian on nonmotorized scooter injured in collision with two- or three-wheeled motor vehicle in nontraffic accident

● New code ▲ Revised code **Excludes1:** Not coded here **Excludes2:** Not included here ⊗ Placeholder required ⑦7th digit required

Pedestrian on sled injured in collision with two- or three-wheeled motor vehicle in nontraffic accident

Pedestrian on snowboard injured in collision with two- or three-wheeled motor vehicle in nontraffic accident

Pedestrian on snow-skis injured in collision with two- or three-wheeled motor vehicle in nontraffic accident

Pedestrian in wheelchair (powered) injured in collision with two- or three-wheeled motor vehicle in nontraffic accident

Pedestrian in motorized mobility scooter injured in collision with two- or three-wheeled motor vehicle in nontraffic accident

V02.1 **Pedestrian injured in collision with two- or three-wheeled motor vehicle in traffic accident**

⊗⑦**V02.10** **Pedestrian on foot injured in collision with two- or three-wheeled motor vehicle in traffic accident**

Pedestrian NOS injured in collision with two- or three-wheeled motor vehicle in traffic accident

⊗⑦**V02.11** **Pedestrian on roller-skates injured in collision with two- or three-wheeled motor vehicle in traffic accident**

⊗⑦**V02.12** **Pedestrian on skateboard injured in collision with two- or three-wheeled motor vehicle in traffic accident**

⊗⑦**V02.19** **Pedestrian with other conveyance injured in collision with two- or three-wheeled motor vehicle in traffic accident**

Pedestrian with babystroller injured in collision with two- or three-wheeled motor vehicle in traffic accident

Pedestrian on ice-skates injured in collision with two- or three-wheeled motor vehicle in traffic accident

Pedestrian on nonmotorized scooter injured in collision with two- or three-wheeled motor vehicle in traffic accident

Pedestrian on sled injured in collision with two- or three-wheeled motor vehicle in traffic accident

Pedestrian on snowboard injured in collision with two- or three-wheeled motor vehicle in traffic accident

Pedestrian on snow-skis injured in collision with two- or three-wheeled motor vehicle in traffic accident

Pedestrian in wheelchair (powered) injured in collision with two- or three-wheeled motor vehicle in traffic accident

Pedestrian in motorized mobility scooter injured in collision with two- or three-wheeled motor vehicle in traffic accident

V02.9 **Pedestrian injured in collision with two- or three-wheeled motor vehicle, unspecified whether traffic or nontraffic accident**

⊗⑦**V02.90** **Pedestrian on foot injured in collision with two- or three-wheeled motor vehicle, unspecified whether traffic or nontraffic accident**

Pedestrian NOS injured in collision with two- or three-wheeled motor vehicle, unspecified whether traffic or nontraffic accident

⊗⑦**V02.91** **Pedestrian on roller-skates injured in collision with two- or three-wheeled motor vehicle, unspecified whether traffic or nontraffic accident**

⊗⑦**V02.92** **Pedestrian on skateboard injured in collision with two- or three-wheeled motor vehicle, unspecified whether traffic or nontraffic accident**

⊗⑦**V02.99** **Pedestrian with other conveyance injured in collision with two- or three-wheeled motor vehicle, unspecified whether traffic or nontraffic accident**

Pedestrian with babystroller injured in collision with two- or three-wheeled motor vehicle, unspecified whether traffic or nontraffic accident

Pedestrian on ice-skates injured in collision with two- or three-wheeled motor vehicle, unspecified whether traffic or nontraffic accident

Pedestrian on nonmotorized scooter injured in collision with two- or three-wheeled motor vehicle, unspecified whether traffic or nontraffic accident

Pedestrian on sled injured in collision with two- or three-wheeled motor vehicle, unspecified whether traffic or nontraffic accident

Pedestrian on snowboard injured in collision with two- or three-wheeled motor vehicle, unspecified whether traffic or nontraffic accident

Pedestrian on snow-skis injured in collision with two- or three-wheeled motor vehicle, unspecified whether traffic or nontraffic accident

Pedestrian in wheelchair (powered) injured in collision with two- or three-wheeled motor vehicle, unspecified whether traffic or nontraffic accident

Pedestrian in motorized mobility scooter injured in collision with two- or three-wheeled motor vehicle, unspecified whether traffic or nontraffic accident

V03 **Pedestrian injured in collision with car, pick-up truck or van**

The appropriate 7th character is to be added to each code from category V03

A - initial encounter

D - subsequent encounter

S - sequela

V03.0 **Pedestrian injured in collision with car, pick-up truck or van in nontraffic accident**

⊗⑦**V03.00** **Pedestrian on foot injured in collision with car, pick-up truck or van in nontraffic accident**

Pedestrian NOS injured in collision with car, pick-up truck or van in nontraffic accident

⊗⑦**V03.01** **Pedestrian on roller-skates injured in collision with car, pick-up truck or van in nontraffic accident**

⊗⑦**V03.02** **Pedestrian on skateboard injured in collision with car, pick-up truck or van in nontraffic accident**

⊗⑦**V03.09** **Pedestrian with other conveyance injured in collision with car, pick-up truck or van in nontraffic accident**

Pedestrian with babystroller injured in collision with car, pick-up truck or van in nontraffic accident

Pedestrian on ice-skates injured in collision with car, pick-up truck or van in nontraffic accident

Pedestrian on nonmotorized scooter injured in collision with car, pick-up truck or van in nontraffic accident

Pedestrian on sled injured in collision with car, pick-up truck or van in nontraffic accident

Pedestrian on snowboard injured in collision with car, pick-up truck or van in nontraffic accident

Pedestrian on snow-skis injured in collision with car, pick-up truck or van in nontraffic accident

Pedestrian in wheelchair (powered) injured in collision with car, pick-up truck or van in nontraffic accident

Pedestrian in motorized mobility scooter injured in collision with car, pick-up truck or van in nontraffic accident

V03.1 **Pedestrian injured in collision with car, pick-up truck or van in traffic accident**

⊗⑦**V03.10** **Pedestrian on foot injured in collision with car, pick-up truck or van in traffic accident**

Pedestrian NOS injured in collision with car, pick-up truck or van in traffic accident

⊗⑦**V03.11** **Pedestrian on roller-skates injured in collision with car, pick-up truck or van in traffic accident**

⊗⑦**V03.12** **Pedestrian on skateboard injured in collision with car, pick-up truck or van in traffic accident**

⊗⑦**V03.19** **Pedestrian with other conveyance injured in collision with car, pick-up truck or van in traffic accident**

Pedestrian with babystroller injured in collision with car, pick-up truck or van in traffic accident

Pedestrian on ice-skates injured in collision with car, pick-up truck or van in traffic accident

Pedestrian on nonmotorized scooter injured in collision with car, pick-up truck or van in traffic accident

Pedestrian on sled injured in collision with car, pick-up truck or van in traffic accident

Pedestrian on snowboard injured in collision with car, pick-up truck or van in traffic accident

Pedestrian on snow-skis injured in collision with car, pick-up truck or van in traffic accident

Pedestrian in wheelchair (powered) injured in collision with car, pick-up truck or van in traffic accident

Pedestrian in motorized mobility scooter injured in collision with car, pick-up truck or van in traffic accident

V03.9 **Pedestrian injured in collision with car, pick-up truck or van, unspecified whether traffic or nontraffic accident**

⊗⑦**V03.90** **Pedestrian on foot injured in collision with car, pick-up truck or van, unspecified whether traffic or nontraffic accident**

Pedestrian NOS injured in collision with car, pick-up truck or van, unspecified whether traffic or nontraffic accident

⊗⑦**V03.91** **Pedestrian on roller-skates injured in collision with car, pick-up truck or van, unspecified whether traffic or nontraffic accident**

⊗⑦**V03.92** **Pedestrian on skateboard injured in collision with car, pick-up truck or van, unspecified whether traffic or nontraffic accident**

⊗⑦**V03.99** **Pedestrian with other conveyance injured in collision with car, pick-up truck or van, unspecified whether traffic or nontraffic accident**

Pedestrian with babystroller injured in collision with car, pick-up truck or van, unspecified whether traffic or nontraffic accident

Pedestrian on ice-skates injured in collision with car, pick-up truck or van, unspecified whether traffic or nontraffic accident

Pedestrian on nonmotorized scooter injured in collision with car, pick-up truck or van, unspecified whether traffic or nontraffic accident

Pedestrian on sled injured in collision with car, pick-up truck or van in nontraffic accident

Pedestrian on snowboard injured in collision with car, pick-up truck or van, unspecified whether traffic or nontraffic accident

Pedestrian on snow-skis injured in collision with car, pick-up truck or van, unspecified whether traffic or nontraffic accident

Pedestrian in wheelchair (powered) injured in collision with car, pick-up truck or van, unspecified whether traffic or nontraffic accident

Pedestrian in motorized mobility scooter injured in collision with car, pick-up truck or van, unspecified whether traffic or nontraffic accident

V04 **Pedestrian injured in collision with heavy transport vehicle or bus**

Excludes1: pedestrian injured in collision with military vehicle (V09.01, V09.21)

The appropriate 7th character is to be added to each code from category V04

A - initial encounter

D - subsequent encounter

S - sequela

V04.0 **Pedestrian injured in collision with heavy transport vehicle or bus in nontraffic accident**

⊗⑦**V04.00** **Pedestrian on foot injured in collision with heavy transport vehicle or bus in nontraffic accident**

Pedestrian NOS injured in collision with heavy transport vehicle or bus in nontraffic accident

⊗⑦**V04.01** **Pedestrian on roller-skates injured in collision with heavy transport vehicle or bus in nontraffic accident**

⊗⑦**V04.02** **Pedestrian on skateboard injured in collision with heavy transport vehicle or bus in nontraffic accident**

⊗⑦**V04.09** **Pedestrian with other conveyance injured in collision with heavy transport vehicle or bus in nontraffic accident**

● New code   ▲ Revised code   **Excludes1:** Not coded here   **Excludes2:** Not included here   ⊗ Placeholder required   ⑦ 7th digit required

Pedestrian with babystroller injured in collision with heavy transport vehicle or bus in nontraffic accident

Pedestrian on ice-skates injured in collision with heavy transport vehicle or bus in nontraffic accident

Pedestrian on nonmotorized scooter injured in collision with heavy transport vehicle or bus in nontraffic accident

Pedestrian on sled injured in collision with heavy transport vehicle or bus in nontraffic accident

Pedestrian on snowboard injured in collision with heavy transport vehicle or bus in nontraffic accident

Pedestrian on snow-skis injured in collision with heavy transport vehicle or bus in nontraffic accident

Pedestrian in wheelchair (powered) injured in collision with heavy transport vehicle or bus in nontraffic accident

Pedestrian in motorized mobility scooter injured in collision with heavy transport vehicle or bus in nontraffic accident

V04.1 Pedestrian injured in collision with heavy transport vehicle or bus in traffic accident

⊗⑦**V04.10 Pedestrian on foot injured in collision with heavy transport vehicle or bus in traffic accident**

Pedestrian NOS injured in collision with heavy transport vehicle or bus in traffic accident

⊗⑦**V04.11 Pedestrian on roller-skates injured in collision with heavy transport vehicle or bus in traffic accident**

⊗⑦**V04.12 Pedestrian on skateboard injured in collision with heavy transport vehicle or bus in traffic accident**

⊗⑦**V04.19 Pedestrian with other conveyance injured in collision with heavy transport vehicle or bus in traffic accident**

Pedestrian with babystroller injured in collision with heavy transport vehicle or bus in traffic accident

Pedestrian on ice-skates injured in collision with heavy transport vehicle or bus in traffic accident

Pedestrian on nonmotorized scooter injured in collision with heavy transport vehicle or bus in traffic accident

Pedestrian on sled injured in collision with heavy transport vehicle or bus in traffic accident

Pedestrian on snowboard injured in collision with heavy transport vehicle or bus in traffic accident

Pedestrian on snow-skis injured in collision with heavy transport vehicle or bus in traffic accident

Pedestrian in wheelchair (powered) injured in collision with heavy transport vehicle or bus in traffic accident

Pedestrian in motorized mobility scooter injured in collision with heavy transport vehicle or bus in traffic accident

V04.9 Pedestrian injured in collision with heavy transport vehicle or bus, unspecified whether traffic or nontraffic accident

⊗⑦**V04.90 Pedestrian on foot injured in collision with heavy transport vehicle or bus, unspecified whether traffic or nontraffic accident**

Pedestrian NOS injured in collision with heavy transport vehicle or bus, unspecified whether traffic or nontraffic accident

⊗⑦**V04.91 Pedestrian on roller-skates injured in collision with heavy transport vehicle or bus, unspecified whether traffic or nontraffic accident**

⊗⑦**V04.92 Pedestrian on skateboard injured in collision with heavy transport vehicle or bus, unspecified whether traffic or nontraffic accident**

⊗⑦**V04.99 Pedestrian with other conveyance injured in collision with heavy transport vehicle or bus, unspecified whether traffic or nontraffic accident**

Pedestrian with babystroller injured in collision with heavy transport vehicle or bus, unspecified whether traffic or nontraffic accident

Pedestrian on ice-skates injured in collision with heavy transport vehicle or bus, unspecified whether traffic or nontraffic accident

Pedestrian on nonmotorized scooter injured in collision with heavy transport vehicle or bus, unspecified whether traffic or nontraffic accident

Pedestrian on sled injured in collision with heavy transport vehicle or bus, unspecified whether traffic or nontraffic accident

Pedestrian on snowboard injured in collision with heavy transport vehicle or bus, unspecified whether traffic or nontraffic accident

Pedestrian on snow-skis injured in collision with heavy transport vehicle or bus, unspecified whether traffic or nontraffic accident

Pedestrian in wheelchair (powered) injured in collision with heavy transport vehicle or bus, unspecified whether traffic or nontraffic accident

Pedestrian in motorized mobility scooter injured in collision with heavy transport vehicle or bus,

unspecified whether traffic or nontraffic accident

V05 Pedestrian injured in collision with railway train or railway vehicle

The appropriate 7th character is to be added to each code from category V05

A - initial encounter

D - subsequent encounter

S - sequela

V05.0 Pedestrian injured in collision with railway train or railway vehicle in nontraffic accident

⊗⑦**V05.00 Pedestrian on foot injured in collision with railway train or railway vehicle in nontraffic accident**

Pedestrian NOS injured in collision with railway train or railway vehicle in nontraffic accident

---

⊗⑦**V05.01** **Pedestrian on roller-skates injured in collision with railway train or railway vehicle in nontraffic accident**

⊗⑦**V05.02** **Pedestrian on skateboard injured in collision with railway train or railway vehicle in nontraffic accident**

⊗⑦**V05.09** **Pedestrian with other conveyance injured in collision with railway train or railway vehicle in nontraffic accident**

Pedestrian with babystroller injured in collision with railway train or railway vehicle in nontraffic accident

Pedestrian on ice-skates injured in collision with railway train or railway vehicle in nontraffic accident

Pedestrian on nonmotorized scooter injured in collision with railway train or railway vehicle in nontraffic accident

Pedestrian on sled injured in collision with railway train or railway vehicle in nontraffic accident

Pedestrian on snowboard injured in collision with railway train or railway vehicle in nontraffic accident

Pedestrian on snow-skis injured in collision with railway train or railway vehicle in nontraffic accident

Pedestrian in wheelchair (powered) injured in collision with railway train or railway vehicle in nontraffic accident

Pedestrian in motorized mobility scooter injured in collision with railway train or railway vehicle in nontraffic accident

V05.1 **Pedestrian injured in collision with railway train or railway vehicle in traffic accident**

⊗⑦**V05.10** **Pedestrian on foot injured in collision with railway train or railway vehicle in traffic accident**

Pedestrian NOS injured in collision with railway train or railway vehicle in traffic accident

⊗⑦**V05.11** **Pedestrian on roller-skates injured in collision with railway train or railway vehicle in traffic accident**

⊗⑦**V05.12** **Pedestrian on skateboard injured in collision with railway train or railway vehicle in traffic accident**

⊗⑦**V05.19** **Pedestrian with other conveyance injured in collision with railway train or railway vehicle in traffic accident**

Pedestrian with babystroller injured in collision with railway train or railway vehicle in traffic accident

Pedestrian on ice-skates injured in collision with railway train or railway vehicle in traffic accident

Pedestrian on nonmotorized scooter injured in collision with railway train or railway vehicle in traffic accident

Pedestrian on sled injured in collision with railway train or railway vehicle in traffic accident

Pedestrian on snowboard injured in collision with railway train or railway vehicle in traffic accident

Pedestrian on snow-skis injured in collision with railway train or railway vehicle in traffic accident

Pedestrian in wheelchair (powered) injured in collision with railway train or railway vehicle in traffic accident

Pedestrian in motorized mobility scooter injured in collision with railway train or railway vehicle in traffic accident

V05.9 **Pedestrian injured in collision with railway train or railway vehicle, unspecified whether traffic or nontraffic accident**

⊗⑦**V05.90** **Pedestrian on foot injured in collision with railway train or railway vehicle, unspecified whether traffic or nontraffic accident**

Pedestrian NOS injured in collision with railway train or railway vehicle, unspecified whether traffic or nontraffic accident

⊗⑦**V05.91** **Pedestrian on roller-skates injured in collision with railway train or railway vehicle, unspecified whether traffic or nontraffic accident**

⊗⑦**V05.92** **Pedestrian on skateboard injured in collision with railway train or railway vehicle, unspecified whether traffic or nontraffic accident**

⊗⑦**V05.99** **Pedestrian with other conveyance injured in collision with railway train or railway vehicle, unspecified whether traffic or nontraffic accident**

Pedestrian with babystroller injured in collision with railway train or railway vehicle, unspecified whether traffic or nontraffic

Pedestrian on ice-skates injured in collision with railway train or railway vehicle, unspecified whether traffic or nontraffic

Pedestrian on nonmotorized scooter injured in collision with railway train or railway vehicle, unspecified whether traffic or nontraffic

Pedestrian on sled injured in collision with railway train or railway vehicle, unspecified whether traffic or nontraffic

Pedestrian on snowboard injured in collision with railway train or railway vehicle, unspecified whether traffic or nontraffic

Pedestrian on snow-skis injured in collision with railway train or railway vehicle, unspecified whether traffic or nontraffic

Pedestrian in wheelchair (powered) injured in collision with railway train or railway vehicle, unspecified whether traffic or nontraffic

Pedestrian in motorized mobility scooter injured in collision with railway train or railway vehicle, unspecified whether traffic or nontraffic

V06 **Pedestrian injured in collision with other nonmotor vehicle**

Includes: collision with animal-drawn vehicle, animal being ridden, nonpowered streetcar

Excludes1: pedestrian injured in collision with pedestrian conveyance (V00.0-)

The appropriate 7th character is to be added to each code from category V06

A - initial encounter

D - subsequent encounter

S - sequela

● New code ▲ Revised code **Excludes1:** Not coded here **Excludes2:** Not included here ⊗ Placeholder required ⑦7th digit required

V06.0 Pedestrian injured in collision with other nonmotor vehicle in nontraffic accident

⊗⑦**V06.00** **Pedestrian on foot injured in collision with other nonmotor vehicle in nontraffic accident**

Pedestrian NOS injured in collision with other nonmotor vehicle in nontraffic accident

⊗⑦**V06.01** **Pedestrian on roller-skates injured in collision with other nonmotor vehicle in nontraffic accident**

⊗⑦**V06.02** **Pedestrian on skateboard injured in collision with other nonmotor vehicle in nontraffic accident**

⊗⑦**V06.09** **Pedestrian with other conveyance injured in collision with other nonmotor vehicle in nontraffic accident**

Pedestrian with babystroller injured in collision with other nonmotor vehicle in nontraffic accident

Pedestrian on ice-skates injured in collision with other nonmotor vehicle in nontraffic accident

Pedestrian on nonmotorized scooter injured in collision with other nonmotor vehicle in nontraffic accident

Pedestrian on sled injured in collision with other nonmotor vehicle in nontraffic accident

Pedestrian on snowboard injured in collision with other nonmotor vehicle in nontraffic accident

Pedestrian on snow-skis injured in collision with other nonmotor vehicle in nontraffic accident

Pedestrian in wheelchair (powered) injured in collision with other nonmotor vehicle in nontraffic accident

Pedestrian in motorized mobility scooter injured in collision with other nonmotor vehicle in nontraffic accident

V06.1 Pedestrian injured in collision with other nonmotor vehicle in traffic accident

⊗⑦**V06.10** **Pedestrian on foot injured in collision with other nonmotor vehicle in traffic accident**

Pedestrian NOS injured in collision with other nonmotor vehicle in traffic accident

⊗⑦**V06.11** **Pedestrian on roller-skates injured in collision with other nonmotor vehicle in traffic accident**

⊗⑦**V06.12** **Pedestrian on skateboard injured in collision with other nonmotor vehicle in traffic accident**

⊗⑦**V06.19** **Pedestrian with other conveyance injured in collision with other nonmotor vehicle in traffic accident**

Pedestrian with babystroller injured in collision with other nonmotor vehicle in nontraffic accident

Pedestrian on ice-skates injured in collision with other nonmotor vehicle in traffic accident

Pedestrian on nonmotorized scooter injured in collision with other nonmotor vehicle in traffic accident

Pedestrian on sled injured in collision with other nonmotor vehicle in traffic accident

Pedestrian on snowboard injured in collision with other nonmotor vehicle in traffic accident

Pedestrian on snow-skis injured in collision with other nonmotor vehicle in traffic accident

Pedestrian in wheelchair (powered) injured in collision with other nonmotor vehicle in traffic accident

Pedestrian in motorized mobility scooter injured in collision with other nonmotor vehicle in traffic accident

V06.9 Pedestrian injured in collision with other nonmotor vehicle, unspecified whether traffic or nontraffic accident

⊗⑦**V06.90** **Pedestrian on foot injured in collision with other nonmotor vehicle, unspecified whether traffic or nontraffic accident**

Pedestrian NOS injured in collision with other nonmotor vehicle, unspecified whether traffic or nontraffic accident

⊗⑦**V06.91** **Pedestrian on roller-skates injured in collision with other nonmotor vehicle, unspecified whether traffic or nontraffic accident**

⊗⑦**V06.92** **Pedestrian on skateboard injured in collision with other nonmotor vehicle, unspecified whether traffic or nontraffic accident**

⊗⑦**V06.99** **Pedestrian with other conveyance injured in collision with other nonmotor vehicle, unspecified whether traffic or nontraffic accident**

Pedestrian with babystroller injured in collision with other nonmotor vehicle, unspecified whether traffic or nontraffic accident

Pedestrian on ice-skates injured in collision with other nonmotor vehicle, unspecified whether traffic or nontraffic accident

Pedestrian on nonmotorized scooter injured in collision with other nonmotor vehicle, unspecified whether traffic or nontraffic accident

Pedestrian on sled injured in collision with other nonmotor vehicle, unspecified whether traffic or nontraffic accident

Pedestrian on snowboard injured in collision with other nonmotor vehicle, unspecified whether traffic or nontraffic accident

Pedestrian on snow-skis injured in collision with other nonmotor vehicle, unspecified whether traffic or nontraffic accident

Pedestrian in wheelchair (powered) injured in collision with other nonmotor vehicle, unspecified whether traffic or nontraffic accident

Pedestrian in motorized mobility scooter injured in collision with other nonmotor vehicle, unspecified whether traffic or nontraffic accident

V09 Pedestrian injured in other and unspecified transport accidents

The appropriate 7th character is to be added to each code from category V09

A - initial encounter

D - subsequent encounter

S - sequela

V09.0 Pedestrian injured in nontraffic accident involving other and unspecified motor vehicles

⊗⑦**V09.00** **Pedestrian injured in nontraffic accident involving unspecified motor vehicles**

Add 4th-7th digits   Nonspecific code   Unspecified code   Manifestation code

⊗⑦V09.01 Pedestrian injured in nontraffic accident involving military vehicle

⊗⑦V09.09 Pedestrian injured in nontraffic accident involving other motor vehicles

Pedestrian injured in nontraffic accident by special vehicle

⊗⑦V09.1 Pedestrian injured in unspecified nontraffic accident

V09.2 Pedestrian injured in traffic accident involving other and unspecified motor vehicles

⊗⑦V09.20 Pedestrian injured in traffic accident involving unspecified motor vehicles

⊗⑦V09.21 Pedestrian injured in traffic accident involving military vehicle

⊗⑦V09.29 Pedestrian injured in traffic accident involving other motor vehicles

⊗⑦V09.3 Pedestrian injured in unspecified traffic accident

⊗⑦V09.9 Pedestrian injured in unspecified transport accident

PEDAL CYCLE RIDER INJURED IN TRANSPORT ACCIDENT (V10-V19)

Includes: any non-motorized vehicle, excluding an animal-drawn vehicle, or a sidecar or trailer attached to the pedal cycle

Excludes2: rupture of pedal cycle tire (W37.0)

V10 Pedal cycle rider injured in collision with pedestrian or animal

Excludes1: pedal cycle rider collision with animal-drawn vehicle or animal being ridden (V16.-)

The appropriate 7th character is to be added to each code from category V10

A - initial encounter

D - subsequent encounter

S - sequela

⊗⑦V10.0 Pedal cycle driver injured in collision with pedestrian or animal in nontraffic accident

⊗⑦V10.1 Pedal cycle passenger injured in collision with pedestrian or animal in nontraffic accident

⊗⑦V10.2 Unspecified pedal cyclist injured in collision with pedestrian or animal in nontraffic accident

⊗⑦V10.3 Person boarding or alighting a pedal cycle injured in collision with pedestrian or animal

⊗⑦V10.4 Pedal cycle driver injured in collision with pedestrian or animal in traffic accident

⊗⑦V10.5 Pedal cycle passenger injured in collision with pedestrian or animal in traffic accident

⊗⑦V10.9 Unspecified pedal cyclist injured in collision with pedestrian or animal in traffic accident

V11 Pedal cycle rider injured in collision with other pedal cycle

The appropriate 7th character is to be added to each code from category V11

A - initial encounter

D - subsequent encounter

S - sequela

⊗⑦V11.0 Pedal cycle driver injured in collision with other pedal cycle in nontraffic accident

⊗⑦V11.1 Pedal cycle passenger injured in collision with other pedal cycle in nontraffic accident

⊗⑦V11.2 Unspecified pedal cyclist injured in collision with other pedal cycle in nontraffic accident

⊗⑦V11.3 Person boarding or alighting a pedal cycle injured in collision with other pedal cycle

⊗⑦V11.4 Pedal cycle driver injured in collision with other pedal cycle in traffic accident

⊗⑦V11.5 Pedal cycle passenger injured in collision with other pedal cycle in traffic accident

⊗⑦V11.9 Unspecified pedal cyclist injured in collision with other pedal cycle in traffic accident

V12 Pedal cycle rider injured in collision with two- or three-wheeled motor vehicle

The appropriate 7th character is to be added to each code from category V12

A - initial encounter

D - subsequent encounter

S - sequela

⊗⑦V12.0 Pedal cycle driver injured in collision with two- or three-wheeled motor vehicle in nontraffic accident

⊗⑦V12.1 Pedal cycle passenger injured in collision with two- or three-wheeled motor vehicle in nontraffic accident

⊗⑦V12.2 Unspecified pedal cyclist injured in collision with two- or three-wheeled motor vehicle in nontraffic accident

⊗⑦V12.3 Person boarding or alighting a pedal cycle injured in collision with two- or three-wheeled motor vehicle

⊗⑦V12.4 Pedal cycle driver injured in collision with two- or three-wheeled motor vehicle in traffic accident

⊗⑦V12.5 Pedal cycle passenger injured in collision with two- or three-wheeled motor vehicle in traffic accident

⊗⑦V12.9 Unspecified pedal cyclist injured in collision with two- or three-wheeled motor vehicle in traffic accident

V13 Pedal cycle rider injured in collision with car, pick-up truck or van

The appropriate 7th character is to be added to each code from category V13

A - initial encounter

D - subsequent encounter

S - sequela

⊗⑦V13.0 Pedal cycle driver injured in collision with car, pick-up truck or van in nontraffic accident

⊗⑦V13.1 Pedal cycle passenger injured in collision with car, pick-up truck or van in nontraffic accident

⊗⑦V13.2 Unspecified pedal cyclist injured in collision with car, pick-up truck or van in nontraffic accident

⊗⑦V13.3 Person boarding or alighting a pedal cycle injured in collision with car, pick-up truck or van

⊗⑦V13.4 Pedal cycle driver injured in collision with car, pick-up truck or van in traffic accident

⊗⑦V13.5 Pedal cycle passenger injured in collision with car, pick-up truck or van in traffic accident

⊗⑦V13.9 Unspecified pedal cyclist injured in collision with car, pick-up truck or van in traffic accident

V14 Pedal cycle rider injured in collision with heavy transport vehicle or bus

Excludes1: pedal cycle rider injured in collision with military vehicle (V19.81)

The appropriate 7th character is to be added to each code from category V14

A - initial encounter

D - subsequent encounter

S - sequela

⊗⑦V14.0 Pedal cycle driver injured in collision with heavy transport vehicle or bus in nontraffic accident

⊗⑦V14.1 Pedal cycle passenger injured in collision with heavy transport vehicle or bus in nontraffic accident

⊗⑦V14.2 Unspecified pedal cyclist injured in collision with heavy transport vehicle or bus in nontraffic accident

⊗⑦V14.3 Person boarding or alighting a pedal cycle injured in collision with heavy transport vehicle or bus

● New code   ▲ Revised code   **Excludes1:** Not coded here   **Excludes2:** Not included here   ⊗ Placeholder required   ⑦7th digit required

⊗⑦**V14.4** Pedal cycle driver injured in collision with heavy transport vehicle or bus in traffic accident

⊗⑦**V14.5** Pedal cycle passenger injured in collision with heavy transport vehicle or bus in traffic accident

⊗⑦**V14.9** Unspecified pedal cyclist injured in collision with heavy transport vehicle or bus in traffic accident

V15 Pedal cycle rider injured in collision with railway train or railway vehicle

The appropriate 7th character is to be added to each code from category V15

A - initial encounter

D - subsequent encounter

S - sequela

⊗⑦**V15.0** Pedal cycle driver injured in collision with railway train or railway vehicle in nontraffic accident

⊗⑦**V15.1** Pedal cycle passenger injured in collision with railway train or railway vehicle in nontraffic accident

⊗⑦**V15.2** Unspecified pedal cyclist injured in collision with railway train or railway vehicle in nontraffic accident

⊗⑦**V15.3** Person boarding or alighting a pedal cycle injured in collision with railway train or railway vehicle

⊗⑦**V15.4** Pedal cycle driver injured in collision with railway train or railway vehicle in traffic accident

⊗⑦**V15.5** Pedal cycle passenger injured in collision with railway train or railway vehicle in traffic accident

⊗⑦**V15.9** Unspecified pedal cyclist injured in collision with railway train or railway vehicle in traffic accident

V16 Pedal cycle rider injured in collision with other nonmotor vehicle

Includes: collision with animal-drawn vehicle, animal being ridden, streetcar

The appropriate 7th character is to be added to each code from category V16

A - initial encounter

D - subsequent encounter

S - sequela

⊗⑦**V16.0** Pedal cycle driver injured in collision with other nonmotor vehicle in nontraffic accident

⊗⑦**V16.1** Pedal cycle passenger injured in collision with other nonmotor vehicle in nontraffic accident

⊗⑦**V16.2** Unspecified pedal cyclist injured in collision with other nonmotor vehicle in nontraffic accident

⊗⑦**V16.3** Person boarding or alighting a pedal cycle injured in collision with other nonmotor vehicle in nontraffic accident

⊗⑦**V16.4** Pedal cycle driver injured in collision with other nonmotor vehicle in traffic accident

⊗⑦**V16.5** Pedal cycle passenger injured in collision with other nonmotor vehicle in traffic accident

⊗⑦**V16.9** Unspecified pedal cyclist injured in collision with other nonmotor vehicle in traffic accident

V17 Pedal cycle rider injured in collision with fixed or stationary object

The appropriate 7th character is to be added to each code from category V17

A - initial encounter

D - subsequent encounter

S - sequela

⊗⑦**V17.0** Pedal cycle driver injured in collision with fixed or stationary object in nontraffic accident

⊗⑦**V17.1** Pedal cycle passenger injured in collision with fixed or stationary object in nontraffic accident

⊗⑦**V17.2** Unspecified pedal cyclist injured in collision with fixed or stationary object in nontraffic accident

⊗⑦**V17.3** Person boarding or alighting a pedal cycle injured in collision with fixed or stationary object

⊗⑦**V17.4** Pedal cycle driver injured in collision with fixed or stationary object in traffic accident

⊗⑦**V17.5** Pedal cycle passenger injured in collision with fixed or stationary object in traffic accident

⊗⑦**V17.9** Unspecified pedal cyclist injured in collision with fixed or stationary object in traffic accident

V18 Pedal cycle rider injured in noncollision transport accident

Includes: fall or thrown from pedal cycle (without antecedent collision)

overturning pedal cycle NOS overturning pedal cycle without collision

The appropriate 7th character is to be added to each code from category V18

A - initial encounter

D - subsequent encounter

S - sequela

⊗⑦**V18.0** Pedal cycle driver injured in noncollision transport accident in nontraffic accident

⊗⑦**V18.1** Pedal cycle passenger injured in noncollision transport accident in nontraffic accident

⊗⑦**V18.2** Unspecified pedal cyclist injured in noncollision transport accident in nontraffic accident

⊗⑦**V18.3** Person boarding or alighting a pedal cycle injured in noncollision transport accident

⊗⑦**V18.4** Pedal cycle driver injured in noncollision transport accident in traffic accident

⊗⑦**V18.5** Pedal cycle passenger injured in noncollision transport accident in traffic accident

⊗⑦**V18.9** Unspecified pedal cyclist injured in noncollision transport accident in traffic accident

V19 Pedal cycle rider injured in other and unspecified transport accidents

The appropriate 7th character is to be added to each code from category V19

A - initial encounter

D - subsequent encounter

S - sequela

V19.0 Pedal cycle driver injured in collision with other and unspecified motor vehicles in nontraffic accident

⊗⑦**V19.00** Pedal cycle driver injured in collision with unspecified motor vehicles in nontraffic accident

⊗⑦**V19.09** Pedal cycle driver injured in collision with other motor vehicles in nontraffic accident

V19.1 Pedal cycle passenger injured in collision with other and unspecified motor vehicles in nontraffic accident

⊗⑦**V19.10** Pedal cycle passenger injured in collision with unspecified motor vehicles in nontraffic accident

⊗⑦**V19.19** Pedal cycle passenger injured in collision with other motor vehicles in nontraffic accident

V19.2 Unspecified pedal cyclist injured in collision with other and unspecified motor vehicles in nontraffic accident

⊗⑦**V19.20** Unspecified pedal cyclist injured in collision with unspecified motor vehicles in nontraffic accident

Pedal cycle collision NOS, nontraffic

⊗⑦**V19.29** ▲ Unspecified pedal cyclist injured in collision with other motor vehicles in nontraffic accident

⊗⑦**V19.3** Pedal cyclist (driver) (passenger) injured in unspecified nontraffic accident

Pedal cycle accident NOS, nontraffic

Pedal cyclist injured in nontraffic accident NOS

V19.4 Pedal cycle driver injured in collision with other and unspecified motor vehicles in traffic accident

⊗⑦**V19.40** Pedal cycle driver injured in collision with unspecified motor vehicles in traffic accident

⊗⑦**V19.49** Pedal cycle driver injured in collision with other motor vehicles in traffic accident

V19.5 Pedal cycle passenger injured in collision with other and unspecified motor vehicles in traffic accident

⊗⑦**V19.50** Pedal cycle passenger injured in collision with unspecified motor vehicles in traffic accident

⊗⑦**V19.59** Pedal cycle passenger injured in collision with other motor vehicles in traffic accident

V19.6 Unspecified pedal cyclist injured in collision with other and unspecified motor vehicles in traffic accident

⊗⑦**V19.60** Unspecified pedal cyclist injured in collision with unspecified motor vehicles in traffic accident

Pedal cycle collision NOS (traffic)

⊗⑦**V19.69** Unspecified pedal cyclist injured in collision with other motor vehicles in traffic accident

V19.8 Pedal cyclist (driver) (passenger) injured in other specified transport accidents

⊗⑦**V19.81** Pedal cyclist (driver) (passenger) injured in transport accident with military vehicle

⊗⑦**V19.88** Pedal cyclist (driver) (passenger) injured in other specified transport accidents

⊗⑦**V19.9** Pedal cyclist (driver) (passenger) injured in unspecified traffic accident

Pedal cycle accident NOS

MOTORCYCLE RIDER INJURED IN TRANSPORT ACCIDENT (V20-V29)

Includes: moped

motorcycle with sidecar motorized bicycle motor scooter

Excludes1: three-wheeled motor vehicle (V30-V39)

V20 Motorcycle rider injured in collision with pedestrian or animal

Excludes1: motorcycle rider collision with animal-drawn vehicle or animal being ridden (V26.-)

The appropriate 7th character is to be added to each code from category V20

A - initial encounter

D - subsequent encounter

S - sequela

⊗⑦**V20.0** Motorcycle driver injured in collision with pedestrian or animal in nontraffic accident

⊗⑦**V20.1** Motorcycle passenger injured in collision with pedestrian or animal in nontraffic accident

⊗⑦**V20.2** Unspecified motorcycle rider injured in collision with pedestrian or animal in nontraffic accident

⊗⑦**V20.3** Person boarding or alighting a motorcycle injured in collision with pedestrian or animal

⊗⑦**V20.4** Motorcycle driver injured in collision with pedestrian or animal in traffic accident

⊗⑦**V20.5** Motorcycle passenger injured in collision with pedestrian or animal in traffic accident

⊗⑦**V20.9** Unspecified motorcycle rider injured in collision with pedestrian or animal in traffic accident

V21 Motorcycle rider injured in collision with pedal cycle

The appropriate 7th character is to be added to each code from category V21

A - initial encounter

D - subsequent encounter

S - sequela

⊗⑦**V21.0** Motorcycle driver injured in collision with pedal cycle in nontraffic accident

⊗⑦**V21.1** Motorcycle passenger injured in collision with pedal cycle in nontraffic accident

⊗⑦**V21.2** Unspecified motorcycle rider injured in collision with pedal cycle in nontraffic accident

⊗⑦**V21.3** Person boarding or alighting a motorcycle injured in collision with pedal cycle

⊗⑦**V21.4** Motorcycle driver injured in collision with pedal cycle in traffic accident

⊗⑦**V21.5** Motorcycle passenger injured in collision with pedal cycle in traffic accident

⊗⑦**V21.9** Unspecified motorcycle rider injured in collision with pedal cycle in traffic accident

V22 Motorcycle rider injured in collision with two- or three-wheeled motor vehicle

The appropriate 7th character is to be added to each code from category V22

A - initial encounter

D - subsequent encounter

S - sequela

⊗⑦**V22.0** Motorcycle driver injured in collision with two- or three-wheeled motor vehicle in nontraffic accident

⊗⑦**V22.1** Motorcycle passenger injured in collision with two- or three-wheeled motor vehicle in nontraffic accident

⊗⑦**V22.2** Unspecified motorcycle rider injured in collision with two- or three-wheeled motor vehicle in nontraffic accident

⊗⑦**V22.3** Person boarding or alighting a motorcycle injured in collision with two- or three-wheeled motor vehicle

⊗⑦**V22.4** Motorcycle driver injured in collision with two- or three-wheeled motor vehicle in traffic accident

⊗⑦**V22.5** Motorcycle passenger injured in collision with two- or three-wheeled motor vehicle in traffic accident

⊗⑦**V22.9** Unspecified motorcycle rider injured in collision with two- or three-wheeled motor vehicle in traffic accident

V23 Motorcycle rider injured in collision with car, pick-up truck or van

The appropriate 7th character is to be added to each code from category V23

A - initial encounter

D - subsequent encounter

S - sequela

⊗⑦**V23.0** Motorcycle driver injured in collision with car, pick-up truck or van in nontraffic accident

⊗⑦**V23.1** Motorcycle passenger injured in collision with car, pick-up truck or van in nontraffic accident

⊗⑦**V23.2** Unspecified motorcycle rider injured in collision with car, pick-up truck or van in nontraffic accident

⊗⑦**V23.3** Person boarding or alighting a motorcycle injured in collision with car, pick-up truck or van

⊗⑦**V23.4** Motorcycle driver injured in collision with car, pick-up truck or van in traffic accident

⊗⑦**V23.5** Motorcycle passenger injured in collision with car, pick-up truck or van in traffic accident

⊗⑦**V23.9** Unspecified motorcycle rider injured in collision with car, pick-up truck or van in traffic accident

V24 Motorcycle rider injured in collision with heavy transport vehicle or bus

Excludes1: motorcycle rider injured in collision with military vehicle (V29.81)

The appropriate 7th character is to be added to each code from category V24

A - initial encounter

D - subsequent encounter

S - sequela

⊗⑦**V24.0** Motorcycle driver injured in collision with heavy transport vehicle or bus in nontraffic accident

⊗⑦**V24.1** Motorcycle passenger injured in collision with heavy transport vehicle or bus in nontraffic accident

⊗⑦**V24.2** Unspecified motorcycle rider injured in collision with heavy transport vehicle or bus in nontraffic accident

⊗⑦**V24.3** Person boarding or alighting a motorcycle injured in collision with heavy transport vehicle or bus

⊗⑦**V24.4** Motorcycle driver injured in collision with heavy transport vehicle or bus in traffic accident

⊗⑦**V24.5** Motorcycle passenger injured in collision with heavy transport vehicle or bus in traffic accident

⊗⑦**V24.9** Unspecified motorcycle rider injured in collision with heavy transport vehicle or bus in traffic accident

V25 Motorcycle rider injured in collision with railway train or railway vehicle

The appropriate 7th character is to be added to each code from category V25

A - initial encounter

D - subsequent encounter

S - sequela

⊗⑦**V25.0** Motorcycle driver injured in collision with railway train or railway vehicle in nontraffic accident

⊗⑦**V25.1** Motorcycle passenger injured in collision with railway train or railway vehicle in nontraffic accident

⊗⑦**V25.2** Unspecified motorcycle rider injured in collision with railway train or railway vehicle in nontraffic accident

⊗⑦**V25.3** Person boarding or alighting a motorcycle injured in collision with railway train or railway vehicle

⊗⑦**V25.4** Motorcycle driver injured in collision with railway train or railway vehicle in traffic accident

⊗⑦**V25.5** Motorcycle passenger injured in collision with railway train or railway vehicle in traffic accident

⊗⑦**V25.9** Unspecified motorcycle rider injured in collision with railway train or railway vehicle in traffic accident

V26 Motorcycle rider injured in collision with other nonmotor vehicle

Includes: collision with animal-drawn vehicle, animal being ridden, streetcar

The appropriate 7th character is to be added to each code from category V26

A - initial encounter

D - subsequent encounter

S - sequela

⊗⑦**V26.0** Motorcycle driver injured in collision with other nonmotor vehicle in nontraffic accident

⊗⑦**V26.1** Motorcycle passenger injured in collision with other nonmotor vehicle in nontraffic accident

⊗⑦**V26.2** Unspecified motorcycle rider injured in collision with other nonmotor vehicle in nontraffic accident

⊗⑦**V26.3** Person boarding or alighting a motorcycle injured in collision with other nonmotor vehicle

⊗⑦**V26.4** Motorcycle driver injured in collision with other nonmotor vehicle in traffic accident

⊗⑦**V26.5** Motorcycle passenger injured in collision with other nonmotor vehicle in traffic accident

⊗⑦**V26.9** Unspecified motorcycle rider injured in collision with other nonmotor vehicle in traffic accident

V27 Motorcycle rider injured in collision with fixed or stationary object

The appropriate 7th character is to be added to each code from category V27

A - initial encounter

D - subsequent encounter

S - sequela

⊗⑦**V27.0** Motorcycle driver injured in collision with fixed or stationary object in nontraffic accident

⊗⑦**V27.1** Motorcycle passenger injured in collision with fixed or stationary object in nontraffic accident

⊗⑦**V27.2** Unspecified motorcycle rider injured in collision with fixed or stationary object in nontraffic accident

⊗⑦**V27.3** Person boarding or alighting a motorcycle injured in collision with fixed or stationary object

⊗⑦**V27.4** Motorcycle driver injured in collision with fixed or stationary object in traffic accident

⊗⑦**V27.5** Motorcycle passenger injured in collision with fixed or stationary object in traffic accident

⊗⑦**V27.9** Unspecified motorcycle rider injured in collision with fixed or stationary object in traffic accident

V28 Motorcycle rider injured in noncollision transport accident

Includes: fall or thrown from motorcycle (without antecedent collision)

overturning motorcycle NOS overturning motorcycle without collision

The appropriate 7th character is to be added to each code from category V28

A - initial encounter

D - subsequent encounter

S - sequela

⊗⑦**V28.0** Motorcycle driver injured in noncollision transport accident in nontraffic accident

⊗⑦**V28.1** Motorcycle passenger injured in noncollision transport accident in nontraffic accident

⊗⑦**V28.2** Unspecified motorcycle rider injured in noncollision transport accident in nontraffic accident

⊗⑦**V28.3** Person boarding or alighting a motorcycle injured in noncollision transport accident

⊗⑦**V28.4** Motorcycle driver injured in noncollision transport accident in traffic accident

⊗⑦**V28.5** Motorcycle passenger injured in noncollision transport accident in traffic accident

⊗⑦**V28.9** Unspecified motorcycle rider injured in noncollision transport accident in traffic accident

V29 Motorcycle rider injured in other and unspecified transport accidents

The appropriate 7th character is to be added to each code from category V29

A - initial encounter

D - subsequent encounter

S - sequela

V29.0 Motorcycle driver injured in collision with other and unspecified motor vehicles in nontraffic accident

⊗⑦V29.00 **Motorcycle driver injured in collision with unspecified motor vehicles in nontraffic accident**

⊗⑦V29.09 **Motorcycle driver injured in collision with other motor vehicles in nontraffic accident**

V29.1 Motorcycle passenger injured in collision with other and unspecified motor vehicles in nontraffic accident

⊗⑦V29.10 **Motorcycle passenger injured in collision with unspecified motor vehicles in nontraffic accident**

⊗⑦V29.19 **Motorcycle passenger injured in collision with other motor vehicles in nontraffic accident**

V29.2 Unspecified motorcycle rider injured in collision with other and unspecified motor vehicles in nontraffic accident

⊗⑦V29.20 **Unspecified motorcycle rider injured in collision with unspecified motor vehicles in nontraffic accident**

Motorcycle collision NOS, nontraffic

⊗⑦V29.29 **Unspecified motorcycle rider injured in collision with other motor vehicles in nontraffic accident**

⊗⑦V29.3 **Motorcycle rider (driver) (passenger) injured in unspecified nontraffic accident**

Motorcycle accident NOS, nontraffic

Motorcycle rider injured in nontraffic accident NOS

V29.4 Motorcycle driver injured in collision with other and unspecified motor vehicles in traffic accident

⊗⑦V29.40 **Motorcycle driver injured in collision with unspecified motor vehicles in traffic accident**

⊗⑦V29.49 **Motorcycle driver injured in collision with other motor vehicles in traffic accident**

V29.5 Motorcycle passenger injured in collision with other and unspecified motor vehicles in traffic accident

⊗⑦V29.50 **Motorcycle passenger injured in collision with unspecified motor vehicles in traffic accident**

⊗⑦V29.59 **Motorcycle passenger injured in collision with other motor vehicles in traffic accident**

V29.6 Unspecified motorcycle rider injured in collision with other and unspecified motor vehicles in traffic accident

⊗⑦V29.60 **Unspecified motorcycle rider injured in collision with unspecified motor vehicles in traffic accident**

Motorcycle collision NOS (traffic)

⊗⑦V29.69 **Unspecified motorcycle rider injured in collision with other motor vehicles in traffic accident**

V29.8 Motorcycle rider (driver) (passenger) injured in other specified transport accidents

⊗⑦V29.81 **Motorcycle rider (driver) (passenger) injured in transport accident with military vehicle**

⊗⑦V29.88 **Motorcycle rider (driver) (passenger) injured in other specified transport accidents**

⊗⑦V29.9 **Motorcycle rider (driver) (passenger) injured in unspecified traffic accident**

Motorcycle accident NOS

OCCUPANT OF THREE-WHEELED MOTOR VEHICLE INJURED IN TRANSPORT ACCIDENT (V30-V39)

Includes: motorized tricycle

motorized rickshaw three-wheeled motor car

Excludes1: all-terrain vehicles (V86.-)

motorcycle with sidecar (V20-V29)

vehicle designed primarily for off-road use (V86.-)

V30 Occupant of three-wheeled motor vehicle injured in collision with pedestrian or animal

Excludes1: three-wheeled motor vehicle collision with animal-drawn vehicle or animal being ridden (V36.-)

The appropriate 7th character is to be added to each code from category V30

A - initial encounter

D - subsequent encounter

S - sequela

⊗⑦V30.0 **Driver of three-wheeled motor vehicle injured in collision with pedestrian or animal in nontraffic accident**

⊗⑦V30.1 **Passenger in three-wheeled motor vehicle injured in collision with pedestrian or animal in nontraffic accident**

⊗⑦V30.2 **Person on outside of three-wheeled motor vehicle injured in collision with pedestrian or animal in nontraffic accident**

⊗⑦V30.3 **Unspecified occupant of three-wheeled motor vehicle injured in collision with pedestrian or animal in nontraffic accident**

⊗⑦V30.4 **Person boarding or alighting a three-wheeled motor vehicle injured in collision with pedestrian or animal**

⊗⑦V30.5 **Driver of three-wheeled motor vehicle injured in collision with pedestrian or animal in traffic accident**

⊗⑦V30.6 **Passenger in three-wheeled motor vehicle injured in collision with pedestrian or animal in traffic accident**

⊗⑦V30.7 **Person on outside of three-wheeled motor vehicle injured in collision with pedestrian or animal in traffic accident**

⊗⑦V30.9 **Unspecified occupant of three-wheeled motor vehicle injured in collision with pedestrian or animal in traffic accident**

V31 Occupant of three-wheeled motor vehicle injured in collision with pedal cycle

The appropriate 7th character is to be added to each code from category V31

A - initial encounter

D - subsequent encounter

S - sequela

⊗⑦V31.0 **Driver of three-wheeled motor vehicle injured in collision with pedal cycle in nontraffic accident**

⊗⑦V31.1 **Passenger in three-wheeled motor vehicle injured in collision with pedal cycle in nontraffic accident**

⊗⑦V31.2 **Person on outside of three-wheeled motor vehicle injured in collision with pedal cycle in nontraffic accident**

⊗⑦V31.3 **Unspecified occupant of three-wheeled motor vehicle injured in collision with pedal cycle in nontraffic accident**

⊗⑦V31.4 **Person boarding or alighting a three-wheeled motor vehicle injured in collision with pedal cycle**

⊗⑦V31.5 **Driver of three-wheeled motor vehicle injured in collision with pedal cycle in traffic accident**

⊗⑦V31.6 **Passenger in three-wheeled motor vehicle injured in collision with pedal cycle in traffic accident**

● New code ▲ Revised code **Excludes1:** Not coded here **Excludes2:** Not included here ⊗ Placeholder required ⑦ 7th digit required

⊗⑦**V31.7** **Person on outside of three-wheeled motor vehicle injured in collision with pedal cycle in traffic accident**

⊗⑦**V31.9** **Unspecified occupant of three-wheeled motor vehicle injured in collision with pedal cycle in traffic accident**

V32 **Occupant of three-wheeled motor vehicle injured in collision with two- or three-wheeled motor vehicle**

The appropriate 7th character is to be added to each code from category V32

A - initial encounter

D - subsequent encounter

S - sequela

⊗⑦**V32.0** **Driver of three-wheeled motor vehicle injured in collision with two- or three-wheeled motor vehicle in nontraffic accident**

⊗⑦**V32.1** **Passenger in three-wheeled motor vehicle injured in collision with two- or three-wheeled motor vehicle in nontraffic accident**

⊗⑦**V32.2** **Person on outside of three-wheeled motor vehicle injured in collision with two- or three-wheeled motor vehicle in nontraffic accident**

⊗⑦**V32.3** **Unspecified occupant of three-wheeled motor vehicle injured in collision with two- or three-wheeled motor vehicle in nontraffic accident**

⊗⑦**V32.4** **Person boarding or alighting a three-wheeled motor vehicle injured in collision with two- or three-wheeled motor vehicle**

⊗⑦**V32.5** **Driver of three-wheeled motor vehicle injured in collision with two- or three-wheeled motor vehicle in traffic accident**

⊗⑦**V32.6** **Passenger in three-wheeled motor vehicle injured in collision with two- or three-wheeled motor vehicle in traffic accident**

⊗⑦**V32.7** **Person on outside of three-wheeled motor vehicle injured in collision with two- or three-wheeled motor vehicle in traffic accident**

⊗⑦**V32.9** **Unspecified occupant of three-wheeled motor vehicle injured in collision with two- or three-wheeled motor vehicle in traffic accident**

V33 **Occupant of three-wheeled motor vehicle injured in collision with car, pick-up truck or van**

The appropriate 7th character is to be added to each code from category V33

A - initial encounter

D - subsequent encounter

S - sequela

⊗⑦**V33.0** **Driver of three-wheeled motor vehicle injured in collision with car, pick-up truck or van in nontraffic accident**

⊗⑦**V33.1** **Passenger in three-wheeled motor vehicle injured in collision with car, pick-up truck or van in nontraffic accident**

⊗⑦**V33.2** **Person on outside of three-wheeled motor vehicle injured in collision with car, pick-up truck or van in nontraffic accident**

⊗⑦**V33.3** **Unspecified occupant of three-wheeled motor vehicle injured in collision with car, pick-up truck or van in nontraffic accident**

⊗⑦**V33.4** **Person boarding or alighting a three-wheeled motor vehicle injured in collision with car, pick-up truck or van**

⊗⑦**V33.5** **Driver of three-wheeled motor vehicle injured in collision with car, pick-up truck or van in traffic accident**

⊗⑦**V33.6** **Passenger in three-wheeled motor vehicle injured in collision with car, pick-up truck or van in traffic accident**

⊗⑦**V33.7** **Person on outside of three-wheeled motor vehicle injured in collision with car, pick-up truck or van in traffic accident**

⊗⑦**V33.9** **Unspecified occupant of three-wheeled motor vehicle injured in collision with car, pick-up truck or van in traffic accident**

V34 **Occupant of three-wheeled motor vehicle injured in collision with heavy transport vehicle or bus**

Excludes1: occupant of three-wheeled motor vehicle injured in collision with military vehicle (V39.81)

The appropriate 7th character is to be added to each code from category V34

A - initial encounter

D - subsequent encounter

S - sequela

⊗⑦**V34.0** **Driver of three-wheeled motor vehicle injured in collision with heavy transport vehicle or bus in nontraffic accident**

⊗⑦**V34.1** **Passenger in three-wheeled motor vehicle injured in collision with heavy transport vehicle or bus in nontraffic accident**

⊗⑦**V34.2** **Person on outside of three-wheeled motor vehicle injured in collision with heavy transport vehicle or bus in nontraffic accident**

⊗⑦**V34.3** **Unspecified occupant of three-wheeled motor vehicle injured in collision with heavy transport vehicle or bus in nontraffic accident**

⊗⑦**V34.4** **Person boarding or alighting a three-wheeled motor vehicle injured in collision with heavy transport vehicle or bus**

⊗⑦**V34.5** **Driver of three-wheeled motor vehicle injured in collision with heavy transport vehicle or bus in traffic accident**

⊗⑦**V34.6** **Passenger in three-wheeled motor vehicle injured in collision with heavy transport vehicle or bus in traffic accident**

⊗⑦**V34.7** **Person on outside of three-wheeled motor vehicle injured in collision with heavy transport vehicle or bus in traffic accident**

⊗⑦**V34.9** **Unspecified occupant of three-wheeled motor vehicle injured in collision with heavy transport vehicle or bus in traffic accident**

V35 **Occupant of three-wheeled motor vehicle injured in collision with railway train or railway vehicle**

The appropriate 7th character is to be added to each code from category V35

A - initial encounter

D - subsequent encounter

S - sequela

⊗⑦**V35.0** **Driver of three-wheeled motor vehicle injured in collision with railway train or railway vehicle in nontraffic accident**

⊗⑦**V35.1** **Passenger in three-wheeled motor vehicle injured in collision with railway train or railway vehicle in nontraffic accident**

⊗⑦**V35.2** **Person on outside of three-wheeled motor vehicle injured in collision with railway train or railway vehicle in nontraffic accident**

⊗⑦**V35.3** **Unspecified occupant of three-wheeled motor vehicle injured in collision with railway train or railway vehicle in nontraffic accident**

⊗⑦**V35.4** **Person boarding or alighting a three-wheeled motor vehicle injured in collision with railway train or railway vehicle**

⊗⑦V35.5 **Driver of three-wheeled motor vehicle injured in collision with railway train or railway vehicle in traffic accident**

⊗⑦V35.6 **Passenger in three-wheeled motor vehicle injured in collision with railway train or railway vehicle in traffic accident**

⊗⑦V35.7 **Person on outside of three-wheeled motor vehicle injured in collision with railway train or railway vehicle in traffic accident**

⊗⑦V35.9 **Unspecified occupant of three-wheeled motor vehicle injured in collision with railway train or railway vehicle in traffic accident**

V36 **Occupant of three-wheeled motor vehicle injured in collision with other nonmotor vehicle**

Includes: collision with animal-drawn vehicle, animal being ridden, streetcar

The appropriate 7th character is to be added to each code from category V36

A - initial encounter

D - subsequent encounter

S - sequela

⊗⑦V36.0 **Driver of three-wheeled motor vehicle injured in collision with other nonmotor vehicle in nontraffic accident**

⊗⑦V36.1 **Passenger in three-wheeled motor vehicle injured in collision with other nonmotor vehicle in nontraffic accident**

⊗⑦V36.2 **Person on outside of three-wheeled motor vehicle injured in collision with other nonmotor vehicle in nontraffic accident**

⊗⑦V36.3 **Unspecified occupant of three-wheeled motor vehicle injured in collision with other nonmotor vehicle in nontraffic accident**

⊗⑦V36.4 **Person boarding or alighting a three-wheeled motor vehicle injured in collision with other nonmotor vehicle**

⊗⑦V36.5 **Driver of three-wheeled motor vehicle injured in collision with other nonmotor vehicle in traffic accident**

⊗⑦V36.6 **Passenger in three-wheeled motor vehicle injured in collision with other nonmotor vehicle in traffic accident**

⊗⑦V36.7 **Person on outside of three-wheeled motor vehicle injured in collision with other nonmotor vehicle in traffic accident**

⊗⑦V36.9 **Unspecified occupant of three-wheeled motor vehicle injured in collision with other nonmotor vehicle in traffic accident**

V37 **Occupant of three-wheeled motor vehicle injured in collision with fixed or stationary object**

The appropriate 7th character is to be added to each code from category V37

A - initial encounter

D - subsequent encounter

S - sequela

⊗⑦V37.0 **Driver of three-wheeled motor vehicle injured in collision with fixed or stationary object in nontraffic accident**

⊗⑦V37.1 **Passenger in three-wheeled motor vehicle injured in collision with fixed or stationary object in nontraffic accident**

⊗⑦V37.2 **Person on outside of three-wheeled motor vehicle injured in collision with fixed or stationary object in nontraffic accident**

⊗⑦V37.3 **Unspecified occupant of three-wheeled motor vehicle injured in collision with fixed or stationary object in nontraffic accident**

⊗⑦V37.4 **Person boarding or alighting a three-wheeled motor vehicle injured in collision with fixed or stationary object**

⊗⑦V37.5 **Driver of three-wheeled motor vehicle injured in collision with fixed or stationary object in traffic accident**

⊗⑦V37.6 **Passenger in three-wheeled motor vehicle injured in collision with fixed or stationary object in traffic accident**

⊗⑦V37.7 **Person on outside of three-wheeled motor vehicle injured in collision with fixed or stationary object in traffic accident**

⊗⑦V37.9 **Unspecified occupant of three-wheeled motor vehicle injured in collision with fixed or stationary object in traffic accident**

V38 **Occupant of three-wheeled motor vehicle injured in noncollision transport accident**

Includes: fall or thrown from three-wheeled motor vehicle

overturning of three-wheeled motor vehicle NOS

overturning of three-wheeled motor vehicle without collision

The appropriate 7th character is to be added to each code from category V38

A - initial encounter

D - subsequent encounter

S - sequela

⊗⑦V38.0 **Driver of three-wheeled motor vehicle injured in noncollision transport accident in nontraffic accident**

⊗⑦V38.1 **Passenger in three-wheeled motor vehicle injured in noncollision transport accident in nontraffic accident**

⊗⑦V38.2 **Person on outside of three-wheeled motor vehicle injured in noncollision transport accident in nontraffic accident**

⊗⑦V38.3 **Unspecified occupant of three-wheeled motor vehicle injured in noncollision transport accident in nontraffic accident**

⊗⑦V38.4 **Person boarding or alighting a three-wheeled motor vehicle injured in noncollision transport accident**

⊗⑦V38.5 **Driver of three-wheeled motor vehicle injured in noncollision transport accident in traffic accident**

⊗⑦V38.6 **Passenger in three-wheeled motor vehicle injured in noncollision transport accident in traffic accident**

⊗⑦V38.7 **Person on outside of three-wheeled motor vehicle injured in noncollision transport accident in traffic accident**

⊗⑦V38.9 **Unspecified occupant of three-wheeled motor vehicle injured in noncollision transport accident in traffic accident**

V39 **Occupant of three-wheeled motor vehicle injured in other and unspecified transport accidents**

The appropriate 7th character is to be added to each code from category V39

A - initial encounter

D - subsequent encounter

S - sequela

V39.0 **Driver of three-wheeled motor vehicle injured in collision with other and unspecified motor vehicles in nontraffic accident**

⊗⑦V39.00 **Driver of three-wheeled motor vehicle injured in collision with unspecified motor vehicles in nontraffic accident**

● New code ▲ Revised code **Excludes1:** Not coded here **Excludes2:** Not included here ⊗ Placeholder required ⑦ 7th digit required

⊗⑦**V39.09** Driver of three-wheeled motor vehicle injured in collision with other motor vehicles in nontraffic accident

V39.1 Passenger in three-wheeled motor vehicle injured in collision with other and unspecified motor vehicles in nontraffic accident

⊗⑦**V39.10** Passenger in three-wheeled motor vehicle injured in collision with unspecified motor vehicles in nontraffic accident

⊗⑦**V39.19** Passenger in three-wheeled motor vehicle injured in collision with other motor vehicles in nontraffic accident

V39.2 Unspecified occupant of three-wheeled motor vehicle injured in collision with other and unspecified motor vehicles in nontraffic accident

⊗⑦**V39.20** Unspecified occupant of three-wheeled motor vehicle injured in collision with unspecified motor vehicles in nontraffic accident

Collision NOS involving three-wheeled motor vehicle, nontraffic

⊗⑦**V39.29** Unspecified occupant of three-wheeled motor vehicle injured in collision with other motor vehicles in nontraffic accident

⊗⑦**V39.3** Occupant (driver) (passenger) of three-wheeled motor vehicle injured in unspecified nontraffic accident

Accident NOS involving three-wheeled motor vehicle, nontraffic

Occupant of three-wheeled motor vehicle injured in nontraffic accident NOS

V39.4 Driver of three-wheeled motor vehicle injured in collision with other and unspecified motor vehicles in traffic accident

⊗⑦**V39.40** Driver of three-wheeled motor vehicle injured in collision with unspecified motor vehicles in traffic accident

⊗⑦**V39.49** Driver of three-wheeled motor vehicle injured in collision with other motor vehicles in traffic accident

V39.5 Passenger in three-wheeled motor vehicle injured in collision with other and unspecified motor vehicles in traffic accident

⊗⑦**V39.50** Passenger in three-wheeled motor vehicle injured in collision with unspecified motor vehicles in traffic accident

⊗⑦**V39.59** Passenger in three-wheeled motor vehicle injured in collision with other motor vehicles in traffic accident

V39.6 Unspecified occupant of three-wheeled motor vehicle injured in collision with other and unspecified motor vehicles in traffic accident

⊗⑦**V39.60** Unspecified occupant of three-wheeled motor vehicle injured in collision with unspecified motor vehicles in traffic accident

Collision NOS involving three-wheeled motor vehicle (traffic)

⊗⑦**V39.69** Unspecified occupant of three-wheeled motor vehicle injured in collision with other motor vehicles in traffic accident

V39.8 Occupant (driver) (passenger) of three-wheeled motor vehicle injured in other specified transport accidents

⊗⑦**V39.81** Occupant (driver) (passenger) of three-wheeled motor vehicle injured in transport accident with military vehicle

⊗⑦**V39.89** Occupant (driver) (passenger) of three-wheeled motor vehicle injured in other specified transport accidents

⊗⑦**V39.9** Occupant (driver) (passenger) of three-wheeled motor vehicle injured in unspecified traffic accident

Accident NOS involving three-wheeled motor vehicle

CAR OCCUPANT INJURED IN TRANSPORT ACCIDENT (V40-V49)

Includes: a four-wheeled motor vehicle designed primarily for carrying passengers

automobile (pulling a trailer or camper)

Excludes1: bus (V50-V59)

minibus (V50-V59)

minivan (V50-V59)

motorcoach (V70-V79)

pick-up truck (V50-V59)

sport utility vehicle (SUV) (V50-V59)

V40 Car occupant injured in collision with pedestrian or animal

Excludes1: car collision with animal-drawn vehicle or animal being ridden (V46.-)

The appropriate 7th character is to be added to each code from category V40

A - initial encounter

D - subsequent encounter

S - sequela

⊗⑦**V40.0** Car driver injured in collision with pedestrian or animal in nontraffic accident

⊗⑦**V40.1** Car passenger injured in collision with pedestrian or animal in nontraffic accident

⊗⑦**V40.2** Person on outside of car injured in collision with pedestrian or animal in nontraffic accident

⊗⑦**V40.3** Unspecified car occupant injured in collision with pedestrian or animal in nontraffic accident

⊗⑦**V40.4** Person boarding or alighting a car injured in collision with pedestrian or animal

⊗⑦**V40.5** Car driver injured in collision with pedestrian or animal in traffic accident

⊗⑦**V40.6** Car passenger injured in collision with pedestrian or animal in traffic accident

⊗⑦**V40.7** Person on outside of car injured in collision with pedestrian or animal in traffic accident

⊗⑦**V40.9** Unspecified car occupant injured in collision with pedestrian or animal in traffic accident

V41 Car occupant injured in collision with pedal cycle

The appropriate 7th character is to be added to each code from category V41

A - initial encounter

D - subsequent encounter

S - sequela

⊗⑦**V41.0** Car driver injured in collision with pedal cycle in nontraffic accident

⊗⑦**V41.1** Car passenger injured in collision with pedal cycle in nontraffic accident

⊗⑦**V41.2** Person on outside of car injured in collision with pedal cycle in nontraffic accident

⊗⑦**V41.3** Unspecified car occupant injured in collision with pedal cycle in nontraffic accident

⊗⑦**V41.4** Person boarding or alighting a car injured in collision with pedal cycle

⊗⑦V41.5 Car driver injured in collision with pedal cycle in traffic accident

⊗⑦V41.6 Car passenger injured in collision with pedal cycle in traffic accident

⊗⑦V41.7 Person on outside of car injured in collision with pedal cycle in traffic accident

⊗⑦V41.9 Unspecified car occupant injured in collision with pedal cycle in traffic accident

V42 Car occupant injured in collision with two- or three-wheeled motor vehicle

The appropriate 7th character is to be added to each code from category V42

A - initial encounter

D - subsequent encounter

S - sequela

⊗⑦V42.0 Car driver injured in collision with two- or three-wheeled motor vehicle in nontraffic accident

⊗⑦V42.1 Car passenger injured in collision with two- or three-wheeled motor vehicle in nontraffic accident

⊗⑦V42.2 Person on outside of car injured in collision with two- or three-wheeled motor vehicle in nontraffic accident

⊗⑦V42.3 Unspecified car occupant injured in collision with two- or three-wheeled motor vehicle in nontraffic accident

⊗⑦V42.4 Person boarding or alighting a car injured in collision with two- or three-wheeled motor vehicle

⊗⑦V42.5 Car driver injured in collision with two- or three-wheeled motor vehicle in traffic accident

⊗⑦V42.6 Car passenger injured in collision with two- or three-wheeled motor vehicle in traffic accident

⊗⑦V42.7 Person on outside of car injured in collision with two- or three-wheeled motor vehicle in traffic accident

⊗⑦V42.9 Unspecified car occupant injured in collision with two- or three-wheeled motor vehicle in traffic accident

V43 Car occupant injured in collision with car, pick-up truck or van

The appropriate 7th character is to be added to each code from category V43

A - initial encounter

D - subsequent encounter

S - sequela

V43.0 Car driver injured in collision with car, pick-up truck or van in nontraffic accident

⊗⑦V43.01 Car driver injured in collision with sport utility vehicle in nontraffic accident

⊗⑦V43.02 Car driver injured in collision with other type car in nontraffic accident

⊗⑦V43.03 Car driver injured in collision with pick-up truck in nontraffic accident

⊗⑦V43.04 Car driver injured in collision with van in nontraffic accident

V43.1 Car passenger injured in collision with car, pick-up truck or van in nontraffic accident

⊗⑦V43.11 Car passenger injured in collision with sport utility vehicle in nontraffic accident

⊗⑦V43.12 Car passenger injured in collision with other type car in nontraffic accident

⊗⑦V43.13 Car passenger injured in collision with pick-up in nontraffic accident

⊗⑦V43.14 Car passenger injured in collision with van in nontraffic accident

V43.2 Person on outside of car injured in collision with car, pick-up truck or van in nontraffic accident

⊗⑦V43.21 Person on outside of car injured in collision with sport utility vehicle in nontraffic accident

⊗⑦V43.22 Person on outside of car injured in collision with other type car in nontraffic accident

⊗⑦V43.23 Person on outside of car injured in collision with pick-up truck in nontraffic accident

⊗⑦V43.24 Person on outside of car injured in collision with van in nontraffic accident

V43.3 Unspecified car occupant injured in collision with car, pick-up truck or van in nontraffic accident

⊗⑦V43.31 Unspecified car occupant injured in collision with sport utility vehicle in nontraffic accident

⊗⑦V43.32 Unspecified car occupant injured in collision with other type car in nontraffic accident

⊗⑦V43.33 Unspecified car occupant injured in collision with pick-up truck in nontraffic accident

⊗⑦V43.34 Unspecified car occupant injured in collision with van in nontraffic accident

V43.4 Person boarding or alighting a car injured in collision with car, pick-up truck or van

⊗⑦V43.41 Person boarding or alighting a car injured in collision with sport utility vehicle

⊗⑦V43.42 Person boarding or alighting a car injured in collision with other type car

⊗⑦V43.43 Person boarding or alighting a car injured in collision with pick-up truck

⊗⑦V43.44 Person boarding or alighting a car injured in collision with van

V43.5 Car driver injured in collision with car, pick-up truck or van in traffic accident

⊗⑦V43.51 Car driver injured in collision with sport utility vehicle in traffic accident

⊗⑦V43.52 Car driver injured in collision with other type car in traffic accident

⊗⑦V43.53 Car driver injured in collision with pick-up truck in traffic accident

⊗⑦V43.54 Car driver injured in collision with van in traffic accident

V43.6 Car passenger injured in collision with car, pick-up truck or van in traffic accident

⊗⑦V43.61 Car passenger injured in collision with sport utility vehicle in traffic accident

⊗⑦V43.62 Car passenger injured in collision with other type car in traffic accident

⊗⑦V43.63 Car passenger injured in collision with pick-up truck in traffic accident

⊗⑦V43.64 Car passenger injured in collision with van in traffic accident

V43.7 Person on outside of car injured in collision with car, pick-up truck or van in traffic accident

⊗⑦V43.71 Person on outside of car injured in collision with sport utility vehicle in traffic accident

⊗⑦V43.72 Person on outside of car injured in collision with other type car in traffic accident

⊗⑦V43.73 Person on outside of car injured in collision with pick-up truck in traffic accident

⊗⑦V43.74 Person on outside of car injured in collision with van in traffic accident

V43.9 Unspecified car occupant injured in collision with car, pick-up truck or van in traffic accident

⊗⑦V43.91 Unspecified car occupant injured in collision with sport utility vehicle in traffic accident

⊗⑦**V43.92** Unspecified car occupant injured in collision with other type car in traffic accident

⊗⑦**V43.93** Unspecified car occupant injured in collision with pick-up truck in traffic accident

⊗⑦**V43.94** Unspecified car occupant injured in collision with van in traffic accident

V44 Car occupant injured in collision with heavy transport vehicle or bus

Excludes1: car occupant injured in collision with military vehicle (V49.81)

The appropriate 7th character is to be added to each code from category V44

A - initial encounter

D - subsequent encounter

S - sequela

⊗⑦**V44.0** Car driver injured in collision with heavy transport vehicle or bus in nontraffic accident

⊗⑦**V44.1** Car passenger injured in collision with heavy transport vehicle or bus in nontraffic accident

⊗⑦**V44.2** Person on outside of car injured in collision with heavy transport vehicle or bus in nontraffic accident

⊗⑦**V44.3** Unspecified car occupant injured in collision with heavy transport vehicle or bus in nontraffic accident

⊗⑦**V44.4** Person boarding or alighting a car injured in collision with heavy transport vehicle or bus

⊗⑦**V44.5** Car driver injured in collision with heavy transport vehicle or bus in traffic accident

⊗⑦**V44.6** Car passenger injured in collision with heavy transport vehicle or bus in traffic accident

⊗⑦**V44.7** Person on outside of car injured in collision with heavy transport vehicle or bus in traffic accident

⊗⑦**V44.9** Unspecified car occupant injured in collision with heavy transport vehicle or bus in traffic accident

V45 Car occupant injured in collision with railway train or railway vehicle

The appropriate 7th character is to be added to each code from category V45

A - initial encounter

D - subsequent encounter

S - sequela

⊗⑦**V45.0** Car driver injured in collision with railway train or railway vehicle in nontraffic accident

⊗⑦**V45.1** Car passenger injured in collision with railway train or railway vehicle in nontraffic accident

⊗⑦**V45.2** Person on outside of car injured in collision with railway train or railway vehicle in nontraffic accident

⊗⑦**V45.3** Unspecified car occupant injured in collision with railway train or railway vehicle in nontraffic accident

⊗⑦**V45.4** Person boarding or alighting a car injured in collision with railway train or railway vehicle

⊗⑦**V45.5** Car driver injured in collision with railway train or railway vehicle in traffic accident

⊗⑦**V45.6** Car passenger injured in collision with railway train or railway vehicle in traffic accident

⊗⑦**V45.7** Person on outside of car injured in collision with railway train or railway vehicle in traffic accident

⊗⑦**V45.9** Unspecified car occupant injured in collision with railway train or railway vehicle in traffic accident

V46 Car occupant injured in collision with other nonmotor vehicle

Includes: collision with animal-drawn vehicle, animal being ridden, streetcar

The appropriate 7th character is to be added to each code from category V46

A - initial encounter

D - subsequent encounter

S - sequela

⊗⑦**V46.0** Car driver injured in collision with other nonmotor vehicle in nontraffic accident

⊗⑦**V46.1** Car passenger injured in collision with other nonmotor vehicle in nontraffic accident

⊗⑦**V46.2** Person on outside of car injured in collision with other nonmotor vehicle in nontraffic accident

⊗⑦**V46.3** Unspecified car occupant injured in collision with other nonmotor vehicle in nontraffic accident

⊗⑦**V46.4** Person boarding or alighting a car injured in collision with other nonmotor vehicle

⊗⑦**V46.5** Car driver injured in collision with other nonmotor vehicle in traffic accident

⊗⑦**V46.6** Car passenger injured in collision with other nonmotor vehicle in traffic accident

⊗⑦**V46.7** Person on outside of car injured in collision with other nonmotor vehicle in traffic accident

⊗⑦**V46.9** Unspecified car occupant injured in collision with other nonmotor vehicle in traffic accident

V47 Car occupant injured in collision with fixed or stationary object

The appropriate 7th character is to be added to each code from category V47

A - initial encounter

D - subsequent encounter

S - sequela

⊗⑦**V47.0** Car driver injured in collision with fixed or stationary object in nontraffic accident

⊗⑦**V47.1** Car passenger injured in collision with fixed or stationary object in nontraffic accident

⊗⑦**V47.2** Person on outside of car injured in collision with fixed or stationary object in nontraffic accident

⊗⑦**V47.3** Unspecified car occupant injured in collision with fixed or stationary object in nontraffic accident

⊗⑦**V47.4** Person boarding or alighting a car injured in collision with fixed or stationary object

⊗⑦**V47.5** Car driver injured in collision with fixed or stationary object in traffic accident

⊗⑦**V47.6** Car passenger injured in collision with fixed or stationary object in traffic accident

⊗⑦**V47.7** Person on outside of car injured in collision with fixed or stationary object in traffic accident

⊗⑦**V47.9** Unspecified car occupant injured in collision with fixed or stationary object in traffic accident

V48 Car occupant injured in noncollision transport accident

Includes: overturning car NOS

overturning car without collision

The appropriate 7th character is to be added to each code from category V48

A - initial encounter

D - subsequent encounter

S - sequela

⊗⑦**V48.0** Car driver injured in noncollision transport accident in nontraffic accident

⊗⑦**V48.1** Car passenger injured in noncollision transport accident in nontraffic accident

⊗⑦**V48.2** Person on outside of car injured in noncollision transport accident in nontraffic accident

⊗⑦**V48.3** Unspecified car occupant injured in noncollision transport accident in nontraffic accident

---

Add 4th-7th digits　　Nonspecific code　　Unspecified code　　Manifestation code

⊗⑦**V48.4** Person boarding or alighting a car injured in noncollision transport accident

⊗⑦**V48.5** Car driver injured in noncollision transport accident in traffic accident

⊗⑦**V48.6** Car passenger injured in noncollision transport accident in traffic accident

⊗⑦**V48.7** Person on outside of car injured in noncollision transport accident in traffic accident

⊗⑦**V48.9** Unspecified car occupant injured in noncollision transport accident in traffic accident

V49 Car occupant injured in other and unspecified transport accidents

The appropriate 7th character is to be added to each code from category V49

A - initial encounter

D - subsequent encounter

S - sequela

V49.0 Driver injured in collision with other and unspecified motor vehicles in nontraffic accident

⊗⑦**V49.00** Driver injured in collision with unspecified motor vehicles in nontraffic accident

⊗⑦**V49.09** Driver injured in collision with other motor vehicles in nontraffic accident

V49.1 Passenger injured in collision with other and unspecified motor vehicles in nontraffic accident

⊗⑦**V49.10** Passenger injured in collision with unspecified motor vehicles in nontraffic accident

⊗⑦**V49.19** Passenger injured in collision with other motor vehicles in nontraffic accident

V49.2 Unspecified car occupant injured in collision with other and unspecified motor vehicles in nontraffic accident

⊗⑦**V49.20** Unspecified car occupant injured in collision with unspecified motor vehicles in nontraffic accident

Car collision NOS, nontraffic

⊗⑦**V49.29** Unspecified car occupant injured in collision with other motor vehicles in nontraffic accident

⊗⑦**V49.3** Car occupant (driver) (passenger) injured in unspecified nontraffic accident

Car accident NOS, nontraffic

Car occupant injured in nontraffic accident NOS

V49.4 Driver injured in collision with other and unspecified motor vehicles in traffic accident

⊗⑦**V49.40** Driver injured in collision with unspecified motor vehicles in traffic accident

⊗⑦**V49.49** Driver injured in collision with other motor vehicles in traffic accident

V49.5 Passenger injured in collision with other and unspecified motor vehicles in traffic accident

⊗⑦**V49.50** Passenger injured in collision with unspecified motor vehicles in traffic accident

⊗⑦**V49.59** Passenger injured in collision with other motor vehicles in traffic accident

V49.6 Unspecified car occupant injured in collision with other and unspecified motor vehicles in traffic accident

⊗⑦**V49.60** Unspecified car occupant injured in collision with unspecified motor vehicles in traffic accident

Car collision NOS (traffic)

⊗⑦**V49.69** Unspecified car occupant injured in collision with other motor vehicles in traffic accident

V49.8 Car occupant (driver) (passenger) injured in other specified transport accidents

⊗⑦**V49.81** Car occupant (driver) (passenger) injured in transport accident with military vehicle

⊗⑦**V49.88** Car occupant (driver) (passenger) injured in other specified transport accidents

⊗⑦**V49.9** Car occupant (driver) (passenger) injured in unspecified traffic accident

Car accident NOS

OCCUPANT OF PICK-UP TRUCK OR VAN INJURED IN TRANSPORT ACCIDENT (V50-V59)

Includes: a four or six wheel motor vehicle designed primarily for carrying passengers and property but weighing less than the local limit for classification as a heavy goods vehicle

minibus

minivan

sport utility vehicle (SUV)

truck

van

Excludes1: heavy transport vehicle (V60-V69)

V50 Occupant of pick-up truck or van injured in collision with pedestrian or animal

Excludes1: pick-up truck or van collision with animal-drawn vehicle or animal being ridden (V56.-)

The appropriate 7th character is to be added to each code from category V50

A - initial encounter

D - subsequent encounter

S - sequela

⊗⑦**V50.0** Driver of pick-up truck or van injured in collision with pedestrian or animal in nontraffic accident

⊗⑦**V50.1** Passenger in pick-up truck or van injured in collision with pedestrian or animal in nontraffic accident

⊗⑦**V50.2** Person on outside of pick-up truck or van injured in collision with pedestrian or animal in nontraffic accident

⊗⑦**V50.3** Unspecified occupant of pick-up truck or van injured in collision with pedestrian or animal in nontraffic accident

⊗⑦**V50.4** Person boarding or alighting a pick-up truck or van injured in collision with pedestrian or animal

⊗⑦**V50.5** Driver of pick-up truck or van injured in collision with pedestrian or animal in traffic accident

⊗⑦**V50.6** Passenger in pick-up truck or van injured in collision with pedestrian or animal in traffic accident

⊗⑦**V50.7** Person on outside of pick-up truck or van injured in collision with pedestrian or animal in traffic accident

⊗⑦**V50.9** Unspecified occupant of pick-up truck or van injured in collision with pedestrian or animal in traffic accident

V51 Occupant of pick-up truck or van injured in collision with pedal cycle

The appropriate 7th character is to be added to each code from category V51

A - initial encounter

D - subsequent encounter

S - sequela

⊗⑦**V51.0** Driver of pick-up truck or van injured in collision with pedal cycle in nontraffic accident

⊗⑦V51.1 **Passenger in pick-up truck or van injured in collision with pedal cycle in nontraffic accident**

⊗⑦V51.2 **Person on outside of pick-up truck or van injured in collision with pedal cycle in nontraffic accident**

⊗⑦V51.3 **Unspecified occupant of pick-up truck or van injured in collision with pedal cycle in nontraffic accident**

⊗⑦V51.4 **Person boarding or alighting a pick-up truck or van injured in collision with pedal cycle**

⊗⑦V51.5 **Driver of pick-up truck or van injured in collision with pedal cycle in traffic accident**

⊗⑦V51.6 **Passenger in pick-up truck or van injured in collision with pedal cycle in traffic accident**

⊗⑦V51.7 **Person on outside of pick-up truck or van injured in collision with pedal cycle in traffic accident**

⊗⑦V51.9 **Unspecified occupant of pick-up truck or van injured in collision with pedal cycle in traffic accident**

V52 **Occupant of pick-up truck or van injured in collision with two- or three-wheeled motor vehicle**

The appropriate 7th character is to be added to each code from category V52

A - initial encounter

D - subsequent encounter

S - sequela

⊗⑦V52.0 **Driver of pick-up truck or van injured in collision with two- or three-wheeled motor vehicle in nontraffic accident**

⊗⑦V52.1 **Passenger in pick-up truck or van injured in collision with two- or three-wheeled motor vehicle in nontraffic accident**

⊗⑦V52.2 **Person on outside of pick-up truck or van injured in collision with two- or three-wheeled motor vehicle in nontraffic accident**

⊗⑦V52.3 **Unspecified occupant of pick-up truck or van injured in collision with two- or three-wheeled motor vehicle in nontraffic accident**

⊗⑦V52.4 **Person boarding or alighting a pick-up truck or van injured in collision with two- or three-wheeled motor vehicle**

⊗⑦V52.5 **Driver of pick-up truck or van injured in collision with two- or three-wheeled motor vehicle in traffic accident**

⊗⑦V52.6 **Passenger in pick-up truck or van injured in collision with two- or three-wheeled motor vehicle in traffic accident**

⊗⑦V52.7 **Person on outside of pick-up truck or van injured in collision with two- or three-wheeled motor vehicle in traffic accident**

⊗⑦V52.9 **Unspecified occupant of pick-up truck or van injured in collision with two- or three-wheeled motor vehicle in traffic accident**

V53 **Occupant of pick-up truck or van injured in collision with car, pick-up truck or van**

The appropriate 7th character is to be added to each code from category V53

A - initial encounter

D - subsequent encounter

S - sequela

⊗⑦V53.0 **Driver of pick-up truck or van injured in collision with car, pick-up truck or van in nontraffic accident**

⊗⑦V53.1 **Passenger in pick-up truck or van injured in collision with car, pick-up truck or van in nontraffic accident**

⊗⑦V53.2 **Person on outside of pick-up truck or van injured in collision with car, pick-up truck or van in nontraffic accident**

⊗⑦V53.3 **Unspecified occupant of pick-up truck or van injured in collision with car, pick-up truck or van in nontraffic accident**

⊗⑦V53.4 **Person boarding or alighting a pick-up truck or van injured in collision with car, pick-up truck or van**

⊗⑦V53.5 **Driver of pick-up truck or van injured in collision with car, pick-up truck or van in traffic accident**

⊗⑦V53.6 **Passenger in pick-up truck or van injured in collision with car, pick-up truck or van in traffic accident**

⊗⑦V53.7 **Person on outside of pick-up truck or van injured in collision with car, pick-up truck or van in traffic accident**

⊗⑦V53.9 **Unspecified occupant of pick-up truck or van injured in collision with car, pick-up truck or van in traffic accident**

V54 **Occupant of pick-up truck or van injured in collision with heavy transport vehicle or bus**

Excludes1: occupant of pick-up truck or van injured in collision with military vehicle (V59.81)

The appropriate 7th character is to be added to each code from category V54

A - initial encounter

D - subsequent encounter

S - sequela

⊗⑦V54.0 **Driver of pick-up truck or van injured in collision with heavy transport vehicle or bus in nontraffic accident**

⊗⑦V54.1 **Passenger in pick-up truck or van injured in collision with heavy transport vehicle or bus in nontraffic accident**

⊗⑦V54.2 **Person on outside of pick-up truck or van injured in collision with heavy transport vehicle or bus in nontraffic accident**

⊗⑦V54.3 **Unspecified occupant of pick-up truck or van injured in collision with heavy transport vehicle or bus in nontraffic accident**

⊗⑦V54.4 **Person boarding or alighting a pick-up truck or van injured in collision with heavy transport vehicle or bus**

⊗⑦V54.5 **Driver of pick-up truck or van injured in collision with heavy transport vehicle or bus in traffic accident**

⊗⑦V54.6 **Passenger in pick-up truck or van injured in collision with heavy transport vehicle or bus in traffic accident**

⊗⑦V54.7 **Person on outside of pick-up truck or van injured in collision with heavy transport vehicle or bus in traffic accident**

⊗⑦V54.9 **Unspecified occupant of pick-up truck or van injured in collision with heavy transport vehicle or bus in traffic accident**

V55 **Occupant of pick-up truck or van injured in collision with railway train or railway vehicle**

The appropriate 7th character is to be added to each code from category V55

A - initial encounter

D - subsequent encounter

S - sequela

⊗⑦V55.0 **Driver of pick-up truck or van injured in collision with railway train or railway vehicle in nontraffic accident**

⊗⑦V55.1 **Passenger in pick-up truck or van injured in collision with railway train or railway vehicle in nontraffic accident**

⊗⑦V55.2 **Person on outside of pick-up truck or van injured in collision with railway train or railway vehicle in nontraffic accident**

| | Add 4th-7th digits | | Nonspecific code | | Unspecified code | | Manifestation code | 1003 |

⊗⑦**V55.3** Unspecified occupant of pick-up truck or van injured in collision with railway train or railway vehicle in nontraffic accident

⊗⑦**V55.4** Person boarding or alighting a pick-up truck or van injured in collision with railway train or railway vehicle

⊗⑦**V55.5** Driver of pick-up truck or van injured in collision with railway train or railway vehicle in traffic accident

⊗⑦**V55.6** Passenger in pick-up truck or van injured in collision with railway train or railway vehicle in traffic accident

⊗⑦**V55.7** Person on outside of pick-up truck or van injured in collision with railway train or railway vehicle in traffic accident

⊗⑦**V55.9** Unspecified occupant of pick-up truck or van injured in collision with railway train or railway vehicle in traffic accident

V56 Occupant of pick-up truck or van injured in collision with other nonmotor vehicle

Includes: collision with animal-drawn vehicle, animal being ridden, streetcar

The appropriate 7th character is to be added to each code from category V56

A - initial encounter

D - subsequent encounter

S - sequela

⊗⑦**V56.0** Driver of pick-up truck or van injured in collision with other nonmotor vehicle in nontraffic accident

⊗⑦**V56.1** Passenger in pick-up truck or van injured in collision with other nonmotor vehicle in nontraffic accident

⊗⑦**V56.2** Person on outside of pick-up truck or van injured in collision with other nonmotor vehicle in nontraffic accident

⊗⑦**V56.3** Unspecified occupant of pick-up truck or van injured in collision with other nonmotor vehicle in nontraffic accident

⊗⑦**V56.4** Person boarding or alighting a pick-up truck or van injured in collision with other nonmotor vehicle

⊗⑦**V56.5** Driver of pick-up truck or van injured in collision with other nonmotor vehicle in traffic accident

⊗⑦**V56.6** Passenger in pick-up truck or van injured in collision with other nonmotor vehicle in traffic accident

⊗⑦**V56.7** Person on outside of pick-up truck or van injured in collision with other nonmotor vehicle in traffic accident

⊗⑦**V56.9** Unspecified occupant of pick-up truck or van injured in collision with other nonmotor vehicle in traffic accident

V57 Occupant of pick-up truck or van injured in collision with fixed or stationary object

The appropriate 7th character is to be added to each code from category V57

A - initial encounter

D - subsequent encounter

S - sequela

⊗⑦**V57.0** Driver of pick-up truck or van injured in collision with fixed or stationary object in nontraffic accident

⊗⑦**V57.1** Passenger in pick-up truck or van injured in collision with fixed or stationary object in nontraffic accident

⊗⑦**V57.2** Person on outside of pick-up truck or van injured in collision with fixed or stationary object in nontraffic accident

⊗⑦**V57.3** Unspecified occupant of pick-up truck or van injured in collision with fixed or stationary object in nontraffic accident

⊗⑦**V57.4** Person boarding or alighting a pick-up truck or van injured in collision with fixed or stationary object

⊗⑦**V57.5** Driver of pick-up truck or van injured in collision with fixed or stationary object in traffic accident

⊗⑦**V57.6** Passenger in pick-up truck or van injured in collision with fixed or stationary object in traffic accident

⊗⑦**V57.7** Person on outside of pick-up truck or van injured in collision with fixed or stationary object in traffic accident

⊗⑦**V57.9** Unspecified occupant of pick-up truck or van injured in collision with fixed or stationary object in traffic accident

V58 Occupant of pick-up truck or van injured in noncollision transport accident

Includes: overturning pick-up truck or van NOS

overturning pick-up truck or van without collision

The appropriate 7th character is to be added to each code from category V58

A - initial encounter

D - subsequent encounter

S - sequela

⊗⑦**V58.0** Driver of pick-up truck or van injured in noncollision transport accident in nontraffic accident

⊗⑦**V58.1** Passenger in pick-up truck or van injured in noncollision transport accident in nontraffic accident

⊗⑦**V58.2** Person on outside of pick-up truck or van injured in noncollision transport accident in nontraffic accident

⊗⑦**V58.3** Unspecified occupant of pick-up truck or van injured in noncollision transport accident in nontraffic accident

⊗⑦**V58.4** Person boarding or alighting a pick-up truck or van injured in noncollision transport accident

⊗⑦**V58.5** Driver of pick-up truck or van injured in noncollision transport accident in traffic accident

⊗⑦**V58.6** Passenger in pick-up truck or van injured in noncollision transport accident in traffic accident

⊗⑦**V58.7** Person on outside of pick-up truck or van injured in noncollision transport accident in traffic accident

⊗⑦**V58.9** Unspecified occupant of pick-up truck or van injured in noncollision transport accident in traffic accident

V59 Occupant of pick-up truck or van injured in other and unspecified transport accidents

The appropriate 7th character is to be added to each code from category V59

A - initial encounter

D - subsequent encounter

S - sequela

V59.0 Driver of pick-up truck or van injured in collision with other and unspecified motor vehicles in nontraffic accident

⊗⑦**V59.00** Driver of pick-up truck or van injured in collision with unspecified motor vehicles in nontraffic accident

⊗⑦**V59.09** Driver of pick-up truck or van injured in collision with other motor vehicles in nontraffic accident

V59.1 Passenger in pick-up truck or van injured in collision with other and unspecified motor vehicles in nontraffic accident

⊗⑦**V59.10** Passenger in pick-up truck or van injured in collision with unspecified motor vehicles in nontraffic accident

⊗⑦**V59.19** Passenger in pick-up truck or van injured in collision with other motor vehicles in nontraffic accident

V59.2 Unspecified occupant of pick-up truck or van injured in collision with other and unspecified motor vehicles in nontraffic accident

⊗⑦**V59.20** Unspecified occupant of pick-up truck or van injured in collision with unspecified motor vehicles in nontraffic accident

Collision NOS involving pick-up truck or van, nontraffic

⊗⑦**V59.29** Unspecified occupant of pick-up truck or van injured in collision with other motor vehicles in nontraffic accident

⊗⑦**V59.3** Occupant (driver) (passenger) of pick-up truck or van injured in unspecified nontraffic accident

Accident NOS involving pick-up truck or van, nontraffic

Occupant of pick-up truck or van injured in nontraffic accident NOS

V59.4 Driver of pick-up truck or van injured in collision with other and unspecified motor vehicles in traffic accident

⊗⑦**V59.40** Driver of pick-up truck or van injured in collision with unspecified motor vehicles in traffic accident

⊗⑦**V59.49** Driver of pick-up truck or van injured in collision with other motor vehicles in traffic accident

V59.5 Passenger in pick-up truck or van injured in collision with other and unspecified motor vehicles in traffic accident

⊗⑦**V59.50** Passenger in pick-up truck or van injured in collision with unspecified motor vehicles in traffic accident

⊗⑦**V59.59** Passenger in pick-up truck or van injured in collision with other motor vehicles in traffic accident

V59.6 Unspecified occupant of pick-up truck or van injured in collision with other and unspecified motor vehicles in traffic accident

⊗⑦**V59.60** Unspecified occupant of pick-up truck or van injured in collision with unspecified motor vehicles in traffic accident

Collision NOS involving pick-up truck or van (traffic)

⊗⑦**V59.69** Unspecified occupant of pick-up truck or van injured in collision with other motor vehicles in traffic accident

V59.8 Occupant (driver) (passenger) of pick-up truck or van injured in other specified transport accidents

⊗⑦**V59.81** Occupant (driver) (passenger) of pick-up truck or van injured in transport accident with military vehicle

⊗⑦**V59.88** Occupant (driver) (passenger) of pick-up truck or van injured in other specified transport accidents

⊗⑦**V59.9** Occupant (driver) (passenger) of pick-up truck or van injured in unspecified traffic accident

Accident NOS involving pick-up truck or van

OCCUPANT OF HEAVY TRANSPORT VEHICLE INJURED IN TRANSPORT ACCIDENT (V60-V69)

Includes: 18 wheeler

armored car panel truck

Excludes1: bus

motorcoach

V60 Occupant of heavy transport vehicle injured in collision with pedestrian or animal

Excludes1: heavy transport vehicle collision with animal-drawn vehicle or animal being ridden (V66.-)

The appropriate 7th character is to be added to each code from category V60

A - initial encounter

D - subsequent encounter

S - sequela

⊗⑦**V60.0** Driver of heavy transport vehicle injured in collision with pedestrian or animal in nontraffic accident

⊗⑦**V60.1** Passenger in heavy transport vehicle injured in collision with pedestrian or animal in nontraffic accident

⊗⑦**V60.2** Person on outside of heavy transport vehicle injured in collision with pedestrian or animal in nontraffic accident

⊗⑦**V60.3** Unspecified occupant of heavy transport vehicle injured in collision with pedestrian or animal in nontraffic accident

⊗⑦**V60.4** Person boarding or alighting a heavy transport vehicle injured in collision with pedestrian or animal

⊗⑦**V60.5** Driver of heavy transport vehicle injured in collision with pedestrian or animal in traffic accident

⊗⑦**V60.6** Passenger in heavy transport vehicle injured in collision with pedestrian or animal in traffic accident

⊗⑦**V60.7** Person on outside of heavy transport vehicle injured in collision with pedestrian or animal in traffic accident

⊗⑦**V60.9** Unspecified occupant of heavy transport vehicle injured in collision with pedestrian or animal in traffic accident

V61 Occupant of heavy transport vehicle injured in collision with pedal cycle

The appropriate 7th character is to be added to each code from category V61

A - initial encounter

D - subsequent encounter

S - sequela

⊗⑦**V61.0** Driver of heavy transport vehicle injured in collision with pedal cycle in nontraffic accident

⊗⑦**V61.1** Passenger in heavy transport vehicle injured in collision with pedal cycle in nontraffic accident

⊗⑦**V61.2** Person on outside of heavy transport vehicle injured in collision with pedal cycle in nontraffic accident

⊗⑦**V61.3** Unspecified occupant of heavy transport vehicle injured in collision with pedal cycle in nontraffic accident

⊗⑦**V61.4** Person boarding or alighting a heavy transport vehicle injured in collision with pedal cycle while boarding or alighting

⊗⑦**V61.5** Driver of heavy transport vehicle injured in collision with pedal cycle in traffic accident

⊗⑦**V61.6** Passenger in heavy transport vehicle injured in collision with pedal cycle in traffic accident

⊗⑦**V61.7** Person on outside of heavy transport vehicle injured in collision with pedal cycle in traffic accident

⊗⑦**V61.9** Unspecified occupant of heavy transport vehicle injured in collision with pedal cycle in traffic accident

V62 Occupant of heavy transport vehicle injured in collision with two- or three-wheeled motor vehicle

The appropriate 7th character is to be added to each code from category V62

A - initial encounter

D - subsequent encounter

S - sequela

⊗⑦**V62.0** Driver of heavy transport vehicle injured in collision with two- or three-wheeled motor vehicle in nontraffic accident

⊗⑦**V62.1** Passenger in heavy transport vehicle injured in collision with two- or three-wheeled motor vehicle in nontraffic accident

⊗⑦**V62.2** Person on outside of heavy transport vehicle injured in collision with two- or three-wheeled motor vehicle in nontraffic accident

⊗⑦**V62.3** Unspecified occupant of heavy transport vehicle injured in collision with two- or three-wheeled motor vehicle in nontraffic accident

⊗⑦**V62.4** Person boarding or alighting a heavy transport vehicle injured in collision with two- or three-way veh vehicle

⊗⑦**V62.5** Driver of heavy transport vehicle injured in collision with two- or three-wheeled motor vehicle in traffic accident

⊗⑦**V62.6** Passenger in heavy transport vehicle injured in collision with two- or three-wheeled motor vehicle in traffic accident

⊗⑦**V62.7** Person on outside of heavy transport vehicle injured in collision with two- or three-wheeled motor vehicle in traffic accident

⊗⑦**V62.9** Unspecified occupant of heavy transport vehicle injured in collision with two- or three-wheeled motor vehicle in traffic accident

V63 Occupant of heavy transport vehicle injured in collision with car, pick-up truck or van

The appropriate 7th character is to be added to each code from category V63

A - initial encounter

D - subsequent encounter

S - sequela

⊗⑦**V63.0** Driver of heavy transport vehicle injured in collision with car, pick-up truck or van in nontraffic accident

⊗⑦**V63.1** Passenger in heavy transport vehicle injured in collision with car, pick-up truck or van in nontraffic accident

⊗⑦**V63.2** Person on outside of heavy transport vehicle injured in collision with car, pick-up truck or van in nontraffic accident

⊗⑦**V63.3** Unspecified occupant of heavy transport vehicle injured in collision with car, pick-up truck or van in nontraffic accident

⊗⑦**V63.4** Person boarding or alighting a heavy transport vehicle injured in collision with car, pick-up truck or van

⊗⑦**V63.5** Driver of heavy transport vehicle injured in collision with car, pick-up truck or van in traffic accident

⊗⑦**V63.6** Passenger in heavy transport vehicle injured in collision with car, pick-up truck or van in traffic accident

⊗⑦**V63.7** Person on outside of heavy transport vehicle injured in collision with car, pick-up truck or van in traffic accident

⊗⑦**V63.9** Unspecified occupant of heavy transport vehicle injured in collision with car, pick-up truck or van in traffic accident

V64 Occupant of heavy transport vehicle injured in collision with heavy transport vehicle or bus

Excludes1: occupant of heavy transport vehicle injured in collision with military vehicle (V69.81)

The appropriate 7th character is to be added to each code from category V64

A - initial encounter

D - subsequent encounter

S - sequela

⊗⑦**V64.0** Driver of heavy transport vehicle injured in collision with heavy transport vehicle or bus in nontraffic accident

⊗⑦**V64.1** Passenger in heavy transport vehicle injured in collision with heavy transport vehicle or bus in nontraffic accident

⊗⑦**V64.2** Person on outside of heavy transport vehicle injured in collision with heavy transport vehicle or bus in nontraffic accident

⊗⑦**V64.3** Unspecified occupant of heavy transport vehicle injured in collision with heavy transport vehicle or bus in nontraffic accident

⊗⑦**V64.4** Person boarding or alighting a heavy transport vehicle injured in collision with heavy transport vehicle or bus while boarding or alighting

⊗⑦**V64.5** Driver of heavy transport vehicle injured in collision with heavy transport vehicle or bus in traffic accident

⊗⑦**V64.6** Passenger in heavy transport vehicle injured in collision with heavy transport vehicle or bus in traffic accident

⊗⑦**V64.7** Person on outside of heavy transport vehicle injured in collision with heavy transport vehicle or bus in traffic accident

⊗⑦**V64.9** Unspecified occupant of heavy transport vehicle injured in collision with heavy transport vehicle or bus in traffic accident

V65 Occupant of heavy transport vehicle injured in collision with railway train or railway vehicle

The appropriate 7th character is to be added to each code from category V65

A - initial encounter

D - subsequent encounter

S - sequela

⊗⑦**V65.0** Driver of heavy transport vehicle injured in collision with railway train or railway vehicle in nontraffic accident

⊗⑦**V65.1** Passenger in heavy transport vehicle injured in collision with railway train or railway vehicle in nontraffic accident

⊗⑦**V65.2** Person on outside of heavy transport vehicle injured in collision with railway train or railway vehicle in nontraffic accident

⊗⑦**V65.3** Unspecified occupant of heavy transport vehicle injured in collision with railway train or railway vehicle in nontraffic accident

⊗⑦**V65.4** Person boarding or alighting a heavy transport vehicle injured in collision with railway train or railway vehicle

⊗⑦**V65.5** Driver of heavy transport vehicle injured in collision with railway train or railway vehicle in traffic accident

● New code ▲ Revised code **Excludes1:** Not coded here **Excludes2:** Not included here ⊗ Placeholder required ⑦ 7th digit required

⊗⑦**V65.6** Passenger in heavy transport vehicle injured in collision with railway train or railway vehicle in traffic accident

⊗⑦**V65.7** Person on outside of heavy transport vehicle injured in collision with railway train or railway vehicle in traffic accident

⊗⑦**V65.9** Unspecified occupant of heavy transport vehicle injured in collision with railway train or railway vehicle in traffic accident

V66 Occupant of heavy transport vehicle injured in collision with other nonmotor vehicle

Includes: collision with animal-drawn vehicle, animal being ridden, streetcar

The appropriate 7th character is to be added to each code from category V66

A - initial encounter

D - subsequent encounter

S - sequela

⊗⑦**V66.0** Driver of heavy transport vehicle injured in collision with other nonmotor vehicle in nontraffic accident

⊗⑦**V66.1** Passenger in heavy transport vehicle injured in collision with other nonmotor vehicle in nontraffic accident

⊗⑦**V66.2** Person on outside of heavy transport vehicle injured in collision with other nonmotor vehicle in nontraffic accident

⊗⑦**V66.3** Unspecified occupant of heavy transport vehicle injured in collision with other nonmotor vehicle in nontraffic accident

⊗⑦**V66.4** Person boarding or alighting a heavy transport vehicle injured in collision with other nonmotor vehicle

⊗⑦**V66.5** Driver of heavy transport vehicle injured in collision with other nonmotor vehicle in traffic accident

⊗⑦**V66.6** Passenger in heavy transport vehicle injured in collision with other nonmotor vehicle in traffic accident

⊗⑦**V66.7** Person on outside of heavy transport vehicle injured in collision with other nonmotor vehicle in traffic accident

⊗⑦**V66.9** Unspecified occupant of heavy transport vehicle injured in collision with other nonmotor vehicle in traffic accident

V67 Occupant of heavy transport vehicle injured in collision with fixed or stationary object

The appropriate 7th character is to be added to each code from category V67

A - initial encounter

D - subsequent encounter

S - sequela

⊗⑦**V67.0** Driver of heavy transport vehicle injured in collision with fixed or stationary object in nontraffic accident

⊗⑦**V67.1** Passenger in heavy transport vehicle injured in collision with fixed or stationary object in nontraffic accident

⊗⑦**V67.2** Person on outside of heavy transport vehicle injured in collision with fixed or stationary object in nontraffic accident

⊗⑦**V67.3** Unspecified occupant of heavy transport vehicle injured in collision with fixed or stationary object in nontraffic accident

⊗⑦**V67.4** Person boarding or alighting a heavy transport vehicle injured in collision with fixed or stationary object vehicle injured in collision with other motor vehicles in nontraffic accident

V69.2 Unspecified occupant of heavy transport vehicle injured in collision with other and unspecified motor vehicles in nontraffic accident

⊗⑦**V69.20** Unspecified occupant of heavy transport vehicle injured in collision with unspecified motor vehicles in nontraffic accident

Collision NOS involving heavy transport vehicle, nontraffic

⊗⑦**V69.29** Unspecified occupant of heavy transport vehicle injured in collision with other motor vehicles in nontraffic accident

⊗⑦**V69.3** Occupant (driver) (passenger) of heavy transport vehicle injured in unspecified nontraffic accident

Accident NOS involving heavy transport vehicle, nontraffic

Occupant of heavy transport vehicle injured in nontraffic accident NOS

V69.4 Driver of heavy transport vehicle injured in collision with other and unspecified motor vehicles in traffic accident

⊗⑦**V69.40** Driver of heavy transport vehicle injured in collision with unspecified motor vehicles in traffic accident

⊗⑦**V69.49** Driver of heavy transport vehicle injured in collision with other motor vehicles in traffic accident

V69.5 Passenger in heavy transport vehicle injured in collision with other and unspecified motor vehicles in traffic accident

⊗⑦**V69.50** Passenger in heavy transport vehicle injured in collision with unspecified motor vehicles in traffic accident

⊗⑦**V69.59** Passenger in heavy transport vehicle injured in collision with other motor vehicles in traffic accident

V69.6 Unspecified occupant of heavy transport vehicle injured in collision with other and unspecified motor vehicles in traffic accident

⊗⑦**V69.60** Unspecified occupant of heavy transport vehicle injured in collision with unspecified motor vehicles in traffic accident

Collision NOS involving heavy transport vehicle (traffic)

⊗⑦**V69.69** Unspecified occupant of heavy transport vehicle injured in collision with other motor vehicles in traffic accident

V69.8 Occupant (driver) (passenger) of heavy transport vehicle injured in other specified transport accidents

⊗⑦**V69.81** Occupant (driver) (passenger) of heavy transport vehicle injured in transport accidents with military vehicle

⊗⑦**V69.88** Occupant (driver) (passenger) of heavy transport vehicle injured in other specified transport accidents

⊗⑦**V69.9** Occupant (driver) (passenger) of heavy transport vehicle injured in unspecified traffic accident

Accident NOS involving heavy transport vehicle

BUS OCCUPANT INJURED IN TRANSPORT ACCIDENT (V70-V79)

Includes: motorcoach

Excludes1: minibus (V50-V59)

V70 Bus occupant injured in collision with pedestrian or animal

The appropriate 7th character is to be added to each code from category V70

A - initial encounter

D - subsequent encounter

S - sequela

Excludes1: bus collision with animal-drawn vehicle or animal being ridden (V76.-)

⊗⑦**V70.0** **Driver of bus injured in collision with pedestrian or animal in nontraffic accident**

⊗⑦**V70.1** **Passenger on bus injured in collision with pedestrian or animal in nontraffic accident**

⊗⑦**V70.2** **Person on outside of bus injured in collision with pedestrian or animal in nontraffic accident**

⊗⑦**V70.3** **Unspecified occupant of bus injured in collision with pedestrian or animal in nontraffic accident**

⊗⑦**V70.4** **Person boarding or alighting from bus injured in collision with pedestrian or animal**

⊗⑦**V70.5** **Driver of bus injured in collision with pedestrian or animal in traffic accident**

⊗⑦**V70.6** **Passenger on bus injured in collision with pedestrian or animal in traffic accident**

⊗⑦**V70.7** **Person on outside of bus injured in collision with pedestrian or animal in traffic accident**

⊗⑦**V70.9** **Unspecified occupant of bus injured in collision with pedestrian or animal in traffic accident**

V71 **Bus occupant injured in collision with pedal cycle**

The appropriate 7th character is to be added to each code from category V71

A - initial encounter

D - subsequent encounter

S - sequela

⊗⑦**V71.0** **Driver of bus injured in collision with pedal cycle in nontraffic accident**

⊗⑦**V71.1** **Passenger on bus injured in collision with pedal cycle in nontraffic accident**

⊗⑦**V71.2** **Person on outside of bus injured in collision with pedal cycle in nontraffic accident**

⊗⑦**V71.3** **Unspecified occupant of bus injured in collision with pedal cycle in nontraffic accident**

⊗⑦**V71.4** **Person boarding or alighting from bus injured in collision with pedal cycle**

⊗⑦**V71.5** **Driver of bus injured in collision with pedal cycle in traffic accident**

⊗⑦**V71.6** **Passenger on bus injured in collision with pedal cycle in traffic accident**

⊗⑦**V71.7** **Person on outside of bus injured in collision with pedal cycle in traffic accident**

⊗⑦**V71.9** **Unspecified occupant of bus injured in collision with pedal cycle in traffic accident**

V72 **Bus occupant injured in collision with two- or three-wheeled motor vehicle**

The appropriate 7th character is to be added to each code from category V72

A - initial encounter

D - subsequent encounter

S - sequela

⊗⑦**V72.0** **Driver of bus injured in collision with two- or three-wheeled motor vehicle in nontraffic accident**

⊗⑦**V72.1** **Passenger on bus injured in collision with two- or three-wheeled motor vehicle in nontraffic accident**

⊗⑦**V72.2** **Person on outside of bus injured in collision with two- or three-wheeled motor vehicle in nontraffic accident**

⊗⑦**V72.3** **Unspecified occupant of bus injured in collision with two- or three-wheeled motor vehicle in nontraffic accident**

⊗⑦**V72.4** **Person boarding or alighting from bus injured in collision with two- or three-wheeled motor vehicle**

⊗⑦**V72.5** **Driver of bus injured in collision with two- or three-wheeled motor vehicle in traffic accident**

⊗⑦**V72.6** **Passenger on bus injured in collision with two- or three-wheeled motor vehicle in traffic accident**

⊗⑦**V72.7** **Person on outside of bus injured in collision with two- or three-wheeled motor vehicle in traffic accident**

⊗⑦**V72.9** **Unspecified occupant of bus injured in collision with two- or three-wheeled motor vehicle in traffic accident**

V73 **Bus occupant injured in collision with car, pick-up truck or van**

The appropriate 7th character is to be added to each code from category V73

A - initial encounter

D - subsequent encounter

S - sequela

⊗⑦**V73.0** **Driver of bus injured in collision with car, pick-up truck or van in nontraffic accident**

⊗⑦**V73.1** **Passenger on bus injured in collision with car, pick-up truck or van in nontraffic accident**

⊗⑦**V73.2** **Person on outside of bus injured in collision with car, pick-up truck or van in nontraffic accident**

⊗⑦**V73.3** **Unspecified occupant of bus injured in collision with car, pick-up truck or van in nontraffic accident**

⊗⑦**V73.4** **Person boarding or alighting from bus injured in collision with car, pick-up truck or van**

⊗⑦**V73.5** **Driver of bus injured in collision with car, pick-up truck or van in traffic accident**

⊗⑦**V73.6** **Passenger on bus injured in collision with car, pick-up truck or van in traffic accident**

⊗⑦**V73.7** **Person on outside of bus injured in collision with car, pick-up truck or van in traffic accident**

⊗⑦**V73.9** **Unspecified occupant of bus injured in collision with car, pick-up truck or van in traffic accident**

V74 **Bus occupant injured in collision with heavy transport vehicle or bus**

Excludes1: bus occupant injured in collision with military vehicle (V79.81)

The appropriate 7th character is to be added to each code from category V74

A - initial encounter

D - subsequent encounter

S - sequela

⊗⑦**V74.0** **Driver of bus injured in collision with heavy transport vehicle or bus in nontraffic accident**

⊗⑦**V74.1** **Passenger on bus injured in collision with heavy transport vehicle or bus in nontraffic accident**

⊗⑦**V74.2** **Person on outside of bus injured in collision with heavy transport vehicle or bus in nontraffic accident**

⊗⑦**V74.3** **Unspecified occupant of bus injured in collision with heavy transport vehicle or bus in nontraffic accident**

⊗⑦**V74.4** **Person boarding or alighting from bus injured in collision with heavy transport vehicle or bus**

⊗⑦**V74.5** **Driver of bus injured in collision with heavy transport vehicle or bus in traffic accident**

⊗⑦**V74.6** **Passenger on bus injured in collision with heavy transport vehicle or bus in traffic accident**

⊗⑦**V74.7** **Person on outside of bus injured in collision with heavy transport vehicle or bus in traffic accident**

⊗⑦**V74.9** **Unspecified occupant of bus injured in collision with heavy transport vehicle or bus in traffic accident**

V75 Bus occupant injured in collision with railway train or railway vehicle

The appropriate 7th character is to be added to each code from category V75

A - initial encounter

D - subsequent encounter

S - sequela

⊗⑦**V75.0** Driver of bus injured in collision with railway train or railway vehicle in nontraffic accident

⊗⑦**V75.1** Passenger on bus injured in collision with railway train or railway vehicle in nontraffic accident

⊗⑦**V75.2** Person on outside of bus injured in collision with railway train or railway vehicle in nontraffic accident

⊗⑦**V75.3** Unspecified occupant of bus injured in collision with railway train or railway vehicle in nontraffic accident

⊗⑦**V75.4** Person boarding or alighting from bus injured in collision with railway train or railway vehicle

⊗⑦**V75.5** Driver of bus injured in collision with railway train or railway vehicle in traffic accident

⊗⑦**V75.6** Passenger on bus injured in collision with railway train or railway vehicle in traffic accident

⊗⑦**V75.7** Person on outside of bus injured in collision with railway train or railway vehicle in traffic accident

⊗⑦**V75.9** Unspecified occupant of bus injured in collision with railway train or railway vehicle in traffic accident

V76 Bus occupant injured in collision with other nonmotor vehicle

Includes: collision with animal-drawn vehicle, animal being ridden, streetcar

The appropriate 7th character is to be added to each code from category V76

A - initial encounter

D - subsequent encounter

S - sequela

⊗⑦**V76.0** Driver of bus injured in collision with other nonmotor vehicle in nontraffic accident

⊗⑦**V76.1** Passenger on bus injured in collision with other nonmotor vehicle in nontraffic accident

⊗⑦**V76.2** Person on outside of bus injured in collision with other nonmotor vehicle in nontraffic accident

⊗⑦**V76.3** Unspecified occupant of bus injured in collision with other nonmotor vehicle in nontraffic accident

⊗⑦**V76.4** Person boarding or alighting from bus injured in collision with other nonmotor vehicle

⊗⑦**V76.5** Driver of bus injured in collision with other nonmotor vehicle in traffic accident

⊗⑦**V76.6** Passenger on bus injured in collision with other nonmotor vehicle in traffic accident

⊗⑦**V76.7** Person on outside of bus injured in collision with other nonmotor vehicle in traffic accident

⊗⑦**V76.9** Unspecified occupant of bus injured in collision with other nonmotor vehicle in traffic accident

V77 Bus occupant injured in collision with fixed or stationary object

The appropriate 7th character is to be added to each code from category V77

A - initial encounter

D - subsequent encounter

S - sequela

⊗⑦**V77.0** Driver of bus injured in collision with fixed or stationary object in nontraffic accident

⊗⑦**V77.1** Passenger on bus injured in collision with fixed or stationary object in nontraffic accident

⊗⑦**V77.2** Person on outside of bus injured in collision with fixed or stationary object in nontraffic accident

⊗⑦**V77.3** Unspecified occupant of bus injured in collision with fixed or stationary object in nontraffic accident

⊗⑦**V77.4** Person boarding or alighting from bus injured in collision with fixed or stationary object

⊗⑦**V77.5** Driver of bus injured in collision with fixed or stationary object in traffic accident

⊗⑦**V77.6** Passenger on bus injured in collision with fixed or stationary object in traffic accident

⊗⑦**V77.7** Person on outside of bus injured in collision with fixed or stationary object in traffic accident

⊗⑦**V77.9** Unspecified occupant of bus injured in collision with fixed or stationary object in traffic accident

V78 Bus occupant injured in noncollision transport accident

Includes: overturning bus NOS

overturning bus without collision

The appropriate 7th character is to be added to each code from category V78

A - initial encounter

D - subsequent encounter

S - sequela

⊗⑦**V78.0** Driver of bus injured in noncollision transport accident in nontraffic accident

⊗⑦**V78.1** Passenger on bus injured in noncollision transport accident in nontraffic accident

⊗⑦**V78.2** Person on outside of bus injured in noncollision transport accident in nontraffic accident

⊗⑦**V78.3** Unspecified occupant of bus injured in noncollision transport accident in nontraffic accident

⊗⑦**V78.4** Person boarding or alighting from bus injured in noncollision transport accident

⊗⑦**V78.5** Driver of bus injured in noncollision transport accident in traffic accident

⊗⑦**V78.6** Passenger on bus injured in noncollision transport accident in traffic accident

⊗⑦**V78.7** Person on outside of bus injured in noncollision transport accident in traffic accident

⊗⑦**V78.9** Unspecified occupant of bus injured in noncollision transport accident in traffic accident

V79 Bus occupant injured in other and unspecified transport accidents

The appropriate 7th character is to be added to each code from category V79

A - initial encounter

D - subsequent encounter

S - sequela

V79.0 Driver of bus injured in collision with other and unspecified motor vehicles in nontraffic accident

⊗⑦**V79.00** Driver of bus injured in collision with unspecified motor vehicles in nontraffic accident

⊗⑦**V79.09** Driver of bus injured in collision with other motor vehicles in nontraffic accident

V79.1 Passenger on bus injured in collision with other and unspecified motor vehicles in nontraffic accident

⊗⑦**V79.10** Passenger on bus injured in collision with unspecified motor vehicles in nontraffic accident

⊗⑦**V79.19** Passenger on bus injured in collision with other motor vehicles in nontraffic accident

V79.2 Unspecified bus occupant injured in collision with other and unspecified motor vehicles in nontraffic accident

---

⊗⑦**V79.20** Unspecified bus occupant injured in collision with unspecified motor vehicles in nontraffic accident

Bus collision NOS, nontraffic

⊗⑦**V79.29** Unspecified bus occupant injured in collision with other motor vehicles in nontraffic accident

V79.3 Bus occupant (driver) (passenger) injured in unspecified nontraffic accident

Bus accident NOS, nontraffic

Bus occupant injured in nontraffic accident NOS

V79.4 Driver of bus injured in collision with other and unspecified motor vehicles in traffic accident

⊗⑦**V79.40** Driver of bus injured in collision with unspecified motor vehicles in traffic accident

⊗⑦**V79.49** Driver of bus injured in collision with other motor vehicles in traffic accident

V79.5 Passenger on bus injured in collision with other and unspecified motor vehicles in traffic accident

⊗⑦**V79.50** Passenger on bus injured in collision with unspecified motor vehicles in traffic accident

⊗⑦**V79.59** Passenger on bus injured in collision with other motor vehicles in traffic accident

V79.6 Unspecified bus occupant injured in collision with other and unspecified motor vehicles in traffic accident

⊗⑦**V79.60** Unspecified bus occupant injured in collision with unspecified motor vehicles in traffic accident

Bus collision NOS (traffic)

⊗⑦**V79.69** Unspecified bus occupant injured in collision with other motor vehicles in traffic accident

V79.8 Bus occupant (driver) (passenger) injured in other specified transport accidents

⊗⑦**V79.81** Bus occupant (driver) (passenger) injured in transport accidents with military vehicle

⊗⑦**V79.88** Bus occupant (driver) (passenger) injured in other specified transport accidents

⊗⑦**V79.9** Bus occupant (driver) (passenger) injured in unspecified traffic accident

Bus accident NOS

OTHER LAND TRANSPORT ACCIDENTS (V80-V89)

V80 Animal-rider or occupant of animal-drawn vehicle injured in transport accident

The appropriate 7th character is to be added to each code from category V80

A - initial encounter

D - subsequent encounter

S - sequela

V80.0 Animal-rider or occupant of animal drawn vehicle injured by fall from or being thrown from animal or animal-drawn vehicle in noncollision accident

V80.01 Animal-rider injured by fall from or being thrown from animal in noncollision accident

⑦**V80.010** Animal-rider injured by fall from or being thrown from horse in noncollision accident

⑦**V80.018** Animal-rider injured by fall from or being thrown from other animal in noncollision accident

⊗⑦**V80.02** Occupant of animal-drawn vehicle injured by fall from or being thrown from animal-drawn vehicle in noncollision accident

Overturning animal-drawn vehicle NOS

Overturning animal-drawn vehicle without collision

V80.1 Animal-rider or occupant of animal-drawn vehicle injured in collision with pedestrian or animal

Excludes1: animal-rider or animal-drawn vehicle collision with animal-drawn vehicle or animal being ridden (V80.7)

⊗⑦**V80.11** Animal-rider injured in collision with pedestrian or animal

⊗⑦**V80.12** Occupant of animal-drawn vehicle injured in collision with pedestrian or animal

V80.2 Animal-rider or occupant of animal-drawn vehicle injured in collision with pedal cycle

⊗⑦**V80.21** Animal-rider injured in collision with pedal cycle

⊗⑦**V80.22** Occupant of animal-drawn vehicle injured in collision with pedal cycle

V80.3 Animal-rider or occupant of animal-drawn vehicle injured in collision with two- or three-wheeled motor vehicle

⊗⑦**V80.31** Animal-rider injured in collision with two- or three-wheeled motor vehicle

⊗⑦**V80.32** Occupant of animal-drawn vehicle injured in collision with two- or three-wheeled motor vehicle

V80.4 Animal-rider or occupant of animal-drawn vehicle injured in collision with car, pick-up truck, van, heavy transport vehicle or bus

Excludes1: animal-rider injured in collision with military vehicle (V80.910)

occupant of animal-drawn vehicle injured in collision with military vehicle (V80.920)

⊗⑦**V80.41** Animal-rider injured in collision with car, pick-up truck, van, heavy transport vehicle or bus

⊗⑦**V80.42** Occupant of animal-drawn vehicle injured in collision with car, pick-up truck, van, heavy transport vehicle or bus

V80.5 Animal-rider or occupant of animal-drawn vehicle injured in collision with other specified motor vehicle

⊗⑦**V80.51** Animal-rider injured in collision with other specified motor vehicle

⊗⑦**V80.52** Occupant of animal-drawn vehicle injured in collision with other specified motor vehicle

V80.6 Animal-rider or occupant of animal-drawn vehicle injured in collision with railway train or railway vehicle

⊗⑦**V80.61** Animal-rider injured in collision with railway train or railway vehicle

⊗⑦**V80.62** Occupant of animal-drawn vehicle injured in collision with railway train or railway vehicle

V80.7 Animal-rider or occupant of animal-drawn vehicle injured in collision with other nonmotor vehicles

V80.71 Animal-rider or occupant of animal-drawn vehicle injured in collision with animal being ridden

⑦**V80.710** Animal-rider injured in collision with other animal being ridden

⑦V80.711 Occupant of animal-drawn vehicle injured in collision with animal being ridden

V80.72 Animal-rider or occupant of animal-drawn vehicle injured in collision with other animal-drawn vehicle

⑦V80.720 Animal-rider injured in collision with animal-drawn vehicle

⑦V80.721 Occupant of animal-drawn vehicle injured in collision with other animal-drawn vehicle

V80.73 Animal-rider or occupant of animal-drawn vehicle injured in collision with streetcar

⑦V80.730 Animal-rider injured in collision with streetcar

⑦V80.731 Occupant of animal-drawn vehicle injured in collision with streetcar

V80.79 Animal-rider or occupant of animal-drawn vehicle injured in collision with other nonmotor vehicles

⑦V80.790 Animal-rider injured in collision with other nonmotor vehicles

⑦V80.791 Occupant of animal-drawn vehicle injured in collision with other nonmotor vehicles

V80.8 Animal-rider or occupant of animal-drawn vehicle injured in collision with fixed or stationary object

⊗⑦V80.81 Animal-rider injured in collision with fixed or stationary object

⊗⑦V80.82 Occupant of animal-drawn vehicle injured in collision with fixed or stationary object

V80.9 Animal-rider or occupant of animal-drawn vehicle injured in other and unspecified transport accidents

V80.91 Animal-rider injured in other and unspecified transport accidents

⑦V80.910 Animal-rider injured in transport accident with military vehicle

⑦V80.918 Animal-rider injured in other transport accident

⑦V80.919 Animal-rider injured in unspecified transport accident

Animal rider accident NOS

V80.92 Occupant of animal-drawn vehicle injured in other and unspecified transport accidents

⑦V80.920 Occupant of animal-drawn vehicle injured in transport accident with military vehicle

⑦V80.928 Occupant of animal-drawn vehicle injured in other transport accident

⑦V80.929 Occupant of animal-drawn vehicle injured in unspecified transport accident

Animal-drawn vehicle accident NOS

V81 Occupant of railway train or railway vehicle injured in transport accident

Includes: derailment of railway train or railway vehicle

person on outside of train

Excludes1: streetcar (V82.-)

The appropriate 7th character is to be added to each code from category V81

A - initial encounter

D - subsequent encounter

S - sequela

⊗⑦V81.0 Occupant of railway train or railway vehicle injured in collision with motor vehicle in nontraffic accident

Excludes1: Occupant of railway train or railway vehicle injured due to collision with military vehicle (V81.83)

⊗⑦V81.1 Occupant of railway train or railway vehicle injured in collision with motor vehicle in traffic accident

Excludes1: Occupant of railway train or railway vehicle injured due to collision with military vehicle (V81.83)

⊗⑦V81.2 Occupant of railway train or railway vehicle injured in collision with or hit by rolling stock

⊗⑦V81.3 Occupant of railway train or railway vehicle injured in collision with other object

Railway collision NOS

⊗⑦V81.4 Person injured while boarding or alighting from railway train or railway vehicle

⊗⑦V81.5 Occupant of railway train or railway vehicle injured by fall in railway train or railway vehicle

⊗⑦V81.6 Occupant of railway train or railway vehicle injured by fall from railway train or railway vehicle

⊗⑦V81.7 Occupant of railway train or railway vehicle injured in derailment without antecedent collision

V81.8 Occupant of railway train or railway vehicle injured in other specified railway accidents

⊗⑦V81.81 Occupant of railway train or railway vehicle injured due to explosion or fire on train

⊗⑦V81.82 Occupant of railway train or railway vehicle injured due to object falling onto train

Occupant of railway train or railway vehicle injured due to falling earth onto train

Occupant of railway train or railway vehicle injured due to falling rocks onto train

Occupant of railway train or railway vehicle injured due to falling snow onto train

Occupant of railway train or railway vehicle injured due to falling trees onto train

⊗⑦V81.83 Occupant of railway train or railway vehicle injured due to collision with military vehicle

⊗⑦V81.89 Occupant of railway train or railway vehicle injured due to other specified railway accident

⊗⑦V81.9 Occupant of railway train or railway vehicle injured in unspecified railway accident

Railway accident NOS

V82 Occupant of powered streetcar injured in transport accident

Includes: interurban electric car

person on outside of streetcar tram (car)

trolley (car)

Excludes1: bus (V70-V79)

motorcoach (V70-V79)

nonpowered streetcar (V76.-) train (V81.-)

The appropriate 7th character is to be added to each code from category V82

A - initial encounter

D - subsequent encounter

S - sequela

⊗⑦V82.0 Occupant of streetcar injured in collision with motor vehicle in nontraffic accident

⊗⑦V82.1 Occupant of streetcar injured in collision with motor vehicle in traffic accident

---

Add 4th-7th digits   Nonspecific code   Unspecified code   Manifestation code

⊗⑦**V82.2** **Occupant of streetcar injured in collision with or hit by rolling stock**

⊗⑦**V82.3** **Occupant of streetcar injured in collision with other object**

Excludes1: collision with animal-drawn vehicle or animal being ridden (V82.8)

⊗⑦**V82.4** **Person injured while boarding or alighting from streetcar**

⊗⑦**V82.5** **Occupant of streetcar injured by fall in streetcar**

Excludes1: fall in streetcar:

while boarding or alighting (V82.4)

with antecedent collision (V82.0-V82.3)

⊗⑦**V82.6** **Occupant of streetcar injured by fall from streetcar**

Excludes1: fall from streetcar:

while boarding or alighting (V82.4)

with antecedent collision (V82.0-V82.3)

⊗⑦**V82.7** **Occupant of streetcar injured in derailment without antecedent collision**

Excludes1: occupant of streetcar injured in derailment with antecedent collision (V82.0-V82.3)

⊗⑦**V82.8** **Occupant of streetcar injured in other specified transport accidents**

Streetcar collision with military vehicle

Streetcar collision with train or nonmotor vehicles

⊗⑦**V82.9** **Occupant of streetcar injured in unspecified traffic accident**

Streetcar accident NOS

V83 **Occupant of special vehicle mainly used on industrial premises injured in transport accident**

Includes: battery-powered airport passenger vehicle

battery-powered truck (baggage) (mail)

coal-car in mine

forklift (truck)

logging car

self-propelled industrial truck

station baggage truck (powered)

tram, truck, or tub (powered) in mine or quarry

Excludes1: special construction vehicles (V85.-)

special industrial vehicle in stationary use or maintenance (W31.-)

The appropriate 7th character is to be added to each code from category V83

A - initial encounter

D - subsequent encounter

S - sequela

⊗⑦**V83.0** **Driver of special industrial vehicle injured in traffic accident**

⊗⑦**V83.1** **Passenger of special industrial vehicle injured in traffic accident**

⊗⑦**V83.2** **Person on outside of special industrial vehicle injured in traffic accident**

⊗⑦**V83.3** **Unspecified occupant of special industrial vehicle injured in traffic accident**

⊗⑦**V83.4** **Person injured while boarding or alighting from special industrial vehicle**

⊗⑦**V83.5** **Driver of special industrial vehicle injured in nontraffic accident**

⊗⑦**V83.6** **Passenger of special industrial vehicle injured in nontraffic accident**

⊗⑦**V83.7** **Person on outside of special industrial vehicle injured in nontraffic accident**

⊗⑦**V83.9** **Unspecified occupant of special industrial vehicle injured in nontraffic accident**

Special-industrial-vehicle accident NOS

V84 **Occupant of special vehicle mainly used in agriculture injured in transport accident**

Includes: self-propelled farm machinery

tractor (and trailer)

Excludes1: animal-powered farm machinery accident (W30.8-)

contact with combine harvester (W30.0)

special agricultural vehicle in stationary use or maintenance (W30.-)

The appropriate 7th character is to be added to each code from category V84

A - initial encounter

D - subsequent encounter

S - sequela

⊗⑦**V84.0** **Driver of special agricultural vehicle injured in traffic accident**

⊗⑦**V84.1** **Passenger of special agricultural vehicle injured in traffic accident**

⊗⑦**V84.2** **Person on outside of special agricultural vehicle injured in traffic accident**

⊗⑦**V84.3** **Unspecified occupant of special agricultural vehicle injured in traffic accident**

⊗⑦**V84.4** **Person injured while boarding or alighting from special agricultural vehicle**

⊗⑦**V84.5** **Driver of special agricultural vehicle injured in nontraffic accident**

⊗⑦**V84.6** **Passenger of special agricultural vehicle injured in nontraffic accident**

⊗⑦**V84.7** **Person on outside of special agricultural vehicle injured in nontraffic accident**

⊗⑦**V84.9** **Unspecified occupant of special agricultural vehicle injured in nontraffic accident**

Special-agricultural vehicle accident NOS

V85 **Occupant of special construction vehicle injured in transport accident**

Includes: bulldozer

digger dump truck

earth-leveller mechanical shovel road-roller

Excludes1: special industrial vehicle (V83.-)

special construction vehicle in stationary use or maintenance (W31.-)

The appropriate 7th character is to be added to each code from category V85

A - initial encounter

D - subsequent encounter

S - sequela

⊗⑦**V85.0** **Driver of special construction vehicle injured in traffic accident**

⊗⑦**V85.1** **Passenger of special construction vehicle injured in traffic accident**

⊗⑦**V85.2** **Person on outside of special construction vehicle injured in traffic accident**

⊗⑦**V85.3** **Unspecified occupant of special construction vehicle injured in traffic accident**

⊗⑦**V85.4** **Person injured while boarding or alighting from special construction vehicle**

⊗⑦**V85.5** **Driver of special construction vehicle injured in nontraffic accident**

⊗⑦**V85.6** **Passenger of special construction vehicle injured in nontraffic accident**

⊗⑦**V85.7** Person on outside of special construction vehicle injured in nontraffic accident

⊗⑦**V85.9** Unspecified occupant of special construction vehicle injured in nontraffic accident

    Special-construction-vehicle accident NOS

V86 Occupant of special all-terrain or other off-road motor vehicle, injured in transport accident

    Excludes1: special all-terrain vehicle in stationary use or maintenance (W31.-)

      sport-utility vehicle (V50-V59)

      three-wheeled motor vehicle designed for on-road use (V30-V39)

The appropriate 7th character is to be added to each code from category V86

A - initial encounter

D - subsequent encounter

S - sequela

V86.0 Driver of special all-terrain or other off-road motor vehicle injured in traffic accident

  ⊗⑦**V86.01** Driver of ambulance or fire engine injured in traffic accident

  ⊗⑦**V86.02** Driver of snowmobile injured in traffic accident

  ⊗⑦**V86.03** Driver of dune buggy injured in traffic accident

  ⊗⑦**V86.04** Driver of military vehicle injured in traffic accident

  •⊗⑦**V86.05** Driver of 3- or 4- wheeled all-terrain vehicle (ATV) injured in traffic accident

  •⊗⑦**V86.06** Driver of dirt bike or motor/cross bike injured in traffic accident

  ⊗⑦**V86.09** Driver of other special all-terrain or other off-road motor vehicle injured in traffic accident

    Driver of dirt bike injured in traffic accident

    Driver of go cart injured in traffic accident

    Driver of golf cart injured in traffic accident

V86.1 Passenger of special all-terrain or other off-road motor vehicle injured in traffic accident

  ⊗⑦**V86.11** Passenger of ambulance or fire engine injured in traffic accident

  ⊗⑦**V86.12** Passenger of snowmobile injured in traffic accident

  ⊗⑦**V86.13** Passenger of dune buggy injured in traffic accident

  ⊗⑦**V86.14** Passenger of military vehicle injured in traffic accident

  •⊗⑦**V86.15** Passenger of 3- or 4- wheeled all-terrain vehicle (ATV) injured in traffic accident

  •⊗⑦**V86.16** Passenger of dirt bike or motor/cross bike injured in traffic accident

  ⊗⑦**V86.19** Passenger of other special all-terrain or other off-road motor vehicle injured in traffic accident

    Passenger of dirt bike injured in traffic accident

    Passenger of go cart injured in traffic accident

    Passenger of golf cart injured in traffic accident

V86.2 Person on outside of special all-terrain or other off-road motor vehicle injured in traffic accident

  ⊗⑦**V86.21** Person on outside of ambulance or fire engine injured in traffic accident

  ⊗⑦**V86.22** Person on outside of snowmobile injured in traffic accident

  ⊗⑦**V86.23** Person on outside of dune buggy injured in traffic accident

  ⊗⑦**V86.24** Person on outside of military vehicle injured in traffic accident

  •⊗⑦**V86.25** Person on outside of 3- or 4- wheeled all-terrain vehicle (ATV) injured in traffic accident

  •⊗⑦**V86.26** Person on outside of dirt bike or motor/cross bike injured in traffic accident

  ⊗⑦**V86.29** Person on outside of other special all-terrain or other off-road motor vehicle injured in traffic accident

    Person on outside of dirt bike injured in traffic accident

    Person on outside of go cart in traffic accident

    Person on outside of golf cart injured in traffic accident

V86.3 Unspecified occupant of special all-terrain or other off-road motor vehicle injured in traffic accident

  ⊗⑦**V86.31** Unspecified occupant of ambulance or fire engine injured in traffic accident

  ⊗⑦**V86.32** Unspecified occupant of snowmobile injured in traffic accident

  ⊗⑦**V86.33** Unspecified occupant of dune buggy injured in traffic accident

  ⊗⑦**V86.34** Unspecified occupant of military vehicle injured in traffic accident

  •⊗⑦**V86.35** Unspecified occupant of 3- or 4- wheeled all-terrain vehicle (ATV) injured in traffic accident

  •⊗⑦**V86.36** Unspecified occupant of dirt bike or motor/cross bike injured in traffic accident

  ⊗⑦**V86.39** Unspecified occupant of other special all-terrain or other off-road motor vehicle injured in traffic accident

    Unspecified occupant of dirt bike injured in traffic accident

    Unspecified occupant of go cart injured in traffic accident

    Unspecified occupant of golf cart injured in traffic accident

V86.4 Person injured while boarding or alighting from special all-terrain or other off-road motor vehicle

  ⊗⑦**V86.41** Person injured while boarding or alighting from ambulance or fire engine

  ⊗⑦**V86.42** Person injured while boarding or alighting from snowmobile

  ⊗⑦**V86.43** Person injured while boarding or alighting from dune buggy

  ⊗⑦**V86.44** Person injured while boarding or alighting from military vehicle

  •⊗⑦**V86.45** Person injured while boarding or alighting from a 3- or 4- wheeled all-terrain vehicle (ATV)

  •⊗⑦**V86.46** Person injured while boarding or alighting from a dirt bike or motor/cross bike

  ⊗⑦**V86.49** Person injured while boarding or alighting from other special all-terrain or other off-road motor vehicle

    Person injured while boarding or alighting from dirt bike

    Person injured while boarding or alighting from go cart

    Person injured while boarding or alighting from golf cart

V86.5 Driver of special all-terrain or other off-road motor vehicle injured in nontraffic accident

⊗⑦**V86.51** Driver of ambulance or fire engine injured in nontraffic accident

⊗⑦**V86.52** Driver of snowmobile injured in nontraffic accident

⊗⑦**V86.53** Driver of dune buggy injured in nontraffic accident

⊗⑦**V86.54** Driver of military vehicle injured in nontraffic accident

•⊗⑦**V86.55** Driver of 3- or 4- wheeled all-terrain vehicle (ATV) injured in nontraffic accident

•⊗⑦**V86.56** Driver of dirt bike or motor/cross bike injured in nontraffic accident

⊗⑦**V86.59** Driver of other special all-terrain or other off-road motor vehicle injured in nontraffic accident

Driver of dirt bike injured in nontraffic accident

Driver of go cart injured in nontraffic accident

Driver of golf cart injured in nontraffic accident

V86.6 Passenger of special all-terrain or other off-road motor vehicle injured in nontraffic accident

⊗⑦**V86.61** Passenger of ambulance or fire engine injured in nontraffic accident

⊗⑦**V86.62** Passenger of snowmobile injured in nontraffic accident

⊗⑦**V86.63** Passenger of dune buggy injured in nontraffic accident

⊗⑦**V86.64** Passenger of military vehicle injured in nontraffic accident

•⊗⑦**V86.65** Passenger of 3- or 4- wheeled all-terrain vehicle (ATV) injured in nontraffic accident

•⊗⑦**V86.66** Passenger of dirt bike or motor/cross bike injured in nontraffic accident

⊗⑦**V86.69** Passenger of other special all-terrain or other off-road motor vehicle injured in nontraffic accident

Passenger of dirt bike injured in nontraffic accident

Passenger of go cart injured in nontraffic accident

Passenger of golf cart injured in nontraffic accident

V86.7 Person on outside of special all-terrain or other off-road motor vehicle injured in nontraffic accident

⊗⑦**V86.71** Person on outside of ambulance or fire engine injured in nontraffic accident

⊗⑦**V86.72** Person on outside of snowmobile injured in nontraffic accident

⊗⑦**V86.73** Person on outside of dune buggy injured in nontraffic accident

⊗⑦**V86.74** Person on outside of military vehicle injured in nontraffic accident

•⊗⑦**V86.75** Person on outside of 3- or 4- wheeled all-terrain vehicle (ATV) injured in nontraffic accident

•⊗⑦**V86.76** Person on outside of dirt bike or motor/cross bike injured in nontraffic accident

⊗⑦**V86.79** Person on outside of other special all-terrain or other off-road motor vehicles injured in nontraffic accident

Person on outside of dirt bike injured in nontraffic accident

Person on outside of go cart injured in nontraffic accident

Person on outside of golf cart injured in nontraffic accident

V86.9 Unspecified occupant of special all-terrain or other off-road motor vehicle injured in nontraffic accident

⊗⑦**V86.91** Unspecified occupant of ambulance or fire engine injured in nontraffic accident

⊗⑦**V86.92** Unspecified occupant of snowmobile injured in nontraffic accident

⊗⑦**V86.93** Unspecified occupant of dune buggy injured in nontraffic accident

⊗⑦**V86.94** Unspecified occupant of military vehicle injured in nontraffic accident

•⊗⑦**V86.95** Unspecified occupant of 3- or 4- wheeled all-terrain vehicle (ATV) injured in nontraffic accident

•⊗⑦**V86.96** Unspecified occupant of dirt bike or motor/cross bike injured in nontraffic accident

⊗⑦**V86.99** Unspecified occupant of other special all-terrain or other off-road motor vehicle injured in nontraffic accident

Off-road motor-vehicle accident NOS

Other motor-vehicle accident NOS

Unspecified occupant of go cart injured in nontraffic accident

Unspecified occupant of golf cart injured in nontraffic accident

V87 Traffic accident of specified type but victim's mode of transport unknown

Excludes1: collision involving:

pedal cycle (V10-V19)

pedestrian (V01-V09)

The appropriate 7th character is to be added to each code from category V87

A - initial encounter

D - subsequent encounter

S - sequela

⊗⑦**V87.0** Person injured in collision between car and two- or three-wheeled powered vehicle (traffic)

⊗⑦**V87.1** Person injured in collision between other motor vehicle and two- or three-wheeled motor vehicle (traffic)

⊗⑦**V87.2** Person injured in collision between car and pick-up truck or van (traffic)

⊗⑦**V87.3** Person injured in collision between car and bus (traffic)

⊗⑦**V87.4** Person injured in collision between car and heavy transport vehicle (traffic)

⊗⑦**V87.5** Person injured in collision between heavy transport vehicle and bus (traffic)

⊗⑦**V87.6** Person injured in collision between railway train or railway vehicle and car (traffic)

⊗⑦**V87.7** Person injured in collision between other specified motor vehicles (traffic)

⊗⑦**V87.8** Person injured in other specified noncollision transport accidents involving motor vehicle (traffic)

⊗⑦**V87.9** Person injured in other specified (collision)(noncollision) transport accidents involving nonmotor vehicle (traffic)

V88 Nontraffic accident of specified type but victim's mode of transport unknown

Excludes1: collision involving:

pedal cycle (V10-V19)

pedestrian (V01-V09)

The appropriate 7th character is to be added to each code from category V88

A - initial encounter

D - subsequent encounter

S - sequela

V88.0 **Person injured in collision between car and two- or three-wheeled motor vehicle, nontraffic**

⊗⑦**V88.1** **Person injured in collision between other motor vehicle and two- or three-wheeled motor vehicle, nontraffic**

⊗⑦**V88.2** **Person injured in collision between car and pick-up truck or van, nontraffic**

⊗⑦**V88.3** **Person injured in collision between car and bus, nontraffic**

⊗⑦**V88.4** **Person injured in collision between car and heavy transport vehicle, nontraffic**

⊗⑦**V88.5** **Person injured in collision between heavy transport vehicle and bus, nontraffic**

⊗⑦**V88.6** **Person injured in collision between railway train or railway vehicle and car, nontraffic**

⊗⑦**V88.7** **Person injured in collision between other specified motor vehicle, nontraffic**

⊗⑦**V88.8** **Person injured in other specified noncollision transport accidents involving motor vehicle, nontraffic**

⊗⑦**V88.9** **Person injured in other specified (collision)(noncollision) transport accidents involving nonmotor vehicle, nontraffic**

V89 **Motor- or nonmotor-vehicle accident, type of vehicle unspecified**

The appropriate 7th character is to be added to each code from category V89

A - initial encounter

D - subsequent encounter

S - sequela

⊗⑦**V89.0** **Person injured in unspecified motor-vehicle accident, nontraffic**

Motor-vehicle accident NOS, nontraffic

⊗⑦**V89.1** **Person injured in unspecified nonmotor-vehicle accident, nontraffic**

Nonmotor-vehicle accident NOS (nontraffic)

⊗⑦**V89.2** **Person injured in unspecified motor-vehicle accident, traffic**

Motor-vehicle accident [MVA] NOS

Road (traffic) accident [RTA] NOS

⊗⑦**V89.3** **Person injured in unspecified nonmotor-vehicle accident, traffic**

Nonmotor-vehicle traffic accident NOS

⊗⑦**V89.9** **Person injured in unspecified vehicle accident**

Collision NOS

WATER TRANSPORT ACCIDENTS (V90-V94)

V90 **Drowning and submersion due to accident to watercraft**

Excludes1: civilian water transport accident involving military watercraft (V94.81-)

fall into water not from watercraft (W16.-)

military watercraft accident in military or war operations (Y36.0-, Y37.0-)

water-transport-related drowning or submersion without accident to watercraft (V92.-)

The appropriate 7th character is to be added to each code from category V90

A - initial encounter

D - subsequent encounter

S - sequela

V90.0 **Drowning and submersion due to watercraft overturning**

⊗⑦**V90.00** **Drowning and submersion due to merchant ship overturning**

⊗⑦**V90.01** **Drowning and submersion due to passenger ship overturning**

Drowning and submersion due to Ferry-boat overturning

Drowning and submersion due to Liner overturning

⊗⑦**V90.02** **Drowning and submersion due to fishing boat overturning**

⊗⑦**V90.03** **Drowning and submersion due to other powered watercraft overturning**

Drowning and submersion due to Hovercraft (on open water) overturning

Drowning and submersion due to Jet ski overturning

⊗⑦**V90.04** **Drowning and submersion due to sailboat overturning**

⊗⑦**V90.05** **Drowning and submersion due to canoe or kayak overturning**

⊗⑦**V90.06** **Drowning and submersion due to (nonpowered) inflatable craft overturning**

⊗⑦**V90.08** **Drowning and submersion due to other unpowered watercraft overturning**

Drowning and submersion due to windsurfer overturning

⊗⑦**V90.09** **Drowning and submersion due to unspecified watercraft overturning**

Drowning and submersion due to boat NOS overturning

Drowning and submersion due to ship NOS overturning

Drowning and submersion due to watercraft NOS overturning

V90.1 **Drowning and submersion due to watercraft sinking**

⊗⑦**V90.10** **Drowning and submersion due to merchant ship sinking**

⊗⑦**V90.11** **Drowning and submersion due to passenger ship sinking**

Drowning and submersion due to Ferry-boat sinking

Drowning and submersion due to Liner sinking

⊗⑦**V90.12** **Drowning and submersion due to fishing boat sinking**

⊗⑦**V90.13** **Drowning and submersion due to other powered watercraft sinking**

Drowning and submersion due to Hovercraft (on open water) sinking

Drowning and submersion due to Jet ski sinking

⊗⑦**V90.14** **Drowning and submersion due to sailboat sinking**

⊗⑦**V90.15** **Drowning and submersion due to canoe or kayak sinking**

⊗⑦**V90.16** **Drowning and submersion due to (nonpowered) inflatable craft sinking**

�| Add 4th-7th digits		Nonspecific code	Unspecified code	Manifestation code

⊗⑦**V90.18** **Drowning and submersion due to other unpowered watercraft sinking**

⊗⑦**V90.19** **Drowning and submersion due to unspecified watercraft sinking**

Drowning and submersion due to boat NOS sinking

Drowning and submersion due to ship NOS sinking

Drowning and submersion due to watercraft NOS sinking

V90.2 **Drowning and submersion due to falling or jumping from burning watercraft**

⊗⑦**V90.20** **Drowning and submersion due to falling or jumping from burning merchant ship**

⊗⑦**V90.21** **Drowning and submersion due to falling or jumping from burning passenger ship**

Drowning and submersion due to falling or jumping from burning Ferry-boat

Drowning and submersion due to falling or jumping from burning Liner

⊗⑦**V90.22** **Drowning and submersion due to falling or jumping from burning fishing boat**

⊗⑦**V90.23** **Drowning and submersion due to falling or jumping from other burning powered watercraft**

Drowning and submersion due to falling and jumping from burning Hovercraft (on open water)

Drowning and submersion due to falling and jumping from burning Jet ski

⊗⑦**V90.24** **Drowning and submersion due to falling or jumping from burning sailboat**

⊗⑦**V90.25** **Drowning and submersion due to falling or jumping from burning canoe or kayak**

⊗⑦**V90.26** **Drowning and submersion due to falling or jumping from burning (nonpowered) inflatable craft**

⊗⑦**V90.27** **Drowning and submersion due to falling or jumping from burning water-skis**

⊗⑦**V90.28** **Drowning and submersion due to falling or jumping from other burning unpowered watercraft**

Drowning and submersion due to falling and jumping from burning surf-board

Drowning and submersion due to falling and jumping from burning windsurfer

⊗⑦**V90.29** **Drowning and submersion due to falling or jumping from unspecified burning watercraft**

Drowning and submersion due to falling or jumping from burning boat NOS

Drowning and submersion due to falling or jumping from burning ship NOS

Drowning and submersion due to falling or jumping from burning watercraft NOS

V90.3 **Drowning and submersion due to falling or jumping from crushed watercraft**

⊗⑦**V90.30** **Drowning and submersion due to falling or jumping from crushed merchant ship**

⊗⑦**V90.31** **Drowning and submersion due to falling or jumping from crushed passenger ship**

Drowning and submersion due to falling and jumping from crushed Ferry boat

Drowning and submersion due to falling and jumping from crushed Liner

⊗⑦**V90.32** **Drowning and submersion due to falling or jumping from crushed fishing boat**

⊗⑦**V90.33** **Drowning and submersion due to falling or jumping from other crushed powered watercraft**

Drowning and submersion due to falling and jumping from crushed Hovercraft

Drowning and submersion due to falling and jumping from crushed Jet ski

⊗⑦**V90.34** **Drowning and submersion due to falling or jumping from crushed sailboat**

⊗⑦**V90.35** **Drowning and submersion due to falling or jumping from crushed canoe or kayak**

⊗⑦**V90.36** **Drowning and submersion due to falling or jumping from crushed (nonpowered) inflatable craft**

⊗⑦**V90.37** **Drowning and submersion due to falling or jumping from crushed water-skis**

⊗⑦**V90.38** **Drowning and submersion due to falling or jumping from other crushed unpowered watercraft**

Drowning and submersion due to falling and jumping from crushed surf-board

Drowning and submersion due to falling and jumping from crushed windsurfer

⊗⑦**V90.39** **Drowning and submersion due to falling or jumping from crushed unspecified watercraft**

Drowning and submersion due to falling and jumping from crushed boat NOS

Drowning and submersion due to falling and jumping from crushed ship NOS

Drowning and submersion due to falling and jumping from crushed watercraft NOS

V90.8 **Drowning and submersion due to other accident to watercraft**

⊗⑦**V90.80** **Drowning and submersion due to other accident to merchant ship**

⊗⑦**V90.81** **Drowning and submersion due to other accident to passenger ship**

Drowning and submersion due to other accident to Ferry-boat

Drowning and submersion due to other accident to Liner

⊗⑦**V90.82** **Drowning and submersion due to other accident to fishing boat**

⊗⑦**V90.83** **Drowning and submersion due to other accident to other powered watercraft**

Drowning and submersion due to other accident to Hovercraft (on open water)

Drowning and submersion due to other accident to Jet ski

⊗⑦**V90.84** **Drowning and submersion due to other accident to sailboat**

⊗⑦**V90.85** **Drowning and submersion due to other accident to canoe or kayak**

⊗⑦**V90.86** **Drowning and submersion due to other accident to (nonpowered) inflatable craft**

⊗⑦**V90.87** **Drowning and submersion due to other accident to water-skis**

⊗⑦**V90.88** **Drowning and submersion due to other accident to other unpowered watercraft**

Drowning and submersion due to other accident to surf-board

● New code   ▲ Revised code   **Excludes1:** Not coded here   **Excludes2:** Not included here   ⊗ Placeholder required   ⑦ 7ᵗʰ digit required

Drowning and submersion due **to other accident to windsurfer**

⊗⑦**V90.89** **Drowning and submersion due to other accident to unspecified watercraft**

Drowning and submersion due **to other accident to boat NOS**

Drowning and submersion due **to other accident to ship NOS**

Drowning and submersion due **to other accident to watercraft NOS**

V91 **Other injury due to accident to watercraft**

Includes: any injury except drowning and submersion as a result of an accident to watercraft

Excludes1: civilian water transport accident involving military watercraft (V94.81-)

military watercraft accident in military or war operations (Y36, Y37.-)

Excludes2: drowning and submersion due to accident to watercraft (V90.-)

The appropriate 7th character is to be added to each code from category V91

A - initial encounter

D - subsequent encounter

S - sequela

V91.0 **Burn due to watercraft on fire**

Excludes1: burn from localized fire or explosion on board ship without accident to watercraft (V93.-)

⊗⑦**V91.00** **Burn due to merchant ship on fire**

⊗⑦**V91.01** **Burn due to passenger ship on fire**

Burn due to Ferry-boat on fire

Burn due to Liner on fire

⊗⑦**V91.02** **Burn due to fishing boat on fire**

⊗⑦**V91.03** **Burn due to other powered watercraft on fire**

Burn due to Hovercraft (on open water) on fire

Burn due to Jet ski on fire

⊗⑦**V91.04** **Burn due to sailboat on fire**

⊗⑦**V91.05** **Burn due to canoe or kayak on fire**

⊗⑦**V91.06** **Burn due to (nonpowered) inflatable craft on fire**

⊗⑦**V91.07** **Burn due to water-skis on fire**

⊗⑦**V91.08** **Burn due to other unpowered watercraft on fire**

⊗⑦**V91.09** **Burn due to unspecified watercraft on fire**

Burn due to boat NOS on fire

Burn due to ship NOS on fire

Burn due to watercraft NOS on fire

V91.1 **Crushed between watercraft and other watercraft or other object due to collision**

Crushed by lifeboat after abandoning ship in a collision

Note: select the specified type of watercraft that the victim was on at the time of the collision

⊗⑦**V91.10** **Crushed between merchant ship and other watercraft or other object due to collision**

⊗⑦**V91.11** **Crushed between passenger ship and other watercraft or other object due to collision**

Crushed between Ferry-boat and other watercraft or other object due to collision

Crushed between Liner and other watercraft or other object due to collision

⊗⑦**V91.12** **Crushed between fishing boat and other watercraft or other object due to collision**

⊗⑦**V91.13** **Crushed between other powered watercraft and other watercraft or other object due to collision**

Crushed between Hovercraft (on open water) and other watercraft or other object due to collision

Crushed between Jet ski and other watercraft or other object due to collision

⊗⑦**V91.14** **Crushed between sailboat and other watercraft or other object due to collision**

⊗⑦**V91.15** **Crushed between canoe or kayak and other watercraft or other object due to collision**

⊗⑦**V91.16** **Crushed between (nonpowered) inflatable craft and other watercraft or other object due to collision**

⊗⑦**V91.18** **Crushed between other unpowered watercraft and other watercraft or other object due to collision**

Crushed between surfboard and other watercraft or other object due to collision

Crushed between windsurfer and other watercraft or other object due to collision

⊗⑦**V91.19** **Crushed between unspecified watercraft and other watercraft or other object due to collision**

Crushed between boat NOS and other watercraft or other object due to collision

Crushed between ship NOS and other watercraft or other object due to collision

Crushed between watercraft NOS and other watercraft or other object due to collision

V91.2 **Fall due to collision between watercraft and other watercraft or other object**

Fall while remaining on watercraft after collision

Note: select the specified type of watercraft that the victim was on at the time of the collision

Excludes1: crushed between watercraft and other watercraft and other object due to collision (V91.1-)

drowning and submersion due to falling from crushed watercraft (V90.3-)

⊗⑦**V91.20** **Fall due to collision between merchant ship and other watercraft or other object**

⊗⑦**V91.21** **Fall due to collision between passenger ship and other watercraft or other object**

Fall due to collision between Ferry-boat and other watercraft or other object

Fall due to collision between Liner and other watercraft or other object

⊗⑦**V91.22** **Fall due to collision between fishing boat and other watercraft or other object**

⊗⑦**V91.23** **Fall due to collision between other powered watercraft and other watercraft or other object**

Fall due to collision between Hovercraft (on open water) and other watercraft or other object

Fall due to collision between Jet ski and other watercraft or other object

⊗⑦**V91.24** **Fall due to collision between sailboat and other watercraft or other object**

⊗⑦**V91.25** **Fall due to collision between canoe or kayak and other watercraft or other object**

⊗⑦**V91.26** Fall due to collision between (nonpowered) inflatable craft and other watercraft or other object

⊗⑦**V91.29** Fall due to collision between unspecified watercraft and other watercraft or other object

Fall due to collision between boat NOS and other watercraft or other object

Fall due to collision between ship NOS and other watercraft or other object

Fall due to collision between watercraft NOS and other watercraft or other object

V91.3 **Hit or struck by falling object due to accident to watercraft**

Hit or struck by falling object (part of damaged watercraft or other object) after falling or jumping from damaged watercraft

Excludes2: drowning or submersion due to fall or jumping from damaged watercraft (V90.2-, V90.3-)

⊗⑦**V91.30** Hit or struck by falling object due to accident to merchant ship

⊗⑦**V91.31** Hit or struck by falling object due to accident to passenger ship

Hit or struck by falling object due to accident to Ferry-boat

Hit or struck by falling object due to accident to Liner

⊗⑦**V91.32** Hit or struck by falling object due to accident to fishing boat

⊗⑦**V91.33** Hit or struck by falling object due to accident to other powered watercraft

Hit or struck by falling object due to accident to Hovercraft (on open water)

Hit or struck by falling object due to accident to Jet ski

⊗⑦**V91.34** Hit or struck by falling object due to accident to sailboat

⊗⑦**V91.35** Hit or struck by falling object due to accident to canoe or kayak

⊗⑦**V91.36** Hit or struck by falling object due to accident to (nonpowered) inflatable craft

⊗⑦**V91.37** Hit or struck by falling object due to accident to water-skis

Hit by water-skis after jumping off of waterskis

⊗⑦**V91.38** Hit or struck by falling object due to accident to other unpowered watercraft

Hit or struck by surf-board after falling off damaged surf-board

Hit or struck by object after falling off damaged windsurfer

⊗⑦**V91.39** Hit or struck by falling object due to accident to unspecified watercraft

Hit or struck by falling object due to accident to boat NOS

Hit or struck by falling object due to accident to ship NOS

Hit or struck by falling object due to accident to watercraft NOS

V91.8 **Other injury due to other accident to watercraft**

⊗⑦**V91.80** Other injury due to other accident to merchant ship

⊗⑦**V91.81** Other injury due to other accident to passenger ship

Other injury due to other accident to Ferry-boat Other injury due to other accident to Liner

⊗⑦**V91.82** Other injury due to other accident to fishing boat

⊗⑦**V91.83** Other injury due to other accident to other powered watercraft

Other injury due to other accident to Hovercraft (on open water)

Other injury due to other accident to Jet ski

⊗⑦**V91.84** Other injury due to other accident to sailboat

⊗⑦**V91.85** Other injury due to other accident to canoe or kayak

⊗⑦**V91.86** Other injury due to other accident to (nonpowered) inflatable craft

⊗⑦**V91.87** Other injury due to other accident to water-skis

⊗⑦**V91.88** Other injury due to other accident to other unpowered watercraft

Other injury due to other accident to surf-board

Other injury due to other accident to windsurfer

⊗⑦**V91.89** Other injury due to other accident to unspecified watercraft

Other injury due to other accident to boat NOS

Other injury due to other accident to ship NOS

Other injury due to other accident to watercraft NOS

V92 **Drowning and submersion due to accident on board watercraft, without accident to watercraft**

Excludes1: civilian water transport accident involving military watercraft (V94.81-)

drowning or submersion due to accident to watercraft (V90-V91)

drowning or submersion of diver who voluntarily jumps from boat not involved in an accident (W16.711, W16.721)

fall into water without watercraft (W16.-)

military watercraft accident in military or war operations (Y36, Y37)

The appropriate 7th character is to be added to each code from category V92

A - initial encounter

D - subsequent encounter

S - sequela

V92.0 **Drowning and submersion due to fall off watercraft**

Drowning and submersion due to fall from gangplank of watercraft

Drowning and submersion due to fall overboard watercraft

Excludes2: hitting head on object or bottom of body of water due to fall from watercraft (V94.0-)

⊗⑦**V92.00** Drowning and submersion due to fall off merchant ship

⊗⑦**V92.01** Drowning and submersion due to fall off passenger ship

Drowning and submersion due to fall off Ferry-boat

Drowning and submersion due to fall off Liner

⊗⑦**V92.02** Drowning and submersion due to fall off fishing boat

⊗⑦**V92.03** **Drowning and submersion due to fall off other powered watercraft**

Drowning and submersion due to fall off Hovercraft (on open water)

Drowning and submersion due to fall off Jet ski

⊗⑦**V92.04** **Drowning and submersion due to fall off sailboat**

⊗⑦**V92.05** **Drowning and submersion due to fall off canoe or kayak**

⊗⑦**V92.06** **Drowning and submersion due to fall off (nonpowered) inflatable craft**

⊗⑦**V92.07** **Drowning and submersion due to fall off water-skis**

Excludes1: drowning and submersion due to falling off burning water-skis (V90.27)

drowning and submersion due to falling off crushed water-skis (V90.37)

hit by boat while water-skiing NOS (V94.X)

⊗⑦**V92.08** **Drowning and submersion due to fall off other unpowered watercraft**

Drowning and submersion due to fall off surf-board

Drowning and submersion due to fall off windsurfer

Excludes1: drowning and submersion due to fall off burning unpowered watercraft (V90.28)

drowning and submersion due to fall off crushed unpowered watercraft (V90.38)

drowning and submersion due to fall off damaged unpowered watercraft (V90.88)

drowning and submersion due to rider of nonpowered watercraft being hit by other watercraft (V94.-)

Other injury due to rider of nonpowered watercraft being hit by other watercraft (V94.-)

⊗⑦**V92.09** **Drowning and submersion due to fall off unspecified watercraft**

Drowning and submersion due to fall off boat NOS

Drowning and submersion due to fall off ship

Drowning and submersion due to fall off watercraft NOS

V92.1 **Drowning and submersion due to being thrown overboard by motion of watercraft**

Excludes1: drowning and submersion due to fall off surf-board (V92.08)

drowning and submersion due to fall off water-skis (V92.07)

drowning and submersion due to fall off windsurfer (V92.08)

⊗⑦**V92.10** **Drowning and submersion due to being thrown overboard by motion of merchant ship**

⊗⑦**V92.11** **Drowning and submersion due to being thrown overboard by motion of passenger ship**

Drowning and submersion due to being thrown overboard by motion of Ferry-boat

Drowning and submersion due to being thrown overboard by motion of Liner

⊗⑦**V92.12** **Drowning and submersion due to being thrown overboard by motion of fishing boat**

⊗⑦**V92.13** **Drowning and submersion due to being thrown overboard by motion of other powered watercraft**

Drowning and submersion due to being thrown overboard by motion of Hovercraft

⊗⑦**V92.14** **Drowning and submersion due to being thrown overboard by motion of sailboat**

⊗⑦**V92.15** **Drowning and submersion due to being thrown overboard by motion of canoe or kayak**

⊗⑦**V92.16** **Drowning and submersion due to being thrown overboard by motion of (nonpowered) inflatable craft**

⊗⑦**V92.19** **Drowning and submersion due to being thrown overboard by motion of unspecified watercraft**

Drowning and submersion due to being thrown overboard by motion of boat NOS

Drowning and submersion due to being thrown overboard by motion of ship NOS

Drowning and submersion due to being thrown overboard by motion of watercraft NOS

V92.2 **Drowning and submersion due to being washed overboard from watercraft**

Code first any associated cataclysm (X37.0-)

⊗⑦**V92.20** **Drowning and submersion due to being washed overboard from merchant ship**

⊗⑦**V92.21** **Drowning and submersion due to being washed overboard from passenger ship**

Drowning and submersion due to being washed overboard from Ferry-boat

Drowning and submersion due to being washed overboard from Liner

⊗⑦**V92.22** **Drowning and submersion due to being washed overboard from fishing boat**

⊗⑦**V92.23** **Drowning and submersion due to being washed overboard from other powered watercraft**

Drowning and submersion due to being washed overboard from Hovercraft (on open water)

Drowning and submersion due to being washed overboard from Jet ski

⊗⑦**V92.24** **Drowning and submersion due to being washed overboard from sailboat**

⊗⑦**V92.25** **Drowning and submersion due to being washed overboard from canoe or kayak**

⊗⑦**V92.26** **Drowning and submersion due to being washed overboard from (nonpowered) inflatable craft**

⊗⑦**V92.27** **Drowning and submersion due to being washed overboard from water-skis**

Excludes1: drowning and submersion due to fall off water-skis (V92.07)

⊗⑦**V92.28** **Drowning and submersion due to being washed overboard from other unpowered watercraft**

Drowning and submersion due to being washed overboard from surf-board

Drowning and submersion due to being washed overboard from windsurfer

▓ Add 4th-7th digits	▓ Nonspecific code	▓ Unspecified code	▓ Manifestation code

⊗⑦**V92.29** **Drowning and submersion due to being washed overboard from unspecified watercraft**

Drowning and submersion due to being washed overboard from boat NOS

Drowning and submersion due to being washed overboard from ship NOS

Drowning and submersion due to being washed overboard from watercraft NOS

V93 **Other injury due to accident on board watercraft, without accident to watercraft**

Excludes1: civilian water transport accident involving military watercraft (V94.81-)

Other injury due to accident to watercraft (V91.-)

military watercraft accident in military or war operations (Y36, Y37.-)

Excludes2: drowning and submersion due to accident on board watercraft, without accident to watercraft (V92.-)

The appropriate 7th character is to be added to each code from category V93

A - initial encounter

D - subsequent encounter

S - sequela

V93.0 **Burn due to localized fire on board watercraft**

Excludes1: burn due to watercraft on fire (V91.0-)

⊗⑦**V93.00** **Burn due to localized fire on board merchant vessel**

⊗⑦**V93.01** **Burn due to localized fire on board passenger vessel**

Burn due to localized fire on board Ferry-boat

Burn due to localized fire on board Liner

⊗⑦**V93.02** **Burn due to localized fire on board fishing boat**

⊗⑦**V93.03** **Burn due to localized fire on board other powered watercraft**

Burn due to localized fire on board Hovercraft

Burn due to localized fire on board Jet ski

⊗⑦**V93.04** **Burn due to localized fire on board sailboat**

⊗⑦**V93.09** **Burn due to localized fire on board unspecified watercraft**

Burn due to localized fire on board boat NOS

Burn due to localized fire on board ship NOS

Burn due to localized fire on board watercraft NOS

V93.1 **Other burn on board watercraft**

Burn due to source **Other** than fire on board watercraft

Excludes1: burn due to watercraft on fire (V91.0-)

⊗⑦**V93.10** **Other burn on board merchant vessel**

⊗⑦**V93.11** **Other burn on board passenger vessel**

Other burn on board Ferry-boat

Other burn on board Liner

⊗⑦**V93.12** **Other burn on board fishing boat**

⊗⑦**V93.13** **Other burn on board other powered watercraft**

Other burn on board Hovercraft

Other burn on board Jet ski

⊗⑦**V93.14** **Other burn on board sailboat**

⊗⑦**V93.19** **Other burn on board unspecified watercraft**

Other burn on board boat NOS

Other burn on board ship NOS

Other burn on board watercraft NOS

V93.2 **Heat exposure on board watercraft**

Excludes1: exposure to man-made heat not aboard watercraft (W92)

exposure to natural heat while on board watercraft (X30)

exposure to sunlight while on board watercraft (X32)

Excludes2: burn due to fire on board watercraft (V93.0-)

⊗⑦**V93.20** **Heat exposure on board merchant ship**

⊗⑦**V93.21** **Heat exposure on board passenger ship**

Heat exposure on board Ferry-boat

Heat exposure on board Liner

⊗⑦**V93.22** **Heat exposure on board fishing boat**

⊗⑦**V93.23** **Heat exposure on board other powered watercraft**

Heat exposure on board hovercraft

⊗⑦**V93.24** **Heat exposure on board sailboat**

⊗⑦**V93.29** **Heat exposure on board unspecified watercraft**

Heat exposure on board boat NOS

Heat exposure on board ship NOS

Heat exposure on board watercraft NOS

V93.3 **Fall on board watercraft**

Excludes1: fall due to collision of watercraft (V91.2-)

⊗⑦**V93.30** **Fall on board merchant ship**

⊗⑦**V93.31** **Fall on board passenger ship**

Fall on board Ferry-boat Fall on board Liner

⊗⑦**V93.32** **Fall on board fishing boat**

⊗⑦**V93.33** **Fall on board other powered watercraft**

Fall on board Hovercraft (on open water)

Fall on board Jet ski

⊗⑦**V93.34** **Fall on board sailboat**

⊗⑦**V93.35** **Fall on board canoe or kayak**

⊗⑦**V93.36** **Fall on board (nonpowered) inflatable craft**

⊗⑦**V93.38** **Fall on board other unpowered watercraft**

⊗⑦**V93.39** **Fall on board unspecified watercraft**

Fall on board boat NOS Fall on board ship NOS

Fall on board watercraft NOS

V93.4 **Struck by falling object on board watercraft**

Hit by falling object on board watercraft

Excludes1: struck by falling object due to accident to watercraft (V91.3)

⊗⑦**V93.40** **Struck by falling object on merchant ship**

⊗⑦**V93.41** **Struck by falling object on passenger ship**

Struck by falling object on Ferry-boat

Struck by falling object on Liner

⊗⑦**V93.42** **Struck by falling object on fishing boat**

⊗⑦**V93.43** **Struck by falling object on other powered watercraft**

Struck by falling object on Hovercraft

⊗⑦**V93.44** **Struck by falling object on sailboat**

⊗⑦**V93.48** **Struck by falling object on other unpowered watercraft**

⊗⑦**V93.49** **Struck by falling object on unspecified watercraft**

V93.5 **Explosion on board watercraft**

Boiler explosion on steamship

● New code ▲ Revised code **Excludes1:** Not coded here **Excludes2:** Not included here ⊗ Placeholder required ⑦ 7th digit required

Excludes2: fire on board watercraft (V93.0-)

⊗⑦**V93.50** **Explosion on board merchant ship**

⊗⑦**V93.51** **Explosion on board passenger ship**

Explosion on board Ferry-boat

Explosion on board Liner

⊗⑦**V93.52** **Explosion on board fishing boat**

⊗⑦**V93.53** **Explosion on board other powered watercraft**

Explosion on board Hovercraft

Explosion on board Jet ski

⊗⑦**V93.54** **Explosion on board sailboat**

⊗⑦**V93.59** **Explosion on board unspecified watercraft**

Explosion on board boat NOS

Explosion on board ship NOS

Explosion on board watercraft NOS

V93.6 Machinery accident on board watercraft

Excludes1: machinery explosion on board watercraft (V93.4-)

machinery fire on board watercraft (V93.0-)

⊗⑦**V93.60** **Machinery accident on board merchant ship**

⊗⑦**V93.61** **Machinery accident on board passenger ship**

Machinery accident on board Ferry-boat

Machinery accident on board Liner

⊗⑦**V93.62** **Machinery accident on board fishing boat**

⊗⑦**V93.63** **Machinery accident on board other powered watercraft**

Machinery accident on board Hovercraft

⊗⑦**V93.64** **Machinery accident on board sailboat**

⊗⑦**V93.69** **Machinery accident on board unspecified watercraft**

Machinery accident on board boat NOS

Machinery accident on board ship NOS

Machinery accident on board watercraft NOS

V93.8 Other injury due to other accident on board watercraft

Accidental poisoning by gases or fumes on watercraft

⊗⑦**V93.80** **Other injury due to other accident on board merchant ship**

⊗⑦**V93.81** **Other injury due to other accident on board passenger ship**

Other injury due to other accident on board Ferry-boat

Other injury due to other accident on board Liner

⊗⑦**V93.82** **Other injury due to other accident on board fishing boat**

⊗⑦**V93.83** **Other injury due to other accident on board other powered watercraft**

Other injury due to other accident on board Hovercraft

Other injury due to other accident on board Jet ski

⊗⑦**V93.84** **Other injury due to other accident on board sailboat**

⊗⑦**V93.85** **Other injury due to other accident on board canoe or kayak**

⊗⑦**V93.86** **Other injury due to other accident on board (nonpowered) inflatable craft**

⊗⑦**V93.87** **Other injury due to other accident on board water-skis**

Hit or struck by object while waterskiing

⊗⑦**V93.88** **Other injury due to other accident on board other unpowered watercraft**

Hit or struck by object while surfing

Hit or struck by object while on board windsurfer

⊗⑦**V93.89** **Other injury due to other accident on board unspecified watercraft**

Other injury due to other accident on board boat NOS

Other injury due to other accident on board ship NOS

Other injury due to other accident on board watercraft NOS

V94 Other and unspecified water transport accidents

Excludes1: military watercraft accidents in military or war operations (Y36, Y37)

The appropriate 7th character is to be added to each code from category V94

A - initial encounter

D - subsequent encounter

S - sequela

⊗⑦**V94.0** **Hitting object or bottom of body of water due to fall from watercraft**

Excludes2: drowning and submersion due to fall from watercraft (V92.0-)

⊗⑦**V94.1** **Bather struck by watercraft**

Swimmer hit by watercraft

⊗⑦**V94.11** **Bather struck by powered watercraft**

⊗⑦**V94.12** **Bather struck by nonpowered watercraft**

V94.2 Rider of nonpowered watercraft struck by other watercraft

⊗⑦**V94.21** **Rider of nonpowered watercraft struck by other nonpowered watercraft**

Canoer hit by other nonpowered watercraft

Surfer hit by other nonpowered watercraft

Windsurfer hit by other nonpowered watercraft

⊗⑦**V94.22** **Rider of nonpowered watercraft struck by powered watercraft**

Canoer hit by motorboat

Surfer hit by motorboat

Windsurfer hit by motorboat

V94.3 Injury to rider of (inflatable) watercraft being pulled behind other watercraft

⊗⑦**V94.31** **Injury to rider of (inflatable) recreational watercraft being pulled behind other watercraft**

Injury to rider of inner-tube pulled behind motor boat

⊗⑦**V94.32** **Injury to rider of non-recreational watercraft being pulled behind other watercraft**

Injury to occupant of dingy being pulled behind boat or ship

Injury to occupant of life-raft being pulled behind boat or ship

⊗⑦**V94.4 Injury to barefoot water-skier**

Injury to person being pulled behind boat or ship

V94.8 Other water transport accident

V94.81 **Water transport accident involving military watercraft**

⑦ **V94.810 Civilian watercraft involved in water transport accident with military watercraft**

Passenger on civilian watercraft injured due to accident with military watercraft

⑦ **V94.811 Civilian in water injured by military watercraft**

⑦ **V94.818 Other water transport accident involving military watercraft**

⊗⑦ **V94.89 Other water transport accident**

⊗⑦ **V94.9 Unspecified water transport accident**

Water transport accident NOS

AIR AND SPACE TRANSPORT ACCIDENTS (V95-V97)

Excludes1: military aircraft accidents in military or war operations (Y36, Y37)

V95 Accident to powered aircraft causing injury to occupant

The appropriate 7th character is to be added to each code from category V95

A - initial encounter

D - subsequent encounter

S - sequela

V95.0 Helicopter accident injuring occupant

⊗⑦ **V95.00 Unspecified helicopter accident injuring occupant**

⊗⑦ **V95.01 Helicopter crash injuring occupant**

⊗⑦ **V95.02 Forced landing of helicopter injuring occupant**

⊗⑦ **V95.03 Helicopter collision injuring occupant**

Helicopter collision with any object, fixed, movable or moving

⊗⑦ **V95.04 Helicopter fire injuring occupant**

⊗⑦ **V95.05 Helicopter explosion injuring occupant**

⊗⑦ **V95.09 Other helicopter accident injuring occupant**

V95.1 Ultralight, microlight or powered-glider accident injuring occupant

⊗⑦ **V95.10 Unspecified ultralight, microlight or powered-glider accident injuring occupant**

⊗⑦ **V95.11 Ultralight, microlight or powered-glider crash injuring occupant**

⊗⑦ **V95.12 Forced landing of ultralight, microlight or powered-glider injuring occupant**

⊗⑦ **V95.13 Ultralight, microlight or powered-glider collision injuring occupant**

Ultralight, microlight or powered-glider collision with any object, fixed, movable or moving

⊗⑦ **V95.14 Ultralight, microlight or powered-glider fire injuring occupant**

⊗⑦ **V95.15 Ultralight, microlight or powered-glider explosion injuring occupant**

⊗⑦ **V95.19 Other ultralight, microlight or powered-glider accident injuring occupant**

V95.2 Other private fixed-wing aircraft accident injuring occupant

⊗⑦ **V95.20 Unspecified accident to other private fixed-wing aircraft, injuring occupant**

⊗⑦ **V95.21 Other private fixed-wing aircraft crash injuring occupant**

⊗⑦ **V95.22 Forced landing of other private fixed-wing aircraft injuring occupant**

⊗⑦ **V95.23 Other private fixed-wing aircraft collision injuring occupant**

Other private fixed-wing aircraft collision with any object, fixed, movable or moving

⊗⑦ **V95.24 Other private fixed-wing aircraft fire injuring occupant**

⊗⑦ **V95.25 Other private fixed-wing aircraft explosion injuring occupant**

⊗⑦ **V95.29 Other accident to other private fixed-wing aircraft injuring occupant**

V95.3 Commercial fixed-wing aircraft accident injuring occupant

⊗⑦ **V95.30 Unspecified accident to commercial fixed-wing aircraft injuring occupant**

⊗⑦ **V95.31 Commercial fixed-wing aircraft crash injuring occupant**

⊗⑦ **V95.32 Forced landing of commercial fixed-wing aircraft injuring occupant**

⊗⑦ **V95.33 Commercial fixed-wing aircraft collision injuring occupant**

Commercial fixed-wing aircraft collision with any object, fixed, movable or moving

⊗⑦ **V95.34 Commercial fixed-wing aircraft fire injuring occupant**

⊗⑦ **V95.35 Commercial fixed-wing aircraft explosion injuring occupant**

⊗⑦ **V95.39 Other accident to commercial fixed-wing aircraft injuring occupant**

V95.4 Spacecraft accident injuring occupant

⊗⑦ **V95.40 Unspecified spacecraft accident injuring occupant**

⊗⑦ **V95.41 Spacecraft crash injuring occupant**

⊗⑦ **V95.42 Forced landing of spacecraft injuring occupant**

⊗⑦ **V95.43 Spacecraft collision injuring occupant**

Spacecraft collision with any object, fixed, moveable or moving

⊗⑦ **V95.44 Spacecraft fire injuring occupant**

⊗⑦ **V95.45 Spacecraft explosion injuring occupant**

⊗⑦ **V95.49 Other spacecraft accident injuring occupant**

⊗⑦ **V95.8 Other powered aircraft accidents injuring occupant**

⊗⑦ **V95.9 Unspecified aircraft accident injuring occupant**

Aircraft accident NOS

Air transport accident NOS

V96 Accident to nonpowered aircraft causing injury to occupant

The appropriate 7th character is to be added to each code from category V96

A - initial encounter

D - subsequent encounter

S - sequela

V96.0 Balloon accident injuring occupant

⊗⑦ **V96.00 Unspecified balloon accident injuring occupant**

⊗⑦ **V96.01 Balloon crash injuring occupant**

⊗⑦ **V96.02 Forced landing of balloon injuring occupant**

⊗⑦ **V96.03 Balloon collision injuring occupant**

Balloon collision with any object, fixed, moveable or moving

⊗⑦ **V96.04 Balloon fire injuring occupant**

⊗⑦ **V96.05 Balloon explosion injuring occupant**

⊗⑦ **V96.09 Other balloon accident injuring occupant**

V96.1　　Hang-glider accident injuring occupant

⊗⑦**V96.10**　Unspecified hang-glider accident injuring occupant

⊗⑦V96.11　Hang-glider crash injuring occupant

⊗⑦V96.12　Forced landing of hang-glider injuring occupant

⊗⑦V96.13　Hang-glider collision injuring occupant

　　　　　Hang-glider collision with any object, fixed, moveable or moving

⊗⑦V96.14　Hang-glider fire injuring occupant

⊗⑦V96.15　Hang-glider explosion injuring occupant

⊗⑦**V96.19**　Other hang-glider accident injuring occupant

V96.2　　Glider (nonpowered) accident injuring occupant

⊗⑦V96.20　Unspecified glider (nonpowered) accident injuring occupant

⊗⑦V96.21　Glider (nonpowered) crash injuring occupant

⊗⑦V96.22　Forced landing of glider (nonpowered) injuring occupant

⊗⑦V96.23　Glider (nonpowered) collision injuring occupant

　　　　　Glider (nonpowered) collision with any object, fixed, moveable or moving

⊗⑦V96.24　Glider (nonpowered) fire injuring occupant

⊗⑦V96.25　Glider (nonpowered) explosion injuring occupant

⊗⑦**V96.29**　Other glider (nonpowered) accident injuring occupant

⊗⑦**V96.8**　Other nonpowered-aircraft accidents injuring occupant

　　　　　Kite carrying a person accident injuring occupant

⊗⑦**V96.9**　Unspecified nonpowered-aircraft accident injuring occupant

　　　　　Nonpowered-aircraft accident NOS

V97　Other specified air transport accidents

The appropriate 7th character is to be added to each code from category V97

A - initial encounter

D - subsequent encounter

S - sequela

⊗⑦**V97.0**　Occupant of aircraft injured in other specified air transport accidents

　　　　　Fall in, on or from aircraft in air transport accident

　　　　　Excludes1: accident while boarding or alighting aircraft (V97.1)

⊗⑦V97.1　Person injured while boarding or alighting from aircraft

V97.2　　Parachutist accident

⊗⑦V97.21　Parachutist entangled in object

　　　　　Parachutist landing in tree

⊗⑦V97.22　Parachutist injured on landing

⊗⑦**V97.29**　Other parachutist accident

V97.3　　Person on ground injured in air transport accident

⊗⑦V97.31　Hit by object falling from aircraft

　　　　　Hit by crashing aircraft

　　　　　Injured by aircraft hitting house

　　　　　Injured by aircraft hitting car

⊗⑦V97.32　Injured by rotating propeller

⊗⑦V97.33　Sucked into jet engine

⊗⑦**V97.39**　Other injury to person on ground due to air transport accident

⊗⑦V97.8　Other air transport accidents, not elsewhere classified

　　　　　Excludes1: aircraft accident NOS (V95.9)

　　　　　　　exposure to changes in air pressure during ascent or descent (W94.-)

V97.81　Air transport accident involving military aircraft

⑦V97.810　Civilian aircraft involved in air transport accident with military aircraft

　　　　　Passenger in civilian aircraft injured due to accident with military aircraft

⑦V97.811　Civilian injured by military aircraft

⑦**V97.818**　Other air transport accident involving military aircraft

⊗⑦**V97.89**　Other air transport accidents, not elsewhere classified

　　　　　Injury from machinery on aircraft

OTHER AND UNSPECIFIED TRANSPORT ACCIDENTS (V98-V99)

Excludes1: vehicle accident, type of vehicle unspecified (V89.-)

V98　Other specified transport accidents

The appropriate 7th character is to be added to each code from category V98

A - initial encounter

D - subsequent encounter

S - sequela

⊗⑦**V98.0**　Accident to, on or involving cable-car, not on rails

　　　　　Caught or dragged by cable-car, not on rails

　　　　　Fall or jump from cable-car, not on rails

　　　　　Object thrown from or in cable-car, not on rails

⊗⑦V98.1　Accident to, on or involving land-yacht

⊗⑦V98.2　Accident to, on or involving ice yacht

⊗⑦V98.3　Accident to, on or involving ski lift

　　　　　Accident to, on or involving ski chair-lift

　　　　　Accident to, on or involving ski-lift with gondola

⊗⑦**V98.8**　Other specified transport accidents

⊗⑦**V99**　Unspecified transport accident

The appropriate 7th character is to be added to code V99

A - initial encounter

D - subsequent encounter

S - sequela

OTHER EXTERNAL CAUSES OF ACCIDENTAL INJURY (W00-X58)

SLIPPING, TRIPPING, STUMBLING AND FALLS (W00-W19)

Excludes1: assault involving a fall (Y01-Y02)

　　　　fall from animal (V80.-)

　　　　fall (in) (from) machinery (in operation) (W28-W31)

　　　　fall (in) (from) transport vehicle (V01-V99)

　　　　intentional self-harm involving a fall (X80-X81)

Excludes2: at risk for fall (history of fall) Z91.81

　　　　fall (in) (from) burning building (X00.-)

　　　　fall into fire (X00-X04, X08)

W00 Fall due to ice and snow

Includes: pedestrian on foot falling (slipping) on ice and snow

Excludes1: fall on (from) ice and snow involving pedestrian conveyance (V00.-)

fall from stairs and steps not due to ice and snow (W10.-)

The appropriate 7th character is to be added to each code from category W00

A - initial encounter

D - subsequent encounter

S - sequela

⊗⑦**W00.0 Fall on same level due to ice and snow**

⊗⑦**W00.1 Fall from stairs and steps due to ice and snow**

⊗⑦**W00.2 Other fall from one level to another due to ice and snow**

⊗⑦**W00.9 Unspecified fall due to ice and snow**

W01 Fall on same level from slipping, tripping and stumbling

Includes: fall on moving sidewalk

Excludes1: fall due to bumping (striking) against object (W18.0-)

fall in shower or bathtub (W18.2-)

fall on same level NOS (W18.30)

fall on same level from slipping, tripping and stumbling due to ice or snow (W00.0)

fall off or from toilet (W18.1-)

slipping, tripping and stumbling NOS (W18.40)

slipping, tripping and stumbling without falling (W18.4-)

The appropriate 7th character is to be added to each code from category W01

A - initial encounter

D - subsequent encounter

S - sequela

⊗⑦**W01.0 Fall on same level from slipping, tripping and stumbling without subsequent striking against object**

Falling over animal

W01.1 Fall on same level from slipping, tripping and stumbling with subsequent striking against object

⊗⑦**W01.10 Fall on same level from slipping, tripping and stumbling with subsequent striking against unspecified object**

W01.11 Fall on same level from slipping, tripping and stumbling with subsequent striking against sharp object

⑦**W01.110 Fall on same level from slipping, tripping and stumbling with subsequent striking against sharp glass**

⑦**W01.111 Fall on same level from slipping, tripping and stumbling with subsequent striking against power tool or machine**

⑦**W01.118 Fall on same level from slipping, tripping and stumbling with subsequent striking against other sharp object**

⑦**W01.119 Fall on same level from slipping, tripping and stumbling with subsequent striking against unspecified sharp object**

W01.19 Fall on same level from slipping, tripping and stumbling with subsequent striking against other object

⑦**W01.190 Fall on same level from slipping, tripping and stumbling with**

subsequent striking against furniture

⑦**W01.198 Fall on same level from slipping, tripping and stumbling with subsequent striking against other object**

⊗⑦**W03 Other fall on same level due to collision with another person**

Fall due to non-transport collision **with other** person

Excludes1: collision with another person without fall (W51)

crushed or pushed by a crowd or human stampede (W52)

fall involving pedestrian conveyance (V00-V09)

fall due to ice or snow (W00)

fall on same level NOS (W18.30)

The appropriate 7th character is to be added to code W03

A - initial encounter

D - subsequent encounter

S - sequela

⊗⑦**W04 Fall while being carried or supported by other persons**

Accidentally dropped while being carried

The appropriate 7th character is to be added to code W04

A - initial encounter

D - subsequent encounter

S - sequela

W05 Fall from non-moving wheelchair, nonmotorized scooter and motorized mobility scooter

Excludes1: fall from moving wheelchair (powered) (V00.811)

fall from moving motorized mobility scooter (V00.831)

fall from nonmotorized scooter (V00.141)

The appropriate 7th character is to be added to each code from category W05

A - initial encounter

D - subsequent encounter

S - sequela

⊗⑦**W05.0 Fall from non-moving wheelchair**

⊗⑦**W05.1 Fall from non-moving nonmotorized scooter**

⊗⑦**W05.2 Fall from non-moving motorized mobility scooter**

⊗⑦**W06 Fall from bed**

The appropriate 7th character is to be added to code W06

A - initial encounter

D - subsequent encounter

S - sequela

⊗⑦**W07 Fall from chair**

The appropriate 7th character is to be added to code W07

A - initial encounter

D - subsequent encounter

S - sequela

⊗⑦**W08 Fall from other furniture**

The appropriate 7th character is to be added to code W08

A - initial encounter

D - subsequent encounter

S - sequela

W09 Fall on and from playground equipment

Excludes1: fall involving recreational machinery (W31)

The appropriate 7th character is to be added to each code from category W09

A - initial encounter

D - subsequent encounter

S - sequela

⊗⑦W09.0 **Fall on or from playground slide**

⊗⑦W09.1 **Fall from playground swing**

⊗⑦W09.2 **Fall on or from jungle gym**

⊗⑦W09.8 **Fall on or from other playground equipment**

W10 **Fall on and from stairs and steps**

Excludes1: Fall from stairs and steps due to ice and snow (W00.1)

The appropriate 7th character is to be added to each code from category W10

A - initial encounter

D - subsequent encounter

S - sequela

⊗⑦W10.0 **Fall (on)(from) escalator**

⊗⑦W10.1 **Fall (on)(from) sidewalk curb**

⊗⑦W10.2 **Fall (on)(from) incline**

Fall (on) (from) ramp

⊗⑦W10.8 **Fall (on) (from) other stairs and steps**

⊗⑦W10.9 **Fall (on) (from) unspecified stairs and steps**

⊗⑦W11 **Fall on and from ladder**

The appropriate 7th character is to be added to code W11

A - initial encounter

D - subsequent encounter

S - sequela

⊗⑦W12 **Fall on and from scaffolding**

The appropriate 7th character is to be added to code W12

A - initial encounter

D - subsequent encounter

S - sequela

W13 **Fall from, out of or through building or structure**

The appropriate 7th character is to be added to each code from category W13

A - initial encounter

D - subsequent encounter

S - sequela

⊗⑦W13.0 **Fall from, out of or through balcony**

Fall from, out of or through railing

⊗⑦W13.1 **Fall from, out of or through bridge**

⊗⑦W13.2 **Fall from, out of or through roof**

⊗⑦W13.3 **Fall through floor**

⊗⑦W13.4 **Fall from, out of or through window**

Excludes2: fall with subsequent striking against sharp glass (W01.110)

⊗⑦W13.8 **Fall from, out of or through other building or structure**

Fall from, out of or through viaduct

Fall from, out of or through wall

Fall from, out of or through flag-pole

⊗⑦W13.9 **Fall from, out of or through building, not otherwise specified**

Excludes1: collapse of a building or structure (W20.-)

fall or jump from burning building or structure (X00.-)

⊗⑦W14 **Fall from tree**

The appropriate 7th character is to be added to code W14

A - initial encounter

D - subsequent encounter

S - sequela

⊗⑦W15 **Fall from cliff**

The appropriate 7th character is to be added to code W15

A - initial encounter

D - subsequent encounter

S - sequela

W16 **Fall, jump or diving into water**

Excludes1: accidental non-watercraft drowning and submersion not involving fall (W65-W74)

effects of air pressure from diving (W94.-)

fall into water from watercraft (V90-V94)

hitting an object or against bottom when falling from watercraft (V94.0)

Excludes2: striking or hitting diving board (W21.4)

The appropriate 7th character is to be added to each code from category W16

A - initial encounter

D - subsequent encounter

S - sequela

W16.0 **Fall into swimming pool**

Fall into swimming pool NOS

Excludes1: fall into empty swimming pool (W17.3)

W16.01 **Fall into swimming pool striking water surface**

⑦W16.011 **Fall into swimming pool striking water surface causing drowning and submersion**

Excludes1: drowning and submersion while in swimming pool without fall (W67)

⑦W16.012 **Fall into swimming pool striking water surface causing other injury**

W16.02 **Fall into swimming pool striking bottom**

⑦W16.021 **Fall into swimming pool striking bottom causing drowning and submersion**

Excludes1: drowning and submersion while in swimming pool without fall (W67)

⑦W16.022 **Fall into swimming pool striking bottom causing other injury**

W16.03 **Fall into swimming pool striking wall**

⑦W16.031 **Fall into swimming pool striking wall causing drowning and submersion**

Excludes1: drowning and submersion while in swimming pool without fall (W67)

⑦W16.032 **Fall into swimming pool striking wall causing other injury**

W16.1 **Fall into natural body of water**

Fall into lake

Fall into open sea Fall into river

Fall into stream

W16.11 **Fall into natural body of water striking water surface**

⑦W16.111 **Fall into natural body of water striking water surface causing drowning and submersion**

Excludes1: drowning and submersion while in natural body of water without fall (W69)

⑦ W16.112 Fall into natural body of water striking water surface causing other injury

W16.12 Fall into natural body of water striking bottom

⑦ W16.121 Fall into natural body of water striking bottom causing drowning and submersion

Excludes1: drowning and submersion while in natural body of water without fall (W69)

⑦ W16.122 Fall into natural body of water striking bottom causing other injury

W16.13 Fall into natural body of water striking side

⊗⑦W16.131 Fall into natural body of water striking side causing drowning and submersion

Excludes1: drowning and submersion while in natural body of water without fall (W69)

⑦ W16.132 Fall into natural body of water striking side causing other injury

W16.2 Fall in (into) filled bathtub or bucket of water

W16.21 Fall in (into) filled bathtub

Excludes1: fall into empty bathtub (W18.2)

⑦ W16.211 Fall in (into) filled bathtub causing drowning and submersion

Excludes1: drowning and submersion while in filled bathtub without fall (W65)

⑦ W16.212 Fall in (into) filled bathtub causing other injury

W16.22 Fall in (into) bucket of water

⑦ W16.221 Fall in (into) bucket of water causing drowning and submersion

⑦ W16.222 Fall in (into) bucket of water causing other injury

W16.3 Fall into other water

Fall into fountain Fall into reservoir

W16.31 Fall into other water striking water surface

⑦ W16.311 Fall into other water striking water surface causing drowning and submersion

Excludes1: drowning and submersion while **in other water** without fall (W73)

⑦ W16.312 Fall into other water striking water surface causing other injury

W16.32 Fall into other water striking bottom

⑦ W16.321 Fall into other water striking bottom causing drowning and submersion

Excludes1: drowning and submersion while **in other water** without fall (W73)

⑦ W16.322 Fall into other water striking bottom causing other injury

W16.33 Fall into other water striking wall

⑦ W16.331 Fall into other water striking wall causing drowning and submersion

Excludes1: drowning and submersion while **in other water** without fall (W73)

⑦ W16.332 Fall into other water striking wall causing other injury

W16.4 Fall into unspecified water

⊗⑦W16.41 Fall into unspecified water causing drowning and submersion

⊗⑦W16.42 Fall into unspecified water causing other injury

W16.5 Jumping or diving into swimming pool

⊗⑦W16.51 Jumping or diving into swimming pool striking water surface

⑦ W16.511 Jumping or diving into swimming pool striking water surface causing drowning and submersion

Excludes1: drowning and submersion while in swimming pool without jumping or diving (W67)

⑦ W16.512 Jumping or diving into swimming pool striking water surface causing other injury

W16.52 Jumping or diving into swimming pool striking bottom

⑦ W16.521 Jumping or diving into swimming pool striking bottom causing drowning and submersion

Excludes1: drowning and submersion while in swimming pool without jumping or diving (W67)

⑦ W16.522 Jumping or diving into swimming pool striking bottom causing other injury

W16.53 Jumping or diving into swimming pool striking wall

⑦ W16.531 Jumping or diving into swimming pool striking wall causing drowning and submersion

Excludes1: drowning and submersion while in swimming pool without jumping or diving (W67)

⑦ W16.532 Jumping or diving into swimming pool striking wall causing other injury

W16.6 Jumping or diving into natural body of water

Jumping or diving into lake

Jumping or diving into open sea

Jumping or diving into river

Jumping or diving into stream

W16.61 Jumping or diving into natural body of water striking water surface

⑦ W16.611 Jumping or diving into natural body of water striking water surface causing drowning and submersion

Excludes1: drowning and submersion while in natural body of water without jumping or diving (W69)

⑦**W16.612** **Jumping or diving into natural body of water striking water surface causing other injury**

W16.62 **Jumping or diving into natural body of water striking bottom**

⑦**W16.621** **Jumping or diving into natural body of water striking bottom causing drowning and submersion**

Excludes1: drowning and submersion while in natural body of water without jumping or diving (W69)

⑦**W16.622** **Jumping or diving into natural body of water striking bottom causing other injury**

W16.7 **Jumping or diving from boat**

Excludes1: Fall from boat into water -see watercraft accident (V90-V94)

W16.71 **Jumping or diving from boat striking water surface**

⑦**W16.711** **Jumping or diving from boat striking water surface causing drowning and submersion**

⑦**W16.712** **Jumping or diving from boat striking water surface causing other injury**

W16.72 **Jumping or diving from boat striking bottom**

⑦**W16.721** **Jumping or diving from boat striking bottom causing drowning and submersion**

⑦**W16.722** **Jumping or diving from boat striking bottom causing other injury**

W16.8 **Jumping or diving into other water**

Jumping or diving into fountain

Jumping or diving into reservoir

W16.81 **Jumping or diving into other water striking water surface**

⑦**W16.811** **Jumping or diving into other water striking water surface causing drowning and submersion**

Excludes1: drowning and submersion while in other water without jumping or diving (W73)

⑦**W16.812** **Jumping or diving into other water striking water surface causing other injury**

W16.82 **Jumping or diving into other water striking bottom**

⑦**W16.821** **Jumping or diving into other water striking bottom causing drowning and submersion**

Excludes1: drowning and submersion while in other water without jumping or diving (W73)

⑦**W16.822** **Jumping or diving into other water striking bottom causing other injury**

W16.83 **Jumping or diving into other water striking wall**

⑦**W16.831** **Jumping or diving into other water striking wall causing drowning and submersion**

Excludes1: drowning and submersion while in other water without jumping or diving (W73)

⑦**W16.832** **Jumping or diving into other water striking wall causing other injury**

W16.9 **Jumping or diving into unspecified water**

⊗⑦**W16.91** **Jumping or diving into unspecified water causing drowning and submersion**

⊗⑦**W16.92** **Jumping or diving into unspecified water causing other injury**

W17 **Other fall from one level to another**

The appropriate 7th character is to be added to each code from category W17

A - initial encounter

D - subsequent encounter

S - sequela

⊗⑦**W17.0** **Fall into well**

⊗⑦**W17.1** **Fall into storm drain or manhole**

⊗⑦**W17.2** **Fall into hole**

Fall into pit

⊗⑦**W17.3** **Fall into empty swimming pool**

Excludes1: fall into filled swimming pool (W16.0-)

⊗⑦**W17.4** **Fall from dock**

W17.8 **Other fall from one level to another**

⊗⑦**W17.81** **Fall down embankment (hill)**

⊗⑦**W17.82** **Fall from (out of) grocery cart**

Fall due to grocery cart tipping over

⊗⑦**W17.89** **Other fall from one level to another**

Fall from cherry picker Fall from lifting device

Fall from mobile elevated work platform [MEWP]

Fall from sky lift

W18 **Other slipping, tripping and stumbling and falls**

The appropriate 7th character is to be added to each code from category W18

A - initial encounter

D - subsequent encounter

S - sequela

W18.0 **Fall due to bumping against object**

Striking against object with subsequent fall

Excludes1: fall on same level due to slipping, tripping, or stumbling with subsequent striking against object (W01.1-)

⊗⑦**W18.00** **Striking against unspecified object with subsequent fall**

⊗⑦**W18.01** **Striking against sports equipment with subsequent fall**

⊗⑦**W18.02** **Striking against glass with subsequent fall**

⊗⑦**W18.09** **Striking against other object with subsequent fall**

W18.1 **Fall from or off toilet**

⊗⑦**W18.11** **Fall from or off toilet without subsequent striking against object**

Fall from (off) toilet NOS

⊗⑦**W18.12** **Fall from or off toilet with subsequent striking against object**

⊗⑦**W18.2** **Fall in (into) shower or empty bathtub**

Excludes1: fall in full bathtub causing drowning or submersion (W16.21-)

W18.3 **Other and unspecified fall on same level**

⊗⑦**W18.30** **Fall on same level, unspecified**

⊗⑦**W18.31** **Fall on same level due to stepping on an object**

Fall on same level due to stepping on an animal

Excludes1: slipping, tripping and stumbling without fall due to stepping on animal (W18.41)

⊗⑦**W18.39** **Other fall on same level**

W18.4 **Slipping, tripping and stumbling without falling**

Excludes1: collision with another person without fall (W51)

⊗⑦**W18.40** **Slipping, tripping and stumbling without falling, unspecified**

⊗⑦**W18.41** **Slipping, tripping and stumbling without falling due to stepping on object**

Slipping, tripping and stumbling without falling due to stepping on animal

Excludes1: slipping, tripping and stumbling with fall due to stepping on animal (W18.31)

⊗⑦**W18.42** **Slipping, tripping and stumbling without falling due to stepping into hole or opening**

⊗⑦**W18.43** **Slipping, tripping and stumbling without falling due to stepping from one level to another**

⊗⑦**W18.49** **Other slipping, tripping and stumbling without falling**

⊗⑦**W19** **Unspecified fall**

Accidental fall NOS

The appropriate 7th character is to be added to code W19

A - initial encounter

D - subsequent encounter

S - sequela

EXPOSURE TO INANIMATE MECHANICAL FORCES (W20-W49)

Excludes1: assault (X92-Y09)

contact or collision with animals or persons (W50-W64)

exposure to inanimate mechanical forces involving military or war operations (Y36.-, Y37.-)

intentional self-harm (X71-X83)

W20 **Struck by thrown, projected or falling object**

Code first any associated:

cataclysm (X34-X39)

lightning strike (T75.00)

Excludes1: falling object in machinery accident (W24, W28-W31)

falling object in transport accident (V01-V99)

object set in motion by explosion (W35-W40)

object set in motion by firearm (W32-W34)

struck by thrown sports equipment (W21.-)

The appropriate 7th character is to be added to each code from categoryW20

A - initial encounter

D - subsequent encounter

S - sequela

⊗⑦**W20.0** **Struck by falling object in cave-in**

Excludes2: asphyxiation due to cave-in (T71.21)

⊗⑦**W20.1** **Struck by object due to collapse of building**

Excludes1: struck by object due to collapse of burning building (X00.2, X02.2)

⊗⑦**W20.8** **Other cause of strike by thrown, projected or falling object**

Excludes1: struck by thrown sports equipment (W21.-)

W21 **Striking against or struck by sports equipment**

Excludes1: assault with sports equipment (Y08.0-)

striking against or struck by sports equipment with subsequent fall (W18.01)

The appropriate 7th character is to be added to each code from category W21

A - initial encounter

D - subsequent encounter

S - sequela

W21.0 **Struck by hit or thrown ball**

⊗⑦**W21.00** **Struck by hit or thrown ball, unspecified type**

⊗⑦**W21.01** **Struck by football**

⊗⑦**W21.02** **Struck by soccer ball**

⊗⑦**W21.03** **Struck by baseball**

⊗⑦**W21.04** **Struck by golf ball**

⊗⑦**W21.05** **Struck by basketball**

⊗⑦**W21.06** **Struck by volleyball**

⊗⑦**W21.07** **Struck by softball**

⊗⑦**W21.09** **Struck by other hit or thrown ball**

W21.1 **Struck by bat, racquet or club**

⊗⑦**W21.11** **Struck by baseball bat**

⊗⑦**W21.12** **Struck by tennis racquet**

⊗⑦**W21.13** **Struck by golf club**

⊗⑦**W21.19** **Struck by other bat, racquet or club**

W21.2 **Struck by hockey stick or puck**

W21.21 **Struck by hockey stick**

⑦**W21.210** **Struck by ice hockey stick**

⑦**W21.211** **Struck by field hockey stick**

W21.22 **Struck by hockey puck**

⑦**W21.220** **Struck by ice hockey puck**

⑦**W21.221** **Struck by field hockey puck**

W21.3 **Struck by sports foot wear**

⊗⑦**W21.31** **Struck by shoe cleats**

Stepped on by shoe cleats

⊗⑦**W21.32** **Struck by skate blades**

Skated over by skate blades

⊗⑦**W21.39** **Struck by other sports foot wear**

⊗⑦**W21.4** **Striking against diving board**

Use additional code for subsequent falling into water, if applicable (W16.-)

W21.8 **Striking against or struck by other sports equipment**

⊗⑦**W21.81** **Striking against or struck by football helmet**

⊗⑦**W21.89** **Striking against or struck by other sports equipment**

⊗⑦**W21.9** **Striking against or struck by unspecified sports equipment**

W22 **Striking against or struck by other objects**

Excludes1: striking against or struck by object with subsequent fall (W18.09)

● New code ▲ Revised code **Excludes1:** Not coded here **Excludes2:** Not included here ⊗ Placeholder required ⑦ 7th digit required

The appropriate 7th character is to be added to each code from category W22

A - initial encounter

D - subsequent encounter

S - sequela

W22.0 Striking against stationary object

> **Excludes1:** striking against stationary sports equipment (W21.8)

⊗⑦**W22.01 Walked into wall**

⊗⑦**W22.02 Walked into lamppost**

⊗⑦**W22.03 Walked into furniture**

W22.04 Striking against wall of swimming pool

⑦**W22.041 Striking against wall of swimming pool causing drowning and submersion**

> **Excludes1:** drowning and submersion while swimming without striking against wall (W67)

⑦**W22.042 Striking against wall of swimming pool causing other injury**

⊗⑦**W22.09 Striking against other stationary object**

W22.1 Striking against or struck by automobile airbag

⊗⑦**W22.10 Striking against or struck by unspecified automobile airbag**

⊗⑦**W22.11 Striking against or struck by driver side automobile airbag**

⊗⑦**W22.12 Striking against or struck by front passenger side automobile airbag**

⊗⑦**W22.19 Striking against or struck by other automobile airbag**

⊗⑦**W22.8 Striking against or struck by other objects**

Striking against or struck by object NOS

> **Excludes1:** struck by thrown, projected or falling object (W20.-)

W23 Caught, crushed, jammed or pinched in or between objects

> **Excludes1:** injury caused by cutting or piercing instruments (W25-W27)
>
> injury caused by firearms malfunction (W32.1, W33.1-, W34.1-)
>
> injury caused by lifting and transmission devices (W24.-)
>
> injury caused by machinery (W28-W31)
>
> injury caused by nonpowered hand tools (W27.-)
>
> injury caused by transport vehicle being used as a means of transportation (V01-V99)
>
> injury caused by struck by thrown, projected or falling object (W20.-)

The appropriate 7th character is to be added to each code from category W23

A - initial encounter

D - subsequent encounter

S - sequela

⊗⑦**W23.0 Caught, crushed, jammed, or pinched between moving objects**

⊗⑦**W23.1 Caught, crushed, jammed, or pinched between stationary objects**

W24 Contact with lifting and transmission devices, not elsewhere classified

> **Excludes1:** transport accidents (V01-V99)

The appropriate 7th character is to be added to each code from category W24

A - initial encounter

D - subsequent encounter

S - sequela

⊗⑦**W24.0 Contact with lifting devices, not elsewhere classified**

Contact with chain hoist

Contact with drive belt

Contact with pulley (block)

⊗⑦**W24.1 Contact with transmission devices, not elsewhere classified**

Contact with transmission belt or cable

⊗⑦**W25 Contact with sharp glass**

> **Code first** any associated:
>
> injury due to flying glass from explosion or firearm discharge (W32-W40)
>
> transport accident (V00-V99)
>
> **Excludes1:** fall on same level due to slipping, tripping and stumbling with subsequent striking against sharp glass (W01.10)
>
> striking against sharp glass with subsequent fall (W18.02)
>
> **Excludes2:** glass embedded in skin (W45)

The appropriate 7th character is to be added to code W25

A - initial encounter

D - subsequent encounter

S - sequela

W26 Contact with other sharp objects

> **Excludes2:** sharp object(s) embedded in skin (W45)

The appropriate 7th character is to be added to each code from category W26

A - initial encounter

D - subsequent encounter

S - sequela

⊗⑦**W26.0 Contact with knife**

> **Excludes1:** contact with electric knife (W29.1)

⊗⑦**W26.1 Contact with sword or dagger**

⊗⑦**W26.2 Contact with edge of stiff paper**

Paper cut

⊗⑦**W26.8 Contact with other sharp object(s), not elsewhere classified**

Contact with tin can lid

⊗⑦**W26.9 Contact with unspecified sharp object(s)**

W27 Contact with nonpowered hand tool

The appropriate 7th character is to be added to each code from category W27

A - initial encounter

D - subsequent encounter

S - sequela

⊗⑦**W27.0 Contact with workbench tool**

Contact with auger

Contact with axe

Contact with chisel

Contact with handsaw

Contact with screwdriver

⊗⑦**W27.1 Contact with garden tool**

Contact with hoe

Contact with nonpowered lawn mower

Contact with pitchfork

Contact with rake

⊗⑦**W27.2 Contact with scissors**

⊗⑦**W27.3   Contact with needle (sewing)**
Excludes1: contact with hypodermic needle (W46.-)

⊗⑦**W27.4   Contact with kitchen utensil**
Contact with fork
Contact with ice-pick
Contact with can-opener NOS

⊗⑦**W27.5   Contact with paper-cutter**

⊗⑦**W27.8   Contact with other nonpowered hand tool**
Contact with nonpowered sewing machine
Contact with shovel

⊗⑦**W28   Contact with powered lawn mower**
Powered lawn mower (commercial) (residential)
Excludes1: contact with nonpowered lawn mower (W27.1)
Excludes2: exposure to electric current (W86.-)
The appropriate 7th character is to be added to code W28
A - initial encounter
D - subsequent encounter
S - sequela

W29   Contact with other powered hand tools and household machinery
Excludes1: contact with commercial machinery (W31.82)
contact with hot household appliance (X15)
contact with nonpowered hand tool (W27.-)
exposure to electric current (W86)
The appropriate 7th character is to be added to each code from category W29
A - initial encounter
D - subsequent encounter
S - sequela

⊗⑦**W29.0   Contact with powered kitchen appliance**
Contact with blender
Contact with can-opener
Contact with garbage disposal
Contact with mixer

⊗⑦**W29.1   Contact with electric knife**

⊗⑦**W29.2   Contact with other powered household machinery**
Contact with electric fan
Contact with powered dryer (clothes) (powered) (spin)
Contact with washing-machine
Contact with sewing machine

⊗⑦**W29.3   Contact with powered garden and outdoor hand tools and machinery**
Contact with chainsaw
Contact with edger
Contact with garden cultivator (tiller)
Contact with hedge trimmer
Contact with other powered garden tool
Excludes1: contact with powered lawn mower (W28)

⊗⑦**W29.4   Contact with nail gun**

▲⊗⑦**W29.8   Contact with other powered hand tools and household machinery**
Contact with do-it-yourself tool NOS

W30   Contact with agricultural machinery
Includes: animal-powered farm machine
Excludes1: agricultural transport vehicle accident (V01-V99)
explosion of grain store (W40.8)
exposure to electric current (W86.-)

The appropriate 7th character is to be added to each code from category W30
A - initial encounter
D - subsequent encounter
S - sequela

⊗⑦**W30.0   Contact with combine harvester**
Contact with reaper
Contact with thresher

⊗⑦**W30.1   Contact with power take-off devices (PTO)**

⊗⑦**W30.2   Contact with hay derrick**

⊗⑦**W30.3   Contact with grain storage elevator**
Excludes1: explosion of grain store (W40.8)

W30.8   Contact with other specified agricultural machinery

⊗⑦**W30.81   Contact with agricultural transport vehicle in stationary use**
Contact with agricultural transport vehicle under repair, not on public roadway
Excludes1: agricultural transport vehicle accident (V01-V99)

⊗⑦**W30.89   Contact with other specified agricultural machinery**

⊗⑦**W30.9   Contact with unspecified agricultural machinery**
Contact with farm machinery NOS

W31   Contact with other and unspecified machinery
Excludes1: contact with agricultural machinery (W30.-)
contact with machinery in transport under own power or being towed by a vehicle (V01-V99)
exposure to electric current (W86)
The appropriate 7th character is to be added to each code from category W31
A - initial encounter
D - subsequent encounter
S - sequela

⊗⑦**W31.0   Contact with mining and earth-drilling machinery**
Contact with bore or drill (land) (seabed)
Contact with shaft hoist
Contact with shaft lift
Contact with under cutter

⊗⑦**W31.1   Contact with metalworking machines**
Contact with abrasive wheel
Contact with forging machine
Contact with lathe
Contact with mechanical shears
Contact with metal drilling machine
Contact with milling machine
Contact with power press
Contact with rolling-mill
Contact with metal sawing machine

⊗⑦**W31.2   Contact with powered woodworking and forming machines**
Contact with band saw
Contact with bench saw
Contact with circular saw
Contact with molding machine
Contact with overhead plane
Contact with powered saw
Contact with radial saw
Contact with sander

Excludes1: nonpowered woodworking tools (W27.0)

⊗⑦**W31.3** **Contact with prime movers**

Contact with gas turbine

Contact with internal combustion engine

Contact with steam engine

Contact with water driven turbine

W31.8 **Contact with other specified machinery**

⊗⑦**W31.81** **Contact with recreational machinery**

Contact with roller coaster

⊗⑦**W31.82** **Contact with other commercial machinery**

Contact with commercial electric fan

Contact with commercial kitchen appliances

Contact with commercial powered dryer (clothes) (powered) (spin)

Contact with commercial washing-machine

Contact with commercial sewing machine

Excludes1: contact with household machinery (W29.-)

contact with powered lawn mower (W28)

⊗⑦**W31.83** **Contact with special construction vehicle in stationary use**

Contact with special construction vehicle under repair, not on public roadway

Excludes1: special construction vehicle accident (V01-V99)

⊗⑦**W31.89** **Contact with other specified machinery**

⊗⑦**W31.9** **Contact with unspecified machinery**

Contact with machinery NOS

W32 **Accidental handgun discharge and malfunction**

Includes: accidental discharge and malfunction of gun for single hand use

accidental discharge and malfunction of pistol accidental discharge and malfunction of revolver

Handgun discharge and malfunction NOS

Excludes1: accidental airgun discharge and malfunction (W34.010, W34.110)

accidental BB gun discharge and malfunction (W34.010, W34.110)

accidental pellet gun discharge and malfunction (W34.010, W34.110)

accidental shotgun discharge and malfunction (W33.01, W33.11)

assault by handgun discharge (X93)

handgun discharge involving legal intervention (Y35.0-)

handgun discharge involving military or war operations (Y36.4-)

intentional self-harm by handgun discharge (X72)

Very pistol discharge and malfunction (W34.09, W34.19)

The appropriate 7th character is to be added to each code from category W32

A - initial encounter

D - subsequent encounter

S - sequela

⊗⑦**W32.0** **Accidental handgun discharge**

⊗⑦**W32.1** **Accidental handgun malfunction**

Injury due to explosion of handgun (parts)

Injury due to malfunction of mechanism or component of handgun

Injury due to recoil of handgun

Powder burn from handgun

W33 **Accidental rifle, shotgun and larger firearm discharge and malfunction**

Includes: rifle, shotgun and larger firearm discharge and malfunction NOS

Excludes1: accidental airgun discharge and malfunction (W34.010, W34.110)

accidental BB gun discharge and malfunction (W34.010, W34.110)

accidental handgun discharge and malfunction (W32.-)

accidental pellet gun discharge and malfunction (W34.010, W34.110)

assault by rifle, shotgun and larger firearm discharge (X94)

firearm discharge involving legal intervention (Y35.0-)

firearm discharge involving military or war operations (Y36.4-)

intentional self-harm by rifle, shotgun and larger firearm discharge (X73)

The appropriate 7th character is to be added to each code from category W33

A - initial encounter

D - subsequent encounter

S - sequela

W33.0 **Accidental rifle, shotgun and larger firearm discharge**

⊗⑦**W33.00** **Accidental discharge of unspecified larger firearm**

Discharge of unspecified larger firearm NOS

⊗⑦**W33.01** **Accidental discharge of shotgun**

Discharge of shotgun NOS

⊗⑦**W33.02** **Accidental discharge of hunting rifle**

Discharge of hunting rifle NOS

⊗⑦**W33.03** **Accidental discharge of machine gun**

Discharge of machine gun NOS

⊗⑦**W33.09** **Accidental discharge of other larger firearm**

Discharge of other larger firearm NOS

W33.1 **Accidental rifle, shotgun and larger firearm malfunction**

Injury due to explosion of rifle, shotgun and larger firearm (parts)

Injury due to malfunction of mechanism or component of rifle, shotgun and larger firearm

Injury due to piercing, cutting, crushing or pinching due to (by) slide trigger mechanism, scope or other gun part

Injury due to recoil of rifle, shotgun and larger firearm

Powder burn from rifle, shotgun and larger firearm

⊗⑦**W33.10** **Accidental malfunction of unspecified larger firearm**

Malfunction of unspecified larger firearm NOS

⊗⑦**W33.11** **Accidental malfunction of shotgun**

Malfunction of shotgun NOS

⊗⑦**W33.12** **Accidental malfunction of hunting rifle**

Malfunction of hunting rifle NOS

⊗⑦**W33.13** **Accidental malfunction of machine gun**

Malfunction of machine gun NOS

⊗⑦**W33.19** **Accidental malfunction of other larger firearm**

Malfunction of other larger firearm NOS

W34 **Accidental discharge and malfunction from other and unspecified firearms and guns**

	Add 4th-7th digits		Nonspecific code		Unspecified code		Manifestation code	**1031**

The appropriate 7th character is to be added to each code from category W34

A - initial encounter

D - subsequent encounter

S - sequela

W34.0 **Accidental discharge from other and unspecified firearms and guns**

⊗⑦**W34.00** **Accidental discharge from unspecified firearms or gun**

Discharge from firearm NOS

Gunshot wound NOS

Shot NOS

W34.01 **Accidental discharge of gas, air or spring-operated guns**

⑦**W34.010** **Accidental discharge of airgun**

Accidental discharge of BB gun

Accidental discharge of pellet gun

⑦**W34.011** **Accidental discharge of paintball gun**

Accidental injury due to paintball discharge

⑦**W34.018** **Accidental discharge of other gas, air or spring-operated gun**

⊗⑦**W34.09** **Accidental discharge from other specified firearms**

Accidental discharge from Very pistol [flare]

W34.1 **Accidental malfunction from other and unspecified firearms and guns**

⊗⑦**W34.10** **Accidental malfunction from unspecified firearms or gun**

Firearm malfunction NOS

W34.11 **Accidental malfunction of gas, air or spring-operated guns**

⑦**W34.110** **Accidental malfunction of airgun**

Accidental malfunction of BB gun

Accidental malfunction of pellet gun

⑦**W34.111** **Accidental malfunction of paintball gun**

Accidental injury due to paintball gun malfunction

⑦**W34.118** **Accidental malfunction of other gas, air or spring-operated gun**

⊗⑦**W34.19** **Accidental malfunction from other specified firearms**

Accidental malfunction from Very pistol [flare]

⊗⑦**W35** **Explosion and rupture of boiler**

Excludes1: explosion and rupture of boiler on watercraft (V93.4)

The appropriate 7th character is to be added to code W35

A - initial encounter

D - subsequent encounter

S - sequela

W36 **Explosion and rupture of gas cylinder**

The appropriate 7th character is to be added to each code from category W36

A - initial encounter

D - subsequent encounter

S - sequela

⊗⑦**W36.1** **Explosion and rupture of aerosol can**

⊗⑦**W36.2** **Explosion and rupture of air tank**

⊗⑦**W36.3** **Explosion and rupture of pressurized-gas tank**

⊗⑦**W36.8** **Explosion and rupture of other gas cylinder**

⊗⑦**W36.9** **Explosion and rupture of unspecified gas cylinder**

W37 **Explosion and rupture of pressurized tire, pipe or hose**

The appropriate 7th character is to be added to each code from category W37

A - initial encounter

D - subsequent encounter

S - sequela

⊗⑦**W37.0** **Explosion of bicycle tire**

⊗⑦**W37.8** **Explosion and rupture of other pressurized tire, pipe or hose**

⊗⑦**W38** **Explosion and rupture of other specified pressurized devices**

The appropriate 7th character is to be added to code W38

A - initial encounter

D - subsequent encounter

S - sequela

⊗⑦**W39** **Discharge of firework**

The appropriate 7th character is to be added to code W39

A - initial encounter

D - subsequent encounter

S - sequela

W40 **Explosion of other materials**

Excludes1: assault by explosive material (X96)

explosion involving legal intervention (Y35.1-)

explosion involving military or war operations (Y36.0-, Y36.2-)

intentional self-harm by explosive material (X75)

The appropriate 7th character is to be added to each code from category W40

A - initial encounter

D - subsequent encounter

S - sequela

⊗⑦**W40.0** **Explosion of blasting material**

Explosion of blasting cap

Explosion of detonator

Explosion of dynamite

Explosion of explosive (any) used in blasting operations

⊗⑦**W40.1** **Explosion of explosive gases**

Explosion of acetylene

Explosion of butane

Explosion of coal gas

Explosion in mine NOS

Explosion of explosive gas

Explosion of fire damp

Explosion of gasoline fumes

Explosion of methane

Explosion of propane

⊗⑦**W40.8** **Explosion of other specified explosive materials**

Explosion in dump NOS

Explosion in factory NOS

Explosion in grain store

Explosion in munitions

Excludes1: explosion involving legal intervention (Y35.1-)

explosion involving military or war operations (Y36.0-, Y36.2-)

⊗⑦**W40.9** **Explosion of unspecified explosive materials**

Explosion NOS

W42   Exposure to noise

The appropriate 7th character is to be added to each code from category W42

A - initial encounter

D - subsequent encounter

S - sequela

⊗⑦**W42.0   Exposure to supersonic waves**

⊗⑦**W42.9   Exposure to other noise**

Exposure to sound waves NOS

W45   Foreign body or object entering through skin

Includes: foreign body or object embedded in skin

nail embedded in skin

Excludes2: contact with hand tools (nonpowered) (powered) (W27-W29)

contact with other sharp object(s) (W26.-)

contact with sharp glass (W25.-)

struck by objects (W20-W22)

The appropriate 7th character is to be added to each code from category W45

A - initial encounter

D - subsequent encounter

S - sequela

⊗⑦**W45.0   Nail entering through skin**

⊗⑦**W45.8   Other foreign body or object entering through skin**

Splinter in skin NOS

W46   Contact with hypodermic needle

The appropriate 7th character is to be added to each code from category W46

A - initial encounter

D - subsequent encounter

S - sequela

⊗⑦**W46.0   Contact with hypodermic needle**

Hypodermic needle stick NOS

⊗⑦**W46.1   Contact with contaminated hypodermic needle**

W49   Exposure to other inanimate mechanical forces

Includes: exposure to abnormal gravitational [G] forces

exposure to inanimate mechanical forces NEC

Excludes1: exposure to inanimate mechanical forces involving military or war operations (Y36.-, Y37.-)

The appropriate 7th character is to be added to each code from category W49

A - initial encounter

D - subsequent encounter

S - sequela

W49.0   Item causing external constriction

⊗⑦**W49.01   Hair causing external constriction**

⊗⑦**W49.02   String or thread causing external constriction**

⊗⑦**W49.03   Rubber band causing external constriction**

⊗⑦**W49.04   Ring or other jewelry causing external constriction**

⊗⑦**W49.09   Other specified item causing external constriction**

⊗⑦**W49.9   Exposure to other inanimate mechanical forces**

EXPOSURE TO ANIMATE MECHANICAL FORCES (W50-W64)

Excludes1: Toxic effect of contact with venomous animals and plants (T63.-)

W50   Accidental hit, strike, kick, twist, bite or scratch by another person

Includes: hit, strike, kick, twist, bite, or scratch by another person NOS

Excludes1: assault by bodily force (Y04)

struck by objects (W20-22)

The appropriate 7th character is to be added to each code from category W50

A - initial encounter

D - subsequent encounter

S - sequela

⊗⑦**W50.0   Accidental hit or strike by another person**

Hit or strike by another person NOS

⊗⑦**W50.1   Accidental kick by another person**

Kick by another person NOS

⊗⑦**W50.2   Accidental twist by another person**

Twist by another person NOS

⊗⑦**W50.3   Accidental bite by another person**

Human bite

Bite by another person NOS

⊗⑦**W50.4   Accidental scratch by another person**

Scratch by another person NOS

⊗⑦**W51   Accidental striking against or bumped into by another person**

Excludes1: assault by striking against or bumping into by another person (Y04.2)

fall due to collision with another person (W03)

The appropriate 7th character is to be added to code W51

A - initial encounter

D - subsequent encounter

S - sequela

⊗⑦**W52   Crushed, pushed or stepped on by crowd or human stampede**

Crushed, pushed or stepped on by crowd or human stampede with or without fall

The appropriate 7th character is to be added to code W52

A - initial encounter

D - subsequent encounter

S - sequela

W53   Contact with rodent

Includes: contact with saliva, feces or urine of rodent

The appropriate 7th character is to be added to each code from category W53

A - initial encounter

D - subsequent encounter

S - sequela

W53.0   Contact with mouse

⊗⑦**W53.01   Bitten by mouse**

⊗⑦**W53.09   Other contact with mouse**

W53.1   Contact with rat

⊗⑦**W53.11   Bitten by rat**

⊗⑦**W53.19   Other contact with rat**

W53.2   Contact with squirrel

⊗⑦**W53.21   Bitten by squirrel**

⊗⑦**W53.29   Other contact with squirrel**

W53.8   Contact with other rodent

⊗⑦**W53.81   Bitten by other rodent**

⊗⑦**W53.89   Other contact with other rodent**

W54   Contact with dog

Includes: contact with saliva, feces or urine of dog

Add 4th-7th digits   Nonspecific code   Unspecified code   Manifestation code

The appropriate 7th character is to be added to each code from category W54

A - initial encounter

D - subsequent encounter

S - sequela

⊗⑦**W54.0 Bitten by dog**

⊗⑦**W54.1 Struck by dog**

Knocked over by dog

⊗⑦**W54.8 Other contact with dog**

W55 **Contact with other mammals**

Includes: contact with saliva, feces or urine of mammal

Excludes1: animal being ridden- see transport accidents

bitten or struck by dog (W54)

bitten or struck by rodent (W53.-)

contact with marine mammals (W56.-)

The appropriate 7th character is to be added to each code from category W55

A - initial encounter

D - subsequent encounter

S - sequela

W55.0 Contact with cat

⊗⑦**W55.01 Bitten by cat**

⊗⑦**W55.03 Scratched by cat**

⊗⑦**W55.09 Other contact with cat**

W55.1 Contact with horse

⊗⑦**W55.11 Bitten by horse**

⊗⑦**W55.12 Struck by horse**

⊗⑦**W55.19 Other contact with horse**

W55.2 Contact with cow

Contact with bull

⊗⑦**W55.21 Bitten by cow**

⊗⑦**W55.22 Struck by cow**

Gored by bull

⊗⑦**W55.29 Other contact with cow**

W55.3 Contact with other hoof stock

Contact with goats

Contact with sheep

⊗⑦**W55.31 Bitten by other hoof stock**

⊗⑦**W55.32 Struck by other hoof stock**

Gored by goat

Gored by ram

⊗⑦**W55.39 Other contact with other hoof stock**

W55.4 Contact with pig

⊗⑦**W55.41 Bitten by pig**

⊗⑦**W55.42 Struck by pig**

⊗⑦**W55.49 Other contact with pig**

W55.5 Contact with raccoon

⊗⑦**W55.51 Bitten by raccoon**

⊗⑦**W55.52 Struck by raccoon**

⊗⑦**W55.59 Other contact with raccoon**

W55.8 Contact with other mammals

⊗⑦**W55.81 Bitten by other mammals**

⊗⑦**W55.82 Struck by other mammals**

⊗⑦**W55.89 Other contact with other mammals**

W56 **Contact with nonvenomous marine animal**

Excludes1: contact with venomous marine animal (T63.-)

The appropriate 7th character is to be added to each code from category W56

A - initial encounter

D - subsequent encounter

S - sequela

W56.0 Contact with dolphin

⊗⑦**W56.01 Bitten by dolphin**

⊗⑦**W56.02 Struck by dolphin**

⊗⑦**W56.09 Other contact with dolphin**

W56.1 Contact with sea lion

⊗⑦**W56.11 Bitten by sea lion**

⊗⑦**W56.12 Struck by sea lion**

⊗⑦**W56.19 Other contact with sea lion**

W56.2 Contact with orca

Contact with killer whale

⊗⑦**W56.21 Bitten by orca**

⊗⑦**W56.22 Struck by orca**

⊗⑦**W56.29 Other contact with orca**

W56.3 Contact with other marine mammals

⊗⑦**W56.31 Bitten by other marine mammals**

⊗⑦**W56.32 Struck by other marine mammals**

⊗⑦**W56.39 Other contact with other marine mammals**

W56.4 Contact with shark

⊗⑦**W56.41 Bitten by shark**

⊗⑦**W56.42 Struck by shark**

⊗⑦**W56.49 Other contact with shark**

W56.5 Contact with other fish

⊗⑦**W56.51 Bitten by other fish**

⊗⑦**W56.52 Struck by other fish**

⊗⑦**W56.59 Other contact with other fish**

W56.8 Contact with other nonvenomous marine animals

⊗⑦**W56.81 Bitten by other nonvenomous marine animals**

⊗⑦**W56.82 Struck by other nonvenomous marine animals**

⊗⑦**W56.89 Other contact with other nonvenomous marine animals**

⊗⑦W57 **Bitten or stung by nonvenomous insect and other nonvenomous arthropods**

Excludes1: contact with venomous insects and arthropods (T63.2-, T63.3-, T63.4-)

The appropriate 7th character is to be added to code W57

A - initial encounter

D - subsequent encounter

S - sequela

W58 **Contact with crocodile or alligator**

The appropriate 7th character is to be added to each code from category W58

A - initial encounter

D - subsequent encounter

S - sequela

W58.0 Contact with alligator

⊗⑦**W58.01 Bitten by alligator**

⊗⑦**W58.02 Struck by alligator**

⊗⑦**W58.03 Crushed by alligator**

⊗⑦**W58.09 Other contact with alligator**

W58.1 Contact with crocodile

⊗⑦**W58.11 Bitten by crocodile**

● New code   ▲ Revised code   **Excludes1:** Not coded here   **Excludes2:** Not included here   ⊗ Placeholder required   ⑦7ᵗʰ digit required

⊗⑦**W58.12**   **Struck by crocodile**

⊗⑦**W58.13**   **Crushed by crocodile**

⊗⑦**W58.19**   **Other contact with crocodile**

W59   **Contact with other nonvenomous reptiles**

Excludes1: contact with venomous reptile (T63.0-, T63.1-)

The appropriate 7th character is to be added to each code from category W59

A - initial encounter

D - subsequent encounter

S - sequela

W59.0   **Contact with nonvenomous lizards**

⊗⑦**W59.01**   **Bitten by nonvenomous lizards**

⊗⑦**W59.02**   **Struck by nonvenomous lizards**

⊗⑦**W59.09**   **Other contact with nonvenomous lizards**

Exposure to nonvenomous lizards

W59.1   **Contact with nonvenomous snakes**

⊗⑦**W59.11**   **Bitten by nonvenomous snake**

⊗⑦**W59.12**   **Struck by nonvenomous snake**

⊗⑦**W59.13**   **Crushed by nonvenomous snake**

⊗⑦**W59.19**   **Other contact with nonvenomous snake**

W59.2   **Contact with turtles**

Excludes1: contact with tortoises (W59.8-)

⊗⑦**W59.21**   **Bitten by turtle**

⊗⑦**W59.22**   **Struck by turtle**

⊗⑦**W59.29**   **Other contact with turtle**

Exposure to turtles

W59.8   **Contact with other nonvenomous reptiles**

⊗⑦**W59.81**   **Bitten by other nonvenomous reptiles**

⊗⑦**W59.82**   **Struck by other nonvenomous reptiles**

⊗⑦**W59.83**   **Crushed by other nonvenomous reptiles**

⊗⑦**W59.89**   **Other contact with other nonvenomous reptiles**

⊗⑦**W60**   **Contact with nonvenomous plant thorns and spines and sharp leaves**

Excludes1: Contact with venomous plants (T63.7-)

The appropriate 7th character is to be added to code W60

A - initial encounter

D - subsequent encounter

S - sequela

W61   **Contact with birds (domestic) (wild)**

Includes: contact with excreta of birds

The appropriate 7th character is to be added to each code from category W61

A - initial encounter

D - subsequent encounter

S - sequela

W61.0   **Contact with parrot**

⊗⑦**W61.01**   **Bitten by parrot**

⊗⑦**W61.02**   **Struck by parrot**

⊗⑦**W61.09**   **Other contact with parrot**

Exposure to parrots

W61.1   **Contact with macaw**

⊗⑦**W61.11**   **Bitten by macaw**

⊗⑦**W61.12**   **Struck by macaw**

⊗⑦**W61.19**   **Other contact with macaw**

Exposure to macaws

W61.2   **Contact with other psittacines**

⊗⑦**W61.21**   **Bitten by other psittacines**

⊗⑦**W61.22**   **Struck by other psittacines**

⊗⑦**W61.29**   **Other contact with other psittacines**

Exposure **to other** psittacines

W61.3   **Contact with chicken**

⊗⑦**W61.32**   **Struck by chicken**

⊗⑦**W61.33**   **Pecked by chicken**

⊗⑦**W61.39**   **Other contact with chicken**

Exposure to chickens

W61.4   **Contact with turkey**

⊗⑦**W61.42**   **Struck by turkey**

⊗⑦**W61.43**   **Pecked by turkey**

⊗⑦**W61.49**   **Other contact with turkey**

W61.5   **Contact with goose**

⊗⑦**W61.51**   **Bitten by goose**

⊗⑦**W61.52**   **Struck by goose**

⊗⑦**W61.59**   **Other contact with goose**

W61.6   **Contact with duck**

⊗⑦**W61.61**   **Bitten by duck**

⊗⑦**W61.62**   **Struck by duck**

⊗⑦**W61.69**   **Other contact with duck**

W61.9   **Contact with other birds**

⊗⑦**W61.91**   **Bitten by other birds**

⊗⑦**W61.92**   **Struck by other birds**

⊗⑦**W61.99**   **Other contact with other birds**

Contact with bird NOS

W62   **Contact with nonvenomous amphibians**

Excludes1: contact with venomous amphibians (T63.81-R63.83)

The appropriate 7th character is to be added to each code from category W62

A - initial encounter

D - subsequent encounter

S - sequela

⊗⑦**W62.0**   **Contact with nonvenomous frogs**

⊗⑦**W62.1**   **Contact with nonvenomous toads**

⊗⑦**W62.9**   **Contact with other nonvenomous amphibians**

⊗⑦**W64**   **Exposure to other animate mechanical forces**

Includes: exposure to nonvenomous animal NOS

Excludes1: contact with venomous animal (T63.-)

The appropriate 7th character is to be added to code ⊗⑦W64

A - initial encounter

D - subsequent encounter

S - sequela

ACCIDENTAL NON-TRANSPORT DROWNING AND SUBMERSION (W65-W74)

Excludes1: accidental drowning and submersion due to fall into water (W16.-)

accidental drowning and submersion due to water transport accident (V90.-, V92.-)

Excludes2: accidental drowning and submersion due to cataclysm (X34-X39)

⊗⑦**W65**   **Accidental drowning and submersion while in bath-tub**

Excludes1: accidental drowning and submersion due to fall in (into) bathtub (W16.211)

The appropriate 7th character is to be added to code W65

A - initial encounter

⊗⑦**W67** **Accidental drowning and submersion while in swimming-pool**

Excludes1: accidental drowning and submersion due to fall into swimming pool (W16.011, W16.021, W16.031)

accidental drowning and submersion due to striking into wall of swimming pool (W22.041)

The appropriate 7th character is to be added to code W67

A - initial encounter

D - subsequent encounter

S - sequela

⊗⑦**W69** **Accidental drowning and submersion while in natural water**

Accidental drowning and submersion while in lake

Accidental drowning and submersion while in open sea

Accidental drowning and submersion while in river

Accidental drowning and submersion while in stream

Excludes1: accidental drowning and submersion due to fall into natural body of water (W16.111, W16.121, W16.131)

The appropriate 7th character is to be added to code W69

A - initial encounter

D - subsequent encounter

S - sequela

⊗⑦**W73** **Other specified cause of accidental non-transport drowning and submersion**

Accidental drowning and submersion while in quenching tank

Accidental drowning and submersion while in reservoir

Excludes1: accidental drowning and submersion due to fall into other water (W16.311, W16.321, W16.331)

The appropriate 7th character is to be added to code W73

A - initial encounter

D - subsequent encounter

S - sequela

⊗⑦**W74** **Unspecified cause of accidental drowning and submersion**

Drowning NOS

The appropriate 7th character is to be added to code W74

A - initial encounter

D - subsequent encounter

S - sequela

EXPOSURE TO ELECTRIC CURRENT, RADIATION AND EXTREME AMBIENT AIR TEMPERATURE AND PRESSURE (W85-W99)

Excludes1: exposure to:

failure in dosage of radiation or temperature during surgical and medical care (Y63.2-Y63.5)

lightning (T75.0-)

natural cold (X31)

natural heat (X30)

natural radiation NOS (X39)

radiological procedure and radiotherapy (Y84.2)

sunlight (X32)

⊗⑦**W85** **Exposure to electric transmission lines**

Broken power line

The appropriate 7th character is to be added to code W85

A - initial encounter

D - subsequent encounter

S - sequela

W86 **Exposure to other specified electric current**

The appropriate 7th character is to be added to each code from category W86

A - initial encounter

D - subsequent encounter

S - sequela

⊗⑦**W86.0** **Exposure to domestic wiring and appliances**

⊗⑦**W86.1** **Exposure to industrial wiring, appliances and electrical machinery**

Exposure to conductors

Exposure to control apparatus

Exposure to electrical equipment and machinery

Exposure to transformers

⊗⑦**W86.8** **Exposure to other electric current**

Exposure to wiring and appliances in or on farm (not farmhouse)

Exposure to wiring and appliances outdoors

Exposure to wiring and appliances in or on public building

Exposure to wiring and appliances in or on residential institutions

Exposure to wiring and appliances in or on schools

W88 **Exposure to ionizing radiation**

Excludes1: exposure to sunlight (X32)

The appropriate 7th character is to be added to each code from category W88

A - initial encounter

D - subsequent encounter

S - sequela

⊗⑦**W88.0** **Exposure to X-rays**

⊗⑦**W88.1** **Exposure to radioactive isotopes**

⊗⑦**W88.8** **Exposure to other ionizing radiation**

W89 **Exposure to man-made visible and ultraviolet light**

Includes: exposure to welding light (arc)

Excludes1: exposure to sunlight (X32)

The appropriate 7th character is to be added to each code from category W89

A - initial encounter

D - subsequent encounter

S - sequela

⊗⑦**W89.0** **Exposure to welding light (arc)**

⊗⑦**W89.1** **Exposure to tanning bed**

⊗⑦**W89.8** **Exposure to other man-made visible and ultraviolet light**

⊗⑦**W89.9** **Exposure to unspecified man-made visible and ultraviolet light**

W90 **Exposure to other nonionizing radiation**

Excludes1: exposure to sunlight (X32)

The appropriate 7th character is to be added to each code from category W90

A - initial encounter

D - subsequent encounter

S - sequela

⊗⑦**W90.0** **Exposure to radiofrequency**

⊗⑦**W90.1** **Exposure to infrared radiation**

⊗⑦**W90.2** **Exposure to laser radiation**

⊗⑦**W90.8** **Exposure to other nonionizing radiation**

⊗⑦**W92** **Exposure to excessive heat of man-made origin**

The appropriate 7th character is to be added to code W92

A - initial encounter

● New code ▲ Revised code **Excludes1:** Not coded here **Excludes2:** Not included here ⊗ Placeholder required ⑦ 7th digit required

W93 Exposure to excessive cold of man-made origin

D - subsequent encounter

S - sequela

The appropriate 7th character is to be added to each code from category W93

A - initial encounter

D - subsequent encounter

S - sequela

W93.0 **Contact with or inhalation of dry ice**

⊗⑦W93.01 **Contact with dry ice**

⊗⑦W93.02 **Inhalation of dry ice**

W93.1 **Contact with or inhalation of liquid air**

⊗⑦W93.11 **Contact with liquid air**

Contact with liquid hydrogen

Contact with liquid nitrogen

⊗⑦W93.12 **Inhalation of liquid air**

Inhalation of liquid hydrogen

Inhalation of liquid nitrogen

⊗⑦W93.2 **Prolonged exposure in deep freeze unit or refrigerator**

⊗⑦W93.8 **Exposure to other excessive cold of man-made origin**

⊗⑦W94 **Exposure to high and low air pressure and changes in air pressure**

The appropriate 7th character is to be added to each code from category W94

A - initial encounter

D - subsequent encounter

S - sequela

⊗⑦W94.0 **Exposure to prolonged high air pressure**

W94.1 **Exposure to prolonged low air pressure**

⊗⑦W94.11 **Exposure to residence or prolonged visit at high altitude**

⊗⑦W94.12 **Exposure to other prolonged low air pressure**

W94.2 **Exposure to rapid changes in air pressure during ascent**

⊗⑦W94.21 **Exposure to reduction in atmospheric pressure while surfacing from deep-water diving**

⊗⑦W94.22 **Exposure to reduction in atmospheric pressure while surfacing from underground**

⊗⑦W94.23 **Exposure to sudden change in air pressure in aircraft during ascent**

⊗⑦W94.29 **Exposure to other rapid changes in air pressure during ascent**

W94.3 **Exposure to rapid changes in air pressure during descent**

⊗⑦W94.31 **Exposure to sudden change in air pressure in aircraft during descent**

⊗⑦W94.32 **Exposure to high air pressure from rapid descent in water**

⊗⑦W94.39 **Exposure to other rapid changes in air pressure during descent**

⊗⑦W99 **Exposure to other man-made environmental factors**

The appropriate 7th character is to be added to code W99

A - initial encounter

D - subsequent encounter

S - sequela

EXPOSURE TO SMOKE, FIRE AND FLAMES (X00-X08)

Excludes1: arson (X97)

Excludes2: explosions (W35-W40)

lightning (T75.0-)

transport accident (V01-V99)

X00 Exposure to uncontrolled fire in building or structure

Includes: conflagration in building or structure

Code first any associated cataclysm

Excludes2: Exposure to ignition or melting of nightwear (X05)

Exposure to ignition or melting of other clothing and apparel (X06.-)

Exposure to other specified smoke, fire and flames (X08.-)

The appropriate 7th character is to be added to each code from category X00

A - initial encounter

D - subsequent encounter

S - sequela

⊗⑦X00.0 **Exposure to flames in uncontrolled fire in building or structure**

⊗⑦X00.1 **Exposure to smoke in uncontrolled fire in building or structure**

⊗⑦X00.2 **Injury due to collapse of burning building or structure in uncontrolled fire**

Excludes1: injury due to collapse of building not on fire (W20.1)

⊗⑦X00.3 **Fall from burning building or structure in uncontrolled fire**

⊗⑦X00.4 **Hit by object from burning building or structure in uncontrolled fire**

⊗⑦X00.5 **Jump from burning building or structure in uncontrolled fire**

⊗⑦X00.8 **Other exposure to uncontrolled fire in building or structure**

X01 Exposure to uncontrolled fire, not in building or structure

Includes: exposure to forest fire

The appropriate 7th character is to be added to each code from category X01

A - initial encounter

D - subsequent encounter

S - sequela

⊗⑦X01.0 **Exposure to flames in uncontrolled fire, not in building or structure**

⊗⑦X01.1 **Exposure to smoke in uncontrolled fire, not in building or structure**

⊗⑦X01.3 **Fall due to uncontrolled fire, not in building or structure**

⊗⑦X01.4 **Hit by object due to uncontrolled fire, not in building or structure**

⊗⑦X01.8 **Other exposure to uncontrolled fire, not in building or structure**

X02 Exposure to controlled fire in building or structure

Includes: exposure to fire in fireplace

exposure to fire in stove

The appropriate 7th character is to be added to each code from category X02

A - initial encounter

D - subsequent encounter

S - sequela

⊗⑦X02.0 **Exposure to flames in controlled fire in building or structure**

⊗⑦**X02.1** **Exposure to smoke in controlled fire in building or structure**

⊗⑦**X02.2** **Injury due to collapse of burning building or structure in controlled fire**

Excludes1: injury due to collapse of building not on fire (W20.1)

⊗⑦**X02.3** **Fall from burning building or structure in controlled fire**

⊗⑦**X02.4** **Hit by object from burning building or structure in controlled fire**

⊗⑦**X02.5** **Jump from burning building or structure in controlled fire**

⊗⑦**X02.8** **Other exposure to controlled fire in building or structure**

X03 **Exposure to controlled fire, not in building or structure**

Includes: exposure to bon fire

exposure to camp-fire

exposure to trash fire

The appropriate 7th character is to be added to each code from category X03

A - initial encounter

D - subsequent encounter

S - sequela

⊗⑦**X03.0** **Exposure to flames in controlled fire, not in building or structure**

⊗⑦**X03.1** **Exposure to smoke in controlled fire, not in building or structure**

⊗⑦**X03.3** **Fall due to controlled fire, not in building or structure**

⊗⑦**X03.4** **Hit by object due to controlled fire, not in building or structure**

⊗⑦**X03.8** **Other exposure to controlled fire, not in building or structure**

X04 **Exposure to ignition of highly flammable material**

Exposure to ignition of gasoline

Exposure to ignition of kerosene

Exposure to ignition of petrol

Excludes2: exposure to ignition or melting of nightwear (X05)

exposure to ignition or melting **of other** clothing and apparel (X06)

The appropriate 7th character is to be added to code X04

A - initial encounter

D - subsequent encounter

S - sequela

⊗⑦**X05** **Exposure to ignition or melting of nightwear**

Excludes2: exposure to uncontrolled fire in building or structure (X00.-)

exposure to uncontrolled fire, not in building or structure (X01.-)

exposure to controlled fire in building or structure (X02.-)

exposure to controlled fire, not in building or structure (X03.-)

exposure to ignition of highly flammable materials (X04.-)

The appropriate 7th character is to be added to code X05

A - initial encounter

D - subsequent encounter

S - sequela

X06 **Exposure to ignition or melting of other clothing and apparel**

Excludes2: exposure to uncontrolled fire in building or structure (X00.-)

exposure to uncontrolled fire, not in building or structure (X01.-)

exposure to controlled fire in building or structure (X02.-)

exposure to controlled fire, not in building or structure (X03.-)

exposure to ignition of highly flammable materials (X04.-)

The appropriate 7th character is to be added to each code from category X06

A - initial encounter

D - subsequent encounter

S - sequela

⊗⑦**X06.0** **Exposure to ignition of plastic jewelry**

⊗⑦**X06.1** **Exposure to melting of plastic jewelry**

⊗⑦**X06.2** **Exposure to ignition of other clothing and apparel**

⊗⑦**X06.3** **Exposure to melting of other clothing and apparel**

X08 **Exposure to other specified smoke, fire and flames**

The appropriate 7th character is to be added to each code from category X08

A - initial encounter

D - subsequent encounter

S - sequela

X08.0 **Exposure to bed fire**

Exposure to mattress fire

⊗⑦**X08.00** **Exposure to bed fire due to unspecified burning material**

⊗⑦**X08.01** **Exposure to bed fire due to burning cigarette**

⊗⑦**X08.09** **Exposure to bed fire due to other burning material**

X08.1 **Exposure to sofa fire**

⊗⑦**X08.10** **Exposure to sofa fire due to unspecified burning material**

⊗⑦**X08.11** **Exposure to sofa fire due to burning cigarette**

⊗⑦**X08.19** **Exposure to sofa fire due to other burning material**

X08.2 **Exposure to other furniture fire**

⊗⑦**X08.20** **Exposure to other furniture fire due to unspecified burning material**

⊗⑦**X08.21** **Exposure to other furniture fire due to burning cigarette**

⊗⑦**X08.29** **Exposure to other furniture fire due to other burning material**

⊗⑦**X08.8** **Exposure to other specified smoke, fire and flames**

CONTACT WITH HEAT AND HOT SUBSTANCES (X10-X19)

Excludes1: exposure to excessive natural heat (X30)

exposure to fire and flames (X00-X08)

X10 **Contact with hot drinks, food, fats and cooking oils**

The appropriate 7th character is to be added to each code from category X10

A - initial encounter

D - subsequent encounter

S - sequela

⊗⑦**X10.0** **Contact with hot drinks**

⊗⑦**X10.1** **Contact with hot food**

⊗⑦**X10.2** **Contact with fats and cooking oils**

X11 **Contact with hot tap-water**

Includes: contact with boiling tap-water

contact with boiling water NOS

Excludes1: contact with water heated on stove (X12)

The appropriate 7th character is to be added to each code from category X11

A - initial encounter

D - subsequent encounter

S - sequela

⊗⑦**X11.0 Contact with hot water in bath or tub**

Excludes1: contact with running hot water in bath or tub (X11.1)

⊗⑦**X11.1 Contact with running hot water**

Contact with hot water running out of hose

Contact with hot water running out of tap

⊗⑦**X11.8 Contact with other hot tap-water**

Contact with hot water in bucket

Contact with hot tap-water NOS

⊗⑦**X12 Contact with other hot fluids**

Contact with water heated on stove

Excludes1: hot (liquid) metals (X18)

The appropriate 7th character is to be added to code X12

A - initial encounter

D - subsequent encounter

S - sequela

X13 Contact with steam and other hot vapors

The appropriate 7th character is to be added to each code from category X13

A - initial encounter

D - subsequent encounter

S - sequela

⊗⑦**X13.0 Inhalation of steam and other hot vapors**

⊗⑦**X13.1 Other contact with steam and other hot vapors**

X14 Contact with hot air and other hot gases

The appropriate 7th character is to be added to each code from category X14

A - initial encounter

D - subsequent encounter

S - sequela

⊗⑦**X14.0 Inhalation of hot air and gases**

⊗⑦**X14.1 Other contact with hot air and other hot gases**

X15 Contact with hot household appliances

Excludes1: contact with heating appliances (X16)

contact with powered household appliances (W29.-)

exposure to controlled fire in building or structure due to household appliance (X02.8)

exposure to household appliances electrical current (W86.0)

The appropriate 7th character is to be added to each code from category X15

A - initial encounter

D - subsequent encounter

S - sequela

⊗⑦**X15.0 Contact with hot stove (kitchen)**

⊗⑦**X15.1 Contact with hot toaster**

⊗⑦**X15.2 Contact with hotplate**

⊗⑦**X15.3 Contact with hot saucepan or skillet**

⊗⑦**X15.8 Contact with other hot household appliances**

Contact with cooker

Contact with kettle

Contact with light bulbs

⊗⑦**X16 Contact with hot heating appliances, radiators and pipes**

Excludes1: contact with powered appliances (W29.-)

exposure to controlled fire in building or structure due to appliance (X02.8)

exposure to industrial appliances electrical current (W86.1)

The appropriate 7th character is to be added to code X16

A - initial encounter

D - subsequent encounter

S - sequela

⊗⑦**X17 Contact with hot engines, machinery and tools**

Excludes1: contact with hot heating appliances, radiators and pipes (X16)

contact with hot household appliances (X15)

The appropriate 7th character is to be added to code X17

A - initial encounter

D - subsequent encounter

S - sequela

⊗⑦**X18 Contact with other hot metals**

Contact with liquid metal

The appropriate 7th character is to be added to code X18

A - initial encounter

D - subsequent encounter

S - sequela

⊗⑦**X19 Contact with other heat and hot substances**

Excludes1: objects that are not normally hot, e.g., an object made hot by a house fire (X00-X08)

The appropriate 7th character is to be added to code X19

A - initial encounter

D - subsequent encounter

S - sequela

EXPOSURE TO FORCES OF NATURE (X30-X39)

⊗⑦**X30 Exposure to excessive natural heat**

Exposure to excessive heat as the cause of sunstroke

Exposure to heat NOS

Excludes1: excessive heat of man-made origin (W92)

exposure to man-made radiation (W89)

exposure to sunlight (X32)

exposure to tanning bed (W89)

The appropriate 7th character is to be added to code X30

A - initial encounter

D - subsequent encounter

S - sequela

⊗⑦**X31 Exposure to excessive natural cold**

Excessive cold as the cause of chilblains NOS

Excessive cold as the cause of immersion foot or hand

Exposure to cold NOS

Exposure to weather conditions

Excludes1: cold of man-made origin (W93.-)

contact with or inhalation of dry ice (W93.-)

contact with or inhalation of liquefied gas (W93.-)

The appropriate 7th character is to be added to code X31

A - initial encounter

D - subsequent encounter

S - sequela

⊗⑦**X32 Exposure to sunlight**

Excludes1: man-made radiation (tanning bed) (W89)

Excludes2: radiation-related disorders of the skin and subcutaneous tissue (L55-L59)

The appropriate 7th character is to be added to code X32

A - initial encounter

D - subsequent encounter

S - sequela

⊗⑦**X34** **Earthquake**

Excludes2: tidal wave (tsunami) due to earthquake (X37.41)

The appropriate 7th character is to be added to code X34

A - initial encounter

D - subsequent encounter

S – sequela

⊗⑦**X35** **Volcanic eruption**

Excludes2: tidal wave (tsunami) due to volcanic eruption (X37.41)

The appropriate 7th character is to be added to code X35

A - initial encounter

D - subsequent encounter

S - sequela

X36 **Avalanche, landslide and other earth movements**

Includes: victim of mudslide of cataclysmic nature

Excludes1: earthquake (X34)

Excludes2: transport accident involving collision with avalanche or landslide not in motion (V01-V99)

The appropriate 7th character is to be added to each code from category X36

A - initial encounter

D - subsequent encounter

S - sequela

⊗⑦**X36.0** **Collapse of dam or man-made structure causing earth movement**

⊗⑦**X36.1** **Avalanche, landslide, or mudslide**

X37 **Cataclysmic storm**

The appropriate 7th character is to be added to each code from category X37

A - initial encounter

D - subsequent encounter

S - sequela

⊗⑦**X37.0** **Hurricane**

Storm surge

Typhoon

⊗⑦**X37.1** **Tornado**

Cyclone

Twister

⊗⑦**X37.2** **Blizzard (snow)(ice)**

⊗⑦**X37.3** **Dust storm**

X37.4 **Tidal wave**

⊗⑦**X37.41** **Tidal wave due to earthquake or volcanic eruption**

Tidal wave NOS

Tsunami

⊗⑦**X37.42** **Tidal wave due to storm**

⊗⑦**X37.43** **Tidal wave due to landslide**

⊗⑦**X37.8** **Other cataclysmic storms**

Cloudburst

Torrential rain

Excludes2: flood (X38)

⊗⑦**X37.9** **Unspecified cataclysmic storm**

Storm NOS

Excludes1: collapse of dam or man-made structure causing earth movement (X39.0)

⊗⑦**X38** **Flood**

Flood arising from remote storm

Flood of cataclysmic nature arising from melting snow

Flood resulting directly from storm

Excludes1: collapse of dam or man-made structure causing earth movement (X39.0)

tidal wave NOS (X37.41)

tidal wave caused by storm (X37.2)

The appropriate 7th character is to be added to code X38

A - initial encounter

D - subsequent encounter

S - sequela

X39 **Exposure to other forces of nature**

The appropriate 7th character is to be added to each code from category X39

A - initial encounter

D - subsequent encounter

S - sequela

⊗⑦**X39.0** **Exposure to natural radiation**

Excludes1: contact with and (suspected) exposure to radon and other naturally occurring radiation (Z77.123)

exposure to man-made radiation (W88-W90)

exposure to sunlight (X32)

⊗⑦**X39.01** **Exposure to radon**

⊗⑦**X39.08** **Exposure to other natural radiation**

⊗⑦**X39.8** **Other exposure to forces of nature**

OVEREXERTION AND STRENUOUS OR REPETITIVE MOVEMENTS (X50)

X50 **Overexertion and strenuous or repetitive movements**

The appropriate 7th character is to be added to each code from category X50

A - initial encounter

D - subsequent encounter

S - sequela

⊗⑦**X50.0** **Overexertion from strenuous movement or load**

Lifting heavy objects

Lifting weights

⊗⑦**X50.1** **Overexertion from prolonged static or awkward postures**

Prolonged bending

Prolonged kneeling

Prolonged reaching

Prolonged sitting

Prolonged standing

Prolonged twisting

Static bending

Static kneeling

Static reaching

Static sitting

Static standing

Static twisting

⊗⑦**X50.3** **Overexertion from repetitive movements**

Use of hand as hammer

Excludes2: Overuse from prolonged static or awkward
postures (X50.1)

⊗⑦**X50.9** **Other and unspecified overexertion or strenuous movements or postures**

Contact pressure

Contact stress

ACCIDENTAL EXPOSURE TO OTHER SPECIFIED FACTORS (X52-X58)

⊗⑦**X52** **Prolonged stay in weightless environment**

Weightlessness in spacecraft (simulator)

The appropriate 7th character is to be added to code X52

A - initial encounter

D - subsequent encounter

S - sequela

⊗⑦**X58** **Exposure to other specified factors**

Accident NOS

Exposure NOS

The appropriate 7th character is to be added to code X58

A - initial encounter

D - subsequent encounter

S - sequela

INTENTIONAL SELF-HARM (X71-X83)

Purposely self-inflicted injury Suicide (attempted)

X71 **Intentional self-harm by drowning and submersion**

The appropriate 7th character is to be added to each code from category X71

A - initial encounter

D - subsequent encounter

S - sequela

⊗⑦**X71.0** **Intentional self-harm by drowning and submersion while in bathtub**

⊗⑦**X71.1** **Intentional self-harm by drowning and submersion while in swimming pool**

⊗⑦**X71.2** **Intentional self-harm by drowning and submersion after jump into swimming pool**

⊗⑦**X71.3** **Intentional self-harm by drowning and submersion in natural water**

⊗⑦**X71.8** **Other intentional self-harm by drowning and submersion**

⊗⑦**X71.9** **Intentional self-harm by drowning and submersion, unspecified**

⊗⑦**X72** **Intentional self-harm by handgun discharge**

Intentional self-harm by gun for single hand use

Intentional self-harm by pistol

Intentional self-harm by revolver

Excludes1: Very pistol (X74.8)

The appropriate 7th character is to be added to code X72

A - initial encounter

D - subsequent encounter

S - sequela

X73 **Intentional self-harm by rifle, shotgun and larger firearm discharge**

Excludes1: airgun (X74.01)

The appropriate 7th character is to be added to each code from category X73

A - initial encounter

D - subsequent encounter

⊗⑦**X73.0** **Intentional self-harm by shotgun discharge**

⊗⑦**X73.1** **Intentional self-harm by hunting rifle discharge**

⊗⑦**X73.2** **Intentional self-harm by machine gun discharge**

⊗⑦**X73.8** **Intentional self-harm by other larger firearm discharge**

⊗⑦**X73.9** **Intentional self-harm by unspecified larger firearm discharge**

X74 **Intentional self-harm by other and unspecified firearm and gun discharge**

The appropriate 7th character is to be added to each code from category X74

A - initial encounter

D - subsequent encounter

S - sequela

X74.0 **Intentional self-harm by gas, air or spring-operated guns**

⊗⑦**X74.01** **Intentional self-harm by airgun**

Intentional self-harm by BB gun discharge

Intentional self-harm by pellet gun discharge

⊗⑦**X74.02** **Intentional self-harm by paintball gun**

⊗⑦**X74.09** **Intentional self-harm by other gas, air or spring-operated gun**

⊗⑦**X74.8** **Intentional self-harm by other firearm discharge**

Intentional self-harm by Very pistol [flare] discharge

⊗⑦**X74.9** **Intentional self-harm by unspecified firearm discharge**

⊗⑦**X75** **Intentional self-harm by explosive material**

The appropriate 7th character is to be added to code X75

A - initial encounter

D - subsequent encounter

S - sequela

⊗⑦**X76** **Intentional self-harm by smoke, fire and flames**

The appropriate 7th character is to be added to code X76

A - initial encounter

D - subsequent encounter

S - sequela

X77 **Intentional self-harm by steam, hot vapors and hot objects**

The appropriate 7th character is to be added to each code from category X77

A - initial encounter

D - subsequent encounter

S - sequela

⊗⑦**X77.0** **Intentional self-harm by steam or hot vapors**

⊗⑦**X77.1** **Intentional self-harm by hot tap water**

⊗⑦**X77.2** **Intentional self-harm by other hot fluids**

⊗⑦**X77.3** **Intentional self-harm by hot household appliances**

⊗⑦**X77.8** **Intentional self-harm by other hot objects**

⊗⑦**X77.9** **Intentional self-harm by unspecified hot objects**

X78 **Intentional self-harm by sharp object**

The appropriate 7th character is to be added to each code from category X78

A - initial encounter

D - subsequent encounter

S - sequela

⊗⑦**X78.0** **Intentional self-harm by sharp glass**

⊗⑦**X78.1** **Intentional self-harm by knife**

⊗⑦**X78.2** **Intentional self-harm by sword or dagger**

⊗⑦**X78.8** **Intentional self-harm by other sharp object**

⊗⑦X78.9   Intentional self-harm by unspecified sharp object

⊗⑦X79   **Intentional self-harm by blunt object**

The appropriate 7th character is to be added to code X79

A - initial encounter

D - subsequent encounter

S - sequela

⊗⑦X80   **Intentional self-harm by jumping from a high place**

Intentional fall from one level to another

The appropriate 7th character is to be added to code X80

A - initial encounter

D - subsequent encounter

S - sequela

X81   **Intentional self-harm by jumping or lying in front of moving object**

The appropriate 7th character is to be added to each code from category X81

A - initial encounter

D - subsequent encounter

S - sequela

⊗⑦X81.0   **Intentional self-harm by jumping or lying in front of motor vehicle**

⊗⑦X81.1   **Intentional self-harm by jumping or lying in front of (subway) train**

⊗⑦X81.8   **Intentional self-harm by jumping or lying in front of other moving object**

X82   **Intentional self-harm by crashing of motor vehicle**

The appropriate 7th character is to be added to each code from category X82

A - initial encounter

D - subsequent encounter

S - sequela

⊗⑦X82.0   **Intentional collision of motor vehicle with other motor vehicle**

⊗⑦X82.1   **Intentional collision of motor vehicle with train**

⊗⑦X82.2   **Intentional collision of motor vehicle with tree**

⊗⑦X82.8   **Other intentional self-harm by crashing of motor vehicle**

X83   **Intentional self-harm by other specified means**

Excludes1: intentional self-harm by poisoning or contact with toxic substance- See Table of Drugs and Chemicals

The appropriate 7th character is to be added to each code from category X83

A - initial encounter

D - subsequent encounter

S - sequela

⊗⑦X83.0   **Intentional self-harm by crashing of aircraft**

⊗⑦X83.1   **Intentional self-harm by electrocution**

⊗⑦X83.2   **Intentional self-harm by exposure to extremes of cold**

⊗⑦X83.8   **Intentional self-harm by other specified means**

ASSAULT (X92-Y09)

Includes: homicide

injuries inflicted by another person with intent to injure or kill, by any means

Excludes1: injuries due to legal intervention (Y35.-)

injuries due to operations of war (Y36.-)

injuries due to terrorism (Y38.-)

X92   **Assault by drowning and submersion**

The appropriate 7th character is to be added to each code from category X92

A - initial encounter

D - subsequent encounter

S - sequela

⊗⑦X92.0   **Assault by drowning and submersion while in bathtub**

⊗⑦X92.1   **Assault by drowning and submersion while in swimming pool**

⊗⑦X92.2   **Assault by drowning and submersion after push into swimming pool**

⊗⑦X92.3   **Assault by drowning and submersion in natural water**

⊗⑦X92.8   **Other assault by drowning and submersion**

⊗⑦X92.9   **Assault by drowning and submersion, unspecified**

⊗⑦X93   **Assault by handgun discharge**

Assault by discharge of gun for single hand use

Assault by discharge of pistol

Assault by discharge of revolver

Excludes1: Very pistol (X95.8)

The appropriate 7th character is to be added to code X93

A - initial encounter

D - subsequent encounter

S - sequela

X94   **Assault by rifle, shotgun and larger firearm discharge**

Excludes1: airgun (X95.01)

The appropriate 7th character is to be added to each code from category X94

A - initial encounter

D - subsequent encounter

S - sequela

⊗⑦X94.0   **Assault by shotgun**

⊗⑦X94.1   **Assault by hunting rifle**

⊗⑦X94.2   **Assault by machine gun**

⊗⑦X94.8   **Assault by other larger firearm discharge**

⊗⑦X94.9   **Assault by unspecified larger firearm discharge**

X95   **Assault by other and unspecified firearm and gun discharge**

The appropriate 7th character is to be added to each code from category X95

A - initial encounter

D - subsequent encounter

S - sequela

X95.0   **Assault by gas, air or spring-operated guns**

⊗⑦X95.01   **Assault by airgun discharge**

Assault by BB gun discharge

Assault by pellet gun discharge

⊗⑦X95.02   **Assault by paintball gun discharge**

⊗⑦X95.09   **Assault by other gas, air or spring-operated gun**

⊗⑦X95.8   **Assault by other firearm discharge**

Assault by very pistol [flare] discharge

⊗⑦X95.9   **Assault by unspecified firearm discharge**

X96   **Assault by explosive material**

Excludes1: incendiary device (X97)

terrorism involving explosive material (Y38.2-)

The appropriate 7th character is to be added to each code from category X96

A - initial encounter

D - subsequent encounter

S - sequela

⊗⑦**X96.0**   **Assault by antipersonnel bomb**

Excludes1: antipersonnel bomb use in military or war (Y36.2-)

⊗⑦**X96.1**   **Assault by gasoline bomb**

⊗⑦**X96.2**   **Assault by letter bomb**

⊗⑦**X96.3**   **Assault by fertilizer bomb**

⊗⑦**X96.4**   **Assault by pipe bomb**

⊗⑦**X96.8**   **Assault by other specified explosive**

⊗⑦**X96.9**   **Assault by unspecified explosive**

⊗⑦**X97**   **Assault by smoke, fire and flames**

Assault by arson

Assault by cigarettes

Assault by incendiary device

The appropriate 7th character is to be added to code X97

A - initial encounter

D - subsequent encounter

S - sequela

X98   **Assault by steam, hot vapors and hot objects**

The appropriate 7th character is to be added to each code from category X98

A - initial encounter

D - subsequent encounter

S - sequela

⊗⑦**X98.0**   **Assault by steam or hot vapors**

⊗⑦**X98.1**   **Assault by hot tap water**

⊗⑦**X98.2**   **Assault by hot fluids**

⊗⑦**X98.3**   **Assault by hot household appliances**

⊗⑦**X98.8**   **Assault by other hot objects**

⊗⑦**X98.9**   **Assault by unspecified hot objects**

X99   **Assault by sharp object**

Excludes1: assault by strike by sports equipment (Y08.0-)

The appropriate 7th character is to be added to each code from category X99

A - initial encounter

D - subsequent encounter

S - sequela

⊗⑦**X99.0**   **Assault by sharp glass**

⊗⑦**X99.1**   **Assault by knife**

⊗⑦**X99.2**   **Assault by sword or dagger**

⊗⑦**X99.8**   **Assault by other sharp object**

⊗⑦**X99.9**   **Assault by unspecified sharp object**

Assault by stabbing NOS

⊗⑦**Y00**   **Assault by blunt object**

Excludes1: assault by strike by sports equipment (Y08.0-)

The appropriate 7th character is to be added to code Y00

A - initial encounter

D - subsequent encounter

S - sequela

⊗⑦**Y01**   **Assault by pushing from high place**

The appropriate 7th character is to be added to code Y01

A - initial encounter

D - subsequent encounter

S - sequela

Y02   **Assault by pushing or placing victim in front of moving object**

The appropriate 7th character is to be added to each code from category Y02

A - initial encounter

D - subsequent encounter

S - sequela

⊗⑦**Y02.0**   **Assault by pushing or placing victim in front of motor vehicle**

⊗⑦**Y02.1**   **Assault by pushing or placing victim in front of (subway) train**

⊗⑦**Y02.8**   **Assault by pushing or placing victim in front of other moving object**

Y03   **Assault by crashing of motor vehicle**

The appropriate 7th character is to be added to each code from category Y03

A - initial encounter

D - subsequent encounter

S - sequela

⊗⑦**Y03.0**   **Assault by being hit or run over by motor vehicle**

⊗⑦**Y03.8**   **Other assault by crashing of motor vehicle**

Y04   **Assault by bodily force**

Excludes1: assault by:

submersion (X92.-)

use of weapon (X93-X95, X99, Y00)

The appropriate 7th character is to be added to each code from category Y04

A - initial encounter

D - subsequent encounter

S - sequela

⊗⑦**Y04.0**   **Assault by unarmed brawl or fight**

⊗⑦**Y04.1**   **Assault by human bite**

⊗⑦**Y04.2**   **Assault by strike against or bumped into by another person**

⊗⑦**Y04.8**   **Assault by other bodily force**

Assault by bodily force NOS

Y07   **Perpetrator of assault, maltreatment and neglect**

Note: Codes from this category are for use only in cases of confirmed abuse (T74.-)

Selection of the correct perpetrator code is based on the relationship between the perpetrator and the victim

Includes: perpetrator of abandonment

perpetrator of emotional neglect perpetrator of mental cruelty

perpetrator of physical abuse perpetrator of physical neglect

perpetrator of sexual abuse perpetrator of torture

Y07.0   **Spouse or partner, perpetrator of maltreatment and neglect**

Spouse or partner, perpetrator of maltreatment and neglect against spouse or partner

Y07.01   **Husband, perpetrator of maltreatment and neglect**

Y07.02   **Wife, perpetrator of maltreatment and neglect**

Y07.03   **Male partner, perpetrator of maltreatment and neglect**

Y07.04   **Female partner, perpetrator of maltreatment and neglect**

Y07.1   **Parent (adoptive) (biological), perpetrator of maltreatment and neglect**

Y07.11   **Biological father, perpetrator of maltreatment and neglect**

Y07.12   Biological mother, perpetrator of maltreatment and neglect

Y07.13   Adoptive father, perpetrator of maltreatment and neglect

Y07.14   Adoptive mother, perpetrator of maltreatment and neglect

Y07.4   Other family member, perpetrator of maltreatment and neglect

Y07.41   Sibling, perpetrator of maltreatment and neglect

Excludes1: stepsibling, perpetrator of maltreatment and neglect (Y07.435, Y07.436)

Y07.410   Brother, perpetrator of maltreatment and neglect

Y07.411   Sister, perpetrator of maltreatment and neglect

Y07.42   Foster parent, perpetrator of maltreatment and neglect

Y07.420   Foster father, perpetrator of maltreatment and neglect

Y07.421   Foster mother, perpetrator of maltreatment and neglect

Y07.43   Stepparent or stepsibling, perpetrator of maltreatment and neglect

Y07.430   Stepfather, perpetrator of maltreatment and neglect

Y07.432   Male friend of parent (co-residing in household), perpetrator of maltreatment and neglect

Y07.433   Stepmother, perpetrator of maltreatment and neglect

Y07.434   Female friend of parent (co-residing in household), perpetrator of maltreatment and neglect

Y07.435   Stepbrother, perpetrator or maltreatment and neglect

Y07.436   Stepsister, perpetrator of maltreatment and neglect

Y07.49   Other family member, perpetrator of maltreatment and neglect

Y07.490   Male cousin, perpetrator of maltreatment and neglect

Y07.491   Female cousin, perpetrator of maltreatment and neglect

Y07.499   Other family member, perpetrator of maltreatment and neglect

Y07.5   Non-family member, perpetrator of maltreatment and neglect

Y07.50   Unspecified non-family member, perpetrator of maltreatment and neglect

Y07.51   Daycare provider, perpetrator of maltreatment and neglect

Y07.510   At-home childcare provider, perpetrator of maltreatment and neglect

Y07.511   Daycare center childcare provider, perpetrator of maltreatment and neglect

Y07.512   At-home adult care provider, perpetrator of maltreatment and neglect

Y07.513   Adult care center provider, perpetrator of maltreatment and neglect

Y07.519   Unspecified daycare provider, perpetrator of maltreatment and neglect

Y07.52   Healthcare provider, perpetrator of maltreatment and neglect

Y07.521   Mental health provider, perpetrator of maltreatment and neglect

Y07.528   Other therapist or healthcare provider, perpetrator of maltreatment and neglect

Nurse perpetrator of maltreatment and neglect

Occupational therapist perpetrator of maltreatment and neglect

Physical therapist perpetrator of maltreatment and neglect

Speech therapist perpetrator of maltreatment and neglect

Y07.529   Unspecified healthcare provider, perpetrator of maltreatment and neglect

Y07.53   Teacher or instructor, perpetrator of maltreatment and neglect

Coach, perpetrator of maltreatment and neglect

Y07.59   Other non-family member, perpetrator of maltreatment and neglect

Y07.9   Unspecified perpetrator of maltreatment and neglect

Y08   Assault by other specified means

The appropriate 7th character is to be added to each code from category Y08

A - initial encounter

D - subsequent encounter

S - sequela

Y08.0   Assault by strike by sport equipment

⊗⑦Y08.01   Assault by strike by hockey stick

⊗⑦Y08.02   Assault by strike by baseball bat

⊗⑦Y08.09   Assault by strike by other specified type of sport equipment

Y08.8   Assault by other specified means

⊗⑦Y08.81   Assault by crashing of aircraft

⊗⑦Y08.89   Assault by other specified means

Y09   Assault by unspecified means

Assassination (attempted) NOS

Homicide (attempted) NOS

Manslaughter (attempted) NOS

Murder (attempted) NOS

EVENT OF UNDETERMINED INTENT (Y21-Y33)

Undetermined intent is only for use when there is specific documentation in the record that the intent of the injury cannot be determined. If no such documentation is present, code to accidental (unintentional)

Y21   Drowning and submersion, undetermined intent

The appropriate 7th character is to be added to each code from category Y21

A - initial encounter

D - subsequent encounter

S - sequela

⊗⑦**Y21.0** **Drowning and submersion while in bathtub, undetermined intent**

⊗⑦**Y21.1** **Drowning and submersion after fall into bathtub, undetermined intent**

⊗⑦**Y21.2** **Drowning and submersion while in swimming pool, undetermined intent**

⊗⑦**Y21.3** **Drowning and submersion after fall into swimming pool, undetermined intent**

⊗⑦**Y21.4** **Drowning and submersion in natural water, undetermined intent**

⊗⑦**Y21.8** **Other drowning and submersion, undetermined intent**

⊗⑦**Y21.9** **Unspecified drowning and submersion, undetermined intent**

⊗⑦**Y22** **Handgun discharge, undetermined intent**

Discharge of gun for single hand use, undetermined intent

Discharge of pistol, undetermined intent

Discharge of revolver, undetermined intent

Excludes2: very pistol (Y24.8)

The appropriate 7th character is to be added to code Y22

A - initial encounter

D - subsequent encounter

S - sequela

Y23 **Rifle, shotgun and larger firearm discharge, undetermined intent**

Excludes2: airgun (Y24.0)

The appropriate 7th character is to be added to each code from category Y23

A - initial encounter

D - subsequent encounter

S - sequela

⊗⑦**Y23.0** **Shotgun discharge, undetermined intent**

⊗⑦**Y23.1** **Hunting rifle discharge, undetermined intent**

⊗⑦**Y23.2** **Military firearm discharge, undetermined intent**

⊗⑦**Y23.3** **Machine gun discharge, undetermined intent**

⊗⑦**Y23.8** **Other larger firearm discharge, undetermined intent**

⊗⑦**Y23.9** **Unspecified larger firearm discharge, undetermined intent**

Y24 **Other and unspecified firearm discharge, undetermined intent**

The appropriate 7th character is to be added to each code from category Y24

A - initial encounter

D - subsequent encounter

S - sequela

⊗⑦**Y24.0** **Airgun discharge, undetermined intent**

BB gun discharge, undetermined intent

Pellet gun discharge, undetermined intent

⊗⑦**Y24.8** **Other firearm discharge, undetermined intent**

Paintball gun discharge, undetermined intent

Very pistol [flare] discharge, undetermined intent

⊗⑦**Y24.9** **Unspecified firearm discharge, undetermined intent**

⊗⑦**Y25** **Contact with explosive material, undetermined intent**

The appropriate 7th character is to be added to code Y25

A - initial encounter

D - subsequent encounter

S - sequela

⊗⑦**Y26** **Exposure to smoke, fire and flames, undetermined intent**

The appropriate 7th character is to be added to code Y26

A - initial encounter

D - subsequent encounter

S - sequela

Y27 **Contact with steam, hot vapors and hot objects, undetermined intent**

The appropriate 7th character is to be added to each code from category Y27

A - initial encounter

D - subsequent encounter

S - sequela

⊗⑦**Y27.0** **Contact with steam and hot vapors, undetermined intent**

⊗⑦**Y27.1** **Contact with hot tap water, undetermined intent**

⊗⑦**Y27.2** **Contact with hot fluids, undetermined intent**

⊗⑦**Y27.3** **Contact with hot household appliance, undetermined intent**

⊗⑦**Y27.8** **Contact with other hot objects, undetermined intent**

⊗⑦**Y27.9** **Contact with unspecified hot objects, undetermined intent**

Y28 **Contact with sharp object, undetermined intent**

The appropriate 7th character is to be added to each code from category Y28

A - initial encounter

D - subsequent encounter

S - sequela

⊗⑦**Y28.0** **Contact with sharp glass, undetermined intent**

⊗⑦**Y28.1** **Contact with knife, undetermined intent**

⊗⑦**Y28.2** **Contact with sword or dagger, undetermined intent**

⊗⑦**Y28.8** **Contact with other sharp object, undetermined intent**

⊗⑦**Y28.9** **Contact with unspecified sharp object, undetermined intent**

⊗⑦**Y29** **Contact with blunt object, undetermined intent**

The appropriate 7th character is to be added to code Y29

A - initial encounter

D - subsequent encounter

S - sequela

⊗⑦**Y30** **Falling, jumping or pushed from a high place, undetermined intent**

Victim falling from one level to another, undetermined intent

The appropriate 7th character is to be added to code Y30

A - initial encounter

D - subsequent encounter

S - sequela

⊗⑦**Y31** **Falling, lying or running before or into moving object, undetermined intent**

The appropriate 7th character is to be added to code Y31

A - initial encounter

D - subsequent encounter

S - sequela

⊗⑦**Y32** **Crashing of motor vehicle, undetermined intent**

The appropriate 7th character is to be added to code Y32

A - initial encounter

D - subsequent encounter

S - sequela

⊗⑦**Y33** **Other specified events, undetermined intent**

The appropriate 7th character is to be added to code Y33

A - initial encounter

D - subsequent encounter

S - sequela

LEGAL INTERVENTION, OPERATIONS OF WAR, MILITARY OPERATIONS, AND TERRORISM (Y35-Y38)

Y35 **Legal intervention**

Includes: any injury sustained as a result of an encounter with any law enforcement official, serving in any capacity at the time of the encounter, whether on-duty or off-duty

Includes: injury to law enforcement official, suspect and bystander

The appropriate 7th character is to be added to each code from category Y35

A - initial encounter

D - subsequent encounter

S - sequela

Y35.0 **Legal intervention involving firearm discharge**

Y35.00 **Legal intervention involving unspecified firearm discharge**

Legal intervention involving gunshot wound

Legal intervention involving shot NOS

⑦**Y35.001** **Legal intervention involving unspecified firearm discharge, law enforcement official injured**

⑦**Y35.002** **Legal intervention involving unspecified firearm discharge, bystander injured**

⑦**Y35.003** **Legal intervention involving unspecified firearm discharge, suspect injured**

Y35.01 **Legal intervention involving injury by machine gun**

⑦**Y35.011** **Legal intervention involving injury by machine gun, law enforcement official injured**

⑦**Y35.012** **Legal intervention involving injury by machine gun, bystander injured**

⑦**Y35.013** **Legal intervention involving injury by machine gun, suspect injured**

Y35.02 **Legal intervention involving injury by handgun**

⑦**Y35.021** **Legal intervention involving injury by handgun, law enforcement official injured**

⑦**Y35.022** **Legal intervention involving injury by handgun, bystander injured**

⑦**Y35.023** **Legal intervention involving injury by handgun, suspect injured**

Y35.03 **Legal intervention involving injury by rifle pellet**

⑦**Y35.031** **Legal intervention involving injury by rifle pellet, law enforcement official injured**

⑦**Y35.032** **Legal intervention involving injury by rifle pellet, bystander injured**

⑦**Y35.033** **Legal intervention involving injury by rifle pellet, suspect injured**

Y35.04 **Legal intervention involving injury by rubber bullet**

⑦**Y35.041** **Legal intervention involving injury by rubber bullet, law enforcement official injured**

⑦**Y35.042** **Legal intervention involving injury by rubber bullet, bystander injured**

⑦**Y35.043** **Legal intervention involving injury by rubber bullet, suspect injured**

Y35.09 **Legal intervention involving other firearm discharge**

⑦**Y35.091** **Legal intervention involving other firearm discharge, law enforcement official injured**

⑦**Y35.092** **Legal intervention involving other firearm discharge, bystander injured**

⑦**Y35.093** **Legal intervention involving other firearm discharge, suspect injured**

Y35.1 **Legal intervention involving explosives**

Y35.10 **Legal intervention involving unspecified explosives**

⑦**Y35.101** **Legal intervention involving unspecified explosives, law enforcement official injured**

⑦**Y35.102** **Legal intervention involving unspecified explosives, bystander injured**

⑦**Y35.103** **Legal intervention involving unspecified explosives, suspect injured**

Y35.11 **Legal intervention involving injury by dynamite**

⑦**Y35.111** **Legal intervention involving injury by dynamite, law enforcement official injured**

⑦**Y35.112** **Legal intervention involving injury by dynamite, bystander injured**

⑦**Y35.113** **Legal intervention involving injury by dynamite, suspect injured**

Y35.12 **Legal intervention involving injury by explosive shell**

⑦**Y35.121** **Legal intervention involving injury by explosive shell, law enforcement official injured**

⑦**Y35.122** **Legal intervention involving injury by explosive shell, bystander injured**

⑦**Y35.123** **Legal intervention involving injury by explosive shell, suspect injured**

Y35.19 **Legal intervention involving other explosives**

Legal intervention involving injury by grenade

Legal intervention involving injury by mortar bomb

⑦**Y35.191** **Legal intervention involving other explosives, law enforcement official injured**

⑦**Y35.192** **Legal intervention involving other explosives, bystander injured**

⑦**Y35.193** **Legal intervention involving other explosives, suspect injured**

Y35.2 **Legal intervention involving gas**

● New code ▲ Revised code **Excludes1:** Not coded here **Excludes2:** Not included here ⊗ Placeholder required ⑦7ᵗʰ digit required

Legal intervention involving asphyxiation by gas

Legal intervention involving poisoning by gas

Y35.20   Legal intervention involving unspecified gas

⑦**Y35.201**   Legal intervention involving unspecified gas, law enforcement official injured

⑦**Y35.202**   Legal intervention involving unspecified gas, bystander injured

⑦**Y35.203**   Legal intervention involving unspecified gas, suspect injured

Y35.21   Legal intervention involving injury by tear gas

⑦**Y35.211**   Legal intervention involving injury by tear gas, law enforcement official injured

⑦**Y35.212**   Legal intervention involving injury by tear gas, bystander injured

⑦**Y35.213**   Legal intervention involving injury by tear gas, suspect injured

Y35.29   Legal intervention involving other gas

⑦**Y35.291**   Legal intervention involving other gas, law enforcement official injured

⑦**Y35.292**   Legal intervention involving other gas, bystander injured

⑦**Y35.293**   Legal intervention involving other gas, suspect injured

Y35.3   Legal intervention involving blunt objects

Legal intervention involving being hit or struck by blunt object

Y35.30   Legal intervention involving unspecified blunt objects

⑦**Y35.301**   Legal intervention involving unspecified blunt objects, law enforcement official injured

⑦**Y35.302**   Legal intervention involving unspecified blunt objects, bystander injured

⑦**Y35.303**   Legal intervention involving unspecified blunt objects, suspect injured

Y35.31   Legal intervention involving baton

⑦**Y35.311**   Legal intervention involving baton, law enforcement official injured

⑦**Y35.312**   Legal intervention involving baton, bystander injured

⑦**Y35.313**   Legal intervention involving baton, suspect injured

Y35.39   Legal intervention involving other blunt objects

⑦**Y35.391**   Legal intervention involving other blunt objects, law enforcement official injured

⑦**Y35.392**   Legal intervention involving other blunt objects, bystander injured

⑦**Y35.393**   Legal intervention involving other blunt objects, suspect injured

Y35.4   Legal intervention involving sharp objects

Legal intervention involving being cut by sharp objects

Legal intervention involving being stabbed by sharp objects

Y35.40   Legal intervention involving unspecified sharp objects

⑦**Y35.401**   Legal intervention involving unspecified sharp objects, law enforcement official injured

⑦**Y35.402**   Legal intervention involving unspecified sharp objects, bystander injured

⑦**Y35.403**   Legal intervention involving unspecified sharp objects, suspect injured

Y35.41   Legal intervention involving bayonet

⑦**Y35.411**   Legal intervention involving bayonet, law enforcement official injured

⑦**Y35.412**   Legal intervention involving bayonet, bystander injured

⑦**Y35.413**   Legal intervention involving bayonet, suspect injured

Y35.49   Legal intervention involving other sharp objects

⑦**Y35.491**   Legal intervention involving other sharp objects, law enforcement official injured

⑦**Y35.492**   Legal intervention involving other sharp objects, bystander injured

⑦**Y35.493**   Legal intervention involving other sharp objects, suspect injured

Y35.8   Legal intervention involving other specified means

Y35.81   Legal intervention involving manhandling

⑦**Y35.811**   Legal intervention involving manhandling, law enforcement official injured

⑦**Y35.812**   Legal intervention involving manhandling, bystander injured

⑦**Y35.813**   Legal intervention involving manhandling, suspect injured

Y35.89   Legal intervention involving other specified means

⑦**Y35.891**   Legal intervention involving other specified means, law enforcement official injured

⑦**Y35.892**   Legal intervention involving other specified means, bystander injured

⑦**Y35.893**   Legal intervention involving other specified means, suspect injured

Y35.9   Legal intervention, means unspecified

⊗⑦**Y35.91**   Legal intervention, means unspecified, law enforcement official injured

⊗⑦**Y35.92**   Legal intervention, means unspecified, bystander injured

⊗⑦**Y35.93**   Legal intervention, means unspecified, suspect injured

Y36   Operations of war

Includes: injuries to military personnel and civilians caused by war, civil insurrection, and peacekeeping missions

Excludes1: injury to military personnel occurring during peacetime military operations (Y37.-)

military vehicles involved in transport accidents with non-military vehicle during peacetime (V09.01, V09.21, V19.81, V29.81, V39.81, V49.81, V59.81, V69.81, V79.81)

The appropriate 7th character is to be added to each code from category Y36

A - initial encounter
D - subsequent encounter
S - sequela

Y36.0 **War operations involving explosion of marine weapons**

    Y36.00 **War operations involving explosion of unspecified marine weapon**

        War operations involving underwater blast NOS

        ⑦**Y36.000** **War operations involving explosion of unspecified marine weapon, military personnel**

        ⑦**Y36.001** **War operations involving explosion of unspecified marine weapon, civilian**

    Y36.01 **War operations involving explosion of depth-charge**

        ⑦**Y36.010** **War operations involving explosion of depth-charge, military personnel**

        ⑦**Y36.011** **War operations involving explosion of depth-charge, civilian**

    Y36.02 **War operations involving explosion of marine mine**

        War operations involving explosion of marine mine, at sea or in harbor

        ⑦**Y36.020** **War operations involving explosion of marine mine, military personnel**

        ⑦**Y36.021** **War operations involving explosion of marine mine, civilian**

    Y36.03 **War operations involving explosion of sea-based artillery shell**

        ⑦**Y36.030** **War operations involving explosion of sea-based artillery shell, military personnel**

        ⑦**Y36.031** **War operations involving explosion of sea-based artillery shell, civilian**

    Y36.04 **War operations involving explosion of torpedo**

        ⑦**Y36.040** **War operations involving explosion of torpedo, military personnel**

        ⑦**Y36.041** **War operations involving explosion of torpedo, civilian**

    Y36.05 **War operations involving accidental detonation of onboard marine weapons**

        ⑦**Y36.050** **War operations involving accidental detonation of onboard marine weapons, military personnel**

        ⑦**Y36.051** **War operations involving accidental detonation of onboard marine weapons, civilian**

    Y36.09 **War operations involving explosion of other marine weapons**

        ⑦**Y36.090** **War operations involving explosion of other marine weapons, military personnel**

        ⑦**Y36.091** **War operations involving explosion of other marine weapons, civilian**

Y36.1 **War operations involving destruction of aircraft**

    Y36.10 **War operations involving unspecified destruction of aircraft**

        ⑦**Y36.100** **War operations involving unspecified destruction of aircraft, military personnel**

        ⑦**Y36.101** **War operations involving unspecified destruction of aircraft, civilian**

    Y36.11 **War operations involving destruction of aircraft due to enemy fire or explosives**

        War operations involving destruction of aircraft due to air to air missile

        War operations involving destruction of aircraft due to explosive placed on aircraft

        War operations involving destruction of aircraft due to rocket propelled grenade [RPG]

        War operations involving destruction of aircraft due to small arms fire

        War operations involving destruction of aircraft due to surface to air missile

        ⑦**Y36.110** **War operations involving destruction of aircraft due to enemy fire or explosives, military personnel**

        ⑦**Y36.111** **War operations involving destruction of aircraft due to enemy fire or explosives, civilian**

    Y36.12 **War operations involving destruction of aircraft due to collision with other aircraft**

        ⑦**Y36.120** **War operations involving destruction of aircraft due to collision with other aircraft, military personnel**

        ⑦**Y36.121** **War operations involving destruction of aircraft due to collision with other aircraft, civilian**

    Y36.13 **War operations involving destruction of aircraft due to onboard fire**

        ⑦**Y36.130** **War operations involving destruction of aircraft due to onboard fire, military personnel**

        ⑦**Y36.131** **War operations involving destruction of aircraft due to onboard fire, civilian**

    Y36.14 **War operations involving destruction of aircraft due to accidental detonation of onboard munitions and explosives**

        ⑦**Y36.140** **War operations involving destruction of aircraft due to accidental detonation of onboard munitions and explosives, military personnel**

        ⑦**Y36.141** **War operations involving destruction of aircraft due to accidental detonation of onboard munitions and explosives, civilian**

    Y36.19 **War operations involving other destruction of aircraft**

        ⑦**Y36.190** **War operations involving other destruction of aircraft, military personnel**

        ⑦**Y36.191** **War operations involving other destruction of aircraft, civilian**

Y36.2 **War operations involving other explosions and fragments**

● New code   ▲ Revised code   **Excludes1:** Not coded here   **Excludes2:** Not included here   ⊗ Placeholder required   ⑦7ᵗʰ digit required

Excludes1: war operations involving explosion of aircraft (Y36.1-)

war operations involving explosion of marine weapons (Y36.0-)

war operations involving explosion of nuclear weapons (Y36.5-)

war operations involving explosion occurring after cessation of hostilities (Y36.8-)

Y36.20 War operations involving unspecified explosion and fragments

War operations involving air blast NOS

War operations involving blast NOS

War operations involving blast fragments NOS

War operations involving blast wave NOS

War operations involving blast wind NOS

War operations involving explosion NOS

War operations involving explosion of bomb NOS

⑦**Y36.200 War operations involving unspecified explosion and fragments, military personnel**

⑦**Y36.201 War operations involving unspecified explosion and fragments, civilian**

Y36.21 War operations involving explosion of aerial bomb

⑦**Y36.210 War operations involving explosion of aerial bomb, military personnel**

⑦**Y36.211 War operations involving explosion of aerial bomb, civilian**

Y36.22 War operations involving explosion of guided missile

⑦**Y36.220 War operations involving explosion of guided missile, military personnel**

⑦**Y36.221 War operations involving explosion of guided missile, civilian**

Y36.23 War operations involving explosion of improvised explosive device [IED]

War operations involving explosion of person-borne improvised explosive device [IED]

War operations involving explosion of vehicle-borne improvised explosive device [IED]

War operations involving explosion of roadside improvised explosive device [IED]

⑦**Y36.230 War operations involving explosion of improvised explosive device [IED], military personnel**

⑦**Y36.231 War operations involving explosion of improvised explosive device [IED], civilian**

Y36.24 War operations involving explosion due to accidental detonation and discharge of own munitions or munitions launch device

⑦**Y36.240 War operations involving explosion due to accidental detonation and discharge of own munitions or munitions launch device, military personnel**

⑦**Y36.241 War operations involving explosion due to accidental detonation and discharge of own**

munitions or munitions launch device, civilian

Y36.25 War operations involving fragments from munitions

⑦**Y36.250 War operations involving fragments from munitions, military personnel**

⑦**Y36.251 War operations involving fragments from munitions, civilian**

Y36.26 War operations involving fragments of improvised explosive device [IED]

War operations involving fragments of person-borne improvised explosive device [IED]

War operations involving fragments of vehicle-borne improvised explosive device [IED]

War operations involving fragments of roadside improvised explosive device [IED]

⑦**Y36.260 War operations involving fragments of improvised explosive device [IED], military personnel**

⑦**Y36.261 War operations involving fragments of improvised explosive device [IED], civilian**

Y36.27 War operations involving fragments from weapons

⑦**Y36.270 War operations involving fragments from weapons, military personnel**

⑦**Y36.271 War operations involving fragments from weapons, civilian**

Y36.29 War operations involving other explosions and fragments

War operations involving explosion of grenade War operations involving explosions of land mine War operations involving shrapnel NOS

⑦**Y36.290 War operations involving other explosions and fragments, military personnel**

⑦**Y36.291 War operations involving other explosions and fragments, civilian**

Y36.3 War operations involving fires, conflagrations and hot substances

War operations involving smoke, fumes, and heat from fires, conflagrations and hot substances

Excludes1: war operations involving fires and conflagrations aboard military aircraft (Y36.1-)

war operations involving fires and conflagrations aboard military watercraft (Y36.0-)

war operations involving fires and conflagrations caused indirectly by conventional weapons (Y36.2-)

war operations involving fires and thermal effects of nuclear weapons (Y36.53-)

Y36.30 War operations involving unspecified fire, conflagration and hot substance

⑦**Y36.300 War operations involving unspecified fire, conflagration and hot substance, military personnel**

⑦**Y36.301 War operations involving unspecified fire, conflagration and hot substance, civilian**

Y36.31 War operations involving gasoline bomb

War operations involving incendiary bomb

War operations involving petrol bomb

⑦**Y36.310** **War operations involving gasoline bomb, military personnel**

⑦**Y36.311** **War operations involving gasoline bomb, civilian**

Y36.32 **War operations involving incendiary bullet**

⑦**Y36.320** **War operations involving incendiary bullet, military personnel**

⑦**Y36.321** **War operations involving incendiary bullet, civilian**

Y36.33 **War operations involving flamethrower**

⑦**Y36.330** **War operations involving flamethrower, military personnel**

⑦**Y36.331** **War operations involving flamethrower, civilian**

Y36.39 **War operations involving other fires, conflagrations and hot substances**

⑦**Y36.390** **War operations involving other fires, conflagrations and hot substances, military personnel**

⑦**Y36.391** **War operations involving other fires, conflagrations and hot substances, civilian**

Y36.4 **War operations involving firearm discharge and other forms of conventional warfare**

Y36.41 **War operations involving rubber bullets**

⑦**Y36.410** **War operations involving rubber bullets, military personnel**

⑦**Y36.411** **War operations involving rubber bullets, civilian**

Y36.42 **War operations involving firearms pellets**

⑦**Y36.420** **War operations involving firearms pellets, military personnel**

⑦**Y36.421** **War operations involving firearms pellets, civilian**

Y36.43 **War operations involving other firearms discharge**

War operations involving bullets NOS

Excludes1: war operations involving munitions fragments (Y36.25-)

war operations involving incendiary bullets (Y36.32-)

⑦**Y36.430** **War operations involving other firearms discharge, military personnel**

⑦**Y36.431** **War operations involving other firearms discharge, civilian**

Y36.44 **War operations involving unarmed hand to hand combat**

Excludes1: war operations involving combat using blunt or piercing object (Y36.45-)

war operations involving intentional restriction of air and airway (Y36.46-)

war operations involving unintentional restriction of air and airway (Y36.47-)

⑦**Y36.440** **War operations involving unarmed hand to hand combat, military personnel**

⑦**Y36.441** **War operations involving unarmed hand to hand combat, civilian**

Y36.45 **War operations involving combat using blunt or piercing object**

⑦**Y36.450** **War operations involving combat using blunt or piercing object, military personnel**

⑦**Y36.451** **War operations involving combat using blunt or piercing object, civilian**

Y36.46 **War operations involving intentional restriction of air and airway**

⑦**Y36.460** **War operations involving intentional restriction of air and airway, military personnel**

⑦**Y36.461** **War operations involving intentional restriction of air and airway, civilian**

Y36.47 **War operations involving unintentional restriction of air and airway**

⑦**Y36.470** **War operations involving unintentional restriction of air and airway, military personnel**

⑦**Y36.471** **War operations involving unintentional restriction of air and airway, civilian**

Y36.49 **War operations involving other forms of conventional warfare**

⑦**Y36.490** **War operations involving other forms of conventional warfare, military personnel**

⑦**Y36.491** **War operations involving other forms of conventional warfare, civilian**

Y36.5 **War operations involving nuclear weapons**

War operations involving dirty bomb NOS

Y36.50 **War operations involving unspecified effect of nuclear weapon**

⑦**Y36.500** **War operations involving unspecified effect of nuclear weapon, military personnel**

⑦**Y36.501** **War operations involving unspecified effect of nuclear weapon, civilian**

Y36.51 **War operations involving direct blast effect of nuclear weapon**

War operations involving blast pressure of nuclear weapon

⑦**Y36.510** **War operations involving direct blast effect of nuclear weapon, military personnel**

⑦**Y36.511** **War operations involving direct blast effect of nuclear weapon, civilian**

Y36.52 **War operations involving indirect blast effect of nuclear weapon**

War operations involving being thrown by blast of nuclear weapon

War operations involving being struck or crushed by blast debris of nuclear weapon

⑦**Y36.520** **War operations involving indirect blast effect of nuclear weapon, military personnel**

⑦Y36.521　**War operations involving indirect blast effect of nuclear weapon, civilian**

Y36.53　**War operations involving thermal radiation effect of nuclear weapon**

War operations involving direct heat from nuclear weapon

War operation involving fireball effects from nuclear weapon

⑦Y36.530　**War operations involving thermal radiation effect of nuclear weapon, military personnel**

⑦Y36.531　**War operations involving thermal radiation effect of nuclear weapon, civilian**

Y36.54　**War operation involving nuclear radiation effects of nuclear weapon**

War operation involving acute radiation exposure from nuclear weapon

War operation involving exposure to immediate ionizing radiation from nuclear weapon

War operation involving fallout exposure from nuclear weapon

War operation involving secondary effects of nuclear weapons

⑦Y36.540　**War operation involving nuclear radiation effects of nuclear weapon, military personnel**

⑦Y36.541　**War operation involving nuclear radiation effects of nuclear weapon, civilian**

Y36.59　**War operation involving other effects of nuclear weapons**

⑦Y36.590　**War operation involving other effects of nuclear weapons, military personnel**

⑦Y36.591　**War operation involving other effects of nuclear weapons, civilian**

Y36.6　**War operations involving biological weapons**

Y36.6X **War operations involving biological weapons**

⑦Y36.6X0　**War operations involving biological weapons, military personnel**

⑦Y36.6X1　**War operations involving biological weapons, civilian**

Y36.7　**War operations involving chemical weapons and other forms of unconventional warfare**

Excludes1: war operations involving incendiary devices (Y36.3-, Y36.5-)

Y36.7X **War operations involving chemical weapons and other forms of unconventional warfare**

⑦Y36.7X0　**War operations involving chemical weapons and other forms of unconventional warfare, military personnel**

⑦Y36.7X1　**War operations involving chemical weapons and other forms of unconventional warfare, civilian**

Y36.8　**War operations occurring after cessation of hostilities**

War operations classifiable to categories Y36.0-Y36.8 but occurring after cessation of hostilities

Y36.81　Explosion of mine placed during war operations but exploding after cessation of hostilities

⑦Y36.810　**Explosion of mine placed during war operations but exploding after cessation of hostilities, military personnel**

⑦Y36.811　**Explosion of mine placed during war operations but exploding after cessation of hostilities, civilian**

Y36.82　Explosion of bomb placed during war operations but exploding after cessation of hostilities

⑦Y36.820　**Explosion of bomb placed during war operations but exploding after cessation of hostilities, military personnel**

⑦Y36.821　**Explosion of bomb placed during war operations but exploding after cessation of hostilities, civilian**

Y36.88　Other war operations occurring after cessation of hostilities

⑦Y36.880　**Other war operations occurring after cessation of hostilities, military personnel**

⑦Y36.881　**Other war operations occurring after cessation of hostilities, civilian**

Y36.89　Unspecified war operations occurring after cessation of hostilities

⑦Y36.890　**Unspecified war operations occurring after cessation of hostilities, military personnel**

⑦Y36.891　**Unspecified war operations occurring after cessation of hostilities, civilian**

Y36.9　**Other and unspecified war operations**

⊗⑦Y36.90　**War operations, unspecified**

⊗⑦Y36.91　**War operations involving unspecified weapon of mass destruction [WMD]**

⊗⑦Y36.92　**War operations involving friendly fire**

Y37　**Military operations**

Includes: injuries to military personnel and civilians occurring during peacetime on military property and during routine military exercises and operations

Excludes1: military aircraft involved in aircraft accident with civilian aircraft (V97.81-)

military vehicles involved in transport accident with civilian vehicle (V09.01, V09.21, V19.81, V29.81, V39.81, V49.81, V59.81, V69.81, V79.81)

military watercraft involved in water transport accident with civilian watercraft (V94.81-) war operations (Y36.-)

The appropriate 7th character is to be added to each code from category Y37

A - initial encounter

D - subsequent encounter

S - sequela

Y37.0　**Military operations involving explosion of marine weapons**

Y37.00　**Military operations involving explosion of unspecified marine weapon**

Military operations involving underwater blast NOS

	Add 4th-7th digits		Nonspecific code		Unspecified code		Manifestation code

⑦ **Y37.000**   **Military operations involving explosion of unspecified marine weapon, military personnel**

⑦ **Y37.001**   **Military operations involving explosion of unspecified marine weapon, civilian**

Y37.01   **Military operations involving explosion of depth-charge**

⑦ **Y37.010**   **Military operations involving explosion of depth-charge, military personnel**

⑦ **Y37.011**   **Military operations involving explosion of depth-charge, civilian**

Y37.02   **Military operations involving explosion of marine mine**

Military operations involving explosion of marine mine, at sea or in harbor

⑦ **Y37.020**   **Military operations involving explosion of marine mine, military personnel**

⑦ **Y37.021**   **Military operations involving explosion of marine mine, civilian**

Y37.03   **Military operations involving explosion of sea-based artillery shell**

⑦ **Y37.030**   **Military operations involving explosion of sea-based artillery shell, military personnel**

⑦ **Y37.031**   **Military operations involving explosion of sea-based artillery shell, civilian**

Y37.04   **Military operations involving explosion of torpedo**

⑦ **Y37.040**   **Military operations involving explosion of torpedo, military personnel**

⑦ **Y37.041**   **Military operations involving explosion of torpedo, civilian**

Y37.05   **Military operations involving accidental detonation of onboard marine weapons**

⑦ **Y37.050**   **Military operations involving accidental detonation of onboard marine weapons, military personnel**

⑦ **Y37.051**   **Military operations involving accidental detonation of onboard marine weapons, civilian**

Y37.09   **Military operations involving explosion of other marine weapons**

⑦ **Y37.090**   **Military operations involving explosion of other marine weapons, military personnel**

⑦ **Y37.091**   **Military operations involving explosion of other marine weapons, civilian**

Y37.1   **Military operations involving destruction of aircraft**

Y37.10   **Military operations involving unspecified destruction of aircraft**

⑦ **Y37.100**   **Military operations involving unspecified destruction of aircraft, military personnel**

⑦ **Y37.101**   **Military operations involving unspecified destruction of aircraft, civilian**

Y37.11   **Military operations involving destruction of aircraft due to enemy fire or explosives**

Military operations involving destruction of aircraft due to air to air missile

Military operations involving destruction of aircraft due to explosive placed on aircraft

Military operations involving destruction of aircraft due to rocket propelled grenade [RPG]

Military operations involving destruction of aircraft due to small arms fire

Military operations involving destruction of aircraft due to surface to air missile

⑦ **Y37.110**   **Military operations involving destruction of aircraft due to enemy fire or explosives, military personnel**

⑦ **Y37.111**   **Military operations involving destruction of aircraft due to enemy fire or explosives, civilian**

Y37.12   **Military operations involving destruction of aircraft due to collision with other aircraft**

⑦ **Y37.120**   **Military operations involving destruction of aircraft due to collision with other aircraft, military personnel**

⑦ **Y37.121**   **Military operations involving destruction of aircraft due to collision with other aircraft, civilian**

Y37.13   **Military operations involving destruction of aircraft due to onboard fire**

⑦ **Y37.130**   **Military operations involving destruction of aircraft due to onboard fire, military personnel**

⑦ **Y37.131**   **Military operations involving destruction of aircraft due to onboard fire, civilian**

Y37.14   **Military operations involving destruction of aircraft due to accidental detonation of onboard munitions and explosives**

⑦ **Y37.140**   **Military operations involving destruction of aircraft due to accidental detonation of onboard munitions and explosives, military personnel**

⑦ **Y37.141**   **Military operations involving destruction of aircraft due to accidental detonation of onboard munitions and explosives, civilian**

Y37.19   **Military operations involving other destruction of aircraft**

⑦ **Y37.190**   **Military operations involving other destruction of aircraft, military personnel**

⑦ **Y37.191**   **Military operations involving other destruction of aircraft, civilian**

Y37.2   **Military operations involving other explosions and fragments**

Excludes1: military operations involving explosion of aircraft (Y37.1-)

military operations involving explosion of marine weapons (Y37.0-)

military operations involving explosion of nuclear weapons (Y37.5-)

Y37.20   **Military operations involving unspecified explosion and fragments**

Military operations involving air blast NOS

Military operations involving blast NOS

Military operations involving blast fragments NOS

Military operations involving blast wave NOS

Military operations involving blast wind NOS

Military operations involving explosion NOS

Military operations involving explosion of bomb NOS

⑦**Y37.200** **Military operations involving unspecified explosion and fragments, military personnel**

⑦**Y37.201** **Military operations involving unspecified explosion and fragments, civilian**

Y37.21 **Military operations involving explosion of aerial bomb**

⑦**Y37.210** **Military operations involving explosion of aerial bomb, military personnel**

⑦**Y37.211** **Military operations involving explosion of aerial bomb, civilian**

Y37.22 **Military operations involving explosion of guided missile**

⑦**Y37.220** **Military operations involving explosion of guided missile, military personnel**

⑦**Y37.221** **Military operations involving explosion of guided missile, civilian**

Y37.23 **Military operations involving explosion of improvised explosive device [IED]**

Military operations involving explosion of person-borne improvised explosive device [IED]

Military operations involving explosion of vehicle-borne improvised explosive device [IED]

Military operations involving explosion of roadside improvised explosive device [IED]

⑦**Y37.230** **Military operations involving explosion of improvised explosive device [IED], military personnel**

⑦**Y37.231** **Military operations involving explosion of improvised explosive device [IED], civilian**

Y37.24 **Military operations involving explosion due to accidental detonation and discharge of own munitions or munitions launch device**

⑦**Y37.240** **Military operations involving explosion due to accidental detonation and discharge of own munitions or munitions launch device, military personnel**

⑦**Y37.241** **Military operations involving explosion due to accidental detonation and discharge of own munitions or munitions launch device, civilian**

Y37.25 **Military operations involving fragments from munitions**

⑦**Y37.250** **Military operations involving fragments from munitions, military personnel**

⑦**Y37.251** **Military operations involving fragments from munitions, civilian**

Y37.26 **Military operations involving fragments of improvised explosive device [IED]**

Military operations involving fragments of person-borne improvised explosive device [IED]

Military operations involving fragments of vehicle-borne improvised explosive device [IED]

Military operations involving fragments of roadside improvised explosive device [IED]

⑦**Y37.260** **Military operations involving fragments of improvised explosive device [IED], military personnel**

⑦**Y37.261** **Military operations involving fragments of improvised explosive device [IED], civilian**

Y37.27 **Military operations involving fragments from weapons**

⑦**Y37.270** **Military operations involving fragments from weapons, military personnel**

⑦**Y37.271** **Military operations involving fragments from weapons, civilian**

Y37.29 **Military operations involving other explosions and fragments**

Military operations involving explosion of grenade

Military operations involving explosions of land mine

Military operations involving shrapnel NOS

⑦**Y37.290** **Military operations involving other explosions and fragments, military personnel**

⑦**Y37.291** **Military operations involving other explosions and fragments, civilian**

Y37.3 **Military operations involving fires, conflagrations and hot substances**

Military operations involving smoke, fumes, and heat from fires, conflagrations and hot substances

Excludes1: military operations involving fires and conflagrations aboard military aircraft (Y37.1-)

military operations involving fires and conflagrations aboard military watercraft (Y37.0-)

military operations involving fires and conflagrations caused indirectly by conventional weapons (Y37.2-)

military operations involving fires and thermal effects of nuclear weapons (Y36.53-)

Y37.30 **Military operations involving unspecified fire, conflagration and hot substance**

⑦**Y37.300** **Military operations involving unspecified fire, conflagration and hot substance, military personnel**

⑦**Y37.301** **Military operations involving unspecified fire, conflagration and hot substance, civilian**

Y37.31 **Military operations involving gasoline bomb**

Military operations involving incendiary bomb

Military operations involving petrol bomb

⑦**Y37.310** **Military operations involving gasoline bomb, military personnel**

⑦ **Y37.311** **Military operations involving gasoline bomb, civilian**

Y37.32 **Military operations involving incendiary bullet**

⑦ **Y37.320** **Military operations involving incendiary bullet, military personnel**

⑦ **Y37.321** **Military operations involving incendiary bullet, civilian**

Y37.33 **Military operations involving flamethrower**

⑦ **Y37.330** **Military operations involving flamethrower, military personnel**

⑦ **Y37.331** **Military operations involving flamethrower, civilian**

Y37.39 **Military operations involving other fires, conflagrations and hot substances**

⑦ **Y37.390** **Military operations involving other fires, conflagrations and hot substances, military personnel**

⑦ **Y37.391** **Military operations involving other fires, conflagrations and hot substances, civilian**

Y37.4 **Military operations involving firearm discharge and other forms of conventional warfare**

Y37.41 **Military operations involving rubber bullets**

⑦ **Y37.410** **Military operations involving rubber bullets, military personnel**

⑦ **Y37.411** **Military operations involving rubber bullets, civilian**

Y37.42 **Military operations involving firearms pellets**

⑦ **Y37.420** **Military operations involving firearms pellets, military personnel**

⑦ **Y37.421** **Military operations involving firearms pellets, civilian**

Y37.43 **Military operations involving other firearms discharge**

Military operations involving bullets NOS

Excludes1: military operations involving munitions fragments (Y37.25-)

military operations involving incendiary bullets (Y37.32-)

⑦ **Y37.430** **Military operations involving other firearms discharge, military personnel**

⑦ **Y37.431** **Military operations involving other firearms discharge, civilian**

Y37.44 **Military operations involving unarmed hand to hand combat**

Excludes1: military operations involving combat using blunt or piercing object (Y37.45-)

military operations involving intentional restriction of air and airway (Y37.46-)

military operations involving unintentional restriction of air and airway (Y37.47-)

⑦ **Y37.440** **Military operations involving unarmed hand to hand combat, military personnel**

⑦ **Y37.441** **Military operations involving unarmed hand to hand combat, civilian**

Y37.45 **Military operations involving combat using blunt or piercing object**

⑦ **Y37.450** **Military operations involving combat using blunt or piercing object, military personnel**

⑦ **Y37.451** **Military operations involving combat using blunt or piercing object, civilian**

Y37.46 **Military operations involving intentional restriction of air and airway**

⑦ **Y37.460** **Military operations involving intentional restriction of air and airway, military personnel**

⑦ **Y37.461** **Military operations involving intentional restriction of air and airway, civilian**

Y37.47 **Military operations involving unintentional restriction of air and airway**

⑦ **Y37.470** **Military operations involving unintentional restriction of air and airway, military personnel**

⑦ **Y37.471** **Military operations involving unintentional restriction of air and airway, civilian**

Y37.49 **Military operations involving other forms of conventional warfare**

⑦ **Y37.490** **Military operations involving other forms of conventional warfare, military personnel**

⑦ **Y37.491** **Military operations involving other forms of conventional warfare, civilian**

Y37.5 **Military operations involving nuclear weapons**

Military operation involving dirty bomb NOS

Y37.50 **Military operations involving unspecified effect of nuclear weapon**

⑦ **Y37.500** **Military operations involving unspecified effect of nuclear weapon, military personnel**

⑦ **Y37.501** **Military operations involving unspecified effect of nuclear weapon, civilian**

Y37.51 **Military operations involving direct blast effect of nuclear weapon**

Military operations involving blast pressure of nuclear weapon

⑦ **Y37.510** **Military operations involving direct blast effect of nuclear weapon, military personnel**

⑦ **Y37.511** **Military operations involving direct blast effect of nuclear weapon, civilian**

Y37.52 **Military operations involving indirect blast effect of nuclear weapon**

Military operations involving being thrown by blast of nuclear weapon

Military operations involving being struck or crushed by blast debris of nuclear weapon

⑦ **Y37.520** **Military operations involving indirect blast effect of nuclear weapon, military personnel**

⑦ **Y37.521** **Military operations involving indirect blast effect of nuclear weapon, civilian**

Y37.53 **Military operations involving thermal radiation effect of nuclear weapon**

● New code   ▲ Revised code   **Excludes1:** Not coded here   **Excludes2:** Not included here   ⊗ Placeholder required   ⑦ 7th digit required

Military operations involving direct heat from nuclear weapon

Military operation involving fireball effects from nuclear weapon

⑦Y37.530 **Military operations involving thermal radiation effect of nuclear weapon, military personnel**

⑦Y37.531 **Military operations involving thermal radiation effect of nuclear weapon, civilian**

Y37.54 **Military operation involving nuclear radiation effects of nuclear weapon**

Military operation involving acute radiation exposure from nuclear weapon

Military operation involving exposure to immediate ionizing radiation from nuclear weapon

Military operation involving fallout exposure from nuclear weapon

Military operation involving secondary effects of nuclear weapons

⑦Y37.540 **Military operation involving nuclear radiation effects of nuclear weapon, military personnel**

⑦Y37.541 **Military operation involving nuclear radiation effects of nuclear weapon, civilian**

Y37.59 **Military operation involving other effects of nuclear weapons**

⑦Y37.590 **Military operation involving other effects of nuclear weapons, military personnel**

⑦Y37.591 **Military operation involving other effects of nuclear weapons, civilian**

Y37.6 **Military operations involving biological weapons**

Y37.6X **Military operations involving biological weapons**

⑦Y37.6X0 **Military operations involving biological weapons, military personnel**

⑦Y37.6X1 **Military operations involving biological weapons, civilian**

Y37.7 **Military operations involving chemical weapons and other forms of unconventional warfare**

Excludes1: military operations involving incendiary devices (Y36.3-, Y36.5-)

Y37.7X **Military operations involving chemical weapons and other forms of unconventional warfare**

⑦Y37.7X0 **Military operations involving chemical weapons and other forms of unconventional warfare, military personnel**

⑦Y37.7X1 **Military operations involving chemical weapons and other forms of unconventional warfare, civilian**

Y37.9 **Other and unspecified military operations**

⊗⑦Y37.90 **Military operations, unspecified**

⊗⑦Y37.91 **Military operations involving unspecified weapon of mass destruction [WMD]**

⊗⑦Y37.92 **Military operations involving friendly fire**

Y38 Terrorism

These codes are for use to identify injuries resulting from the unlawful use of force or violence against persons or property to intimidate or coerce a Government, the civilian population, or any segment thereof, in furtherance of political or social objective

Use additional code for place of occurrence (Y92.-)

The appropriate 7th character is to be added to each code from category Y38

A - initial encounter

D - subsequent encounter

S - sequela

Y38.0 **Terrorism involving explosion of marine weapons**

Terrorism involving depth-charge

Terrorism involving marine mine

Terrorism involving mine NOS, at sea or in harbor

Terrorism involving sea-based artillery shell

Terrorism involving torpedo

Terrorism involving underwater blast

Y38.0X **Terrorism involving explosion of marine weapons**

⑦Y38.0X1 **Terrorism involving explosion of marine weapons, public safety official injured**

⑦Y38.0X2 **Terrorism involving explosion of marine weapons, civilian injured**

⑦Y38.0X3 **Terrorism involving explosion of marine weapons, terrorist injured**

Y38.1 **Terrorism involving destruction of aircraft**

Terrorism involving aircraft burned

Terrorism involving aircraft exploded

Terrorism involving aircraft being shot down

Terrorism involving aircraft used as a weapon

Y38.1X **Terrorism involving destruction of aircraft**

⑦Y38.1X1 **Terrorism involving destruction of aircraft, public safety official injured**

⑦Y38.1X2 **Terrorism involving destruction of aircraft, civilian injured**

⑦Y38.1X3 **Terrorism involving destruction of aircraft, terrorist injured**

Y38.2 **Terrorism involving other explosions and fragments**

Terrorism involving antipersonnel (fragments) bomb

Terrorism involving blast NOS

Terrorism involving explosion NOS

Terrorism involving explosion of breech block

Terrorism involving explosion of cannon block

Terrorism involving explosion (fragments) of artillery shell

Terrorism involving explosion (fragments) of bomb

Terrorism involving explosion (fragments) of grenade

Terrorism involving explosion (fragments) of guided missile

Terrorism involving explosion (fragments) of land mine

Terrorism involving explosion of mortar bomb

Terrorism involving explosion of munitions

Terrorism involving explosion (fragments) of rocket

Terrorism involving explosion (fragments) of shell

Terrorism involving shrapnel

Terrorism involving mine NOS, on land

Excludes1: terrorism involving explosion of nuclear weapon (Y38.5)

| | Add 4th-7th digits | | Nonspecific code | | Unspecified code | | Manifestation code |

terrorism involving suicide bomber (Y38.81)

Y38.2X Terrorism involving other explosions and fragments

⑦ Y38.2X1 **Terrorism involving other explosions and fragments, public safety official injured**

⑦ Y38.2X2 **Terrorism involving other explosions and fragments, civilian injured**

⑦ Y38.2X3 **Terrorism involving other explosions and fragments, terrorist injured**

Y38.3 Terrorism involving fires, conflagration and hot substances

Terrorism involving conflagration NOS

Terrorism involving fire NOS

Terrorism involving petrol bomb

Excludes1: terrorism involving fire or heat of nuclear weapon (Y38.5)

Y38.3X Terrorism involving fires, conflagration and hot substances

⑦ Y38.3X1 **Terrorism involving fires, conflagration and hot substances, public safety official injured**

⑦ Y38.3X2 **Terrorism involving fires, conflagration and hot substances, civilian injured**

⑦ Y38.3X3 **Terrorism involving fires, conflagration and hot substances, terrorist injured**

Y38.4 Terrorism involving firearms

Terrorism involving carbine bullet

Terrorism involving machine gun bullet

Terrorism involving pellets (shotgun)

Terrorism involving pistol bullet

Terrorism involving rifle bullet

Terrorism involving rubber (rifle) bullet

Y38.4X Terrorism involving firearms

⑦ Y38.4X1 **Terrorism involving firearms, public safety official injured**

⑦ Y38.4X2 **Terrorism involving firearms, civilian injured**

⑦ Y38.4X3 **Terrorism involving firearms, terrorist injured**

Y38.5 Terrorism involving nuclear weapons

Terrorism involving blast effects of nuclear weapon

Terrorism involving exposure to ionizing radiation from nuclear weapon

Terrorism involving fireball effect of nuclear weapon

Terrorism involving heat from nuclear weapon

Y38.5X Terrorism involving nuclear weapons

⑦ Y38.5X1 **Terrorism involving nuclear weapons, public safety official injured**

⑦ Y38.5X2 **Terrorism involving nuclear weapons, civilian injured**

⑦ Y38.5X3 **Terrorism involving nuclear weapons, terrorist injured**

Y38.6 Terrorism involving biological weapons

Terrorism involving anthrax

Terrorism involving cholera

Terrorism involving smallpox

Y38.6X Terrorism involving biological weapons

⑦ Y38.6X1 **Terrorism involving biological weapons, public safety official injured**

⑦ Y38.6X2 **Terrorism involving biological weapons, civilian injured**

⑦ Y38.6X3 **Terrorism involving biological weapons, terrorist injured**

Y38.7 Terrorism involving chemical weapons

Terrorism involving gases, fumes, chemicals

Terrorism involving hydrogen cyanide

Terrorism involving phosgene

Terrorism involving sarin

Y38.7X Terrorism involving chemical weapons

⑦ Y38.7X1 **Terrorism involving chemical weapons, public safety official injured**

⑦ Y38.7X2 **Terrorism involving chemical weapons, civilian injured**

⑦ Y38.7X3 **Terrorism involving chemical weapons, terrorist injured**

Y38.8 Terrorism involving other and unspecified means

⊗⑦ Y38.80 **Terrorism involving unspecified means**

Terrorism NOS

Y38.81 Terrorism involving suicide bomber

⑦ Y38.811 **Terrorism involving suicide bomber, public safety official injured**

⑦ Y38.812 **Terrorism involving suicide bomber, civilian injured**

Y38.89 Terrorism involving other means

Terrorism involving drowning and submersion

Terrorism involving lasers

Terrorism involving piercing or stabbing instruments

⑦ Y38.891 **Terrorism involving other means, public safety official injured**

⑦ Y38.892 **Terrorism involving other means, civilian injured**

⑦ Y38.893 **Terrorism involving other means, terrorist injured**

Y38.9 Terrorism, secondary effects

Note: This code is for use to identify conditions occurring subsequent to a terrorist attack not those that are due to the initial terrorist attack

Y38.9X Terrorism, secondary effects

⑦ Y38.9X1 **Terrorism, secondary effects, public safety official injured**

⑦ Y38.9X2 **Terrorism, secondary effects, civilian injured**

COMPLICATIONS OF MEDICAL AND SURGICAL CARE (Y62-Y84)

Includes: complications of medical devices

surgical and medical procedures as the cause of abnormal reaction of the patient, or of later complication, without mention of misadventure at the time of the procedure

MISADVENTURES TO PATIENTS DURING SURGICAL AND MEDICAL CARE (Y62-Y69)

Excludes1: surgical and medical procedures as the cause of abnormal reaction of the patient, without mention of misadventure at the time of the procedure (Y83-Y84)

Excludes2: breakdown or malfunctioning of medical device (during procedure) (after implantation) (ongoing use) (Y70-Y82)

Y62 **Failure of sterile precautions during surgical and medical care**

Y62.0 **Failure of sterile precautions during surgical operation**

Y62.1 **Failure of sterile precautions during infusion or transfusion**

Y62.2 **Failure of sterile precautions during kidney dialysis and other perfusion**

Y62.3 **Failure of sterile precautions during injection or immunization**

Y62.4 **Failure of sterile precautions during endoscopic examination**

Y62.5 **Failure of sterile precautions during heart catheterization**

Y62.6 **Failure of sterile precautions during aspiration, puncture and other catheterization**

Y62.8 **Failure of sterile precautions during other surgical and medical care**

Y62.9 **Failure of sterile precautions during unspecified surgical and medical care**

Y63 **Failure in dosage during surgical and medical care**

Excludes2: accidental overdose of drug or wrong drug given in error (T36-T50)

Y63.0 **Excessive amount of blood or other fluid given during transfusion or infusion**

Y63.1 **Incorrect dilution of fluid used during infusion**

Y63.2 **Overdose of radiation given during therapy**

Y63.3 **Inadvertent exposure of patient to radiation during medical care**

Y63.4 **Failure in dosage in electroshock or insulin-shock therapy**

Y63.5 **Inappropriate temperature in local application and packing**

Y63.6 **Underdosing and nonadministration of necessary drug, medicament or biological substance**

Y63.8 **Failure in dosage during other surgical and medical care**

Y63.9 **Failure in dosage during unspecified surgical and medical care**

Y64 **Contaminated medical or biological substances**

Y64.0 **Contaminated medical or biological substance, transfused or infused**

Y64.1 **Contaminated medical or biological substance, injected or used for immunization**

Y64.8 **Contaminated medical or biological substance administered by other means**

Y64.9 **Contaminated medical or biological substance administered by unspecified means**

Administered contaminated medical or biological substance NOS

Y65 **Other misadventures during surgical and medical care**

Y65.0 **Mismatched blood in transfusion**

Y65.1 **Wrong fluid used in infusion**

Y65.2 **Failure in suture or ligature during surgical operation**

Y65.3 **Endotracheal tube wrongly placed during anesthetic procedure**

Y65.4 **Failure to introduce or to remove other tube or instrument**

Y65.5 **Performance of wrong procedure (operation)**

Y65.51 **Performance of wrong procedure (operation) on correct patient**

Wrong device implanted into correct surgical site

Excludes1: performance of correct procedure (operation) on wrong side or body part (Y65.53)

Y65.52 **Performance of procedure (operation) on patient not scheduled for surgery**

Performance of procedure (operation) intended for another patient

Performance of procedure (operation) on wrong patient

Y65.53 **Performance of correct procedure (operation) on wrong side or body part**

Performance of correct procedure (operation) on wrong side

Performance of correct procedure (operation) on wrong site

Y65.8 **Other specified misadventures during surgical and medical care**

Y66 **Nonadministration of surgical and medical care**

Premature cessation of surgical and medical care

Excludes1: DNR status (Z66)

palliative care (Z51.5)

Y69 **Unspecified misadventure during surgical and medical care**

MEDICAL DEVICES ASSOCIATED WITH ADVERSE INCIDENTS IN DIAGNOSTIC AND THERAPEUTIC USE (Y70-Y82)

Includes: breakdown or malfunction of medical devices (during use) (after implantation) (ongoing use)

Excludes2: breakdown or malfunctioning of medical device (after implantation) (during procedure) (ongoing use) (Y70-Y82)

later complications following use of medical devices without breakdown or malfunctioning of device (Y83-Y84)

misadventure to patients during surgical and medical care, classifiable to (Y62-Y69)

surgical and other medical procedures as the cause of abnormal reaction of the patient, or of later complication, without mention of misadventure at the time of the procedure (Y83-Y84)

Y70 **Anesthesiology devices associated with adverse incidents**

Y70.0 **Diagnostic and monitoring anesthesiology devices associated with adverse incidents**

Y70.1 **Therapeutic (nonsurgical) and rehabilitative anesthesiology devices associated with adverse incidents**

Y70.2 **Prosthetic and other implants, materials and accessory anesthesiology devices associated with adverse incidents**

Y70.3 **Surgical instruments, materials and anesthesiology devices (including sutures) associated with adverse incidents**

Y70.8 **Miscellaneous anesthesiology devices associated with adverse incidents, not elsewhere classified**

Y71 **Cardiovascular devices associated with adverse incidents**

Y71.0 **Diagnostic and monitoring cardiovascular devices associated with adverse incidents**

Y71.1 **Therapeutic (nonsurgical) and rehabilitative cardiovascular devices associated with adverse incidents**

Y71.2 **Prosthetic and other implants, materials and accessory cardiovascular devices associated with adverse incidents**

Y71.3 Surgical instruments, materials and cardiovascular devices (including sutures) associated with adverse incidents

Y71.8 Miscellaneous cardiovascular devices associated with adverse incidents, not elsewhere classified

Y72 Otorhinolaryngological devices associated with adverse incidents

Y72.0 Diagnostic and monitoring otorhinolaryngological devices associated with adverse incidents

Y72.1 Therapeutic (nonsurgical) and rehabilitative otorhinolaryngological devices associated with adverse incidents

Y72.2 **Prosthetic and other implants, materials and accessory otorhinolaryngological devices associated with adverse incidents**

Y72.3 Surgical instruments, materials and otorhinolaryngological devices (including sutures) associated with adverse incidents

Y72.8 Miscellaneous otorhinolaryngological devices associated with adverse incidents, not elsewhere classified

Y73 Gastroenterology and urology devices associated with adverse incidents

Y73.0 Diagnostic and monitoring gastroenterology and urology devices associated with adverse incidents

Y73.1 Therapeutic (nonsurgical) and rehabilitative gastroenterology and urology devices associated with adverse incidents

Y73.2 **Prosthetic and other implants, materials and accessory gastroenterology and urology devices associated with adverse incidents**

Y73.3 Surgical instruments, materials and gastroenterology and urology devices (including sutures) associated with adverse incidents

Y73.8 Miscellaneous gastroenterology and urology devices associated with adverse incidents, not elsewhere classified

Y74 General hospital and personal-use devices associated with adverse incidents

Y74.0 Diagnostic and monitoring general hospital and personal-use devices associated with adverse incidents

Y74.1 Therapeutic (nonsurgical) and rehabilitative general hospital and personal-use devices associated with adverse incidents

Y74.2 **Prosthetic and other implants, materials and accessory general hospital and personal-use devices associated with adverse incidents**

Y74.3 Surgical instruments, materials and general hospital and personal-use devices (including sutures) associated with adverse incidents

Y74.8 Miscellaneous general hospital and personal-use devices associated with adverse incidents, not elsewhere classified

Y75 Neurological devices associated with adverse incidents

Y75.0 Diagnostic and monitoring neurological devices associated with adverse incidents

Y75.1 Therapeutic (nonsurgical) and rehabilitative neurological devices associated with adverse incidents

Y75.2 **Prosthetic and other implants, materials and neurological devices associated with adverse incidents**

Y75.3 Surgical instruments, materials and neurological devices (including sutures) associated with adverse incidents

Y75.8 Miscellaneous neurological devices associated with adverse incidents, not elsewhere classified

Y76 Obstetric and gynecological devices associated with adverse incidents

Y76.0 Diagnostic and monitoring obstetric and gynecological devices associated with adverse incidents

Y76.1 Therapeutic (nonsurgical) and rehabilitative obstetric and gynecological devices associated with adverse incidents

Y76.2 **Prosthetic and other implants, materials and accessory obstetric and gynecological devices associated with adverse incidents**

Y76.3 Surgical instruments, materials and obstetric and gynecological devices (including sutures) associated with adverse incidents

Y76.8 Miscellaneous obstetric and gynecological devices associated with adverse incidents, not elsewhere classified

Y77 Ophthalmic devices associated with adverse incidents

Y77.0 Diagnostic and monitoring ophthalmic devices associated with adverse incidents

Y77.1 Therapeutic (nonsurgical) and rehabilitative ophthalmic devices associated with adverse incidents

Y77.2 **Prosthetic and other implants, materials and accessory ophthalmic devices associated with adverse incidents**

Y77.3 Surgical instruments, materials and ophthalmic devices (including sutures) associated with adverse incidents

Y77.8 Miscellaneous ophthalmic devices associated with adverse incidents, not elsewhere classified

Y78 Radiological devices associated with adverse incidents

Y78.0 Diagnostic and monitoring radiological devices associated with adverse incidents

Y78.1 Therapeutic (nonsurgical) and rehabilitative radiological devices associated with adverse incidents

Y78.2 **Prosthetic and other implants, materials and accessory radiological devices associated with adverse incidents**

Y78.3 Surgical instruments, materials and radiological devices (including sutures) associated with adverse incidents

Y78.8 Miscellaneous radiological devices associated with adverse incidents, not elsewhere classified

Y79 Orthopedic devices associated with adverse incidents

Y79.0 Diagnostic and monitoring orthopedic devices associated with adverse incidents

Y79.1 Therapeutic (nonsurgical) and rehabilitative orthopedic devices associated with adverse incidents

Y79.2 **Prosthetic and other implants, materials and accessory orthopedic devices associated with adverse incidents**

Y79.3 Surgical instruments, materials and orthopedic devices (including sutures) associated with adverse incidents

Y79.8 Miscellaneous orthopedic devices associated with adverse incidents, not elsewhere classified

Y80 Physical medicine devices associated with adverse incidents

Y80.0 Diagnostic and monitoring physical medicine devices associated with adverse incidents

Y80.1 Therapeutic (nonsurgical) and rehabilitative physical medicine devices associated with adverse incidents

Y80.2 Prosthetic and other implants, materials and accessory physical medicine devices associated with adverse incidents

Y80.3 Surgical instruments, materials and physical medicine devices (including sutures) associated with adverse incidents

Y80.8 Miscellaneous physical medicine devices associated with adverse incidents, not elsewhere classified

Y81 General- and plastic-surgery devices associated with adverse incidents

Y81.0 Diagnostic and monitoring general- and plastic-surgery devices associated with adverse incidents

Y81.1 Therapeutic (nonsurgical) and rehabilitative general- and plastic-surgery devices associated with adverse incidents

Y81.2 Prosthetic and other implants, materials and accessory general- and plastic-surgery devices associated with adverse incidents

Y81.3 Surgical instruments, materials and general- and plastic-surgery devices (including sutures) associated with adverse incidents

Y81.8 Miscellaneous general- and plastic-surgery devices associated with adverse incidents, not elsewhere classified

Y82 Other and unspecified medical devices associated with adverse incidents

Y82.8 Other medical devices associated with adverse incidents

Y82.9 Unspecified medical devices associated with adverse incidents

SURGICAL AND OTHER MEDICAL PROCEDURES AS THE CAUSE OF ABNORMAL REACTION OF THE PATIENT, OR OF LATER COMPLICATION, WITHOUT MENTION OF MISADVENTURE AT THE TIME OF THE PROCEDURE (Y83-Y84)

Excludes1: misadventures to patients during surgical and medical care, classifiable to (Y62-Y69)

Excludes2: breakdown or malfunctioning of medical device (after implantation) (during procedure) (ongoing use) (Y70-Y82)

Y83 Surgical operation and other surgical procedures as the cause of abnormal reaction of the patient, or of later complication, without mention of misadventure at the time of the procedure

Y83.0 Surgical operation with transplant of whole organ as the cause of abnormal reaction of the patient, or of later complication, without mention of misadventure at the time of the procedure

Y83.1 Surgical operation with implant of artificial internal device as the cause of abnormal reaction of the patient, or of later complication, without mention of misadventure at the time of the procedure

Y83.2 Surgical operation with anastomosis, bypass or graft as the cause of abnormal reaction of the patient, or of later complication, without mention of misadventure at the time of the procedure

Y83.3 Surgical operation with formation of external stoma as the cause of abnormal reaction of the patient, or of later complication, without mention of misadventure at the time of the procedure

Y83.4 Other reconstructive surgery as the cause of abnormal reaction of the patient, or of later complication, without mention of misadventure at the time of the procedure

Y83.5 Amputation of limb(s) as the cause of abnormal reaction of the patient, or of later complication, without mention of misadventure at the time of the procedure

Y83.6 Removal of other organ (partial) (total) as the cause of abnormal reaction of the patient, or of later complication, without mention of misadventure at the time of the procedure

Y83.8 Other surgical procedures as the cause of abnormal reaction of the patient, or of later complication, without mention of misadventure at the time of the procedure

Y83.9 Surgical procedure, unspecified as the cause of abnormal reaction of the patient, or of later complication, without mention of misadventure at the time of the procedure

Y84 Other medical procedures as the cause of abnormal reaction of the patient, or of later complication, without mention of misadventure at the time of the procedure

Y84.0 Cardiac catheterization as the cause of abnormal reaction of the patient, or of later complication, without mention of misadventure at the time of the procedure

Y84.1 Kidney dialysis as the cause of abnormal reaction of the patient, or of later complication, without mention of misadventure at the time of the procedure

Y84.2 Radiological procedure and radiotherapy as the cause of abnormal reaction of the patient, or of later complication, without mention of misadventure at the time of the procedure

Y84.3 Shock therapy as the cause of abnormal reaction of the patient, or of later complication, without mention of misadventure at the time of the procedure

Y84.4 Aspiration of fluid as the cause of abnormal reaction of the patient, or of later complication, without mention of misadventure at the time of the procedure

Y84.5 Insertion of gastric or duodenal sound as the cause of abnormal reaction of the patient, or of later complication, without mention of misadventure at the time of the procedure

Y84.6 Urinary catheterization as the cause of abnormal reaction of the patient, or of later complication, without mention of misadventure at the time of the procedure

Y84.7 Blood-sampling as the cause of abnormal reaction of the patient, or of later complication, without mention of misadventure at the time of the procedure

Y84.8 Other medical procedures as the cause of abnormal reaction of the patient, or of later complication, without mention of misadventure at the time of the procedure

Y84.9 Medical procedure, unspecified as the cause of abnormal reaction of the patient, or of later complication, without mention of misadventure at the time of the procedure

SUPPLEMENTARY FACTORS RELATED TO CAUSES OF MORBIDITY CLASSIFIED ELSEWHERE (Y90-Y99)

Note: These categories may be used to provide supplementary information concerning causes of morbidity. They are not to be used for single-condition coding.

Y90 Evidence of alcohol involvement determined by blood alcohol level

Code first any associated alcohol related disorders (F10)

Y90.0 Blood alcohol level of less than 20 mg/100 ml

Y90.1 Blood alcohol level of 20-39 mg/100 ml

Y90.2 Blood alcohol level of 40-59 mg/100 ml

Y90.3 Blood alcohol level of 60-79 mg/100 ml

Y90.4 Blood alcohol level of 80-99 mg/100 ml

Y90.5 Blood alcohol level of 100-119 mg/100 ml

	Add 4th-7th digits	Nonspecific code	Unspecified code	Manifestation code

Y90.6   Blood alcohol level of 120-199 mg/100 ml

Y90.7   Blood alcohol level of 200-239 mg/100 ml

Y90.8   Blood alcohol level of 240 mg/100 ml or more

Y90.9   Presence of alcohol in blood, level not specified

Y92   Place of occurrence of the external cause

The following category is for use, when relevant, to identify the place of occurrence of the external cause. Use in conjunction with an activity code.

Place of occurrence should be recorded only at the initial encounter for treatment

Y92.0   Non-institutional (private) residence as the place of occurrence of the external cause

> **Excludes1:** abandoned or derelict house (Y92.89)
>
> home under construction but not yet occupied (Y92.6-)
>
> institutional place of residence (Y92.1-)

Y92.00   Unspecified non-institutional (private) residence as the place of occurrence of the external cause

Y92.000   Kitchen of unspecified non-institutional (private) residence as the place of occurrence of the external cause

Y92.001   Dining room of unspecified non-institutional (private) residence as the place of occurrence of the external cause

Y92.002   Bathroom of unspecified non-institutional (private) residence single-family (private) house as the place of occurrence of the external cause

Y92.003   Bedroom of unspecified non-institutional (private) residence as the place of occurrence of the external cause

Y92.007   Garden or yard of unspecified non-institutional (private) residence as the place of occurrence of the external cause

Y92.008   Other place in unspecified non-institutional (private) residence as the place of occurrence of the external cause

Y92.009   Unspecified place in unspecified non-institutional (private) residence as the place of occurrence of the external cause

> Home (NOS) as the place of occurrence of the external cause

Y92.01   Single-family non-institutional (private) house as the place of occurrence of the external cause

> Farmhouse as the place of occurrence of the external cause
>
> **Excludes1:** barn (Y92.71)
>
> chicken coop or hen house (Y92.72)
>
> farm field (Y92.73)
>
> orchard (Y92.74)
>
> single family mobile home or trailer (Y92.02-)
>
> slaughter house (Y92.86)

Y92.010   Kitchen of single-family (private) house as the place of occurrence of the external cause

Y92.011   Dining room of single-family (private) house as the place of occurrence of the external cause

Y92.012   Bathroom of single-family (private) house as the place of occurrence of the external cause

Y92.013   Bedroom of single-family (private) house as the place of occurrence of the external cause

Y92.014   Private driveway to single-family (private) house as the place of occurrence of the external cause

Y92.015   Private garage of single-family (private) house as the place of occurrence of the external cause

Y92.016   Swimming-pool in single-family (private) house or garden as the place of occurrence of the external cause

Y92.017   Garden or yard in single-family (private) house as the place of occurrence of the external cause

Y92.018   Other place in single-family (private) house as the place of occurrence of the external cause

Y92.019   Unspecified place in single-family (private) house as the place of occurrence of the external cause

Y92.02   Mobile home as the place of occurrence of the external cause

Y92.020   Kitchen in mobile home as the place of occurrence of the external cause

Y92.021   Dining room in mobile home as the place of occurrence of the external cause

Y92.022   Bathroom in mobile home as the place of occurrence of the external cause

Y92.023   Bedroom in mobile home as the place of occurrence of the external cause

Y92.024   Driveway of mobile home as the place of occurrence of the external cause

Y92.025   Garage of mobile home as the place of occurrence of the external cause

Y92.026   Swimming-pool of mobile home as the place of occurrence of the external cause

Y92.027   Garden or yard of mobile home as the place of occurrence of the external cause

Y92.028   Other place in mobile home as the place of occurrence of the external cause

Y92.029   Unspecified place in mobile home as the place of occurrence of the external cause

Y92.03   Apartment as the place of occurrence of the external cause

> Condominium as the place of occurrence of the external cause
>
> Co-op apartment as the place of occurrence of the external cause

Y92.030 Kitchen in apartment as the place of occurrence of the external cause

Y92.031 Bathroom in apartment as the place of occurrence of the external cause

Y92.032 Bedroom in apartment as the place of occurrence of the external cause

Y92.038 Other place in apartment as the place of occurrence of the external cause

Y92.039 Unspecified place in apartment as the place of occurrence of the external cause

Y92.04 Boarding-house as the place of occurrence of the external cause

Y92.040 Kitchen in boarding-house as the place of occurrence of the external cause

Y92.041 Bathroom in boarding-house as the place of occurrence of the external cause

Y92.042 Bedroom in boarding-house as the place of occurrence of the external cause

Y92.043 Driveway of boarding-house as the place of occurrence of the external cause

Y92.044 Garage of boarding-house as the place of occurrence of the external cause

Y92.045 Swimming-pool of boarding-house as the place of occurrence of the external cause

Y92.046 Garden or yard of boarding-house as the place of occurrence of the external cause

Y92.048 Other place in boarding-house as the place of occurrence of the external cause

Y92.049 Unspecified place in boarding-house as the place of occurrence of the external cause

Y92.09 Other non-institutional residence as the place of occurrence of the external cause

Y92.090 Kitchen in other non-institutional residence as the place of occurrence of the external cause

Y92.091 Bathroom in other non-institutional residence as the place of occurrence of the external cause

Y92.092 Bedroom in other non-institutional residence as the place of occurrence of the external cause

Y92.093 Driveway of other non-institutional residence as the place of occurrence of the external cause

Y92.094 Garage of other non-institutional residence as the place of occurrence of the external cause

Y92.095 Swimming-pool of other non-institutional residence as the place of occurrence of the external cause

Y92.096 Garden or yard of other non-institutional residence as the place of occurrence of the external cause

Y92.098 Other place in other non-institutional residence as the place of occurrence of the external cause

Y92.099 Unspecified place in other non-institutional residence as the place of occurrence of the external cause

Y92.1 Institutional (nonprivate) residence as the place of occurrence of the external cause

Y92.10 Unspecified residential institution as the place of occurrence of the external cause

Y92.11 Children's home and orphanage as the place of occurrence of the external cause

Y92.110 Kitchen in children's home and orphanage as the place of occurrence of the external cause

Y92.111 Bathroom in children's home and orphanage as the place of occurrence of the external cause

Y92.112 Bedroom in children's home and orphanage as the place of occurrence of the external cause

Y92.113 Driveway of children's home and orphanage as the place of occurrence of the external cause

Y92.114 Garage of children's home and orphanage as the place of occurrence of the external cause

Y92.115 Swimming-pool of children's home and orphanage as the place of occurrence of the external cause

Y92.116 Garden or yard of children's home and orphanage as the place of occurrence of the external cause

Y92.118 Other place in children's home and orphanage as the place of occurrence of the external cause

Y92.119 Unspecified place in children's home and orphanage as the place of occurrence of the external cause

Y92.12 Nursing home as the place of occurrence of the external cause

Home for the sick as the place of occurrence of the external cause

Hospice as the place of occurrence of the external cause

Y92.120 Kitchen in nursing home as the place of occurrence of the external cause

Y92.121 Bathroom in nursing home as the place of occurrence of the external cause

Y92.122 Bedroom in nursing home as the place of occurrence of the external cause

Y92.123 Driveway of nursing home as the place of occurrence of the external cause

Y92.124 **Garage of nursing home as the place of occurrence of the external cause**

Y92.125 **Swimming-pool of nursing home as the place of occurrence of the external cause**

Y92.126 **Garden or yard of nursing home as the place of occurrence of the external cause**

Y92.128 **Other place in nursing home as the place of occurrence of the external cause**

Y92.129 **Unspecified place in nursing home as the place of occurrence of the external cause**

Y92.13 **Military base as the place of occurrence of the external cause**

Excludes1: military training grounds (Y92.83)

Y92.130 **Kitchen on military base as the place of occurrence of the external cause**

Y92.131 **Mess hall on military base as the place of occurrence of the external cause**

Y92.133 **Barracks on military base as the place of occurrence of the external cause**

Y92.135 **Garage on military base as the place of occurrence of the external cause**

Y92.136 **Swimming-pool on military base as the place of occurrence of the external cause**

Y92.137 **Garden or yard on military base as the place of occurrence of the external cause**

Y92.138 **Other place on military base as the place of occurrence of the external cause**

Y92.139 **Unspecified place military base as the place of occurrence of the external cause**

Y92.14 **Prison as the place of occurrence of the external cause**

Y92.140 **Kitchen in prison as the place of occurrence of the external cause**

Y92.141 **Dining room in prison as the place of occurrence of the external cause**

Y92.142 **Bathroom in prison as the place of occurrence of the external cause**

Y92.143 **Cell of prison as the place of occurrence of the external cause**

Y92.146 **Swimming-pool of prison as the place of occurrence of the external cause**

Y92.147 **Courtyard of prison as the place of occurrence of the external cause**

Y92.148 **Other place in prison as the place of occurrence of the external cause**

Y92.149 **Unspecified place in prison as the place of occurrence of the external cause**

Y92.15 **Reform school as the place of occurrence of the external cause**

Y92.150 **Kitchen in reform school as the place of occurrence of the external cause**

Y92.151 **Dining room in reform school as the place of occurrence of the external cause**

Y92.152 **Bathroom in reform school as the place of occurrence of the external cause**

Y92.153 **Bedroom in reform school as the place of occurrence of the external cause**

Y92.154 **Driveway of reform school as the place of occurrence of the external cause**

Y92.155 **Garage of reform school as the place of occurrence of the external cause**

Y92.156 **Swimming-pool of reform school as the place of occurrence of the external cause**

Y92.157 **Garden or yard of reform school as the place of occurrence of the external cause**

Y92.158 **Other place in reform school as the place of occurrence of the external cause**

Y92.159 **Unspecified place in reform school as the place of occurrence of the external cause**

Y92.16 **School dormitory as the place of occurrence of the external cause**

Excludes1: reform school as the place of occurrence of the external cause (Y92.15-)

school buildings and grounds as the place of occurrence of the external cause (Y92.2-)

school sports and athletic areas as the place of occurrence of the external cause (Y92.3-)

Y92.160 **Kitchen in school dormitory as the place of occurrence of the external cause**

Y92.161 **Dining room in school dormitory as the place of occurrence of the external cause**

Y92.162 **Bathroom in school dormitory as the place of occurrence of the external cause**

Y92.163 **Bedroom in school dormitory as the place of occurrence of the external cause**

Y92.168 **Other place in school dormitory as the place of occurrence of the external cause**

Y92.169 **Unspecified place in school dormitory as the place of occurrence of the external cause**

Y92.19 **Other specified residential institution as the place of occurrence of the external cause**

Y92.190 **Kitchen in other specified residential institution as the place of occurrence of the external cause**

● New code   ▲ Revised code   **Excludes1:** Not coded here   **Excludes2:** Not included here   ⊗ Placeholder required   ⑦ 7th digit required

Y92.191 Dining room in other specified residential institution as the place of occurrence of the external cause

Y92.192 Bathroom in other specified residential institution as the place of occurrence of the external cause

Y92.193 Bedroom in other specified residential institution as the place of occurrence of the external cause

Y92.194 Driveway of other specified residential institution as the place of occurrence of the external cause

Y92.195 Garage of other specified residential institution as the place of occurrence of the external cause

Y92.196 Pool of other specified residential institution as the place of occurrence of the external cause

Y92.197 Garden or yard of other specified residential institution as the place of occurrence of the external cause

Y92.198 Other place in other specified residential institution as the place of occurrence of the external cause

Y92.199 Unspecified place in other specified residential institution as the place of occurrence of the external cause

Y92.2 School, other institution and public administrative area as the place of occurrence of the external cause

Building and adjacent grounds used by the general public or by a particular group of the public

Excludes1: building under construction as the place of occurrence of the external cause (Y92.6)

residential institution as the place of occurrence of the external cause (Y92.1)

school dormitory as the place of occurrence of the external cause (Y92.16-)

sports and athletics area of schools as the place of occurrence of the external cause (Y92.3-)

Y92.21 School (private) (public) (state) as the place of occurrence of the external cause

Y92.210 Daycare center as the place of occurrence of the external cause

Y92.211 Elementary school as the place of occurrence of the external cause

Kindergarten as the place of occurrence of the external cause

Y92.212 Middle school as the place of occurrence of the external cause

Y92.213 High school as the place of occurrence of the external cause

Y92.214 College as the place of occurrence of the external cause

University as the place of occurrence of the external cause

Y92.215 Trade school as the place of occurrence of the external cause

Y92.218 Other school as the place of occurrence of the external cause

Y92.219 Unspecified school as the place of occurrence of the external cause

Y92.22 Religious institution as the place of occurrence of the external cause

Church as the place of occurrence of the external cause

Mosque as the place of occurrence of the external cause

Synagogue as the place of occurrence of the external cause

Y92.23 Hospital as the place of occurrence of the external cause

Excludes1: ambulatory (outpatient) health services establishments (Y92.53-)

home for the sick as the place of occurrence of the external cause (Y92.12-)

hospice as the place of occurrence of the external cause (Y92.12-)

nursing home as the place of occurrence of the external cause (Y92.12-)

Y92.230 Patient room in hospital as the place of occurrence of the external cause

Y92.231 Patient bathroom in hospital as the place of occurrence of the external cause

Y92.232 Corridor of hospital as the place of occurrence of the external cause

Y92.233 Cafeteria of hospital as the place of occurrence of the external cause

Y92.234 Operating room of hospital as the place of occurrence of the external cause

Y92.238 Other place in hospital as the place of occurrence of the external cause

Y92.239 Unspecified place in hospital as the place of occurrence of the external cause

Y92.24 Public administrative building as the place of occurrence of the external cause

Y92.240 Courthouse as the place of occurrence of the external cause

Y92.241 Library as the place of occurrence of the external cause

Y92.242 Post office as the place of occurrence of the external cause

Y92.243 City hall as the place of occurrence of the external cause

Y92.248 Other public administrative building as the place of occurrence of the external cause

Y92.25 Cultural building as the place of occurrence of the external cause

Y92.250 Art Gallery as the place of occurrence of the external cause

Y92.251 Museum as the place of occurrence of the external cause

Y92.252 Music hall as the place of occurrence of the external cause

Y92.253 Opera house as the place of occurrence of the external cause

Y92.254 Theater (live) as the place of occurrence of the external cause

Y92.258 Other cultural public building as the place of occurrence of the external cause

Y92.26 Movie house or cinema as the place of occurrence of the external cause

Y92.29 Other specified public building as the place of occurrence of the external cause

Assembly hall as the place of occurrence of the external cause

Clubhouse as the place of occurrence of the external cause

Y92.3 Sports and athletics area as the place of occurrence of the external cause

Y92.31 Athletic court as the place of occurrence of the external cause

Excludes1: tennis court in private home or garden (Y92.09)

Y92.310 Basketball court as the place of occurrence of the external cause

Y92.311 Squash court as the place of occurrence of the external cause

Y92.312 Tennis court as the place of occurrence of the external cause

Y92.318 Other athletic court as the place of occurrence of the external cause

Y92.32 Athletic field as the place of occurrence of the external cause

Y92.320 Baseball field as the place of occurrence of the external cause

Y92.321 Football field as the place of occurrence of the external cause

Y92.322 Soccer field as the place of occurrence of the external cause

Y92.328 Other athletic field as the place of occurrence of the external cause

Cricket field as the place of occurrence of the external cause

Hockey field as the place of occurrence of the external cause

Y92.33 Skating rink as the place of occurrence of the external cause

Y92.330 Ice skating rink (indoor) (outdoor) as the place of occurrence of the external cause

Y92.331 Roller skating rink as the place of occurrence of the external cause

Y92.34 Swimming pool (public) as the place of occurrence of the external cause

Excludes1: swimming pool in private home or garden (Y92.016)

Y92.39 Other specified sports and athletic area as the place of occurrence of the external cause

Golf-course as the place of occurrence of the external cause

Gymnasium as the place of occurrence of the external cause

Riding-school as the place of occurrence of the external cause

Stadium as the place of occurrence of the external cause

Y92.4 Street, highway and other paved roadways as the place of occurrence of the external cause

Excludes1: private driveway of residence (Y92.014, Y92.024, Y92.043, Y92.093, Y92.113, Y92.123, Y92.154, Y92.194)

Y92.41 Street and highway as the place of occurrence of the external cause

Y92.410 Unspecified street and highway as the place of occurrence of the external cause

Road NOS as the place of occurrence of the external cause

Y92.411 Interstate highway as the place of occurrence of the external cause

Freeway as the place of occurrence of the external cause

Motorway as the place of occurrence of the external cause

Y92.412 Parkway as the place of occurrence of the external cause

Y92.413 State road as the place of occurrence of the external cause

Y92.414 Local residential or business street as the place of occurrence of the external cause

Y92.415 Exit ramp or entrance ramp of street or highway as the place of occurrence of the external cause

Y92.48 Other paved roadways as the place of occurrence of the external cause

Y92.480 Sidewalk as the place of occurrence of the external cause

Y92.481 Parking lot as the place of occurrence of the external cause

Y92.482 Bike path as the place of occurrence of the external cause

Y92.488 Other paved roadways as the place of occurrence of the external cause

Y92.5 Trade and service area as the place of occurrence of the external cause

Excludes1: garage in private home (Y92.015)

schools and other public administration buildings (Y92.2-)

Y92.51 Private commercial establishments as the place of occurrence of the external cause

Y92.510 Bank as the place of occurrence of the external cause

Y92.511 Restaurant or café as the place of occurrence of the external cause

Y92.512 Supermarket, store or market as the place of occurrence of the external cause

Y92.513 Shop (commercial) as the place of occurrence of the external cause

Y92.52 Service areas as the place of occurrence of the external cause

Y92.520 Airport as the place of occurrence of the external cause

Y92.521 Bus station as the place of occurrence of the external cause

Y92.522 Railway station as the place of occurrence of the external cause

Y92.523 Highway rest stop as the place of occurrence of the external cause

Y92.524 Gas station as the place of occurrence of the external cause

Petroleum station as the place of occurrence of the external cause

Service station as the place of occurrence of the external cause

Y92.53 Ambulatory health services establishments as the place of occurrence of the external cause

Y92.530 Ambulatory surgery center as the place of occurrence of the external cause

Outpatient surgery center, including that connected with a hospital as the place of occurrence of the external cause

Same day surgery center, including that connected with a hospital as the place of occurrence of the external cause

Y92.531 Health care provider office as the place of occurrence of the external cause

Physician office as the place of occurrence of the external cause

Y92.532 Urgent care center as the place of occurrence of the external cause

Y92.538 Other ambulatory health services establishments as the place of occurrence of the external cause

Y92.59 Other trade areas as the place of occurrence of the external cause

Office building as the place of occurrence of the external cause

Casino as the place of occurrence of the external cause

Garage (commercial) as the place of occurrence of the external cause

Hotel as the place of occurrence of the external cause

Radio or television station as the place of occurrence of the external cause

Shopping mall as the place of occurrence of the external cause

Warehouse as the place of occurrence of the external cause

Y92.6 Industrial and construction area as the place of occurrence of the external cause

Y92.61 Building [any] under construction as the place of occurrence of the external cause

Y92.62 Dock or shipyard as the place of occurrence of the external cause

Dockyard as the place of occurrence of the external cause

Dry dock as the place of occurrence of the external cause

Shipyard as the place of occurrence of the external cause

Y92.63 Factory as the place of occurrence of the external cause

Factory building as the place of occurrence of the external cause

Factory premises as the place of occurrence of the external cause

Industrial yard as the place of occurrence of the external cause

Y92.64 Mine or pit as the place of occurrence of the external cause

Mine as the place of occurrence of the external cause

Y92.65 Oil rig as the place of occurrence of the external cause

Pit (coal) (gravel) (sand) as the place of occurrence of the external cause

Y92.69 Other specified industrial and construction area as the place of occurrence of the external cause

Gasworks as the place of occurrence of the external cause

Power-station (coal) (nuclear) (oil) as the place of occurrence of the external cause

Tunnel under construction as the place of occurrence of the external cause

Workshop as the place of occurrence of the external cause

Y92.7 Farm as the place of occurrence of the external cause

Ranch as the place of occurrence of the external cause

Excludes1: farmhouse and home premises of farm (Y92.01-)

Y92.71 Barn as the place of occurrence of the external cause

Y92.72 Chicken coop as the place of occurrence of the external cause

Hen house as the place of occurrence of the external cause

Y92.73 Farm field as the place of occurrence of the external cause

Y92.74 Orchard as the place of occurrence of the external cause

Y92.79 Other farm location as the place of occurrence of the external cause

Y92.8 Other places as the place of occurrence of the external cause

Y92.81 Transport vehicle as the place of occurrence of the external cause

Excludes1: transport accidents (V00-V99)

Y92.810 Car as the place of occurrence of the external cause

Y92.811 Bus as the place of occurrence of the external cause

Y92.812 Truck as the place of occurrence of the external cause

Y92.813 Airplane as the place of occurrence of the external cause

Y92.814 Boat as the place of occurrence of the external cause

Y92.815 Train as the place of occurrence of the external cause

Y92.816 Subway car as the place of occurrence of the external cause

Y92.818 Other transport vehicle as the place of occurrence of the external cause

Y92.82 Wilderness area

Y92.820 Desert as the place of occurrence of the external cause

Y92.821 Forest as the place of occurrence of the external cause

Y92.828 **Other wilderness area as the place of occurrence of the external cause**

Swamp as the place of occurrence of the external cause

Mountain as the place of occurrence of the external cause

Marsh as the place of occurrence of the external cause

Prairie as the place of occurrence of the external cause

Y92.83 **Recreation area as the place of occurrence of the external cause**

Y92.830 **Public park as the place of occurrence of the external cause**

Y92.831 **Amusement park as the place of occurrence of the external cause**

Y92.832 **Beach as the place of occurrence of the external cause**

Seashore as the place of occurrence of the external cause

Y92.833 **Campsite as the place of occurrence of the external cause**

Y92.834 **Zoological garden (Zoo) as the place of occurrence of the external cause**

Y92.838 **Other recreation area as the place of occurrence of the external cause**

Y92.84 **Military training ground as the place of occurrence of the external cause**

Y92.85 **Railroad track as the place of occurrence of the external cause**

Y92.86 **Slaughter house as the place of occurrence of the external cause**

Y92.89 **Other specified places as the place of occurrence of the external cause**

Derelict house as the place of occurrence of the external cause

Y92.9 **Unspecified place or not applicable**

Y93 **Activity codes**

Note: Category Y93 is provided for use to indicate the activity of the person seeking healthcare for an injury or health condition, such as a heart attack while shoveling snow, which resulted from, or was contributed to, by the activity. These codes are appropriate for use for both acute injuries, such as those from chapter 19, and conditions that are due to the long-term, cumulative effects of an activity, such as those from chapter 13. They are also appropriate for use with external cause codes for cause and intent if identifying the activity provides additional information on the event. These codes should be used in conjunction with codes for external cause status (Y99) and place of occurrence (Y92).

This section contains the following broad activity categories: Y93.0

Activities involving walking and running Y93.1

Activities involving water and water craft Y93.2

Activities involving ice and snow Y93.3

Activities involving climbing, rappelling, and jumping off Y93.4

Activities involving dancing and other rhythmic movement Y93.5

Activities involving other sports and athletics played individually Y93.6

Activities involving other sports and athletics played as a team or group Y93.7

Activities involving other specified sports and athletics Y93.A

Activities involving other cardiorespiratory exercise Y93.B

Activities involving other muscle strengthening exercises Y93.C

Activities involving computer technology and electronic devices Y93.D

Activities involving arts and handcrafts Y93.E

Activities involving personal hygiene and interior property and clothing maintenance Y93.F

Activities involving caregiving Y93.G

Activities involving food preparation, cooking and grilling Y93.H

Activities involving exterior property and land maintenance, building and construction Y93.I

Activities involving roller coasters and other types of external motion Y93.J

Activities involving playing musical instrument Y93.K

Activities involving animal care Y93.8

Activities, other specified Y93.9

Activity, unspecified

Y93.0 **Activities involving walking and running**

Excludes1: activity, walking an animal (Y93.K1)

activity, walking or running on a treadmill (Y93.A1)

Y93.01 **Activity, walking, marching and hiking**

Activity, walking, marching and hiking on level or elevated terrain

Excludes1: activity, mountain climbing (Y93.31)

Y93.02 **Activity, running**

Y93.1 **Activities involving water and water craft**

Excludes1: activities involving ice (Y93.2-)

Y93.11 **Activity, swimming**

Y93.12 **Activity, springboard and platform diving**

Y93.13 **Activity, water polo**

Y93.14 **Activity, water aerobics and water exercise**

Y93.15 **Activity, underwater diving and snorkeling**

Activity, SCUBA diving

Y93.16 **Activity, rowing, canoeing, kayaking, rafting and tubing**

Activity, canoeing, kayaking, rafting and tubing in calm and turbulent water

Y93.17 **Activity, water skiing and wake boarding**

Y93.18 **Activity, surfing, windsurfing and boogie boarding**

Activity, water sliding

Y93.19 **Activity, other involving water and watercraft**

Activity involving water NOS

Activity, parasailing

Activity, water survival training and testing

Y93.2 **Activities involving ice and snow**

Excludes1: activity, shoveling ice and snow (Y93.H1)

Y93.21 **Activity, ice skating**

Activity, figure skating (singles) (pairs)

Activity, ice dancing

Excludes1: activity, ice hockey (Y93.22)

Y93.22 **Activity, ice hockey**

Y93.23 **Activity, snow (alpine) (downhill) skiing, snow boarding, sledding, tobogganing and snow**

tubing

Excludes1: activity, cross country skiing

(Y93.24)

Y93.24 **Activity, cross country skiing**

Activity, Nordic skiing

Y93.29 **Activity, other involving ice and snow**

Activity involving ice and snow NOS

Y93.3 **Activities involving climbing, rappelling and jumping off**

Excludes1: activity, hiking on level or elevated terrain (Y93.01)

activity, jumping rope (Y93.56)

activity, trampoline jumping (Y93.44)

Y93.31 **Activity, mountain climbing, rock climbing and wall climbing**

Y93.32 **Activity, rappelling**

Y93.33 **Activity, BASE jumping**

Activity, Building, Antenna, Span, Earth jumping

Y93.34 **Activity, bungee jumping**

Y93.35 **Activity, hang gliding**

Y93.39 **Activity, other involving climbing, rappelling and jumping off**

Y93.4 **Activities involving dancing and other rhythmic movement**

Excludes1: activity, martial arts (Y93.75)

Y93.41 **Activity, dancing**

Y93.42 **Activity, yoga**

Y93.43 **Activity, gymnastics**

Activity, rhythmic gymnastics

Excludes1: activity, trampolining (Y93.44)

Y93.44 **Activity, trampolining**

Y93.45 **Activity, cheerleading**

Y93.49 **Activity, other involving dancing and other rhythmic movements**

Y93.5 **Activities involving other sports and athletics played individually**

Excludes1: activity, dancing (Y93.41)

activity, gymnastic (Y93.43)

activity, trampolining (Y93.44)

activity, yoga (Y93.42)

Y93.51 **Activity, roller skating (inline) and skateboarding**

Y93.52 **Activity, horseback riding**

Y93.53 **Activity, golf**

Y93.54 **Activity, bowling**

Y93.55 **Activity, bike riding**

Y93.56 **Activity, jumping rope**

Y93.57 **Activity, non-running track and field events**

Excludes1: activity, running (any form) (Y93.02)

Y93.59 **Activity, other involving other sports and athletics played individually**

Excludes1: activities involving climbing, rappelling, and jumping (Y93.3-)

activities involving ice and snow (Y93.2-)

activities involving walking and running (Y93.0-)

activities involving water and watercraft (Y93.1-)

Y93.6 **Activities involving other sports and athletics played as a team or group**

Excludes1: activity, ice hockey (Y93.22)

activity, water polo (Y93.13)

Y93.61 **Activity, American tackle football**

Activity, football NOS

Y93.62 **Activity, American flag or touch football**

Y93.63 **Activity, rugby**

Y93.64 **Activity, baseball**

Activity, softball

Y93.65 **Activity, lacrosse and field hockey**

Y93.66 **Activity, soccer**

Y93.67 **Activity, basketball**

Y93.68 **Activity, volleyball (beach) (court)**

Y93.6A **Activity, physical games generally associated with school recess, summer camp and children**

Activity, capture the flag

Activity, dodge ball

Activity, four square

Activity, kickball

Y93.69 **Activity, other involving other sports and athletics played as a team or group**

Activity, cricket

Y93.7 **Activities involving other specified sports and athletics**

Y93.71 **Activity, boxing**

Y93.72 **Activity, wrestling**

Y93.73 **Activity, racquet and hand sports**

Activity, handball

Activity, racquetball

Activity, squash

Activity, tennis

Y93.74 **Activity, frisbee**

Activity, ultimate frisbee

Y93.75 **Activity, martial arts**

Activity, combatives

Y93.79 **Activity, other specified sports and athletics**

Excludes1: sports and athletics activities specified in categories Y93.0-Y93.6

Y93.A **Activities involving other cardiorespiratory exercise**

Activities involving physical training

Y93.A1 **Activity, exercise machines primarily for cardiorespiratory conditioning**

Activity, elliptical and stepper machines

Activity, stationary bike

Activity, treadmill

Y93.A2 **Activity, calisthenics**

Activity, jumping jacks

Activity, warm up and cool down

Y93.A3 **Activity, aerobic and step exercise**

Y93.A4 **Activity, circuit training**

Y93.A5 **Activity, obstacle course**

Activity, challenge course

Activity, confidence course

Y93.A6 **Activity, grass drills**

Activity, guerilla drills

Y93.A9 Activity, other involving cardiorespiratory exercise

> Excludes1: activities involving cardiorespiratory exercise specified in categories Y93.0-Y93.7

Y93.B Activities involving other muscle strengthening exercises

Y93.B1 Activity, exercise machines primarily for muscle strengthening

Y93.B2 Activity, push-ups, pull-ups, sit-ups

Y93.B3 Activity, free weights

Activity, barbells

Activity, dumbbells

Y93.B4 Activity, pilates

Y93.B9 Activity, other involving muscle strengthening exercises

> Excludes1: activities involving muscle strengthening specified in categories Y93.0-Y93.A

Y93.C Activities involving computer technology and electronic devices

> Excludes1: activity, electronic musical keyboard or instruments (Y93.J-)

Y93.C1 Activity, computer keyboarding

Activity, electronic game playing using keyboard or other stationary device

Y93.C2 Activity, hand held interactive electronic device

Activity, cellular telephone and communication device

Activity, electronic game playing using interactive device

> Excludes1: activity, electronic game playing using keyboard or other stationary device (Y93.C1)

Y93.C9 Activity, other involving computer technology and electronic devices

Y93.D Activities involving arts and handcrafts

> Excludes1: activities involving playing musical instrument (Y93.J-)

Y93.D1 Activity, knitting and crocheting

Y93.D2 Activity, sewing

Y93.D3 Activity, furniture building and finishing

Activity, furniture repair

Y93.D9 Activity, other involving arts and handcrafts

Y93.E Activities involving personal hygiene and interior property and clothing maintenance

> Excludes1: activities involving cooking and grilling (Y93.G-)
>
> activities involving exterior property and land maintenance, building and construction (Y93.H-)
>
> activities involving caregiving (Y93.F-)
>
> activity, dishwashing (Y93.G1)
>
> activity, food preparation (Y93.G1)
>
> activity, gardening (Y93.H2)

Y93.E1 Activity, personal bathing and showering

Y93.E2 Activity, laundry

Y93.E3 Activity, vacuuming

Y93.E4 Activity, ironing

Y93.E5 Activity, floor mopping and cleaning

Y93.E6 Activity, residential relocation

Activity, packing up and unpacking involved in moving to a new residence

Y93.E8 Activity, other personal hygiene

Y93.E9 Activity, other interior property and clothing maintenance

Y93.F Activities involving caregiving

Activity involving the provider of caregiving

Y93.F1 Activity, caregiving, bathing

Y93.F2 Activity, caregiving, lifting

Y93.F9 Activity, other caregiving

Y93.G Activities involving food preparation, cooking and grilling

Y93.G1 Activity, food preparation and clean up

Activity, dishwashing

Y93.G2 Activity, grilling and smoking food

Y93.G3 Activity, cooking and baking

Activity, use of stove, oven and microwave oven

Y93.G9 Activity, other involving cooking and grilling

Y93.H Activities involving exterior property and land maintenance, building and construction

Y93.H1 Activity, digging, shoveling and raking

Activity, dirt digging

Activity, raking leaves

Activity, snow shoveling

Y93.H2 Activity, gardening and landscaping

Activity, pruning, trimming shrubs, weeding

Y93.H3 Activity, building and construction

Y93.H9 Activity, other involving exterior property and land maintenance, building and construction

Y93.I Activities involving roller coasters and other types of external motion

Y93.I1 Activity, roller coaster riding

Y93.I9 Activity, other involving external motion

Y93.J Activities involving playing musical instrument

Activity involving playing electric musical instrument

Y93.J1 Activity, piano playing

Activity, musical keyboard (electronic) playing

Y93.J2 Activity, drum and other percussion instrument playing

Y93.J3 Activity, string instrument playing

Y93.J4 Activity, winds and brass instrument playing

Y93.K Activities involving animal care

> Excludes1: activity, horseback riding (Y93.52)

Y93.K1 Activity, walking an animal

Y93.K2 Activity, milking an animal

Y93.K3 Activity, grooming and shearing an animal

Y93.K9 Activity, other involving animal care

Y93.8 Activities, other specified

Y93.81 Activity, refereeing a sports activity

Y93.82 Activity, spectator at an event

Y93.83 Activity, rough housing and horseplay

Y93.84 Activity, sleeping

Y93.85 Activity, choking game

Activity, blackout game

Activity, fainting game

Activity, pass out game

Y93.89 **Activity, other specified**

Y93.9 **Activity, unspecified**

Y95 **Nosocomial condition**

Y99 **External cause status**

Note: A single code from category Y99 should be used in conjunction with the external cause code(s) assigned to a record to indicate the status of the person at the time the event occurred.

Y99.0 **Civilian activity done for income or pay**

Civilian activity done for financial or other compensation

Excludes1: military activity (Y99.1)

volunteer activity (Y99.2)

Y99.1 **Military activity**

Excludes1: activity of off duty military personnel (Y99.8)

Y99.2 **Volunteer activity**

Excludes1: activity of child or other family member assisting in compensated work **of other** family member (Y99.8)

Y99.8 **Other external cause status**

Activity NEC

Activity of child or other family member assisting in compensated work of other family member

Hobby not done for income

Leisure activity

Off-duty activity of military personnel

Recreation or sport not for income or while a student

Student activity

Excludes1: civilian activity done for income or compensation (Y99.0)

military activity (Y99.1)

Y99.9 **Unspecified external cause status**

Add 4th-7th digits   Nonspecific code   Unspecified code   Manifestation code

● New code ▲ Revised code **Excludes1:** Not coded here **Excludes2:** Not included here ⊗ Placeholder required ⑦ 7th digit required

Chapter 21: Factors Influencing Health Status And Contact With Health Services (Z00-Z99)

DEFINITIONS

This chapter includes definitions of selected key words, terms and phrases and coding alerts for adding points to the clinical domain, and references to coding late effects where appropriate. An example from this chapter is as follows:

Z14   Genetic carrier

Definition: A genetic carrier (or just carrier), is a person who has inherited a genetic trait or mutation but does not display that trait or show symptoms of the disease. Carriers are, however, able to pass the gene onto their offspring, who may then express the gene.

MULTIPLE CODING FOR A SINGLE CONDITION

In addition to the etiology/manifestation convention that requires two codes to fully describe a single condition that affects multiple body systems, there are other single conditions that also require more than one code. "Use additional code" notes are found in the Tabular List at codes that are not part of an etiology/manifestation pair where a secondary code is useful to fully describe a condition. The sequencing rule is the same as the etiology/manifestation pair, "use additional code" indicates that a secondary code should be added.

For example, for bacterial infections that are not included in chapter 1, a secondary code from category B95, Streptococcus, Staphylococcus, and Enterococcus, as the cause of diseases classified elsewhere, or B96, Other bacterial agents as the cause of diseases classified elsewhere, may be required to identify the bacterial organism causing the infection. A "use additional code" note will normally be found at the infectious disease code, indicating a need for the organism code to be added as a secondary code.

 "Code first" notes are also under certain codes that are not specifically manifestation codes but may be due to an underlying cause. When there is a "code first" note and an underlying condition is present, the underlying condition should be sequenced first.

"Code, if applicable, any causal condition first", notes indicate that this code may be assigned as a principal diagnosis when the causal condition is unknown or not applicable. If a causal condition is known, then the code for that condition should be sequenced as the principal or first-listed diagnosis.

Multiple codes may be needed for sequela, complication codes and obstetric codes to more fully describe a condition. See the specific guidelines for these conditions for further instruction.

COMBINATION CODE

A combination code is a single code used to classify: Two diagnoses, or a diagnosis with an associated secondary process (manifestation) A diagnosis with an associated complication

Combination codes are identified by referring to subterm entries in the Alphabetic Index and by reading the inclusion and exclusion notes in the Tabular List.

Assign only the combination code when that code fully identifies the diagnostic conditions involved or when the Alphabetic Index so directs. Multiple coding should not be used when the classification provides a combination code that clearly identifies all of the elements documented in the diagnosis. When the combination code lacks necessary specificity in describing the manifestation or complication, an additional code should be used as a secondary code.

SEQUELA (LATE EFFECTS)

A sequela is the residual effect (condition produced) after the acute phase of an illness or injury has terminated. There is no time limit on when a sequela code can be used. The residual may be apparent early, such as in cerebral infarction, or it may occur months or years later, such as that due to a previous injury. Coding of sequela generally requires two codes sequenced in the following order: The condition or nature of the sequela is sequenced first.

The sequela code is sequenced second.

An exception to the above guidelines are those instances where the code for the sequela is followed by a manifestation code identified in the Tabular List and title, or the sequela code has been expanded (at the fourth, fifth or sixth character levels) to include the manifestation(s). The code for the acute phase of an illness or injury that led to the sequela is never used with a code for the late effect.

Note: The chapter specific guidelines provide additional information about the use of Z codes for specified encounters.

USE OF Z CODES IN ANY HEALTHCARE SETTING

Z codes are for use in any healthcare setting. Z codes may be used as either a first-listed (principal diagnosis code in the inpatient setting) or secondary code, depending on the circumstances of the encounter. Certain Z codes may only be used as first-listed or principal diagnosis.

Z CODES INDICATE A REASON FOR AN ENCOUNTER

Z codes are not procedure codes. A corresponding procedure code must accompany a Z code to describe any procedure performed.

CATEGORIES OF Z CODES

1)   **Contact/Exposure**

Category Z20 indicates contact with, and suspected exposure to, communicable diseases. These codes are for patients who do not show any sign or symptom of a disease but are suspected to have been exposed to it by close personal contact with an infected individual or are in an area where a disease is epidemic.

Category Z77, Other contact with and (suspected) exposures hazardous to health, indicates contact with and suspected exposures hazardous to health.

Contact/exposure codes may be used as a first-listed code to explain an encounter for testing, or, more commonly, as a secondary code to identify a potential risk.

2) Inoculations and vaccinations

Code Z23 is for encounters for inoculations and vaccinations. It indicates that a patient is being seen to receive a prophylactic inoculation against a disease. Procedure codes are required to identify the actual administration of the injection and the type(s) of immunizations given. Code Z23 may be used as a secondary code if the inoculation is given as a routine part of preventive health care, such as a well-baby visit.

3) Status

Status codes indicate that a patient is either a carrier of a disease or has the sequelae or residual of a past disease or condition. This includes such things as the presence of prosthetic or mechanical devices resulting from past treatment. A status code is informative, because the status may affect the course of treatment and its outcome. A status code is distinct from a history code. The history code indicates that the patient no longer has the condition.

A status code should not be used with a diagnosis code from one of the body system chapters, if the diagnosis code includes the information provided by the status code. For example, code Z94.1, Heart transplant status, should not be used with a code from subcategory T86.2, Complications of heart transplant. The status code does not provide additional information. The complication code indicates that the patient is a heart transplant patient.

For encounters for weaning from a mechanical ventilator, assign a code from subcategory J96.1, Chronic respiratory failure, followed by code Z99.11, Dependence on respirator [ventilator] status.

The status Z codes/categories are:

Z14   Genetic carrier

Genetic carrier status indicates that a person carries a gene, associated with a particular disease, which may be passed to offspring who may develop that disease. The person does not have the disease and is not at risk of developing the disease.

Z15   Genetic susceptibility to disease

Genetic susceptibility indicates that a person has a gene that increases the risk of that person developing the disease.

Codes from category Z15 should not be used as principal or first-listed codes. If the patient has the condition to which he/she is susceptible, and that condition is the reason for the encounter, the code for the current condition should be sequenced first. If the patient is being seen for follow-up after completed treatment for this condition, and the condition no longer exists, a follow-up code should be sequenced first, followed by the appropriate personal history and genetic susceptibility codes. If the purpose of the encounter is genetic counseling associated with procreative management, code Z31.5, Encounter for genetic counseling, should be assigned as the first-listed code, followed by a code from category Z15. Additional codes should be assigned for any applicable family or personal history.

Z16   Resistance to antimicrobial drugs

This code indicates that a patient has a condition that is resistant to antimicrobial drug treatment. Sequence the infection code first.

Z17   Estrogen receptor status

Z18   Retained foreign body fragments

Z19   Hormone sensitivity malignancy status

Z21   Asymptomatic HIV infection status

This code indicates that a patient has tested positive for HIV but has manifested no signs or symptoms of the disease.

Z22   Carrier of infectious disease

Carrier status indicates that a person harbors the specific organisms of a disease without manifest symptoms and is capable of transmitting the infection.

Z28.3   Underimmunization status

Z33.1   Pregnant state, incidental

This code is a secondary code only for use when the pregnancy is in no way complicating the reason for visit. Otherwise, a code from the obstetric chapter is required.

Z66   Do not resuscitate

This code may be used when it is documented by the provider that a patient is on do not resuscitate status at any time during the stay.

Z67   Blood type

Z68   Body mass index (BMI)

> As with all other secondary diagnosis codes, the BMI codes should only be assigned when they meet the definition of a reportable diagnosis (see Section III, Reporting Additional Diagnoses).

Z74.01   Bed confinement status

Z76.82   Awaiting organ transplant status

Z78   Other specified health status

> Code Z78.1, Physical restraint status, may be used when it is documented by the provider that a patient has been put in restraints during the current encounter. Please note that this code should not be reported when it is documented by the provider that a patient is temporarily restrained during a procedure.

Z79   Long-term (current) drug therapy

> Codes from this category indicate a patient's continuous use of a prescribed drug (including such things as aspirin therapy) for the long-term treatment of a condition or for prophylactic use. It is not for use for patients who have addictions to drugs. This subcategory is not for use of medications for detoxification or maintenance programs to prevent withdrawal symptoms in patients with drug dependence (e.g., methadone maintenance for opiate dependence). Assign the appropriate code for the drug dependence instead.

> Assign a code from Z79 if the patient is receiving a medication for an extended period as a prophylactic measure (such as for the prevention of deep vein thrombosis) or as treatment of a chronic condition (such as arthritis) or a disease requiring a lengthy course of treatment (such as cancer). Do not assign a code from category Z79 for medication being administered for a brief period of time to treat an acute illness or injury (such as a course of antibiotics to treat acute bronchitis).

Z88   Allergy status to drugs, medicaments and biological substances

> Except: Z88.9, Allergy status to unspecified drugs, medicaments and biological substances status

Z89   Acquired absence of limb

Z90   Acquired absence of organs, not elsewhere classified

Z91.0-   Allergy status, other than to drugs and biological substances

Z92.82   Status post administration of tPA (rtPA) in a different facility within the last 24 hours prior to admission to a current facility

> Assign code Z92.82, Status post administration of tPA (rtPA) in a different facility within the last 24 hours prior to admission to current facility, as a secondary diagnosis when a patient is received by transfer into a facility and documentation indicates they were administered tissue plasminogen activator (tPA) within the last 24 hours prior to admission to the current facility.

> This guideline applies even if the patient is still receiving the tPA at the time they are received into the current facility.

> The appropriate code for the condition for which the tPA was administered (such as cerebrovascular disease or myocardial infarction) should be assigned first.

> Code Z92.82 is only applicable to the receiving facility record and not to the transferring facility record.

Z93   Artificial opening status

Z94   Transplanted organ and tissue status

Z95   Presence of cardiac and vascular implants and grafts

Z96   Presence of other functional implants

Z97   Presence of other devices

Z98   Other postprocedural states

> Assign code Z98.85, Transplanted organ removal status, to indicate that a transplanted organ has been previously removed. This code should not be assigned for the encounter in which the transplanted organ is removed. The complication necessitating removal of the transplant organ should be assigned for that encounter.

> *See section I.C19. for information on the coding of organ transplant complications.*

Z99   Dependence on enabling machines and devices, not elsewhere classified

---

Note: Categories Z89-Z90 and Z93-Z99 are for use only if there are no complications or malfunctions of the organ or tissue replaced, the amputation site or the equipment on which the patient is dependent.

4) History (of)

There are two types of history Z codes, personal and family. Personal history codes explain a patient's past medical condition that no longer exists and is not receiving any treatment, but that has the potential for recurrence, and therefore may require continued monitoring.

Family history codes are for use when a patient has a family member(s) who has had a particular disease that causes the patient to be at higher risk of also contracting the disease.

Personal history codes may be used in conjunction with follow-up codes and family history codes may be used in conjunction with screening codes to explain the need for a test or procedure. History codes are also acceptable on any medical record regardless of the reason for visit. A history of an illness, even if no longer present, is important information that may alter the type of treatment ordered.

The history Z code categories are:

Z80   Family history of primary malignant neoplasm

Z81   Family history of mental and behavioral disorders

Z82   Family history of certain disabilities and chronic diseases (leading to disablement)

Z83   Family history of other specific disorders

Z84   Family history of other conditions

Z85   Personal history of malignant neoplasm

Z86   Personal history of certain other diseases

Z87   Personal history of other diseases and conditions

Z91.4- Personal history of psychological trauma, not elsewhere classified

Z91.5   Personal history of self-harm

Z91.8- Other specified personal risk factors, not elsewhere classified Exception:

Z91.83 Wandering in diseases classified elsewhere

Z92   Personal history of medical treatment

Except: Z92.0, Personal history of contraception Except: Z92.82, Status post administration of tPA (rtPA) in a different facility within the last 24 hours prior to admission to a current facility

5) Screening

Screening is the testing for disease or disease precursors in seemingly well individuals so that early detection and treatment can be provided for those who test positive for the disease (e.g., screening mammogram).

The testing of a person to rule out or confirm a suspected diagnosis because the patient has some sign or symptom is a diagnostic examination, not a screening. In these cases, the sign or symptom is used to explain the reason for the test.

A screening code may be a first-listed code if the reason for the visit is specifically the screening exam. It may also be used as an additional code if the screening is done during an office visit for other health problems. A screening code is not necessary if the screening is inherent to a routine examination, such as a pap smear done during a routine pelvic examination.

Should a condition be discovered during the screening then the code for the condition may be assigned as an additional diagnosis.

The Z code indicates that a screening exam is planned. A procedure code is required to confirm that the screening was performed.

The screening Z codes/categories:

Z11   Encounter for screening for infectious and parasitic diseases

Z12   Encounter for screening for malignant neoplasms

Z13   Encounter for screening for other diseases and disorders

Except: Z13.9, Encounter for screening, unspecified

Z36   Encounter for antenatal screening for mother

● New code   ▲ Revised code   **Excludes1:** Not coded here   **Excludes2:** Not included here   ⊗ Placeholder required   ⑦7ᵗʰ digit required

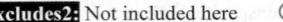

6) Observation

There are three observation Z code categories. They are for use in very limited circumstances when a person is being observed for a suspected condition that is ruled out. The observation codes are not for use if an injury or illness or any signs or symptoms related to the suspected condition are present. In such cases the diagnosis/symptom code is used with the corresponding external cause code.

The observation codes are to be used as principal diagnosis only. The only exception to this is when the principal diagnosis is required to be a code from category Z38, Liveborn infants according to place of birth and type of delivery. Then a code from category Z05, Encounter for observation and evaluation of newborn for suspected diseases and conditions ruled out, is sequenced after the Z38 code. Additional codes may be used in addition to the observation code, but only if they are unrelated to the suspected condition being observed.

Codes from subcategory Z03.7, Encounter for suspected maternal and fetal conditions ruled out, may either be used as a first-listed or as an additional code assignment depending on the case. They are for use in very limited circumstances on a maternal record when an encounter is for a suspected maternal or fetal condition that is ruled out during that encounter (for example, a maternal or fetal condition may be suspected due to an abnormal test result). These codes should not be used when the condition is confirmed. In those cases, the confirmed condition should be coded. In addition, these codes are not for use if an illness or any signs or symptoms related to the suspected condition or problem are present. In such cases the diagnosis/symptom code is used.

Additional codes may be used in addition to the code from subcategory Z03.7, but only if they are unrelated to the suspected condition being evaluated.

Codes from subcategory Z03.7 may not be used for encounters for antenatal screening of mother. *See Section I.C.21. Screening.*

For encounters for suspected fetal condition that are inconclusive following testing and evaluation, assign the appropriate code from category O35, O36, O40 or O41.

The observation Z code categories:

Z03   Encounter for medical observation for suspected diseases and conditions ruled out

Z04   Encounter for examination and observation for other reasons

   Except: Z04.9, Encounter for examination and observation for unspecified reason

Z05   Encounter for observation and evaluation of newborn for suspected diseases and conditions ruled out

7) Aftercare

Aftercare visit codes cover situations when the initial treatment of a disease has been performed and the patient requires continued care during the healing or recovery phase, or for the long-term consequences of the disease. The aftercare Z code should not be used if treatment is directed at a current, acute disease. The diagnosis code is to be used in these cases. Exceptions to this rule are codes Z51.0, Encounter for antineoplastic radiation therapy, and codes from subcategory Z51.1, Encounter for antineoplastic chemotherapy and immunotherapy. These codes are to be first-listed, followed by the diagnosis code when a patient's encounter is solely to receive radiation therapy, chemotherapy, or immunotherapy for the treatment of a neoplasm. If the reason for the encounter is more than one type of antineoplastic therapy, code Z51.0 and a code from subcategory Z51.1 may be assigned together, in which case one of these codes would be reported as a secondary diagnosis.

The aftercare Z codes should also not be used for aftercare for injuries. For aftercare of an injury, assign the acute injury code with the appropriate 7th character (for subsequent encounter).

The aftercare codes are generally first-listed to explain the specific reason for the encounter. An aftercare code may be used as an additional code when some type of aftercare is provided in addition to the reason for admission and no diagnosis code is applicable. An example of this would be the closure of a colostomy during an encounter for treatment of another condition.

Aftercare codes should be used in conjunction with other aftercare codes or diagnosis codes to provide better detail on the specifics of an aftercare encounter visit, unless otherwise directed by the classification. Should a patient receive multiple types of antineoplastic therapy during the same encounter, code Z51.0, Encounter for antineoplastic radiation therapy, and codes from subcategory Z51.1, Encounter for antineoplastic chemotherapy and immunotherapy, may be used together on a record. The sequencing of multiple aftercare codes depends on the circumstances of the encounter.

Certain aftercare Z code categories need a secondary diagnosis code to describe the resolving condition or sequelae. For others, the condition is included in the code title.

Additional Z code aftercare category terms include fitting and adjustment, and attention to artificial openings.

Status Z codes may be used with aftercare Z codes to indicate the nature of the aftercare. For example code Z95.1, Presence of aortocoronary bypass graft, may be used with code Z48.812, Encounter for surgical aftercare following surgery on the circulatory system, to indicate the surgery for which the aftercare is being performed. A status code should not be used when the aftercare code indicates the type of status, such as using Z43.0, Encounter for attention to tracheostomy, with Z93.0, Tracheostomy status.

The aftercare Z category/codes:

Z42   Encounter for plastic and reconstructive surgery following medical procedure or healed injury

Z43   Encounter for attention to artificial openings Z44 Encounter for fitting and adjustment of external prosthetic device

Z45   Encounter for adjustment and management of implanted device
Z46   Encounter for fitting and adjustment of other devices

Z47	Orthopedic aftercare
Z48	Encounter for other postprocedural aftercare
Z49	Encounter for care involving renal dialysis
Z51	Encounter for other aftercare and medical care

8) Follow-up

The follow-up codes are used to explain continuing surveillance following completed treatment of a disease, condition, or injury. They imply that the condition has been fully treated and no longer exists. They should not be confused with aftercare codes, or injury codes with a 7th character for subsequent encounter, that explain ongoing care of a healing condition or its sequelae. Follow-up codes may be used in conjunction with history codes to provide the full picture of the healed condition and its treatment. The follow-up code is sequenced first, followed by the history code.

A follow-up code may be used to explain multiple visits. Should a condition be found to have recurred on the follow-up visit, then the diagnosis code for the condition should be assigned in place of the follow-up code.

The follow-up Z code categories:

Z08	Encounter for follow-up examination after completed treatment for malignant neoplasm
Z09	Encounter for follow-up examination after completed treatment for conditions other than malignant neoplasm
Z39	Encounter for maternal postpartum care and examination

9) Donor

Codes in category Z52, Donors of organs and tissues, are used for living individuals who are donating blood or other body tissue. These codes are only for individuals donating for others, not for self-donations. They are not used to identify cadaveric donations.

10) Counseling

Counseling Z codes are used when a patient or family member receives assistance in the aftermath of an illness or injury, or when support is required in coping with family or social problems. They are not used in conjunction with a diagnosis code when the counseling component of care is considered integral to standard treatment.

The counseling Z codes/categories:

Z30.0-	Encounter for general counseling and advice on contraception
Z31.5	Encounter for genetic counseling
Z31.6-	Encounter for general counseling and advice on procreation
Z32.2	Encounter for childbirth instruction
Z32.3	Encounter for childcare instruction
Z69	Encounter for mental health services for victim and perpetrator of abuse
Z70	Counseling related to sexual attitude, behavior and orientation
Z71	Persons encountering health services for other counseling and medical advice, not elsewhere classified
Z76.81	Expectant mother prebirth pediatrician visit

11) Encounters for Obstetrical and Reproductive Services

See Section I.C.15. Pregnancy, Childbirth, and the Puerperium, for further instruction on the use of these codes.

Z codes for pregnancy are for use in those circumstances when none of the problems or complications included in the codes from the Obstetrics chapter exist (a routine prenatal visit or postpartum care). Codes in category Z34, Encounter for supervision of normal pregnancy, are always first-listed and are not to be used with any other code from the OB chapter.

Codes in category Z3A, Weeks of gestation, may be assigned to provide additional information about the pregnancy. Category Z3A codes should not be assigned for pregnancies with abortive outcomes (categories O00-O08), elective termination of pregnancy (code Z33.32), nor for postpartum conditions, as category Z3A is not applicable to these conditions. The date of the admission should be used to determine weeks of gestation for inpatient admissions that encompass more than one gestational week.

The outcome of delivery, category Z37, should be included on all maternal delivery records. It is always a secondary code. Codes in category Z37 should not be used on the newborn record.

● New code ▲ Revised code **Excludes1:** Not coded here **Excludes2:** Not included here ⊗ Placeholder required ⑦7th digit required

Z codes for family planning (contraceptive) or procreative management and counseling should be included on an obstetric record either during the pregnancy or the postpartum stage, if applicable.

Z codes/categories for obstetrical and reproductive services:

Z30   Encounter for contraceptive management

Z31   Encounter for procreative management

Z32.2   Encounter for childbirth instruction

Z32.3   Encounter for childcare instruction

Z33   Pregnant state

Z34   Encounter for supervision of normal pregnancy

Z36   Encounter for antenatal screening of mother

Z3A   Weeks of gestation

Z37   Outcome of delivery

Z39   Encounter for maternal postpartum care and examination

Z76.81   Expectant mother prebirth pediatrician visit

12) Newborns and Infants

See Section I.C.16. Newborn (Perinatal) Guidelines, for further instruction on the use of these codes.

Newborn Z codes/categories:

Z76.1   Encounter for health supervision and care of foundling

Z00.1-   Encounter for routine child health examination

Z38   Liveborn infants according to place of birth and type of delivery

13) Routine and administrative examinations

The Z codes allow for the description of encounters for routine examinations, such as, a general check-up, or, examinations for administrative purposes, such as, a pre-employment physical. The codes are not to be used if the examination is for diagnosis of a suspected condition or for treatment purposes. In such cases the diagnosis code is used. During a routine exam, should a diagnosis or condition be discovered, it should be coded as an additional code. Pre-existing and chronic conditions and history codes may also be included as additional codes as long as the examination is for administrative purposes and not focused on any particular condition.

Some of the codes for routine health examinations distinguish between "with" and "without" abnormal findings. Code assignment depends on the information that is known at the time the encounter is being coded. For example, if no abnormal findings were found during the examination, but the encounter is being coded before test results are back, it is acceptable to assign the code for "without abnormal findings." When assigning a code for "with abnormal findings," additional code(s) should be assigned to identify the specific abnormal finding(s).

Pre-operative examination and pre-procedural laboratory examination Z codes are for use only in those situations when a patient is being cleared for a procedure or surgery and no treatment is given.

The Z codes/categories for routine and administrative examinations:

Z00   Encounter for general examination without complaint, suspected or reported diagnosis

Z01   Encounter for other special examination without complaint, suspected or reported diagnosis

Z02   Encounter for administrative examination

        Except: Z02.9, Encounter for administrative examinations, unspecified

Z32.0-   Encounter for pregnancy test

14) Miscellaneous Z codes

The miscellaneous Z codes capture a number of other health care encounters that do not fall into one of the other categories. Certain of these codes identify the reason for the encounter; others are for use as additional codes that provide useful information on circumstances that may affect a patient's care and treatment.

Prophylactic Organ Removal

For encounters specifically for prophylactic removal of an organ (such as prophylactic removal of breasts due to a genetic susceptibility to cancer or a family history of cancer), the principal or first-listed code should be a code from category Z40, Encounter for prophylactic surgery, followed by the appropriate codes to identify the associated risk factor (such as genetic susceptibility or family history).

If the patient has a malignancy of one site and is having prophylactic removal at another site to prevent either a new primary malignancy or metastatic disease, a code for the malignancy should also be assigned in addition to a code from subcategory Z40.0, Encounter for prophylactic surgery for risk factors related to malignant neoplasms. A Z40.0 code should not be assigned if the patient is having organ removal for treatment of a malignancy, such as the removal of the testes for the treatment of prostate cancer.

Miscellaneous Z codes/categories:

Z28   Immunization not carried out

     Except: Z28.3, Underimmunization status

Z29   Encounter for other prophylactic measures

Z40   Encounter for prophylactic surgery

Z41   Encounter for procedures for purposes other than remedying health state

     Except: Z41.9, Encounter for procedure for purposes other than remedying health state, unspecified

Z53   Persons encountering health services for specific procedures and treatment, not carried out

Z55   Problems related to education and literacy

Z56   Problems related to employment and unemployment

Z57   Occupational exposure to risk factors

Z58   Problems related to physical environment

Z59   Problems related to housing and economic circumstances

Z60   Problems related to social environment

Z62   Problems related to upbringing

Z63   Other problems related to primary support group, including family circumstances

Z64   Problems related to certain psychosocial circumstances

Z65   Problems related to other psychosocial circumstances

Z72   Problems related to lifestyle

     Note: These codes should be assigned only when the documentation specifies that the patient has an associated problem

Z73   Problems related to life management difficulty

Z74   Problems related to care provider dependency

     Except: Z74.01, Bed confinement status

Z75   Problems related to medical facilities and other health care

Z76.0   Encounter for issue of repeat prescription

Z76.3   Healthy person accompanying sick person

Z76.4   Other boarder to healthcare facility

Z76.5   Malingerer [conscious simulation]

Z91.1- Patient's noncompliance with medical treatment and regimen

Z91.83 Wandering in diseases classified elsewhere

Z91.89 Other specified personal risk factors, not elsewhere classified

15)   Nonspecific Z codes

Certain Z codes are so non-specific, or potentially redundant with other codes in the classification, that there can be little justification for their use in the inpatient setting. Their use in the outpatient setting should be limited to those instances when there is no further documentation to permit more precise coding. Otherwise, any sign or symptom or any other reason for visit that is captured in another code should be used.

Nonspecific Z codes/categories:

Z02.9   Encounter for administrative examinations, unspecified

Z04.9   Encounter for examination and observation for unspecified reason

Z13.9   Encounter for screening, unspecified

Z41.9   Encounter for procedure for purposes other than remedying health state, unspecified

Z52.9   Donor of unspecified organ or tissue

Z86.59   Personal history of other mental and behavioral disorders

Z88.9   Allergy status to unspecified drugs, medicaments and biological substances status

Z92.0   Personal history of contraception

16) Z Codes That May Only be Principal/First-Listed Diagnosis

The following Z codes/categories may only be reported as the principal/first-listed diagnosis, except when there are multiple encounters on the same day and the medical records for the encounters are combined:

Z00   Encounter for general examination without complaint, suspected or reported diagnosis

     Except: Z00.6

Z01   Encounter for other special examination without complaint, suspected or reported diagnosis

Z02   Encounter for administrative examination

Z03   Encounter for medical observation for suspected diseases and conditions ruled out

Z04   Encounter for examination and observation for other reasons

Z33.2   Encounter for elective termination of pregnancy

Z31.81   Encounter for male factor infertility in female patient

Z31.83   Encounter for assisted reproductive fertility procedure cycle

Z31.84   Encounter for fertility preservation procedure

Z34   Encounter for supervision of normal pregnancy

Z39   Encounter for maternal postpartum care and examination

Z38   Liveborn infants according to place of birth and type of delivery

Z42   Encounter for plastic and reconstructive surgery following medical procedure or healed injury

Z51.0   Encounter for antineoplastic radiation therapy

Z51.1-   Encounter for antineoplastic chemotherapy and immunotherapy

Z52   Donors of organs and tissues

     Except: Z52.9, Donor of unspecified organ or tissue

Z76.1   Encounter for health supervision and care of foundling

Z76.2   Encounter for health supervision and care of other healthy infant and child

Z99.12   Encounter for respirator [ventilator] dependence during power failure

Chapter 21

Factors Influencing Health Status And Contact With Health Services (Z00-Z99)

Note: Z codes represent reasons for encounters. A corresponding procedure code must accompany a Z code if a procedure is performed. Categories Z00-Z99 are provided for occasions when circumstances other than a disease, injury or external cause classifiable to categories A00-Y89 are recorded as 'diagnoses' or 'problems'. This can arise in two main ways: (a) When a person who may or may not be sick encounters the health services for some specific purpose, such as to receive limited care or service for a current condition, to donate an organ or tissue, to receive prophylactic vaccination (immunization), or to discuss a problem which is in itself not a disease or injury. (b) When some circumstance or problem is present which influences the person's health status but is not in itself a current illness or injury.

This chapter contains the following blocks:

Z00-Z13	Persons encountering health services for examinations
Z14-Z15	Genetic carrier and genetic susceptibility to disease
Z16	Resistance to antimicrobial drugs
Z17	Estrogen receptor status
Z18	Retained foreign body fragments
Z20-Z29	Persons with potential health hazards related to communicable diseases
Z30-Z39	Persons encountering health services in circumstances related to reproduction
Z40-Z53	Encounters for other specific health care
Z55-Z65	Persons with potential health hazards related to socioeconomic and psychosocial circumstances
Z66	Do not resuscitate status
Z67	Blood type
Z68	Body mass index (BMI)
Z69-Z76	Persons encountering health services **in other** circumstances
Z77-Z99	Persons with potential health hazards related to family and personal history and certain conditions influencing health status

PERSONS ENCOUNTERING HEALTH SERVICES FOR EXAMINATIONS (Z00-Z13)

Note: Nonspecific abnormal findings disclosed at the time of these examinations are classified to categories R70-R94.

Excludes1: examinations related to pregnancy and reproduction (Z30-Z36, Z39.-)

Z00 **Encounter for general examination without complaint, suspected or reported diagnosis**

Excludes1: encounter for examination for administrative purposes (Z02.-)

Excludes2: encounter for pre-procedural examinations (Z01.81-)

special screening examinations (Z11-Z13)

Z00.0 **Encounter for general adult medical examination**

Encounter for adult periodic examination (annual) (physical) and any associated laboratory and radiologic examinations

Excludes1: encounter for examination of sign or symptom-code to sign or symptom

general health check-up of infant or child (Z00.12.-)

Z00.00 **Encounter for general adult medical examination without abnormal findings**

Encounter for adult health check-up NOS

Z00.01 **Encounter for general adult medical examination with abnormal findings**

Use additional code to identify abnormal findings

Z00.1 **Encounter for newborn, infant and child health examinations**

Z00.11 **Newborn health examination**

Health check for child under 29 days old

Use additional code to identify any abnormal findings

Excludes1: health check for child over 28 days old (Z00.12-)

Z00.110 **Health examination for newborn under 8 days old**

Health check for newborn under 8 days old

Z00.111 **Health examination for newborn 8 to 28 days old**

Health check for newborn 8 to 28 days old Newborn weight check

Z00.12 **Encounter for routine child health examination**

Encounter for development testing of infant or child

Health check (routine) for child over 28 days old

Excludes1: health check for child under 29 days old (Z00.11-)

health supervision of foundling or other healthy infant or child (Z76.1-Z76.2)

newborn health examination (Z00.11-)

Z00.121 **Encounter for routine child health examination with abnormal findings**

Use additional code to identify abnormal findings

Z00.129 **Encounter for routine child health examination without abnormal findings**

Encounter for routine child health examination NOS

Z00.2 **Encounter for examination for period of rapid growth in childhood**

Z00.3 **Encounter for examination for adolescent development state**

Encounter for puberty development state

Z00.5 **Encounter for examination of potential donor of organ and tissue**

Z00.6 **Encounter for examination for normal comparison and control in clinical research program**

Examination of participant or control in clinical research program

Z00.7 **Encounter for examination for period of delayed growth in childhood**

Z00.70 **Encounter for examination for period of delayed growth in childhood without abnormal findings**

Z00.71 **Encounter for examination for period of delayed growth in childhood with abnormal findings**

Use additional code to identify abnormal findings

Z00.8 **Encounter for other general examination**

Encounter for health examination in population surveys

Z01 **Encounter for other special examination without complaint, suspected or reported diagnosis**

Includes: routine examination of specific system

Note: Codes from category Z01 represent the reason for the encounter. A separate procedure code is required to identify any examinations or procedures performed

Excludes1: encounter for examination for administrative purposes (Z02.-)

encounter for examination for suspected conditions, proven not to exist (Z03.-)

encounter for laboratory and radiologic examinations as a component of general medical examinations (Z00.0-)

encounter for laboratory, radiologic and imaging examinations for sign(s) and symptom(s) - code to the sign(s) or symptom(s)

Excludes2: screening examinations (Z11-Z13)

Z01.0 Encounter for examination of eyes and vision

Excludes1: examination for driving license (Z02.4)

Z01.00 Encounter for examination of eyes and vision without abnormal findings

Encounter for examination of eyes and vision NOS

Z01.01 Encounter for examination of eyes and vision with abnormal findings

Use additional code to identify abnormal findings

Z01.1 Encounter for examination of ears and hearing

Z01.10 Encounter for examination of ears and hearing without abnormal findings

Encounter for examination of ears and hearing NOS

Z01.11 Encounter for examination of ears and hearing with abnormal findings

Z01.110 Encounter for hearing examination following failed hearing screening

Z01.118 Encounter for examination of ears and hearing with other abnormal findings

Use additional code to identify abnormal findings

Z01.12 Encounter for hearing conservation and treatment

Z01.2 Encounter for dental examination and cleaning

Z01.20 Encounter for dental examination and cleaning without abnormal findings

Encounter for dental examination and cleaning NOS

Z01.21 Encounter for dental examination and cleaning with abnormal findings

Use additional code to identify abnormal findings

Z01.3 Encounter for examination of blood pressure

Z01.30 Encounter for examination of blood pressure without abnormal findings

Encounter for examination of blood pressure NOS

Z01.31 Encounter for examination of blood pressure with abnormal findings

Use additional code to identify abnormal findings

Z01.4 Encounter for gynecological examination

Excludes2: pregnancy examination or test (Z32.0-)

routine examination for contraceptive maintenance (Z30.4-)

Z01.41 Encounter for routine gynecological examination

Encounter for general gynecological examination with or without cervical smear

Encounter for gynecological examination (general) (routine) NOS

Encounter for pelvic examination (annual) (periodic)

Use additional code:

for screening for human papillomavirus, if applicable, (Z11.51)

for screening vaginal pap smear, if applicable (Z12.72)

to identify acquired absence of uterus, if applicable (Z90.71-)

Excludes1: gynecologic examination status-post hysterectomy for malignant condition (Z08)

screening cervical pap smear not a part of a routine gynecological examination (Z12.4)

Z01.411 Encounter for gynecological examination (general) (routine) with abnormal findings

Use additional code to identify abnormal findings

Z01.419 Encounter for gynecological examination (general) (routine) without abnormal findings

Z01.42 Encounter for cervical smear to confirm findings of recent normal smear following initial abnormal smear

Z01.8 Encounter for other specified special examinations

Z01.81 Encounter for preprocedural examinations

Encounter for preoperative examinations

Encounter for radiological and imaging examinations as part of preprocedural examination

Z01.810 Encounter for preprocedural cardiovascular examination

Z01.811 Encounter for preprocedural respiratory examination

Z01.812 Encounter for preprocedural laboratory examination

Blood and urine tests prior to treatment or procedure

Z01.818 Encounter for other preprocedural examination

Encounter for preprocedural examination NOS

Encounter for examinations prior to antineoplastic chemotherapy

Z01.82 Encounter for allergy testing

Excludes1: encounter for antibody response examination (Z01.84)

Z01.83 Encounter for blood typing

Encounter for Rh typing

Z01.84 Encounter for antibody response examination

Encounter for immunity status testing

Excludes1: encounter for allergy testing (Z01.82)

Z01.89 Encounter for other specified special examinations

Z02 Encounter for administrative examination

Z02.0 Encounter for examination for admission to educational institution

Encounter for examination for admission to preschool (education)

Encounter for examination for re-admission to school following illness or medical treatment

Z02.1 Encounter for pre-employment examination

Z02.2 Encounter for examination for admission to residential institution

Excludes1: examination for admission to prison (Z02.89)

Z02.3 Encounter for examination for recruitment to armed forces

Z02.4 Encounter for examination for driving license

Z02.5 Encounter for examination for participation in sport

Excludes1: blood-alcohol and blood-drug test (Z02.83)

Z02.6 **Encounter for examination for insurance purposes**

Z02.7 **Encounter for issue of medical certificate**

Excludes1: encounter for general medical examination (Z00-Z01, Z02.0-Z02.6, Z02.8-Z02.9,)

Z02.71 **Encounter for disability determination**

Encounter for issue of medical certificate of incapacity

Encounter for issue of medical certificate of invalidity

Z02.79 **Encounter for issue of other medical certificate**

Z02.8 **Encounter for other administrative examinations**

Z02.81 **Encounter for paternity testing**

Z02.82 **Encounter for adoption services**

Z02.83 **Encounter for blood-alcohol and blood-drug test**

Use additional code for findings of alcohol or drugs in blood (R78.-)

Z02.89 **Encounter for other administrative examinations**

Encounter for examination for admission to prison

Encounter for examination for admission to summer camp

Encounter for immigration examination

Encounter for naturalization examination

Encounter for premarital examination

Excludes1: health supervision of foundling or other healthy infant or child (Z76.1-Z76.2)

Z02.9 **Encounter for administrative examinations, unspecified**

Z03 **Encounter for medical observation for suspected diseases and conditions ruled out**

This category is to be used when a person without a diagnosis is suspected of having an abnormal condition, without signs or symptoms, which requires study, but after examination and observation, is ruled out. This category is also for use for administrative and legal observation status.

Excludes1: contact with and (suspected) exposures hazardous to health (Z77.-)

encounter for observation and evaluation of newborn for suspected diseases and conditions ruled out (Z05.0-)

person with feared complaint in whom no diagnosis is made (Z71.1) signs or symptoms under study- code to signs or symptoms

Z03.6 **Encounter for observation for suspected toxic effect from ingested substance ruled out**

Encounter for observation for suspected adverse effect from drug

Encounter for observation for suspected poisoning

Z03.7 **Encounter for suspected maternal and fetal conditions ruled out**

Encounter for suspected maternal and fetal conditions not found

Excludes1: known or suspected fetal anomalies affecting management of mother, not ruled out (O26.-, O35.-, O36.-, O40.-, O41.-)

Z03.71 **Encounter for suspected problem with amniotic cavity and membrane ruled out**

Encounter for suspected oligohydramnios ruled out

Encounter for suspected polyhydramnios ruled out

Z03.72 **Encounter for suspected placental problem ruled out**

Z03.73 **Encounter for suspected fetal anomaly ruled out**

Z03.74 **Encounter for suspected problem with fetal growth ruled out**

Z03.75 **Encounter for suspected cervical shortening ruled out**

Z03.79 **Encounter for other suspected maternal and fetal conditions ruled out**

Z03.8 **Encounter for observation for other suspected diseases and conditions ruled out**

Z03.81 **Encounter for observation for suspected exposure to biological agents ruled out**

Z03.810 **Encounter for observation for suspected exposure to anthrax ruled out**

Z03.818 **Encounter for observation for suspected exposure to other biological agents ruled out**

Z03.89 **Encounter for observation for other suspected diseases and conditions ruled out**

Z04 **Encounter for examination and observation for other reasons**

Includes: encounter for examination for medicolegal reasons

This category is to be used when a person without a diagnosis is suspected of having an abnormal condition, without signs or symptoms, which requires study, but after examination and observation, is ruled-out. This category is also for use for administrative and legal observation status.

Z04.1 **Encounter for examination and observation following transport accident**

Excludes1: encounter for examination and observation following work accident (Z04.2)

Z04.2 **Encounter for examination and observation following work accident**

Z04.3 **Encounter for examination and observation following other accident**

Z04.4 **Encounter for examination and observation following alleged rape**

Encounter for examination and observation of victim following alleged rape

Encounter for examination and observation of victim following alleged sexual abuse

Z04.41 **Encounter for examination and observation following alleged adult rape**

Suspected adult rape, ruled out

Suspected adult sexual abuse, ruled out

Z04.42 **Encounter for examination and observation following alleged child rape**

Suspected child rape, ruled out

Suspected child sexual abuse, ruled out

Z04.6 **Encounter for general psychiatric examination, requested by authority**

Z04.7 **Encounter for examination and observation following alleged physical abuse**

Z04.71 **Encounter for examination and observation following alleged adult physical abuse**

Suspected adult physical abuse, ruled out

Excludes1: confirmed case of adult physical abuse (T74.-)

encounter for examination and observation following alleged adult sexual abuse (Z04.41)

suspected case of adult physical abuse, not ruled out (T76.-)

Z04.72 **Encounter for examination and observation following alleged child physical abuse**

Suspected child physical abuse, ruled out

Excludes1: confirmed case of child physical abuse (T74.-)

encounter for examination and observation following alleged child sexual abuse (Z04.42)

suspected case of child physical abuse, not ruled out (T76.-)

Z04.8 **Encounter for examination and observation for other specified reasons**

Encounter for examination and observation for request for expert evidence

Z04.9 **Encounter for examination and observation for unspecified reason**

Encounter for observation NOS

Z05 **Encounter for observation and evaluation of newborn for suspected diseases and conditions ruled out**

This category is to be used for newborns, within the neonatal period (the first 28 days of life), who are suspected of having an abnormal condition, but without signs or symptoms, and which, after examination and observation, is ruled out.

Z05.0 **Observation and evaluation of newborn for suspected cardiac condition ruled out**

Z05.1 **Observation and evaluation of newborn for suspected infectious condition ruled out**

Z05.2 **Observation and evaluation of newborn for suspected neurological condition ruled out**

Z05.3 **Observation and evaluation of newborn for suspected respiratory condition ruled out**

Z05.4 **Observation and evaluation of newborn for suspected genetic, metabolic or immunologic condition ruled out**

Z05.41 **Observation and evaluation of newborn for suspected genetic condition ruled out**

Z05.42 **Observation and evaluation of newborn for suspected metabolic condition ruled out**

Z05.43 **Observation and evaluation of newborn for suspected immunologic condition ruled out**

Z05.5 **Observation and evaluation of newborn for suspected gastrointestinal condition ruled out**

Z05.6 **Observation and evaluation of newborn for suspected genitourinary condition ruled out**

Z05.7 **Observation and evaluation of newborn for suspected skin, subcutaneous, musculoskeletal and connective tissue condition ruled out**

Z05.71 **Observation and evaluation of newborn for suspected skin and subcutaneous tissue condition ruled out**

Z05.72 **Observation and evaluation of newborn for suspected musculoskeletal condition ruled out**

Z05.73 **Observation and evaluation of newborn for suspected connective tissue condition ruled out**

Z05.8 **Observation and evaluation of newborn for other specified suspected condition ruled out**

Z05.9 **Observation and evaluation of newborn for unspecified suspected condition ruled out**

Z08 **Encounter for follow-up examination after completed treatment for malignant neoplasm**

Medical surveillance following completed treatment

Use additional code to identify any acquired absence of organs (Z90.-)

Use additional code to identify the personal history of malignant neoplasm (Z85.-)

Excludes1: aftercare following medical care (Z43-Z49, Z51)

Z09 **Encounter for follow-up examination after completed treatment for conditions other than malignant neoplasm**

Medical surveillance following completed treatment

Use additional code to identify any applicable history of disease code (Z86.-. Z87.-)

Excludes1: aftercare following medical care (Z43-Z49, Z51)

surveillance of contraception (Z30.4-)

surveillance of prosthetic and other medical devices (Z44-Z46)

Z11 **Encounter for screening for infectious and parasitic diseases**

Screening is the testing for disease or disease precursors in asymptomatic individuals so that early detection and treatment can be provided for those who test positive for the disease.

Excludes1: encounter for diagnostic examination-code to sign or symptom

Z11.0 **Encounter for screening for intestinal infectious diseases**

Z11.1 **Encounter for screening for respiratory tuberculosis**

Z11.2 **Encounter for screening for other bacterial diseases**

Z11.3 **Encounter for screening for infections with a predominantly sexual mode of transmission**

Excludes2: encounter for screening for human immunodeficiency virus [HIV] (Z11.4)

encounter for screening for human papillomavirus (Z11.51)

Z11.4 **Encounter for screening for human immunodeficiency virus [HIV]**

Z11.5 **Encounter for screening for other viral diseases**

Excludes2: encounter for screening for viral intestinal disease (Z11.0)

Z11.51 **Encounter for screening for human papillomavirus (HPV)**

Z11.59 **Encounter for screening for other viral diseases**

Z11.6 **Encounter for screening for other protozoal diseases and helminthiases**

Excludes2: encounter for screening for protozoal intestinal disease (Z11.0)

Z11.8 **Encounter for screening for other infectious and parasitic diseases**

Encounter for screening for chlamydia

Encounter for screening for rickettsial

Encounter for screening for spirochetal

Encounter for screening for mycoses

Z11.9 **Encounter for screening for infectious and parasitic diseases, unspecified**

Z12 **Encounter for screening for malignant neoplasms**

Screening is the testing for disease or disease precursors in asymptomatic individuals so that early detection and treatment can be provided for those who test positive for the disease.

Use additional code to identify any family history of malignant neoplasm (Z80.-)

Excludes1: encounter for diagnostic examination-code to sign or symptom

Z12.0 **Encounter for screening for malignant neoplasm of stomach**

Z12.1 **Encounter for screening for malignant neoplasm of intestinal tract**

Z12.10 **Encounter for screening for malignant neoplasm of intestinal tract, unspecified**

Z12.11 **Encounter for screening for malignant neoplasm of colon**

Encounter for screening colonoscopy NOS

Z12.12 **Encounter for screening for malignant neoplasm of rectum**

Z12.13 Encounter for screening for malignant neoplasm of small intestine

Z12.2 Encounter for screening for malignant neoplasm of respiratory organs

Z12.3 Encounter for screening for malignant neoplasm of breast

Z12.31 Encounter for screening mammogram for malignant neoplasm of breast

Excludes1: inconclusive mammogram (R92.2)

Z12.39 Encounter for other screening for malignant neoplasm of breast

Z12.4 Encounter for screening for malignant neoplasm of cervix

Encounter for screening pap smear for malignant neoplasm of cervix

Excludes1: when screening is part of general gynecological examination (Z01.4-)

Excludes2: encounter for screening for human papillomavirus (Z11.51)

Z12.5 Encounter for screening for malignant neoplasm of prostate

Z12.6 Encounter for screening for malignant neoplasm of bladder

Z12.7 Encounter for screening for malignant neoplasm of other genitourinary organs

Z12.71 Encounter for screening for malignant neoplasm of testis

Z12.72 Encounter for screening for malignant neoplasm of vagina

Vaginal pap smear status-post hysterectomy for non-malignant condition

Use additional code to identify acquired absence of uterus (Z90.71-)

Excludes1: vaginal pap smear status-post hysterectomy for malignant conditions (Z08)

Z12.73 Encounter for screening for malignant neoplasm of ovary

Z12.79 Encounter for screening for malignant neoplasm of other genitourinary organs

Z12.8 Encounter for screening for malignant neoplasm of other sites

Z12.81 Encounter for screening for malignant neoplasm of oral cavity

Z12.82 Encounter for screening for malignant neoplasm of nervous system

Z12.83 Encounter for screening for malignant neoplasm of skin

Z12.89 Encounter for screening for malignant neoplasm of other sites

Z12.9 Encounter for screening for malignant neoplasm, site unspecified

Z13 Encounter for screening for other diseases and disorders

Screening is the testing for disease or disease precursors in asymptomatic individuals so that early detection and treatment can be provided for those who test positive for the disease.

Excludes1: encounter for diagnostic examination-code to sign or symptom

Z13.0 Encounter for screening for diseases of the blood and blood-forming organs and certain disorders involving the immune mechanism

Z13.1 Encounter for screening for diabetes mellitus

Z13.2 Encounter for screening for nutritional, metabolic and other endocrine disorders

Z13.21 Encounter for screening for nutritional disorder

Z13.22 Encounter for screening for metabolic disorder

Z13.220 Encounter for screening for lipoid disorders

Encounter for screening for cholesterol level

Encounter for screening for hypercholesterolemia

Encounter for screening for hyperlipidemia

Z13.228 Encounter for screening for other metabolic disorders

Z13.29 Encounter for screening for other suspected endocrine disorder

Excludes1: encounter for screening for diabetes mellitus (Z13.1)

Z13.4 Encounter for screening for certain developmental disorders in childhood

Encounter for screening for developmental handicaps in early childhood

Excludes1: routine development testing of infant or child (Z00.1-)

Z13.5 Encounter for screening for eye and ear disorders

Excludes2: encounter for general hearing examination (Z01.1-)

encounter for general vision examination (Z01.0-)

Z13.6 Encounter for screening for cardiovascular disorders

Z13.7 Encounter for screening for genetic and chromosomal anomalies

Excludes1: genetic testing for procreative management (Z31.4-)

Z13.71 Encounter for nonprocreative screening for genetic disease carrier status

Z13.79 Encounter for other screening for genetic and chromosomal anomalies

Z13.8 Encounter for screening for other specified diseases and disorders

Excludes2: screening for malignant neoplasms (Z12.-)

Z13.81 Encounter for screening for digestive system disorders

Z13.810 Encounter for screening for upper gastrointestinal disorder

Z13.811 Encounter for screening for lower gastrointestinal disorder

Excludes1: encounter for screening for intestinal infectious disease (Z11.0)

Z13.818 Encounter for screening for other digestive system disorders

Z13.82 Encounter for screening for musculoskeletal disorder

Z13.820 Encounter for screening for osteoporosis

Z13.828 Encounter for screening for other musculoskeletal disorder

Z13.83 Encounter for screening for respiratory disorder NEC

Excludes1: encounter for screening for respiratory tuberculosis (Z11.1)

Z13.84 Encounter for screening for dental disorders

Z13.85 Encounter for screening for nervous system disorders

Z13.850 Encounter for screening for traumatic brain injury

Z13.858   **Encounter for screening for other nervous system disorders**

Z13.88   **Encounter for screening for disorder due to exposure to contaminants**

> **Excludes1:** those exposed to contaminants without suspected disorders (Z57.-, Z77.-)

Z13.89   **Encounter for screening for other disorder**

Encounter for screening for genitourinary disorders

Z13.9   **Encounter for screening, unspecified**

GENETIC CARRIER AND GENETIC SUSCEPTIBILITY TO DISEASE (Z14-Z15)

Z14   **Genetic carrier**

Definition: A genetic carrier is a person who has inherited a genetic trait or mutation but does not display that trait or show symptoms of the disease. Genetic carriers are, however, able to pass the gene onto their offspring, who may then express the gene.

Z14.0   **Hemophilia A carrier**

Z14.01   **Asymptomatic hemophilia A carrier**

Z14.02   **Symptomatic hemophilia A carrier**

Z14.1   **Cystic fibrosis carrier**

Z14.8   **Genetic carrier of other disease**

Z15   **Genetic susceptibility to disease**

Includes: confirmed abnormal gene

> **Use additional code**, if applicable, for any associated family history of the disease (Z80-Z84)

> **Excludes1:** chromosomal anomalies (Q90-Q99)

Z15.0   **Genetic susceptibility to malignant neoplasm**

> **Code first**, if applicable, any current malignant neoplasm (C00-C75, C81-C96)

> **Use additional code**, if applicable, for any personal history of malignant neoplasm (Z85.-)

Z15.01   **Genetic susceptibility to malignant neoplasm of breast**

Z15.02   **Genetic susceptibility to malignant neoplasm of ovary**

Z15.03   **Genetic susceptibility to malignant neoplasm of prostate**

Z15.04   **Genetic susceptibility to malignant neoplasm of endometrium**

Z15.09   **Genetic susceptibility to other malignant neoplasm**

Z15.8   **Genetic susceptibility to other disease**

Z15.81   **Genetic susceptibility to multiple endocrine neoplasia [MEN]**

> **Excludes1:** multiple endocrine neoplasia [MEN] syndromes (E31.2-)

Z15.89   **Genetic susceptibility to other disease**

RESISTANCE TO ANTIMICROBIAL DRUGS (Z16)

Definition: An antimicrobial is an agent that kills microorganisms or inhibits their growth. Antimicrobial drugs can be grouped according to the microorganisms they act primarily against.

Z16   **Resistance to antimicrobial drugs**

Note: The codes in this category are provided for use as additional codes to identify the resistance and non-responsiveness of a condition to antimicrobial drugs.

Code first the infection

> **Excludes1:** Methicillin resistant Staphylococcus aureus infection (A49.02)

Methicillin resistant Staphylococcus aureus infection in diseases classified elsewhere (B95.62)

Methicillin resistant Staphylococcus aureus pneumonia (J15.212)

Sepsis due to Methicillin resistant Staphylococcus aureus (A41.02)

Z16.1   **Resistance to beta lactam antibiotics**

Z16.10   **Resistance to unspecified beta lactam antibiotics**

Z16.11   **Resistance to penicillins**

Resistance to amoxicillin

Resistance to ampicillin

Z16.12   **Extended spectrum beta lactamase (ESBL) resistance**

> **Excludes2:** Methicillin resistant Staphylococcus aureus infection in diseases classified elsewhere (B95.62)

Z16.19   **Resistance to other specified beta lactam antibiotics**

Resistance to cephalosporins

Z16.2   **Resistance to other antibiotics**

Z16.20   **Resistance to unspecified antibiotic**

Resistance to antibiotics NOS

Z16.21   **Resistance to vancomycin**

Z16.22   **Resistance to vancomycin related antibiotics**

Z16.23   **Resistance to quinolones and fluoroquinolones**

Z16.24   **Resistance to multiple antibiotics**

Z16.29   **Resistance to other single specified antibiotic**

Resistance to aminoglycosides

Resistance to macrolides

Resistance to sulfonamides

Resistance to tetracyclines

Z16.3   **Resistance to other antimicrobial drugs**

> **Excludes1:** resistance to antibiotics (Z16.1-, Z16.2-)

Z16.30   **Resistance to unspecified antimicrobial drugs**

Drug resistance NOS

Z16.31   **Resistance to antiparasitic drug(s)**

Resistance to quinine and related compounds

Z16.32   **Resistance to antifungal drug(s)**

Z16.33   **Resistance to antiviral drug(s)**

Z16.34   **Resistance to antimycobacterial drug(s)**

Resistance to tuberculostatics

Z16.341   **Resistance to single antimycobacterial drug**

Resistance to antimycobacterial drug NOS

Z16.342   **Resistance to multiple antimycobacterial drugs**

Z16.35   **Resistance to multiple antimicrobial drugs**

> **Excludes1:** Resistance to multiple antibiotics only (Z16.24)

Z16.39   **Resistance to other specified antimicrobial drug**

ESTROGEN RECEPTOR STATUS (Z17)

Z17   **Estrogen receptor status**

> **Code first** malignant neoplasm of breast (C50.-)

Z17.0   **Estrogen receptor positive status [ER+]**

Z17.1   **Estrogen receptor negative status [ER-]**

RETAINED FOREIGN BODY FRAGMENTS (Z18)

Z18   **Retained foreign body fragments**

Includes: embedded fragment (status)

embedded splinter (status) retained foreign body status

Excludes1: artificial joint prosthesis status (Z96.6-)

foreign body accidentally left during a procedure (T81.5-)

foreign body entering through orifice (T15-T19)

in situ cardiac device (Z95.-)

organ or tissue replaced by means other than transplant (Z96.-, Z97.-)

organ or tissue replaced by transplant (Z94.-)

personal history of retained foreign body fully removed Z87.821

superficial foreign body (non-embedded splinter) - code to superficial foreign body, by site

Z18.0 **Retained radioactive fragments**

Z18.01 **Retained depleted uranium fragments**

Z18.09 **Other retained radioactive fragments**

Other retained depleted isotope fragments

Retained nontherapeutic radioactive fragments

Z18.1 **Retained metal fragments**

Excludes1: retained radioactive metal fragments (Z18.01-Z18.09)

Z18.10 **Retained metal fragments, unspecified**

Retained metal fragment NOS

Z18.11 **Retained magnetic metal fragments**

Z18.12 **Retained nonmagnetic metal fragments**

Z18.2 **Retained plastic fragments**

Acrylics fragments

Diethylhexylphthalates fragments

Isocyanate fragments

Z18.3 **Retained organic fragments**

Z18.31 **Retained animal quills or spines**

Z18.32 **Retained tooth**

Z18.33 **Retained wood fragments**

Z18.39 **Other retained organic fragments**

Z18.8 **Other specified retained foreign body**

Z18.81 **Retained glass fragments**

Z18.83 **Retained stone or crystalline fragments**

Retained concrete or cement fragments

Z18.89 **Other specified retained foreign body fragments**

Z18.9 **Retained foreign body fragments, unspecified material**

HORMONE SENSITIVITY MALIGNANCY STATUS (Z19)

Z19 **Hormone sensitivity malignancy status**

Code first malignant neoplasm - see Table of Neoplasms, by site, malignant

Z19.1 **Hormone sensitive malignancy status**

Z19.2 **Hormone resistant malignancy status**

Castrate resistant prostate malignancy status

PERSONS WITH POTENTIAL HEALTH HAZARDS RELATED TO COMMUNICABLE DISEASES (Z20-Z29)

Z20 **Contact with and (suspected) exposure to communicable diseases**

Excludes1: carrier of infectious disease (Z22.-)

diagnosed current infectious or parasitic disease -see Alphabetic Index

Excludes2: personal history of infectious and parasitic diseases (Z86.1-)

Z20.0 **Contact with and (suspected) exposure to intestinal infectious diseases**

Z20.01 **Contact with and (suspected) exposure to intestinal infectious diseases due to Escherichia coli (E. coli)**

Z20.09 **Contact with and (suspected) exposure to other intestinal infectious diseases**

Z20.1 **Contact with and (suspected) exposure to tuberculosis**

Z20.2 **Contact with and (suspected) exposure to infections with a predominantly sexual mode of transmission**

Z20.3 **Contact with and (suspected) exposure to rabies**

Z20.4 **Contact with and (suspected) exposure to rubella**

Z20.5 **Contact with and (suspected) exposure to viral hepatitis**

Z20.6 **Contact with and (suspected) exposure to human immunodeficiency virus [HIV]**

Excludes1: asymptomatic human immunodeficiency virus [HIV]

HIV infection status (Z21)

Z20.7 **Contact with and (suspected) exposure to pediculosis, acariasis and other infestations**

Z20.8 **Contact with and (suspected) exposure to other communicable diseases**

Z20.81 **Contact with and (suspected) exposure to other bacterial communicable diseases**

Z20.810 **Contact with and (suspected) exposure to anthrax**

Z20.811 **Contact with and (suspected) exposure to meningococcus**

Z20.818 **Contact with and (suspected) exposure to other bacterial communicable diseases**

Z20.82 **Contact with and (suspected) exposure to other viral communicable diseases**

Z20.820 **Contact with and (suspected) exposure to varicella**

Z20.828 **Contact with and (suspected) exposure to other viral communicable diseases**

Z20.89 **Contact with and (suspected) exposure to other communicable diseases**

Z20.9 **Contact with and (suspected) exposure to unspecified communicable disease**

Z21 **Asymptomatic human immunodeficiency virus [HIV] infection status**

HIV positive NOS

Code first Human immunodeficiency virus [HIV] disease complicating pregnancy, childbirth and the puerperium, if applicable (O98.7-)

Excludes1: acquired immunodeficiency syndrome (B20)

contact with human immunodeficiency virus [HIV] (Z20.6)

exposure to human immunodeficiency virus [HIV] (Z20.6)

human immunodeficiency virus [HIV] disease (B20)

inconclusive laboratory evidence of human immunodeficiency virus [HIV] (R75)

Z22 **Carrier of infectious disease**

Includes: colonization status

suspected carrier

Excludes2: carrier of viral hepatitis (B18.-)

Z22.0 **Carrier of typhoid**

Z22.1 **Carrier of other intestinal infectious diseases**

Z22.2 **Carrier of diphtheria**

Z22.3 **Carrier of other specified bacterial diseases**

Z22.31 **Carrier of bacterial disease due to meningococci**

Z22.32 **Carrier of bacterial disease due to staphylococci**

	Add 4th-7th digits	Nonspecific code	Unspecified code	Manifestation code

Z22.321 Carrier or suspected carrier of Methicillin susceptible Staphylococcus aureus

MSSA colonization

Z22.322 Carrier or suspected carrier of Methicillin resistant Staphylococcus aureus

MRSA colonization

Z22.33 Carrier of bacterial disease due to streptococci

Z22.330 Carrier of Group B streptococcus

Excludes1: Carrier of streptococcus group B (GBS) complicating pregnancy, childbirth and the puerperium (O99.82-)

Z22.338 Carrier of other streptococcus

Z22.39 Carrier of other specified bacterial diseases

Z22.4 Carrier of infections with a predominantly sexual mode of transmission

Z22.6 Carrier of human T-lymphotropic virus type-1 [HTLV-1] infection

Z22.8 Carrier of other infectious diseases

Z22.9 Carrier of infectious disease, unspecified

Z23 Encounter for immunization

<u>Code first</u> any routine childhood examination

Note: procedure codes are required to identify the types of immunizations given

Z28 Immunization not carried out and underimmunization status

Includes: vaccination not carried out

Z28.0 Immunization not carried out because of contraindication

Z28.01 Immunization not carried out because of acute illness of patient

Z28.02 Immunization not carried out because of chronic illness or condition of patient

Z28.03 Immunization not carried out because of immune compromised state of patient

Z28.04 Immunization not carried out because of patient allergy to vaccine or component

Z28.09 Immunization not carried out because of other contraindication

Z28.1 Immunization not carried out because of patient decision for reasons of belief or group pressure

Immunization not carried out because of religious belief

Z28.2 Immunization not carried out because of patient decision for other and unspecified reason

Z28.20 Immunization not carried out because of patient decision for unspecified reason

Z28.21 Immunization not carried out because of patient refusal

Z28.29 Immunization not carried out because of patient decision for other reason

Z28.3 Underimmunization status

Delinquent immunization status Lapsed immunization schedule status

Z28.8 Immunization not carried out for other reason

Z28.81 Immunization not carried out due to patient having had the disease

Z28.82 Immunization not carried out because of caregiver refusal

Immunization not carried out because of guardian refusal

Immunization not carried out because of parent refusal

Excludes1: immunization not carried out because of caregiver refusal because of religious belief (Z28.1)

Z28.89 Immunization not carried out for other reason

Z28.9 Immunization not carried out for unspecified reason

Z29 Encounter for other prophylactic measures

Excludes 1: desensitization to allergens (Z51.6)

prophylactic surgery (Z40.-)

Z29.1 Encounter for prophylactic immunotherapy

Encounter for administration of immunoglobulin

Z29.11 Encounter for prophylactic immunotherapy for respiratory syncytial virus (RSV)

Z29.12 Encounter for prophylactic antivenin

Z29.13 Encounter for prophylactic Rho(D) immune globulin

Z29.14 Encounter for prophylactic rabies immune globin

Z29.3 Encounter for prophylactic fluoride administration

Z29.8 Encounter for other specified prophylactic measures

Z29.9 Encounter for prophylactic measures, unspecified

PERSONS ENCOUNTERING HEALTH SERVICES IN CIRCUMSTANCES RELATED TO REPRODUCTION (Z30-Z39)

Z30 Encounter for contraceptive management

Z30.0 Encounter for general counseling and advice on contraception

Z30.01 Encounter for initial prescription of contraceptives

Excludes1: encounter for surveillance of contraceptives (Z30.4-)

Z30.011 Encounter for initial prescription of contraceptive pills

Z30.012 Encounter for prescription of emergency contraception

Encounter for postcoital contraception

Z30.013 Encounter for initial prescription of injectable contraceptive

Z30.014 Encounter for initial prescription of intrauterine contraceptive device

Excludes1: encounter for insertion of intrauterine contraceptive device (Z30.430, Z30.432)

Z30.015 Encounter for initial prescription of vaginal ring hormonal contraceptive

Z30.016 Encounter for initial prescription of transdermal patch hormonal contraceptive device

Z30.017 Encounter for initial prescription of implantable subdermal contraceptive

Z30.018 Encounter for initial prescription of other contraceptives

Encounter for initial prescription of barrier contraception

Encounter for initial prescription of diaphragm

Z30.019 Encounter for initial prescription of contraceptives, unspecified

Z30.02 Counseling and instruction in natural family planning to avoid pregnancy

Z30.09 Encounter for other general counseling and advice on contraception

Encounter for family planning advice NOS

● New code ▲ Revised code **Excludes1:** Not coded here **Excludes2:** Not included here ⊗ Placeholder required ⑦7th digit required

Z30.2 Encounter for sterilization

Z30.4 Encounter for surveillance of contraceptives

Z30.40 Encounter for surveillance of contraceptives, unspecified

Z30.41 Encounter for surveillance of contraceptive pills

Encounter for repeat prescription for contraceptive pill

Z30.42 Encounter for surveillance of injectable contraceptive

Z30.43 Encounter for surveillance of intrauterine contraceptive device

Z30.430 Encounter for insertion of intrauterine contraceptive device

Z30.431 Encounter for routine checking of intrauterine contraceptive device

Z30.432 Encounter for removal of intrauterine contraceptive device

Z30.433 Encounter for removal and reinsertion of intrauterine contraceptive device

Encounter for replacement of intrauterine contraceptive device

Z30.44 Encounter for surveillance of vaginal ring hormonal contraceptive device

Z30.45 Encounter for surveillance of transdermal patch hormonal contraceptive device

Z30.46 Encounter for surveillance of implantable subdermal contraceptive

Encounter for checking, reinsertion or removal of implantable subdermal contraceptive

Z30.49 Encounter for surveillance of other contraceptives

Encounter for surveillance of barrier contraception

Encounter for surveillance of diaphragm

Z30.8 Encounter for other contraceptive management

Encounter for postvasectomy sperm count

Encounter for routine examination for contraceptive maintenance

Excludes1: sperm count following sterilization reversal (Z31.42)

sperm count for fertility testing (Z31.41)

Z30.9 Encounter for contraceptive management, unspecified

Z31 Encounter for procreative management

Excludes1: complications associated with artificial fertilization (N98.-)

female infertility (N97.-)

male infertility (N46.-)

Z31.0 Encounter for reversal of previous sterilization

Z31.4 Encounter for procreative investigation and testing

Excludes1: postvasectomy sperm count (Z30.8)

Z31.41 Encounter for fertility testing

Encounter for fallopian tube patency testing

Encounter for sperm count for fertility testing

Z31.42 Aftercare following sterilization reversal

Sperm count following sterilization reversal

Z31.43 Encounter for genetic testing of female for procreative management

Use additional code for recurrent pregnancy loss, if applicable (N96, O26.2-)

Excludes1: nonprocreative genetic testing (Z13.7-)

Z31.430 Encounter of female for testing for genetic disease carrier status for procreative management

Z31.438 Encounter for other genetic testing of female for procreative management

Z31.44 Encounter for genetic testing of male for procreative management

Excludes1: nonprocreative genetic testing (Z13.7-)

Z31.440 Encounter of male for testing for genetic disease carrier status for procreative management

Z31.441 Encounter for testing of male partner of patient with recurrent pregnancy loss

Z31.448 Encounter for other genetic testing of male for procreative management

Z31.49 Encounter for other procreative investigation and testing

▲**Z31.5** Encounter for procreative genetic counseling

Z31.6 Encounter for general counseling and advice on procreation

Z31.61 Procreative counseling and advice using natural family planning

Z31.62 Encounter for fertility preservation counseling

Encounter for fertility preservation counseling prior to cancer therapy

Encounter for fertility preservation counseling prior to surgical removal of gonads

Z31.69 Encounter for other general counseling and advice on procreation

Z31.7 Encounter for procreative management and counseling for gestational carrier

Excludes1: pregnant state, gestational carrier (Z33.3)

Z31.8 Encounter for other procreative management

Z31.81 Encounter for male factor infertility in female patient

Z31.82 Encounter for Rh incompatibility status

Z31.83 Encounter for assisted reproductive fertility procedure cycle

Patient undergoing in vitro fertilization cycle

Use additional code to identify the type of infertility

Excludes1: pre-cycle diagnosis and testing - code to reason for encounter

Z31.84 Encounter for fertility preservation procedure

Encounter for fertility preservation procedure prior to cancer therapy

Encounter for fertility preservation procedure prior to surgical removal of gonads

Z31.89 Encounter for other procreative management

Z31.9 Encounter for procreative management, unspecified

Z32 Encounter for pregnancy test and childbirth and childcare instruction

Z32.0 Encounter for pregnancy test

Z32.00 Encounter for pregnancy test, result unknown

Encounter for pregnancy test NOS

Z32.01 Encounter for pregnancy test, result positive

Z32.02 Encounter for pregnancy test, result negative

Z32.2 Encounter for childbirth instruction

Z32.3 Encounter for childcare instruction

Encounter for prenatal or postpartum childcare instruction

Z33 Pregnant state

Add 4th-7th digits   Nonspecific code   Unspecified code   Manifestation code

Z33.1 Pregnant state, incidental

Pregnant state NOS

Excludes1: complications of pregnancy (O00-O9A)

pregnant state, gestational carrier (Z33.3)

Z33.2 Encounter for elective termination of pregnancy

Excludes1: early fetal death with retention of dead fetus (O02.1)

late fetal death (O36.4) spontaneous abortion (O03)

Z33.3 Pregnant state, gestational carrier

Excludes1: encounter for procreative management and counseling for gestational carrier (Z31.7)

Z34 Encounter for supervision of normal pregnancy

Excludes1: any complication of pregnancy (O00-O9A)

encounter for pregnancy test (Z32.0-)

encounter for supervision of high risk pregnancy (O09.-)

Z34.0 Encounter for supervision of normal first pregnancy

Z34.00 Encounter for supervision of normal first pregnancy, unspecified trimester

Z34.01 Encounter for supervision of normal first pregnancy, first trimester

Z34.02 Encounter for supervision of normal first pregnancy, second trimester

Z34.03 Encounter for supervision of normal first pregnancy, third trimester

Z34.8 Encounter for supervision of other normal pregnancy

Z34.80 Encounter for supervision of other normal pregnancy, unspecified trimester

Z34.81 Encounter for supervision of other normal pregnancy, first trimester

Z34.82 Encounter for supervision of other normal pregnancy, second trimester

Z34.83 Encounter for supervision of other normal pregnancy, third trimester

Z34.9 Encounter for supervision of normal pregnancy, unspecified

Z34.90 Encounter for supervision of normal pregnancy, unspecified, unspecified trimester

Z34.91 Encounter for supervision of normal pregnancy, unspecified, first trimester

Z34.92 Encounter for supervision of normal pregnancy, unspecified, second trimester

Z34.93 Encounter for supervision of normal pregnancy, unspecified, third trimester

Z36 Encounter for antenatal screening of mother

Includes: Encounter for placental sample (taken vaginally)

Screening is the testing for disease or disease precursors in asymptomatic individuals so that early detection and treatment can be provided for those who test positive for the disease.

Excludes1: diagnostic examination- code to sign or symptom

encounter for suspected maternal and fetal conditions ruled out (Z03.7-)

suspected fetal condition affecting management of pregnancy - code to condition in Chapter 15

Excludes2: abnormal findings on antenatal screening of mother (O28.-)

genetic counseling and testing (Z31.43-, Z31.5)

routine prenatal care (Z34)

●**Z36.0 Encounter for antenatal screening for chromosomal anomalies**

●**Z36.1 Encounter for antenatal screening for raised alphafetoprotein level**

Encounter for antenatal screening for elevated maternal serum alphafetoprotein level

●**Z36.2 Encounter for other antenatal screening follow-up**

Non-visualized anatomy on a previous scan

●**Z36.3 Encounter for antenatal screening for malformations**

Screening for a suspected anomaly

●**Z36.4 Encounter for antenatal screening for fetal growth retardation**

Intrauterine growth restriction (IUGR)/small-for-dates

●**Z36.5 Encounter for antenatal screening for isoimmunization**

●**Z36.8 Encounter for other antenatal screening**

●**Z36.81 Encounter for antenatal screening for hydrops fetalis**

●**Z36.82 Encounter for antenatal screening for nuchal translucency**

●**Z36.83 Encounter for fetal screening for congenital cardiac abnormalities**

●**Z36.84 Encounter for antenatal screening for fetal lung maturity**

●**Z36.85 Encounter for antenatal screening for Streptococcus B**

●**Z36.86 Encounter for antenatal screening for cervical length**

Screening for risk of pre-term labor

●**Z36.87 Encounter for antenatal screening for uncertain dates**

●**Z36.88 Encounter for antenatal screening for fetal macrosomia**

Screening for large-for-dates

●**Z36.89 Encounter for other specified antenatal screening**

●**Z36.8A Encounter for antenatal screening for other genetic defects**

●**Z36.9 Encounter for antenatal screening, unspecified**

Z3A Weeks of gestation

Note: Codes from category Z3A are for use, only on the maternal record, to indicate the weeks of gestation of the pregnancy, if known.

Code first complications of pregnancy, childbirth and the puerperium (O09-O9A)

Z3A.0 Weeks of gestation of pregnancy, unspecified or less than 10 weeks

Z3A.00 Weeks of gestation of pregnancy not specified

Z3A.01 Less than 8 weeks gestation of pregnancy

Z3A.08 8 weeks gestation of pregnancy

Z3A.09 9 weeks gestation of pregnancy

Z3A.1 Weeks of gestation of pregnancy, weeks 10-19

Z3A.10 10 weeks gestation of pregnancy

Z3A.11 11 weeks gestation of pregnancy

Z3A.12 12 weeks gestation of pregnancy

Z3A.13 13 weeks gestation of pregnancy

Z3A.14 14 weeks gestation of pregnancy

Z3A.15 15 weeks gestation of pregnancy

Z3A.16 16 weeks gestation of pregnancy

Z3A.17 17 weeks gestation of pregnancy

Z3A.18 18 weeks gestation of pregnancy

Z3A.19 19 weeks gestation of pregnancy

Z3A.2 Weeks of gestation of pregnancy, weeks 20-29

Z3A.20 20 weeks gestation of pregnancy

Z3A.21 21 weeks gestation of pregnancy

Z3A.22 22 weeks gestation of pregnancy

Z3A.23   23 weeks gestation of pregnancy
Z3A.24   24 weeks gestation of pregnancy
Z3A.25   25 weeks gestation of pregnancy
Z3A.26   26 weeks gestation of pregnancy
Z3A.27   27 weeks gestation of pregnancy
Z3A.28   28 weeks gestation of pregnancy
Z3A.29   29 weeks gestation of pregnancy

Z3A.3   Weeks of gestation of pregnancy, weeks 30-39

Z3A.30   30 weeks gestation of pregnancy
Z3A.31   31 weeks gestation of pregnancy
Z3A.32   32 weeks gestation of pregnancy
Z3A.33   33 weeks gestation of pregnancy
Z3A.34   34 weeks gestation of pregnancy
Z3A.35   35 weeks gestation of pregnancy
Z3A.36   36 weeks gestation of pregnancy
Z3A.37   37 weeks gestation of pregnancy
Z3A.38   38 weeks gestation of pregnancy
Z3A.39   39 weeks gestation of pregnancy

Z3A.4   Weeks of gestation of pregnancy, weeks 40 or greater

Z3A.40   40 weeks gestation of pregnancy
Z3A.41   41 weeks gestation of pregnancy
Z3A.42   42 weeks gestation of pregnancy
Z3A.49   Greater than 42 weeks gestation of pregnancy

Z37   Outcome of delivery

This category is intended for use as an additional code to identify the outcome of delivery on the mother's record. It is not for use on the newborn record.

Excludes1: stillbirth (P95)

Z37.0   Single live birth

Z37.1   Single stillbirth

Z37.2   Twins, both liveborn

Z37.3   Twins, one liveborn and one stillborn

Z37.4   Twins, both stillborn

Z37.5   Other multiple births, all liveborn

Z37.50   Multiple births, unspecified, all liveborn

Z37.51   Triplets, all liveborn

Z37.52   Quadruplets, all liveborn

Z37.53   Quintuplets, all liveborn

Z37.54   Sextuplets, all liveborn

Z37.59   Other multiple births, all liveborn

Z37.6   Other multiple births, some liveborn

Z37.60   Multiple births, unspecified, some liveborn

Z37.61   Triplets, some liveborn

Z37.62   Quadruplets, some liveborn

Z37.63   Quintuplets, some liveborn

Z37.64   Sextuplets, some liveborn

Z37.69   Other multiple births, some liveborn

Z37.7   Other multiple births, all stillborn

Z37.9   Outcome of delivery, unspecified

Multiple birth NOS

Single birth NOS

Z38   Liveborn infants according to place of birth and type of delivery

This category is for use as the principal code on the initial record of a newborn baby. It is to be used for the initial birth record only. It is not to be used on the mother's record.

Z38.0   Single liveborn infant, born in hospital

Single liveborn infant, born in birthing center **or other** health care facility

Z38.00   Single liveborn infant, delivered vaginally

Z38.01   Single liveborn infant, delivered by cesarean

Z38.1   Single liveborn infant, born outside hospital

Z38.2   Single liveborn infant, unspecified as to place of birth

Single liveborn infant NOS

Z38.3   Twin liveborn infant, born in hospital

Z38.30   Twin liveborn infant, delivered vaginally

Z38.31   Twin liveborn infant, delivered by cesarean

Z38.4   Twin liveborn infant, born outside hospital

Z38.5   Twin liveborn infant, unspecified as to place of birth

Z38.6   Other multiple liveborn infant, born in hospital

Z38.61   Triplet liveborn infant, delivered vaginally

Z38.62   Triplet liveborn infant, delivered by cesarean

Z38.63   Quadruplet liveborn infant, delivered vaginally

Z38.64   Quadruplet liveborn infant, delivered by cesarean

Z38.65   Quintuplet liveborn infant, delivered vaginally

Z38.66   Quintuplet liveborn infant, delivered by cesarean

Z38.68   Other multiple liveborn infant, delivered vaginally

Z38.69   Other multiple liveborn infant, delivered by cesarean

Z38.7   Other multiple liveborn infant, born outside hospital

Z38.8   Other multiple liveborn infant, unspecified as to place of birth

Z39   Encounter for maternal postpartum care and examination

Z39.0   Encounter for care and examination of mother immediately after delivery

Care and observation in uncomplicated cases when the delivery occurs outside a healthcare facility

Excludes1: care for postpartum complication- see Alphabetic index

Z39.1   Encounter for care and examination of lactating mother

Encounter for supervision of lactation

Excludes1: disorders of lactation (O92.-)

Z39.2   Encounter for routine postpartum follow-up

ENCOUNTERS FOR OTHER SPECIFIC HEALTH CARE (Z40-Z53)

Categories Z40-Z53 are intended for use to indicate a reason for care. They may be used for patients who have already been treated for a disease or injury, but who are receiving aftercare or prophylactic care, or care to consolidate the treatment, or to deal with a residual state

Excludes2: follow-up examination for medical surveillance after treatment (Z08-Z09)

Z40   Encounter for prophylactic surgery

Excludes1: organ donations (Z52.-)

therapeutic organ removal-code to condition

Z40.0   Encounter for prophylactic surgery for risk factors related to malignant neoplasms

Admission for prophylactic organ removal

Use additional code to identify risk factor

Z40.00   Encounter for prophylactic removal of unspecified organ

Z40.01   Encounter for prophylactic removal of breast

▲Z40.02   Encounter for prophylactic removal of ovary(s)

Encounter for prophylactic removal of ovary(s) and fallopian tube(s)

•Z40.03   Encounter for prophylactic removal of fallopian tube(s)

Z40.09 Encounter for prophylactic removal of other organ

Z40.8 Encounter for other prophylactic surgery

Z40.9 Encounter for prophylactic surgery, unspecified

Z41 Encounter for procedures for purposes other than remedying health state

    Z41.1 Encounter for cosmetic surgery

      Encounter for cosmetic breast implant

      Encounter for cosmetic procedure

      Excludes1: encounter for plastic and reconstructive surgery following medical procedure or healed injury (Z42.-)

        encounter for post-mastectomy breast implantation (Z42.1)

    Z41.2 Encounter for routine and ritual male circumcision

    Z41.3 Encounter for ear piercing

    Z41.8 Encounter for other procedures for purposes other than remedying health state

    Z41.9 Encounter for procedure for purposes other than remedying health state, unspecified

Z42 Encounter for plastic and reconstructive surgery following medical procedure or healed injury

    Excludes1: encounter for cosmetic plastic surgery (Z41.1)

      encounter for plastic surgery for treatment of current injury - code to relevant injury

    Z42.1 Encounter for breast reconstruction following mastectomy

      Excludes1: deformity and disproportion of reconstructed breast (N65.1-)

    Z42.8 Encounter for other plastic and reconstructive surgery following medical procedure or healed injury

Z43 Encounter for attention to artificial openings

    Includes: closure of artificial openings

      passage of sounds or bougies through artificial openings

      reforming artificial openings

      removal of catheter from artificial openings toilet or cleansing of artificial openings

    Excludes1: complications of external stoma (J95.0-, K94.-, N99.5-)

    Excludes2: artificial opening status only, without need for care (Z93.-)

      fitting and adjustment of prosthetic and other devices (Z44-Z46)

    Z43.0 Encounter for attention to tracheostomy

    Z43.1 Encounter for attention to gastrostomy

    Z43.2 Encounter for attention to ileostomy

    Z43.3 Encounter for attention to colostomy

    Z43.4 Encounter for attention to other artificial openings of digestive tract

    Z43.5 Encounter for attention to cystostomy

    Z43.6 Encounter for attention to other artificial openings of urinary tract

      Encounter for attention to nephrostomy

      Encounter for attention to ureterostomy

      Encounter for attention to urethrostomy

    Z43.7 Encounter for attention to artificial vagina

    Z43.8 Encounter for attention to other artificial openings

    Z43.9 Encounter for attention to unspecified artificial opening

Z44 Encounter for fitting and adjustment of external prosthetic device

    Includes: removal or replacement of external prosthetic device

    Excludes1: malfunction **or other** complications of device - see Alphabetical Index

    presence of prosthetic device (Z97.-)

    Z44.0 Encounter for fitting and adjustment of artificial arm

      Z44.00 Encounter for fitting and adjustment of unspecified artificial arm

        Z44.001 Encounter for fitting and adjustment of unspecified right artificial arm

        Z44.002 Encounter for fitting and adjustment of unspecified left artificial arm

        Z44.009 Encounter for fitting and adjustment of unspecified artificial arm, unspecified arm

      Z44.01 Encounter for fitting and adjustment of complete artificial arm

        Z44.011 Encounter for fitting and adjustment of complete right artificial arm

        Z44.012 Encounter for fitting and adjustment of complete left artificial arm

        Z44.019 Encounter for fitting and adjustment of complete artificial arm, unspecified arm

      Z44.02 Encounter for fitting and adjustment of partial artificial arm

        Z44.021 Encounter for fitting and adjustment of partial artificial right arm

        Z44.022 Encounter for fitting and adjustment of partial artificial left arm

        Z44.029 Encounter for fitting and adjustment of partial artificial arm, unspecified arm

    Z44.1 Encounter for fitting and adjustment of artificial leg

      Z44.10 Encounter for fitting and adjustment of unspecified artificial leg

        Z44.101 Encounter for fitting and adjustment of unspecified right artificial leg

        Z44.102 Encounter for fitting and adjustment of unspecified left artificial leg

        Z44.109 Encounter for fitting and adjustment of unspecified artificial leg, unspecified leg

      Z44.11 Encounter for fitting and adjustment of complete artificial leg

        Z44.111 Encounter for fitting and adjustment of complete right artificial leg

        Z44.112 Encounter for fitting and adjustment of complete left artificial leg

        Z44.119 Encounter for fitting and adjustment of complete artificial leg, unspecified leg

      Z44.12 Encounter for fitting and adjustment of partial artificial leg

        Z44.121 Encounter for fitting and adjustment of partial artificial right leg

        Z44.122 Encounter for fitting and adjustment of partial artificial left leg

        Z44.129 Encounter for fitting and adjustment of partial artificial leg, unspecified leg

    Z44.2 Encounter for fitting and adjustment of artificial eye

      Excludes1: mechanical complication of ocular prosthesis (T85.3)

      Z44.20 Encounter for fitting and adjustment of artificial eye, unspecified

Z44.21 Encounter for fitting and adjustment of artificial right eye

Z44.22 Encounter for fitting and adjustment of artificial left eye

Z44.3 Encounter for fitting and adjustment of external breast prosthesis

> **Excludes1:** complications of breast implant (T85.4-)
>
> encounter for adjustment or removal of breast implant (Z45.81-)
>
> encounter for initial breast implant insertion for cosmetic breast augmentation (Z41.1)
>
> encounter for breast reconstruction following mastectomy (Z42.1)

Z44.30 Encounter for fitting and adjustment of external breast prosthesis, unspecified breast

Z44.31 Encounter for fitting and adjustment of external right breast prosthesis

Z44.32 Encounter for fitting and adjustment of external left breast prosthesis

Z44.8 Encounter for fitting and adjustment of other external prosthetic devices

Z44.9 Encounter for fitting and adjustment of unspecified external prosthetic device

Z45 Encounter for adjustment and management of implanted device

> **Includes:** removal or replacement of implanted device
>
> **Excludes1:** malfunction or other complications of device - see Alphabetical Index
>
> **Excludes2:** encounter for fitting and adjustment of non-implanted device (Z46.-)

Z45.0 Encounter for adjustment and management of cardiac device

Z45.01 Encounter for adjustment and management of cardiac pacemaker

> Encounter for adjustment and management of cardiac resynchronization therapy pacemaker (CRT-P)
>
> **Excludes1:** encounter for adjustment and management of automatic implantable cardiac defibrillator with synchronous cardiac pacemaker (Z45.02)

Z45.010 Encounter for checking and testing of cardiac pacemaker pulse generator [battery]

> Encounter for replacing cardiac pacemaker pulse generator [battery]

Z45.018 Encounter for adjustment and management of other part of cardiac pacemaker

> **Excludes2:** presence of prosthetic and other devices (Z95-Z97)

Z45.02 Encounter for adjustment and management of automatic implantable cardiac defibrillator

> Encounter for adjustment and management of automatic implantable cardiac defibrillator with synchronous cardiac pacemaker
>
> Encounter for adjustment and management of cardiac resynchronization therapy defibrillator (CRT-D)

Z45.09 Encounter for adjustment and management of other cardiac device

Z45.1 Encounter for adjustment and management of infusion pump

Z45.2 Encounter for adjustment and management of vascular access device

Encounter for adjustment and management of vascular catheters

> **Excludes1:** encounter for adjustment and management of renal dialysis catheter (Z49.01)

Z45.3 Encounter for adjustment and management of implanted devices of the special senses

Z45.31 Encounter for adjustment and management of implanted visual substitution device

Z45.32 Encounter for adjustment and management of implanted hearing device

> **Excludes1:** Encounter for fitting and adjustment of hearing aide (Z46.1)

Z45.320 Encounter for adjustment and management of bone conduction device

Z45.321 Encounter for adjustment and management of cochlear device

Z45.328 Encounter for adjustment and management of other implanted hearing device

Z45.4 Encounter for adjustment and management of implanted nervous system device

Z45.41 Encounter for adjustment and management of cerebrospinal fluid drainage device

> Encounter for adjustment and management of cerebral ventricular (communicating) shunt

Z45.42 Encounter for adjustment and management of neuropacemaker (brain) (peripheral nerve) (spinal cord)

Z45.49 Encounter for adjustment and management of other implanted nervous system device

Z45.8 Encounter for adjustment and management of other implanted devices

Z45.81 Encounter for adjustment or removal of breast implant

> Encounter for elective implant exchange (different material) (different size)
>
> Encounter removal of tissue expander without synchronous insertion of permanent implant
>
> **Excludes1:** complications of breast implant (T85.4-)
>
> encounter for initial breast implant insertion for cosmetic breast augmentation (Z41.1)
>
> encounter for breast reconstruction following mastectomy (Z42.1)

Z45.811 Encounter for adjustment or removal of right breast implant

Z45.812 Encounter for adjustment or removal of left breast implant

Z45.819 Encounter for adjustment or removal of unspecified breast implant

Z45.82 Encounter for adjustment or removal of myringotomy device (stent) (tube)

Z45.89 Encounter for adjustment and management of other implanted devices

Z45.9 Encounter for adjustment and management of unspecified implanted device

Z46 Encounter for fitting and adjustment of other devices

> **Includes:** removal or replacement of other device
>
> **Excludes1:** malfunction or other complications of device - see Alphabetical Index
>
> **Excludes2:** encounter for fitting and management of implanted devices (Z45.-)
>
> issue of repeat prescription only (Z76.0)
>
> presence of prosthetic and other devices (Z95-Z97)

Add 4th-7th digits   Nonspecific code   Unspecified code   Manifestation code

Z46.0 **Encounter for fitting and adjustment of spectacles and contact lenses**

Z46.1 **Encounter for fitting and adjustment of hearing aid**

> **Excludes1:** encounter for adjustment and management of implanted hearing device (Z45.32-)

Z46.2 **Encounter for fitting and adjustment of other devices related to nervous system and special senses**

> **Excludes2:** encounter for adjustment and management of implanted nervous system device (Z45.4-)
>
> encounter for adjustment and management of implanted visual substitution device (Z45.31)

Z46.3 **Encounter for fitting and adjustment of dental prosthetic device**

Encounter for fitting and adjustment of dentures

Z46.4 **Encounter for fitting and adjustment of orthodontic device**

Z46.5 **Encounter for fitting and adjustment of other gastrointestinal appliance and device**

> **Excludes1:** encounter for attention to artificial openings of digestive tract (Z43.1-Z43.4)

Z46.51 **Encounter for fitting and adjustment of gastric lap band**

Z46.59 **Encounter for fitting and adjustment of other gastrointestinal appliance and device**

Z46.6 **Encounter for fitting and adjustment of urinary device**

> **Excludes2:** attention to artificial openings of urinary tract (Z43.5, Z43.6)

Z46.8 **Encounter for fitting and adjustment of other specified devices**

Z46.81 **Encounter for fitting and adjustment of insulin pump**

Encounter for insulin pump instruction and training

Encounter for insulin pump titration

Z46.82 **Encounter for fitting and adjustment of non-vascular catheter**

Z46.89 **Encounter for fitting and adjustment of other specified devices**

Encounter for fitting and adjustment of wheelchair

Z46.9 **Encounter for fitting and adjustment of unspecified device**

Z47 **Orthopedic aftercare**

> **Excludes1:** aftercare for healing fracture-code to fracture with 7th character D

Z47.1 **Aftercare following joint replacement surgery**

Use additional code to identify the joint (Z96.6-)

Z47.2 **Encounter for removal of internal fixation device**

> **Excludes1:** encounter for adjustment of internal fixation device for fracture treatment- code to fracture with appropriate 7th character
>
> encounter for removal of external fixation device-code to fracture with 7th character D infection or inflammatory reaction to internal fixation device (T84.6-)
>
> mechanical complication of internal fixation device (T84.1-)

Z47.3 **Aftercare following explantation of joint prosthesis**

Aftercare following explantation of joint prosthesis, staged procedure

Encounter for joint prosthesis insertion following prior explantation of joint prosthesis

Z47.31 **Aftercare following explantation of shoulder joint prosthesis**

> **Excludes1:** acquired absence of shoulder joint following prior explantation of shoulder joint prosthesis (Z89.23-)
>
> shoulder joint prosthesis explantation status (Z89.23-)

Z47.32 **Aftercare following explantation of hip joint prosthesis**

> **Excludes1:** acquired absence of hip joint following prior explantation of hip joint prosthesis (Z89.62-)
>
> hip joint prosthesis explantation status (Z89.62-)

Z47.33 **Aftercare following explantation of knee joint prosthesis**

> **Excludes1:** acquired absence of knee joint following prior explantation of knee prosthesis (Z89.52-
>
> knee joint prosthesis explantation status (Z89.52-)

Z47.8 **Encounter for other orthopedic aftercare**

Z47.81 **Encounter for orthopedic aftercare following surgical amputation**

Use additional code to identify the limb amputated (Z89.-)

Z47.82 **Encounter for orthopedic aftercare following scoliosis surgery**

Z47.89 **Encounter for other orthopedic aftercare**

Z48 **Encounter for other postprocedural aftercare**

> **Excludes1:** encounter for follow-up examination after completed treatment (Z08-Z09)
>
> **Excludes2:** encounter for attention to artificial openings (Z43.-)
>
> encounter for fitting and adjustment of prosthetic **and** other devices (Z44-Z46)

Z48.0 **Encounter for attention to dressings, sutures and drains**

> **Excludes1:** encounter for aftercare following injury - code to Injury, by site, with appropriate 7th character for subsequent encounter
>
> encounter for planned postprocedural wound closure (Z48.1)

Z48.00 **Encounter for change or removal of nonsurgical wound dressing**

Encounter for change or removal of wound dressing NOS

Z48.01 **Encounter for change or removal of surgical wound dressing**

Z48.02 **Encounter for removal of sutures**

Encounter for removal of staples

Z48.03 **Encounter for change or removal of drains**

Z48.1 **Encounter for planned postprocedural wound closure**

> **Excludes1:** encounter for attention to dressings and sutures (Z48.0-)

Z48.2 **Encounter for aftercare following organ transplant**

Z48.21 **Encounter for aftercare following heart transplant**

Z48.22 **Encounter for aftercare following kidney transplant**

Z48.23 **Encounter for aftercare following liver transplant**

Z48.24 **Encounter for aftercare following lung transplant**

Z48.28 **Encounter for aftercare following multiple organ transplant**

Z48.280 Encounter for aftercare following heart-lung transplant

Z48.288 Encounter for aftercare following multiple organ transplant

Z48.29 Encounter for aftercare following other organ transplant

Z48.290 Encounter for aftercare following bone marrow transplant

Z48.298 Encounter for aftercare following other organ transplant

Z48.3 Aftercare following surgery for neoplasm

Use additional code to identify the neoplasm

Z48.8 Encounter for other specified postprocedural aftercare

Z48.81 Encounter for surgical aftercare following surgery on specified body systems

These codes identify the body system requiring aftercare. They are for use in conjunction **with** **other** aftercare codes to fully explain the aftercare encounter. The condition treated should also be coded if still present.

Excludes1: aftercare for injury- code the injury with 7th character D

aftercare following surgery for neoplasm (Z48.3)

Excludes2: aftercare following organ transplant (Z48.2-)

orthopedic aftercare (Z47.-)

Z48.810 Encounter for surgical aftercare following surgery on the sense organs

Z48.811 Encounter for surgical aftercare following surgery on the nervous system

Excludes2: encounter for surgical aftercare following surgery on the sense organs (Z48.810)

Z48.812 Encounter for surgical aftercare following surgery on the circulatory system

Z48.813 Encounter for surgical aftercare following surgery on the respiratory system

Z48.814 Encounter for surgical aftercare following surgery on the teeth or oral cavity

Z48.815 Encounter for surgical aftercare following surgery on the digestive system

Z48.816 Encounter for surgical aftercare following surgery on the genitourinary system

Excludes1: encounter for aftercare following sterilization reversal (Z31.42)

Z48.817 Encounter for surgical aftercare following surgery on the skin and subcutaneous tissue

Z48.89 Encounter for other specified surgical aftercare

Z49 **Encounter for care involving renal dialysis**

Code also associated end stage renal disease (N18.6)

Z49.0 Preparatory care for renal dialysis

Encounter for dialysis instruction and training

Z49.01 Encounter for fitting and adjustment of extracorporeal dialysis catheter

Removal or replacement of renal dialysis catheter

Toilet or cleansing of renal dialysis catheter

Z49.02 Encounter for fitting and adjustment of peritoneal dialysis catheter

Z49.3 Encounter for adequacy testing for dialysis

Z49.31 Encounter for adequacy testing for hemodialysis

Z49.32 Encounter for adequacy testing for peritoneal dialysis

Encounter for peritoneal equilibration test

Z51 **Encounter for other aftercare and medical care**

Code also condition requiring care

Excludes1: follow-up examination after treatment (Z08-Z09)

Z51.0 Encounter for antineoplastic radiation therapy

Z51.1 Encounter for antineoplastic chemotherapy and immunotherapy

Excludes2: encounter for chemotherapy and immunotherapy for nonneoplastic condition - code to condition

Z51.11 Encounter for antineoplastic chemotherapy

Z51.12 Encounter for antineoplastic immunotherapy

Z51.5 Encounter for palliative care

Z51.6 Encounter for desensitization to allergens

Z51.8 Encounter for other specified aftercare

Excludes1: holiday relief care (Z75.5)

Z51.81 Encounter for therapeutic drug level monitoring

Code also any long-term (current) drug therapy (Z79.-)

Excludes1: encounter for blood-drug test for administrative or medicolegal reasons (Z02.83)

Z51.89 Encounter for other specified aftercare

Z52 **Donors of organs and tissues**

Includes: autologous and other living donors

Excludes1: cadaveric donor - omit code

examination of potential donor (Z00.5)

Z52.0 Blood donor

Z52.00 Unspecified blood donor

Z52.000 Unspecified donor, whole blood

Z52.001 Unspecified donor, stem cells

Z52.008 Unspecified donor, other blood

Z52.01 Autologous blood donor

Z52.010 Autologous donor, whole blood

Z52.011 Autologous donor, stem cells

Z52.018 Autologous donor, other blood

Z52.09 Other blood donor Volunteer donor

Z52.090 Other blood donor, whole blood

Z52.091 Other blood donor, stem cells

Z52.098 Other blood donor, other blood

Z52.1 Skin donor

Z52.10 Skin donor, unspecified

Z52.11 Skin donor, autologous

Z52.19 Skin donor, other

Z52.2 Bone donor

Z52.20 Bone donor, unspecified

Z52.21 Bone donor, autologous

Z52.29 Bone donor, other

Z52.3 Bone marrow donor

Z52.4 Kidney donor

Z52.5 Cornea donor

Z52.6 Liver donor

▓ Add 4th-7th digits	▓ Nonspecific code	▓ Unspecified code	▓ Manifestation code

Z52.8 Donor of other specified organs or tissues

    Z52.81 Egg (Oocyte) donor

        Z52.810 Egg (Oocyte) donor under age 35, anonymous recipient

            Egg donor under age 35 NOS

        Z52.811 Egg (Oocyte) donor under age 35, designated recipient

        Z52.812 Egg (Oocyte) donor age 35 and over, anonymous recipient

            Egg donor age 35 and over NOS

        Z52.813 Egg (Oocyte) donor age 35 and over, designated recipient

        Z52.819 Egg (Oocyte) donor, unspecified

    Z52.89 Donor of other specified organs or tissues

Z52.9 Donor of unspecified organ or tissue

    Donor NOS

Z53 Persons encountering health services for specific procedures and treatment, not carried out

Z53.0 Procedure and treatment not carried out because of contraindication

    Z53.01 Procedure and treatment not carried out due to patient smoking

    Z53.09 Procedure and treatment not carried out because of other contraindication

Z53.1 Procedure and treatment not carried out because of patient's decision for reasons of belief and group pressure

Z53.2 Procedure and treatment not carried out because of patient's decision for other and unspecified reasons

    Z53.20 Procedure and treatment not carried out because of patient's decision for unspecified reasons

    Z53.21 Procedure and treatment not carried out due to patient leaving prior to being seen by health care provider

    Z53.29 Procedure and treatment not carried out because of patient's decision for other reasons

Z53.3 Procedure converted to open procedure

    Z53.31 Laparoscopic surgical procedure converted to open procedure

    Z53.32 Thoracoscopic surgical procedure converted to open procedure

    Z53.33 Arthroscopic surgical procedure converted to open procedure

    Z53.39 Other specified procedure converted to open procedure

Z53.8 Procedure and treatment not carried out for other reasons

Z53.9 Procedure and treatment not carried out, unspecified reason

PERSONS WITH POTENTIAL HEALTH HAZARDS RELATED TO SOCIOECONOMIC AND PSYCHOSOCIAL CIRCUMSTANCES (Z55-Z65)

Z55 Problems related to education and literacy

    Excludes1: disorders of psychological development (F80-F89)

Z55.0 Illiteracy and low-level literacy

Z55.1 Schooling unavailable and unattainable

Z55.2 Failed school examinations

Z55.3 Underachievement in school

Z55.4 Educational maladjustment and discord with teachers and classmates

Z55.8 Other problems related to education and literacy

    Problems related to inadequate teaching

Z55.9 Problems related to education and literacy, unspecified

    Academic problems NOS

Z56 Problems related to employment and unemployment

    Excludes2: occupational exposure to risk factors (Z57.-)

    problems related to housing and economic circumstances (Z59.-)

Z56.0 Unemployment, unspecified

Z56.1 Change of job

Z56.2 Threat of job loss

Z56.3 Stressful work schedule

Z56.4 Discord with boss and workmates

Z56.5 Uncongenial work environment

    Difficult conditions at work

Z56.6 Other physical and mental strain related to work

Z56.8 Other problems related to employment

    Z56.81 Sexual harassment on the job

    Z56.82 Military deployment status

        Individual (civilian or military) currently deployed in theater or in support of military war, peacekeeping and humanitarian operations

    Z56.89 Other problems related to employment

Z56.9 Unspecified problems related to employment

    Occupational problems NOS

Z57 Occupational exposure to risk factors

Z57.0 Occupational exposure to noise

Z57.1 Occupational exposure to radiation

Z57.2 Occupational exposure to dust

Z57.3 Occupational exposure to other air contaminants

    Z57.31 Occupational exposure to environmental tobacco smoke

        Excludes2: exposure to environmental tobacco smoke (Z77.22)

    Z57.39 Occupational exposure to other air contaminants

Z57.4 Occupational exposure to toxic agents in agriculture

    Occupational exposure to solids, liquids, gases or vapors in agriculture

Z57.5 Occupational exposure to toxic agents in other industries

    Occupational exposure to solids, liquids, gases or vapors in other industries

Z57.6 Occupational exposure to extreme temperature

Z57.7 Occupational exposure to vibration

Z57.8 Occupational exposure to other risk factors

Z57.9 Occupational exposure to unspecified risk factor

Z59 Problems related to housing and economic circumstances

    Excludes2: problems related to upbringing (Z62.-)

Z59.0 Homelessness

Z59.1 Inadequate housing

    Lack of heating

    Restriction of space

    Technical defects in home preventing adequate care

    Unsatisfactory surroundings

    Excludes1: problems related to the natural and physical environment (Z77.1-)

Z59.2 Discord with neighbors, lodgers and landlord

Z59.3 Problems related to living in residential institution

    Boarding-school resident

Excludes1: institutional upbringing (Z62.2)

Z59.4 **Lack of adequate food and safe drinking water**

Inadequate drinking water supply

Excludes1: effects of hunger (T73.0)

inappropriate diet or eating habits (Z72.4)

malnutrition (E40-E46)

Z59.5 **Extreme poverty**

Z59.6 **Low income**

Z59.7 **Insufficient social insurance and welfare support**

Z59.8 **Other problems related to housing and economic circumstances**

Foreclosure on loan

Isolated dwelling

Problems with creditors

Z59.9 **Problem related to housing and economic circumstances, unspecified**

Z60 **Problems related to social environment**

Z60.0 **Problems of adjustment to life-cycle transitions**

Empty nest syndrome

Phase of life problem

Problem with adjustment to retirement [pension]

Z60.2 **Problems related to living alone**

Z60.3 **Acculturation difficulty**

Problem with migration

Problem with social transplantation

Z60.4 **Social exclusion and rejection**

Exclusion and rejection on the basis of personal characteristics, such as unusual physical appearance, illness or behavior.

Excludes1: target of adverse discrimination such as for racial or religious reasons (Z60.5)

Z60.5 **Target of (perceived) adverse discrimination and persecution**

Excludes1: social exclusion and rejection (Z60.4)

Z60.8 **Other problems related to social environment**

Z60.9 **Problem related to social environment, unspecified**

Z62 **Problems related to upbringing**

Includes: current and past negative life events in childhood

current and past problems of a child related to upbringing

Excludes2: maltreatment syndrome (T74.-)

problems related to housing and economic circumstances (Z59.-)

Z62.0 **Inadequate parental supervision and control**

Z62.1 **Parental overprotection**

Z62.2 **Upbringing away from parents**

Excludes1: problems with boarding school (Z59.3)

Z62.21 **Child in welfare custody**

Child in care of non-parental family member

Child in foster care

Excludes2: problem for parent due to child in welfare custody (Z63.5)

Z62.22 **Institutional upbringing**

Child living in orphanage or group home

Z62.29 **Other upbringing away from parents**

Z62.3 **Hostility towards and scapegoating of child**

Z62.6 **Inappropriate (excessive) parental pressure**

Z62.8 **Other specified problems related to upbringing**

Z62.81 **Personal history of abuse in childhood**

Z62.810 **Personal history of physical and sexual abuse in childhood**

Excludes1: current child physical abuse (T74.12, T76.12)

current child sexual abuse (T74.22, T76.22)

Z62.811 **Personal history of psychological abuse in childhood**

Excludes1: current child psychological abuse (T74.32, T76.32)

Z62.812 **Personal history of neglect in childhood**

Excludes1: current child neglect (T74.02, T76.02)

Z62.819 **Personal history of unspecified abuse in childhood**

Excludes1: current child abuse NOS (T74.92, T76.92)

Z62.82 **Parent-child conflict**

Z62.820 **Parent-biological child conflict**

Parent-child problem NOS

Z62.821 **Parent-adopted child conflict**

Z62.822 **Parent-foster child conflict**

Z62.89 **Other specified problems related to upbringing**

Z62.890 **Parent-child estrangement NEC**

Z62.891 **Sibling rivalry**

Z62.898 **Other specified problems related to upbringing**

Z62.9 **Problem related to upbringing, unspecified**

Z63 **Other problems related to primary support group, including family circumstances**

Excludes2: maltreatment syndrome (T74.-, T76)

parent-child problems (Z62.-)

problems related to negative life events in childhood (Z62.-)

problems related to upbringing (Z62.-)

Z63.0 **Problems in relationship with spouse or partner**

Relationship distress with spouse or intimate partner

Excludes1: counseling for spousal or partner abuse problems (Z69.1)

counseling related to sexual attitude, behavior, and orientation (Z70.-)

Z63.1 **Problems in relationship with in-laws**

Z63.3 **Absence of family member**

Excludes1: absence of family member due to disappearance and death (Z63.4)

absence of family member due to separation and divorce (Z63.5)

Z63.31 **Absence of family member due to military deployment**

Individual or family affected by other family member being on military deployment

Excludes1: family disruption due to return of family member from military deployment (Z63.71)

Z63.32 **Other absence of family member**

Z63.4 **Disappearance and death of family member**

Assumed death of family member

Bereavement

Z63.5 **Disruption of family by separation and divorce**

Marital estrangement

Z63.6   Dependent relative needing care at home

Z63.7   Other stressful life events affecting family and household

Z63.71   Stress on family due to return of family member from military deployment

Individual or family affected by family member having returned from military deployment (current or past conflict)

Z63.72   Alcoholism and drug addiction in family

Z63.79   Other stressful life events affecting family and household

Anxiety (normal) about sick person in family

Health problems within family

Ill or disturbed family member

Isolated family

Z63.8   Other specified problems related to primary support group

Family discord NOS Family estrangement NOS

High expressed emotional level within family

Inadequate family support NOS

Inadequate or distorted communication within family

Z63.9   Problem related to primary support group, unspecified

Relationship disorder NOS

Z64   Problems related to certain psychosocial circumstances

Z64.0   Problems related to unwanted pregnancy

Z64.1   Problems related to multiparity

Z64.4   Discord with counselors

Discord with probation officer

Discord with social worker

Z65   Problems related to other psychosocial circumstances

Z65.0   Conviction in civil and criminal proceedings without imprisonment

Z65.1   Imprisonment and other incarceration

Z65.2   Problems related to release from prison

Z65.3   Problems related to other legal circumstances

Arrest

Child custody or support proceedings Litigation

Prosecution

Z65.4   Victim of crime and terrorism

Victim of torture

Z65.5   Exposure to disaster, war and other hostilities

Excludes1: target of perceived discrimination or persecution (Z60.5)

Z65.8   Other specified problems related to psychosocial circumstances

Religious or spiritual problem

Z65.9   Problem related to unspecified psychosocial circumstances

DO NOT RESUSCITATE STATUS (Z66)

Z66   Do not resuscitate

DNR status

BLOOD TYPE (Z67)

Z67   Blood type

Z67.1   Type A blood

Z67.10   Type A blood, Rh positive

Z67.11   Type A blood, Rh negative

Z67.2   Type B blood

Z67.20   Type B blood, Rh positive

Z67.21   Type B blood, Rh negative

Z67.3   Type AB blood

Z67.30   Type AB blood, Rh positive

Z67.31   Type AB blood, Rh negative

Z67.4   Type O blood

Z67.40   Type O blood, Rh positive

Z67.41   Type O blood, Rh negative

Z67.9   Unspecified blood type

Z67.90   Unspecified blood type, Rh positive

Z67.91   Unspecified blood type, Rh negative

BODY MASS INDEX [BMI] (Z68)

Definition: Body Mass Index is a measure of body fat that is the ratio of the weight of the body in kilograms to the square of its height in meters.

Z68   Body mass index [BMI]

Kilograms per meters squared

Note: BMI adult codes are for use for persons 21 years of age or older

BMI pediatric codes are for use for persons 2-20 years of age. These percentiles are based on the growth charts published by the Centers for Disease Control and Prevention (CDC)

▲Z68.1   Body mass index (BMI) 19.9 or less, adult

Z68.2   Body mass index (BMI) 20-29, adult

Z68.20   Body mass index (BMI) 20.0-20.9, adult

Z68.21   Body mass index (BMI) 21.0-21.9, adult

Z68.22   Body mass index (BMI) 22.0-22.9, adult

Z68.23   Body mass index (BMI) 23.0-23.9, adult

Z68.24   Body mass index (BMI) 24.0-24.9, adult

Z68.25   Body mass index (BMI) 25.0-25.9, adult

Z68.26   Body mass index (BMI) 26.0-26.9, adult

Z68.27   Body mass index (BMI) 27.0-27.9, adult

Z68.28   Body mass index (BMI) 28.0-28.9, adult

Z68.29   Body mass index (BMI) 29.0-29.9, adult

Z68.3   Body mass index (BMI) 30-39, adult

Z68.30   Body mass index (BMI) 30.0-30.9, adult

Z68.31   Body mass index (BMI) 31.0-31.9, adult

Z68.32   Body mass index (BMI) 32.0-32.9, adult

Z68.33   Body mass index (BMI) 33.0-33.9, adult

Z68.34   Body mass index (BMI) 34.0-34.9, adult

Z68.35   Body mass index (BMI) 35.0-35.9, adult

Z68.36   Body mass index (BMI) 36.0-36.9, adult

Z68.37   Body mass index (BMI) 37.0-37.9, adult

Z68.38   Body mass index (BMI) 38.0-38.9, adult

Z68.39   Body mass index (BMI) 39.0-39.9, adult

Z68.4   Body mass index (BMI) 40 or greater, adult

Z68.41   Body mass index (BMI) 40.0-44.9, adult

Z68.42   Body mass index (BMI) 45.0-49.9, adult

Z68.43   Body mass index (BMI) 50-59.9, adult

Z68.44   Body mass index (BMI) 60.0-69.9, adult

Z68.45   Body mass index (BMI) 70 or greater, adult

Z68.5   Body mass index (BMI) pediatric

Z68.51   Body mass index (BMI) pediatric, less than 5th percentile for age

Z68.52   Body mass index (BMI) pediatric, 5th percentile to less than 85th percentile for age

Z68.53   Body mass index (BMI) pediatric, 85th percentile to less than 95th percentile for age

Z68.54   **Body mass index (BMI) pediatric, greater than or equal to 95th percentile for age**

PERSONS ENCOUNTERING HEALTH SERVICES IN OTHER CIRCUMSTANCES (Z69-Z76)

Z69   **Encounter for mental health services for victim and perpetrator of abuse**

   Includes: counseling for victims and perpetrators of abuse

   Z69.0   **Encounter for mental health services for child abuse problems**

      Z69.01   **Encounter for mental health services for parental child abuse**

         Z69.010   **Encounter for mental health services for victim of parental child abuse**

            Encounter for mental health services for victim of child abuse by parent

            Encounter for mental health services for victim of child neglect by parent

            Encounter for mental health services for victim of child psychological abuse by parent

            Encounter for mental health services for victim of child sexual abuse by parent

         Z69.011   **Encounter for mental health services for perpetrator of parental child abuse**

            Encounter for mental health services for perpetrator of parental child neglect

            Encounter for mental health services for perpetrator of parental child psychological abuse

            Encounter for mental health services for perpetrator of parental child sexual abuse

            Excludes1: encounter for mental health services for non-parental child abuse (Z69.02-)

      Z69.02   **Encounter for mental health services for non-parental child abuse**

         Z69.020   **Encounter for mental health services for victim of non-parental child abuse**

            Encounter for mental health services for victim of non-parental child neglect

            Encounter for mental health services for victim of non-parental child psychological abuse

            Encounter for mental health services for victim of non-parental child sexual abuse

         Z69.021   **Encounter for mental health services for perpetrator of non-parental child abuse**

            Encounter for mental health services for perpetrator of non-parental child neglect

            Encounter for mental health services for perpetrator of non-parental child psychological abuse

            Encounter for mental health services for perpetrator of non-parental child sexual abuse

   Z69.1   **Encounter for mental health services for spousal or partner abuse problems**

      Z69.11   **Encounter for mental health services for victim of spousal or partner abuse**

         Encounter for mental health services for victim of spouse or partner neglect

         Encounter for mental health services for victim of spouse or partner psychological abuse

         Encounter for mental health services for victim of spouse or partner violence, physical

      Z69.12   **Encounter for mental health services for perpetrator of spousal or partner abuse**

         Encounter for mental health services for perpetrator of spouse or partner neglect

         Encounter for mental health services for perpetrator of spouse or partner psychological abuse

         Encounter for mental health services for perpetrator of spouse or partner violence, physical

         Encounter for mental health services for perpetrator of spouse or partner violence, sexual

   Z69.8   **Encounter for mental health services for victim or perpetrator of other abuse**

      Z69.81   **Encounter for mental health services for victim of other abuse**

         Encounter for mental health services for perpetrator of non-spousal adult abuse Encounter for mental health services for victim of non-spousal adult abuse

         Encounter for mental health services for victim of spouse or partner violence, sexual

         Encounter for rape victim counseling

      Z69.82   **Encounter for mental health services for perpetrator of other abuse**

Z70   **Counseling related to sexual attitude, behavior and orientation**

   Includes: encounter for mental health services for sexual attitude, behavior and orientation

   Excludes2: contraceptive or procreative counseling (Z30-Z31)

   Z70.0   **Counseling related to sexual attitude**

   Z70.1   **Counseling related to patient's sexual behavior and orientation**

      Patient concerned regarding impotence

      Patient concerned regarding non-responsiveness

      Patient concerned regarding promiscuity

      Patient concerned regarding sexual orientation

   Z70.2   **Counseling related to sexual behavior and orientation of third party**

      Advice sought regarding sexual behavior and orientation of child

      Advice sought regarding sexual behavior and orientation of partner

      Advice sought regarding sexual behavior and orientation of spouse

   Z70.3   **Counseling related to combined concerns regarding sexual attitude, behavior and orientation**

   Z70.8   **Other sex counseling**

      Encounter for sex education

   Z70.9   **Sex counseling, unspecified**

Z71   **Persons encountering health services for other counseling and medical advice, not elsewhere classified**

   Excludes2: contraceptive or procreation counseling (Z30-Z31)

      sex counseling (Z70.-)

   Z71.0   **Person encountering health services to consult on behalf of another person**

      Person encountering health services to seek advice or treatment for non-attending third party

      Excludes2: anxiety (normal) about sick person in family (Z63.7)

   Add 4th-7th digits   Nonspecific code   Unspecified code   Manifestation code

expectant (adoptive) parent(s) pre-birth pediatrician visit (Z76.81)

Z71.1 **Person with feared health complaint in whom no diagnosis is made**

Person encountering health services with feared condition which was not demonstrated

Person encountering health services in which problem was normal state

'Worried well'

Excludes1: medical observation for suspected diseases and conditions proven not to exist (Z03.-)

Z71.2 **Person consulting for explanation of examination or test findings**

Z71.3 **Dietary counseling and surveillance**

Use additional code for any associated underlying medical condition

Use additional code to identify body mass index (BMI), if known (Z68.-)

Z71.4 **Alcohol abuse counseling and surveillance**

Use additional code for alcohol abuse or dependence (F10.-)

Z71.41 **Alcohol abuse counseling and surveillance of alcoholic**

Z71.42 **Counseling for family member of alcoholic**

Counseling for significant other, partner, or friend of alcoholic

Z71.5 **Drug abuse counseling and surveillance**

Use additional code for drug abuse or dependence (F11-F16, F18-F19)

Z71.51 **Drug abuse counseling and surveillance of drug abuser**

Z71.52 **Counseling for family member of drug abuser**

Counseling for significant Other, partner, or friend of drug abuser

Z71.6 **Tobacco abuse counseling**

Use additional code for nicotine dependence (F17.-)

Z71.7 **Human immunodeficiency virus [HIV] counseling**

Z71.8 **Other specified counseling**

Excludes2: counseling for contraception (Z30.0-)

Z71.81 **Spiritual or religious counseling**

●**Z71.82** **Exercise counseling**

●**Z71.83** **Encounter for nonprocreative genetic counseling**

Excludes1: counseling for procreative genetics (Z31.5)

counseling for procreative management (Z31.6)

Z71.89 **Other specified counseling**

Z71.9 **Counseling, unspecified**

Encounter for medical advice NOS

Z72 **Problems related to lifestyle**

Excludes2: problems related to life-management difficulty (Z73.-)

problems related to socioeconomic and psychosocial circumstances (Z55-Z65)

Z72.0 **Tobacco use**

Tobacco use NOS

Excludes1: history of tobacco dependence (Z87.891)

nicotine dependence (F17.2-)

tobacco dependence (F17.2-)

tobacco use during pregnancy (O99.33-)

Z72.3 **Lack of physical exercise**

Z72.4 **Inappropriate diet and eating habits**

Excludes1: behavioral eating disorders of infancy or childhood (F98.2.-F98.3)

eating disorders (F50.-)

lack of adequate food (Z59.4)

malnutrition and other nutritional deficiencies (E40-E64)

Z72.5 **High risk sexual behavior**

Promiscuity

Excludes1: paraphilias (F65)

Z72.51 **High risk heterosexual behavior**

Z72.52 **High risk homosexual behavior**

Z72.53 **High risk bisexual behavior**

Z72.6 **Gambling and betting**

Excludes1: compulsive or pathological gambling (F63.0)

Z72.8 **Other problems related to lifestyle**

Z72.81 **Antisocial behavior**

Excludes1: conduct disorders (F91.-)

Z72.810 **Child and adolescent antisocial behavior** Antisocial behavior (child) (adolescent) without manifest psychiatric disorder

Delinquency NOS

Group delinquency

Offenses in the context of gang membership

Stealing in company with others

Truancy from school

Z72.811 **Adult antisocial behavior** Adult antisocial behavior without manifest psychiatric disorder

Z72.82 **Problems related to sleep**

Z72.820 **Sleep deprivation**

Lack of adequate sleep

Excludes1: insomnia (G47.0-)

Z72.821 **Inadequate sleep hygiene**

Bad sleep habits

Irregular sleep habits

Unhealthy sleep wake schedule

Excludes1: insomnia (F51.0-, G47.0-)

Z72.89 **Other problems related to lifestyle**

Self-damaging behavior

Z72.9 **Problem related to lifestyle, unspecified**

Z73 **Problems related to life management difficulty**

Excludes2: problems related to socioeconomic and psychosocial circumstances (Z55-Z65)

Z73.0 **Burn-out**

Z73.1 **Type A behavior pattern**

Z73.2 **Lack of relaxation and leisure**

Z73.3 **Stress, not elsewhere classified**

Physical and mental strain NOS

Excludes1: stress related to employment or unemployment (Z56.-)

Z73.4 **Inadequate social skills, not elsewhere classified**

Z73.5 **Social role conflict, not elsewhere classified**

Z73.6 **Limitation of activities due to disability**

Excludes1: care-provider dependency (Z74.-)

Z73.8 **Other problems related to life management difficulty**

Z73.81 **Behavioral insomnia of childhood**

Z73.810   **Behavioral insomnia of childhood, sleep-onset association type**

Z73.811   **Behavioral insomnia of childhood, limit setting type**

Z73.812   **Behavioral insomnia of childhood, combined type**

Z73.819   **Behavioral insomnia of childhood, unspecified type**

Z73.82   **Dual sensory impairment**

Z73.89   **Other problems related to life management difficulty**

Z73.9   **Problem related to life management difficulty, unspecified**

Z74   **Problems related to care provider dependency**

Excludes2: dependence on enabling machines or devices NEC (Z99.-)

Z74.0   **Reduced mobility**

Z74.01   **Bed confinement status**

Bedridden

Z74.09   **Other reduced mobility**

Chair ridden

Reduced mobility NOS

Excludes2: wheelchair dependence (Z99.3)

Z74.1   **Need for assistance with personal care**

Z74.2   **Need for assistance at home and no other household member able to render care**

Z74.3   **Need for continuous supervision**

Z74.8   **Other problems related to care provider dependency**

Z74.9   **Problem related to care provider dependency, unspecified**

Z75   **Problems related to medical facilities and other health care**

Z75.0   **Medical services not available in home**

Excludes1: no **Other** household member able to render care (Z74.2)

Z75.1   **Person awaiting admission to adequate facility elsewhere**

Z75.2   **Other waiting period for investigation and treatment**

Z75.3   **Unavailability and inaccessibility of health-care facilities**

Excludes1: bed unavailable (Z75.1)

Z75.4   **Unavailability and inaccessibility of other helping agencies**

Z75.5   **Holiday relief care**

Z75.8   **Other problems related to medical facilities and other health care**

Z75.9   **Unspecified problem related to medical facilities and other health care**

Z76   **Persons encountering health services in other circumstances**

Z76.0   **Encounter for issue of repeat prescription**

Encounter for issue of repeat prescription for appliance

Encounter for issue of repeat prescription for medicaments

Encounter for issue of repeat prescription for spectacles

Excludes2: issue of medical certificate (Z02.7)

repeat prescription for contraceptive (Z30.4-)

Z76.1   **Encounter for health supervision and care of foundling**

Z76.2   **Encounter for health supervision and care of other healthy infant and child**

Encounter for medical or nursing care or supervision of healthy infant under circumstances such as adverse socioeconomic conditions at home

Encounter for medical or nursing care or supervision of healthy infant under circumstances such as awaiting foster or adoptive placement

Encounter for medical or nursing care or supervision of healthy infant under circumstances such as maternal illness

Encounter for medical or nursing care or supervision of healthy infant under circumstances such as number of children at home preventing or interfering with normal care

Z76.3   **Healthy person accompanying sick person**

Z76.4   **Other boarder to healthcare facility**

Excludes1: homelessness (Z59.0)

Z76.5   **Malingerer [conscious simulation]**

Person feigning illness (with obvious motivation)

Excludes1: factitious disorder (F68.1-)

peregrinating patient (F68.1-)

Z76.8   **Persons encountering health services in other specified circumstances**

Z76.81   **Expectant parent(s) prebirth pediatrician visit**

Pre-adoption pediatrician visit for adoptive parent(s)

Z76.82   **Awaiting organ transplant status**

Patient waiting for organ availability

Z76.89   **Persons encountering health services in other specified circumstances**

Persons encountering health services NOS

PERSONS WITH POTENTIAL HEALTH HAZARDS RELATED TO FAMILY AND PERSONAL HISTORY AND CERTAIN CONDITIONS INFLUENCING HEALTH STATUS (Z77-Z99)

Code also any follow-up examination (Z08-Z09)

Z77   **Other contact with and (suspected) exposures hazardous to health**

Includes: contact with and (suspected) exposures to potential hazards to health

Excludes2: contact with and (suspected) exposure to communicable diseases (Z20.-)

exposure to (parental) (environmental) tobacco smoke in the perinatal period (P96.81)

newborn affected by noxious substances transmitted via placenta or breast milk (P04.-)

occupational exposure to risk factors (Z57.-)

retained foreign body (Z18.-)

retained foreign body fully removed (Z87.821)

toxic effects of substances chiefly nonmedicinal as to source (T51-T65)

Z77.0   **Contact with and (suspected) exposure to hazardous, chiefly nonmedicinal, chemicals**

Z77.01   **Contact with and (suspected) exposure to hazardous metals**

Z77.010   **Contact with and (suspected) exposure to arsenic**

Z77.011   **Contact with and (suspected) exposure to lead**

Z77.012   **Contact with and (suspected) exposure to uranium**

Excludes1: retained depleted uranium fragments (Z18.01)

Z77.018   **Contact with and (suspected) exposure to other hazardous metals**

Contact with and (suspected) exposure to chromium compounds

Contact with and (suspected) exposure to nickel dust

Z77.02   **Contact with and (suspected) exposure to hazardous aromatic compounds**

Z77.020 **Contact with and (suspected) exposure to aromatic amines**

Z77.021 **Contact with and (suspected) exposure to benzene**

Z77.028 **Contact with and (suspected) exposure to other hazardous aromatic compounds**

Aromatic dyes NOS

Polycyclic aromatic hydrocarbons

Z77.09 **Contact with and (suspected) exposure to other hazardous, chiefly nonmedicinal, chemicals**

Z77.090 **Contact with and (suspected) exposure to asbestos**

Z77.098 **Contact with and (suspected) exposure to other hazardous, chiefly nonmedicinal, chemicals** Dyes NOS

Z77.1 **Contact with and (suspected) exposure to environmental pollution and hazards in the physical environment**

Z77.11 **Contact with and (suspected) exposure to environmental pollution**

Z77.110 **Contact with and (suspected) exposure to air pollution**

Z77.111 **Contact with and (suspected) exposure to water pollution**

Z77.112 **Contact with and (suspected) exposure to soil pollution**

Z77.118 **Contact with and (suspected) exposure to other environmental pollution**

Z77.12 **Contact with and (suspected) exposure to hazards in the physical environment**

Z77.120 **Contact with and (suspected) exposure to mold (toxic)**

Z77.121 **Contact with and (suspected) exposure to harmful algae and algae toxins**

Contact with and (suspected) exposure to (harmful) algae bloom NOS

Contact with and (suspected) exposure to blue-green algae bloom

Contact with and (suspected) exposure to brown tide

Contact with and (suspected) exposure to cyanobacteria bloom

Contact with and (suspected) exposure to Florida red tide

Contact with and (suspected) exposure to pfiesteria piscicida

Contact with and (suspected) exposure to red tide

Z77.122 **Contact with and (suspected) exposure to noise**

Z77.123 **Contact with and (suspected) exposure to radon and other naturally occurring radiation**

Excludes2: radiation exposure as the cause of a confirmed condition (W88-W90, X39.0-)

radiation sickness NOS (T66)

Z77.128 **Contact with and (suspected) exposure to other hazards in the physical environment**

Z77.2 **Contact with and (suspected) exposure to other hazardous substances**

Z77.21 **Contact with and (suspected) exposure to potentially hazardous body fluids**

Z77.22 **Contact with and (suspected) exposure to environmental tobacco smoke (acute) (chronic)**

Exposure to second hand tobacco smoke (acute) (chronic)

Passive smoking (acute) (chronic)

Excludes1: nicotine dependence (F17.-)

tobacco use (Z72.0)

Excludes2: occupational exposure to environmental tobacco smoke (Z57.31)

Z77.29 **Contact with and (suspected) exposure to other hazardous substances**

Z77.9 **Other contact with and (suspected) exposures hazardous to health**

Z78 **Other specified health status**

Excludes2: asymptomatic human immunodeficiency virus [HIV] infection status (Z21)

postprocedural status (Z93-Z99)

sex reassignment status (Z87.890)

Z78.0 **Asymptomatic menopausal state**

Menopausal state NOS

Postmenopausal status NOS

Excludes2: symptomatic menopausal state (N95.1)

Z78.1 **Physical restraint status**

Excludes1: physical restraint due to a procedure - omit code

Z78.9 **Other specified health status**

Z79 **Long term (current) drug therapy**

Includes: long term (current) drug use for prophylactic purposes

Code also any therapeutic drug level monitoring (Z51.81)

Excludes2: drug abuse and dependence (F11-F19)

drug use complicating pregnancy, childbirth, and the puerperium (O99.32-)

long term (current) use of oral antidiabetic drugs (Z79.84)

long term (current) use of oral hypoglycemic drugs (Z79.84)

Z79.0 **Long term (current) use of anticoagulants and antithrombotics/antiplatelets**

Excludes2: long term (current) use of aspirin (Z79.82)

Z79.01 **Long term (current) use of anticoagulants**

Z79.02 **Long term (current) use of antithrombotics/antiplatelets**

Z79.1 **Long term (current) use of non-steroidal anti-inflammatories (NSAID)**

Excludes2: long term (current) use of aspirin (Z79.82)

Z79.2 **Long term (current) use of antibiotics**

Z79.3 **Long term (current) use of hormonal contraceptives**

Long term (current) use of birth control pill or patch

Z79.4 **Long term (current) use of insulin**

Z79.5 **Long term (current) use of steroids**

Z79.51 **Long term (current) use of inhaled steroids**

Z79.52 **Long term (current) use of systemic steroids**

Z79.8 **Other long term (current) drug therapy**

Z79.81 **Long term (current) use of agents affecting estrogen receptors and estrogen levels**

Code first, if applicable:

malignant neoplasm of breast (C50.-)

malignant neoplasm of prostate (C61)

Use additional code, if applicable, to identify:

estrogen receptor positive status (Z17.0)

family history of breast cancer (Z80.3)

genetic susceptibility to malignant neoplasm (cancer) (Z15.0-)

personal history of breast cancer (Z85.3)

personal history of prostate cancer (Z85.46)

postmenopausal status (Z78.0)

Excludes1: hormone replacement therapy (Z79.890)

Z79.810 Long term (current) use of selective estrogen receptor modulators (SERMs)

Long term (current) use of raloxifene (Evista)

Long term (current) use of tamoxifen (Nolvadex)

Long term (current) use of toremifene (Fareston)

Z79.811 Long term (current) use of aromatase inhibitors

Long term (current) use of anastrozole (Arimidex)

Long term (current) use of exemestane (Aromasin)

Long term (current) use of letrozole (Femara)

Z79.818 Long term (current) use of other agents affecting estrogen receptors and estrogen levels

Long term (current) use of estrogen receptor downregulators

Long term (current) use of fulvestrant (Faslodex)

Long term (current) use of gonadotropin-releasing hormone (GnRH) agonist

Long term (current) use of goserelin acetate (Zoladex)

Long term (current) use of leuprolide acetate (leuprorelin) (Lupron)

Long term (current) use of megestrol acetate (Megace)

Z79.82 Long term (current) use of aspirin

Z79.83 Long term (current) use of bisphosphonates

Z79.84 Long term (current) use of oral hypoglycemic drugs

Long term (current) use of oral antidiabetic drugs

Excludes2: long term (current) use of insulin (Z79.4)

Z79.89 Other long term (current) drug therapy

▲**Z79.890 Hormone replacement therapy**

Z79.891 Long term (current) use of opiate analgesic

Long term (current) use of methadone for pain management

Excludes1: methadone use NOS (F11.9-)

use of methadone for treatment of heroin addiction (F11.2-)

Z79.899 Other long term (current) drug therapy

Z80 Family history of primary malignant neoplasm

Z80.0 Family history of malignant neoplasm of digestive organs

Conditions classifiable to C15-C26

Z80.1 Family history of malignant neoplasm of trachea, bronchus and lung

Conditions classifiable to C33-C34

Z80.2 Family history of malignant neoplasm of other respiratory and intrathoracic organs

Conditions classifiable to C30-C32, C37-C39

Z80.3 Family history of malignant neoplasm of breast

Conditions classifiable to C50.-

Z80.4 Family history of malignant neoplasm of genital organs

Conditions classifiable to C51-C63

Z80.41 Family history of malignant neoplasm of ovary

Z80.42 Family history of malignant neoplasm of prostate

Z80.43 Family history of malignant neoplasm of testis

Z80.49 Family history of malignant neoplasm of other genital organs

Z80.5 Family history of malignant neoplasm of urinary tract

Conditions classifiable to C64-C68

Z80.51 Family history of malignant neoplasm of kidney

Z80.52 Family history of malignant neoplasm of bladder

Z80.59 Family history of malignant neoplasm of other urinary tract organ

Z80.6 Family history of leukemia

Conditions classifiable to C91-C95

Z80.7 Family history of other malignant neoplasms of lymphoid, hematopoietic and related tissues

Conditions classifiable to C81-C90, C96.-

Z80.8 Family history of malignant neoplasm of other organs or systems

Conditions classifiable to C00-C14, C40-C49, C69-C79

Z80.9 Family history of malignant neoplasm, unspecified

Conditions classifiable to C80.1

Z81 Family history of mental and behavioral disorders

Z81.0 Family history of intellectual disabilities

Conditions classifiable to F70-F79

Z81.1 Family history of alcohol abuse and dependence

Conditions classifiable to F10.-

Z81.2 Family history of tobacco abuse and dependence

Conditions classifiable to F17.-

Z81.3 Family history of other psychoactive substance abuse and dependence

Conditions classifiable to F11-F16, F18-F19

Z81.4 Family history of other substance abuse and dependence

Conditions classifiable to F55

Z81.8 Family history of other mental and behavioral disorders

Conditions classifiable elsewhere in F01-F99

Z82 Family history of certain disabilities and chronic diseases (leading to disablement)

Z82.0 Family history of epilepsy and other diseases of the nervous system

Conditions classifiable to G00-G99

Z82.1 Family history of blindness and visual loss

Conditions classifiable to H54.-

Z82.2 Family history of deafness and hearing loss

Conditions classifiable to H90-H91

Z82.3 Family history of stroke

Conditions classifiable to I60-I64

Z82.4 **Family history of ischemic heart disease and other diseases of the circulatory system**

Conditions classifiable to I00-I52, I65-I99

Z82.41 **Family history of sudden cardiac death**

Z82.49 **Family history of ischemic heart disease and other diseases of the circulatory system**

Z82.5 **Family history of asthma and other chronic lower respiratory diseases**

Conditions classifiable to J40-J47

Excludes2: family history of other diseases of the respiratory system (Z83.6)

Z82.6 **Family history of arthritis and other diseases of the musculoskeletal system and connective tissue**

Conditions classifiable to M00-M99

Z82.61 **Family history of arthritis**

Z82.62 **Family history of osteoporosis**

Z82.69 **Family history of other diseases of the musculoskeletal system and connective tissue**

Z82.7 **Family history of congenital malformations, deformations and chromosomal abnormalities**

Conditions classifiable to Q00-Q99

Z82.71 **Family history of polycystic kidney**

Z82.79 **Family history of other congenital malformations, deformations and chromosomal abnormalities**

Z82.8 **Family history of other disabilities and chronic diseases leading to disablement, not elsewhere classified**

Z83 **Family history of other specific disorders**

Excludes2: contact with and (suspected) exposure to communicable disease in the family (Z20.-)

Z83.0 **Family history of human immunodeficiency virus [HIV] disease**

Conditions classifiable to B20

Z83.1 **Family history of other infectious and parasitic diseases**

Conditions classifiable to A00-B19, B25-B94, B99

Z83.2 **Family history of diseases of the blood and blood-forming organs and certain disorders involving the immune mechanism**

Conditions classifiable to D50-D89

Z83.3 **Family history of diabetes mellitus**

Conditions classifiable to E08-E13

Z83.4 **Family history of other endocrine, nutritional and metabolic diseases**

Conditions classifiable to E00-E07, E15-E88

Z83.41 **Family history of multiple endocrine neoplasia [MEN] syndrome**

Z83.42 **Family history of familial hypercholesterolemia**

Z83.49 **Family history of other endocrine, nutritional and metabolic diseases**

Z83.5 **Family history of eye and ear disorders**

Z83.51 **Family history of eye disorders**

Conditions classifiable to H00-H53, H55-H59

Excludes2: family history of blindness and visual loss (Z82.1)

Z83.511 **Family history of glaucoma**

Z83.518 **Family history of other specified eye disorder**

Z83.52 **Family history of ear disorders**

Conditions classifiable to H60-H83, H92-H95

Excludes2: family history of deafness and hearing

loss (Z82.2)

Z83.6 **Family history of other diseases of the respiratory system**

Conditions classifiable to J00-J39, J60-J99

Excludes2: family history of asthma **and other** chronic lower respiratory diseases (Z82.5)

Z83.7 **Family history of diseases of the digestive system**

Conditions classifiable to K00-K93

Z83.71 **Family history of colonic polyps**

Excludes2: family history of malignant neoplasm of digestive organs (Z80.0)

Z83.79 **Family history of other diseases of the digestive system**

Z84 **Family history of other conditions**

Z84.0 **Family history of diseases of the skin and subcutaneous tissue**

Conditions classifiable to L00-L99

Z84.1 **Family history of disorders of kidney and ureter**

Conditions classifiable to N00-N29

Z84.2 **Family history of other diseases of the genitourinary system**

Conditions classifiable to N30-N99

Z84.3 **Family history of consanguinity**

Z84.8 **Family history of other specified conditions**

Z84.81 **Family history of carrier of genetic disease**

Z84.82 **Family history of sudden infant death syndrome**

Family history of SIDS

Z84.89 **Family history of other specified conditions**

Z85 **Personal history of malignant neoplasm**

Code first any follow-up examination after treatment of malignant neoplasm (Z08)

Use additional code to identify:

alcohol use and dependence (F10.-)

exposure to environmental tobacco smoke (Z77.22)

history of tobacco dependence (Z87.891)

occupational exposure to environmental tobacco smoke (Z57.31)

tobacco dependence (F17.-)

tobacco use (Z72.0)

Excludes2: personal history of benign neoplasm (Z86.01-)

personal history of carcinoma-in-situ (Z86.00-)

Z85.0 **Personal history of malignant neoplasm of digestive organs**

Z85.00 **Personal history of malignant neoplasm of unspecified digestive organ**

Z85.01 **Personal history of malignant neoplasm of esophagus**

Conditions classifiable to C15

Z85.02 **Personal history of malignant neoplasm of stomach**

Z85.020 **Personal history of malignant carcinoid tumor of stomach**

Conditions classifiable to C7A.092

Z85.028 **Personal history of other malignant neoplasm of stomach**

Conditions classifiable to C16

Z85.03 **Personal history of malignant neoplasm of large intestine**

Z85.030 **Personal history of malignant carcinoid tumor of large intestine**

Conditions classifiable to C7A.022-
C7A.025, C7A.029

Z85.038 **Personal history of other malignant neoplasm of large intestine**

Conditions classifiable to C18

Z85.04 **Personal history of malignant neoplasm of rectum, rectosigmoid junction, and anus**

Z85.040 **Personal history of malignant carcinoid tumor of rectum**

Conditions classifiable to C7A.026

Z85.048 **Personal history of other malignant neoplasm of rectum, rectosigmoid junction, and anus**

Conditions classifiable to C19-C21

Z85.05 **Personal history of malignant neoplasm of liver**

Conditions classifiable to C22

Z85.06 **Personal history of malignant neoplasm of small intestine**

Z85.060 **Personal history of malignant carcinoid tumor of small intestine**

Conditions classifiable to C7A.01-

Z85.068 **Personal history of other malignant neoplasm of small intestine**

Conditions classifiable to C17

Z85.07 **Personal history of malignant neoplasm of pancreas**

Conditions classifiable to C25

Z85.09 **Personal history of malignant neoplasm of other digestive organs**

Z85.1 **Personal history of malignant neoplasm of trachea, bronchus and lung**

Z85.11 **Personal history of malignant neoplasm of bronchus and lung**

Z85.110 **Personal history of malignant carcinoid tumor of bronchus and lung**
Conditions classifiable to C7A.090

Z85.118 **Personal history of other malignant neoplasm of bronchus and lung**
Conditions classifiable to C34

Z85.12 **Personal history of malignant neoplasm of trachea**

Conditions classifiable to C33

Z85.2 **Personal history of malignant neoplasm of other respiratory and intrathoracic organs**

Z85.20 **Personal history of malignant neoplasm of unspecified respiratory organ**

Z85.21 **Personal history of malignant neoplasm of larynx**

Conditions classifiable to C32

Z85.22 **Personal history of malignant neoplasm of nasal cavities, middle ear, and accessory sinuses**

Conditions classifiable to C30-C31

Z85.23 **Personal history of malignant neoplasm of thymus**

Z85.230 **Personal history of malignant carcinoid tumor of thymus**

Conditions classifiable to C7A.091

Z85.238 **Personal history of other malignant neoplasm of thymus**

Conditions classifiable to C37

Z85.29 **Personal history of malignant neoplasm of other respiratory and intrathoracic organs**

Z85.3 **Personal history of malignant neoplasm of breast**

Conditions classifiable to C50.-

Z85.4 **Personal history of malignant neoplasm of genital organs**

Conditions classifiable to C51-C63

Z85.40 **Personal history of malignant neoplasm of unspecified female genital organ**

Z85.41 **Personal history of malignant neoplasm of cervix uteri**

Z85.42 **Personal history of malignant neoplasm of other parts of uterus**

Z85.43 **Personal history of malignant neoplasm of ovary**

Z85.44 **Personal history of malignant neoplasm of other female genital organs**

Z85.45 **Personal history of malignant neoplasm of unspecified male genital organ**

Z85.46 **Personal history of malignant neoplasm of prostate**

Z85.47 **Personal history of malignant neoplasm of testis**

Z85.48 **Personal history of malignant neoplasm of epididymis**

Z85.49 **Personal history of malignant neoplasm of other male genital organs**

Z85.5 **Personal history of malignant neoplasm of urinary tract**

Conditions classifiable to C64-C68

Z85.50 **Personal history of malignant neoplasm of unspecified urinary tract organ**

Z85.51 **Personal history of malignant neoplasm of bladder**

Z85.52 **Personal history of malignant neoplasm of kidney**

Excludes1: personal history of malignant neoplasm of renal pelvis (Z85.53)

Z85.520 **Personal history of malignant carcinoid tumor of kidney**

Conditions classifiable to C7A.093

Z85.528 **Personal history of other malignant neoplasm of kidney**

Conditions classifiable to C64

Z85.53 **Personal history of malignant neoplasm of renal pelvis**

Z85.54 **Personal history of malignant neoplasm of ureter**

Z85.59 **Personal history of malignant neoplasm of other urinary tract organ**

Z85.6 **Personal history of leukemia**

Conditions classifiable to C91-C95

Excludes1: leukemia in remission C91.0-C95.9 with 5th character 1

Z85.7 **Personal history of other malignant neoplasms of lymphoid, hematopoietic and related tissues**

Z85.71 **Personal history of Hodgkin lymphoma**

Conditions classifiable to C81

Z85.72 **Personal history of non-Hodgkin lymphomas**

Conditions classifiable to C82-C85

Z85.79 **Personal history of other malignant neoplasms of lymphoid, hematopoietic and related tissues**

Conditions classifiable to C88-C90, C96

Excludes1: multiple myeloma in remission (C90.01)

plasma cell leukemia in remission (C90.11)

plasmacytoma in remission (C90.21)

Z85.8 **Personal history of malignant neoplasms of other organs and systems**

Conditions classifiable to C00-C14, C40-C49, C69-C75, C7A.098, C76-C79

Z85.81 **Personal history of malignant neoplasm of lip, oral cavity, and pharynx**

Z85.810 **Personal history of malignant neoplasm of tongue**

Z85.818 **Personal history of malignant neoplasm of other sites of lip, oral cavity, and pharynx**

Z85.819 **Personal history of malignant neoplasm of unspecified site of lip, oral cavity, and pharynx**

Z85.82 **Personal history of malignant neoplasm of skin**

Z85.820 **Personal history of malignant melanoma of skin**

Conditions classifiable to C43

Z85.821 **Personal history of Merkel cell carcinoma**

Conditions classifiable to C4A

Z85.828 **Personal history of other malignant neoplasm of skin**

Conditions classifiable to C44

Z85.83 **Personal history of malignant neoplasm of bone and soft tissue**

Z85.830 **Personal history of malignant neoplasm of bone**

Z85.831 **Personal history of malignant neoplasm of soft tissue**

Excludes2: personal history of malignant neoplasm of skin (Z85.82-)

Z85.84 **Personal history of malignant neoplasm of eye and nervous tissue**

Z85.840 **Personal history of malignant neoplasm of eye**

Z85.841 **Personal history of malignant neoplasm of brain**

Z85.848 **Personal history of malignant neoplasm of other parts of nervous tissue**

Z85.85 **Personal history of malignant neoplasm of endocrine glands**

Z85.850 **Personal history of malignant neoplasm of thyroid**

Z85.858 **Personal history of malignant neoplasm of other endocrine glands**

Z85.89 **Personal history of malignant neoplasm of other organs and systems**

Z85.9 **Personal history of malignant neoplasm, unspecified**

Conditions classifiable to C7A.00, C80.1

Z86 **Personal history of certain other diseases**

Code first any follow-up examination after treatment (Z09)

Z86.0 **Personal history of in-situ and benign neoplasms and neoplasms of uncertain behavior**

Excludes2: personal history of malignant neoplasms (Z85.-)

Z86.00 **Personal history of in-situ neoplasm**

Conditions classifiable to D00-D09

Z86.000 **Personal history of in-situ neoplasm of breast**

Z86.001 **Personal history of in-situ neoplasm of cervix uteri**

Personal history of cervical intraepithelial neoplasia III [CIN III]

Z86.008 **Personal history of in-situ neoplasm of other site**

Personal history of vaginal intraepithelial neoplasia III [VAIN III]

Personal history of vulvar intraepithelial neoplasia III [VIN III]

Z86.01 **Personal history of benign neoplasm**

Z86.010 **Personal history of colonic polyps**

Z86.011 **Personal history of benign neoplasm of the brain**

Z86.012 **Personal history of benign carcinoid tumor**

Z86.018 **Personal history of other benign neoplasm**

Z86.03 **Personal history of neoplasm of uncertain behavior**

Z86.1 **Personal history of infectious and parasitic diseases**

Conditions classifiable to A00-B89, B99

Excludes1: personal history of infectious diseases specific to a body system

sequelae of infectious and parasitic diseases (B90-B94)

Z86.11 **Personal history of tuberculosis**

Z86.12 **Personal history of poliomyelitis**

Z86.13 **Personal history of malaria**

Z86.14 **Personal history of Methicillin resistant Staphylococcus aureus infection**

Personal history of MRSA infection

Z86.19 **Personal history of other infectious and parasitic diseases**

Z86.2 **Personal history of diseases of the blood and blood-forming organs and certain disorders involving the immune mechanism**

Conditions classifiable to D50-D89

Z86.3 **Personal history of endocrine, nutritional and metabolic diseases**

Conditions classifiable to E00-E88

Z86.31 **Personal history of diabetic foot ulcer**

Excludes2: current diabetic foot ulcer (E08.621, E09.621, E10.621, E11.621, E13.621)

Z86.32 **Personal history of gestational diabetes**

Personal history of conditions classifiable to O24.4-

Excludes1: gestational diabetes mellitus in current pregnancy (O24.4-)

Z86.39 **Personal history of other endocrine, nutritional and metabolic disease**

Z86.5 **Personal history of mental and behavioral disorders**

Conditions classifiable to F40-F59

Z86.51 **Personal history of combat and operational stress reaction**

Z86.59 **Personal history of other mental and behavioral disorders**

Z86.6 **Personal history of diseases of the nervous system and sense organs**

Conditions classifiable to G00-G99, H00-H95

Z86.61 **Personal history of infections of the central nervous system**

Personal history of encephalitis

Personal history of meningitis

Z86.69 **Personal history of other diseases of the nervous system and sense organs**

Z86.7 **Personal history of diseases of the circulatory system**

Conditions classifiable to I00-I99

Excludes2: old myocardial infarction (I25.2)

personal history of anaphylactic shock (Z87.892)

postmyocardial infarction syndrome (I24.1)

Z86.71 **Personal history of venous thrombosis and embolism**

Z86.711 **Personal history of pulmonary embolism**

Z86.718 **Personal history of other venous thrombosis and embolism**

Z86.72 **Personal history of thrombophlebitis**

Z86.73 **Personal history of transient ischemic attack (TIA), and cerebral infarction without residual deficits**

Personal history of prolonged reversible ischemic neurological deficit (PRIND)

Personal history of stroke NOS without residual deficits

Excludes1: personal history of traumatic brain injury (Z87.820)

sequelae of cerebrovascular disease (I69.-)

Z86.74 **Personal history of sudden cardiac arrest**

Personal history of sudden cardiac death successfully resuscitated

Z86.79 **Personal history of other diseases of the circulatory system**

Z87 **Personal history of other diseases and conditions**

Code first any follow-up examination after treatment (Z09)

Z87.0 **Personal history of diseases of the respiratory system**

Conditions classifiable to J00-J99

Z87.01 **Personal history of pneumonia (recurrent)**

Z87.09 **Personal history of other diseases of the respiratory system**

Z87.1 **Personal history of diseases of the digestive system**

Conditions classifiable to K00-K93

Z87.11 **Personal history of peptic ulcer disease**

Z87.19 **Personal history of other diseases of the digestive system**

Z87.2 **Personal history of diseases of the skin and subcutaneous tissue**

Conditions classifiable to L00-L99

Excludes2: personal history of diabetic foot ulcer (Z86.31)

Z87.3 **Personal history of diseases of the musculoskeletal system and connective tissue**

Conditions classifiable to M00-M99

Excludes2: personal history of (healed) traumatic fracture (Z87.81)

Z87.31 **Personal history of (healed) nontraumatic fracture**

Z87.310 **Personal history of (healed) osteoporosis fracture**

Personal history of (healed) fragility fracture

Personal history of (healed) collapsed vertebra due to osteoporosis

Z87.311 **Personal history of (healed) other pathological fracture**

Personal history of (healed) collapsed vertebra NOS

Excludes2: personal history of osteoporosis fracture (Z87.310)

Z87.312 **Personal history of (healed) stress fracture**

Personal history of (healed) fatigue fracture

Z87.39 **Personal history of other diseases of the musculoskeletal system and connective tissue**

Z87.4 **Personal history of diseases of genitourinary system**

Conditions classifiable to N00-N99

Z87.41 **Personal history of dysplasia of the female genital tract**

Excludes1: personal history of intraepithelial neoplasia III of female genital tract (Z86.001, Z87.008)

personal history of malignant neoplasm of female genital tract (Z85.40-Z85.44)

Z87.410 **Personal history of cervical dysplasia**

Z87.411 **Personal history of vaginal dysplasia**

Z87.412 **Personal history of vulvar dysplasia**

Z87.42 **Personal history of other diseases of the female genital tract**

Z87.43 **Personal history of diseases of male genital organs**

Z87.430 **Personal history of prostatic dysplasia**

Excludes1: personal history of malignant neoplasm of prostate (Z85.46)

Z87.438 **Personal history of other diseases of male genital organs**

Z87.44 **Personal history of diseases of urinary system**

Excludes1: personal history of malignant neoplasm of cervix uteri (Z85.41)

Z87.440 **Personal history of urinary (tract) infections**

Z87.441 **Personal history of nephrotic syndrome**

Z87.442 **Personal history of urinary calculi**

Personal history of kidney stones

Z87.448 **Personal history of other diseases of urinary system**

Z87.5 **Personal history of complications of pregnancy, childbirth and the puerperium**

Conditions classifiable to O00-O9A

Excludes2: recurrent pregnancy loss (N96)

Z87.51 **Personal history of pre-term labor**

Excludes1: current pregnancy with history of pre-term labor (O09.21-)

Z87.59 **Personal history of other complications of pregnancy, childbirth and the puerperium**

Personal history of trophoblastic disease

Z87.7 **Personal history of (corrected) congenital malformations**

Conditions classifiable to Q00-Q89 that have been repaired or corrected

Excludes1: congenital malformations that have been partially corrected or repair but which still require medical treatment - code to condition

Excludes2: Other postprocedural states (Z98.-)

Add 4th-7th digits   Nonspecific code   Unspecified code   Manifestation code

personal history of medical treatment (Z92.-)

presence of cardiac and vascular implants and grafts (Z95.-) presence of other devices (Z97.-)

presence of other functional implants (Z96.-) transplanted organ and tissue status (Z94.-)

Z87.71   Personal history of (corrected) congenital malformations of genitourinary system

   Z87.710   Personal history of (corrected) hypospadias

   Z87.718   Personal history of other specified (corrected) congenital malformations of genitourinary system

Z87.72   Personal history of (corrected) congenital malformations of nervous system and sense organs

   Z87.720   Personal history of (corrected) congenital malformations of eye

   Z87.721   Personal history of (corrected) congenital malformations of ear

   Z87.728   Personal history of other specified (corrected) congenital malformations of nervous system and sense organs

Z87.73   Personal history of (corrected) congenital malformations of digestive system

   Z87.730   Personal history of (corrected) cleft lip and palate

   Z87.738   Personal history of other specified (corrected) congenital malformations of digestive system

Z87.74   Personal history of (corrected) congenital malformations of heart and circulatory system

Z87.75   Personal history of (corrected) congenital malformations of respiratory system

Z87.76   Personal history of (corrected) congenital malformations of integument, limbs and musculoskeletal system

Z87.79   Personal history of other (corrected) congenital malformations

   Z87.790   Personal history of (corrected) congenital malformations of face and neck

   Z87.798   Personal history of other (corrected) congenital malformations

Z87.8   Personal history of other specified conditions

   Excludes2: personal history of self harm (Z91.5)

Z87.81   Personal history of (healed) traumatic fracture

   Excludes2: personal history of (healed) nontraumatic fracture (Z87.31-)

Z87.82   Personal history of other (healed) physical injury and trauma

   Conditions classifiable to S00-T88, except traumatic fractures

   Z87.820   Personal history of traumatic brain injury

      Excludes1: personal history of transient ischemic attack (TIA), and cerebral infarction without residual deficits (Z86.73)

   Z87.821   Personal history of retained foreign body fully removed

   Z87.828   Personal history of other (healed) physical injury and trauma

Z87.89   Personal history of other specified conditions

   Z87.890   Personal history of sex reassignment

   Z87.891   Personal history of nicotine dependence

      Excludes1: current nicotine dependence (F17.2-)

   Z87.892   Personal history of anaphylaxis

      <u>Code also</u> allergy status such as:

      allergy status to drugs, medicaments and biological substances (Z88.-)

      allergy status, other than to drugs and biological substances (Z91.0-)

   Z87.898   Personal history of other specified conditions

Z88   Allergy status to drugs, medicaments and biological substances

   Excludes2: Allergy status, **other** than to drugs and biological substances (Z91.0-)

Z88.0   Allergy status to penicillin

Z88.1   Allergy status to other antibiotic agents status

Z88.2   Allergy status to sulfonamides status

Z88.3   Allergy status to other anti-infective agents status

Z88.4   Allergy status to anesthetic agent status

Z88.5   Allergy status to narcotic agent status

Z88.6   Allergy status to analgesic agent status

Z88.7   Allergy status to serum and vaccine status

Z88.8   Allergy status to other drugs, medicaments and biological substances status

Z88.9   Allergy status to unspecified drugs, medicaments and biological substances status

Z89   Acquired absence of limb

   Includes: amputation status

      postprocedural loss of limb

      post-traumatic loss of limb

   Excludes1: acquired deformities of limbs (M20-M21)

      congenital absence of limbs (Q71-Q73)

Z89.0   Acquired absence of thumb and other finger(s)

   Z89.01   Acquired absence of thumb

      Z89.011   Acquired absence of right thumb

      Z89.012   Acquired absence of left thumb

      Z89.019   Acquired absence of unspecified thumb

   Z89.02   Acquired absence of other finger(s)

      Excludes2: acquired absence of thumb (Z89.01-)

      Z89.021   Acquired absence of right finger(s)

      Z89.022   Acquired absence of left finger(s)

      Z89.029   Acquired absence of unspecified finger(s)

Z89.1   Acquired absence of hand and wrist

   Z89.11   Acquired absence of hand

      Z89.111   Acquired absence of right hand

      Z89.112   Acquired absence of left hand

      Z89.119   Acquired absence of unspecified hand

   Z89.12   Acquired absence of wrist

      Disarticulation at wrist

      Z89.121   Acquired absence of right wrist

      Z89.122   Acquired absence of left wrist

      Z89.129   Acquired absence of unspecified wrist

Z89.2   Acquired absence of upper limb above wrist

   Z89.20   Acquired absence of upper limb, unspecified level

● New code   ▲ Revised code   **Excludes1:** Not coded here   **Excludes2:** Not included here   ⊗ Placeholder required   ⑦ 7th digit required

Z89.201   **Acquired absence of right upper limb, unspecified level**

Z89.202   **Acquired absence of left upper limb, unspecified level**

Z89.209   **Acquired absence of unspecified upper limb, unspecified level**

Acquired absence of arm NOS

Z89.21   **Acquired absence of upper limb below elbow**

Z89.211   **Acquired absence of right upper limb below elbow**

Z89.212   **Acquired absence of left upper limb below elbow**

Z89.219   **Acquired absence of unspecified upper limb below elbow**

Z89.22   **Acquired absence of upper limb above elbow**

Disarticulation at elbow

Z89.221   **Acquired absence of right upper limb above elbow**

Z89.222   **Acquired absence of left upper limb above elbow**

Z89.229   **Acquired absence of unspecified upper limb above elbow**

Z89.23   **Acquired absence of shoulder**

Acquired absence of shoulder joint following explantation of shoulder joint prosthesis, with or without presence of antibiotic-impregnated cement spacer

Z89.231   **Acquired absence of right shoulder**

Z89.232   **Acquired absence of left shoulder**

Z89.239   **Acquired absence of unspecified shoulder**

Z89.4   **Acquired absence of toe(s), foot, and ankle**

Z89.41   **Acquired absence of great toe**

Z89.411   **Acquired absence of right great toe**

Z89.412   **Acquired absence of left great toe**

Z89.419   **Acquired absence of unspecified great toe**

Z89.42   **Acquired absence of other toe(s)**

Excludes2: acquired absence of great toe (Z89.41-)

Z89.421   **Acquired absence of other right toe(s)**

Z89.422   **Acquired absence of other left toe(s)**

Z89.429   **Acquired absence of other toe(s), unspecified side**

Z89.43   **Acquired absence of foot**

Z89.431   **Acquired absence of right foot**

Z89.432   **Acquired absence of left foot**

Z89.439   **Acquired absence of unspecified foot**

Z89.44   **Acquired absence of ankle**

Disarticulation of ankle

Z89.441   **Acquired absence of right ankle**

Z89.442   **Acquired absence of left ankle**

Z89.449   **Acquired absence of unspecified ankle**

Z89.5   **Acquired absence of leg below knee**

Z89.51   **Acquired absence of leg below knee**

Z89.511   **Acquired absence of right leg below knee**

Z89.512   **Acquired absence of left leg below knee**

Z89.519   **Acquired absence of unspecified leg below knee**

Z89.52   **Acquired absence of knee**

Acquired absence of knee joint following explantation of knee joint prosthesis, with or without presence of antibiotic-impregnated cement spacer

Z89.521   **Acquired absence of right knee**

Z89.522   **Acquired absence of left knee**

Z89.529   **Acquired absence of unspecified knee**

Z89.6   **Acquired absence of leg above knee**

Z89.61   **Acquired absence of leg above knee**

Acquired absence of leg NOS

Disarticulation at knee

Z89.611   **Acquired absence of right leg above knee**

Z89.612   **Acquired absence of left leg above knee**

Z89.619   **Acquired absence of unspecified leg above knee**

Z89.62   **Acquired absence of hip**

Acquired absence of hip joint following explantation of hip joint prosthesis, with or without presence of antibiotic-impregnated cement spacer

Disarticulation at hip

Z89.621   **Acquired absence of right hip joint**

Z89.622   **Acquired absence of left hip joint**

Z89.629   **Acquired absence of unspecified hip joint**

Z89.9   **Acquired absence of limb, unspecified**

Z90   **Acquired absence of organs, not elsewhere classified**

Includes: postprocedural or post-traumatic loss of body part NEC

Excludes1: congenital absence - see Alphabetical Index

Excludes2: postprocedural absence of endocrine glands (E89.-)

Z90.0   **Acquired absence of part of head and neck**

Z90.01   **Acquired absence of eye**

Z90.02   **Acquired absence of larynx**

Z90.09   **Acquired absence of other part of head and neck**

Acquired absence of nose

Excludes2: teeth (K08.1)

Z90.1   **Acquired absence of breast and nipple**

Z90.10   **Acquired absence of unspecified breast and nipple**

Z90.11   **Acquired absence of right breast and nipple**

Z90.12   **Acquired absence of left breast and nipple**

Z90.13   **Acquired absence of bilateral breasts and nipples**

Z90.2   **Acquired absence of lung [part of]**

Z90.3   **Acquired absence of stomach [part of]**

Z90.4   **Acquired absence of other specified parts of digestive tract**

Z90.41   **Acquired absence of pancreas**

Code also exocrine pancreatic insufficiency (K86.81)

Use additional code to identify any associated:

insulin use (Z79.4)

diabetes mellitus, postpancreatectomy (E13.-)

Z90.410   **Acquired total absence of pancreas**

Acquired absence of pancreas NOS

Z90.411   **Acquired partial absence of pancreas**

Z90.49   **Acquired absence of other specified parts of digestive tract**

Z90.5 Acquired absence of kidney

Z90.6 Acquired absence of other parts of urinary tract

Acquired absence of bladder

Z90.7 Acquired absence of genital organ(s)

Excludes1: personal history of sex reassignment (Z87.890)

Excludes2: female genital mutilation status (N90.81-)

Z90.71 Acquired absence of cervix and uterus

Z90.710 Acquired absence of both cervix and uterus

Acquired absence of uterus NOS

Status post total hysterectomy

Z90.711 Acquired absence of uterus with remaining cervical stump

Status post partial hysterectomy with remaining cervical stump

Z90.712 Acquired absence of cervix with remaining uterus

Z90.72 Acquired absence of ovaries

Z90.721 Acquired absence of ovaries, unilateral

Z90.722 Acquired absence of ovaries, bilateral

Z90.79 Acquired absence of other genital organ(s)

Z90.8 Acquired absence of other organs

Z90.81 Acquired absence of spleen

Z90.89 Acquired absence of other organs

Z91 Personal risk factors, not elsewhere classified

Excludes2: contact with and (suspected) exposures hazardous to health (Z77.-)

exposure to pollution and other problems related to physical environment (Z77.1-)

female genital mutilation status (N90.81-)

personal history of physical injury and trauma (Z87.81, Z87.82-)

occupational exposure to risk factors (Z57.-)

Z91.0 Allergy status, other than to drugs and biological substances

Excludes2: Allergy status to drugs, medicaments, and biological substances (Z88.-)

Z91.01 Food allergy status

Excludes2: food additives allergy status (Z91.02)

Z91.010 Allergy to peanuts

Z91.011 Allergy to milk products

Excludes1: lactose intolerance (E73.-)

Z91.012 Allergy to eggs

Z91.013 Allergy to seafood

Allergy to shellfish

Allergy to octopus or squid ink

Z91.018 Allergy to other foods

Allergy to nuts other than peanuts

Z91.02 Food additives allergy status

Z91.03 Insect allergy status

Z91.030 Bee allergy status

Z91.038 Other insect allergy status

Z91.04 Nonmedicinal substance allergy status

Z91.040 Latex allergy status

Latex sensitivity status

Z91.041 Radiographic dye allergy status

Allergy status to contrast media used for diagnostic X-ray procedure

Z91.048 Other nonmedicinal substance allergy status

Z91.09 Other allergy status, other than to drugs and biological substances

Z91.1 Patient's noncompliance with medical treatment and regimen

Z91.11 Patient's noncompliance with dietary regimen

Z91.12 Patient's intentional underdosing of medication regimen

Code first underdosing of medication (T36-T50) with fifth or sixth character 6

Excludes1: adverse effect of prescribed drug taken as directed- code to adverse effect poisoning (overdose) -code to poisoning

Z91.120 Patient's intentional underdosing of medication regimen due to financial hardship

Z91.128 Patient's intentional underdosing of medication regimen for other reason

Z91.13 Patient's unintentional underdosing of medication regimen

Code first underdosing of medication (T36-T50) with fifth or sixth character 6

Excludes1: adverse effect of prescribed drug taken as directed- code to adverse effect poisoning (overdose) -code to poisoning

Z91.130 Patient's unintentional underdosing of medication regimen due to age-related debility

Z91.138 Patient's unintentional underdosing of medication regimen for other reason

Z91.14 Patient's other noncompliance with medication regimen

Patient's underdosing of medication NOS

Z91.15 Patient's noncompliance with renal dialysis

Z91.19 Patient's noncompliance with other medical treatment and regimen

Nonadherence to medical treatment

Z91.4 Personal history of psychological trauma, not elsewhere classified

Z91.41 Personal history of adult abuse

Excludes2: personal history of abuse in childhood (Z62.81-)

Z91.410 Personal history of adult physical and sexual abuse

Excludes1: current adult physical abuse (T74.11, T76.11)

current adult sexual abuse (T74.21, T76.11)

Z91.411 Personal history of adult psychological abuse

Z91.412 Personal history of adult neglect

Excludes1: current adult neglect (T74.01, T76.01)

Z91.419 Personal history of unspecified adult abuse

Z91.49 Other personal history of psychological trauma, not elsewhere classified

Z91.5 Personal history of self-harm

Personal history of parasuicide

Personal history of self-poisoning

Personal history of suicide attempt

Z91.8 **Other specified personal risk factors, not elsewhere classified**

   Z91.81 **History of falling**

      At risk for falling

   Z91.82 **Personal history of military deployment**

      Individual (civilian or military) with past history of military war, peacekeeping and humanitarian deployment (current or past conflict)

      Returned from military deployment

   Z91.83 **Wandering in diseases classified elsewhere**

      <u>Code first</u> underlying disorder such as:

      Alzheimer's disease (G30.-)

      autism or pervasive developmental disorder (F84.-)

      intellectual disabilities (F70-F79)

      unspecified dementia with behavioral disturbance (F03.9-)

   •**Z91.84** **Oral health risk factors**

     •**Z91.841** **Risk for dental caries, low**

     •**Z91.842** **Risk for dental caries, moderate**

     •**Z91.843** **Risk for dental caries, high**

     •**Z91.849** **Unspecified risk for dental caries**

   Z91.89 **Other specified personal risk factors, not elsewhere classified**

Z92 **Personal history of medical treatment**

  Excludes2: postprocedural states (Z98.-)

  Z92.0 **Personal history of contraception**

    Excludes1: counseling or management of current contraceptive practices (Z30.-)

      long term (current) use of contraception (Z79.3)

      presence of (intrauterine) contraceptive device (Z97.5)

  Z92.2 **Personal history of drug therapy**

    Excludes2: long term (current) drug therapy (Z79.-)

   Z92.21 **Personal history of antineoplastic chemotherapy**

   Z92.22 **Personal history of monoclonal drug therapy**

   Z92.23 **Personal history of estrogen therapy**

   Z92.24 **Personal history of steroid therapy**

   Z92.240 **Personal history of inhaled steroid therapy**

   Z92.241 **Personal history of systemic steroid therapy**

      Personal history of steroid therapy NOS

   Z92.25 **Personal history of immunosuppression therapy**

     Excludes2: personal history of steroid therapy (Z92.24)

   Z92.29 **Personal history of other drug therapy**

  Z92.3 **Personal history of irradiation**

    Personal history of exposure to therapeutic radiation

    Excludes1: exposure to radiation in the physical environment (Z77.12)

      occupational exposure to radiation (Z57.1)

  Z92.8 **Personal history of other medical treatment**

   Z92.81 **Personal history of extracorporeal membrane oxygenation (ECMO)**

   Z92.82 **Status post administration of tPA (rtPA) in a different facility within the last 24 hours prior to admission to current facility**

     <u>Code first</u> condition requiring tPA administration, such as:

     acute cerebral infarction (I63.-)

     acute myocardial infarction (I21.-, I22.-)

   Z92.83 **Personal history of failed moderate sedation**

     Personal history of failed conscious sedation

     Excludes2: failed moderate sedation during procedure (T88.52)

   Z92.84 **Personal history of unintended awareness under general anesthesia**

     Excludes2: unintended awareness under general anesthesia during procedure (T88.53)

   Z92.89 **Personal history of other medical treatment**

Z93 **Artificial opening status**

  Excludes1: artificial openings requiring attention or management (Z43.-)

    complications of external stoma (J95.0-, K94.-, N99.5-)

  Z93.0 **Tracheostomy status**

  Z93.1 **Gastrostomy status**

  Z93.2 **Ileostomy status**

  Z93.3 **Colostomy status**

  Z93.4 **Other artificial openings of gastrointestinal tract status**

  Z93.5 **Cystostomy status**

   Z93.50 **Unspecified cystostomy status**

   Z93.51 **Cutaneous-vesicostomy status**

   Z93.52 **Appendico-vesicostomy status**

   Z93.59 **Other cystostomy status**

  Z93.6 **Other artificial openings of urinary tract status**

    Nephrostomy status

    Ureterostomy status

    Urethrostomy status

  Z93.8 **Other artificial opening status**

  Z93.9 **Artificial opening status, unspecified**

Z94 **Transplanted organ and tissue status**

  Includes: organ or tissue replaced by heterogenous or homogenous transplant

  Excludes1: complications of transplanted organ or tissue - see Alphabetical Index

  Excludes2: presence of vascular grafts (Z95.-)

  Z94.0 **Kidney transplant status**

  Z94.1 **Heart transplant status**

    Excludes1: artificial heart status (Z95.812)

      heart-valve replacement status (Z95.2-Z95.4)

  Z94.2 **Lung transplant status**

  Z94.3 **Heart and lungs transplant status**

  Z94.4 **Liver transplant status**

  Z94.5 **Skin transplant status**

    Autogenous skin transplant status

  Z94.6 **Bone transplant status**

  Z94.7 **Corneal transplant status**

  Z94.8 **Other transplanted organ and tissue status**

   Z94.81 **Bone marrow transplant status**

   Z94.82 **Intestine transplant status**

   Z94.83 **Pancreas transplant status**

   Z94.84 **Stem cells transplant status**

   Z94.89 **Other transplanted organ and tissue status**

  Z94.9 **Transplanted organ and tissue status, unspecified**

Z95 **Presence of cardiac and vascular implants and grafts**

  Excludes2: complications of cardiac and vascular devices, implants and grafts (T82.-)

  Z95.0 **Presence of cardiac pacemaker**

Presence of cardiac resynchronization therapy (CRT-P) pacemaker

Excludes1: adjustment or management of cardiac device (Z45.0-)

adjustment or management of cardiac pacemaker (Z45.0)

presence of automatic (implantable) cardiac defibrillator with synchronous cardiac pacemaker (Z95.810)

Z95.1 **Presence of aortocoronary bypass graft**

Presence of coronary artery bypass graft

Z95.2 **Presence of prosthetic heart valve**

Presence of heart valve NOS

Z95.3 **Presence of xenogenic heart valve**

Z95.4 **Presence of other heart-valve replacement**

Z95.5 **Presence of coronary angioplasty implant and graft**

Excludes1: coronary angioplasty status without implant and graft (Z98.61)

Z95.8 **Presence of other cardiac and vascular implants and grafts**

Z95.81 **Presence of other cardiac implants and grafts**

Z95.810 **Presence of automatic (implantable) cardiac defibrillator**

Presence of automatic (implantable) cardiac defibrillator with synchronous cardiac pacemaker

Presence of cardiac resynchronization therapy defibrillator (CRT-D)

Presence of cardioverter-defibrillator (ICD)

Z95.811 **Presence of heart assist device**

Z95.812 **Presence of fully implantable artificial heart**

Z95.818 **Presence of other cardiac implants and grafts**

Z95.82 **Presence of other vascular implants and grafts**

Z95.820 **Peripheral vascular angioplasty status with implants and grafts**

Excludes1: peripheral vascular angioplasty without implant and graft (Z98.62)

Z95.828 **Presence of other vascular implants and grafts**

Presence of intravascular prosthesis NEC

Z95.9 **Presence of cardiac and vascular implant and graft, unspecified**

Z96 **Presence of other functional implants**

Excludes2: complications of internal prosthetic devices, implants and grafts (T82-T85)

fitting and adjustment of prosthetic and other devices (Z44-Z46)

Z96.0 **Presence of urogenital implants**

Z96.1 **Presence of intraocular lens**

Presence of pseudophakia

Z96.2 **Presence of otological and audiological implants**

Z96.20 **Presence of otological and audiological implant, unspecified**

Z96.21 **Cochlear implant status**

Z96.22 **Myringotomy tube(s) status**

Z96.29 **Presence of other otological and audiological implants**

Presence of bone-conduction hearing device

Presence of eustachian tube stent

Stapes replacement

Z96.3 **Presence of artificial larynx**

Z96.4 **Presence of endocrine implants**

Z96.41 **Presence of insulin pump (external) (internal)**

Z96.49 **Presence of other endocrine implants**

Z96.5 **Presence of tooth-root and mandibular implants**

Z96.6 **Presence of orthopedic joint implants**

Z96.60 **Presence of unspecified orthopedic joint implant**

Z96.61 **Presence of artificial shoulder joint**

Z96.611 **Presence of right artificial shoulder joint**

Z96.612 **Presence of left artificial shoulder joint**

Z96.619 **Presence of unspecified artificial shoulder joint**

Z96.62 **Presence of artificial elbow joint**

Z96.621 **Presence of right artificial elbow joint**

Z96.622 **Presence of left artificial elbow joint**

Z96.629 **Presence of unspecified artificial elbow joint**

Z96.63 **Presence of artificial wrist joint**

Z96.631 **Presence of right artificial wrist joint**

Z96.632 **Presence of left artificial wrist joint**

Z96.639 **Presence of unspecified artificial wrist joint**

Z96.64 **Presence of artificial hip joint**

Hip-joint replacement (partial) (total)

Z96.641 **Presence of right artificial hip joint**

Z96.642 **Presence of left artificial hip joint**

Z96.643 **Presence of artificial hip joint, bilateral**

Z96.649 **Presence of unspecified artificial hip joint**

Z96.65 **Presence of artificial knee joint**

Z96.651 **Presence of right artificial knee joint**

Z96.652 **Presence of left artificial knee joint**

Z96.653 **Presence of artificial knee joint, bilateral**

Z96.659 **Presence of unspecified artificial knee joint**

Z96.66 **Presence of artificial ankle joint**

Z96.661 **Presence of right artificial ankle joint**

Z96.662 **Presence of left artificial ankle joint**

Z96.669 **Presence of unspecified artificial ankle joint**

Z96.69 **Presence of other orthopedic joint implants**

Z96.691 **Finger-joint replacement of right hand**

Z96.692 **Finger-joint replacement of left hand**

Z96.693 **Finger-joint replacement, bilateral**

Z96.698 **Presence of other orthopedic joint implants**

Z96.7 **Presence of other bone and tendon implants**

Presence of skull plate

Z96.8 **Presence of other specified functional implants**

Z96.81 **Presence of artificial skin**

Z96.89 **Presence of other specified functional implants**

Z96.9 **Presence of functional implant, unspecified**

Z97 **Presence of other devices**

● New code ▲ Revised code **Excludes1:** Not coded here **Excludes2:** Not included here ⊗ Placeholder required ⑦ 7th digit required

Excludes1: complications of internal prosthetic devices, implants and grafts (T82-T85)

fitting and adjustment of prosthetic **and other** devices (Z44-Z46)

Excludes2: presence of cerebrospinal fluid drainage device (Z98.2)

Z97.0   Presence of artificial eye

Z97.1   Presence of artificial limb (complete) (partial)

    Z97.10   Presence of artificial limb (complete) (partial), unspecified

    Z97.11   Presence of artificial right arm (complete) (partial)

    Z97.12   Presence of artificial left arm (complete) (partial)

    Z97.13   Presence of artificial right leg (complete) (partial)

    Z97.14   Presence of artificial left leg (complete) (partial)

    Z97.15   Presence of artificial arms, bilateral (complete) (partial)

    Z97.16   Presence of artificial legs, bilateral (complete) (partial)

Z97.2   Presence of dental prosthetic device (complete) (partial)

Presence of dentures (complete) (partial)

Z97.3   Presence of spectacles and contact lenses

Z97.4   Presence of external hearing-aid

Z97.5   Presence of (intrauterine) contraceptive device

    Excludes1: checking, reinsertion or removal of implantable subdermal contraceptive (Z30.46)

    checking, reinsertion or removal of intrauterine contraceptive device (Z30.43-)

Z97.8   Presence of other specified devices

Z98   Other postprocedural states

Excludes2: aftercare (Z43-Z49, Z51)

follow-up medical care (Z08-Z09)

postprocedural complication - see Alphabetical Index

Z98.0   Intestinal bypass and anastomosis status

    Excludes2: bariatric surgery status (Z98.84)

    gastric bypass status (Z98.84)

    obesity surgery status (Z98.84)

Z98.1   Arthrodesis status

Z98.2   Presence of cerebrospinal fluid drainage device

Presence of CSF shunt

Z98.3   Post therapeutic collapse of lung status

Code first underlying disease

Z98.4   Cataract extraction status

Use additional code to identify intraocular lens implant status (Z96.1)

Excludes1: aphakia (H27.0)

    Z98.41   Cataract extraction status, right eye

    Z98.42   Cataract extraction status, left eye

    Z98.49   Cataract extraction status, unspecified eye

Z98.5   Sterilization status

    Excludes1: female infertility (N97.-)

    male infertility (N46.-)

    Z98.51   Tubal ligation status

    Z98.52   Vasectomy status

Z98.6   Angioplasty status

    Z98.61   Coronary angioplasty status

    Excludes1: coronary angioplasty status with implant and graft (Z95.5)

    Z98.62   Peripheral vascular angioplasty status

    Excludes1: peripheral vascular angioplasty status with implant and graft (Z95.820)

Z98.8   Other specified postprocedural states

    Z98.81   Dental procedure status

    Z98.810   Dental sealant status

    Z98.811   Dental restoration status

    Dental crown status

    Dental fillings status

    Z98.818   Other dental procedure status

    Z98.82   Breast implant status

    Excludes1: breast implant removal status (Z98.86)

    Z98.83   Filtering (vitreous) bleb after glaucoma surgery status

    Excludes1: Inflammation (infection) of postprocedural bleb (H59.4-)

    Z98.84   Bariatric surgery status

    Gastric banding status

    Gastric bypass status for obesity

    Obesity surgery status

    Excludes1: bariatric surgery status complicating pregnancy, childbirth, or the puerperium (O99.84)

    Excludes2: intestinal bypass and anastomosis status (Z98.0)

    Z98.85   Transplanted organ removal status

    Transplanted organ previously removed due to complication, failure, rejection or infection

    Excludes1: encounter for removal of transplanted organ -code to complication of transplanted organ (T86.-)

    Z98.86   Personal history of breast implant removal

    Z98.87   Personal history of in utero procedure

    Z98.870   Personal history of in utero procedure during pregnancy

    Excludes2: complications from in utero procedure for current pregnancy (O35.7)

    supervision of current pregnancy with history of in utero procedure during previous pregnancy (O09.82-)

    Z98.871   Personal history of in utero procedure while a fetus

    Z98.89   Other specified postprocedural states

    Z98.890   Other specified postprocedural states

    Personal history of surgery, not elsewhere classified

    Z98.891   History of uterine scar from previous surgery

    Excludes1: Maternal care due to uterine scar from previous surgery (O34.2-)

Z99   Dependence on enabling machines and devices, not elsewhere classified

Excludes1: cardiac pacemaker status (Z95.0)

Z99.0   Dependence on aspirator

Z99.1   Dependence on respirator Dependence on ventilator

    Z99.11   Dependence on respirator [ventilator] status

    Z99.12   Encounter for respirator [ventilator] dependence during power failure

---

Excludes1: mechanical complication of respirator
[ventilator] (J95.850)

Z99.2 **Dependence on renal dialysis**
Hemodialysis status
Peritoneal dialysis status
Presence of arteriovenous shunt for dialysis
Renal dialysis status NOS
Excludes1: encounter for fitting and adjustment of dialysis
catheter (Z49.0-)
Excludes2: noncompliance with renal dialysis (Z91.15)

Z99.3 **Dependence on wheelchair**
Wheelchair confinement status
Code first cause of dependence, such as:
muscular dystrophy (G71.0) obesity (E66.-)

Z99.8 **Dependence on other enabling machines and devices**

Z99.81 **Dependence on supplemental oxygen**
Dependence on long-term oxygen

Z99.89 **Dependence on other enabling machines and
devices**
Dependence on machine or device NOS

● New code   ▲ Revised code   **Excludes1:** Not coded here   **Excludes2:** Not included here   ⊗ Placeholder required   ⑦ 7ᵗʰ digit required

Alphabetic Index To Diseases And Injuries

The Alphabetic Index is an alphabetical list of ICD-10-CM terms and their corresponding code that helps determine which section to refer to in the Tabular List. The Alphabetic Index has two parts; the Index to Diseases and Injuries; and the Index to External Causes of Injury. The Alphabetic Index is followed by the Table of Neoplasms and the Table of Drugs and Chemicals. The ICD-10-CM Official Guidelines for Coding and Reporting include important references to the proper use of the Alphabetic Index which are listed below.

LOCATING A CODE IN THE ICD-10-CM

To select a code in the classification that corresponds to a diagnosis or reason for visit documented in a medical record, first locate the term in the Alphabetic Index, and then verify the code in the Tabular List. Read and be guided by instructional notations that appear in both the Alphabetic Index and the Tabular List.

It is essential to use both the Alphabetic Index and Tabular List when locating and assigning a code. The Alphabetic Index does not always provide the full code. Selection of the full code, including laterality and any applicable 7th character can only be done in the Tabular List. A dash (-) at the end of an Alphabetic Index entry indicates that additional characters are required. Even if a dash is not included at the Alphabetic Index entry, it is necessary to refer to the Tabular List to verify that no 7th character is required.

ALPHABETIC INDEX ABBREVIATIONS

NEC "Not elsewhere classifiable"

This abbreviation in the Alphabetic Index represents "other specified." When a specific code is not available for a condition, the Alphabetic Index directs the coder to the "other specified" code in the Tabular List.

NOS "Not otherwise specified"

This abbreviation is the equivalent of unspecified.

PUNCTUATION

[ ]   Brackets are used in the Alphabetic Index to identify manifestation codes.

( )   Parentheses are used in the Alphabetic Index to enclose supplementary words that may be present or absent in the statement of a disease or procedure without affecting the code number to which it is assigned. The terms within the parentheses are referred to as nonessential modifiers. The nonessential modifiers in the Alphabetic Index to Diseases apply to subterms following a main term except when a nonessential modifier and a subentry are mutually exclusive, the subentry takes precedence.

OTHER CODES

Codes titled "other" or "other specified" are for use when the information in the medical record provides detail for which a specific code does not exist. Alphabetic Index entries with NEC in the line designate "other" codes in the Tabular List. These Alphabetic Index entries represent specific disease entities for which no specific code exists so the term is included within an "other" code.

ETIOLOGY/MANIFESTATION CONVENTION

Certain conditions have both an underlying etiology and multiple body system manifestations due to the underlying etiology. For such conditions, the ICD-10-CM has a coding convention that requires the underlying condition be sequenced first, if applicable, followed by the manifestation.

In addition to the notes in the Tabular List, these conditions also have a specific Alphabetic Index entry structure. In the Alphabetic Index both conditions are listed together with the etiology code first followed by the manifestation codes in brackets. The code in brackets is always to be sequenced second.

WITH

The word "with" should be interpreted to mean "associated with" or "due to" when it appears in a code title, the Alphabetic Index, or an instructional note in the Tabular List. The classification presumes a causal relationship between the two conditions linked by these terms in the Alphabetic Index or Tabular List.

SEE AND SEE ALSO

The "see" instruction following a main term in the Alphabetic Index indicates that another term should be referenced. It is necessary to go to the main term referenced with the "see" note to locate the correct code.

A "see also" instruction following a main term in the Alphabetic Index instructs that there is another main term that may also be referenced that may provide additional Alphabetic Index entries that may be useful. It is not necessary to follow the "see also" note when the original main term provides the necessary code.

DEFAULT CODES

A code listed next to a main term in the ICD-10-CM Alphabetic Index is referred to as a default code. The default code represents that condition that is most commonly associated with the main term, or is the unspecified code for the condition. If a condition is documented in a medical record without any additional information, such as acute or chronic, the default code should be assigned.

ACUTE AND CHRONIC CONDITIONS

If the same condition is described as both acute (subacute) and chronic, and separate subentries exist in the Alphabetic Index at the same indentation level, code both and sequence the acute (subacute) code first.

COMBINATION CODE

A combination code is a single code used to classify:

- Two diagnoses, or
- A diagnosis with an associated secondary process (manifestation)
- A diagnosis with an associated complication

Combination codes are identified by referring to subterm entries in the Alphabetic Index and by reading the inclusion and exclusion notes in the Tabular List.

Assign only the combination code when that code fully identifies the diagnostic conditions involved or when the Alphabetic Index so directs.

SYNDROMES

Follow the Alphabetic Index guidance when coding syndromes. In the absence of Alphabetic Index guidance, assign codes for the documented manifestations of the syndrome.

NEOPLASMS

The Table of Neoplasms provides the proper code based on histology of the neoplasm and site. The neoplasm table following the Alphabetic Index should be referenced first. However, if the histological term is documented, that term should be referenced first, rather than going immediately to the Neoplasm Table, in order to determine which column in the Neoplasm Table is appropriate. For example, if the documentation indicates "adenoma," refer to the term in the Alphabetic Index to review the entries under this term and the instructional note to "see also neoplasm, by site, benign." The table provides the proper code based on the type of neoplasm and the site. It is important to select the proper column in the table that corresponds to the type of neoplasm. The Tabular List should then be referenced to verify that the correct code has been selected from the table and that a more specific site code does not exist.

A

Aarskog's syndrome Q87.1
Abandonment - *see* Maltreatment
Abasia (-astasia) (hysterical) F44.4
Abderhalden-kaufmann-lignac syndrome (cystinosis) E72.04
Abdomen, abdominal - *see also* condition
  acute R10.0
  angina K55.1
  muscle deficiency syndrome Q79.4
Abdominalgia - *see* Pain, abdominal
Abduction contracture, hip or other joint - *see* Contraction, joint
Aberrant (congenital) - *see also* Malposition, congenital
  adrenal gland Q89.1
  artery (peripheral) Q27.8
    basilar NEC Q28.1
    cerebral Q28.3
    coronary Q24.5
    digestive system Q27.8
    eye Q15.8
    lower limb Q27.8
    precerebral Q28.1
    pulmonary Q25.79
    renal Q27.2
    retina Q14.1
    specified site NEC Q27.8
    subclavian Q27.8
    upper limb Q27.8
    vertebral Q28.1
  breast Q83.8
  endocrine gland NEC Q89.2
  hepatic duct Q44.5
  pancreas Q45.3
  parathyroid gland Q89.2
  pituitary gland Q89.2
  sebaceous glands, mucous membrane, mouth, congenital Q38.6
  spleen Q89.09
  subclavian artery Q27.8
  thymus (gland) Q89.2
  thyroid gland Q89.2
  vein (peripheral) NEC Q27.8
    cerebral Q28.3
    digestive system Q27.8
    lower limb Q27.8
    precerebral Q28.1
    specified site NEC Q27.8
    upper limb Q27.8
Aberration
  distantial - *see* Disturbance, visual
  mental F99
Abetalipoproteinemia E78.6
Abiotrophy R68.89
Ablatio, ablation
  retinae - *see* Detachment, retina
Ablepharia, ablepharon Q10.3
Abnormal, abnormality, abnormalities - *see also* Anomaly
  acid-base balance (mixed) E87.4
  albumin R77.0
  alphafetoprotein R77.2
  alveolar ridge K08.9
  anatomical relationship Q89.9
  apertures, congenital, diaphragm Q79.1
  auditory perception H93.29-
    diplacusis - *see* Diplacusis
    hyperacusis - *see* Hyperacusis
    recruitment - *see* Recruitment, auditory
    threshold shift - *see* Shift, auditory threshold
  autosomes Q99.9
    fragile site Q95.5
  basal metabolic rate R94.8

Abnormal, abnormality, abnormalities - *continued*
  biosynthesis, testicular androgen E29.1
  bleeding time R79.1
  blood-gas level R79.81
  blood level (of)
    cobalt R79.0
    copper R79.0
    iron R79.0
    lithium R78.89
    magnesium R79.0
    mineral NEC R79.0
    zinc R79.0
  blood pressure
    elevated R03.0
    low reading (nonspecific) R03.1
  blood sugar R73.09
  bowel sounds R19.15
    absent R19.11
    hyperactive R19.12
  brain scan R94.02
  breathing R06.9
  caloric test R94.138
  cerebrospinal fluid R83.9
    cytology R83.6
    drug level R83.2
    enzyme level R83.0
    hormones R83.1
    immunology R83.4
    microbiology R83.5
    nonmedicinal level R83.3
    specified type NEC R83.8
  chemistry, blood R79.9
    C-reactive protein R79.82
    drugs - *see* Findings, abnormal, in blood
    gas level R79.81
    minerals R79.0
    pancytopenia D61.818
    PTT R79.1
    specified NEC R79.89
    toxins - *see* Findings, abnormal, in blood
  chest sounds (friction) (rales) R09.89
  chromosome, chromosomal Q99.9
    with more than three X chromosomes, female Q97.1
    analysis result R89.8
      bronchial washings R84.8
      cerebrospinal fluid R83.8
      cervix uteri NEC R87.89
      nasal secretions R84.8
      nipple discharge R89.8
      peritoneal fluid R85.89
      pleural fluid R84.8
      prostatic secretions R86.8
      saliva R85.89
      seminal fluid R86.8
      sputum R84.8
      synovial fluid R89.8
      throat scrapings R84.8
      vagina R87.89
      vulva R87.89
      wound secretions R89.8
    dicentric replacement Q93.2
    ring replacement Q93.2
    sex Q99.8
      female phenotype Q97.9
        specified NEC Q97.8
      male phenotype Q98.9
        specified NEC Q98.8
      structural male Q98.6
    specified NEC Q99.8
  clinical findings NEC R68.89
  coagulation D68.9
    newborn, transient P61.6

Abnormal, abnormality, abnormalities - *continued*
    profile R79.1
    time R79.1
  communication - *see* Fistula
  conjunctiva, vascular H11.41-
  coronary artery Q24.5
  cortisol-binding globulin E27.8
  course, eustachian tube Q17.8
  creatinine clearance R94.4
  cytology
    anus R85.619
      atypical squamous cells cannot exclude high grade squamous intraepithelial lesion (ASC-h) R85.611
      atypical squamous cells of undetermined significance (ASC-US) R85.610
      cytologic evidence of malignancy R85.614
      high grade squamous intraepithelial lesion (HGSIL) R85.613
      human papillomavirus (HPV) DNA test high risk positive R85.81
      low risk positive R85.82
      inadequate smear R85.615
      low grade squamous intraepithelial lesion (LGSIL) R85.612
      satisfactory anal smear but lacking transformation zone R85.616
      specified NEC R85.618
      unsatisfactory smear R85.615
    female genital organs - *see* Abnormal, Papanicolaou (smear)
  dark adaptation curve H53.61
  dentofacial NEC - *see* Anomaly, dentofacial
  development, developmental Q89.9
    central nervous system Q07.9
  diagnostic imaging
    abdomen, abdominal region NEC R93.5
    biliary tract R93.2
    bladder R93.41
    breast R92.8
    central nervous system NEC R90.89
    cerebrovascular NEC R90.89
    coronary circulation R93.1
    digestive tract NEC R93.3
    gastrointestinal (tract) R93.3
    genitourinary organs R93.8
    head R93.0
    heart R93.1
    intrathoracic organ NEC R93.8
    kidney R93.42-
    limbs R93.6
    liver R93.2
    lung (field) R91.8
    musculoskeletal system NEC R93.7
    renal pelvis R93.41
    retroperitoneum R93.5
    site specified NEC R93.8
    skin and subcutaneous tissue R93.8
    skull R93.0
    urinary organs specified NEC R93.49
    ureter R93.41
  direction, teeth, fully erupted M26.30
  ear ossicles, acquired NEC H74.39
    ankylosis - *see* Ankylosis, ear ossicles
    discontinuity - *see* Discontinuity, ossicles, ear
    partial loss - *see* Loss, ossicles, ear (partial)
  Ebstein Q22.5
  echocardiogram R93.1
  echoencephalogram R90.81
  echogram - *see* Abnormal, diagnostic imaging
  electrocardiogram [ECG] [EKG] R94.31
  electroencephalogram [EEG] R94.01

Abnormal, abnormality, abnormalities - *continued*

electrolyte - *see* Imbalance, electrolyte
electromyogram [EMG] R94.131
electro-oculogram [EOG] R94.110
electrophysiological intracardiac studies R94.39
electroretinogram [ERG] R94.111
erythrocytes
  congenital, with perinatal jaundice D58.9
feces (color) (contents) (mucus) R19.5
finding - *see* Findings, abnormal, without diagnosis
fluid
  amniotic - *see* Abnormal, specimen, specified
  cerebrospinal - *see* Abnormal, cerebrospinal fluid
  peritoneal - *see* Abnormal, specimen, digestive organs
  pleural - *see* Abnormal, specimen, respiratory organs
  synovial - *see* Abnormal, specimen, specified
  thorax (bronchial washings) (pleural fluid) - *see* Abnormal, specimen, respiratory organs
  vaginal - *see* Abnormal, specimen, female genital organs
form
  teeth K00.2
  uterus - *see* Anomaly, uterus
function studies
  auditory R94.120
  bladder R94.8
  brain R94.09
  cardiovascular R94.30
  ear R94.128
  endocrine NEC R94.7
  eye NEC R94.118
  kidney R94.4
  liver R94.5
  nervous system
    central NEC R94.09
    peripheral NEC R94.138
  pancreas R94.8
  placenta R94.8
  pulmonary R94.2
  special senses NEC R94.128
  spleen R94.8
  thyroid R94.6
  vestibular R94.121
gait - *see* Gait
  hysterical F44.4
gastrin secretion E16.4
globulin R77.1
  cortisol-binding E27.8
  thyroid-binding E07.89
glomerular, minor - *see also* N00-N07 with fourth character .0 N05.0
glucagon secretion E16.3
glucose tolerance (test) (non-fasting) R73.09
gravitational (G) forces or states (effect of) T75.81
hair (color) (shaft) L67.9
  specified NEC L67.8
hard tissue formation in pulp (dental) K04.3
head movement R25.0
heart
  rate R00.9
    specified NEC R00.8
  shadow R93.1
  sounds NEC R01.2
hemoglobin (disease) - *see also* Disease, hemoglobin D58.2
  trait - *see* Trait, hemoglobin, abnormal
histology NEC R89.7

Abnormal, abnormality, abnormalities - *continued*

immunological findings R89.4
  in serum R76.9
    specified NEC R76.8
increase in appetite R63.2
involuntary movement - *see* Abnormal, movement, involuntary
jaw closure M26.51
karyotype R89.8
kidney function test R94.4
knee jerk R29.2
leukocyte (cell) (differential) NEC D72.9
liver function test R94.5
loss of
  height R29.890
  weight R63.4
mammogram NEC R92.8
  calcification (calculus) R92.1
  microcalcification R92.0
Mantoux test R76.11
movement (disorder) - *see also* Disorder, movement
  head R25.0
  involuntary R25.9
    fasciculation R25.3
    of head R25.0
    spasm R25.2
    specified type NEC R25.8
    tremor R25.1
myoglobin (Aberdeen) (Annapolis) R89.7
neonatal screening P09
oculomotor study R94.113
palmar creases Q82.8
Papanicolaou (smear)
  anus R85.619
    atypical squamous cells cannot exclude high grade squamous intraepithelial lesion (ASC-h) R85.611
    atypical squamous cells of undetermined significance (ASC-US) R85.610
    cytologic evidence of malignancy R85.614
    high grade squamous intraepithelial lesion (HGSIL) R85.613
    human papillomavirus (HPV) DNA test
      high risk positive R85.81
      low risk positive R85.82
    inadequate smear R85.615
    low grade squamous intraepithelial lesion (LGSIL) R85.612
    satisfactory anal smear but lacking transformation zone R85.616
    specified NEC R85.618
    unsatisfactory smear R85.615
  bronchial washings R84.6
  cerebrospinal fluid R83.6
  cervix R87.619
    atypical squamous cells cannot exclude high grade squamous intraepithelial lesion (ASC-h) R87.611
    atypical squamous cells of undetermined significance (ASC-US) R87.610
    cytologic evidence of malignancy R87.614
    high grade squamous intraepithelial lesion (HGSIL) R87.613
    inadequate smear R87.615
    low grade squamous intraepithelial lesion (LGSIL) R87.612
    non-atypical endometrial cells R87.618
    satisfactory cervical smear but lacking transformation zone R87.616
    specified NEC R87.618
    thin preparation R87.619
    unsatisfactory smear R87.615

Abnormal, abnormality, abnormalities - *continued*

nasal secretions R84.6
nipple discharge R89.6
peritoneal fluid R85.69
pleural fluid R84.6
prostatic secretions R86.6
saliva R85.69
seminal fluid R86.6
sites NEC R89.6
sputum R84.6
synovial fluid R89.6
throat scrapings R84.6
vagina R87.629
  atypical squamous cells cannot exclude high grade squamous intraepithelial lesion (ASC-h) R87.621
  atypical squamous cells of undetermined significance (ASC-US) R87.620
  cytologic evidence of malignancy R87.624
  high grade squamous intraepithelial lesion (HGSIL) R87.623
  inadequate smear R87.625
  low grade squamous intraepithelial lesion (LGSIL) R87.622
  specified NEC R87.628
  thin preparation R87.629
  unsatisfactory smear R87.625
vulva R87.69
wound secretions R89.6
partial thromboplastin time (PTT) R79.1
pelvis (bony) - *see* Deformity, pelvis
percussion, chest (tympany) R09.89
periods (grossly) - *see* Menstruation
phonocardiogram R94.39
plantar reflex R29.2
plasma
  protein R77.9
    specified NEC R77.8
  viscosity R70.1
pleural (folds) Q34.0
posture R29.3
product of conception O02.9
  specified type NEC O02.89
prothrombin time (PT) R79.1
pulmonary
  artery, congenital Q25.79
  function, newborn P28.89
  test results R94.2
pulsations in neck R00.2
pupillary H21.56-
  function (reaction) (reflex) - *see* Anomaly, pupil, function
radiological examination - *see* Abnormal, diagnostic imaging
red blood cell(s) (morphology) (volume) R71.8
reflex - *see* Reflex
renal function test R94.4
response to nerve stimulation R94.130
retinal correspondence H53.31
retinal function study R94.111
rhythm, heart - *see also* Arrhythmia
saliva - *see* Abnormal, specimen, digestive organs
scan
  kidney R94.4
  liver R93.2
  thyroid R94.6
secretion
  gastrin E16.4
  glucagon E16.3

Abnormal, abnormality, abnormalities -
continued
serum level (of)
  acid phosphatase R74.8
  alkaline phosphatase R74.8
  amylase R74.8
  enzymes R74.9
    specified NEC R74.8
  lipase R74.8
  triacylglycerol lipase R74.8
shape
  gravid uterus - *see* Anomaly, uterus
sinus venosus Q21.1
size, tooth, teeth K00.2
spacing, tooth, teeth, fully erupted M26.30
specimen
  digestive organs (peritoneal fluid) (saliva) R85.9
    cytology R85.69
    drug level R85.2
    enzyme level R85.0
    histology R85.7
    hormones R85.1
    immunology R85.4
    microbiology R85.5
    nonmedicinal level R85.3
    specified type NEC R85.89
  female genital organs (secretions) (smears) R87.9
    cytology R87.69
      cervix R87.619
        human papillomavirus (HPV) DNA test
          high risk positive R87.810
          low risk positive R87.820
        inadequate (unsatisfactory) smear R87.615
        non-atypical endometrial cells R87.618
        specified NEC R87.618
      vagina R87.629
        human papillomavirus (HPV) DNA test
          high risk positive R87.811
          low risk positive R87.821
        inadequate (unsatisfactory) smear R87.625
      vulva R87.69
    drug level R87.2
    enzyme level R87.0
    histological R87.7
    hormones R87.1
    immunology R87.4
    microbiology R87.5
    nonmedicinal level R87.3
    specified type NEC R87.89
  male genital organs (prostatic secretions) (semen) R86.9
    cytology R86.6
    drug level R86.2
    enzyme level R86.0
    histological R86.7
    hormones R86.1
    immunology R86.4
    microbiology R86.5
    nonmedicinal level R86.3
    specified type NEC R86.8
  nipple discharge - *see* Abnormal, specimen, specified
  respiratory organs (bronchial washings) (nasal secretions) (pleural fluid) (sputum) R84.9
    cytology R84.6
    drug level R84.2
    enzyme level R84.0
    histology R84.7
    hormones R84.1

Abnormal, abnormality, abnormalities -
continued
    immunology R84.4
    microbiology R84.5
    nonmedicinal level R84.3
    specified type NEC R84.8
  specified organ, system and tissue NOS R89.9
    cytology R89.6
    drug level R89.2
    enzyme level R89.0
    histology R89.7
    hormones R89.1
    immunology R89.4
    microbiology R89.5
    nonmedicinal level R89.3
    specified type NEC R89.8
  synovial fluid - *see* Abnormal, specimen, specified
  thorax (bronchial washings) (pleural fluids) - *see* Abnormal, specimen, respiratory organs
  vagina (secretion) (smear) R87.629
  vulva (secretion) (smear) R87.69
  wound secretion - *see* Abnormal, specimen, specified
spermatozoa - *see* Abnormal, specimen, male genital organs
sputum (amount) (color) (odor) R09.3
stool (color) (contents) (mucus) R19.5
  bloody K92.1
  guaiac positive R19.5
synchondrosis Q78.8
thermography - *see also* Abnormal, diagnostic imaging R93.8
thyroid-binding globulin E07.89
tooth, teeth (form) (size) K00.2
toxicology (findings) R78.9
transport protein E88.09
tumor marker NEC R97.8
ultrasound results - *see* Abnormal, diagnostic imaging
umbilical cord complicating delivery O69.9
urination NEC R39.198
urine (constituents) R82.90
  bile R82.2
  cytological examination R82.8
  drugs R82.5
  fat R82.0
  glucose R81
  heavy metals R82.6
  hemoglobin R82.3
  histological examination R82.8
  ketones R82.4
  microbiological examination (culture) R82.79
  myoglobin R82.1
  positive culture R82.79
  protein - *see* Proteinuria
  specified substance NEC R82.99
    chromoabnormality NEC R82.91
  substances nonmedical R82.6
uterine hemorrhage - *see* Hemorrhage, uterus
vectorcardiogram R94.39
visually evoked potential (VEP) R94.112
white blood cells D72.9
  specified NEC D72.89
X-ray examination - *see* Abnormal, diagnostic imaging
Abnormity (any organ or part) - *see* Anomaly
Abocclusion M26.29
hemolytic disease (newborn) P55.1
incompatibility reaction ABO - *see*
Complication(s), transfusion, incompatibility reaction, ABO

Abolition, language R48.8
Aborter, habitual or recurrent - *see* Loss (of), pregnancy, recurrent
Abortion (complete) (spontaneous) O03.9
with
  retained products of conception - *see* Abortion, incomplete
attempted (elective) (failed) O07.4
  complicated by O07.30
    afibrinogenemia O07.1
    cardiac arrest O07.36
    chemical damage of pelvic organ(s) O07.34
    circulatory collapse O07.31
    cystitis O07.38
    defibrination syndrome O07.1
    electrolyte imbalance O07.33
    embolism (air) (amniotic fluid) (blood clot) (fat) (pulmonary) (septic) (soap) O07.2
    endometritis O07.0
    genital tract and pelvic infection O07.0
    hemolysis O07.1
    hemorrhage (delayed) (excessive) O07.1
    infection
      genital tract or pelvic O07.0
      urinary tract O07.38
    intravascular coagulation O07.1
    laceration of pelvic organ(s) O07.34
    metabolic disorder O07.33
    oliguria O07.32
    oophoritis O07.0
    parametritis O07.0
    pelvic peritonitis O07.0
    perforation of pelvic organ(s) O07.34
    renal failure or shutdown O07.32
    salpingitis or salpingo-oophoritis O07.0
    sepsis O07.37
    shock O07.31
    specified condition NEC O07.39
    tubular necrosis (renal) O07.32
    uremia O07.32
    urinary tract infection O07.38
    venous complication NEC O07.35
      embolism (air) (amniotic fluid) (blood clot) (fat) (pulmonary) (septic) (soap) O07.2
complicated (by) (following) O03.80
  afibrinogenemia O03.6
  cardiac arrest O03.86
  chemical damage of pelvic organ(s) O03.84
  circulatory collapse O03.81
  cystitis O03.88
  defibrination syndrome O03.6
  electrolyte imbalance O03.83
  embolism (air) (amniotic fluid) (blood clot) (fat) (pulmonary) (septic) (soap) O03.7
  endometritis O03.5
  genital tract and pelvic infection O03.5
  hemolysis O03.6
  hemorrhage (delayed) (excessive) O03.6
  infection
    genital tract or pelvic O03.5
    urinary tract O03.88
  intravascular coagulation O03.6
  laceration of pelvic organ(s) O03.84
  metabolic disorder O03.83
  oliguria O03.82
  oophoritis O03.5
  parametritis O03.5
  pelvic peritonitis O03.5
  perforation of pelvic organ(s) O03.84
  renal failure or shutdown O03.82
  salpingitis or salpingo-oophoritis O03.5
  sepsis O03.87
  shock O03.81
  specified condition NEC O03.89

Abortion (complete) (spontaneous) -
continued
  tubular necrosis (renal) O03.82
  uremia O03.82
  urinary tract infection O03.88
  venous complication NEC O03.85
    embolism (air) (amniotic fluid) (blood clot)
      (fat) (pulmonary) (septic) (soap) O03.7
  failed - *see* Abortion, attempted
  habitual or recurrent N96
    with current abortion - *see* categories O03-
      o04
    without current pregnancy N96
    care in current pregnancy O26.2-
  incomplete (spontaneous) O03.4
  complicated (by) (following) O03.30
    afibrinogenemia O03.1
    cardiac arrest O03.36
    chemical damage of pelvic organ(s) O03.34
    circulatory collapse O03.31
    cystitis O03.38
    defibrination syndrome O03.1
    electrolyte imbalance O03.33
    embolism (air) (amniotic fluid) (blood clot)
      (fat) (pulmonary) (septic) (soap) O03.2
    endometritis O03.0
    genital tract and pelvic infection O03.0
    hemolysis O03.1
    hemorrhage (delayed) (excessive) O03.1
    infection
      genital tract or pelvic O03.0
      urinary tract O03.38
    intravascular coagulation O03.1
    laceration of pelvic organ(s) O03.34
    metabolic disorder O03.33
    oliguria O03.32
    oophoritis O03.0
    parametritis O03.0
    pelvic peritonitis O03.0
    perforation of pelvic organ(s) O03.34
    renal failure or shutdown O03.32
    salpingitis or salpingo-oophoritis O03.0
    sepsis O03.37
    shock O03.31
    specified condition NEC O03.39
    tubular necrosis (renal) O03.32
    uremia O03.32
    urinary infection O03.38
    venous complication NEC O03.35
      embolism (air) (amniotic fluid) (blood
      clot) (fat) (pulmonary) (septic) (soap)
      O03.2
  induced (encounter for) Z33.2
  complicated by O04.80
    afibrinogenemia O04.6
    cardiac arrest O04.86
    chemical damage of pelvic organ(s) O04.84
    circulatory collapse O04.81
    cystitis O04.88
    defibrination syndrome O04.6
    electrolyte imbalance O04.83
    embolism (air) (amniotic fluid) (blood clot)
      (fat) (pulmonary) (septic) (soap) O04.7
    endometritis O04.5
    genital tract and pelvic infection O04.5
    hemolysis O04.6
    hemorrhage (delayed) (excessive) O04.6
    infection
      genital tract or pelvic O04.5
      urinary tract O04.88
    intravascular coagulation O04.6
    laceration of pelvic organ(s) O04.84
    metabolic disorder O04.83
    oliguria O04.82

Abortion (complete) (spontaneous) -
continued
    oophoritis O04.5
    parametritis O04.5
    pelvic peritonitis O04.5
    perforation of pelvic organ(s) O04.84
    renal failure or shutdown O04.82
    salpingitis or salpingo-oophoritis O04.5
    sepsis O04.87
    shock O04.81
    specified condition NEC O04.89
    tubular necrosis (renal) O04.82
    uremia O04.82
    urinary tract infection O04.88
    venous complication NEC O04.85
      embolism (air) (amniotic fluid) (blood
      clot) (fat) (pulmonary) (septic) (soap)
      O04.7
  missed O02.1
  spontaneous - *see* Abortion (complete)
  (spontaneous)
    threatened O20.0
  threatened (spontaneous) O20.0
  tubal O00.10-
    with intrauterine pregnancy O00.11-
Abortus fever A23.1
Aboulomania F60.7
Abrami's disease D59.8
Abramov-Fiedler myocarditis (acute isolated
  myocarditis) I40.1
Abrasion T14.8
  abdomen, abdominal (wall) S30.811
  alveolar process S00.512
  ankle S90.51-
  antecubital space - *see* Abrasion, elbow
  anus S30.817
  arm (upper) S40.81-
  auditory canal - *see* Abrasion, ear
  auricle - *see* Abrasion, ear
  axilla - *see* Abrasion, arm
  back, lower S30.810
  breast S20.11-
  brow S00.81
  buttock S30.810
  calf - *see* Abrasion, leg
  canthus - *see* Abrasion, eyelid
  cheek S00.81
    internal S00.512
  chest wall - *see* Abrasion, thorax
  chin S00.81
  clitoris S30.814
  cornea S05.0-
  costal region - *see* Abrasion, thorax
  dental K03.1
  digit(s)
    foot - *see* Abrasion, toe
    hand - *see* Abrasion, finger
  ear S00.41-
  elbow S50.31-
  epididymis S30.813
  epigastric region S30.811
  epiglottis S10.11
  esophagus (thoracic) S27.818
    cervical S10.11
  eyebrow - *see* Abrasion, eyelid
  eyelid S00.21-
  face S00.81
  finger(s) S60.41-
    index S60.41-
    little S60.41-
    middle S60.41-
    ring S60.41-
  flank S30.811
  foot (except toe(s) alone) S90.81-

Abrasion - *continued*
  toe - *see* Abrasion, toe
  forearm S50.81-
    elbow only - *see* Abrasion, elbow
  forehead S00.81
  genital organs, external
    female S30.816
    male S30.815
  groin S30.811
  gum S00.512
  hand S60.51-
  head S00.91
    ear - *see* Abrasion, ear
    eyelid - *see* Abrasion, eyelid
    lip S00.511
    nose S00.31
    oral cavity S00.512
    scalp S00.01
    specified site NEC S00.81
  heel - *see* Abrasion, foot
  hip S70.21-
  inguinal region S30.811
  interscapular region S20.419
  jaw S00.81
  knee S80.21-
  labium (majus) (minus) S30.814
  larynx S10.11
  leg (lower) S80.81-
    knee - *see* Abrasion, knee
    upper - *see* Abrasion, thigh
  lip S00.511
  lower back S30.810
  lumbar region S30.810
  malar region S00.81
  mammary - *see* Abrasion, breast
  mastoid region S00.81
  mouth S00.512
  nail
    finger - *see* Abrasion, finger
    toe - *see* Abrasion, toe
  nape S10.81
  nasal S00.31
  neck S10.91
    specified site NEC S10.81
    throat S10.11
  nose S00.31
  occipital region S00.01
  oral cavity S00.512
  orbital region - *see* Abrasion, eyelid
  palate S00.512
  palm - *see* Abrasion, hand
  parietal region S00.01
  pelvis S30.810
  penis S30.812
  perineum
    female S30.814
    male S30.810
  periocular area - *see* Abrasion, eyelid
  phalanges
    finger - *see* Abrasion, finger
    toe - *see* Abrasion, toe
  pharynx S10.11
  pinna - *see* Abrasion, ear
  popliteal space - *see* Abrasion, knee
  prepuce S30.812
  pubic region S30.810
  pudendum
    female S30.816
    male S30.815
  sacral region S30.810
  scalp S00.01
  scapular region - *see* Abrasion, shoulder
  scrotum S30.813
  shin - *see* Abrasion, leg

Abrasion - *continued*
shoulder S40.21-
skin NEC T14.8
sternal region S20.319
submaxillary region S00.81
submental region S00.81
subungual
finger(s) - *see* Abrasion, finger
toe(s) - *see* Abrasion, toe
supraclavicular fossa S10.81
supraorbital S00.81
temple S00.81
temporal region S00.81
testis S30.813
thigh S70.31-
thorax, thoracic (wall) S20.91
back S20.41-
front S20.31-
throat S10.11
thumb S60.31
toe(s) (lesser) S90.416
great S90.41-
tongue S00.512
tooth, teeth (dentifrice) (habitual) (hard
tissues) (occupational) (ritual) (traditional)
K03.1
trachea S10.11
tunica vaginalis S30.813
tympanum, tympanic membrane - *see*
Abrasion, ear
uvula S00.512
vagina S30.814
vocal cords S10.11
vulva S30.814
wrist S60.81-
Abrism - *see* Poisoning, food, noxious, plant
Abruptio placentae O45.9-
with
afibrinogenemia O45.01-
coagulation defect O45.00-
specified NEC O45.09-
disseminated intravascular coagulation
O45.02-
hypofibrinogenemia O45.01-
specified NEC O45.8-
Abruption, placenta - *see* Abruptio placentae
Abscess (connective tissue) (embolic)
(fistulous) (infective) (metastatic) (multiple)
(pernicious) (pyogenic) (septic) L02.91
with
diverticular disease (intestine) K57.80
with bleeding K57.81
large intestine K57.20
with
bleeding K57.21
small intestine K57.40
with bleeding K57.41
small intestine K57.00
with
bleeding K57.01
large intestine K57.40
with bleeding K57.41
lymphangitis
code by site under Abscess
abdomen, abdominal
cavity K65.1
wall L02.211
abdominopelvic K65.1
accessory sinus - *see* Sinusitis
adrenal (capsule) (gland) E27.8
alveolar K04.7
with sinus K04.6
amebic A06.4
brain (and liver or lung abscess) A06.6

Abscess - *continued*
genitourinary tract A06.82
liver (without mention of brain or lung
abscess) A06.4
lung (and liver) (without mention of brain
abscess) A06.5
specified site NEC A06.89
spleen A06.89
anaerobic A48.0
ankle - *see* Abscess, lower limb
anorectal K61.2
antecubital space - *see* Abscess, upper limb
antrum (chronic) (Highmore) - *see* Sinusitis,
maxillary
anus K61.0
apical (tooth) K04.7
with sinus (alveolar) K04.6
appendix K35.3
areola (acute) (chronic) (nonpuerperal) N61.1
puerperal, postpartum or gestational - *see*
Infection, nipple
arm (any part) - *see* Abscess, upper limb
artery (wall) I77.89
atheromatous I77.2
auricle, ear - *see* Abscess, ear, external
axilla (region) L02.41-
lymph gland or node L04.2
back (any part, except buttock) L02.212
Bartholin's gland N75.1
with
abortion - *see* Abortion, by type
complicated by, sepsis
ectopic or molar pregnancy O08.0
following ectopic or molar pregnancy O08.0
Bezold's - *see* Mastoiditis, acute
bilharziasis B65.1
bladder (wall) - *see* Cystitis, specified type
NEC
bone (subperiosteal) - *see also* Osteomyelitis,
specified type NEC
accessory sinus (chronic) - *see* Sinusitis
chronic or old - *see* Osteomyelitis, chronic
jaw (lower) (upper) M27.2
mastoid - *see* Mastoiditis, acute,
subperiosteal
petrous - *see* Petrositis
spinal (tuberculous) A18.01
nontuberculous - *see* Osteomyelitis,
vertebra
bowel K63.0
brain (any part) (cystic) (otogenic) G06.0
amebic (with abscess of any other site) A06.6
gonococcal A54.82
pheomycotic (chromomycotic) B43.1
tuberculous A17.81
breast (acute) (chronic) (nonpuerperal) N61.1
newborn P39.0
puerperal, postpartum, gestational - *see*
Mastitis, obstetric, purulent
broad ligament N73.2
acute N73.0
chronic N73.1
Brodie's (localized) (chronic) M86.8X-
bronchi J98.09
buccal cavity K12.2
bulbourethral gland N34.0
bursa M71.00
ankle M71.07-
elbow M71.02-
foot M71.07-
hand M71.04-
hip M71.05-
knee M71.06-
multiple sites M71.09

Abscess - *continued*
pharyngeal J39.1
shoulder M71.01-
specified site NEC M71.08
wrist M71.03-
buttock L02.31
canthus - *see* Blepharoconjunctivitis
cartilage - *see* Disorder, cartilage, specified
type NEC
cecum K35.3
cerebellum, cerebellar G06.0
sequelae G09
cerebral (embolic) G06.0
sequelae G09
cervical (meaning neck) L02.11
lymph gland or node L04.0
cervix (stump) (uteri) - *see* Cervicitis
cheek (external) L02.01
inner K12.2
chest J86.9
with fistula J86.0
wall L02.213
chin L02.01
choroid - *see* Inflammation, chorioretinal
circumtonsillar J36
cold (lung) (tuberculous) - *see also*
Tuberculosis, abscess, lung
articular - *see* Tuberculosis, joint
colon (wall) K63.0
colostomy K94.02
conjunctiva - *see* Conjunctivitis, acute
cornea H16.31-
corpus
cavernosum N48.21
luteum - *see* Oophoritis
Cowper's gland N34.0
cranium G06.0
cul-de-sac (Douglas') (posterior) - *see*
Peritonitis, pelvic, female
cutaneous - *see* Abscess, by site
dental K04.7
with sinus (alveolar) K04.6
dentoalveolar K04.7
with sinus K04.6
diaphragm, diaphragmatic K65.1
Douglas' cul-de-sac or pouch - *see* Peritonitis,
pelvic, female
Dubois A50.59
ear (middle) - *see also* Otitis, media,
suppurative
acute - *see* Otitis, media, suppurative, acute
external H60.0-
entamebic - *see* Abscess, amebic
enterostomy K94.12
epididymis N45.4
epidural G06.2
brain G06.0
spinal cord G06.1
epiglottis J38.7
epiploon, epiploic K65.1
erysipelatous - *see* Erysipelas
esophagus K20.8
ethmoid (bone) (chronic) (sinus) J32.2
external auditory canal - *see* Abscess, ear,
external
extradural G06.2
brain G06.0
sequelae G09
spinal cord G06.1
extraperitoneal K68.19
eye - *see* Endophthalmitis, purulent
eyelid H00.03-
face (any part, except ear, eye and nose)
L02.01

Abscess - *continued*
fallopian tube - *see* Salpingitis
fascia M72.8
fauces J39.1
fecal K63.0
femoral (region) - *see* Abscess, lower limb
filaria, filarial - *see* Infestation, filarial
finger (any) - *see also* Abscess, hand
  nail - *see* Cellulitis, finger
foot L02.61-
forehead L02.01
frontal sinus (chronic) J32.1
gallbladder K81.0
genital organ or tract
  female (external) N76.4
  male N49.9
    multiple sites N49.8
    specified NEC N49.8
gestational mammary O91.11-
gestational subareolar O91.11-
gingival - *see* Periodontitis, aggressive,
  localized
gland, glandular (lymph) (acute) - *see*
  Lymphadenitis, acute
gluteal (region) L02.31
gonorrheal - *see* Gonococcus
groin L02.214
gum - *see* Periodontitis, aggressive, localized
hand L02.51-
head NEC L02.811
  face (any part, except ear, eye and nose)
  L02.01
heart - *see* Carditis
heel - *see* Abscess, foot
helminthic - *see* Infestation, helminth
hepatic (cholangitic) (hematogenic)
  (lymphogenic) (pylephlebitic) K75.0
  amebic A06.4
hip (region) - *see* Abscess, lower limb
ileocecal K35.3
ileostomy (bud) K94.12
iliac (region) L02.214
  fossa K35.3
infraclavicular (fossa) - *see* Abscess, upper
  limb
inguinal (region) L02.214
  lymph gland or node L04.1
intestine, intestinal NEC K63.0
  rectal K61.1
intra-abdominal - *see also* Abscess,
  peritoneum K65.1
  postprocedural T81.4
  retroperitoneal K68.11
intracranial G06.0
intramammary - *see* Abscess, breast
intraorbital - *see* Abscess, orbit
intraperitoneal K65.1
intrasphincteric (anus) K61.4
intraspinal G06.1
intratonsillar J36
ischiorectal (fossa) K61.3
jaw (bone) (lower) (upper) M27.2
joint - *see* Arthritis, pyogenic or pyemic
  spine (tuberculous) A18.01
    nontuberculous - *see* Spondylopathy,
    infective
kidney N15.1
  with calculus N20.0
    with hydronephrosis N13.6
  puerperal (postpartum) O86.21
knee - *see also* Abscess, lower limb
  joint M00.9
labium (majus) (minus) N76.4

Abscess - *continued*
lacrimal
  caruncle - *see* Inflammation, lacrimal,
  passages, acute
  gland - *see* Dacryoadenitis
  passages (duct) (sac) - *see* Inflammation,
  lacrimal, passages, acute
lacunar N34.0
larynx J38.7
lateral (alveolar) K04.7
  with sinus K04.6
leg (any part) - *see* Abscess, lower limb
lens H27.8
lingual K14.0
  tonsil J36
lip K13.0
Littre's gland N34.0
liver (cholangitic) (hematogenic)
(lymphogenic) (pylephlebitic) (pyogenic)
K75.0
  amebic (due to Entamoeba histolytica)
  (dysenteric) (tropical) A06.4
    with
      brain abscess (and liver or lung abscess)
      A06.6
      lung abscess A06.5
loin (region) L02.211
lower limb L02.41-
lumbar (tuberculous) A18.01
  nontuberculous L02.212
lung (miliary) (putrid) J85.2
  with pneumonia J85.1
    due to specified organism (see Pneumonia,
    in (due to))
  amebic (with liver abscess) A06.5
    with
      brain abscess A06.6
      pneumonia A06.5
lymph, lymphatic, gland or node (acute) - *see*
  also Lymphadenitis, acute
  mesentery I88.0
malar M27.2
mammary gland - *see* Abscess, breast
marginal, anus K61.0
mastoid - *see* Mastoiditis, acute
maxilla, maxillary M27.2
  molar (tooth) K04.7
    with sinus K04.6
  premolar K04.7
  sinus (chronic) J32.0
mediastinum J85.3
meibomian gland - *see* Hordeolum
meninges G06.2
mesentery, mesenteric K65.1
mesosalpinx - *see* Salpingitis
mons pubis L02.215
mouth (floor) K12.2
muscle - *see* Myositis, infective
myocardium I40.0
nabothian (follicle) - *see* Cervicitis
nasal J32.9
nasopharyngeal J39.1
navel L02.216
  newborn P38.9
    with mild hemorrhage P38.1
    without hemorrhage P38.9
neck (region) L02.11
  lymph gland or node L04.0
nephritic - *see* Abscess, kidney   nipple N61.1
  associated with
    lactation - *see* Pregnancy, complicated by
    pregnancy - *see* Pregnancy, complicated by

Abscess - *continued*
nose (external) (fossa) (septum) J34.0
  sinus (chronic) - *see* Sinusitis
omentum K65.1
operative wound T81.4
orbit, orbital - *see* Cellulitis, orbit
otogenic G06.0
ovary, ovarian (corpus luteum) - *see*
  Oophoritis
oviduct - *see* Oophoritis
palate (soft) K12.2
  hard M27.2
palmar (space) - *see* Abscess, hand
pancreas (duct) - *see* Pancreatitis, acute
parafrenal N48.21
parametric, parametrium N73.2
  acute N73.0
  chronic N73.1
paranephric N15.1
parapancreatic - *see* Pancreatitis, acute
parapharyngeal J39.0
pararectal K61.1
parasinus - *see* Sinusitis
parauterine - *see also* Disease, pelvis,
  inflammatory N73.2
paravaginal - *see* Vaginitis
parietal region (scalp) L02.811
parodontal - *see* Periodontitis, aggressive,
  localized
parotid (duct) (gland) K11.3
  region K12.2
Abscess - *continued*
pectoral (region) L02.213
pelvis, pelvic
  female - *see* Disease, pelvis, inflammatory
  male, peritoneal K65.1
penis N48.21
  gonococcal (accessory gland) (periurethral)
  A54.1
perianal K61.0
periapical K04.7
  with sinus (alveolar) K04.6
periappendicular K35.3
pericardial I30.1
pericecal K35.3
pericemental - *see* Periodontitis, aggressive,
  localized
pericholecystic - *see* Cholecystitis, acute
pericoronal - *see* Periodontitis, aggressive,
  localized
peridental - *see* Periodontitis, aggressive,
  localized
perimetric - *see also* Disease, pelvis,
  inflammatory N73.2
perinephric, perinephritic - *see* Abscess,
  kidney
perineum, perineal (superficial) L02.215
  urethra N34.0
periodontal (parietal) - *see* Periodontitis,
  aggressive, localized
  apical K04.7
periosteum, periosteal - *see also* Osteomyelitis,
  specified type NEC
  with osteomyelitis - *see also* Osteomyelitis,
  specified type NEC
    acute - *see* Osteomyelitis, acute
    chronic - *see* Osteomyelitis, chronic
peripharyngeal J39.0
peripleuritic J86.9
  with fistula J86.0
periprostatic N41.2
perirectal K61.1
perirenal (tissue) - *see* Abscess, kidney
perisinuous (nose) - *see* Sinusitis

Abscess - *continued*

peritoneum, peritoneal (perforated) (ruptured) K65.1
  with appendicitis K35.3
  pelvic
    female - *see* Peritonitis, pelvic, female
    male K65.1
  postoperative T81.4
  puerperal, postpartum, childbirth O85
  tuberculous A18.31
peritonsillar J36
perityphlic K35.3
periureteral N28.89
periurethral N34.0
  gonococcal (accessory gland) (periurethral) A54.1
periuterine - *see also* Disease, pelvis, inflammatory N73.2
perivesical - *see* Cystitis, specified type NEC
petrous bone - *see* Petrositis
phagedenic NOS L02.91
  chancroid A57
pharynx, pharyngeal (lateral) J39.1
pilonidal L05.01
pituitary (gland) E23.6
pleura J86.9
  with fistula J86.0
popliteal - *see* Abscess, lower limb
postcecal K35.3
postlaryngeal J38.7
postnasal J34.0
postoperative (any site) T81.4
  retroperitoneal K68.11
postpharyngeal J39.0
posttonsillar J36
post-typhoid A01.09
pouch of Douglas - *see* Peritonitis, pelvic, female
premammary - *see* Abscess, breast
prepatellar - *see* Abscess, lower limb
prostate N41.2
  gonococcal (acute) (chronic) A54.22
psoas muscle K68.12
puerperal
  code by site under Puerperal, abscess
pulmonary - *see* Abscess, lung
pulp, pulpal (dental) K04.01
  irreversible K04.02
  reversible K04.01
rectovaginal septum K63.0
rectovesical - *see* Cystitis, specified type NEC
rectum K61.1
renal - *see* Abscess, kidney
retina - *see* Inflammation, chorioretinal
retrobulbar - *see* Abscess, orbit
retrocecal K65.1
retrolaryngeal J38.7
retromammary - *see* Abscess, breast
retroperitoneal NEC K68.19
  postprocedural K68.11
retropharyngeal J39.0
retrouterine - *see* Peritonitis, pelvic, female
retrovesical - *see* Cystitis, specified type NEC
root, tooth K04.7
  with sinus (alveolar) K04.6
round ligament - *see also* Disease, pelvis, inflammatory N73.2
rupture (spontaneous) NOS L02.91
sacrum (tuberculous) A18.01
  nontuberculous M46.28
salivary (duct) (gland) K11.3
scalp (any part) L02.811
scapular - *see* Osteomyelitis, specified type NEC

Abscess - *continued*

sclera - *see* Scleritis
scrofulous (tuberculous) A18.2
scrotum N49.2
seminal vesicle N49.0
septal, dental K04.7
  with sinus (alveolar) K04.6
serous - *see* Periostitis
shoulder (region) - *see* Abscess, upper limb
sigmoid K63.0
sinus (accessory) (chronic) (nasal) - *see also* Sinusitis
  intracranial venous (any) G06.0
Skene's duct or gland N34.0
skin - *see* Abscess, by site
specified site NEC L02.818
spermatic cord N49.1
sphenoidal (sinus) (chronic) J32.3
spinal cord (any part) (staphylococcal) G06.1
  tuberculous A17.81
spine (column) (tuberculous) A18.01
  epidural G06.1
  nontuberculous - *see* Osteomyelitis, vertebra
spleen D73.3
  amebic A06.89
stitch T81.4
subarachnoid G06.2
  brain G06.0
  spinal cord G06.1
subareolar - *see* Abscess, breast
subcecal K35.3
subcutaneous - *see also* Abscess, by site
  pheomycotic (chromomycotic) B43.2
subdiaphragmatic K65.1
subdural G06.2
  brain G06.0
    sequelae G09
  spinal cord G06.1
subgaleal L02.811
subhepatic K65.1
sublingual K12.2
  gland K11.3
submammary - *see* Abscess, breast
submandibular (region) (space) (triangle) K12.2
  gland K11.3
submaxillary (region) L02.01
  gland K11.3
submental L02.01
  gland K11.3
subperiosteal - *see* Osteomyelitis, specified type NEC
subphrenic K65.1
  postoperative T81.4
suburethral N34.0
sudoriparous L75.8
supraclavicular (fossa) - *see* Abscess, upper limb
suprapelvic, acute N73.0
suprapelvic, acute N73.0
suprarenal (capsule) (gland) E27.8
sweat gland L74.8
tear duct - *see* Inflammation, lacrimal, passages, acute
temple L02.01
temporal region L02.01
temporosphenoidal G06.0
tendon (sheath) M65.00
  ankle M65.07-
  foot M65.07-
  forearm M65.03-
  hand M65.04-
  lower leg M65.06-
  pelvic region M65.05-
  shoulder region M65.01-

Abscess - *continued*

specified site NEC M65.08
thigh M65.05-
  upper arm M65.02-
testis N45.4
thigh - *see* Abscess, lower limb
thorax J86.9
  with fistula J86.0
throat J39.1
thumb - *see also* Abscess, hand
  nail - *see* Cellulitis, finger
thymus (gland) E32.1
thyroid (gland) E06.0
toe (any) - *see also* Abscess, foot
  nail - *see* Cellulitis, toe
tongue (staphylococcal) K14.0
tonsil(s) (lingual) J36
tonsillopharyngeal J36
tooth, teeth (root) K04.7
  with sinus (alveolar) K04.6
  supporting structures NEC - *see* Periodontitis, aggressive, localized
trachea J39.8
trunk L02.219
  abdominal wall L02.211
  back L02.212
  chest wall L02.213
  groin L02.214
  perineum L02.215
  umbilicus L02.216
tubal - *see* Salpingitis
tuberculous - *see* Tuberculosis, abscess
tubo-ovarian - *see* Salpingo-oophoritis
tunica vaginalis N49.1
umbilicus L02.216
upper
  limb L02.41-
  respiratory J39.8
urethral (gland) N34.0
urinary N34.0
uterus, uterine (wall) - *see also* Endometritis
  ligament - *see also* Disease, pelvis, inflammatory N73.2
  neck - *see* Cervicitis
uvula K12.2
vagina (wall) - *see* Vaginitis
vaginorectal - *see* Vaginitis
vas deferens N49.1
vermiform appendix K35.3
vertebra (column) (tuberculous) A18.01
  nontuberculous - *see* Osteomyelitis, vertebra
vesical - *see* Cystitis, specified type NEC
vesico-uterine pouch - *see* Peritonitis, pelvic, female
vitreous (humor) - *see* Endophthalmitis, purulent
vocal cord J38.3
von Bezold's - *see* Mastoiditis, acute
vulva N76.4
vulvovaginal gland N75.1
web space - *see* Abscess, hand
wound T81.4
wrist - *see* Abscess, upper limb

Absence (of) (organ or part) (complete or partial)

adrenal (gland) (congenital) Q89.1
  acquired E89.6
albumin in blood E88.09
alimentary tract (congenital) Q45.8
  upper Q40.8
alveolar process (acquired) - *see* Anomaly, alveolar
ankle (acquired) Z89.44-
anus (congenital) Q42.3

Absence (of) (organ or part) (complete or partial) - *continued*
  with fistula Q42.2
  aorta (congenital) Q25.41
  appendix, congenital Q42.8
  arm (acquired) Z89.20-
    above elbow Z89.22-
      congenital (with hand present) - *see*
        Agenesis, arm, with hand present
        and hand - *see* Agenesis, forearm, and
        hand
    below elbow Z89.21-
      congenital (with hand present) - *see*
        Agenesis, arm, with hand present
        and hand - *see* Agenesis, forearm, and
        hand
    congenital - *see* Defect, reduction, upper limb
    shoulder (following explanation of shoulder
      joint prosthesis) (joint) (with or without
      presence of antibiotic-impregnated cement
      spacer) Z89.23-
        congenital (with hand present) - *see*
          Agenesis, arm, with hand present
  artery (congenital) (peripheral) Q27.8
    brain Q28.3
    coronary Q24.5
    pulmonary Q25.79
    specified NEC Q27.8
    umbilical Q27.0
  atrial septum (congenital) Q21.1
  auditory canal (congenital) (external) Q16.1
  auricle (ear), congenital Q16.0
  bile, biliary duct, congenital Q44.5
  bladder (acquired) Z90.6
    congenital Q64.5
  bowel sounds R19.11
  brain Q00.0
    part of Q04.3
  breast(s) (and nipple(s)) (acquired) Z90.1-
    congenital Q83.8
  broad ligament Q50.6
  bronchus (congenital) Q32.4
  canaliculus lacrimalis, congenital Q10.4
  cerebellum (vermis) Q04.3
  cervix (acquired) (with uterus) Z90.710
    with remaining uterus Z90.712
    congenital Q51.5
  chin, congenital Q18.8
  cilia (congenital) Q10.3
    acquired - *see* Madarosis
  clitoris (congenital) Q52.6
  coccyx, congenital Q76.49
  cold sense R20.8
  congenital
    lumen - *see* Atresia
    organ or site NEC - *see* Agenesis
    septum - *see* Imperfect, closure
  corpus callosum Q04.0
  cricoid cartilage, congenital Q31.8
  diaphragm (with hernia), congenital Q79.1
  digestive organ(s) or tract, congenital Q45.8
    acquired NEC Z90.49
    upper Q40.8
  ductus arteriosus Q28.8
  duodenum (acquired) Z90.49
    congenital Q41.0
  ear, congenital Q16.9
    acquired H93.8-
    auricle Q16.0
    external Q16.0
    inner Q16.5
    lobe, lobule Q17.8
    middle, except ossicles Q16.4
      ossicles Q16.3

Absence (of) (organ or part) (complete or partial) - *continued*
  ossicles Q16.3
  ejaculatory duct (congenital) Q55.4
  endocrine gland (congenital) NEC Q89.2
    acquired E89.89
  epididymis (congenital) Q55.4
    acquired Q90.79
  epiglottis, congenital Q31.8
  esophagus (congenital) Q39.8
    acquired (partial) Z90.49
  eustachian tube (congenital) Q16.2
  extremity (acquired) Z89.9
    congenital Q73.0
    knee (following explanation of knee joint
      prosthesis) (joint) (with or without presence
      of antibiotic-impregnated cement spacer)
      Z89.52-
    lower (above knee) Z89.619
      below knee Z89.51-
    upper - *see* Absence, arm
  eye (acquired) Z90.01
    congenital Q11.1
    muscle (congenital) Q10.3
  eyeball (acquired) Z90.01
  eyelid (fold) (congenital) Q10.3
    acquired Z90.01
  face, specified part NEC Q18.8
  fallopian tube(s) (acquired) Z90.79
    congenital Q50.6
  family member (causing problem in home)
    NEC - *see also* Disruption, family Z63.32
  femur, congenital - *see* Defect, reduction,
    lower limb, longitudinal, femur
  fibrinogen (congenital) D68.2
    acquired D65
  finger(s) (acquired) Z89.02-
    congenital - *see* Agenesis, hand
  foot (acquired) Z89.43-
    congenital - *see* Agenesis, foot
  forearm (acquired) - *see* Absence, arm, below
    elbow
  gallbladder (acquired) Z90.49
    congenital Q44.0
  gamma globulin in blood D80.1
    hereditary D80.0
  genital organs
    acquired (female) (male) Z90.79
    female, congenital Q52.8
      external Q52.71
      internal NEC Q52.8
    male, congenital Q55.8
  genitourinary organs, congenital NEC
    female Q52.8
    male Q55.8
  globe (acquired) Z90.01
    congenital Q11.1
  glottis, congenital Q31.8
  hand and wrist (acquired) Z89.11-
    congenital - *see* Agenesis, hand
  head, part (acquired) NEC Z90.09
  heat sense R20.8
  hip (following explanation of hip joint
    prosthesis) (joint) (with or without presence
    of antibiotic-impregnated cement spacer)
    Z89.62-
  hymen (congenital) Q52.4
  ileum (acquired) Z90.49
    congenital Q41.2
  immunoglobulin, isolated NEC D80.3
    IgA D80.2
    IgG D80.3
    IgM D80.4
  incus (acquired) - *see* Loss, ossicles, ear

Absence (of) (organ or part) (complete or partial) - *continued*
  congenital Q16.3
  inner ear, congenital Q16.5
  intestine (acquired) (small) Z90.49
    congenital Q41.9
    specified NEC Q41.8
    large Z90.49
      congenital Q42.9
      specified NEC Q42.8
  iris, congenital Q13.1
  jejunum (acquired) Z90.49
    congenital Q41.1
  joint
    acquired
      hip (following explanation of hip joint
        prosthesis) (with or without presence of
        antibiotic-impregnated cement spacer)
        Z89.62-
      knee (following explanation of knee joint
        prosthesis) (with or without presence of
        antibiotic-impregnated cement spacer)
        Z89.52-
      shoulder (following explanation of
        shoulder joint prosthesis) (with or without
        presence of antibiotic-impregnated cement
        spacer) Z89.23-
    congenital NEC Q74.8
  kidney(s) (acquired) Z90.5
    congenital Q60.2
      bilateral Q60.1
      unilateral Q60.0
  knee (following explanation of knee joint
    prosthesis) (joint) (with or without presence
    of antibiotic-impregnated cement spacer)
    Z89.52-
  labyrinth, membranous Q16.5
  larynx (congenital) Q31.8
    acquired Z90.02
  leg (acquired) (above knee) Z89.61-
    below knee (acquired) Z89.51-
    congenital - *see* Defect, reduction, lower limb
  lens (acquired) - *see also* Aphakia
    congenital Q12.3
    post cataract extraction Z98.4-
  limb (acquired) - *see* Absence, extremity
  lip Q38.6
  liver (congenital) Q44.7
  lung (fissure) (lobe) (bilateral) (unilateral)
    (congenital) Q33.3
    acquired (any part) Z90.2
  menstruation - *see* Amenorrhea
  muscle (congenital) (pectoral) Q79.8
    ocular Q10.3
  neck, part Q18.8
  neutrophil - *see* Agranulocytosis
  nipple(s) (with breast(s)) (acquired) Z90.1-
    congenital Q83.2
  nose (congenital) Q30.1
    acquired Z90.09
  organ
    of Corti, congenital Q16.5
    or site, congenital NEC Q89.8
      acquired NEC Z90.89
  osseous meatus (ear) Q16.4
  ovary (acquired)
    bilateral Z90.722
    congenital
      bilateral Q50.02
      unilateral Q50.01
    unilateral Z90.721
  oviduct (acquired)
    bilateral Z90.722
    congenital Q50.6

Absence (of) (organ or part) (complete or partial) - *continued*
unilateral Z90.721
pancreas (congenital) Q45.0
acquired Z90.410
complete Z90.410
partial Z90.411
total Z90.410
parathyroid gland (acquired) E89.2
congenital Q89.2
patella, congenital Q74.1
penis (congenital) Q55.5
acquired Z90.79
pericardium (congenital) Q24.8
pituitary gland (congenital) Q89.2
acquired E89.3
prostate (acquired) Z90.79
congenital Q55.4
pulmonary valve Q22.0
punctum lacrimale (congenital) Q10.4
radius, congenital - *see* Defect, reduction, upper limb, longitudinal, radius
rectum (congenital) Q42.1
with fistula Q42.0
acquired Z90.49
respiratory organ NOS Q34.9
rib (acquired) Z90.89
congenital Q76.6
sacrum, congenital Q76.49
salivary gland(s), congenital Q38.4
scrotum, congenital Q55.29
seminal vesicles (congenital) Q55.4
acquired Z90.79
septum
atrial (congenital) Q21.1
between aorta and pulmonary artery Q21.4
ventricular (congenital) Q20.4
sex chromosome
female phenotype Q97.8
male phenotype Q98.8
skull bone (congenital) Q75.8
with
anencephaly Q00.0
encephalocele - *see* Encephalocele
hydrocephalus Q03.9
with spina bifida - *see* Spina bifida, by site, with hydrocephalus
microcephaly Q02
spermatic cord, congenital Q55.4
spine, congenital Q76.49
spleen (congenital) Q89.01
acquired Z90.81
sternum, congenital Q76.7
stomach (acquired) (partial) Z90.3
congenital Q40.2
superior vena cava, congenital Q26.8
teeth, tooth (congenital) K00.0
acquired (complete) K08.109
class I K08.101
class II K08.102
class III K08.103
class IV K08.104
due to
caries K08.139
class I K08.131
class II K08.132
class III K08.133
class IV K08.134
periodontal disease K08.129
class I K08.121
class II K08.122
class III K08.123
class IV K08.124
specified NEC K08.199

Absence (of) (organ or part) (complete or partial) - *continued*
class I K08.191
class II K08.192
class III K08.193
class IV K08.194
trauma K08.119
class I K08.111
class II K08.112
class III K08.113
class IV K08.114
partial K08.409
class I K08.401
class II K08.402
class III K08.403
class IV K08.404
due to
caries K08.439
class I K08.431
class II K08.432
class III K08.433
class IV K08.434
periodontal disease K08.429
class I K08.421
class II K08.422
class III K08.423
class IV K08.424
specified NEC K08.499
class I K08.491
class II K08.492
class III K08.493
class IV K08.494
trauma K08.419
class I K08.411
class II K08.412
class III K08.413
class IV K08.414
tendon (congenital) Q79.8
testis (congenital) Q55.0
acquired Z90.79
thumb (acquired) Z89.01-
congenital - *see* Agenesis, hand
thymus gland Q89.2
thyroid (gland) (acquired) E89.0
cartilage, congenital Q31.8
congenital E03.1
toe(s) (acquired) Z89.42-
with foot - *see* Absence, foot and ankle
congenital - *see* Agenesis, foot
great Z89.41-
tongue, congenital Q38.3
trachea (cartilage), congenital Q32.1
transverse aortic arch, congenital Q25.49
tricuspid valve Q22.4
umbilical artery, congenital Q27.0
upper arm and forearm with hand present, congenital - *see* Agenesis, arm, with hand present
ureter (congenital) Q62.4
acquired Z90.6
urethra, congenital Q64.5
uterus (acquired) Z90.710
with cervix Z90.710
with remaining cervical stump Z90.711
congenital Q51.0
uvula, congenital Q38.5
vagina, congenital Q52.0
vas deferens (congenital) Q55.4
acquired Z90.79
vein (peripheral) congenital NEC Q27.8
cerebral Q28.3
digestive system Q27.8
great Q26.8
lower limb Q27.8

Absence (of) (organ or part) (complete or partial) - *continued*
portal Q26.5
precerebral Q28.1
specified site NEC Q27.8
upper limb Q27.8
vena cava (inferior) (superior), congenital Q26.8
ventricular septum Q20.4
vertebra, congenital Q76.49
vulva, congenital Q52.71
wrist (acquired) Z89.12-
Absorbent system disease I87.8
Absorption
carbohydrate, disturbance K90.49
chemical - *see* Table of Drugs and Chemicals
through placenta (newborn) P04.9
environmental substance P04.6
nutritional substance P04.5
obstetric anesthetic or analgesic drug P04.0
drug NEC - *see* Table of Drugs and Chemicals
addictive
through placenta (newborn) P04.49
cocaine P04.41
medicinal
through placenta (newborn) P04.1
through placenta (newborn) P04.1
obstetric anesthetic or analgesic drug P04.0
fat, disturbance K90.49
pancreatic K90.3
noxious substance - *see* Table of Drugs and Chemicals
protein, disturbance K90.49
starch, disturbance K90.49
toxic substance - *see* Table of Drugs and Chemicals
uremic - *see* Uremia
Abstinence symptoms, syndrome
alcohol F10.239
with delirium F10.231
cocaine F14.23
neonatal P96.1
nicotine - *see* Dependence, drug, nicotine, with, withdrawal
opioid F11.93
with dependence F11.23
psychoactive NEC F19.939
with
delirium F19.931
dependence F19.239
with
delirium F19.231
perceptual disturbance F19.232
uncomplicated F19.230
perceptual disturbance F19.932
uncomplicated F19.930
sedative F13.939
with
delirium F13.931
dependence F13.239
with
delirium F13.231
perceptual disturbance F13.232
uncomplicated F13.230
perceptual disturbance F13.932
uncomplicated F13.930
stimulant NEC F15.93
with dependence F15.23
Abulia R68.89
Abulomania F60.7
Abuse
adult - *see* Maltreatment, adult

Abuse - *continued*
  as reason for
    couple seeking advice (including offender)
    Z63.0
  alcohol (non-dependent) F10.10
    in remission (early) (sustained) F10.11
    with
      anxiety disorder F10.180
      intoxication F10.129
        with delirium F10.121
        uncomplicated F10.120
      mood disorder F10.14
      other specified disorder F10.188
      psychosis F10.159
        delusions F10.150
        hallucinations F10.151
      sexual dysfunction F10.181
      sleep disorder F10.182
      unspecified disorder F10.19
    counseling and surveillance Z71.41
  amphetamine (or related substance) - *see*
    Abuse, drug, stimulant NEC
  analgesics (non-prescribed) (over the counter)
    F55.8
  antacids F55.0
  antidepressants - *see* Abuse, drug,
    psychoactive NEC
  anxiolytic - *see* Abuse, drug, sedative
  barbiturates - *see* Abuse, drug, sedative
  caffeine - *see* Abuse, drug, stimulant NEC
  cannabis, cannabinoids - *see* Abuse, drug,
    cannabis
  child - *see* Maltreatment, child
  cocaine - *see* Abuse, drug, cocaine
  drug NEC (non-dependent) F19.10
    with sleep disorder F19.182
    amphetamine type - *see* Abuse, drug,
      stimulant NEC
    analgesics (non-prescribed) (over the
      counter) F55.8
    antacids F55.0
    antidepressants - *see* Abuse, drug,
      psychoactive NEC
    anxiolytics - *see* Abuse, drug, sedative
    barbiturates - *see* Abuse, drug, sedative
    caffeine - *see* Abuse, drug, stimulant NEC
    cannabis F12.10
      in remission (early) (sustained) F12.11
      with
        anxiety disorder F12.180
        intoxication F12.129
          with
            delirium F12.121
            perceptual disturbance F12.122
          uncomplicated F12.120
        other specified disorder F12.188
        psychosis F12.159
          delusions F12.150
          hallucinations F12.151
        unspecified disorder F12.19
    cocaine F14.10
      in remission (early) (sustained) F14.11
      with
        anxiety disorder F14.180
        intoxication F14.129
          with
            delirium F14.121
            perceptual disturbance F14.122
          uncomplicated F14.120
        mood disorder F14.14
        other specified disorder F14.188
        psychosis F14.159
          delusions F14.150
          hallucinations F14.151

Abuse - *continued*
      sexual dysfunction F14.181
      sleep disorder F14.182
      unspecified disorder F14.19
  counseling and surveillance Z71.51
  hallucinogen F16.10
    in remission (early) (sustained) F16.11
    with
      anxiety disorder F16.180
      flashbacks F16.183
      intoxication F16.129
        with
          delirium F16.121
          perceptual disturbance F16.122
        uncomplicated F16.120
      mood disorder F16.14
      other specified disorder F16.188
      perception disorder, persisting F16.183
      psychosis F16.159
        delusions F16.150
        hallucinations F16.151
      unspecified disorder F16.19
  hashish - *see* Abuse, drug, cannabis
  herbal or folk remedies F55.1
  hormones F55.3
  hypnotics - *see* Abuse, drug, sedative
  inhalant F18.10
    in remission (early) (sustained) F18.11
  in remission (early) (sustained) F19.11
    with
      anxiety disorder F18.180
      dementia, persisting F18.17
      intoxication F18.129
        with delirium F18.121
        uncomplicated F18.120
      mood disorder F18.14
      other specified disorder F18.188
      psychosis F18.159
        delusions F18.150
        hallucinations F18.151
      unspecified disorder F18.19
  laxatives F55.2
  LSD - *see* Abuse, drug, hallucinogen
  marihuana - *see* Abuse, drug, cannabis
  morphine type (opioids) - *see* Abuse, drug,
    opioid
  opioid F11.10
    in remission (early) (sustained) F11.11
    with
      intoxication F11.129
        with
          delirium F11.121
          perceptual disturbance F11.122
        uncomplicated F11.120
      mood disorder F11.14
      other specified disorder F11.188
      psychosis F11.159
        delusions F11.150
        hallucinations F11.151
      sexual dysfunction F11.181
      sleep disorder F11.182
      unspecified disorder F11.19
  PCP (phencyclidine) (or related substance) -
    see Abuse, drug, hallucinogen
  psychoactive NEC F19.10
    with
      amnestic disorder F19.16
      anxiety disorder F19.180
      dementia F19.17
      intoxication F19.129
        with
          delirium F19.121
          perceptual disturbance F19.122
        uncomplicated F19.120

Abuse - *continued*
      mood disorder F19.14
      other specified disorder F19.188
      psychosis F19.159
        delusions F19.150
        hallucinations F19.151
      sexual dysfunction F19.181
      sleep disorder F19.182
      unspecified disorder F19.19
  sedative, hypnotic or anxiolytic F13.10
    in remission (early) (sustained) F13.11
    with
      anxiety disorder F13.180
      intoxication F13.129
        with delirium F13.121
        uncomplicated F13.120
      mood disorder F13.14
      other specified disorder F13.188
      psychosis F13.159
        delusions F13.150
        hallucinations F13.151
      sexual dysfunction F13.181
      sleep disorder F13.182
      unspecified disorder F13.19
  solvent - *see* Abuse, drug, inhalant
  steroids F55.3
  stimulant NEC F15.10
    in remission (early) (sustained) F15.11
    with
      anxiety disorder F15.180
      intoxication F15.129
        with
          delirium F15.121
          perceptual disturbance F15.122
        uncomplicated F15.120
      mood disorder F15.14
      other specified disorder F15.188
      psychosis F15.159
        delusions F15.150
        hallucinations F15.151
      sexual dysfunction F15.181
      sleep disorder F15.182
      unspecified disorder F15.19
  tranquilizers - *see* Abuse, drug, sedative
  vitamins F55.4
  hallucinogens - *see* Abuse, drug, hallucinogen
  hashish - *see* Abuse, drug, cannabis
  herbal or folk remedies F55.1
  hormones F55.3
  hypnotic - *see* Abuse, drug, sedative
  inhalant - *see* Abuse, drug, inhalant
  laxatives F55.2
  LSD - *see* Abuse, drug, hallucinogen
  marihuana - *see* Abuse, drug, cannabis
  morphine type (opioids) - *see* Abuse, drug,
    opioid
  non-psychoactive substance NEC F55.8
    antacids F55.0
    folk remedies F55.1
    herbal remedies F55.1
    hormones F55.3
    laxatives F55.2
    steroids F55.3
    vitamins F55.4
  opioids - *see* Abuse, drug, opioid
  PCP (phencyclidine) (or related substance) -
    see Abuse, drug, hallucinogen
  physical (adult) (child) - *see* Maltreatment
  psychoactive substance - *see* Abuse, drug,
    psychoactive NEC
  psychological (adult) (child) - *see*
    Maltreatment
  sedative - *see* Abuse, drug, sedative
  sexual - *see* Maltreatment

Abuse - *continued*
  solvent - *see* Abuse, drug, inhalant
  steroids F55.3
  vitamins F55.4
Acalculia R48.8
  developmental F81.2
Acanthamebiasis (with) B60.10
  conjunctiva B60.12
  keratoconjunctivitis B60.13
  meningoencephalitis B60.11
  other specified B60.19
Acanthocephaliasis B83.8
Acanthocheilonemiasis B74.4
Acanthocytosis E78.6
Acantholysis L11.9
Acanthosis (acquired) (nigricans) L83
  benign Q82.8
  congenital Q82.8
  seborrheic L82.1
    inflamed L82.0
  tongue K14.3
Acapnia E87.3
Acarbia E87.2
Acardia, acardius Q89.8
Acardiacus amorphus Q89.8
Acardiotrophia I51.4
Acariasis B88.0
  scabies B86
Acarodermatitis (urticarioides) B88.0
Acarophobia F40.218
Acatalasemia, acatalasia E80.3
Acathisia (drug induced) G25.71
Accelerated atrioventricular conduction I45.6
Accentuation of personality traits (type A)
  Z73.1
Accessory (congenital)
  adrenal gland Q89.1
  anus Q43.4
  appendix Q43.4
  atrioventricular conduction I45.6
  auditory ossicles Q16.3
  auricle (ear) Q17.0
  biliary duct or passage Q44.5
  bladder Q64.79
  blood vessels NEC Q27.9
    coronary Q24.5
  bone NEC Q79.8
  breast tissue, axilla Q83.1
  carpal bones Q74.0
  cecum Q43.4
  chromosome(s) NEC (nonsex) Q92.9
    with complex rearrangements NEC Q92.5
      seen only at prometaphase Q92.8
    partial Q92.9
    sex
      female phenotype Q97.8
    13 - *see* Trisomy, 13
    18 - *see* Trisomy, 18
    21 - *see* Trisomy, 21
  coronary artery Q24.5
  cusp(s), heart valve NEC Q24.8
    pulmonary Q22.3
  cystic duct Q44.5
  digit(s) Q69.9
  ear (auricle) (lobe) Q17.0
  endocrine gland NEC Q89.2
  eye muscle Q10.3
  eyelid Q10.3
  face bone(s) Q75.8
  fallopian tube (fimbria) (ostium) Q50.6
  finger(s) Q69.0
  foreskin N47.8
  frontonasal process Q75.8
  gallbladder Q44.1

Accessory (congenital) - *continued*
  genital organ(s)
    female Q52.8
      external Q52.79
      internal NEC Q52.8
    male Q55.8
    genitourinary organs NEC Q89.8
      female Q52.8
      male Q55.8
  hallux Q69.2
  heart Q24.8
    valve NEC Q24.8
      pulmonary Q22.3
  hepatic ducts Q44.5
  hymen Q52.4
  intestine (large) (small) Q43.4
  kidney Q63.0
  lacrimal canal Q10.6
  leaflet, heart valve NEC Q24.8
  ligament, broad Q50.6
  liver Q44.7
    duct Q44.5
  lobule (ear) Q17.0
  lung (lobe) Q33.1
  muscle Q79.8
  navicular of carpus Q74.0
  nervous system, part NEC Q07.8
  nipple Q83.3
  nose Q30.8
  organ or site not listed - *see* Anomaly, by site
  ovary Q50.31
  oviduct Q50.6
  pancreas Q45.3
  parathyroid gland Q89.2
  parotid gland (and duct) Q38.4
  pituitary gland Q89.2
  preauricular appendage Q17.0
  prepuce N47.8
  renal arteries (multiple) Q27.2
  rib Q76.6
    cervical Q76.5
  roots (teeth) K00.2
  salivary gland Q38.4
  sesamoid bones Q74.8
    foot Q74.2
    hand Q74.0
  skin tags Q82.8
  spleen Q89.09
  sternum Q76.7
  submaxillary gland Q38.4
  tarsal bones Q74.2
  teeth, tooth K00.1
  tendon Q79.8
  thumb Q69.1
  thymus gland Q89.2
  thyroid gland Q89.2
  toes Q69.2
  tongue Q38.3
  tooth, teeth K00.1
  tragus Q17.0
  ureter Q62.5
  urethra Q64.79
  urinary organ or tract NEC Q64.8
  uterus Q51.2
  vagina Q52.10
  valve, heart NEC Q24.8
    pulmonary Q22.3
  vertebra Q76.49
  vocal cords Q31.8
  vulva Q52.79
Accident
  birth - *see* Birth, injury
  cardiac - *see* Infarct, myocardium

Accident - *continued*
  cerebral I63.9
  cerebrovascular (embolic) (ischemic)
    (thrombotic) I63.9
    aborted I63.9
    hemorrhagic - *see* Hemorrhage, intracranial,
      intracerebral
    old (without sequelae) Z86.73
      with sequelae (of) - *see* Sequelae,
        infarction, cerebral
  coronary - *see* Infarct, myocardium
  craniovascular I63.9
  vascular, brain I63.9
Accidental - *see* condition
Accommodation (disorder) - *see also*
  condition
  hysterical paralysis of F44.89
  insufficiency of H52.4
  paresis - *see* Paresis, of accommodation
  spasm - *see* Spasm, of accommodation
Accouchement - *see* Delivery
Accreta placenta O43.21-
Accretio cordis (nonrheumatic) I31.0
Accretions, tooth, teeth K03.6
Acculturation difficulty Z60.3
Accumulation secretion, prostate N42.89
Acephalia, acephalism, acephalus, acephaly
  Q00.0
Acephalobrachia monster Q89.8
Acephalochirus monster Q89.8
Acephalogaster Q89.8
Acephalostomus monster Q89.8
Acephalothorax Q89.8
Acerophobia F40.298
Acetonemia R79.89
  in Type 1 diabetes E10.10
    with coma E10.11
Acetonuria R82.4
Achalasia (cardia) (esophagus) K22.0
  congenital Q39.5
  pylorus Q40.0
  sphincteral NEC K59.8
Ache(s) - *see* Pain
Acheilia Q38.6
Achillobursitis - *see* Tendinitis, Achilles
Achillodynia - *see* Tendinitis, Achilles
Achlorhydria, achlorhydric (neurogenic)
  K31.83
  anemia D50.8
  diarrhea K31.83
  psychogenic F45.8
  secondary to vagotomy K91.1
Achluophobia F40.228
Acholia K82.8
Acholuric jaundice (familial) (splenomegalic)
  - *see also* Spherocytosis
  acquired D59.8
Achondrogenesis Q77.0
Achondroplasia (osteosclerosis congenita)
  Q77.4
Achroma, cutis L80
Achromat (ism), achromatopsia (acquired)
  (congenital) H53.51
Achromia, congenital - *see* Albinism
Achromia parasitica B36.0
Achylia gastrica K31.89
  psychogenic F45.8
Acid
  burn - *see* Corrosion
  deficiency
    amide nicotinic E52
    ascorbic E54
    folic E53.8
    nicotinic E52

Acid - *continued*
  pantothenic E53.8
  intoxication E87.2
  peptic disease K30
  phosphatase deficiency E83.39
  stomach K30
    psychogenic F45.8
Acidemia E87.2
  argininosuccinic E72.22
  isovaleric E71.110
  metabolic (newborn) P19.9
    first noted before onset of labor P19.0
    first noted during labor P19.1
    noted at birth P19.2
  methylmalonic E71.120
  pipecolic E72.3
  propionic E71.121
Acidity, gastric (high) K30
  psychogenic F45.8
Acidocytopenia - *see* Agranulocytosis
Acidocytosis D72.1
Acidopenia - *see* Agranulocytosis
Acidosis (lactic) (respiratory) E87.2
  in Type 1 diabetes E10.10
    with coma E10.11
  kidney, tubular N25.89
  lactic E87.2
  metabolic NEC E87.2
    with respiratory acidosis E87.4
    late, of newborn P74.0
  mixed metabolic and respiratory, newborn P84
  newborn P84
  renal (hyperchloremic) (tubular) N25.89
  respiratory E87.2
    complicated by
      metabolic
        acidosis E87.4
        alkalosis E87.4
Aciduria
  argininosuccinic E72.22
  glutaric (type I) E72.3
    type II E71.313
    type III E71.5-
  orotic (congenital) (hereditary) (pyrimidine deficiency) E79.8
    anemia D53.0
Acladiosis (skin) B36.0
Aclasis, diaphyseal Q78.6
Acleistocardia Q21.1
Aclusion - *see* Anomaly, dentofacial, malocclusion
Acne L70.9
  artificialis L70.8
  atrophica L70.2
  cachecticorum (Hebra) L70.8
  conglobata L70.1
  cystic L70.0
  decalvans L66.2
  excoriée (des jeunes filles) L70.5
  frontalis L70.2
  indurata L70.0
  infantile L70.4
  keloid L73.0
  lupoid L70.2
  necrotic, necrotica (miliaris) L70.2
  neonatal L70.4
  nodular L70.0
  occupational L70.8
  picker's L70.5
  pustular L70.0
  rodens L70.2
  rosacea L71.9
  specified NEC L70.8

Acne - *continued*
  tropica L70.3
  varioliformis L70.2
  vulgaris L70.0
Acnitis (primary) A18.4
Acosta's disease T70.29
Acoustic - *see* condition
Acousticophobia F40.298
Acquired - *see also* condition
  immunodeficiency syndrome (AIDS) B20
Acrania Q00.0
Acroangiodermatitis I78.9
Acroasphyxia, chronic I73.89
Acrobystitis N47.7
Acrocephalopolysyndactyly Q87.0
Acrocephalosyndactyly Q87.0
Acrocephaly Q75.0
Acrochondrohyperplasia - *see* Syndrome, Marfan's
Acrocyanosis I73.8
  newborn P28.2
    meaning transient blue hands and feet omit code
Acrodermatitis L30.8
  atrophicans (chronica) L90.4
  continua (Hallopeau) L40.2
  enteropathica (hereditary) E83.2
  Hallopeau's L40.2
  infantile papular L44.4
  perstans L40.2
  pustulosa continua L40.2
  recalcitrant pustular L40.2
Acrodynia - *see* Poisoning, mercury
Acromegaly, acromegalia E22.0
Acromelalgia I73.81
Acromicria, acromicria Q79.8
Acronyx L60.0
Acropachy, thyroid - *see* Thyrotoxicosis
Acroparesthesia (simple) (vasomotor) I73.89
Acropathy, thyroid - *see* Thyrotoxicosis
Acrophobia F40.241
Acroposthitis N47.7
Acroscleriasis, acroscleroderma, acrosclerosis - *see* Sclerosis, systemic
Acrosphacelus I96
Acrospiroma, eccrine - *see* Neoplasm, skin, benign
Acrostealgia - *see* Osteochondropathy
Acrotrophodynia - *see* Immersion
ACTH ectopic syndrome E24.3
Actinic - *see* condition
Actinobacillosis, actinobacillus A28.8
  mallei A24.0
  muris A25.1
Actinomyces israelii (infection) - *see* Actinomycosis
Actinomycetoma (foot) B47.1
Actinomycosis, actinomycotic A42.9
  with pneumonia A42.0
  abdominal A42.1
  cervicofacial A42.2
  cutaneous A42.89
  gastrointestinal A42.1
  pulmonary A42.0
  sepsis A42.7
  specified site NEC A42.89
Actinoneuritis G62.82
Action, heart
  disorder I49.9
  irregular I49.9
    psychogenic F45.8
Activated protein C resistance D68.51
Activation
  mast cell (disorder) (syndrome) D89.40

Activation - *continued*
  idiopathic D89.42
  monoclonal D89.41
  secondary D89.43
  specified type NEC D89.49
Active - *see* condition
Acute - *see also* condition
  abdomen R10.0
  gallbladder - *see* Cholecystitis, acute
Acyanotic heart disease (congenital) Q24.9
Acystia Q64.5
Adair-Dighton syndrome (brittle bones and blue sclera, deafness) Q78.0
Adamantinoblastoma - *see* Ameloblastoma
Adamantinoma - *see also* Cyst, calcifying odontogenic
  long bones C40.90
    lower limb C40.2-
    upper limb C40.0-
  malignant C41.1
    jaw (bone) (lower) C41.1
    upper C41.0
  tibial C40.2-
Adamantoblastoma - *see* Ameloblastoma
Adams-stokes (-Morgagni) disease or syndrome I45.9
Adaption reaction - *see* Disorder, adjustment
Addiction - *see also* Dependence F19.20
  alcohol, alcoholic (ethyl) (methyl) (wood) (without remission) F10.20
    with remission F10.21
  drug - *see* Dependence, drug
  ethyl alcohol (without remission) F10.20
    with remission F10.21
  heroin - *see* Dependence, drug, opioid
  methyl alcohol (without remission) F10.20
    with remission F10.21
  methylated spirit (without remission) F10.20
    with remission F10.21
  morphine (-like substances) - *see* Dependence, drug, opioid
  nicotine - *see* Dependence, drug, nicotine
  opium and opioids - *see* Dependence, drug, opioid
  tobacco - *see* Dependence, drug, nicotine
Addisonian crisis E27.2
Addison's
  anemia (pernicious) D51.0
  disease (bronze) or syndrome E27.1
    tuberculous A18.7
  keloid L94.0
Addison-Biermer anemia (pernicious) D51.0
Addison-Schilder complex E71.528
Additional - *see also* Accessory
  chromosome(s) Q99.8
  sex - *see* Abnormal, chromosome, sex 21
- *see* Trisomy, 21
Adduction contracture, hip or other joint - *see* Contraction, joint
Adenitis - *see also* Lymphadenitis
  acute, unspecified site L04.9
  axillary I88.9
    acute L04.2
    chronic or subacute I88.1
  Bartholin's gland N75.8
  bulbourethral gland - *see* Urethritis
  cervical I88.9
    acute L04.0
    chronic or subacute I88.1
  chancroid (Hemophilus ducreyi) A57
  chronic, unspecified site I88.1
  Cowper's gland - *see* Urethritis

Adenitis - *continued*
  due to Pasteurella multocida (P. septica) A28.0
  epidemic, acute B27.09
  gangrenous L04.9
  gonorrheal NEC A54.89
  groin I88.9
    acute L04.1
    chronic or subacute I88.1
  infectious (acute) (epidemic) B27.09
  inguinal I88.9
    acute L04.1
    chronic or subacute I88.1
  lymph gland or node, except mesenteric I88.9
    acute - *see* Lymphadenitis, acute
    chronic or subacute I88.1
  mesenteric (acute) (chronic) (nonspecific)
    (subacute) I88.0
  parotid gland (suppurative) - *see* Sialoadenitis
  salivary gland (any) (suppurative) - *see*
    Sialoadenitis
  scrofulous (tuberculous) A18.2
  Skene's duct or gland - *see* Urethritis
  strumous, tuberculous A18.2
  subacute, unspecified site I88.1
  sublingual gland (suppurative) - *see*
    Sialoadenitis
  submandibular gland (suppurative) - *see*
  Sialoadenitis
  submaxillary gland (suppurative) - *see*
  Sialoadenitis
  tuberculous - *see* Tuberculosis, lymph gland
  urethral gland - *see* Urethritis
  Wharton's duct (suppurative) - *see*
    Sialoadenitis
Adenoacanthoma - *see* Neoplasm, malignant,
  by site
Adenoameloblastoma - *see* Cyst, calcifying
  odontogenic
Adenocarcinoid (tumor) - *see* Neoplasm,
  malignant, by site
Adenocarcinoma - *see also* Neoplasm,
  malignant, by site
  acidophil
    specified site - *see* Neoplasm, malignant, by
      site
    unspecified site C75.1
  adrenal cortical C74.0-
  alveolar - *see* Neoplasm, lung, malignant
  apocrine
    breast - *see* Neoplasm, breast, malignant
    in situ
      breast D05.8-
      specified site NEC - *see* Neoplasm, skin, in
        situ
      unspecified site D04.9
    specified site NEC - *see* Neoplasm, skin,
      malignant
    unspecified site C44.99
  basal cell
    specified site - *see* Neoplasm, skin, malignant
    unspecified site C08.9
  basophil
    specified site - *see* Neoplasm, malignant, by
      site
    unspecified site C75.1
  bile duct type C22.1
    liver C22.1
    specified site NEC - *see* Neoplasm,
      malignant, by site
    unspecified site C22.1
  bronchiolar - *see* Neoplasm, lung, malignant
  bronchioloalveolar - *see* Neoplasm, lung,
    malignant
  ceruminous C44.29-

Adenocarcinoma - *continued*
  cervix, in situ - *see also* Carcinoma, cervix
    uteri, in situ D06.9
  chromophobe
    specified site - *see* Neoplasm, malignant, by
      site
    unspecified site C75.1
  diffuse type
    specified site - *see* Neoplasm, malignant, by
      site
    unspecified site C16.9
  duct
    infiltrating
      with Paget's disease - *see* Neoplasm, breast,
        malignant
      specified site - *see* Neoplasm, malignant, by
        site
      unspecified site (female) C50.91-
        male C50.92-
    specified site - *see* Neoplasm, malignant,
      by site
    unspecified site
      female C56.9
      male C61
  eosinophil
    specified site - *see* Neoplasm, malignant, by
      site
    unspecified site C75.1
  follicular
    with papillary C73
    moderately differentiated C73
    specified site - *see* Neoplasm, malignant, by
      site
    trabecular C73
    unspecified site C73
    well differentiated C73
  Hürthle cell C73
  in
    adenomatous
      polyposis coli C18.9
  infiltrating duct
    with Paget's disease - *see* Neoplasm, breast,
      malignant
    specified site - *see* Neoplasm, by site,
      malignant
    unspecified site (female) C50.91-
      male C50.92-
  inflammatory
    specified site - *see* Neoplasm, by site,
      malignant
    unspecified site (female) C50.91-
      male C50.92-
  intestinal type
    specified site - *see* Neoplasm, by site,
      malignant
    unspecified site C16.9
  intracystic papillary
  intraductal
    breast D05.1-
    noninfiltrating
      breast D05.1-
      papillary
        with invasion
          specified site - *see* Neoplasm, by site,
            malignant
          unspecified site (female) C50.91-
            male C50.92-
        breast D05.1-
        specified site NEC - *see* Neoplasm, in situ,
          by site
        unspecified site D05.1-
    specified site NEC - *see* Neoplasm, in situ,
      by site
    unspecified site D05.1-

Adenocarcinoma - *continued*
  papillary
    with invasion
      specified site - *see* Neoplasm, malignant,
        by site
      unspecified site (female) C50.91-
        male C50.92-
    breast D05.1-
    specified site - *see* Neoplasm, in situ, by
      site
    unspecified site D05.1-
    specified site NEC - *see* Neoplasm, in situ,
      by site
    unspecified site D05.1-
  islet cell
    with exocrine, mixed
      specified site - *see* Neoplasm, malignant, by
        site
      unspecified site C25.9
    pancreas C25.4
    specified site NEC - *see* Neoplasm,
      malignant, by site
    unspecified site C25.4
  lobular
    in situ
      breast D05.0-
      specified site NEC - *see* Neoplasm, in situ,
        by site
      unspecified site D05.0-
    specified site - *see* Neoplasm, malignant, by
      site
    unspecified site (female) C50.91-
      male C50.92-
  mucoid - *see also* Neoplasm, malignant, by
    site
    cell
      specified site - *see* Neoplasm, malignant, by
        site
      unspecified site C75.1
  nonencapsulated sclerosing C73
  papillary
    with follicular C73
    follicular variant C73
    intraductal (noninfiltrating)
      with invasion
        specified site - *see* Neoplasm, malignant,
          by site
        unspecified site (female) C50.91-
          male C50.92-
      breast D05.1-
      specified site NEC - *see* Neoplasm, in situ,
        by site
      unspecified site D05.1-
    serous
      specified site - *see* Neoplasm, malignant, by
        site
      unspecified site C56.9
  papillocystic
    specified site - *see* Neoplasm, malignant, by
      site
    unspecified site C56.9
  pseudomucinous
    specified site - *see* Neoplasm, malignant, by
      site
    unspecified site C56.9
  renal cell C64-
  sebaceous - *see* Neoplasm, skin, malignant
  serous - *see also* Neoplasm, malignant, by site
    papillary
      specified site - *see* Neoplasm, malignant, by
        site
      unspecified site C56.9
  sweat gland - *see* Neoplasm, skin, malignant
  water-clear cell C75.0

Adenocarcinoma-in-situ - *see also* Neoplasm,
  in situ, by site
  breast D05.9-
Adenofibroma
  clear cell - *see* Neoplasm, benign, by site
  endometrioid D27.9
    borderline malignancy D39.10
    malignant C56-
  mucinous
    specified site - *see* Neoplasm, benign, by site
    unspecified site D27.9
  papillary
    specified site - *see* Neoplasm, benign, by site
    unspecified site D27.9
  prostate - *see* Enlargement, enlarged, prostate
  serous
    specified site - *see* Neoplasm, benign, by site
    unspecified site D27.9
  specified site - *see* Neoplasm, benign, by site
  unspecified site D27.9
Adenofibrosis
  breast - *see* Fibroadenosis, breast
  endometrioid N80.0
Adenoiditis (chronic) J35.02
  with tonsillitis J35.03
  acute J03.90
    recurrent J03.91
    specified organism NEC J03.80
      recurrent J03.81
    staphylococcal J03.80
      recurrent J03.81
    streptococcal J03.00
      recurrent J03.01
Adenoids - *see* condition
Adenolipoma - *see* Neoplasm, benign, by site
Adenolipomatosis, Launois-Bensaude E88.89
Adenolymphoma
  specified site - *see* Neoplasm, benign, by site
  unspecified site D11.9
Adenoma - *see also* Neoplasm, benign, by site
  acidophil
    specified site - *see* Neoplasm, benign, by site
    unspecified site D35.2
  acidophil-basophil, mixed
    specified site - *see* Neoplasm, benign, by site
    unspecified site D35.2
  adrenal (cortical) D35.00
    clear cell D35.00
    compact cell D35.00
    glomerulosa cell D35.00
    heavily pigmented variant D35.00
    mixed cell D35.00
  alpha-cell
    pancreas D13.7
    specified site NEC - *see* Neoplasm, benign,
      by site
    unspecified site D13.7
  alveolar D14.30
  apocrine
    breast D24-
    specified site NEC - *see* Neoplasm, skin,
      benign, by site
    unspecified site D23.9
  basal cell D11.9
  basophil
    specified site - *see* Neoplasm, benign, by site
    unspecified site D35.2
  basophil-acidophil, mixed
    specified site - *see* Neoplasm, benign, by site
    unspecified site D35.2
  beta-cell
    pancreas D13.7
    specified site NEC - *see* Neoplasm, benign,
      by site

Adenoma - *continued*
  unspecified site D13.7
  bile duct D13.4
    common D13.5
    extrahepatic D13.5
    intrahepatic D13.4
    specified site NEC - *see* Neoplasm, benign,
      by site
    unspecified site D13.4
  black D35.00
  bronchial D38.1
    cylindroid type - *see* Neoplasm, lung,
  malignant
  ceruminous D23.2-
  chief cell D35.1
  chromophobe
    specified site - *see* Neoplasm, benign, by site
    unspecified site D35.2
  colloid
    specified site - *see* Neoplasm, benign, by site
    unspecified site D34
  duct
  eccrine, papillary - *see* Neoplasm, skin, benign
  endocrine, multiple
    single specified site - *see* Neoplasm,
      uncertain behavior, by site
    two or more specified sites D44-
    unspecified site D44.9
  endometrioid - *see also* Neoplasm, benign
    borderline malignancy - *see* Neoplasm,
      uncertain behavior, by site
  eosinophil
    specified site - *see* Neoplasm, benign, by site
    unspecified site D35.2
  fetal
    specified site - *see* Neoplasm, benign, by site
    unspecified site D34
  follicular
    specified site - *see* Neoplasm, benign, by site
    unspecified site D34
  hepatocellular D13.4
  Hürthle cell D34
  islet cell
    pancreas D13.7
    specified site NEC - *see* Neoplasm, benign,
      by site
    unspecified site D13.7
  liver cell D13.4
  macrofollicular
    specified site - *see* Neoplasm, benign, by site
    unspecified site D34
  malignant, malignum - *see* Neoplasm,
    malignant, by site
  microcystic
    pancreas D13.6
    specified site NEC - *see* Neoplasm, benign,
      by site
    unspecified site D13.6
  microfollicular
    specified site - *see* Neoplasm, benign, by site
    unspecified site D34
  mucoid cell
    specified site - *see* Neoplasm, benign, by site
    unspecified site D35.2
  multiple endocrine
    single specified site - *see* Neoplasm,
      uncertain behavior, by site
    two or more specified sites D44-
    unspecified site D44.9
  nipple D24-
  papillary - *see also* Neoplasm, benign, by site
    eccrine - *see* Neoplasm, skin, benign, by site
  Pick's tubular
    specified site - *see* Neoplasm, benign, by site

Adenoma - *continued*
  unspecified site
    female D27.9
    male D29.20
  pleomorphic
    carcinoma in - *see* Neoplasm, salivary gland,
      malignant
      specified site - *see* Neoplasm, malignant, by
        site
    unspecified site C08.9
  polypoid - *see also* Neoplasm, benign
    adenocarcinoma in - *see* Neoplasm,
      malignant, by site
    adenocarcinoma in situ - *see* Neoplasm, in
      situ, by site
  prostate - *see* Neoplasm, benign, prostate
  rete cell D29.20
  sebaceous - *see* Neoplasm, skin, benign
  Sertoli cell
    specified site - *see* Neoplasm, benign, by site
    unspecified site
      female D27.9
      male D29.20
  skin appendage - *see* Neoplasm, skin, benign
  sudoriferous gland - *see* Neoplasm, skin,
    benign
  sweat gland - *see* Neoplasm, skin, benign
  testicular
    specified site - *see* Neoplasm, benign, by site
    unspecified site
      female D27.9
      male D29.20
  tubular - *see also* Neoplasm, benign, by site
    adenocarcinoma in - *see* Neoplasm,
      malignant, by site
    adenocarcinoma in situ - *see* Neoplasm, in
      situ, by site
  Pick's
    specified site - *see* Neoplasm, benign, by
      site
    unspecified site
      female D27.9
      male D29.20
  tubulovillous - *see also* Neoplasm, benign, by
    site
    adenocarcinoma in - *see* Neoplasm,
      malignant, by site
    adenocarcinoma in situ - *see* Neoplasm, in
      situ, by site
  villous - *see* Neoplasm, uncertain behavior, by
    site
    adenocarcinoma in - *see* Neoplasm,
      malignant, by site
    adenocarcinoma in situ - *see* Neoplasm, in
      situ, by site
  water-clear cell D35.1
Adenomatosis
  endocrine (multiple) E31.20
    single specified site - *see* Neoplasm,
      uncertain behavior, by site
  erosive of nipple D24-
  pluriendocrine - *see* Adenomatosis, endocrine
  pulmonary D38.1
    malignant - *see* Neoplasm, lung, malignant
  specified site - *see* Neoplasm, benign, by site
  unspecified site D12.6
Adenomatous
  goiter (nontoxic) E04.9
    with hyperthyroidism - *see* Hyperthyroidism,
      with, goiter, nodular
    toxic - *see* Hyperthyroidism, with, goiter,
  nodular
Adenomyoma - *see also* Neoplasm, benign, by
  site

Adenomyoma - *continued- continued*
 prostate - *see* Enlarged, prostate
Adenomyometritis N80.0
Adenomyosis N80.0
Adenopathy (lymph gland) R59.9
 generalized R59.1
 inguinal R59.0
 localized R59.0
 mediastinal R59.0
 mesentery R59.0
 syphilitic (secondary) A51.49
 tracheobronchial R59.0
  tuberculous A15.4
   primary (progressive) A15.7
 tuberculous - *see also* Tuberculosis, lymph
 gland
  tracheobronchial A15.4
   primary (progressive) A15.7
Adenosalpingitis - *see* Salpingitis
Adenosarcoma - *see* Neoplasm, malignant, by
site
Adenosclerosis I88.8
Adenosis (sclerosing) breast - *see*
Fibroadenosis, breast
**Adenovirus, as cause of disease classified
elsewhere** B97.0
Adentia (complete) (partial) - *see* Absence,
teeth
Adherent - *see also* Adhesions
 labia (minora) N90.89
 pericardium (nonrheumatic) I31.0
  rheumatic I09.2
 placenta (with hemorrhage) O72.0
  without hemorrhage O73.0
 prepuce, newborn N47.0
 scar (skin) L90.5
 tendon in scar L90.5
Adhesions, adhesive (postinfective) K66.0
 with intestinal obstruction K56.50
  complete K56.52
  incomplete K56.51
  partial K56.51
 abdominal (wall) - *see* Adhesions, peritoneum
 appendix K38.8
 bile duct (common) (hepatic) K83.8
 bladder (sphincter) N32.89
 bowel - *see* Adhesions, peritoneum
 cardiac I31.0
  rheumatic I09.2
 cecum - *see* Adhesions, peritoneum
 cervicovaginal N88.1
  congenital Q52.8
  postpartal O90.89
   old N88.1
 cervix N88.1
 ciliary body NEC - *see* Adhesions, iris
 clitoris N90.89
 colon - *see* Adhesions, peritoneum
 common duct K83.8
 congenital - *see also* Anomaly, by site
  fingers - *see* Syndactylism, complex, fingers
  omental, anomalous Q43.3
  peritoneal Q43.3
  tongue (to gum or roof of mouth) Q38.3
 conjunctiva (acquired) H11.21-
  congenital Q15.8
 cystic duct K82.8
 diaphragm - *see* Adhesions, peritoneum
 due to foreign body - *see* Foreign body
 duodenum - *see* Adhesions, peritoneum
 ear
  middle H74.1-
 epididymis N50.89

Adhesions, adhesive (postinfective) -
continued
 epidural - *see* Adhesions, meninges
 epiglottis J38.7
 eyelid H02.59
 female pelvis N73.6
 gallbladder K82.8
 globe H44.89
 heart I31.0
  rheumatic I09.2
 ileocecal (coil) - *see* Adhesions, peritoneum
 ileum - *see* Adhesions, peritoneum
 intestine - *see also* Adhesions, peritoneum
  with obstruction K56.50
   complete K56.52
   incomplete K56.51
   partial K56.51
 intra-abdominal - *see* Adhesions, peritoneum
 iris H21.50-
  anterior H21.51-
  goniosynechiae H21.52-
  posterior H21.54-
  to corneal graft T85.898
 joint - *see* Ankylosis
  knee M23.8X
  temporomandibular M26.61-
 labium (majus) (minus), congenital Q52.5
 liver - *see* Adhesions, peritoneum
 lung J98.4
 mediastinum J98.59
 meninges (cerebral) (spinal) G96.12
  congenital Q07.8
  tuberculous (cerebral) (spinal) A17.0
 mesenteric - *see* Adhesions, peritoneum
 nasal (septum) (to turbinates) J34.89
 ocular muscle - *see* Strabismus, mechanical
 omentum - *see* Adhesions, peritoneum
 ovary N73.6
  congenital (to cecum, kidney or omentum)
  Q50.39
 paraovarian N73.6
 pelvic (peritoneal)
  female N73.6
   postprocedural N99.4
  male - *see* Adhesions, peritoneum
  postpartal (old) N73.6
  tuberculous A18.17
 penis to scrotum (congenital) Q55.8
 periappendiceal - *see also* Adhesions,
  peritoneum
 pericardium (nonrheumatic) I31.0
  focal I31.8
  rheumatic I09.2
  tuberculous A18.84
 pericholecystic K82.8
 perigastric - *see* Adhesions, peritoneum
 periovarian N73.6
 periprostatic N42.89
 perirectal - *see* Adhesions, peritoneum
 perirenal N28.89
 peritoneum, peritoneal (postinfective)
  with obstruction (intestinal) K56.50
   complete K56.52
   incomplete K56.51
   partial K56.51
  congenital Q43.3
  pelvic, female N73.6
   postprocedural N99.4
  postpartal, pelvic N73.6
  postprocedural K66.0
  to uterus N73.6
 peritubal N73.6
 periureteral N28.89
 periuterine N73.6

Adhesions, adhesive (postinfective) -
continued
 perivesical N32.89
 perivesicular (seminal vesicle) N50.89
 pleura, pleuritic J94.8
  tuberculous NEC A15.6
 pleuropericardial J94.8
 postoperative (gastrointestinal tract) K66.0
  due to foreign body accidentally left in
   wound - *see* Foreign body, accidentally left
   during a procedure
  pelvic peritoneal N99.4
  urethra - *see* Stricture, urethra,
   postprocedural
  vagina N99.2
  with obstruction (see also Obstruction,
  intestine, postoperative) K91.30
 postpartal, old (vulva or perineum) N90.89
 preputial, prepuce N47.5
 pulmonary J98.4
 pylorus - *see* Adhesions, peritoneum
 sciatic nerve - *see* Lesion, nerve, sciatic
 seminal vesicle N50.89
 shoulder (joint) - *see* Capsulitis, adhesive
 sigmoid flexure - *see* Adhesions, peritoneum
 spermatic cord (acquired) N50.89
  congenital Q55.4
 spinal canal G96.12
 stomach - *see* Adhesions, peritoneum
 subscapular - *see* Capsulitis, adhesive
 temporomandibular M26.61-
 tendinitis - *see also* Tenosynovitis, specified
  type NEC
  shoulder - *see* Capsulitis, adhesive
 testis N44.8
 tongue, congenital (to gum or roof of mouth)
  Q38.3
  acquired K14.8
 trachea J39.8
 tubo-ovarian N73.6
 tunica vaginalis N44.8
 uterus N73.6
  internal N85.6
  to abdominal wall N73.6
 vagina (chronic) N89.5
  postoperative N99.2
 vitreomacular H43.82-
 vitreous H43.89
 vulva N90.89
Adiaspiromycosis B48.8
Adie (-Holmes) pupil or syndrome - *see*
Anomaly, pupil, function, tonic pupil
Adiponecrosis neonatorum P83.88
Adiposis - *see also* Obesity cerebralis E23.6
 dolorosa E88.2
Adiposity - *see also* Obesity
 heart - *see* Degeneration, myocardial
 localized E65
Adiposogenital dystrophy E23.6
Adjustment
 disorder - *see* Disorder, adjustment
 implanted device - *see* Encounter (for),
  adjustment (of)
 prosthesis, external - *see* Fitting
 reaction - *see* Disorder, adjustment
**Administration of tPA (rtPA) in a different
facility within the last 24 hours prior to
admission to current facility** Z92.82
Admission (for) - *see also* Encounter (for)
 adjustment (of)
  artificial
   arm Z44.00-
    complete Z44.01-
    partial Z44.02-

Admission (for) - *continued*
  eye Z44.2
  leg Z44.10-
    complete Z44.11-
    partial Z44.12-
  brain neuropacemaker Z46.2
    implanted Z45.42
  breast
    implant Z45.81
    prosthesis (external) Z44.3
  colostomy belt Z46.89
  contact lenses Z46.0
  cystostomy device Z46.6
  dental prosthesis Z46.3
  device NEC
    abdominal Z46.89
    implanted Z45.89
      cardiac Z45.09
        defibrillator (with synchronous cardiac pacemaker) Z45.02
        pacemaker (cardiac resynchronization therapy (CRT-p)) Z45.018
          pulse generator Z45.010
        resynchronization therapy defibrillator (CRT-d) Z45.02
      hearing device Z45.328
        bone conduction Z45.320
        cochlear Z45.321
      infusion pump Z45.1
      nervous system Z45.49
        CSF drainage Z45.41
        hearing device - *see* Admission, adjustment, device, implanted, hearing device
        neuropacemaker Z45.42
        visual substitution Z45.31
      specified NEC Z45.89
      vascular access Z45.2
      visual substitution Z45.31
    nervous system Z46.2
      implanted - *see* Admission, adjustment, device, implanted, nervous system
    orthodontic Z46.4
    prosthetic Z44.9
      arm - *see* Admission, adjustment, artificial, arm
      breast Z44.3
      dental Z46.3
      eye Z44.2
      leg - *see* Admission, adjustment, artificial, leg
      specified type NEC Z44.8
    substitution
      auditory Z46.2
        implanted - *see* Admission, adjustment, device, implanted, hearing device
      nervous system Z46.2
        implanted - *see* Admission, adjustment, device, implanted, nervous system
      visual Z46.2
        implanted Z45.31
      urinary Z46.6
  hearing aid Z46.1
    implanted - *see* Admission, adjustment, device, implanted, hearing device
  ileostomy device Z46.89
  intestinal appliance or device NEC Z46.89
  neuropacemaker (brain) (peripheral nerve) (spinal cord) Z46.2
    implanted Z45.42
  orthodontic device Z46.4
  orthopedic (brace) (cast) (device) (shoes) Z46.89
  pacemaker (cardiac resynchronization

Admission (for) - *continued*
  therapy (CRT-p))
    cardiac Z45.018
      pulse generator Z45.010
    nervous system Z46.2
      implanted Z45.42
  portacath (port-a-cath) Z45.2
  prosthesis Z44.9
    arm - *see* Admission, adjustment, artificial, arm
    breast Z44.3
    dental Z46.3
    eye Z44.2
    leg - *see* Admission, adjustment, artificial, leg
    specified NEC Z44.8
  spectacles Z46.0
aftercare - *see also* Aftercare Z51.89
  postpartum
    immediately after delivery Z39.0
    routine follow-up Z39.2
  radiation therapy (antineoplastic) Z51.0
attention to artificial opening (of) Z43.9
  artificial vagina Z43.7
  colostomy Z43.3
  cystostomy Z43.5
  enterostomy Z43.4
  gastrostomy Z43.1
  ileostomy Z43.2
  jejunostomy Z43.4
  nephrostomy Z43.6
  specified site NEC Z43.8
    intestinal tract Z43.4
    urinary tract Z43.6
  tracheostomy Z43.0
  ureterostomy Z43.6
  urethrostomy Z43.6
breast augmentation or reduction Z41.1
breast reconstruction following mastectomy Z42.1
change of
  dressing (nonsurgical) Z48.00
  neuropacemaker device (brain) (peripheral nerve) (spinal cord) Z46.2
    implanted Z45.42
  surgical dressing Z48.01
circumcision, ritual or routine (in absence of diagnosis) Z41.2
clinical research investigation (control) (normal comparison) (participant) Z00.6
contraceptive management Z30.9
cosmetic surgery NEC Z41.1
counseling - *see also* Counseling
  dietary Z71.3
  gestational carrier Z31.7
  HIV Z71.7
  human immunodeficiency virus Z71.7
  nonattending third party Z71.0
  procreative management NEC Z31.69
delivery, full-term, uncomplicated O80
  cesarean, without indication O82
desensitization to allergens Z51.6
dietary surveillance and counseling Z71.3
ear piercing Z41.3
examination at health care facility (adult) - *see also* Examination Z00.00
  with abnormal findings Z00.01
  clinical research investigation (control) (normal comparison) (participant) Z00.6
  dental Z01.20
    with abnormal findings Z01.21
  donor (potential) Z00.5
  ear Z01.10
    with abnormal findings NEC Z01.118

Admission (for) - *continued*
  eye Z01.00
    with abnormal findings Z01.01
  general, specified reason NEC Z00.8
  hearing Z01.10
    with abnormal findings NEC Z01.118
  postpartum checkup Z39.2
  psychiatric (general) Z00.8
    requested by authority Z04.6
  vision Z01.00
    with abnormal findings Z01.01
fitting (of)
  artificial
    arm - *see* Admission, adjustment, artificial, arm
    eye Z44.2
    leg - *see* Admission, adjustment, artificial, leg
  brain neuropacemaker Z46.2
    implanted Z45.42
  breast prosthesis (external) Z44.3
  colostomy belt Z46.89
  contact lenses Z46.0
  cystostomy device Z46.6
  dental prosthesis Z46.3
  dentures Z46.3
  device NEC
    abdominal Z46.89
    nervous system Z46.2
      implanted - *see* Admission, adjustment, device, implanted, nervous system
    orthodontic Z46.4
    prosthetic Z44.9
      breast Z44.3
      dental Z46.3
      eye Z44.2
    substitution
      auditory Z46.2
        implanted - *see* Admission, adjustment, device, implanted, hearing device
      nervous system Z46.2
        implanted - *see* Admission, adjustment, device, implanted, nervous system
      visual Z46.2
        implanted Z45.31
  hearing aid Z46.1
  ileostomy device Z46.89
  intestinal appliance or device NEC Z46.89
  neuropacemaker (brain) (peripheral nerve) (spinal cord) Z46.2
    implanted Z45.42
  orthodontic device Z46.4
  orthopedic device (brace) (cast) (shoes) Z46.89
  prosthesis Z44.9
    arm - *see* Admission, adjustment, artificial, arm
    breast Z44.3
    dental Z46.3
    eye Z44.2
    leg - *see* Admission, adjustment, artificial, leg
    specified type NEC Z44.8
  spectacles Z46.0
follow-up examination Z09
intrauterine device management Z30.431
  initial prescription Z30.014
mental health evaluation Z00.8
  requested by authority Z04.6
observation - *see* Observation
Papanicolaou smear, cervix Z12.4
  for suspected malignant neoplasm Z12.4
plastic and reconstructive surgery following medical procedure or healed injury NEC

Admission (for) - *continued*
Z42.8
plastic surgery, cosmetic NEC Z41.1
postpartum observation
immediately after delivery Z39.0
routine follow-up Z39.2
poststerilization (for restoration) Z31.0
aftercare Z31.42
procreative management Z31.9
prophylactic (measure) - *see also* Encounter,
prophylactic measures
organ removal Z40.00
breast Z40.01
fallopian tube(s) Z40.03
with ovary(s) Z40.02
ovary(s) Z40.02
specified organ NEC Z40.09
testes Z40.09
vaccination Z23
psychiatric examination (general) Z00.8
requested by authority Z04.6
radiation therapy (antineoplastic) Z51.0
reconstructive surgery following medical
procedure or healed injury NEC Z42.8
removal of
cystostomy catheter Z43.5
drains Z48.03
dressing (nonsurgical) Z48.00
implantable subdermal contraceptive Z30.46
intrauterine contraceptive device Z30.432
neuropacemaker (brain) (peripheral nerve)
(spinal cord) Z46.2
implanted Z45.42
staples Z48.02
surgical dressing Z48.01
sutures Z48.02
ureteral stent Z46.6
respirator [ventilator] use during power failure
Z99.12
restoration of organ continuity
(poststerilization) Z31.0
aftercare Z31.42
sensitivity test - *see also* Test, skin
allergy NEC Z01.82
Mantoux Z11.1
tuboplasty following previous sterilization
Z31.0
aftercare Z31.42
vasoplasty following previous sterilization
Z31.0
aftercare Z31.42
vision examination Z01.00
with abnormal findings Z01.01
waiting period for admission to other facility
Z75.1
Adnexitis (suppurative) - *see* Salpingo-
oophoritis
Adolescent X-linked adrenoleukodystrophy
E71.521
Adrenal (gland) - *see* condition
Adrenalism, tuberculous A18.7
Adrenalitis, adrenitis E27.8
autoimmune E27.1
meningococcal, hemorrhagic A39.1
Adrenarche, premature E27.0
Adrenocortical syndrome - *see* Cushing's,
syndrome
Adrenogenital syndrome E25.9
acquired E25.8
congenital E25.0
salt loss E25.0
Adrenogenitalism, congenital E25.0
Adrenoleukodystrophy E71.529
neonatal E71.511

Adrenoleukodystrophy - *continued*
X-linked E71.529
Addison only phenotype E71.528
Addison-Schilder E71.528
adolescent E71.521
adrenomyeloneuropathy E71.522
childhood cerebral E71.520
other specified E71.528
Adrenomyeloneuropathy E71.522
Adventitious bursa - *see* Bursopathy, specified
type NEC
Adverse effect - *see* Table of Drugs and
Chemicals, categories T36-t50, with 6th
character 5
Advice - *see* Counseling
Adynamia (episodica) (hereditary) (periodic)
G72.3
Aeration lung imperfect, newborn - *see*
Atelectasis
Aerobullosis T70.3
Aerocele - *see* Embolism, air
Aerodermectasia
subcutaneous (traumatic) T79.7
Aerodontalgia T70.29
Aeroembolism T70.3
Aerogenes capsulatus infection A48.0
Aero-otitis media T70.0
Aerophagy, aerophagia (psychogenic) F45.8
Aerophobia F40.228
Aerosinusitis T70.1
Aerotitis T70.0
Affection - *see* Disease
Afibrinogenemia - *see also* Defect, coagulation
D68.8
acquired D65
congenital D68.2
following ectopic or molar pregnancy O08.1
in abortion - *see* Abortion, by type,
complicated by, afibrinogenemia
puerperal O72.3
African
sleeping sickness B56.9
tick fever A68.1
trypanosomiasis B56.9
Gambian B56.0
Rhodesian B56.1
Aftercare - *see also* Care Z51.89
following surgery (for) (on)
amputation Z47.81
attention to
drains Z48.03
dressings (nonsurgical) Z48.00
surgical Z48.01
sutures Z48.02
circulatory system Z48.812
delayed (planned) wound closure Z48.1
digestive system Z48.815
explantation of joint prosthesis (staged
procedure)
hip Z47.32
knee Z47.33
shoulder Z47.31
genitourinary system Z48.816
joint replacement Z47.1
neoplasm Z48.3
nervous system Z48.811
oral cavity Z48.814
organ transplant
bone marrow Z48.290
heart Z48.21
heart-lung Z48.280
kidney Z48.22
liver Z48.23

Aftercare - *continued*
lung Z48.24
multiple organs NEC Z48.288
specified NEC Z48.298
orthopedic NEC Z47.89
planned wound closure Z48.1
removal of internal fixation device Z47.2
respiratory system Z48.813
scoliosis Z47.82
sense organs Z48.810
skin and subcutaneous tissue Z48.817
specified body system
circulatory Z48.812
digestive Z48.815
genitourinary Z48.816
nervous Z48.811
oral cavity Z48.814
respiratory Z48.813
sense organs Z48.810
skin and subcutaneous tissue Z48.817
teeth Z48.814
specified NEC Z48.89
spinal Z47.89
teeth Z48.814
fracture
code to fracture with seventh character D
involving
removal of
drains Z48.03
dressings (nonsurgical) Z48.00
staples Z48.02
surgical dressings Z48.01
sutures Z48.02
neuropacemaker (brain) (peripheral nerve)
(spinal cord) Z46.2
implanted Z45.42
orthopedic NEC Z47.89
postprocedural - *see* Aftercare, following
surgery
After-cataract - *see* Cataract, secondary
Agalactia (primary) O92.3
elective, secondary or therapeutic O92.5
Agammaglobulinemia (acquired (secondary))
(nonfamilial) D80.1
with
immunoglobulin-bearing B-lymphocytes
D80.1
lymphopenia D81.9
autosomal recessive (Swiss type) D80.0
Bruton's X-linked D80.0
common variable (CVA gamma) D80.1
congenital sex-linked D80.0
hereditary D80.0
lymphopenic D81.9
Swiss type (autosomal recessive) D80.0
X-linked (with growth hormone deficiency)
(Bruton) D80.0
Aganglionosis (bowel) (colon) Q43.1
Age (old) - *see* Senility
Agenesis
adrenal (gland) Q89.1
alimentary tract (complete) (partial) NEC
Q45.8
upper Q40.8
anus, anal (canal) Q42.3
with fistula Q42.2
aorta Q25.41
appendix Q42.8
arm (complete) Q71.0-
with hand present Q71.1-
artery (peripheral) Q27.9
brain Q28.3
coronary Q24.5
pulmonary Q25.79

Agenesis - *continued*
  specified NEC Q27.8
  umbilical Q27.0
  auditory (canal) (external) Q16.1
  auricle (ear) Q16.0
  bile duct or passage Q44.5
  bladder Q64.5
  bone Q79.9
  brain Q00.0
    part of Q04.3
  breast (with nipple present) Q83.8
    with absent nipple Q83.0
  bronchus Q32.4
  canaliculus lacrimalis Q10.4
  carpus - *see* Agenesis, hand
  cartilage Q79.9
  cecum Q42.8
  cerebellum Q04.3
  cervix Q51.5
  chin Q18.8
  cilia Q10.3
  circulatory system, part NOS Q28.9
  clavicle Q74.0
  clitoris Q52.6
  coccyx Q76.49
  colon Q42.9
    specified NEC Q42.8
  corpus callosum Q04.0
  cricoid cartilage Q31.8
  diaphragm (with hernia) Q79.1
  digestive organ(s) or tract (complete) (partial)
    NEC Q45.8
    upper Q40.8
  ductus arteriosus Q28.8
  duodenum Q41.0
  ear Q16.9
    auricle Q16.0
    lobe Q17.8
  ejaculatory duct Q55.4
  endocrine (gland) NEC Q89.2
  epiglottis Q31.8
  esophagus Q39.8
  eustachian tube Q16.2
  eye Q11.1
    adnexa Q15.8
  eyelid (fold) Q10.3
  face
    bones NEC Q75.8
    specified part NEC Q18.8
  fallopian tube Q50.6
  femur - *see* Defect, reduction, lower limb,
    longitudinal, femur
  fibula - *see* Defect, reduction, lower limb,
    longitudinal, fibula
  finger (complete) (partial) - *see* Agenesis, hand
  foot (and toes) (complete) (partial) Q72.3-
  forearm (with hand present) - *see* Agenesis,
    arm, with hand present
    and hand Q71.2-
  gallbladder Q44.0
  gastric Q40.2
  genitalia, genital (organ(s))
    female Q52.8
      external Q52.71
      internal NEC Q52.8
    male Q55.8
  glottis Q31.8
  hair Q84.0
  hand (and fingers) (complete) (partial) Q71.3-
  heart Q24.8
    valve NEC Q24.8
      pulmonary Q22.0
  hepatic Q44.7
  humerus - *see* Defect, reduction, upper limb

Agenesis - *continued*
  hymen Q52.4
  ileum Q41.2
  incus Q16.3
  intestine (small) Q41.9
    large Q42.9
      specified NEC Q42.8
  iris (dilator fibers) Q13.1
  jaw M26.09
  jejunum Q41.1
  kidney(s) (partial) Q60.2
    bilateral Q60.1
    unilateral Q60.0
  labium (majus) (minus) Q52.71
  labyrinth, membranous Q16.5
  lacrimal apparatus Q10.4
  larynx Q31.8
  leg (complete) Q72.0-
    with foot present Q72.1-
    lower leg (with foot present) - *see* Agenesis,
      leg, with foot present
      and foot Q72.2-
  lens Q12.3
  limb (complete) Q73.0
    lower - *see* Agenesis, leg
    upper - *see* Agenesis, arm
  lip Q38.0
  liver Q44.7
  lung (fissure) (lobe) (bilateral) (unilateral)
    Q33.3
  mandible, maxilla M26.09
  metacarpus - *see* Agenesis, hand
  metatarsus - *see* Agenesis, foot
  muscle Q79.8
    eyelid Q10.3
    ocular Q15.8
  musculoskeletal system NEC Q79.8
  nail(s) Q84.3
  neck, part Q18.8
  nerve Q07.8
  nervous system, part NEC Q07.8
  nipple Q83.2
  nose Q30.1
  nuclear Q07.8
  organ
    of Corti Q16.5
    or site not listed - *see* Anomaly, by site
  osseous meatus (ear) Q16.1
  ovary
    bilateral Q50.02
    unilateral Q50.01
  oviduct Q50.6
  pancreas Q45.0
  parathyroid (gland) Q89.2
  parotid gland(s) Q38.4
  patella Q74.1
  pelvic girdle (complete) (partial) Q74.2
  penis Q55.5
  pericardium Q24.8
  pituitary (gland) Q89.2
  prostate Q55.4
  punctum lacrimale Q10.4
  radioulnar - *see* Defect, reduction, upper limb
  radius - *see* Defect, reduction, upper limb,
    longitudinal, radius
  rectum Q42.1
    with fistula Q42.0
  renal Q60.2
    bilateral Q60.1
    unilateral Q60.0
  respiratory organ NEC Q34.8
  rib Q76.6
  roof of orbit Q75.8
  round ligament Q52.8

Agenesis - *continued*
  sacrum Q76.49
  salivary gland Q38.4
  scapula Q74.0
  scrotum Q55.29
  seminal vesicles Q55.4
  septum
    atrial Q21.1
    between aorta and pulmonary artery Q21.4
    ventricular Q20.4
  shoulder girdle (complete) (partial) Q74.0
  skull (bone) Q75.8
    with
      anencephaly Q00.0
      encephalocele - *see* Encephalocele
      hydrocephalus Q03.9
        with spina bifida - *see* Spina bifida, by
          site, with hydrocephalus
      microcephaly Q02
  spermatic cord Q55.4
  spinal cord Q06.0
  spine Q76.49
  spleen Q89.01
  sternum Q76.7
  stomach Q40.2
  submaxillary gland(s) (congenital) Q38.4
  tarsus - *see* Agenesis, foot
  tendon Q79.8
  testicle Q55.0
  thymus (gland) Q89.2
  thyroid (gland) E03.1
    cartilage Q31.8
  tibia - *see* Defect, reduction, lower limb,
    longitudinal, tibia
  tibiofibular - *see* Defect, reduction, lower limb,
    specified type NEC
  toe (and foot) (complete) (partial) - *see*
    Agenesis, foot
  tongue Q38.3
  trachea (cartilage) Q32.1
  ulna - *see* Defect, reduction, upper limb,
    longitudinal, ulna
  upper limb - *see* Agenesis, arm
  ureter Q62.4
  urethra Q64.5
  urinary tract NEC Q64.8
  uterus Q51.0
  uvula Q38.5
  vagina Q52.0
  vas deferens Q55.4
  vein(s) (peripheral) Q27.9
    brain Q28.3
    great NEC Q26.8
    portal Q26.5
  vena cava (inferior) (superior) Q26.8
  vermis of cerebellum Q04.3
  vertebra Q76.49
  vulva Q52.71
Ageusia R43.2
Agitated - *see* condition **Agitation** R45.1
Aglossia (congenital) Q38.3
Aglossia-adactylia syndrome Q87.0
Aglycogenosis E74.00
Agnosia (body image) (other senses) (tactile)
  R48.1
  developmental F88
  verbal R48.1
    auditory R48.1
      developmental F80.2
  developmental F80.2
  visual (object) R48.3
Agoraphobia F40.00
  with panic disorder F40.01
  without panic disorder F40.02

Agrammatism R48.8
Agranulocytopenia - *see* Agranulocytosis
Agranulocytosis (chronic) (cyclical) (genetic)
(infantile) (periodic) (pernicious) - *see also*
Neutropenia D70.9
congenital D70.0
cytoreductive cancer chemotherapy sequela
D70.1
drug-induced D70.2
due to cytoreductive cancer chemotherapy
D70.1
due to infection D70.3
secondary D70.4
drug-induced D70.2
due to cytoreductive cancer chemotherapy
D70.1
Agraphia (absolute) R48.8
with alexia R48.0
developmental F81.81
Ague (dumb) - *see* Malaria
Agyria Q04.3
Ahumada-del Castillo syndrome E23.0
Aichmophobia F40.298
AIDS (related complex) B20
Ailment heart - *see* Disease, heart
Ailurophobia F40.218
Ainhum (disease) L94.6
AIN - *see* Neoplasia, intraepithelial, anal
AIPHI (acute idiopathic pulmonary
hemorrhage in infants (over 28 days old))
R04.81
Air
anterior mediastinum J98.2
compressed, disease T70.3
conditioner lung or pneumonitis J67.7
embolism (artery) (cerebral) (any site) T79.0
with ectopic or molar pregnancy O08.2
due to implanted device NEC - *see*
Complications, by site and type, specified
NEC
following
abortion - *see* Abortion by type,
complicated by, embolism
ectopic or molar pregnancy O08.2
infusion, therapeutic injection or transfusion
T80.0
in pregnancy, childbirth or puerperium - *see*
Embolism, obstetric
traumatic T79.0
hunger, psychogenic F45.8
rarefied, effects of - *see* Effect, adverse, high
altitude
sickness T75.3
Airplane sickness T75.3
Akathisia (drug-induced) (treatment-
induced) G25.71
neuroleptic induced (acute) G25.71
tardive G25.71
Akinesia R29.898
Akinetic mutism R41.89
Akureyri's disease G93.3
Alactasia, congenital E73.0
Alagille's syndrome Q44.7
Alastrim B03
Albers-Schonberg syndrome Q78.2
Albert's syndrome - *see* Tendinitis, Achilles
Albinism, albino E70.30
with hematologic abnormality E70.339
Chédiak-Higashi syndrome E70.330
Hermansky-Pudlak syndrome E70.331
other specified E70.338
I E70.320
II E70.321
ocular E70.319

Albinism, albino - *continued*
autosomal recessive E70.311
other specified E70.318
X-linked E70.310
oculocutaneous E70.329
other specified E70.328
tyrosinase (ty) negative E70.320
tyrosinase (ty) positive E70.321
other specified E70.39
Albinismus E70.30
Albright (-McCune)(-Sternberg) syndrome
Q78.1
Albuminous - *see* condition
Albuminuria, albuminuric (acute) (chronic)
(subacute) - *see also* Proteinuria R80.9
complicating pregnancy - *see* Proteinuria,
gestational
with
gestational hypertension - *see* Pre-
eclampsia
pre-existing hypertension - *see*
Hypertension, complicating pregnancy, pre-
existing, with, pre-eclampsia
gestational - *see* Proteinuria, gestational
with
gestational hypertension - *see* Pre-
eclampsia
pre-existing hypertension - *see*
Hypertension, complicating pregnancy, pre-
existing, with, pre-eclampsia
orthostatic R80.2
postural R80.2
pre-eclamptic - *see* Pre-eclampsia
scarlatinal A38.8
Albuminurophobia F40.298
Alcaptonuria E70.29
Alcohol, alcoholic, alcohol-induced addiction
(without remission) F10.20
with remission F10.21
amnestic disorder, persisting F10.96
with dependence F10.26
anxiety disorder F10.980
bipolar and related disorder F10.94
depressive disorder F10.94
major neurocognitive disorder, amnestic-
confabulatory type F10.96
major neurocognitive disorder, non-amnestic-
confabulatory type F10.97
mild neurocognitive disorder F10.988
psychotic disorder F10.959
sexual dysfunction F10.981
sleep disorder F10.982
brain syndrome, chronic F10.97
with dependence F10.27
cardiopathy I42.6
counseling and surveillance Z71.41
family member Z71.42
delirium (acute) (tremens) (withdrawal)
F10.231
with intoxication F10.921
in
abuse F10.121
dependence F10.221
dementia F10.97
with dependence F10.27
deterioration F10.97
with dependence F10.27
hallucinosis (acute) F10.951
in
abuse F10.151
dependence F10.251
insanity F10.959
intoxication (acute) (without dependence)
F10.129

Alcohol, alcoholic, alcohol - *continued*
with
delirium F10.121
dependence F10.229
with delirium F10.221
uncomplicated F10.220
uncomplicated F10.120
jealousy F10.988
Korsakoff's, Korsakov's, Korsakow's F10.26
liver K70.9
acute - *see* Disease, liver, alcoholic, hepatitis
mania (acute) (chronic) F10.959
paranoia, paranoid (type) psychosis F10.950
pellagra E52
poisoning, accidental (acute) NEC - *see* Table
of Drugs and Chemicals, alcohol, poisoning
psychosis - *see* Psychosis, alcoholic
withdrawal (without convulsions) F10.239
with delirium F10.231
Alcoholism (chronic) (without remission)
F10.20
with
psychosis - *see* Psychosis, alcoholic
remission F10.21
Korsakov's F10.96
with dependence F10.26
Alder (-Reilly) anomaly or syndrome
(leukocyte granulation) D72.0
Aldosteronism E26.9
familial (type I) E26.02
glucocorticoid-remediable E26.02
primary (due to (bilateral) adrenal hyperplasia)
E26.09
primary NEC E26.09
secondary E26.1
specified NEC E26.89
Aldosteronoma D44.10
Aldrich (-Wiskott) syndrome (eczema-
thrombocytopenia) D82.0
Alektorophobia F40.218
Aleppo boil B55.1
Aleukemic - *see* condition
Aleukia
congenital D70.0
hemorrhagica D61.9
congenital D61.09
splenica D73.1
Alexia R48.0
developmental F81.0
secondary to organic lesion R48.0
Algoneurodystrophy M89.00
ankle M89.07-
foot M89.07-
forearm M89.03-
hand M89.04-
Algoneurodystrophy - *continued*
lower leg M89.06-
multiple sites M89.0-
shoulder M89.01-
specified site NEC M89.08
thigh M89.05-
upper arm M89.02-
Algophobia F40.298
Alienation, mental - *see* Psychosis
Alkalemia E87.3
Alkalosis E87.3
metabolic E87.3
with respiratory acidosis E87.4
respiratory E87.3
Alkaptonuria E70.29
Allen-masters syndrome N83.8
Allergy, allergic (reaction) (to) T78.40
air-borne substance NEC (rhinitis) J30.89
alveolitis (extrinsic) J67.9

Allergy, allergic (reaction) (to) - *continued*
due to
Aspergillus clavatus J67.4
Cryptostroma corticale J67.6
organisms (fungal, thermophilic actinomycete) growing in ventilation (air conditioning) systems J67.7
specified type NEC J67.8
anaphylactic reaction or shock T78.2
angioneurotic edema T78.3
animal (dander) (epidermal) (hair) (rhinitis) J30.81
bee sting (anaphylactic shock) - *see* Toxicity, venom, arthropod, bee
biological - *see* Allergy, drug
colitis - *see also* Colitis, allergic K52.29
dander (animal) (rhinitis) J30.81
dandruff (rhinitis) J30.81
dental restorative material (existing) K08.55
dermatitis - *see* Dermatitis, contact, allergic
diathesis - *see* History, allergy
drug, medicament & biological (any) (external) (internal) T78.40
correct substance properly administered - *see* Table of Drugs and Chemicals, by drug, adverse effect
wrong substance given or taken NEC (by accident) - *see* Table of Drugs and Chemicals, by drug, poisoning
due to pollen J30.1
dust (house) (stock) (rhinitis) J30.89
with asthma - *see* Asthma, allergic extrinsic
eczema - *see* Dermatitis, contact, allergic
epidermal (animal) (rhinitis) J30.81
feathers (rhinitis) J30.89
food (any) (ingested) NEC T78.1
anaphylactic shock - *see* Shock, anaphylactic, due to food
dermatitis - *see* Dermatitis, due to, food
dietary counseling and surveillance Z71.3
in contact with skin L23.6
rhinitis J30.5
status (without reaction) Z91.018
eggs Z91.012
milk products Z91.011
peanuts Z91.010
seafood Z91.013
specified NEC Z91.018
gastrointestinal - *see also* specific type of allergic reaction
meaning colitis - *see also* Colitis, allergic K52.29
meaning gastroenteritis - *see also* Gastroenteritis, allergic K52.29
meaning other adverse food reaction not elsewhere classified T78.1
grain J30.1
grass (hay fever) (pollen) J30.1
asthma - *see* Asthma, allergic extrinsic
hair (animal) (rhinitis) J30.81
history (of) - *see* History, allergy
horse serum - *see* Allergy, serum
inhalant (rhinitis) J30.89
pollen J30.1
kapok (rhinitis) J30.89
medicine - *see* Allergy, drug
milk protein - *see also* Allergy, food Z91.011
anaphylactic reaction T78.07
dermatitis L27.2
enterocolitis syndrome K52.21
enteropathy K52.22
gastroenteritis K52.29
gastroesophageal reflux - *see also* Reaction, adverse, food K21.9

Allergy, allergic (reaction) (to) - *continued*
with esophagitis K21.0
proctocolitis K52.82
nasal, seasonal due to pollen J30.1
pneumonia J82
pollen (any) (hay fever) J30.1
asthma - *see* Asthma, allergic extrinsic
primrose J30.1
primula J30.1
proctocolitis K52.82
purpura D69.0
ragweed (hay fever) (pollen) J30.1
asthma - *see* Asthma, allergic extrinsic
rose (pollen) J30.1
seasonal NEC J30.2
Senecio jacobae (pollen) J30.1
serum - *see also* Reaction, serum T80.69
anaphylactic shock T80.59
shock (anaphylactic) T78.2
due to
administration of blood and blood products T80.51
adverse effect of correct medicinal substance properly administered T88.6
immunization T80.52
serum NEC T80.59
vaccination T80.52
specific NEC T78.49
tree (any) (hay fever) (pollen) J30.1
asthma - *see* Asthma, allergic extrinsic
upper respiratory J30.9
urticaria L50.0
vaccine - *see* Allergy, serum
wheat - *see* Allergy, food
Allescheriasis B48.2
Alligator skin disease Q80.9
Allocheiria, allochiria R20.8
Almeida's disease - *see* Paracoccidioidomycosis
Alopecia (hereditaria) (seborrheica) L65.9
androgenic L64.9
drug-induced L64.0
specified NEC L64.8
areata L63.9
ophiasis L63.2
specified NEC L63.8
totalis L63.0
universalis L63.1
cicatricial L66.9
specified NEC L66.8
circumscripta L63.9
congenital, congenitalis Q84.0
due to cytotoxic drugs NEC L65.8
mucinosa L65.2
postinfective NEC L65.8
postpartum L65.0
premature L64.8
specific (syphilitic) A51.32
specified NEC L65.8
syphilitic (secondary) A51.32
totalis (capitis) L63.0
universalis (entire body) L63.1
X-ray L58.1
Alpers' disease G31.81
Alpine sickness T70.29
Alport syndrome Q87.81
ALTE (apparent life threatening event) in newborn and infant R68.13
Alteration (of), Altered
awareness
transient R40.4
unintended under general anesthesia, during procedure T88.53

Alteration (of), Altered - *continued*
mental status R41.82
pattern of family relationships affecting child Z62.898
sensation
following
cerebrovascular disease I69.998
cerebral infarction I69.398
intracerebral hemorrhage I69.198
nontraumatic intracranial hemorrhage NEC I69.298
specified disease NEC I69.898
subarachnoid hemorrhage I69.098
Alternating - *see* condition
Altitude, high (effects) - *see* Effect, adverse, high altitude
Aluminosis (of lung) J63.0
Alveolitis
allergic (extrinsic) - *see* Pneumonitis, hypersensitivity due to
Aspergillus clavatus J67.4
Cryptostroma corticale J67.6
fibrosing (cryptogenic) (idiopathic) J84.112
jaw M27.3
sicca dolorosa M27.3
Alveolus, alveolar - *see* condition
Alymphocytosis D72.810
thymic (with immunodeficiency) D82.1
Alymphoplasia, thymic D82.1
Alzheimer's disease or sclerosis - *see* Disease, Alzheimer's
Amastia (with nipple present) Q83.8
with absent nipple Q83.0
Amathophobia F40.228
Amaurosis (acquired) (congenital) - *see also* Blindness
fugax G45.3
hysterical F44.6
Leber's congenital H35.50
uremic - *see* Uremia
Amaurotic idiocy (infantile) (juvenile) (late) E75.4
Amaxophobia F40.248
Ambiguous genitalia Q56.4
Amblyopia (congenital) (ex anopsia) (partial) (suppression) H53.00-
anisometropic - *see* Amblyopia, refractive
deprivation H53.01-
hysterical F44.6
nocturnal - *see also* Blindness, night
vitamin A deficiency E50.5
refractive H53.02-
strabismic H53.03-
suspect H53.04-
tobacco H53.8
toxic NEC H53.8
uremic - *see* Uremia
Ameba, amebic (histolytica) - *see also* Amebiasis
abscess (liver) A06.4
Amebiasis A06.9
with abscess - *see* Abscess, amebic
acute A06.0
chronic (intestine) A06.1
with abscess - *see* Abscess, amebic
cutaneous A06.7
cutis A06.7
cystitis A06.81
genitourinary tract NEC A06.82
hepatic - *see* Abscess, liver, amebic
intestine A06.0
nondysenteric colitis A06.2
skin A06.7

Amebiasis - *continued*
specified site NEC A06.89
Ameboma (of intestine) A06.3
Amelia Q73.0
lower limb - *see* Agenesis, leg
upper limb - *see* Agenesis, arm
Ameloblastoma - *see also* Cyst, calcifying
odontogenic
long bones C40.9-
lower limb C40.2-
upper limb C40.0-
malignant C41.1
jaw (bone) (lower) C41.1
upper C41.0
tibial C40.2-
Amelogenesis imperfecta K00.5
nonhereditaria (segmentalis) K00.4
Amenorrhea N91.2
hyperhormonal E28.8
primary N91.0
secondary N91.1
Amentia - *see* Disability, intellectual
Meynert's (nonalcoholic) F04
American
leishmaniasis B55.2
mountain tick fever A93.2
Ametropia - *see* Disorder, refraction
AMH (asymptomatic microscopic hematuria)
R31.21
Amianthosis J61
Amimia R48.8
Amino-acid disorder E72.9
anemia D53.0
Aminoacidopathy E72.9
Aminoaciduria E72.9
Amnes (t)ic syndrome (post-traumatic) F04
induced by
alcohol F10.96
with dependence F10.26
psychoactive NEC F19.96
with
abuse F19.16
dependence F19.26
sedative F13.96
with dependence F13.26
Amnesia R41.3
anterograde R41.1
auditory R48.8
dissociative F44.0
with dissociative fugue F44.1
hysterical F44.0
postictal in epilepsy - *see* Epilepsy
psychogenic F44.0
retrograde R41.2
transient global G45.4
Amnion, amniotic - *see* condition
Amnionitis - *see* Pregnancy, complicated by
Amok F68.8
Amoral traits F60.89
Amphetamine (or other stimulant) -induced
anxiety disorder F15.980
bipolar and related disorder F15.94
delirium F15.921
depressive disorder F15.94
obsessive-compulsive and related disorder
F15.988
psychotic disorder F15.959
sexual dysfunction F15.981
sleep disorder F15.982
stimulant withdrawal F15.23
Ampulla
lower esophagus K22.8
phrenic K22.8

Amputation - *see also* Absence, by site,
acquired
neuroma (postoperative) (traumatic) - *see*
Complications, amputation stump, neuroma
stump (surgical)
abnormal, painful, or with complication (late)
- *see* Complications, amputation stump
healed or old NOS Z89.9
traumatic (complete) (partial)
arm (upper) (complete) S48.91-
at
elbow S58.01-
partial S58.02-
shoulder joint (complete) S48.01-
partial S48.02-
between
elbow and wrist (complete) S58.11-
partial S58.12-
shoulder and elbow (complete) S48.11-
partial S48.12-
partial S48.92-
breast (complete) S28.21-
partial S28.22-
clitoris (complete) S38.211
partial S38.212
ear (complete) S08.11-
partial S08.12-
finger (complete) (metacarpophalangeal)
S68.11-
index S68.11-
little S68.11-
middle S68.11-
partial S68.12-
index S68.12-
little S68.12-
middle S68.12-
ring S68.12-
ring S68.11-
thumb - *see* Amputation, traumatic, thumb
transphalangeal (complete) S68.61-
index S68.61-
little S68.61-
middle S68.61-
partial S68.62-
index S68.62-
little S68.62-
middle S68.62-
ring S68.62-
ring S68.61-
foot (complete) S98.91-
at ankle level S98.01-
partial S98.02-
midfoot S98.31-
partial S98.32-
partial S98.92-
forearm (complete) S58.91-
at elbow level (complete) S58.01-
partial S58.02-
between elbow and wrist (complete)
S58.11-
partial S58.12-
partial S58.92-
genital organ(s) (external)
female (complete) S38.211
partial S38.212
male
penis (complete) S38.221
partial S38.222
scrotum (complete) S38.231
partial S38.232
testes (complete) S38.231
partial S38.232
hand (complete) (wrist level) S68.41-
finger(s) alone - *see* Amputation, traumatic,

Amputation - *continued*
finger
partial S68.42-
thumb alone - *see* Amputation, traumatic,
thumb
transmetacarpal (complete) S68.71-
partial S68.72-
head
ear - *see* Amputation, traumatic, ear
nose (partial) S08.812
complete S08.811
part S08.89
scalp S08.0
hip (and thigh) (complete) S78.91-
at hip joint (complete) S78.01-
partial S78.02-
between hip and knee (complete) S78.11-
partial S78.12-
partial S78.92-
labium (majus) (minus) (complete) S38.21-
partial S38.21-
leg (lower) S88.91-
at knee level S88.01-
partial S88.02-
between knee and ankle S88.11-
partial S88.12-
partial S88.92-
nose (partial) S08.812
complete S08.811
penis (complete) S38.221
partial S38.222
scrotum (complete) S38.231
partial S38.232
shoulder - *see* Amputation, traumatic, arm
at shoulder joint - *see* Amputation,
traumatic, arm, at shoulder joint
testes (complete) S38.231
partial S38.232
thigh - *see* Amputation, traumatic, hip
thorax, part of S28.1
breast - *see* Amputation, traumatic, breast
thumb (complete) (metacarpophalangeal)
S68.01-
partial S68.02-
transphalangeal (complete) S68.51-
partial S68.52-
toe (lesser) S98.13-
great S98.11-
partial S98.12-
more than one S98.21-
partial S98.22-
partial S98.14-
vulva (complete) S38.211
partial S38.212
Amputee (bilateral) (old) Z89.9
Amsterdam dwarfism Q87.1
Amusia R48.8
developmental F80.89
Amyelencephalus, amyelencephaly Q00.0
Amyelia Q06.0
Amygdalitis - *see* Tonsillitis
Amygdalolith J35.8
Amyloid heart (disease) E85.4 [*I43*]
Amyloidosis (generalized) (primary) E85.9
with lung involvement E85.4 [*J99*]
familial E85.2
genetic E85.2
heart E85.4 [*I43*]
hemodialysis-associated E85.3
light chain (AL) E85.81
liver E85.4 [*K77*]
localized E85.4
neuropathic heredofamilial E85.1
non neuropathic heredofamilial E85.0

Amyloidosis - *continued*
organ limited E85.4
Portuguese E85.1
pulmonary E85.4 [*J99*]
secondary systemic E85.3
senile systemic (SSA) E85.82
skin (lichen) (macular) E85.4 [*L99*]
specified NEC E85.89
subglottic E85.4 [*J99*]
wild-type transthyretin-related (ATTR) E85.82
Amylopectinosis (brancher enzyme deficiency) E74.03
Amylophagia - *see* Pica
Amyoplasia congenita Q79.8
Amyotonia M62.89
congenita G70.2
Amyotrophia, amyotrophy, amyotrophic G71.8
congenita Q79.8
diabetic - *see* Diabetes, amyotrophy
lateral sclerosis G12.21
neuralgic G54.5
spinal progressive G12.25
Anacidity, gastric K31.83
psychogenic F45.8
Anaerosis of newborn P28.89
Analbuminemia E88.09
Analgesia - *see* Anesthesia
Analphalipoproteinemia E78.6
Anaphylactic
purpura D69.0
shock or reaction - *see* Shock, anaphylactic
Anaphylactoid shock or reaction - *see* Shock, anaphylactic
Anaphylactoid syndrome of pregnancy O88.01-
Anaphylaxis - *see* Shock, anaphylactic
Anaplasia cervix - *see also* Dysplasia, cervix N87.9
Anaplasmosis, human A77.49
Anarthria R47.1
Anasarca R60.1
cardiac - *see* Failure, heart, congestive
lung J18.2
newborn P83.2
nutritional E43
pulmonary J18.2
renal N04.9
Anastomosis
aneurysmal - *see* Aneurysm
arteriovenous ruptured brain I60.8
intestinal K63.89
complicated NEC K91.89
involving urinary tract N99.89
retinal and choroidal vessels (congenital) Q14.8
Anatomical narrow angle H40.03-
Ancylostoma, ancylostomiasis (braziliense) (caninum) (ceylanicum) (duodenale) B76.0
Necator americanus B76.1
Andersen's disease (glycogen storage) E74.09
Anderson-Fabry disease E75.21
Andes disease T70.29
Andrews' disease (bacterid) L08.89
Androblastoma
benign
specified site - *see* Neoplasm, benign, by site
unspecified site
female D27.9
male D29.20
malignant
specified site - *see* Neoplasm, malignant, by site
unspecified site

Androblastoma - *continued*
female C56.9
male C62.90
specified site - *see* Neoplasm, uncertain behavior, by site
tubular
with lipid storage
specified site - *see* Neoplasm, benign, by site
unspecified site
female D27.9
male D29.20
specified site - *see* Neoplasm, benign, by site
unspecified site
female D27.9
male D29.20
unspecified site
female D39.10
male D40.10
Androgen insensitivity syndrome - *see also* Syndrome, androgen insensitivity E34.50
Androgen resistance syndrome - *see also* Syndrome, androgen insensitivity E34.50
Android pelvis Q74.2
with disproportion (fetopelvic) O33.3
causing obstructed labor O65.3
Androphobia F40.290
Anectasis, pulmonary (newborn) - *see* Atelectasis
Anemia (essential) (general) (hemoglobin deficiency) (infantile) (primary) (profound) D64.9
with (due to) (in)
disorder of
anaerobic glycolysis D55.2
pentose phosphate pathway D55.1
koilonychia D50.9
achlorhydric D50.8
achrestic D53.1
Addison (-Biermer) (pernicious) D51.0
agranulocytic - *see* Agranulocytosis
amino-acid-deficiency D53.0
aplastic D61.9
congenital D61.09
drug-induced D61.1
due to
drugs D61.1
external agents NEC D61.2
infection D61.2
radiation D61.2
idiopathic D61.3
red cell (pure) D60.9
chronic D60.0
congenital D61.01
specified type NEC D60.8
transient D60.1
specified type NEC D61.89
toxic D61.2
aregenerative
congenital D61.09
asiderotic D50.9
atypical (primary) D64.9
Baghdad spring D55.0
Balantidium coli A07.0
Biermer's (pernicious) D51.0
blood loss (chronic) D50.0
acute D62
bothriocephalus B70.0 [*D63.8*]
brickmaker's B76.9 [*D63.8*]
cerebral I67.89
childhood D58.9
chlorotic D50.8
chronic
blood loss D50.0

Anemia - *continued*
hemolytic D58.9
idiopathic D59.9
simple D53.9
chronica congenita aregenerativa D61.09
combined system disease NEC D51.0 [*G32.0*]
due to dietary vitamin B12 deficiency D51.3 [*G32.0*]
complicating pregnancy, childbirth or puerperium - *see* Pregnancy, complicated by (management affected by), anemia
congenital P61.4
aplastic D61.09
due to isoimmunization NOS P55.9
dyserythropoietic, dyshematopoietic D64.4
following fetal blood loss P61.3
Heinz body D58.2
hereditary hemolytic NOS D58.9
pernicious D51.0
spherocytic D58.0
Cooley's (erythroblastic) D56.1
cytogenic D51.0
deficiency D53.9
2, 3 diphosphoglycerate mutase D55.2
2, 3 PG D55.2
6 phosphogluconate dehydrogenase D55.1
6-pGD D55.1
amino-acid D53.0
combined B12 and folate D53.1
enzyme D55.9
drug-induced (hemolytic) D59.2
glucose 6-phosphate dehydrogenase (G6PD) D55.0
glycolytic D55.2
nucleotide metabolism D55.3
related to hexose monophosphate (HMP) shunt pathway NEC D55.1
specified type NEC D55.8
erythrocytic glutathione D55.1
folate D52.9
dietary D52.0
drug-induced D52.1
folic acid D52.9
dietary D52.0
drug-induced D52.1
G SH D55.1
GGS-r D55.1
glucose 6-phosphate dehydrogenase D55.0
glutathione reductase D55.1
glyceraldehyde phosphate dehydrogenase D55.2
G6PD D55.0
hexokinase D55.2
iron D50.9
secondary to blood loss (chronic) D50.0
nutritional D53.9
with
poor iron absorption D50.8
specified deficiency NEC D53.8
phosphofructo-aldolase D55.2
phosphoglycerate kinase D55.2
PK D55.2
protein D53.0
pyruvate kinase D55.2
transcobalamin II D51.2
triose-phosphate isomerase D55.2
vitamin B12 NOS D51.9
dietary D51.3
due to
intrinsic factor deficiency D51.0
selective vitamin B12 malabsorption with proteinuria D51.1
pernicious D51.0
specified type NEC D51.8

Anemia - *continued*
Diamond-Blackfan (congenital hypoplastic) D61.01
Dibothriocephalus B70.0 [*D63.8*]
dimorphic D53.1
diphasic D53.1
Diphyllobothrium (Dibothriocephalus) B70.0 [*D63.8*]
due to (in) (with)
  antineoplastic chemotherapy D64.81
  blood loss (chronic) D50.0
    acute D62
  chemotherapy, antineoplastic D64.81
  chronic disease classified elsewhere NEC D63.8
  chronic kidney disease D63.1
  deficiency
    amino-acid D53.0
    copper D53.8
    folate (folic acid) D52.9
      dietary D52.0
      drug-induced D52.1
    molybdenum D53.8
    protein D53.0
    zinc D53.8
  dietary vitamin B12 deficiency D51.3
  disorder of
    glutathione metabolism D55.1
    nucleotide metabolism D55.3
  drug - *see* Anemia, by type - *see also* Table of Drugs and Chemicals
  end stage renal disease D63.1
  enzyme disorder D55.9
  fetal blood loss P61.3
  fish tapeworm (D. Latum) infestation B70.0 [*D63.8*]
  hemorrhage (chronic) D50.0
    acute D62
  impaired absorption D50.9
  loss of blood (chronic) D50.0
    acute D62
  myxedema E03.9 [*D63.8*]
  Necator americanus B76.1 [*D63.8*]
  prematurity P61.2
  selective vitamin B12 malabsorption with proteinuria D51.1
  transcobalamin II deficiency D51.2
Dyke-Young type (secondary) (symptomatic) D59.1
dyserythropoietic (congenital) D64.4
dyshematopoietic (congenital) D64.4
Egyptian B76.9 [*D63.8*]
elliptocytosis - *see* Elliptocytosis
enzyme-deficiency, drug-induced D59.2
epidemic - *see also* Ancylostomiasis B76.9 [*D63.8*]
erythroblastic
  familial D56.1
  newborn - *see also* Disease, hemolytic P55.9
  of childhood D56.1
erythrocytic glutathione deficiency D55.1
erythropoietin-resistant anemia (EPO resistant anemia) D63.1
Faber's (achlorhydric anemia) D50.9
factitious (self-induced blood letting) D50.0
familial erythroblastic D56.1
Fanconi's (congenital pancytopenia) D61.09
favism D55.0
fish tapeworm (D. latum) infestation B70.0 [*D63.8*]
folate (folic acid) deficiency D52.9
glucose 6-phosphate dehydrogenase (G6PD) deficiency D55.0
glutathione-reductase deficiency D55.1

Anemia - *continued*
goat's milk D52.0
granulocytic - *see* Agranulocytosis
Heinz body, congenital D58.2
hemolytic D58.9
  acquired D59.9
    with hemoglobinuria NEC D59.6
    autoimmune NEC D59.1
    infectious D59.4
    specified type NEC D59.8
    toxic D59.4
  acute D59.9
    due to enzyme deficiency specified type NEC D55.8
    Lederer's D59.1
  autoimmune D59.1
    drug-induced D59.0
  chronic D58.9
    idiopathic D59.9
  cold type (secondary) (symptomatic) D59.1
  congenital (spherocytic) - *see* Spherocytosis
  due to
    cardiac conditions D59.4
    drugs (nonautoimmune) D59.2
      autoimmune D59.0
    enzyme disorder D55.9
      drug-induced D59.2
    presence of shunt or other internal prosthetic device D59.4
  familial D58.9
  hereditary D58.9
    due to enzyme disorder D55.9
      specified type NEC D55.8
    specified type NEC D58.8
  idiopathic (chronic) D59.9
  mechanical D59.4
  microangiopathic D59.4
  nonautoimmune D59.4
    drug-induced D59.2
  nonspherocytic
    congenital or hereditary NEC D55.8
      glucose 6-phosphate dehydrogenase deficiency D55.0
      pyruvate kinase deficiency D55.2
      type
        I D55.1
        II D55.2
    type
        I D55.1
        II D55.2
  secondary D59.4
    autoimmune D59.1
  specified (hereditary) type NEC D58.8
  Stransky-Regala type - *see also* Hemoglobinopathy D58.8
  symptomatic D59.4
    autoimmune D59.1
  toxic D59.4
  warm type (secondary) (symptomatic) D59.1
hemorrhagic (chronic) D50.0
  acute D62
Herrick's D57.1
hexokinase deficiency D55.2
hookworm B76.9 [*D63.8*]
hypochromic (idiopathic) (microcytic) (normoblastic) D50.9
  due to blood loss (chronic) D50.0
    acute D62
  familial sex-linked D64.0
  pyridoxine-responsive D64.3
  sideroblastic, sex-linked D64.0
hypoplasia, red blood cells D61.9
  congenital or familial D61.01
hypoplastic (idiopathic) D61.9

Anemia - *continued*
congenital or familial (of childhood) D61.01
hypoproliferative (refractive) D61.9
idiopathic D64.9
  aplastic D61.3
  hemolytic, chronic D59.9
in (due to) (with)
  chronic kidney disease D63.1
  end stage renal disease D63.1
  failure, kidney (renal) D63.1
  neoplastic disease - *see also* Neoplasm D63.0
intertropical - *see also* Ancylostomiasis D63.8
iron deficiency D50.9
  secondary to blood loss (chronic) D50.0
    acute D62
  specified type NEC D50.8
Joseph-diamond-Blackfan (congenital hypoplastic) D61.01
Lederer's (hemolytic) D59.1
leukoerythroblastic D61.82
macrocytic D53.9
  nutritional D52.0
  tropical D52.8
malarial - *see also* Malaria B54 [*D63.8*]
malignant (progressive) D51.0
malnutrition D53.9
marsh - *see also* Malaria B54 [*D63.8*]
Mediterranean (with other hemoglobinopathy) D56.9
megaloblastic D53.1
  combined B12 and folate deficiency D53.1
  hereditary D51.1
  nutritional D52.0
  orotic aciduria D53.0
  refractory D53.1
  specified type NEC D53.1
megalocytic D53.1
microcytic (hypochromic) D50.9
  due to blood loss (chronic) D50.0
    acute D62
  familial D56.8
microdrepanocytosis D57.40
microelliptopoikilocytic (Rietti-grippe Micheli) D56.9
miner's B76.9 [*D63.8*]
myelodysplastic D46.9
myelofibrosis D75.81
myelogenous D64.89
myelopathic D64.89
myelophthisic D61.82
myeloproliferative D47.Z9
newborn P61.4
  due to
    ABO (antibodies, isoimmunization, maternal/fetal incompatibility) P55.1
    Rh (antibodies, isoimmunization, maternal/fetal incompatibility) P55.0
    following fetal blood loss P61.3
    posthemorrhagic (fetal) P61.3
nonspherocytic hemolytic - *see* Anemia, hemolytic, nonspherocytic
normocytic (infectional) D64.9
  due to blood loss (chronic) D50.0
    acute D62
  myelophthisic D61.82
nutritional (deficiency) D53.9
  with
    poor iron absorption D50.8
    specified deficiency NEC D53.8
  megaloblastic D52.0
  of prematurity P61.2
orotaciduric (congenital) (hereditary) D53.0
osteosclerotic D64.89
ovalocytosis (hereditary) - *see* Elliptocytosis

Anemia - *continued*
paludal - *see also* Malaria B54 [*D63.8*]
pernicious (congenital) (malignant)
  (progressive) D51.0
pleochromic D64.89
  of sprue D52.8
posthemorrhagic (chronic) D50.0
  acute D62
  newborn P61.3
postoperative (postprocedural)
  due to (acute) blood loss D62
    chronic blood loss D50.0
  specified NEC D64.9
postpartum O90.81
pressure D64.89
progressive D64.9
  malignant D51.0
  pernicious D51.0
protein-deficiency D53.0
pseudoleukemica infantum D64.89
pure red cell D60.9
  congenital D61.01
pyridoxine-responsive D64.3
pyruvate kinase deficiency D55.2
refractory D46.4
  with
    excess of blasts D46.20
      1 (RAEB 1) D46.21
      2 (RAEB 2) D46.22
      in transformation (RAEB T) - *see*
        Leukemia, acute myeloblastic
      hemochromatosis D46.1
      sideroblasts (ring) (RARS) D46.1
    megaloblastic D53.1
    sideroblastic D46.1
    sideropenic D50.9
  without ring sideroblasts, so stated D46.0
  without sideroblasts without excess of blasts
    D46.0
Rietti-grippe-Micheli D56.9
scorbutic D53.2
secondary to
  blood loss (chronic) D50.0
    acute D62
  hemorrhage (chronic) D50.0
    acute D62
semiplastic D61.89
sickle-cell - *see* Disease, sickle-cell
sideroblastic D64.3
  hereditary D64.0
  hypochromic, sex-linked D64.0
  pyridoxine-responsive NEC D64.3
  refractory D46.1
  secondary (due to)
    disease D64.1
    drugs and toxins D64.2
  specified type NEC D64.3
sideropenic (refractory) D50.9
  due to blood loss (chronic) D50.0
    acute D62
simple chronic D53.9
specified type NEC D64.89
spherocytic (hereditary) - *see* Spherocytosis
splenic D64.89
splenomegalic D64.89
stomatocytosis D58.8
syphilitic (acquired) (late) A52.79 [*D63.8*]
target cell D64.89
thalassemia D56.9
thrombocytopenic - *see* Thrombocytopenia
toxic D61.2
tropical B76.9 [*D63.8*]
  macrocytic D52.8
tuberculous A18.89 [*D63.8*]

Anemia - *continued*
vegan D51.3
vitamin
  B6-responsive D64.3
  B12 deficiency (dietary) pernicious D51.0
von Jaksch's D64.89
Witts' (achlorhydric anemia) D50.8
Anemophobia F40.228
Anencephalus, anencephaly Q00.0
Anergasia - *see* Psychosis, organic
Anesthesia, anesthetic R20.0
complication or reaction NEC - *see also*
Complications, anesthesia T88.59
  due to
    correct substance properly administered -
  see Table of Drugs and Chemicals, by drug,
  adverse effect
    overdose or wrong substance given - *see*
    Table of Drugs and Chemicals, by drug,
    poisoning
  unintended awareness under general
  anesthesia during procedure T88.53
    personal history of Z92.84
cornea H18.81-
dissociative F44.6
functional (hysterical) F44.6
hyperesthetic, thalamic G89.0
hysterical F44.6
local skin lesion R20.0
sexual (psychogenic) F52.1
shock (due to) T88.2
skin R20.0
testicular N50.9
Anetoderma (maculosum) (of) L90.8
Jadassohn-Pellizzari L90.2
Schweniger-Buzzi L90.1
Aneurin deficiency E51.9
Aneurysm (anastomotic) (artery) (cirsoid)
(diffuse) (false) (fusiform) (multiple)
(saccular) I72.9
abdominal (aorta) I71.4
  ruptured I71.3
  syphilitic A52.01
aorta, aortic (nonsyphilitic) I71.9
  abdominal I71.4
    ruptured I71.3
  arch I71.2
    ruptured I71.1
  arteriosclerotic I71.9
    ruptured I71.8
  ascending I71.2
    ruptured I71.1
  congenital Q25.43
  descending I71.9
    abdominal I71.4
      ruptured I71.3
      ruptured I71.8
    thoracic I71.2
      ruptured I71.1
  root Q25.43
  ruptured I71.8
  sinus, congenital Q25.43
  syphilitic A52.01
  thoracic I71.2
    ruptured I71.1
  thoracoabdominal I71.6
    ruptured I71.5
  thorax, thoracic (arch) I71.2
    ruptured I71.1
  transverse I71.2
    ruptured I71.1
  valve (heart) - *see also* Endocarditis, aortic
    I35.8
arteriosclerotic I72.9

Aneurysm - *continued*
cerebral I67.1
  ruptured - *see* Hemorrhage, intracranial,
  subarachnoid
arteriovenous (congenital) - *see also*
Malformation, arteriovenous
  acquired I77.0
    brain I67.1
    coronary I25.41
    pulmonary I28.0
  brain Q28.2
    ruptured I60.8
  peripheral - *see* Malformation, arteriovenous,
    peripheral
  precerebral vessels Q28.0
  specified site NEC - *see also* Malformation,
  arteriovenous
    acquired I77.0
basal - *see* Aneurysm, brain
basilar (trunk) I72.5
berry (congenital) (nonruptured) I67.1
  ruptured I60.7
brain I67.1
  arteriosclerotic I67.1
    ruptured - *see* Hemorrhage, intracranial,
    subarachnoid
  arteriovenous (congenital) (nonruptured)
    Q28.2
    acquired I67.1
      ruptured I60.8
    ruptured I60.8
  berry (congenital) (nonruptured) I67.1
    ruptured - *see also* Hemorrhage,
    intracranial, subarachnoid I60.7
  congenital Q28.3
    ruptured I60.7
  meninges I67.1
    ruptured I60.8
  miliary (congenital) (nonruptured) I67.1
    ruptured - *see also* Hemorrhage,
    intracranial, subarachnoid I60.7
  mycotic I33.0
    ruptured - *see* Hemorrhage, intracranial,
    subarachnoid
  syphilitic (hemorrhage) A52.05
cardiac (false) - *see also* Aneurysm, heart
  I25.3
carotid artery (common) (external) I72.0
  internal (intracranial) I67.1
    extracranial portion I72.0
  ruptured into brain I60.0-
  syphilitic A52.09
    intracranial A52.05
cavernous sinus I67.1
  arteriovenous (congenital) (nonruptured)
    Q28.3
    ruptured I60.8
celiac I72.8
central nervous system, syphilitic A52.05
cerebral - *see* Aneurysm, brain
chest - *see* Aneurysm, thorax   circle of Willis
  I67.1
  congenital Q28.3
    ruptured I60.6
  ruptured I60.6
common iliac artery I72.3
congenital (peripheral) Q27.8
  aorta (root) (sinus) Q25.43
  brain Q28.3
    ruptured I60.7
  coronary Q24.5
  digestive system Q27.8
  lower limb Q27.8
  pulmonary Q25.79

Aneurysm - *continued*
  retina Q14.1
    specified site NEC Q27.8
    upper limb Q27.8
  conjunctiva - *see* Abnormality, conjunctiva, vascular
  conus arteriosus - *see* Aneurysm, heart
  coronary (arteriosclerotic) (artery) I25.41
    arteriovenous, congenital Q24.5
    congenital Q24.5
    ruptured - *see* Infarct, myocardium
    syphilitic A52.06
    vein I25.89
  cylindroid (aorta) I71.9
    ruptured I71.8
    syphilitic A52.01
  ductus arteriosus Q25.0
  endocardial, infective (any valve) I33.0
  femoral (artery) (ruptured) I72.4
  gastroduodenal I72.8
  gastroepiploic I72.8
  heart (wall) (chronic or with a stated duration of over 4 weeks) I25.3
    valve - *see* Endocarditis
  hepatic I72.8
  iliac (common) (artery) (ruptured) I72.3
  infective I72.9
    endocardial (any valve) I33.0
  innominate (nonsyphilitic) I72.8
    syphilitic A52.09
  interauricular septum - *see* Aneurysm, heart
  interventricular septum - *see* Aneurysm, heart
  intrathoracic (nonsyphilitic) I71.2
    ruptured I71.1
    syphilitic A52.01
  lower limb I72.4
  lung (pulmonary artery) I28.1
  mediastinal (nonsyphilitic) I72.8
    syphilitic A52.09
  miliary (congenital) I67.1
    ruptured - *see* Hemorrhage, intracerebral, subarachnoid, intracranial
  mitral (heart) (valve) I34.8
  mural - *see* Aneurysm, heart
  mycotic I72.9
    endocardial (any valve) I33.0
    ruptured, brain - *see* Hemorrhage, intracerebral, subarachnoid
  myocardium - *see* Aneurysm, heart
  neck I72.0
  pancreaticoduodenal I72.8
  patent ductus arteriosus Q25.0
  peripheral NEC I72.8
    congenital Q27.8
      digestive system Q27.8
      lower limb Q27.8
      specified site NEC Q27.8
      upper limb Q27.8
  popliteal (artery) (ruptured) I72.4
  precerebral
    congenital (nonruptured) Q28.1
    specified site, NEC I72.5
  pulmonary I28.1
    arteriovenous Q25.72
      acquired I28.0
    syphilitic A52.09
    valve (heart) - *see* Endocarditis, pulmonary
  racemose (peripheral) I72.9
    congenital - *see* Aneurysm, congenital
  radial I72.1
  Rasmussen NEC A15.0
  renal (artery) I72.2
  retina - *see also* Disorder, retina, microaneurysms

Aneurysm - *continued*
  congenital Q14.1
  diabetic - *see* Diabetes, microaneurysms, retinal
  sinus of Valsalva Q25.49
  specified NEC I72.8
  spinal (cord) I72.8
    syphilitic (hemorrhage) A52.09
  splenic I72.8
  subclavian (artery) (ruptured) I72.8
    syphilitic A52.09
  superior mesenteric I72.8
  syphilitic (aorta) A52.01
    central nervous system A52.05
    congenital (late) A50.54 [*179.0*]
    spine, spinal A52.09
  thoracoabdominal (aorta) I71.6
    ruptured I71.5
    syphilitic A52.01
  thorax, thoracic (aorta) (arch) (nonsyphilitic) I71.2
    ruptured I71.1
    syphilitic A52.01
  traumatic (complication) (early), specified site - *see* Injury, blood vessel
  tricuspid (heart) (valve) I07.8
  ulnar I72.1
  upper limb (ruptured) I72.1
  valve, valvular - *see* Endocarditis
  venous - *see also* Varix I86.8
    congenital Q27.8
      digestive system Q27.8
      lower limb Q27.8
      specified site NEC Q27.8
      upper limb Q27.8
  ventricle - *see* Aneurysm, heart
  vertebral artery I72.6
  visceral NEC I72.8
Angelman syndrome Q93.5
Anger R45.4
Angiectasis, angiectopia I99.8
Angiitis I77.6
  allergic granulomatous M30.1
  hypersensitivity M31.0
  necrotizing M31.9
    specified NEC M31.8
  nervous system, granulomatous I67.7
Angina (attack) (cardiac) (chest) (heart) (pectoris) (syndrome) (vasomotor) I20.9
  with
    atherosclerotic heart disease - *see* Arteriosclerosis, coronary (artery), documented spasm I20.1
  abdominal K55.1
  accelerated - *see* Angina, unstable
  agranulocytic - *see* Agranulocytosis
  angiospastic - *see* Angina, with documented spasm
  aphthous B08.5
  crescendo - *see* Angina, unstable
  croupous J05.0
  cruris I73.9
  de novo effort - *see* Angina, unstable
  diphtheritic, membranous A36.0
  equivalent I20.8
  exudative, chronic J37.0
  following acute myocardial infarction I23.7
  gangrenous diphtheritic A36.0
  intestinal K55.1
  Ludovici K12.2
  Ludwig's K12.2
  malignant diphtheritic A36.0
  membranous J05.0
    diphtheritic A36.0

Angina - *continued*
  Vincent's A69.1
  mesenteric K55.1
  monocytic - *see* Mononucleosis, infectious
  of effort - *see* Angina, specified NEC
  phlegmonous J36
    diphtheritic A36.0
  post-infarctional I23.7
  pre-infarctional - *see* Angina, unstable
  Prinzmetal - *see* Angina, with documented spasm
  progressive - *see* Angina, unstable
  pseudomembranous A69.1
  pultaceous, diphtheritic A36.0
  spasm-induced - *see* Angina, with documented spasm
  specified NEC I20.8
  stable I20.8
  stenocardia - *see* Angina, specified NEC
  stridulous, diphtheritic A36.2
  tonsil J36
  trachealis J05.0
  unstable I20.0
  variant - *see* Angina, with documented spasm
  Vincent's A69.1
  worsening effort - *see* Angina, unstable
Angioblastoma - *see* Neoplasm, connective tissue, uncertain behavior
Angiocholecystitis - *see* Cholecystitis, acute
Angiocholitis - *see also* Cholecystitis, acute K83.0
Angiodysgenesis spinalis G95.19
Angiodysplasia (cecum) (colon) K55.20
  with bleeding K55.21
  duodenum (and stomach) K31.819
    with bleeding K31.811
  stomach (and duodenum) K31.819
    with bleeding K31.811
Angioedema (allergic) (any site) (with urticaria) T78.3
  hereditary D84.1
Angioendothelioma - *see* Neoplasm, uncertain behavior, by site
  benign D18.00
    intra-abdominal D18.03
    intracranial D18.02
    skin D18.01
    specified site NEC D18.09
  bone - *see* Neoplasm, bone, malignant
  Ewing's - *see* Neoplasm, bone, malignant
Angioendotheliomatosis C85.8-
Angiofibroma - *see also* Neoplasm, benign, by site
  juvenile
    specified site - *see* Neoplasm, benign, by site
    unspecified site D10.6
Angiohemophilia (A) (B) D68.0
Angioid streaks (choroid) (macula) (retina) H35.33
Angiokeratoma - *see* Neoplasm, skin, benign
  corporis diffusum E75.21
Angioleiomyoma - *see* Neoplasm, connective tissue, benign
Angiolipoma - *see also* Lipoma
  infiltrating - *see* Lipoma
Angioma - *see also* Hemangioma, by site
  capillary I78.1
  hemorrhagicum hereditaria I78.0
  intra-abdominal D18.03
  intracranial D18.02
  malignant - *see* Neoplasm, connective tissue, malignant
  plexiform D18.00
    intra-abdominal D18.03

Angioma – *continued*
  intracranial D18.02
    skin D18.01
    specified site NEC D18.09
  senile I78.1
  serpiginosum L81.7
  skin D18.01
  specified site NEC D18.09
  spider I78.1
  stellate I78.1
  venous Q28.3
Angiomatosis Q82.8
  bacillary A79.89
  encephalotrigeminal Q85.8
  hemorrhagic familial I78.0
  hereditary familial I78.0
  liver K76.4
Angiomyolipoma - *see* Lipoma
Angiomyoliposarcoma - *see* Neoplasm,
  connective tissue, malignant
Angiomyoma - *see* Neoplasm, connective
  tissue, benign
Angiomyosarcoma - *see* Neoplasm, connective
  tissue, malignant
Angiomyxoma - *see* Neoplasm, connective
  tissue, uncertain behavior
Angioneurosis F45.8
Angioneurotic edema (allergic) (any site)
  (with urticaria) T78.3
  hereditary D84.1
Angiopathia, angiopathy I99.9
  cerebral I67.9
    amyloid E85.4 [*I68.0*]
  diabetic (peripheral) - *see* Diabetes,
    angiopathy
  peripheral I73.9
    diabetic - *see* Diabetes, angiopathy
    specified type NEC I73.89
  retinae syphilitica A52.05
  retinalis (juvenilis)
    diabetic - *see* Diabetes, retinopathy
    proliferative - *see* Retinopathy, proliferative
Angiosarcoma - *see also* Neoplasm, connective
  tissue, malignant
  liver C22.3
Angiosclerosis - *see* Arteriosclerosis
Angiospasm (peripheral) (traumatic) (vessel)
  I73.9
  brachial plexus G54.0
  cerebral G45.9
  cervical plexus G54.2
  nerve
    arm - *see* Mononeuropathy, upper limb
      axillary G54.0
      median - *see* Lesion, nerve, median
      ulnar - *see* Lesion, nerve, ulnar
    axillary G54.0
    leg - *see* Mononeuropathy, lower limb
    median - *see* Lesion, nerve, median
    plantar - *see* Lesion, nerve, plantar
    ulnar - *see* Lesion, nerve, ulnar
Angiospastic disease or edema I73.9
Angiostrongyliasis
  due to
    Parastrongylus
      cantonensis B83.2
      costaricensis B81.3
  intestinal B81.3
Anguillulosis - *see* Strongyloidiasis
Angulation
  cecum - *see* Obstruction, intestine
  coccyx (acquired) - *see also* subcategory
    M43.8
      congenital NEC Q76.49

Angulation - *continued*
  femur (acquired) - *see also* Deformity, limb,
    specified type NEC, thigh
      congenital Q74.2
  intestine (large) (small) - *see* Obstruction,
    intestine
  sacrum (acquired) - *see also* subcategory
    M43.8
      congenital NEC Q76.49
  sigmoid (flexure) - *see* Obstruction, intestine
  spine - *see* Dorsopathy, deforming, specified
    NEC
  tibia (acquired) - *see also* Deformity, limb,
    specified type NEC, lower leg
      congenital Q74.2
  ureter N13.5
    with infection N13.6
  wrist (acquired) - *see also* Deformity, limb,
    specified type NEC, forearm
      congenital Q74.0
Angulus infectiosus (lips) K13.0
Anhedonia R45.84
  sexual F52.0
Anhidrosis L74.4
Anhydration E86.0
Anhydremia E86.0
Anidrosis L74.4
Aniridia (congenital) Q13.1
Anisakiasis (infection) (infestation) B81.0
Anisakis larvae infestation B81.0
Aniseikonia H52.32
Anisocoria (pupil) H57.02
  congenital Q13.2
Anisocytosis R71.8
Anisometropia (congenital) H52.31
Ankle - *see* condition
Ankyloblepharon (eyelid) (acquired) - *see*
  also Blepharophimosis
  filiforme (adnatum) (congenital) Q10.3
  total Q10.3
Ankyloglossia Q38.1
Ankylosis (fibrous) (osseous) (joint) M24.60
  ankle M24.67-
  arthrodesis status Z98.1
  cricoarytenoid (cartilage) (joint) (larynx) J38.7
  dental K03.5
  ear ossicles H74.31-
  elbow M24.62-
  foot M24.67-
  hand M24.64-
  hip M24.65-
  incostapedial joint (infectional) - *see*
    Ankylosis, ear ossicles
  jaw (temporomandibular) M26.61-
  knee M24.66-
  lumbosacral (joint) M43.27
  postoperative (status) Z98.1
  produced by surgical fusion, status Z98.1
  sacro-iliac (joint) M43.28
  shoulder M24.61-
  spine (joint) - *see also* Fusion, spine
    spondylitic - *see* Spondylitis, ankylosing
  surgical Z98.1
  temporomandibular M26.61-
  tooth, teeth (hard tissues) K03.5
  wrist M24.63-
Ankylostoma - *see* Ancylostoma
Ankylostomiasis - *see* Ancylostomiasis
Ankylurethria - *see* Stricture, urethra
Annular - *see also* condition
  detachment, cervix N88.8
  organ or site, congenital NEC - *see* Distortion
  pancreas (congenital) Q45.1

Anodontia (complete) (partial) (vera) K00.0
  acquired K08.10
Anomaly, anomalous (congenital) (unspecified
  type) Q89.9
  abdominal wall NEC Q79.59
  acoustic nerve Q07.8
  adrenal (gland) Q89.1
  Alder (-Reilly) (leukocyte granulation) D72.0
  alimentary tract Q45.9
    upper Q40.9
  alveolar M26.70
    hyperplasia M26.79
      mandibular M26.72
      maxillary M26.71
    hypoplasia M26.79
      mandibular M26.74
      maxillary M26.73
    ridge (process) M26.79
    specified NEC M26.79
  ankle (joint) Q74.2
  anus Q43.9
  aorta (arch) NEC Q25.40
    coarctation (preductal) (postductal) Q25.1
  aortic cusp or valve Q23.9
  appendix Q43.8
  apple peel syndrome Q41.1
  aqueduct of Sylvius Q03.0
    with spina bifida - *see* Spina bifida, with
      hydrocephalus
  arm Q74.0
  arteriovenous NEC
    coronary Q24.5
    gastrointestinal Q27.33
      acquired - *see* Angiodysplasia
  artery (peripheral) Q27.9
    basilar NEC Q28.1
    cerebral Q28.3
    coronary Q24.5
    digestive system Q27.8
    eye Q15.8
    great Q25.9
      specified NEC Q25.8
    lower limb Q27.8
    peripheral Q27.9
      specified NEC Q27.8
    pulmonary NEC Q25.79
    renal Q27.2
    retina Q14.1
    specified site NEC Q27.8
    subclavian Q27.8
      origin Q25.48
    umbilical Q27.0
    upper limb Q27.8
    vertebral NEC Q28.1
  aryteno-epiglottic folds Q31.8
  atrial
    bands or folds Q20.8
    septa Q21.1
  atrioventricular
    excitation I45.6
    septum Q21.0
  auditory canal Q17.8
  auricle
    ear Q17.8
      causing impairment of hearing Q16.9
    heart Q20.8
  Axenfeld's Q15.0
  back Q89.9
  band
    atrial Q20.8
    heart Q24.8
    ventricular Q24.8
  Bartholin's duct Q38.4
  biliary duct or passage Q44.5

Anomaly, anomalous - *continued*

bladder Q64.70
  absence Q64.5
  diverticulum Q64.6
  exstrophy Q64.10
    cloacal Q64.12
    extroversion Q64.19
    specified type NEC Q64.19
    supravesical fissure Q64.11
  neck obstruction Q64.31
  specified type NEC Q64.79
bone Q79.9
  arm Q74.0
  face Q75.9
  leg Q74.2
  pelvic girdle Q74.2
  shoulder girdle Q74.0
  skull Q75.9
    with
      anencephaly Q00.0
      encephalocele - *see* Encephalocele
      hydrocephalus Q03.9
        with spina bifida - *see* Spina bifida, by
site, with hydrocephalus
      microcephaly Q02
brain (multiple) Q04.9
  vessel Q28.3
breast Q83.9
broad ligament Q50.6
bronchus Q32.4
bulbus cordis Q21.9
bursa Q79.9
canal of Nuck Q52.4
canthus Q10.3
capillary Q27.9
cardiac Q24.9
  chambers Q20.9
    specified NEC Q20.8
  septal closure Q21.9
    specified NEC Q21.8
  valve NEC Q24.8
    pulmonary Q22.3
cardiovascular system Q28.8
carpus Q74.0
caruncle, lacrimal Q10.6
cascade stomach Q40.2
cauda equina Q06.3
cecum Q43.9
cerebral Q04.9
  vessels Q28.3
cervix Q51.9
Chédiak-Higashi (-Steinbrinck) (congenital
  gigantism of peroxidase granules) E70.330
cheek Q18.9
chest wall Q67.8
  bones Q76.9
chin Q18.9
chordae tendineae Q24.8
choroid Q14.3
  plexus Q07.8
chromosomes, chromosomal Q99.9
  D (1) - *see* condition, chromosome 13
  E (3) - *see* condition, chromosome 18
  G - *see* condition, chromosome 21
  sex
    female phenotype Q97.8
    gonadal dysgenesis (pure) Q99.1
    Klinefelter's Q98.4
    male phenotype Q98.9
    Turner's Q96.9
  specified NEC Q99.8
cilia Q10.3
circulatory system Q28.9
clavicle Q74.0

Anomaly, anomalous - *continued*

clitoris Q52.6
coccyx Q76.49
colon Q43.9
common duct Q44.5
communication
  coronary artery Q24.5
  left ventricle with right atrium Q21.0
concha (ear) Q17.3
connection
  portal vein Q26.5
  pulmonary venous Q26.4
    partial Q26.3
    total Q26.2
  renal artery with kidney Q27.2
cornea (shape) Q13.4
coronary artery or vein Q24.5
cranium - *see* Anomaly, skull
cricoid cartilage Q31.8
cystic duct Q44.5
dental
  alveolar - *see* Anomaly, alveolar
  arch relationship M26.20
    specified NEC M26.29
dentofacial M26.9
  alveolar - *see* Anomaly, alveolar
  dental arch relationship M26.20
    specified NEC M26.29
  functional M26.50
    specified NEC M26.59
  jaw-cranial base relationship M26.10
    asymmetry M26.12
      maxillary M26.11
    specified type NEC M26.19
  jaw size M26.00
    macrogenia M26.05
    mandibular
      hyperplasia M26.03
      hypoplasia M26.04
    maxillary
      hyperplasia M26.01
      hypoplasia M26.02
    microgenia M26.06
    specified type NEC M26.09
  malocclusion M26.4
    dental arch relationship NEC M26.29
    jaw-cranial base relationship - *see*
      Anomaly, dentofacial, jaw-cranial base
      relationship
    jaw size - *see* Anomaly, dentofacial, jaw
      size
    specified type NEC M26.89
  temporomandibular joint M26.60-
    adhesions M26.61-
    ankylosis M26.61-
    arthralgia M26.62-
    articular disc M26.63-
    specified type NEC M26.69
  tooth position, fully erupted M26.30
    specified NEC M26.39
dermatoglyphic Q82.8
diaphragm (apertures) NEC Q79.1
digestive organ(s) or tract Q45.9
  lower Q43.9
  upper Q40.9
distance, interarch (excessive) (inadequate)
  M26.25
distribution, coronary artery Q24.5
ductus
  arteriosus Q25.0
  botalli Q25.0
duodenum Q43.9
dura (brain) Q04.9
  spinal cord Q06.9

Anomaly, anomalous - *continued*

ear (external) Q17.9
  causing impairment of hearing Q16.9
  inner Q16.5
  middle (causing impairment of hearing)
    Q16.4
    ossicles Q16.3
Ebstein's (heart) (tricuspid valve) Q22.5
ectodermal Q82.9
Eisenmenger's (ventricular septal defect)
  Q21.8
ejaculatory duct Q55.4
elbow Q74.0
endocrine gland NEC Q89.2
epididymis Q55.4
epiglottis Q31.8
esophagus Q39.9
eustachian tube Q17.8
eye Q15.9
  anterior segment Q13.9
    specified NEC Q13.89
  posterior segment Q14.9
    specified NEC Q14.8
  ptosis (eyelid) Q10.0
  specified NEC Q15.8
eyebrow Q18.8
eyelid Q10.3
  ptosis Q10.0
face Q18.9
  bone(s) Q75.9
fallopian tube Q50.6
fascia Q79.9
femur NEC Q74.2
fibula NEC Q74.2
finger Q74.0
fixation, intestine Q43.3
flexion (joint) NOS Q74.9
  hip or thigh Q65.89
foot NEC Q74.2
  varus (congenital) Q66.3
foramen
  Botalli Q21.1
  ovale Q21.1
forearm Q74.0
forehead Q75.8
form, teeth K00.2
fovea centralis Q14.1
frontal bone - *see* Anomaly, skull
gallbladder (position) (shape) (size) Q44.1
Gartner's duct Q52.4
gastrointestinal tract Q45.9
genitalia, genital organ(s) or system
  female Q52.9
    external Q52.70
    internal NOS Q52.9
  male Q55.9
    hydrocele P83.5
    specified NEC Q55.8
genitourinary NEC
  female Q52.9
  male Q55.9
Gerbode Q21.0
glottis Q31.8
granulation or granulocyte, genetic
  (constitutional) (leukocyte) D72.0
gum Q38.6
gyri Q07.9
hair Q84.2
hand Q74.0
hard tissue formation in pulp K04.3
head - *see* Anomaly, skull
heart Q24.9
  auricle Q20.8
  bands or folds Q24.8

Anomaly, anomalous - *continued*
fibroelastosis cordis I42.4
obstructive NEC Q22.6
patent ductus arteriosus (Botalli) Q25.0
septum Q21.9
  auricular Q21.1
  interatrial Q21.1
  interventricular Q21.0
  with pulmonary stenosis or atresia,
dextroposition of aorta and hypertrophy of
right ventricle Q21.3
  specified NEC Q21.8
  ventricular Q21.0
  with pulmonary stenosis or atresia,
dextroposition of aorta and hypertrophy of
right ventricle Q21.3
  tetralogy of Fallot Q21.3
valve NEC Q24.8
  aortic
    bicuspid valve Q23.1
    insufficiency Q23.1
    stenosis Q23.0
      subaortic Q24.4
  mitral
    insufficiency Q23.3
    stenosis Q23.2
  pulmonary Q22.3
    atresia Q22.0
    insufficiency Q22.2
    stenosis Q22.1
      infundibular Q24.3
      subvalvular Q24.3
  tricuspid
    atresia Q22.4
    stenosis Q22.4
ventricle Q20.8
heel NEC Q74.2
Hegglin's D72.0
hemianencephaly Q00.0
hemicephaly Q00.0
hemicrania Q00.0
hepatic duct Q44.5
hip NEC Q74.2
hourglass stomach Q40.2
humerus Q74.0
hydatid of Morgagni
  female Q50.5
  male (epididymal) Q55.4
    testicular Q55.29
hymen Q52.4
hypersegmentation of neutrophils, hereditary
D72.0
hypophyseal Q89.2
ileocecal (coil) (valve) Q43.9
ileum Q43.9
ilium NEC Q74.2
integument Q84.9
  specified NEC Q84.8
interarch distance (excessive) (inadequate)
M26.25
intervertebral cartilage or disc Q76.49
intestine (large) (small) Q43.9
  with anomalous adhesions, fixation or
malrotation Q43.3
iris Q13.2
ischium NEC Q74.2
jaw - *see* Anomaly, dentofacial
  alveolar - *see* Anomaly, alveolar
jaw-cranial base relationship - *see* Anomaly,
dentofacial, jaw-cranial base relationship
jejunum Q43.8
joint Q74.9
  specified NEC Q74.8
Jordan's D72.0

Anomaly, anomalous - *continued*
kidney(s) (calyx) (pelvis) Q63.9
  artery Q27.2
  specified NEC Q63.8
Klippel-Feil (brevicollis) Q76.1
knee Q74.1
labium (majus) (minus) Q52.70
labyrinth, membranous Q16.5
lacrimal apparatus or duct Q10.6
larynx, laryngeal (muscle) Q31.9
  web (bed) Q31.0
lens Q12.9
leukocytes, genetic D72.0
  granulation (constitutional) D72.0
lid (fold) Q10.3
ligament Q79.9
  broad Q50.6
  round Q52.8
limb Q74.9
  lower NEC Q74.2
    reduction deformity - *see* Defect, reduction,
lower limb
  upper Q74.0
lip Q38.0
liver Q44.7
  duct Q44.5
lower limb NEC Q74.2
lumbosacral (joint) (region) Q76.49
  kyphosis - *see* Kyphosis, congenital
  lordosis - *see* Lordosis, congenital
lung (fissure) (lobe) Q33.9
mandible - *see* Anomaly, dentofacial
maxilla - *see* Anomaly, dentofacial
May (-Hegglin) D72.0
meatus urinarius NEC Q64.79
meningeal bands or folds Q07.9
  constriction of Q07.8
  spinal Q06.9
meninges Q07.9
  cerebral Q04.8
  spinal Q06.9
meningocele Q05.9
mesentery Q45.9
metacarpus Q74.0
metatarsus NEC Q74.2
middle ear Q16.4
  ossicles Q16.3
mitral (leaflets) (valve) Q23.9
  insufficiency Q23.3
  specified NEC Q23.8
  stenosis Q23.2
mouth Q38.6
Müllerian - *see also* Anomaly, by site
  uterus NEC Q51.818
multiple NEC Q89.7
muscle Q79.9
  eyelid Q10.3
musculoskeletal system, except limbs Q79.9
myocardium Q24.8
nail Q84.6
narrowness, eyelid Q10.3
nasal sinus (wall) Q30.8
neck (any part) Q18.9
nerve Q07.9
  acoustic Q07.8
  optic Q07.8
nervous system (central) Q07.9
nipple Q83.9
nose, nasal (bones) (cartilage) (septum) (sinus)
Q30.9
  specified NEC Q30.8
ocular muscle Q15.8
omphalomesenteric duct Q43.0
opening, pulmonary veins Q26.4

Anomaly, anomalous - *continued*
optic
  disc Q14.2
  nerve Q07.8
opticociliary vessels Q13.2
orbit (eye) Q10.7
organ Q89.9
  of Corti Q16.5
origin
  artery
    innominate Q25.8
    pulmonary Q25.79
    renal Q27.2
    subclavian Q25.48
osseous meatus (ear) Q16.1
ovary Q50.39
oviduct Q50.6
palate (hard) (soft) NEC Q38.5
pancreas or pancreatic duct Q45.3
papillary muscles Q24.8
parathyroid gland Q89.2
paraurethral ducts Q64.79
parotid (gland) Q38.4
patella Q74.1
Pelger-Huët (hereditary hyposegmentation)
D72.0
pelvic girdle NEC Q74.2
pelvis (bony) NEC Q74.2
  rachitic E64.3
penis (glans) Q55.69
pericardium Q24.8
peripheral vascular system Q27.9
Peter's Q13.4
pharynx Q38.8
pigmentation L81.9
  congenital Q82.8
pituitary (gland) Q89.2
pleural (folds) Q34.0
portal vein Q26.5
  connection Q26.5
position, tooth, teeth, fully erupted M26.30
  specified NEC M26.39
precerebral vessel Q28.1
prepuce Q55.69
prostate Q55.4
pulmonary Q33.9
  artery NEC Q25.79
  valve Q22.3
    atresia Q22.0
    insufficiency Q22.2
    specified type NEC Q22.3
    stenosis Q22.1
      infundibular Q24.3
      subvalvular Q24.3
  venous connection Q26.4
    partial Q26.3
    total Q26.2
pupil Q13.2
  function H57.00
    anisocoria H57.02
    Argyll Robertson pupil H57.01
    miosis H57.03
    mydriasis H57.04
    specified type NEC H57.09
    tonic pupil H57.05-
pylorus Q40.3
radius Q74.0
rectum Q43.9
reduction (extremity) (limb)
  femur (longitudinal) - *see* Defect, reduction,
lower limb, longitudinal, femur
  fibula (longitudinal) - *see* Defect, reduction,
lower limb, longitudinal, fibula
  lower limb - *see* Defect, reduction, lower

Anomaly, anomalous - *continued*
- limb
  - radius (longitudinal) - *see* Defect, reduction, upper limb, longitudinal, radius
  - tibia (longitudinal) - *see* Defect, reduction, lower limb, longitudinal, tibia
  - ulna (longitudinal) - *see* Defect, reduction, upper limb, longitudinal, ulna
  - upper limb - *see* Defect, reduction, upper limb
- refraction - *see* Disorder, refraction
- renal Q63.9
  - artery Q27.2
  - pelvis Q63.9
    - specified NEC Q63.8
- respiratory system Q34.9
  - specified NEC Q34.8
- retina Q14.1
- rib Q76.6
  - cervical Q76.5
- Rieger's Q13.81
- rotation - *see* Malrotation
  - hip or thigh Q65.89
- round ligament Q52.8
- sacroiliac (joint) NEC Q74.2
- sacrum NEC Q76.49
  - kyphosis - *see* Kyphosis, congenital
  - lordosis - *see* Lordosis, congenital
- saddle nose, syphilitic A50.57
- salivary duct or gland Q38.4
- scapula Q74.0
- scrotum - *see* Malformation, testis and scrotum
- sebaceous gland Q82.9
- seminal vesicles Q55.4
- sense organs NEC Q07.8
- sex chromosomes NEC - *see also* Anomaly, chromosomes
  - female phenotype Q97.8
  - male phenotype Q98.9
- shoulder (girdle) (joint) Q74.0
- sigmoid (flexure) Q43.9
- simian crease Q82.8
- sinus of Valsalva Q25.49
- skeleton generalized Q78.9
- skin (appendage) Q82.9
- skull Q75.9
  - with
    - anencephaly Q00.0
    - encephalocele - *see* Encephalocele
    - hydrocephalus Q03.9
      - with spina bifida - *see* Spina bifida, by site, with hydrocephalus
    - microcephaly Q02
  - specified organ or site NEC Q89.8
- spermatic cord Q55.4
- spine, spinal NEC Q76.49
  - column NEC Q76.49
    - kyphosis - *see* Kyphosis, congenital
    - lordosis - *see* Lordosis, congenital
  - cord Q06.9
    - nerve root Q07.8
- spleen Q89.09
  - agenesis Q89.01
- stenonian duct Q38.4
- sternum NEC Q76.7
- stomach Q40.3
- submaxillary gland Q38.4
- tarsus NEC Q74.2
- tendon Q79.9
- testis - *see* Malformation, testis and scrotum
- thigh NEC Q74.2
- thorax (wall) Q67.8
  - bony Q76.9
- throat Q38.8

Anomaly, anomalous - *continued*
- thumb Q74.0
- thymus gland Q89.2
- thyroid (gland) Q89.2
  - cartilage Q31.8
- tibia NEC Q74.2
  - saber A50.56
- toe Q74.2
- tongue Q38.3
- tooth, teeth K00.9
  - eruption K00.6
  - position, fully erupted M26.30
  - spacing, fully erupted M26.30
- trachea (cartilage) Q32.1
- tragus Q17.9
- tricuspid (leaflet) (valve) Q22.9
  - atresia or stenosis Q22.4
  - Ebstein's Q22.5
- Uhl's (hypoplasia of myocardium, right ventricle) Q24.8
- ulna Q74.0
- umbilical artery Q27.0
- union
  - cricoid cartilage and thyroid cartilage Q31.8
  - thyroid cartilage and hyoid bone Q31.8
  - trachea with larynx Q31.8
- upper limb Q74.0
- urachus Q64.4
- ureter Q62.8
  - obstructive NEC Q62.39
    - cecoureterocele Q62.32
    - orthotopic ureterocele Q62.31
- urethra Q64.70
  - absence Q64.5
  - double Q64.74
  - fistula to rectum Q64.73
  - obstructive Q64.39
    - stricture Q64.32
  - prolapse Q64.71
  - specified type NEC Q64.79
- urinary tract Q64.9
- uterus Q51.9
  - with only one functioning horn Q51.4
- uvula Q38.5
- vagina Q52.4
- valleculae Q31.8
- valve (heart) NEC Q24.8
  - coronary sinus Q24.5
  - inferior vena cava Q24.8
  - pulmonary Q22.3
  - sinus coronario Q24.5
  - venae cavae inferioris Q24.8
- vas deferens Q55.4
- vascular Q27.9
  - brain Q28.3
  - ring Q25.45
- vein(s) (peripheral) Q27.9
  - brain Q28.3
  - cerebral Q28.3
  - coronary Q24.5
  - developmental Q28.3
  - great Q26.9
    - specified NEC Q26.8
- vena cava (inferior) (superior) Q26.9
- venous - *see* Anomaly, vein(s)
- venous return Q26.8
- ventricular
  - bands or folds Q24.8
  - septa Q21.0
- vertebra Q76.49
  - kyphosis - *see* Kyphosis, congenital
  - lordosis - *see* Lordosis, congenital
- vesicourethral orifice Q64.79
- vessel(s) Q27.9

Anomaly, anomalous - *continued*
- optic papilla Q14.2
- precerebral Q28.1
- vitelline duct Q43.0
- vitreous body or humor Q14.0
- vulva Q52.70
- wrist (joint) Q74.0

Anomia R48.8

Anonychia (congenital) Q84.3
- acquired L60.8

Anophthalmos, anophthalmus (congenital) (globe) Q11.1
- acquired Z90.01

Anopia, anopsia H53.46-
- quadrant H53.46-

Anorchia, anorchism, anorchidism Q55.0

Anorexia R63.0
- hysterical F44.89
- nervosa F50.00
  - atypical F50.9
  - binge-eating type F50.2
    - with purging F50.02
  - restricting type F50.01

Anorgasmy, psychogenic (female) F52.31
- male F52.32

Anosmia R43.0
- hysterical F44.6
- postinfectional J39.8

Anosognosia R41.89

Anosteoplasia Q78.9

Anovulatory cycle N97.0

Anoxemia R09.02
- newborn P84

Anoxia (pathological) R09.02
- altitude T70.29
- cerebral G93.1
  - complicating
    - anesthesia (general) (local) or other sedation T88.59
      - in labor and delivery O74.3
      - in pregnancy O29.21-
      - postpartum, puerperal O89.2
    - delivery (cesarean) (instrumental) O75.4
  - during a procedure G97.81
  - newborn P84
  - resulting from a procedure G97.82
- due to
  - drowning T75.1
  - high altitude T70.29
- heart - *see* Insufficiency, coronary
- intrauterine P84
- myocardial - *see* Insufficiency, coronary
- newborn P84
- spinal cord G95.11
- systemic (by suffocation) (low content in atmosphere) - *see* Asphyxia, traumatic

Anteflexion - *see* Anteversion

Antenatal
- care (normal pregnancy) Z34.90
- screening (encounter for) of mother (see also Encounter, antenatal screening) Z36.9

Antepartum - *see* condition

Anterior - *see* condition

Antero-occlusion M26.220

Anteversion
- cervix - *see* Anteversion, uterus
- femur (neck), congenital Q65.89
- uterus, uterine (cervix) (postinfectional) (postpartal, old) N85.4
  - congenital Q51.818
  - in pregnancy or childbirth - *see* Pregnancy, complicated by

Anthophobia F40.228

Anthracosilicosis J60
Anthracosis (lung) (occupational) J60
  lingua K14.3
Anthrax A22.9
  with pneumonia A22.1
  cerebral A22.8
  colitis A22.2
  cutaneous A22.0
  gastrointestinal A22.2
  inhalation A22.1
  intestinal A22.2
  meningitis A22.8
  pulmonary A22.1
  respiratory A22.1
  sepsis A22.7
  specified manifestation NEC A22.8
Anthropoid pelvis Q74.2
  with disproportion (fetopelvic) O33.0
Anthropophobia F40.10
  generalized F40.11
Antibodies, maternal (blood group) - *see*
  Isoimmunization, affecting management of
  pregnancy anti-d - *see* Isoimmunization,
  affecting management of pregnancy, Rh
  newborn P55.0
Antibody
  anticardiolipin R76.0
    with
      hemorrhagic disorder D68.312
      hypercoagulable state D68.61
  antiphosphatidylglycerol R76.0
    with
      hemorrhagic disorder D68.312
      hypercoagulable state D68.61
  antiphosphatidylinositol R76.0
    with
      hemorrhagic disorder D68.312
      hypercoagulable state D68.61
  antiphosphatidylserine R76.0
    with
      hemorrhagic disorder D68.312
      hypercoagulable state D68.61
  antiphospholipid R76.0
    with
      hemorrhagic disorder D68.312
      hypercoagulable state D68.61
Anticardiolipin syndrome D68.61
Anticoagulant, circulating (intrinsic) - *see
  also* Disorder, hemorrhagic D68.318
  drug-induced (extrinsic) - *see also* Disorder,
  hemorrhagic D68.32
  iatrogenic D68.32
Antidiuretic hormone syndrome E22.2
Antimonial cholera - *see* Poisoning, antimony
Antiphospholipid
  antibody
    with hemorrhagic disorder D68.312
  syndrome D68.61
Antisocial personality F60.2
Antithrombinemia - *see* Circulating
  anticoagulants
Antithromboplastinemia D68.318
Antithromboplastinogenemia D68.318
Antitoxin complication or reaction - *see*
  Complications, vaccination
Antlophobia F40.228
Antritis J32.0
  maxilla J32.0
  acute J01.00
    recurrent J01.01
  stomach K29.60
    with bleeding K29.61
Antrum, antral - *see* condition

Anuria R34
  calculous (impacted) (recurrent) - *see also*
  Calculus, urinary N20.9
  following
    abortion - *see* Abortion by type complicated
      by, renal failure
    ectopic or molar pregnancy O08.4
  newborn P96.0
  postprocedural N99.0
  postrenal N13.8
  traumatic (following crushing) T79.5
Anus, anal - *see* condition
Anusitis K62.89
Anxiety F41.9
  depression F41.8
  episodic paroxysmal F41.0
  generalized F41.1
  hysteria F41.8
  neurosis F41.1
  panic type F41.0
  reaction F41.1
  separation, abnormal (of childhood) F93.0
  specified NEC F41.8
  state F41.1
Aorta, aortic - *see* condition
Aortectasia - *see* Ectasia, aorta
  with aneurysm - *see* Aneurysm, aorta
Aortitis (nonsyphilitic) (calcific) I77.6
  arteriosclerotic I70.0
  Doehle-Heller A52.02
  luetic A52.02
  rheumatic - *see* Endocarditis, acute, rheumatic
  specific (syphilitic) A52.02
  syphilitic A52.02
    congenital A50.54 [*I79.1*]
Apathetic thyroid storm - *see* Thyrotoxicosis
Apathy R45.3
Apeirophobia F40.228
Apepsia K30
  psychogenic F45.8
Aperistalsis, esophagus K22.0
Apertognathia M26.29
Apert's syndrome Q87.0
Aphagia R13.0
  psychogenic F50.9
Aphakia (acquired) (postoperative) H27.0-
  congenital Q12.3
**Aphasia (amnestic) (global) (nominal)
  (semantic) (syntactic)** R47.01
  acquired, with epilepsy (Landau-Kleffner
    syndrome) - *see* Epilepsy, specified NEC
  auditory (developmental) F80.2
  developmental (receptive type) F80.2
    expressive type F80.1
    Wernicke's F80.2
  following
    cerebrovascular disease I69.920
      cerebral infarction I69.320
      intracerebral hemorrhage I69.120
      nontraumatic intracranial hemorrhage NEC
        I69.220
      specified disease NEC I69.820
      subarachnoid hemorrhage I69.020
  primary progressive G31.01 [*F02.80]*
    with behavioral disturbance G31.01
      [*F02.81]*
  progressive isolated G31.01 [*F02.80]*
    with behavioral disturbance G31.01
      [*F02.81]*
  sensory F80.2
  syphilis, tertiary A52.19
  Wernicke's (developmental) F80.2

Aphonia (organic) R49.1
  hysterical F44.4
  psychogenic F44.4
  Bednar's K12.0
  cachectic K14.0
  epizootic B08.8
  fever B08.8
  oral (recurrent) K12.0
  stomatitis (major) (minor) K12.0
  thrush B37.0
  ulcer (oral) (recurrent) K12.0
  genital organ(s) NEC
    female N76.6
    male N50.89
  larynx J38.7
Apical - *see* condition
Apiphobia F40.218
Aplasia - *see also* Agenesis
  abdominal muscle syndrome Q79.4
  alveolar process (acquired) - *see* Anomaly,
    alveolar
    congenital Q38.6
  aorta (congenital) Q25.41
  axialis extracorticalis (congenita) E75.29
  bone marrow (myeloid) D61.9
    congenital D61.01
  brain Q00.0
    part of Q04.3
  bronchus Q32.4
  cementum K00.4
  cerebellum Q04.3
  cervix (congenital) Q51.5
  congenital pure red cell D61.01
  corpus callosum Q04.0
  cutis congenita Q84.8
  erythrocyte congenital D61.01
  extracortical axial E75.29
  eye Q11.1
  fovea centralis (congenital) Q14.1
  gallbladder, congenital Q44.0
  iris Q13.1
  labyrinth, membranous Q16.5
  limb (congenital) Q73.8
    lower - *see* Defect, reduction, lower limb
    upper - *see* Agenesis, arm
  lung, congenital (bilateral) (unilateral) Q33.3
  pancreas Q45.0
  parathyroid-thymic D82.1
  Pelizaeus-Merzbacher E75.29
  penis Q55.5
  prostate Q55.4
  red cell (with thymoma) D60.9
    acquired D60.9
      due to drugs D60.9
    adult D60.9
    chronic D60.0
    congenital D61.01
    constitutional D61.01
    due to drugs D60.9
    hereditary D61.01
    of infants D61.01
    primary D61.01
    pure D61.01
      due to drugs D60.9
    specified type NEC D60.8
    transient D60.1
  round ligament Q52.8
  skin Q84.8
  spermatic cord Q55.4
  spleen Q89.01
  testicle Q55.0
  thymic, with immunodeficiency D82.1
  thyroid (congenital) (with myxedema) E03.1
  uterus Q51.0

Aplasia - *continued*
ventral horn cell Q06.1
Apnea, apneic (of) (spells) R06.81
newborn NEC P28.4
obstructive P28.4
sleep (central) (obstructive) (primary) P28.3
prematurity P28.4
sleep G47.30
central (primary) G47.31
idiopathic G47.31
in conditions classified elsewhere G47.37
obstructive (adult) (pediatric) G47.33
hypopnea G47.33
primary central G47.31
specified NEC G47.39
Apneumatosis, newborn P28.0
Apocrine metaplasia (breast) - *see* Dysplasia, mammary, specified type NEC
Apophysitis (bone) - *see also* Osteochondropathy
calcaneus M92.8
juvenile M92.9
Apoplectiform convulsions (cerebral ischemia) I67.82
Apoplexia, apoplexy, apoplectic
adrenal A39.1
heart (auricle) (ventricle) - *see* Infarct, myocardium
heat T67.0
hemorrhagic (stroke) - *see* Hemorrhage, intracranial
meninges, hemorrhagic - *see* Hemorrhage, intracranial, subarachnoid
uremic N18.9 [*I68.8*]
Appearance
bizarre R46.1
specified NEC R46.89
very low level of personal hygiene R46.0
Appendage
epididymal (organ of Morgagni) Q55.4
intestine (epiploic) Q43.8
preauricular Q17.0
testicular (organ of Morgagni) Q55.29
Appendicitis (pneumococcal) (retrocecal) K37
with
perforation or rupture K35.2
peritoneal abscess K35.3
peritonitis NEC K35.3
generalized (with perforation or rupture) K35.2
localized (with perforation or rupture) K35.3
acute (catarrhal) (fulminating) (gangrenous) (obstructive) (retrocecal) (suppurative) K35.80
with
peritoneal abscess K35.3
peritonitis NEC K35.3
generalized (with perforation or rupture) K35.2
localized (with perforation or rupture) K35.3
specified NEC K35.89
amebic A06.89
chronic (recurrent) K36
exacerbation - *see* Appendicitis, acute
gangrenous - *see* Appendicitis, acute
healed (obliterative) K36
interval K36
neurogenic K36
obstructive K36
recurrent K36

Appendicitis - *continued*
relapsing K36
subacute (adhesive) K36
subsiding K36
suppurative - *see* Appendicitis, acute
tuberculous A18.32
Appendicopathia oxyurica B80
Appendix, appendicular - *see also* condition
epididymis Q55.4
Morgagni
female Q50.5
male (epididymal) Q55.4
testicular Q55.29
testis Q55.29
Appetite
depraved - *see* Pica
excessive R63.2
lack or loss - *see also* Anorexia R63.0
nonorganic origin F50.89
psychogenic F50.89
perverted (hysterical) - *see* Pica
Apple peel syndrome Q41.1
Apprehension state F41.1
Apprehensiveness, abnormal F41.9
Approximal wear K03.0
Apraxia (classic) (ideational) (ideokinetic) (ideomotor) (motor) (verbal) R48.2
following
cerebrovascular disease I69.990
cerebral infarction I69.390
intracerebral hemorrhage I69.190
nontraumatic intracranial hemorrhage NEC I69.290
specified disease NEC I69.890
subarachnoid hemorrhage I69.090
oculomotor, congenital H51.8
Aptyalism K11.7
Apudoma - *see* Neoplasm, uncertain behavior, by site
Aqueous misdirection H40.83-
Arabicum elephantiasis - *see* Infestation, filarial
Arachnitis - *see* Meningitis
Arachnodactyly - *see* Syndrome, Marfan's
Arachnoiditis (acute) (adhesive) (basal) (brain) (cerebrospinal) - *see* Meningitis
Arachnophobia F40.210
Arboencephalitis, Australian A83.4
Arborization block (heart) I45.5
ARC (AIDS-related complex) B20
Arch
aortic Q25.49
bovine Q25.49
Arches - *see* condition
Arcuate uterus Q51.810
Arcuatus uterus Q51.810
Arcus (cornea) senilis - *see* Degeneration, cornea, senile
Arc-welder's lung J63.4
Areflexia R29.2
Areola - *see* condition
Argentaffinoma - *see also* Neoplasm, uncertain behavior, by site
malignant - *see* Neoplasm, malignant, by site
syndrome E34.0
Argininemia E72.21
Arginosuccinic aciduria E72.22
Argyll Robertson phenomenon, pupil or syndrome (syphilitic) A52.19
atypical H57.09
nonsyphilitic H57.09
Argyria, argyriasis
conjunctival H11.13-

Argyria, argyriasis
from drug or medicament - *see* Table of Drugs and Chemicals, by substance
Argyrosis, conjunctival H11.13-
Arhinencephaly Q04.1
Ariboflavinosis E53.0
Arm - *see* condition
Arnold-Chiari disease, obstruction or syndrome (type II) Q07.00
with
hydrocephalus Q07.02
with spina bifida Q07.03
spina bifida Q07.01
with hydrocephalus Q07.03
type III - *see* Encephalocele
type IV Q04.8
Aromatic amino-acid metabolism disorder E70.9
specified NEC E70.8
Arousals, confusional G47.51
Arrest, arrested
cardiac I46.9
complicating
abortion - *see* Abortion, by type, complicated by, cardiac arrest
anesthesia (general) (local) or other sedation - *see* Table of Drugs and Chemicals, by drug,
in labor and delivery O74.2
in pregnancy O29.11-
postpartum, puerperal O89.1
delivery (cesarean) (instrumental) O75.4
due to
cardiac condition I46.2
specified condition NEC I46.8
intraoperative I97.71-
newborn P29.81
postprocedural I97.12-
obstetric procedure O75.4
cardiorespiratory - *see* Arrest, cardiac
circulatory - *see* Arrest, cardiac
deep transverse O64.0
development or growth
bone - *see* Disorder, bone, development or growth
child R62.50
tracheal rings Q32.1
epiphyseal
complete
femur M89.15-
humerus M89.12-
tibia M89.16-
ulna M89.13-
forearm M89.13-
specified NEC M89.13-
ulna - *see* Arrest, epiphyseal, by type, ulna
lower leg M89.16-
specified NEC M89.168
tibia - *see* Arrest, epiphyseal, by type, tibia
partial
femur M89.15-
humerus M89.12-
tibia M89.16-
ulna M89.13-
personal history, successfully resuscitated Z86.74
specified NEC M89.18
granulopoiesis - *see* Agranulocytosis
growth plate - *see* Arrest, epiphyseal
heart - *see* Arrest, cardiac
legal, anxiety concerning Z65.3
physeal - *see* Arrest, epiphyseal
respiratory R09.2
newborn P28.81

Arrest, arrested - *continued*
  sinus I45.5
  spermatogenesis (complete) - *see* Azoospermia
    incomplete - *see* Oligospermia
  transverse (deep) O64.0
Arrhenoblastoma
  benign
    specified site - *see* Neoplasm, benign, by site
    unspecified site
      female D27.9
      male D29.20
  malignant
    specified site - *see* Neoplasm, malignant, by
site
    unspecified site
      female C56.9
      male C62.90
  specified site - *see* Neoplasm, uncertain
    behavior, by site
  unspecified site
    female D39.10
    male D40.10
Arrhythmia (auricle) (cardiac)
  (juvenile)(nodal) (reflex) (sinus)
  (supraventricular)(transitory)(ventricle) I49.9
  block I45.9
  extrasystolic I49.49
  newborn
    bradycardia P29.12
    occurring before birth P03.819
      before onset of labor P03.810
      during labor P03.811
    tachycardia P29.11
  psychogenic F45.8
  specified NEC I49.8
  vagal R55
  ventricular re-entry I47.0
**Arrillaga-Ayerza syndrome (pulmonary
  sclerosis with pulmonary hypertension)**
  I27.0
Arsenical pigmentation L81.8
  from drug or medicament - *see* Table of Drugs
  and Chemicals
Arsenism - *see* Poisoning, arsenic
Arterial - *see* condition
Arteriofibrosis - *see* Arteriosclerosis
Arteriolar sclerosis - *see* Arteriosclerosis
Arteriolith - *see* Arteriosclerosis
Arteriolitis I77.6
  necrotizing, kidney I77.5
  renal - *see* Hypertension, kidney
Arteriolosclerosis - *see* Arteriosclerosis
Arterionephrosclerosis - *see* Hypertension,
  kidney
Arteriopathy I77.9
Arteriosclerosis, arteriosclerotic (diffuse)
  (obliterans) (of) (senile) (with calcification)
  I70.90
  aorta I70.0
  arteries of extremities - *see* Arteriosclerosis,
    extremities
  brain I67.2
  bypass graft
    coronary - *see* Arteriosclerosis, coronary,
    bypass graft
    extremities - *see* Arteriosclerosis, extremities,
    bypass graft
  cardiac - *see* Disease, heart, ischemic,
    atherosclerotic
  cardiopathy - *see* Disease, heart, ischemic,
    atherosclerotic
  cardiorenal - *see* Hypertension, cardiorenal
  cardiovascular - *see* Disease, heart, ischemic,
    atherosclerotic

Arteriosclerosis, arteriosclerotic - *continued*
  carotid - *see also* Occlusion, artery, carotid
    I65.2-
  central nervous system I67.2
  cerebral I67.2
  cerebrovascular I67.2
  coronary (artery) I25.10
    due to
      calcified coronary lesion (severely) I25.84
      lipid rich plaque I25.83
    bypass graft I25.810
      with
        angina pectoris I25.709
          with documented spasm I25.701
          specified type NEC I25.708
          unstable I25.700
        ischemic chest pain I25.709
      autologous artery I25.810
        with
          angina pectoris I25.729
            with documented spasm I25.721
            specified type I25.728
            unstable I25.720
          ischemic chest pain I25.729
      autologous vein I25.810
        with
          angina pectoris I25.719
            with documented spasm I25.711
            specified type I25.718
            unstable I25.710
          ischemic chest pain I25.719
      nonautologous biological I25.810
        with
          angina pectoris I25.739
            with documented spasm I25.731
            specified type I25.738
            unstable I25.730
          ischemic chest pain I25.739
      specified type NEC I25.810
        with
          angina pectoris I25.799
            with documented spasm I25.791
            specified type I25.798
            unstable I25.790
          ischemic chest pain I25.799
    native vessel
      with
        angina pectoris I25.119
          with documented spasm I25.111
          specified type NEC I25.118
          unstable I25.110
        ischemic chest pain I25.119
    transplanted heart I25.811
      bypass graft I25.812
        with
          angina pectoris I25.769
            with documented spasm I25.761
            specified type I25.768
            unstable I25.760
          ischemic chest pain I25.769
      native coronary artery I25.811
        with
          angina pectoris I25.759
            with documented spasm I25.751
            specified type I25.758
            unstable I25.750
          ischemic chest pain I25.759
  extremities (native arteries) I70.209
    bypass graft I70.309
      autologous vein graft I70.409
        leg I70.409
          with
            gangrene (and intermittent claudication,
            rest pain and ulcer) I70.469

Arteriosclerosis, arteriosclerotic - *continued*
        intermittent claudication I70.419
        rest pain (and intermittent claudication)
        I70.429
        bilateral I70.403
          with
            gangrene (and intermittent
            claudication, rest pain and ulcer)
            I70.463
            intermittent claudication I70.413
            rest pain (and intermittent
            claudication) I70.423
            specified type NEC I70.493
        left I70.402
          with
            gangrene (and intermittent
            claudication, rest pain and ulcer)
            I70.462
            intermittent claudication I70.412
            rest pain (and intermittent
            claudication) I70.422
            ulceration (and intermittent
            claudication and rest pain) I70.449
              ankle I70.443
              calf I70.442
              foot site NEC I70.445
              heel I70.444
              lower leg NEC I70.448
              midfoot I70.444
              thigh I70.441
            specified type NEC I70.492
        right I70.401
          with
            gangrene (and intermittent
            claudication, rest pain and ulcer)
            I70.461
            intermittent claudication I70.411
            rest pain (and intermittent
            claudication) I70.421
            ulceration (and intermittent
            claudication and rest pain) I70.439
              ankle I70.433
              calf I70.432
              foot site NEC I70.435
              heel I70.434
              lower leg NEC I70.438
              midfoot I70.434
              thigh I70.431
            specified type NEC I70.491
        specified type NEC I70.499
      specified NEC I70.408
        with
          gangrene (and intermittent claudication,
          rest pain and ulcer) I70.468
          intermittent claudication I70.418
          rest pain (and intermittent claudication)
          I70.428
          ulceration (and intermittent
          claudication and rest pain) I70.45
          specified type NEC I70.498
      leg I70.309
        with
          gangrene (and intermittent claudication,
          rest pain and ulcer) I70.369
          intermittent claudication I70.319
          rest pain (and intermittent claudication)
          I70.329
        bilateral I70.303
          with
            gangrene (and intermittent claudication,
            rest pain and ulcer) I70.363
            intermittent claudication I70.313
            rest pain (and intermittent claudication)
            I70.323

Arteriosclerosis, arteriosclerotic - *continued*
    specified type NEC I70.393
    left I70.302
      with
        gangrene (and intermittent claudication, rest pain and ulcer) I70.362
        intermittent claudication I70.312
        rest pain (and intermittent claudication) I70.322
        ulceration (and intermittent claudication and rest pain) I70.349
          ankle I70.343
          calf I70.342
          foot site NEC I70.345
          heel I70.344
          lower leg NEC I70.348
          midfoot I70.344
          thigh I70.341
        specified type NEC I70.392
    right I70.301
      with
        gangrene (and intermittent claudication, rest pain and ulcer) I70.361
        intermittent claudication I70.311
        rest pain (and intermittent claudication) I70.321
        ulceration (and intermittent claudication and rest pain) I70.339
          ankle I70.333
          calf I70.332
          foot site NEC I70.335
          heel I70.334
          lower leg NEC I70.338
          midfoot I70.334
          thigh I70.331
        specified type NEC I70.391
    specified type NEC I70.399
    nonautologous biological graft I70.509
    leg I70.509
      with
        gangrene (and intermittent claudication, rest pain and ulcer) I70.569
        intermittent claudication I70.519
        rest pain (and intermittent claudication) I70.529
        bilateral I70.503
          with
            gangrene (and intermittent claudication, rest pain and ulcer) I70.563
            intermittent claudication I70.513
            rest pain (and intermittent claudication) I70.523
            specified type NEC I70.593
        left I70.502
          with
            gangrene (and intermittent claudication, rest pain and ulcer) I70.562
            intermittent claudication I70.512
            rest pain (and intermittent claudication) I70.522
            ulceration (and intermittent claudication and rest pain) I70.549
              ankle I70.543
              calf I70.542
              foot site NEC I70.545
               heel I70.544
              lower leg NEC I70.548
              midfoot I70.544
              thigh I70.541
          specified type NEC I70.592
        right I70.501
          with

Arteriosclerosis, arteriosclerotic - *continued*
        gangrene (and intermittent claudication, rest pain and ulcer) I70.561
        intermittent claudication I70.511
        rest pain (and intermittent claudication) I70.521
        ulceration (and intermittent claudication and rest pain) I70.539
          ankle I70.533
          calf I70.532
          foot site NEC I70.535
          heel I70.534
          lower leg NEC I70.538
          midfoot I70.534
          thigh I70.531
      specified type NEC I70.591
    specified type NEC I70.599
    specified NEC I70.508
      with
        gangrene (and intermittent claudication, rest pain and ulcer) I70.568
        intermittent claudication I70.518
        rest pain (and intermittent claudication) I70.528
        ulceration (and intermittent claudication and rest pain) I70.55
        specified type NEC I70.598
    nonbiological graft I70.609
    leg I70.609
      with
        gangrene (and intermittent claudication, rest pain and ulcer) I70.669
        intermittent claudication I70.619
        rest pain (and intermittent claudication) I70.629
        bilateral I70.603
          with
            gangrene (and intermittent claudication, rest pain and ulcer) I70.663
            intermittent claudication I70.613
            rest pain (and intermittent claudication) I70.623
            specified type NEC I70.693
        left I70.602
          with
            gangrene (and intermittent claudication, rest pain and ulcer) I70.662
            intermittent claudication I70.612
            rest pain (and intermittent claudication) I70.622
            ulceration (and intermittent claudication and rest pain) I70.649
              ankle I70.643
              calf I70.642
              foot site NEC I70.645
              heel I70.644
              lower leg NEC I70.648
              midfoot I70.644
              thigh I70.641
          specified type NEC I70.692
        right I70.601
          with
            gangrene (and intermittent claudication, rest pain and ulcer) I70.661
            intermittent claudication I70.611
            rest pain (and intermittent claudication) I70.621
            ulceration (and intermittent claudication and rest pain) I70.639
              ankle I70.633

Arteriosclerosis, arteriosclerotic - *continued*
              calf I70.632
              foot site NEC I70.635
              heel I70.634
              lower leg NEC I70.638
              midfoot I70.634
              thigh I70.631
          specified type NEC I70.691
      specified type NEC I70.699
    specified NEC I70.608
      with
        gangrene (and intermittent claudication, rest pain and ulcer) I70.668
        intermittent claudication I70.618
        rest pain (and intermittent claudication) I70.628
        ulceration (and intermittent claudication and rest pain) I70.65
        specified type NEC I70.698
    specified graft NEC I70.709
    leg I70.709
      with
        gangrene (and intermittent claudication, rest pain and ulcer) I70.769
        intermittent claudication I70.719
        rest pain (and intermittent claudication) I70.729
        bilateral I70.703
          with
            gangrene (and intermittent claudication, rest pain and ulcer) I70.763
            intermittent claudication I70.713
            rest pain (and intermittent claudication) I70.723
            specified type NEC I70.793
        left I70.702
          with
            gangrene (and intermittent claudication, rest pain and ulcer) I70.762
            intermittent claudication I70.712
            rest pain (and intermittent claudication) I70.722
            ulceration (and intermittent claudication and rest pain) I70.749
              ankle I70.743
              calf I70.742
              foot site NEC I70.745
              heel I70.744
              lower leg NEC I70.748
              midfoot I70.744
              thigh I70.741
          specified type NEC I70.792
        right I70.701
          with
            gangrene (and intermittent claudication, rest pain and ulcer) I70.761
            intermittent claudication I70.711
            rest pain (and intermittent claudication) I70.721
            ulceration (and intermittent claudication and rest pain) I70.739
              ankle I70.733
              calf I70.732
              foot site NEC I70.735
              heel I70.734
              lower leg NEC I70.738
              midfoot I70.734
              thigh I70.731
          specified type NEC I70.791
      specified type NEC I70.799
    specified NEC I70.708

Arteriosclerosis, arteriosclerotic - *continued*
  with
    gangrene (and intermittent claudication, rest pain and ulcer) I70.768
    intermittent claudication I70.718
    rest pain (and intermittent claudication) I70.728
    ulceration (and intermittent claudication and rest pain) I70.75
    specified type NEC I70.798
  specified NEC I70.308
    with
      gangrene (and intermittent claudication, rest pain and ulcer) I70.368
      intermittent claudication I70.318
      rest pain (and intermittent claudication) I70.328
      ulceration (and intermittent claudication and rest pain) I70.35
      specified type NEC I70.398
  leg I70.209
    with
      gangrene (and intermittent claudication, rest pain and ulcer) I70.269
      intermittent claudication I70.219
      rest pain (and intermittent claudication) I70.229
    bilateral I70.203
      with
        gangrene (and intermittent claudication, rest pain and ulcer) I70.263
        intermittent claudication I70.213
        rest pain (and intermittent claudication) I70.223
      specified type NEC I70.293
    left I70.202
      with
        gangrene (and intermittent claudication, rest pain and ulcer) I70.262
        intermittent claudication I70.212
        rest pain (and intermittent claudication) I70.222
        ulceration (and intermittent claudication and rest pain) I70.249
        ankle I70.243
        calf I70.242
        foot site NEC I70.245
        heel I70.244
        lower leg NEC I70.248
        midfoot I70.244
        thigh I70.241
      specified type NEC I70.292
    right I70.201
      with
        gangrene (and intermittent claudication, rest pain and ulcer) I70.261
        intermittent claudication I70.211
        rest pain (and intermittent claudication) I70.221
        ulceration (and intermittent claudication and rest pain) I70.239
        ankle I70.233
        calf I70.232
        foot site NEC I70.235
        heel I70.234
        lower leg NEC I70.238
        midfoot I70.234
        thigh I70.231
      specified type NEC I70.291
    specified type NEC I70.299
  specified site NEC I70.208
    with
      gangrene (and intermittent claudication, rest pain and ulcer) I70.268

Arteriosclerosis, arteriosclerotic - *continued*
      intermittent claudication I70.218
      rest pain (and intermittent claudication) I70.228
      ulceration (and intermittent claudication and rest pain) I70.25
      specified type NEC I70.298
  generalized I70.91
  heart (disease) - *see* Arteriosclerosis, coronary (artery), kidney - *see* Hypertension, kidney
  medial - *see* Arteriosclerosis, extremities
  mesenteric (artery) K55.1
  Mönckeberg's - *see* Arteriosclerosis, extremities
  myocarditis I51.4
  peripheral (of extremities) - *see* Arteriosclerosis, extremities
  pulmonary (idiopathic) I27.0
  renal (arterioles) - *see also* Hypertension, kidney
    artery I70.1
  retina (vascular) I70.8 [*H35.0-*]
  specified artery NEC I70.8
  spinal (cord) G95.19
  vertebral (artery) I67.2
Arteriospasm I73.9
Arteriovenous - *see* condition
Arteritis I77.6
  allergic M31.0
  aorta (nonsyphilitic) I77.6
    syphilitic A52.02
  aortic arch M31.4
  brachiocephalic M31.4
  brain I67.7
    syphilitic A52.04
  cerebral I67.7
    in
      diseases classified elsewhere I68.2
      systemic lupus erythematosus M32.19
    listerial A32.89
    syphilitic A52.04
    tuberculous A18.89
  coronary (artery) I25.89
    rheumatic I01.8
      chronic I09.89
    syphilitic A52.06
  cranial (left) (right), giant cell M31.6
  deformans - *see* Arteriosclerosis
  giant cell NEC M31.6
    with polymyalgia rheumatica M31.5
  necrosing or necrotizing M31.9
    specified NEC M31.8
  nodosa M30.0
  obliterans - *see* Arteriosclerosis
  pulmonary I28.8
  rheumatic - *see* Fever, rheumatic
  senile - *see* Arteriosclerosis
  suppurative I77.2
  syphilitic (general) A52.09
    brain A52.04
    coronary A52.06
    spinal A52.09
  temporal, giant cell M31.6
  young female aortic arch syndrome M31.4
Artery, arterial - *see also* condition
  abscess I77.89
  single umbilical Q27.0
Arthralgia (allergic) - *see also* Pain, joint
  in caisson disease T70.3
  temporomandibular M26.62-
Arthritis, arthritic (acute) (chronic) (nonpyogenic) (subacute) M19.90
  allergic - *see* Arthritis, specified form NEC

Arthritis, arthritic - *continued*
  ankylosing (crippling) (spine) - *see also* Spondylitis, ankylosing
    sites other than spine - *see* Arthritis, specified form NEC
  atrophic - *see* Osteoarthritis
    spine - *see* Spondylitis, ankylosing
  back - *see* Spondylopathy, inflammatory
  blennorrhagic (gonococcal) A54.42
  Charcot's - *see* Arthropathy, neuropathic
    diabetic - *see* Diabetes, arthropathy, neuropathic
    syringomyelic G95.0
  chylous (filarial) - *see also* category M01 B74.9
  climacteric (any site) NEC - *see* Arthritis, specified form NEC
  crystal (-induced) - *see* Arthritis, in, crystals
  deformans - *see* Osteoarthritis
  degenerative - *see* Osteoarthritis
  due to or associated with
    acromegaly E22.0
    brucellosis - *see* Brucellosis
    caisson disease T70.3
    diabetes - *see* Diabetes, arthropathy
    dracontiasis - *see also* category M01 B72
    enteritis NEC
      regional - *see* Enteritis, regional
    erysipelas - *see also* category M01 A46
    erythema
      epidemic A25.1
      nodosum L52
    filariasis NOS B74.9
    glanders A24.0
    helminthiasis - *see also* category M01 B83.9
    hemophilia D66 [*M36.2*]
    Henoch (Schönlein) purpura D69.0 [*M36.4*]
    human parvovirus - *see also* category M01 B97.6
    infectious disease NEC - *see* category M01
    leprosy (see also category M01) - *see also* Leprosy A30.9
    Lyme disease A69.23
    mycobacteria - *see also* category M01 A31.8
    parasitic disease NEC - *see also* category M01 B89
    paratyphoid fever (see also category M01) - *see also* Fever, paratyphoid A01.4
    rat bite fever - *see also* category M01 A25.1
    regional enteritis - *see* Enteritis, regional
    respiratory disorder NOS J98.9
    serum sickness - *see also* Reaction, serum T80.69
    syringomyelia G95.0
    typhoid fever A01.04
  epidemic erythema A25.1
  febrile - *see* Fever, rheumatic
  gonococcal A54.42
  gouty (acute) - *see* Gout
  in (due to)
    acromegaly - *see also* subcategory M14.8 E22.0
    amyloidosis - *see also* subcategory M14.8 E85.4
    bacterial disease - *see also* subcategory M01 A49.9
    Behçet's syndrome M35.2
    caisson disease - *see also* subcategory M14.8 T70.3
    coliform bacilli (Escherichia coli) - *see* Arthritis, in, pyogenic organism NEC
    crystals M11.9
      dicalcium phosphate - *see* Arthritis, in, crystals, specified type NEC

Arthritis, arthritic - *continued*

hydroxyapatite M11.0-
pyrophosphate - *see* Arthritis, in, crystals, specified type NEC
specified type NEC M11.80
ankle M11.87-
elbow M11.82-
foot joint M11.87-
hand joint M11.84-
hip M11.85-
knee M11.86-
multiple sites M11.8-
shoulder M11.81-
vertebrae M11.88
wrist M11.83-
dermatoarthritis, lipoid E78.81
dracontiasis (dracunculiasis) - *see also* category M01 B72
endocrine disorder NEC - *see also* subcategory M14.8 E34.9
enteritis, infectious NEC - *see also* category M01 A09
specified organism NEC - *see also* category M01 A08.8
erythema
multiforme - *see also* subcategory M14.8 L51.9
nodosum - *see also* subcategory M14.8 L52
gout - *see* Gout
helminthiasis NEC - *see also* category M01 B83.9
hemochromatosis - *see also* subcategory M14.8 E83.118
hemoglobinopathy NEC D58.2 [*M36.3*]
hemophilia NEC D66 [*M36.2*]
Hemophilus influenzae M00.8 [*B96.3*]
Henoch (-Schönlein) purpura D69.0 [*M36.4*]
hyperparathyroidism NEC - *see also* subcategory M14.8 E21.3
hypersensitivity reaction NEC T78.49 [*M36.4*]
hypogammaglobulinemia - *see also* subcategory M14.8 D80.1
hypothyroidism NEC - *see also* subcategory M14.8 E03.9
infection - *see* Arthritis, pyogenic or pyemic
spine - *see* Spondylopathy, infective
infectious disease NEC - *see* category M01
leprosy - *see also* category M01 A30.9
leukemia NEC C95.9 [*M36.1*]
lipoid dermatoarthritis E78.81
Lyme disease A69.23
Mediterranean fever, familial - *see also* subcategory M14.8 M04.1
Meningococcus A39.83
metabolic disorder NEC - *see also* subcategory M14.8 E88.9
multiple myelomatosis C90.0- [*M36.1*]
mumps B26.85
mycosis NEC - *see also* category M01 B49
myelomatosis (multiple) C90.0- [*M36.1*]
neurological disorder NEC G98.0
ochronosis - *see also* subcategory M14.8 E70.29
O'nyong nyong - *see also* category M01 A92.1
parasitic disease NEC - *see also* category M01 B89
paratyphoid fever - *see also* category M01 A01.4
Pseudomonas - *see* Arthritis, pyogenic, bacterial NEC
psoriasis L40.50

Arthritis, arthritic - *continued*

pyogenic organism NEC - *see* Arthritis, pyogenic, bacterial NEC
Reiter's disease - *see* Reiter's disease
respiratory disorder NEC - *see also* subcategory M14.8 J98.9
reticulosis, malignant - *see also* subcategory M14.8 C86.0
rubella B06.82
Salmonella (arizonae) (cholerae-suis) (enteritidis) (typhimurium) A02.23
sarcoidosis D86.86
specified bacteria NEC - *see* Arthritis, pyogenic, bacterial NEC
sporotrichosis B42.82
syringomyelia G95.0
thalassemia NEC D56.9 [*M36.3*]
tuberculosis - *see* Tuberculosis, arthritis
typhoid fever A01.04
urethritis, Reiter's - *see* Reiter's disease
viral disease NEC - *see also* category M01 B34.9
infectious or infective - *see also* Arthritis, pyogenic or pyemic
spine - *see* Spondylopathy, infective
juvenile M08.90
with systemic onset - *see* Still's disease
ankle M08.97-
elbow M08.92-
foot joint M08.97-
hand joint M08.94-
hip M08.95-
knee M08.96-
multiple site M08.99
pauciarticular M08.40
ankle M08.47-
elbow M08.42-
foot joint M08.47-
hand joint M08.44-
hip M08.45-
knee M08.46-
shoulder M08.41-
vertebrae M08.48
wrist M08.43-
psoriatic L40.54
rheumatoid - *see* Arthritis, rheumatoid, juvenile
shoulder M08.91
vertebra M08.98
specified type NEC M08.80
ankle M08.87-
elbow M08.82-
foot joint M08.87-
hand joint M08.84-
hip M08.85-
knee M08.86-
multiple site M08.89
shoulder M08.81-
specified joint NEC M08.88
vertebrae M08.88
wrist M08.83-
wrist M08.93-
meaning osteoarthritis - *see* Osteoarthritis
meningococcal A39.83
menopausal (any site) NEC - *see* Arthritis, specified form NEC
mutilans (psoriatic) L40.52
mycotic NEC - *see also* category M01 B49
neuropathic (Charcot) - *see* Arthropathy, neuropathic
diabetic - *see* Diabetes, arthropathy, neuropathic
nonsyphilitic NEC G98.0
syringomyelic G95.0

Arthritis, arthritic - *continued*

ochronotic - *see also* subcategory M14.8 E70.29
palindromic (any site) - *see* Rheumatism, palindromic
pneumococcal M00.10
ankle M00.17-
elbow M00.12-
foot joint - *see* Arthritis, pneumococcal, ankle
hand joint M00.14-
hip M00.15-
knee M00.16-
multiple site M00.19
shoulder M00.11-
vertebra M00.18
wrist M00.13-
postdysenteric - *see* Arthropathy, postdysenteric
postmeningococcal A39.84
postrheumatic, chronic - *see* Arthropathy, postrheumatic, chronic
primary progressive - *see also* Arthritis, specified form NEC
spine - *see* Spondylitis, ankylosing
psoriatic L40.50
purulent (any site except spine) - *see* Arthritis, pyogenic or pyemic
spine - *see* Spondylopathy, infective
pyogenic or pyemic (any site except spine) M00.9
bacterial NEC M00.80
ankle M00.87-
elbow M00.82-
foot joint - *see* Arthritis, pyogenic, bacterial NEC, ankle
hand joint M00.84-
hip M00.85-
knee M00.86-
multiple site M00.89
shoulder M00.81-
vertebra M00.88
wrist M00.83-
pneumococcal - *see* Arthritis, pneumococcal
spine - *see* Spondylopathy, infective
staphylococcal - *see* Arthritis, staphylococcal
streptococcal - *see* Arthritis, streptococcal NEC
pneumococcal - *see* Arthritis, pneumococcal
reactive - *see* Reiter's disease
rheumatic - *see also* Arthritis, rheumatoid
acute or subacute - *see* Fever, rheumatic
rheumatoid M06.9
with
carditis - *see* Rheumatoid, carditis
endocarditis - *see* Rheumatoid, carditis
heart involvement NEC - *see* Rheumatoid, carditis
lung involvement - *see* Rheumatoid, lung
myocarditis - *see* Rheumatoid, carditis
myopathy - *see* Rheumatoid, myopathy
pericarditis - *see* Rheumatoid, carditis
polyneuropathy - *see* Rheumatoid, polyneuropathy
rheumatoid factor - *see* Arthritis, rheumatoid, seropositive
splenoadenomegaly and leukopenia - *see* Felty's syndrome
vasculitis - *see* Rheumatoid, vasculitis
visceral involvement NEC - *see* Rheumatoid, arthritis, with involvement of organs NEC
juvenile (with or without rheumatoid factor)

Arthropathy - *continued*
  foot joint M14.67-
  hand joint M14.64-
  hip M14.65-
  knee M14.66-
  multiple site M14.69
  nonsyphilitic NEC G98.0
  shoulder M14.61-
  syringomyelic G95.0
  vertebra M14.68
  wrist M14.63-
  osteopulmonary - *see* Osteoarthropathy,
    hypertrophic, specified NEC
  postdysenteric M02.10
    ankle M02.17-
    elbow M02.12-
    foot joint M02.17-
    hand joint M02.14-
    hip M02.15-
    knee M02.16-
    multiple site M02.19
    shoulder M02.11-
    vertebra M02.18
    wrist M02.13-
  postimmunization M02.20
    ankle M02.27-
    elbow M02.22-
    foot joint M02.27-
    hand joint M02.24-
    hip M02.25-
    knee M02.26-
    multiple site M02.29
    shoulder M02.21-
    vertebra M02.28
    wrist M02.23-
  postinfectious NEC B99 [*M12.80*]
    in (due to)
      enteritis due to Yersinia enterocolitica
      A04.6 [*M12.80*]
      syphilis A52.77
      viral hepatitis NEC B19.9 [*M12.80*]
  postrheumatic, chronic (Jaccoud) M12.00
    ankle M12.07-
    elbow M12.02-
    foot joint M12.07-
    hand joint M12.04-
    hip M12.05-
    knee M12.06-
    multiple site M12.09
    shoulder M12.01-
    specified joint NEC M12.08
    vertebrae M12.08
    wrist M12.03-
  psoriatic NEC L40.59
    interphalangeal, distal L40.51
  reactive M02.9
    in (due to)
      infective endocarditis I33.0 [*M02.9*]
    specified type NEC M02.80
      ankle M02.87-
      elbow M02.82-
      foot joint M02.87-
      hand joint M02.84-
      hip M02.85-
      knee M02.86-
      multiple site M02.89
      shoulder M02.81-
      vertebra M02.88
      wrist M02.83-
  specified form NEC M12.80
    ankle M12.87-
    elbow M12.82-
    foot joint M12.87-
    hand joint M12.84-

Arthropathy - *continued*
  hip M12.85-
  knee M12.86-
  multiple site M12.89
  shoulder M12.81-
  specified joint NEC M12.88
  vertebrae M12.88
  wrist M12.83-
  syringomyelic G95.0
  tabes dorsalis A52.16
  tabetic A52.16
  transient - *see* Arthropathy, specified form
    NEC
  traumatic M12.50
    ankle M12.57-
    elbow M12.52-
    foot joint M12.57-
    hand joint M12.54-
    hip M12.55-
    knee M12.56-
    multiple site M12.59
    shoulder M12.51-
    specified joint NEC M12.58
    vertebrae M12.58
    wrist M12.53-
Arthropyosis - *see* Arthritis, pyogenic or
  pyemic
Arthrosis (deformans) (degenerative)
  (localized) - *see also* Osteoarthritis M19.90
  spine - *see* Spondylosis
Arthus' phenomenon or reaction T78.41
  due to
    drug - *see* Table of Drugs and Chemicals, by
    drug
Articular - *see* condition
Articulation, reverse (teeth) M26.24
Artificial
  insemination complication - *see*
  Complications, artificial, fertilization
  opening status (functioning) (without
  complication) Z93.9
    anus (colostomy) Z93.3
    colostomy Z93.3
    cystostomy Z93.50
      appendico-vesicostomy Z93.52
      cutaneous Z93.51
      specified NEC Z93.59
    enterostomy Z93.4
    gastrostomy Z93.1
    ileostomy Z93.2
    intestinal tract NEC Z93.4
    jejunostomy Z93.4
    nephrostomy Z93.6
    specified site NEC Z93.8
    tracheostomy Z93.0
    ureterostomy Z93.6
    urethrostomy Z93.6
    urinary tract NEC Z93.6
    vagina Z93.8
  vagina status Z93.8
Arytenoid - *see* condition
Asbestosis (occupational) J61
ASC-h (atypical squamous cells cannot
  exclude high grade squamous intraepithelial
  lesion on cytologic smear)
  anus R85.611
  cervix R87.611
  vagina R87.621
ASC-US (atypical squamous cells of
  undetermined significance on cytologic
  smear)
  anus R85.610
  cervix R87.610
  vagina R87.620

Ascariasis B77.9
  with
    complications NEC B77.89
    intestinal complications B77.0
    pneumonia, pneumonitis B77.81
Ascaridosis, ascaridiasis - *see* Ascariasis
Ascaris (infection) (infestation)
  (lumbricoides) - *see* Ascariasis
Ascending - *see* condition
Aschoff's bodies - *see* Myocarditis, rheumatic
Ascites (abdominal) R18.8
  cardiac (see also Failure, heart, right) I50.810
  chylous (nonfilarial) I89.8
    filarial - *see* Infestation, filarial
  due to
    cirrhosis, alcoholic K70.31
    hepatitis
      alcoholic K70.11
      chronic active K71.51
    S. japonicum B65.2
  heart (see also Failure, heart, right) I50.810
  malignant R18.0
  pseudochylous R18.8
  syphilitic A52.74
  tuberculous A18.31
Aseptic - *see* condition
Asherman's syndrome N85.6
Asialia K11.7
Asiatic cholera - *see* Cholera
Asimultagnosia (simultanagnosia) R48.3
Askin's tumor - *see* Neoplasm, connective
  tissue, malignant
Asocial personality F60.2
Asomatognosia R41.4
Aspartylglucosaminuria E77.1
Asperger's disease or syndrome F84.5
Aspergilloma - *see* Aspergillosis
Aspergillosis (with pneumonia) B44.9
  bronchopulmonary, allergic B44.81
  disseminated B44.7
  generalized B44.7
  pulmonary NEC B44.1
    allergic B44.81
    invasive B44.0
  specified NEC B44.89
  tonsillar B44.2
Aspergillus (flavus) (fumigatus) (infection)
  (terreus) - *see* Aspergillosis
Aspermatogenesis - *see* Azoospermia
Aspermia (testis) - *see* Azoospermia
Asphyxia, asphyxiation (by) R09.01
  antenatal P84
  birth P84
  bunny bag - *see* Asphyxia, due to, mechanical
    threat to breathing, trapped in bed clothes
  crushing S28.0
  drowning T75.1
  gas, fumes, or vapor - *see* Table of Drugs and
    Chemicals
  inhalation - *see* Inhalation
  intrauterine P84
  local I73.00
    with gangrene I73.01
  mucus - *see also* Foreign body, respiratory
    tract, causing asphyxia
  newborn P84
  pathological R09.01
  postnatal P84
    mechanical - *see* Asphyxia, due to,
    mechanical threat to breathing
  prenatal P84
  reticularis R23.1
  strangulation - *see* Asphyxia, due to,
    mechanical threat to breathing

Asphyxia, asphyxiation - *continued*
 submersion T75.1
 traumatic T71.9
  due to
   crushed chest S28.0
   foreign body (in) - *see* Foreign body,
  respiratory tract, causing asphyxia
   low oxygen content of ambient air T71.20
    due to
     being trapped in
      low oxygen environment T71.29
       in car trunk T71.221
        circumstances undetermined
         T71.224
        done with intent to harm by
         another person T71.223
         self T71.222
       in refrigerator T71.231
        circumstances undetermined
         T71.234
        done with intent to harm by
         another person T71.233
         self T71.232
   cave-in T71.21
   mechanical threat to breathing (accidental)
    T71.191
    circumstances undetermined T71.194
    done with intent to harm by
     another person T71.193
     self T71.192
   hanging T71.161
    circumstances undetermined T71.164
    done with intent to harm by
     another person T71.163
     self T71.162
   plastic bag T71.121
    circumstances undetermined T71.124
    done with intent to harm by
     another person T71.123
     self T71.122
   smothering
    in furniture T71.151
     circumstances undetermined T71.154
     done with intent to harm by
      another person T71.153
      self T71.152
    under
     another person's body T71.141
      circumstances undetermined T71.144
      done with intent to harm T71.143
     pillow T71.111
      circumstances undetermined T71.114
      done with intent to harm by
       another person T71.113
       self T71.112
    trapped in bed clothes T71.131
     circumstances undetermined T71.134
     done with intent to harm by
      another person T71.133
      self T71.132
 vomiting, vomitus - *see* Foreign body,
  respiratory tract, causing asphyxia
Aspiration
 amniotic (clear) fluid (newborn) P24.10
  with
   pneumonia (pneumonitis) P24.11
   respiratory symptoms P24.11
 blood
  newborn (without respiratory symptoms)
   P24.20
   with
    pneumonia (pneumonitis) P24.21
    respiratory symptoms P24.21
  specified age NEC - *see* Foreign body,

Aspiration - *continued*
 respiratory tract
 bronchitis J69.0
 food or foreign body (with asphyxiation) - *see*
  Asphyxia, food liquor (amnii) (newborn)
   P24.10
   with
    pneumonia (pneumonitis) P24.11
    respiratory symptoms P24.11
 meconium (newborn) (without respiratory
  symptoms) P24.00
  with
   pneumonitis (pneumonitis) P24.01
   respiratory symptoms P24.01
 milk (newborn) (without respiratory
  symptoms) P24.30
  with
   pneumonia (pneumonitis) P24.31
   respiratory symptoms P24.31
  specified age NEC - *see* Foreign body,
 respiratory tract

 mucus - *see also* Foreign body, by site,
  causing asphyxia
  newborn P24.10
   with
    pneumonia (pneumonitis) P24.11
    respiratory symptoms P24.11
  neonatal P24.9
  specific NEC (without respiratory symptoms)
   P24.80
   with
    pneumonia (pneumonitis) P24.81
    respiratory symptoms P24.81
  newborn P24.9
  specific NEC (without respiratory symptoms)
   P24.80
   with
    pneumonia (pneumonitis) P24.81
    respiratory symptoms P24.81
 pneumonia J69.0
 pneumonitis J69.0
 syndrome of newborn - *see* Aspiration, by
  substance, with pneumonia
 vernix caseosa (newborn) P24.80
  with
   pneumonia (pneumonitis) P24.81
   respiratory symptoms P24.81
 vomitus - *see also* Foreign body, respiratory
  tract
  newborn (without respiratory symptoms)
   P24.30
   with
    pneumonia (pneumonitis) P24.31
    respiratory symptoms P24.31
Asplenia (congenital) Q89.01
 postsurgical Z90.81
Assam fever B55.0
Assault, sexual - *see* Maltreatment
Assmann's focus NEC A15.0
Astasia (-abasia) (hysterical) F44.4
Asteatosis cutis L85.3
Astereognosia, astereognosis R48.1
Asterixis R27.8
 in liver disease K71.3
Asteroid hyalitis - *see* Deposit, crystalline
Asthenia, asthenic R53.1
 cardiac - *see also* Failure, heart I50.9
  psychogenic F45.8
 cardiovascular - *see also* Failure, heart I50.9
  psychogenic F45.8
 heart - *see also* Failure, heart I50.9
  psychogenic F45.8
 hysterical F44.4

Asthenia, asthenic
 myocardial - *see also* Failure, heart I50.9
  psychogenic F45.8
 nervous F48.8
 neurocirculatory F45.8
 neurotic F48.8
 psychogenic F48.8
 psychoneurotic F48.8
 psychophysiologic F48.8
 reaction (psychophysiologic) F48.8
 senile R54
Asthenopia - *see also* Discomfort, visual
 hysterical F44.6
 psychogenic F44.6
Asthenospermia - *see* Abnormal, specimen,
 male genital organs
Asthma, asthmatic (bronchial) (catarrh)
 (spasmodic) J45.909
 with
  chronic obstructive bronchitis J44.9
   with
    acute lower respiratory infection J44.0
    exacerbation (acute) J44.1
  chronic obstructive pulmonary disease J44.9
   with
    acute lower respiratory infection J44.0
    exacerbation (acute) J44.1
  exacerbation (acute) J45.901
 hay fever - *see* Asthma, allergic extrinsic
  rhinitis, allergic - *see* Asthma, allergic
   extrinsic
  status asthmaticus J45.902
 allergic extrinsic J45.909
  with
   exacerbation (acute) J45.901
   status asthmaticus J45.902
 atopic - *see* Asthma, allergic extrinsic
 cardiac - *see* Failure, ventricular, left
 cardiobronchial I50.1
 childhood J45.909
  with
   exacerbation (acute) J45.901
   status asthmaticus J45.902
 chronic obstructive J44.9
  with
   acute lower respiratory infection J44.0
   exacerbation (acute) J44.1
 collier's J60
 cough variant J45.991
 detergent J69.8
 due to
  detergent J69.8
  inhalation of fumes J68.3
 eosinophilic J82
 extrinsic, allergic - *see* Asthma, allergic
  extrinsic
 grinder's J62.8
 hay - *see* Asthma, allergic extrinsic
 heart I50.1
 idiosyncratic - *see* Asthma, nonallergic
 intermittent (mild) J45.20
  with
   exacerbation (acute) J45.21
   status asthmaticus J45.22
 intrinsic, nonallergic - *see* Asthma, nonallergic
 Kopp's E32.8
 late-onset J45.909
  with
   exacerbation (acute) J45.901
   status asthmaticus J45.902
 mild intermittent J45.20
  with
   exacerbation (acute) J45.21
   status asthmaticus J45.22

Asthma, asthmatic - *continued*
  mild persistent J45.30
    with
      exacerbation (acute) J45.31
      status asthmaticus J45.32
    Millar's (laryngismus stridulus) J38.5
  miner's J60
  mixed J45.909
    with
      exacerbation (acute) J45.901
      status asthmaticus J45.902
  moderate persistent J45.40
    with
      exacerbation (acute) J45.41
      status asthmaticus J45.42
  nervous - *see* Asthma, nonallergic
  nonallergic (intrinsic) J45.909
    with
      exacerbation (acute) J45.901
      status asthmaticus J45.902
  persistent
    mild J45.30
      with
        exacerbation (acute) J45.31
        status asthmaticus J45.32
    moderate J45.40
      with
        exacerbation (acute) J45.41
        status asthmaticus J45.42
    severe J45.50
      with
        exacerbation (acute) J45.51
        status asthmaticus J45.52
  platinum J45.998
  pneumoconiotic NEC J64
  potter's J62.8
  predominantly allergic J45.909
  psychogenic F54
  pulmonary eosinophilic J82
  red cedar J67.8
  Rostan's I50.1
  sandblaster's J62.8
  sequoiosis J67.8
  severe persistent J45.50
    with
      exacerbation (acute) J45.51
      status asthmaticus J45.52
  specified NEC J45.998
  stonemason's J62.8
  thymic E32.8
  tuberculous - *see* Tuberculosis, pulmonary
  Wichmann's (laryngismus stridulus) J38.5
  wood J67.8
Astigmatism (compound) (congenital)
  H52.20-
  irregular H52.21-
  regular H52.22-
Astraphobia F40.220
Astroblastoma
  specified site - *see* Neoplasm, malignant, by
    site
  unspecified site C71.9
Astrocytoma (cystic)
  anaplastic
    specified site - *see* Neoplasm, malignant,
      site
    unspecified site C71.9
  fibrillary
    specified site - *see* Neoplasm, malignant,
      by site
    unspecified site C71.9
  fibrous
    specified site - *see* Neoplasm, malignant,
      site

Astrocytoma (cystic) - *continued*
  unspecified site C71.9
  gemistocytic
    specified site - *see* Neoplasm, malignant, by
      site
    unspecified site C71.9
  juvenile
    specified site - *see* Neoplasm, malignant, by
      site
    unspecified site C71.9
  pilocytic
    specified site - *see* Neoplasm, malignant, by
      site
    unspecified site C71.9
  piloid
    specified site - *see* Neoplasm, malignant, by
      site
    unspecified site C71.9
  protoplasmic
    specified site - *see* Neoplasm, malignant, by
      site
    unspecified site C71.9
  specified site NEC - *see* Neoplasm, malignant,
    by site
  subependymal D43.2
    giant cell
      specified site - *see* Neoplasm, uncertain
        behavior, by site
      unspecified site D43.2
    specified site - *see* Neoplasm, uncertain
      behavior, by site
    unspecified site D43.2
  unspecified site C71.9
Astroglioma
  specified site - *see* Neoplasm, malignant, by
    site
  unspecified site C71.9
Asymbolia R48.8
Asymmetry - *see also* Distortion
  between native and reconstructed breast N65.1
  face Q67.0
  jaw (lower) - *see* Anomaly, dentofacial, jaw-
    cranial base relationship, asymmetry
Asynergia, asynergy R27.8
  ventricular I51.89
Asystole (heart) - *see* Arrest, cardiac
At risk
  for
    dental caries Z91.849
      high Z91.843
      low Z91.841
      moderate Z91.842   falling Z91.81
Ataxia, ataxy, ataxic R27.0
  acute R27.8
  brain (hereditary) G11.9
  cerebellar (hereditary) G11.9
    with defective DNA repair G11.3
    alcoholic G31.2
    early-onset G11.1
    in
      alcoholism G31.2
      myxedema E03.9 [*G13.2*]
      neoplastic disease - *see also* Neoplasm
        D49.9 [*G32.81*]
      specified disease NEC G32.81
    late-onset (Marie's) G11.2
  cerebral (hereditary) G11.9
  congenital nonprogressive G11.0
  family, familial - *see* Ataxia, hereditary
  following
    cerebrovascular disease I69.993
      cerebral infarction I69.393
      intracerebral hemorrhage I69.193
      nontraumatic intracranial hemorrhage NEC

Ataxia, ataxy, ataxic - *continued*
        I69.293
      specified disease NEC I69.893
      subarachnoid hemorrhage I69.093
  Friedreich's (heredofamilial) (cerebellar)
    (spinal) G11.1
  gait R26.0
    hysterical F44.4
  general R27.8
  gluten M35.9 [*G32.81*]
    with celiac disease K90.0 [*G32.81*]
  hereditary G11.9
    with neuropathy G60.2
    cerebellar - *see* Ataxia, cerebellar
    spastic G11.4
    specified NEC G11.8
    spinal (Friedreich's) G11.1
  heredofamilial - *see* Ataxia, hereditary
  Hunt's G11.1
  hysterical F44.4
  locomotor (progressive) (syphilitic) (partial)
    (spastic) A52.11
    diabetic - *see* Diabetes, ataxia
  Marie's (cerebellar) (heredofamilial) (late
    onset) G11.2
  nonorganic origin F44.4
  nonprogressive, congenital G11.0
  psychogenic F44.4
  Roussy-Lévy G60.0
  Sanger-brown's (hereditary) G11.2
  spastic hereditary G11.4
  spinal
    hereditary (Friedreich's) G11.1
    progressive (syphilitic) A52.11
  spinocerebellar, X-linked recessive G11.1
  telangiectasia (Louis-bar) G11.3
Ataxia-telangiectasia (Louis-bar) G11.3
Atelectasis (massive) (partial) (pressure)
  (pulmonary) J98.11
  newborn P28.10
    due to resorption P28.11
    partial P28.19
    primary P28.0
    secondary P28.19
  primary (newborn) P28.0
  tuberculous - *see* Tuberculosis, pulmonary
Atelocardia Q24.9
Atelomyelia Q06.1
Atheroembolism
  of
    extremities
      lower I75.02-
      upper I75.01-
    kidney I75.81
    specified NEC I75.89
Atheroma, atheromatous - *see also*
  Arteriosclerosis I70.90
  aorta, aortic I70.0
    valve - *see also* Endocarditis, aortic I35.8
  aorto-iliac I70.0
  artery - *see* Arteriosclerosis
  basilar (artery) I67.2
  carotid (artery) (common) (internal) I67.2
  cerebral (arteries) I67.2
  coronary (artery) I25.10
    with angina pectoris - *see* Arteriosclerosis,
      coronary (artery),
  degeneration - *see* Arteriosclerosis
  heart, cardiac - *see* Disease, heart, ischemic,
    atherosclerotic
  mitral (valve) I34.8
  myocardium, myocardial - *see* Disease, heart,
    ischemic, atherosclerotic

Atheroma, atheromatous - *continued*
  pulmonary valve (heart) - *see also*
  Endocarditis, pulmonary I37.8
  tricuspid (heart) (valve) I36.8
  valve, valvular - *see* Endocarditis
  vertebral (artery) I67.2
Atheromatosis - *see* Arteriosclerosis
Atherosclerosis - *see also* Arteriosclerosis
  coronary
    artery I25.10
      with angina pectoris - *see* Arteriosclerosis,
        coronary (artery),
        due to
          calcified coronary lesion (severely) I25.84
          lipid rich plaque I25.83
    transplanted heart I25.811
      bypass graft I25.812
        with angina pectoris - *see* Arteriosclerosis,
        coronary (artery),
        native coronary artery I25.811
          with angina pectoris - *see* Arteriosclerosis,
          coronary (artery),
Athetosis (acquired) R25.8
  bilateral (congenital) G80.3
  congenital (bilateral) (double) G80.3
  double (congenital) G80.3
  unilateral R25.8
Athlete's
  foot B35.3
  heart I51.7
Athrepsia E41
Athyrea (acquired) - *see also* Hypothyroidism
  congenital E03.1
Atonia, atony, atonic
  bladder (sphincter) (neurogenic) N31.2
  capillary I78.8
  cecum K59.8
    psychogenic F45.8
  colon - *see* Atony, intestine
  congenital P94.2
  esophagus K22.8
  intestine K59.8
    psychogenic F45.8
  stomach K31.89
    neurotic or psychogenic F45.8
  uterus (during labor) O62.2
    with hemorrhage (postpartum) O72.1
    postpartum (with hemorrhage) O72.1
      without hemorrhage O75.89
Atopy - *see* History, allergy
Atransferrinemia, congenital E88.09
Atresia, atretic
  alimentary organ or tract NEC Q45.8
    upper Q40.8
  ani, anus, anal (canal) Q42.3
    with fistula Q42.2
  aorta (ring) Q25.29
  aortic (orifice) (valve) Q23.0
    arch Q25.21
    congenital with hypoplasia of ascending
      aorta and defective development of left
      ventricle (with mitral stenosis) Q23.4
    in hypoplastic left heart syndrome Q23.4
  aqueduct of Sylvius Q03.0
    with spina bifida - *see* Spina bifida, with
      hydrocephalus
  artery NEC Q27.8
    cerebral Q28.3
    coronary Q24.5
    digestive system Q27.8
    eye Q15.8
    lower limb Q27.8
    pulmonary Q25.5
    specified site NEC Q27.8

Atresia, atretic - *continued*
  umbilical Q27.0
  upper limb Q27.8
  auditory canal (external) Q16.1
  bile duct (common) (congenital) (hepatic)
    Q44.2
    acquired - *see* Obstruction, bile duct
  bladder (neck) Q64.39
    obstruction Q64.31
  bronchus Q32.4
  cecum Q42.8
  cervix (acquired) N88.2
    congenital Q51.828
    in pregnancy or childbirth - *see* Anomaly,
    cervix, in pregnancy or childbirth
      causing obstructed labor O65.5
  choana Q30.0
  colon Q42.9
    specified NEC Q42.8
  common duct Q44.2
  cricoid cartilage Q31.8
  cystic duct Q44.2
    acquired K82.8
      with obstruction K82.0
  digestive organs NEC Q45.8
  duodenum Q41.0
  ear canal Q16.1
  ejaculatory duct Q55.4
  epiglottis Q31.8
  esophagus Q39.0
    with tracheoesophageal fistula Q39.1
  eustachian tube Q17.8
  fallopian tube (congenital) Q50.6
    acquired N97.1
  follicular cyst N83.0-
  foramen of
    Luschka Q03.1
      with spina bifida - *see* Spina bifida, with
        hydrocephalus
    Magendie Q03.1
      with spina bifida - *see* Spina bifida, with
        hydrocephalus
  gallbladder Q44.1
  genital organ
    external
      female Q52.79
      male Q55.8
    internal
      female Q52.8
      male Q55.8
  glottis Q31.8
  gullet Q39.0
    with tracheoesophageal fistula Q39.1
  heart valve NEC Q24.8
    pulmonary Q22.0
    tricuspid Q22.4
  hymen Q52.3
    acquired (postinfective) N89.6
  ileum Q41.2
  intestine (small) Q41.9
    large Q42.9
      specified NEC Q42.8
  iris, filtration angle Q15.0
  jejunum Q41.1
  lacrimal apparatus Q10.4
  larynx Q31.8
  meatus urinarius Q64.33
  mitral valve Q23.2
    in hypoplastic left heart syndrome Q23.4
  nares (anterior) (posterior) Q30.0
  nasopharynx Q34.8
  nose, nostril Q30.0
    acquired J34.89
  organ or site NEC Q89.8

Atresia, atretic - *continued*
  osseous meatus (ear) Q16.1
  oviduct (congenital) Q50.6
    acquired N97.1
  parotid duct Q38.4
    acquired K11.8
  pulmonary (artery) Q25.5
    valve Q22.0
  pulmonic Q22.0
  pupil Q13.2
  rectum Q42.1
    with fistula Q42.0
  salivary duct Q38.4
    acquired K11.8
  sublingual duct Q38.4
    acquired K11.8
  submandibular duct Q38.4
    acquired K11.8
  submaxillary duct Q38.4
    acquired K11.8
  thyroid cartilage Q31.8
  trachea Q32.1
  tricuspid valve Q22.4
  ureter Q62.10
    pelvic junction Q62.11
    vesical orifice Q62.12
  ureteropelvic junction Q62.11
  ureterovesical orifice Q62.12
  urethra (valvular) Q64.39
    stricture Q64.32
  urinary tract NEC Q64.8
  uterus Q51.818
    acquired N85.8
  vagina (congenital) Q52.4
    acquired (postinfectional) (senile) N89.5
  vas deferens Q55.3
  vascular NEC Q27.8
    cerebral Q28.3
    digestive system Q27.8
    lower limb Q27.8
    specified site NEC Q27.8
    upper limb Q27.8
  vein NEC Q27.8
    digestive system Q27.8
    great Q26.8
    lower limb Q27.8
    portal Q26.5
    pulmonary Q26.4
      partial Q26.3
      total Q26.2
    specified site NEC Q27.8
    upper limb Q27.8
  vena cava (inferior) (superior) Q26.8
  vesicourethral orifice Q64.31
  vulva Q52.79
    acquired N90.5
Atrichia, atrichosis - *see* Alopecia
Atrophia - *see also* Atrophy
  cutis senilis L90.8
    due to radiation L57.8
  gyrata of choroid and retina H31.23
  senilis R54
    dermatological L90.8
      due to radiation (nonionizing) (solar) L57.8
  unguium L60.3
    congenita Q84.6
Atrophie blanche (en plaque) (de Milian)
  L95.0
Atrophoderma, atrophoderma (of) L90.9
  diffusum (idiopathic) L90.4
  maculatum L90.8
    et striatum L90.8
      due to syphilis A52.79
    syphilitic A51.39

Atrophoderma, atrophoderma (of) - continued

neuriticum L90.8
Pasini and Pierini L90.3
pigmentosum Q82.1
reticulatum symmetricum faciei L66.4
senile L90.8
  due to radiation (nonionizing) (solar) L57.8
vermiculata (cheeks) L66.4

Atrophy, atrophic (of)

adrenal (capsule) (gland) E27.49
  primary (autoimmune) E27.1
alveolar process or ridge (edentulous) K08.20
anal sphincter (disuse) N81.84
appendix K38.8
arteriosclerotic - see Arteriosclerosis
bile duct (common) (hepatic) K83.8
bladder N32.89
  neurogenic N31.8
blanche (en plaque) (of Milian) L95.0
bone (senile) NEC - see also Disorder, bone,
specified type NEC
  due to
    tabes dorsalis (neurogenic) A52.11
brain (cortex) (progressive) G31.9
  frontotemporal circumscribed G31.01
    [F02.80]
    with behavioral disturbance G31.01
    [F02.81]
  senile NEC G31.1
breast N64.2
  obstetric - see Disorder, breast, specified type
NEC
buccal cavity K13.79
cardiac - see Degeneration, myocardial
cartilage (infectional) (joint) - see Disorder,
cartilage, specified NEC
cerebellar - see Atrophy, brain
cerebral - see Atrophy, brain
cervix (mucosa) (senile) (uteri) N88.8
  menopausal N95.8
Charcot-Marie-tooth G60.0
choroid (central) (macular) (myopic) (retina)
H31.10-
  diffuse secondary H31.12-
  gyrate H31.23
  senile H31.11-
ciliary body - see Atrophy, iris
conjunctiva (senile) H11.89
corpus cavernosum N48.89
cortical - see Atrophy, brain
cystic duct K82.8
Déjérine-Thomas G23.8
disuse NEC - see Atrophy, muscle
Duchenne-Aran G12.21
ear H93.8-
edentulous alveolar ridge K08.20
endometrium (senile) N85.8
  cervix N88.8
enteric K63.89
epididymis N50.89
eyeball - see Disorder, globe, degenerated
condition, atrophy
eyelid (senile) - see Disorder, eyelid,
degenerative
facial (skin) L90.9
fallopian tube (senile) N83.32-
  with ovary N83.33-
fascioscapulohumeral (Landouzy Déjérine)
G71.0
fatty, thymus (gland) E32.8
gallbladder K82.8
gastric K29.40
  with bleeding K29.41

Atrophy, atrophic (of) - continued

gastrointestinal K63.89
glandular I89.8
globe H44.52-
gum see Recession, gingival
hair L67.8
heart (brown) - see Degeneration, myocardial
hemifacial Q67.4
  Romberg G51.8
infantile E41
  paralysis, acute - see Poliomyelitis, paralytic
intestine K63.89
iris (essential) (progressive) H21.26-
  specified NEC H21.29
kidney (senile) (terminal) - see also Sclerosis,
renal N26.1
  congenital or infantile Q60.5
    bilateral Q60.4
    unilateral Q60.3
  hydronephrotic - see Hydronephrosis
lacrimal gland (primary) H04.14-
  secondary H04.15-
Landouzy-Dejerine G71.0
laryngitis, infective J37.0
larynx J38.7
Leber's optic (hereditary) H47.22
lip K13.0
liver (yellow) K72.90
  with coma K72.91
  acute, subacute K72.00
    with coma K72.01
  chronic K72.10
    with coma K72.11
lung (senile) J98.4
macular (dermatological) L90.8
  syphilitic, skin A51.39
    striated A52.79
mandible (edentulous) K08.20
  minimal K08.21
  moderate K08.22
  severe K08.23
maxilla K08.20
  minimal K08.24
  moderate K08.25
  severe K08.26
muscle, muscular (diffuse) (general)
(idiopathic) (primary) M62.50
  ankle M62.57-
  Duchenne-Aran G12.21
  foot M62.57-
  forearm M62.53-
  hand M62.54-
  infantile spinal G12.0
  lower leg M62.56-
  multiple sites M62.59
  myelopathic - see Atrophy, muscle, spinal
  myotonic G71.11
  neuritic G58.9
  neuropathic (peroneal) (progressive) G60.0
  pelvic (disuse) N81.84
  peroneal G60.0
  progressive (bulbar) G12.25
    adult G12.1
    infantile (spinal) G12.0
    spinal G12.25
      adult G12.1
      infantile G12.0
  pseudohypertrophic G71.0
  shoulder region M62.51-
  specified site NEC M62.58
  spinal G12.9
    adult form G12.1
    Aran-Duchenne G12.21
    childhood form, type II G12.1

Atrophy, atrophic (of) - continued

distal G12.1
  hereditary NEC G12.1
  infantile, type I (Werdnig-Hoffmann) G12.0
  juvenile form, type III (Kugelberg
    Welander) G12.1
  progressive G12.21
  scapuloperoneal form G12.1
  specified NEC G12.8
  syphilitic A52.78
  thigh M62.55-
  upper arm M62.52-
myocardium - see Degeneration, myocardial
myometrium (senile) N85.8
  cervix N88.8
myopathic NEC - see Atrophy, muscle
myotonia G71.11
nail L60.3
nasopharynx J31.1
nerve - see also Disorder, nerve
  abducens - see Strabismus, paralytic, sixth
    nerve
  accessory G52.8
  acoustic or auditory - see subcategory H93.3
  cranial G52.9
    eighth (auditory) - see subcategory H93.3
    eleventh (accessory) G52.8
    fifth (trigeminal) G50.8
    first (olfactory) G52.0
    fourth (trochlear) - see Strabismus,
      paralytic, fourth nerve
    second (optic) H47.20
    sixth (abducens) - see Strabismus, paralytic,
      sixth nerve
    tenth (pneumogastric) (vagus) G52.2
    third (oculomotor) - see Strabismus,
      paralytic, third nerve
    twelfth (hypoglossal) G52.3
  hypoglossal G52.3
  oculomotor - see Strabismus, paralytic, third
    nerve
  olfactory G52.0
  optic (papillomacular bundle)
    syphilitic (late) A52.15
      congenital A50.44
  pneumogastric G52.2
  trigeminal G50.8
  trochlear - see Strabismus, paralytic, fourth
    nerve
  vagus (pneumogastric) G52.2
neurogenic, bone, tabetic A52.11
nutritional E41
old age R54
olivopontocerebellar G23.8
optic (nerve) H47.20
  glaucomatous H47.23-
  hereditary H47.22
  primary H47.21-
  specified type NEC H47.29-
  syphilitic (late) A52.15
    congenital A50.44
orbit H05.31-
ovary (senile) N83.31-
  with fallopian tube N83.33-
oviduct (senile) - see Atrophy, fallopian tube
palsy, diffuse (progressive) G12.22
pancreas (duct) (senile) K86.89
parotid gland K11.0
pelvic muscle N81.84
penis N48.89
pharynx J39.2
pluriglandular E31.8
  autoimmune E31.0
polyarthritis M15.9

Atrophy, atrophic (of) - *continued*
  prostate N42.89
  pseudohypertrophic (muscle) G71.0
  renal - *see also* Sclerosis, renal N26.1
  retina, retinal (postinfectional) H35.89
  rhinitis J31.0
  salivary gland K11.0
  scar L90.5
  sclerosis, lobar (of brain) G31.09 *[F02.80]*
    with behavioral disturbance G31.09
      [F02.81]
  scrotum N50.89
  seminal vesicle N50.89
  senile R54
    due to radiation (nonionizing) (solar) L57.8
  skin (patches) (spots) L90.9
    degenerative (senile) L90.8
    due to radiation (nonionizing) (solar) L57.8
    senile L90.8
  spermatic cord N50.89
  spinal (acute) (cord) G95.89
    muscular - *see* Atrophy, muscle, spinal
    paralysis G12.20
      acute - *see* Poliomyelitis, paralytic
      meaning progressive muscular atrophy
        G12.21
  spine (column) - *see* Spondylopathy, specified
    NEC
  spleen (senile) D73.0
  stomach K29.40
    with bleeding K29.41
  striate (skin) L90.6
    syphilitic A52.79
  subcutaneous L90.9
  sublingual gland K11.0
  submandibular gland K11.0
  submaxillary gland K11.0
  Sudeck's - *see* Algoneurodystrophy
  suprarenal (capsule) (gland) E27.49
    primary E27.1
  systemic affecting central nervous system
    in
      myxedema E03.9 *[G13.2]*
      neoplastic disease - *see also* Neoplasm
        D49.9 *[G13.1]*
      specified disease NEC G13.8
  tarso-orbital fascia, congenital Q10.3
  testis N50.0
  thenar, partial - *see* Syndrome, carpal tunnel
  thymus (fatty) E32.8
  thyroid (gland) (acquired) E03.4
    with cretinism E03.1
    congenital (with myxedema) E03.1
  tongue (senile) K14.8
    papillae K14.4
  trachea J39.8
  tunica vaginalis N50.89
  turbinate J34.89
  tympanic membrane (nonflaccid) H73.82-
    flaccid H73.81-
  upper respiratory tract J39.8
  uterus, uterine (senile) N85.8
    cervix N88.8
    due to radiation (intended effect) N85.8
      adverse effect or misadventure N99.89
  vagina (senile) N95.2
  vas deferens N50.89
  vascular I99.8
  vertebra (senile) - *see* Spondylopathy,
    specified NEC
  vulva (senile) N90.5
  Werdnig-Hoffmann G12.0
  yellow - *see* Failure, hepatic

Attack, attacks
  with alteration of consciousness (with
    automatisms) - *see* Epilepsy, localization-
    related, symptomatic, with complex
  partial seizures
    Adams-stokes I45.9
    akinetic - *see* Epilepsy, generalized, specified
      NEC
    angina - *see* Angina
    atonic - *see* Epilepsy, generalized, specified
      NEC
    benign shuddering G25.83
    cataleptic - *see* Catalepsy
    coronary - *see* Infarct, myocardium
    cyanotic, newborn P28.2
    drop NEC R55
    epileptic - *see* Epilepsy
    heart - *see* infarct, myocardium
    hysterical F44.9
    jacksonian - *see* Epilepsy, localization-related,
      symptomatic, with simple partial seizures
    myocardium, myocardial - *see* Infarct,
      myocardium
    myoclonic - *see* Epilepsy, generalized,
      specified NEC
    panic F41.0
    psychomotor - *see* Epilepsy, localization-
      related, symptomatic, with complex partial
      seizures
    salaam - *see* Epilepsy, spasms
    schizophreniform, brief F23
    shuddering, benign G25.83
    Stokes-Adams I45.9
    syncope R55
    transient ischemic (TIA) G45.9
      specified NEC G45.8
    unconsciousness R55
      hysterical F44.89
    vasomotor R55
    vasovagal (paroxysmal) (idiopathic) R55
    without alteration of consciousness - *see*
      Epilepsy, localization-related, symptomatic,
      with simple partial seizures

Attention (to)
  artificial
    opening (of) Z43.9
      digestive tract NEC Z43.4
        colon Z43.3
        ilium Z43.2
        stomach Z43.1
      specified NEC Z43.8
      trachea Z43.0
      urinary tract NEC Z43.6
        cystostomy Z43.5
        nephrostomy Z43.6
        ureterostomy Z43.6
        urethrostomy Z43.6
      vagina Z43.7
  colostomy Z43.3
  cystostomy Z43.5
  deficit disorder or syndrome F98.8
    with hyperactivity - *see* Disorder, attention-
    deficit hyperactivity   gastrostomy Z43.1
  ileostomy Z43.2
  jejunostomy Z43.4
  nephrostomy Z43.6
  surgical dressings Z48.01
  sutures Z48.02
  tracheostomy Z43.0
  ureterostomy Z43.6
  urethrostomy Z43.6

Attrition
  gum *see* Recession, gingival
  tooth, teeth (excessive) (hard tissues) K03.0
Atypical, atypism - *see also* condition
  cells (on cytological smear) (endocervical)
    (endometrial) (glandular)
    cervix R87.619
    vagina R87.629
  cervical N87.9
  endometrium N85.9
    hyperplasia N85.00
  parenting situation Z62.9
Auditory - *see* condition
Aujeszky's disease B33.8
Aurantiasis, cutis E67.1
Auricle, auricular - *see also* condition
  cervical Q18.2
Auriculotemporal syndrome G50.8
Austin Flint murmur (aortic insufficiency)
  I35.1
Australian
  Q fever A78
  X disease A83.4
Autism, autistic (childhood) (infantile) F84.0
  atypical F84.9
  spectrum disorder F84.0
Autodigestion R68.89
Autoerythrocyte sensitization (syndrome)
  D69.2
Autographism L50.3
Autoimmune
  disease (systemic) M35.9
  inhibitors to clotting factors D68.311
  lymphoproliferative syndrome [ALPS] D89.82
  thyroiditis E06.3
Autointoxication R68.89
Automatism G93.89
  with temporal sclerosis G93.81
  epileptic - *see* Epilepsy, localization-related,
    symptomatic, with complex partial seizures
  paroxysmal, idiopathic - *see* Epilepsy,
    localization-related, symptomatic, with
    complex partial seizures
Autonomic, autonomous
  bladder (neurogenic) N31.2
  hysteria seizure F44.5
Autosensitivity, erythrocyte D69.2
Autosensitization, cutaneous L30.2
Autosome - *see* condition by chromosome
  involved
Autotopagnosia R48.1
Autotoxemia R68.89
Autumn - *see* condition
Avellis' syndrome G46.8
Aversion
  oral R63.3
    newborn P92.-
    nonorganic origin F98.2
  sexual F52.1
Aviator's
  disease or sickness - *see* Effect, adverse, high
    altitude
  ear T70.0
Avitaminosis (multiple) - *see also* Deficiency,
  vitamin E56.9
  B E53.9
    with
      beriberi E51.11
      pellagra E52
  B2 E53.0
  B6 E53.1
  B12 E53.8
  D E55.9
    with rickets E55.0

Avitaminosis (multiple) - *continued*
G E53.0
K E56.1
nicotinic acid E52

AVNRT (atrioventricular nodal re-entrant tachycardia) I47.1

AVRT (atrioventricular nodal re-entrant tachycardia) I47.1

Avulsion (traumatic)
blood vessel - *see* Injury, blood vessel
bone - *see* Fracture, by site
cartilage - *see also* Dislocation, by site
  symphyseal (inner), complicating delivery O71.6
external site other than limb - *see* Wound, open, by site
eye S05.7-
head (intracranial)
  external site NEC S08.89
  scalp S08.0
internal organ or site - *see* Injury, by site
joint - *see also* Dislocation, by site
  capsule - *see* Sprain, by site
kidney S37.06-
ligament - *see* Sprain, by site
limb - *see also* Amputation, traumatic, by site
  skin and subcutaneous tissue - *see* Wound, open, by site
muscle - *see* Injury, muscle
nerve (root) - *see* Injury, nerve
scalp S08.0
skin and subcutaneous tissue - *see* Wound, open, by site
spleen S36.032
symphyseal cartilage (inner), complicating delivery O71.6
tendon - *see* Injury, muscle
tooth S03.2

Awareness of heart beat R00.2

Axenfeld's
anomaly or syndrome Q15.0
degeneration (calcareous) Q13.4

Axilla, axillary - *see also* condition
breast Q83.1

Axonotmesis - *see* Injury, nerve

Ayerza's disease or syndrome (pulmonary artery sclerosis with pulmonary hypertension) I27.0

Azoospermia (organic) N46.01
due to
  drug therapy N46.021
  efferent duct obstruction N46.023

Azoospermia (organic) - *continued*
  infection N46.022
  radiation N46.024
  specified cause NEC N46.029
  systemic disease N46.025

Azotemia R79.89
meaning uremia N19

Aztec ear Q17.3

Azygos
continuation inferior vena cava Q26.8
lobe (lung) Q33.1

B

Baastrup's disease - *see* Kissing spine
Babesiosis B60.0
Babington's disease (familial hemorrhagic telangiectasia) I78.0
Babinski's syndrome A52.79
Baby
crying constantly R68.11
floppy (syndrome) P94.2

Bacillary - *see* condition
Bacilluria R82.71
Bacillus - *see also* Infection, bacillus
abortus infection A23.1
anthracis infection A22.9
coli infection - *see also* Escherichia coli B96.20
Flexner's A03.1
mallei infection A24.0
Shiga's A03.0
suipestifer infection - *see* Infection, salmonella
Back - *see* condition
Backache (postural) M54.9
sacroiliac M53.3
specified NEC M54.89
Backflow - *see* Reflux
Backward reading (dyslexia) F81.0
Bacteremia R78.81
with sepsis - *see* Sepsis
Bactericholia - *see* Cholecystitis, acute
Bacterid, bacteride (pustular) L40.3
Bacterium, bacteria, bacterial
agent NEC, as cause of disease classified elsewhere B96.89
in blood - *see* Bacteremia
in urine - *see* Bacteriuria
Bacteriuria, bacteruria R82.71
asymptomatic R82.71
Bacteroides
fragilis, as cause of disease classified elsewhere B96.6
Bad
heart - *see* Disease, heart
trip
  due to drug abuse - *see* Abuse, drug, hallucinogen
  due to drug dependence - *see* Dependence, drug, hallucinogen
Baelz's disease (cheilitis glandularis apostematosa) K13.0
Baerensprung's disease (eczema marginatum) B35.6
Bagasse disease or pneumonitis J67.1
Bagassosis J67.1
Baker's cyst - *see* Cyst, Baker's
Bakwin-Krida syndrome (metaphyseal dysplasia) Q78.5
Balancing side interference M26.56
Balanitis (circinata) (erosiva) (gangrenosa) (phagedenic) (vulgaris) N48.1
amebic A06.82
candidal B37.42
due to Haemophilus ducreyi A57
gonococcal (acute) (chronic) A54.09
xerotica obliterans N48.0
Balanoposthitis N47.6
gonococcal (acute) (chronic) A54.09
ulcerative (specific) A63.8
Balanorrhagia - *see* Balanitis
Balantidiasis, balantidiosis A07.0
Bald tongue K14.4
Baldness - *see also* Alopecia
male-pattern - *see* Alopecia, androgenic
Balkan grippe A78
Balloon disease - *see* Effect, adverse, high altitude
Balo's disease (concentric sclerosis) G37.5
Bamberger-Marie disease - *see* Osteoarthropathy, hypertrophic, specified type NEC
Bancroft's filariasis B74.0
Band(s)
adhesive - *see* Adhesions, peritoneum
anomalous or congenital - *see also* Anomaly,

Band(s) - *continued*
by site
  heart (atrial) (ventricular) Q24.8
  intestine Q43.3
  omentum Q43.3
cervix N88.1
constricting, congenital Q79.8
gallbladder (congenital) Q44.1
intestinal (adhesive) - *see* Adhesions, peritoneum
obstructive
  intestine K56.50
    complete K56.52
    incomplete K56.51
    partial K56.51
  peritoneum K56.50
    complete K56.52
    incomplete K56.51
    partial K56.51
periappendiceal, congenital Q43.3
peritoneal (adhesive) - *see* Adhesions, peritoneum
uterus N73.6
  internal N85.6
vagina N89.5
Bandemia D72.825
Bandl's ring (contraction), complicating delivery O62.4
Bangkok hemorrhagic fever A91
Bang's disease (brucella abortus) A23.1
Bankruptcy, anxiety concerning Z59.8
Bannister's disease T78.3
hereditary D84.1
Banti's disease or syndrome (with cirrhosis) (with portal hypertension) K76.6
Bar, median, prostate - *see* Enlargement, enlarged, prostate
Barcoo disease or rot - *see* Ulcer, skin
Barlow's disease E54
Barodontalgia T70.29
Baron Münchausen syndrome - *see* Disorder, factitious
Barosinusitis T70.1
Barotitis T70.0
Barotrauma T70.29
odontalgia T70.29
otitic T70.0
sinus T70.1
Barraquer (-Simons) disease or syndrome (progressive lipodystrophy) E88.1
Barré-Guillain disease or syndrome G61.0

Barré-Liéou syndrome (posterior cervical sympathetic) M53.0
Barrel chest M95.4
Barrett's
disease - *see* Barrett's, esophagus
esophagus K22.70
  with dysplasia K22.719
    high grade K22.711
    low grade K22.710
  without dysplasia K22.70
syndrome - *see* Barrett's, esophagus
ulcer K22.10
  with bleeding K22.11
  without bleeding K22.10
Bársony (-Polgár) (-Teschendorf) syndrome (corkscrew esophagus) K22.4
Bartholinitis (suppurating) N75.8
gonococcal (acute) (chronic) (with abscess) A54.1
Barth syndrome E78.71
Bartonellosis A44.9
cutaneous A44.1

Bartonellosis - *continued*
  mucocutaneous A44.1
  specified NEC A44.8
  systemic A44.0
Barton's fracture S52.56-
Bartter's syndrome E26.81
Basal - *see* condition
Basan's (hidrotic) ectodermal dysplasia
  Q82.4
Baseball finger - *see* Dislocation, finger
Basedow's disease (exophthalmic goiter) - *see*
  Hyperthyroidism, with, goiter
Basic - *see* condition
Basilar - *see* condition
Bason's (hidrotic) ectodermal dysplasia
  Q82.4
Basopenia - *see* Agranulocytosis
Basophilia D72.824
Basophilism (cortico-adrenal) (Cushing's)
  (pituitary) E24.0
Bassen-Kornzweig disease or syndrome E78.6
Bat ear Q17.5
Bateman's
  disease B08.1
  purpura (senile) D69.2
Bathing cramp T75.1
Bathophobia F40.248
Batten (-Mayou) disease E75.4
  retina E75.4 [*H36*]
Batten-Steinert syndrome G71.11
Battered - *see* Maltreatment
Battey Mycobacterium infection A31.0
Battle exhaustion F43.0
Battledore placenta O43.19-
Baumgarten-Cruveilhier cirrhosis, disease or
  syndrome K74.69
Bauxite fibrosis (of lung) J63.1
Bayle's disease (general paresis) A52.17
Bazin's disease (primary) (tuberculous)
  A18.4
Beach ear - *see* Swimmer's, ear
Beaded hair (congenital) Q84.1
Béal conjunctivitis or syndrome B30.2
Beard's disease (neurasthenia) F48.8
Beat(s)
  atrial, premature I49.1
  ectopic I49.49
  elbow - *see* Bursitis, elbow
  escaped, heart I49.49
  hand - *see* Bursitis, hand
  knee - *see* Bursitis, knee   premature I49.40
    atrial I49.1
    auricular I49.1
    supraventricular I49.1
Beau's
  disease or syndrome - *see* Degeneration,
    myocardial
  lines (transverse furrows on fingernails) L60.4
Beck's syndrome (anterior spinal artery
  occlusion) I65.8
Becker's
  cardiomyopathy I42.8
  disease
    idiopathic mural endomyocardial disease
      I42.3
    myotonia congenita, recessive form G71.12
  dystrophy G71.0
  pigmented hairy nevus D22.5
Beckwith-Wiedemann syndrome Q87.3
Bed confinement status Z74.01
Bed sore - *see* Ulcer, pressure, by site
Bedbug bite(s) - *see* Bite(s), by site, superficial,
  insect

Bedclothes, asphyxiation or suffocation by -
  see Asphyxia, traumatic, due to, mechanical,
    trapped
Bednar's
  aphthae K12.0
  tumor - *see* Neoplasm, malignant, by site
Bedridden Z74.01
Bedsore - *see* Ulcer, pressure, by site
Bedwetting - *see* Enuresis
Bee sting (with allergic or anaphylactic
  shock) - *see* Toxicity, venom, arthropod, bee
Beer drinker's heart (disease) I42.6
Begbie's disease (exophthalmic goiter) - *see*
  Hyperthyroidism, with, goiter
Behavior
  antisocial
    adult Z72.811
    child or adolescent Z72.810
  disorder, disturbance - *see* Disorder, conduct
  disruptive - *see* Disorder, conduct
  drug seeking Z76.5
  inexplicable R46.2
  marked evasiveness R46.5
  obsessive-compulsive R46.81
  overactivity R46.3
  poor responsiveness R46.4
  self-damaging (life-style) Z72.89
  sleep-incompatible Z72.821
  slowness R46.4
  specified NEC R46.89
  strange (and inexplicable) R46.2
  suspiciousness R46.5
  type A pattern Z73.1
  undue concern or preoccupation with stressful
    events R46.6
  verbosity and circumstantial detail obscuring
    reason for contact R46.7
Behçet's disease or syndrome M35.2
Behr's disease - *see* Degeneration, macula
Beigel's disease or morbus (white piedra)
  B36.2
Bejel A65
Bekhterev's syndrome - *see* Spondylitis,
  ankylosing
Belching - *see* Eructation
Bell's
  mania F30.8
  palsy, paralysis G51.0
    infant or newborn P11.3
  spasm G51.3
Bence Jones albuminuria or proteinuria NEC
  R80.3
Bends T70.3
Benedikt's paralysis or syndrome G46.3
Benign - *see also* condition
  prostatic hyperplasia - *see* Hyperplasia,
    prostate
Bennett's fracture (displaced) S62.21-
Benson's disease - *see* Deposit, crystalline
Bent
  back (hysterical) F44.4
  nose M95.0
    congenital Q67.4
Bereavement (uncomplicated) Z63.4
Bergeron's disease (hysterical chorea) F44.4
Berger's disease - *see* Nephropathy, IgA
Beriberi (dry) E51.11
  heart (disease) E51.12
  polyneuropathy E51.11
  wet E51.12
    involving circulatory system E51.11
Berlin's disease or edema (traumatic)
  S05.8X-
Berlock (berloque) dermatitis L56.2

Bernard-Horner syndrome G90.2
Bernard-Soulier disease or thrombopathia
  D69.1
Bernhardt (-Roth) disease - *see*
  Mononeuropathy, lower limb, meralgia
  paresthetica
Bernheim's syndrome - *see* Failure, heart, right
Bertielliasis B71.8
Berylliosis (lung) J63.2
Besnier-Boeck (-Schaumann) disease - *see*
  Sarcoidosis
Besnier's
  lupus pernio D86.3
  prurigo L20.0
Bestiality F65.89
Best's disease H35.50
Beta-mercaptolactate-cysteine disulfiduria
  E72.09
Betalipoproteinemia, broad or floating E78.2
Betting and gambling Z72.6
  pathological (compulsive) F63.0
Bezoar T18.9
  intestine T18.3
  stomach T18.2
Bezold's abscess - *see* Mastoiditis, acute
Bianchi's syndrome R48.8
Bicornate or bicornis uterus Q51.3
  in pregnancy or childbirth O34.00
    causing obstructed labor O65.5
Bicuspid aortic valve Q23.1
Biedl-Bardet syndrome Q87.89
Bielschowsky (-Jansky) disease E75.4
Biermer's (pernicious) anemia or disease
  D51.0
Biett's disease L93.0
Bifid (congenital)
  apex, heart Q24.8
  clitoris Q52.6
  kidney Q63.8
  nose Q30.2
  patella Q74.1
  scrotum Q55.29
  toe NEC Q74.2
  tongue Q38.3
  ureter Q62.8
  uterus Q51.3
  uvula Q35.7
Biforis uterus (suprasimplex) Q51.3
Bifurcation (congenital)
  gallbladder Q44.1
  kidney pelvis Q63.8
  renal pelvis Q63.8
  rib Q76.6
  tongue, congenital Q38.3
  trachea Q32.1
  ureter Q62.8
  urethra Q64.74
  vertebra Q76.49
Big spleen syndrome D73.1
Bigeminal pulse R00.8
Bilateral - *see* condition
Bile
  duct - *see* condition
  pigments in urine R82.2
Bilharziasis - *see also* Schistosomiasis
  chyluria B65.0
  cutaneous B65.3
  galacturia B65.0
  hematochyluria B65.0
  intestinal B65.1
  lipemia B65.9
  lipuria B65.0
  oriental B65.2

Bilharziasis - *continued*
  piarhemia B65.9
  pulmonary NOS B65.9 *[J99]*
    pneumonia B65.9 *[J17]*
  tropical hematuria B65.0
  vesical B65.0
Biliary - *see* condition
Bilirubin metabolism disorder E80.7
  specified NEC E80.6
Bilirubinemia, familial nonhemolytic E80.4
Bilirubinuria R82.2
Biliuria R82.2
Bilocular stomach K31.2
Binswanger's disease I67.3
Biparta, bipartite
  carpal scaphoid Q74.0
  patella Q74.1
  vagina Q52.10
Bird
  face Q75.8
  fancier's disease or lung J67.2
Birt-Hogg-Dube syndrome Q87.89
Birth
  complications in mother - *see* Delivery,
    complicated
  compression during NOS P15.9
  defect - *see* Anomaly
  immature (less than 37
    completed weeks) - *see* Preterm, newborn
      extremely (less than 28 completed weeks) -
      see Immaturity, extreme
  inattention, at or after - *see* Maltreatment,
    child, neglect
  injury NOS P15.9
    basal ganglia P11.1
    brachial plexus NEC P14.3
    brain (compression) (pressure) P11.2
    central nervous system NOS P11.9
    cerebellum P11.1
    cerebral hemorrhage P10.1
    external genitalia P15.5
    eye P15.3
    face P15.4
    fracture
      bone P13.9
        specified NEC P13.8
      clavicle P13.4
      femur P13.2
      humerus P13.3
      long bone, except femur P13.3
      radius and ulna P13.3
      skull P13.0
      spine P11.5
      tibia and fibula P13.3
    intracranial P11.2
      laceration or hemorrhage P10.9
        specified NEC P10.8
    intraventricular hemorrhage P10.2
    laceration
      brain P10.1
      by scalpel P15.8
      peripheral nerve P14.9
    liver P15.0
    meninges
      brain P11.1
      spinal cord P11.5
    nerve
      brachial plexus P14.3
      cranial NEC (except facial) P11.4
      facial P11.3
      peripheral P14.9
      phrenic (paralysis) P14.2
    paralysis
      facial nerve P11.3

Birth - *continued*
    spinal P11.5
    penis P15.5
    rupture
      spinal cord P11.5
    scalp P12.9
    scalpel wound P15.8
    scrotum P15.5
    skull NEC P13.1
      fracture P13.0
    specified type NEC P15.8
    spinal cord P11.5
    spine P11.5
    spleen P15.1
    sternomastoid (hematoma) P15.2
    subarachnoid hemorrhage P10.3
    subcutaneous fat necrosis P15.6
    subdural hemorrhage P10.0
    tentorial tear P10.4
    testes P15.5
    vulva P15.5
  lack of care, at or after - *see* Maltreatment,
    child, neglect
  neglect, at or after - *see* Maltreatment, child,
    neglect
  palsy or paralysis, newborn, NOS (birth
    injury) P14.9
  premature (infant) - *see* Preterm, newborn
  shock, newborn P96.89
  trauma - *see* Birth, injury weight
    low (2499 grams or less) - *see* Low,
    birthweight
      extremely (999 grams or less) - *see* Low,
      birthweight, extreme
    4000 grams to 4499 grams P08.1
    4500 grams or more P08.0
Birthmark Q82.5
Bisalbuminemia E88.09
Biskra's button B55.1
Bite(s) (animal) (human)
  abdomen, abdominal
    wall S31.159
      with penetration into peritoneal cavity
      S31.659
      epigastric region S31.152
        with penetration into peritoneal cavity
        S31.652
      left
        lower quadrant S31.154
          with penetration into peritoneal cavity
          S31.654
        upper quadrant S31.151
          with penetration into peritoneal cavity
          S31.651
      periumbilic region S31.155
        with penetration into peritoneal cavity
        S31.655
      right
        lower quadrant S31.153
          with penetration into peritoneal cavity
          S31.653
        upper quadrant S31.150
          with penetration into peritoneal cavity
          S31.650
      superficial NEC S30.871
        insect S30.861
  alveolar (process) - *see* Bite, oral cavity
  amphibian (venomous) - *see* Venom, bite,
    amphibian
  animal - *see also* Bite, by site
    venomous - *see* Venom
  ankle S91.05-
    superficial NEC S90.57-
      insect S90.56-

Bite(s) (animal) (human) - *continued*
  antecubital space - *see* Bite, elbow
  anus S31.835
    superficial NEC S30.877
      insect S30.867
  arm (upper) S41.15-
    lower - *see* Bite, forearm
    superficial NEC S40.87-
      insect S40.86-
  arthropod NEC - *see* Venom, bite, arthropod
  auditory canal (external) (meatus) - *see* Bite,
    ear
  auricle, ear - *see* Bite, ear
  axilla - *see* Bite, arm
  back - *see also* Bite, thorax, back
    lower S31.050
      with penetration into retroperitoneal space
      S31.051
      superficial NEC S30.870
        insect S30.860
  bedbug - *see* Bite(s), by site, superficial, insect
  breast S21.05-
    superficial NEC S20.17-
      insect S20.16-
  brow - *see* Bite, head, specified site NEC
  buttock S31.805
    left S31.825
    right S31.815
    superficial NEC S30.870
      insect S30.860
  calf - *see* Bite, leg
  canaliculus lacrimalis - *see* Bite, eyelid
  canthus, eye - *see* Bite, eyelid
  centipede - *see* Toxicity, venom, arthropod,
    centipede
  cheek (external) S01.45-
    superficial NEC S00.87
      insect S00.86
    internal - *see* Bite, oral cavity chest wall -
    see Bite, thorax
  chigger B88.0
  chin - *see* Bite, head, specified site NEC
  clitoris - *see* Bite, vulva
  costal region - *see* Bite, thorax digit(s)
    hand - *see* Bite, finger
    toe - *see* Bite, toe
  ear (canal) (external) S01.35-
    superficial NEC S00.47-
      insect S00.46-
  elbow S51.05-
    superficial NEC S50.37-
      insect S50.36-
  epididymis - *see* Bite, testis
  epigastric region - *see* Bite, abdomen
  epiglottis - *see* Bite, neck, specified site NEC
  esophagus, cervical S11.25
    superficial NEC S10.17
      insect S10.16
  eyebrow - *see* Bite, eyelid
  eyelid S01.15-
    superficial NEC S00.27-
      insect S00.26-
  face NEC - *see* Bite, head, specified site NEC
  finger(s) S61.259
    with
      damage to nail S61.359
    index S61.258
      with
        damage to nail S61.358
      left S61.251
        with
          damage to nail S61.351
      right S61.250
        with

Bite(s) (animal) (human) - *continued*
  superficial NEC S20.97
    back S20.47-
    front S20.37-
    insect S20.96
      back S20.46-
      front S20.36-
  throat - *see* Bite, neck, throat
  thumb S61.05-
    with
      damage to nail S61.15-
    superficial NEC S60.37-
      insect S60.36-
  thyroid S11.15
    superficial NEC S10.87
      insect S10.86
  toe(s) S91.15-
    with
      damage to nail S91.25-
    great S91.15
      with
        damage to nail S91.25-
    lesser S91.15-
      with
        damage to nail S91.25-
    superficial NEC S90.47-
      great S90.47-
      insect S90.46-
        great S90.46-
  tongue S01.552
  trachea S11.025
    superficial NEC S10.17
      insect S10.16
  tunica vaginalis - *see* Bite, testis
  tympanum, tympanic membrane - *see* Bite, ear
  umbilical region S31.155
  uvula - *see* Bite, oral cavity vagina - *see* Bite,
  vulva
  venomous - *see* Venom
  vocal cords S11.035
    superficial NEC S10.17
      insect S10.16
  vulva S31.45
    superficial NEC S30.874
      insect S30.864
  wrist S61.55-
    superficial NEC S60.87-
      insect S60.86-
Biting, cheek or lip K13.1
Biventricular failure (heart) I50.82
Björck (-Thorson) syndrome (malignant carcinoid) E34.0
Black
  death A20.9
  eye S00.1-
  hairy tongue K14.3
  heel (foot) S90.3-
  lung (disease) J60
  palm (hand) S60.22-
Blackfan-diamond anemia or syndrome (congenital hypoplastic anemia) D61.01
Blackhead L70.0
Blackout R55
Bladder - *see* condition
Blast (air) (hydraulic) (immersion) (underwater)
  blindness S05.8X-
  injury
    abdomen or thorax - *see* Injury, by site
    ear (acoustic nerve trauma) - *see* Injury,
    nerve, acoustic, specified type NEC
    syndrome NEC T70.8
Blastoma - *see* Neoplasm, malignant, by site
  pulmonary - *see* Neoplasm, lung, malignant

Blastomycosis, blastomycotic B40.9
  Brazilian - *see* Paracoccidioidomycosis
  cutaneous B40.3
  disseminated B40.7
  European - *see* Cryptococcosis
  generalized B40.7
  keloidal B48.0
  North American B40.9
  primary pulmonary B40.0
  pulmonary B40.2
    acute B40.0
    chronic B40.1
  skin B40.3
  South American - *see* Paracoccidioidomycosis
  specified NEC B40.89
Bleb(s) R23.8
  emphysematous (lung) (solitary) J43.9
  endophthalmitis H59.43
  filtering (vitreous), after glaucoma surgery Z98.83
  inflamed (infected), postprocedural H59.40
    stage 1 H59.41
    stage 2 H59.42
    stage 3 H59.43
  lung (ruptured) J43.9
    congenital - *see* Atelectasis
    newborn P25.8
  subpleural (emphysematous) J43.9
Blebitis, postprocedural H59.40
  stage 1 H59.41
  stage 2 H59.42
  stage 3 H59.43
Bleeder (familial) (hereditary) - *see* Hemophilia
Bleeding - *see also* Hemorrhage
  anal K62.5
  anovulatory N97.0
  atonic, following delivery O72.1
  capillary I78.8
    puerperal O72.2
  contact (postcoital) N93.0
  due to uterine subinvolution N85.3
  ear - *see* Otorrhagia
  excessive, associated with menopausal onset N92.4
  familial - *see* Defect, coagulation
  following intercourse N93.0
  gastrointestinal K92.2
  hemorrhoids - *see* Hemorrhoids
  intermenstrual (regular) N92.3
    irregular N92.1
  intraoperative - *see* Complication, intraoperative, hemorrhage
  irregular N92.6
  menopausal N92.4
  newborn, intraventricular - *see* Newborn, affected by, hemorrhage, intraventricular
  nipple N64.59
  nose R04.0
  ovulation N92.3
  postclimacteric N95.0
  postcoital N93.0
  postmenopausal N95.0
  postoperative - *see* Complication, postprocedural, hemorrhage
  preclimacteric N92.4
  pre-pubertal vaginal N93.1
  puberty (excessive, with onset of menstrual periods) N92.2
  rectum, rectal K62.5
    newborn P54.2
  tendencies - *see* Defect, coagulation
  throat R04.1
  tooth socket (post-extraction) K91.840

Bleeding - *continued*
  umbilical stump P51.9
  uterus, uterine NEC N93.9
    climacteric N92.4
    dysfunctional or functional N93.8
    menopausal N92.4
    preclimacteric or premenopausal N92.4
    unrelated to menstrual cycle N93.9
  vagina, vaginal (abnormal) N93.9
    dysfunctional or functional N93.8
    newborn P54.6
    pre-pubertal N93.1
  vicarious N94.89
Blennorrhagia, blennorrhagic - *see* Gonorrhea
Blennorrhea (acute) (chronic) - *see also* Gonorrhea
  inclusion (neonatal) (newborn) P39.1
  lower genitourinary tract (gonococcal) A54.00
  neonatorum (gonococcal ophthalmia) A54.31
Blepharelosis - *see* Entropion
Blepharitis (angularis) (ciliaris) (eyelid) (marginal) (nonulcerative) H01.009
  herpes zoster B02.39
  left H01.006
    lower H01.005
    upper H01.004
  right H01.003
    lower H01.002
    upper H01.001
  squamous H01.029
    left H01.026
      lower H01.025
      upper H01.024
    right H01.023
      lower H01.022
      upper H01.021
  ulcerative H01.019
    left H01.016
      lower H01.015
      upper H01.014
    right H01.013
      lower H01.012
      upper H01.011
Blepharochalasis H02.30
  congenital Q10.0
  left H02.36
    lower H02.35
    upper H02.34
  right H02.33
    lower H02.32
    upper H02.31
Blepharoclonus H02.59
Blepharoconjunctivitis H10.50-
  angular H10.52-
  contact H10.53-
  ligneous H10.51-
Blepharophimosis (eyelid) H02.529
  congenital Q10.3
  left H02.526
    lower H02.525
    upper H02.524
  right H02.523
    lower H02.522
    upper H02.521
Blepharoptosis H02.40-
  congenital Q10.0
  mechanical H02.41-
  myogenic H02.42-
  neurogenic H02.43-
  paralytic H02.43-
Blepharopyorrhea, gonococcal A54.39
Blepharospasm G24.5
  drug induced G24.01
Blighted ovum O02.0

Blind - *see also* Blindness
  bronchus (congenital) Q32.4
  loop syndrome K90.2
    congenital Q43.8
  sac, fallopian tube (congenital) Q50.6
  spot, enlarged - *see* Defect, visual field,
    localized, scotoma, blind spot area
  tract or tube, congenital NEC - *see* Atresia, by
site
Blindness (acquired) (congenital) (both eyes)
H54.0X-
  blast S05.8X-
  color - *see* Deficiency, color vision
  concussion S05.8X-
  cortical H47.619
    left brain H47.612
    right brain H47.611
  day H53.11
  due to injury (current episode) S05.9-
    sequelae   code to injury with seventh
    character S
  eclipse (total) - *see* Retinopathy, solar
  emotional (hysterical) F44.6
  face H53.16
  hysterical F44.6
  legal (both eyes) (USA definition) H54.8
  mind R48.8
  night H53.60
    abnormal dark adaptation curve H53.61
    acquired H53.62
    congenital H53.63
    specified type NEC H53.69
    vitamin A deficiency E50.5
  one eye (other eye normal) H54.40
    left (normal vision on right) H54.42-
      low vision on right H54.12-
    low vision, other eye H54.10
    right (normal vision on left) H54.41-
      low vision on left H54.11-
  psychic R48.8
  river B73.01
  snow - *see* Photokeratitis
  sun, solar - *see* Retinopathy, solar
  transient - *see* Disturbance, vision, subjective,
    loss, transient
  traumatic (current episode) S05.9-
  word (developmental) F81.0
    acquired R48.0
    secondary to organic lesion R48.0
Blister (nonthermal)
  abdominal wall S30.821
  alveolar process S00.522
  ankle S90.52-
  antecubital space - *see* Blister, elbow
  anus S30.827
  arm (upper) S40.82-
  auditory canal - *see* Blister, ear
  auricle - *see* Blister, ear
  axilla - *see* Blister, arm
  back, lower S30.820
  beetle dermatitis L24.89
  breast S20.12-
  brow S00.82
  calf - *see* Blister, leg
  canthus - *see* Blister, eyelid
  cheek S00.82
    internal S00.522
  chest wall - *see* Blister, thorax   chin S00.82
  costal region - *see* Blister, thorax   digit(s)
    foot - *see* Blister, toe
    hand - *see* Blister, finger
  due to burn - *see* Burn, by site, second degree
    ear S00.42-
  elbow S50.32-

Blister (nonthermal) - *continued*
  epiglottis S10.12
  esophagus, cervical S10.12
  eyebrow - *see* Blister, eyelid
  eyelid S00.22-
  face S00.82
  fever B00.1
  finger(s) S60.429
    index S60.42-
    little S60.42-
    middle S60.42-
    ring S60.42-
  foot (except toe(s) alone) S90.82-
    toe - *see* Blister, toe
  forearm S50.82-
    elbow only - *see* Blister, elbow
  forehead S00.82
  fracture
  omit code
  genital organ
    female S30.826
    male S30.825
  gum S00.522
  hand S60.52-
  head S00.92
    ear - *see* Blister, ear
    eyelid - *see* Blister, eyelid
    lip S00.521
    nose S00.32
    oral cavity S00.522
    scalp S00.02
    specified site NEC S00.82
  heel - *see* Blister, foot
  hip S70.22-
  interscapular region S20.429
  jaw S00.82
  knee S80.22-
  larynx S10.12
  leg (lower) S80.82-
    knee - *see* Blister, knee
    upper - *see* Blister, thigh
  lip S00.521
  malar region S00.82
  mammary - *see* Blister, breast
  mastoid region S00.82
  mouth S00.522
  multiple, skin, nontraumatic R23.8
  nail
    finger - *see* Blister, finger
    toe - *see* Blister, toe
  nasal S00.32
  neck S10.92
    specified site NEC S10.82
    throat S10.12
  nose S00.32
  occipital region S00.02
  oral cavity S00.522
  orbital region - *see* Blister, eyelid
  palate S00.522
  palm - *see* Blister, hand
  parietal region S00.02
  pelvis S30.820
  penis S30.822
  periocular area - *see* Blister, eyelid
  phalanges
    finger - *see* Blister, finger
    toe - *see* Blister, toe
  pharynx S10.12
  pinna - *see* Blister, ear
  popliteal space - *see* Blister, knee   scalp
    S00.02
  scapular region - *see* Blister, shoulder
  scrotum S30.823
  shin - *see* Blister, leg

Blister (nonthermal) - *continued*
  shoulder S40.22-
  sternal region S20.329
  submaxillary region S00.82
  submental region S00.82
  subungual
    finger(s) - *see* Blister, finger
    toe(s) - *see* Blister, toe
  supraclavicular fossa S10.82
  supraorbital S00.82
  temple S00.82
  temporal region S00.82
  testis S30.823
  thermal - *see* Burn, second degree, by site
  thigh S70.32-
  thorax, thoracic (wall) S20.92
    back S20.42-
    front S20.32-
  throat S10.12
  thumb S60.32-
  toe(s) S90.42-
    great S90.42-
  tongue S00.522
  trachea S10.12
  tympanum, tympanic membrane - *see* Blister,
    ear
  upper arm - *see* Blister, arm (upper)
  uvula S00.522
  vagina S30.824
  vocal cords S10.12
  vulva S30.824
  wrist S60.82-
Bloating R14.0
Bloch-Sulzberger disease or syndrome Q82.3
Block, blocked
  alveolocapillary J84.10
  arborization (heart) I45.5
  arrhythmic I45.9
  atrioventricular (incomplete) (partial) I44.30
    with atrioventricular dissociation I44.2
    complete I44.2
      congenital Q24.6
    congenital Q24.6
    first degree I44.0
    second degree (types I and II) I44.1
    specified NEC I44.39
    third degree I44.2
    types I and II I44.1
  auriculoventricular - *see* Block,
    atrioventricular
  bifascicular (cardiac) I45.2
  bundle-branch (complete) (false) (incomplete)
    I45.4
    bilateral I45.2
    left I44.7
      with right bundle branch block I45.2
      hemiblock I44.60
        anterior I44.4
        posterior I44.5
      incomplete I44.7
        with right bundle branch block I45.2
    right I45.10
      with
        left bundle branch block I45.2
        left fascicular block I45.2
      specified NEC I45.19
    Wilson's type I45.19
  cardiac I45.9
  conduction I45.9
    complete I44.2
  fascicular (left) I44.60
    anterior I44.4
    posterior I44.5
    right I45.0

Block, blocked - *continued*

specified NEC I44.69
foramen Magendie (acquired) G91.1
  congenital Q03.1
  with spina bifida - *see* Spina bifida, by site,
with hydrocephalus
heart I45.9
  bundle branch I45.4
    bilateral I45.2
  complete (atrioventricular) I44.2
  congenital Q24.6
  first degree (atrioventricular) I44.0
  second degree (atrioventricular) I44.1
  specified type NEC I45.5
  third degree (atrioventricular) I44.2
hepatic vein I82.0
intraventricular (nonspecific) I45.4
  bundle branch
    bilateral I45.2
kidney N28.9
  postcystoscopic or postprocedural N99.0
Mobitz (types I and II) I44.1
myocardial - *see* Block, heart
nodal I45.5
organ or site, congenital NEC - *see* Atresia, by
site
portal (vein) I81
second degree (types I and II) I44.1
sinoatrial I45.5
sinoauricular I45.5
third degree I44.2
trifascicular I45.3
tubal N97.1
vein NOS I82.90
Wenckebach (types I and II) I44.1
Blockage - *see* Obstruction
Blocq's disease F44.4
Blood
constituents, abnormal R78.9
disease D75.9
donor - *see* Donor, blood dyscrasia D75.9
with
  abortion - *see* Abortion, by type,
complicated by, hemorrhage
  ectopic pregnancy O08.1
  molar pregnancy O08.1
following ectopic or molar pregnancy O08.1
newborn P61.9
puerperal, postpartum O72.3
flukes NEC - *see* Schistosomiasis
in
  feces K92.1
    occult R19.5
  urine - *see* Hematuria
mole O02.0
occult in feces R19.5
pressure
  decreased, due to shock following injury
  T79.4
  examination only Z01.30
  fluctuating I99.8
  high - *see* Hypertension
    borderline R03.0
    incidental reading, without diagnosis of
    hypertension R03.0
  low - *see also* Hypotension
    incidental reading, without diagnosis of
    hypotension R03.1
spitting - *see* Hemoptysis
staining cornea - *see* Pigmentation, cornea,
stromal
transfusion
  reaction or complication - *see* Complications,
  transfusion

Blood – *continued*

type
  A (Rh positive) Z67.10
    Rh negative Z67.11
  AB (Rh positive) Z67.30
    Rh negative Z67.31
  B (Rh positive) Z67.20
    Rh negative Z67.21
  O (Rh positive) Z67.40
    Rh negative Z67.41
  Rh (positive) Z67.90
    negative Z67.91
vessel rupture - *see* Hemorrhage
vomiting - *see* Hematemesis
Blood-forming organs, disease D75.9
Bloodgood's disease - *see* Mastopathy, cystic
Bloom (-Machacek)(-Torre) syndrome Q82.8
Blount's disease or osteochondrosis - *see*
Osteochondrosis, juvenile, tibia
Blue
baby Q24.9
diaper syndrome E72.09
dome cyst (breast) - *see* Cyst, breast
dot cataract Q12.0
nevus D22.9
sclera Q13.5
  with fragility of bone and deafness Q78.0
toe syndrome I75.02-
Blueness - *see* Cyanosis
Blues, postpartal O90.6
baby O90.6
Blurring, visual H53.8
Blushing (abnormal) (excessive) R23.2
BMI - *see* Body, mass index
Boarder, hospital NEC Z76.4
accompanying sick person Z76.3
healthy infant or child Z76.2
foundling Z76.1
Bockhart's impetigo L01.02
**Bodechtel-Guttman disease (subacute
sclerosing panencephalitis)** A81.1
**Boder-Sedgwick syndrome (ataxia-
telangiectasia)** G11.3
Body, bodies
Aschoff's - *see* Myocarditis, rheumatic
asteroid, vitreous - *see* Deposit, crystalline
cytoid (retina) - *see* Occlusion, artery, retina
drusen (degenerative) (macula) (retinal) - *see
also* Degeneration, macula, drusen
  optic disc - *see* Drusen, optic disc
foreign - *see* Foreign body
loose
  joint, except knee - *see* Loose, body, joint
    knee M23.4-
  sheath, tendon - *see* Disorder, tendon,
  specified type NEC
mass index (BMI)
  adult
    19.9 or less Z68.1
    20.0-20.9 Z68.20
    21.0-21.9 Z68.21
    22.0-22.9 Z68.22
    23.0-23.9 Z68.23
    24.0-24.9 Z68.24
    25.0-25.9 Z68.25
    26.0-26.9 Z68.26
    27.0-27.9 Z68.27
    28.0-28.9 Z68.28
    29.0-29.9 Z68.29
    30.0-30.9 Z68.30
    31.0-31.9 Z68.31
    32.0-32.9 Z68.32
    33.0-33.9 Z68.33
    34.0-34.9 Z68.34

Blood – *continued*

35.0-35.9 Z68.35
36.0-36.9 Z68.36
37.0-37.9 Z68.37
38.0-38.9 Z68.38
39.0-39.9 Z68.39
40.0-44.9 Z68.41
45.0-49.9 Z68.42
50.0-59.9 Z68.43
60.0-69.9 Z68.44
70 and over Z68.45
pediatric
  5th percentile to less than 85th percentile
  for age Z68.52
  85th percentile to less than 95th percentile
  for age Z68.53
  greater than or equal to ninety-fifth
  percentile for age Z68.54
  less than fifth percentile for age Z68.51
Mooser's A75.2
rice - *see also* Loose, body, joint
  knee M23.4-
rocking F98.4
Boeck's
disease or sarcoid - *see* Sarcoidosis
lupoid (miliary) D86.3
**Boerhaave's syndrome (spontaneous
esophageal rupture)** K22.3
Boggy
cervix N88.8
uterus N85.8
Boil - *see also* Furuncle, by site
Aleppo B55.1
Baghdad B55.1
Delhi B55.1
lacrimal
  gland - *see* Dacryoadenitis
  passages (duct) (sac) - *see* Inflammation,
  lacrimal, passages, acute
Natal B55.1
orbit, orbital - *see* Abscess, orbit
tropical B55.1
Bold hives - *see* Urticaria
Bombé, iris - *see* Membrane, pupillary
Bone - *see* condition
Bonnevie-Ullrich syndrome - *see also* Turner's
syndrome Q87.1
Bonnier's syndrome - *see* subcategory H81.8
Bonvale dam fever T73.3
Bony block of joint - *see* Ankylosis
**BOOP (bronchiolitis obliterans organized
pneumonia)** J84.89
Borderline
diabetes mellitus R73.03
hypertension R03.0
osteopenia M85.8-
pelvis, with obstruction during labor O65.1
personality F60.3
Borna disease A83.9
Bornholm disease B33.0
Boston exanthem A88.0
Botalli, ductus (patent) (persistent) Q25.0
Bothriocephalus latus infestation B70.0
Botulism (foodborne intoxication) A05.1
infant A48.51
non-foodborne A48.52
wound A48.52
Bouba - *see* Yaws
Bouchard's nodes (with arthropathy) M15.2
Bouffée délirante F23
**Bouillaud's disease or syndrome (rheumatic
heart disease)** I01.9
Bourneville's disease Q85.1

Boutonniere deformity (finger) - *see*
  Deformity, finger, boutonniere
Bouveret (-Hoffmann) syndrome
  (paroxysmal tachycardia) I47.9
Bovine heart - *see* Hypertrophy, cardiac
Bowel - *see* condition
Bowen's
  dermatosis (precancerous) - *see* Neoplasm,
    skin, in situ
  disease - *see* Neoplasm, skin, in situ
  epithelioma - *see* Neoplasm, skin, in situ
  type
    epidermoid carcinoma-in-situ - *see*
      Neoplasm, skin, in situ
    intraepidermal squamous cell carcinoma - *see*
      Neoplasm, skin, in situ
Bowing
  femur - *see also* Deformity, limb, specified
    type NEC, thigh
    congenital Q68.3
  fibula - *see also* Deformity, limb, specified
    type NEC, lower leg
    congenital Q68.4
  forearm - *see* Deformity, limb, specified type
    NEC, forearm
  leg(s), long bones, congenital Q68.5
  radius - *see* Deformity, limb, specified type
    NEC, forearm
  tibia - *see also* Deformity, limb, specified type
    NEC, lower leg
    congenital Q68.4
Bowleg(s) (acquired) M21.16-
  congenital Q68.5
  rachitic E64.3
Boyd's dysentery A03.2
Brachial - *see* condition
Brachycardia R00.1
Brachycephaly Q75.0
Bradley's disease A08.19
Bradyarrhythmia, cardiac I49.8
Bradycardia (sinoatrial) (sinus) (vagal) R00.1
  neonatal P29.12
  reflex G90.09
  tachycardia syndrome I49.5
Bradykinesia R25.8
Bradypnea R06.89
Bradytachycardia I49.5
Brailsford's disease or osteochondrosis - *see*
  Osteochondrosis, juvenile, radius
Brain - *see also* condition
  death G93.82
  syndrome - *see* Syndrome, brain
Branched-chain amino-acid disorder E71.2
Branchial - *see* condition
  cartilage, congenital Q18.2
Branchiogenic remnant (in neck) Q18.0
Brandt's syndrome (acrodermatitis
  enteropathica) E83.2
Brash (water) R12

Bravais-jacksonian epilepsy - *see* Epilepsy,
  localization-related, symptomatic, with simple
  partial seizures
Braxton Hicks contractions - *see* False, labor
Brazilian leishmaniasis B55.2
BRBPR K62.5
Break, retina (without detachment) H33.30-
  with retinal detachment - *see* Detachment,
    retina
  horseshoe tear H33.31-
  multiple H33.33-
  round hole H33.32-

Breakdown
  device, graft or implant - *see also*
  Complications, by site and type, mechanical
  T85.618
    arterial graft NEC - *see* Complication,
      cardiovascular device, mechanical, vascular
    breast (implant) T85.41
    catheter NEC T85.618
      cystostomy T83.010
      Hopkins T83.018
      ileostomy T83.018
      dialysis (renal) T82.41
        intraperitoneal T85.611
      infusion NEC T82.514
        cranial T85.610
        epidural T85.610
        intrathecal T85.610
        spinal T85.610
        subarachnoid T85.610
        subdural T85.610
      nephrostomy T83.012
      urethral indwelling T83.011
      urinary NEC T83.018
      urostomy T83.018
    electronic (electrode) (pulse generator)
    (stimulator)
      bone T84.310
      cardiac T82.119
        electrode T82.110
        pulse generator T82.111
        specified type NEC T82.118
      nervous system - *see* Complication,
        prosthetic device, mechanical, electronic
        nervous system stimulator
      urinary - *see* Complication, genitourinary,
        device, urinary, mechanical
    fixation, internal (orthopedic) NEC - *see*
    Complication, fixation device, mechanical
    gastrointestinal - *see* Complications,
    prosthetic device, mechanical,
    gastrointestinal device
    genital NEC T83.418
      intrauterine contraceptive device T83.31
      penile prosthesis (cylinder) (implanted)
        (pump) (reservoir) T83.410
      testicular prosthesis T83.411
    heart NEC - *see* Complication,
    cardiovascular device, mechanical
    intrathecal infusion pump T85.615
    joint prosthesis - *see* Complications..., joint
    prosthesis, internal, mechanical, by site
    nervous system, specified device NEC
    T85.615
    ocular NEC - *see* Complications, prosthetic
    device, mechanical, ocular device
    orthopedic NEC - *see* Complication,
    orthopedic, device, mechanical
    specified NEC T85.618
    subcutaneous device pocket
      nervous system prosthetic device, implant,
        or graft T85.890
      other internal prosthetic device, implant, or
        graft T85.898
    sutures, permanent T85.612
    used in bone repair - *see* Complications,
    fixation device, internal (orthopedic),
    mechanical
    urinary NEC T83.118
      graft T83.21
      sphincter, implanted T83.111
      stent (ileal conduit) (nephroureteral)
        T83.113
      ureteral indwelling T83.112
    vascular NEC - *see* Complication,

Breakdown - *continued*
    cardiovascular device, mechanical
    ventricular intracranial shunt T85.01
  nervous F48.8
  perineum O90.1
  respirator J95.850
    specified NEC J95.859
  ventilator J95.850
    specified NEC J95.859
Breast - *see also* condition
  buds E30.1
    in newborn P96.89
  dense R92.2
  nodule (see also Lump, breast) N63.0
Breath
  foul R19.6
  holder, child R06.89
  holding spell R06.89
  shortness R06.02
Breathing
  labored - *see* Hyperventilation
  mouth R06.5
    causing malocclusion M26.5
  periodic R06.3
    high altitude G47.32
Breathlessness R06.81
Breda's disease - *see* Yaws
Breech presentation (mother) O32.1
  causing obstructed labor O64.1
  footling O32.8
    causing obstructed labor O64.8
  incomplete O32.8
    causing obstructed labor O64.8
Breisky's disease N90.4
Brennemann's syndrome I88.0
Brenner
  tumor (benign) D27.9
    borderline malignancy D39.1-
    malignant C56
    proliferating D39.1-
Bretonneau's disease or angina A36.0
Breus' mole O02.0
Brevicollis Q76.49
Brickmakers' anemia B76.9 *[D63.8]*
Bridge, myocardial Q24.5
Bright red blood per rectum (BRBPR) K62.5
Bright's disease - *see also* Nephritis
  arteriosclerotic - *see* Hypertension, kidney
Brill (-Zinsser) disease (recrudescent typhus)
  A75.1
  flea-borne A75.2
  louse-borne A75.1
Brill-Symmers' disease C82.90
Brion-Kayser disease - *see* Fever, parathyroid
Briquet's disorder or syndrome F45.0
Brissaud's
  infantilism or dwarfism E23.0
  motor-verbal tic F95.2
Brittle
  bones disease Q78.0
  nails L60.3
    congenital Q84.6
Broad - *see also* condition
  beta disease E78.2
  ligament laceration syndrome N83.8
Broad or floating-betalipoproteinemia E78.2
Brock's syndrome (atelectasis due to
  enlarged lymph nodes) J98.19
Brocq-Duhring disease (dermatitis
  herpetiformis) L13.0
Brodie's abscess or disease M86.8X-
Broken
  arches - *see also* Deformity, limb, flat foot
  arm (meaning upper limb) - *see* Fracture, arm

Broken - *continued*
back - *see* Fracture, vertebra
bone - *see* Fracture
implant or internal device - *see* Complications, by site and type, mechanical
leg (meaning lower limb) - *see* Fracture, leg
nose S02.2
tooth, teeth - *see* Fracture, tooth
Bromhidrosis, bromidrosis L75.0
Bromidism, bromism G92
due to
correct substance properly administered - *see* Table of Drugs and Chemicals, by drug, adverse effect
overdose or wrong substance given or taken - *see* Table of Drugs and Chemicals, by drug, poisoning
chronic (dependence) F13.20
Bromidrosiphobia F40.298
Bronchi, bronchial - *see* condition
Bronchiectasis (cylindrical) (diffuse) (fusiform) (localized) (saccular) J47.9
with
acute
bronchitis J47.0
lower respiratory infection J47.0
exacerbation (acute) J47.1
congenital Q33.4
tuberculous NEC - *see* Tuberculosis, pulmonary
Bronchiolectasis - *see* Bronchiectasis
Bronchiolitis (acute) (infective) (subacute) J21.9
with
bronchospasm or obstruction J21.9
influenza, flu or grippe - *see* Influenza, with, respiratory manifestations NEC
chemical (chronic) J68.4
acute J68.0
chronic (fibrosing) (obliterative) J44.9
due to
external agent - *see* Bronchitis, acute, due to
human metapneumovirus J21.1
respiratory syncytial virus J21.0
specified organism NEC J21.8
fibrosa obliterans J44.9
influenzal - *see* Influenza, with, respiratory manifestations NEC
obliterans J42
with organizing pneumonia (BOOP) J84.89
obliterative (chronic) (subacute) J44.9
due to fumes or vapors J68.4
due to chemicals, gases, fumes or vapors (inhalation) J68.4
respiratory, interstitial lung disease J84.115
Bronchitis (diffuse) (fibrinous) (hypostatic) (infective) (membranous) J40
with
influenza, flu or grippe - *see* Influenza, with, respiratory manifestations NEC
obstruction (airway) (lung) J44.9
tracheitis (15 years of age and above) J40
acute or subacute J20.9
chronic J42
under 15 years of age J20.9
acute or subacute (with bronchospasm or obstruction) J20.9
with
bronchiectasis J47.0
chronic obstructive pulmonary disease J44.0
chemical (due to gases, fumes or vapors) J68.0

Bronchitis - *continued*
due to
fumes or vapors J68.0
Haemophilus influenzae J20.1
Mycoplasma pneumoniae J20.0
radiation J70.0
specified organism NEC J20.8
Streptococcus J20.2
virus
coxsackie J20.3
echovirus J20.7
parainfluenzae J20.4
respiratory syncytial J20.5
rhinovirus J20.6
viral NEC J20.8
allergic (acute) J45.909
with
exacerbation (acute) J45.901
status asthmaticus J45.902
arachidic T17.528
aspiration (due to fumes or vapors) J68.0
asthmatic J45.9
chronic J44.9
with
acute lower respiratory infection J44.0
exacerbation (acute) J44.1
capillary - *see* Pneumonia, broncho
caseous (tuberculous) A15.5
Castellani's A69.8
catarrhal (15 years of age and above) J40
acute - *see* Bronchitis, acute
chronic J41.0
under 15
years of age J20.9
chemical (acute) (subacute) J68.0
chronic J68.4
due to fumes or vapors J68.0
chronic J68.4
chronic J42
with
airways obstruction J44.9
tracheitis (chronic) J42
asthmatic (obstructive) J44.9
catarrhal J41.0
chemical (due to fumes or vapors) J68.4
due to
chemicals, gases, fumes or vapors (inhalation) J68.4
radiation J70.1
tobacco smoking J41.0
emphysematous J44.9
mucopurulent J41.1
non-obstructive J41.0
obliterans J44.9
obstructive J44.9
purulent J41.1
simple J41.0
croupous - *see* Bronchitis, acute
due to gases, fumes or vapors (chemical) J68.0
emphysematous (obstructive) J44.9
exudative - *see* Bronchitis, acute
fetid J41.1
grippal - *see* Influenza, with, respiratory manifestations NEC
in those under 15 years age - *see* Bronchitis, acute
chronic - *see* Bronchitis, chronic
influenzal - *see* Influenza, with, respiratory manifestations NEC
mixed simple and mucopurulent J41.8
moulder's J62.8
mucopurulent (chronic) (recurrent) J41.1
acute or subacute J20.9
simple (mixed) J41.8

Bronchitis - *continued*
obliterans (chronic) J44.9
obstructive (chronic) (diffuse) J44.9
pituitous J41.1
pneumococcal, acute or subacute J20.2
pseudomembranous, acute or subacute - *see* Bronchitis, acute
purulent (chronic) (recurrent) J41.1
acute or subacute - *see* Bronchitis, acute
putrid J41.1
senile (chronic) J42
simple and mucopurulent (mixed) J41.8
smokers' J41.0
spirochetal NEC A69.8
subacute - *see* Bronchitis, acute
suppurative (chronic) J41.1
acute or subacute - *see* Bronchitis, acute
tuberculous A15.5
under 15 years of age - *see* Bronchitis, acute
chronic - *see* Bronchitis, chronic
viral NEC, acute or subacute - *see also* Bronchitis, acute J20.8
Bronchoalveolitis J18.0
Bronchoaspergillosis B44.1
Bronchocele meaning goiter E04.0
Broncholithiasis J98.09
tuberculous NEC A15.5
Bronchomalacia J98.09
congenital Q32.2
Bronchomycosis NOS B49 [*J99*]
candidal B37.1
Bronchopleuropneumonia - *see* Pneumonia, broncho
Bronchopneumonia - *see* Pneumonia, broncho
Bronchopneumonitis - *see* Pneumonia, broncho
Bronchopulmonary - *see* condition
Bronchopulmonitis - *see* Pneumonia, broncho
Bronchorrhagia (see Hemoptysis)
Bronchorrhea J98.09
acute J20.9
chronic (infective) (purulent) J42
Bronchospasm (acute) J98.01
with
bronchiolitis, acute J21.9
bronchitis, acute (conditions in J20) - *see* Bronchitis, acute
due to external agent - *see* condition, respiratory, acute, due to
exercise induced J45.990
Bronchospirochetosis A69.8
Castellani A69.8
Bronchostenosis J98.09
Bronchus - *see* condition
Brontophobia F40.220
Bronze baby syndrome P83.88
Brooke's tumor - *see* Neoplasm, skin, benign
Brown enamel of teeth (hereditary) K00.5
Brown's sheath syndrome H50.61-
Brown-Séquard disease, paralysis or syndrome G83.81
Bruce sepsis A23.0
Brucellosis (infection) A23.9
abortus A23.1
canis A23.3
dermatitis A23.9
melitensis A23.0
mixed A23.8
sepsis A23.9
melitensis A23.0
specified NEC A23.8
suis A23.2
Bruck-de Lange disease Q87.1
Bruck's disease - *see* Deformity, limb

BRUE (brief resolved unexplained event)
R68.13
Brugsch's syndrome Q82.8
Bruise (skin surface intact) - *see also*
Contusion
with
open wound - *see* Wound, open
internal organ - *see* Injury, by site
newborn P54.5
scalp, due to birth injury, newborn P12.3
umbilical cord O69.5
Bruit (arterial) R09.89
cardiac R01.1
Brush burn - *see* Abrasion, by site
Bruton's X-linked agammaglobulinemia
D80.0
Bruxism
psychogenic F45.8
sleep related G47.63
Bubbly lung syndrome P27.0
Bubo I88.8
blennorrhagic (gonococcal) A54.89
chancroidal A57
climatic A55
due to Haemophilus ducreyi A57
gonococcal A54.89
indolent (nonspecific) I88.8
inguinal (nonspecific) I88.8
chancroidal A57
climatic A55
due to H. ducreyi A57
infective I88.8
scrofulous (tuberculous) A18.2
soft chancre A57
suppurating - *see* Lymphadenitis, acute
syphilitic (primary) A51.0
congenital A50.07
tropical A55
virulent (chancroidal) A57
Bubonic plague A20.0
Bubonocele - *see* Hernia, inguinal
Buccal - *see* condition
Buchanan's disease or osteochondrosis M91.0
Buchem's syndrome (hyperostosis corticalis)
M85.2
Bucket-handle fracture or tear (semilunar
cartilage) - *see* Tear, meniscus
Budd-Chiari syndrome (hepatic vein
thrombosis) I82.0
Budgerigar fancier's disease or lung J67.2
Buds
breast E30.1
in newborn P96.89
Buerger's disease (thromboangiitis
obliterans) I73.1
Bulbar - *see* condition
Bulbus cordis (left ventricle) (persistent)
Q21.8
Bulimia (nervosa) F50.2
atypical F50.9
normal weight F50.9
Bulky
stools R19.5
uterus N85.2
Bulla (e) R23.8
lung (emphysematous) (solitary) J43.9
newborn P25.8
Bullet wound - *see also* Wound, open
fracture
code as Fracture, by site
internal organ - *see* Injury, by site
Bundle
branch block (complete) (false) (incomplete) -
see Block, bundle-branch

Bundle - *continued*
of His - *see* condition
Bunion M21.61-
tailor's M21.62-
Bunionette M21.62-
Buphthalmia, buphthalmos (congenital)
Q15.0
Burdwan fever B55.0
Bürger-Grütz disease or syndrome E78.3
Buried
penis (congenital) Q55.64
acquired N48.83
roots K08.3
Burke's syndrome K86.89
Burkitt
cell leukemia C91.0-
lymphoma (malignant) C83.7-
small noncleaved, diffuse C83.7-
spleen C83.77
undifferentiated C83.7-
tumor C83.7-
type
acute lymphoblastic leukemia C91.0-
undifferentiated C83.7-
Burn (electricity) (flame) (hot gas, liquid or hot
object) (radiation) (steam) (thermal) T30.0
abdomen, abdominal (muscle) (wall) T21.02
first degree T21.12
second degree T21.22
third degree T21.32
above elbow T22.039
first degree T22.139
left T22.032
first degree T22.132
second degree T22.232
third degree T22.332
right T22.031
first degree T22.131
second degree T22.231
third degree T22.331
second degree T22.239
third degree T22.339
acid (caustic) (external) (internal) - *see*
Corrosion, by site
alimentary tract NEC T28.2
esophagus T28.1
mouth T28.0
pharynx T28.0
alkaline (caustic) (external) (internal) - *see*
Corrosion, by site
ankle T25.019
first degree T25.119
left T25.012
first degree T25.112
second degree T25.212
third degree T25.312
multiple with foot - *see* Burn, lower, limb,
multiple, ankle and foot
right T25.011
first degree T25.111
second degree T25.211
third degree T25.311
second degree T25.219
third degree T25.319
anus - *see* Burn, buttock
arm (lower) (upper) - *see* Burn, upper, limb
axilla T22.049
first degree T22.149
left T22.042
first degree T22.142
second degree T22.242
third degree T22.342
right T22.041
first degree T22.141

Burn - *continued*
second degree T22.241
third degree T22.341
second degree T22.249
third degree T22.349
back (lower) T21.04
first degree T21.14
second degree T21.24
third degree T21.34
upper T21.03
first degree T21.13
second degree T21.23
third degree T21.33
blisters
code as Burn, second degree, by site
breast(s) - *see* Burn, chest wall
buttock(s) T21.05
first degree T21.15
second degree T21.25
third degree T21.35
calf T24.039
first degree T24.139
left T24.032
first degree T24.132
second degree T24.232
third degree T24.332
right T24.031
first degree T24.131
second degree T24.231
third degree T24.331
second degree T24.239
third degree T24.339
canthus (eye) - *see* Burn, eyelid
caustic acid or alkaline - *see* Corrosion, by site
cervix T28.3
cheek T20.06
first degree T20.16
second degree T20.26
third degree T20.36
chemical (acids) (alkalines) (caustics)
(external) (internal) - *see* Corrosion, by site
chest wall T21.01
first degree T21.11
second degree T21.21
third degree T21.31
chin T20.03
first degree T20.13
second degree T20.23
third degree T20.33
colon T28.2
conjunctiva (and cornea) - *see* Burn, cornea
cornea (and conjunctiva) T26.1-
chemical - *see* Corrosion, cornea
corrosion (external) (internal) - *see* Corrosion,
by site
deep necrosis of underlying tissue   code as
Burn, third degree, by site
dorsum of hand T23.069
first degree T23.169
left T23.062
first degree T23.162
second degree T23.262
third degree T23.362
right T23.061
first degree T23.161
second degree T23.261
third degree T23.361
second degree T23.269
third degree T23.369
due to ingested chemical agent - *see*
Corrosion, by site
ear (auricle) (external) (canal) T20.01
first degree T20.11
second degree T20.21

Burn - *continued*
  third degree T20.31
  elbow T22.029
    first degree T22.129
    left T22.022
      first degree T22.122
      second degree T22.222
      third degree T22.322
    right T22.021
      first degree T22.121
      second degree T22.221
      third degree T22.321
    second degree T22.229
    third degree T22.329
  epidermal loss
  code as Burn, second degree, by site
  erythema, erythematous
  code as Burn, first degree, by site
  esophagus T28.1
  extent (percentage of body surface)
    less than 10 percent T31.0
    10-19 percent T31.10
      with 0-9 percent third degree burns T31.10
      with 10-19 percent third degree burns T31.11
    20-29 percent T31.20
      with 0-9 percent third degree burns T31.20
      with 10-19 percent third degree burns T31.21
      with 20-29 percent third degree burns T31.22
    30-39 percent T31.30
      with 0-9 percent third degree burns T31.30
      with 10-19 percent third degree burns T31.31
      with 20-29 percent third degree burns T31.32
      with 30-39 percent third degree burns T31.33
    40-49 percent T31.40
      with 0-9 percent third degree burns T31.40
      with 10-19 percent third degree burns T31.41
      with 20-29 percent third degree burns T31.42
      with 30-39 percent third degree burns T31.43
      with 40-49 percent third degree burns T31.44
    50-59 percent T31.50
      with 0-9 percent third degree burns T31.50
      with 10-19 percent third degree burns T31.51
      with 20-29 percent third degree burns T31.52
      with 30-39 percent third degree burns T31.53
      with 40-49 percent third degree burns T31.54
      with 50-59 percent third degree burns T31.55
    60-69 percent T31.60
      with 0-9 percent third degree burns T31.60
      with 10-19 percent third degree burns T31.61
      with 20-29 percent third degree burns T31.62
      with 30-39 percent third degree burns T31.63
      with 40-49 percent third degree burns T31.64
      with 50-59 percent third degree burns T31.65
      with 60-69 percent third degree burns

Burn - *continued*
      T31.66
    70-79 percent T31.70
      with 0-9 percent third degree burns T31.70
      with 10-19 percent third degree burns T31.71
      with 20-29 percent third degree burns T31.72
      with 30-39 percent third degree burns T31.73
      with 40-49 percent third degree burns T31.74
      with 50-59 percent third degree burns T31.75
      with 60-69 percent third degree burns T31.76
      with 70-79 percent third degree burns T31.77
    80-89 percent T31.80
      with 0-9 percent third degree burns T31.80
      with 10-19 percent third degree burns T31.81
      with 20-29 percent third degree burns T31.82
      with 30-39 percent third degree burns T31.83
      with 40-49 percent third degree burns T31.84
      with 50-59 percent third degree burns T31.85
      with 60-69 percent third degree burns T31.86
      with 70-79 percent third degree burns T31.87
      with 80-89 percent third degree burns T31.88
    90 percent or more T31.90
      with 0-9 percent third degree burns T31.90
      with 10-19 percent third degree burns T31.91
      with 20-29 percent third degree burns T31.92
      with 30-39 percent third degree burns T31.93
      with 40-49 percent third degree burns T31.94
      with 50-59 percent third degree burns T31.95
      with 60-69 percent third degree burns T31.96
      with 70-79 percent third degree burns T31.97
      with 80-89 percent third degree burns T31.98
      with 90 percent or more third degree burns T31.99
  extremity - *see* Burn, limb
  eye(s) and adnexa T26.4-
    with resulting rupture and destruction of eyeball T26.2-
    conjunctival sac - *see* Burn, cornea
    cornea - *see* Burn, cornea
    lid - *see* Burn, eyelid
    periocular area - *see* Burn, eyelid
    specified site NEC T26.3-
  eyeball - *see* Burn, eye eyelid(s) T26.0-
    chemical - *see* Corrosion, eyelid
  face - *see* Burn, head
  finger T23.029
    first degree T23.129
    left T23.022
      first degree T23.122
      second degree T23.222
      third degree T23.322

Burn - *continued*
    multiple sites (without thumb) T23.039
      with thumb T23.049
        first degree T23.149
        left T23.042
          first degree T23.142
          second degree T23.242
          third degree T23.342
        right T23.041
          first degree T23.141
          second degree T23.241
          third degree T23.341
        second degree T23.249
        third degree T23.349
      first degree T23.139
      left T23.032
        first degree T23.132
        second degree T23.232
        third degree T23.332
      right T23.031
        first degree T23.131
        second degree T23.231
        third degree T23.331
      second degree T23.239
      third degree T23.339
    right T23.021
      first degree T23.121
      second degree T23.221
      third degree T23.321
    second degree T23.229
    third degree T23.329
  flank - *see* Burn, abdominal wall
  foot T25.029
    first degree T25.129
    left T25.022
      first degree T25.122
      second degree T25.222
      third degree T25.322
    multiple with ankle - *see* Burn, lower, limb, multiple, ankle and foot
    right T25.021
      first degree T25.121
      second degree T25.221
      third degree T25.321
    second degree T25.229
    third degree T25.329
  forearm T22.019
    first degree T22.119
    left T22.012
      first degree T22.112
      second degree T22.212
      third degree T22.312
    right T22.011
      first degree T22.111
      second degree T22.211
      third degree T22.311
    second degree T22.219
    third degree T22.319
  forehead T20.06
    first degree T20.16
    second degree T20.26
    third degree T20.36
  fourth degree   code as Burn, third degree, by site
  friction - *see* Burn, by site
  from swallowing caustic or corrosive substance NEC - *see* Corrosion, by site
  full thickness skin loss
  code as Burn, third degree, by site
  gastrointestinal tract NEC T28.2
    from swallowing caustic or corrosive substance T28.7
  genital organs
    external

Burn - *continued*
- female T21.07
  - first degree T21.17
  - second degree T21.27
  - third degree T21.37
  - male T21.06
    - first degree T21.16
    - second degree T21.26
    - third degree T21.36
  - internal T28.3
    - from caustic or corrosive substance T28.8
- groin - *see* Burn, abdominal wall
- hand(s) T23.009
  - back - *see* Burn, dorsum of hand
  - finger - *see* Burn, finger
  - first degree T23.109
  - left T23.002
    - first degree T23.102
    - second degree T23.202
    - third degree T23.302
  - multiple sites with wrist T23.099
    - first degree T23.199
    - left T23.092
      - first degree T23.192
      - second degree T23.292
      - third degree T23.392
    - right T23.091
      - first degree T23.191
      - second degree T23.291
      - third degree T23.391
    - second degree T23.299
    - third degree T23.399
  - palm - *see* Burn, palm
  - right T23.001
    - first degree T23.101
    - second degree T23.201
    - third degree T23.301
  - second degree T23.209
  - third degree T23.309
  - thumb - *see* Burn, thumb
- head (and face) (and neck) T20.00
  - cheek - *see* Burn, cheek
  - chin - *see* Burn, chin
  - ear - *see* Burn, ear
  - eye(s) only - *see* Burn, eye
  - first degree T20.10
  - forehead - *see* Burn, forehead
  - lip - *see* Burn, lip
  - multiple sites T20.09
    - first degree T20.19
    - second degree T20.29
    - third degree T20.39
  - neck - *see* Burn, neck
  - nose - *see* Burn, nose
  - scalp - *see* Burn, scalp
  - second degree T20.20
  - third degree T20.30
- hip(s) - *see* Burn, thigh
- inhalation - *see* Burn, respiratory tract
  - caustic or corrosive substance (fumes) - *see* Corrosion, respiratory tract
- internal organ(s) T28.40
  - alimentary tract T28.2
    - esophagus T28.1
  - eardrum T28.41
  - esophagus T28.1
  - from caustic or corrosive substance (swallowing) NEC - *see* Corrosion, by site
  - genitourinary T28.3
  - mouth T28.0
  - pharynx T28.0
  - respiratory tract - *see* Burn, respiratory tract
  - specified organ NEC T28.49
- interscapular region - *see* Burn, back, upper

Burn - *continued*
- intestine (large) (small) T28.2
- knee T24.029
  - first degree T24.129
  - left T24.022
    - first degree T24.122
    - second degree T24.222
    - third degree T24.322
  - right T24.021
    - first degree T24.121
    - second degree T24.221
    - third degree T24.321
  - second degree T24.229
  - third degree T24.329
- labium (majus) (minus) - *see* Burn, genital organs, external, female
- lacrimal apparatus, duct, gland or sac - *see* Burn, eye, specified site NEC
- larynx T27.0
  - with lung T27.1
- leg(s) (lower) (upper) - *see* Burn, lower, limb
- lightning - *see* Burn, by site
- limb(s)
  - lower (except ankle or foot alone) - *see* Burn, lower, limb
  - upper - *see* Burn, upper limb
- lip(s) T20.02
  - first degree T20.12
  - second degree T20.22
  - third degree T20.32
- lower
  - back - *see* Burn, back
  - limb T24.009
    - ankle - *see* Burn, ankle
    - calf - *see* Burn, calf
    - first degree T24.109
    - foot - *see* Burn, foot
    - hip - *see* Burn, thigh
    - knee - *see* Burn, knee
    - left T24.002
      - first degree T24.102
      - second degree T24.202
      - third degree T24.302
    - multiple sites, except ankle and foot T24.099
      - ankle and foot T25.099
        - first degree T25.199
        - left T25.092
          - first degree T25.192
          - second degree T25.292
          - third degree T25.392
        - right T25.091
          - first degree T25.191
          - second degree T25.291
          - third degree T25.391
        - second degree T25.299
        - third degree T25.399
      - first degree T24.199
      - left T24.092
        - first degree T24.192
        - second degree T24.292
        - third degree T24.392
      - right T24.091
        - first degree T24.191
        - second degree T24.291
        - third degree T24.391
      - second degree T24.299
      - third degree T24.399
    - right T24.001
      - first degree T24.101
      - second degree T24.201
      - third degree T24.301
    - second degree T24.209
  - thigh - *see* Burn, thigh

Burn - *continued*
- third degree T24.309
- toe - *see* Burn, toe
- lung (with larynx and trachea) T27.1
- mouth T28.0
- neck T20.07
  - first degree T20.17
  - second degree T20.27
  - third degree T20.37
- nose (septum) T20.04
  - first degree T20.14
  - second degree T20.24
  - third degree T20.34
- ocular adnexa - *see* Burn, eye   orbit region - *see* Burn, eyelid
- palm T23.059
  - first degree T23.159
  - left T23.052
    - first degree T23.152
    - second degree T23.252
    - third degree T23.352
  - right T23.051
    - first degree T23.151
    - second degree T23.251
    - third degree T23.351
  - second degree T23.259
  - third degree T23.359
- partial thickness
- code as Burn, unspecified degree, by site
- pelvis - *see* Burn, trunk
- penis - *see* Burn, genital organs, external, male
- perineum
  - female - *see* Burn, genital organs, external, female
  - male - *see* Burn, genital organs, external, male
- periocular area - *see* Burn, eyelid
- pharynx T28.0
- rectum T28.2
- respiratory tract T27.3
  - larynx - *see* Burn, larynx
  - specified part NEC T27.2
  - trachea - *see* Burn, trachea
- sac, lacrimal - *see* Burn, eye, specified site NEC
- scalp T20.05
  - first degree T20.15
  - second degree T20.25
  - third degree T20.35
- scapular region T22.069
  - first degree T22.169
  - left T22.062
    - first degree T22.162
    - second degree T22.262
    - third degree T22.362
  - right T22.061
    - first degree T22.161
    - second degree T22.261
    - third degree T22.361
  - second degree T22.269
  - third degree T22.369
- sclera - *see* Burn, eye, specified site NEC
- scrotum - *see* Burn, genital organs, external, male
- shoulder T22.059
  - first degree T22.159
  - left T22.052
    - first degree T22.152
    - second degree T22.252
    - third degree T22.352
  - right T22.051
    - first degree T22.151
    - second degree T22.251
    - third degree T22.351

Burn - *continued*
    second degree T23.299
      third degree T23.399
    right T23.071
      first degree T23.171
      second degree T23.271
      third degree T23.371
    second degree T23.279
    third degree T23.379
Burnett's syndrome E83.52
Burning
  feet syndrome E53.9
  sensation R20.8
  tongue K14.6
Burn-out (state) Z73.0
Burns' disease or osteochondrosis - *see*
  Osteochondrosis, juvenile, ulna
Bursa - *see* condition
Bursitis M71.9
  Achilles - *see* Tendinitis, Achilles
  adhesive - *see* Bursitis, specified NEC
  ankle - *see* Enthesopathy, lower limb, ankle,
    specified type NEC
  calcaneal - *see* Enthesopathy, foot, specified
    type NEC
  collateral ligament, tibial - *see* Bursitis, tibial
    collateral
  due to use, overuse, pressure - *see also*
    Disorder, soft tissue, due to use, specified
    type NEC
    specified NEC - *see* Disorder, soft tissue, due
    to use, specified NEC
  Duplay's M75.0
  elbow NEC M70.3-
    olecranon M70.2-
  finger - *see* Disorder, soft tissue, due to use,
    specified type NEC, hand
  foot - *see* Enthesopathy, foot, specified type
    NEC
  gonococcal A54.49
  gouty - *see* Gout
  hand M70.1-
  hip NEC M70.7-
    trochanteric M70.6-
  infective NEC M71.10
    abscess - *see* Abscess, bursa
    ankle M71.17-
    elbow M71.12-
    foot M71.17-
    hand M71.14-
    hip M71.15-
    knee M71.16-
    multiple sites M71.19
    shoulder M71.11-
    specified site NEC M71.18
    wrist M71.13-
  ischial - *see* Bursitis, hip
  knee NEC M70.5-
    prepatellar M70.4-
  occupational NEC - *see also* Disorder, soft
    tissue, due to, use
  olecranon - *see* Bursitis, elbow, olecranon
  pharyngeal J39.1
  popliteal - *see* Bursitis, knee prepatellar
    M70.4-
  radiohumeral M77.8
  rheumatoid M06.20
    ankle M06.27-
    elbow M06.22-
    foot joint M06.27-
    hand joint M06.24-
    hip M06.25-
    knee M06.26-
    multiple site M06.29

Bursitis - *continued*
    shoulder M06.21-
    vertebra M06.28
    wrist M06.23-
  scapulohumeral - *see* Bursitis, shoulder
  semimembranous muscle (knee) - *see* Bursitis,
    knee
  shoulder M75.5-
    adhesive - *see* Capsulitis, adhesive
  specified NEC M71.50
    ankle M71.57-
    due to use, overuse or pressure - *see*
      Disorder, soft tissue, due to, use
    elbow M71.52-
    foot M71.57-
    hand M71.54-
    hip M71.55-
    knee M71.56-
    shoulder - *see* Bursitis, shoulder
    specified site NEC M71.58
    tibial collateral M76.4-
    wrist M71.53-
  subacromial - *see* Bursitis, shoulder
  subcoracoid - *see* Bursitis, shoulder
  subdeltoid - *see* Bursitis, shoulder
  syphilitic A52.78
  Thornwaldt, Tornwaldt J39.2
  tibial collateral M76.4-
  toe - *see* Enthesopathy, foot, specified type
    NEC
  trochanteric (area) - *see* Bursitis, hip,
    trochanteric
  wrist - *see* Bursitis, hand
Bursopathy M71.9
  specified type NEC M71.80
    ankle M71.87-
    elbow M71.82-
    foot M71.87-
    hand M71.84-
    hip M71.85-
    knee M71.86-
    multiple sites M71.89
    shoulder M71.81-
    specified site NEC M71.88
    wrist M71.83-
Burst stitches or sutures (complication of
surgery) T81.31
  external operation wound T81.31
  internal operation wound T81.32
Buruli ulcer A31.1
Bury's disease L95.1
Buschke's
  disease B45.3
  scleredema - *see* Sclerosis, systemic
Busse-Buschke disease B45.3
Buttock - *see* condition
Button
  Biskra B55.1
  Delhi B55.1
  oriental B55.1
Buttonhole deformity (finger) - *see* Deformity,
  finger, boutonniere
Bwamba fever A92.8
Byssinosis J66.0
Bywaters' syndrome T79.5

C

Cachexia R64
  cancerous R64
  cardiac - *see* Disease, heart
  dehydration E86.0
  due to malnutrition R64
  exophthalmic - *see* Hyperthyroidism

Cachexia - *continued*
  heart - *see* Disease, heart
  hypophyseal E23.0
  hypopituitary E23.0
  lead - *see* Poisoning, lead
  malignant R64
  marsh - *see* Malaria
  nervous F48.8
  old age R54
  paludal - *see* Malaria
  pituitary E23.0
  renal N28.9
  saturnine - *see* Poisoning, lead
  senile R54
  Simmonds' E23.0
  splenica D73.0
  strumipriva E03.4
  tuberculous NEC - *see* Tuberculosis
Café, au lait spots L81.3
Caffeine-induced
  anxiety disorder F15.980
  sleep disorder F15.982
Caffey's syndrome Q78.8
Caisson disease T70.3
Cake kidney Q63.1
Caked breast (puerperal, postpartum)
  O92.79
Calabar swelling B74.3
Calcaneal spur - *see* Spur, bone, calcaneal
Calcaneo-apophysitis M92.8
Calcareous - *see* condition
Calcicosis J62.8
Calciferol (vitamin D) deficiency E55.9
  with rickets E55.0
Calcification
  adrenal (capsule) (gland) E27.49
    tuberculous E35 [*B90.8*]
  aorta I70.0
  artery (annular) - *see* Arteriosclerosis
  auricle (ear) - *see* Disorder, pinna, specified
    type NEC
  basal ganglia G23.8
  bladder N32.89
    due to Schistosoma hematobium B65.0
  brain (cortex) - *see* Calcification, cerebral
  bronchus J98.09
  bursa M71.40
    ankle M71.47-
    elbow M71.42-
    foot M71.47-
    hand M71.44-
    hip M71.45-
    knee M71.46-
    multiple sites M71.49
    shoulder M75.3-
    specified site NEC M71.48
    wrist M71.43-
  cardiac - *see* Degeneration, myocardial
  cerebral (cortex) G93.89
    artery I67.2
  cervix (uteri) N88.8
  choroid plexus G93.89
  conjunctiva - *see* Concretion, conjunctiva
  corpora cavernosa (penis) N48.89
  cortex (brain) - *see* Calcification, cerebral
  dental pulp (nodular) K04.2
  dentinal papilla K00.4
  fallopian tube N83.8
  falx cerebri G96.19
  gallbladder K82.8
  general E83.59
  heart - *see also* Degeneration, myocardial
    valve - *see* Endocarditis
  idiopathic infantile arterial (IIAC) Q28.8

Calcification - *continued*
intervertebral cartilage or disc (postinfective) - *see* Disorder, disc, specified NEC
intracranial - *see* Calcification, cerebral
joint - *see* Disorder, joint, specified type NEC
kidney N28.89
tuberculous N29 *[B90.1]*
larynx (senile) J38.7
lens - *see* Cataract, specified NEC
lung (active) (postinfectional) J98.4
tuberculous B90.9
lymph gland or node (postinfectional) I89.8
tuberculous - *see also* Tuberculosis, lymph gland B90.8
mammographic R92.1
massive (paraplegic) - *see* Myositis, ossificans, in, quadriplegia
medial - *see* Arteriosclerosis, extremities
meninges (cerebral) (spinal) G96.19
metastatic E83.59
Mönckeberg's - *see* Arteriosclerosis, extremities
muscle M61.9
due to burns - *see* Myositis, ossificans, in, burns
paralytic - *see* Myositis, ossificans, in, quadriplegia
specified type NEC M61.40
ankle M61.47-
foot M61.47-
forearm M61.43-
hand M61.44-
lower leg M61.46-
multiple sites M61.49
pelvic region M61.45-
shoulder region M61.41-
specified site NEC M61.48
thigh M61.45-
upper arm M61.42-
myocardium, myocardial - *see* Degeneration, myocardial
ovary N83.8
pancreas K86.89
penis N48.89
periarticular - *see* Disorder, joint, specified type NEC
pericardium - *see also* Pericarditis I31.1
pineal gland E34.8
pleura J94.8
postinfectional J94.8
tuberculous NEC B90.9
pulpal (dental) (nodular) K04.2
sclera H15.89
spleen D73.89
subcutaneous L94.2
suprarenal (capsule) (gland) E27.49
tendon (sheath) - *see also* Tenosynovitis, specified type NEC
with bursitis, synovitis or tenosynovitis - *see* Tendinitis, calcific
trachea J39.8
ureter N28.89
uterus N85.8
vitreous - *see* Deposit, crystalline
Calcified - *see* Calcification
Calcinosis (interstitial) (tumoral) (universalis) E83.59
with Raynaud's phenomenon, esophageal dysfunction, sclerodactyly, telangiectasia (CREST syndrome) M34.1
circumscripta (skin) L94.2
cutis L94.2
Calciphylaxis - *see also* Calcification, by site E83.59

Calcium
deposits - *see* Calcification, by site
metabolism disorder E83.50
salts or soaps in vitreous - *see* Deposit, crystalline
Calciuria R82.99
Calculi - *see* Calculus
Calculosis, intrahepatic - *see* Calculus, bile duct
Calculus, calculi, calculous
ampulla of Vater - *see* Calculus, bile duct
anuria (impacted) (recurrent) - *see also* Calculus, urinary N20.9
appendix K38.1
bile duct (common) (hepatic) K80.50
with
calculus of gallbladder - *see* Calculus, gallbladder and bile duct
cholangitis K80.30
with
cholecystitis - *see* Calculus, bile duct, with cholecystitis
obstruction K80.31
acute K80.32
with
chronic cholangitis K80.36
with obstruction K80.37
obstruction K80.33
chronic K80.34
with
acute cholangitis K80.36
with obstruction K80.37
obstruction K80.35
cholecystitis (with cholangitis) K80.40
with obstruction K80.41
acute K80.42
with
chronic cholecystitis K80.46
with obstruction K80.47
obstruction K80.43
chronic K80.44
with
acute cholecystitis K80.46
with obstruction K80.47
obstruction K80.45
obstruction K80.51
biliary - *see also* Calculus, gallbladder
specified NEC K80.80
with obstruction K80.81
bilirubin, multiple - *see* Calculus, gallbladder
bladder (encysted) (impacted) (urinary) (diverticulum) N21.0
bronchus J98.09
calyx (kidney) (renal) - *see* Calculus, kidney
cholesterol (pure) (solitary) - *see* Calculus, gallbladder
common duct (bile) - *see* Calculus, bile duct
conjunctiva - *see* Concretion, conjunctiva
cystic N21.0
duct - *see* Calculus, gallbladder
dental (subgingival) (supragingival) K03.6
diverticulum
bladder N21.0
kidney N20.0
epididymis N50.89
gallbladder K80.20
with
bile duct calculus - *see* Calculus, gallbladder and bile duct
cholecystitis K80.10
with obstruction K80.11
acute K80.00
with
chronic cholecystitis K80.12

Calculus, calculi, calculous - *continued*
with obstruction K80.13
obstruction K80.01
chronic K80.10
with
acute cholecystitis K80.12
with obstruction K80.13
obstruction K80.11
specified NEC K80.18
with obstruction K80.19
obstruction K80.21
gallbladder and bile duct K80.70
with
cholecystitis K80.60
with obstruction K80.61
acute K80.62
with
chronic cholecystitis K80.66
with obstruction K80.67
obstruction K80.63
chronic K80.64
with
acute cholecystitis K80.66
with obstruction K80.67
obstruction K80.65
obstruction K80.71
hepatic (duct) - *see* Calculus, bile duct
hepatobiliary K80.80
with obstruction K80.81
ileal conduit N21.8
intestinal (impaction) (obstruction) K56.49
kidney (impacted) (multiple) (pelvis) (recurrent) (staghorn) N20.0
with calculus, ureter N20.2
congenital Q63.8
lacrimal passages - *see* Dacryolith
liver (impacted) - *see* Calculus, bile duct
lung J98.4
mammographic R92.1
nephritic (impacted) (recurrent) - *see* Calculus, kidney nose J34.89
pancreas (duct) K86.89
parotid duct or gland K11.5
pelvis, encysted - *see* Calculus, kidney
prostate N42.0
pulmonary J98.4
pyelitis (impacted) (recurrent) N20.0
with hydronephrosis N13.2
pyelonephritis (impacted) (recurrent) - *see* category N20
with hydronephrosis N13.2
renal (impacted) (recurrent) - *see* Calculus, kidney salivary (duct) (gland) K11.5
seminal vesicle N50.89
staghorn - *see* Calculus, kidney Stensen's duct K11.5
stomach K31.89
sublingual duct or gland K11.5
congenital Q38.4
submandibular duct, gland or region K11.5
submaxillary duct, gland or region K11.5
suburethral N21.8
tonsil J35.8
tooth, teeth (subgingival) (supragingival) K03.6
tunica vaginalis N50.89
ureter (impacted) (recurrent) N20.1
with calculus, kidney N20.2
with hydronephrosis N13.2
with infection N13.6
urethra (impacted) N21.1
urinary (duct) (impacted) (passage) (tract) N20.9
with hydronephrosis N13.2

Calculus, calculi, calculous - *continued*
  with infection N13.6
  in (due to)
    lower N21.9
      specified NEC N21.8
    vagina N89.8
    vesical (impacted) N21.0
    Wharton's duct K11.5
    xanthine E79.8 [*N22*]
Caliectasis N28.89
Caliectasis N28.89
California
  disease B38.9
  encephalitis A83.5
Caligo cornea - *see* Opacity, cornea, central
Callositas, callosity (infected) L84
Callus (infected) L84
  bone - *see* Osteophyte
    excessive, following fracture
    code as Sequelae of fracture
CALME (childhood asymmetric labium majus enlargement) N90.61
Calorie deficiency or malnutrition - *see also* Malnutrition E46
Calvé-Perthes disease - *see* Legg-Calvé-Perthes disease
Calvé's disease - *see* Osteochondrosis, juvenile, spine
Calvities - *see* Alopecia, androgenic
Cameroon fever - *see* Malaria
Camptocormia (hysterical) F44.4
Camurati-Engelmann syndrome Q78.3
Canal - *see also* condition
  atrioventricular common Q21.2
Canaliculitis (lacrimal) (acute) (subacute) H04.33-
  Actinomyces A42.89
  chronic H04.42-**canavan's disease** E75.29
Canceled procedure (surgical) Z53.9
  because of
    contraindication Z53.09
      smoking Z53.01
    left against medical advice (AMA) Z53.21
    patient's decision Z53.20
      for reasons of belief or group pressure Z53.1
      specified reason NEC Z53.29
    specified reason NEC Z53.8
Cancer - *see also* Neoplasm, by site, malignant
  bile duct type liver C22.1
  blood - *see* Leukemia
  breast - *see also* Neoplasm, breast, malignant C50.91-
  hepatocellular C22.0
  lung - *see also* Neoplasm, lung, malignant C34.90-
  ovarian - *see also* Neoplasm ovary, malignant C56.9-
  unspecified site (primary) C80.1
Cancer (o) phobia F45.29
Cancerous - *see* Neoplasm, malignant, by site
Cancrum oris A69.0
Candidiasis, candidal B37.9
  balanitis B37.42
  bronchitis B37.1
  cheilitis B37.83
  congenital P37.5
  cystitis B37.41
  disseminated B37.7
  endocarditis B37.6
  enteritis B37.82
  esophagitis B37.81
  intertrigo B37.2

Candidiasis, candidal - *continued*
  lung B37.1
  meningitis B37.5
  mouth B37.0
  nails B37.2
  neonatal P37.5
  onychia B37.2
  oral B37.0
  osteomyelitis B37.89
  otitis externa B37.84
  paronychia B37.2
  perionyxis B37.2
  pneumonia B37.1
  proctitis B37.82
  pulmonary B37.1
  pyelonephritis B37.49
  sepsis B37.7
  skin B37.2
  specified site NEC B37.89
  stomatitis B37.0
  systemic B37.7
  urethritis B37.41
  urogenital site NEC B37.49
  vagina B37.3
  vulva B37.3
  vulvovaginitis B37.3
Candidid L30.2
Candidosis - *see* Candidiasis
Candiru infection or infestation B88.8
Canities (premature) L67.1
  congenital Q84.2
Canker (mouth) (sore) K12.0
  rash A38.9
Cannabinosis J66.2
Cannabis induced
  anxiety disorder F12.980
  psychotic disorder F12.959
  sleep disorder F12.988
Canton fever A75.9
Cantrell's syndrome Q87.89
Capillariasis (intestinal) B81.1
  hepatic B83.8
Capillary - *see* condition
Caplan's syndrome - *see* Rheumatoid, lung
Capsule - *see* condition
Capsulitis (joint) - *see also* Enthesopathy
  adhesive (shoulder) M75.0-
  hepatic K65.8
  labyrinthine - *see* Otosclerosis, specified NEC
  thyroid E06.9
Caput
  crepitus Q75.8
  medusae I86.8
  succedaneum P12.81
Car sickness T75.3
Carapata (disease) A68.0
Carate - *see* Pinta
Carbon lung J60
Carbuncle L02.93
  abdominal wall L02.231
  anus K61.0
  auditory canal, external - *see* Abscess, ear, external
  auricle ear - *see* Abscess, ear, external
  axilla L02.43-
  back (any part) L02.232
  breast N61.1
  buttock L02.33
  cheek (external) L02.03
  chest wall L02.233
  chin L02.03
  corpus cavernosum N48.21
  ear (any part) (external) (middle) - *see* Abscess, ear, external

Carbuncle - *continued*
  external auditory canal - *see* Abscess, ear, external
  eyelid - *see* Abscess, eyelid
  face NEC L02.03
  femoral (region) - *see* Carbuncle, lower limb
  finger - *see* Carbuncle, hand
  flank L02.231
  foot L02.63-
  forehead L02.03
  genital - *see* Abscess, genital
  gluteal (region) L02.33
  groin L02.234
  hand L02.53-
  head NEC L02.831
  heel - *see* Carbuncle, foot
  hip - *see* Carbuncle, lower limb
  kidney - *see* Abscess, kidney
  knee - *see* Carbuncle, lower limb
  labium (majus) (minus) N76.4
  lacrimal
    gland - *see* Dacryoadenitis
    passages (duct) (sac) - *see* Inflammation, lacrimal, passages, acute
  leg - *see* Carbuncle, lower limb
  lower limb L02.43-
  malignant A22.0
  navel L02.236
  neck L02.13
  nose (external) (septum) J34.0
  orbit, orbital - *see* Abscess, orbit
  palmar (space) - *see* Carbuncle, hand
  partes posteriores L02.33
  pectoral region L02.233
  penis N48.21
  perineum L02.235
  pinna - *see* Abscess, ear, external
  popliteal - *see* Carbuncle, lower limb
  scalp L02.831
  seminal vesicle N49.0
  shoulder - *see* Carbuncle, upper limb
  specified site NEC L02.838
  temple (region) L02.03
  thumb - *see* Carbuncle, hand
  toe - *see* Carbuncle, foot
  trunk L02.239
    abdominal wall L02.231
    back L02.232
    chest wall L02.233
    groin L02.234
    perineum L02.235
    umbilicus L02.236
  umbilicus L02.236
  upper limb L02.43-
  urethra N34.0
  vulva N76.4
Carbunculus - *see* Carbuncle
Carcinoid (tumor) - *see* Tumor, carcinoid
Carcinoidosis E34.0
Carcinoma (malignant) - *see also* Neoplasm, by site, malignant
  acidophil
    specified site - *see* Neoplasm, malignant, by site
    unspecified site C75.1
  acidophil-basophil, mixed
    specified site - *see* Neoplasm, malignant, by site
    unspecified site C75.1
  adnexal (skin) - *see* Neoplasm, skin, malignant
  adrenal cortical C74.0-
  alveolar - *see* Neoplasm, lung, malignant
    cell - *see* Neoplasm, lung, malignant
  ameloblastic C41.1

Carcinoma - *continued*

upper jaw (bone) C41.0

apocrine

breast - *see* Neoplasm, breast, malignant

specified site NEC - *see* Neoplasm, skin, malignant

unspecified site C44.99

basal cell (pigmented) (see also Neoplasm, skin, malignant) C44.91

fibro-epithelial - *see* Neoplasm, skin, malignant

morphea - *see* Neoplasm, skin, malignant

multicentric - *see* Neoplasm, skin, malignant

basaloid

basal-squamous cell, mixed - *see* Neoplasm, skin, malignant

basophil

specified site - *see* Neoplasm, malignant, by site

unspecified site C75.1

basophil-acidophil, mixed

specified site - *see* Neoplasm, malignant, by site

unspecified site C75.1

basosquamous - *see* Neoplasm, skin, malignant

bile duct

with hepatocellular, mixed C22.0

liver C22.1

specified site NEC - *see* Neoplasm, malignant, by site

unspecified site C22.1

branchial or branchiogenic C10.4

bronchial or bronchogenic - *see* Neoplasm, lung, malignant

bronchiolar - *see* Neoplasm, lung, malignant

bronchioloalveolar - *see* Neoplasm, lung, malignant

C cell

specified site - *see* Neoplasm, malignant, by site

unspecified site C73

ceruminous C44.29-

cervix uteri

in situ D06.9

endocervix D06.0

exocervix D06.1

specified site NEC D06.7

chorionic

specified site - *see* Neoplasm, malignant, by site

unspecified site

female C58

male C62.90

chromophobe

specified site - *see* Neoplasm, malignant, by site

unspecified site C75.1

cloacogenic

specified site - *see* Neoplasm, malignant, by site

unspecified site C21.2

diffuse type

specified site - *see* Neoplasm, malignant, by site

unspecified site C16.9

duct (cell)

with Paget's disease - *see* Neoplasm, breast, malignant

infiltrating

with lobular carcinoma (in situ)

specified site - *see* Neoplasm, malignant, by site

unspecified site (female) C50.91-

male C50.92-

Carcinoma - *continued*

specified site - *see* Neoplasm, malignant, by site

unspecified site (female) C50.91-

male C50.92-

ductal

with lobular

specified site - *see* Neoplasm, malignant, by site

unspecified site (female) C50.91-

male C50.92-

ductular, infiltrating

specified site - *see* Neoplasm, malignant, by site

unspecified site (female) C50.91-

male C50.92-

embryonal

liver C22.7

endometrioid

specified site - *see* Neoplasm, malignant, by site

unspecified site

female C56.9

male C61

eosinophil

specified site - *see* Neoplasm, malignant, by site

unspecified site C75.1

epidermoid - *see also* Neoplasm, skin malignant

in situ, Bowen's type - *see* Neoplasm, skin, in situ

fibroepithelial, basal cell - *see* Neoplasm, skin, malignant

follicular

with papillary (mixed) C73

moderately differentiated C73

pure follicle C73

specified site - *see* Neoplasm, malignant, by site

trabecular C73

unspecified site C73

well differentiated C73

generalized, with unspecified primary site C80.0

glycogen-rich - *see* Neoplasm, breast, malignant

granulosa cell C56-

hepatic cell C22.0

hepatocellular C22.0

with bile duct, mixed C22.0

fibrolamellar C22.0

hepatocholangiolitic C22.0

Hürthle cell C73

in

adenomatous

polyposis coli C18.9

pleomorphic adenoma - *see* Neoplasm, salivary glands, malignant

situ - *see* Carcinoma-in-situ

infiltrating

duct

with lobular

specified site - *see* Neoplasm, malignant, by site

unspecified site (female) C50.91-

male C50.92-

with Paget's disease - *see* Neoplasm, breast, malignant

specified site - *see* Neoplasm, malignant

unspecified site (female) C50.91-

male C50.92-

ductular

specified site - *see* Neoplasm, malignant

Carcinoma - *continued*

unspecified site (female) C50.91-

male C50.92-

lobular

specified site - *see* Neoplasm, malignant

unspecified site (female) C50.91-

male C50.92-

inflammatory

specified site - *see* Neoplasm, malignant

unspecified site (female) C50.91-

male C50.92-

intestinal type

specified site - *see* Neoplasm, malignant, by site

unspecified site C16.9

intracystic

noninfiltrating - *see* Neoplasm, in situ, by site

intraductal (noninfiltrating)

with Paget's disease - *see* Neoplasm, breast, malignant

breast D05.1-

papillary

with invasion

specified site - *see* Neoplasm, malignant, by site

unspecified site (female) C50.91-

male C50.92-

breast D05.1-

specified site NEC - *see* Neoplasm, in situ, by site

unspecified site (female) D05.1-

specified site NEC - *see* Neoplasm, in situ, by site

unspecified site (female) D05.1-

intraepidermal - *see* Neoplasm, in situ

squamous cell, Bowen's type - *see* Neoplasm, skin, in situ

intraepithelial - *see* Neoplasm, in situ, by site

squamous cell - *see* Neoplasm, in situ, by site

intraosseous C41.1

upper jaw (bone) C41.0

islet cell

with exocrine, mixed

specified site - *see* Neoplasm, malignant, by site

unspecified site C25.9

pancreas C25.4

specified site NEC - *see* Neoplasm, malignant, by site

unspecified site C25.4

juvenile, breast - *see* Neoplasm, breast, malignant

large cell

small cell

specified site - *see* Neoplasm, malignant, by site

unspecified site C34.90

Leydig cell (testis)

specified site - *see* Neoplasm, malignant, by site

unspecified site

female C56.9

male C62.90

lipid-rich (female) C50.91-

male C50.92-

liver cell C22.0

liver NEC C22.7

lobular (infiltrating)

with intraductal

specified site - *see* Neoplasm, malignant, by site

unspecified site (female) C50.91-

male C50.92-

noninfiltrating

Carcinoma - *continued*
 breast D05.0-
  specified site NEC - *see* Neoplasm, in situ,
   by site
  unspecified site D05.0-
 specified site - *see* Neoplasm, malignant, by
  site
 unspecified site (female) C50.91-
  male C50.92-
 medullary
  with
   amyloid stroma
    specified site - *see* Neoplasm, malignant,
     by site
    unspecified site C73
   lymphoid stroma
    specified site - *see* Neoplasm, malignant,
     by site
    unspecified site (female) C50.91-
     male C50.92-
 Merkel cell C4A.9
  anal margin C4A.51
  anal skin C4A.51
  canthus C4A.1-
  ear and external auricular canal C4A.2-
  external auricular canal C4A.2-
  eyelid, including canthus C4A.1-
  face C4A.30
   specified NEC C4A.39
  hip C4A.7-
  lip C4A.0
  lower limb, including hip C4A.7-
  neck C4A.4
  nodal presentation C7B.1
  nose C4A.31
  overlapping sites C4A.8
  perianal skin C4A.51
  scalp C4A.4
  secondary C7B.1
  shoulder C4A.6-
  skin of breast C4A.52
  trunk NEC C4A.59
  upper limb, including shoulder C4A.6-
  visceral metastatic C7B.1
 metastatic - *see* Neoplasm, secondary, by site
 metatypical - *see* Neoplasm, skin, malignant
 morphea, basal cell - *see* Neoplasm, skin,
  malignant
 mucoid
  cell
   specified site - *see* Neoplasm, malignant, by
    site
   unspecified site C75.1
 neuroendocrine - *see also* Tumor,
  neuroendocrine
  high grade, any site C7A.1
  poorly differentiated, any site C7A.1
 nonencapsulated sclerosing C73
 noninfiltrating
  intracystic - *see* Neoplasm, in situ, by site
  intraductal
   breast D05.1-
   papillary
    breast D05.1-
    specified site NEC - *see* Neoplasm, in situ,
     by site
    unspecified site D05.1-
   specified site - *see* Neoplasm, in situ, by
    site
   unspecified site D05.1-
  lobular
   breast D05.0-
   specified site NEC - *see* Neoplasm, in situ,
    by site

Carcinoma - *continued*
  unspecified site (female) D05.0-
 oat cell
  specified site - *see* Neoplasm, malignant, by
   site
  unspecified site C34.90
 odontogenic C41.1
  upper jaw (bone) C41.0
 papillary
  with follicular (mixed) C73
  follicular variant C73
  intraductal (noninfiltrating)
   with invasion
    specified site - *see* Neoplasm, malignant,
     by site
    unspecified site (female) C50.91-
     male C50.92-
   breast D05.1-
   specified site NEC - *see* Neoplasm, in situ,
    by site
   unspecified site D05.1-
  serous
   specified site - *see* Neoplasm, malignant, by
    site
   surface
    specified site - *see* Neoplasm, malignant,
     by site
    unspecified site C56.9
   unspecified site C56.9
 papillocystic
  specified site - *see* Neoplasm, malignant, by
   site
  unspecified site C56.9
 parafollicular cell
  specified site - *see* Neoplasm, malignant, by
   site
  unspecified site C73
 pilomatrix - *see* Neoplasm, skin, malignant
 pseudomucinous
  specified site - *see* Neoplasm, malignant, by
   site
  unspecified site C56.9
 renal cell C64-
 Schmincke - *see* Neoplasm, nasopharynx,
  malignant
 Schneiderian
  specified site - *see* Neoplasm, malignant, by
   site
  unspecified site C30.0
 sebaceous - *see* Neoplasm, skin, malignant
 secondary - *see also* Neoplasm, secondary, by
  site
  Merkel cell C7B.1
 secretory, breast - *see* Neoplasm, breast,
  malignant
 serous
  papillary
   specified site - *see* Neoplasm, malignant, by
    site
   unspecified site C56.9
  surface, papillary
   specified site - *see* Neoplasm, malignant, by
    site
   unspecified site C56.9
 Sertoli cell
  specified site - *see* Neoplasm, malignant, by
   site
  unspecified site C62.90
   female C56.9
   male C62.90
 skin appendage - *see* Neoplasm, skin,
  malignant
 small cell
  fusiform cell

Carcinoma - *continued*
  specified site - *see* Neoplasm, malignant, by
   site
  unspecified site C34.90
 intermediate cell
  specified site - *see* Neoplasm, malignant, by
   site
  unspecified site C34.90
 large cell
  specified site - *see* Neoplasm, malignant, by
   site
  unspecified site C34.90
 solid
  with amyloid stroma
   specified site - *see* Neoplasm, malignant, by
    site
   unspecified site C73
 microinvasive
  specified site - *see* Neoplasm, malignant, by
   site
  unspecified site C53.9
 sweat gland - *see* Neoplasm, skin, malignant
 theca cell C56.-
 thymic C37
 unspecified site (primary) C80.1
 water-clear cell C75.0
Carcinoma-in-situ - *see also* Neoplasm, in situ,
 by site
 breast NOS D05.9-
  specified type NEC D05.8-
 epidermoid - *see also* Neoplasm, in situ, by
  site
  with questionable stromal invasion
   cervix D06.9
   specified site NEC - *see* Neoplasm, in situ,
    by site
   unspecified site D06.9
 Bowen's type - *see* Neoplasm, skin, in situ
 intraductal
  breast D05.1-
  specified site NEC - *see* Neoplasm, in situ,
   by site
  unspecified site D05.1-
 lobular
  with
   infiltrating duct
    breast (female) C50.91-
     male C50.92-
    specified site NEC - *see* Neoplasm,
     malignant
    unspecified site (female) C50.91-
     male C50.92-
   intraductal
    breast D05.8-
    specified site NEC - *see* Neoplasm, in situ,
     by site
    unspecified site (female) D05.8-
  breast D05.0-
  specified site NEC - *see* Neoplasm, in situ,
   by site
  unspecified site D05.0-
 squamous cell - *see also* Neoplasm, in situ, by
  site
  with questionable stromal invasion
   cervix D06.9
   specified site NEC - *see* Neoplasm, in situ,
    by site
   unspecified site D06.9
Carcinomaphobia F45.29
Carcinomatosis C80.0
 peritonei C78.6
 unspecified site (primary) (secondary) C80.0

Carcinosarcoma - *see* Neoplasm, malignant, by site
  embryonal - *see* Neoplasm, malignant, by site
Cardia, cardial - *see* condition
Cardiac - *see also* condition
  death, sudden - *see* Arrest, cardiac
  pacemaker
    in situ Z95.0
      management or adjustment Z45.018
  tamponade I31.4
Cardialgia - *see* Pain, precordial
Cardiectasis - *see* Hypertrophy, cardiac
Cardiochalasia K21.9
Cardiomalacia I51.5
Cardiomegalia glycogenica diffusa E74.02 [I43]
Cardiomegaly - *see also* Hypertrophy, cardiac
  congenital Q24.8
  glycogen E74.02 [I43]
  idiopathic I51.7
Cardiomyoliposis I51.5
Cardiomyopathy (familial) (idiopathic) I42.9
  alcoholic I42.6
  amyloid E85.4 [I43]
    transthyretin-related (ATTR) familial E85.4
  arteriosclerotic - *see* Disease, heart, ischemic, atherosclerotic
  beriberi E51.12
  cobalt-beer I42.6
  congenital I42.4
  congestive I42.0
  constrictive NOS I42.5
  dilated I42.0
  due to
    alcohol I42.6
    beriberi E51.12
    cardiac glycogenosis E74.02 [I43]
    drugs I42.7
    external agents NEC I42.7
    Friedreich's ataxia G11.1
    myotonia atrophica G71.11 [I43]
    progressive muscular dystrophy G71.0 [I43]
  glycogen storage E74.02 [I43]
  hypertensive - *see* Hypertension, heart
  hypertrophic (nonobstructive) I42.2
    obstructive I42.1
      congenital Q24.8
  in
    Chagas' disease (chronic) B57.2
      acute B57.0
    sarcoidosis D86.85
  ischemic I25.5
  metabolic E88.9 [I43]
    thyrotoxic E05.90 [I43]
      with thyroid storm E05.91 [I43]
  newborn I42.8
    congenital I42.4
  nutritional E63.9 [I43]
    beriberi E51.12
  obscure of Africa I42.8
  peripartum O90.3
  postpartum O90.3
  restrictive NEC I42.5
  rheumatic I09.0
  secondary I42.9
  stress induced I51.81
  takotsubo I51.81
  thyrotoxic E05.90 [I43]
    with thyroid storm E05.91 [I43]
  toxic NEC I42.7
  transthyretin-related (ATTR) familial amyloid E85.4
  tuberculous A18.84
  viral B33.24

Cardionephritis - *see* Hypertension, cardiorenal
Cardionephropathy - *see* Hypertension, cardiorenal
Cardionephrosis - *see* Hypertension, cardiorenal
Cardiopathia nigra I27.0
Cardiopathy - *see also* Disease, heart I51.9
  idiopathic I42.9
  mucopolysaccharidosis E76.3 [I52]
Cardiopericarditis - *see* Pericarditis
Cardiophobia F45.29
Cardiorenal - *see* condition
Cardiorrhexis - *see* Infarct, myocardium
Cardiosclerosis - *see* Disease, heart, ischemic, atherosclerotic
Cardiosis - *see* Disease, heart
Cardiospasm (esophagus) (reflex) (stomach) K22.0
  congenital Q39.5
    with megaesophagus Q39.5
Cardiostenosis - *see* Disease, heart
Cardiosymphysis I31.0
Cardiovascular - *see* condition
Carditis (acute) (bacterial) (chronic) (subacute) I51.89
  meningococcal A39.50
  rheumatic - *see* Disease, heart, rheumatic
  rheumatoid - *see* Rheumatoid, carditis
  viral B33.20
Care (of) (for) (following)
  child (routine) Z76.2
  family member (handicapped) (sick)
    creating problem for family Z63.6
    provided away from home for holiday relief Z75.5
    unavailable, due to
      absence (person rendering care) (sufferer) Z74.2
      inability (any reason) of person rendering care Z74.2
  foundling Z76.1
  holiday relief Z75.5
  improper - *see* Maltreatment
  lack of (at or after birth) (infant) - *see* Maltreatment, child, neglect
  lactating mother Z39.1
  palliative Z51.5
  postpartum
    immediately after delivery Z39.0
    routine follow-up Z39.2
  respite Z75.5
  unavailable, due to
    absence of person rendering care Z74.2
    inability (any reason) of person rendering care Z74.2
  well-baby Z76.2
Caries
  bone NEC A18.03
  dental (dentino enamel junction) (early childhood) (of dentine) (pre-eruptive) (recurrent) (to the pulp) K02.9
    arrested (coronal) (root) K02.3
    chewing surface
      limited to enamel K02.51
      penetrating into dentin K02.52
      penetrating into pulp K02.53
    coronal surface
      chewing surface
        limited to enamel K02.51
        penetrating into dentin K02.52
        penetrating into pulp K02.53
      pit and fissure surface

Caries - *continued*
      limited to enamel K02.51
      penetrating into dentin K02.52
      penetrating into pulp K02.53
      smooth surface
        limited to enamel K02.61
        penetrating into dentin K02.62
        penetrating into pulp K02.63
    pit and fissure surface
      limited to enamel K02.51
      penetrating into dentin K02.52
      penetrating into pulp K02.53
    primary, cervical origin K02.52
    root K02.7
    smooth surface
      limited to enamel K02.61
      penetrating into dentin K02.62
      penetrating into pulp K02.63
  external meatus - *see* Disorder, ear, external, specified type NEC
  hip (tuberculous) A18.02
  initial (tooth)
    chewing surface K02.51
    pit and fissure surface K02.51
    smooth surface K02.61
  knee (tuberculous) A18.02
  labyrinth - *see* subcategory H83.8
  limb NEC (tuberculous) A18.03
  mastoid process (chronic) - *see* Mastoiditis, chronic
    tuberculous A18.03
  middle ear - *see* subcategory H74.8
  nose (tuberculous) A18.03
  orbit (tuberculous) A18.03
  ossicles, ear - *see* Abnormal, ear ossicles
  petrous bone - *see* Petrositis
  root (dental) (tooth) K02.7
  sacrum (tuberculous) A18.01
  spine, spinal (column) (tuberculous) A18.01
  syphilitic A52.77
    congenital (early) A50.02 [M90.80]
  tooth, teeth - *see* Caries, dental
  tuberculous A18.03
  vertebra (column) (tuberculous) A18.01
Carious teeth - *see* Caries, dental
Carneous mole O02.0
Carnitine insufficiency E71.40
Carotid body or sinus syndrome G90.01
Carotidynia G90.01
Carotinemia (dietary) E67.1
Carotinosis (cutis) (skin) E67.1
Carpal tunnel syndrome - *see* Syndrome, carpal tunnel
Carpenter's syndrome Q87.0
Carpopedal spasm - *see* Tetany
Carr-Barr-Plunkett syndrome Q97.1
Carrier (suspected) of
  amebiasis Z22.1
  bacterial disease NEC Z22.39
    diphtheria Z22.2
    intestinal infectious NEC Z22.1
      typhoid Z22.0
    meningococcal Z22.31
    sexually transmitted Z22.4
    specified NEC Z22.39
    staphylococcal (Methicillin susceptible) Z22.321
      Methicillin resistant Z22.322
    streptococcal Z22.338
      group B Z22.330
        complicating pregnancy or delivery O99.82-
    typhoid Z22.0
  cholera Z22.1

Carrier (suspected) of - *continued*
diphtheria Z22.2
gastrointestinal pathogens NEC Z22.1
genetic Z14.8
  cystic fibrosis Z14.1
  hemophilia A (asymptomatic) Z14.01
    symptomatic Z14.02
gestational, pregnant Z33.1
gonorrhea Z22.4
HAA (hepatitis Australian-antigen) B18.8
HB (c)(s) -aG B18.1
hepatitis (viral) B18.9
  Australia-antigen (HAA) B18.8
  B surface antigen (HBsAg) B18.1
    with acute delta (super) infection B17.0
  C B18.2
  specified NEC B18.8
human T-cell lymphotropic virus type 1
  (HTLV 1) infection Z22.6
infectious organism Z22.9
  specified NEC Z22.8
meningococci Z22.31
Salmonella typhosa Z22.0
serum hepatitis - *see* Carrier, hepatitis
staphylococci (Methicillin susceptible)
  Z22.321
  Methicillin resistant Z22.322
streptococci Z22.338
  group B Z22.330
    complicating pregnancy or delivery
    O99.82-
syphilis Z22.4
typhoid Z22.0
venereal disease NEC Z22.4
Carrion's disease A44.0
Carter's relapsing fever (Asiatic) A68.1
Cartilage - *see* condition
Caruncle (inflamed)
conjunctiva (acute) - *see* Conjunctivitis, acute
labium (majus) (minus) N90.89
lacrimal - *see* Inflammation, lacrimal, passages
myrtiform N89.8
urethral (benign) N36.2
Cascade stomach K31.2
Caseation lymphatic gland (tuberculous)
  A18.2
Cassidy (-Scholte) syndrome (malignant
  carcinoid) E34.0
Castellani's disease A69.8
Castration, traumatic, male S38.231
Casts in urine R82.99
Cat
cry syndrome Q93.4
ear Q17.3
eye syndrome Q92.8
Catabolism, senile R54
Catalepsy (hysterical) F44.2
schizophrenic F20.2
Cataplexy (idiopathic) - *see* Narcolepsy
Cataract (cortical) (immature) (incipient)
  H26.9
with
  neovascularization - *see* Cataract,
    complicated
age-related - *see* Cataract, senile
anterior
  and posterior axial embryonal Q12.0
  pyramidal Q12.0
associated with
  galactosemia E74.21 [*H28*]
  myotonic disorders G71.19 [*H28*]
blue Q12.0
central Q12.0
cerulean Q12.0

Cataract - *continued*
complicated H26.20
with
  neovascularization H26.21-
    ocular disorder H26.22-
  glaucomatous flecks H26.23-
congenital Q12.0
coralliform Q12.0
coronary Q12.0
crystalline Q12.0
diabetic - *see* Diabetes, cataract
drug-induced H26.3-
due to
  ocular disorder - *see* Cataract, complicated
  radiation H26.8
electric H26.8
extraction status Z98.4-
glass-blower's H26.8
heat ray H26.8
heterochromic - *see* Cataract, complicated
hypermature - *see* Cataract, senile, morgagnian
type   in (due to)
  chronic iridocyclitis - *see* Cataract,
    complicated
  diabetes - *see* Diabetes, cataract
  endocrine disease E34.9 [*H28*]
  eye disease - *see* Cataract, complicated
  hypoparathyroidism E20.9 [*H28*]
  malnutrition-dehydration E46 [*H28*]
  metabolic disease E88.9 [*H28*]
  myotonic disorders G71.19 [*H28*]
  nutritional disease E63.9 [*H28*]
infantile - *see* Cataract, presenile
irradiational - *see* Cataract, specified NEC
juvenile - *see* Cataract, presenile
malnutrition-dehydration E46 [*H28*]
morgagnian - *see* Cataract, senile, morgagnian
type   myotonic G71.19 [*H28*]
myxedema E03.9 [*H28*]
nuclear
  embryonal Q12.0
  sclerosis - *see* Cataract, senile, nuclear
presenile H26.00-
  combined forms H26.06-
  cortical H26.01-
  lamellar - *see* Cataract, presenile, cortical
  nuclear H26.03-
  specified NEC H26.09
  subcapsular polar (anterior) H26.04-
    posterior H26.05-
  zonular - *see* Cataract, presenile, cortical
secondary H26.40
  Soemmering's ring H26.41-
  specified NEC H26.49-
  to eye disease - *see* Cataract, complicated
senile H25.9
  brunescens - *see* Cataract, senile, nuclear
  combined forms H25.81-
  coronary - *see* Cataract, senile, incipient
  cortical H25.01-
  hypermature - *see* Cataract, senile,
    morgagnian type
  incipient (mature) (total) H25.09-
    cortical - *see* Cataract, senile, cortical
    subcapsular - *see* Cataract, senile,
      subcapsular
  morgagnian type (hypermature) H25.2-
  nuclear (sclerosis) H25.1-
  polar subcapsular (anterior) (posterior) - *see*
    Cataract, senile, incipient
  punctate - *see* Cataract, senile, incipient
  specified NEC H25.89
  subcapsular polar (anterior) H25.03-
    posterior H25.04-

Cataract - *continued*
snowflake - *see* Diabetes, cataract
specified NEC H26.8
toxic - *see* Cataract, drug-induced   traumatic
  H26.10-
  localized H26.11-
  partially resolved H26.12-
  total H26.13-
zonular (perinuclear) Q12.0
Cataracta - *see also* Cataract
brunescens - *see* Cataract, senile, nuclear
centralis pulverulenta Q12.0
cerulea Q12.0
complicata - *see* Cataract, complicated
congenita Q12.0
coralliformis Q12.0
coronaria Q12.0
diabetic - *see* Diabetes, cataract
membranacea
  accreta - *see* Cataract, secondary
  congenita Q12.0
nigra - *see* Cataract, senile, nuclear
sunflower - *see* Cataract, complicated
Catarrh, catarrhal (acute) (febrile)
  (infectious) (inflammation) - *see also*
  condition J00
bronchial - *see* Bronchitis
chest - *see* Bronchitis
chronic J31.0
due to congenital syphilis A50.03
enteric - *see* Enteritis
eustachian H68.009
fauces - *see* Pharyngitis
gastrointestinal - *see* Enteritis
gingivitis K05.00
  nonplaque induced K05.01
  plaque induced K05.00
hay - *see* Fever, hay
intestinal - *see* Enteritis
larynx, chronic J37.0
liver B15.9
  with hepatic coma B15.0
lung - *see* Bronchitis
middle ear, chronic - *see* Otitis, media,
  nonsuppurative, chronic, serous
mouth K12.1
nasal (chronic) - *see* Rhinitis
nasobronchial J31.1
nasopharyngeal (chronic) J31.1
  acute J00
pulmonary - *see* Bronchitis
spring (eye) (vernal) - *see* Conjunctivitis,
  acute, atopic
summer (hay) - *see* Fever, hay
throat J31.2
tubotympanal - *see also* Otitis, media,
  nonsuppurative
  chronic - *see* Otitis, media, nonsuppurative,
    chronic, serous
Catatonia (schizophrenic) F20.2
Catatonic
disorder due to known physiologic condition
  F06.1
schizophrenia F20.2
stupor R40.1
Cat-scratch - *see also* Abrasion
disease or fever A28.1
Cauda equina - *see* condition
Cauliflower ear M95.1-
Causalgia (upper limb) G56.4-
lower limb G57.7-
Cause
external, general effects T75.89

Caustic burn - see Corrosion, by site
Cavare's disease (familial periodic paralysis)
G72.3
Cave-in, injury
  crushing (severe) - see Crush
  suffocation - see Asphyxia, traumatic, due to
  low oxygen, due to cave-in
Cavernitis (penis) N48.29
Cavernositis N48.29
Cavernous - see condition
Cavitation of lung - see also Tuberculosis,
  pulmonary
  nontuberculous J98.4
Cavities, dental - see Caries, dental
Cavity
  lung - see Cavitation of lung
  optic papilla Q14.2
  pulmonary - see Cavitation of lung
Cavovarus foot, congenital Q66.1
Cavus foot (congenital) Q66.7
  acquired - see Deformity, limb, foot, specified
  NEC
Cazenave's disease L10.2
Cecitis K52.9
  with perforation, peritonitis, or rupture K65.8
Cecum - see condition
Celiac
  artery compression syndrome I77.4
  disease (with steatorrhea) K90.0
  infantilism K90.0
Cell(s), cellular - see also condition
  in urine R82.99
Cellulitis (diffuse) (phlegmonous) (septic)
  (suppurative) L03.90
  abdominal wall L03.311
  anaerobic A48.0
  ankle - see Cellulitis, lower limb
  anus K61.0
  arm - see Cellulitis, upper limb
  auricle (ear) - see Cellulitis, ear
  axilla L03.11-
  back (any part) L03.312
  breast (acute) (nonpuerperal) (subacute) N61.0
    nipple N61.0
  broad ligament
    acute N73.0
  buttock L03.317
  cervical (meaning neck) L03.221
  cervix (uteri) - see Cervicitis
  cheek (external) L03.211
    internal K12.2
  chest wall L03.313
  chronic L03.90
  clostridial A48.0
  corpus cavernosum N48.22
  digit
    finger - see Cellulitis, finger
    toe - see Cellulitis, toe
  Douglas' cul-de-sac or pouch
    acute N73.0
  drainage site (following operation) T81.4
  ear (external) H60.1-
  eosinophilic (granulomatous) L98.3
  erysipelatous - see Erysipelas
  external auditory canal - see Cellulitis, ear
  eyelid - see Abscess, eyelid
  face NEC L03.211
  finger (intrathecal) (periosteal) (subcutaneous)
    (subcuticular) L03.01-
  foot - see Cellulitis, lower limb
  gangrenous - see Gangrene
  genital organ NEC
    female (external) N76.4
    male N49.9

Cellulitis - continued
  multiple sites N49.8
    specified NEC N49.8
  gluteal (region) L03.317
  gonococcal A54.89
  groin L03.314
  hand - see Cellulitis, upper limb
  head NEC L03.811
    face (any part, except ear, eye and nose)
  L03.211
  heel - see Cellulitis, lower limb
  hip - see Cellulitis, lower limb
  jaw (region) L03.211
  knee - see Cellulitis, lower limb
  labium (majus) (minus) - see Vulvitis
  lacrimal passages - see Inflammation, lacrimal,
    passages
  larynx J38.7
  leg - see Cellulitis, lower limb
  lip K13.0
  lower limb L03.11-
    toe - see Cellulitis, toe   mouth (floor) K12.2
  multiple sites, so stated L03.90
  nasopharynx J39.1
  navel L03.316
    newborn P38.9
      with mild hemorrhage P38.1
      without hemorrhage P38.9
  neck (region) L03.221
  nipple (acute) (nonpuerperal) (subacute) N61.0
  nose (septum) (external) J34.0
  orbit, orbital H05.01-
  palate (soft) K12.2
  pectoral (region) L03.313
  pelvis, pelvic (chronic)
    female - see also Disease, pelvis,
      inflammatory N73.2
      acute N73.0
    following ectopic or molar pregnancy O08.0
    male K65.0
  penis N48.22
  perineal, perineum L03.315
  periorbital L03.213
  perirectal K61.1
  peritonsillar J36
  periurethral N34.0
  periuterine - see also Disease, pelvis,
    inflammatory N73.2
    acute N73.0
  pharynx J39.1
  preseptal L03.213
  rectum K61.1
  retroperitoneal K68.9
  round ligament
    acute N73.0
  scalp (any part) L03.811
  scrotum N49.2
  seminal vesicle N49.0
  shoulder - see Cellulitis, upper limb
  specified site NEC L03.818
  submandibular (region) (space) (triangle)
    K12.2
    gland K11.3
  submaxillary (region) K12.2
    gland K11.3
  thigh - see Cellulitis, lower limb
  thumb (intrathecal) (periosteal) (subcutaneous)
    (subcuticular) - see Cellulitis, finger
  toe (intrathecal) (periosteal) (subcutaneous)
    (subcuticular) L03.03-
  tonsil J36
  trunk L03.319
    abdominal wall L03.311
    back (any part) L03.312

Cellulitis - continued
  buttock L03.317
  chest wall L03.313
  groin L03.314
  perineal, perineum L03.315
  umbilicus L03.316
  tuberculous (primary) A18.4
  umbilicus L03.316
  upper limb L03.11-
    axilla - see Cellulitis, axilla
    finger - see Cellulitis, finger
    thumb - see Cellulitis, finger
  vaccinal T88.0
  vocal cord J38.3
  vulva - see Vulvitis
  wrist - see Cellulitis, upper limb
Cementoblastoma, benign - see Cyst,
  calcifying odontogenic
Cementoma - see Cyst, calcifying odontogenic
Cementoperiostitis - see Periodontitis
Cementosis K03.4
Central auditory processing disorder H93.25
Central pain syndrome G89.0
Cephalematocele, cephal (o) hematocele
  newborn P52.8
    birth injury P10.8
  traumatic - see Hematoma, brain
Cephalematoma, cephalhematoma (calcified)
  newborn (birth injury) P12.0
  traumatic - see Hematoma, brain
Cephalgia, cephalalgia - see also Headache
  histamine G44.009
    intractable G44.001
    not intractable G44.009
  trigeminal autonomic (TAC) NEC G44.099
    intractable G44.091
    not intractable G44.099
Cephalic - see condition
Cephalitis - see Encephalitis
Cephalocele - see Encephalocele
Cephalomenia N94.89
Cephalopelvic - see condition
Cerclage (with cervical incompetence) in
  pregnancy - see Incompetence, cervix, in
  pregnancy
Cerebellitis - see Encephalitis
Cerebellum, cerebellar - see condition
Cerebral - see condition
Cerebritis - see Encephalitis
Cerebro-hepato-renal syndrome Q87.89
Cerebromalacia - see Softening, brain
  sequelae of cerebrovascular disease I69.398
Cerebroside lipidosis E75.22
Cerebrospasticity (congenital) G80.1
Cerebrospinal - see condition
Cerebrum - see condition
Ceroid-lipofuscinosis, neuronal E75.4
Cerumen (accumulation) (impacted) H61.2-
Cervical - see also condition
  auricle Q18.2
  dysplasia in pregnancy - see Abnormal, cervix,
    in pregnancy or childbirth
  erosion in pregnancy - see Abnormal, cervix,
    in pregnancy or childbirth
  fibrosis in pregnancy - see Abnormal, cervix,
    in pregnancy or childbirth
  fusion syndrome Q76.1
  rib Q76.5
  shortening (complicating pregnancy) O26.87-
Cervicalgia M54.2
Cervicitis (acute) (chronic) (nonvenereal)
  (senile (atrophic)) (subacute) (with ulceration)
  N72
  with

Cervicitis - *continued*
abortion - *see* Abortion, by type complicated
by genital tract and pelvic infection
ectopic pregnancy O08.0
molar pregnancy O08.0
chlamydial A56.09
gonococcal A54.03
herpesviral A60.03
puerperal (postpartum) O86.11
syphilitic A52.76
trichomonal A59.09
tuberculous A18.16
Cervicocolpitis (emphysematosa) (see also
Cervicitis) N72
Cervix - *see* condition
**Cesarean delivery, previous, affecting
management of pregnancy** O34.219
classical (vertical) scar O34.212
low transverse scar O34.211
Céstan (-Chenais) paralysis or syndrome
G46.3
Céstan-Raymond syndrome I65.8
Cestode infestation B71.9
specified type NEC B71.8
Cestodiasis B71.9
Chabert's disease A22.9
Chacaleh E53.8
Chafing L30.4
Chagas' (-Mazza) disease (chronic) B57.2
with
cardiovascular involvement NEC B57.2
digestive system involvement B57.30
megacolon B57.32
megaesophagus B57.31
other specified B57.39
megacolon B57.32
megaesophagus B57.31
myocarditis B57.2
nervous system involvement B57.40
meningitis B57.41
meningoencephalitis B57.42
other specified B57.49
specified organ involvement NEC B57.5
acute (with) B57.1
cardiovascular NEC B57.0
myocarditis B57.0
Chagres fever B50.9
Chair ridden Z74.09
Chalasia (cardiac sphincter) K21.9
Chalazion H00.19
left H00.16
lower H00.15
upper H00.14
right H00.13
lower H00.12
upper H00.11
Chalcosis - *see also* Disorder, globe,
degenerative, chalcosis
cornea - *see* Deposit, cornea
crystalline lens - *see* Cataract, complicated
retina H35.89
Chalicosis (pulmonum) J62.8
Chancre (any genital site) (hard) (hunterian)
(mixed) (primary) (seronegative)
(seropositive) (syphilitic) A51.0
congenital A50.07
conjunctiva NEC A51.2
Ducrey's A57
extragenital A51.2
eyelid A51.2
lip A51.2
nipple A51.2
Nisbet's A57
of

Chancre - *continued*
carate A67.0
pinta A67.0
yaws A66.0
palate, soft A51.2
phagedenic A57
simple A57
soft A57
bubo A57
palate A51.2
urethra A51.0
yaws A66.0
Chancroid (anus) (genital) (penis) (perineum)
(rectum) (urethra) (vulva) A57
Chandler's disease (osteochondritis dissecans,
hip) - *see* Osteochondritis, dissecans, hip
Change(s) (in) (of) - *see also* Removal
arteriosclerotic - *see* Arteriosclerosis
bone - *see also* Disorder, bone
diabetic - *see* Diabetes, bone change
bowel habit R19.4
cardiorenal (vascular) - *see* Hypertension,
cardiorenal
cardiovascular - *see* Disease, cardiovascular
circulatory I99.9
cognitive (mild) (organic) R41.89
color, tooth, teeth
during formation K00.8
posteruptive K03.7
contraceptive device Z30.433
corneal membrane H18.30
Bowman's membrane fold or rupture H18.31-
Descemet's membrane
fold H18.32-
rupture H18.33-
coronary - *see* Disease, heart, ischemic
degenerative, spine or vertebra - *see*
Spondylosis
dental pulp, regressive K04.2
dressing (nonsurgical) Z48.00
surgical Z48.01
heart - *see* Disease, heart
hip joint - *see* Derangement, joint, hip
hyperplastic larynx J38.7
hypertrophic
nasal sinus J34.89
turbinate, nasal J34.3
upper respiratory tract J39.8
indwelling catheter Z46.6
inflammatory - *see also* Inflammation
sacroiliac M46.1
job, anxiety concerning Z56.1
joint - *see* Derangement, joint
life - *see* Menopause
mental status R41.82
minimal (glomerular) - *see also* N00-N07 with
fourth character .0 N05.0
myocardium, myocardial - *see* Degeneration,
myocardial
of life - *see* Menopause   pacemaker Z45.018
pulse generator Z45.010
personality (enduring) F68.8
due to (secondary to)
general medical condition F07.0
secondary (nonspecific) F60.89
regressive, dental pulp K04.2
renal - *see* Disease, renal
retina H35.9
myopic (see also Myopia, degenerative)
H44.2-
sacroiliac joint M53.3
senile - *see also* condition R54
sensory R20.8
skin R23.9

Change(s) (in) (of) - *continued*
acute, due to ultraviolet radiation L56.9
specified NEC L56.8
chronic, due to nonionizing radiation L57.9
specified NEC L57.8
cyanosis R23.0
flushing R23.2
pallor R23.1
petechiae R23.3
specified change NEC R23.8
swelling - *see* Mass, localized
texture R23.4
trophic
arm - *see* Mononeuropathy, upper limb
leg - *see* Mononeuropathy, lower limb
vascular I99.9
vasomotor I73.9
voice R49.9
psychogenic F44.4
specified NEC R49.8
**Changing sleep-work schedule, affecting
sleep** G47.26
Changuinola fever A93.1
Chapping skin T69.8
**Charcot-Marie-tooth disease, paralysis or
syndrome** G60.0
Charcot's
arthropathy - *see* Arthropathy, neuropathic
cirrhosis K74.3
disease (tabetic arthropathy) A52.16
joint (disease) (tabetic) A52.16
diabetic - *see* Diabetes, with, arthropathy
syringomyelic G95.0
syndrome (intermittent claudication) I73.9
CHARGE association Q89.8
Charley-horse (quadriceps) M62.831
traumatic (quadriceps) S76.11-
Charlouis' disease - *see* Yaws
Cheadle's disease E54
Checking (of)
cardiac pacemaker (battery) (electrode(s))
Z45.018
pulse generator Z45.010
implantable subdermal contraceptive Z30.46
intrauterine contraceptive device Z30.431
wound Z48.0-
due to injury   code to Injury, by site, using
appropriate seventh character for subsequent
encounter
Check-up - *see* Examination
**Chédiak-Higashi (-Steinbrinck) syndrome
(congenital gigantism of peroxidase
granules)** E70.330
Cheek - *see* condition
Cheese itch B88.0
Cheese-washer's lung J67.8
Cheese-worker's lung J67.8
**Cheilitis (acute) (angular) (catarrhal)
(chronic) (exfoliative) (gangrenous)
(glandular) (infectional) (suppurative)
(ulcerative) (vesicular)** K13.0
actinic (due to sun) L56.8
other than from sun L59.8
candidal B37.83
Cheilodynia K13.0
Cheiloschisis - *see* Cleft, lip
Cheilosis (angular) K13.0
with pellagra E52
due to
vitamin B2 (riboflavin) deficiency E53.0
Cheiromegaly M79.89
Cheiropompholyx L30.1
Cheloid - *see* Keloid
Chemical burn - *see* Corrosion, by site

Chemodectoma - *see* Paraganglioma, nonchromaffin
Chemosis, conjunctiva - *see* Edema, conjunctiva
Chemotherapy (session) (for)
cancer Z51.11
neoplasm Z51.11
Cherubism M27.8
Chest - *see* condition
Cheyne-stokes breathing (respiration) R06.3
Chiari's
disease or syndrome (hepatic vein thrombosis) I82.0
malformation
type I G93.5
type II - *see* Spina bifida
net Q24.8
Chicago disease B40.9
Chickenpox - *see* Varicella
Chiclero ulcer or sore B55.1
Chigger (infestation) B88.0
Chignon (disease) B36.8
newborn (from vacuum extraction) (birth injury) P12.1
Chilaiditi's syndrome (subphrenic displacement, colon) Q43.3
Chilblain(s) (lupus) T69.1
Child
custody dispute Z65.3
Childbirth - *see* Delivery
Childhood
cerebral X-linked adrenoleukodystrophy E71.520
period of rapid growth Z00.2
Chill(s) R68.83
with fever R50.9
congestive in malarial regions B54
without fever R68.83
Chilomastigiasis A07.8
Chimera 46,XX/46,XY Q99.0
Chin - *see* condition
Chinese dysentery A03.9
Chionophobia F40.228
Chitral fever A93.1
Chlamydia, chlamydial A74.9
cervicitis A56.09
conjunctivitis A74.0
cystitis A56.01
endometritis A56.11
epididymitis A56.19
female
pelvic inflammatory disease A56.11
pelviperitonitis A56.11
orchitis A56.19
peritonitis A74.81
pharyngitis A56.4
proctitis A56.3
psittaci (infection) A70
salpingitis A56.11
sexually-transmitted infection NEC A56.8
specified NEC A74.89
urethritis A56.01
vulvovaginitis A56.02
Chlamydiosis - *see* Chlamydia
Chloasma (skin) (idiopathic) (symptomatic) L81.1
eyelid H02.719
hyperthyroid E05.90 [*H02.719*]
with thyroid storm E05.91 [*H02.719*]
left H02.716
lower H02.715
upper H02.714
right H02.713
lower H02.712

Chloasma - *continued*
upper H02.711
Chloroma C92.3-
Chlorosis D50.9
Egyptian B76.9 [*D63.8*]
miner's B76.9 [*D63.8*]
Chlorotic anemia D50.8
Chocolate cyst (ovary) N80.1
Choked
disc or disk - *see* Papilledema
on food, phlegm, or vomitus NOS - *see* Foreign body, by site
while vomiting NOS - *see* Foreign body, by site
Chokes (resulting from bends) T70.3
Choking sensation R09.89
Cholangiectasis K83.8
Cholangiocarcinoma
with hepatocellular carcinoma, combined C22.0
liver C22.1
specified site NEC - *see* Neoplasm, malignant, by site
unspecified site C22.1
Cholangiohepatitis K83.8
due to fluke infestation B66.1
Cholangiohepatoma C22.0
Cholangiolitis (acute) (chronic) (extrahepatic) (gangrenous) (intrahepatic) K83.0
paratyphoidal - *see* Fever, paratyphoid
typhoidal A01.09
Cholangioma D13.4
malignant - *see* Cholangiocarcinoma
Cholangitis (ascending) (primary) (recurrent) (sclerosing) (secondary) (stenosing) (suppurative) K83.0
with calculus, bile duct - *see* Calculus, bile duct, with cholangitis
chronic nonsuppurative destructive K74.3
Cholecystectasia K82.8
Cholecystitis K81.9
with
calculus, stones in
bile duct (common) (hepatic) - *see* Calculus, bile duct, with cholecystitis
cystic duct - *see* Calculus, gallbladder, with cholecystitis
gallbladder - *see* Calculus, gallbladder, with cholecystitis
choledocholithiasis - *see* Calculus, bile duct, with cholecystitis
cholelithiasis - *see* Calculus, gallbladder, with cholecystitis
acute (emphysematous) (gangrenous) (suppurative) K81.0
with
calculus, stones in
cystic duct - *see* Calculus, gallbladder, with cholecystitis, acute
gallbladder - *see* Calculus, gallbladder, with cholecystitis, acute
choledocholithiasis - *see* Calculus, bile duct, with cholecystitis, acute
cholelithiasis - *see* Calculus, gallbladder, with cholecystitis, acute
chronic cholecystitis K81.2
with gallbladder calculus K80.12
with obstruction K80.13
chronic K81.1
with acute cholecystitis K81.2
with gallbladder calculus K80.12
with obstruction K80.13
emphysematous (acute) - *see* Cholecystitis, acute

Cholecystitis - *continued*
gangrenous - *see* Cholecystitis, acute
paratyphoidal, current A01.4
suppurative - *see* Cholecystitis, acute
typhoidal A01.09
Cholecystolithiasis - *see* Calculus, gallbladder
Choledochitis (suppurative) K83.0
Choledocholith - *see* Calculus, bile duct
Choledocholithiasis (common duct) (hepatic duct) - *see* Calculus, bile duct
cystic - *see* Calculus, gallbladder
typhoidal A01.09
Cholelithiasis (cystic duct) (gallbladder) (impacted) (multiple) - *see* Calculus, gallbladder
bile duct (common) (hepatic) - *see* Calculus, bile duct
hepatic duct - *see* Calculus, bile duct
specified NEC K80.80
with obstruction K80.81
Cholemia - *see also* Jaundice
familial (simple) (congenital) E80.4
Gilbert's E80.4
Choleperitoneum, choleperitonitis K65.3
Cholera (Asiatic) (epidemic) (malignant) A00.9
antimonial - *see* Poisoning, antimony
classical A00.0
due to Vibrio cholerae 01 A00.9
biovar cholerae A00.0
biovar eltor A00.1
el tor A00.1
el tor A00.1
Cholerine - *see* Cholera
Cholestasis NEC K83.1
with hepatocyte injury K71.0
due to total parenteral nutrition (TPN) K76.89
pure K71.0
Cholesteatoma (ear) (middle) (with reaction) H71.9-
attic H71.0-
external ear (canal) H60.4-
mastoid H71.2-
postmastoidectomy cavity (recurrent) - *see* Complications, postmastoidectomy, recurrent cholesteatoma
recurrent (postmastoidectomy) - *see* Complications, postmastoidectomy, recurrent cholesteatoma
tympanum H71.1-
Cholesteatosis, diffuse H71.3-
Cholesteremia E78.00
Cholesterin in vitreous - *see* Deposit, crystalline
Cholesterol
deposit
retina H35.89
vitreous - *see* Deposit, crystalline
elevated (high) E78.00
with elevated (high) triglycerides E78.2
Cholesterol - *continued*
screening for Z13.220
imbibition of gallbladder K82.4
Cholesterolemia (essential) (pure) E78.00
familial E78.01
hereditary E78.01
Cholesterolosis, cholesterosis (gallbladder) K82.4
cerebrotendinous E75.5
Cholocolic fistula K82.3
Choluria R82.2
Chondritis M94.8X9
auricle H61.03-
costal (Tietze's) M94.0
external ear H61.03-

Chondritis - *continued*
  patella, posttraumatic - *see* Chondromalacia,
    patella
  pinna H61.03-
  purulent M94.8X-
  tuberculous NEC A18.02
    intervertebral A18.01
Chondroblastoma - *see also* Neoplasm, bone,
  benign
  malignant - *see* Neoplasm, bone, malignant
Chondrocalcinosis M11.20
  ankle M11.27-
  elbow M11.22-
  familial M11.10
    ankle M11.17-
    elbow M11.12-
    foot joint M11.17-
    hand joint M11.14-
    hip M11.15-
    knee M11.16-
    multiple site M11.19
    shoulder M11.11-
    vertebrae M11.18
    wrist M11.13-
  foot joint M11.27-
  hand joint M11.24-
  hip M11.25-
  knee M11.26-
  multiple site M11.29
  shoulder M11.21-
  vertebrae M11.28
  specified type NEC M11.20
    ankle M11.27-
    elbow M11.22-
    foot joint M11.27-
    hand joint M11.24-
    hip M11.25-
    knee M11.26-
    multiple site M11.29
    shoulder M11.21-
    vertebrae M11.28
    wrist M11.23-
  wrist M11.23-
Chondrodermatitis nodularis helicis or
  anthelicis - *see* Perichondritis, ear
Chondrodysplasia Q78.9
  with hemangioma Q78.4
  calcificans congenita Q77.3
  fetalis Q77.4
  metaphyseal (Jansen's) (McKusick's)
    (Schmid's) Q78.8
  punctata Q77.3
Chondrodystrophy, chondrodystrophia
  (familial) (fetalis) (hypoplastic) Q78.9
  calcificans congenita Q77.3
  myotonic (congenital) G71.13
  punctata Q77.3
Chondroectodermal dysplasia Q77.6
Chondrogenesis imperfecta Q77.4
Chondrolysis M94.35-
Chondroma - *see also* Neoplasm, cartilage,
  benign
  juxtacortical - *see* Neoplasm, bone, benign
  periosteal - *see* Neoplasm, bone, benign
Chondromalacia (systemic) M94.20
  acromioclavicular joint M94.21-
  ankle M94.27-
  elbow M94.22-
  foot joint M94.27-
  glenohumeral joint M94.21-
  hand joint M94.24-
  hip M94.25-
  knee M94.26-
  patella M22.4-

Chondromalacia (systemic) - *continued*
  multiple sites M94.29
  patella M22.4-
  rib M94.28
  sacroiliac joint M94.259
  shoulder M94.21-
  sternoclavicular joint M94.21-
  vertebral joint M94.28
  wrist M94.23-
Chondromatosis - *see also* Neoplasm,
  cartilage, uncertain behavior
  internal Q78.4
Chondromyxosarcoma - *see* Neoplasm,
  cartilage, malignant
Chondro-osteodysplasia (Morquio-Brailsford
  type) E76.219
Chondro-osteodystrophy E76.29
Chondro-osteoma - *see* Neoplasm, bone,
  benign
Chondropathia tuberosa M94.0
Chondrosarcoma - *see* Neoplasm, cartilage,
  malignant
  juxtacortical - *see* Neoplasm, bone, malignant
  mesenchymal - *see* Neoplasm, connective
    tissue, malignant
  myxoid - *see* Neoplasm, cartilage, malignant
Chordee (nonvenereal) N48.89
  congenital Q54.4
  gonococcal A54.09
Chorditis (fibrinous) (nodosa) (tuberosa) J38.2
Chordoma - *see* Neoplasm, vertebral (column),
  malignant
Chorea (chronic) (gravis) (posthemiplegic)
  (senile) (spasmodic) G25.5
  with
    heart involvement I02.0
      active or acute (conditions in I01) I02.0
        rheumatic I02.9
          with valvular disorder I02.0
    rheumatic heart disease (chronic)
  (inactive)(quiescent)   code to rheumatic heart
  condition involved   drug-induced G25.4
  habit F95.8
  hereditary G10
  Huntington's G10
  hysterical F44.4
  minor I02.9
    with heart involvement I02.0
  progressive G25.5
    hereditary G10
  rheumatic (chronic) I02.9
    with heart involvement I02.0
  Sydenham's I02.9
    with heart involvement - *see* Chorea, with
      rheumatic heart disease
  nonrheumatic G25.5
Choreoathetosis (paroxysmal) G25.5
Chorioadenoma (destruens) D39.2
Chorioamnionitis O41.12-
Chorioangioma D26.7
Choriocarcinoma - *see* Neoplasm, malignant,
  by site
  combined with
    embryonal carcinoma - *see* Neoplasm,
      malignant, by site
    other germ cell elements - *see* Neoplasm,
      malignant, by site
    teratoma - *see* Neoplasm, malignant, by site
  specified site - *see* Neoplasm, malignant, by
  site
  unspecified site
    female C58
    male C62.90

Chorioencephalitis (acute) (lymphocytic)
  (serous) A87.2
Chorioepithelioma - *see* Choriocarcinoma
Choriomeningitis (acute) (lymphocytic)
  (serous) A87.2
Chorionepithelioma - *see* Choriocarcinoma
Chorioretinitis - *see also* Inflammation,
  chorioretinal
  disseminated - *see also* Inflammation,
    chorioretinal, disseminated
    in neurosyphilis A52.19
  Egyptian B76.9 [D63.8]
  focal - *see also* Inflammation, chorioretinal,
    focal
  histoplasmic B39.9 [H32]
  in (due to)
    histoplasmosis B39.9 [H32]
    syphilis (secondary) A51.43
      late A52.71
    toxoplasmosis (acquired) B58.01
      congenital (active) P37.1 [H32]
    tuberculosis A18.53
  juxtapapillary, juxtapapillaris - *see*
    Inflammation, chorioretinal, focal,
    juxtapapillary
  leprous A30.9 [H32]
  miner's B76.9 [D63.8]
  progressive myopia (degeneration) (see also
    Myopia, degenerative) H44.2-
  syphilitic (secondary) A51.43
    congenital (early) A50.01 [H32]
    late A50.32
    late A52.71
  tuberculous A18.53
Chorioretinopathy, central serous H35.71-
Choroid - *see* condition
Choroideremia H31.21
Choroiditis - *see* Chorioretinitis
Choroidopathy - *see* Disorder, choroid
Choroidoretinitis - *see* Chorioretinitis
Choroidoretinopathy, central serous - *see*
  Chorioretinopathy, central serous
Christian-weber disease M35.6
Christmas disease D67
Chromaffinoma - *see also* Neoplasm, benign,
  by site
  malignant - *see* Neoplasm, malignant, by site
Chromatopsia - *see* Deficiency, color vision
Chromhidrosis, chromidrosis L75.1
Chromoblastomycosis - *see* Chromomycosis
Chromoconversion R82.91
Chromomycosis B43.9
  brain abscess B43.1
  cerebral B43.1
  cutaneous B43.0
  skin B43.0
  specified NEC B43.8
  subcutaneous abscess or cyst B43.2
Chromophytosis B36.0
Chromosome - *see* condition by chromosome
  involved
  D (1) - *see* condition, chromosome 13
  E (3) - *see* condition, chromosome 18
  G - *see* condition, chromosome 21
Chromotrichomycosis B36.8
Chronic - *see* condition
  fracture - *see* Fracture, pathological
Churg-Strauss syndrome M30.1
Chyle cyst, mesentery I89.8
Chylocele (nonfilarial) I89.8
  filarial - *see also* Infestation, filarial B74.9
    [N51]
  tunica vaginalis N50.89

Chylocele (nonfilarial) - *continued*
  filarial - *see also* Infestation, filarial B74.9
    [*N51*]
Chylomicronemia (fasting) (with
  hyperprebetalipoproteinemia) E78.3
Chylopericardium I31.3
  acute I30.9
Chylothorax (nonfilarial) I89.8
  filarial - *see also* Infestation, filarial B74.9
    [*J91.8*]
Chylous - *see* condition
Chyluria (nonfilarial) R82.0
  due to
    bilharziasis B65.0
    Brugia (malayi) B74.1
      timori B74.2
    schistosomiasis (bilharziasis) B65.0
    Wuchereria (bancrofti) B74.0
  filarial - *see* Infestation, filarial
Cicatricial (deformity) - *see* Cicatrix
Cicatrix (adherent) (contracted) (painful)
  (vicious) - *see also* Scar L90.5
  adenoid (and tonsil) J35.8
  alveolar process M26.79
  anus K62.89
  auricle - *see* Disorder, pinna, specified type
    NEC
  bile duct (common) (hepatic) K83.8
  bladder N32.89
  bone - *see* Disorder, bone, specified type NEC
  brain G93.89
  cervix (postoperative) (postpartal) N88.1
  common duct K83.8
  cornea H17.9
    tuberculous A18.59
  duodenum (bulb), obstructive K31.5
  esophagus K22.2
  eyelid - *see* Disorder, eyelid function
  hypopharynx J39.2
  lacrimal passages - *see* Obstruction, lacrimal
  larynx J38.7
  lung J98.4
  middle ear - *see* subcategory H74.8
  mouth K13.79
  muscle M62.89
    with contracture - *see* Contraction, muscle
    NEC
  nasopharynx J39.2
  palate (soft) K13.79
  penis N48.89
  pharynx J39.2
  prostate N42.89
  rectum K62.89
  retina - *see* Scar, chorioretinal
  semilunar cartilage - *see* Derangement,
    meniscus
  seminal vesicle N50.89
  skin L90.5
    infected L08.89
    postinfective L90.5
    tuberculous B90.8
  specified site NEC L90.5
  throat J39.2
  tongue K14.8
  tonsil (and adenoid) J35.8
  trachea J39.8
  tuberculous NEC B90.9
  urethra N36.8
  uterus N85.8
  vagina N89.8
    postoperative N99.2
  vocal cord J38.3
  wrist, constricting (annular) L90.5

CIDP (chronic inflammatory demyelinating
  polyneuropathy) G61.81
CIN - *see* Neoplasia, intraepithelial, cervix
CINCA (chronic infantile neurological,
  cutaneous and articular syndrome) M04.2
Cinchonism - *see* Deafness, ototoxic
  correct substance properly administered - *see*
    Table of Drugs and Chemicals, by drug,
    adverse effect
  overdose or wrong substance given or taken -
    see Table of Drugs and Chemicals, by drug,
    poisoning
Circle of Willis - *see* condition
Circular - *see* condition
Circulating anticoagulants - *see also*
  Disorder, hemorrhagic D68.318
  due to drugs - *see also* Disorder, hemorrhagic
    D68.32
  following childbirth O72.3
Circulation
  collateral, any site I99.8
  defective (lower extremity) I99.9
    congenital Q28.9
  embryonic Q28.9
  failure (peripheral) R57.9
    newborn P29.89
  fetal, persistent P29.38
  heart, incomplete Q28.9
Circulatory system - *see* condition
Circulus senilis (cornea) - *see* Degeneration,
  cornea, senile
Circumcision (in absence of medical
  indication) (ritual) (routine) Z41.2
Circumscribed - *see* condition
Circumvallate placenta O43.11-
Cirrhosis, cirrhotic (hepatic) (liver) K74.60
  alcoholic K70.30
    with ascites K70.31
  atrophic - *see* Cirrhosis, liver
  Baumgarten-Cruveilhier K74.69
  biliary (cholangiolitic) (cholangitic)
    (hypertrophic) (obstructive)
    (pericholangiolitic) K74.5
    due to
      Clonorchiasis B66.1
      flukes B66.3
    primary K74.3
    secondary K74.4
  cardiac (of liver) K76.1
  Charcot's K74.3
  cholangiolitic, cholangitic, cholestatic
    (primary) K74.3
  congestive K76.1
  Cruveilhier-Baumgarten K74.69
  cryptogenic (liver) K74.69
  due to
    hepatolenticular degeneration E83.01
    Wilson's disease E83.01
    xanthomatosis E78.2
  fatty K76.0
    alcoholic K70.0
  Hanot's (hypertrophic) K74.3
  hepatic - *see* Cirrhosis, liver
  hypertrophic K74.3
  Indian childhood K74.69
  kidney - *see* Sclerosis, renal
  Laennec's K70.30
    with ascites K70.31
    alcoholic K70.30
      with ascites K70.31
    nonalcoholic K74.69
  liver K74.60
    alcoholic K70.30
      with ascites K70.31

Cirrhosis, cirrhotic - *continued*
  fatty K70.0
  congenital P78.81
  syphilitic A52.74
  lung (chronic) J84.10
  macronodular K74.69
    alcoholic K70.30
      with ascites K70.31
  micronodular K74.69
    alcoholic K70.30
      with ascites K70.31
  mixed type K74.69
  monolobular K74.3
  nephritis - *see* Sclerosis, renal
  nutritional K74.69
    alcoholic K70.30
      with ascites K70.31
  obstructive - *see* Cirrhosis, biliary
  ovarian N83.8
  pancreas (duct) K86.89
  pigmentary E83.110
  portal K74.69
    alcoholic K70.30
      with ascites K70.31
  postnecrotic K74.69
    alcoholic K70.30
      with ascites K70.31
  pulmonary J84.10
  renal - *see* Sclerosis, renal
  spleen D73.2
  stasis K76.1
  Todd's K74.3
  unilobar K74.3
  xanthomatous (biliary) K74.5
    due to xanthomatosis (familial) (metabolic)
      (primary) E78.2
Cistern, subarachnoid R93.0
Citrullinemia E72.23
Citrullinuria E72.23
Civatte's disease or poikiloderma L57.3
Clam digger's itch B65.3
Clammy skin R23.1
Clap - *see* Gonorrhea
Clarke-Hadfield syndrome (pancreatic
  infantilism) K86.89
Clark's paralysis G80.9
Clastothrix L67.8
Claude Bernard-Horner syndrome G90.2
  traumatic - *see* Injury, nerve, cervical
    sympathetic
Claude's disease or syndrome G46.3
Claudication (intermittent) I73.9
  cerebral (artery) G45.9
  spinal cord (arteriosclerotic) G95.19
    syphilitic A52.09
  venous (axillary) I87.8
Claudication venosa intermittens I87.8
Claustrophobia F40.240
Clavus (infected) L84
Clawfoot (congenital) Q66.89
  acquired - *see* Deformity, limb, clawfoot
Clawhand (acquired) - *see also* Deformity,
  limb, clawhand
  congenital Q68.1
Claw toe (congenital) Q66.89
  acquired - *see* Deformity, toe, specified NEC
Clay eating - *see* Pica
Cleansing of artificial opening - *see* Attention
  to, artificial, opening
Cleft (congenital) - *see also* Imperfect, closure
  alveolar process M26.79
  branchial (persistent) Q18.2
    cyst Q18.0
    fistula Q18.0

Cleft (congenital) - *continued*
  sinus Q18.0
  cricoid cartilage, posterior Q31.8
  foot Q72.7
  hand Q71.6
  lip (unilateral) Q36.9
   with cleft palate Q37.9
    hard Q37.1
     with soft Q37.5
    soft Q37.3
     with hard Q37.5
   bilateral Q36.0
    with cleft palate Q37.8
     hard Q37.0
      with soft Q37.4
     soft Q37.2
      with hard Q37.4
   median Q36.1
  nose Q30.2
  palate Q35.9
   with cleft lip (unilateral) Q37.9
    bilateral Q37.8
   hard Q35.1
    with
     cleft lip (unilateral) Q37.1
      bilateral Q37.0
     soft Q35.5
      with cleft lip (unilateral) Q37.5
       bilateral Q37.4
   medial Q35.5
   soft Q35.3
    with
     cleft lip (unilateral) Q37.3
      bilateral Q37.2
     hard Q35.5
      with cleft lip (unilateral) Q37.5
       bilateral Q37.4
  penis Q55.69
  scrotum Q55.29
  thyroid cartilage Q31.8
  uvula Q35.7
Cleidocranial dysostosis Q74.0
Cleptomania F63.2
Clicking hip (newborn) R29.4
Climacteric (female) - *see also* Menopause
  arthritis (any site) NEC - *see* Arthritis,
  specified form NEC
  depression (single episode) F32.89
   recurrent episode F33.8
  melancholia (single episode) F32.89
   recurrent episode F33.8
  male (symptoms) (syndrome) NEC N50.89
  paranoid state F22
  polyarthritis NEC - *see* Arthritis, specified
  form NEC
  symptoms (female) N95.1
Clinical research investigation (clinical trial)
  (control subject) (normal comparison)
  (participant) Z00.6
Clitoris - *see* condition
Cloaca (persistent) Q43.7
Clonorchiasis, Clonorchis infection (liver)
  B66.1
Clonus R25.8
Closed bite M26.29
Clostridium (C.) perfringens, as cause of
  disease classified elsewhere B96.7
Closure
  congenital, nose Q30.0
  cranial sutures, premature Q75.0
  defective or imperfect NEC - *see* Imperfect,
  closure
  fistula, delayed - *see* Fistula

Closure - *continued*
  foramen ovale, imperfect Q21.1
  hymen N89.6
  interauricular septum, defective Q21.1
  interventricular septum, defective Q21.0
  lacrimal duct - *see also* Stenosis, lacrimal, duct
   congenital Q10.5
  nose (congenital) Q30.0
   acquired M95.0
  of artificial opening - *see* Attention to,
   artificial, opening
  primary angle, without glaucoma damage
   H40.06-
  vagina N89.5
  valve - *see* Endocarditis
  vulva N90.5
Clot (blood) - *see also* Embolism
  artery (obstruction) (occlusion) - *see*
   Embolism
  bladder N32.89
  brain (intradural or extradural) - *see* Occlusion,
   artery, cerebral
  circulation I74.9
  heart - *see also* Infarct, myocardium
   not resulting in infarction I51.3
  vein - *see* Thrombosis
Clouded state R40.1
  epileptic - *see* Epilepsy, specified NEC
  paroxysmal - *see* Epilepsy, specified NEC
Cloudy antrum, antra J32.0
Clouston's (hidrotic) ectodermal dysplasia
  Q82.4
Clubbed nail pachydermoperiostosis M89.40
  [L62]
Clubbing of finger(s) (nails) R68.3
Club finger R68.3
  congenital Q68.1
Clubfoot (congenital) Q66.89
  acquired - *see* Deformity, limb, clubfoot
  equinovarus Q66.0
  paralytic - *see* Deformity, limb, clubfoot
Clubhand (congenital) (radial) Q71.4-
  acquired - *see* Deformity, limb, clubhand
Club nail R68.3
  congenital Q84.6
Clump, kidney Q63.1
Clumsiness, clumsy child syndrome F82
Cluttering F80.81
Clutton's joints A50.51 *[M12.80]*
Coagulation, intravascular (diffuse)
  (disseminated) - *see also* Defibrination
  syndrome
  complicating abortion - *see* Abortion, by type,
   complicated by, intravascular coagulation
  following ectopic or molar pregnancy O08.1
Coagulopathy - *see also* Defect, coagulation
  consumption D65
  intravascular D65
   newborn P60
Coalition
  calcaneo-scaphoid Q66.89
  tarsal Q66.89
Coalminer's
  elbow - *see* Bursitis, elbow, olecranon
  lung or pneumoconiosis J60
Coalworker's lung or pneumoconiosis J60
Coarctation
  aorta (preductal) (postductal) Q25.1
  pulmonary artery Q25.71
Coated tongue K14.3
Coats' disease (exudative retinopathy) - *see*
  Retinopathy, exudative
Cocaine-induced
  anxiety disorder F14.980

Cocaine-induced - *continued*
  bipolar and related disorder F14.94
  depressive disorder F14.94
  obsessive-compulsive and related disorder
   F14.988
  psychotic disorder F14.959
  sleep disorder F14.982
  sexual dysfunction F14.981
Cocainism - *see* Disorder, cocaine use
Coccidioidomycosis B38.9
  cutaneous B38.3
  disseminated B38.7
  generalized B38.7
  meninges B38.4
  prostate B38.81
  pulmonary B38.2
   acute B38.0
   chronic B38.1
  skin B38.3
  specified NEC B38.89
Coccidioidosis - *see* Coccidioidomycosis
Coccidiosis (intestinal) A07.3
Coccydynia, coccygodynia M53.3
Coccyx - *see* condition
Cochin-china diarrhea K90.1
Cockayne's syndrome Q87.1
Cocked up toe - *see* Deformity, toe, specified
  NEC
Cock's peculiar tumor L72.3
Codman's tumor - *see* Neoplasm, bone, benign
Coenurosis B71.8
Coffee-worker's lung J67.8
Cogan's syndrome H16.32-
  oculomotor apraxia H51.8
Coitus, painful (female) N94.10
  male N53.12
  psychogenic F52.6
Cold J00
  agglutinin disease or hemoglobinuria (chronic)
   D59.1
  bronchial - *see* Bronchitis
  chest - *see* Bronchitis
  common (head) J00
  effects of T69.9
   specified effect NEC T69.8
  excessive, effects of T69.9
   specified effect NEC T69.8
  exhaustion from T69.8
  exposure to T69.9
   specified effect NEC T69.8
  head J00
  injury syndrome (newborn) P80.0
  on lung - *see* Bronchitis
  rose J30.1
  sensitivity, auto-immune D59.1
  symptoms J00
  virus J00
  with influenza, flu, or grippe - *see* Influenza,
   with, respiratory manifestations NEC
Cold sore B00.1
Colibacillosis A49.8
  as the cause of other disease - *see also*
   Escherichia coli B96.20
  generalized A41.50
Colic (bilious) (infantile) (intestinal) (recurrent)
  (spasmodic) R10.83
  abdomen R10.83
   psychogenic F45.8
  appendix, appendicular K38.8
  bile duct - *see* Calculus, bile duct
  biliary - *see* Calculus, bile duct
  common duct - *see* Calculus, bile duct
  cystic duct - *see* Calculus, gallbladder

Colic - *continued*
  Devonshire NEC - *see* Poisoning, lead
  gallbladder - *see* Calculus, gallbladder
  gallstone - *see* Calculus, gallbladder
    gallbladder or cystic duct - *see* Calculus,
    gallbladder
  hepatic (duct) - *see* Calculus, bile duct
  hysterical F45.8
  kidney N23
  lead NEC - *see* Poisoning, lead
  mucous K58.9
    with diarrhea K58.0
    psychogenic F54
  nephritic N23
  painter's NEC - *see* Poisoning, lead
  pancreas K86.89
  psychogenic F45.8
  renal N23
  saturnine NEC - *see* Poisoning, lead
  ureter N23
  urethral N36.8
    due to calculus N21.1
  uterus NEC N94.89
    menstrual - *see* Dysmenorrhea
  worm NOS B83.9
Colicystitis - *see* Cystitis
Colitis (acute) (catarrhal) (chronic)
    (noninfective) (hemorrhagic) - *see also*
    Enteritis K52.9
  allergic K52.29
    with
      food protein-induced enterocolitis
        syndrome K52.21
      proctocolitis K52.82
  amebic (acute) - *see also* Amebiasis A06.0
    nondysenteric A06.2
  anthrax A22.2
  bacillary - *see* Infection, Shigella
  balantidial A07.0
  Clostridium difficile
    not specified as recurrent A04.72
    recurrent A04.71
  coccidial A07.3
  collagenous K52.831
  cystica superficialis K52.89
  dietary counseling and surveillance (for) Z71.3
  dietetic - *see also* Colitis, allergic K52.29
  drug-induced K52.1
  due to radiation K52.0
  eosinophilic K52.82
  food hypersensitivity - *see also* Colitis, allergic
    K52.29
  giardial A07.1
  granulomatous - *see* Enteritis, regional, large
    intestine
  indeterminate, so stated K52.3
  infectious - *see* Enteritis, infectious
  ischemic K55.9
    acute (subacute) - *see also* Ischemia,
      intestine, acute K55.039
    chronic K55.1
    due to mesenteric artery insufficiency K55.1
    fulminant (acute) - *see also* Ischemia,
  intestine, acute K55.039
  left sided K51.50
    with
      abscess K51.514
      complication K51.519
        specified NEC K51.518
      fistula K51.513
      obstruction K51.512
      rectal bleeding K51.511
  lymphocytic K52.832
  membranous

Colitis - *continued*
    psychogenic F54
  microscopic K52.839
    specified NEC K52.838
  mucous - *see* Syndrome, irritable, bowel
    psychogenic F54
  noninfective K52.9
    specified NEC K52.89
  polyposa - *see* Polyp, colon, inflammatory
  protozoal A07.9
  pseudomembranous
    not specified as recurrent A04.72
    recurrent A04.71
  pseudomucinous - *see* Syndrome, irritable,
    bowel
  regional - *see* Enteritis, regional, large
    intestine
    infectious A09
  segmental - *see* Enteritis, regional, large
    intestine
  septic - *see* Enteritis, infectious
  spastic K58.9
    with diarrhea K58.0
    psychogenic F54
  staphylococcal A04.8
    foodborne A05.0
  subacute ischemic - *see also* Ischemia,
    intestine, acute K55.039
  thromboulcerative - *see also* Ischemia,
    intestine, acute K55.039
  toxic NEC K52.1
    due to Clostridium difficile
      not specified as recurrent A04.72
      recurrent A04.71
  transmural - *see* Enteritis, regional, large
    intestine
  trichomonal A07.8
  tuberculous (ulcerative) A18.32
  ulcerative (chronic) K51.90
    with
      complication K51.919
        abscess K51.914
        fistula K51.913
        obstruction K51.912
        rectal bleeding K51.911
        specified complication NEC K51.918
    enterocolitis - *see* Enterocolitis, ulcerative
    ileocolitis - *see* Ileocolitis, ulcerative
    mucosal proctocolitis - *see* Proctocolitis,
      mucosal
    proctitis - *see* Proctitis, ulcerative
    pseudopolyposis - *see* Polyp, colon,
  inflammatory
    psychogenic F54
    rectosigmoiditis - *see* Rectosigmoiditis,
  ulcerative
    specified type NEC K51.80
      with
        complication K51.819
          abscess K51.814
          fistula K51.813
          obstruction K51.812
          rectal bleeding K51.811
          specified complication NEC K51.818
Collagenosis, collagen disease (nonvascular)
    (vascular) M35.9
  cardiovascular I42.8
  reactive perforating L87.1
  specified NEC M35.8
Collapse R55
  adrenal E27.2
  cardiorespiratory R57.0
  cardiovascular R57.0
    newborn P29.89

Collapse - *continued*
  circulatory (peripheral) R57.9
    during or after labor and delivery O75.1
    following ectopic or molar pregnancy O08.3
    newborn P29.89
  during or
    after labor and delivery O75.1
    resulting from a procedure, not elsewhere
    classified T81.10
  external ear canal - *see* Stenosis, external ear
  canal
  general R55
  heart - *see* Disease, heart
  heat T67.1
  hysterical F44.89
  labyrinth, membranous (congenital) Q16.5
  lung (massive) - *see also* Atelectasis J98.19
    pressure due to anesthesia (general) (local) or
  other sedation T88.2
      during labor and delivery O74.1
      in pregnancy O29.02-
      postpartum, puerperal O89.09
  myocardial - *see* Disease, heart
  nervous F48.8
  neurocirculatory F45.8
  nose M95.0
  postoperative T81.10
  pulmonary - *see also* Atelectasis J98.19
    newborn - *see* Atelectasis
  trachea J39.8
  tracheobronchial J98.09
  valvular - *see* Endocarditis
  vascular (peripheral) R57.9
    during or after labor and delivery O75.1
    following ectopic or molar pregnancy O08.3
    newborn P29.89
  vertebra M48.50-
    cervical region M48.52-
    cervicothoracic region M48.53-
    in (due to)
      metastasis - *see* Collapse, vertebra, in,
        specified disease NEC
      osteoporosis - *see also* Osteoporosis
        M80.88
        cervical region M80.88
        cervicothoracic region M80.88
        lumbar region M80.88
        lumbosacral region M80.88
        multiple sites M80.88
        occipito-atlanto-axial region M80.88
        sacrococcygeal region M80.88
        thoracic region M80.88
        thoracolumbar region M80.88
      specified disease NEC M48.50-
        cervical region M48.52-
        cervicothoracic region M48.53-
        lumbar region M48.56-
        lumbosacral region M48.57-
        occipito-atlanto-axial region M48.51-
        sacrococcygeal region M48.58-
        thoracic region M48.54-
        thoracolumbar region M48.55-
    lumbar region M48.56-
    lumbosacral region M48.57-
    occipito-atlanto-axial region M48.51-
    sacrococcygeal region M48.58-
    thoracic region M48.54-
    thoracolumbar region M48.55-
Collateral - *see also* condition
  circulation (venous) I87.8
  dilation, veins I87.8
Colles' fracture S52.53-
Collet (-Sicard) syndrome G52.7
Collier's asthma or lung J60

Collodion baby Q80.2
Colloid nodule (of thyroid) (cystic) E04.1
Coloboma (iris) Q13.0
　eyelid Q10.3
　fundus Q14.8
　lens Q12.2
　optic disc (congenital) Q14.2
　　acquired H47.31-
Coloenteritis - see Enteritis
Colon - see condition
Colonization
　MRSA (Methicillin resistant Staphylococcus
　　aureus) Z22.322
　MSSA (Methicillin susceptible
　　Staphylococcus aureus) Z22.321
　status - see Carrier (suspected) of
Coloptosis K63.4
Color blindness - see Deficiency, color vision
Colostomy
　attention to Z43.3
　fitting or adjustment Z46.89
　malfunctioning K94.03
　status Z93.3
Colpitis (acute) - see Vaginitis
Colpocele N81.5
Colpocystitis - see Vaginitis
Colpospasm N94.2
Column, spinal, vertebral - see condition
Coma R40.20
　with
　　motor response (none) R40.231
　　　abnormal R40.233
　　　abnormal extensor posturing to pain or
　　　　noxious stimuli (< 2 years of age)
　　　　R40.232
　　　abnormal flexure posturing to pain or
　　　　noxious stimuli (0-5 years of age)
　　　　R40.233
　　　extension R40.232
　　　extensor posturing to pain or noxious
　　　　stimuli (2 5 years of age) R40.232
　　　flexion withdrawal R40.234
　　　flexion/decorticate posturing (< 2 years of
　　　　age) R40.233
　　　localizes pain (2 5 years of age) R40.235
　　　normal or spontaneous movement (< 2
　　　　years of age) R40.236
　　　obeys commands (2 5 years of age)
　　　　R40.236
　　　withdraws from pain or noxious stimuli (0-
　　　　5 years of age) R40.234
　　　withdraws to touch (< 2 years of age)
　　　　R40.235
　　opening of eyes (never) R40.211
　　　in response to
　　　　pain R40.212
　　　　sound R40.213
　　　spontaneous R40.214
　　verbal response (none) R40.221
　　　cooing or babbling or crying appropriately
　　　　(< 2 years of age) R40.225
　　　inappropriate crying or screaming (< 2
　　　　years of age) R40.223
　　　confused conversation R40.224
　　　inappropriate words (2 5 years of age)
　　　　R40.224
　　　incomprehensible words R40.222
　　　oriented R40.225
　　　incomprehensible sounds (2 5 years of age)
　　　　R40.222
　　　irritable cries (< 2 years of age) R40.224
　　　moans/grunts to pain; restless (< 2 years
　　　　old) R40.222
　　　screaming (2 5 years of age) R40.223

Coma - continued
　　uses appropriate words (2 5 years of age)
　　　R40.225
　eclamptic - see Eclampsia
　epileptic - see Epilepsy
　Glasgow, scale score - see Glasgow coma
　　scale
　hepatic - see Failure, hepatic, by type, with
　　coma
　hyperglycemic (diabetic) - see Diabetes, by
　　type, with hyperosmolarity, with coma
　hyperosmolar (diabetic) - see Diabetes, by
　　type, with hyperosmolarity, with coma
　hypoglycemic (diabetic) - see Diabetes, by
　　type, with hypoglycemia, with coma
　　nondiabetic E15
　in diabetes - see Diabetes, coma
　insulin-induced - see Coma, hypoglycemic
　ketoacidotic (diabetic) - see Diabetes, by type,
　　with ketoacidosis, with coma
　myxedematous E03.5
　newborn P91.5
　persistent vegetative state R40.3
　specified NEC, without documented Glasgow
　　coma scale score, or with partial Glasgow
　　coma scale score reported R40.244
Comatose - see Coma
Combat fatigue F43.0
Combined - see condition
Comedo, comedones (giant) L70.0
Comedocarcinoma - see also Neoplasm,
　breast, malignant
　noninfiltrating
　　breast D05.8-
　　specified site - see Neoplasm, in situ, by site
　　unspecified site D05.8-
Comedomastitis - see Ectasia, mammary duct
Comminuted fracture   code as Fracture,
　closed Common
　arterial trunk Q20.0
　atrioventricular canal Q21.2
　atrium Q21.1
　cold (head) J00
　truncus (arteriosus) Q20.0
　variable immunodeficiency - see
　　Immunodeficiency, common variable
　ventricle Q20.4
Commotio, commotion (current)
　brain - see Injury, intracranial, concussion
　cerebri - see Injury, intracranial, concussion
　retinae S05.8X-
　spinal cord - see Injury, spinal cord, by region
　spinalis - see Injury, spinal cord, by region
Communication
　between
　　base of aorta and pulmonary artery Q21.4
　　left ventricle and right atrium Q20.5
　　pericardial sac and pleural sac Q34.8
　　pulmonary artery and pulmonary vein,
　　　congenital Q25.72
　congenital between uterus and digestive or
　　urinary tract Q51.7
Compartment syndrome (deep) (posterior)
　(traumatic) T79.A0
　abdomen T79.A3
　lower extremity (hip, buttock, thigh, leg, foot,
　　toes) T79.A2
　nontraumatic
　　abdomen M79.A3
　　lower extremity (hip, buttock, thigh, leg,
　　　foot, toes) M79.A2-
　　specified site NEC M79.A9
　　upper extremity (shoulder, arm, forearm,
　　　wrist, hand, fingers) M79.A1-

Compartment syndrome - continued
　specified site NEC T79.A9
　upper extremity (shoulder, arm, forearm, wrist,
　　hand, fingers) T79.A1
Compensation
　failure - see Disease, heart
　neurosis, psychoneurosis - see Disorder,
　　factitious
Complaint - see also Disease
　bowel, functional K59.9
　　psychogenic F45.8
　intestine, functional K59.9
　　psychogenic F45.8
　kidney - see Disease, renal
　miners' J60
Complete - see condition
Complex
　Addison-Schilder E71.528
　cardiorenal - see Hypertension, cardiorenal
　Costen's M26.69
　disseminated mycobacterium avium
　　intracellulare (DMAC) A31.2
　Eisenmenger's (ventricular septal defect)
　　I27.83
　hypersexual F52.8
　jumped process, spine - see Dislocation,
　　vertebra
　primary, tuberculous A15.7
　Schilder-Addison E71.528
　subluxation (vertebral) M99.19
　　abdomen M99.19
　　acromioclavicular M99.17
　　cervical region M99.11
　　cervicothoracic M99.11
　　costochondral M99.18
　　costovertebral M99.18
　　head region M99.10
　　hip M99.15
　　lower extremity M99.16
　　lumbar region M99.13
　　lumbosacral M99.13
　　occipitocervical M99.10
　　pelvic region M99.15
　　pubic M99.15
　　rib cage M99.18
　　sacral region M99.14
　　sacrococcygeal M99.14
　　sacroiliac M99.14
　　specified NEC M99.19
　　sternochondral M99.18
　　sternoclavicular M99.17
　　thoracic region M99.12
　　thoracolumbar M99.12
　　upper extremity M99.17
　Taussig-bing (transposition, aorta and
　　overriding pulmonary artery) Q20.1
Complication(s) (from) (of)
　accidental puncture or laceration during a
　　procedure (of) - see Complications,
　　intraoperative (intraprocedural), puncture or
　　laceration
　amputation stump (surgical) (late) NEC T87.9
　　dehiscence T87.81
　　infection or inflammation T87.40
　　　lower limb T87.4-
　　　upper limb T87.4-
　　necrosis T87.50
　　　lower limb T87.5-
　　　upper limb T87.5-
　　neuroma T87.30
　　　lower limb T87.3-
　　　upper limb T87.3-
　　specified type NEC T87.89
　anastomosis (and bypass) - see also

Complication(s) (from) (of) - *continued*
  Complications, prosthetic device or implant
    intestinal (internal) NEC K91.89
      involving urinary tract N99.89
    urinary tract (involving intestinal tract)
      N99.89
    vascular - *see* Complications, cardiovascular
      device or implant
  anesthesia, anesthetic - *see also* Anesthesia,
    complication T88.59
  brain, postpartum, puerperal O89.2
  cardiac
    in
      labor and delivery O74.2
      pregnancy O29.19-
    postpartum, puerperal O89.1
  central nervous system
    in
      labor and delivery O74.3
      pregnancy O29.29-
    postpartum, puerperal O89.2
  difficult or failed intubation T88.4
    in pregnancy O29.6-
  failed sedation (conscious) (moderate) during
    procedure T88.52
  general, unintended awareness during
    procedure T88.53
  hyperthermia, malignant T88.3
  hypothermia T88.51
  intubation failure T88.4
  malignant hyperthermia T88.3
  pulmonary
    in
      labor and delivery O74.1
      pregnancy NEC O29.09-
    postpartum, puerperal O89.09
  shock T88.2
  spinal and epidural
    in
      labor and delivery NEC O74.6
        headache O74.5
      pregnancy NEC O29.5X-
    postpartum, puerperal NEC O89.5
      headache O89.4
  unintended awareness under general
    anesthesia during procedure T88.53
anti-reflux device - *see* Complications,
  esophageal anti-reflux device
aortic (bifurcation) graft - *see* Complications,
  graft, vascular
aortocoronary (bypass) graft - *see*
  Complications, coronary artery (bypass) graft
aortofemoral (bypass) graft - *see*
  Complications, extremity artery (bypass)
  graft
arteriovenous
  fistula, surgically created T82.9
    embolism T82.818
    fibrosis T82.828
    hemorrhage T82.838
    infection or inflammation T82.7
    mechanical
      breakdown T82.510
      displacement T82.520
      leakage T82.530
      malposition T82.520
      obstruction T82.590
      perforation T82.590
      protrusion T82.590
    pain T82.848
    specified type NEC T82.898
    stenosis T82.858
    thrombosis T82.868
  shunt, surgically created T82.9

Complication(s) (from) (of) - *continued*
    embolism T82.818
    fibrosis T82.828
    hemorrhage T82.838
    infection or inflammation T82.7
    mechanical
      breakdown T82.511
      displacement T82.521
      leakage T82.531
      malposition T82.521
      obstruction T82.591
      perforation T82.591
      protrusion T82.591
    pain T82.848
    specified type NEC T82.898
    stenosis T82.858
    thrombosis T82.868
  arthroplasty - *see* Complications, joint
prosthesis
  artificial
    fertilization or insemination N98.9
      attempted introduction (of)
        embryo in embryo transfer N98.3
        ovum following in vitro fertilization
          N98.2
      hyperstimulation of ovaries N98.1
      infection N98.0
      specified NEC N98.8
    heart T82.9
      embolism T82.817
      fibrosis T82.827
      hemorrhage T82.837
      infection or inflammation T82.7
      mechanical
        breakdown T82.512
        displacement T82.522
        leakage T82.532
        malposition T82.522
        obstruction T82.592
        perforation T82.592
        protrusion T82.592
      pain T82.847
      specified type NEC T82.897
      stenosis T82.857
      thrombosis T82.867
    opening
      cecostomy - *see* Complications, colostomy
      colostomy - *see* Complications, colostomy
      cystostomy - *see* Complications,
        cystostomy
      enterostomy - *see* Complications,
        enterostomy
      gastrostomy - *see* Complications,
        gastrostomy
      ileostomy - *see* Complications, enterostomy
      jejunostomy - *see* Complications,
        enterostomy
      nephrostomy - *see* Complications, stoma,
        urinary tract
      tracheostomy - *see* Complications,
        tracheostomy
      ureterostomy - *see* Complications, stoma,
        urinary tract
      urethrostomy - *see* Complications, stoma,
        urinary tract
  balloon implant or device
    gastrointestinal T85.9
      embolism T85.818
      fibrosis T85.828
      hemorrhage T85.838
      infection and inflammation T85.79
      pain T85.848
      specified type NEC T85.898
      stenosis T85.858

Complication(s) (from) (of) - *continued*
    thrombosis T85.868
  vascular (counterpulsation) T82.9
    embolism T82.818
    fibrosis T82.828
    hemorrhage T82.838
    infection or inflammation T82.7
    mechanical
      breakdown T82.513
      displacement T82.523
      leakage T82.533
      malposition T82.523
      obstruction T82.593
      perforation T82.593
      protrusion T82.593
    pain T82.848
    specified type NEC T82.898
    stenosis T82.858
    thrombosis T82.868
bariatric procedure
  gastric band procedure K95.09
    infection K95.01
  specified procedure NEC K95.89
    infection K95.81
bile duct implant (prosthetic) T85.9
  embolism T85.818
  fibrosis T85.828
  hemorrhage T85.838
  infection and inflammation T85.79
  mechanical
    breakdown T85.510
    displacement T85.520
    malfunction T85.510
    malposition T85.520
    obstruction T85.590
    perforation T85.590
    protrusion T85.590
    specified NEC T85.590
  pain T85.848
  specified type NEC T85.898
  stenosis T85.858
  thrombosis T85.868
bladder device (auxiliary) - *see* Complications,
  genitourinary, device or implant, urinary
  system
bleeding (postoperative) - *see* Complication,
  postoperative, hemorrhage
  intraoperative - *see* Complication,
    intraoperative, hemorrhage
blood vessel graft - *see* Complications, graft,
  vascular
bone
  device NEC T84.9
    embolism T84.81
    fibrosis T84.82
    hemorrhage T84.83
    infection or inflammation T84.7
    mechanical
      breakdown T84.318
      displacement T84.328
      malposition T84.328
      obstruction T84.398
      perforation T84.398
      protrusion T84.398
    pain T84.84
    specified type NEC T84.89
    stenosis T84.85
    thrombosis T84.86
  graft - *see* Complications, graft, bone
  growth stimulator (electrode) - *see*
    Complications, electronic stimulator device,
    bone
  marrow transplant - *see* Complications,
    transplant, bone, marrow

Complication(s) (from) (of) - *continued*
 brain neurostimulator (electrode) - *see*
  Complications, electronic stimulator device,
  brain
 breast implant (prosthetic) T85.9
  capsular contracture T85.44
  embolism T85.818
  fibrosis T85.828
  hemorrhage T85.838
  infection and inflammation T85.79
  mechanical
   breakdown T85.41
   displacement T85.42
   leakage T85.43
   malposition T85.42
   obstruction T85.49
   perforation T85.49
   protrusion T85.49
   specified NEC T85.49
  pain T85.848
  specified type NEC T85.898
  stenosis T85.858
  thrombosis T85.868
 bypass - *see also* Complications, prosthetic
 device or implant
  aortocoronary - *see* Complications, coronary
   artery (bypass) graft
  arterial - *see also* Complications, graft,
   vascular
  extremity - *see* Complications, extremity
   artery (bypass) graft
 cardiac - *see also* Disease, heart
  device, implant or graft T82.9
   embolism T82.817
   fibrosis T82.827
   hemorrhage T82.837
   infection or inflammation T82.7
    valve prosthesis T82.6
   mechanical
    breakdown T82.519
     specified device NEC T82.518
    displacement T82.529
     specified device NEC T82.528
    leakage T82.539
     specified device NEC T82.538
    malposition T82.529
     specified device NEC T82.528
    obstruction T82.599
     specified device NEC T82.598
    perforation T82.599
     specified device NEC T82.598
    protrusion T82.599
     specified device NEC T82.598
   pain T82.847
   specified type NEC T82.897
   stenosis T82.857
   thrombosis T82.867
 cardiovascular device, graft or implant T82.9
  aortic graft - *see* Complications, graft,
   vascular
  arteriovenous
   fistula, artificial - *see* Complication,
    arteriovenous, fistula, surgically created
   shunt - *see* Complication, arteriovenous,
    shunt, surgically created
  artificial heart - *see* Complication, artificial,
   heart
  balloon (counterpulsation) device - *see*
   Complication, balloon implant, vascular
  carotid artery graft - *see* Complications, graft,
   vascular
  coronary bypass graft - *see* Complication,
   coronary artery (bypass) graft
  dialysis catheter (vascular) - *see*

Complication(s) (from) (of) - *continued*
 Complication, catheter, dialysis
 electronic T82.9
  electrode T82.9
   embolism T82.817
   fibrosis T82.827
   hemorrhage T82.837
   infection T82.7
   mechanical
    breakdown T82.110
    displacement T82.120
    leakage T82.190
    obstruction T82.190
    perforation T82.190
    protrusion T82.190
    specified type NEC T82.190
   pain T82.847
   specified NEC T82.897
   stenosis T82.857
   thrombosis T82.867
  embolism T82.817
  fibrosis T82.827
  hemorrhage T82.837
  infection T82.7
  mechanical
   breakdown T82.119
   displacement T82.129
   leakage T82.199
   obstruction T82.199
   perforation T82.199
   protrusion T82.199
   specified type NEC T82.199
  pain T82.847
  pulse generator T82.9
   embolism T82.817
   fibrosis T82.827
   hemorrhage T82.837
   infection T82.7
   mechanical
    breakdown T82.111
    displacement T82.121
    leakage T82.191
    obstruction T82.191
    perforation T82.191
    protrusion T82.191
    specified type NEC T82.191
   pain T82.847
   specified NEC T82.897
   stenosis T82.857
   thrombosis T82.867
  specified condition NEC T82.897
  specified device NEC T82.9
   embolism T82.817
   fibrosis T82.827
   hemorrhage T82.837
   infection T82.7
   mechanical
    breakdown T82.118
    displacement T82.128
    leakage T82.198
    obstruction T82.198
    perforation T82.198
    protrusion T82.198
    specified type NEC T82.198
   pain T82.847
   specified NEC T82.897
   stenosis T82.857
   thrombosis T82.867
  stenosis T82.857
  thrombosis T82.867
 extremity artery graft - *see* Complication,
  extremity artery (bypass) graft
 femoral artery graft - *see* Complication,
  extremity artery (bypass) graft

Complication(s) (from) (of) - *continued*
 heart-lung transplant - *see* Complication,
  transplant, heart, with lung
 heart
  transplant - *see* Complication, transplant,
   heart
  valve - *see* Complication, prosthetic device,
   heart valve
   graft - *see* Complication, heart, valve,
    graft
  infection or inflammation T82.7
  umbrella device - *see* Complication, umbrella
   device, vascular
  vascular graft (or anastomosis) - *see*
   Complication, graft, vascular
 carotid artery (bypass) graft - *see*
  Complications, graft, vascular
 catheter (device) NEC - *see also*
 Complications, prosthetic device or implant
  cranial infusion
   infection and inflammation T85.735
   mechanical
    breakdown T85.610
    displacement T85.620
    leakage T85.630
    malfunction T85.690
    malposition T85.620
    obstruction T85.690
    perforation T85.690
    protrusion T85.690
    specified NEC T85.690
  cystostomy T83.9
   embolism T83.81
   fibrosis T83.82
   hemorrhage T83.83
   infection and inflammation T83.510
   mechanical
    breakdown T83.010
    displacement T83.020
    leakage T83.030
    malposition T83.020
    obstruction T83.090
    perforation T83.090
    protrusion T83.090
    specified NEC T83.090
   pain T83.84
   specified type NEC T83.89
   stenosis T83.85
   thrombosis T83.86
  dialysis (vascular) T82.9
   embolism T82.818
   fibrosis T82.828
   hemorrhage T82.838
   infection and inflammation T82.7
   intraperitoneal - *see* Complications,
    catheter, intraperitoneal
   mechanical
    breakdown T82.41
    displacement T82.42
    leakage T82.43
    malposition T82.42
    obstruction T82.49
    perforation T82.49
    protrusion T82.49
   pain T82.848
   specified type NEC T82.898
   stenosis T82.858
   thrombosis T82.868
  epidural infusion T85.9
   embolism T85.810
   fibrosis T85.820
   hemorrhage T85.830
   infection and inflammation T85.735
   mechanical

Complication(s) (from) (of) - *continued*
   breakdown T85.610
      displacement T85.620
      leakage T85.630
      malfunction T85.610
      malposition T85.620
      obstruction T85.690
      perforation T85.690
      protrusion T85.690
      specified NEC T85.690
   pain T85.840
   specified type NEC T85.890
   stenosis T85.850
   thrombosis T85.860
   intraperitoneal dialysis T85.9
      embolism T85.818
      fibrosis T85.828
      hemorrhage T85.838
      infection and inflammation T85.71
      mechanical
         breakdown T85.611
         displacement T85.621
         leakage T85.631
         malfunction T85.611
         malposition T85.621
         obstruction T85.691
         perforation T85.691
         protrusion T85.691
         specified NEC T85.691
      pain T85.848
      specified type NEC T85.898
      stenosis T85.858
      thrombosis T85.868
   intrathecal infusion
      infection and inflammation T85.735
      mechanical
         breakdown T85.610
         displacement T85.620
         leakage T85.630
         malfunction T85.690
         malposition T85.620
         obstruction T85.690
         perforation T85.690
         protrusion T85.690
         specified NEC T85.690
   intravenous infusion T82.9
      embolism T82.818
      fibrosis T82.828
      hemorrhage T82.838
      infection or inflammation T82.7
      mechanical
         breakdown T82.514
         displacement T82.524
         leakage T82.534
         malposition T82.524
         obstruction T82.594
         perforation T82.594
         protrusion T82.594
      pain T82.848
      specified type NEC T82.898
      stenosis T82.858
      thrombosis T82.868
   spinal infusion
      infection and inflammation T85.735
      mechanical
         breakdown T85.610
         displacement T85.620
         leakage T85.630
         malfunction T85.690
         malposition T85.620
         obstruction T85.690
         perforation T85.690
         protrusion T85.690
         specified NEC T85.690

Complication(s) (from) (of) - *continued*
   subarachnoid infusion
      infection and inflammation T85.735-
      mechanical
         breakdown T85.610
         displacement T85.620
         leakage T85.630
         malfunction T85.690
         malposition T85.620
         obstruction T85.690
         perforation T85.690
         protrusion T85.690
         specified NEC T85.690
   subdural infusion T85.9
      embolism T85.810
      fibrosis T85.820
      hemorrhage T85.830
      infection and inflammation T85.735
      mechanical
         breakdown T85.610
         displacement T85.620
         leakage T85.630
         malfunction T85.610
         malposition T85.620
         obstruction T85.690
         perforation T85.690
         protrusion T85.690
         specified NEC T85.690
      pain T85.840
      specified type NEC T85.890
      stenosis T85.850
      thrombosis T85.860
   urethral T83.9
      displacement T83.028
      embolism T83.81
      fibrosis T83.82
      hemorrhage T83.83
      indwelling
         breakdown T83.011
         displacement T83.021
         infection and inflammation T83.511
         leakage T83.031
         specified complication NEC T83.091
      infection and inflammation T83.511
      leakage T83.038
      malposition T83.028
      mechanical
         breakdown T83.011
      obstruction (mechanical) T83.091
      pain T83.84
      perforation T83.091
      protrusion T83.091
      specified type NEC T83.091
      stenosis T83.85
      thrombosis T83.86
   urinary NEC
      breakdown T83.018
      displacement T83.028
      infection and inflammation T83.518
      leakage T83.038
      specified complication NEC T83.098
   cecostomy (stoma) - *see* Complications,
   colostomy
   cesarean delivery wound NEC O90.89
      disruption O90.0
      hematoma O90.2
      infection (following delivery) O86.0
   chemotherapy (antineoplastic) NEC T88.7
   chin implant (prosthetic) - *see* Complication,
   prosthetic device or implant, specified NEC
   circulatory system I99.8
      intraoperative I97.88
      postprocedural I97.89
         following cardiac surgery (see also Infarct,

Complication(s) (from) (of) - *continued*
   myocardium, associated with revascularization
   procedure) I97.19-
         postcardiotomy syndrome I97.0
      hypertension I97.3
      lymphedema after mastectomy I97.2
      postcardiotomy syndrome I97.0
      specified NEC I97.89
   colostomy (stoma) K94.00
      hemorrhage K94.01
      infection K94.02
      malfunction K94.03
      mechanical K94.03
      specified complication NEC K94.09
   contraceptive device, intrauterine - *see*
      Complications, intrauterine, contraceptive
      device
   cord (umbilical) - *see* Complications,
      umbilical cord
   corneal graft - *see* Complications, graft, cornea
   coronary artery (bypass) graft T82.9
      atherosclerosis - *see* Arteriosclerosis,
      coronary (artery), embolism T82.818
      fibrosis T82.828
      hemorrhage T82.838
      infection and inflammation T82.7
      mechanical
         breakdown T82.211
         displacement T82.212
         leakage T82.213
         malposition T82.212
         obstruction T82.218
         perforation T82.218
         protrusion T82.218
         specified NEC T82.218
      pain T82.848
      specified type NEC T82.898
      stenosis T82.858
      thrombosis T82.868
   counterpulsation device (balloon), intra aortic
      - *see* Complications, balloon implant,
      vascular
   cystostomy (stoma) N99.518
      catheter - *see* Complications, catheter,
         cystostomy
      hemorrhage N99.510
      infection N99.511
      malfunction N99.512
      specified type NEC N99.518
   delivery - *see also* Complications, obstetric
      O75.9
      procedure (instrumental) (manual) (surgical)
         O75.4
      specified NEC O75.89
   dialysis (peritoneal) (renal) - *see also*
      Complications, infusion
      catheter (vascular) - *see* Complication,
         catheter, dialysis
      peritoneal, intraperitoneal - *see*
         Complications, catheter, intraperitoneal
   dorsal column (spinal) neurostimulator - *see*
      Complications, electronic stimulator device,
      spinal cord
   drug NEC T88.7
   ear procedure - *see also* Disorder, ear
      intraoperative H95.88
      hematoma - *see* Complications,
         intraoperative, hemorrhage (hematoma)
         (of), ear
      hemorrhage - *see* Complications,
         intraoperative, hemorrhage (hematoma)
         (of), ear
      laceration - *see* Complications,
         intraoperative, puncture or laceration...,

Complication(s) (from) (of) - *continued*
ear
  specified NEC H95.88
postoperative H95.89
  external ear canal stenosis H95.81-
  hematoma - *see* Complications,
    postprocedural, hematoma (of), ear
  hemorrhage - *see* Complications,
    postprocedural, hemorrhage (of), ear
  postmastoidectomy - *see* Complications,
    postmastoidectomy
  seroma - *see* Complications,
    postprocedural, seroma (of), mastoid
    process
  specified NEC H95.89
ectopic pregnancy O08.9
  damage to pelvic organs O08.6
  embolism O08.2
  genital infection O08.0
  hemorrhage (delayed) (excessive) O08.1
  metabolic disorder O08.5
  renal failure O08.4
  shock O08.3
  specified type NEC O08.0
  venous complication NEC O08.7
electronic stimulator device
  bladder (urinary) - *see* Complications,
    electronic stimulator device, urinary
  bone T84.9
    breakdown T84.310
    displacement T84.320
    embolism T84.81
    fibrosis T84.82
    hemorrhage T84.83
    infection or inflammation T84.7
    malfunction T84.310
    malposition T84.320
    mechanical NEC T84.390
    obstruction T84.390
    pain T84.84
    perforation T84.390
    protrusion T84.390
    specified type NEC T84.89
    stenosis T84.85
    thrombosis T84.86
  brain T85.9
    embolism T85.810
    fibrosis T85.820
    hemorrhage T85.830
    infection and inflammation T85.731
    mechanical
      breakdown T85.110
      displacement T85.120
      leakage T85.190
      malposition T85.120
      obstruction T85.190
      perforation T85.190
      protrusion T85.190
      specified NEC T85.190
    pain T85.840
    specified type NEC T85.890
    stenosis T85.850
    thrombosis T85.860
  cardiac (defibrillator) (pacemaker) - *see*
  Complications, cardiovascular device or
  implant, electronic
  generator (brain) (gastric) (peripheral)
  (sacral) (spinal)
    breakdown T85.113
    displacement T85.123
    leakage T85.193
    malposition T85.123
    obstruction T85.193
    perforation T85.193

Complication(s) (from) (of) - *continued*
    protrusion T85.193
    specified type NEC T85.193
  muscle T84.9
    breakdown T84.418
    displacement T84.428
    embolism T84.81
    fibrosis T84.82
    hemorrhage T84.83
    infection or inflammation T84.7
    mechanical NEC T84.498
    pain T84.84
    specified type NEC T84.89
    stenosis T84.85
    thrombosis T84.86
  nervous system T85.9
    brain - *see* Complications, electronic
      stimulator device, brain
    cranial nerve - *see* Complications,
      electronic stimulator device, peripheral
      nerve
    embolism T85.810
    fibrosis T85.820
    gastric nerve - *see* Complications,
      electronic stimulator device, peripheral
      nerve
    hemorrhage T85.830
    infection and inflammation T85.738
    mechanical
      breakdown T85.118
      displacement T85.128
      leakage T85.199
      malposition T85.128
      obstruction T85.199
      perforation T85.199
      protrusion T85.199
      specified NEC T85.199
    pain T85.840
    peripheral nerve - *see* Complications,
      electronic stimulator device, peripheral
      nerve
    sacral nerve - *see* Complications, electronic
      stimulator device, peripheral nerve
    specified type NEC T85.890
    spinal cord - *see* Complications, electronic
      stimulator device, spinal cord
    stenosis T85.850
    thrombosis T85.860
    vagal nerve - *see* Complications, electronic
      stimulator device, peripheral nerve
  peripheral nerve T85.9
    embolism T85.810
    fibrosis T85.820
    hemorrhage T85.830
    infection and inflammation T85.732
    mechanical
      breakdown T85.111
      displacement T85.121
      leakage T85.191
      malposition T85.121
      obstruction T85.191
      perforation T85.191
      protrusion T85.191
      specified NEC T85.191
    pain T85.840
    specified type NEC T85.890
    stenosis T85.850
    thrombosis T85.860
  spinal cord T85.9
    embolism T85.810
    fibrosis T85.820
    hemorrhage T85.830
    infection and inflammation T85.733
    mechanical

Complication(s) (from) (of) - *continued*
    breakdown T85.112
    displacement T85.122
    leakage T85.192
    malposition T85.122
    obstruction T85.192
    perforation T85.192
    protrusion T85.192
    specified NEC T85.192
    pain T85.840
    specified type NEC T85.890
    stenosis T85.850
    thrombosis T85.860
  urinary T83.9
    embolism T83.81
    fibrosis T83.82
    hemorrhage T83.83
    infection and inflammation T83.598
    mechanical
      breakdown T83.110
      displacement T83.120
      malposition T83.120
      perforation T83.190
      protrusion T83.190
      specified NEC T83.190
    pain T83.84
    specified type NEC T83.89
    stenosis T83.85
    thrombosis T83.86
electroshock therapy T88.9
  specified NEC T88.8
endocrine E34.9
  postprocedural
    adrenal hypofunction E89.6
    hypoinsulinemia E89.1
    hypoparathyroidism E89.2
    hypopituitarism E89.3
    hypothyroidism E89.0
    ovarian failure E89.40
      asymptomatic E89.40
      symptomatic E89.41
    specified NEC E89.89
    testicular hypofunction E89.5
endodontic treatment NEC M27.59
enterostomy (stoma) K94.10
  hemorrhage K94.11
  infection K94.12
  malfunction K94.13
  mechanical K94.13
  specified complication NEC K94.19
episiotomy, disruption O90.1
esophageal anti-reflux device T85.9
  embolism T85.818
  fibrosis T85.828
  hemorrhage T85.838
  infection and inflammation T85.79
  mechanical
    breakdown T85.511
    displacement T85.521
    malfunction T85.511
    malposition T85.521
    obstruction T85.591
    perforation T85.591
    protrusion T85.591
    specified NEC T85.591
  pain T85.848
  specified type NEC T85.898
  stenosis T85.858
  thrombosis T85.868
esophagostomy K94.30
  hemorrhage K94.31
  infection K94.32
  malfunction K94.33
  mechanical K94.33

Complication(s) (from) (of) - *continued*
  specified complication NEC K94.39
  extracorporeal circulation T80.90
  extremity artery (bypass) graft T82.9
    arteriosclerosis - *see* Arteriosclerosis,
      extremities, bypass graft
    embolism T82.818
    fibrosis T82.828
    hemorrhage T82.838
    infection and inflammation T82.7
    mechanical
      breakdown T82.318
        femoral artery T82.312
      displacement T82.328
        femoral artery T82.322
      leakage T82.338
        femoral artery T82.332
      malposition T82.328
        femoral artery T82.322
      obstruction T82.398
        femoral artery T82.392
      perforation T82.398
        femoral artery T82.392
      protrusion T82.398
        femoral artery T82.392
    pain T82.848
    specified type NEC T82.898
    stenosis T82.858
    thrombosis T82.868
  eye H57.9
  corneal graft - *see* Complications, graft,
    cornea
    implant (prosthetic) T85.9
      embolism T85.818
      fibrosis T85.828
      hemorrhage T85.838
      infection and inflammation T85.79
      mechanical
        breakdown T85.318
        displacement T85.328
        leakage T85.398
        malposition T85.328
        obstruction T85.398
        perforation T85.398
        protrusion T85.398
        specified NEC T85.398
      pain T85.848
      specified type NEC T85.898
      stenosis T85.858
      thrombosis T85.868
    intraocular lens - *see* Complications,
      intraocular lens
    orbital prosthesis - *see* Complications, orbital
      prosthesis
  female genital N94.9
  device, implant or graft NEC - *see*
    Complications, genitourinary, device or
    implant, genital tract
  femoral artery (bypass) graft - *see*
    Complication, extremity artery (bypass) graft
  fixation device, internal (orthopedic) T84.9
    infection and inflammation T84.60
      arm T84.61-
        humerus T84.61-
        radius T84.61-
        ulna T84.61-
      leg T84.629
        femur T84.62-
        fibula T84.62-
        tibia T84.62-
      specified site NEC T84.69
      spine T84.63
    mechanical
      breakdown

Complication(s) (from) (of) - *continued*
    limb T84.119
      carpal T84.210
      femur T84.11-
      fibula T84.11-
      humerus T84.11-
      metacarpal T84.210
      metatarsal T84.213
      phalanx
        foot T84.213
        hand T84.210
      radius T84.11-
      tarsal T84.213
      tibia T84.11-
      ulna T84.11-
    specified bone NEC T84.218
    spine T84.216
    displacement
      limb T84.129
      carpal T84.220
      femur T84.12-
      fibula T84.12-
      humerus T84.12-
      metacarpal T84.220
      metatarsal T84.223
      phalanx
        foot T84.223
        hand T84.220
      radius T84.12-
      tarsal T84.223
      tibia T84.12-
      ulna T84.12-
    specified bone NEC T84.228
    spine T84.226
    malposition - *see* Complications, fixation
      device, internal, mechanical, displacement
    obstruction - *see* Complications, fixation
      device, internal, mechanical, specified
      type NEC
    perforation - *see* Complications, fixation
      device, internal, mechanical, specified
      type NEC
    protrusion - *see* Complications, fixation
      device, internal, mechanical, specified
      type NEC
    specified type NEC
      limb T84.199
      carpal T84.290
      femur T84.19-
      fibula T84.19-
      humerus T84.19-
      metacarpal T84.290
      metatarsal T84.293
      phalanx
        foot T84.293
        hand T84.290
      radius T84.19-
      tarsal T84.293
      tibia T84.19-
      ulna T84.19-
    specified bone NEC T84.298
    vertebra T84.296
  specified type NEC T84.89
    embolism T84.81
    fibrosis T84.82
    hemorrhage T84.83
    pain T84.84
    specified complication NEC T84.89
    stenosis T84.85
    thrombosis T84.86
  following
    acute myocardial infarction NEC I23.8
    aneurysm (false) (of cardiac wall) (of heart
      wall) (ruptured) I23.3

Complication(s) (from) (of) - *continued*
    angina I23.7
    atrial
      septal defect I23.1
      thrombosis I23.6
    cardiac wall rupture I23.3
    chordae tendinae rupture I23.4
    defect
      septal
        atrial (heart) I23.1
        ventricular (heart) I23.2
    hemopericardium I23.0
    papillary muscle rupture I23.5
    rupture
      cardiac wall I23.3
        with hemopericardium I23.0
      chordae tendineae I23.4
      papillary muscle I23.5
    specified NEC I23.8
    thrombosis
      atrium I23.6
      auricular appendage I23.6
      ventricle (heart) I23.6
    ventricular
      septal defect I23.2
      thrombosis I23.6
  ectopic or molar pregnancy O08.9
    cardiac arrest O08.81
    sepsis O08.82
    specified type NEC O08.89
    urinary tract infection O08.83
  termination of pregnancy - *see* Abortion
  gastrointestinal K92.9
    bile duct prosthesis - *see* Complications, bile
      duct implant
    esophageal anti-reflux device - *see*
      Complications, esophageal anti-reflux
      device
    postoperative
      colostomy - *see* Complications, colostomy
      dumping syndrome K91.1
      enterostomy - *see* Complications,
        enterostomy
      gastrostomy - *see* Complications,
        gastrostomy
      malabsorption NEC K91.2
      obstruction (see also Obstruction, intestine,
      postoperative) K91.30
      postcholecystectomy syndrome K91.5
      specified NEC K91.89
      vomiting after GI surgery K91.0
    prosthetic device or implant
      bile duct prosthesis - *see* Complications,
        bile duct implant
      esophageal anti-reflux device - *see*
        Complications, esophageal anti-reflux
        device
      specified type NEC
        embolism T85.818
        fibrosis T85.828
        hemorrhage T85.838
        mechanical
          breakdown T85.518
          displacement T85.528
          malfunction T85.518
          malposition T85.528
          obstruction T85.598
          perforation T85.598
          protrusion T85.598
          specified NEC T85.598
        pain T85.848
        specified complication NEC T85.898
        stenosis T85.858
        thrombosis T85.868

Complication(s) (from) (of) - *continued*

gastrostomy (stoma) K94.20
- hemorrhage K94.21
- infection K94.22
- malfunction K94.23
- mechanical K94.23
- specified complication NEC K94.29

genitourinary
- device or implant T83.9
  - genital tract T83.9
    - infection or inflammation T83.69
    - intrauterine contraceptive device - *see* Complications, intrauterine, contraceptive device
    - mechanical - *see* Complications, by device, mechanical
    - mesh - *see* Complications, mesh
    - penile prosthesis - *see* Complications, prosthetic device, penile
    - specified type NEC T83.89
      - embolism T83.81
      - fibrosis T83.82
      - hemorrhage T83.83
      - pain T83.84
      - specified complication NEC T83.89
      - stenosis T83.85
      - thrombosis T83.86
    - vaginal mesh - *see* Complications, mesh
  - urinary system T83.9
    - cystostomy catheter - *see* Complication, catheter, cystostomy
    - electronic stimulator - *see* Complications, electronic stimulator device, urinary
    - indwelling urethral catheter - *see* Complications, catheter, urethral, indwelling
    - infection or inflammation T83.598
      - indwelling urethral catheter T83.511
    - kidney transplant - *see* Complication, transplant, kidney
    - organ graft - *see* Complication, graft, urinary organ
    - specified type NEC T83.89
      - embolism T83.81
      - fibrosis T83.82
      - hemorrhage T83.83
      - mechanical T83.198
        - breakdown T83.118
        - displacement T83.128
        - malfunction T83.118
        - malposition T83.128
        - obstruction T83.198
        - perforation T83.198
        - protrusion T83.198
        - specified NEC T83.198
      - sphincter, implanted T83.191
      - stent (ileal conduit) (nephroureteral) T83.193
        - ureteral indwelling T83.192
      - pain T83.84
      - specified complication NEC T83.89
      - stenosis T83.85
      - thrombosis T83.86
    - sphincter implant - *see* Complications, implant, urinary sphincter
  - postprocedural
    - pelvic peritoneal adhesions N99.4
    - renal failure N99.0
    - specified NEC N99.89
    - stoma - *see* Complications, stoma, urinary tract
    - urethral stricture - *see* Stricture, urethra, postprocedural
  - vaginal

Complication(s) (from) (of) - *continued*

- adhesions N99.2
- vault prolapse N99.3

graft (bypass) (patch) - *see also* Complications, prosthetic device or implant
- aorta - *see* Complications, graft, vascular
- arterial - *see* Complication, graft, vascular
- bone T86.839
  - failure T86.831
  - infection T86.832
  - mechanical T84.318
    - breakdown T84.318
    - displacement T84.328
    - protrusion T84.398
    - specified type NEC T84.398
  - rejection T86.830
  - specified type NEC T86.838
- carotid artery - *see* Complications, graft, vascular
- cornea T86.849
  - failure T86.841
  - infection T86.842
  - mechanical T85.398
    - breakdown T85.318
    - displacement T85.328
    - protrusion T85.398
    - specified type NEC T85.398
  - rejection T86.840
  - retroprosthetic membrane T85.398
  - specified type NEC T86.848
- femoral artery (bypass) - *see* Complication, extremity artery (bypass) graft
- genital organ or tract - *see* Complications, genitourinary, device or implant, genital tract
- muscle T84.9
  - breakdown T84.410
  - displacement T84.420
  - embolism T84.81
  - fibrosis T84.82
  - hemorrhage T84.83
  - infection and inflammation T84.7
  - mechanical NEC T84.490
  - pain T84.84
  - specified type NEC T84.89
  - stenosis T84.85
  - thrombosis T84.86
- nerve - *see* Complication, prosthetic device or implant, specified NEC
- skin - *see* Complications, prosthetic device or implant, skin graft
- tendon T84.9
  - breakdown T84.410
  - displacement T84.420
  - embolism T84.81
  - fibrosis T84.82
  - hemorrhage T84.83
  - infection and inflammation T84.7
  - mechanical NEC T84.490
  - pain T84.84
  - specified type NEC T84.89
  - stenosis T84.85
  - thrombosis T84.86
- urinary organ T83.9
  - embolism T83.81
  - fibrosis T83.82
  - hemorrhage T83.83
  - infection and inflammation T83.598
    - indwelling urethral catheter T83.511
  - mechanical
    - breakdown T83.21
    - displacement T83.22
    - erosion T83.24
    - exposure T83.25

Complication(s) (from) (of) - *continued*

- leakage T83.23
- malposition T83.22
- obstruction T83.29
- perforation T83.29
- protrusion T83.29
- specified NEC T83.29
- pain T83.84
- specified type NEC T83.89
- stenosis T83.85
- thrombosis T83.86

vascular T82.9
- embolism T82.818
- femoral artery - *see* Complication, extremity artery (bypass) graft
- fibrosis T82.828
- hemorrhage T82.838
- mechanical
  - breakdown T82.319
    - aorta (bifurcation) T82.310
    - carotid artery T82.311
    - specified vessel NEC T82.318
  - displacement T82.329
    - aorta (bifurcation) T82.320
    - carotid artery T82.321
    - specified vessel NEC T82.328
  - leakage T82.339
    - aorta (bifurcation) T82.330
    - carotid artery T82.331
    - specified vessel NEC T82.338
  - malposition T82.329
    - aorta (bifurcation) T82.320
    - carotid artery T82.321
    - specified vessel NEC T82.328
  - obstruction T82.399
    - aorta (bifurcation) T82.390
    - carotid artery T82.391
    - specified vessel NEC T82.398
  - perforation T82.399
    - aorta (bifurcation) T82.390
    - carotid artery T82.391
    - specified vessel NEC T82.398
  - protrusion T82.399
    - aorta (bifurcation) T82.390
    - carotid artery T82.391
    - specified vessel NEC T82.398
- pain T82.848
- specified complication NEC T82.898
- stenosis T82.858
- thrombosis T82.868

heart I51.9
- assist device
  - infection and inflammation T82.7
- following acute myocardial infarction - *see* Complications, following, acute myocardial infarction
- postoperative - *see* Complications, circulatory system
- transplant - *see* Complication, transplant, heart
- and lung(s) - *see* Complications, transplant, heart, with lung
- valve
  - graft (biological) T82.9
    - embolism T82.817
    - fibrosis T82.827
    - hemorrhage T82.837
    - infection and inflammation T82.7
    - mechanical T82.228
      - breakdown T82.221
      - displacement T82.222
      - leakage T82.223
      - malposition T82.222
      - obstruction T82.228

Complication(s) (from) (of) - *continued*

    perforation T82.228
    protrusion T82.228
    pain T82.847
    specified type NEC T82.897
    stenosis T82.857
    thrombosis T82.867
  prosthesis T82.9
    embolism T82.817
    fibrosis T82.827
    hemorrhage T82.837
    infection or inflammation T82.6
    mechanical T82.09
      breakdown T82.01
      displacement T82.02
      leakage T82.03
      malposition T82.02
      obstruction T82.09
      perforation T82.09
      protrusion T82.09
    pain T82.847
    specified type NEC T82.897
      mechanical T82.09
    stenosis T82.857
    thrombosis T82.867
  hematoma
    intraoperative - *see* Complication,
      intraoperative, hemorrhage
    postprocedural - *see* Complication,
      postprocedural, hematoma
  hemodialysis - *see* Complications, dialysis
  hemorrhage
    intraoperative - *see* Complication,
      intraoperative, hemorrhage
    postprocedural - *see* Complication,
      postprocedural, hemorrhage
  ileostomy (stoma) - *see* Complications,
    enterostomy
  immunization (procedure) - *see* Complications,
    vaccination
  implant - *see also* Complications, by site and
  type
    urinary sphincter T83.9
      embolism T83.81
      fibrosis T83.82
      hemorrhage T83.83
      infection and inflammation T83.591
      mechanical
        breakdown T83.111
        displacement T83.121
        leakage T83.191
        malposition T83.121
        obstruction T83.191
        perforation T83.191
        protrusion T83.191
        specified NEC T83.191
      pain T83.84
      specified type NEC T83.89
      stenosis T83.85
      thrombosis T83.86
  infusion (procedure) T80.90
    air embolism T80.0
    blood - *see* Complications, transfusion
    catheter - *see* Complications, catheter
    infection T80.29
    pump - *see* Complications, cardiovascular,
      device or implant
    sepsis T80.29
    serum reaction - *see also* Reaction, serum
    T80.69
      anaphylactic shock - *see also* Shock,
      anaphylactic T80.59
    specified type NEC T80.89
  inhalation therapy NEC T81.81

Complication(s) (from) (of) - *continued*

  injection (procedure) T80.90
    drug reaction - *see* Reaction, drug
    infection T80.29
    sepsis T80.29
    serum (prophylactic) (therapeutic) - *see*
      Complications, vaccination
    specified type NEC T80.89
    vaccine (any) - *see* Complications,
      vaccination
  inoculation (any) - *see* Complications,
    vaccination
  insulin pump
    infection and inflammation T85.72
    mechanical
      breakdown T85.614
      displacement T85.624
      leakage T85.633
      malposition T85.624
      obstruction T85.694
      perforation T85.694
      protrusion T85.694
      specified NEC T85.694
  intestinal pouch NEC K91.858
  intraocular lens (prosthetic) T85.9
    embolism T85.818
    fibrosis T85.828
    hemorrhage T85.838
    infection and inflammation T85.79
    mechanical
      breakdown T85.21
      displacement T85.22
      malposition T85.22
      obstruction T85.29
      perforation T85.29
      protrusion T85.29
      specified NEC T85.29
    pain T85.848
    specified type NEC T85.898
    stenosis T85.858
    thrombosis T85.868
  intraoperative (intraprocedural)
    cardiac arrest *see also* Infarct, myocardium,
  associated with revascularization procedure
      during cardiac surgery I97.710
      during other surgery I97.711
    cardiac functional disturbance NEC *see also*
      Infarct, myocardium, associated with
      revascularization procedure
      during cardiac surgery I97.790
      during other surgery I97.791
    hemorrhage (hematoma) (of)
      circulatory system organ or structure
        during cardiac bypass I97.411
        during cardiac catheterization I97.410
        during other circulatory system procedure
         I97.418
        during other procedure I97.42
      digestive system organ
        during procedure on digestive system
         K91.61
        during procedure on other organ K91.62
      ear
        during procedure on ear and mastoid
         process H95.21
        during procedure on other organ H95.22
      endocrine system organ or structure
        during procedure on endocrine system
         organ or structure E36.01
        during procedure on other organ E36.02
      eye and adnexa
        during ophthalmic procedure H59.11-
        during other procedure H59.12-
      genitourinary organ or structure

Complication(s) (from) (of) - *continued*

    during procedure on genitourinary organ
      or structure N99.61
    during procedure on other organ N99.62
    mastoid process
      during procedure on ear and mastoid
        process H95.21
      during procedure on other organ H95.22
    musculoskeletal structure
      during musculoskeletal surgery M96.810
      during non-orthopedic surgery M96.811
      during orthopedic surgery M96.810
    nervous system
      during a nervous system procedure
        G97.31
      during other procedure G97.32
    respiratory system
      during other procedure J95.62
      during procedure on respiratory system
        organ or structure J95.61
    skin and subcutaneous tissue
      during a dermatologic procedure L76.01
      during a procedure on other organ L76.02
    spleen
      during a procedure on other organ D78.02
      during a procedure on the spleen D78.01
  puncture or laceration (accidental)
  (unintentional) (of)
    brain
      during a nervous system procedure
        G97.48
      during other procedure G97.49
    circulatory system organ or structure
      during circulatory system procedure
        I97.51
      during other procedure I97.52
    digestive system
      during procedure on digestive system
        K91.71
      during procedure on other organ K91.72
    ear
      during procedure on ear and mastoid
        process H95.31
      during procedure on other organ H95.32
    endocrine system organ or structure
      during procedure on endocrine system
        organ or structure E36.11
      during procedure on other organ E36.12
    eye and adnexa
      during ophthalmic procedure H59.21-
      during other procedure H59.22-
    genitourinary organ or structure
      during procedure on genitourinary organ
        or structure N99.71
      during procedure on other organ N99.72
    mastoid process
      during procedure on ear and mastoid
        process H95.31
      during procedure on other organ H95.32
    musculoskeletal structure
      during musculoskeletal surgery M96.820
      during non-orthopedic surgery M96.821
      during orthopedic surgery M96.820
    nervous system
      during a nervous system procedure
        G97.48
      during other procedure G97.49
    respiratory system
      during other procedure J95.72
      during procedure on respiratory system
        organ or structure J95.71
    skin and subcutaneous tissue
      during a dermatologic procedure L76.11
      during a procedure on other organ L76.12

spleen
during a procedure on other organ D78.12
during a procedure on the spleen D78.11
specified NEC
circulatory system I97.88
digestive system K91.81
ear H95.88
endocrine system E36.8
eye and adnexa H59.88
genitourinary system N99.81
mastoid process H95.88
musculoskeletal structure M96.89
nervous system G97.81
respiratory system J95.88
skin and subcutaneous tissue L76.81
spleen D78.81
intraperitoneal catheter (dialysis) (infusion) -
see Complications, catheter, intraperitoneal
intrathecal infusion pump
infection and inflammation T85.738
mechanical
breakdown T85.615
displacement T85.625
leakage T85.635
malfunction T85.695
malposition T85.625
obstruction T85.695
perforation T85.695
protrusion T85.695
specified NEC T85.695
intrauterine
contraceptive device
embolism T83.81
fibrosis T83.82
hemorrhage T83.83
infection and inflammation T83.69
mechanical
breakdown T83.31
displacement T83.32
malposition T83.32
obstruction T83.39
perforation T83.39
protrusion T83.39
specified NEC T83.39
pain T83.84
specified type NEC T83.89
stenosis T83.85
thrombosis T83.86
procedure (fetal), to newborn P96.5
jejunostomy (stoma) - *see* Complications,
enterostomy
joint prosthesis, internal T84.9
breakage (fracture) T84.01-
dislocation T84.02-
fracture T84.01-
infection or inflammation T84.50
hip T84.5-
knee T84.5-
specified joint NEC T84.59
instability T84.02-
malposition - *see* Complications, joint
prosthesis, mechanical, displacement
mechanical
breakage, broken T84.01-
dislocation T84.02-
fracture T84.01-
instability T84.02-
leakage - *see* Complications, joint
prosthesis, mechanical, specified NEC
loosening T84.039
hip T84.03-
knee T84.03-
specified joint NEC T84.038

obstruction - *see* Complications, joint
prosthesis, mechanical, specified NEC
perforation - *see* Complications, joint
prosthesis, mechanical, specified NEC
osteolysis T84.059
hip T84.05-
knee T84.05-
other specified joint T84.058
protrusion - *see* Complications, joint
prosthesis, mechanical, specified NEC
specified complication NEC T84.099
hip T84.09-
knee T84.09-
other specified joint T84.098
subluxation T84.02-
wear of articular bearing surface T84.069
hip T84.06-
knee T84.06-
other specified joint T84.068
specified joint NEC T84.89
embolism T84.81
fibrosis T84.82
hemorrhage T84.83
pain T84.84
specified complication NEC T84.89
stenosis T84.85
thrombosis T84.86
subluxation T84.02-
kidney transplant - *see* Complications,
transplant, kidney   labor O75.9
specified NEC O75.89
liver transplant (immune or nonimmune) - *see*
Complications, transplant, liver
lumbar puncture G97.1
cerebrospinal fluid leak G97.0
headache or reaction G97.1
lung transplant - *see* Complications, transplant,
lung
and heart - *see* Complications, transplant,
lung, with heart
male genital N50.9
device, implant or graft - *see* Complications,
genitourinary, device or implant, genital
tract
postprocedural or postoperative - *see*
Complications, genitourinary, postprocedural
specified NEC N99.89
mastoid (process) procedure
intraoperative H95.88
hematoma - *see* Complications,
intraoperative, hemorrhage (hematoma)
(of), mastoid process
hemorrhage - *see* Complications,
intraoperative, hemorrhage (hematoma)
(of), mastoid process
laceration - *see* Complications,
intraoperative, puncture or laceration...,
mastoid process
specified NEC H95.88
postmastoidectomy - *see* Complications,
postmastoidectomy
postoperative H95.89
external ear canal stenosis H95.81-
hematoma - *see* Complications...,
postprocedural, hematoma (of), mastoid
process
hemorrhage - *see* Complications...,
postprocedural, hemorrhage (of), mastoid
process
postmastoidectomy - *see* Complications,
postmastoidectomy
seroma - *see* Complications,
postprocedural, seroma (of), mastoid

process
specified NEC H95.89
mastoidectomy cavity - *see* Complications,
postmastoidectomy
mechanical - *see* Complications, by site and
type, mechanical
medical procedures - *see also* Complication(s),
intraoperative T88.9
metabolic E88.9
postoperative E89.89
specified NEC E89.89
molar pregnancy NOS O08.9
damage to pelvic organs O08.6
embolism O08.2
genital infection O08.0
hemorrhage (delayed) (excessive) O08.1
metabolic disorder O08.5
renal failure O08.4
shock O08.3
specified type NEC O08.0
venous complication NEC O08.7
musculoskeletal system - *see also*
Complication, intraoperative (intraprocedural),
by site
device, implant or graft NEC - *see*
Complications, orthopedic, device or
implant
internal fixation (nail) (plate) (rod) - *see*
Complications, fixation device, internal
joint prosthesis - *see* Complications, joint
prosthesis
postoperative (postprocedural) M96.89
with osteoporosis - *see* Osteoporosis
fracture following insertion of device - *see*
Fracture, following insertion of orthopedic
implant, joint prosthesis or bone plate
joint instability after prosthesis removal
M96.89
lordosis M96.4
postlaminectomy syndrome NEC M96.1
kyphosis M96.3
pseudarthrosis M96.0
specified complication NEC M96.89
post radiation M96.89
kyphosis M96.2
scoliosis M96.5
specified complication NEC M96.89
nephrostomy (stoma) - *see* Complications,
stoma, urinary tract, external NEC
nervous system G98.8
central G96.9
device, implant or graft - *see also*
Complication, prosthetic device or implant,
specified NEC
electronic stimulator (electrode(s)) - *see*
Complications, electronic stimulator device
specified NEC
infection and inflammation T85.738
mechanical T85.695
breakdown T85.615
displacement T85.625
leakage T85.635
malfunction T85.695
malposition T85.625
obstruction T85.695
perforation T85.695
protrusion T85.695
specified NEC T85.695
ventricular shunt - *see* Complications,
ventricular shunt
electronic stimulator (electrode(s)) - *see*
Complications, electronic stimulator device
postprocedural G97.82

Complication(s) (from) (of) - *continued*
  intracranial hypotension G97.2
    specified NEC G97.82
    spinal fluid leak G97.0
  newborn, due to intrauterine (fetal) procedure P96.5
  nonabsorbable (permanent) sutures - *see* Complication, sutures, permanent
  obstetric O75.9
    procedure (instrumental) (manual) (surgical)
      specified NEC O75.4
    specified NEC O75.89
    surgical wound NEC O90.89
      hematoma O90.2
      infection O86.0
  ocular lens implant - *see* Complications, intraocular lens
  ophthalmologic
    postprocedural bleb - *see* Blebitis
  orbital prosthesis T85.9
    embolism T85.818
    fibrosis T85.828
    hemorrhage T85.838
    infection and inflammation T85.79
    mechanical
      breakdown T85.31-
      displacement T85.32-
      malposition T85.32-
      obstruction T85.39-
      perforation T85.39-
      protrusion T85.39-
      specified NEC T85.39-
    pain T85.848
    specified type NEC T85.898
    stenosis T85.858
    thrombosis T85.868
  organ or tissue transplant (partial) (total) - *see* Complications, transplant
  orthopedic - *see also* Disorder, soft tissue
    device or implant T84.9
      bone
        device or implant - *see* Complication, bone, device NEC
        graft - *see* Complication, graft, bone
      breakdown T84.418
      displacement T84.428
      electronic bone stimulator - *see* Complications, electronic stimulator device, bone
      embolism T84.81
      fibrosis T84.82
      fixation device - *see* Complication, fixation device, internal
      hemorrhage T84.83
      infection or inflammation T84.7
      joint prosthesis - *see* Complication, joint prosthesis, internal
      malfunction T84.418
      malposition T84.428
      mechanical NEC T84.498
      muscle graft - *see* Complications, graft, muscle
      obstruction T84.498
      pain T84.84
      perforation T84.498
      protrusion T84.498
      specified complication NEC T84.89
      stenosis T84.85
      tendon graft - *see* Complications, graft, tendon
      thrombosis T84.86
    fracture (following insertion of device) - *see* Fracture, following insertion of orthopedic implant, joint prosthesis or bone plate

Complication(s) (from) (of) - *continued*
  postprocedural M96.89
    fracture - *see* Fracture, following insertion of orthopedic implant, joint prosthesis or bone plate
    postlaminectomy syndrome NEC M96.1
      kyphosis M96.3
      lordosis M96.4
    postradiation
      kyphosis M96.2
      scoliosis M96.5
    pseudarthrosis post-fusion M96.0
    specified type NEC M96.89
  pacemaker (cardiac) - *see* Complications, cardiovascular device or implant, electronic
  pancreas transplant - *see* Complications, transplant, pancreas
  penile prosthesis (implant) - *see* Complications, prosthetic device, penile
  perfusion NEC T80.90
  perineal repair (obstetrical) NEC O90.89
    disruption O90.1
    hematoma O90.2
    infection (following delivery) O86.0
  phototherapy T88.9
    specified NEC T88.8
  postmastoidectomy NEC H95.19-
    cyst, mucosal H95.13-
    granulation H95.12-
    inflammation, chronic H95.11-
    recurrent cholesteatoma H95.0-
  postoperative - *see* Complications, postprocedural
    circulatory - *see* Complications, circulatory system
    ear - *see* Complications, ear
    endocrine - *see* Complications, endocrine
    eye - *see* Complications, eye
    lumbar puncture G97.1
      cerebrospinal fluid leak G97.0
    nervous system (central) (peripheral) - *see* Complications, nervous system
    respiratory system - *see* Complications, respiratory system
  postprocedural - *see also* Complications, surgical procedure
    cardiac arrest *see also* Infarct, myocardium, associated with revascularization procedure
      following cardiac surgery I97.120
      following other surgery I97.121
    cardiac functional disturbance NEC *see* also Infarct, myocardium, associated with revascularization procedure
      following cardiac surgery I97.190
      following other surgery I97.191
    cardiac insufficiency
      following cardiac surgery I97.110
      following other surgery I97.111
    chorioretinal scars following retinal surgery H59.81-
    following cataract surgery
      cataract (lens) fragments H59.02-
      cystoid macular edema H59.03-
      specified NEC H59.09-
      vitreous (touch) syndrome H59.01-
    heart failure
      following cardiac surgery I97.130
      following other surgery I97.131
    hematoma (of)
      circulatory system organ or structure
        following cardiac bypass I97.631
        following cardiac catheterization I97.630
        following other circulatory system

Complication(s) (from) (of) - *continued*
        procedure I97.638
        following other procedure I97.621
      digestive system
        following procedure on digestive system K91.870
        following procedure on other organ K91.871
      ear
        following other procedure H95.52
        following procedure on ear and mastoid process H95.51
      endocrine system
        following endocrine system procedure E89.820
        following other procedure E89.821
      eye and adnexa
        following ophthalmic procedure H59.33-
        following other procedure H59.34-
      genitourinary organ or structure
        following procedure on genitourinary organ or structure N99.840
        following procedure on other organ N99.841
      mastoid process
        following other procedure H95.52
        following procedure on ear and mastoid process H95.51
      musculoskeletal structure
        following musculoskeletal surgery M96.840
        following non-orthopedic surgery M96.841
        following orthopedic surgery M96.840
      nervous system
        following nervous system procedure G97.61
        following other procedure G97.62
      respiratory system
        following other procedure J95.861
        following procedure on respiratory system organ or structure J95.860
      skin and subcutaneous tissue
        following dermatologic procedure L76.31
        following procedure on other organ L76.32
      spleen
        following procedure on other organ D78.32
        following procedure on the spleen D78.31
    hemorrhage (of)
      circulatory system organ or structure
        following cardiac bypass I97.611
        following cardiac catheterization I97.610
        following other circulatory system procedure I97.618
        following other procedure I97.620
      digestive system
        following procedure on digestive system K91.840
        following procedure on other organ K91.841
      ear
        following other procedure H95.42
        following procedure on ear and mastoid process H95.41
      endocrine system
        following endocrine system procedure E89.810
        following other procedure E89.811
      eye and adnexa
        following ophthalmic procedure H59.31-
        following other procedure H59.32-
      genitourinary organ or structure

Complication(s) (from) (of) - *continued*
  following procedure on genitourinary
    organ or structure N99.820
  following procedure on other organ
    N99.821
  mastoid process
    following other procedure H95.42
    following procedure on ear and mastoid
      process H95.41
  musculoskeletal structure
    following musculoskeletal surgery
      M96.830
    following non-orthopedic surgery
      M96.831
    following orthopedic surgery M96.830
  nervous system
    following nervous system procedure
      G97.51
    following other procedure G97.52
  respiratory system
    following other procedure J95.831
    following procedure on respiratory system
      organ or structure J95.830
  skin and subcutaneous tissue
    following dermatologic procedure L76.21
    following a procedure on other organ
      L76.22
  spleen
    following procedure on other organ
      D78.22
    following procedure on the spleen D78.21
  seroma (of)
    circulatory system organ or structure
      following cardiac bypass I97.641
      following cardiac catheterization I97.640
      following other circulatory system
        procedure I97.648
      following other procedure I97.622
    digestive system
      following procedure on digestive system
        K91.872
      following procedure on other organ
        K91.873
    ear
      following other procedure H95.54
      following procedure on ear and mastoid
        process H95.53
    endocrine system
      following endocrine system procedure
        E89.822
      following other procedure E89.823
    eye and adnexa
      following ophthalmic procedure H59.35-
      following other procedure H59.36-
    genitourinary organ or structure
      following procedure on genitourinary
        organ or structure N99.842
      following procedure on other organ
        N99.843
    mastoid process
      following other procedure H95.54
      following procedure on ear and mastoid
        process H95.53
    musculoskeletal structure
      following musculoskeletal surgery
        M96.842
      following non-orthopedic surgery
        M96.843
      following orthopedic surgery M96.842
    nervous system
      following nervous system procedure
        G97.63
      following other procedure G97.64
    respiratory system

Complication(s) (from) (of) - *continued*
    following other procedure J95.863
    following procedure on respiratory system
      organ or structure J95.862
  skin and subcutaneous tissue
    following dermatologic procedure L76.33
    following procedure on other organ
      L76.34
  spleen
    following procedure on other organ
      D78.34
    following procedure on the spleen D78.33
  specified NEC
    circulatory system I97.89
    digestive K91.89
    ear H95.89
    endocrine E89.89
    eye and adnexa H59.89
    genitourinary N99.89
    mastoid process H95.89
    metabolic E89.89
    musculoskeletal structure M96.89
    nervous system G97.82
    respiratory system J95.89
    skin and subcutaneous tissue L76.82
    spleen D78.89
  pregnancy NEC - *see* Pregnancy, complicated
    by
  prosthetic device or implant T85.9
    bile duct - *see* Complications, bile duct
      implant
    breast - *see* Complications, breast implant
    bulking agent
      ureteral
        erosion T83.714
        exposure T83.724
      urethral
        erosion T83.713
        exposure T83.723
    cardiac and vascular NEC - *see*
      Complications, cardiovascular device or
      implant
    corneal transplant - *see* Complications, graft,
      cornea
    electronic nervous system stimulator - *see*
      Complications, electronic stimulator device
    epidural infusion catheter - *see*
      Complications, catheter, epidural
    esophageal anti-reflux device - *see*
      Complications, esophageal anti-reflux
      device
    genital organ or tract - *see* Complications,
      genitourinary, device or implant, genital
      tract
      specified NEC T83.79
    heart valve - *see* Complications, heart, valve,
      prosthesis
    infection or inflammation T85.79
      intestine transplant T86.892
      liver transplant T86.43
      lung transplant T86.812
      pancreas transplant T86.892
      skin graft T86.822
    intraocular lens - *see* Complications,
      intraocular lens
    intraperitoneal (dialysis) catheter - *see*
      Complications, catheter, intraperitoneal
    joint - *see* Complications, joint prosthesis,
      internal
    mechanical NEC T85.698
      dialysis catheter (vascular) - *see also*
        Complication, catheter, dialysis, mechanical
        peritoneal - *see* Complication, catheter,
        intraperitoneal, mechanical

Complication(s) (from) (of) - *continued*
    gastrointestinal device T85.598
    ocular device T85.398
    subdural (infusion) catheter T85.690
    suture, permanent T85.692
      that for bone repair - *see* Complications,
        fixation device, internal (orthopedic),
        mechanical
    ventricular shunt
      breakdown T85.01
      displacement T85.02
      leakage T85.03
      malposition T85.02
      obstruction T85.09
      perforation T85.09
      protrusion T85.09
      specified NEC T85.09
  mesh
    erosion (to surrounding organ or tissue)
      T83.718
      urethral (into pelvic floor muscles)
        T83.712
      vaginal (into pelvic floor muscles)
        T83.711
    exposure (into surrounding organ or tissue)
      T83.728
      urethral (through urethral wall) T83.722
      vaginal (into vagina) (through vaginal
        wall) T83.721
  orbital - *see* Complications, orbital prosthesis
  penile T83.9
    embolism T83.81
    fibrosis T83.82
    hemorrhage T83.83
    infection and inflammation T83.61
    mechanical
      breakdown T83.410
      displacement T83.420
      leakage T83.490
      malposition T83.420
      obstruction T83.490
      perforation T83.490
      protrusion T83.490
      specified NEC T83.490
    pain T83.84
    specified type NEC T83.89
    stenosis T83.85
    thrombosis T83.86
  prosthetic materials NEC
    erosion (to surrounding organ or tissue)
      T83.718
    exposure (into surrounding organ or tissue)
      T83.728
  skin graft T86.829
    artificial skin or decellularized allodermis
      embolism T85.818
      fibrosis T85.828
      hemorrhage T85.838
      infection and inflammation T85.79
      mechanical
        breakdown T85.613
        displacement T85.623
        malfunction T85.613
        malposition T85.623
        obstruction T85.693
        perforation T85.693
        protrusion T85.693
        specified NEC T85.693
      pain T85.848
      specified type NEC T85.898
      stenosis T85.858
      thrombosis T85.868
    failure T86.821
    infection T86.822

Complication(s) (from) (of) - *continued*
  rejection T86.820
  specified NEC T86.828
  sling
    urethral (female) (male)
      erosion T83.712
      exposure T83.722
  specified NEC T85.9
    embolism T85.818
    fibrosis T85.828
    hemorrhage T85.838
    infection and inflammation T85.79
    mechanical
      breakdown T85.618
      displacement T85.628
      leakage T85.638
      malfunction T85.618
      malposition T85.628
      obstruction T85.698
      perforation T85.698
      protrusion T85.698
      specified NEC T85.698
    pain T85.848
    specified type NEC T85.898
    stenosis T85.858
    thrombosis T85.868
  subdural infusion catheter - *see*
    Complications, catheter, subdural
  sutures - *see* Complications, sutures
  urinary organ or tract NEC - *see*
    Complications, genitourinary, device or
    implant, urinary system
  vascular - *see* Complications, cardiovascular
    device or implant
  ventricular shunt - *see* Complications,
    ventricular shunt (device)
  puerperium - *see* Puerperal
  puncture, spinal G97.1
    cerebrospinal fluid leak G97.0
    headache or reaction G97.1
  pyelogram N99.89
  radiation
    kyphosis M96.2
    scoliosis M96.5
  reattached
    extremity (infection) (rejection)
      lower T87.1X-
      upper T87.0X-
    specified body part NEC T87.2
  reconstructed breast
    asymmetry between native and reconstructed
      breast N65.1
    deformity N65.0
    disproportion between native and
      reconstructed breast N65.1
    excess tissue N65.0
    misshapen N65.0
  reimplant NEC - *see also* Complications,
    prosthetic device or implant
    limb (infection) (rejection) - *see*
      Complications, reattached, extremity
    organ (partial) (total) - *see* Complications,
      transplant
    prosthetic device NEC - *see* Complications,
      prosthetic device
  renal N28.9
    allograft - *see* Complications, transplant,
      kidney
    dialysis - *see* Complications, dialysis
  respirator
    mechanical J95.850
      specified NEC J95.859
  respiratory system J98.9
    device, implant or graft - *see* Complication,

Complication(s) (from) (of) - *continued*
    prosthetic device or implant, specified NEC
  lung transplant - *see* Complications,
    prosthetic device or implant, lung transplant
  postoperative J95.89
    air leak J95.812
    Mendelson's syndrome (chemical
      pneumonitis) J95.4
    pneumothorax J95.811
    pulmonary insufficiency (acute) (after
      nonthoracic surgery) J95.2
      chronic J95.3
      following thoracic surgery J95.1
    respiratory failure (acute) J95.821
      acute and chronic J95.822
    specified NEC J95.89
    subglottic stenosis J95.5
    tracheostomy complication - *see*
      Complications, tracheostomy
  therapy T81.89
  sedation during labor and delivery O74.9
    cardiac O74.2
    central nervous system O74.3
    pulmonary NEC O74.1
  shunt - *see also* Complications, prosthetic
    device or implant
    arteriovenous - *see* Complications,
      arteriovenous, shunt
    ventricular (communicating) - *see*
      Complications, ventricular shunt
  skin
    graft T86.829
      failure T86.821
      infection T86.822
      rejection T86.820
      specified type NEC T86.828
  spinal
    anesthesia - *see* Complications, anesthesia,
      spinal
    catheter (epidural) (subdural) - *see*
      Complications, catheter
    puncture or tap G97.1
      cerebrospinal fluid leak G97.0
      headache or reaction G97.1
  stent
    bile duct - *see* Complications, bile duct
      prosthesis
    ureteral indwelling
      breakdown T83.112
      displacement T83.122
      leakage T83.192
      malposition T83.122
      obstruction T83.192
      perforation T83.192
      protrusion T83.192
      specified NEC T83.192
    urinary NEC (ileal conduit) (nephroureteral)
      T83.193
      embolism T83.81
      fibrosis T83.82
      hemorrhage T83.83
      infection and inflammation T83.593
      mechanical
        breakdown T83.113
        displacement T83.123
        leakage T83.193
        malposition T83.123
        obstruction T83.193
        perforation T83.193
        protrusion T83.193
        specified NEC T83.193
      pain T83.84
      specified type NEC T83.89
      stenosis T83.85

Complication(s) (from) (of) - *continued*
    thrombosis T83.86
  vascular
    end stent stenosis - *see* Restenosis, stent
    in stent stenosis - *see* Restenosis, stent
  stoma
    digestive tract
      colostomy - *see* Complications, colostomy
      enterostomy - *see* Complications,
        enterostomy
      esophagostomy - *see* Complications,
        esophagostomy
      gastrostomy - *see* Complications,
        gastrostomy
    urinary tract N99.528
      continent N99.538
        hemorrhage N99.530
        herniation N99.533
        infection N99.531
        malfunction N99.532
        specified type NEC N99.538
        stenosis N99.534
      cystostomy - *see* Complications,
        cystostomy
      external NOS N99.528
        hemorrhage N99.520
        herniation N99.523
        incontinent N99.528
          hemorrhage N99.520
          herniation N99.523
          infection N99.521
          malfunction N99.522
          specified type NEC N99.528
          stenosis N99.524
        infection N99.521
        malfunction N99.522
        specified type NEC N99.528
        stenosis N99.524
  stomach banding - *see* Complication(s),
    bariatric procedure
  stomach stapling - *see* Complication(s),
    bariatric procedure
  surgical material, nonabsorbable - *see*
    Complication, suture, permanent
  surgical procedure (on) T81.9
    amputation stump (late) - *see* Complications,
      amputation stump
    cardiac - *see* Complications, circulatory
      system
    cholesteatoma, recurrent - *see* Complications,
      postmastoidectomy, recurrent
      cholesteatoma
    circulatory (early) - *see* Complications,
      circulatory system
    digestive system - *see* Complications,
      gastrointestinal
    dumping syndrome (postgastrectomy) K91.1
    ear - *see* Complications, ear
    elephantiasis or lymphedema I97.89
      postmastectomy I97.2
    emphysema (surgical) T81.82
    endocrine - *see* Complications, endocrine
    eye - *see* Complications, eye
    fistula (persistent postoperative) T81.83
    foreign body inadvertently left in wound
      (sponge) (suture) (swab) - *see* Foreign body,
      accidentally left during a procedure
    gastrointestinal - *see* Complications,
      gastrointestinal
    genitourinary NEC N99.89
    hematoma
      intraoperative - *see* Complication,
        intraoperative, hemorrhage
      postprocedural - *see* Complication,

Complication(s) (from) (of) - *continued*
    postprocedural, hematoma
    hemorrhage
      intraoperative - *see* Complication,
        intraoperative, hemorrhage
      postprocedural - *see* Complication,
        postprocedural, hemorrhage
    hepatic failure K91.82
    hyperglycemia (postpancreatectomy) E89.1
    hypoinsulinemia (postpancreatectomy) E89.1
    hypoparathyroidism (postparathyroidectomy)
      E89.2
    hypopituitarism (posthypophysectomy)
      E89.3
    hypothyroidism (post-thyroidectomy) E89.0
    intestinal obstruction (see also Obstruction,
      intestine, postoperative) K91.30
    intracranial hypotension following
      ventricular shunting (ventriculostomy)
      G97.2
    lymphedema I97.89
      postmastectomy I97.2
    malabsorption (postsurgical) NEC K91.2
      osteoporosis - *see* Osteoporosis,
        postsurgical malabsorption
    mastoidectomy cavity NEC - *see*
    Complications, postmastoidectomy
    metabolic E89.89
      specified NEC E89.89
    musculoskeletal - *see* Complications,
      musculoskeletal system
    nervous system (central) (peripheral) - *see*
      Complications, nervous system
    ovarian failure E89.40
      asymptomatic E89.40
      symptomatic E89.41
    peripheral vascular - *see* Complications,
      surgical procedure, vascular
    postcardiotomy syndrome I97.0
    postcholecystectomy syndrome K91.5
    postcommissurotomy syndrome I97.0
    postgastrectomy dumping syndrome K91.1
    postlaminectomy syndrome NEC M96.1
      kyphosis M96.3
    postmastectomy lymphedema syndrome
      I97.2
    postmastoidectomy cholesteatoma - *see*
      Complications, postmastoidectomy,
      recurrent cholesteatoma
    postvagotomy syndrome K91.1
    postvalvulotomy syndrome I97.0
    pulmonary insufficiency (acute) J95.2
      chronic J95.3
      following thoracic surgery J95.1
    reattached body part - *see* Complications,
      reattached
    respiratory - *see* Complications, respiratory
      system
    shock (hypovolemic) T81.19
    spleen (postoperative) D78.89
      intraoperative D78.81
    stitch abscess T81.4
    subglottic stenosis (postsurgical) J95.5
    testicular hypofunction E89.5
    transplant - *see* Complications, organ or
      tissue transplant
    urinary NEC N99.89
    vaginal vault prolapse (posthysterectomy)
      N99.3
    vascular (peripheral)
      artery T81.719
        mesenteric T81.710
        renal T81.711
        specified NEC T81.718

Complication(s) (from) (of) - *continued*
      vein T81.72
    wound infection T81.4
    suture, permanent (wire) NEC T85.9
      with repair of bone - *see* Complications,
        fixation device, internal
      embolism T85.818
      fibrosis T85.828
      hemorrhage T85.838
      infection and inflammation T85.79
      mechanical
        breakdown T85.612
        displacement T85.622
        malfunction T85.612
        malposition T85.622
        obstruction T85.692
        perforation T85.692
        protrusion T85.692
        specified NEC T85.692
      pain T85.848
      specified type NEC T85.898
      stenosis T85.858
      thrombosis T85.868
    tracheostomy J95.00
      granuloma J95.09
      hemorrhage J95.01
      infection J95.02
      malfunction J95.03
      mechanical J95.03
      obstruction J95.03
      specified type NEC J95.09
      tracheo-esophageal fistula J95.04
    transfusion (blood) (lymphocytes) (plasma)
      T80.92
      air embolism T80.0
      circulatory overload E87.71
      febrile nonhemolytic transfusion reaction
        R50.84
      hemolysis T80.89
      hemochromatosis E83.111
      hemolytic reaction (antigen unspecified)
        T80.919
      incompatibility reaction (antigen unspecified)
        T80.919
      ABO T80.30
        delayed serologic (DSTR) T80.39
        hemolytic transfusion reaction (HTR)
        (unspecified time after transfusion)
        T80.319
          acute (AHTR) (less than 24 hours after
            transfusion) T80.310
          delayed (DHTR) (24 hours or more after
            transfusion) T80.311
        specified NEC T80.39
      acute (antigen unspecified) T80.910
      delayed (antigen unspecified) T80.911
      delayed serologic (DSTR) T80.89
      Non-aBO (minor antigens (Duffy) (Kell)
        (Kidd) (Lewis) (M) (N) (P) (S)) T80.A0
        delayed serologic (DSTR) T80.A9
        hemolytic transfusion reaction (HTR)
        (unspecified time after transfusion)
        T80.A19
          acute (AHTR) (less than 24 hours after
            transfusion) T80.A10
          delayed (DHTR) (24 hours or more after
            transfusion) T80.A11
        specified NEC T80.A9
      Rh (antigens (C) (c) (D) (E) (e)) (factor)
        T80.40
        delayed serologic (DSTR) T80.49
        hemolytic transfusion reaction (HTR)
        (unspecified time after transfusion)
        T80.419

Complication(s) (from) (of) - *continued*
          acute (AHTR) (less than 24 hours after
            transfusion) T80.410
          delayed (DHTR) (24 hours or more after
            transfusion) T80.411
        specified NEC T80.49
      infection T80.29
        acute T80.22
      reaction NEC T80.89
      sepsis T80.29
      shock T80.89
    transplant T86.90
      bone T86.839
        failure T86.831
        infection T86.832
        rejection T86.830
        specified type NEC T86.838
      bone marrow T86.00
        failure T86.02
        infection T86.03
        rejection T86.01
        specified type NEC T86.09
      cornea T86.849
        failure T86.841
        infection T86.842
        rejection T86.840
        specified type NEC T86.848
      failure T86.92
      heart T86.20
        with lung T86.30
        cardiac allograft vasculopathy T86.290
        failure T86.32
        infection T86.33
        rejection T86.31
        specified type NEC T86.39
        failure T86.22
        infection T86.23
        rejection T86.21
        specified type NEC T86.298
      infection T86.93
      intestine T86.859
        failure T86.851
        infection T86.852
        rejection T86.850
        specified type NEC T86.858
      kidney T86.10
        failure T86.12
        infection T86.13
        rejection T86.11
        specified type NEC T86.19
      liver T86.40
        failure T86.42
        infection T86.43
        rejection T86.41
        specified type NEC T86.49
      lung T86.819
        with heart T86.30
        failure T86.32
        infection T86.33
        rejection T86.31
        specified type NEC T86.39
        failure T86.811
        infection T86.812
        rejection T86.810
        specified type NEC T86.818
      malignant neoplasm C80.2
      pancreas T86.899
        failure T86.891
        infection T86.892
        rejection T86.890
        specified type NEC T86.898
      peripheral blood stem cells T86.5
      post-transplant lymphoproliferative disorder
        (PTLD) D47.Z1

rejection T86.91
skin T86.829
 failure T86.821
 infection T86.822
 rejection T86.820
 specified type NEC T86.828
specified
 tissue T86.899
  failure T86.891
  infection T86.892
  rejection T86.890
  specified type NEC T86.898
 type NEC T86.99
stem cell (from peripheral blood) (from umbilical cord) T86.5
umbilical cord stem cells T86.5
trauma (early) T79.9
 specified NEC T79.8
ultrasound therapy NEC T88.9
umbilical cord NEC
 complicating delivery O69.9
 specified NEC O69.89
umbrella device, vascular T82.9
 embolism T82.818
 fibrosis T82.828
 hemorrhage T82.838
 infection or inflammation T82.7
 mechanical
  breakdown T82.515
  displacement T82.525
  leakage T82.535
  malposition T82.525
  obstruction T82.595
  perforation T82.595
  protrusion T82.595
 pain T82.848
 specified type NEC T82.898
 stenosis T82.858
 thrombosis T82.868
urethral catheter - *see* Complications, catheter, urethral, indwelling
vaccination T88.1
 anaphylaxis NEC T80.52
 arthropathy - *see* Arthropathy, postimmunization
 cellulitis T88.0
 encephalitis or encephalomyelitis G04.02
 infection (general) (local) NEC T88.0
 meningitis G03.8
 myelitis G04.02
 protein sickness T80.62
 rash T88.1
 reaction (allergic) T88.1
  serum T80.62
 sepsis T88.0
 serum intoxication, sickness, rash, or other serum reaction NEC T80.62
  anaphylactic shock T80.52
 shock (allergic) (anaphylactic) T80.52
 vaccinia (generalized) (localized) T88.1
vas deferens device or implant - *see* Complications, genitourinary, device or implant, genital tract
vascular I99.9
 device or implant T82.9
  embolism T82.818
  fibrosis T82.828
  hemorrhage T82.838
  infection or inflammation T82.7
  mechanical
   breakdown T82.519
    specified device NEC T82.518
   displacement T82.529

    specified device NEC T82.528
   leakage T82.539
    specified device NEC T82.538
   malposition T82.529
    specified device NEC T82.528
   obstruction T82.599
    specified device NEC T82.598
   perforation T82.599
    specified device NEC T82.598
   protrusion T82.599
    specified device NEC T82.598
  pain T82.848
  specified type NEC T82.898
  stenosis T82.858
  thrombosis T82.868
 dialysis catheter - *see* Complication, catheter, dialysis
 following infusion, therapeutic injection or transfusion T80.1
 graft T82.9
  embolism T82.818
  fibrosis T82.828
  hemorrhage T82.838
  mechanical
   breakdown T82.319
    aorta (bifurcation) T82.310
    carotid artery T82.311
    specified vessel NEC T82.318
   displacement T82.329
    aorta (bifurcation) T82.320
    carotid artery T82.321
    specified vessel NEC T82.328
   leakage T82.339
    aorta (bifurcation) T82.330
    carotid artery T82.331
    specified vessel NEC T82.338
   malposition T82.329
    aorta (bifurcation) T82.320
    carotid artery T82.321
    specified vessel NEC T82.328
   obstruction T82.399
    aorta (bifurcation) T82.390
    carotid artery T82.391
    specified vessel NEC T82.398
   perforation T82.399
    aorta (bifurcation) T82.390
    carotid artery T82.391
    specified vessel NEC T82.398
   protrusion T82.399
    aorta (bifurcation) T82.390
    carotid artery T82.391
    specified vessel NEC T82.398
  pain T82.848
  specified complication NEC T82.898
  stenosis T82.858
  thrombosis T82.868
 postoperative - *see* Complications, postoperative, circulatory
 vena cava device (filter) (sieve) (umbrella) - *see* Complications, umbrella device, vascular
ventilation therapy NEC T81.81
ventilator
 mechanical J95.850
  specified NEC J95.859
ventricular (communicating) shunt (device) T85.9
 embolism T85.810
 fibrosis T85.820
 hemorrhage T85.830
 infection and inflammation T85.730
 mechanical
  breakdown T85.01
  displacement T85.02

   leakage T85.03
   malposition T85.02
   obstruction T85.09
   perforation T85.09
   protrusion T85.09
   specified NEC T85.09
  pain T85.840
  specified type NEC T85.890
  stenosis T85.850
  thrombosis T85.860
 wire suture, permanent (implanted) - *see* Complications, suture, permanent
Compressed air disease T70.3
Compression
 with injury code by Nature of injury artery I77.1
 celiac, syndrome I77.4
 brachial plexus G54.0
 brain (stem) G93.5
  due to
   contusion (diffuse) - *see* Injury, intracranial, diffuse
    focal - *see* Injury, intracranial, focal
   injury NEC - *see* Injury, intracranial, diffuse
   traumatic - *see* Injury, intracranial, diffuse
 bronchus J98.09
 cauda equina G83.4
 celiac (artery) (axis) I77.4
 cerebral - *see* Compression, brain
 cervical plexus G54.2
 cord
  spinal - *see* Compression, spinal
  umbilical - *see* Compression, umbilical cord
 cranial nerve G52.9
  eighth - *see* subcategory H93.3
  eleventh G52.8
  fifth G50.8
  first G52.0
  fourth - *see* Strabismus, paralytic, fourth nerve
  ninth G52.1
  second - *see* Disorder, nerve, optic
  seventh G51.8
  sixth - *see* Strabismus, paralytic, sixth nerve
  tenth G52.2
  third - *see* Strabismus, paralytic, third nerve
  twelfth G52.3
 diver's squeeze T70.3
 during birth (newborn) P15.9
 esophagus K22.2
 eustachian tube - *see* Obstruction, eustachian tube, cartilaginous
 facies Q67.1
 fracture
  nontraumatic NOS - *see* Collapse, vertebra
  pathological - *see* Fracture, pathological
  traumatic - *see* Fracture, traumatic
 heart - *see* Disease, heart
 intestine - *see* Obstruction, intestine
 laryngeal nerve, recurrent G52.2
  with paralysis of vocal cords and larynx J38.00
   bilateral J38.02
   unilateral J38.01
 lumbosacral plexus G54.1
 lung J98.4
 lymphatic vessel I89.0
 medulla - *see* Compression, brain
 nerve - *see also* Disorder, nerve G58.9
  arm NEC - *see* Mononeuropathy, upper limb
  axillary G54.0
  cranial - *see* Compression, cranial nerve

Compression - *continued*
  leg NEC - *see* Mononeuropathy, lower limb
  median (in carpal tunnel) - *see* Syndrome, carpal tunnel
  optic - *see* Disorder, nerve, optic
  plantar - *see* Lesion, nerve, plantar
  posterior tibial (in tarsal tunnel) - *see* Syndrome, tarsal tunnel
  root or plexus NOS (in) G54.9
    intervertebral disc disorder NEC - *see* Disorder, disc, with, radiculopathy
      with myelopathy - *see* Disorder, disc, with, myelopathy
    neoplastic disease - *see also* Neoplasm D49.9 [G55]
    spondylosis - *see* Spondylosis, with radiculopathy
  sciatic (acute) - *see* Lesion, nerve, sciatic
  sympathetic G90.8
  traumatic - *see* Injury, nerve
  ulnar - *see* Lesion, nerve, ulnar
  upper extremity NEC - *see* Mononeuropathy, upper limb
  spinal (cord) G95.20
    by displacement of intervertebral disc NEC - *see also* Disorder, disc, with, myelopathy
    nerve root NOS G54.9
      due to displacement of intervertebral disc NEC - *see* Disorder, disc, with, radiculopathy
        with myelopathy - *see* Disorder, disc, with, myelopathy
    specified NEC G95.29
    spondylogenic (cervical) (lumbar, lumbosacral) (thoracic) - *see* Spondylosis, with myelopathy NEC
      anterior - *see* Syndrome, anterior, spinal artery, compression
    traumatic - *see* Injury, spinal cord, by region
  subcostal nerve (syndrome) - *see* Mononeuropathy, upper limb, specified NEC
  sympathetic nerve NEC G90.8
  syndrome T79.5
  trachea J39.8
  ulnar nerve (by scar tissue) - *see* Lesion, nerve, ulnar
  umbilical cord
    complicating delivery O69.2
      cord around neck O69.1
      prolapse O69.0
      specified NEC O69.2
  ureter N13.5
  vein I87.1
  vena cava (inferior) (superior) I87.1
Compulsion, compulsive
  gambling F63.0
  neurosis F42.8
  personality F60.5
  states F42.8
  swearing F42.8
    in Gilles de la Tourette's syndrome F95.2
  tics and spasms F95.9
Concato's disease (pericardial polyserositis) A19.9
  nontubercular I31.1
  pleural - *see* Pleurisy, with effusion
Concavity chest wall M95.4
Concealed penis Q55.69
Concern (normal) about sick person in family Z63.6
Concrescence (teeth) K00.2
Concretio cordis I31.1
  rheumatic I09.2

Concretion - *see also* Calculus
  appendicular K38.1
  canaliculus - *see* Dacryolith
  clitoris N90.89
  conjunctiva H11.12-
  eyelid - *see* Disorder, eyelid, specified type NEC
  lacrimal passages - *see* Dacryolith
  prepuce (male) N47.8
  salivary gland (any) K11.5
  seminal vesicle N50.89
  tonsil J35.8
Concussion (brain) (cerebral) (current) S06.0X9
  with
    loss of consciousness of 30 minutes or less S06.0X1
    loss of consciousness of unspecified duration S06.0X9
  blast (air) (hydraulic) (immersion) (underwater)
    abdomen or thorax - *see* Injury, blast, by site
    ear with acoustic nerve injury - *see* Injury, nerve, acoustic, specified type NEC
  cauda equina S34.3
  conus medullaris S34.02
  ocular S05.8X-
  spinal (cord)
    cervical S14.0
    lumbar S34.01
    sacral S34.02
    thoracic S24.0
  syndrome F07.81
  without loss of consciousness S06.0X0
Condition - *see* Disease
Conditions arising in the perinatal period - *see* Newborn, affected by
Conduct disorder - *see* Disorder, conduct
Condyloma A63.0
  acuminatum A63.0
  gonorrheal A54.09
  latum A51.31
  syphilitic A51.31
    congenital A50.07
  venereal, syphilitic A51.31
Conflagration - *see also* Burn
  asphyxia (by inhalation of gases, fumes or vapors) - *see also* Table of Drugs and Chemicals T59.9-
Conflict (with) - *see also* Discord
  family Z73.9
  marital Z63.0
    involving divorce or estrangement Z63.5
  parent-child Z62.820
    parent-adopted child Z62.821
    parent-biological child Z62.820
    parent-foster child Z62.822
  social role NEC Z73.5
Confluent - *see* condition
Confusion, confused R41.0
  epileptic F05
  mental state (psychogenic) F44.89
  psychogenic F44.89
  reactive (from emotional stress, psychological trauma) F44.89
Confusional arousals G47.51
Congelation T69.9
Congenital - *see also* condition
  aortic septum Q25.49
  intrinsic factor deficiency D51.0
  malformation - *see* Anomaly
Congestion, congestive
  bladder N32.89
  bowel K63.89

Congestion, congestive
  brain G93.89
  breast N64.59
  bronchial J98.09
  catarrhal J31.0
  chest R09.89
  chill, malarial - *see* Malaria
  circulatory NEC I99.8
  duodenum K31.89
  eye - *see* Hyperemia, conjunctiva
  facial, due to birth injury P15.4
  general R68.89
  glottis J37.0
  heart - *see* Failure, heart, congestive
  hepatic K76.1
  hypostatic (lung) - *see* Edema, lung
  intestine K63.89
  kidney N28.89
  labyrinth - *see* subcategory H83.8
  larynx J37.0
  liver K76.1
  lung R09.89
    active or acute - *see* Pneumonia
  malaria, malarial - *see* Malaria
  nasal R09.81
  nose R09.81
  orbit, orbital - *see also* Exophthalmos
    inflammatory (chronic) - *see* Inflammation, orbit
  ovary N83.8
  pancreas K86.89
  pelvic, female N94.89
  pleural J94.8
  prostate (active) N42.1
  pulmonary - *see* Congestion, lung
  renal N28.89
  retina H35.81
  seminal vesicle N50.1
  spinal cord G95.19
  spleen (chronic) D73.2
  stomach K31.89
  trachea - *see* Tracheitis
  urethra N36.8
  uterus N85.8
    with subinvolution N85.3
  venous (passive) I87.8
  viscera R68.89
Congestive - *see* Congestion
Conical
  cervix (hypertrophic elongation) N88.4
  cornea - *see* Keratoconus
  teeth K00.2
Conjoined twins Q89.4
Conjugal maladjustment Z63.0
  involving divorce or estrangement Z63.5
Conjunctiva - *see* condition
Conjunctivitis (staphylococcal) (streptococcal) NOS H10.9
  Acanthamoeba B60.12
  acute H10.3-
    atopic H10.1-
    mucopurulent H10.02-
      follicular H10.01-
    chemical - *see also* Corrosion, cornea H10.21-
    pseudomembranous H10.22-
    serous except viral H10.23-
      viral - *see* Conjunctivitis, viral
    toxic H10.21-
  adenoviral (acute) (follicular) B30.1
  allergic (acute) - *see* Conjunctivitis, acute, atopic
    chronic H10.45
    vernal H10.44

Conjunctivitis - *continued*
  anaphylactic - *see* Conjunctivitis, acute, atopic
  Apollo B30.3
  atopic (acute) - *see* Conjunctivitis, acute, atopic
  Béal's B30.2
  blennorrhagic (gonococcal) (neonatorum) A54.31
  chemical (acute) - *see also* Corrosion, cornea H10.21-
  chlamydial A74.0 - *continued*
    due to trachoma A71.1
    neonatal P39.1
  chronic (nodosa) (petrificans) (phlyctenular) H10.40-
    allergic H10.45
      vernal H10.44
    follicular H10.43-
    giant papillary H10.41-
    simple H10.42-
    vernal H10.44
  coxsackievirus 24 B30.3
  diphtheritic A36.86
  due to
    dust - *see* Conjunctivitis, acute, atopic
    filariasis B74.9
    mucocutaneous leishmaniasis B55.2
  enterovirus type 70 (hemorrhagic) B30.3
  epidemic (viral) B30.9
    hemorrhagic B30.3
  gonococcal (neonatorum) A54.31
  granular (trachomatous) A71.1
    sequelae (late effect) B94.0
  hemorrhagic (acute) (epidemic) B30.3
  herpes zoster B02.31
  in (due to)
    Acanthamoeba B60.12
    adenovirus (acute) (follicular) B30.1
    Chlamydia A74.0
    coxsackievirus 24 B30.3
    diphtheria A36.86
    enterovirus type 70 (hemorrhagic) B30.3
    filariasis B74.9
    gonococci A54.31
    herpes (simplex) virus B00.53
      zoster B02.31
    infectious disease NEC B99
    meningococci A39.89
    mucocutaneous leishmaniasis B55.2
    rosacea L71.9
    syphilis (late) A52.71
    zoster B02.31
  inclusion A74.0
  infantile P39.1
    gonococcal A54.31
  Koch-Weeks' - *see* Conjunctivitis, acute, mucopurulent
  light - *see* Conjunctivitis, acute, atopic
  ligneous - *see* Blepharoconjunctivitis, ligneous
  meningococcal A39.89
  mucopurulent - *see* Conjunctivitis, acute, mucopurulent
  neonatal P39.1
    gonococcal A54.31
  Newcastle B30.8
  of Béal B30.2
  parasitic
    filariasis B74.9
    mucocutaneous leishmaniasis B55.2
  Parinaud's H10.89
  petrificans H10.89
  rosacea L71.9
  specified NEC H10.89
  swimming-pool B30.1

Conjunctivitis - *continued*
  trachomatous A71.1
    acute A71.0
    sequelae (late effect) B94.0
  traumatic NEC H10.89
  tuberculous A18.59
  tularemic A21.1
  tularensis A21.1
  viral B30.9
    due to
      adenovirus B30.1
      enterovirus B30.3
    specified NEC B30.8
Conjunctivochalasis H11.82-
Connective tissue - *see* condition
Conn's syndrome E26.01
Conradi (-Hunermann) disease Q77.3
Consanguinity Z84.3
  counseling Z71.89
Conscious simulation (of illness) Z76.5
Consecutive - *see* condition
Consolidation lung (base) - *see* Pneumonia, lobar
Constipation (atonic) (neurogenic) (simple) (spastic) K59.00
  chronic K59.09
    idiopathic K59.04
  drug-induced K59.03
  functional K59.04
  outlet dysfunction K59.02
  psychogenic F45.8
  slow transit K59.01
  specified NEC K59.09
Constitutional - *see also* condition
  substandard F60.7
Constitutionally substandard F60.7
Constriction - *see also* Stricture
  auditory canal - *see* Stenosis, external ear canal
  bronchial J98.09
  duodenum K31.5
  esophagus K22.2
  external
    abdomen, abdominal (wall) S30.841
    alveolar process S00.542
    ankle S90.54-
    antecubital space - *see* Constriction, external, forearm
    arm (upper) S40.84-
    auricle - *see* Constriction, external, ear
    axilla - *see* Constriction, external, arm
    back, lower S30.840
    breast S20.14-
    brow S00.84
    buttock S30.840
    calf - *see* Constriction, external, leg
    canthus - *see* Constriction, external, eyelid
    cheek S00.84
      internal S00.542
    chest wall - *see* Constriction, external, thorax
    chin S00.84
    clitoris S30.844
    costal region - *see* Constriction, external, thorax
    digit(s)
      foot - *see* Constriction, external, toe
      hand - *see* Constriction, external, finger
    ear S00.44-
    elbow S50.34-
    epididymis S30.843
    epigastric region S30.841
    esophagus, cervical S10.14
    eyebrow - *see* Constriction, external, eyelid
    eyelid S00.24-

Constriction - *continued*
    face S00.84
    finger(s) S60.44-
      index S60.44
      little S60.44-
      middle S60.44-
      ring S60.44-
    flank S30.841
    foot (except toe(s) alone) S90.84-
      toe - *see* Constriction, external, toe
    forearm S50.84-
      elbow only - *see* Constriction, external, elbow
    forehead S00.84
    genital organs, external
      female S30.846
      male S30.845
    groin S30.841
    gum S00.542
    hand S60.54-
    head S00.94
      ear - *see* Constriction, external, ear
      eyelid - *see* Constriction, external, eyelid
      lip S00.541
      nose S00.34
      oral cavity S00.542
      scalp S00.04
      specified site NEC S00.84
    heel - *see* Constriction, external, foot
    hip S70.24-
    inguinal region S30.841
    interscapular region S20.449
    jaw S00.84
    knee S80.24-
    labium (majus) (minus) S30.844
    larynx S10.14
    leg (lower) S80.84-
      knee - *see* Constriction, external, knee
      upper - *see* Constriction, external, thigh
    lip S00.541
    lower back S30.840
    lumbar region S30.840
    malar region S00.84
    mammary - *see* Constriction, external, breast
    mastoid region S00.84
    mouth S00.542
    nail
      finger - *see* Constriction, external, finger
      toe - *see* Constriction, external, toe
    nasal S00.34
    neck S10.94
      specified site NEC S10.84
      throat S10.14
    nose S00.34
    occipital region S00.04
    oral cavity S00.542
    orbital region - *see* Constriction, external, eyelid
    palate S00.542
    palm - *see* Constriction, external, hand
    parietal region S00.04
    pelvis S30.840
    penis S30.842
    perineum
      female S30.844
      male S30.840
    periocular area - *see* Constriction, external, eyelid
    phalanges
      finger - *see* Constriction, external, finger
      toe - *see* Constriction, external, toe
    pharynx S10.14
    pinna - *see* Constriction, external, ear

Constriction - *continued*
  popliteal space - *see* Constriction, external,
    knee
  prepuce S30.842
  pubic region S30.840
  pudendum
    female S30.846
    male S30.845
  sacral region S30.840
  scalp S00.04
  scapular region - *see* Constriction, external,
    shoulder
  scrotum S30.843
  shin - *see* Constriction, external, leg
  shoulder S40.24-
  sternal region S20.349
  submaxillary region S00.84
  submental region S00.84
  subungual
    finger(s) - *see* Constriction, external, finger
    toe(s) - *see* Constriction, external, toe
  supraclavicular fossa S10.84
  supraorbital S00.84
  temple S00.84
  temporal region S00.84
  testis S30.843
  thigh S70.34-
  thorax, thoracic (wall) S20.94
    back S20.44-
    front S20.34-
  throat S10.14
  thumb S60.34-
  toe(s) (lesser) S90.44-
    great S90.44-
  tongue S00.542
  trachea S10.14
  tunica vaginalis S30.843
  uvula S00.542
  vagina S30.844
  vulva S30.844
  wrist S60.84-
  gallbladder - *see* Obstruction, gallbladder
  intestine - *see* Obstruction, intestine
  larynx J38.6
    congenital Q31.8
      specified NEC Q31.8
      subglottic Q31.1
  organ or site, congenital NEC - *see* Atresia, by
    site
  prepuce (acquired) (congenital) N47.1
  pylorus (adult hypertrophic) K31.1
    congenital or infantile Q40.0
    newborn Q40.0
  ring dystocia (uterus) O62.4
  spastic - *see also* Spasm
    ureter N13.5
  ureter N13.5
    with infection N13.6
  urethra - *see* Stricture, urethra
  visual field (peripheral) (functional) - *see*
    Defect, visual field
Constrictive - *see* condition
Consultation
  medical - *see* Counseling, medical
  religious Z71.81
  specified reason NEC Z71.89
  spiritual Z71.81
  without complaint or sickness Z71.9
    feared complaint unfounded Z71.1
    specified reason NEC Z71.89
Consumption - *see* Tuberculosis
Contact (with) - *see also* Exposure (to)
  acariasis Z20.7
  AIDS virus Z20.6

Contact (with) - *continued*
  air pollution Z77.110
  algae and algae toxins Z77.121
  algae bloom Z77.121
  anthrax Z20.810
  aromatic amines Z77.020
  aromatic (hazardous) compounds NEC
    Z77.028
  aromatic dyes NOS Z77.028
  arsenic Z77.010
  asbestos Z77.090
  bacterial disease NEC Z20.818
  benzene Z77.021
  blue-green algae bloom Z77.121
  body fluids (potentially hazardous) Z77.21
  brown tide Z77.121
  chemicals (chiefly nonmedicinal) (hazardous)
    NEC Z77.098
  cholera Z20.09
  chromium compounds Z77.018
  communicable disease Z20.9
    bacterial NEC Z20.818
    specified NEC Z20.89
    viral NEC Z20.828
  cyanobacteria bloom Z77.121
  dyes Z77.098
  Escherichia coli (E. coli) Z20.01
  fiberglass - *see* Table of Drugs and Chemicals,
    fiberglass
  German measles Z20.4
  gonorrhea Z20.2
  hazardous metals NEC Z77.018
  hazardous substances NEC Z77.29
  hazards in the physical environment NEC
    Z77.128
  hazards to health NEC Z77.9
  HIV Z20.6
  HTLV-III/LAV Z20.6
  human immunodeficiency virus (HIV) Z20.6
  infection Z20.9
    specified NEC Z20.89
  infestation (parasitic) NEC Z20.7
  intestinal infectious disease NEC Z20.09
    Escherichia coli (E. coli) Z20.01
  lead Z77.011
  meningococcus Z20.811
  mold (toxic) Z77.120
  nickel dust Z77.018
  noise Z77.122
  parasitic disease Z20.7
  pediculosis Z20.7
  pfiesteria piscicida Z77.121
  poliomyelitis Z20.89
  pollution
    air Z77.110
    environmental NEC Z77.118
    soil Z77.112
    water Z77.111
  polycyclic aromatic hydrocarbons Z77.028
  rabies Z20.3
  radiation, naturally occurring NEC Z77.123
  radon Z77.123
  red tide (Florida) Z77.121
  rubella Z20.4
  sexually-transmitted disease Z20.2
  smallpox (laboratory) Z20.89
  syphilis Z20.2
  tuberculosis Z20.1
  uranium Z77.012
  varicella Z20.820
  venereal disease Z20.2
  viral disease NEC Z20.828
  viral hepatitis Z20.5
  water pollution Z77.111

Contamination, food - *see* Intoxication,
  foodborne
Contraception, contraceptive
  advice Z30.09
  counseling Z30.09
  device (intrauterine) (in situ) Z97.5
    causing menorrhagia T83.83
    checking Z30.431
    complications - *see* Complications,
    intrauterine, contraceptive device
    in place Z97.5
    initial prescription Z30.014
    reinsertion Z30.433
    removal Z30.432
    replacement Z30.433
  emergency (postcoital) Z30.012
  initial prescription Z30.019
    barrier Z30.018
    diaphragm Z30.018
    injectable Z30.013
    intrauterine device Z30.014
    pills Z30.011
    postcoital (emergency) Z30.012
    specified type NEC Z30.018
    subdermal implantable Z30.017
    transdermal patch hormonal Z30.016
    vaginal ring hormonal Z30.015
  maintenance Z30.40
    barrier Z30.49
    diaphragm Z30.49
    examination Z30.8
    injectable Z30.42
    intrauterine device Z30.431
    pills Z30.41
    specified type NEC Z30.49
    subdermal implantable Z30.46
    transdermal patch hormonal Z30.45
    vaginal ring hormonal Z30.44
  management Z30.9
    specified NEC Z30.8
  postcoital (emergency) Z30.012
  prescription Z30.019
    repeat Z30.40
  sterilization Z30.2
  surveillance (drug) - *see* Contraception,
    maintenance
Contraction(s), contracture, contracted
  Achilles tendon - *see also* Short, tendon,
    Achilles
    congenital Q66.89
  amputation stump (surgical) (flexion) (late)
    (next proximal joint) T87.89
  anus K59.8
  bile duct (common) (hepatic) K83.8
  bladder N32.89
    neck or sphincter N32.0
  bowel, cecum, colon or intestine, any part - *see*
    Obstruction, intestine
  Braxton Hicks - *see* False, labor
  breast implant, capsular T85.44
  bronchial J98.09
  burn (old) - *see* Cicatrix
  cervix - *see* Stricture, cervix
  cicatricial - *see* Cicatrix
  conjunctiva, trachomatous, active A71.1
    sequelae (late effect) B94.0
  Dupuytren's M72.0
  eyelid - *see* Disorder, eyelid function
  fascia (lata) (postural) M72.8
    Dupuytren's M72.0
    palmar M72.0
    plantar M72.2
  finger NEC - *see also* Deformity, finger
    congenital Q68.1

Contraction(s), contracture, contracted
- *continued*
    joint - *see* Contraction, joint, hand
    flaccid - *see* Contraction, paralytic
    gallbladder K82.0
    heart valve - *see* Endocarditis
    hip - *see* Contraction, joint, hip
    hourglass
      bladder N32.89
        congenital Q64.79
      gallbladder K82.0
        congenital Q44.1
      stomach K31.89
        congenital Q40.2
        psychogenic F45.8
      uterus (complicating delivery) O62.4
    hysterical F44.4
    internal os - *see* Stricture, cervix
    joint (abduction) (acquired) (adduction)
    (flexion) (rotation) M24.50
      ankle M24.57-
      congenital NEC Q68.8
        hip Q65.89
      elbow M24.52-
      foot joint M24.57-
      hand joint M24.54-
      hip M24.55-
        congenital Q65.89
      hysterical F44.4
      knee M24.56-
      shoulder M24.51-
      wrist M24.53-
    kidney (granular) (secondary) N26.9
      congenital Q63.8
      hydronephrotic - *see* Hydronephrosis
      Page N26.2
      pyelonephritic - *see* Pyelitis, chronic
      tuberculous A18.11
    ligament - *see also* Disorder, ligament
      congenital Q79.8
    muscle (postinfective) (postural) NEC M62.40
      with contracture of joint - *see* Contraction,
      joint
      ankle M62.47-
      congenital Q79.8
        sternocleidomastoid Q68.0
      extraocular - *see* Strabismus
      eye (extrinsic) - *see* Strabismus
      foot M62.47-
      forearm M62.43-
      hand M62.44-
      hysterical F44.4
      ischemic (Volkmann's) T79.6
      lower leg M62.46-
      multiple sites M62.49
      pelvic region M62.45-
      posttraumatic - *see* Strabismus, paralytic
      psychogenic F45.8
        conversion reaction F44.4
      shoulder region M62.41-
      specified site NEC M62.48
      thigh M62.45-
      upper arm M62.42-
    neck - *see* Torticollis
    ocular muscle - *see* Strabismus
    organ or site, congenital NEC - *see* Atresia, by
    site
    outlet (pelvis) - *see* Contraction, pelvis
    palmar fascia M72.0
    paralytic
      joint - *see* Contraction, joint
      muscle - *see also* Contraction, muscle NEC
        ocular - *see* Strabismus, paralytic
    pelvis (acquired) (general) M95.5

Contraction(s), contracture, contracted
- *continued*
    with disproportion (fetopelvic) O33.1
      causing obstructed labor O65.1
      inlet O33.2
      mid-cavity O33.3
      outlet O33.3
    plantar fascia M72.2
    premature
      atrium I49.1
      auriculoventricular I49.49
      heart I49.49
      junctional I49.2
      supraventricular I49.1
      ventricular I49.3
    prostate N42.89
    pylorus NEC - *see also* Pylorospasm
      psychogenic F45.8
    rectum, rectal (sphincter) K59.8
    ring (Bandl's) (complicating delivery) O62.4
    scar - *see* Cicatrix
    spine - *see* Dorsopathy, deforming
    sternocleidomastoid (muscle), congenital
    Q68.0
    stomach K31.89
      hourglass K31.89
        congenital Q40.2
        psychogenic F45.8
      psychogenic F45.8
    tendon (sheath) M62.40
      with contracture of joint - *see* Contraction,
      joint
      Achilles - *see* Short, tendon, Achilles
      ankle M62.47-
        Achilles - *see* Short, tendon, Achilles
      foot M62.47-
      forearm M62.43-
      hand M62.44-
      lower leg M62.46-
      multiple sites M62.49
      neck M62.48
      pelvic region M62.45-
      shoulder region M62.41-
      specified site NEC M62.48
      thigh M62.45-
      thorax M62.48
      trunk M62.48
      upper arm M62.42-
    toe - *see* Deformity, toe, specified NEC
    ureterovesical orifice (postinfectional) N13.5
      with infection N13.6
    urethra - *see also* Stricture, urethra
      orifice N32.0
    uterus N85.8
      abnormal NEC O62.9
      clonic (complicating delivery) O62.4
      dyscoordinate (complicating delivery) O62.4
      hourglass (complicating delivery) O62.4
      hypertonic O62.4
      hypotonic NEC O62.2
      inadequate
        primary O62.0
        secondary O62.1
      incoordinate (complicating delivery) O62.4
      poor O62.2
      tetanic (complicating delivery) O62.4
    vagina (outlet) N89.5
    vesical N32.89
      neck or urethral orifice N32.0
    visual field - *see* Defect, visual field,
    generalized
    Volkmann's (ischemic) T79.6

Contusion (skin surface intact) T14.8
    abdomen, abdominal (muscle) (wall) S30.1
    adnexa, eye NEC S05.8X-
    adrenal gland S37.812
    alveolar process S00.532
    ankle S90.0-
    antecubital space - *see* Contusion, forearm
    anus S30.3
    arm (upper) S40.02-
      lower (with elbow) - *see* Contusion, forearm
    auditory canal - *see* Contusion, ear
    auricle - *see* Contusion, ear
    axilla - *see* Contusion, arm, upper
    back - *see also* Contusion, thorax, back
      lower S30.0
    bile duct S36.13
    bladder S37.22
    bone NEC T14.8
    brain (diffuse) - *see* Injury, intracranial, diffuse
      focal - *see* Injury, intracranial, focal
    brainstem S06.38-
    breast S20.0-
    broad ligament S37.892
    brow S00.83
    buttock S30.0
    canthus, eye S00.1-
    cauda equina S34.3
    cerebellar, traumatic S06.37-
    cerebral S06.33-
      left side S06.32-
      right side S06.31-
    cheek S00.83
      internal S00.532
    chest (wall) - *see* Contusion, thorax chin
    S00.83
    clitoris S30.23
    colon - *see* Injury, intestine, large, contusion
    common bile duct S36.13
    conjunctiva S05.1-
      with foreign body (in conjunctival sac) - *see*
      Foreign body, conjunctival sac
    conus medullaris (spine) S34.139
    cornea - *see* Contusion, eyeball
      with foreign body - *see* Foreign body, cornea
    corpus cavernosum S30.21
    cortex (brain) (cerebral) - *see* Injury,
    intracranial, diffuse
      focal - *see* Injury, intracranial, focal
    costal region - *see* Contusion, thorax cystic
    duct S36.13
    diaphragm S27.802
    duodenum S36.420
    ear S00.43-
    elbow S50.0-
      with forearm - *see* Contusion, forearm
    epididymis S30.22
    epigastric region S30.1
    epiglottis S10.0
    esophagus (thoracic) S27.812
      cervical S10.0
    eyeball S05.1-
    eyebrow S00.1-
    eyelid (and periocular area) S00.1-
    face NEC S00.83
    fallopian tube S37.529
      bilateral S37.522
      unilateral S37.521
    femoral triangle S30.1
    finger(s) S60.00
      with damage to nail (matrix) S60.10
      index S60.02-
        with damage to nail S60.12-
      little S60.05-
        with damage to nail S60.15-

Contusion - *continued*
  middle S60.03-
    with damage to nail S60.13-
  ring S60.04-
    with damage to nail S60.14-
  thumb - *see* Contusion, thumb
flank S30.1
foot (except toe(s) alone) S90.3-
  toe - *see* Contusion, toe
forearm S50.1-
  elbow only - *see* Contusion, elbow
forehead S00.83
gallbladder S36.122
genital organs, external
  female S30.202
  male S30.201
globe (eye) - *see* Contusion, eyeball
groin S30.1
gum S00.532
hand S60.22-
  finger(s) - *see* Contusion, finger
  wrist - *see* Contusion, wrist
head S00.93
  ear - *see* Contusion, ear
  eyelid - *see* Contusion, eyelid
  lip S00.531
  nose S00.33
  oral cavity S00.532
  scalp S00.03
  specified part NEC S00.83
heart - *see also* Injury, heart S26.91
heel - *see* Contusion, foot
hepatic duct S36.13
hip S70.0-
ileum S36.428
iliac region S30.1
inguinal region S30.1
interscapular region S20.229
intra-abdominal organ S36.92
  colon - *see* Injury, intestine, large, contusion
  liver S36.112
  pancreas - *see* Contusion, pancreas
  rectum S36.62
  small intestine - *see* Injury, intestine, small, contusion
  specified organ NEC S36.892
  spleen - *see* Contusion, spleen
  stomach S36.32
iris (eye) - *see* Contusion, eyeball
jaw S00.83
jejunum S36.428
kidney S37.01-
  major (greater than 2 cm) S37.02-
  minor (less than 2 cm) S37.01-
knee S80.0-
labium (majus) (minus) S30.23
lacrimal apparatus, gland or sac S05.8X
larynx S10.0
leg (lower) S80.1-
  knee - *see* Contusion, knee   lens - *see*
  Contusion, eyeball
lip S00.531
liver S36.112
lower back S30.0
lumbar region S30.0
lung S27.329
  bilateral S27.322
  unilateral S27.321
malar region S00.83
mastoid region S00.83
membrane, brain - *see* Injury, intracranial, diffuse
  focal - *see* Injury, intracranial, focal
mesentery S36.892

Contusion - *continued*
  mesosalpinx S37.892
mouth S00.532
muscle - *see* Contusion, by site
nail
  finger - *see* Contusion, finger, with damage to nail
  toe - *see* Contusion, toe, with damage to nail
nasal S00.33
neck S10.93
  specified site NEC S10.83
  throat S10.0
nerve - *see* Injury, nerve
newborn P54.5
nose S00.33
occipital
  lobe (brain) - *see* Injury, intracranial, diffuse
    focal - *see* Injury, intracranial, focal
  region (scalp) S00.03
orbit (region) (tissues) S05.1-
ovary S37.429
  bilateral S37.422
  unilateral S37.421
palate S00.532
pancreas S36.229
  body S36.221
  head S36.220
  tail S36.222
parietal
  lobe (brain) - *see* Injury, intracranial, diffuse
    focal - *see* Injury, intracranial, focal
  region (scalp) S00.03
pelvic organ S37.92
  adrenal gland S37.812
  bladder S37.22
  fallopian tube - *see* Contusion, fallopian tube
  kidney - *see* Contusion, kidney
  ovary - *see* Contusion, ovary
  prostate S37.822
  specified organ NEC S37.892
  ureter S37.12
  urethra S37.32
  uterus S37.62
pelvis S30.0
penis S30.21
perineum
  female S30.23
  male S30.0
periocular area S00.1-
peritoneum S36.81
periurethral tissue - *see* Contusion, urethra
pharynx S10.0
pinna - *see* Contusion, ear
popliteal space - *see* Contusion, knee   prepuce
S30.21
prostate S37.822
pubic region S30.1
pudendum
  female S30.202
  male S30.201
quadriceps femoris - *see* Contusion, thigh
rectum S36.62
retroperitoneum S36.892
round ligament S37.892
sacral region S30.0
scalp S00.03
  due to birth injury P12.3
scapular region - *see* Contusion, shoulder
sclera - *see* Contusion, eyeball
scrotum S30.22
seminal vesicle S37.892
shoulder S40.01-
skin NEC T14.8
small intestine - *see* Injury, intestine, small,

Contusion - *continued*
  contusion
spermatic cord S30.22
spinal cord - *see* Injury, spinal cord, by region
  cauda equina S34.3
  conus medullaris S34.139
spleen S36.029
  major S36.021
  minor S36.020
sternal region S20.219
stomach S36.32
subconjunctival S05.1-
subcutaneous NEC T14.8
submaxillary region S00.83
submental region S00.83
subperiosteal NEC T14.8
subungual
  finger - *see* Contusion, finger, with damage to nail
  toe - *see* Contusion, toe, with damage to nail
supraclavicular fossa S10.83
supraorbital S00.83
suprarenal gland S37.812
temple (region) S00.83
temporal
  lobe (brain) - *see* Injury, intracranial, diffuse
    focal - *see* Injury, intracranial, focal
  region S00.83
testis S30.22
thigh S70.1-
thorax (wall) S20.20
  back S20.22-
  front S20.21-
throat S10.0
thumb S60.01-
  with damage to nail S60.11-
toe(s) (lesser) S90.12-
  with damage to nail S90.22-
  great S90.11-
    with damage to nail S90.21-
tongue S00.532
trachea (cervical) S10.0
  thoracic S27.52
tunica vaginalis S30.22
tympanum, tympanic membrane - *see*
  Contusion, ear
ureter S37.12
urethra S37.32
urinary organ NEC S37.892
uterus S37.62
uvula S00.532
vagina S30.23
vas deferens S37.892
vesical S37.22
vocal cord(s) S10.0
vulva S30.23
wrist S60.21-
Conus (congenital) (any type) Q14.8
  cornea - *see* Keratoconus
  medullaris syndrome G95.81
Conversion hysteria, neurosis or reaction
F44.9
Converter, tuberculosis (test reaction) R76.11
Conviction (legal), anxiety concerning Z65.0
  with imprisonment Z65.1
Convulsions (idiopathic) - *see also* Seizure(s)
R56.9
  apoplectiform (cerebral ischemia) I67.82
  dissociative F44.5
  epileptic - *see* Epilepsy
  epileptiform, epileptoid - *see* Seizure,
    epileptiform
  ether (anesthetic) - *see* Table of Drugs and
    Chemicals, by drug

Corrosion - *continued*
  with
    10-19 percent third degree T32.31
    20-29 percent third degree T32.32
    30-39 percent third degree T32.33
  40-49 percent (0-9 percent third degree) T32.40
  with
    10-19 percent third degree T32.41
    20-29 percent third degree T32.42
    30-39 percent third degree T32.43
    40-49 percent third degree T32.44
  50-59 percent (0-9 percent third degree) T32.50
  with
    10-19 percent third degree T32.51
    20-29 percent third degree T32.52
    30-39 percent third degree T32.53
    40-49 percent third degree T32.54
    50-59 percent third degree T32.55
  60-69 percent (0-9 percent third degree) T32.60
  with
    10-19 percent third degree T32.61
    20-29 percent third degree T32.62
    30-39 percent third degree T32.63
    40-49 percent third degree T32.64
    50-59 percent third degree T32.65
    60-69 percent third degree T32.66
  70-79 percent (0-9 percent third degree) T32.70
  with
    10-19 percent third degree T32.71
    20-29 percent third degree T32.72
    30-39 percent third degree T32.73
    40-49 percent third degree T32.74
    50-59 percent third degree T32.75
    60-69 percent third degree T32.76
    70-79 percent third degree T32.77
  80-89 percent (0-9 percent third degree) T32.80
  with
    10-19 percent third degree T32.81
    20-29 percent third degree T32.82
    30-39 percent third degree T32.83
    40-49 percent third degree T32.84
    50-59 percent third degree T32.85
    60-69 percent third degree T32.86
    70-79 percent third degree T32.87
    80-89 percent third degree T32.88
  90 percent or more (0-9 percent third degree) T32.90
  with
    10-19 percent third degree T32.91
    20-29 percent third degree T32.92
    30-39 percent third degree T32.93
    40-49 percent third degree T32.94
    50-59 percent third degree T32.95
    60-69 percent third degree T32.96
    70-79 percent third degree T32.97
    80-89 percent third degree T32.98
    90-99 percent third degree T32.99
extremity - *see* Corrosion, limb
eye(s) and adnexa T26.9-
  with resulting rupture and destruction of eyeball T26.7-
  conjunctival sac - *see* Corrosion, cornea
  cornea - *see* Corrosion, cornea
  lid - *see* Corrosion, eyelid
  periocular area - *see* Corrosion eyelid
  specified site NEC T26.8-
  eyeball - *see* Corrosion, eye eyelid(s) T26.5-
face - *see* Corrosion, head finger T23.429
  first degree T23.529

Corrosion - *continued*
  left T23.422
    first degree T23.522
    second degree T23.622
    third degree T23.722
  multiple sites (without thumb) T23.439
    with thumb T23.449
      first degree T23.549
      left T23.442
        first degree T23.542
        second degree T23.642
        third degree T23.742
      right T23.441
        first degree T23.541
        second degree T23.641
        third degree T23.741
      second degree T23.649
      third degree T23.749
    first degree T23.539
    left T23.432
      first degree T23.532
      second degree T23.632
      third degree T23.732
    right T23.431
      first degree T23.531
      second degree T23.631
      third degree T23.731
    second degree T23.639
    third degree T23.739
  right T23.421
    first degree T23.521
    second degree T23.621
    third degree T23.721
  second degree T23.629
  third degree T23.729
flank - *see* Corrosion, abdomen
foot T25.429
  first degree T25.529
  left T25.422
    first degree T25.522
    second degree T25.622
    third degree T25.722
  multiple with ankle - *see* Corrosion, lower, limb, multiple, ankle and foot
  right T25.421
    first degree T25.521
    second degree T25.621
    third degree T25.721
  second degree T25.629
  third degree T25.729
forearm T22.419
  first degree T22.519
  left T22.412
    first degree T22.512
    second degree T22.612
    third degree T22.712
  right T22.411
    first degree T22.511
    second degree T22.611
    third degree T22.711
  second degree T22.619
  third degree T22.719
forehead T20.46
  first degree T20.56
  second degree T20.66
  third degree T20.76
fourth degree code as Corrosion, third degree, by site
full thickness skin loss
code as Corrosion, third degree, by site
gastrointestinal tract NEC T28.7
genital organs
  external
    female T21.47

Corrosion - *continued*
    first degree T21.57
    second degree T21.67
    third degree T21.77
    male T21.46
      first degree T21.56
      second degree T21.66
      third degree T21.76
  internal T28.8
groin - *see* Corrosion, abdominal wall
hand(s) T23.409
  back - *see* Corrosion, dorsum of hand
  finger - *see* Corrosion, finger
  first degree T23.509
  left T23.402
    first degree T23.502
    second degree T23.602
    third degree T23.702
  multiple sites with wrist T23.499
    first degree T23.599
    left T23.492
      first degree T23.592
      second degree T23.692
      third degree T23.792
    right T23.491
      first degree T23.591
      second degree T23.691
      third degree T23.791
    second degree T23.699
    third degree T23.799
  palm - *see* Corrosion, palm
  right T23.401
    first degree T23.501
    second degree T23.601
    third degree T23.701
  second degree T23.609
  third degree T23.709
  thumb - *see* Corrosion, thumb
head (and face) (and neck) T20.40
  cheek - *see* Corrosion, cheek
  chin - *see* Corrosion, chin
  ear - *see* Corrosion, ear
  eye(s) only - *see* Corrosion, eye
  first degree T20.50
  forehead - *see* Corrosion, forehead
  lip - *see* Corrosion, lip
  multiple sites T20.49
    first degree T20.59
    second degree T20.69
    third degree T20.79
  neck - *see* Corrosion, neck
  nose - *see* Corrosion, nose
  scalp - *see* Corrosion, scalp
  second degree T20.60
  third degree T20.70
hip(s) - *see* Corrosion, lower, limb
inhalation - *see* Corrosion, respiratory tract
internal organ(s) - *see also* Corrosion, by site T28.90
  alimentary tract T28.7
    esophagus T28.6
  esophagus T28.6
  genitourinary T28.8
  mouth T28.5
  pharynx T28.5
  specified organ NEC T28.99
interscapular region - *see* Corrosion, back, upper
intestine (large) (small) T28.7
knee T24.429
  first degree T24.529
  left T24.422
    first degree T24.522
    second degree T24.622

Corrosion - *continued*

third degree T24.722
  right T24.421
    first degree T24.521
    second degree T24.621
    third degree T24.721
  second degree T24.629
  third degree T24.729
labium (majus) (minus) - *see* Corrosion, genital organs, external, female
lacrimal apparatus, duct, gland or sac - *see* Corrosion, eye, specified site NEC
larynx T27.4
  with lung T27.5
leg(s) (meaning lower limb(s)) - *see* Corrosion, lower limb
limb(s)
  lower - *see* Corrosion, lower, limb
  upper - *see* Corrosion, upper limb
lip(s) T20.42
  first degree T20.52
  second degree T20.62
  third degree T20.72
lower
  back - *see* Corrosion, back
  limb T24.409
    ankle - *see* Corrosion, ankle
    calf - *see* Corrosion, calf
    first degree T24.509
    foot - *see* Corrosion, foot
    knee - *see* Corrosion, knee
    left T24.402
      first degree T24.502
      second degree T24.602
      third degree T24.702
    multiple sites, except ankle and foot T24.499
      ankle and foot T25.499
        first degree T25.599
        left T25.492
          first degree T25.592
          second degree T25.692
          third degree T25.792
        right T25.491
          first degree T25.591
          second degree T25.691
          third degree T25.791
        second degree T25.699
        third degree T25.799
      first degree T24.599
      left T24.492
        first degree T24.592
        second degree T24.692
        third degree T24.792
      right T24.491
        first degree T24.591
        second degree T24.691
        third degree T24.791
      second degree T24.699
      third degree T24.799
    right T24.401
      first degree T24.501
      second degree T24.601
      third degree T24.701
    second degree T24.609
    hip - *see* Corrosion, thigh
    thigh - *see* Corrosion, thigh
    third degree T24.709
lung (with larynx and trachea) T27.5
mouth T28.5
neck T20.47
  first degree T20.57
  second degree T20.67
  third degree T20.77

Corrosion - *continued*

nose (septum) T20.44
  first degree T20.54
  second degree T20.64
  third degree T20.74
ocular adnexa - *see* Corrosion, eye orbit
region - *see* Corrosion, eyelid
palm T23.459
  first degree T23.559
  left T23.452
    first degree T23.552
    second degree T23.652
    third degree T23.752
  right T23.451
    first degree T23.551
    second degree T23.651
    third degree T23.751
  second degree T23.659
  third degree T23.759
partial thickness
  code as Corrosion, unspecified degree, by site
pelvis - *see* Corrosion, trunk
penis - *see* Corrosion, genital organs, external, male
perineum
  female - *see* Corrosion, genital organs, external, female
  male - *see* Corrosion, genital organs, external, male
periocular area - *see* Corrosion, eyelid
pharynx T28.5
rectum T28.7
respiratory tract T27.7
  larynx - *see* Corrosion, larynx
  specified part NEC T27.6
  trachea - *see* Corrosion, larynx
sac, lacrimal - *see* Corrosion, eye, specified site NEC
scalp T20.45
  first degree T20.55
  second degree T20.65
  third degree T20.75
scapular region T22.469
  first degree T22.569
  left T22.462
    first degree T22.562
    second degree T22.662
    third degree T22.762
  right T22.461
    first degree T22.561
    second degree T22.661
    third degree T22.761
  second degree T22.669
  third degree T22.769
sclera - *see* Corrosion, eye, specified site NEC
scrotum - *see* Corrosion, genital organs, external, male
shoulder T22.459
  first degree T22.559
  left T22.452
    first degree T22.552
    second degree T22.652
    third degree T22.752
  right T22.451
    first degree T22.551
    second degree T22.651
    third degree T22.751
  second degree T22.659
  third degree T22.759
stomach T28.7
temple - *see* Corrosion, head
testis - *see* Corrosion, genital organs, external, male
thigh T24.419

Corrosion - *continued*

first degree T24.519
  left T24.412
    first degree T24.512
    second degree T24.612
    third degree T24.712
  right T24.411
    first degree T24.511
    second degree T24.611
    third degree T24.711
  second degree T24.619
  third degree T24.719
thorax (external) - *see* Corrosion, trunk
throat (meaning pharynx) T28.5
thumb(s) T23.419
  first degree T23.519
  left T23.412
    first degree T23.512
    second degree T23.612
    third degree T23.712
  multiple sites with fingers T23.449
    first degree T23.549
    left T23.442
      first degree T23.542
      second degree T23.642
      third degree T23.742
    right T23.441
      first degree T23.541
      second degree T23.641
      third degree T23.741
    second degree T23.649
    third degree T23.749
  right T23.411
    first degree T23.511
    second degree T23.611
    third degree T23.711
  second degree T23.619
  third degree T23.719
toe T25.439
  first degree T25.539
  left T25.432
    first degree T25.532
    second degree T25.632
    third degree T25.732
  right T25.431
    first degree T25.531
    second degree T25.631
    third degree T25.731
  second degree T25.639
  third degree T25.739
tongue T28.5
tonsil(s) T28.5
total body - *see* Corrosion, multiple body regions
trachea T27.4
  with lung T27.5
trunk T21.40
  abdominal wall - *see* Corrosion, abdominal wall
  anus - *see* Corrosion, buttock
  axilla - *see* Corrosion, upper limb
  back - *see* Corrosion, back
  breast - *see* Corrosion, chest wall
  buttock - *see* Corrosion, buttock
  chest wall - *see* Corrosion, chest wall
  first degree T21.50
  flank - *see* Corrosion, abdominal wall
  genital
    female - *see* Corrosion, genital organs, external, female
    male - *see* Corrosion, genital organs, external, male
  groin - *see* Corrosion, abdominal wall
  interscapular region - *see* Corrosion, back,

Corrosion - *continued*
upper
labia - *see* Corrosion, genital organs,
external, female
lower back - *see* Corrosion, back
penis - *see* Corrosion, genital organs,
external, male
perineum
female - *see* Corrosion, genital organs,
external, female
male - *see* Corrosion, genital organs,
external, male
scapular region - *see* Corrosion, upper limb
scrotum - *see* Corrosion, genital organs,
external, male
second degree T21.60
shoulder - *see* Corrosion, upper limb
specified site NEC T21.49
first degree T21.59
second degree T21.69
third degree T21.79
testes - *see* Corrosion, genital organs,
external, male
third degree T21.70
upper back - *see* Corrosion, back, upper
vagina T28.8
vulva - *see* Corrosion, genital organs,
external, female
unspecified site with extent of body surface
involved specified
less than 10 percent T32.0
10-19 percent (0-9 percent third degree)
T32.10
with 10-19 percent third degree T32.11
20-29 percent (0-9 percent third degree)
T32.20
with
10-19 percent third degree T32.21
20-29 percent third degree T32.22
30-39 percent (0-9 percent third degree)
T32.30
with
10-19 percent third degree T32.31
20-29 percent third degree T32.32
30-39 percent third degree T32.33
40-49 percent (0-9 percent third degree)
T32.40
with
10-19 percent third degree T32.41
20-29 percent third degree T32.42
30-39 percent third degree T32.43
40-49 percent third degree T32.44
50-59 percent (0-9 percent third degree)
T32.50
with
10-19 percent third degree T32.51
20-29 percent third degree T32.52
30-39 percent third degree T32.53
40-49 percent third degree T32.54
50-59 percent third degree T32.55
60-69 percent (0-9 percent third degree)
T32.60
with
10-19 percent third degree T32.61
20-29 percent third degree T32.62
30-39 percent third degree T32.63
40-49 percent third degree T32.64
50-59 percent third degree T32.65
60-69 percent third degree T32.66
70-79 percent (0-9 percent third degree)
T32.70
with
10-19 percent third degree T32.71
20-29 percent third degree T32.72

Corrosion - *continued*
30-39 percent third degree T32.73
40-49 percent third degree T32.74
50-59 percent third degree T32.75
60-69 percent third degree T32.76
70-79 percent third degree T32.77
80-89 percent (0-9 percent third degree)
T32.80
with
10-19 percent third degree T32.81
20-29 percent third degree T32.82
30-39 percent third degree T32.83
40-49 percent third degree T32.84
50-59 percent third degree T32.85
60-69 percent third degree T32.86
70-79 percent third degree T32.87
80-89 percent third degree T32.88
90 percent or more (0-9 percent third
degree) T32.90
with
10-19 percent third degree T32.91
20-29 percent third degree T32.92
30-39 percent third degree T32.93
40-49 percent third degree T32.94
50-59 percent third degree T32.95
60-69 percent third degree T32.96
70-79 percent third degree T32.97
80-89 percent third degree T32.98
90-99 percent third degree T32.99
upper limb (axilla) (scapular region) T22.40
above elbow - *see* Corrosion, above elbow
axilla - *see* Corrosion, axilla
elbow - *see* Corrosion, elbow
first degree T22.50
forearm - *see* Corrosion, forearm
hand - *see* Corrosion, hand
interscapular region - *see* Corrosion, back,
upper
multiple sites T22.499
first degree T22.599
left T22.492
first degree T22.592
second degree T22.692
third degree T22.792
right T22.491
first degree T22.591
second degree T22.691
third degree T22.791
second degree T22.699
third degree T22.799
scapular region - *see* Corrosion, scapular
region
second degree T22.60
shoulder - *see* Corrosion, shoulder
third degree T22.70
wrist - *see* Corrosion, hand
uterus T28.8
vagina T28.8
vulva - *see* Corrosion, genital organs, external,
female
wrist T23.479
first degree T23.579
left T23.472
first degree T23.572
second degree T23.672
third degree T23.772
multiple sites with hand T23.499
first degree T23.599
left T23.492
first degree T23.592
second degree T23.692
third degree T23.792
right T23.491
first degree T23.591

Corrosion - *continued*
second degree T23.691
third degree T23.791
second degree T23.699
third degree T23.799
right T23.471
first degree T23.571
second degree T23.671
third degree T23.771
second degree T23.679
third degree T23.779
Corrosive burn - *see* Corrosion
Corsican fever - *see* Malaria
Cortical - *see* condition
Cortico-adrenal - *see* condition
Coryza (acute) J00
with grippe or influenza - *see* Influenza, with,
respiratory manifestations NEC
syphilitic
congenital (chronic) A50.05
Costen's syndrome or complex M26.69
Costiveness - *see* Constipation
Costochondritis M94.0
Cotard's syndrome F22
Cot death R99
Cotia virus B08.8
Cotton wool spots (retinal) H35.81
Cotugno's disease - *see* Sciatica
Cough (affected) (chronic) (epidemic)
(nervous) R05
with hemorrhage - *see* Hemoptysis
bronchial R05
with grippe or influenza - *see* Influenza, with,
respiratory manifestations NEC
functional F45.8
hysterical F45.8
laryngeal, spasmodic R05
psychogenic F45.8
smokers' J41.0
tea taster's B49
Counseling (for) Z71.9
abuse NEC
perpetrator Z69.82
victim Z69.81
alcohol abuser Z71.41
family Z71.42
child abuse
nonparental
perpetrator Z69.021
victim Z69.020
parental
perpetrator Z69.011
victim Z69.010
consanguinity Z71.89
contraceptive Z30.09
dietary Z71.3
drug abuser Z71.51
family member Z71.52
exercise Z71.82
family Z71.89
fertility preservation (prior to cancer therapy)
(prior to removal of gonads) Z31.62
for non-attending third party Z71.0
related to sexual behavior or orientation
Z70.2
genetic
nonprocreative Z71.83
procreative NEC Z31.5
gestational carrier Z31.7
health (advice) (education) (instruction) - *see*
Counseling, medical
human immunodeficiency virus (HIV) Z71.7
impotence Z70.1
insulin pump use Z46.81

Counseling - *continued*
  medical (for) Z71.9
    boarding school resident Z59.3
    consanguinity Z71.89
    feared complaint and no disease found Z71.1
    human immunodeficiency virus (HIV) Z71.7
    institutional resident Z59.3
    on behalf of another Z71.0
      related to sexual behavior or orientation Z70.2
    person living alone Z60.2
    specified reason NEC Z71.89
  natural family planning
    procreative Z31.61
    to avoid pregnancy Z30.02
  perpetrator (of)
    abuse NEC Z69.82
    child abuse
      non-parental Z69.021
      parental Z69.011
    rape NEC Z69.82
    spousal abuse Z69.12
  procreative NEC Z31.69
    fertility preservation (prior to cancer therapy) (prior to removal of gonads) Z31.62
    using natural family planning Z31.61
  promiscuity Z70.1
  rape victim Z69.81
  religious Z71.81
  sex, sexual (related to) Z70.9
    attitude(s) Z70.0
    behavior or orientation Z70.1
    combined concerns Z70.3
    non-responsiveness Z70.1
    on behalf of third party Z70.2
    specified reason NEC Z70.8
  specified reason NEC Z71.89
  spiritual Z71.81
  spousal abuse (perpetrator) Z69.12
    victim Z69.11
  substance abuse Z71.89
    alcohol Z71.41
    drug Z71.51
    tobacco Z71.6
  tobacco use Z71.6
  use (of)
    insulin pump Z46.81
  victim (of)
    abuse Z69.81
    child abuse
      by parent Z69.010
      non-parental Z69.020
    rape NEC Z69.81
Coupled rhythm R00.8
Couvelaire syndrome or uterus (complicating delivery) O45.8X-
Cowperitis - *see* Urethritis
Cowper's gland - *see* condition
Cowpox B08.010
  due to vaccination T88.1
Coxa
  magna M91.4-
  plana M91.2-
  valga (acquired) - *see also* Deformity, limb, specified type NEC, thigh
    congenital Q65.81
    sequelae (late effect) of rickets E64.3
  vara (acquired) - *see also* Deformity, limb, specified type NEC, thigh
    congenital Q65.82
    sequelae (late effect) of rickets E64.3
Coxalgia, coxalgic (nontuberculous) - *see also* Pain, joint, hip
  tuberculous A18.02

Coxitis - *see* Monoarthritis, hip
Coxsackie (virus) (infection) B34.1
  as cause of disease classified elsewhere B97.11
  carditis B33.20
  central nervous system NEC A88.8
  endocarditis B33.21
  enteritis A08.39
  meningitis (aseptic) A87.0
  myocarditis B33.22
  pericarditis B33.23
  pharyngitis B08.5
  pleurodynia B33.0
  specific disease NEC B33.8
Crabs, meaning pubic lice B85.3
Crack baby P04.41
Cracked nipple N64.0
  associated with
    lactation O92.13
    pregnancy O92.11-
    puerperium O92.12
Cracked tooth K03.81
Cradle cap L21.0
Craft neurosis F48.8
Cramp(s) R25.2
  abdominal - *see* Pain, abdominal
  bathing T75.1
  colic R10.83
    psychogenic F45.8
  due to immersion T75.1
  fireman T67.2
  heat T67.2
  immersion T75.1
  intestinal - *see* Pain, abdominal
    psychogenic F45.8
  leg, sleep related G47.62
  limb (lower) (upper) NEC R25.2
    sleep related G47.62
  linotypist's F48.8
    organic G25.89
  muscle (limb) (general) R25.2
    due to immersion T75.1
    psychogenic F45.8
  occupational (hand) F48.8
    organic G25.89
  salt-depletion E87.1
  sleep related, leg G47.62
  stoker's T67.2
  swimmer's T75.1
  telegrapher's F48.8
    organic G25.89
  typist's F48.8
    organic G25.89
  uterus N94.89
    menstrual - *see* Dysmenorrhea
  writer's F48.8
    organic G25.89
Cranial - *see* condition
Craniocleidodysostosis Q74.0
Craniofenestria (skull) Q75.8
Craniolacunia (skull) Q75.8
Craniopagus Q89.4
Craniopathy, metabolic M85.2
Craniopharyngeal - *see* condition
Craniopharyngioma D44.4
Craniorachischisis (totalis) Q00.1
Cranioschisis Q75.8
Craniostenosis Q75.0
Craniosynostosis Q75.0
Craniotabes (cause unknown) M83.8
  neonatal P96.3
  rachitic E64.3
  syphilitic A50.56

Cranium - *see* condition
Craw-craw - *see* Onchocerciasis
Creaking joint - *see* Derangement, joint, specified type NEC
Creeping
  eruption B76.9
  palsy or paralysis G12.22
Crenated tongue K14.8
Creotoxism A05.9
Crepitus
  caput Q75.8
  joint - *see* Derangement, joint, specified type NEC
Crescent or conus choroid, congenital Q14.3
CREST syndrome M34.1
Cretin, cretinism (congenital) (endemic) (nongoitrous) (sporadic) E00.9
  pelvis
    with disproportion (fetopelvic) O33.0
      causing obstructed labor O65.0
  type
    hypothyroid E00.1
    mixed E00.2
    myxedematous E00.1
    neurological E00.0
Creutzfeldt-Jakob disease or syndrome (with dementia) A81.00
  familial A81.09
  iatrogenic A81.09
  specified NEC A81.09
  sporadic A81.09
  variant (vCJD) A81.01
Crib death R99
Cribriform hymen Q52.3
Cri-du-chat syndrome Q93.4
Crigler Najjar disease or syndrome E80.5
Crime, victim of Z65.4
Crimean hemorrhagic fever A98.0
Criminalism F60.2
Crisis
  abdomen R10.0
  acute reaction F43.0
  addisonian E27.2
  adrenal (cortical) E27.2
  celiac K90.0
  Dietl's N13.8
  emotional - *see also* Disorder, adjustment
    acute reaction to stress F43.0
    specific to childhood and adolescence F93.8
  glaucomatocyclitic - *see* Glaucoma, secondary, inflammation
  heart - *see* Failure, heart
  nitritoid I95.2
    correct substance properly administered - *see* Table of Drugs and Chemicals, by drug, adverse effect
    overdose or wrong substance given or taken - *see* Table of Drugs and Chemicals, by drug, poisoning
  oculogyric H51.8
    psychogenic F45.8
  Pel's (tabetic) A52.11
  psychosexual identity F64.2
  renal N28.0
  sickle-cell D57.00
    with
      acute chest syndrome D57.01
      splenic sequestration D57.02
  state (acute reaction) F43.0
  tabetic A52.11
  thyroid - *see* Thyrotoxicosis with thyroid storm
  thyrotoxic - *see* Thyrotoxicosis with thyroid storm

Crocq's disease (acrocyanosis) I73.89
Crohn's disease - see Enteritis, regional
Crooked septum, nasal J34.2
Cross syndrome E70.328
Crossbite (anterior) (posterior) M26.24
Cross-eye - see Strabismus, convergent
  concomitant
Croup, croupous (catarrhal) (infectious)
  (inflammatory) (non diphtheritic) J05.0
  bronchial J20.9
  diphtheritic A36.2
  false J38.5
  spasmodic J38.5
    diphtheritic A36.2
  stridulous J38.5
    diphtheritic A36.2
Crouzon's disease Q75.1
Crowding, tooth, teeth, fully erupted M26.31
CRST syndrome M34.1
Cruchet's disease A85.8
Cruelty in children - see also Disorder,
  conduct
Crural ulcer - see Ulcer, lower limb
Crush, crushed, crushing T14.8
  abdomen S38.1
  ankle S97.0-
  arm (upper) (and shoulder) S47.   axilla - see
    Crush, arm
  back, lower S38.1
  buttock S38.1
  cheek S07.0
  chest S28.0
  cranium S07.1
  ear S07.0
  elbow S57.0-
  extremity
    lower
      ankle - see Crush, ankle
      below knee - see Crush, leg
      foot - see Crush, foot
      hip - see Crush, hip
      knee - see Crush, knee
      thigh - see Crush, thigh
      toe - see Crush, toe
    upper
      below elbow S67.9-
      elbow - see Crush, elbow
      finger - see Crush, finger
      forearm - see Crush, forearm
      hand - see Crush, hand
      thumb - see Crush, thumb
      upper arm - see Crush, arm
      wrist - see Crush, wrist
  face S07.0
  finger(s) S67.1-
    with hand (and wrist) - see Crush, hand,
      specified site NEC
    index S67.19-
    little S67.19-
    middle S67.19-
    ring S67.19-
    thumb - see Crush, thumb
  foot S97.8-
    toe - see Crush, toe   forearm S57.8-
  genitalia, external
    female S38.002
      vagina S38.03
      vulva S38.03
    male S38.001
      penis S38.01
      scrotum S38.02
      testis S38.02
  hand (except fingers alone) S67.2-
    with wrist S67.4-

Crush, crushed, crushing - continued
  head S07.9
    specified NEC S07.8
  heel - see Crush, foot
  hip S77.0-
    with thigh S77.2-
  internal organ (abdomen, chest, or pelvis)
    NEC T14.8
  knee S87.0-
  labium (majus) (minus) S38.03
  larynx S17.0
  leg (lower) S87.8-
    knee - see Crush, knee   lip S07.0
  lower
    back S38.1
    leg - see Crush, leg
  neck S17.9
  nerve - see Injury, nerve
  nose S07.0
  pelvis S38.1
  penis S38.01
  scalp S07.8
  scapular region - see Crush, arm
  scrotum S38.02
  severe, unspecified site T14.8
  shoulder (and upper arm) - see Crush, arm
  skull S07.1
  syndrome (complication of trauma) T79.5
  testis S38.02
  thigh S77.1-
    with hip S77.2-
  throat S17.8
  thumb S67.0-
    with hand (and wrist) - see Crush, hand,
      specified site NEC
  toe(s) S97.10-
    great S97.11-
    lesser S97.12-
  trachea S17.0
  vagina S38.03
  vulva S38.03
  wrist S67.3-
    with hand S67.4-
Crusta lactea L21.0
Crusts R23.4
Crutch paralysis - see Injury, brachial plexus
Cruveilhier-Baumgarten cirrhosis, disease or
  syndrome K74.69
Cruveilhier's atrophy or disease G12.8
Crying (constant) (continuous) (excessive)
  child, adolescent, or adult R45.83
  infant (baby) (newborn) R68.11
Cryofibrinogenemia D89.2
Cryoglobulinemia (essential) (idiopathic)
  (mixed) (primary) (purpura) (secondary)
  (vasculitis) D89.1
  with lung involvement D89.1 [J99]
Cryptitis (anal) (rectal) K62.89
Cryptococcosis, cryptococcus (infection)
  (neoformans) B45.9
  bone B45.3
  cerebral B45.1
  cutaneous B45.2
  disseminated B45.7
  generalized B45.7
  meningitis B45.1
  meningocerebralis B45.1
  osseous B45.3
  pulmonary B45.0
  skin B45.2
  specified NEC B45.8
Cryptopapillitis (anus) K62.89

Cryptophthalmos Q11.2
  syndrome Q87.0
Cryptorchid, cryptorchism, cryptorchidism
  Q53.9
  bilateral Q53.20
    abdominal Q53.211
    perineal Q53.22
  unilateral Q53.10
    abdominal Q53.111
    perineal Q53.12
Cryptosporidiosis A07.2
  hepatobiliary B88.8
  respiratory B88.8
Cryptostromosis J67.6
Crystalluria R82.99
Cubitus
  congenital Q68.8
  valgus (acquired) M21.0-
    congenital Q68.8
    sequelae (late effect) of rickets E64.3
  varus (acquired) M21.1-
    congenital Q68.8
    sequelae (late effect) of rickets E64.3
Cultural deprivation or shock Z60.3
Curling esophagus K22.4
Curling's ulcer - see Ulcer, peptic, acute
Curschmann (-batten) (-Steinert) disease or
  syndrome G71.11
Curse, Ondine's - see Apnea, sleep
Curvature
  organ or site, congenital NEC - see Distortion
  penis (lateral) Q55.61
  Pott's (spinal) A18.01
  radius, idiopathic, progressive (congenital)
    Q74.0
  spine (acquired) (angular) (idiopathic)
    (incorrect) (postural) - see Dorsopathy,
    deforming
    congenital Q67.5
    due to or associated with
      Charcot-Marie-tooth disease - see also
        subcategory M49.8 G60.0
      osteitis
        deformans M88.88
        fibrosa cystica - see also subcategory
          M49.8 E21.0
      tuberculosis (Pott's curvature) A18.01
    sequelae (late effect) of rickets E64.3
    tuberculous A18.01
Cushingoid due to steroid therapy E24.2
  correct substance properly administered - see
    Table of Drugs and Chemicals, by drug,
    adverse effect
  overdose or wrong substance given or taken -
    see Table of Drugs and Chemicals, by drug,
    poisoning
Cushing's
  syndrome or disease E24.9
    drug-induced E24.2
    iatrogenic E24.2
    pituitary-dependent E24.0
    specified NEC E24.8
  ulcer - see Ulcer, peptic, acute
Cusp, Carabelli   omit code
Cut (external) - see also Laceration
  muscle - see Injury, muscle
Cutaneous - see also condition
  hemorrhage R23.3
  larva migrans B76.9
Cutis - see also condition
  hyperelastica Q82.8
    acquired L57.4
  laxa (hyperelastica) - see Dermatolysis
  marmorata R23.8

Cutis - *continued*
osteosis L94.2
pendula - *see* Dermatolysis
rhomboidalis nuchae L57.2
verticis gyrata Q82.8
acquired L91.8
Cyanosis R23.0
due to
patent foramen botalli Q21.1
persistent foramen ovale Q21.1
enterogenous D74.8
paroxysmal digital - *see* Raynaud's disease
with gangrene I73.01
retina, retinal H35.89
Cyanotic heart disease I24.9
congenital Q24.9
Cycle
anovulatory N97.0
menstrual, irregular N92.6
Cyclencephaly Q04.9
Cyclical vomiting - *see also* Vomiting, cyclical
G43.A0
psychogenic F50.89
Cyclitis - *see also* Iridocyclitis H20.9
chronic - *see* Iridocyclitis, chronic
Fuchs' heterochromic H20.81-
granulomatous - *see* Iridocyclitis, chronic
lens-induced - *see* Iridocyclitis, lens-induced
posterior H30.2-
Cycloid personality F34.0
Cyclophoria H50.54
Cyclopia, cyclops Q87.0
Cyclopism Q87.0
Cyclosporiasis A07.4
Cyclothymia F34.0
Cyclothymic personality F34.0
Cyclotropia H50.41-
Cylindroma - *see also* Neoplasm, malignant, by
site
eccrine dermal - *see* Neoplasm, skin, benign
skin - *see* Neoplasm, skin, benign
Cylindruria R82.99
Cynanche
diphtheritic A36.2
tonsillaris J36
Cynophobia F40.218
Cynorexia R63.2
Cyphosis - *see* Kyphosis
Cyprus fever - *see* Brucellosis
Cyst (colloid) (mucous) (simple) (retention)
adenoid (infected) J35.8
adrenal gland E27.8
congenital Q89.1
air, lung J98.4
allantoic Q64.4
alveolar process (jaw bone) M27.40
amnion, amniotic O41.8X-
aneurysmal M27.49
anterior
chamber (eye) - *see* Cyst, iris
nasopalatine K09.1
antrum J34.1
anus K62.89
apical (tooth) (periodontal) K04.8
appendix K38.8
arachnoid, brain (acquired) G93.0
congenital Q04.6
arytenoid J38.7
Baker's M71.2-
ruptured M66.0
tuberculous A18.02
Bartholin's gland N75.0
bile duct (common) (hepatic) K83.5
bladder (multiple) (trigone) N32.89

Cyst - *continued*
blue dome (breast) - *see* Cyst, breast
bone (local) NEC M85.60
aneurysmal M85.50
ankle M85.57-
foot M85.57-
forearm M85.53-
hand M85.54-
jaw M27.49
lower leg M85.56-
multiple site M85.59
neck M85.58
rib M85.58
shoulder M85.51-
skull M85.58
specified site NEC M85.58
thigh M85.55-
toe M85.57-
upper arm M85.52-
vertebra M85.58
solitary M85.40
ankle M85.47-
fibula M85.46-
foot M85.47-
hand M85.44-
humerus M85.42-
jaw M27.49
neck M85.48
pelvis M85.45-
radius M85.43-
rib M85.48
shoulder M85.41-
skull M85.48
specified site NEC M85.48
tibia M85.46-
toe M85.47-
ulna M85.43-
vertebra M85.48
specified type NEC M85.60
ankle M85.67-
foot M85.67-
forearm M85.63-
hand M85.64-
jaw M27.40
developmental (nonodontogenic) K09.1
odontogenic K09.0
latent M27.0
lower leg M85.66-
multiple site M85.69
neck M85.68
rib M85.68
shoulder M85.61-
skull M85.68
specified site NEC M85.68
thigh M85.65-
toe M85.67-
upper arm M85.62-
vertebra M85.68
brain (acquired) G93.0
congenital Q04.6
hydatid B67.99 [*G94*]
third ventricle (colloid), congenital Q04.6
branchial (cleft) Q18.0
branchiogenic Q18.0
breast (benign) (blue dome) (pedunculated)
(solitary) N60.0-
involution - *see* Dysplasia, mammary,
specified type NEC
sebaceous - *see* Dysplasia, mammary,
specified type NEC
broad ligament (benign) N83.8
bronchogenic (mediastinal) (sequestration)
J98.4
congenital Q33.0

Cyst - *continued*
buccal K09.8
bulbourethral gland N36.8
bursa, bursal NEC M71.30
with rupture - *see* Rupture, synovium
ankle M71.37-
elbow M71.32-
foot M71.37-
hand M71.34-
hip M71.35-
multiple sites M71.39
pharyngeal J39.2
popliteal space - *see* Cyst, Baker's
shoulder M71.31-
specified site NEC M71.38
wrist M71.33-
calcifying odontogenic D16.5
upper jaw (bone) (maxilla) D16.4
canal of Nuck (female) N94.89
congenital Q52.4
canthus - *see* Cyst, conjunctiva
carcinomatous - *see* Neoplasm, malignant, by
site
cauda equina G95.89
cavum septi pellucidi - *see* Cyst, brain
celomic (pericardium) Q24.8
cerebellopontine (angle) - *see* Cyst, brain
cerebellum - *see* Cyst, brain
cerebral - *see* Cyst, brain
cervical lateral Q18.0
cervix NEC N88.8
embryonic Q51.6
nabothian N88.8
chiasmal optic NEC - *see* Disorder, optic,
chiasm
chocolate (ovary) N80.1
choledochus, congenital Q44.4
chorion O41.8X-
choroid plexus G93.0
ciliary body - *see* Cyst, iris
clitoris N90.7
colon K63.89
common (bile) duct K83.5
congenital NEC Q89.8
adrenal gland Q89.1
epiglottis Q31.8
esophagus Q39.8
fallopian tube Q50.4
kidney Q61.00
more than one (multiple) Q61.02
specified as polycystic Q61.3
adult type Q61.2
infantile type NEC Q61.19
collecting duct dilation Q61.11
solitary Q61.01
larynx Q31.8
liver Q44.6
lung Q33.0
mediastinum Q34.1
ovary Q50.1
oviduct Q50.4
periurethral (tissue) Q64.79
prepuce Q55.69
salivary gland (any) Q38.4
sublingual Q38.6
submaxillary gland Q38.6
thymus (gland) Q89.2
tongue Q38.3
ureterovesical orifice Q62.8
vulva Q52.79
conjunctiva H11.44-
cornea H18.89-
corpora quadrigemina G93.0
corpus

Cyst - *continued*
  albicans N83.29-
    luteum (hemorrhagic) (ruptured) N83.1-
  Cowper's gland (benign) (infected) N36.8
  cranial meninges G93.0
  craniobuccal pouch E23.6
  craniopharyngeal pouch E23.6
  cystic duct K82.8
  Cysticercus - *see* Cysticercosis
  Dandy-Walker Q03.1
    with spina bifida - *see* Spina bifida
  dental (root) K04.8
    developmental K09.0
    eruption K09.0
    primordial K09.0
  dentigerous (mandible) (maxilla) K09.0
  dermoid - *see* Neoplasm, benign, by site
    with malignant transformation C56.-
    implantation
      external area or site (skin) NEC L72.0
      iris - *see* Cyst, iris, implantation
      vagina N89.8
      vulva N90.7
    mouth K09.8
    oral soft tissue K09.8
    sacrococcygeal - *see* Cyst, pilonidal
  developmental K09.1
    odontogenic K09.0
    oral region (nonodontogenic) K09.1
    ovary, ovarian Q50.1
  dura (cerebral) G93.0
    spinal G96.19
  ear (external) Q18.1
  echinococcal - *see* Echinococcus
  embryonic
    cervix uteri Q51.6
    fallopian tube Q50.4
    vagina Q52.4
  endometrium, endometrial (uterus) N85.8
    ectopic - *see* Endometriosis
  enterogenous Q43.8
  epidermal, epidermoid (inclusion) (see also
    Cyst, skin) L72.0
    mouth K09.8
    oral soft tissue K09.8
  epididymis N50.3
  epiglottis J38.7
  epiphysis cerebri E34.8
  epithelial (inclusion) L72.0
  epoophoron Q50.5
  eruption K09.0
  esophagus K22.8
  ethmoid sinus J34.1
  external female genital organs NEC N90.7
  eye NEC H57.8
    congenital Q15.8
  eyelid (sebaceous) H02.829
    infected - *see* Hordeolum
    left H02.826
      lower H02.825
      upper H02.824
    right H02.823
      lower H02.822
      upper H02.821
  fallopian tube N83.8
    congenital Q50.4
  fimbrial (twisted) Q50.4
  fissural (oral region) K09.1
  follicle (graafian) (hemorrhagic) N83.0-
    nabothian N88.8
  follicular (atretic) (hemorrhagic) (ovarian)
    N83.0-
    dentigerous K09.0
    odontogenic K09.0

Cyst - *continued*
  skin L72.9
    specified NEC L72.8
  frontal sinus J34.1
  gallbladder K82.8
  ganglion - *see* Ganglion
  Gartner's duct Q52.4
  gingiva K09.0
  gland of Moll - *see* Cyst, eyelid
  globulomaxillary K09.1
  graafian follicle (hemorrhagic) N83.0-
  granulosal lutein (hemorrhagic) N83.1-
  hemangiomatous D18.00
    intra-abdominal D18.03
    intracranial D18.02
    skin D18.01
    specified site NEC D18.09
  hemorrhagic M27.49
  hydatid - *see also* Echinococcus B67.90
    brain B67.99 [*G94*]
    liver - *see also* Cyst, liver, hydatid B67.8
    lung NEC B67.99 [*J99*]
    Morgagni
      female Q50.5
      male (epididymal) Q55.4
        testicular Q55.29
    specified site NEC B67.99
  hymen N89.8
    embryonic Q52.4
  hypopharynx J39.2
  hypophysis, hypophyseal (duct) (recurrent)
    E23.6
    cerebri E23.6
  implantation (dermoid)
    external area or site (skin) NEC L72.0
    iris - *see* Cyst, iris, implantation
    vagina N89.8
    vulva N90.7
  incisive canal K09.1
  inclusion (epidermal) (epithelial) (epidermoid)
    (squamous) L72.0
    not of skin
    code under Cyst, by site
  intestine (large) (small) K63.89
  intracranial - *see* Cyst, brain
  intraligamentous - *see also* Disorder, ligament
    knee - *see* Derangement, knee
  intrasellar E23.6
  iris H21.309
    exudative H21.31-
    idiopathic H21.30-
    implantation H21.32-
    parasitic H21.33-
    pars plana (primary) H21.34-
      exudative H21.35-
  jaw (bone) M27.40
    aneurysmal M27.49
    hemorrhagic M27.49
    traumatic M27.49
    developmental (odontogenic) K09.0
    fissural K09.1
  joint NEC - *see* Disorder, joint, specified type
    NEC
  kidney (acquired) N28.1
    calyceal - *see* Hydronephrosis
    congenital Q61.00
    more than one (multiple) Q61.02
      specified as polycystic Q61.3
        adult type (autosomal dominant) Q61.2
        infantile type (autosomal recessive) NEC
          Q61.19
            collecting duct dilation Q61.11
    pyelogenic - *see* Hydronephrosis
    simple N28.1

Cyst - *continued*
  solitary (single) Q61.01
    acquired N28.1
  labium (majus) (minus) N90.7
    sebaceous N90.7
  lacrimal - *see also* Disorder, lacrimal system,
    specified NEC
    gland H04.13-
    passages or sac - *see* Disorder, lacrimal
  system, specified NEC
  larynx J38.7
  lateral periodontal K09.0
  lens H27.8
    congenital Q12.8
  lip (gland) K13.0
  liver (idiopathic) (simple) K76.89
    congenital Q44.6
    hydatid B67.8
      granulosus B67.0
      multilocularis B67.5
  lung J98.4
    congenital Q33.0
    giant bullous J43.9
  lutein N83.1-
  lymphangiomatous D18.1
  lymphoepithelial, oral soft tissue K09.8
  macula - *see* Degeneration, macula, hole
  malignant - *see* Neoplasm, malignant, by site
  mammary gland - *see* Cyst, breast
  mandible M27.40
    dentigerous K09.0
    radicular K04.8
  maxilla M27.40
    dentigerous K09.0
    radicular K04.8
  medial, face and neck Q18.8
  median
    anterior maxillary K09.1
    palatal K09.1
  mediastinum, congenital Q34.1
  meibomian (gland) - *see* Chalazion
    infected - *see* Hordeolum
  membrane, brain G93.0
  meninges (cerebral) G93.0
    spinal G96.19
  meniscus, knee - *see* Derangement, knee,
    meniscus, cystic
  mesentery, mesenteric K66.8
    chyle I89.8
  mesonephric duct
    female Q50.5
    male Q55.4
  milk N64.89
  Morgagni (hydatid)
    female Q50.5
    male (epididymal) Q55.4
      testicular Q55.29
  mouth K09.8
  Müllerian duct Q50.4
    appendix testis Q55.29
    cervix Q51.6
    fallopian tube Q50.4
    female Q50.4
    male Q55.29
    prostatic utricle Q55.4
    vagina (embryonal) Q52.4
  multilocular (ovary) D39.10
    benign - *see* Neoplasm, benign, by site
  myometrium N85.8
  nabothian (follicle) (ruptured) N88.8
  nasoalveolar K09.1
  nasolabial K09.1
  nasopalatine (anterior) (duct) K09.1
  nasopharynx J39.2

Cyst - *continued*
  neoplastic - *see* Neoplasm, uncertain behavior, by site
    benign - *see* Neoplasm, benign, by site
  nervous system NEC G96.8
  neuroenteric (congenital) Q06.8
  nipple - *see* Cyst, breast
  nose (turbinates) J34.1
    sinus J34.1
  odontogenic, developmental K09.0
  omentum (lesser) K66.8
    congenital Q45.8
  ora serrata - *see* Cyst, retina, ora serrata
  oral
    region K09.9
      developmental (nonodontogenic) K09.1
        specified NEC K09.8
      soft tissue K09.9
        specified NEC K09.8
  orbit H05.81-
  ovary, ovarian (twisted) N83.20-
    adherent N83.20-
    chocolate N80.1
    corpus
      albicans N83.29-
      luteum (hemorrhagic) N83.1-
    dermoid D27.9
    developmental Q50.1
    due to failure of involution NEC N83.20-
    endometrial N80.1
    follicular (graafian) (hemorrhagic) N83.0-
    hemorrhagic N83.20-
    in pregnancy or childbirth O34.8-
      with obstructed labor O65.5
    multilocular D39.10
    pseudomucinous D27.9
    retention N83.29-
    serous N83.20-
    specified NEC N83.29-
    theca lutein (hemorrhagic) N83.1-
    tuberculous A18.18
  oviduct N83.8
  palate (median) (fissural) K09.1
  palatine papilla (jaw) K09.1
  pancreas, pancreatic (hemorrhagic) (true) K86.2
    congenital Q45.2
    false K86.3
  paralabral
    hip M24.85-
    shoulder S43.43-
  paramesonephric duct Q50.4
    female Q50.4
    male Q55.29
  paranephric N28.1
  paraphysis, cerebri, congenital Q04.6
  parasitic B89
  parathyroid (gland) E21.4
  paratubal N83.8
  paraurethral duct N36.8
  paroophoron Q50.5
  parotid gland K11.6
  parovarian Q50.5
  pelvis, female N94.89
    in pregnancy or childbirth O34.8-
      causing obstructed labor O65.5
  penis (sebaceous) N48.89
  periapical K04.8
  pericardial (congenital) Q24.8
    acquired (secondary) I31.8
  pericoronal K09.0
  periodontal K04.8
    lateral K09.0
  peripelvic (lymphatic) N28.1

Cyst - *continued*
  peritoneum K66.8
    chylous I89.8
  periventricular, acquired, newborn P91.1
  pharynx (wall) J39.2
  pilar L72.11
  pilonidal (infected) (rectum) L05.91
    with abscess L05.01
    malignant C44.59-
  pituitary (duct) (gland) E23.6
  placenta O43.19-
  pleura J94.8
  popliteal - *see* Cyst, Baker's
  porencephalic Q04.6
    acquired G93.0
  postanal (infected) - *see* Cyst, pilonidal
  postmastoidectomy cavity (mucosal) - *see*
  Complications, postmastoidectomy, cyst
  preauricular Q18.1
  prepuce N47.4
    congenital Q55.69
  primordial (jaw) K09.0
  prostate N42.83
  pseudomucinous (ovary) D27.9
  pupillary, miotic H21.27-
  radicular (residual) K04.8
  radiculodental K04.8
  ranular K11.8
  Rathke's pouch E23.6
  rectum (epithelium) (mucous) K62.89
  renal - *see* Cyst, kidney
  residual (radicular) K04.8
  retention (ovary) N83.29-
    salivary gland K11.6
  retina H33.19-
    ora serrata H33.11-
    parasitic H33.12-
  retroperitoneal K68.9
  sacrococcygeal (dermoid) - *see* Cyst, pilonidal
  salivary gland or duct (mucous extravasation or retention) K11.6
  Sampson's N80.1
  sclera H15.89
  scrotum L72.9
    sebaceous L72.3
  sebaceous (duct) (gland) L72.3
    breast - *see* Dysplasia, mammary, specified type NEC
    eyelid - *see* Cyst, eyelid
    genital organ NEC
      female N94.89
      male N50.89
    scrotum L72.3
  semilunar cartilage (knee) (multiple) - *see*
  Derangement, knee, meniscus, cystic
  seminal vesicle N50.89
  serous (ovary) N83.20-
  sinus (accessory) (nasal) J34.1
  Skene's gland N36.8
  skin L72.9
    breast - *see* Dysplasia, mammary, specified type NEC
    epidermal, epidermoid L72.0
    epithelial L72.0
    eyelid - *see* Cyst, eyelid
    genital organ NEC
      female N90.7
      male N50.89
    inclusion L72.0
    scrotum L72.9
    sebaceous L72.3
    sweat gland or duct L74.8
  solitary
    bone - *see* Cyst, bone, solitary

Cyst - *continued*
  jaw M27.40
  kidney N28.1
  spermatic cord N50.89
  sphenoid sinus J34.1
  spinal meninges G96.19
  spleen NEC D73.4
    congenital Q89.09
    hydatid - *see also* Echinococcus B67.99 [*D77*]
  Stafne's M27.0
  subarachnoid intrasellar R93.0
  subcutaneous, pheomycotic (chromomycotic) B43.2
  subdural (cerebral) G93.0
    spinal cord G96.19
  sublingual gland K11.6
  submandibular gland K11.6
  submaxillary gland K11.6
  suburethral N36.8
  suprarenal gland E27.8
  suprasellar - *see* Cyst, brain
  sweat gland or duct L74.8
  synovial - *see also* Cyst, bursa
    ruptured - *see* Rupture, synovium
  tarsal - *see* Chalazion
  tendon (sheath) - *see* Disorder, tendon, specified type NEC
  testis N44.2
    tunica albuginea N44.1
  theca lutein (ovary) N83.1-
  Thornwaldt's J39.2
  thymus (gland) E32.8
  thyroglossal duct (infected) (persistent) Q89.2
  thyrolingual duct (infected) (persistent) Q89.2
  thyroid (gland) E04.1
  tongue K14.8
  tonsil J35.8
  tooth - *see* Cyst, dental
  Tornwaldt's J39.2
  trichilemmal (proliferating) L72.12
  trichodermal L72.12
  tubal (fallopian) N83.8
    inflammatory - *see* Salpingitis, chronic
  tubo-ovarian N83.8
    inflammatory N70.13
  tunica
    albuginea testis N44.1
    vaginalis N50.89
  turbinate (nose) J34.1
  Tyson's gland N48.89
  urachus, congenital Q64.4
  ureter N28.89
  ureterovesical orifice N28.89
  urethra, urethral (gland) N36.8
  uterine ligament N83.8
  uterus (body) (corpus) (recurrent) N85.8
    embryonic Q51.818
    cervix Q51.6
  vagina, vaginal (implantation) (inclusion) (squamous cell) (wall) N89.8
    embryonic Q52.4
  vallecula, vallecular (epiglottis) J38.7
  vesical (orifice) N32.89
  vitreous body H43.89
  vulva (implantation) (inclusion) N90.7
    congenital Q52.79
    sebaceous gland N90.7
  vulvovaginal gland N90.7
  wolffian
    female Q50.5
    male Q55.4

Cystadenocarcinoma - *see* Neoplasm, malignant, by site
  bile duct C22.1
  endometrioid - *see* Neoplasm, malignant, by site
    specified site - *see* Neoplasm, malignant, by site
    unspecified site
      female C56.9
      male C61
  mucinous
    papillary
      specified site - *see* Neoplasm, malignant, by site
      unspecified site C56.9
    specified site - *see* Neoplasm, malignant, by site
    unspecified site C56.9
  papillary
    mucinous
      specified site - *see* Neoplasm, malignant, by site
      unspecified site C56.9
    pseudomucinous
      specified site - *see* Neoplasm, malignant, by site
      unspecified site C56.9
    serous
      specified site - *see* Neoplasm, malignant, by site
      unspecified site C56.9
    specified site - *see* Neoplasm, malignant, by site
    unspecified site C56.9
  pseudomucinous
    papillary
      specified site - *see* Neoplasm, malignant, by site
      unspecified site C56.9
    specified site - *see* Neoplasm, malignant, by site
    unspecified site C56.9
  serous
    papillary
      specified site - *see* Neoplasm, malignant, by site
      unspecified site C56.9
    specified site - *see* Neoplasm, malignant, by site
    unspecified site C56.9
Cystadenofibroma
  clear cell - *see* Neoplasm, benign, by site
  endometrioid D27.9
    borderline malignancy D39.1-
    malignant C56.-
  mucinous
    specified site - *see* Neoplasm, benign, by site
    unspecified site D27.9
  serous
    specified site - *see* Neoplasm, benign, by site
    unspecified site D27.9
  specified site - *see* Neoplasm, benign, by site
  unspecified site D27.9
Cystadenoma - *see also* Neoplasm, benign, by site
  bile duct D13.4
  endometrioid - *see* Neoplasm, benign, by site
    borderline malignancy - *see* Neoplasm, uncertain behavior, by site
  malignant - *see* Neoplasm, malignant, by site
  mucinous
    borderline malignancy
      ovary C56.-
      specified site NEC - *see* Neoplasm,

Cystadenoma - *continued*
  uncertain behavior, by site
    unspecified site C56.9
  papillary
    borderline malignancy
      ovary C56.-
      specified site NEC - *see* Neoplasm, uncertain behavior, by site
      unspecified site C56.9
    specified site - *see* Neoplasm, benign, by site
    unspecified site D27.9
  specified site - *see* Neoplasm, benign, by site
  unspecified site D27.9
  papillary
    borderline malignancy
      ovary C56.-
      specified site NEC - *see* Neoplasm, uncertain behavior, by site
      unspecified site C56.9
    lymphomatosum
      specified site - *see* Neoplasm, benign, by site
      unspecified site D11.9
    mucinous
      borderline malignancy
        ovary C56.-
        specified site NEC - *see* Neoplasm, uncertain behavior, by site
        unspecified site C56.9
      specified site - *see* Neoplasm, benign, by site
      unspecified site D27.9
    pseudomucinous
      borderline malignancy
        ovary C56.-
        specified site NEC - *see* Neoplasm, uncertain behavior, by site
        unspecified site C56.9
      specified site - *see* Neoplasm, benign, by site
      unspecified site D27.9
    serous
      borderline malignancy
        ovary C56.-
        specified site NEC - *see* Neoplasm, uncertain behavior, by site
        unspecified site C56.9
      specified site - *see* Neoplasm, benign, by site
      unspecified site D27.9
    specified site - *see* Neoplasm, benign, by site
    unspecified site D27.9
  pseudomucinous
    borderline malignancy
      ovary C56.-
      specified site NEC - *see* Neoplasm, uncertain behavior, by site
      unspecified site C56.9
    papillary
      borderline malignancy
        ovary C56.-
        specified site NEC - *see* Neoplasm, uncertain behavior, by site
        unspecified site C56.9
      specified site - *see* Neoplasm, benign, by site
      unspecified site D27.9
    specified site - *see* Neoplasm, benign, by site
    unspecified site D27.9
  serous
    borderline malignancy
      ovary C56.-
      specified site NEC - *see* Neoplasm,

Cystadenoma - *continued*
  uncertain behavior, by site
    unspecified site C56.9
  papillary
    borderline malignancy
      ovary C56.-
      specified site NEC - *see* Neoplasm, uncertain behavior, by site
      unspecified site C56.9
    specified site - *see* Neoplasm, benign, by site
    unspecified site D27.9
  specified site - *see* Neoplasm, benign, by site
  unspecified site D27.9
Cystathionine synthase deficiency E72.11
Cystathioninemia E72.19
Cystathioninuria E72.19
Cystic - *see also* condition
  breast (chronic) - *see* Mastopathy, cystic
  corpora lutea (hemorrhagic) N83.1-
  duct - *see* condition
  eyeball (congenital) Q11.0
  fibrosis - *see* Fibrosis, cystic
  kidney (congenital) Q61.9
    adult type Q61.2
    infantile type NEC Q61.19
      collecting duct dilatation Q61.11
    medullary Q61.5
  liver, congenital Q44.6
  lung disease J98.4
    congenital Q33.0
  mastitis, chronic - *see* Mastopathy, cystic
  medullary, kidney Q61.5
  meniscus - *see* Derangement, knee, meniscus, cystic
  ovary N83.20-
Cysticercosis, cysticerciasis B69.9
  with
    epileptiform fits B69.0
    myositis B69.81
  brain B69.0
  central nervous system B69.0
  cerebral B69.0
  ocular B69.1
  specified NEC B69.89
Cysticercus cellulose infestation - *see* Cysticercosis
Cystinosis (malignant) E72.04
Cystinuria E72.01
Cystitis (exudative) (hemorrhagic) (septic) (suppurative) N30.90
  with
    fibrosis - *see* Cystitis, chronic, interstitial
    hematuria N30.91
    leukoplakia - *see* Cystitis, chronic, interstitial
    malakoplakia - *see* Cystitis, chronic, interstitial
    metaplasia - *see* Cystitis, chronic, interstitial
    prostatitis N41.3
  acute N30.00
    with hematuria N30.01
    of trigone N30.30
      with hematuria N30.31
  allergic - *see* Cystitis, specified type NEC
  amebic A06.81
  bilharzial B65.9 [*N33*]
  blennorrhagic (gonococcal) A54.01
  bullous - *see* Cystitis, specified type NEC
  calculous N21.0
  chlamydial A56.01
  chronic N30.20
    with hematuria N30.21
    interstitial N30.10

Cystitis - *continued*
>with hematuria N30.11
>of trigone N30.30
>>with hematuria N30.31
>>specified NEC N30.20
>>>with hematuria N30.21
>cystic (a) - *see* Cystitis, specified type NEC
>diphtheritic A36.85
>echinococcal
>>granulosus B67.39
>>multilocularis B67.69
>emphysematous - *see* Cystitis, specified type NEC
>encysted - *see* Cystitis, specified type NEC
>eosinophilic - *see* Cystitis, specified type NEC
>follicular - *see* Cystitis, of trigone
>gangrenous - *see* Cystitis, specified type NEC
>glandularis - *see* Cystitis, specified type NEC
>gonococcal A54.01
>incrusted - *see* Cystitis, specified type NEC
>interstitial (chronic) - *see* Cystitis, chronic, interstitial
>irradiation N30.40
>>with hematuria N30.41
>irritation - *see* Cystitis, specified type NEC
>malignant - *see* Cystitis, specified type NEC
>of trigone N30.30
>>with hematuria N30.31
>panmural - *see* Cystitis, chronic, interstitial
>polyposa - *see* Cystitis, specified type NEC
>prostatic N41.3
>puerperal (postpartum) O86.22
>radiation - *see* Cystitis, irradiation
>specified type NEC N30.80
>>with hematuria N30.81
>subacute - *see* Cystitis, chronic
>submucous - *see* Cystitis, chronic, interstitial
>syphilitic (late) A52.76
>trichomonal A59.03
>tuberculous A18.12
>ulcerative - *see* Cystitis, chronic, interstitial
Cystocele (-urethrocele)
>female N81.10
>>with prolapse of uterus - *see* Prolapse, uterus
>>lateral N81.12
>>midline N81.11
>>paravaginal N81.12
>in pregnancy or childbirth O34.8-
>>causing obstructed labor O65.5
>male N32.89
Cystolithiasis N21.0
Cystoma - *see also* Neoplasm, benign, by site
>endometrial, ovary N80.1
>mucinous
>>specified site - *see* Neoplasm, benign, by site
>>unspecified site D27.9
>serous
>>specified site - *see* Neoplasm, benign, by site
>>unspecified site D27.9
>simple (ovary) N83.29-
Cystoplegia N31.2
Cystoptosis N32.89
Cystopyelitis - *see* Pyelonephritis
Cystorrhagia N32.89
Cystosarcoma phyllodes D48.6-
>benign D24-
>malignant - *see* Neoplasm, breast, malignant
Cystostomy
>attention to Z43.5
>complication - *see* Complications, cystostomy
>status Z93.50
>>appendico-vesicostomy Z93.52
>>cutaneous Z93.51
>>specified NEC Z93.59

Cystourethritis - *see* Urethritis
Cystourethrocele - *see also* Cystocele
>female N81.10
>>with uterine prolapse - *see* Prolapse, uterus
>>lateral N81.12
>>midline N81.11
>>paravaginal N81.12
>male N32.89
Cytomegalic inclusion disease congenital P35.1
Cytomegalovirus infection B25.9
Cytomycosis (reticuloendothelial) B39.4
Cytopenia D75.9
>refractory
>>with multilineage dysplasia D46.A
>>>and ring sideroblasts (RCMD RS) D46.B
Czerny's disease (periodic hydrarthrosis of the knee) - *see* Effusion, joint, knee

D

Daae (-finsen) disease (epidemic pleurodynia) B33.0
Da Costa's syndrome F45.8
Dabney's grip B33.0
Dacryoadenitis, dacryadenitis H04.00-
>acute H04.01-
>chronic H04.02-
Dacryocystitis H04.30-
>acute H04.32-
>chronic H04.41-
>neonatal P39.1
>phlegmonous H04.31-
>syphilitic A52.71
>>congenital (early) A50.01
>trachomatous, active A71.1
>>sequelae (late effect) B94.0
Dacryocystoblennorrhea - *see* Inflammation, lacrimal, passages, chronic
Dacryocystocele - *see* Disorder, lacrimal system, changes
Dacryolith, dacryolithiasis H04.51-
Dacryoma - *see* Disorder, lacrimal system, changes
Dacryopericystitis - *see* Dacryocystitis
Dacryops H04.11-
Dacryostenosis - *see also* Stenosis, lacrimal
>congenital Q10.5
Dactylitis
>bone - *see* Osteomyelitis
>sickle-cell D57.00
>>Hb C D57.219
>>Hb SS D57.00
>>specified NEC D57.819
>skin L08.9
>syphilitic A52.77
>tuberculous A18.03
Dactylolysis spontanea (ainhum) L94.6
Dactylosymphysis Q70.9
>fingers - *see* Syndactylism, complex, fingers
>toes - *see* Syndactylism, complex, toes
Damage
>arteriosclerotic - *see* Arteriosclerosis
>brain (nontraumatic) G93.9
>>anoxic, hypoxic G93.1
>>>resulting from a procedure G97.82
>>child NEC G80.9
>>due to birth injury P11.2
>cardiorenal (vascular) - *see* Hypertension, cardiorenal
>cerebral NEC - *see* Damage, brain
>coccyx, complicating delivery O71.6
>coronary - *see* Disease, heart, ischemic
>eye, birth injury P15.3

Damage - *continued*
>liver (nontraumatic) K76.9
>>alcoholic K70.9
>>due to drugs - *see* Disease, liver, toxic
>>toxic - *see* Disease, liver, toxic
>medication T88.7
>pelvic
>>joint or ligament, during delivery O71.6
>>organ NEC
>>>during delivery O71.5
>>>following ectopic or molar pregnancy O08.6
>renal - *see* Disease, renal
>subendocardium, subendocardial - *see* Degeneration, myocardial
>vascular I99.9
Dana-Putnam syndrome (subacute combined sclerosis with pernicious anemia) - *see* Degeneration, combined
Danbolt (-cross) syndrome (acrodermatitis enteropathica) E83.2
Dandruff L21.0
Dandy-Walker syndrome Q03.1
>with spina bifida - *see* Spina bifida
Danlos' syndrome Q79.6
Darier (-White) disease (congenital) Q82.8
>meaning erythema annulare centrifugum L53.1
Darier-Roussy sarcoid D86.3
Darling's disease or histoplasmosis B39.4
Darwin's tubercle Q17.8
Dawson's (inclusion body) encephalitis A81.1
De Beurmanni (-Gougerot) disease B42.1
De la Tourette's syndrome F95.2
De Lange's syndrome Q87.1
De Morgan's spots (senile angiomas) I78.1
De Quervain's
>disease (tendon sheath) M65.4
>syndrome E34.51
>thyroiditis (subacute granulomatous thyroiditis) E06.1
De Toni-Fanconi (-Debre) syndrome E72.09
>with cystinosis E72.04
Dead
>fetus, retained (mother) O36.4
>>early pregnancy O02.1
>labyrinth - *see* subcategory H83.2
>ovum, retained O02.0
Deaf nonspeaking NEC H91.3
Deafmutism (acquired) (congenital) NEC H91.3
>hysterical F44.6
>syphilitic, congenital - *see also* subcategory H94.8 A50.09
Deafness (acquired) (complete) (hereditary) (partial) H91.9-
>with blue sclera and fragility of bone Q78.0
>auditory fatigue - *see* Deafness, specified type NEC
>aviation T70.0
>>nerve injury - *see* Injury, nerve, acoustic, specified type NEC
>boilermaker's - *see* subcategory H83.3
>central - *see* Deafness, sensorineural
>conductive H90.2
>>and sensorineural
>>>mixed H90.8
>>>>bilateral H90.6
>>bilateral H90.0
>>unilateral H90.1-
>>>with restricted hearing on the contralateral side H90.A congenital H90.5
>with blue sclera and fragility of bone Q78.0
>due to toxic agents - *see* Deafness, ototoxic
>emotional (hysterical) F44.6

Deafness - *continued*
  functional (hysterical) F44.6
  high frequency H91.9-
  hysterical F44.6
  low frequency H91.9-
  mental R48.8
  mixed conductive and sensorineural H90.8
    bilateral H90.6
    unilateral H90.7-
  nerve - *see* Deafness, sensorineural
  neural - *see* Deafness, sensorineural
  noise-induced - *see also* subcategory H83.3
    nerve injury - *see* Injury, nerve, acoustic,
    specified type NEC
  nonspeaking H91.3
  ototoxic - *see* subcategory H91.0
  perceptive - *see* Deafness, sensorineural
  psychogenic (hysterical) F44.6
  sensorineural H90.5
    and conductive
      mixed H90.8
        bilateral H90.6
    bilateral H90.3
    unilateral H90.4-
      with restricted hearing on the contralateral
      side H90.A   sensory - *see* Deafness,
      sensorineural
  specified type NEC - *see* subcategory H91.8
  sudden (idiopathic) H91.2-
  syphilitic A52.15
  transient ischemic H93.01-
  traumatic - *see* Injury, nerve, acoustic,
  specified type NEC
  word (developmental) H93.25
Death (cause unknown) (of) (unexplained)
(unspecified cause) R99
  brain G93.82
  cardiac (sudden) (with successful
  resuscitation)
  code to underlying disease
    family history of Z82.41
    personal history of Z86.74
  family member (assumed) Z63.4
Debility (chronic) (general) (nervous) R53.81
  congenital or neonatal NOS P96.9
  nervous R53.81
  old age R54
  senile R54
Debove's disease (splenomegaly) R16.1
Decalcification
  bone - *see* Osteoporosis
  teeth K03.89
Decapsulation, kidney N28.89
Decay
  dental - *see* Caries, dental
  senile R54
  tooth, teeth - *see* Caries, dental **Deciduitis**
(acute)
  following ectopic or molar pregnancy O08.0
Decline (general) - *see* Debility
  cognitive, age-associated R41.81
Decompensation
  cardiac (acute) (chronic) - *see* Disease, heart
  cardiovascular - *see* Disease, cardiovascular
  heart - *see* Disease, heart
  hepatic - *see* Failure, hepatic
  myocardial (acute) (chronic) - *see* Disease,
  heart
  respiratory J98.8
Decompression sickness T70.3
Decrease(d)
  absolute neutrophile count - *see* Neutropenia
  blood
    platelets - *see* Thrombocytopenia

Decrease(d) - *continued*
  pressure R03.1
    due to shock following
      injury T79.4
      operation T81.19
  estrogen E28.39
    postablative E89.40
      asymptomatic E89.40
      symptomatic E89.41
  fragility of erythrocytes D58.8
  function
    lipase (pancreatic) K90.3
    ovary in hypopituitarism E23.0
    parenchyma of pancreas K86.89
    pituitary (gland) (anterior) (lobe) E23.0
      posterior (lobe) E23.0
  functional activity R68.89
  glucose R73.09
  hematocrit R71.0
  hemoglobin R71.0
  leukocytes D72.819
    specified NEC D72.818
  libido R68.82
  lymphocytes D72.810
  platelets D69.6
  respiration, due to shock following injury
  T79.4
  sexual desire R68.82
  tear secretion NEC - *see* Syndrome, dry eye
  tolerance
    fat K90.49
    glucose R73.09
    pancreatic K90.3
    salt and water E87.8
  vision NEC H54.7
  white blood cell count D72.819
    specified NEC D72.818
Decubitus (ulcer) - *see* Ulcer, pressure, by site
  cervix N86
Deepening acetabulum - *see* Derangement,
joint, specified type NEC, hip
Defect, defective Q89.9
  3-beta-hydroxysteroid dehydrogenase E25.0
  11-hydroxylase E25.0
  21-hydroxylase E25.0
  abdominal wall, congenital Q79.59
  antibody immunodeficiency D80.9
  aorticopulmonary septum Q21.4
  atrial septal (ostium secundum type) Q21.1
    following acute myocardial infarction
    (current complication) I23.1
    ostium primum type Q21.2
  atrioventricular
    canal Q21.2
    septum Q21.2
  auricular septal Q21.1
  bilirubin excretion NEC E80.6
  biosynthesis, androgen (testicular) E29.1
  bulbar septum Q21.0
  catalase E80.3
  cell membrane receptor complex (CR3) D71
  circulation I99.9
    congenital Q28.9
    newborn Q28.9
  coagulation (factor) - *see also* Deficiency,
  factor D68.9
    with
      ectopic pregnancy O08.1
      molar pregnancy O08.1
    acquired D68.4
    antepartum with hemorrhage - *see*
  Hemorrhage, antepartum, with coagulation
  defect
    due to

Defect, defective - *continued*
    liver disease D68.4
      vitamin K deficiency D68.4
    hereditary NEC D68.2
    intrapartum O67.0
    newborn, transient P61.6
    postpartum O99.13
      with hemorrhage O72.3
    specified type NEC D68.8
  complement system D84.1
  conduction (heart) I45.9
    bone - *see* Deafness, conductive
  congenital, organ or site not listed - *see*
    Anomaly, by site
  coronary sinus Q21.1
  cushion, endocardial Q21.2
  degradation, glycoprotein E77.1
  dental bridge, crown, fillings - *see* Defect,
    dental restoration
  dental restoration K08.50
    specified NEC K08.59
  dentin (hereditary) K00.5
  Descemet's membrane, congenital Q13.89
  developmental - *see also* Anomaly
    cauda equina Q06.3
  diaphragm
    with elevation, eventration or hernia - *see*
    Hernia, diaphragm
    congenital Q79.1
      with hernia Q79.0
      gross (with hernia) Q79.0
  ectodermal, congenital Q82.9
  Eisenmenger's Q21.8
  enzyme
    catalase E80.3
    peroxidase E80.3
  esophagus, congenital Q39.9
  extensor retinaculum M62.89
  fibrin polymerization D68.2
  filling
    bladder R93.41
    kidney R93.42-
    renal pelvis R93.41
    stomach R93.3
    ureter R93.41
    urinary organs, specified NEC R93.49
  Gerbode Q21.0
  glycoprotein degradation E77.1
  Hageman (factor) D68.2
  hearing - *see* Deafness
  high grade F70
  interatrial septal Q21.1
  interauricular septal Q21.1
  interventricular septal Q21.0
    with dextroposition of aorta, pulmonary
    stenosis and hypertrophy of right ventricle
    Q21.3
    in tetralogy of Fallot Q21.3
  learning (specific) - *see* Disorder, learning
  lymphocyte function antigen 1 (LFA 1) D84.0
  lysosomal enzyme, post-translational
    modification E77.0
  major osseous M89.70
    ankle M89.77-
    carpus M89.74-
    clavicle M89.71-
    femur M89.75-
    fibula M89.76-
    fingers M89.74-
    foot M89.77-
    forearm M89.73-
    hand M89.74-
    humerus M89.72-
    lower leg M89.76-

Deficiency, deficient - *continued*
    vitamin K deficiency D68.4
      newborn, transient P61.6
      postpartum O72.3
      specified NEC D68.8
  cognitive F09
  color vision H53.50
    achromatopsia H53.51
    acquired H53.52
    deuteranomaly H53.53
    protanomaly H53.54
    specified type NEC H53.59
    tritanomaly H53.55
  combined glucocorticoid and
    mineralocorticoid E27.49
  contact factor D68.2
  copper (nutritional) E61.0
  corticoadrenal E27.40
    primary E27.1
  craniofacial axis Q75.0
  cyanocobalamin E53.8
  C1 esterase inhibitor (C1-iNH) D84.1
  debrancher enzyme (limit dextrinosis) E74.03
  dehydrogenase
    long chain/very long chain acyl CoA
      E71.310
    medium chain acyl CoA E71.311
    short chain acyl CoA E71.312
  diet E63.9
  dihydropyrimidine dehydrogenase (DPD)
    E88.89
  disaccharidase E73.9
  edema - *see* Malnutrition, severe
  endocrine E34.9
  energy-supply - *see* Malnutrition
  enzymes, circulating NEC E88.09
  ergosterol E55.9
    with
      adult osteomalacia M83.8
      rickets - *see* Rickets
  essential fatty acid (EFA) E63.0
  factor - *see also* Deficiency, coagulation
    Hageman D68.2
    I (congenital) (hereditary) D68.2
    II (congenital) (hereditary) D68.2
    IX (congenital) (functional) (hereditary)
      (with functional defect) D67
    multiple (congenital) D68.8
      acquired D68.4
    V (congenital) (hereditary) D68.2
    VII (congenital) (hereditary) D68.2
    VIII (congenital) (functional) (hereditary)
      (with functional defect) D66
      with vascular defect D68.0
    X (congenital) (hereditary) D68.2
    XI (congenital) (hereditary) D68.1
    XII (congenital) (hereditary) D68.2
    XIII (congenital) (hereditary) D68.2
  femoral, proximal focal (congenital) - *see*
    Defect, reduction, lower limb, longitudinal,
    femur
  fibrin-stabilizing factor (congenital)
    (hereditary) D68.2
    acquired D68.4
  fibrinase D68.2
  fibrinogen (congenital) (hereditary) D68.2
    acquired D65
  folate E53.8
  folic acid E53.8
  foreskin N47.3
  fructokinase E74.11
  fructose 1,6-diphosphatase E74.19
  fructose 1-phosphate aldolase E74.19
  galactokinase E74.29

Deficiency, deficient - *continued*
  galactose 1-phosphate uridyl transferase
    E74.29
  gammaglobulin in blood D80.1
    hereditary D80.0
  glass factor D68.2
  glucocorticoid E27.49
    mineralocorticoid E27.49
  glucose 6-phosphatase E74.01
  glucose 6-phosphate dehydrogenase anemia
    D55.0
  glucuronyl transferase E80.5
  glycogen synthetase E74.09
  gonadotropin (isolated) E23.0
  growth hormone (idiopathic) (isolated) E23.0
  Hageman factor D68.2
  hemoglobin D64.9
  hepatophosphorylase E74.09
  homogentisate 1,2-dioxygenase E70.29
  hormone
    anterior pituitary (partial) NEC E23.0
      growth E23.0
    growth (isolated) E23.0
    pituitary E23.0
    testicular E29.1
  hypoxanthine (guanine)-
    phosphoribosyltransferase (HG PRT) (total
    H-pRT) E79.1
  immunity D84.9
    cell-mediated D84.8
      with thrombocytopenia and eczema D82.0
    combined D81.9
    humoral D80.9
    IgA (secretory) D80.2
    IgG D80.3
    IgM D80.4
  immuno - *see* Immunodeficiency
  immunoglobulin, selective
    A (IgA) D80.2
    G (IgG) (subclasses) D80.3
    M (IgM) D80.4
  inositol (B complex) E53.8
  intrinsic
    factor (congenital) D51.0
    sphincter N36.42
      with urethral hypermobility N36.43
  iodine E61.8
    congenital syndrome - *see* Syndrome, iodine-
    deficiency, congenital
  iron E61.1
    anemia D50.9
  kalium E87.6
  kappa-light chain D80.8
  labile factor (congenital) (hereditary) D68.2
    acquired D68.4
  lacrimal fluid (acquired) - *see also* Syndrome,
  dry eye
    congenital Q10.6
    congenital E73.0
    secondary E73.1
  lactase
  Laki-Lorand factor D68.2
  lecithin cholesterol acyltransferase E78.6
  lipocaic K86.89
  lipoprotein (familial) (high density) E78.6
  liver phosphorylase E74.09
  lysosomal alpha 1, 4 glucosidase E74.02
  magnesium E61.2
  major histocompatibility complex
    class I D81.6
    class II D81.7
  manganese E61.3
  menadione (vitamin K) E56.1
    newborn P53

Deficiency, deficient - *continued*
  mental (familial) (hereditary) - *see* Disability,
    intellectual
  methylenetetrahydrofolate reductase
    (MTHFR) E72.12
  mevalonate kinase M04.1
  mineral NEC E61.8
  mineralocorticoid E27.49
    with glucocorticoid E27.49
  molybdenum (nutritional) E61.5
  moral F60.2
  multiple nutrient elements E61.7
  muscle
    carnitine (palmitoyltransferase) E71.314
    phosphofructokinase E74.09
  myoadenylate deaminase E79.2
  myocardial - *see* Insufficiency, myocardial
  myophosphorylase E74.04
  NADH diaphorase or reductase (congenital)
    D74.0
  NADH-methemoglobin reductase (congenital)
    D74.0
  natrium E87.1
  niacin (amide) (-tryptophan) E52
  nicotinamide E52
  nicotinic acid E52
  number of teeth - *see* Anodontia
  nutrient element E61.9
    multiple E61.7
    specified NEC E61.8
  nutrition, nutritional E63.9
    sequelae - *see* Sequelae, nutritional
    deficiency
    specified NEC E63.8
  of interleukin 1
  receptor antagonist [DIRA] M04.8
  ornithine transcarbamylase E72.4
  ovarian E28.39
  oxygen - *see* Anoxia
  pantothenic acid E53.8
  parathyroid (gland) E20.9
  perineum (female) N81.89
  phenylalanine hydroxylase E70.1
  phosphoenolpyruvate carboxykinase E74.4
  phosphofructokinase E74.19
  phosphomannomutase E74.8
  phosphomannose isomerase E74.8
  phosphomannosyl mutase E74.8
  phosphorylase kinase, liver E74.09
  pituitary hormone (isolated) E23.0
  plasma thromboplastin
    antecedent (PTA) D68.1
    component (PTC) D67
  platelet NEC D69.1
    constitutional D68.0
  polyglandular E31.8
    autoimmune E31.0
  potassium (K) E87.6
  prepuce N47.3
  proaccelerin (congenital) (hereditary) D68.2
    acquired D68.4
  proconvertin factor (congenital) (hereditary)
    D68.2
    acquired D68.4
  protein - *see also* Malnutrition E46
    anemia D53.0
    C D68.59
    S D68.59
  prothrombin (congenital) (hereditary) D68.2
    acquired D68.4
  Prower factor D68.2
  pseudocholinesterase E88.09
  PTA (plasma thromboplastin antecedent)
    D68.1

Deficiency, deficient - *continued*
  PTC (plasma thromboplastin component) D67
  purine nucleoside phosphorylase (PNP) D81.5
  pyracin (alpha) (beta) E53.1
  pyridoxal E53.1
  pyridoxamine E53.1
  pyridoxine (derivatives) E53.1
  pyruvate
    carboxylase E74.4
    dehydrogenase E74.4
  riboflavin (vitamin B2) E53.0
  salt E87.1
  secretion
    ovary E28.39
    salivary gland (any) K11.7
    urine R34
  selenium (dietary) E59
  serum antitrypsin, familial E88.01
  short stature homeobox gene (SHOX)
    with
      dyschondrosteosis Q78.8
      short stature (idiopathic) E34.3
      Turner's syndrome Q96.9
  sodium (Na) E87.1
  SPCA (factor VII) D68.2
  sphincter, intrinsic N36.42
    with urethral hypermobility N36.43
  stable factor (congenital) (hereditary) D68.2
    acquired D68.4
  Stuart-Prower (factor X) D68.2
  sucrase E74.39
  sulfatase E75.29
  sulfite oxidase E72.19
  thiamin, thiaminic (chloride) E51.9
    beriberi (dry) E51.11
      wet E51.12
  thrombokinase D68.2
    newborn P53
  thyroid (gland) - *see* Hypothyroidism
  tocopherol E56.0
  tooth bud K00.0
  transcobalamine II (anemia) D51.2
  vanadium E61.6
  vascular I99.9
  vasopressin E23.2
  vertical ridge K06.8
  viosterol - *see* Deficiency, calciferol
  vitamin (multiple) NOS E56.9
    A E50.9
      with
        Bitot's spot (corneal) E50.1
        follicular keratosis E50.8
        keratomalacia E50.4
        manifestations NEC E50.8
        night blindness E50.5
        scar of cornea, xerophthalmic E50.6
        xeroderma E50.8
        xerophthalmia E50.7
        xerosis
          conjunctival E50.0
            and Bitot's spot E50.1
          cornea E50.2
            and ulceration E50.3
      sequelae E64.1
    B (complex) NOS E53.9
      with
        beriberi (dry) E51.11
          wet E51.12
        pellagra E52
    B1 NOS E51.9
      beriberi (dry) E51.11
        with circulatory system manifestations
          E51.11
        wet E51.12

Deficiency, deficient - *continued*
  B12 E53.8
  B2 (riboflavin) E53.0
  B6 E53.1
  C E54
    sequelae E64.2
  D E55.9
    with
      adult osteomalacia M83.8
      rickets - *see* Rickets
      25-hydroxylase E83.32
  E E56.0
  folic acid E53.8
  G E53.0
  group B E53.9
    specified NEC E53.8
  H (biotin) E53.8
  K E56.1
    of newborn P53
  nicotinic E52
  P E56.8
  PP (pellagra-preventing) E52
  specified NEC E56.8
  thiamin E51.9
    beriberi - *see* Beriberi
  zinc, dietary E60
Deficit - *see also* Deficiency
  attention and concentration R41.840
    following
      cerebral infarction I69.310
      cerebrovascular disease I69.910
        specified disease NEC I69.810
      nontraumatic
        intracerebral hemorrhage I69.110
        specified intracranial hemorrhage NEC
          I69.210
        subarachnoid hemorrhage I69.010
  disorder - *see* Attention, deficit
  cognitive
    communication R41.841
    emotional
      following
        cerebral infarction I69.315
        cerebrovascular disease I69.915
          specified disease NEC I69.815
        nontraumatic
          intracerebral hemorrhage I69.115
          specified intracranial hemorrhage NEC
            I69.215
      cerebral infarction I69.319
      cerebrovascular disease I69.919
        subarachnoid hemorrhage I69.015
    following
      specified disease NEC I69.819
      nontraumatic
        intracerebral hemorrhage I69.119
        specified intracranial hemorrhage NEC
          I69.219
        subarachnoid hemorrhage I69.019
    social
      following
        cerebral infarction I69.315
        cerebrovascular disease I69.915
          specified disease NEC I69.815
        nontraumatic
          intracerebral hemorrhage I69.115
          specified intracranial hemorrhage NEC
            I69.215
          subarachnoid hemorrhage I69.015
  cognitive NEC R41.89
    following
      cerebral infarction I69.318
      cerebrovascular disease I69.918
        specified disease NEC I69.818

Deficit - *continued*
  nontraumatic
    intracerebral hemorrhage I69.118
    specified intracranial hemorrhage NEC
      I69.218
    subarachnoid hemorrhage I69.018
  concentration R41.840
  executive function R41.844
    following
      cerebral infarction I69.314
      cerebrovascular disease I69.914
        specified disease NEC I69.814
      nontraumatic
        intracerebral hemorrhage I69.114
        specified intracranial hemorrhage NEC
          I69.214
        subarachnoid hemorrhage I69.014
  frontal lobe R41.844
    following
      cerebral infarction I69.314
      cerebrovascular disease I69.914
        specified disease NEC I69.814
      nontraumatic
        intracerebral hemorrhage I69.114
        specified intracranial hemorrhage NEC
          I69.214
        subarachnoid hemorrhage I69.014
  memory
    following
      cerebral infarction I69.311
      cerebrovascular disease I69.911
        specified disease NEC I69.811
      nontraumatic
        intracerebral hemorrhage I69.111
        specified intracranial hemorrhage NEC
          I69.211
        subarachnoid hemorrhage I69.011
  neurologic NEC R29.818
    ischemic
      reversible (RIND) I63.9
      prolonged (PRIND) I63.9
  oxygen R09.02
  prolonged reversible ischemic neurologic
    (PRIND) I63.9
  psychomotor R41.843
    following
      cerebral infarction I69.313
      cerebrovascular disease I69.913
        specified disease NEC I69.813
      nontraumatic
        intracerebral hemorrhage I69.113
        specified intracranial hemorrhage NEC
          I69.213
        subarachnoid hemorrhage I69.013
  visuospatial R41.842
    following
      cerebral infarction I69.312
      cerebrovascular disease I69.912
        specified disease NEC I69.812
      nontraumatic
        intracerebral hemorrhage I69.112
        specified intracranial hemorrhage NEC
          I69.212
        subarachnoid hemorrhage I69.012
Deflection
  radius - *see* Deformity, limb, specified type
    NEC, forearm
  septum (acquired) (nasal) (nose) J34.2
  spine - *see* Curvature, spine
  turbinate (nose) J34.2
Defluvium
  capillorum - *see* Alopecia
  ciliorum - *see* Madarosis
  unguium L60.8

Deformity Q89.9
- abdomen, congenital Q89.9
- abdominal wall
  - acquired M95.8
  - congenital Q79.59
- acquired (unspecified site) M95.9
- adrenal gland Q89.1
- alimentary tract, congenital Q45.9
  - upper Q40.9
- ankle (joint) (acquired) - *see also* Deformity, limb, lower leg
  - abduction - *see* Contraction, joint, ankle
  - congenital Q68.8
  - contraction - *see* Contraction, joint, ankle
  - specified type NEC - *see* Deformity, limb, foot, specified NEC
- anus (acquired) K62.89
  - congenital Q43.9
- aorta (arch) (congenital) Q25.40
  - acquired I77.89
- aortic
  - arch, acquired I77.89
  - cusp or valve (congenital) Q23.8
    - acquired - *see also* Endocarditis, aortic I35.8
- arm (acquired) (upper) - *see also* Deformity, limb, upper arm
  - congenital Q68.8
  - forearm - *see* Deformity, limb, forearm
- artery (congenital) (peripheral) NOS Q27.9
  - acquired I77.89
  - coronary (acquired) I25.9
    - congenital Q24.5
  - umbilical Q27.0
- atrial septal Q21.1
- auditory canal (external) (congenital) - *see also* Malformation, ear, external
  - acquired - *see* Disorder, ear, external, specified type NEC
- auricle
  - ear (congenital) - *see also* Malformation, ear, external
    - acquired - *see* Disorder, pinna, deformity
- bile duct (common) (congenital) (hepatic) Q44.5
- back - *see* Dorsopathy, deforming
  - acquired K83.8
- biliary duct or passage (congenital) Q44.5
  - acquired K83.8
- bladder (neck) (trigone) (sphincter) (acquired) N32.89
  - congenital Q64.79
- bone (acquired) NOS M95.9
  - congenital Q79.9
  - turbinate M95.0
- brain (congenital) Q04.9
  - acquired G93.89
  - reduction Q04.3
- breast (acquired) N64.89
  - congenital Q83.9
  - reconstructed N65.0
- bronchus (congenital) Q32.4
  - acquired NEC J98.09
- bursa, congenital Q79.9
- canaliculi (lacrimalis) (acquired) - *see also* Disorder, lacrimal system, changes
  - congenital Q10.6
- canthus, acquired - *see* Disorder, eyelid, specified type NEC
- capillary (acquired) I78.8
- cardiovascular system, congenital Q28.9
- caruncle, lacrimal (acquired) - *see also* Disorder, lacrimal system, changes
  - congenital Q10.6

Deformity - *continued*
- cascade, stomach K31.2
- cecum (congenital) Q43.9
  - acquired K63.89
- cerebral, acquired G93.89
  - congenital Q04.9
- cervix (uterus) (acquired) NEC N88.8
  - congenital Q51.9
- cheek (acquired) M95.2
  - congenital Q18.9
- chest (acquired) (wall) M95.4
  - congenital Q67.8
  - sequelae (late effect) of rickets E64.3
- chin (acquired) M95.2
  - congenital Q18.9
- choroid (congenital) Q14.3
  - acquired H31.8
  - plexus Q07.8
    - acquired G96.19
- cicatricial - *see* Cicatrix
- cilia, acquired - *see* Disorder, eyelid, specified type NEC
- clavicle (acquired) M95.8
  - congenital Q68.8
- clitoris (congenital) Q52.6
  - acquired N90.89
- clubfoot - *see* Clubfoot
- coccyx (acquired) - *see* subcategory M43.8
- colon (congenital) Q43.9
  - acquired K63.89
- concha (ear), congenital - *see also* Malformation, ear, external
  - acquired - *see* Disorder, pinna, deformity
- cornea (acquired) H18.70
  - congenital Q13.4
  - descemetocele - *see* Descemetocele
  - ectasia - *see* Ectasia, cornea
  - specified NEC H18.79-
  - staphyloma - *see* Staphyloma, cornea
- coronary artery (acquired) I25.9
- cranium (acquired) - *see* Deformity, skull
- cricoid cartilage (congenital) Q31.8
  - congenital Q24.5
  - acquired J38.7
- cystic duct (congenital) Q44.5
  - acquired K82.8
- Dandy-Walker Q03.1
  - with spina bifida - *see* Spina bifida
- diaphragm (congenital) Q79.1
  - acquired J98.6
- digestive organ NOS Q45.9
- ductus arteriosus Q25.0
- duodenal bulb K31.89
- duodenum (congenital) Q43.9
  - acquired K31.89
- dura - *see* Deformity, meninges
- ear (acquired) - *see also* Disorder, pinna, deformity
  - congenital (external) Q17.9
    - internal Q16.5
    - middle Q16.4
      - ossicles Q16.3
    - ossicles Q16.3
- ectodermal (congenital) NEC Q84.9
- ejaculatory duct (congenital) Q55.4
  - acquired N50.89
- elbow (joint) (acquired) - *see also* Deformity, limb, upper arm
  - congenital Q68.8
  - contraction - *see* Contraction, joint, elbow
- endocrine gland NEC Q89.2
- epididymis (congenital) Q55.4
  - acquired N50.89
- epiglottis (congenital) Q31.8

Deformity - *continued*
- acquired J38.7
- esophagus (congenital) Q39.9
  - acquired K22.8
- eustachian tube (congenital) NEC Q17.8
- eye, congenital Q15.9
- eyebrow (congenital) Q18.8
- eyelid (acquired) - *see also* Disorder, eyelid, specified type NEC
  - congenital Q10.3
- face (acquired) M95.2
  - congenital Q18.9
- fallopian tube, acquired N83.8
- femur (acquired) - *see* Deformity, limb, specified type NEC, thigh
- fetal
  - with fetopelvic disproportion O33.7
  - causing obstructed labor O66.3
- finger (acquired) M20.00-
  - boutonniere M20.02-
  - congenital Q68.1
  - flexion contracture - *see* Contraction, joint, hand
  - mallet finger M20.01-
  - specified NEC M20.09-
  - swan neck M20.03-
- flexion (joint) (acquired) - *see also* Deformity, limb, flexion M21.20
  - congenital NOS Q74.9
  - hip Q65.89
- foot (acquired) - *see also* Deformity, limb, lower leg
  - cavovarus (congenital) Q66.1
  - congenital NOS Q66.9
    - specified type NEC Q66.89
  - specified type NEC - *see* Deformity, limb, foot, specified NEC
  - varus (congenital) NEC Q66.3
    - acquired - *see* Deformity, varus, ankle
- forearm (acquired) - *see also* Deformity, limb, forearm
  - congenital Q68.8
- forehead (acquired) M95.2
  - congenital Q75.8
- frontal bone (acquired) M95.2
  - congenital Q75.8
- gallbladder (congenital) Q44.1
  - acquired K82.8
- gastrointestinal tract (congenital) NOS Q45.9
  - acquired K63.89
- genitalia, genital organ(s) or system NEC
  - female (congenital) Q52.9
    - acquired N94.89
    - external Q52.70
  - male (congenital) Q55.9
    - acquired N50.89
- globe (eye) (congenital) Q15.8
  - acquired H44.89
- gum, acquired NEC K06.8
- hand (acquired) - *see* Deformity, limb, hand
  - congenital Q68.1
- head (acquired) M95.2
  - congenital Q75.8
- heart (congenital) Q24.9
  - septum Q21.9
    - auricular Q21.1
    - ventricular Q21.0
  - valve (congenital) NEC Q24.8
    - acquired - *see* Endocarditis
- heel (acquired) - *see* Deformity, foot
- hepatic duct (congenital) Q44.5
  - acquired K83.8
- hip (joint) (acquired) - *see also* Deformity, limb, thigh

Deformity - *continued*
congenital Q65.9
due to (previous) juvenile osteochondrosis -
see Coxa, plana
flexion - *see* Contraction, joint, hip
hourglass - *see* Contraction, hourglass
humerus (acquired) M21.82-
congenital Q74.0
hypophyseal (congenital) Q89.2
ileocecal (coil) (valve) (acquired) K63.89
congenital Q43.9
ileum (congenital) Q43.9
acquired K63.89
ilium (acquired) M95.5
congenital Q74.2
integument (congenital) Q84.9
intervertebral cartilage or disc (acquired) - *see*
Disorder, disc, specified NEC
intestine (large) (small) (congenital) NOS
Q43.9
acquired K63.89
intrinsic minus or plus (hand) - *see* Deformity,
limb, specified type NEC, forearm
iris (acquired) H21.89
congenital Q13.2
ischium (acquired) M95.5
congenital Q74.2
jaw (acquired) (congenital) M26.9
joint (acquired) NEC M21.90
congenital Q68.8
elbow M21.92-
hand M21.94-
shoulder M21.92-
wrist M21.93-
hip M21.95-
knee M21.96-
kidney(s) (calyx) (pelvis) (congenital) Q63.9
acquired N28.89
artery (congenital) Q27.2
acquired I77.89
Klippel-Feil (brevicollis) Q76.1
knee (acquired) NEC - *see also* Deformity,
limb, lower leg
congenital Q68.2
labium (majus) (minus) (congenital) Q52.79
acquired N90.89
lacrimal passages or duct (congenital) NEC
Q10.6
acquired - *see* Disorder, lacrimal system,
changes
larynx (muscle) (congenital) Q31.8
acquired J38.7
web (glottic) Q31.0
leg (upper) (acquired) NEC - *see also*
Deformity, limb, thigh
congenital Q68.8
lower leg - *see* Deformity, limb, lower leg
lens (acquired) H27.8
congenital Q12.9
lid (fold) (acquired) - *see also* Disorder, eyelid,
specified type NEC
congenital Q10.3
ligament (acquired) - *see* Disorder, ligament
congenital Q79.9
limb (acquired) M21.90
clawfoot M21.53-
clawhand M21.51-
clubfoot M21.54-
clubhand M21.52-
congenital, except reduction deformity Q74.9
flat foot M21.4-
flexion M21.20
ankle M21.27-
elbow M21.22-

Deformity - *continued*
finger M21.24-
hip M21.25-
knee M21.26-
shoulder M21.21-
toe M21.27-
wrist M21.23-
foot
claw - *see* Deformity, limb, clawfoot
club - *see* Deformity, limb, clubfoot
drop M21.37-
flat - *see* Deformity, limb, flat foot
specified NEC M21.6X-
forearm M21.93-
hand M21.94-
lower leg M21.96-
specified type NEC M21.80
forearm M21.83-
lower leg M21.86-
thigh M21.85-
upper arm M21.82-
thigh M21.95-
unequal length M21.70
short site is
femur M21.75-
fibula M21.76-
humerus M21.72-
radius M21.73-
upper arm M21.92-
valgus - *see* Deformity, valgus
varus - *see* Deformity, varus
tibia M21.76-
ulna M21.73-
wrist drop M21.33-
lip (acquired) NEC K13.0
congenital Q38.0
liver (congenital) Q44.7
acquired K76.89
lumbosacral (congenital) (joint) (region)
Q76.49
acquired - *see* subcategory M43.8
kyphosis - *see* Kyphosis, congenital
lordosis - *see* Lordosis, congenital
lung (congenital) Q33.9
acquired J98.4
lymphatic system, congenital Q89.9
Madelung's (radius) Q74.0
mandible (acquired) (congenital) M26.9
maxilla (acquired) (congenital) M26.9
meninges or membrane (congenital) Q07.9
cerebral Q04.8
acquired G96.19
spinal cord (congenital) G96.19
acquired G96.19
metacarpus (acquired) - *see* Deformity, limb,
forearm
congenital Q74.0
metatarsus (acquired) - *see* Deformity, foot
congenital Q66.9
middle ear (congenital) Q16.4
ossicles Q16.3
mitral (leaflets) (valve) I05.8
parachute Q23.2
stenosis, congenital Q23.2
mouth (acquired) K13.79
congenital Q38.6
multiple, congenital NEC Q89.7
muscle (acquired) M62.89
congenital Q79.9
sternocleidomastoid Q68.0
musculoskeletal system (acquired) M95.9
congenital Q79.9
specified NEC M95.8
nail (acquired) L60.8

Deformity - *continued*
congenital Q84.6
nasal - *see* Deformity, nose   neck (acquired)
M95.3
congenital Q18.9
sternocleidomastoid Q68.0
nervous system (congenital) Q07.9
nipple (congenital) Q83.9
acquired N64.89
nose (acquired) (cartilage) M95.0
bone (turbinate) M95.0
congenital Q30.9
bent or squashed Q67.4
saddle M95.0
syphilitic A50.57
septum (acquired) J34.2
congenital Q30.8
sinus (wall) (congenital) Q30.8
acquired M95.0
syphilitic (congenital) A50.57
late A52.73
ocular muscle (congenital) Q10.3
acquired - *see* Strabismus, mechanical
opticociliary vessels (congenital) Q13.2
orbit (eye) (acquired) H05.30
atrophy - *see* Atrophy, orbit
congenital Q10.7
due to
bone disease NEC H05.32-
trauma or surgery H05.33-
enlargement - *see* Enlargement, orbit
exostosis - *see* Exostosis, orbit
organ of Corti (congenital) Q16.5
ovary (congenital) Q50.39
acquired N83.8
oviduct, acquired N83.8
palate (congenital) Q38.5
acquired M27.8
cleft (congenital) - *see* Cleft, palate
pancreas (congenital) Q45.3
acquired K86.89
parathyroid (gland) Q89.2
parotid (gland) (congenital) Q38.4
acquired K11.8
patella (acquired) - *see* Disorder, patella,
specified NEC
pelvis, pelvic (acquired) (bony) M95.5
with disproportion (fetopelvic) O33.0
causing obstructed labor O65.0
congenital Q74.2
rachitic sequelae (late effect) E64.3
penis (glans) (congenital) Q55.69
acquired N48.89
pericardium (congenital) Q24.8
acquired - *see* Pericarditis
pharynx (congenital) Q38.8
acquired J39.2
pinna, acquired - *see also* Disorder, pinna,
deformity
congenital Q17.9
pituitary (congenital) Q89.2
posture - *see* Dorsopathy, deforming
prepuce (congenital) Q55.69
acquired N47.8
prostate (congenital) Q55.4
acquired N42.89
pupil (congenital) Q13.2
acquired - *see* Abnormality, pupillary
pylorus (congenital) Q40.3
acquired K31.89
rachitic (acquired), old or healed E64.3
radius (acquired) - *see also* Deformity, limb,
forearm
congenital Q68.8

Deformity - *continued*

rectum (congenital) Q43.9
  acquired K62.89
reduction (extremity) (limb), congenital - *see also* condition and site Q73.8
  brain Q04.3
  lower - *see* Defect, reduction, lower limb
  upper - *see* Defect, reduction, upper limb
renal - *see* Deformity, kidney
respiratory system (congenital) Q34.9
rib (acquired) M95.4
  congenital Q76.6
    cervical Q76.5
rotation (joint) (acquired) - *see* Deformity, limb, specified site NEC
  congenital Q74.9
  hip - *see* Deformity, limb, specified type NEC, thigh
    congenital Q65.89
sacroiliac joint (congenital) Q74.2
  acquired - *see* subcategory M43.8
sacrum (acquired) - *see* subcategory M43.8
  nose M95.0
    syphilitic A50.57
saddle
  back - *see* Lordosis
salivary gland or duct (congenital) Q38.4
  acquired K11.8
scapula (acquired) M95.8
  congenital Q68.8
scrotum (congenital) - *see also* Malformation, testis and scrotum
  acquired N50.89
seminal vesicles (congenital) Q55.4
  acquired N50.89
septum, nasal (acquired) J34.2
shoulder (joint) (acquired) - *see* Deformity, limb, upper arm
  congenital Q74.0
  contraction - *see* Contraction, joint, shoulder
sigmoid (flexure) (congenital) Q43.9
  acquired K63.89
skin (congenital) Q82.9
skull (acquired) M95.2
  congenital Q75.8
    with
      anencephaly Q00.0
      encephalocele - *see* Encephalocele
      hydrocephalus Q03.9
        with spina bifida - *see* Spina bifida, by site, with hydrocephalus
      microcephaly Q02
soft parts, organs or tissues (of pelvis)
  in pregnancy or childbirth NEC O34.8-
    causing obstructed labor O65.5
spermatic cord (congenital) Q55.4
  acquired N50.89
  torsion - *see* Torsion, spermatic cord
spinal - *see* Dorsopathy, deforming
  column (acquired) - *see* Dorsopathy, deforming
    congenital Q67.5
  cord (congenital) Q06.9
    acquired G95.89
  nerve root (congenital) Q07.9
spine (acquired) - *see also* Dorsopathy, deforming
  congenital Q67.5
  rachitic E64.3
  specified NEC - *see* Dorsopathy, deforming, specified NEC
spleen
  acquired D73.89
  congenital Q89.09

Deformity - *continued*

Sprengel's (congenital) Q74.0
sternocleidomastoid (muscle), congenital Q68.0
sternum (acquired) M95.4
  congenital NEC Q76.7
stomach (congenital) Q40.3
  acquired K31.89
submandibular gland (congenital) Q38.4
submaxillary gland (congenital) Q38.4
  acquired K11.8
talipes - *see* Talipes
testis (congenital) - *see also* Malformation, testis and scrotum
  acquired N44.8
    torsion - *see* Torsion, testis
thigh (acquired) - *see also* Deformity, limb, thigh
  congenital NEC Q68.8
  sequelae of rickets E64.3
thumb (acquired) - *see* Deformity, finger
  congenital NEC Q68.1
thorax (acquired) (wall) M95.4
  congenital Q67.8
thymus (tissue) (congenital) Q89.2
thyroid (gland) (congenital) Q89.2
  cartilage Q31.8
    acquired J38.7
tibia (acquired) - *see also* Deformity, limb, specified type NEC, lower leg
  congenital NEC Q68.8
  saber (syphilitic) A50.56
toe (acquired) M20.6-
  congenital Q66.9
  hallux rigidus M20.2-
  hallux valgus M20.1-
  hallux varus M20.3-
  hammer toe M20.4-
  specified NEC M20.5X-
tongue (congenital) Q38.3
  acquired K14.8
tooth, teeth K00.2
trachea (rings) (congenital) Q32.1
  acquired J39.8
transverse aortic arch (congenital) Q25.49
tricuspid (leaflets) (valve) I07.8
  atresia or stenosis Q22.4
  Ebstein's Q22.5
trunk (acquired) M95.8
  congenital Q89.9
ulna (acquired) - *see also* Deformity, limb, forearm
  congenital NEC Q68.8
urachus, congenital Q64.4
ureter (opening) (congenital) Q62.8
  acquired N28.89
urethra (congenital) Q64.79
  acquired N36.8
urinary tract (congenital) Q64.9
  urachus Q64.4
uterus (congenital) Q51.9
  acquired N85.8
uvula (congenital) Q38.5
vagina (acquired) N89.8
  congenital Q52.4
valgus NEC M21.00
  ankle M21.07-
  elbow M21.02-
  hip M21.05-
  knee M21.06-
valve, valvular (congenital) (heart) Q24.8
  acquired - *see* Endocarditis
varus NEC M21.10
  ankle M21.17-

Deformity - *continued*

  elbow M21.12-
  hip M21.15
  knee M21.16-
  tibia - *see* Osteochondrosis, juvenile, tibia
vas deferens (congenital) Q55.4
  acquired N50.89
vein (congenital) Q27.9
  great Q26.9
vertebra - *see* Dorsopathy, deforming
vertical talus (congenital) Q66.80
  left foot Q66.82
  right foot Q66.81
vesicourethral orifice (acquired) N32.89
  congenital NEC Q64.79
vessels of optic papilla (congenital) Q14.2
visual field (contraction) - *see* Defect, visual field
vitreous body, acquired H43.89
vulva (congenital) Q52.79
  acquired N90.89
wrist (joint) (acquired) - *see also* Deformity, limb, forearm
  congenital Q68.8
  contraction - *see* Contraction, joint, wrist

Degeneration, degenerative

adrenal (capsule) (fatty) (gland) (hyaline) (infectional) E27.8
amyloid - *see also* Amyloidosis E85.9
anterior cornua, spinal cord G12.29
anterior labral S43.49-
aorta, aortic I70.0
  fatty I77.89
aortic valve (heart) - *see* Endocarditis, aortic
arteriovascular - *see* Arteriosclerosis
artery, arterial (atheromatous) (calcareous) - *see also* Arteriosclerosis
  cerebral, amyloid E85.4 [*I68.0*]
  medial - *see* Arteriosclerosis, extremities
articular cartilage NEC - *see* Derangement, joint, articular cartilage, by site
atheromatous - *see* Arteriosclerosis
basal nuclei or ganglia G23.9
  specified NEC G23.8
bone NEC - *see* Disorder, bone, specified type NEC
brachial plexus G54.0
brain (cortical) (progressive) G31.9
  alcoholic G31.2
  arteriosclerotic I67.2
  childhood G31.9
    specified NEC G31.89
  cystic G31.89
    congenital Q04.6
  in
    alcoholism G31.2
    beriberi E51.2
    cerebrovascular disease I67.9
    congenital hydrocephalus Q03.9
      with spina bifida - *see also* Spina bifida
    Fabry-Anderson disease E75.21
    Gaucher's disease E75.22
    Hunter's syndrome E76.1
    lipidosis
      cerebral E75.4
      generalized E75.6
    mucopolysaccharidosis - *see* Mucopolysaccharidosis
    myxedema E03.9 [*G32.89*]
    neoplastic disease - *see also* Neoplasm D49.6 [*G32.89*]
    Niemann-pick disease E75.249 [*G32.89*]
    sphingolipidosis E75.3 [*G32.89*]
    vitamin B12 deficiency E53.8 [*G32.89*]

Degeneration, degenerative - *continued*

senile NEC G31.1
breast N64.89
Bruch's membrane - *see* Degeneration, choroid
capillaries (fatty) I78.8
amyloid E85.89 [*I79.8*]
cardiac - *see also* Degeneration, myocardial
valve, valvular - *see* Endocarditis
cardiorenal - *see* Hypertension, cardiorenal
cardiovascular - *see also* Disease, cardiovascular
renal - *see* Hypertension, cardiorenal
cerebellar NOS G31.9
cerebral - *see* Degeneration, brain
cerebrovascular I67.9
due to hypertension I67.4
alcoholic G31.2
primary (hereditary) (sporadic) G11.9
cervical plexus G54.2
cervix N88.8
due to radiation (intended effect) N88.8
adverse effect or misadventure N99.89
chamber angle H21.21-
changes, spine or vertebra - *see* Spondylosis
chorioretinal - *see also* Degeneration, choroid
hereditary H31.20
choroid (colloid) (drusen) H31.10-
atrophy - *see* Atrophy, choroidal
hereditary - *see* Dystrophy, choroidal, hereditary
ciliary body H21.22-
cochlear - *see* subcategory H83.8
combined (spinal cord) (subacute) E53.8 [*G32.0*]
with anemia (pernicious) D51.0 [*G32.0*]
due to dietary vitamin B12 deficiency D51.3 [*G32.0*]
in (due to)
vitamin B12 deficiency E53.8 [*G32.0*]
anemia D51.9 [*G32.0*]
conjunctiva H11.10
concretions - *see* Concretion, conjunctiva
deposits - *see* Deposit, conjunctiva
pigmentations - *see* Pigmentation, conjunctiva
pinguecula - *see* Pinguecula
xerosis - *see* Xerosis, conjunctiva
cornea H18.40
calcereous H18.43
band keratopathy H18.42-
familial, hereditary - *see* Dystrophy, cornea
hyaline (of old scars) H18.49
keratomalacia - *see* Keratomalacia
nodular H18.45-
peripheral H18.46-
senile H18.41-
specified type NEC H18.49
cortical (cerebellar) (parenchymatous) G31.89
alcoholic G31.2
diffuse, due to arteriopathy I67.2
corticobasal G31.85
cutis L98.8
amyloid E85.4 [*L99*]
dental pulp K04.2
disc disease - *see* Degeneration, intervertebral disc NEC
dorsolateral (spinal cord) - *see* Degeneration, combined
extrapyramidal G25.9
eye, macular - *see also* Degeneration, macula
congenital or hereditary - *see* Dystrophy, retina
facet joints - *see* Spondylosis
fatty

Degeneration, degenerative - *continued*

liver NEC K76.0
alcoholic K70.0
grey matter (brain) (Alpers') G31.81
heart - *see also* Degeneration, myocardial
amyloid E85.4 [*I43*]
atheromatous - *see* Disease, heart, ischemic, atherosclerotic
ischemic - *see* Disease, heart, ischemic
hepatolenticular (Wilson's) E83.01
localized - *see* Degeneration, by site
infrapatellar fat pad M79.4
intervertebral disc NOS
hepatorenal K76.7
hyaline (diffuse) (generalized)
with
myelopathy - *see* Disorder, disc, with, myelopathy
radiculitis or radiculopathy - *see* Disorder, disc, with, radiculopathy
cervical, cervicothoracic - *see* Disorder, disc, cervical, degeneration
with
myelopathy - *see* Disorder, disc, cervical, with myelopathy
neuritis, radiculitis or radiculopathy - *see* Disorder, disc, cervical, with neuritis
lumbar region M51.36
with
myelopathy M51.06
neuritis, radiculitis, radiculopathy or sciatica M51.16
lumbosacral region M51.37
with
neuritis, radiculitis, radiculopathy or sciatica M51.17
sacrococcygeal region M53.3
thoracic region M51.34
with
myelopathy M51.04
neuritis, radiculitis, radiculopathy M51.14
thoracolumbar region M51.35
with
myelopathy M51.05
neuritis, radiculitis, radiculopathy M51.15
intestine, amyloid E85.4
iris (pigmentary) H21.23-
ischemic - *see* Ischemia
joint disease - *see* Osteoarthritis
kidney N28.89
amyloid E85.4 [*N29*]
cystic, congenital Q61.9
fatty N28.89
polycystic Q61.3
adult type (autosomal dominant) Q61.2
infantile type (autosomal recessive) NEC Q61.19
collecting duct dilatation Q61.11
Kuhnt-Junius - *see also* Degeneration, macula H35.32-
lens - *see* Cataract
lenticular (familial) (progressive) (Wilson's) (with cirrhosis of liver) E83.01
liver (diffuse) NEC K76.89
amyloid E85.4 [*K77*]
cystic K76.89
congenital Q44.6
fatty NEC K76.0
alcoholic K70.0
hypertrophic K76.89
parenchymatous, acute or subacute K72.00
with coma K72.01
pigmentary K76.89
toxic (acute) K71.9

Degeneration, degenerative - *continued*

lung J98.4
lymph gland I89.8
hyaline I89.8
macula, macular (acquired) (age-related) (senile) H35.30
angioid streaks H35.33
atrophic age-related H35.31-
congenital or hereditary - *see* Dystrophy, retina
cystoid H35.35-
drusen H35.36-
dry age-related H35.31-
exudative H35.32-
hole H35.34-
nonexudative H35.31-
puckering H35.37-
toxic H35.38-
wet age-related H35.32-
membranous labyrinth, congenital (causing impairment of hearing) Q16.5
meniscus - *see* Derangement, meniscus
mitral - *see* Insufficiency, mitral
Mönckeberg's - *see* Arteriosclerosis, extremities
motor centers, senile G31.1
multi-system G90.3
mural - *see* Degeneration, myocardial
muscle (fatty) (fibrous) (hyaline) (progressive) M62.89
heart - *see* Degeneration, myocardial
myelin, central nervous system G37.9
myocardial, myocardium (fatty) (hyaline) (senile) I51.5
with rheumatic fever (conditions in I00) I09.0
active, acute or subacute I01.2
with chorea I02.0
inactive or quiescent (with chorea) I09.0
hypertensive - *see* Hypertension, heart
rheumatic - *see* Degeneration, myocardial, with rheumatic fever
syphilitic A52.06
nasal sinus (mucosa) J32.9
frontal J32.1
maxillary J32.0
nerve - *see* Disorder, nerve
nervous system G31.9
alcoholic G31.2
amyloid E85.4 [*G99.8*]
autonomic G90.9
fatty G31.89
specified NEC G31.89
nipple N64.89
olivopontocerebellar (hereditary) (familial) G23.8
osseous labyrinth - *see* subcategory H83.8
ovary N83.8
cystic N83.20-
microcystic N83.20-
pallidal pigmentary (progressive) G23.0
pancreas K86.89
tuberculous A18.83
penis N48.89
pigmentary (diffuse) (general)
localized - *see* Degeneration, by site
pallidal (progressive) G23.0
pineal gland E34.8
pituitary (gland) E23.6
popliteal fat pad M79.4
posterolateral (spinal cord) - *see* Degeneration, combined
pulmonary valve (heart) I37.8
pulp (tooth) K04.2

Degeneration, degenerative - *continued*
  pupillary margin H21.24-
  renal - *see* Degeneration, kidney   retina H35.9
    hereditary (cerebroretinal) (congenital)
    (juvenile) (macula) (peripheral) (pigmentary) -
      see Dystrophy, retina
    Kuhnt-Junius - *see also* Degeneration,
      macula H35.32-
    macula (cystic) (exudative) (hole)
    (nonexudative) (pseudohole) (senile) (toxic) -
      see Degeneration, macula
    peripheral H35.40
      lattice H35.41-
      microcystoid H35.42-
      paving stone H35.43-
      secondary
        pigmentary H35.45-
        vitreoretinal H35.46-
      senile reticular H35.44-
    pigmentary (primary) - *see also* Dystrophy,
      retina
      secondary - *see* Degeneration, retina,
        peripheral, secondary
    posterior pole - *see* Degeneration, macula
  saccule, congenital (causing impairment of
    hearing) Q16.5
  senile R54
    brain G31.1
    cardiac, heart or myocardium - *see*
      Degeneration, myocardial
      motor centers G31.1
      vascular - *see* Arteriosclerosis
  sinus (cystic) - *see also* Sinusitis
    polypoid J33.1
  skin L98.8
    amyloid E85.4 [L99]
    colloid L98.8
  spinal (cord) G31.89
    amyloid E85.4 [G32.89]
    combined (subacute) - *see* Degeneration,
      combined
      dorsolateral - *see* Degeneration, combined
      familial NEC G31.89
      fatty G31.89
      funicular - *see* Degeneration, combined
      posterolateral - *see* Degeneration, combined
      subacute combined - *see* Degeneration,
        combined
      tuberculous A17.81
  spleen D73.0
    amyloid E85.4 [D77]
  stomach K31.89
  striatonigral G23.2
  suprarenal (capsule) (gland) E27.8
  synovial membrane (pulpy) - *see* Disorder,
    synovium, specified type NEC
  tapetoretinal - *see* Dystrophy, retina
  thymus (gland) E32.8
    fatty E32.8
  thyroid (gland) E07.89
  tricuspid (heart) (valve) I07.9
  tuberculous NEC - *see* Tuberculosis
  turbinate J34.89
  uterus (cystic) N85.8
  vascular (senile) - *see* Arteriosclerosis
    hypertensive - *see* Hypertension
  vitreoretinal, secondary - *see* Degeneration,
    retina, peripheral, secondary, vitreoretinal
  vitreous (body) H43.81-
  Wallerian - *see* Disorder, nerve
  Wilson's hepatolenticular E83.01
Deglutition
  paralysis R13.0
    hysterical F44.4

Deglutition - *continued*
  pneumonia J69.0
Degos' disease I77.89
Dehiscence (of)
  amputation stump T87.81
  cesarean wound O90.0
  closure of
    cornea T81.31
    craniotomy T81.32
    fascia (muscular) (superficial) T81.32
    internal organ or tissue T81.32
    laceration (external) (internal) T81.33
    ligament T81.32
    mucosa T81.31
    muscle or muscle flap T81.32
    ribs or rib cage T81.32
    skin and subcutaneous tissue (full-thickness)
      (superficial) T81.31
    skull T81.32
    sternum (sternotomy) T81.32
    tendon T81.32
    traumatic laceration (external) (internal)
      T81.33
  episiotomy O90.1
  operation wound NEC T81.31
    external operation wound (superficial)
      T81.31
    internal operation wound (deep) T81.32
  perineal wound (postpartum) O90.1
  traumatic injury wound repair T81.33
  wound T81.30
    traumatic repair T81.33
Dehydration E86.0
  newborn P74.1
Déjérine-Roussy syndrome G89.0
Déjérine-Sottas disease or neuropathy
  (hypertrophic) G60.0
Déjérine-Thomas atrophy G23.8
Delay, delayed
  any plane in pelvis
    complicating delivery O66.9
  birth or delivery NOS O63.9
  closure, ductus arteriosus (Botalli) P29.38
  coagulation - *see* Defect, coagulation
  conduction (cardiac) (ventricular) I45.9
  delivery, second twin, triplet, etc O63.2
  development R62.50
    global F88
    intellectual (specific) F81.9
    language F80.9
      due to hearing loss F80.4
    learning F81.9
    pervasive F84.9
    physiological R62.50
      specified stage NEC R62.0
    reading F81.0
    sexual E30.0
    speech F80.9
      due to hearing loss F80.4
    spelling F81.81
  ejaculation F52.32
  gastric emptying K30
  menarche E30.0
  menstruation (cause unknown) N91.0
  milestone R62.0
  passage of meconium (newborn) P76.0
  primary respiration P28.9
  puberty (constitutional) E30.0
  separation of umbilical cord P96.82 sexual
    maturation, female E30.0
  sleep phase syndrome G47.21
  union, fracture - *see* Fracture, by site
  vaccination Z28.9

Deletion(s)
  autosome Q93.9
    identified by fluorescence in situ
      hybridization (FISH) Q93.89
    identified by in situ hybridization (ISH)
      Q93.89
  chromosome
    with complex rearrangements NEC Q93.7
    part of NEC Q93.5
    seen only at prometaphase Q93.89
    short arm
      4 Q93.3
      5p Q93.4
      22q11.2 Q93.81
    specified NEC Q93.89
  long arm chromosome 18 or 21 Q93.89
    with complex rearrangements NEC Q93.7
  microdeletions NEC Q93.88
Delhi boil or button B55.1
Delinquency (juvenile) (neurotic) F91.8
  group Z72.810
Delinquent immunization status Z28.3
Delirium, delirious (acute or subacute) (not
  alcohol or drug-induced) (with dementia)
  R41.0
  alcoholic (acute) (tremens) (withdrawal)
    F10.921
    with intoxication F10.921
      in
        abuse F10.121
        dependence F10.221
  due to (secondary to)
    alcohol
      intoxication F10.921
        in
          abuse F10.121
          dependence F10.221
      withdrawal F10.231
    amphetamine intoxication F15.921
      in
        abuse F15.121
        dependence F15.221
    anxiolytic
      intoxication F13.921
        in
          abuse F13.121
          dependence F13.221
      withdrawal F13.231
    cannabis intoxication (acute) F12.921
      in
        abuse F12.121
        dependence F12.221
    cocaine intoxication (acute) F14.921
      in
        abuse F14.121
        dependence F14.221
    general medical condition F05
    hallucinogen intoxication F16.921
      in
        abuse F16.121
        dependence F16.221
    hypnotic
      intoxication F13.921
        in
          abuse F13.121
          dependence F13.221
      withdrawal F13.231
    inhalant intoxication (acute) F18.921
      in
        abuse F18.121
        dependence F18.221
    multiple etiologies F05
    opioid intoxication (acute) F11.921
      in

Delirium, delirious - *continued*
    abuse F11.121
    dependence F11.221
  other (or unknown) substance F19.921
  phencyclidine intoxication (acute) F16.921
    in
      abuse F16.121
      dependence F16.221
  psychoactive substance NEC intoxication
  (acute) F19.921
    in
      abuse F19.121
      dependence F19.221
  sedative
    intoxication F13.921
      in
        abuse F13.121
        dependence F13.221
    withdrawal F13.231
  unknown etiology F05
  exhaustion F43.0
  hysterical F44.89
  postprocedural (postoperative) F05
  puerperal F05
  thyroid - *see* Thyrotoxicosis with thyroid
  storm
  traumatic - *see* Injury, intracranial
  tremens (alcohol-induced) F10.231
    sedative-induced F13.231
Delivery (childbirth) (labor)
  arrested active phase O62.1
  cesarean (for)
    abnormal
      pelvis (bony) (deformity) (major) NEC with
      disproportion (fetopelvic) O33.0
        with obstructed labor O65.0
      presentation or position O32.9
    abruptio placentae - *see also* Abruptio
    placentae O45.9-
    acromion presentation O32.2
    atony, uterus O62.2
    breech presentation O32.1
      incomplete O32.8
    brow presentation O32.3
    cephalopelvic disproportion O33.9
    cerclage O34.3-
    chin presentation O32.3
    cicatrix of cervix O34.4-
    contracted pelvis (general)
      inlet O33.2
      outlet O33.3
    cord presentation or prolapse O69.0
    cystocele O34.8-
    deformity (acquired) (congenital)
      pelvic organs or tissues NEC O34.8-
      pelvis (bony) NEC O33.0
    disproportion NOS O33.9
    eclampsia - *see* Eclampsia
    face presentation O32.3
    failed
      forceps O66.5
      induction of labor O61.9
        instrumental O61.1
        mechanical O61.1
        medical O61.0
        specified NEC O61.8
        surgical O61.1
      trial of labor NOS O66.40
        following previous cesarean delivery
        O66.41
    vacuum extraction O66.5
    ventouse O66.5
    fetal-maternal hemorrhage O43.01-
    hemorrhage (intrapartum) O67.9

Delivery (childbirth) (labor) - *continued*
    with coagulation defect O67.0
      specified cause NEC O67.8
    high head at term O32.4
    hydrocephalic fetus O33.6
    incarceration of uterus O34.51-
    incoordinate uterine action O62.4
    increased size, fetus O33.5
    inertia, uterus O62.2
      primary O62.0
      secondary O62.1
    lateroversion, uterus O34.59-
    mal lie O32.9
    malposition
      fetus O32.9
      pelvic organs or tissues NEC O34.8-
      uterus NEC O34.59-
    malpresentation NOS O32.9
    oblique presentation O32.2
    occurring after 37 completed weeks of
    gestation but before 39 completed weeks
    gestation due to (spontaneous) onset of labor
    O75.82
    oversize fetus O33.5
    pelvic tumor NEC O34.8-
    placenta previa O44.0-
      complete O44.0-
        with hemorrhage O44.1-
    placental insufficiency O36.51-
    planned, occurring after 37 completed weeks
    of gestation but before 39 completed weeks
    gestation due to (spontaneous) onset of labor
    O75.82
    polyp, cervix O34.4-
      causing obstructed labor O65.5
    poor dilatation, cervix O62.0
    pre-eclampsia O14.94
      mild O14.04
      moderate O14.04
      severe O14.14
        with hemolysis, elevated liver enzymes
        and low platelet count (HELLP) O14.24
    previous
      cesarean delivery O34.219
        classical (vertical) scar O34.212
        low transverse scar O34.211
      surgery (to)
        cervix O34.4-
        gynecological NEC O34.8-
        rectum O34.7-
        uterus O34.29
        vagina O34.6-
    prolapse
      arm or hand O32.2
      uterus O34.52-
    prolonged labor NOS O63.9
    rectocele O34.8-
    retroversion
      uterus O34.53-
    rigid   cervix O34.4-
      pelvic floor O34.8-
      perineum O34.7-
      vagina O34.6-
      vulva O34.7-
    sacculation, pregnant uterus O34.59-
    scar(s)
      cervix O34.4-
      cesarean delivery O34.219
        classical (vertical) O34.212
        low transverse O34.211
      transmural uterine O34.29
      uterus O34.29
    Shirodkar suture in situ O34.3-
    shoulder presentation O32.2

Delivery (childbirth) (labor) - *continued*
    stenosis or stricture, cervix O34.4-
    streptococcus group B (GBS) carrier state
    O99.824
    transmural uterine scar O34.29
    transverse presentation or lie O32.2
    tumor, pelvic organs or tissues NEC O34.8-
      cervix O34.4-
    umbilical cord presentation or prolapse
    O69.0
    without indication O82
  completely normal case O80
  complicated O75.9
    by
      abnormal, abnormality (of)
        forces of labor O62.9
          specified type NEC O62.8
        glucose O99.814
        uterine contractions NOS O62.9
      abruptio placentae - *see also* Abruptio
      placentae O45.9-
      abuse
        physical O9A.32
        psychological O9A.52
        sexual O9A.42
      adherent placenta O72.0
        without hemorrhage O73.0
      alcohol use O99.314
      anemia (pre-existing) O99.02
      anesthetic death O74.8
      annular detachment of cervix O71.3
      atony, uterus O62.2
      attempted vacuum extraction and forceps
      O66.5
      Bandl's ring O62.4
      bariatric surgery status O99.844
      biliary tract disorder O26.62
      bleeding - *see* Delivery, complicated by,
      hemorrhage
      blood disorder NEC O99.12
      cervical dystocia (hypotonic) O62.2
        primary O62.0
        secondary O62.1
      circulatory system disorder O99.42
      compression of cord (umbilical) NEC
      O69.2
      condition NEC O99.89
      contraction, contracted ring O62.4
      cord (umbilical)
        around neck
          with compression O69.1
          without compression O69.81
        bruising O69.5
        complication O69.9
          specified NEC O69.89
        compression NEC O69.2
        entanglement O69.2
          without compression O69.82
        hematoma O69.5
        presentation O69.0
        prolapse O69.0
        short O69.3
        thrombosis (vessels) O69.5
        vascular lesion O69.5
      Couvelaire uterus O45.8X-
      damage to (injury to) NEC
        perineum O71.82
        periurethral tissue O71.82
        vulva O71.82
      delay following rupture of membranes
      (spontaneous) - *see* Pregnancy,
      complicated by, premature rupture of
      membranes
      depressed fetal heart tones O76

Delivery (childbirth) (labor) - *continued*
  diabetes O24.92
    gestational O24.429
      diet controlled O24.420
      insulin controlled O24.424
      oral drug controlled (antidiabetic)
        (hypoglycemic) O24.425
    pre-existing O24.32
      specified NEC O24.82
      type 1 O24.02
      type 2 O24.12
  diastasis recti (abdominis) O71.89
  dilatation
    bladder O66.8
    cervix incomplete, poor or slow O62.0
  disease NEC O99.89
  disruptio uteri - *see* Delivery, complicated
    by, rupture, uterus
  drug use O99.324
  dysfunction, uterus NOS O62.9
    hypertonic O62.4
    hypotonic O62.2
      primary O62.0
      secondary O62.1
    incoordinate O62.4
  eclampsia O15.1
  embolism (pulmonary) - *see* Embolism,
    obstetric
  endocrine, nutritional or metabolic disease
    NEC O99.284
  failed
    attempted vaginal birth after previous
      cesarean delivery O66.41
    induction of labor O61.9
      instrumental O61.1
      mechanical O61.1
      medical O61.0
      specified NEC O61.8
      surgical O61.1
    trial of labor O66.40
  female genital mutilation O65.5
  fetal
    abnormal acid-base balance O68
    acidemia O68
    acidosis O68
    alkalosis O68
    death, early O02.1
    deformity O66.3
    heart rate or rhythm (abnormal) (non-
      reassuring) O76
    hypoxia O77.8
    stress O77.9
      due to drug administration O77.1
      electrocardiographic evidence of O77.8
      specified NEC O77.8
      ultrasound evidence of O77.8
  fever during labor O75.2
  gastric banding status O99.844
  gastric bypass status O99.844
  gastrointestinal disease NEC O99.62
  gestational
    diabetes O24.429
      diet controlled O24.420
      insulin (and diet) controlled O24.424
      oral drug controlled (antidiabetic)
        (hypoglycemic) O24.425
    edema O12.04
      with proteinuria O12.24
    proteinuria O12.14
  gonorrhea O98.22
  hematoma O71.7
    ischial spine O71.7
    pelvic O71.7
    vagina O71.7

Delivery (childbirth) (labor) - *continued*
    vulva or perineum O71.7
  hemorrhage (uterine) O67.9
    associated with
      afibrinogenemia O67.0
      coagulation defect O67.0
      hyperfibrinolysis O67.0
      hypofibrinogenemia O67.0
    due to
      low implantation of placenta O44.5-
      low lying placenta O44.5-
      placenta previa O44.1-
        marginal O44.3-
        partial O44.3-
      premature separation of placenta
        (normally implanted) - *see also* Abruptio
        placentae O45.9-
      retained placenta O72.0
      uterine leiomyoma O67.8
    placenta NEC O67.8
    postpartum NEC (atonic) (immediate)
      O72.1
      with retained or trapped placenta O72.0
      delayed O72.2
      secondary O72.2
      third stage O72.0
  hourglass contraction, uterus O62.4
  hypertension, hypertensive (pre-existing) -
    see Hypertension, complicated by,
    childbirth (labor)
  hypotension O26.5-
  incomplete dilatation (cervix) O62.0
  incoordinate uterus contractions O62.4
  inertia, uterus O62.2
    during latent phase of labor O62.0
    primary O62.0
    secondary O62.1
  infection (maternal) O98.92
    carrier state NEC O99.834
    gonorrhea O98.22
    human immunodeficiency virus (HIV)
      O98.72
    sexually transmitted NEC O98.32
    specified NEC O98.82
    syphilis O98.12
    tuberculosis O98.02
    viral hepatitis O98.42
    viral NEC O98.52
  injury (to mother) - *see also* Delivery,
    complicated, by, damage to O71.9
    nonobstetric O9A.22
      caused by abuse - *see* Delivery,
        complicated, by, abuse
  intrauterine fetal death, early O02.1
  inversion, uterus O71.2
  laceration (perineal) O70.9
    anus (sphincter) O70.4
      with third degree laceration - *see also*
        Delivery, complicated, by, laceration,
        perineum, third degree O70.20
          with mucosa O70.3
      without third degree laceration O70.4
    bladder (urinary) O71.5
    bowel O71.5
    cervix (uteri) O71.3
    fourchette O70.0
    hymen O70.0
    labia O70.0
    pelvic
      floor O70.1
      organ NEC O71.5
    perineum, perineal O70.9
      first degree O70.0
      fourth degree O70.3

Delivery (childbirth) (labor) - *continued*
    muscles O70.1
    second degree O70.1
    skin O70.0
    slight O70.0
    third degree O70.20
      with
        both external anal sphincter (EAS)
          and internal anal sphincter (IAS) torn
          (IIIc) O70.23
        less than 50% of external anal
          sphincter (EAS) thickness torn (IIIa)
          O70.21
        more than 50% external anal sphincter
          (EAS) thickness torn (IIIb) O70.22
      IIIa O70.21
      IIIb O70.22
      IIIc O70.23
    peritoneum (pelvic) O71.5
    rectovaginal (septum) (without perineal
      laceration) O71.4
      with perineum - *see also* Delivery,
        complicated, by, laceration, perineum,
        third degree O70.20
        with anal or rectal mucosa O70.3
    specified NEC O71.89
    sphincter ani - *see* Delivery, complicated,
      by, laceration, anus (sphincter)
    urethra O71.5
    uterus O71.81
      before labor O71.81
    vagina, vaginal (deep) (high) (without
      perineal laceration) O71.4
      with perineum O70.0
      muscles, with perineum O70.1
    vulva O70.0
  liver disorder O26.62
  malignancy O9A.12
  malnutrition O25.2
  malposition, malpresentation
    placenta O44.0-
      with hemorrhage O44.1-
    uterus or cervix O65.5
    without obstruction - *see also* Delivery,
      complicated by, obstruction O32.9
      breech O32.1
      compound O32.6
      face (brow) (chin) O32.3
      footling O32.8
      high head O32.4
      oblique O32.2
      specified NEC O32.8
      transverse O32.2
      unstable lie O32.0
  meconium in amniotic fluid O77.0
  mental disorder NEC O99.344
  metrorrhexis - *see* Delivery, complicated
    by, rupture, uterus
  nervous system disorder O99.354
  obesity (pre-existing) O99.214
  obesity surgery status O99.844
  obstetric trauma O71.9
    specified NEC O71.89
  obstructed labor
    due to
      breech (complete) (frank) presentation
        O64.1
        incomplete O64.8
      brow presentation O64.3
      buttock presentation O64.1
      chin presentation O64.2
      compound presentation O64.5
      contracted pelvis O65.1
      deep transverse arrest O64.0

Delivery (childbirth) (labor) - *continued*
- deformed pelvis O65.0
- dystocia (fetal) O66.9
  - due to
    - conjoined twins O66.3
    - fetal
      - abnormality NEC O66.3
      - ascites O66.3
      - hydrops O66.3
      - meningomyelocele O66.3
      - sacral teratoma O66.3
      - tumor O66.3
    - hydrocephalic fetus O66.3
    - shoulder O66.0
  - face presentation O64.2
  - fetopelvic disproportion O65.4
  - footling presentation O64.8
  - impacted shoulders O66.0
  - incomplete rotation of fetal head O64.0
  - large fetus O66.2
  - locked twins O66.1
  - malposition O64.9
    - specified NEC O64.8
  - malpresentation O64.9
    - specified NEC O64.8
  - multiple fetuses NEC O66.6
  - pelvic
    - abnormality (maternal) O65.9
      - organ O65.5
      - specified NEC O65.8
    - contraction
      - inlet O65.2
      - mid-cavity O65.3
      - outlet O65.3
  - persistent (position)
    - occipitoiliac O64.0
    - occipitoposterior O64.0
    - occipitosacral O64.0
    - occipitotransverse O64.0
  - prolapsed arm O64.4
  - shoulder presentation O64.4
  - specified NEC O66.8
- pathological retraction ring, uterus O62.4
- penetration, pregnant uterus by instrument O71.1
- perforation - *see* Delivery, complicated by, laceration
- placenta, placental
  - ablatio - *see also* Abruptio placentae O45.9-
  - abnormality O43.9-
    - specified NEC O43.89-
  - abruptio - *see also* Abruptio placentae O45.9-
  - accreta O43.21-
  - adherent (with hemorrhage) O72.0
    - without hemorrhage O73.0
  - detachment (premature) - *see also* Abruptio placentae O45.9-
  - disorder O43.9-
    - specified NEC O43.89-
  - hemorrhage NEC O67.8
  - increta O43.22-
  - low (implantation) (lying) O44.4-
    - with hemorrhage O44.5-
  - malformation O43.10-
  - malposition O44.0-
    - without hemorrhage O44.1-
  - percreta O43.23-
  - previa (central) (complete) (lateral) (total) O44.0-
    - with hemorrhage O44.1-
    - marginal O44.2-
      - with hemorrhage O44.3-

Delivery (childbirth) (labor) - *continued*
- partial O44.2-
  - with hemorrhage O44.3-
- retained (with hemorrhage) O72.0
  - without hemorrhage O73.0
- separation (premature) O45.9-
  - specified NEC O45.8X-
- vicious insertion O44.1-
- precipitate labor O62.3
- premature rupture, membranes - *see also* Pregnancy, complicated by, premature rupture of membranes O42.90
- prolapse
  - arm or hand O32.2
  - cord (umbilical) O69.0
  - foot or leg O32.8
  - uterus O34.52-
- prolonged labor O63.9
  - first stage O63.0
  - second stage O63.1
- protozoal disease (maternal) O98.62
- respiratory disease NEC O99.52
- retained membranes or portions of placenta O72.2
  - without hemorrhage O73.1
- retarded birth O63.9
- retention of secundines (with hemorrhage) O72.0
  - without hemorrhage O73.0
  - partial O72.2
    - without hemorrhage O73.1
- rupture
  - bladder (urinary) O71.5
  - cervix O71.3
  - pelvic organ NEC O71.5
  - urethra O71.5
  - uterus (during or after labor) O71.1
    - before labor O71.0-
- separation, pubic bone (symphysis pubis) O71.6   shock O75.1
- shoulder presentation O64.4
- skin disorder NEC O99.72
- spasm, cervix O62.4
- stenosis or stricture, cervix O65.5
- streptococcus group B (GBS) carrier state O99.824
- subluxation of symphysis (pubis) O26.72
- syphilis (maternal) O98.12
- tear - *see* Delivery, complicated by, laceration
- tetanic uterus O62.4
- trauma (obstetrical) - *see also* Delivery, complicated, by, damage to O71.9
  - non-obstetric O9A.22
  - periurethral O71.82
  - specified NEC O71.89
- tuberculosis (maternal) O98.02
- tumor, pelvic organs or tissues NEC O65.5
- umbilical cord around neck
  - with compression O69.1
  - without compression O69.81
- uterine inertia O62.2
  - during latent phase of labor O62.0
  - primary O62.0
  - secondary O62.1
- vasa previa O69.4
- velamentous insertion of cord O43.12-
- specified complication NEC O75.89
- delayed NOS O63.9
- following rupture of membranes
  - artificial O75.5
  - second twin, triplet, etc. O63.2
- forceps, low following failed vacuum extraction O66.5

Delivery (childbirth) (labor) - *continued*
- missed (at or near term) O36.4
- normal O80
- obstructed - *see* Delivery, complicated by, obstructed labor
- precipitate O62.3
- preterm - *see also* Pregnancy, complicated by, preterm labor O60.10
- spontaneous O80
- term pregnancy NOS O80
- uncomplicated O80
- vaginal, following previous cesarean delivery O34.219
  - classical (vertical) scar O34.212
  - low transverse scar O34.211

Delusions (paranoid) - *see* Disorder, delusional

Dementia (degenerative (primary)) (old age) (persisting) F03.90
- with
  - aggressive behavior F03.91
  - behavioral disturbance F03.91
  - combative behavior F03.91
  - Lewy bodies G31.83 [*F02.80*]
    - with behavioral disturbance G31.83 [*F02.81*]
  - Parkinsonism G31.83 [*F02.80*]
    - with behavioral disturbance G31.83 [*F02.81*]
  - Parkinson's disease G20- [*F02.80*]
    - with behavioral disturbance G20- [*F02.81*]
  - violent behavior F03.91
- alcoholic F10.97
  - with dependence F10.27
- Alzheimer's type - *see* Disease, Alzheimer's
- arteriosclerotic - *see* Dementia, vascular
- atypical, Alzheimer's type - *see* Disease, Alzheimer's, specified NEC
- congenital - *see* Disability, intellectual
- frontal (lobe) G31.09 [*F02.80*]
  - with behavioral disturbance G31.09 [*F02.81*]
- frontotemporal G31.09 [*F02.80*]
  - with behavioral disturbance G31.09 [*F02.81*]
  - specified NEC G31.09 [*F02.80*]
    - with behavioral disturbance G31.09 [*F02.81*]
- in (due to)
  - alcohol F10.97
    - with dependence F10.27
  - Alzheimer's disease - *see* Disease, Alzheimer's
  - arteriosclerotic brain disease - *see* Dementia, vascular
  - cerebral lipidoses E75. [*F02.80*]
    - with behavioral disturbance E75. [*F02.81*]
  - Creutzfeldt-Jakob disease - *see also* Creutzfeldt-Jakob disease or syndrome (with dementia) A81.00
  - epilepsy G40. [*F02.80*]
    - with behavioral disturbance G40. [*F02.81*]
  - hepatolenticular degeneration E83.01 [*F02.80*]
    - with behavioral disturbance E83.01 [*F02.81*]
  - human immunodeficiency virus (HIV) disease B20- [*F02.80*]
    - with behavioral disturbance B20- [*F02.81*]
  - Huntington's disease or chorea G10 [*F02.80*]
    - with behavioral disturbance G10 [*F02.81*]
  - hypercalcemia E83.52 [*F02.80*]
    - with behavioral disturbance E83.52 [*F02.81*]
  - hypothyroidism, acquired E03.9 [*F02.80*]

Dementia - *continued*
  with behavioral disturbance E03.9 [*F02.81*]
    due to iodine deficiency E01.8 [*F02.80*]
      with behavioral disturbance E01.8
      [*F02.81*]
  inhalants F18.97
    with dependence F18.27
  multiple
    etiologies F03
    sclerosis G35 [*F02.80*]
      with behavioral disturbance G35
      [*F02.81*]
  neurosyphilis A52.17 [*F02.80*]
    with behavioral disturbance A52.17
    [*F02.81*]
    juvenile A50.49 [*F02.80*]
      with behavioral disturbance A50.49
      [*F02.81*]
  niacin deficiency E52 [*F02.80*]
    with behavioral disturbance E52 [*F02.81*]
  paralysis agitans G20- [*F02.80*]
    with behavioral disturbance G20- [*F02.81*]
  Parkinson's disease G20- [*F02.80*]
  pellagra E52 [*F02.80*]
    with behavioral disturbance E52 [*F02.81*]
  Pick's G31.01 [*F02.80*]
    with behavioral disturbance G31.01
    [*F02.81*]
  polyarteritis nodosa M30.0- [*F02.80*]
    with behavioral disturbance M30.0-
    [*F02.81*]
  psychoactive drug F19.97
    with dependence F19.27
    inhalants F18.97
      with dependence F18.27
    sedatives, hypnotics or anxiolytics F13.97
      with dependence F13.27
  sedatives, hypnotics or anxiolytics F13.97
    with dependence F13.27
  systemic lupus erythematosus M32.
  [*F02.80*]
    with behavioral disturbance M32. [*F02.81*]
  trypanosomiasis
    African B56.9 [*F02.80*]
      with behavioral disturbance B56.9
      [*F02.81*]
  unknown etiology F03
  vitamin B12
  deficiency E53.8 [*F02.80*]
    with behavioral disturbance E53.8
    [*F02.81*]
  volatile solvents F18.97
    with dependence F18.27
  with behavioral disturbance G31.83
  [*F02.81*]
  infantile, infantilis F84.3
  Lewy body G31.83 [*F02.80*]
    with behavioral disturbance G31.83
    [*F02.81*]
  multi-infarct - *see* Dementia, vascular
  paralytica, paralytic (syphilitic) A52.17
  [*F02.80*]
    with behavioral disturbance A52.17
    [*F02.81*]
    juvenilis A50.45
  paretic A52.17
  praecox - *see* Schizophrenia
  presenile F03
    Alzheimer's type - *see* Disease, Alzheimer's,
    early onset
  primary degenerative F03
  progressive, syphilitic A52.17
  senile F03
    with acute confusional state F05

Dementia - *continued*
  Alzheimer's type - *see* Disease, Alzheimer's,
  late onset
    depressed or paranoid type F03
  vascular (acute onset) (mixed) (multi-infarct)
  (subcortical) F01.50
    with behavioral disturbance F01.51
Demineralization, bone - *see* Osteoporosis
Demodex folliculorum (infestation) B88.0
Demophobia F40.248
Demoralization R45.3
Demyelination, demyelinization
  central nervous system G37.9
    specified NEC G37.8
  corpus callosum (central) G37.1
  disseminated, acute G36.9
    specified NEC G36.8
  global G35
  in optic neuritis G36.0
Dengue (classical) (fever) A90
  hemorrhagic A91
  sandfly A93.1
Dennie-Marfan syphilitic syndrome A50.45
Dens evaginatus, in dente or invaginatus
  K00.2
Dense breasts R92.2
Density
  increased, bone (disseminated) (generalized)
  (spotted) - *see* Disorder, bone, density and
  structure, specified type NEC
  lung (nodular) J98.4
Dental - *see also* condition
  examination Z01.20
    with abnormal findings Z01.21
  restoration
    aesthetically inadequate or displeasing
    K08.56
    defective K08.50
      specified NEC K08.59
    failure of marginal integrity K08.51
    failure of periodontal anatomical integrity
    K08.54
Dentia praecox K00.6
Denticles (pulp) K04.2
Dentigerous cyst K09.0
Dentin
  irregular (in pulp) K04.3
  opalescent K00.5
  secondary (in pulp) K04.3
  sensitive K03.89
Dentinogenesis imperfecta K00.5
Dentinoma - *see* Cyst, calcifying odontogenic
Dentition (syndrome) K00.7
  delayed K00.6
  difficult K00.7
  precocious K00.6
  premature K00.6
  retarded K00.6
Dependence (on) (syndrome) F19.20
  with remission F19.21
  alcohol (ethyl) (methyl) (without remission)
  F10.20
    with
      amnestic disorder, persisting F10.26
      anxiety disorder F10.280
      dementia, persisting F10.27
      intoxication F10.229
        with delirium F10.221
        uncomplicated F10.220
      mood disorder F10.24
      psychotic disorder F10.259
        with
          delusions F10.250
          hallucinations F10.251

Dependence (on) (syndrome) - *continued*
  remission F10.21
    sexual dysfunction F10.281
    sleep disorder F10.282
    specified disorder NEC F10.288
    withdrawal F10.239
      with
        delirium F10.231
        perceptual disturbance F10.232
      uncomplicated F10.230
  counseling and surveillance Z71.41
  amobarbital - *see* Dependence, drug, sedative
  amphetamine(s) (type) - *see* Dependence,
  drug, stimulant NEC
  amytal (sodium) - *see* Dependence, drug,
  sedative
  analgesic NEC F55.8
  anesthetic (agent) (gas) (general) (local) NEC -
  see Dependence, drug, psychoactive NEC
  anxiolytic NEC - *see* Dependence, drug,
  sedative
  barbital(s) - *see* Dependence, drug, sedative
  barbiturate(s) (compounds) (drugs classifiable
  to T42) - *see* Dependence, drug, sedative
  benzedrine - *see* Dependence, drug, stimulant
  NEC
  bhang - *see* Dependence, drug, cannabis
  bromide(s) NEC - *see* Dependence, drug,
  sedative
  caffeine - *see* Dependence, drug, stimulant
  NEC
  cannabis (sativa) (indica) (resin) (derivatives)
  (type) - *see* Dependence, drug, cannabis
  chloral (betaine) (hydrate) - *see* Dependence,
  drug, sedative
  chlordiazepoxide - *see* Dependence, drug,
  sedative
  coca (leaf) (derivatives) - *see* Dependence,
  drug, cocaine
  cocaine - *see* Dependence, drug, cocaine
  codeine - *see* Dependence, drug, opioid
  combinations of drugs F19.20
  dagga - *see* Dependence, drug, cannabis
  demerol - *see* Dependence, drug, opioid
  dexamphetamine - *see* Dependence, drug,
  stimulant NEC
  dexedrine - *see* Dependence, drug, stimulant
  NEC
  dextromethorphan - *see* Dependence, drug,
  opioid
  dextromoramide - *see* Dependence, drug,
  opioid
  dextro nor-pseudo-ephedrine - *see*
  Dependence, drug, stimulant NEC
  dextrorphan - *see* Dependence, drug, opioid
  diazepam - *see* Dependence, drug, sedative
  dilaudid - *see* Dependence, drug, opioid
  D-lysergic acid diethylamide - *see*
  Dependence, drug, hallucinogen
  drug NEC F19.20
    with sleep disorder F19.282
    cannabis F12.20
      with
        anxiety disorder F12.280
        intoxication F12.229
          with
            delirium F12.221
            perceptual disturbance F12.222
          uncomplicated F12.220
        other specified disorder F12.288
        psychosis F12.259
          delusions F12.250
          hallucinations F12.251
        unspecified disorder F12.29

Dependence (on) (syndrome) - *continued*
in remission F12.21
  cocaine F14.20
    with
      anxiety disorder F14.280
      intoxication F14.229
        with
          delirium F14.221
            perceptual disturbance F14.222
        uncomplicated F14.220
      mood disorder F14.24
      other specified disorder F14.288
      psychosis F14.259
        delusions F14.250
        hallucinations F14.251
      sexual dysfunction F14.281
      sleep disorder F14.282
      unspecified disorder F14.29
      withdrawal F14.23
    in remission F14.21
    withdrawal symptoms in newborn P96.1
  counseling and surveillance Z71.51
  hallucinogen F16.20
    with
      anxiety disorder F16.280
      flashbacks F16.283
      intoxication F16.229
        with delirium F16.221
        uncomplicated F16.220
      mood disorder F16.24
      other specified disorder F16.288
      perception disorder, persisting F16.283
      psychosis F16.259
        delusions F16.250
        hallucinations F16.251
      unspecified disorder F16.29
    in remission F16.21
  in remission F19.21
  inhalant F18.20
    with
      anxiety disorder F18.280
      dementia, persisting F18.27
      intoxication F18.229
        with delirium F18.221
        uncomplicated F18.220
      mood disorder F18.24
      other specified disorder F18.288
      psychosis F18.259
        delusions F18.250
        hallucinations F18.251
      unspecified disorder F18.29
    in remission F18.21
  nicotine F17.200
    with disorder F17.209
      in remission F17.201
      specified disorder NEC F17.208
      withdrawal F17.203
    chewing tobacco F17.220
      with disorder F17.229
        in remission F17.221
      specified disorder NEC F17.228
      withdrawal F17.223
    cigarettes F17.210
      with disorder F17.219
        in remission F17.211
      specified disorder NEC F17.218
      withdrawal F17.213
    specified product NEC F17.290
      with disorder F17.299
        remission F17.291
      specified disorder NEC F17.298
      withdrawal F17.293
  opioid F11.20
    with

Dependence (on) (syndrome) - *continued*
  intoxication F11.229
    with
      delirium F11.221
      perceptual disturbance F11.222
    uncomplicated F11.220
  mood disorder F11.24
  other specified disorder F11.288
  psychosis F11.259
    delusions F11.250
    hallucinations F11.251
  sexual dysfunction F11.281
  sleep disorder F11.282
  unspecified disorder F11.29
  withdrawal F11.23
  in remission F11.21
  psychoactive NEC F19.20
    with
      amnestic disorder F19.26
      anxiety disorder F19.280
      dementia F19.27
      intoxication F19.229
        with
          delirium F19.221
          perceptual disturbance F19.222
        uncomplicated F19.220
      mood disorder F19.24
      other specified disorder F19.288
      psychosis F19.259
        delusions F19.250
        hallucinations F19.251
      sexual dysfunction F19.281
      sleep disorder F19.282
      unspecified disorder F19.29
      withdrawal F19.239
        with
          delirium F19.231
          perceptual disturbance F19.232
        uncomplicated F19.230
  sedative, hypnotic or anxiolytic F13.20
    with
      amnestic disorder F13.26
      anxiety disorder F13.280
      dementia, persisting F13.27
      intoxication F13.229
        with delirium F13.221
        uncomplicated F13.220
      mood disorder F13.24
      other specified disorder F13.288
      psychosis F13.259
        delusions F13.250
        hallucinations F13.251
      sexual dysfunction F13.281
      sleep disorder F13.282
      unspecified disorder F13.29
      withdrawal F13.239
        with
          delirium F13.231
          perceptual disturbance F13.232
        uncomplicated F13.230
    in remission F13.21
  stimulant NEC F15.20
    with
      anxiety disorder F15.280
      intoxication F15.229
        with
          delirium F15.221
          perceptual disturbance F15.222
        uncomplicated F15.220
      mood disorder F15.24
      other specified disorder F15.288
      psychosis F15.259
        delusions F15.250
        hallucinations F15.251

Dependence (on) (syndrome) - *continued*
  sexual dysfunction F15.281
    sleep disorder F15.282
    unspecified disorder F15.29
    withdrawal F15.23
  in remission F15.21
  ethyl
    alcohol (without remission) F10.20
      with remission F10.21
    bromide - *see* Dependence, drug, sedative
    carbamate F19.20
    chloride F19.20
    morphine - *see* Dependence, drug, opioid
  ganja - *see* Dependence, drug, cannabis
  glue (airplane) (sniffing) - *see* Dependence,
    drug, inhalant
  glutethimide - *see* Dependence, drug, sedative
  hallucinogenics - *see* Dependence, drug,
    hallucinogen
  hashish - *see* Dependence, drug, cannabis
  hemp - *see* Dependence, drug, cannabis
  heroin (salt) (any) - *see* Dependence, drug,
    opioid
  hypnotic NEC - *see* Dependence, drug,
    sedative
  Indian hemp - *see* Dependence, drug, cannabis
  inhalants - *see* Dependence, drug, inhalant
  khat - *see* Dependence, drug, stimulant NEC
  laudanum - *see* Dependence, drug, opioid
  LSD (25) (derivatives) - *see* Dependence,
    drug, hallucinogen
  luminal - *see* Dependence, drug, sedative
  lysergic acid - *see* Dependence, drug,
    hallucinogen
  maconha - *see* Dependence, drug, cannabis
  marihuana - *see* Dependence, drug, cannabis
  meprobamate - *see* Dependence, drug, sedative
  mescaline - *see* Dependence, drug,
    hallucinogen
  methadone - *see* Dependence, drug, opioid
  methamphetamine(s) - *see* Dependence, drug,
    stimulant NEC
  methaqualone - *see* Dependence, drug,
    sedative
  methyl
    alcohol (without remission) F10.20
      with remission F10.21
    bromide - *see* Dependence, drug, sedative
    morphine - *see* Dependence, drug, opioid
    phenidate - *see* Dependence, drug, stimulant
      NEC
    sulfonal - *see* Dependence, drug, sedative
  morphine (sulfate) (sulfite) (type) - *see*
    Dependence, drug, opioid
  narcotic (drug) NEC - *see* Dependence, drug,
    opioid
  nembutal - *see* Dependence, drug, sedative
  neraval - *see* Dependence, drug, sedative
  neravan - *see* Dependence, drug, sedative
  neurobarb - *see* Dependence, drug, sedative
  nicotine - *see* Dependence, drug, nicotine
  nitrous oxide F19.20
  nonbarbiturate sedatives and tranquilizers with
    similar effect - *see* Dependence, drug,
    sedative
  on
    artificial heart (fully implantable)
    (mechanical) Z95.812
    aspirator Z99.0
    care provider (because of) Z74.9
      impaired mobility Z74.09
      need for
        assistance with personal care Z74.1
        continuous supervision Z74.3

Dependence (on) (syndrome) - *continued*
no other household member able to render
care Z74.2
specified reason NEC Z74.8
machine Z99.89
enabling NEC Z99.89
specified type NEC Z99.89
renal dialysis (hemodialysis) (peritoneal)
Z99.2
respirator Z99.11
ventilator Z99.11
wheelchair Z99.3
opiate - *see* Dependence, drug, opioid
opioids - *see* Dependence, drug, opioid
opium (alkaloids) (derivatives) (tincture) - *see*
Dependence, drug, opioid
oxygen (long-term) (supplemental) Z99.81
paraldehyde - *see* Dependence, drug, sedative
paregoric - *see* Dependence, drug, opioid
PCP (phencyclidine) (or related substance) -
see Dependence, drug, hallucinogen
pentobarbital - *see* Dependence, drug, sedative
pentobarbitone (sodium) - *see* Dependence,
drug, sedative
pentothal - *see* Dependence, drug, sedative
peyote - *see* Dependence, drug, hallucinogen
phencyclidine (PCP) (or related substance) -
see Dependence, drug, hallucinogen
phenmetrazine - *see* Dependence, drug,
stimulant NEC
phenobarbital - *see* Dependence, drug, sedative
polysubstance F19.20
psilocybin, psilocin, psilocin, psilocyline - *see*
Dependence, drug, hallucinogen
psychostimulant NEC - *see* Dependence, drug,
stimulant NEC
secobarbital - *see* Dependence, drug, sedative
seconal - *see* Dependence, drug, sedative
sedative NEC - *see* Dependence, drug,
sedative
specified drug NEC - *see* Dependence, drug
stimulant NEC - *see* Dependence, drug,
stimulant NEC
substance NEC - *see* Dependence, drug
supplemental oxygen Z99.81
tobacco - *see* Dependence, drug, nicotine
counseling and surveillance Z71.6
tranquilizer NEC - *see* Dependence, drug,
sedative
vitamin B6 E53.1
volatile solvents - *see* Dependence, drug,
inhalant
Dependency
care-provider Z74.9
passive F60.7
reactions (persistent) F60.7
Depersonalization (in neurotic state)
(neurotic) (syndrome) F48.1
Depletion
extracellular fluid E86.9
plasma E86.1
potassium E87.6
nephropathy N25.89
salt or sodium E87.1
causing heat exhaustion or prostration T67.4
nephropathy N28.9
volume NOS E86.9
Deployment (current) (military) status
Z56.82
in theater or in support of military war,
peacekeeping and humanitarian operations
Z56.82
personal history of Z91.82
military war, peacekeeping and humanitarian

Deployment (current) (military) - *continued*
deployment (current or past conflict) Z91.82
returned from Z91.82
Depolarization, premature I49.40
atrial I49.1
junctional I49.2
specified NEC I49.49
ventricular I49.3
Deposit
bone in Boeck's sarcoid D86.89
calcareous, calcium - *see* Calcification
cholesterol
retina H35.89
vitreous (body) (humor) - *see* Deposit,
crystalline
conjunctiva H11.11-
cornea H18.00-
argentous H18.02-
due to metabolic disorder H18.03-
Kayser-Fleischer ring H18.04-
pigmentation - *see* Pigmentation, cornea
crystalline, vitreous (body) (humor) H43.2-
hemosiderin in old scars of cornea - *see*
Pigmentation, cornea, stromal
metallic in lens - *see* Cataract, specified NEC
skin R23.8
tooth, teeth (betel) (black) (green) (materia
alba) (orange) (tobacco) K03.6
urate, kidney - *see* Calculus, kidney
Depraved appetite - *see* Pica
Depressed
HDL cholesterol E78.6
Depression (acute) (mental) F32.9
agitated (single episode) F32.2
anaclitic - *see* Disorder, adjustment
anxiety F41.8
persistent F34.1
arches - *see also* Deformity, limb, flat foot
atypical (single episode) F32.89
recurrent episode F33.8
basal metabolic rate R94.8
bone marrow D75.89
central nervous system R09.2
cerebral R29.818
newborn P91.4
cerebrovascular I67.9
chest wall M95.4
climacteric (single episode) F32.89
recurrent episode F33.8
endogenous (without psychotic symptoms)
F33.2
with psychotic symptoms F33.3
functional activity R68.89
hysterical F44.89
involutional (single episode) F32.89
recurrent episode F33.8
major F32.9
with psychotic symptoms F32.3
recurrent - *see* Disorder, depressive, recurrent
manic-depressive - *see* Disorder, depressive,
recurrent
masked (single episode) F32.89
medullary G93.89
menopausal (single episode) F32.89
recurrent episode F33.8
metatarsus - *see* Depression, arches
monopolar F33.9
nervous F34.1
neurotic F34.1
nose M95.0
postnatal F53
postpartum F53
post-psychotic of schizophrenia F32.89
post-schizophrenic F32.89

Depression - *continued*
psychogenic (reactive) (single episode) F32.9
psychoneurotic F34.1
psychotic (single episode) F32.3
recurrent F33.3
reactive (psychogenic) (single episode) F32.9
psychotic (single episode) F32.3
recurrent - *see* Disorder, depressive, recurrent
respiratory center G93.89
seasonal - *see* Disorder, depressive, recurrent
senile F03
severe, single episode F32.2
situational F43.21
skull Q67.4
specified NEC (single episode) F32.89
sternum M95.4
visual field - *see* Defect, visual field
vital (recurrent) (without psychotic symptoms)
F33.2
with psychotic symptoms F33.3
single episode F32.2
Deprivation
cultural Z60.3
effects NOS T73.9
specified NEC T73.8
emotional NEC Z65.8
affecting infant or child - *see* Maltreatment,
child, psychological
food T73.0
protein - *see* Malnutrition
sleep Z72.820
social Z60.4
affecting infant or child - *see* Maltreatment,
child, psychological
specified NEC T73.8
vitamins - *see* Deficiency, vitamin
water T73.1
Derangement
ankle (internal) - *see* Derangement, joint, ankle
cartilage (articular) NEC - *see* Derangement,
joint, articular cartilage, by site
recurrent - *see* Dislocation, recurrent
cruciate ligament, anterior, current injury - *see*
Sprain, knee, cruciate, anterior
elbow (internal) - *see* Derangement, joint,
elbow
hip (joint) (internal) (old) - *see* Derangement,
joint, hip
joint (internal) M24.9
ankylosis - *see* Ankylosis
articular cartilage M24.10
ankle M24.17-
elbow M24.12-
foot M24.17-
hand M24.14-
hip M24.15-
knee NEC M23.9-
loose body - *see* Loose, body
shoulder M24.11-
wrist M24.13-
contracture - *see* Contraction, joint
current injury - *see also* Dislocation
knee, meniscus or cartilage - *see* Tear,
meniscus
dislocation
pathological - *see* Dislocation, pathological
recurrent - *see* Dislocation, recurrent
knee - *see* Derangement, knee
ligament - *see* Disorder, ligament
loose body - *see* Loose, body
recurrent - *see* Dislocation, recurrent
specified type NEC M24.80
ankle M24.87-
elbow M24.82-

Derangement - *continued*
    foot joint M24.87-
    hand joint M24.84-
    hip M24.85-
    shoulder M24.81-
    wrist M24.83-
    temporomandibular M26.69
  knee (recurrent) M23.9-
    ligament disruption, spontaneous M23.60-
      anterior cruciate M23.61-
      capsular M23.67-
      instability, chronic M23.5-
      lateral collateral M23.64-
      medial collateral M23.63-
      posterior cruciate M23.62-
    loose body M23.4-
    meniscus M23.30-
      cystic M23.00-
        lateral M23.002
          anterior horn M23.04-
          posterior horn M23.05-
          specified NEC M23.06-
        medial M23.005
          anterior horn M23.01-
          posterior horn M23.02-
          specified NEC M23.03-
      degenerate - *see* Derangement, knee,
  meniscus, specified NEC
      detached - *see* Derangement, knee,
  meniscus, specified NEC
      due to old tear or injury M23.20-
        lateral M23.20-
          anterior horn M23.24-
          posterior horn M23.25-
          specified NEC M23.26-
        medial M23.20-
          anterior horn M23.21-
          posterior horn M23.22-
          specified NEC M23.23-
      retained - *see* Derangement, knee,
  meniscus, specified NEC
      specified NEC M23.30-
        lateral M23.30-
          anterior horn M23.34-
          posterior horn M23.35-
          specified NEC M23.36-
        medial M23.30-
          anterior horn M23.31-
          posterior horn M23.32-
          specified NEC M23.33-
    old M23.8X-
    specified NEC - *see* subcategory M23.8
  low back NEC - *see* Dorsopathy, specified
NEC
  meniscus - *see* Derangement, knee, meniscus
  mental - *see* Psychosis
  patella, specified NEC - *see* Disorder, patella,
derangement NEC
  semilunar cartilage (knee) - *see* Derangement,
knee, meniscus, specified NEC
  shoulder (internal) - *see* Derangement, joint,
shoulder
Dercum's disease E88.2
Derealization (neurotic) F48.1
Dermal - *see* condition **Dermaphytid** - *see*
Dermatophytosis
Dermatitis (eczematous) L30.9
  ab igne L59.0
  acarine B88.0
  actinic (due to sun) L57.8
    other than from sun L59.8 allergic - *see*
  Dermatitis, contact, allergic
  ambustionis, due to burn or scald - *see* Burn
  amebic A06.7

Dermatitis - *continued*
  ammonia L22
  arsenical (ingested) L27.8
  artefacta L98.1
    psychogenic F54
  atopic L20.9
    psychogenic F54
    specified NEC L20.89
  autoimmune progesterone L30.8
  berlock, berloque L56.2
  blastomycotic B40.3
  blister beetle L24.89
  bullous, bullosa L13.9
    mucosynechial, atrophic L12.1
    seasonal L30.8
    specified NEC L13.8
  calorica L59.0
    due to burn or scald - *see* Burn
  caterpillar L24.89
  cercarial B65.3
  combustionis L59.0
    due to burn or scald - *see* Burn
  congelationis T69.1
  contact (occupational) L25.9
    allergic L23.9
      due to
        adhesives L23.1
        cement L23.5
        chemical products NEC L23.5
        chromium L23.0
        cosmetics L23.2
        dander (cat) (dog) L23.81
        drugs in contact with skin L23.3
        dyes L23.4
        food in contact with skin L23.6
        hair (cat) (dog) L23.81
        insecticide L23.5
        metals L23.0
        nickel L23.0
        plants, non-food L23.7
        plastic L23.5
        rubber L23.5
        specified agent NEC L23.89
    due to
      cement L25.3
      chemical products NEC L25.3
      cosmetics L25.0
      dander (cat) (dog) L23.81
      drugs in contact with skin L25.1
      dyes L25.2
      food in contact with skin L25.4
      hair (cat) (dog) L23.81
      plants, non-food L25.5
      specified agent NEC L25.8
    irritant L24.9
      due to
        cement L24.5
        chemical products NEC L24.5
        cosmetics L24.3
        detergents L24.0
        drugs in contact with skin L24.4
        food in contact with skin L24.6
        oils and greases L24.1
        plants, non-food L24.7
        solvents L24.2
        specified agent NEC L24.89
  contusiformis L52
  diabetic - *see* E08-e13 with .620
  diaper L22
  diphtheritica A36.3
  dry skin L85.3
  due to
    acetone (contact) (irritant) L24.2
    acids (contact) (irritant) L24.5

Dermatitis - *continued*
  adhesive(s) (allergic) (contact) (plaster)
L23.1
    irritant L24.5
  alcohol (irritant) (skin contact) (substances in
category T51) L24.2
    taken internally L27.8
  alkalis (contact) (irritant) L24.5
  arsenic (ingested) L27.8
  carbon disulfide (contact) (irritant) L24.2
  caustics (contact) (irritant) L24.5
  cement (contact) L25.3
  cereal (ingested) L27.2
  chemical(s) NEC L25.3
    taken internally L27.8
  chlorocompounds L24.2
  chromium (contact) (irritant) L24.81
  coffee (ingested) L27.2
  cold weather L30.8
  cosmetics (contact) L25.0
    allergic L23.2
    irritant L24.3
  cyclohexanes L24.2
  dander (cat) (dog) L23.81
  Demodex species B88.0
  Dermanyssus gallinae B88.0
  detergents (contact) (irritant) L24.0
  dichromate L24.81
  drugs and medicaments (generalized)
(internal use) L27.0
    external - *see* Dermatitis, due to, drugs, in
  contact with skin
    in contact with skin L25.1
      allergic L23.3
      irritant L24.4
    localized skin eruption L27.1
    specified substance - *see* Table of Drugs
  and Chemicals
  dyes (contact) L25.2
    allergic L23.4
    irritant L24.89
  epidermophytosis - *see* Dermatophytosis
  esters L24.2
  external irritant NEC L24.9
  fish (ingested) L27.2
  flour (ingested) L27.2
  food (ingested) L27.2
    in contact with skin L25.4
  fruit (ingested) L27.2
  furs (allergic) (contact) L23.81
  glues - *see* Dermatitis, due to, adhesives
  glycols L24.2
  greases NEC (contact) (irritant) L24.1
  hair (cat) (dog) L23.81
  hot
    objects and materials - *see* Burn
    weather or places L59.0
  hydrocarbons L24.2
  infrared rays L59.8
  ingestion, ingested substance L27.9
    chemical NEC L27.8
    drugs and medicaments - *see* Dermatitis,
  due to, drugs
    food L27.2
    specified NEC L27.8
  insecticide in contact with skin L24.5
  internal agent L27.9
    drugs and medicaments (generalized) - *see*
  Dermatitis, due to, drugs
    food L27.2
  irradiation - *see* Dermatitis, due to,
radioactive substance
  ketones L24.2
  lacquer tree (allergic) (contact) L23.7

Dermatitis - *continued*
  light (sun) NEC L57.8
    acute L56.8
    other L59.8
  Liponyssoides sanguineus B88.0
  low temperature L30.8
  meat (ingested) L27.2
  metals, metal salts (contact) (irritant) L24.81
  milk (ingested) L27.2
  nickel (contact) (irritant) L24.81
  nylon (contact) (irritant) L24.5
  oils NEC (contact) (irritant) L24.1
  paint solvent (contact) (irritant) L24.2
  petroleum products (contact) (irritant)
    (substances in T52.0) L24.2
  plants NEC (contact) L25.5
    allergic L23.7
    irritant L24.7
  plasters (adhesive) (any) (allergic) (contact)
    L23.1
    irritant L24.5
  plastic (contact) L25.3
  preservatives (contact) - *see* Dermatitis, due
    to, chemical, in contact with skin
  primrose (allergic) (contact) L23.7
  primula (allergic) (contact) L23.7
  radiation L59.8
    nonionizing (chronic exposure) L57.8
    sun NEC L57.8
      acute L56.8
  radioactive substance L58.9
    acute L58.0
    chronic L58.1
  radium L58.9
    acute L58.0
    chronic L58.1
  ragweed (allergic) (contact) L23.7
  Rhus (allergic) (contact) (diversiloba)
    (radicans) (toxicodendron) (venenata)
    (verniciflua) L23.7
  rubber (contact) L24.5
  Senecio jacobaea (allergic) (contact) L23.7
  solvents (contact) (irritant) (substances in
    categories T52) L24.2
  specified agent NEC (contact) L25.8
    allergic L23.89
    irritant L24.89
  sunshine NEC L57.8
    acute L56.8
  tetrachlorethylene (contact) (irritant) L24.2
  toluene (contact) (irritant) L24.2
  turpentine (contact) L24.2
  ultraviolet rays (sun NEC) (chronic
    exposure) L57.8
    acute L56.8
  vaccine or vaccination L27.0
    specified substance - *see* Table of Drugs
      and Chemicals
  varicose veins - *see* Varix, leg, with,
    inflammation   X-rays L58.9
    acute L58.0
    chronic L58.1
  dyshidrotic L30.1
  dysmenorrheica N94.6
  escharotica - *see* Burn
  exfoliative, exfoliativa (generalized) L26
    neonatorum L00
  eyelid - *see also* Dermatosis, eyelid
    allergic H01.119
      left H01.116
        lower H01.115
        upper H01.114
      right H01.113
        lower H01.112

Dermatitis - *continued*
    upper H01.111
  contact - *see* Dermatitis, eyelid, allergic
  due to
    Demodex species B88.0
    herpes (zoster) B02.39
      simplex B00.59
  eczematous H01.139
    left H01.136
      lower H01.135
      upper H01.134
    right H01.133
      lower H01.132
      upper H01.131
  facta, factitia, factitial L98.1
    psychogenic F54
  flexural NEC L20.82
  friction L30.4
  fungus B36.9
    specified type NEC B36.8
  gangrenosa, gangrenous infantum L08.0
  harvest mite B88.0
  heat L59.0
  herpesviral, vesicular (ear) (lip) B00.1
  herpetiformis (bullous) (erythematous)
    (pustular) (vesicular) L13.0
    juvenile L12.2
    senile L12.0
  hiemalis L30.8
  hypostatic, hypostatica - *see* Varix, leg, with,
    inflammation
  infectious eczematoid L30.3
  infective L30.3
  irritant - *see* Dermatitis, contact, irritant
  Jacquet's (diaper dermatitis) L22
  Leptus B88.0
  lichenified NEC L28.0
  medicamentosa (generalized) (internal use) -
    see Dermatitis, due to drugs
  mite B88.0
  multiformis L13.0
    juvenile L12.2
  napkin L22
  neurotica L13.0
  nummular L30.0
  papillaris capillitii L73.0
  pellagrous E52
  perioral L71.0
  photocontact L56.2
  polymorpha dolorosa L13.0
  pruriginosa L13.0
  pruritic NEC L30.8
  psychogenic F54
  purulent L08.0
  pustular
    contagious B08.02
    subcorneal L13.1
  pyococcal L08.0
  pyogenica L08.0
  repens L40.2
  Ritter's (exfoliativa) L00
  Schamberg's L81.7
  schistosome B65.3
  seasonal bullous L30.8
  seborrheic L21.9
    infantile L21.1
    specified NEC L21.8
  sensitization NOS L23.9
  septic L08.0
  solare L57.8
  specified NEC L30.8
  stasis I87.2
    with
      varicose ulcer - *see* Varix, leg, with ulcer,

Dermatitis - *continued*
    with inflammation
      varicose veins - *see* Varix, leg, with,
        inflammation
    due to postthrombotic syndrome - *see*
      Syndrome, postthrombotic
  suppurative L08.0
  traumatic NEC L30.4
  trophoneurotica L13.0
  ultraviolet (sun) (chronic exposure) L57.8
    acute L56.8
  varicose - *see* Varix, leg, with, inflammation
  vegetans L10.1
  verrucosa B43.0
  vesicular, herpesviral B00.1
Dermatoarthritis, lipoid E78.81
Dermatochalasis, eyelid H02.839
  left H02.836
    lower H02.835
    upper H02.834
  right H02.833
    lower H02.832
    upper H02.831
Dermatofibroma (lenticulare) - *see* Neoplasm,
  skin, benign
  protuberans - *see* Neoplasm, skin, uncertain
  behavior
Dermatofibrosarcoma (pigmented)
  (protuberans) - *see* Neoplasm, skin,
  malignant
Dermatographia L50.3
Dermatolysis (exfoliativa) (congenital) Q82.8
  acquired L57.4
  eyelids - *see* Blepharochalasis
  palpebrarum - *see* Blepharochalasis
  senile L57.4
Dermatomegaly NEC Q82.8
Dermatomucosomyositis M33.10
  with
    myopathy M33.12
    respiratory involvement M33.11
    specified organ involvement NEC M33.19
Dermatomycosis B36.9
  furfuracea B36.0
  specified type NEC B36.8
Dermatomyositis (acute) (chronic) - *see also*
  Dermatopolymyositis
  adult (see also Dermatomyositis, specified
  NEC) M33.10
  in (due to) neoplastic disease - *see also*
    Neoplasm D49.9 [*M36.0*]
  juvenile M33.00
    with
      myopathy M33.02
      respiratory involvement M33.01
      specified organ involvement NEC M33.09
    without myopathy M33.03
  specified NEC M33.10
    with
      myopathy M33.12
      respiratory involvement M33.11
      specified organ involvement NEC M33.19
    without myopathy M33.13
Dermatoneuritis of children - *see* Poisoning,
  mercury
Dermatophilosis A48.8
Dermatophytid L30.2
Dermatophytid - *see* Dermatophytosis
Dermatophytosis (epidermophyton)
  (infection) (Microsporum) (tinea)
  (Trichophyton) B35.9
  beard B35.0
  body B35.4
  capitis B35.0

Dermatophytosis - *continued*
  corporis B35.4
  deep-seated B35.8
  disseminated B35.8
  foot B35.3
  granulomatous B35.8
  groin B35.6
  hand B35.2
  nail B35.1
  perianal (area) B35.6
  scalp B35.0
  specified NEC B35.8
Dermatopolymyositis M33.90
  with
    myopathy M33.92
    respiratory involvement M33.91
    specified organ involvement NEC M33.99
  in neoplastic disease - *see also* Neoplasm
  D49.9 [*M36.0*]
  juvenile M33.00
    with
      myopathy M33.02
      respiratory involvement M33.01
      specified organ involvement NEC M33.09
    specified NEC M33.10
    myopathy M33.12
    respiratory involvement M33.11
    specified organ involvement NEC M33.19
  without myopathy M33.93
Dermatopolyneuritis - *see* Poisoning, mercury
Dermatorrhexis Q79.6
  acquired L57.4
Dermatosclerosis - *see also* Scleroderma
  localized L94.0
Dermatosis L98.9
  Andrews' L08.89
  Bowen's - *see* Neoplasm, skin, in situ
  bullous L13.9
    specified NEC L13.8
  exfoliativa L26
  eyelid (noninfectious)
    dermatitis - *see* Dermatitis, eyelid
    discoid lupus erythematosus - *see* Lupus,
    erythematosus, eyelid
    xeroderma - *see* Xeroderma, acquired, eyelid
  factitial L98.1
  febrile neutrophilic L98.2
  gonococcal A54.89
  herpetiformis L13.0
    juvenile L12.2
  linear IgA L13.8
  menstrual NEC L98.8
  neutrophilic, febrile L98.2
  occupational - *see* Dermatitis, contact
  papulosa nigra L82.1
  pigmentary L81.9
    progressive L81.7
    Schamberg's L81.7
  psychogenic F54
  purpuric, pigmented L81.7
  pustular, subcorneal L13.1
  transient acantholytic L11.1
Dermographia, dermographism L50.3
Dermoid (cyst) - *see also* Neoplasm, benign, by
  site
  with malignant transformation C56-
  due to radiation (nonionizing) L57.8
Dermopathy
  infiltrative with thyrotoxicosis - *see*
  Thyrotoxicosis
  nephrogenic fibrosing L90.8
Dermophytosis - *see* Dermatophytosis
Descemetocele H18.73-
Descemet's membrane - *see* condition

Descending - *see* condition
Descensus uteri - *see* Prolapse, uterus
Desert
  rheumatism B38.0
  sore - *see* Ulcer, skin
Desertion (newborn) - *see* Maltreatment
Desmoid (extra-abdominal) (tumor) - *see*
  Neoplasm, connective tissue, uncertain
  behavior
  abdominal D48.1
Despondency F32.9
Desquamation, skin R23.4
Destruction, destructive - *see also* Damage
  articular facet - *see also* Derangement, joint,
  specified type NEC
    knee M23.8X-
    vertebra - *see* Spondylosis
  bone - *see also* Disorder, bone, specified type
  NEC
    syphilitic A52.77
  joint - *see also* Derangement, joint, specified
  type NEC
    sacroiliac M53.3
  rectal sphincter K62.89
  septum (nasal) J34.89
  tuberculous NEC - *see* Tuberculosis
  tympanum, tympanic membrane
  (nontraumatic) - *see* Disorder, tympanic
  membrane, specified NEC
  vertebral disc - *see* Degeneration,
  intervertebral disc
Destructiveness - *see also* Disorder, conduct
  adjustment reaction - *see* Disorder, adjustment
Desultory labor O62.2
Detachment
  cartilage - *see* Sprain
  cervix, annular N88.8
    complicating delivery O71.3
  choroid (old) (postinfectional) (simple)
  (spontaneous) H31.40-
    hemorrhagic H31.41-
    serous H31.42-
  ligament - *see* Sprain
  meniscus (knee) - *see also* Derangement, knee,
  meniscus, specified NEC
    current injury - *see* Tear, meniscus
    due to old tear or injury - *see* Derangement,
  knee, meniscus, due to old tear
  retina (without retinal break) (serous) H33.2-
    with retinal:
      break H33.00-
        giant H33.03-
        multiple H33.02-
        single H33.01-
      dialysis H33.04-
    pigment epithelium - *see* Degeneration,
  retina, separation of layers, pigment epithelium
  detachment
    rhegmatogenous - *see* Detachment, retina,
  with retinal, break
    specified NEC H33.8
    total H33.05-
    traction H33.4-
  vitreous (body) H43.81
Detergent asthma J69.8
Deterioration
  epileptic F06.8
  general physical R53.81
  heart, cardiac - *see* Degeneration, myocardial
  mental - *see* Psychosis
  myocardial, myocardium - *see* Degeneration,
  myocardial
  senile (simple) R54

Deuteranomaly (anomalous trichromat)
  H53.53
Deuteranopia (complete) (incomplete) H53.53
Development
  abnormal, bone Q79.9
  arrested R62.50
    bone - *see* Arrest, development or growth,
    bone
    child R62.50
    due to malnutrition E45
  defective, congenital - *see also* Anomaly, by
  site
    cauda equina Q06.3
    left ventricle Q24.8
      in hypoplastic left heart syndrome Q23.4
    valve Q24.8
    pulmonary Q22.3
  delayed - *see also* Delay, development R62.50
    arithmetical skills F81.2
    language (skills) (expressive) F80.1
    learning skill F81.9
    mixed skills F88
    motor coordination F82
    reading F81.0
    specified learning skill NEC F81.89
    speech F80.9
    spelling F81.81
    written expression F81.81
  imperfect, congenital - *see also* Anomaly, by
  site
    heart Q24.9
    lungs Q33.6
  incomplete
    bronchial tree Q32.4
    organ or site not listed - *see* Hypoplasia, by
    site
    respiratory system Q34.9
  sexual, precocious NEC E30.1
  tardy, mental - *see also* Disability, intellectual
  F79
Developmental - *see* condition
  testing, infant or child - *see* Examination, child
Devergie's disease (pityriasis rubra pilaris)
  L44.0
Deviation (in)
  conjugate palsy (eye) (spastic) H51.0
  esophagus (acquired) K22.8
  eye, skew H51.8
  midline (jaw) (teeth) (dental arch) M26.29
    specified site NEC - *see* Malposition
  nasal septum J34.2
    congenital Q67.4
  opening and closing of the mandible M26.53
  organ or site, congenital NEC - *see*
  Malposition, congenital
  septum (nasal) (acquired) J34.2
    congenital Q67.4
  sexual F65.9
    bestiality F65.89
    erotomania F52.8
    exhibitionism F65.2
    fetishism, fetishistic F65.0
      transvestism F65.1
    frotteurism F65.81
    masochism F65.51
    multiple F65.89
    necrophilia F65.89
    nymphomania F52.8
    pederosis F65.4
    pedophilia F65.4
    sadism, sadomasochism F65.52
    satyriasis F52.8
    specified type NEC F65.89
    transvestism F64.1

Deviation (in) - *continued*
  voyeurism F65.3
  teeth, midline M26.29
  trachea J39.8
  ureter, congenital Q62.61
Device
  cerebral ventricle (communicating) in situ Z98.2
  contraceptive - *see* Contraceptive, device
  drainage, cerebrospinal fluid, in situ Z98.2
Devic's disease G36.0
Devil's
  grip B33.0
  pinches (purpura simplex) D69.2
Devitalized tooth K04.99
Devonshire colic - *see* Poisoning, lead
Dextrinosis, limit (debrancher enzyme deficiency) E74.03
Dextrocardia (true) Q24.0
  with
    complete transposition of viscera Q89.3
    situs inversus Q89.3
Dextroposition, aorta Q20.3
  in tetralogy of Fallot Q21.3
Dextrotransposition, aorta Q20.3
d-glycericacidemia E72.59
Dhat syndrome F48.8
Dhobi itch B35.6
Di George's syndrome D82.1
Di Guglielmo's disease C94.0-
Diabetes, diabetic (mellitus) (sugar) E11.9
  with
    amyotrophy E11.44
    arthropathy NEC E11.618
    autonomic (poly) neuropathy E11.43
    cataract E11.36
    Charcot's joints E11.610
    chronic kidney disease E11.22
    circulatory complication NEC E11.59
    complication E11.8
      specified NEC E11.69
    dermatitis E11.620
    foot ulcer E11.621
    gangrene E11.52
    gastroparalysis E11.43
    gastroparesis E11.43
    glomerulonephrosis, intracapillary E11.21
    glomerulosclerosis, intercapillary E11.21
    hyperglycemia E11.65
    hyperosmolarity E11.00
      with coma E11.01
    hypoglycemia E11.649
      with coma E11.641
    ketoacidosis E11.10
      with coma E11.11
    kidney complications NEC E11.29
    Kimmelstiel-Wilson disease E11.21
    loss of protective sensation (LOPS) - *see* Diabetes, by type, with neuropathy
    mononeuropathy E11.41
    myasthenia E11.44
    necrobiosis lipoidica E11.620
    nephropathy E11.21
    neuralgia E11.42
    neurologic complication NEC E11.49
    neuropathic arthropathy E11.610
    neuropathy E11.40
    ophthalmic complication NEC E11.39
    oral complication NEC E11.638
    osteomyelitis E11.69
    periodontal disease E11.630
    peripheral angiopathy E11.51
      with gangrene E11.52
    polyneuropathy E11.42

Diabetes, diabetic - *continued*
    renal complication NEC E11.29
    renal tubular degeneration E11.29
    retinopathy E11.319
      with macular edema E11.311
        resolved following treatment E11.37
      nonproliferative E11.329
        with macular edema E11.321
        mild E11.329
          with macular edema E11.321
        moderate E11.339
          with macular edema E11.331
        severe E11.349
          with macular edema E11.341
      proliferative E11.359
        with
          combined traction retinal detachment and rhegmatogenous retinal detachment E11.354
          macular edema E11.351
          stable proliferative diabetic retinopathy E11.355
          traction retinal detachment involving the macula E11.352
          traction retinal detachment not involving the macula E11.353
    skin complication NEC E11.628
    skin ulcer NEC E11.622
  brittle - *see* Diabetes, type 1
  bronzed E83.110
  complicating pregnancy - *see* Pregnancy, complicated by, diabetes
  dietary counseling and surveillance Z71.3
  due to
    autoimmune process - *see* Diabetes, type 1
    immune mediated pancreatic islet beta-cell destruction - *see* Diabetes, type 1
  due to drug or chemical E09.9
    with
      amyotrophy E09.44
      arthropathy NEC E09.618
      autonomic (poly) neuropathy E09.43
      cataract E09.36
      Charcot's joints E09.610
      chronic kidney disease E09.22
      circulatory complication NEC E09.59
      complication E09.8
        specified NEC E09.69
      dermatitis E09.620
      foot ulcer E09.621
      gangrene E09.52
      gastroparalysis E09.43
      gastroparesis E09.43
      glomerulonephrosis, intracapillary E09.21
      glomerulosclerosis, intercapillary E09.21
      hyperglycemia E09.65
      hyperosmolarity E09.00
        with coma E09.01
      hypoglycemia E09.649
        with coma E09.641
      ketoacidosis E09.10
        with coma E09.11
      kidney complications NEC E09.29
      Kimmelstiel-Wilson disease E09.21
      mononeuropathy E09.41
      myasthenia E09.44
      necrobiosis lipoidica E09.620
      nephropathy E09.21
      neuralgia E09.42
      neurologic complication NEC E09.49
      neuropathic arthropathy E09.610
      neuropathy E09.40
      ophthalmic complication NEC E09.39
      oral complication NEC E09.638

Diabetes, diabetic - *continued*
      periodontal disease E09.630
      peripheral angiopathy E09.51
        with gangrene E09.52
      polyneuropathy E09.42
      renal complication NEC E09.29
      renal tubular degeneration E09.29
      retinopathy E09.319
        with macular edema E09.311
          resolved following treatment E09.37
        nonproliferative E09.329
          with macular edema E09.321
          mild E09.329
            with macular edema E09.321
          moderate E09.339
            with macular edema E09.331
          severe E09.349
            with macular edema E09.341
        proliferative E09.359
          with
            combined traction retinal detachment and rhegmatogenous retinal detachment E09.354
            macular edema E09.351
            stable proliferative diabetic retinopathy E09.355
            traction retinal detachment involving the macula E09.352
            traction retinal detachment not involving the macula E09.353
      skin complication NEC E09.628
      skin ulcer NEC E09.622
  due to underlying condition E08.9
    with
      amyotrophy E08.44
      arthropathy NEC E08.618
      autonomic (poly) neuropathy E08.43
      cataract E08.36
      Charcot's joints E08.610
      chronic kidney disease E08.22
      circulatory complication NEC E08.59
      complication E08.8
        specified NEC E08.69
      dermatitis E08.620
      foot ulcer E08.621
      gangrene E08.52
      gastroparalysis E08.43
      gastroparesis E08.43
      glomerulonephrosis, intracapillary E08.21
      glomerulosclerosis, intercapillary E08.21
      hyperglycemia E08.65
      hyperosmolarity E08.00
        with coma E08.01
      hypoglycemia E08.649
        with coma E08.641
      ketoacidosis E08.10
        with coma E08.11
      kidney complications NEC E08.29
      Kimmelstiel-Wilson disease E08.21
      mononeuropathy E08.41
      myasthenia E08.44
      necrobiosis lipoidica E08.620
      nephropathy E08.21
      neuralgia E08.42
      neurologic complication NEC E08.49
      neuropathic arthropathy E08.610
      neuropathy E08.40
      ophthalmic complication NEC E08.39
      oral complication NEC E08.638
      periodontal disease E08.630
      peripheral angiopathy E08.51
        with gangrene E08.52
      polyneuropathy E08.42
      renal complication NEC E08.29

Diabetes, diabetic - *continued*
   renal tubular degeneration E08.29
   retinopathy E08.319
     with macular edema E08.311
     resolved following treatment E08.37
     nonproliferative E08.329
      with macular edema E08.321
      mild E08.329
       with macular edema E08.321
      moderate E08.339
       with macular edema E08.331
      severe E08.349
       with macular edema E08.341
     proliferative E08.359
      with
       combined traction retinal detachment and rhegmatogenous retinal detachment E08.354
       macular edema E08.351
       stable proliferative diabetic retinopathy E08.355
       traction retinal detachment involving the macula E08.352
       traction retinal detachment not involving the macula E08.353
   skin complication NEC E08.628
   skin ulcer NEC E08.622
  gestational (in pregnancy) O24.419
   affecting newborn P70.0
   diet controlled O24.410
   in childbirth O24.429
    diet controlled O24.420
    insulin (and diet) controlled O24.424
    oral drug controlled (antidiabetic) (hypoglycemic) O24.425
   insulin (and diet) controlled O24.414
   oral drug controlled (antidiabetic) (hypoglycemic) O24.415
   puerperal O24.439
    diet controlled O24.430
    insulin (and diet) controlled O24.434
    oral drug controlled (antidiabetic) (hypoglycemic) O24.435
  hepatogenous E13.9
  idiopathic - *see* Diabetes, type 1
  inadequately controlled code to Diabetes, by type, with hyperglycemia
  insipidus E23.2
   nephrogenic N25.1
   pituitary E23.2
   vasopressin resistant N25.1
  insulin dependent code to type of diabetes
  juvenile-onset - *see* Diabetes, type 1
  ketosis-prone - *see* Diabetes, type 1
  latent R73.03
  neonatal (transient) P70.2
  non-insulin dependent
  code to type of diabetes
  out of control
  code to Diabetes, by type, with hyperglycemia
  phosphate E83.39
  poorly controlled code to Diabetes, by type, with hyperglycemia
  postpancreatectomy - *see* Diabetes, specified type NEC
  postprocedural - *see* Diabetes, specified type NEC
  secondary diabetes mellitus NEC - *see* Diabetes, specified type NEC
  specified type NEC E13.9
   with
    amyotrophy E13.44
    arthropathy NEC E13.618
    autonomic (poly) neuropathy E13.43

Diabetes, diabetic - *continued*
   cataract E13.36
   Charcot's joints E13.610
   chronic kidney disease E13.22
   circulatory complication NEC E13.59
   complication E13.8
    specified NEC E13.69
   dermatitis E13.620
   foot ulcer E13.621
   gangrene E13.52
   gastroparalysis E13.43
   gastroparesis E13.43
   glomerulonephrosis, intracapillary E13.21
   glomerulosclerosis, intercapillary E13.21
   hyperglycemia E13.65
   hyperosmolarity E13.00
    with coma E13.01
   hypoglycemia E13.649
    with coma E13.641
   ketoacidosis E13.10
    with coma E13.11
   kidney complications NEC E13.29
   Kimmelstiel-Wilson disease E13.21
   mononeuropathy E13.41
   myasthenia E13.44
   necrobiosis lipoidica E13.620
   nephropathy E13.21
   neuralgia E13.42
   neurologic complication NEC E13.49
   neuropathic arthropathy E13.610
   neuropathy E13.40
   ophthalmic complication NEC E13.39
   oral complication NEC E13.638
   periodontal disease E13.630
   peripheral angiopathy E13.51
    with gangrene E13.52
   polyneuropathy E13.42
   renal complication NEC E13.29
   renal tubular degeneration E13.29
   retinopathy E13.319
    with macular edema E13.311
    resolved following treatment E13.37
    nonproliferative E13.329
     with macular edema E13.321
     mild E13.329
      with macular edema E13.321
     moderate E13.339
      with macular edema E13.331
     severe E13.349
      with macular edema E13.341
    proliferative E13.359
     with
      combined traction retinal detachment and rhegmatogenous retinal detachment E13.354
      macular edema E13.351
      stable proliferative diabetic retinopathy E13.355
      traction retinal detachment involving the macula E13.352
      traction retinal detachment not involving the macula E13.353
   skin complication NEC E13.628
   skin ulcer NEC E13.622
  steroid-induced - *see* Diabetes, due to, drug or chemical
  type 1 E10.9
   with
    amyotrophy E10.44
    arthropathy NEC E10.618
    autonomic (poly) neuropathy E10.43
    cataract E10.36
    Charcot's joints E10.610
    chronic kidney disease E10.22

Diabetes, diabetic - *continued*
   circulatory complication NEC E10.59
   complication E10.8
    specified NEC E10.69
   dermatitis E10.620
   foot ulcer E10.621
   gangrene E10.52
   gastroparalysis E10.43
   gastroparesis E10.43
   glomerulonephrosis, intracapillary E10.21
   glomerulosclerosis, intercapillary E10.21
   hyperglycemia E10.65
   hypoglycemia E10.649
    with coma E10.641
   ketoacidosis E10.10
    with coma E10.11
   kidney complications NEC E10.29
   Kimmelstiel-Wilson disease E10.21
   mononeuropathy E10.41
   myasthenia E10.44
   necrobiosis lipoidica E10.620
   nephropathy E10.21
   neuralgia E10.42
   neurologic complication NEC E10.49
   neuropathic arthropathy E10.610
   neuropathy E10.40
   ophthalmic complication NEC E10.39
   oral complication NEC E10.638
   osteomyelitis E10.69
   periodontal disease E10.630
   peripheral angiopathy E10.51
    with gangrene E10.52
   polyneuropathy E10.42
   renal complication NEC E10.29
   renal tubular degeneration E10.29
   retinopathy E10.319
    with macular edema E10.311
    resolved following treatment E10.37
    nonproliferative E10.329
     with macular edema E10.321
     mild E10.329
      with macular edema E10.321
     moderate E10.339
      with macular edema E10.331
     severe E10.349
      with macular edema E10.341
    proliferative E10.359
     with
      combined traction retinal detachment and rhegmatogenous retinal detachment E10.354
      macular edema E10.351
      stable proliferative diabetic retinopathy E10.355
      traction retinal detachment involving the macula E10.352
      traction retinal detachment not involving the macula E10.353
   skin complication NEC E10.628
   skin ulcer NEC E10.622
  type 2 E11.9
   with
    amyotrophy E11.44
    arthropathy NEC E11.618
    autonomic (poly) neuropathy E11.43
    cataract E11.36
    Charcot's joints E11.610
    chronic kidney disease E11.22
    circulatory complication NEC E11.59
    complication E11.8
     specified NEC E11.69
    dermatitis E11.620
    foot ulcer E11.621
    gangrene E11.52

Diabetes, diabetic - *continued*
- gastroparalysis E11.43
- gastroparesis E11.43
- glomerulonephrosis, intracapillary E11.21
- glomerulosclerosis, intercapillary E11.21
- hyperglycemia E11.65
- hyperosmolarity E11.00
  - with coma E11.01
- hypoglycemia E11.649
  - with coma E11.641
- ketoacidosis E11.10
  - with coma E11.11
- kidney complications NEC E11.29
- Kimmelstiel-Wilson disease E11.21
- mononeuropathy E11.41
- myasthenia E11.44
- necrobiosis lipoidica E11.620
- nephropathy E11.21
- neuralgia E11.42
- neurologic complication NEC E11.49
- neuropathic arthropathy E11.610
- neuropathy E11.40
- ophthalmic complication NEC E11.39
- oral complication NEC E11.638
- osteomyelitis E11.69
- periodontal disease E11.630
- peripheral angiopathy E11.51
  - with gangrene E11.52
- polyneuropathy E11.42
- renal complication NEC E11.29
- renal tubular degeneration E11.29
- retinopathy E11.319
  - with macular edema E11.311
  - resolved following treatment E11.37
  - nonproliferative E11.329
    - with macular edema E11.321
    - mild E11.329
      - with macular edema E11.321
    - moderate E11.339
      - with macular edema E11.331
    - severe E11.349
      - with macular edema E11.341
  - proliferative E11.359
    - with
      - combined traction retinal detachment and rhegmatogenous retinal detachment E11.354
      - macular edema E11.351
      - stable proliferative diabetic retinopathy E11.355
      - traction retinal detachment involving the macula E11.352
      - traction retinal detachment not involving the macula E11.353
- skin complication NEC E11.628
- skin ulcer NEC E11.622
- uncontrolled
- meaning
  - hyperglycemia - *see* Diabetes, by type, with, hyperglycemia
  - hypoglycemia - *see* Diabetes, by type, with, hypoglycemia

Diacyclothrombopathia D69.1
Diagnosis deferred R69
Dialysis (intermittent) (treatment)
- noncompliance (with) Z91.15
- renal (hemodialysis) (peritoneal), status Z99.2
- retina, retinal - *see* Detachment, retina, with, retinal, dialysis
Diamond-Blackfan anemia (congenital hypoplastic) D61.01
Diamond-gardener syndrome (autoerythrocyte sensitization) D69.2
Diaper rash L22

Diaphoresis (excessive) R61
Diaphragm - *see* condition
Diaphragmalgia R07.1
Diaphragmatitis, diaphragmitis J98.6
Diaphysial aclasis Q78.6
Diaphysitis - *see* Osteomyelitis, specified type NEC
Diarrhea, diarrheal (disease) (infantile) (inflammatory) R19.7
- achlorhydric K31.83
- allergic K52.29
  - due to
    - colitis - *see* Colitis, allergic
    - enteritis - *see* Enteritis, allergic
- amebic - *see also* Amebiasis A06.0
  - with abscess - *see* Abscess, amebic
  - acute A06.0
  - chronic A06.1
  - nondysenteric A06.2
- bacillary - *see* Dysentery, bacillary
- balantidial A07.0
- cachectic NEC K52.89
- Chilomastix A07.8
- choleriformis A00.1
- chronic (noninfectious) K52.9
- coccidial A07.3
- Cochin-china K90.1
  - strongyloidiasis B78.0
- Dientamoeba A07.8
- dietetic - *see also* Diarrhea, allergic K52.29
- drug-induced K52.1
- due to
  - bacteria A04.9
    - specified NEC A04.8
  - Campylobacter A04.5
  - Capillaria philippinensis B81.1
  - Clostridium difficile
    - not specified as recurrent A04.72
    - recurrent A04.71
  - Clostridium perfringens (C) (F) A04.8
  - Cryptosporidium A07.2
  - drugs K52.1
  - Escherichia coli A04.4
    - enteroaggregative A04.4
    - enterohemorrhagic A04.3
    - enteroinvasive A04.2
    - enteropathogenic A04.0
    - enterotoxigenic A04.1
    - specified NEC A04.4
  - food hypersensitivity - *see also* Diarrhea, allergic K52.29
  - Necator americanus B76.1
  - S. japonicum B65.2
  - specified organism NEC A08.8
    - bacterial A04.8
    - viral A08.39
  - Staphylococcus A04.8
  - Trichuris trichiura B79
  - virus - *see* Enteritis, viral
  - Yersinia enterocolitica A04.6
- dysenteric A09
- endemic A09
- epidemic A09
- flagellate A07.9
- Flexner's (ulcerative) A03.1
- functional K59.1
  - following gastrointestinal surgery K91.89
  - psychogenic F45.8
- Giardia lamblia A07.1
- giardial A07.1
- hill K90.1
- infectious A09
- malarial - *see* Malaria
- mite B88.0

Diarrhea, diarrheal - *continued*
- mycotic NEC B49
- neonatal (noninfectious) P78.3
- nervous F45.8
- neurogenic K59.1
- noninfectious K52.9
- postgastrectomy K91.1
- postvagotomy K91.1
- protozoal A07.9
  - specified NEC A07.8
- psychogenic F45.8
- specified
  - bacterium NEC A04.8
  - virus NEC A08.39
- strongyloidiasis B78.0
- toxic K52.1
- trichomonal A07.8
- tropical K90.1
- tuberculous A18.32
- viral - *see* Enteritis, viral
Diastasis
- cranial bones M84.88
  - congenital NEC Q75.8
- joint (traumatic) - *see* Dislocation
- muscle M62.00
  - ankle M62.07-
  - congenital Q79.8
  - foot M62.07-
  - forearm M62.03-
  - hand M62.04-
  - lower leg M62.06-
  - pelvic region M62.05-
  - shoulder region M62.01-
  - specified site NEC M62.08
  - thigh M62.05-
  - upper arm M62.02-
- recti (abdomen)
  - complicating delivery O71.89
  - congenital Q79.59
Diastema, tooth, teeth, fully erupted M26.32
Diastematomyelia Q06.2
Diataxia, cerebral G80.4
Diathesis
- allergic - *see* History, allergy   bleeding (familial) D69.9
- cystine (familial) E72.00
- gouty - *see* Gout
- hemorrhagic (familial) D69.9
  - newborn P53
- spasmophilic R29.0
Diaz's disease or osteochondrosis (juvenile) (talus) - *see* Osteochondrosis, juvenile, tarsus
Dibothriocephalus, dibothriocephaliasis (latus) (infection) (infestation) B70.0
- larval B70.1
Dicephalus, dicephaly Q89.4
Dichotomy, teeth K00.2
Dichromat, dichromatopsia (congenital) - *see* Deficiency, color vision
Dichuchwa A65
Dicroceliasis B66.2
Didelphia, didelphys - *see* Double uterus
Didymitis N45.1
- with orchitis N45.3
Dietary
- inadequacy or deficiency E63.9
- surveillance and counseling Z71.3
Dietl's crisis N13.8
Dieulafoy lesion (hemorrhagic)
- duodenum K31.82
- esophagus K22.8
- intestine (colon) K63.81
- stomach K31.82

Difficult, difficulty (in)
acculturation Z60.3
feeding R63.3
  newborn P92.9
    breast P92.5
    specified NEC P92.8
  nonorganic (infant or child) F98.29
intubation, in anesthesia T88.4
mechanical, gastroduodenal stoma K91.89
  causing obstruction (see also Obstruction, intestine, postoperative) K91.30
micturition
  need to immediately re-void R39.191
  position dependent R39.192
  specified NEC R39.198
reading (developmental) F81.0
  secondary to emotional disorders F93.9
spelling (specific) F81.81
  with reading disorder F81.89
  due to inadequate teaching Z55.8
swallowing - see Dysphagia
walking R26.2
work
  conditions NEC Z56.5
  schedule Z56.3
Diffuse - see condition
Digeorge's syndrome (thymic hypoplasia) D82.1
Digestive - see condition
Dihydropyrimidine dehydrogenase disease (DPD) E88.89
Diktyoma - see Neoplasm, malignant, by site
Dilaceration, tooth K00.4
Dilatation
anus K59.8
  venule - see Hemorrhoids
aorta (focal) (general) - see Ectasia, aorta
  with aneurysm - see Aneurysm, aorta
  congenital Q25.44
artery - see Aneurysm
bladder (sphincter) N32.89
  congenital Q64.79
blood vessel I99.8
bronchial J47.9
  with
    exacerbation (acute) J47.1
    lower respiratory infection J47.0
calyx (due to obstruction) - see Hydronephrosis
capillaries I78.8
cardiac (acute) (chronic) - see also Hypertrophy, cardiac
  congenital Q24.8
    valve NEC Q24.8
    pulmonary Q22.3
  valve - see Endocarditis
cavum septi pellucidi Q06.8
cervix (uteri) - see also Incompetency, cervix
  incomplete, poor, slow complicating delivery O62.0
colon K59.39
  congenital Q43.1
  psychogenic F45.8
  toxic K59.31
common duct (acquired) K83.8
  congenital Q44.5
cystic duct (acquired) K82.8
  congenital Q44.5
duct, mammary - see Ectasia, mammary duct
duodenum K59.8
esophagus K22.8
  congenital Q39.5
  due to achalasia K22.0
eustachian tube, congenital Q17.8

Dilatation - continued
gallbladder K82.8
gastric - see Dilatation, stomach
heart (acute) (chronic) - see also Hypertrophy, cardiac
  congenital Q24.8
  valve - see Endocarditis
ileum K59.8
  psychogenic F45.8
jejunum K59.8
  psychogenic F45.8
kidney (calyx) (collecting structures) (cystic) (parenchyma) (pelvis) (idiopathic) N28.89
lacrimal passages or duct - see Disorder, lacrimal system, changes
lymphatic vessel I89.0
mammary duct - see Ectasia, mammary duct
Meckel's diverticulum (congenital) Q43.0
  malignant - see Table of Neoplasms, small intestine, malignant
myocardium (acute) (chronic) - see Hypertrophy, cardiac
organ or site, congenital NEC - see Distortion
pancreatic duct K86.89
pericardium - see Pericarditis
pharynx J39.2
prostate N42.89
pulmonary
  artery (idiopathic) I28.8
  valve, congenital Q22.3
pupil H57.04
rectum K59.39
saccule, congenital Q16.5
salivary gland (duct) K11.8
sphincter ani K62.89
stomach K31.89
  acute K31.0
  psychogenic F45.8
submaxillary duct K11.8
trachea, congenital Q32.1
ureter (idiopathic) N28.82
  congenital Q62.2
  due to obstruction N13.4
urethra (acquired) N36.8
vasomotor I73.9
vein I86.8
ventricular, ventricle (acute) (chronic) - see also Hypertrophy, cardiac
  cerebral, congenital Q04.8
venule NEC I86.8
vesical orifice N32.89
Dilated, dilation - see Dilatation
Diminished, diminution
hearing (acuity) - see Deafness
sense or sensation (cold) (heat) (tactile) (vibratory) R20.8
vision NEC H54.7
vital capacity R94.2
Diminuta taenia B71.0
Dimitri-Sturge-Weber disease Q85.8
Dimple
congenital sacral Q82.6
parasacral Q82.6
pilonidal or postanal - see Cyst, pilonidal
Dioctophyma renalis (infection) (infestation) B83.8
Dipetalonemiasis B74.4
Diphallus Q55.69
Diphtheria, diphtheritic (gangrenous) (hemorrhagic) A36.9
carrier (suspected) Z22.2
cutaneous A36.3
faucial A36.0
infection of wound A36.3

Diphtheria, diphtheritic - continued
laryngeal A36.2
myocarditis A36.81
nasal, anterior A36.89
nasopharyngeal A36.1
neurological complication A36.89
pharyngeal A36.0
specified site NEC A36.89
tonsillar A36.0
Diphyllobothriasis (intestine) B70.0
larval B70.1
Diplacusis H93.22-
Diplegia (upper limbs) G83.0
congenital (cerebral) G80.8
facial G51.0
lower limbs G82.20
spastic G80.1
Diplococcus, diplococcal - see condition
Diplopia H53.2
Dipsomania F10.20
with
  psychosis - see Psychosis, alcoholic
  remission F10.21
Dipylidiasis B71.1
DIRA (deficiency of interleukin 1 receptor antagonist) M04.8
Direction, teeth, abnormal, fully erupted M26.30
Dirofilariasis B74.8
Dirt-eating child F98.3
Disability, disabilities
heart - see Disease, heart
intellectual F79
  with
    autistic features F84.9
  mild (I.Q.50-69) F70
  moderate (I.Q.35 49) F71
  profound (I.Q. under 20) F73
  severe (I.Q.20-34) F72
  specified level NEC F78
knowledge acquisition F81.9
learning F81.9
limiting activities Z73.6
spelling, specific F81.81
Disappearance of family member Z63.4
Disarticulation - see Amputation
meaning traumatic amputation - see Amputation, traumatic
Discharge (from)
abnormal finding in - see Abnormal, specimen
breast (female) (male) N64.52
diencephalic autonomic idiopathic - see Epilepsy, specified NEC
ear - see also Otorrhea
  blood - see Otorrhagia
excessive urine R35.8
nipple N64.52
penile R36.9
postnasal R09.82
prison, anxiety concerning Z65.2
urethral R36.9
  without blood R36.0
  hematospermia R36.1
vaginal N89.8
Discitis, diskitis M46.40
cervical region M46.42
cervicothoracic region M46.43
lumbar region M46.46
lumbosacral region M46.47
multiple sites M46.49
occipito-atlanto-axial region M46.41
pyogenic - see Infection, intervertebral disc, pyogenic
sacrococcygeal region M46.48

Discitis, diskitis - *continued*
  thoracic region M46.44
  thoracolumbar region M46.45
Discoid
  meniscus (congenital) Q68.6
  semilunar cartilage (congenital) - *see*
    Derangement, knee, meniscus, specified NEC
Discoloration
  nails L60.8
  teeth (posteruptive) K03.7
    during formation K00.8
Discomfort
  chest R07.89
  visual H53.14-
Discontinuity, ossicles, ear H74.2-
Discord (with)
  boss Z56.4
  classmates Z55.4
  counselor Z64.4
  employer Z56.4
  family Z63.8
  fellow employees Z56.4
  in-laws Z63.1
  landlord Z59.2
  lodgers Z59.2
  neighbors Z59.2
  probation officer Z64.4
  social worker Z64.4
  teachers Z55.4
  workmates Z56.4
Discordant connection
  atrioventricular (congenital) Q20.5
  ventriculoarterial Q20.3
Discrepancy
  centric occlusion maximum intercuspation
    M26.55
  leg length (acquired) - *see* Deformity, limb,
    unequal length
    congenital - *see* Defect, reduction, lower limb
  uterine size date O26.84-
Discrimination
  ethnic Z60.5
  political Z60.5
  racial Z60.5
  religious Z60.5
  sex Z60.5
Disease, diseased - *see also* Syndrome
  absorbent system I87.8
  acid-peptic K30
  Acosta's T70.29
  Adams-stokes (-Morgagni) (syncope with
    heart block) I45.9
  Addison's anemia (pernicious) D51.0
  adenoids (and tonsils) J35.9
  adrenal (capsule) (cortex) (gland) (medullary)
    E27.9
    hyperfunction E27.0
    specified NEC E27.8
  ainhum L94.6
  airway
    obstructive, chronic J44.9
      due to
        cotton dust J66.0
        specific organic dusts NEC J66.8
    reactive - *see* Asthma
  akamushi (scrub typhus) A75.3
  Albers-Schonberg (marble bones) Q78.2
  Albert's - *see* Tendinitis, Achilles
  alimentary canal K63.9
  alligator-skin Q80.9
    acquired L85.0
  alpha heavy chain C88.3
  alpine T70.29
  altitude T70.20

Disease, diseased - *continued*
  alveolar ridge
    edentulous K06.9
      specified NEC K06.8
  alveoli, teeth K08.9
  Alzheimer's G30.9 [*F02.80*]
    with behavioral disturbance G30.9 [*F02.81*]
    early onset G30.0- [*F02.80*]
      with behavioral disturbance G30.0-
        [*F02.81*]
    late onset G30.1 [*F02.80*]
      with behavioral disturbance G30.1
        [*F02.81*]
    specified NEC G30.8 [*F02.80*]
      with behavioral disturbance G30.8
        [*F02.81*]
  amyloid - *see* Amyloidosis
  Andersen's (glycogenosis IV) E74.09
  Andes T70.29
  Andrews' (bacterid) L08.89
  angiospastic I73.9
    cerebral G45.9
    vein I87.8
  anterior
    chamber H21.9
    horn cell G12.29
  antiglomerular basement membrane (anti
    GBM) antibody M31.0
    tubulo-interstitial nephritis N12
  antral - *see* Sinusitis, maxillary
  anus K62.9
    specified NEC K62.89
  aorta (nonsyphilitic) I77.9
    syphilitic NEC A52.02
  aortic (heart) (valve) I35.9
    rheumatic I06.9
  Apollo B30.3
  aponeuroses - *see* Enthesopathy
  appendix K38.9
    specified NEC K38.8
  aqueous (chamber) H21.9
  Arnold-Chiari - *see* Arnold-Chiari disease
  arterial I77.9
    occlusive - *see* Occlusion, by site
    due to stricture or stenosis I77.1
  arteriocardiorenal - *see* Hypertension,
    cardiorenal
  arteriolar (generalized) (obliterative) I77.9
  arteriorenal - *see* Hypertension, kidney
  arteriosclerotic - *see also* Arteriosclerosis
    cardiovascular - *see* Disease, heart, ischemic,
      atherosclerotic
    coronary (artery) - *see* Disease, heart,
      ischemic, atherosclerotic
    heart - *see* Disease, heart, ischemic,
      atherosclerotic
  artery I77.9
    cerebral I67.9
    coronary I25.10
      with angina pectoris - *see* Arteriosclerosis,
        coronary (artery),
  arthropod-borne NOS (viral) A94
    specified type NEC A93.8
  atticoantral, chronic H66.20
    left H66.22
      with right H66.23
    right H66.21
      with left H66.23
  auditory canal - *see* Disorder, ear, external
  auricle, ear NEC - *see* Disorder, pinna
  Australian X A83.4
  autoimmune (systemic) NOS M35.9
    hemolytic (cold type) (warm type) D59.1
      drug-induced D59.0

Disease, diseased - *continued*
  thyroid E06.3
  aviator's - *see* Effect, adverse, high altitude
  Ayerza's (pulmonary artery sclerosis with
    pulmonary hypertension) I27.0
  Babington's (familial hemorrhagic
    telangiectasia) I78.0
  bacterial A49.9
    specified NEC A48.8
    zoonotic A28.9
      specified type NEC A28.8
  Baelz's (cheilitis glandularis apostematosa)
    K13.0
  bagasse J67.1
  balloon - *see* Effect, adverse, high altitude
  Bang's (brucella abortus) A23.1
  Bannister's T78.3
  barometer makers' - *see* Poisoning, mercury
  Barraquer (-Simons') (progressive
    lipodystrophy) E88.1
  Barrett's - *see* Barrett's, esophagus
  Bartholin's gland N75.9
  basal ganglia G25.9
    degenerative G23.9
      specified NEC G23.8
    specified NEC G25.89
  Basedow's (exophthalmic goiter) - *see*
    Hyperthyroidism, with, goiter (diffuse)
  Bateman's B08.1
  Batten-Steinert G71.11
  Battey A31.0
  Beard's (neurasthenia) F48.8
  Becker
    idiopathic mural endomyocardial I42.3
    myotonia congenita G71.12
  Begbie's (exophthalmic goiter) - *see*
    Hyperthyroidism, with, goiter (diffuse)
  behavioral, organic F07.9
  Beigel's (white piedra) B36.2
  Benson's - *see* Deposit, crystalline
  Bernard-Soulier (thrombopathy) D69.1
  Bernhardt (-Roth) - *see* Mononeuropathy,
    lower limb, meralgia paresthetica
  Biermer's (pernicious anemia) D51.0
  bile duct (common) (hepatic) K83.9
    with calculus, stones - *see* Calculus, bile duct
    specified NEC K83.8
  biliary (tract) K83.9
    specified NEC K83.8
  Billroth's - *see* Spina bifida
  bird fancier's J67.2
  black lung J60
  bladder N32.9
    in (due to)
      schistosomiasis (bilharziasis) B65.0 [*N33*]
    specified NEC N32.89
  bleeder's D66
  blood D75.9
    forming organs D75.9
    vessel I99.9
  Bloodgood's - *see* Mastopathy, cystic
  Bodechtel-Guttmann (subacute sclerosing
    panencephalitis) A81.1
  bone - *see also* Disorder, bone
    aluminum M83.4
    fibrocystic NEC
      jaw M27.49
  bone-marrow D75.9
  Borna A83.9
  Bornholm (epidemic pleurodynia) B33.0
  Bouchard's (myopathic dilatation of the
    stomach) K31.0
  Bouillaud's (rheumatic heart disease) I01.9

Disease, diseased - *continued*

Bourneville (-Brissaud) (tuberous sclerosis)
  Q85.1
Bouveret (-Hoffmann) (paroxysmal
  tachycardia) I47.9
bowel K63.9
  functional K59.9
    psychogenic F45.8
brain G93.9
  arterial, artery I67.9
  arteriosclerotic I67.2
  congenital Q04.9
  degenerative - *see* Degeneration, brain
  inflammatory - *see* Encephalitis
  organic G93.9
    arteriosclerotic I67.2
  parasitic NEC B71.9 [*G94*]
  senile NEC G31.1
  specified NEC G93.89
breast - *see also* Disorder, breast N64.9
  cystic (chronic) - *see* Mastopathy, cystic
  fibrocystic - *see* Mastopathy, cystic
  Paget's
    female, unspecified side C50.91-
    male, unspecified side C50.92-
  specified NEC N64.89
Breda's - *see* Yaws
Bretonneau's (diphtheritic malignant angina)
  A36.0
Bright's - *see* Nephritis
  arteriosclerotic - *see* Hypertension, kidney
Brill's (recrudescent typhus) A75.1
Brill-Zinsser (recrudescent typhus) A75.1
Brion-Kayser - *see* Fever, paratyphoid
broad
  beta E78.2
  ligament (noninflammatory) N83.9
    inflammatory - *see* Disease, pelvis,
    inflammatory
    specified NEC N83.8
Brocq-Duhring (dermatitis herpetiformis)
  L13.0
Brocq's
  meaning
    dermatitis herpetiformis L13.0
    prurigo L28.2
bronchopulmonary J98.4
bronchus NEC J98.09
bronze Addison's E27.1
  tuberculous A18.7
budgerigar fancier's J67.2
bullous L13.9
  chronic of childhood L12.2
  specified NEC L13.8
Buerger's (thromboangiitis obliterans) I73.1
Bürger-Grütz (essential familial hyperlipemia)
  E78.3
bursa - *see* Bursopathy
caisson T70.3
California - *see* Coccidioidomycosis
capillaries I78.9
  specified NEC I78.8
Carapata A68.0
cardiac - *see* Disease, heart
cardiopulmonary, chronic I27.9
cardiorenal (hepatic) (hypertensive) (vascular)
  - *see* Hypertension, cardiorenal
cardiovascular (atherosclerotic) I25.10
  with angina pectoris - *see* Arteriosclerosis,
    coronary (artery),   congenital Q28.9
  newborn P29.9
    specified NEC P29.89
  hypertensive - *see* Hypertension, heart
  renal (hypertensive) - *see* Hypertension,

Disease, diseased - *continued*

cardiorenal
  syphilitic (asymptomatic) A52.00
cartilage - *see* Disorder, cartilage
Castellani's A69.8
Castleman (unicentric) (multicentric) D47.Z2
  HHV 8-associated - *see also* Herpesvirus,
    human, 8 D47.Z2
cat-scratch A28.1
Cavare's (familial periodic paralysis) G72.3
cecum K63.9
celiac (adult) (infantile) (with steatorrhea)
  K90.0
cellular tissue L98.9
central core G71.2
cerebellar, cerebellum - *see* Disease, brain
cerebral - *see also* Disease, brain
  degenerative - *see* Degeneration, brain
cerebrospinal G96.9
cerebrovascular I67.9
  acute I67.89
    embolic I63.4-
    thrombotic I63.3-
  arteriosclerotic I67.2
  specified NEC I67.89
cervix (uteri) (noninflammatory) N88.9
  inflammatory - *see* Cervicitis
  specified NEC N88.8
Chabert's A22.9
Chandler's (osteochondritis dissecans, hip) -
  see Osteochondritis, dissecans, hip
Charlouis - *see* Yaws
Chédiak-Steinbrinck (-Higashi) (congenital
  gigantism of peroxidase granules) E70.330
chest J98.9
Chiari's (hepatic vein thrombosis) I82.0
Chicago B40.9
Chignon B36.8
chigo, chigoe B88.1
childhood granulomatous D71
Chinese liver fluke B66.1
chlamydial A74.9
  specified NEC A74.89
cholecystic K82.9
choroid H31.9
  specified NEC H31.8
Christmas D67
chronic bullous of childhood L12.2
chylomicron retention E78.3
ciliary body H21.9
  specified NEC H21.89
circulatory (system) NEC I99.8
  newborn P29.9
  syphilitic A52.00
    congenital A50.54
coagulation factor deficiency (congenital) - *see*
  Defect, coagulation
coccidioidal - *see* Coccidioidomycosis
cold
  agglutinin or hemoglobinuria D59.1
    paroxysmal D59.6
  hemagglutinin (chronic) D59.1
collagen NOS (nonvascular) (vascular) M35.9
  specified NEC M35.8
colon K63.9
  functional K59.9
    congenital Q43.2
  ischemic - *see also* Ischemia, intestine, acute
    K55.039
colonic inflammatory bowel, unclassified
  (IBDU) K52.3
combined system - *see* Degeneration,
  combined
compressed air T70.3

Disease, diseased - *continued*

Concato's (pericardial polyserositis) A19.9
  nontubercular I31.1
  pleural - *see* Pleurisy, with effusion
conjunctiva H11.9
  chlamydial A74.0
  specified NEC H11.89
  viral B30.9
    specified NEC B30.8
connective tissue, systemic (diffuse) M35.9
  in (due to)
    hypogammaglobulinemia D80.1 [*M36.8*]
    ochronosis E70.29 [*M36.8*]
  specified NEC M35.8
Conor and Bruch's (boutonneuse fever) A77.1
Cooper's - *see* Mastopathy, cystic
Cori's (glycogenosis III) E74.03
cork handler's or cork worker's J67.3
cornea H18.9
  specified NEC H18.89-
coronary (artery) - *see* Disease, heart,
  ischemic, atherosclerotic
  congenital Q24.5
  ostial, syphilitic (aortic) (mitral) (pulmonary)
    A52.03
corpus cavernosum N48.9
  specified NEC N48.89
Cotugno's - *see* Sciatica
coxsackie (virus) NEC B34.1
cranial nerve NOS G52.9
Creutzfeldt-Jakob - *see* Creutzfeldt-Jakob
  disease or syndrome   Crocq's (acrocyanosis)
    I73.89
Crohn's - *see* Enteritis, regional
Curschmann's G71.11
cystic
  breast (chronic) - *see* Mastopathy, cystic
  kidney, congenital Q61.9
  liver, congenital Q44.6
  lung J98.4
    congenital Q33.0
cytomegalic inclusion (generalized) B25.9
  with pneumonia B25.0
  congenital P35.1
cytomegaloviral B25.9
  specified NEC B25.8
Czerny's (periodic hydrarthrosis of the knee) -
  see Effusion, joint, knee   Daae (-finsen)
    (epidemic pleurodynia) B33.0
Darling's - *see* Histoplasmosis capsulati
Debove's (splenomegaly) R16.1
deer fly - *see* Tularemia
Degos' I77.89
demyelinating, demyelinizating (nervous
  system) G37.9
  multiple sclerosis G35
  specified NEC G37.8
dense deposit - *see also* N00-N07 with fourth
  character .6 N05.6
deposition, hydroxyapatite - *see* Disease,
  hydroxyapatite deposition
de Quervain's (tendon sheath) M65.4
  thyroid (subacute granulomatous thyroiditis)
    E06.1
Devergie's (pityriasis rubra pilaris) L44.0
Devic's G36.0
diaphorase deficiency D74.0
diaphragm J98.6
diarrheal, infectious NEC A09
digestive system K92.9
  specified NEC K92.89
disc, degenerative - *see* Degeneration,
  intervertebral disc
discogenic - *see also* Displacement,

Disease, diseased - *continued*
intervertebral disc NEC
   with myelopathy - *see* Disorder, disc, with,
    myelopathy
   diverticular - *see* Diverticula
   Dubois (thymus) A50.59 [E35]
   Duchenne-Griesinger G71.0
   Duchenne's
    muscular dystrophy G71.0
    pseudohypertrophy, muscles G71.0
   ductless glands E34.9
   Duhring's (dermatitis herpetiformis) L13.0
   duodenum K31.9
    specified NEC K31.89
   Dupré's (meningism) R29.1
   Dupuytren's (muscle contracture) M72.0
   Durand Nicholas-Favre (climatic bubo) A55
   Duroziez's (congenital mitral stenosis) Q23.2
   ear - *see* Disorder, ear
   Eberth's - *see* Fever, typhoid
   Ebola (virus) A98.4
   Ebstein's heart Q22.5
   Echinococcus - *see* Echinococcus
   echovirus NEC B34.1
   Eddowes' (brittle bones and blue sclera) Q78.0
   edentulous (alveolar) ridge K06.9
    specified NEC K06.8
   Edsall's T67.2
   Eichstedt's (pityriasis versicolor) B36.0
   Eisenmenger's (irreversible) I27.83
   Ellis-van Creveld (chondroectodermal
    dysplasia) Q77.6
   end stage renal (ESRD) N18.6
    due to hypertension I12.0
   endocrine glands or system NEC E34.9
   endomyocardial (eosinophilic) I42.3
   English (rickets) E55.0
   enteroviral, enterovirus NEC B34.1
    central nervous system NEC A88.8
   epidemic B99.9
    specified NEC B99.8
   epididymis N50.9
   Erb (-Landouzy) G71.0
   Erdheim-Chester (ECD) E88.89
   esophagus K22.9
    functional K22.4
    psychogenic F45.8
    specified NEC K22.8
   Eulenburg's (congenital paramyotonia) G71.19
   eustachian tube - *see* Disorder, eustachian tube
    external
     auditory canal - *see* Disorder, ear, external
    ear - *see* Disorder, ear, external
   extrapyramidal G25.9
    specified NEC G25.89
   eye H57.9
    anterior chamber H21.9
    inflammatory NEC H57.8
    muscle (external) - *see* Strabismus
    specified NEC H57.8
    syphilitic - *see* Oculopathy, syphilitic
   eyeball H44.9
    specified NEC H44.89
   eyelid - *see* Disorder, eyelid
    specified NEC - *see* Disorder, eyelid,
     specified type NEC
   eyeworm of Africa B74.3
   facial nerve (seventh) G51.9
    newborn (birth injury) P11.3
   Fahr (of brain) G23.8
   Fahr Volhard (of kidney) I12.-
   fallopian tube (noninflammatory) N83.9
    inflammatory - *see* Salpingo-oophoritis
    specified NEC N83.8

Disease, diseased - *continued*
   familial periodic paralysis G72.3
   Fanconi's (congenital pancytopenia) D61.09
   fascia NEC - *see also* Disorder, muscle
    inflammatory - *see* Myositis
    specified NEC M62.89
   Fauchard's (periodontitis) - *see* Periodontitis
   Favre-Durand Nicolas (climatic bubo) A55
   Fede's K14.0
   Feer's - *see* Poisoning, mercury
   female pelvic inflammatory - *see also* Disease,
    pelvis, inflammatory N73.9
    syphilitic (secondary) A51.42
    tuberculous A18.17
   Fernels' (aortic aneurysm) I71.9
   fibrocaseous of lung - *see* Tuberculosis,
    pulmonary
   fibrocystic - *see* Fibrocystic disease
   Fiedler's (leptospiral jaundice) A27.0
   fifth B08.3
   file-cutter's - *see* Poisoning, lead   fish-skin
    Q80.9
    acquired L85.0
   Flajani (-Basedow) (exophthalmic goiter) - *see*
    Hyperthyroidism, with, goiter (diffuse)
   flax-dresser's J66.1
   fluke - *see* Infestation, fluke   foot and mouth
    B08.8
   foot process N04.9
   Forbes' (glycogenosis III) E74.03
   Fordyce-fox (apocrine miliaria) L75.2
   Fordyce's (ectopic sebaceous glands) (mouth)
    Q38.6
   Forestier's (rhizomelic pseudopolyarthritis)
    M35.3
    meaning ankylosing hyperostosis - *see*
     Hyperostosis, ankylosing
   Fothergill's
    neuralgia - *see* Neuralgia, trigeminal
    scarlatina anginosa A38.9
   Fournier (gangrene) N49.3
    female N76.89
   fourth B08.8
   Fox (-Fordyce) (apocrine miliaria) L75.2
   Francis' - *see* Tularemia
   Franklin C88.2
   Frei's (climatic bubo) A55
   Friedreich's
    combined systemic or ataxia G11.1
    myoclonia G25.3
   frontal sinus - *see* Sinusitis, frontal
   fungus NEC B49
   Gaisböck's (polycythemia hypertonica) D75.1
   gallbladder K82.9
    calculus - *see* Calculus, gallbladder
    cholecystitis - *see* Cholecystitis
    cholesterolosis K82.4
    fistula - *see* Fistula, gallbladder
    hydrops K82.1
    obstruction - *see* Obstruction, gallbladder
    perforation K82.2
    specified NEC K82.8
   gamma heavy chain C88.2
   Gamna's (siderotic splenomegaly) D73.2
   Gamstorp's (adynamia episodica hereditaria)
    G72.3
   Gandy Nanta (siderotic splenomegaly) D73.2
   ganister J62.8
   gastric - *see* Disease, stomach
   gastroesophageal reflux (GERD) K21.9
    with esophagitis K21.0
   gastrointestinal (tract) K92.9
    amyloid E85.4
    functional K59.9

Disease, diseased - *continued*
    psychogenic F45.8
    specified NEC K92.89
   Gee (-Herter) (-Heubner) (-Thaysen)
    (nontropical sprue) K90.0
   genital organs
    female N94.9
    male N50.9
   Gerhardt's (erythromelalgia) I73.81
   Gibert's (pityriasis rosea) L42
   Gierke's (glycogenosis I) E74.01
   Gilles de la Tourette's (motor-verbal tic) F95.2
   gingiva K06.9
    plaque induced K05.00
    specified NEC K06.8
   gland (lymph) I89.9
   Glanzmann's (hereditary hemorrhagic
    thrombasthenia) D69.1
   glass-blower's (cataract) - *see* Cataract,
    specified NEC
    salivary gland hypertrophy K11.1
   Glisson's - *see* Rickets
   globe H44.9
    specified NEC H44.89
   glomerular - *see also* Glomerulonephritis
    with edema - *see* Nephrosis
    acute - *see* Nephritis, acute
    chronic - *see* Nephritis, chronic
    minimal change N05.0
    rapidly progressive N01.9
   glycogen storage E74.00
    Andersen's E74.09
    Cori's E74.03
    Forbes' E74.03
    generalized E74.00
    glucose 6-phosphatase deficiency E74.01
    heart E74.02 [143]
    hepatorenal E74.09
    Hers' E74.09
    liver and kidney E74.09
    McArdle's E74.04
    muscle phosphofructokinase E74.09
    myocardium E74.02 [143]
    Pompe's E74.02
    Tauri's E74.09
    type 0 E74.09
    type I E74.01
    type II E74.02
    type III E74.03
    type IV E74.09
    type V E74.04
    type VI-XI E74.09
    Von Gierke's E74.01
   Goldstein's (familial hemorrhagic
    telangiectasia) I78.0
   gonococcal NOS A54.9
   graft-versus-host (GVH) D89.813
    acute D89.810
    acute on chronic D89.812
    chronic D89.811
   grain handler's J67.8
   granulomatous (childhood) (chronic) D71
   Graves' (exophthalmic goiter) - *see*
    Hyperthyroidism, with, goiter (diffuse)
   Griesinger's - *see* Ancylostomiasis
   Grisel's M43.6
   Gruby's (tinea tonsurans) B35.0
   Guillain-Barré G61.0
   Guinon's (motor-verbal tic) F95.2
   gum K06.9
   gynecological N94.9
   H (Hartnup's) E72.02
   Haff - *see* Poisoning, mercury

Disease, diseased - *continued*

Hageman (congenital factor XII deficiency) D68.2

hair (color) (shaft) L67.9
  follicles L73.9
    specified NEC L73.8

Hamman's (spontaneous mediastinal emphysema) J98.2

hand, foot and mouth B08.4

Hansen's - *see* Leprosy

Hantavirus, with pulmonary manifestations B33.4
  with renal manifestations A98.5

Harada's H30.81-

Hartnup (pellagra-cerebellar ataxia-renal aminoaciduria) E72.02

Hart's (pellagra-cerebellar ataxia-renal aminoaciduria) E72.02

Hashimoto's (struma lymphomatosa) E06.3

Hb - *see* Disease, hemoglobin

heart (organic) I51.9
  with
    pulmonary edema (acute) - *see also* Failure, ventricular, left I50.1
    rheumatic fever (conditions in I00)
      active I01.9
        with chorea I02.0
        specified NEC I01.8
      inactive or quiescent (with chorea) I09.9
        specified NEC I09.89
  amyloid E85.4 [143]
  aortic (valve) I35.9
  arteriosclerotic or sclerotic (senile) - *see* Disease, heart, ischemic, atherosclerotic
  artery, arterial - *see* Disease, heart, ischemic, atherosclerotic
  beer drinkers' I42.6
  beriberi (wet) E51.12
  black I27.0
  congenital Q24.9
    cyanotic Q24.9
    specified NEC Q24.8
  coronary - *see* Disease, heart, ischemic
  cryptogenic I51.9
  fibroid - *see* Myocarditis
  functional I51.89
    psychogenic F45.8
  glycogen storage E74.02 [143]
  gonococcal A54.83
  hypertensive - *see* Hypertension, heart
  hyperthyroid - *see also* Hyperthyroidism E05.90 [143]
    with thyroid storm E05.91 [143]
  ischemic (chronic or with a stated duration of over 4 weeks) I25.9
    atherosclerotic (of) I25.10
      with angina pectoris - *see* Arteriosclerosis, coronary (artery)
      coronary artery bypass graft - *see* Arteriosclerosis, coronary (artery), cardiomyopathy I25.5
    diagnosed on ECG or other special investigation, but currently presenting no symptoms I25.6
    silent I25.6
    specified form NEC I25.89
  kyphoscoliotic I27.1
  meningococcal A39.50
    endocarditis A39.51
    myocarditis A39.52
    pericarditis A39.53
  mitral I05.9
    specified NEC I05.8
  muscular - *see* Degeneration, myocardial

Disease, diseased - *continued*

psychogenic (functional) F45.8

pulmonary (chronic) I27.9
  in schistosomiasis B65.9 [152]
  specified NEC I27.89

rheumatic (chronic) (inactive) (old) (quiescent) (with chorea) I09.9
  active or acute I01.9
    with chorea (acute) (rheumatic) (Sydenham's) I02.0
  specified NEC I09.89

senile - *see* Myocarditis

syphilitic A52.06
  aortic A52.03
    aneurysm A52.01
  congenital A50.54 [152]

thyrotoxic - *see also* Thyrotoxicosis E05.90 [143]
  with thyroid storm E05.91 [143]

valve, valvular (obstructive) (regurgitant) - *see also* Endocarditis
  congenital NEC Q24.8
    pulmonary Q22.3

vascular - *see* Disease, cardiovascular

heavy chain NEC C88.2
  alpha C88.3
  gamma C88.2
  mu C88.2

Hebra's
  pityriasis
    maculata et circinata L42
    rubra pilaris L44.0
  prurigo L28.2

hematopoietic organs D75.9

hemoglobin or Hb
  abnormal (mixed) NEC D58.2
    with thalassemia D56.9
  AS genotype D57.3
  Bart's D56.0
  C (Hb-c) D58.2
    with other abnormal hemoglobin NEC D58.2
    elliptocytosis D58.1
    Hb-s D57.2-
    sickle-cell D57.2-
    thalassemia D56.8
  Constant Spring D58.2
  D (Hb-d) D58.2
  E (Hb-e) D58.2
  E-beta thalassemia D56.5
  elliptocytosis D58.1
  H (Hb-h) (thalassemia) D56.0
    with other abnormal hemoglobin NEC D56.9
    Constant Spring D56.0
  I thalassemia D56.9
  M D74.0
  S or SS D57.1
  SC D57.2-
  SD D57.8-
  SE D57.8-
  spherocytosis D58.0
  unstable, hemolytic D58.2

hemolytic (newborn) P55.9
  autoimmune (cold type) (warm type) D59.1
  drug-induced D59.0
  due to or with
    incompatibility
      ABO (blood group) P55.1
      blood (group) (Duffy) (K(ell)) (Kidd) (Lewis) (M) (S) NEC P55.8
      Rh (blood group) (factor) P55.0
    Rh negative mother P55.0
  specified type NEC P55.8

Disease, diseased - *continued*

unstable hemoglobin D58.2

hemorrhagic D69.9
  newborn P53

Henoch (-Schönlein) (purpura nervosa) D69.0

hepatic - *see* Disease, liver

hepatobiliary K83.9
  toxic K71.9

hepatolenticular E83.01

heredodegenerative NEC
  spinal cord G95.89

herpesviral, disseminated B00.7

Hers' (glycogenosis VI) E74.09

Herter (-gee) (-Heubner) (nontropical sprue) K90.0

Heubner-Herter (nontropical sprue) K90.0

high fetal gene or hemoglobin thalassemia D56.9

Hildebrand's - *see* Typhus

hip (joint) M25.9
  congenital Q65.89
  suppurative M00.9
  tuberculous A18.02

His (-Werner) (trench fever) A79.0

Hodgson's I71.2
  ruptured I71.1

Holla - *see* Spherocytosis

hookworm B76.9
  specified NEC B76.8

host-versus-graft D89.813
  acute D89.810
  acute on chronic D89.812
  chronic D89.811

human immunodeficiency virus (HIV) B20

Huntington's G10
  with dementia G10 [F02.80]

Hutchinson's (cheiropompholyx) - *see* Hutchinson's disease hyaline (diffuse) (generalized)
  membrane (lung) (newborn) P22.0
    adult J80

hydatid - *see* Echinococcus

hydroxyapatite deposition M11.00
  ankle M11.07-
  elbow M11.02-
  foot joint M11.07-
  hand joint M11.04-
  hip M11.05-
  knee M11.06-
  multiple site M11.09
  shoulder M11.01-
  vertebra M11.08
  wrist M11.03-

hyperkinetic - *see* Hyperkinesia

hypertensive - *see* Hypertension

hypophysis E23.7

Iceland G93.3

I-cell E77.0

immune D89.9

immunoproliferative (malignant) C88.9
  small intestinal C88.3
  specified NEC C88.8

inclusion B25.9
  salivary gland B25.9

infectious, infective B99.9
  congenital P37.9
    specified NEC P37.8
    viral P35.9
      specified type NEC P35.8
  specified NEC B99.8

inflammatory
  penis N48.29
    abscess N48.21
    cellulitis N48.22

Disease, diseased - *continued*
prepuce N47.7
  balanoposthitis N47.6
tubo-ovarian - *see* Salpingo-oophoritis
intervertebral disc - *see also* Disorder, disc
  with myelopathy - *see* Disorder, disc, with, myelopathy
  cervical, cervicothoracic - *see* Disorder, disc, cervical
    with
      myelopathy - *see* Disorder, disc, cervical, with myelopathy
      neuritis, radiculitis or radiculopathy - *see* Disorder, disc, cervical, with neuritis
      specified NEC - *see* Disorder, disc, cervical, specified type NEC
  lumbar (with)
    myelopathy M51.06
    neuritis, radiculitis, radiculopathy or sciatica M51.16
    specified NEC M51.86
  lumbosacral (with)
    neuritis, radiculitis, radiculopathy or sciatica M51.17
    specified NEC M51.87
  specified NEC - *see* Disorder, disc, specified NEC
  thoracic (with)
    myelopathy M51.04
    neuritis, radiculitis or radiculopathy M51.14
    specified NEC M51.84
  thoracolumbar (with)
    myelopathy M51.05
    neuritis, radiculitis or radiculopathy M51.15
    specified NEC M51.85
intestine K63.9
  functional K59.9
    psychogenic F45.8
    specified NEC K59.8
  organic K63.9
  protozoal A07.9
  specified NEC K63.89
iris H21.9
  specified NEC H21.89
iron metabolism or storage E83.10
island (scrub typhus) A75.3
itai-itai - *see* Poisoning, cadmium
Jakob-Creutzfeldt - *see* Creutzfeldt-Jakob
disease or syndrome jaw M27.9
  fibrocystic M27.49
  specified NEC M27.8
jigger B88.1
joint - *see also* Disorder, joint
  Charcot's - *see* Arthropathy, neuropathic (Charcot)
  degenerative - *see* Osteoarthritis
    multiple M15.9
    spine - *see* Spondylosis
  hypertrophic - *see* Osteoarthritis
  sacroiliac M53.3
  specified NEC - *see* Disorder, joint, specified type NEC
  spine NEC - *see* Dorsopathy
  suppurative - *see* Arthritis, pyogenic or pyemic
Jourdain's (acute gingivitis) K05.00
  nonplaque induced K05.01
  plaque induced K05.00
Kaschin-beck (endemic polyarthritis) M12.10
  ankle M12.17-
  elbow M12.12-
  foot joint M12.17-
  hand joint M12.14-
  hip M12.15-

Disease, diseased - *continued*
  knee M12.16-
  multiple site M12.19
  shoulder M12.11-
  vertebra M12.18
  wrist M12.13-
Katayama B65.2
Kedani (scrub typhus) A75.3
Keshan E59
kidney (functional) (pelvis) N28.9
  chronic N18.9
    hypertensive - *see* Hypertension, kidney
    stage 1 N18.1
    stage 2(mild) N18.2
    stage 3(moderate) N18.3
    stage 4(severe) N18.4
    stage 5 N18.5
  complicating pregnancy - *see* Pregnancy, complicated by, renal disease
  cystic (congenital) Q61.9
  diabetic - *see* E08-e13 with .22
  fibrocystic (congenital) Q61.8
  hypertensive - *see* Hypertension, kidney
  in (due to)
    schistosomiasis (bilharziasis) B65.9 *[N29]*
  multicystic Q61.4
  polycystic Q61.3
    adult type Q61.2
    childhood type NEC Q61.19
      collecting duct dilatation Q61.11
Kimmelstiel (-Wilson) (intercapillary polycystic (congenital) glomerulosclerosis) - *see* E08-e13 with .21
Kimura D21.9
  specified site (see Neoplasm, connective tissue benign)
Kinnier Wilson's (hepatolenticular degeneration) E83.01
kissing - *see* Mononucleosis, infectious
Klebs' - *see also* Glomerulonephritis N05.
Klippel-Feil (brevicollis) Q76.1
Köhler-Pellegrini-Stieda (calcification, knee joint) - *see* Bursitis, tibial collateral
Kok Q89.8
Koenig's (osteochondritis dissecans) - *see* Osteochondritis, dissecans
Korsakoff's (nonalcoholic) F04
  alcoholic F10.96
    with dependence F10.26
Kostmann's (infantile genetic agranulocytosis) D70.0
kuru A81.81
Kyasanur Forest A98.2
labyrinth, ear - *see* Disorder, ear, inner
lacrimal system - *see* Disorder, lacrimal system
Lafora's - *see* Epilepsy, generalized, idiopathic
Lancereaux-Mathieu (leptospiral jaundice) A27.0
Landry's G61.0
Larrey-Weil (leptospiral jaundice) A27.0
larynx J38.7
legionnaires' A48.1
  nonpneumonic A48.2
Lenegre's I44.2
lens H27.9
  specified NEC H27.8
Lev's (acquired complete heart block) I44.2
Lewy body (dementia) G31.83 *[F02.80]*
  with behavioral disturbance G31.83 *[F02.81]*
Lichtheim's (subacute combined sclerosis with pernicious anemia) D51.0
Lightwood's (renal tubular acidosis) N25.89

Disease, diseased - *continued*
Lignac's (cystinosis) E72.04
lip K13.0
lipid-storage E75.6
  specified NEC E75.5
Lipschütz's N76.6
liver (chronic) (organic) K76.9
  alcoholic (chronic) K70.9
    acute - *see* Disease, liver, alcoholic, hepatitis
    cirrhosis K70.30
      with ascites K70.31
    failure K70.40
      with coma K70.41
    fatty liver K70.0
    fibrosis K70.2
    hepatitis K70.10
      with ascites K70.11
    sclerosis K70.2
  cystic, congenital Q44.6
  drug-induced (idiosyncratic) (toxic) (predictable) (unpredictable) - *see* Disease, liver, toxic
  end stage K72.90
    due to hepatitis - *see* Hepatitis
  fatty, nonalcoholic (NAFLD) K76.0
    alcoholic K70.0
  fibrocystic (congenital) Q44.6
  fluke
    Chinese B66.1
    oriental B66.1
    sheep B66.3
  gestational alloimmune (GALD) P78.84
  glycogen storage E74.09 *[K77]*
  in (due to)
    schistosomiasis (bilharziasis) B65.9 *[K77]*
  inflammatory K75.9
    alcoholic K70.1
    specified NEC K75.89
  polycystic (congenital) Q44.6
  toxic K71.9
    with
      cholestasis K71.0
      cirrhosis (liver) K71.7
      fibrosis (liver) K71.7
      focal nodular hyperplasia K71.8
      hepatic granuloma K71.8
      hepatic necrosis K71.10
        with coma K71.11
      hepatitis NEC K71.6
        acute K71.2
        chronic
          active K71.50
            with ascites K71.51
          lobular K71.4
          persistent K71.3
          lupoid K71.50
            with ascites K71.51
      peliosis hepatis K71.8
      veno-occlusive disease (VOD) of liver K71.8
  veno-occlusive K76.5
Lobo's (keloid blastomycosis) B48.0
Lobstein's (brittle bones and blue sclera) Q78.0
Ludwig's (submaxillary cellulitis) K12.2
lumbosacral region M53.87
lung J98.4
  black J60
  congenital Q33.9
  cystic J98.4
    congenital Q33.0
  fibroid (chronic) - *see* Fibrosis, lung
  fluke B66.4

Disease, diseased - *continued*
  oriental B66.4
  in
    amyloidosis E85.4 *[J99]*
    sarcoidosis D86.0
    Sjögren's syndrome M35.02
    systemic
      lupus erythematosus M32.13
      sclerosis M34.81
  interstitial J84.9
    of childhood, specified NEC J84.848
    respiratory bronchiolitis J84.115
    specified NEC J84.89
  obstructive (chronic) J44.9
    with
      acute
        bronchitis J44.0
        exacerbation NEC J44.1
        lower respiratory infection J44.0
      alveolitis, allergic J67.9
      asthma J44.9
      bronchiectasis J47.9
        with
          exacerbation (acute) J47.1
          lower respiratory infection J47.0
      bronchitis J44.9
        with
          exacerbation (acute) J44.1
          lower respiratory infection J44.0
      emphysema J43.9
      hypersensitivity pneumonitis J67.9
    decompensated J44.1
      with
        exacerbation (acute) J44.1
  polycystic J98.4
    congenital Q33.0
  rheumatoid (diffuse) (interstitial) - *see*
    Rheumatoid, lung
  Lutembacher's (atrial septal defect with mitral
    stenosis) Q21.1
  Lyme A69.20
  lymphatic (gland) (system) (channel) (vessel)
    I89.9
  lymphoproliferative D47.9
    specified NEC D47.Z9
    T-gamma D47.Z9
    X-linked D82.3
  Magitot's M27.2
  malarial - *see* Malaria
  malignant - *see also* Neoplasm, malignant, by
    site
  Manson's B65.1
  maple bark J67.6
  maple-syrup-urine E71.0
  Marburg (virus) A98.3
  Marion's (bladder neck obstruction) N32.0
  Marsh's (exophthalmic goiter) - *see*
    Hyperthyroidism, with, goiter (diffuse)
  mastoid (process) - *see* Disorder, ear, middle
  Mathieu's (leptospiral jaundice) A27.0
  Maxcy's A75.2
  McArdle (-Schmid-Pearson) (glycogenosis V)
    E74.04
  mediastinum J98.59
  medullary center (idiopathic) (respiratory)
    G93.89
  Meige's (chronic hereditary edema) Q82.0
  meningococcal - *see* Infection, meningococcal
  mental F99
    organic F09
  mesenchymal M35.9
  mesenteric embolic - *see also* Ischemia,
    intestine, acute K55.039
  metabolic, metabolism E88.9

Disease, diseased - *continued*
  bilirubin E80.7
  metal-polisher's J62.8
  metastatic - *see also* Neoplasm, secondary, by
    site C79.9
  microvascular
    code to condition
  microvillus
    atrophy Q43.8
    inclusion (MVD) Q43.8
  middle ear - *see* Disorder, ear, middle
  Mikulicz' (dryness of mouth, absent or
    decreased lacrimation) K11.8
  Milroy's (chronic hereditary edema) Q82.0
  Minamata - *see* Poisoning, mercury   minicore
    G71.2
  Minor's G95.19
  Minot's (hemorrhagic disease, newborn) P53
  Minot-von Willebrand-Jurgens
    (angiohemophilia) D68.0
  Mitchell's (erythromelalgia) I73.81
  mitral (valve) I05.9
    nonrheumatic I34.9
  mixed connective tissue M35.1
  moldy hay J67.0
  Monge's T70.29
  Morgagni-Adams-stokes (syncope with heart
    block) I45.9
  Morgagni's (syndrome) (hyperostosis frontalis
    interna) M85.2
  Morton's (with metatarsalgia) - *see* Lesion,
    nerve, plantar
  Morvan's G60.8
  motor neuron (bulbar) (mixed type) (spinal)
    G12.20
    amyotrophic lateral sclerosis G12.21
    familial G12.24
    progressive bulbar palsy G12.22
    specified NEC G12.29
  moyamoya I67.5
  mu heavy chain disease C88.2
  multicore G71.2
  muscle - *see also* Disorder, muscle
    inflammatory - *see* Myositis
    ocular (external) - *see* Strabismus
  musculoskeletal system, soft tissue - *see also*
    Disorder, soft tissue
    specified NEC - *see* Disorder, soft tissue,
    specified type NEC
  mushroom workers' J67.5
  mycotic B49
  myelodysplastic, not classified C94.6
  myeloproliferative, not classified C94.6
    chronic D47.1
  myocardium, myocardial - *see also*
    Degeneration, myocardial I51.5
    primary (idiopathic) I42.9
  myoneural G70.9
  Naegeli's D69.1
  nails L60.9
    specified NEC L60.8
  Nairobi (sheep virus) A93.8
  nasal J34.9
  nemaline body G71.2
  nerve - *see* Disorder, nerve
  nervous system G98.8
    autonomic G90.9
    central G96.9
      specified NEC G96.8
    congenital Q07.9
    parasympathetic G90.9
    specified NEC G98.8
    sympathetic G90.9
    vegetative G90.9

Disease, diseased - *continued*
  neuromuscular system G70.9
  Newcastle B30.8
  Nicolas (-Durand)-Favre (climatic bubo) A55
  nipple N64.9
    Paget's C50.01-
      female C50.01-
      male C50.02-
  Nishimoto (-Takeuchi) I67.5
  nonarthropod-borne NOS (viral) B34.9
    enterovirus NEC B34.1
  nonautoimmune hemolytic D59.4
    drug-induced D59.2
  Nonne-Milroy-Meige (chronic hereditary
    edema) Q82.0
  nose J34.9
  nucleus pulposus - *see* Disorder, disc
  nutritional E63.9
  oast-house-urine E72.19
    ocular
      herpesviral B00.50
      zoster B02.30
  obliterative vascular I77.1
  Ohara's - *see* Tularemia
  Opitz's (congestive splenomegaly) D73.2
  Oppenheim-Urbach (necrobiosis lipoidica
    diabeticorum) - *see* E08-e13 with .620
  optic nerve NEC - *see* Disorder, nerve, optic
  orbit - *see* Disorder, orbit
  Oriental liver fluke B66.1
  Oriental lung fluke B66.4
  Ormond's N13.5
  Oropouche virus A93.0
  Osler-Rendu (familial hemorrhagic
    telangiectasia) I78.0
  osteofibrocystic E21.0
  Otto's M24.7
  outer ear - *see* Disorder, ear, external
  ovary (noninflammatory) N83.9
    cystic N83.20-
    inflammatory - *see* Salpingo-oophoritis
    polycystic E28.2
    specified NEC N83.8
  Owren's (congenital) - *see* Defect, coagulation
  pancreas K86.9
    cystic K86.2
    fibrocystic E84.9
    specified NEC K86.89
  panvalvular I08.9
    specified NEC I08.8
  parametrium (noninflammatory) N83.9
  parasitic B89
    cerebral NEC B71.9 *[G94]*
    intestinal NOS B82.9
    mouth B37.0
    skin NOS B88.9
    specified type - *see* Infestation
    tongue B37.0
  parathyroid (gland) E21.5
    specified NEC E21.4
  Parkinson's G20
  parodontal K05.6
  Parrot's (syphilitic osteochondritis) A50.02
  Parry's (exophthalmic goiter) - *see*
    Hyperthyroidism, with, goiter (diffuse)
  Parson's (exophthalmic goiter) - *see*
    Hyperthyroidism, with, goiter (diffuse)
  Paxton's (white piedra) B36.2
  pearl-worker's - *see* Osteomyelitis, specified
    type NEC
  Pellegrini-Stieda (calcification, knee joint) -
    see Bursitis, tibial collateral
  pelvis, pelvic
    female NOS N94.9

Disease, diseased - *continued*
  specified NEC N94.89
  gonococcal (acute) (chronic) A54.24
  inflammatory (female) N73.9
    acute N73.0
    chlamydial A56.11
    chronic N73.1
    specified NEC N73.8
    syphilitic (secondary) A51.42
      late A52.76
    tuberculous A18.17
  organ, female N94.9
  peritoneum, female NEC N94.89
  penis N48.9
    inflammatory N48.29
      abscess N48.21
      cellulitis N48.22
    specified NEC N48.89
  periapical tissues NOS K04.90
  periodontal K05.6
    specified NEC K05.5
  periosteum - *see* Disorder, bone, specified type
    NEC
  peripheral
    arterial I73.9
    autonomic nervous system G90.9
    nerves - *see* Polyneuropathy
    vascular NOS I73.9
  peritoneum K66.9
    pelvic, female NEC N94.89
    specified NEC K66.8
  persistent mucosal (middle ear) H66.20
    left H66.22
      with right H66.23
    right H66.21
      with left H66.23
  Petit's - *see* Hernia, abdomen, specified site
    NEC
  pharynx J39.2
    specified NEC J39.2
  Phocas' - *see* Mastopathy, cystic
  photochromogenic (acid-fast bacilli)
    (pulmonary) A31.0
    nonpulmonary A31.9
  Pick's G31.01 [*F02.80*]
    with behavioral disturbance G31.01
    [*F02.81*]
    brain G31.01 [*F02.80*]
      with behavioral disturbance G31.01
      [*F02.81*]
    of pericardium (pericardial pseudocirrhosis
    of liver) I31.1
  pigeon fancier's J67.2
  pineal gland E34.8
  pink - *see* Poisoning, mercury Pinkus' (lichen
    nitidus) L44.1
  pinworm B80
  Piry virus A93.8
  pituitary (gland) E23.7
  pituitary-snuff-taker's J67.8
  pleura (cavity) J94.9
    specified NEC J94.8
  pneumatic drill (hammer) T75.21
  Pollitzer's (hidradenitis suppurativa) L73.2
  polycystic
    kidney or renal Q61.3
      adult type Q61.2
      childhood type NEC Q61.19
        collecting duct dilatation Q61.11
    liver or hepatic Q44.6
    lung or pulmonary J98.4
      congenital Q33.0
    ovary, ovaries E28.2
    spleen Q89.09

Disease, diseased - *continued*
  polyethylene T84.05-
  Pompe's (glycogenosis II) E74.02
  Posadas-Wernicke B38.9
  Potain's (pulmonary edema) - *see* Edema, lung
  prepuce N47.8
    inflammatory N47.7
      balanoposthitis N47.6
  Pringle's (tuberous sclerosis) Q85.1
  prion, central nervous system A81.9
    specified NEC A81.89
  prostate N42.9
    specified NEC N42.89
  protozoal B64
    acanthamebiasis - *see* Acanthamebiasis
    African trypanosomiasis - *see* African
      trypanosomiasis
    babesiosis B60.0
    Chagas disease - *see* Chagas disease
    intestine, intestinal A07.9
    leishmaniasis - *see* Leishmaniasis
    malaria - *see* Malaria
    naegleriasis B60.2
    pneumocystosis B59
    specified organism NEC B60.8
    toxoplasmosis - *see* Toxoplasmosis
  pseudo-hurler's E77.0
  psychiatric F99
  psychotic - *see* Psychosis
  Puente's (simple glandular cheilitis) K13.0
  puerperal - *see also* Puerperal O90.89
  pulmonary - *see also* Disease, lung
    artery I28.9
    chronic obstructive J44.9
      with
        acute bronchitis J44.0
        exacerbation (acute) J44.1
        lower respiratory infection (acute) J44.0
      decompensated J44.1
        with
          exacerbation (acute) J44.1
    heart I27.9
      specified NEC I27.89
    hypertensive (vascular) (see also
      Hypertension, pulmonary) I27.20
      primary (idiopathic) I27.0
    valve I37.9
      rheumatic I09.89
  pulp (dental) NOS K04.90
  pulseless M31.4
  Putnam's (subacute combined sclerosis with
    pernicious anemia) D51.0
  Pyle (-Cohn) (metaphyseal dysplasia) Q78.5
  ragpicker's or ragsorter's A22.1
  Raynaud's - *see* Raynaud's disease reactive
    airway - *see* Asthma
  Reclus' (cystic) - *see* Mastopathy, cystic
  rectum K62.9
    specified NEC K62.89
  Refsum's (heredopathia atactica
    polyneuritiformis) G60.1
  renal (functional) (pelvis) - *see also* Disease,
    kidney N28.9
    with
      edema - *see* Nephrosis
      glomerular lesion - *see* Glomerulonephritis
        with edema - *see* Nephrosis
      interstitial nephritis N12
    acute N28.9
    chronic - *see also* Disease, kidney, chronic
    N18.9
    cystic, congenital Q61.9
    diabetic - *see* E08-e13 with .22
    end-stage (failure) N18.6

Disease, diseased - *continued*
    due to hypertension I12.0
    fibrocystic (congenital) Q61.8
    hypertensive - *see* Hypertension, kidney
    lupus M32.14
    phosphate-losing (tubular) N25.0
    polycystic (congenital) Q61.3
      adult type Q61.2
      childhood type NEC Q61.19
        collecting duct dilatation Q61.11
    rapidly progressive N01.9
    subacute N01.9
  Rendu-Osler-weber (familial hemorrhagic
    telangiectasia) I78.0
  renovascular (arteriosclerotic) - *see*
    Hypertension, kidney
  respiratory (tract) J98.9
    acute or subacute NOS J06.9
      due to
        chemicals, gases, fumes or vapors
          (inhalation) J68.3
        external agent J70.9
          specified NEC J70.8
        radiation J70.0
        smoke inhalation J70.5
      noninfectious J39.8
    chronic NOS J98.9
      due to
        chemicals, gases, fumes or vapors J68.4
        external agent J70.9
          specified NEC J70.8
        radiation J70.1
      newborn P27.9
        specified NEC P27.8
    due to
      chemicals, gases, fumes or vapors J68.9
        acute or subacute NEC J68.3
        chronic J68.4
      external agent J70.9
        specified NEC J70.8
      newborn P28.9
        specified type NEC P28.89
    upper J39.9
      acute or subacute J06.9
      noninfectious NEC J39.8
      specified NEC J39.8
      streptococcal J06.9
  retina, retinal H35.9
    Batten's or Batten-Mayou E75.4 [*H36*]
    specified NEC H35.89
  rheumatoid - *see* Arthritis, rheumatoid
  rickettsial NOS A79.9
    specified type NEC A79.89
  Riga (-Fede) (cachectic aphthae) K14.0
  Riggs' (compound periodontitis) - *see*
    Periodontitis
  Ritter's L00
  Rivalta's (cervicofacial actinomycosis) A42.2
  Robles' (onchocerciasis) B73.01
  Roger's (congenital interventricular septal
    defect) Q21.0
  Rosenthal's (factor XI deficiency) D68.1
  Rossbach's (hyperchlorhydria) K30
  Ross River B33.1
  Rotes Quérol - *see* Hyperostosis, ankylosing
  Roth (-Bernhardt) - *see* Mononeuropathy,
    lower limb, meralgia paresthetica
  Runeberg's (progressive pernicious anemia)
    D51.0
  sacroiliac NEC M53.3
  salivary gland or duct K11.9
    inclusion B25.9
    specified NEC K11.8
    virus B25.9

Disease, diseased - *continued*
  sandworm B76.9
  Schimmelbusch's - *see* Mastopathy, cystic
  Schmorl's - *see* Schmorl's disease or nodes
  Schönlein (-Henoch) (purpura rheumatica)
    D69.0
  Schottmüller's - *see* Fever, paratyphoid
  Schultz's (agranulocytosis) - *see*
    Agranulocytosis
  Schwalbe-Ziehen-Oppenheim G24.1
  Schwartz-Jampel G71.13
  sclera H15.9
    specified NEC H15.89
  scrofulous (tuberculous) A18.2
  scrotum N50.9
  sebaceous glands L73.9
  semilunar cartilage, cystic - *see also*
    Derangement, knee, meniscus, cystic
  seminal vesicle N50.9
  serum NEC - *see also* Reaction, serum T80.69
  sexually transmitted A64
    anogenital
      herpesviral infection - *see* Herpes,
        anogenital
      warts A63.0
    chancroid A57
    chlamydial infection - *see* Chlamydia
    gonorrhea - *see* Gonorrhea
    granuloma inguinale A58
    specified organism NEC A63.8
    syphilis - *see* Syphilis
    trichomoniasis - *see* Trichomoniasis
  Sézary C84.1-
  shimamushi (scrub typhus) A75.3
  shipyard B30.0
  sickle-cell D57.1
    with crisis (vasoocclusive pain) D57.00
      with
        acute chest syndrome D57.01
        splenic sequestration D57.02
    elliptocytosis D57.8-
    Hb-c D57.20
      with crisis (vasoocclusive pain) D57.219
        with
          acute chest syndrome D57.211
          splenic sequestration D57.212
      without crisis D57.20
    Hb-sD D57.80
      with crisis D57.819
        with
          acute chest syndrome D57.811
          splenic sequestration D57.812
    Hb-sE D57.80
      with crisis D57.819
        with
          acute chest syndrome D57.811
          splenic sequestration D57.812
    specified NEC D57.80
      with crisis D57.819
        with
          acute chest syndrome D57.811
          splenic sequestration D57.812
    spherocytosis D57.80
      with crisis D57.819
        with
          acute chest syndrome D57.811
          splenic sequestration D57.812
    thalassemia D57.40
      with crisis (vasoocclusive pain) D57.419
        with
          acute chest syndrome D57.411
          splenic sequestration D57.412
      without crisis D57.40
  silo-filler's J68.8

Disease, diseased - *continued*
    bronchitis J68.0
    pneumonitis J68.0
    pulmonary edema J68.1
  simian B B00.4
  Simons' (progressive lipodystrophy) E88.1
  sin nombre virus B33.4
  sinus - *see* Sinusitis
  Sirkari's B55.0
  sixth B08.20
    due to human herpesvirus 6 B08.21
    due to human herpesvirus 7 B08.22
  skin L98.9
    due to metabolic disorder NEC E88.9 [*L99*]
    specified NEC L98.8
  slim (HIV) B20
  small vessel I73.9
  Sneddon-Wilkinson (subcorneal pustular
    dermatosis) L13.1
  South African creeping B88.0
  spinal (cord) G95.9
    congenital Q06.9
    specified NEC G95.89
  spine - *see also* Spondylopathy
    joint - *see* Dorsopathy
    tuberculous A18.01
  spinocerebellar (hereditary) G11.9
    specified NEC G11.8
  spleen D73.9
    amyloid E85.4 [*D77*]
    organic D73.9
    polycystic Q89.09
    postinfectional D73.89
  sponge-diver's - *see* Toxicity, venom, marine
    animal, sea anemone
  Startle Q89.8
  Steinert's G71.11
  Sticker's (erythema infectiosum) B08.3
  Stieda's (calcification, knee joint) - *see*
    Bursitis, tibial collateral
  Stokes' (exophthalmic goiter) - *see*
    Hyperthyroidism, with, goiter (diffuse)
  Stokes-Adams (syncope with heart block)
    I45.9
  stomach K31.9
    functional, psychogenic F45.8
    specified NEC K31.89
  stonemason's J62.8
  storage
    glycogen - *see* Disease, glycogen storage
    mucopolysaccharide - *see*
      Mucopolysaccharidosis
  striatopallidal system NEC G25.89
  Stuart-Prower (congenital factor X deficiency)
    D68.2
  Stuart's (congenital factor X deficiency) D68.2
  subcutaneous tissue - *see* Disease, skin
  supporting structures of teeth K08.9
    specified NEC K08.89
  suprarenal (capsule) (gland) E27.9
    hyperfunction E27.0
    specified NEC E27.8
  sweat glands L74.9
    specified NEC L74.8
  Sweeley-Klionsky E75.21
  Swift (-Feer) - *see* Poisoning, mercury
    swimming-pool granuloma A31.1
  Sylvest's (epidemic pleurodynia) B33.0
  sympathetic nervous system G90.9
  syphilitic - *see* Syphilis
  synovium - *see* Disorder, synovium
  systemic tissue mast cell C96.20
  tanapox (virus) B08.71
  Tangier E78.6

Disease, diseased - *continued*
  Tarral-Besnier (pityriasis rubra pilaris) L44.0
  Tauri's E74.09
  tear duct - *see* Disorder, lacrimal system
  tendon, tendinous - *see also* Disorder, tendon
    nodular - *see* Trigger finger
  terminal vessel I73.9
  testis N50.9
  thalassemia Hb-s - *see* Disease, sickle-cell,
    thalassemia
  Thaysen-gee (nontropical sprue) K90.0
  Thomsen G71.12
  throat J39.2
    septic J02.0
  thromboembolic - *see* Embolism
  thymus (gland) E32.9
    specified NEC E32.8
  thyroid (gland) E07.9
    heart - *see also* Hyperthyroidism E05.90
      [*143*]
      with thyroid storm E05.91 [*143*]
    specified NEC E07.89
  Tietze's M94.0
  tongue K14.9
    specified NEC K14.8
  tonsils, tonsillar (and adenoids) J35.9
  tooth, teeth K08.9
    hard tissues K03.9
      specified NEC K03.89
    pulp NEC K04.99
    specified NEC K08.89
  Tourette's F95.2
  trachea NEC J39.8
  tricuspid I07.9
    nonrheumatic I36.9
  triglyceride-storage E75.5
  trophoblastic - *see* Mole, hydatidiform
  tsutsugamushi A75.3
  tube (fallopian) (noninflammatory) N83.9
    inflammatory - *see* Salpingitis
    specified NEC N83.8
  tuberculous NEC - *see* Tuberculosis
  tubo-ovarian (noninflammatory) N83.9
    inflammatory - *see* Salpingo-oophoritis
    specified NEC N83.8
  tubotympanic, chronic - *see* Otitis, media,
    suppurative, chronic, tubotympanic
  tubulo-interstitial N15.9
    specified NEC N15.8
  tympanum - *see* Disorder, tympanic membrane
  Uhl's Q24.8
  Underwood's (sclerema neonatorum) P83.0
  Unverricht (-Lundborg) - *see* Epilepsy,
    generalized, idiopathic
  Urbach-Oppenheim (necrobiosis lipoidica
    diabeticorum) - *see* E08-e13 with .620
  ureter N28.9
    in (due to)
      schistosomiasis (bilharziasis) B65.0 [*N29*]
  urethra N36.9
    specified NEC N36.8
  urinary (tract) N39.9
    bladder N32.9
      specified NEC N32.89
    specified NEC N39.8
  uterus (noninflammatory) N85.9
    infective - *see* Endometritis
    inflammatory - *see* Endometritis
    specified NEC N85.8
  uveal tract (anterior) H21.9
    posterior H31.9
  vagabond's B85.1
  vagina, vaginal (noninflammatory) N89.9
    inflammatory NEC N76.89

Disease, diseased - *continued*
 specified NEC N89.8
 valve, valvular I38
  multiple I08.9
   specified NEC I08.8
 van Creveld-von Gierke (glycogenosis I)
  E74.01
 vas deferens N50.9
 vascular I99.9
  arteriosclerotic - *see* Arteriosclerosis
  ciliary body NEC - *see* Disorder, iris,
 vascular
  hypertensive - *see* Hypertension
  iris NEC - *see* Disorder, iris, vascular
  obliterative I77.1
   peripheral I73.9
  occlusive I99.8
  peripheral (occlusive) I73.9
   in diabetes mellitus - *see* E08-e13 with .51
 vasomotor I73.9
 vasospastic I73.9
 vein I87.9
 venereal - *see also* Disease, sexually
 transmitted A64
  chlamydial NEC A56.8
   anus A56.3
   genitourinary NOS A56.2
   pharynx A56.4
   rectum A56.3
  fifth A55
  sixth A55
  specified nature or type NEC A63.8
 vertebra, vertebral - *see also* Spondylopathy
  disc - *see* Disorder, disc
 vibration - *see* Vibration, adverse effects
 viral, virus - *see also* Disease, by type of virus
  B34.9
  arbovirus NOS A94
  arthropod-borne NOS A94
  congenital P35.9
   specified NEC P35.8
  Hanta (with renal manifestations) (Dobrava)
   (Puumala) (Seoul) A98.5
    with pulmonary manifestations (Andes)
     (Bayou) (Bermejo) (Black Creek Canal)
     (Choclo) (Juquitiba) (Laguna
     negra)(Lechiguanas) (New York) (Oran)
     (Sin nombre) B33.4
  Hantaan (Korean hemorrhagic fever) A98.5
  human immunodeficiency (HIV) B20
  Kunjin A83.4
  nonarthropod-borne NOS B34.9
  Powassan A84.8
  Rocio (encephalitis) A83.6
  Sin nombre (Hantavirus) (cardio)-pulmonary
   syndrome) B33.4
  Tahyna B33.8
  vesicular stomatitis A93.8
 vitreous H43.9
  specified NEC H43.89
 vocal cord J38.3
 Volkmann's, acquired T79.6
 von Eulenburg's (congenital paramyotonia)
  G71.19
 von Gierke's (glycogenosis I) E74.01
 von Graefe's - *see* Strabismus, paralytic,
  ophthalmoplegia, progressive
 von Willebrand (-Jurgens) (angiohemophilia)
  D68.0
 Vrolik's (osteogenesis imperfecta) Q78.0
 vulva (noninflammatory) N90.9
  inflammatory NEC N76.89
  specified NEC N90.89
 Wallgren's (obstruction of splenic vein with

Disease, diseased - *continued*
  collateral circulation) I87.8
 Wassilieff's (leptospiral jaundice) A27.0
 wasting NEC R64
  due to malnutrition E41
 Waterhouse-Friderichsen A39.1
 Wegner's (syphilitic osteochondritis) A50.02
 Weil's (leptospiral jaundice of lung) A27.0
 Weir Mitchell's (erythromelalgia) I73.81
 Werdnig-Hoffmann G12.0
 Wermer's E31.21
 Werner-his (trench fever) A79.0
 Werner-Schultz (neutropenic splenomegaly)
  D73.81
 Wernicke-Posadas B38.9
 whipworm B79
 white blood cells D72.9
  specified NEC D72.89
 white matter R90.82
 white-spot, meaning lichen sclerosus et
  atrophicus L90.0
  penis N48.0
  vulva N90.4
 Wilkie's K55.1
 Wilkinson-Sneddon (subcorneal pustular
  dermatosis) L13.1
 Willis' - *see* Diabetes
 Wilson's (hepatolenticular degeneration)
  E83.01
 woolsorter's A22.1
 yaba monkey tumor B08.72
 yaba pox (virus) B08.72
 Zika virus A92.5
 zoonotic, bacterial A28.9
  specified type NEC A28.8
Disfigurement (due to scar) L90.5
Disgerminoma - *see* Dysgerminoma
DISH (diffuse idiopathic skeletal
 hyperostosis) - *see* Hyperostosis, ankylosing
Disinsertion, retina - *see* Detachment, retina
Dislocatable hip, congenital Q65.6
Dislocation (articular)
 with fracture - *see* Fracture
 acromioclavicular (joint) S43.10-
  with displacement
   100% 200% S43.12-
   more than 200% S43.13-
  inferior S43.14-
  posterior S43.15-
 ankle S93.0-
 astragalus - *see* Dislocation, ankle
 atlantoaxial S13.121
 atlantooccipital S13.111
 atloido-occipital S13.111
 breast bone S23.29
 capsule, joint
  code by site under Dislocation
 carpal (bone) - *see* Dislocation, wrist
 carpometacarpal (joint) NEC S63.05-
  thumb S63.04-
 cartilage (joint)
  code by site under Dislocation
 cervical spine (vertebra) - *see* Dislocation,
  vertebra, cervical
 chronic - *see* Dislocation, recurrent
 clavicle - *see* Dislocation, acromioclavicular
  joint
 coccyx S33.2
 congenital NEC Q68.8
 coracoid - *see* Dislocation, shoulder
 costal cartilage S23.29
 costochondral S23.29
 cricoarytenoid articulation S13.29
 cricothyroid articulation S13.29

Dislocation (articular) - *continued*
 dorsal vertebra - *see* Dislocation, vertebra,
  thoracic
 ear ossicle - *see* Discontinuity, ossicles, ear
 elbow S53.10-
  congenital Q68.8
  pathological - *see* Dislocation, pathological
   NEC, elbow
  radial head alone - *see* Dislocation, radial
   head
  recurrent - *see* Dislocation, recurrent, elbow
  traumatic S53.10-
   anterior S53.11-
   lateral S53.14-
   medial S53.13-
   posterior S53.12-
   specified type NEC S53.19-
 eye, nontraumatic - *see* Luxation, globe
 eyeball, nontraumatic - *see* Luxation, globe
 femur
  distal end - *see* Dislocation, knee
  proximal end - *see* Dislocation, hip
 fibula
  distal end - *see* Dislocation, ankle
  proximal end - *see* Dislocation, knee finger
 S63.25-
  index S63.25-
  interphalangeal S63.27-
   distal S63.29-
    index S63.29-
    little S63.29-
    middle S63.29-
    ring S63.29-
   index S63.27-
   little S63.27-
   middle S63.27-
   proximal S63.28-
    index S63.28-
    little S63.28-
    middle S63.28-
    ring S63.28-
   ring S63.27-
  little S63.25-
  metacarpophalangeal S63.26-
   index S63.26-
   little S63.26-
   middle S63.26-
   ring S63.26-
  middle S63.25-
  recurrent - *see* Dislocation, recurrent, finger
  ring S63.25-
  thumb - *see* Dislocation, thumb
 foot S93.30-
  recurrent - *see* Dislocation, recurrent, foot
  specified site NEC S93.33-
  tarsal joint S93.31-
  tarsometatarsal joint S93.32-
  toe - *see* Dislocation, toe
 fracture - *see* Fracture
 glenohumeral (joint) - *see* Dislocation,
  shoulder
 glenoid - *see* Dislocation, shoulder
 habitual - *see* Dislocation, recurrent
 hip S73.00-
  anterior S73.03-
   obturator S73.02-
  central S73.04-
  congenital (total) Q65.2
   bilateral Q65.1
   partial Q65.5
    bilateral Q65.4
    unilateral Q65.3-
   unilateral Q65.0-
  developmental M24.85-

Dislocation (articular) - *continued*
  pathological - *see* Dislocation, pathological
    NEC, hip
    posterior S73.01-
    recurrent - *see* Dislocation, recurrent, hip
  humerus, proximal end - *see* Dislocation,
    shoulder
  incomplete - *see* Subluxation, by site
  incus - *see* Discontinuity, ossicles, ear
  infracoracoid - *see* Dislocation, shoulder
  innominate (pubic junction) (sacral junction)
    S33.39
    acetabulum - *see* Dislocation, hip
  interphalangeal (joint(s))
    finger S63.279
      distal S63.29-
        index S63.29-
        little S63.29-
        middle S63.29-
        ring S63.29-
      index S63.27-
      little S63.27-
      middle S63.27-
      proximal S63.28-
        index S63.28-
        little S63.28-
        middle S63.28-
        ring S63.28-
      ring S63.27-
    foot or toe - *see* Dislocation, toe
    thumb S63.12-
      distal joint S63.14-
      proximal joint S63.13-
  jaw (cartilage) (meniscus) S03.0-
  joint prosthesis - *see* Complications, joint
    prosthesis, mechanical, displacement, by site
  knee S83.106
    cap - *see* Dislocation, patella
    congenital Q68.2
    old M23.8X-
    patella - *see* Dislocation, patella
    pathological - *see* Dislocation, pathological
      NEC, knee
    proximal tibia
      anteriorly S83.11-
      laterally S83.14-
      medially S83.13-
      posteriorly S83.12-
    recurrent - *see also* Derangement, knee,
      specified NEC
    specified type NEC S83.19-
  lacrimal gland H04.16-
  lens (complete) H27.10
    anterior H27.12-
    congenital Q12.1
    ocular implant - *see* Complications,
      intraocular lens
    partial H27.11-
    posterior H27.13-
    traumatic S05.8X-
  ligament
  code by site under Dislocation
  lumbar (vertebra) - *see* Dislocation, vertebra,
    lumbar
  lumbosacral (vertebra) - *see also* Dislocation,
    vertebra, lumbar
    congenital Q76.49
  mandible S03.0-
  meniscus (knee) - *see* Tear, meniscus
    other sites
  code by site under Dislocation
  metacarpal (bone)
    distal end - *see* Dislocation, finger
    proximal end S63.06-

Dislocation (articular) - *continued*
  metacarpophalangeal (joint)
    finger S63.26-
      index S63.26-
      little S63.26-
      middle S63.26-
      ring S63.26-
      thumb S63.11-
  metatarsal (bone) - *see* Dislocation, foot
  metatarsophalangeal (joint(s)) - *see*
    Dislocation, toe midcarpal (joint) S63.03-
  midtarsal (joint) - *see* Dislocation, foot
  neck S13.20
    specified site NEC S13.29
    vertebra - *see* Dislocation, vertebra, cervical
  nose (septal cartilage) S03.1
  occipitoatloid S13.111
  old - *see* Derangement, joint, specified type
    NEC
  ossicles, ear - *see* Discontinuity, ossicles, ear
  partial - *see* Subluxation, by site
  patella S83.006
    congenital Q74.1
    lateral S83.01-
    recurrent (nontraumatic) M22.0-
      incomplete M22.1-
    specified type NEC S83.09-
  pathological NEC M24.30
    ankle M24.37-
    elbow M24.32-
    foot joint M24.37-
    hand joint M24.34-
    hip M24.35-
    knee M24.36-
    lumbosacral joint - *see* subcategory M53.2
    pelvic region - *see* Dislocation, pathological,
      hip
    sacroiliac - *see* subcategory M53.2
    shoulder M24.31-
    wrist M24.33-
  pelvis NEC S33.30
    specified NEC S33.39
  phalanx
    finger or hand - *see* Dislocation, finger
    foot or toe - *see* Dislocation, toe
  prosthesis, internal - *see* Complications,
    prosthetic device, by site, mechanical
  radial head S53.006
    anterior S53.01-
    posterior S53.02-
    specified type NEC S53.09-
  radiocarpal (joint) S63.02-
  radiohumeral (joint) - *see* Dislocation, radial
    head radioulnar (joint)
    distal S63.01-
    proximal - *see* Dislocation, elbow
  radius
    distal end - *see* Dislocation, wrist
    proximal end - *see* Dislocation, radial head
  recurrent M24.40
    ankle M24.47-
    elbow M24.42-
    finger M24.44-
    foot joint M24.47-
    hand joint M24.44-
    hip M24.45-
    knee M24.46-
      patella - *see* Dislocation, patella, recurrent
    patella - *see* Dislocation, patella, recurrent
    sacroiliac - *see* subcategory M53.2
    shoulder M24.41-
    toe M24.47-
    vertebra - *see also* subcategory M43.5
      atlantoaxial M43.4

Dislocation (articular) - *continued*
    with myelopathy M43.3
      wrist M24.43-
  rib (cartilage) S23.29
  sacrococcygeal S33.2
  sacroiliac (joint) (ligament) S33.2
    congenital Q74.2
    recurrent - *see* subcategory M53.2
  sacrum S33.2
  scaphoid (bone) (hand) (wrist) - *see*
    Dislocation, wrist
    foot - *see* Dislocation, foot
  scapula - *see* Dislocation, shoulder, girdle,
    scapula
  semilunar cartilage, knee - *see* Tear, meniscus
  septal cartilage (nose) S03.1
  septum (nasal) (old) J34.2
  sesamoid bone
  code by site under Dislocation
  shoulder (blade) (ligament) (joint) (traumatic)
    S43.006
    acromioclavicular - *see* Dislocation,
      acromioclavicular
    chronic - *see* Dislocation, recurrent, shoulder
    congenital Q68.8
    girdle S43.30-
      scapula S43.31-
      specified site NEC S43.39-
    humerus S43.00-
      anterior S43.01-
      inferior S43.03-
      posterior S43.02-
    pathological - *see* Dislocation, pathological
      NEC, shoulder
    recurrent - *see* Dislocation, recurrent,
  shoulder
    specified type NEC S43.08-
  spine
    cervical - *see* Dislocation, vertebra, cervical
    congenital Q76.49
    due to birth trauma P11.5
    lumbar - *see* Dislocation, vertebra, lumbar
    thoracic - *see* Dislocation, vertebra, thoracic
  spontaneous - *see* Dislocation, pathological
  sternoclavicular (joint) S43.206
    anterior S43.21-
    posterior S43.22-
  sternum S23.29
  subglenoid - *see* Dislocation, shoulder
  symphysis pubis S33.4
  talus - *see* Dislocation, ankle
  tarsal (bone(s)) (joint(s)) - *see* Dislocation,
    foot
  tarsometatarsal (joint(s)) - *see* Dislocation,
    foot
  temporomandibular (joint) S03.0-
  thigh, proximal end - *see* Dislocation, hip
  thorax S23.20
    specified site NEC S23.29
    vertebra - *see* Dislocation, vertebra
  thumb S63.10-
    interphalangeal joint - *see* Dislocation,
      interphalangeal (joint), thumb
    metacarpophalangeal joint - *see* Dislocation,
      metacarpophalangeal (joint), thumb
  thyroid cartilage S13.29
  tibia
    distal end - *see* Dislocation, ankle
    proximal end - *see* Dislocation, knee
  tibiofibular (joint)
    distal - *see* Dislocation, ankle
    superior - *see* Dislocation, knee toe(s)
    S93.106
    great S93.10-

Dislocation (articular) - *continued*
interphalangeal joint S93.11-
metatarsophalangeal joint S93.12-
interphalangeal joint S93.119
lesser S93.106
interphalangeal joint S93.11-
metatarsophalangeal joint S93.12-
metatarsophalangeal joint S93.12-
tooth S03.2
trachea S23.29
ulna
distal end S63.07-
proximal end - *see* Dislocation, elbow
ulnohumeral (joint) - *see* Dislocation, elbow
vertebra (articular process) (body) (traumatic)
cervical S13.101
atlantoaxial joint S13.121
atlantooccipital joint S13.111
atloido-occipital joint S13.111
joint between
C0 and C1 S13.111
C1 and C2 S13.121
C2 and C3 S13.131
C3 and C4 S13.141
C4 and C5 S13.151
C5 and C6 S13.161
C6 and C7 S13.171
C7 and T1 S13.181
occipitoatloid joint S13.111
congenital Q76.49
lumbar S33.101
joint between
L1 and L2 S33.111
L2 and L3 S33.121
L3 and L4 S33.131
L4 and L5 S33.141
nontraumatic - *see* Displacement,
intervertebral disc
partial - *see* Subluxation, by site
recurrent NEC - *see* subcategory M43.5
thoracic S23.101
joint between
T1 and T2 S23.111
T2 and T3 S23.121
T3 and T4 S23.123
T4 and T5 S23.131
T5 and T6 S23.133
T6 and T7 S23.141
T7 and T8 S23.143
T8 and T9 S23.151
T9 and T10 S23.153
T10 and T11 S23.161
T11 and T12 S23.163
T12 and L1 S23.171
wrist (carpal bone) S63.006
carpometacarpal joint - *see* Dislocation,
carpometacarpal (joint)
distal radioulnar joint - *see* Dislocation,
radioulnar (joint), distal
metacarpal bone, proximal - *see* Dislocation,
metacarpal (bone), proximal end
midcarpal - *see* Dislocation, midcarpal (joint)
radiocarpal joint - *see* Dislocation,
radiocarpal (joint)
recurrent - *see* Dislocation, recurrent, wrist
specified site NEC S63.09-
ulna - *see* Dislocation, ulna, distal end
xiphoid cartilage S23.29
Disorder (of) - *see also* Disease   acantholytic
L11.9
specified NEC L11.8
acute
psychotic - *see* Psychosis, acute
stress F43.0

Disorder (of) - *continued*
adjustment (grief) F43.20
with
anxiety F43.22
with depressed mood F43.23
conduct disturbance F43.24
with emotional disturbance F43.25
depressed mood F43.21
with anxiety F43.23
other specified symptom F43.29
adrenal (capsule) (gland) (medullary) E27.9
specified NEC E27.8
adrenogenital E25.9
drug-induced E25.8
iatrogenic E25.8
idiopathic E25.8
adult personality (and behavior) F69
specified NEC F68.8
affective (mood) - *see* Disorder, mood
aggressive, unsocialized F91.1
alcohol-related F10.99
with
amnestic disorder, persisting F10.96
anxiety disorder F10.980
dementia, persisting F10.97
intoxication F10.929
with delirium F10.921
uncomplicated F10.920
mood disorder F10.94
other specified F10.988
psychotic disorder F10.959
with
delusions F10.950
hallucinations F10.951
sexual dysfunction F10.981
sleep disorder F10.982
alcohol use
mild F10.10
in remission (early) (sustained) F10.11
with
alcohol-induced
anxiety disorder F10.180
bipolar and related disorder F10.14
depressive disorder F10.14
psychotic disorder F10.159
sexual dysfunction F10.181
sleep disorder F10.182
alcohol intoxication F10.129
delirium F10.121
moderate or severe F10.20
in remission (early) (sustained) F10.21
with
alcohol-induced
anxiety disorder F10.280
bipolar and related disorder F10.24
depressive disorder F10.24
major neurocognitive disorder, amnestic-
confabulatory type F10.26
major neurocognitive disorder, non-
amnestic-confabulatory type F10.27
mild neurocognitive disorder F10.288
psychotic disorder F10.259
sexual dysfunction F10.281
sleep disorder F10.282
alcohol intoxication F10.229
delirium F10.221
allergic - *see* Allergy
alveolar NEC J84.09
amino-acid
cystathioninuria E72.19
cystinosis E72.04
cystinuria E72.01
glycinuria E72.09
homocystinuria E72.11

Disorder (of) - *continued*
metabolism - *see* Disturbance, metabolism,
amino-acid
specified NEC E72.8
neonatal, transitory P74.8
renal transport NEC E72.09
transport NEC E72.09
amnesic, amnestic
alcohol-induced F10.96
with dependence F10.26
due to (secondary to) general medical
condition F04
psychoactive NEC-induced F19.96
with
abuse F19.16
dependence F19.26
sedative, hypnotic or anxiolytic-induced
F13.96
with dependence F13.26
amphetamine-type substance use
mild F15.10
in remission (early) (sustained) F15.11
moderate F15.20
in remission (early) (sustained) F15.21
severe F15.20
in remission (early) (sustained) F15.21
amphetamine (or other stimulant) use
mild
with
amphetamine (or other stimulant) -induced
anxiety disorder F15.180
bipolar and related disorder F15.14
depressive disorder F15.14
obsessive-compulsive and related
disorder F15.188
psychotic disorder F15.159
sexual dysfunction F15.181
amphetamine, cocaine, or other stimulant
intoxication
with perceptual disturbances F15.122
without perceptual disturbances F15.129
intoxication delirium F15.121
moderate or severe
with
amphetamine (or other stimulant) -induced
anxiety disorder F15.280
obsessive-compulsive and related
disorder F15.288
sexual dysfunction F15.281
bipolar and related disorder F15.24
depressive disorder F15.24
psychotic disorder F15.259
amphetamine, cocaine, or other stimulant
intoxication
with perceptual disturbances F15.222
without perceptual disturbances F15.229
intoxication delirium F15.221
anaerobic glycolysis with anemia D55.2
anxiety F41.9
due to (secondary to)
alcohol F10.980
amphetamine F15.980
in
abuse F15.180
dependence F15.280
anxiolytic F13.980
in
abuse F13.180
dependence F13.280
caffeine F15.980
in
abuse F15.180
dependence F15.280

Disorder (of) - *continued*
cannabis F12.980
  in
    abuse F12.180
    dependence F12.280
  cocaine F14.980
  in
    abuse F14.180
    dependence F14.180
  general medical condition F06.4
  hallucinogen F16.980
  in
    abuse F16.180
    dependence F16.280
  hypnotic F13.980
  in
    abuse F13.180
    dependence F13.280
  inhalant F18.980
  in
    abuse F18.180
    dependence F18.280
  phencyclidine F16.980
  in
    abuse F16.180
    dependence F16.280
  psychoactive substance NEC F19.980
  in
    abuse F19.180
    dependence F19.280
  sedative F13.980
  in
    abuse F13.180
    dependence F13.280
  volatile solvents F18.980
  in
    abuse F18.180
    dependence F18.280
generalized F41.1
illness F45.21
mixed
  with depression (mild) F41.8
  specified NEC F41.3
organic F06.8
phobic F40.9
  of childhood F40.8
  specified NEC F41.8
aortic valve - *see* Endocarditis, aortic
aromatic amino-acid metabolism E70.9
  specified NEC E70.8
arteriole NEC I77.89
artery NEC I77.89
articulation - *see* Disorder, joint
attachment (childhood)
  disinhibited F94.2
  reactive F94.1
attention-deficit hyperactivity (adolescent)
  (adult) (child) F90.9
  combined
    presentation F90.2
    type F90.2
  hyperactive
    impulsive presentation F90.1
    type F90.1
  inattentive
    presentation F90.0
    type F90.0
  specified type NEC F90.8
attention-deficit without hyperactivity
  (adolescent) (adult) (child) F98.8
auditory processing (central) H93.25
autistic F84.0
autism spectrum F84.0
autoimmune D89.89

Disorder (of) - *continued*
autonomic nervous system G90.9
  specified NEC G90.8
avoidant
  child or adolescent F40.10
  restrictive food intake F50.82
balance
  acid-base E87.8
    mixed E87.4
  electrolyte E87.8
  fluid NEC E87.8
behavioral (disruptive) - *see* Disorder, conduct
beta-amino-acid metabolism E72.8
bile acid and cholesterol metabolism E78.70
  Barth syndrome E78.71
  other specified E78.79
  Smith-Lemli-Opitz syndrome E78.72
bilirubin excretion E80.6
binge eating F50.81
binocular
  movement H51.9
    convergence
      excess H51.12
      insufficiency H51.11
    internuclear ophthalmoplegia - *see*
      Ophthalmoplegia, internuclear
    palsy of conjugate gaze H51.0
    specified type NEC H51.8
  vision NEC - *see* Disorder, vision, binocular
bipolar (I) (type 1) F31.9
  and related due to a known physiological
    condition
  with
    manic features F06.33
    manic or hypomanic-like episodes F06.33
    mixed features F06.34
  current (or most recent) episode
    depressed F31.9
      with psychotic features F31.5
      without psychotic features F31.30
        mild F31.31
        moderate F31.32
        severe (without psychotic features) F31.4
          with psychotic features F31.5
    hypomanic F31.0
    manic F31.9
      with psychotic features F31.2
      without psychotic features F31.10
        mild F31.11
        moderate F31.12
        severe (without psychotic features)
          F31.13
          with psychotic features F31.2
    mixed F31.60
      mild F31.61
      moderate F31.62
      severe (without psychotic features) F31.63
        with psychotic features F31.64
      severe depression (without psychotic
        features) F31.4
        with psychotic features F31.5
  in remission (currently) F31.70
  in full remission
    most recent episode
      depressed F31.76
      hypomanic F31.72
      manic F31.74
      mixed F31.78
  in partial remission
    most recent episode
      depressed F31.75
      hypomanic F31.71
      manic F31.73
      mixed F31.77

Disorder (of) - *continued*
  specified NEC F31.89
  II (type 2) F31.81
  organic F06.30
  single manic episode F30.9
    mild F30.11
    moderate F30.12
    severe (without psychotic symptoms)
      F30.13
      with psychotic symptoms F30.2
bladder N32.9
  functional NEC N31.9
  in schistosomiasis B65.0 [*N33*]
  specified NEC N32.89
bleeding D68.9
blood D75.9
  in congenital early syphilis A50.09 [*D77*]
body dysmorphic F45.22
bone M89.9
  continuity M84.9
    specified type NEC M84.80
      ankle M84.87-
      fibula M84.86-
      foot M84.87-
      hand M84.84-
      humerus M84.82-
      neck M84.88
      pelvis M84.859
      radius M84.83-
      rib M84.88
      shoulder M84.81-
      skull M84.88
      thigh M84.85-
      tibia M84.86-
      ulna M84.83-
      vertebra M84.88
  density and structure M85.9
    cyst - *see also* Cyst, bone, specified type
      NEC
      aneurysmal - *see* Cyst, bone, aneurysmal
      solitary - *see* Cyst, bone, solitary
    diffuse idiopathic skeletal hyperostosis - *see*
      Hyperostosis, ankylosing
    fibrous dysplasia (monostotic) - *see*
      Dysplasia, fibrous, bone
    fluorosis - *see* Fluorosis, skeletal
    hyperostosis of skull M85.2
    osteitis condensans - *see* Osteitis,
      condensans
    specified type NEC M85.8-
      ankle M85.87-
      foot M85.87-
      forearm M85.83-
      hand M85.84-
      lower leg M85.86-
      multiple sites M85.89
      neck M85.88
      rib M85.88
      shoulder M85.81-
      skull M85.88
      thigh M85.85-
      upper arm M85.82-
      vertebra M85.88
  development and growth NEC M89.20
    carpus M89.24-
    clavicle M89.21-
    femur M89.25-
    fibula M89.26-
    finger M89.24-
    humerus M89.22-
    ilium M89.259
    ischium M89.259
    metacarpus M89.24-
    metatarsus M89.27-

Disorder (of) - *continued*

multiple sites M89.29
neck M89.28
radius M89.23-
rib M89.28
scapula M89.21-
skull M89.28
tarsus M89.27-
tibia M89.26-
toe M89.27-
ulna M89.23-
vertebra M89.28
specified type NEC M89.8X   brachial
plexus G54.0
branched-chain amino-acid metabolism E71.2
specified NEC E71.19
breast N64.9
agalactia - *see* Agalactia
associated with
lactation O92.70
specified NEC O92.79
pregnancy O92.20
specified NEC O92.29
puerperium O92.20
specified NEC O92.29
cracked nipple - *see* Cracked nipple
galactorrhea - *see* Galactorrhea
hypogalactia O92.4
lactation disorder NEC O92.79
mastitis - *see* Mastitis
nipple infection - *see* Infection, nipple
retracted nipple - *see* Retraction, nipple
specified type NEC N64.89
Briquet's F45.0
bullous, in diseases classified elsewhere L14
caffeine use
mild
with
caffeine-induced
anxiety disorder F15.180
sleep disorder F15.182
moderate or severe
with
caffeine-induced
anxiety disorder F15.280
sleep disorder F15.282
cannabis use
mild F12.10
in remission (early) (sustained) F12.11
with
cannabis-induced
anxiety disorder F12.180
psychotic disorder F12.159
sleep disorder F12.188
cannabis intoxication delirium F12.121
with perceptual disturbances F12.122
without perceptual disturbances F12.129
moderate or severe F12.20
in remission (early) (sustained) F12.21
with
cannabis-induced
anxiety disorder F12.280
psychotic disorder F12.259
sleep disorder F12.288
cannabis intoxication
with perceptual disturbances F12.222
without perceptual disturbances F12.229
delirium F12.221
carbohydrate
absorption, intestinal NEC E74.39
metabolism (congenital) E74.9
specified NEC E74.8
cardiac, functional I51.89
carnitine metabolism E71.40

Disorder (of) - *continued*

cartilage M94.9
articular NEC - *see* Derangement, joint,
articular cartilage
chondrocalcinosis - *see* Chondrocalcinosis
specified type NEC M94.8X-
articular - *see* Derangement, joint, articular
cartilage
multiple sites M94.8X0
catatonia (due to known physiological
condition) (with another mental disorder)
F06.1
catatonic
due to (secondary to) known physiological
condition F06.1
organic F06.1
central auditory processing H93.25
cervical
region NEC M53.82
root (nerve) NEC G54.2
character NOS F60.9
childhood disintegrative NEC F84.3
cholesterol and bile acid metabolism E78.70
Barth syndrome E78.71
other specified E78.79
Smith-Lemli-Opitz syndrome E78.72
choroid H31.9
atrophy - *see* Atrophy, choroid
degeneration - *see* Degeneration, choroid
detachment - *see* Detachment, choroid
dystrophy - *see* Dystrophy, choroid
hemorrhage - *see* Hemorrhage, choroid
rupture - *see* Rupture, choroid
scar - *see* Scar, chorioretinal
solar retinopathy - *see* Retinopathy, solar
specified type NEC H31.8
ciliary body - *see* Disorder, iris
degeneration - *see* Degeneration, ciliary body
coagulation (factor) - *see also* Defect,
coagulation D68.9
newborn, transient P61.6
cocaine use
mild F14.10
in remission (early) (sustained) F14.11
with
amphetamine, cocaine, or other stimulant
intoxication
with perceptual disturbances F14.122
without perceptual disturbances F14.129
cocaine-induced
anxiety disorder F14.180
bipolar and related disorder F14.14
depressive disorder F14.14
obsessive-compulsive and related
disorder F14.188
psychotic disorder F14.159
sexual dysfunction F14.181
sleep disorder F14.182
cocaine intoxication delirium F14.121
moderate or severe F14.20
in remission (early) (sustained) F14.21
with
amphetamine, cocaine, or other stimulant
intoxication
with perceptual disturbances F14.222
without perceptual disturbances F14.229
cocaine-induced
anxiety disorder F14.280
bipolar and related disorder F14.24
depressive disorder F14.24
obsessive-compulsive and related
disorder F14.288
psychotic disorder F14.259
sexual dysfunction F14.281

Disorder (of) - *continued*

sleep disorder F14.282
cocaine intoxication delirium F14.221
coccyx NEC M53.3
cognitive F09
due to (secondary to) general medical
condition F09
persisting R41.89
due to
alcohol F10.97
with dependence F10.27
anxiolytics F13.97
with dependence F13.27
hypnotics F13.97
with dependence F13.27
sedatives F13.97
with dependence F13.27
specified substance NEC F19.97
with
abuse F19.17
dependence F19.27
communication F80.9
social pragmatic F80.82
conduct (childhood) F91.9
adjustment reaction - *see* Disorder,
adjustment
adolescent onset type F91.2
childhood onset type F91.1
compulsive F63.9
confined to family context F91.0
depressive F91.8
group type F91.2
hyperkinetic - *see* Disorder, attention-deficit
hyperactivity
oppositional defiance F91.3
socialized F91.2
solitary aggressive type F91.1
specified NEC F91.8
unsocialized (aggressive) F91.1
conduction, heart I45.9
congenital glycosylation (CDG) E74.8
conjunctiva H11.9
infection - *see* Conjunctivitis
connective tissue, localized L94.9
specified NEC L94.8
conversion (functional neurological symptom
disorder)
with
abnormal movement F44.4
anesthesia or sensory loss F44.6
attacks or seizures F44.5
mixed symptoms F44.7
special sensory symptoms F44.6
speech symptoms F44.4
swallowing symptoms F44.4
weakness or paralysis F44.4
convulsive (secondary) - *see* Convulsions
cornea H18.9
deformity - *see* Deformity, cornea
degeneration - *see* Degeneration, cornea
deposits - *see* Deposit, cornea
due to contact lens H18.82-
specified as edema - *see* Edema, cornea
edema - *see* Edema, cornea
keratitis - *see* Keratitis
keratoconjunctivitis - *see*
Keratoconjunctivitis
membrane change - *see* Change, corneal
membrane
neovascularization - *see* Neovascularization,
cornea
scar - *see* Opacity, cornea
specified type NEC H18.89-
ulcer - *see* Ulcer, cornea

Disorder (of) - *continued*
corpus cavernosum N48.9
cranial nerve - *see* Disorder, nerve, cranial
cyclothymic F34.0
defiant oppositional F91.3
delusional (persistent) (systematized) F22
  induced F24
depersonalization F48.1
depressive F32.9
  due to known physiological condition
    with
      depressive features F06.31
      major depressive-like episode F06.32
      mixed features F06.34
    major F32.9
      with psychotic symptoms F32.3
      in remission (full) F32.5
        partial F32.4
      recurrent F33.9
        with psychotic features F33.3
      single episode F32.9
        mild F32.0
        moderate F32.1
        severe (without psychotic symptoms)
          F32.2
          with psychotic symptoms F32.3
    organic F06.31
    persistent F34.1
    recurrent F33.9
      current episode
        mild F33.0
        moderate F33.1
        severe (without psychotic symptoms)
          F33.2
          with psychotic symptoms F33.3
      in remission F33.40
        full F33.42
        partial F33.41
      specified NEC F33.8
    single episode - *see* Episode, depressive
    specified NEC F32.89
developmental F89
  arithmetical skills F81.2
  coordination (motor) F82
  expressive writing F81.81
  language F80.9
    expressive F80.1
    mixed receptive and expressive F80.2
    receptive type F80.2
    specified NEC F80.89
  learning F81.9
    arithmetical F81.2
    reading F81.0
  mixed F88
  motor coordination or function F82
  pervasive F84.9
    specified NEC F84.8
  phonological F80.0
  reading F81.0
  scholastic skills - *see also* Disorder, learning
    mixed F81.89
  specified NEC F88
  speech F80.9
    articulation F80.0
    specified NEC F80.89
  written expression F81.81
diaphragm J98.6
digestive (system) K92.9
  newborn P78.9
    specified NEC P78.89
  postprocedural - *see* Complication,
    gastrointestinal
  psychogenic F45.8
disc (intervertebral) M51.9

Disorder (of) - *continued*
  with
    myelopathy
      cervical region M50.00
      cervicothoracic region M50.03
      high cervical region M50.01
      lumbar region M51.06
      mid-cervical region M50.020
      sacrococcygeal region M53.3
      thoracic region M51.04
      thoracolumbar region M51.05
    radiculopathy
      cervical region M50.10
      cervicothoracic region M50.13
      high cervical region M50.11
      lumbar region M51.16
      lumbosacral region M51.17
      mid-cervical region M50.120
      sacrococcygeal region M53.3
      thoracic region M51.14
      thoracolumbar region M51.15
  cervical M50.90
    with
      myelopathy M50.00
        C2-C3 M50.01
        C3-C4 M50.01
        C4-C5 M50.021
        C5-C6 M50.022
        C6-C7 M50.023
        C7-T1 M50.03
      cervicothoracic region M50.03
      high cervical region M50.01
      mid-cervical region M50.020
      neuritis, radiculitis or radiculopathy
        M50.10
        C2-C3 M50.11
        C3-C4 M50.11
        C4-C5 M50.121
        C5-C6 M50.122
        C6-C7 M50.123
        C7-T1 M50.13
      cervicothoracic region M50.13
      high cervical region M50.11
      mid-cervical region M50.120
        C2-C3 M50.91
        C3-C4 M50.91
        C4-C5 M50.921
        C5-C6 M50.922
        C6-C7 M50.923
        C7-T1 M50.93
    cervicothoracic region M50.93
    degeneration M50.30
      C2-C3 M50.31
      C3-C4 M50.31
      C4-C5 M50.321
      C5-C6 M50.322
      C6-C7 M50.323
      C7-T1 M50.33
    cervicothoracic region M50.33
    high cervical region M50.31
    mid-cervical region M50.320
    displacement M50.20
      C2-C3 M50.21
      C3-C4 M50.21
      C4-C5 M50.221
      C5-C6 M50.222
      C6-C7 M50.223
      C7-T1 M50.23
    cervicothoracic region M50.23
    high cervical region M50.21
    mid-cervical region M50.220
    high cervical region M50.91
    mid-cervical region M50.920
    specified type NEC M50.80

Disorder (of) - *continued*
      C2-C3 M50.81
      C3-C4 M50.81
      C4-C5 M50.821
      C5-C6 M50.822
      C6-C7 M50.823
      C7-T1 M50.83
    cervicothoracic region M50.83
    high cervical region M50.81
    mid-cervical region M50.820
  specified NEC
    lumbar region M51.86
    lumbosacral region M51.87
    sacrococcygeal region M53.3
    thoracic region M51.84
    thoracolumbar region M51.85
disinhibited attachment (childhood) F94.2
disintegrative, childhood NEC F84.3
disruptive F91.9
  mood dysregulation F34.81
  specified NEC F91.8
disruptive behavior   *see* Disorder, conduct
dissocial personality F60.2
dissociative F44.9
  affecting
    motor function F44.4
      and sensation F44.7
    sensation F44.6
      and motor function F44.7
  brief reactive F43.0
  due to (secondary to) general medical
    condition F06.8
  mixed F44.7
  organic F06.8
  other specified NEC F44.89
double heterozygous sickling - *see* Disease,
  sickle-cell
dream anxiety F51.5
drug induced hemorrhagic D68.32
drug related F19.99
  abuse - *see* Abuse, drug
  dependence - *see* Dependence, drug
dysmorphic body F45.22
dysthymic F34.1
ear H93.9-
  bleeding - *see* Otorrhagia
  deafness - *see* Deafness
  degenerative H93.09-
  discharge - *see* Otorrhea
  external H61.9-
    auditory canal stenosis - *see* Stenosis,
      external ear canal
    exostosis - *see* Exostosis, external ear canal
    impacted cerumen - *see* Impaction, cerumen
    otitis - *see* Otitis, externa
    perichondritis - *see* Perichondritis, ear
    pinna - *see* Disorder, pinna
    specified type NEC H61.89-
      in diseases classified elsewhere H62.8X-
  inner H83.9-
    vestibular dysfunction - *see* Disorder,
      vestibular function
  middle H74.9-
    adhesive H74.1-
    ossicle - *see* Abnormal, ear ossicles
    polyp - *see* Polyp, ear (middle)
    specified NEC, in diseases classified
      elsewhere H75.8-
  postprocedural - *see* Complications, ear,
    procedure
  specified NEC, in diseases classified
    elsewhere H94.8-
eating (adult) (psychogenic) F50.9
  anorexia - *see* Anorexia

Disorder (of) - *continued*

binge F50.81
bulimia F50.2
child F98.29
  pica F98.3
  rumination disorder F98.21
pica F50.89
  childhood F98.3
electrolyte (balance) NEC E87.8
  with
    abortion - *see* Abortion by type complicated
      by specified condition NEC
    ectopic pregnancy O08.5
    molar pregnancy O08.5
  acidosis (metabolic) (respiratory) E87.2
  alkalosis (metabolic) (respiratory) E87.3
elimination, transepidermal L87.9
  specified NEC L87.8
emotional (persistent) F34.9
  of childhood F93.9
    specified NEC F93.8
endocrine E34.9
  postprocedural E89.89
  specified NEC E89.89
erectile (male) (organic) - *see also*
Dysfunction, sexual, male, erectile N52.9
  nonorganic F52.21
erythematous - *see* Erythema
esophagus K22.9
  functional K22.4
  psychogenic F45.8
eustachian tube H69.9-
  infection - *see* Salpingitis, eustachian
  obstruction - *see* Obstruction, eustachian tube
  patulous - *see* Patulous, eustachian tube
  specified NEC H69.8-
exhibitionistic F65.2
extrapyramidal G25.9
  in diseases classified elsewhere *see*
category G26
  specified type NEC G25.89
eye H57.9
  postprocedural - *see* Complication,
postprocedural, eye eyelid H02.9
  cyst - *see* Cyst, eyelid
  degenerative H02.70
    chloasma - *see* Chloasma, eyelid
    madarosis - *see* Madarosis
    specified type NEC H02.79
    vitiligo - *see* Vitiligo, eyelid
    xanthelasma - *see* Xanthelasma
  dermatochalasis - *see* Dermatochalasis
  edema - *see* Edema, eyelid
  elephantiasis - *see* Elephantiasis, eyelid
  foreign body, retained - *see* Foreign body,
retained, eyelid
  function H02.59
    abnormal innervation syndrome - *see*
Syndrome, abnormal innervation
    blepharochalasis - *see* Blepharochalasis
    blepharoclonus - *see* Blepharoclonus
    blepharophimosis - *see* Blepharophimosis
    blepharoptosis - *see* Blepharoptosis
    lagophthalmos - *see* Lagophthalmos
    lid retraction - *see* Retraction, lid
  hypertrichosis - *see* Hypertrichosis, eyelid
  specified type NEC H02.89
  vascular H02.879
    left H02.876
      lower H02.875
      upper H02.874
    right H02.873
      lower H02.872
      upper H02.871

Disorder (of) - *continued*

factitious F68.10
  with predominantly
    psychological symptoms F68.11
      with physical symptoms F68.13
    physical symptoms F68.12
      with psychological symptoms F68.13
factor, coagulation - *see* Defect, coagulation
fatty acid
  metabolism E71.30
    specified NEC E71.39
  oxidation
    LCAD E71.310
    MCAD E71.311
    SCAD E71.312
    specified deficiency NEC E71.318
feeding (infant or child) - *see also* Disorder,
eating R63.3
  or eating disorder F50.9
  specified NEC F50.9
feigned (with obvious motivation) Z76.5
  without obvious motivation - *see* Disorder,
factitious
female
  hypoactive sexual desire F52.0
  orgasmic F52.31
  sexual interest/arousal F52.22
fetishistic F65.0
fibroblastic M72.9
  specified NEC M72.8
fluency
  adult onset F98.5
  childhood onset F80.81
  following
    cerebral infarction I69.323
    cerebrovascular disease I69.923
      specified disease NEC I69.823
    intracerebral hemorrhage I69.123
    nontraumatic intracranial hemorrhage NEC
I69.223
    subarachnoid hemorrhage I69.023
  in conditions classified elsewhere R47.82
fluid balance E87.8
follicular (skin) L73.9
  specified NEC L73.8
frotteuristic F65.81
fructose metabolism E74.10
  essential fructosuria E74.11
  fructokinase deficiency E74.11
  fructose 1, 6-diphosphatase deficiency
E74.19
  hereditary fructose intolerance E74.12
  other specified E74.19
functional polymorphonuclear neutrophils D71
gallbladder, biliary tract and pancreas in
diseases classified elsewhere K87
gambling F63.0
gamma-glutamyl cycle E72.8
gastric (functional) K31.9
  motility K30
  psychogenic F45.8
  secretion K30
gastrointestinal (functional) NOS K92.9
  newborn P78.9
  psychogenic F45.8
gender-identity or -role F64.9
  childhood F64.2
  effect on relationship F66
  of adolescence or adulthood F64.0
    nontranssexual F64.8
  specified NEC F64.8
  uncertainty F66
genito-pelvic pain penetration F52.6
genitourinary system

Disorder (of) - *continued*

  female N94.9
  male N50.9
  psychogenic F45.8
globe H44.9
  degenerated condition H44.50
    absolute glaucoma H44.51-
    atrophy H44.52-
    leucocoria H44.53-
  degenerative H44.30
    chalcosis H44.31-
    myopia (see also Myopia, degenerative)
H44.2-
    siderosis H44.32-
    specified type NEC H44.39-
  endophthalmitis - *see* Endophthalmitis
  foreign body, retained - *see* Foreign body,
intraocular, old, retained
  hemophthalmos - *see* Hemophthalmos
  hypotony H44.40
    due to
      ocular fistula H44.42-
      specified disorder NEC H44.43-
    flat anterior chamber H44.41-
    primary H44.44-
  luxation - *see* Luxation, globe
  specified type NEC H44.89
glomerular (in) N05.9
  amyloidosis E85.4 [*N08*]
  cryoglobulinemia D89.1 [*N08*]
  disseminated intravascular coagulation D65
[*N08*]
  Fabry's disease E75.21 [*N08*]
  familial lecithin cholesterol acyltransferase
deficiency E78.6 [*N08*]
  Goodpasture's syndrome M31.0
  hemolytic-uremic syndrome D59.3
  Henoch (-Schönlein) purpura D69.0 [*N08*]
  malariae malaria B52.0
  microscopic polyangiitis M31.7 [*N08*]
  multiple myeloma C90.0- [*N08*]
  mumps B26.83
  schistosomiasis B65.9 [*N08*]
  sepsis NEC A41. [*N08*]
    streptococcal A40. [*N08*]
  sickle-cell disorders D57. [*N08*]
  strongyloidiasis B78.9 [*N08*]
  subacute bacterial endocarditis I33.0 [*N08*]
  syphilis A52.75
  systemic lupus erythematosus M32.14
  thrombotic thrombocytopenic purpura M31.1
[*N08*]
  Waldenström macroglobulinemia C88.0
[*N08*]
  Wegener's granulomatosis M31.31
gluconeogenesis E74.4
glucosaminoglycan metabolism - *see* Disorder,
metabolism, glucosaminoglycan
glycine metabolism E72.9
  d-glycericacidemia E72.59
  hyperhydroxyprolinemia E72.59
  hyperoxaluria E72.53
  hyperprolinemia E72.59
  non-ketotic hyperglycinemia E72.51
  oxalosis E72.53
  oxaluria E72.53
  sarcosinemia E72.59
  trimethylaminuria E72.52
glycoprotein metabolism E77.9
  specified NEC E77.8
habit (and impulse) F63.9
  involving sexual behavior NEC F65.9
  specified NEC F63.89
hallucinogen use

Disorder (of) - *continued*
  mild F16.10
    in remission (early) (sustained) F16.11
    with
      hallucinogen-induced
        anxiety disorder F16.180
        bipolar and related disorder F16.14
        depressive disorder F16.14
        psychotic disorder F16.159
      hallucinogen intoxication delirium
        F16.121
      other hallucinogen intoxication F16.129
  moderate or severe F16.20
    in remission (early) (sustained) F16.21
    with
      hallucinogen-induced
        anxiety disorder F16.280
        bipolar and related disorder F16.24
        depressive disorder F16.24
        psychotic disorder F16.259
      hallucinogen intoxication delirium
        F16.221
      other hallucinogen intoxication F16.229
  heart action I49.9
  hematological D75.9
    newborn (transient) P61.9
    specified NEC P61.8
  hematopoietic organs D75.9
  hemorrhagic NEC D69.9
    drug-induced D68.32
    due to
      extrinsic circulating anticoagulants D68.32
      increase in
        anti-iIa D68.32
        anti-Xa D68.32
      intrinsic
        circulating anticoagulants D68.318
        increase in
          antithrombin D68.318
          anti-VIIIa D68.318
          anti-iXa D68.318
          anti-XIa D68.318
    following childbirth O72.3
  hemostasis - *see* Defect, coagulation
  histidine metabolism E70.40
    histidinemia E70.41
    other specified E70.49
  hoarding F42.3
  hyperkinetic - *see* Disorder, attention-deficit
    hyperactivity hyperleucine-isoleucinemia
      E71.19
  hypervalinemia E71.19
  hypoactive sexual desire F52.0
  hypochondriacal F45.20
    body dysmorphic F45.22
    neurosis F45.21
    other specified F45.29
  identity
    dissociative F44.81
    of childhood F93.8
    illness anxiety F45.21
  immune mechanism (immunity) D89.9
    specified type NEC D89.89
  impaired renal tubular function N25.9
    specified NEC N25.89
  impulse (control) F63.9
  inflammatory
    pelvic, in diseases classified elsewhere *see*
  category N74
    penis N48.29
      abscess N48.21
      cellulitis N48.22
  inhalant use
    mild F18.10

Disorder (of) - *continued*
  in remission (early) (sustained) F18.11
  with
    inhalant-induced
      anxiety disorder F18.180
      depressive disorder F18.14
      major neurocognitive disorder F18.17
      mild neurocognitive disorder F18.188
      psychotic disorder F18.159
    inhalant intoxication F18.129
    inhalant intoxication delirium F18.121
  moderate or severe F18.20
    in remission (early) (sustained) F18.21
    with
      inhalant-induced
        anxiety disorder F18.280
        depressive disorder F18.24
        major neurocognitive disorder F18.27
        mild neurocognitive disorder F18.288
        psychotic disorder F18.259
      inhalant intoxication F18.229
      inhalant intoxication delirium F18.221
  integument, newborn P83.9
    specified NEC P83.88
  intermittent explosive F63.81
  internal secretion pancreas - *see* Increased,
    secretion, pancreas, endocrine
  intestine, intestinal
    carbohydrate absorption NEC E74.39
      postoperative K91.2
    functional NEC K59.9
      postoperative K91.89
    psychogenic F45.8
    vascular K55.9
      chronic K55.1
      specified NEC K55.8
  intraoperative (intraprocedural) - *see*
    Complications, intraoperative
  involuntary emotional expression (IEED)
    F48.2
  iris H21.9
    adhesions - *see* Adhesions, iris
    atrophy - *see* Atrophy, iris
    chamber angle recession - *see* Recession,
      chamber angle
    cyst - *see* Cyst, iris
    degeneration - *see* Degeneration, iris
    in diseases classified elsewhere H22
    iridodialysis - *see* Iridodialysis
    iridoschisis - *see* Iridoschisis
    miotic pupillary cyst - *see* Cyst, pupillary
    pupillary
      abnormality - *see* Abnormality, pupillary
      membrane - *see* Membrane, pupillary
    specified type NEC H21.89
    vascular NEC H21.1X-
  iron metabolism E83.10
    specified NEC E83.19
  isovaleric acidemia E71.110
  jaw, developmental M27.0
    temporomandibular - *see also* Anomaly,
  dentofacial, temporomandibular joint M26.60-
  joint M25.9
    derangement - *see* Derangement, joint
    effusion - *see* Effusion, joint
    fistula - *see* Fistula, joint
    hemarthrosis - *see* Hemarthrosis
    instability - *see* Instability, joint
    osteophyte - *see* Osteophyte
    pain - *see* Pain, joint
    psychogenic F45.8
    specified type NEC M25.80
      ankle M25.87-
      elbow M25.82-

Disorder (of) - *continued*
    foot joint M25.87-
    hand joint M25.84-
    hip M25.85-
    knee M25.86-
    shoulder M25.81-
    wrist M25.83-
  stiffness - *see* Stiffness, joint
  ketone metabolism E71.32
  kidney N28.9
    functional (tubular) N25.9
    in
      schistosomiasis B65.9 [*N29*]
    tubular function N25.9
    specified NEC N25.89
  lacrimal system H04.9
    changes H04.69
    fistula - *see* Fistula, lacrimal
    gland H04.19
      atrophy - *see* Atrophy, lacrimal gland
      cyst - *see* Cyst, lacrimal, gland
      dacryops - *see* Dacryops
      dislocation - *see* Dislocation, lacrimal gland
      dry eye syndrome - *see* Syndrome, dry eye
      infection - *see* Dacryoadenitis
      granuloma - *see* Granuloma, lacrimal
      inflammation - *see* Inflammation, lacrimal
      obstruction - *see* Obstruction, lacrimal
    specified NEC H04.89
  lactation NEC O92.79
  language (developmental) F80.9
    expressive F80.1
    mixed receptive and expressive F80.2
    receptive F80.2
  late luteal phase dysphoric N94.89
  learning (specific) F81.9
    acalculia R48.8
    alexia R48.0
    mathematics F81.2
    reading F81.0
    specified
      with impairment in
        mathematics F81.2
        reading F81.0
        written expression F81.81
    specified NEC F81.89
    spelling F81.81
    written expression F81.81
  lens H27.9
    aphakia - *see* Aphakia
    cataract - *see* Cataract
    dislocation - *see* Dislocation, lens
    specified type NEC H27.8
  ligament M24.20
    ankle M24.27-
    attachment, spine - *see* Enthesopathy, spinal
    elbow M24.22-
    foot joint M24.27-
    hand joint M24.24-
    hip M24.25-
    knee - *see* Derangement, knee, specified
  NEC
    shoulder M24.21-
    vertebra M24.28
    wrist M24.23-
  ligamentous attachments - *see also*
  Enthesopathy
    spine - *see* Enthesopathy, spinal
  lipid
    metabolism, congenital E78.9
    storage E75.6
    specified NEC E75.5
  lipoprotein
    deficiency (familial) E78.6

Disorder (of) - *continued*
  metabolism E78.9
    specified NEC E78.89
  liver K76.9
    malarial B54 [*K77*]
  low back - *see also* Dorsopathy, specified
    NEC
  lumbosacral
    plexus G54.1
    root (nerve) NEC G54.4
  lung, interstitial, drug-induced J70.4
    acute J70.2
    chronic J70.3
  lymphoproliferative, post-transplant (PTLD)
    D47.Z1
  lysine and hydroxylysine metabolism E72.3
  major neurocognitive - *see* Dementia, in (due
    to)
  male
    erectile (organic) - *see also* Dysfunction,
      sexual, male, erectile N52.9
      nonorganic F52.21
    hypoactive sexual desire F52.0
    orgasmic F52.32
  manic F30.9
    organic F06.33
  mast cell activation - *see* Activation, mast cell
  mastoid - *see also* Disorder, ear, middle
    postprocedural - *see* Complications, ear,
    procedure
  meniscus - *see* Derangement, knee, meniscus
  menopausal N95.9
    specified NEC N95.8
  menstrual N92.6
    psychogenic F45.8
    specified NEC N92.5
  mental (or behavioral) (nonpsychotic) F99
    due to (secondary to)
      amphetamine
        due to drug abuse - *see* Abuse, drug,
        stimulant
        due to drug dependence - *see* Dependence,
        drug, stimulant
      brain disease, damage and dysfunction F09
      caffeine use
        due to drug abuse - *see* Abuse, drug,
        stimulant
        due to drug dependence - *see* Dependence,
        drug, stimulant
      cannabis use
        due to drug abuse - *see* Abuse, drug,
        cannabis
        due to drug dependence - *see* Dependence,
        drug, cannabis
      general medical condition F09
      sedative or hypnotic use
        due to drug abuse - *see* Abuse, drug,
        sedative
        due to drug dependence - *see* Dependence,
        drug, sedative
      tobacco (nicotine) use - *see* Dependence,
      drug, nicotine
    following organic brain damage F07.9
      frontal lobe syndrome F07.0
      personality change F07.0
      postconcussional syndrome F07.81
      specified NEC F07.89
    infancy, childhood or adolescence F98.9
    neurotic - *see* Neurosis
    organic or symptomatic F09
    presenile, psychotic F03
    problem NEC
    psychoneurotic - *see* Neurosis
    psychotic - *see* Psychosis

Disorder (of) - *continued*
  puerperal F53
  senile, psychotic NEC F03
  metabolic, amino acid, transitory, newborn
    P74.8
  metabolism NOS E88.9
    amino-acid E72.9
      aromatic E70.9
        albinism - *see* Albinism
        histidine E70.40
          histidinemia E70.41
          other specified E70.49
        hyperphenylalaninemia E70.1
          classical phenylketonuria E70.0
        other specified E70.8
        tryptophan E70.5
        tyrosine E70.20
          hypertyrosinemia E70.21
          other specified E70.29
      branched chain E71.2
        3-methylglutaconic aciduria E71.111
        hyperleucine-isoleucinemia E71.19
        hypervalinemia E71.19
        isovaleric acidemia E71.110
        maple syrup urine disease E71.0
        methylmalonic acidemia E71.120
        organic aciduria NEC E71.118
        other specified E71.19
        propionate NEC E71.128
        propionic acidemia E71.121
      glycine E72.50
        d-glycericacidemia E72.59
        hyperhydroxyprolinemia E72.59
        hyperoxaluria E72.53
        hyperprolinemia E72.59
        non-ketotic hyperglycinemia E72.51
        other specified E72.59
        sarcosinemia E72.59
        trimethylaminuria E72.52
      hydroxylysine E72.3
      lysine E72.3
      ornithine E72.4
      other specified E72.8
        beta-amino acid E72.8
        gamma-glutamyl cycle E72.8
        straight-chain E72.8
      sulfur-bearing E72.10
        homocystinuria E72.11
        methylenetetrahydrofolate reductase
        deficiency E72.12
        other specified E72.19
    bile acid and cholesterol metabolism E78.70
    bilirubin E80.7
      specified NEC E80.6
    calcium E83.50
      hypercalcemia E83.52
      hypocalcemia E83.51
      other specified E83.59
    carbohydrate E74.9
      specified NEC E74.8
    cholesterol and bile acid metabolism E78.70
    congenital E88.9
    copper E83.00
      Wilson's disease E83.01
      specified type NEC E83.09
    cystinuria E72.01
    fructose E74.10
    galactose E74.20
    glucosaminoglycan E76.9
      mucopolysaccharidosis - *see*
      Mucopolysaccharidosis
      specified NEC E76.8
    glutamine E72.8
    glycine E72.50

Disorder (of) - *continued*
    glycogen storage (hepatorenal) E74.09
    glycoprotein E77.9
      specified NEC E77.8
    glycosaminoglycan E76.9
      specified NEC E76.8
    in labor and delivery O75.89
    iron E83.10
    isoleucine E71.19
    leucine E71.19
    lipoid E78.9
    lipoprotein E78.9
      specified NEC E78.89
    magnesium E83.40
      hypermagnesemia E83.41
      hypomagnesemia E83.42
      other specified E83.49
    mineral E83.9
      specified NEC E83.89
    mitochondrial E88.40
      MELAS syndrome E88.41
      MERRF syndrome (myoclonic epilepsy
      associated with ragged-red fibers) E88.42
      other specified E88.49
    ornithine E72.4
    phosphatases E83.30
    phosphorus E83.30
      acid phosphatase deficiency E83.39
      hypophosphatasia E83.39
      hypophosphatemia E83.39
        familial E83.31
      other specified E83.39
      pseudovitamin D deficiency E83.32
    plasma protein NEC E88.09
    porphyrin - *see* Porphyria
    postprocedural E89.89
      specified NEC E89.89
    purine E79.9
      specified NEC E79.8
    pyrimidine E79.9
      specified NEC E79.8
    pyruvate E74.4
    serine E72.8
    sodium E87.8
    specified NEC E88.89
    threonine E72.8
    valine E71.19
    zinc E83.2
  methylmalonic acidemia E71.120
  micturition NEC - *see also* Difficulty,
  micturition R39.198
    feeling of incomplete emptying R39.14
    hesitancy R39.11
    poor stream R39.12
    psychogenic F45.8
    split stream R39.13
    straining R39.16
    urgency R39.15
  mild neurocognitive G31.84
  mitochondrial metabolism E88.40
  mitral (valve) - *see* Endocarditis, mitral
  mixed
    anxiety and depressive F41.8
    of scholastic skills (developmental) F81.89
    receptive expressive language F80.2
  mood F39
    bipolar - *see* Disorder, bipolar
    depressive - *see* Disorder, depressive
    due to (secondary to)
      alcohol F10.94
      amphetamine F15.94
      in
        abuse F15.14
        dependence F15.24

Disorder (of) - *continued*
  anxiolytic F13.94
    in
      abuse F13.14
      dependence F13.24
  cocaine F14.94
    in
      abuse F14.14
      dependence F14.24
  general medical condition F06.30
  hallucinogen F16.94
    in
      abuse F16.14
      dependence F16.24
  hypnotic F13.94
    in
      abuse F13.14
      dependence F13.24
  inhalant F18.94
    in
      abuse F18.14
      dependence F18.24
  opioid F11.94
    in
      abuse F11.14
      dependence F11.24
  phencyclidine (PCP) F16.94
    in
      abuse F16.14
      dependence F16.24
  physiological condition F06.30
    with
      depressive features F06.31
      major depressive-like episode F06.32
      manic features F06.33
      mixed features F06.34
  psychoactive substance NEC F19.94
    in
      abuse F19.14
      dependence F19.24
  sedative F13.94
    in
      abuse F13.14
      dependence F13.24
  volatile solvents F18.94
    in
      abuse F18.14
      dependence F18.24
  manic episode F30.9
    with psychotic symptoms F30.2
    in remission (full) F30.4
      partial F30.3
    specified type NEC F30.8
    without psychotic symptoms F30.10
      mild F30.11
      moderate F30.12
      severe F30.13
  organic F06.30
    right hemisphere F07.89
  persistent F34.9
    cyclothymia F34.0
    dysthymia F34.1
    specified type NEC F34.89
  recurrent F39
  right hemisphere organic F07.89
  movement G25.9
    drug-induced G25.70
      akathisia G25.71
      specified NEC G25.79
    hysterical F44.4
    in diseases classified elsewhere *see*
    category G26
    periodic limb G47.61
      sleep related G47.61

Disorder (of) - *continued*
    specified NEC G25.89
    sleep related NEC G47.69
    stereotyped F98.4
    treatment-induced G25.9
  multiple personality F44.81
  muscle M62.9
    attachment, spine - *see* Enthesopathy, spinal
    in trichinellosis - *see* Trichinellosis, with
      muscle disorder
    psychogenic F45.8
    specified type NEC M62.89
    tone, newborn P94.9
      specified NEC P94.8
  muscular
    attachments - *see also* Enthesopathy
      spine - *see* Enthesopathy, spinal
    urethra N36.44
  musculoskeletal system, soft tissue - *see*
  Disorder, soft tissue
    postprocedural M96.89
    psychogenic F45.8
  myoneural G70.9
    due to lead G70.1
    specified NEC G70.89
    toxic G70.1
  myotonic NEC G71.19
  nail, in diseases classified elsewhere L62
  neck region NEC - *see* Dorsopathy, specified
  NEC
  neonatal onset multisystemic inflammatory
    (NOMID) M04.2
  nerve G58.9
    abducent NEC - *see* Strabismus, paralytic,
  sixth nerve
    accessory G52.8
    acoustic - *see* subcategory H93.3
    auditory - *see* subcategory H93.3
    auriculotemporal G50.8
    axillary G54.0
    cerebral - *see* Disorder, nerve, cranial
    cranial G52.9
      eighth - *see* subcategory H93.3
      eleventh G52.8
      fifth G50.9
      first G52.0
      fourth NEC - *see* Strabismus, paralytic,
        fourth nerve
      multiple G52.7
      ninth G52.1
      second NEC - *see* Disorder, nerve, optic
      seventh NEC G51.8
      sixth NEC - *see* Strabismus, paralytic, sixth
        nerve
      specified NEC G52.8
      tenth G52.2
      third NEC - *see* Strabismus, paralytic, third
        nerve
      twelfth G52.3
    entrapment - *see* Neuropathy, entrapment
    facial G51.9
      specified NEC G51.8
    femoral - *see* Lesion, nerve, femoral
    glossopharyngeal NEC G52.1
    hypoglossal G52.3
    intercostal G58.0
    lateral
      cutaneous of thigh - *see* Mononeuropathy,
        lower limb, meralgia paresthetica
      popliteal - *see* Lesion, nerve, popliteal
    lower limb - *see* Mononeuropathy, lower
      limb
    medial popliteal - *see* Lesion, nerve,
      popliteal, medial

Disorder (of) - *continued*
    median NEC - *see* Lesion, nerve, median
    multiple G58.7
    oculomotor NEC - *see* Strabismus, paralytic,
      third nerve
    olfactory G52.0
    optic NEC H47.09-
      hemorrhage into sheath - *see* Hemorrhage,
        optic nerve
      ischemic H47.01-
    peroneal - *see* Lesion, nerve, popliteal
    phrenic G58.8
    plantar - *see* Lesion, nerve, plantar
    pneumogastric G52.2
    posterior tibial - *see* Syndrome, tarsal tunnel
    radial - *see* Lesion, nerve, radial
    recurrent laryngeal G52.2
    root G54.9
      cervical G54.2
      lumbosacral G54.1
      specified NEC G54.8
      thoracic G54.3
    sciatic NEC - *see* Lesion, nerve, sciatic
    specified NEC G58.8
      lower limb - *see* Mononeuropathy, lower
        limb, specified NEC
      upper limb - *see* Mononeuropathy, upper
        limb, specified NEC
    sympathetic G90.9
    tibial - *see* Lesion, nerve, popliteal, medial
    trigeminal G50.9
      specified NEC G50.8
    trochlear NEC - *see* Strabismus, paralytic,
      fourth nerve
    ulnar - *see* Lesion, nerve, ulnar
    upper limb - *see* Mononeuropathy, upper
      limb
    vagus G52.2
  nervous system G98.8
    autonomic (peripheral) G90.9
      specified NEC G90.8
    central G96.9
      specified NEC G96.8
    parasympathetic G90.9
    specified NEC G98.8
    sympathetic G90.9
    vegetative G90.9
  neurocognitive R41.9
    major
      with
        aggressive behavior F01.51
        combative behavior F01.51
        violent behavior F01.51
      due to vascular disease, with behavioral
        disturbance F01.51
      in (due to) (other diseases classified
        elsewhere) - *see also* Dementia, in (due to)
        F02.80
        with
          aggressive behavior F02.81
          combative behavior F02.81
          violent behavior F02.81
        without behavioral disturbance F01.50
      mild G31.84
  neurodevelopmental F89
    specified NEC F88
  neurohypophysis NEC E23.3
  neurological NEC R29.818
  neuromuscular G70.9
    hereditary NEC G71.9
    specified NEC G70.89
    toxic G70.1
  neurotic F48.9
    specified NEC F48.8

Disorder (of) - *continued*
 neutrophil, polymorphonuclear D71
 nicotine use - *see* Dependence, drug, nicotine
 nightmare F51.5
 non-rapid eye movement sleep arousal
  sleep terror type F51.4
  sleepwalking type F51.3
 nose J34.9
  specified NEC J34.89
 obsessive-compulsive F42.9
  and related disorder due to a known
   physiological condition F06.8
 odontogenesis NOS K00.9
 opioid use
  with
   opioid-induced psychotic disorder F11.959
    with
     delusions F11.950
     hallucinations F11.951
  due to drug abuse - *see* Abuse, drug, opioid
  due to drug dependence - *see* Dependence,
   drug, opioid
  mild F11.10
   in remission (early) (sustained) F11.11
    with
     opioid-induced
      anxiety disorder F11.188
      depressive disorder F11.14
      sexual dysfunction F11.181
     opioid intoxication
      with perceptual disturbances F11.122
      delirium F11.121
      without perceptual disturbances F11.129
  moderate or severe F11.20
   in remission (early) (sustained) F11.21
    with
     opioid-induced
      anxiety disorder F11.288
      anxiety disorder F11.988
      depressive disorder F11.24
      depressive disorder F11.94
      sexual dysfunction F11.281
      sexual dysfunction F11.981
     opioid intoxication
      with perceptual disturbances F11.222
      delirium F11.221
      without perceptual disturbances F11.229
 oppositional defiant F91.3
 optic
  chiasm H47.49
   due to
    inflammatory disorder H47.41
    neoplasm H47.42
    vascular disorder H47.43
  disc H47.39-
   coloboma - *see* Coloboma, optic disc
   drusen - *see* Drusen, optic disc
   pseudopapilledema - *see*
    Pseudopapilledema
  radiations - *see* Disorder, visual, pathway
  tracts - *see* Disorder, visual, pathway   orbit
   H05.9
  cyst - *see* Cyst, orbit
  deformity - *see* Deformity, orbit
  edema - *see* Edema, orbit
  enophthalmos - *see* Enophthalmos
  exophthalmos - *see* Exophthalmos
  hemorrhage - *see* Hemorrhage, orbit
  inflammation - *see* Inflammation, orbit
  myopathy - *see* Myopathy, extraocular
   muscles
  retained foreign body - *see* Foreign body,
   orbit, old
  specified type NEC H05.89

Disorder (of) - *continued*
 organic
  anxiety F06.4
  catatonic F06.1
  delusional F06.2
  dissociative F06.8
  emotionally labile (asthenic) F06.8
  mood (affective) F06.30
  schizophrenia-like F06.2
 orgasmic (female) F52.31
  male F52.32
 ornithine metabolism E72.4
 overanxious F41.1
  of childhood F93.8
 pain
  with related psychological factors F45.42
  exclusively related to psychological factors
   F45.41
  genito-pelvic penetration disorder F52.6
 pancreatic internal secretion E16.9
  specified NEC E16.8
 panic F41.0
  with agoraphobia F40.01
 papulosquamous L44.9
  in diseases classified elsewhere L45
  specified NEC L44.8
 paraphilic F65.9
  specified NEC F65.89
 paranoid F22
  induced F24
  shared F24
 parathyroid (gland) E21.5
  specified NEC E21.4
 parietoalveolar NEC J84.09
 paroxysmal, mixed R56.9
 patella M22.9-
  chondromalacia - *see* Chondromalacia,
   patella
  derangement NEC M22.3X-
  recurrent
   dislocation - *see* Dislocation, patella,
    recurrent
   subluxation - *see* Dislocation, patella,
    recurrent, incomplete
  specified NEC M22.8X-
 patellofemoral M22.2X
 pedophilic F65.4
 pentose phosphate pathway with anemia D55.1
 perception, due to hallucinogens F16.983
  in
   abuse F16.183
   dependence F16.283
 peripheral nervous system NEC G64
 peroxisomal E71.50
  biogenesis
   neonatal adrenoleukodystrophy E71.511
   specified disorder NEC E71.518
   Zellweger syndrome E71.510
  rhizomelic chondrodysplasia punctata
   E71.540
  specified form NEC E71.548
   group 1 E71.518
   group 2 E71.53
   group 3 E71.542
  X-linked adrenoleukodystrophy E71.529
   adolescent E71.521
   adrenomyeloneuropathy E71.522
   childhood E71.520
   specified form NEC E71.528
  Zellweger-like syndrome E71.541
 persistent
  (somatoform) pain F45.41
  affective (mood) F34.9
 personality - *see also* Personality F60.9

Disorder (of) - *continued*
 affective F34.0
 aggressive F60.3
 amoral F60.2
 anankastic F60.5
 antisocial F60.2
 anxious F60.6
 asocial F60.2
 asthenic F60.7
 avoidant F60.6
 borderline F60.3
 change (secondary) due to general medical
  condition F07.0
 compulsive F60.5
 cyclothymic F34.0
 dependent (passive) F60.7
 depressive F34.1
 dissocial F60.2
 emotional instability F60.3
 expansive paranoid F60.0
 explosive F60.3
 following organic brain damage F07.9
 histrionic F60.4
 hyperthymic F34.0
 hypothymic F34.1
 hysterical F60.4
 immature F60.89
 inadequate F60.7
 labile F60.3
 mixed (nonspecific) F60.89
 moral deficiency F60.2
 narcissistic F60.81
 negativistic F60.89
 obsessional F60.5
 obsessive (-compulsive) F60.5
 organic F07.9
 overconscientious F60.5
 paranoid F60.0
 passive (-dependent) F60.7
 passive-aggressive F60.89
 pathological NEC F60.9
 pseudosocial F60.2
 psychopathic F60.2
 schizoid F60.1
 schizotypal F21
 self-defeating F60.7
 specified NEC F60.89
 type A F60.5
 unstable (emotional) F60.3
 pervasive, developmental F84.9
 phencyclidine use
  mild F16.10
   in remission (early) (sustained) F16.11
    with
     phencyclidine-induced
      anxiety disorder F16.180
      bipolar and related disorder F16.14
      depressive disorder F16.14
      psychotic disorder F16.159
     phencyclidine intoxication F16.129
     phencyclidine intoxication delirium
      F16.121
  moderate or severe F16.20
   in remission (early) (sustained) F16.21
    with
     phencyclidine-induced
      anxiety disorder F16.280
      bipolar and related disorder F16.24
      depressive disorder F16.24
      psychotic disorder F16.259
     phencyclidine intoxication F16.229
     phencyclidine intoxication delirium
      F16.221
 phobic anxiety, childhood F40.8

Disorder (of) - *continued*
  phosphate-losing tubular N25.0
  pigmentation L81.9
    choroid, congenital Q14.3
    diminished melanin formation L81.6
    iron L81.8
    specified NEC L81.8
  pinna (noninfective) H61.10-
    deformity, acquired H61.11-
    hematoma H61.12-
    perichondritis - *see* Perichondritis, ear
    specified type NEC H61.19-
  pituitary gland E23.7
    iatrogenic (postprocedural) E89.3
    specified NEC E23.6
  platelets D69.1
  plexus G54.9
    specified NEC G54.8
  polymorphonuclear neutrophils D71
  porphyrin metabolism - *see* Porphyria
  postconcussional F07.81
  posthallucinogen perception F16.983
    in
      abuse F16.183
      dependence F16.283
  postmenopausal N95.9
    specified NEC N95.8
  postprocedural (postoperative) - *see*
Complications, postprocedural
  post-transplant lymphoproliferative D47.Z1
  post-traumatic stress (PTSD) F43.10
    acute F43.11
    chronic F43.12
  premenstrual dysphoric (PMDD) F32.81
  prepuce N47.8
  propionic acidemia E71.121
  prostate N42.9
    specified NEC N42.89
  psychogenic NOS - *see also* condition F45.9
    anxiety F41.8
    appetite F50.9
    asthenic F48.8
    cardiovascular (system) F45.8
    compulsive F42.8
    cutaneous F54
    depressive F32.9
    digestive (system) F45.8
    dysmenorrheic F45.8
    dyspneic F45.8
    endocrine (system) F54
    eye NEC F45.8
    feeding - *see* Disorder, eating
    functional NEC F45.8
    gastric F45.8
    gastrointestinal (system) F45.8
    genitourinary (system) F45.8
    heart (function) (rhythm) F45.8
    hyperventilatory F45.8
    hypochondriacal - *see* Disorder,
    hypochondriacal
    intestinal F45.8
    joint F45.8
    learning F81.9
    limb F45.8
    lymphatic (system) F45.8
    menstrual F45.8
    micturition F45.8
    monoplegic NEC F44.4
    motor F44.4
    muscle F45.8
    musculoskeletal F45.8
    neurocirculatory F45.8
    obsessive F42.8
    occupational F48.8

Disorder (of) - *continued*
  organ or part of body NEC F45.8
  paralytic NEC F44.4
  phobic F40.9
  physical NEC F45.8
  rectal F45.8
  respiratory (system) F45.8
  rheumatic F45.8
  sexual (function) F52.9
  skin (allergic) (eczematous) F54
  sleep F51.9
  specified part of body NEC F45.8
  stomach F45.8
  psychological F99
    associated with
      disease classified elsewhere F54
      sexual
        development F66
        relationship F66
      uncertainty about gender identity F64.9
  psychomotor NEC F44.4
    hysterical F44.4
  psychoneurotic - *see also* Neurosis
    mixed NEC F48.8
  psychophysiologic - *see* Disorder, somatoform
  psychosexual F65.9
    development F66
    identity of childhood F64.2
  psychosomatic NOS - *see* Disorder,
somatoform
    multiple F45.0
    undifferentiated F45.1
  psychotic - *see* Psychosis
    transient (acute) F23
  puberty E30.9
    specified NEC E30.8
  pulmonary (valve) - *see* Endocarditis,
pulmonary
  purine metabolism E79.9
  pyrimidine metabolism E79.9
  pyruvate metabolism E74.4
  reactive attachment (childhood) F94.1
  reading R48.0
    developmental (specific) F81.0
  receptive language F80.2
  receptor, hormonal, peripheral - *see also*
  Syndrome, androgen insensitivity E34.50
  recurrent brief depressive F33.8
  reflex R29.2
  refraction H52.7
    aniseikonia H52.32
    anisometropia H52.31
    astigmatism - *see* Astigmatism
    hypermetropia - *see* Hypermetropia
    myopia - *see* Myopia
    presbyopia H52.4
    specified NEC H52.6
  relationship F68.8
    due to sexual orientation F66
  REM sleep behavior G47.52
  renal function, impaired (tubular) N25.9
  resonance R49.9
    specified NEC R49.8
  respiratory function, impaired - *see also*
  Failure, respiration
    postprocedural - *see* Complication,
    postoperative, respiratory system
    psychogenic F45.8
  retina H35.9
    angioid streaks H35.33
    changes in vascular appearance H35.01-
    degeneration - *see* Degeneration, retina
    dystrophy (hereditary) - *see* Dystrophy, retina
    edema H35.81

Disorder (of) - *continued*
  hemorrhage - *see* Hemorrhage, retina
  ischemia H35.82
  macular degeneration - *see* Degeneration,
  macula
  microaneurysms H35.04-
  microvascular abnormality NEC H35.09
  neovascularization - *see* Neovascularization,
retina
  retinopathy - *see* Retinopathy
  separation of layers H35.70
    central serous chorioretinopathy H35.71-
    pigment epithelium detachment (serous)
H35.72-
      hemorrhagic H35.73-
  specified type NEC H35.89
  telangiectasis - *see* Telangiectasis, retina
  vasculitis - *see* Vasculitis, retina
  retroperitoneal K68.9
  right hemisphere organic affective F07.89
  rumination (infant or child) F98.21
  sacrum, sacrococcygeal NEC M53.3
  schizoaffective F25.9
    bipolar type F25.0
    depressive type F25.1
    manic type F25.0
    mixed type F25.0
    specified NEC F25.8
  schizoid of childhood F84.5
  schizophrenia spectrum and other psychotic
disorder F29
    specified NEC F28
  schizophreniform F20.81
    brief F23
  schizotypal (personality) F21
  secretion, thyrocalcitonin E07.0
  sedative, hypnotic, or anxiolytic use
    mild F13.10
      in remission (early) (sustained) F13.11
      with
        sedative, hypnotic, or anxiolytic-induced
          anxiety disorder F13.180
          bipolar and related disorder F13.14
          depressive disorder F13.14
          psychotic disorder F13.159
          sexual dysfunction F13.181
        sedative, hypnotic, or anxiolytic
        intoxication F13.129
        sedative, hypnotic, or anxiolytic
        intoxication delirium F13.121
    moderate or severe F13.20
      in remission (early) (sustained) F13.21
      with
        sedative, hypnotic, or anxiolytic-induced
          anxiety disorder F13.280
          bipolar and related disorder F13.24
          depressive disorder F13.24
          major neurocognitive disorder F13.27
          mild neurocognitive disorder F13.288
          psychotic disorder F13.259
          sexual dysfunction F13.281
        sedative, hypnotic, or anxiolytic
        intoxication F13.229
        sedative, hypnotic, or anxiolytic
        intoxication delirium F13.221
  seizure - *see also* Epilepsy G40.909
    intractable G40.919
      with status epilepticus G40.911
  semantic pragmatic F80.89
    with autism F84.0
  sense of smell R43.1
    psychogenic F45.8
  separation anxiety, of childhood F93.0
  sexual

Disorder (of) - *continued*

arousal, female F52.22
aversion F52.1
function, psychogenic F52.9
interest/arousal, female F52.22
masochism F65.51
maturation F66
nonorganic F52.9
preference - *see also* Deviation, sexual F65.9
fetishistic transvestism F65.1
relationship F66
sadism F65.52
shyness, of childhood and adolescence F40.10
sibling rivalry F93.8
sickle-cell (sickling) (homozygous) - *see*
Disease, sickle-cell
heterozygous D57.3
specified type NEC D57.8-
trait D57.3
sinus (nasal) J34.9
specified NEC J34.89
skin L98.9
atrophic L90.9
specified NEC L90.88
granulomatous L92.9
specified NEC L92.8
hypertrophic L91.9
specified NEC L91.8
infiltrative NEC L98.6
newborn P83.9
specified NEC P83.8
picking F42.4
psychogenic (allergic) (eczematous) F54
sleep G47.9
breathing-related - *see* Apnea, sleep
circadian rhythm G47.20
advance sleep phase type G47.22
delayed sleep phase type G47.21
due to
alcohol
abuse F10.182
dependence F10.282
use F10.982
amphetamines
abuse F15.182
dependence F15.282
use F15.982
caffeine
abuse F15.182
dependence F15.282
use F15.982
cocaine
abuse F14.182
dependence F14.282
use F14.982
drug NEC
abuse F19.182
dependence F19.282
use F19.982
opioid
abuse F11.182
dependence F11.282
use F11.982
psychoactive substance NEC
abuse F19.182
dependence F19.282
use F19.982
sedative, hypnotic, or anxiolytic
abuse F13.182
dependence F13.282
use F13.982
stimulant NEC
abuse F15.182
dependence F15.282

Disorder (of) - *continued*

use F15.982
free running type G47.24
in conditions classified elsewhere G47.27
irregular sleep wake type G47.23
jet lag type G47.25
non 24-hour sleep-wake type G47.24
shift work type G47.26
specified NEC G47.29
due to
alcohol
abuse F10.182
dependence F10.282
use F10.982
amphetamine
abuse F15.182
dependence F15.282
use F15.982
anxiolytic
abuse F13.182
dependence F13.282
use F13.982
caffeine
abuse F15.182
dependence F15.282
use F15.982
cocaine
abuse F14.182
dependence F14.282
use F14.982
drug NEC
abuse F19.182
dependence F19.282
use F19.982
hypnotic
abuse F13.182
dependence F13.282
use F13.982
opioid
abuse F11.182
dependence F11.282
use F11.982
psychoactive substance NEC
abuse F19.182
dependence F19.282
use F19.982
sedative
abuse F13.182
dependence F13.282
use F13.982
stimulant NEC
abuse F15.182
dependence F15.282
use F15.982
emotional F51.9
excessive somnolence - *see* Hypersomnia
hypersomnia type - *see* Hypersomnia
initiating or maintaining - *see* Insomnia
nightmares F51.5
nonorganic F51.9
specified NEC F51.8
parasomnia type G47.50
specified NEC G47.8
terrors F51.4
walking F51.3
sleep-wake pattern or schedule (see also
Disorder, sleep, circadian rhythm) G47.9
specified NEC G47.8
social
anxiety (of childhood) F40.10
generalized F40.11
functioning in childhood F94.9
specified NEC F94.8
pragmatic F80.82

Disorder (of) - *continued*

soft tissue M79.9
ankle M79.9
due to use, overuse and pressure M70.90
ankle M70.97-
bursitis - *see* Bursitis
foot M70.97-
forearm M70.93-
hand M70.94-
lower leg M70.96-
multiple sites M70.99
pelvic region M70.95-
shoulder region M70.91-
specified site NEC M70.98
specified type NEC M70.80
ankle M70.87-
foot M70.87-
forearm M70.83-
hand M70.84-
lower leg M70.86-
multiple sites M70.89
pelvic region M70.85-
shoulder region M70.81-
specified site NEC M70.88
thigh M70.85-
upper arm M70.82-
thigh M70.95-
upper arm M70.92-
foot M79.9
forearm M79.9
hand M79.9
lower leg M79.9
multiple sites M79.9
occupational - *see* Disorder, soft tissue, due
to use, overuse and pressure
pelvic region M79.9
shoulder region M79.9
specified type NEC M79.89
thigh M79.9
upper arm M79.9
somatic symptom F45.1
somatization F45.0
somatoform F45.9
pain (persistent) F45.41
somatization (multiple) (long-lasting) F45.0
specified NEC F45.8
undifferentiated F45.1
somnolence, excessive - *see* Hypersomnia
specific
arithmetical F81.2
developmental, of motor F82
reading F81.0
speech and language F80.9
spelling F81.81
written expression F81.81
speech R47.9
articulation (functional) (specific) F80.0
developmental F80.9
specified NEC R47.89
speech-sound F80.0
spelling (specific) F81.81
spine - *see also* Dorsopathy
ligamentous or muscular attachments,
peripheral - *see* Enthesopathy, spinal
specified NEC - *see* Dorsopathy, specified
NEC
stereotyped, habit or movement F98.4
stimulant use (other) (unspecified)
mild F15.10
in remission (early) (sustained) F15.11
moderate or severe F15.20
in remission (early) (sustained) F15.21
stomach (functional) - *see* Disorder, gastric
stress F43.9

Disorder (of) - *continued*

acute F43.0
post-traumatic F43.10
acute F43.11
chronic F43.12
substance use (other) (unknown)
mild F19.10
with substance-induced
anxiety disorder F19.180
bipolar and related disorder F19.14
depressive disorder F19.14
major neurocognitive disorder F19.17
mild neurocognitive disorder F19.188
obsessive-compulsive and related disorder F19.188
sexual dysfunction F19.181
substance intoxication F19.129
substance intoxication delirium F19.121
moderate or severe F19.20
in remission (early) (sustained) F19.21
with substance-induced
anxiety disorder F19.280
bipolar and related disorder F19.24
depressive disorder F19.24
major neurocognitive disorder F19.27
mild neurocognitive disorder F19.288
obsessive-compulsive and related disorder F19.288
sexual dysfunction F19.281
substance intoxication F19.229
substance intoxication delirium F19.221
sulfur-bearing amino-acid metabolism E72.10
sweat gland (eccrine) L74.9
apocrine L75.9
specified NEC L75.8
specified NEC L74.8
synovium M67.90
acromioclavicular M67.91-
ankle M67.97-
elbow M67.92-
foot M67.97-
forearm M67.93-
hand M67.94-
hip M67.95-
knee M67.96-
multiple sites M67.99
rupture - *see* Rupture, synovium
shoulder M67.91-
specified type NEC M67.80
acromioclavicular M67.81-
ankle M67.87-
elbow M67.82-
foot M67.87-
hand M67.84-
hip M67.85-
knee M67.86-
multiple sites M67.89
wrist M67.83-
synovitis - *see* Synovitis
upper arm M67.92-
wrist M67.93-
temperature regulation, newborn P81.9
specified NEC P81.8
temporomandibular joint M26.60-
tendon M67.90
acromioclavicular M67.91-
ankle M67.97-
contracture - *see* Contracture, tendon
elbow M67.92-
foot M67.97-
forearm M67.93-
hand M67.94-
hip M67.95-
knee M67.96-

Disorder (of) - *continued*

multiple sites M67.99
rupture - *see* Rupture, tendon
shoulder M67.91-
specified type NEC M67.80
acromioclavicular M67.81-
ankle M67.87-
elbow M67.82-
foot M67.87-
hand M67.84-
hip M67.85-
knee M67.86-
multiple sites M67.89
trunk M67.88
wrist M67.83-
synovitis - *see* Synovitis
tendinitis - *see* Tendinitis
tenosynovitis - *see* Tenosynovitis
trunk M67.98
upper arm M67.92-
wrist M67.93-
thoracic root (nerve) NEC G54.3
thyrocalcitonin hypersecretion E07.0
thyroid (gland) E07.9
function NEC, neonatal, transitory P72.2
iodine-deficiency related E01.8
specified NEC E07.89
tic - *see* Tic
tobacco use
chewing tobacco (mild) (moderate) (severe)
in remission (early) (sustained) F17.221
cigarettes (mild) (moderate) (severe)
in remission (early) (sustained) F17.211
mild Z72.0
in remission (early) (sustained) F17.201
moderate F17.200
in remission (early) (sustained) F17.201
severe F17.200
in remission (early) (sustained) F17.201
specified product NEC (mild) (moderate) (severe)
in remission (early) (sustained) F17.291
tooth K08.9
development K00.9
transvestic F65.1
voyeuristic F65.3
specified NEC K00.8
eruption K00.6
Tourette's F95.2
trance and possession F44.89
trauma and stressor-related F43.9
other specified F43.8
tricuspid (valve) - *see* Endocarditis, tricuspid
tryptophan metabolism E70.5
tubular, phosphate-losing N25.0
tubulo-interstitial (in)
brucellosis A23.9 [N16]
cystinosis E72.04
diphtheria A36.84
glycogen storage disease E74.00 [N16]
leukemia NEC C95.9 [N16]
lymphoma NEC C85.9 [N16]
mixed cryoglobulinemia D89.1 [N16]
multiple myeloma C90.0- [N16]
Salmonella infection A02.25
sarcoidosis D86.84
sepsis A41.9 [N16]
streptococcal A40.9 [N16]
systemic lupus erythematosus M32.15
toxoplasmosis B58.83
transplant rejection T86.91 [N16]
Wilson's disease E83.01 [N16]
tubulo-renal function, impaired N25.9
specified NEC N25.89

Disorder (of) - *continued*

tympanic membrane H73.9-
atrophy - *see* Atrophy, tympanic membrane
infection - *see* Myringitis
perforation - *see* Perforation, tympanum
specified NEC H73.89-
unsocialized aggressive F91.1
urea cycle metabolism E72.20
argininemia E72.21
arginosuccinic aciduria E72.22
citrullinemia E72.23
ornithine transcarbamylase deficiency E72.4
other specified E72.29
ureter (in) N28.9
schistosomiasis B65.0 [N29]
tuberculosis A18.11
urethra N36.9
specified NEC N36.8
urinary system N39.9
specified NEC N39.8
valve, heart
aortic - *see* Endocarditis, aortic
mitral - *see* Endocarditis, mitral
pulmonary - *see* Endocarditis, pulmonary
rheumatic
aortic - *see* Endocarditis, aortic, rheumatic
mitral - *see* Endocarditis, mitral
pulmonary - *see* Endocarditis, pulmonary, rheumatic
tricuspid - *see* Endocarditis, tricuspid
tricuspid - *see* Endocarditis, tricuspid
vestibular function H81.9-
specified NEC - *see* subcategory H81.8
in diseases classified elsewhere H82.-
vertigo - *see* Vertigo
vision, binocular H53.30
abnormal retinal correspondence H53.31
diplopia H53.2
fusion with defective stereopsis H53.32
simultaneous perception H53.33
suppression H53.34
visual
cortex
blindness H47.619
left brain H47.612
right brain H47.611
due to
inflammatory disorder H47.629
left brain H47.622
right brain H47.621
neoplasm H47.639
left brain H47.632
right brain H47.631
vascular disorder H47.649
left brain H47.642
right brain H47.641
pathway H47.9
due to
inflammatory disorder H47.51-
neoplasm H47.52-
vascular disorder H47.53-
optic chiasm - *see* Disorder, optic, chiasm
vitreous body H43.9
crystalline deposits - *see* Deposit, crystalline
degeneration - *see* Degeneration, vitreous
hemorrhage - *see* Hemorrhage, vitreous
opacities - *see* Opacity, vitreous
prolapse - *see* Prolapse, vitreous
specified type NEC H43.89
voice R49.9
specified type NEC R49.8
volatile solvent use
due to drug abuse - *see* Abuse, drug, inhalant
due to drug dependence - *see* Dependence,

Disorder (of) - *continued*
drug, inhalant
  white blood cells D72.9
    specified NEC D72.89
  withdrawing, child or adolescent F40.10
Disorientation R41.0
Displacement, displaced
acquired traumatic of bone, cartilage, joint, tendon NEC - *see* Dislocation
adrenal gland (congenital) Q89.1
appendix, retrocecal (congenital) Q43.8
auricle (congenital) Q17.4
bladder (acquired) N32.89
  congenital Q64.19
brachial plexus (congenital) Q07.8
brain stem, caudal (congenital) Q04.8
canaliculus (lacrimalis), congenital Q10.6
cardia through esophageal hiatus (congenital) Q40.1
cerebellum, caudal (congenital) Q04.8
cervix - *see* Malposition, uterus
colon (congenital) Q43.3
device, implant or graft - *see also* Complications, by site and type, mechanical T85.628
  arterial graft NEC - *see* Complication, cardiovascular device, mechanical, vascular
  breast (implant) T85.42
  catheter NEC T85.628
    dialysis (renal) T82.42
      intraperitoneal T85.621
    infusion NEC T82.524
      spinal (epidural) (subdural) T85.620
    urinary
      cystostomy T83.020
      Hopkins T83.028
      ileostomy T83.028
      indwelling T83.021
      nephrostomy T83.022
      specified NEC T83.028
      urostomy T83.028
  electronic (electrode) (pulse generator) (stimulator) - *see* Complication, electronic stimulator
  fixation, internal (orthopedic) NEC - *see* Complication, fixation device, mechanical
  gastrointestinal - *see* Complications, prosthetic device, mechanical, gastrointestinal device
  genital NEC T83.428
    intrauterine contraceptive device (string) T83.32
    penile prosthesis (cylinder) (implanted) (pump) (reservoir) T83.420
    testicular prosthesis T83.421
  heart NEC - *see* Complication, cardiovascular device, mechanical
  joint prosthesis - *see* Complications, joint prosthesis, mechanical
  ocular - *see* Complications, prosthetic device, mechanical, ocular device
  orthopedic NEC - *see* Complication, orthopedic, device or graft, mechanical
  specified NEC T85.628
  urinary NEC T83.128
    graft T83.22
    sphincter, implanted T83.121
    stent (ileal conduit) (nephroureteral) T83.123
      ureteral indwelling T83.122
  vascular NEC - *see* Complication, cardiovascular device, mechanical
  ventricular intracranial shunt T85.02
electronic stimulator

Displacement, displaced - *continued*
bone T84.320
cardiac - *see* Complications, cardiac device, electronic
nervous system - *see* Complication, prosthetic device, mechanical, electronic nervous system stimulator
urinary - *see* Complications, electronic stimulator, urinary
esophageal mucosa into cardia of stomach, congenital Q39.8
esophagus (acquired) K22.8
  congenital Q39.8
eyeball (acquired) (lateral) (old) - *see* Displacement, globe
  congenital Q15.8
  current - *see* Avulsion, eye
fallopian tube (acquired) N83.4-
  congenital Q50.6
  opening (congenital) Q50.6
gallbladder (congenital) Q44.1
gastric mucosa (congenital) Q40.2
globe (acquired) (old) (lateral) H05.21-
  current - *see* Avulsion, eye
heart (congenital) Q24.8
  acquired I51.89
hymen (upward) (congenital) Q52.4
intervertebral disc NEC
  with myelopathy - *see* Disorder, disc, with, myelopathy
  cervical, cervicothoracic (with) M50.20
    myelopathy - *see* Disorder, disc, cervical, with myelopathy
    neuritis, radiculitis or radiculopathy - *see* Disorder, disc, cervical, with neuritis
  due to trauma - *see* Dislocation, vertebra
  lumbar region M51.26
    with
      myelopathy M51.06
      neuritis, radiculitis, radiculopathy or sciatica M51.16
  lumbosacral region M51.27
    with
      neuritis, radiculitis, radiculopathy or sciatica M51.17
  sacrococcygeal region M53.3
  thoracic region M51.24
    with
      myelopathy M51.04
      neuritis, radiculitis, radiculopathy M51.14
  thoracolumbar region M51.25
    with
      myelopathy M51.05
      neuritis, radiculitis, radiculopathy M51.15
intrauterine device (string) T83.32
kidney (acquired) N28.83
  congenital Q63.2
lachrymal, lacrimal apparatus or duct (congenital) Q10.6
lens, congenital Q12.1
macula (congenital) Q14.1
Meckel's diverticulum Q43.0
  malignant - *see* Table of Neoplasms, small intestine, malignant
nail (congenital) Q84.6
  acquired L60.8
opening of Wharton's duct in mouth Q38.4
organ or site, congenital NEC - *see* Malposition, congenital
ovary (acquired) N83.4-
  congenital Q50.39
  free in peritoneal cavity (congenital) Q50.39
  into hernial sac N83.4-
oviduct (acquired) N83.4-

Displacement, displaced - *continued*
congenital Q50.6
parathyroid (gland) E21.4
parotid gland (congenital) Q38.4
punctum lacrimale (congenital) Q10.6
sacro-iliac (joint) (congenital) Q74.2
  current injury S33.2
  old - *see* subcategory M53.2
salivary gland (any) (congenital) Q38.4
spleen (congenital) Q89.09
stomach, congenital Q40.2
sublingual duct Q38.4
tongue (downward) (congenital) Q38.3
tooth, teeth, fully erupted M26.30
  horizontal M26.33
  vertical M26.34
trachea (congenital) Q32.1
ureter or ureteric opening or orifice (congenital) Q62.62
uterine opening of oviducts or fallopian tubes Q50.6
uterus, uterine - *see* Malposition, uterus
ventricular septum Q21.0
  with rudimentary ventricle Q20.4
Disproportion
between native and reconstructed breast N65.1
fiber-type G71.2
Disruptio uteri - *see* Rupture, uterus
Disruption (of)
ciliary body NEC H21.89
closure of
  cornea T81.31
  craniotomy T81.32
  fascia (muscular) (superficial) T81.32
  internal organ or tissue T81.32
  laceration (external) (internal) T81.33
  ligament T81.32
  mucosa T81.31
  muscle or muscle flap T81.32
  ribs or rib cage T81.32
  skin and subcutaneous tissue (full-thickness) (superficial) T81.31
  skull T81.32
  sternum (sternotomy) T81.32
  tendon T81.32
  traumatic laceration (external) (internal) T81.33
family Z63.8
  due to
    absence of family member due to military deployment Z63.31
    absence of family member NEC Z63.32
    alcoholism and drug addiction in family Z63.72
    bereavement Z63.4
    death (assumed) or disappearance of family member Z63.4
    divorce or separation Z63.5
    drug addiction in family Z63.72
    return of family member from military deployment (current or past conflict) Z63.71
    stressful life events NEC Z63.79
iris NEC H21.89
ligament(s) - *see also* Sprain
  knee
    current injury - *see* Dislocation, knee
    old (chronic) - *see* Derangement, knee, ligament, instability, chronic
    spontaneous NEC - *see* Derangement, knee, disruption ligament
ossicular chain - *see* Discontinuity, ossicles, ear
pelvic ring (stable) S32.810

Disruption (of) - *continued*
   unstable S32.811
   wound T81.30
     episiotomy O90.1
     operation T81.31
       cesarean O90.0
       external operation wound (superficial)
         T81.31
       internal operation wound (deep) T81.32
       perineal (obstetric) O90.1
       traumatic injury repair T81.33
     traumatic injury wound repair T81.33
Dissatisfaction with
   employment Z56.9
   school environment Z55.4
Dissecting - *see* condition
Dissection
   aorta I71.00
     abdominal I71.02
     thoracic I71.01
     thoracoabdominal I71.03
   artery I77.70
     basilar (trunk) I77.75
     carotid I77.71
     cerebral (nonruptured) I67.0
       ruptured - *see* Hemorrhage, intracranial,
         subarachnoid
     coronary I25.42
     extremity
       lower I77.77
       upper I77.76
     iliac I77.72
     precerebral
       congenital (nonruptured) Q28.1
       specified site NEC I77.75
     renal I77.73
     specified NEC I77.79
     vertebral I77.74
   precerebral artery, congential (nonruptured)
   Q28.1
     Heartland A93.8
   traumatic - *see* Wound, open, by site
   vascular I99.8
   wound - *see* Wound, open
Disseminated - *see* condition
Dissociation
   auriculoventricular or atrioventricular (AV)
   (any degree) (isorhythmic) I45.89
     with heart block I44.2
   interference I45.89
Dissociative reaction, state F44.9
Dissolution, vertebra - *see* Osteoporosis
Distension, distention
   abdomen R14.0
   bladder N32.89
   cecum K63.89
   colon K63.89
   gallbladder K82.8
   intestine K63.89
   kidney N28.89
   liver K76.89
   seminal vesicle N50.89
   stomach K31.89
     acute K31.0
     psychogenic F45.8
   ureter - *see* Dilatation, ureter
   uterus N85.8
Distoma hepaticum infestation B66.3
Distomiasis B66.9
   bile passages B66.3
   hemic B65.9
   hepatic B66.3
     due to Clonorchis sinensis B66.1
   intestinal B66.5

Dissection - *continued*
   liver B66.3
     due to Clonorchis sinensis B66.1
   lung B66.4
   pulmonary B66.4
Distomolar (fourth molar) K00.1
Disto-occlusion (Division I) (Division II)
   M26.212
Distortion(s) (congenital)
   adrenal (gland) Q89.1
   arm NEC Q68.8
   bile duct or passage Q44.5
   bladder Q64.79
   brain Q04.9
   cervix (uteri) Q51.9
   chest (wall) Q67.8
     bones Q76.8
   clavicle Q74.0
   clitoris Q52.6
   coccyx Q76.49
   common duct Q44.5
   coronary Q24.5
   cystic duct Q44.5
   ear (auricle) (external) Q17.3
     inner Q16.5
     middle Q16.4
       ossicles Q16.3
   endocrine NEC Q89.2
   eustachian tube Q17.8
   eye (adnexa) Q15.8
   face bone(s) NEC Q75.8
   fallopian tube Q50.6
   femur NEC Q68.8
   fibula NEC Q68.8
   finger(s) Q68.1
   foot Q66.9
   genitalia, genital organ(s)
     female Q52.8
       external Q52.79
       internal NEC Q52.8
   gyri Q04.8
   hand bone(s) NEC Q68.1
   heart (auricle) (ventricle) Q24.8
     valve (cusp) Q24.8
   hepatic duct Q44.5
   humerus NEC Q68.8
   hymen Q52.4
   intrafamilial communications Z63.8
   jaw NEC M26.89
   labium (majus) (minus) Q52.79
   leg NEC Q68.8
   lens Q12.8
   liver Q44.7
   lumbar spine Q76.49
     with disproportion O33.8
       causing obstructed labor O65.0
   lumbosacral (joint) (region) Q76.49
     kyphosis - *see* Kyphosis, congenital
     lordosis - *see* Lordosis, congenital
   nerve Q07.8
   nose Q30.8
   organ
     of Corti Q16.5
     or site not listed - *see* Anomaly, by site
   ossicles, ear Q16.3
   oviduct Q50.6
   pancreas Q45.3
   parathyroid (gland) Q89.2
   pituitary (gland) Q89.2
   radius NEC Q68.8
   sacroiliac joint Q74.2
   sacrum Q76.49
   scapula Q74.0
   shoulder girdle Q74.0

Distortion(s) (congenital) - *continued*
   skull bone(s) NEC Q75.8
     with
       anencephalus Q00.0
       encephalocele - *see* Encephalocele
       hydrocephalus Q03.9
         with spina bifida - *see* Spina bifida, with
          hydrocephalus
       microcephaly Q02
   spinal cord Q06.8
   spine Q76.49
     kyphosis - *see* Kyphosis, congenital
     lordosis - *see* Lordosis, congenital
   spleen Q89.09
   sternum NEC Q76.7
   thorax (wall) Q67.8
     bony Q76.8
   thymus (gland) Q89.2
   thyroid (gland) Q89.2
   tibia NEC Q68.8
   toe(s) Q66.9
   tongue Q38.3
   trachea (cartilage) Q32.1
   ulna NEC Q68.8
   ureter Q62.8
   urethra Q64.79
     causing obstruction Q64.39
   uterus Q51.9
   vagina Q52.4
   vertebra Q76.49
     kyphosis - *see* Kyphosis, congenital
     lordosis - *see* Lordosis, congenital
   visual - *see also* Disturbance, vision
     shape and size H53.15
   vulva Q52.79
   wrist (bones) (joint) Q68.8
Distress
   abdomen - *see* Pain, abdominal
   acute respiratory R06.03
     syndrome (adult) (child) J80
   epigastric R10.13
   fetal P84
     complicating pregnancy - *see* Stress, fetal
   gastrointestinal (functional) K30
     psychogenic F45.8
   intestinal (functional) NOS K59.9
     psychogenic F45.8
   maternal, during labor and delivery O75.0
   relationship, with spouse or intimate partner
   Z63.0
   respiratory (adult) (child) R06.03
     newborn P22.9
       specified NEC P22.8
     orthopnea R06.01
     psychogenic F45.8
     shortness of breath R06.02
     specified type NEC R06.09
Distribution vessel, atypical Q27.9
   coronary artery Q24.5
   precerebral Q28.1
Districhiasis L68.8
Disturbance(s) - *see also* Disease   absorption
   K90.9
     calcium E58
     carbohydrate K90.49
     fat K90.49
       pancreatic K90.3
     protein K90.49
     starch K90.49
     vitamin - *see* Deficiency, vitamin
   acid-base equilibrium E87.8
     mixed E87.4
   activity and attention (with hyperkinesis) - *see*
   Disorder, attention-deficit hyperactivity

Disturbance(s) - *continued*
amino acid transport E72.00
  assimilation, food K90.9
  auditory nerve, except deafness - *see*
    subcategory H93.3
  behavior - *see* Disorder, conduct
  blood clotting (mechanism) - *see also* Defect,
    coagulation D68.9
  cerebral
    nerve - *see* Disorder, nerve, cranial
    status, newborn P91.9
      specified NEC P91.88
  circulatory I99.9
  conduct - *see also* Disorder, conduct F91.9
    adjustment reaction - *see* Disorder,
      adjustment
    compulsive F63.9
    disruptive F91.9
    hyperkinetic - *see* Disorder, attention-deficit
      hyperactivity
    socialized F91.2
    specified NEC F91.8
    unsocialized F91.1
  coordination R27.8
  cranial nerve - *see* Disorder, nerve, cranial
  deep sensibility - *see* Disturbance, sensation
  digestive K30
    psychogenic F45.8
  electrolyte - *see also* Imbalance, electrolyte
    newborn, transitory P74.4
      hyperammonemia P74.6
      potassium balance P74.3
      sodium balance P74.2
      specified type NEC P74.4
  emotions specific to childhood and
  adolescence F93.9
    with
      anxiety and fearfulness NEC F93.8
      elective mutism F94.0
      oppositional disorder F91.3
      sensitivity (withdrawal) F40.10
      shyness F40.10
      social withdrawal F40.10
    involving relationship problems F93.8
    mixed F93.8
    specified NEC F93.8
  endocrine (gland) E34.9
    neonatal, transitory P72.9
      specified NEC P72.8
  equilibrium R42
  fructose metabolism E74.10
  gait - *see* Gait
    hysterical F44.4
    psychogenic F44.4
  gastrointestinal (functional) K30
    psychogenic F45.8
  habit, child F98.9
  hearing, except deafness and tinnitus - *see*
    Abnormal, auditory perception
  heart, functional (conditions in I44-i50)
    due to presence of (cardiac) prosthesis
      I97.19-
    postoperative I97.89
      cardiac surgery (see also Infarct,
  myocardium, associated with revascularization
  procedure) I97.19-
  hormones E34.9
  innervation uterus (parasympathetic)
    (sympathetic) N85.8
  keratinization NEC
    gingiva K05.10
      nonplaque induced K05.11
      plaque induced K05.10
    lip K13.0

Disturbance(s) - *continued*
  oral (mucosa) (soft tissue) K13.29
    tongue K13.29
  learning (specific) - *see* Disorder, learning
  memory - *see* Amnesia
    mild, following organic brain damage F06.8
  mental F99
    associated with diseases classified elsewhere
      F54
  metabolism E88.9
    with
      abortion - *see* Abortion, by type with other
        specified complication
      ectopic pregnancy O08.5
      molar pregnancy O08.5
    amino-acid E72.9
      aromatic E70.9
      branched-chain E71.2
      straight-chain E72.8
      sulfur-bearing E72.10
    ammonia E72.20
    arginine E72.21
    arginosuccinic acid E72.22
    carbohydrate E74.9
    cholesterol E78.9
    citrulline E72.23
    cystathionine E72.19
    general E88.9
    glutamine E72.8
    histidine E70.40
    homocystine E72.19
    hydroxylysine E72.3
    in labor or delivery O75.89
    iron E83.10
    lipoid E78.9
    lysine E72.3
    methionine E72.19
    neonatal, transitory P74.9
      calcium and magnesium P71.9
        specified type NEC P71.8
      carbohydrate metabolism P70.9
        specified type NEC P70.8
      specified NEC P74.8
    ornithine E72.4
    phosphate E83.39
    sodium NEC E87.8
    threonine E72.8
    tryptophan E70.5
    tyrosine E70.20
    urea cycle E72.20
  motor R29.2
  nervous, functional R45.0
  neuromuscular mechanism (eye), due to
  syphilis A52.15
  nutritional E63.9
    nail L60.3
  ocular motion H51.9
    psychogenic F45.8
  oculogyric H51.8
    psychogenic F45.8
  oculomotor H51.9
    psychogenic F45.8
  olfactory nerve R43.1
  optic nerve NEC - *see* Disorder, nerve, optic
  oral epithelium, including tongue NEC K13.29
  perceptual due to
    alcohol withdrawal F10.232
    amphetamine intoxication F15.922
      in
        abuse F15.122
        dependence F15.222
    anxiolytic withdrawal F13.232
    cannabis intoxication (acute) F12.922
      in

Disturbance(s) - *continued*
        abuse F12.122
        dependence F12.222
    cocaine intoxication (acute) F14.922
      in
        abuse F14.122
        dependence F14.222
    hypnotic withdrawal F13.232
    opioid intoxication (acute) F11.922
      in
        abuse F11.122
        dependence F11.222
    phencyclidine intoxication (acute) F16.122
    sedative withdrawal F13.232
  personality (pattern) (trait) - *see also* Disorder,
  personality F60.9
    following organic brain damage F07.9
  polyglandular E31.9
    specified NEC E31.8
  potassium balance, newborn P74.3
  psychogenic F45.9
  psychomotor F44.4
  psychophysical visual H53.16
  pupillary - *see* Anomaly, pupil, function
  reflex R29.2
  rhythm, heart I49.9
  salivary secretion K11.7
  sensation (cold) (heat) (localization) (tactile
    discrimination) (texture) (vibratory) NEC
    R20.9
    hysterical F44.6
    skin R20.9
      anesthesia R20.0
      hyperesthesia R20.3
      hypoesthesia R20.1
      paresthesia R20.2
      specified type NEC R20.8
    smell R43.9
      and taste (mixed) R43.8
      anosmia R43.0
      parosmia R43.1
      specified NEC R43.8
    taste R43.9
      and smell (mixed) R43.8
      parageusia R43.2
      specified NEC R43.8
  sensory - *see* Disturbance, sensation
  situational (transient) - *see also* Disorder,
  adjustment
    acute F43.0
  sleep G47.9
    nonorganic origin F51.9
  smell - *see* Disturbance, sensation, smell
  sociopathic F60.2
  sodium balance, newborn P74.2
  speech R47.9
    developmental F80.9
    specified NEC R47.89
  stomach (functional) K31.9
  sympathetic (nerve) G90.9
  taste - *see* Disturbance, sensation, taste
  temperature
    regulation, newborn P81.9
      specified NEC P81.8
    sense R20.8
      hysterical F44.6
  tooth
    eruption K00.6
    formation K00.4
    structure, hereditary NEC K00.5
  touch - *see* Disturbance, sensation
  vascular I99.9
    arteriosclerotic - *see* Arteriosclerosis
  vasomotor I73.9

Disturbance(s) - *continued*
vasospastic I73.9
vision, visual H53.9
following
cerebral infarction I69.398
cerebrovascular disease I69.998
specified NEC I69.898
intracerebral hemorrhage I69.198
nontraumatic intracranial hemorrhage NEC
I69.298
specified disease NEC I69.898
subarachnoid hemorrhage I69.098
psychophysical H53.16
specified NEC H53.8
subjective H53.10
day blindness H53.11
discomfort H53.14-
distortions of shape and size H53.15
loss
sudden H53.13-
transient H53.12-
specified type NEC H53.19
voice R49.9
psychogenic F44.4
specified NEC R49.8
Diuresis R35.8
Diver's palsy, paralysis or squeeze T70.3
Diverticulitis (acute) K57.92
bladder - *see* Cystitis
ileum - *see* Diverticulitis, intestine, small
intestine K57.92
with
abscess, perforation or peritonitis K57.80
with bleeding K57.81
bleeding K57.93
congenital Q43.8
large K57.32
with
abscess, perforation or peritonitis K57.20
with bleeding K57.21
bleeding K57.33
small intestine K57.52
with
abscess, perforation or peritonitis
K57.40
with bleeding K57.41
bleeding K57.53
small K57.12
with
abscess, perforation or peritonitis K57.00
with bleeding K57.01
bleeding K57.13
large intestine K57.52
with
abscess, perforation or peritonitis
K57.40
with bleeding K57.41
bleeding K57.53
Diverticulosis K57.90
with bleeding K57.91
large intestine K57.30
with
bleeding K57.31
small intestine K57.50
with bleeding K57.51
small intestine K57.10
with
bleeding K57.11
large intestine K57.50
with bleeding K57.51
Diverticulum, diverticula (multiple) K57.90
appendix (noninflammatory) K38.2
bladder (sphincter) N32.3
congenital Q64.6

Diverticulum, diverticula - *continued*
bronchus (congenital) Q32.4
acquired J98.09
calyx, calyceal (kidney) N28.89
cardia (stomach) K31.4
cecum - *see* Diverticulosis, intestine, large
congenital Q43.8
colon - *see* Diverticulosis, intestine, large
congenital Q43.8
duodenum - *see* Diverticulosis, intestine, small
congenital Q43.8
epiphrenic (esophagus) K22.5
esophagus (congenital) Q39.6
acquired (epiphrenic) (pulsion) (traction)
K22.5
eustachian tube - *see* Disorder, eustachian
tube, specified NEC
fallopian tube N83.8
gastric K31.4
heart (congenital) Q24.8
ileum - *see* Diverticulosis, intestine, small
jejunum - *see* Diverticulosis, intestine, small
kidney (pelvis) (calyces) N28.89
with calculus - *see* Calculus, kidney
Meckel's (displaced) (hypertrophic) Q43.0
malignant - *see* Table of Neoplasms, small
intestine, malignant
midthoracic K22.5
organ or site, congenital NEC - *see* Distortion
pericardium (congenital) (cyst) Q24.8
acquired I31.8
pharyngoesophageal (congenital) Q39.6
acquired K22.5
pharynx (congenital) Q38.7
rectosigmoid - *see* Diverticulosis, intestine,
large
congenital Q43.8
rectum - *see* Diverticulosis, intestine, large
Rokitansky's K22.5
seminal vesicle N50.89
sigmoid - *see* Diverticulosis, intestine, large
congenital Q43.8
stomach (acquired) K31.4
congenital Q40.2
trachea (acquired) J39.8
ureter (acquired) N28.89
congenital Q62.8
ureterovesical orifice N28.89
urethra (acquired) N36.1
congenital Q64.79
ventricle, left (congenital) Q24.8
vesical N32.3
congenital Q64.6
Zenker's (esophagus) K22.5
Division
cervix uteri (acquired) N88.8
glans penis Q55.69
labia minora (congenital) Q52.79
ligament (partial or complete) (current) - *see
also* Sprain
with open wound - *see* Wound, open
muscle (partial or complete) (current) - *see
also* Injury, muscle
with open wound - *see* Wound, open
nerve (traumatic) - *see* Injury, nerve
spinal cord - *see* Injury, spinal cord, by region
vein I87.8
Divorce, causing family disruption Z63.5
Dix-Hallpike neurolabyrinthitis - *see*
Neuronitis, vestibular
Dizziness R42
hysterical F44.89
psychogenic F45.8

DMAC (disseminated mycobacterium avium intracellulare complex) A31.2
DNR (do not resuscitate) Z66
Doan-Wiseman syndrome (primary splenic neutropenia) - *see* Agranulocytosis
Doehle-Heller aortitis A52.02
Dog bite - *see* Bite
Dohle body panmyelopathic syndrome D72.0
Dolichocephaly Q67.2
Dolichocolon Q43.8
Dolichostenomelia - *see* Syndrome, Marfan's
Donohue's syndrome E34.8
Donor (organ or tissue) Z52.9
blood (whole) Z52.000
autologous Z52.010
specified component (lymphocytes)
(platelets) NEC Z52.008
autologous Z52.018
specified donor NEC Z52.098
specified donor NEC Z52.090
stem cells Z52.001
autologous Z52.011
specified donor NEC Z52.091
bone Z52.20
autologous Z52.21
marrow Z52.3
specified type NEC Z52.29
cornea Z52.5
egg (Oocyte) Z52.819
age 35 and over Z52.812
anonymous recipient Z52.812
designated recipient Z52.813
under age 35 Z52.810
anonymous recipient Z52.810
designated recipient Z52.811
kidney Z52.4
liver Z52.6
lung Z52.89
lymphocyte - *see* Donor, blood, specified
components NEC
Oocyte - *see* Donor, egg
platelets Z52.008
potential, examination of Z00.5
semen Z52.89
skin Z52.10
autologous Z52.11
specified type NEC Z52.19
specified organ or tissue NEC Z52.89
sperm Z52.89
Donovanosis A58
Dorsalgia M54.9
psychogenic F45.41
specified NEC M54.89
Dorsopathy M53.9
deforming M43.9
specified NEC - *see* subcategory M43.8
specified NEC M53.80
cervical region M53.82
cervicothoracic region M53.83
lumbar region M53.86
lumbosacral region M53.87
occipito-atlanto-axial region M53.81
sacrococcygeal region M53.88
thoracic region M53.84
thoracolumbar region M53.85
Double
albumin E88.09
aortic arch Q25.45
auditory canal Q17.8
auricle (heart) Q20.8
bladder Q64.79
cervix Q51.820
with doubling of uterus (and vagina) Q51.10
with obstruction Q51.11

Double - *continued*
  inlet ventricle Q20.4
  kidney with double pelvis (renal) Q63.0
  meatus urinarius Q64.75
  monster Q89.4
  outlet
    left ventricle Q20.2
    right ventricle Q20.1
  pelvis (renal) with double ureter Q62.5
  tongue Q38.3
  ureter (one or both sides) Q62.5
    with double pelvis (renal) Q62.5
  urethra Q64.74
  urinary meatus Q64.75
  uterus Q51.2
    with
      doubling of cervix (and vagina) Q51.10
        with obstruction Q51.11
      in pregnancy or childbirth O34.59-
        causing obstructed labor O65.5
    vagina Q52.10
      with doubling of uterus (and cervix) Q51.10
        with obstruction Q51.11
  vision H53.2
  vulva Q52.79
Douglas' pouch, cul-de-sac - *see* condition
Down syndrome Q90.9
  meiotic nondisjunction Q90.0
  mitotic nondisjunction Q90.1
  mosaicism Q90.1
  translocation Q90.2
DPD (dihydropyrimidine dehydrogenase deficiency) E88.89
Dracontiasis B72
Dracunculiasis, dracunculosis B72
Dream state, hysterical F44.89
Dreschlera (hawaiiensis) (infection) B43.8
Drepanocytic anemia - *see* Disease, sickle-cell
Dresbach's syndrome (elliptocytosis) D58.1
Dressler's syndrome I24.1
Drift, ulnar - *see* Deformity, limb, specified
  type NEC, forearm
Drinking (alcohol)
  excessive, to excess NEC (without dependence) F10.10
    habitual (continual) (without remission) F10.20
      with remission F10.21
Drip, postnasal (chronic) R09.82
  due to
    allergic rhinitis - *see* Rhinitis, allergic
    common cold J00
    gastroesophageal reflux - *see* Reflux, gastroesophageal
    nasopharyngitis - *see* Nasopharyngitis
    other know condition
  code to condition
    sinusitis - *see* Sinusitis
Droop
  facial R29.810
  cerebrovascular disease I69.992
    cerebral infarction I69.392
    intracerebral hemorrhage I69.192
    nontraumatic intracranial hemorrhage NEC I69.292
    specified disease NEC I69.892
    subarachnoid hemorrhage I69.092
Drop (in)
  attack NEC R55
  finger - *see* Deformity, finger
  foot - *see* Deformity, limb, foot, drop
  hematocrit (precipitous) R71.0
  hemoglobin R71.0
  toe - *see* Deformity, toe, specified NEC

Drop (in) - *continued*
  wrist - *see* Deformity, limb, wrist drop
Dropped heart beats I45.9
Dropsy, dropsical - *see also* Hydrops
  abdomen R18.8
  brain - *see* Hydrocephalus
  cardiac, heart - *see* Failure, heart, congestive
  gangrenous - *see* Gangrene
  heart - *see* Failure, heart, congestive
  kidney - *see* Nephrosis
  lung - *see* Edema, lung
  newborn due to isoimmunization P56.0
  pericardium - *see* Pericarditis
Drowned, drowning (near) T75.1
Drowsiness R40.0
Drug
  abuse counseling and surveillance Z71.51
  addiction - *see* Dependence
  dependence - *see* Dependence
  habit - *see* Dependence
  harmful use - *see* Abuse, drug
  induced fever R50.2
  overdose - *see* Table of Drugs and Chemicals, by drug, poisoning
  poisoning - *see* Table of Drugs and Chemicals, by drug, poisoning
  resistant organism infection - *see also* Resistant, organism, to, drug Z16.30
  therapy
    long term (current) (prophylactic) - *see* Therapy, drug long-term (current) (prophylactic)
    short term
  omit code
  wrong substance given or taken in error - *see* Table of Drugs and Chemicals, by drug, poisoning
Drunkenness (without dependence) F10.129
  acute in alcoholism F10.229
  chronic (without remission) F10.20
    with remission F10.21
  pathological (without dependence) F10.129
    with dependence F10.229
  sleep F51.9
Drusen
  macula (degenerative) (retina) - *see* Degeneration, macula, drusen
  optic disc H47.32-
Dry, dryness - *see also* condition
  larynx J38.7
  mouth R68.2
    due to dehydration E86.0
  nose J34.89
  socket (teeth) M27.3
  throat J39.2
DSAP L56.5
Duane's syndrome H50.81-
Dubin-Johnson disease or syndrome E80.6
Dubois' disease (thymus gland) A50.59 [*E35*]
Dubowitz' syndrome Q87.1
Duchenne-Aran muscular atrophy G12.21
Duchenne-Griesinger disease G71.0
Duchenne's
  disease or syndrome
    motor neuron disease G12.22
    muscular dystrophy G71.0
  locomotor ataxia (syphilitic) A52.11
  paralysis
    birth injury P14.0
    due to or associated with
      motor neuron disease G12.22
      muscular dystrophy G71.0
Ducrey's chancre A57
Duct, ductus - *see* condition

Duhring's disease (dermatitis herpetiformis) L13.0
Dullness, cardiac (decreased) (increased) R01.2
Dumb ague - *see* Malaria
Dumbness - *see* Aphasia
Dumdum fever B55.0
Dumping syndrome (postgastrectomy) K91.1
Duodenitis (nonspecific) (peptic) K29.80
  with bleeding K29.81
Duodenocholangitis - *see* Cholangitis
Duodenum, duodenal - *see* condition
Duplay's bursitis or periarthritis - *see* Tendinitis, calcific, shoulder
Duplication, duplex - *see also* Accessory
  alimentary tract Q45.8
  anus Q43.4
  appendix (and cecum) Q43.4
  biliary duct (any) Q44.5
  bladder Q64.79
  cecum (and appendix) Q43.4
  cervix Q51.820
  chromosome NEC
    with complex rearrangements NEC Q92.5
    seen only at prometaphase Q92.8
  cystic duct Q44.5
  digestive organs Q45.8
  esophagus Q39.8
  frontonasal process Q75.8
  intestine (large) (small) Q43.4
  kidney Q63.0
  liver Q44.7
  pancreas Q45.3
  penis Q55.69
  respiratory organs NEC Q34.8
  salivary duct Q38.4
  spinal cord (incomplete) Q06.2
  stomach Q40.2
Dupré's disease (meningism) R29.1
Dupuytren's contraction or disease M72.0
Durand Nicolas-Favre disease A55
Durotomy (inadvertent) (incidental) G97.41
Duroziez's disease (congenital mitral stenosis) Q23.2
Dutton's relapsing fever (West African) A68.1
Dwarfism E34.3
  achondroplastic Q77.4
  congenital E34.3
  constitutional E34.3
  hypochondroplastic Q77.4
  hypophyseal E23.0
  infantile E34.3
  Laron-type E34.3
  Lorain (-Lévi) type E23.0
  metatropic Q77.8
  nephrotic-glycosuric (with hypophosphatemic rickets) E72.09
  nutritional E45
  pancreatic K86.89
  pituitary E23.0
  renal N25.0
  thanatophoric Q77.1
Dyke-Young anemia (secondary) (symptomatic) D59.1
Dysacusis - *see* Abnormal, auditory perception
Dysadrenocortism E27.9
  hyperfunction E27.0
Dysarthria R47.1
  following
    cerebral infarction I69.322
    cerebrovascular disease I69.922
      specified disease NEC I69.822
    intracerebral hemorrhage I69.122

Dysarthria - *continued*
  nontraumatic intracranial hemorrhage NEC
    I69.222
  subarachnoid hemorrhage I69.022
Dysautonomia (familial) G90.1
Dysbarism T70.3
Dysbasia R26.2
  angiosclerotica intermittens I73.9
  hysterical F44.4
  lordotica (progressiva) G24.1
  nonorganic origin F44.4
  psychogenic F44.4
Dysbetalipoproteinemia (familial) E78.2
Dyscalculia R48.8
  developmental F81.2
Dyschezia K59.00
Dyschondroplasia (with hemangiomata)
  Q78.4
Dyschromia (skin) L81.9
Dyscollagenosis M35.9
Dyscranio-pygo-phalangy Q87.0
Dyscrasia
  blood (with) D75.9
    antepartum hemorrhage - *see* Hemorrhage,
      antepartum, with coagulation defect
    newborn P61.9
      specified type NEC P61.8
    intrapartum hemorrhage O67.0
    puerperal, postpartum O72.3
  polyglandular, pluriglandular E31.9
Dysendocrinism E34.9
Dysentery, dysenteric (catarrhal) (diarrhea)
  (epidemic) (hemorrhagic) (infectious)
  (sporadic) (tropical) A09
  abscess, liver A06.4
  amebic - *see also* Amebiasis A06.0
    with abscess - *see* Abscess, amebic
    acute A06.0
    chronic A06.1
  arthritis - *see also* category M01 A09
    bacillary - *see also* category M01 A03.9
  bacillary A03.9
    arthritis - *see also* category M01 A03.9
    Boyd A03.2
    Flexner A03.1
    Schmitz (-Stutzer) A03.0
    Shiga (-Kruse) A03.0
    Shigella A03.9
      boydii A03.2
      dysenteriae A03.0
      flexneri A03.1
      group A A03.0
      group B A03.1
      group C A03.2
      group D A03.3
      sonnei A03.3
      specified type NEC A03.8
    Sonne A03.3
    specified type NEC A03.8
  balantidial A07.0
  Balantidium coli A07.0
  Boyd's A03.2
  candidal B37.82
  Chilomastix A07.8
  Chinese A03.9
  coccidial A07.3
  Dientamoeba (fragilis) A07.8
  Embadomonas A07.8
  Entamoeba, entamebic - *see* Dysentery,
    amebic
  Flexner-Boyd A03.2
  Flexner's A03.1
  Giardia lamblia A07.1
  Hiss-Russell A03.1

Dysarthria - *continued*
  Lamblia A07.1
  leishmanial B55.0
  malarial - *see* Malaria
  metazoal B82.0
  monilial B37.82
  protozoal A07.9
  Salmonella A02.0
  schistosomal B65.1
  Schmitz (-Stutzer) A03.0
  Shiga (-Kruse) A03.0
  Shigella NOS - *see* Dysentery, bacillary
  Sonne A03.3
  strongyloidiasis B78.0
  trichomonal A07.8
  viral - *see also* Enteritis, viral A08.4
Dysequilibrium R42
Dysesthesia R20.8
  hysterical F44.6
Dysfibrinogenemia (congenital) D68.2
Dysfunction
  adrenal E27.9
    hyperfunction E27.0
  autonomic
    due to alcohol G31.2
    somatoform F45.8
  bladder N31.9
    neurogenic NOS - *see* Dysfunction, bladder,
    neuromuscular
      neuromuscular NOS N31.9
        atonic (motor) (sensory) N31.2
        autonomous N31.2
        flaccid N31.2
        nonreflex N31.2
        reflex N31.1
        specified NEC N31.8
        uninhibited N31.0
  bleeding, uterus N93.8
  cerebral G93.89
  colon K59.9
    psychogenic F45.8
  colostomy K94.03
  cystic duct K82.8
  cystostomy (stoma) - *see* Complications,
    cystostomy
  ejaculatory N53.19
    anejaculatory orgasm N53.13
    painful N53.12
    premature F52.4
    retarded N53.11
  endocrine NOS E34.9
  endometrium N85.8
  enterostomy K94.13
  erectile - *see* Dysfunction, sexual, male,
    erectile
  gallbladder K82.8
  gastrostomy (stoma) K94.23
  gland, glandular NOS E34.9
  heart I51.89
  hemoglobin D75.89
  hepatic K76.89
  hypophysis E23.7
  hypothalamic NEC E23.3
  ileostomy (stoma) K94.13
  jejunostomy (stoma) K94.13
  kidney - *see* Disease, renal
  labyrinthine   *see* subcategory H83.2
  left ventricular, following sudden emotional
    stress I51.81
  liver K76.89
  male - *see* Dysfunction, sexual, male
  orgasmic (female) F52.31
    male F52.32
  ovary E28.9

Dysfunction - *continued*
  specified NEC E28.8
  papillary muscle I51.89
  parathyroid E21.4
  physiological NEC R68.89
    psychogenic F59
  pineal gland E34.8
  pituitary (gland) E23.3
  platelets D69.1
  polyglandular E31.9
    specified NEC E31.8
  psychophysiologic F59
  psychosexual F52.9
    with
      dyspareunia F52.6
      premature ejaculation F52.4
      vaginismus F52.5
  pylorus K31.9
  rectum K59.9
    psychogenic F45.8
  reflex (sympathetic) - *see* Syndrome, pain,
  complex regional I
  segmental - *see* Dysfunction, somatic
  senile R54
  sexual (due to) R37
    alcohol F10.981
    amphetamine F15.981
      in
        abuse F15.181
        dependence F15.281
    anxiolytic F13.981
      in
        abuse F13.181
        dependence F13.281
    cocaine F14.981
      in
        abuse F14.181
        dependence F14.281
    excessive sexual drive F52.8
    failure of genital response (male) F52.21
      female F52.22
    female N94.9
      aversion F52.1
      dyspareunia N94.10
        psychogenic F52.6
      frigidity F52.22
      nymphomania F52.8
      orgasmic F52.31
      psychogenic F52.9
        aversion F52.1
        dyspareunia F52.6
        frigidity F52.22
        nymphomania F52.8
        orgasmic F52.31
        vaginismus F52.5
      vaginismus N94.2
        psychogenic F52.5
    hypnotic F13.981
      in
        abuse F13.181
        dependence F13.281
    inhibited orgasm (female) F52.31
      male F52.32
    lack
      of sexual enjoyment F52.1
      or loss of sexual desire F52.0
    male N53.9
      anejaculatory orgasm N53.13
      ejaculatory N53.19
        painful N53.12
        premature F52.4
        retarded N53.11
      erectile N52.9
        drug induced N52.2

Dysfunction - *continued*
  due to
    disease classified elsewhere N52.1
    drug N52.2
    postoperative (postprocedural) N52.39
    following
      cryotherapy N52.37
      interstitial seed therapy N52.36
      prostate ablative therapy N52.37
      prostatectomy N52.34
        radical N52.31
      radiation therapy N52.35
      radical cystectomy N52.32
      ultrasound ablative therapy N52.37
      urethral surgery N52.33
    psychogenic F52.21
    specified cause NEC N52.8
    vasculogenic
      arterial insufficiency N52.01
        with corporo-venous occlusive N52.03
      corporo-venous occlusive N52.02
        with arterial insufficiency N52.03
  impotence - *see* Dysfunction, sexual, male,
    erectile
  psychogenic F52.9
    aversion F52.1
    erectile F52.21
    orgasmic F52.32
    premature ejaculation F52.4
    satyriasis F52.8
    specified type NEC F52.8
    specified type NEC N53.8
  nonorganic F52.9
    specified NEC F52.8
  opioid F11.981
    in
      abuse F11.181
      dependence F11.281
  orgasmic dysfunction (female) F52.31
    male F52.32
  premature ejaculation F52.4
  psychoactive substances NEC F19.981
    in
      abuse F19.181
      dependence F19.281
  psychogenic F52.9
  sedative F13.981
    in
      abuse F13.181
      dependence F13.281
  sexual aversion F52.1
  vaginismus (nonorganic) (psychogenic)
    F52.5
sinoatrial node I49.5
somatic M99.09
  abdomen M99.09
  acromioclavicular M99.07
  cervical region M99.01
  cervicothoracic M99.01
  costochondral M99.08
  costovertebral M99.08
  head region M99.00
  hip M99.05
  lower extremity M99.06
  lumbar region M99.03
  lumbosacral M99.03
  occipitocervical M99.00
  pelvic region M99.05
  pubic M99.05
  rib cage M99.08
  sacral region M99.04
  sacrococcygeal M99.04
  sacroiliac M99.04
  specified NEC M99.09

Dysfunction - *continued*
  sternochondral M99.08
  sternoclavicular M99.07
  thoracic region M99.02
  thoracolumbar M99.02
  upper extremity M99.07
  somatoform autonomic F45.8
  stomach K31.89
    psychogenic F45.8
  suprarenal E27.9
    hyperfunction E27.0
  symbolic R48.9
    specified type NEC R48.8
  temporomandibular (joint) M26.69
    joint-pain syndrome M26.62-
  testicular (endocrine) E29.9
    specified NEC E29.8
  thymus E32.9
  thyroid E07.9
  ureterostomy (stoma) - *see* Complications,
  stoma, urinary tract
  uterus, complicating delivery O62.9
    hypertonic O62.4
    hypotonic O62.2
      primary O62.0
      secondary O62.1
  ventricular I51.9
    with congestive heart failure (see also
      Failure, heart) I50.9
    left, reversible, following sudden emotional
    stress I51.81
Dysgenesis
  gonadal (due to chromosomal anomaly) Q96.9
    pure Q99.1
  renal Q60.5
    bilateral Q60.4
    unilateral Q60.3
  reticular D72.0
  tidal platelet D69.3
Dysgerminoma
  specified site - *see* Neoplasm, malignant, by
  site
  unspecified site
    female C56.9
    male C62.90
Dysgeusia R43.2
Dysgraphia R27.8
Dyshidrosis, dysidrosis L30.1
Dyskaryotic cervical smear R87.619
Dyskeratosis L85.8
  cervix - *see* Dysplasia, cervix
  congenital Q82.8
  uterus NEC N85.8
Dyskinesia G24.9
  biliary (cystic duct or gallbladder) K82.8
  drug induced
    orofacial G24.01
  esophagus K22.4
  hysterical F44.4
  intestinal K59.8
  nonorganic origin F44.4
  orofacial (idiopathic) G24.4
    drug induced G24.01
  psychogenic F44.4
  subacute, drug induced G24.01
  tardive G24.01
    neuroleptic induced G24.01
  trachea J39.8
  tracheobronchial J98.09
Dyslalia (developmental) F80.0
Dyslexia R48.0
  developmental F81.0

Dyslipidemia E78.5
  depressed HDL cholesterol E78.6
  elevated fasting triglycerides E78.1
Dysmaturity - *see also* Light for dates
  pulmonary (newborn) (Wilson-Mikity) P27.0
Dysmenorrhea (essential) (exfoliative) N94.6
  congestive (syndrome) N94.6
  primary N94.4
  psychogenic F45.8
  secondary N94.5
Dysmetabolic syndrome X E88.81
Dysmetria R27.8
Dysmorphism (due to)
  alcohol Q86.0
  exogenous cause NEC Q86.8
  hydantoin Q86.1
  warfarin Q86.2
Dysmorphophobia (nondelusional) F45.22
  delusional F22
Dysnomia R47.01
Dysorexia R63.0
  psychogenic F50.89
Dysostosis
  cleidocranial, cleidocranialis Q74.0
  craniofacial Q75.1
  Fairbank's (idiopathic familial generalized
    osteophytosis) Q78.9
  mandibulofacial (incomplete) Q75.4
  multiplex E76.01
  oculomandibular Q75.5
Dyspareunia (female) N94.10
  deep N94.12
  male N53.12
  nonorganic F52.6
  psychogenic F52.6
  secondary N94.19
  specified NEC N94.19
  superficial (introital) N94.11
Dyspepsia R10.13
  atonic K30
  functional (allergic) (congenital)
    (gastrointestinal) (occupational) (reflex) K30
  intestinal K59.8
  nervous F45.8
  neurotic F45.8
  psychogenic F45.8
Dysphagia R13.10
  cervical R13.19
  following
    cerebral infarction I69.391
    cerebrovascular disease I69.991
      specified NEC I69.891
    intracerebral hemorrhage I69.191
    nontraumatic intracranial hemorrhage NEC
      I69.291
    specified disease NEC I69.891
    subarachnoid hemorrhage I69.091
  functional (hysterical) F45.8
  hysterical F45.8
  nervous (hysterical) F45.8
  neurogenic R13.19
  oral phase R13.11
  oropharyngeal phase R13.12
  pharyngeal phase R13.13
  pharyngoesophageal phase R13.14
  psychogenic F45.8
  sideropenic D50.1
  spastica K22.4
  specified NEC R13.19
Dysphagocytosis, congenital D71
Dysphasia R47.02
  developmental
    expressive type F80.1
    receptive type F80.2

Dysphasia - *continued*
following
cerebrovascular disease I69.921
cerebral infarction I69.321
intracerebral hemorrhage I69.121
nontraumatic intracranial hemorrhage NEC I69.221
specified disease NEC I69.821
subarachnoid hemorrhage I69.021
Dysphonia R49.0
functional F44.4
hysterical F44.4
psychogenic F44.4
spastica J38.3
Dysphoria
gender F64.9
specified NEC F64.8
in
adolescence and adulthood F64.0
children F64.2
postpartal O90.6
Dyspituitarism E23.3
Dysplasia - *see also* Anomaly
acetabular, congenital Q65.89
alveolar capillary, with vein misalignment J84.843
anus (histologically confirmed) (mild) (moderate) K62.82
severe D01.3
arrhythmogenic right ventricular I42.8
arterial, fibromuscular I77.3
asphyxiating thoracic (congenital) Q77.2
brain Q07.9
bronchopulmonary, perinatal P27.1
cervix (uteri) N87.9
mild N87.0
moderate N87.1
severe D06.9
chondroectodermal Q77.6
colon D12.6
craniometaphyseal Q78.8
dentinal K00.5
diaphyseal, progressive Q78.3
dystrophic Q77.5
ectodermal (anhidrotic) (congenital) (hereditary) Q82.4
hidrotic Q82.8
epithelial, uterine cervix - *see* Dysplasia, cervix
eye (congenital) Q11.2
fibrous
bone NEC (monostotic) M85.00
ankle M85.07-
foot M85.07-
forearm M85.03-
hand M85.04-
lower leg M85.06-
multiple site M85.09
neck M85.08
rib M85.08
shoulder M85.01-
skull M85.08
specified site NEC M85.08
thigh M85.05-
toe M85.07-
upper arm M85.02-
vertebra M85.08
diaphyseal, progressive Q78.3
jaw M27.8
polyostotic Q78.1
florid osseous - *see also* Cyst, calcifying odontogenic
high grade, focal D12.6
hip, congenital Q65.89

Dysplasia - *continued*
joint, congenital Q74.8
kidney Q61.4
multicystic Q61.4
leg Q74.2
lung, congenital (not associated with short gestation) Q33.6
mammary (gland) (benign) N60.9-
cyst (solitary) - *see* Cyst, breast
cystic - *see* Mastopathy, cystic
duct ectasia - *see* Ectasia, mammary duct
fibroadenosis - *see* Fibroadenosis, breast
fibrosclerosis - *see* Fibrosclerosis, breast
specified type NEC N60.8-
metaphyseal Q78.5
muscle Q79.8
oculodentodigital Q87.0
periapical (cemental) (cemento-osseous) - *see* Cyst, calcifying odontogenic
periosteum - *see* Disorder, bone, specified type NEC
polyostotic fibrous Q78.1
prostate - *see also* Neoplasia, intraepithelial, prostate N42.30
severe D07.5
specified NEC N42.39
renal Q61.4
multicystic Q61.4
retinal, congenital Q14.1
right ventricular, arrhythmogenic I42.8
septo-optic Q04.4
skin L98.8
spinal cord Q06.1
spondyloepiphyseal Q77.7
thymic, with immunodeficiency D82.1
vagina N89.3
mild N89.0
moderate N89.1
severe NEC D07.2
vulva N90.3
mild N90.0
moderate N90.1
severe NEC D07.1
Dyspnea (nocturnal) (paroxysmal) R06.00
asthmatic (bronchial) J45.909
with
exacerbation (acute) J45.901
bronchitis J45.909
with
exacerbation (acute) J45.901
status asthmaticus J45.902
chronic J44.9
status asthmaticus J45.902
cardiac - *see* Failure, ventricular, left
cardiac - *see* Failure, ventricular, left
functional F45.8
hyperventilation R06.4
hysterical F45.8
newborn P28.89
orthopnea R06.01
psychogenic F45.8
shortness of breath R06.02
specified type NEC R06.09
Dyspraxia R27.8
developmental (syndrome) F82
Dysproteinemia E88.09
Dysreflexia, autonomic G90.4
Dysrhythmia
cardiac I49.9
newborn
bradycardia P29.12
occurring before birth P03.819
before onset of labor P03.810
during labor P03.811

Dysrhythmia - *continued*
tachycardia P29.11
postoperative I97.89
cerebral or cortical - *see* Epilepsy
Dyssomnia - *see* Disorder, sleep
Dyssynergia
biliary K83.8
bladder sphincter N36.44
cerebellaris myoclonica (Hunt's ataxia) G11.1
Dysthymia F34.1
Dysthyroidism E07.9
Dystocia O66.9
affecting newborn P03.1
cervical (hypotonic) O62.2
affecting newborn P03.6
primary O62.0
secondary O62.1
contraction ring O62.4
fetal O66.9
abnormality NEC O66.3
conjoined twins O66.3
oversize O66.2
maternal O66.9
positional O64.9
shoulder (girdle) O66.0
causing obstructed labor O66.0
uterine NEC O62.4
Dystonia G24.9
deformans progressiva G24.1
drug induced NEC G24.09
acute G24.02
specified NEC G24.09
familial G24.1
idiopathic G24.1
familial G24.1
nonfamilial G24.2
orofacial G24.4
lenticularis G24.8
musculorum deformans G24.1
neuroleptic induced (acute) G24.02
orofacial (idiopathic) G24.4
oromandibular G24.4
due to drug G24.01
specified NEC G24.8
torsion (familial) (idiopathic) G24.1
acquired G24.8
genetic G24.1
symptomatic (nonfamilial) G24.2
Dystonic movements R25.8
Dystrophy, dystrophia
adiposogenital E23.6
Becker's type G71.0
cervical sympathetic G90.2
choroid (hereditary) H31.20
central areolar H31.22
choroideremia H31.21
gyrate atrophy H31.23
specified type NEC H31.29
cornea (hereditary) H18.50
endothelial H18.51
epithelial H18.52
granular H18.53
lattice H18.54
macular H18.55
specified type NEC H18.59
Duchenne's type G71.0
due to malnutrition E45
Erb's G71.0
Fuchs' H18.51
Gower's muscular G71.0
hair L67.8
infantile neuraxonal G31.89
Landouzy-Déjérine G71.0
Leyden-Mobius G71.0

Dystrophy, dystrophia - *continued*
  muscular G71.0
    benign (Becker type) G71.0
    congenital (hereditary) (progressive) (with
      specific morphological abnormalities of
      the muscle fiber) G71.0
      myotonic G71.11
    distal G71.0
    Duchenne type G71.0
    Emery-Dreifuss G71.0
    Erb type G71.0
    facioscapulohumeral G71.0
    Gower's G71.0
    hereditary (progressive) G71.0
    Landouzy-Déjérine type G71.0
    limb-girdle G71.0
    myotonic G71.11
    progressive (hereditary) G71.0
      Charcot-Marie (-tooth) type G60.0
    pseudohypertrophic (infantile) G71.0
    severe (Duchenne type) G71.0
  myocardium, myocardial - *see* Degeneration,
    myocardial
  myotonic, myotonica G71.11
  nail L60.3
    congenital Q84.6
  nutritional E45
  ocular G71.0
  oculocerebrorenal E72.03
  oculopharyngeal G71.0
  ovarian N83.8
  polyglandular E31.8
  reflex (neuromuscular) (sympathetic) - *see*
    Syndrome, pain, complex regional I
  retinal (hereditary) H35.50
    in
      lipid storage disorders E75.6 [*H36*]
      systemic lipidoses E75.6 [*H36*]
    involving
      pigment epithelium H35.54
      sensory area H35.53
    pigmentary H35.52
    vitreoretinal H35.51
  Salzmann's nodular - *see* Degeneration,
    cornea, nodular
  scapuloperoneal G71.0
  skin NEC L98.8
  sympathetic (reflex) - *see* Syndrome, pain,
    complex regional I
    cervical G90.2
  tapetoretinal H35.54
  thoracic, asphyxiating Q77.2
  unguium L60.3
    congenital Q84.6
  vitreoretinal H35.51
  vulva N90.4
  yellow (liver) - *see* Failure, hepatic
Dysuria R30.0
  psychogenic F45.8

E

Eales' disease H35.06-
Ear - *see also* condition
  piercing Z41.3
  tropical NEC B36.9 [*H62.40*]
    in
      aspergillosis B44.89
      candidiasis B37.84
      moniliasis B37.84
  wax (impacted) H61.20
    left H61.22
      with right H61.23
    right H61.21

Ear - *continued*
    with left H61.23
Earache - *see* subcategory H92.0
Early satiety R68.81
Eaton-lambert syndrome - *see* Syndrome,
  Lambert-Eaton
Eberth's disease (typhoid fever) A01.00
Ebola virus disease A98.4
Ebstein's anomaly or syndrome (heart) Q22.5
Eccentro-osteochondrodysplasia E76.29
Ecchondroma - *see* Neoplasm, bone, benign
Ecchondrosis D48.0
Ecchymosis R58
  conjunctiva - *see* Hemorrhage, conjunctiva
  eye (traumatic) - *see* Contusion, eyeball
  eyelid (traumatic) - *see* Contusion, eyelid
  newborn P54.5
  spontaneous R23.3
  traumatic - *see* Contusion
Echinococciasis - *see* Echinococcus
Echinococcosis - *see* Echinococcus
Echinococcus (infection) B67.90
  granulosus B67.4
    bone B67.2
    liver B67.0
    lung B67.1
    multiple sites B67.32
    specified site NEC B67.39
    thyroid B67.31
  liver NOS B67.8
    granulosus B67.0
    multilocularis B67.5
  lung NEC B67.99
    granulosus B67.1
    multilocularis B67.69
  multilocularis B67.7
    liver B67.5
    multiple sites B67.61
    specified site NEC B67.69
  specified site NEC B67.99
    granulosus B67.39
    multilocularis B67.69
  thyroid NEC B67.99
    granulosus B67.31
    multilocularis B67.69 [*E35*]
Echinorhynchiasis B83.8
Echinostomiasis B66.8
Echolalia R48.8
Echovirus, as cause of disease classified
  elsewhere B97.12
Eclampsia, eclamptic (coma) (convulsions)
  (delirium) (with hypertension) NEC O15.9
  complicating
    labor and delivery O15.1
    postpartum O15.2
    pregnancy O15.0-
    puerperium O15.2
Economic circumstances affecting care Z59.9
Economo's disease A85.8
Ectasia, ectasis
  annuloaortic I35.8
  aorta I77.819
    with aneurysm - *see* Aneurysm, aorta
    abdominal I77.811
    thoracic I77.810
    thoracoabdominal I77.812
  breast - *see* Ectasia, mammary duct
  capillary I78.8
  cornea H18.71-
  gastric antral vascular (GAVE) K31.819
    with hemorrhage K31.811
    without hemorrhage K31.819
  mammary duct N60.4-
  salivary gland (duct) K11.8

Ectasia, ectasis - *continued*
  sclera - *see* Sclerectasia
Ecthyma L08.0
  contagiosum B08.02
  gangrenosum L08.0
  infectiosum B08.02
Ectocardia Q24.8
Ectodermal dysplasia (anhidrotic) Q82.4
Ectodermosis erosiva pluriorificialis L51.1
Ectopic, ectopia (congenital)
  abdominal viscera Q45.8
    due to defect in anterior abdominal wall
      Q79.59
  ACTH syndrome E24.3
  adrenal gland Q89.1
  anus Q43.5
  atrial beats I49.1
  beats I49.49
    atrial I49.1
    ventricular I49.3
  bladder Q64.10
  bone and cartilage in lung Q33.5
  brain Q04.8
  breast tissue Q83.8
  cardiac Q24.8
  cerebral Q04.8
  cordis Q24.8
  endometrium - *see* Endometriosis
  gastric mucosa Q40.2
  gestation - *see* Pregnancy, by site
  heart Q24.8
  hormone secretion NEC E34.2
  kidney (crossed) (pelvis) Q63.2
  lens, lentis Q12.1
  mole - *see* Pregnancy, by site
  organ or site NEC - *see* Malposition,
    congenital
  pancreas Q45.3
  pregnancy - *see* Pregnancy, ectopic
  pupil - *see* Abnormality, pupillary
  renal Q63.2
  sebaceous glands of mouth Q38.6
  spleen Q89.09
  testis Q53.00
    bilateral Q53.02
    unilateral Q53.01
  thyroid Q89.2
  tissue in lung Q33.5
  ureter Q62.63
  ventricular beats I49.3
  vesicae Q64.10
Ectromelia Q73.8
  lower limb - *see* Defect, reduction, limb,
    lower, specified type NEC
  upper limb - *see* Defect, reduction, limb,
    upper, specified type NEC
Ectropion H02.109
  cervix N86
    with cervicitis N72
  congenital Q10.1
  eyelid (paralytic) H02.109
    cicatricial H02.119
      left H02.116
        lower H02.115
        upper H02.114
      right H02.113
        lower H02.112
        upper H02.111
    congenital Q10.1
    left H02.106
      lower H02.105
      upper H02.104
    mechanical H02.129
      left H02.126

Ectropion - *continued*
- lower H02.125
- upper H02.124
- right H02.123
  - lower H02.122
  - upper H02.121
- right H02.103
  - lower H02.102
  - upper H02.101
- senile H02.139
  - left H02.136
    - lower H02.135
    - upper H02.134
  - right H02.133
    - lower H02.132
    - upper H02.131
- spastic H02.149
  - left H02.146
    - lower H02.145
    - upper H02.144
  - right H02.143
    - lower H02.142
    - upper H02.141
- iris H21.89
- lip (acquired) K13.0
  - congenital Q38.0
- urethra N36.8
- uvea H21.89

Eczema (acute) (chronic) (erythematous) (fissum) (rubrum) (squamous) - *see also*
Dermatitis L30.9
- contact - *see* Dermatitis, contact
- dyshidrotic L30.1
- external ear - *see* Otitis, externa, acute, eczematoid
- flexural L20.82
- herpeticum B00.0
- hypertrophicum L28.0
- hypostatic - *see* Varix, leg, with, inflammation
- impetiginous L01.1
- infantile (due to any substance) L20.83
  - intertriginous L21.1
  - seborrheic L21.1
- intertriginous NEC L30.4
  - infantile L21.1
- intrinsic (allergic) L20.84
- lichenified NEC L28.0
- marginatum (hebrae) B35.6
- pustular L30.3
- stasis I87.2
  - with varicose veins - *see* Varix, leg, with, inflammation
- vaccination, vaccinatum T88.1
- varicose - *see* Varix, leg, with, inflammation

Eczematid L30.2
Eddowes (-Spurway) syndrome Q78.0
Edema, edematous (infectious) (pitting) (toxic) R60.9
- with nephritis - *see* Nephrosis
- allergic T78.3
- amputation stump (surgical) (sequelae (late effect)) T87.89
- angioneurotic (allergic) (any site) (with urticaria) T78.3
  - hereditary D84.1
- angiospastic I73.9
- Berlin's (traumatic) S05.8X-
- brain (cytotoxic) (vasogenic) G93.6
  - due to birth injury P11.0
  - newborn (anoxia or hypoxia) P52.4
    - birth injury P11.0
  - traumatic - *see* Injury, intracranial, cerebral edema
- cardiac - *see* Failure, heart, congestive

Edema, edematous - *continued*
- cardiovascular - *see* Failure, heart, congestive
- cerebral - *see* Edema, brain
- cerebrospinal - *see* Edema, brain
- cervix (uteri) (acute) N88.8
  - puerperal, postpartum O90.89
- chronic hereditary Q82.0
- circumscribed, acute T78.3
  - hereditary D84.1
- conjunctiva H11.42-
- cornea H18.2-
  - idiopathic H18.22-
  - secondary H18.23-
    - due to contact lens H18.21-
- due to
  - lymphatic obstruction I89.0
  - salt retention E87.0
- epiglottis - *see* Edema, glottis
- essential, acute T78.3
  - hereditary D84.1
- extremities, lower - *see* Edema, legs
- eyelid NEC H02.849
  - left H02.846
    - lower H02.845
    - upper H02.844
  - right H02.843
    - lower H02.842
    - upper H02.841
- familial, hereditary Q82.0
- famine - *see* Malnutrition, severe
- generalized R60.1
- glottis, glottic, glottidis (obstructive) (passive) J38.4
  - allergic T78.3
    - hereditary D84.1
- heart - *see* Failure, heart, congestive
- heat T67.7
- hereditary Q82.0
- inanition - *see* Malnutrition, severe
- intracranial G93.6
- iris H21.89
- joint - *see* Effusion, joint
- larynx - *see* Edema, glottis
- legs R60.0
  - due to venous obstruction I87.1
  - hereditary Q82.0
- localized R60.0
  - due to venous obstruction I87.1
- lower limbs - *see* Edema, legs
- lung J81.1
  - with heart condition or failure - *see* Failure, ventricular, left
  - acute J81.0
  - chemical (acute) J68.1
    - chronic J68.1
  - chronic J81.1
  - due to
    - chemicals, gases, fumes or vapors (inhalation) J68.1
    - external agent J70.9
      - specified NEC J70.8
    - radiation J70.1
  - due to
    - chemicals, fumes or vapors (inhalation) J68.1
    - external agent J70.9
      - specified NEC J70.8
    - high altitude T70.29
    - near drowning T75.1
    - radiation J70.0
  - meaning failure, left ventricle I50.1
- lymphatic I89.0
  - due to mastectomy I97.2
- macula H35.81

Edema, edematous - *continued*
- cystoid, following cataract surgery - *see* Complications, postprocedural, following cataract surgery
- diabetic - *see* Diabetes, by type, with, retinopathy, with macular edema
- malignant - *see* Gangrene, gas
- Milroy's Q82.0
- nasopharynx J39.2
- newborn P83.30
  - hydrops fetalis - *see* Hydrops, fetalis
  - specified NEC P83.39
- nutritional - *see also* Malnutrition, severe
  - with dyspigmentation, skin and hair E40
- optic disc or nerve - *see* Papilledema
- orbit H05.22-
- pancreas K86.89
- papilla, optic - *see* Papilledema
- penis N48.89
- periodic T78.3
  - hereditary D84.1
- pharynx J39.2
- pulmonary - *see* Edema, lung
- Quincke's T78.3
  - hereditary D84.1
- renal - *see* Nephrosis
- retina H35.81
  - diabetic - *see* Diabetes, by type, with, retinopathy, with macular edema
- salt E87.0
- scrotum N50.89
- seminal vesicle N50.89
- spermatic cord N50.89
- spinal (cord) (vascular) (nontraumatic) G95.19
- starvation - *see* Malnutrition, severe
- stasis - *see* Hypertension, venous, (chronic)
- subglottic - *see* Edema, glottis
- supraglottic - *see* Edema, glottis
- testis N44.8
- tunica vaginalis N50.89
- vas deferens N50.89
- vulva (acute) N90.89

Edentulism - *see* Absence, teeth, acquired
Edsall's disease T67.2
Educational handicap Z55.9
- specified NEC Z55.8
Edward's syndrome - *see* Trisomy, 18
Effect, adverse
- abnormal gravitational (G) forces or states T75.81
- abuse - *see* Maltreatment
- air pressure T70.9
  - specified NEC T70.8
- altitude (high) - *see* Effect, adverse, high altitude
- anesthesia - *see also* Anesthesia T88.59
  - in labor and delivery O74.9
  - local, toxic
    - in labor and delivery O74.4
    - in pregnancy NEC O29.3-
    - postpartum, puerperal O89.3
  - postpartum, puerperal O89.9
  - specified NEC T88.59
    - in labor and delivery O74.8
    - postpartum, puerperal O89.8
  - spinal and epidural T88.59
    - headache T88.59
      - in labor and delivery O74.5
      - postpartum, puerperal O89.4
    - specified NEC
      - in labor and delivery O74.6
      - postpartum, puerperal O89.5
- antitoxin - *see* Complications, vaccination
- atmospheric pressure T70.9

Effect, adverse - *continued*
due to explosion T70.8
high T70.3
low - *see* Effect, adverse, high altitude
specified effect NEC T70.8
biological, correct substance properly
administered - *see* Effect, adverse, drug
blood (derivatives) (serum) (transfusion) - *see*
Complications, transfusion
chemical substance - *see* Table of Drugs and
Chemicals
cold (temperature) (weather) T69.9
chilblains T69.1
frostbite - *see* Frostbite
specified effect NEC T69.8
drugs and medicaments T88.7
specified drug - *see* Table of Drugs and
Chemicals, by drug, adverse effect
specified effect
code to condition
electric current, electricity (shock) T75.4
burn - *see* Burn
exertion (excessive) T73.3
exposure - *see* Exposure
external cause NEC T75.89
foodstuffs T78.1
allergic reaction - *see* Allergy, food
causing anaphylaxis - *see* Shock,
anaphylactic, due to food
noxious - *see* Poisoning, food, noxious
gases, fumes, or vapors T59.9-
specified agent - *see* Table of Drugs and
Chemicals
glue (airplane) sniffing
due to drug abuse - *see* Abuse, drug, inhalant
due to drug dependence - *see* Dependence,
drug, inhalant
heat - *see* Heat
high altitude NEC T70.29
anoxia T70.29
on
ears T70.0
sinuses T70.1
polycythemia D75.1
high pressure fluids T70.4
hot weather - *see* Heat
hunger T73.0
immersion, foot - *see* Immersion
immunization - *see* Complications, vaccination
immunological agents - *see* Complications,
vaccination
infrared (radiation) (rays) NOS T66
dermatitis or eczema L59.8
infusion - *see* Complications, infusion
lack of care of infants - *see* Maltreatment,
child
lightning - *see* Lightning
medical care T88.9
specified NEC T88.8
medicinal substance, correct, properly
administered - *see* Effect, adverse, drug
motion T75.3
noise, on inner ear - *see* subcategory H83.3
overheated places - *see* Heat
psychosocial, of work environment Z56.5
radiation (diagnostic) (infrared) (natural
source) (therapeutic) (ultraviolet) (X-ray) NOS
T66
dermatitis or eczema - *see* Dermatitis, due to,
radiation
fibrosis of lung J70.1
pneumonitis J70.0
pulmonary manifestations
acute J70.0

Effect, adverse - *continued*
chronic J70.1
skin L59.9
radioactive substance NOS
dermatitis or eczema - *see* Radiodermatitis
reduced temperature T69.9
immersion foot or hand - *see* Immersion
specified effect NEC T69.8
serum NEC - *see also* Reaction, serum T80.69
specified NEC T78.8
external cause NEC T75.89
strangulation - *see* Asphyxia, traumatic
submersion T75.1
thirst T73.1
toxic - *see* Toxicity
transfusion - *see* Complications, transfusion
ultraviolet (radiation) (rays) NOS T66
burn - *see* Burn
dermatitis or eczema - *see* Dermatitis, due to,
ultraviolet rays
acute L56.8
vaccine (any) - *see* Complications, vaccination
vibration - *see* Vibration, adverse effects
water pressure NEC T70.9
specified NEC T70.8
weightlessness T75.82
whole blood - *see* Complications, transfusion
work environment Z56.5
Effect(s) (of) (from) - *see* Effect, adverse NEC
Effects, late - *see* Sequelae
Effluvium
anagen L65.1
telogen L65.0
Effort syndrome (psychogenic) F45.8
Effusion
amniotic fluid - *see* Pregnancy, complicated
by, premature rupture of membranes
brain (serous) G93.6
bronchial - *see* Bronchitis
cerebral G93.6
cerebrospinal - *see also* Meningitis
vessel G93.6
chest - *see* Effusion, pleura
chylous, chyliform (pleura) J94.0
intracranial G93.6
joint M25.40
ankle M25.47-
elbow M25.42-
foot joint M25.47-
hand joint M25.44-
hip M25.45-
knee M25.46-
shoulder M25.41-
specified joint NEC M25.48
wrist M25.43-
malignant pleural J91.0
meninges - *see* Meningitis
pericardium, pericardial (noninflammatory)
I31.3
acute - *see* Pericarditis, acute
peritoneal (chronic) R18.8
pleura, pleurisy, pleuritic, pleuropericardial
J90
chylous, chyliform J94.0
due to systemic lupus erythematosus M32.13
in conditions classified elsewhere J91.8
influenzal - *see* Influenza, with, respiratory
manifestations NEC
malignant J91.0
newborn P28.89
tuberculous NEC A15.6
primary (progressive) A15.7
spinal - *see* Meningitis
thorax, thoracic - *see* Effusion, pleura

Egg shell nails L60.3
congenital Q84.6
Egyptian splenomegaly B65.1
Ehrlichiosis A77.40
due to
E. chafeensis A77.41
E. sennetsu A79.81
specified organism NEC A77.49
Ehlers-Danlos syndrome Q79.6
Eichstedt's disease B36.0
Eisenmenger's
complex or syndrome I27.83
defect Q21.8
Ejaculation
delayed F52.32
painful N53.12
premature F52.4
retarded N53.11
retrograde N53.14
semen, painful N53.12
psychogenic F52.6
Ekbom's syndrome (restless legs) G25.81
**Ekman's syndrome (brittle bones and blue
sclera)** Q78.0
Elastic skin Q82.8
acquired L57.4
Elastofibroma - *see* Neoplasm, connective
tissue, benign
Elastoma (juvenile) Q82.8
Miescher's L87.2
Elastomyofibrosis I42.4
Elastosis
actinic, solar L57.8
atrophicans (senile) L57.4
perforans serpiginosa L87.2
senilis L57.4
Elbow - *see* condition
**Electric current, electricity, effects
(concussion) (fatal) (nonfatal) (shock)** T75.4
burn - *see* Burn
Electric feet syndrome E53.8
Electrocution T75.4
from electroshock gun (taser) T75.4
Electrolyte imbalance E87.8
with
abortion - *see* Abortion by type, complicated
by, electrolyte imbalance
ectopic pregnancy O08.5
molar pregnancy O08.5
Elephantiasis (nonfilarial) I89.0
arabicum - *see* Infestation, filarial
bancroftian B74.0
congenital (any site) (hereditary) Q82.0
due to
Brugia (malayi) B74.1
timori B74.2
mastectomy I97.2
Wuchereria (bancrofti) B74.0
eyelid H02.859
left H02.856
lower H02.855
upper H02.854
right H02.853
lower H02.852
upper H02.851
filarial, filariensis - *see* Infestation, filarial
glandular I89.0
graecorum A30.9
lymphangiectatic I89.0
lymphatic vessel I89.0
due to mastectomy I97.2
scrotum (nonfilarial) I89.0
streptococcal I89.0
surgical I97.89

Elephantiasis (nonfilarial) - *continued*
  postmastectomy I97.2
  telangiectodes I89.0
  vulva (nonfilarial) N90.89
Elevated, elevation
  antibody titer R76.0
  basal metabolic rate R94.8
  blood pressure - *see also* Hypertension
    reading (incidental) (isolated) (nonspecific),
      no diagnosis of hypertension R03.0
  blood sugar R73.9
  body temperature (of unknown origin) R50.9
  C-reactive protein (CRP) R79.82
  cancer antigen 125 [CA 125] R97.1
  carcinoembryonic antigen [CEA] R97.0
  cholesterol E78.00
    with high triglycerides E78.2
  conjugate, eye H51.0
  diaphragm, congenital Q79.1
  erythrocyte sedimentation rate R70.0
  fasting glucose R73.01
  fasting triglycerides E78.1
  finding on laboratory examination - *see*
    Findings, abnormal, inconclusive, without
      diagnosis, by type of exam
  GFR (glomerular filtration rate) - *see* Findings,
    abnormal, inconclusive, without diagnosis,
    by type of exam
  glucose tolerance (oral) R73.02
  immunoglobulin level R76.8
  indoleacetic acid R82.5
  lactic acid dehydrogenase (LDH) level R74.0
  leukocytes D72.829
  lipoprotein a level E78.8
  liver function
    study R94.5
    test R79.89
      alkaline phosphatase R74.8
      aminotransferase R74.0
      bilirubin R17
      hepatic enzyme R74.8
      lactate dehydrogenase R74.0
  lymphocytes D72.820
  prostate specific antigen [PSA] R97.20
  Rh titer - *see* Complication(s), transfusion,
    incompatibility reaction, Rh (factor)
  scapula, congenital Q74.0
  sedimentation rate R70.0
  SGOT R74.0
  SGPT R74.0
  transaminase level R74.0
  triglycerides E78.1
    with high cholesterol E78.2
  tumor associated antigens [TAA] NEC R97.8
  tumor specific antigens [TSA] NEC R97.8
  urine level of
    catecholamine R82.5
    indoleacetic acid R82.5
    17-ketosteroids R82.5
    steroids R82.5
    vanillylmandelic acid (VMA) R82.5
  venous pressure I87.8
  white blood cell count D72.829
    specified NEC D72.828
Elliptocytosis (congenital) (hereditary) D58.1
  Hb C (disease) D58.1
  hemoglobin disease D58.1
  sickle-cell (disease) D57.8-
    trait D57.3
Ellison-Zollinger syndrome E16.4
**Ellis-van Creveld syndrome
  (chondroectodermal dysplasia)** Q77.6

Elongated, elongation (congenital) - *see also*
  Distortion
  bone Q79.9
  cervix (uteri) Q51.828
    acquired N88.4
    hypertrophic N88.4
  colon Q43.8
  common bile duct Q44.5
  cystic duct Q44.5
  frenulum, penis Q55.69
  labia minora (acquired) N90.69
  ligamentum patellae Q74.1
  petiolus (epiglottidis) Q31.8
  tooth, teeth K00.2
  uvula Q38.6
Eltor cholera A00.1
Emaciation (due to malnutrition) E41
Embadomoniasis A07.8
Embedded tooth, teeth K01.0
  root only K08.3
Embolic - *see* condition
Embolism (multiple) (paradoxical) I74.9
  air (any site) (traumatic) T79.0
    following
      abortion - *see* Abortion by type complicated
        by embolism
      ectopic pregnancy O08.2
      infusion, therapeutic injection or transfusion
        T80.0
      molar pregnancy O08.2
      procedure NEC
        artery T81.719
          mesenteric T81.710
          renal T81.711
          specified NEC T81.718
        vein T81.72
    in pregnancy, childbirth or puerperium - *see*
      Embolism, obstetric
  amniotic fluid (pulmonary) - *see also*
    Embolism, obstetric
    following
      abortion - *see* Abortion by type complicated
        by embolism
      ectopic pregnancy O08.2
      molar pregnancy O08.2
  aorta, aortic I74.10
    abdominal I74.09
      saddle I74.01
    bifurcation I74.09
      saddle I74.01
    thoracic I74.11
  artery I74.9
    auditory, internal I65.8
    basilar - *see* Occlusion, artery, basilar
    carotid (common) (internal) - *see* Occlusion,
      artery, carotid
    cerebellar (anterior inferior) (posterior
      inferior) (superior) I66.3
    cerebral - *see* Occlusion, artery, cerebral
    choroidal (anterior) I65.8
    communicating posterior I65.8
    coronary - *see also* Infarct, myocardium
      not resulting in infarction I24.0
    extremity I74.4
      lower I74.3
      upper I74.2
    hypophyseal I65.8
    iliac I74.5
    limb I74.4
      lower I74.3
      upper I74.2
    mesenteric (with gangrene) - *see also*
      Ischemia, intestine, acute K55.059
    ophthalmic - *see* Occlusion, artery, retina

Embolism - *continued*
  peripheral I74.4
  pontine I65.8
  precerebral - *see* Occlusion, artery,
    precerebral
  pulmonary - *see* Embolism, pulmonary
  renal N28.0
  retinal - *see* Occlusion, artery, retina
  septic I76
  specified NEC I74.8
  vertebral - *see* Occlusion, artery, vertebral
  basilar (artery) I65.1
  blood clot
    following
      abortion - *see* Abortion by type complicated
        by embolism
      ectopic or molar pregnancy O08.2
    in pregnancy, childbirth or puerperium - *see*
      Embolism, obstetric
  brain - *see also* Occlusion, artery, cerebral
    following
      abortion - *see* Abortion by type complicated
        by embolism
      ectopic or molar pregnancy O08.2
    puerperal, postpartum, childbirth - *see*
      Embolism, obstetric
  capillary I78.8
  cardiac - *see also* Infarct, myocardium
    not resulting in infarction I51.3
  carotid (artery) (common) (internal) - *see*
    Occlusion, artery, carotid
  cavernous sinus (venous) - *see* Embolism,
    intracranial venous sinus
  cerebral - *see* Occlusion, artery, cerebral
  cholesterol - *see* Atheroembolism
  coronary (artery or vein) (systemic) - *see*
    Occlusion, coronary
  due to device, implant or graft - *see also*
  Complications, by site and type, specified
  NEC
    arterial graft NEC T82.818
    breast (implant) T85.818
    catheter NEC T85.818
      dialysis (renal) T82.818
        intraperitoneal T85.818
      infusion NEC T82.818
        spinal (epidural) (subdural) T85.810
      urinary (indwelling) T83.81
    electronic (electrode) (pulse generator)
      (stimulator)
      bone T84.81
      cardiac T82.817
      nervous system (brain) (peripheral nerve)
        (spinal) T85.810
      urinary T83.81
    fixation, internal (orthopedic) NEC T84.81
    gastrointestinal (bile duct) (esophagus)
      T85.818
    genital NEC T83.81
    heart (graft) (valve) T82.817
    joint prosthesis T84.81
    ocular (corneal graft) (orbital implant)
      T85.818
    orthopedic (bone graft) NEC T86.838
    specified NEC T85.818
    urinary (graft) NEC T83.81
    vascular NEC T82.818
    ventricular intracranial shunt T85.810
  extremities
    lower - *see* Embolism, vein, lower extremity
      arterial I74.3
    upper I74.2
  eye H34.9
  fat (cerebral) (pulmonary) (systemic) T79.1

Embolism - *continued*
following
abortion - *see* Abortion by type complicated
by embolism
ectopic or molar pregnancy O08.2
complicating delivery - *see* Embolism,
obstetric
following
abortion - *see* Abortion by type complicated
by embolism
ectopic or molar pregnancy O08.2
infusion, therapeutic injection or transfusion
air T80.0
heart (fatty) - *see also* Infarct, myocardium
not resulting in infarction I51.3
hepatic (vein) I82.0
in pregnancy, childbirth or puerperium - *see*
Embolism, obstetric
intestine (artery) (vein) (with gangrene) - *see*
also Ischemia, intestine, acute K55.039
intracranial - *see also* Occlusion, artery,
cerebral
venous sinus (any) G08
nonpyogenic I67.6
intraspinal venous sinuses or veins G08
nonpyogenic G95.19
kidney (artery) N28.0
lateral sinus (venous) - *see* Embolism,
intracranial, venous sinus
leg - *see* Embolism, vein, lower extremity
arterial I74.3
longitudinal sinus (venous) - *see* Embolism,
intracranial, venous sinus
lung (massive) - *see* Embolism, pulmonary
meninges I66.8
mesenteric (artery) (vein) (with gangrene) -
see also Ischemia, intestine, acute K55.059
obstetric (in) (pulmonary)
childbirth O88.22
air O88.02
amniotic fluid O88.12
blood clot O88.22
fat O88.82
pyemic O88.32
septic O88.32
specified type NEC O88.82
pregnancy O88.21-
air O88.01-
amniotic fluid O88.11-
blood clot O88.21-
fat O88.81-
pyemic O88.31-
septic O88.31-
specified type NEC O88.81-
puerperal O88.23
air O88.03
amniotic fluid O88.13
blood clot O88.23
fat O88.83
pyemic O88.33
septic O88.33
specified type NEC O88.83
ophthalmic - *see* Occlusion, artery, retina
penis N48.81
peripheral artery NOS I74.4
pituitary E23.6
popliteal (artery) I74.3
portal (vein) I81
postoperative, postprocedural
artery T81.719
mesenteric T81.710
renal T81.711
specified NEC T81.718
vein T81.72

Embolism - *continued*
precerebral artery - *see* Occlusion, artery,
precerebral
puerperal - *see* Embolism, obstetric
pulmonary (acute) (artery) (vein) I26.99
with acute cor pulmonale I26.09
chronic I27.82
following
abortion - *see* Abortion by type complicated
by embolism
ectopic or molar pregnancy O08.2
healed or old Z86.711
in pregnancy, childbirth or puerperium - *see*
Embolism, obstetric
personal history of Z86.711
saddle I26.92
with acute cor pulmonale I26.02
septic I26.90
with acute cor pulmonale I26.01
pyemic (multiple) I76
following
abortion - *see* Abortion by type complicated
by embolism
ectopic or molar pregnancy O08.2
Hemophilus influenzae A41.3
pneumococcal A40.3
with pneumonia J13
puerperal, postpartum, childbirth (any
organism) - *see* Embolism, obstetric
specified organism NEC A41.89
staphylococcal A41.2
streptococcal A40.9
renal (artery) N28.0
vein I82.3
retina, retinal - *see* Occlusion, artery, retina
saddle
abdominal aorta I74.01
pulmonary artery I26.92
with acute cor pulmonale I26.02
septic (arterial) I76
complicating abortion - *see* Abortion, by
type, complicated by, embolism
sinus - *see* Embolism, intracranial, venous
sinus
soap complicating abortion - *see* Abortion, by
type, complicated by, embolism
spinal cord G95.19
pyogenic origin G06.1
spleen, splenic (artery) I74.8
upper extremity I74.2
vein (acute) I82.90
antecubital I82.61-
chronic I82.71-
axillary I82.A1-
chronic I82.A2-
basilic I82.61-
chronic I82.71-
brachial I82.62-
chronic I82.72-
brachiocephalic (innominate) I82.290
chronic I82.291
cephalic I82.61-
chronic I82.71-
chronic I82.91
deep (DVT) I82.40-
calf I82.4Z-
chronic I82.5Z-
lower leg I82.4Z-
chronic I82.5Z-
thigh I82.4Y-
chronic I82.5Y-
upper leg I82.4Y
chronic I82.5Y-
femoral I82.41-

Embolism - *continued*
chronic I82.51-
iliac (iliofemoral) I82.42-
chronic I82.52-
innominate I82.290
chronic I82.291
internal jugular I82.C1-
chronic I82.C2-
lower extremity
deep I82.40-
chronic I82.50-
specified NEC I82.49-
chronic NEC I82.59-
distal
deep I82.4Z-
proximal
deep I82.4Y-
chronic I82.5Y-
superficial I82.81-
popliteal I82.43-
chronic I82.53-
radial I82.62-
chronic I82.72-
renal I82.3
saphenous (greater) (lesser) I82.81-
specified NEC I82.890
chronic NEC I82.891
subclavian I82.B1-
chronic I82.B2-
thoracic NEC I82.290
chronic I82.291
tibial I82.44-
chronic I82.54-
ulnar I82.62-
chronic I82.72-
upper extremity I82.60-
chronic I82.70-
deep I82.62-
chronic I82.72-
superficial I82.61-
chronic I82.71-
vena cava
inferior (acute) I82.220
chronic I82.221
superior (acute) I82.210
chronic I82.211
venous sinus G08
vessels of brain - *see* Occlusion, artery,
cerebral
Embolus - *see* Embolism
Embryoma - *see also* Neoplasm, uncertain
behavior, by site
benign - *see* Neoplasm, benign, by site
kidney C64.-
liver C22.0
malignant - *see also* Neoplasm, malignant, by
site
kidney C64.-
liver C22.0
testis C62.9-
descended (scrotal) C62.1-
undescended C62.0-
testis C62.9-
descended (scrotal) C62.1-
undescended C62.0-
Embryonic
circulation Q28.9
heart Q28.9
vas deferens Q55.4
Embryopathia NOS Q89.9
Embryotoxon Q13.4
Emesis - *see* Vomiting
Emotional lability R45.86
Emotionality, pathological F60.3

Emotogenic disease - *see* Disorder, psychogenic

Emphysema (atrophic) (bullous) (chronic) (interlobular) (lung) (obstructive) (pulmonary) (senile) (vesicular) J43.9
- cellular tissue (traumatic) T79.7
  - surgical T81.82
- centrilobular J43.2
- compensatory J98.3
- congenital (interstitial) P25.0
- conjunctiva H11.89
- connective tissue (traumatic) T79.7
  - surgical T81.82
- due to chemicals, gases, fumes or vapors J68.4
- eyelid(s) - *see* Disorder, eyelid, specified type NEC
  - surgical T81.82
  - traumatic T79.7
- interstitial J98.2
  - congenital P25.0
  - perinatal period P25.0
- laminated tissue T79.7
  - surgical T81.82
- mediastinal J98.2
  - newborn P25.2
- orbit, orbital - *see* Disorder, orbit, specified type NEC
- panacinar J43.1
- panlobular J43.1
- specified NEC J43.8
- subcutaneous (traumatic) T79.7
  - nontraumatic J98.2
  - postprocedural T81.82
  - surgical T81.82
- surgical T81.82
- thymus (gland) (congenital) E32.8
- traumatic (subcutaneous) T79.7
- unilateral J43.0

Empty nest syndrome Z60.0

Empyema (acute) (chest) (double) (pleura) (supradiaphragmatic) (thorax) J86.9
- with fistula J86.0
- accessory sinus (chronic) - *see* Sinusitis
- antrum (chronic) - *see* Sinusitis, maxillary
- brain (any part) - *see* Abscess, brain
- ethmoidal (chronic) (sinus) - *see* Sinusitis, ethmoidal
- extradural - *see* Abscess, extradural
- frontal (chronic) (sinus) - *see* Sinusitis, frontal
- gallbladder K81.0
- mastoid (process) (acute) - *see* Mastoiditis, acute
- maxilla, maxillary M27.2
  - sinus (chronic) - *see* Sinusitis, maxillary
- nasal sinus (chronic) - *see* Sinusitis
- sinus (accessory) (chronic) (nasal) - *see* Sinusitis
- sphenoidal (sinus) (chronic) - *see* Sinusitis, sphenoidal
- subarachnoid - *see* Abscess, extradural
- subdural - *see* Abscess, subdural
- tuberculous A15.6
- ureter - *see* Ureteritis
- ventricular - *see* Abscess, brain

En coup de sabre lesion L94.1

Enamel pearls K00.2

Enameloma K00.2

Enanthema, viral B09

Encephalitis (chronic) (hemorrhagic) (idiopathic) (nonepidemic) (spurious) (subacute) G04.90
- acute - *see also* Encephalitis, viral A86
  - disseminated G04.00
    - infectious G04.01

Encephalitis - *continued*
- noninfectious G04.81
  - postimmunization (postvaccination) G04.02
  - postinfectious G04.01
- inclusion body A85.8
- necrotizing hemorrhagic G04.30
  - postimmunization G04.32
  - postinfectious G04.31
  - specified NEC G04.39
- arboviral, arbovirus NEC A85.2
- arthropod-borne NEC (viral) A85.2
- Australian A83.4
- California (virus) A83.5
- Central European (tick-borne) A84.1
- Czechoslovakian A84.1
- Dawson's (inclusion body) A81.1
- diffuse sclerosing A81.1
- disseminated, acute G04.00
- due to
  - cat scratch disease A28.1
  - human immunodeficiency virus (HIV) disease B20 [*G05.3*]
  - malaria - *see* Malaria
  - rickettsiosis - *see* Rickettsiosis
  - smallpox inoculation G04.02
  - typhus - *see* Typhus
- Eastern equine A83.2
- endemic (viral) A86
- epidemic NEC (viral) A86
- equine (acute) (infectious) (viral) A83.9
  - Eastern A83.2
  - Venezuelan A92.2
  - Western A83.1
- Far Eastern (tick-borne) A84.0
- following vaccination or other immunization procedure G04.02
- herpes zoster B02.0
- herpesviral B00.4
  - due to herpesvirus 6 B10.01
  - due to herpesvirus 7 B10.09
  - specified NEC B10.09
- Ilhéus (virus) A83.8
- inclusion body A81.1
- in (due to)
  - actinomycosis A42.82
  - adenovirus A85.1
  - African trypanosomiasis B56.9 [*G05.3*]
  - Chagas' disease (chronic) B57.42
  - cytomegalovirus B25.8
  - enterovirus A85.0
  - herpes (simplex) virus B00.4
    - due to herpesvirus 6 B10.01
    - due to herpesvirus 7 B10.09
    - specified NEC B10.09
  - infectious disease NEC B99 [*G05.3*]
  - influenza - *see* Influenza, with, encephalopathy
  - listeriosis A32.12
  - measles B05.0
  - mumps B26.2
  - naegleriasis B60.2
  - parasitic disease NEC B89 [*G05.3*]
  - poliovirus A80.9 [*G05.3*]
  - rubella B06.01
  - syphilis
    - congenital A50.42
    - late A52.14
  - systemic lupus erythematosus M32.19
  - toxoplasmosis (acquired) B58.2
    - congenital P37.1
  - tuberculosis A17.82
  - zoster B02.0
- infectious (acute) (virus) NEC A86
- Japanese (B type) A83.0

Encephalitis - *continued*
- La Crosse A83.5
- lead - *see* Poisoning, lead
- lethargica (acute) (infectious) A85.8
- louping ill A84.8
- lupus erythematosus, systemic M32.19
- lymphatica A87.2
- Mengo A85.8
- meningococcal A39.81
- Murray Valley A83.4
- otitic NEC H66.40 [*G05.3*]
- parasitic NOS B71.9
- periaxial G37.0
- periaxialis (concentrica) (diffuse) G37.5
- post chickenpox B01.11
- postexanthematous NEC B09
- postimmunization G04.02
- postinfectious NEC G04.01
- postmeasles B05.0
- postvaccinal G04.02
- post varicella B01.11
- postviral NEC A86
- Powassan A84.8
- Rasmussen G04.81
- Rio Bravo A85.8
- Russian
  - autumnal A83.0
  - spring-summer (taiga) A84.0
- saturnine - *see* Poisoning, lead   specified NEC G04.81
- St. Louis A83.3
- subacute sclerosing A81.1
- summer A83.0
- suppurative G04.81
- tick-borne A84.9
- Torula, torular (cryptococcal) B45.1
- toxic NEC G92
- trichinosis B75 [*G05.3*]
- type
  - B A83.0
  - C A83.3
- van Bogaert's A81.1
- Venezuelan equine A92.2
- Vienna A85.8
- viral, virus A86
  - arthropod-borne NEC A85.2
    - mosquito-borne A83.9
      - Australian X disease A83.4
      - California virus A83.5
      - Eastern equine A83.2
      - Japanese (B type) A83.0
      - Murray Valley A83.4
      - specified NEC A83.8
      - St. Louis A83.3
      - type B A83.0
      - type C A83.3
      - Western equine A83.1
    - tick-borne A84.9
      - biundulant A84.1
      - central European A84.1
      - Czechoslovakian A84.1
      - diphasic meningoencephalitis A84.1
      - Far Eastern A84.0
      - Russian spring-summer (taiga) A84.0
      - specified NEC A84.8
    - specified type NEC A85.8
- Western equine A83.1

Encephalocele Q01.9
- frontal Q01.0
- nasofrontal Q01.1
- occipital Q01.2
- specified NEC Q01.8

Encephalocystocele - *see* Encephalocele

Encephaloduroarteriomyosynangiosis (EDAMS) I67.5
Encephalomalacia (brain) (cerebellar) (cerebral) - *see* Softening, brain
Encephalomeningitis - *see* Meningoencephalitis
Encephalomeningocele - *see* Encephalocele
Encephalomeningomyelitis - *see* Meningoencephalitis
Encephalomyelitis - *see also* Encephalitis G04.90
  acute disseminated G04.00
    infectious G04.01
    noninfectious G04.81
    postimmunization G04.02
    postinfectious G04.01
  acute necrotizing hemorrhagic G04.30
    postimmunization G04.32
    postinfectious G04.31
    specified NEC G04.39
  benign myalgic G93.3
  equine A83.9
    Eastern A83.2
    Venezuelan A92.2
    Western A83.1
  in diseases classified elsewhere G05.3
  myalgic, benign G93.3
  post chickenpox B01.11
  postinfectious NEC G04.01
  postmeasles B05.0
  postvaccinal G04.02
  post varicella B01.11
  rubella B06.01
  specified NEC G04.81
  Venezuelan equine A92.2
Encephalomyelocele - *see* Encephalocele
Encephalomyelomeningitis - *see* Meningoencephalitis
Encephalomyelopathy G96.9
Encephalomyeloradiculitis (acute) G61.0
Encephalomyeloradiculoneuritis (acute) (Guillain-Barré) G61.0
Encephalomyeloradiculopathy G96.9
Encephalopathia hyperbilirubinemic, newborn P57.9
  due to isoimmunization (conditions in P55) P57.0
Encephalopathy (acute) G93.40
  acute necrotizing hemorrhagic G04.30
    postimmunization G04.32
    postinfectious G04.31
    specified NEC G04.39
  alcoholic G31.2
  anoxic - *see* Damage, brain, anoxic
  arteriosclerotic I67.2
  centrolobar progressive (Schilder) G37.0
  congenital Q07.9
  degenerative, in specified disease NEC G32.89
  demyelinating callosal G37.1
  due to
    drugs - *see also* Table of Drugs and Chemicals G92
  hepatic - *see* Failure, hepatic
  hyperbilirubinemic, newborn P57.9
    due to isoimmunization (conditions in P55) P57.0
  hypertensive I67.4
  hypoglycemic E16.2
  hypoxic - *see* Damage, brain, anoxic
  hypoxic ischemic P91.60
    mild P91.61
    moderate P91.62
    severe P91.63
  in (due to) (with)

Encephalopathy (acute) - *continued*
  birth injury P11.1
  hyperinsulinism E16.1 [*G94*]
  influenza - *see* Influenza, with, encephalopathy
  lack of vitamin - *see also* Deficiency, vitamin E56.9 [*G32.89*]
  neoplastic disease (see also Neoplasm) D49.9 [*G13.1*]
  serum - *see also* Reaction, serum T80.69
  syphilis A52.17
  trauma (postconcussional) F07.81
    current injury - *see* Injury, intracranial
  vaccination G04.02
  lead - *see* Poisoning, lead metabolic G93.41
  drug induced G92
  toxic G92
  myoclonic, early, symptomatic - *see* Epilepsy, generalized, specified NEC
  necrotizing, subacute (Leigh) G31.82
  neonatal P91.819
    in diseases classified elsewhere P91.811
  pellagrous E52 [*G32.89*]
  portosystemic - *see* Failure, hepatic
  postcontusional F07.81
    current injury - *see* Injury, intracranial, diffuse posthypoglycemic (coma) E16.1 [*G94*]
  postradiation G93.89
  saturnine - *see* Poisoning, lead septic G93.41
  specified NEC G93.49
  spongiform, subacute (viral) A81.09
  toxic G92
    metabolic G92
  traumatic (postconcussional) F07.81
    current injury - *see* Injury, intracranial
  vitamin B deficiency NEC E53.9 [*G32.89*]
    vitamin B1 E51.2
  Wernicke's E51.2
Encephalorrhagia - *see* Hemorrhage, intracranial, intracerebral
Encephalosis, posttraumatic F07.81
Enchondroma - *see also* Neoplasm, bone, benign
Enchondromatosis (cartilaginous) (multiple) Q78.4
Encopresis R15.9
  functional F98.1
  nonorganic origin F98.1
  psychogenic F98.1
Encounter (with health service) (for) Z76.89
  adjustment and management (of)
    breast implant Z45.81
    implanted device NEC Z45.89
    myringotomy device (stent) (tube) Z45.82
  administrative purpose only Z02.9
    examination for
      adoption Z02.82
      armed forces Z02.3
      disability determination Z02.71
      driving license Z02.4
      employment Z02.1
      insurance Z02.6
      medical certificate NEC Z02.79
      paternity testing Z02.81
      residential institution admission Z02.2
      school admission Z02.0
      sports Z02.5
    specified reason NEC Z02.89
  aftercare - *see* Aftercare
  antenatal screening Z36.9
    cervical length Z36.86
    chromosomal anomalies Z36.0
    congenital cardiac abnormalities Z36.83

Encounter (with health service) (for) – *continued*
  elevated maternal serum alphafetoprotein level Z36.1
  fetal growth retardation Z36.4
  fetal lung maturity Z36.84
  fetal macrosomia Z36.88
  hydrops fetalis Z36.81
  intrauterine growth restriction (IUGR) /small-for-dates Z36.4
  isoimmunization Z36.5
  large-for-dates Z36.88
  malformations Z36.3
  non-visualized anatomy on a previous scan Z36.2
  nuchal translucency Z36.82
  raised alphafetoprotein level Z36.1
  risk of pre-term labor Z36.86
  specified type NEC Z36.89
  specified follow-up NEC Z36.2
  specified genetic defects NEC Z36.8A
  Streptococcus B Z36.85
  suspected anomaly Z36.3
  uncertain dates Z36.87
  assisted reproductive fertility procedure cycle Z31.83
  blood typing Z01.83
    Rh typing Z01.83
  breast augmentation or reduction Z41.1
  breast implant exchange (different material) (different size) Z45.81
  breast reconstruction following mastectomy Z42.1
  check-up - *see* Examination
  chemotherapy for neoplasm Z51.11
  colonoscopy, screening Z12.11
  counseling - *see* Counseling
  delivery, full-term, uncomplicated O80
    cesarean, without indication O82
  desensitization to allergens Z51.6
  ear piercing Z41.3
  examination - *see* Examination
  expectant parent(s) (adoptive) pre-birth pediatrician visit Z76.81
  fertility preservation procedure (prior to cancer therapy) (prior to removal of gonads) Z31.84
  fitting (of) - *see* Fitting (and adjustment) (of)
  genetic
    counseling
      nonprocreative Z71.83
      procreative Z31.5
    testing - *see* Test, genetic
  hearing conservation and treatment Z01.12
  immunotherapy for neoplasm Z51.12
  in vitro fertilization cycle Z31.83
  instruction (in)
    childbirth Z32.2
    child care (postpartal) (prenatal) Z32.3
    natural family planning
      procreative Z31.61
      to avoid pregnancy Z30.02
  insulin pump titration Z46.81
  joint prosthesis insertion following prior explantation of joint prosthesis (staged procedure)
    hip Z47.32
    knee Z47.33
    shoulder Z47.31
  laboratory (as part of a general medical examination) Z00.00
    with abnormal findings Z00.01
  mental health services (for)
    abuse NEC
      perpetrator Z69.82

Encounter (with health service) (for) – continued
    victim Z69.81
  child abuse
    nonparental
  child neglect
    nonparental
      perpetrator Z69.021
      victim Z69.020
    parental
      perpetrator Z69.011
      victim Z69.010
  child psychological abuse
    nonparental
      perpetrator Z69.021
      victim Z69.020
    parental
      perpetrator Z69.011
      victim Z69.010
  child sexual abuse
    nonparental
      perpetrator Z69.021
      victim Z69.020
    parental
      perpetrator Z69.011
      victim Z69.010
  non-spousal adult abuse (perpetrator) (victim) Z69.81
  spousal or partner
    abuse
      perpetrator Z69.12
      victim Z69.11
    neglect
      perpetrator Z69.12
      victim Z69.11
    psychological abuse
      perpetrator Z69.12
      victim Z69.11
    violence
      perpetrator (physical) (sexual) Z69.12
      victim (physical) Z69.11
      sexual Z69.81
  placental sample (taken vaginally) (see also Encounter, antenatal screening) Z36.9
    perpetrator Z69.021
    victim Z69.020
    parental
      perpetrator Z69.011
      victim Z69.010
  observation (for) (ruled out)
    exposure to (suspected)
      anthrax Z03.810
      biological agent NEC Z03.818
  pediatrician visit, by expectant parent(s) (adoptive) Z76.81
  plastic and reconstructive surgery following medical procedure or healed injury NEC Z42.8
  pregnancy
    supervision of - see Pregnancy, supervision of
    test Z32.00
      result negative Z32.02
      result positive Z32.01
  procreative management and counseling for gestational carrier Z31.7
  prophylactic measures Z29.9
    antivenin Z29.12
    fluoride administration Z29.3
    immunotherapy for respiratory syncytial virus (RSV) Z29.11
    rabies immune globin Z29.14
    Rho (D) immune globulin Z29.13
    specified NEC Z29.8

Encounter (with health service) (for) - continued
  radiation therapy (antineoplastic) Z51.0
  radiological (as part of a general medical examination) Z00.00
    with abnormal findings Z00.01
  reconstructive surgery following medical procedure or healed injury NEC Z42.8
  removal (of) - see also Removal
    artificial
      arm Z44.00-
        complete Z44.01-
        partial Z44.02-
      eye Z44.2-
      leg Z44.10-
        complete Z44.11-
        partial Z44.12-
    breast implant Z45.81
      tissue expander (without synchronous insertion of permanent implant) Z45.81
    device Z46.9
      specified NEC Z46.89
    external
      fixation device
        code to fracture with seventh character D
    prosthesis, prosthetic device Z44.9
      breast Z44.3-
        specified NEC Z44.8
    implanted device NEC Z45.89
    insulin pump Z46.81
    internal fixation device Z47.2
    myringotomy device (stent) (tube) Z45.82
    nervous system device NEC Z46.2
      brain neuropacemaker Z46.2
      visual substitution device Z46.2
        implanted Z45.31
    non-vascular catheter Z46.82
    orthodontic device Z46.4
    stent
      ureteral Z46.6
    urinary device Z46.6
  repeat cervical smear to confirm findings of recent normal smear following initial abnormal smear Z01.42
  respirator [ventilator] use during power failure Z99.12
  Rh typing Z01.83
  screening - see Screening
  specified NEC Z76.89
  sterilization Z30.2
  suspected condition, ruled out
    amniotic cavity and membrane Z03.71
    cervical shortening Z03.75
    fetal anomaly Z03.73
    fetal growth Z03.74
    maternal and fetal conditions NEC Z03.79
    oligohydramnios Z03.71
    placental problem Z03.72
    polyhydramnios Z03.71
  suspected exposure (to), ruled out
    anthrax Z03.810
    biological agents NEC Z03.818
  termination of pregnancy, elective Z33.2
  testing - see Test
  therapeutic drug level monitoring Z51.81
  titration, insulin pump Z46.81
  to determine fetal viability of pregnancy O36.80
  training
    insulin pump Z46.81
  X-ray of chest (as part of a general medical examination) Z00.00
    with abnormal findings Z00.01

Encystment - see Cyst
Endarteritis (bacterial, subacute) (infective) I77.6
  brain I67.7
  cerebral or cerebrospinal I67.7
  deformans - see Arteriosclerosis
  embolic - see Embolism
  obliterans - see also Arteriosclerosis
    pulmonary I28.8
  pulmonary I28.8
  retina - see Vasculitis, retina
  senile - see Arteriosclerosis
  syphilitic A52.09
    brain or cerebral A52.04
    congenital A50.54 [I79.8]
  tuberculous A18.89
Endemic - see condition
Endocarditis (chronic) (marantic) (nonbacterial) (thrombotic) (valvular) I38
  with rheumatic fever (conditions in I00)
    active - see Endocarditis, acute, rheumatic
    inactive or quiescent (with chorea) I09.1
  acute or subacute I33.9
    infective I33.0
    rheumatic (aortic) (mitral) (pulmonary) (tricuspid) I01.1
      with chorea (acute) (rheumatic) (Sydenham's) I02.0
  aortic (heart) (nonrheumatic) (valve) I35.8
    with
      mitral disease I08.0
        with tricuspid (valve) disease I08.3
        active or acute I01.1
          with chorea (acute) (rheumatic) (Sydenham's) I02.0
      rheumatic fever (conditions in I00)
        active - see Endocarditis, acute, rheumatic
        inactive or quiescent (with chorea) I06.9
      tricuspid (valve) disease I08.2
        with mitral (valve) disease I08.3
    acute or subacute I33.9
    arteriosclerotic I35.8
    rheumatic I06.9
      with mitral disease I08.0
        with tricuspid (valve) disease I08.3
      active or acute I01.1
        with chorea (acute) (rheumatic) (Sydenham's) I02.0
      active or acute I01.1
        with chorea (acute) (rheumatic) (Sydenham's) I02.0
      specified NEC I06.8
    specified cause NEC I35.8
    syphilitic A52.03
  arteriosclerotic I38
  atypical verrucous (Libman-sacks) M32.11
  bacterial (acute) (any valve) (subacute) I33.0
  candidal B37.6
  congenital Q24.8
  constrictive I33.0
  Coxiella burnetii A78 [I39]
  Coxsackie B33.21
  due to
    prosthetic cardiac valve T82.6
    Q fever A78 [I39]
    Serratia marcescens I33.0
    typhoid (fever) A01.02
  gonococcal A54.83
  infectious or infective (acute) (any valve) (subacute) I33.0
  lenta (acute) (any valve) (subacute) I33.0
  Libman-sacks M32.11
  listerial A32.82
  Löffler's I42.3

Endocarditis - *continued*
  malignant (acute) (any valve) (subacute) I33.0
  meningococcal A39.51
  mitral (chronic) (double) (fibroid) (heart)
   (inactive) (valve) (with chorea) I05.9
   with
    aortic (valve) disease I08.0
     with tricuspid (valve) disease I08.3
     active or acute I01.1
      with chorea (acute) (rheumatic)
       (Sydenham's) I02.0
    rheumatic fever (conditions in I00)
     active - *see* Endocarditis, acute, rheumatic
     inactive or quiescent (with chorea) I05.9
    tricuspid (valve) disease I08.1
     with aortic (valve) disease I08.3
   active or acute I01.1
    with chorea (acute) (rheumatic)
     (Sydenham's) I02.0
   bacterial I33.0
   arteriosclerotic I34.8
   nonrheumatic I34.8
    acute or subacute I33.9
   specified NEC I05.8
  monilial B37.6
  multiple valves I08.9
   specified disorders I08.8
  mycotic (acute) (any valve) (subacute) I33.0
  pneumococcal (acute) (any valve) (subacute)
   I33.0
  pulmonary (chronic) (heart) (valve) I37.8
   with rheumatic fever (conditions in I00)
    active - *see* Endocarditis, acute, rheumatic
    inactive or quiescent (with chorea) I09.89
     with aortic, mitral or tricuspid disease
     I08.8
   acute or subacute I33.9
    rheumatic I01.1
     with chorea (acute) (rheumatic)
      (Sydenham's) I02.0
   arteriosclerotic I37.8
   congenital Q22.2
   rheumatic (chronic) (inactive) (with chorea)
   I09.89
    active or acute I01.1
     with chorea (acute) (rheumatic)
      (Sydenham's) I02.0
   syphilitic A52.03
  purulent (acute) (any valve) (subacute) I33.0
  Q fever A78 *[139]*
  rheumatic (chronic) (inactive) (with chorea)
   I09.1
   active or acute (aortic) (mitral) (pulmonary)
   (tricuspid) I01.1
    with chorea (acute) (rheumatic)
     (Sydenham's) I02.0
  rheumatoid - *see* Rheumatoid, carditis
  septic (acute) (any valve) (subacute) I33.0
  streptococcal (acute) (any valve) (subacute)
   I33.0
  subacute - *see* Endocarditis, acute
  suppurative (acute) (any valve) (subacute)
   I33.0
  syphilitic A52.03
  toxic I33.9
  tricuspid (chronic) (heart) (inactive)
   (rheumatic) (valve) (with chorea) I07.9
   with
    aortic (valve) disease I08.2
     mitral (valve) disease I08.3
    mitral (valve) disease I08.1
     aortic (valve) disease I08.3
    rheumatic fever (conditions in I00)
     active - *see* Endocarditis, acute, rheumatic

Endocarditis - *continued*
   inactive or quiescent (with chorea) I07.8
   active or acute I01.1
    with chorea (acute) (rheumatic)
     (Sydenham's) I02.0
  arteriosclerotic I36.8
  nonrheumatic I36.8
   acute or subacute I33.9
  specified cause, except rheumatic I36.8
  tuberculous - *see* Tuberculosis, endocarditis
  typhoid A01.02
  ulcerative (acute) (any valve) (subacute) I33.0
  vegetative (acute) (any valve) (subacute) I33.0
  verrucous (atypical) (nonbacterial)
   (nonrheumatic) M32.11
Endocardium, endocardial - *see also* condition
  cushion defect Q21.2
Endocervicitis - *see also* Cervicitis
  due to intrauterine (contraceptive) device
   T83.69
  hyperplastic N72
Endocrine - *see* condition
Endocrinopathy, pluriglandular E31.9
Endodontic
  overfill M27.52
  underfill M27.53
Endodontitis K04.01
  irreversible K04.02
  reversible K04.01
Endomastoiditis - *see* Mastoiditis
Endometrioma N80.9
Endometriosis N80.9
  appendix N80.5
  bladder N80.8
  bowel N80.5
  broad ligament N80.3
  cervix N80.0
  colon N80.5
  cul-de-sac (Douglas') N80.3
  exocervix N80.0
  fallopian tube N80.2
  female genital organ NEC N80.8
  gallbladder N80.8
  in scar of skin N80.6
  internal N80.0
  intestine N80.5
  lung N80.8
  myometrium N80.0
  ovary N80.1
  parametrium N80.3
  pelvic peritoneum N80.3
  peritoneal (pelvic) N80.3
  rectovaginal septum N80.4
  rectum N80.5
  round ligament N80.3
  skin (scar) N80.6
  specified site NEC N80.8
  stromal D39.0
  thorax N80.8
  umbilicus N80.8
  uterus (internal) N80.0
  vagina N80.4
  vulva N80.8
Endometritis (decidual) (nonspecific)
(purulent) (senile) (atrophic) (suppurative)
N71.9
  with ectopic pregnancy O08.0
  acute N71.0
  blenorrhagic (gonococcal) (acute) (chronic)
   A54.24
  cervix, cervical (with erosion or ectropion) -
  see also Cervicitis
   hyperplastic N72
  chlamydial A56.11

Endometritis - *continued*
  chronic N71.1
  following
   abortion - *see* Abortion by type complicated
   by genital infection
   ectopic or molar pregnancy O08.0
  gonococcal, gonorrheal (acute) (chronic)
   A54.24
  hyperplastic - *see also* Hyperplasia,
   endometrial N85.00-
    cervix N72
  puerperal, postpartum, childbirth O86.12
  subacute N71.0
  tuberculous A18.17
Endometrium - *see* condition
Endomyocardiopathy, South African I42.3
Endomyocarditis - *see* Endocarditis
Endomyofibrosis I42.3
Endomyometritis - *see* Endometritis
Endopericarditis - *see* Endocarditis
Endoperineuritis - *see* Disorder, nerve
Endophlebitis - *see* Phlebitis
Endophthalmia - *see* Endophthalmitis, purulent
Endophthalmitis (acute) (infective)
(metastatic) (subacute) H44.009
  bleb associated H59.4 - *see also* Bleb,
   inflamed (infected), postprocedural
  gonorrheal A54.39
  in (due to)
   cysticercosis B69.1
   onchocerciasis B73.01
   toxocariasis B83.0
  panuveitis - *see* Panuveitis
  parasitic H44.12-
  purulent H44.00-
   panophthalmitis - *see* Panophthalmitis
   vitreous abscess H44.02-
  specified NEC H44.19
  sympathetic - *see* Uveitis, sympathetic
Endosalpingoma D28.2
Endosalpingiosis N94.89
Endosteitis - *see* Osteomyelitis
Endothelioma, bone - *see* Neoplasm, bone,
  malignant
Endotheliosis (hemorrhagic infectional)
  D69.8
Endotoxemia   code to condition
Endotrachelitis - *see* Cervicitis
Engelmann (-Camurati) syndrome Q78.3
English disease - *see* Rickets
Engman's disease L30.3
Engorgement
  breast N64.59
   newborn P83.4
   puerperal, postpartum O92.79
  lung (passive) - *see* Edema, lung
  pulmonary (passive) - *see* Edema, lung
  stomach K31.89
  venous, retina - *see* Occlusion, retina, vein,
   engorgement
Enlargement, enlarged - *see also* Hypertrophy
  adenoids J35.2
   with tonsils J35.3
  alveolar ridge K08.89
   congenital - *see* Anomaly, alveolar
  apertures of diaphragm (congenital) Q79.1
  gingival K06.1
  heart, cardiac - *see* Hypertrophy, cardiac
  labium majus, childhood asymmetric
   (CALME) N90.61
  lacrimal gland, chronic H04.03-
  liver - *see* Hypertrophy, liver
  lymph gland or node R59.9
   generalized R59.1

Enlargement, enlarged - *continued*
  localized R59.0
  orbit H05.34-
  organ or site, congenital NEC - *see* Anomaly, by site
  parathyroid (gland) E21.0
  pituitary fossa R93.0
  prostate N40.0
    with lower urinary tract symptoms (LUTS) N40.1
    without lower urinary tract symptoms (LUTS) N40.0
  sella turcica R93.0
  spleen - *see* Splenomegaly
  thymus (gland) (congenital) E32.0
  thyroid (gland) - *see* Goiter
  tongue K14.8
  tonsils J35.1
    with adenoids J35.3
  uterus N85.2
  vestibular aqueduct Q16.5
Enophthalmos H05.40-
  due to
    orbital tissue atrophy H05.41-
    trauma or surgery H05.42-
Enostosis M27.8
Entamebic, entamebiasis - *see* Amebiasis
Entanglement
  umbilical cord(s) O69.82
    with compression O69.2
    around neck (with compression) O69.81
      with compression O69.1
    without compression O69.82
    without compression O69.81
  of twins in monoamniotic sac O69.2
Enteralgia - *see* Pain, abdominal
Enteric - *see* condition
Enteritis (acute) (diarrheal) (hemorrhagic) (noninfective) K52.9
  adenovirus A08.2
  aertrycke infection A02.0
  allergic K52.29
    with
      eosinophilic gastritis or gastroenteritis K52.81
      food protein-induced enterocolitis syndrome K52.21
      food protein-induced enteropathy K52.22
  amebic (acute) A06.0
    with abscess - *see* Abscess, amebic
    chronic A06.1
      with abscess - *see* Abscess, amebic
      nondysenteric A06.2
    nondysenteric A06.2
  astrovirus A08.32
  bacillary NOS A03.9
  bacterial A04.9
    specified NEC A04.8
  calicivirus A08.31
  candidal B37.82
  Chilomastix A07.8
  choleriformis A00.1
  chronic (noninfectious) K52.9
    ulcerative - *see* Colitis, ulcerative
  cicatrizing (chronic) - *see* Enteritis, regional, small intestine
  Clostridium
    botulinum (food poisoning) A05.1
    difficile
      not specified as recurrent A04.72
      recurrent A04.71
  coccidial A07.3
  coxsackie virus A08.39
  dietetic - *see also* Enteritis, allergic K52.29

Enteritis - *continued*
  drug-induced K52.1
  due to
    astrovirus A08.32
    calicivirus A08.31
    coxsackie virus A08.39
    drugs K52.1
    echovirus A08.39
    enterovirus NEC A08.39
    food hypersensitivity - *see also* Enteritis, allergic K52.29
    infectious organism (bacterial) (viral) - *see* Enteritis, infectious
    torovirus A08.39
    Yersinia enterocolitica A04.6
  echovirus A08.39
  eltor A00.1
  enterovirus NEC A08.39
  eosinophilic K52.81
  epidemic (infectious) A09
  fulminant - *see also* Ischemia, intestine, acute K55.019
  gangrenous - *see* Enteritis, infectious
  giardial A07.1
  infectious NOS A09
    due to
      adenovirus A08.2
      Aerobacter aerogenes A04.8
      Arizona (bacillus) A02.0
      bacteria NOS A04.9
        specified NEC A04.8
      Campylobacter A04.5
      Clostridium difficile
        not specified as recurrent A04.72
        recurrent A04.71
      Clostridium perfringens A04.8
      Enterobacter aerogenes A04.8
      enterovirus A08.39
      Escherichia coli A04.4
        enteroaggregative A04.4
        enterohemorrhagic A04.3
        enteroinvasive A04.2
        enteropathogenic A04.0
        enterotoxigenic A04.1
        specified NEC A04.4
      specified
        bacteria NEC A04.8
        virus NEC A08.39
      Staphylococcus A04.8
      virus NEC A08.4
        specified type NEC A08.39
      Yersinia enterocolitica A04.6
    specified organism NEC A08.8
  influenzal - *see* Influenza, with, digestive manifestations
  ischemic K55.9
    acute - *see also* Ischemia, intestine, acute K55.019
    chronic K55.1
  microsporidial A07.8
  mucomembranous, myxomembranous - *see* Syndrome, irritable bowel
  mucous - *see* Syndrome, irritable bowel
  necroticans A05.2
  necrotizing of newborn - *see* Enterocolitis, necrotizing, in newborn
  neurogenic - *see* Syndrome, irritable bowel
  newborn necrotizing - *see* Enterocolitis, necrotizing, in newborn
  noninfectious K52.9
  norovirus A08.11
  parasitic NEC B82.9
  paratyphoid (fever) - *see* Fever, paratyphoid
  protozoal A07.9

Enteritis - *continued*
  specified NEC A07.8
  radiation K52.0
  regional (of) K50.90
    with
      complication K50.919
        abscess K50.914
        fistula K50.913
        intestinal obstruction K50.912
        rectal bleeding K50.911
        specified complication NEC K50.918
    colon - *see* Enteritis, regional, large intestine
    duodenum - *see* Enteritis, regional, small intestine
    ileum - *see* Enteritis, regional, small intestine
    jejunum - *see* Enteritis, regional, small intestine
    large bowel - *see* Enteritis, regional, large intestine
    large intestine (colon) (rectum) K50.10
      with
        complication K50.119
          abscess K50.114
          fistula K50.113
          intestinal obstruction K50.112
          rectal bleeding K50.111
          small intestine (duodenum) (ileum) (jejunum) involvement K50.80
            with
              complication K50.819
                abscess K50.814
                fistula K50.813
                intestinal obstruction K50.812
                rectal bleeding K50.811
                specified complication NEC K50.818
          specified complication NEC K50.118
    rectum - *see* Enteritis, regional, large intestine
    small intestine (duodenum) (ileum) (jejunum) K50.00
      with
        complication K50.019
          abscess K50.014
          fistula K50.013
          intestinal obstruction K50.012
          large intestine (colon) (rectum) involvement K50.80
            with
              complication K50.819
                abscess K50.814
                fistula K50.813
                intestinal obstruction K50.812
                rectal bleeding K50.811
                specified complication NEC K50.818
          rectal bleeding K50.011
          specified complication NEC K50.018
  Rotaviral A08.0
  Salmonella, salmonellosis (arizonae) (cholerae-suis) (enteritidis) (typhimurium) A02.0
  segmental - *see* Enteritis, regional
  septic A09
  Shigella - *see* Infection, Shigella
  small round structured NEC A08.19
  spasmodic, spastic - *see* Syndrome, irritable bowel
  staphylococcal A04.8
    due to food A05.0
  torovirus A08.39
  toxic NEC K52.1
    due to Clostridium difficile
      not specified as recurrent A04.72

Enteritis - *continued*
    recurrent A04.71
    trichomonal A07.8
    tuberculous A18.32
    typhosa A01.00
    ulcerative (chronic) - *see* Colitis, ulcerative
    viral A08.4
      adenovirus A08.2
      enterovirus A08.39
      Rotavirus A08.0
      small round structured NEC A08.19
      specified NEC A08.39
      virus specified NEC A08.39
Enterobiasis B80
Enterobius vermicularis (infection) (infestation) B80
Enterocele - *see also* Hernia, abdomen
    pelvic, pelvis (acquired) (congenital) N81.5
    vagina, vaginal (acquired) (congenital) NEC N81.5
Enterocolitis - *see also* Enteritis K52.9
    due to Clostridium difficile
      not specified as recurrent A04.72
      recurrent A04.71
    fulminant ischemic - *see also* Ischemia, intestine, acute K55.059
    granulomatous - *see* Enteritis, regional
    hemorrhagic (acute) - *see also* Ischemia, intestine, acute K55.059
      chronic K55.1
    infectious NEC A09
    ischemic K55.9
    necrotizing K55.30
      with
        perforation K55.33
        pneumatosis K55.32
          and perforation K55.33
      due to Clostridium difficile
        not specified as recurrent A04.72
        recurrent A04.71
      in non newborn K55.30
        stage 1 (without pneumatosis, without perforation) K55.31
        stage 2 (with pneumatosis, without perforation) K55.32
        stage 3 (with pneumatosis, with perforation) K55.33
      in newborn P77.9
        stage 1 (without pneumatosis, without perforation) P77.1
        stage 2 (with pneumatosis, without perforation) P77.2
        stage 3 (with pneumatosis, with perforation) P77.3
      without pneumatosis or perforation K55.31
    noninfectious K52.9
    newborn - *see* Enterocolitis, necrotizing, in newborn
    pseudomembranous (newborn)
      not specified as recurrent A04.72
      recurrent A04.71
    radiation K52.0
    newborn - *see* Enterocolitis, necrotizing, in newborn
    ulcerative (chronic) - *see* Pancolitis, ulcerative (chronic)
Enterogastritis - *see* Enteritis
Enteropathy K63.9
    celiac-gluten-sensitive K90.0
      non-celiac K90.41
    food protein-induced enterocolitis K52.22
    hemorrhagic, terminal - *see also* Ischemia, intestine, acute K55.059
    protein-losing K90.49

Enteroperitonitis - *see* Peritonitis
Enteroptosis K63.4
Enterorrhagia K92.2
Enterospasm - *see also* Syndrome, irritable, bowel
    psychogenic F45.8
Enterostenosis (see also Obstruction, intestine, specified NEC) K56.699
Enterostomy
    complication - *see* Complication, enterostomy
    status Z93.4
Enterovirus, as cause of disease classified elsewhere B97.10
    coxsackievirus B97.11
    echovirus B97.12
    other specified B97.19
Enthesopathy (peripheral) M77.9
    Achilles tendinitis - *see* Tendinitis, Achilles
    ankle and tarsus M77.9
      specified type NEC - *see* Enthesopathy, foot, specified type NEC
    anterior tibial syndrome M76.81-
    calcaneal spur - *see* Spur, bone, calcaneal
    elbow region M77.8
      lateral epicondylitis - *see* Epicondylitis, lateral
      medial epicondylitis - *see* Epicondylitis, medial
    foot NEC M77.9
      metatarsalgia - *see* Metatarsalgia
      specified type NEC M77.5-
    forearm M77.9
    gluteal tendinitis - *see* Tendinitis, gluteal
    hand M77.9
    hip - *see* Enthesopathy, lower limb, specified type NEC
    iliac crest spur - *see* Spur, bone, iliac crest
    iliotibial band syndrome - *see* Syndrome, iliotibial band
    knee - *see* Enthesopathy, lower limb, lower leg, specified type NEC
    lateral epicondylitis - *see* Epicondylitis, lateral
    lower limb (excluding foot) M76.9
      Achilles tendinitis - *see* Tendinitis, Achilles
      anterior tibial syndrome M76.81-
      gluteal tendinitis - *see* Tendinitis, gluteal
      iliac crest spur - *see* Spur, bone, iliac crest
      iliotibial band syndrome - *see* Syndrome, iliotibial band
      patellar tendinitis - *see* Tendinitis, patellar
      pelvic region - *see* Enthesopathy, lower limb, specified type NEC
      peroneal tendinitis - *see* Tendinitis, peroneal
      posterior tibial syndrome M76.82-
      psoas tendinitis - *see* Tendinitis, psoas
      shoulder M77.9
      specified type NEC M76.89-
      tibial collateral bursitis - *see* Bursitis, tibial collateral
    medial epicondylitis - *see* Epicondylitis, medial
    metatarsalgia - *see* Metatarsalgia
    multiple sites M77.9
    patellar tendinitis - *see* Tendinitis, patellar
    pelvis M77.9
    periarthritis of wrist - *see* Periarthritis, wrist
    peroneal tendinitis - *see* Tendinitis, peroneal
    posterior tibial syndrome M76.82-
    psoas tendinitis - *see* Tendinitis, psoas
    shoulder region - *see* Lesion, shoulder
    specified site NEC M77.9
    specified type NEC M77.8
    spinal M46.00
      cervical region M46.02

Enthesopathy - *continued*
    cervicothoracic region M46.03
    lumbar region M46.06
    lumbosacral region M46.07
    multiple sites M46.09
    occipito-atlanto-axial region M46.01
    sacrococcygeal region M46.08
    thoracic region M46.04
    thoracolumbar region M46.05
    tibial collateral bursitis - *see* Bursitis, tibial collateral
    upper arm M77.9
    wrist and carpus NEC M77.8
      calcaneal spur - *see* Spur, bone, calcaneal
      periarthritis of wrist - *see* Periarthritis, wrist
Entomophobia F40.218
Entomophthoromycosis B46.8
Entrance, air into vein - *see* Embolism, air
Entrapment, nerve - *see* Neuropathy, entrapment
Entropion (eyelid) (paralytic) H02.009
    cicatricial H02.019
      left H02.016
        lower H02.015
        upper H02.014
      right H02.013
        lower H02.012
        upper H02.011
    congenital Q10.2
    left H02.006
      lower H02.005
      upper H02.004
    mechanical H02.029
      left H02.026
        lower H02.025
        upper H02.024
      right H02.023
        lower H02.022
        upper H02.021
    right H02.003
      lower H02.002
      upper H02.001
    senile H02.039
      left H02.036
        lower H02.035
        upper H02.034
      right H02.033
        lower H02.032
        upper H02.031
    spastic H02.049
      left H02.046
        lower H02.045
        upper H02.044
      right H02.043
        lower H02.042
        upper H02.041
Enucleated eye (traumatic, current) S05.7-
Enuresis R32
    functional F98.0
    habit disturbance F98.0
    nocturnal N39.44
      psychogenic F98.0
    nonorganic origin F98.0
    psychogenic F98.0
Eosinopenia - *see* Agranulocytosis
Eosinophilia (allergic) (hereditary) (idiopathic) (secondary) D72.1
    with
      angiolymphoid hyperplasia (ALHE) D18.01
    infiltrative J82
    Löffler's J82
    peritoneal - *see* Peritonitis, eosinophilic
    pulmonary NEC J82
    tropical (pulmonary) J82

Eosinophilia-myalgia syndrome M35.8
Ependymitis (acute) (cerebral) (chronic)
  (granular) - *see* Encephalomyelitis
Ependymoblastoma
  specified site - *see* Neoplasm, malignant, by
    site
  unspecified site C71.9
Ependymoma (epithelial) (malignant)
  anaplastic
    specified site - *see* Neoplasm, malignant, by
      site
    unspecified site C71.9
  benign
    specified site - *see* Neoplasm, benign, by site
    unspecified site D33.2
  myxopapillary D43.2
    specified site - *see* Neoplasm, uncertain
      behavior, by site
    unspecified site D43.2
  papillary D43.2
    specified site - *see* Neoplasm, uncertain
      behavior, by site
    unspecified site D43.2
  specified site - *see* Neoplasm, malignant, by
    site
  unspecified site C71.9
Ependymopathy G93.89
Ephelis, ephelides L81.2
Epiblepharon (congenital) Q10.3
Epicanthus, epicanthic fold (eyelid)
  (congenital) Q10.3
Epicondylitis (elbow)
  lateral M77.1-
  medial M77.0-
Epicystitis - *see* Cystitis
Epidemic - *see* condition
Epidermidalization, cervix - *see* Dysplasia,
  cervix
Epidermis, epidermal - *see* condition
Epidermodysplasia verruciformis B07.8
Epidermolysis
  bullosa (congenital) Q81.9
    acquired L12.30
      drug-induced L12.31
      specified cause NEC L12.35
    dystrophica Q81.2
    letalis Q81.1
    simplex Q81.0
    specified NEC Q81.8
  necroticans combustiformis L51.2
  due to drug - *see* Table of Drugs and
    Chemicals, by drug
Epidermophytid - *see* Dermatophytosis
Epidermophytosis (infected) - *see*
  Dermatophytosis
Epididymis - *see* condition
Epididymitis (acute) (nonvenereal)
  (recurrent) (residual) N45.1
  with orchitis N45.3
  blennorrhagic (gonococcal) A54.23
  caseous (tuberculous) A18.15
  chlamydial A56.19
  filarial - *see also* Infestation, filarial B74.9
    [*N51*]
  gonococcal A54.23
  syphilitic A52.76
  tuberculous A18.15
Epididymo-orchitis - *see also* Epididymitis
  N45.3
Epidural - *see* condition
Epigastrium, epigastric - *see* condition
Epigastrocele - *see* Hernia, ventral
Epiglottis - *see* condition

Epiglottitis, epiglottiditis (acute) J05.10
  with obstruction J05.11
  chronic J37.0
Epignathus Q89.4
Epilepsia partialis continua - *see also*
  Kozhevnikov's epilepsy G40.1-
Epilepsy, epileptic, epilepsia (attack)
  (cerebral) (convulsion) (fit) (seizure)
  G40.909
Note: the following terms are to be considered
equivalent to intractable: pharmacoresistent
(pharmacologically resistant), treatment
resistant, refractory (medically) and poorly
controlled
  with
    complex partial seizures - *see* Epilepsy,
      localization-related, symptomatic, with
      complex partial seizures
    grand mal seizures on awakening - *see*
      Epilepsy, generalized, specified NEC
    myoclonic absences - *see* Epilepsy,
      generalized, specified NEC
    myoclonic-astatic seizures - *see* Epilepsy,
      generalized, specified NEC
    simple partial seizures - *see* Epilepsy,
      localization-related, symptomatic, with
      simple partial seizures
  akinetic - *see* Epilepsy, generalized, specified
    NEC
  benign childhood with centrotemporal EEG
    spikes - *see* Epilepsy, localization-related,
    idiopathic
  benign myoclonic in infancy G40.80-
  Bravais-jacksonian - *see* Epilepsy,
    localization-related, symptomatic, with
    simple partial seizures
  childhood
    with occipital EEG paroxysms - *see*
      Epilepsy, localization-related, idiopathic
    absence G40.A09
      intractable G40.A19
        with status epilepticus G40.A11
        without status epilepticus G40.A19
      not intractable G40.A09
        with status epilepticus G40.A01
        without status epilepticus G40.A09
  climacteric - *see* Epilepsy, specified NEC
  cysticercosis B69.0
  deterioration (mental) F06.8
  due to syphilis A52.19
  focal - *see* Epilepsy, localization-related,
    symptomatic, with simple partial seizures
  generalized
    idiopathic G40.309
      intractable G40.319
        with status epilepticus G40.311
        without status epilepticus G40.319
      not intractable G40.309
        with status epilepticus G40.301
        without status epilepticus G40.309
    specified NEC G40.409
      intractable G40.419
        with status epilepticus G40.411
        without status epilepticus G40.419
      not intractable G40.409
        with status epilepticus G40.401
        without status epilepticus G40.409
  impulsive petit mal - *see* Epilepsy, juvenile
    myoclonic
  intractable G40.919
    with status epilepticus G40.911
    without status epilepticus G40.919
  juvenile absence G40.A09
    intractable G40.A19

Epilepsy, epileptic, epilepsia - *continued*
  with status epilepticus G40.A11
  without status epilepticus G40.A19
  not intractable G40.A09
    with status epilepticus G40.A01
    without status epilepticus G40.A09
  juvenile myoclonic G40.B09
    intractable G40.B19
      with status epilepticus G40.B11
      without status epilepticus G40.B19
    not intractable G40.B09
      with status epilepticus G40.B01
      without status epilepticus G40.B09
  localization-related (focal) (partial)
    idiopathic G40.009
      with seizures of localized onset G40.009
        intractable G40.019
          with status epilepticus G40.011
          without status epilepticus G40.019
        not intractable G40.009
          with status epilepticus G40.001
          without status epilepticus G40.009
    symptomatic
      with complex partial seizures G40.209
        intractable G40.219
          with status epilepticus G40.211
          without status epilepticus G40.219
        not intractable G40.209
          with status epilepticus G40.201
          without status epilepticus G40.209
      with simple partial seizures G40.109
        intractable G40.119
          with status epilepticus G40.111
          without status epilepticus G40.119
        not intractable G40.109
          with status epilepticus G40.101
          without status epilepticus G40.109
  myoclonus, myoclonic - *see* Epilepsy,
    generalized, specified NEC
  progressive - *see* Epilepsy, generalized,
    idiopathic
  not intractable G40.909
    with status epilepticus G40.901
    without status epilepticus G40.909
  on awakening - *see* Epilepsy, generalized,
    specified NEC
  parasitic NOS B71.9 [*G94*]
  partialis continua - *see also* Kozhevnikov's
    epilepsy G40.1-
  peripheral - *see* Epilepsy, specified NEC
  procursiva - *see* Epilepsy, localization-related,
    symptomatic, with simple partial seizures
  progressive (familial) myoclonic - *see*
    Epilepsy, generalized, idiopathic
  reflex - *see* Epilepsy, specified NEC
  related to
    alcohol G40.509
      not intractable G40.509
        with status epilepticus G40.501
        without status epilepticus G40.509
    drugs G40.509
      not intractable G40.509
        with status epilepticus G40.501
        without status epilepticus G40.509
    external causes G40.509
      not intractable G40.509
        with status epilepticus G40.501
        without status epilepticus G40.509
    hormonal changes G40.509
      not intractable G40.509
        with status epilepticus G40.501
        without status epilepticus G40.509
    sleep deprivation G40.509
      not intractable G40.509

Epilepsy, epileptic, epilepsia - *continued*
with status epilepticus G40.501
without status epilepticus G40.509
stress G40.509
not intractable G40.509
with status epilepticus G40.501
without status epilepticus G40.509
somatomotor - *see* Epilepsy, localization-related, symptomatic, with simple partial seizures
somatosensory - *see* Epilepsy, localization-related, symptomatic, with simple partial seizures
spasms G40.822
intractable G40.824
with status epilepticus G40.823
without status epilepticus G40.824
not intractable G40.822
with status epilepticus G40.821
without status epilepticus G40.822
specified NEC G40.802
intractable G40.804
with status epilepticus G40.803
without status epilepticus G40.804
not intractable G40.802
with status epilepticus G40.801
without status epilepticus G40.802
syndromes
generalized
idiopathic G40.309
intractable G40.319
with status epilepticus G40.311
without status epilepticus G40.319
not intractable G40.309
with status epilepticus G40.301
without status epilepticus G40.309
specified NEC G40.409
intractable G40.419
with status epilepticus G40.411
without status epilepticus G40.419
not intractable G40.409
with status epilepticus G40.401
without status epilepticus G40.409
localization-related (focal) (partial)
idiopathic G40.009
with seizures of localized onset G40.009
intractable G40.019
with status epilepticus G40.011
without status epilepticus G40.019
not intractable G40.009
with status epilepticus G40.001
without status epilepticus G40.009
symptomatic
with complex partial seizures G40.209
intractable G40.219
with status epilepticus G40.211
without status epilepticus G40.219
not intractable G40.209
with status epilepticus G40.201
without status epilepticus G40.209
with simple partial seizures G40.109
intractable G40.119
with status epilepticus G40.111
without status epilepticus G40.119
not intractable G40.109
with status epilepticus G40.101
without status epilepticus G40.109
specified NEC G40.802
intractable G40.804
with status epilepticus G40.803
without status epilepticus G40.804
not intractable G40.802
with status epilepticus G40.801
without status epilepticus G40.802

Epilepsy, epileptic, epilepsia - *continued*
tonic (-clonic) - *see* Epilepsy, generalized, specified NEC
twilight F05
uncinate (gyrus) - *see* Epilepsy, localization-related, symptomatic, with complex partial seizures
Unverricht (-Lundborg) (familial myoclonic) - *see* Epilepsy, generalized, idiopathic
visceral - *see* Epilepsy, specified NEC
visual - *see* Epilepsy, specified NEC
Epiloia Q85.1
Epimenorrhea N92.0
Epipharyngitis - *see* Nasopharyngitis
Epiphora H04.20-
due to
excess lacrimation H04.21-
insufficient drainage H04.22-
Epiphyseal arrest - *see* Arrest, epiphyseal
Epiphyseolysis, epiphysiolysis - *see* Osteochondropathy
Epiphysitis - *see also* Osteochondropathy
juvenile M92.9
syphilitic (congenital) A50.02
Epiplocele - *see* Hernia, abdomen
Epiploitis - *see* Peritonitis
Epiplosarcomphalocele - *see* Hernia, umbilicus
Episcleritis (suppurative) H15.10-
in (due to)
syphilis A52.71
tuberculosis A18.51
nodular H15.12-
periodica fugax H15.11-
angioneurotic - *see* Edema, angioneurotic
syphilitic (late) A52.71
tuberculous A18.51
Episode
affective, mixed F39
depersonalization (in neurotic state) F48.1
depressive F32.9
major F32.9
mild F32.0
moderate F32.1
severe (without psychotic symptoms) F32.2
with psychotic symptoms F32.3
recurrent F33.9
brief F33.8
specified NEC F32.89
hypomanic F30.8
manic F30.9
with
psychotic symptoms F30.2
remission (full) F30.4
partial F30.3
other specified F30.8
recurrent F31.89
without psychotic symptoms F30.10
mild F30.11
moderate F30.12
severe (without psychotic symptoms) F30.13
with psychotic symptoms F30.2
psychotic F23
organic F06.8
schizophrenic (acute) NEC, brief F23
Epispadias (female) (male) Q64.0
Episplenitis D73.89
Epistaxis (multiple) R04.0
hereditary I78.0
vicarious menstruation N94.89
Epithelioma (malignant) - *see also* Neoplasm, malignant, by site
adenoides cysticum - *see* Neoplasm, skin, benign

Epithelioma (malignant) - *continued*
basal cell - *see* Neoplasm, skin, malignant
benign - *see* Neoplasm, benign, by site
Bowen's - *see* Neoplasm, skin, in situ
calcifying, of Malherbe - *see* Neoplasm, skin, benign
external site - *see* Neoplasm, skin, malignant
intraepidermal, Jadassohn - *see* Neoplasm, skin, benign
squamous cell - *see* Neoplasm, malignant, by site
Epitheliomatosis pigmented Q82.1
Epitheliopathy, multifocal placoid pigment H30.14-
Epithelium, epithelial - *see* condition
Epituberculosis (with atelectasis) (allergic) A15.7
Eponychia Q84.6
Epstein's
nephrosis or syndrome - *see* Nephrosis
pearl K09.8
Epulis (gingiva) (fibrous) (giant cell) K06.8
Equinia A24.0
Equinovarus (congenital) (talipes) Q66.0
acquired - *see* Deformity, limb, clubfoot
Equivalent
convulsive (abdominal) - *see* Epilepsy, specified NEC
epileptic (psychic) - *see* Epilepsy, localization-related, symptomatic, with complex partial seizures
Erb (-Duchenne) paralysis (birth injury) (newborn) P14.0
Erb-Goldflam disease or syndrome G70.00
with exacerbation (acute) G70.01
in crisis G70.01
Erb's
disease G71.0
palsy, paralysis (brachial) (birth) (newborn) P14.0
spinal (spastic) syphilitic A52.17
pseudohypertrophic muscular dystrophy G71.0
Erdheim's syndrome (acromegalic macrospondylitis) E22.0
Erection, painful (persistent) - *see* Priapism
Ergosterol deficiency (vitamin D) E55.9
with
adult osteomalacia M83.8
rickets - *see* Rickets
Ergotism - *see also* Poisoning, food, noxious, plant
from ergot used as drug (migraine therapy) - *see* Table of Drugs and Chemicals
Erosio interdigitalis blastomycetica B37.2
Erosion
artery I77.2
without rupture I77.89
bone - *see* Disorder, bone, density and structure, specified NEC
bronchus J98.09
cartilage (joint) - *see* Disorder, cartilage, specified type NEC
cervix (uteri) (acquired) (chronic) (congenital) N86
with cervicitis N72
cornea (nontraumatic) - *see* Ulcer, cornea
recurrent H18.83
traumatic - *see* Abrasion, cornea
dental (idiopathic) (occupational) (due to diet, drugs or vomiting) K03.2
duodenum, postpyloric - *see* Ulcer, duodenum
esophagus K22.10
with bleeding K22.11
gastric - *see* Ulcer, stomach

Erosion - *continued*
gastrojejunal - *see* Ulcer, gastrojejunal
implanted mesh - *see* Complications, mesh
intestine K63.3
lymphatic vessel I89.8
pylorus, pyloric (ulcer) - *see* Ulcer, stomach
spine, aneurysmal A52.09
stomach - *see* Ulcer, stomach
subcutaneous device pocket
  nervous system prosthetic device, implant, or
    graft T85.890
  other internal prosthetic device, implant, or
    graft T85.898
teeth (idiopathic) (occupational) (due to diet,
  drugs or vomiting) K03.2
urethra N36.8
uterus N85.8
Erotomania F52.8
Error
metabolism, inborn se Disorder, metabolism
refractive - *see* Disorder, refraction
Eructation R14.2
nervous or psychogenic F45.8
Eruption
creeping B76.9
drug (generalized) (taken internally) L27.0
  fixed L27.1
  in contact with skin - *see* Dermatitis, due to
  drugs
    localized L27.1
Hutchinson, summer L56.4
Kaposi's varicelliform B00.0
napkin L22
polymorphous light (sun) L56.4
recalcitrant pustular L13.8
ringed R23.8
skin (nonspecific) R21
  creeping (meaning hookworm) B76.9
  due to inoculation/vaccination (generalized) -
  see also Dermatitis, due to, vaccine L27.0
    localized L27.1
  erysipeloid A26.0
  feigned L98.1
  Kaposi's varicelliform B00.0
  lichenoid L28.0
  meaning dermatitis - *see* Dermatitis
  toxic NEC L53.0
tooth, teeth, abnormal (incomplete) (late)
  (premature) (sequence) K00.6
vesicular R23.8
Erysipelas (gangrenous) (infantile) (newborn)
(phlegmonous) (suppurative) A46
external ear A46 [H62.40]
puerperal, postpartum O86.89
Erysipeloid A26.9
cutaneous (Rosenbach's) A26.0
disseminated A26.8
sepsis A26.7
specified NEC A26.8
Erythema, erythematous (infectional)
(inflammation) L53.9
ab igne L59.0
annulare (centrifugum) (rheumaticum) L53.1
arthriticum epidemicum A25.1
brucellum - *see* Brucellosis
chronic figurate NEC L53.3
chronicum migrans (Borrelia burgdorferi)
  A69.20
diaper L22
due to
  chemical NEC L53.0
    in contact with skin L24.5
  drug (internal use) - *see* Dermatitis, due to,
  drugs

Erythema, erythematous - *continued*
elevatum diutinum L95.1
endemic E52
epidemic, arthritic A25.1
figuratum perstans L53.3
gluteal L22
heat
  code by site under Burn, first degree
  ichthyosiforme congenitum bullous Q80.3
in diseases classified elsewhere L54
induratum (nontuberculous) L52
  tuberculous A18.4
infectiosum B08.3
intertrigo L30.4
iris L51.9
marginatum L53.2
  in (due to) acute rheumatic fever I00
medicamentosum - *see* Dermatitis, due to,
  drugs
migrans A26.0
  chronicum A69.20
  tongue K14.1
multiforme (major) (minor) L51.9
  bullous, bullosum L51.1
  conjunctiva L51.1
  nonbullous L51.0
  pemphigoides L12.0
  specified NEC L51.8
napkin L22
neonatorum P83.88
  toxic P83.1
nodosum L52
  tuberculous A18.4
palmar L53.8
pernio T69.1
rash, newborn P83.88
scarlatiniform (recurrent) (exfoliative) L53.8
solare L55.0
specified NEC L53.8
toxic, toxicum NEC L53.0
  newborn P83.1
tuberculous (primary) A18.4
Erythematous, erythematosus - *see* condition
Erythermalgia (primary) I73.81
Erythralgia I73.81
Erythrasma L08.1
Erythredema (polyneuropathy) - *see*
Poisoning, mercury
Erythremia (acute) C94.0-
chronic D45
secondary D75.1
Erythroblastopenia - *see also* Aplasia, red cell
D60.9
congenital D61.01
Erythroblastophthisis D61.09
Erythroblastosis (fetalis) (newborn) P55.9
due to
  ABO (antibodies) (incompatibility)
    (isoimmunization) P55.1
  Rh (antibodies) (incompatibility)
    (isoimmunization) P55.0
Erythrocyanosis (crurum) I73.89
Erythrocythemia - *see* Erythremia
Erythrocytosis (megalosplenic) (secondary)
D75.1
familial D75.0
oval, hereditary - *see* Elliptocytosis
secondary D75.1
stress D75.1
Erythroderma (secondary) - *see also*
Erythema L53.9
bullous ichthyosiform, congenital Q80.3
desquamativum L21.1
ichthyosiform, congenital (bullous) Q80.3

Erythroderma - *continued*
neonatorum P83.88
psoriaticum L40.8
Erythrodysesthesia, palmar plantar (PPE)
L27.1
Erythrogenesis imperfecta D61.09
Erythroleukemia C94.0-
Erythromelalgia I73.81
Erythrophagocytosis D75.89
Erythrophobia F40.298
Erythroplakia, oral epithelium, and tongue
K13.29
Erythroplasia (Queyrat) D07.4
specified site - *see* Neoplasm, skin, in situ
unspecified site D07.4
Escherichia coli (E. coli), as cause of disease
classified elsewhere B96.20
non-o157 Shiga toxin-producing (with known
  O group) B96.22
non-shiga toxin-producing B96.29
O157 with confirmation of Shiga toxin when
  H antigen is unknown, or is not H7 B96.21
O157:H (nonmotile) with confirmation of
  Shiga toxin B96.21
Shiga toxin-producing (with unspecified O
  group) (STEC) B96.23
O157 B96.21
O157:H7 with or without confirmation of
  Shiga toxin-production B96.21
specified NEC B96.29
Esophagismus K22.4
Esophagitis (acute) (alkaline) (chemical)
(chronic) (infectional) (necrotic) (peptic)
(postoperative) K20.9
candidal B37.81
due to gastrointestinal reflux disease K21.0
eosinophilic K20.0
reflux K21.0
specified NEC K20.8
tuberculous A18.83
ulcerative K22.10
  with bleeding K22.11
Esophagocele K22.5
Esophagomalacia K22.8
Esophagospasm K22.4
Esophagostenosis K22.2
Esophagostomiasis B81.8
Esophagotracheal - *see* condition
Esophagus - *see* condition
Esophoria H50.51
convergence, excess H51.12
divergence, insufficiency H51.8
Esotropia - *see* Strabismus, convergent
concomitant
Espundia B55.2
Essential - *see* condition
Esthesioneuroblastoma C30.0
Esthesioneurocytoma C30.0
Esthesioneuroepithelioma C30.0
Esthiomene A55
Estivo-autumnal malaria (fever) B50.9
Estrangement (marital) Z63.5
parent-child NEC Z62.890
Estriasis - *see* Myiasis
Ethanolism - *see* Alcoholism
Etherism - *see* Dependence, drug, inhalant
Ethmoid, ethmoidal - *see* condition
Ethmoiditis (chronic) (nonpurulent)
(purulent) - *see also* Sinusitis, ethmoidal
influenzal - *see* Influenza, with, respiratory
  manifestations NEC
Woakes' J33.1
Ethylism - *see* Alcoholism

Eulenburg's disease (congenital paramyotonia) G71.19
Eumycetoma B47.0
Eunuchoidism E29.1
  hypogonadotropic E23.0
European blastomycosis - see Cryptococcosis
Eustachian - see condition
Evaluation (for) (of)
  development state
    adolescent Z00.3
    period of
      delayed growth in childhood Z00.70
        with abnormal findings Z00.71
      rapid growth in childhood Z00.2
    puberty Z00.3
  growth and developmental state (period of rapid growth) Z00.2
    delayed growth Z00.70
      with abnormal findings Z00.71
  mental health (status) Z00.8
    requested by authority Z04.6
  period of
    delayed growth in childhood Z00.70
      with abnormal findings Z00.71
    rapid growth in childhood Z00.2
  suspected condition - see Observation
Evans syndrome D69.41
Event
  apparent life threatening in newborn and infant (ALTE) R68.13
  brief resolved unexplained event (BRUE) R68.13
Eventration - see also Hernia, ventral
  colon into chest - see Hernia, diaphragm
  diaphragm (congenital) Q79.1
Eversion
  bladder N32.89
  cervix (uteri) N86
    with cervicitis N72
  foot NEC - see also Deformity, valgus, ankle
    congenital Q66.6
  punctum lacrimale (postinfectional) (senile) H04.52-
  ureter (meatus) N28.89
  urethra (meatus) N36.8
  uterus N81.4
Evidence
  cytologic
    of malignancy on anal smear R85.614
    of malignancy on cervical smear R87.614
    of malignancy on vaginal smear R87.624
Evisceration
  birth injury P15.8
  traumatic NEC
    eye - see Enucleated eye
Evulsion - see Avulsion
Ewing's sarcoma or tumor
  - see Neoplasm, bone, malignant
Examination (for) (following) (general) (of) (routine) Z00.00
  with abnormal findings Z00.01
  abuse, physical (alleged), ruled out
    adult Z04.71
    child Z04.72
  adolescent (development state) Z00.3
  alleged rape or sexual assault (victim), ruled out
    adult Z04.41
    child Z04.42
  allergy Z01.82
  annual (adult) (periodic) (physical) Z00.00
    with abnormal findings Z00.01
  gynecological Z01.419

Examination - continued
  with abnormal findings Z01.411
  antibody response Z01.84
  blood - see Examination, laboratory   blood
    pressure Z01.30
    with abnormal findings Z01.31
  cancer staging - see Neoplasm, malignant, by site
  cervical Papanicolaou smear Z12.4
    as part of routine gynecological examination Z01.419
      with abnormal findings Z01.411
  child (over 28 days old) Z00.129
    with abnormal findings Z00.121
    under 28 days old - see Newborn, examination
  clinical research control or normal comparison (control) (participant) Z00.6
  contraceptive (drug) maintenance (routine) Z30.8
    device (intrauterine) Z30.431
  dental Z01.20
    with abnormal findings Z01.21
  developmental - see Examination, child
    donor (potential) Z00.5
  ear Z01.10
    with abnormal findings NEC Z01.118
  eye Z01.00
    with abnormal findings Z01.01
  following
    accident NEC Z04.3
      transport Z04.1
      work Z04.2
    assault, alleged, ruled out
      adult Z04.71
      child Z04.72
    motor vehicle accident Z04.1
    treatment (for) Z09
      combined NEC Z09
        fracture Z09
        malignant neoplasm Z08
      malignant neoplasm Z08
      mental disorder Z09
      specified condition NEC Z09
  follow-up (routine) (following) Z09
    chemotherapy NEC Z09
      malignant neoplasm Z08
    fracture Z09
    malignant neoplasm Z08
    postpartum Z39.2
    psychotherapy Z09
    radiotherapy NEC Z09
      malignant neoplasm Z08
    surgery NEC Z09
      malignant neoplasm Z08
  gynecological Z01.419
    with abnormal findings Z01.411
    for contraceptive maintenance Z30.8
  health - see Examination, medical
  hearing Z01.10
    with abnormal findings NEC Z01.118
    following failed hearing screening Z01.110
  immunity status testing Z01.84
  laboratory (as part of a general medical examination) Z00.00
    with abnormal findings Z00.01
    preprocedural Z01.812
  lactating mother Z39.1
  medical (adult) (for) (of) Z00.00
    with abnormal findings Z00.01
    administrative purpose only Z02.9
      specified NEC Z02.89
    admission to
      armed forces Z02.3

Examination - continued
  old age home Z02.2
  prison Z02.89
  residential institution Z02.2
  school Z02.0
    following illness or medical treatment Z02.0
    summer camp Z02.89
  adoption Z02.82
  blood alcohol or drug level Z02.83
  camp (summer) Z02.89
  clinical research, normal subject (control) (participant) Z00.6
  control subject in clinical research (normal comparison) (participant) Z00.6
  donor (potential) Z00.5
  driving license Z02.4
  general (adult) Z00.00
    with abnormal findings Z00.01
  immigration Z02.89
  insurance purposes Z02.6
  marriage Z02.89
  medicolegal reasons NEC Z04.8
  naturalization Z02.89
  participation in sport Z02.5
  paternity testing Z02.81
  population survey Z00.8
  pre-employment Z02.1
  pre-operative - see Examination, pre-procedural
  pre-procedural
    cardiovascular Z01.810
    respiratory Z01.811
    specified NEC Z01.818
  preschool children
    for admission to school Z02.0
  prisoners
    for entrance into prison Z02.89
  recruitment for armed forces Z02.3
  specified NEC Z00.8
  sport competition Z02.5
  medicolegal reason NEC Z04.8
  newborn - see Newborn, examination
  pelvic (annual) (periodic) Z01.419
    with abnormal findings Z01.411
  period of rapid growth in childhood Z00.2
  periodic (adult) (annual) (routine) Z00.00
    with abnormal findings Z00.01
  physical (adult) - see also Examination, medical Z00.00
  sports Z02.5
  postpartum
    immediately after delivery Z39.0
    routine follow-up Z39.2
  prenatal (normal pregnancy) - see also Pregnancy, normal Z34.9-
  pre-chemotherapy (antineoplastic) Z01.818
  pre-procedural (pre-operative)
    cardiovascular Z01.810
    laboratory Z01.812
    respiratory Z01.811
    specified NEC Z01.818
  prior to chemotherapy (antineoplastic) Z01.818
  psychiatric NEC Z00.8
    follow-up not needing further care Z09
    requested by authority Z04.6
  radiological (as part of a general medical examination) Z00.00
    with abnormal findings Z00.01
  repeat cervical smear to confirm findings of recent normal smear following initial abnormal smear Z01.42
  skin (hypersensitivity) Z01.82

Examination - *continued*
  special - *see also* Examination, by type Z01.89
    specified type NEC Z01.89
  specified type or reason NEC Z04.8
  teeth Z01.20
    with abnormal findings Z01.21
  urine - *see* Examination, laboratory   vision
    Z01.00
    with abnormal findings Z01.01
Exanthem, exanthema - *see also* Rash
  with enteroviral vesicular stomatitis B08.4
  Boston A88.0
  epidemic with meningitis A88.0 [*G02*]
  subitum B08.20
    due to human herpesvirus 6 B08.21
    due to human herpesvirus 7 B08.22
  viral, virus B09
    specified type NEC B08.8
Excess, excessive, excessively   alcohol level in
    blood R78.0
  androgen (ovarian) E28.1
  attrition, tooth, teeth K03.0
  carotene, carotin (dietary) E67.1
  cold, effects of T69.9
    specified effect NEC T69.8
  convergence H51.12
  crying
    in child, adolescent, or adult R45.83
    in infant R68.11
  development, breast N62
  divergence H51.8
  drinking (alcohol) NEC (without dependence)
    F10.10
    habitual (continual) (without remission)
      F10.20
  eating R63.2
  estrogen E28.0
  fat - *see also* Obesity
    in heart - *see* Degeneration, myocardial
    localized E65
  foreskin N47.8
  gas R14.0
  glucagon E16.3
  heat - *see* Heat
  intermaxillary vertical dimension of fully
    erupted teeth M26.37
  interocclusal distance of fully erupted teeth
    M26.37
  kalium E87.5
  large
    colon K59.39
      congenital Q43.8
    infant P08.0
    organ or site, congenital NEC - *see* Anomaly,
      by site
  long
    organ or site, congenital NEC - *see* Anomaly,
      by site
  menstruation (with regular cycle) N92.0
    with irregular cycle N92.1
  napping Z72.821
  natrium E87.0
  number of teeth K00.1
  nutrient (dietary) NEC R63.2
  potassium (K) E87.5
  salivation K11.7
  secretion - *see also* Hypersecretion
    milk O92.6
    sputum R09.3
    sweat R61
  sexual drive F52.8
  short
    organ or site, congenital NEC - *see* Anomaly,
      by site

Excess, excessive, excessively - *continued*
  umbilical cord in labor or delivery O69.3
  skin L98.7
    and subcutaneous tissue L98.7
    eyelid (acquired) - *see* Blepharochalasis
      congenital Q10.3
  sodium (Na) E87.0
  spacing of fully erupted teeth M26.32
  sputum R09.3
  sweating R61
  thirst R63.1
    due to deprivation of water T73.1
  tuberosity of jaw M26.07
  vitamin
    A (dietary) E67.0
      administered as drug (prolonged intake) -
        see Table of Drugs and Chemicals,
        vitamins, adverse effect
      overdose or wrong substance given or taken
        - *see* Table of Drugs and Chemicals,
        vitamins, poisoning
    D (dietary) E67.3
      administered as drug (prolonged intake) -
        see Table of Drugs and Chemicals,
        vitamins, adverse effect
      overdose or wrong substance given or taken
        - *see* Table of Drugs and Chemicals,
        vitamins, poisoning
  weight
    gain R63.5
    loss R63.4
**Excitability, abnormal, under minor stress
  (personality disorder)** F60.3
Excitation
  anomalous atrioventricular I45.6
  psychogenic F30.8
  reactive (from emotional stress, psychological
    trauma) F30.8
Excitement
  hypomanic F30.8
  manic F30.9
  mental, reactive (from emotional stress,
    psychological trauma) F30.8
  state, reactive (from emotional stress,
    psychological trauma) F30.8
Excoriation (traumatic) - *see also* Abrasion
  neurotic L98.1
  skin picking disorder F42.4
Exfoliation
  due to erythematous conditions according to
    extent of body surface involved L49.0
    10-19 percent of body surface L49.1
    20-29 percent of body surface L49.2
    30-39 percent of body surface L49.3
    40-49 percent of body surface L49.4
    50-59 percent of body surface L49.5
    60-69 percent of body surface L49.6
    70-79 percent of body surface L49.7
    80-89 percent of body surface L49.8
    90-99 percent of body surface L49.9
    less than 10 percent of body surface L49.0
  teeth, due to systemic causes K08.0
Exfoliative - *see* condition
Exhaustion, exhaustive (physical NEC)
  R53.83
  battle F43.0
  cardiac - *see* Failure, heart
  delirium F43.0
  due to
    cold T69.8
    excessive exertion T73.3
    exposure T73.2
    neurasthenia F48.8
  heart - *see* Failure, heart

Exhaustion, exhaustive - *continued*
  heat - *see also* Heat, exhaustion T67.5
    due to
      salt depletion T67.4
      water depletion T67.3
  maternal, complicating delivery O75.81
  mental F48.8
  myocardium, myocardial - *see* Failure, heart
  nervous F48.8
  old age R54
  psychogenic F48.8
  psychosis F43.0
  senile R54
  vital NEC Z73.0
Exhibitionism F65.2
Exocervicitis - *see* Cervicitis
Exomphalos Q79.2
  meaning hernia - *see* Hernia, umbilicus
Exophoria H50.52
  convergence, insufficiency H51.11
  divergence, excess H51.8
Exophthalmos H05.2-
  congenital Q15.8
  constant NEC H05.24-
  displacement, globe - *see* Displacement, globe
  due to thyrotoxicosis (hyperthyroidism) - *see*
    Hyperthyroidism, with, goiter (diffuse)
  dysthyroid - *see* Hyperthyroidism, with, goiter
    (diffuse)
  goiter - *see* Hyperthyroidism, with, goiter
    (diffuse)
  intermittent NEC H05.25-
  malignant - *see* Hyperthyroidism, with, goiter
    (diffuse)
  orbital
    edema - *see* Edema, orbit
    hemorrhage - *see* Hemorrhage, orbit
  pulsating NEC H05.26-
  thyrotoxic, thyrotropic - *see* Hyperthyroidism,
    with, goiter (diffuse)
Exostosis - *see also* Disorder, bone
  cartilaginous - *see* Neoplasm, bone, benign
  congenital (multiple) Q78.6
  external ear canal H61.81-
  gonococcal A54.49
  jaw (bone) M27.8
  multiple, congenital Q78.6
  orbit H05.35-
  osteocartilaginous - *see* Neoplasm, bone,
    benign
  syphilitic A52.77
Exotropia - *see* Strabismus, divergent
  concomitant
Explanation of
  investigation finding Z71.2
  medication Z71.89
Exposure (to) - *see also* Contact, with T75.89
  acariasis Z20.7
  AIDS virus Z20.6
  air pollution Z77.110
  algae and algae toxins Z77.121
  algae bloom Z77.121
  anthrax Z20.810
  aromatic amines Z77.020
  aromatic (hazardous) compounds NEC
    Z77.028
  aromatic dyes NOS Z77.028
  arsenic Z77.010
  asbestos Z77.090
  bacterial disease NEC Z20.818
  benzene Z77.021
  blue-green algae bloom Z77.121
  body fluids (potentially hazardous) Z77.21
  brown tide Z77.121

Exposure (to) - *continued*

chemicals (chiefly nonmedicinal) (hazardous) NEC Z77.098

cholera Z20.09

chromium compounds Z77.018

cold, effects of T69.9

specified effect NEC T69.8

communicable disease Z20.9

bacterial NEC Z20.818

specified NEC Z20.89

viral NEC Z20.828

cyanobacteria bloom Z77.121

disaster Z65.5

discrimination Z60.5

dyes Z77.098

effects of T73.9

environmental tobacco smoke (acute) (chronic) Z77.22

Escherichia coli (E. coli) Z20.01

exhaustion due to T73.2

fiberglass - *see* Table of Drugs and Chemicals, fiberglass

German measles Z20.4

gonorrhea Z20.2

hazardous metals NEC Z77.018

hazardous substances NEC Z77.29

hazards in the physical environment NEC Z77.128

hazards to health NEC Z77.9

human immunodeficiency virus (HIV) Z20.6

human T-lymphotropic virus type 1 (HTLV 1) Z20.89

implanted

mesh - *see* Complications, mesh

prosthetic materials NEC - *see* Complications, prosthetic materials NEC

infestation (parasitic) NEC Z20.7

intestinal infectious disease NEC Z20.09

Escherichia coli (E. coli) Z20.01

lead Z77.011

meningococcus Z20.811

mold (toxic) Z77.120

nickel dust Z77.018

noise Z77.122

occupational

air contaminants NEC Z57.39

dust Z57.2

environmental tobacco smoke Z57.31

extreme temperature Z57.6

noise Z57.0

radiation Z57.1

risk factors Z57.9

specified NEC Z57.8

toxic agents (gases) (liquids) (solids) (vapors) in agriculture Z57.4

toxic agents (gases) (liquids) (solids) (vapors) in industry NEC Z57.5

vibration Z57.7

parasitic disease NEC Z20.7

pediculosis Z20.7

persecution Z60.5

pfiesteria piscicida Z77.121

poliomyelitis Z20.89

polycyclic aromatic hydrocarbons Z77.028

pollution

air Z77.110

environmental NEC Z77.118

soil Z77.112

water Z77.111

prenatal (drugs) (toxic chemicals) - *see* Newborn, affected by, noxious substances transmitted via placenta or breast milk

rabies Z20.3

radiation, naturally occurring NEC Z77.123

Exposure (to) - *continued*

radon Z77.123

red tide (Florida) Z77.121

rubella Z20.4

second hand tobacco smoke (acute) (chronic) Z77.22

in the perinatal period P96.81

sexually-transmitted disease Z20.2

smallpox (laboratory) Z20.89

syphilis Z20.2

terrorism Z65.4

torture Z65.4

tuberculosis Z20.1

uranium Z77.012

varicella Z20.820

venereal disease Z20.2

viral disease NEC Z20.828

war Z65.5

water pollution Z77.111

Exsanguination - *see* Hemorrhage

Exstrophy

abdominal contents Q45.8

bladder Q64.10

cloacal Q64.12

specified type NEC Q64.19

supravesical fissure Q64.11

Extensive - *see* condition

Extra - *see also* Accessory

marker chromosomes (normal individual) Q92.61

in abnormal individual Q92.62

rib Q76.6

cervical Q76.5

Extrasystoles (supraventricular) I49.49

atrial I49.1

auricular I49.1

junctional I49.2

ventricular I49.3

Extrauterine gestation or pregnancy - *see* Pregnancy, by site

Extravasation

blood R58

chyle into mesentery I89.8

pelvicalyceal N13.8

pyelosinus N13.8

urine (from ureter) R39.0

vesicant agent

antineoplastic chemotherapy T80.810

other agent NEC T80.818

Extremity - *see* condition, limb

Extrophy - *see* Exstrophy

Extroversion

bladder Q64.19

uterus N81.4

complicating delivery O71.2

postpartal (old) N81.4

Extruded tooth (teeth) M26.34

Extrusion

breast implant (prosthetic) T85.42

eye implant (globe) (ball) T85.328

intervertebral disc - *see* Displacement, intervertebral disc

ocular lens implant (prosthetic) - *see* Complications, intraocular lens

vitreous - *see* Prolapse, vitreous

Exudate

pleural - *see* Effusion, pleura

retina H35.89

Exudative - *see* condition

Eye, eyeball, eyelid - *see* condition

Eyestrain - *see* Disturbance, vision, subjective

Eyeworm disease of Africa B74.3

F

Faber's syndrome (achlorhydric anemia) D50.9

Fabry (-Anderson) disease E75.21

Faciocephalalgia, autonomic - *see also* Neuropathy, peripheral, autonomic G90.09

Factor(s)

psychic, associated with diseases classified elsewhere F54

psychological

affecting physical conditions F54

or behavioral

affecting general medical condition F54

associated with disorders or diseases classified elsewhere F54

Fahr disease (of brain) G23.8

Fahr Volhard disease (of kidney) I12.

Failure, failed

abortion - *see* Abortion, attempted

aortic (valve) I35.8

rheumatic I06.8

attempted abortion - *see* Abortion, attempted

biventricular I50.82

due to left heart failure I50.814

bone marrow - *see* Anemia, aplastic

cardiac - *see* Failure, heart

cardiorenal (chronic) (see also Failure, renal, and Failure, heart) I50.9

hypertensive I13.2

cardiorespiratory - *see also* Failure, heart R09.2

cardiovascular (chronic) - *see* Failure, heart

cerebrovascular I67.9

cervical dilatation in labor O62.0

circulation, circulatory (peripheral) R57.9

newborn P29.89

compensation - *see* Disease, heart

compliance with medical treatment or regimen - *see* Noncompliance

congestive - *see* Failure, heart, congestive

dental implant (endosseous) M27.69

due to

failure of dental prosthesis M27.63

lack of attached gingiva M27.62

occlusal trauma (poor prosthetic design) M27.62

parafunctional habits M27.62

periodontal infection (peri-implantitis) M27.62

poor oral hygiene M27.62

osseointegration M27.61

due to

complications of systemic disease M27.61

poor bone quality M27.61

iatrogenic M27.61

post-osseointegration

biological M27.62

due to complications of systemic disease M27.62

iatrogenic M27.62

mechanical M27.63

pre-integration M27.61

pre-osseointegration M27.61

specified NEC M27.69

descent of head (at term) of pregnancy (mother) O32.4

endosseous dental implant - *see* Failure, dental implant

engagement of head (term of pregnancy) (mother) O32.4

erection (penile) - *see also* Dysfunction, sexual, male, erectile N52.9

nonorganic F52.21

Failure, failed - *continued*

examination(s), anxiety concerning Z55.2
expansion terminal respiratory units (newborn)
   (primary) P28.0
forceps NOS (with subsequent cesarean
   delivery) O66.5
gain weight (child over 28 days old) R62.51
   adult R62.7
   newborn P92.6
genital response (male) F52.21
   female F52.22
heart (acute) (senile) (sudden) I50.9
   with
      acute pulmonary edema - *see* Failure,
         ventricular, left
      decompensation (see also Failure, heart, by
         type as diastolic or systolic, acute and
         chronic) I50.9
      dilatation - *see* Disease, heart
      normal ejection fraction   *see* Failure, heart,
         diastolic
      preserved ejection fraction   *see* Failure,
         heart, diastolic
      reduced ejection fraction   *see* Failure,
         heart, systolic
   arteriosclerotic I70.90
   biventricular I50.82
      due to left heart failure I50.814
   combined left-right sided I50.82
      due to left heart failure I50.814
   compensated (see also Failure, heart, by type
      as diastolic or systolic, chronic) I50.9
   complicating
      anesthesia (general) (local) or other
         sedation
            in labor and delivery O74.2
            in pregnancy O29.12-
            postpartum, puerperal O89.1
      delivery (cesarean) (instrumental) O75.4
   congestive I50.9
      with rheumatic fever (conditions in I00)
            active I01.8
            inactive or quiescent (with chorea) I09.81
      newborn P29.0
      rheumatic (chronic) (inactive) (with chorea)
         I09.81
            active or acute I01.8
               with chorea I02.0
   decompensated (see also Failure, heart, by
      type as diastolic or systolic, acute and chronic)
      I50.9
   degenerative - *see* Degeneration, myocardial
   diastolic (congestive) (left ventricular) I50.30
      acute (congestive) I50.31
         and (on) chronic (congestive) I50.33
      chronic (congestive) I50.32
         and (on) acute (congestive) I50.33
      combined with systolic (congestive) I50.40
         acute (congestive) I50.41
            and (on) chronic (congestive) I50.43
         chronic (congestive) I50.42
            and (on) acute (congestive) I50.43
   due to presence of cardiac prosthesis I97.13-
   end stage (see also Failure, heart, by type as
      diastolic or systolic, chronic) I50.84
   following cardiac surgery I97.13-
   high output NOS I50.83
   hypertensive - *see* Hypertension, heart
   left (ventricular)   *see also* Failure,
      ventricular, left
         combined diastolic and systolic   *see*
            Failure, heart, diastolic, combined with
            systolic
         diastolic   *see* Failure, heart, diastolic

Failure, failed - *continued*

   systolic   *see* Failure, heart, systolic
   low output (syndrome) NOS I50.9
      newborn P29.0
   organic - *see* Disease, heart
   peripartum O90.3
   postprocedural I97.13-
   rheumatic (chronic) (inactive) I09.9
   right (isolated) (ventricular) I50.810
      acute I50.811
         and (on) chronic I50.813
      chronic I50.812
         and acute I50.813
      secondary to left heart failure I50.814
   specified NEC I50.89
Note: heart failure stages A, B, C, and D are
based on the American College of Cardiology
and American Heart Association stages of
heart failure, which complement and should
not be confused with the New York Heart
Association Classification of Heart Failure,
into Class I, Class II, Class III, and Class IV
   stage A Z91.89
      stage B (see also Failure, heart, by type as
         diastolic or systolic) I50.9
      stage C (see also Failure, heart, by type as
         diastolic or systolic) I50.9
      stage D (see also Failure, heart, by type as
         diastolic or systolic, chronic) I50.84
   systolic (congestive) (left ventricular) I50.20
      acute (congestive) I50.21
         and (on) chronic (congestive) I50.23
      chronic (congestive) I50.22
         and (on) acute (congestive) I50.23
      combined with diastolic (congestive) I50.40
         acute (congestive) I50.41
            and (on) chronic (congestive) I50.43
         chronic (congestive) I50.42
            and (on) acute (congestive) I50.43
   thyrotoxic (see also Thyrotoxicosis) E05.90
      [143]
      with
         high output (see also Thyrotoxicosis)
            I50.83
         thyroid storm E05.91 [143]
            high output (see also Thyrotoxicosis)
               I50.83
   valvular   *see* Endocarditis
hepatic K72.90
   with coma K72.91
   acute or subacute K72.00
      with coma K72.01
      due to drugs K71.10
         with coma K71.11
   alcoholic (acute) (chronic) (subacute) K70.40
      with coma K70.41
   chronic K72.10
      with coma K72.11
      due to drugs (acute) (subacute) (chronic)
         K71.10
         with coma K71.11
   due to drugs (acute) (subacute) (chronic)
      K71.10
      with coma K71.11
   postprocedural K91.82
hepatorenal K76.7
induction (of labor) O61.9
   abortion - *see* Abortion, attempted
   by
      oxytocic drugs O61.0
      prostaglandins O61.0
   instrumental O61.1
   mechanical O61.1
   medical O61.0

Failure, failed - *continued*

   specified NEC O61.8
   surgical O61.1
intubation during anesthesia T88.4
   in pregnancy O29.6-
   labor and delivery O74.7
   postpartum, puerperal O89.6
involution, thymus (gland) E32.0
kidney - *see also* Disease, kidney, chronic N19
   acute - *see also* Failure, renal, acute N17.9-
   diabetic - *see* E08-e13 with .22
lactation (complete) O92.3
   partial O92.4
Leydig's cell, adult E29.1
liver - *see* Failure, hepatic
menstruation at puberty N91.0
mitral I05.8
myocardial, myocardium - *see also* Failure,
   heart I50.9
   chronic - *see also* Failure, heart, congestive
      I50.9
   congestive - *see also* Failure, heart,
      congestive I50.9
orgasm (female) (psychogenic) F52.31
   male F52.32
ovarian (primary) E28.39
   iatrogenic E89.40
      asymptomatic E89.40
      symptomatic E89.41
   postprocedural (postablative)
      (postirradiation) (postsurgical) E89.40
         asymptomatic E89.40
         symptomatic E89.41
ovulation causing infertility N97.0
polyglandular, autoimmune E31.0
prosthetic joint implant - *see* Complications,
   joint prosthesis, mechanical, breakdown, by
   site
renal N19
   with
      tubular necrosis (acute) N17.0
   acute N17.9
      with
         cortical necrosis N17.1
         medullary necrosis N17.2
         tubular necrosis N17.0
      specified NEC N17.8
   chronic N18.9
      hypertensive - *see* Hypertension, kidney
   congenital P96.0
   end stage (chronic) N18.6
      due to hypertension I12.0
   following
      abortion - *see* Abortion by type complicated
         by specified condition NEC
      crushing T79.5
      ectopic or molar pregnancy O08.4
      labor and delivery (acute) O90.4
   hypertensive - *see* Hypertension, kidney
   postprocedural N99.0
respiration, respiratory J96.90
   with
      hypercapnia J96.92
      hypercarbia J96.02
      hypoxia J96.91
   acute J96.00
      with
         hypercapnia J96.02
         hypercarbia J96.02
         hypoxia J96.01
   center G93.89
   acute and (on) chronic J96.20
      with
         hypercapnia J96.22

Failure, failed - *continued*
   hypercarbia J96.22
   hypoxia J96.21
   chronic J96.10
     with
       hypercapnia J96.12
       hypercarbia J96.12
       hypoxia J96.11
   newborn P28.5
   postprocedural (acute) J95.821
     acute and chronic J95.822
   rotation
     cecum Q43.3
     colon Q43.3
     intestine Q43.3
     kidney Q63.2
   sedation (conscious) (moderate) during
   procedure T88.52
     history of Z92.83
   segmentation - *see also* Fusion
     fingers - *see* Syndactylism, complex, fingers
     vertebra Q76.49
       with scoliosis Q76.3
   seminiferous tubule, adult E29.1
   senile (general) R54
   sexual arousal (male) F52.21
     female F52.22
   testicular endocrine function E29.1
   to thrive (child over 28 days old) R62.51
     adult R62.7
     newborn P92.6
   transplant T86.92
     bone T86.831
       marrow T86.02
     cornea T86.841
     heart T86.22
       with lung(s) T86.32
     intestine T86.851
     kidney T86.12
     liver T86.42
     lung(s) T86.811
       with heart T86.32
     pancreas T86.891
     skin (allograft) (autograft) T86.821
     specified organ or tissue NEC T86.891
     stem cell (peripheral blood) (umbilical cord)
     T86.5
   trial of labor (with subsequent cesarean
   delivery) O66.40
     following previous cesarean delivery O66.41
   tubal ligation N99.89
   urinary - *see* Disease, kidney, chronic
   vacuum extraction NOS (with subsequent
   cesarean delivery) O66.5
   vasectomy N99.89
   ventouse NOS (with subsequent cesarean
   delivery) O66.5
   ventricular - *see also* Failure, heart I50.9
     left (see also Failure, heart, left) I50.1
       with rheumatic fever (conditions in I00)
         active I01.8
           with chorea I02.0
         inactive or quiescent (with chorea) I09.81
         rheumatic (chronic) (inactive) (with chorea)
         I09.81
           active or acute I01.8
             with chorea I02.0
     right see Failure, heart, right
   vital centers, newborn P91.88
Fainting (fit) R55
Fallen arches - *see* Deformity, limb, flat foot

Falling, falls (repeated) R29.6
   any organ or part - *see* Prolapse
Fallopian
   insufflation Z31.41
   tube - *see* condition
Fallot's
   pentalogy Q21.8
   tetrad or tetralogy Q21.3
   triad or trilogy Q22.3
False - *see also* condition
   croup J38.5
   joint - *see* Nonunion, fracture
   labor (pains) O47.9
     at or after 37 completed weeks of gestation
       O47.1
     before 37 completed weeks of gestation
       O47.0-
   passage, urethra (prostatic) N36.5
   pregnancy F45.8
Family, familial - *see also* condition
   disruption Z63.8
     involving divorce or separation Z63.5
   Li-Fraumeni (syndrome) Z15.01
   planning advice Z30.09
   problem Z63.9
     specified NEC Z63.8
   retinoblastoma C69.2-
Famine (effects of) T73.0
   edema - *see* Malnutrition, severe
Fanconi (-de Toni)(-Debre) syndrome E72.09
   with cystinosis E72.04
Fanconi's anemia (congenital pancytopenia)
   D61.09
Farber's disease or syndrome E75.29
Farcy A24.0
Farmer's
   lung J67.0
   skin L57.8
Farsightedness - *see* Hypermetropia
Fascia - *see* condition
Fasciculation R25.3
Fasciitis M72.9
   diffuse (eosinophilic) M35.4
   infective M72.8
     necrotizing M72.6
   necrotizing M72.6
   nodular M72.4
   perirenal (with ureteral obstruction) N13.5
     with infection N13.6
   plantar M72.2
   specified NEC M72.8
   traumatic (old) M72.8
     current
     code by site under Sprain
Fascioliasis B66.3
Fasciolopsis, fasciolopsiasis (intestinal) B66.5
Fascioscapulohumeral myopathy G71.0
Fast pulse R00.0
Fat
   embolism - *see* Embolism, fat
   excessive - *see also* Obesity
     in heart - *see* Degeneration, myocardial
   in stool R19.5
   localized (pad) E65
     heart - *see* Degeneration, myocardial
     knee M79.4
     retropatellar M79.4
   necrosis
     breast N64.1
     mesentery K65.4
     omentum K65.4
   pad E65
     knee M79.4

Fatigue R53.83
   auditory deafness - *see* Deafness
   chronic R53.82
   combat F43.0
   general R53.83
     psychogenic F48.8
   heat (transient) T67.6
   muscle M62.89
   myocardium - *see* Failure, heart
   neoplasm-related R53.0
   nervous, neurosis F48.8
   operational F48.8
   psychogenic (general) F48.8
   senile R54
   voice R49.8
Fatness - *see* Obesity
Fatty - *see also* condition
   apron E65
   degeneration - *see* Degeneration, fatty
   heart (enlarged) - *see* Degeneration,
     myocardial
   liver NEC K76.0
     alcoholic K70.0
     nonalcoholic K76.0
   necrosis - *see* Degeneration, fatty
Fauces - *see* condition
Fauchard's disease (periodontitis) - *see*
   Periodontitis
Faucitis J02.9
Favism (anemia) D55.0
Favus - *see* Dermatophytosis
Fazio-Londe disease or syndrome G12.1
Fear complex or reaction F40.9
Fear of - *see* Phobia
Feared complaint unfounded Z71.1
Febris, febrile - *see also* Fever
   flava - *see also* Fever, yellow A95.9
   melitensis A23.0
   pestis - *see* Plague
   recurrens - *see* Fever, relapsing
   rubra A38.9
Fecal
   incontinence R15.9
   smearing R15.1
   soiling R15.1
   urgency R15.2
Fecalith (impaction) K56.41
   appendix K38.1
   congenital P76.8
Fede's disease K14.0
**Feeble rapid pulse due to shock following
injury** T79.4
Feeble-minded F70
Feeding
   difficulties R63.3
   problem R63.3
     newborn P92.9
       specified NEC P92.8
     nonorganic (adult) - *see* Disorder, eating
Feeling (of)
   foreign body in throat R09.89
Feer's disease - *see* Poisoning, mercury
Feet - *see* condition
Feigned illness Z76.5
Feil-Klippel syndrome (brevicollis) Q76.1
Feinmesser's (hidrotic) ectodermal dysplasia
   Q82.4
Felinophobia F40.218
Felon - *see also* Cellulitis, digit
   with lymphangitis - *see* Lymphangitis, acute,
     digit
Felty's syndrome M05.00
   ankle M05.07-
   elbow M05.02-

Felty's syndrome - *continued*
  foot joint M05.07-
  hand joint M05.04-
  hip M05.05-
  knee M05.06-
  multiple site M05.09
  shoulder M05.01-
  vertebra - *see* Spondylitis, ankylosing
  wrist M05.03-
Female genital cutting status - *see* Female
  genital mutilation status (FGM)
Female genital mutilation status (FGM)
  N90.810
  specified NEC N90.818
  type I (clitorectomy status) N90.811
  type II (clitorectomy with excision of labia
    minora status) N90.812
  type III (infibulation status) N90.813
  type IV N90.818
Femur, femoral - *see* condition
Fenestration, fenestrated - *see also* Imperfect,
  closure
  aortico-pulmonary Q21.4
  cusps, heart valve NEC Q24.8
    pulmonary Q22.3
  pulmonic cusps Q22.3
Fernell's disease (aortic aneurysm) I71.9
Fertile eunuch syndrome E23.0
Fetid
  breath R19.6
  sweat L75.0
Fetishism F65.0
  transvestic F65.1
Fetus, fetal - *see also* condition
  alcohol syndrome (dysmorphic) Q86.0
  compressus O31.0-
  hydantoin syndrome Q86.1
  lung tissue P28.0
  papyraceous O31.0-
Fever (inanition) (of unknown origin)
(persistent) (with chills) (with rigor) R50.9
  abortus A23.1
  Aden (dengue) A90
  African tick-borne A68.1
  American
    mountain (tick) A93.2
    spotted A77.0
  aphthous B08.8
  arbovirus, arboviral A94
    hemorrhagic A94
    specified NEC A93.8
  Argentinian hemorrhagic A96.0
  Assam B55.0
  Australian Q A78
  Bangkok hemorrhagic A91
  Barmah forest A92.8
  Bartonella A44.0
  bilious, hemoglobinuric B50.8
  blackwater B50.8
  blister B00.1
  Bolivian hemorrhagic A96.1
  Bonvale dam T73.3
  boutonneuse A77.1
  brain - *see* Encephalitis
  Brazilian purpuric A48.4
  breakbone A90
  Bullis A77.0
  Bunyamwera A92.8
  Burdwan B55.0
  Bwamba A92.8
  Cameroon - *see* Malaria
  Canton A75.9
  catarrhal (acute) J00
    chronic J31.0

Fever - *continued*
  cat-scratch A28.1
  Central Asian hemorrhagic A98.0
  cerebral - *see* Encephalitis
  cerebrospinal meningococcal A39.0
  Chagres B50.9
  Chandipura A92.8
  Changuinola A93.1
  Charcot's (biliary) (hepatic) (intermittent) *see*
    Calculus, bile duct
  Chikungunya (viral) (hemorrhagic) A92.0
  Chitral A93.1
  Colombo - *see* Fever, paratyphoid
  Colorado tick (virus) A93.2
  congestive (remittent) - *see* Malaria
  Congo virus A98.0
    malarial B50.9
  Corsican - *see* Malaria
  Crimean-congo hemorrhagic A98.0
  Cyprus - *see* Brucellosis
  dandy A90
  deer fly - *see* Tularemia
  dengue (virus) A90
    hemorrhagic A91
    sandfly A93.1
  desert B38.0
  drug induced R50.2
  due to
    conditions classified elsewhere R50.81
    heat T67.0
  enteric A01.00
  enteroviral exanthematous (Boston exanthem)
    A88.0
  ephemeral (of unknown origin) R50.9
  epidemic hemorrhagic A98.5
  erysipelatous - *see* Erysipelas
  estivo-autumnal (malarial) B50.9
  famine A75.0
  five day A79.0
  following delivery O86.4
  Fort Bragg A27.89
  gastroenteric A01.00
  gastromalarial - *see* Malaria
  Gibraltar - *see* Brucellosis
  glandular - *see* Mononucleosis, infectious
  Guama (viral) A92.8
  Haverhill A25.1
  hay (allergic) J30.1
    with asthma (bronchial) J45.909
      with
        exacerbation (acute) J45.901
        status asthmaticus J45.902
    due to
      allergen other than pollen J30.89
      pollen, any plant or tree J30.1
  heat (effects) T67.0
  hematuric, bilious B50.8
  hemoglobinuric (malarial) (bilious) B50.8
  hemorrhagic (arthropod-borne) NOS A94
    with renal syndrome A98.5
    arenaviral A96.9
      specified NEC A96.8
    Argentinian A96.0
    Bangkok A91
    Bolivian A96.1
    Central Asian A98.0
    Chikungunya A92.0
    Crimean-congo A98.0
    dengue (virus) A91
    epidemic A98.5
    Junin (virus) A96.0
    Korean A98.5
    Kyasanur forest A98.2
    Machupo (virus) A96.1
    mite-borne A93.8

Fever - *continued*
    mosquito-borne A92.8
    Omsk A98.1
    Philippine A91
    Russian A98.5
    Singapore A91
    Southeast Asia A91
    Thailand A91
    tick-borne NEC A93.8
    viral A99
      specified NEC A98.8
  hepatic - *see* Cholecystitis
  herpetic - *see* Herpes
  icterohemorrhagic A27.0
  Indiana A93.8
  infective B99.9
    specified NEC B99.8
  intermittent (bilious) - *see also* Malaria
    of unknown origin R50.9
    pernicious B50.9
  iodide R50.2
  Japanese river A75.3
  jungle - *see also* Malaria
    yellow A95.0
  Junin (virus) hemorrhagic A96.0
  Katayama B65.2
  kedani A75.3
  Kenya (tick) A77.1
  Kew Garden A79.1
  Korean hemorrhagic A98.5
  Lassa A96.2
  Lone Star A77.0
  Machupo (virus) hemorrhagic A96.1
  malaria, malarial - *see* Malaria
  Malta A23.9
  Marseilles A77.1
  marsh - *see* Malaria
  Mayaro (viral) A92.8
  Mediterranean - *see also* Brucellosis A23.9
    familial M04.1
    tick A77.1
  meningeal - *see* Meningitis
  Meuse A79.0
  Mexican A75.2
  mianeh A68.1
  miasmatic - *see* Malaria
  mosquito-borne (viral) A92.9
    hemorrhagic A92.8
  mountain - *see also* Brucellosis
    meaning Rocky Mountain spotted fever
      A77.0
    tick (American) (Colorado) (viral) A93.2
  Mucambo (viral) A92.8
  mud A27.9
  Neapolitan - *see* Brucellosis
  neutropenic D70.9
  newborn P81.9
    environmental P81.0
  Nine-mile A78
  non-exanthematous tick A93.2
  North Asian tick-borne A77.2
  Omsk hemorrhagic A98.1
  O'nyong nyong (viral) A92.1
  Oropouche (viral) A93.0
  Oroya A44.0
  paludal - *see* Malaria
  Panama (malarial) B50.9
  Pappataci A93.1
  paratyphoid A01.4
    A A01.1
    B A01.2
    C A01.3
  parrot A70
  periodic (Mediterranean) M04.1
  persistent (of unknown origin) R50.9

Fever - *continued*
  petechial A39.0
  pharyngoconjunctival B30.2
  Philippine hemorrhagic A91
  phlebotomus A93.1
  Piry (virus) A93.8
  Pixuna (viral) A92.8
  Plasmodium ovale B53.0
  polioviral (nonparalytic) A80.4
  Pontiac A48.2
  postimmunization R50.83
  postoperative R50.82
    due to infection T81.4
  posttransfusion R50.84
  postvaccination R50.83
  presenting with conditions classified elsewhere
    R50.81
  pretibial A27.89
  puerperal O86.4
  Q A78
  quadrilateral A78
  quartan (malaria) B52.9
  Queensland (coastal) (tick) A77.3
  quintan A79.0
  rabbit - *see* Tularemia
  rat-bite A25.9
    due to
      Spirillum A25.0
      Streptobacillus moniliformis A25.1
  recurrent - *see* Fever, relapsing
  relapsing (Borrelia) A68.9
    Carter's (Asiatic) A68.1
    Dutton's (West African) A68.1
    Koch's A68.9
    louse-borne A68.0
    Novy's
      louse-borne A68.0
      tick-borne A68.1
    Obermeyer's (European) A68.0
    tick-borne A68.1
  remittent (bilious) (congestive) (gastric) - *see*
    Malaria
  rheumatic (active) (acute) (chronic) (subacute)
    I00
    with central nervous system involvement
      I02.9
    active with heart involvement - *see* category
      I01
    inactive or quiescent with
      cardiac hypertrophy I09.89
      carditis I09.9
      endocarditis I09.1
        aortic (valve) I06.9
          with mitral (valve) disease I08.0
        mitral (valve) I05.9
          with aortic (valve) disease I08.0
        pulmonary (valve) I09.89
        tricuspid (valve) I07.8
      heart disease NEC I09.89
      heart failure (congestive) (conditions in
        I50.) I09.81
      left ventricular failure (conditions in I50.1
        I50.4) I09.81
      myocarditis, myocardial degeneration
        (conditions in I51.4) I09.0
      pancarditis I09.9
      pericarditis I09.2
  Rift Valley (viral) A92.4
  Rocky Mountain spotted A77.0
  rose J30.1
  Ross River B33.1
  Russian hemorrhagic A98.5
  San Joaquin (Valley) B38.0
  sandfly A93.1

Fever - *continued*
  Sao Paulo A77.0
  scarlet A38.9
  seven day (leptospirosis) (autumnal)
    (Japanese) A27.89
    dengue A90
  shin-bone A79.0
  Singapore hemorrhagic A91
  solar A90
  Songo A98.5
  sore B00.1
  South African tick-bite A68.1
  Southeast Asia hemorrhagic A91
  spinal - *see* Meningitis
  spirillary A25.0
  splenic - *see* Anthrax spotted A77.9
    American A77.0
    Brazilian A77.0
    cerebrospinal meningitis A39.0
    Colombian A77.0
    due to Rickettsia
      australis A77.3
      conorii A77.1
      rickettsii A77.0
      sibirica A77.2
      specified type NEC A77.8
    Ehrlichiosis A77.40
      due to
        E. chafeensis A77.41
        specified organism NEC A77.49
    Rocky Mountain A77.0
  steroid R50.2
  streptobacillary A25.1
  subtertian B50.9
  Sumatran mite A75.3
  sun A90
  swamp A27.9
  swine A02.8
  sylvatic, yellow A95.0
  Tahyna B33.8
  tertian - *see* Malaria, tertian
  Thailand hemorrhagic A91
  thermic T67.0
  three-day A93.1
  tick
    American mountain A93.2
    Colorado A93.2
    Kemerovo A93.8
    Mediterranean A77.1
    mountain A93.2
    nonexanthematous A93.2
    Quaranfil A93.8
  tick-bite NEC A93.8
  tick-borne (hemorrhagic) NEC A93.8
  trench A79.0
  tsutsugamushi A75.3
  typhogastric A01.00
  typhoid (abortive) (hemorrhagic) (intermittent)
    (malignant) A01.00
    complicated by
      arthritis A01.04
      heart involvement A01.02
      meningitis A01.01
      osteomyelitis A01.05
      pneumonia A01.03
      specified NEC A01.09
  typhomalarial - *see* Malaria
  typhus - *see* Typhus (fever)
  undulant - *see* Brucellosis
  unknown origin R50.9
  uveoparotid D86.89
  valley B38.0
  Venezuelan equine A92.2
  vesicular stomatitis A93.8

Fever - *continued*
  viral hemorrhagic - *see* Fever, hemorrhagic, by
    type of virus
  Volhynian A79.0
  Wesselsbron (viral) A92.8
  West
    African B50.8
    Nile (viral) A92.30
      with
        complications NEC A92.39
        cranial nerve disorders A92.32
        encephalitis A92.31
        encephalomyelitis A92.31
        neurologic manifestation NEC A92.32
        optic neuritis A92.32
        polyradiculitis A92.32
  Whitmore's - *see* Melioidosis
  Wolhynian A79.0
  worm B83.9
  yellow A95.9
    jungle A95.0
    sylvatic A95.0
    urban A95.1
  Zika virus A92.5
Fibrillation
  atrial or auricular (established) I48.91
    chronic I48.2
    paroxysmal I48.0
    permanent I48.2
    persistent I48.1
  cardiac I49.8
  heart I49.8
  muscular M62.89
  ventricular I49.01
Fibrin
  ball or bodies, pleural (sac) J94.1
  chamber, anterior (eye) (gelatinous exudate) -
    see Iridocyclitis, acute
Fibrinogenolysis - *see* Fibrinolysis
Fibrinogenopenia D68.8
  acquired D65
  congenital D68.2
Fibrinolysis (hemorrhagic) (acquired) D65
  antepartum hemorrhage - *see* Hemorrhage,
    antepartum, with coagulation defect
  following
    abortion - *see* Abortion by type complicated
      by hemorrhage
    ectopic or molar pregnancy O08.1
  intrapartum O67.0
  newborn, transient P60
  postpartum O72.3
Fibrinopenia (hereditary) D68.2
  acquired D68.4
Fibrinopurulent - *see* condition
Fibrinous - *see* condition
Fibroadenoma
  cellular intracanalicular D24-
  giant D24-
  intracanalicular
    cellular D24-
    giant D24-
    specified site - *see* Neoplasm, benign, by site
    unspecified site D24-
  juvenile D24-
  pericanalicular
    specified site - *see* Neoplasm, benign, by site
    unspecified site D24-
  phyllodes D24-
  prostate D29.1
  specified site NEC - *see* Neoplasm, benign, by
    site
  unspecified site D24-

Fibroadenosis, breast (chronic) (cystic) (diffuse) (periodic) (segmental) N60.2-
Fibroangioma - *see also* Neoplasm, benign, by site
  juvenile
    specified site - *see* Neoplasm, benign, by site
    unspecified site D10.6
Fibrochondrosarcoma - *see* Neoplasm, cartilage, malignant
Fibrocystic
  disease - *see also* Fibrosis, cystic
    breast - *see* Mastopathy, cystic
    jaw M27.49
    kidney (congenital) Q61.8
    liver Q44.6
    pancreas E84.9
  kidney (congenital) Q61.8
Fibrodysplasia ossificans progressiva - *see* Myositis, ossificans, progressiva
Fibroelastosis (cordis) (endocardial) (endomyocardial) I42.4
Fibroid (tumor) - *see also* Neoplasm, connective tissue, benign
  disease, lung (chronic) - *see* Fibrosis, lung
  heart (disease) - *see* Myocarditis
  in pregnancy or childbirth O34.1-
    causing obstructed labor O65.5
  induration, lung (chronic) - *see* Fibrosis, lung
  lung - *see* Fibrosis, lung
  pneumonia (chronic) - *see* Fibrosis, lung
  uterus (see also Leiomyoma, uterus) D25.9
Fibrolipoma - *see* Lipoma
Fibroliposarcoma - *see* Neoplasm, connective tissue, malignant
Fibroma - *see also* Neoplasm, connective tissue, benign
  ameloblastic - *see* Cyst, calcifying odontogenic
  bone (nonossifying) - *see* Disorder, bone, specified type NEC
    ossifying - *see* Neoplasm, bone, benign
  cementifying - *see* Neoplasm, bone, benign
  chondromyxoid - *see* Neoplasm, bone, benign
  desmoplastic - *see* Neoplasm, connective tissue, uncertain behavior
  durum - *see* Neoplasm, connective tissue, benign
  fascial - *see* Neoplasm, connective tissue, benign
  invasive - *see* Neoplasm, connective tissue, uncertain behavior
  molle - *see* Lipoma
  myxoid - *see* Neoplasm, connective tissue, benign
  nasopharynx, nasopharyngeal (juvenile) D10.6
  nonosteogenic (nonossifying) - *see* Dysplasia, fibrous
  odontogenic (central) - *see* Cyst, calcifying odontogenic
  ossifying - *see* Neoplasm, bone, benign
  periosteal - *see* Neoplasm, bone, benign
  soft - *see* Lipoma
Fibromatosis M72.9
  abdominal - *see* Neoplasm, connective tissue, uncertain behavior
  aggressive - *see* Neoplasm, connective tissue, uncertain behavior
  congenital generalized - *see* Neoplasm, connective tissue, uncertain behavior
  Dupuytren's M72.0
  gingival K06.1
  palmar (fascial) M72.0
  plantar (fascial) M72.2
  pseudosarcomatous (proliferative)

Fibromatosis - *continued*
  (subcutaneous) M72.4
  retroperitoneal D48.3
  specified NEC M72.8
Fibromyalgia M79.7
Fibromyoma - *see also* Neoplasm, connective tissue, benign
  uterus (corpus) - *see also* Leiomyoma, uterus
    in pregnancy or childbirth - *see* Fibroid, in pregnancy or childbirth
      causing obstructed labor O65.5
Fibromyositis M79.7
Fibromyxolipoma D17.9
Fibromyxoma - *see* Neoplasm, connective tissue, benign
Fibromyxosarcoma - *see* Neoplasm, connective tissue, malignant
Fibro-odontoma, ameloblastic - *see* Cyst, calcifying odontogenic
Fibro-osteoma - *see* Neoplasm, bone, benign
Fibroplasia, retrolental H35.17-
Fibropurulent - *see* condition
Fibrosarcoma - *see also* Neoplasm, connective tissue, malignant
  ameloblastic C41.1
    upper jaw (bone) C41.0
  congenital - *see* Neoplasm, connective tissue, malignant
  fascial - *see* Neoplasm, connective tissue, malignant
  infantile - *see* Neoplasm, connective tissue, malignant
  odontogenic C41.1
    upper jaw (bone) C41.0
  periosteal - *see* Neoplasm, bone, malignant
Fibrosclerosis
  breast N60.3-
  multifocal M35.5
  penis (corpora cavernosa) N48.6
Fibrosis, fibrotic
  adrenal (gland) E27.8
  amnion O41.8X-
  anal papillae K62.89
  arteriocapillary - *see* Arteriosclerosis
  bladder N32.89
    interstitial - *see* Cystitis, chronic, interstitial
    localized submucosal - *see* Cystitis, chronic, interstitial
    panmural - *see* Cystitis, chronic, interstitial
  breast - *see* Fibrosclerosis, breast
  capillary - *see also* Arteriosclerosis I70.90
    lung (chronic) - *see* Fibrosis, lung
  cardiac - *see* Myocarditis
  cervix N88.8
  chorion O41.8X-
  corpus cavernosum (sclerosing) N48.6
  cystic (of pancreas) E84.9
    with
      distal intestinal obstruction syndrome E84.19
      fecal impaction E84.19
      intestinal manifestations NEC E84.19
      pulmonary manifestations E84.0
      specified manifestations NEC E84.8
  due to device, implant or graft - *see also* Complications, by site and type, specified NEC T85.828
    arterial graft NEC T82.828
    breast (implant) T85.828
    catheter NEC T85.828
      dialysis (renal) T82.828
        intraperitoneal T85.828
      infusion NEC T82.828
        spinal (epidural) (subdural) T85.820

Fibrosis, fibrotic - *continued*
  urinary (indwelling) T83.82
  electronic (electrode) (pulse generator) (stimulator)
    bone T84.82
    cardiac T82.827
    nervous system (brain) (peripheral nerve) (spinal) T85.820
    urinary T83.82
  fixation, internal (orthopedic) NEC T84.82
  gastrointestinal (bile duct) (esophagus) T85.828
  genital NEC T83.82
  heart NEC T82.827
  joint prosthesis T84.82
  ocular (corneal graft) (orbital implant) NEC T85.828
  orthopedic NEC T84.82
  specified NEC T85.828
  urinary NEC T83.82
  vascular NEC T82.828
  ventricular intracranial shunt T85.820
  ejaculatory duct N50.89
  endocardium - *see* Endocarditis
  endomyocardial (tropical) I42.3
  epididymis N50.89
  eye muscle - *see* Strabismus, mechanical
  heart - *see* Myocarditis
  hepatic - *see* Fibrosis, liver
  hepatolienal (portal hypertension) K76.6
  hepatosplenic (portal hypertension) K76.6
  infrapatellar fat pad M79.4
  intrascrotal N50.89
  kidney N26.9
  liver K74.0
    with sclerosis K74.2
    alcoholic K70.2
  lung (atrophic) (chronic) (confluent) (massive) (perialveolar) (peribronchial) J84.10
    with
      anthracosilicosis J60
      anthracosis J60
      asbestosis J61
      bagassosis J67.1
      bauxite J63.1
      berylliosis J63.2
      byssinosis J66.0
      calcicosis J62.8
      chalicosis J62.8
      dust reticulation J64
      farmer's lung J67.0
      ganister disease J62.8
      graphite J63.3
      pneumoconiosis NOS J64
      siderosis J63.4
      silicosis J62.8
    capillary J84.10
    congenital P27.8
    diffuse (idiopathic) J84.10
      chemicals, gases, fumes or vapors (inhalation) J68.4
      interstitial J84.10
        acute J84.114
      talc J62.0
    following radiation J70.1
    idiopathic J84.112
    postinflammatory J84.10
    silicotic J62.8
    tuberculous - *see* Tuberculosis, pulmonary
  lymphatic gland I89.8
  median bar - *see* Hyperplasia, prostate
  mediastinum (idiopathic) J98.59
  meninges G96.19
  myocardium, myocardial - *see* Myocarditis

Fibrosis, fibrotic - *continued*
- ovary N83.8
- oviduct N83.8
- pancreas K86.89
- penis NEC N48.6
- pericardium I31.0
- perineum, in pregnancy or childbirth O34.7-
  - causing obstructed labor O65.5
- pleura J94.1
- popliteal fat pad M79.4
- prostate (chronic) - *see* Hyperplasia, prostate
- pulmonary - *see also* Fibrosis, lung J84.10
  - congenital P27.8
  - idiopathic J84.112
- rectal sphincter K62.89
- retroperitoneal, idiopathic (with ureteral obstruction) N13.5
  - with infection N13.6
- sclerosing mesenteric (idiopathic) K65.4
- scrotum N50.89
- seminal vesicle N50.89
- senile R54
- skin L90.5
- spermatic cord N50.89
- spleen D73.89
  - in schistosomiasis (bilharziasis) B65.9 *[D77]*
- subepidermal nodular - *see* Neoplasm, skin, benign
- submucous (oral) (tongue) K13.5
- testis N44.8
  - chronic, due to syphilis A52.76
- thymus (gland) E32.8
- tongue, submucous K13.5
- tunica vaginalis N50.89
- uterus (non neoplastic) N85.8
- vagina N89.8
- valve, heart - *see* Endocarditis
- vas deferens N50.89
- vein I87.8

Fibrositis (periarticular) M79.7
- nodular, chronic (Jaccoud's) (rheumatoid) - *see* Arthropathy, postrheumatic, chronic

Fibrothorax J94.1

Fibrotic - *see* Fibrosis

Fibrous - *see* condition

Fibroxanthoma - *see also* Neoplasm, connective tissue, benign
- atypical - *see* Neoplasm, connective tissue, uncertain behavior
- malignant - *see* Neoplasm, connective tissue, malignant

Fibroxanthosarcoma - *see* Neoplasm, connective tissue, malignant

Fiedler's
- disease (icterohemorrhagic leptospirosis) A27.0
- myocarditis (acute) I40.1

Fifth disease B08.3
- venereal A55

Filaria, filarial, filariasis - *see* Infestation, filarial

Filatov's disease - *see* Mononucleosis, infectious

File-cutter's disease - *see* Poisoning, lead

Filling defect
- biliary tract R93.2
- bladder R93.41
- duodenum R93.3
- gallbladder R93.2
- gastrointestinal tract R93.3
- intestine R93.3
- kidney R93.42-
- stomach R93.3
- ureter R93.41
- urinary organs, specified NEC R93.49

Fimbrial cyst Q50.4

Financial problem affecting care NOS Z59.9
- bankruptcy Z59.8
- foreclosure on loan Z59.8

Findings, abnormal, inconclusive, without diagnosis - *see also* Abnormal
- 17-ketosteroids, elevated R82.5
- acetonuria R82.4
- alcohol in blood R78.0
- anisocytosis R71.8
- antenatal screening of mother O28.9
  - biochemical O28.1
  - chromosomal O28.5
  - cytological O28.2
  - genetic O28.5
  - hematological O28.0
  - radiological O28.4
  - specified NEC O28.8
  - ultrasonic O28.3
- antibody titer, elevated R76.0
- anticardiolipin antibody R76.0
- antiphosphatidylglycerol antibody R76.0
- antiphosphatidylinositol antibody R76.0
- antiphosphatidylserine antibody R76.0
- antiphospholipid antibody R76.0
- bacteriuria R82.71
- bicarbonate E87.8
- bile in urine R82.2
- blood sugar R73.09
  - high R73.9
  - low (transient) E16.2
- body fluid or substance, specified NEC R88.8
- casts, urine R82.99
- catecholamines R82.5
- cells, urine R82.99
- chloride E87.8
- cholesterol E78.9
  - high E78.00
    - with high triglycerides E78.2
- chyluria R82.0
- cloudy
  - dialysis effluent R88.0
  - urine R82.90
- creatinine clearance R94.4
- crystals, urine R82.99
- culture
  - blood R78.81
  - positive - *see* Positive, culture
- echocardiogram R93.1
- electrolyte level, urinary R82.99
- function study NEC R94.8
  - bladder R94.8
  - endocrine NEC R94.7
    - thyroid R94.6
  - kidney R94.4
  - liver R94.5
  - pancreas R94.8
  - placenta R94.8
  - pulmonary R94.2
  - spleen R94.8
- gallbladder, nonvisualization R93.2
- glucose (tolerance test) (non-fasting) R73.09
- glycosuria R81
- heart
  - shadow R93.1
  - sounds R01.2
- hematinuria R82.3
- hematocrit drop (precipitous) R71.0
- hemoglobinuria R82.3
- human papillomavirus (HPV) DNA test positive
  - cervix
    - high risk R87.810
    - low risk R87.820

Findings - *continued*
- vagina
  - high risk R87.811
  - low risk R87.821
- in blood (of substance not normally found in blood) R78.9
  - addictive drug NEC R78.4
  - alcohol (excessive level) R78.0
  - cocaine R78.2
  - hallucinogen R78.3
  - heavy metals (abnormal level) R78.79
  - lead R78.71
  - lithium (abnormal level) R78.89
  - opiate drug R78.1
  - psychotropic drug R78.5
  - specified substance NEC R78.89
  - steroid agent R78.6
- indoleacetic acid, elevated R82.5
- ketonuria R82.4
- lactic acid dehydrogenase (LDH) R74.0
- liver function test R79.89
- mammogram NEC R92.8
  - calcification (calculus) R92.1
  - inconclusive result (due to dense breasts) R92.2
  - microcalcification R92.0
- mediastinal shift R93.8
- melanin, urine R82.99
- myoglobinuria R82.1
- neonatal screening P09
- nonvisualization of gallbladder R93.2
- odor of urine NOS R82.90
- Papanicolaou cervix R87.619
  - non-atypical endometrial cells R87.618
- pneumoencephalogram R93.0
- poikilocytosis R71.8
- potassium (deficiency) E87.6
  - excess E87.5
- PPD R76.11
- radiologic (X-ray) R93.8
  - abdomen R93.5
  - biliary tract R93.2
  - breast R92.8
  - gastrointestinal tract R93.3
  - genitourinary organs R93.8
  - head R93.0
  - inconclusive due to excess body fat of patient R93.9
  - intrathoracic organs NEC R93.1
  - placenta R93.8
  - retroperitoneum R93.5
  - skin R93.8
  - skull R93.0
  - subcutaneous tissue R93.8
- red blood cell (count) (morphology) (sickling) (volume) R71.8
- scan NEC R94.8
  - bladder R94.8
  - bone R94.8
  - kidney R94.4
  - liver R93.2
  - lung R94.2
  - pancreas R94.8
  - placental R94.8
  - spleen R94.8
  - thyroid R94.6
- sedimentation rate, elevated R70.0
- SGOT R74.0
- SGPT R74.0
- sodium (deficiency) E87.1
  - excess E87.0
- specified body fluid NEC R88.8
- stress test R94.39
- thyroid (function) (metabolic rate) (scan)

Findings - *continued*
  (uptake) R94.6
  transaminase (level) R74.0
  triglycerides E78.9
    high E78.1
      with high cholesterol E78.2
  tuberculin skin test (without active
  tuberculosis) R76.11
  urine R82.90
    acetone R82.4
    bacteria R82.71
    bile R82.2
    casts or cells R82.99
    chyle R82.0
    culture positive R82.79
    glucose R81
    hemoglobin R82.3
    ketone R82.4
    sugar R81
  vanillylmandelic acid (VMA), elevated R82.5
  vectorcardiogram (VCG) R94.39
  ventriculogram R93.0
  white blood cell (count) (differential)
  (morphology) D72.9
  xerography R92.8
Finger - *see* condition
Fire, Saint Anthony's - *see* Erysipelas
Fire-setting
  pathological (compulsive) F63.1
Fish hook stomach K31.89
Fishmeal-worker's lung J67.8
Fissure, fissured
  anus, anal K60.2
    acute K60.0
    chronic K60.1
    congenital Q43.8
  ear, lobule, congenital Q17.8
  epiglottis (congenital) Q31.8
  larynx J38.7
    congenital Q31.8
  lip K13.0
    congenital - *see* Cleft, lip
  nipple N64.0
    associated with
      lactation O92.13
      pregnancy O92.11-
      puerperium O92.12
  nose Q30.2
  palate (congenital) - *see* Cleft, palate
  skin R23.4
  spine (congenital) - *see also* Spina bifida
    with hydrocephalus - *see* Spina bifida, by
    site, with hydrocephalus
  tongue (acquired) K14.5
    congenital Q38.3
Fistula (cutaneous) L98.8
  abdomen (wall) K63.2
    bladder N32.2
    intestine NEC K63.2
    ureter N28.89
    uterus N82.5
  abdominorectal K63.2
  abdominosigmoidal K63.2
  abdominothoracic J86.0
  abdominouterine N82.5
    congenital Q51.7
  abdominovesical N32.2
  accessory sinuses - *see* Sinusitis
  actinomycotic - *see* Actinomycosis
  alveolar antrum - *see* Sinusitis, maxillary
  alveolar process K04.6
  anorectal K60.5
  antrobuccal - *see* Sinusitis, maxillary

Fistula (cutaneous) - *continued*
  antrum - *see* Sinusitis, maxillary
  anus, anal (recurrent) (infectional) K60.3
    congenital Q43.6
      with absence, atresia and stenosis Q42.2
    tuberculous A18.32
  aorta-duodenal I77.2
  appendix, appendicular K38.3
  arteriovenous (acquired) (nonruptured) I77.0
    brain I67.1
      congenital Q28.2
        ruptured I60.8
      ruptured I60.8
    cerebral - *see* Fistula, arteriovenous, brain
    congenital (peripheral) - *see also*
    Malformation, arteriovenous
      brain Q28.2
        ruptured I60.8
      coronary Q24.5
      pulmonary Q25.72
    coronary I25.41
      congenital Q24.5
    pulmonary I28.0
      congenital Q25.72
    surgically created (for dialysis) Z99.2
      complication - *see* Complication,
      arteriovenous, fistula, surgically created
    traumatic - *see* Injury, blood vessel
  artery I77.2
  aural (mastoid) - *see* Mastoiditis, chronic
  auricle - *see also* Disorder, pinna, specified
  type NEC
    congenital Q18.1
  Bartholin's gland N82.8
  bile duct (common) (hepatic) K83.3
    with calculus, stones - *see* Calculus, bile duct
  biliary (tract) - *see* Fistula, bile duct
  bladder (sphincter) NEC - *see also* Fistula,
  vesico N32.2
    into seminal vesicle N32.2
  bone - *see also* Disorder, bone, specified type
  NEC
    with osteomyelitis, chronic - *see*
    Osteomyelitis, chronic, with draining sinus
  brain G93.89
    arteriovenous (acquired) I67.1
      congenital Q28.2
  branchial (cleft) Q18.0
  branchiogenous Q18.0
  breast N61.0
    puerperal, postpartum or gestational, due to
    mastitis (purulent) - *see* Mastitis, obstetric,
    purulent
  bronchial J86.0
  bronchocutaneous, bronchomediastinal,
    bronchopleural, bronchopleuromediastinal
    (infective) J86.0
    tuberculous NEC A15.5
  bronchoesophageal J86.0
    congenital Q39.2
      with atresia of esophagus Q39.1
  bronchovisceral J86.0
  buccal cavity (infective) K12.2
  cecosigmoidal K63.2
  cecum K63.2
  cerebrospinal (fluid) G96.0
  cervical, lateral Q18.1
  cervicoaural Q18.1
  cervicosigmoidal N82.4
  cervicovesical N82.1
  cervix N82.8
  chest (wall) J86.0
  cholecystenteric - *see* Fistula, gallbladder
  cholecystocolic - *see* Fistula, gallbladder

Fistula (cutaneous) - *continued*
  cholecystocolonic - *see* Fistula, gallbladder
  cholecystoduodenal - *see* Fistula, gallbladder
  cholecystogastric - *see* Fistula, gallbladder
  cholecystointestinal - *see* Fistula, gallbladder
  choledochoduodenal - *see* Fistula, bile duct
  cholocolic K82.3
  coccyx - *see* Sinus, pilonidal
  colon K63.2
  colostomy K94.09
  common duct - *see* Fistula, bile duct
  congenital, site not listed - *see* Anomaly, by
  site
  coronary, arteriovenous I25.41
    congenital Q24.5
  costal region J86.0
  cul-de-sac, Douglas' N82.8
  cystic duct - *see also* Fistula, gallbladder
    congenital Q44.5
  dental K04.6
  diaphragm J86.0
  duodenum K31.6
  ear (external) (canal) - *see* Disorder, ear,
  external, specified type NEC
  enterocolic K63.2
  enterocutaneous K63.2
  enterouterine N82.4
    congenital Q51.7
  enterovaginal N82.4
    congenital Q52.2
    large intestine N82.3
    small intestine N82.2
  enterovesical N32.1
  epididymis N50.89
    tuberculous A18.15
  esophagobronchial J86.0
    congenital Q39.2
      with atresia of esophagus Q39.1
  esophagocutaneous K22.8
  esophagopleural-cutaneous J86.0
  esophagotracheal J86.0
    congenital Q39.2
      with atresia of esophagus Q39.1
  esophagus K22.8
    congenital Q39.2
      with atresia of esophagus Q39.1
  ethmoid - *see* Sinusitis, ethmoidal
  eyeball (cornea) (sclera) - *see* Disorder, globe,
  hypotony eyelid H01.8
  fallopian tube, external N82.5
  fecal K63.2
    congenital Q43.6
  from periapical abscess K04.6
  frontal sinus - *see* Sinusitis, frontal
  gallbladder K82.3
    with calculus, cholelithiasis, stones - *see*
    Calculus, gallbladder
  gastric K31.6
  gastrocolic K31.6
    congenital Q40.2
    tuberculous A18.32
  gastroenterocolic K31.6
  gastroesophageal K31.6
  gastrojejunal K31.6
  gastrojejunocolic K31.6
  genital tract (female) N82.9
    specified NEC N82.8
    to intestine NEC N82.4
    to skin N82.5
  hepatic artery-portal vein, congenital Q26.6
  hepatopleural J86.0
  hepatopulmonary J86.0
  ileorectal or ileosigmoidal K63.2
  ileovaginal N82.2

Fistula (cutaneous) - *continued*
  ileovesical N32.1
  ileum K63.2
  in ano K60.3
    tuberculous A18.32
  inner ear (labyrinth) - *see* subcategory H83.1
  intestine NEC K63.2
  intestinocolonic (abdominal) K63.2
  intestinoureteral N28.89
  intestinouterine N82.4
  intestinovaginal N82.4
    large intestine N82.3
    small intestine N82.2
  intestinovesical N32.1
  ischiorectal (fossa) K61.3
  jejunum K63.2
  joint M25.10
    ankle M25.17-
    elbow M25.12-
    foot joint M25.17-
    hand joint M25.14-
    hip M25.15-
    knee M25.16-
    shoulder M25.11-
    specified joint NEC M25.18
    tuberculous - *see* Tuberculosis, joint
    vertebrae M25.18
    wrist M25.13-
  kidney N28.89
  labium (majus) (minus) N82.8
  labyrinth - *see* subcategory H83.1
  lacrimal (gland) (sac) H04.61-
  lacrimonasal duct - *see* Fistula, lacrimal
  laryngotracheal, congenital Q34.8
  larynx J38.7
  lip K13.0
    congenital Q38.0
  lumbar, tuberculous A18.01
  lung J86.0
  lymphatic I89.8
  mammary (gland) N61.0
  mastoid (process) (region) - *see* Mastoiditis,
    chronic
  maxillary J32.0
  medial, face and neck Q18.8
  mediastinal J86.0
  mediastinobronchial J86.0
  mediastinocutaneous J86.0
  middle ear - *see* subcategory H74.8
  mouth K12.2
  nasal J34.89
    sinus - *see* Sinusitis
  nasopharynx J39.2
  nipple N64.0
  nose J34.89
  oral (cutaneous) K12.2
    maxillary J32.0
    nasal (with cleft palate) - *see* Cleft, palate
  orbit, orbital - *see* Disorder, orbit, specified
    type NEC
  oroantral J32.0
  oviduct, external N82.5
  palate (hard) M27.8
  pancreatic K86.89
  pancreaticoduodenal K86.89
  parotid (gland) K11.4
    region K12.2
  penis N48.89
  perianal K60.3
  pericardium (pleura) (sac) - *see* Pericarditis
  pericecal K63.2
  perineorectal K60.4
  perineosigmoidal K63.2
  perineum, perineal (with urethral involvement)

Fistula (cutaneous) - *continued*
NEC N36.0
    tuberculous A18.13
    ureter N28.89
  perirectal K60.4
    tuberculous A18.32
  peritoneum K65.9
  pharyngoesophageal J39.2
  pharynx J39.2
    branchial cleft (congenital) Q18.0
  pilonidal (infected) (rectum) - *see* Sinus,
    pilonidal
  pleura, pleural, pleurocutaneous,
    pleuroperitoneal J86.0
    tuberculous NEC A15.6
  pleuropericardial I31.8
  portal vein-hepatic artery, congenital Q26.6
  postauricular H70.81-
  postoperative, persistent T81.83
    specified site - *see* Fistula, by site
  preauricular (congenital) Q18.1
  prostate N42.89
  pulmonary J86.0
    arteriovenous I28.0
      congenital Q25.72
    tuberculous - *see* Tuberculosis, pulmonary
  pulmonoperitoneal J86.0
  rectolabial N82.4
  rectosigmoid (intercommunicating) K63.2
  rectoureteral N28.89
  rectourethral N36.0
    congenital Q64.73
  rectouterine N82.4
    congenital Q51.7
  rectovaginal N82.3
    congenital Q52.2
    tuberculous A18.18
  rectovesical N32.1
    congenital Q64.79
  rectovesicovaginal N82.3
  rectovulval N82.4
    congenital Q52.79
  rectum (to skin) K60.4
    congenital Q43.6
      with absence, atresia and stenosis Q42.0
    tuberculous A18.32
  renal N28.89
  retroauricular - *see* Fistula, postauricular
  salivary duct or gland (any) K11.4
    congenital Q38.4
  scrotum (urinary) N50.89
    tuberculous A18.15
  semicircular canals - *see* subcategory H83.1
  sigmoid K63.2
    to bladder N32.1
  sinus - *see* Sinusitis
  skin L98.8
    to genital tract (female) N82.5
  splenocolic D73.89
  stercoral K63.2
  stomach K31.6
  sublingual gland K11.4
  submandibular gland K11.4
  submaxillary (gland) K11.4
    region K12.2
  thoracic J86.0
    duct I89.8
  thoracoabdominal J86.0
  thoracogastric J86.0
  thoracointestinal J86.0
  thorax J86.0
  thyroglossal duct Q89.2
  thyroid E07.89
  trachea, congenital (external) (internal) Q32.1

Fistula (cutaneous) - *continued*
  tracheoesophageal J86.0
    congenital Q39.2
      with atresia of esophagus Q39.1
    following tracheostomy J95.04
  traumatic arteriovenous - *see* Injury, blood
    vessel, by site
  tuberculous
  code by site under Tuberculosis
  typhoid A01.09
  umbilicourinary Q64.8
  urachus, congenital Q64.4
  ureter (persistent) N28.89
  ureteroabdominal N28.89
  ureterorectal N28.89
  ureterosigmoido-abdominal N28.89
  ureterovaginal N82.1
  ureterovesical N32.2
  urethra N36.0
    congenital Q64.79
    tuberculous A18.13
  urethroperineal N36.0
  urethroperineovesical N32.2
  urethrorectal N36.0
    congenital Q64.73
  urethroscrotal N50.89
  urethrovaginal N82.1
  urethrovesical N32.2
  urinary (tract) (persistent) (recurrent) N36.0
  uteroabdominal N82.5
    congenital Q51.7
  uteroenteric, uterointestinal N82.4
    congenital Q51.7
  uterorectal N82.4
    congenital Q51.7
  uteroureteric N82.1
  uterourethral Q51.7
  uterovaginal N82.8
  uterovesical N82.1
    congenital Q51.7
  uterus N82.8
  vagina (postpartal) (wall) N82.8
  vaginocutaneous (postpartal) N82.5
  vaginointestinal NEC N82.4
    large intestine N82.3
    small intestine N82.2
  vaginoperineal N82.5
  vasocutaneous, congenital Q55.7
  vesical NEC N32.2
  vesicoabdominal N32.2
  vesicocervicovaginal N82.1
  vesicocolic N32.1
  vesicocutaneous N32.2
  vesicoenteric N32.1
  vesicointestinal N32.1
  vesicometrorectal N82.4
  vesicoperineal N32.2
  vesicorectal N32.1
    congenital Q64.79
  vesicosigmoidal N32.1
  vesicosigmoidovaginal N82.3
  vesicoureteral N32.2
  vesicourethrovaginal N82.1
  vesicourethral N32.2
  vesicourethrorectal N32.1
  vesicouterine N82.1
    congenital Q51.7
  vesicovaginal N82.0
  vulvorectal N82.4
    congenital Q52.79

Fit R56.9
  epileptic - *see* Epilepsy
  fainting R55
  hysterical F44.5
  newborn P90

Fitting (and adjustment) (of)
  artificial
    arm - *see* Admission, adjustment, artificial, arm
    breast Z44.3
    eye Z44.2
    leg - *see* Admission, adjustment, artificial, leg
  automatic implantable cardiac defibrillator (with synchronous cardiac pacemaker) Z45.02
  brain neuropacemaker Z46.2
    implanted Z45.42
  cardiac defibrillator - *see* Fitting (and adjustment) (of), automatic implantable cardiac defibrillator
  catheter, non-vascular Z46.82
  colostomy belt Z46.89
  contact lenses Z46.0
  CRT-d (resynchronization therapy defibrillator) Z45.02
  CRT-p (cardiac resynchronization therapy pacemaker) Z45.018
    pulse generator Z45.010
  cystostomy device Z46.6
  defibrillator, cardiac - *see* Fitting (and adjustment) (of), automatic implantable cardiac defibrillator
  dentures Z46.3
  device NOS Z46.9
    abdominal Z46.89
    gastrointestinal NEC Z46.59
    implanted NEC Z45.89
    nervous system Z46.2
      implanted - *see* Admission, adjustment, device, implanted, nervous system
    orthodontic Z46.4
    orthoptic Z46.0
    orthotic Z46.89
    prosthetic (external) Z44.9
      breast Z44.3
      dental Z46.3
      eye Z44.2
      specified NEC Z44.8
    specified NEC Z46.89
  substitution
    auditory Z46.2
      implanted - *see* Admission, adjustment, device, implanted, hearing device
    nervous system Z46.2
      implanted - *see* Admission, adjustment, device, implanted, nervous system
    visual Z46.2
      implanted Z45.31
    urinary Z46.6
  gastric lap band Z46.51
  gastrointestinal appliance NEC Z46.59
  glasses (reading) Z46.0
  hearing aid Z46.1
  ileostomy device Z46.89
  insulin pump Z46.81
  intestinal appliance NEC Z46.89
  myringotomy device (stent) (tube) Z45.82
  neuropacemaker Z46.2
    implanted Z45.42
  non-vascular catheter Z46.82
  orthodontic device Z46.4
  orthopedic device (brace) (cast) (corset) (shoes) Z46.89
  pacemaker (cardiac) (cardiac resynchronization therapy (CRT-p)) Z45.018
    nervous system (brain) (peripheral nerve) (spinal cord) Z46.2
      implanted Z45.42

Fitting (and adjustment) (of) - *continued*
  pulse generator Z45.010
  portacath (port-a-cath) Z45.2
  prosthesis (external) Z44.9
    arm - *see* Admission, adjustment, artificial, arm
    breast Z44.3
    dental Z46.3
    eye Z44.2
    leg - *see* Admission, adjustment, artificial, leg
    specified NEC Z44.8
  spectacles Z46.0
  wheelchair Z46.89
Fitzhugh-Curtis syndrome
  due to
    Chlamydia trachomatis A74.81
    Neisseria gonorrhorea (gonococcal peritonitis) A54.85
Fitz's syndrome (acute hemorrhagic pancreatitis) - *see also* Pancreatitis, acute K85.80
Fixation
  joint - *see* Ankylosis
  larynx J38.7
  stapes - *see* Ankylosis, ear ossicles
    deafness - *see* Deafness, conductive
  uterus (acquired) - *see* Malposition, uterus
  vocal cord J38.3
Flabby ridge K06.8
Flaccid - *see also* condition
  palate, congenital Q38.5
Flail
  chest S22.5
    newborn (birth injury) P13.8
  joint (paralytic) M25.20
    ankle M25.27-
    elbow M25.22-
    foot joint M25.27-
    hand joint M25.24-
    hip M25.25-
    knee M25.26-
    shoulder M25.21-
    specified joint NEC M25.28
    wrist M25.23-
Flajani's disease - *see* Hyperthyroidism, with, goiter (diffuse)
Flap, liver K71.3
Flashbacks (residual to hallucinogen use) F16.283
Flat
  chamber (eye) - *see* Disorder, globe, hypotony, flat anterior chamber
  chest, congenital Q67.8
  foot (acquired) (fixed type) (painful) (postural) - *see also* Deformity, limb, flat foot
    congenital (rigid) (spastic (everted)) Q66.5-
    rachitic sequelae (late effect) E64.3
  organ or site, congenital NEC - *see* Anomaly, by site
  pelvis M95.5
    with disproportion (fetopelvic) O33.0
      causing obstructed labor O65.0
    congenital Q74.2
Flatau-Schilder disease G37.0
Flatback syndrome M40.30
  lumbar region M40.36
  lumbosacral region M40.37
  thoracolumbar region M40.35
Flattening
  head, femur M89.8X5
  hip - *see* Coxa, plana
  lip (congenital) Q18.8
  nose (congenital) Q67.4
    acquired M95.0

Flatulence R14.3
  psychogenic F45.8
Flatus R14.3
  vaginalis N89.8
Flax-dresser's disease J66.1
Flea bite - *see* Injury, bite, by site, superficial, insect
Flecks, glaucomatous (subcapsular) - *see* Cataract, complicated
Fleischer (-Kayser) ring (cornea) H18.04-
Fleshy mole O02.0
Flexibilitas cerea - *see* Catalepsy
Flexion
  amputation stump (surgical) T87.89
  cervix - *see* Malposition, uterus
  contracture, joint - *see* Contraction, joint
  deformity, joint - *see also* Deformity, limb, flexion M21.20
    hip, congenital Q65.89
  uterus - *see also* Malposition, uterus
    lateral - *see* Lateroversion, uterus
Flexner-Boyd dysentery A03.2
Flexner's dysentery A03.1
Flexure - *see* Flexion
Flint murmur (aortic insufficiency) I35.1
Floater, vitreous - *see* Opacity, vitreous
Floating
  cartilage (joint) - *see also* Loose, body, joint
    knee - *see* Derangement, knee, loose body
  gallbladder, congenital Q44.1
  kidney N28.89
    congenital Q63.8
  spleen D73.89
Flooding N92.0
Floor - *see* condition
Floppy
  baby syndrome (nonspecific) P94.2
  iris syndrome (intraoperative) (IFIS) H21.81
  nonrheumatic mitral valve syndrome I34.1
Flu - *see also* Influenza
  avian - *see also* Influenza, due to, identified novel influenza A virus J09.X2
  bird - *see also* Influenza, due to, identified novel influenza A virus J09.X2
  intestinal NEC A08.4
  swine (viruses that normally cause infections in pigs) - *see also* Influenza, due to, identified novel influenza A virus J09.X2
Fluctuating blood pressure I99.8
Fluid
  abdomen R18.8
  chest J94.8
  heart - *see* Failure, heart, congestive
  joint - *see* Effusion, joint
  loss (acute) E86.9
  lung - *see* Edema, lung
  overload E87.70
    specified NEC E87.79
  peritoneal cavity R18.8
  pleural cavity J94.8
  retention R60.9
Flukes NEC - *see also* Infestation, fluke blood NEC - *see* Schistosomiasis
  liver B66.3
Fluor (vaginalis) N89.8
  trichomonal or due to Trichomonas (vaginalis) A59.00
Fluorosis
  dental K00.3
  skeletal M85.10
    ankle M85.17-
    foot M85.17-
    forearm M85.13-
    hand M85.14-

Fluorosis - *continued*
  lower leg M85.16-
  multiple site M85.19
  neck M85.18
  rib M85.18
  shoulder M85.11-
  skull M85.18
  specified site NEC M85.18
  thigh M85.15-
  toe M85.17-
  upper arm M85.12-
  vertebra M85.18
Flush syndrome E34.0
Flushing R23.2
  menopausal N95.1
Flutter
  atrial or auricular I48.92
   atypical I48.4
   type I I48.3
   type II I48.4
   typical I48.3
  heart I49.8
   atrial or auricular I48.92
    atypical I48.4
    type I I48.3
    type II I48.4
    typical I48.3
   ventricular I49.02
  ventricular I49.02
FNHTR (febrile nonhemolytic transfusion reaction) R50.84
Fochier's abscess   code by site under Abscess
Focus, Assmann's - *see* Tuberculosis, pulmonary
Fogo selvagem L10.3
Foix-Alajouanine syndrome G95.19
Fold, folds (anomalous) - *see also* Anomaly, by site
  Descemet's membrane - *see* Change, corneal membrane, Descemet's, fold
  epicanthic Q10.3
  heart Q24.8
Folie à deux F24
Follicle
  cervix (nabothian) (ruptured) N88.8
  graafian, ruptured, with hemorrhage N83.0-
  nabothian N88.8
Follicular - *see* condition
Folliculitis (superficial) L73.9
  abscedens et suffodiens L66.3
  cyst N83.0-
  decalvans L66.2
  deep - *see* Furuncle, by site
  gonococcal (acute) (chronic) A54.01
  keloid, keloidalis L73.0
  pustular L01.02
  ulerythematosa reticulata L66.4
Folliculome lipidique
  specified site - *see* Neoplasm, benign, by site
  unspecified site
   female D27.9
   male D29.20
Følling's disease E70.0
Follow-up - *see* Examination, follow-up
Fong's syndrome (hereditary osteo-onychodysplasia) Q87.2
Food
  allergy L27.2
  asphyxia (from aspiration or inhalation) - *see* Foreign body, by site
  choked on - *see* Foreign body, by site
  deprivation T73.0
   specified kind of food NEC E63.8
  intoxication - *see* Poisoning, food

Food - *continued*
  lack of T73.0
  poisoning - *see* Poisoning, food
  rejection NEC - *see* Disorder, eating
  strangulation or suffocation - *see* Foreign body, by site
  toxemia - *see* Poisoning, food
Foot - *see* condition
Foramen ovale (nonclosure) (patent) (persistent) Q21.1
Forbes' glycogen storage disease E74.03
Fordyce-fox disease L75.2
Fordyce's disease (mouth) Q38.6
Forearm - *see* condition
Foreign body
  with
   laceration - *see* Laceration, by site, with foreign body
   puncture wound - *see* Puncture, by site, with foreign body
  accidentally left following a procedure T81.509
   aspiration T81.506
    resulting in
     adhesions T81.516
     obstruction T81.526
     perforation T81.536
     specified complication NEC T81.596
   cardiac catheterization T81.505
    resulting in
     acute reaction T81.60
      aseptic peritonitis T81.61
      specified NEC T81.69
     adhesions T81.515
     obstruction T81.525
     perforation T81.535
     specified complication NEC T81.595
   causing
    acute reaction T81.60
     aseptic peritonitis T81.61
     specified complication NEC T81.69
    adhesions T81.519
    aseptic peritonitis T81.61
    obstruction T81.529
    perforation T81.539
    specified complication NEC T81.599
   endoscopy T81.504
    resulting in
     adhesions T81.514
     obstruction T81.524
     perforation T81.534
     specified complication NEC T81.594
   immunization T81.503
    resulting in
     adhesions T81.513
     obstruction T81.523
     perforation T81.533
     specified complication NEC T81.593
   infusion T81.501
    resulting in
     adhesions T81.511
     obstruction T81.521
     perforation T81.531
     specified complication NEC T81.591
   injection T81.503
    resulting in
     adhesions T81.513
     obstruction T81.523
     perforation T81.533
     specified complication NEC T81.593
   kidney dialysis T81.502
    resulting in
     adhesions T81.512
     obstruction T81.522

Foreign body - *continued*
     perforation T81.532
     specified complication NEC T81.592
   packing removal T81.507
    resulting in
     acute reaction T81.60
      aseptic peritonitis T81.61
      specified NEC T81.69
     adhesions T81.517
     obstruction T81.527
     perforation T81.537
     specified complication NEC T81.597
   puncture T81.506
    resulting in
     adhesions T81.516
     obstruction T81.526
     perforation T81.536
     specified complication NEC T81.596
   specified procedure NEC T81.508
    resulting in
     acute reaction T81.60
      aseptic peritonitis T81.61
      specified NEC T81.69
     adhesions T81.518
     obstruction T81.528
     perforation T81.538
     specified complication NEC T81.598
   surgical operation T81.500
    resulting in
     acute reaction T81.60
      aseptic peritonitis T81.61
      specified NEC T81.69
     adhesions T81.510
     obstruction T81.520
     perforation T81.530
     specified complication NEC T81.590
   transfusion T81.501
    resulting in
     adhesions T81.511
     obstruction T81.521
     perforation T81.531
     specified complication NEC T81.591
  alimentary tract T18.9
  anus T18.5
  colon T18.4
  esophagus - *see* Foreign body, esophagus
  mouth T18.0
  multiple sites T18.8
  rectosigmoid (junction) T18.5
  rectum T18.5
  small intestine T18.3
  specified site NEC T18.8
  stomach T18.2
  anterior chamber (eye) S05.5-
  auditory canal - *see* Foreign body, entering through orifice, ear
  bronchus T17.508
   causing
    asphyxiation T17.500
     food (bone) (seed) T17.520
     gastric contents (vomitus) T17.510
     specified type NEC T17.590
    injury NEC T17.508
     food (bone) (seed) T17.528
     gastric contents (vomitus) T17.518
     specified type NEC T17.598
  canthus - *see* Foreign body, conjunctival sac
  ciliary body (eye) S05.5-
  conjunctival sac T15.1-
  cornea T15.0-
  entering through orifice
   accessory sinus T17.0
   alimentary canal T18.9
    multiple parts T18.8

Foreign body - *continued*
- specified part NEC T18.8
- alveolar process T18.0
- antrum (Highmore's) T17.0
- anus T18.5
- appendix T18.4
- auditory canal - *see* Foreign body, entering through orifice, ear
- auricle - *see* Foreign body, entering through orifice, ear
- bladder T19.1
- bronchioles - *see* Foreign body, respiratory tract, specified site NEC
- bronchus (main) - *see* Foreign body, bronchus
- buccal cavity T18.0
- canthus (inner) - *see* Foreign body, conjunctival sac
- cecum T18.4
- cervix (canal) (uteri) T19.3
- colon T18.4
- conjunctival sac - *see* Foreign body, conjunctival sac
- cornea - *see* Foreign body, cornea
- digestive organ or tract NOS T18.9
  - multiple parts T18.8
  - specified part NEC T18.8
- duodenum T18.3
- ear (external) T16.-
- esophagus - *see* Foreign body, esophagus
- eye (external) NOS T15.9-
  - conjunctival sac - *see* Foreign body, conjunctival sac
  - cornea - *see* Foreign body, cornea
  - specified part NEC T15.8-
- eyeball - *see also* Foreign body, entering through orifice, eye, specified part NEC
  - with penetrating wound - *see* Puncture, eyeball
- eyelid - *see also* Foreign body, conjunctival sac
  - with
    - laceration - *see* Laceration, eyelid, with foreign body
    - puncture - *see* Puncture, eyelid, with foreign body
    - superficial injury - *see* Foreign body, superficial, eyelid
- gastrointestinal tract T18.9
  - multiple parts T18.8
  - specified part NEC T18.8
- genitourinary tract T19.9
  - multiple parts T19.8
  - specified part NEC T19.8
- globe - *see* Foreign body, entering through orifice, eyeball
- gum T18.0
- Highmore's antrum T17.0
- hypopharynx - *see* Foreign body, pharynx
- ileum T18.3
- intestine (small) T18.3
  - large T18.4
- lacrimal apparatus (punctum) - *see* Foreign body, entering through orifice, eye, specified part NEC
- large intestine T18.4
- larynx - *see* Foreign body, larynx
- lung - *see* Foreign body, respiratory tract, specified site NEC
- maxillary sinus T17.0
- mouth T18.0
- nasal sinus T17.0
- nasopharynx - *see* Foreign body, pharynx
- nose (passage) T17.1

Foreign body - *continued*
- nostril T17.1
- oral cavity T18.0
- palate T18.0
- penis T19.4
- pharynx - *see* Foreign body, pharynx
- piriform sinus - *see* Foreign body, pharynx
- rectosigmoid (junction) T18.5
- rectum T18.5
- respiratory tract - *see* Foreign body, respiratory tract
- sinus (accessory) (frontal) (maxillary) (nasal) T17.0
  - piriform - *see* Foreign body, pharynx
- small intestine T18.3
- stomach T18.2
- suffocation by - *see* Foreign body, by site
- tear ducts or glands - *see* Foreign body, entering through orifice, eye, specified part NEC
- throat - *see* Foreign body, pharynx
- tongue T18.0
- tonsil, tonsillar (fossa) - *see* Foreign body, pharynx
- trachea - *see* Foreign body, trachea
- ureter T19.8
- urethra T19.0
- uterus (any part) T19.3
- vagina T19.2
- vulva T19.2
- esophagus T18.108
  - causing
    - injury NEC T18.108
      - food (bone) (seed) T18.128
      - gastric contents (vomitus) T18.118
      - specified type NEC T18.198
    - tracheal compression T18.100
      - food (bone) (seed) T18.120
      - gastric contents (vomitus) T18.110
      - specified type NEC T18.190
- feeling of, in throat R09.89
- fragment - *see* Retained, foreign body fragments (type of)
- genitourinary tract T19.9
  - bladder T19.1
  - multiple parts T19.8
  - penis T19.4
  - specified site NEC T19.8
  - urethra T19.0
  - uterus T19.3
    - IUD Z97.5
  - vagina T19.2
    - contraceptive device Z97.5
  - vulva T19.2
- granuloma (old) (soft tissue) - *see also* Granuloma, foreign body
  - skin L92.3
- in
  - laceration - *see* Laceration, by site, with foreign body
  - puncture wound - *see* Puncture, by site, with foreign body
  - soft tissue (residual) M79.5
- inadvertently left in operation wound - *see* Foreign body, accidentally left during a procedure
- ingestion, ingested NOS T18.9
- inhalation or inspiration - *see* Foreign body, by site
- internal organ, not entering through a natural orifice
  - code as specific injury with foreign body
- intraocular S05.5-
  - old, retained (nonmagnetic) H44.70-

Foreign body - *continued*
- anterior chamber H44.71-
- ciliary body H44.72-
- iris H44.72-
- lens H44.73-
- magnetic H44.60-
  - anterior chamber H44.61-
  - ciliary body H44.62-
  - iris H44.62-
  - lens H44.63-
  - posterior wall H44.64-
  - specified site NEC H44.69-
  - vitreous body H44.65-
- posterior wall H44.74-
- specified site NEC H44.79-
- vitreous body H44.75-
- iris - *see* Foreign body, intraocular
- lacrimal punctum - *see* Foreign body, entering through orifice, eye, specified part NEC
- larynx T17.308
  - causing
    - asphyxiation T17.300
      - food (bone) (seed) T17.320
      - gastric contents (vomitus) T17.310
      - specified type NEC T17.390
    - injury NEC T17.308
      - food (bone) (seed) T17.328
      - gastric contents (vomitus) T17.318
      - specified type NEC T17.398
- lens - *see* Foreign body, intraocular
- ocular muscle S05.4-
  - old, retained - *see* Foreign body, orbit, old
- old or residual
  - soft tissue (residual) M79.5
- operation wound, left accidentally - *see* Foreign body, accidentally left during a procedure
- orbit S05.4-
  - old, retained H05.5-
- pharynx T17.208
  - causing
    - asphyxiation T17.200
      - food (bone) (seed) T17.220
      - gastric contents (vomitus) T17.210
      - specified type NEC T17.290
    - injury NEC T17.208
      - food (bone) (seed) T17.228
      - gastric contents (vomitus) T17.218
      - specified type NEC T17.298
- respiratory tract T17.908
  - bronchioles - *see* Foreign body, respiratory tract, specified site NEC
  - bronchus - *see* Foreign body, bronchus
  - causing
    - asphyxiation T17.900
      - food (bone) (seed) T17.920
      - gastric contents (vomitus) T17.910
      - specified type NEC T17.990
    - injury NEC T17.908
      - food (bone) (seed) T17.928
      - gastric contents (vomitus) T17.918
      - specified type NEC T17.998
  - larynx - *see* Foreign body, larynx
  - lung - *see* Foreign body, respiratory tract, specified site NEC
  - multiple parts - *see* Foreign body, respiratory tract, specified site NEC
  - nasal sinus T17.0
  - nasopharynx - *see* Foreign body, pharynx
  - nose T17.1
  - nostril T17.1
  - pharynx - *see* Foreign body, pharynx
  - specified site NEC T17.808
    - causing

Foreign body - *continued*

asphyxiation T17.800
    food (bone) (seed) T17.820
    gastric contents (vomitus) T17.810
    specified type NEC T17.890
    injury NEC T17.808
       food (bone) (seed) T17.828
       gastric contents (vomitus) T17.818
       specified type NEC T17.898
throat - *see* Foreign body, pharynx
trachea - *see* Foreign body, trachea
retained (old) (nonmagnetic) (in)
anterior chamber (eye) - *see* Foreign body, intraocular, old, retained, anterior chamber
    magnetic - *see* Foreign body, intraocular, old, retained, magnetic, anterior chamber
ciliary body - *see* Foreign body, intraocular, old, retained, ciliary body
    magnetic - *see* Foreign body, intraocular, old, retained, magnetic, ciliary body
eyelid H02.819
    left H02.816
       lower H02.815
       upper H02.814
    right H02.813
       lower H02.812
       upper H02.811
fragments - *see* Retained, foreign body fragments (type of)
globe - *see* Foreign body, intraocular, old, retained
    magnetic - *see* Foreign body, intraocular, old, retained, magnetic
intraocular - *see* Foreign body, intraocular, old, retained
    magnetic - *see* Foreign body, intraocular, old, retained, magnetic
iris - *see* Foreign body, intraocular, old, retained, iris
    magnetic - *see* Foreign body, intraocular, old, retained, magnetic, iris
lens - *see* Foreign body, intraocular, old, retained, lens
    magnetic - *see* Foreign body, intraocular, old, retained, magnetic, lens
muscle - *see* Foreign body, retained, soft tissue
orbit - *see* Foreign body, orbit, old
posterior wall of globe - *see* Foreign body, intraocular, old, retained, posterior wall
    magnetic - *see* Foreign body, intraocular, old, retained, magnetic, posterior wall
retrobulbar - *see* Foreign body, orbit, old, retrobulbar
soft tissue M79.5
vitreous - *see* Foreign body, intraocular, old, retained, vitreous body
    magnetic - *see* Foreign body, intraocular, old, retained, magnetic, vitreous body
retina S05.5-
superficial, without open wound
abdomen, abdominal (wall) S30.851
alveolar process S00.552
ankle S90.55-
antecubital space - *see* Foreign body, superficial, forearm
anus S30.857
arm (upper) S40.85-
auditory canal - *see* Foreign body, superficial, ear
auricle - *see* Foreign body, superficial, ear
axilla - *see* Foreign body, superficial, arm
back, lower S30.850
breast S20.15-

Foreign body - *continued*

brow S00.85
buttock S30.850
calf - *see* Foreign body, superficial, leg
canthus - *see* Foreign body, superficial, eyelid
cheek S00.85
    internal S00.552
chest wall - *see* Foreign body, superficial, thorax
chin S00.85
clitoris S30.854
costal region - *see* Foreign body, superficial, thorax
digit(s)
    hand - *see* Foreign body, superficial, finger
    foot - *see* Foreign body, superficial, toe
ear S00.45-
elbow S50.35-
epididymis S30.853
epigastric region S30.851
epiglottis S10.15
esophagus, cervical S10.15
eyebrow - *see* Foreign body, superficial, eyelid
eyelid S00.25-
face S00.85
finger(s) S60.459
    index S60.45-
    little S60.45-
    middle S60.45-
    ring S60.45-
flank S30.851
foot (except toe(s) alone) S90.85-
    toe - *see* Foreign body, superficial, toe
forearm S50.85-
    elbow only - *see* Foreign body, superficial, elbow
forehead S00.85
genital organs, external
    female S30.856
    male S30.855
groin S30.851
gum S00.552
hand S60.55-
head S00.95
    ear - *see* Foreign body, superficial, ear
    eyelid - *see* Foreign body, superficial, eyelid
    lip S00.551
    nose S00.35
    oral cavity S00.552
    scalp S00.05
    specified site NEC S00.85
heel - *see* Foreign body, superficial, foot
hip S70.25-
inguinal region S30.851
interscapular region S20.459
jaw S00.85
knee S80.25-
labium (majus) (minus) S30.854
larynx S10.15
leg (lower) S80.85-
    knee - *see* Foreign body, superficial, knee
    upper - *see* Foreign body, superficial, thigh
lip S00.551
lower back S30.850
lumbar region S30.850
malar region S00.85
mammary - *see* Foreign body, superficial, breast
mastoid region S00.85
mouth S00.552
nail

Foreign body - *continued*

finger - *see* Foreign body, superficial, finger
toe - *see* Foreign body, superficial, toe
nape S10.85
nasal S00.35
neck S10.95
    specified site NEC S10.85
    throat S10.15
nose S00.35
occipital region S00.05
oral cavity S00.552
orbital region - *see* Foreign body, superficial, eyelid
palate S00.552
palm - *see* Foreign body, superficial, hand
parietal region S00.05
pelvis S30.850
penis S30.852
perineum
    female S30.854
    male S30.850
periocular area - *see* Foreign body, superficial, eyelid
phalanges
    finger - *see* Foreign body, superficial, finger
    toe - *see* Foreign body, superficial, toe
pharynx S10.15
pinna - *see* Foreign body, superficial, ear
popliteal space - *see* Foreign body, superficial, knee
prepuce S30.852
pubic region S30.850
pudendum
    female S30.856
    male S30.855
sacral region S30.850
scalp S00.05
scapular region - *see* Foreign body, superficial, shoulder
scrotum S30.853
shin - *see* Foreign body, superficial, leg
shoulder S40.25-
sternal region S20.359
submaxillary region S00.85
submental region S00.85
subungual
    finger(s) - *see* Foreign body, superficial, finger
    toe(s) - *see* Foreign body, superficial, toe
supraclavicular fossa S10.85
supraorbital S00.85
temple S00.85
temporal region S00.85
testis S30.853
thigh S70.35-
thorax, thoracic (wall) S20.95
    back S20.45-
    front S20.35-
throat S10.15
thumb S60.35-
toe(s) (lesser) S90.456
    great S90.45-
tongue S00.552
trachea S10.15
tunica vaginalis S30.853
tympanum, tympanic membrane - *see* Foreign body, superficial, ear
uvula S00.552
vagina S30.854
vocal cords S10.15
vulva S30.854
wrist S60.85-
swallowed T18.9
trachea T17.408

Foreign body - *continued*
  causing
    asphyxiation T17.400
      food (bone) (seed) T17.420
      gastric contents (vomitus) T17.410
      specified type NEC T17.490
    injury NEC T17.408
      food (bone) (seed) T17.428
      gastric contents (vomitus) T17.418
      specified type NEC T17.498
  type of fragment - *see* Retained, foreign body
    fragments (type of)
  vitreous (humor) S05.5-
Forestier's disease (rhizomelic pseudopolyarthritis) M35.3
  meaning ankylosing hyperostosis - *see* Hyperostosis, ankylosing
Formation
  hyalin in cornea - *see* Degeneration, cornea
  sequestrum in bone (due to infection) - *see* Osteomyelitis, chronic
  valve
    colon, congenital Q43.8
    ureter (congenital) Q62.39
Formication R20.2
Fort Bragg fever A27.89
Fossa - *see also* condition
  pyriform - *see* condition
Foster-Kennedy syndrome H47.14-
Fothergill's
  disease (trigeminal neuralgia) - *see also* Neuralgia, trigeminal
  scarlatina anginosa A38.9
Foul breath R19.6
Foundling Z76.1
Fournier disease or gangrene N49.3
  female N76.89
Fourth
  cranial nerve - *see* condition
  molar K00.1
Foville's (peduncular) disease or syndrome G46.3
Fox (-Fordyce) disease (apocrine miliaria) L75.2
Fracture, burst - *see* Fracture, traumatic, by site
Fracture, chronic *see* Fracture, pathological, by site
Fracture, nontraumatic, NEC
  atypical
    femur M84.750-
      complete
        oblique M84.759
          left side M84.758
          right side M84.757
        transverse M84.756
          left side M84.755
          right side M84.754
      incomplete M84.753
        left side M84.752
        right side M84.751
Fracture, pathological (pathologic) - *see also* Fracture, traumatic M84.40
  ankle M84.47-
  carpus M84.44-
  clavicle M84.41-
  compression (not due to trauma) - *see also* Collapse, vertebra M48.50-
  dental implant M27.63
  dental restorative material K08.539
    with loss of material K08.531
    without loss of material K08.530
  due to

Fracture, pathological - *continued*
  neoplastic disease NEC - *see also* Neoplasm M84.50
    ankle M84.57
    carpus M84.54-
    clavicle M84.51-
    femur M84.55-
    fibula M84.56-
    finger M84.54-
    hip M84.559
    humerus M84.52-
    ilium M84.550
    ischium M84.550
    metacarpus M84.54-
    metatarsus M84.57-
    neck M84.58
    pelvis M84.550
    radius M84.53-
    rib M84.58
    scapula M84.51-
    skull M84.58
    specified site NEC M84.58
    tarsus M84.57-
    tibia M84.56-
    toe M84.57-
    ulna M84.53-
    vertebra M84.58
  osteoporosis M80.00
    disuse - *see* Osteoporosis, specified type NEC, with pathological fracture
    drug-induced - *see* Osteoporosis, drug induced, with pathological fracture
    idiopathic - *see* Osteoporosis, specified type NEC, with pathological fracture
    postmenopausal - *see* Osteoporosis, postmenopausal, with pathological fracture
    postoophorectomy - *see* Osteoporosis, postoophorectomy, with pathological fracture
    postsurgical malabsorption - *see* Osteoporosis, specified type NEC, with pathological fracture
    specified cause NEC - *see* Osteoporosis, specified type NEC, with pathological fracture
  specified disease NEC M84.60
    ankle M84.67-
    carpus M84.64-
    clavicle M84.61-
    femur M84.65-
    fibula M84.66-
    finger M84.64-
    hip M84.65-
    humerus M84.62-
    ilium M84.650
    ischium M84.650
    metacarpus M84.64-
    metatarsus M84.67-
    neck M84.68
    radius M84.63-
    rib M84.68
    scapula M84.61-
    skull M84.68
    tarsus M84.67-
    tibia M84.66-
    toe M84.67-
    ulna M84.63-
    vertebra M84.68
  femur M84.45-
  fibula M84.46-
  finger M84.44-
  hip M84.459
  humerus M84.42-

Fracture, pathological - *continued*
  ilium M84.454
  ischium M84.454
  joint prosthesis - *see* Complications, joint prosthesis, mechanical, breakdown, by site
    periprosthetic - *see* Fracture, pathological, periprosthetic
  metacarpus M84.44-
  metatarsus M84.47-
  neck M84.48
  pelvis M84.454
  periprosthetic M97.9
    ankle M97.2-
    elbow M97.4-
    finger M97.8
    hip M97.0-
    knee M97.1-
    other specified joint M97.8
    shoulder M97.3-
    spinal joint M97.8
    toe joint M97.8
    wrist joint M97.8
  radius M84.43-
  restorative material (dental) K08.539
    with loss of material K08.531
    without loss of material K08.530
  rib M84.48
  scapula M84.41-
  skull M84.48
  tarsus M84.47-
  tibia M84.46-
  toe M84.47-
  ulna M84.43-
  vertebra M84.48
Fracture, traumatic (abduction) (adduction) (separation) - *see also* Fracture, pathological T14.8
  acetabulum S32.40-
    column
      anterior (displaced) (iliopubic) S32.43-
        nondisplaced S32.436
      posterior (displaced) (ilioischial) S32.443
        nondisplaced S32.44-
    dome (displaced) S32.48-
      nondisplaced S32.48
    specified NEC S32.49-
    transverse (displaced) S32.45-
      with associated posterior wall fracture (displaced) S32.46-
        nondisplaced S32.46-
      nondisplaced S32.45-
    wall
      anterior (displaced) S32.41-
        nondisplaced S32.41-
      medial (displaced) S32.47-
        nondisplaced S32.47-
      posterior (displaced) S32.42-
        with associated transverse fracture (displaced) S32.46-
          nondisplaced S32.46-
        nondisplaced S32.42-
  acromion - *see* Fracture, scapula, acromial process
  ankle S82.899
    bimalleolar (displaced) S82.84-
      nondisplaced S82.84-
    lateral malleolus only (displaced) S82.6-
      nondisplaced S82.6-
    medial malleolus (displaced) S82.5-
      associated with Maisonneuve's fracture - *see* Fracture, Maisonneuve's
      nondisplaced S82.5-
    talus - *see* Fracture, tarsal, talus
    trimalleolar (displaced) S82.85-

Fracture, traumatic - *continued*
  nondisplaced S82.85-
  arm (upper) - *see also* Fracture, humerus, shaft
    humerus - *see* Fracture, humerus
    radius - *see* Fracture, radius
    ulna - *see* Fracture, ulna
  astragalus - *see* Fracture, tarsal, talus
  atlas - *see* Fracture, neck, cervical vertebra,
    first
  axis - *see* Fracture, neck, cervical vertebra,
    second
  back - *see* Fracture, vertebra
  Barton's - *see* Barton's fracture
  base of skull - *see* Fracture, skull, base
  basicervical (basal) (femoral) S72.0
  Bennett's - *see* Bennett's fracture
  bimalleolar - *see* Fracture, ankle, bimalleolar
  blow-out S02.3-
  bone NEC T14.8
    birth injury P13.9
    following insertion of orthopedic implant,
      joint prosthesis or bone plate - *see* Fracture,
      following insertion of orthopedic implant,
      joint prosthesis or bone plate
    in (due to) neoplastic disease NEC - *see*
      Fracture, pathological, due to, neoplastic
      disease
    pathological (cause unknown) - *see* Fracture,
      pathological
  breast bone - *see* Fracture, sternum
  bucket handle (semilunar cartilage) - *see* Tear,
    meniscus
  burst - *see* Fracture, traumatic, by site
  calcaneus - *see* Fracture, tarsal, calcaneus
  carpal bone(s) S62.10-
    capitate (displaced) S62.13-
      nondisplaced S62.13-
    cuneiform - *see* Fracture, carpal bone,
    triquetrum
    hamate (body) (displaced) S62.143
      hook process (displaced) S62.15-
        nondisplaced S62.15-
      nondisplaced S62.14-
    larger multangular - *see* Fracture, carpal
      bones, trapezium
    lunate (displaced) S62.12-
      nondisplaced S62.12-
    navicular S62.00-
      distal pole (displaced) S62.01-
        nondisplaced S62.01-
      middle third (displaced) S62.02-
        nondisplaced S62.02-
      proximal third (displaced) S62.03-
        nondisplaced S62.03-
      volar tuberosity - *see* Fracture, carpal
      bones, navicular, distal pole
    os magnum - *see* Fracture, carpal bones,
    capitate
    pisiform (displaced) S62.16-
      nondisplaced S62.16-
    semilunar - *see* Fracture, carpal bones, lunate
    smaller multangular - *see* Fracture, carpal
      bones, trapezoid
    trapezium (displaced) S62.17-
      nondisplaced S62.17-
    trapezoid (displaced) S62.18-
      nondisplaced S62.18-
    triquetrum (displaced) S62.11-
      nondisplaced S62.11-
    unciform - *see* Fracture, carpal bones, hamate
  cervical - *see* Fracture, vertebra, cervical
  clavicle S42.00-
    acromial end (displaced) S42.03-
      nondisplaced S42.03-

Fracture, traumatic - *continued*
  birth injury P13.4
  lateral end - *see* Fracture, clavicle, acromial
    end
  shaft (displaced) S42.02-
    nondisplaced S42.02-
  sternal end (anterior) (displaced) S42.01-
    nondisplaced S42.01-
    posterior S42.01-
  coccyx S32.2
  collapsed - *see* Collapse, vertebra
  collar bone - *see* Fracture, clavicle
  Colles' - *see* Colles' fracture
  coronoid process - *see* Fracture, ulna, upper
    end, coronoid process
  corpus cavernosum penis S39.840
  costochondral cartilage S23.41
  costochondral, costosternal junction - *see*
    Fracture, rib
  cranium - *see* Fracture, skull
  cricoid cartilage S12.8
  cuboid (ankle) - *see* Fracture, tarsal, cuboid
  cuneiform
    foot - *see* Fracture, tarsal, cuneiform
    wrist - *see* Fracture, carpal, triquetrum
  delayed union - *see* Delay, union, fracture
  dental restorative material K08.539
    with loss of material K08.531
    without loss of material K08.530
  due to
    birth injury - *see* Birth, injury, fracture
    osteoporosis - *see* Osteoporosis, with fracture
  Dupuytren's - *see* Fracture, ankle, lateral
    malleolus
  elbow S42.40-
  ethmoid (bone) (sinus) - *see* Fracture, skull,
    base
  face bone S02.92
  fatigue - *see also* Fracture, stress
    vertebra M48.40
      cervical region M48.42
      cervicothoracic region M48.43
      lumbar region M48.46
      lumbosacral region M48.47
      occipito-atlanto-axial region M48.41
      sacrococcygeal region M48.48
      thoracic region M48.44
      thoracolumbar region M48.45
  femur, femoral S72.9-
    basicervical (basal) S72.0
    birth injury P13.2
    capital epiphyseal S79.01-
    condyles, epicondyles - *see* Fracture, femur,
      lower end
    distal end - *see* Fracture, femur, lower end
    epiphysis
      head - *see* Fracture, femur, upper end,
        epiphysis
      lower - *see* Fracture, femur, lower end,
        epiphysis
      upper - *see* Fracture, femur, upper end,
        epiphysis
    following insertion of implant, prosthesis or
      plate M96.66-
    head - *see* Fracture, femur, upper end, head
    intertrochanteric - *see* Fracture, femur,
      trochanteric
    intratrochanteric - *see* Fracture, femur,
      trochanteric
    lower end S72.40-
      condyle (displaced) S72.41-
      lateral (displaced) S72.42-
        nondisplaced S72.42-
      medial (displaced) S72.43-

Fracture, traumatic - *continued*
    nondisplaced S72.43-
    nondisplaced S72.41-
    epiphysis (displaced) S72.44-
      nondisplaced S72.44-
    physeal S79.10-
      Salter-Harris
        Type I S79.11-
        Type II S79.12-
        Type III S79.13-
        Type IV S79.14-
      specified NEC S79.19-
    specified NEC S72.49-
    supracondylar (displaced) S72.45-
      with intracondylar extension (displaced)
      S72.46-
        nondisplaced S72.46-
      nondisplaced S72.45-
    torus S72.47-
  neck - *see* Fracture, femur, upper end, neck
  pertrochanteric - *see* Fracture, femur,
    trochanteric
  shaft (lower third) (middle third) (upper
    third) S72.30-
    comminuted (displaced) S72.35-
      nondisplaced S72.35-
    oblique (displaced) S72.33-
      nondisplaced S72.33-
    segmental (displaced) S72.36-
      nondisplaced S72.36-
    specified NEC S72.39-
    spiral (displaced) S72.34-
      nondisplaced S72.34-
    transverse (displaced) S72.32-
      nondisplaced S72.32-
  specified site NEC - *see* subcategory S72.8
  subcapital (displaced) S72.01-
  subtrochanteric (region) (section) (displaced)
    S72.2-
    nondisplaced S72.2-
  transcervical - *see* Fracture, femur, upper
    end, neck
  transtrochanteric - *see* Fracture, femur,
    trochanteric
  trochanteric S72.10-
    apophyseal (displaced) S72.13-
      nondisplaced S72.13-
    greater trochanter (displaced) S72.11-
      nondisplaced S72.11-
    intertrochanteric (displaced) S72.14-
      nondisplaced S72.14-
    lesser trochanter (displaced) S72.12-
      nondisplaced S72.12-
  upper end S72.00-
    apophyseal (displaced) S72.13-
      nondisplaced S72.13-
    cervicotrochanteric - *see* Fracture, femur,
      upper end, neck, base
    epiphysis (displaced) S72.02-
      nondisplaced S72.02-
    head S72.05-
      articular (displaced) S72.06-
        nondisplaced S72.06-
      specified NEC S72.09-
    intertrochanteric (displaced) S72.14-
      nondisplaced S72.14-
    intracapsular S72.01-
    midcervical (displaced) S72.03-
      nondisplaced S72.03-
    neck S72.00-
      base (displaced) S72.04-
        nondisplaced S72.04-
      specified NEC S72.09-
    pertrochanteric - *see* Fracture, femur, upper

Fracture, traumatic - *continued*
  end, trochanteric
  physeal S79.00-
    Salter-Harris type I S79.01-
    specified NEC S79.09-
  subcapital (displaced) S72.01-
  subtrochanteric (displaced) S72.2-
    nondisplaced S72.2-
  transcervical - *see* Fracture, femur, upper
    end, midcervical
  trochanteric S72.10-
    greater (displaced) S72.11-
      nondisplaced S72.11-
    lesser (displaced) S72.12-
      nondisplaced S72.12-
fibula (shaft) (styloid) S82.40-
  comminuted (displaced) S82.45-
    nondisplaced S82.45-
  following insertion of implant, prosthesis or
    plate M96.67-
  involving ankle or malleolus - *see* Fracture,
    fibula, lateral malleolus
  lateral malleolus (displaced) S82.6-
    nondisplaced S82.6-
  lower end
    physeal S89.30-
      Salter-Harris
        Type I S89.31-
        Type II S89.32-
      specified NEC S89.39-
    specified NEC S82.83-
    torus S82.82-
  oblique (displaced) S82.43-
    nondisplaced S82.43-
  segmental (displaced) S82.46-
    nondisplaced S82.46-
  specified NEC S82.49-
  spiral (displaced) S82.44-
    nondisplaced S82.44-
  transverse (displaced) S82.42-
    nondisplaced S82.42-
  upper end
    physeal S89.20-
      Salter-Harris
        Type I S89.21-
        Type II S89.22-
      specified NEC S89.29-
    specified NEC S82.83-
    torus S82.81-
finger (except thumb) S62.60-
  distal phalanx (displaced) S62.63-
    nondisplaced S62.66-
  index S62.60-
    distal phalanx (displaced) S62.63-
      nondisplaced S62.66-
    medial phalanx (displaced) S62.62-
      nondisplaced S62.65-
    proximal phalanx (displaced) S62.61-
      nondisplaced S62.64
  little S62.60-
    distal phalanx (displaced) S62.63-
      nondisplaced S62.66-
    medial phalanx (displaced) S62.62-
      nondisplaced S62.65-
    proximal phalanx (displaced) S62.61-
      nondisplaced S62.64-
  medial phalanx (displaced) S62.62-
    nondisplaced S62.65-
  middle S62.60-
    distal phalanx (displaced) S62.63-
      nondisplaced S62.66-
    medial phalanx (displaced) S62.62-
      nondisplaced S62.65-
    proximal phalanx (displaced) S62.61-

Fracture, traumatic - *continued*
    nondisplaced S62.64-
  proximal phalanx (displaced) S62.61-
    nondisplaced S62.64-
  ring S62.60-
    distal phalanx (displaced) S62.63-
      nondisplaced S62.66-
    medial phalanx (displaced) S62.62-
      nondisplaced S62.65-
    proximal phalanx (displaced) S62.61-
      nondisplaced S62.64-
  thumb - *see* Fracture, thumb
following insertion (intraoperative)
(postoperative) of orthopedic implant, joint
prosthesis or bone plate M96.69
  femur M96.66-
  fibula M96.67-
  humerus M96.62-
  pelvis M96.65
  radius M96.63-
  specified bone NEC M96.69
  tibia M96.67-
  ulna M96.63-
foot S92.90-
  astragalus - *see* Fracture, tarsal, talus
  calcaneus - *see* Fracture, tarsal, calcaneus
  cuboid - *see* Fracture, tarsal, cuboid
  cuneiform - *see* Fracture, tarsal, cuneiform
  metatarsal - *see* Fracture, metatarsal
  navicular - *see* Fracture, tarsal, navicular
  sesamoid S92.81-
  specified NEC S92.81-
  talus - *see* Fracture, tarsal, talus
  tarsal - *see* Fracture, tarsal
  toe - *see* Fracture, toe
forearm S52.9-
  radius - *see* Fracture, radius
  ulna - *see* Fracture, ulna
fossa (anterior) (middle) (posterior) S02.19
frontal (bone) (skull) S02.0
  sinus S02.19
glenoid (cavity) (scapula) - *see* Fracture,
  scapula, glenoid cavity   greenstick - *see*
  Fracture, by site
hallux - *see* Fracture, toe, great
hand S62.9-
  carpal - *see* Fracture, carpal bone
  finger (except thumb) - *see* Fracture, finger
  metacarpal - *see* Fracture, metacarpal
  navicular (scaphoid) (hand) - *see* Fracture,
    carpal bone, navicular
  thumb - *see* Fracture, thumb
healed or old
  with complications
code by Nature of the complication
heel bone - *see* Fracture, tarsal, calcaneus
Hill-Sachs S42.29-
hip - *see* Fracture, femur, neck
humerus S42.30-
  anatomical neck - *see* Fracture, humerus,
    upper end
  articular process - *see* Fracture, humerus,
    lower end
  capitellum - *see* Fracture, humerus, lower
    end, condyle, lateral
  distal end - *see* Fracture, humerus, lower end
  epiphysis
    lower - *see* Fracture, humerus, lower end,
      physeal
    upper - *see* Fracture, humerus, upper end,
      physeal
  external condyle - *see* Fracture, humerus,
    lower end, condyle, lateral

Fracture, traumatic - *continued*
  following insertion of implant, prosthesis or
    plate M96.62-
  great tuberosity - *see* Fracture, humerus,
    upper end, greater tuberosity
  intercondylar - *see* Fracture, humerus, lower
    end
  internal epicondyle - *see* Fracture, humerus,
    lower end, epicondyle, medial
  lesser tuberosity - *see* Fracture, humerus,
    upper end, lesser tuberosity
  lower end S42.40-
    condyle
      lateral (displaced) S42.45-
        nondisplaced S42.45-
      medial (displaced) S42.46-
        nondisplaced S42.46-
    epicondyle
      lateral (displaced) S42.43-
        nondisplaced S42.43-
      medial (displaced) S42.44-
        incarcerated S42.44-
        nondisplaced S42.44-
    physeal S49.10-
      Salter-Harris
        Type I S49.11-
        Type II S49.12-
        Type III S49.13-
        Type IV S49.14-
      specified NEC S49.19-
    specified NEC (displaced) S42.49-
      nondisplaced S42.49-
    supracondylar (simple) (displaced) S42.41-
      with intercondylar fracture - *see* Fracture,
        humerus, lower end
      comminuted (displaced) S42.42-
        nondisplaced S42.42-
      nondisplaced S42.41-
    torus S42.48-
    transcondylar (displaced) S42.47-
      nondisplaced S42.47-
  proximal end - *see* Fracture, humerus, upper
    end
  shaft S42.30-
    comminuted (displaced) S42.35-
      nondisplaced S42.35-
    greenstick S42.31-
    oblique (displaced) S42.33-
      nondisplaced S42.33-
    segmental (displaced) S42.36-
      nondisplaced S42.36-
    specified NEC S42.39-
    spiral (displaced) S42.34-
      nondisplaced S42.34-
    transverse (displaced) S42.32-
      nondisplaced S42.32-
  supracondylar - *see* Fracture, humerus, lower
    end
  surgical neck - *see* Fracture, humerus, upper
    end, surgical neck
  trochlea - *see* Fracture, humerus, lower end,
    condyle, medial
  tuberosity - *see* Fracture, humerus, upper end
  upper end S42.20-
    anatomical neck - *see* Fracture, humerus,
      upper end, specified NEC
    articular head - *see* Fracture, humerus,
      upper end, specified NEC
    epiphysis - *see* Fracture, humerus, upper
      end, physeal
    greater tuberosity (displaced) S42.25-
      nondisplaced S42.25-
    lesser tuberosity (displaced) S42.26-
      nondisplaced S42.26-
    physeal S49.00-

Fracture, traumatic - *continued*

    Salter-Harris
        Type I S49.01-
        Type II S49.02-
        Type III S49.03-
        Type IV S49.04-
        specified NEC S49.09-
    specified NEC (displaced) S42.29-
        nondisplaced S42.29-
    surgical neck (displaced) S42.21-
        four-part S42.24-
        nondisplaced S42.21-
        three-part S42.23-
        two-part (displaced) S42.22-
        nondisplaced S42.22-
    torus S42.27-
    transepiphyseal - *see* Fracture, humerus, upper end, physeal
hyoid bone S12.8
ilium S32.30-
  with disruption of pelvic ring - *see* Disruption, pelvic ring
  avulsion (displaced) S32.31-
    nondisplaced S32.31-
  specified NEC S32.39-
impaction, impacted   code as Fracture, by site
innominate bone - *see* Fracture, ilium
instep - *see* Fracture, foot
ischium S32.60-
  with disruption of pelvic ring - *see* Disruption, pelvic ring
  avulsion (displaced) S32.61-
    nondisplaced S32.61-
  specified NEC S32.69-
jaw (bone) (lower) - *see* Fracture, mandible
  upper - *see* Fracture, maxilla
joint prosthesis - *see* Complications, joint prosthesis, mechanical, breakdown, by site
  periprosthetic - *see* Fracture, traumatic, periprosthetic
knee cap - *see* Fracture, patella
larynx S12.8
late effects - *see* Sequelae, fracture
leg (lower) S82.9-
  ankle - *see* Fracture, ankle
  femur - *see* Fracture, femur
  fibula - *see* Fracture, fibula
  malleolus - *see* Fracture, ankle
  patella - *see* Fracture, patella
  specified site NEC S82.89-
  tibia - *see* Fracture, tibia
lumbar spine - *see* Fracture, vertebra, lumbar
lumbosacral spine S32.9
Maisonneuve's (displaced) S82.86-
  nondisplaced S82.86-
malar bone - *see also* Fracture, maxilla S02.400
  left side S02.40B
  right side S02.40A
malleolus - *see* Fracture, ankle
malunion - *see* Fracture, by site
mandible (lower jaw (bone)) S02.609
  alveolus S02.67-
  angle (of jaw) S02.65-
  body, unspecified S02.600
    left side S02.602
    right side S02.601
  condylar process S02.61-
  coronoid process S02.63-
  ramus, unspecified S02.64-
  specified site NEC S02.69
  subcondylar process S02.62-
  symphysis S02.66
manubrium (sterni) S22.21

Fracture, traumatic - *continued*

  dissociation from sternum S22.23
march - *see* Fracture, traumatic, stress, by site
maxilla, maxillary (bone) (sinus) (superior) (upper jaw) S02.401
  alveolus S02.42
  inferior - *see* Fracture, mandible
  LeFort I S02.411
  LeFort II S02.412
  LeFort III S02.413
  left side S02.40D
  right side S02.40C metacarpal S62.309
  base (displaced) S62.319
    nondisplaced S62.349
  fifth S62.30-
    base (displaced) S62.31-
      nondisplaced S62.34-
    neck (displaced) S62.33-
      nondisplaced S62.36-
    shaft (displaced) S62.32-
      nondisplaced S62.35-
    specified NEC S62.398
  first S62.20-
    base NEC (displaced) S62.23-
      nondisplaced S62.23-
    Bennett's - *see* Bennett's fracture
    neck (displaced) S62.25-
      nondisplaced S62.25-
    shaft (displaced) S62.24-
      nondisplaced S62.24-
    specified NEC S62.29-
  fourth S62.30-
    base (displaced) S62.31-
      nondisplaced S62.34-
    neck (displaced) S62.33-
      nondisplaced S62.36-
    shaft (displaced) S62.32-
      nondisplaced S62.35-
    specified NEC S62.39-
    neck (displaced) S62.33-
      nondisplaced S62.36-
  Rolando's - *see* Rolando's fracture
  second S62.30-
    base (displaced) S62.31-
      nondisplaced S62.34-
    neck (displaced) S62.33-
      nondisplaced S62.36-
    shaft (displaced) S62.32-
      nondisplaced S62.35-
    specified NEC S62.39-
    shaft (displaced) S62.32-
      nondisplaced S62.35-
  third S62.30-
    base (displaced) S62.31-
      nondisplaced S62.34-
    neck (displaced) S62.33-
      nondisplaced S62.36-
    shaft (displaced) S62.32-
      nondisplaced S62.35-
    specified NEC S62.39-
  specified NEC S62.399
metastatic - *see* Fracture, pathological, due to, neoplastic disease - *see also* Neoplasm
metatarsal bone S92.30-
  fifth (displaced) S92.35-
    nondisplaced S92.35-
  first (displaced) S92.31-
    nondisplaced S92.31-
  fourth (displaced) S92.34-
    nondisplaced S92.34-
  physeal S99.10-
    Salter-Harris
      Type I S99.11-
      Type II S99.12-

Fracture, traumatic - *continued*

      Type III S99.13-
      Type IV S99.14-
    specified NEC S99.19-
  second (displaced) S92.32-
    nondisplaced S92.32-
  third (displaced) S92.33-
    nondisplaced S92.33-
Monteggia's - *see* Monteggia's fracture
multiple
  hand (and wrist) NEC - *see* Fracture, by site
  ribs - *see* Fracture, rib, multiple
nasal (bone(s)) S02.2
navicular (scaphoid) (foot) - *see also* Fracture, tarsal, navicular
  hand - *see* Fracture, carpal, navicular
neck S12.9
  cervical vertebra S12.9
    fifth (displaced) S12.400
      nondisplaced S12.401
      specified type NEC (displaced) S12.490
        nondisplaced S12.491
    first (displaced) S12.000
      burst (stable) S12.01
        unstable S12.02
      lateral mass (displaced) S12.040
        nondisplaced S12.041
      nondisplaced S12.001
      posterior arch (displaced) S12.030
        nondisplaced S12.031
      specified type NEC (displaced) S12.090
        nondisplaced S12.091
    fourth (displaced) S12.300
      nondisplaced S12.301
      specified type NEC (displaced) S12.390
        nondisplaced S12.391
    second (displaced) S12.100
      nondisplaced S12.101
      dens (anterior) (displaced) (type II) S12.110
        nondisplaced S12.112
        posterior S12.111
      specified type NEC (displaced) S12.120
        nondisplaced S12.121
      specified type NEC (displaced) S12.190
        nondisplaced S12.191
    seventh (displaced) S12.600
      nondisplaced S12.601
      specified type NEC (displaced) S12.690
        nondisplaced S12.691
    sixth (displaced) S12.500
      nondisplaced S12.501
      specified type NEC (displaced) S12.590
        nondisplaced S12.591
    third (displaced) S12.200
      nondisplaced S12.201
      specified type NEC (displaced) S12.290
        nondisplaced S12.291
  hyoid bone S12.8
  larynx S12.8
  specified site NEC S12.8
  thyroid cartilage S12.8
  trachea S12.8
neoplastic NEC - *see* Fracture, pathological, due to, neoplastic disease
neural arch - *see* Fracture, vertebra
newborn - *see* Birth, injury, fracture
nontraumatic - *see* Fracture, pathological
nonunion - *see* Nonunion, fracture
nose, nasal (bone) (septum) S02.2
occiput - *see* Fracture, skull, base, occiput
odontoid process - *see* Fracture, neck, cervical vertebra, second
olecranon (process) (ulna) - *see* Fracture, ulna,

Fracture, traumatic - *continued*
upper end, olecranon process
  orbit, orbital (bone) (region) S02.8-
    floor (blow-out) S02.3-
      roof S02.19
  os
    calcis - *see* Fracture, tarsal, calcaneus
    magnum - *see* Fracture, carpal, capitate
    pubis - *see* Fracture, pubis
  palate S02.8-
  parietal bone (skull) S02.0
  patella S82.00-
    comminuted (displaced) S82.04-
      nondisplaced S82.04-
    longitudinal (displaced) S82.02-
      nondisplaced S82.02-
    osteochondral (displaced) S82.01-
      nondisplaced S82.01-
    specified NEC S82.09-
    transverse (displaced) S82.03-
      nondisplaced S82.03-
  pedicle (of vertebral arch) - *see* Fracture,
    vertebra
  pelvis, pelvic (bone) S32.9
    acetabulum - *see* Fracture, acetabulum
    circle - *see* Disruption, pelvic ring
    following insertion of implant, prosthesis or
      plate M96.65
    ilium - *see* Fracture, ilium
    ischium - *see* Fracture, ischium
    multiple
      with disruption of pelvic ring (circle) - *see*
        Disruption, pelvic ring
      without disruption of pelvic ring (circle)
        S32.82
    pubis - *see* Fracture, pubis
    specified site NEC S32.89
    sacrum - *see* Fracture, sacrum
  periprosthetic, around internal prosthetic joint
    M97.9
    ankle M97.2-
    elbow M97.4-
    finger M97.8
    hip M97.0-
    knee M97.1-
    shoulder M97.3-
    specified joint NEC M97.8
    spine M97.8
    toe M97.8
    wrist M97.8
  phalanx
    foot - *see* Fracture, toe
    hand - *see* Fracture, finger
  pisiform - *see* Fracture, carpal, pisiform
  pond - *see* Fracture, skull
  prosthetic device, internal - *see* Complications,
    prosthetic device, by site, mechanical
  pubis S32.50-
    with disruption of pelvic ring - *see*
      Disruption, pelvic ring
    specified site NEC S32.59-
    superior rim S32.51-
  radius S52.9-
    distal end - *see* Fracture, radius, lower end
    following insertion of implant, prosthesis or
      plate M96.63-
    head - *see* Fracture, radius, upper end, head
    lower end S52.50-
      Barton's - *see* Barton's fracture
      Colles' - *see* Colles' fracture
      extraarticular NEC S52.55-
      intraarticular NEC S52.57-
      physeal S59.20-
        Salter-Harris

Fracture, traumatic - *continued*
          Type I S59.21-
          Type II S59.22-
          Type III S59.23-
          Type IV S59.24-
          specified NEC S59.29-
      Smith's - *see* Smith's fracture
      specified NEC S52.59-
      styloid process (displaced) S52.51-
        nondisplaced S52.51-
      torus S52.52-
    neck - *see* Fracture, radius, upper end
    proximal end - *see* Fracture, radius, upper
      end
    shaft S52.30-
      bent bone S52.38-
      comminuted (displaced) S52.35-
        nondisplaced S52.35-
      Galeazzi's - *see* Galeazzi's fracture
      greenstick S52.31-
      oblique (displaced) S52.33-
        nondisplaced S52.33-
      segmental (displaced) S52.36-
        nondisplaced S52.36-
      specified NEC S52.39-
      spiral (displaced) S52.34-
        nondisplaced S52.34-
      transverse (displaced) S52.32-
        nondisplaced S52.32-
    upper end S52.10-
      head (displaced) S52.12-
        nondisplaced S52.12-
      neck (displaced) S52.13-
        nondisplaced S52.13-
      specified NEC S52.18-
      physeal S59.10-
        Salter-Harris
          Type I S59.11-
          Type II S59.12-
          Type III S59.13-
          Type IV S59.14-
          specified NEC S59.19-
      torus S52.11-
  ramus
    inferior or superior, pubis - *see* Fracture,
      pubis
    mandible - *see* Fracture, mandible
  restorative material (dental) K08.539
    with loss of material K08.531
    without loss of material K08.530
  rib S22.3-
    with flail chest - *see* Flail, chest
    multiple S22.4-
      with flail chest - *see* Flail, chest
  root, tooth - *see* Fracture, tooth
  sacrum S32.10
    specified NEC S32.19
    Type
      1 S32.14
      2 S32.15
      3 S32.16
      4 S32.17
    Zone
      I S32.119
        displaced (minimally) S32.111
          severely S32.112
        nondisplaced S32.110
      II S32.129
        displaced (minimally) S32.121
          severely S32.122
        nondisplaced S32.120
      III S32.139
        displaced (minimally) S32.131
          severely S32.132

Fracture, traumatic - *continued*
        nondisplaced S32.130
  scaphoid (hand) - *see also* Fracture, carpal,
    navicular
    foot - *see* Fracture, tarsal, navicular
  scapula S42.10-
    acromial process (displaced) S42.12-
      nondisplaced S42.12-
    body (displaced) S42.11-
      nondisplaced S42.11-
    coracoid process (displaced) S42.13-
      nondisplaced S42.13-
    glenoid cavity (displaced) S42.14-
      nondisplaced S42.14-
    neck (displaced) S42.15-
      nondisplaced S42.15-
    specified NEC S42.19-
  semilunar bone, wrist - *see* Fracture, carpal,
    lunate
  sequelae - *see* Sequelae, fracture
  sesamoid bone
    foot S92.81-
    hand - *see* Fracture, carpal
    other - *see* Fracture, traumatic, by site
  shepherd's - *see* Fracture, tarsal, talus
  shoulder (girdle) S42.9-
    blade - *see* Fracture, scapula
  sinus (ethmoid) (frontal) S02.19
  skull S02.91
    base S02.10-
      occiput S02.119
        condyle S02.113
          type I S02.110
            left side S02.11B
            right side S02.11A
          type II S02.111
            left side S02.11D
            right side S02.11C
          type III S02.112
            left side S02.11F
            right side S02.11E
          specified NEC S02.118
            left side S02.11H
            right side S02.11G
      specified NEC S02.19
    birth injury P13.0
    frontal bone S02.0
    parietal bone S02.0
    specified site NEC S02.8-
    temporal bone S02.19
    vault S02.0
  Smith's - *see* Smith's fracture
  sphenoid (bone) (sinus) S02.19
  spine - *see* Fracture, vertebra
  spinous process - *see* Fracture, vertebra
  spontaneous (cause unknown) - *see* Fracture,
    pathological
  stave (of thumb) - *see* Fracture, metacarpal,
    first
  sternum S22.20
    with flail chest - *see* Flail, chest
    body S22.22
    manubrium S22.21
    xiphoid (process) S22.24
  stress M84.30
    ankle M84.37-
    carpus M84.34-
    clavicle M84.31-
    femoral neck M84.359
    femur M84.35-
    fibula M84.36-
    finger M84.34-
    hip M84.359
    humerus M84.32-

Fracture, traumatic - *continued*
  ilium M84.350
  ischium M84.350
  metacarpus M84.34-
  metatarsus M84.37-
  neck - *see* Fracture, fatigue, vertebra
  pelvis M84.350
  radius M84.33-
  rib M84.38
  scapula M84.31-
  skull M84.38
  tarsus M84.37-
  tibia M84.36-
  toe M84.37-
  ulna M84.33-
  vertebra - *see* Fracture, fatigue, vertebra
  supracondylar, elbow - *see* Fracture, humerus, lower end, supracondylar
  symphysis pubis - *see* Fracture, pubis
  talus (ankle bone) - *see* Fracture, tarsal, talus
  tarsal bone(s) S92.20-
    astragalus - *see* Fracture, tarsal, talus
    calcaneus S92.00-
      anterior process (displaced) S92.02-
        nondisplaced S92.02-
      body (displaced) S92.01-
        nondisplaced S92.01-
      extraarticular NEC (displaced) S92.05-
        nondisplaced S92.05-
      intraarticular (displaced) S92.06-
        nondisplaced S92.06
      physeal S99.00-
        Salter-Harris
          Type I S99.01-
          Type II S99.02-
          Type III S99.03-
          Type IV S99.04-
        specified NEC S99.09-
      tuberosity (displaced) S92.04-
        avulsion (displaced) S92.03-
          nondisplaced S92.03-
        nondisplaced S92.04-
    cuboid (displaced) S92.21-
      nondisplaced S92.21-
    cuneiform
      intermediate (displaced) S92.23-
        nondisplaced S92.23-
      lateral (displaced) S92.22-
        nondisplaced S92.22-
      medial (displaced) S92.24-
        nondisplaced S92.24-
    navicular (displaced) S92.25-
      nondisplaced S92.25-
    scaphoid - *see* Fracture, tarsal, navicular
    talus S92.10-
      avulsion (displaced) S92.15-
        nondisplaced S92.15-
      body (displaced) S92.12-
        nondisplaced S92.12-
      dome (displaced) S92.14-
        nondisplaced S92.14-
      head (displaced) S92.12-
        nondisplaced S92.12-
      lateral process (displaced) S92.14-
        nondisplaced S92.14-
      neck (displaced) S92.11-
        nondisplaced S92.11-
      posterior process (displaced) S92.13-
        nondisplaced S92.13-
      specified NEC S92.19-
  temporal bone (styloid) S02.19
  thorax (bony) S22.9
    with flail chest - *see* Flail, chest
    rib S22.3-

Fracture, traumatic - *continued*
  multiple S22.4-
    with flail chest - *see* Flail, chest
  sternum S22.20
    body S22.22
    manubrium S22.21
    xiphoid process S22.24
  vertebra (displaced) S22.009
    burst (stable) S22.001
      unstable S22.002
    eighth S22.069
      burst (stable) S22.061
        unstable S22.062
      specified type NEC S22.068
      wedge compression S22.060
    eleventh S22.089
      burst (stable) S22.081
        unstable S22.082
      specified type NEC S22.088
      wedge compression S22.080
    fifth S22.059
      burst (stable) S22.051
        unstable S22.052
      specified type NEC S22.058
      wedge compression S22.050
    first S22.019
      burst (stable) S22.011
        unstable S22.012
      specified type NEC S22.018
      wedge compression S22.010
    fourth S22.049
      burst (stable) S22.041
        unstable S22.042
      specified type NEC S22.048
      wedge compression S22.040
    ninth S22.079
      burst (stable) S22.071
        unstable S22.072
      specified type NEC S22.078
      wedge compression S22.070
    nondisplaced S22.001
    second S22.029
      burst (stable) S22.021
        unstable S22.022
      specified type NEC S22.028
      wedge compression S22.020
    seventh S22.069
      burst (stable) S22.061
        unstable S22.062
      specified type NEC S22.068
      wedge compression S22.060
    sixth S22.059
      burst (stable) S22.051
        unstable S22.052
      specified type NEC S22.058
      wedge compression S22.050
    specified type NEC S22.008
    tenth S22.079
      burst (stable) S22.071
        unstable S22.072
      specified type NEC S22.078
      wedge compression S22.070
    third S22.039
      burst (stable) S22.031
        unstable S22.032
      specified type NEC S22.038
      wedge compression S22.030
    twelfth S22.089
      burst (stable) S22.081
        unstable S22.082
      specified type NEC S22.088
      wedge compression S22.080
    wedge compression S22.000
  thumb S62.50-

Fracture, traumatic - *continued*
  distal phalanx (displaced) S62.52-
    nondisplaced S62.52-
  proximal phalanx (displaced) S62.51-
    nondisplaced S62.51-
  thyroid cartilage S12.8
  tibia (shaft) S82.20-
    comminuted (displaced) S82.25-
      nondisplaced S82.25-
    condyles - *see* Fracture, tibia, upper end
    distal end - *see* Fracture, tibia, lower end
    epiphysis
      lower - *see* Fracture, tibia, lower end
      upper - *see* Fracture, tibia, upper end
    following insertion of implant, prosthesis or plate M96.67-
    head (involving knee joint) - *see* Fracture, tibia, upper end
    intercondyloid eminence - *see* Fracture, tibia, upper end
    involving ankle or malleolus - *see* Fracture, ankle, medial malleolus
    lower end S82.30-
      physeal S89.10-
        Salter-Harris
          Type I S89.11-
          Type II S89.12-
          Type III S89.13-
          Type IV S89.14-
        specified NEC S89.19-
      pilon (displaced) S82.87-
        nondisplaced S82.87-
      specified NEC S82.39-
      torus S82.31-
    malleolus - *see* Fracture, ankle, medial malleolus
    oblique (displaced) S82.23-
      nondisplaced S82.23-
    pilon - *see* Fracture, tibia, lower end, pilon
    proximal end - *see* Fracture, tibia, upper end
    segmental (displaced) S82.26-
      nondisplaced S82.26-
    specified NEC S82.29-
    spine *see* Fracture, tibia, upper end, spine
    spiral (displaced) S82.24-
      nondisplaced S82.24-
    transverse (displaced) S82.22-
      nondisplaced S82.22-
    tuberosity - *see* Fracture, tibia, upper end, tuberosity
    upper end S82.10-
      bicondylar (displaced) S82.14-
        nondisplaced S82.14-
      lateral condyle (displaced) S82.12-
        nondisplaced S82.12-
      medial condyle (displaced) S82.13-
        nondisplaced S82.13-
      physeal S89.00-
        Salter-Harris
          Type I S89.01-
          Type II S89.02-
          Type III S89.03-
          Type IV S89.04-
        specified NEC S89.09-
      plateau - *see* Fracture, tibia, upper end, bicondylar
      spine (displaced) S82.11-
        nondisplaced S82.11-
      torus S82.16-
      specified NEC S82.19-
      tuberosity (displaced) S82.15-
        nondisplaced S82.15-
  toe S92.91-
    great (displaced) S92.40-

Fracture, traumatic - *continued*
distal phalanx (displaced) S92.42-
nondisplaced S92.42-
nondisplaced S92.40-
proximal phalanx (displaced) S92.41-
nondisplaced S92.41-
specified NEC S92.49-
lesser (displaced) S92.50-
distal phalanx (displaced) S92.53-
nondisplaced S92.53-
medial phalanx (displaced) S92.52-
nondisplaced S92.52-
nondisplaced S92.50-
proximal phalanx (displaced) S92.51-
nondisplaced S92.51-
specified NEC S92.59-
physeal
phalanx S99.20-
Salter-Harris
Type I S99.21-
Type II S99.22-
Type III S99.23-
Type IV S99.24-
specified NEC S99.29-
tooth (root) S02.5
trachea (cartilage) S12.8
transverse process - *see* Fracture, vertebra
trapezium or trapezoid bone - *see* Fracture, carpal
trimalleolar - *see* Fracture, ankle, trimalleolar
triquetrum (cuneiform of carpus) - *see* Fracture, carpal, triquetrum
trochanter - *see* Fracture, femur, trochanteric
tuberosity (external) - *see* Fracture, traumatic, by site
ulna (shaft) S52.20-
bent bone S52.28-
coronoid process - *see* Fracture, ulna, upper end, coronoid process
distal end - *see* Fracture, ulna, lower end
following insertion of implant, prosthesis or plate M96.63-
head S52.60-
lower end S52.60-
physeal S59.00-
Salter-Harris
Type I S59.01-
Type II S59.02-
Type III S59.03-
Type IV S59.04-
specified NEC S59.09-
specified NEC S52.69-
styloid process (displaced) S52.61-
nondisplaced S52.61-
torus S52.62-
proximal end - *see* Fracture, ulna, upper end
shaft S52.20-
comminuted (displaced) S52.25-
nondisplaced S52.25-
greenstick S52.21-
Monteggia's - *see* Monteggia's fracture
oblique (displaced) S52.23-
nondisplaced S52.23-
segmental (displaced) S52.26-
nondisplaced S52.26-
specified NEC S52.29-
spiral (displaced) S52.24-
nondisplaced S52.24-
transverse (displaced) S52.22-
nondisplaced S52.22-
upper end S52.00-
coronoid process (displaced) S52.04-
nondisplaced S52.04-
olecranon process (displaced) S52.02-

Fracture, traumatic - *continued*
with intraarticular extension S52.03-
nondisplaced S52.02-
with intraarticular extension S52.03-
specified NEC S52.09-
torus S52.01-
unciform - *see* Fracture, carpal, hamate
vault of skull S02.0
vertebra, vertebral (arch) (body) (column) (neural arch) (pedicle) (spinous process) (transverse process)
atlas - *see* Fracture, neck, cervical vertebra, first
axis - *see* Fracture, neck, cervical vertebra, second
cervical (teardrop) S12.9
axis - *see* Fracture, neck, cervical vertebra, second
first (atlas) - *see* Fracture, neck, cervical vertebra, first
second (axis) - *see* Fracture, neck, cervical vertebra, second
chronic M84.48
coccyx S32.2
dorsal - *see* Fracture, thorax, vertebra
lumbar S32.009
burst (stable) S32.001
unstable S32.002
fifth S32.059
burst (stable) S32.051
unstable S32.052
specified type NEC S32.058
wedge compression S32.050
first S32.019
burst (stable) S32.011
unstable S32.012
specified type NEC S32.018
wedge compression S32.010
fourth S32.049
burst (stable) S32.041
unstable S32.042
specified type NEC S32.048
wedge compression S32.040
second S32.029
burst (stable) S32.021
unstable S32.022
specified type NEC S32.028
wedge compression S32.020
specified type NEC S32.008
third S32.039
burst (stable) S32.031
unstable S32.032
specified type NEC S32.038
wedge compression S32.030
wedge compression S32.000
metastatic - *see* Collapse, vertebra, in,
specified disease NEC - *see also* Neoplasm
newborn (birth injury) P11.5
sacrum S32.10
specified NEC S32.19
Type
1 S32.14
2 S32.15
3 S32.16
4 S32.17
Zone
I S32.119
displaced (minimally) S32.111
severely S32.112
nondisplaced S32.110
II S32.129
displaced (minimally) S32.121
severely S32.122
nondisplaced S32.120

Fracture, traumatic - *continued*
III S32.139
displaced (minimally) S32.131
severely S32.132
nondisplaced S32.130
thoracic - *see* Fracture, thorax, vertebra
vertex S02.0
vomer (bone) S02.2
wrist S62.10-
carpal - *see* Fracture, carpal bone
navicular (scaphoid) (hand) - *see* Fracture, carpal, navicular
xiphisternum, xiphoid (process) S22.24
zygoma S02.402
left side S02.40F
right side S02.40E
Fragile, fragility
autosomal site Q95.5
bone, congenital (with blue sclera) Q78.0
capillary (hereditary) D69.8
hair L67.8
nails L60.3
non-sex chromosome site Q95.5
X chromosome Q99.2
Fragilitas
crinium L67.8
ossium (with blue sclerae) (hereditary) Q78.0
unguium L60.3
congenital Q84.6
Fragments, cataract (lens), following cataract surgery H59.02-
retained foreign body - *see* Retained, foreign body fragments (type of)
Frailty (frail) R54
mental R41.81
Frambesia, frambesial (tropica) - *see also* Yaws
initial lesion or ulcer A66.0
primary A66.0
Frambeside
gummatous A66.4
of early yaws A66.2
Frambesioma A66.1
Franceschetti-Klein (-Wildervanck) disease or syndrome Q75.4
Francis' disease - *see* Tularemia
Franklin disease C88.2
Frank's essential thrombocytopenia D69.3
Fraser's syndrome Q87.0
Freckle(s) L81.2
malignant melanoma in - *see* Melanoma
melanotic (Hutchinson's) - *see* Melanoma, in situ
retinal D49.81
Frederickson's hyperlipoproteinemia, type I and V E78.3
IIA E78.00
IIB and III E78.2
IV E78.1
Freeman Sheldon syndrome Q87.0
Freezing - *see also* Effect, adverse, cold T69.9
Freiberg's disease (infraction of metatarsal head or osteochondrosis) - *see* Osteochondrosis, juvenile, metatarsus
Frei's disease A55
Fremitus, friction, cardiac R01.2
Frenum, frenulum
external os Q51.828
tongue (shortening) (congenital) Q38.1
Frequency micturition (nocturnal) R35.0
psychogenic F45.8
Frey's syndrome
auriculotemporal G50.8
hyperhidrosis L74.52

Friction
burn - *see* Burn, by site
fremitus, cardiac R01.2
precordial R01.2
sounds, chest R09.89
Friderichsen-Waterhouse syndrome or
disease A39.1
Friedländer's B (bacillus) NEC - *see also*
condition A49.8
Friedreich's
ataxia G11.1
combined systemic disease G11.1
facial hemihypertrophy Q67.4
sclerosis (cerebellum) (spinal cord) G11.1
Frigidity F52.22
Fröhlich's syndrome E23.6
Frontal - *see also* condition
lobe syndrome F07.0
Frostbite (superficial) T33.90
with
partial thickness skin loss - *see* Frostbite
(superficial), by site
tissue necrosis T34.90
abdominal wall T33.3
with tissue necrosis T34.3
ankle T33.81-
with tissue necrosis T34.81-
arm T33.4-
with tissue necrosis T34.4-
finger(s) - *see* Frostbite, finger
hand - *see* Frostbite, hand
wrist - *see* Frostbite, wrist
ear T33.01-
with tissue necrosis T34.01-
face T33.09
with tissue necrosis T34.09
finger T33.53-
with tissue necrosis T34.53-
foot T33.82-
with tissue necrosis T34.82-
hand T33.52-
with tissue necrosis T34.52-
head T33.09
with tissue necrosis T34.09
ear - *see* Frostbite, ear
nose - *see* Frostbite, nose   hip (and thigh)
T33.6-
with tissue necrosis T34.6-
knee T33.7-
with tissue necrosis T34.7-
leg T33.9-
with tissue necrosis T34.9-
ankle - *see* Frostbite, ankle
foot - *see* Frostbite, foot
knee - *see* Frostbite, knee
lower T33.7-
with tissue necrosis T34.7-
thigh - *see* Frostbite, hip
toe - *see* Frostbite, toe
limb
lower T33.99
with tissue necrosis T34.99
upper - *see* Frostbite, arm
neck T33.1
with tissue necrosis T34.1
nose T33.02
with tissue necrosis T34.02
pelvis T33.3
with tissue necrosis T34.3
specified site NEC T33.99
with tissue necrosis T34.99
thigh - *see* Frostbite, hip
thorax T33.2
with tissue necrosis T34.2

Frostbite (superficial) - *continued*
toes T33.83-
with tissue necrosis T34.83-
trunk T33.99
with tissue necrosis T34.99
wrist T33.51-
with tissue necrosis T34.51-
Frotteurism F65.81
Frozen - *see also* Effect, adverse, cold T69.9
pelvis (female) N94.89
male K66.8
shoulder - *see* Capsulitis, adhesive
Fructokinase deficiency E74.11
Fructose 1,6
diphosphatase deficiency E74.19
Fructosemia (benign) (essential) E74.12
Fructosuria (benign) (essential) E74.11
Fuchs'
black spot (myopic) (see also Myopia,
degenerative) H44.2-
dystrophy (corneal endothelium) H18.51
heterochromic cyclitis - *see* Cyclitis, Fuchs'
heterochromic
Fucosidosis E77.1
Fugue R68.89
dissociative F44.1
hysterical (dissociative) F44.1
postictal in epilepsy - *see* Epilepsy
reaction to exceptional stress (transient) F43.0
Fulminant, fulminating - *see* condition
Functional - *see also* condition
bleeding (uterus) N93.8
Functioning, intellectual, borderline R41.83
Fundus - *see* condition
Fungemia NOS B49
Fungus, fungous
cerebral G93.89
disease NOS B49
infection - *see* Infection, fungus
Funiculitis (acute) (chronic) (endemic) N49.1
gonococcal (acute) (chronic) A54.23
tuberculous A18.15
Funnel
breast (acquired) M95.4
congenital Q67.6
sequelae (late effect) of rickets E64.3
chest (acquired) M95.4
congenital Q67.6
sequelae (late effect) of rickets E64.3
pelvis (acquired) M95.5
with disproportion (fetopelvic) O33.3
causing obstructed labor O65.3
congenital Q74.2
FUO (fever of unknown origin) R50.9
Furfur L21.0
microsporon B36.0
Furrier's lung J67.8
Furrowed K14.5
nail(s) (transverse) L60.4
congenital Q84.6
tongue K14.5
congenital Q38.3
Furuncle L02.92
abdominal wall L02.221
ankle - *see* Furuncle, lower limb
anus K61.0
antecubital space - *see* Furuncle, upper limb
arm - *see* Furuncle, upper limb
auditory canal, external - *see* Abscess, ear,
external
auricle (ear) - *see* Abscess, ear, external
axilla (region) L02.42-
back (any part) L02.222
breast N61.1

Furuncle - *continued*
buttock L02.32
cheek (external) L02.02
chest wall L02.223
chin L02.02
corpus cavernosum N48.21
ear, external - *see* Abscess, ear, external
external auditory canal - *see* Abscess, ear,
external
eyelid - *see* Abscess, eyelid
face L02.02
femoral (region) - *see* Furuncle, lower limb
finger - *see* Furuncle, hand
flank L02.221
foot L02.62-
forehead L02.02
gluteal (region) L02.32
groin L02.224
hand L02.52-
head L02.821
face L02.02
hip - *see* Furuncle, lower limb
kidney - *see* Abscess, kidney
knee - *see* Furuncle, lower limb
labium (majus) (minus) N76.4
lacrimal
gland - *see* Dacryoadenitis
passages (duct) (sac) - *see* Inflammation,
lacrimal, passages, acute
leg (any part) - *see* Furuncle, lower limb
lower limb L02.42-
malignant A22.0
mouth K12.2
navel L02.226
neck L02.12
nose J34.0
orbit, orbital - *see* Abscess, orbit
palmar (space) - *see* Furuncle, hand
partes posteriores L02.32
pectoral region L02.223
penis N48.21
perineum L02.225
pinna - *see* Abscess, ear, external
popliteal - *see* Furuncle, lower limb
prepatellar - *see* Furuncle, lower limb
scalp L02.821
seminal vesicle N49.0
shoulder - *see* Furuncle, upper limb
specified site NEC L02.828
submandibular K12.2
temple (region) L02.02
thumb - *see* Furuncle, hand
toe - *see* Furuncle, foot
trunk L02.229
abdominal wall L02.221
back L02.222
chest wall L02.223
groin L02.224
perineum L02.225
umbilicus L02.226
umbilicus L02.226
upper limb L02.42-
vulva N76.4
Furunculosis - *see* Furuncle
Fused - *see* Fusion, fused
Fusion, fused (congenital)
astragaloscaphoid Q74.2
atria Q21.1
auditory canal Q16.1
auricles, heart Q21.1
binocular with defective stereopsis H53.32
bone Q79.8
cervical spine M43.22
choanal Q30.0

Fusion, fused - *continued*
  commissure, mitral valve Q23.2
  cusps, heart valve NEC Q24.8
    mitral Q23.2
    pulmonary Q22.1
    tricuspid Q22.4
  ear ossicles Q16.3
  fingers Q70.0-
  hymen Q52.3
  joint (acquired) - *see also* Ankylosis
    congenital Q74.8
  kidneys (incomplete) Q63.1
  labium (majus) (minus) Q52.5
  larynx and trachea Q34.8
  limb, congenital Q74.8
    lower Q74.2
    upper Q74.0
  lobes, lung Q33.8
  lumbosacral (acquired) M43.27
    arthrodesis status Z98.1
    congenital Q76.49
    postprocedural status Z98.1
  nares, nose, nasal, nostril(s) Q30.0
  organ or site not listed - *see* Anomaly, by site
  ossicles Q79.9
    auditory Q16.3
  pulmonic cusps Q22.1
  ribs Q76.6
  sacroiliac (joint) (acquired) M43.28
    arthrodesis status Z98.1
    congenital Q74.2
    postprocedural status Z98.1
  spine (acquired) NEC M43.20
    arthrodesis status Z98.1
    cervical region M43.22
    cervicothoracic region M43.23
    congenital Q76.49
    lumbar M43.26
    lumbosacral region M43.27
    occipito-atlanto-axial region M43.21
    postoperative status Z98.1
    sacrococcygeal region M43.28
    thoracic region M43.24
    thoracolumbar region M43.25
  sublingual duct with submaxillary duct at opening in mouth Q38.4
  testes Q55.1
  toes Q70.2-
  tooth, teeth K00.2
  trachea and esophagus Q39.8
  twins Q89.4
  vagina Q52.4
  ventricles, heart Q21.0
  vertebra (arch) - *see* Fusion, spine
  vulva Q52.5
Fusospirillosis (mouth) (tongue) (tonsil) A69.1
Fussy baby R68.12

G

Gain in weight (abnormal) (excessive) - *see also* Weight, gain
Gaisböck's disease (polycythemia hypertonica) D75.1
Gait abnormality R26.9
  ataxic R26.0
  falling R29.6
  hysterical (ataxic) (staggering) F44.4
  paralytic R26.1
  spastic R26.1
  specified type NEC R26.89
  staggering R26.0
  unsteadiness R26.81
  walking difficulty NEC R26.2

Galactocele (breast) N64.89
  puerperal, postpartum O92.79
Galactokinase deficiency E74.29
Galactophoritis N61.0
  gestational, puerperal, postpartum O91.2-
Galactorrhea O92.6
  not associated with childbirth N64.3
Galactosemia (classic) (congenital) E74.21
Galactosuria E74.29
Galacturia R82.0
  schistosomiasis (bilharziasis) B65.0
GALD (gestational alloimmune liver disease) P78.84
Galeazzi's fracture S52.37-
Galen's vein - *see* condition
Galeophobia F40.218
Gall duct - *see* condition
Gallbladder - *see also* condition
  acute K81.0
Gallop rhythm R00.8
Gallstone (colic) (cystic duct) (gallbladder) (impacted) (multiple) - *see also* Calculus, gallbladder
  with
    cholecystitis - *see* Calculus, gallbladder, with cholecystitis
  bile duct (common) (hepatic) - *see* Calculus, bile duct
  causing intestinal obstruction K56.3
  specified NEC K80.80
    with obstruction K80.81
Gambling Z72.6
  pathological (compulsive) F63.0
Gammopathy (of undetermined significance [MGUS]) D47.2
  associated with lymphoplasmacytic dyscrasia D47.2
  monoclonal D47.2
  polyclonal D89.0
Gamna's disease (siderotic splenomegaly) D73.1
Gamophobia F40.298
Gampsodactylia (congenital) Q66.7
Gamstorp's disease (adynamia episodica hereditaria) G72.3
Gandy Nanta disease (siderotic splenomegaly) D73.1
Gang
  membership offenses Z72.810
Gangliocytoma D36.10
Ganglioglioma - *see* Neoplasm, uncertain behavior, by site
Ganglion (compound) (diffuse) (joint) (tendon (sheath)) M67.40
  ankle M67.47-
  foot M67.47-
  forearm M67.43-
  hand M67.44-
  lower leg M67.46-
  multiple sites M67.49
  of yaws (early) (late) A66.6
  pelvic region M67.45-
  periosteal - *see* Periostitis
  shoulder region M67.41-
  specified site NEC M67.48
  thigh region M67.45-
  tuberculous A18.09
  upper arm M67.42-
  wrist M67.43-
Ganglioneuroblastoma - *see* Neoplasm, nerve, malignant
Ganglioneuroma D36.10
  malignant - *see* Neoplasm, nerve, malignant
Ganglioneuromatosis D36.10

Ganglionitis
  fifth nerve - *see* Neuralgia, trigeminal
  gasserian (postherpetic) (postzoster) B02.21
  geniculate G51.1
    newborn (birth injury) P11.3
    postherpetic, postzoster B02.21
  herpes zoster B02.21
  postherpetic geniculate B02.21
Gangliosidosis E75.10
  GM1 E75.19
  GM2 E75.00
    other specified E75.09
    Sandhoff disease E75.01
    Tay-Sachs disease E75.02
  GM3 E75.19
  mucolipidosis IV E75.11
Gangosa A66.5
Gangrene, gangrenous (connective tissue) (dropsical) (dry) (moist) (skin) (ulcer) - *see also* Necrosis I96
  with diabetes (mellitus) - *see* Diabetes, gangrene
  abdomen (wall) I96
  alveolar M27.3
  appendix K35.80
    with
      perforation or rupture K35.2
      peritoneal abscess K35.3
      peritonitis NEC K35.3
        generalized (with perforation or rupture) K35.2
        localized (with perforation or rupture) K35.3
  arteriosclerotic (general) (senile) - *see* Arteriosclerosis, extremities, with, gangrene
  auricle I96
  Bacillus welchii A48.0
  bladder (infectious) - *see* Cystitis, specified type NEC
  bowel, cecum, or colon - *see* Gangrene, intestine
  Clostridium perfringens or welchii A48.0
  cornea H18.89-
  corpora cavernosa N48.29
    noninfective N48.89
  cutaneous, spreading I96
  decubital - *see* Ulcer, pressure, by site
  diabetic (any site) - *see* Diabetes, gangrene
  epidemic - *see* Poisoning, food, noxious, plant
  epididymis (infectional) N45.1
  erysipelas - *see* Erysipelas
  emphysematous - *see* Gangrene, gas
  extremity (lower) (upper) I96
  Fournier N49.3
    female N76.89
  fusospirochetal A69.0
  gallbladder - *see* Cholecystitis, acute
  gas (bacillus) A48.0
    following
      abortion - *see* Abortion by type complicated by infection
      ectopic or molar pregnancy O08.0
  glossitis K14.0
  hernia - *see* Hernia, by site, with gangrene
  intestine, intestinal (hemorrhagic) (massive) - *see also* Infarct, intestine K55.069
    with
      mesenteric embolism - *see also* Infarct, intestine K55.069
      obstruction - *see* Obstruction, intestine
  laryngitis J04.0
  limb (lower) (upper) I96
  lung J85.0
    spirochetal A69.8

Gangrene, gangrenous - *continued*
lymphangitis I89.1
Meleney's (synergistic) - *see* Ulcer, skin
mesentery - *see also* Infarct, intestine K55.069
with
embolism - *see also* Infarct, intestine
K55.069
intestinal obstruction - *see* Obstruction,
intestine
mouth A69.0
ovary - *see* Oophoritis
pancreas - *see* Pancreatitis, acute
penis N48.29
noninfective N48.89
perineum I96
pharynx - *see also* Pharyngitis
Vincent's A69.1
presenile I73.1
progressive synergistic - *see* Ulcer, skin
pulmonary J85.0
pulpal (dental) K04.1
quinsy J36
Raynaud's (symmetric gangrene) I73.01
retropharyngeal J39.2
scrotum N49.3
noninfective N50.89
senile (atherosclerotic) - *see* Arteriosclerosis,
extremities, with, gangrene
spermatic cord N49.1
noninfective N50.89
spine I96
spirochetal NEC A69.8
spreading cutaneous I96
stomatitis A69.0
symmetrical I73.01
testis (infectional) N45.2
noninfective N44.8
throat - *see also* Pharyngitis
diphtheritic A36.0
Vincent's A69.1
thyroid (gland) E07.89
tooth (pulp) K04.1
tuberculous NEC - *see* Tuberculosis
tunica vaginalis N49.1
noninfective N50.89
umbilicus I96
uterus - *see* Endometritis
uvulitis K12.2
vas deferens N49.1
noninfective N50.89
vulva N76.89
Ganister disease J62.8
Ganser's syndrome (hysterical) F44.89
Gardner-diamond syndrome
(autoerythrocyte sensitization) D69.2
Gargoylism E76.01
Garré's disease, osteitis (sclerosing),
osteomyelitis - *see* Osteomyelitis, specified
type NEC
Garrod's pad, knuckle M72.1
Gartner's duct
cyst Q52.4
persistent Q50.6
Gas R14.3
asphyxiation, inhalation, poisoning,
suffocation NEC - *see* Table of Drugs and
Chemicals
excessive R14.0
gangrene A48.0
following
abortion - *see* Abortion by type complicated
by infection
ectopic or molar pregnancy O08.0
on stomach R14.0
pains R14.1

Gastralgia - *see also* Pain, abdominal
Gastrectasis K31.0
psychogenic F45.8
Gastric - *see* condition
Gastrinoma
malignant
pancreas C25.4
specified site NEC - *see* Neoplasm,
malignant, by site
unspecified site C25.4
specified site - *see* Neoplasm, uncertain
behavior
unspecified site D37.9
Gastritis (simple) K29.70
with bleeding K29.71
acute (erosive) K29.00
with bleeding K29.01
alcoholic K29.20
with bleeding K29.21
allergic K29.60
with bleeding K29.61
atrophic (chronic) K29.40
with bleeding K29.41
chronic (antral) (fundal) K29.50
with bleeding K29.51
atrophic K29.40
with bleeding K29.41
superficial K29.30
with bleeding K29.31
dietary counseling and surveillance Z71.3
due to diet deficiency E63.9
eosinophilic K52.81
giant hypertrophic K29.60
with bleeding K29.61
granulomatous K29.60
with bleeding K29.61
hypertrophic (mucosa) K29.60
with bleeding K29.61
nervous F54
spastic K29.60
with bleeding K29.61
specified NEC K29.60
with bleeding K29.61
superficial chronic K29.30
with bleeding K29.31
tuberculous A18.83
viral NEC A08.4
Gastrocarcinoma - *see* Neoplasm, malignant,
stomach
Gastrocolic - *see* condition
Gastrodisciasis, gastrodiscoidiasis B66.8
Gastroduodenitis K29.90
with bleeding K29.91
virus, viral A08.4
specified type NEC A08.39
Gastrodynia - *see* Pain, abdominal
Gastroenteritis (acute) (chronic)
(noninfectious) - *see also* Enteritis K52.9
allergic K52.29
with
eosinophilic gastritis or gastroenteritis
K52.81
food protein-induced enterocolitis
syndrome K52.21
food protein-induced enteropathy K52.22
dietetic - *see also* Gastroenteritis, allergic
K52.29
drug-induced K52.1
due to
Cryptosporidium A07.2
drugs K52.1
food poisoning - *see* Intoxication, foodborne
radiation K52.0
eosinophilic K52.81

Gastroenteritis - *continued*
epidemic (infectious) A09
food hypersensitivity - *see also* Gastroenteritis,
allergic K52.29
infectious - *see* Enteritis, infectious
influenzal - *see* Influenza, with gastroenteritis
noninfectious K52.9
specified NEC K52.89
Rotaviral A08.0
Salmonella A02.0
toxic K52.1
viral NEC A08.4
acute infectious A08.39
type Norwalk A08.11
infantile (acute) A08.39
Norwalk agent A08.11
Rotaviral A08.0
severe of infants A08.39
specified type NEC A08.39
Gastroenteropathy - *see also* Gastroenteritis
K52.9
acute, due to Norwalk agent A08.11
acute, due to Norovirus A08.11
infectious A09
Gastroenteroptosis K63.4
Gastroesophageal laceration hemorrhage
syndrome K22.6
Gastrointestinal - *see* condition
Gastrojejunal - *see* condition
Gastrojejunitis - *see also* Enteritis K52.9
Gastrojejunocolic - *see* condition
Gastroliths K31.89
Gastromalacia K31.89
Gastroparalysis K31.84
diabetic - *see* Diabetes, gastroparalysis
Gastroparesis K31.84
diabetic - *see* Diabetes, by type, with
gastroparesis
Gastropathy K31.9
congestive portal K31.89
erythematous K29.70
exudative K90.89
portal hypertensive K31.89
Gastroptosis K31.89
Gastrorrhagia K92.2
psychogenic F45.8
Gastroschisis (congenital) Q79.3
Gastrospasm (neurogenic) (reflex) K31.89
neurotic F45.8
psychogenic F45.8
Gastrostaxis - *see* Gastritis, with bleeding
Gastrostenosis K31.89
Gastrostomy
attention to Z43.1
status Z93.1
Gastrosuccorrhea (continuous) (intermittent)
K31.89
neurotic F45.8
psychogenic F45.8
Gatophobia F40.218
Gaucher's disease or splenomegaly (adult)
(infantile) E75.22
Gee (-Herter)(-Thaysen) disease (nontropical
sprue) K90.0
Gélineau's syndrome G47.419
with cataplexy G47.411
Gemination, tooth, teeth K00.2
Gemistocytoma
specified site - *see* Neoplasm, malignant, by
site
unspecified site C71.9
General, generalized - *see* condition
Genetic
carrier (status)

Genetic - *continued*
cystic fibrosis Z14.1
hemophilia A (asymptomatic) Z14.01
symptomatic Z14.02
specified NEC Z14.8
susceptibility to disease NEC Z15.89
malignant neoplasm Z15.09
breast Z15.01
endometrium Z15.04
ovary Z15.02
prostate Z15.03
specified NEC Z15.09
multiple endocrine neoplasia Z15.81
Genital - *see* condition
Genito-anorectal syndrome A55
Genitourinary system - *see* condition
Genu
congenital Q74.1
extrorsum (acquired) - *see also* Deformity, varus, knee
congenital Q74.1
sequelae (late effect) of rickets E64.3
introrsum (acquired) - *see also* Deformity, valgus, knee
congenital Q74.1
sequelae (late effect) of rickets E64.3
rachitic (old) E64.3
recurvatum (acquired) - *see also* Deformity, limb, specified type NEC, lower leg
congenital Q68.2
sequelae (late effect) of rickets E64.3
valgum (acquired) (knock-knee) M21.06-
congenital Q74.1
sequelae (late effect) of rickets E64.3
varum (acquired) (bowleg) M21.16-
congenital Q74.1
sequelae (late effect) of rickets E64.3
Geographic tongue K14.1
Geophagia - *see* Pica **Geotrichosis** B48.3
stomatitis B48.3
Gephyrophobia F40.242
Gerbode defect Q21.0
GERD (gastroesophageal reflux disease) K21.9
Gerhardt's
disease (erythromelalgia) I73.81
syndrome (vocal cord paralysis) J38.00
bilateral J38.02
unilateral J38.01
German measles - *see also* Rubella
exposure to Z20.4
Germinoblastoma (diffuse) C85.9-
follicular C82.9-
Germinoma - *see* Neoplasm, malignant, by site
Gerontoxon - *see* Degeneration, cornea, senile
Gerstmann-Sträussler-Scheinker syndrome (GSS) A81.82
Gerstmann's syndrome R48.8
developmental F81.2
Gestation (period) - *see also* Pregnancy
ectopic - *see* Pregnancy, by site
multiple O30.9-
greater than quadruplets - *see* Pregnancy, multiple (gestation), specified NEC
specified NEC - *see* Pregnancy, multiple (gestation), specified NEC
Gestational
mammary abscess O91.11-
purulent mastitis O91.11-
subareolar abscess O91.11-
Ghon tubercle, primary infection A15.7
Ghost
teeth K00.4
vessels (cornea) H16.41
-ghoul hand A66.3

Gianotti-Crosti disease L44.4
Giant
cell
epulis K06.8
peripheral granuloma K06.8
esophagus, congenital Q39.5
kidney, congenital Q63.3
urticaria T78.3
hereditary D84.1
Giardiasis A07.1
Gibert's disease or pityriasis L42
Giddiness R42
hysterical F44.89
psychogenic F45.8
Gierke's disease (glycogenosis I) E74.01
Gigantism (cerebral) (hypophyseal) (pituitary) E22.0
constitutional E34.4
Gilbert's disease or syndrome E80.4
Gilchrist's disease B40.9
Gilford-Hutchinson disease E34.8
Gilles de la Tourette's disease or syndrome (motor-verbal tic) F95.2
Gingivitis K05.10
acute (catarrhal) K05.00
necrotizing A69.1
nonplaque induced K05.01
plaque induced K05.00
chronic (desquamative) (hyperplastic) (simple marginal) (pregnancy associated) (ulcerative) K05.10
nonplaque induced K05.11
plaque induced K05.10
expulsiva - *see* Periodontitis
necrotizing ulcerative (acute) A69.1
pellagrous E52
acute necrotizing A69.1
Vincent's A69.1
Gingivoglossitis K14.0
Gingivopericementitis - *see* Periodontitis
Gingivosis - *see* Gingivitis, chronic
Gingivostomatitis K05.10
herpesviral B00.2
necrotizing ulcerative (acute) A69.1
Gland, glandular - *see* condition
Glanders A24.0
Glanzmann (Naegeli) disease or thrombasthenia D69.1
Glasgow coma scale
total score
3-8 R40.243
9-12 R40.242
13-15 R40.241
Glass-blower's disease (cataract) - *see* Cataract, specified NEC
Glaucoma H40.9
with
increased episcleral venous pressure H40.81-
pseudoexfoliation of lens - *see* Glaucoma, open angle, primary, capsular
absolute H44.51-
angle-closure (primary) H40.20-
acute (attack) (crisis) H40.21-
chronic H40.22-
intermittent H40.23-
residual stage H40.24-
borderline H40.00-
capsular (with pseudoexfoliation of lens) - *see* Glaucoma, open angle, primary, capsular
childhood Q15.0
closed angle - *see* Glaucoma, angle-closure
congenital Q15.0
corticosteroid-induced - *see* Glaucoma, secondary, drugs

Glaucoma- *continued*
hypersecretion H40.82-
in (due to)
amyloidosis E85.4 [*H42*]
aniridia Q13.1 [*H42*]
concussion of globe - *see* Glaucoma, secondary, trauma
dislocation of lens - *see* Glaucoma, secondary
disorder of lens NEC - *see* Glaucoma, secondary
drugs - *see* Glaucoma, secondary, drugs
endocrine disease NOS E34.9 [*H42*]
eye
inflammation - *see* Glaucoma, secondary, inflammation
trauma - *see* Glaucoma, secondary, trauma
hypermature cataract - *see* Glaucoma, secondary
iridocyclitis - *see* Glaucoma, secondary, inflammation
lens disorder - *see* Glaucoma, secondary, Lowe's syndrome E72.03 [*H42*]
metabolic disease NOS E88.9 [*H42*]
ocular disorders NEC - *see* Glaucoma, secondary
onchocerciasis B73.02
pupillary block - *see* Glaucoma, secondary
retinal vein occlusion - *see* Glaucoma, secondary
Rieger's anomaly Q13.81 [*H42*]
rubeosis of iris - *see* Glaucoma, secondary
tumor of globe - *see* Glaucoma, secondary
infantile Q15.0
low tension - *see* Glaucoma, open angle, primary, low-tension
malignant H40.83-
narrow angle - *see* Glaucoma, angle-closure
newborn Q15.0
noncongestive (chronic) - *see* Glaucoma, open angle
nonobstructive - *see* Glaucoma, open angle
obstructive - *see also* Glaucoma, angle-closure
due to lens changes - *see* Glaucoma, secondary
open angle H40.10-
primary H40.11-
capsular (with pseudoexfoliation of lens) H40.14-
low-tension H40.12
pigmentary H40.13-
residual stage H40.15-
phacolytic - *see* Glaucoma, secondary
pigmentary - *see* Glaucoma, open angle, primary, pigmentary
postinfectious - *see* Glaucoma, secondary, inflammation
secondary (to) H40.5-
drugs H40.6-
inflammation H40.4-
trauma H40.3-
simple (chronic) H40.11-
simplex H40.11-
specified type NEC H40.89
suspect H40.00-
syphilitic A52.71
traumatic - *see also* Glaucoma, secondary, trauma
newborn (birth injury) P15.3
tuberculous A18.59
Glaucomatous flecks (subcapsular) - *see* Cataract, complicated
Glazed tongue K14.4
Gleet (gonococcal) A54.01

Glénard's disease K63.4
Glioblastoma (multiforme)
with sarcomatous component
specified site - *see* Neoplasm, malignant, by site
unspecified site C71.9
giant cell
specified site - *see* Neoplasm, malignant, by site
unspecified site C71.9
specified site - *see* Neoplasm, malignant, by site
unspecified site C71.9
Glioma (malignant)
astrocytic
specified site - *see* Neoplasm, malignant, by site
unspecified site C71.9
mixed
specified site - *see* Neoplasm, malignant, by site
unspecified site C71.9
nose Q30.8
specified site NEC - *see* Neoplasm, malignant, by site
subependymal D43.2
specified site - *see* Neoplasm, uncertain behavior, by site
unspecified site D43.2
unspecified site C71.9
Gliomatosis cerebri C71.0
Glioneuroma - *see* Neoplasm, uncertain behavior, by site
Gliosarcoma
specified site - *see* Neoplasm, malignant, by site
unspecified site C71.9
Gliosis (cerebral) G93.89
spinal G95.89
Glisson's disease - *see* Rickets
Globinuria R82.3
Globus (hystericus) F45.8
Glomangioma D18.00
intra-abdominal D18.03
intracranial D18.02
skin D18.01
specified site NEC D18.09
Glomangiomyoma D18.00
intra-abdominal D18.03
intracranial D18.02
skin D18.01
specified site NEC D18.09
Glomangiosarcoma - *see* Neoplasm, connective tissue, malignant
Glomerular
disease in syphilis A52.75
nephritis - *see* Glomerulonephritis
Glomerulitis - *see* Glomerulonephritis
Glomerulonephritis - *see also* Nephritis N05.9
with
edema - *see* Nephrosis
minimal change N05.0
minor glomerular abnormality N05.0
acute N00.9
chronic N03.9
crescentic (diffuse) NEC - *see also* N00-N07 with fourth character .7 N05.7
dense deposit - *see also* N00-N07 with fourth character .6 N05.6
diffuse
crescentic - *see also* N00-N07 with fourth character .7 N05.7
endocapillary proliferative - *see also* N00-N07 with fourth character .4 N05.4

Glomerulonephritis - *continued*
membranous - *see also* N00-N07 with fourth character .2 N05.2
mesangial proliferative - *see also* N00-N07 with fourth character .3 N05.3
mesangiocapillary - *see also* N00-N07 with fourth character .5 N05.5
sclerosing N18.9
endocapillary proliferative (diffuse) NEC - *see also* N00-N07 with fourth character .4 N05.4
extracapillary NEC - *see also* N00-N07 with fourth character .7 N05.7
focal (and segmental) - *see also* N00-N07 with fourth character .1 N05.1
hypocomplementemic - *see* Glomerulonephritis, membranoproliferative
IgA - *see* Nephropathy, IgA
immune complex (circulating) NEC N05.8
in (due to)
amyloidosis E85.4 [N08]
bilharziasis B65.9 [N08]
cryoglobulinemia D89.1 [N08]
defibrination syndrome D65 [N08]
diabetes mellitus - *see* Diabetes, glomerulosclerosis
disseminated intravascular coagulation D65 [N08]
Fabry (-Anderson) disease E75.21 [N08]
Goodpasture's syndrome M31.0
hemolytic-uremic syndrome D59.3
Henoch (-Schönlein) purpura D69.0 [N08]
lecithin cholesterol acyltransferase deficiency E78.6 [N08]
microscopic polyangiitis M31.7 [N08]
multiple myeloma C90.0- [N08]
Plasmodium malariae B52.0
schistosomiasis B65.9 [N08]
sepsis A41.9 [N08]
streptococcal A40- [N08]
sickle-cell disorders D57. [N08]
strongyloidiasis B78.9 [N08]
subacute bacterial endocarditis I33.0 [N08]
syphilis (late) congenital A50.59 [N08]
systemic lupus erythematosus M32.14
thrombotic thrombocytopenic purpura M31.1 [N08]
typhoid fever A01.09
Waldenström macroglobulinemia C88.0 [N08]
Wegener's granulomatosis M31.31
latent or quiescent N03.9
lobular, lobulonodular - *see* Glomerulonephritis, membranoproliferative
membranoproliferative (diffuse)(type 1 or 3) - *see also* N00-N07 with fourth character .5 N05.5
dense deposit (type 2) NEC - *see also* N00-N07 with fourth character .6 N05.6
membranous (diffuse) NEC - *see also* N00-N07 with fourth character .2 N05.2
mesangial
IgA/IgG - *see* Nephropathy, IgA
proliferative (diffuse) NEC - *see also* N00-N07 with fourth character .3 N05.3
mesangiocapillary (diffuse) NEC - *see also* N00-N07 with fourth character .5 N05.5
necrotic, necrotizing NEC - *see also* N00-N07 with fourth character .8 N05.8
nodular - *see* Glomerulonephritis, membranoproliferative
poststreptococcal NEC N05.9
acute N00.9
chronic N03.9
rapidly progressive N01.9

Glomerulonephritis - *continued*
proliferative NEC - *see also* N00-N07 with fourth character .8 N05.8
diffuse (lupus) M32.14
rapidly progressive N01.9
sclerosing, diffuse N18.9
specified pathology NEC - *see also* N00-N07 with fourth character .8 N05.8
subacute N01.9
Glomerulopathy - *see* Glomerulonephritis
Glomerulosclerosis - *see also* Sclerosis, renal
intercapillary (nodular) (with diabetes) - *see* Diabetes, glomerulosclerosis
intracapillary - *see* Diabetes, glomerulosclerosis
Glossagra K14.6
Glossalgia K14.6
Glossitis (chronic superficial) (gangrenous) (Moeller's) K14.0
areata exfoliativa K14.1
atrophic K14.4
benign migratory K14.1
cortical superficial, sclerotic K14.0
Hunter's D51.0
interstitial, sclerous K14.0
median rhomboid K14.2
pellagrous E52
superficial, chronic K14.0
Glossocele K14.8
Glossodynia K14.6
exfoliativa K14.4
Glossoncus K14.8
Glossopathy K14.9
Glossophytia K14.3
Glossoplegia K14.8
Glossoptosis K14.8
Glossopyrosis K14.6
Glossotrichia K14.3
Glossy skin L90.8
Glottis - *see* condition
Glottitis - *see also* Laryngitis J04.0
Glucagonoma
pancreas
benign D13.7
malignant C25.4
uncertain behavior D37.8
specified site NEC
benign - *see* Neoplasm, benign, by site
malignant - *see* Neoplasm, malignant, by site
uncertain behavior - *see* Neoplasm, uncertain behavior, by site
unspecified site
benign D13.7
malignant C25.4
uncertain behavior D37.8
Glucoglycinuria E72.51
Glucose-galactose malabsorption E74.39
Glue
ear - *see* Otitis, media, nonsuppurative, chronic, mucoid
sniffing (airplane) - *see* Abuse, drug, inhalant
dependence - *see* Dependence, drug, inhalant
Glutaric aciduria E72.3
Glycinemia E72.51
Glycinuria (renal) (with ketosis) E72.09
Glycogen
infiltration - *see* Disease, glycogen storage
storage disease - *see* Disease, glycogen storage
Glycogenosis (diffuse) (generalized) - *see also* Disease, glycogen storage
cardiac E74.02 [I43]
diabetic, secondary - *see* Diabetes, glycogenosis, secondary
pulmonary interstitial J84.842

Glycopenia E16.2
Glycosuria R81
  renal E74.8
Gnathostoma spinigerum (infection) (infestation), gnathostomiasis (wandering swelling) B83.1
Goiter (plunging) (substernal) E04.9
  with
    hyperthyroidism (recurrent) - *see* Hyperthyroidism, with, goiter
    thyrotoxicosis - *see* Hyperthyroidism, with, goiter
  adenomatous - *see* Goiter, nodular
  cancerous C73
  congenital (nontoxic) E03.0
    diffuse E03.0
    parenchymatous E03.0
    transitory, with normal functioning P72.0
  cystic E04.2
    due to iodine-deficiency E01.1
  due to
    enzyme defect in synthesis of thyroid hormone E07.1
    iodine-deficiency (endemic) E01.2
  dyshormonogenetic (familial) E07.1
  endemic (iodine-deficiency) E01.2
    diffuse E01.0
    multinodular E01.1
  exophthalmic - *see* Hyperthyroidism, with, goiter
  iodine-deficiency (endemic) E01.2
    diffuse E01.0
    multinodular E01.1
    nodular E01.1
  lingual Q89.2
  lymphadenoid E06.3
  malignant C73
  multinodular (cystic) (nontoxic) E04.2
    toxic or with hyperthyroidism E05.20
      with thyroid storm E05.21
  neonatal NEC P72.0
  nodular (nontoxic) (due to) E04.9
    with
      hyperthyroidism E05.20
        with thyroid storm E05.21
      thyrotoxicosis E05.20
        with thyroid storm E05.21
    endemic E01.1
    iodine-deficiency E01.1
    sporadic E04.9
    toxic E05.20
      with thyroid storm E05.21
  nontoxic E04.9
    diffuse (colloid) E04.0
    multinodular E04.2
    simple E04.0
    specified NEC E04.8
    uninodular E04.1
  simple E04.0
  toxic - *see* Hyperthyroidism, with, goiter
  uninodular (nontoxic) E04.1
    toxic or with hyperthyroidism E05.10
      with thyroid storm E05.11
Goiter-deafness syndrome E07.1
Goldberg syndrome Q89.8
Goldberg-maxwell syndrome E34.51
Goldblatt's hypertension or kidney I70.1
Goldenhar (-Gorlin) syndrome Q87.0
Goldflam-erb disease or syndrome G70.00
  with exacerbation (acute) G70.01
  in crisis G70.01
Goldscheider's disease Q81.8
Goldstein's disease (familial hemorrhagic telangiectasia) I78.0

Golfer's elbow - *see* Epicondylitis, medial
Gonadoblastoma
  specified site - *see* Neoplasm, uncertain behavior, by site
  unspecified site
    female D39.10
    male D40.10
Gonecystitis - *see* Vesiculitis
Gongylonemiasis B83.8
Goniosynechiae - *see* Adhesions, iris, goniosynechiae
Gonococcemia A54.86
Gonococcus, gonococcal (disease) (infection) - *see also* condition A54.9
  anus A54.6
  bursa, bursitis A54.49
  conjunctiva, conjunctivitis (neonatorum) A54.31
  endocardium A54.83
  eye A54.30
    conjunctivitis A54.31
    iridocyclitis A54.32
    keratitis A54.33
    newborn A54.31
    other specified A54.39
  fallopian tubes (acute) (chronic) A54.24
  genitourinary (organ) (system) (tract) (acute)
    lower A54.00
      with abscess (accessory gland) (periurethral) A54.1
    upper - *see also* condition A54.29
  heart A54.83
  iridocyclitis A54.32
  joint A54.42
  lymphatic (gland) (node) A54.89
  meninges, meningitis A54.81
  musculoskeletal A54.40
    arthritis A54.42
    osteomyelitis A54.43
    other specified A54.49
    spondylopathy A54.41
  pelviperitonitis A54.24
  pelvis (acute) (chronic) A54.24
  pharynx A54.5
  proctitis A54.6
  pyosalpinx (acute) (chronic) A54.24
  rectum A54.6
  skin A54.89
  specified site NEC A54.89
  tendon sheath A54.49
  throat A54.5
  urethra (acute) (chronic) A54.01
    with abscess (accessory gland) (periurethral) A54.1
  vulva (acute) (chronic) A54.02
Gonocytoma
  specified site - *see* Neoplasm, uncertain behavior, by site
  unspecified site
    female D39.10
    male D40.10
Gonorrhea (acute) (chronic) A54.9
  Bartholin's gland (acute) (chronic) (purulent) A54.02
    with abscess (accessory gland) (periurethral) A54.1
  bladder A54.01
  cervix A54.03
  conjunctiva, conjunctivitis (neonatorum) A54.31
  contact Z20.2
  Cowper's gland (with abscess) A54.1
  exposure to Z20.2
  fallopian tube (acute) (chronic) A54.24

Gonorrhea - *continued*
  kidney (acute) (chronic) A54.21
  lower genitourinary tract A54.00
    with abscess (accessory gland) (periurethral) A54.1
  ovary (acute) (chronic) A54.24
  pelvis (acute) (chronic) A54.24
    female pelvic inflammatory disease A54.24
  penis A54.09
  prostate (acute) (chronic) A54.22
  seminal vesicle (acute) (chronic) A54.23
  specified site not listed - *see also* Gonococcus A54.89
  spermatic cord (acute) (chronic) A54.23
  urethra A54.01
    with abscess (accessory gland) (periurethral) A54.1
  vagina A54.02
  vas deferens (acute) (chronic) A54.23
  vulva A54.02
Goodall's disease A08.19
Goodpasture's syndrome M31.0
Gopalan's syndrome (burning feet) E53.0
Gorlin-Chaudry-moss syndrome Q87.0
Gottron's papules L94.4
Gougerot's syndrome (trisymptomatic) L81.7
Gougerot-Blum syndrome (pigmented purpuric lichenoid dermatitis) L81.7
Gougerot-Carteaud disease or syndrome (confluent reticulate papillomatosis) L83
Gouley's syndrome (constrictive pericarditis) I31.1
Goundou A66.6
Gout, gouty (acute) (attack) (flare) - *see also* Gout, chronic M10.9
  drug-induced M10.20
    ankle M10.27-
    elbow M10.22-
    foot joint M10.27-
    hand joint M10.24-
    hip M10.25-
    knee M10.26-
    multiple site M10.29
    shoulder M10.21-
    vertebrae M10.28
    wrist M10.23-
  idiopathic M10.00
    ankle M10.07-
    elbow M10.02-
    foot joint M10.07-
    hand joint M10.04-
    hip M10.05-
    knee M10.06-
    multiple site M10.09
    shoulder M10.01-
    vertebrae M10.08
    wrist M10.03-
  in (due to) renal impairment M10.30
    ankle M10.37-
    elbow M10.32-
    foot joint M10.37-
    hand joint M10.34-
    hip M10.35-
    knee M10.36-
    multiple site M10.39
    shoulder M10.31-
    vertebrae M10.38
    wrist M10.33-
  lead-induced M10.10
    ankle M10.17-
    elbow M10.12-
    foot joint M10.17-
    hand joint M10.14-
    hip M10.15-
    knee M10.16-

Gout, gouty - *continued*

multiple site M10.19
shoulder M10.11-
vertebrae M10.18
wrist M10.13-
primary - *see* Gout, idiopathic
saturnine - *see* Gout, lead-induced   secondary
NEC M10.40
ankle M10.47-
elbow M10.42-
foot joint M10.47-
hand joint M10.44-
hip M10.45-
knee M10.46-
multiple site M10.49
shoulder M10.41-
vertebrae M10.48
wrist M10.43-
syphilitic - *see also* subcategory M14.8
A52.77
tophi - *see* Gout, chronic
Gout, chronic - *see also* Gout, gouty M1A.9
drug-induced M1A.20
ankle M1A.27-
elbow M1A.22-
foot joint M1A.27-
hand joint M1A.24-
hip M1A.25-
knee M1A.26-
multiple site M1A.29-
shoulder M1A.21-
vertebrae M1A.28
wrist M1A.23-
idiopathic M1A.00
ankle M1A.07-
elbow M1A.02-
foot joint M1A.07-
hand joint M1A.04-
hip M1A.05-
knee M1A.06-
multiple site M1A.09
shoulder M1A.01-
vertebrae M1A.08
wrist M1A.03-
in (due to) renal impairment M1A.30
ankle M1A.37-
elbow M1A.32-
foot joint M1A.37-
hand joint M1A.34-
hip M1A.35-
knee M1A.36-
multiple site M1A.39
shoulder M1A.31-
vertebrae M1A.38
wrist M1A.33-
lead-induced M1A.10
ankle M1A.17-
elbow M1A.12-
foot joint M1A.17-
hand joint M1A.14-
hip M1A.15-
knee M1A.16-
multiple site M1A.19
shoulder M1A.11-
vertebrae M1A.18
wrist M1A.13-
primary - *see* Gout, chronic, idiopathic
saturnine - *see* Gout, chronic, lead-induced
secondary NEC M1A.40
ankle M1A.47-
elbow M1A.42-
foot joint M1A.47-
hand joint M1A.44-
hip M1A.45-

Gout, chronic - *continued*

knee M1A.46-
multiple site M1A.49
shoulder M1A.41-
vertebrae M1A.48
wrist M1A.43-
syphilitic - *see also* subcategory M14.8
A52.77
tophi M1A.9
Gower's
muscular dystrophy G71.0
syndrome (vasovagal attack) R55
Gradenigo's syndrome - *see* Otitis, media,
suppurative, acute
Graefe's disease - *see* Strabismus, paralytic,
ophthalmoplegia, progressive
Graft-versus-host disease D89.813
acute D89.810
acute on chronic D89.812
chronic D89.811
Grain handler's disease or lung J67.8
Grain mite (itch) B88.0
Grand mal - *see* Epilepsy, generalized,
specified NEC
Grand multipara status only (not pregnant)
Z64.1
pregnant - *see* Pregnancy, complicated by,
grand multiparity
Granite worker's lung J62.8
Granular - *see also* condition
inflammation, pharynx J31.2
kidney (contracting) - *see* Sclerosis, renal
liver K74.69
Granulation tissue (abnormal) (excessive)
L92.9
postmastoidectomy cavity - *see* Complications,
postmastoidectomy, granulation
Granulocytopenia (primary) (malignant) -
see Agranulocytosis
Granuloma L92.9
abdomen K66.8
from residual foreign body L92.3
pyogenicum L98.0
actinic L57.5
annulare (perforating) L92.0
apical K04.5
aural - *see* Otitis, externa, specified NEC
beryllium (skin) L92.3
bone
eosinophilic C96.6
from residual foreign body - *see*
Osteomyelitis, specified type NEC
lung C96.6
brain (any site) G06.0
schistosomiasis B65.9 [G07]
canaliculus lacrimalis - *see* Granuloma,
lacrimal
candidal (cutaneous) B37.2
cerebral (any site) G06.0
coccidioidal (primary) (progressive) B38.7
lung B38.1
meninges B38.4
colon K63.89
conjunctiva H11.22-
dental K04.5
ear, middle - *see* Cholesteatoma
eosinophilic C96.6
bone C96.6
lung C96.6
oral mucosa K13.4
skin L92.2
eyelid H01.8
facial (e) L92.2
foreign body (in soft tissue) NEC M60.20

Granuloma - *continued*

ankle M60.27-
foot M60.27-
forearm M60.23-
hand M60.24-
in operation wound - *see* Foreign body,
accidentally left during a procedure
lower leg M60.26-
pelvic region M60.25-
shoulder region M60.21-
skin L92.3
specified site NEC M60.28
subcutaneous tissue L92.3
thigh M60.25-
upper arm M60.22-
gangraenescens M31.2
genito-inguinale A58
giant cell (central) (reparative) (jaw) M27.1
gingiva (peripheral) K06.8
gland (lymph) I88.8
hepatic NEC K75.3
in (due to)
berylliosis J63.2 [K77]
sarcoidosis D86.89
Hodgkin C81.9
ileum K63.89
infectious B99.9
specified NEC B99.8
inguinale (Donovan) (venereal) A58
intestine NEC K63.89
intracranial (any site) G06.0
intraspinal (any part) G06.1
iridocyclitis - *see* Iridocyclitis, chronic
jaw (bone) (central) M27.1
reparative giant cell M27.1
kidney - *see also* Infection, kidney N15.8
lacrimal H04.81-
larynx J38.7
lethal midline (faciale(e)) M31.2
liver NEC - *see* Granuloma, hepatic
lung (infectious) - *see also* Fibrosis, lung
coccidioidal B38.1
eosinophilic C96.6
Majocchi's B35.8
malignant (facial(e)) M31.2
mandible (central) M27.1
midline (lethal) M31.2
monilial (cutaneous) B37.2
nasal sinus - *see* Sinusitis
operation wound T81.89
foreign body - *see* Foreign body, accidentally
left during a procedure
stitch T81.89
talc - *see* Foreign body, accidentally left
during a procedure
oral mucosa K13.4
orbit, orbital H05.11-
paracoccidioidal B41.8
penis, venereal A58
periapical K04.5
peritoneum K66.8
due to ova of helminths NOS - *see also*
Helminthiasis B83.9 [K67]
postmastoidectomy cavity - *see* Complications,
postmastoidectomy, recurrent cholesteatoma
prostate N42.89
pudendi (ulcerating) A58
pulp, internal (tooth) K03.3
pyogenic, pyogenicum (of) (skin) L98.0
gingiva K06.8
maxillary alveolar ridge K04.5
oral mucosa K13.4
rectum K62.89
reticulohistiocytic D76.3

Granuloma - *continued*
rubrum nasi L74.8
Schistosoma - *see* Schistosomiasis
septic (skin) L98.0
silica (skin) L92.3
sinus (accessory) (infective) (nasal) - *see*
Sinusitis
skin L92.9
from residual foreign body L92.3
pyogenicum L98.0
spine
syphilitic (epidural) A52.19
tuberculous A18.01
stitch (postoperative) T81.89
suppurative (skin) L98.0
swimming pool A31.1
talc - *see also* Granuloma, foreign body
in operation wound - *see* Foreign body,
accidentally left during a procedure
telangiectaticum (skin) L98.0
tracheostomy J95.09
trichophyticum B35.8
tropicum A66.4
umbilical P83.81
umbilicus P83.81
urethra N36.8
uveitis - *see* Iridocyclitis, chronic
vagina A58
venereum A58
vocal cord J38.3
Granulomatosis L92.9
lymphoid C83.8-
miliary (listerial) A32.89
necrotizing, respiratory M31.30
progressive septic D71
specified NEC L92.8
Wegener's M31.30
with renal involvement M31.31
Granulomatous tissue (abnormal) (excessive)
L92.9
Granulosis rubra nasi L74.8
Graphite fibrosis (of lung) J63.3
Graphospasm F48.8
organic G25.89
Grating scapula M89.8X1
Gravel (urinary) - *see* Calculus, urinary
Graves' disease - *see* Hyperthyroidism, with,
goiter
Gravis - *see* condition
Grawitz tumor C64.-
Gray syndrome (newborn) P93.0
Grayness, hair (premature) L67.1
congenital Q84.2
Green sickness D50.8
Greenfield's disease
meaning
concentric sclerosis (encephalitis periaxialis
concentrica) G37.5
metachromatic leukodystrophy E75.25
Greenstick fracture
code as Fracture, by site Grey syndrome
(newborn) P93.0
Grief F43.21
prolonged F43.29
reaction - *see also* Disorder, adjustment
F43.20
Griesinger's disease B76.9
Grinder's lung or pneumoconiosis J62.8
Grinding, teeth
psychogenic F45.8
sleep related G47.63
Grip
Dabney's B33.0
devil's B33.0

Grippe, grippal - *see also* Influenza
Balkan A78
summer, of Italy A93.1
Grisel's disease M43.6
Groin - *see* condition
Grooved tongue K14.5
Ground itch B76.9
Grover's disease or syndrome L11.1
Growing pains, children R29.898
Growth (fungoid) (neoplastic) (new) - *see also*
Neoplasm
adenoid (vegetative) J35.8
benign - *see* Neoplasm, benign, by site
malignant - *see* Neoplasm, malignant, by site
rapid, childhood Z00.2
secondary - *see* Neoplasm, secondary, by site
Gruby's disease B35.0
Gubler-Millard paralysis or syndrome G46.3
Guerin-stern syndrome Q74.3
Guidance, insufficient anterior (occlusal)
M26.54
Guillain-Barré disease or syndrome G61.0
sequelae G65.0
Guinea worms (infection) (infestation) B72
Guinon's disease (motor-verbal tic) F95.2
Gull's disease E03.4
Gum - *see* condition
Gumboil K04.7
with sinus K04.6
Gumma (syphilitic) A52.79
artery A52.09
cerebral A52.04
bone A52.77
of yaws (late) A66.6
brain A52.19
cauda equina A52.19
central nervous system A52.3
ciliary body A52.71
congenital A50.59
eyelid A52.71
heart A52.06
intracranial A52.19
iris A52.71
kidney A52.75
larynx A52.73
leptomeninges A52.19
liver A52.74
meninges A52.19
myocardium A52.06
nasopharynx A52.73
neurosyphilitic A52.3
nose A52.73
orbit A52.71
palate (soft) A52.79
penis A52.76
pericardium A52.06
pharynx A52.73
pituitary A52.79
scrofulous (tuberculous) A18.4
skin A52.79
specified site NEC A52.79
spinal cord A52.19
tongue A52.79
tonsil A52.73
trachea A52.73
tuberculous A18.4
ulcerative due to yaws A66.4
ureter A52.75
yaws A66.4
bone A66.6
Gunn's syndrome Q07.8
Gunshot wound - *see also* Wound, open
fracture
code as Fracture, by site
internal organs - *see* Injury, by site

Gynandrism Q56.0
Gynandroblastoma
specified site - *see* Neoplasm, uncertain
behavior, by site
unspecified site
female D39.10
male D40.10
Gynecological examination (periodic)
(routine) Z01.419
with abnormal findings Z01.411
Gynecomastia N62
Gynephobia F40.291
Gyrate scalp Q82.8

H

H (Hartnup's) disease E72.02
Haas' disease or osteochondrosis (juvenile)
(head of humerus) - *see* Osteochondrosis,
juvenile, humerus
Habit, habituation
bad sleep Z72.821
chorea F95.8
disturbance, child F98.9
drug - *see* Dependence, drug
irregular sleep Z72.821
laxative F55.2
spasm - *see* Tic
tic - *see* Tic
Haemophilus (H.) influenzae, as cause of
disease classified elsewhere B96.3
Haff disease - *see* Poisoning, mercury
Hageman's factor defect, deficiency or
disease D68.2
Haglund's disease or osteochondrosis
(juvenile) (os tibiale externum) - *see*
Osteochondrosis, juvenile, tarsus
Hailey-Hailey disease Q82.8
Hair - *see also* condition
plucking F63.3
in stereotyped movement disorder F98.4
tourniquet syndrome - *see also* Constriction,
external, by site
finger S60.44-
penis S30.842
thumb S60.34-
toe S90.44-
Hairball in stomach T18.2
Hair-pulling, pathological (compulsive) F63.3
Hairy black tongue K14.3
Half vertebra Q76.49
Halitosis R19.6
Hallerman-Streiff syndrome Q87.0
Hallervorden-Spatz disease G23.0
Hallopeau's acrodermatitis or disease L40.2
Hallucination R44.3
auditory R44.0
gustatory R44.2
olfactory R44.2
specified NEC R44.2
tactile R44.2
visual R44.1
Hallucinosis (chronic) F28
alcoholic (acute) F10.951
in
abuse F10.151
dependence F10.251
drug-induced F19.951
cannabis F12.951
cocaine F14.951
hallucinogen F16.151
in
abuse F19.151
cannabis F12.151

Hallucinosis - *continued*
  cocaine F14.151
    hallucinogen F16.151
    inhalant F18.151
    opioid F11.151
    sedative, anxiolytic or hypnotic F13.151
    stimulant NEC F15.151
  dependence F19.251
    cannabis F12.251
    hallucinogen F16.251
    inhalant F18.251
    cocaine F14.251
    opioid F11.251
    sedative, anxiolytic or hypnotic F13.251
    stimulant NEC F15.251
  inhalant F18.951
  opioid F11.951
  sedative, anxiolytic or hypnotic F13.951
  stimulant NEC F15.951
  organic F06.0
Hallux
  deformity (acquired) NEC M20.5X   limitus M20.5X-
  malleus (acquired) NEC M20.3-
  rigidus (acquired) M20.2-
    congenital Q74.2
    sequelae (late effect) of rickets E64.3
  valgus (acquired) M20.1-
    congenital Q66.6
  varus (acquired) M20.3-
    congenital Q66.3
Halo, visual H53.19
Hamartoma, hamartoblastoma Q85.9
  epithelial (gingival), odontogenic, central or peripheral - *see* Cyst, calcifying odontogenic
Hamartoses Q85.9
Hamman-rich syndrome J84.114
Hammer toe (acquired) NEC - *see also* Deformity, toe, hammer toe
  congenital Q66.89
  sequelae (late effect) of rickets E64.3
Hand - *see* condition
Hand-foot syndrome L27.1
Handicap, handicapped
  educational Z55.9
    specified NEC Z55.8
Hand-Schüller-Christian disease or syndrome C96.5
Hanging (asphyxia) (strangulation) (suffocation) - *see* Asphyxia, traumatic, due to mechanical threat
Hangnail - *see also* Cellulitis, digit
  with lymphangitis - *see* Lymphangitis, acute, digit
Hangover (alcohol) F10.129
Hanhart's syndrome Q87.0
Hanot-Chauffard (-Troisier) syndrome E83.19
Hanot's cirrhosis or disease K74.3
Hansen's disease - *see* Leprosy
Hantaan virus disease (Korean hemorrhagic fever) A98.5
Hantavirus disease (with renal manifestations) (Dobrava) (Puumala) (Seoul) A98.5
  with pulmonary manifestations (Andes) (Bayou) (Bermejo) (Black Creek Canal) (Choclo) (Juquitiba) (Laguna negra) (Lechiguanas) (New York) (Oran) (Sin nombre) B33.4
Happy puppet syndrome Q93.5
Harada's disease or syndrome H30.81-
Hardening
  artery - *see* Arteriosclerosis
  brain G93.89

Harelip (complete) (incomplete) - *see* Cleft, lip
Harlequin (newborn) Q80.4
Harley's disease D59.6
Harmful use (of)
  alcohol F10.10
  anxiolytics - *see* Abuse, drug, sedative
  cannabinoids - *see* Abuse, drug, cannabis
  cocaine - *see* Abuse, drug, cocaine
  drug - *see* Abuse, drug
  hallucinogens - *see* Abuse, drug, hallucinogen
  hypnotics - *see* Abuse, drug, sedative
  opioids - *see* Abuse, drug, opioid
  PCP (phencyclidine) - *see* Abuse, drug, hallucinogen
  sedatives - *see* Abuse, drug, sedative
  stimulants NEC - *see* Abuse, drug, stimulant
Harris' lines - *see* Arrest, epiphyseal
Hartnup's disease E72.02
Harvester's lung J67.0
Harvesting ovum for in vitro fertilization Z31.83
Hashimoto's disease or thyroiditis E06.3
Hashitoxicosis (transient) E06.3
Hassal-Henle bodies or warts (cornea) H18.49
Haut mal - *see* Epilepsy, generalized, specified NEC
Haverhill fever A25.1
Hay fever - *see also* Fever, hay J30.1
Hayem-Widal syndrome D59.8
Haygarth's nodes M15.8
Haymaker's lung J67.0
Hb (abnormal)
  Bart's disease D56.0
  disease - *see* Disease, hemoglobin
  trait - *see* Trait
Head - *see* condition
Headache R51
  allergic NEC G44.89
  associated with sexual activity G44.82
  chronic daily R51
  cluster G44.009
    chronic G44.029
      intractable G44.021
      not intractable G44.029
    episodic G44.019
      intractable G44.011
      not intractable G44.019
    intractable G44.001
    not intractable G44.009
  cough (primary) G44.83
  daily chronic R51
  drug-induced NEC G44.40
    intractable G44.41
    not intractable G44.40
  exertional (primary) G44.84
  histamine G44.009
    intractable G44.001
    not intractable G44.009
  hypnic G44.81
  lumbar puncture G97.1
  medication overuse G44.40
    intractable G44.41
    not intractable G44.40
  menstrual - *see* Migraine, menstrual
  migraine (type) - *see also* Migraine G43.909
  nasal septum R51
  neuralgiform, short lasting unilateral, with conjunctival injection and tearing (SUNCT) G44.059
    intractable G44.051
    not intractable G44.059
  new daily persistent (NDPH) G44.52
  orgasmic G44.82

Headache - *continued*
  periodic syndromes in adults and children G43.C0
    with refractory migraine G43.C1
      intractable G43.C1
      not intractable G43.C0
    without refractory migraine G43.C0
  postspinal puncture G97.1
  post-traumatic G44.309
    acute G44.319
      intractable G44.311
      not intractable G44.319
    chronic G44.329
      intractable G44.321
      not intractable G44.329
    intractable G44.301
    not intractable G44.309
  pre-menstrual - *see* Migraine, menstrual
  preorgasmic G44.82
  primary
    cough G44.83
    exertional G44.84
    stabbing G44.85
    thunderclap G44.53
  rebound G44.40
    intractable G44.41
    not intractable G44.40
  short lasting unilateral neuralgiform, with conjunctival injection and tearing (SUNCT) G44.059
    intractable G44.051
    not intractable G44.059
  specified syndrome NEC G44.89
  spinal and epidural anesthesia induced T88.59
    in labor and delivery O74.5
    in pregnancy O29.4-
    postpartum, puerperal O89.4
  spinal fluid loss (from puncture) G97.1
  stabbing (primary) G44.85
  tension (-type) G44.209
    chronic G44.229
      intractable G44.221
      not intractable G44.229
    episodic G44.219
      intractable G44.211
      not intractable G44.219
    intractable G44.201
    not intractable G44.209
  thunderclap (primary) G44.53
  vascular NEC G44.1
Healthy
  infant
    accompanying sick mother Z76.3
    receiving care Z76.2
  person accompanying sick person Z76.3
Hearing examination Z01.10
  with abnormal findings NEC Z01.118
  following failed hearing screening Z01.110
  for hearing conservation and treatment Z01.12
Heart - *see* condition
Heart beat
  abnormality R00.9
    specified NEC R00.8
  awareness R00.2
  rapid R00.0
  slow R00.1
Heartburn R12
  psychogenic F45.8
Heartland virus disease A93.8
Heat (effects) T67.9
  apoplexy T67.0
  burn - *see also* Burn L55.9
  collapse T67.1

Heat (effects) - *continued*
cramps T67.2
dermatitis or eczema L59.0
edema T67.7
erythem*a* code by site under Burn, first degree
excessive T67.9
specified effect NEC T67.8
exhaustion T67.5
anhydrotic T67.3
due to
salt (and water) depletion T67.4
water depletion T67.3
with salt depletion T67.4
fatigue (transient) T67.6
fever T67.0
hyperpyrexia T67.0
prickly L74.0
prostration - *see* Heat, exhaustion
pyrexia T67.0
rash L74.0
specified effect NEC T67.8
stroke T67.0
sunburn - *see* Sunburn
syncope T67.1
Heavy-for-dates NEC (infant) (4000g to 4499g) P08.1
exceptionally (4500g or more) P08.0
Hebephrenia, hebephrenic (schizophrenia) F20.1
Heberden's disease or nodes (with arthropathy) M15.1
Hebra's
pityriasis L26
prurigo L28.2
Heel - *see* condition **Heerfordt's disease** D86.89
Hegglin's anomaly or syndrome D72.0
Heilmeyer-Schoner disease D45
Heine-Medin disease A80.9
Heinz body anemia, congenital D58.2
Heliophobia F40.228
Heller's disease or syndrome F84.3
HELLP syndrome (hemolysis, elevated liver enzymes and low platelet count) O14.2-
complicating
childbirth O14.24
puerperium O14.25
Helminthiasis - *see also* Infestation, helminth
Ancylostoma B76.0
intestinal B82.0
mixed types (types classifiable to more than one of the titles B65.0-b81.3 and B81.8) B81.4
specified type NEC B81.8
mixed types (intestinal) (types classifiable to more than one of the titles B65.0-b81.3 and B81.8) B81.4
Necator (americanus) B76.1
specified type NEC B83.8
Heloma L84
Hemangioblastoma - *see* Neoplasm, connective tissue, uncertain behavior
malignant - *see* Neoplasm, connective tissue, malignant
Hemangioendothelioma - *see also* Neoplasm, uncertain behavior, by site
benign D18.00
intra-abdominal D18.03
intracranial D18.02
skin D18.01
specified site NEC D18.09
bone (diffuse) - *see* Neoplasm, bone, malignant

Hemangioendothelioma - *continued*
epithelioid - *see also* Neoplasm, uncertain behavior, by site
malignant - *see* Neoplasm, malignant, by site
malignant - *see* Neoplasm, connective tissue, malignant
Hemangiofibroma - *see* Neoplasm, benign, by site
Hemangiolipoma - *see* Lipoma
Hemangioma D18.00
arteriovenous D18.00
intra-abdominal D18.03
intracranial D18.02
skin D18.01
specified site NEC D18.09
capillary D18.00
intra-abdominal D18.03
intracranial D18.02
skin D18.01
specified site NEC D18.09
cavernous D18.00
intra-abdominal D18.03
intracranial D18.02
skin D18.01
specified site NEC D18.09
epithelioid D18.00
intra-abdominal D18.03
intracranial D18.02
skin D18.01
specified site NEC D18.09
histiocytoid D18.00
intra-abdominal D18.03
intracranial D18.02
skin D18.01
specified site NEC D18.09
infantile D18.00
intra-abdominal D18.03
intracranial D18.02
skin D18.01
specified site NEC D18.09
intra-abdominal D18.03
intracranial D18.02
intramuscular D18.00
intra-abdominal D18.03
intracranial D18.02
skin D18.01
specified site NEC D18.09
intrathoracic structures D18.09
juvenile D18.00
malignant - *see* Neoplasm, connective tissue, malignant
plexiform D18.00
intra-abdominal D18.03
intracranial D18.02
skin D18.01
specified site NEC D18.09
racemose D18.00
intra-abdominal D18.03
intracranial D18.02
skin D18.01
specified site NEC D18.09
sclerosing - *see* Neoplasm, skin, benign
simplex D18.00
intra-abdominal D18.03
intracranial D18.02
skin D18.01
specified site NEC D18.09
skin D18.01
specified site NEC D18.09
venous D18.00
intra-abdominal D18.03
intracranial D18.02
skin D18.01
specified site NEC D18.09

Hemangioma - *continued*
verrucous keratotic D18.00
intra-abdominal D18.03
intracranial D18.02
skin D18.01
specified site NEC D18.09
Hemangiomatosis (systemic) I78.8
involving single site - *see* Hemangioma
Hemangiopericytoma - *see also* Neoplasm, connective tissue, uncertain behavior
benign - *see* Neoplasm, connective tissue, benign
malignant - *see* Neoplasm, connective tissue, malignant
Hemangiosarcoma - *see* Neoplasm, connective tissue, malignant
Hemarthrosis (nontraumatic) M25.00
ankle M25.07-
elbow M25.02-
foot joint M25.07-
hand joint M25.04-
hip M25.05-
in hemophilic arthropathy - *see* Arthropathy, hemophilic
knee M25.06-
shoulder M25.01-
specified joint NEC M25.08
traumatic - *see* Sprain, by site
vertebrae M25.08
wrist M25.03-
Hematemesis K92.0
with ulcer
code by site under Ulcer, with hemorrhage K27.4
newborn, neonatal P54.0
due to swallowed maternal blood P78.2
Hematidrosis L74.8
Hematinuria - *see also* Hemoglobinuria
malarial B50.8
Hematobilia K83.8
Hematocele
female NEC N94.89
with ectopic pregnancy O00.90
with intrauterine pregnancy O00.91
ovary N83.8
male N50.1
Hematochezia - *see also* Melena K92.1
Hematochyluria - *see also* Infestation, filarial
schistosomiasis (bilharziasis) B65.0
Hematocolpos (with hematometra or hematosalpinx) N89.7
Hematocornea - *see* Pigmentation, cornea, stromal
Hematogenous - *see* condition
Hematoma (traumatic) (skin surface intact) - *see also* Contusion
with
injury of internal organs - *see* Injury, by site
open wound - *see* Wound, open
amputation stump (surgical) (late) T87.89
aorta, dissecting I71.00
abdominal I71.02
thoracic I71.01
thoracoabdominal I71.03
aortic intramural - *see* Dissection, aorta
arterial (complicating trauma) - *see* Injury, blood vessel, by site
auricle - *see* Contusion, ear
nontraumatic - *see* Disorder, pinna, hematoma
birth injury NEC P15.8
brain (traumatic)
with
cerebral laceration or contusion (diffuse) -

Hematoma - *continued*
  see Injury, intracranial, diffuse
  focal - *see* Injury, intracranial, focal
    cerebellar, traumatic S06.37-
    newborn NEC P52.4
      birth injury P10.1
  intracerebral, traumatic - *see* Injury,
  intracranial, intracerebral hemorrhage
    nontraumatic - *see* Hemorrhage, intracranial
    subarachnoid, arachnoid, traumatic - *see*
  Injury, intracranial, subarachnoid hemorrhage
    subdural, traumatic - *see* Injury, intracranial,
  subdural hemorrhage
  breast (nontraumatic) N64.89
  broad ligament (nontraumatic) N83.7
    traumatic S37.892
  cerebellar, traumatic S06.37-
  cerebral - *see* Hematoma, brain
  cerebrum S06.36-
    left S06.35-
    right S06.34-
  cesarean delivery wound O90.2
  complicating delivery (perineal) (pelvic)
  (vagina) (vulva) O71.7
  corpus cavernosum (nontraumatic) N48.89
  epididymis (nontraumatic) N50.1
  epidural (traumatic) - *see* Injury, intracranial,
  epidural hemorrhage
    spinal - *see* Injury, spinal cord, by region
  episiotomy O90.2
  face, birth injury P15.4
  genital organ NEC (nontraumatic)
    female (nonobstetric) N94.89
      traumatic S30.202
    male N50.1
      traumatic S30.201
  internal organs - *see* Injury, by site
  intracerebral, traumatic - *see* Injury,
  intracranial, intracerebral hemorrhage
  intraoperative - *see* Complications,
  intraoperative, hemorrhage
  labia (major) (minor) (nonobstetric) N90.89
  liver (subcapsular) (nontraumatic) K76.89
    birth injury P15.0
  mediastinum - *see* Injury, intrathoracic
  mesosalpinx (nontraumatic) N83.7
    traumatic S37.898
  muscle
  code by site under Contusion
  nontraumatic
    muscle M79.81
    soft tissue M79.81
  obstetrical surgical wound O90.2
  orbit, orbital (nontraumatic) - *see also*
  Hemorrhage, orbit
    traumatic - *see* Contusion, orbit
  pelvis (female) (nontraumatic) (nonobstetric)
  N94.89
    obstetric O71.7
    traumatic - *see* Injury, by site
  penis (nontraumatic) N48.89
    birth injury P15.5
  perianal (nontraumatic) K64.5
  perineal S30.23
    complicating delivery O71.7
  perirenal - *see* Injury, kidney
  pinna - *see* Contusion, ear
    nontraumatic - *see* Disorder, pinna,
  hematoma
  placenta O43.89-
  postoperative (postprocedural) - *see*
  Complication, postprocedural, hematoma
  retroperitoneal (nontraumatic) K66.1
    traumatic S36.892

Hematoma - *continued*
  scrotum, superficial S30.22
    birth injury P15.5
  seminal vesicle (nontraumatic) N50.1
    traumatic S37.892
  spermatic cord (traumatic) S37.892
    nontraumatic N50.1
  spinal (cord) (meninges) - *see also* Injury,
  spinal cord, by region
    newborn (birth injury) P11.5
  spleen D73.5
    intraoperative - *see* Complications,
    intraoperative, hemorrhage, spleen
    postprocedural (postoperative) - *see*
    Complications, postprocedural, hemorrhage,
    spleen
  sternocleidomastoid, birth injury P15.2
  sternomastoid, birth injury P15.2
  subarachnoid (traumatic) - *see* Injury,
  intracranial, subarachnoid hemorrhage
    newborn (nontraumatic) P52.5
    due to birth injury P10.3
    nontraumatic - *see* Hemorrhage, intracranial,
    subarachnoid
  subdural (traumatic) - *see* Injury, intracranial,
  subdural hemorrhage
    newborn (localized) P52.8
      birth injury P10.0
    nontraumatic - *see* Hemorrhage, intracranial,
    subdural
    superficial, newborn P54.5
  testis (nontraumatic) N50.1
    birth injury P15.5
  tunica vaginalis (nontraumatic) N50.1
  umbilical cord, complicating delivery O69.5
  uterine ligament (broad) (nontraumatic) N83.7
    traumatic S37.892
  vagina (ruptured) (nontraumatic) N89.8
    complicating delivery O71.7
  vas deferens (nontraumatic) N50.1
    traumatic S37.892
  vitreous - *see* Hemorrhage, vitreous
  vulva (nontraumatic) (nonobstetric) N90.89
    complicating delivery O71.7
    newborn (birth injury) P15.5
Hematometra N85.7
  with hematocolpos N89.7
Hematomyelia (central) G95.19
  newborn (birth injury) P11.5
  traumatic T14.8
Hematomyelitis G04.90
Hematoperitoneum - *see* Hemoperitoneum
Hematophobia F40.230
Hematopneumothorax (see Hemothorax)
Hematopoiesis, cyclic D70.4
Hematoporphyria - *see* Porphyria
Hematorachis, hematorrhachis G95.19
  newborn (birth injury) P11.5
Hematosalpinx N83.6
  with
    hematocolpos N89.7
    hematometra N85.7
      with hematocolpos N89.7
  infectional - *see* Salpingitis
Hematospermia R36.1
Hematothorax (see Hemothorax)
Hematuria R31.9
  due to sulphonamide, sulfonamide - *see* Table
  of Drugs and Chemicals, by drug
  benign (familial) (of childhood) - *see also*
  Hematuria, idiopathic
    essential microscopic R31.1
  endemic - *see also* Schistosomiasis B65.0
  gross R31.0

Hematuria - *continued*
  idiopathic N02.9
    with glomerular lesion
      crescentic (diffuse) glomerulonephritis
      N02.7
      dense deposit disease N02.6
      endocapillary proliferative
      glomerulonephritis N02.4
      focal and segmental hyalinosis or sclerosis
      N02.1
      membranoproliferative (diffuse) N02.5
      membranous (diffuse) N02.2
      mesangial proliferative (diffuse) N02.3
      mesangiocapillary (diffuse) N02.5
      minor abnormality N02.0
      proliferative NEC N02.8
      specified pathology NEC N02.8
  intermittent - *see* Hematuria, idiopathic
  malarial B50.8
  microscopic NEC (with symptoms) R31.29
    asymptomatic R31.21
    benign essential R31.1
  paroxysmal - *see also* Hematuria, idiopathic
    nocturnal D59.5
  persistent - *see* Hematuria, idiopathic
  recurrent - *see* Hematuria, idiopathic
  tropical - *see also* Schistosomiasis B65.0
  tuberculous A18.13
Hemeralopia (day blindness) H53.11
  vitamin A deficiency E50.5
Hemi-akinesia R41.4
Hemianalgesia R20.0
Hemianencephaly Q00.0
Hemianesthesia R20.0
Hemianopia, hemianopsia (heteronymous)
  H53.47
  homonymous H53.46-
  syphilitic A52.71
Hemiathetosis R25.8
Hemiatrophy R68.89
  cerebellar G31.9
  face, facial, progressive (Romberg) G51.8
  tongue K14.8
Hemiballism (us) G25.5
Hemicardia Q24.8
Hemicephalus, hemicephaly Q00.0
Hemichorea G25.5
Hemicolitis, left - *see* Colitis, left sided
Hemicrania
  congenital malformation Q00.0
  continua G44.51
  meaning migraine - *see also* Migraine G43.909
  paroxysmal G44.039
    chronic G44.049
      intractable G44.041
      not intractable G44.049
    episodic G44.039
      intractable G44.031
      not intractable G44.039
    intractable G44.031
    not intractable G44.039
Hemidystrophy - *see* Hemiatrophy
Hemiectromelia Q73.8
Hemihypalgesia R20.8
Hemihypesthesia R20.1
Hemi-inattention R41.4
Hemimelia Q73.8
  lower limb - *see* Defect, reduction, lower limb,
  specified type NEC
  upper limb - *see* Defect, reduction, upper limb,
  specified type NEC
Hemiparalysis - *see* Hemiplegia
Hemiparesis - *see* Hemiplegia
Hemiparesthesia R20.2

Hemiparkinsonism G20
Hemiplegia G81.9-
  alternans facialis G83.89
  ascending NEC G81.90
    spinal G95.89
  congenital (cerebral) G80.8
    spastic G80.2
  embolic (current episode) I63.4-
  flaccid G81.0-
  following
    cerebrovascular disease I69.959
      cerebral infarction I69.35-
      intracerebral hemorrhage I69.15-
      nontraumatic intracranial hemorrhage NEC
        I69.25-
      specified disease NEC I69.85-
      stroke NOS I69.35-
      subarachnoid hemorrhage I69.05-
  hysterical F44.4
  newborn NEC P91.88
    birth injury P11.9
  spastic G81.1-
    congenital G80.2
  thrombotic (current episode) I63.3-
Hemisection, spinal cord - see Injury, spinal
  cord, by region
Hemispasm (facial) R25.2
Hemisporosis B48.8
Hemitremor R25.1
Hemivertebra Q76.49
  failure of segmentation with scoliosis Q76.3
  fusion with scoliosis Q76.3
Hemochromatosis E83.119
  with refractory anemia D46.1
  due to repeated red blood cell transfusion
    E83.111
  hereditary (primary) E83.110
  neonatal P78.84
  primary E83.110
  specified NEC E83.118
Hemoglobin - see also condition
  abnormal (disease) - see Disease, hemoglobin
  AS genotype D57.3
  Constant Spring D58.2
  E-beta thalassemia D56.5
  fetal, hereditary persistence (HPFH) D56.4
  H Constant Spring D56.0
  low NOS D64.9
  S (Hb S), heterozygous D57.3
Hemoglobinemia D59.9
  due to blood transfusion T80.89
  paroxysmal D59.6
    nocturnal D59.5
Hemoglobinopathy (mixed) D58.2
  with thalassemia D56.8
  sickle-cell D57.1
    with thalassemia D57.40
      with crisis (vasoocclusive pain) D57.419
        with
          acute chest syndrome D57.411
          splenic sequestration D57.412
      without crisis D57.40
Hemoglobinuria R82.3
  with anemia, hemolytic, acquired (chronic)
    NEC D59.6
  cold (agglutinin) (paroxysmal) (with
    Raynaud's syndrome) D59.6
  due to exertion or hemolysis NEC D59.6
  intermittent D59.6
  malarial B50.8
  march D59.6
  nocturnal (paroxysmal) D59.5
  paroxysmal (cold) D59.6
    nocturnal D59.5

Hemolymphangioma D18.1
Hemolysis
  intravascular
    with
      abortion - see Abortion, by type,
      complicated by, hemorrhage
      ectopic or molar pregnancy O08.1
      hemorrhage
        antepartum - see Hemorrhage, antepartum,
          with coagulation defect
        intrapartum - see also Hemorrhage,
          complicating, delivery O67.0
      postpartum O72.3
  neonatal (excessive) P58.9
    specified NEC P58.8
Hemolytic - see condition
Hemopericardium I31.2
  following acute myocardial infarction (current
    complication) I23.0
  newborn P54.8
  traumatic - see Injury, heart, with
    hemopericardium
Hemoperitoneum K66.1
  infectional K65.9
  traumatic S36.899
    with open wound - see Wound, open, with
      penetration into peritoneal cavity
Hemophilia (classical) (familial) (hereditary)
  D66
  A D66
  B D67
  C D68.1
  acquired D68.311
  autoimmune D68.311
  calcipriva - see also Defect, coagulation D68.4
  nonfamilial - see also Defect, coagulation
    D68.4
  secondary D68.311
  vascular D68.0
Hemophthalmos H44.81-
Hemopneumothorax - see also Hemothorax
  traumatic S27.2
Hemoptysis R04.2
  newborn P26.9
  tuberculous - see Tuberculosis, pulmonary
Hemorrhage, hemorrhagic (concealed) R58
  abdomen R58
  accidental antepartum - see Hemorrhage,
    antepartum
  acute idiopathic pulmonary, in infants R04.81
  adenoid J35.8
  adrenal (capsule) (gland) E27.49
    medulla E27.8
    newborn P54.4
  after delivery - see Hemorrhage, postpartum
  alveolar
    lung, newborn P26.8
    process K08.89
  alveolus K08.89
  amputation stump (surgical) T87.89
  anemia (chronic) D50.0
    acute D62
  antepartum (with) O46.90
    with coagulation defect O46.00-
      afibrinogenemia O46.01-
      disseminated intravascular coagulation
        O46.02-
      hypofibrinogenemia O46.01-
      specified defect NEC O46.09-
    before 20 weeks gestation O20.9
      specified type NEC O20.8
      threatened abortion O20.0
    due to
      abruptio placenta - see also Abruptio

Hemorrhage, hemorrhagic - continued
  placentae O45.9-
    leiomyoma, uterus - see Hemorrhage,
  antepartum, specified cause NEC
    placenta previa O44.1-
    specified cause NEC - see subcategory
      O46.8X-
  anus (sphincter) K62.5
  apoplexy (stroke) - see Hemorrhage,
    intracranial, intracerebral
  arachnoid - see Hemorrhage, intracranial,
    subarachnoid
  artery R58
  brain - see Hemorrhage, intracranial,
    intracerebral
  basilar (ganglion) I61.0
  bladder N32.89
  bowel K92.2
    newborn P54.3
  brain (miliary) (nontraumatic) - see
  Hemorrhage, intracranial, intracerebral
    due to
      birth injury P10.1
      syphilis A52.05
    epidural or extradural (traumatic) - see
  Injury, intracranial, epidural hemorrhage
    newborn P52.4
      birth injury P10.1
    subarachnoid - see Hemorrhage, intracranial,
      subarachnoid
    subdural - see Hemorrhage, intracranial,
      subdural
  brainstem (nontraumatic) I61.3
    traumatic S06.38-
  breast N64.59
  bronchial tube - see Hemorrhage, lung
  bronchopulmonary - see Hemorrhage, lung
  bronchus - see Hemorrhage, lung
  bulbar I61.5
  capillary I78.8
    primary D69.8
  cecum K92.2
  cerebellar, cerebellum (nontraumatic) I61.4
    newborn P52.6
    traumatic S06.37-
  cerebral, cerebrum - see also Hemorrhage,
    intracranial, intracerebral
    newborn (anoxic) P52.4
      birth injury P10.1
    lobe I61.1
  cerebromeningeal I61.8
  cerebrospinal - see Hemorrhage, intracranial,
    intracerebral
  cervix (uteri) (stump) NEC N88.8
  chamber, anterior (eye) - see Hyphema
  childbirth - see Hemorrhage, complicating,
    delivery   choroid H31.30-
    expulsive H31.31-
  ciliary body - see Hyphema
  cochlea - see subcategory H83.8
  colon K92.2
  complicating
    abortion - see Abortion, by type, complicated
      by, hemorrhage
    delivery O67.9
      associated with coagulation defect
        (afibrinogenemia) (DIC)
        (hyperfibrinolysis) O67.0
      specified cause NEC O67.8
    surgical procedure - see Hemorrhage,
  intraoperative
  conjunctiva H11.3-
    newborn P54.8
  cord, newborn (stump) P51.9

Hemorrhage, hemorrhagic - *continued*
corpus luteum (ruptured) cyst N83.1-
cortical (brain) I61.1
cranial - *see* Hemorrhage, intracranial
cutaneous R23.3
  due to autosensitivity, erythrocyte D69.2
  newborn P54.5
delayed
  following ectopic or molar pregnancy O08.1
  postpartum O72.2
diathesis (familial) D69.9
disease D69.9
  newborn P53
  specified type NEC D69.8
due to or associated with
  afibrinogenemia or other coagulation defect
    (conditions in categories D65-d69)
    antepartum - *see* Hemorrhage, antepartum,
      with coagulation defect
    intrapartum O67.0
dental implant M27.61
device, implant or graft - *see also*
  Complications, by site and type, specified
  NEC T85.838
  arterial graft NEC T82.838
  breast T85.838
  catheter NEC T85.838
    dialysis (renal) T82.838
      intraperitoneal T85.838
    infusion NEC T82.838
      spinal (epidural) (subdural) T85.830
    urinary (indwelling) T83.83
  electronic (electrode) (pulse generator)
    (stimulator)
    bone T84.83
    cardiac T82.837
    nervous system (brain) (peripheral nerve)
      (spinal) T85.830
    urinary T83.83
  fixation, internal (orthopedic) NEC T84.83
  gastrointestinal (bile duct) (esophagus)
    T85.838
  genital NEC T83.83
  heart NEC T82.837
  joint prosthesis T84.83
  ocular (corneal graft) (orbital implant) NEC
    T85.838
  orthopedic NEC T84.83
    bone graft T86.838
  specified NEC T85.838
  urinary NEC T83.83
  vascular NEC T82.838
  ventricular intracranial shunt T85.830
duodenum, duodenal K92.2
  ulcer - *see* Ulcer, duodenum, with
  hemorrhage
dura mater - *see* Hemorrhage, intracranial,
subdural
endotracheal - *see* Hemorrhage, lung
epicranial subaponeurotic (massive), birth
injury P12.2
epidural (traumatic) - *see also* Injury,
intracranial, epidural hemorrhage
  nontraumatic I62.1
esophagus K22.8
  varix I85.01
    secondary I85.11
excessive, following ectopic gestation
  (subsequent episode) O08.1
extradural (traumatic) - *see* Injury, intracranial,
  epidural hemorrhage
  birth injury P10.8
  newborn (anoxic) (nontraumatic) P52.8
  nontraumatic I62.1

Hemorrhage, hemorrhagic - *continued*
eye NEC H57.8
  fundus - *see* Hemorrhage, retina
  lid - *see* Disorder, eyelid, specified type NEC
fallopian tube N83.6
fibrinogenolysis - *see* Fibrinolysis
fibrinolytic (acquired) - *see* Fibrinolysis
from
  ear (nontraumatic) - *see* Otorrhagia
  tracheostomy stoma J95.01
fundus, eye - *see* Hemorrhage, retina
funis - *see* Hemorrhage, umbilicus, cord
gastric - *see* Hemorrhage, stomach
gastroenteric K92.2
  newborn P54.3
gastrointestinal (tract) K92.2
  newborn P54.3
genital organ, male N50.1
genitourinary (tract) NOS R31.9
gingiva K06.8
globe (eye) - *see* Hemophthalmos
graafian follicle cyst (ruptured) N83.0-
gum K06.8
heart I51.89
hypopharyngeal (throat) R04.1
intermenstrual (regular) N92.3
  irregular N92.1
internal (organs) NEC R58
  capsule I61.0
  ear - *see* subcategory H83.8
  newborn P54.8
intestine K92.2
  newborn P54.3
intra-abdominal R58
intra-alveolar (lung), newborn P26.8
intracerebral (nontraumatic) - *see* Hemorrhage,
intracranial, intracerebral
intracranial (nontraumatic) I62.9
  birth injury P10.9
  epidural, nontraumatic I62.1
  extradural, nontraumatic I62.1
  newborn P52.9
    specified NEC P52.8
  intracerebral (nontraumatic) (in) I61.9
    brain stem I61.3
    cerebellum I61.4
    newborn P52.4
      birth injury P10.1
    hemisphere I61.2
      cortical (superficial) I61.1
      subcortical (deep) I61.0
    intraoperative
      during a nervous system procedure
        G97.31
      during other procedure G97.32
    intraventricular I61.5
    multiple localized I61.6
    postprocedural
      following a nervous system procedure
        G97.51
      following other procedure G97.52
    specified NEC I61.8
    superficial I61.1
    traumatic (diffuse) - *see* Injury, intracranial,
    diffuse
      focal - *see* Injury, intracranial, focal
  subarachnoid (nontraumatic) (from) I60.9
    newborn P52.5
      birth injury P10.3
    intracranial (cerebral) artery I60.7
      anterior communicating I60.2
      basilar I60.4
      carotid siphon and bifurcation I60.0-
      communicating I60.7

Hemorrhage, hemorrhagic - *continued*
      anterior I60.2
        posterior I60.3-
      middle cerebral I60.1-
      posterior communicating I60.3-
      specified artery NEC I60.6
      vertebral I60.5-
    specified NEC I60.8
    traumatic S06.6X-
  subdural (nontraumatic) I62.00
    acute I62.01
    birth injury P10.0
    chronic I62.03
    newborn (anoxic) (hypoxic) P52.8
      birth injury P10.0
    spinal G95.19
    subacute I62.02
    traumatic - *see* Injury, intracranial, subdural
hemorrhage
  traumatic - *see* Injury, intracranial, focal
brain injury
intramedullary NEC G95.19
intraocular - *see* Hemophthalmos
intraoperative, intraprocedural - *see*
  Complication, hemorrhage (hematoma),
  intraoperative (intraprocedural), by site
intrapartum - *see* Hemorrhage, complicating,
delivery
intrapelvic
  female N94.89
  male K66.1
intraperitoneal K66.1
intrapontine I61.3
intraprocedural - *see* Complication,
hemorrhage (hematoma), intraoperative
(intraprocedural), by site
intrauterine N85.7
  complicating delivery - *see also* Hemorrhage,
    complicating, delivery O67.9
  postpartum - *see* Hemorrhage, postpartum
intraventricular I61.5
  newborn (nontraumatic) - *see also* Newborn,
    affected by, hemorrhage P52.3
    due to birth injury P10.2
    grade
      1 P52.0
      2 P52.1
      3 P52.21
      4 P52.22
intravesical N32.89
iris (postinfectional) (postinflammatory)
  (toxic) - *see* Hyphema
joint (nontraumatic) - *see* Hemarthrosis
kidney N28.89
knee (joint) (nontraumatic) - *see* Hemarthrosis,
  knee
labyrinth - *see* subcategory H83.8
lenticular striate artery I61.0
ligature, vessel - *see* Hemorrhage,
  postoperative
liver K76.89
lung R04.89
  newborn P26.9
    massive P26.1
    specified NEC P26.8
  tuberculous - *see* Tuberculosis, pulmonary
massive umbilical, newborn P51.0
mediastinum - *see* Hemorrhage, lung
medulla I61.3
membrane (brain) I60.8
  spinal cord - *see* Hemorrhage, spinal cord
meninges, meningeal (brain) (middle) I60.8
  spinal cord - *see* Hemorrhage, spinal cord
mesentery K66.1

Hemorrhage, hemorrhagic - *continued*
metritis - *see* Endometritis
mouth K13.79
mucous membrane NEC R58
  newborn P54.8
muscle M62.89
nail (subungual) L60.8
nasal turbinate R04.0
  newborn P54.8
navel, newborn P51.9
newborn P54.9
  specified NEC P54.8
nipple N64.59
nose R04.0
  newborn P54.8
omentum K66.1
optic nerve (sheath) H47.02-
orbit, orbital H05.23-
ovary NEC N83.8
oviduct N83.6
pancreas K86.89
parathyroid (gland) (spontaneous) E21.4
parturition - *see* Hemorrhage, complicating,
  delivery   penis N48.89
pericardium, pericarditis I31.2
peritoneum, peritoneal K66.1
peritonsillar tissue J35.8
  due to infection J36
petechial R23.3
  due to autosensitivity, erythrocyte D69.2
pituitary (gland) E23.6
pleura - *see* Hemorrhage, lung
polioencephalitis, superior E51.2
polymyositis - *see* Polymyositis
pons, pontine I61.3
posterior fossa (nontraumatic) I61.8
  newborn P52.6
postmenopausal N95.0
postnasal R04.0
postoperative - *see* Complications,
  postprocedural, hemorrhage, by site
postpartum NEC (following delivery of
  placenta) O72.1
  delayed or secondary O72.2
  retained placenta O72.0
  third stage O72.0
pregnancy - *see* Hemorrhage, antepartum
preretinal - *see* Hemorrhage, retina
prostate N42.1
puerperal - *see* Hemorrhage, postpartum
  delayed or secondary O72.2
pulmonary R04.89
  newborn P26.9
    massive P26.1
    specified NEC P26.8
  tuberculous - *see* Tuberculosis, pulmonary
purpura (primary) D69.3
rectum (sphincter) K62.5
  newborn P54.2
recurring, following initial hemorrhage at time
  of injury T79.2
renal N28.89
respiratory passage or tract R04.9
  specified NEC R04.89
retina, retinal (vessels) H35.6-
  diabetic - *see* Diabetes, retinal, hemorrhage
retroperitoneal R58
scalp R58
scrotum N50.1
secondary (nontraumatic) R58
  following initial hemorrhage at time of injury
  T79.2
seminal vesicle N50.1
skin R23.3

Hemorrhage, hemorrhagic - *continued*
newborn P54.5
slipped umbilical ligature P51.8
spermatic cord N50.1
spinal (cord) G95.19
  newborn (birth injury) P11.5
spleen D73.5
  intraoperative - *see* Complications,
    intraoperative, hemorrhage, spleen
  postprocedural - *see* Complications,
    postprocedural, hemorrhage, spleen
stomach K92.2
  newborn P54.3
  ulcer - *see* Ulcer, stomach, with hemorrhage
subarachnoid (nontraumatic) - *see*
  Hemorrhage, intracranial, subarachnoid
subconjunctival - *see also* Hemorrhage,
conjunctiva
  birth injury P15.3
subcortical (brain) I61.0
subcutaneous R23.3
subdiaphragmatic R58
subdural (acute) (nontraumatic) - *see*
  Hemorrhage, intracranial, subdural
subependymal
  newborn P52.0
    with intraventricular extension P52.1
      and intracerebral extension P52.22
subgaleal P12.2
subhyaloid - *see* Hemorrhage, retina
subperiosteal - *see* Disorder, bone, specified
  type NEC
subretinal - *see* Hemorrhage, retina
subtentorial - *see* Hemorrhage, intracranial,
  subdural
subungual L60.8
suprarenal (capsule) (gland) E27.49
  newborn P54.4
tentorium (traumatic) NEC - *see* Hemorrhage,
  brain
  newborn (birth injury) P10.4
testis N50.1
third stage (postpartum) O72.0
thorax - *see* Hemorrhage, lung
throat R04.1
thymus (gland) E32.8
thyroid (cyst) (gland) E07.89
tongue K14.8
tonsil J35.8
trachea - *see* Hemorrhage, lung
tracheobronchial R04.89
  newborn P26.0
traumatic
code to specific injury
  cerebellar - *see* Hemorrhage, brain
  intracranial - *see* Hemorrhage, brain
  recurring or secondary (following initial
    hemorrhage at time of injury) T79.2
  tuberculous NEC - *see also* Tuberculosis,
    pulmonary A15.0
tunica vaginalis N50.1
ulcer
code by site under Ulcer, with hemorrhage
  K27.4
umbilicus, umbilical
  cord
    after birth, newborn P51.9
    complicating delivery O69.5
  newborn P51.9
    massive P51.0
    slipped ligature P51.8
  stump P51.9
urethra (idiopathic) N36.8
uterus, uterine (abnormal) N93.9

Hemorrhage, hemorrhagic - *continued*
climacteric N92.4
complicating delivery - *see* Hemorrhage,
complicating, delivery
dysfunctional or functional N93.8
intermenstrual (regular) N92.3
  irregular N92.1
postmenopausal N95.0
postpartum - *see* Hemorrhage, postpartum
preclimacteric or premenopausal N92.4
prepubertal N93.8
pubertal N92.2
vagina (abnormal) N93.9
  newborn P54.6
vas deferens N50.1
vasa previa O69.4
ventricular I61.5
vesical N32.89
viscera NEC R58
  newborn P54.8
vitreous (humor) (intraocular) H43.1-
vulva N90.89
**Hemorrhoids (bleeding) (without mention of
degree) K64.9**
1st degree (grade/stage I) (without prolapse
  outside of anal canal) K64.0
2nd degree (grade/stage II) (that prolapse with
  straining but retract spontaneously) K64.1
3rd degree (grade/stage III) (that prolapse with
  straining and require manual replacement
  back inside anal canal) K64.2
4th degree (grade/stage IV) (with prolapsed
  tissue that cannot be manually replaced)
  K64.3
complicating
  pregnancy O22.4
  puerperium O87.2
external K64.4
  with
    thrombosis K64.5
internal (without mention of degree) K64.8
prolapsed K64.8
skin tags
  anus K64.4
  residual K64.4
specified NEC K64.8
strangulated - *see also* Hemorrhoids, by degree
  K64.8
thrombosed - *see also* Hemorrhoids, by degree
  K64.5
ulcerated - *see also* Hemorrhoids, by degree
  K64.8
Hemosalpinx N83.6
with
  hematocolpos N89.7
  hematometra N85.7
    with hematocolpos N89.7
Hemosiderosis (dietary) E83.19
pulmonary, idiopathic E83.1 *[J84.03]*
transfusion T80.89
Hemothorax (bacterial) (nontuberculous)
J94.2
newborn P54.8
traumatic S27.1
  with pneumothorax S27.2
tuberculous NEC A15.6
**Henoch (-Schönlein) disease or syndrome
(purpura) D69.0**
Henpue, henpuye A66.6
Hepar lobatum (syphilitic) A52.74
Hepatalgia K76.89
Hepatitis K75.9
acute B17.9
  with coma K72.01

Hepatitis - *continued*
 with hepatic failure - *see* Failure, hepatic
 alcoholic - *see* Hepatitis, alcoholic
 infectious B17.9
 non-viral K72.0
 viral B17.9
 alcoholic (acute) (chronic) K70.10
 with ascites K70.11
 amebic - *see* Abscess, liver, amebic
 anicteric, (viral) - *see* Hepatitis, viral
 antigen-associated (HAA) - *see* Hepatitis, B
 Australia-antigen (positive) - *see* Hepatitis, B
 autoimmune K75.4
 B B19.10
 with hepatic coma B19.11
 acute B16.9
 with
 delta-agent (coinfection) (without hepatic coma) B16.1
 with hepatic coma B16.0
 hepatic coma (without delta-agent coinfection) B16.2
 chronic B18.1
 with delta-agent B18.0
 bacterial NEC K75.89
 C (viral) B19.20
 with hepatic coma B19.21
 acute B17.10
 with hepatic coma B17.11
 chronic B18.2
 catarrhal (acute) B15.9
 with hepatic coma B15.0
 cholangiolitic K75.89
 cholestatic K75.89
 chronic K73.9
 active NEC K73.2
 lobular NEC K73.1
 persistent NEC K73.0
 specified NEC K73.8
 cytomegaloviral B25.1
 due to ethanol (acute) (chronic) - *see* Hepatitis, alcoholic
 epidemic B15.9
 with hepatic coma B15.0
 fulminant NEC (viral) - *see* Hepatitis, viral
 neonatal giant cell P59.29
 granulomatous NEC K75.3
 herpesviral B00.81
 history of
 B Z86.19
 C Z86.19
 homologous serum - *see* Hepatitis, viral, type B
 in (due to)
 mumps B26.81
 toxoplasmosis (acquired) B58.1
 congenital (active) P37.1 [K77]
 infectious, infective B15.9
 acute (subacute) B17.9
 chronic B18.9
 inoculation - *see* Hepatitis, viral, type B
 interstitial (chronic) K74.69
 lupoid NEC K75.4
 malignant NEC (with hepatic failure) K72.90
 with coma K72.91
 neonatal (idiopathic) (toxic) P59.29
 newborn P59.29
 postimmunization - *see* Hepatitis, viral, type B
 post-transfusion - *see* Hepatitis, viral, type B
 reactive, nonspecific K75.2
 serum - *see* Hepatitis, viral, type B
 specified type NEC
 with hepatic failure - *see* Failure, hepatic
 syphilitic (late) A52.74

Hepatitis - *continued*
 congenital (early) A50.08 [K77]
 late A50.59 [K77]
 secondary A51.45
 toxic - *see also* Disease, liver, toxic K71.6
 tuberculous A18.83
 viral, virus B19.9
 with hepatic coma B19.0
 acute B17.9
 chronic B18.9
 specified NEC B18.8
 type
 B B18.1
 with delta-agent B18.0
 C B18.2
 congenital P35.3
 coxsackie B33.8 [K77]
 cytomegalic inclusion B25.1
 in remission, any type   code to Hepatitis, chronic, by type
 non-a, non-b B17.8
 specified type NEC (with or without coma) B17.8
 type
 A B15.9
 with hepatic coma B15.0
 B B19.10
 with hepatic coma B19.11
 acute B16.9
 with
 delta-agent (coinfection) (without hepatic coma) B16.1
 with hepatic coma B16.0
 hepatic coma (without delta-agent coinfection) B16.2
 chronic B18.1
 with delta-agent B18.0
 C B19.20
 with hepatic coma B19.21
 acute B17.10
 with hepatic coma B17.11
 chronic B18.2
 E B17.2
 non-a, non-b B17.8
Hepatization lung (acute) - *see* Pneumonia, lobar
Hepatoblastoma C22.2
Hepatocarcinoma C22.0
Hepatocholangiocarcinoma C22.0
Hepatocholangioma, benign D13.4
Hepatocholangitis K75.89
Hepatolenticular degeneration E83.01
Hepatoma (malignant) C22.0
 benign D13.4
 embryonal C22.0
Hepatomegaly - *see also* Hypertrophy, liver
 with splenomegaly R16.2
 congenital Q44.7
 in mononucleosis
 gammaherpesviral B27.09
 infectious specified NEC B27.89
Hepatoptosis K76.89
Hepatorenal syndrome following labor and delivery O90.4
Hepatosis K76.89
Hepatosplenomegaly R16.2
 hyperlipemic (Bürger-Grütz type) E78.3 [K77]
Hereditary - *see* condition
Heredodegeneration, macular - *see* Dystrophy, retina
Heredopathia atactica polyneuritiformis G60.1
Heredosyphilis - *see* Syphilis, congenital
Herlitz' syndrome Q81.1

Hermansky-Pudlak syndrome E70.331
Hermaphrodite, hermaphroditism (true) Q56.0
 46,XX with streak gonads Q99.1
 46,XX/46,XY Q99.0
 46,XY with streak gonads Q99.1
 chimera 46,XX/46,XY Q99.0
Hernia, hernial (acquired) (recurrent) K46.9
 with
 gangrene - *see* Hernia, by site, with, gangrene
 incarceration - *see* Hernia, by site, with, obstruction
 irreducible - *see* Hernia, by site, with, obstruction
 obstruction - *see* Hernia, by site, with, obstruction
 strangulation - *see* Hernia, by site, with, obstruction
 abdomen, abdominal K46.9
 with
 gangrene (and obstruction) K46.1
 obstruction K46.0
 femoral - *see* Hernia, femoral
 incisional - *see* Hernia, incisional
 inguinal - *see* Hernia, inguinal
 specified site NEC K45.8
 with
 gangrene (and obstruction) K45.1
 obstruction K45.0
 umbilical - *see* Hernia, umbilical
 wall - *see* Hernia, ventral
 appendix - *see* Hernia, abdomen
 bladder (mucosa) (sphincter)
 congenital (female) (male) Q79.51
 female - *see* Cystocele
 male N32.89
 brain, congenital - *see* Encephalocele
 cartilage, vertebra - *see* Displacement, intervertebral disc   cerebral, congenital - *see also* Encephalocele
 endaural Q01.8
 ciliary body (traumatic) S05.2-
 colon - *see* Hernia, abdomen
 Cooper's - *see* Hernia, abdomen, specified site NEC
 crural - *see* Hernia, femoral
 diaphragm, diaphragmatic K44.9
 with
 gangrene (and obstruction) K44.1
 obstruction K44.0
 congenital Q79.0
 direct (inguinal) - *see* Hernia, inguinal
 diverticulum, intestine - *see* Hernia, abdomen
 double (inguinal) - *see* Hernia, inguinal, bilateral
 due to adhesions (with obstruction) K56.50
 epigastric - *see also* Hernia, ventral K43.9
 esophageal hiatus - *see* Hernia, hiatal
 external (inguinal) - *see* Hernia, inguinal
 fallopian tube N83.4-
 fascia M62.89
 femoral K41.90
 with
 gangrene (and obstruction) K41.40
 not specified as recurrent K41.40
 recurrent K41.41
 obstruction K41.30
 not specified as recurrent K41.30
 recurrent K41.31
 bilateral K41.20
 with
 gangrene (and obstruction) K41.10
 not specified as recurrent K41.10
 recurrent K41.11

Hernia, hernial - *continued*
obstruction K41.00
not specified as recurrent K41.00
recurrent K41.01
not specified as recurrent K41.20
recurrent K41.21
unilateral K41.90
with
gangrene (and obstruction) K41.40
not specified as recurrent K41.40
recurrent K41.41
obstruction K41.30
not specified as recurrent K41.30
recurrent K41.31
not specified as recurrent K41.90
recurrent K41.91
not specified as recurrent K41.90
recurrent K41.91
foramen magnum G93.5
congenital Q01.8
funicular (umbilical) - *see also* Hernia, umbilicus
spermatic (cord) - *see* Hernia, inguinal
gastrointestinal tract - *see* Hernia, abdomen
Hesselbach's - *see* Hernia, femoral, specified site NEC
hiatal (esophageal) (sliding) K44.9
with
gangrene (and obstruction) K44.1
obstruction K44.0
congenital Q40.1
hypogastric - *see* Hernia, ventral
incarcerated - *see also* Hernia, by site, with obstruction
with gangrene - *see* Hernia, by site, with gangrene
incisional K43.2
with
gangrene (and obstruction) K43.1
obstruction K43.0
indirect (inguinal) - *see* Hernia, inguinal
inguinal (direct) (external) (funicular) (indirect) (internal) (oblique) (scrotal) (sliding) K40.90
with
gangrene (and obstruction) K40.40
not specified as recurrent K40.40
recurrent K40.41
obstruction K40.30
not specified as recurrent K40.30
recurrent K40.31
not specified as recurrent K40.90
recurrent K40.91
bilateral K40.20
with
gangrene (and obstruction) K40.10
not specified as recurrent K40.10
recurrent K40.11
obstruction K40.00
not specified as recurrent K40.00
recurrent K40.01
not specified as recurrent K40.20
recurrent K40.21
unilateral K40.90
with
gangrene (and obstruction) K40.40
not specified as recurrent K40.40
recurrent K40.41
obstruction K40.30
not specified as recurrent K40.30
recurrent K40.31
not specified as recurrent K40.90
recurrent K40.91
internal - *see also* Hernia, abdomen

Hernia, hernial - *continued*
inguinal - *see* Hernia, inguinal
interstitial - *see* Hernia, abdomen
intervertebral cartilage or disc - *see* Displacement, intervertebral disc intestine, intestinal - *see* Hernia, by site
intra-abdominal - *see* Hernia, abdomen
iris (traumatic) S05.2-
irreducible - *see also* Hernia, by site, with obstruction
with gangrene - *see* Hernia, by site, with gangrene
ischiatic - *see* Hernia, abdomen, specified site NEC
ischiorectal - *see* Hernia, abdomen, specified site NEC
lens (traumatic) S05.2-
linea (alba) (semilunaris) - *see* Hernia, ventral
Littre's - *see* Hernia, abdomen
lumbar - *see* Hernia, abdomen, specified site NEC
lung (subcutaneous) J98.4
mediastinum J98.59
mesenteric (internal) - *see* Hernia, abdomen
midline - *see* Hernia, ventral
muscle (sheath) M62.89
nucleus pulposus - *see* Displacement, intervertebral disc oblique (inguinal) - *see* Hernia, inguinal
obstructive - *see also* Hernia, by site, with obstruction
with gangrene - *see* Hernia, by site, with gangrene
obturator - *see* Hernia, abdomen, specified site NEC
omental - *see* Hernia, abdomen
ovary N83.4-
oviduct N83.4-
paraesophageal - *see also* Hernia, diaphragm
congenital Q40.1
parastomal K43.5
with
gangrene (and obstruction) K43.4
obstruction K43.3
paraumbilical - *see* Hernia, umbilicus
perineal - *see* Hernia, abdomen, specified site NEC
Petit's - *see* Hernia, abdomen, specified site NEC
postoperative - *see* Hernia, incisional
pregnant uterus - *see* Abnormal, uterus in pregnancy or childbirth
prevesical N32.89
properitoneal - *see* Hernia, abdomen, specified site NEC
pudendal - *see* Hernia, abdomen, specified site NEC
rectovaginal N81.6
retroperitoneal - *see* Hernia, abdomen, specified site NEC
Richter's - *see* Hernia, abdomen, with obstruction
Rieux's, Riex's - *see* Hernia, abdomen, specified site NEC
sac condition (adhesion) (dropsy) (inflammation) (laceration) (suppuration) code by site under Hernia
sciatic - *see* Hernia, abdomen, specified site NEC
scrotum, scrotal - *see* Hernia, inguinal
sliding (inguinal) - *see also* Hernia, inguinal
hiatus - *see* Hernia, hiatal
spigelian - *see* Hernia, ventral
spinal - *see* Spina bifida

Hernia, hernial - *continued*
strangulated - *see also* Hernia, by site, with obstruction
with gangrene - *see* Hernia, by site, with gangrene
subxiphoid - *see* Hernia, ventral
supra-umbilicus - *see* Hernia, ventral
tendon - *see* Disorder, tendon, specified type NEC
Treitz's (fossa) - *see* Hernia, abdomen, specified site NEC
tunica vaginalis Q55.29
umbilicus, umbilical K42.9
with
gangrene (and obstruction) K42.1
obstruction K42.0
ureter N28.89
urethra, congenital Q64.79
urinary meatus, congenital Q64.79
uterus N81.4
pregnant - *see* Abnormal, uterus in pregnancy or childbirth
vaginal (anterior) (wall) - *see* Cystocele
Velpeau's - *see* Hernia, femoral
ventral K43.9
with
gangrene (and obstruction) K43.7
obstruction K43.6
recurrent - *see* Hernia, incisional
incisional K43.2
with
gangrene (and obstruction) K43.1
obstruction K43.0
specified NEC K43.9
with
gangrene (and obstruction) K43.7
obstruction K43.6
vesical
congenital (female) (male) Q79.51
female - *see* Cystocele
male N32.89
vitreous (into wound) S05.2-
into anterior chamber - *see* Prolapse, vitreous
Herniation - *see also* Hernia
brain (stem) G93.5
cerebral G93.5
mediastinum J98.59
nucleus pulposus - *see* Displacement, intervertebral disc
Herpangina B08.5
Herpes, herpesvirus, herpetic B00.9
anogenital A60.9
perianal skin A60.1
rectum A60.1
urogenital tract A60.00
cervix A60.03
male genital organ NEC A60.02
penis A60.01
specified site NEC A60.09
vagina A60.04
vulva A60.04
blepharitis (zoster) B02.39
simplex B00.59
circinatus B35.4
bullosus L12.0
conjunctivitis (simplex) B00.53
zoster B02.31
cornea B02.33
encephalitis B00.4
due to herpesvirus 6 B10.01
due to herpesvirus 7 B10.09
specified NEC B10.09
eye (zoster) B02.30
simplex B00.50

Herpes, herpesvirus, herpetic - *continued*
  eyelid (zoster) B02.39
    simplex B00.59
  facialis B00.1
  febrilis B00.1
  geniculate ganglionitis B02.21
  genital, genitalis A60.00
    female A60.09
    male A60.02
  gestational, gestationis O26.4-
  gingivostomatitis B00.2
  human B00.9
    1 - *see* Herpes, simplex
    2 - *see* Herpes, simplex
    3 - *see* Varicella
    4 - *see* Mononucleosis, Epstein-Barr (virus)
    5 - *see* Disease, cytomegalic inclusion
      (generalized)
    6
      encephalitis B10.01
      specified NEC B10.81
    7
      encephalitis B10.09
      specified NEC B10.82
    8 B10.89
  infection NEC B10.89
    Kaposi's sarcoma associated B10.89
  iridocyclitis (simplex) B00.51
    zoster B02.32
  iris (vesicular erythema multiforme) L51.9
  iritis (simplex) B00.51
  Kaposi's sarcoma associated B10.89
  keratitis (simplex) (dendritic) (disciform)
    (interstitial) B00.52
    zoster (interstitial) B02.33
  keratoconjunctivitis (simplex) B00.52
    zoster B02.33
  labialis B00.1
  lip B00.1
  meningitis (simplex) B00.3
    zoster B02.1
  ophthalmicus (zoster) NEC B02.30
    simplex B00.50
  penis A60.01
  perianal skin A60.1
  pharyngitis, pharyngotonsillitis B00.2
  rectum A60.1
  scrotum A60.02
  sepsis B00.7
  simplex B00.9
    complicated NEC B00.89
    congenital P35.2
    conjunctivitis B00.53
    external ear B00.1
    eyelid B00.59
    hepatitis B00.81
    keratitis (interstitial) B00.52
    myelitis B00.82
    specified complication NEC B00.89
    visceral B00.89
  stomatitis B00.2
  tonsurans B35.0
  visceral B00.89
  vulva A60.04
  whitlow B00.89
  zoster - *see also* condition B02.9
    auricularis B02.21
    complicated NEC B02.8
    conjunctivitis B02.31
    disseminated B02.7
    encephalitis B02.0
    eye (lid) B02.39
    geniculate ganglionitis B02.21
    keratitis (interstitial) B02.33

Herpes, herpesvirus, herpetic - *continued*
  meningitis B02.1
  myelitis B02.24
  neuritis, neuralgia B02.29
  ophthalmicus NEC B02.30
  oticus B02.21
  polyneuropathy B02.23
  specified complication NEC B02.8
  trigeminal neuralgia B02.22
Herpesvirus (human) - *see* Herpes
Herpetophobia F40.218
Herrick's anemia - *see* Disease, sickle-cell
Hers' disease E74.09
Herter-gee syndrome K90.0
Herxheimer's reaction R68.89
Hesitancy
  of micturition R39.11
  urinary R39.11
Hesselbach's hernia - *see* Hernia, femoral,
  specified site NEC
Heterochromia (congenital) Q13.2
  cataract - *see* Cataract, complicated
  cyclitis (Fuchs) - *see* Cyclitis, Fuchs'
    heterochromic
  hair L67.1
  iritis - *see* Cyclitis, Fuchs' heterochromic
  retained metallic foreign body (nonmagnetic) -
    see Foreign body, intraocular, old, retained
      magnetic - *see* Foreign body, intraocular, old,
      retained, magnetic
  uveitis - *see* Cyclitis, Fuchs' heterochromic
Heterophoria - *see* Strabismus, heterophoria
Heterophyes, heterophyiasis (small intestine)
  B66.8
Heterotopia, heterotopic - *see also*
  Malposition, congenital
  cerebralis Q04.8
Heterotropia - *see* Strabismus
Heubner-Herter disease K90.0
Hexadactylism Q69.9
HGSIL (cytology finding) (high grade
  squamous intraepithelial lesion on cytologic
  smear) (Pap smear finding)
  anus R85.613
  cervix R87.613
    biopsy (histology) finding - *see* Neoplasia,
    intraepithelial, cervix, grade II or grade III
  vagina R87.623
    biopsy (histology) finding - *see* Neoplasia,
    intraepithelial, vagina, grade II or grade III
Hibernoma - *see* Lipoma
Hiccup, hiccough R06.6
  epidemic B33.0
  psychogenic F45.8
Hidden penis (congenital) Q55.64
  acquired N48.83
Hidradenitis (axillaris) (suppurative) L73.2
Hidradenoma (nodular) - *see also* Neoplasm,
  skin, benign
  clear cell - *see* Neoplasm, skin, benign
  papillary - *see* Neoplasm, skin, benign
Hidrocystoma - *see* Neoplasm, skin, benign
High
  altitude effects T70.20
    anoxia T70.29
    on
      ears T70.0
      sinuses T70.1
    polycythemia D75.1
  arch
    foot Q66.7
    palate, congenital Q38.5
  arterial tension - *see* Hypertension
  basal metabolic rate R94.8

High - *continued*
  blood pressure - *see also* Hypertension
    borderline R03.0
    reading (incidental) (isolated) (nonspecific),
  without diagnosis of hypertension R03.0
  cholesterol E78.00
    with high triglycerides E78.2
  diaphragm (congenital) Q79.1
  expressed emotional level within family Z63.8
  head at term O32.4
  palate, congenital Q38.5
  risk
    infant NEC Z76.2
    sexual behavior (heterosexual) Z72.51
      bisexual Z72.53
      homosexual Z72.52
  scrotal testis, testes
    bilateral Q53.23
    unilateral Q53.13
  temperature (of unknown origin) R50.9
  thoracic rib Q76.6
  triglycerides E78.1
    with high cholesterol E78.2
Hildebrand's disease A75.0
Hilum - *see* condition
Hip - *see* condition
Hippel's disease Q85.8
Hippophobia F40.218
Hippus H57.09
Hirschsprung's disease or megacolon Q43.1
Hirsutism, hirsuties L68.0
Hirudiniasis
  external B88.3
  internal B83.4
Hiss-Russell dysentery A03.1
Histidinemia, histidinuria E70.41
Histiocytoma - *see also* Neoplasm, skin, benign
  fibrous - *see also* Neoplasm, skin, benign
    atypical - *see* Neoplasm, connective tissue,
  uncertain behavior
    malignant - *see* Neoplasm, connective tissue,
  malignant
Histiocytosis D76.3
  acute differentiated progressive C96.0
  Langerhans' cell NEC C96.6
    multifocal X
      multisystemic (disseminated) C96.0
      unisystemic C96.5
    pulmonary, adult (adult PLCH) J84.82
    unifocal (X) C96.6
  lipid, lipoid D76.3
    essential E75.29
  malignant C96.A
  mononuclear phagocytes NEC D76.1
    Langerhans' cells C96.6
  non-Langerhans cell D76.3
  polyostotic sclerosing D76.3
  sinus, with massive lymphadenopathy D76.3
  syndrome NEC D76.3
  X NEC C96.6
    acute (progressive) C96.0
    chronic C96.6
    multifocal C96.5
    multisystemic C96.0
    unifocal C96.6
Histoplasmosis B39.9
  with pneumonia NEC B39.2
  African B39.5
  American - *see* Histoplasmosis, capsulati
  capsulati B39.4
    disseminated B39.3
    generalized B39.3
    pulmonary B39.2
      acute B39.0

Histoplasmosis - *continued*
    chronic B39.1
    Darling's B39.4
    duboisii B39.5
    lung NEC B39.2

History
    family (of) - *see also* History, personal (of)
      alcohol abuse Z81.1
      allergy NEC Z84.89
      anemia Z83.2
      arthritis Z82.61
      asthma Z82.5
      blindness Z82.1
      cardiac death (sudden) Z82.41
      carrier of genetic disease Z84.81
      chromosomal anomaly Z82.79
      chronic
        disabling disease NEC Z82.8
        lower respiratory disease Z82.5
      colonic polyps Z83.71
      congenital malformations and deformations Z82.79
        polycystic kidney Z82.71
      consanguinity Z84.3
      deafness Z82.2
      diabetes mellitus Z83.3
      disability NEC Z82.8
      disease or disorder (of)
        allergic NEC Z84.89
        behavioral NEC Z81.8
        blood and blood-forming organs Z83.2
        cardiovascular NEC Z82.49
        chronic disabling NEC Z82.8
        digestive Z83.79
        ear NEC Z83.52
        endocrine NEC Z83.49
        eye NEC Z83.518
          glaucoma Z83.511
        familial hypercholesterolemia Z83.42
        genitourinary NEC Z84.2
        glaucoma Z83.511
        hematological Z83.2
        immune mechanism Z83.2
        infectious NEC Z83.1
        ischemic heart Z82.49
        kidney Z84.1
        mental NEC Z81.8
        metabolic Z83.49
        musculoskeletal NEC Z82.69
        neurological NEC Z82.0
        nutritional Z83.49
        parasitic NEC Z83.1
        psychiatric NEC Z81.8
        respiratory NEC Z83.6
        skin and subcutaneous tissue NEC Z84.0
        specified NEC Z84.89
      drug abuse NEC Z81.3
      epilepsy Z82.0
      familial hypercholesterolemia Z83.42
      genetic disease carrier Z84.81
      glaucoma Z83.511
      hearing loss Z82.2
      human immunodeficiency virus (HIV) infection Z83.0
      Huntington's chorea Z82.0
      intellectual disability Z81.0
      leukemia Z80.6
      malignant neoplasm (of) NOS Z80.9
        bladder Z80.52
        breast Z80.3
        bronchus Z80.1
        digestive organ Z80.0
        gastrointestinal tract Z80.0
        genital organ Z80.49

History - *continued*
        ovary Z80.41
        prostate Z80.42
        specified organ NEC Z80.49
        testis Z80.43
        hematopoietic NEC Z80.7
        intrathoracic organ NEC Z80.2
        kidney Z80.51
        lung Z80.1
        lymphatic NEC Z80.7
        ovary Z80.41
        prostate Z80.42
        respiratory organ NEC Z80.2
        specified site NEC Z80.8
        testis Z80.43
        trachea Z80.1
        urinary organ or tract Z80.59
          bladder Z80.52
          kidney Z80.51
      mental
        disorder NEC Z81.8
      multiple endocrine neoplasia (MEN) syndrome Z83.41
      osteoporosis Z82.62
      polycystic kidney Z82.71
      polyps (colon) Z83.71
      psychiatric disorder Z81.8
      psychoactive substance abuse NEC Z81.3
      respiratory condition NEC Z83.6
        asthma and other lower respiratory conditions Z82.5
      self-harmful behavior Z81.8
      SIDS (sudden infant death syndrome) Z84.82
      skin condition Z84.0
      specified condition NEC Z84.89
      stroke (cerebrovascular) Z82.3
      substance abuse NEC Z81.4
        alcohol Z81.1
        drug NEC Z81.3
        psychoactive NEC Z81.3
        tobacco Z81.2
      sudden
        cardiac death Z82.41
        infant death syndrome (SIDS) Z84.82
      tobacco abuse Z81.2
      violence, violent behavior Z81.8
      visual loss Z82.1
    personal (of) - *see also* History, family (of)
      abuse
        childhood Z62.819
          physical Z62.810
          psychological Z62.811
          sexual Z62.810
        adult Z91.419
          physical and sexual Z91.410
          psychological Z91.411
      alcohol dependence F10.21
      allergy (to) Z88.9
        analgesic agent NEC Z88.6
        anesthetic Z88.4
        antibiotic agent NEC Z88.1
        anti-infective agent NEC Z88.3
        contrast media Z91.041
        drugs, medicaments and biological substances Z88.9
          specified NEC Z88.8
        food Z91.018
          additives Z91.02
          eggs Z91.012
          milk products Z91.011
          peanuts Z91.010
          seafood Z91.013
          specified food NEC Z91.018
        insect Z91.038

History - *continued*
        bee Z91.030
        latex Z91.040
        medicinal agents Z88.9
          specified NEC Z88.8
        narcotic agent NEC Z88.5
        nonmedicinal agents Z91.048
        penicillin Z88.0
        serum Z88.7
        specified NEC Z91.09
        sulfonamides Z88.2
        vaccine Z88.7
      anaphylactic shock Z87.892
      anaphylaxis Z87.892
      behavioral disorders Z86.59
      benign carcinoid tumor Z86.012
      benign neoplasm Z86.018
        carcinoid Z86.012
        brain Z86.011
        colonic polyps Z86.010
      brain injury (traumatic) Z87.820
      breast implant removal Z98.86
      calculi, renal Z87.442
      cancer - *see* History, personal (of), malignant neoplasm (of)
      cardiac arrest (death), successfully resuscitated Z86.74
      cerebral infarction without residual deficit Z86.73
      cervical dysplasia Z87.410
      chemotherapy for neoplastic condition Z92.21
      childhood abuse - *see* History, personal (of), abuse
      cleft lip (corrected) Z87.730
      cleft palate (corrected) Z87.730
      collapsed vertebra (healed) Z87.311
        due to osteoporosis Z87.310
      combat and operational stress reaction Z86.51
      congenital malformation (corrected) Z87.798
        circulatory system (corrected) Z87.74
        digestive system (corrected) NEC Z87.738
        ear (corrected) Z87.721
        eye (corrected) Z87.720
        face and neck (corrected) Z87.790
        genitourinary system (corrected) NEC Z87.718
        heart (corrected) Z87.74
        integument (corrected) Z87.76
        limb(s) (corrected) Z87.76
        musculoskeletal system (corrected) Z87.76
        neck (corrected) Z87.790
        nervous system (corrected) NEC Z87.728
        respiratory system (corrected) Z87.75
        sense organs (corrected) NEC Z87.728
        specified NEC Z87.798
      contraception Z92.0
      deployment (military) Z91.82
      diabetic foot ulcer Z86.31
      disease or disorder (of) Z87.898
        blood and blood-forming organs Z86.2
        circulatory system Z86.79
          specified condition NEC Z86.79
        connective tissue NEC Z87.39
        digestive system Z87.19
          colonic polyp Z86.010
          peptic ulcer disease Z87.11
          specified condition NEC Z87.19
        ear Z86.69
        endocrine Z86.39
          diabetic foot ulcer Z86.31
          gestational diabetes Z86.32
          specified type NEC Z86.39

History - *continued*
- eye Z86.69
- genital (track) system NEC
  - female Z87.42
  - male Z87.438
- hematological Z86.2
- Hodgkin Z85.71
- immune mechanism Z86.2
- infectious Z86.19
  - malaria Z86.13
  - Methicillin resistant Staphylococcus aureus (MRSA) Z86.14
  - poliomyelitis Z86.12
  - specified NEC Z86.19
  - tuberculosis Z86.11
- mental NEC Z86.59
- metabolic Z86.39
  - diabetic foot ulcer Z86.31
  - gestational diabetes Z86.32
  - specified type NEC Z86.39
- musculoskeletal NEC Z87.39
- nervous system Z86.69
- nutritional Z86.39
- parasitic Z86.19
- respiratory system NEC Z87.09
- sense organs Z86.69
- skin Z87.2
- specified site or type NEC Z87.898
- subcutaneous tissue Z87.2
- trophoblastic Z87.59
- urinary system NEC Z87.448
- drug dependence - *see* Dependence, drug, by type, in remission
- drug therapy
  - antineoplastic chemotherapy Z92.21
  - estrogen Z92.23
  - immunosuppression Z92.25
  - inhaled steroids Z92.240
  - monoclonal drug Z92.22
  - specified NEC Z92.29
  - steroid Z92.241
  - systemic steroids Z92.241
- dysplasia
  - cervical (mild) (moderate) Z87.410
    - severe (grade III) Z86.001
  - prostatic Z87.430
  - vaginal (mild) (moderate) Z87.411
    - severe (grade III) Z86.008
  - vulvar (mild) (moderate) Z87.412
    - severe (grade III) Z86.008
- embolism (venous) Z86.718
  - pulmonary Z86.711
- encephalitis Z86.61
- estrogen therapy Z92.23
- extracorporeal membrane oxygenation (ECMO) Z92.81
- failed moderate sedation Z92.83
- failed conscious sedation Z92.83
- fall, falling Z91.81
- fracture (healed)
  - fatigue Z87.312
  - fragility Z87.310
  - osteoporosis Z87.310
  - pathological NEC Z87.311
  - stress Z87.312
  - traumatic Z87.81
- gestational diabetes Z86.32
- hepatitis
  - B Z86.19
  - C Z86.19
- Hodgkin disease Z85.71
- hyperthermia, malignant Z88.4
- hypospadias (corrected) Z87.710
- hysterectomy Z90.710

History - *continued*
- immunosuppression therapy Z92.25
- in situ neoplasm
  - breast Z86.000
  - cervix uteri Z86.001
  - specified NEC Z86.008
- infection NEC Z86.19
  - central nervous system Z86.61
  - Methicillin resistant Staphylococcus aureus (MRSA) Z86.14
  - urinary (recurrent) (tract) Z87.440
- injury NEC Z87.828
- in utero procedure during pregnancy Z98.870
- in utero procedure while a fetus Z98.871
- irradiation Z92.3
- kidney stones Z87.442
- leukemia Z85.6
- lymphoma (non-Hodgkin) Z85.72
- malignant melanoma (skin) Z85.820
- malignant neoplasm (of) Z85.9
  - accessory sinuses Z85.22
  - anus NEC Z85.048
    - carcinoid Z85.040
  - bladder Z85.51
  - bone Z85.830
  - brain Z85.841
  - breast Z85.3
  - bronchus NEC Z85.118
    - carcinoid Z85.110
  - carcinoid - *see* History, personal (of), malignant neoplasm, by site, carcinoid
  - cervix Z85.41
  - colon NEC Z85.038
    - carcinoid Z85.030
  - digestive organ Z85.00
    - specified NEC Z85.09
  - endocrine gland NEC Z85.858
  - epididymis Z85.48
  - esophagus Z85.01
  - eye Z85.840
  - gastrointestinal tract - *see* History, malignant neoplasm, digestive organ
  - genital organ
    - female Z85.40
      - specified NEC Z85.44
    - male Z85.45
      - specified NEC Z85.49
  - hematopoietic NEC Z85.79
  - intrathoracic organ Z85.20
  - kidney NEC Z85.528
    - carcinoid Z85.520
  - large intestine NEC Z85.038
    - carcinoid Z85.030
  - larynx Z85.21
  - liver Z85.05
  - lung NEC Z85.118
    - carcinoid Z85.110
  - mediastinum Z85.29
  - Merkel cell Z85.821
  - middle ear Z85.22
  - nasal cavities Z85.22
  - nervous system NEC Z85.848
  - oral cavity Z85.819
    - specified site NEC Z85.818
  - ovary Z85.43
  - pancreas Z85.07
  - pharynx Z85.819
    - specified site NEC Z85.818
  - pelvis Z85.53
  - pleura Z85.29
  - prostate Z85.46
  - rectosigmoid junction NEC Z85.048
    - carcinoid Z85.040
  - rectum NEC Z85.048

History - *continued*
  - carcinoid Z85.040
  - respiratory organ Z85.20
  - sinuses, accessory Z85.22
  - skin NEC Z85.828
    - melanoma Z85.820
    - Merkel cell Z85.821
  - small intestine NEC Z85.068
    - carcinoid Z85.060
  - soft tissue Z85.831
  - specified site NEC Z85.89
  - stomach NEC Z85.028
    - carcinoid Z85.020
  - testis Z85.47
  - thymus NEC Z85.238
    - carcinoid Z85.230
  - thyroid Z85.850
  - tongue Z85.810
  - trachea Z85.12
  - ureter Z85.54
  - urinary organ or tract Z85.50
    - specified NEC Z85.59
  - uterus Z85.42
- maltreatment Z91.89
- medical treatment NEC Z92.89
- melanoma (malignant) (skin) Z85.820
- meningitis Z86.61
- mental disorder Z86.59
- Merkel cell carcinoma (skin) Z85.821
- Methicillin resistant Staphylococcus aureus (MRSA) Z86.14
- military deployment Z91.82
- military war, peacekeeping and humanitarian deployment (current or past conflict) Z91.82
- myocardial infarction (old) I25.2
- neglect (in)
  - adult Z91.412
  - childhood Z62.812
- neoplasm
  - benign Z86.018
    - brain Z86.011
    - colon polyp Z86.010
  - in situ
    - breast Z86.000
    - cervix uteri Z86.001
    - specified NEC Z86.008
  - malignant - *see* History of, malignant neoplasm
  - uncertain behavior Z86.03
- nephrotic syndrome Z87.441
- nicotine dependence Z87.891
- noncompliance with medical treatment or regimen - *see* Noncompliance
- nutritional deficiency Z86.39
- obstetric complications Z87.59
  - childbirth Z87.59
  - pregnancy Z87.59
  - pre-term labor Z87.51
  - puerperium Z87.59
- osteoporosis fractures Z87.31
- parasuicide (attempt) Z91.5
- physical trauma NEC Z87.828
  - self-harm or suicide attempt Z91.5
- poisoning NEC Z91.89
  - self-harm or suicide attempt Z91.5
- poor personal hygiene Z91.89
- pneumonia (recurrent) Z87.01
- preterm labor Z87.51
- prolonged reversible ischemic neurologic deficit (PRIND) Z86.73
- procedure during pregnancy Z98.870
- procedure while a fetus Z98.871
- prostatic dysplasia Z87.430

History - *continued*
  psychological
    abuse
      adult Z91.411
      child Z62.811
      trauma, specified NEC Z91.49
  radiation therapy Z92.3
  removal
    implant
      breast Z98.86
  renal calculi Z87.442
  respiratory condition NEC Z87.09
  retained foreign body fully removed Z87.821
  risk factors NEC Z91.89
  self-harm Z91.5
  self-poisoning attempt Z91.5
  sex reassignment Z87.890
  sleep-wake cycle problem Z72.821
  specified NEC Z87.898
  steroid therapy (systemic) Z92.241
    inhaled Z92.240
  stroke without residual deficits Z86.73
  substance abuse NEC F10-f19
  sudden cardiac arrest Z86.74
  sudden cardiac death successfully
    resuscitated Z86.74
  suicide attempt Z91.5
  surgery NEC Z98.890
    with uterine scar Z98.891
    sex reassignment Z87.890
    transplant - *see* Transplant
  thrombophlebitis Z86.72
  thrombosis (venous) Z86.718
    pulmonary Z86.711
  tobacco dependence Z87.891
  transient ischemic attack (TIA) without
  residual deficits Z86.73
  trauma (physical) NEC Z87.828
    psychological NEC Z91.49
    self-harm Z91.5
  traumatic brain injury Z87.820
  unhealthy sleep-wake cycle Z72.821
  unintended awareness under general
    anesthesia Z92.84
  urinary calculi Z87.442
  urinary (recurrent) (tract) infection(s)
    Z87.440
  uterine scar from previous surgery Z98.891
  vaginal dysplasia Z87.411
  venous thrombosis or embolism Z86.718
    pulmonary Z86.711
  vulvar dysplasia Z87.412
His-Werner disease A79.0
HIV - *see also* Human, immunodeficiency virus
  B20
  laboratory evidence (nonconclusive) R75
  positive, seropositive Z21
  nonconclusive test (in infants) R75
Hives (bold) - *see* Urticaria
Hoarseness R49.0
Hobo Z59.0
Hodgkin disease - *see* Lymphoma, Hodgkin
Hodgson's disease I71.2
  ruptured I71.1
Hoffa-Kastert disease E88.89
Hoffa's disease E88.89
Hoffmann-Bouveret syndrome I47.9
Hoffmann's syndrome E03.9 [*G73.7*]
Hole (round)
  macula H35.34-
  retina (without detachment) - *see* Break, retina,
  round hole
    with detachment - *see* Detachment, retina,
    with retinal, break

Holiday relief care Z75.5
Hollenhorst's plaque - *see* Occlusion, artery,
  retina
Hollow foot (congenital) Q66.7
  acquired - *see* Deformity, limb, foot, specified
  NEC
Holoprosencephaly Q04.2
Holt-Oram syndrome Q87.2
Homelessness Z59.0
Homesickness - *see* Disorder, adjustment
Homocystinemia, homocystinuria E72.11
Homogentisate 1,2-dioxygenase deficiency
  E70.29
Homologous serum hepatitis (prophylactic)
  (therapeutic) - *see* Hepatitis, viral, type B
Honeycomb lung J98.4
  congenital Q33.0
Hooded
  clitoris Q52.6
  penis Q55.69
Hookworm (anemia) (disease) (infection)
  (infestation) B76.9
  specified NEC B76.8
Hordeolum (eyelid) (externum) (recurrent)
  H00.019
  internum H00.029
    left H00.026
      lower H00.025
      upper H00.024
    right H00.023
      lower H00.022
      upper H00.021
    left H00.016
      lower H00.015
      upper H00.014
    right H00.013
      lower H00.012
      upper H00.011
Horn
  cutaneous L85.8
  nail L60.2
    congenital Q84.6
Horner (-Claude Bernard) syndrome G90.2
  traumatic - *see* Injury, nerve, cervical
  sympathetic
Horseshoe kidney (congenital) Q63.1
Horton's headache or neuralgia G44.099
  intractable G44.091
  not intractable G44.099
Hospital hopper syndrome - *see* Disorder,
  factitious
Hospitalism in children - *see* Disorder,
  adjustment
Hostility R45.5
  towards child Z62.3
Hot flashes
  menopausal N95.1
Hourglass (contracture) - *see also* Contraction,
  hourglass
  stomach K31.89
    congenital Q40.2
    stricture K31.2
Household, housing circumstance affecting
  care Z59.9
  specified NEC Z59.8
Housemaid's knee - *see* Bursitis, prepatellar
Hudson (-Stähli) line (cornea) - *see*
  Pigmentation, cornea, anterior
Human
  bite (open wound) - *see also* Bite
    intact skin surface - *see* Bite, superficial
  herpesvirus - *see* Herpes
  immunodeficiency virus (HIV) disease
  (infection) B20

Human - *continued*
  asymptomatic status Z21
  contact Z20.6
  counseling Z71.7
  dementia B20- [*F02.80*]
    with behavioral disturbance B20- [*F02.81*]
  exposure to Z20.6
  laboratory evidence R75
  type 2 (HIV 2) as cause of disease classified
  elsewhere B97.35
  papillomavirus (HPV)
    DNA test positive
      high risk
        cervix R87.810
        vagina R87.811
      low risk
        cervix R87.820
        vagina R87.821
    screening for Z11.51
  T-cell lymphotropic virus
    type 1(HTLV-i) infection B33.3
      as cause of disease classified elsewhere
      B97.33
      carrier Z22.6
    type 2 (HTLV-II) as cause of disease
    classified elsewhere B97.34
Humidifier lung or pneumonitis J67.7
Humiliation (experience) in childhood
  Z62.898
Humpback (acquired) - *see* Kyphosis
Hunchback (acquired) - *see* Kyphosis
Hunger T73.0
  air, psychogenic F45.8
Hungry bone syndrome E83.81
Hunner's ulcer - *see* Cystitis, chronic,
  interstitial
Hunter's
  glossitis D51.0
  syndrome E76.1
Huntington's disease or chorea G10
  with dementia G10- [*F02.80*]
    with behavioral disturbance G10- [*F02.81*]
Hunt's
  disease or syndrome (herpetic geniculate
  ganglionitis) B02.21
  dyssynergia cerebellaris myoclonica G11.1
  neuralgia B02.21
Hurler (-Scheie) disease or syndrome E76.02
Hurst's disease G36.1
Hürthle cell
  adenocarcinoma C73
  adenoma D34
  carcinoma C73
  tumor D34
Hutchinson-Boeck disease or syndrome - *see*
  Sarcoidosis
Hutchinson-Gilford disease or syndrome
  E34.8
Hutchinson's
  disease, meaning
    angioma serpiginosum L81.7
    pompholyx (cheiropompholyx) L30.1
    prurigo estivalis L56.4
    summer eruption or summer prurigo L56.4
  melanotic freckle - *see* Melanoma, in situ
    malignant melanoma in - *see* Melanoma
  teeth or incisors (congenital syphilis) A50.52
  triad (congenital syphilis) A50.53
Hyalin plaque, sclera, senile H15.89
Hyaline membrane (disease) (lung)
  (pulmonary) (newborn) P22.0
Hyalinosis
  cutis (et mucosae) E78.89
  focal and segmental (glomerular) - *see also*
  N00-N07 with fourth character .1N05.1

Hyalitis, hyalosis, asteroid - *see also* Deposit, crystalline
  syphilitic (late) A52.71
Hydatid
  cyst or tumor - *see* Echinococcus
  mole - *see* Hydatidiform mole
  Morgagni
    female Q50.5
    male (epididymal) Q55.4
      testicular Q55.29
Hydatidiform mole (benign) (complicating pregnancy) (delivered) (undelivered) O01.9
  classical O01.0
  complete O01.0
  incomplete O01.1
  invasive D39.2
  malignant D39.2
  partial O01.1
Hydatidosis - *see* Echinococcus
Hydradenitis (axillaris) (suppurative) L73.2
Hydradenoma - *see* Hidradenoma
Hydramnios O40.-
Hydrancephaly, hydranencephaly Q04.3
  with spina bifida - *see* Spina bifida, with hydrocephalus
Hydrargyrism NEC - *see* Poisoning, mercury
Hydrarthrosis - *see also* Effusion, joint
  gonococcal A54.42
  intermittent M12.40
    ankle M12.47-
    elbow M12.42-
    foot joint M12.47-
    hand joint M12.44-
    hip M12.45-
    knee M12.46-
    multiple site M12.49
    shoulder M12.41-
    specified joint NEC M12.48
    wrist M12.43-
  of yaws (early) (late) - *see also* subcategory M14.8 A66.6
  syphilitic (late) A52.77
    congenital A50.55 [*M12.80*]
Hydremia D64.89
Hydrencephalocele (congenital) - *see* Encephalocele
Hydrencephalomeningocele (congenital) - *see* Encephalocele
Hydroa R23.8
  aestivale L56.4
  vacciniforme L56.4
Hydroadenitis (axillaris) (suppurative) L73.2
Hydrocalycosis - *see* Hydronephrosis
Hydrocele (spermatic cord) (testis) (tunica vaginalis) N43.3
  canal of Nuck N94.89
  communicating N43.2
    congenital P83.5
  congenital P83.5
  encysted N43.0
  female NEC N94.89
  infected N43.1
  newborn P83.5
  round ligament N94.89
  specified NEC N43.2
  spinalis - *see* Spina bifida
  vulva N90.89
Hydrocephalus (acquired) (external) (internal) (malignant) (recurrent) G91.9
  aqueduct Sylvius stricture Q03.0
  causing disproportion O33.6
    with obstructed labor O66.3
  communicating G91.0
  congenital (external) (internal) Q03.9

Hydrocephalus - *continued*
  with spina bifida Q05.4
    cervical Q05.0
    dorsal Q05.1
    lumbar Q05.2
    lumbosacral Q05.2
    sacral Q05.3
    thoracic Q05.1
    thoracolumbar Q05.1
    specified NEC Q03.8
  due to toxoplasmosis (congenital) P37.1
  foramen Magendie block (acquired) G91.1
    congenital - *see also* Hydrocephalus, congenital Q03.1
  in (due to)
    infectious disease NEC B89 [*G91.4*]
    neoplastic disease NEC (see also Neoplasm) G91.4
    parasitic disease B89 [*G91.4*]
  newborn Q03.9
    with spina bifida - *see* Spina bifida, with hydrocephalus
  noncommunicating G91.1
  normal pressure G91.2
    secondary G91.0
  obstructive G91.1
  otitic G93.2
  post-traumatic NEC G91.3
  secondary G91.4
    post-traumatic G91.3
  specified NEC G91.8
  syphilitic, congenital A50.49
Hydrocolpos (congenital) N89.8
Hydrocystoma - *see* Neoplasm, skin, benign
Hydroencephalocele (congenital) - *see* Encephalocele
Hydroencephalomeningocele (congenital) - *see* Encephalocele
Hydrohematopneumothorax - *see* Hemothorax
Hydromeningitis - *see* Meningitis
Hydromeningocele (spinal) - *see also* Spina bifida
  cranial - *see* Encephalocele
Hydrometra N85.8
Hydrometrocolpos N89.8
Hydromicrocephaly Q02
Hydromphalus (since birth) Q45.8
Hydromyelia Q06.4
Hydromyelocele - *see* Spina bifida
Hydronephrosis (atrophic) (early) (functionless) (intermittent) (primary) (secondary) NEC N13.30
  with
    infection N13.6
    obstruction (by) (of)
      renal calculus N13.2
        with infection N13.6
      ureteral NEC N13.1
        with infection N13.6
        calculus N13.2
          with infection N13.6
      ureteropelvic junction (congenital) Q62.11
        acquired N13.0
          with infection N13.6
      ureteral stricture NEC N13.1
        with infection N13.6
  congenital Q62.0
    due to acquired occlusion of ureteropelvic junction N13.0
  specified type NEC N13.39
  tuberculous A18.11
Hydropericarditis - *see* Pericarditis
Hydropericardium - *see* Pericarditis

Hydroperitoneum R18.8
Hydrophobia - *see* Rabies
Hydrophthalmos Q15.0
Hydropneumohemothorax - *see* Hemothorax
Hydropneumopericarditis - *see* Pericarditis
Hydropneumopericardium - *see* Pericarditis
Hydropneumothorax J94.8
  traumatic - *see* Injury, intrathoracic, lung
  tuberculous NEC A15.6
Hydrops R60.9
  abdominis R18.8
  articulorum intermittens - *see* Hydrarthrosis, intermittent
  cardiac - *see* Failure, heart, congestive
    causing obstructed labor (mother) O66.3
  endolymphatic H81.0-
  fetal - *see* Pregnancy, complicated by, hydrops, fetalis
  fetalis P83.2
    due to
      ABO isoimmunization P56.0
      alpha thalassemia D56.0
      hemolytic disease P56.90
        specified NEC P56.99
      isoimmunization (ABO) (Rh) P56.0
      other specified nonhemolytic disease NEC P83.2
      Rh incompatibility P56.0
  during pregnancy - *see* Pregnancy, complicated by, hydrops, fetalis
  gallbladder K82.1
  joint - *see* Effusion, joint
  labyrinth H81.0-
  newborn (idiopathic) P83.2
    due to
      ABO isoimmunization P56.0
      alpha thalassemia D56.0
      hemolytic disease P56.90
        specified NEC P56.99
      isoimmunization (ABO) (Rh) P56.0
      Rh incompatibility P56.0
  nutritional - *see* Malnutrition, severe
  pericardium - *see* Pericarditis
  pleura - *see* Hydrothorax
  spermatic cord - *see* Hydrocele
Hydropyonephrosis N13.6
Hydrorachis Q06.4
Hydrorrhea (nasal) J34.89
  pregnancy - *see* Rupture, membranes, premature
Hydrosadenitis (axillaris) (suppurative) L73.2
Hydrosalpinx (fallopian tube) (follicularis) N70.11
Hydrothorax (double) (pleura) J94.8
  chylous (nonfilarial) I89.8
    filarial - *see also* Infestation, filarial B74.9 [*J91.8*]
  traumatic - *see* Injury, intrathoracic
  tuberculous NEC (non primary) A15.6
Hydroureter - *see also* Hydronephrosis N13.4
  with infection N13.6
  congenital Q62.39
Hydroureteronephrosis - *see* Hydronephrosis
Hydrourethra N36.8
Hydroxykynureninuria E70.8
Hydroxylysinemia E72.3
Hydroxyprolinemia E72.59
Hygiene, sleep
  abuse Z72.821
  inadequate Z72.821
  poor Z72.821
Hygroma (congenital) (cystic) D18.1
  praepatellare, prepatellar - *see* Bursitis, prepatellar

Hymen - *see* condition
**Hymenolepis, hymenolepiasis (diminuta)
(infection) (infestation) (nana)** B71.0
Hypalgesia R20.8
Hyperacidity (gastric) K31.89
  psychogenic F45.8
Hyperactive, hyperactivity F90.9
  basal cell, uterine cervix - *see* Dysplasia,
    cervix
  bowel sounds R19.12
  cervix epithelial (basal) - *see* Dysplasia, cervix
  child F90.9
    attention deficit - *see* Disorder, attention-
    deficit hyperactivity detrusor muscle N32.81
  gastrointestinal K31.89
    psychogenic F45.8
  nasal mucous membrane J34.3
  stomach K31.89
  thyroid (gland) - *see* Hyperthyroidism
Hyperacusis H93.23-
Hyperadrenalism E27.5
Hyperadrenocorticism E24.9
  congenital E25.0
  iatrogenic E24.2
    correct substance properly administered - *see*
      Table of Drugs and Chemicals, by drug,
      adverse effect
    overdose or wrong substance given or taken -
      see Table of Drugs and Chemicals, by drug,
      poisoning
  not associated with Cushing's syndrome E27.0
  pituitary-dependent E24.0
Hyperaldosteronism E26.9
  familial (type I) E26.02
  glucocorticoid-remediable E26.02
  primary (due to (bilateral) adrenal hyperplasia)
    E26.09
  primary NEC E26.09
  secondary E26.1
  specified NEC E26.89
Hyperalgesia R20.8
Hyperalimentation R63.2
  carotene, carotin E67.1
  specified NEC E67.8
  vitamin
    A E67.0
    D E67.3
Hyperaminoaciduria arginine E72.21
  cystine E72.01
  lysine E72.3
  ornithine E72.4
Hyperammonemia (congenital) E72.20
Hyperazotemia - *see* Uremia
Hyperbetalipoproteinemia (familial) E78.00
  with prebetalipoproteinemia E78.2
Hyperbilirubinemia
  constitutional E80.6
  familial conjugated E80.6
  neonatal (transient) - *see* Jaundice, newborn
Hypercalcemia, hypocalciuric, familial
  E83.52
Hypercalciuria, idiopathic E83.52
Hypercapnia R06.89
  newborn P84
**Hypercarotenemia, hypercarotenemia
  (dietary)** E67.1
Hypercementosis K03.4
Hyperchloremia E87.8
Hyperchlorhydria K31.89
  neurotic F45.8
  psychogenic F45.8
Hypercholesterinemia - *see*
  Hypercholesterolemia

**Hypercholesterolemia (essential) (primary)
  (pure)** E78.00
  with hyperglyceridemia, endogenous E78.2
  dietary counseling and surveillance Z71.3
  familial E78.01
  hereditary E78.01
Hyperchylia gastrica, psychogenic F45.8
Hyperchylomicronemia (familial) (primary)
  E78.3
  with hyperbetalipoproteinemia E78.3
Hypercoagulable (state) D68.59
  activated protein C resistance D68.51
  antithrombin (III) deficiency D68.59
  factor V Leiden mutation D68.51
  primary NEC D68.59
  protein C deficiency D68.59
  protein S deficiency D68.59
  prothrombin gene mutation D68.52
  secondary D68.69
  specified NEC D68.69
Hypercoagulation (state) D68.59
Hypercorticalism, pituitary-dependent E24.0
Hypercorticosolism - *see* Cushing's, syndrome
Hypercorticosteronism E24.2
  correct substance properly administered - *see*
    Table of Drugs and Chemicals, by drug,
    adverse effect
  overdose or wrong substance given or taken -
    see Table of Drugs and Chemicals, by drug,
    poisoning
Hypercortisonism E24.2
  correct substance properly administered - *see*
    Table of Drugs and Chemicals, by drug,
    adverse effect
  overdose or wrong substance given or taken -
    see Table of Drugs and Chemicals, by drug,
    poisoning **H**
hyperekplexia Q89.8
Hyperelectrolytemia E87.8
Hyperemesis R11.10
  with nausea R11.2
  gravidarum (mild) O21.0
    with
      carbohydrate depletion O21.1
      dehydration O21.1
      electrolyte imbalance O21.1
      metabolic disturbance O21.1
    severe (with metabolic disturbance) O21.1
  projectile R11.12
  psychogenic F45.8
Hyperemia (acute) (passive) R68.89
  anal mucosa K62.89
  bladder N32.89
  cerebral I67.89
  conjunctiva H11.43-
  ear internal, acute *see* subcategory H83.0
  enteric K59.8
  eye - *see* Hyperemia, conjunctiva
  eyelid (active) (passive) - *see* Disorder, eyelid,
    specified type NEC
  intestine K59.8
  iris - *see* Disorder, iris, vascular
  kidney N28.89
  labyrinth - *see* subcategory H83.0
  liver (active) K76.89
  lung (passive) - *see* Edema, lung
  pulmonary (passive) - *see* Edema, lung
  renal N28.89
  retina H35.89
  stomach K31.89
Hyperesthesia (body surface) R20.3
  larynx (reflex) J38.7
    hysterical F44.89
  pharynx (reflex) J39.2
    hysterical F44.89

**Hyperestrogenism (drug-induced)
  (iatrogenic)** E28.0
Hyperexplexia Q89.8
Hyperfibrinolysis - *see* Fibrinolysis
Hyperfructosemia E74.19
Hyperfunction
  adrenal cortex, not associated with Cushing's
    syndrome E27.0
    medulla E27.5
      adrenomedullary E27.5
    virilism E25.9
      congenital E25.0
  ovarian E28.8
  pancreas K86.89
  parathyroid (gland) E21.3
  pituitary (gland) (anterior) E22.9
    specified NEC E22.8
  polyglandular E31.1
  testicular E29.0
Hypergammaglobulinemia D89.2
  polyclonal D89.0
  Waldenström D89.0
Hypergastrinemia E16.4
Hyperglobulinemia R77.1
Hyperglycemia, hyperglycemic (transient)
  R73.9
  coma - *see* Diabetes, by type, with coma
  postpancreatectomy E89.1
**Hyperglyceridemia (endogenous) (essential)
  (familial) (hereditary) (pure)** E78.1
  mixed E78.3
Hyperglycinemia (non-ketotic) E72.51
Hypergonadism
  ovarian E28.8
  testicular (primary) (infantile) E29.0
Hyperheparinemia D68.32
Hyperhidrosis, hyperidrosis R61
  focal
    primary L74.519
      axilla L74.510
      face L74.511
      palms L74.512
      soles L74.513
    secondary L74.52
  generalized R61
  localized
    primary L74.519
      axilla L74.510
      face L74.511
      palms L74.512
      soles L74.513
    secondary L74.52
  psychogenic F45.8
  secondary R61
    focal L74.52
Hyperhistidinemia E70.41
Hyperhomocysteinemia E72.11
Hyperhydroxyprolinemia E72.59
Hyperinsulinism (functional) E16.1
  with
    coma (hypoglycemic) E15
    encephalopathy E16.1 *[G94]*
  ectopic E16.1
  therapeutic misadventure (from administration
    of insulin) - *see* subcategory T38.3
Hyperkalemia E87.5
Hyperkeratosis - *see also* Keratosis L85.9
  cervix N88.0
  due to yaws (early) (late) (palmar or plantar)
    A66.3
  follicularis Q82.8
    penetrans (in cutem) L87.0
  palmoplantaris climacterica L85.1
  pinta A67.1

Hyperkeratosis - *continued*
  senile (with pruritus) L57.0
  universalis congenita Q80.8
  vocal cord J38.3
  vulva N90.4
Hyperkinesia, hyperkinetic (disease)
  (reaction) (syndrome) (childhood)
  (adolescence) - *see also* Disorder, attention-
    deficit hyperactivity
  heart I51.89
Hyperleucine-isoleucinemia E71.19
Hyperlipemia, hyperlipidemia E78.5
  combined E78.2
    familial E78.4
  group
    A E78.00
    B E78.1
    C E78.2
    D E78.3
  mixed E78.2
  specified NEC E78.4
Hyperlipidosis E75.6
  hereditary NEC E75.5
Hyperlipoproteinemia E78.5
  Fredrickson's type
    I E78.3
    IIa E78.00
    IIb E78.2
    III E78.2
    IV E78.1
    V E78.3
  low-density-lipoprotein-type (LDL) E78.00
  very-low-density-lipoprotein-type (VLDL)
    E78.1
Hyperlucent lung, unilateral J43.0
Hyperlysinemia E72.3
Hypermagnesemia E83.41
  neonatal P71.8
Hypermenorrhea N92.0
Hypermethioninemia E72.19
Hypermetropia (congenital) H52.0-
Hypermobility, hypermotility
  cecum - *see* Syndrome, irritable bowel
  coccyx - *see* subcategory M53.2
  colon - *see* Syndrome, irritable bowel
    psychogenic F45.8
  ileum K58.9
  intestine - *see also* Syndrome, irritable bowel
    K58.9
    psychogenic F45.8
  meniscus (knee) - *see* Derangement, knee,
    meniscus
  scapula - *see* Instability, joint, shoulder
  stomach K31.89
    psychogenic F45.8
  syndrome M35.7
  urethra N36.41
    with intrinsic sphincter deficiency N36.43
Hypernasality R49.21
Hypernatremia E87.0
Hypernephroma C64.-**hyperopia** - *see*
  Hypermetropia
Hyperorexia nervosa F50.2
Hyperornithinemia E72.4
Hyperosmia R43.1
Hyperosmolality E87.0
Hyperostosis (monomelic) - *see also* Disorder,
  bone, density and structure, specified NEC
  ankylosing (spine) M48.10
    cervical region M48.12
    cervicothoracic region M48.13
    lumbar region M48.16
    lumbosacral region M48.17
    multiple sites M48.19

Hyperostosis - *continued*
    occipito-atlanto-axial region M48.11
    sacrococcygeal region M48.18
    thoracic region M48.14
    thoracolumbar region M48.15
  cortical (skull) M85.2
    infantile M89.8X-
  frontal, internal of skull M85.2
  interna frontalis M85.2
  skeletal, diffuse idiopathic - *see* Hyperostosis,
    ankylosing
  skull M85.2
    congenital Q75.8
  vertebral, ankylosing - *see* Hyperostosis,
    ankylosing
Hyperovarism E28.8
Hyperoxaluria (primary) E72.53
Hyperparathyroidism E21.3
  primary E21.0
  secondary (renal) N25.81
    non-renal E21.1
  specified NEC E21.2
  tertiary E21.2
Hyperpathia R20.8
Hyperperistalsis R19.2
  psychogenic F45.8
Hyperpermeability, capillary I78.8
Hyperphagia R63.2
Hyperphenylalaninemia NEC E70.1
Hyperphoria (alternating) H50.53
Hyperphosphatemia E83.39
Hyperpiesis, hyperpiesia - *see* Hypertension
Hyperpigmentation - *see also* Pigmentation
  melanin NEC L81.4
  postinflammatory L81.0
Hyperpinealism E34.8
Hyperpituitarism E22.9
Hyperplasia, hyperplastic
  adenoids J35.2
  adrenal (capsule) (cortex) (gland) E27.8
    with
      sexual precocity (male) E25.9
        congenital E25.0
      virilism, adrenal E25.9
        congenital E25.0
      virilization (female) E25.9
        congenital E25.0
    congenital E25.0
    salt-losing E25.0
  adrenomedullary E27.5
  angiolymphoid, eosinophilia (ALHE) D18.01
  appendix (lymphoid) K38.0
  artery, fibromuscular I77.3
  bone - *see also* Hypertrophy, bone
    marrow D75.89
  breast - *see also* Hypertrophy, breast
    ductal (atypical) N60.9-
  C-cell, thyroid E07.0
  cementation (tooth) (teeth) K03.4
  cervical gland R59.0
  cervix (uteri) (basal cell) (endometrium)
    (polypoid) - *see also* Dysplasia, cervix
    congenital Q51.828
  clitoris, congenital Q52.6
  denture K06.2
  endocervicitis N72
  endometrium, endometrial (adenomatous)
    (benign) (cystic) (glandular) (glandular-cystic)
    (polypoid) N85.00
    with atypia N85.02
    cervix - *see* Dysplasia, cervix
    complex (without atypia) N85.01
    simple (without atypia) N85.01
  epithelial L85.9

Hyperplasia, hyperplastic - *continued*
    focal, oral, including tongue K13.29
  nipple N62
  skin L85.9
  tongue K13.29
  vaginal wall N89.3
  erythroid D75.89
  fibromuscular of artery (carotid) (renal) I77.3
  genital
    female NEC N94.89
    male N50.89
  gingiva K06.1
  glandularis cystica uteri (interstitialis) - *see
    also* Hyperplasia, endometrial N85.00-
  gum K06.1
  hymen, congenital Q52.4
  irritative, edentulous (alveolar) K06.2
  jaw M26.09
    alveolar M26.79
      lower M26.03
        alveolar M26.72
      upper M26.01
        alveolar M26.71
  kidney (congenital) Q63.3
  labia N90.69
    epithelial N90.3
  liver (congenital) Q44.7
    nodular, focal K76.89
  lymph gland or node R59.9
  mandible, mandibular M26.03
    alveolar M26.72
    unilateral condylar M27.8
  maxilla, maxillary M26.01
    alveolar M26.71
  myometrium, myometrial N85.2
  neuroendocrine cell, of infancy J84.841
  nose
    lymphoid J34.89
    polypoid J33.9
  oral mucosa (irritative) K13.6
  organ or site, congenital NEC - *see* Anomaly,
    by site
  ovary N83.8
  palate, papillary (irritative) K13.6
  pancreatic islet cells E16.9
    alpha E16.8
      with excess
        gastrin E16.4
        glucagon E16.3
    beta E16.1
  parathyroid (gland) E21.0
  pharynx (lymphoid) J39.2
  prostate (adenofibromatous) (nodular) N40.0
    with lower urinary tract symptoms (LUTS)
      N40.1
    without lower urinary tract symptoms
      (LUTS) N40.0
  renal artery I77.89
  reticulo-endothelial (cell) D75.89
  salivary gland (any) K11.1
  Schimmelbusch's - *see* Mastopathy, cystic
  suprarenal capsule (gland) E27.8
  thymus (gland) (persistent) E32.0
  thyroid (gland) - *see* Goiter
  tonsils (faucial) (infective) (lingual)
    (lymphoid) J35.1
    with adenoids J35.3
  unilateral condylar M27.8
  uterus, uterine N85.2
    endometrium (glandular) - *see also*
      Hyperplasia, endometrial N85.00-
  vulva N90.69
    epithelial N90.3
Hyperpnea - *see* Hyperventilation

Hyperpotassemia E87.5
Hyperprebetalipoproteinemia (familial)
E78.1
Hyperprolactinemia E22.1
Hyperprolinemia (type I) (type II) E72.59
Hyperproteinemia E88.09
Hyperprothrombinemia, causing coagulation factor deficiency D68.4
Hyperpyrexia R50.9
  heat (effects) T67.0
  malignant, due to anesthetic T88.3
  rheumatic - *see* Fever, rheumatic
  unknown origin R50.9
Hyper-reflexia R29.2
Hypersalivation K11.7
Hypersecretion
  ACTH (not associated with Cushing's syndrome) E27.0
    pituitary E24.0
  adrenaline E27.5
  adrenomedullary E27.5
  androgen (testicular) E29.0
    ovarian (drug-induced) (iatrogenic) E28.1
  calcitonin E07.0
  catecholamine E27.5
  corticoadrenal E24.9
  cortisol E24.9
  epinephrine E27.5
  estrogen E28.0
  gastric K31.89
    psychogenic F45.8
  gastrin E16.4
  glucagon E16.3
  hormone(s)
    ACTH (not associated with Cushing's syndrome) E27.0
      pituitary E24.0
    antidiuretic E22.2
    growth E22.0
    intestinal NEC E34.1
    ovarian androgen E28.1
    pituitary E22.9
    testicular E29.0
    thyroid stimulating E05.80
      with thyroid storm E05.81
  insulin - *see* Hyperinsulinism
  lacrimal glands - *see* Epiphora
  medulloadrenal E27.5
  milk O92.6
  ovarian androgens E28.1
  salivary gland (any) K11.7
  thyrocalcitonin E07.0
  upper respiratory J39.8
Hypersegmentation, leukocytic, hereditary
D72.0
Hypersensitive, hypersensitiveness, hypersensitivity - *see also* Allergy carotid
  sinus G90.01
  colon - *see* Irritable, colon
  drug T88.7
  gastrointestinal K52.29
    immediate K52.29
    psychogenic F45.8
  labyrinth - *see* subcategory H83.2
  pain R20.8
  pneumonitis - *see* Pneumonitis, allergic
  reaction T78.40
    upper respiratory tract NEC J39.3
Hypersomnia (organic) G47.10
  due to
    alcohol
      abuse F10.182
      dependence F10.282
      use F10.982

Hypersomnia (organic) - *continued*
  amphetamines
    abuse F15.182
    dependence F15.282
    use F15.982
  caffeine
    abuse F15.182
    dependence F15.282
    use F15.982
  cocaine
    abuse F14.182
    dependence F14.282
    use F14.982
  drug NEC
    abuse F19.182
    dependence F19.282
    use F19.982
  medical condition G47.14
  mental disorder F51.13
  opioid
    abuse F11.182
    dependence F11.282
    use F11.982
  psychoactive substance NEC
    abuse F19.182
    dependence F19.282
    use F19.982
  sedative, hypnotic, or anxiolytic
    abuse F13.182
    dependence F13.282
    use F13.982
  stimulant NEC
    abuse F15.182
    dependence F15.282
    use F15.982
  idiopathic G47.11
    with long sleep time G47.11
    without long sleep time G47.12
  menstrual related G47.13
  nonorganic origin F51.11
    specified NEC F51.19
  not due to a substance or known physiological condition F51.11
    specified NEC F51.19
  primary F51.11
  recurrent G47.13
  specified NEC G47.19
Hypersplenia, hypersplenism D73.1
Hyperstimulation, ovaries (associated with induced ovulation) N98.1
Hypersusceptibility - *see* Allergy
Hypertelorism (ocular) (orbital) Q75.2
Hypertension, hypertensive (accelerated) (benign) (essential) (idiopathic) (malignant) (systemic) I10
  with
    heart failure (congestive) I11.0
    heart involvement (conditions in I50. , I51.4 I51.9 due to hypertension) *see* Hypertension, heart
    kidney involvement - *see* Hypertension, kidney
  benign, intracranial G93.2
  borderline R03.0
  cardiorenal (disease) I13.10
    with heart failure I13.0
      with stage 1 through stage 4 chronic kidney disease I13.0
      with stage 5 or end stage renal disease I13.2
    without heart failure I13.10
      with stage 1 through stage 4 chronic kidney disease I13.10
      with stage 5 or end stage renal disease I13.11

Hypertension, hypertensive - *continued*
  cardiovascular
    disease (arteriosclerotic) (sclerotic) - *see* Hypertension, heart
    renal (disease) - *see* Hypertension, cardiorenal
  chronic venous - *see* Hypertension, venous (chronic)
  complicating
    childbirth (labor) O16.4
      pre-existing O10.92
        with
          heart disease O10.12
            with renal disease O10.32
          pre-eclampsia O11.4
          renal disease O10.22
            with heart disease O10.32
        essential O10.02
        secondary O10.42
    pregnancy O16.-
      with edema - *see also* Pre-eclampsia O14.9-
      gestational (pregnancy induced) (without proteinuria) O13.-
        with proteinuria O14.9-
          mild pre-eclampsia O14.0-
          moderate pre-eclampsia O14.0-
          severe pre-eclampsia O14.1-
            with hemolysis, elevated liver enzymes and low platelet count (HELLP) O14.2-
      pre-existing O10.91-
        with
          heart disease O10.11-
            with renal disease O10.31-
          pre-eclampsia - *see* category O11
          renal disease O10.21-
            with heart disease O10.31-
        essential O10.01-
        secondary O10.41-
        transient O13.-
    puerperium, pre-existing O16.5
      pre-existing
        with
          heart disease O10.13
            with renal disease O10.33
          pre-eclampsia O11.5
          renal disease O10.23
            with heart disease O10.33
        essential O10.03
      pregnancy-induced O13.9
      secondary O10.43
  crisis I16.9
  due to
    endocrine disorders I15.2
    pheochromocytoma I15.2
    renal disorders NEC I15.1
      arterial I15.0
    renovascular disorders I15.0
    specified disease NEC I15.8
  emergency I16.1
  encephalopathy I67.4
  gestational (without significant proteinuria) (pregnancy-induced) (transient) O13.-
    with significant proteinuria - *see* Pre-eclampsia
    complicating
      delivery O13.4
      puerperium O13.5
  Goldblatt's I70.1
  heart (disease) (conditions in I51.4-i51.9 due to hypertension) I11.9
    with
      heart failure (congestive) I11.0
      kidney disease (chronic) - *see* Hypertension, cardiorenal

Hypertension, hypertensive - *continued*
  intracranial (benign) G93.2
  kidney I12.9
    with
      heart disease - *see* Hypertension,
        cardiorenal
      stage 5 chronic kidney disease (CKD) or
        end stage renal disease (ESRD) I12.0
      stage 1 through stage 4 chronic kidney
        disease I12.9
  lesser circulation I27.0
  maternal O16.-
  newborn P29.2
    pulmonary (persistent) P29.30
  ocular H40.05-
  pancreatic duct
    code to underlying condition
      with chronic pancreatitis K86.1
  portal (due to chronic liver disease)
    (idiopathic) K76.6
    gastropathy K31.89
    in (due to) schistosomiasis (bilharziasis)
      B65.9 [*K77*]
  postoperative I97.3
  psychogenic F45.8
  pulmonary I27.20
    with
      cor pulmonale (chronic) I27.29
        acute I26.09
      right heart ventricular strain/failure I27.29
        acute I26.09
      right to left shunt related to congenital heart
        disease I27.83
      unclear multifactorial mechanisms I27.29
    arterial (associated) (drug-induced) (toxin-
      induced) I27.21
    chronic thromboembolic I27.24
    due to
      hematologic disorders I27.29
      left heart disease I27.22
      lung diseases and hypoxia I27.23
      metabolic disorders I27.29
      specified systemic disorders NEC I27.29
    group 1 (associated) (drug-induced) (toxin-
      induced) I27.21
    group 2 I27.22
    group 3 I27.23
    group 4 I27.24
    group 5 I27.29
    of newborn (persistent) P29.30
    primary (idiopathic) I27.0
    secondary
      arterial I27.21
      specified NEC I27.29
  renal - *see* Hypertension, kidney
  renovascular I15.0
  secondary NEC I15.9
    due to
      endocrine disorders I15.2
      pheochromocytoma I15.2
      renal disorders NEC I15.1
        arterial I15.0
      renovascular disorders I15.0
    specified NEC I15.8
  transient, of pregnancy O13.
  urgency I16.0
  venous (chronic)
    due to
      deep vein thrombosis - *see* Syndrome,
    postthrombotic
    idiopathic I87.309
      with
        inflammation I87.32-
          with ulcer I87.33-

Hypertension, hypertensive - *continued*
    specified complication NEC I87.39-
      ulcer I87.31-
        with inflammation I87.33-
      asymptomatic I87.30-
Hypertensive urgency - *see* Hypertension
Hyperthecosis ovary E28.8
Hyperthermia (of unknown origin) - *see also*
  Hyperpyrexia
  malignant, due to anesthesia T88.3
  newborn P81.9
    environmental P81.0
Hyperthyroid (recurrent) - *see*
  Hyperthyroidism
Hyperthyroidism (latent) (pre-adult)
  (recurrent) E05.90
  with
    goiter (diffuse) E05.00
      with thyroid storm E05.01
      nodular (multinodular) E05.20
        with thyroid storm E05.21
        uninodular E05.10
          with thyroid storm E05.11
    storm E05.91
  due to ectopic thyroid tissue E05.30
    with thyroid storm E05.31
  neonatal, transitory P72.1
  specified NEC E05.80
    with thyroid storm E05.81
Hypertony, hypertonia, hypertonicity
  bladder N31.8
  congenital P94.1
  stomach K31.89
    psychogenic F45.8
  uterus, uterine (contractions) (complicating
    delivery) O62.4
Hypertrichosis L68.9
  congenital Q84.2
  eyelid H02.869
    left H02.866
      lower H02.865
      upper H02.864
    right H02.863
      lower H02.862
      upper H02.861
  lanuginosa Q84.2
    acquired L68.1
  localized L68.2
  specified NEC L68.8
Hypertriglyceridemia, essential E78.1
Hypertrophy, hypertrophic
  adenofibromatous, prostate - *see* Enlargement,
  enlarged, prostate
  adenoids (infective) J35.2
    with tonsils J35.3
  adrenal cortex E27.8
  alveolar process or ridge - *see* Anomaly,
  alveolar
  anal papillae K62.89
  artery I77.89
    congenital NEC Q27.8
      digestive system Q27.8
      lower limb Q27.8
      specified site NEC Q27.8
      upper limb Q27.8
  auricular - *see* Hypertrophy, cardiac
  Bartholin's gland N75.8
  bile duct (common) (hepatic) K83.8
  bladder (sphincter) (trigone) N32.89
  bone M89.30
    carpus M89.34-
    clavicle M89.31-
    femur M89.35-
    fibula M89.36-

Hypertrophy, hypertrophic - *continued*
    finger M89.34-
    humerus M89.32-
    ilium M89.359
    ischium M89.359
    metacarpus M89.34-
    metatarsus M89.37-
    multiple sites M89.39
    neck M89.38
    radius M89.33-
    rib M89.38
    scapula M89.31-
    skull M89.38
    tarsus M89.37-
    tibia M89.36-
    toe M89.37-
    ulna M89.33-
    vertebra M89.38
  brain G93.89
  breast N62
    cystic - *see* Mastopathy, cystic
    newborn P83.4
    pubertal, massive N62
    puerperal, postpartum - *see* Disorder, breast,
  specified type NEC
    senile (parenchymatous) N62
  cardiac (chronic) (idiopathic) I51.7
    with rheumatic fever (conditions in I00)
      active I01.8
      inactive or quiescent (with chorea) I09.89
    congenital NEC Q24.8
    fatty - *see* Degeneration, myocardial
    hypertensive - *see* Hypertension, heart
    rheumatic (with chorea) I09.89
      active or acute I01.8
        with chorea I02.0
    valve - *see* Endocarditis
  cartilage - *see* Disorder, cartilage, specified
  type NEC
  cecum - *see* Megacolon
  cervix (uteri) N88.8
    congenital Q51.828
    elongation N88.4
  clitoris (cirrhotic) N90.89
    congenital Q52.6
  colon - *see also* Megacolon
    congenital Q43.2
  conjunctiva, lymphoid H11.89
  corpora cavernosa N48.89
  cystic duct K82.8
  duodenum K31.89
  endometrium (glandular) - *see also*
  Hyperplasia, endometrial N85.00-
    cervix N88.8
  epididymis N50.89
  esophageal hiatus (congenital) Q79.1
    with hernia - *see* Hernia, hiatal
  eyelid - *see* Disorder, eyelid, specified type
  NEC
  fat pad E65
    knee (infrapatellar) (popliteal) (prepatellar)
  (retropatellar) M79.4
  foot (congenital) Q74.2
  frenulum, frenum (tongue) K14.8
    lip K13.0
  gallbladder K82.8
  gastric mucosa K29.60
    with bleeding K29.61
  gland, glandular R59.9
    generalized R59.1
    localized R59.0
  gum (mucous membrane) K06.1
  heart (idiopathic) - *see also* Hypertrophy,
  cardiac

Hypertrophy, hypertrophic - *continued*
valve - *see also* Endocarditis I38
hemifacial Q67.4
hepatic - *see* Hypertrophy, liver
hiatus (esophageal) Q79.1
hilus gland R59.0
hymen, congenital Q52.4
ileum K63.89
intestine NEC K63.89
jejunum K63.89
kidney (compensatory) N28.81
  congenital Q63.3
labium (majus) (minus) N90.60
ligament - *see* Disorder, ligament
lingual tonsil (infective) J35.1
  with adenoids J35.3
lip K13.0
  congenital Q18.6
liver R16.0
  acute K76.89
  congenital Q44.7
  cirrhotic - *see* Cirrhosis, liver
  fatty - *see* Fatty, liver
lymph, lymphatic gland R59.9
  generalized R59.1
  localized R59.0
  tuberculous - *see* Tuberculosis, lymph gland
mammary gland - *see* Hypertrophy, breast
Meckel's diverticulum (congenital) Q43.0
  malignant - *see* Table of Neoplasms, small intestine, malignant
median bar - *see* Hyperplasia, prostate
meibomian gland - *see* Chalazion
meniscus, knee, congenital Q74.1
metatarsal head - *see* Hypertrophy, bone, metatarsus
metatarsus - *see* Hypertrophy, bone, metatarsus
mucous membrane
  alveolar ridge K06.2
  gum K06.1
  nose (turbinate) J34.3
muscle M62.89
muscular coat, artery I77.89
myocardium - *see also* Hypertrophy, cardiac
  idiopathic I42.2
myometrium N85.2
nail L60.2
  congenital Q84.5
nasal J34.89
  alae J34.89
  bone J34.89
  cartilage J34.89
  mucous membrane (septum) J34.3
  sinus J34.89
  turbinate J34.3
nasopharynx, lymphoid (infectional) (tissue) (wall) J35.2
nipple N62
organ or site, congenital NEC - *see* Anomaly, by site
ovary N83.8
palate (hard) M27.8
  soft K13.79
pancreas, congenital Q45.3
parathyroid (gland) E21.0
parotid gland K11.1
penis N48.89
pharyngeal tonsil J35.2
pharynx J39.2
  lymphoid (infectional) (tissue) (wall) J35.2
pituitary (anterior) (fossa) (gland) E23.6
prepuce (congenital) N47.8
  female N90.89

Hypertrophy, hypertrophic - *continued*
prostate - *see* Enlargement, enlarged, prostate
  congenital Q55.4
pseudomuscular G71.0
pylorus (adult) (muscle) (sphincter) K31.1
  congenital or infantile Q40.0
rectal, rectum (sphincter) K62.89
rhinitis (turbinate) J31.0
salivary gland (any) K11.1
  congenital Q38.4
scaphoid (tarsal) - *see* Hypertrophy, bone, tarsus
scar L91.0
scrotum N50.89
seminal vesicle N50.89
sigmoid - *see* Megacolon
skin L91.9
  specified NEC L91.8
spermatic cord N50.89
spleen - *see* Splenomegaly
spondylitis - *see* Spondylosis
stomach K31.89
sublingual gland K11.1
submandibular gland K11.1
suprarenal cortex (gland) E27.8
synovial NEC M67.20
  acromioclavicular M67.21-
  ankle M67.27-
  elbow M67.22-
  foot M67.27-
  hand M67.24-
  hip M67.25-
  knee M67.26-
  multiple sites M67.29
  specified site NEC M67.28
  wrist M67.23-
tendon - *see* Disorder, tendon, specified type NEC
testis N44.8
  congenital Q55.29
thymic, thymus (gland) (congenital) E32.0
thyroid (gland) - *see* Goiter
toe (congenital) Q74.2
  acquired - *see also* Deformity, toe, specified NEC
tongue K14.8
  congenital Q38.2
  papillae (foliate) K14.3
tonsils (faucial) (infective) (lingual) (lymphoid) J35.1
  with adenoids J35.3
tunica vaginalis N50.89
ureter N28.89
urethra N36.8
uterus N85.2
  neck (with elongation) N88.4
  puerperal O90.89
uvula K13.79
vagina N89.8
vas deferens N50.89
vein I87.8
ventricle, ventricular (heart) - *see also* Hypertrophy, cardiac
  congenital Q24.8
  in tetralogy of Fallot Q21.3
verumontanum N36.8
vocal cord J38.3
vulva N90.60
  stasis (nonfilarial) N90.69
Hypertropia H50.2-
Hypertyrosinemia E70.21
Hyperuricemia (asymptomatic) E79.0
Hypervalinemia E71.19

Hyperventilation (tetany) R06.4
hysterical F45.8
psychogenic F45.8
syndrome F45.8
Hypervitaminosis (dietary) NEC E67.8
A E67.0
  administered as drug (prolonged intake) - *see* Table of Drugs and Chemicals, vitamins, adverse effect
  overdose or wrong substance given or taken - *see* Table of Drugs and Chemicals, vitamins, poisoning
B6 E67.2
D E67.3
  administered as drug (prolonged intake) - *see* Table of Drugs and Chemicals, vitamins, adverse effect
  overdose or wrong substance given or taken - *see* Table of Drugs and Chemicals, vitamins, poisoning
K E67.8
  administered as drug (prolonged intake) - *see* Table of Drugs and Chemicals, vitamins, adverse effect
  overdose or wrong substance given or taken - *see* Table of Drugs and Chemicals, vitamins, poisoning
Hypervolemia E87.70
specified NEC E87.79
Hypesthesia R20.1
cornea - *see* Anesthesia, cornea
Hyphema H21.0-
traumatic S05.1-
Hypoacidity, gastric K31.89
psychogenic F45.8
Hypoadrenalism, hypoadrenia E27.40
primary E27.1
tuberculous A18.7
Hypoadrenocorticism E27.40
pituitary E23.0
primary E27.1
Hypoalbuminemia E88.09
Hypoaldosteronism E27.40
Hypoalphalipoproteinemia E78.6
Hypobarism T70.29
Hypobaropathy T70.29
Hypobetalipoproteinemia (familial) E78.6
Hypocalcemia E83.51
dietary E58
neonatal P71.1
  due to cow's milk P71.0
  phosphate-loading (newborn) P71.1
Hypochloremia E87.8
Hypochlorhydria K31.89
neurotic F45.8
psychogenic F45.8
Hypochondria, hypochondriac, hypochondriasis (reaction) F45.21
sleep F51.03
Hypochondrogenesis Q77.0
Hypochondroplasia Q77.4
Hypochromasia, blood cells D50.8
Hypodontia - *see* Anodontia
Hypoeosinophilia D72.89
Hypoesthesia R20.1
Hypofibrinogenemia D68.8
acquired D65
congenital (hereditary) D68.2
Hypofunction
adrenocortical E27.40
  drug-induced E27.3
  postprocedural E89.6
  primary E27.1
adrenomedullary, postprocedural E89.6

Hypofunction - *continued*
cerebral R29.818
corticoadrenal NEC E27.40
intestinal K59.8
labyrinth - *see* subcategory H83.2
ovary E28.39
pituitary (gland) (anterior) E23.0
testicular E29.1
postprocedural (postsurgical)
(postirradiation) (iatrogenic) E89.5
Hypogalactia O92.4
Hypogammaglobulinemia - *see also*
Agammaglobulinemia D80.1
hereditary D80.0
nonfamilial D80.1
transient, of infancy D80.7
Hypogenitalism (congenital) - *see*
Hypogonadism
Hypoglossia Q38.3
Hypoglycemia (spontaneous) E16.2
coma E15
diabetic *see* Diabetes, by type, with
hypoglycemia, with coma
diabetic - *see* Diabetes, hypoglycemia
dietary counseling and surveillance Z71.3
drug-induced E16.0
with coma (nondiabetic) E15
due to insulin E16.0
with coma (nondiabetic) E15
therapeutic misadventure *see* subcategory
T38.3
functional, nonhyperinsulinemic E16.1
iatrogenic E16.0
with coma (nondiabetic) E15
in infant of diabetic mother P70.1
gestational diabetes P70.0
infantile E16.1
leucine-induced E71.19
neonatal (transitory) P70.4
iatrogenic P70.3
reactive (not drug-induced) E16.1
transitory neonatal P70.4
Hypogonadism
female E28.39
hypogonadotropic E23.0
male E29.1
ovarian (primary) E28.39
pituitary E23.0
testicular (primary) E29.1
Hypohidrosis, hypoidrosis L74.4
Hypoinsulinemia, postprocedural E89.1
Hypokalemia E87.6
Hypoleukocytosis - *see* Agranulocytosis
Hypolipoproteinemia (alpha) (beta) E78.6
Hypomagnesemia E83.42
neonatal P71.2
Hypomania, hypomanic reaction F30.8
Hypomenorrhea - *see* Oligomenorrhea
Hypometabolism R63.8
Hypomotility
gastrointestinal (tract) K31.89
psychogenic F45.8
intestine K59.8
psychogenic F45.8
stomach K31.89
psychogenic F45.8
Hyponasality R49.22
Hyponatremia E87.1
Hypo-osmolality E87.1
Hypo-ovarianism, hypo-ovarism E28.39
Hypoparathyroidism E20.9
familial E20.8
idiopathic E20.0
neonatal, transitory P71.4

Hypoparathyroidism - *continued*
postprocedural E89.2
specified NEC E20.8
Hypoperfusion (in)
newborn P96.89
Hypopharyngitis - *see* Laryngopharyngitis
Hypophoria H50.53
**Hypophosphatemia, hypophosphatasia
(acquired) (congenital) (renal)** E83.39
familial E83.31
Hypophyseal, hypophysis - *see also* condition
dwarfism E23.0
gigantism E22.0
Hypopiesis - *see* Hypotension
Hypopinealism E34.8
Hypopituitarism (juvenile) E23.0
drug-induced E23.1
due to
hypophysectomy E89.3
radiotherapy E89.3
iatrogenic NEC E23.1
postirradiation E89.3
postpartum O99.285
postprocedural E89.3
Hypoplasia, hypoplastic
adrenal (gland), congenital Q89.1
alimentary tract, congenital Q45.8
upper Q40.8
anus, anal (canal) Q42.3
with fistula Q42.2
aorta, aortic Q25.42
ascending, in hypoplastic left heart syndrome
Q23.4
valve Q23.1
in hypoplastic left heart syndrome Q23.4
areola, congenital Q83.8
arm (congenital) - *see* Defect, reduction, upper
limb
artery (peripheral) Q27.8
brain (congenital) Q28.3
coronary Q24.5
digestive system Q27.8
lower limb Q27.8
pulmonary Q25.79
functional, unilateral J43.0
retinal (congenital) Q14.1
specified site NEC Q27.8
umbilical Q27.0
upper limb Q27.8
auditory canal Q17.8
causing impairment of hearing Q16.9
biliary duct or passage Q44.5
bone NOS Q79.9
face Q75.8
marrow D61.9
megakaryocytic D69.49
skull - *see* Hypoplasia, skull
brain Q02
gyri Q04.3
part of Q04.3
breast (areola) N64.82
bronchus Q32.4
cardiac Q24.8
carpus - *see* Defect, reduction, upper limb,
specified type NEC
cartilage hair Q78.8
cecum Q42.8
cementum K00.4
cephalic Q02
cerebellum Q04.3
cervix (uteri), congenital Q51.821
clavicle (congenital) Q74.0
coccyx Q76.49
colon Q42.9

Hypoplasia, hypoplastic - *continued*
specified NEC Q42.8
corpus callosum Q04.0
cricoid cartilage Q31.2
digestive organ(s) or tract NEC Q45.8
upper (congenital) Q40.8
ear (auricle) (lobe) Q17.2
middle Q16.4
enamel of teeth (neonatal) (postnatal)
(prenatal) K00.4
endocrine (gland) NEC Q89.2
endometrium N85.8
epididymis (congenital) Q55.4
epiglottis Q31.2
erythroid, congenital D61.01
esophagus (congenital) Q39.8
eustachian tube Q17.8
eye Q11.2
eyelid (congenital) Q10.3
face Q18.8
bone(s) Q75.8
femur (congenital) - *see* Defect, reduction,
lower limb, specified type NEC
fibula (congenital) - *see* Defect, reduction,
lower limb, specified type NEC
finger (congenital) - *see* Defect, reduction,
upper limb, specified type NEC
focal dermal Q82.8
foot - *see* Defect, reduction, lower limb,
specified type NEC
gallbladder Q44.0
genitalia, genital organ(s)
female, congenital Q52.8
external Q52.79
internal NEC Q52.8
in adiposogenital dystrophy E23.6
glottis Q31.2
hair Q84.2
hand (congenital) - *see* Defect, reduction,
upper limb, specified type NEC
heart Q24.8
humerus (congenital) - *see* Defect, reduction,
upper limb, specified type NEC
intestine (small) Q41.9
large Q42.9
specified NEC Q42.8
jaw M26.09
alveolar M26.79
lower M26.04
alveolar M26.74
upper M26.02
alveolar M26.73
kidney(s) Q60.5
bilateral Q60.4
unilateral Q60.3
labium (majus) (minus), congenital Q52.79
larynx Q31.2
left heart syndrome Q23.4
leg (congenital) - *see* Defect, reduction, lower
limb
limb Q73.8
lower (congenital) - *see* Defect, reduction,
lower limb
upper (congenital) - *see* Defect, reduction,
upper limb
liver Q44.7
lung (lobe) (not associated with short
gestation) Q33.6
associated with immaturity, low birth weight,
prematurity, or short gestation P28.0
mammary (areola), congenital Q83.8
mandible, mandibular M26.04
alveolar M26.74
unilateral condylar M27.8

Hypoplasia, hypoplastic - *continued*
  maxillary M26.02
    alveolar M26.73
  medullary D61.9
  megakaryocytic D69.49
  metacarpus - *see* Defect, reduction, upper limb, specified type NEC
  metatarsus - *see* Defect, reduction, lower limb, specified type NEC
  muscle Q79.8
  nail(s) Q84.6
  nose, nasal Q30.1
  optic nerve H47.03-
  osseous meatus (ear) Q17.8
  ovary, congenital Q50.39
  pancreas Q45.0
  parathyroid (gland) Q89.2
  parotid gland Q38.4
  patella Q74.1
  pelvis, pelvic girdle Q74.2
  penis (congenital) Q55.62
  peripheral vascular system Q27.8
    digestive system Q27.8
    lower limb Q27.8
    specified site NEC Q27.8
    upper limb Q27.8
  pituitary (gland) (congenital) Q89.2
  pulmonary (not associated with short gestation) Q33.6
    artery, functional J43.0
    associated with short gestation P28.0
  radioulnar - *see* Defect, reduction, upper limb, specified type NEC
  radius - *see* Defect, reduction, upper limb
  rectum Q42.1
    with fistula Q42.0
  respiratory system NEC Q34.8
  rib Q76.6
  right heart syndrome Q22.6
  sacrum Q76.49
  scapula Q74.0
  scrotum Q55.1
  shoulder girdle Q74.0
  skin Q82.8
  skull (bone) Q75.8
    with
      anencephaly Q00.0
      encephalocele - *see* Encephalocele
      hydrocephalus Q03.9
        with spina bifida - *see* Spina bifida, by site, with hydrocephalus
      microcephaly Q02
  spinal (cord) (ventral horn cell) Q06.1
  spine Q76.49
  sternum Q76.7
  tarsus - *see* Defect, reduction, lower limb, specified type NEC
  testis Q55.1
  thymic, with immunodeficiency D82.1
  thymus (gland) Q89.2
    with immunodeficiency D82.1
  thyroid (gland) E03.1
    cartilage Q31.2
  tibiofibular (congenital) - *see* Defect, reduction, lower limb, specified type NEC
  toe - *see* Defect, reduction, lower limb, specified type NEC
  tongue Q38.3
  Turner's K00.4
  ulna (congenital) - *see* Defect, reduction, upper limb
  umbilical artery Q27.0
  unilateral condylar M27.8
  ureter Q62.8

Hypoplasia, hypoplastic - *continued*
  uterus, congenital Q51.811
  vagina Q52.4
  vascular NEC peripheral Q27.8
    brain Q28.3
    digestive system Q27.8
    lower limb Q27.8
    specified site NEC Q27.8
    upper limb Q27.8
  vein(s) (peripheral) Q27.8
    brain Q28.3
    digestive system Q27.8
    great Q26.8
    lower limb Q27.8
    specified site NEC Q27.8
    upper limb Q27.8
  vena cava (inferior) (superior) Q26.8
  vertebra Q76.49
  vulva, congenital Q52.79
  zonule (ciliary) Q12.8
Hypopnea, obstructive sleep apnea G47.33
Hypopotassemia E87.6
Hypoproconvertinemia, congenital (hereditary) D68.2
Hypoproteinemia E77.8
Hypoprothrombinemia (congenital) (hereditary) (idiopathic) D68.2
  acquired D68.4
  newborn, transient P61.6
Hypoptyalism K11.7
Hypopyon (eye) (anterior chamber) - *see* Iridocyclitis, acute, hypopyon
Hypopyrexia R68.0
Hyporeflexia R29.2
Hyposecretion
  ACTH E23.0
  antidiuretic hormone E23.2
  ovary E28.39
  salivary gland (any) K11.7
  vasopressin E23.2
Hyposegmentation, leukocytic, hereditary D72.0
Hyposiderinemia D50.9
Hypospadias Q54.9
  balanic Q54.0
  coronal Q54.0
  glandular Q54.0
  penile Q54.1
  penoscrotal Q54.2
  perineal Q54.3
  specified NEC Q54.8
Hypospermatogenesis - *see* Oligospermia
Hyposplenism D73.0
Hypostasis pulmonary, passive - *see* Edema, lung
Hypostatic - *see* condition
Hyposthenuria N28.89
Hypotension (arterial) (constitutional) I95.9
  chronic I95.89
  due to (of) hemodialysis I95.3
  drug-induced I95.2
  iatrogenic I95.89
  idiopathic (permanent) I95.0
  intracranial, following ventricular shunting (ventriculostomy) G97.2
  intra-dialytic I95.3
  maternal, syndrome (following labor and delivery) O26.5-
  neurogenic, orthostatic G90.3
  orthostatic (chronic) I95.1
    due to drugs I95.2
    neurogenic G90.3
  postoperative I95.81
  postural I95.1
  specified NEC I95.89

Hypothermia (accidental) T68
  due to anesthesia, anesthetic T88.51
  low environmental temperature T68
  neonatal P80.9
    environmental (mild) NEC P80.8
    mild P80.8
    severe (chronic) (cold injury syndrome) P80.0
    specified NEC P80.8
  not associated with low environmental temperature R68.0
Hypothyroidism (acquired) E03.9
  autoimmune *see* Thyroiditis, autoimmune
  congenital (without goiter) E03.1
    with goiter (diffuse) E03.0
  due to
    exogenous substance NEC E03.2
    iodine-deficiency, acquired E01.8
      subclinical E02
    irradiation therapy E89.0
    medicament NEC E03.2
    P-aminosalicylic acid (PAS) E03.2
    phenylbutazone E03.2
    resorcinol E03.2
    sulfonamide E03.2
    surgery E89.0
    thiourea group drugs E03.2
  iatrogenic NEC E03.2
  iodine-deficiency (acquired) E01.8
    congenital - *see* Syndrome, iodine deficiency, congenital
    subclinical E02
  neonatal, transitory P72.2
  postinfectious E03.3
  postirradiation E89.0
  postprocedural E89.0
  postsurgical E89.0
  specified NEC E03.8
  subclinical, iodine-deficiency related E02
Hypotonia, hypotonicity, hypotony
  bladder N31.2
  congenital (benign) P94.2
  eye - *see* Disorder, globe, hypotony
Hypotrichosis - *see* Alopecia
Hypotropia H50.2-
Hypoventilation R06.89
  congenital central alveolar G47.35
  sleep related
    idiopathic nonobstructive alveolar G47.34
    in conditions classified elsewhere G47.36
Hypovitaminosis - *see* Deficiency, vitamin
Hypovolemia E86.1
  surgical shock T81.19
  traumatic (shock) T79.4
Hypoxemia R09.02
  newborn P84
  sleep related, in conditions classified elsewhere G47.36
Hypoxia - *see also* Anoxia R09.02
  cerebral, during a procedure NEC G97.81
    postprocedural NEC G97.82
  intrauterine P84
  myocardial - *see* Insufficiency, coronary
  newborn P84
  sleep-related G47.34
Hypsarrhythmia - *see* Epilepsy, generalized, specified NEC
Hysteralgia, pregnant uterus O26.89-
Hysteria, hysterical (conversion) (dissociative state) F44.9
  anxiety F41.8
  convulsions F44.5
  psychosis, acute F44.9
Hysteroepilepsy F44.5

I

IBDU (colonic inflammatory bowel disease unclassified) K52.3
Ichthyoparasitism due to Vandellia cirrhosa B88.8
Ichthyosis (congenital) Q80.9
  acquired L85.0
  fetalis Q80.4
  hystrix Q80.8
  lamellar Q80.2
  lingual K13.29
  palmaris and plantaris Q82.8
  simplex Q80.0
  vera Q80.8
  vulgaris Q80.0
  X-linked Q80.1
Ichthyotoxism - *see* Poisoning, fish
  bacterial - *see* Intoxication, foodborne
Icteroanemia, hemolytic (acquired) D59.9
  congenital - *see* Spherocytosis
Icterus - *see also* Jaundice
  conjunctiva R17
  newborn P59.9
  gravis, newborn P55.0
  hematogenous (acquired) D59.9
  hemolytic (acquired) D59.9
    congenital - *see* Spherocytosis
  hemorrhagic (acute) (leptospiral) (spirochetal) A27.0
    newborn P53
  infectious B15.9
    with hepatic coma B15.0
    leptospiral A27.0
    spirochetal A27.0
  neonatorum - *see* Jaundice, newborn
  spirochetal A27.0
Ictus solaris, solis T67.0
Ideation
  homicidal R45.850
  suicidal R45.851
Identity disorder (child) F64.9
  gender role F64.2
  psychosexual F64.2
Id reaction (due to bacteria) L30.2
Idioglossia F80.0
Idiopathic - *see* condition
Idiot, idiocy (congenital) F73
  amaurotic (Bielschowsky(-Jansky)) (family) (infantile (late)) (juvenile (late)) (Vogt-Spielmeyer) E75.4
  microcephalic Q02
IgE asthma J45.909
IIAC (idiopathic infantile arterial calcification) Q28.8
Ileitis (chronic) (noninfectious) - *see also* Enteritis K52.9
  backwash - *see* Pancolitis, ulcerative (chronic)
  infectious A09
  regional (ulcerative) - *see* Enteritis, regional, small intestine
  segmental - *see* Enteritis, regional
  terminal (ulcerative) - *see* Enteritis, regional, small intestine
Ileocolitis - *see also* Enteritis K52.9
  regional - *see* Enteritis, regional
  infectious A09
  ulcerative K51.0-
Ileostomy
  attention to Z43.2
  malfunctioning K94.13
  status Z93.2
    with complication - *see* Complications, enterostomy

Ileotyphus - *see* Typhoid
Ileum - *see* condition
Ileus (bowel) (colon) (inhibitory) (intestine) K56.7
  adynamic K56.0
  due to gallstone (in intestine) K56.3
  duodenal (chronic) K31.5
  gallstone K56.3
  mechanical NEC (see also Obstruction, intestine, specified NEC) K56.699
  meconium P76.0
    in cystic fibrosis E84.11
    meaning meconium plug (without cystic fibrosis) P76.0
  myxedema K59.8
  neurogenic K56.0
    Hirschsprung's disease or megacolon Q43.1
  newborn
    due to meconium P76.0
      in cystic fibrosis E84.11
      meaning meconium plug (without cystic fibrosis) P76.0
    transitory P76.1
  obstructive (see also Obstruction, intestine, specified NEC) K56.699
  postoperative K91.89
  paralytic K56.0
Iliac - *see* condition
Iliotibial band syndrome M76.3-
Illiteracy Z55.0
Illness - *see also* Disease R69
  manic-depressive - *see* Disorder, bipolar
Imbalance R26.89
  autonomic G90.8
  constituents of food intake E63.1
  electrolyte E87.8
    with
      abortion - *see* Abortion by type, complicated by, electrolyte imbalance
      molar pregnancy O08.5
    due to hyperemesis gravidarum O21.1
    following ectopic or molar pregnancy O08.5
    neonatal, transitory NEC P74.4
      potassium P74.3
      sodium P74.2
  endocrine E34.9
  eye muscle NOS H50.9
  hormone E34.9
  hysterical F44.4
  labyrinth - *see* subcategory H83.2
  posture R29.3
  protein-energy - *see* Malnutrition
  sympathetic G90.8
Imbecile, imbecility (I.Q.35 49) F71
Imbedding, intrauterine device T83.39
Imbibition, cholesterol (gallbladder) K82.4
Imbrication, teeth,, fully erupted M26.30
Imerslund (-Grasbeck) syndrome D51.1
Immature - *see also* Immaturity
  birth (less than 37
  completed weeks) - *see* Preterm, newborn
    extremely (less than 28
  completed weeks) - *see* Immaturity, extreme
  personality F60.89
Immaturity (less than 37 completed weeks) - *see also* Preterm, newborn
  extreme of newborn (less than 28
  completed weeks of gestation) (less than 196
  completed days of gestation)
  (unspecified weeks of gestation) P07.20
    gestational age
      23 completed weeks (23 weeks, 0 days through 23 weeks, 6 days) P07.22
      24 completed weeks (24 weeks, 0 days

Immaturity - *continued*
      through 24 weeks, 6 days) P07.23
      25 completed weeks (25 weeks, 0 days through 25 weeks, 6 days) P07.24
      26 completed weeks (26 weeks, 0 days through 26 weeks, 6 days) P07.25
      27 completed weeks (27 weeks, 0 days through 27 weeks, 6 days) P07.26
      less than 23 completed weeks P07.21
  fetus or infant light-for-dates - *see* Light-for-dates
  lung, newborn P28.0
  organ or site NEC - *see* Hypoplasia
  pulmonary, newborn P28.0
  reaction F60.89
  sexual (female) (male), after puberty E30.0
Immersion T75.1
  hand T69.01-
  foot T69.02-
Immobile, immobility
  complete, due to severe physical disability or frailty R53.2
  intestine K59.8
  syndrome (paraplegic) M62.3
Immune reconstitution (inflammatory) syndrome [IRIS] D89.3
Immunization - *see also* Vaccination
  ABO - *see* Incompatibility, ABO
    in newborn P55.1
  complication - *see* Complications, vaccination
  encounter for Z23
  not done (not carried out) Z28.9
    because (of)
      acute illness of patient Z28.01
      allergy to vaccine (or component) Z28.04
      caregiver refusal Z28.82
      chronic illness of patient Z28.02
      contraindication NEC Z28.09
      group pressure Z28.1
      guardian refusal Z28.82
      immune compromised state of patient Z28.03
      parent refusal Z28.82
      patient's belief Z28.1
      patient had disease being vaccinated against Z28.81
      patient refusal Z28.21
      religious beliefs of patient Z28.1
      specified reason NEC Z28.89
        of patient Z28.29
      unspecified patient reason Z28.20
  Rh factor
    affecting management of pregnancy NEC O36.09-
      anti-d antibody O36.01-
    from transfusion - *see* Complication(s), transfusion, incompatibility reaction, Rh (factor)
Immunocytoma C83.0-
Immunodeficiency D84.9
  with
    adenosine-deaminase deficiency D81.3
    antibody defects D80.9
      specified type NEC D80.8
    hyperimmunoglobulinemia D80.6
    increased immunoglobulin M (IgM) D80.5
    major defect D82.9
      specified type NEC D82.8
    partial albinism D82.8
    short-limbed stature D82.2
    thrombocytopenia and eczema D82.0
  antibody with
    hyperimmunoglobulinemia D80.6
    near normal immunoglobulins D80.6

Immunodeficiency - *continued*
 autosomal recessive, Swiss type D80.0
 combined D81.9
  biotin-dependent carboxylase D81.819
   biotinidase D81.810
   holocarboxylase synthetase D81.818
   specified type NEC D81.818
  severe (SCID) D81.9
   with
    low or normal B-cell numbers D81.2
    low T and B-cell numbers D81.1
    reticular dysgenesis D81.0
  specified type NEC D81.89
 common variable D83.9
  with
   abnormalities of B-cell numbers and
    function D83.0
   autoantibodies to B or T-cells D83.2
   immunoregulatory T-cell disorders D83.1
  specified type NEC D83.8
 following hereditary defective response to
  Epstein-Barr virus (EBV) D82.3
 selective, immunoglobulin
  A (IgA) D80.2
  G (IgG) (subclasses) D80.3
  M (IgM) D80.4
 severe combined (SCID) D81.9
 specified type NEC D84.8
 X-linked, with increased IgM D80.5
Immunotherapy (encounter for)
 antineoplastic Z51.12
Impaction, impacted
 bowel, colon, rectum - *see also* Impaction,
  fecal K56.49
  by gallstone K56.3
 calculus - *see* Calculus
 cerumen (ear) (external) H61.2-
 cuspid - *see* Impaction, tooth
 dental (same or adjacent tooth) K01.1
 fecal, feces K56.41
 fracture - *see* Fracture, by site
 gallbladder - *see* Calculus, gallbladder
 gallstone(s) - *see* Calculus, gallbladder
  bile duct (common) (hepatic) - *see* Calculus,
   bile duct
  cystic duct - *see* Calculus, gallbladder
  in intestine, with obstruction (any part) K56.3
 intestine (calculous) NEC - *see also* Impaction,
  fecal K56.49
  gallstone, with ileus K56.3
 intrauterine device (IUD) T83.39
 molar - *see* Impaction, tooth
 shoulder, causing obstructed labor O66.0
 tooth, teeth K01.1
 turbinate J34.89
Impaired, impairment (function)
 auditory discrimination - *see* Abnormal,
  auditory perception
 cognitive, mild, so stated G31.84
 dual sensory Z73.82
 fasting glucose R73.01
 glucose tolerance (oral) R73.02
 hearing - *see* Deafness
 heart - *see* Disease, heart
 kidney N28.9
  disorder resulting from N25.9
   specified NEC N25.89
 liver K72.90
  with coma K72.91
 mastication K08.89
 mild cognitive, so stated G31.84
 mobility
  ear ossicles - *see* Ankylosis, ear ossicles
  requiring care provider Z74.09

Impaired, impairment - *continued*
 myocardium, myocardial - *see* Insufficiency,
  myocardial
 rectal sphincter R19.8
 renal (acute) (chronic) N28.9
  disorder resulting from N25.9
   specified NEC N25.89
 vision NEC H54.7
  both eyes H54.3
Impediment, speech R47.9
 psychogenic (childhood) F98.8
 slurring R47.81
 specified NEC R47.89
Impending
 coronary syndrome I20.0
 delirium tremens F10.239
 myocardial infarction I20.0
Imperception auditory (acquired) - *see also*
 Deafness
 congenital H93.25
Imperfect
 aeration, lung (newborn) NEC - *see* Atelectasis
 closure (congenital)
  alimentary tract NEC Q45.8
   lower Q43.8
   upper Q40.8
  atrioventricular ostium Q21.2
  atrium (secundum) Q21.1
  branchial cleft NOS Q18.2
   cyst Q18.0
   fistula Q18.0
   sinus Q18.0
  choroid Q14.3
  cricoid cartilage Q31.8
  cusps, heart valve NEC Q24.8
   pulmonary Q22.3
  ductus
   arteriosus Q25.0
   Botalli Q25.0
  ear drum (causing impairment of hearing)
   Q16.4
  esophagus with communication to bronchus
   or trachea Q39.1
  eyelid Q10.3
  foramen
   botalli Q21.1
   ovale Q21.1
  genitalia, genital organ(s) or system
   female Q52.8
    external Q52.79
    internal NEC Q52.8
   male Q55.8
  glottis Q31.8
  interatrial ostium or septum Q21.1
  interauricular ostium or septum Q21.1
  interventricular ostium or septum Q21.0
  larynx Q31.8
  lip - *see* Cleft, lip
  nasal septum Q30.3
  nose Q30.2
  omphalomesenteric duct Q43.0
  optic nerve entry Q14.2
  organ or site not listed - *see* Anomaly, by site
  ostium
   interatrial Q21.1
   interauricular Q21.1
   interventricular Q21.0
  palate - *see* Cleft, palate
  preauricular sinus Q18.1
  retina Q14.1
  roof of orbit Q75.8
  sclera Q13.5
  septum
   aorticopulmonary Q21.4

Imperfect - *continued*
  atrial (secundum) Q21.1
  between aorta and pulmonary artery Q21.4
  heart Q21.9
  interatrial (secundum) Q21.1
  interauricular (secundum) Q21.1
  interventricular Q21.0
   in tetralogy of Fallot Q21.3
  nasal Q30.3
  ventricular Q21.0
   with pulmonary stenosis or atresia,
    dextroposition of aorta, and hypertrophy
    of right ventricle Q21.3
   in tetralogy of Fallot Q21.3
  skull Q75.0
   with
    anencephaly Q00.0
    encephalocele - *see* Encephalocele
    hydrocephalus Q03.9
     with spina bifida - *see* Spina bifida, by
      site, with hydrocephalus
    microcephaly Q02
  spine (with meningocele) - *see* Spina bifida
  trachea Q32.1
  tympanic membrane (causing impairment of
   hearing) Q16.4
  uterus Q51.818
  vitelline duct Q43.0
 erection - *see* Dysfunction, sexual, male,
  erectile
 fusion - *see* Imperfect, closure
 inflation, lung (newborn) - *see* Atelectasis
 posture R29.3
 rotation, intestine Q43.3
 septum, ventricular Q21.0
Imperfectly descended testis - *see* Cryptorchid
Imperforate (congenital) - *see also* Atresia
 anus Q42.3
  with fistula Q42.2
 cervix (uteri) Q51.828
 esophagus Q39.0
  with tracheoesophageal fistula Q39.1
 hymen Q52.3
 jejunum Q41.1
 pharynx Q38.8
 rectum Q42.1
  with fistula Q42.0
 urethra Q64.39
 vagina Q52.4
Impervious (congenital) - *see also* Atresia
 anus Q42.3
  with fistula Q42.2
 bile duct Q44.2
 esophagus Q39.0
  with tracheoesophageal fistula Q39.1
 intestine (small) Q41.9
  large Q42.9
   specified NEC Q42.8
 rectum Q42.1
  with fistula Q42.0
 ureter - *see* Atresia, ureter
 urethra Q64.39
Impetiginization of dermatoses L01.1
Impetigo (any organism) (any site) (circinate)
(contagiosa) (simplex) (vulgaris) L01.00
 Bockhart's L01.02
 bullous, bullosa L01.03
 external ear L01.00 [*H62.40*]
 follicularis L01.02
 furfuracea L30.5
 herpetiformis L40.1
  nonobstetrical L40.1
 neonatorum L01.03
 nonbullous L01.01

Impetigo - *continued*
specified type NEC L01.09
ulcerative L01.09
Impingement (on teeth)
soft tissue
anterior M26.81
posterior M26.82
Implant, endometrial N80.9
Implantation
anomalous - *see* Anomaly, by site
ureter Q62.63
cyst
external area or site (skin) NEC L72.0
iris - *see* Cyst, iris, implantation
vagina N89.8
vulva N90.7
dermoid (cyst) - *see* Implantation, cyst
Impotence (sexual) N52.9
counseling Z70.1
organic origin - *see also* Dysfunction, sexual,
male, erectile N52.9
psychogenic F52.21
Impression, basilar Q75.8
Imprisonment, anxiety concerning Z65.1
Improper care (child) (newborn) - *see*
Maltreatment
**Improperly tied umbilical cord (causing
hemorrhage)** P51.8
Impulsiveness (impulsive) R45.87
Inability to swallow - *see* Aphagia
Inaccessible, inaccessibility
health care NEC Z75.3
due to
waiting period Z75.2
for admission to facility elsewhere Z75.1
other helping agencies Z75.4
Inactive - *see* condition
Inadequate, inadequacy
aesthetics of dental restoration K08.56
biologic, constitutional, functional, or social
F60.7
development
child R62.50
genitalia
after puberty NEC E30.0
congenital
female Q52.8
external Q52.79
internal Q52.8
male Q55.8
lungs Q33.6
associated with short gestation P28.0
organ or site not listed - *see* Anomaly, by site
diet (causing nutritional deficiency) E63.9
eating habits Z72.4
environment, household Z59.1
family support Z63.8
food (supply) NEC Z59.4
hunger effects T73.0
functional F60.7
household care, due to
family member
handicapped or ill Z74.2
on vacation Z75.5
temporarily away from home Z74.2
technical defects in home Z59.1
temporary absence from home of person
rendering care Z74.2
housing (heating) (space) Z59.1
income (financial) Z59.6
intrafamilial communication Z63.8
material resources Z59.9
mental - *see* Disability, intellectual
parental supervision or control of child Z62.0

Inadequate, inadequacy - *continued*
personality F60.7
pulmonary
function R06.89
newborn P28.5
ventilation, newborn P28.5
sample of cytologic smear
anus R85.615
cervix R87.615
vagina R87.625
social F60.7
insurance Z59.7
skills NEC Z73.4
supervision of child by parent Z62.0
teaching affecting education Z55.8
welfare support Z59.7
Inanition R64
with edema - *see* Malnutrition, severe
due to
deprivation of food T73.0
malnutrition - *see* Malnutrition
fever R50.9
Inappropriate
change in quantitative human chorionic
gonadotropin (hCG) in early pregnancy
O02.81
diet or eating habits Z72.4
level of quantitative human chorionic
gonadotropin (hCG) for gestational age in
early pregnancy O02.81
secretion
antidiuretic hormone (ADH) (excessive)
E22.2
deficiency E23.2
pituitary (posterior) E22.2
Inattention at or after birth - *see* Neglect
Incarceration, incarcerated
enterocele K46.0
gangrenous K46.1
epiplocele K46.0
gangrenous K46.1
exomphalos K42.0
gangrenous K42.1
hernia - *see also* Hernia, by site, with
obstruction
with gangrene - *see* Hernia, by site, with
gangrene
iris, in wound - *see* Injury, eye, laceration,
with prolapse
lens, in wound - *see* Injury, eye, laceration,
with prolapse
omphalocele K42.0
prison, anxiety concerning Z65.1
rupture - *see* Hernia, by site
sarcoepiplocele K46.0
gangrenous K46.1
sarcoepiplomphalocele K42.0
with gangrene K42.1
uterus N85.8
gravid O34.51-
causing obstructed labor O65.5
Incised wound
external - *see* Laceration
internal organs - *see* Injury, by site
Incision, incisional
hernia K43.2
with
gangrene (and obstruction) K43.1
obstruction K43.0
surgical, complication - *see* Complications,
surgical procedure
traumatic
external - *see* Laceration
internal organs - *see* Injury, by site

Inclusion
azurophilic leukocytic D72.0
blennorrhea (neonatal) (newborn) P39.1
gallbladder in liver (congenital) Q44.1
Incompatibility
ABO
affecting management of pregnancy O36.11-
anti-a sensitization O36.11-
anti-b sensitization O36.19-
specified NEC O36.19-
infusion or transfusion reaction - *see*
Complication(s), transfusion, incompatibility
reaction, ABO
newborn P55.1
blood (group) (Duffy) (K(ell)) (Kidd) (Lewis)
(M) (S) NEC
affecting management of pregnancy O36.11-
anti-a sensitization O36.11-
anti-b sensitization O36.19
infusion or transfusion reaction T80.89
newborn P55.8
divorce or estrangement Z63.5
Rh (blood group) (factor) Z31.82
affecting management of pregnancy NEC
O36.09-
anti-d antibody O36.01-
infusion or transfusion reaction - *see*
Complication(s), transfusion,
incompatibility reaction, Rh (factor)
newborn P55.0
rhesus - *see* Incompatibility, Rh
Incompetency, incompetent, incompetence
annular
aortic (valve) - *see* Insufficiency, aortic
mitral (valve) I34.0
pulmonary valve (heart) I37.1
aortic (valve) - *see* Insufficiency, aortic
cardiac valve - *see* Endocarditis
cervix, cervical (os) N88.3
in pregnancy O34.3-
chronotropic I45.89
with
autonomic dysfunction G90.8
ischemic heart disease I25.89
left ventricular dysfunction I51.89
sinus node dysfunction I49.8
esophagogastric (junction) (sphincter) K22.0
mitral (valve) - *see* Insufficiency, mitral
pelvic fundus N81.89
pubocervical tissue N81.82
pulmonary valve (heart) I37.1
congenital Q22.3
rectovaginal tissue N81.83
tricuspid (annular) (valve) - *see* Insufficiency,
tricuspid
valvular - *see* Endocarditis
congenital Q24.8
vein, venous (saphenous) (varicose) - *see*
Varix, leg
Incomplete - *see also* condition
bladder, emptying R33.9
defecation R15.0
expansion lungs (newborn) NEC - *see*
Atelectasis
rotation, intestine Q43.3
Inconclusive
diagnostic imaging due to excess body fat of
patient R93.9
findings on diagnostic imaging of breast NEC
R92.8
mammogram (due to dense breasts) R92.2
Incontinence R32
anal sphincter R15.9
coital N39.491

Incontinence - *continued*
  feces R15.9
    nonorganic origin F98.1
  insensible (urinary) N39.42
  overflow N39.490
  postural (urinary) N39.492
  psychogenic F45.8
  rectal R15.9
  reflex N39.498
  stress (female) (male) N39.3
    and urge N39.46
  urethral sphincter R32
  urge N39.41
    and stress (female) (male) N39.46
  urine (urinary) R32
    continuous N39.45
    due to cognitive impairment, or severe
    physical disability or immobility R39.81
    functional R39.81
    insensible N39.42
    mixed (stress and urge) N39.46
    nocturnal N39.44
    nonorganic origin F98.0
    overflow N39.490
    post dribbling N39.43
    postural N39.492
    reflex N39.498
    specified NEC N39.498
    stress (female) (male) N39.3
      and urge N39.46
    total N39.498
    unaware N39.42
    urge N39.41
      and stress (female) (male) N39.46
Incontinentia pigmenti Q82.3
Incoordinate, incoordination
  esophageal-pharyngeal (newborn) - *see*
    Dysphagia
  muscular R27.8
  uterus (action) (contractions) (complicating
    delivery) O62.4
Increase, increased
  abnormal, in development R63.8
  androgens (ovarian) E28.1
  anticoagulants (antithrombin) (anti-VIIIa)
    (anti-iXa) (anti-Xa) (anti-XIa) - *see*
    Circulating anticoagulants
  cold sense R20.8
  estrogen E28.0
  function
    adrenal
      cortex - *see* Cushing's, syndrome
      medulla E27.5
    pituitary (gland) (anterior) (lobe) E22.9
      posterior E22.2
  heat sense R20.8
  intracranial pressure (benign) G93.2
  permeability, capillaries I78.8
  pressure, intracranial G93.2
  secretion
    gastrin E16.4
    glucagon E16.3
    pancreas, endocrine E16.9
      growth hormone-releasing hormone E16.8
      pancreatic polypeptide E16.8
      somatostatin E16.8
      vasoactive-intestinal polypeptide E16.8
  sphericity, lens Q12.4
  splenic activity D73.1
  venous pressure I87.8
    portal K76.6
Increta placenta O43.22-
Incrustation, cornea, foreign body
  (lead)(zinc) - *see* Foreign body, cornea

Incyclophoria H50.54
Incyclotropia - *see* Cyclotropia **Indeterminate**
  sex Q56.4
India rubber skin Q82.8
Indigestion (acid) (bilious) (functional) K30
  catarrhal K31.89
  due to decomposed food NOS A05.9
  nervous F45.8
  psychogenic F45.8
Indirect - *see* condition
Induration penis plastica N48.6
Induration, indurated
  brain G93.89
  breast (fibrous) N64.51
    puerperal, postpartum O92.29
  broad ligament N83.8
  chancre
    anus A51.1
    congenital A50.07
    extragenital NEC A51.2
  corpora cavernosa (penis) (plastic) N48.6
  liver (chronic) K76.89
  lung (black) (chronic) (fibroid) - *see also*
    Fibrosis, lung J84.10
    essential brown J84.03
  penile (plastic) N48.6
  phlebitic - *see* Phlebitis
  skin R23.4
Inebriety (without dependence) - *see* Alcohol,
  intoxication
Inefficiency, kidney N28.9
Inelasticity, skin R23.4
Inequality, leg (length) (acquired) - *see also*
  Deformity, limb, unequal length
  congenital - *see* Defect, reduction, lower limb
  lower leg - *see* Deformity, limb, unequal
    length
Inertia
  bladder (neurogenic) N31.2
  stomach K31.89
    psychogenic F45.8
  uterus, uterine during labor O62.2
    during latent phase of labor O62.0
    primary O62.0
    secondary O62.1
  vesical (neurogenic) N31.2
Infancy, infantile, infantilism - *see also*
  condition
  celiac K90.0
  genitalia, genitals (after puberty) E30.0
  Herter's (nontropical sprue) K90.0
  intestinal K90.0
  Lorain E23.0
  pancreatic K86.89
  pelvis M95.5
    with disproportion (fetopelvic) O33.1
      causing obstructed labor O65.1
  pituitary E23.0
  renal N25.0
  uterus - *see* Infantile, genitalia
Infant(s) - *see also* Infancy
  excessive crying R68.11
  irritable child R68.12
  lack of care - *see* Neglect
  liveborn (singleton) Z38.2
    born in hospital Z38.00
      by cesarean Z38.01
    born outside hospital Z38.1
    multiple NEC Z38.8
      born in hospital Z38.68
        by cesarean Z38.69
      born outside hospital Z38.7
    quadruplet Z38.8
      born in hospital Z38.63

Infant(s) - *continued*
    by cesarean Z38.64
    born outside hospital Z38.7
  quintuplet Z38.8
    born in hospital Z38.65
      by cesarean Z38.66
    born outside hospital Z38.7
  triplet Z38.8
    born in hospital Z38.61
      by cesarean Z38.62
    born outside hospital Z38.7
  twin Z38.5
    born in hospital Z38.30
      by cesarean Z38.31
    born outside hospital Z38.4
  of diabetic mother (syndrome of) P70.1
    gestational diabetes P70.0
Infantile - *see also* condition
  genitalia, genitals E30.0
  os, uterine E30.0
  penis E30.0
  testis E29.1
  uterus E30.0
Infantilism - *see* Infancy
Infarct, infarction
  adrenal (capsule) (gland) E27.49
  appendices epiploicae - *see also* Infarct,
    intestine K55.069
  bowel - *see also* Infarct, intestine K55.069
  brain (stem) - *see* Infarct, cerebral
  breast N64.89
  brewer's (kidney) N28.0
  cardiac - *see* Infarct, myocardium
  cerebellar - *see* Infarct, cerebral
  cerebral - *see also* Occlusion, artery cerebral
    or precerebral, with infarction I63.9-
      aborted I63.9
      cortical I63.9
      due to
        cerebral venous thrombosis, nonpyogenic
          I63.6
        embolism
          cerebral arteries I63.4-
          precerebral arteries I63.1-
        occlusion NEC
          cerebral arteries I63.5-
          precerebral arteries I63.2-
        stenosis NEC
          cerebral arteries I63.5-
          precerebral arteries I63.2-
        thrombosis
          cerebral artery I63.3-
          precerebral artery I63.0-
      intraoperative
        during cardiac surgery I97.810
        during other surgery I97.811
      postprocedural
        following cardiac surgery I97.820
        following other surgery I97.821
      specified NEC I63.8
  colon (acute) (agnogenic) (embolic)
    (hemorrhagic) (nonocclusive)
    (nonthrombotic) (occlusive) (segmental)
    (thrombotic)(with gangrene) - *see also*
    Infarct, intestine K55.049
  coronary artery - *see* Infarct, myocardium
  embolic - *see* Embolism
  fallopian tube N83.8
  gallbladder K82.8
  heart - *see* Infarct, myocardium
  hepatic K76.3
  hypophysis (anterior lobe) E23.6
  impending (myocardium) I20.0
  intestine (acute) (agnogenic) (embolic)

Infarct, infarction - *continued*
(hemorrhagic) (nonocclusive) (nonthrombotic)
　(occlusive) (thrombotic) (with
gangrene) K55.069
　diffuse K55.062
　　focal K55.061
　　large K55.049
　　　diffuse K55.042
　　　focal K55.041
　　small K55.029
　　　diffuse K55.022
　　　focal K55.021
　kidney N28.0
　liver K76.3
　lung (embolic) (thrombotic) - *see* Embolism,
　　pulmonary
　lymph node I89.8
　mesentery, mesenteric (embolic) (thrombotic)
　　(with gangrene) - *see also* Infarct, intestine
　　K55.069
　muscle (ischemic) M62.20
　　ankle M62.27-
　　foot M62.27-
　　forearm M62.23-
　　hand M62.24-
　　lower leg M62.26-
　　pelvic region M62.25-
　　shoulder region M62.21-
　　specified site NEC M62.28
　　thigh M62.25-
　　upper arm M62.22-
　myocardium, myocardial (acute) (with stated
　　duration of 4weeks or less) I21.9
　　　associated with revascularization procedure
　　　　I21.A9
　　　diagnosed on ECG, but presenting no
　　　　symptoms I25.2
　　　due to
　　　　demand ischemia I21.A1
　　　　ischemic imbalance I21.A1
　　　healed or old I25.2
　　intraoperative　*see also* Infarct, myocardium,
　　associated with revascularization procedure
　　　during cardiac surgery I97.790
　　　during other surgery I97.791
　　non-Q wave I21.4
　　non-ST elevation (NSTEMI) I21.4
　　　subsequent I22.2
　　nontransmural I21.4
　　past (diagnosed on ECG or other
　　　investigation, but currently presenting no
　　　symptoms) I25.2
　　postprocedural　*see also* Infarct,
　　myocardium, associated with revascularization
　　procedure
　　　following cardiac surgery (see also Infarct,
　　myocardium, type 4 or type 5) I97.190
　　　following other surgery I97.191
　　Q wave (see also, Infarct, myocardium, by
　　　site) I21.3
　　secondary to
　　　demand ischemia I21.A1
　　　ischemic imbalance I21.A1
　　ST elevation (STEMI) I21.3
　　　anterior (anteroapical) (anterolateral)
　　　　(anteroseptal) (Q wave) (wall) I21.09
　　　　subsequent I22.0
　　　inferior (diaphragmatic) (inferolateral)
　　　　(inferoposterior) (wall) NEC I21.19
　　　　subsequent I22.1
　　　inferoposterior transmural (Q wave) I21.11
　　　involving
　　　　coronary artery of anterior wall NEC
　　　　　I21.09

Infarct, infarction - *continued*
　　　coronary artery of inferior wall NEC
　　　　I21.19
　　　diagonal coronary artery I21.02
　　　left anterior descending coronary artery
　　　　I21.02
　　　left circumflex coronary artery I21.21
　　　left main coronary artery I21.01
　　　oblique marginal coronary artery I21.21
　　　right coronary artery I21.11
　　　lateral (apical-lateral) (basal-lateral) (high)
　　　　I21.29
　　　　subsequent I22.8
　　　posterior (posterobasal) (posterolateral)
　　　　(posteroseptal) (true) I21.29
　　　　subsequent I22.8
　　　septal I21.29
　　　　subsequent I22.8
　　　specified NEC I21.29
　　　　subsequent I22.8
　　　subsequent I22.9
　　subsequent (recurrent) (reinfarction) I22.9
　　　anterior (anteroapical) (anterolateral)
　　　　(anteroseptal) (wall) I22.0
　　　diaphragmatic (wall) I22.1
　　　inferior (diaphragmatic) (inferolateral)
　　　　(inferoposterior) (wall) I22.1
　　　lateral (apical-lateral) (basal-lateral) (high)
　　　　I22.8
　　　non-ST elevation (NSTEMI) I22.2
　　　posterior (posterobasal) (posterolateral)
　　　　(posteroseptal) (true) I22.8
　　　septal I22.8
　　　specified NEC I22.8
　　ST elevation I22.9
　　　anterior (anteroapical) (anterolateral)
　　　　(anteroseptal) (wall) I22.0
　　　inferior (diaphragmatic) (inferolateral)
　　　　(inferoposterior) (wall) I22.1
　　　specified NEC I22.8
　　subendocardial I22.2
　　transmural I22.9
　　　anterior (anteroapical) (anterolateral)
　　　　(anteroseptal) (wall) I22.0
　　　diaphragmatic (wall) I22.1
　　　inferior (diaphragmatic) (inferolateral)
　　　　(inferoposterior) (wall) I22.1
　　　lateral (apical-lateral) (basal-lateral) (high)
　　　　I22.8
　　　posterior (posterobasal) (posterolateral)
　　　　(posteroseptal) (true) I22.8
　　　specified NEC I22.8
　　type 1 (see also Infarction, myocardial,
　　　subsequent, by site, or by ST elevation or
　　　non-ST elevation) I22.9
　　type 2 I21.A1
　　type 3 I21.A9
　　type 4 I21.A9
　　type 5 I21.A9
　syphilitic A52.06
　transmural I21.9
　　anterior (anteroapical) (anterolateral)
　　　(anteroseptal) (Q wave) (wall) NEC I21.09
　　inferior (diaphragmatic) (inferolateral)
　　　(inferoposterior) (Q wave) (wall) NEC
　　　I21.19
　　inferoposterior (Q wave) I21.11
　　lateral (apical-lateral) (basal-lateral) (high)
　　　NEC I21.29
　　posterior (posterobasal) (posterolateral)
　　　(posteroseptal) (true) NEC I21.29
　　septal NEC I21.29
　　specified NEC I21.29

Infarct, infarction - *continued*
　　type 1 (see also Infarction, myocardial, by
　　　site, or by ST elevation or non-ST elevation)
　　　I21.9
　　type 2 I21.A1
　　type 3 I21.A9
　　type 4 (a) (b) (c) I21.A9
　　type 5 I21.A9
　nontransmural I21.4
　omentum - *see also* Infarct, intestine K55.069
　ovary N83.8
　pancreas K86.89
　papillary muscle - *see* Infarct, myocardium
　parathyroid gland E21.4
　pituitary (gland) E23.6
　placenta O43.81-
　prostate N42.89
　pulmonary (artery) (vein) (hemorrhagic) - *see*
　　Embolism, pulmonary
　renal (embolic) (thrombotic) N28.0
　retina, retinal (artery) - *see* Occlusion, artery,
　　retina
　spinal (cord) (acute) (embolic) (nonembolic)
　　G95.11
　spleen D73.5
　　embolic or thrombotic I74.8
　subendocardial (acute) (nontransmural) I21.4
　suprarenal (capsule) (gland) E27.49
　testis N50.1
　thrombotic - *see also* Thrombosis
　　artery, arterial - *see* Embolism
　thyroid (gland) E07.89
　ventricle (heart) - *see* Infarct, myocardium
Infecting - *see* condition
Infection, infected, infective (opportunistic)
　B99.9
　with
　　drug resistant organism - *see* Resistance (to),
　　　drug - *see also* specific organism
　　lymphangitis - *see* Lymphangitis
　　organ dysfunction (acute) R65.20
　　　with septic shock R65.21
　abscess (skin)
　code by site under Abscess
　Absidia - *see* Mucormycosis
　Acanthamoeba - *see* Acanthamebiasis
　Acanthocheilonema (perstans) (streptocerca)
　　B74.4
　accessory sinus (chronic) - *see* Sinusitis
　achorion - *see* Dermatophytosis
　Acremonium falciforme B47.0
　acromioclavicular M00.9
　Actinobacillus (actinomycetem-comitans)
　　A28.8
　　mallei A24.0
　　muris A25.1
　Actinomadura B47.1
　Actinomyces (israelii) - *see also*
　　Actinomycosis A42.9
　Actinomycetales - *see* Actinomycosis
　actinomycotic NOS - *see* Actinomycosis
　adenoid (and tonsil) J03.90
　　chronic J35.02
　adenovirus NEC
　　as cause of disease classified elsewhere
　　　B97.0
　　unspecified nature or site B34.0
　aerogenes capsulatus A48.0
　aertrycke - *see* Infection, salmonella
　alimentary canal NOS - *see* Enteritis,
　　infectious
　Allescheria boydii B48.2
　Alternaria B48.8
　alveolus, alveolar (process) K04.7

Infection, infected, infective - *continued*
Ameba, amebic (histolytica) - *see* Amebiasis
amniotic fluid, sac or cavity O41.10-
    chorioamnionitis O41.12-
    placentitis O41.14-
amputation stump (surgical) - *see*
    Complication, amputation stump, infection
Ancylostoma (duodenalis) B76.0
Anisakiasis, Anisakis larvae B81.0
anthrax - *see* Anthrax
antrum (chronic) - *see* Sinusitis, maxillary
anus, anal (papillae) (sphincter) K62.89
arbovirus (arbor virus) A94
    specified type NEC A93.8
artificial insemination N98.0
Ascaris lumbricoides - *see* Ascariasis
Ascomycetes B47.0
Aspergillus (flavus) (fumigatus) (terreus) - *see*
    Aspergillosis
atypical
    acid-fast (bacilli) - *see* Mycobacterium,
    atypical
    mycobacteria - *see* Mycobacterium, atypical
    virus A81.9
        specified type NEC A81.89
auditory meatus (external) - *see* Otitis, externa,
    infective
auricle (ear) - *see* Otitis, externa, infective
axillary gland (lymph) L04.2
Bacillus A49.9
    abortus A23.1
    anthracis - *see* Anthrax
    Ducrey's (any location) A57
    Flexner's A03.1
    Friedländer's NEC A49.8
    gas (gangrene) A48.0
    mallei A24.0
    melitensis A23.0
    paratyphoid, paratyphosus A01.4
        A A01.1
        B A01.2
        C A01.3
    Shiga (-Kruse) A03.0
    suipestifer - *see* Infection, salmonella
    swimming pool A31.1
    typhosa A01.00
    welchii - *see* Gangrene, gas
bacterial NOS A49.9
    as cause of disease classified elsewhere
    B96.89
        Clostridium perfringens [C. perfringens]
        B96.7
        Bacteroides fragilis [B. fragilis] B96.6
        Enterobacter sakazakii B96.89
        Enterococcus B95.2
        Escherichia coli [E. coli] - *see also*
        Escherichia coli B96.20
        Helicobacter pylori [H. pylori] B96.81
        Hemophilus influenzae [H. influenzae]
        B96.3
        Klebsiella pneumoniae [K. pneumoniae]
        B96.1
        Mycoplasma pneumoniae [M. pneumoniae]
        B96.0
        Proteus (mirabilis) (morganii) B96.4
        Pseudomonas (aeruginosa) (mallei)
        (pseudomallei) B96.5
        Staphylococcus B95.8
            aureus (methicillin susceptible) (MSSA)
            B95.61
                methicillin resistant (MRSA) B95.62
            specified NEC B95.7
        Streptococcus B95.5
            group A B95.0

Infection, infected, infective - *continued*
    group B B95.1
    pneumoniae B95.3
    specified NEC B95.4
    Vibrio vulnificus B96.82
    specified NEC A48.8
Bacterium
    paratyphosum A01.4
        A A01.1
        B A01.2
        C A01.3
    typhosum A01.00
Bacteroides NEC A49.8
    fragilis, as cause of disease classified
    elsewhere B96.6
Balantidium coli A07.0
Bartholin's gland N75.8
Basidiobolus B46.8
bile duct (common) (hepatic) - *see* Cholangitis
bladder - *see* Cystitis
Blastomyces, blastomycotic - *see also*
Blastomycosis
    brasiliensis - *see* Paracoccidioidomycosis
    dermatitidis - *see* Blastomycosis
    European - *see* Cryptococcosis
    Loboi B48.0
    North American B40.9
    South American - *see*
    Paracoccidioidomycosis
bleb, postprocedure - *see* Blebitis
bone - *see* Osteomyelitis
Bordetella - *see* Whooping cough
Borrelia bergdorfi A69.20
brain - *see also* Encephalitis G04.90
    membranes - *see* Meningitis
    septic G06.0
        meninges - *see* Meningitis, bacterial
branchial cyst Q18.0
breast - *see* Mastitis
bronchus - *see* Bronchitis
Brucella A23.9
    abortus A23.1
    canis A23.3
    melitensis A23.0
    mixed A23.8
    specified NEC A23.8
    suis A23.2
Brugia (malayi) B74.1
    timori B74.2
bursa - *see* Bursitis, infective
buttocks (skin) L08.9
Campylobacter, intestinal A04.5
    as cause of disease classified elsewhere
    B96.81
Candida (albicans) (tropicalis) - *see*
Candidiasis
candiru B88.8
Capillaria (intestinal) B81.1
    hepatica B83.8
    philippinensis B81.1
cartilage - *see* Disorder, cartilage, specified
    type NEC
catheter-related bloodstream (CRBSI) T80.211
cat liver fluke B66.0
cellulitis
code by site under Cellulitis
central line-associated T80.219
    bloodstream (CLABSI) T80.211
    specified NEC T80.218
Cephalosporium falciforme B47.0
cerebrospinal - *see* Meningitis
cervical gland (lymph) L04.0
cervix - *see* Cervicitis
cesarean delivery wound (puerperal) O86.0

Infection, infected, infective - *continued*
cestodes - *see* Infestation, cestodes
chest J22
Chilomastix (intestinal) A07.8
Chlamydia, chlamydial A74.9
    anus A56.3
    genitourinary tract A56.2
        lower A56.00
        specified NEC A56.19
    lymphogranuloma A55
    pharynx A56.4
    psittaci A70
    rectum A56.3
    sexually transmitted NEC A56.8
cholera - *see* Cholera
Cladosporium
    bantianum (brain abscess) B43.1
    carrionii B43.0
    castellanii B36.1
    trichoides (brain abscess) B43.1
    werneckii B36.1
Clonorchis (sinensis) (liver) B66.1
Clostridium NEC
    bifermentans A48.0
    botulinum (food poisoning) A05.1
        infant A48.51
        wound A48.52
    difficile
    as cause of disease classified elsewhere
    B96.89
        foodborne (disease)
            not specified as recurrent A04.72
            recurrent A04.71
        gas gangrene A48.0
        necrotizing enterocolitis
            not specified as recurrent A04.72
            recurrent A04.71
        sepsis A41.4
    gas-forming NEC A48.0
    histolyticum A48.0
    novyi, causing gas gangrene A48.0
    oedematiens A48.0
    perfringens
        as cause of disease classified elsewhere
        B96.7
        due to food A05.2
        foodborne (disease) A05.2
        gas gangrene A48.0
        sepsis A41.4
    septicum, causing gas gangrene A48.0
    sordellii, causing gas gangrene A48.0
    welchii
        as cause of disease classified elsewhere
        B96.7
        foodborne (disease) A05.2
        gas gangrene A48.0
        necrotizing enteritis A05.2
        sepsis A41.4
Coccidioides (immitis) - *see*
    Coccidioidomycosis
colon - *see* Enteritis, infectious
colostomy K94.02
common duct - *see* Cholangitis
congenital P39.9
    Candida (albicans) P37.5
    cytomegalovirus P35.1
    hepatitis, viral P35.3
    herpes simplex P35.2
    infectious or parasitic disease P37.9
        specified NEC P37.8
    listeriosis (disseminated) P37.2
    malaria NEC P37.4
        falciparum P37.3
    Plasmodium falciparum P37.3

Infection, infected, infective - *continued*
  poliomyelitis P35.8
  rubella P35.0
  skin P39.4
  toxoplasmosis (acute) (subacute) (chronic)
    P37.1
  tuberculosis P37.0
  urinary (tract) P39.3
  vaccinia P35.8
  virus P35.9
    specified type NEC P35.8
  Conidiobolus B46.8
  coronavirus NEC B34.2
    as cause of disease classified elsewhere
      B97.29
    severe acute respiratory syndrome (SARS
    associated) B97.21
  corpus luteum - *see* Salpingo-oophoritis
  Corynebacterium diphtheriae - *see* Diphtheria
  cotia virus B08.8
  Coxiella burnetii A78
  coxsackie - *see* Coxsackie
  Cryptococcus neoformans - *see*
    Cryptococcosis
  Cryptosporidium A07.2
  Cunninghamella - *see* Mucormycosis
  cyst - *see* Cyst
  cystic duct - *see also* Cholecystitis K81.9
  Cysticercus cellulosae - *see* Cysticercosis
  cytomegalovirus, cytomegaloviral B25.9
    congenital P35.1
    maternal, maternal care for (suspected)
      damage to fetus O35.3
    mononucleosis B27.10
      with
        complication NEC B27.19
        meningitis B27.12
        polyneuropathy B27.11
  delta-agent (acute), in hepatitis B carrier B17.0
  dental (pulpal origin) K04.7
  Deuteromycetes B47.0
  Dicrocoelium dendriticum B66.2
  Dipetalonema (perstans) (streptocerca) B74.4
  diphtherial - *see* Diphtheria
  Diphyllobothrium (adult) (latum) (pacificum)
    B70.0
    larval B70.1
  Diplogonoporus (grandis) B71.8
  Dipylidium caninum B67.4
  Dirofilaria B74.8
  Dracunculus medinensis B72
  Drechslera (hawaiiensis) B43.8
  Ducrey Haemophilus (any location) A57
  due to or resulting from
    artificial insemination N98.0
    central venous catheter T80.219
      bloodstream T80.211
      exit or insertion site T80.212
      localized T80.212
      port or reservoir T80.212
      specified NEC T80.218
      tunnel T80.212
    device, implant or graft - *see also*
    Complications, by site and type, infection or
    inflammation T85.79
      arterial graft NEC T82.7
      breast (implant) T85.79
      catheter NEC T85.79
        dialysis (renal) T82.7
          intraperitoneal T85.71
        infusion NEC T82.7
          cranial T85.735
          intrathecal T85.735
          spinal (epidural) (subdural) T85.735

Infection, infected, infective - *continued*
        subarachnoid T85.735
      urinary T83.518
        cystostomy T83.510
        Hopkins T83.518
        ileostomy T83.518
        nephrostomy T83.512
        specified NEC T83.518
        urethral indwelling T83.511
        urostomy T83.518
    electronic (electrode) (pulse generator)
    (stimulator)
      bone T84.7
      cardiac T82.7
      nervous system T85.738
        brain T85.731
        cranial nerve T85.732
        gastric nerve T85.732
        generator pocket T85.734
        neurostimulator generator T85.734
        peripheral nerve T85.732
        sacral nerve T85.732
        spinal cord T85.733
        vagal nerve T85.732
      urinary T83.590
    fixation, internal (orthopedic) NEC - *see*
      Complication, fixation device, infection
    gastrointestinal (bile duct) (esophagus)
    T85.79
      neurostimulator electrode (lead) T85.732
    genital NEC T83.69
    heart NEC T82.7
      valve (prosthesis) T82.6
      graft T82.7
    joint prosthesis - *see* Complication, joint
      prosthesis, infection
    ocular (corneal graft) (orbital implant) NEC
    T85.79
    orthopedic NEC T84.7
    penile (cylinder) (pump) (reservoir) T83.61
    specified NEC T85.79
    testicular T83.62
    urinary NEC T83.598
      ileal conduit stent T83.593
      implanted neurostimulation T83.590
      implanted sphincter T83.591
      indwelling ureteral stent T83.592
      nephroureteral stent T83.593
      specified stent NEC T83.593
    vascular NEC T82.7
    ventricular intracranial (communicating)
    shunt T85.730
    Hickman catheter T80.219
      bloodstream T80.211
      localized T80.212
      specified NEC T80.218
    immunization or vaccination T88.0
    infusion, injection or transfusion NEC
    T80.29
      acute T80.22
    injury NEC
  code by site under Wound, open
    peripherally inserted central catheter (PICC)
    T80.219
      bloodstream T80.211
      localized T80.212
      specified NEC T80.218
    portacath (port-a-cath) T80.219
      bloodstream T80.211
      localized T80.212
      specified NEC T80.218
    pulmonary artery catheter - *see* Infection, due
      to or resulting from, central venous catheter
    surgery T81.4

Infection, infected, infective - *continued*
    Swan Ganz catheter - *see* Infection, due to or
      resulting from, central venous catheter
    triple lumen catheter T80.219
      bloodstream T80.211
      localized T80.212
      specified NEC T80.218
    umbilical venous catheter T80.219
      bloodstream T80.211
      localized T80.212
      specified NEC T80.218
  during labor NEC O75.3
  ear (middle) - *see also* Otitis media
    external - *see* Otitis, externa, infective
    inner - *see* subcategory H83.0
  Eberthella typhosa A01.00
  Echinococcus - *see* Echinococcus
  echovirus
    as cause of disease classified elsewhere
      B97.12
    unspecified nature or site B34.1
  endocardium I33.0
  endocervix - *see* Cervicitis
  Entamoeba - *see* Amebiasis
  enteric - *see* Enteritis, infectious
  Enterobacter sakazakii B96.89
  Enterobius vermicularis B80
  enterostomy K94.12
  enterovirus B34.1
    as cause of disease classified elsewhere
      B97.10
      coxsackievirus B97.11
      echovirus B97.12
      specified NEC B97.19
  Entomophthora B46.8
  Epidermophyton - *see* Dermatophytosis
  epididymis - *see* Epididymitis
  episiotomy (puerperal) O86.0
  Erysipelothrix (insidiosa) (rhusiopathiae) - *see*
    Erysipeloid
  erythema infectiosum B08.3
  Escherichia (E.) coli NEC A49.8
    as cause of disease classified elsewhere - *see*
      also Escherichia coli B96.20
    congenital P39.8
      sepsis P36.4
    generalized A41.51
    intestinal - *see* Enteritis, infectious, due to,
      Escherichia coli
  ethmoidal (chronic) (sinus) - *see* Sinusitis,
    ethmoidal
  eustachian tube (ear) - *see* Salpingitis,
    eustachian
  external auditory canal (meatus) NEC - *see*
    Otitis, externa, infective
  eye (purulent) - *see* Endophthalmitis, purulent
  eyelid - *see* Inflammation, eyelid
  fallopian tube - *see* Salpingo-oophoritis
  Fasciola (gigantica) (hepatica) (indica) B66.3
  Fasciolopsis (buski) B66.5
  filarial - *see* Infestation, filarial
  finger (skin) L08.9
    nail L03.01-
      fungus B35.1
  fish tapeworm B70.0
    larval B70.1
  flagellate, intestinal A07.9
  fluke - *see* Infestation, fluke
  focal
    teeth (pulpal origin) K04.7
    tonsils J35.01
  Fonsecaea (compactum) (pedrosoi) B43.0
  food - *see* Intoxication, foodborne
  foot (skin) L08.9

Infection, infected, infective - *continued*
  dermatophytic fungus B35.3
  Francisella tularensis - *see* Tularemia
  frontal (sinus) (chronic) - *see* Sinusitis, frontal
  fungus NOS B49
    beard B35.0
    dermatophytic - *see* Dermatophytosis
    foot B35.3
    groin B35.6
    hand B35.2
    nail B35.1
    pathogenic to compromised host only B48.8
    perianal (area) B35.6
    scalp B35.0
    skin B36.9
      foot B35.3
      hand B35.2
      toenails B35.1
  Fusarium B48.8
  gallbladder - *see* Cholecystitis
  gas bacillus - *see* Gangrene, gas
  gastrointestinal - *see* Enteritis, infectious
  generalized NEC - *see* Sepsis
  generator pocket, implanted electronic
    neurostimulator T85.734
  genital organ or tract
    female - *see* Disease, pelvis, inflammatory
    male N49.9
      multiple sites N49.8
      specified NEC N49.8
  Ghon tubercle, primary A15.7
  Giardia lamblia A07.1
  gingiva (chronic) K05.10
    acute K05.00
      nonplaque induced K05.01
      plaque induced K05.00
    nonplaque induced K05.11
    plaque induced K05.10
  glanders A24.0
  glenosporosis B48.0
  Gnathostoma (spinigerum) B83.1
  Gongylonema B83.8
  gonococcal - *see* Gonococcus
  gram negative bacilli NOS A49.9
  guinea worm B72
  gum (chronic) K05.10
    acute K05.00
      nonplaque induced K05.01
      plaque induced K05.00
    nonplaque induced K05.11
    plaque induced K05.10
  Haemophilus - *see* Infection, Hemophilus
  heart - *see* Carditis
  Helicobacter pylori A04.8
    as cause of disease classified elsewhere
    B96.81
  helminths B83.9
    intestinal B82.0
      mixed (types classifiable to more than one
        of the titles B65.0-b81.3 and B81.8) B81.4
      specified type NEC B81.8
    specified type NEC B83.8
  Hemophilus
    aegyptius, systemic A48.4
    Ducrey (any location) A57
    influenzae NEC A49.2
      as cause of disease classified elsewhere
      B96.3
    generalized A41.3
  herpes (simplex) - *see also* Herpes
    congenital P35.2
    disseminated B00.7
    zoster B02.9
  herpesvirus, herpesviral - *see* Herpes

Infection, infected, infective - *continued*
  hip (joint) NEC M00.9
    due to internal joint prosthesis
      left T84.52
      right T84.51
    skin NEC L08.9
  Heterophyes (heterophyes) B66.8
  Histoplasma - *see* Histoplasmosis
    American B39.4
    capsulatum B39.4
  hookworm B76.9
  human
    papilloma virus A63.0
    T-cell lymphotropic virus type 1(HTLV 1)
    B33.3
  hydrocele N43.0
  Hymenolepis B71.0
  hypopharynx - *see* Pharyngitis
  inguinal (lymph) glands L04.1
    due to soft chancre A57
  intervertebral disc, pyogenic M46.30
    cervical region M46.32
    cervicothoracic region M46.33
    lumbar region M46.36
    lumbosacral region M46.37
    multiple sites M46.39
    occipito-atlanto-axial region M46.31
    sacrococcygeal region M46.38
    thoracic region M46.34
    thoracolumbar region M46.35
  intestine, intestinal - *see* Enteritis, infectious
    specified NEC A08.8
  intra-amniotic affecting newborn NEC P39.2
  Isospora belli or hominis A07.3
  Japanese B encephalitis A83.0
  jaw (bone) (lower) (upper) M27.2
  joint NEC M00.9
    due to internal joint prosthesis T84.50
  kidney (cortex) (hematogenous) N15.9
    with calculus N20.0
      with hydronephrosis N13.6
    following ectopic gestation O08.83
    pelvis and ureter (cystic) N28.85
    puerperal (postpartum) O86.21
    specified NEC N15.8
  Klebsiella (K.) pneumoniae NEC A49.8
    as cause of disease classified elsewhere
    B96.1
  knee (joint) NEC M00.9
    joint M00.9
    due to internal joint prosthesis
      left T84.54
      right T84.53
    skin L08.9
  Koch's - *see* Tuberculosis
  labia (majora) (minora) (acute) - *see* Vulvitis
  lacrimal
    gland - *see* Dacryoadenitis
    passages (duct) (sac) - *see* Inflammation,
  lacrimal, passages
  lancet fluke B66.2
  larynx NEC J38.7
  leg (skin) NOS L08.9
  Legionella pneumophila A48.1
    nonpneumonic A48.2
  Leishmania - *see also* Leishmaniasis
    aethiopica B55.1
    braziliensis B55.2
    chagasi B55.0
    donovani B55.0
    infantum B55.0
    major B55.1
    mexicana B55.1
    tropica B55.1

Infection, infected, infective - *continued*
  lentivirus, as cause of disease classified
    elsewhere B97.31
  Leptosphaeria senagalensis B47.0
  Leptospira interrogans A27.9
    autumnalis A27.89
    canicola A27.89
    hebdomadis A27.89
    icterohaemorrhagiae A27.0
    pomona A27.89
    specified type NEC A27.89
  leptospirochetal NEC - *see* Leptospirosis
  Listeria monocytogenes - *see also* Listeriosis
    congenital P37.2
  Loa Loa B74.3
    with conjunctival infestation B74.3
    eyelid B74.3
  Loboa loboi B48.0
  local, skin (staphylococcal) (streptococcal)
    L08.9
    abscess
  code by site under Abscess
    cellulitis
  code by site under Cellulitis
    specified NEC L08.89
    ulcer - *see* Ulcer, skin
  Loefflerella mallei A24.0
  lung - *see also* Pneumonia J18.9
    atypical Mycobacterium A31.0
    spirochetal A69.8
    tuberculous - *see* Tuberculosis, pulmonary
    virus - *see* Pneumonia, viral
  lymph gland - *see also* Lymphadenitis, acute
    mesenteric I88.0
  lymphoid tissue, base of tongue or posterior
    pharynx, NEC (chronic) J35.03
  Madurella (grisea) (mycetomii) B47.0
  major
    following ectopic or molar pregnancy O08.0
    puerperal, postpartum, childbirth O85
  Malassezia furfur B36.0
  Malleomyces
    mallei A24.0
    pseudomallei (whitmori) - *see* Melioidosis
  mammary gland N61.0
  Mansonella (ozzardi) (perstans) (streptocerca)
    B74.4
  mastoid - *see* Mastoiditis
  maxilla, maxillary M27.2
    sinus (chronic) - *see* Sinusitis, maxillary
  mediastinum J98.51
  Medina (worm) B72
  meibomian cyst or gland - *see* Hordeolum
  meninges - *see* Meningitis, bacterial
  meningococcal - *see also* condition A39.9
    adrenals A39.1
    brain A39.81
    cerebrospinal A39.0
    conjunctiva A39.89
    endocardium A39.51
    heart A39.50
      endocardium A39.51
      myocardium A39.52
      pericardium A39.53
    joint A39.83
    meninges A39.0
    meningococcemia A39.4
      acute A39.2
      chronic A39.3
    myocardium A39.52
    pericardium A39.53
    retrobulbar neuritis A39.82
    specified site NEC A39.89
  mesenteric lymph nodes or glands NEC I88.0

Infection, infected, infective - *continued*

Metagonimus B66.8
metatarsophalangeal M00.9
methicillin
  resistant Staphylococcus aureus (MRSA) A49.02
  susceptible Staphylococcus aureus (MSSA) A49.01
Microsporum, microsporic - *see* Dermatophytosis
mixed flora (bacterial) NEC A49.8
Monilia - *see* Candidiasis
Monosporium apiospermum B48.2
mouth, parasitic B37.0
Mucor - *see* Mucormycosis
muscle NEC - *see* Myositis, infective
mycelium NOS B49
mycetoma B47.9
  actinomycotic NEC B47.1
  mycotic NEC B47.0
Mycobacterium, mycobacterial - *see* Mycobacterium
Mycoplasma NEC A49.3
  pneumoniae, as cause of disease classified elsewhere B96.0
mycotic NOS B49
  pathogenic to compromised host only B48.8
  skin NOS B36.9
myocardium NEC I40.0
nail (chronic)
  with lymphangitis - *see* Lymphangitis, acute, digit
  finger L03.01-
    fungus B35.1
  ingrowing L60.0
  toe L03.03-
    fungus B35.1
nasal sinus (chronic) - *see* Sinusitis
nasopharynx - *see* Nasopharyngitis
navel L08.82
Necator americanus B76.1
Neisseria - *see* Gonococcus
Neotestudina rosati B47.0
newborn P39.9
  intra-amniotic NEC P39.2
  skin P39.4
  specified type NEC P39.8
nipple N61.0
  associated with
    lactation O91.03
    pregnancy O91.01-
    puerperium O91.02
Nocardia - *see* Nocardiosis
obstetrical surgical wound (puerperal) O86.0
Oesophagostomum (apiostomum) B81.8
Oestrus ovis - *see* Myiasis
Oidium albicans B37.9
Onchocerca (volvulus) - *see* Onchocerciasis
oncovirus, as cause of disease classified elsewhere B97.32
operation wound T81.4
Opisthorchis (felineus) (viverrini) B66.0
orbit, orbital - *see* Inflammation, orbit
orthopoxvirus NEC B08.09
ovary - *see* Salpingo-oophoritis
Oxyuris vermicularis B80
pancreas (acute) - *see* Pancreatitis, acute
  abscess - *see* Pancreatitis, acute
  specified NEC - *see also* Pancreatitis, acute K85.80
papillomavirus, as cause of disease classified elsewhere B97.7
papovavirus NEC B34.4

Infection, infected, infective - *continued*

Paracoccidioides brasiliensis - *see* Paracoccidioidomycosis
Paragonimus (westermani) B66.4
parainfluenza virus B34.8
parameningococcus NOS A39.9
parapoxvirus B08.60
  specified NEC B08.69
parasitic B89
Parastrongylus
  cantonensis B83.2
  costaricensis B81.3
  paratyphoid A01.4
    Type A A01.1
    Type B A01.2
    Type C A01.3
paraurethral ducts N34.2
parotid gland - *see* Sialoadenitis
parvovirus NEC B34.3
  as cause of disease classified elsewhere B97.6
Pasteurella NEC A28.0
  multocida A28.0
  pestis - *see* Plague
  pseudotuberculosis A28.0
  septica (cat bite) (dog bite) A28.0
  tularensis - *see* Tularemia
pelvic, female - *see* Disease, pelvis, inflammatory Penicillium (marneffei) B48.4
penis (glans) (retention) NEC N48.29
periapical K04.5
peridental, periodontal K05.20
  generalized - *see* Periodontitis, aggressive, generalized
  localized - *see* Periodontitis, aggressive, localized
perinatal period P39.9
  specified type NEC P39.8
perineal repair (puerperal) O86.0
periorbital - *see* Inflammation, orbit
perirectal K62.89
perirenal - *see* Infection, kidney peritoneal - *see* Peritonitis
periureteral N28.89
Petriellidium boydii B48.2
pharynx - *see also* Pharyngitis
  coxsackievirus B08.5
  posterior, lymphoid (chronic) J35.03
Phialophora
  gougerotii (subcutaneous abscess or cyst) B43.2
  jeanselmei (subcutaneous abscess or cyst) B43.2
  verrucosa (skin) B43.0
Piedraia hortae B36.3
pinta A67.9
  intermediate A67.1
  late A67.2
  mixed A67.3
  primary A67.0
pinworm B80
Pityrosporum furfur B36.0
pleuro-pneumonia-like organism (PPLO) NEC A49.3
  as cause of disease classified elsewhere B96.0
pneumococcus, pneumococcal NEC A49.1
  as cause of disease classified elsewhere B95.3
  generalized (purulent) A40.3
    with pneumonia J13
Pneumocystis carinii (pneumonia) B59
Pneumocystis jiroveci (pneumonia) B59
port or reservoir T80.212

Infection, infected, infective - *continued*

postoperative T81.4
postoperative wound T81.4
postprocedural T81.4
postvaccinal T88.0
prepuce NEC N47.7
  with penile inflammation N47.6
prion - *see* Disease, prion, central nervous system
prostate (capsule) - *see* Prostatitis
Proteus (mirabilis) (morganii) (vulgaris) NEC A49.8
  as cause of disease classified elsewhere B96.4
protozoal NEC B64
  intestinal A07.9
    specified NEC A07.8
  specified NEC B60.8
Pseudoallescheria boydii B48.2
Pseudomonas NEC A49.8
  as cause of disease classified elsewhere B96.5
  mallei A24.0
  pneumonia J15.1
  pseudomallei - *see* Melioidosis
puerperal O86.4
  genitourinary tract NEC O86.89
  major or generalized O85
  minor O86.4
  specified NEC O86.89
pulmonary - *see* Infection, lung
purulent - *see* Abscess
Pyrenochaeta romeroi B47.0
Q fever A78
rectum (sphincter) K62.89
renal - *see also* Infection, kidney
  pelvis and ureter (cystic) N28.85
reovirus, as cause of disease classified elsewhere B97.5
respiratory (tract) NEC J98.8
  acute J22
  chronic J98.8
  influenzal (upper) (acute) - *see* Influenza, with, respiratory manifestations NEC
  lower (acute) J22
    chronic - *see* Bronchitis, chronic
  rhinovirus J00
  syncytial virus, as cause of disease classified elsewhere B97.4
  upper (acute) NOS J06.9
    chronic J39.8
    streptococcal J06.9
    viral NOS J06.9
resulting from
  presence of internal prosthesis, implant, graft - *see* Complications, by site and type, infection
retortamoniasis A07.8
retroperitoneal NEC K68.9
retrovirus B33.3
  as cause of disease classified elsewhere B97.30
    human
      immunodeficiency, type 2 (HIV 2) B97.35
      T-cell lymphotropic
        type I (HTLV-i) B97.33
        type II (HTLV-II) B97.34
    lentivirus B97.31
    oncovirus B97.32
    specified NEC B97.39
Rhinosporidium (seeberi) B48.1
rhinovirus
  as cause of disease classified elsewhere B97.89
  unspecified nature or site B34.8

Infection, infected, infective - *continued*
  Rhizopus - *see* Mucormycosis
  rickettsial NOS A79.9
  roundworm (large) NEC B82.0
    Ascariasis - *see also* Ascariasis B77.9
  rubella - *see* Rubella
  Saccharomyces - *see* Candidiasis
  salivary duct or gland (any) - *see* Sialoadenitis
  Salmonella (aertrycke) (arizonae) (gallinarum)
    (cholerae-suis) (enteritidis) (suipestifer)
    (typhimurium) A02.9
    with
      (gastro) enteritis A02.0
      sepsis A02.1
      specified manifestation NEC A02.8
    due to food (poisoning) A02.9
    hirschfeldii A01.3
    localized A02.20
      arthritis A02.23
      meningitis A02.21
      osteomyelitis A02.24
      pneumonia A02.22
      pyelonephritis A02.25
      specified NEC A02.29
    paratyphi A01.4
      A A01.1
      B A01.2
      C A01.3
    schottmuelleri A01.2
    typhi, typhosa - *see* Typhoid
  Sarcocystis A07.8
  scabies B86
  Schistosoma - *see* Infestation, Schistosoma
  scrotum (acute) NEC N49.2
  seminal vesicle - *see* Vesiculitis
  septic
    localized, skin - *see* Abscess
  sheep liver fluke B66.3
  Shigella A03.9
    boydii A03.2
    dysenteriae A03.0
    flexneri A03.1
    group
      A A03.0
      B A03.1
      C A03.2
      D A03.3
    Schmitz (-Stutzer) A03.0
    schmitzii A03.0
    shigae A03.0
    sonnei A03.3
    specified NEC A03.8
  shoulder (joint) NEC M00.9
    due to internal joint prosthesis T84.59
    skin NEC L08.9
  sinus (accessory) (chronic) (nasal) - *see also*
    Sinusitis
    pilonidal - *see* Sinus, pilonidal
    skin NEC L08.89
  Skene's duct or gland - *see* Urethritis
  skin (local) (staphylococcal) (streptococcal)
    L08.9
    abscess
    code by site under Abscess
    cellulitis
    code by site under Cellulitis
    due to fungus B36.9
      specified type NEC B36.8
    mycotic B36.9
      specified type NEC B36.8
    newborn P39.4
    ulcer - *see* Ulcer, skin
  slow virus A81.9
    specified NEC A81.89

Infection, infected, infective - *continued*
  Sparganum (mansoni) (proliferum) (baxteri)
    B70.1
  specific - *see also* Syphilis
    to perinatal period - *see* Infection, congenital
  specified NEC B99.8
  spermatic cord NEC N49.1
  sphenoidal (sinus) - *see* Sinusitis, sphenoidal
  spinal cord NOS - *see also* Myelitis G04.91
    abscess G06.1
    meninges - *see* Meningitis
    streptococcal G04.89
  Spirillum A25.0
  spirochetal NOS A69.9
    lung A69.8
    specified NEC A69.8
  Spirometra larvae B70.1
  spleen D73.89
  Sporotrichum, Sporothrix (schenckii) - *see*
    Sporotrichosis
  staphylococcal, unspecified site
    aureus (methicillin susceptible) (MSSA)
      A49.01
      methicillin resistant (MRSA) A49.02
    as cause of disease classified elsewhere
      B95.8
      aureus (methicillin susceptible) (MSSA)
        B95.61
        methicillin resistant (MRSA) B95.62
      specified NEC B95.7
    food poisoning A05.0
    generalized (purulent) A41.2
    pneumonia - *see* Pneumonia, staphylococcal
  Stellantchasmus falcatus B66.8
  streptobacillus moniliformis A25.1
  streptococcal NEC A49.1
    as cause of disease classified elsewhere
      B95.5
    B genitourinary complicating
      childbirth O98.82
      pregnancy O98.81-
      puerperium O98.83
    congenital
      sepsis P36.10
        group B P36.0
        specified NEC P36.19
    generalized (purulent) A40.9
  Streptomyces B47.1
  Strongyloides (stercoralis) - *see*
    Strongyloidiasis
  stump (amputation) (surgical) - *see*
    Complication, amputation stump, infection
  subcutaneous tissue, local L08.9
  suipestifer - *see* Infection, salmonella
  swimming pool bacillus A31.1
  Taenia - *see* Infestation, Taenia
  Taeniarhynchus saginatus B68.1
  tapeworm - *see* Infestation, tapeworm
  tendon (sheath) - *see* Tenosynovitis, infective
    NEC
  Ternidens diminutus B81.8
  testis - *see* Orchitis
  threadworm B80
  throat - *see* Pharyngitis
  thyroglossal duct K14.8
  toe (skin) L08.9
    cellulitis L03.03-
      fungus B35.1
    nail L03.03-
      fungus B35.1
  tongue NEC K14.0
    parasitic B37.0
  tonsil (and adenoid) (faucial) (lingual)
    (pharyngeal) - *see* Tonsillitis

Infection, infected, infective - *continued*
  tooth, teeth K04.7
    periapical K04.7
    peridental, periodontal K05.20
      generalized - *see* Periodontitis, aggressive,
        generalized
      localized - *see* Periodontitis, aggressive,
        localized
    pulp K04.01
      irreversible K04.02
      reversible K04.01
    socket M27.3
  TORCH - *see* Infection, congenital
    without active infection P00.2
  Torula histolytica - *see* Cryptococcosis
  Toxocara (canis) (cati) (felis) B83.0
  Toxoplasma gondii - *see* Toxoplasma
  trachea, chronic J42
  trematode NEC - *see* Infestation, fluke
  trench fever A79.0
  Treponema pallidum - *see* Syphilis
  Trichinella (spiralis) B75
  Trichomonas A59.9
    cervix A59.09
    intestine A07.8
    prostate A59.02
    specified site NEC A59.8
    urethra A59.03
    urogenitalis A59.00
    vagina A59.01
    vulva A59.01
  Trichophyton, trichophytic - *see*
    Dermatophytosis
  Trichosporon (beigelii) cutaneum B36.2
  Trichostrongylus B81.2
  Trichuris (trichiura) B79
  Trombicula (irritans) B88.0
  Trypanosoma
    brucei
      gambiense B56.0
      rhodesiense B56.1
    cruzi - *see* Chagas' disease
  tubal - *see* Salpingo-oophoritis
  tuberculous NEC - *see* Tuberculosis
  tubo-ovarian - *see* Salpingo-oophoritis
  tunnel T80.212
  tunica vaginalis N49.1
  tympanic membrane NEC - *see* Myringitis
  typhoid (abortive) (ambulant) (bacillus) - *see*
    Typhoid
  typhus A75.9
    flea-borne A75.2
    mite-borne A75.3
    recrudescent A75.1
    tick-borne A77.9
      African A77.1
      North Asian A77.2
  umbilicus L08.82
  ureter N28.86
  urethra - *see* Urethritis
  urinary (tract) N39.0
    bladder - *see* Cystitis
    complicating
      pregnancy O23.4-
        specified type NEC O23.3-
    kidney - *see* Infection, kidney
    newborn P39.3
    puerperal (postpartum) O86.20
    tuberculous A18.13
    urethra - *see* Urethritis
  uterus, uterine - *see* Endometritis
  vaccination T88.0
  vaccinia not from vaccination B08.011
  vagina (acute) - *see* Vaginitis

Infection, infected, infective - *continued*
  varicella B01.9
  varicose veins - *see* Varix
  vas deferens NEC N49.1
  vesical - *see* Cystitis
  Vibrio
    cholerae A00.0
      El Tor A00.1
    parahaemolyticus (food poisoning) A05.3
    vulnificus
      as cause of disease classified elsewhere
        B96.82
      foodborne intoxication A05.5
  Vincent's (gum) (mouth) (tonsil) A69.1
  virus, viral NOS B34.9
    adenovirus
      as cause of disease classified elsewhere
        B97.0
      unspecified nature or site B34.0
    arborvirus, arbovirus arthropod-borne A94
    as cause of disease classified elsewhere
      B97.89
      adenovirus B97.0
      coronavirus B97.29
        SARS-associated B97.21
      coxsackievirus B97.11
      echovirus B97.12
      enterovirus B97.10
        coxsackievirus B97.11
        echovirus B97.12
        specified NEC B97.19
      human
        immunodeficiency, type 2 (HIV 2) B97.35
        T-cell lymphotropic,
          type I (HTLV-i) B97.33
          type II (HTLV-II) B97.34
        metapneumovirus B97.81
      papillomavirus B97.7
      parvovirus B97.6
      reovirus B97.5
      respiratory syncytial B97.4
      retrovirus B97.30
        human
          immunodeficiency, type 2 (HIV 2)
            B97.35
          T-cell lymphotropic,
            type I (HTLV-i) B97.33
            type II (HTLV-II) B97.34
        lentivirus B97.31
        oncovirus B97.32
        specified NEC B97.39
      specified NEC B97.89
    central nervous system A89
      atypical A81.9
        specified NEC A81.89
      enterovirus NEC A88.8
        meningitis A87.0
      slow virus A81.9
        specified NEC A81.89
      specified NEC A88.8
    chest J98.8
    cotia B08.8
    coxsackie - *see also* Infection, coxsackie
      B34.1
      as cause of disease classified elsewhere
        B97.11
    ECHO
      as cause of disease classified elsewhere
        B97.12
      unspecified nature or site B34.1
    encephalitis, tick-borne A84.9
    enterovirus, as cause of disease classified
      elsewhere B97.10
      coxsackievirus B97.11

Infection, infected, infective - *continued*
    echovirus B97.12
      specified NEC B97.19
    exanthem NOS B09
    human papilloma as cause of disease
      classified elsewhere B97.7
    human metapneumovirus as cause of disease
      classified elsewhere B97.81
    intestine - *see* Enteritis, viral
    respiratory syncytial
      as cause of disease classified elsewhere
        B97.4
      bronchopneumonia J12.1
      common cold syndrome J00
      nasopharyngitis (acute) J00
    rhinovirus
      as cause of disease classified elsewhere
        B97.89
      unspecified nature or site B34.8
    slow A81.9
      specified NEC A81.89
    specified type NEC B33.8
      as cause of disease classified elsewhere
        B97.89
      unspecified nature or site B34.8
    unspecified nature or site B34.9
    West Nile - *see* Virus, West Nile
  vulva (acute) - *see* Vulvitis
  West Nile - *see* Virus, West Nile
  whipworm B79
  worms B83.9
    specified type NEC B83.8
  Wuchereria (bancrofti) B74.0
    malayi B74.1
  yatapoxvirus B08.70
    specified NEC B08.79
  yeast - *see also* Candidiasis B37.9
  yellow fever - *see* Fever, yellow
  Yersinia
    enterocolitica (intestinal) A04.6
    pestis - *see* Plague
    pseudotuberculosis A28.2
  Zeis' gland - *see* Hordeolum
  Zika virus A92.5
  zoonotic bacterial NOS A28.9
  Zofia senagalensis B47.0
Infective, infectious - *see* condition
Infertility N97.9
  female N97.9
    age-related N97.8
    associated with
      anovulation N97.0
      cervical (mucus) disease or anomaly N88.3
      congenital anomaly
        cervix N88.3
        fallopian tube N97.1
        uterus N97.2
        vagina N97.8
      dysmucorrhea N88.3
      fallopian tube disease or anomaly N97.1
      pituitary-hypothalamic origin E23.0
      specified origin NEC N97.8
      Stein-Leventhal syndrome E28.2
      uterine disease or anomaly N97.2
      vaginal disease or anomaly N97.8
    due to
      cervical anomaly N88.3
      fallopian tube anomaly N97.1
      ovarian failure E28.39
      Stein-Leventhal syndrome E28.2
      uterine anomaly N97.2
      vaginal anomaly N97.8
    nonimplantation N97.2
  origin

Infertility - *continued*
    cervical N88.3
    tubal (block) (occlusion) (stenosis) N97.1
    uterine N97.2
    vaginal N97.8
  male N46.9
    azoospermia N46.01
      extratesticular cause N46.029
        drug therapy N46.021
        efferent duct obstruction N46.023
        infection N46.022
        radiation N46.024
        specified cause NEC N46.029
        systemic disease N46.025
    oligospermia N46.11
      extratesticular cause N46.129
        drug therapy N46.121
        efferent duct obstruction N46.123
        infection N46.122
        radiation N46.124
        specified cause NEC N46.129
        systemic disease N46.125
    specified type NEC N46.8
Infestation B88.9
  Acanthocheilonema (perstans) (streptocerca)
    B74.4
  Acariasis B88.0
    demodex folliculorum B88.0
    sarcoptes scabiei B86
    trombiculae B88.0
  Agamofilaria streptocerca B74.4
  Ancylostoma, ankylostoma (braziliense)
    (caninum) (ceylanicum) (duodenale) B76.0
    americanum B76.1
    new world B76.1
  Anisakis larvae, anisakiasis B81.0
  arthropod NEC B88.2
  Ascaris lumbricoides - *see* Ascariasis
  Balantidium coli A07.0
  beef tapeworm B68.1
  Bothriocephalus (latus) B70.0
    larval B70.1
  broad tapeworm B70.0
    larval B70.1
  Brugia (malayi) B74.1
    timori B74.2
  candiru B88.8
  Capillaria
    hepatica B83.8
    philippinensis B81.1
  cat liver fluke B66.0
  cestodes B71.9
    diphyllobothrium - *see* Infestation,
      diphyllobothrium
    dipylidiasis B71.1
    hymenolepiasis B71.0
    specified type NEC B71.8
  chigger B88.0
  chigo, chigoe B88.1
  Clonorchis (sinensis) (liver) B66.1
  coccidial A07.3
  crab-lice B85.3
  Cysticercus cellulosae - *see* Cysticercosis
  Demodex (folliculorum) B88.0
  Dermanyssus gallinae B88.0
  Dermatobia (hominis) - *see* Myiasis
  Dibothriocephalus (latus) B70.0
    larval B70.1
  Dicrocoelium dendriticum B66.2
  Diphyllobothrium (adult) (latum) (intestinal)
    (pacificum) B70.0
    larval B70.1
  Diplogonoporus (grandis) B71.8
  Dipylidium caninum B67.4

Infestation - *continued*
- Distoma hepaticum B66.3
- dog tapeworm B67.4
- Dracunculus medinensis B72
- dragon worm B72
- dwarf tapeworm B71.0
- Echinococcus - *see* Echinococcus
- Echinostomum ilocanum B66.8
- Entamoeba (histolytica) - *see* Infection, Ameba
- Enterobius vermicularis B80
- eyelid
  - in (due to)
    - leishmaniasis B55.1
    - loiasis B74.3
    - onchocerciasis B73.09
    - phthiriasis B85.3
  - parasitic NOS B89
- eyeworm B74.3
- Fasciola (gigantica) (hepatica) (indica) B66.3
- Fasciolopsis (buski) (intestine) B66.5
- filarial B74.9
  - bancroftian B74.0
  - conjunctiva B74.9
  - due to
    - Acanthocheilonema (perstans) (streptocerca) B74.4
    - Brugia (malayi) B74.1
      - timori B74.2
    - Dracunculus medinensis B72
    - guinea worm B72
    - Loa Loa B74.3
    - Mansonella (ozzardi) (perstans) (streptocerca) B74.4
    - Onchocerca volvulus B73.00
      - eye B73.00
      - eyelid B73.09
    - Wuchereria (bancrofti) B74.0
  - Malayan B74.1
  - ozzardi B74.4
  - specified type NEC B74.8
- fish tapeworm B70.0
  - larval B70.1
- fluke B66.9
  - blood NOS - *see* Schistosomiasis
  - cat liver B66.0
  - intestinal B66.5
  - liver (sheep) B66.3
    - cat B66.0
    - Chinese B66.1
    - due to clonorchiasis B66.1
    - oriental B66.1
  - lancet B66.2
  - lung (oriental) B66.4
  - sheep liver B66.3
  - specified type NEC B66.8
- fly larvae - *see* Myiasis
- Gasterophilus (intestinalis) - *see* Myiasis
- Gastrodiscoides hominis B66.8
- Giardia lamblia A07.1
- Gnathostoma (spinigerum) B83.1
- Gongylonema B83.8
- guinea worm B72
- helminth B83.9
  - angiostrongyliasis B83.2
    - intestinal B81.3
  - gnathostomiasis B83.1
  - hirudiniasis, internal B83.4
  - intestinal B82.0
    - angiostrongyliasis B81.3
    - anisakiasis B81.0
    - ascariasis - *see* Ascariasis
    - capillariasis B81.1
    - cysticercosis - *see* Cysticercosis

Infestation - *continued*
- diphyllobothriasis - *see* Infestation, diphyllobothriasis
  - dracunculiasis B72
  - echinococcus - *see* Echinococcosis
  - enterobiasis B80
  - filariasis - *see* Infestation, filarial
  - fluke - *see* Infestation, fluke
  - hookworm - *see* Infestation, hookworm
  - mixed (types classifiable to more than one of the titles B65.0-b81.3 and B81.8) B81.4
  - onchocerciasis - *see* Onchocerciasis
  - schistosomiasis - *see* Infestation, Schistosoma
  - specified
    - cestode NEC - *see* Infestation, cestode type NEC B81.8
    - strongyloidiasis - *see* Strongyloidiasis
    - taenia - *see* Infestation, taenia
    - trichinellosis B75
    - trichostrongyliasis B81.2
    - trichuriasis B79
  - specified type NEC B83.8
  - syngamiasis B83.3
  - visceral larva migrans B83.0
- Heterophyes (heterophyes) B66.8
- hookworm B76.9
  - ancylostomiasis B76.0
  - necatoriasis B76.1
  - specified type NEC B76.8
- Hymenolepis (diminuta) (nana) B71.0
- intestinal NEC B82.9
- leeches (aquatic) (land) - *see* Hirudiniasis
- Leishmania - *see* Leishmaniasis
- lice, louse - *see* Infestation, Pediculus
- Linguatula B88.8
- Liponyssoides sanguineus B88.0
- Loa Loa B74.3
  - conjunctival B74.3
  - eyelid B74.3
- louse - *see* Infestation, Pediculus
- maggots - *see* Myiasis
- Mansonella (ozzardi) (perstans) (streptocerca) B74.4
- Medina (worm) B72
- Metagonimus (yokogawai) B66.8
- microfilaria streptocerca - *see* Onchocerciasis
  - eye B73.00
  - eyelid B73.09
- mites B88.9
  - scabic B86
- Monilia (albicans) - *see* Candidiasis
- mouth B37.0
- Necator americanus B76.1
- nematode NEC (intestinal) B82.0
  - Ancylostoma B76.0
  - conjunctiva NEC B83.9
  - Enterobius vermicularis B80
  - Gnathostoma spinigerum B83.1
  - physaloptera B80
  - specified NEC B81.8
  - trichostrongylus B81.2
  - trichuris (trichuria) B79
- Oesophagostomum (apiostomum) B81.8
- Oestrus ovis - *see also* Myiasis B87.9
- Onchocerca (volvulus) - *see* Onchocerciasis
- Opisthorchis (felineus) (viverrini) B66.0
- orbit, parasitic NOS B89
- Oxyuris vermicularis B80
- Paragonimus (westermani) B66.4
- parasite, parasitic B89
  - eyelid B89
  - intestinal NOS B82.9
  - mouth B37.0

Infestation - *continued*
- skin B88.9
- tongue B37.0
- Parastrongylus
  - cantonensis B83.2
  - costaricensis B81.3
- Pediculus B85.2
  - body B85.1
  - capitis (humanus) (any site) B85.0
  - corporis (humanus) (any site) B85.1
  - head B85.0
  - mixed (classifiable to more than one of the titles B85.0-b85.3) B85.4
  - pubis (any site) B85.3
- Pentastoma B88.8
- Phthirus (pubis) (any site) B85.3
  - with any infestation classifiable to B85.0-b85.2 B85.4
- pinworm B80
- pork tapeworm (adult) B68.0
- protozoal NEC B64
  - intestinal A07.9
    - specified NEC A07.8
  - specified NEC B60.8
- pubic, louse B85.3
- rat tapeworm B71.0
- red bug B88.0
- roundworm (large) NEC B82.0
  - Ascariasis - *see also* Ascariasis B77.9
- sandflea B88.1
- Sarcoptes scabiei B86
- scabies B86
- Schistosoma B65.9
  - bovis B65.8
  - cercariae B65.3
  - haematobium B65.0
  - intercalatum B65.8
  - japonicum B65.2
  - mansoni B65.1
  - mattheei B65.8
  - mekongi B65.8
  - specified type NEC B65.8
  - spindale B65.8
- screw worms - *see* Myiasis
- skin NOS B88.9
- Sparganum (mansoni) (proliferum) (baxteri) B70.1
  - larval B70.1
- specified type NEC B88.8
- Spirometra larvae B70.1
- Stellantchasmus falcatus B66.8
- Strongyloides stercoralis - *see* Strongyloidiasis
- Taenia B68.9
  - diminuta B71.0
  - echinococcus - *see* Echinococcus
  - mediocanellata B68.1
  - nana B71.0
  - saginata B68.1
  - solium (intestinal form) B68.0
    - larval form - *see* Cysticercosis
- Taeniarhynchus saginatus B68.1
- tapeworm B71.9
  - beef B68.1
  - broad B70.0
    - larval B70.1
  - dog B67.4
  - dwarf B71.0
  - fish B70.0
    - larval B70.1
  - pork B68.0
  - rat B71.0
- Ternidens diminutus B81.8
- Tetranychus molestissimus B88.0
- threadworm B80

Infestation - *continued*
tongue B37.0
Toxocara (canis) (cati) (felis) B83.0
trematode(s) NEC - *see* Infestation, fluke
Trichinella (spiralis) B75
Trichocephalus B79
Trichomonas - *see* Trichomoniasis
Trichostrongylus B81.2
Trichuris (trichiura) B79
Trombicula (irritans) B88.0
Tunga penetrans B88.1
Uncinaria americana B76.1
Vandellia cirrhosa B88.8
whipworm B79
worms B83.9
   intestinal B82.0
Wuchereria (bancrofti) B74.0

Infiltrate, infiltration
amyloid (generalized) (localized) - *see*
   Amyloidosis
calcareous NEC R89.7
   localized - *see* Degeneration, by site
calcium salt R89.7
cardiac
   fatty - *see* Degeneration, myocardial
   glycogenic E74.02 [143]
corneal - *see* Edema, cornea
eyelid - *see* Inflammation, eyelid
glycogen, glycogenic - *see* Disease, glycogen
   storage
heart, cardiac
   fatty - *see* Degeneration, myocardial
   glycogenic E74.02 [143]
inflammatory in vitreous H43.89
kidney N28.89
leukemic - *see* Leukemia
liver K76.89
   fatty - *see* Fatty, liver NEC
   glycogen - *see also* Disease, glycogen
   storage E74.03 [K77]
lung R91.8
   eosinophilic J82
lymphatic - *see also* Leukemia, lymphatic
   C91.9-
   gland I88.9
muscle, fatty M62.89
myocardium, myocardial
   fatty - *see* Degeneration, myocardial
   glycogenic E74.02 [143]
on chest x-ray R91.8
pulmonary R91.8
   with eosinophilia J82
skin (lymphocytic) L98.6
thymus (gland) (fatty) E32.8
urine R39.0
vesicant agent
   antineoplastic chemotherapy T80.810
   other agent NEC T80.818
vitreous body H43.89

Infirmity R68.89
senile R54

Inflammation, inflamed, inflammatory (with exudation)
abducent (nerve) - *see* Strabismus, paralytic,
   sixth nerve
accessory sinus (chronic) - *see* Sinusitis
adrenal (gland) E27.8
alveoli, teeth M27.3
   scorbutic E54
anal canal, anus K62.89
antrum (chronic) - *see* Sinusitis, maxillary
appendix - *see* Appendicitis
arachnoid - *see* Meningitis
areola N61.0

Inflammation - *continued*
puerperal, postpartum or gestational - *see*
   Infection, nipple
areolar tissue NOS L08.9
artery - *see* Arteritis
auditory meatus (external) - *see* Otitis, externa
Bartholin's gland N75.8
bile duct (common) (hepatic) or passage - *see*
   Cholangitis
bladder - *see* Cystitis
bone - *see* Osteomyelitis
brain - *see also* Encephalitis
   membrane - *see* Meningitis
breast N61.0
   puerperal, postpartum, gestational - *see*
   Mastitis, obstetric
broad ligament - *see* Disease, pelvis,
   inflammatory
bronchi - *see* Bronchitis
catarrhal J00
cecum - *see* Appendicitis
cerebral - *see also* Encephalitis
   membrane - *see* Meningitis
cerebrospinal
   meningococcal A39.0
cervix (uteri) - *see* Cervicitis
chest J98.8
chorioretinal H30.9-
   cyclitis - *see* Cyclitis
   disseminated H30.10-
      generalized H30.13-
      peripheral H30.12-
      posterior pole H30.11-
   epitheliopathy - *see* Epitheliopathy
   focal H30.00-
      juxtapapillary H30.01-
      macular H30.04-
      paramacular - *see* Inflammation,
         chorioretinal, focal, macular
      peripheral H30.03-
      posterior pole H30.02-
   specified type NEC H30.89-
choroid - *see* Inflammation, chorioretinal
chronic, postmastoidectomy cavity - *see*
   Complications, postmastoidectomy,
   inflammation
colon - *see* Enteritis
connective tissue (diffuse) NEC - *see* Disorder,
   soft tissue, specified type NEC
cornea - *see* Keratitis
corpora cavernosa N48.29
cranial nerve - *see* Disorder, nerve, cranial
Douglas' cul-de-sac or pouch (chronic) N73.0
due to device, implant or graft - *see also*
   Complications, by site and type, infection or
   inflammation
   arterial graft T82.7
   breast (implant) T85.79
   catheter T85.79
      dialysis (renal) T82.7
         intraperitoneal T85.71
      infusion T82.7
         cranial T85.735
         intrathecal T85.735
         spinal (epidural) (subdural) T85.735
         subarachnoid T85.735
      urinary T83.518
         cystostomy T83.510
         Hopkins T83.518
         ileostomy T83.518
         nephrostomy T83.512
         specified NEC T83.518
         urethral indwelling T83.511
         urostomy T83.518

Inflammation - *continued*
electronic (electrode) (pulse generator)
   (stimulator)
   bone T84.7
   cardiac T82.7
   nervous system T85.738
      brain T85.731
      cranial nerve T85.732
      gastric nerve T85.732
      neurostimulator generator T85.734
      peripheral nerve T85.732
      sacral nerve T85.732
      spinal cord T85.733
      vagal nerve T85.732
   urinary T83.590
fixation, internal (orthopedic) NEC - *see*
   Complication, fixation device, infection
gastrointestinal (bile duct) (esophagus)
   T85.79
   neurostimulator electrode (lead) T85.732
genital NEC T83.69
heart NEC T82.7
   valve (prosthesis) T82.6
      graft T82.7
joint prosthesis - *see* Complication, joint
   prosthesis, infection
ocular (corneal graft) (orbital implant) NEC
   T85.79
orthopedic NEC T84.7
penile (cylinder) (pump) (reservoir) T83.61
specified NEC T85.79
testicular T83.62
urinary NEC T83.598
   ileal conduit stent T83.593
   implanted neurostimulation T83.590
   implanted sphincter T83.591
   indwelling ureteral stent T83.592
   nephroureteral stent T83.593
   specified stent NEC T83.593
vascular NEC T82.7
ventricular intracranial (communicating)
   shunt T85.730
duodenum K29.80
   with bleeding K29.81
dura mater - *see* Meningitis
ear (middle) - *see also* Otitis, media
   external - *see* Otitis, externa
   inner - *see* subcategory H83.0
epididymis - *see* Epididymitis
esophagus K20.9
ethmoidal (sinus) (chronic) - *see* Sinusitis,
   ethmoidal
eustachian tube (catarrhal) - *see* Salpingitis,
   eustachian
eyelid H01.9
   abscess - *see* Abscess, eyelid
   blepharitis - *see* Blepharitis
   chalazion - *see* Chalazion
   dermatosis (noninfectious) - *see* Dermatosis,
      eyelid
   hordeolum - *see* Hordeolum
   specified NEC H01.8
fallopian tube - *see* Salpingo-oophoritis
fascia - *see* Myositis
follicular, pharynx J31.2
frontal (sinus) (chronic) - *see* Sinusitis, frontal
gallbladder - *see* Cholecystitis
gastric - *see* Gastritis
gastrointestinal - *see* Enteritis
genital organ (internal) (diffuse)
   female - *see* Disease, pelvis, inflammatory
   male N49.9
      multiple sites N49.8
      specified NEC N49.8

Inflammation - *continued*
gland (lymph) - *see* Lymphadenitis
glottis - *see* Laryngitis
granular, pharynx J31.2
gum K05.10
  nonplaque induced K05.11
  plaque induced K05.10
heart - *see* Carditis
hepatic duct - *see* Cholangitis
ileoanal (internal) pouch K91.850
ileum - *see also* Enteritis
  regional or terminal - *see* Enteritis, regional
intestine (any part) - *see* Enteritis
intestinal pouch K91.850
jaw (acute) (bone) (chronic) (lower)
  (suppurative) (upper) M27.2
joint NEC - *see* Arthritis
  sacroiliac M46.1
kidney - *see* Nephritis
knee (joint) M13.169
  tuberculous A18.02
labium (majus) (minus) - *see* Vulvitis
lacrimal
  gland - *see* Dacryoadenitis
  passages (duct) (sac) - *see also*
  Dacryocystitis
    canaliculitis - *see* Canaliculitis, lacrimal
larynx - *see* Laryngitis
leg NOS L08.9
lip K13.0
liver (capsule) - *see also* Hepatitis
  chronic K73.9
  suppurative K75.0
lung (acute) - *see also* Pneumonia
  chronic J98.4
lymph gland or node - *see* Lymphadenitis
lymphatic vessel - *see* Lymphangitis
maxilla, maxillary M27.2
  sinus (chronic) - *see* Sinusitis, maxillary
membranes of brain or spinal cord - *see*
  Meningitis
meninges - *see* Meningitis
mouth K12.1
muscle - *see* Myositis
myocardium - *see* Myocarditis
nasal sinus (chronic) - *see* Sinusitis
nasopharynx - *see* Nasopharyngitis
navel L08.82
nerve NEC - *see* Neuralgia
nipple N61.0
  puerperal, postpartum or gestational - *see*
  Infection, nipple
nose - *see* Rhinitis
oculomotor (nerve) - *see* Strabismus, paralytic,
  third nerve
optic nerve - *see* Neuritis, optic
orbit (chronic) H05.10
  acute H05.00
    abscess - *see* Abscess, orbit
    cellulitis - *see* Cellulitis, orbit
    osteomyelitis - *see* Osteomyelitis, orbit
    periostitis - *see* Periostitis, orbital
    tenonitis - *see* Tenonitis, eye
    granuloma - *see* Granuloma, orbit
    myositis - *see* Myositis, orbital
ovary - *see* Salpingo-oophoritis
oviduct - *see* Salpingo-oophoritis
pancreas (acute) - *see* Pancreatitis
parametrium N73.0
parotid region L08.9
pelvis, female - *see* Disease, pelvis,
  inflammatory   penis (corpora cavernosa)
  N48.29
perianal K62.89

Inflammation - *continued*
pericardium - *see* Pericarditis
perineum (female) (male) L08.9
perirectal K62.89
peritoneum - *see* Peritonitis
periuterine - *see* Disease, pelvis, inflammatory
  perivesical - *see* Cystitis
petrous bone (acute) (chronic) - *see* Petrositis
pharynx (acute) - *see* Pharyngitis
pia mater - *see* Meningitis
pleura - *see* Pleurisy
polyp, colon - *see also* Polyp, colon,
  inflammatory K51.40
prostate - *see also* Prostatitis
  specified type NEC N41.8
rectosigmoid - *see* Rectosigmoiditis
rectum - *see also* Proctitis K62.89
respiratory, upper - *see also* Infection,
  respiratory, upper J06.9
  acute, due to radiation J70.0
  chronic, due to external agent - *see* condition,
  respiratory, chronic, due to
  due to
    chemicals, gases, fumes or vapors
    (inhalation) J68.2
    radiation J70.1
retina - *see* Chorioretinitis
retrocecal - *see* Appendicitis
retroperitoneal - *see* Peritonitis
salivary duct or gland (any) (suppurative) - *see*
  Sialoadenitis
scorbutic, alveoli, teeth E54
scrotum N49.2
seminal vesicle - *see* Vesiculitis
sigmoid - *see* Enteritis
sinus - *see* Sinusitis
Skene's duct or gland - *see* Urethritis
skin L08.9
spermatic cord N49.1
sphenoidal (sinus) - *see* Sinusitis, sphenoidal
spinal
  cord - *see* Encephalitis
  membrane - *see* Meningitis
  nerve - *see* Disorder, nerve
  spine - *see* Spondylopathy, inflammatory
  spleen (capsule) D73.89
stomach - *see* Gastritis
subcutaneous tissue L08.9
suprarenal (gland) E27.8
synovial - *see* Tenosynovitis
tendon (sheath) NEC - *see* Tenosynovitis
testis - *see* Orchitis
throat (acute) - *see* Pharyngitis
thymus (gland) E32.8
thyroid (gland) - *see* Thyroiditis
tongue K14.0
tonsil - *see* Tonsillitis
trachea - *see* Tracheitis
trochlear (nerve) - *see* Strabismus, paralytic,
  fourth nerve
tubal - *see* Salpingo-oophoritis
tuberculous NEC - *see* Tuberculosis
tubo-ovarian - *see* Salpingo-oophoritis
tunica vaginalis N49.1
tympanic membrane - *see* Tympanitis
umbilicus, umbilical L08.82
uterine ligament - *see* Disease, pelvis,
  inflammatory   uterus (catarrhal) - *see*
  Endometritis
uveal tract (anterior) NOS - *see also*
Iridocyclitis
  posterior - *see* Chorioretinitis
vagina - *see* Vaginitis
vas deferens N49.1

Inflammation - *continued*
vein - *see also* Phlebitis
  intracranial or intraspinal (septic) G08
  thrombotic I80.9
    leg - *see* Phlebitis, leg
    lower extremity - *see* Phlebitis, leg
vocal cord J38.3
vulva - *see* Vulvitis
Wharton's duct (suppurative) - *see*
Sialoadenitis
Inflation, lung, imperfect (newborn) - *see*
Atelectasis
**Influenza (bronchial) (epidemic) (respiratory
(upper)) (unidentified influenza virus)** J11.1
  with
    digestive manifestations J11.2
    encephalopathy J11.81
    enteritis J11.2
    gastroenteritis J11.2
    gastrointestinal manifestations J11.2
    laryngitis J11.1
    myocarditis J11.82
    otitis media J11.83
    pharyngitis J11.1
    pneumonia J11.00
      specified type J11.08
    respiratory manifestations NEC J11.1
    specified manifestation NEC J11.89
A/H5N1
- *see also* Influenza, due to, identified novel
  influenza A virus J09.X2
  avian - *see also* Influenza, due to, identified
    novel influenza A virus J09.X2
  bird - *see also* Influenza, due to, identified
    novel influenza A virus J09.X2
  novel (2009) H1N1
influenza - *see also* Influenza, due to, identified
  influenza virus NEC J10.1
  novel influenza A/H1N1
- *see also* Influenza, due to, identified influenza
  virus NEC J10.1
  due to
    avian - *see also* Influenza, due to, identified
    novel influenza A virus J09.X2
    identified influenza virus NEC J10.1
      with
        digestive manifestations J10.2
        encephalopathy J10.81
        enteritis J10.2
        gastroenteritis J10.2
        gastrointestinal manifestations J10.2
        laryngitis J10.1
        myocarditis J10.82
        otitis media J10.83
        pharyngitis J10.1
        pneumonia (unspecified type) J10.00
          with same identified influenza virus
          J10.01
          specified type NEC J10.08
        respiratory manifestations NEC J10.1
        specified manifestation NEC J10.89
    identified novel influenza A virus J09.X2
      with
        digestive manifestations J09.X3
        encephalopathy J09.X9
        enteritis J09.X3
        gastroenteritis J09.X3
        gastrointestinal manifestations J09.X3
        laryngitis J09.X2
        myocarditis J09.X9
        otitis media J09.X9
        pharyngitis J09.X2
        pneumonia J09.X1
        respiratory manifestations NEC J09.X2

Influenza - *continued*
 specified manifestation NEC J09.X9
 upper respiratory symptoms J09.X2
  of other animal origin, not bird or swine
  – *see also* Influenza, due to, identified
  novel influenza A virus J09.X2
 swine (viruses that normally cause infections
  in pigs) - *see also* Influenza, due to,
  identified novel influenza A virus J09.X2
Influenza-like disease - *see* Influenza
Influenzal - *see* Influenza
Infraction, Freiberg's (metatarsal head) - *see*
 Osteochondrosis, juvenile, metatarsus
Infraeruption of tooth (teeth) M26.34
**Infusion complication, misadventure, or
reaction** - *see* Complications, infusion
Ingestion
 chemical - *see* Table of Drugs and Chemicals,
  by substance, poisoning
 drug or medicament
  correct substance properly administered - *see*
   Table of Drugs and Chemicals, by drug,
   adverse effect
  overdose or wrong substance given or taken -
   see Table of Drugs and Chemicals, by drug,
   poisoning
 foreign body - *see* Foreign body, alimentary
  tract
 tularemia A21.3
Ingrowing
 hair (beard) L73.1
 nail (finger) (toe) L60.0
Inguinal - *see also* condition
 testicle Q53.9
  bilateral Q53.212
  unilateral Q53.112
Inhalant-induced
 anxiety disorder F18.980
 depressive disorder F18.94
 major neurocognitive disorder F18.97
 mild neurocognitive disorder F18.988
 psychotic disorder F18.959
Inhalation
 anthrax A22.1
 flame T27.3
 food or foreign body - *see* Foreign body, by
  site
 gases, fumes, or vapors NEC T59.9-
  specified agent - *see* Table of Drugs and
   Chemicals, by substance
 liquid or vomitus - *see* Asphyxia
 meconium (newborn) P24.00
  with
   pneumonia (pneumonitis) P24.01
   with respiratory symptoms P24.01
 mucus - *see* Asphyxia, mucus
 oil or gasoline (causing suffocation) - *see*
  Foreign body, by site
 smoke J70.5
  due to chemicals, gases, fumes and vapors
   J68.9
 steam - *see* Toxicity, vapors
 stomach contents or secretions - *see* Foreign
  body, by site
  due to anesthesia (general) (local) or other
   sedation T88.59
   in labor and delivery O74.0
   in pregnancy O29.01-
   postpartum, puerperal O89.01
Inhibition, orgasm
 female F52.31
 male F52.32
**Inhibitor, systemic lupus erythematosus
(presence of)** D68.62

Iniencephalus, iniencephaly Q00.2
**Injection, traumatic jet (air) (industrial)
(water) (paint or dye)** T70.4
Injury - *see also* specified injury type T14.90
 abdomen, abdominal S39.91
  blood vessel - *see* Injury, blood vessel,
   abdomen
  cavity - *see* Injury, intra-abdominal
  contusion S30.1
  internal - *see* Injury, intra-abdominal
  intra-abdominal organ - *see* Injury, intra-
   abdominal
  nerve - *see* Injury, nerve, abdomen
  open - *see* Wound, open, abdomen
  specified NEC S39.81
  superficial - *see* Injury, superficial, abdomen
 Achilles tendon S86.00-
  laceration S86.02-
  specified type NEC S86.09-
  strain S86.01-
 acoustic, resulting in deafness - *see* Injury,
  nerve, acoustic
 adrenal (gland) S37.819
  contusion S37.812
  laceration S37.813
  specified type NEC S37.818
 alveolar (process) S09.93
 ankle S99.91-
  contusion - *see* Contusion, ankle
  dislocation - *see* Dislocation, ankle
  fracture - *see* Fracture, ankle
  nerve - *see* Injury, nerve, ankle
  open - *see* Wound, open, ankle
  specified type NEC S99.81-
  sprain - *see* Sprain, ankle
  superficial - *see* Injury, superficial, ankle
 anterior chamber, eye - *see* Injury, eye,
  specified site NEC
 anus - *see* Injury, abdomen
 aorta (thoracic) S25.00
  abdominal S35.00
   laceration (minor) (superficial) S35.01
    major S35.02
   specified type NEC S35.09
  laceration (minor) (superficial) S25.01
   major S25.02
  specified type NEC S25.09
 arm (upper) S49.9-
  blood vessel - *see* Injury, blood vessel, arm
  contusion - *see* Contusion, arm, upper
  fracture - *see* Fracture, humerus
  lower - *see* Injury, forearm
  muscle - *see* Injury, muscle, shoulder
  nerve - *see* Injury, nerve, arm
  open - *see* Wound, open, arm
  specified type NEC S49.8-
  superficial - *see* Injury, superficial, arm
 artery (complicating trauma) - *see also* Injury,
  blood vessel, by site
  cerebral or meningeal - *see* Injury,
   intracranial
 auditory canal (external) (meatus) S09.91
 auricle, auris, ear S09.91
 axilla - *see* Injury, shoulder
 back - *see* Injury, back, lower
 bile duct S36.13
 birth - *see also* Birth, injury P15.9
 bladder (sphincter) S37.20
  at delivery O71.5
  contusion S37.22
  laceration S37.23
  obstetrical trauma O71.5
  specified type NEC S37.29

Injury - *continued*
 blast (air) (hydraulic) (immersion)
  (underwater) NEC T14.8
  acoustic nerve trauma - *see* Injury, nerve,
   acoustic
  bladder - *see* Injury, bladder
  brain - *see* Concussion
  colon - *see* Injury, intestine, large, blast
   injury
  ear (primary) S09.31-
   secondary S09.39-
  generalized T70.8
  lung - *see* Injury, intrathoracic, lung, blast
   injury
  multiple body organs T70.8
  peritoneum S36.81
  rectum S36.61
  retroperitoneum S36.898
  small intestine S36.419
   duodenum S36.410
   specified site NEC S36.418
  specified
   intra-abdominal organ NEC S36.898
   pelvic organ NEC S37.899
 blood vessel NEC T14.8
  abdomen S35.9-
   aorta - *see* Injury, aorta, abdominal
   celiac artery - *see* Injury, blood vessel,
    celiac artery
   iliac vessel - *see* Injury, blood vessel, iliac
   laceration S35.91
   mesenteric vessel - *see* Injury, mesenteric
   portal vein - *see* Injury, blood vessel, portal
    vein
   renal vessel - *see* Injury, blood vessel, renal
   specified vessel NEC S35.8X-
   splenic vessel - *see* Injury, blood vessel,
    splenic
   vena cava - *see* Injury, vena cava, inferior
  ankle - *see* Injury, blood vessel, foot
  aorta (abdominal) (thoracic) - *see* Injury,
   aorta
  arm (upper) NEC S45.90-
   forearm - *see* Injury, blood vessel, forearm
   laceration S45.91-
   specified
    site NEC S45.80-
     laceration S45.81-
     specified type NEC S45.89-
    type NEC S45.99-
   superficial vein S45.30-
    laceration S45.31-
    specified type NEC S45.39-
  axillary
   artery S45.00-
    laceration S45.01-
    specified type NEC S45.09-
   vein S45.20-
    laceration S45.21-
    specified type NEC S45.29-
  azygos vein - *see* Injury, blood vessel,
   thoracic, specified site NEC
  brachial
   artery S45.10-
    laceration S45.11-
    specified type NEC S45.19-
   vein S45.20-
    laceration S45.219
    specified type NEC S45.29-
  carotid artery (common) (external) (internal,
   extracranial) S15.00-
   internal, intracranial S06.8-
   laceration (minor) (superficial) S15.01-

Injury - *continued*
    major S15.02-
    specified type NEC S15.09-
  celiac artery S35.219
    branch S35.299
      laceration (minor) (superficial) S35.291
        major S35.292
      specified NEC S35.298
    laceration (minor) (superficial) S35.211
      major S35.212
    specified type NEC S35.218
  cerebral - *see* Injury, intracranial
  deep plantar - *see* Injury, blood vessel,
    plantar artery
  digital (hand) - *see* Injury, blood vessel,
    finger
  dorsal
    artery (foot) S95.00-
      laceration S95.01-
      specified type NEC S95.09-
    vein (foot) S95.20-
      laceration S95.21-
      specified type NEC S95.29-
  due to accidental laceration during procedure
    - *see* Laceration, accidental complicating
    surgery
  extremity - *see* Injury, blood vessel, limb
  femoral
    artery (common) (superficial) S75.00-
      laceration (minor) (superficial) S75.01-
        major S75.02-
      specified type NEC S75.09-
    vein (hip level) (thigh level) S75.10-
      laceration (minor) (superficial) S75.11-
        major S75.12-
      specified type NEC S75.19-
  finger S65.50-
    index S65.50-
      laceration S65.51-
      specified type NEC S65.59-
    laceration S65.51-
    little S65.50-
      laceration S65.51-
      specified type NEC S65.59-
    middle S65.50-
      laceration S65.51-
      specified type NEC S65.59-
    specified type NEC S65.59-
    thumb - *see* Injury, blood vessel, thumb
  foot S95.90-
    dorsal
      artery - *see* Injury, blood vessel, dorsal,
      artery
      vein - *see* Injury, blood vessel, dorsal, vein
    laceration S95.91-
    plantar artery - *see* Injury, blood vessel,
      plantar artery
    specified
      site NEC S95.80-
        laceration S95.81-
        specified type NEC S95.89-
      specified type NEC S95.99-
  forearm S55.90-
    laceration S55.91-
    radial artery - *see* Injury, blood vessel,
      radial artery
    specified
      site NEC S55.80-
        laceration S55.81-
        specified type NEC S55.89-
      type NEC S55.99-
    ulnar artery - *see* Injury, blood vessel, ulnar
      artery
    vein S55.20-

Injury - *continued*
    laceration S55.21-
    specified type NEC S55.29-
  gastric
    artery - *see* Injury, mesenteric, artery,
    branch
    vein - *see* Injury, blood vessel, abdomen
  gastroduodenal artery - *see* Injury,
    mesenteric, artery, branch
  greater saphenous vein (lower leg level)
    S85.30-
    hip (and thigh) level S75.20-
      laceration (minor) (superficial) S75.21-
        major S75.22-
      specified type NEC S75.29-
    laceration S85.31-
    specified type NEC S85.39-
  hand (level) S65.90-
    finger - *see* Injury, blood vessel, finger
    laceration S65.91-
    palmar arch - *see* Injury, blood vessel,
      palmar arch
    radial artery - *see* Injury, blood vessel,
      radial artery, hand
    specified
      site NEC S65.80-
        laceration S65.81-
        specified type NEC S65.89-
      type NEC S65.99-
    thumb - *see* Injury, blood vessel, thumb
    ulnar artery - *see* Injury, blood vessel, ulnar
      artery, hand
  head S09.0
    intracranial - *see* Injury, intracranial
    multiple S09.0
  hepatic
    artery - *see* Injury, mesenteric, artery
    vein - *see* Injury, vena cava, inferior
  hip S75.90-
    femoral artery - *see* Injury, blood vessel,
      femoral, artery
    femoral vein - *see* Injury, blood vessel,
      femoral, vein
    greater saphenous vein - *see* Injury, blood
      vessel, greater saphenous, hip level
    laceration S75.91-
    specified
      site NEC S75.80-
        laceration S75.81-
        specified type NEC S75.89-
      type NEC S75.99-
  hypogastric (artery) (vein) - *see* Injury, blood
    vessel, iliac
  iliac S35.5-
    artery S35.51-
    specified vessel NEC S35.5-
    uterine vessel - *see* Injury, blood vessel,
      uterine
    vein S35.51-
  innominate - *see* Injury, blood vessel,
    thoracic, innominate
  intercostal (artery) (vein) - *see* Injury, blood
    vessel, thoracic, intercostal
  jugular vein (external) S15.20-
    internal S15.30-
      laceration (minor) (superficial) S15.31-
        major S15.32-
      specified type NEC S15.39-
    laceration (minor) (superficial) S15.21-
      major S15.22-
    specified type NEC S15.29-
  leg (level) (lower) S85.90-
    greater saphenous - *see* Injury, blood vessel,
      greater saphenous

Injury - *continued*
    laceration S85.91-
    lesser saphenous - *see* Injury, blood vessel,
      lesser saphenous
    peroneal artery - *see* Injury, blood vessel,
      peroneal artery
    popliteal
      artery - *see* Injury, blood vessel, popliteal,
      artery
      vein - *see* Injury, blood vessel, popliteal,
      vein
    specified
      site NEC S85.80-
        laceration S85.81-
        specified type NEC S85.89-
      type NEC S85.99-
    thigh - *see* Injury, blood vessel, hip
    tibial artery - *see* Injury, blood vessel, tibial
      artery
  lesser saphenous vein (lower leg level)
    S85.40-
    laceration S85.41-
    specified type NEC S85.49-
  limb
    lower - *see* Injury, blood vessel, leg
    upper - *see* Injury, blood vessel, arm
  lower back - *see* Injury, blood vessel,
    abdomen
    specified NEC - *see* Injury, blood vessel,
    abdomen, specified, site NEC
  mammary (artery) (vein) - *see* Injury, blood
    vessel, thoracic, specified site NEC
  mesenteric (inferior) (superior)
    artery - *see* Injury, mesenteric, artery
    vein - *see* Injury, mesenteric, vein
  neck S15.9
    specified site NEC S15.8
  ovarian (artery) (vein) - *see* subcategory
    S35.8
  palmar arch (superficial) S65.20-
    deep S65.30-
      laceration S65.31-
      specified type NEC S65.39-
    laceration S65.21-
    specified type NEC S65.29-
  pelvis - *see* Injury, blood vessel, abdomen
    specified NEC - *see* Injury, blood vessel,
  abdomen, specified, site NEC
  peroneal artery S85.20-
    laceration S85.21-
    specified type NEC S85.29-
  plantar artery (deep) (foot) S95.10-
    laceration S95.11-
    specified type NEC S95.19-
  popliteal
    artery S85.00-
      laceration S85.01-
      specified type NEC S85.09-
    vein S85.50-
      laceration S85.51-
      specified type NEC S85.59-
  portal vein S35.319
    laceration S35.311
    specified type NEC S35.318
  precerebral - *see* Injury, blood vessel, neck
  pulmonary (artery) (vein) - *see* Injury, blood
    vessel, thoracic, pulmonary
  radial artery (forearm level) S55.10-
    hand and wrist (level) S65.10-
      laceration S65.11-
      specified type NEC S65.19-
    laceration S55.11-
    specified type NEC S55.19-
  renal

Injury - *continued*
artery S35.40-
   laceration S35.41-
   specified NEC S35.49-
vein S35.40-
   laceration S35.41-
   specified NEC S35.49-
saphenous vein (greater) (lower leg level) -
   see Injury, blood vessel, greater saphenous
hip and thigh level - *see* Injury, blood
   vessel, greater saphenous, hip level
lesser - *see* Injury, blood vessel, lesser
   saphenous
shoulder
   specified NEC - *see* Injury, blood vessel,
     arm, specified site NEC
   superficial vein - *see* Injury, blood vessel,
     arm, superficial vein
specified NEC T14.8
splenic
   artery - *see* Injury, blood vessel, celiac
     artery, branch
   vein S35.329
     laceration S35.321
     specified NEC S35.328
subclavian - *see* Injury, blood vessel,
   thoracic, innominate
thigh - *see* Injury, blood vessel, hip
thoracic S25.90
   aorta S25.00
     laceration (minor) (superficial) S25.01
       major S25.02
     specified type NEC S25.09
   azygos vein - *see* Injury, blood vessel,
     thoracic, specified, site NEC
   innominate
     artery S25.10-
       laceration (minor) (superficial) S25.11-
         major S25.12-
       specified type NEC S25.19-
     vein S25.30-
       laceration (minor) (superficial) S25.31-
         major S25.32
       specified type NEC S25.39-
   intercostal S25.50-
     laceration S25.51-
     specified type NEC S25.59-
   laceration S25.91
   mammary vessel - *see* Injury, blood vessel,
thoracic, specified, site NEC
   pulmonary S25.40-
     laceration (minor) (superficial) S25.41-
       major S25.42-
     specified type NEC S25.49-
   specified
     site NEC S25.80-
       laceration S25.81-
       specified type NEC S25.89-
     type NEC S25.99
   subclavian - *see* Injury, blood vessel,
     thoracic, innominate
   vena cava (superior) S25.20
     laceration (minor) (superficial) S25.21
       major S25.22
     specified type NEC S25.29
thumb S65.40-
   laceration S65.41-
   specified type NEC S65.49-
tibial artery S85.10-
   anterior S85.13-
     laceration S85.14-
     specified injury NEC S85.15-
   laceration S85.11-
   posterior S85.16-

Injury - *continued*
     laceration S85.17-
     specified injury NEC S85.18-
   specified injury NEC S85.12-
ulnar artery (forearm level) S55.00-
   hand and wrist (level) S65.00-
     laceration S65.01-
     specified type NEC S65.09-
   laceration S55.01-
   specified type NEC S55.09-
upper arm (level) - *see* Injury, blood vessel,
   arm
   superficial vein - *see* Injury, blood vessel,
     arm, superficial vein
uterine S35.5-
   artery S35.53-
   vein S35.53-
vena cava - *see* Injury, vena cava
vertebral artery S15.10-
   laceration (minor) (superficial) S15.11-
     major S15.12-
   specified type NEC S15.19-
wrist (level) - *see* Injury, blood vessel, hand
brachial plexus S14.3
   newborn P14.3
brain (traumatic) S06.9-
   diffuse (axonal) S06.2X-
   focal S06.30-
   brainstem S06.38-
breast NOS S29.9
broad ligament - *see* Injury, pelvic organ,
specified site NEC
bronchus, bronchi - *see* Injury, intrathoracic,
bronchus
brow S09.90
buttock S39.92
canthus, eye S05.90
cardiac plexus - *see* Injury, nerve, thorax,
   sympathetic
cauda equina S34.3
cavernous sinus - *see* Injury, intracranial
cecum - *see* Injury, colon
celiac ganglion or plexus - *see* Injury, nerve,
   lumbosacral, sympathetic
cerebellum - *see* Injury, intracranial
cerebral - *see* Injury, intracranial
cervix (uteri) - *see* Injury, uterus
cheek (wall) S09.93
chest - *see* Injury, thorax
childbirth (newborn) - *see also* Birth, injury
   maternal NEC O71.9
chin S09.93
choroid (eye) - *see* Injury, eye, specified site
   NEC
clitoris S39.94
coccyx - *see also* Injury, back, lower
   complicating delivery O71.6
colon - *see* Injury, intestine, large
common bile duct - *see* Injury, liver
conjunctiva (superficial) - *see* Injury, eye,
   conjunctiva
conus medullaris - *see* Injury, spinal, sacral
cord
   spermatic (pelvic region) S37.898
     scrotal region S39.848
   spinal - *see* Injury, spinal cord, by region
cornea - *see* Injury, eye, specified site NEC
   abrasion - *see* Injury, eye, cornea, abrasion
cortex (cerebral) - *see also* Injury, intracranial
   visual - *see* Injury, nerve, optic
costal region NEC S29.9
costochondral NEC S29.9
cranial
   cavity - *see* Injury, intracranial

Injury - *continued*
nerve - *see* Injury, nerve, cranial
crushing - *see* Crush
cutaneous sensory nerve
cystic duct - *see* Injury, liver
deep tissue - *see* Contusion, by site
   meaning pressure ulcer - *see* Ulcer, pressure,
   unstageable, by site
delivery (newborn) P15.9
   maternal NEC O71.9
Descemet's membrane - *see* Injury, eyeball,
   penetrating
diaphragm - *see* Injury, intrathoracic,
   diaphragm
duodenum - *see* Injury, intestine, small,
   duodenum
ear (auricle) (external) (canal) S09.91
   abrasion - *see* Abrasion, ear
   bite - *see* Bite, ear
   blister - *see* Blister, ear
   bruise - *see* Contusion, ear
   contusion - *see* Contusion, ear
   external constriction - *see* Constriction,
     external, ear
   hematoma - *see* Hematoma, ear
   inner - *see* Injury, ear, middle
   laceration - *see* Laceration, ear
   middle S09.30-
     blast - *see* Injury, blast, ear
     specified NEC S09.39-
   puncture - *see* Puncture, ear
   superficial - *see* Injury, superficial, ear
eighth cranial nerve (acoustic or auditory) - *see*
   Injury, nerve, acoustic
elbow S59.90-
   contusion - *see* Contusion, elbow
   dislocation - *see* Dislocation, elbow
   fracture - *see* Fracture, ulna, upper end
   open - *see* Wound, open, elbow
   specified NEC S59.80-
   sprain - *see* Sprain, elbow
   superficial - *see* Injury, superficial, elbow
eleventh cranial nerve (accessory) - *see* Injury,
   nerve, accessory   epididymis S39.94
epigastric region S39.91
epiglottis NEC S19.89
esophageal plexus - *see* Injury, nerve, thorax,
   sympathetic
esophagus (thoracic part) - *see also* Injury,
   intrathoracic, esophagus
   cervical NEC S19.85
eustachian tube S09.30-
eye S05.9-
   avulsion S05.7-
   ball - *see* Injury, eyeball
   conjunctiva S05.0-
   cornea
     abrasion S05.0-
     laceration S05.3-
     with prolapse S05.2-
   lacrimal apparatus S05.8X-
   orbit penetration S05.4-
   specified site NEC S05.8X   eyeball S05.8X-
   contusion S05.1-
   penetrating S05.6-
     with
       foreign body S05.5-
       prolapse or loss of intraocular tissue
         S05.2-
       without prolapse or loss of intraocular
         tissue S05.3-
   specified type NEC S05.8-
eyebrow S09.93
eyelid S09.93

Injury - *continued*

abrasion - *see* Abrasion, eyelid
contusion - *see* Contusion, eyelid
open - *see* Wound, open, eyelid
face S09.93
fallopian tube S37.509
  bilateral S37.502
    blast injury S37.512
    contusion S37.522
    laceration S37.532
    specified type NEC S37.592
  blast injury (primary) S37.519
    bilateral S37.512
    secondary - *see* Injury, fallopian tube,
      specified type NEC
    unilateral S37.511
  contusion S37.529
    bilateral S37.522
    unilateral S37.521
  laceration S37.539
    bilateral S37.532
    unilateral S37.531
  specified type NEC S37.599
    bilateral S37.592
    unilateral S37.591
  unilateral S37.501
    blast injury S37.511
    contusion S37.521
    laceration S37.531
    specified type NEC S37.591
fascia - *see* Injury, muscle
fifth cranial nerve (trigeminal) - *see* Injury,
  nerve, trigeminal
finger (nail) S69.9-
  blood vessel - *see* Injury, blood vessel, finger
  contusion - *see* Contusion, finger
  dislocation - *see* Dislocation, finger
  fracture - *see* Fracture, finger
  muscle - *see* Injury, muscle, finger
  nerve - *see* Injury, nerve, digital, finger
  open - *see* Wound, open, finger
  specified NEC S69.8-
  sprain - *see* Sprain, finger
  superficial - *see* Injury, superficial, finger
first cranial nerve (olfactory) - *see* Injury,
  nerve, olfactory   flank - *see* Injury, abdomen
foot S99.92-
  blood vessel - *see* Injury, blood vessel, foot
  contusion - *see* Contusion, foot
  dislocation - *see* Dislocation, foot
  fracture - *see* Fracture, foot
  muscle - *see* Injury, muscle, foot
  open - *see* Wound, open, foot
  specified type NEC S99.82-
  sprain - *see* Sprain, foot
  superficial - *see* Injury, superficial, foot
forceps NOS P15.9
forearm S59.91-
  blood vessel - *see* Injury, blood vessel,
    forearm
  contusion - *see* Contusion, forearm
  fracture - *see* Fracture, forearm
  muscle - *see* Injury, muscle, forearm
  nerve - *see* Injury, nerve, forearm
  open - *see* Wound, open, forearm
  specified NEC S59.81-
  superficial - *see* Injury, superficial, forearm
forehead S09.90
fourth cranial nerve (trochlear) - *see* Injury,
  nerve, trochlear
gallbladder S36.129
  contusion S36.122
  laceration S36.123
  specified NEC S36.128

Injury - *continued*

ganglion
  celiac, coeliac - *see* Injury, nerve,
    lumbosacral, sympathetic
  gasserian - *see* Injury, nerve, trigeminal
  stellate - *see* Injury, nerve, thorax,
    sympathetic
  thoracic sympathetic - *see* Injury, nerve,
    thorax, sympathetic
gasserian ganglion - *see* Injury, nerve,
  trigeminal
gastric artery - *see* Injury, blood vessel, celiac
  artery, branch
gastroduodenal artery - *see* Injury, blood
  vessel, celiac artery, branch
gastrointestinal tract - *see* Injury, intra-
  abdominal
  with open wound into abdominal cavity - *see*
    Wound, open, with penetration into
    peritoneal cavity
  colon - *see* Injury, intestine, large
  rectum - *see* Injury, intestine, large, rectum
    with open wound into abdominal cavity
    S36.61
  specified site NEC - *see* Injury, intra-
    abdominal, specified, site NEC
  stomach - *see* Injury, stomach
  small intestine - *see* Injury, intestine, small
genital organ(s)
  external S39.94
    specified NEC S39.848
  internal S37.90
    fallopian tube - *see* Injury, fallopian tube
    ovary - *see* Injury, ovary
    prostate - *see* Injury, prostate
    seminal vesicle - *see* Injury, pelvis, organ,
      specified site NEC
    uterus - *see* Injury, uterus
    vas deferens - *see* Injury, pelvis, organ,
      specified site NEC
    obstetrical trauma O71.9
gland
  lacrimal laceration - *see* Injury, eye, specified
    site NEC
  salivary S09.93
  thyroid NEC S19.84
globe (eye) S05.90
  specified NEC S05.8X-
groin - *see* Injury, abdomen
gum S09.90
hand S69.9-
  blood vessel - *see* Injury, blood vessel, hand
  contusion - *see* Contusion, hand
  fracture - *see* Fracture, hand
  muscle - *see* Injury, muscle, hand
  nerve - *see* Injury, nerve, hand
  open - *see* Wound, open, hand
  specified NEC S69.8-
  sprain - *see* Sprain, hand
  superficial - *see* Injury, superficial, hand
head S09.90
  with loss of consciousness S06.9-
  specified NEC S09.8
heart S26.90
  with hemopericardium S26.00
    contusion S26.01
    laceration (mild) S26.020
      moderate S26.021
      major S26.022
    specified type NEC S26.09
  contusion S26.91
  laceration S26.92
  specified type NEC S26.99
  without hemopericardium S26.10

Injury - *continued*

  contusion S26.11
  laceration S26.12
  specified type NEC S26.19
heel - *see* Injury, foot
hepatic
  artery - *see* Injury, blood vessel, celiac artery,
    branch
  duct - *see* Injury, liver
  vein - *see* Injury, vena cava, inferior
hip S79.91-
  blood vessel - *see* Injury, blood vessel, hip
  contusion - *see* Contusion, hip
  dislocation - *see* Dislocation, hip
  fracture - *see* Fracture, femur, neck
  muscle - *see* Injury, muscle, hip
  nerve - *see* Injury, nerve, hip
  open - *see* Wound, open, hip
  sprain - *see* Sprain, hip
  superficial - *see* Injury, superficial, hip
  specified NEC S79.81-
hymen S39.94
hypogastric
  blood vessel - *see* Injury, blood vessel, iliac
  plexus - *see* Injury, nerve, lumbosacral,
    sympathetic
ileum - *see* Injury, intestine, small
iliac region S39.91
instrumental (during surgery) - *see* Laceration,
accidental complicating surgery
  birth injury - *see* Birth, injury
  nonsurgical - *see* Injury, by site
  obstetrical O71.9
    bladder O71.5
    cervix O71.3
    high vaginal O71.4
    perineal NOS O70.9
    urethra O71.5
    uterus O71.5
      with rupture or perforation O71.1
internal T14.8
  aorta - *see* Injury, aorta
  bladder (sphincter) - *see* Injury, bladder
    with
      ectopic or molar pregnancy O08.6
      following ectopic or molar pregnancy
        O08.6
      obstetrical trauma O71.5
  bronchus, bronchi - *see* Injury, intrathoracic,
    bronchus
  cecum - *see* Injury, intestine, large
  cervix (uteri) - *see also* Injury, uterus
    with ectopic or molar pregnancy O08.6
    following ectopic or molar pregnancy
      O08.6
    obstetrical trauma O71.3
  chest - *see* Injury, intrathoracic
  gastrointestinal tract - *see* Injury, intra-
    abdominal
  heart - *see* Injury, heart
  intestine NEC - *see* Injury, intestine
  intrauterine - *see* Injury, uterus
  mesentery - *see* Injury, intra-abdominal,
    specified, site NEC
  pelvis, pelvic (organ) S37.90
    following ectopic or molar pregnancy
      (subsequent episode) O08.6
    obstetrical trauma NEC O71.5
      rupture or perforation O71.1
    specified NEC S39.83
  rectum - *see* Injury, intestine, large, rectum
  stomach - *see* Injury, stomach
  ureter - *see* Injury, ureter
  urethra (sphincter) following ectopic or

Injury - *continued*
  molar pregnancy O08.6
  uterus - *see* Injury, uterus
 interscapular area - *see* Injury, thorax
 intestine
  large S36.509
   ascending (right) S36.500
    blast injury (primary) S36.510
     secondary S36.590
    contusion S36.520
    laceration S36.530
    specified type NEC S36.590
   blast injury (primary) S36.519
    ascending (right) S36.510
    descending (left) S36.512
    rectum S36.61
    sigmoid S36.513
    specified site NEC S36.518
    transverse S36.511
   contusion S36.529
    ascending (right) S36.520
    descending (left) S36.522
    rectum S36.62
    sigmoid S36.523
    specified site NEC S36.528
    transverse S36.521
   descending (left) S36.502
    blast injury (primary) S36.512
     secondary S36.592
    contusion S36.522
    laceration S36.532
    specified type NEC S36.592
   laceration S36.539
    ascending (right) S36.530
    descending (left) S36.532
    rectum S36.63
    sigmoid S36.533
    specified site NEC S36.538
    transverse S36.531
   rectum S36.60
    blast injury (primary) S36.61
     secondary S36.69
    contusion S36.62
    laceration S36.63
    specified type NEC S36.69
   sigmoid S36.503
    blast injury (primary) S36.513
     secondary S36.593
    contusion S36.523
    laceration S36.533
    specified type NEC S36.593
   specified
    site NEC S36.508
     blast injury (primary) S36.518
      secondary S36.598
     contusion S36.528
     laceration S36.538
     specified type NEC S36.598
    type NEC S36.599
     ascending (right) S36.590
     descending (left) S36.592
     rectum S36.69
     sigmoid S36.593
     specified site NEC S36.598
     transverse S36.591
   transverse S36.501
    blast injury (primary) S36.511
     secondary S36.591
    contusion S36.521
    laceration S36.531
    specified type NEC S36.591
  small S36.409
   blast injury (primary) S36.419
   duodenum S36.410

Injury - *continued*
    secondary S36.499
     duodenum S36.490
     specified site NEC S36.498
    specified site NEC S36.418
   contusion S36.429
    duodenum S36.420
    specified site NEC S36.428
   duodenum S36.400
    blast injury (primary) S36.410
     secondary S36.490
    contusion S36.420
    laceration S36.430
    specified site NEC S36.490
   laceration S36.439
    duodenum S36.430
    specified site NEC S36.438
   specified
    type NEC S36.499
     duodenum S36.490
     specified site NEC S36.498
    site NEC S36.408
 intra-abdominal S36.90
  adrenal gland - *see* Injury, adrenal gland
  bladder - *see* Injury, bladder
  colon - *see* Injury, intestine, large
  contusion S36.92
  fallopian tube - *see* Injury, fallopian tube
  gallbladder - *see* Injury, gallbladder
  intestine - *see* Injury, intestine
  laceration S36.93
  liver - *see* Injury, liver
  kidney - *see* Injury, kidney
  ovary - *see* Injury, ovary
  pancreas - *see* Injury, pancreas
  pelvic NOS S37.90
  peritoneum - *see* Injury, intra-abdominal,
   specified, site NEC
  prostate - *see* Injury, prostate
  rectum - *see* Injury, intestine, large, rectum
  retroperitoneum - *see* Injury, intra-
   abdominal, specified, site NEC
  seminal vesicle - *see* Injury, pelvis, organ,
   specified site NEC
  small intestine - *see* Injury, intestine, small
  specified
   site NEC S36.899
    contusion S36.892
    laceration S36.893
    specified type NEC S36.898
   type NEC S36.99
  pelvic S37.90
   specified
    site NEC S37.899
     specified type NEC S37.898
    type NEC S37.99
  spleen - *see* Injury, spleen
  stomach - *see* Injury, stomach
  ureter - *see* Injury, ureter
  urethra - *see* Injury, urethra
  uterus - *see* Injury, uterus
  vas deferens - *see* Injury, pelvis, organ,
   specified site NEC
 intracranial (traumatic) S06.9-
  cerebellar hemorrhage, traumatic - *see* Injury,
   intracranial, focal
  cerebral edema, traumatic S06.1X-
   diffuse S06.1X-
   focal S06.1X-
  diffuse (axonal) S06.2X-
  epidural hemorrhage (traumatic) S06.4X-
  focal brain injury S06.30-
   contusion - *see* Contusion, cerebral
   laceration - *see* Laceration, cerebral

Injury - *continued*
  intracerebral hemorrhage, traumatic S06.36-
   left side S06.35-
   right side S06.34-
  subarachnoid hemorrhage, traumatic S06.6X-
  subdural hemorrhage, traumatic S06.5X-
 intraocular - *see* Injury, eyeball, penetrating
 intrathoracic S27.9
  bronchus S27.409
   bilateral S27.402
   blast injury (primary) S27.419
    bilateral S27.412
    secondary - *see* Injury, intrathoracic,
     bronchus, specified type NEC
    unilateral S27.411
   contusion S27.429
    bilateral S27.422
    unilateral S27.421
   laceration S27.439
    bilateral S27.432
    unilateral S27.431
   specified type NEC S27.499
    bilateral S27.492
    unilateral S27.491
   unilateral S27.401
  diaphragm S27.809
   contusion S27.802
   laceration S27.803
   specified type NEC S27.808
  esophagus (thoracic) S27.819
   contusion S27.812
   laceration S27.813
   specified type NEC S27.818
  heart - *see* Injury, heart
  hemopneumothorax S27.2
  hemothorax S27.1
  lung S27.309
   aspiration J69.0
   bilateral S27.302
   blast injury (primary) S27.319
    bilateral S27.312
    secondary - *see* Injury, intrathoracic, lung,
     specified type NEC
    unilateral S27.311
   contusion S27.329
    bilateral S27.322
    unilateral S27.321
   laceration S27.339
    bilateral S27.332
    unilateral S27.331
   specified type NEC S27.399
    bilateral S27.392
    unilateral S27.391
   unilateral S27.301
  pleura S27.60
   laceration S27.63
   specified type NEC S27.69
  pneumothorax S27.0
  specified organ NEC S27.899
   contusion S27.892
   laceration S27.893
   specified type NEC S27.898
  thoracic duct - *see* Injury, intrathoracic,
   specified organ NEC
  thymus gland - *see* Injury, intrathoracic,
   specified organ NEC
  trachea, thoracic S27.50
   blast (primary) S27.51
   contusion S27.52
   laceration S27.53
   specified type NEC S27.59
 iris - *see* Injury, eye, specified site NEC
  penetrating - *see* Injury, eyeball, penetrating
 jaw S09.93

Injury - *continued*
    specified type NEC S56.49-
    strain S56.41-
   flexor (forearm level)
    hand level S66.10-
     laceration S66.12-
     specified type NEC S66.19-
     strain S66.11-
    laceration S56.12-
    specified type NEC S56.19-
    strain S56.11-
    intrinsic S66.50-
     laceration S66.52-
     specified type NEC S66.59-
     strain S66.51-
  flexor
   finger(s) (other than thumb) - *see* Injury,
    muscle, finger
   forearm level, specified NEC - *see* Injury,
    muscle, forearm, flexor
   thumb - *see* Injury, muscle, thumb, flexor
   toe (long) (ankle level) (foot level) - *see*
    Injury, muscle, toe, flexor
  foot S96.90-
   intrinsic S96.20-
    laceration S96.22-
    specified type NEC S96.29-
    strain S96.21-
   laceration S96.92-
   long extensor, toe - *see* Injury, muscle, toe,
    extensor
   long flexor, toe - *see* Injury, muscle, toe,
    flexor
   specified
    site NEC S96.80-
     laceration S96.82-
     specified type NEC S96.89-
     strain S96.81-
    type NEC S96.99-
    strain S96.91-
  forearm (level) S56.90-
   extensor S56.50-
    laceration S56.52-
    specified type NEC S56.59-
    strain S56.51-
   flexor S56.20-
    laceration S56.22-
    specified type NEC S56.29-
    strain S56.21-
   laceration S56.92-
   specified S56.99-
    site NEC S56.80-
     laceration S56.82-
     strain S56.81-
     type NEC S56.89-
    strain S56.91-
  hand (level) S66.90-
   laceration S66.92-
   specified
    site NEC S66.80-
     laceration S66.82-
     specified type NEC S66.89-
     strain S66.81-
    type NEC S66.99-
    strain S66.91-
  head S09.10
   laceration S09.12
   specified type NEC S09.19
   strain S09.11
  hip NEC S76.00-
   laceration S76.02-
   specified type NEC S76.09-
   strain S76.01-
  intrinsic

Injury - *continued*
   ankle and foot level - *see* Injury, muscle,
    foot, intrinsic
   finger (other than thumb) - *see* Injury,
    muscle, finger by site, intrinsic
   foot (level) - *see* Injury, muscle, foot,
    intrinsic
   thumb - *see* Injury, muscle, thumb, intrinsic
  leg (level) (lower) S86.90-
   Achilles tendon - *see* Injury, Achilles
    tendon
   anterior muscle group - *see* Injury, muscle,
    anterior muscle group
   laceration S86.92-
   peroneal muscle group - *see* Injury, muscle,
    peroneal muscle group
   posterior muscle group - *see* Injury, muscle,
    posterior muscle group, leg level
   specified
    site NEC S86.80-
     laceration S86.82-
     specified type NEC S86.89-
     strain S86.81-
    type NEC S86.99-
   strain S86.91-
  long
   extensor toe, at ankle and foot level - *see*
    Injury, muscle, toe, extensor
   flexor, toe, at ankle and foot level - *see*
    Injury, muscle, toe, flexor
   head, biceps - *see* Injury, muscle, biceps,
    long head
  lower back S39.002
   laceration S39.022
   specified type NEC S39.092
   strain S39.012
  neck (level) S16.9
   laceration S16.2
   specified type NEC S16.8
   strain S16.1
  pelvis S39.003
   laceration S39.023
   specified type NEC S39.093
   strain S39.013
  peroneal muscle group, at leg level (lower)
    S86.30-
   laceration S86.32-
   specified type NEC S86.39-
   strain S86.31-
  posterior muscle (group)
   leg level (lower) S86.10-
    laceration S86.12-
    specified type NEC S86.19-
    strain S86.11-
   thigh level S76.30-
    laceration S76.32-
    specified type NEC S76.39-
    strain S76.31-
  quadriceps (thigh) S76.10-
   laceration S76.12-
   specified type NEC S76.19-
   strain S76.11-
  shoulder S46.90-
   laceration S46.92-
   rotator cuff - *see* Injury, rotator cuff
   specified site NEC S46.80-
    laceration S46.82-
    strain S46.81-
    specified type NEC S46.89-
   strain S46.91-
   specified type NEC S46.99-
  thigh NEC (level) S76.90-
   adductor - *see* Injury, muscle, adductor,
    thigh

Injury - *continued*
   laceration S76.92-
   posterior muscle (group) - *see* Injury,
    muscle, posterior muscle, thigh level
   quadriceps - *see* Injury, muscle, quadriceps
   specified
    site NEC S76.80-
     laceration S76.82-
     specified type NEC S76.89-
     strain S76.81-
    type NEC S76.99-
   strain S76.91-
  thorax (level) S29.009
   back wall S29.002
   front wall S29.001
   laceration S29.029
    back wall S29.022
    front wall S29.021
   specified type NEC S29.099
    back wall S29.092
    front wall S29.091
   strain S29.019
    back wall S29.012
    front wall S29.011
  thumb
   abductor (forearm level) S56.30-
    laceration S56.32-
    specified type NEC S56.39-
    strain S56.31-
   extensor (forearm level) S56.30-
    hand level S66.20-
     laceration S66.22-
     specified type NEC S66.29-
     strain S66.21-
    laceration S56.32-
    specified type NEC S56.39-
    strain S56.31-
   flexor (forearm level) S56.00-
    hand level S66.00-
     laceration S66.02-
     specified type NEC S66.09-
     strain S66.01-
    laceration S56.02-
    specified type NEC S56.09-
    strain S56.01-
    wrist level - *see* Injury, muscle, thumb,
     flexor, hand level
   intrinsic S66.40-
    laceration S66.42-
    specified type NEC S66.49-
    strain S66.41-
  toe - *see also* Injury, muscle, foot
   extensor, long S96.10-
    laceration S96.12-
    specified type NEC S96.19-
    strain S96.11-
   flexor, long S96.00-
    laceration S96.02-
    specified type NEC S96.09-
    strain S96.01-
  triceps S46.30-
   laceration S46.32-
   specified type NEC S46.39-
   strain S46.31-
  wrist (and hand) level - *see* Injury, muscle,
   hand
  musculocutaneous nerve - *see* Injury, nerve,
   musculocutaneous
  myocardium - *see* Injury, heart
  nape - *see* Injury, neck
  nasal (septum) (sinus) S09.92
  nasopharynx S09.92
  neck S19.9
   specified NEC S19.80

Injury - *continued*
  specified site NEC S19.89
nerve NEC T14.8
  abdomen S34.9
    peripheral S34.6
    specified site NEC S34.8
  abducens S04.4-
    contusion S04.4-
    laceration S04.4-
    specified type NEC S04.4-
  abducent - *see* Injury, nerve, abducens
  accessory S04.7-
    contusion S04.7-
    laceration S04.7-
    specified type NEC S04.7-
  acoustic S04.6-
    contusion S04.6-
    laceration S04.6-
    specified type NEC S04.6-
  ankle S94.9-
    cutaneous sensory S94.3-
    specified site NEC - *see* subcategory S94.8
  anterior crural, femoral - *see* Injury, nerve,
    femoral
  arm (upper) S44.9-
    axillary - *see* Injury, nerve, axillary
    cutaneous - *see* Injury, nerve, cutaneous,
      arm
    median - *see* Injury, nerve, median, upper
      arm
    musculocutaneous - *see* Injury, nerve,
      musculocutaneous
    radial - *see* Injury, nerve, radial, upper arm
    specified site NEC - *see* subcategory S44.8
    ulnar - *see* Injury, nerve, ulnar, arm
  auditory - *see* Injury, nerve, acoustic
  axillary S44.3-
  brachial plexus - *see* Injury, brachial plexus
  cervical sympathetic S14.5
  cranial S04.9
    contusion S04.9
    eighth (acoustic or auditory) - *see* Injury,
      nerve, acoustic
    eleventh (accessory) - *see* Injury, nerve,
      accessory
    fifth (trigeminal) - *see* Injury, nerve,
      trigeminal
    first (olfactory) - *see* Injury, nerve,
      olfactory
    fourth (trochlear) - *see* Injury, nerve,
      trochlear
    laceration S04.9
    ninth (glossopharyngeal) - *see* Injury, nerve,
      glossopharyngeal
    second (optic) - *see* Injury, nerve, optic
    seventh (facial) - *see* Injury, nerve, facial
    sixth (abducent) - *see* Injury, nerve,
      abducens
    specified
      nerve NEC S04.89-
        contusion S04.89-
        laceration S04.89-
        specified type NEC S04.89-
      type NEC S04.9
    tenth (pneumogastric or vagus) - *see* Injury,
      nerve, vagus
    third (oculomotor) - *see* Injury, nerve,
      oculomotor
    twelfth (hypoglossal) - *see* Injury, nerve,
      hypoglossal
  cutaneous sensory
    ankle (level) S94.3-
    arm (upper) (level) S44.5-

Injury - *continued*
    foot (level) - *see* Injury, nerve, cutaneous
      ensory, ankle
    forearm (level) S54.3-
    hip (level) S74.2-
    leg (lower level) S84.2-
    shoulder (level) - *see* Injury, nerve,
      cutaneous sensory, arm
    thigh (level) - *see* Injury, nerve, cutaneous
      sensory, hip
  deep peroneal - *see* Injury, nerve, peroneal,
    foot
  digital
    finger S64.4-
      index S64.49-
      little S64.49-
      middle S64.49-
      ring S64.49-
      thumb S64.3-
    toe - *see* Injury, nerve, ankle, specified site
      NEC
  eighth cranial (acoustic or auditory) - *see*
    Injury, nerve, acoustic
  eleventh cranial (accessory) - *see* Injury,
    nerve, accessory
  facial S04.5-
    contusion S04.5-
    laceration S04.5-
    newborn P11.3
    specified type NEC S04.5-
  femoral (hip level) (thigh level) S74.1-
  fifth cranial (trigeminal) - *see* Injury, nerve,
    trigeminal
  finger (digital) - *see* Injury, nerve, digital,
    finger
  first cranial (olfactory) - *see* Injury, nerve,
    olfactory
  foot S94.9-
    cutaneous sensory S94.3-
    deep peroneal S94.2-
    lateral plantar S94.0-
    medial plantar S94.1-
    specified site NEC - *see* subcategory S94.8
  forearm (level) S54.9-
    cutaneous sensory - *see* Injury, nerve,
      cutaneous sensory, forearm
    median - *see* Injury, nerve, median
    radial - *see* Injury, nerve, radial
    specified site NEC - *see* subcategory S54.8
    ulnar - *see* Injury, nerve, ulnar
  fourth cranial (trochlear) - *see* Injury, nerve,
    trochlear
  glossopharyngeal S04.89-
    specified type NEC S04.89-
  hand S64.9-
    median - *see* Injury, nerve, median, hand
    radial - *see* Injury, nerve, radial, hand
    specified NEC - *see* subcategory S64.8
    ulnar - *see* Injury, nerve, ulnar, hand
  hip (level) S74.9-
    cutaneous sensory - *see* Injury, nerve,
      cutaneous sensory, hip
    femoral - *see* Injury, nerve, femoral
    sciatic - *see* Injury, nerve, sciatic
    specified site NEC - *see* subcategory S74.8
  hypoglossal S04.89-
    specified type NEC S04.89-
  lateral plantar S94.0-
  leg (lower) S84.9-
    cutaneous sensory - *see* Injury, nerve,
      cutaneous sensory, leg
    peroneal - *see* Injury, nerve, peroneal
    specified site NEC - *see* subcategory S84.8
    tibial - *see* Injury, nerve, tibial

Injury - *continued*
    upper - *see* Injury, nerve, thigh
  lower
    back - *see* Injury, nerve, abdomen, specified
      site NEC
      peripheral - *see* Injury, nerve, abdomen,
        peripheral
    limb - *see* Injury, nerve, leg
  lumbar spinal - *see* Injury, nerve, spinal,
    lumbar
  lumbar plexus - *see* Injury, nerve,
    lumbosacral, sympathetic
  lumbosacral
    plexus - *see* Injury, nerve, lumbosacral,
      sympathetic
    sympathetic S34.5
  medial plantar S94.1-
  median (forearm level) S54.1-
    hand (level) S64.1-
    upper arm (level) S44.1-
    wrist (level) - *see* Injury, nerve, median,
      hand
  musculocutaneous S44.4-
  musculospiral (upper arm level) - *see* Injury,
    nerve, radial, upper arm
  neck S14.9
    peripheral S14.4
    specified site NEC S14.8
    sympathetic S14.5
  ninth cranial (glossopharyngeal) - *see* Injury,
    nerve, glossopharyngeal
  oculomotor S04.1-
    contusion S04.1-
    laceration S04.1-
    specified type NEC S04.1-
  olfactory S04.81-
    specified type NEC S04.81-
  optic S04.01-
    contusion S04.01-
    laceration S04.01-
    specified type NEC S04.01-
  pelvic girdle - *see* Injury, nerve, hip
  pelvis - *see* Injury, nerve, abdomen, specified
    site NEC
    peripheral - *see* Injury, nerve, abdomen,
      peripheral
  peripheral NEC T14.8
    abdomen - *see* Injury, nerve, abdomen,
      peripheral
    lower back - *see* Injury, nerve, abdomen,
      peripheral
    neck - *see* Injury, nerve, neck, peripheral
    pelvis - *see* Injury, nerve, abdomen,
      peripheral
    specified NEC T14.8
  peroneal (lower leg level) S84.1-
    foot S94.2-
  plexus
    brachial - *see* Injury, brachial plexus
    celiac, coeliac - *see* Injury, nerve,
      lumbosacral, sympathetic
    mesenteric, inferior - *see* Injury, nerve,
      lumbosacral, sympathetic
    sacral - *see* Injury, lumbosacral plexus
    spinal
      brachial - *see* Injury, brachial plexus
      lumbosacral - *see* Injury, lumbosacral
        plexus
  pneumogastric - *see* Injury, nerve, vagus
  radial (forearm level) S54.2-
    hand (level) S64.2-
    upper arm (level) S44.2-
    wrist (level) - *see* Injury, nerve, radial, hand
  root - *see* Injury, nerve, spinal, root

Injury - *continued*

sacral plexus - *see* Injury, lumbosacral plexus
sacral spinal - *see* Injury, nerve, spinal, sacral
sciatic (hip level) (thigh level) S74.0-
second cranial (optic) - *see* Injury, nerve,
   optic
seventh cranial (facial) - *see* Injury, nerve,
   facial
shoulder - *see* Injury, nerve, arm
sixth cranial (abducent) - *see* Injury, nerve,
   abducens
spinal
   plexus - *see* Injury, nerve, plexus, spinal
   root
      cervical S14.2
      dorsal S24.2
      lumbar S34.21
      sacral S34.22
      thoracic - *see* Injury, nerve, spinal, root,
         dorsal
splanchnic - *see* Injury, nerve, lumbosacral,
   sympathetic
sympathetic NEC - *see* Injury, nerve,
   lumbosacral, sympathetic
   cervical - *see* Injury, nerve, cervical
   sympathetic
tenth cranial (pneumogastric or vagus) - *see*
   Injury, nerve, vagus
thigh (level) - *see* Injury, nerve, hip
   cutaneous sensory - *see* Injury, nerve,
      cutaneous sensory, hip
   femoral - *see* Injury, nerve, femoral
   sciatic - *see* Injury, nerve, sciatic
   specified NEC - *see* Injury, nerve, hip
third cranial (oculomotor) - *see* Injury, nerve,
   oculomotor
thorax S24.9
   peripheral S24.3
   specified site NEC S24.8
   sympathetic S24.4
thumb, digital - *see* Injury, nerve, digital,
   thumb
tibial (lower leg level) (posterior) S84.0-
toe - *see* Injury, nerve, ankle
trigeminal S04.3-
   contusion S04.3-
   laceration S04.3-
   specified type NEC S04.3-
trochlear S04.2-
   contusion S04.2-
   laceration S04.2-
   specified type NEC S04.2-
twelfth cranial (hypoglossal) - *see* Injury,
   nerve, hypoglossal
ulnar (forearm level) S54.0-
   arm (upper) (level) S44.0-
   hand (level) S64.0-
   wrist (level) - *see* Injury, nerve, ulnar, hand
vagus S04.89-
   specified type NEC S04.89-
wrist (level) - *see* Injury, nerve, hand
ninth cranial nerve (glossopharyngeal) - *see*
   Injury, nerve, glossopharyngeal
nose (septum) S09.92
obstetrical O71.9
   specified NEC O71.89
occipital (region) (scalp) S09.90
   lobe - *see* Injury, intracranial
optic chiasm S04.02
optic radiation S04.03-
optic tract and pathways S04.03-
orbit, orbital (region) - *see* Injury, eye
   penetrating (with foreign body) - *see* Injury,
      eye, orbit, penetrating

Injury - *continued*

specified NEC - *see* Injury, eye, specified site
   NEC
ovary, ovarian S37.409
   bilateral S37.402
      contusion S37.422
      laceration S37.432
      specified type NEC S37.492
   blood vessel - *see* Injury, blood vessel,
      ovarian
   contusion S37.429
      bilateral S37.422
      unilateral S37.421
   laceration S37.439
      bilateral S37.432
      unilateral S37.431
   specified type NEC S37.499
      bilateral S37.492
      unilateral S37.491
   unilateral S37.401
      contusion S37.421
      laceration S37.431
      specified type NEC S37.491
palate (hard) (soft) S09.93
pancreas S36.209
   body S36.201
      contusion S36.221
      laceration S36.231
         major S36.261
         minor S36.241
         moderate S36.251
      specified type NEC S36.291
   contusion S36.229
   head S36.200
      contusion S36.220
      laceration S36.230
         major S36.260
         minor S36.240
         moderate S36.250
      specified type NEC S36.290
   laceration S36.239
      major S36.269
      minor S36.249
      moderate S36.259
   specified type NEC S36.299
   tail S36.202
      contusion S36.222
      laceration S36.232
         major S36.262
         minor S36.242
         moderate S36.252
      specified type NEC S36.292
parietal (region) (scalp) S09.90
   lobe - *see* Injury, intracranial
patellar ligament (tendon) S76.10-
   laceration S76.12-
   specified NEC S76.19-
   strain S76.11-
pelvis, pelvic (floor) S39.93
   complicating delivery O70.1
   joint or ligament, complicating delivery
      O71.6
   organ S37.90
      with ectopic or molar pregnancy O08.6
      complication of abortion - *see* Abortion
      contusion S37.92
      following ectopic or molar pregnancy
         O08.6
      laceration S37.93
      obstetrical trauma NEC O71.5
      specified
         site NEC S37.899
            contusion S37.892
            laceration S37.893

Injury - *continued*

         specified type NEC S37.898
         type NEC S37.99
      specified NEC S39.83
penis S39.94
perineum S39.94
peritoneum S36.81
   laceration S36.893
periurethral tissue - *see* Injury, urethra
   complicating delivery O71.82
phalanges
   foot - *see* Injury, foot
   hand - *see* Injury, hand
pharynx NEC S19.85
pleura - *see* Injury, intrathoracic, pleura
plexus
   brachial - *see* Injury, brachial plexus
   cardiac - *see* Injury, nerve, thorax,
      sympathetic
   celiac, coeliac - *see* Injury, nerve,
      lumbosacral, sympathetic
   esophageal - *see* Injury, nerve, thorax,
      sympathetic
   hypogastric - *see* Injury, nerve, lumbosacral,
      sympathetic
   lumbar, lumbosacral - *see* Injury,
      lumbosacral plexus
   mesenteric - *see* Injury, nerve, lumbosacral,
      sympathetic
   pulmonary - *see* Injury, nerve, thorax,
      sympathetic
postcardiac surgery (syndrome) I97.0
prepuce S39.94
prostate S37.829
   contusion S37.822
   laceration S37.823
   specified type NEC S37.828
pubic region S39.94
pudendum S39.94
pulmonary plexus - *see* Injury, nerve, thorax,
   sympathetic
rectovaginal septum NEC S39.83
rectum - *see* Injury, intestine, large, rectum
retina - *see* Injury, eye, specified site NEC
   penetrating - *see* Injury, eyeball, penetrating
retroperitoneal - *see* Injury, intra-abdominal,
   specified site NEC
rotator cuff (muscle(s)) (tendon(s)) S46.00-
   laceration S46.02-
   specified type NEC S46.09
   strain S46.01-
round ligament - *see* Injury, pelvic organ,
   specified site NEC
sacral plexus - *see* Injury, lumbosacral plexus
salivary duct or gland S09.93
scalp S09.90
   newborn (birth injury) P12.9
      due to monitoring (electrode) (sampling
         incision) P12.4
      specified NEC P12.89
      caput succedaneum P12.81
scapular region - *see* Injury, shoulder
sclera - *see* Injury, eye, specified site NEC
   penetrating - *see* Injury, eyeball, penetrating
scrotum S39.94
second cranial nerve (optic) - *see* Injury, nerve,
   optic
seminal vesicle - *see* Injury, pelvic organ,
   specified site NEC
seventh cranial nerve (facial) - *see* Injury,
   nerve, facial
shoulder S49.9-
   blood vessel - *see* Injury, blood vessel, arm
   contusion - *see* Contusion, shoulder

Injury - *continued*

back - *see also* Injury, superficial, thorax, back
  lower S30.91
    abrasion S30.810
    contusion S30.0
    external constriction S30.840
    superficial
      bite NEC S30.870
        insect S30.860
      foreign body S30.850
bite NEC - *see* Bite, superficial NEC, by site
blister - *see* Blister, by site
breast S20.10-
  abrasion - *see* Abrasion, breast
  bite - *see* Bite, superficial, breast
  contusion - *see* Contusion, breast
  external constriction - *see* Constriction, external, breast
  foreign body - *see* Foreign body, superficial, breast
brow - *see* Injury, superficial, head, specified NEC
buttock S30.91
calf - *see* Injury, superficial, leg
canthus, eye - *see* Injury, superficial, periocular area
cheek (external) - *see* Injury, superficial, head, specified NEC
  internal - *see* Injury, superficial, oral cavity
chest wall - *see* Injury, superficial, thorax
chin - *see* Injury, superficial, head NEC
clitoris S30.95
conjunctiva - *see* Injury, eye, conjunctiva
  with foreign body (in conjunctival sac) - *see* Foreign body, conjunctival sac
contusion - *see* Contusion, by site
costal region - *see* Injury, superficial, thorax
digit(s)
  hand - *see* Injury, superficial, finger
ear (auricle) (canal) (external) S00.40-
  abrasion - *see* Abrasion, ear
  bite - *see* Bite, superficial, ear
  contusion - *see* Contusion, ear
  external constriction - *see* Constriction, external, ear
  foreign body - *see* Foreign body, superficial, ear
elbow S50.90-
  abrasion - *see* Abrasion, elbow
  bite - *see* Bite, superficial, elbow
  blister - *see* Blister, elbow
  contusion - *see* Contusion, elbow
  external constriction - *see* Constriction, external, elbow
  foreign body - *see* Foreign body, superficial, elbow
epididymis S30.94
epigastric region S30.92
epiglottis - *see* Injury, superficial, throat
esophagus
  cervical - *see* Injury, superficial, throat
external constriction - *see* Constriction, external, by site
extremity NEC T14.8
eyeball NEC - *see* Injury, eye, specified site NEC
eyebrow - *see* Injury, superficial, periocular area
eyelid S00.20-
  abrasion - *see* Abrasion, eyelid
  bite - *see* Bite, superficial, eyelid
  contusion - *see* Contusion, eyelid
  external constriction - *see* Constriction,

Injury - *continued*

  external, eyelid
  foreign body - *see* Foreign body, superficial, eyelid
face NEC - *see* Injury, superficial, head, specified NEC
finger(s) S60.949
  abrasion - *see* Abrasion, finger
  bite - *see* Bite, superficial, finger
  blister - *see* Blister, finger
  contusion - *see* Contusion, finger
  external constriction - *see* Constriction, external, finger
  foreign body - *see* Foreign body, superficial, finger
  insect bite - *see* Bite, by site, superficial, insect
  index S60.94-
  little S60.94-
  middle S60.94-
  ring S60.94-
flank S30.92
foot S90.92-
  abrasion - *see* Abrasion, foot
  bite - *see* Bite, foot
  blister - *see* Blister, foot
  contusion - *see* Contusion, foot
  external constriction - *see* Constriction, external, foot
  foreign body - *see* Foreign body, superficial, foot
forearm S50.91-
  abrasion - *see* Abrasion, forearm
  bite - *see* Bite, forearm, superficial
  blister - *see* Blister, forearm
  contusion - *see* Contusion, forearm
  elbow only - *see* Injury, superficial, elbow
  external constriction - *see* Constriction, external, forearm
  foreign body - *see* Foreign body, superficial, forearm
forehead - *see* Injury, superficial, head NEC
foreign body - *see* Foreign body, superficial
genital organs, external
  female S30.97
  male S30.96
globe (eye) - *see* Injury, eye, specified site NEC
groin S30.92
gum - *see* Injury, superficial, oral cavity
hand S60.92-
  abrasion - *see* Abrasion, hand
  bite - *see* Bite, superficial, hand
  contusion - *see* Contusion, hand
  external constriction - *see* Constriction, external, hand
  foreign body - *see* Foreign body, superficial, hand
head S00.90
  ear - *see* Injury, superficial, ear
  eyelid - *see* Injury, superficial, eyelid
  nose S00.30
  oral cavity S00.502
  scalp S00.00
  specified site NEC S00.80
heel - *see* Injury, superficial, foot
hip S70.91-
  abrasion - *see* Abrasion, hip
  bite - *see* Bite, superficial, hip
  blister - *see* Blister, hip
  contusion - *see* Contusion, hip
  external constriction - *see* Constriction, external, hip

Injury - *continued*

  foreign body - *see* Foreign body, superficial, hip
iliac region - *see* Injury, superficial, abdomen
inguinal region - *see* Injury, superficial, abdomen
insect bite - *see* Bite, by site, superficial, insect
interscapular region - *see* Injury, superficial, thorax, back
jaw - *see* Injury, superficial, head, specified NEC
knee S80.91-
  abrasion - *see* Abrasion, knee
  bite - *see* Bite, superficial, knee
  blister - *see* Blister, knee
  contusion - *see* Contusion, knee
  external constriction - *see* Constriction, external, knee
  foreign body - *see* Foreign body, superficial, knee
labium (majus) (minus) S30.95
lacrimal (apparatus) (gland) (sac) - *see* Injury, eye, specified site NEC
larynx - *see* Injury, superficial, throat
leg (lower) S80.92-
  abrasion - *see* Abrasion, leg
  bite - *see* Bite, superficial, leg
  contusion - *see* Contusion, leg
  external constriction - *see* Constriction, external, leg
  foreign body - *see* Foreign body, superficial, leg
  knee - *see* Injury, superficial, knee
limb NEC T14.8
lip S00.501
lower back S30.91
lumbar region S30.91
malar region - *see* Injury, superficial, head, specified NEC
mammary - *see* Injury, superficial, breast
mastoid region - *see* Injury, superficial, head, specified NEC
mouth - *see* Injury, superficial, oral cavity
muscle NEC T14.8
nail NEC T14.8
  finger - *see* Injury, superficial, finger
  toe - *see* Injury, superficial, toe
nasal (septum) - *see* Injury, superficial, nose
neck S10.90
  specified site NEC S10.80
nose (septum) S00.30
occipital region - *see* Injury, superficial, scalp
oral cavity S00.502
orbital region - *see* Injury, superficial, periocular area
palate - *see* Injury, superficial, oral cavity
palm - *see* Injury, superficial, hand
parietal region - *see* Injury, superficial, scalp
pelvis S30.91
  girdle - *see* Injury, superficial, hip
penis S30.93
perineum
  female S30.95
  male S30.91
periocular area S00.20-
  abrasion - *see* Abrasion, eyelid
  bite - *see* Bite, superficial, eyelid
  contusion - *see* Contusion, eyelid
  external constriction - *see* Constriction, external, eyelid
  foreign body - *see* Foreign body, superficial, eyelid
phalanges

Injury - *continued*

    finger - *see* Injury, superficial, finger
    toe - *see* Injury, superficial, toe
  pharynx - *see* Injury, superficial, throat
  pinna - *see* Injury, superficial, ear
  popliteal space - *see* Injury, superficial, knee
  prepuce S30.93
  pubic region S30.91
  pudendum
    female S30.97
    male S30.96
  sacral region S30.91
  scalp S00.00
  scapular region - *see* Injury, superficial, shoulder
  sclera - *see* Injury, eye, specified site NEC
  scrotum S30.94
  shin - *see* Injury, superficial, leg
  shoulder S40.91-
    abrasion - *see* Abrasion, shoulder
    bite - *see* Bite, superficial, shoulder
    blister - *see* Blister, shoulder
    contusion - *see* Contusion, shoulder
    external constriction - *see* Constriction, external, shoulder
    foreign body - *see* Foreign body, superficial, shoulder
  skin NEC T14.8
  sternal region - *see* Injury, superficial, thorax, front
  subconjunctival - *see* Injury, eye, specified site NEC
  subcutaneous NEC T14.8
  submaxillary region - *see* Injury, superficial, head, specified NEC
  submental region - *see* Injury, superficial, head, specified NEC
  subungual
    finger(s) - *see* Injury, superficial, finger
    toe(s) - *see* Injury, superficial, toe
  supraclavicular fossa - *see* Injury, superficial, neck
  supraorbital - *see* Injury, superficial, head, specified NEC
  temple - *see* Injury, superficial, head, specified NEC
  temporal region - *see* Injury, superficial, head, specified NEC
  testis S30.94
  thigh S70.92-
    abrasion - *see* Abrasion, thigh
    bite - *see* Bite, superficial, thigh
    blister - *see* Blister, thigh
    contusion - *see* Contusion, thigh
    external constriction - *see* Constriction, external, thigh
    foreign body - *see* Foreign body, superficial, thigh
  thorax, thoracic (wall) S20.90
    abrasion - *see* Abrasion, thorax
    back S20.40-
    bite - *see* Bite, thorax, superficial
    blister - *see* Blister, thorax
    contusion - *see* Contusion, thorax
    external constriction - *see* Constriction, external, thorax
    foreign body - *see* Foreign body, superficial, thorax
    front S20.30-
  throat S10.10
    abrasion S10.11
    bite S10.17
      insect S10.16
    blister S10.12

Injury - *continued*

    contusion S10.0
    external constriction S10.14
    foreign body S10.15
  thumb S60.93-
    abrasion - *see* Abrasion, thumb
    bite - *see* Bite, superficial, thumb
    blister - *see* Blister, thumb
    contusion - *see* Contusion, thumb
    external constriction - *see* Constriction, external, thumb
    foreign body - *see* Foreign body, superficial, thumb
    insect bite - *see* Bite, by site, superficial, insect
    specified type NEC S60.39-
  toe(s) S90.93-
    abrasion - *see* Abrasion, toe
    bite - *see* Bite, toe
    blister - *see* Blister, toe
    contusion - *see* Contusion, toe
    external constriction - *see* Constriction, external, toe
    foreign body - *see* Foreign body, superficial, toe
    great S90.93-
  tongue - *see* Injury, superficial, oral cavity
  tooth, teeth - *see* Injury, superficial, oral cavity
  trachea S10.10
  tunica vaginalis S30.94
  tympanum, tympanic membrane - *see* Injury, superficial, ear
  uvula - *see* Injury, superficial, oral cavity
  vagina S30.95
  vocal cords - *see* Injury, superficial, throat
  vulva S30.95
  wrist S60.91-
  supraclavicular region - *see* Injury, neck
  supraorbital S09.93
  suprarenal gland (multiple) - *see* Injury, adrenal
  surgical complication (external or internal site) - *see* Laceration, accidental complicating surgery   temple S09.90
  temporal region S09.90
  tendon - *see also* Injury, muscle, by site
    abdomen - *see* Injury, muscle, abdomen
    Achilles - *see* Injury, Achilles tendon
    lower back - *see* Injury, muscle, lower back
    pelvic organs - *see* Injury, muscle, pelvis
  tenth cranial nerve (pneumogastric or vagus) - *see* Injury, nerve, vagus
  testis S39.94
  thigh S79.92-
    blood vessel - *see* Injury, blood vessel, hip
    contusion - *see* Contusion, thigh
    fracture - *see* Fracture, femur
    muscle - *see* Injury, muscle, thigh
    nerve - *see* Injury, nerve, thigh
    open - *see* Wound, open, thigh
    specified NEC S79.82-
    superficial - *see* Injury, superficial, thigh
  third cranial nerve (oculomotor) - *see* Injury, nerve, oculomotor
  thorax, thoracic S29.9
    blood vessel - *see* Injury, blood vessel, thorax
    cavity - *see* Injury, intrathoracic
    dislocation - *see* Dislocation, thorax
    external (wall) S29.9
      contusion - *see* Contusion, thorax
      nerve - *see* Injury, nerve, thorax
      open - *see* Wound, open, thorax
    specified NEC S29.8

Injury - *continued*

    sprain - *see* Sprain, thorax
    superficial - *see* Injury, superficial, thorax
    fracture - *see* Fracture, thorax
    internal - *see* Injury, intrathoracic
    intrathoracic organ - *see* Injury, intrathoracic
    sympathetic ganglion - *see* Injury, nerve, thorax, sympathetic
  throat - *see also* Injury, neck S19.9
  thumb S69.9-
    blood vessel - *see* Injury, blood vessel, thumb
    contusion - *see* Contusion, thumb
    dislocation - *see* Dislocation, thumb
    fracture - *see* Fracture, thumb
    muscle - *see* Injury, muscle, thumb
    nerve - *see* Injury, nerve, digital, thumb
    open - *see* Wound, open, thumb
    specified NEC S69.8
    sprain - *see* Sprain, thumb
    superficial - *see* Injury, superficial, thumb
  thymus (gland) - *see* Injury, intrathoracic, specified organ NEC
  thyroid (gland) NEC S19.84
  toe S99.92-
    contusion - *see* Contusion, toe
    dislocation - *see* Dislocation, toe
    fracture - *see* Fracture, toe
    muscle - *see* Injury, muscle, toe
    open - *see* Wound, open, toe
    specified type NEC S99.82-
    sprain - *see* Sprain, toe
    superficial - *see* Injury, superficial, toe
  tongue S09.93
  tonsil S09.93
  tooth S09.93
  trachea (cervical) NEC S19.82
    thoracic - *see* Injury, intrathoracic, trachea, thoracic
  transfusion-related acute lung (TRALI) J95.84
  tunica vaginalis S39.94
  twelfth cranial nerve (hypoglossal) - *see* Injury, nerve, hypoglossal
  ureter S37.10
    contusion S37.12
    laceration S37.13
    specified type NEC S37.19
  urethra (sphincter) S37.30
    at delivery O71.5
    contusion S37.32
    laceration S37.33
    specified type NEC S37.39
  urinary organ S37.90
    contusion S37.92
    laceration S37.93
    specified
      site NEC S37.899
        contusion S37.892
        laceration S37.893
        specified type NEC S37.898
      type NEC S37.99
  uterus, uterine S37.60
    with ectopic or molar pregnancy O08.6
    blood vessel - *see* Injury, blood vessel, iliac
    contusion S37.62
    laceration S37.63
      cervix at delivery O71.3
    rupture associated with obstetrics - *see* Rupture, uterus
    specified type NEC S37.69
  uvula S09.93
  vagina S39.93
    abrasion S30.814
    bite S31.45
      insect S30.864

Insufficiency, insufficient - *continued*
  basilar G45.0
  carotid (hemispheric) G45.1
  cerebral I67.81
  coronary (acute or subacute) I24.8
  mesenteric K55.1
  peripheral I73.9
  precerebral (multiple) (bilateral) G45.2
  vertebral G45.0
  arteriovenous I99.8
  biliary K83.8
  cardiac - *see also* Insufficiency, myocardial
    due to presence of (cardiac) prosthesis
    I97.11-
    postprocedural I97.11-
  cardiorenal, hypertensive I13.2
  cardiovascular - *see* Disease, cardiovascular
  cerebrovascular (acute) I67.81
    with transient focal neurological signs and
    symptoms G45.8
  circulatory NEC I99.8
    newborn P29.89
  clinical crown length K08.89
  convergence H51.11
  coronary (acute or subacute) I24.8
    chronic or with a stated duration of over 4
    weeks I25.89
  corticoadrenal E27.40
    primary E27.1
  dietary E63.9
  divergence H51.8
  food T73.0
  gastroesophageal K22.8
  gonadal
    ovary E28.39
    testis E29.1
  heart - *see also* Insufficiency, myocardial
    newborn P29.0
    valve - *see* Endocarditis
  hepatic - *see* Failure, hepatic
  idiopathic autonomic G90.09
  interocclusal distance of fully erupted teeth
    (ridge) M26.36
  kidney N28.9
    acute N28.9
    chronic N18.9
  lacrimal (secretion) H04.12-
    passages - *see* Stenosis, lacrimal
  liver - *see* Failure, hepatic
  lung - *see* Insufficiency, pulmonary
  mental (congenital) - *see* Disability,
  intellectual
  mesenteric K55.1
  mitral (valve) I34.0
    with
      aortic valve disease I08.0
        with tricuspid (valve) disease I08.3
      obstruction or stenosis I05.2
        with aortic valve disease I08.0
      tricuspid (valve) disease I08.1
        with aortic (valve) disease I08.3
    congenital Q23.3
    rheumatic I05.1
      with
        aortic valve disease I08.0
          with tricuspid (valve) disease I08.3
        obstruction or stenosis I05.2
          with aortic valve disease I08.0
            with tricuspid (valve) disease I08.3
        tricuspid (valve) disease I08.1
          with aortic (valve) disease I08.3
    active or acute I01.1
      with chorea, rheumatic (Sydenham's)
      I02.0

Insufficiency, insufficient - *continued*
    specified cause, except rheumatic I34.0
  muscle - *see also* Disease, muscle
    heart - *see* Insufficiency, myocardial
    ocular NEC H50.9
  myocardial, myocardium (with
    arteriosclerosis) (see also Failure, heart)
    I50.9
    with
      rheumatic fever (conditions in I00) I09.0
        active, acute or subacute I01.2
          with chorea I02.0
        inactive or quiescent (with chorea) I09.0
    congenital Q24.8
    hypertensive - *see* Hypertension, heart
    newborn P29.0
    rheumatic I09.0
      active, acute, or subacute I01.2
    syphilitic A52.06
  nourishment T73.0
  pancreatic K86.89
    exocrine K86.81
  parathyroid (gland) E20.9
  peripheral vascular (arterial) I73.9
  pituitary E23.0
  placental (mother) O36.51-
  platelets D69.6
  prenatal care affecting management of
  pregnancy O09.3-
  progressive pluriglandular E31.0
  pulmonary J98.4
    acute, following surgery (nonthoracic) J95.2
      thoracic J95.1
    chronic, following surgery J95.3
    following
      shock J98.4
      trauma J98.4
    newborn P28.5
    valve I37.1
      with stenosis I37.2
      congenital Q22.2
      rheumatic I09.89
        with aortic, mitral or tricuspid (valve)
    disease I08.8
  pyloric K31.89
  renal (acute) N28.9
    chronic N18.9
  respiratory R06.89
    newborn P28.5
  rotation - *see* Malrotation
  sleep syndrome F51.12
  social insurance Z59.7
  suprarenal E27.40
    primary E27.1
  tarso-orbital fascia, congenital Q10.3
  testis E29.1
  thyroid (gland) (acquired) E03.9
    congenital E03.1
  tricuspid (valve) (rheumatic) I07.1
    with
      aortic (valve) disease I08.2
        with mitral (valve) disease I08.3
      mitral (valve) disease I08.1
        with aortic (valve) disease I08.3
      obstruction or stenosis I07.2
        with aortic (valve) disease I08.2
        with mitral (valve) disease I08.3
    congenital Q22.8
    nonrheumatic I36.1
      with stenosis I36.2
  urethral sphincter R32
  valve, valvular (heart) I38
    mitral *see* Insufficiency, mitral (valve)

Insufficiency, insufficient - *continued*
  pulmonary *see* Insufficiency, pulmonary,
    valve
  tricuspid *see* Insufficiency, tricuspid (valve)
  aortic *see* Insufficiency, aortic (valve)
  congenital Q24.8
  vascular I99.8
    intestine K55.9
      acute - *see also* Ischemia, intestine, acute
      K55.059
    mesenteric K55.1
    peripheral I73.9
    renal - *see* Hypertension, kidney
  velopharyngeal
    acquired K13.79
    congenital Q38.8
  venous (chronic) (peripheral) I87.2
  ventricular - *see* Insufficiency, myocardial
  welfare support Z59.7
Insufflation, fallopian Z31.41
Insular - *see condition* **Insulinoma**
  pancreas
    benign D13.7
    malignant C25.4
    uncertain behavior D37.8
  specified site
    benign - *see* Neoplasm, by site, benign
    malignant - *see* Neoplasm, by site, malignant
    uncertain behavior - *see* Neoplasm, by site,
    uncertain behavior
  unspecified site
    benign D13.7
    malignant C25.4
    uncertain behavior D37.8
Insuloma - *see* Insulinoma
Interference
  balancing side M26.56
  non-working side M26.56
Intermenstrual - *see condition*
Intermittent - *see condition*
Internal - *see condition*
Interrogation
  cardiac defibrillator (automatic) (implantable)
    Z45.02
  cardiac pacemaker Z45.018
  cardiac (event) (loop) recorder Z45.09
  infusion pump (implanted) (intrathecal) Z45.1
  neurostimulator Z46.2
Interruption
  aortic arch Q25.21
  bundle of His I44.30
  phase-shift, sleep cycle - *see* Disorder, sleep,
    circadian rhythm
  sleep phase-shift, or 24
  hour sleep-wake cycle - *see* Disorder, sleep,
    circadian rhythm
Interstitial - *see condition*
Intertrigo L30.4
  labialis K13.0
Intervertebral disc - *see condition*
Intestine, intestinal - *see condition*
Intolerance
  carbohydrate K90.49
  disaccharide, hereditary E73.0
  fat NEC K90.49
    pancreatic K90.3
  food K90.49
    dietary counseling and surveillance Z71.3
  fructose E74.10
    hereditary E74.12
  glucose (-galactose) E74.39
  gluten K90.41
  lactose E73.9
    specified NEC E73.8

Intolerance - *continued*
- lysine E72.3
- milk NEC K90.49
- lactose E73.9
- protein K90.49
- starch NEC K90.49
- sucrose (-isomaltose) E74.31

Intoxicated NEC (without dependence) - *see* Alcohol, intoxication

Intoxication
- acid E87.2
- alcoholic (acute) (without dependence) - *see* Alcohol, intoxication
- alimentary canal K52.1
- amphetamine (without dependence) - *see* Abuse, drug, stimulant, with intoxication
  - with dependence - *see* Dependence, drug, stimulant, with intoxication
- anxiolytic (acute) (without dependence) - *see* Abuse, drug, sedative, with intoxication
  - with dependence - *see* Dependence, drug, sedative, with intoxication
- caffeine F15.929
  - with dependence - *see* Dependence, drug, stimulant, with intoxication
- cannabinoids (acute) (without dependence) - *see* Use, cannabis, with intoxication
  - with
    - abuse - *see* Abuse, drug, cannabis, with intoxication
    - dependence - *see* Dependence, drug, cannabis, with intoxication
- chemical - *see* Table of Drugs and Chemicals
  - via placenta or breast milk - *see* Absorption, chemical, through placenta
- cocaine (acute) (without dependence) - *see* Abuse, drug, cocaine, with intoxication
  - with dependence - *see* Dependence, drug, cocaine, with intoxication
- drug
  - acute (without dependence) - *see* Abuse, drug, by type with intoxication
    - with dependence - *see* Dependence, drug, by type with intoxication
  - addictive
    - via placenta or breast milk - *see* Absorption, drug, addictive, through placenta
  - newborn P93.8
    - gray baby syndrome P93.0
  - overdose or wrong substance given or taken - *see* Table of Drugs and Chemicals, by drug, poisoning
- enteric K52.1
- foodborne A05.9
  - bacterial A05.9
  - classical (Clostridium botulinum) A05.1
  - due to
    - Bacillus cereus A05.4
    - bacterium A05.9
      - specified NEC A05.8
    - Clostridium
      - botulinum A05.1
      - perfringens A05.2
      - welchii A05.2
    - Salmonella A02.9
      - with
        - (gastro) enteritis A02.0
        - localized infection(s) A02.20
          - arthritis A02.23
          - meningitis A02.21
          - osteomyelitis A02.24
          - pneumonia A02.22
          - pyelonephritis A02.25
          - specified NEC A02.29

Intoxication - *continued*
- sepsis A02.1
  - specified manifestation NEC A02.8
- Staphylococcus A05.0
- Vibrio
  - parahaemolyticus A05.3
  - vulnificus A05.5
- enterotoxin, staphylococcal A05.0
- noxious - *see* Poisoning, food, noxious
- gastrointestinal K52.1
- hallucinogenic (without dependence) - *see* Abuse, drug, hallucinogen, with intoxication
  - with dependence - *see* Dependence, drug, hallucinogen, with intoxication
- hypnotic (acute) (without dependence) - *see* Abuse, drug, sedative, with intoxication
  - with dependence - *see* Dependence, drug, sedative, with intoxication
- inhalant (acute) (without dependence) - *see* Abuse, drug, inhalant, with intoxication
  - with dependence - *see* Dependence, drug, inhalant, with intoxication
- meaning
  - inebriation - *see* category F10
  - poisoning - *see* Table of Drugs and Chemicals
- methyl alcohol (acute) (without dependence) - *see* Alcohol, intoxication
- opioid (acute) (without dependence) - *see* Abuse, drug, opioid, with intoxication
  - with dependence - *see* Dependence, drug, opioid, with intoxication
- pathologic NEC (without dependence) - *see* Alcohol, intoxication
- phencyclidine (without dependence) - *see* Abuse, drug, hallucinogen, with intoxication
  - with dependence - *see* Dependence, drug, hallucinogen, with intoxication
- potassium (K) E87.5
- psychoactive substance NEC (without dependence) - *see* Abuse, drug, psychoactive NEC, with intoxication
  - with dependence - *see* Dependence, drug, psychoactive NEC, with intoxication
- sedative (acute) (without dependence) - *see* Abuse, drug, sedative, with intoxication
  - with dependence - *see* Dependence, drug, sedative, with intoxication
- serum - *see also* Reaction, serum T80.69
- uremic - *see* Uremia
- volatile solvents (acute) (without dependence) - *see* Abuse, drug, inhalant, with intoxication
  - with dependence - *see* Dependence, drug, inhalant, with intoxication
- water E87.79

Intraabdominal testis, testes
- bilateral Q53.211
- unilateral Q53.111

Intracranial - *see* condition
Intrahepatic gallbladder Q44.1
Intraligamentous - *see* condition
Intrathoracic - *see also* condition
- kidney Q63.2
Intrauterine contraceptive device
- checking Z30.431
- insertion Z30.430
  - immediately following removal Z30.433
- in situ Z97.5
- management Z30.431
- reinsertion Z30.433
- removal Z30.432
- replacement Z30.433
- retention in pregnancy O26.3
Intraventricular - *see* condition

Intrinsic deformity - *see* Deformity
Intubation, difficult or failed T88.4
Intumescence, lens (eye) (cataract) - *see* Cataract
Intussusception (bowel) (colon) (enteric) (ileocecal) (ileocolic) (intestine) (rectum) K56.1
- appendix K38.8
- congenital Q43.8
- ureter (with obstruction) N13.5
Invagination (bowel, colon, intestine or rectum) K56.1
Inversion
- albumin-globulin (A-g) ratio E88.09
- bladder N32.89
- cecum - *see* Intussusception
- cervix N88.8
- chromosome in normal individual Q95.1
- circadian rhythm - *see* Disorder, sleep, circadian rhythm
- nipple N64.59
  - congenital Q83.8
  - gestational - *see* Retraction, nipple
  - puerperal, postpartum - *see* Retraction, nipple
- nyctohemeral rhythm - *see* Disorder, sleep, circadian rhythm
- optic papilla Q14.2
- organ or site, congenital NEC - *see* Anomaly, by site
- sleep rhythm - *see* Disorder, sleep, circadian rhythm
- testis (congenital) Q55.29
- uterus (chronic) (postinfectional) (postpartal, old) N85.5
  - postpartum O71.2
- vagina (posthysterectomy) N99.3
- ventricular Q20.5
Investigation - *see also* Examination Z04.9
- clinical research subject (control) (normal comparison) (participant) Z00.6
Involuntary movement, abnormal R25.9
Involution, involutional - *see also* condition
- breast, cystic - *see* Dysplasia, mammary, specified type NEC
- depression (single episode) F32.89
  - recurrent episode F33.9
- melancholia (single episode) F32.89
  - recurrent episode F33.8
- ovary, senile - *see* Atrophy, ovary
- thymus failure E32.8
I.Q.
- under 20 F73
- 20-34 F72
- 35 49 F71
- 50-69 F70
IRDS (type I) P22.0
- type II P22.1
Irideremia Q13.1
Iridis rubeosis - *see* Disorder, iris, vascular
Iridochoroiditis (panuveitis) - *see* Panuveitis
Iridocyclitis H20.9
- acute H20.0-
  - hypopyon H20.05-
  - primary H20.01-
  - recurrent H20.02-
  - secondary (noninfectious) H20.04-
    - infectious H20.03-
- chronic H20.1-
- due to allergy - *see* Iridocyclitis, acute, secondary
- endogenous - *see* Iridocyclitis, acute, primary
- Fuchs' - *see* Cyclitis, Fuchs' heterochromic
- gonococcal A54.32
- granulomatous - *see* Iridocyclitis, chronic

Iridocyclitis - *continued*
herpes, herpetic (simplex) B00.51
  zoster B02.32
hypopyon - *see* Iridocyclitis, acute, hypopyon
in (due to)
  ankylosing spondylitis M45.9
  gonococcal infection A54.32
  herpes (simplex) virus B00.51
    zoster B02.32
  infectious disease NOS B99
  parasitic disease NOS B89 [*H22*]
  sarcoidosis D86.83
  syphilis A51.43
  tuberculosis A18.54
  zoster B02.32
lens-induced H20.2-
nongranulomatous - *see* Iridocyclitis, acute
recurrent - *see* Iridocyclitis, acute, recurrent
rheumatic - *see* Iridocyclitis, chronic
subacute - *see* Iridocyclitis, acute
sympathetic - *see* Uveitis, sympathetic
syphilitic (secondary) A51.43
tuberculous (chronic) A18.54
Vogt-Koyanagi H20.82-
Iridocyclochoroiditis (panuveitis) - *see*
Panuveitis
Iridodialysis H21.53-
Iridodonesis H21.89
Iridoplegia (complete) (partial) (reflex)
H57.09
Iridoschisis H21.25-
Iris - *see also* condition
bombé - *see* Membrane, pupillary
Iritis - *see also* Iridocyclitis
chronic - *see* Iridocyclitis, chronic
diabetic - *see* E08-e13 with .39
due to
  herpes simplex B00.51
  leprosy A30.9 [*H22*]
gonococcal A54.32
gouty - *see also* Gout, by type M10.9 [*H22*]
granulomatous - *see* Iridocyclitis, chronic
lens induced - *see* Iridocyclitis, lens-induced
papulosa (syphilitic) A52.71
rheumatic - *see* Iridocyclitis, chronic
syphilitic (secondary) A51.43
  congenital (early) A50.01
  late A52.71
tuberculous A18.54
Iron - *see* condition
Iron-miner's lung J63.4
Irradiated enamel (tooth, teeth) K03.89
Irradiation effects, adverse T66
Irreducible, irreducibility - *see* condition
Irregular, irregularity
action, heart I49.9
alveolar process K08.89
bleeding N92.6
breathing R06.89
contour of cornea (acquired) - *see* Deformity,
cornea
  congenital Q13.4
contour, reconstructed breast N65.0
dentin (in pulp) K04.3
eye movements H55.89
  nystagmus - *see* Nystagmus
  saccadic H55.81
labor O62.2
menstruation (cause unknown) N92.6
periods N92.6
prostate N42.9
pupil - *see* Abnormality, pupillary
reconstructed breast N65.0
respiratory R06.89

Iridocyclitis - *continued*
septum (nasal) J34.2
shape, organ or site, congenital NEC - *see*
Distortion
sleep-wake pattern (rhythm) G47.23
Irritable, irritability R45.4
bladder N32.89
bowel (syndrome) K58.9
  with
    constipation K58.1
    diarrhea K58.0
  mixed K58.2
  psychogenic F45.8
  specified NEC K58.8
bronchial - *see* Bronchitis
cerebral, in newborn P91.3
colon - *see also* Irritable, bowel K58.9
  with diarrhea K58.0
  psychogenic F45.8
duodenum K59.8
heart (psychogenic) F45.8
hip - *see* Derangement, joint, specified type
  NEC, hip
ileum K59.8
infant R68.12
jejunum K59.8
rectum K59.8
stomach K31.89
  psychogenic F45.8
sympathetic G90.8
urethra N36.8
Irritation
anus K62.89
axillary nerve G54.0
bladder N32.89
brachial plexus G54.0
bronchial - *see* Bronchitis
cervical plexus G54.2
cervix - *see* Cervicitis
choroid, sympathetic - *see* Endophthalmitis
cranial nerve - *see* Disorder, nerve, cranial
gastric K31.89
  psychogenic F45.8
globe, sympathetic - *see* Uveitis, sympathetic
labyrinth - *see* subcategory H83.2
lumbosacral plexus G54.1
meninges (traumatic) - *see* Injury, intracranial
  nontraumatic - *see* Meningismus
nerve - *see* Disorder, nerve
nervous R45.0
penis N48.89
perineum NEC L29.3
peripheral autonomic nervous system G90.8
peritoneum - *see* Peritonitis
pharynx J39.2
plantar nerve - *see* Lesion, nerve, plantar
spinal (cord) (traumatic) - *see also* Injury,
spinal cord, by region
  nerve G58.9
    root NEC - *see* Radiculopathy
    nontraumatic - *see* Myelopathy
stomach K31.89
  psychogenic F45.8
sympathetic nerve NEC G90.8
ulnar nerve - *see* Lesion, nerve, ulnar
vagina N89.8
Ischemia, ischemic I99.8
brain - *see* Ischemia, cerebral
bowel (transient)
  acute - *see also* Ischemia, intestine, acute
    K55.059
  chronic K55.1
  due to mesenteric artery insufficiency K55.1
cardiac (see Disease, heart, ischemic)

Ischemia, ischemic - *continued*
cardiomyopathy I25.5
cerebral (chronic) (generalized) I67.82
  arteriosclerotic I67.2
  intermittent G45.9
  newborn P91.0
  recurrent focal G45.8
  transient G45.9
colon chronic (due to mesenteric artery
  insufficiency) K55.1
coronary - *see* Disease, heart, ischemic
demand (coronary) - *see also* Angina I24.8
  with myocardial infarction I21.A1
  resulting in myocardial infarction I21.A1
heart (chronic or with a stated duration of over
  4weeks) I25.9
  acute or with a stated duration of 4
weeks or less I24.9
  subacute I24.9
infarction, muscle - *see* Infarct, muscle
intestine (large) (small) (transient) K55.9
  acute K55.059
    diffuse K55.052
    focal K55.051
    large K55.039
      diffuse K55.032
      focal K55.031
    small K55.019
      diffuse K55.012
      focal K55.011
  chronic K55.1
  due to mesenteric artery insufficiency K55.1
kidney N28.0
mesenteric, acute - *see also* Ischemia,
  intestine, acute K55.059
muscle, traumatic T79.6
myocardium, myocardial (chronic or with a
  stated duration of over 4 weeks) I25.9
  acute, without myocardial infarction I51.3
  silent (asymptomatic) I25.6
  transient of newborn P29.4
renal N28.0
retina, retinal - *see* Occlusion, artery, retina
small bowel
  acute K55.019
    diffuse K55.012
    focal K55.011
  chronic K55.1
  due to mesenteric artery insufficiency K55.1
spinal cord G95.11
subendocardial - *see* Insufficiency, coronary
supply (coronary) - *see also* Angina I25.9
  due to vasospasm I20.1
Ischial spine - *see* condition
Ischialgia - *see* Sciatica
Ischiopagus Q89.4
Ischium, ischial - *see* condition
Ischuria R34
Iselin's disease or osteochondrosis - *see*
Osteochondrosis, juvenile, metatarsus
Islands of
parotid tissue in
  lymph nodes Q38.6
  neck structures Q38.6
submaxillary glands in
  fascia Q38.6
  lymph nodes Q38.6
  neck muscles Q38.6
Islet cell tumor, pancreas D13.7
Isoimmunization NEC - *see also*
Incompatibility
affecting management of pregnancy (ABO)
(with hydrops fetalis) O36.11-
  anti-a sensitization O36.11-

Isoimmunization NEC - *continued*
  anti-b sensitization O36.19-
  anti-c sensitization O36.09-
  anti-c sensitization O36.09-
  anti-e sensitization O36.09-
  anti-e sensitization O36.09-
  Rh NEC O36.09-
    anti-d antibody O36.01-
  specified NEC O36.19-
  newborn P55.9
    with
      hydrops fetalis P56.0
      kernicterus P57.0
    ABO (blood groups) P55.1
    Rhesus (Rh) factor P55.0
    specified type NEC P55.8
Isolation, isolated
  dwelling Z59.8
  family Z63.79
  social Z60.4
Isoleucinosis E71.19
Isomerism atrial appendages (with asplenia or polysplenia) Q20.6
Isosporiasis, isosporosis A07.3
Isovaleric acidemia E71.110
Issue of
  medical certificate Z02.79
    for disability determination Z02.71
  repeat prescription (appliance) (glasses) (medicinal substance, medicament, medicine) Z76.0
    contraception - *see* Contraception
Itch, itching - *see also* Pruritus
  baker's L23.6
  barber's B35.0
  bricklayer's L24.5
  cheese B88.0
  clam digger's B65.3
  coolie B76.9
  copra B88.0
  dew B76.9
  dhobi B35.6
  filarial - *see* Infestation, filarial
  grain B88.0
  grocer's B88.0
  ground B76.9
  harvest B88.0
  jock B35.6
  Malabar B35.5
    beard B35.0
    foot B35.3
    scalp B35.0
  meaning scabies B86
  Norwegian B86
  perianal L29.0
  poultry men's B88.0
  sarcoptic B86
  scabies B86
  scrub B88.0
  straw B88.0
  swimmer's B65.3
  water B76.9
  winter L29.8
Ivemark's syndrome (asplenia with congenital heart disease) Q89.01
Ivory bones Q78.2
Ixodiasis NEC B88.8

J

Jaccoud's syndrome - *see* Arthropathy, postrheumatic, chronic
Jackson's
  membrane Q43.3

Jackson's - *continued*
  paralysis or syndrome G83.89
  veil Q43.3
Jacquet's dermatitis (diaper dermatitis) L22
Jadassohn-Pellizari's disease or anetoderma L90.2
Jadassohn's
  blue nevus - *see* Nevus
  intraepidermal epithelioma - *see* Neoplasm, skin, benign
Jaffe-Lichtenstein (-Uehlinger) syndrome - *see* Dysplasia, fibrous, bone NEC
Jakob-Creutzfeldt disease or syndrome - *see* Creutzfeldt-Jakob disease or syndrome
Jaksch-Luzet disease D64.89
Jamaican
  neuropathy G92
  paraplegic tropical ataxic-spastic syndrome G92
Janet's disease F48.8
Janiceps Q89.4
Jansky-Bielschowsky amaurotic idiocy E75.4
Japanese
  B-type encephalitis A83.0
  river fever A75.3
Jaundice (yellow) R17
  acholuric (familial) (splenomegalic) - *see also* Spherocytosis
    acquired D59.8
  breast-milk (inhibitor) P59.3
  catarrhal (acute) B15.9
    with hepatic coma B15.0
  cholestatic (benign) R17
  due to or associated with
    delayed conjugation P59.8
      associated with (due to) preterm delivery P59.0
    preterm delivery P59.0
  epidemic (catarrhal) B15.9
    with hepatic coma B15.0
    leptospiral A27.0
    spirochetal A27.0
  familial nonhemolytic (congenital) (Gilbert) E80.4
    Crigler Najjar E80.5
  febrile (acute) B15.9
    with hepatic coma B15.0
    leptospiral A27.0
    spirochetal A27.0
  hematogenous D59.9
  hemolytic (acquired) D59.9
    congenital - *see* Spherocytosis
  hemorrhagic (acute) (leptospiral) (spirochetal) A27.0
  infectious (acute) (subacute) B15.9
    with hepatic coma B15.0
    leptospiral A27.0
    spirochetal A27.0
  leptospiral (hemorrhagic) A27.0
  malignant (without coma) K72.90
    with coma K72.91
  newborn P59.9
    due to or associated with
      ABO
        antibodies P55.1
        incompatibility, maternal/fetal P55.1
        isoimmunization P55.1
      absence or deficiency of enzyme system for bilirubin conjugation (congenital) P59.8
      bleeding P58.1
      breast milk inhibitors to conjugation P59.3
        associated with preterm delivery P59.0
      bruising P58.0
      Crigler Najjar syndrome E80.5

Jaundice (yellow) - *continued*
  delayed conjugation P59.8
    associated with preterm delivery P59.0
  drugs or toxins
    given to newborn P58.42
    transmitted from mother P58.41
  excessive hemolysis P58.9
    due to
      bleeding P58.1
      bruising P58.0
      drugs or toxins
        given to newborn P58.42
        transmitted from mother P58.41
      infection P58.2
      polycythemia P58.3
      swallowed maternal blood P58.5
    specified type NEC P58.8
  galactosemia E74.21
  Gilbert syndrome E80.4
  hemolytic disease P55.9
    ABO isoimmunization P55.1
    Rh isoimmunization P55.0
    specified NEC P55.8
  hepatocellular damage P59.20
    specified NEC P59.29
  hereditary hemolytic anemia P58.8
  hypothyroidism, congenital E03.1
  incompatibility, maternal/fetal NOS P55.9
  infection P58.2
  inspissated bile syndrome P59.1
  isoimmunization NOS P55.9
  mucoviscidosis E84.9
  polycythemia P58.3
  preterm delivery P59.0
  Rh
    antibodies P55.0
    incompatibility, maternal/fetal P55.0
    isoimmunization P55.0
  specified cause NEC P59.8
  swallowed maternal blood P58.5
  spherocytosis (congenital) D58.0
  neonatal - *see* Jaundice, newborn
  nonhemolytic congenital familial (Gilbert) E80.4
  nuclear, newborn - *see also* Kernicterus of newborn P57.9
  obstructive - *see also* Obstruction, bile duct K83.1
  post-immunization - *see* Hepatitis, viral, type, B
  post-transfusion - *see* Hepatitis, viral, type, B
  regurgitation - *see also* Obstruction, bile duct K83.1
  serum (homologous) (prophylactic) (therapeutic) - *see* Hepatitis, viral, type, B
  spirochetal (hemorrhagic) A27.0
  symptomatic R17
    newborn P59.9
Jaw - *see* condition
Jaw-winking phenomenon or syndrome Q07.8
Jealousy
  alcoholic F10.988
  childhood F93.8
  sibling F93.8
Jejunitis - *see* Enteritis
Jejunostomy status Z93.4
Jejunum, jejunal - *see* condition
Jensen's disease - *see* Inflammation, chorioretinal, focal, juxtapapillary
Jerks, myoclonic G25.3
Jervell-Lange Nielsen syndrome I45.81
Jeune's disease Q77.2
Jigger disease B88.1

Job's syndrome (chronic granulomatous disease) D71
Joint - *see also* condition
mice - *see* Loose, body, joint
knee M23.4-
Jordan's anomaly or syndrome D72.0
Joseph-diamond-Blackfan anemia (congenital hypoplastic) D61.01
Jungle yellow fever A95.0
Jüngling's disease - *see* Sarcoidosis
Juvenile - *see* condition

K

Kahler's disease C90.0-
Kakke E51.11
Kala-azar B55.0
Kallmann's syndrome E23.0
Kanner's syndrome (autism) - *see* Psychosis, childhood
Kaposi's
dermatosis (xeroderma pigmentosum) Q82.1
lichen ruber L44.0
acuminatus L44.0
sarcoma
colon C46.4
connective tissue C46.1
gastrointestinal organ C46.4
lung C46.5-
lymph node (multiple) C46.3
palate (hard) (soft) C46.2
rectum C46.4
skin (multiple sites) C46.0
specified site NEC C46.7
stomach C46.4
unspecified site C46.9
varicelliform eruption B00.0
vaccinia T88.1
Kartagener's syndrome or triad (sinusitis, bronchiectasis, situs inversus) Q89.3
Karyotype
with abnormality except iso (Xq) Q96.2
45,X Q96.0
46,X
iso (Xq) Q96.1
46,XX Q98.3
with streak gonads Q50.32
hermaphrodite (true) Q99.1
male Q98.3
46,XY
with streak gonads Q56.1
female Q97.3
hermaphrodite (true) Q99.1
47,XXX Q97.0
47,XXY Q98.0
47,XYY Q98.5
Kaschin-beck disease - *see* Disease, Kaschin-beck
Katayama's disease or fever B65.2
Kawasaki's syndrome M30.3
Kayser-Fleischer ring (cornea) (pseudosclerosis) H18.04-
Kaznelson's syndrome (congenital hypoplastic anemia) D61.01
Kearns-Sayre syndrome H49.81-
Kedani fever A75.3
Kelis L91.0
Kelly (-Patterson) syndrome (sideropenic dysphagia) D50.1
Keloid, cheloid L91.0
acne L73.0
Addison's L94.0
cornea - *see* Opacity, cornea
Hawkin's L91.0
scar L91.0

Keloma L91.0
Kenya fever A77.1
Keratectasia - *see also* Ectasia, cornea
congenital Q13.4
Keratinization of alveolar ridge mucosa
excessive K13.23
minimal K13.22
Keratinized residual ridge mucosa excessive K13.23
minimal K13.22
Keratitis (nodular) (nonulcerative) (simple) (zonular) H16.9
with ulceration (central) (marginal) (perforated) (ring) - *see* Ulcer, cornea
actinic - *see* Photokeratitis
arborescens (herpes simplex) B00.52
areolar H16.11-
bullosa H16.8
deep H16.309
specified type NEC H16.399
dendritic (a) (herpes simplex) B00.52
disciform (is) (herpes simplex) B00.52
varicella B01.81
filamentary H16.12-
gonococcal (congenital or prenatal) A54.33
herpes, herpetic (simplex) B00.52
zoster B02.33
in (due to)
acanthamebiasis B60.13
adenovirus B30.0
exanthema - *see also* Exanthem B09
herpes (simplex) virus B00.52
measles B05.81
syphilis A50.31
tuberculosis A18.52
zoster B02.33
interstitial (nonsyphilitic) H16.30-
diffuse H16.32-
herpes, herpetic (simplex) B00.52
zoster B02.33
sclerosing H16.33-
specified type NEC H16.39
syphilitic (congenital) (late) A50.31
tuberculous A18.52
macular H16.11-
nummular H16.11-
oyster shuckers' H16.8
parenchymatous - *see* Keratitis, interstitial
petrificans H16.8
postmeasles B05.81
punctata
leprosa A30.9 [*H16.14*]
syphilitic (profunda) A50.31
punctate H16.14-
purulent H16.8
rosacea L71.8
sclerosing H16.33-
specified type NEC H16.8
stellate H16.11-
striate H16.11-
superficial H16.10-
with conjunctivitis - *see* Keratoconjunctivitis
due to light - *see* Photokeratitis
suppurative H16.8
syphilitic (congenital) (prenatal) A50.31
trachomatous A71.1
sequelae B94.0
tuberculous A18.52
vesicular H16.8
xerotic - *see also* Keratomalacia H16.8
vitamin A deficiency E50.4
Keratoacanthoma L85.8
Keratocele - *see* Descemetocele

Keratoconjunctivitis H16.20-
Acanthamoeba B60.13
adenoviral B30.0
epidemic B30.0
exposure H16.21-
herpes, herpetic (simplex) B00.52
zoster B02.33
in exanthema - *see also* Exanthem B09
infectious B30.0
lagophthalmic - *see* Keratoconjunctivitis, specified type NEC
neurotrophic H16.23-
phlyctenular H16.25-
postmeasles B05.81
shipyard B30.0
sicca (Sjogren's) M35.0-
not Sjogren's H16.22-
specified type NEC H16.29-
tuberculous (phlyctenular) A18.52
vernal H16.26-
Keratoconus H18.60-
congenital Q13.4
stable H18.61-
unstable H18.62-
Keratocyst (dental) (odontogenic) - *see* Cyst, calcifying odontogenic
Keratoderma, keratodermia (congenital) (palmaris et plantaris) (symmetrical) Q82.8
acquired L85.1
in diseases classified elsewhere L86
climactericum L85.1
gonococcal A54.89
gonorrheal A54.89
punctata L85.2
Reiter's - *see* Reiter's disease
Keratodermatocele - *see* Descemetocele
Keratoglobus H18.79
congenital Q15.8
with glaucoma Q15.0
Keratohemia - *see* Pigmentation, cornea, stromal
Keratoiritis - *see also* Iridocyclitis
syphilitic A50.39
tuberculous A18.54
Keratoma L57.0
palmaris and plantaris hereditarium Q82.8
senile L57.0
Keratomalacia H18.44-
vitamin A deficiency E50.4
Keratomegaly Q13.4
Keratomycosis B49
nigrans, nigricans (palmaris) B36.1
Keratopathy H18.9
band H18.42-
bullous H18.1-
bullous (aphakic), following cataract surgery H59.01-
Keratoscleritis, tuberculous A18.52
Keratosis L57.0
actinic L57.0
arsenical L85.8
congenital, specified NEC Q80.8
female genital NEC N94.89
follicularis Q82.8
acquired L11.0
congenita Q82.8
et parafollicularis in cutem penetrans L87.0
spinulosa (decalvans) Q82.8
vitamin A deficiency E50.8
gonococcal A54.89
male genital (external) N50.89
nigricans L83
obturans, external ear (canal) - *see* Cholesteatoma, external ear

Keratosis - *continued*
  palmaris et plantaris (inherited) (symmetrical)
    Q82.8
    acquired L85.1
  penile N48.89
  pharynx J39.2
  pilaris, acquired L85.8
  punctata (palmaris et plantaris) L85.2
  scrotal N50.89
  seborrheic L82.1
    inflamed L82.0
  senile L57.0
  solar L57.0
  tonsillaris J35.8
  vagina N89.4
  vegetans Q82.8
  vitamin A deficiency E50.8
  vocal cord J38.3
Kerato-uveitis - *see* Iridocyclitis
Keraunoparalysis T75.09
Kerion (celsi) B35.0
**Kernicterus of newborn (not due to
  isoimmunization)** P57.9
  due to isoimmunization (conditions in P55.0-
    p55.9) P57.0
  specified type NEC P57.8
Keshan disease E59
Ketoacidosis E87.2
  diabetic - *see* Diabetes, by type, with
    ketoacidosis
Ketonuria R82.4
Ketosis NEC E88.89
  diabetic - *see* Diabetes, by type, with
    ketoacidosis
Kew Garden fever A79.1
Kidney - *see* condition
Kienböck's disease - *see also* Osteochondrosis,
  juvenile, hand, carpal lunate
  adult M93.1
Kimmelstiel (-Wilson) disease - *see* Diabetes,
  Kimmelstiel (-Wilson) disease
Kimura disease D21.9
  specified site (see Neoplasm, connective tissue
  benign)
Kink, kinking
  artery I77.1
  hair (acquired) L67.8
  ileum or intestine - *see* Obstruction, intestine
  Lane's - *see* Obstruction, intestine
  organ or site, congenital NEC - *see* Anomaly,
    by site
  ureter (pelvic junction) N13.5
    with
      hydronephrosis N13.1
        with infection N13.6
      pyelonephritis (chronic) N11.1
    congenital Q62.39
  vein(s) I87.8
    caval I87.1
    peripheral I87.1
**Kinnier Wilson's disease (hepatolenticular
  degeneration)** E83.01
Kissing spine M48.20
  cervical region M48.22
  cervicothoracic region M48.23
  lumbar region M48.26
  lumbosacral region M48.27
  occipito-atlanto-axial region M48.21
  thoracic region M48.24
  thoracolumbar region M48.25
Klatskin's tumor C24.0
Klauder's disease A26.8
Klebs' disease - *see also* Glomerulonephritis
  N05.-

**Klebsiella (K.) pneumoniae, as cause of
  disease classified elsewhere** B96.1
Klein (e) -levin syndrome G47.13
Kleptomania F63.2
Klinefelter's syndrome Q98.4
  karyotype 47,XXY Q98.0
  male with more than two X chromosomes
    Q98.1
**Klippel-Feil deficiency, disease, or syndrome
  (brevicollis)** Q76.1
Klippel's disease I67.2
Klippel-Trenaunay (-Weber) syndrome
  Q87.2
**Klumpke (-Déjérine) palsy, paralysis (birth)
  (newborn)** P14.1
Knee - *see* condition
Knock knee (acquired) M21.06-
  congenital Q74.1
Knot(s)
  intestinal, syndrome (volvulus) K56.2
  surfer S89.8-
  umbilical cord (true) O69.2
Knotting (of)
  hair L67.8
  intestine K56.2
Knuckle pad (Garrod's) M72.1
Koch's
  infection - *see* Tuberculosis
  relapsing fever A68.9
Koch-Weeks' conjunctivitis - *see*
  Conjunctivitis, acute, mucopurulent
Köebner's syndrome Q81.8
Köenig's disease (osteochondritis dissecans) -
  see Osteochondritis, dissecans
**Köhler-Pellegrini-Steida disease or syndrome
  (calcification, knee joint)** - *see* Bursitis, tibial
  collateral
Köhler's disease
  patellar - *see* Osteochondrosis, juvenile, patella
  tarsal navicular - *see* Osteochondrosis,
    juvenile, tarsus
Koilonychia L60.3
  congenital Q84.6
Kojevnikov's, epilepsy - *see* Kozhevnikov's
  epilepsy
Koplik's spots B05.9
Kopp's asthma E32.8
**Korsakoff's (Wernicke) disease, psychosis or
  syndrome (alcoholic)** F10.96
  with dependence F10.26
  drug-induced
    due to drug abuse - *see* Abuse, drug, by type,
      with amnestic disorder
    due to drug dependence - *see* Dependence,
      drug, by type, with amnestic disorder
  nonalcoholic F04
Korsakov's disease, psychosis or syndrome -
  see Korsakoff's disease
Korsakow's disease, psychosis or syndrome -
  see Korsakoff's disease
**Kostmann's disease or syndrome (infantile
  genetic agranulocytosis)** - *see*
  Agranulocytosis
Kozhevnikov's epilepsy G40.109
  intractable G40.119
    with status epilepticus G40.111
    without status epilepticus G40.119
  not intractable G40.109
    with status epilepticus G40.101
    without status epilepticus G40.109
Krabbe's
  disease E75.23
  syndrome, congenital muscle hypoplasia
    Q79.8

Kraepelin-morel disease - *see* Schizophrenia
Kraft-Weber-Dimitri disease Q85.8
Kraurosis
  ani K62.89
  penis N48.0
  vagina N89.8
  vulva N90.4
Kreotoxism A05.9
Krukenberg's
  spindle - *see* Pigmentation, cornea, posterior
  tumor C79.6-
Kufs' disease E75.4
Kugelberg-Welander disease G12.1
Kuhnt-Junius degeneration - *see also*
  Degeneration, macula H35.32-
Kümmell's disease or spondylitis - *see*
  Spondylopathy, traumatic
Kupffer cell sarcoma C22.3
Kuru A81.81
Kussmaul's
  disease M30.0
  respiration E87.2
    in diabetic acidosis - *see* Diabetes, by type,
      with ketoacidosis
Kwashiorkor E40
  marasmic, marasmus type E42
Kyasanur Forest disease A98.2
Kyphoscoliosis, kyphoscoliotic (acquired) -
  see also Scoliosis M41.9
  congenital Q67.5
  heart (disease) I27.1
  sequelae of rickets E64.3
  tuberculous A18.01
Kyphosis, kyphotic (acquired) M40.209
  cervical region M40.202
  cervicothoracic region M40.203
  congenital Q76.419
    cervical region Q76.412
    cervicothoracic region Q76.413
    occipito-atlanto-axial region Q76.411
    thoracic region Q76.414
    thoracolumbar region Q76.415
  Morquio-Brailsford type (spinal) - *see also*
    subcategory M49.8 E76.219
  postlaminectomy M96.3
  postradiation therapy M96.2
  postural (adolescent) M40.00
    cervicothoracic region M40.03
    thoracic region M40.04
    thoracolumbar region M40.05
  secondary NEC M40.10
    cervical region M40.12
    cervicothoracic region M40.13
    thoracic region M40.14
    thoracolumbar region M40.15
  sequelae of rickets E64.3
  specified type NEC M40.299
    cervical region M40.292
    cervicothoracic region M40.293
    thoracic region M40.294
    thoracolumbar region M40.295
  syphilitic, congenital A50.56
  thoracic region M40.204
  thoracolumbar region M40.205
  tuberculous A18.01
Kyrle disease L87.0

L

Labia, labium - *see* condition
Labile
  blood pressure R09.89
  vasomotor system I73.9
Labioglossal paralysis G12.29

Labium leporinum - *see* Cleft, lip
Labor - *see* Delivery
Labored breathing - *see* Hyperventilation
Labyrinthitis (circumscribed) (destructive)
   (diffuse) (inner ear) (latent) (purulent)
   (suppurative) - *see also* subcategory H83.0
   syphilitic A52.79
Laceration
   with abortion - *see* Abortion, by type,
      complicated by laceration of pelvic organs
   abdomen, abdominal
      wall S31.119
         with
            foreign body S31.129
            penetration into peritoneal cavity S31.619
               with foreign body S31.629
         epigastric region S31.112
            with
               foreign body S31.122
               penetration into peritoneal cavity
                  S31.612
                  with foreign body S31.622
         left
            lower quadrant S31.114
               with
                  foreign body S31.124
                  penetration into peritoneal cavity
                     S31.614
                     with foreign body S31.624
            upper quadrant S31.111
               with
                  foreign body S31.121
                  penetration into peritoneal cavity
                     S31.611
                     with foreign body S31.621
         periumbilic region S31.115
            with
               foreign body S31.125
               penetration into peritoneal cavity
                  S31.615
                  with foreign body S31.625
         right
            lower quadrant S31.113
               with
                  foreign body S31.123
                  penetration into peritoneal cavity
                     S31.613
                     with foreign body S31.623
            upper quadrant S31.110
               with
                  foreign body S31.120
                  penetration into peritoneal cavity
                     S31.610
                     with foreign body S31.620
   accidental, complicating surgery - *see*
      Complications, surgical, accidental puncture
      or laceration
   Achilles tendon S86.02-
   adrenal gland S37.813
   alveolar (process) - *see* Laceration, oral cavity
   ankle S91.01-
      with
         foreign body S91.02-
   antecubital space - *see* Laceration, elbow
   anus (sphincter) S31.831
      with
         ectopic or molar pregnancy O08.6
         foreign body S31.832
      complicating delivery - *see* Delivery,
         complicated, by, laceration, anus (sphincter)
      following ectopic or molar pregnancy O08.6
      nontraumatic, nonpuerperal - *see* Fissure,
         anus
   arm (upper) S41.11-

Laceration - *continued*
   with foreign body S41.12-
      lower - *see* Laceration, forearm
   auditory canal (external) (meatus) - *see*
      Laceration, ear
   auricle, ear - *see* Laceration, ear
   axilla - *see* Laceration, arm
   back - *see also* Laceration, thorax, back
      lower S31.010
         with
            foreign body S31.020
               with penetration into retroperitoneal
                  space S31.021
               penetration into retroperitoneal space
                  S31.011
   bile duct S36.13
   bladder S37.23
      with ectopic or molar pregnancy O08.6
      following ectopic or molar pregnancy O08.6
      obstetrical trauma O71.5
   blood vessel - *see* Injury, blood vessel
   bowel - *see also* Laceration, intestine
      with ectopic or molar pregnancy O08.6
      complicating abortion - *see* Abortion, by
         type, complicated by, specified condition
         NEC
      following ectopic or molar pregnancy O08.6
      obstetrical trauma O71.5
   brain (any part) (cortex) (diffuse) (membrane)
      - *see also* Injury, intracranial, diffuse
      during birth P10.8
         with hemorrhage P10.1
      focal - *see* Injury, intracranial, focal brain
         injury   brainstem S06.38-
   breast S21.01-
      with foreign body S21.02-
   broad ligament S37.893
      with ectopic or molar pregnancy O08.6
      following ectopic or molar pregnancy O08.6
      laceration syndrome N83.8
      obstetrical trauma O71.6
      syndrome (laceration) N83.8
   buttock S31.801
      with foreign body S31.802
      left S31.821
         with foreign body S31.822
      right S31.811
         with foreign body S31.812
   calf - *see* Laceration, leg
   canaliculus lacrimalis - *see* Laceration, eyelid
   canthus, eye - *see* Laceration, eyelid
   capsule, joint - *see* Sprain
   causing eversion of cervix uteri (old) N86
   central (perineal), complicating delivery O70.9
   cerebellum, traumatic S06.37-
   cerebral S06.33-
      left side S06.32-
      during birth P10.8
         with hemorrhage P10.1
      right side S06.31-
   cervix (uteri)
      with ectopic or molar pregnancy O08.6
      following ectopic or molar pregnancy O08.6
      nonpuerperal, nontraumatic N88.1
      obstetrical trauma (current) O71.3
      old (postpartal) N88.1
      traumatic S37.63
   cheek (external) S01.41-
      with foreign body S01.42-
      internal - *see* Laceration, oral cavity   chest
         wall - *see* Laceration, thorax
   chin - *see* Laceration, head, specified site NEC
   chordae tendinae NEC I51.1

Laceration - *continued*
   concurrent with acute myocardial infarction -
      see Infarct, myocardium
      following acute myocardial infarction
         (current complication) I23.4
   clitoris - *see* Laceration, vulva
   colon - *see* Laceration, intestine, large, colon
   common bile duct S36.13
   cortex (cerebral) - *see* Injury, intracranial,
      diffuse
   costal region - *see* Laceration, thorax
   cystic duct S36.13
   diaphragm S27.803
   digit(s)
      hand - *see* Laceration, finger
      foot - *see* Laceration, toe
   duodenum S36.430
   ear (canal) (external) S01.31-
      with foreign body S01.32-
      drum S09.2-
   elbow S51.01-
      with
         foreign body S51.02-
   epididymis - *see* Laceration, testis
   epigastric region - *see* Laceration, abdomen,
      wall, epigastric region
   esophagus K22.8
      traumatic
         cervical S11.21
            with foreign body S11.22
         thoracic S27.813
   eye (ball) S05.3-
      with prolapse or loss of intraocular tissue
         S05.2-
      penetrating S05.6-
   eyebrow - *see* Laceration, eyelid
   eyelid S01.11-
      with foreign body S01.12-
   face NEC - *see* Laceration, head, specified site
      NEC
   fallopian tube S37.539
      bilateral S37.532
      unilateral S37.531
   finger(s) S61.219
      with
         damage to nail S61.319
            with
               foreign body S61.329
         foreign body S61.229
      index S61.218
         with
            damage to nail S61.318
               with
                  foreign body S61.328
            foreign body S61.228
      left S61.211
         with
            damage to nail S61.311
               with
                  foreign body S61.321
            foreign body S61.221
      right S61.210
         with
            damage to nail S61.310
               with
                  foreign body S61.320
            foreign body S61.220
      little S61.218
         with
            damage to nail S61.318
               with
                  foreign body S61.328
            foreign body S61.228
      left S61.217

Laceration - *continued*
 with
  damage to nail S61.317
   with
    foreign body S61.327
  foreign body S61.227
  right S61.216
   with
    damage to nail S61.316
     with
      foreign body S61.326
    foreign body S61.226
 middle S61.218
  with
   damage to nail S61.318
    with
     foreign body S61.328
   foreign body S61.228
  left S61.213
   with
    damage to nail S61.313
     with
      foreign body S61.323
    foreign body S61.223
  right S61.212
   with
    damage to nail S61.312
     with
      foreign body S61.322
    foreign body S61.222
 ring S61.218
  with
   damage to nail S61.318
    with
     foreign body S61.328
   foreign body S61.228
  left S61.215
   with
    damage to nail S61.315
     with
      foreign body S61.325
    foreign body S61.225
  right S61.214
   with
    damage to nail S61.314
     with
      foreign body S61.324
    foreign body S61.224
 flank S31.119
  with foreign body S31.129
 foot (except toe(s) alone) S91.319
  with foreign body S91.329
  left S91.312
   with foreign body S91.322
  right S91.311
   with foreign body S91.321
  toe - *see* Laceration, toe
 forearm S51.819
  with
   foreign body S51.829
  elbow only - *see* Laceration, elbow
  left S51.812
   with
    foreign body S51.822
  right S51.811
   with
    foreign body S51.821
 forehead S01.81
  with foreign body S01.82
 fourchette O70.0
  with ectopic or molar pregnancy O08.6
  complicating delivery O70.0
  following ectopic or molar pregnancy O08.6
 gallbladder S36.123

Laceration - *continued*
 genital organs, external
  female S31.512
   with foreign body S31.522
   vagina - *see* Laceration, vagina
   vulva - *see* Laceration, vulva
  male S31.511
   with foreign body S31.521
   penis - *see* Laceration, penis
   scrotum - *see* Laceration, scrotum
   testis - *see* Laceration, testis
 groin - *see* Laceration, abdomen, wall
 gum - *see* Laceration, oral cavity
 hand S61.419
  with
   foreign body S61.429
  finger - *see* Laceration, finger
  left S61.412
   with
    foreign body S61.422
  right S61.411
   with
    foreign body S61.421
  thumb - *see* Laceration, thumb
 head S01.91
  with foreign body S01.92
  cheek - *see* Laceration, cheek
  ear - *see* Laceration, ear
  eyelid - *see* Laceration, eyelid
  lip - *see* Laceration, lip
  nose - *see* Laceration, nose
  oral cavity - *see* Laceration, oral cavity
  scalp S01.01
   with foreign body S01.02
  specified site NEC S01.81
   with foreign body S01.82
  temporomandibular area - *see* Laceration,
   cheek
 heart - *see* Injury, heart, laceration
 heel - *see* Laceration, foot
 hepatic duct S36.13
 hip S71.019
  with foreign body S71.029
  left S71.012
   with foreign body S71.022
  right S71.011
   with foreign body S71.021
 hymen - *see* Laceration, vagina
 hypochondrium - *see* Laceration, abdomen,
  wall
 hypogastric region - *see* Laceration, abdomen,
  wall
 ileum S36.438
 inguinal region - *see* Laceration, abdomen,
  wall
 instep - *see* Laceration, foot
 internal organ - *see* Injury, by site
 interscapular region - *see* Laceration, thorax,
  back
 intestine
  large
   colon S36.539
    ascending S36.530
    descending S36.532
    sigmoid S36.533
    specified site NEC S36.538
   rectum S36.63
   transverse S36.531
  small S36.439
   duodenum S36.430
   specified site NEC S36.438
 intra-abdominal organ S36.93
 intestine - *see* Laceration, intestine
 liver - *see* Laceration, liver

Laceration - *continued*
 pancreas - *see* Laceration, pancreas
 peritoneum S36.81
 specified site NEC S36.893
 spleen - *see* Laceration, spleen
 stomach - *see* Laceration, stomach
 intracranial NEC - *see also* Injury, intracranial,
  diffuse
  birth injury P10.9
 jaw - *see* Laceration, head, specified site NEC
 jejunum S36.438
 joint capsule - *see* Sprain, by site
 kidney S37.03-
  major (greater than 3 cm) (massive) (stellate)
   S37.06-
  minor (less than 1 cm) S37.04-
  moderate (1 to 3 cm) S37.05-
  multiple S37.06-
 knee S81.01-
  with foreign body S81.02-
 labium (majus) (minus) - *see* Laceration, vulva
 lacrimal duct - *see* Laceration, eyelid
 large intestine - *see* Laceration, intestine, large
 larynx S11.011
  with foreign body S11.012
 leg (lower) S81.819
  with foreign body S81.829
  foot - *see* Laceration, foot
  knee - *see* Laceration, knee
  left S81.812
   with foreign body S81.822
  right S81.811
   with foreign body S81.821
  upper - *see* Laceration, thigh
 ligament - *see* Sprain
 lip S01.511
  with foreign body S01.521
 liver S36.113
  major (stellate) S36.116
  minor S36.114
  moderate S36.115
 loin - *see* Laceration, abdomen, wall
 lower back - *see* Laceration, back, lower
 lumbar region - *see* Laceration, back, lower
 lung S27.339
  bilateral S27.332
  unilateral S27.331
 malar region - *see* Laceration, head, specified
  site NEC
 mammary - *see* Laceration, breast
 mastoid region - *see* Laceration, head,
  specified site NEC
 meninges - *see* Injury, intracranial, diffuse
 meniscus - *see* Tear, meniscus
 mesentery S36.893
 mesosalpinx S37.893
 mouth - *see* Laceration, oral cavity
 muscle - *see* Injury, muscle, by site, laceration
 nail
  finger - *see* Laceration, finger, with damage
   to nail
  toe - *see* Laceration, toe, with damage to nail
 nasal (septum) (sinus) - *see* Laceration, nose
 nasopharynx - *see* Laceration, head, specified
  site NEC
 neck S11.91
  with foreign body S11.92
  involving
   cervical esophagus S11.21
    with foreign body S11.22
   larynx - *see* Laceration, larynx
   pharynx - *see* Laceration, pharynx
   thyroid gland - *see* Laceration, thyroid
    gland

Laceration - *continued*
  trachea - *see* Laceration, trachea
  specified site NEC S11.81
    with foreign body S11.82
  nerve - *see* Injury, nerve
  nose (septum) (sinus) S01.21
    with foreign body S01.22
  ocular NOS S05.3-
    adnexa NOS S01.11-
  oral cavity S01.512
    with foreign body S01.522
  orbit (eye) - *see* Wound, open, ocular, orbit
  ovary S37.439
    bilateral S37.432
    unilateral S37.431
  palate - *see* Laceration, oral cavity   palm - *see*
Laceration, hand
  pancreas S36.239
    body S36.231
      major S36.261
      minor S36.241
      moderate S36.251
    head S36.230
      major S36.260
      minor S36.240
      moderate S36.250
    major S36.269
    minor S36.249
    moderate S36.259
    tail S36.232
      major S36.262
      minor S36.242
      moderate S36.252
  pelvic S31.010
    with
      foreign body S31.020
        penetration into retroperitoneal cavity
          S31.021
      penetration into retroperitoneal cavity
        S31.011
  floor - *see also* Laceration, back, lower
    with ectopic or molar pregnancy O08.6
    complicating delivery O70.1
    following ectopic or molar pregnancy
      O08.6
    old (postpartal) N81.89
  organ S37.93
    with ectopic or molar pregnancy O08.6
    adrenal gland S37.813
    bladder S37.23
    fallopian tube - *see* Laceration, fallopian
      tube
    following ectopic or molar pregnancy
      O08.6
    kidney - *see* Laceration, kidney
    obstetrical trauma O71.5
    ovary - *see* Laceration, ovary
    prostate S37.823
    specified site NEC S37.893
    ureter S37.13
    urethra S37.33
    uterus S37.63
  penis S31.21
    with foreign body S31.22
  perineum
    female S31.41
      with
        ectopic or molar pregnancy O08.6
        foreign body S31.42
      during delivery O70.9
        first degree O70.0
        fourth degree O70.3
        second degree O70.1
        third degree - *see also* Delivery,

Laceration - *continued*
  complicated, by, laceration, perineum,
    third degree O70.20
  old (postpartal) N81.89
  postpartal N81.89
  secondary (postpartal) O90.1
  male S31.119
    with foreign body S31.129
  periocular area (with or without lacrimal
    passages) - *see* Laceration, eyelid
  peritoneum S36.893
  periumbilic region - *see* Laceration, abdomen,
    wall, periumbilic
  periurethral tissue - *see* Laceration, urethra
  phalanges
    finger - *see* Laceration, finger
    toe - *see* Laceration, toe
  pharynx S11.21
    with foreign body S11.22
  pinna - *see* Laceration, ear
  popliteal space - *see* Laceration, knee
  prepuce - *see* Laceration, penis
  prostate S37.823
  pubic region S31.119
    with foreign body S31.129
  pudendum - *see* Laceration, genital organs,
    external
  rectovaginal septum - *see* Laceration, vagina
  rectum S36.63
  retroperitoneum S36.893
  round ligament S37.893
  sacral region - *see* Laceration, back, lower
  sacroiliac region - *see* Laceration, back, lower
  salivary gland - *see* Laceration, oral cavity
  scalp S01.01
    with foreign body S01.02
  scapular region - *see* Laceration, shoulder
  scrotum S31.31
    with foreign body S31.32
  seminal vesicle S37.893
  shin - *see* Laceration, leg
  shoulder S41.019
    with foreign body S41.029
    left S41.012
      with foreign body S41.022
    right S41.011
      with foreign body S41.021
  small intestine - *see* Laceration, intestine,
    small
  spermatic cord - *see* Laceration, testis
  spinal cord (meninges) - *see also* Injury, spinal
    cord, by region
    due to injury at birth P11.5
    newborn (birth injury) P11.5
  spleen S36.039
    major (massive) (stellate) S36.032
    moderate S36.031
    superficial (minor) S36.030
  sternal region - *see* Laceration, thorax, front
  stomach S36.33
  submaxillary region - *see* Laceration, head,
    specified site NEC
  submental region - *see* Laceration, head,
    specified site NEC
  subungual
    finger(s) - *see* Laceration, finger, with
      damage to nail
    toe(s) - *see* Laceration, toe, with damage to
      nail
  suprarenal gland - *see* Laceration, adrenal
    gland
  temple, temporal region - *see* Laceration, head,
    specified site NEC
  temporomandibular area - *see* Laceration,

Laceration - *continued*
  cheek
  tendon - *see* Injury, muscle, by site, laceration
    Achilles S86.02-
  tentorium cerebelli - *see* Injury, intracranial,
    diffuse
  testis S31.31
    with foreign body S31.32
  thigh S71.11-
    with foreign body S71.12-
  thorax, thoracic (wall) S21.91
    with foreign body S21.92
    back S21.22-
      with penetration into thoracic cavity
        S21.42-
    front S21.12-
      with penetration into thoracic cavity
        S21.32-
    back S21.21-
      with
        foreign body S21.22-
          with penetration into thoracic cavity
            S21.42-
        penetration into thoracic cavity S21.41-
    breast - *see* Laceration, breast
    front S21.11-
      with
        foreign body S21.12-
          with penetration into thoracic cavity
            S21.32-
        penetration into thoracic cavity S21.31-
  thumb S61.019
    with
      damage to nail S61.119
        with
          foreign body S61.129
      foreign body S61.029
    left S61.012
      with
        damage to nail S61.112
          with
            foreign body S61.122
        foreign body S61.022
    right S61.011
      with
        damage to nail S61.111
          with
            foreign body S61.121
        foreign body S61.021
  thyroid gland S11.11
    with foreign body S11.12
  toe(s) S91.119
    with
      damage to nail S91.219
        with
          foreign body S91.229
      foreign body S91.129
    great S91.113
      with
        damage to nail S91.213
          with
            foreign body S91.223
        foreign body S91.123
      left S91.112
        with
          damage to nail S91.212
            with
              foreign body S91.222
          foreign body S91.122
        right S91.111
          with
            damage to nail S91.211
              with
                foreign body S91.221

Laceration - *continued*
    foreign body S91.121
  lesser S91.116
    with
      damage to nail S91.216
        with
          foreign body S91.226
      foreign body S91.126
  left S91.115
    with
      damage to nail S91.215
        with
          foreign body S91.225
      foreign body S91.125
  right S91.114
    with
      damage to nail S91.214
        with
          foreign body S91.224
      foreign body S91.124
  tongue - *see* Laceration, oral cavity trachea S11.021
    with foreign body S11.022
  tunica vaginalis - *see* Laceration, testis
  tympanum, tympanic membrane - *see* Laceration, ear, drum
  umbilical region S31.115
    with foreign body S31.125
  ureter S37.13
  urethra S37.33
    with or following ectopic or molar pregnancy O08.6
    obstetrical trauma O71.5
  urinary organ NEC S37.893
  uterus S37.63
    with ectopic or molar pregnancy O08.6
    following ectopic or molar pregnancy O08.6
    nonpuerperal, nontraumatic N85.8
    obstetrical trauma NEC O71.81
    old (postpartal) N85.8
  uvula - *see* Laceration, oral cavity vagina S31.41
    with
      ectopic or molar pregnancy O08.6
      foreign body S31.42
    during delivery O71.4
      with perineal laceration - *see* Laceration, perineum, female, during delivery
    following ectopic or molar pregnancy O08.6
    nonpuerperal, nontraumatic N89.8
    old (postpartal) N89.8
  vas deferens S37.893
  vesical - *see* Laceration, bladder
  vocal cords S11.031
    with foreign body S11.032
  vulva S31.41
    with
      ectopic or molar pregnancy O08.6
      foreign body S31.42
    complicating delivery O70.0
    following ectopic or molar pregnancy O08.6
    nonpuerperal, nontraumatic N90.89
    old (postpartal) N90.89
  wrist S61.519
    with
      foreign body S61.529
    left S61.512
      with
        foreign body S61.522
    right S61.511
      with
        foreign body S61.521
Lack of
  achievement in school Z55.3

Lack of - *continued*
  adequate
    food Z59.4
    intermaxillary vertical dimension of fully erupted teeth M26.36
    sleep Z72.820
  appetite (see Anorexia) R63.0
  awareness R41.9
  care
    in home Z74.2
    of infant (at or after birth) T76.02
      confirmed T74.02
  cognitive functions R41.9
  coordination R27.9
    ataxia R27.0
    specified type NEC R27.8
  development (physiological) R62.50
    failure to thrive (child over 28 days old) R62.51
    adult R62.7
    newborn P92.6
    short stature R62.52
    specified type NEC R62.59
  energy R53.83
  financial resources Z59.6
  food T73.0
  growth R62.52
  heating Z59.1
  housing (permanent) (temporary) Z59.0
    adequate Z59.1
  learning experiences in childhood Z62.898
  leisure time (affecting life-style) Z73.2
  material resources Z59.9
  memory - *see also* Amnesia
    mild, following organic brain damage F06.8
  ovulation N97.0
  parental supervision or control of child Z62.0
  person able to render necessary care Z74.2
  physical exercise Z72.3
  play experience in childhood Z62.898
  posterior occlusal support M26.57
  relaxation (affecting life-style) Z73.2
  sexual
    desire F52.0
    enjoyment F52.1
  shelter Z59.0
  sleep (adequate) Z72.820
  supervision of child by parent Z62.0
  support, posterior occlusal M26.57
  water T73.1
Lacrimal - *see* condition
Lacrimation, abnormal - *see* Epiphora
Lacrimonasal duct - *see* condition
Lactation, lactating (breast) (puerperal, postpartum)
  associated
    cracked nipple O92.13
    retracted nipple O92.03
  defective O92.4
Lactation disorder NEC O92.79
  excessive O92.6
  failed (complete) O92.3
    partial O92.4
  mastitis NEC - *see* Mastitis, obstetric
  mother (care and/or examination) Z39.1
  nonpuerperal N64.3
Lacticemia, excessive E87.2
Lacunar skull Q75.8
Laennec's cirrhosis K70.30
  with ascites K70.31
  nonalcoholic K74.69
Lafora's disease - *see* Epilepsy, generalized, idiopathic
Lag, lid (nervous) - *see* Retraction, lid

Lagophthalmos (eyelid) (nervous) H02.209
  cicatricial H02.219
    left H02.216
      lower H02.215
      upper H02.214
    right H02.213
      lower H02.212
      upper H02.211
  keratoconjunctivitis - *see* Keratoconjunctivitis
    left H02.206
      lower H02.205
      upper H02.204
  mechanical H02.229
    left H02.226
      lower H02.225
      upper H02.224
    right H02.223
      lower H02.222
      upper H02.221
  paralytic H02.239
    left H02.236
      lower H02.235
      upper H02.234
    right H02.233
      lower H02.232
      upper H02.231
    right H02.203
      lower H02.202
      upper H02.201
Laki-Lorand factor deficiency - *see* Defect, coagulation, specified type NEC
Lalling F80.0
Lambert-Eaton syndrome - *see* Syndrome, Lambert-Eaton
Lambliasis, lambliosis A07.1
Landau-Kleffner syndrome - *see* Epilepsy, specified NEC
Landouzy-Déjérine dystrophy or facioscapulohumeral atrophy G71.0
Landouzy's disease (icterohemorrhagic leptospirosis) A27.0
Landry-Guillain-Barré, syndrome or paralysis G61.0
Landry's disease or paralysis G61.0
Lane's
  band Q43.3
  kink - *see* Obstruction, intestine
  syndrome K90.2
Langdon Down syndrome - *see* Trisomy, 21
Lapsed immunization schedule status Z28.3
Large
  baby (regardless of gestational age) (4000g to 4499g) P08.1
  ear, congenital Q17.1
  physiological cup Q14.2
  stature R68.89
Large-for-dates NEC (infant) (4000g to 4499g) P08.1
  affecting management of pregnancy O36.6-
  exceptionally (4500g or more) P08.0
Larsen-Johansson disease or osteochondrosis - *see* Osteochondrosis, juvenile, patella
Larsen's syndrome (flattened facies and multiple congenital dislocations) Q74.8
Larva migrans
  cutaneous B76.9
    Ancylostoma B76.0
  visceral B83.0
Laryngeal - *see* condition
Laryngismus (stridulus) J38.5
  congenital P28.89
  diphtheritic A36.2

Laryngitis (acute) (edematous) (fibrinous) (infective) (infiltrative) (malignant) (membranous) (phlegmonous) (pneumococcal) (pseudomembranous) (septic) (subglottic) (suppurative) (ulcerative) J04.0
  with
    influenza, flu, or grippe - *see* Influenza, with, laryngitis
    tracheitis (acute) - *see* Laryngotracheitis
  atrophic J37.0
  catarrhal J37.0
  chronic J37.0
    with tracheitis (chronic) J37.1
  diphtheritic A36.2
  due to external agent - *see* Inflammation, respiratory, upper, due to
  Hemophilus influenzae J04.0
  H. influenzae J04.0
  hypertrophic J37.0
  influenzal - *see* Influenza, with, respiratory manifestations NEC
  obstructive J05.0
  sicca J37.0
  spasmodic J05.0
    acute J04.0
  streptococcal J04.0
  stridulous J05.0
  syphilitic (late) A52.73
    congenital A50.59 [*J99*]
    early A50.03 [*J99*]
  tuberculous A15.5
  Vincent's A69.1
Laryngocele (congenital) (ventricular) Q31.3
Laryngofissure J38.7
  congenital Q31.8
Laryngomalacia (congenital) Q31.5
Laryngopharyngitis (acute) J06.0
  chronic J37.0
  due to external agent - *see* Inflammation, respiratory, upper, due to
Laryngoplegia J38.00
  bilateral J38.02
  unilateral J38.01
Laryngoptosis J38.7
Laryngospasm J38.5
Laryngostenosis J38.6
Laryngotracheitis (acute) (Infectional) (infective) (viral) J04.2
  atrophic J37.1
  catarrhal J37.1
  chronic J37.1
  diphtheritic A36.2
  due to external agent - *see* Inflammation, respiratory, upper, due to
  Hemophilus influenzae J04.2
  hypertrophic J37.1
  influenzal - *see* Influenza, with, respiratory manifestations NEC
  pachydermic J38.7
  sicca J37.1
  spasmodic J38.5
    acute J05.0
  streptococcal J04.2
  stridulous J38.5
  syphilitic (late) A52.73
    congenital A50.59 [*J99*]
    early A50.03 [*J99*]
  tuberculous A15.5
  Vincent's A69.1
Laryngotracheobronchitis - *see* Bronchitis
Larynx, laryngeal - *see* condition
Lassa fever A96.2
Lassitude - *see* Weakness

Late
  talker R62.0
  walker R62.0
Late effect(s) - *see* Sequelae
Latent - *see* condition
Laterocession - *see* Lateroversion
Lateroflexion - *see* Lateroversion
Lateroversion
  cervix - *see* Lateroversion, uterus
  uterus, uterine (cervix) (postinfectional) (postpartal, old) N85.4
    congenital Q51.818
    in pregnancy or childbirth O34.59-**lathyrism** - *see* Poisoning, food, noxious, plant
Launois' syndrome (pituitary gigantism) E22.0
Launois-Bensaude adenolipomatosis E88.89
Laurence-moon (-Bardet) -Biedl syndrome Q87.89
Lax, laxity - *see also* Relaxation
  ligament (ous) - *see also* Disorder, ligament
    familial M35.7
    knee - *see* Derangement, knee
  skin (acquired) L57.4
    congenital Q82.8
Laxative habit F55.2
Lazy leukocyte syndrome D70.8
Lead miner's lung J63.6
Leak, leakage
  air NEC J93.82
    postprocedural J95.812
  amniotic fluid - *see* Rupture, membranes, premature
  blood (microscopic), fetal, into maternal circulation affecting management of pregnancy - *see* Pregnancy, complicated by
  cerebrospinal fluid G96.0
    from spinal (lumbar) puncture G97.0
  device, implant or graft - *see also* Complications, by site and type, mechanical
    arterial graft NEC - *see* Complication, cardiovascular device, mechanical, vascular
    breast (implant) T85.43
    catheter NEC T85.638
      urinary T83.038
        cystostomy T83.030
        Hopkins T83.038
        ileostomy T83.038
        indwelling T83.031
        nephrostomy T83.032
        specified NEC T83.038
        urostomy T83.038
    dialysis (renal) T82.43
      intraperitoneal T85.631
    infusion NEC T82.534
      spinal (epidural) (subdural) T85.630
    gastrointestinal - *see* Complications, prosthetic device, mechanical, gastrointestinal device
    genital NEC T83.498
      penile prosthesis (cylinder) (implanted) (pump) (reservoir) T83.490
      testicular prosthesis T83.491
    heart NEC - *see* Complication, cardiovascular device, mechanical
    joint prosthesis - *see* Complications, joint prosthesis, mechanical, specified NEC, by site
    ocular NEC - *see* Complications, prosthetic device, mechanical, ocular device
    orthopedic NEC - *see* Complication, orthopedic, device, mechanical
    persistent air J93.82
    specified NEC T85.638

Leak, leakage - *continued*
    urinary NEC - *see also* Complication, genitourinary, device, urinary, mechanical graft T83.23
    vascular NEC - *see* Complication, cardiovascular device, mechanical ventricular intracranial shunt T85.03
  urine - *see* Incontinence
Leaky heart - *see* Endocarditis
Learning defect (specific) F81.9
Leather bottle stomach C16.9
Leber's
  congenital amaurosis H35.50
  optic atrophy (hereditary) H47.22
Lederer's anemia D59.1
Leeches (external) - *see* Hirudiniasis
Leg - *see* condition
Legg (-Calvé) -Perthes disease, syndrome or osteochondrosis M91.1-
Legionellosis A48.1
  nonpneumonic A48.2
Legionnaires'
  disease A48.1
    nonpneumonic A48.2
  pneumonia A48.1
Leigh's disease G31.82
Leiner's disease L21.1
Leiofibromyoma - *see* Leiomyoma
Leiomyoblastoma - *see* Neoplasm, connective tissue, benign
Leiomyofibroma - *see also* Neoplasm, connective tissue, benign
  uterus (cervix) (corpus) D25.9
Leiomyoma - *see also* Neoplasm, connective tissue, benign
  bizarre - *see* Neoplasm, connective tissue, benign
  cellular - *see* Neoplasm, connective tissue, benign
  epithelioid - *see* Neoplasm, connective tissue, benign
  uterus (cervix) (corpus) D25.9
    intramural D25.1
    submucous D25.0
    subserosal D25.2
  vascular - *see* Neoplasm, connective tissue, benign
Leiomyoma, leiomyomatosis (intravascular) - *see* Neoplasm, connective tissue, uncertain behavior
Leiomyosarcoma - *see also* Neoplasm, connective tissue, malignant
  epithelioid - *see* Neoplasm, connective tissue, malignant
  myxoid - *see* Neoplasm, connective tissue, malignant
Leishmaniasis B55.9
  American (mucocutaneous) B55.2
    cutaneous B55.1
  Asian Desert B55.1
  Brazilian B55.2
  cutaneous (any type) B55.1
  dermal - *see also* Leishmaniasis, cutaneous
    post-kala-azar B55.0
  eyelid B55.1
  infantile B55.0
  Mediterranean B55.0
  mucocutaneous (American) (New World) B55.2
  naso-oral B55.2
  nasopharyngeal B55.2
  old world B55.1
  tegumentaria diffusa B55.1
  visceral B55.0

Leishmanoid, dermal - *see also* Leishmaniasis, cutaneous
  post-kala-azar B55.0
Lenegre's disease I44.2
Lengthening, leg - *see* Deformity, limb, unequal length
Lennert's lymphoma - *see* Lymphoma, Lennert's
Lennox-Gastaut syndrome G40.812
  intractable G40.814
    with status epilepticus G40.813
    without status epilepticus G40.814
  not intractable G40.812
    with status epilepticus G40.811
    without status epilepticus G40.812
Lens - *see* condition
Lenticonus (anterior) (posterior) (congenital) Q12.8
Lenticular degeneration, progressive E83.01
Lentiglobus (posterior) (congenital) Q12.8
Lentigo (congenital) L81.4
  maligna - *see also* Melanoma, in situ
    melanoma - *see* Melanoma
Lentivirus, as cause of disease classified elsewhere B97.31
Leontiasis
  ossium M85.2
  syphilitic (late) A52.78
    congenital A50.59
Lepothrix A48.8
Lepra - *see* Leprosy
Leprechaunism E34.8
Leprosy A30.-
  with muscle disorder A30.9 *[M63.80]*
    ankle A30.9 *[M63.87]*
    foot A30.9 *[M63.87]*
    forearm A30.9 *[M63.83]*
    hand A30.9 *[M63.84]*
    lower leg A30.9 *[M63.86]*
    multiple sites A30.9 *[M63.89]*
    pelvic region A30.9 *[M63.85]*
    shoulder region A30.9 *[M63.81]*
    specified site NEC A30.9 *[M63.88]*
    thigh A30.9 *[M63.85]*
    upper arm A30.9 *[M63.82]*
  anesthetic A30.9
  BB A30.3
  BL A30.4
  borderline (infiltrated) (neuritic) A30.3
    lepromatous A30.4
    tuberculoid A30.2
  BT A30.2
  dimorphous (infiltrated) (neuritic) A30.3
  I A30.0
  indeterminate (macular) (neuritic) A30.0
  lepromatous (diffuse) (infiltrated) (macular) (neuritic) (nodular) A30.5
  LL A30.5
  macular (early) (neuritic) (simple) A30.9
  maculoanesthetic A30.9
  mixed A30.3
  neural A30.9
  nodular A30.5
  primary neuritic A30.3
  specified type NEC A30.8
  TT A30.1
  tuberculoid (major) (minor) A30.1
Leptocytosis, hereditary D56.9
Leptomeningitis (chronic) (circumscribed) (hemorrhagic) (nonsuppurative) - *see* Meningitis
Leptomeningopathy G96.19
Leptospiral - *see* condition

Leptospirochetal - *see* condition **Leptospirosis** A27.9
  canicola A27.89
  due to Leptospira interrogans serovar icterohaemorrhagiae A27.0
  icterohemorrhagica A27.0
  pomona A27.89
  Weil's disease A27.0
Leptus dermatitis B88.0
Leriche's syndrome (aortic bifurcation occlusion) I74.09
Leri's pleonosteosis Q78.8
Leri-Weill syndrome Q77.8
Lermoyez' syndrome - *see* Vertigo, peripheral NEC
Lesch Nyhan syndrome E79.1
Leser-Trélat disease L82.1
  inflamed L82.0
Lesion(s) (nontraumatic)
  abducens nerve - *see* Strabismus, paralytic, sixth nerve
  alveolar process K08.9
  angiocentric immunoproliferative D47.Z9
  anorectal K62.9
  aortic (valve) I35.9
  auditory nerve - *see* subcategory H93.3
  basal ganglion G25.9
  bile duct - *see* Disease, bile duct
  biomechanical M99.9
    specified type NEC M99.89
      abdomen M99.89
      acromioclavicular M99.87
      cervical region M99.81
      cervicothoracic M99.81
      costochondral M99.88
      costovertebral M99.88
      head region M99.80
      hip M99.85
      lower extremity M99.86
      lumbar region M99.83
      lumbosacral M99.83
      occipitocervical M99.80
      pelvic region M99.85
      pubic M99.85
      rib cage M99.88
      sacral region M99.84
      sacrococcygeal M99.84
      sacroiliac M99.84
      specified NEC M99.89
      sternochondral M99.88
      sternoclavicular M99.87
      thoracic region M99.82
      thoracolumbar M99.82
      upper extremity M99.87
  bladder N32.9
  bone - *see* Disorder, bone
  brachial plexus G54.0
  brain G93.9
    congenital Q04.9
    vascular I67.9
      degenerative I67.9
      hypertensive I67.4
  buccal cavity K13.79
  calcified - *see* Calcification
  canthus - *see* Disorder, eyelid
  carate - *see* Pinta, lesions
  cardia K31.9
  cardiac - *see also* Disease, heart I51.9
    congenital Q24.9
    valvular - *see* Endocarditis
  cauda equina G83.4
  cecum K63.9
  cerebral - *see* Lesion, brain
  cerebrovascular I67.9

Lesion(s) (nontraumatic) - *continued*
  degenerative I67.9
    hypertensive I67.4
  cervical (nerve) root NEC G54.2
  chiasmal - *see* Disorder, optic, chiasm
  chorda tympani G51.8
  coin, lung R91.1
  colon K63.9
  combined periodontic endodontic K05.5
  congenital - *see* Anomaly, by site
  conjunctiva H11.9
  conus medullaris - *see* Injury, conus medullaris
  coronary artery - *see* Ischemia, heart
  cranial nerve G52.9
    eighth - *see* Disorder, ear
    eleventh G52.9
    fifth G50.9
    first G52.0
    fourth - *see* Strabismus, paralytic, fourth nerve
    seventh G51.9
    sixth - *see* Strabismus, paralytic, sixth nerve
    tenth G52.2
    twelfth G52.3
  cystic - *see* Cyst
  degenerative - *see* Degeneration
  duodenum K31.9
  edentulous (alveolar) ridge, associated with trauma, due to traumatic occlusion K06.2
  en coup de sabre L94.1
  eyelid - *see* Disorder, eyelid
  gasserian ganglion G50.8
  gastric K31.9
  gastroduodenal K31.9
  gastrointestinal K63.9
  gingiva, associated with trauma K06.2
  glomerular
    focal and segmental - *see also* N00-N07 with fourth character .1 N05.1
    minimal change - *see also* N00-N07 with fourth character .0 N05.0
  heart (organic) - *see* Disease, heart
  hyperchromic, due to pinta (carate) A67.1
  hyperkeratotic - *see* Hyperkeratosis
  hypothalamic E23.7
  ileocecal K63.9
  ileum K63.9
  iliohypogastric nerve G57.8-
  inflammatory - *see* Inflammation
  intestine K63.9
  intracerebral - *see* Lesion, brain
  intrachiasmal (optic) - *see* Disorder, optic, chiasm
  intracranial, space-occupying R90.0
  joint - *see* Disorder, joint
    sacroiliac (old) M53.3
  keratotic - *see* Keratosis
  kidney - *see* Disease, renal
  laryngeal nerve (recurrent) G52.2
  lip K13.0
  liver K76.9
  lumbosacral
    plexus G54.1
    root (nerve) NEC G54.4
  lung (coin) R91.1
  maxillary sinus J32.0
  mitral I05.9
  Morel-Lavallée - *see* Hematoma, by site
  motor cortex NEC G93.89
  mouth K13.79
  nerve G58.9
    femoral G57.2-
    median G56.1-

Lesion(s) (nontraumatic) - *continued*
　　carpal tunnel syndrome - *see* Syndrome,
　　　carpal tunnel
　　plantar G57.6-
　　popliteal (lateral) G57.3-
　　　medial G57.4-
　　radial G56.3-
　　sciatic G57.0-
　　spinal - *see* Injury, nerve, spinal
　　ulnar G56.2-
　nervous system, congenital Q07.9
　nonallopathic - *see* Lesion, biomechanical
　nose (internal) J34.89
　obstructive - *see* Obstruction
　obturator nerve G57.8-
　oral mucosa K13.70
　organ or site NEC - *see* Disease, by site
　osteolytic - *see* Osteolysis
　peptic K27.9
　periodontal, due to traumatic occlusion K05.5
　pharynx J39.2
　pigment, pigmented (skin) L81.9
　pinta - *see* Pinta, lesions
　polypoid - *see* Polyp
　prechiasmal (optic) - *see* Disorder, optic,
　　chiasm
　primary - *see also* Syphilis, primary A51.0
　　carate A67.0
　　pinta A67.0
　　yaws A66.0
　pulmonary J98.4
　　valve I37.9
　pylorus K31.9
　rectosigmoid K63.9
　retina, retinal H35.9
　sacroiliac (joint) (old) M53.3
　salivary gland K11.9
　　benign lymphoepithelial K11.8
　saphenous nerve G57.8-
　sciatic nerve G57.0-
　secondary - *see* Syphilis, secondary
　shoulder (region) M75.9-
　　specified NEC M75.8-
　sigmoid K63.9
　sinus (accessory) (nasal) J34.89
　skin L98.9
　　suppurative L08.0
　SLAP S43.43-
　spinal cord G95.9
　　congenital Q06.9
　spleen D73.89
　stomach K31.9
　superior glenoid labrum S43.43-
　syphilitic - *see* Syphilis
　tertiary - *see* Syphilis, tertiary
　thoracic root (nerve) NEC G54.3
　tonsillar fossa J35.9
　tooth, teeth K08.9
　　white spot
　　　chewing surface K02.51
　　　pit and fissure surface K02.51
　　　smooth surface K02.61
　traumatic - *see* specific type of injury by site
　tricuspid (valve) I07.9
　　nonrheumatic I36.9
　trigeminal nerve G50.9
　ulcerated or ulcerative - *see* Ulcer, skin
　uterus N85.9
　vagus nerve G52.2
　valvular - *see* Endocarditis
　vascular I99.9
　　affecting central nervous system I67.9
　　following trauma NEC T14.8
　　umbilical cord, complicating delivery O69.5

Lesion(s) (nontraumatic) - *continued*
　warty - *see* Verruca
　white spot (tooth)
　　chewing surface K02.51
　　pit and fissure surface K02.51
　　smooth surface K02.61
Lethargic - *see* condition
Lethargy R53.83
Letterer-Siwe's disease C96.0
Leukemia, leukemic C95.9-
　acute basophilic C94.8-
　acute bilineal C95.0-
　acute erythroid C94.0-
　acute lymphoblastic C91.0-
　acute megakaryoblastic C94.2-
　acute megakaryocytic C94.2-
　acute mixed lineage C95.0-
　acute monoblastic (monoblastic/monocytic)
　　C93.0-
　acute monocytic (monoblastic/monocytic)
　　C93.0-
　acute myeloblastic (minimal differentiation)
　　(with maturation) C92.0-
　acute myeloid
　　with
　　　11q23-abnormality C92.6-
　　　dysplasia of remaining hematopoesis and/or
　　　　myelodysplastic disease in its history
　　　　C92.A-
　　　multilineage dysplasia C92.A-
　　　variation of MLL-gene C92.6-
　　M6 (a)(b) C94.0-
　　M7 C94.2-
　acute myelomonocytic C92.5-
　acute promyelocytic C92.4-
　adult T-cell (HTLV 1-associated) (acute
　　variant) (chronic variant) (lymphomatoid
　　variant) (smouldering variant) C91.5-
　aggressive NK-cell C94.8-
　AML (1/ETO) (M0) (M1) (M2) (without a
　　FAB classification) C92.0-
　AML M3 C92.4-
　AML M4 (EO with inv(16) or t(16;16)) C92.5-
　AML M5 C93.0-
　AML M5a C93.0-
　AML M5b C93.0-
　AML Me with t (15;17) and variants C92.4-
　atypical chronic myeloid, BCR/ABL negative
　　C92.2-
　biphenotypic acute C95.0-
　blast cell C95.0-
　Burkitt-type, mature B-cell C91.A-
　chronic lymphocytic, of B-cell type C91.1-
　chronic monocytic C93.1-
　chronic myelogenous (Philadelphia
　　chromosome (Ph1) positive) (t(9;22))
　　(q34;q11) (with crisis of blast cells) C92.1-
　chronic myeloid, BCR/ABL-positive C92.1-
　　atypical, BCR/ABL negative C92.2-
　chronic myelomonocytic C93.1-
　chronic neutrophilic D47.1
　CMML (1) (2) (with eosinophilia) C93.1-
　granulocytic - *see also* Category C92 C92.9-
　hairy cell C91.4-
　juvenile myelomonocytic C93.3-
　lymphoid C91.9-
　　specified NEC C91.Z　mast cell C94.3-
　mature B-cell, Burkitt-type C91.A　monocytic
　　(subacute) C93.9-
　　specified NEC C93.Z-
　myelogenous - *see also* Category C92 C92.9-
　myeloid C92.9-
　　specified NEC C92.Z　plasma cell C90.1-
　plasmacytic C90.1-

Leukemia, leukemic - *continued*
　prolymphocytic
　　of B-cell type C91.3-
　　of T-cell type C91.6-
　specified NEC C94.8-
　stem cell, of unclear lineage C95.0-
　subacute lymphocytic C91.9-
　T-cell large granular lymphocytic C91.Z
　unspecified cell type C95.9-
　　acute C95.0-
　　chronic C95.1-
Leukemoid reaction - *see also* Reaction,
　leukemoid D72.823-
Leukoaraiosis (hypertensive) I67.81
Leukoariosis - *see* Leukoaraiosis
Leukocoria - *see* Disorder, globe, degenerative
　condition, leucocoria
Leukocytopenia D72.819
Leukocytosis D72.829
　eosinophilic D72.1
Leukoderma, leukodermia NEC L81.5
　syphilitic A51.39
　　late A52.79
Leukodystrophy E75.29
Leukoedema, oral epithelium K13.29
Leukoencephalitis G04.81
　acute (subacute) hemorrhagic G36.1
　　postimmunization or postvaccinal G04.02
　postinfectious G04.01
　subacute sclerosing A81.1
　van Bogaert's (sclerosing) A81.1
Leukoencephalopathy - *see also*
　Encephalopathy G93.49
　Binswanger's I67.3
　heroin vapor G92
　metachromatic E75.25
　multifocal (progressive) A81.2
　postimmunization and postvaccinal G04.02
　progressive multifocal A81.2
　reversible, posterior G93.6
　van Bogaert's (sclerosing) A81.1
　vascular, progressive I67.3
Leukoerythroblastosis D75.9
Leukokeratosis - *see also* Leukoplakia
　mouth K13.21
　nicotina palati K13.24
　oral mucosa K13.21
　tongue K13.21
　vocal cord J38.3
Leukokraurosis vulva (e) N90.4
Leukoma (cornea) - *see also* Opacity, cornea
　adherent H17.0-
　interfering with central vision - *see* Opacity,
　　cornea, central
Leukomalacia, cerebral, newborn P91.2
　periventricular P91.2
Leukomelanopathy, hereditary D72.0
Leukonychia (punctata) (striata) L60.8
　congenital Q84.4
Leukopathia unguium L60.8
　congenital Q84.4
Leukopenia D72.819
　basophilic D72.818
　chemotherapy (cancer) induced D70.1
　congenital D70.0
　cyclic D70.0
　drug induced NEC D70.2
　　due to cytoreductive cancer chemotherapy
　　　D70.1
　eosinophilic D72.818
　familial D70.0
　infantile genetic D70.0
　malignant D70.9
　periodic D70.0
　transitory neonatal P61.5

Leukopenic - *see* condition
Leukoplakia
  anus K62.89
  bladder (postinfectional) N32.89
  buccal K13.21
  cervix (uteri) N88.0
  esophagus K22.8
  gingiva K13.21
  hairy (oral mucosa) (tongue) K13.3
  kidney (pelvis) N28.89
  larynx J38.7
  lip K13.21
  mouth K13.21
  oral epithelium, including tongue (mucosa)
    K13.21
  palate K13.21
  pelvis (kidney) N28.89
  penis (infectional) N48.0
  rectum K62.89
  syphilitic (late) A52.79
  tongue K13.21
  ureter (postinfectional) N28.89
  urethra (postinfectional) N36.8
  uterus N85.8
  vagina N89.4
  vocal cord J38.3
  vulva N90.4
Leukorrhea N89.8
  due to Trichomonas (vaginalis) A59.00
  trichomonal A59.00
Leukosarcoma C85.9-
Levocardia (isolated) Q24.1
  with situs inversus Q89.3
Levotransposition Q20.5
Lev's disease or syndrome (acquired
  complete heart block) I44.2
Levulosuria - *see* Fructosuria
Levurid L30.2
Lewy body (ies) (dementia) (disease) G31.83
Leyden-Moebius dystrophy G71.0
Leydig cell
  carcinoma
    specified site - *see* Neoplasm, malignant, by
      site
    unspecified site
      female C56.9
      male C62.9-
  tumor
    benign
      specified site - *see* Neoplasm, benign, by
        site
      unspecified site
        female D27.-
        male D29.2-
    malignant
      specified site - *see* Neoplasm, malignant, by
        site
      unspecified site
        female C56.-
        male C62.9-
    specified site - *see* Neoplasm, uncertain
      behavior, by site
    unspecified site
      female D39.1-
      male D40.1-
Leydig-Sertoli cell tumor
  specified site - *see* Neoplasm, benign, by site
  unspecified site
    female D27.-
    male D29.2-
LGSIL (Low grade squamous intraepithelial
  lesion on cytologic smear of)
  anus R85.612
  cervix R87.612
  vagina R87.622

Liar, pathologic F60.2
Libido
  decreased R68.82
Libman-sacks disease M32.11
Lice (infestation) B85.2
  body (Pediculus corporis) B85.1
  crab B85.3
  head (Pediculus capitis) B85.0
  mixed (classifiable to more than one of the
    titles B85.0-b85.3) B85.4
  pubic (Phthirus pubis) B85.3
Lichen L28.0
  albus L90.0
    penis N48.0
    vulva N90.4
  amyloidosis E85.4 [*L99*]
  atrophicus L90.0
    penis N48.0
    vulva N90.4
  congenital Q82.8
  myxedematosus L98.5
  nitidus L44.1
  pilaris Q82.8
    acquired L85.8
  planopilaris L66.1
  planus (chronicus) L43.9
    annularis L43.8
    bullous L43.1
    follicular L66.1
    hypertrophic L43.0
    moniliformis L44.3
    of Wilson L43.9
    specified NEC L43.8
    subacute (active) L43.3
    tropicus L43.3
  ruber
    acuminatus L44.0
    moniliformis L44.3
    planus L43.9
  sclerosus (et atrophicus) L90.0
    penis N48.0
    vulva N90.4
  scrofulosus (primary) (tuberculous) A18.4
  simplex (chronicus) (circumscriptus) L28.0
  striatus L44.2
  urticatus L28.2
Lichenification L28.0
Lichenoides tuberculosis (primary) A18.4
Lichtheim's disease or syndrome - *see*
  Degeneration, combined
Lien migrans D73.89
Ligament - *see* condition
Light
  for gestational age - *see* Light for dates
  headedness R42
Light-for-dates (infant) P05.00
  with weight of
    499 grams or less P05.01
    500-749 grams P05.02
    750-999 grams P05.03
    1000-1249 grams P05.04
    1250-1499 grams P05.05
    1500-1749 grams P05.06
    1750-1999 grams P05.07
    2000-2499 grams P05.08
    2500 grams and over P05.09
  specified NEC P05.09
  and small-for-dates - *see* Small for dates
  affecting management of pregnancy O36.59-
Lightning (effects) (stroke) (struck by) T75.00
  burn - *see* Burn
  foot E53.8
  shock T75.01
  specified effect NEC T75.09

Lightwood-Albright syndrome N25.89
Lightwood's disease or syndrome (renal
  tubular acidosis) N25.89
Lignac (-de Toni) (-Fanconi) (-Debre) disease
  or syndrome E72.09
  with cystinosis E72.04
Ligneous thyroiditis E06.5
Likoff's syndrome I20.8
Limb - *see* condition
Limbic epilepsy personality syndrome F07.0
Limitation, limited
  activities due to disability Z73.6
  cardiac reserve - *see* Disease, heart
  eye muscle duction, traumatic - *see*
    Strabismus, mechanical
  mandibular range of motion M26.52
Lindau (-von Hippel) disease Q85.8
Line(s)
  Beau's L60.4
  Harris' - *see* Arrest, epiphyseal
  Hudson's (cornea) - *see* Pigmentation, cornea,
    anterior
  Stähli's (cornea) - *see* Pigmentation, cornea,
    anterior
Linea corneae senilis - *see* Change, cornea,
  senile
Lingua
  geographica K14.1
  nigra (villosa) K14.3
  plicata K14.5
  tylosis K13.29
Lingual - *see* condition
Linguatulosis B88.8
Linitis (gastric) plasticaC16.9
Lip - *see* condition
Lipedema - *see* Edema
Lipemia - *see also* Hyperlipidemia
  retina, retinalis E78.3
Lipidosis E75.6
  cerebral (infantile) (juvenile) (late) E75.4
  cerebroretinal E75.4
  cerebroside E75.22
  cholesterol (cerebral) E75.5
  glycolipid E75.21
  hepatosplenomegalic E78.3
  sphingomyelin - *see* Niemann-pick disease or
    syndrome
  sulfatide E75.29
Lipoadenoma - *see* Neoplasm, benign, by site
Lipoblastoma - *see* Lipoma
Lipoblastomatosis - *see* Lipoma
Lipochondrodystrophy E76.01
Lipodermatosclerosis - *see* Varix, leg, with,
  inflammation
  ulcerated - *see* Varix, leg, with, ulcer, with
    inflammation by site
Lipochrome histiocytosis (familial) D71
Lipodystrophia progressiva E88.1
Lipodystrophy (progressive) E88.1
  insulin E88.1
  intestinal K90.81
  mesenteric K65.4
Lipofibroma - *see* Lipoma
Lipofuscinosis, neuronal (with ceroidosis)
  E75.4
Lipogranuloma, sclerosing L92.8
Lipogranulomatosis E78.89
Lipoid - *see also* condition
  histiocytosis D76.3
    essential E75.29
  nephrosis N04.9
  proteinosis of Urbach E78.89
Lipoidemia - *see* Hyperlipidemia
Lipoidosis - *see* Lipidosis

Lipoma D17.9
  fetal D17.9
    fat cell D17.9
  infiltrating D17.9
  intramuscular D17.9
  pleomorphic D17.9
  site classification
    arms (skin) (subcutaneous) D17.2-
    connective tissue D17.30
      intra-abdominal D17.5
      intrathoracic D17.4
      peritoneum D17.79
      retroperitoneum D17.79
      specified site NEC D17.39
      spermatic cord D17.6
    face (skin) (subcutaneous) D17.0
    genitourinary organ NEC D17.72
    head (skin) (subcutaneous) D17.0
    intra-abdominal D17.5
    intrathoracic D17.4
    kidney D17.71
    legs (skin) (subcutaneous) D17.2-
    neck (skin) (subcutaneous) D17.0
    peritoneum D17.79
    retroperitoneum D17.79
    skin D17.30
      specified site NEC D17.39
    specified site NEC D17.79
    spermatic cord D17.6
    subcutaneous D17.30
      specified site NEC D17.39
    trunk (skin) (subcutaneous) D17.1
    unspecified D17.9
  spindle cell D17.9
Lipomatosis E88.2
  dolorosa (Dercum) E88.2
  fetal - see Lipoma
  Launois-Bensaude E88.89
Lipomyoma - see Lipoma
Lipomyxoma - see Lipoma
Lipomyxosarcoma - see Neoplasm, connective
  tissue, malignant
Lipoprotein metabolism disorder E78.9
Lipoproteinemia E78.5
  broad-beta E78.2
  floating-beta E78.2
  hyper-pre-beta E78.1
Liposarcoma - see also Neoplasm, connective
  tissue, malignant
  dedifferentiated - see Neoplasm, connective
    tissue, malignant
  differentiated type - see Neoplasm, connective
    tissue, malignant
  embryonal - see Neoplasm, connective tissue,
    malignant
  mixed type - see Neoplasm, connective tissue,
    malignant
  myxoid - see Neoplasm, connective tissue,
    malignant
  pleomorphic - see Neoplasm, connective
    tissue, malignant
  round cell - see Neoplasm, connective tissue,
    malignant
  well differentiated type - see Neoplasm,
    connective tissue, malignant
Liposynovitis prepatellaris E88.89
Lipping, cervix N86
Lipschütz disease or ulcer N76.6
Lipuria R82.0
  schistosomiasis (bilharziasis) B65.0
Lisping F80.0
Lissauer's paralysis A52.17
Lissencephalia, lissencephaly Q04.3

Listeriosis, listerellosis A32.9
  congenital (disseminated) P37.2
  cutaneous A32.0
  neonatal, newborn (disseminated) P37.2
  oculoglandular A32.81
  specified NEC A32.89
Lithemia E79.0
Lithiasis - see Calculus
Lithosis J62.8
Lithuria R82.99
Litigation, anxiety concerning Z65.3
Little leaguer's elbow - see Epicondylitis,
  medial
Little's disease G80.9
Littre's
  gland - see condition
  hernia - see Hernia, abdomen
Littritis - see Urethritis
Livedo (annularis) (racemosa) (reticularis)
  R23.1
Liver - see condition
Living alone (problems with) Z60.2
  with handicapped person Z74.2
Lloyd's syndrome - see Adenomatosis,
  endocrine
Loa Loa, loaiasis, loiasis B74.3
Lobar - see condition
Lobomycosis B48.0
Lobo's disease B48.0
Lobotomy syndrome F07.0
Lobstein (-Ekman) disease or syndrome
  Q78.0
Lobster-claw hand Q71.6-
Lobulation (congenital) - see also Anomaly,
  by site
  kidney, Q63.1
  liver, abnormal Q44.7
  spleen Q89.09
Lobule, lobular - see condition
Local, localized - see condition
Locked-in state G83.5
Locked twins causing obstructed labor O66.1
Locking
  joint - see Derangement, joint, specified type
    NEC
    knee - see Derangement, knee
Lockjaw - see Tetanus
Löffler's
  endocarditis I42.3
  eosinophilia J82
  pneumonia J82
  syndrome (eosinophilic pneumonitis) J82
Loiasis (with conjunctival infestation) (eyelid)
  B74.3
Lone Star fever A77.0
Long
  labor O63.9
    first stage O63.0
    second stage O63.1
  QT syndrome I45.81
Long-term (current) (prophylactic) drug
  therapy (use of)
  agents affecting estrogen receptors and
    estrogen levels NEC Z79.818
  anastrozole (Arimidex) Z79.811
  antibiotics Z79.2
    short-term use omit code
  anticoagulants Z79.01
  anti-inflammatory, non-steroidal (NSAID)
    Z79.1
  antiplatelet Z79.02
  antithrombotics Z79.02
  aromatase inhibitors Z79.811
  aspirin Z79.82

Long-term drug therapy - continued
  birth control pill or patch Z79.3
  bisphosphonates Z79.83
  contraceptive, oral Z79.3
  drug, specified NEC Z79.899
  estrogen receptor downregulators Z79.818
  Evista Z79.810
  exemestane (Aromasin) Z79.811
  Fareston Z79.810
  fulvestrant (Faslodex) Z79.818
  gonadotropin-releasing hormone (GnRH)
    agonist Z79.818
  goserelin acetate (Zoladex) Z79.818
  hormone replacement Z79.890
  insulin Z79.4
  letrozole (Femara) Z79.811
  leuprolide acetate (leuprorelin) (Lupron)
    Z79.818
  megestrol acetate (Megace) Z79.818
  methadone for pain management Z79.891
  Nolvadex Z79.810
  non-steroidal anti-inflammatories (NSAID)
    Z79.1
  opiate analgesic Z79.891
  oral
    antidiabetic Z79.84
    contraceptive Z79.3
    hypoglycemic Z79.84
  raloxifene (Evista) Z79.810
  selective estrogen receptor modulators
    (SERMs) Z79.810
  steroids
    inhaled Z79.51
    systemic Z79.52
  tamoxifen (Nolvadex) Z79.810
  toremifene (Fareston) Z79.810
Longitudinal stripes or grooves, nails L60.8
  congenital Q84.6
Loop
  intestine - see Volvulus
  vascular on papilla (optic) Q14.2
Loose - see also condition
  body
    joint M24.00
      ankle M24.07-
      elbow M24.02-
      hand M24.04-
      hip M24.05-
      knee M23.4-
      shoulder (region) M24.01-
      specified site NEC M24.08
      vertebra M24.08
      toe M24.07-
      wrist M24.03-
    knee M23.4-
    sheath, tendon - see Disorder, tendon,
      specified type NEC
  cartilage - see Loose, body, joint
  skin and subcutaneous tissue (following
    bariatric surgery weight loss) (following
    dietary weight loss) L98.7
  tooth, teeth K08.89
Loosening
  aseptic
    joint prosthesis - see Complications, joint
      prosthesis, mechanical, loosening, by site
    epiphysis - see Osteochondropathy
  mechanical
    joint prosthesis - see Complications, joint
      prosthesis, mechanical, loosening, by site
Looser-milkman (-Debray) syndrome M83.8
Lop ear (deformity) Q17.3
Lorain (-Lévi) short stature syndrome E23.0

Lordosis M40.50
 acquired - *see* Lordosis, specified type NEC
 congenital Q76.429
  lumbar region Q76.426
  lumbosacral region Q76.427
  sacral region Q76.428
  sacrococcygeal region Q76.428
  thoracolumbar region Q76.425
 lumbar region M40.56
 lumbosacral region M40.57
 postsurgical M96.4
 postural - *see* Lordosis, specified type NEC
 rachitic (late effect) (sequelae) E64.3
 sequelae of rickets E64.3
 specified type NEC M40.40
  lumbar region M40.46
  lumbosacral region M40.47
  thoracolumbar region M40.45
 thoracolumbar region M40.55
 tuberculous A18.01

Loss (of)
 appetite (see Anorexia) R63.0
  hysterical F50.89
  nonorganic origin F50.89
  psychogenic F50.89
 blood - *see* Hemorrhage
 bone - *see* Loss, substance of, bone
 control, sphincter, rectum R15.9
  nonorganic origin F98.1
 consciousness, transient R55
  traumatic - *see* Injury, intracranial
 elasticity, skin R23.4
 family (member) in childhood Z62.898
 fluid (acute) E86.9
 function of labyrinth - *see* subcategory H83.2
 hair, nonscarring - *see* Alopecia
 hearing - *see also* Deafness
  central NOS H90.5
  conductive H90.2
   bilateral H90.0
   unilateral
    with
     restricted hearing on the contralateral
      side H90.A1-
     unrestricted hearing on the contralateral
      side H90.1-
  mixed conductive and sensorineural hearing
   loss H90.8
   bilateral H90.6
   unilateral
    with
     restricted hearing on the contralateral
      side H90.A3-
     unrestricted hearing on the contralateral
      side H90.7-
  neural NOS H90.5
  perceptive NOS H90.5
  sensorineural NOS H90.5
   bilateral H90.3
   unilateral
    with
     restricted hearing on the contralateral
      side H90.A2-
     unrestricted hearing on the contralateral
      side H90.4-
  sensory NOS H90.5
 height R29.890
 limb or member, traumatic, current - *see*
  Amputation, traumatic
 love relationship in childhood Z62.898
 memory - *see also* Amnesia
  mild, following organic brain damage F06.8
 mind - *see* Psychosis
 occlusal vertical dimension of fully erupted

Loss (of) - *continued*
 teeth M26.37
  organ or part - *see* Absence, by site, acquired
  ossicles, ear (partial) H74.32-
 parent in childhood Z63.4
 pregnancy, recurrent N96
  care in current pregnancy O26.2-
  without current pregnancy N96
 recurrent pregnancy - *see* Loss, pregnancy,
  recurrent
 self-esteem, in childhood Z62.898
 sense of
  smell - *see* Disturbance, sensation, smell
  taste - *see* Disturbance, sensation, taste
  touch R20.8
 sensory R44.9
  dissociative F44.6
 sexual desire F52.0
 sight (acquired) (complete) (congenital) - *see*
  Blindness
 substance of
  bone - *see* Disorder, bone, density and
   structure, specified NEC
   horizontal alveolar K06.3
  cartilage - *see* Disorder, cartilage, specified
   type NEC
   auricle (ear) - *see* Disorder, pinna, specified
    type NEC
  vitreous (humor) H15.89
 tooth, teeth - *see* Absence, teeth, acquired
 vision, visual H54.7
  both eyes H54.3
  one eye H54.60
   left (normal vision on right) H54.62
   right (normal vision on left) H54.61
  specified as blindness - *see* Blindness
  subjective
   sudden H53.13-
   transient H53.12-
 vitreous - *see* Prolapse, vitreous
 voice - *see* Aphonia
 weight (abnormal) (cause unknown) R63.4
Louis-bar syndrome (ataxia-telangiectasia)
 G11.3
Louping ill (encephalitis) A84.8
Louse, lousiness - *see* Lice
Low
 achiever, school Z55.3
 back syndrome M54.5
 basal metabolic rate R94.8
 birthweight (2499 grams or less) P07.10
  with weight of
   1000-1249 grams P07.14
   1250-1499 grams P07.15
   1500-1749 grams P07.16
   1750-1999 grams P07.17
   2000-2499 grams P07.18
  extreme (999 grams or less) P07.00
   with weight of
    499 grams or less P07.01
    500-749 grams P07.02
    750-999 grams P07.03
  for gestational age - *see* Light for dates
 blood pressure - *see also* Hypotension
  reading (incidental) (isolated) (nonspecific)
   R03.1
 cardiac reserve - *see* Disease, heart
 function - *see also* Hypofunction
  kidney N28.9
 hematocrit D64.9
 hemoglobin D64.9
 income Z59.6
 level of literacy Z55.0
 lying

Loss (of) - *continued*
 kidney N28.89
  organ or site, congenital - *see* Malposition,
   congenital
 output syndrome (cardiac) - *see* Failure, heart
 platelets (blood) - *see* Thrombocytopenia
  reserve, kidney N28.89
 salt syndrome E87.1
 self esteem R45.81
 set ears Q17.4
 vision H54.2X-
  one eye (other eye normal) H54.50
   left (normal vision on right) H54.52A-
   other eye blind - *see* Blindness
   right (normal vision on left) H54.511-
Low-density-lipoprotein-type (LDL)
 hyperlipoproteinemia E78.00
Lowe's syndrome E72.03
Lown-Ganong-Levine syndrome I45.6
LSD reaction (acute) (without dependence)
 F16.90
 with dependence F16.20
L-shaped kidney Q63.8
Ludwig's angina or disease K12.2
Lues (venerea), luetic - *see* Syphilis
Luetscher's syndrome (dehydration) E86.0
Lumbago, lumbalgia M54.5
 with sciatica M54.4-
  due to intervertebral disc disorder M51.17
 due to displacement, intervertebral disc
  M51.27
  with sciatica M51.17
Lumbar - *see* condition
Lumbarization, vertebra, congenital Q76.49
Lumbermen's itch B88.0
Lump   *see also* Mass
 breast N63.0
  axillary tail
   left N63.32
   right N63.31
  left
   lower inner quadrant N63.24
   lower outer quadrant N63.23
   unspecified quadrant N63.20
   upper inner quadrant N63.22
   upper outer quadrant N63.21
  right
   lower inner quadrant N63.14
   lower outer quadrant N63.13
   unspecified quadrant N63.10
   upper inner quadrant N63.12
   upper outer quadrant N63.11
  subareolar
   left N63.42
   right N63.41
Lunacy - *see* Psychosis
Lung - *see* condition
Lupoid (miliary) of Boeck D86.3
Lupus
 anticoagulant D68.62
  with
   hemorrhagic disorder D68.312
   hypercoagulable state D68.62
  finding without diagnosis R76.0
 discoid (local) L93.0
 erythematosus (discoid) (local) L93.0
  disseminated - *see* Lupus, erythematosus,
   systemic
 eyelid H01.129
  left H01.126
   lower H01.125
   upper H01.124
  right H01.123
   lower H01.122

Lupus - *continued*
upper H01.121
profundus L93.2
specified NEC L93.2
subacute cutaneous L93.1
systemic M32.9
with organ or system involvement M32.10
endocarditis M32.11
lung M32.13
pericarditis M32.12
renal (glomerular) M32.14
tubulo-interstitial M32.15
specified organ or system NEC M32.19
drug-induced M32.0
inhibitor (presence of) D68.62
with
hemorrhagic disorder D68.312
hypercoagulable state D68.62
finding without diagnosis R76.0
specified NEC M32.8
exedens A18.4
hydralazine M32.0
correct substance properly administered - *see*
Table of Drugs and Chemicals, by drug,
adverse effect
overdose or wrong substance given or taken -
see Table of Drugs and Chemicals, by drug,
poisoning
nephritis (chronic) M32.14
nontuberculous, not disseminated L93.0
panniculitis L93.2
pernio (Besnier) D86.3
systemic - *see* Lupus, erythematosus, systemic
tuberculous A18.4
eyelid A18.4
vulgaris A18.4
eyelid A18.4
Luteinoma D27.-
Lutembacher's disease or syndrome (atrial
septal defect with mitral stenosis) Q21.1
Luteoma D27.-
Lutz (-Splendore-de Almeida) disease - *see*
Paracoccidioidomycosis
Luxation - *see also* Dislocation
eyeball (nontraumatic) - *see* Luxation, globe
birth injury P15.3
globe, nontraumatic H44.82-
lacrimal gland - *see* Dislocation, lacrimal
gland
lens (old) (partial) (spontaneous)
congenital Q12.1
syphilitic A50.39
Lycanthropy F22
Lyell's syndrome L51.2
due to drug L51.2
correct substance properly administered - *see*
Table of Drugs and Chemicals, by drug,
adverse effect
overdose or wrong substance given or taken -
see Table of Drugs and Chemicals, by drug,
poisoning
Lyme disease A69.20
Lymph
gland or node - *see* condition
scrotum - *see* Infestation, filarial
Lymphadenitis I88.9
with ectopic or molar pregnancy O08.0
acute L04.9
axilla L04.2
face L04.0
head L04.0
hip L04.3
limb
lower L04.3

Lymphadenitis - *continued*
upper L04.2
neck L04.0
shoulder L04.2
specified site NEC L04.8
trunk L04.1
anthracosis (occupational) J60
any site, except mesenteric I88.9
chronic I88.1
subacute I88.1
breast
gestational - *see* Mastitis, obstetric
puerperal, postpartum (nonpurulent) O91.22
chancroidal (congenital) A57
chronic I88.1
mesenteric I88.0
due to
Brugia (malayi) B74.1
timori B74.2
chlamydial lymphogranuloma A55
diphtheria (toxin) A36.89
lymphogranuloma venereum A55
Wuchereria bancrofti B74.0
following ectopic or molar pregnancy O08.0
gonorrheal A54.89
infective - *see* Lymphadenitis, acute
mesenteric (acute) (chronic) (nonspecific)
(subacute) I88.0
due to Salmonella typhi A01.09
tuberculous A18.39
mycobacterial A31.8
purulent - *see* Lymphadenitis, acute
pyogenic - *see* Lymphadenitis, acute
regional, nonbacterial I88.8
septic - *see* Lymphadenitis, acute
subacute, unspecified site I88.1
suppurative - *see* Lymphadenitis, acute
syphilitic (early) (secondary) A51.49
late A52.79
tuberculous - *see* Tuberculosis, lymph gland
venereal (chlamydial) A55
Lymphadenoid goiter E06.3
Lymphadenopathy (generalized) R59.1
angioimmunoblastic, with dysproteinemia
(AILD) C86.5
due to toxoplasmosis (acquired) B58.89
congenital (acute) (subacute) (chronic) P37.1
localized R59.0
syphilitic (early) (secondary) A51.49
Lymphadenosis R59.1
Lymphangiectasis I89.0
conjunctiva H11.89
postinfectional I89.0
scrotum I89.0
Lymphangiectatic elephantiasis, nonfilarial
I89.0
Lymphangioendothelioma D18.1
malignant - *see* Neoplasm, connective tissue,
malignant
Lymphangioleiomyomatosis J84.81
Lymphangioma D18.1
capillary D18.1
cavernous D18.1
cystic D18.1
malignant - *see* Neoplasm, connective tissue,
malignant
Lymphangiomyoma D18.1
Lymphangiomyomatosis J84.81
Lymphangiosarcoma - *see* Neoplasm,
connective tissue, malignant
Lymphangitis I89.1
with
abscess
code by site under Abscess

Lymphangitis - *continued*
cellulitis
code by site under Cellulitis
ectopic or molar pregnancy O08.0
acute L03.91
abdominal wall L03.321
ankle - *see* Lymphangitis, acute, lower limb
arm - *see* Lymphangitis, acute, upper limb
auricle (ear) - *see* Lymphangitis, acute, ear
axilla L03.12-
back (any part) L03.322
buttock L03.327
cervical (meaning neck) L03.222
cheek (external) L03.212
chest wall L03.323
digit
finger - *see* Lymphangitis, acute, finger
toe - *see* Lymphangitis, acute, toe
ear (external) H60.1-
external auditory canal - *see* Lymphangitis,
acute, ear
eyelid - *see* Abscess, eyelid
face NEC L03.212
finger (intrathecal) (periosteal)
(subcutaneous) (subcuticular) L03.02-
foot - *see* Lymphangitis, acute, lower limb
gluteal (region) L03.327
groin L03.324
hand - *see* Lymphangitis, acute, upper limb
head NEC L03.891
face (any part, except ear, eye and nose)
L03.212
heel - *see* Lymphangitis, acute, lower limb
hip - *see* Lymphangitis, acute, lower limb
jaw (region) L03.212
knee - *see* Lymphangitis, acute, lower limb
leg - *see* Lymphangitis, acute, lower limb
lower limb L03.12-
toe - *see* Lymphangitis, acute, toe
navel L03.326
neck (region) L03.222
orbit, orbital - *see* Cellulitis, orbit
pectoral (region) L03.323
perineal, perineum L03.325
scalp (any part) L03.891
shoulder - *see* Lymphangitis, acute, upper
limb
specified site NEC L03.898
thigh - *see* Lymphangitis, acute, lower limb
thumb (intrathecal) (periosteal)
(subcutaneous) (subcuticular) - *see*
Lymphangitis, acute, finger
toe (intrathecal) (periosteal) (subcutaneous)
(subcuticular) L03.04-
trunk L03.329
abdominal wall L03.321
back (any part) L03.322
buttock L03.327
chest wall L03.323
groin L03.324
perineal, perineum L03.325
umbilicus L03.326
umbilicus L03.326
upper limb L03.12-
axilla - *see* Lymphangitis, acute, axilla
finger - *see* Lymphangitis, acute, finger
thumb - *see* Lymphangitis, acute, finger
wrist - *see* Lymphangitis, acute, upper limb
breast
gestational - *see* Mastitis, obstetric
chancroidal A57
chronic (any site) I89.1
due to
Brugia (malayi) B74.1

Lymphangitis - *continued*
  timori B74.2
  Wuchereria bancrofti B74.0
 following ectopic or molar pregnancy O08.89
 penis
  acute N48.29
  gonococcal (acute) (chronic) A54.09
 puerperal, postpartum, childbirth O86.89
 strumous, tuberculous A18.2
 subacute (any site) I89.1
 tuberculous - *see* Tuberculosis, lymph gland
Lymphatic (vessel) - *see* condition
Lymphatism E32.8
Lymphectasia I89.0
Lymphedema (acquired) - *see also*
 Elephantiasis
 congenital Q82.0
 hereditary (chronic) (idiopathic) Q82.0
 postmastectomy I97.2
 praecox I89.0
 secondary I89.0
 surgical NEC I97.89
  postmastectomy (syndrome) I97.2
Lymphoblastic - *see* condition
Lymphoblastoma (diffuse) - *see* Lymphoma,
 lymphoblastic (diffuse)
 giant follicular - *see* Lymphoma,
  lymphoblastic (diffuse)
 macrofollicular - *see* Lymphoma,
  lymphoblastic (diffuse)
Lymphocele I89.8
Lymphocytic
 chorioencephalitis (acute) (serous) A87.2
 choriomeningitis (acute) (serous) A87.2
 meningoencephalitis A87.2
Lymphocytoma, benign cutis L98.8
Lymphocytopenia D72.810
Lymphocytosis (symptomatic) D72.820
 infectious (acute) B33.8
Lymphoepithelioma - *see* Neoplasm,
 malignant, by site
Lymphogranuloma (malignant) - *see also*
 Lymphoma, Hodgkin
 chlamydial A55
 inguinale A55
 venereum (any site) (chlamydial) (with
  stricture of rectum) A55
Lymphogranulomatosis (malignant) - *see also*
 Lymphoma, Hodgkin
 benign (Boeck's sarcoid) (Schaumann's) D86.1
**Lymphohistiocytosis, hemophagocytic
(familial)** D76.1
Lymphoid - *see* condition
Lymphoma (of) (malignant) C85.90
 adult T-cell (HTLV 1-associated) (acute
  variant) (chronic variant) (lymphomatoid
  variant) (smouldering variant) C91.5-
 anaplastic large cell
  ALK negative C84.7-
  ALK-positive C84.6-
  CD30-positive C84.6-
  primary cutaneous C86.6
 angioimmunoblastic T-cell C86.5
 BALT C88.4
 B-cell C85.1-
 B-precursor C83.5-
 blastic NK-cell C86.4
 blastic plasmacytoid dendritic cell neoplasm
  (BPDCN) C86.4
 bronchial-associated lymphoid tissue [BALT-
  lymphoma] C88.4
 Burkitt (atypical) C83.7-
 Burkitt-like C83.7-
 centrocytic C83.1-

Lymphoma - *continued*
 cutaneous follicle center C82.6-
 cutaneous T-cell C84.A-
 diffuse follicle center C82.5-
 diffuse large cell C83.3-
  anaplastic C83.3-
  B-cell C83.3-
  CD30-positive C83.3-
  centroblastic C83.3-
  immunoblastic C83.3-
  plasmablastic C83.3-
  subtype not specified C83.3-
  T-cell rich C83.3-
 enteropathy-type (associated) (intestinal) T-
  cell C86.2
 extranodal NK/T-cell, nasal type C86.0
 extranodal marginal zone B-cell lymphoma of
  mucosa-associated lymphoid tissue [MALT-
  lymphoma] C88.4
 follicular C82.9-
  grade
   I C82.0-
   II C82.1-
   III C82.2-
   IIIa C82.3-
   IIIb C82.4-
  specified NEC C82.8-
 hepatosplenic T-cell (alpha-beta) (gamma-
  delta) C86.1
 histiocytic C85.9-
  true C96.A
 Hodgkin C81.9
  lymphocyte-rich (classical) C81.4-
  lymphocyte depleted (classical) C81.3-
  mixed cellularity (classical) C81.2-
  nodular sclerosis (classical) C81.1-
  specified NEC (classical) C81.7-
  lymphocyte-rich classical C81.4-
  lymphocyte depleted classical C81.3-
  mixed cellularity classical C81.2-
  nodular
   lymphocyte predominant C81.0-
   sclerosis (classical) C81.1-
 intravascular large B-cell C83.8-
 Lennert's C84.4-
 lymphoblastic B-cell C83.5-
 lymphoblastic (diffuse) C83.5-
 lymphoblastic T-cell C83.5-
 lymphoepithelioid C84.4-
 lymphoplasmacytic C83.0-
  with IgM-production C88.0
 MALT C88.4
 mantle cell C83.1-
 mature T-cell NEC C84.4-
 mature T/NK-cell C84.9-
  specified NEC C84.Z-
 mediastinal (thymic) large B-cell C85.2-
 Mediterranean C88.3
 mucosa-associated lymphoid tissue [MALT-
  lymphoma] C88.4
 NK/T cell C84.9-
 nodal marginal zone C83.0-
 non-follicular (diffuse) C83.9-
  specified NEC C83.8-
 non-Hodgkin - *see also* Lymphoma, by type
  C85.9-
  specified NEC C85.8-
 non-leukemic variant of B-cLL C83.0-
 peripheral T-cell, not classified C84.4-
 primary cutaneous
  anaplastic large cell C86.6
  CD30-positive large T-cell C86.6
 primary effusion B-cell C83.8-
 SALT C88.4

Lymphoma - *continued*
 skin-associated lymphoid tissue [SALT-
  lymphoma] C88.4
 small cell B-cell C83.0-
 splenic marginal zone C83.0-
 subcutaneous panniculitis-like T-cell C86.3
 T-precursor C83.5-
 true histiocytic C96.A
Lymphomatosis - *see* Lymphoma
Lymphopathia venereum, veneris A55
Lymphopenia D72.810
Lymphoplasmacytic leukemia - *see* Leukemia,
 chronic lymphocytic, B-cell type
Lymphoproliferation, X-linked disease D82.3
Lymphoreticulosis, benign (of inoculation)
 A28.1
Lymphorrhea I89.8
Lymphosarcoma (diffuse) - *see also*
 Lymphoma C85.9-
Lymphostasis I89.8
Lypemania - *see* Melancholia
**Lysine and hydroxylysine metabolism
disorder** E72.3
Lyssa - *see* Rabies

M

Macacus ear Q17.3
Maceration, wet feet, tropical (syndrome)
 T69.02-
MacLeod's syndrome J43.0
Macrocephalia, macrocephaly Q75.3
Macrocheilia, macrochilia (congenital) Q18.6
Macrocolon - *see also* Megacolon Q43.1
Macrocornea Q15.8
 with glaucoma Q15.0
Macrocytic - *see* condition **Macrocytosis**
 D75.89
**Macrodactylia, macrodactylism (fingers)
(thumbs)** Q74.0
 toes Q74.2
Macrodontia K00.2
Macrogenia M26.05
Macrogenitosomia (adrenal) (male) (praecox)
 E25.9
 congenital E25.0
Macroglobulinemia (idiopathic) (primary)
 C88.0
 monoclonal (essential) D47.2
 Waldenström C88.0
Macroglossia (congenital) Q38.2
 acquired K14.8
**Macrognathia, macrognathism (congenital)
(mandibular) (maxillary)** M26.09
Macrogyria (congenital) Q04.8
Macrohydrocephalus - *see* Hydrocephalus
Macromastia - *see* Hypertrophy, breast
Macrophthalmos Q11.3
 in congenital glaucoma Q15.0
Macropsia H53.15
Macrosigmoid K59.39
 congenital Q43.2
Macrospondylitis , acromegalic E22.0
Macrostomia (congenital) Q18.4
Macrotia (external ear) (congenital) Q17.1
Macula
 cornea, corneal - *see* Opacity, cornea
 degeneration (atrophic) (exudative) (senile) -
  see also Degeneration, macula
  hereditary - *see* Dystrophy, retina
Maculae ceruleae B85.1
Maculopathy, toxic - *see* Degeneration,
 macula, toxic

Madarosis (eyelid) H02.729
  left H02.726
    lower H02.725
    upper H02.724
  right H02.723
    lower H02.722
    upper H02.721
Madelung's
  deformity (radius) Q74.0
  disease
    radial deformity Q74.0
    symmetrical lipomas, neck E88.89
Madness - *see* Psychosis
Madura
  foot B47.9
    actinomycotic B47.1
    mycotic B47.0
Maduromycosis B47.0
Maffucci's syndrome Q78.4
Magnesium metabolism disorder - *see*
  Disorder, metabolism, magnesium
Main en griffe (acquired) - *see also* Deformity,
  limb, clawhand
  congenital Q74.0
Maintenance (encounter for)
  antineoplastic chemotherapy Z51.11
  antineoplastic radiation therapy Z51.0
  methadone F11.20
Majocchi's
  disease L81.7
  granuloma B35.8
Major - *see* condition
Malabar itch (any site) B35.5
Malabsorption K90.9
  calcium K90.89
  carbohydrate K90.49
  disaccharide E73.9
  fat K90.49
  galactose E74.20
  glucose (-galactose) E74.39
  intestinal K90.9
    specified NEC K90.89
  isomaltose E74.31
  lactose E73.9
  methionine E72.19
  monosaccharide E74.39
  postgastrectomy K91.2
  postsurgical K91.2
  protein K90.49
  starch K90.49
  sucrose E74.39
  syndrome K90.9
    postsurgical K91.2
Malacia, bone (adult) M83.9
  juvenile - *see* Rickets
Malacoplakia
  bladder N32.89
  pelvis (kidney) N28.89
  ureter N28.89
  urethra N36.8
Malacosteon, juvenile - *see* Rickets
Maladaptation - *see* Maladjustment
Maladie de Roger Q21.0
Maladjustment
  conjugal Z63.0
    involving divorce or estrangement Z63.5
  educational Z55.4
  family Z63.9
  marital Z63.0
    involving divorce or estrangement Z63.5
  occupational NEC Z56.89
  simple, adult - *see* Disorder, adjustment
  situational - *see* Disorder, adjustment
  social Z60.9

Maladjustment - *continued*
  due to
    acculturation difficulty Z60.3
    discrimination and persecution (perceived)
      Z60.5
    exclusion and isolation Z60.4
    life-cycle (phase of life) transition Z60.0
    rejection Z60.4
    specified reason NEC Z60.8
Malaise R53.81
Malakoplakia - *see* Malacoplakia
Malaria, malarial (fever) B54
  with
    blackwater fever B50.8
      hemoglobinuric (bilious) B50.8
    hemoglobinuria B50.8
  accidentally induced (therapeutically)
  code by type under Malaria algid B50.9
  cerebral B50.0 *[G94]*
  clinically diagnosed (without parasitological
    confirmation) B54
  congenital NEC P37.4
    falciparum P37.3
  congestion, congestive B54
  continued (fever) B50.9
  estivo-autumnal B50.9
  falciparum B50.9
    with complications NEC B50.8
      cerebral B50.0 *[G94]*
    severe B50.8
  hemorrhagic B54
  malariae B52.9
    with
      complications NEC B52.8
      glomerular disorder B52.0
  malignant (tertian) - *see* Malaria, falciparum
  mixed infections
  code to first listed type in B50-b53
  ovale B53.0
  parasitologically confirmed NEC B53.8
  pernicious, acute - *see* Malaria, falciparum
  Plasmodium (P.)
    falciparum NEC - *see* Malaria, falciparum
    malariae NEC B52.9
      with Plasmodium
        falciparum (and or vivax) - *see* Malaria,
          falciparum
        vivax - *see also* Malaria, vivax
          and falciparum - *see* Malaria, falciparum
    ovale B53.0
      with Plasmodium malariae - *see also*
        Malaria, malariae
        and vivax - *see also* Malaria, vivax
          and falciparum - *see* Malaria, falciparum
    simian B53.1
      with Plasmodium malariae - *see also*
        Malaria, malariae
        and vivax - *see also* Malaria, vivax
          and falciparum - *see* Malaria, falciparum
    vivax NEC B51.9
      with Plasmodium falciparum - *see* Malaria,
        falciparum
  quartan - *see* Malaria, malariae
  quotidian - *see* Malaria, falciparum
  recurrent B54
  remittent B54
  specified type NEC (parasitologically
    confirmed) B53.8
  spleen B54
  subtertian (fever) - *see* Malaria, falciparum
  tertian (benign) - *see also* Malaria, vivax
    malignant B50.9
  tropical B50.9
  typhoid B54

Malaria, malarial - *continued*
  vivax B51.9
    with
      complications NEC B51.8
      ruptured spleen B51.0
Malassimilation K90.9
Malassez's disease (cystic) N50.89
Mal de los pintos - *see* Pinta
Mal de mer T75.3
Maldescent, testis Q53.9
  bilateral Q53.20
    abdominal Q53.211
    perineal Q53.22
  unilateral Q53.10
    abdominal Q53.111
    perineal Q53.12
Maldevelopment - *see also* Anomaly   brain
  Q07.9
  colon Q43.9
  hip Q74.2
    congenital dislocation Q65.2
      bilateral Q65.1
      unilateral Q65.0-
  mastoid process Q75.8
  middle ear Q16.4
    except ossicles Q16.4
    ossicles Q16.3
  ossicles Q16.3
  spine Q76.49
  toe Q74.2
Male type pelvis Q74.2
  with disproportion (fetopelvic) O33.3
    causing obstructed labor O65.3
Malformation (congenital) - *see also* Anomaly
  adrenal gland Q89.1
  affecting multiple systems with skeletal
    changes NEC Q87.5
  alimentary tract Q45.9
    specified type NEC Q45.8
    upper Q40.9
      specified type NEC Q40.8
  aorta Q25.40
    absence Q25.41
    aneurysm, congenital Q25.43
    aplasia Q25.41
    atresia Q25.29
      aortic arch Q25.21
    coarctation (preductal) (postductal) Q25.1
    dilatation, congenital Q25.44
    hypoplasia Q25.42
    patent ductus arteriosus Q25.0
    specified type NEC Q25.49
    stenosis Q25.1
      supravalvular Q25.3
  aortic valve Q23.9
    specified NEC Q23.8
  arteriovenous, aneurysmatic (congenital)
    Q27.30
    brain Q28.2
    cerebral Q28.2
    peripheral Q27.30
      digestive system Q27.33
      lower limb Q27.32
      other specified site Q27.39
      renal vessel Q27.34
      upper limb Q27.31
    precerebral vessels (nonruptured) Q28.0
  auricle
    ear (congenital) Q17.3
      acquired H61.119
        left H61.112
          with right H61.113
        right H61.111
          with left H61.113

Malformation - *continued*
- bile duct Q44.5
- bladder Q64.79
  - aplasia Q64.5
  - diverticulum Q64.6
  - exstrophy - *see* Exstrophy, bladder
  - neck obstruction Q64.31
- bone Q79.9
  - face Q75.9
    - specified type NEC Q75.8
  - skull Q75.9
    - specified type NEC Q75.8
- brain (multiple) Q04.9
  - arteriovenous Q28.2
  - specified type NEC Q04.8
- branchial cleft Q18.2
- breast Q83.9
  - specified type NEC Q83.8
- broad ligament Q50.6
- bronchus Q32.4
- bursa Q79.9
- cardiac
  - chambers Q20.9
    - specified type NEC Q20.8
  - septum Q21.9
    - specified type NEC Q21.8
- cerebral Q04.9
  - vessels Q28.3
- cervix uteri Q51.9
  - specified type NEC Q51.828
- Chiari
  - Type I G93.5
  - Type II Q07.01
- choroid (congenital) Q14.3
  - plexus Q07.8
- circulatory system Q28.9
- cochlea Q16.5
- cornea Q13.4
- coronary vessels Q24.5
- corpus callosum (congenital) Q04.0
- diaphragm Q79.1
- digestive system NEC, specified type NEC Q45.8
- dura Q07.9
  - brain Q04.9
  - spinal Q06.9
- ear Q17.9
  - causing impairment of hearing Q16.9
  - external Q17.9
    - accessory auricle Q17.0
    - causing impairment of hearing Q16.9
      - absence of
        - auditory canal Q16.1
        - auricle Q16.0
    - macrotia Q17.1
    - microtia Q17.2
    - misplacement Q17.4
    - misshapen NEC Q17.3
    - prominence Q17.5
    - specified type NEC Q17.8
  - inner Q16.5
  - middle Q16.4
    - absence of eustachian tube Q16.2
    - ossicles (fusion) Q16.3
  - ossicles Q16.3
  - specified type NEC Q17.8
- epididymis Q55.4
- esophagus Q39.9
  - specified type NEC Q39.8
- eye Q15.9
  - lid Q10.3
  - specified NEC Q15.8
- fallopian tube Q50.6
- genital organ - *see* Anomaly, genitalia

Malformation - *continued*
- great
  - artery Q25.9
    - aorta - *see* Malformation, aorta
    - pulmonary artery - *see* Malformation, pulmonary, artery
    - specified type NEC Q25.8
  - vein Q26.9
    - anomalous
      - portal venous connection Q26.5
      - pulmonary venous connection Q26.4
        - partial Q26.3
        - total Q26.2
    - persistent left superior vena cava Q26.1
    - portal vein-hepatic artery fistula Q26.6
    - specified type NEC Q26.8
    - vena cava stenosis, congenital Q26.0
- gum Q38.6
- hair Q84.2
- heart Q24.9
  - specified type NEC Q24.8
- integument Q84.9
  - specified type NEC Q84.8
- internal ear Q16.5
- intestine Q43.9
  - specified type NEC Q43.8
- iris Q13.2
- joint Q74.9
  - ankle Q74.2
  - lumbosacral Q76.49
  - sacroiliac Q74.2
  - specified type NEC Q74.8
- kidney Q63.9
  - accessory Q63.0
  - giant Q63.3
  - horseshoe Q63.1
  - hydronephrosis Q62.0
  - malposition Q63.2
  - specified type NEC Q63.8
- lacrimal apparatus Q10.6
- lip Q38.0
- lingual Q38.3
- liver Q44.7
- lung Q33.9
- meninges or membrane (congenital) Q07.9
  - cerebral Q04.8
  - spinal (cord) Q06.9
- middle ear Q16.4
  - ossicles Q16.3
- mitral valve Q23.9
  - specified NEC Q23.8
- Mondini's (congenital) (malformation, cochlea) Q16.5
- mouth (congenital) Q38.6
- multiple types NEC Q89.7
- musculoskeletal system Q79.9
- myocardium Q24.8
- nail Q84.6
- nervous system (central) Q07.9
- nose Q30.9
  - specified type NEC Q30.8
- optic disc Q14.2
- orbit Q10.7
- ovary Q50.39
- palate Q38.5
- parathyroid gland Q89.2
- pelvic organs or tissues NEC
  - in pregnancy or childbirth O34.8-
    - causing obstructed labor O65.5
- penis Q55.69
  - aplasia Q55.5
  - curvature (lateral) Q55.61
  - hypoplasia Q55.62
- pericardium Q24.8

Malformation - *continued*
- peripheral vascular system Q27.9
  - specified type NEC Q27.8
- pharynx Q38.8
- precerebral vessels Q28.1
- prostate Q55.4
- pulmonary
  - arteriovenous Q25.72
  - artery Q25.9
    - atresia Q25.5
    - specified type NEC Q25.79
    - stenosis Q25.6
  - valve Q22.3
- renal artery Q27.2
- respiratory system Q34.9
- retina Q14.1
- scrotum - *see* Malformation, testis and scrotum
- seminal vesicles Q55.4
- sense organs NEC Q07.9
- skin Q82.9
  - specified NEC Q89.8
- spinal
  - cord Q06.9
  - nerve root Q07.8
- spine Q76.49
  - kyphosis - *see* Kyphosis, congenital
  - lordosis - *see* Lordosis, congenital
- spleen Q89.09
- stomach Q40.3
  - specified type NEC Q40.2
- teeth, tooth K00.9
- tendon Q79.9
- testis and scrotum Q55.20
  - aplasia Q55.0
  - hypoplasia Q55.1
  - polyorchism Q55.21
  - retractile testis Q55.22
  - scrotal transposition Q55.23
  - specified NEC Q55.29
- throat Q38.8
- thorax, bony Q76.9
- thyroid gland Q89.2
- tongue (congenital) Q38.3
  - hypertrophy Q38.2
  - tie Q38.1
- trachea Q32.1
- tricuspid valve Q22.9
  - specified type NEC Q22.8
- umbilical cord NEC (complicating delivery) O69.89
- umbilicus Q89.9
- ureter Q62.8
  - agenesis Q62.4
  - duplication Q62.5
  - malposition - *see* Malposition, congenital, ureter
  - obstructive defect - *see* Defect, obstructive, ureter
  - vesico-uretero-renal reflux Q62.7
- urethra Q64.79
  - aplasia Q64.5
  - duplication Q64.74
  - posterior valves Q64.2
  - prolapse Q64.71
  - stricture Q64.32
- urinary system Q64.9
- uterus Q51.9
  - specified type NEC Q51.818
- vagina Q52.4
- vascular system, peripheral Q27.9
- vas deferens Q55.4
  - atresia Q55.3
- venous - *see* Anomaly, vein(s)
- vulva Q52.70

Malfunction - *see also* Dysfunction
  cardiac electronic device T82.119
    electrode T82.110
    pulse generator T82.111
    specified type NEC T82.118
  catheter device NEC T85.618
    cystostomy T83.010
    dialysis (renal) (vascular) T82.41
      intraperitoneal T85.611
    infusion NEC T82.514
      cranial T85.610
      epidural T85.610
      intrathecal T85.610
      spinal T85.610
      subarachnoid T85.610
      subdural T85.610
    urinary - *see also* Breakdown, device,
      catheter T83.018
  colostomy K94.03
    valve K94.03
  cystostomy (stoma) N99.512
    catheter T83.010
  enteric stoma K94.13
  enterostomy K94.13
  esophagostomy K94.33
  gastroenteric K31.89
  gastrostomy K94.23
  ileostomy K94.13
    valve K94.13
  intrathecal infusion pump T85.615
  jejunostomy K94.13
  nervous system device, implant or graft,
    specified NEC T85.615
  pacemaker - *see* Malfunction, cardiac
    electronic device
  prosthetic device, internal - *see* Complications,
    prosthetic device, by site, mechanical
  tracheostomy J95.03
  urinary device NEC - *see* Complication,
    genitourinary, device, urinary, mechanical
  valve
    colostomy K94.03
    heart T82.09
    ileostomy K94.13
  vascular graft or shunt NEC - *see*
    Complication, cardiovascular device,
    mechanical, vascular
  ventricular (communicating shunt) T85.01
Malherbe's tumor - *see* Neoplasm, skin,
  benign
Malibu disease L98.8
Malignancy - *see also* Neoplasm, malignant, by
  site
  unspecified site (primary) C80.1
Malignant - *see* condition
Malingerer, malingering Z76.5
Mallet finger (acquired) - *see* Deformity,
  finger, mallet finger
  congenital Q74.0
  sequelae of rickets E64.3
Malleus A24.0
Mallory's bodies R89.7
Mallory-Weiss syndrome K22.6
Malnutrition E46
  degree
    first E44.1
    mild (protein) E44.1
    moderate (protein) E44.0
    second E44.0
    severe (protein-energy) E43
      intermediate form E42
        with
          kwashiorkor (and marasmus) E42
          marasmus E41

Malnutrition - *continued*
  third E43
  following gastrointestinal surgery K91.2
  intrauterine
    light-for-dates - *see* Light for dates
    small-for-dates - *see* Small for dates
  lack of care, or neglect (child) (infant) T76.02
    confirmed T74.02
  malignant E40
  protein E46
    calorie E46
      mild E44.1
      moderate E44.0
      severe E43
        intermediate form E42
          with
            kwashiorkor (and marasmus) E42
            marasmus E41
  energy E46
    mild E44.1
    moderate E44.0
    severe E43
      intermediate form E42
        with
          kwashiorkor (and marasmus) E42
          marasmus E41
  severe (protein-energy) E43
    with
      kwashiorkor (and marasmus) E42
      marasmus E41
Malocclusion (teeth) M26.4
  Angle's M26.219
    class I M26.211
    class II M26.212
    class III M26.213
  due to
    abnormal swallowing M26.59
    mouth breathing M26.59
    tongue, lip or finger habits M26.59
  temporomandibular (joint) M26.69
Malposition
  cervix - *see* Malposition, uterus
  congenital
    adrenal (gland) Q89.1
    alimentary tract Q45.8
      lower Q43.8
      upper Q40.8
    aorta Q25.49
    appendix Q43.8
    arterial trunk Q20.0
    artery (peripheral) Q27.8
      coronary Q24.5
      digestive system Q27.8
      lower limb Q27.8
      pulmonary Q25.79
      specified site NEC Q27.8
      upper limb Q27.8
    auditory canal Q17.8
      causing impairment of hearing Q16.9
    auricle (ear) Q17.4
      causing impairment of hearing Q16.9
    cervical Q18.2
    biliary duct or passage Q44.5
    bladder (mucosa) - *see* Exstrophy, bladder
    brachial plexus Q07.8
    brain tissue Q04.8
    breast Q83.8
    bronchus Q32.4
    cecum Q43.8
    clavicle Q74.0
    colon Q43.8
    digestive organ or tract NEC Q45.8
      lower Q43.8
      upper Q40.8

Malposition - *continued*
  ear (auricle) (external) Q17.4
    ossicles Q16.3
  endocrine (gland) NEC Q89.2
  epiglottis Q31.8
  eustachian tube Q17.8
  eye Q15.8
  facial features Q18.8
  fallopian tube Q50.6
  finger(s) Q68.1
    supernumerary Q69.0
  foot Q66.9
  gallbladder Q44.1
  gastrointestinal tract Q45.8
  genitalia, genital organ(s) or tract
    female Q52.8
      external Q52.79
      internal NEC Q52.8
    male Q55.8
  glottis Q31.8
  hand Q68.1
  heart Q24.8
    dextrocardia Q24.0
      with complete transposition of viscera
        Q89.3
  hepatic duct Q44.5
  hip (joint) Q65.89
  intestine (large) (small) Q43.8
    with anomalous adhesions, fixation or
      malrotation Q43.3
  joint NEC Q68.8
  kidney Q63.2
  larynx Q31.8
  limb Q68.8
    lower Q68.8
    upper Q68.8
  liver Q44.7
  lung (lobe) Q33.8
  nail(s) Q84.6
  nerve Q07.8
  nervous system NEC Q07.8
  nose, nasal (septum) Q30.8
  organ or site not listed - *see* Anomaly, by site
  ovary Q50.39
  pancreas Q45.3
  parathyroid (gland) Q89.2
  patella Q74.1
  peripheral vascular system Q27.8
  pituitary (gland) Q89.2
  respiratory organ or system NEC Q34.8
  rib (cage) Q76.6
    supernumerary in cervical region Q76.5
  scapula Q74.0
  shoulder Q74.0
  spinal cord Q06.8
  spleen Q89.09
  sternum NEC Q76.7
  stomach Q40.2
  symphysis pubis Q74.2
  thymus (gland) Q89.2
  thyroid (gland) (tissue) Q89.2
    cartilage Q31.8
  toe(s) Q66.9
    supernumerary Q69.2
  tongue Q38.3
  trachea Q32.1
  ureter Q62.60
    deviation Q62.61
    displacement Q62.62
    ectopia Q62.63
    specified type NEC Q62.69
  uterus Q51.818
  vein(s) (peripheral) Q27.8
    great Q26.8

Malposition - *continued*
  vena cava (inferior) (superior) Q26.8
  device, implant or graft - *see also*
    Complications, by site and type, mechanical
    T85.628
    arterial graft NEC - *see* Complication,
  cardiovascular device, mechanical, vascular
    breast (implant) T85.42
    catheter NEC T85.628
     cystostomy T83.020
     dialysis (renal) T82.42
      intraperitoneal T85.621
     infusion NEC T82.524
      spinal (epidural) (subdural) T85.620
     urinary - *see also* Displacement, device,
    catheter, urinary T83.028
    electronic (electrode) (pulse generator)
    (stimulator)
     bone T84.320
     cardiac T82.129
      electrode T82.120
      pulse generator T82.121
      specified type NEC T82.128
     nervous system - *see* Complication,
    prosthetic device, mechanical, electronic
    nervous system stimulator
     urinary - *see* Complication, genitourinary,
    device, urinary, mechanical
  fixation, internal (orthopedic) NEC - *see*
    Complication, fixation device, mechanical
  gastrointestinal - *see* Complications,
    prosthetic device, mechanical,
    gastrointestinal device
  genital NEC T83.428
    intrauterine contraceptive device (string)
    T83.32
    penile prosthesis (cylinder) (implanted)
    (pump) (reservoir) T83.420
    testicular prosthesis T83.421
  heart NEC - *see* Complication,
    cardiovascular device, mechanical
  joint prosthesis - *see* Complication, joint
    prosthesis, mechanical
  ocular NEC - *see* Complications, prosthetic
    device, mechanical, ocular device
  orthopedic NEC - *see* Complication,
    orthopedic, device, mechanical
  specified NEC T85.628
  urinary NEC - *see also* Complication,
    genitourinary, device, urinary, mechanical
    graft T83.22
  vascular NEC - *see* Complication,
    cardiovascular device, mechanical
  ventricular intracranial shunt T85.02
  fetus - *see* Pregnancy, complicated by
    (management affected by), presentation, fetal
  gallbladder K82.8
  gastrointestinal tract, congenital Q45.8
  heart, congenital NEC Q24.8
  joint prosthesis - *see* Complications, joint
    prosthesis, mechanical, displacement, by site
  stomach K31.89
    congenital Q40.2
  tooth, teeth, fully erupted M26.30
  uterus (acute) (acquired) (adherent)
    (asymptomatic) (postinfectional) (postpartal,
    old) N85.4
    anteflexion or anteversion N85.4
     congenital Q51.818
    flexion N85.4
     lateral - *see* Lateroversion, uterus
    inversion N85.5
    lateral (flexion) (version) - *see* Lateroversion,
    uterus

Malposition - *continued*
  in pregnancy or childbirth - *see* subcategory
    O34.5
  retroflexion or retroversion - *see*
    Retroversion, uterus
Malposture R29.3
Malrotation
  cecum Q43.3
  colon Q43.3
  intestine Q43.3
  kidney Q63.2
Maltreatment
  adult
    abandonment
     confirmed T74.01
     suspected T76.01
    confirmed T74.91
    history of Z91.419
    neglect
     confirmed T74.01
     suspected T76.01
    physical abuse
     confirmed T74.11
     suspected T76.11
    psychological abuse
     confirmed T74.31
     suspected T76.31
     history of Z91.411
    sexual abuse
     confirmed T74.21
     suspected T76.21
    suspected T76.91
  child
    abandonment
     confirmed T74.02
     suspected T76.02
    confirmed T74.92
    history of - *see* History, personal (of), abuse
    neglect
     confirmed T74.02
     history of - *see* History, personal (of), abuse
     suspected T76.02
    physical abuse
     confirmed T74.12
     history of - *see* History, personal (of), abuse
     suspected T76.12
    psychological abuse
     confirmed T74.32
     history of - *see* History, personal (of), abuse
     suspected T76.32
    sexual abuse
     confirmed T74.22
     history of - *see* History, personal (of), abuse
     suspected T76.22
     suspected T76.92
  personal history of Z91.89
Malta fever - *see* Brucellosis
Maltworker's lung J67.4
Malunion, fracture - *see* Fracture, by site
Mammillitis N61.0
  puerperal, postpartum O91.02
Mammitis - *see* Mastitis
Mammogram (examination) Z12.39
  routine Z12.31
Mammoplasia N62
Management (of)
  bone conduction hearing device (implanted)
    Z45.320
  cardiac pacemaker NEC Z45.018
  cerebrospinal fluid drainage device Z45.41
  cochlear device (implanted) Z45.321
  contraceptive Z30.9
    specified NEC Z30.8
  implanted device Z45.9

Management (of) - *continued*
    specified NEC Z45.89
  infusion pump Z45.1
  procreative Z31.9
    male factor infertility in female Z31.81
    specified NEC Z31.89
  prosthesis (external) - *see also* Fitting Z44.9
    implanted Z45.9
     specified NEC Z45.89
  renal dialysis catheter Z49.01
  vascular access device Z45.2
Mangled - *see* specified injury by site
Mania (monopolar) - *see also* Disorder, mood,
  manic episode
  with psychotic symptoms F30.2
  without psychotic symptoms F30.10
    mild F30.11
    moderate F30.12
    severe F30.13
  Bell's F30.8
  chronic (recurrent) F31.89
  hysterical F44.89
  puerperal F30.8
  recurrent F31.89
Manic depression F31.9
Manic-depressive insanity, psychosis, or
  syndrome - *see* Disorder, bipolar
Mannosidosis E77.1
Mansonelliasis, mansonellosis B74.4
Manson's
  disease B65.1
  schistosomiasis B65.1
Manual - *see* condition
Maple-bark-stripper's lung (disease) J67.6
Maple-syrup-urine disease E71.0
Marable's syndrome (celiac artery
  compression) I77.4
Marasmus E41
  due to malnutrition E41
  intestinal E41
  nutritional E41
  senile R54
  tuberculous NEC - *see* Tuberculosis
Marble
  bones Q78.2
  skin R23.8
Marburg virus disease A98.3
March
  fracture - *see* Fracture, traumatic, stress, by
    site
  hemoglobinuria D59.6
Marchesani (-Weill) syndrome Q87.0
Marchiafava (-Bignami) syndrome or disease
  G37.1
Marchiafava-Micheli syndrome D59.5
Marcus Gunn's syndrome Q07.8
Marfan's syndrome - *see* Syndrome, Marfan's
Marie-Bamberger disease - *see*
  Osteoarthropathy, hypertrophic, specified NEC
Marie-Charcot-tooth neuropathic muscular
  atrophy G60.0
Marie's
  cerebellar ataxia (late-onset) G11.2
  disease or syndrome (acromegaly) E22.0
Marie-Strumpell arthritis, disease or
  spondylitis - *see* Spondylitis, ankylosing
Marion's disease (bladder neck obstruction)
  N32.0
Marital conflict Z63.0
Mark
  port wine Q82.5
  raspberry Q82.5
  strawberry Q82.5
  stretch L90.6
  tattoo L81.8

Marker heterochromatin - see Extra, marker chromosomes

Maroteaux-Lamy syndrome (mild) (severe) E76.29

Marrow (bone)
  arrest D61.9
  poor function D75.89

Marseilles fever A77.1

Marsh fever - see Malaria

Marshall's (hidrotic) ectodermal dysplasia Q82.4

Marsh's disease (exophthalmic goiter) E05.00
  with storm E05.01

Masculinization (female) with adrenal hyperplasia E25.9
  congenital E25.0

Masculinovoblastoma D27.-

Masochism (sexual) F65.51

Mason's lung J62.8

Mass
  abdominal R19.00
    epigastric R19.06
    generalized R19.07
    left lower quadrant R19.04
    left upper quadrant R19.02
    periumbilic R19.05
    right lower quadrant R19.03
    right upper quadrant R19.01
    specified site NEC R19.09
  breast (see also Lump, breast) N63.0
  chest R22.2
  cystic - see Cyst
  ear H93.8-
  head R22.0
  intra-abdominal (diffuse) (generalized) - see Mass, abdominal
  kidney N28.89
  liver R16.0
  localized (skin) R22.9
    chest R22.2
    head R22.0
    limb
      lower R22.4-
      upper R22.3-
    neck R22.1
    trunk R22.2
  lung R91.8
  malignant - see Neoplasm, malignant, by site
  neck R22.1
  pelvic (diffuse) (generalized) - see Mass, abdominal
  specified organ NEC - see Disease, by site
  splenic R16.1
  substernal thyroid - see Goiter
  superficial (localized) R22.9
  umbilical (diffuse) (generalized) R19.09

Massive - see condition

Mast cell
  disease, systemic tissue D47.02
  leukemia C94.3-
  neoplasm
    malignant C96.20
      specified type NEC C96.29
    of uncertain behavior NEC D47.09
  sarcoma C96.22
  tumor D47.09

Mastalgia N64.4

Masters-Allen syndrome N83.8

Mastitis (acute) (diffuse) (nonpuerperal) (subacute) N61.0
  with abscess N61.1
  chronic (cystic) - see Mastopathy, cystic
  cystic (Schimmelbusch's type) - see Mastopathy, cystic

Mastitis - continued
  fibrocystic - see Mastopathy, cystic
  infective N61.0
    newborn P39.0
  interstitial, gestational or puerperal - see Mastitis, obstetric
  neonatal (noninfective) P83.4
    infective P39.0
  obstetric (interstitial) (nonpurulent)
    associated with
      lactation O91.23
      pregnancy O91.21-
      puerperium O91.22
    purulent
      associated with
        lactation O91.13
        pregnancy O91.11-
        puerperium O91.12
  periductal - see Ectasia, mammary duct
  phlegmonous - see Mastopathy, cystic
  plasma cell - see Ectasia, mammary duct
  without abscess N61.0

Mastocytoma (extracutaneous) D47.09
  malignant C96.2
  solitary D47.01

Mastocytosis D47.09
  aggressive systemic C96.21
  cutaneous (diffuse) (maculopapular) D47.01
    congenital Q82.2
    of neonatal onset Q82.2
    of newborn onset Q82.2
  indolent systemic D47.02
  isolated bone marrow D47.02

  malignant C96.29
  systemic (indolent) (smoldering)
    with an associated hematological non-mast cell lineage disease (SM-AHNMD) D47.02

Mastodynia N64.4

Mastoid - see condition

Mastoidalgia - see subcategory H92.0

Mastoiditis (coalescent) (hemorrhagic) (suppurative) H70.9-
  acute, subacute H70.00-
    complicated NEC H70.09-
    subperiosteal H70.01-
  chronic (necrotic) (recurrent) H70.1-
  in (due to)
    infectious disease NEC B99 [H75.0-]
    parasitic disease NEC B89 [H75.0-]
    tuberculosis A18.03
  petrositis - see Petrositis
  postauricular fistula - see Fistula, postauricular
  specified NEC H70.89-
  tuberculous A18.03

Mastopathy, mastopathia N64.9
  chronica cystica - see Mastopathy, cystic
  cystic (chronic) (diffuse) N60.1-
    with epithelial proliferation N60.3-
  diffuse cystic - see Mastopathy, cystic
  estrogenic, oestrogenica N64.89
  ovarian origin N64.89

Mastoplasia, mastoplastia N62

Masturbation (excessive) F98.8

Maternal care (for) - see Pregnancy (complicated by) (management affected by)

Matheiu's disease (leptospiral jaundice) A27.0

Mauclaire's disease or osteochondrosis - see Osteochondrosis, juvenile, hand, metacarpal

Maxcy's disease A75.2

Maxilla, maxillary - see condition

May (-Hegglin) anomaly or syndrome D72.0

McArdle (-Schmid)(-Pearson) disease (glycogen storage) E74.04

McCune-Albright syndrome Q78.1

McQuarrie's syndrome (idiopathic familial hypoglycemia) E16.2

Meadow's syndrome Q86.1

Measles (black) (hemorrhagic) (suppressed) B05.9
  with
    complications NEC B05.89
    encephalitis B05.0
    intestinal complications B05.4
    keratitis (keratoconjunctivitis) B05.81
    meningitis B05.1
    otitis media B05.3
    pneumonia B05.2
  French - see Rubella
  German - see Rubella
  Liberty - see Rubella

Meatitis, urethral - see Urethritis

Meatus, meatal - see condition

Meat-wrappers' asthma J68.9

Meckel-Gruber syndrome Q61.9

Meckel's diverticulitis, diverticulum (displaced) (hypertrophic) Q43.0
  malignant - see Table of Neoplasms, small intestine, malignant

Meconium
  ileus, newborn P76.0
    in cystic fibrosis E84.11
    meaning meconium plug (without cystic fibrosis) P76.0
  obstruction, newborn P76.0
    due to fecaliths P76.0
    in mucoviscidosis E84.11
  peritonitis P78.0
  plug syndrome (newborn) NEC P76.0

Median - see also condition
  arcuate ligament syndrome I77.4
  bar (prostate) (vesical orifice) - see Hyperplasia, prostate
  rhomboid glossitis K14.2

Mediastinal shift R93.8

Mediastinitis (acute) (chronic) J98.51
  syphilitic A52.73
  tuberculous A15.8

Mediastinopericarditis - see also Pericarditis
  acute I30.9
  adhesive I31.0
  chronic I31.8
  rheumatic I09.2

Mediastinum, mediastinal - see condition

Medicine poisoning - see Table of Drugs and Chemicals, by drug, poisoning

Mediterranean
  fever - see Brucellosis
    familial M04.1
    tick A77.1
  kala-azar B55.0
  leishmaniasis B55.0
  tick fever A77.1

Medulla - see condition

Medullary cystic kidney Q61.5

Medullated fibers
  optic (nerve) Q14.8
  retina Q14.1

Medulloblastoma
  desmoplastic C71.6
  specified site - see Neoplasm, malignant, by site
  unspecified site C71.6

Medulloepithelioma - see also Neoplasm, malignant, by site
  teratoid - see Neoplasm, malignant, by site

Medullomyoblastoma
  specified site - *see* Neoplasm, malignant, by
    site
  unspecified site C71.6
Meekeren-Ehlers-Danlos syndrome Q79.6
Megacolon (acquired) (functional) (not
  Hirschsprung's disease) (in) K59.39
  Chagas' disease B57.32
  congenital, congenitum (aganglionic) Q43.1
  Hirschsprung's (disease) Q43.1
  toxic NEC K59.31
    due to Clostridium difficile
      not specified as recurrent A04.72
      recurrent A04.71
Megaesophagus (functional) K22.0
  congenital Q39.5
  in (due to) Chagas' disease B57.31
Megalencephaly Q04.5
Megalerythema (epidemic) B08.3
Megaloappendix Q43.8
Megalocephalous, megalocephaly NEC Q75.3
Megalocornea Q15.8
  with glaucoma Q15.0
Megalocytic anemia D53.1
Megalodactylia (fingers) (thumbs)
  (congenital) Q74.0
  toes Q74.2
Megaloduodenum Q43.8
Megaloesophagus (functional) K22.0
  congenital Q39.5
Megalogastria (acquired) K31.89
  congenital Q40.2
Megalophthalmos Q11.3
Megalopsia H53.15
Megalosplenia - *see* Splenomegaly
 Megaloureter N28.82
  congenital Q62.2
Megarectum K62.89
Megasigmoid K59.39
  congenital Q43.2
Megaureter N28.82
  congenital Q62.2
Megavitamin-b6
syndrome E67.2
Megrim - *see* Migraine
Meibomian
  cyst, infected - *see* Hordeolum
  gland - *see* condition
  sty, stye - *see* Hordeolum **Meibomitis** - *see*
    Hordeolum
Meige-Milroy disease (chronic hereditary
  edema) Q82.0
Meige's syndrome Q82.0
Melalgia, nutritional E53.8
Melancholia F32.9
  climacteric (single episode) F32.89
    recurrent episode F33.8
  hypochondriac F45.29
  intermittent (single episode) F32.89
    recurrent episode F33.8
  involutional (single episode) F32.89
    recurrent episode F33.8
  menopausal (single episode) F32.89
    recurrent episode F33.8
  puerperal F32.89
  reactive (emotional stress or trauma) F32.3
  recurrent F33.9
  senile F03
  stuporous (single episode) F32.89
    recurrent episode F33.8
Melanemia R79.89
Melanoameloblastoma - *see* Neoplasm, bone,
  benign
Melanoblastoma - *see* Melanoma

Melanocarcinoma - *see* Melanoma
Melanocytoma, eyeball D31.9-
Melanocytosis, neurocutaneous Q82.8
Melanoderma, melanodermia L81.4
Melanodontia, infantile K03.89
Melanodontoclasia K03.89
Melanoepithelioma - *see* Melanoma
  (malignant) C43.9
Melanoma (malignant) C43.9
  acral lentiginous, malignant - *see* Melanoma,
    skin, by site
  amelanotic - *see* Melanoma, skin, by site
  balloon cell - *see* Melanoma, skin, by site
  benign - *see* Nevus
  desmoplastic, malignant - *see* Melanoma, skin,
    by site
  epithelioid cell - *see* Melanoma, skin, by site
    with spindle cell, mixed - *see* Melanoma,
      skin, by site
  in
    giant pigmented nevus - *see* Melanoma, skin,
      by site
    Hutchinson's melanotic freckle - *see*
      Melanoma, skin, by site
    junctional nevus - *see* Melanoma, skin, by
      site
    precancerous melanosis - *see* Melanoma,
      skin, by site
  in situ D03.9
    abdominal wall D03.59
    ala nasi D03.39
    ankle D03.7-
    anus, anal (margin) (skin) D03.51
    arm D03.6-
    auditory canal D03.2-
    auricle (ear) D03.2-
    auricular canal (external) D03.2-
    axilla, axillary fold D03.59
    back D03.59
    breast D03.52
    brow D03.39
    buttock D03.59
    canthus (eye) D03.1-
    cheek (external) D03.39
    chest wall D03.59
    chin D03.39
    choroid D03.8
    conjunctiva D03.8
    ear (external) D03.2-
    external meatus (ear) D03.2-
    eye D03.8
    eyebrow D03.39
    eyelid (lower) (upper) D03.1-
    face D03.30
      specified NEC D03.39
    female genital organ (external) NEC D03.8
    finger D03.6-
    flank D03.59
    foot D03.7-
    forearm D03.6-
    forehead D03.39
    foreskin D03.8
    gluteal region D03.59
    groin D03.59
    hand D03.6-
    heel D03.7-
    helix D03.2-
    hip D03.7-
    interscapular region D03.59
    iris D03.8
    jaw D03.39
    knee D03.7-
    labium (majus) (minus) D03.8
    lacrimal gland D03.8

Melanoma (malignant) - *continued*
  leg D03.7-
  lip (lower) (upper) D03.0
  lower limb NEC D03.7-
  male genital organ (external) NEC D03.8
  nail D03.9
    finger D03.6-
    toe D03.7-
  neck D03.4
  nose (external) D03.39
  orbit D03.8
  penis D03.8
  perianal skin D03.51
  perineum D03.51
  pinna D03.2-
  popliteal fossa or space D03.7-
  prepuce D03.8
  pudendum D03.8
  retina D03.8
  retrobulbar D03.8
  scalp D03.4
  scrotum D03.8
  shoulder D03.6
  specified site NEC D03.8
  submammary fold D03.52
  temple D03.39
  thigh D03.7-
  toe D03.7-
  trunk NEC D03.59
  umbilicus D03.59
  upper limb NEC D03.6-
  vulva D03.8
  juvenile - *see* Nevus
  malignant, of soft parts except skin - *see*
    Neoplasm, connective tissue, malignant
  metastatic
    breast C79.81
    genital organ C79.82
    specified site NEC C79.89
  neurotropic, malignant - *see* Melanoma, skin,
    by site
  nodular - *see* Melanoma, skin, by site
  regressing, malignant - *see* Melanoma, skin, by
    site
  skin C43.9
    abdominal wall C43.59
    ala nasi C43.31
    ankle C43.7-
    anus, anal (skin) C43.51
    arm C43.6-
    auditory canal (external) C43.2-
    auricle (ear) C43.2-
    auricular canal (external) C43.2-
    axilla, axillary fold C43.59
    back C43.59
    breast (female) (male) C43.52
    brow C43.39
    buttock C43.59
    canthus (eye) C43.1-
    cheek (external) C43.39
    chest wall C43.59
    chin C43.39
    ear (external) C43.2-
    elbow C43.6-
    external meatus (ear) C43.2-
    eyebrow C43.39
    eyelid (lower) (upper) C43.1-
    face C43.30
      specified NEC C43.39
    female genital organ (external) NEC C51.9
    finger C43.6-
    flank C43.59
    foot C43.7-
    forearm C43.6-

Melanoma (malignant) - *continued*
  forehead C43.39
  foreskin C60.0
  glabella C43.39
  gluteal region C43.59
  groin C43.59
  hand C43.6-
  heel C43.7-
  helix C43.2-
  hip C43.7-
  interscapular region C43.59
  jaw (external) C43.39
  knee C43.7-
  labium C51.9
    majus C51.0
    minus C51.1
  leg C43.7-
  lip (lower) (upper) C43.0
  lower limb NEC C43.7-
  male genital organ (external) NEC C63.9
  nail
    finger C43.6-
    toe C43.7-
  nasolabial groove C43.39
  nates C43.59
  neck C43.4
  nose (external) C43.31
  overlapping site C43.8
  palpebra C43.1-
  penis C60.9
  perianal skin C43.51
  perineum C43.51
  pinna C43.2-
  popliteal fossa or space C43.7-
  prepuce C60.0
  pudendum C51.9
  scalp C43.4
  scrotum C63.2
  shoulder C43.6-
  skin NEC C43.9
  submammary fold C43.52
  temple C43.39
  thigh C43.7-
  toe C43.7-
  trunk NEC C43.59
  umbilicus C43.59
  upper limb NEC C43.6-
  vulva C51.9
    overlapping sites C51.8
  spindle cell
    with epithelioid, mixed - *see* Melanoma,
    skin, by site
    type A C69.4-
    type B C69.4-
  superficial spreading - *see* Melanoma, skin, by
  site
Melanosarcoma - *see also* Melanoma
  epithelioid cell - *see* Melanoma
Melanosis L81.4
  addisonian E27.1
    tuberculous A18.7
  adrenal E27.1
  colon K63.89
  conjunctiva - *see* Pigmentation, conjunctiva
    congenital Q13.89
  cornea (presenile) (senile) - *see also*
  Pigmentation, cornea
    congenital Q13.4
  eye NEC H57.8
    congenital Q15.8
  lenticularis progressiva Q82.1
  liver K76.89
  precancerous - *see also* Melanoma, in situ
    malignant melanoma in - *see* Melanoma

Melanosis - *continued*
  Riehl's L81.4
  sclera H15.89
    congenital Q13.89
  suprarenal E27.1
  tar L81.4
  toxic L81.4
Melanuria R82.99
MELAS syndrome E88.41
Melasma L81.1
  adrenal (gland) E27.1
  suprarenal (gland) E27.1
Melena K92.1
  with ulcer
  code by site under Ulcer, with hemorrhage
    K27.4
  due to swallowed maternal blood P78.2
  newborn, neonatal P54.1
    due to swallowed maternal blood P78.2
Meleney's
  gangrene (cutaneous) - *see* Ulcer, skin
  ulcer (chronic undermining) - *see* Ulcer, skin
Melioidosis A24.9
  acute A24.1
  chronic A24.2
  fulminating A24.1
  pneumonia A24.1
  pulmonary (chronic) A24.2
    acute A24.1
    subacute A24.2
  sepsis A24.1
  specified NEC A24.3
  subacute A24.2
Melitensis, febris A23.0
Melkersson (-Rosenthal) syndrome G51.2
Mellitus, diabetes - *see* Diabetes
Melorheostosis (bone) - *see* Disorder, bone,
  density and structure, specified NEC
Meloschisis Q18.4
Melotia Q17.4
Membrana
  capsularis lentis posterior Q13.89
  epipapillaris Q14.2
Membranacea placenta O43.19-
Membranaceous uterus N85.8
Membrane(s), membranous - *see also*
  condition
  cyclitic - *see* Membrane, pupillary
  folds, congenital - *see* Web   Jackson's Q43.3
  over face of newborn P28.9
  premature rupture - *see* Rupture, membranes,
    premature
  pupillary H21.4-
    persistent Q13.89
  retained (with hemorrhage) (complicating
    delivery) O72.2
    without hemorrhage O73.1
  secondary cataract - *see* Cataract, secondary
  unruptured (causing asphyxia) - *see* Asphyxia,
    newborn
  vitreous - *see* Opacity, vitreous, membranes
    and strands
Membranitis - *see* Chorioamnionitis
Memory disturbance, lack or loss - *see also*
  Amnesia
  mild, following organic brain damage F06.8
Menadione deficiency E56.1
Menarche
  delayed E30.0
  precocious E30.1
Mendacity, pathologic F60.2
Mendelson's syndrome (due to anesthesia)
  J95.4
  in labor and delivery O74.0

Mendelson's syndrome - *continued*
  in pregnancy O29.01-
  obstetric O74.0
  postpartum, puerperal O89.01
Ménétrier's disease or syndrome K29.60
  with bleeding K29.61
Ménière's disease, syndrome or vertigo
  H81.0-
Meninges, meningeal - *see* condition
Meningioma - *see also* Neoplasm, meninges,
  benign
  angioblastic - *see* Neoplasm, meninges, benign
  angiomatous - *see* Neoplasm, meninges,
    benign
  endotheliomatous - *see* Neoplasm, meninges,
    benign
  fibroblastic - *see* Neoplasm, meninges, benign
  fibrous - *see* Neoplasm, meninges, benign
  hemangioblastic - *see* Neoplasm, meninges,
    benign
  hemangiopericytic - *see* Neoplasm, meninges,
    benign
  malignant - *see* Neoplasm, meninges,
    malignant
  meningothelial - *see* Neoplasm, meninges,
    benign
  meningotheliomatous - *see* Neoplasm,
    meninges, benign
  mixed - *see* Neoplasm, meninges, benign
  multiple - *see* Neoplasm, meninges, uncertain
    behavior
  papillary - *see* Neoplasm, meninges, uncertain
    behavior
  psammomatous - *see* Neoplasm, meninges,
    benign
  syncytial - *see* Neoplasm, meninges, benign
  transitional - *see* Neoplasm, meninges, benign
Meningiomatosis (diffuse) - *see* Neoplasm,
  meninges, uncertain behavior
Meningism - *see* Meningismus
Meningismus (infectional) (pneumococcal)
  R29.1
  due to serum or vaccine R29.1
  influenzal - *see* Influenza, with, manifestations
  NEC
Meningitis (basal) (basic) (brain) (cerebral)
  (cervical) (congestive) (diffuse)
  (hemorrhagic) (infantile) (membranous)
  (metastatic) (nonspecific) (pontine)
  (progressive) (simple) (spinal) (subacute)
  (sympathetic) (toxic) G03.9
  abacterial G03.0
  actinomycotic A42.81
  adenoviral A87.1
  arboviral A87.8
  aseptic (acute) G03.0
  bacterial G00.9
    Escherichia coli (E. coli) G00.8
    Friedländer (bacillus) G00.8
    gram negative G00.9
    H. influenzae G00.0
    Klebsiella G00.8
    pneumococcal G00.1
    specified organism NEC G00.8
    staphylococcal G00.3
    streptococcal (acute) G00.2
  benign recurrent (Mollaret) G03.2
  candidal B37.5
  caseous (tuberculous) A17.0
  cerebrospinal A39.0
  chronic NEC G03.1
  clear cerebrospinal fluid NEC G03.0
  coxsackievirus A87.0
  cryptococcal B45.1

Meningitis - *continued*
  diplococcal (gram positive) A39.0
  echovirus A87.0
  enteroviral A87.0
  eosinophilic B83.2
  epidemic NEC A39.0
  Escherichia coli (E. coli) G00.8
  fibrinopurulent G00.9
    specified organism NEC G00.8
  Friedländer (bacillus) G00.8
  gonococcal A54.81
  gram negative cocci G00.9
  gram-positive cocci G00.9
  Haemophilus (influenzae) G00.0
  H. influenzae G00.0
  in (due to)
    adenovirus A87.1
    African trypanosomiasis B56.9 [G02]
    anthrax A22.8
    bacterial disease NEC A48.8 [G01]
    Chagas' disease (chronic) B57.41
    chickenpox B01.0
    coccidioidomycosis B38.4
    Diplococcus pneumoniae G00.1
    enterovirus A87.0
    herpes (simplex) virus B00.3
      zoster B02.1
    infectious mononucleosis B27.92
    leptospirosis A27.81
    Listeria monocytogenes A32.11
    Lyme disease A69.21
    measles B05.1
    mumps (virus) B26.1
    neurosyphilis (late) A52.13
    parasitic disease NEC B89 [G02]
    poliovirus A80.9 [G02]
    preventive immunization, inoculation or
  vaccination G03.8
    rubella B06.02
    Salmonella infection A02.21
    specified cause NEC G03.8
    Streptococcal pneumoniae G00.1
    typhoid fever A01.01
    varicella B01.0
    viral disease NEC A87.8
    whooping cough A37.90
    zoster B02.1
  infectious G00.9
  influenzal (H. influenzae) G00.0
  Klebsiella G00.8
  leptospiral (aseptic) A27.81
  lymphocytic (acute) (benign) (serous) A87.2
  meningococcal A39.0
  Mima polymorpha G00.8
  Mollaret (benign recurrent) G03.2
  monilial B37.5
  mycotic NEC B49 [G02]
  Neisseria A39.0
  nonbacterial G03.0
  nonpyogenic NEC G03.0
  ossificans G96.19
  pneumococcal streptococcus pneumoniae
    G00.1
  poliovirus A80.9 [G02]
  postmeasles B05.1
  purulent G00.9
    specified organism NEC G00.8
  pyogenic G00.9
    specified organism NEC G00.8
  Salmonella (arizonae) (Cholerae-suis)
    (enteritidis) (typhimurium) A02.21
  septic G00.9
    specified organism NEC G00.8
  serosa circumscripta NEC G03.0

Meningitis - *continued*
  serous NEC G93.2
  specified organism NEC G00.8
  sporotrichosis B42.81
  staphylococcal G00.3
  sterile G03.0
  Streptococcal (acute) G00.2
    pneumoniae G00.1
  suppurative G00.9
    specified organism NEC G00.8
  syphilitic (late) (tertiary) A52.13
    acute A51.41
    congenital A50.41
    secondary A51.41
  Torula histolytica (cryptococcal) B45.1
  traumatic (complication of injury) T79.8
  tuberculous A17.0
  typhoid A01.01
  viral NEC A87.9
  Yersinia pestis A20.3
Meningocele (spinal) - *see also* Spina bifida
  with hydrocephalus - *see* Spina bifida, by site,
    with hydrocephalus
  acquired (traumatic) G96.19
  cerebral - *see* Encephalocele
Meningocerebritis - *see* Meningoencephalitis
Meningococcemia A39.4
  acute A39.2
  chronic A39.3
Meningococcus, meningococcal - *see also*
  condition A39.9
  adrenalitis, hemorrhagic A39.1
  carrier (suspected) of Z22.31
  meningitis (cerebrospinal) A39.0
Meningoencephalitis - *see also* Encephalitis
  G04.90
  acute NEC - *see also* Encephalitis, viral A86
  bacterial NEC G04.2
  California A83.5
  diphasic A84.1
  eosinophilic B83.2
  epidemic A39.81
  herpesviral, herpetic B00.4
    due to herpesvirus 6 B10.01
    due to herpesvirus 7 B10.09
    specified NEC B10.09
  in (due to)
    blastomycosis NEC B40.81
    diseases classified elsewhere G05.3
    free-living amebae B60.2
    Hemophilus influenzae (H .influenzae) G00.0
    herpes B00.4
      due to herpesvirus 6B10.01
      due to herpesvirus 7 B10.09
      specified NEC B10.09
    H. influenzae G00.0
    Lyme disease A69.22
    mercury - *see* subcategory T56.1
    mumps B26.2
    Naegleria (amebae) (organisms) (fowleri)
      B60.2
    Parastrongylus cantonensis B83.2
    toxoplasmosis (acquired) B58.2
      congenital P37.1
  infectious (acute) (viral) A86
  influenzal (H. influenzae) G00.0
  Listeria monocytogenes A32.12
  lymphocytic (serous) A87.2
  mumps B26.2
  parasitic NEC B89 [G05.3]
  pneumococcal G04.2
  primary amebic B60.2
  specific (syphilitic) A52.14
  specified organism NEC G04.81

Meningoencephalitis - *continued*
  staphylococcal G04.2
  streptococcal G04.2
  syphilitic A52.14
  toxic NEC G92
    due to mercury - *see* subcategory T56.1
  tuberculous A17.82
  virus NEC A86
Meningoencephalocele - *see also*
  Encephalocele
  syphilitic A52.19
    congenital A50.49
Meningoencephalomyelitis - *see also*
  Meningoencephalitis
  acute NEC (viral) A86
    disseminated G04.00
      postimmunization or postvaccination
        G04.02
      postinfectious G04.01
  due to
    actinomycosis A42.82
    Torula B45.1
    Toxoplasma or toxoplasmosis (acquired)
      B58.2
    congenital P37.1
  postimmunization or postvaccination G04.02
Meningoencephalomyelopathy G96.9
Meningoencephalopathy G96.9
Meningomyelitis - *see also*
  Meningoencephalitis
  bacterial NEC G04.2
  blastomycotic NEC B40.81
  cryptococcal B45.1
  in diseases classified elsewhere G05.4
  meningococcal A39.81
  syphilitic A52.14
  tuberculous A17.82
Meningomyelocele - *see also* Spina bifida
  syphilitic A52.19
Meningomyeloneuritis - *see*
  Meningoencephalitis
Meningoradiculitis - *see* Meningitis
Meningovascular - *see* condition
Menkes' disease or syndrome E83.09
  meaning maple-syrup-urine disease E71.0
Menometrorrhagia N92.1
**Menopause, menopausal (asymptomatic)
(state)** Z78.0
  arthritis (any site) NEC - *see* Arthritis,
  specified form NEC
  bleeding N92.4
  depression (single episode) F32.89
    agitated (single episode) F32.2
      recurrent episode F33.9
    psychotic (single episode) F32.89
      recurrent episode F33.9
    recurrent episode F33.8
  melancholia (single episode) F32.89
    recurrent episode F33.8
  paranoid state F22
  premature E28.319
    asymptomatic E28.319
      postirradiation E89.40
      postsurgical E89.40
    symptomatic E28.310
      postirradiation E89.41
      postsurgical E89.41
  psychosis NEC F28
  symptomatic N95.1
  toxic polyarthritis NEC - *see* Arthritis,
  specified form NEC
Menorrhagia (primary) N92.0
  climacteric N92.4
    menopausal N92.4

Menorrhagia (primary) - *continued*
  menopausal N92.4
  postclimacteric N95.0
  postmenopausal N95.0
  preclimacteric or premenopausal N92.4
  pubertal (menses retained) N92.2
Menostaxis N92.0
Menses, retention N94.89
Menstrual - *see* Menstruation
  absent - *see* Amenorrhea
  anovulatory N97.0
  cycle, irregular N92.6
  delayed N91.0
  disorder N93.9
    psychogenic F45.8
  during pregnancy O20.8
  excessive (with regular cycle) N92.0
    with irregular cycle N92.1
    at puberty N92.2
  frequent N92.0
  infrequent - *see* Oligomenorrhea
  irregular N92.6
    specified NEC N92.5
  latent N92.5
  membranous N92.5
  painful - *see also* Dysmenorrhea N94.6
    primary N94.4
    psychogenic F45.8
    secondary N94.5
  passage of clots N92.0
  precocious E30.1
  protracted N92.5
  rare - *see* Oligomenorrhea
  retained N94.89
  retrograde N92.5
  scanty - *see* Oligomenorrhea
  suppression N94.89
  vicarious (nasal) N94.89
Mental - *see also* condition
  deficiency - *see* Disability, intellectual
  deterioration - *see* Psychosis
  disorder - *see* Disorder, mental
  exhaustion F48.8
  insufficiency (congenital) - *see* Disability,
    intellectual
  observation without need for further medical
    care Z03.89
  retardation - *see* Disability, intellectual
  subnormality - *see* Disability, intellectual
  upset - *see* Disorder, mental
Meralgia paresthetica G57.1-
Mercurial - *see* condition
Mercurialism - *see* subcategory T56.1
MERRF syndrome (myoclonic epilepsy
  associated with ragged-red fiber) E88.42
Merkel cell tumor - *see* Carcinoma, Merkel
  cell
Merocele - *see* Hernia, femoral
Meromelia
  lower limb - *see* Defect, reduction, lower limb
    intercalary
      femur - *see* Defect, reduction, lower limb,
      specified type NEC
        tibiofibular (complete) (incomplete) - *see*
        Defect, reduction, lower limb
  upper limb - *see* Defect, reduction, upper limb
    intercalary, humeral, radioulnar - *see*
    Agenesis, arm, with hand present
Merzbacher-Pelizaeus disease E75.29
Mesaortitis - *see* Aortitis
Mesarteritis - *see* Arteritis
Mesencephalitis - *see* Encephalitis
Mesenchymoma - *see also* Neoplasm,
  connective tissue, uncertain behavior

Mesenchymoma - *continued*
  benign - *see* Neoplasm, connective tissue,
    benign
  malignant - *see* Neoplasm, connective tissue,
    malignant
Mesenteritis
  retractile K65.4
  sclerosing K65.4
Mesentery, mesenteric - *see* condition
Mesiodens, mesiodentes K00.1
Mesio-occlusion M26.213
Mesocolon - *see* condition
Mesonephroma (malignant) - *see* Neoplasm,
  malignant, by site
  benign - *see* Neoplasm, benign, by site
Mesophlebitis - *see* Phlebitis
Mesostromal dysgenesia Q13.89
Mesothelioma (malignant) C45.9
  benign
    mesentery D19.1
    mesocolon D19.1
    omentum D19.1
    peritoneum D19.1
    pleura D19.0
    specified site NEC D19.7
    unspecified site D19.9
  biphasic C45.9
    benign
      mesentery D19.1
      mesocolon D19.1
      omentum D19.1
      peritoneum D19.1
      pleura D19.0
      specified site NEC D19.7
      unspecified site D19.9
  cystic D48.4
  epithelioid C45.9
    benign
      mesentery D19.1
      mesocolon D19.1
      omentum D19.1
      peritoneum D19.1
      pleura D19.0
      specified site NEC D19.7
      unspecified site D19.9
  fibrous C45.9
    benign
      mesentery D19.1
      mesocolon D19.1
      omentum D19.1
      peritoneum D19.1
      pleura D19.0
      specified site NEC D19.7
      unspecified site D19.9
  site classification
    liver C45.7
    lung C45.7
    mediastinum C45.7
    mesentery C45.1
    mesocolon C45.1
    omentum C45.1
    pericardium C45.2
    peritoneum C45.1
    pleura C45.0
      parietal C45.0
    retroperitoneum C45.7
    specified site NEC C45.7
    unspecified C45.9
Metabolic syndrome E88.81
Metagonimiasis B66.8
Metagonimus infestation (intestine) B66.8
Metal
  pigmentation L81.8
  polisher's disease J62.8

Metamorphopsia H53.15
Metaplasia
  apocrine (breast) - *see* Dysplasia, mammary,
    specified type NEC
  cervix (squamous) - *see* Dysplasia, cervix
  endometrium (squamous) (uterus) N85.8
  esophagus K22.7-
  kidney (pelvis) (squamous) N28.89
  myelogenous D73.1
  myeloid (agnogenic) (megakaryocytic) D73.1
  spleen D73.1
  squamous cell, bladder N32.89
Metastasis, metastatic
  abscess - *see* Abscess
  calcification E83.59
  cancer
    from specified site - *see* Neoplasm,
      malignant, by site
    to specified site - *see* Neoplasm, secondary,
      by site
  deposits (in) - *see* Neoplasm, secondary, by
    site
  disease - *see also* Neoplasm, secondary, by site
    C79.9
  spread (to) - *see* Neoplasm, secondary, by site
Metastrongyliasis B83.8
Metatarsalgia M77.4-
  anterior G57.6-
  Morton's G57.6-
Metatarsus, metatarsal - *see also* condition
  adductus, congenital Q66.22
  valgus (abductus), congenital Q66.6
  varus (congenital) Q66.22
    primus Q66.21
Methadone use - *see* Use, opioid
Methemoglobinemia D74.9
  acquired (with sulfhemoglobinemia) D74.8
  congenital D74.0
  enzymatic (congenital) D74.0
  Hb M disease D74.0
  hereditary D74.0
  toxic D74.8
Methemoglobinuria - *see* Hemoglobinuria
Methioninemia E72.19
Methylmalonic acidemia E71.120
Metritis (catarrhal) (hemorrhagic) (septic)
  (suppurative) - *see also* Endometritis
  cervical - *see* Cervicitis
Metropathia hemorrhagica N93.8
Metroperitonitis - *see* Peritonitis, pelvic,
  female
Metrorrhagia N92.1
  climacteric N92.4
  menopausal N92.4
  postpartum NEC (atonic) (following delivery
    of placenta) O72.1
    delayed or secondary O72.2
  preclimacteric or premenopausal N92.4
  psychogenic F45.8
Metrorrhexis - *see* Rupture, uterus
Metrosalpingitis N70.91
Metrostaxis N93.8
Metrovaginitis - *see* Endometritis
Meyer-Schwickerath and Weyers syndrome
  Q87.0
Meynert's amentia (nonalcoholic) F04
  alcoholic F10.96
    with dependence F10.26
Mibelli's disease (porokeratosis) Q82.8
Mice, joint - *see* Loose, body, joint
  knee M23.4-
Micrencephalon, micrencephaly Q02
Microalbuminuria R80.9

Microaneurysm, retinal - *see also* Disorder, retina, microaneurysms
  diabetic - *see* E08-e13 with .31
Microangiopathy (peripheral) I73.9
  thrombotic M31.1
Microcalcifications, breast R92.0
Microcephalus, microcephalic, microcephaly Q02
  due to toxoplasmosis (congenital) P37.1
Microcheilia Q18.7
Microcolon (congenital) Q43.8
Microcornea (congenital) Q13.4
Microcytic - *see* condition **Microdeletions NEC** Q93.88
Microdontia K00.2
Microdrepanocytosis D57.40
  with crisis (vasoocclusive pain) D57.419
    with
      acute chest syndrome D57.411
      splenic sequestration D57.412
Microembolism
  atherothrombotic - *see* Atheroembolism
  retinal - *see* Occlusion, artery, retina
Microencephalon Q02
Microfilaria streptocerca infestation - *see* Onchocerciasis
Microgastria (congenital) Q40.2
Microgenia M26.06
Microgenitalia, congenital
  female Q52.8
  male Q55.8
Microglioma - *see* Lymphoma, non-Hodgkin, specified NEC **Microglossia (congenital)** Q38.3
Micrognathia, micrognathism (congenital) (mandibular) (maxillary) M26.09
Microgyria (congenital) Q04.3
Microinfarct of heart - *see* Insufficiency, coronary
Microlentia (congenital) Q12.8
Microlithiasis, alveolar, pulmonary J84.02
Micromastia N64.82
Micromyelia (congenital) Q06.8
Micropenis Q55.62
Microphakia (congenital) Q12.8
Microphthalmos, microphthalmia (congenital) Q11.2
  due to toxoplasmosis P37.1
Micropsia H53.15
Microscopic polyangiitis (polyarteritis) M31.7
Microsporidiosis B60.8
  intestinal A07.8
Microsporon furfur infestation B36.0
Microsporosis - *see also* Dermatophytosis
  nigra B36.1
Microstomia (congenital) Q18.5
Microtia (congenital) (external ear) Q17.2
Microtropia H50.40
Microvillus inclusion disease (MVD) (MVID) Q43.8
Micturition
  disorder NEC - *see also* Difficulty, micturition R39.198
    psychogenic F45.8
  frequency R35.0
    psychogenic F45.8
  hesitancy R39.11
  incomplete emptying R39.14
  nocturnal R35.1
  painful R30.9
    dysuria R30.0
    psychogenic F45.8
    tenesmus R30.1
  poor stream R39.12

Micturition - *continued*
  position dependent R39.192
  split stream R39.13
  straining R39.16
  urgency R39.15
Mid plane - *see* condition
Middle
  ear - *see* condition
  lobe (right) syndrome J98.19
Miescher's elastoma L87.2
Mietens' syndrome Q87.2
Migraine (idiopathic) G43.909
  with refractory migraine G43.919
    with status migrainosus G43.911
    without status migrainosus G43.919
  with aura (acute-onset) (prolonged) (typical) (without headache) G43.109
    with refractory migraine G43.119
      with status migrainosus G43.111
      without status migrainosus G43.119
    intractable G43.119
      with status migrainosus G43.111
      without status migrainosus G43.119
    not intractable G43.109
      with status migrainosus G43.101
      without status migrainosus G43.109
    persistent G43.509
      with cerebral infarction G43.609
        with refractory migraine G43.619
          with status migrainosus G43.611
          without status migrainosus G43.619
        intractable G43.619
          with status migrainosus G43.611
          without status migrainosus G43.619
        not intractable G43.609
          with status migrainosus G43.601
          without status migrainosus G43.609
        without refractory migraine G43.609
          with status migrainosus G43.601
          without status migrainosus G43.609
      without cerebral infarction G43.509
        with refractory migraine G43.519
          with status migrainosus G43.511
          without status migrainosus G43.519
        intractable G43.519
          with status migrainosus G43.511
          without status migrainosus G43.519
        not intractable G43.509
          with status migrainosus G43.501
          without status migrainosus G43.509
        without refractory migraine G43.509
          with status migrainosus G43.501
          without status migrainosus G43.509
    without mention of refractory migraine G43.109
      with status migrainosus G43.101
      without status migrainosus G43.109
  abdominal G43.D0
    with refractory migraine G43.D1
    intractable G43.D1
    not intractable G43.D0
    without refractory migraine G43.D0
  basilar - *see* Migraine, with aura
  classical - *see* Migraine, with aura
  common - *see* Migraine, without aura
  complicated G43.109
  equivalents - *see* Migraine, with aura
  familiar - *see* Migraine, hemiplegic
  hemiplegic G43.409
    with refractory migraine G43.419
      with status migrainosus G43.411
      without status migrainosus G43.419
    intractable G43.419
      with status migrainosus G43.411

Migraine - *continued*
    without status migrainosus G43.419
    not intractable G43.409
      with status migrainosus G43.401
      without status migrainosus G43.409
    without refractory migraine G43.409
      with status migrainosus G43.401
      without status migrainosus G43.409
  intractable G43.919
    with status migrainosus G43.911
    without status migrainosus G43.919
  menstrual G43.829
    with refractory migraine G43.839
      with status migrainosus G43.831
      without status migrainosus G43.839
    intractable G43.839
      with status migrainosus G43.831
      without status migrainosus G43.839
    not intractable 4G43.829
      with status migrainosus G43.821
      without status migrainosus G43.829
    without refractory migraine G43.829
      with status migrainosus G43.821
      without status migrainosus G43.829
  menstrually related - *see* Migraine, menstrual
  not intractable G43.909
    with status migrainosus G43.901
    without status migrainosus G43.919
  ophthalmoplegic G43.B0
    with refractory migraine G43.B1
    intractable G43.B1
    not intractable G43.B0
    without refractory migraine G43.B0
  persistent aura (with, without) cerebral infarction - *see* Migraine, with aura, persistent
  preceded or accompanied by transient focal neurological phenomena - *see* Migraine, with aura
  pre-menstrual - *see* Migraine, menstrual
  pure menstrual - *see* Migraine, menstrual
  retinal - *see* Migraine, with aura
  specified NEC G43.809
    intractable G43.819
      with status migrainosus G43.811
      without status migrainosus G43.819
    not intractable G43.809
      with status migrainosus G43.801
      without status migrainosus G43.809
  sporadic - *see* Migraine, hemiplegic
  transformed - *see* Migraine, without aura, chronic
  triggered seizures - *see* Migraine, with aura
  without aura G43.009
    with refractory migraine G43.019
      with status migrainosus G43.011
      without status migrainosus G43.019
    chronic G43.709
      with refractory migraine G43.719
        with status migrainosus G43.711
        without status migrainosus G43.719
      intractable
        with status migrainosus G43.711
        without status migrainosus G43.719
      not intractable
        with status migrainosus G43.701
        without status migrainosus G43.709
      without refractory migraine G43.709
        with status migrainosus G43.701
        without status migrainosus G43.709
    intractable
      with status migrainosus G43.011
      without status migrainosus G43.019
    not intractable
      with status migrainosus G43.001

Migraine - *continued*
   without status migrainosus G43.009
   without mention of refractory migraine
    G43.009
     with status migrainosus G43.001
     without status migrainosus G43.009
   without refractory migraineG43.909
    with status migrainosus G43.901
    without status migrainosus G43.919
Migrant, social Z59.0
Migration, anxiety concerning Z60.3
Migratory, migrating - *see also* condition
   person Z59.0
   testis Q55.29
Mikity-Wilson disease or syndrome P27.0
Mikulicz' disease or syndrome K11.8
Miliaria L74.3
   alba L74.1
   apocrine L75.2
   crystallina L74.1
   profunda L74.2
   rubra L74.0
   tropicalis L74.2
Miliary - *see* condition **Milium** L72.0
   colloid L57.8
Milk
   crust L21.0
   excessive secretion O92.6
   poisoning - *see* Poisoning, food, noxious
   retention O92.79
   sickness - *see* Poisoning, food, noxious
   spots I31.0
Milk-alkali disease or syndrome E83.52
Milk-leg (deep vessels) (nonpuerperal) - *see*
   Embolism, vein, lower extremity
   complicating pregnancy O22.3-
   puerperal, postpartum, childbirth O87.1
Milkman's disease or syndrome M83.8
Milky urine - *see* Chyluria
Millard-Gubler (-Foville) paralysis or
   syndrome G46.3
Millar's asthma J38.5
Miller Fisher syndrome G61.0
Mills' disease - *see* Hemiplegia
Millstone maker's pneumoconiosis J62.8
Milroy's disease (chronic hereditary edema)
   Q82.0
Minamata disease T56.1
Miners' asthma or lung J60
Minkowski-Chauffard syndrome - *see*
   Spherocytosis
Minor - *see* condition
Minor's disease (hematomyelia) G95.19
Minot's disease (hemorrhagic disease),
   newborn P53
Minot-von Willebrand-Jurgens disease or
   syndrome (angiohemophilia) D68.0
Minus (and plus) hand (intrinsic) - *see*
   Deformity, limb, specified type NEC, forearm
Miosis (pupil) H57.03
Mirizzi's syndrome (hepatic duct stenosis)
   K83.1
Mirror writing F81.0
Misadventure (of) (prophylactic)
   (therapeutic) - *see also* Complications T88.9
   administration of insulin (by accident) - *see*
    subcategory T38.3
   infusion - *see* Complications, infusion
   local applications (of fomentations, plasters,
    etc.) T88.9
    burn or scald - *see* Burn
    specified NEC T88.8
   medical care (early) (late) T88.9
    adverse effect of drugs or chemicals - *see*

Misadventure - *continued*
   Table of Drugs and Chemicals
   medical care (early) (late)
    burn or scald - *see* Burn
    specified NEC T88.8
   specified NEC T88.8
   surgical procedure (early) (late) - *see*
    Complications, surgical procedure
   transfusion - *see* Complications, transfusion
   vaccination or other immunological procedure
    - *see* Complications, vaccination
Miscarriage O03.9
Misdirection, aqueous H40.83-
Misperception, sleep state F51.02
Misplaced, misplacement
   ear Q17.4
   kidney (acquired) N28.89
    congenital Q63.2
   organ or site, congenital NEC - *see*
   Malposition, congenital
Missed
   abortion O02.1
   delivery O36.4
Missing - *see also* Absence
   string of intrauterine contraceptive device
    T83.32
Misuse of drugs F19.99
Mitchell's disease (erythromelalgia) I73.81
Mite(s) (infestation) B88.9
   diarrhea B88.0
   grain (itch) B88.0
   hair follicle (itch) B88.0
   in sputum B88.0
Mitral - *see* condition **Mittelschmerz** N94.0
Mixed - *see* condition
MMN (multifocal motor neuropathy) G61.82
MNGIE (Mitochondrial
   Neurogastrointestinal Encephalopathy)
   syndrome E88.49
Mobile, mobility
   cecum Q43.3
   excessive - *see* Hypermobility   gallbladder,
    congenital Q44.1
   kidney N28.89
   organ or site, congenital NEC - *see*
   Malposition, congenital
Mobitz heart block (atrioventricular) I44.1
Moebius, Möbius
   disease (ophthalmoplegic migraine) - *see*
    Migraine, ophthalmoplegic
   syndrome Q87.0
    congenital oculofacial paralysis (with other
     anomalies) Q87.0
    ophthalmoplegic migraine - *see* Migraine,
    ophthalmoplegic
Moeller's glossitis K14.0
Mohr's syndrome (Types I and II) Q87.0
Mola destruens D39.2
Molar pregnancy O02.0
Molarization of premolars K00.2
Molding, head (during birth) - omit code
Mole (pigmented) - *see also* Nevus
   blood O02.0
   Breus' O02.0
   cancerous - *see* Melanoma
   carneous O02.0
   destructive D39.2
   fleshy O02.0
   hydatid, hydatidiform (benign) (complicating
    pregnancy) (delivered) (undelivered) O01.9
    classical O01.0
    complete O01.0
    incomplete O01.1
    invasive D39.2

Mole (pigmented) - *continued*
   malignant D39.2
   partial O01.1
   intrauterine O02.0
   invasive (hydatidiform) D39.2
   malignant
    meaning
     malignant hydatidiform mole D39.2
     melanoma - *see* Melanoma
   nonhydatidiform O02.0
   nonpigmented - *see* Nevus
   pregnancy NEC O02.0
   skin - *see* Nevus
   tubal O00.10-
    with intrauterine pregnancy O00.11-
   vesicular - *see* Mole, hydatidiform
Molimen, molimina (menstrual) N94.3
Molluscum contagiosum (epitheliale) B08.1
Mönckeberg's arteriosclerosis, disease, or
   sclerosis - *see* Arteriosclerosis, extremities
Mondini's malformation (cochlea) Q16.5
Mondor's disease I80.8
Monge's disease T70.29
Monilethrix (congenital) Q84.1
Moniliasis - *see also* Candidiasis B37.9
   neonatal P37.5
Monitoring (encounter for)
   therapeutic drug level Z51.81
Monkey malaria B53.1
Monkeypox B04
Monoarthritis M13.10
   ankle M13.17-
   elbow M13.12-
   foot joint M13.17-
   hand joint M13.14-
   hip M13.15-
   knee M13.16-
   shoulder M13.11-
   wrist M13.13-
Monoblastic - *see* condition
Monochromat (ism), monochromatopsia
   (acquired) (congenital) H53.51
Monocytic - *see* condition
Monocytopenia D72.818
Monocytosis (symptomatic) D72.821
Monomania - *see* Psychosis
Mononeuritis G58.9
   cranial nerve - *see* Disorder, nerve, cranial
   femoral nerve G57.2-
   lateral
    cutaneous nerve of thigh G57.1-
    popliteal nerve G57.3-
   lower limb G57.9-
    specified nerve NEC G57.8-
   medial popliteal nerve G57.4-
   median nerve G56.1-
   multiplex G58.7
   plantar nerve G57.6-
   posterior tibial nerve G57.5-
   radial nerve G56.3-
   sciatic nerve G57.0-
   specified NEC G58.8
   tibial nerve G57.4-
   ulnar nerve G56.2-
   upper limb G56.9-
    specified nerve NEC G56.8-
   vestibular - *see* subcategory H93.3
Mononeuropathy G58.9
   carpal tunnel syndrome - *see* Syndrome, carpal
    tunnel
   diabetic NEC - *see* E08-e13with .41
   femoral nerve - *see* Lesion, nerve, femoral
   ilioinguinal nerve G57.8-

Mononeuropathy - *continued*
in diseases classified elsewhere *see category* G59
intercostal G58.0
lower limb G57.9-
  causalgia - *see* Causalgia, lower limb
  femoral nerve - *see* Lesion, nerve, femoral
  meralgia paresthetica G57.1-
  plantar nerve - *see* Lesion, nerve, plantar
  popliteal nerve - *see* Lesion, nerve, popliteal
  sciatic nerve - *see* Lesion, nerve, sciatic
  specified NEC G57.8-
  tarsal tunnel syndrome - *see* Syndrome, tarsal tunnel
median nerve - *see* Lesion, nerve, median
multiplex G58.7
obturator nerve G57.8-
popliteal nerve - *see* Lesion, nerve, popliteal
radial nerve - *see* Lesion, nerve, radial
saphenous nerve G57.8-
specified NEC G58.8
tarsal tunnel syndrome - *see* Syndrome, tarsal tunnel
tuberculous A17.83
ulnar nerve - *see* Lesion, nerve, ulnar
upper limb G56.9-
  carpal tunnel syndrome - *see* Syndrome, carpal tunnel
  causalgia - *see* Causalgia
  median nerve - *see* Lesion, nerve, median
  radial nerve - *see* Lesion, nerve, radial
  specified site NEC G56.8-
  ulnar nerve - *see* Lesion, nerve, ulnar
Mononucleosis, infectious B27.90
with
  complication NEC B27.99
  meningitis B27.92
  polyneuropathy B27.91
cytomegaloviral B27.10
with
  complication NEC B27.19
  meningitis B27.12
  polyneuropathy B27.11
Epstein-Barr (virus) B27.00
with
  complication NEC B27.09
  meningitis B27.02
  polyneuropathy B27.01
gammaherpesviral B27.00
with
  complication NEC B27.09
  meningitis B27.02
  polyneuropathy B27.01
specified NEC B27.80
with
  complication NEC B27.89
  meningitis B27.82
  polyneuropathy B27.81
Monoplegia G83.3-
congenital (cerebral) G80.8
  spastic G80.1
embolic (current episode) I63.4-
following
  cerebrovascular disease
    cerebral infarction
      lower limb I69.34-
      upper limb I69.33-
    intracerebral hemorrhage
      lower limb I69.14-
      upper limb I69.13-
    lower limb I69.94-
    nontraumatic intracranial hemorrhage NEC
      lower limb I69.24-
      upper limb I69.23-

Monoplegia - *continued*
specified disease NEC
  lower limb I69.84-
  upper limb I69.83-
stroke NOS
  lower limb I69.34-
  upper limb I69.33-
subarachnoid hemorrhage
  lower limb I69.04-
  upper limb I69.03-
  upper limb I69.93-
hysterical (transient) F44.4
lower limb G83.1-
psychogenic (conversion reaction) F44.4
thrombotic (current episode) I63.3-
transient R29.818
upper limb G83.2-
Monorchism, monorchidism Q55.0
Monosomy - *see also* Deletion, chromosome Q93.9
specified NEC Q93.89
whole chromosome
  meiotic nondisjunction Q93.0
  mitotic nondisjunction Q93.1
  mosaicism Q93.1
X Q96.9
Monster, monstrosity (single) Q89.7
acephalic Q00.0
twin Q89.4
Monteggia's fracture (-dislocation) S52.27-
Mooren's ulcer (cornea) - *see* Ulcer, cornea, Mooren's
Moore's syndrome - *see* Epilepsy, specified NEC
Mooser Neill reaction A75.2
Mooser's bodies A75.2
Morbidity not stated or unknown R69
Morbilli - *see* Measles
Morbus - *see also* Disease
angelicus, anglorum E55.0
Beigel B36.2
caducus - *see* Epilepsy
celiacus K90.0
comitialis - *see* Epilepsy
cordis - *see also* Disease, heart I51.9
  valvulorum - *see* Endocarditis
coxae senilis M16.9
  tuberculous A18.02
hemorrhagicus neonatorum P53
maculosus neonatorum P54.5

Morel (-Stewart)(-Morgagni) syndrome M85.2
Morel-Kraepelin disease - *see* Schizophrenia
Morel-Moore syndrome M85.2
Morgagni's
cyst, organ, hydatid, or appendage
  female Q50.5
  male (epididymal) Q55.4
    testicular Q55.29
syndrome M85.2
Morgagni-stokes-Adams syndrome I45.9
Morgagni-Stewart-morel syndrome M85.2
Morgagni-turner (-Albright) syndrome Q96.9
Moria F07.0
Moron (I.Q.50-69) F70
Morphea L94.0
Morphinism (without remission) F11.20
with remission F11.21
Morphinomania (without remission) F11.20
with remission F11.21
Morquio (-Ullrich)(-Brailsford) disease or syndrome - *see* Mucopolysaccharidosis
Mortification (dry) (moist) - *see* Gangrene

Morton's metatarsalgia (neuralgia)(neuroma) (syndrome) G57.6-
Morvan's disease or syndrome G60.8
Mosaicism, mosaic (autosomal) (chromosomal)
45,X/other cell lines NEC with abnormal sex chromosome Q96.4
45,X/46,XX Q96.3
sex chromosome
  female Q97.8
  lines with various numbers of X chromosomes Q97.2
  male Q98.7
XY Q96.3
Moschowitz' disease M31.1
Mother yaw A66.0
Motion sickness (from travel, any vehicle) (from roundabouts or swings) T75.3
Mottled, mottling, teeth (enamel) (endemic) (nonendemic) K00.3
Mounier-Kuhn syndrome Q32.4
with bronchiectasis J47.9
  exacerbation (acute) J47.1
  lower respiratory infection J47.0
acquired J98.09
  with bronchiectasis J47.9
  with
    exacerbation (acute) J47.1
    lower respiratory infection J47.0
Mountain
sickness T70.29
  with polycythemia , acquired (acute) D75.1
tick fever A93.2
Mouse, joint - *see* Loose, body, joint
knee M23.4-
Mouth - *see* condition **Movable**
coccyx - *see* subcategory M53.2
kidney N28.89
  congenital Q63.8
spleen D73.89
Movements, dystonic R25.8
Moyamoya disease I67.5
MRSA (Methicillin resistant Staphylococcus aureus)
infection A49.02
  as the cause of diseases classified elsewhere B95.62
sepsis A41.02
MSSA (Methicillin susceptible Staphylococcus aureus)
infection A49.01
  as the cause of diseases classified elsewhere B95.61
sepsis A41.01
Mucha-Habermann disease L41.0
Mucinosis (cutaneous) (focal) (papular) (reticular erythematosus) (skin) L98.5
oral K13.79
Mucocele
appendix K38.8
buccal cavity K13.79
gallbladder K82.1
lacrimal sac, chronic H04.43-
nasal sinus J34.1
nose J34.1
salivary gland (any) K11.6
sinus (accessory) (nasal) J34.1
turbinate (bone) (middle) (nasal) J34.1
uterus N85.8
Mucolipidosis
I E77.1
II, III E77.0
IV E75.11

Mucopolysaccharidosis E76.3
  beta-gluduronidase deficiency E76.29
  cardiopathy E76.3 [152]
  Hunter's syndrome E76.1
  Hurler's syndrome E76.01
  Hurler-Scheie syndrome E76.02
  Maroteaux-Lamy syndrome E76.29
  Morquio syndrome E76.219
    A E76.210
    B E76.211
    classic E76.210
  Sanfilippo syndrome E76.22
  Scheie's syndrome E76.03
  specified NEC E76.29
  type
    I
      Hurler's syndrome E76.01
      Hurler-Scheie syndrome E76.02
      Scheie's syndrome E76.03
    II E76.1
    III E76.22
    IV E76.219
    IVA E76.210
    IVB E76.211
    VI E76.29
    VII E76.29
Mucormycosis B46.5
  cutaneous B46.3
  disseminated B46.4
  gastrointestinal B46.2
  generalized B46.4
  pulmonary B46.0
  rhinocerebral B46.1
  skin B46.3
  subcutaneous B46.3
Mucositis (ulcerative) K12.30
  due to drugs NEC K12.32
  gastrointestinal K92.81
  mouth (oral) (oropharyngeal) K12.30
    due to antineoplastic therapy K12.31
    due to drugs NEC K12.32
    due to radiation K12.33
    specified NEC K12.39
    viral K12.39
  nasal J34.81
  oral cavity - *see* Mucositis, mouth
  oral soft tissues - *see* Mucositis, mouth
  vagina and vulva N76.81
Mucositis necroticans agranulocytica - *see*
  Agranulocytosis
Mucous - *see also* condition
  patches (syphilitic) A51.39
    congenital A50.07
Mucoviscidosis E84.9
  with meconium obstruction E84.11
Mucus
  asphyxia or suffocation - *see* Asphyxia, mucus
  in stool R19.5
  plug - *see* Asphyxia, mucus
Muguet B37.0
Mulberry molars (congenital syphilis) A50.52
Müllerian mixed tumor
  specified site - *see* Neoplasm, malignant, by
    site
  unspecified site C54.9
Multicystic kidney (development) Q61.4
Multiparity (grand) Z64.1
  affecting management of pregnancy, labor and
    delivery (supervision only) O09.4-
  requiring contraceptive management - *see*
    Contraception
Multipartita placenta O43.19-
Multiple, multiplex - *see also* condition
  digits (congenital) Q69.9

Multiple, multiplex - *continued*
  endocrine neoplasia - *see* Neoplasia,
    endocrine, multiple (MEN)
  personality F44.81
Mumps B26.9
  arthritis B26.85
  complication NEC B26.89
  encephalitis B26.2
  hepatitis B26.81
  meningitis (aseptic) B26.1
  meningoencephalitis B26.2
  myocarditis B26.82
  oophoritis B26.89
  orchitis B26.0
  pancreatitis B26.3
  polyneuropathy B26.84
Mumu - *see also* Infestation, filarial B74.9
  [N51]
Münchhausen's syndrome - *see* Disorder,
  factitious
Münchmeyer's syndrome - *see* Myositis,
  ossificans, progressiva
Mural - *see* condition
Murmur (cardiac) (heart) (organic) R01.1
  abdominal R19.15
  aortic (valve) - *see* Endocarditis, aortic
  benign R01.0
  diastolic - *see* Endocarditis
  Flint I35.1
  functional R01.0
  Graham Steell I37.1
  innocent R01.0
  mitral (valve) - *see* Insufficiency, mitral
  nonorganic R01.0
  presystolic, mitral - *see* Insufficiency, mitral
  pulmonic (valve) I37.8
  systolic R01.1
  tricuspid (valve) I07.9
  valvular - *see* Endocarditis
Murri's disease (intermittent
  hemoglobinuria) D59.6
Muscle, muscular - *see also* condition
  carnitine (palmitoyltransferase) deficiency
    E71.314
Musculoneuralgia - *see* Neuralgia
Mushroom-workers' (pickers') disease or
  lung J67.5
Mushrooming hip - *see* Derangement, joint,
  specified NEC, hip
Mutation(s)
  factor V Leiden D68.51
  surfactant, of lung J84.83
  prothrombin gene D68.52
Mutism - *see also* Aphasia
  deaf (acquired) (congenital) NEC H91.3
  elective (adjustment reaction) (childhood)
    F94.0
  hysterical F44.4
  selective (childhood) F94.0
MVD (microvillus inclusion disease) Q43.8
MVID (microvillus inclusion disease) Q43.8
Myalgia M79.1
  epidemic (cervical) B33.0
  traumatic NEC T14.8
Myasthenia G70.9
  congenital G70.2
  cordis - *see* Failure, heart
  developmental G70.2
  gravis G70.00
    with exacerbation (acute) G70.01
    in crisis G70.01
  neonatal, transient P94.0
  pseudoparalytica G70.00
    with exacerbation (acute) G70.01

Myasthenia - *continued*
  in crisis G70.01
  stomach, psychogenic F45.8
  syndrome
    in
      diabetes mellitus - *see* E08-e13 with .44
      neoplastic disease - *see also* Neoplasm
        D49.9 [G73.3]
      pernicious anemia D51.0 [G73.3]
      thyrotoxicosis E05.90 [G73.3]
        with thyroid storm E05.91 [G73.3]
Myasthenic M62.81
Mycelium infection B49
Mycetismus - *see* Poisoning, food, noxious,
  mushroom
Mycetoma B47.9
  actinomycotic B47.1
  bone (mycotic) B47.9 [M90.80]
  eumycotic B47.0
  foot B47.9
    actinomycotic B47.1
    mycotic B47.0
  madurae NEC B47.9
    mycotic B47.0
  maduromycotic B47.0
  mycotic B47.0
  nocardial B47.1
Mycobacteriosis - *see* Mycobacterium
Mycobacterium, mycobacterial (infection)
  A31.9
  anonymous A31.9
  atypical A31.9
    cutaneous A31.1
    pulmonary A31.0
      tuberculous - *see* Tuberculosis, pulmonary
    specified site NEC A31.8
  avium (intracellulare complex) A31.0
  balnei A31.1
  Battey A31.0
  chelonei A31.8
  cutaneous A31.1
  extrapulmonary systemic A31.8
  fortuitum A31.8
  intracellulare (Battey bacillus) A31.0
  kansasii (yellow bacillus) A31.0
  kakaferifu A31.8
  kasongo A31.8
  leprae - *see also* Leprosy A30.9
  luciflavum A31.1
  marinum (M. balnei) A31.1
  nonspecific - *see* Mycobacterium, atypical
  pulmonary (atypical) A31.0
    tuberculous - *see* Tuberculosis, pulmonary
  scrofulaceum A31.8
  simiae A31.8
  systemic, extrapulmonary A31.8
  szulgai A31.8
  terrae A31.8
  triviale A31.8
  tuberculosis (human, bovine) *see* Tuberculosis
  ulcerans A31.1
  xenopi A31.8
Mycoplasma (M.) pneumoniae, as cause of
  disease classified elsewhere B96.0
Mycosis, mycotic B49
  cutaneous NEC B36.9
  ear B36.9
  in
    aspergillosis B44.89
    candidiasis B37.84
    moniliasis B37.84
  fungoides (extranodal) (solid organ) C84.0-
  mouth B37.0
  nails B35.1

Mycosis, mycotic - *continued*
  opportunistic B48.8
  skin NEC B36.9
  specified NEC B48.8
  stomatitis B37.0
  vagina, vaginitis (candidal) B37.3
Mydriasis (pupil) H57.04
Myelatelia Q06.1
Myelinolysis, pontine, central G37.2
Myelitis (acute) (ascending) (childhood)
  (chronic) (descending) (diffuse)
  (disseminated) (idiopathic) (pressure)
  (progressive) (spinal cord) (subacute) - *see*
    also Encephalitis G04.91
  herpes simplex B00.82
  herpes zoster B02.24
  in diseases classified elsewhere G05.4
  necrotizing, subacute G37.4
  optic neuritis in G36.0
  post chickenpox B01.12
  postherpetic B02.24
  postimmunization G04.02
  postinfectious NEC G04.89
  postvaccinal G04.02
  specified NEC G04.89
  syphilitic (transverse) A52.14
  toxic G92
  transverse (in demyelinating diseases of
    central nervous system) G37.3
  tuberculous A17.82
  varicella B01.12
Myeloblastic - *see* condition
Myeloblastoma
  granular cell - *see also* Neoplasm, connective
    tissue
    malignant - *see* Neoplasm, connective tissue,
      malignant
    tongue D10.1
Myelocele - *see* Spina bifida
Myelocystocele - *see* Spina bifida
Myelocytic - *see* condition
Myelodysplasia D46.9
  specified NEC D46.Z
  spinal cord (congenital) Q06.1
Myelodysplastic syndrome D46.9
  with
    5q deletion D46.C
    isolated del (5q) chromosomal abnormality
      D46.C specified NEC D46.Z
Myeloencephalitis - *see* Encephalitis
Myelofibrosis D75.81
  with myeloid metaplasia D47.4
  acute C94.4-
  idiopathic (chronic) D47.4
  primary D47.1
  secondary D75.81
    in myeloproliferative disease D47.4
Myelogenous - *see* condition
Myeloid - *see* condition
Myelokathexis D70.9
Myeloleukodystrophy E75.29
Myelolipoma - *see* Lipoma
Myeloma (multiple) C90.0-
  monostotic C90.3
    plasma cell C90.0-
  plasma cell C90.0-
  solitary - *see also* Plasmacytoma, solitary
    C90.3-
Myelomalacia G95.89
Myelomatosis C90.0-
Myelomeningitis - *see* Meningoencephalitis
Myelomeningocele (spinal cord) - *see* Spina
  bifida

Myelo-osteo-musculodysplasia hereditaria
  Q79.8
Myelopathic
  anemia D64.89
  muscle atrophy - *see* Atrophy, muscle, spinal
  pain syndrome G89.0
Myelopathy (spinal cord) G95.9
  drug-induced G95.89
  in (due to)
    degeneration or displacement, intervertebral
      disc NEC - *see* Disorder, disc, with,
      myelopathy
    infection - *see* Encephalitis
    intervertebral disc disorder - *see also*
      Disorder, disc, with, myelopathy
    mercury - *see* subcategory T56.1
    neoplastic disease - *see also* Neoplasm D49.9
      [G99.2]
    pernicious anemia D51.0 [G99.2]
    spondylosis - *see* Spondylosis, with
      myelopathy NEC
  necrotic (subacute) (vascular) G95.19
  radiation-induced G95.89
  spondylogenic NEC - *see* Spondylosis, with
    myelopathy NEC
  toxic G95.89
  transverse, acute G37.3
  vascular G95.19
  vitamin B12 E53.8 [G32.0]
Myelophthisis D61.82
Myeloradiculitis G04.91
Myeloradiculodysplasia (spinal) Q06.1
Myelosarcoma C92.3-
Myelosclerosis D75.89
  with myeloid metaplasia D47.4
  disseminated, of nervous system G35
  megakaryocytic D47.4
    with myeloid metaplasia D47.4
Myelosis
  acute C92.0-
  aleukemic C92.9-
  chronic D47.1
  erythremic (acute) C94.0-
  megakaryocytic C94.2-
  nonleukemic D72.828
  subacute C92.9-
Myiasis (cavernous) B87.9
  aural B87.4
  creeping B87.0
  cutaneous B87.0
  dermal B87.0
  ear (external) (middle) B87.4
  eye B87.2
  genitourinary B87.81
  intestinal B87.82
  laryngeal B87.3
  nasopharyngeal B87.3
  ocular B87.2
  orbit B87.2
  skin B87.0
  specified site NEC B87.89
  traumatic B87.1
  wound B87.1
Myoadenoma, prostate - *see* Hyperplasia,
  prostate
Myoblastoma
  granular cell - *see also* Neoplasm, connective
    tissue, benign
    malignant - *see* Neoplasm, connective tissue,
      malignant
    tongue D10.1
Myocardial - *see* condition

Myocardiopathy (congestive) (constrictive)
  (familial) (hypertrophic nonobstructive)
  (idiopathic) (infiltrative) (obstructive)
  (primary) (restrictive) (sporadic) - *see also*
    Cardiomyopathy I42.9
  alcoholic I42.6
  cobalt-beer I42.6
  glycogen storage E74.02 [I43]
  hypertrophic obstructive I42.1
  in (due to)
    beriberi E51.12
    cardiac glycogenosis E74.02 [I43]
    Friedreich's ataxia G11.1 [I43]
    myotonia atrophica G71.11 [I43]
    progressive muscular dystrophy G71.0 [I43]
  obscure (African) I42.8
  secondary I42.9
  thyrotoxic E05.90 [I43]
    with storm E05.91 [I43]
  toxic NEC I42.7
Myocarditis (with
  arteriosclerosis)(chronic)(fibroid)
  (interstitial) (old) (progressive) (senile) I51.4
  with
    rheumatic fever (conditions in I00) I09.0
      active - *see* Myocarditis, acute, rheumatic
    inactive or quiescent (with chorea) I09.0
  active I40.9
    rheumatic I01.2
      with chorea (acute) (rheumatic)
        (Sydenham's) I02.0
  acute or subacute (interstitial) I40.9
    due to
      streptococcus (beta-hemolytic) I01.2
    idiopathic I40.1
    rheumatic I01.2
      with chorea (acute) (rheumatic)
        (Sydenham's) I02.0
    specified NEC I40.8
  aseptic of newborn B33.22
  bacterial (acute) I40.0
  Coxsackie (virus) B33.22
  diphtheritic A36.81
  eosinophilic I40.1
  epidemic of newborn (Coxsackie) B33.22
  Fiedler's (acute) (isolated) I40.1
  giant cell (acute) (subacute) I40.1
  gonococcal A54.83
  granulomatous (idiopathic) (isolated)
    (nonspecific) I40.1
  hypertensive - *see* Hypertension, heart
  idiopathic (granulomatous) I40.1
  in (due to)
    diphtheria A36.81
    epidemic louse-borne typhus A75.0 [I41]
    Lyme disease A69.29
    sarcoidosis D86.85
    scarlet fever A38.1
    toxoplasmosis (acquired) B58.81
    typhoid A01.02
    typhus NEC A75.9 [I41]
  infective I40.0
  influenzal - *see* Influenza, with, myocarditis
  isolated (acute) I40.1
  meningococcal A39.52
  mumps B26.82
  nonrheumatic, active I40.9
  parenchymatous I40.9
  pneumococcal I40.0
  rheumatic (chronic) (inactive) (with chorea)
    I09.0
    active or acute I01.2
      with chorea (acute) (rheumatic)
        (Sydenham's) I02.0

Myocarditis - *continued*
 rheumatoid - *see* Rheumatoid, carditis
 septic I40.0
 staphylococcal I40.0
 suppurative I40.0
 syphilitic (chronic) A52.06
 toxic I40.8
  rheumatic - *see* Myocarditis, acute, rheumatic
 tuberculous A18.84
 typhoid A01.02
 valvular - *see* Endocarditis
 virus, viral I40.0
  of newborn (Coxsackie) B33.22
Myocardium, myocardial - *see* condition
Myocardosis - *see* Cardiomyopathy
Myoclonus, myoclonic, myoclonia (familial)
 (essential) (multifocal) (simplex) G25.3
 drug-induced G25.3
 epilepsy - *see also* Epilepsy, generalized,
  specified NEC G40.4-
  familial (progressive) G25.3
 epileptica G40.409
  with status epilepticus G40.401
 facial G51.3
 familial progressive G25.3
 Friedreich's G25.3
 jerks G25.3
 massive G25.3
 palatal G25.3
 pharyngeal G25.3
Myocytolysis I51.5
Myodiastasis - *see* Diastasis, muscle
Myoendocarditis - *see* Endocarditis
Myoepithelioma - *see* Neoplasm, benign, by
 site
Myofasciitis (acute) - *see* Myositis
Myofibroma - *see also* Neoplasm, connective
 tissue, benign
 uterus (cervix) (corpus) - *see* Leiomyoma
Myofibromatosis D48.1
 infantile Q89.8
Myofibrosis M62.89
 heart - *see* Myocarditis
 scapulohumeral - *see* Lesion, shoulder,
  specified NEC
Myofibrositis M79.7
 scapulohumeral - *see* Lesion, shoulder,
  specified NEC
Myoglobulinuria, myoglobinuria (primary)
 R82.1
Myokymia, facial G51.4
Myolipoma - *see* Lipoma
Myoma - *see also* Neoplasm, connective tissue,
 benign
 malignant - *see* Neoplasm, connective tissue,
  malignant
 prostate D29.1
 uterus (cervix) (corpus) - *see* Leiomyoma
Myomalacia M62.89
Myometritis - *see* Endometritis
Myometrium - *see* condition
Myonecrosis, clostridial A48.0
Myopathy G72.9
 acute
  necrotizing G72.81
   quadriplegic G72.81
 alcoholic G72.1
 benign congenital G71.2
 central core G71.2
 centronuclear G71.2
 congenital (benign) G71.2
 critical illness G72.81
 distal G71.0
 drug-induced G72.0

Myopathy - *continued*
 endocrine NEC E34.9 [*G73.7*]
 extraocular muscles H05.82-
 facioscapulohumeral G71.0
 hereditary G71.9
  specified NEC G71.8
 immune NEC G72.49
 in (due to)
  Addison's disease E27.1 [*G73.7*]
  alcohol G72.1
  amyloidosis E85.0 [*G73.7*]
  cretinism E00.9 [*G73.7*]
  Cushing's syndrome E24.9 [*G73.7*]
  drugs G72.0
  endocrine disease NEC E34.9 [*G73.7*]
  giant cell arteritis M31.6 [*G73.7*]
  glycogen storage disease E74.00 [*G73.7*]
  hyperadrenocorticism E24.9 [*G73.7*]
  hyperparathyroidism NEC E21.3 [*G73.7*]
  hypoparathyroidism E20.9 [*G73.7*]
  hypopituitarism E23.0 [*G73.7*]
  hypothyroidism E03.9 [*G73.7*]
  infectious disease NEC B99 [*G73.7*]
  lipid storage disease E75.6 [*G73.7*]
  metabolic disease NEC E88.9 [*G73.7*]
  myxedema E03.9 [*G73.7*]
  parasitic disease NEC B89 [*G73.7*]
  polyarteritis nodosa M30.0 [*G73.7*]
  rheumatoid arthritis - *see* Rheumatoid,
  myopathy
  sarcoidosis D86.87
  scleroderma M34.82
  sicca syndrome M35.03
  Sjögren's syndrome M35.03
  systemic lupus erythematosus M32.19
  thyrotoxicosis (hyperthyroidism) E05.90
   [*G73.7*]
   with thyroid storm E05.91 [*G73.7*]
  toxic agent NEC G72.2
 inflammatory NEC G72.49
 intensive care (ICU) G72.81
 limb-girdle G71.0
 mitochondrial NEC G71.3
 mytonic, proximal (PROMM) G71.11
 myotubular G71.2
 nemaline G71.2
 ocular G71.0
 oculopharyngeal G71.0
 of critical illness G72.81
 primary G71.9
  specified NEC G71.8
 progressive NEC G72.89
 proximal myotonic (PROMM) G71.11
 rod G71.2
 scapulohumeral G71.0
 specified NEC G72.89
 toxic G72.2
Myopericarditis - *see also* Pericarditis
 chronic rheumatic I09.2
Myopia (axial) (congenital) H52.1-
 degenerative (malignant) H44.20-
  with
   choroidal neovascularization H44.2A-
   foveoschisis H44.2D-
   macular hole H44.2B-
   retinal detachment H44.2C-
   specified maculopathy NEC H44.2E-
  bilateral H44.23
  left eye H44.22
  right eye H44.21
 malignant (see also Myopia, degenerative)
  H44.2-
 pernicious (see also Myopia, degenerative)
  H44.2-

Myopia - *continued*
 progressive high (degenerative) (see also
  Myopia, degenerative) H44.2-
Myosarcoma - *see* Neoplasm, connective
 tissue, malignant
Myosis (pupil) H57.03
 stromal (endolymphatic) D39.0
Myositis M60.9
 clostridial A48.0
 due to posture - *see* Myositis, specified type
  NEC
 epidemic B33.0
 fibrosa or fibrous (chronic), Volkmann's T79.6
 foreign body granuloma - *see* Granuloma,
  foreign body
 in (due to)
  bilharziasis B65.9 [*M63.8*]
  cysticercosis B69.81
  leprosy A30.9 [*M63.8*]
  mycosis B49 [*M63.8*]
  sarcoidosis D86.87
  schistosomiasis B65.9 [*M63.8*]
  syphilis
   late A52.78
   secondary A51.49
  toxoplasmosis (acquired) B58.82
  trichinellosis B75 [*M63.8*]
  tuberculosis A18.09
 inclusion body [IBM] G72.41
 infective M60.009
  arm M60.002
   left M60.001
   right M60.000
  leg M60.005
   left M60.004
   right M60.003
  lower limb M60.005
   ankle M60.07-
   foot M60.07-
   lower leg M60.06-
   thigh M60.05-
   toe M60.07-
  multiple sites M60.09
  specified site NEC M60.08
  upper limb M60.002
   finger M60.04-
   forearm M60.03-
   hand M60.04-
   shoulder region M60.01-
   upper arm M60.02-
 interstitial M60.10
  ankle M60.17-
  foot M60.17-
  forearm M60.13-
  hand M60.14-
  lower leg M60.16-
  multiple sites M60.19
  shoulder region M60.11-
  specified site NEC M60.18
  thigh M60.15-
  upper arm M60.12-
 mycotic B49 [*M63.8*]
 orbital, chronic H05.12-
 ossificans or ossifying (circumscripta) - *see*
  also Ossification, muscle, specified NEC
  in (due to)
   burns M61.30
    ankle M61.37-
    foot M61.37-
    forearm M61.33-
    hand M61.34-
    lower leg M61.36-
    multiple sites M61.39
    pelvic region M61.35-

Myositis - *continued*
    shoulder region M61.31-
    specified site NEC M61.38
    thigh M61.35-
    upper arm M61.32-
  quadriplegia or paraplegia M61.20
    ankle M61.27-
    foot M61.27-
    forearm M61.23-
    hand M61.24-
    lower leg M61.26-
    multiple sites M61.29
    pelvic region M61.25-
    shoulder region M61.21-
    specified site NEC M61.28
    thigh M61.25-
    upper arm M61.22-
  progressiva M61.10
    ankle M61.17-
    finger M61.14-
    foot M61.17-
    forearm M61.13-
    hand M61.14-
    lower leg M61.16-
    multiple sites M61.19
    pelvic region M61.15-
    shoulder region M61.11-
    specified site NEC M61.18
    thigh M61.15-
    toe M61.17-
    upper arm M61.12-
  traumatica M61.00
    ankle M61.07-
    foot M61.07-
    forearm M61.03-
    hand M61.04-
    lower leg M61.06-
    multiple sites M61.09
    pelvic region M61.05-
    shoulder region M61.01-
    specified site NEC M61.08
    thigh M61.05-
    upper arm M61.02-
  purulent - *see* Myositis, infective
  specified type NEC M60.80
    ankle M60.87-
    foot M60.87-
    forearm M60.83-
    hand M60.84-
    lower leg M60.86-
    multiple sites M60.89
    pelvic region M60.85-
    shoulder region M60.81-
    specified site NEC M60.88
    thigh M60.85-
    upper arm M60.82-
  suppurative - *see* Myositis, infective
  traumatic (old) - *see* Myositis, specified type
  NEC
Myospasia impulsiva F95.2
Myotonia (acquisita) (intermittens) M62.89
  atrophica G71.11
  chondrodystrophic G71.13
  congenita (acetazolamide responsive)
    (dominant) (recessive) G71.12
  drug-induced G71.14
  dystrophica G71.11
  fluctuans G71.19
  levior G71.12
  permanens G71.19
  symptomatic G71.19
Myotonic pupil - *see* Anomaly, pupil, function,
  tonic pupil
Myriapodiasis B88.2

Myringitis H73.2-
  with otitis media - *see* Otitis, media
  acute H73.00-
    bullous H73.01-
    specified NEC H73.09-
  bullous - *see* Myringitis, acute, bullous
  chronic H73.1-
Mysophobia F40.228
Mytilotoxism - *see* Poisoning, fish
Myxadenitis labialis K13.0
Myxedema (adult) (idiocy) (infantile)
  (juvenile) - *see also* Hypothyroidism E03.9
  circumscribed E05.90
    with storm E05.91
  coma E03.5
  congenital E00.1
  cutis L98.5
  localized (pretibial) E05.90
    with storm E05.91
  papular L98.5
Myxochondrosarcoma - *see* Neoplasm,
  cartilage, malignant
Myxofibroma - *see* Neoplasm, connective
  tissue, benign
  odontogenic - *see* Cyst, calcifying odontogenic
Myxofibrosarcoma - *see* Neoplasm, connective
  tissue, malignant
Myxolipoma D17.9
Myxoliposarcoma - *see* Neoplasm, connective
  tissue, malignant

Myxoma - *see also* Neoplasm, connective
  tissue, benign
  nerve sheath - *see* Neoplasm, nerve, benign
  odontogenic - *see* Cyst, calcifying odontogenic
Myxosarcoma - *see* Neoplasm, connective
  tissue, malignant

N

Naegeli's
  disease Q82.8
  leukemia, monocytic C93.1-
Naegleriasis (with meningoencephalitis)
  B60.2
Naffziger's syndrome G54.0
Naga sore - *see* Ulcer, skin
Nägele's pelvis M95.5
  with disproportion (fetopelvic) O33.0
    causing obstructed labor O65.0
Nail - *see also* condition
  biting F98.8
  patella syndrome Q87.2
Nanism, nanosomia - *see* Dwarfism
Nanophyetiasis B66.8
Nanukayami A27.89
Napkin rash L22
Narcolepsy G47.419
  with cataplexy G47.411
  in conditions classified elsewhere G47.429
    with cataplexy G47.421
Narcosis R06.89
Narcotism - *see* Dependence
NARP (Neuropathy, Ataxia and Retinitis
  pigmentosa) syndrome E88.49
Narrow
  anterior chamber angle H40.03-
  gingival width (of periodontal soft tissue)
    K05.5
  pelvis - *see* Contraction, pelvis
Narrowing - *see also* Stenosis
  artery I77.1
    auditory, internal I65.8
    basilar - *see* Occlusion, artery, basilar

Narrowing - *continued*
    carotid - *see* Occlusion, artery, carotid
    cerebellar - *see* Occlusion, artery, cerebellar
    cerebral - *see* Occlusion artery, cerebral
    choroidal - *see* Occlusion, artery, cerebral,
    specified NEC
    communicating posterior - *see* Occlusion,
    artery, cerebral, specified NEC
    coronary - *see also* Disease, heart, ischemic,
    atherosclerotic
      congenital Q24.5
      syphilitic A50.54 [152]
      due to syphilis NEC A52.06
    hypophyseal - *see* Occlusion, artery, cerebral,
    specified NEC
    pontine - *see* Occlusion, artery, cerebral,
    specified NEC
    precerebral - *see* Occlusion, artery,
    precerebral
    vertebral - *see* Occlusion, artery, vertebral
  auditory canal (external) - *see* Stenosis,
    external ear canal
  eustachian tube - *see* Obstruction, eustachian
    tube
  eyelid - *see* Disorder, eyelid function
  larynx J38.6
  mesenteric artery - *see also* Ischemia,
    intestine, acute K55.059
  palate M26.89
  palpebral fissure - *see* Disorder, eyelid
  function
  ureter N13.5
    with infection N13.6
  urethra - *see* Stricture, urethra
Narrowness, abnormal, eyelid Q10.3
Nasal - *see* condition
Nasolachrymal, nasolacrimal - *see* condition
Nasopharyngeal - *see also* condition
  pituitary gland Q89.2
  torticollis M43.6
Nasopharyngitis (acute) (infective)
  (streptococcal) (subacute) J00
  chronic (suppurative) (ulcerative) J31.1
Nasopharynx, nasopharyngeal - *see* condition
Natal tooth, teeth K00.6
Nausea (without vomiting) R11.0
  with vomiting R11.2
  gravidarum - *see* Hyperemesis, gravidarum
  marina T75.3
  navalis T75.3
Navel - *see* condition
Neapolitan fever - *see* Brucellosis
Near drowning T75.1
Nearsightedness - *see* Myopia
Near-syncope R55
Nebula, cornea - *see* Opacity, cornea
Necator americanus infestation B76.1
Necatoriasis B76.1
Neck - *see* condition **Necrobiosis** R68.89
  lipoidica NEC L92.1
    with diabetes - *see* E08-e13 with .620
Necrolysis, toxic epidermal L51.2
  due to drug
    correct substance properly administered - *see*
    Table of Drugs and Chemicals, by drug,
    adverse effect
    overdose or wrong substance given or taken -
    see Table of Drugs and Chemicals, by drug,
    poisoning
Necrophilia F65.89
Necrosis, necrotic (ischemic) - *see also*
  Gangrene
  adrenal (capsule) (gland) E27.49
  amputation stump (surgical) (late) T87.50

Necrosis, necrotic - *continued*
  arm T87.5-
  leg T87.5-
  antrum J32.0
  aorta (hyaline) - *see also* Aneurysm, aorta
    cystic medial - *see* Dissection, aorta
  artery I77.5
  bladder (aseptic) (sphincter) N32.89
  bone - *see also* Osteonecrosis M87.9
    aseptic or avascular - *see* Osteonecrosis
      idiopathic M87.00
    ethmoid J32.2
    jaw M27.2
    tuberculous - *see* Tuberculosis, bone
  brain I67.89
  breast (aseptic) (fat) (segmental) N64.1
  bronchus J98.09
  central nervous system NEC I67.89
  cerebellar I67.89
  cerebral I67.89
  colon - *see also* Infarct, intestine K55.049
  cornea H18.89-
  cortical (acute) (renal) N17.1
  cystic medial (aorta) - *see* Dissection, aorta
  dental pulp K04.1
  esophagus K22.8
  ethmoid (bone) J32.2
  eyelid - *see* Disorder, eyelid, degenerative
  fat, fatty (generalized) - *see also* Disorder, soft
  tissue, specified type NEC
    abdominal wall K65.4
    breast (aseptic) (segmental) N64.1
    localized - *see* Degeneration, by site, fatty
    mesentery K65.4
    omentum K65.4
    pancreas K86.89
    peritoneum K65.4
    skin (subcutaneous), newborn P83.0
    subcutaneous, due to birth injury P15.6
  gallbladder - *see* Cholecystitis, acute
  heart - *see* Infarct, myocardium
  hip, aseptic or avascular - *see* Osteonecrosis,
  by type, femur
  intestine (acute) (hemorrhagic) (massive) - *see*
  also Infarct, intestine K55.069
  jaw M27.2
  kidney (bilateral) N28.0
    acute N17.9
    cortical (acute) (bilateral) N17.1
      with ectopic or molar pregnancy O08.4
    medullary (bilateral) (in acute renal failure)
    (papillary) N17.2
    papillary (bilateral) (in acute renal failure)
    N17.2
    tubular N17.0
      with ectopic or molar pregnancy O08.4
      complicating
        abortion - *see* Abortion, by type,
        complicated by, tubular necrosis
        ectopic or molar pregnancy O08.4
        pregnancy - *see* Pregnancy, complicated
        by, diseases of, specified type or system
        NEC
      following ectopic or molar pregnancy
      O08.4
      traumatic T79.5
  larynx J38.7
  liver (with hepatic failure) (cell) - *see* Failure,
  hepatic
    hemorrhagic, central K76.2
  lung J85.0
  lymphatic gland - *see* Lymphadenitis, acute
  mammary gland (fat) (segmental) N64.1
  mastoid (chronic) - *see* Mastoiditis, chronic

Necrosis, necrotic - *continued*
  medullary (acute) (renal) N17.2
  mesentery - *see also* Infarct, intestine K55.069
    fat K65.4
  mitral valve - *see* Insufficiency, mitral
  myocardium, myocardial - *see* Infarct,
  myocardium
  nose J34.0
  omentum (with mesenteric infarction) - *see*
  also Infarct, intestine K55.069
    fat K65.4
  orbit, orbital - *see* Osteomyelitis, orbit
  ossicles, ear - *see* Abnormal, ear ossicles
  ovary N70.92
  pancreas (aseptic) (duct) (fat) K86.89
    acute (infective) - *see* Pancreatitis, acute
    infective - *see* Pancreatitis, acute
  papillary (acute) (renal) N17.2
  perineum N90.89
  peritoneum (with mesenteric infarction) - *see*
  also Infarct, intestine K55.069
    fat K65.4
  pharynx J02.9
    in granulocytopenia - *see* Neutropenia
    Vincent's A69.1
  phosphorus - *see* subcategory T54.2
  pituitary (gland) E23.0
    postpartum O99.285
    Sheehan O99.285
  pressure - *see* Ulcer, pressure, by site
  pulmonary J85.0
  pulp (dental) K04.1
  radiation - *see* Necrosis, by site
  radium - *see* Necrosis, by site
  renal - *see* Necrosis, kidney   sclera H15.89
  scrotum N50.89
  skin or subcutaneous tissue NEC I96
  spine, spinal (column) - *see also*
  Osteonecrosis, by type, vertebra
    cord G95.19
  spleen D73.5
  stomach K31.89
  stomatitis (ulcerative) A69.0
  subcutaneous fat, newborn P83.88
  subendocardial (acute) I21.4
    chronic I25.89
  suprarenal (capsule) (gland) E27.49
  testis N50.89
  thymus (gland) E32.8
  tonsil J35.8
  trachea J39.8
  tuberculous NEC - *see* Tuberculosis
  tubular (acute) (anoxic) (renal) (toxic) N17.0
    postprocedural N99.0
  vagina N89.8
  vertebra - *see also* Osteonecrosis, by type,
  vertebra
    tuberculous A18.01
  vulva N90.89
  X-ray - *see* Necrosis, by site
Necrospermia - *see* Infertility, male
Need (for)
  care provider because (of)
    assistance with personal care Z74.1
    continuous supervision required Z74.3
    impaired mobility Z74.09
    no other household member able to render
  care Z74.2
    specified reason NEC Z74.8
  immunization - *see* Vaccination
  vaccination - *see* Vaccination
Neglect
  adult
    confirmed T74.01

Neglect - *continued*
    history of Z91.412
    suspected T76.01
  child (childhood)
    confirmed T74.02
    history of Z62.812
    suspected T76.02
  emotional, in childhood Z62.898
  hemispatial R41.4
  left-sided R41.4
  sensory R41.4
  visuospatial R41.4
Neisserian infection NEC - *see* Gonococcus
Nélaton's syndrome G60.8
Nelson's syndrome E24.1
Nematodiasis (intestinal) B82.0
  Ancylostoma B76.0
Neonatal - *see also* Newborn
  acne L70.4
  bradycardia P29.12
  tachycardia P29.11
  screening, abnormal findings on P09
  tooth, teeth K00.6
Neonatorum - *see* condition
Neoplasia
  endocrine, multiple (MEN) E31.20
    type I E31.21
    type IIA E31.22
    type IIB E31.23
  intraepithelial (histologically confirmed)
    anal (AIN) (histologically confirmed) K62.82
      grade I K62.82
      grade II K62.82
      severe D01.3
    cervical glandular (histologically confirmed)
    D06.9
    cervix (uteri) (CIN) (histologically
    confirmed) N87.9
      glandular D06.9
      grade I N87.0
      grade II N87.1
      grade III (severe dysplasia) - *see also*
      Carcinoma, cervix uteri, in situ D06.9
    prostate (histologically confirmed) (PIN)
    N42.31
      grade I N42.31
      grade II N42.31
      grade III (severe dysplasia) D07.5
    vagina (histologically confirmed) (VAIN)
    N89.3
      grade I N89.0
      grade II N89.1
      grade III (severe dysplasia) D07.2
    vulva (histologically confirmed) (VIN)
    N90.3
      grade I N90.0
      grade II N90.1
      grade III (severe dysplasia) D07.1
Neoplasm, neoplastic - *see also* Table of
Neoplasms
  malignant mast cell C96.20
    specified type NEC C96.29
  mast cell, of uncertain behavior NEC D47.09
  lipomatous, benign - *see* Lipoma
Neovascularization
  ciliary body - *see* Disorder, iris, vascular
  cornea H16.40-
    deep H16.44-
    ghost vessels - *see* Ghost, vessels
    localized H16.43-
    pannus - *see* Pannus
  iris - *see* Disorder, iris, vascular
  retina H35.05-
Nephralgia N23

Nephritis, nephritic (albuminuric) (azotemic) (congenital) (disseminated) (epithelial) (familial) (focal) (granulomatous) (hemorrhagic) (infantile) (nonsuppurative, excretory) (uremic) N05.9
 with
  dense deposit disease N05.6
  diffuse
   crescentic glomerulonephritis N05.7
   endocapillary proliferative glomerulonephritis N05.4
   membranous glomerulonephritis N05.2
   mesangial proliferative glomerulonephritis N05.3
   mesangiocapillary glomerulonephritis N05.5
  edema - see Nephrosis
  focal and segmental glomerular lesions N05.1
  foot process disease N04.9
  glomerular lesion
   diffuse sclerosing N05.8
   hypocomplementemic - see Nephritis, membranoproliferative
   IgA - see Nephropathy, IgA
   lobular, lobulonodular - see Nephritis, membranoproliferative
   nodular - see Nephritis, membranoproliferative
  lesion of
   glomerulonephritis, proliferative N05.8
   renal necrosis N05.9
  minor glomerular abnormality N05.0
  specified morphological changes NEC N05.8
 acute N00.9
  with
   dense deposit disease N00.6
   diffuse
    crescentic glomerulonephritis N00.7
    endocapillary proliferative glomerulonephritis N00.4
    membranous glomerulonephritis N00.2
    mesangial proliferative glomerulonephritis N00.3
    mesangiocapillary glomerulonephritis N00.5
   focal and segmental glomerular lesions N00.1
   minor glomerular abnormality N00.0
   specified morphological changes NEC N00.8
  amyloid E85.4 [N08]
  antiglomerular basement membrane (anti-gBM) antibody NEC
   in Goodpasture's syndrome M31.0
  antitubular basement membrane (tubulo-interstitial) NEC N12
  toxic - see Nephropathy, toxic
  arteriolar - see Hypertension, kidney
  arteriosclerotic - see Hypertension, kidney
  ascending - see Nephritis, tubulo-interstitial
  atrophic N03.9
  Balkan (endemic) N15.0
  calculous, calculus - see Calculus, kidney
  cardiac - see Hypertension, kidney
  cardiovascular - see Hypertension, kidney
  chronic N03.9
   with
    dense deposit disease N03.6
    diffuse
     crescentic glomerulonephritis N03.7
     endocapillary proliferative glomerulonephritis N03.4
     membranous glomerulonephritis N03.2

Nephritis, nephritic - *continued*
     mesangial proliferative glomerulonephritis N03.3
     mesangiocapillary glomerulonephritis N03.5
     focal and segmental glomerular lesions N03.1
     minor glomerular abnormality N03.0
     specified morphological changes NEC N03.8
   arteriosclerotic - see Hypertension, kidney
  cirrhotic N26.9
  complicating pregnancy O26.83
  croupous N00.9
  degenerative - see Nephrosis
  diffuse sclerosing N05.8
  due to
   diabetes mellitus - see E08-e13 with .21
   subacute bacterial endocarditis I33.0
   systemic lupus erythematosus (chronic) M32.14
   typhoid fever A01.09
  gonococcal (acute) (chronic) A54.21
  hypocomplementemic - see Nephritis, membranoproliferative
  IgA - see Nephropathy, IgA
  immune complex (circulating) NEC N05.8
  infective - see Nephritis, tubulo-interstitial
  interstitial - see Nephritis, tubulo-interstitial
  lead N14.3
  membranoproliferative (diffuse) (type 1 or 3) - see also N00-N07 with fourth character .5 N05.5
   type 2 - see also N00-N07 with fourth character .6 N05.6
  minimal change N05.0
  necrotic, necrotizing NEC - see also N00-N07 with fourth character .8 N05.8
  nephrotic - see Nephrosis
  nodular - see Nephritis, membranoproliferative
  polycystic Q61.3
   adult type Q61.2
   autosomal
    dominant Q61.2
    recessive NEC Q61.19
   childhood type NEC Q61.19
   infantile type NEC Q61.19
  poststreptococcal N05.9
   acute N00.9
   chronic N03.9
   rapidly progressive N01.9
  proliferative NEC - see also N00-N07 with fourth character .8 N05.8
  purulent - see Nephritis, tubulo-interstitial
  rapidly progressive N01.9
   with
    dense deposit disease N01.6
    diffuse
     crescentic glomerulonephritis N01.7
     endocapillary proliferative glomerulonephritis N01.4
     membranous glomerulonephritis N01.2
     mesangial proliferative glomerulonephritis N01.3
     mesangiocapillary glomerulonephritis N01.5
    focal and segmental glomerular lesions N01.1
    minor glomerular abnormality N01.0
    specified morphological changes NEC N01.8
  salt losing or wasting NEC N28.89
  saturnine N14.3
  sclerosing, diffuse N05.8

Nephritis, nephritic - *continued*
  septic - see Nephritis, tubulo-interstitial
  specified pathology NEC - see also N00-N07 with fourth character .8 N05.8
  subacute N01.9
  suppurative - see Nephritis, tubulo-interstitial
  syphilitic (late) A52.75
   congenital A50.59 [N08]
   early (secondary) A51.44
  toxic - see Nephropathy, toxic
  tubal, tubular - see Nephritis, tubulo-interstitial
  tuberculous A18.11
  tubulo-interstitial (in) N12
   acute (infectious) N10
   chronic (infectious) N11.9
    nonobstructive N11.8
     reflux-associated N11.0
    obstructive N11.1
    specified NEC N11.8
   due to
    brucellosis A23.9 [N16]
    cryoglobulinemia D89.1 [N16]
    glycogen storage disease E74.00 [N16]
    Sjögren's syndrome M35.04
  vascular - see Hypertension, kidney   war N00.9
Nephroblastoma (epithelial) (mesenchymal) C64-
Nephrocalcinosis E83.59 [N29]
Nephrocystitis, pustular - see Nephritis, tubulo-interstitial
Nephrolithiasis (congenital) (pelvis) (recurrent) - see also Calculus, kidney
Nephroma C64-
  mesoblastic D41.0-**Nephronephritis** - see Nephrosis
Nephronophthisis Q61.5
Nephropathia epidemica A98.5
Nephropathy - see also Nephritis N28.9
 with
  edema - see Nephrosis
  glomerular lesion - see Glomerulonephritis
  amyloid, hereditary E85.0
  analgesic N14.0
   with medullary necrosis, acute N17.2
  Balkan (endemic) N15.0
  chemical - see Nephropathy, toxic
  diabetic - see E08-e13 with .21
  drug-induced N14.2
   specified NEC N14.1
  focal and segmental hyalinosis or sclerosis N02.1
  heavy metal-induced N14.3
  hereditary NEC N07.9
   with
    dense deposit disease N07.6
    diffuse
     crescentic glomerulonephritis N07.7
     endocapillary proliferative glomerulonephritis N07.4
     membranous glomerulonephritis N07.2
     mesangial proliferative glomerulonephritis N07.3
     mesangiocapillary glomerulonephritis N07.5
    focal and segmental glomerular lesions N07.1
    minor glomerular abnormality N07.0
    specified morphological changes NEC N07.8
  hypercalcemic N25.89
  hypertensive - see Hypertension, kidney
  hypokalemic (vacuolar) N25.89
  IgA N02.8

Nephropathy - *continued*
  with glomerular lesion N02.9
    focal and segmental hyalinosis or sclerosis
      N02.1
    membranoproliferative (diffuse) N02.5
    membranous (diffuse) N02.2
    mesangial proliferative (diffuse) N02.3
    mesangiocapillary (diffuse) N02.5
    proliferative NEC N02.8
    specified pathology NEC N02.8
  lead N14.3
  membranoproliferative (diffuse) N02.5
  membranous (diffuse) N02.2
  mesangial (IgA/IgG) - *see* Nephropathy, IgA
    proliferative (diffuse) N02.3
  mesangiocapillary (diffuse) N02.5
  obstructive N13.8
  phenacetin N17.2
  phosphate-losing N25.0
  potassium depletion N25.89
  pregnancy-related O26.83-
  proliferative NEC - *see also* N00-N07 with
    fourth character .8 N05.8
  protein-losing N25.89
  saturnine N14.3
  sickle-cell D57. *[N08]*
  toxic NEC N14.4
    due to
      drugs N14.2
        analgesic N14.0
        specified NEC N14.1
      heavy metals N14.3
  vasomotor N17.0
  water-losing N25.89
Nephroptosis N28.83
Nephropyosis - *see* Abscess, kidney
Nephrorrhagia N28.89
Nephrosclerosis (arteriolar)(arteriosclerotic)
  (chronic) (hyaline) - *see also* Hypertension,
  kidney   hyperplastic - *see* Hypertension,
  kidney   senile N26.9
Nephrosis, nephrotic (Epstein's) (syndrome)
  (congenital) N04.9
  with
    foot process disease N04.9
    glomerular lesion N04.1
    hypocomplementemic N04.5
  acute N04.9
  anoxic - *see* Nephrosis, tubular
  chemical - *see* Nephrosis, tubular
  cholemic K76.7
  diabetic - *see* E08-e13 with .21
  Finnish type (congenital) Q89.8
  hemoglobin N10
  hemoglobinuric - *see* Nephrosis, tubular
  in
    amyloidosis E85.4 *[N08]*
    diabetes mellitus - *see* E08-e13 with .21
    epidemic hemorrhagic fever A98.5
    malaria (malariae) B52.0
  ischemic - *see* Nephrosis, tubular
  lipoid N04.9
  lower nephron - *see* Nephrosis, tubular
  malarial (malariae) B52.0
  minimal change N04.0
  myoglobin N10
  necrotizing - *see* Nephrosis, tubular
  osmotic (sucrose) N25.89
  radiation N04.9
  syphilitic (late) A52.75
  toxic - *see* Nephrosis, tubular
  tubular (acute) N17.0
    postprocedural N99.0
    radiation N04.9

Nephrosonephritis, hemorrhagic (endemic)
  A98.5
Nephrostomy
  attention to Z43.6
  status Z93.6
Nerve - *see also* condition
  injury - *see* Injury, nerve, by body site **Nerves**
    R45.0
Nervous - *see also* condition R45.0
  heart F45.8
  stomach F45.8
  tension R45.0
Nervousness R45.0
Nesidioblastoma
  pancreas D13.7
  specified site NEC - *see* Neoplasm, benign, by
    site
  unspecified site D13.7
Nettleship's syndrome   *see* Urticaria
  pigmentosa
Neumann's disease or syndrome L10.1
Neuralgia, neuralgic (acute) M79.2
  accessory (nerve) G52.8
  acoustic (nerve) - *see* subcategory H93.3
  auditory (nerve) - *see* subcategory H93.3
  ciliary G44.009
    intractable G44.001
    not intractable G44.009
  cranial
    nerve - *see also* Disorder, nerve, cranial
      fifth or trigeminal - *see* Neuralgia,
        trigeminal
    postherpetic, postzoster B02.29
  ear - *see* subcategory H92.0
  facialis vera G51.1
  Fothergill's - *see* Neuralgia, trigeminal
  glossopharyngeal (nerve) G52.1
  Horton's G44.099
    intractable G44.091
    not intractable G44.099
  Hunt's B02.21
  hypoglossal (nerve) G52.3
  infraorbital - *see* Neuralgia, trigeminal
  malarial - *see* Malaria
  migrainous G44.009
    intractable G44.001
    not intractable G44.009
  Morton's G57.6-
  nerve, cranial - *see* Disorder, nerve, cranial
  nose G52.0
  occipital M54.81
  olfactory G52.0
  penis N48.9
  perineum R10.2
  postherpetic NEC B02.29
    trigeminal B02.22
  pubic region R10.2
  scrotum R10.2
  Sluder's G44.89
  specified nerve NEC G58.8
  spermatic cord R10.2
  sphenopalatine (ganglion) G90.09
  trifacial - *see* Neuralgia, trigeminal
  trigeminal G50.0
    postherpetic, postzoster B02.22
  vagus (nerve) G52.2
  writer's F48.8
    organic G25.89
Neurapraxia - *see* Injury, nerve
Neurasthenia F48.8
  cardiac F45.8
  gastric F45.8
  heart F45.8

Neurilemmoma - *see also* Neoplasm, nerve,
  benign
  acoustic (nerve) D33.3
  malignant - *see also* Neoplasm, nerve,
  malignant
    acoustic (nerve) C72.4-
Neurilemmosarcoma - *see* Neoplasm, nerve,
  malignant
Neurinoma - *see* Neoplasm, nerve, benign
Neurinomatosis - *see* Neoplasm, nerve,
  uncertain behavior
Neuritis (rheumatoid) M79.2
  abducens (nerve) - *see* Strabismus, paralytic,
    sixth nerve
  accessory (nerve) G52.8
  acoustic (nerve) - *see also* subcategory H93.3
    in (due to)
      infectious disease NEC B99 *[H94.0-]*
      parasitic disease NEC B89 *[H94.0-]*
    syphilitic A52.15
  alcoholic G62.1
    with psychosis - *see* Psychosis, alcoholic
  amyloid, any site E85.4 *[G63]*
  auditory (nerve) - *see* subcategory H93.3
  brachial - *see* Radiculopathy
    due to displacement, intervertebral disc - *see*
      Disorder, disc, cervical, with neuritis
  cranial nerve
    due to Lyme disease A69.22
    eighth or acoustic or auditory - *see*
      subcategory H93.3
    eleventh or accessory G52.8
    fifth or trigeminal G51.0
    first or olfactory G52.0
    fourth or trochlear - *see* Strabismus,
      paralytic, fourth nerve
    second or optic - *see* Neuritis, optic
    seventh or facial G51.8
      newborn (birth injury) P11.3
    sixth or abducent - *see* Strabismus, paralytic,
      sixth nerve
    tenth or vagus G52.2
    third or oculomotor - *see* Strabismus,
      paralytic, third nerve
    twelfth or hypoglossal G52.3
  Déjérine-Sottas G60.0
  diabetic (mononeuropathy) - *see* E08-e13 with
    .41
    polyneuropathy - *see* E08-e13 with .42
  due to
    beriberi E51.11
    displacement, prolapse or rupture,
      intervertebral disc - *see* Disorder, disc, with,
      radiculopathy
    herniation, nucleus pulposus M51.9 *[G55]*
  endemic E51.11
  facial G51.8
    newborn (birth injury) P11.3
  general - *see* Polyneuropathy
  geniculate ganglion G51.1
    due to herpes (zoster) B02.21
  gouty - *see also* Gout, by type M10.9 *[G63]*
  hypoglossal (nerve) G52.3
  ilioinguinal (nerve) G57.9-
  infectious (multiple) NEC G61.0
  interstitial hypertrophic progressive G60.0
  lumbar M54.16
  lumbosacral M54.17
  multiple - *see also* Polyneuropathy
    endemic E51.11
    infective, acute G61.0
  multiplex endemica E51.11
  nerve root - *see* Radiculopathy
  oculomotor (nerve) - *see* Strabismus, paralytic,

Neuritis - *continued*
third nerve
  olfactory nerve G52.0
  optic (nerve) (hereditary) (sympathetic) H46.9
    with demyelination G36.0
    in myelitis G36.0
    nutritional H46.2
    papillitis - *see* Papillitis, optic
    retrobulbar H46.1-
    specified type NEC H46.8
    toxic H46.3
peripheral (nerve) G62.9
  multiple - *see* Polyneuropathy
  single - *see* Mononeuritis
pneumogastric (nerve) G52.2
postherpetic, postzoster B02.29
progressive hypertrophic interstitial G60.0
retrobulbar - *see also* Neuritis, optic, retrobulbar
  in (due to)
    late syphilis A52.15
    meningococcal infection A39.82
    meningococcal A39.82
    syphilitic A52.15
sciatic (nerve) - *see also* Sciatica
  due to displacement of intervertebral disc - *see* Disorder, disc, with, radiculopathy
serum - *see also* Reaction, serum T80.69
shoulder-girdle G54.5
specified nerve NEC G58.8
spinal (nerve) root - *see* Radiculopathy
syphilitic A52.15
thenar (median) G56.1-
thoracic M54.14
toxic NEC G62.2
trochlear (nerve) - *see* Strabismus, paralytic, fourth nerve
vagus (nerve) G52.2
Neuroastrocytoma - *see* Neoplasm, uncertain behavior, by site
Neuroavitaminosis E56.9 [*G99.8*]
Neuroblastoma olfactory C30.0
specified site - *see* Neoplasm, malignant, by site
unspecified site C74.90
Neurochorioretinitis - *see* Chorioretinitis
Neurocirculatory asthenia F45.8
Neurocysticercosis B69.0
Neurocytoma - *see* Neoplasm, benign, by site
Neurodermatitis (circumscribed) (circumscripta) (local) L28.0
atopic L20.81
diffuse (Brocq) L20.81
disseminated L20.81
Neuroencephalomyelopathy, optic G36.0
Neuroepithelioma - *see also* Neoplasm, malignant, by site
olfactory C30.0
Neurofibroma - *see also* Neoplasm, nerve, benign
melanotic - *see* Neoplasm, nerve, benign
multiple - *see* Neurofibromatosis
plexiform - *see* Neoplasm, nerve, benign
Neurofibromatosis (multiple) (nonmalignant) Q85.00
acoustic Q85.02
malignant - *see* Neoplasm, nerve, malignant
specified NEC Q85.09
type 1(von Recklinghausen) Q85.01
type 2Q85.02
Neurofibrosarcoma - *see* Neoplasm, nerve, malignant
Neurogenic - *see also* condition
bladder - *see also* Dysfunction, bladder,

Neurogenic - *continued*
neuromuscular N31.9
  cauda equina syndrome G83.4
bowel NEC K59.2
heart F45.8
Neuroglioma - *see* Neoplasm, uncertain behavior, by site
Neurolabyrinthitis (of Dix and Hallpike) - *see* Neuronitis, vestibular
Neurolathyrism - *see* Poisoning, food, noxious, plant
Neuroleprosy A30.9
Neuroma - *see also* Neoplasm, nerve, benign
acoustic (nerve) D33.3
amputation (stump) (traumatic) (surgical complication) (late) T87.3-
  arm T87.3-
  leg T87.3-
digital (toe) G57.6-
interdigital G58.8
  lower limb (toe) G57.8-
  upper limb G56.8-
intermetatarsal G57.8-
Morton's G57.6-
nonneoplastic
  arm G56.9-
  leg G57.9-
  lower extremity G57.9-
  upper extremity G56.9-
optic (nerve) D33.3
plantar G57.6-
plexiform - *see* Neoplasm, nerve, benign
surgical (nonneoplastic)
  arm G56.9-
  leg G57.9-
  lower extremity G57.9-
  upper extremity G56.9-
Neuromyalgia - *see* Neuralgia
Neuromyasthenia (epidemic) (postinfectious) G93.3
Neuromyelitis G36.9
ascending G61.0
optica G36.0
Neuromyopathy G70.9
paraneoplastic D49.9 [*G13.0*]
Neuromyotonia (Isaacs) G71.19
Neuronevus - *see* Nevus
Neuronitis G58.9
ascending (acute) G57.2-
vestibular H81.2-
Neuroparalytic - *see* condition
Neuropathy, neuropathic G62.9
acute motor G62.81
alcoholic G62.1
  with psychosis - *see* Psychosis, alcoholic
arm G56.9-
autonomic, peripheral - *see* Neuropathy, peripheral, autonomic
axillary G56.9-
bladder N31.9
  atonic (motor) (sensory) N31.2
  autonomous N31.2
  flaccid N31.2
  nonreflex N31.2
  reflex N31.1
  uninhibited N31.0
brachial plexus G54.0
cervical plexus G54.2
chronic
  progressive segmentally demyelinating G62.89
  relapsing demyelinating G62.89
Déjérine-Sottas G60.0
diabetic - *see* E08-e13 with .40

Neuropathy, neuropathic - *continued*
mononeuropathy - *see* E08-e13 with .41
polyneuropathy - *see* E08-e13 with .42
entrapment G58.9
  iliohypogastric nerve G57.8-
  ilioinguinal nerve G57.8-
  lateral cutaneous nerve of thigh G57.1-
  median nerve G56.0-
  obturator nerve G57.8-
  peroneal nerve G57.3-
  posterior tibial nerve G57.5-
  saphenous nerve G57.8-
  ulnar nerve G56.2-
facial nerve G51.9
hereditary G60.9
  motor and sensory (types I-IV) G60.0
  sensory G60.8
  specified NEC G60.8
hypertrophic G60.0
  Charcot-Marie-tooth G60.0
  Déjérine-Sottas G60.0
  interstitial progressive G60.0
  of infancy G60.0
  Refsum G60.1
idiopathic G60.9
  progressive G60.3
  specified NEC G60.8
in association with hereditary ataxia G60.2
intercostal G58.0
ischemic - *see* Disorder, nerve
Jamaica (ginger) G62.2
leg NEC G57.9-
lower extremity G57.9-
lumbar plexus G54.1
median nerve G56.1-
motor and sensory - *see also* Polyneuropathy
  hereditary (types I-IV) G60.0
multifocal motor (MMN) G61.82
multiple (acute) (chronic) - *see* Polyneuropathy
optic (nerve) - *see also* Neuritis, optic
  ischemic H47.01-
paraneoplastic (sensorial) (Denny Brown) D49.9 [*G13.0*]
peripheral (nerve) - *see also* Polyneuropathy G62.9
  autonomic G90.9
    idiopathic G90.09
    in (due to)
      amyloidosis E85.4 [*G99.0*]
      diabetes mellitus - *see* E08-e13 with .43
      endocrine disease NEC E34.9 [*G99.0*]
      gout M10.00 [*G99.0*]
      hyperthyroidism E05.90 [*G99.0*]
        with thyroid storm E05.91 [*G99.0*]
      metabolic disease NEC E88.9 [*G99.0*]
idiopathic G60.9
  progressive G60.3
in (due to)
  antitetanus serum G62.0
  arsenic G62.2
  drugs NEC G62.0
  lead G62.2
  organophosphate compounds G62.2
  toxic agent NEC G62.2
plantar nerves G57.6-
progressive
  hypertrophic interstitial G60.0
  inflammatory G62.81
radicular NEC - *see* Radiculopathy
sacral plexus G54.1
sciatic G57.0-
serum G61.1
toxic NEC G62.2

Neuropathy, neuropathic - *continued*
  trigeminal sensory G50.8
  ulnar nerve G56.2-
  uremic N18.9 [*G63*]
  vitamin B12 E53.8 [*G63*]
    with anemia (pernicious) D51.0 [*G63*]
    due to dietary deficiency D51.3 [*G63*]
Neurophthisis - *see also* Disorder, nerve
  peripheral, diabetic - *see* E08-e13 with .42
Neuroretinitis - *see* Chorioretinitis
Neuroretinopathy, hereditary optic H47.22
Neurosarcoma - *see* Neoplasm, nerve,
  malignant
Neurosclerosis - *see* Disorder, nerve
Neurosis, neurotic F48.9
  anankastic F42.8
  anxiety (state) F41.1
    panic type F41.0
  asthenic F48.8
  bladder F45.8
  cardiac (reflex) F45.8
  cardiovascular F45.8
  character F60.9
  colon F45.8
  compensation F68.1
  compulsive, compulsion F42.8
  conversion F44.9
  craft F48.8
  cutaneous F45.8
  depersonalization F48.1
  depressive (reaction) (type) F34.1
  environmental F48.8
  excoriation L98.1
  fatigue F48.8
  functional - *see* Disorder, somatoform
  gastric F45.8
  gastrointestinal F45.8
  heart F45.8
  hypochondriacal F45.21
  hysterical F44.9
  incoordination F45.8
    larynx F45.8
    vocal cord F45.8
  intestine F45.8
  larynx (sensory) F45.8
    hysterical F44.4
  mixed NEC F48.8
  musculoskeletal F45.8
  obsessional F42.8
  obsessive-compulsive F42.8
  occupational F48.8
  ocular NEC F45.8
  organ - *see* Disorder, somatoform
  pharynx F45.8
  phobic F40.9
  posttraumatic (situational) F43.10
    acute F43.11
    chronic F43.12
  psychasthenic (type) F48.8
  railroad F48.8
  rectum F45.8
  respiratory F45.8
  rumination F45.8
  sexual F65.9
  situational F48.8
  social F40.10
    generalized F40.11
  specified type NEC F48.8
  state F48.9
    with depersonalization episode F48.1
  stomach F45.8
  traumatic F43.10
    acute F43.11
    chronic F43.12

Neurosis, neurotic - *continued*
  vasomotor F45.8
  visceral F45.8
  war F48.8
Neurospongioblastosis diffusa Q85.1
Neurosyphilis (arrested) (early) (gumma)
  (late) (latent) (recurrent) (relapse) A52.3
  with ataxia (cerebellar) (locomotor) (spastic)
    (spinal) A52.19
  aneurysm (cerebral) A52.05
  arachnoid (adhesive) A52.13
  arteritis (any artery) (cerebral) A52.04
  asymptomatic A52.2
  congenital A50.40
  dura (mater) A52.13
  general paresis A52.17
  hemorrhagic A52.05
  juvenile (asymptomatic) (meningeal) A50.40
  leptomeninges (aseptic) A52.13
  meningeal, meninges (adhesive) A52.13
  meningitis A52.13
  meningovascular (diffuse) A52.13
  optic atrophy A52.15
  parenchymatous (degenerative) A52.19
  paresis, paretic A52.17
    juvenile A50.45
  remission in (sustained) A52.3
  serological (without symptoms) A52.2
  specified nature or site NEC A52.19
  tabes, tabetic (dorsalis) A52.11
    juvenile A50.45
  taboparesis A52.17
    juvenile A50.45
  thrombosis (cerebral) A52.05
  vascular (cerebral) NEC A52.05
Neurothekeoma - *see* Neoplasm, nerve, benign
Neurotic - *see* Neurosis
Neurotoxemia - *see* Toxemia
Neutroclusion M26.211
Neutropenia, neutropenic (chronic) (genetic)
  (idiopathic) (immune) (infantile)
  (malignant) (pernicious) (splenic) D70.9
  congenital (primary) D70.0
  cyclic D70.4
  cytoreductive cancer chemotherapy sequela
    D70.1
  drug-induced D70.2
    due to cytoreductive cancer chemotherapy
      D70.1
  due to infection D70.3
  fever D70.9
  neonatal, transitory (isoimmune) (maternal
    transfer) P61.5
  periodic D70.4
  secondary (cyclic) (periodic) (splenic) D70.4
    drug-induced D70.2
      due to cytoreductive cancer chemotherapy
        D70.1
  toxic D70.8
Neutrophilia, hereditary giant D72.0
Nevocarcinoma - *see* Melanoma
Nevus D22.9
  achromic - *see* Neoplasm, skin, benign
  amelanotic - *see* Neoplasm, skin, benign
  angiomatous D18.00
    intra-abdominal D18.03
    intracranial D18.02
    skin D18.01
    specified site NEC D18.09
  araneus I78.1
  balloon cell - *see* Neoplasm, skin, benign
  bathing trunk D48.5
  blue - *see* Neoplasm, skin, benign
    cellular - *see* Neoplasm, skin, benign

Nevus - *continued*
  giant - *see* Neoplasm, skin, benign
  Jadassohn's - *see* Neoplasm, skin, benign
  malignant - *see* Melanoma
  capillary D18.00
    intra-abdominal D18.03
    intracranial D18.02
    skin D18.01
    specified site NEC D18.09
  cavernous D18.00
    intra-abdominal D18.03
    intracranial D18.02
    skin D18.01
    specified site NEC D18.09
  cellular - *see* Neoplasm, skin, benign
    blue - *see* Neoplasm, skin, benign
  choroid D31.3-
  comedonicus Q82.5
  conjunctiva D31.0-
  dermal - *see* Neoplasm, skin, benign
    with epidermal nevus - *see* Neoplasm, skin,
      benign
  dysplastic - *see* Neoplasm, skin, benign
  eye D31.9-
  flammeus Q82.5
  hemangiomatous D18.00
    intra-abdominal D18.03
    intracranial D18.02
    skin D18.01
    specified site NEC D18.09
  iris D31.4-
  lacrimal gland D31.5-
  lymphatic D18.1
  magnocellular
    specified site - *see* Neoplasm, benign, by site
    unspecified site D31.40
  malignant - *see* Melanoma
  meaning hemangioma D18.00
    intra-abdominal D18.03
    intracranial D18.02
    skin D18.01
    specified site NEC D18.09
  mouth (mucosa) D10.30
    specified site NEC D10.39
    white sponge Q38.6
  multiplex Q85.1
  non neoplastic I78.1
  oral mucosa D10.30
    specified site NEC D10.39
    white sponge Q38.6
  orbit D31.6-
  pigmented
    giant - *see also* Neoplasm, skin, uncertain
      behavior D48.5
      malignant melanoma in - *see* Melanoma
  portwine Q82.5
  retina D31.2-
  retrobulbar D31.6-
  sanguineous Q82.5
  senile I78.1
  skin D22.9
    abdominal wall D22.5
    ala nasi D22.39
    ankle D22.7-
    anus, anal D22.5
    arm D22.6-
    auditory canal (external) D22.2-
    auricle (ear) D22.2-
    auricular canal (external) D22.2-
    axilla, axillary fold D22.5
    back D22.5
    breast D22.5
    brow D22.39
    buttock D22.5

Nevus - *continued*
- canthus (eye) D22.1-
- cheek (external) D22.39
- chest wall D22.5
- chin D22.39
- ear (external) D22.2-
- external meatus (ear) D22.2-
- eyebrow D22.39
- eyelid (lower) (upper) D22.1-
- face D22.30
  - specified NEC D22.39
- female genital organ (external) NEC D28.0
- finger D22.6-
- flank D22.5
- foot D22.7-
- forearm D22.6-
- forehead D22.39
- foreskin D29.0
- genital organ (external) NEC
  - female D28.0
  - male D29.9
- gluteal region D22.5
- groin D22.5
- hand D22.6-
- heel D22.7-
- helix D22.2-
- hip D22.7-
- interscapular region D22.5
- jaw D22.39
- knee D22.7-
- labium (majus) (minus) D28.0
- leg D22.7-
- lip (lower) (upper) D22.0
- lower limb D22.7-
- male genital organ (external) D29.9
- nail D22.9
  - finger D22.6-
  - toe D22.7-
- nasolabial groove D22.39
- nates D22.5
- neck D22.4
- nose (external) D22.39
- palpebra D22.1-
- penis D29.0
- perianal skin D22.5
- perineum D22.5
- pinna D22.2-
- popliteal fossa or space D22.7-
- prepuce D29.0
- pudendum D28.0
- scalp D22.4
- scrotum D29.4
- shoulder D22.6-
- submammary fold D22.5
- temple D22.39
- thigh D22.7-
- toe D22.7-
- trunk NEC D22.5
- umbilicus D22.5
- upper limb D22.6-
- vulva D28.0
- specified site NEC - *see* Neoplasm, by site, benign
- spider I78.1
- stellar I78.1
- strawberry Q82.5
- Sutton's benign D22.9
- unius lateris Q82.5
- Unna's Q82.5
- vascular Q82.5
- verrucous Q82.5

Newborn (infant) (liveborn) (singleton) Z38.2
- acne L70.4
- abstinence syndrome P96.1

Newborn - *continued*
- affected by
  - abnormalities of membranes P02.9
    - specified NEC P02.8
  - abruptio placenta P02.1
  - amino-acid metabolic disorder, transitory P74.8
  - amniocentesis (while in utero) P00.6
  - amnionitis P02.7
  - apparent life threatening event (ALTE) R68.13
  - bleeding (into)
    - cerebral cortex P52.22
    - germinal matrix P52.0
    - ventricles P52.1
  - breech delivery P03.0
  - cardiac arrest P29.81
  - cardiomyopathy I42.8
    - congenital I42.4
  - cerebral ischemia P91.0
  - Cesarean delivery P03.4
  - chemotherapy agents P04.1
  - chorioamnionitis P02.7
  - cocaine (crack) P04.41
  - complications of labor and delivery P03.9
    - specified NEC P03.89
  - compression of umbilical cord NEC P02.5
  - contracted pelvis P03.1
  - delivery P03.9
    - Cesarean P03.4
    - forceps P03.2
    - vacuum extractor P03.3
  - environmental chemicals P04.6
  - entanglement (knot) in umbilical cord P02.5
  - fetal (intrauterine)
    - growth retardation P05.9
    - malnutrition not light or small for gestational age P05.2
  - forceps delivery P03.2
  - heart rate abnormalities
    - bradycardia P29.12
    - intrauterine P03.819
      - before onset of labor P03.810
      - during labor P03.811
    - tachycardia P29.11
  - hemorrhage (antepartum) P02.1
    - cerebellar (nontraumatic) P52.6
    - intracerebral (nontraumatic) P52.4
    - intracranial (nontraumatic) P52.9
      - specified NEC P52.8
    - intraventricular (nontraumatic) P52.3
      - grade 1 P52.0
      - grade 2 P52.1
      - grade 3 P52.21
      - grade 4 P52.22
    - posterior fossa (nontraumatic) P52.6
    - subarachnoid (nontraumatic) P52.5
    - subependymal P52.0
      - with intracerebral extension P52.22
      - with intraventricular extension P52.1
        - with enlargement of ventricles P52.21
      - without intraventricular extension P52.0
  - hypoxic ischemic encephalopathy [HIE] P91.60
    - mild P91.61
    - moderate P91.62
    - severe P91.63
  - induction of labor P03.89
  - intestinal perforation P78.0
  - intrauterine (fetal) blood loss P50.9
    - due to (from)
      - cut end of co-twin cord P50.5
      - hemorrhage into
        - co-twin P50.3

Newborn - *continued*
- maternal circulation P50.4
- placenta P50.2
- ruptured cord blood P50.1
- vasa previa P50.0
- specified NEC P50.8
- intrauterine (fetal) hemorrhage P50.9
- intrauterine (in utero) procedure P96.5
- malpresentation (malposition) NEC P03.1
- maternal (complication of) (use of)
  - alcohol P04.3
  - analgesia (maternal) P04.0
  - anesthesia (maternal) P04.0
  - blood loss P02.1
  - circulatory disease P00.3
  - condition P00.9
    - specified NEC P00.89
  - delivery P03.9
    - Cesarean P03.4
    - forceps P03.2
    - vacuum extractor P03.3
  - diabetes mellitus (pre-existing) P70.1
  - disorder P00.9
    - specified NEC P00.89
  - drugs (addictive) (illegal) NEC P04.49
  - ectopic pregnancy P01.4
  - gestational diabetes P70.0
  - hemorrhage P02.1
  - hypertensive disorder P00.0
  - incompetent cervix P01.0
  - infectious disease P00.2
  - injury P00.5
  - labor and delivery P03.9
  - malpresentation before labor P01.7
  - maternal death P01.6
  - medical procedure P00.7
  - medication P04.1
  - multiple pregnancy P01.5
  - nutritional disorder P00.4
  - oligohydramnios P01.2
  - parasitic disease P00.2
  - periodontal disease P00.81
  - placenta previa P02.0
  - polyhydramnios P01.3
  - precipitate delivery P03.5
  - pregnancy P01.9
    - specified P01.8
  - premature rupture of membranes P01.1
  - renal disease P00.1
  - respiratory disease P00.3
  - surgical procedure P00.6
  - urinary tract disease P00.1
  - uterine contraction (abnormal) P03.6
- meconium peritonitis P78.0
- medication (legal) (maternal use) (prescribed) P04.1
- membrane abnormalities P02.9
  - specified NEC P02.8
- membranitis P02.7
- methamphetamine(s) P04.49
- mixed metabolic and respiratory acidosis P84
- neonatal abstinence syndrome P96.1
- noxious substances transmitted via placenta or breast milk P04.9
  - specified NEC P04.8
- nutritional supplements P04.5
- placenta previa P02.0
- placental
  - abnormality (functional) (morphological) P02.20
    - specified NEC P02.29
  - dysfunction P02.29
  - infarction P02.29
  - insufficiency P02.29

Newborn - *continued*
  separation NEC P02.1
  transfusion syndromes P02.3
placentitis P02.7
precipitate delivery P03.5
prolapsed cord P02.4
respiratory arrest P28.81
slow intrauterine growth P05.9
tobacco P04.2
twin to twin transplacental transfusion P02.3
umbilical cord (tightly) around neck P02.5
umbilical cord condition P02.60
  short cord P02.69
  specified NEC P02.69
uterine contractions (abnormal) P03.6
vasa previa P02.69
  from intrauterine blood loss P50.0
apnea P28.4
  primary P28.3
  obstructive P28.4
  sleep (central) (obstructive) (primary) P28.3
born in hospital Z38.00
  by cesarean Z38.01
born outside hospital Z38.1
breast buds P96.89
breast engorgement P83.4
check-up - *see* Newborn, examination
convulsion P90
dehydration P74.1
examination
  8 to 28 days old Z00.111
  under 8 days old Z00.110
fever P81.9
  environmentally-induced P81.0
hyperbilirubinemia P59.9
  of prematurity P59.0
hypernatremia P74.2
hyponatremia P74.2
infection P39.9
  candidal P37.5
  specified NEC P39.8
  urinary tract P39.3
jaundice P59.9
  due to
    breast milk inhibitor P59.3
    hepatocellular damage P59.20
      specified NEC P59.29
    preterm delivery P59.0
  of prematurity P59.0
  specified NEC P59.8
late metabolic acidosis P74.0
mastitis P39.0
  infective P39.0
  noninfective P83.4
multiple born NEC Z38.8
  born in hospital Z38.68
    by cesarean Z38.69
  born outside hospital Z38.7
omphalitis P38.9
  with mild hemorrhage P38.1
  without hemorrhage P38.9
post-term P08.21
prolonged gestation (over 42 completed
  weeks) P08.22
quadruplet Z38.8
  born in hospital Z38.63
    by cesarean Z38.64
  born outside hospital Z38.7
quintuplet Z38.8
  born in hospital Z38.65
    by cesarean Z38.66
  born outside hospital Z38.7
seizure P90
sepsis (congenital) P36.9

Newborn - *continued*
  due to
    anaerobes NEC P36.5
    Escherichia coli P36.4
    Staphylococcus P36.30
      aureus P36.2
      specified NEC P36.39
    Streptococcus P36.10
      group B P36.0
      specified NEC P36.19
    specified NEC P36.8
  triplet Z38.8
    born in hospital Z38.61
      by cesarean Z38.62
    born outside hospital Z38.7
  twin Z38.5
    born in hospital Z38.30
      by cesarean Z38.31
    born outside hospital Z38.4
  vomiting P92.09
    bilious P92.01
  weight check Z00.111
Newcastle conjunctivitis or disease B30.8
Nezelof's syndrome (pure alymphocytosis)
  D81.4
Niacin (amide) deficiency E52
Nicolas (-Durand) -Favre disease A55
Nicotine - *see* Tobacco
Nicotinic acid deficiency E52
Niemann-pick disease or syndrome E75.249
  specified NEC E75.248
  type
    A E75.240
    B E75.241
    C E75.242
    D E75.243
Night
  blindness - *see* Blindness, night
  sweats R61
  terrors (child) F51.4
Nightmares (REM sleep type) F51.5
NIHSS (National Institutes of Health Stroke
  Scale) score R29.7-
Nipple - *see* condition
Nisbet's chancre A57
Nishimoto (-Takeuchi) disease I67.5
Nitritoid crisis or reaction - *see* Crisis,
  nitritoid
Nitrosohemoglobinemia D74.8
Njovera A65
Nocardiosis, nocardiasis A43.9
  cutaneous A43.1
  lung A43.0
  pneumonia A43.0
  pulmonary A43.0
  specified site NEC A43.8
Nocturia R35.1
  psychogenic F45.8
Nocturnal - *see* condition
Nodal rhythm I49.8
Node(s) - *see also* Nodule
  Bouchard's (with arthropathy) M15.2
  Haygarth's M15.8
  Heberden's (with arthropathy) M15.1
  larynx J38.7
  lymph - *see* condition
  milker's B08.03
  Osler's I33.0
  Schmorl's - *see* Schmorl's disease
  singer's J38.2
  teacher's J38.2
  tuberculous - *see* Tuberculosis, lymph gland
  vocal cord J38.2

Nodule(s), nodular
actinomycotic - *see* Actinomycosis
breast NEC (see also Lump, breast) N63.0
colloid (cystic), thyroid E04.1
cutaneous - *see* Swelling, localized
endometrial (stromal) D26.1
Haygarth's M15.8
inflammatory - *see* Inflammation
juxta-articular
  syphilitic A52.77
  yaws A66.7
larynx J38.7
lung, solitary (subsegmental branch of the
  bronchial tree) R91.1
  multiple R91.8
milker's B08.03
prostate N40.2
  with lower urinary tract symptoms (LUTS)
    N40.3
  without lower urinary tract symptoms
    (LUTS) N40.2
pulmonary, solitary (subsegmental branch of
  the bronchial tree) R91.1
retrocardiac R09.89
rheumatoid M06.30
  ankle M06.37-
  elbow M06.32-
  foot joint M06.37-
  hand joint M06.34-
  hip M06.35-
  knee M06.36-
  multiple site M06.39
  shoulder M06.31-
  vertebra M06.38
  wrist M06.33-
scrotum (inflammatory) N49.2
singer's J38.2
solitary, lung (subsegmental branch of the
  bronchial tree) R91.1
  multiple R91.8
subcutaneous - *see* Swelling, localized
teacher's J38.2
thyroid (cold) (gland) (nontoxic) E04.1
  with thyrotoxicosis E05.20
    with thyroid storm E05.21
  toxic or with hyperthyroidism E05.20
    with thyroid storm E05.21
  vocal cord J38.2
Noma (gangrenous) (hospital) (infective)
  A69.0
  auricle I96
  mouth A69.0
  pudendi N76.89
  vulvae N76.89
Nomad, nomadism Z59.0
NOMID (neonatal onset multisystemic
  inflammatory disorder) M04.2
Nonadherence to medical treatment Z91.19
Nonautoimmune hemolytic anemia D59.4
  drug-induced D59.2
Nonclosure - *see also* Imperfect, closure
  ductus arteriosus (Botallo's) Q25.0
  foramen
    botalli Q21.1
    ovale Q21.1
Noncompliance Z91.19
  with
    dietary regimen Z91.11
    dialysis Z91.15
    medical treatment Z91.19
    medication regimen NEC Z91.14
      underdosing - *see also* Table of Drugs and
        Chemicals, categories T36-t50, with final
        character 6 Z91.14

Noncompliance - *continued*
  intentional NEC Z91.128
    due to financial hardship of patient
     Z91.120
  unintentional NEC Z91.138
    due to patient's age related debility
     Z91.130
  renal dialysis Z91.15
Nondescent (congenital) - *see also*
 Malposition, congenital
  cecum Q43.3
  colon Q43.3
  testicle Q53.9
   bilateral Q53.20
    abdominal Q53.211
    perineal Q53.22
   unilateral Q53.10
    abdominal Q53.111
    perineal Q53.12
Nondevelopment
 brain Q02
  part of Q04.3
 heart Q24.8
 organ or site, congenital NEC - *see* Hypoplasia
Nonengagement
 head NEC O32.4
  in labor, causing obstructed labor O64.8
Nonexanthematous tick fever A93.2
Nonexpansion, lung (newborn) P28.0
Nonfunctioning
 cystic duct - *see also* Disease, gallbladder
  K82.8
 gallbladder - *see also* Disease, gallbladder
  K82.8
 kidney N28.9
 labyrinth - *see* subcategory H83.2
Non-Hodgkin lymphoma NEC - *see*
 Lymphoma, non-Hodgkin
Nonimplantation, ovum N97.2
Noninsufflation, fallopian tube N97.1
Non-ketotic hyperglycinemia E72.51
Nonne-Milroy syndrome Q82.0
Nonovulation N97.0
Non-palpable testicle(s)
 bilateral R39.84
 unilateral R39.83
Nonpatent fallopian tube N97.1
Nonpneumatization, lung NEC P28.0
Nonrotation - *see* Malrotation
Nonsecretion, urine - *see* Anuria
Nonunion
 fracture - *see* Fracture, by site
 joint, following fusion or arthrodesis M96.0
 organ or site, congenital NEC - *see* Imperfect,
  closure
 symphysis pubis, congenital Q74.2
Nonvisualization, gallbladder R93.2
Nonvital, nonvitalized tooth K04.99
Non-working side interference M26.56
Noonan's syndrome Q87.1
Normocytic anemia (infectional) due to blood
loss (chronic) D50.0
 acute D62
Norrie's disease (congenital) Q15.8
North American blastomycosis B40.9
Norwegian itch B86
Nose, nasal - *see* condition
Nosebleed R04.0
Nose-picking F98.8
Nosomania F45.21
Nosophobia F45.22
Nostalgia F43.20
Notch of iris Q13.2
Notching nose, congenital (tip) Q30.2

Nothnagel's
 syndrome - *see* Strabismus, paralytic, third
  nerve
 vasomotor acroparesthesia I73.89
Novy's relapsing fever A68.9
 louse-borne A68.0
 tick-borne A68.1
Noxious
 foodstuffs, poisoning by - *see* Poisoning, food,
  noxious, plant
 substances transmitted through placenta or
  breast milk P04.9
Nucleus pulposus - *see* condition
Numbness R20.0
Nuns' knee - *see* Bursitis, prepatellar
Nursemaid's elbow S53.03-
Nutcracker esophagus K22.4
Nutmeg liver K76.1
Nutrient element deficiency E61.9
 specified NEC E61.8
Nutrition deficient or insufficient - *see also*
 Malnutrition E46
 due to
  insufficient food T73.0
  lack of
   care (child) T76.02
    adult T76.01
   food T73.0
Nutritional stunting E45
Nyctalopia (night blindness) - *see* Blindness,
 night
Nycturia R35.1
 psychogenic F45.8
Nymphomania F52.8
Nystagmus H55.00
 benign paroxysmal - *see* Vertigo, benign
  paroxysmal
 central positional H81.4-
 congenital H55.01
 dissociated H55.04
 latent H55.02
 miners' H55.09
 positional
  benign paroxysmal H81.4-
  central H81.4-
 specified form NEC H55.09
 visual deprivation H55.03

O

Obermeyer's relapsing fever (European)
 A68.0
Obesity E66.9
 with alveolar hypoventilation E66.2
 adrenal E27.8
 complicating
  childbirth O99.214
  pregnancy O99.21-
  puerperium O99.215
 constitutional E66.8
 dietary counseling and surveillance Z71.3
 drug-induced E66.1
 due to
  drug E66.1
  excess calories E66.09
   morbid E66.01
   severe E66.01
 endocrine E66.8
 endogenous E66.8
 exogenous E66.09
 familial E66.8
 glandular E66.8
 hypothyroid - *see* Hypothyroidism
 hypoventilation syndrome (OHS) E66.2

Obesity - *continued*
 morbid E66.01
  with
   alveolar hypoventilation E66.2
   obesity hypoventilation syndrome (OHS)
    E66.2
  due to excess calories E66.01
 nutritional E66.09
 pituitary E23.6
 severe E66.01
 specified type NEC E66.8
Oblique - *see* condition
Obliteration
 appendix (lumen) K38.8
 artery I77.1
 bile duct (noncalculous) K83.1
 common duct (noncalculous) K83.1
 cystic duct - *see* Obstruction, gallbladder
 disease, arteriolar I77.1
 endometrium N85.8
 eye, anterior chamber - *see* Disorder, globe,
  hypotony   fallopian tube N97.1
 lymphatic vessel I89.0
  due to mastectomy I97.2
 organ or site, congenital NEC - *see* Atresia, by
  site
 ureter N13.5
  with infection N13.6
 urethra - *see* Stricture, urethra
 vein I87.8
 vestibule (oral) K08.89
Observation (following) (for) (without need
for further medical care) Z04.9
 accident NEC Z04.3
  at work Z04.2
  transport Z04.1
 adverse effect of drug Z03.6
 alleged rape or sexual assault (victim), ruled
  out
  adult Z04.41
  child Z04.42
 criminal assault Z04.8
 development state
  adolescent Z00.3
  period of rapid growth in childhood Z00.2
  puberty Z00.3
 disease, specified NEC Z03.89
 following work accident Z04.2
 growth and development state - *see*
  Observation, development state
 injuries (accidental) NEC - *see also*
  Observation, accident
 newborn (for)
  suspected condition, related to exposure from
  the mother or birth process - *see*   Newborn,
  affected by, maternal
   ruled out Z05.9
    cardiac Z05.0
    connective tissue Z05.73
    gastrointestinal Z05.5
    genetic Z05.41
    genitourinary Z05.6
    immunologic Z05.43
    infectious Z05.1
    metabolic Z05.42
    musculoskeletal Z05.72
    neurological Z05.2
    respiratory Z05.3
    skin and subcutaneous tissue Z05.71
    specified condition NEC Z05.8
 postpartum
  immediately after delivery Z39.0
  routine follow-up Z39.2

Observation - *continued*
pregnancy (normal) (without complication)
Z34.9-
 high risk O09.9-
suicide attempt, alleged NEC Z03.89
 self-poisoning Z03.6
suspected, ruled out - *see also* Suspected
condition, ruled out
 abuse, physical
  adult Z04.71
  child Z04.72
 accident at work Z04.2
 adult battering victim Z04.71
 child battering victim Z04.72
 condition NEC Z03.89
  newborn - *see also* Observation, newborn
   (for), suspected condition, ruled out Z05.9
 drug poisoning or adverse effect Z03.6
 exposure (to)
  anthrax Z03.810
  biological agent NEC Z03.818
 inflicted injury NEC Z04.8
 suicide attempt, alleged Z03.89
  self-poisoning Z03.6
 toxic effects from ingested substance (drug)
  (poison) Z03.6
 toxic effects from ingested substance (drug)
  (poison) Z03.6
Obsession, obsessional state F42.8
 mixed thoughts and acts F42.2
Obsessive-compulsive neurosis or reaction
 F42.8
Obstetric embolism, septic - *see* Embolism,
 obstetric, septic
Obstetrical trauma (complicating delivery)
 O71.9
 with or following ectopic or molar pregnancy
  O08.6
 specified type NEC O71.89
Obstipation - *see* Constipation
Obstruction, obstructed, obstructive
 airway J98.8
 with
  allergic alveolitis J67.9
  asthma J45.909
   with
    exacerbation (acute) J45.901
    status asthmaticus J45.902
  bronchiectasis J47.9
   with
    exacerbation (acute) J47.1
    lower respiratory infection J47.0
  bronchitis (chronic) J44.9
  emphysema J43.9
 chronic J44.9
  with
   allergic alveolitis - *see* Pneumonitis,
    hypersensitivity
   bronchiectasis J47.9
    with
     exacerbation (acute) J47.1
     lower respiratory infection J47.0
 due to
  foreign body - *see* Foreign body, by site,
   causing asphyxia
  inhalation of fumes or vapors J68.9
  laryngospasm J38.5
 ampulla of Vater K83.1
 aortic (heart) (valve) - *see* Stenosis, aortic
 aortoiliac I74.09
 aqueduct of Sylvius G91.1
  congenital Q03.0
   with spina bifida - *see* Spina bifida, by site,
    with hydrocephalus

Obstruction - *continued*
 Arnold-Chiari - *see* Arnold-Chiari disease
 artery (see also Atherosclerosis, artery) I70.9
  stent - *see* Restenosis, stent
  basilar (complete) (partial) - *see* Occlusion,
   artery, basilar
  carotid (complete) (partial) - *see* Occlusion,
   artery, carotid
  cerebellar - *see* Occlusion, artery, cerebellar
  cerebral (anterior) (middle) (posterior) - *see*
   Occlusion, artery, cerebral
  precerebral - *see* Occlusion, artery,
   precerebral
  renal N28.0
  retinal NEC - *see* Occlusion, artery, retina
  vertebral (complete) (partial) - *see* Occlusion,
   artery, vertebral
 band (intestinal) (see also Obstruction,
  intestine, specified NEC) K56.699
 bile duct or passage (common) (hepatic)
  (noncalculous) K83.1
  with calculus K80.51
  congenital (causing jaundice) Q44.3
 biliary (duct) (tract) K83.1
  gallbladder K82.0
 bladder neck (acquired) N32.0
  congenital Q64.31
  due to hyperplasia (hypertrophy) of prostate -
   see Hyperplasia, prostate
 bowel - *see* Obstruction, intestine
 bronchus J98.09
 canal, ear - *see* Stenosis, external ear canal
 cardia K22.2
 caval veins (inferior) (superior) I87.1
 cecum - *see* Obstruction, intestine
 circulatory I99.8
 colon - *see* Obstruction, intestine
 common duct (noncalculous) K83.1
 coronary (artery) - *see* Occlusion, coronary
 cystic duct - *see also* Obstruction, gallbladder
  with calculus K80.21
 device, implant or graft - *see also*
 Complications, by site and type, mechanical
 T85.698
  arterial graft NEC - *see* Complication,
   cardiovascular device, mechanical, vascular
  catheter NEC T85.628
   cystostomy T83.090
   dialysis (renal) T82.49
    intraperitoneal T85.691
   Hopkins T83.098
   ileostomy T83.098
   infusion NEC T82.594
    spinal (epidural) (subdural) T85.690
   nephrostomy T83.092
   urethral indwelling T83.091
   urinary T83.098
   urostomy T83.098
  due to infection T85.79
  gastrointestinal - *see* Complications,
   prosthetic device, mechanical,
   gastrointestinal device
  genital NEC T83.498
   intrauterine contraceptive device T83.39
   penile prosthesis (cylinder) (implanted)
    (pump) (reservoir) T83.490
   testicular prosthesis T83.491
  heart NEC - *see* Complication,
   cardiovascular device, mechanical
  joint prosthesis - *see* Complications, joint
   prosthesis, mechanical, specified NEC, by
   site
  orthopedic NEC - *see* Complication,
   orthopedic, device, mechanical

Obstruction - *continued*
 specified NEC T85.628
 urinary NEC - *see also* Complication,
  genitourinary, device, urinary, mechanical
  graft T83.29
 vascular NEC - *see* Complication,
  cardiovascular device, mechanical
 ventricular intracranial shunt T85.09
 due to foreign body accidentally left in
  operative wound T81.529
 duodenum K31.5
 ejaculatory duct N50.89
 esophagus K22.2
 eustachian tube (complete) (partial) H68.10-
  cartilaginous (extrinsic) H68.13-
   intrinsic H68.12-
  osseous H68.11-
 fallopian tube (bilateral) N97.1
 fecal K56.41
  with hernia - *see* Hernia, by site, with
   obstruction
 foramen of Monro (congenital) Q03.8
  with spina bifida - *see* Spina bifida, by site,
   with hydrocephalus
 foreign body - *see* Foreign body
 gallbladder K82.0
  with calculus, stones K80.21
  congenital Q44.1
 gastric outlet K31.1
 gastrointestinal - *see* Obstruction, intestine
 hepatic K76.89
  duct (noncalculous) K83.1
 hepatobiliary K83.1
 ileum - *see* Obstruction, intestine
 iliofemoral (artery) I74.5
 intestine K56.609
  complete K56.601
  incomplete K56.600
  partial K56.600
  with
   adhesions (intestinal) (peritoneal) K56.50
    complete K56.52
    incomplete K56.51
    partial K56.51
  adynamic K56.0
  by gallstone K56.3
  congenital (small) Q41.9
   large Q42.9
    specified part NEC Q42.8
  neurogenic K56.0
   Hirschsprung's disease or megacolon Q43.1
  newborn P76.9
   due to
    fecaliths P76.8
    inspissated milk P76.2
    meconium (plug) P76.0
     in mucoviscidosis E84.11
   specified NEC P76.8
  postoperative K91.30
   complete K91.32
   incomplete K91.31
   partial K91.31
  reflex K56.0
  specified NEC K56.699
   complete K56.691
   incomplete K56.690
   partial K56.690
  volvulus K56.2
 intracardiac ball valve prosthesis T82.09
 jejunum - *see* Obstruction, intestine
 joint prosthesis - *see* Complications, joint
  prosthesis, mechanical, specified NEC, by site
 kidney (calices) N28.89
 labor - *see* Delivery

Obstruction - *continued*
  lacrimal (passages) (duct)
    by
      dacryolith - *see* Dacryolith
      stenosis - *see* Stenosis, lacrimal
    congenital Q10.5
    neonatal H04.53-
  lacrimonasal duct - *see* Obstruction, lacrimal
  lacteal, with steatorrhea K90.2
  laryngitis - *see* Laryngitis
  larynx NEC J38.6
    congenital Q31.8
  lung J98.4
    disease, chronic J44.9
  lymphatic I89.0
  meconium (plug)
    newborn P76.0
      due to fecaliths P76.0
    in mucoviscidosis E84.11
  mitral - *see* Stenosis, mitral
  nasal J34.89
  nasolacrimal duct - *see also* Obstruction, lacrimal
    congenital Q10.5
  nasopharynx J39.2
  nose J34.89
  organ or site, congenital NEC - *see* Atresia, by site
  pancreatic duct K86.89
  parotid duct or gland K11.8
  pelviureteral junction N13.5
    with hydronephrosis N13.0
    congenital Q62.39
  pharynx J39.2
  portal (circulation) (vein) I81
  prostate - *see also* Hyperplasia, prostate
    valve (urinary) N32.0
  pulmonary valve (heart) I37.0
  pyelonephritis (chronic) N11.1
  pylorus
    adult K31.1
    congenital or infantile Q40.0
  rectosigmoid - *see* Obstruction, intestine
  rectum K62.4
  renal N28.89
    outflow N13.8
    pelvis, congenital Q62.39
  respiratory J98.8
    chronic J44.9
  retinal (vessels) H34.9
  salivary duct (any) K11.8
    with calculus K11.5
  sigmoid - *see* Obstruction, intestine
  sinus (accessory) (nasal) J34.89
  Stensen's duct K11.8
  stomach NEC K31.89
    acute K31.0
    congenital Q40.2
    due to pylorospasm K31.3
  submandibular duct K11.8
  submaxillary gland K11.8
    with calculus K11.5
  thoracic duct I89.0
  thrombotic - *see* Thrombosis
  trachea J39.8
  tracheostomy airway J95.03
  tricuspid (valve) - *see* Stenosis, tricuspid
  upper respiratory, congenital Q34.8
  ureter (functional) (pelvic junction) NEC N13.5
    with
      hydronephrosis N13.1
        with infection N13.6
      pyelonephritis (chronic) N11.1

Obstruction - *continued*
  congenital Q62.39
    due to calculus - *see* Calculus, ureter
  urethra NEC N36.8
    congenital Q64.39
  urinary (moderate) N13.9
    due to hyperplasia (hypertrophy) of prostate - *see* Hyperplasia, prostate
    organ or tract (lower) N13.9
    prostatic valve N32.0
    specified NEC N13.8
  uropathy N13.9
  uterus N85.8
  vagina N89.5
  valvular - *see* Endocarditis
  vein, venous I87.1
    caval (inferior) (superior) I87.1
    thrombotic - *see* Thrombosis
  vena cava (inferior) (superior) I87.1
  vesical NEC N32.0
  vesicourethral orifice N32.0
    congenital Q64.31
  vessel NEC I99.8
  stent - *see* Restenosis, stent
Obturator - *see* condition
Occlusal wear, teeth K03.0
Occlusio pupillae - *see* Membrane, pupillary
Occlusion, occluded
  anus K62.4
    congenital Q42.3
      with fistula Q42.2
  aortoiliac (chronic) I74.09
  aqueduct of Sylvius G91.1
    congenital Q03.0
      with spina bifida - *see* Spina bifida, by site, with hydrocephalus
  artery (see also Atherosclerosis, artery) I70.9
    auditory, internal I65.8
    basilar I65.1
      with
        infarction I63.22
          due to
            embolism I63.12
            thrombosis I63.02
    brain or cerebral I66.9
      with infarction (due to) I63.5-
        embolism I63.4-
        thrombosis I63.3-
    carotid I65.2-
      with
        infarction I63.23-
          due to
            embolism I63.13-
            thrombosis I63.03-
    cerebellar (anterior inferior) (posterior inferior) (superior) I66.3
      with infarction I63.54-
        due to
          embolism I63.44-
          thrombosis I63.34-
    cerebral I66.9
      with infarction I63.50
        due to
          embolism I63.40
            specified NEC I63.49
          thrombosis I63.30
            specified NEC I63.39
    anterior I66.1-
      with infarction I63.52-
        due to
          embolism I63.42-
          thrombosis I63.32-
    middle I66.0-
      with infarction I63.51-

Occlusion, occluded - *continued*
      due to
        embolism I63.41-
        thrombosis I63.31-
    posterior I66.2-
      with infarction I63.53-
        due to
          embolism I63.43-
          thrombosis I63.33-
    specified NEC I66.8
      with infarction I63.59
        due to
          embolism I63.4-
          thrombosis I63.3-
  choroidal (anterior) - *see* Occlusion, artery, precerebral, specified NEC
  communicating posterior   *see* Occlusion, artery, precerebral, specified NEC
  complete
    coronary I25.82
    extremities I70.92
  coronary (acute) (thrombotic) (without myocardial infarction) I24.0
    with myocardial infarction - *see* Infarction, myocardium
    chronic total I25.82
    complete I25.82
    healed or old I25.2
    total (chronic) I25.82
  hypophyseal - *see* Occlusion, artery, precerebral, specified NEC
  iliac I74.5
  lower extremities due to stenosis or stricture I77.1
  mesenteric (embolic) (thrombotic) - *see also* Infarct, intestine K55.069
  perforating - *see* Occlusion, artery, cerebral, specified NEC
  peripheral I77.9
    thrombotic or embolic I74.4
  pontine   *see* Occlusion, artery, precerebral, specified NEC
  precerebral I65.9
    with infarction I63.20
      specified NEC I63.29
      due to
        embolism I63.10
          specified NEC I63.19
        thrombosis I63.00
          specified NEC I63.09
    basilar - *see* Occlusion, artery, basilar
    carotid - *see* Occlusion, artery, carotid
    puerperal O88.23
    specified NEC I65.8
      with infarction I63.29
        due to
          embolism I63.19
          thrombosis I63.09
    vertebral - *see* Occlusion, artery, vertebral
  renal N28.0
  retinal
    central H34.1-
    partial H34.21-
    branch H34.23-
    transient H34.0-
  spinal - *see* Occlusion, artery, precerebral, vertebral
  total (chronic)
    coronary I25.82
    extremities I70.92
  vertebral I65.0-
    with
      infarction I63.21-
        due to

Occlusion, occluded - *continued*
    embolism I63.11-
      thrombosis I63.01-
  basilar artery - *see* Occlusion, artery, basilar
  bile duct (common) (hepatic) (noncalculous)
    K83.1
  bowel - *see* Obstruction, intestine
  carotid (artery) (common) (internal) - *see*
    Occlusion, artery, carotid
  centric (of teeth) M26.59
    maximum intercuspation discrepancy
    M26.55
  cerebellar (artery) - *see* Occlusion, artery,
    cerebellar
  cerebral (artery) - *see* Occlusion, artery,
    cerebral
  cerebrovascular - *see also* Occlusion, artery,
    cerebral
    with infarction I63.5-
  cervical canal - *see* Stricture, cervix
  cervix (uteri) - *see* Stricture, cervix
  choanal Q30.0
  choroidal (artery) - *see* Occlusion, artery,
    precerebral, specified NEC
  colon - *see* Obstruction, intestine
  communicating posterior artery - *see*
    Occlusion, artery, precerebral, specified NEC
  coronary (artery) (vein) (thrombotic) - *see also*
    Infarct, myocardium
    chronic total I25.82
    healed or old I25.2
    not resulting in infarction I24.0
    total (chronic) I25.82
  cystic duct - *see* Obstruction, gallbladder
  embolic - *see* Embolism
  fallopian tube N97.1
    congenital Q50.6
  gallbladder - *see also* Obstruction, gallbladder
    congenital (causing jaundice) Q44.1
  gingiva, traumatic K06.2
  hymen N89.6
    congenital Q52.3
  hypophyseal (artery) - *see* Occlusion, artery,
    precerebral, specified NEC
  iliac artery I74.5
  intestine - *see* Obstruction, intestine
  lacrimal passages - *see* Obstruction, lacrimal
  lung J98.4
  lymph or lymphatic channel I89.0
  mammary duct N64.89
  mesenteric artery (embolic) (thrombotic) - *see*
    also Infarct, intestine K55.069
  nose J34.89
    congenital Q30.0
  organ or site, congenital NEC - *see* Atresia, by
    site
  oviduct N97.1
    congenital Q50.6
  peripheral arteries
    due to stricture or stenosis I77.1
    upper extremity I74.2
  pontine (artery) - *see* Occlusion, artery,
    precerebral, specified NEC
  posterior lingual, of mandibular teeth M26.29
  precerebral artery - *see* Occlusion, artery,
    precerebral
  punctum lacrimale - *see* Obstruction, lacrimal
  pupil - *see* Membrane, pupillary
  pylorus, adult - *see also* Stricture, pylorus
    K31.1
  renal artery N28.0
  retina, retinal
    artery - *see* Occlusion, artery, retinal
    vein (central) H34.81-

Occlusion, occluded - *continued*
    engorgement H34.82-
      tributary H34.83-
    vessels H34.9
  spinal artery - *see* Occlusion, artery,
    precerebral, vertebral
  teeth (mandibular) (posterior lingual) M26.29
  thoracic duct I89.0
  thrombotic - *see* Thrombosis, artery
  traumatic
    edentulous (alveolar) ridge K06.2
    gingiva K06.2
    periodontal K05.5
  tubal N97.1
  ureter (complete) (partial) N13.5
    congenital Q62.10
  ureteropelvic junction N13.5
    congenital Q62.11
  ureterovesical orifice N13.5
    congenital Q62.12
  urethra - *see* Stricture, urethra
  uterus N85.8
  vagina N89.5
  vascular NEC I99.8
  vein - *see* Thrombosis
    retinal - *see* Occlusion, retinal, vein
  vena cava (inferior) (superior) - *see* Embolism,
    vena cava
  ventricle (brain) NEC G91.1
  vertebral (artery) - *see* Occlusion, artery,
    vertebral
  vessel (blood) I99.8
  vulva N90.5
Occult
  blood in feces (stools) R19.5
Occupational
  problems NEC Z56.89
Ochlophobia - *see* Agoraphobia
Ochronosis (endogenous) E70.29
Ocular muscle - *see* condition
Oculogyric crisis or disturbance H51.8
  psychogenic F45.8
Oculomotor syndrome H51.9
Oculopathy
  syphilitic NEC A52.71
    congenital
      early A50.01
      late A50.30
    early (secondary) A51.43
    late A52.71
Oddi's sphincter spasm K83.4
Odontalgia K08.89
Odontoameloblastoma - *see* Cyst, calcifying
  odontogenic
Odontoclasia K03.89
Odontodysplasia, regional K00.4
Odontogenesis imperfecta K00.5
Odontoma (ameloblastic) (complex)
  (compound) (fibroameloblastic) - *see* Cyst,
  calcifying odontogenic
Odontomyelitis (closed) (open) K04.01
  irreversible K04.02
  reversible K04.01
Odontorrhagia K08.89
Odontosarcoma, ameloblastic C41.1
  upper jaw (bone) C41.0
Oestriasis - *see* Myiasis
Oguchi's disease H53.63
Ohara's disease - *see* Tularemia
OHS (obesity hypoventilation syndrome)
  E66.2
Oidiomycosis - *see* Candidiasis
Oidium albicans infection - *see* Candidiasis

Old age (without mention of debility) R54
  dementia F03
Old (previous) myocardial infarction I25.2
Olfactory - *see* condition
Oligemia - *see* Anemia
Oligoastrocytoma
  specified site - *see* Neoplasm, malignant, by
    site
  unspecified site C71.9
Oligocythemia D64.9
Oligodendroblastoma
  specified site - *see* Neoplasm, malignant
  unspecified site C71.9
Oligodendroglioma
  anaplastic type
    specified site - *see* Neoplasm, malignant, by
    site
    unspecified site C71.9
  specified site - *see* Neoplasm, malignant, by
    site
  unspecified site C71.9
Oligodontia - *see* Anodontia
Oligoencephalon Q02
Oligohidrosis L74.4
Oligohydramnios O41.0-
Oligohidrosis L74.4
Oligomenorrhea N91.5
  primary N91.3
  secondary N91.4
Oligophrenia - *see also* Disability, intellectual
  phenylpyruvic E70.0
Oligospermia N46.11
  due to
    drug therapy N46.121
    efferent duct obstruction N46.123
    infection N46.122
    radiation N46.124
    specified cause NEC N46.129
    systemic disease N46.125
Oligotrichia - *see* Alopecia
Oliguria R34
  with, complicating or following ectopic or
    molar pregnancy O08.4
  postprocedural N99.0
Ollier's disease Q78.4
Omentitis - *see* Peritonitis
Omenotocele - *see* Hernia, abdomen, specified
  site NEC
Omentum, omental - *see* condition
Omphalitis (congenital) (newborn) P38.9
  with mild hemorrhage P38.1
  without hemorrhage P38.9
  not of newborn L08.82
  tetanus A33
Omphalocele Q79.2
Omphalomesenteric duct, persistent Q43.0
Omphalorrhagia, newborn P51.9
Omsk hemorrhagic fever A98.1
Onanism (excessive) F98.8
Onchocerciasis, onchocercosis B73.1
  with
    eye disease B73.00
      endophthalmitis B73.01
      eyelid B73.09
      glaucoma B73.02
      specified NEC B73.09
    eye NEC B73.00
    eyelid B73.09
Oncocytoma - *see* Neoplasm, benign, by site
Oncovirus, as cause of disease classified
  elsewhere B97.32
Ondine's curse - *see* Apnea, sleep
Oneirophrenia F23

Onychauxis L60.2
  congenital Q84.5
Onychia - *see also* Cellulitis, digit
  with lymphangitis - *see* Lymphangitis, acute, digit
  candidal B37.2
  dermatophytic B35.1
Onychitis - *see also* Cellulitis, digit
  with lymphangitis - *see* Lymphangitis, acute, digit
Onychocryptosis L60.0
Onychodystrophy L60.3
  congenital Q84.6
Onychogryphosis, onychogryposis L60.2
Onycholysis L60.1
Onychomadesis L60.8
Onychomalacia L60.3
Onychomycosis (finger) (toe) B35.1
Onycho-osteodysplasia Q87.2
Onychophagia F98.8
Onychophosis L60.8
Onychoptosis L60.8
Onychorrhexis L60.3
  congenital Q84.6
Onychoschizia L60.3
Onyxis (finger) (toe) L60.0
Onyxitis - *see also* Cellulitis, digit
  with lymphangitis - *see* Lymphangitis, acute, digit
Oophoritis (cystic) (infectional) (interstitial) N70.92
  with salpingitis N70.93
  acute N70.02
    with salpingitis N70.03
  chronic N70.12
    with salpingitis N70.13
  complicating abortion - *see* Abortion, by type, complicated by, oophoritis
Oophorocele N83.4-
Opacity, opacities cornea H17.-
  central H17.1-
  congenital Q13.3
  degenerative - *see* Degeneration, cornea
  hereditary - *see* Dystrophy, cornea
  inflammatory - *see* Keratitis
  minor H17.81-
  peripheral H17.82-
  sequelae of trachoma (healed) B94.0
  specified NEC H17.89
  enamel (teeth) (fluoride) (nonfluoride) K00.3
  lens - *see* Cataract
  snowball - *see* Deposit, crystalline
  vitreous (humor) NEC H43.39-
  congenital Q14.0
  membranes and strands H43.31-
Opalescent dentin (hereditary) K00.5
Open, opening
  abnormal, organ or site, congenital - *see* Imperfect, closure
  angle with
    borderline
      findings
        high risk H40.02-
        low risk H40.01-
      intraocular pressure H40.00-
    cupping of discs H40.01-
    glaucoma (primary) - *see* Glaucoma, open angle
  bite
    anterior M26.220
    posterior M26.221
  false - *see* Imperfect, closure
  margin on tooth restoration K08.51
  restoration margins of tooth K08.51
  wound - *see* Wound, open

Operational fatigue F48.8
Operative - *see* condition
Operculitis - *see* Periodontitis
Operculum - *see* Break, retina
Ophiasis L63.2
Ophthalmia - *see also* Conjunctivitis H10.9
  actinic rays - *see* Photokeratitis
  allergic (acute) - *see* Conjunctivitis, acute, atopic
  blennorrhagic (gonococcal) (neonatorum) A54.31
  diphtheritic A36.86
  Egyptian A71.1
  electrica - *see* Photokeratitis
  gonococcal (neonatorum) A54.31
  metastatic - *see* Endophthalmitis, purulent
  migraine - *see* Migraine, ophthalmoplegic
  neonatorum, newborn P39.1
    gonococcal A54.31
  nodosa H16.24-
  purulent - *see* Conjunctivitis, acute, mucopurulent
  spring - *see* Conjunctivitis, acute, atopic
  sympathetic - *see* Uveitis, sympathetic
Ophthalmitis - *see* Ophthalmia
Ophthalmocele (congenital) Q15.8
Ophthalmoneuromyelitis G36.0
Ophthalmoplegia - *see also* Strabismus, paralytic
  anterior internuclear - *see* Ophthalmoplegia, internuclear
  ataxia-areflexia G61.0
  diabetic - *see* E08-e13 with .39
  exophthalmic E05.00
    with thyroid storm E05.01
  external H49.88-
    progressive H49.4-
      with pigmentary retinopathy - *see* Kearns-Sayre syndrome
    total H49.3-
  internal (complete) (total) H52.51-
  internuclear H51.2-
  migraine - *see* Migraine, ophthalmoplegic
  Parinaud's H49.88-
  progressive external - *see* Ophthalmoplegia, external, progressive
  supranuclear, progressive G23.1
  total (external) - *see* Ophthalmoplegia, external, total
Opioid(s)
  abuse - *see* Abuse, drug, opioids
  dependence - *see* Dependence, drug, opioids
  induced, without use disorder
    anxiety disorder F11.988
    delirium F11.921
    depressive disorder F11.94
    sexual dysfunction F11.981
    sleep disorder F11.982
Opisthognathism M26.09
Opisthorchiasis (felineus) (viverrini) B66.0
Opitz' disease D73.2
Opiumism - *see* Dependence, drug, opioid
Oppenheim's disease G70.2
Oppenheim-Urbach disease (necrobiosis lipoidica diabeticorum) - *see* E08-e13 with .620
Optic nerve - *see* condition
Orbit - *see* condition
Orchioblastoma C62.9-
Orchitis (gangrenous) (nonspecific) (septic) (suppurative) N45.2
  blennorrhagic (gonococcal) (acute) (chronic) A54.23
  chlamydial A56.19

Orchitis - *continued*
  filarial - *see also* Infestation, filarial B74.9 [N51]
  gonococcal (acute) (chronic) A54.23
  mumps B26.0
  syphilitic A52.76
  tuberculous A18.15
ORF (virus disease) B08.02
Organic - *see also* condition
  brain syndrome F09
  heart - *see* Disease, heart
  mental disorder F09
  psychosis F09
Orgasm
  anejaculatory N53.13
Oriental
  bilharziasis B65.2
  schistosomiasis B65.2
Orifice - *see* condition
Origin of both great vessels from right ventricle Q20.1
Ormond's disease (with ureteral obstruction) N13.5
  with infection N13.6
Ornithine metabolism disorder E72.4
Ornithinemia (Type I) (Type II) E72.4
Ornithosis A70
Orotaciduria, oroticaciduria (congenital) (hereditary) (pyrimidine deficiency) E79.8
  anemia D53.0
Orthodontics
  adjustment Z46.4
  fitting Z46.4
Orthopnea R06.01
Orthopoxvirus B08.09
  specified NEC B08.09
Os, uterus - *see* condition
Osgood-Schlatter disease or osteochondrosis - *see* Osteochondrosis, juvenile, tibia
Osler (-Weber) -Rendu disease I78.0
Osler's nodes I33.0
Osmidrosis L75.0
Osseous - *see* condition
Ossification
  artery - *see* Arteriosclerosis
  auricle (ear) - *see* Disorder, pinna, specified type NEC
  bronchial J98.09
  cardiac - *see* Degeneration, myocardial
  cartilage (senile) - *see* Disorder, cartilage, specified type NEC
  coronary (artery) - *see* Disease, heart, ischemic, atherosclerotic
  diaphragm J98.6
  ear, middle - *see* Otosclerosis
  falx cerebri G96.19
  fontanel, premature Q75.0
  heart - *see also* Degeneration, myocardial
    valve - *see* Endocarditis
  larynx J38.7
  ligament - *see* Disorder, tendon, specified type NEC
    posterior longitudinal - *see* Spondylopathy, specified NEC
  meninges (cerebral) (spinal) G96.19
  multiple, eccentric centers - *see* Disorder, bone, development or growth
  muscle - *see also* Calcification, muscle
    due to burns - *see* Myositis, ossificans, in, burns
    paralytic - *see* Myositis, ossificans, in, quadriplegia
    progressive - *see* Myositis, ossificans, progressiva

Osteochondroarthrosis deformans endemica
- *see* Disease, Kaschin-beck
Osteochondritis - *see also* Osteochondropathy,
by site
Brailsford's - *see* Osteochondrosis, juvenile,
radius
dissecans M93.20
ankle M93.27-
elbow M93.22-
foot M93.27-
hand M93.24-
hip M93.25-
knee M93.26-
multiple sites M93.29
shoulder joint M93.21-
specified site NEC M93.28
wrist M93.23-
juvenile M92.9
patellar - *see* Osteochondrosis, juvenile,
patella
syphilitic (congenital) (early) A50.02
[*M90.80*]
ankle A50.02 [*M90.87*]
elbow A50.02 [*M90.82*]
foot A50.02 [*M90.87*]
forearm A50.02 [*M90.83*]
hand A50.02 [*M90.84*]
hip A50.02 [*M90.85*]
knee A50.02 [*M90.86*]
multiple sites A50.02 [*M90.89*]
shoulder joint A50.02 [*M90.81*]
specified site NEC A50.02 [*M90.88*]
Osteochondrodysplasia Q78.9
with defects of growth of tubular bones and
spine Q77.9
specified NEC Q77.8
specified NEC Q78.8
Osteochondrodystrophy E78.9
Osteochondrolysis - *see* Osteochondritis,
dissecans
Osteochondroma - *see* Neoplasm, bone, benign
Osteochondromatosis D48.0
syndrome Q78.4
Osteochondromyxosarcoma - *see* Neoplasm,
bone, malignant
Osteochondropathy M93.90
ankle M93.97-
elbow M93.92-
foot M93.97-
hand M93.94-
hip M93.95-
Kienböck's disease of adults M93.1
knee M93.96-
multiple joints M93.99
osteochondritis dissecans - *see*
Osteochondritis, dissecans
osteochondrosis - *see* Osteochondrosis
shoulder region M93.91-
slipped upper femoral epiphysis - *see* Slipped,
epiphysis, upper femoral
specified joint NEC M93.98
specified type NEC M93.80
ankle M93.87-
elbow M93.82-
foot M93.87-
hand M93.84-
hip M93.85-
knee M93.86-
multiple joints M93.89
shoulder region M93.81-
specified joint NEC M93.88
wrist M93.83-
syphilitic, congenital
early A50.02 [*M90.80*]

Osteochondropathy - *continued*
late A50.56 [*M90.80*]
wrist M93.93-
Osteochondrosarcoma - *see* Neoplasm, bone,
malignant
Osteochondrosis - *see also* Osteochondropathy,
by site
acetabulum (juvenile) M91.0
adult - *see* Osteochondropathy, specified type
NEC, by site
astragalus (juvenile) - *see* Osteochondrosis,
juvenile, tarsus
Blount's - *see* Osteochondrosis, juvenile, tibia
Buchanan's M91.0
Burns' - *see* Osteochondrosis, juvenile, ulna
calcaneus (juvenile) - *see* Osteochondrosis,
juvenile, tarsus
capitular epiphysis (femur) (juvenile) - *see*
Legg-Calvé-Perthes disease
carpal (juvenile) (lunate) (scaphoid) - *see*
Osteochondrosis, juvenile, hand, carpal
lunate
adult M93.1
coxa juvenilis - *see* Legg-Calvé-Perthes
disease
deformans juvenilis, coxae - *see* Legg-Calvé-
Perthes disease
Diaz's - *see* Osteochondrosis, juvenile, tarsus
dissecans (knee) (shoulder) - *see*
Osteochondritis, dissecans
femoral capital epiphysis (juvenile) - *see*
Legg-Calvé-Perthes disease
femur (head), juvenile - *see* Legg-Calvé-
Perthes disease
fibula (juvenile) - *see* Osteochondrosis,
juvenile, fibula
foot NEC (juvenile) M92.8
Freiberg's - *see* Osteochondrosis, juvenile,
metatarsus
Haas' (juvenile) - *see* Osteochondrosis,
juvenile, humerus
Haglund's - *see* Osteochondrosis, juvenile,
tarsus
hip (juvenile) - *see* Legg-Calvé-Perthes disease
humerus (capitulum) (head) (juvenile) - *see*
Osteochondrosis, juvenile, humerus
ilium, iliac crest (juvenile) M91.0
ischiopubic synchondrosis M91.0
Iselin's - *see* Osteochondrosis, juvenile,
metatarsus
juvenile, juvenilis M92.9
after congenital dislocation of hip reduction -
see Osteochondrosis, juvenile, hip, specified
NEC
arm - *see* Osteochondrosis, juvenile, upper
limb NEC
capitular epiphysis (femur) - *see* Legg-Calvé-
Perthes disease
clavicle, sternal epiphysis - *see*
Osteochondrosis, juvenile, upper limb NEC
coxae - *see* Legg-Calvé-Perthes disease
deformans M92.9
fibula M92.5-
foot NEC M92.8
hand M92.20-
carpal lunate M92.21-
metacarpal head M92.22-
specified site NEC M92.29-
head of femur - *see* Legg-Calvé-Perthes
disease
hip and pelvis M91.9-
coxa plana - *see* Coxa, plana
femoral head - *see* Legg-Calvé-Perthes
disease

Osteochondrosis - *continued*
pelvis M91.0
pseudocoxalgia - *see* Pseudocoxalgia
specified NEC M91.8-
humerus M92.0-
limb
lower NEC M92.8
upper NEC - *see* Osteochondrosis, juvenile,
upper limb NEC
medial cuneiform bone - *see*
Osteochondrosis, juvenile, tarsus
metatarsus M92.7-
patella M92.4-
radius M92.1-
specified site NEC M92.8
spine M42.00
cervical region M42.02
cervicothoracic region M42.03
lumbar region M42.06
lumbosacral region M42.07
multiple sites M42.09
occipito-atlanto-axial region M42.01
sacrococcygeal region M42.08
thoracic region M42.04
thoracolumbar region M42.05
tarsus M92.6-
tibia M92.5-
ulna M92.1-
upper limb NEC M92.3-
vertebra (body) (epiphyseal plates) (Calvé's)
(Scheuermann's) - *see* Osteochondrosis,
juvenile, spine
Kienböck's - *see* Osteochondrosis, juvenile,
hand, carpal lunate
adult M93.1
Köhler's
patellar - *see* Osteochondrosis, juvenile,
patella
tarsal navicular - *see* Osteochondrosis,
juvenile, tarsus
Legg-Perthes (-Calvé)(-Waldenström) - *see*
Legg-Calvé-Perthes disease
limb
lower NEC (juvenile) M92.8
upper NEC (juvenile) - *see* Osteochondrosis,
juvenile, upper limb NEC
lunate bone (carpal) (juvenile) - *see also*
Osteochondrosis, juvenile, hand, carpal lunate
adult M93.1
Mauclaire's - *see* Osteochondrosis, juvenile,
hand, metacarpal
metacarpal (head) (juvenile) - *see*
Osteochondrosis, juvenile, hand, metacarpal
metatarsus (fifth) (head) (juvenile) (second) -
see Osteochondrosis, juvenile, metatarsus
navicular (juvenile) - *see* Osteochondrosis,
juvenile, tarsus
os
calcis (juvenile) - *see* Osteochondrosis,
juvenile, tarsus
tibiale externum (juvenile) - *see*
Osteochondrosis, juvenile, tarsus
Osgood-Schlatter - *see* Osteochondrosis,
juvenile, tibia
Panner's - *see* Osteochondrosis, juvenile,
humerus
patellar center (juvenile) (primary) (secondary)
- *see* Osteochondrosis, juvenile, patella
pelvis (juvenile) M91.0
Pierson's M91.0
radius (head) (juvenile) - *see* Osteochondrosis,
juvenile, radius
Scheuermann's - *see* Osteochondrosis,
juvenile, spine

Osteochondrosis - *continued*
   Sever's - *see* Osteochondrosis, juvenile, tarsus
   Sinding-Larsen - *see* Osteochondrosis,
     juvenile, patella
   spine M42.9
     adult M42.10
       cervical region M42.12
       cervicothoracic region M42.13
       lumbar region M42.16
       lumbosacral region M42.17
       multiple sites M42.19
       occipito-atlanto-axial region M42.11
       sacrococcygeal region M42.18
       thoracic region M42.14
       thoracolumbar region M42.15
     juvenile - *see* Osteochondrosis, juvenile,
     spine
   symphysis pubis (juvenile) M91.0
   syphilitic (congenital) A50.02
   talus (juvenile) - *see* Osteochondrosis,
     juvenile, tarsus
   tarsus (navicular) (juvenile) - *see*
     Osteochondrosis, juvenile, tarsus
   tibia (proximal) (tubercle) (juvenile) - *see*
     Osteochondrosis, juvenile, tibia
   tuberculous - *see* Tuberculosis, bone
   ulna (lower) (juvenile) - *see* Osteochondrosis,
     juvenile, ulna
   van Neck's M91.0
   vertebral - *see* Osteochondrosis, spine
Osteoclastoma D48.0
   malignant - *see* Neoplasm, bone, malignant
Osteodynia - *see* Disorder, bone, specified type
   NEC
Osteodystrophy Q78.9
   azotemic N25.0
   congenital Q78.9
   parathyroid, secondary E21.1
   renal N25.0
Osteofibroma - *see* Neoplasm, bone, benign
Osteofibrosarcoma - *see* Neoplasm, bone,
   malignant
Osteogenesis imperfecta Q78.0
Osteogenic - *see* condition
Osteolysis M89.50
   carpus M89.54-
   clavicle M89.51-
   femur M89.55-
   fibula M89.56-
   finger M89.54-
   humerus M89.52-
   ilium M89.559
   ischium M89.559
   joint prosthesis (periprosthetic) - *see*
     Complications, joint prosthesis, mechanical,
     periprosthetic, osteolysis, by site
   metacarpus M89.54-
   metatarsus M89.57-
   multiple sites M89.59
   neck M89.58
   periprosthetic - *see* Complications, joint
     prosthesis, mechanical, periprosthetic,
     osteolysis, by site
   radius M89.53-
   rib M89.58
   scapula M89.51-
   skull M89.58
   tarsus M89.57-
   tibia M89.56-
   toe M89.57-
   ulna M89.53-
   vertebra M89.58
Osteoma - *see also* Neoplasm, bone, benign
   osteoid - *see also* Neoplasm, bone, benign
     giant - *see* Neoplasm, bone, benign

Osteomalacia M83.9
   adult M83.9
     drug-induced NEC M83.5
     due to
       malabsorption (postsurgical) M83.2
       malnutrition M83.3
     specified NEC M83.8
   aluminium-induced M83.4
   infantile - *see* Rickets
   juvenile - *see* Rickets
   oncogenic E83.89
   pelvis M83.8
   puerperal M83.0
   senile M83.1
   vitamin-d-resistant in adults E83.31 [*M90.8*]
     carpus E83.31 [*M90.84*]
     clavicle E83.31 [*M90.81*]
     femur E83.31 [*M90.85*]
     fibula E83.31 [*M90.86*]
     finger E83.31 [*M90.84*]
     humerus E83.31 [*M90.82*]
     ilium E83.31 [*M90.859*]
     ischium E83.31 [*M90.859*]
     metacarpus E83.31 [*M90.84*]
     metatarsus E83.31 [*M90.87*]
     multiple sites E83.31 [*M90.89*]
     neck E83.31 [*M90.88*]
     radius E83.31 [*M90.83*]
     rib E83.31 [*M90.88*]
     scapula E83.31 [*M90.819*]
     skull E83.31 [*M90.88*]
     tarsus E83.31 [*M90.879*]
     tibia E83.31 [*M90.869*]
     toe E83.31 [*M90.879*]
     ulna E83.31 [*M90.839*]
     vertebra E83.31 [*M90.88*]
Osteomyelitis (general) (infective) (localized)
(neonatal) (purulent) (septic)
(staphylococcal) (streptococcal)
(suppurative) (with periostitis) M86.9
   acute M86.10
     carpus M86.14-
     clavicle M86.11-
     femur M86.15-
     fibula M86.16-
     finger M86.14-
     hematogenous M86.00
       carpus M86.04-
       clavicle M86.01-
       femur M86.05-
       fibula M86.06-
       finger M86.04-
       humerus M86.02-
       ilium M86.059
       ischium M86.059
       mandible M27.2
       metacarpus M86.04-
       metatarsus M86.07-
       multiple sites M86.09
       neck M86.08
       orbit H05.02-
       petrous bone - *see* Petrositis
       radius M86.03-
       rib M86.08
       scapula M86.01-
       skull M86.08
       tarsus M86.07-
       tibia M86.06-
       toe M86.07-
       ulna M86.03-
       vertebra - *see* Osteomyelitis, vertebra
     humerus M86.12-
     ilium M86.159
     ischium M86.159

Osteomyelitis - *continued*
     mandible M27.2
     metacarpus M86.14-
     metatarsus M86.17-
     multiple sites M86.19
     neck M86.18
     orbit H05.02-
     petrous bone - *see* Petrositis
     radius M86.13-
     rib M86.18
     scapula M86.11-
     skull M86.18
     tarsus M86.17-
     tibia M86.16-
     toe M86.17-
     ulna M86.13-
     vertebra - *see* Osteomyelitis, vertebra
   chronic (or old) M86.60
     with draining sinus M86.40
       carpus M86.44-
       clavicle M86.41-
       femur M86.45-
       fibula M86.46-
       finger M86.44-
       humerus M86.42-
       ilium M86.459
       ischium M86.459
       mandible M27.2
       metacarpus M86.44-
       metatarsus M86.47-
       multiple sites M86.49
       neck M86.48
       orbit H05.02-
       petrous bone - *see* Petrositis
       radius M86.43-
       rib M86.48
       scapula M86.41-
       skull M86.48
       tarsus M86.47-
       tibia M86.46-
       toe M86.47-
       ulna M86.43-
       vertebra - *see* Osteomyelitis, vertebra
     carpus M86.64-
     clavicle M86.61-
     femur M86.65-
     fibula M86.66-
     finger M86.64-
     hematogenous NEC M86.50
       carpus M86.54-
       clavicle M86.51-
       femur M86.55-
       fibula M86.56-
       finger M86.54-
       humerus M86.52-
       ilium M86.559
       ischium M86.559
       mandible M27.2
       metacarpus M86.54-
       metatarsus M86.57-
       multifocal M86.30
         carpus M86.34-
         clavicle M86.31-
         femur M86.35-
         fibula M86.36-
         finger M86.34-
         humerus M86.32-
         ilium M86.359
         ischium M86.359
         metacarpus M86.34-
         metatarsus M86.37-
         multiple sites M86.39
         neck M86.38
         radius M86.33-

Osteomyelitis - *continued*
- rib M86.38
  - scapula M86.31-
  - skull M86.38
  - tarsus M86.37-
  - tibia M86.36-
  - toe M86.37-
  - ulna M86.33-
  - vertebra - *see* Osteomyelitis, vertebra
- multiple sites M86.59
- neck M86.58
- orbit H05.02-
- petrous bone - *see* Petrositis
- radius M86.53-
- rib M86.58
- scapula M86.51-
- skull M86.58
- tarsus M86.57-
- tibia M86.56-
- toe M86.57-
- ulna M86.53-
- vertebra - *see* Osteomyelitis, vertebra
- humerus M86.62-
- ilium M86.659
- ischium M86.659
- mandible M27.2
- metacarpus M86.64-
- metatarsus M86.67-
- multifocal - *see* Osteomyelitis, chronic, hematogenous, multifocal
- multiple sites M86.69
- neck M86.68
- orbit H05.02-
- petrous bone - *see* Petrositis
- radius M86.63-
- rib M86.68
- scapula M86.61-
- skull M86.68
- tarsus M86.67-
- tibia M86.66-
- toe M86.67-
- ulna M86.63-
- vertebra - *see* Osteomyelitis, vertebra
- echinococcal B67.2
- Garr's - *see* Osteomyelitis, specified type NEC
- in diabetes mellitus - *see* E08-e13 with .69
- jaw (acute) (chronic) (lower) (neonatal) (suppurative) (upper) M27.2
- nonsuppurating - *see* Osteomyelitis, specified type NEC
- orbit H05.02-
- petrous bone - *see* Petrositis
- Salmonella (arizonae) (cholerae-suis) (enteritidis) (typhimurium) A02.24
- sclerosing, nonsuppurative - *see* Osteomyelitis, specified type NEC
- specified type NEC - *see also* subcategory M86.8X-
  - mandible M27.2
  - orbit H05.02-
  - petrous bone - *see* Petrositis
  - vertebra - *see* Osteomyelitis, vertebra
- subacute M86.20
  - carpus M86.24-
  - clavicle M86.21-
  - femur M86.25-
  - fibula M86.26-
  - finger M86.24-
  - humerus M86.22-
  - mandible M27.2
  - metacarpus M86.24-
  - metatarsus M86.27-
  - multiple sites M86.29
  - neck M86.28

Osteomyelitis - *continued*
- orbit H05.02-
- petrous bone - *see* Petrositis
- radius M86.23-
- rib M86.28
- scapula M86.21-
- skull M86.28
- tarsus M86.27-
- tibia M86.26-
- toe M86.27-
- ulna M86.23-
- vertebra - *see* Osteomyelitis, vertebra
- syphilitic A52.77
  - congenital (early) A50.02 [*M90.80*]
- tuberculous - *see* Tuberculosis, bone
- typhoid A01.05
- vertebra M46.20
  - cervical region M46.22
  - cervicothoracic region M46.23
  - lumbar region M46.26
  - lumbosacral region M46.27
  - occipito-atlanto-axial region M46.21
  - sacrococcygeal region M46.28
  - thoracic region M46.24
  - thoracolumbar region M46.25

Osteomyelofibrosis D47.4

Osteomyelosclerosis D75.89

Osteonecrosis M87.9
- due to
  - drugs - *see* Osteonecrosis, secondary, due to, drugs
  - trauma - *see* Osteonecrosis, secondary, due to, trauma
- idiopathic aseptic M87.00
  - ankle M87.07-
  - carpus M87.03-
  - clavicle M87.01-
  - femur M87.05-
  - fibula M87.06-
  - finger M87.04-
  - humerus M87.02-
  - ilium M87.050
  - ischium M87.050
  - metacarpus M87.04-
  - metatarsus M87.07-
  - multiple sites M87.09
  - neck M87.08
  - pelvis M87.050
  - radius M87.03-
  - rib M87.08
  - scapula M87.01-
  - skull M87.08
  - tarsus M87.07-
  - tibia M87.06-
  - toe M87.07-
  - ulna M87.03-
  - vertebra M87.08
- secondary NEC M87.30
  - carpus M87.33-
  - clavicle M87.31-
  - due to
    - drugs M87.10
      - carpus M87.13-
      - clavicle M87.11-
      - femur M87.15-
      - fibula M87.16-
      - finger M87.14-
      - humerus M87.12-
      - ilium M87.159
      - ischium M87.159
      - jaw M87.180
      - metacarpus M87.14-
      - metatarsus M87.17-
      - multiple sites M87.19

Osteonecrosis - *continued*
- neck M87.18
- radius M87.13-
- rib M87.18
- scapula M87.11-
- skull M87.18
- tarsus M87.17-
- tibia M87.16-
- toe M87.17-
- ulna M87.13-
- vertebra M87.18
- hemoglobinopathy NEC D58.2 [*M90.50*]
  - carpus D58.2 [*M90.54*]
  - clavicle D58.2 [*M90.51*]
  - femur D58.2 [*M90.55*]
  - fibula D58.2 [*M90.56*]
  - finger D58.2 [*M90.54*]
  - humerus D58.2 [*M90.52*]
  - ilium D58.2 [*M90.55*]
  - ischium D58.2 [*M90.55*]
  - metacarpus D58.2 [*M90.54*]
  - metatarsus D58.2 [*M90.57*]
  - multiple sites D58.2 [*M90.58*]
  - neck D58.2 [*M90.58*]
  - radius D58.2 [*M90.53*]
  - rib D58.2 [*M90.58*]
  - scapula D58.2 [*M90.51*]
  - skull D58.2 [*M90.58*]
  - tarsus D58.2 [*M90.57*]
  - tibia D58.2 [*M90.56*]
  - toe D58.2 [*M90.57*]
  - ulna D58.2 [*M90.53*]
  - vertebra D58.2 [*M90.58*]
- trauma (previous) M87.20
  - carpus M87.23-
  - clavicle M87.21-
  - femur M87.25-
  - fibula M87.26-
  - finger M87.24-
  - humerus M87.22-
  - ilium M87.25-
  - ischium M87.25-
  - metacarpus M87.24-
  - metatarsus M87.27-
  - multiple sites M87.29
  - neck M87.28
  - radius M87.23-
  - rib M87.28
  - scapula M87.21-
  - skull M87.28
  - tarsus M87.27-
  - tibia M87.26-
  - toe M87.27-
  - ulna M87.23-
  - vertebra M87.28
- femur M87.35-
- fibula M87.36-
- finger M87.34-
- humerus M87.32-
- ilium M87.350
- in
  - caisson disease T70.3 [*M90.50*]
    - carpus T70.3 [*M90.54*]
    - clavicle T70.3 [*M90.51*]
    - femur T70.3 [*M90.55*]
    - fibula T70.3 [*M90.56*]
    - finger T70.3 [*M90.54*]
    - humerus T70.3 [*M90.52*]
    - ilium T70.3 [*M90.55*]
    - ischium T70.3 [*M90.55*]
    - metacarpus T70.3 [*M90.54*]
    - metatarsus T70.3 [*M90.57*]
    - multiple sites T70.3 [*M90.59*]
    - neck T70.3 [*M90.58*]

Osteonecrosis - *continued*
    radius T70.3 [*M90.53*]
    rib T70.3 [*M90.58]*
    scapula T70.3 [*M90.51*]
    skull T70.3 [*M90.58]*
    tarsus T70.3 [*M90.57*]
    tibia T70.3 [*M90.56*]
    toe T70.3 [*M90.57*]
    ulna T70.3 [*M90.53*]
    vertebra T70.3 [*M90.58]*
  ischium M87.350
  metacarpus M87.34-
  metatarsus M87.37-
  multiple site M87.39
  neck M87.38
  radius M87.33-
  rib M87.38
  scapula M87.319
  skull M87.38
  tarsus M87.379
  tibia M87.366
  toe M87.379
  ulna M87.33-
  vertebra M87.38
  specified type NEC M87.80
    carpus M87.83-
    clavicle M87.81-
    femur M87.85-
    fibula M87.86-
    finger M87.84-
    humerus M87.82-
    ilium M87.85-
    ischium M87.85-
    metacarpus M87.84-
    metatarsus M87.87-
    multiple sites M87.89
    neck M87.88
    radius M87.83-
    rib M87.88
    scapula M87.81-
    skull M87.88
    tarsus M87.87-
    tibia M87.86-
    toe M87.87-
    ulna M87.83-
    vertebra M87.88
Osteo-onycho-arthro-dysplasia Q87.2
Osteo-onychodysplasia, hereditary Q87.2
Osteopathia condensans disseminata Q78.8
Osteopathy - *see also* Osteomyelitis,
  Osteonecrosis, Osteoporosis
  after poliomyelitis M89.60
    carpus M89.64-
    clavicle M89.61-
    femur M89.65-
    fibula M89.66-
    finger M89.64-
    humerus M89.62-
    ilium M89.659
    ischium M89.659
    metacarpus M89.64-
    metatarsus M89.67-
    multiple sites M89.69
    neck M89.68
    radius M89.63-
    rib M89.68
    scapula M89.61-
    skull M89.68
    tarsus M89.67-
    tibia M89.66-
    toe M89.67-
    ulna M89.63-
    vertebra M89.68
  in (due to)

Osteopathy - *continued*
  renal osteodystrophy N25.0
  specified diseases classified elsewhere *see*
  subcategory M90.8
Osteopenia M85.8-
  borderline M85.8-
Osteoperiostitis - *see* Osteomyelitis, specified
  type NEC
Osteopetrosis (familial) Q78.2
Osteophyte M25.70
  ankle M25.77-
  elbow M25.72-
  foot joint M25.77-
  hand joint M25.74-
  hip M25.75-
  knee M25.76-
  shoulder M25.71-
  spine M25.78
  vertebrae M25.78
  wrist M25.73-
Osteopoikilosis Q78.8
Osteoporosis (female) (male) M81.0
  with current pathological fracture M80.00
  age-related M81.0
    with current pathologic fracture M80.00
      carpus M80.04-
      clavicle M80.01-
      fibula M80.06-
      finger M80.04-
      humerus M80.02-
      ilium M80.05-
      ischium M80.05-
      metacarpus M80.04-
      metatarsus M80.07-
      pelvis M80.05-
      radius M80.03-
      scapula M80.01-
      tarsus M80.07-
      tibia M80.06-
      toe M80.07-
      ulna M80.03-
      vertebra M80.08
  disuse M81.8
    with current pathological fracture M80.80
      carpus M80.84-
      clavicle M80.81-
      fibula M80.86-
      finger M80.84-
      humerus M80.82-
      ilium M80.85-
      ischium M80.85-
      metacarpus M80.84-
      metatarsus M80.87-
      pelvis M80.85-
      radius M80.83-
      scapula M80.81-
      tarsus M80.87-
      tibia M80.86-
      toe M80.87-
      ulna M80.83-
      vertebra M80.88
  drug-induced - *see* Osteoporosis, specified
    type NEC
  idiopathic - *see* Osteoporosis, specified type
    NEC
  involutional - *see* Osteoporosis, age-related
  Lequesne M81.6
  localized M81.6
  postmenopausal M81.0
    with pathological fracture M80.00
      carpus M80.04-
      clavicle M80.01-
      fibula M80.06-
      finger M80.04-

Osteoporosis - *continued*
    humerus M80.02-
    ilium M80.05-
    ischium M80.05-
    metacarpus M80.04-
    metatarsus M80.07-
    pelvis M80.05-
    radius M80.03-
    scapula M80.01-
    tarsus M80.07-
    tibia M80.06-
    toe M80.07-
    ulna M80.03-
    vertebra M80.08
  postoophorectomy - *see* Osteoporosis,
    specified type NEC
  postsurgical malabsorption - *see* Osteoporosis,
    specified type NEC
  post-traumatic - *see* Osteoporosis, specified
    type NEC
  senile - *see* Osteoporosis, age-related
  specified type NEC M81.8
    with pathological fracture M80.80
      carpus M80.84-
      clavicle M80.81-
      fibula M80.86-
      finger M80.84-
      humerus M80.82-
      ilium M80.85-
      ischium M80.85-
      metacarpus M80.84-
      metatarsus M80.87-
      pelvis M80.85-
      radius M80.83-
      scapula M80.81-
      tarsus M80.87-
      tibia M80.86-
      toe M80.87-
      ulna M80.83-
      vertebra M80.88
Osteopsathyrosis (idiopathica) Q78.0
Osteoradionecrosis, jaw (acute) (chronic)
  (lower) (suppurative) (upper) M27.2
Osteosarcoma (any form) - *see* Neoplasm,
  bone, malignant
Osteosclerosis Q78.2
  acquired M85.8-
  congenita Q77.4
  fragilitas (generalisata) Q78.2
  myelofibrosis D75.81
Osteosclerotic anemia D64.89
Osteosis
  cutis L94.2
  renal fibrocystic N25.0
Österreicher-turner syndrome Q87.2
Ostium
  atrioventriculare commune Q21.2
  primum (arteriosum) (defect) (persistent)
    Q21.2
  secundum (arteriosum) (defect) (patent)
    (persistent) Q21.1
Ostrum-Furst syndrome Q75.8
Otalgia - *see* subcategory H92.0
Otitis (acute) H66.90
  with effusion - *see also* Otitis, media,
    nonsuppurative
    purulent - *see* Otitis, media, suppurative
  adhesive *see* subcategory H74.1
  chronic - *see also* Otitis, media, chronic
    with effusion - *see also* Otitis, media,
    nonsuppurative, chronic
  externa H60.9-
    abscess - *see* Abscess, ear, external
    acute (noninfective) H60.50-

Otitis (acute) - *continued*
actinic H60.51-
chemical H60.52-
contact H60.53-
eczematoid H60.54-
infective - *see* Otitis, externa, infective
reactive H60.55-
specified NEC H60.59-
cellulitis - *see* Cellulitis, ear
chronic H60.6-
diffuse - *see* Otitis, externa, infective, diffuse
hemorrhagic - *see* Otitis, externa, infective,
hemorrhagic
in (due to)
aspergillosis B44.89
candidiasis B37.84
erysipelas A46 [*H62.40*]
herpes (simplex) virus infection B00.1
zoster B02.8
impetigo L01.00 [*H62.40*]
infectious disease NEC B99 [*H62.4*]
mycosis NEC B36.9 [*H62.40*]
parasitic disease NEC B89 [*H62.40*]
viral disease NEC B34.9 [*H62.40*]
zoster B02.8
infective NEC H60.39-
abscess - *see* Abscess, ear, external
cellulitis - *see* Cellulitis, ear
diffuse H60.31-
hemorrhagic H60.32-
swimmer's ear - *see* Swimmer's, ear
malignant H60.2-
mycotic NEC B36.9 [*H62.40*]
in
aspergillosis B44.89
candidiasis B37.84
moniliasis B37.84
necrotizing - *see* Otitis, externa, malignant
Pseudomonas aeruginosa - *see* Otitis,
externa, malignant
reactive - *see* Otitis, externa, acute, reactive
specified NEC - *see* subcategory H60.8
tropical NEC B36.9 [*H62.40*]
in
aspergillosis B44.89
candidiasis B37.84
moniliasis B37.84
insidiosa - *see* Otosclerosis
interna - *see* subcategory H83.0
media (hemorrhagic) (staphylococcal)
(streptococcal) H66.9-
with effusion (nonpurulent) - *see* Otitis,
media, nonsuppurative
acute, subacute H66.90
allergic - *see* Otitis, media, nonsuppurative,
acute, allergic
exudative - *see* Otitis, media, suppurative,
acute
mucoid - *see* Otitis, media, nonsuppurative,
acute
necrotizing - *see also* Otitis, media,
suppurative, acute
in
measles B05.3
scarlet fever A38.0
nonsuppurative NEC - *see* Otitis, media,
nonsuppurative, acute
purulent - *see* Otitis, media, suppurative,
acute
sanguinous - *see* Otitis, media,
nonsuppurative, acute
secretory - *see* Otitis, media,
nonsuppurative, acute, serous
seromucinous - *see* Otitis, media,

Otitis (acute) - *continued*
nonsuppurative, acute
serous - *see* Otitis, media, nonsuppurative,
acute, serous
suppurative - *see* Otitis, media, suppurative,
acute
allergic - *see* Otitis, media, nonsuppurative
catarrhal - *see* Otitis, media, nonsuppurative
chronic H66.90
with effusion (nonpurulent) - *see* Otitis,
media, nonsuppurative, chronic
allergic - *see* Otitis, media, nonsuppurative,
chronic, allergic
benign suppurative - *see* Otitis, media,
suppurative, chronic, tubotympanic
catarrhal - *see* Otitis, media,
nonsuppurative, chronic, serous
exudative - *see* Otitis, media,
nonsuppurative, chronic
mucinous - *see* Otitis, media,
nonsuppurative, chronic, mucoid
mucoid - *see* Otitis, media, nonsuppurative,
chronic, mucoid
nonsuppurative NEC - *see* Otitis, media,
nonsuppurative, chronic
purulent - *see* Otitis, media, suppurative,
chronic
secretory - *see* Otitis, media,
nonsuppurative, chronic, mucoid
seromucinous - *see* Otitis, media,
nonsuppurative, chronic
serous - *see* Otitis, media, nonsuppurative,
chronic, serous
suppurative - *see* Otitis, media, suppurative,
chronic
transudative - *see* Otitis, media,
nonsuppurative, chronic, mucoid
exudative - *see* Otitis, media, suppurative
in (due to) (with)
influenza - *see* Influenza, with, otitis media
measles B05.3
scarlet fever A38.0
tuberculosis A18.6
viral disease NEC B34. [*H67.*]
mucoid - *see* Otitis, media, nonsuppurative
nonsuppurative H65.9-
acute or subacute NEC H65.19-
allergic H65.11-
recurrent H65.11-
recurrent H65.19-
secretory - *see* Otitis, media,
nonsuppurative, serous
serous H65.0-
recurrent H65.0-
chronic H65.49-
allergic H65.41-
mucoid H65.3-
serous H65.2-
postmeasles B05.3
purulent - *see* Otitis, media, suppurative
secretory - *see* Otitis, media, nonsuppurative
seromucinous - *see* Otitis, media,
nonsuppurative
serous - *see* Otitis, media, nonsuppurative
suppurative H66.4-
acute H66.00-
with rupture of ear drum H66.01-
recurrent H66.00-
with rupture of ear drum H66.01-
chronic - *see also* subcategory H66.3
atticoantral H66.2-
benign - *see* Otitis, media, suppurative,
chronic, tubotympanic
tubotympanic H66.1-

Otitis (acute) - *continued*
transudative - *see* Otitis, media,
nonsuppurative
tuberculous A18.6
Otocephaly Q18.2
Otolith syndrome - *see* subcategory H81.8
Otomycosis (diffuse) NEC B36.9 [*H62.40*]
in
aspergillosis B44.89
candidiasis B37.84
moniliasis B37.84
Otoporosis - *see* Otosclerosis
Otorrhagia (nontraumatic) H92.2-
traumatic
code by Type of injury
Otorrhea H92.1-
cerebrospinal G96.0
Otosclerosis (general) H80.9-
cochlear (endosteal) H80.2-
involving
otic capsule - *see* Otosclerosis, cochlear
oval window
nonobliterative H80.0-
obliterative H80.1-
round window - *see* Otosclerosis, cochlear
nonobliterative - *see* Otosclerosis, involving,
oval window, nonobliterative
obliterative - *see* Otosclerosis, involving, oval
window, obliterative
specified NEC H80.8-
Otospongiosis - *see* Otosclerosis
Otto's disease or pelvis M24.7
Outcome of delivery Z37.9
multiple births Z37.9
all liveborn Z37.50
quadruplets Z37.52
quintuplets Z37.53
sextuplets Z37.54
specified number NEC Z37.59
triplets Z37.51
all stillborn Z37.7
some liveborn Z37.60
quadruplets Z37.62
quintuplets Z37.63
sextuplets Z37.64
specified number NEC Z37.69
triplets Z37.61
single NEC Z37.9
liveborn Z37.0
stillborn Z37.1
twins NEC Z37.9
both liveborn Z37.2
both stillborn Z37.4
one liveborn, one stillborn Z37.3
Outlet - *see* condition
Ovalocytosis (congenital) (hereditary) - *see*
Elliptocytosis
Ovarian - *see* Condition
Ovariocele N83.4-
Ovaritis (cystic) - *see* Oophoritis
Ovary, ovarian - *see also* condition
resistant syndrome E28.39
vein syndrome N13.8
Overactive - *see also* Hyperfunction
adrenal cortex NEC E27.0
bladder N32.81
hypothalamus E23.3
thyroid - *see* Hyperthyroidism
Overactivity R46.3
child - *see* Disorder, attention-deficit
hyperactivity
Overbite (deep) (excessive) (horizontal)
(vertical) M26.29
Overbreathing - *see* Hyperventilation

Overconscientious personality F60.5
Overdevelopment - *see* Hypertrophy
Overdistension - *see* Distension
Overdose, overdosage (drug) - *see* Table of
   Drugs and Chemicals, by drug, poisoning
Overeating R63.2
   nonorganic origin F50.89
   psychogenic F50.89
Overexertion (effects) (exhaustion) T73.3
Overexposure (effects) T73.9
   exhaustion T73.2
Overfeeding - *see* Overeating
   newborn P92.4
Overfill, endodontic M27.52
Overgrowth, bone - *see* Hypertrophy, bone
Overhanging of dental restorative material
   (unrepairable) K08.52
Overheated (places) (effects) - *see* Heat
Overjet (excessive horizontal) M26.23
Overlaid, overlying (suffocation) - *see*
   Asphyxia, traumatic, due to mechanical threat
Overlap, excessive horizontal (teeth) M26.23
Overlapping toe (acquired) - *see also*
   Deformity, toe, specified NEC
   congenital (fifth toe) Q66.89
Overload
   circulatory, due to transfusion (blood) (blood
     components) (TACO) E87.71
   fluid E87.70
     due to transfusion (blood) (blood
      components) E87.71
     specified NEC E87.79
   iron, due to repeated red blood cell
     transfusions E83.111
   potassium (K) E87.5
   sodium (Na) E87.0
Overnutrition - *see* Hyperalimentation
Overproduction - *see also* Hypersecretion
   ACTH E27.0
   catecholamine E27.5
   growth hormone E22.0
Overprotection, child by parent Z62.1
Overriding
   aorta Q25.49
   finger (acquired) - *see* Deformity, finger
     congenital Q68.1
   toe (acquired) - *see also* Deformity, toe,
     specified NEC
     congenital Q66.89
Overstrained R53.83
   heart - *see* Hypertrophy, cardiac
Overuse, muscle NEC M70.8-
Overweight E66.3
Overworked R53.83
Oviduct - *see* condition
Ovotestis Q56.0
Ovulation (cycle)
   failure or lack of N97.0
   pain N94.0
Ovum - *see* condition
Owren's disease or syndrome
   (parahemophilia) D68.2
Ox heart - *see* Hypertrophy, cardiac
Oxalosis E72.53
Oxaluria E72.53
Oxycephaly, oxycephalic Q75.0
   syphilitic, congenital A50.02
Oxyuriasis B80
Oxyuris vermicularis (infestation) B80
Ozena J31.0

P

Pachyderma, pachydermia L85.9
   larynx (verrucosa) J38.7

Pachydermatocele (congenital) Q82.8
Pachydermoperiostosis - *see also*
   Osteoarthropathy, hypertrophic, specified type
   NEC
   clubbed nail M89.40 [*L62*]
Pachygyria Q04.3
Pachymeningitis (adhesive) (basal) (brain)
   (cervical) (chronic)(circumscribed)
   (external) (fibrous) (hemorrhagic)
   (hypertrophic) (internal) (purulent) (spinal)
   (suppurative) - *see* Meningitis
Pachyonychia (congenital) Q84.5
Pacinian tumor - *see* Neoplasm, skin, benign
Pad, knuckle or Garrod's M72.1
Paget-Schroetter syndrome I82.890
Paget's disease
   with infiltrating duct carcinoma - *see*
     Neoplasm, breast, malignant
   bone M88.9
     carpus M88.84-
     clavicle M88.81-
     femur M88.85-
     fibula M88.86-
     finger M88.84-
     humerus M88.82-
     ilium M88.85-
     in neoplastic disease - *see* Osteitis,
      deformans, in neoplastic disease
     ischium M88.85-
     metacarpus M88.84-
     metatarsus M88.87-
     multiple sites M88.89
     neck M88.88
     radius M88.83-
     rib M88.88
     scapula M88.81-
     skull M88.0
     tarsus M88.87-
     tibia M88.86-
     toe M88.87-
     ulna M88.83-
     vertebra M88.88
   breast (female) C50.01-
     male C50.02-
   extramammary - *see also* Neoplasm, skin,
   malignant
     anus C21.0
      margin C44.590
      skin C44.590
   intraductal carcinoma - *see* Neoplasm, breast,
   malignant
   malignant - *see* Neoplasm, skin, malignant
     breast (female) C50.01-
      male C50.02-
     unspecified site (female) C50.01-
      male C50.02-
   mammary - *see* Paget's disease, breast
   nipple - *see* Paget's disease, breast
   osteitis deformans - *see* Paget's disease, bone
Pain(s) - *see also* Painful R52
   abdominal R10.9
     colic R10.83
     generalized R10.84
      with acute abdomen R10.0
     lower R10.30
      left quadrant R10.32
      pelvic or perineal R10.2
      periumbilical R10.33
      right quadrant R10.31
     rebound - *see* Tenderness, abdominal,
   rebound
     severe with abdominal rigidity R10.0
     tenderness - *see* Tenderness, abdominal
     upper R10.10

Pain(s) - *continued*
     epigastric R10.13
      left quadrant R10.12
      right quadrant R10.11
   acute R52
     due to trauma G89.11
     neoplasm related G89.3
     postprocedural NEC G89.18
     post-thoracotomy G89.12
     specified by site
      code to Pain, by site
   adnexa (uteri) R10.2
   anginoid - *see* Pain, precordial
   anus K62.89
   arm - *see* Pain, limb, upper
   axillary (axilla) M79.62-
   back (postural) M54.9
   bladder R39.89
     associated with micturition - *see* Micturition,
     painful
     chronic R39.82
   bone - *see* Disorder, bone, specified type NEC
   breast N64.4
   broad ligament R10.2
   cancer associated (acute) (chronic) G89.3
   cecum - *see* Pain, abdominal
   cervicobrachial M53.1
   chest (central) R07.9
     anterior wall R07.89
     atypical R07.89
     ischemic I20.9
     musculoskeletal R07.89
     non-cardiac R07.89
     on breathing R07.1
     pleurodynia R07.81
     precordial R07.2
     wall (anterior) R07.89
   chronic G89.29
     associated with significant psychosocial
     dysfunction G89.4
     due to trauma G89.21
     neoplasm related G89.3
     postoperative NEC G89.28
     postprocedural NEC G89.28
     post-thoracotomy G89.22
     specified NEC G89.29
   coccyx M53.3
   colon - *see* Pain, abdominal
   coronary - *see* Angina
   costochondral R07.1
   diaphragm R07.1
   due to cancer G89.3
   due to device, implant or graft - *see also*
     Complications, by site and type, specified
     NEC T85.848
     arterial graft NEC T82.848
     breast (implant) T85.848
     catheter NEC T85.848
      dialysis (renal) T82.848
       intraperitoneal T85.848
      infusion NEC T82.848
       spinal (epidural) (subdural) T85.840
      urinary (indwelling) T83.84
     electronic (electrode) (pulse generator)
     (stimulator)
      bone T84.84
      cardiac T82.847
      nervous system (brain) (peripheral nerve)
       (spinal) T85.840
      urinary T83.84
     fixation, internal (orthopedic) NEC T84.84
     gastrointestinal (bile duct) (esophagus)
      T85.848
     genital NEC T83.84

Pain(s) - *continued*
  heart NEC T82.847
  infusion NEC T85.848
  joint prosthesis T84.84
  ocular (corneal graft) (orbital implant) NEC
    T85.848
  orthopedic NEC T84.84
  specified NEC T85.848
  urinary NEC T83.84
  vascular NEC T82.848
  ventricular intracranial shunt T85.840
  due to malignancy (primary) (secondary)
    G89.3
  ear - *see* subcategory H92.0
  epigastric, epigastrium R10.13
  eye - *see* Pain, ocular
  face, facial R51
    atypical G50.1
  female genital organs NEC N94.89
  finger - *see* Pain, limb, upper
  flank - *see* Pain, abdominal
  foot - *see* Pain, limb, lower
  gallbladder K82.9
  gas (intestinal) R14.1
  gastric - *see* Pain, abdominal
  generalized NOS R52
  genital organ
    female N94.89
    male N50.89
  groin - *see* Pain, abdominal, lower
  hand - *see* Pain, limb, upper
  head - *see* Headache
  heart - *see* Pain, precordial
  infra-orbital - *see* Neuralgia, trigeminal
  intercostal R07.82
  intermenstrual N94.0
  jaw R68.84
  joint M25.50
    ankle M25.57-
    elbow M25.52-
    finger M25.54-
    foot M25.57-
    hand M25.54-
    hip M25.55-
    knee M25.56-
    shoulder M25.51-
    toe M25.57-
    wrist M25.53-
  kidney N23
  laryngeal R07.0
  leg - *see* Pain, limb, lower
  limb M79.609
    lower M79.60-
      foot M79.67-
      lower leg M79.66-
      thigh M79.65-
      toe M79.67-
    upper M79.60-
      axilla M79.62-
      finger M79.64-
      forearm M79.63-
      hand M79.64-
      upper arm M79.62-
  loin M54.5
  low back M54.5
  lumbar region M54.5
  mandibular R68.84
  mastoid - *see* subcategory H92.0
  maxilla R68.84
  menstrual - *see also* Dysmenorrhea N94.6
  metacarpophalangeal (joint) - *see* Pain, joint,
    hand
  metatarsophalangeal (joint) - *see* Pain, joint,
    foot

Pain(s) - *continued*
  mouth K13.79
  muscle - *see* Myalgia
  musculoskeletal - *see also* Pain, by site M79.1
  myofascial M79.1
  nasal J34.89
  nasopharynx J39.2
  neck NEC M54.2
  nerve NEC - *see* Neuralgia
  neuromuscular - *see* Neuralgia
  nose J34.89
  ocular H57.1-
  ophthalmic - *see* Pain, ocular
  orbital region - *see* Pain, ocular
  ovary N94.89
  over heart - *see* Pain, precordial
  ovulation N94.0
  pelvic (female) R10.2
  penis N48.89
  pericardial - *see* Pain, precordial
  perineal, perineum R10.2
  pharynx J39.2
  pleura, pleural, pleuritic R07.81
  postoperative NOS G89.18
  postprocedural NOS G89.18
  post-thoracotomy G89.12
  precordial (region) R07.2
  premenstrual N94.3
  psychogenic (persistent) (any site) F45.41
  radicular (spinal) - *see* Radiculopathy
  rectum K62.89
  respiration R07.1
  retrosternal R07.2
  rheumatoid, muscular - *see* Myalgia
  rib R07.81
  root (spinal) - *see* Radiculopathy
  round ligament (stretch) R10.2
  sacroiliac M53.3
  sciatic - *see* Sciatica
  scrotum N50.82
  seminal vesicle N50.89
  shoulder M25.51-
  spermatic cord N50.89
  spinal root - *see* Radiculopathy
  spine M54.9
    cervical M54.2
    low back M54.5
      with sciatica M54.4-
    thoracic M54.6
  stomach - *see* Pain, abdominal
  substernal R07.2
  temporomandibular (joint) M26.62-
  testis N50.81-
  thoracic spine M54.6
    with radicular and visceral pain M54.14
  throat R07.0
  tibia - *see* Pain, limb, lower
  toe - *see* Pain, limb, lower
  tongue K14.6
  tooth K08.89
  trigeminal - *see* Neuralgia, trigeminal
  tumor associated G89.3
  ureter N23
  urinary (organ) (system) N23
  uterus NEC N94.89
  vagina R10.2
  vertebrogenic (syndrome) M54.89
  vesical R39.89
    associated with micturition - *see* Micturition,
    painful
  vulva R10.2
Painful - *see also* Pain
  coitus
    female N94.10

Painful - *continued*
    male N53.12
      psychogenic F52.6
  ejaculation (semen) N53.12
    psychogenic F52.6
  erection - *see* Priapism
  feet syndrome E53.8
  joint replacement (hip) (knee) T84.84
  menstruation - *see* Dysmenorrhea
    psychogenic F45.8
  micturition - *see* Micturition, painful
  respiration R07.1
  scar NEC L90.5
  wire sutures T81.89
Painter's colic - *see* subcategory T56.0
Palate - *see* condition
Palatoplegia K13.79
Palatoschisis - *see* Cleft, palate
Palilalia R48.8
Palliative care Z51.5
Pallor R23.1
  optic disc, temporal - *see* Atrophy, optic
Palmar - *see also* condition
  fascia - *see* condition
Palpable
  cecum K63.89
  kidney N28.89
  ovary N83.8
  prostate N42.9
  spleen - *see* Splenomegaly
Palpitations (heart) R00.2
  psychogenic F45.8
Palsy - *see also* Paralysis G83.9
  atrophic diffuse (progressive) G12.22
  Bell's - *see also* Palsy, facial
    newborn P11.3
  brachial plexus NEC G54.0
    newborn (birth injury) P14.3
  brain - *see* Palsy, cerebral
  bulbar (progressive) (chronic) G12.22
    of childhood (Fazio-Londe) G12.1
    pseudo NEC G12.29
    supranuclear (progressive) G23.1
  cerebral (congenital) G80.9
    ataxic G80.4
    athetoid G80.3
    choreoathetoid G80.3
    diplegic G80.8
      spastic G80.1
    dyskinetic G80.3
      athetoid G80.3
      choreoathetoid G80.3
      dystonic G80.3
    dystonic G80.3
    hemiplegic G80.8
      spastic G80.2
    mixed G80.8
    monoplegic G80.8
      spastic G80.1
    paraplegic G80.8
      spastic G80.1
    quadriplegic G80.8
      spastic G80.0
    spastic G80.1
      diplegic G80.1
      hemiplegic G80.2
      monoplegic G80.1
      quadriplegic G80.0
      specified NEC G80.1
      tetraplegic G80.0
    specified NEC G80.8
    syphilitic A52.12
      congenital A50.49
    tetraplegic G80.8

Palsy - *continued*
spastic G80.0
cranial nerve - *see also* Disorder, nerve, cranial
multiple G52.7
in
infectious disease B99 *[G53]*
neoplastic disease - *see also* Neoplasm
D49.9 *[G53]*
parasitic disease B89 *[G53]*
sarcoidosis D86.82
creeping G12.22
diver's T70.3
Erb's P14.0
facial G51.0
newborn (birth injury) P11.3
glossopharyngeal G52.1
Klumpke (-Déjérine) P14.1
lead - *see* subcategory T56.0
median nerve (tardy) G56.1-
nerve G58.9
specified NEC G58.8
peroneal nerve (acute) (tardy) G57.3-
progressive supranuclear G23.1
pseudobulbar NEC G12.29
radial nerve (acute) G56.3-
seventh nerve - *see also* Palsy, facial
newborn P11.3
shaking - *see* Parkinsonism
spastic (cerebral) (spinal) G80.1
ulnar nerve (tardy) G56.2-
wasting G12.29
Paludism - *see* Malaria
Panangiitis M30.0
Panaris, panaritium - *see also* Cellulitis, digit
with lymphangitis - *see* Lymphangitis, acute,
digit
Panarteritis nodosa M30.0
brain or cerebral I67.7
Pancake heart R93.1
with cor pulmonale (chronic) I27.81
Pancarditis (acute) (chronic) I51.89
rheumatic I09.89
active or acute I01.8
Pancoast's syndrome or tumor C34.1-
Pancolitis, ulcerative (chronic) K51.00
with
complication K51.019
abscess K51.014
fistula K51.013
obstruction K51.012
rectal bleeding K51.011
specified complication NEC K51.018
Pancreas, pancreatic - *see* condition
Pancreatitis (annular) (apoplectic)
(calcareous) (edematous) (hemorrhagic)
(malignant) (recurrent) (subacute)
(suppurative) K85.90
with necrosis (uninfected) K85.91
infected K85.92
acute (without necrosis or infection) K85.90
with necrosis (uninfected) K85.91
infected K85.92
alcohol induced (without necrosis or
infection) K85.20
with necrosis (uninfected) K85.21
infected K85.22
biliary (without necrosis or infection) K85.10
with necrosis (uninfected) K85.11
infected K85.12
drug induced (without necrosis or infection)
K85.30
with necrosis (uninfected) K85.31
infected K85.32

Pancreatitis - *continued*
with necrosis (uninfected) K85.11
infected K85.12
idiopathic (without necrosis or infection)
K85.00
with necrosis (uninfected) K85.01
infected K85.02
specified NEC (without necrosis or infection)
K85.80
with necrosis (uninfected) K85.81
infected K85.82
chronic (infectious) K86.1
alcohol-induced K86.0
recurrent K86.1
relapsing K86.1
cystic (chronic) K86.1
cytomegaloviral B25.2
fibrous (chronic) K86.1
gangrenous - *see* Pancreatitis, acute
gallstone (without necrosis or infection)
K85.10
with necrosis (uninfected) K85.11
infected K85.12
interstitial (chronic) K86.1
acute - *see also* Pancreatitis, acute K85.80
mumps B26.3
recurrent (chronic) K86.1
relapsing, chronic K86.1
syphilitic A52.74
Pancreatoblastoma - *see* Neoplasm, pancreas,
malignant
Pancreolithiasis K86.89
Pancytolysis D75.89
Pancytopenia (acquired) D61.818
with
malformations D61.09
myelodysplastic syndrome - *see* Syndrome,
myelodysplastic
antineoplastic chemotherapy induced D61.810
congenital D61.09
drug-induced NEC D61.811
PANDAS (pediatric autoimmune
neuropsychiatric disorders associated with
streptococcal infections
syndrome) D89.89
Panencephalitis, subacute, sclerosing A81.1
Panhematopenia D61.9
congenital D61.09
constitutional D61.09
splenic, primary D73.1
Panhemocytopenia D61.9
congenital D61.09
constitutional D61.09
Panhypogonadism E29.1
Panhypopituitarism E23.0
prepubertal E23.0
Panic (attack) (state) F41.0
reaction to exceptional stress (transient) F43.0
Panmyelopathy, familial, constitutional
D61.09
Panmyelophthisis D61.82
congenital D61.09
Panmyelosis (acute) (with myelofibrosis)
C94.4-
Panner's disease - *see* Osteochondrosis,
juvenile, humerus
Panneuritis endemica E51.11
Panniculitis (nodular) (nonsuppurative)
M79.3
back M54.00
cervical region M54.02
cervicothoracic region M54.03
lumbar region M54.06
lumbosacral region M54.07

Panniculitis - *continued*
multiple sites M54.09
occipito-atlanto-axial region M54.01
sacrococcygeal region M54.08
thoracic region M54.04
thoracolumbar region M54.05
lupus L93.2
mesenteric K65.4
neck M54.02
cervicothoracic region M54.03
occipito-atlanto-axial region M54.01
relapsing M35.6
Panniculus adiposus (abdominal) E65
Pannus (allergic) (cornea) (degenerativus)
(keratic) H16.42-
abdominal (symptomatic) E65
trachomatosus, trachomatous (active) A71.1
Panophthalmitis H44.01-
Pansinusitis (chronic) (hyperplastic)
(nonpurulent) (purulent) J32.4
acute J01.40
recurrent J01.41
tuberculous A15.8
Panuveitis (sympathetic) H44.11-
Panvalvular disease I08.9
specified NEC I08.8
PAPA (pyogenic arthritis, pyoderma
gangrenosum, and acne syndrome) M04.8
Papanicolaou smear, cervix Z12.4
as part of routine gynecological examination
Z01.419
with abnormal findings Z01.411
for suspected neoplasm Z12.4
nonspecific abnormal finding R87.619
routine Z01.419
with abnormal findings Z01.411
Papilledema (choked disc) H47.10
associated with
decreased ocular pressure H47.12
increased intracranial pressure H47.11
retinal disorder H47.13
Foster-Kennedy syndrome H47.14-
Papillitis H46.00
anus K62.89
chronic lingual K14.4
necrotizing, kidney N17.2
optic H46.0-
rectum K62.89
renal, necrotizing N17.2
tongue K14.0
Papilloma - *see also* Neoplasm, benign, by site
acuminatum (female) (male) (anogenital)
A63.0
basal cell L82.1
inflamed L82.0
benign pinta (primary) A67.0
bladder (urinary) (transitional cell) D41.4
choroid plexus (lateral ventricle) (third
ventricle) D33.0
anaplastic C71.5
fourth ventricle D33.1
malignant C71.5
renal pelvis (transitional cell) D41.1-
benign D30.1-
Schneiderian
specified site - *see* Neoplasm, benign, by site
unspecified site D14.0
serous surface
borderline malignancy
specified site - *see* Neoplasm, uncertain
behavior, by site
unspecified site D39.10
specified site - *see* Neoplasm, benign, by site
unspecified site D27.9

Papilloma - *continued*
 transitional (cell)
  bladder (urinary) D41.4
   inverted type - *see* Neoplasm, uncertain
    behavior, by site
  renal pelvis D41.1-
  ureter D41.2-
 ureter (transitional cell) D41.2-
  benign D30.2-
 urothelial - *see* Neoplasm, uncertain behavior,
  by site
 villous - *see* Neoplasm, uncertain behavior, by
  site
  adenocarcinoma in - *see* Neoplasm,
   malignant, by site
  in situ - *see* Neoplasm, in situ
 yaws, plantar or palmar A66.1
Papillomata, multiple, of yaws A66.1
Papillomatosis - *see also* Neoplasm, benign, by
  site
 confluent and reticulated L83
 cystic, breast - *see* Mastopathy, cystic
 ductal, breast - *see* Mastopathy, cystic
 intraductal (diffuse) - *see* Neoplasm, benign,
  by site
 subareolar duct D24-
**Papillomavirus, as cause of disease classified
 elsewhere** B97.7
Papillon-Léage and Psaume syndrome Q87.0
Papule(s) R23.8
 carate (primary) A67.0
 fibrous, of nose D22.39
 Gottron's L94.4
 pinta (primary) A67.0
Papulosis
 lymphomatoid C86.6
 malignant I77.89
Papyraceous fetus O31.0-
Para-albuminemia E88.09
Paracephalus Q89.7
Parachute mitral valve Q23.2
Paracoccidioidomycosis B41.9
 disseminated B41.7
 generalized B41.7
 mucocutaneous-lymphangitic B41.8
 pulmonary B41.0
 specified NEC B41.8
 visceral B41.8
Paradentosis K05.4
Paraffinoma T88.8
Paraganglioma D44.7
 adrenal D35.0-
  malignant C74.1-
 aortic body D44.7
  malignant C75.5
 carotid body D44.6
  malignant C75.4
 chromaffin - *see also* Neoplasm, benign, by
  site
  malignant - *see* Neoplasm, malignant, by site
 extra-adrenal D44.7
  malignant C75.5
   specified site - *see* Neoplasm, malignant, by
    site
   unspecified site C75.5
  specified site - *see* Neoplasm, uncertain
   behavior, by site
  unspecified site D44.7
 gangliocytic D13.2
  specified site - *see* Neoplasm, benign, by site
  unspecified site D13.2
 glomus jugulare D44.7
  malignant C75.5
 jugular D44.7

Paraganglioma - *continued*
 malignant C75.5
  specified site - *see* Neoplasm, malignant, by
   site
  unspecified site C75.5
 nonchromaffin D44.7
  malignant C75.5
   specified site - *see* Neoplasm, malignant, by
    site
   unspecified site C75.5
  specified site - *see* Neoplasm, uncertain
   behavior, by site
  unspecified site D44.7
 parasympathetic D44.7
  specified site - *see* Neoplasm, uncertain
   behavior, by site
  unspecified site D44.7
 specified site - *see* Neoplasm, uncertain
  behavior, by site
 sympathetic D44.7
  specified site - *see* Neoplasm, uncertain
   behavior, by site
  unspecified site D44.7
 unspecified site D44.7
Parageusia R43.2
 psychogenic F45.8
Paragonimiasis B66.4
Paragranuloma, Hodgkin - *see* Lymphoma,
 Hodgkin, specified NEC
Parahemophilia - *see also* Defect, coagulation
 D68.2
Parakeratosis R23.4
 variegata L41.0
Paralysis, paralytic (complete) (incomplete)
 G83.9
 with
  syphilis A52.17
 abducens, abducent (nerve) - *see* Strabismus,
  paralytic, sixth nerve
 abductor, lower extremity G57.9-
 accessory nerve G52.8
 accommodation - *see also* Paresis, of
  accommodation
  hysterical F44.89
 acoustic nerve (except Deafness) - *see*
  subcategory H93.3
 agitans - *see also* Parkinsonism G20
  arteriosclerotic G21.4
 alternating (oculomotor) G83.89
 amyotrophic G12.21
 ankle G57.9-
 anus (sphincter) K62.89
 arm - *see* Monoplegia, upper limb
 ascending (spinal), acute G61.0
 association G12.29
 asthenic bulbar G70.00
  with exacerbation (acute) G70.01
  in crisis G70.01
 ataxic (hereditary) G11.9
  general (syphilitic) A52.17
 atrophic G58.9
  infantile, acute - *see* Poliomyelitis, paralytic
  progressive G12.22
  spinal (acute) - *see* Poliomyelitis, paralytic
 axillary G54.0
 Babinski Nageotte's G83.89
 Bell's G51.0
  newborn P11.3
 Benedikt's G46.3
 birth injury P14.9
  spinal cord P11.5
 bladder (neurogenic) (sphincter) N31.2
 bowel, colon or intestine K56.0
 brachial plexus G54.0

Paralysis, paralytic - *continued*
 birth injury P14.3
  newborn (birth injury) P14.3
 brain G83.9
  diplegia G83.0
  triplegia G83.89
 bronchial J98.09
 Brown-Séquard G83.81
 bulbar (chronic) (progressive) G12.22
  infantile - *see* Poliomyelitis, paralytic
  poliomyelitic - *see* Poliomyelitis, paralytic
  pseudo G12.29
 bulbospinal G70.00
  with exacerbation (acute) G70.01
  in crisis G70.01
 cardiac - *see also* Failure, heart I50.9
 cerebrocerebellar, diplegic G80.1
 cervical
  plexus G54.2
  sympathetic G90.09
 Céstan-Chenais G46.3
 Charcot-Marie-tooth type G60.0
 Clark's G80.9
 colon K56.0
 compressed air T70.3
 compression
  arm G56.9-
  leg G57.9-
  lower extremity G57.9-
  upper extremity G56.9-
 congenital (cerebral) - *see* Palsy, cerebral
 conjugate movement (gaze) (of eye) H51.0
  cortical (nuclear) (supranuclear) H51.0
 cordis - *see* Failure, heart
 cranial or cerebral nerve G52.9
 creeping G12.22
 crossed leg G83.89
 crutch - *see* Injury, brachial plexus
 deglutition R13.0
  hysterical F44.4
 dementia A52.17
 descending (spinal) NEC G12.29
 diaphragm (flaccid) J98.6
  due to accidental dissection of phrenic nerve
   during procedure - *see* Puncture, accidental
   complicating surgery digestive organs NEC
   K59.8
 diplegic - *see* Diplegia
 divergence (nuclear) H51.8
 diver's T70.3
 Duchenne's
  birth injury P14.0
  due to or associated with
   motor neuron disease G12.22
   muscular dystrophy G71.0
  due to intracranial or spinal birth injury - *see*
   Palsy, cerebral
 embolic (current episode) I63.4-
 Erb (-Duchenne) (birth) (newborn) P14.0
 Erb's syphilitic spastic spinal A52.17
 esophagus K22.8
 eye muscle (extrinsic) H49.9
  intrinsic - *see also* Paresis, of
   accommodation
 facial (nerve) G51.0
  birth injury P11.3
  congenital P11.3
  following operation NEC - *see* Puncture,
   accidental complicating surgery
   newborn (birth injury) P11.3
 familial (recurrent) (periodic) G72.3
  spastic G11.4
 fauces J39.2
 finger G56.9-

Paralysis, paralytic - *continued*
gait R26.1
gastric nerve (nondiabetic) G52.2
gaze, conjugate H51.0
general (progressive) (syphilitic) A52.17
  juvenile A50.45
glottis J38.00
  bilateral J38.02
  unilateral J38.01
gluteal G54.1
Gubler (-Millard) G46.3
hand - *see* Monoplegia, upper limb
heart - *see* Arrest, cardiac
hemiplegic - *see* Hemiplegia
hyperkalemic periodic (familial) G72.3
hypoglossal (nerve) G52.3
hypokalemic periodic G72.3
hysterical F44.4
ileus K56.0
infantile - *see also* Poliomyelitis, paralytic
  A80.30
  bulbar - *see* Poliomyelitis, paralytic
  cerebral - *see* Palsy, cerebral
  spastic - *see* Palsy, cerebral, spastic
infective - *see* Poliomyelitis, paralytic
inferior nuclear G83.9
internuclear - *see* Ophthalmoplegia,
internuclear
intestine K56.0
iris H57.09
  due to diphtheria (toxin) A36.89
ischemic, Volkmann's (complicating trauma)
  T79.6
Jackson's G83.89
jake - *see* Poisoning, food, noxious, plant
Jamaica ginger (jake) G62.2
juvenile general A50.45
Klumpke (-Déjérine) (birth) (newborn) P14.1
labioglossal (laryngeal) (pharyngeal) G12.29
Landry's G61.0
laryngeal nerve (recurrent) (superior)
(unilateral) J38.00
  bilateral J38.02
  unilateral J38.01
larynx J38.00
  bilateral J38.02
  due to diphtheria (toxin) A36.2
  unilateral J38.01
lateral G12.23
lead - *see* subcategory T56.0
left side - *see* Hemiplegia
leg G83.1-
  both - *see* Paraplegia
  crossed G83.89
  hysterical F44.4
  psychogenic F44.4
  transient or transitory R29.818
    traumatic NEC - *see* Injury, nerve, leg
levator palpebrae superioris - *see*
  Blepharoptosis, paralytic
limb - *see* Monoplegia
lip K13.0
Lissauer's A52.17
lower limb - *see* Monoplegia, lower limb
  both - *see* Paraplegia
lung J98.4
median nerve G56.1-
medullary (tegmental) G83.89
mesencephalic NEC G83.89
  tegmental G83.89
middle alternating G83.89
Millard-Gubler-Foville G46.3
monoplegic - *see* Monoplegia
motor G83.9

Paralysis, paralytic - *continued*
muscle, muscular NEC G72.89
  due to nerve lesion G58.9
  eye (extrinsic) H49.9
    intrinsic - *see* Paresis, of accommodation
    oblique - *see* Strabismus, paralytic, fourth
nerve
  iris sphincter H21.9
  ischemic (Volkmann's) (complicating
    trauma) T79.6
  progressive G12.21
  pseudohypertrophic G71.0
musculocutaneous nerve G56.9-
musculospiral G56.9-
nerve - *see also* Disorder, nerve
  abducent - *see* Strabismus, paralytic, sixth
  nerve
  accessory G52.8
  auditory (except Deafness) - *see* subcategory
    H93.3
  birth injury P14.9
  cranial or cerebral G52.9
  facial G51.0
    birth injury P11.3
    congenital P11.3
    newborn (birth injury) P11.3
  fourth or trochlear - *see* Strabismus,
    paralytic, fourth nerve
  newborn (birth injury) P14.9
  oculomotor - *see* Strabismus, paralytic, third
    nerve
  phrenic (birth injury) P14.2
  radial G56.3-
  seventh or facial G51.0
    newborn (birth injury) P11.3
  sixth or abducent - *see* Strabismus, paralytic,
  sixth nerve
  syphilitic A52.15
  third or oculomotor - *see* Strabismus,
    paralytic, third nerve
  trigeminal G50.9
  trochlear - *see* Strabismus, paralytic, fourth
    nerve
  ulnar G56.2-
normokalemic periodic G72.3
ocular H49.9
  alternating G83.89
oculofacial, congenital (Moebius) Q87.0
oculomotor (external bilateral) (nerve) - *see*
  Strabismus, paralytic, third nerve
palate (soft) K13.79
paratrigeminal G50.9
periodic (familial) (hyperkalemic)
  (hypokalemic) (myotonic) (normokalemic)
  (potassium sensitive) (secondary) G72.3
peripheral autonomic nervous system - *see*
  Neuropathy, peripheral, autonomic
peroneal (nerve) G57.3-
pharynx J39.2
phrenic nerve G56.8-
plantar nerve(s) G57.6-
pneumogastric nerve G52.2
poliomyelitis (current) - *see* Poliomyelitis,
  paralytic
popliteal nerve G57.3-
postepileptic transitory G83.84
progressive (atrophic) (bulbar) (spinal) G12.22
  general A52.17
  infantile acute - *see* Poliomyelitis, paralytic
  supranuclear G23.1
pseudobulbar G12.29
pseudohypertrophic (muscle) G71.0
psychogenic F44.4
quadriceps G57.9-

Paralysis, paralytic - *continued*
quadriplegic - *see* Tetraplegia
radial nerve G56.3-
rectus muscle (eye) H49.9
recurrent isolated sleep G47.53
respiratory (muscle) (system) (tract) R06.81
  center NEC G93.89
  congenital P28.89
  newborn P28.89
right side - *see* Hemiplegia
saturnine *see* subcategory T56.0
sciatic nerve G57.0-
senile G83.9
shaking - *see* Parkinsonism
shoulder G56.9-
sleep, recurrent isolated G47.53
spastic G83.9
  cerebral - *see* Palsy, cerebral, spastic
  congenital (cerebral) - *see* Palsy, cerebral,
    spastic
  familial G11.4
  hereditary G11.4
  quadriplegic G80.0
  syphilitic (spinal) A52.17
sphincter, bladder - *see* Paralysis, bladder
spinal (cord) G83.9
  accessory nerve G52.8
  acute - *see* Poliomyelitis, paralytic
  ascending acute G61.0
  atrophic (acute) - *see also* Poliomyelitis,
    paralytic
    spastic, syphilitic A52.17
  congenital NEC - *see* Palsy, cerebral
  infantile - *see* Poliomyelitis, paralytic
  hereditary G95.89
  progressive G12.21
  sequelae NEC G83.89
sternomastoid G52.8
stomach K31.84
  diabetic - *see* Diabetes, by type, with
    gastroparesis
  nerve G52.2
    diabetic - *see* Diabetes, by type, with
    gastroparesis
stroke - *see* Infarct, brain
subcapsularis G56.8-
supranuclear (progressive) G23.1
sympathetic G90.8
  cervical G90.09
  nervous system - *see* Neuropathy, peripheral,
    autonomic
syndrome G83.9
  specified NEC G83.89
syphilitic spastic spinal (Erb's) A52.17
thigh G57.9-
throat J39.2
  diphtheritic A36.0
  muscle J39.2
thrombotic (current episode) I63.3-
thumb G56.9-
tick - *see* Toxicity, venom, arthropod,
  specified NEC
Todd's (postepileptic transitory paralysis)
  G83.84
toe G57.6-
tongue K14.8
transient R29.5
  arm or leg NEC R29.818
  traumatic NEC - *see* Injury, nerve
trapezius G52.8
traumatic, transient NEC - *see* Injury, nerve
trembling - *see* Parkinsonism
triceps brachii G56.9-
trigeminal nerve G50.9

Paralysis, paralytic - *continued*
trochlear (nerve) - *see* Strabismus, paralytic, fourth nerve
ulnar nerve G56.2-
upper limb - *see* Monoplegia, upper limb
uremic N18.9 [*G99.8*]
uveoparotitic D86.89
uvula K13.79
postdiphtheritic A36.0
vagus nerve G52.2
vasomotor NEC G90.8
velum palati K13.79
vesical - *see* Paralysis, bladder
vestibular nerve (except Vertigo) - *see* subcategory H93.3
vocal cords J38.00
bilateral J38.02
unilateral J38.01
Volkmann's (complicating trauma) T79.6
wasting G12.29
Weber's G46.3
wrist G56.9-
Paramedial urethrovesical orifice Q64.79
Paramenia N92.6
Parametritis - *see also* Disease, pelvis, inflammatory N73.2
acute N73.0
complicating abortion - *see* Abortion, by type, complicated by, parametritis
Parametrium, parametric - *see* condition
Paramnesia - *see* Amnesia
Paramolar K00.1
Paramyloidosis E85.89
Paramyoclonus multiplex G25.3
Paramyotonia (congenita) G71.19
Parangi - *see* Yaws
Paranoia (querulans) F22
senile F03
Paranoid
dementia (senile) F03
praecox - *see* Schizophrenia
personality F60.0
psychosis (climacteric) (involutional) (menopausal) F22
psychogenic (acute) F23
senile F03
reaction (acute) F23
chronic F22
schizophrenia F20.0
state (climacteric) (involutional) (menopausal) (simple) F22
senile F03
tendencies F60.0
traits F60.0
trends F60.0
type, psychopathic personality F60.0
Paraparesis - *see* Paraplegia
Paraphasia R47.02
Paraphilia F65.9
Paraphimosis (congenital) N47.2
chancroidal A57
Paraphrenia, paraphrenic (late) F22
schizophrenia F20.0
Paraplegia (lower) G82.20
ataxic - *see* Degeneration, combined, spinal cord
complete G82.21
congenital (cerebral) G80.8
spastic G80.1
familial spastic G11.4
functional (hysterical) F44.4
hereditary, spastic G11.4
hysterical F44.4
incomplete G82.22

Paraplegia - *continued*
Pott's A18.01
psychogenic F44.4
spastic
Erb's spinal, syphilitic A52.17
hereditary G11.4
tropical G04.1
syphilitic (spastic) A52.17
tropical spastic G04.1
Parapoxvirus B08.60
specified NEC B08.69
Paraproteinemia D89.2
benign (familial) D89.2
monoclonal D47.2
secondary to malignant disease D47.2
Parapsoriasis L41.9
en plaques L41.4
guttata L41.1
large plaque L41.4
retiform, retiformis L41.5
small plaque L41.3
specified NEC L41.8
varioliformis (acuta) L41.0
Parasitic - *see also* condition
disease NEC B89
stomatitis B37.0
sycosis (beard) (scalp) B35.0
twin Q89.4
Parasitism B89
intestinal B82.9
skin B88.9
specified - *see* Infestation
Parasitophobia F40.218
Parasomnia G47.50
due to
alcohol
abuse F10.182
dependence F10.282
use F10.982
amphetamines
abuse F15.182
dependence F15.282
use F15.982
caffeine
abuse F15.182
dependence F15.282
use F15.982
cocaine
abuse F14.182
dependence F14.282
use F14.982
drug NEC
abuse F19.182
dependence F19.282
use F19.982
opioid
abuse F11.182
dependence F11.282
use F11.982
psychoactive substance NEC
abuse F19.182
dependence F19.282
use F19.982
sedative, hypnotic, or anxiolytic
abuse F13.182
dependence F13.282
use F13.982
stimulant NEC
abuse F15.182
dependence F15.282
use F15.982
in conditions classified elsewhere G47.54
nonorganic origin F51.8
organic G47.50
specified NEC G47.59

Paraspadias Q54.9
Paraspasmus facialis G51.8
Parasuicide (attempt)
history of (personal) Z91.5
in family Z81.8
Parathyroid gland - *see* condition
Parathyroid tetany E20.9
Paratrachoma A74.0
Paratyphlitis - *see* Appendicitis
Paratyphoid (fever) - *see* Fever, paratyphoid
Paratyphus - *see* Fever, paratyphoid
Paraurethral duct Q64.79
nonorganic origin F51.5
Paraurethritis - *see also* Urethritis
gonococcal (acute) (chronic) (with abscess) A54.1
Paravaccinia NEC B08.04
Paravaginitis - *see* Vaginitis
Parencephalitis - *see also* Encephalitis
sequelae G09
Parent-child conflict - *see* Conflict, parent-child estrangement NEC Z62.890
Paresis - *see also* Paralysis
accommodation - *see* Paresis, of accommodation
Bernhardt's G57.1-
bladder (sphincter) - *see also* Paralysis, bladder
tabetic A52.17
bowel, colon or intestine K56.0
extrinsic muscle, eye H49.9
general (progressive) (syphilitic) A52.17
juvenile A50.45
heart - *see* Failure, heart
insane (syphilitic) A52.17
juvenile (general) A50.45
of accommodation H52.52-
peripheral progressive (idiopathic) G60.3
pseudohypertrophic G71.0
senile G83.9
syphilitic (general) A52.17
congenital A50.45
vesical NEC N31.2
Paresthesia (see also Disturbance, sensation, skin) R20.2
Bernhardt G57.1-
Paretic - *see* condition
Parinaud's
conjunctivitis H10.89
oculoglandular syndrome H10.89
ophthalmoplegia H49.88-
Parkinsonism (idiopathic) (primary) G20
with neurogenic orthostatic hypotension (symptomatic) G90.3
arteriosclerotic G21.4
dementia G31.83 [*F02.80*]
with behavioral disturbance G31.83 [*F02.81*]
due to
drugs NEC G21.19
neuroleptic G21.11
medication-induced NEC G21.19
neuroleptic induced G21.11
postencephalitic G21.3
secondary G21.9
due to
arteriosclerosis G21.4
drugs NEC G21.19
neuroleptic G21.11
encephalitis G21.3
external agents NEC G21.2
syphilis A52.19
specified NEC G21.8
syphilitic A52.19

Parkinsonism - *continued*
  treatment-induced NEC G21.19
  vascular G21.4
Parkinson's disease, syndrome or tremor -
  see Parkinsonism
Parodontitis - *see* Periodontitis
Parodontosis K05.4
Paronychia - *see also* Cellulitis, digit
  with lymphangitis - *see* Lymphangitis, acute,
    digit
  candidal (chronic) B37.2
  tuberculous (primary) A18.4
Parorexia (psychogenic) F50.89
Parosmia R43.1
  psychogenic F45.8
Parotid gland - *see* condition
Parotitis, parotiditis (allergic)(nonspecific
  toxic) (purulent) (septic) (suppurative) - *see*
  also Sialoadenitis
  epidemic - *see* Mumps
  infectious - *see* Mumps
  postoperative K91.89
  surgical K91.89
Parrot fever A70
Parrot's disease (early congenital syphilitic
  pseudoparalysis) A50.02
Parry-Romberg syndrome G51.8
Parry's disease or syndrome E05.00
  with thyroid storm E05.01
Pars planitis - *see* Cyclitis
Parsonage (-Aldren) -turner syndrome G54.5
Parson's disease (exophthalmic goiter) E05.00
  with thyroid storm E05.01
Particolored infant Q82.8
Parturition - *see* Delivery **Parulis** K04.7
  with sinus K04.6
Parvovirus, as cause of disease classified
  elsewhere B97.6
Pasini and Pierini's atrophoderma L90.3
Passage
  false, urethra N36.5
  meconium (newborn) during delivery P03.82
  of sounds or bougies - *see* Attention to,
    artificial, opening
Passive - *see* condition
  smoking Z77.22
Pasteurella septica A28.0
Pasteurellosis - *see* Infection, Pasteurella
PAT (paroxysmal atrial tachycardia) I47.1
Patau's syndrome - *see* Trisomy, 13
Patches
  mucous (syphilitic) A51.39
    congenital A50.07
  smokers' (mouth) K13.24
Patellar - *see* condition
Patent - *see also* Imperfect, closure
  canal of Nuck Q52.4
  cervix N88.3
  ductus arteriosus or Botallo's Q25.0
  foramen
    botalli Q21.1
    ovale Q21.1
  interauricular septum Q21.1
  interventricular septum Q21.0
  omphalomesenteric duct Q43.0
  os (uteri) - *see* Patent, cervix
  ostium secundum Q21.1
  urachus Q64.4
  vitelline duct Q43.0
Paterson (-Brown)(-Kelly) syndrome or web
  D50.1
Pathologic, pathological - *see also* condition
  asphyxia R09.01
  fire-setting F63.1

Pathologic, pathological - *continued*
  gambling F63.0
  ovum O02.0
  resorption, tooth K03.3
  stealing F63.2
Pathology (of) - *see* Disease
  periradicular, associated with previous
    endodontic treatment NEC M27.59
Pattern, sleep-wake, irregular G47.23
Patulous - *see also* Imperfect, closure
  (congenital)
  alimentary tract Q45.8
    lower Q43.8
    upper Q40.8
  eustachian tube H69.0-
Pause, sinoatrial I49.5
Paxton's disease B36.2
Pearl(s)
  enamel K00.2
  Epstein's K09.8
Pearl-worker's disease - *see* Osteomyelitis,
  specified type NEC
Pectenosis K62.4
Pectoral - *see* condition
Pectus
  carinatum (congenital) Q67.7
    acquired M95.4
    rachitic sequelae (late effect) E64.3
  excavatum (congenital) Q67.6
    acquired M95.4
    rachitic sequelae (late effect) E64.3
  recurvatum (congenital) Q67.6
Pedatrophia E41
Pederosis F65.4
Pediculosis (infestation) B85.2
  capitis (head-louse) (any site) B85.0
  corporis (body-louse) (any site) B85.1
  eyelid B85.0
  mixed (classifiable to more than one of the
    titles B85.0-b85.3) B85.4
  pubis (pubic louse) (any site) B85.3
  vestimenti B85.1
  vulvae B85.3
Pediculus (infestation) - *see* Pediculosis
Pedophilia F65.4
Peg-shaped teeth K00.2
Pelade - *see* Alopecia, areata
Pelger-Huët anomaly or syndrome D72.0
Peliosis (rheumatica) D69.0
  hepatis K76.4
    with toxic liver disease K71.8
Pelizaeus-Merzbacher disease E75.29
Pellagra (alcoholic) (with polyneuropathy)
  E52
Pellagra-cerebellar-ataxia-renal
  aminoaciduria syndrome E72.02
Pellegrini (-Stieda) disease or syndrome - *see*
  Bursitis, tibial collateral
Pellizzi's syndrome E34.8
Pel's crisis A52.11
Pelvic - *see also* condition
  examination (periodic) (routine) Z01.419
    with abnormal findings Z01.411
  kidney, congenital Q63.2
Pelviolithiasis - *see* Calculus, kidney
Pelviperitonitis - *see also* Peritonitis, pelvic
  gonococcal A54.24
  puerperal O85
Pelvis - *see* condition or type
Pemphigoid L12.9
  benign, mucous membrane L12.1
  bullous L12.0
  cicatricial L12.1
  juvenile L12.2

Pemphigoid - *continued*
  ocular L12.1
  specified NEC L12.8
Pemphigus L10.9
  benign familial (chronic) Q82.8
  Brazilian L10.3
  circinatus L13.0
  conjunctiva L12.1
  drug-induced L10.5
  erythematosus L10.4
  foliaceous L10.2
  gangrenous - *see* Gangrene
  neonatorum L01.03
  ocular L12.1
  paraneoplastic L10.81
  specified NEC L10.89
  syphilitic (congenital) A50.06
  vegetans L10.1
  vulgaris L10.0
  wildfire L10.3
Pendred's syndrome E07.1
Pendulous
  abdomen, in pregnancy - *see* Pregnancy,
    complicated by, abnormal, pelvic organs or
    tissues NEC
  breast N64.89
Penetrating wound - *see also* Puncture
  with internal injury - *see* Injury, by site
  eyeball - *see* Puncture, eyeball
  orbit (with or without foreign body) - *see*
    Puncture, orbit
  uterus by instrument with or following ectopic
    or molar pregnancy O08.6
Penicillosis B48.4
Penis - *see* condition
Penitis N48.29
Pentalogy of Fallot Q21.8
Pentasomy X syndrome Q97.1
Pentosuria (essential) E74.8
Percreta placenta O43.23-
Peregrinating patient - *see* Disorder, factitious
Perforation, perforated (nontraumatic) (of)
  accidental during procedure (blood vessel)
    (nerve) (organ) - *see* Complication,
    accidental puncture or laceration
  antrum - *see* Sinusitis, maxillary
  appendix K35.2
    with localized peritonitis K35.3
  atrial septum, multiple Q21.1
  attic, ear - *see* Perforation, tympanum, attic
  bile duct (common) (hepatic) K83.2
    cystic K82.2
  bladder (urinary)
    with or following ectopic or molar pregnancy
      O08.6
    obstetrical trauma O71.5
    traumatic S37.29
      at delivery O71.5
  bowel K63.1
    with or following ectopic or molar pregnancy
      O08.6
    newborn P78.0
    obstetrical trauma O71.5
    traumatic - *see* Laceration, intestine
  broad ligament N83.8
    with or following ectopic or molar pregnancy
      O08.6
    obstetrical trauma O71.6
  by
    device, implant or graft - *see also*
      Complications, by site and type, mechanical
      T85.628
      arterial graft NEC - *see* Complication,
        cardiovascular device, mechanical,

Perforation, perforated - *continued*
  vascular
    breast (implant) T85.49
    catheter NEC T85.698
      cystostomy T83.090
      dialysis (renal) T82.49
        intraperitoneal T85.691
      infusion NEC T82.594
        spinal (epidural) (subdural) T85.690
      urinary - *see also* Complications, catheter,
      urinary T83.098
    electronic (electrode) (pulse generator)
    (stimulator)
      bone T84.390
      cardiac T82.199
        electrode T82.190
        pulse generator T82.191
        specified type NEC T82.198
      nervous system - *see* Complication,
      prosthetic device, mechanical, electronic
      nervous system stimulator
      urinary - *see* Complication, genitourinary,
      device, urinary, mechanical
    fixation, internal (orthopedic) NEC - *see*
    Complication, fixation device, mechanical
    gastrointestinal - *see* Complications,
    prosthetic device, mechanical,
    gastrointestinal device
    genital NEC T83.498
      intrauterine contraceptive device T83.39
      penile prosthesis T83.490
    heart NEC - *see* Complication,
    cardiovascular device, mechanical
    joint prosthesis - *see* Complications, joint
    prosthesis, mechanical, specified NEC, by
    site
    ocular NEC - *see* Complications, prosthetic
    device, mechanical, ocular device
    orthopedic NEC - *see* Complication,
    orthopedic, device, mechanical
    specified NEC T85.628
    urinary NEC - *see also* Complication,
    genitourinary, device, urinary, mechanical
    graft T83.29
    vascular NEC - *see* Complication,
    cardiovascular device, mechanical
    ventricular intracranial shunt T85.09
  foreign body left accidentally in operative
  wound T81.539
  instrument (any) during a procedure,
  accidental - *see* Puncture, accidental
  complicating surgery　cecum K35.2
    with localized peritonitis K35.3
  cervix (uteri) N88.8
    with or following ectopic or molar pregnancy
    O08.6
    obstetrical trauma O71.3
  colon K63.1
    newborn P78.0
    obstetrical trauma O71.5
    traumatic - *see* Laceration, intestine, large
  common duct (bile) K83.2
  cornea (due to ulceration) - *see* Ulcer, cornea,
  perforated
  cystic duct K82.2
  diverticulum (intestine) K57.80
    with bleeding K57.81
    large intestine K57.20
      with
        bleeding K57.21
        small intestine K57.40
          with bleeding K57.41
    small intestine K57.00
      with

Perforation, perforated - *continued*
    bleeding K57.01
    large intestine K57.40
      with bleeding K57.41
  ear drum - *see* Perforation, tympanum
  esophagus K22.3
  ethmoidal sinus - *see* Sinusitis, ethmoidal
  frontal sinus - *see* Sinusitis, frontal
  gallbladder K82.2
  heart valve - *see* Endocarditis
  ileum K63.1
    newborn P78.0
    obstetrical trauma O71.5
    traumatic - *see* Laceration, intestine, small
  instrumental, surgical (accidental) (blood
  vessel) (nerve) (organ) - *see* Puncture,
  accidental complicating surgery　intestine
  NEC K63.1
    with ectopic or molar pregnancy O08.6
    newborn P78.0
    obstetrical trauma O71.5
    traumatic - *see* Laceration, intestine
    ulcerative NEC K63.1
      newborn P78.0
  jejunum, jejunal K63.1
    obstetrical trauma O71.5
    traumatic - *see* Laceration, intestine, small
    ulcer - *see* Ulcer, gastrojejunal, with
    perforation
  joint prosthesis - *see* Complications, joint
  prosthesis, mechanical, specified NEC, by
  site
  mastoid (antrum) (cell) - *see* Disorder,
  mastoid, specified NEC
  maxillary sinus - *see* Sinusitis, maxillary
  membrana tympani - *see* Perforation,
  tympanum
  nasal
    septum J34.89
      congenital Q30.3
      syphilitic A52.73
    sinus J34.89
      congenital Q30.8
      due to sinusitis - *see* Sinusitis
  palate - *see also* Cleft, palate Q35.9
    syphilitic A52.79
  palatine vault - *see also* Cleft, palate, hard
  Q35.1
    syphilitic A52.79
    congenital A50.59
  pars flaccida (ear drum) - *see* Perforation,
  tympanum, attic
  pelvic
    floor S31.030
      with
        ectopic or molar pregnancy O08.6
        penetration into retroperitoneal space
        S31.031
        retained foreign body S31.040
          with penetration into retroperitoneal
          space S31.041
      following ectopic or molar pregnancy
      O08.6
      obstetrical trauma O70.1
    organ S37.99
      adrenal gland S37.818
      bladder - *see* Perforation, bladder
      fallopian tube S37.599
        bilateral S37.592
        unilateral S37.591
      kidney S37.09-
        obstetrical trauma O71.5
      ovary S37.499
        bilateral S37.492

Perforation, perforated - *continued*
      unilateral S37.491
    prostate S37.828
    specified organ NEC S37.898
    ureter - *see* Perforation, ureter
    urethra - *see* Perforation, urethra
    uterus - *see* Perforation, uterus
  perineum - *see* Laceration, perineum
  pharynx J39.2
  rectum K63.1
    newborn P78.0
    obstetrical trauma O71.5
    traumatic S36.63
  root canal space due to endodontic treatment
  M27.51
  sigmoid K63.1
    newborn P78.0
    obstetrical trauma O71.5
    traumatic S36.533
  sinus (accessory) (chronic) (nasal) J34.89
  sphenoidal sinus - *see* Sinusitis, sphenoidal
  surgical (accidental) (by instrument) (blood
  vessel) (nerve) (organ) - *see* Puncture,
  accidental complicating surgery　traumatic
    external - *see* Puncture
    eye - *see* Puncture, eyeball
    internal organ - *see* Injury, by site
  tympanum, tympanic (membrane) (persistent
  post-traumatic) (postinflammatory) H72.9-
    attic H72.1-
      multiple - *see* Perforation, tympanum,
    multiple
      total - *see* Perforation, tympanum, total
    central H72.0-
      multiple - *see* Perforation, tympanum,
    multiple
      total - *see* Perforation, tympanum, total
    marginal NEC - *see* subcategory H72.2
    multiple H72.81-
    pars flaccida - *see* Perforation, tympanum,
    attic
    total H72.82-
    traumatic, current episode S09.2-
  typhoid, gastrointestinal - *see* Typhoid
  ulcer - *see* Ulcer, by site, with perforation
  ureter N28.89
    traumatic S37.19
  urethra N36.8
    with ectopic or molar pregnancy O08.6
    following ectopic or molar pregnancy O08.6
    obstetrical trauma O71.5
    traumatic S37.39
      at delivery O71.5
  uterus
    with ectopic or molar pregnancy O08.6
    by intrauterine contraceptive device T83.39
    following ectopic or molar pregnancy O08.6
    obstetrical trauma O71.1
    traumatic S37.69
      obstetric O71.1
  uvula K13.79
    syphilitic A52.79
  vagina
    obstetrical trauma O71.4
    other trauma - *see* Puncture, vagina
Periadenitis mucosa necrotica recurrens
K12.0
Periappendicitis (acute) - *see* Appendicitis
Periarteritis nodosa (disseminated)
  (infectious) (necrotizing) M30.0
Periarthritis (joint) - *see also* Enthesopathy
  Duplay's M75.0-
  gonococcal A54.42
  humeroscapularis - *see* Capsulitis, adhesive

Periarthritis (joint) - *continued*
  scapulohumeral - *see* Capsulitis, adhesive
  shoulder - *see* Capsulitis, adhesive
  wrist M77.2-
Periarthrosis (angioneural) - *see* Enthesopathy
Pericapsulitis, adhesive (shoulder) - *see*
  Capsulitis, adhesive
**Pericarditis (with decompensation) (with
  effusion)** I31.9
  with rheumatic fever (conditions in I00)
    active - *see* Pericarditis, rheumatic
    inactive or quiescent I09.2
  acute (hemorrhagic) (nonrheumatic) (Sicca)
    I30.9
    with chorea (acute) (rheumatic)
      (Sydenham's) I02.0
    benign I30.8
    nonspecific I30.0
    rheumatic I01.0
      with chorea (acute) (Sydenham's) I02.0
  adhesive or adherent (chronic) (external)
    (internal) I31.0
    acute - *see* Pericarditis, acute
    rheumatic I09.2
  bacterial (acute) (subacute) (with serous or
    seropurulent effusion) I30.1
  calcareous I31.1
  cholesterol (chronic) I31.8
    acute I30.9
  chronic (nonrheumatic) I31.9
    rheumatic I09.2
  constrictive (chronic) I31.1
  coxsackie B33.23
  fibrinocaseous (tuberculous) A18.84
  fibrinopurulent I30.1
  fibrinous I30.8
  fibrous I31.0
  gonococcal A54.83
  idiopathic I30.0
  in systemic lupus erythematosus M32.12
  infective I30.1
  meningococcal A39.53
  neoplastic (chronic) I31.8
    acute I30.9
  obliterans, obliterating I31.0
  plastic I31.0
  pneumococcal I30.1
  postinfarction I24.1
  purulent I30.1
  rheumatic (active) (acute) (with effusion) (with
    pneumonia) I01.0
    with chorea (acute) (rheumatic)
      (Sydenham's) I02.0
    chronic or inactive (with chorea) I09.2
  rheumatoid - *see* Rheumatoid, carditis
  septic I30.1
  serofibrinous I30.8
  staphylococcal I30.1
  streptococcal I30.1
  suppurative I30.1
  syphilitic A52.06
  tuberculous A18.84
  uremic N18.9 [*I32*]
  viral I30.1
Pericardium, pericardial - *see* condition
Pericellulitis - *see* Cellulitis
Pericementitis (chronic) (suppurative) - *see
  also* Periodontitis
  acute K05.20
    generalized - *see* Periodontitis, aggressive,
    generalized
    localized - *see* Periodontitis, aggressive,
    localized

Perichondritis
  auricle - *see* Perichondritis, ear
  bronchus J98.09
  ear (external) H61.00-
    acute H61.01
    chronic H61.02-
  external auditory canal - *see* Perichondritis, ear
  larynx J38.7
    syphilitic A52.73
    typhoid A01.09
  nose J34.89
  pinna - *see* Perichondritis, ear
  trachea J39.8
Periclasia K05.4
Pericoronitis - *see* Periodontitis
Pericystitis N30.90
  with hematuria N30.91
Peridiverticulitis (intestine) K57.92
  cecum - *see* Diverticulitis, intestine, large
  colon - *see* Diverticulitis, intestine, large
  duodenum - *see* Diverticulitis, intestine, small
  intestine - *see* Diverticulitis, intestine
  jejunum - *see* Diverticulitis, intestine, small
  rectosigmoid - *see* Diverticulitis, intestine,
  large
  rectum - *see* Diverticulitis, intestine, large
  sigmoid - *see* Diverticulitis, intestine, large
Periendocarditis - *see* Endocarditis
Periepididymitis N45.1
Perifolliculitis L01.02
  abscedens, caput, scalp L66.3
  capitis, abscedens (et suffodiens) L66.3
  superficial pustular L01.02
Perihepatitis K65.8
Perilabyrinthitis (acute) - *see* subcategory
  H83.0
Perimeningitis - *see* Meningitis
Perimetritis - *see* Endometritis
Perimetrosalpingitis - *see* Salpingo-oophoritis
Perineocele N81.81
Perinephric, perinephritic - *see* condition
Perinephritis - *see also* Infection, kidney
  purulent - *see* Abscess, kidney
Perineum, perineal - *see* condition
Perineuritis NEC - *see* Neuralgia **Periodic** -
  see condition
**Periodontitis (chronic) (complex)
  (compound) (local) (simplex)** K05.30
  acute K05.20
    generalized K05.229
      moderate K05.222
      severe K05.223
      slight K05.221
    localized K05.219
      moderate K05.212
      severe K05.213
      slight K05.211
  apical K04.5
    acute (pulpal origin) K04.4
  generalized K05.329
    moderate K05.322
    severe K05.323
    slight K05.321
  localized K05.319
    moderate K05.312
    severe K05.313
    slight K05.311
Periodontoclasia K05.4
Periodontosis (juvenile) K05.4
Periods - *see also* Menstruation
  heavy N92.0
  irregular N92.6
  shortened intervals (irregular) N92.1

Perionychia - *see also* Cellulitis, digit
  with lymphangitis - *see* Lymphangitis, acute,
  digit
Perioophoritis - *see* Salpingo-oophoritis
Periorchitis N45.2
Periosteum, periosteal - *see* condition
**Periostitis (albuminosa) (circumscribed)
  (diffuse) (infective) (monomelic)** - *see also*
  Osteomyelitis
  alveolar M27.3
  alveolodental M27.3
  dental M27.3
  gonorrheal A54.43
  jaw (lower) (upper) M27.2
  orbit H05.03-
  syphilitic A52.77
    congenital (early) A50.02 [*M90.80*]
    secondary A51.46
  tuberculous - *see* Tuberculosis, bone
  yaws (hypertrophic) (early) (late) A66.6
    [*M90.80*]
Periostosis (hyperplastic) - *see also* Disorder,
  bone, specified type NEC
  with osteomyelitis - *see* Osteomyelitis,
  specified type NEC
Peripartum
  cardiomyopathy O90.3
Periphlebitis - *see* Phlebitis
Periproctitis K62.89
Periprostatitis - *see* Prostatitis
Perirectal - *see* condition
Perirenal - *see* condition
Perisalpingitis - *see* Salpingo-oophoritis
Perisplenitis (infectional) D73.89
Peristalsis, visible or reversed R19.2
Peritendinitis - *see* Enthesopathy
Peritoneum, peritoneal - *see* condition
**Peritonitis (adhesive) (bacterial) (fibrinous)
  (hemorrhagic) (idiopathic) (localized)
  (perforative) (primary) (with adhesions)
  (with effusion)** K65.9
  with or following
    abscess K65.1
    appendicitis K35.3
      with perforation or rupture K35.2
      generalized K35.2
      localized K35.3
    diverticular disease (intestine) K57.80
      with bleeding K57.81
      large intestine K57.20
      with
        bleeding K57.21
        small intestine K57.40
          with bleeding K57.41
      small intestine K57.00
      with
        bleeding K57.01
        large intestine K57.40
          with bleeding K57.41
    ectopic or molar pregnancy O08.0
  acute (generalized) K65.0
  aseptic T81.61
  bile, biliary K65.3
  chemical T81.61
  chlamydial A74.81
  complicating abortion - *see* Abortion, by type,
  complicated by, pelvic peritonitis
  congenital P78.1
  chronic proliferative K65.8
  diaphragmatic K65.0
  diffuse K65.0
  diphtheritic A36.89
  disseminated K65.0
  due to

Peritonitis - *continued*
- bile K65.3
- foreign
  - body or object accidentally left during a procedure (instrument) (sponge) (swab) T81.599
  - substance accidentally left during a procedure (chemical) (powder) (talc) T81.61
  - talc T81.61
  - urine K65.8
- eosinophilic K65.8
  - acute K65.0
- fibrocaseous (tuberculous) A18.31
- fibropurulent K65.0
- following ectopic or molar pregnancy O08.0
- general (ized) K65.0
- gonococcal A54.85
- meconium (newborn) P78.0
- neonatal P78.1
  - meconium P78.0
- pancreatic K65.0
- paroxysmal, familial E85.0
  - benign E85.0
- pelvic
  - female N73.5
    - acute N73.3
    - chronic N73.4
      - with adhesions N73.6
  - male K65.0
- periodic, familial E85.0
- proliferative, chronic K65.8
- puerperal, postpartum, childbirth O85
- purulent K65.0
- septic K65.0
- specified NEC K65.8
- spontaneous bacterial K65.2
- subdiaphragmatic K65.0
- subphrenic K65.0
- suppurative K65.0
- syphilitic A52.74
  - congenital (early) A50.08 [*K67*]
- talc T81.61
- tuberculous A18.31
- urine K65.8

Peritonsillar - *see* condition
Peritonsillitis J36
Perityphlitis K37
Periureteritis N28.89
Periurethral - *see* condition
Periurethritis (gangrenous) - *see* Urethritis
Periuterine - *see* condition
Perivaginitis - *see* Vaginitis
Perivasculitis, retinal H35.06-
Perivasitis (chronic) N49.1
Perivesiculitis (seminal) - *see* Vesiculitis
Perlèche NEC K13.0
- due to
  - candidiasis B37.83
  - moniliasis B37.83
  - riboflavin deficiency E53.0
  - vitamin B2 (riboflavin) deficiency E53.0

Pernicious - *see* condition
Pernio, perniosis T69.1
Perpetrator (of abuse) - *see* Index to External Causes of Injury, Perpetrator
Persecution
- delusion F22
- social Z60.5

Perseveration (tonic) R48.8
Persistence, persistent (congenital)
- anal membrane Q42.3
  - with fistula Q42.2
- arteria stapedia Q16.3

Persistence, persistent - *continued*
- atrioventricular canal Q21.2
- branchial cleft NOS Q18.2
  - cyst Q18.0
  - fistula Q18.0
  - sinus Q18.0
- bulbus cordis in left ventricle Q21.8
- canal of Cloquet Q14.0
- capsule (opaque) Q12.8
- cilioretinal artery or vein Q14.8
- cloaca Q43.7
- communication - *see* Fistula, congenital
- convolutions
  - aortic arch Q25.46
  - fallopian tube Q50.6
  - oviduct Q50.6
  - uterine tube Q50.6
- double aortic arch Q25.45
- ductus arteriosus (Botalli) Q25.0
- fetal
  - circulation P29.38
  - form of cervix (uteri) Q51.828
  - hemoglobin, hereditary (HPFH) D56.4
- foramen
  - Botalli Q21.1
  - ovale Q21.1
- Gartner's duct Q52.4
- hemoglobin, fetal (hereditary) (HPFH) D56.4
- hyaloid
  - artery (generally incomplete) Q14.0
  - system Q14.8
- hymen, in pregnancy or childbirth - *see* Pregnancy, complicated by, abnormal, vulva
- lanugo Q84.2
- left
  - posterior cardinal vein Q26.8
  - root with right arch of aorta Q25.49
  - superior vena cava Q26.1
- Meckel's diverticulum Q43.0
  - malignant - *see* Table of Neoplasms, small intestine, malignant
- mucosal disease (middle ear) - *see* Otitis, media, suppurative, chronic, tubotympanic
- nail(s), anomalous Q84.6
- omphalomesenteric duct Q43.0
- organ or site not listed - *see* Anomaly, by site
- ostium
  - atrioventriculare commune Q21.2
  - primum Q21.2
  - secundum Q21.1
- ovarian rests in fallopian tube Q50.6
- pancreatic tissue in intestinal tract Q43.8
- primary (deciduous)
  - teeth K00.6
  - vitreous hyperplasia Q14.0
- pupillary membrane Q13.89
- right aortic arch Q25.47
- rhesus (Rh) titer - *see* Complication(s), transfusion, incompatibility reaction, Rh (factor)
- sinus
  - urogenitalis
    - female Q52.8
    - male Q55.8
  - venosus with imperfect incorporation in right auricle Q26.8
- thymus (gland) (hyperplasia) E32.0
- thyroglossal duct Q89.2
- thyrolingual duct Q89.2
- truncus arteriosus or communis Q20.0
- tunica vasculosa lentis Q12.2
- umbilical sinus Q64.4
- urachus Q64.4
- vitelline duct Q43.0

Person (with)
- admitted for clinical research, as a control subject (normal comparison) (participant) Z00.6
- awaiting admission to adequate facility elsewhere Z75.1
- concern (normal) about sick person in family Z63.6
- consulting on behalf of another Z71.0
- feigning illness Z76.5
- living (in)
  - alone Z60.2
  - boarding school Z59.3
  - residential institution Z59.3
  - without
    - adequate housing (heating) (space) Z59.1
    - housing (permanent) (temporary) Z59.0
    - person able to render necessary care Z74.2
    - shelter Z59.0
- on waiting list Z75.1
- sick or handicapped in family Z63.6

Personality (disorder) F60.9
- accentuation of traits (type A pattern) Z73.1
- affective F34.0
- aggressive F60.3
- amoral F60.2
- anancastic, anankastic F60.5
- antisocial F60.2
- anxious F60.6
- asocial F60.2
- asthenic F60.7
- avoidant F60.6
- borderline F60.3
- change due to organic condition (enduring) F07.0
- compulsive F60.5
- cycloid F34.0
- cyclothymic F34.0
- dependent F60.7
- depressive F34.1
- dissocial F60.2
- dual F44.81
- eccentric F60.89
- emotionally unstable F60.3
- expansive paranoid F60.0
- explosive F60.3
- fanatic F60.0
- haltlose type F60.89
- histrionic F60.4
- hyperthymic F34.0
- hypothymic F34.1
- hysterical F60.4
- immature F60.89
- inadequate F60.7
- labile (emotional) F60.3
- mixed (nonspecific) F60.89
- morally defective F60.2
- multiple F44.81
- narcissistic F60.81
- obsessional F60.5
- obsessive (-compulsive) F60.5
- organic F07.0
- overconscientious F60.5
- paranoid F60.0
- passive (-dependent) F60.7
- passive-aggressive F60.89
- pathologic F60.9
- pattern defect or disturbance F60.9
- pseudopsychopathic (organic) F07.0
- pseudoretarded (organic) F07.0
- psychoinfantile F60.4
- psychoneurotic NEC F60.89
- psychopathic F60.2

Personality (disorder) - *continued*
 querulant F60.0
 sadistic F60.89
 schizoid F60.1
 self-defeating F60.7
 sensitive paranoid F60.0
 sociopathic (amoral) (antisocial) (asocial)
  (dissocial) F60.2
 specified NEC F60.89
 type A Z73.1
 unstable (emotional) F60.3
Perthes' disease - *see* Legg-Calvé-Perthes
 disease
Pertussis - *see also* Whooping cough A37.90
Perversion, perverted appetite F50.89
 psychogenic F50.89
 function
  pituitary gland E23.2
   posterior lobe E22.2
 sense of smell and taste R43.8
  psychogenic F45.8
 sexual - *see* Deviation, sexual
Pervious, congenital - *see also* Imperfect,
 closure
 ductus arteriosus Q25.0
Pes (congenital) - *see also* Talipes
 acquired - *see also* Deformity, limb, foot,
  specified NEC
  planus - *see* Deformity, limb, flat foot
 adductus Q66.89
 cavus Q66.7
 deformity NEC, acquired - *see* Deformity,
  limb, foot, specified NEC
 planus (acquired) (any degree) - *see also*
  Deformity, limb, flat foot
  rachitic sequelae (late effect) E64.3
 valgus Q66.6
Pest, pestis - *see* Plague
Petechia, petechiae R23.3
 newborn P54.5
Petechial typhus A75.9
Peter's anomaly Q13.4
Petit mal seizure - *see* Epilepsy, generalized,
 specified NEC
Petit's hernia - *see* Hernia, abdomen, specified
 site NEC
Petriellidiosis B48.2
Petrositis H70.20-
 acute H70.21-
 chronic H70.22-
Peutz-Jeghers disease or syndrome Q85.8
Peyronie's disease N48.6
PFAPA (periodic fever, aphthous stomatitis,
 pharyngitis, and adenopathy syndrome)
 M04.8
Pfeiffer's disease - *see* Mononucleosis,
 infectious
Phagedena (dry) (moist) (sloughing) - *see also*
 Gangrene
 geometric L88
 penis N48.29
 tropical - *see* Ulcer, skin
 vulva N76.6
Phagedenic - *see* condition
Phakoma H35.89
Phakomatosis - *see also* specific eponymous
 syndromes Q85.9
 Bourneville's Q85.1
 specified NEC Q85.8
Phantom limb syndrome (without pain)
 G54.7
 with pain G54.6
Pharyngeal pouch syndrome D82.1

Pharyngitis (acute) (catarrhal)(gangrenous)
 (infective) (malignant) (membranous)
 (phlegmonous) (pseudomembranous)
 (simple) (subacute) (suppurative)
 (ulcerative) (viral) J02.9
 with influenza, flu, or grippe - *see* Influenza,
  with, pharyngitis
 aphthous B08.5
 atrophic J31.2
 chlamydial A56.4
 chronic (atrophic) (granular) (hypertrophic)
  J31.2
 coxsackievirus B08.5
 diphtheritic A36.0
 enteroviral vesicular B08.5
 follicular (chronic) J31.2
 fusospirochetal A69.1
 gonococcal A54.5
 granular (chronic) J31.2
 herpesviral B00.2
 hypertrophic J31.2
 infectional, chronic J31.2
 influenzal - *see* Influenza, with, respiratory
  manifestations NEC
 lymphonodular, acute (enteroviral) B08.8
 pneumococcal J02.8
 purulent J02.9
 putrid J02.9
 septic J02.0
 sicca J31.2
 specified organism NEC J02.8
 staphylococcal J02.8
 streptococcal J02.0
 syphilitic, congenital (early) A50.03
 tuberculous A15.8
 vesicular, enteroviral B08.5
 viral NEC J02.8
Pharyngoconjunctivitis, viral B30.2
Pharyngolaryngitis (acute) J06.0
 chronic J37.0
Pharyngoplegia J39.2
Pharyngotonsillitis, herpesviral B00.2
Pharyngotracheitis, chronic J42
Pharynx, pharyngeal - *see* condition
Phencyclidine-induced
 anxiety disorder F16.980
 bipolar and related disorder F16.94
 depressive disorder F16.94
 psychotic disorder F16.959
Phenomenon
 Arthus' - *see* Arthus' phenomenon
 jaw-winking Q07.8
 lupus erythematosus (LE) cell M32.9
 Raynaud's (secondary) I73.00
  with gangrene I73.01
 vasomotor R55
 vasospastic I73.9
 vasovagal R55
 Wenckebach's I44.1
Phenylketonuria E70.1
 classical E70.0
 maternal E70.1
Pheochromoblastoma
 specified site - *see* Neoplasm, malignant, by
  site
 unspecified site C74.10
Pheochromocytoma malignant
 specified site - *see* Neoplasm, malignant, by
  site
  unspecified site C74.10
 specified site - *see* Neoplasm, benign, by site
 unspecified site D35.00
Phaeohyphomycosis - *see* Chromomycosis
Pheomycosis - *see* Chromomycosis

Phimosis (congenital) (due to infection) N47.1
 chancroidal A57
Phlebectasia - *see also* Varix
 congenital Q27.4
Phlebitis (infective) (pyemic) (septic)
 (suppurative) I80.9
 antepartum - *see* Thrombophlebitis,
  antepartum
 blue - *see* Phlebitis, leg, deep
 breast, superficial I80.8
 cavernous (venous) sinus - *see* Phlebitis,
  intracranial (venous) sinus
 cerebral (venous) sinus - *see* Phlebitis,
  intracranial (venous) sinus
 chest wall, superficial I80.8
 cranial (venous) sinus - *see* Phlebitis,
  intracranial (venous) sinus
 deep (vessels) - *see* Phlebitis, leg, deep
 due to implanted device - *see* Complications,
  by site and type, specified NEC
 during or resulting from a procedure T81.72
 femoral vein (superficial) I80.1-
 femoropopliteal vein I80.0-
 gestational - *see* Phlebopathy, gestational
 hepatic veins I80.8
 iliofemoral - *see* Phlebitis, femoral vein
 intracranial (venous) sinus (any) G08
  nonpyogenic I67.6
 intraspinal venous sinuses and veins G08
  nonpyogenic G95.19
 lateral (venous) sinus - *see* Phlebitis,
  intracranial (venous) sinus
 leg I80.3
  antepartum - *see* Thrombophlebitis,
 antepartum
  deep (vessels) NEC I80.20-
   iliac I80.21-
   popliteal vein I80.22-
   specified vessel NEC I80.29-
   tibial vein I80.23-
  femoral vein (superficial) I80.1-
  superficial (vessels) I80.0-
 longitudinal sinus - *see* Phlebitis, intracranial
  (venous) sinus
 lower limb - *see* Phlebitis, leg
 migrans, migrating (superficial) I82.1
 pelvic
  with ectopic or molar pregnancy O08.0
  following ectopic or molar pregnancy O08.0
  puerperal, postpartum O87.1
 popliteal vein - *see* Phlebitis, leg, deep,
  popliteal
 portal (vein) K75.1
 postoperative T81.72
 pregnancy - *see* Thrombophlebitis, antepartum
 puerperal, postpartum, childbirth O87.0
  deep O87.1
  pelvic O87.1
  superficial O87.0
 retina - *see* Vasculitis, retina
 saphenous (accessory) (great) (long) (small) -
  see Phlebitis, leg, superficial
 sinus (meninges) - *see* Phlebitis, intracranial
  (venous) sinus
 specified site NEC I80.8
 syphilitic A52.09
 tibial vein - *see* Phlebitis, leg, deep, tibial
 ulcerative I80.9
  leg - *see* Phlebitis, leg
 umbilicus I80.8
 uterus (septic) - *see* Endometritis
 varicose (leg) (lower limb) - *see* Varix, leg,
  with, inflammation
Phlebofibrosis I87.8

Phleboliths I87.8
Phlebopathy,
  gestational O22.9-
  puerperal O87.9
Phlebosclerosis I87.8
Phlebothrombosis - see also Thrombosis
  antepartum - see Thrombophlebitis,
    antepartum
  pregnancy - see Thrombophlebitis, antepartum
  puerperal - see Thrombophlebitis, puerperal
Phlebotomus fever A93.1
Phlegmasia
  alba dolens O87.1
    nonpuerperal - see Phlebitis, femoral vein
  cerulea dolens - see Phlebitis, leg, deep
Phlegmon - see Abscess
Phlegmonous - see condition
Phlyctenulosis (allergic)
  (keratoconjunctivitis) (nontuberculous) - see
  also Keratoconjunctivitis
  cornea - see Keratoconjunctivitis
  tuberculous A18.52
Phobia, phobic F40.9
  animal F40.218
    spiders F40.210
  examination F40.298
  reaction F40.9
  simple F40.298
  social F40.10
    generalized F40.11
  specific (isolated) F40.298
    animal F40.218
      spiders F40.210
    blood F40.230
    injection F40.231
    injury F40.233
    men F40.290
    natural environment F40.228
      thunderstorms F40.220
    situational F40.248
      bridges F40.242
      closed in spaces F40.240
      flying F40.243
      heights F40.241
    specified focus NEC F40.298
    transfusion F40.231
    women F40.291
  specified NEC F40.8
    medical care NEC F40.232
  state F40.9
Phocas' disease - see Mastopathy, cystic
Phocomelia Q73.1
  lower limb - see Agenesis, leg, with foot
    present
  upper limb - see Agenesis, arm, with hand
    present
Phoria H50.50
Phosphate-losing tubular disorder N25.0
Phosphatemia E83.39
Phosphaturia E83.39
Photodermatitis (sun) L56.8
  chronic L57.8
  due to drug L56.8
  light other than sun L59.8
Photokeratitis H16.13-
Photophobia H53.14-
Photophthalmia - see Photokeratitis
Photopsia H53.19
Photoretinitis - see Retinopathy, solar
Photosensitivity, photosensitization (sun) skin
  L56.8
  light other than sun L59.8
Phrenitis - see Encephalitis
Phrynoderma (vitamin A deficiency) E50.8

Phthiriasis (pubis) B85.3
  with any infestation classifiable to B85.0-
  b85.2
  B85.4
Phthirus infestation - see Phthiriasis
Phthisis - see also Tuberculosis
  bulbi (infectional) - see Disorder, globe,
    degenerated condition, atrophy
  eyeball (due to infection) - see Disorder, globe,
    degenerated condition, atrophy
Phycomycosis - see Zygomycosis
Physalopteriasis B81.8
Physical restraint status Z78.1
Phytobezoar T18.9
  intestine T18.3
  stomach T18.2
Pian - see Yaws
Pianoma A66.1
Pica F50.89
  in adults F50.89
  infant or child F98.3
Picking, nose F98.8
Pick Niemann disease - see Niemann-pick
  disease or syndrome
Pick's
  cerebral atrophy G31.01 [F02.80]
    with behavioral disturbance G31.01
    [F02.81]
  disease or syndrome (brain) G31.01 [F02.80]
    with behavioral disturbance G31.01
    [F02.81]
    brain G31.01 [F02.80]
      with behavioral disturbance G31.01
      [F02.81]
    pericardium (pericardial pseudocirrhosis of
      liver) I31.1
  syndrome
    brain G31.01 [F02.80]
      with behavioral disturbance G31.01
      [F02.81]
    of heart (pericardial pseudocirrhosis of liver)
      I31.1
Pickwickian syndrome E66.2
Piebaldism E70.39
Piedra (beard) (scalp) B36.8
  black B36.3
  white B36.2
Pierre Robin deformity or syndrome Q87.0
Pierson's disease or osteochondrosis M91.0
Pig-bel A05.2
Pigeon
  breast or chest (acquired) M95.4
    congenital Q67.7
    rachitic sequelae (late effect) E64.3
  breeder's disease or lung J67.2
  fancier's disease or lung J67.2
  toe - see Deformity, toe, specified NEC
Pigmentation (abnormal) (anomaly) L81.9
  conjunctiva H11.13-
  cornea (anterior) H18.01-
    posterior H18.05-
    stromal H18.06-
  diminished melanin formation NEC L81.6
  iron L81.8
  lids, congenital Q82.8
  limbus corneae - see Pigmentation, cornea
  metals L81.8
  optic papilla, congenital Q14.2
  retina, congenital (grouped) (nevoid) Q14.1
  scrotum, congenital Q82.8
  tattoo L81.8
Piles - see also Hemorrhoids K64.9
Pili
  annulati or torti (congenital) Q84.1
  incarnati L73.1

Pill roller hand (intrinsic) - see Parkinsonism
Pilomatrixoma - see Neoplasm, skin, benign
  malignant - see Neoplasm, skin, malignant
Pilonidal - see condition
Pimple R23.8
PIN - see Neoplasia, intraepithelial, prostate
Pinched nerve - see Neuropathy, entrapment
Pindborg tumor - see Cyst, calcifying
  odontogenic
Pineal body or gland - see condition
Pinealoblastoma C75.3
Pinealoma D44.5
  malignant C75.3
Pineoblastoma C75.3
Pineocytoma D44.5
Pinguecula H11.15-
Pingueculitis H10.81-
Pinhole meatus - see also Stricture, urethra
  N35.9
Pink
  disease see subcategory T56.1
  eye - see Conjunctivitis, acute, mucopurulent
Pinkus' disease (lichen nitidus) L44.1
Pinpoint
  meatus - see Stricture, urethra
  os (uteri) - see Stricture, cervix
Pins and needles R20.2
Pinta A67.9
  cardiovascular lesions A67.2
  chancre (primary) A67.0
  erythematous plaques A67.1
  hyperchromic lesions A67.1
  hyperkeratosis A67.1
  lesions A67.9
    cardiovascular A67.2
    hyperchromic A67.1
    intermediate A67.1
    late A67.2
    mixed A67.3
    primary A67.0
    skin (achromic) (cicatricial) (dyschromic)
      A67.2
      hyperchromic A67.1
      mixed (achromic and hyperchromic) A67.3
  papule (primary) A67.0
  skin lesions (achromic) (cicatricial)
    (dyschromic) A67.2
    hyperchromic A67.1
    mixed (achromic and hyperchromic) A67.3
  vitiligo A67.2
Pintids A67.1
Pinworm (disease) (infection) (infestation)
  B80
Piroplasmosis B60.0
Pistol wound - see Gunshot wound
Pitchers' elbow - see Derangement, joint,
  specified type NEC, elbow
Pithecoid pelvis Q74.2
  with disproportion (fetopelvic) O33.0
    causing obstructed labor O65.0
Pithiatism F48.8
Pitted - see Pitting
Pitting - see also Edema R60.9
  lip R60.0
  nail L60.8
  teeth K00.4
Pituitary gland - see condition
Pituitary-snuff-taker's disease J67.8
Pityriasis (capitis) L21.0
  alba L30.5
  circinata (et maculata) L42
  furfuracea L21.0
  Hebra's L26
  lichenoides L41.0

Pityriasis (capitis) - *continued*
　chronica L41.1
　　et varioliformis (acuta) L41.0
　maculata (et circinata) L30.5
　nigra B36.1
　pilaris, Hebra's L44.0
　rosea L42
　rotunda L44.8
　rubra (Hebra) pilaris L44.0
　simplex L30.5
　specified type NEC L30.5
　streptogenes L30.5
　versicolor (scrotal) B36.0
Placenta, placental - *see* Pregnancy,
　complicated by (care of) (management
　affected by), specified condition
Placentitis O41.14-
Plagiocephaly Q67.3
Plague A20.9
　abortive A20.8
　ambulatory A20.8
　asymptomatic A20.8
　bubonic A20.0
　cellulocutaneous A20.1
　cutaneobubonic A20.1
　lymphatic gland A20.0
　meningitis A20.3
　pharyngeal A20.8
　pneumonic (primary) (secondary) A20.2
　pulmonary, pulmonic A20.2
　septicemic A20.7
　tonsillar A20.8
　　septicemic A20.7
Planning, family
　contraception Z30.9
　procreation Z31.69
Plaque(s)
　artery, arterial - *see* Arteriosclerosis
　calcareous - *see* Calcification
　coronary, lipid rich I25.83
　epicardial I31.8
　erythematous, of pinta A67.1
　Hollenhorst's - *see* Occlusion, artery, retina
　lipid rich, coronary I25.83
　pleural (without asbestos) J92.9
　　with asbestos J92.0
　tongue K13.29
Plasmacytoma C90.3-
　extramedullary C90.2-
　medullary C90.0-
　solitary C90.3-
Plasmacytopenia D72.818
Plasmacytosis D72.822
Plaster ulcer - *see* Ulcer, pressure, by site
Plateau iris syndrome (post-iridectomy)
　(postprocedural) (without glaucoma)
　H21.82
　with glaucoma H40.22-
Platybasia Q75.8
Platyonychia (congenital) Q84.6
　acquired L60.8
Platypelloid pelvis M95.5
　with disproportion (fetopelvic) O33.0
　　causing obstructed labor O65.0
　congenital Q74.2
Platyspondylisis Q76.49
Plaut (-Vincent) disease - *see also* Vincent's
　A69.1
Plethora R23.2
　newborn P61.1
Pleura, pleural - *see* condition
Pleuralgia R07.81

Pleurisy (acute) (adhesive) (chronic) (costal)
　(diaphragmatic) (double) (dry) (fibrinous)
　(fibrous) (interlobar) (latent) (plastic)
　(primary) (residual) (sicca) (sterile)
　(subacute) (unresolved) R09.1
　with
　　adherent pleura J86.0
　　effusion J90
　　　chylous, chyliform J94.0
　　　tuberculous (non primary) A15.6
　　　　primary (progressive) A15.7
　　tuberculosis - *see* Pleurisy, tuberculous (non
　primary)
　encysted - *see* Pleurisy, with effusion
　exudative - *see* Pleurisy, with effusion
　fibrinopurulent, fibropurulent - *see* Pyothorax
　hemorrhagic - *see* Hemothorax
　pneumococcal J90
　purulent - *see* Pyothorax　septic - *see*
　Pyothorax
　serofibrinous - *see* Pleurisy, with effusion
　seropurulent - *see* Pyothorax
　serous - *see* Pleurisy, with effusion
　staphylococcal J86.9
　streptococcal J90
　suppurative - *see* Pyothorax
　traumatic (post) (current) - *see* Injury,
　intrathoracic, pleura
　tuberculous (with effusion) (non primary)
　A15.6
　　primary (progressive) A15.7
Pleuritis sicca - *see* Pleurisy
Pleurobronchopneumonia - *see* Pneumonia,
　broncho-
Pleurodynia R07.81
　epidemic B33.0
　viral B33.0
Pleuropericarditis - *see also* Pericarditis
　acute I30.9
Pleuropneumonia (acute) (bilateral) (double)
　(septic) - *see also* Pneumonia J18.8
　chronic - *see* Fibrosis, lung
Pleuro-pneumonia-like-organism (PPLO), as
　cause of disease classified elsewhere B96.0
Pleurorrhea - *see* Pleurisy, with effusion
Plexitis, brachial G54.0
Plica
　polonica B85.0
　syndrome, knee M67.5-
　tonsil J35.8
Plicated tongue K14.5
Plug
　bronchus NEC J98.09
　meconium (newborn) NEC syndrome P76.0
　mucus - *see* Asphyxia, mucus
Plumbism - *see* subcategory T56.0
Plummer's disease E05.20
　with thyroid storm E05.21
Plummer-Vinson syndrome D50.1
Pluricarential syndrome of infancy E40
Plus (and minus) hand (intrinsic) - *see*
　Deformity, limb, specified type NEC, forearm
Pneumathemia - *see* Air, embolism
Pneumatic hammer (drill) syndrome T75.21
Pneumatocele (lung) J98.4
　intracranial G93.89
　tension J44.9
Pneumatosis
　cystoides intestinalis K63.89
　intestinalis K63.89
　peritonei K66.8
Pneumaturia R39.89
Pneumoblastoma - *see* Neoplasm, lung,
　malignant

Pneumocephalus G93.89
Pneumococcemia A40.3
Pneumococcus, pneumococcal - *see* condition
Pneumoconiosis (due to) (inhalation of) J64
　with tuberculosis (any type in A15) J65
　aluminum J63.0
　asbestos J61
　bagasse, bagassosis J67.1
　bauxite J63.1
　beryllium J63.2
　coal miners' (simple) J60
　Coalworker's' (simple) J60
　collier's J60
　cotton dust J66.0
　diatomite (diatomaceous earth) J62.8
　dust
　　inorganic NEC J63.6
　　lime J62.8
　　marble J62.8
　　organic NEC J66.8
　fumes or vapors (from silo) J68.9
　graphite J63.3
　grinder's J62.8
　kaolin J62.8
　mica J62.8
　millstone maker's J62.8
　mineral fibers NEC J61
　miner's J60
　moldy hay J67.0
　potter's J62.8
　rheumatoid - *see* Rheumatoid, lung
　sandblaster's J62.8
　silica, silicate NEC J62.8
　　with carbon J60
　stonemason's J62.8
　talc (dust) J62.0
Pneumocystis carinii pneumonia B59
Pneumocystis jiroveci (pneumonia) B59
Pneumocystosis (with pneumonia) B59
Pneumohemopericardium I31.2
Pneumohemothorax J94.2
　traumatic S27.2
Pneumohydropericardium - *see* Pericarditis
Pneumohydrothorax - *see* Hydrothorax
Pneumomediastinum J98.2
　congenital or perinatal P25.2
Pneumomycosis B49 [*J99*]
Pneumonia (acute) (double) (migratory)
　(purulent) (septic) (unresolved) J18.9
　with
　　lung abscess J85.1
　　due to specified organism - *see* Pneumonia,
　in (due to)
　　influenza - *see* Influenza, with, pneumonia
　adenoviral J12.0
　adynamic J18.2
　alba A50.04
　allergic (eosinophilic) J82
　alveolar - *see* Pneumonia, lobar
　anaerobes J15.8
　anthrax A22.1
　apex, apical - *see* Pneumonia, lobar
　Ascaris B77.81
　aspiration J69.0
　　due to
　　　aspiration of microorganisms
　　　　bacterial J15.9
　　　　viral J12.9
　　　food (regurgitated) J69.0
　　　gastric secretions J69.0
　　　milk (regurgitated) J69.0
　　　oils, essences J69.1
　　　solids, liquids NEC J69.8
　　　vomitus J69.0

Pneumonia - *continued*
  newborn P24.81
    amniotic fluid (clear) P24.11
    blood P24.21
    liquor (amnii) P24.11
    meconium P24.01
    milk P24.31
    mucus P24.11
    food (regurgitated) P24.31
    specified NEC P24.81
    stomach contents P24.31
  postprocedural J95.4
  atypical NEC J18.9
  bacillus J15.9
    specified NEC J15.8
  bacterial J15.9
    specified NEC J15.8
  Bacteroides (fragilis) (oralis)
    (melaninogenicus) J15.8
  basal, basic, basilar - *see* Pneumonia, by type
  bronchiolitis obliterans organized (BOOP)
    J84.89
  broncho , bronchial (confluent) (croupous)
    (diffuse) (disseminated) (hemorrhagic)
    (involving lobes) (lobar) (terminal) J18.0
    allergic (eosinophilic) J82
    aspiration - *see* Pneumonia, aspiration
    bacterial J15.9
      specified NEC J15.8
    chronic - *see* Fibrosis, lung
    diplococcal J13
    Eaton's agent J15.7
    Escherichia coli (E. coli) J15.5
    Friedländer's bacillus J15.0
    Hemophilus influenzae J14
    hypostatic J18.2
    inhalation - *see also* Pneumonia, aspiration
      due to fumes or vapors (chemical) J68.0
      of oils or essences J69.1
    Klebsiella (pneumoniae) J15.0
    lipid, lipoid J69.1
      endogenous J84.89
    Mycoplasma (pneumoniae) J15.7
    pleuro-pneumonia-like-organisms (PPLO)
      J15.7
    pneumococcal J13
    Proteus J15.6
    Pseudomonas J15.1
    Serratia marcescens J15.6
    specified organism NEC J16.8
    staphylococcal - *see* Pneumonia,
      staphylococcal
    streptococcal NEC J15.4
      group B J15.3
      pneumoniae J13
    viral, virus - *see* Pneumonia, viral
  Butyrivibrio (fibriosolvens) J15.8
  Candida B37.1
  caseous - *see* Tuberculosis, pulmonary
  catarrhal - *see* Pneumonia, broncho
  chlamydial J16.0
    congenital P23.1
  cholesterol J84.89
  cirrhotic (chronic) - *see* Fibrosis, lung
  Clostridium (haemolyticum) (novyi) J15.8
  confluent - *see* Pneumonia, broncho
  congenital (infective) P23.9
    due to
      bacterium NEC P23.6
      Chlamydia P23.1
      Escherichia coli P23.4
      Haemophilus influenzae P23.6
      infective organism NEC P23.8
      Klebsiella pneumoniae P23.6

Pneumonia - *continued*
    Mycoplasma P23.6
    Pseudomonas P23.5
    Staphylococcus P23.2
    Streptococcus (except group B) P23.6
      group B P23.3
    viral agent P23.0
    specified NEC P23.8
  croupous - *see* Pneumonia, lobar
  cryptogenic organizing J84.116
  cytomegalic inclusion B25.0
  cytomegaloviral B25.0
  deglutition - *see* Pneumonia, aspiration
  desquamative interstitial J84.117
  diffuse - *see* Pneumonia, broncho
  diplococcal, diplococcus (broncho) (lobar)
    J13
  disseminated (focal) - *see* Pneumonia, broncho
  Eaton's agent J15.7
  embolic, embolism - *see* Embolism,
    pulmonary
  Enterobacter J15.6
  eosinophilic J82
  Escherichia coli (E. coli) J15.5
  Eubacterium J15.8
  fibrinous - *see* Pneumonia, lobar
  fibroid, fibrous (chronic) - *see* Fibrosis, lung
  Friedländer's bacillus J15.0
  Fusobacterium (nucleatum) J15.8
  gangrenous J85.0
  giant cell (measles) B05.2
  gonococcal A54.84
  gram negative bacteria NEC J15.6
    anaerobic J15.8
  Hemophilus influenzae (broncho) (lobar) J14
  human metapneumovirus J12.3
  hypostatic (broncho) (lobar) J18.2
  in (due to)
    actinomycosis A42.0
    adenovirus J12.0
    anthrax A22.1
    ascariasis B77.81
    aspergillosis B44.9
    Bacillus anthracis A22.1
    Bacterium anitratum J15.6
    candidiasis B37.1
    chickenpox B01.2
    Chlamydia J16.0
      neonatal P23.1
    coccidioidomycosis B38.2
      acute B38.0
      chronic B38.1
    cytomegalovirus disease B25.0
    Diplococcus (pneumoniae) J13
    Eaton's agent J15.7
    Enterobacter J15.6
    Escherichia coli (E. coli) J15.5
    Friedländer's bacillus J15.0
    fumes and vapors (chemical) (inhalation)
      J68.0
    gonorrhea A54.84
    Hemophilus influenzae (H. influenzae) J14
    Herellea J15.6
    histoplasmosis B39.2
      acute B39.0
      chronic B39.1
    human metapneumovirus J12.3
    Klebsiella (pneumoniae) J15.0
    measles B05.2
    Mycoplasma (pneumoniae) J15.7
    nocardiosis, nocardiasis A43.0
    ornithosis A70
    parainfluenza virus J12.2

Pneumonia - *continued*
    pleuro-pneumonia-like-organism (PPLO)
      J15.7
    pneumococcus J13
    pneumocystosis (Pneumocystis carinii)
      (Pneumocystis jiroveci) B59
    Proteus J15.6
    Pseudomonas NEC J15.1
      pseudomallei A24.1
    psittacosis A70
    Q fever A78
    respiratory syncytial virus J12.1
    rheumatic fever I00 [*J17*]
    rubella B06.81
    Salmonella (infection) A02.22
      typhi A01.03
    schistosomiasis B65.9 [*J17*]
    Serratia marcescens J15.6
    specified
      bacterium NEC J15.8
      organism NEC J16.8
    spirochetal NEC A69.8
    Staphylococcus J15.20
      aureus (methicillin susceptible) (MSSA)
        J15.211
        methicillin resistant (MRSA) J15.212
      specified NEC J15.29
    Streptococcus J15.4
      group B J15.3
      pneumoniae J13
      specified NEC J15.4
    toxoplasmosis B58.3
    tularemia A21.2
    typhoid (fever) A01.03
    varicella B01.2
    virus - *see* Pneumonia, viral
    whooping cough A37.91
      due to
        Bordetella parapertussis A37.11
        Bordetella pertussis A37.01
        specified NEC A37.81
    Yersinia pestis A20.2
  inhalation of food or vomit - *see* Pneumonia,
    aspiration
  interstitial J84.9
    chronic J84.111
    desquamative J84.117
    due to
      collagen vascular disease J84.17
      known underlying cause J84.17
    idiopathic NOS J84.111
    in disease classified elsewhere J84.17
    lymphocytic (due to collagen vascular
      disease) (in diseases classified elsewhere)
      J84.17
    lymphoid J84.2
    non-specific J84.89
      due to
        collagen vascular disease J84.17
        known underlying cause J84.17
      idiopathic J84.113
      in diseases classified elsewhere J84.17
    plasma cell B59
    pseudomonas J15.1
    usual J84.112
      due to collagen vascular disease J84.17
      idiopathic J84.112
      in diseases classified elsewhere J84.17
  Klebsiella (pneumoniae) J15.0
  lipid, lipoid (exogenous) J69.1
    endogenous J84.89
  lobar (disseminated) (double) (interstitial)
    J18.1
    bacterial J15.9

Pneumonia - *continued*
  specified NEC J15.8
chronic - *see* Fibrosis, lung
Escherichia coli (E. coli) J15.5
Friedländer's bacillus J15.0
Hemophilus influenzae J14
hypostatic J18.2
Klebsiella (pneumoniae) J15.0
pneumococcal J13
Proteus J15.6
Pseudomonas J15.1
specified organism NEC J16.8
staphylococcal - *see* Pneumonia,
  staphylococcal
streptococcal NEC J15.4
Streptococcus pneumoniae J13
viral, virus - *see* Pneumonia, viral
lobular - *see* Pneumonia, broncho
Löffler's J82
lymphoid interstitial J84.2
massive - *see* Pneumonia, lobar
meconium P24.01
MRSA (Methicillin resistant Staphylococcus
  aureus) J15.212
MSSA (methicillin susceptible Staphylococcus
  aureus) J15.211
multilobar - *see* Pneumonia, by type
Mycoplasma (pneumoniae) J15.7
necrotic J85.0
neonatal P23.9
  aspiration - *see* Aspiration, by substance,
    with pneumonia
nitrogen dioxide J68.0
organizing J84.89
  due to
    collagen vascular disease J84.17
    known underlying cause J84.17
  in diseases classified elsewhere J84.17
orthostatic J18.2
parainfluenza virus J12.2
parenchymatous - *see* Fibrosis, lung
passive J18.2
patchy - *see* Pneumonia, broncho
Peptococcus J15.8
Peptostreptococcus J15.8
plasma cell (of infants) B59
pleurolobar - *see* Pneumonia, lobar
pleuro-pneumonia-like organism (PPLO) J15.7
pneumococcal (broncho) (lobar) J13
Pneumocystis (carinii) (jiroveci) B59
postinfectional NEC B99 *[J17]*
postmeasles B05.2
Proteus J15.6
Pseudomonas J15.1
psittacosis A70
radiation J70.0
respiratory syncytial virus J12.1
resulting from a procedure J95.89
rheumatic I00 *[J17]*
Salmonella (arizonae) (cholerae-suis)
  (enteritidis) (typhimurium) A02.22
  typhi A01.03
  typhoid fever A01.03
SARS-associated coronavirus J12.81
segmented, segmental - *see* Pneumonia,
  broncho   Serratia marcescens J15.6
specified NEC J18.8
  bacterium NEC J15.8
  organism NEC J16.8
  virus NEC J12.89
spirochetal NEC A69.8
staphylococcal (broncho) (lobar) J15.20
  aureus (methicillin susceptible) (MSSA)
    J15.211

Pneumonia - *continued*
  methicillin resistant (MRSA) J15.212
  specified NEC J15.29
static, stasis J18.2
streptococcal NEC (broncho) (lobar) J15.4
  group
    A J15.4
    B J15.3
    specified NEC J15.4
Streptococcus pneumoniae J13
syphilitic, congenital (early) A50.04
traumatic (complication) (early) (secondary)
  T79.8
tuberculous (any) - *see* Tuberculosis,
  pulmonary
tularemic A21.2
varicella B01.2
Veillonella J15.8
ventilator associated J95.851
viral, virus (broncho) (interstitial) (lobar) J12.9
  adenoviral J12.0
  congenital P23.0
  human metapneumovirus J12.3
  parainfluenza J12.2
  respiratory syncytial J12.1
  SARS-associated coronavirus J12.81
  specified NEC J12.89
white (congenital) A50.04
Pneumonic - *see* condition
Pneumonitis (acute) (primary) - *see also*
  Pneumonia
air-conditioner J67.7
allergic (due to) J67.9
  organic dust NEC J67.8
  red cedar dust J67.8
  sequoiosis J67.8
  wood dust J67.8
aspiration J69.0
  due to
    anesthesia J95.4
      during
        labor and delivery O74.0
        pregnancy O29.01-
        puerperium O89.01
    fumes or gases J68.0
  obstetric O74.0
chemical (due to gases, fumes or vapors)
  (inhalation) J68.0
  due to anesthesia J95.4
cholesterol J84.89
crack (cocaine) J68.0
chronic - *see* Fibrosis, lung
congenital rubella P35.0
due to
  beryllium J68.0
  cadmium J68.0
  crack (cocaine) J68.0
  detergent J69.8
  fluorocarbon-polymer J68.0
  food, vomit (aspiration) J69.0
  fumes or vapors J68.0
  gases, fumes or vapors (inhalation) J68.0
  inhalation
    blood J69.8
    essences J69.1
    food (regurgitated), milk, vomit J69.0
    oils, essences J69.1
    saliva J69.0
    solids, liquids NEC J69.8
  manganese J68.0
  nitrogen dioxide J68.0
  oils, essences J69.1
  solids, liquids NEC J69.8
toxoplasmosis (acquired) B58.3

Pneumonitis (acute) (primary) - *continued*
  congenital P37.1
vanadium J68.0
ventilator J95.851
eosinophilic J82
hypersensitivity J67.9
  air conditioner lung J67.7
  bagassosis J67.1
  bird fancier's lung J67.2
  farmer's lung J67.0
  Maltworker's lung J67.4
  maple bark-stripper's lung J67.6
  mushroom worker's lung J67.5
  specified organic dust NEC J67.8
  suberosis J67.3
interstitial (chronic) J84.89
  acute J84.114
  lymphoid J84.2
  non-specific J84.89
    idiopathic J84.113
lymphoid, interstitial J84.2
meconium P24.01
postanesthetic J95.4
  correct substance properly administered - *see*
    Table of Drugs and Chemicals, by drug,
    adverse effect
  in labor and delivery O74.0
  in pregnancy O29.01-
  obstetric O74.0
  overdose or wrong substance given or taken
    (by accident) - *see* Table of Drugs and
    Chemicals, by drug, poisoning
postpartum, puerperal O89.01
postoperative J95.4
  obstetric O74.0
radiation J70.0
rubella, congenital P35.0
ventilation (air-conditioning) J67.7
ventilator associated J95.851
wood-dust J67.8
Pneumonoconiosis - *see* Pneumoconiosis
Pneumoparotid K11.8
Pneumopathy NEC J98.4
alveolar J84.09
due to organic dust NEC J66.8
parietoalveolar J84.09
Pneumopericarditis - *see also* Pericarditis
acute I30.9
Pneumopericardium - *see also* Pericarditis
congenital P25.3
newborn P25.3
traumatic (post) - *see* Injury, heart
Pneumophagia (psychogenic) F45.8
Pneumopleurisy, pneumopleuritis - *see also*
  Pneumonia J18.8
Pneumopyopericardium I30.1
Pneumopyothorax - *see* Pyopneumothorax
with fistula J86.0
Pneumorrhagia - *see also* Hemorrhage, lung
tuberculous - *see* Tuberculosis, pulmonary
Pneumothorax NOS J93.9
acute J93.83
chronic J93.81
congenital P25.1
perinatal period P25.1
postprocedural J95.811
specified NEC J93.83
spontaneous NOS J93.83
  newborn P25.1
  primary J93.11
  secondary J93.12
  tension J93.0
tense valvular, infectional J93.0
tension (spontaneous) J93.0

Pneumothorax - *continued*
  traumatic S27.0
    with hemothorax S27.2
  tuberculous - *see* Tuberculosis, pulmonary
Podagra - *see also* Gout M10.9
Podencephalus Q01.9
Poikilocytosis R71.8
Poikiloderma L81.6
  Civatte's L57.3
  congenital Q82.8
  vasculare atrophicans L94.5
Poikilodermatomyositis M33.10
  with
    myopathy M33.12
    respiratory involvement M33.11
    specified organ involvement NEC M33.19
Pointed ear (congenital) Q17.3
**Poison ivy, oak, sumac or other plant
  dermatitis (allergic) (contact)** L23.7
Poisoning (acute) - *see also* Table of Drugs and
  Chemicals
  algae and toxins T65.82-
  Bacillus B (aertrycke) (cholerae (suis))
    (paratyphosus) (suipestifer) A02.9
    botulinus A05.1
  bacterial toxins A05.9
  berries, noxious - *see* Poisoning, food,
    noxious, berries
  botulism A05.1
  ciguatera fish T61.0-
  Clostridium botulinum A05.1
  death-cap (Amanita phalloides) (Amanita
    verna) - *see* Poisoning, food, noxious,
    mushrooms
  drug - *see* Table of Drugs and Chemicals, by
    drug, poisoning
  epidemic, fish (noxious) - *see* Poisoning,
    seafood
    bacterial A05.9
  fava bean D55.0
  fish (noxious) T61.9-
    bacterial - *see* Intoxication, foodborne, by
      agent
    ciguatera fish - *see* Poisoning, ciguatera fish
    scombroid fish - *see* Poisoning, scombroid
      fish
    specified type NEC T61.77-
  food (acute) (diseased) (infected) (noxious)
    NEC T62.9-
    bacterial - *see* Intoxication, foodborne, by
      agent
    due to
      Bacillus (aertrycke) (choleraesuis)
        (paratyphosus) (suipestifer) A02.9
        botulinus A05.1
      Clostridium (perfringens) (Welchii) A05.2
      salmonella (aertrycke) (gallinarum)
        (choleraesuis) (enteritidis) (paratyphi)
        (suipestifer) A02.9
        with
          gastroenteritis A02.0
          sepsis A02.1
      staphylococcus A05.0
      Vibrio
        parahaemolyticus A05.3
        vulnificus A05.5
    noxious or naturally toxic T62.9-
      berries - *see* subcategory T62.1-
      fish - *see* Poisoning, seafood
      mushrooms - *see* subcategory T62.0X-
      plants NEC - *see* subcategory T62.2X-
      seafood - *see* Poisoning, seafood
      specified NEC - *see* subcategory T62.8X
    ichthyotoxism - *see* Poisoning, seafood

Poisoning (acute) - *continued*
  kreotoxism, food A05.9
  latex T65.81-
  lead T56.0-
  mushroom - *see* Poisoning, food, noxious,
    mushroom
  mussels - *see also* Poisoning, shellfish
    bacterial - *see* Intoxication, foodborne, by
      agent
  nicotine (tobacco) T65.2-
  noxious foodstuffs - *see* Poisoning, food,
    noxious
  plants, noxious - *see* Poisoning, food, noxious,
    plants NEC
  ptomaine - *see* Poisoning, food
  radiation J70.0
  Salmonella (arizonae) (cholerae-suis)
    (enteritidis) (typhimurium) A02.9
  scombroid fish T61.1-
  seafood (noxious) T61.9-
    bacterial - *see* Intoxication, foodborne, by
      agent
    fish - *see* Poisoning, fish
    shellfish - *see* Poisoning, shellfish
    specified NEC - *see* subcategory T61.8X-
  shellfish (amnesic) (azaspiracid) (diarrheic)
    (neurotoxic) (noxious) (paralytic) T61.78-
    bacterial - *see* Intoxication, foodborne, by
      agent
    ciguatera mollusk - *see* Poisoning, ciguatera
      fish
  specified substance NEC T65.891
  Staphylococcus, food A05.0
  tobacco (nicotine) T65.2-
  water E87.79
Poker spine - *see* Spondylitis, ankylosing
Poland syndrome Q79.8
Polioencephalitis (acute) (bulbar) A80.9
  inferior G12.22
  influenzal - *see* Influenza, with,
    encephalopathy
  superior hemorrhagic (acute) (Wernicke's)
    E51.2
  Wernicke's E51.2
Polioencephalomyelitis (acute) (anterior)
  A80.9
  with beriberi E51.2
Polioencephalopathy, superior hemorrhagic
  E51.2
  with
    beriberi E51.11
    pellagra E52
Poliomeningoencephalitis - *see*
  Meningoencephalitis
Poliomyelitis (acute) (anterior) (epidemic)
  A80.9
  with paralysis (bulbar) - *see* Poliomyelitis,
    paralytic
  abortive A80.4
  ascending (progressive) - *see* Poliomyelitis,
    paralytic
  bulbar (paralytic) - *see* Poliomyelitis, paralytic
  congenital P35.8
  nonepidemic A80.9
  nonparalytic A80.4
  paralytic A80.30
    specified NEC A80.39
    vaccine-associated A80.0
    wild virus
      imported A80.1
      indigenous A80.2
  spinal, acute A80.9
Poliosis (eyebrow) (eyelashes) L67.1
  circumscripta, acquired L67.1

Pollakiuria R35.0
  psychogenic F45.8
Pollinosis J30.1
Pollitzer's disease L73.2
Polyadenitis - *see also* Lymphadenitis
  malignant A20.0
Polyalgia M79.89
Polyangiitis M30.0
  microscopic M31.7
  overlap syndrome M30.8
Polyarteritis
  microscopic M31.7
  nodosa M30.0
    with lung involvement M30.1
    juvenile M30.2
    related condition NEC M30.8
Polyarthralgia - *see* Pain, joint
Polyarthritis, polyarthropathy - *see also*
  Arthritis M13.0
  due to or associated with other specified
    conditions - *see* Arthritis
  epidemic (Australian) (with exanthema) B33.1
  infective - *see* Arthritis, pyogenic or pyemic
  inflammatory M06.4
  juvenile (chronic) (seronegative) M08.3
  migratory - *see* Fever, rheumatic
  rheumatic, acute - *see* Fever, rheumatic
Polyarthrosis M15.9
  post-traumatic M15.3
  primary M15.0
  specified NEC M15.8
Polycarential syndrome of infancy E40
Polychondritis (atrophic) (chronic) - *see also*
  Disorder, cartilage, specified type NEC
  relapsing M94.1
Polycoria Q13.2
Polycystic (disease)
  degeneration, kidney Q61.3
    autosomal dominant (adult type) Q61.2
    autosomal recessive (infantile type) NEC
      Q61.19
  kidney Q61.3
    autosomal
      dominant Q61.2
      recessive NEC Q61.19
    autosomal dominant (adult type) Q61.2
    autosomal recessive (childhood type) NEC
      Q61.19
    infantile type NEC Q61.19
  liver Q44.6
  lung J98.4
    congenital Q33.0
  ovary, ovaries E28.2
  spleen Q89.09
Polycythemia (secondary) D75.1
  acquired D75.1
  benign (familial) D75.0
  due to
    donor twin P61.1
    erythropoietin D75.1
    fall in plasma volume D75.1
    high altitude D75.1
    maternal-fetal transfusion P61.1
    stress D75.1
  emotional D75.1
  erythropoietin D75.1
  familial (benign) D75.0
  Gaisböck's (hypertonica) D75.1
  high altitude D75.1
  hypertonica D75.1
  hypoxemic D75.1
  neonatorum P61.1
  nephrogenous D75.1
  relative D75.1

Polycythemia - *continued*
secondary D75.1
spurious D75.1
stress D75.1
vera D45
Polycytosis cryptogenica D75.1
Polydactylism, polydactyly Q69.9
toes Q69.2
Polydipsia R63.1
Polydystrophy, pseudo-hurler E77.0
Polyembryoma - *see* Neoplasm, malignant, by site
Polyglandular
deficiency E31.0
dyscrasia E31.9
dysfunction E31.9
syndrome E31.8
Polyhydramnios O40.-
Polymastia Q83.1
Polymenorrhea N92.0
Polymyalgia M35.3
arteritica, giant cell M31.5
rheumatica M35.3
with giant cell arteritis M31.5
Polymyositis (acute) (chronic) (hemorrhagic) M33.20
with
myopathy M33.22
respiratory involvement M33.21
skin involvement - *see* Dermatopolymyositis
specified organ involvement NEC M33.29
ossificans (generalisata) (progressiva) - *see* Myositis, ossificans, progressiva
Polyneuritis, polyneuritic - *see also* Polyneuropathy
acute (post) infective G61.0
alcoholic G62.1
cranialis G52.7
demyelinating, chronic inflammatory (CIDP) G61.81
diabetic - *see* Diabetes, polyneuropathy
diphtheritic A36.83
due to lack of vitamin NEC E56.9 [*G63*]
endemic E51.11
erythredem*a* - *see* subcategory T56.1
febrile, acute G61.0
hereditary ataxic G60.1
idiopathic, acute G61.0
infective (acute) G61.0
inflammatory, chronic demyelinating (CIDP) G61.81
nutritional E63.9 [*G63*]
postinfective (acute) G61.0
specified NEC G62.89
Polyneuropathy (peripheral) G62.9
alcoholic G62.1
amyloid (Portuguese) E85.1 [*G63*]
transthyretin-related (ATTR) familial E85.1
arsenical G62.2
critical illness G62.81
demyelinating, chronic inflammatory (CIDP) G61.81
diabetic - *see* Diabetes, polyneuropathy
drug-induced G62.0
hereditary G60.9
specified NEC G60.8
idiopathic G60.9
progressive G60.3
in (due to)
alcohol G62.1
sequelae G65.2
amyloidosis, familial (Portuguese) E85.1 [*G63*]
antitetanus serum G61.1

Polyneuropathy - *continued*
arsenic G62.2
sequelae G65.2
avitaminosis NEC E56.9 [*G63*]
beriberi E51.11
collagen vascular disease NEC M35.9 [*G63*]
deficiency (of)
B (-complex) vitamins E53.9 [*G63*]
vitamin B6 E53.1 [*G63*]
diabetes - *see* Diabetes, polyneuropathy
diphtheria A36.83
drug or medicament G62.0
correct substance properly administered - *see* Table of Drugs and Chemicals, by drug, adverse effect
overdose or wrong substance given or taken - *see* Table of Drugs and Chemicals, by drug, poisoning
endocrine disease NEC E34.9 [*G63*]
herpes zoster B02.23
hypoglycemia E16.2 [*G63*]
infectious
disease NEC B99 [*G63*]
mononucleosis B27.91
lack of vitamin NEC E56.9 [*G63*]
lead G62.2
sequelae G65.2
leprosy A30.9 [*G63*]
Lyme disease A69.22
metabolic disease NEC E88.9 [*G63*]
microscopic polyangiitis M31.7 [*G63*]
mumps B26.84
neoplastic disease - *see also* Neoplasm D49.9 [*G63*]
nutritional deficiency NEC E63.9 [*G63*]
organophosphate compounds G62.2
sequelae G65.2
parasitic disease NEC B89 [*G63*]
pellagra E52 [*G63*]
polyarteritis nodosa M30.0
porphyria E80.20 [*G63*]
radiation G62.82
rheumatoid arthritis - *see* Rheumatoid, polyneuropathy
sarcoidosis D86.89
serum G61.1
syphilis (late) A52.15
congenital A50.43
systemic
connective tissue disorder M35.9 [*G63*]
lupus erythematosus M32.19
toxic agent NEC G62.2
sequelae G65.2
transthyretin-related (ATTR) familial amyloid E85.1
triorthocresyl phosphate G62.2
sequelae G65.2
tuberculosis A17.89
uremia N18.9 [*G63*]
vitamin B12 deficiency E53.8 [*G63*]
with anemia (pernicious) D51.0 [*G63*]
due to dietary deficiency D51.3 [*G63*]
zoster B02.23
inflammatory G61.9
chronic demyelinating (CIDP) G61.81
sequelae G65.1
specified NEC G61.89
lead G62.2
sequelae G65.2
nutritional NEC E63.9 [*G63*]
postherpetic (zoster) B02.23
progressive G60.3
radiation-induced G62.82
sensory (hereditary) (idiopathic) G60.8

Polyneuropathy - *continued*
specified NEC G62.89
syphilitic (late) A52.15
congenital A50.43
Polyopia H53.8
Polyorchism, polyorchidism Q55.21
Polyosteoarthritis - *see also* Osteoarthritis, generalized M15.9-
post-traumatic M15.3
specified NEC M15.8
Polyostotic fibrous dysplasia Q78.1
Polyotia Q17.0
Polyp, polypus
accessory sinus J33.8
adenocarcinoma in - *see* Neoplasm, malignant, by site
adenocarcinoma in situ in - *see* Neoplasm, in situ, by site
adenoid tissue J33.0
adenomatous - *see also* Neoplasm, benign, by site
adenocarcinoma in - *see* Neoplasm, malignant, by site
adenocarcinoma in situ in - *see* Neoplasm, in situ, by site
carcinoma in - *see* Neoplasm, malignant, by site
carcinoma in situ in - *see* Neoplasm, in situ, by site
multiple - *see* Neoplasm, benign
adenocarcinoma in - *see* Neoplasm, malignant, by site
adenocarcinoma in situ in - *see* Neoplasm, in situ, by site
antrum J33.8
anus, anal (canal) K62.0
Bartholin's gland N84.3
bladder D41.4
carcinoma in - *see* Neoplasm, malignant, by site
carcinoma in situ in - *see* Neoplasm, in situ, by site
cecum D12.0
cervix (uteri) N84.1
in pregnancy or childbirth - *see* Pregnancy, complicated by, abnormal, cervix
mucous N84.1
nonneoplastic N84.1
choanal J33.0
cholesterol K82.4
clitoris N84.3
colon K63.5
adenomatous D12.6
ascending D12.2
cecum D12.0
descending D12.4
inflammatory K51.40
with
abscess K51.414
complication K51.419
specified NEC K51.418
fistula K51.413
intestinal obstruction K51.412
rectal bleeding K51.411
sigmoid D12.5
transverse D12.3
corpus uteri N84.0
dental K04.01
irreversible K04.02
reversible K04.01
duodenum K31.7
ear (middle) H74.4-
endometrium N84.0
ethmoidal (sinus) J33.8

Polyp, polypus - *continued*
  fallopian tube N84.8
  female genital tract N84.9
    specified NEC N84.8
  frontal (sinus) J33.8
  gallbladder K82.8
  gingiva, gum K06.8
  labia, labium (majus) (minus) N84.3
  larynx (mucous) J38.1
    adenomatous D14.1
  malignant - *see* Neoplasm, malignant, by site
  maxillary (sinus) J33.8
  middle ear - *see* Polyp, ear (middle)
  myometrium N84.0
  nares
    anterior J33.9
    posterior J33.0
  nasal (mucous) J33.9
    cavity J33.0
    septum J33.0
  nasopharyngeal J33.0
  nose (mucous) J33.9
  oviduct N84.8
  pharynx J39.2
  placenta O90.89
  prostate - *see* Enlargement, enlarged, prostate
  pudenda, pudendum N84.3
  pulpal (dental) K04.01
    irreversible K04.02
    reversible K04.01
  rectum (nonadenomatous) K62.1
    adenomatous - *see* Polyp, adenomatous
  septum (nasal) J33.0
  sinus (accessory) (ethmoidal) (frontal)
    (maxillary) (sphenoidal) J33.8-
  sphenoidal (sinus) J33.8
  stomach K31.7
    adenomatous D13.1
  tube, fallopian N84.8
  turbinate, mucous membrane J33.8
  umbilical, newborn P83.6
  ureter N28.89
  urethra N36.2
  uterus (body) (corpus) (mucous) N84.0
    cervix N84.1
    in pregnancy or childbirth - *see* Pregnancy,
    complicated by, tumor, uterus
  vagina N84.2
  vocal cord (mucous) J38.1
  vulva N84.3
Polyphagia R63.2
Polyploidy Q92.7
Polypoid - *see* condition
Polyposis - *see also* Polyp
  coli (adenomatous) D12.6
    adenocarcinoma in C18.9
    adenocarcinoma in situ in - *see* Neoplasm, in
    situ, by site
    carcinoma in C18.9
  colon (adenomatous) D12.6
  familial D12.6
    adenocarcinoma in situ in - *see* Neoplasm, in
    situ, by site
  intestinal (adenomatous) D12.6
  malignant lymphomatous C83.1-
  multiple, adenomatous - *see also* Neoplasm,
    benign D36.9
Polyradiculitis - *see* Polyneuropathy
Polyradiculoneuropathy (acute)
  (postinfective) (segmentally demyelinating)
  G61.0
Polyserositis
  due to pericarditis I31.1
  pericardial I31.1

Polyserositis - *continued*
  periodic, familial E85.0
  tuberculous A19.9
    acute A19.1
    chronic A19.8
Polysplenia syndrome Q89.09
Polysyndactyly - *see also* Syndactylism,
  syndactyly Q70.4
Polytrichia L68.3
Polyunguia Q84.6
Polyuria R35.8
  nocturnal R35.1
  psychogenic F45.8
Pompe's disease (glycogen storage) E74.02
Pompholyx L30.1
Poncet's disease (tuberculous rheumatism)
  A18.09
Pond fracture - *see* Fracture, skull
Ponos B55.0
Pons, pontine - *see* condition **Poor**
  aesthetic of existing restoration of tooth
    K08.56
  contractions, labor O62.2
  gingival margin to tooth restoration K08.51
  personal hygiene R46.0
  prenatal care, affecting management of
    pregnancy - *see* Pregnancy, complicated by,
    insufficient, prenatal care
  sucking reflex (newborn) R29.2
  urinary stream R39.12
  vision NEC H54.7
Poradenitis, nostras inguinalis or venerea
  A55
Porencephaly (congenital) (developmental)
  (true) Q04.6
  acquired G93.0
  nondevelopmental G93.0
  traumatic (post) F07.89
Porocephaliasis B88.8
Porokeratosis Q82.8
Poroma, eccrine - *see* Neoplasm, skin, benign
Porphyria (South African) E80.20
  acquired E80.20
  acute intermittent (hepatic) (Swedish) E80.21
  cutanea tarda (hereditary) (symptomatic)
    E80.1
  due to drugs E80.20
    correct substance properly administered - *see*
    Table of Drugs and Chemicals, by drug,
    adverse effect
    overdose or wrong substance given or taken -
    see Table of Drugs and Chemicals, by drug,
    poisoning
  erythropoietic (congenital) (hereditary) E80.0
  hepatocutaneous type E80.1
  secondary E80.20
  toxic NEC E80.20
  variegata E80.20
Porphyrinuria - *see* Porphyria
Porphyruria - *see* Porphyria
Portal - *see* condition
Port wine nevus, mark, or stain Q82.5
Posadas-Wernicke disease B38.9
Positive
  culture (nonspecific)
    blood R78.81
    bronchial washings R84.5
    cerebrospinal fluid R83.5
    cervix uteri R87.5
    nasal secretions R84.5
    nipple discharge R89.5
    nose R84.5
      staphylococcus (Methicillin susceptible)
      Z22.321

Positive - *continued*
    Methicillin resistant Z22.322
  peritoneal fluid R85.5
  pleural fluid R84.5
  prostatic secretions R86.5
  saliva R85.5
  seminal fluid R86.5
  sputum R84.5
  synovial fluid R89.5
  throat scrapings R84.5
  urine R82.79
  vagina R87.5
  vulva R87.5
  wound secretions R89.5
  PPD (skin test) R76.11
  serology for syphilis A53.0
    false R76.8
    with signs or symptoms
    code as Syphilis, by site and stage
  skin test, tuberculin (without active
    tuberculosis) R76.11
  test, human immunodeficiency virus (HIV)
    R75
  VDRL A53.0
    with signs or symptoms
    code by site and stage under Syphilis A53.9
  Wassermann reaction A53.0
Postcardiotomy syndrome I97.0
Postcaval ureter Q62.62
Postcholecystectomy syndrome K91.5
Postclimacteric bleeding N95.0
Postcommissurotomy syndrome I97.0
Postconcussional syndrome F07.81
Postcontusional syndrome F07.81
Postcricoid region - *see* condition
Post-dates (40-42
  weeks) (pregnancy) (mother) O48.0
  more than 42
  weeks gestation O48.1
Postencephalitic syndrome F07.89
Posterior - *see* condition
Posterolateral sclerosis (spinal cord) - *see*
  Degeneration, combined
Postexanthematous - *see* condition
Postfebrile - *see* condition
Postgastrectomy dumping syndrome K91.1
Posthemiplegic chorea - *see* Monoplegia
Posthemorrhagic anemia (chronic) D50.0
  acute D62
  newborn P61.3
Postherpetic neuralgia (zoster) B02.29
  trigeminal B02.22
Posthitis N47.7
Postimmunization complication or reaction -
  see Complications, vaccination
Postinfectious - *see* condition
Postlaminectomy syndrome NEC M96.1
Postleukotomy syndrome F07.0
Postmastectomy lymphedema (syndrome)
  I97.2
Postmaturity, postmature (over 42 weeks)
  maternal (over 42weeks gestation) O48.1
  newborn P08.22
Postmeasles complication NEC - *see also*
  condition B05.89
Postmenopausal
  endometrium (atrophic) N95.8
    suppurative - *see also* Endometritis N71.9
  osteoporosis - *see* Osteoporosis,
    postmenopausal
Postnasal drip R09.82
  due to
    allergic rhinitis - *see* Rhinitis, allergic
    common cold J00

Postnasal drip - *continued*
gastroesophageal reflux - *see* Reflux, gastroesophageal
nasopharyngitis - *see* Nasopharyngitis
other know condition
code to condition
sinusitis - *see* Sinusitis
Postnatal - *see* condition
Postoperative (postprocedural) - *see* Complication, postoperative
pneumothorax, therapeutic Z98.3
state NEC Z98.890
Postpancreatectomy hyperglycemia E89.1
Postpartum - *see* Puerperal
Postphlebitic syndrome - *see* Syndrome, postthrombotic
Postpoliomyelitic - *see also* condition
osteopathy - *see* Osteopathy, after poliomyelitis
Postpolio (myelitic) syndrome G14
Postprocedural - *see also* Postoperative
hypoinsulinemia E89.1
Postschizophrenic depression F32.89
Postsurgery status - *see also* Status (post)
pneumothorax, therapeutic Z98.3
Post-term (40-42
weeks) (pregnancy) (mother) O48.0
infant P08.21
more than 42
weeks gestation (mother) O48.1
Post-traumatic brain syndrome,
nonpsychotic F07.81
Post-typhoid abscess A01.09
Postures, hysterical F44.2
Postvaccinal reaction or complication - *see* Complications, vaccination
Postvalvulotomy syndrome I97.0
Potain's
disease (pulmonary edema) - *see* Edema, lung
syndrome (gastrectasis with dyspepsia) K31.0
Potter's
asthma J62.8
facies Q60.6
lung J62.8
syndrome (with renal agenesis) Q60.6
Pott's
curvature (spinal) A18.01
disease or paraplegia A18.01
spinal curvature A18.01
tumor, puffy - *see* Osteomyelitis, specified type NEC
Pouch
bronchus Q32.4
Douglas' - *see* condition
esophagus, esophageal, congenital Q39.6
acquired K22.5
gastric K31.4
Hartmann's K82.8
pharynx, pharyngeal (congenital) Q38.7
Pouchitis K91.850
Poultry men's itch B88.0
Poverty NEC Z59.6
extreme Z59.5
Poxvirus NEC B08.8
Prader-Willi syndrome Q87.1
Preauricular appendage or tag Q17.0
Prebetalipoproteinemia (acquired) (essential)
(familial) (hereditary) (primary)
(secondary) E78.1
with chylomicronemia E78.3
Precipitate labor or delivery O62.3
Preclimacteric bleeding (menorrhagia) N92.4
Precocious
adrenarche E30.1

Precocious - *continued*
menarche E30.1
menstruation E30.1
pubarche E30.1
puberty E30.1
central E22.8
sexual development NEC E30.1
thelarche E30.8
Precocity, sexual (constitutional)
(cryptogenic) (female) (idiopathic) (male)
E30.1
with adrenal hyperplasia E25.9
congenital E25.0
Precordial pain R07.2
Predeciduous teeth K00.2
Prediabetes, prediabetic R73.03
complicating
pregnancy - *see* Pregnancy, complicated by, diseases of, specified type or system NEC
puerperium O99.89
Predislocation status of hip at birth Q65.6
Pre-eclampsia O14.9-
with pre-existing hypertension - *see* Hypertension, complicating pregnancy, pre-existing, with, pre-eclampsia
complicating
childbirth O14.94
puerperium O14.95
mild O14.0-
complicating
childbirth O14.04
puerperium O14.05
moderate O14.0-
complicating
childbirth O14.04
puerperium O14.05
severe O14.1-
with hemolysis, elevated liver enzymes and low platelet count (HELLP) O14.2-
complicating
childbirth O14.24
puerperium O14.25
complicating
childbirth O14.14
puerperium O14.15
Pre-eruptive color change, teeth, tooth K00.8
Pre-excitation atrioventricular conduction
I45.6
Preglaucoma H40.00-
Pregnancy (single) (uterine) - *see also*
Delivery and Puerperal
Note: The Tabular must be reviewed for assignment of the appropriate character indicating the trimester of the pregnancy
Note: The Tabular must be reviewed for assignment of appropriate seventh character for multiple gestation codes in Chapter 15
abdominal (ectopic) O00.00
with intrauterine pregnancy O00.01
with viable fetus O36.7-
ampullar O00.10-
with intrauterine pregnancy O00.11-
biochemical O02.81
broad ligament O00.80
with intrauterine pregnancy O00.81
cervical O00.80
with intrauterine pregnancy O00.81
chemical O02.81
complicated NOS O26.9-
complicated by (care of) (management affected by)
abnormal, abnormality
cervix O34.4-
causing obstructed labor O65.5

Pregnancy - *continued*
cord (umbilical) O69.9
fetal heart rate or rhythm O36.83-
findings on antenatal screening of mother O28.9
biochemical O28.1
cytological O28.2
chromosomal O28.5
genetic O28.5
hematological O28.0
radiological O28.4
specified NEC O28.8
ultrasonic O28.3
glucose (tolerance) NEC O99.810
pelvic organs O34.9-
specified NEC O34.8-
causing obstructed labor O65.5
pelvis (bony) (major) NEC O33.0
perineum O34.7-
position
placenta O44.0-
with hemorrhage O44.1-
uterus O34.59-
uterus O34.59-
causing obstructed labor O65.5
congenital O34.0-
vagina O34.6-
causing obstructed labor O65.5
vulva O34.7-
causing obstructed labor O65.5
abruptio placentae - *see* Abruptio placentae
abscess or cellulitis
bladder O23.1-
breast O91.11-
genital organ or tract O23.9-
abuse
physical O9A.31-
psychological O9A.51-
sexual O9A.41-
adverse effect anesthesia O29.9-
aspiration pneumonitis O29.01-
cardiac arrest O29.11-
cardiac complication NEC O29.19-
cardiac failure O29.12-
central nervous system complication NEC O29.29-
cerebral anoxia O29.21-
failed or difficult intubation O29.6-
inhalation of stomach contents or secretions NOS O29.01-
local, toxic reaction O29.3X
Mendelson's syndrome O29.01-
pressure collapse of lung O29.02-
pulmonary complications NEC O29.09-
specified NEC O29.8X-
spinal and epidural type NEC O29.5X
induced headache O29.4-
albuminuria - *see also* Proteinuria, gestational O12.1-
alcohol use O99.31-
amnionitis O41.12
anaphylactoid syndrome of pregnancy O88.01-
anemia (conditions in D50-d64) (pre-existing) O99.01-
complicating the puerperium O99.03
antepartum hemorrhage O46.9-
with coagulation defect - *see* Hemorrhage, antepartum, with coagulation defect
specified NEC O46.8X-
appendicitis O99.61-
atrophy (yellow) (acute) liver (subacute) O26.61-
bariatric surgery status O99.84-

Pregnancy - *continued*
  bicornis or bicornuate uterus O34.0-
  biliary tract problems O26.61-
  breech presentation O32.1
  cardiovascular diseases (conditions in I00-
    i09, I20-i52, I70-i99) O99.41-
  cerebrovascular disorders (conditions in I60-
    i69) O99.41-
  cervical shortening O26.87-
  cervicitis O23.51-
  chloasma (gravidarum) O26.89-
  cholestasis (intrahepatic) O26.61-
  cholecystitis O99.61-
  chorioamnionitis O41.12-
  circulatory system disorder (conditions in
    I00-i09, I20-i99, O99.41)
  compound presentation O32.6
  conjoined twins O30.02-
  connective system disorders (conditions in
    M00-m99) O99.89
  contracted pelvis (general) O33.1
    inlet O33.2
    outlet O33.3
  convulsions (eclamptic) (uremic) - *see also*
    Eclampsia O15.9-
  cracked nipple O92.11-
  cystitis O23.1-
  cystocele O34.8-
  death of fetus (near term) O36.4
    early pregnancy O02.1
    of one fetus or more in multiple gestation
      O31.2-
  deciduitis O41.14-
  decreased fetal movement O36.81-
  dental problems O99.61-
  diabetes (mellitus) O24.91-
    gestational (pregnancy induced) - *see*
  Diabetes, gestational
    pre-existing O24.31-
      specified NEC O24.81-
      type 1 O24.01-
      type 2 O24.11-
  digestive system disorders (conditions in
    K00-k93) O99.61-
  diseases of - *see* Pregnancy, complicated by,
    specified body system disease
    biliary tract O26.61-
    blood NEC (conditions in D65-d77)
      O99.11-
    liver O26.61-
    specified NEC O99.89
  disorders of - *see* Pregnancy, complicated by,
    specified body system disorder
    amniotic fluid and membranes O41.9-
      specified NEC O41.8X-
    biliary tract O26.61-
    ear and mastoid process (conditions in H60-
      h95) O99.89
    eye and adnexa (conditions in H00-h59)
      O99.89
    liver O26.61-
    skin (conditions in L00-l99) O99.71-
    specified NEC O99.89
  displacement, uterus NEC O34.59-
    causing obstructed labor O65.5
  disproportion (due to) O33.9
    fetal (ascites) (hydrops)
      (meningomyelocele) (sacral teratoma)
      (tumor) deformities NEC O33.7
    generally contracted pelvis O33.1
    hydrocephalic fetus O33.6
    inlet contraction of pelvis O33.2
    mixed maternal and fetal origin O33.4
    specified NEC O33.8

Pregnancy - *continued*
  double uterus O34.0-
    causing obstructed labor O65.5
  drug use (conditions in F11-f19) O99.32-
  eclampsia, eclamptic (coma) (convulsions)
    (delirium) (nephritis) (uremia) - *see also*
    Eclampsia O15.-
  ectopic pregnancy - *see* Pregnancy, ectopic
  edema O12.0-
    with
      gestational hypertension, mild - *see also*
        Pre-eclampsia O14.0-
      proteinuria O12.2-
  effusion, amniotic fluid - *see* Pregnancy,
    complicated by, premature rupture of
    membranes
  elderly
    multigravida O09.52-
    primigravida O09.51-
  embolism - *see also* Embolism, obstetric,
    pregnancy O88.-
  endocrine diseases NEC O99.28-
  endometritis O86.12
  excessive weight gain O26.0-
  exhaustion O26.81-
    during labor and delivery O75.81
  face presentation O32.3
  failed induction of labor O61.9
    instrumental O61.1
    mechanical O61.1
    medical O61.0
    specified NEC O61.8
    surgical O61.1
  failed or difficult intubation for anesthesia
    O29.6-
  false labor (pains) O47.9
    at or after 37 completed weeks of
      pregnancy O47.1
    before 37 completed weeks of pregnancy
      O47.0-
  fatigue O26.81-
    during labor and delivery O75.81
  fatty metamorphosis of liver O26.61-
  female genital mutilation O34.8 *[N90.81]*
  fetal (maternal care for)
    abnormality or damage O35.9
      acid-base balance O68
      specified type NEC O35.8
    acidemia O68
    acidosis O68
    alkalosis O68
    anemia and thrombocytopenia O36.82-
    anencephaly O35.0
    chromosomal abnormality (conditions in
      Q90-Q99) O35.1
    conjoined twins O30.02-
    damage from
      amniocentesis O35.7
      biopsy procedures O35.7
      drug addiction O35.5
      hematological investigation O35.7
      intrauterine contraceptive device O35.7
      maternal
        alcohol addiction O35.4
        cytomegalovirus infection O35.3
        disease NEC O35.8
        drug addiction O35.5
        listeriosis O35.8
        rubella O35.3
        toxoplasmosis O35.8
        viral infection O35.3
      medical procedure NEC O35.7
      radiation O35.6
    death (near term) O36.4

Pregnancy - *continued*
  early pregnancy O02.1
  decreased movement O36.81-
  disproportion due to deformity (fetal) O33.7
  excessive growth (large for dates) O36.6-
  growth retardation O36.59-
    light for dates O36.59-
    small for dates O36.59-
  heart rate irregularity (bradycardia)
    (decelerations) (tachycardia) O76
  hereditary disease O35.2
  hydrocephalus O35.0
  intrauterine death O36.4
  poor growth O36.59-
    light for dates O36.59-
    small for dates O36.59-
  problem O36.9-
    specified NEC O36.89-
  reduction (elective) O31.3-
  selective termination O31.3-
  spina bifida O35.0
  thrombocytopenia O36.82-
  fibroid (tumor) (uterus) O34.1-
  fissure of nipple O92.11-
  gallstones O99.61-
  gastric banding status O99.84-
  gastric bypass status O99.84-
  genital herpes (asymptomatic) (history of)
    (inactive) O98.3-
  genital tract infection O23.9-
  glomerular diseases (conditions in N00-N07)
    O26.83-
    with hypertension, pre-existing - *see*
      Hypertension, complicating, pregnancy,
      pre-existing, with, renal disease
  gonorrhea O98.21-
  grand multiparity O09.4
  habitual aborter - *see* Pregnancy, complicated
    by, recurrent pregnancy loss
  HELLP syndrome (hemolysis, elevated liver
    enzymes and low platelet count) O14.2-
  hemorrhage
    antepartum - *see* Hemorrhage, antepartum
    before 20 completed weeks gestation O20.9
      specified NEC O20.8
    due to premature separation, placenta - *see
      also* Abruptio placentae O45.9-
    early O20.9
      specified NEC O20.8
    threatened abortion O20.0
  hemorrhoids O22.4-
  hepatitis (viral) O98.41-
  herniation of uterus O34.59-
  high
    head at term O32.4
    risk - *see* Supervision (of) (for), high-risk
  history of in utero procedure during previous
    pregnancy O09.82-
  HIV O98.71-
  human immunodeficiency virus (HIV)
    disease O98.71-
  hydatidiform mole - *see also* Mole,
    hydatidiform O01.9-
  hydramnios O40.-
  hydrocephalic fetus (disproportion) O33.6
  hydrops
    amnii O40.-
    fetalis O36.2-
      associated with isoimmunization - *see also*
        Pregnancy, complicated by,
        isoimmunization O36.11-
  hydrorrhea O42.90
  hyperemesis (gravidarum) (mild) - *see also*
    Hyperemesis, gravidarum O21.0-

Pregnancy - *continued*

hypertension - *see* Hypertension, complicating pregnancy

hypertensive

heart and renal disease, pre-existing - *see* Hypertension, complicating, pregnancy, pre-existing, with, heart disease, with renal disease

heart disease, pre-existing - *see* Hypertension, complicating, pregnancy, pre-existing, with, heart disease

renal disease, pre-existing - *see* Hypertension, complicating, pregnancy, pre-existing, with, renal disease

hypotension O26.5-

immune disorders NEC (conditions in D80-d89) O99.11-

incarceration, uterus O34.51-

incompetent cervix O34.3-

inconclusive fetal viability O36.80

infection(s) O98.91-

amniotic fluid or sac O41.10-

bladder O23.1-

carrier state NEC O99.830

streptococcus B O99.820

genital organ or tract O23.9-

specified NEC O23.59-

genitourinary tract O23.9-

gonorrhea O98.21-

hepatitis (viral) O98.41-

HIV O98.71-

human immunodeficiency virus (HIV) O98.71-

kidney O23.0-

nipple O91.01-

parasitic disease O98.91-

specified NEC O98.81-

protozoal disease O98.61-

sexually transmitted NEC O98.31-

specified type NEC O98.81-

syphilis O98.11-

tuberculosis O98.01-

urethra O23.2-

urinary (tract) O23.4-

specified NEC O23.3-

viral disease O98.51-

injury or poisoning (conditions in S00-t88) O9A.21-

due to abuse

physical O9A.31-

psychological O9A.51-

sexual O9A.41-

insufficient

prenatal care O09.3-

weight gain O26.1-

insulin resistance O26.89

intrauterine fetal death (near term) O36.4

early pregnancy O02.1

multiple gestation (one fetus or more) O31.2-

isoimmunization O36.11-

anti-a sensitization O36.11-

anti-b sensitization O36.19-

Rh O36.09-

anti-d antibody O36.01-

specified NEC O36.19-

laceration of uterus NEC O71.81

malformation

placenta, placental (vessel) O43.10-

specified NEC O43.19-

uterus (congenital) O34.0-

malnutrition (conditions in E40-e46) O25.1-

maternal hypotension syndrome O26.5-

Pregnancy - *continued*

mental disorders (conditions in F01-f09, F20-f99) O99.34-

alcohol use O99.31-

drug use O99.32-

smoking O99.33-

mentum presentation O32.3

metabolic disorders O99.28-

missed

abortion O02.1

delivery O36.4

multiple gestations O30.9-

conjoined twins O30.02-

specified number of multiples NEC - *see* Pregnancy, multiple (gestation), specified NEC

quadruplet - *see* Pregnancy, quadruplet

specified complication NEC O31.8X-

triplet - *see* Pregnancy, triplet

twin - *see* Pregnancy, twin

musculoskeletal condition (conditions is M00-m99) O99.89

necrosis, liver (conditions in K72) O26.61-

neoplasm

benign

cervix O34.4-

corpus uteri O34.1-

uterus O34.1-

malignant O9A.11-

nephropathy NEC O26.83-

nervous system condition (conditions in G00-g99) O99.35-

nutritional diseases NEC O99.28-

obesity (pre-existing) O99.21-

obesity surgery status O99.84-

oblique lie or presentation O32.2

older mother - *see* Pregnancy, complicated by, elderly

oligohydramnios O41.0-

with premature rupture of membranes - *see also* Pregnancy, complicated by, premature rupture of membranes O42.-

onset (spontaneous) of labor after 37 completed weeks of gestation but before 39 completed weeks gestation, with delivery by (planned) cesarean section O75.82

oophoritis O23.52-

overdose, drug - *see also* Table of Drugs and Chemicals, by drug, poisoning O9A.21-

oversize fetus O33.5

papyraceous fetus O31.0-

pelvic inflammatory disease O99.89

periodontal disease O99.61-

peripheral neuritis O26.82-

peritoneal (pelvic) adhesions O99.89

phlebitis O22.9-

phlebopathy O22.9-

phlebothrombosis (superficial) O22.2-

deep O22.3-

placenta accreta O43.21-

placenta increta O43.22-

placenta percreta O43.23-

placenta previa O44.0-

complete O44.0-

with hemorrhage O44.1-

marginal O44.2-

with hemorrhage O44.3-

partial O44.2-

with hemorrhage O44.3-

placental disorder O43.9-

specified NEC O43.89-

placental dysfunction O43.89-

placental infarction O43.81-

placental insufficiency O36.51-

Pregnancy - *continued*

placental transfusion syndromes

fetomaternal O43.01-

fetus to fetus O43.02-

maternofetal O43.01-

placentitis O41.14-

pneumonia O99.51-

poisoning - *see also* Table of Drugs and Chemicals O9A.21-

polyhydramnios O40-

polymorphic eruption of pregnancy O26.86

poor obstetric history NEC O09.29-

postmaturity (post-term) (40 to 42 weeks) O48.0

more than 42 completed weeks gestation (prolonged) O48.1

pre-eclampsia O14.9-

mild O14.0-

moderate O14.0-

severe O14.1-

with hemolysis, elevated liver enzymes and low platelet count (HELLP) O14.2-

premature labor - *see* Pregnancy, complicated by, preterm labor

premature rupture of membranes O42.90

full-term, unspecified as to length of time between rupture and onset of labor O42.92

with onset of labor

within 24 hours O42.00

at or after 37 weeks gestation, onset of labor within 24 hours of rupture O42.02

pre-term (before 37 completed weeks of gestation) O42.01

after 24 hours O42.10

at or after 37 weeks gestation, onset of labor more than 24 hours following rupture O42.12

pre-term (before 37 completed weeks of gestation) O42.11-

at or after 37 weeks gestation, unspecified as to length of time between rupture and onset of labor O42.92

pre-term (before 37 completed weeks of gestation) O42.91-

premature separation of placenta - *see also* Abruptio placentae O45.9-

presentation, fetal - *see* Delivery, complicated by, malposition

preterm delivery O60.10

preterm labor

with delivery O60.10

preterm O60.10

term O60.20

second trimester

with term delivery O60.22

without delivery O60.02

with preterm delivery

second trimester O60.12

third trimester O60.13

third trimester

with term delivery O60.23

without delivery O60.03

with third trimester preterm delivery O60.14

without delivery O60.00

second trimester O60.02

third trimester O60.03

previous history of - *see* Pregnancy, supervision of, high-risk

prolapse, uterus O34.52-

proteinuria (gestational) - *see also* Proteinuria, gestational O12.1-

with edema O12.2-

pruritic urticarial papules and plaques of

Pregnancy - *continued*
　　pregnancy (PUPPP) O26.86
　　pruritus (neurogenic) O26.89-
　　psychosis or psychoneurosis (puerperal) F53
　　ptyalism O26.89-
　　PUPPP (pruritic urticarial papules and
　　　plaques of pregnancy) O26.86
　　pyelitis O23.0-
　　recurrent pregnancy loss O26.2-
　　renal disease or failure NEC O26.83-
　　　with secondary hypertension, pre-existing -
　　　　see Hypertension, complicating,
　　　　pregnancy, pre-existing, secondary
　　　hypertensive, pre-existing - *see*
　　　　Hypertension, complicating, pregnancy,
　　　　pre-existing, with, renal disease
　　respiratory condition (conditions in J00-j99)
　　　O99.51-
　　retained, retention
　　　dead ovum O02.0
　　　intrauterine contraceptive device O26.3-
　　retroversion, uterus O34.53-
　　Rh immunization, incompatibility or
　　　sensitization NEC O36.09-
　　　anti-d antibody O36.01-
　　rupture
　　　amnion (premature) - *see also* Pregnancy,
　　　　complicated by, premature rupture of
　　　　membranes O42-
　　　membranes (premature) - *see also*
　　　　Pregnancy, complicated by, premature
　　　　rupture of membranes O42-
　　　uterus (during labor) O71.1
　　　　before onset of labor O71.0-
　　salivation (excessive) O26.89-
　　salpingitis O23.52-
　　salpingo-oophoritis O23.52-
　　sepsis (conditions in A40, A41) O98.81-
　　size date discrepancy (uterine) O26.84-
　　skin condition (conditions in L00-l99)
　　　O99.71-
　　smoking (tobacco) O99.33-
　　social problem O09.7-
　　specified condition NEC O26.89-
　　spotting O26.85-
　　streptococcus group B (GBS) carrier state
　　　O99.820
　　subluxation of symphysis (pubis) O26.71-
　　syphilis (conditions in A50-a53) O98.11-
　　threatened
　　　abortion O20.0
　　　labor O47.9
　　　　at or after 37 completed weeks of
　　　　　gestation O47.1
　　　　before 37 completed weeks of gestation
　　　　　O47.0-
　　thrombophlebitis (superficial) O22.2-
　　thrombosis O22.9-
　　　cerebral venous O22.5-
　　　cerebrovenous sinus O22.5-
　　　deep O22.3-
　　tobacco use disorder (smoking) O99.33-
　　torsion of uterus O34.59-
　　toxemia O14.9-
　　transverse lie or presentation O32.2
　　tuberculosis (conditions in A15-a19) O98.01-
　　tumor (benign)
　　　cervix O34.4-
　　　malignant O9A.11-
　　　uterus O34.1-
　　unstable lie O32.0
　　upper respiratory infection O99.51-
　　urethritis O23.2-
　　uterine size date discrepancy O26.84-

Pregnancy - *continued*
　　vaginitis or vulvitis O23.59-
　　varicose veins (lower extremities) O22.0-
　　　genitals O22.1-
　　　legs O22.0-
　　　perineal O22.1-
　　　vaginal or vulval O22.1-
　　venereal disease NEC (conditions in A63.8)
　　　O98.31-
　　venous disorders O22.9-
　　　specified NEC O22.8X-
　　viral diseases (conditions in A80-b09, B25-
　　　b34) O98.51-
　　very young mother - *see* Pregnancy,
　　　complicated by, young mother
　　vomiting O21.9
　　　due to diseases classified elsewhere O21.8
　　　hyperemesis gravidarum (mild) - *see also*
　　　　Hyperemesis, gravidarum O21.0-
　　　late (occurring after 20 weeks of gestation)
　　　　O21.2
　　young mother
　　　multigravida O09.62-
　　　primigravida O09.61-
　concealed O09.3-
　continuing following
　　elective fetal reduction of one or more fetus
　　　O31.3-
　　intrauterine death of one or more fetus
　　　O31.2-
　　spontaneous abortion of one or more fetus
　　　O31.1-
　cornual O00.80
　　with intrauterine pregnancy O00.81
　ectopic (ruptured) O00.90
　　with intrauterine pregnancy O00.91
　　abdominal O00.00
　　　with
　　　　intrauterine pregnancy O00.01
　　　　viable fetus O36.7-
　　cervical O00.80
　　　with intrauterine pregnancy O00.81
　　complicated (by) O08.9
　　　afibrinogenemia O08.1
　　　cardiac arrest O08.81
　　　chemical damage of pelvic organ(s) O08.6
　　　circulatory collapse O08.3
　　　defibrination syndrome O08.1
　　　electrolyte imbalance O08.5
　　　embolism (amniotic fluid) (blood clot)
　　　　(pulmonary) (septic) O08.2
　　　endometritis O08.0
　　　genital tract and pelvic infection O08.0
　　　hemorrhage (delayed) (excessive) O08.1
　　　infection
　　　　genital tract or pelvic O08.0
　　　　kidney 008.83
　　　　urinary tract O08.83
　　　intravascular coagulation O08.1
　　　laceration of pelvic organ(s) O08.6
　　　metabolic disorder O08.5
　　　oliguria O08.4
　　　oophoritis O08.0
　　　parametritis O08.0
　　　pelvic peritonitis O08.0
　　　perforation of pelvic organ(s) O08.6
　　　renal failure or shutdown O08.4
　　　salpingitis or salpingo-oophoritis O08.0
　　　sepsis O08.82
　　　shock O08.83
　　　　septic O08.82
　　　specified condition NEC O08.89
　　　tubular necrosis (renal) O08.4
　　　uremia O08.4

Pregnancy - *continued*
　　urinary infection O08.83
　　venous complication NEC O08.7
　　　embolism O08.2
　cornual O00.80
　　with intrauterine pregnancy O00.81
　intraligamentous O00.80
　　with intrauterine pregnancy O00.81
　mural O00.80
　　with intrauterine pregnancy O00.81
　ovarian O00.20-
　　with intrauterine pregnancy O00.21-
　specified site NEC O00.80
　　with intrauterine pregnancy O00.81
　tubal (ruptured) O00.10-
　　with intrauterine pregnancy O00.11-
　examination (normal) Z34.9-
　　high-risk - *see* Pregnancy, supervision of,
　　　high-risk
　　first Z34.0-
　　specified Z34.8-
　extrauterine - *see* Pregnancy, ectopic
　fallopian O00.10-
　　with intrauterine pregnancy O00.11-
　false F45.8
　gestational carrier Z33.3
　hidden O09.3-
　high-risk - *see* Pregnancy, supervision of,
　　high-risk
　incidental finding Z33.1
　interstitial O00.80
　　with intrauterine pregnancy O00.81
　intraligamentous O00.80
　　with intrauterine pregnancy O00.81
　intramural O00.80
　　with intrauterine pregnancy O00.81
　intraperitoneal O00.00
　　with intrauterine pregnancy O00.01
　isthmian O00.10-
　　with intrauterine pregnancy O00.11-
　mesometric (mural) O00.80
　　with intrauterine pregnancy O00.81
　molar NEC O02.0
　　complicated (by) O08.9
　　　afibrinogenemia O08.1
　　　cardiac arrest O08.81
　　　chemical damage of pelvic organ(s) O08.6
　　　circulatory collapse O08.3
　　　defibrination syndrome O08.1
　　　electrolyte imbalance O08.5
　　　embolism (amniotic fluid) (blood clot)
　　　　(pulmonary) (septic) O08.2
　　　endometritis O08.0
　　　genital tract and pelvic infection O08.0
　　　hemorrhage (delayed) (excessive) O08.1
　　　infection
　　　　genital tract or pelvic O08.0
　　　　kidney O08.83
　　　　urinary tract O08.83
　　　intravascular coagulation O08.1
　　　laceration of pelvic organ(s) O08.6
　　　metabolic disorder O08.5
　　　oliguria O08.4
　　　oophoritis O08.0
　　　parametritis O08.0
　　　pelvic peritonitis O08.0
　　　perforation of pelvic organ(s) O08.6
　　　renal failure or shutdown O08.4
　　　salpingitis or salpingo-oophoritis O08.0
　　　sepsis O08.82
　　　shock O08.3
　　　　septic O08.82
　　　specified condition NEC O08.89
　　　tubular necrosis (renal) O08.4

Pregnancy - *continued*
 uremia O08.4
 urinary infection O08.83
 venous complication NEC O08.7
  embolism O08.2
 hydatidiform - *see also* Mole, hydatidiform
  O01.9-
 multiple (gestation) O30.9-
  greater than quadruplets - *see* Pregnancy,
   multiple (gestation), specified NEC
  specified NEC O30.80-
   with
    two or more monoamniotic fetuses
     O30.82-
    two or more monochorionic fetuses
     O30.81-
   two or more monoamniotic fetuses O30.82-
   two or more monochorionic fetuses
    O30.81-
   unable to determine number of placenta and
    number of amniotic sacs O30.89-
   unspecified number of placenta and
    unspecified number of amniotic sacs
    O30.80-
 mural O00.80
  with intrauterine pregnancy O00.81
 normal (supervision of) Z34.9-
  high-risk - *see* Pregnancy, supervision of,
   high-risk
  first Z34.0-
  specified Z34.8-
 ovarian O00.20-
  with intrauterine pregnancy O00.21-
 postmature (40 to 42 weeks) O48.0
  more than 42 weeks gestation O48.1
 post-term (40 to 42 weeks) O48.0
 prenatal care only Z34.9-
  high-risk - *see* Pregnancy, supervision of,
   high-risk
  first Z34.0-
  specified Z34.8-
 prolonged (more than 42 weeks gestation)
  O48.1
 quadruplet O30.20-
  with
   two or more monoamniotic fetuses O30.22-
   two or more monochorionic fetuses
    O30.21-
  two or more monoamniotic fetuses O30.22-
  two or more monochorionic fetuses O30.21-
  unable to determine number of placenta and
   number of amniotic sacs O30.29-
  unspecified number of placenta and
   unspecified number of amniotic sacs
   O30.20-
 quintuplet - *see* Pregnancy, multiple
  (gestation), specified NEC
 sextuplet - *see* Pregnancy, multiple (gestation),
  specified NEC
 supervision of
  concealed pregnancy O09.3-
  elderly mother
   multigravida O09.52-
   primigravida O09.51-
  hidden pregnancy O09.3-
  high-risk O09.9-
   due to (history of)
    ectopic pregnancy O09.1-
    elderly - *see* Pregnancy, supervision,
     elderly mother
    grand multiparity O09.4
    infertility O09.0-
    insufficient prenatal care O09.3-
    in utero procedure during previous

Pregnancy - *continued*
    pregnancy O09.82-
    in vitro fertilization O09.81-
    molar pregnancy O09.A-
    multiple previous pregnancies O09.4-
    older mother - *see* Pregnancy, supervision
     of, elderly mother
    poor reproductive or obstetric history
     NEC O09.29-
    pre-term labor O09.21-
    previous
     neonatal death O09.29-
    social problems O09.7-
    specified NEC O09.89-
    very young mother - *see* Pregnancy,
     supervision, young mother
   resulting from in vitro fertilization O09.81-
  normal Z34.9-
   first Z34.0-
   specified NEC Z34.8-
  young mother
   multigravida O09.62-
   primigravida O09.61-
 triplet O30.10-
  with
   two or more monoamniotic fetuses O30.12-
   two or more monochorionic fetuses
    O30.11-
  two or more monoamniotic fetuses O30.12-
  two or more monochorionic fetuses O30.11-
  unable to determine number of placenta and
   number of amniotic sacs O30.19-
  unspecified number of placenta and
   unspecified number of amniotic sacs
   O30.10-
 tubal (with abortion) (with rupture) O00.10-
  with intrauterine pregnancy O00.11-
 twin O30.00-
  conjoined O30.02-
  dichorionic/diamniotic (two placenta, two
   amniotic sacs) O30.04-
  monochorionic/diamniotic (one placenta, two
   amniotic sacs) O30.03-
  monochorionic/monoamniotic (one placenta,
   one amniotic sac) O30.01-
  unable to determine number of placenta and
   number of amniotic sacs O30.09-
  unspecified number of placenta and
   unspecified number of amniotic sacs
   O30.00-
 unwanted Z64.0
 weeks of gestation
  8 weeks Z3A.08
  9 weeks Z3A.09
  10 weeks Z3A.10
  11 weeks Z3A.11
  12 weeks Z3A.12
  13 weeks Z3A.13
  14 weeks Z3A.14
  15 weeks Z3A.15
  16 weeks Z3A.16
  17 weeks Z3A.17
  18 weeks Z3A.18
  19 weeks Z3A.19
  20 weeks Z3A.20
  21 weeks Z3A.21
  22 weeks Z3A.22
  23 weeks Z3A.23
  24 weeks Z3A.24
  25 weeks Z3A.25
  26 weeks Z3A.26
  27 weeks Z3A.27
  28 weeks Z3A.28
  29 weeks Z3A.29

Pregnancy - *continued*
  30 weeks Z3A.30
  31 weeks Z3A.31
  32 weeks Z3A.32
  33 weeks Z3A.33
  34 weeks Z3A.34
  35 weeks Z3A.35
  36 weeks Z3A.36
  37 weeks Z3A.37
  38 weeks Z3A.38
  39 weeks Z3A.39
  40 weeks Z3A.40
  41 weeks Z3A.41
  42 weeks Z3A.42
  greater than 42 weeks Z3A.49
  less than 8 weeks Z3A.01
  not specified Z3A.00
Preiser's disease - *see* Osteonecrosis,
 secondary, due to, trauma, metacarpus
Pre-kwashiorkor - *see* Malnutrition, severe
Preleukemia (syndrome) D46.9
Preluxation, hip, congenital Q65.6
Premature - *see also* condition
 adrenarche E27.0
 aging E34.8
 beats I49.40
  atrial I49.1
  auricular I49.1
  supraventricular I49.1
 birth NEC - *see* Preterm, newborn
 closure, foramen ovale Q21.8
 contraction
  atrial I49.1
  atrioventricular I49.2
  auricular I49.1
  auriculoventricular I49.49
  heart (extrasystole) I49.49
  junctional I49.2
  ventricular I49.3
 delivery - *see also* Pregnancy, complicated by,
  preterm labor O60.10
 ejaculation F52.4
 infant NEC - *see* Preterm, newborn
  light-for-dates - *see* Light for dates
 labor - *see* Pregnancy, complicated by, preterm
  labor
 lungs P28.0
 menopause E28.319
  asymptomatic E28.319
  symptomatic E28.310
 newborn
  extreme (less than 28 completed weeks) - *see*
   Immaturity, extreme
  less than 37 completed weeks - *see* Preterm,
   newborn
 puberty E30.1
 rupture membranes or amnion - *see* Pregnancy,
  complicated by, premature rupture of
  membranes
 senility E34.8
 thelarche E30.8
 ventricular systole I49.3
Prematurity NEC (less than 37 completed
 weeks) - *see* Preterm, newborn
 extreme (less than 28 completed weeks) - *see*
  Immaturity, extreme
Premenstrual
 dysphoric disorder (PMDD) F32.81
 tension (syndrome) N94.3
Premolarization, cuspids K00.2
Prenatal
 care, normal pregnancy - *see* Pregnancy,
  normal

Prenatal - *continued*
  screening of mother (see also Encounter, antenatal screening) Z36.9
  teeth K00.6
Preparatory care for subsequent treatment NEC
  for dialysis Z49.01
    peritoneal Z49.02
Prepartum - *see* condition
Preponderance, left or right ventricular I51.7
Prepuce - *see* condition
PRES (posterior reversible encephalopathy syndrome) I67.83
Presbycardia R54
Presbycusis, presbyacusia H91.1-
Presbyesophagus K22.8
Presbyophrenia F03
Presbyopia H52.4
Prescription of contraceptives (initial)
  Z30.019
  barrier Z30.018
  diaphragm Z30.018
  emergency (postcoital) Z30.012
  implantable subdermal Z30.017
  injectable Z30.013
  intrauterine contraceptive device Z30.014
  pills Z30.011
  postcoital (emergency) Z30.012
  repeat Z30.40
    barrier Z30.49
    diaphragm Z30.49
    implantable subdermal Z30.46
    injectable Z30.42
    pills Z30.41
    specified type NEC Z30.49
    transdermal patch hormonal Z30.45
    vaginal ring hormonal Z30.44
  specified type NEC Z30.018
    transdermal patch hormonal Z30.016
    vaginal ring hormonal Z30.015
Presence (of)
  ankle-joint implant (functional) (prosthesis) Z96.66-
  aortocoronary (bypass) graft Z95.1
  arterial-venous shunt (dialysis) Z99.2
  artificial
    eye (globe) Z97.0
    heart (fully implantable) (mechanical) Z95.812
      valve Z95.2
    larynx Z96.3
    lens (intraocular) Z96.1
    limb (complete) (partial) Z97.1-
      arm Z97.1-
        bilateral Z97.15
      leg Z97.1-
        bilateral Z97.16
  audiological implant (functional) Z96.29
  bladder implant (functional) Z96.0
  bone
    conduction hearing device Z96.29
    implant (functional) NEC Z96.7
    joint (prosthesis) - *see* Presence, joint implant
  cardiac
    defibrillator (functional) (with synchronous cardiac pacemaker) Z95.810
    implant or graft Z95.9
      specified type NEC Z95.818
    pacemaker Z95.0
    resynchronization therapy
      defibrillator Z95.810
      pacemaker Z95.0
  cerebrospinal fluid drainage device Z98.2
  cochlear implant (functional) Z96.21

Presence (of) - *continued*
  contact lens (es) Z97.3
  coronary artery graft or prosthesis Z95.5
  CRT-d (cardiac resynchronization therapy defibrillator) Z95.810
  CRT-p (cardiac resynchronization therapy pacemaker) Z95.0
  cardioverter-defibrillator (ICD) Z95.810
  CSF shunt Z98.2
  dental prosthesis device Z97.2
  dentures Z97.2
  device (external) NEC Z97.8
    cardiac NEC Z95.818
    heart assist Z95.811
    implanted (functional) Z96.9
      specified NEC Z96.89
    prosthetic Z97.8
  ear implant Z96.20
    cochlear implant Z96.21
    myringotomy tube Z96.22
    specified type NEC Z96.29
  elbow-joint implant (functional) (prosthesis) Z96.62-
  endocrine implant (functional) NEC Z96.49
  eustachian tube stent or device (functional) Z96.29
  external hearing-aid or device Z97.4
  finger-joint implant (functional) (prosthetic) Z96.69-
  functional implant Z96.9
    specified NEC Z96.89
  graft
    cardiac NEC Z95.818
    vascular NEC Z95.828
  hearing-aid or device (external) Z97.4
    implant (bone) (cochlear) (functional) Z96.21
  heart assist device Z95.811
  heart valve implant (functional) Z95.2
    prosthetic Z95.2
    specified type NEC Z95.4
    xenogenic Z95.3
  hip-joint implant (functional) (prosthesis) Z96.64-
  ICD (cardioverter-defibrillator) Z95.810
  implanted device (artificial) (functional) (prosthetic) Z96.9
    automatic cardiac defibrillator (with synchronous cardiac pacemaker) Z95.810
    cardiac pacemaker Z95.0
    cochlear Z96.21
    dental Z96.5
    heart Z95.812
    heart valve Z95.2
      prosthetic Z95.2
      specified NEC Z95.4
      xenogenic Z95.3
    insulin pump Z96.41
    intraocular lens Z96.1
    joint Z96.60
      ankle Z96.66-
      elbow Z96.62-
      finger Z96.69-
      hip Z96.64-
      knee Z96.65-
      shoulder Z96.61-
      specified NEC Z96.698
      wrist Z96.63-
    larynx Z96.3
    myringotomy tube Z96.22
    otological Z96.20
      cochlear Z96.21
      eustachian stent Z96.29
      myringotomy Z96.22
      specified NEC Z96.29

Presence (of) - *continued*
    stapes Z96.29
  skin Z96.81
  skull plate Z96.7
  specified NEC Z96.89
  urogenital Z96.0
  insulin pump (functional) Z96.41
  intestinal bypass or anastomosis Z98.0
  intraocular lens (functional) Z96.1
  intrauterine contraceptive device (IUD) Z97.5
  intravascular implant (functional) (prosthetic) NEC Z95.9
    coronary artery Z95.5
    defibrillator (with synchronous cardiac pacemaker) Z95.810
    peripheral vessel (with angioplasty) Z95.820
  joint implant (prosthetic) (any) Z96.60
    ankle - *see* Presence, ankle joint implant
    elbow - *see* Presence, elbow joint implant
    finger - *see* Presence, finger joint implant
    hip - *see* Presence, hip joint implant
    knee - *see* Presence, knee joint implant
    shoulder - *see* Presence, shoulder joint implant
    specified joint NEC Z96.698
    wrist - *see* Presence, wrist joint implant
  knee-joint implant (functional) (prosthesis) Z96.65-
  laryngeal implant (functional) Z96.3
  mandibular implant (dental) Z96.5
  myringotomy tube(s) Z96.22
  orthopedic-joint implant (prosthetic) (any) - *see* Presence, joint implant
  otological implant (functional) Z96.29
  shoulder-joint implant (functional) (prosthesis) Z96.61-
  skull-plate implant Z96.7
  spectacles Z97.3
  stapes implant (functional) Z96.29
  systemic lupus erythematosus [SLE] inhibitor D68.62
  tendon implant (functional) (graft) Z96.7
  tooth root(s) implant Z96.5
  ureteral stent Z96.0
  urethral stent Z96.0
  urogenital implant (functional) Z96.0
  vascular implant or device Z95.9
    access port device Z95.828
    specified type NEC Z95.828
  wrist-joint implant (functional) (prosthesis) Z96.63-
Presenile - *see also* condition
  dementia F03
  premature aging E34.8
Presentation, fetal - *see* Delivery , complicated by, malposition
Prespondylolisthesis (congenital) Q76.2
Pressure
  area, skin - *see* Ulcer, pressure, by site
  brachial plexus G54.0
  brain G93.5
    injury at birth NEC P11.1
  cerebral - *see* Pressure, brain
  chest R07.89
  cone, tentorial G93.5
  hyposystolic - *see also* Hypotension
    incidental reading, without diagnosis of hypotension R03.1
  increased
    intracranial (benign) G93.2
      injury at birth P11.0
    intraocular H40.05-
  lumbosacral plexus G54.1
  mediastinum J98.59

Pressure - *continued*
  necrosis (chronic) - *see* Ulcer, pressure, by site
  parental, inappropriate (excessive) Z62.6
  sore (chronic) - *see* Ulcer, pressure, by site
  spinal cord G95.20
  ulcer (chronic) - *see* Ulcer, pressure, by site
  venous, increased I87.8
Pre-syncope R55
Preterm
  delivery - *see also* Pregnancy, complicated by,
    preterm labor O60.10
  labor - *see* Pregnancy, complicated by, preterm
    labor
  newborn (infant) P07.30
    gestational age
      28 completed weeks (28 weeks, 0 days
        through 28 weeks, 6 days) P07.31
      29 completed weeks (29 weeks, 0 days
        through 29 weeks, 6 days) P07.32
      30 completed weeks (30 weeks, 0 days
        through 30 weeks, 6 days) P07.33
      31 completed weeks (31 weeks, 0 days
        through 31 weeks, 6 days) P07.34
      32 completed weeks (32 weeks, 0 days
        through 32 weeks, 6 days) P07.35
      33 completed weeks (33 weeks, 0 days
        through 33 weeks, 6 days) P07.36
      34 completed weeks (34 weeks, 0 days
        through 34 weeks, 6 days) P07.37
      35 completed weeks (35 weeks, 0 days
        through 35 weeks, 6 days) P07.38
      36 completed weeks (36 weeks, 0 days
        through 36 weeks, 6 days) P07.39
Previa
  placenta (total) (without hemorrhage) O44.0-
    with hemorrhage O44.1-
    complete O44.0-
      with hemorrhage O44.1-
    low - *see also* Delivery, complicated, by,
      placenta, low O44.4-
      with hemorrhage O44.5-
    marginal O44.2-
      with hemorrhage O44.3-
    partial O44.2-
      with hemorrhage O44.3-
  vasa O69.4
Priapism N48.30
  due to
    disease classified elsewhere N48.32
    drug N48.33
  specified cause NEC N48.39
  trauma N48.31
Prickling sensation (skin) R20.2
Prickly heat L74.0
Primary - *see* condition **Primigravida**
  elderly, affecting management of pregnancy,
    labor and delivery (supervision only) - *see*
    Pregnancy, complicated by, elderly,
    primigravida
  older, affecting management of pregnancy,
    labor and delivery (supervision only) - *see*
    Pregnancy, complicated by,
  elderly, primigravida
  very young, affecting management of
    pregnancy, labor and delivery (supervision
    only) - *see* Pregnancy, complicated by, young
    mother, primigravida
Primipara
  elderly, affecting management of pregnancy,
    labor and delivery (supervision only) - *see*
    Pregnancy, complicated by, elderly,
    primigravida
  older, affecting management of pregnancy,
    labor and delivery (supervision only) - *see*

Primipara - *continued*
  Pregnancy, complicated by, elderly,
    primigravida
  very young, affecting management of
    pregnancy, labor and delivery (supervision
    only) - *see* Pregnancy, complicated by,
    young mother, primigravida
Primus varus (bilateral) Q66.2
PRIND (Prolonged reversible ischemic
  neurologic deficit) I63.9
Pringle's disease (tuberous sclerosis) Q85.1
Prinzmetal angina I20.1
Prizefighter ear - *see* Cauliflower ear
Problem (with) (related to)
  academic Z55.8
  acculturation Z60.3
  adjustment (to)
    change of job Z56.1
    life-cycle transition Z60.0
    pension Z60.0
    retirement Z60.0
  adopted child Z62.821
  alcoholism in family Z63.72
  atypical parenting situation Z62.9
  bankruptcy Z59.8
  behavioral (adult) F69
    drug seeking Z76.5
  birth of sibling affecting child Z62.898
  care (of)
    provider dependency Z74.9
      specified NEC Z74.8
    sick or handicapped person in family or
      household Z63.6
  child
    abuse (affecting the child) - *see*
      Maltreatment, child
    custody or support proceedings Z65.3
    in welfare custody Z62.21
    in care of non-parental family member
      Z62.21
    in foster care Z62.21
    living in orphanage or group home Z62.22
  child-rearing Z62.9
    specified NEC Z62.898
  communication (developmental) F80.9
  conflict or discord (with)
    boss Z56.4
    classmates Z55.4
    counselor Z64.4
    employer Z56.4
    family Z63.9
      specified NEC Z63.8
    probation officer Z64.4
    social worker Z64.4
    teachers Z55.4
    workmates Z56.4
  conviction in legal proceedings Z65.0
    with imprisonment Z65.1
  counselor Z64.4
  creditors Z59.8
  digestive K92.9
  drug addict in family Z63.72
  ear - *see* Disorder, ear
  economic Z59.9
    affecting care Z59.9
    specified NEC Z59.8
  education Z55.9
    specified NEC Z55.8
  employment Z56.9
    change of job Z56.1
    discord Z56.4
    environment Z56.5
    sexual harassment Z56.81
    specified NEC Z56.89

Problem (with) (related to) - *continued*
    stress NEC Z56.6
    stressful schedule Z56.3
    threat of job loss Z56.2
    unemployment Z56.0
  enuresis, child F98.0
  eye H57.9
  failed examinations (school) Z55.2
  falling Z91.81
  family - *see also* Disruption, family Z63.9-
    specified NEC Z63.8
  feeding (elderly) (infant) R63.3
    newborn P92.9
      breast P92.5
      overfeeding P92.4
      slow P92.2
      specified NEC P92.8
      underfeeding P92.3
    nonorganic F50.89
  finance Z59.9
    specified NEC Z59.8
  foreclosure on loan Z59.8
  foster child Z62.822
  frightening experience(s) in childhood
    Z62.898
  genital NEC
    female N94.9
    male N50.9
  health care Z75.9
    specified NEC Z75.8
  hearing - *see* Deafness
  homelessness Z59.0
  housing Z59.9
    inadequate Z59.1
    isolated Z59.8
    specified NEC Z59.8
  identity (of childhood) F93.8
  illegitimate pregnancy (unwanted) Z64.0
  illiteracy Z55.0
  impaired mobility Z74.09
  imprisonment or incarceration Z65.1
  inadequate teaching affecting education Z55.8
  inappropriate (excessive) parental pressure
    Z62.6
  influencing health status NEC Z78.9
  in-law Z63.1
  institutionalization, affecting child Z62.22
  intrafamilial communication Z63.8
  jealousy, child F93.8
  landlord Z59.2
  language (developmental) F80.9
  learning (developmental) F81.9
  legal Z65.3
    conviction without imprisonment Z65.0
    imprisonment Z65.1
    release from prison Z65.2
  life-management Z73.9
    specified NEC Z73.89
  life-style Z72.9
    gambling Z72.6
    high-risk sexual behavior (heterosexual)
      Z72.51
      bisexual Z72.53
      homosexual Z72.52
    inappropriate eating habits Z72.4
    self-damaging behavior NEC Z72.89
    specified NEC Z72.89
    tobacco use Z72.0
  literacy Z55.9
    low level Z55.0
    specified NEC Z55.8
  living alone Z60.2
  lodgers Z59.2
  loss of love relationship in childhood Z62.898

Problem (with) (related to) - *continued*
marital Z63.0
  involving
    divorce Z63.5
    estrangement Z63.5
    gender identity F66
mastication K08.89
medical
  care, within family Z63.6
  facilities Z75.9
    specified NEC Z75.8
mental F48.9
multiparity Z64.1
negative life events in childhood Z62.9
  altered pattern of family relationships Z62.898
  frightening experience Z62.898
  loss of
    love relationship Z62.898
    self-esteem Z62.898
  physical abuse (alleged) - *see* Maltreatment, child
  removal from home Z62.29
  specified event NEC Z62.898
neighbor Z59.2
neurological NEC R29.818
new step-parent affecting child Z62.898
none (feared complaint unfounded) Z71.1
occupational NEC Z56.89
parent-child - *see* Conflict, parent-child
personal hygiene Z91.89
personality F69
phase-of-life transition, adjustment Z60.0
presence of sick or disabled person in family or household Z63.79
  needing care Z63.6
primary support group (family) Z63.9
  specified NEC Z63.8
probation officer Z64.4
psychiatric F99
psychosexual (development) F66
psychosocial Z65.9
  religious or spiritual Z65.8
  specified NEC Z65.8
relationship Z63.9
  childhood F93.8
release from prison Z65.2
  religious or spiritual Z65.8
removal from home affecting child Z62.29
seeking and accepting known hazardous and harmful
  behavioral or psychological interventions Z65.8
  chemical, nutritional or physical interventions Z65.8
sexual function (nonorganic) F52.9
sight H54.7
sleep disorder, child F51.9
smell - *see* Disturbance, sensation, smell
social
  environment Z60.9
    specified NEC Z60.8
  exclusion and rejection Z60.4
  worker Z64.4
speech R47.9
  developmental F80.9
  specified NEC R47.89
swallowing - *see* Dysphagia
taste - *see* Disturbance, sensation, taste
tic, child F95.0
underachievement in school Z55.3
unemployment Z56.0
  threatened Z56.2
unwanted pregnancy Z64.0

Problem (with) (related to) - *continued*
upbringing Z62.9
  specified NEC Z62.898
urinary N39.9
voice production R47.89
work schedule (stressful) Z56.3
Procedure (surgical)
converted
  arthroscopic to open Z53.33
  laparoscopic to open Z53.31
  specified procedure NEC to open Z53.39
  thoracoscopic to open Z53.32
for purpose other than remedying health state Z41.9
  specified NEC Z41.8
not done Z53.9
  because of
    administrative reasons Z53.8
    contraindication Z53.09
      smoking Z53.01
    patient's decision Z53.20
      for reasons of belief or group pressure Z53.1
      left against medical advice (AMA) Z53.21
      specified reason NEC Z53.29
    specified reason NEC Z53.8
Procidentia (uteri) N81.3
Proctalgia K62.89
fugax K59.4
spasmodic K59.4
Proctitis K62.89
amebic (acute) A06.0
chlamydial A56.3
gonococcal A54.6
granulomatous - *see* Enteritis, regional, large intestine
herpetic A60.1
radiation K62.7
tuberculous A18.32
ulcerative (chronic) K51.20
  with
    complication K51.219
      abscess K51.214
      fistula K51.213
      obstruction K51.212
      rectal bleeding K51.211
      specified NEC K51.218
Proctocele
female (without uterine prolapse) N81.6
  with uterine prolapse N81.2
    complete N81.3
male K62.3
Proctocolitis
food-induced eosinophilic K52.82
food protein-induced K52.82
milk protein-induced K52.82
mucosal - *see* Rectosigmoiditis, ulcerative
Proctoptosis K62.3
Proctorrhagia K62.5
Proctosigmoiditis K63.89
ulcerative (chronic) - *see* Rectosigmoiditis, ulcerative
Proctospasm K59.4
psychogenic F45.8
Profichet's disease - *see* Disorder, soft tissue, specified type NEC
Progeria E34.8
Prognathism (mandibular) (maxillary) M26.19
Progonoma (melanotic) - *see* Neoplasm, benign, by site
Progressive - *see* condition
Prolactinoma
specified site - *see* Neoplasm, benign, by site
unspecified site D35.2

Prolapse, prolapsed
anus, anal (canal) (sphincter) K62.2
arm or hand O32.2
  causing obstructed labor O64.4
bladder (mucosa) (sphincter) (acquired)
  congenital Q79.4
  female - *see* Cystocele
  male N32.89
breast implant (prosthetic) T85.49
cecostomy K94.09
cecum K63.4
cervix, cervical (hypertrophied) N81.2
  anterior lip, obstructing labor O65.5
  congenital Q51.828
  postpartal, old N81.2
  stump N81.85
ciliary body (traumatic) - *see* Laceration, eye(ball), with prolapse or loss of interocular tissue
colon (pedunculated) K63.4
colostomy K94.09
disc (intervertebral) - *see* Displacement, intervertebral disc eye implant (orbital) T85.398
  lens (ocular) - *see* Complications, intraocular lens
fallopian tube N83.4-
gastric (mucosa) K31.89
genital, female N81.9
  specified NEC N81.89
globe, nontraumatic - *see* Luxation, globe
ileostomy bud K94.19
intervertebral disc - *see* Displacement, intervertebral disc
intestine (small) K63.4
iris (traumatic) - *see* Laceration, eye(ball), with prolapse or loss of interocular tissue
  nontraumatic H21.89
kidney N28.83
  congenital Q63.2
laryngeal muscles or ventricle J38.7
liver K76.89
meatus urinarius N36.8
mitral (valve) I34.1
ocular lens implant - *see* Complications, intraocular lens
organ or site, congenital NEC - *see* Malposition, congenital
ovary N83.4-
pelvic floor, female N81.89
perineum, female N81.89
rectum (mucosa) (sphincter) K62.3
  due to trichuris trichuria B79
spleen D73.89
stomach K31.89
umbilical cord
  complicating delivery O69.0
urachus, congenital Q64.4
ureter N28.89
  with obstruction N13.5
    with infection N13.6
ureterovesical orifice N28.89
urethra (acquired) (infected) (mucosa) N36.8
  congenital Q64.71
urinary meatus N36.8
  congenital Q64.72
uterovaginal N81.4
  complete N81.3
  incomplete N81.2
uterus (with prolapse of vagina) N81.4
  complete N81.3
  congenital Q51.818
  first degree N81.2
  in pregnancy or childbirth - *see* Pregnancy,

Prolapse, prolapsed - continued
  complicated by, abnormal, uterus
    incomplete N81.2
    postpartal (old) N81.4
    second degree N81.2
    third degree N81.3
  uveal (traumatic) - see Laceration, eye(ball),
    with prolapse or loss of interocular tissue
  vagina (anterior) (wall) - see Cystocele
    with prolapse of uterus N81.4
      complete N81.3
      incomplete N81.2
    posterior wall N81.6
    posthysterectomy N99.3
  vitreous (humor) H43.0-
    in wound - see Laceration, eye(ball), with
    prolapse or loss of interocular tissue
  womb - see Prolapse, uterus
Prolapsus, female N81.9
  specified NEC N81.89
Proliferation(s)
  prostate, atypical small acinar N42.32
  primary cutaneous CD30-positive large T-cell
    C86.6
Proliferative - see condition
Prolonged, prolongation (of)
  bleeding (time) (idiopathic) R79.1
  coagulation (time) R79.1
  gestation (over 42 completed weeks)
    mother O48.1
    newborn P08.22
  interval I44.0
  labor O63.9
    first stage O63.0
    second stage O63.1
  partial thromboplastin time (PTT) R79.1
  pregnancy (more than 42 weeks gestation)
    O48.1
  prothrombin time R79.1
  QT interval I45.81
  uterine contractions in labor O62.4
Prominence, prominent
  auricle (congenital) (ear) Q17.5
  ischial spine or sacral promontory
    with disproportion (fetopelvic) O33.0
      causing obstructed labor O65.0
  nose (congenital) acquired M95.0
Promiscuity - see High, risk, sexual behavior
Pronation
  ankle - see Deformity, limb, foot, specified
    NEC
  foot - see also Deformity, limb, foot, specified
    NEC
    congenital Q74.2
Prophylactic
  administration of
    antibiotics, long-term Z79.2
      short-term use omit code
    drug - see also Long-term (current) drug
      therapy (use of) Z79.899-
    medication Z79.899
  organ removal (for neoplasia management)
    Z40.00
    breast Z40.01
    fallopian tube(s) Z40.03
      with ovary(s) Z40.02
    ovary(s) Z40.02
    specified site NEC Z40.09
  surgery Z40.9
    for risk factors related to malignant neoplasm
    - see Prophylactic, organ removal
    specified NEC Z40.8
  vaccination Z23

Propionic acidemia E71.121
Proptosis (ocular) - see also Exophthalmos
  thyroid - see Hyperthyroidism, with goiter
Prosecution, anxiety concerning Z65.3
Prosopagnosia R48.3
Prostadynia N42.81
Prostate, prostatic - see condition
Prostatism - see Hyperplasia, prostate
**Prostatitis (congestive) (suppurative) (with
cystitis)** N41.9
  acute N41.0
  cavitary N41.8
  chronic N41.1
  diverticular N41.8
  due to Trichomonas (vaginalis) A59.02
  fibrous N41.1
  gonococcal (acute) (chronic) A54.22
  granulomatous N41.4
  hypertrophic N41.1
  subacute N41.1
  trichomonal A59.02
  tuberculous A18.14
Prostatocystitis N41.3
Prostatorrhea N42.89
Prostatosis N42.82
Prostration R53.83
  heat - see also Heat, exhaustion
    anhydrotic T67.3
    due to
      salt (and water) depletion T67.4
      water depletion T67.3
  nervous F48.8
  senile R54
Protanomaly (anomalous trichromat) H53.54
Protanopia (complete) (incomplete) H53.54
Protection (against) (from) - see Prophylactic
Protein
  deficiency NEC - see Malnutrition
  malnutrition - see Malnutrition
  sickness - see also Reaction, serum T80.69
Proteinemia R77.9
Proteinosis
  alveolar (pulmonary) J84.01
  lipid or lipoid (of Urbach) E78.89
Proteinuria R80.9
  Bence Jones R80.3
  complicating pregnancy - see Proteinuria,
    gestational
  gestational
    complicating
      childbirth O12.14
      pregnancy O12.1-
        with edema O12.2-
      puerperium O12.15
  idiopathic R80.0
  isolated R80.0
    with glomerular lesion N06.9
      dense deposit disease N06.6
      diffuse
        crescentic glomerulonephritis N06.7
        endocapillary proliferative
          glomerulonephritis N06.4
        mesangiocapillary glomerulonephritis
          N06.5
      focal and segmental hyalinosis or sclerosis
        N06.1
      membranous (diffuse) N06.2
      mesangial proliferative (diffuse) N06.3
      minimal change N06.0
      specified pathology NEC N06.8
  orthostatic R80.2
    with glomerular lesion - see Proteinuria,
      isolated, with glomerular lesion
  persistent R80.1

Proteinuria - continued
  with glomerular lesion - see Proteinuria,
    isolated, with glomerular lesion
  postural R80.2
    with glomerular lesion - see Proteinuria,
      isolated, with glomerular lesion
  pre-eclamptic - see Pre-eclampsia
  puerperal O12.15
  specified type NEC R80.8
Proteolysis, pathologic D65
**Proteus (mirabilis) (morganii), as cause of
disease classified elsewhere** B96.4
Prothrombin gene mutation D68.52
Protoporphyria, erythropoietic E80.0
Protozoal - see also condition
  disease B64
    specified NEC B60.8
Protrusion, protrusio acetabuli M24.7
  acetabulum (into pelvis) M24.7
  device, implant or graft - see also
    Complications, by site and type, mechanical
    T85.698
    arterial graft NEC - see Complication,
      cardiovascular device, mechanical, vascular
    breast (implant) T85.49
    catheter NEC T85.698
      cystostomy T83.090
      dialysis (renal) T82.49
        intraperitoneal T85.691
      infusion NEC T82.594
        spinal (epidural) (subdural) T85.690
      urinary - see also Complications, catheter,
    urinary T83.098
    electronic (electrode) (pulse generator)
    (stimulator)
      bone T84.390
      nervous system - see Complication,
        prosthetic device, mechanical, electronic
        nervous system stimulator
    fixation, internal (orthopedic) NEC - see
      Complication, fixation device, mechanical
    gastrointestinal - see Complications,
      prosthetic device, mechanical,
      gastrointestinal device
    genital NEC T83.498
      intrauterine contraceptive device T83.39
      penile prosthesis (cylinder) (implanted)
        (pump) (reservoir) T83.490
      testicular prosthesis T83.491
    heart NEC - see Complication,
      cardiovascular device, mechanical
    joint prosthesis - see Complications, joint
      prosthesis, mechanical, specified NEC, by
      site
    ocular NEC - see Complications, prosthetic
      device, mechanical, ocular device
    orthopedic NEC - see Complication,
      orthopedic, device, mechanical
    specified NEC T85.628
    urinary NEC - see also Complication,
      genitourinary, device, urinary, mechanical
      graft T83.29
    vascular NEC - see Complication,
      cardiovascular device, mechanical
    ventricular intracranial shunt T85.09
  intervertebral disc - see Displacement,
    intervertebral disc
  joint prosthesis - see Complications, joint
    prosthesis, mechanical, specified NEC, by
    site
  nucleus pulposus - see Displacement,
    intervertebral disc
Prune belly (syndrome) Q79.4

Prurigo (ferox) (gravis) (Hebrae) (Hebra's) (mitis) (simplex) L28.2
  Besnier's L20.0
  estivalis L56.4
  nodularis L28.1
  psychogenic F45.8
Pruritus, pruritic (essential) L29.9
  ani, anus L29.0
    psychogenic F45.8
  anogenital L29.3
    psychogenic F45.8
  due to onchocerca volvulus B73.1
  gravidarum - *see* Pregnancy, complicated by, specified pregnancy-related condition NEC
  hiemalis L29.8
  neurogenic (any site) F45.8
  perianal L29.0
  psychogenic (any site) F45.8
  scroti, scrotum L29.1
    psychogenic F45.8
  senile, senilis L29.8
  specified NEC L29.8
    psychogenic F45.8
  Trichomonas A59.9
  vulva, vulvae L29.2
    psychogenic F45.8
Pseudarthrosis, pseudoarthrosis (bone) - *see* Nonunion, fracture
  clavicle, congenital Q74.0
  joint, following fusion or arthrodesis M96.0
Pseudoaneurysm - *see* Aneurysm
Pseudoangioma I81
Pseudoangina (pectoris) - *see* Angina
Pseudoarteriosus Q28.8
Pseudoarthrosis - *see* Pseudarthrosis
Pseudobulbar affect (PBA) F48.2
Pseudochromhidrosis L67.8
Pseudocirrhosis, liver, pericardial I31.1
Pseudocowpox B08.03
Pseudocoxalgia M91.3-
Pseudocroup J38.5
Pseudo-Cushing's syndrome, alcohol-induced E24.4
Pseudocyesis F45.8
Pseudocyst
  lung J98.4
  pancreas K86.3
  retina - *see* Cyst, retina
Pseudoelephantiasis neuroarthritica Q82.0
Pseudoexfoliation, capsule (lens) - *see* Cataract, specified NEC
Pseudofolliculitis barbae L73.1
Pseudoglioma H44.89
Pseudohemophilia (Bernuth's) (hereditary) (type B) D68.0
  Type A D69.8
  vascular D69.8
Pseudohermaphroditism Q56.3
  adrenal E25.8
  female Q56.2
    with adrenocortical disorder E25.8
    without adrenocortical disorder Q56.2
    adrenal (congenital) E25.0
    unspecified E25.9
  male Q56.1
    with
      adrenocortical disorder E25.8
      androgen resistance E34.51
      cleft scrotum Q56.1
      feminizing testis E34.51
      5-alpha-reductase deficiency E29.1
    without gonadal disorder Q56.1
    adrenal E25.8
    unspecified E25.9

Pseudo-hurler's polydystrophy E77.0
Pseudohydrocephalus G93.2
Pseudohypertrophic muscular dystrophy (Erb's) G71.0
Pseudohypertrophy, muscle G71.0
Pseudohypoparathyroidism E20.1
Pseudoinsomnia F51.03
Pseudoleukemia, infantile D64.89
Pseudomembranous - *see* condition
Pseudomenses (newborn) P54.6
Pseudomenstruation (newborn) P54.6
Pseudomeningocele (cerebral) (infective) (post-traumatic) G96.19
  postprocedural (spinal) G97.82
Pseudomonas
  aeruginosa, as cause of disease classified elsewhere B96.5
  mallei infection A24.0
    as cause of disease classified elsewhere B96.5
  pseudomallei, as cause of disease classified elsewhere B96.5
Pseudomyotonia G71.19
Pseudomyxoma peritonei C78.6
Pseudoneuritis, optic (nerve) (disc) (papilla), congenital Q14.2
Pseudo-obstruction intestine (acute) (chronic) (idiopathic) (intermittent secondary) (primary) K59.8
Pseudopapilledema H47.33-
  congenital Q14.2
Pseudoparalysis
  arm or leg R29.818
  atonic, congenital P94.2
Pseudopelade L66.0
Pseudophakia Z96.1
Pseudopolyarthritis, rhizomelic M35.3
Pseudopolycythemia D75.1
Pseudopseudohypoparathyroidism E20.1
Pseudopterygium H11.81-
Pseudoptosis (eyelid) - *see* Blepharochalasis
Pseudopuberty, precocious
  female heterosexual E25.8
  male isosexual E25.8
Pseudorickets (renal) N25.0
Pseudorubella B08.20
Pseudosclerema, newborn P83.88
Pseudosclerosis (brain)
  of Westphal (Strümpell) E83.01
  Jakob's - *see* Creutzfeldt-Jakob disease or syndrome
  spastic - *see* Creutzfeldt-Jakob disease or syndrome
Pseudotetanus - *see* Convulsions
Pseudotetany R29.0
  hysterical F44.5
Pseudotruncus arteriosus Q25.49
Pseudotuberculosis A28.2
  enterocolitis A04.8
  pasteurella (infection) A28.0
Pseudotumor
  cerebri G93.2
  orbital H05.11-
Pseudoxanthoma elasticum Q82.8
Psilosis (sprue) (tropical) K90.1
  nontropical K90.0
Psittacosis A70
Psoitis M60.88
Psoriasis L40.9
  arthropathic L40.50
    arthritis mutilans L40.52
    distal interphalangeal L40.51
    juvenile L40.54
    other specified L40.59

Psoriasis - *continued*
  spondylitis L40.53
  buccal K13.29
  flexural L40.8
  guttate L40.4
  mouth K13.29
  nummular L40.0
  plaque L40.0
  psychogenic F54
  pustular (generalized) L40.1
    palmaris et plantaris L40.3
  specified NEC L40.8
  vulgaris L40.0
Psychasthenia F48.8
Psychiatric disorder or problem F99
Psychogenic - *see also* condition
  factors associated with physical conditions F54
Psychological and behavioral factors affecting medical condition F59
Psychoneurosis, psychoneurotic - *see also* Neurosis
  anxiety (state) F41.1
  depersonalization F48.1
  hypochondriacal F45.21
  hysteria F44.9
  neurasthenic F48.8
  personality NEC F60.89
Psychopathy, psychopathic
  affectionless F94.2
  autistic F84.5
  constitution, post-traumatic F07.81
  personality - *see* Disorder, personality sexual - *see* Deviation, sexual
  state F60.2
Psychosexual identity disorder of childhood F64.2
Psychosis, psychotic F29
  acute (transient) F23
    hysterical F44.9
  affective - *see* Disorder, mood   alcoholic F10.959
    with
      abuse F10.159
      anxiety disorder F10.980
        with
          abuse F10.180
          dependence F10.280
      delirium tremens F10.231
      delusions F10.950
        with
          abuse F10.150
          dependence F10.250
      dementia F10.97
        with dependence F10.27
      dependence F10.259
      hallucinosis F10.951
        with
          abuse F10.151
          dependence F10.251
      mood disorder F10.94
        with
          abuse F10.14
          dependence F10.24
      paranoia F10.950
        with
          abuse F10.150
          dependence F10.250
      persisting amnesia F10.96
        with dependence F10.26
    amnestic confabulatory F10.96
      with dependence F10.26
    delirium tremens F10.231
    Korsakoff's, Korsakov's, Korsakow's F10.26
    paranoid type F10.950

Psychosis, psychotic - *continued*
  with
    abuse F10.150
    dependence F10.250
  anergastic - *see* Psychosis, organic
  arteriosclerotic (simple type) (uncomplicated)
    F01.50
    with behavioral disturbance F01.51
  childhood F84.0
    atypical F84.8
  climacteric - *see* Psychosis, involutional
  confusional F29
    acute or subacute F05
    reactive F23
  cycloid F23
  depressive - *see* Disorder, depressive
  disintegrative (childhood) F84.3
  drug-induced - *see* F11-f19 with .x59
    paranoid and hallucinatory states - *see* F11-
      f19 with .x50 or .x51
  due to or associated with
    addiction, drug - *see* F11-f19 with .x59
    dependence
      alcohol F10.259
      drug - *see* F11-f19 with .x59
    epilepsy F06.8
    Huntington's chorea F06.8
    ischemia, cerebrovascular (generalized)
      F06.8
    multiple sclerosis F06.8
    physical disease F06.8
    presenile dementia F03
    senile dementia F03
    vascular disease (arteriosclerotic) (cerebral)
      F01.50
      with behavioral disturbance F01.51
  epileptic F06.8
  episode F23
    due to or associated with physical condition
      F06.8
  exhaustive F43.0
  hallucinatory, chronic F28
  hypomanic F30.8
  hysterical (acute) F44.9
  induced F24
  infantile F84.0
    atypical F84.8
  infective (acute) (subacute) F05
  involutional F28
    depressive - *see* Disorder, depressive
    melancholic - *see* Disorder, depressive
    paranoid (state) F22
  Korsakoff's, Korsakov's, Korsakow's
    (nonalcoholic) F04
    alcoholic F10.96
      in dependence F10.26
    induced by other psychoactive substance -
      see categories F11-f19 with .x5x   mania,
      manic (single episode) F30.2
    recurrent type F31.89
  manic-depressive - *see* Disorder, bipolar
  menopausal - *see* Psychosis, involutional
  mixed schizophrenic and affective F25.8
  multi-infarct (cerebrovascular) F01.50
    with behavioral disturbance F01.51
  nonorganic F29
    specified NEC F28
  organic F09
    due to or associated with
      arteriosclerosis (cerebral) - *see* Psychosis,
        arteriosclerotic
      cerebrovascular disease, arteriosclerotic -
        see Psychosis, arteriosclerotic
      childbirth - *see* Psychosis, puerperal

Psychosis, psychotic - *continued*
    Creutzfeldt-Jakob disease or syndrome - *see*
      Creutzfeldt-Jakob disease or syndrome
    dependence, alcohol F10.259
    disease
      alcoholic liver F10.259
      brain, arteriosclerotic - *see* Psychosis,
        arteriosclerotic
      cerebrovascular F01.50
        with behavioral disturbance F01.51
      Creutzfeldt-Jakob - *see* Creutzfeldt-Jakob
        disease or syndrome
      endocrine or metabolic F06.8
        acute or subacute F05
      liver, alcoholic F10.259
    epilepsy transient (acute) F05
    infection
      brain (intracranial) F06.8
        acute or subacute F05
    intoxication
      alcoholic (acute) F10.259
      drug F19 with .x59 F11-
    ischemia, cerebrovascular (generalized) -
      see Psychosis, arteriosclerotic
    puerperium - *see* Psychosis, puerperal
    trauma, brain (birth) (from electric current)
      (surgical) F06.8
      acute or subacute F05
  infective F06.8
    acute or subacute F05
  post-traumatic F06.8
    acute or subacute F05
  paranoiac F22
  paranoid (climacteric) (involutional)
    (menopausal) F22
    psychogenic (acute) F23
    schizophrenic F20.0
    senile F03
  postpartum F53
  presbyophrenic (type) F03
  presenile F03
  psychogenic (paranoid) F23
    depressive F32.3
  puerperal F53
    specified type - *see* Psychosis, by type
  reactive (brief) (transient) (emotional stress)
    (psychological trauma) F23
    depressive F32.3
      recurrent F33.3
  excitative type F30.8
  schizoaffective F25.9
    depressive type F25.1
    manic type F25.0
  schizophrenia, schizophrenic - *see*
    Schizophrenia
  schizophrenia-like, in epilepsy F06.2
  schizophreniform F20.81
    affective type F25.9
    brief F23
    confusional type F23
    mixed type F25.0
  senile NEC F03
    depressed or paranoid type F03
    simple deterioration F03
    specified type   code to condition
  shared F24
  situational (reactive) F23
  symbiotic (childhood) F84.3
  symptomatic F09
Psychosomatic - *see* Disorder, psychosomatic
Psychosyndrome, organic F07.9
Psychotic episode due to or associated with
  physical condition F06.8

Pterygium (eye) H11.00-
  amyloid H11.01-
  central H11.02-
  colli Q18.3
  double H11.03-
  peripheral
    progressive H11.05-
    stationary H11.04-
  recurrent H11.06-
Ptilosis (eyelid) - *see* Madarosis
Ptomaine (poisoning) - *see* Poisoning, food
Ptosis - *see also* Blepharoptosis
  adiposa (false) - *see* Blepharoptosis
  breast N64.81
  cecum K63.4
  colon K63.4
  congenital (eyelid) Q10.0
    specified site NEC - *see* Anomaly, by site
  eyelid - *see* Blepharoptosis
    congenital Q10.0
  gastric K31.89
  intestine K63.4
  kidney N28.83
  liver K76.89
  renal N28.83
  splanchnic K63.4
  spleen D73.89
  stomach K31.89
  viscera K63.4
PTP D69.51
Ptyalism (periodic) K11.7
  hysterical F45.8
  pregnancy - *see* Pregnancy, complicated by,
    specified pregnancy-related condition NEC
  psychogenic F45.8
Ptyalolithiasis K11.5
Pubarche, precocious E30.1
Pubertas praecox E30.1
Puberty (development state) Z00.3
  bleeding (excessive) N92.2
  delayed E30.0
  precocious (constitutional) (cryptogenic)
    (idiopathic) E30.1
    central E22.8
    due to
      ovarian hyperfunction E28.1
        estrogen E28.0
      testicular hyperfunction E29.0
  premature E30.1
    due to
      adrenal cortical hyperfunction E25.8
      pineal tumor E34.8
      pituitary (anterior) hyperfunction E22.8
Puckering, macula - *see* Degeneration, macula,
  puckering
Pudenda, pudendum - *see* condition
Puente's disease (simple glandular cheilitis)
  K13.0
Puerperal, puerperium (complicated by,
  complications)
  abnormal glucose (tolerance test) O99.815
  abscess
    areola O91.02
      associated with lactation O91.03
    Bartholin's gland O86.19
    breast O91.12
      associated with lactation O91.13
    cervix (uteri) O86.11
    genital organ NEC O86.19
    kidney O86.21
    mammary O91.12
      associated with lactation O91.13
    nipple O91.02
      associated with lactation O91.03

Puerperal, puerperium - *continued*
  peritoneum O85
  subareolar O91.12
    associated with lactation O91.13
  urinary tract - *see* Puerperal, infection, urinary
  uterus O86.12
  vagina (wall) O86.13
  vaginorectal O86.13
  vulvovaginal gland O86.13
  adnexitis O86.19
  afibrinogenemia, or other coagulation defect O72.3
  albuminuria (acute) (subacute) - *see* Proteinuria, gestational
  alcohol use O99.315
  anemia O90.81
    pre-existing (pre-pregnancy) O99.03
  anesthetic death O89.8
  apoplexy O99.43
  bariatric surgery status O99.845
  blood disorder NEC O99.13
  blood dyscrasia O72.3
  cardiomyopathy O90.3
  cerebrovascular disorder (conditions in I60-i69) O99.43
  cervicitis O86.11
  circulatory system disorder O99.43
  coagulopathy (any) O99.13
    with hemorrhage O72.3
  complications O90.9
    specified NEC O90.89
  convulsions - *see* Eclampsia
  cystitis O86.22
  cystopyelitis O86.29
  delirium NEC F05
  diabetes O24.93
    gestational - *see* Puerperal, gestational diabetes
    pre-existing O24.33
      specified NEC O24.83
      type 1 O24.03
      type 2 O24.13
  digestive system disorder O99.63
  disease O90.9
    breast NEC O92.29
    cerebrovascular (acute) O99.43
    nonobstetric NEC O99.89
    tubo-ovarian O86.19
    Valsuani's O99.03
  disorder O90.9
    biliary tract O26.63
    lactation O92.70
    liver O26.63
    nonobstetric NEC O99.89
  disruption
    cesarean wound O90.0
    episiotomy wound O90.1
    perineal laceration wound O90.1
  drug use O99.325
  eclampsia (with pre-existing hypertension) O15.2
  embolism (pulmonary) (blood clot) - *see* Embolism, obstetric, puerperal
  endocrine, nutritional or metabolic disease NEC O99.285
  endophlebitis - *see* Puerperal, phlebitis
  endotrachelitis O86.11
  failure
    lactation (complete) O92.3
      partial O92.4
    renal, acute O90.4
  fever (of unknown origin) O86.4
    septic O85

Puerperal, puerperium - *continued*
  fissure, nipple O92.12
    associated with lactation O92.13
  fistula
    breast (due to mastitis) O91.12
      associated with lactation O91.13
    nipple O91.02
      associated with lactation O91.03
  galactophoritis O91.22
    associated with lactation O91.23
  galactorrhea O92.6
  gastric banding status O99.845
  gastric bypass status O99.845
  gastrointestinal disease NEC O99.63
  gestational
    diabetes O24.439
      diet controlled O24.430
      insulin (and diet) controlled O24.434
      oral drug controlled (antidiabetic) (hypoglycemic) O24.435
    edema O12.05
      with proteinuria O12.25
    proteinuria O12.15
  gonorrhea O98.23
  hematoma, subdural O99.43
  hemiplegia, cerebral O99.355
    due to cerebrovascular disorder O99.43
  hemorrhage O72.1
    brain O99.43
    bulbar O99.43
    cerebellar O99.43
    cerebral O99.43
    cortical O99.43
    delayed or secondary O72.2
    extradural O99.43
    internal capsule O99.43
    intracranial O99.43
    intrapontine O99.43
    meningeal O99.43
    pontine O99.43
    retained placenta O72.0
    subarachnoid O99.43
    subcortical O99.43
    subdural O99.43
    third stage O72.0
    uterine, delayed O72.2
    ventricular O99.43
  hemorrhoids O87.2
  hepatorenal syndrome O90.4
  hypertension - *see* Hypertension, complicating, puerperium
  hypertrophy, breast O92.29
  induration breast (fibrous) O92.29
  infection O86.4
    cervix O86.11
    generalized O85
    genital tract NEC O86.19
      obstetric surgical wound O86.0
    kidney (bacillus coli) O86.21
    maternal O98.93
      carrier state NEC O99.835
      gonorrhea O98.23
      human immunodeficiency virus (HIV) O98.73
      protozoal O98.63
      sexually transmitted NEC O98.33
      specified NEC O98.83
      streptococcus group B (GBS) carrier state O99.825
      syphilis O98.13
      tuberculosis O98.03
      viral hepatitis O98.43
      viral NEC O98.53
    nipple O91.02

Puerperal, puerperium - *continued*
    associated with lactation O91.03
    peritoneum O85
    renal O86.21
    specified NEC O86.89
    urinary (asymptomatic) (tract) NEC O86.20
      bladder O86.22
      kidney O86.21
      specified site NEC O86.29
      urethra O86.22
    vagina O86.13
    vein - *see* Puerperal, phlebitis
  ischemia, cerebral O99.43
  lymphangitis O86.89
    breast O91.22
      associated with lactation O91.23
  malignancy O9A.13
  malnutrition O25.3
  mammillitis O91.02
    associated with lactation O91.03
  mammitis O91.22
    associated with lactation O91.23
  mania F30.8
  mastitis O91.22
    associated with lactation O91.23
    purulent O91.12
      associated with lactation O91.13
  melancholia - *see* Disorder, depressive
  mental disorder NEC O99.345
  metroperitonitis O85
  metrorrhagia - *see* Hemorrhage, postpartum
  metrosalpingitis O86.19
  metrovaginitis O86.13
  milk leg O87.1
  monoplegia, cerebral O99.43
  mood disturbance O90.6
  necrosis, liver (acute) (subacute) (conditions in subcategory K72.0) O26.63
    with renal failure O90.4
  nervous system disorder O99.355
  neuritis O90.89
  obesity (pre-existing prior to pregnancy) O99.215
  obesity surgery status O99.845
  occlusion, precerebral artery O99.43
  paralysis
    bladder (sphincter) O90.89
    cerebral O99.43
  paralytic stroke O99.43
  parametritis O85
  paravaginitis O86.13
  pelviperitonitis O85
  perimetritis O86.12
  perimetrosalpingitis O86.19
  perinephritis O86.21
  periphlebitis - *see* Puerperal phlebitis
  peritoneal infection O85
  peritonitis (pelvic) O85
  perivaginitis O86.13
  phlebitis O87.0
    deep O87.1
    pelvic O87.1
    superficial O87.0
  phlebothrombosis, deep O87.1
  phlegmasia alba dolens O87.1
  placental polyp O90.89
  pneumonia, embolic - *see* Embolism, obstetric, puerperal
  pre-eclampsia - *see* Pre-eclampsia
  psychosis F53
  pyelitis O86.21
  pyelocystitis O86.29
  pyelonephritis O86.21
  pyelonephrosis O86.21

Puerperal, puerperium - *continued*
  pyemia O85
  pyocystitis O86.29
  pyohemia O85
  pyometra O86.12
  pyonephritis O86.21
  pyosalpingitis O86.19
  pyrexia (of unknown origin) O86.4
  renal
    disease NEC O90.89
    failure O90.4
  respiratory disease NEC O99.53
  retention
    decidua - *see* Retention, decidua
    placenta O72.0
    secundines - *see* Retention, secundines
  retracted nipple O92.02
  salpingo-ovaritis O86.19
  salpingoperitonitis O85
  secondary perineal tear O90.1
  sepsis (pelvic) O85
  sepsis O85
  septic thrombophlebitis O86.81
  skin disorder NEC O99.73
  specified condition NEC O99.89
  stroke O99.43
  subinvolution (uterus) O90.89
  subluxation of symphysis (pubis) O26.73
  suppuration - *see* Puerperal, abscess
  tetanus A34
  thelitis O91.02
    associated with lactation O91.03
  thrombocytopenia O72.3
  thrombophlebitis (superficial) O87.0
    deep O87.1
    pelvic O87.1
    septic O86.81
  thrombosis (venous) - *see* Thrombosis,
    puerperal
  thyroiditis O90.5
  toxemia (eclamptic) (pre-eclamptic) (with
    convulsions) O15.2
  trauma, non-obstetric O9A.23
    caused by abuse (physical) (suspected)
      O9A.33
      confirmed O9A.33
      psychological (suspected) O9A.53
        confirmed O9A.53
      sexual (suspected) O9A.43
        confirmed O9A.43
  uremia (due to renal failure) O90.4
  urethritis O86.22
  vaginitis O86.13
  varicose veins (legs) O87.4
    vulva or perineum O87.8
  venous O87.9
  vulvitis O86.19
  vulvovaginitis O86.13
  white leg O87.1
Puerperium - *see* Puerperal
Pulmolithiasis J98.4
Pulmonary - *see* condition
**Pulpitis (acute) (anachoretic) (chronic)
  (hyperplastic) (putrescent) (suppurative)
  (ulcerative)** K04.01
  irreversible K04.02
  reversible K04.01
Pulpless tooth K04.99
Pulse
  alternating R00.8
  bigeminal R00.8
  fast R00.0
  feeble, rapid due to shock following injury
    T79.4

Pulse - *continued*
  rapid R00.0
  weak R09.89
Pulsus alternans or trigeminus R00.8
Punch drunk F07.81
Punctum lacrimale occlusion - *see*
  Obstruction, lacrimal
Puncture
  abdomen, abdominal
    wall S31.139
      with
        foreign body S31.149
        penetration into peritoneal cavity S31.639
          with foreign body S31.649
      epigastric region S31.132
        with
          foreign body S31.142
          penetration into peritoneal cavity
            S31.632
            with foreign body S31.642
      left
        lower quadrant S31.134
          with
            foreign body S31.144
            penetration into peritoneal cavity
              S31.634
              with foreign body S31.644
        upper quadrant S31.131
          with
            foreign body S31.141
            penetration into peritoneal cavity
              S31.631
              with foreign body S31.641
      periumbilic region S31.135
        with
          foreign body S31.145
          penetration into peritoneal cavity
            S31.635
            with foreign body S31.645
      right
        lower quadrant S31.133
          with
            foreign body S31.143
            penetration into peritoneal cavity
              S31.633
              with foreign body S31.643
        upper quadrant S31.130
          with
            foreign body S31.140
            penetration into peritoneal cavity
              S31.630
              with foreign body S31.640
  accidental, complicating surgery - *see*
    Complication, accidental puncture or
    laceration
  alveolar (process) - *see* Puncture, oral cavity
  ankle S91.039
    with
      foreign body S91.049
    left S91.032
      with
        foreign body S91.042
    right S91.031
      with
        foreign body S91.041
  anus S31.833
    with foreign body S31.834
  arm (upper) S41.139
    with foreign body S41.149
    left S41.132
      with foreign body S41.142
    lower - *see* Puncture, forearm
    right S41.131
      with foreign body S41.141

Puncture - *continued*
  auditory canal (external) (meatus) - *see*
  Puncture, ear
  auricle, ear - *see* Puncture, ear
  axilla - *see* Puncture, arm
  back - *see also* Puncture, thorax, back
    lower S31.030
      with
        foreign body S31.040
          with penetration into retroperitoneal
            space S31.041
        penetration into retroperitoneal space
          S31.031
  bladder (traumatic) S37.29
    nontraumatic N32.89
  breast S21.039
    with foreign body S21.049
    left S21.032
      with foreign body S21.042
    right S21.031
      with foreign body S21.041
  buttock S31.803
    with foreign body S31.804
    left S31.823
      with foreign body S31.824
    right S31.813
      with foreign body S31.814
  by
    device, implant or graft - *see* Complications,
      by site and type, mechanical
    foreign body left accidentally in operative
      wound T81.539
    instrument (any) during a procedure,
      accidental - *see* Puncture, accidental
      complicating surgery   calf - *see* Puncture,
      leg
  canaliculus lacrimalis - *see* Puncture, eyelid
  canthus, eye - *see* Puncture, eyelid
  cervical esophagus S11.23
    with foreign body S11.24
  cheek (external) S01.439
    with foreign body S01.449
    left S01.432
      with foreign body S01.442
    right S01.431
      with foreign body S01.441
    internal - *see* Puncture, oral cavity   chest
    wall - *see* Puncture, thorax
  chin - *see* Puncture, head, specified site NEC
  clitoris - *see* Puncture, vulva
  costal region - *see* Puncture, thorax   digit(s)
    hand - *see* Puncture, finger
    foot - *see* Puncture, toe
  ear (canal) (external) S01.339
    with foreign body S01.349
    left S01.332
      with foreign body S01.342
    right S01.331
      with foreign body S01.341
    drum S09.2-
  elbow S51.039
    with
      foreign body S51.049
    left S51.032
      with
        foreign body S51.042
    right S51.031
      with
        foreign body S51.041
  epididymis - *see* Puncture, testis
  epigastric region - *see* Puncture, abdomen,
    wall, epigastric
  epiglottis S11.83
    with foreign body S11.84

Puncture - *continued*
esophagus
  cervical S11.23
   with foreign body S11.24
  thoracic S27.818
eyeball S05.6-
  with foreign body S05.5-
eyebrow - *see* Puncture, eyelid
eyelid S01.13-
  with foreign body S01.14-
  left S01.132
   with foreign body S01.142
  right S01.131
   with foreign body S01.141
face NEC - *see* Puncture, head, specified site
  NEC
finger(s) S61.239
  with
   damage to nail S61.339
    with
     foreign body S61.349
   foreign body S61.249
  index S61.238
   with
    damage to nail S61.338
     with
      foreign body S61.348
    foreign body S61.248
   left S61.231
    with
     damage to nail S61.331
      with
       foreign body S61.341
     foreign body S61.241
   right S61.230
    with
     damage to nail S61.330
      with
       foreign body S61.340
     foreign body S61.240
  little S61.238
   with
    damage to nail S61.338
     with
      foreign body S61.348
    foreign body S61.248
   left S61.237
    with
     damage to nail S61.337
      with
       foreign body S61.347
     foreign body S61.247
   right S61.236
    with
     damage to nail S61.336
      with
       foreign body S61.346
     foreign body S61.246
  middle S61.238
   with
    damage to nail S61.338
     with
      foreign body S61.348
    foreign body S61.248
   left S61.233
    with
     damage to nail S61.333
      with
       foreign body S61.343
     foreign body S61.243
   right S61.232
    with
     damage to nail S61.332
      with

Puncture - *continued*
    foreign body S61.342
   foreign body S61.242
  ring S61.238
   with
    damage to nail S61.338
     with
      foreign body S61.348
    foreign body S61.248
   left S61.235
    with
     damage to nail S61.335
      with
       foreign body S61.345
     foreign body S61.245
   right S61.234
    with
     damage to nail S61.334
      with
       foreign body S61.344
     foreign body S61.244
flank S31.139
  with foreign body S31.149
foot (except toe(s) alone) S91.339
  with foreign body S91.349
  left S91.332
   with foreign body S91.342
  right S91.331
   with foreign body S91.341
  toe - *see* Puncture, toe
forearm S51.839
  with
   foreign body S51.849
  elbow only - *see* Puncture, elbow
  left S51.832
   with
    foreign body S51.842
  right S51.831
   with
    foreign body S51.841
forehead - *see* Puncture, head, specified site
  NEC
genital organs, external
  female S31.532
   with foreign body S31.542
   vagina - *see* Puncture, vagina
   vulva - *see* Puncture, vulva
  male S31.531
   with foreign body S31.541
   penis - *see* Puncture, penis
   scrotum - *see* Puncture, scrotum
   testis - *see* Puncture, testis
groin - *see* Puncture, abdomen, wall
gum - *see* Puncture, oral cavity
hand S61.439
  with
   foreign body S61.449
  finger - *see* Puncture, finger
  left S61.432
   with
    foreign body S61.442
  right S61.431
   with
    foreign body S61.441
  thumb - *see* Puncture, thumb
head S01.93
  with foreign body S01.94
  cheek - *see* Puncture, cheek
  ear - *see* Puncture, ear
  eyelid - *see* Puncture, eyelid
  lip - *see* Puncture, oral cavity
  nose - *see* Puncture, nose
  oral cavity - *see* Puncture, oral cavity
  scalp S01.03

Puncture - *continued*
   with foreign body S01.04
  specified site NEC S01.83
   with foreign body S01.84
  temporomandibular area - *see* Puncture,
  cheek
heart S26.99
  with hemopericardium S26.09
  without hemopericardium S26.19
heel - *see* Puncture, foot
hip S71.039
  with foreign body S71.049
  left S71.032
   with foreign body S71.042
  right S71.031
   with foreign body S71.041
hymen - *see* Puncture, vagina
hypochondrium - *see* Puncture, abdomen, wall
hypogastric region - *see* Puncture, abdomen,
  wall
inguinal region - *see* Puncture, abdomen, wall
instep - *see* Puncture, foot
internal organs - *see* Injury, by site
interscapular region - *see* Puncture, thorax,
  back
intestine
  large
   colon S36.599
    ascending S36.590
    descending S36.592
    sigmoid S36.593
    specified site NEC S36.598
    transverse S36.591
   rectum S36.69
  small S36.499
   duodenum S36.490
   specified site NEC S36.498
intra-abdominal organ S36.99
  gallbladder S36.128
  intestine - *see* Puncture, intestine
  liver S36.118
  pancreas - *see* Puncture, pancreas
  peritoneum S36.81
  specified site NEC S36.898
  spleen S36.09
  stomach S36.39
jaw - *see* Puncture, head, specified site NEC
knee S81.039
  with foreign body S81.049
  left S81.032
   with foreign body S81.042
  right S81.031
   with foreign body S81.041
labium (majus) (minus) - *see* Puncture, vulva
lacrimal duct - *see* Puncture, eyelid
larynx S11.013
  with foreign body S11.014
leg (lower) S81.839
  with foreign body S81.849
  foot - *see* Puncture, foot
  knee - *see* Puncture, knee
  left S81.832
   with foreign body S81.842
  right S81.831
   with foreign body S81.841
  upper - *see* Puncture, thigh
lip S01.531
  with foreign body S01.541
loin - *see* Puncture, abdomen, wall
lower back - *see* Puncture, back, lower
lumbar region - *see* Puncture, back, lower
malar region - *see* Puncture, head, specified
  site NEC
mammary - *see* Puncture, breast

Puncture - *continued*

mastoid region - *see* Puncture, head, specified site NEC
mouth - *see* Puncture, oral cavity
nail
  finger - *see* Puncture, finger, with damage to nail
  toe - *see* Puncture, toe, with damage to nail
nasal (septum) (sinus) - *see* Puncture, nose
nasopharynx - *see* Puncture, head, specified site NEC
neck S11.93
  with foreign body S11.94
  involving
    cervical esophagus - *see* Puncture, cervical esophagus
    larynx - *see* Puncture, larynx
    pharynx - *see* Puncture, pharynx
    thyroid gland - *see* Puncture, thyroid gland
    trachea - *see* Puncture, trachea
  specified site NEC S11.83
    with foreign body S11.84
nose (septum) (sinus) S01.23
  with foreign body S01.24
ocular - *see* Puncture, eyeball
oral cavity S01.532
  with foreign body S01.542
orbit S05.4-
palate - *see* Puncture, oral cavity palm - *see* Puncture, hand
pancreas S36.299
  body S36.291
  head S36.290
  tail S36.292
pelvis - *see* Puncture, back, lower
penis S31.23
  with foreign body S31.24
perineum
  female S31.43
    with foreign body S31.44
  male S31.139
    with foreign body S31.149
periocular area (with or without lacrimal passages) - *see* Puncture, eyelid
phalanges
  finger - *see* Puncture, finger
  toe - *see* Puncture, toe
pharynx S11.23
  with foreign body S11.24
pinna - *see* Puncture, ear
popliteal space - *see* Puncture, knee
prepuce - *see* Puncture, penis
pubic region S31.139
  with foreign body S31.149
pudendum - *see* Puncture, genital organs, external
rectovaginal septum - *see* Puncture, vagina
sacral region - *see* Puncture, back, lower
sacroiliac region - *see* Puncture, back, lower
salivary gland - *see* Puncture, oral cavity
scalp S01.03
  with foreign body S01.04
scapular region - *see* Puncture, shoulder
scrotum S31.33
  with foreign body S31.34
shin - *see* Puncture, leg
shoulder S41.039
  with foreign body S41.049
  left S41.032
    with foreign body S41.042
  right S41.031
    with foreign body S41.041
spermatic cord - *see* Puncture, testis
sternal region - *see* Puncture, thorax, front

Puncture - *continued*

submaxillary region - *see* Puncture, head, specified site NEC
submental region - *see* Puncture, head, specified site NEC
subungual
  finger(s) - *see* Puncture, finger, with damage to nail
  toe - *see* Puncture, toe, with damage to nail
supraclavicular fossa - *see* Puncture, neck, specified site NEC
temple, temporal region - *see* Puncture, head, specified site NEC
temporomandibular area - *see* Puncture, cheek
testis S31.33
  with foreign body S31.34
thigh S71.139
  with foreign body S71.149
  left S71.132
    with foreign body S71.142
  right S71.131
    with foreign body S71.141
thorax, thoracic (wall) S21.93
  with foreign body S21.94
  back S21.23-
    with
      foreign body S21.24-
        with penetration S21.44
      penetration S21.43
  breast - *see* Puncture, breast
  front S21.13-
    with
      foreign body S21.14-
        with penetration S21.34
      penetration S21.33
throat - *see* Puncture, neck
thumb S61.039
  with
    damage to nail S61.139
      with
        foreign body S61.149
    foreign body S61.049
  left S61.032
    with
      damage to nail S61.132
        with
          foreign body S61.142
      foreign body S61.042
  right S61.031
    with
      damage to nail S61.131
        with
          foreign body S61.141
      foreign body S61.041
thyroid gland S11.13
  with foreign body S11.14
toe(s) S91.139
  with
    damage to nail S91.239
      with
        foreign body S91.249
    foreign body S91.149
  great S91.133
    with
      damage to nail S91.233
        with
          foreign body S91.243
      foreign body S91.143
    left S91.132
      with
        damage to nail S91.232
          with
            foreign body S91.242
      foreign body S91.142

Puncture - *continued*

  right S91.131
    with
      damage to nail S91.231
        with
          foreign body S91.241
      foreign body S91.141
  lesser S91.136
    with
      damage to nail S91.236
        with
          foreign body S91.246
      foreign body S91.146
  left S91.135
    with
      damage to nail S91.235
        with
          foreign body S91.245
      foreign body S91.145
  right S91.134
    with
      damage to nail S91.234
        with
          foreign body S91.244
      foreign body S91.144
tongue - *see* Puncture, oral cavity trachea S11.023
  with foreign body S11.024
tunica vaginalis - *see* Puncture, testis
tympanum, tympanic membrane S09.2-
umbilical region S31.135
  with foreign body S31.145
uvula - *see* Puncture, oral cavity vagina S31.43
  with foreign body S31.44
vocal cords S11.033
  with foreign body S11.034
vulva S31.43
  with foreign body S31.44
wrist S61.539
  with
    foreign body S61.549
  left S61.532
    with
      foreign body S61.542
  right S61.531
    with
      foreign body S61.541
PUO (pyrexia of unknown origin) R50.9
Pupillary membrane (persistent) Q13.89
Pupillotonia - *see* Anomaly, pupil, function, tonic pupil
Purpura D69.2
  abdominal D69.0
  allergic D69.0
  anaphylactoid D69.0
  annularis telangiectodes L81.7
  arthritic D69.0
  autoerythrocyte sensitization D69.2
  autoimmune D69.0
  bacterial D69.0
  Bateman's (senile) D69.2
  capillary fragility (hereditary) (idiopathic) D69.8
  cryoglobulinemic D89.1
  Devil's pinches D69.2
  fibrinolytic - *see* Fibrinolysis
  fulminans, fulminous D65
  gangrenous D65
  hemorrhagic, hemorrhagica D69.3
    not due to thrombocytopenia D69.0
  Henoch (-Schönlein) (allergic) D69.0
  hypergammaglobulinemic (benign) (Waldenström) D89.0

Purpura - *continued*
  idiopathic (thrombocytopenic) D69.3
    nonthrombocytopenic D69.0
  immune thrombocytopenic D69.3
  infectious D69.0
  malignant D69.0
  neonatorum P54.5
  nervosa D69.0
  newborn P54.5
  nonthrombocytopenic D69.2
    hemorrhagic D69.0
    idiopathic D69.0
  nonthrombopenic D69.2
  peliosis rheumatica D69.0
  posttransfusion (post-transfusion) (from (fresh)
    whole blood or blood products) D69.51
  primary D69.49
  red cell membrane sensitivity D69.2
  rheumatica D69.0
  Schönlein (-Henoch) (allergic) D69.0
  scorbutic E54 [D77]
  senile D69.2
  simplex D69.2
  symptomatica D69.0
  telangiectasia annularis L81.7
  thrombocytopenic D69.49
    congenital D69.42
    hemorrhagic D69.3
    hereditary D69.42
    idiopathic D69.3
    immune D69.3
    neonatal, transitory P61.0
    thrombotic M31.1
  thrombohemolytic - *see* Fibrinolysis
  thrombolytic - *see* Fibrinolysis
  thrombopenic D69.49
  thrombotic, thrombocytopenic M31.1
  toxic D69.0
  vascular D69.0
  visceral symptoms D69.0
Purpuric spots R23.3
Purulent - *see* condition
Pus
  in
    stool R19.5
    urine N39.0
  tube (rupture) - *see* Salpingo-oophoritis
Pustular rash L08.0
Pustule (nonmalignant) L08.9
  malignant A22.0
Pustulosis palmaris et plantaris L40.3
Putnam (-Dana) disease or syndrome - *see*
  Degeneration, combined
Putrescent pulp (dental) K04.1
Pyarthritis, pyarthrosis - *see* Arthritis,
  pyogenic or pyemic
  tuberculous - *see* Tuberculosis, joint
Pyelectasis - *see* Hydronephrosis
Pyelitis (congenital) (uremic) - *see also*
  Pyelonephritis
  with
    calculus - *see* category N20
      with hydronephrosis N13.2
    contracted kidney N11.9
  acute N10
  chronic N11.9
    with calculus - *see* category N20
      with hydronephrosis N13.2
  cystica N28.84
  puerperal (postpartum) O86.21
  tuberculous A18.11
Pyelocystitis - *see* Pyelonephritis
Pyelonephritis - *see also* Nephritis, tubulo-
  interstitial

Pyelonephritis - *continued*
  with
    calculus - *see* category N20
      with hydronephrosis N13.2
    contracted kidney N11.9
  acute N10
  calculous - *see* category N20
    with hydronephrosis N13.2
  chronic N11.9
    with calculus - *see* category N20
      with hydronephrosis N13.2
    associated with ureteral obstruction or
    stricture N11.1
    nonobstructive N11.8
      with reflux (vesicoureteral) N11.0
    obstructive N11.1
    specified NEC N11.8
  in (due to)
    brucellosis A23.9 [N16]
    cryoglobulinemia (mixed) D89.1 [N16]
    cystinosis E72.04
    diphtheria A36.84
    glycogen storage disease E74.09 [N16]
    leukemia NEC C95.9 [N16]
    lymphoma NEC C85.90 [N16]
    multiple myeloma C90.0- [N16]
    obstruction N11.1
    Salmonella infection A02.25
    sarcoidosis D86.84
    sepsis A41.9 [N16]
    Sjögren's disease M35.04
    toxoplasmosis B58.83
    transplant rejection T86.91 [N16]
    Wilson's disease E83.01 [N16]
  nonobstructive N12
    with reflux (vesicoureteral) N11.0
    chronic N11.8
  syphilitic A52.75
Pyelonephrosis (obstructive) N11.1
  chronic N11.9
Pyelophlebitis I80.8
Pyeloureteritis cystica N28.85
Pyemia, pyemic (fever) (infection) (purulent)
  - *see also* Sepsis
  joint - *see* Arthritis, pyogenic or pyemic
  liver K75.1
  pneumococcal A40.3
  portal K75.1
  postvaccinal T88.0
  puerperal, postpartum, childbirth O85
  specified organism NEC A41.89
  tuberculous - *see* Tuberculosis, miliary
Pygopagus Q89.4
Pyknoepilepsy (idiopathic) - *see* Pyknolepsy
Pyknolepsy G40.A09
  intractable G40.A19
    with status epilepticus G40.A11
    without status epilepticus G40.A19
  not intractable G40.A09
    with status epilepticus G40.A01
    without status epilepticus G40.A09
Pylephlebitis K75.1
Pyle's syndrome Q78.5
Pylethrombophlebitis K75.1
Pylethrombosis K75.1
Pyloritis K29.90
  with bleeding K29.91
Pylorospasm (reflex) NEC K31.3
  congenital or infantile Q40.0
  newborn Q40.0
  neurotic F45.8
  psychogenic F45.8
Pylorus, pyloric - *see* condition

Pyoarthrosis - *see* Arthritis, pyogenic or
  pyemic
Pyocele
  mastoid - *see* Mastoiditis, acute
  sinus (accessory) - *see* Sinusitis
  turbinate (bone) J32.9
  urethra - *see also* Urethritis N34.0
Pyocolpos - *see* Vaginitis
Pyocystitis N30.80
  with hematuria N30.81
Pyoderma, pyodermia L08.0
  gangrenosum L88
  newborn P39.4
  phagedenic L88
  vegetans L08.81
Pyodermatitis L08.0
  vegetans L08.81
Pyogenic - *see* condition
Pyohydronephrosis N13.6
Pyometra, pyometrium, pyometritis - *see*
  Endometritis
Pyomyositis (tropical) - *see* Myositis, infective
Pyonephritis N12
Pyonephrosis N13.6
  tuberculous A18.11
Pyo-oophoritis - *see* Salpingo-oophoritis
Pyo-ovarium - *see* Salpingo-oophoritis
Pyopericarditis, pyopericardium I30.1
Pyophlebitis - *see* Phlebitis
Pyopneumopericardium I30.1
Pyopneumothorax (infective) J86.9
  with fistula J86.0
  tuberculous NEC A15.6
Pyosalpinx, pyosalpingitis - *see also* Salpingo-
  oophoritis
Pyothorax J86.9
  with fistula J86.0
  tuberculous NEC A15.6
Pyoureter N28.89
  tuberculous A18.11
Pyramidopallidonigral syndrome G20
Pyrexia (of unknown origin) R50.9
  atmospheric T67.0
  during labor NEC O75.2
  heat T67.0
  newborn P81.9
    environmentally-induced P81.0
  persistent R50.9
  puerperal O86.4
Pyroglobulinemia NEC E88.09
Pyromania F63.1
Pyrosis R12
Pyuria (bacterial) N39.0

Q

Q fever A78
  with pneumonia A78
Quadricuspid aortic valve Q23.8
Quadrilateral fever A78
Quadriparesis - *see* Quadriplegia
  meaning muscle weakness M62.81
Quadriplegia G82.50
  complete
    C1-C4 level G82.51
    C5-C7 level G82.53
  congenital (cerebral) (spinal) G80.8
    spastic G80.0
  embolic (current episode) I63.4-
  functional R53.2
  incomplete
    C1-C4 level G82.52
    C5-C7 level G82.54
  thrombotic (current episode) I63.3-

Quadriplegia - *continued*
traumatic code to injury with seventh character S
current episode - *see* Injury, spinal (cord), cervical
Quadruplet, pregnancy - *see* Pregnancy, quadruplet
Quarrelsomeness F60.3
Queensland fever A77.3
Quervain's disease M65.4
thyroid E06.1
Queyrat's erythroplasia D07.4
penis D07.4
specified site - *see* Neoplasm, skin, in situ
unspecified site D07.4
Quincke's disease or edema T78.3
hereditary D84.1
Quinsy (gangrenous) J36
Quintan fever A79.0
Quintuplet, pregnancy - *see* Pregnancy, quintuplet

R

Rabbit fever - *see* Tularemia
Rabies A82.9
contact Z20.3
exposure to Z20.3
inoculation reaction - *see* Complications, vaccination
sylvatic A82.0
urban A82.1
Rachischisis - *see* Spina bifida
Rachitic - *see also* condition
deformities of spine (late effect) (sequelae) E64.3
pelvis (late effect) (sequelae) E64.3
with disproportion (fetopelvic) O33.0
causing obstructed labor O65.0
Rachitis, rachitism (acute) (tarda) - *see also* Rickets
renalis N25.0
sequelae E64.3
Radial nerve - *see* condition
Radiation
burn - *see* Burn
effects NOS T66
sickness NOS T66
therapy, encounter for Z51.0
Radiculitis (pressure) (vertebrogenic) - *see* Radiculopathy
Radiculomyelitis - *see also* Encephalitis
toxic, due to
Clostridium tetani A35
Corynebacterium diphtheriae A36.82
Radiculopathy M54.10
cervical region M54.12
cervicothoracic region M54.13
due to
disc disorder
Radiculopathy
C3 M50.11
C4 M50.11
C5 M50.121
C6 M50.122
C7 M50.123
C8 M50.13
displacement of intervertebral disc - *see* Disorder, disc, with, radiculopathy
leg M54.1-
lumbar region M54.16
lumbosacral region M54.17
occipito-atlanto-axial region M54.11
postherpetic B02.29

Radiculopathy - *continued*
sacrococcygeal region M54.18
syphilitic A52.11
thoracic region (with visceral pain) M54.14
thoracolumbar region M54.15
Radiodermal burns (acute, chronic, or occupational) - *see* Burn
Radiodermatitis L58.9
acute L58.0
chronic L58.1
Radiotherapy session Z51.0
RAEB (refractory anemia with excess blasts) D46.2-
Rage, meaning rabies - *see* Rabies
Ragpicker's disease A22.1
Ragsorter's disease A22.1
Raillietiniasis B71.8
Railroad neurosis F48.8
Railway spine F48.8
Raised - *see also* Elevated
antibody titer R76.0
Rake teeth, tooth M26.39
Rales R09.89
Ramifying renal pelvis Q63.8
Ramsay-hunt disease or syndrome - *see also* Hunt's disease B02.21
meaning dyssynergia cerebellaris myoclonica G11.1
Ranula K11.6
congenital Q38.4
Rape
adult
confirmed T74.21
suspected T76.21
alleged, observation or examination, ruled out
adult Z04.41
child Z04.42
child
confirmed T74.22
suspected T76.22
Rapid
feeble pulse, due to shock, following injury T79.4
heart (beat) R00.0
psychogenic F45.8
second stage (delivery) O62.3
time-zone change syndrome - *see* Disorder, sleep, circadian rhythm, psychogenic
Rarefaction, bone - *see* Disorder, bone, density and structure, specified NEC
Rash (toxic) R21
canker A38.9
diaper L22
drug (internal use) L27.0
contact - *see also* Dermatitis, due to, drugs, external L25.1
following immunization T88.1
food - *see* Dermatitis, due to, food
heat L74.0
napkin (psoriasiform) L22
nettle - *see* Urticaria
pustular L08.0
rose R21
epidemic B06.9
scarlet A38.9
serum - *see also* Reaction, serum T80.69
wandering tongue K14.1
Rasmussen aneurysm - *see* Tuberculosis, pulmonary
Rasmussen encephalitis G04.81
Rat-bite fever A25.9
due to Streptobacillus moniliformis A25.1
spirochetal (morsus muris) A25.0
Rathke's pouch tumor D44.3

Raymond (-Cestan) syndrome I65.8
Raynaud's disease, phenomenon or syndrome (secondary) I73.00
with gangrene (symmetric) I73.01
RDS (newborn) (type I) P22.0
type II P22.1
Reaction - *see also* Disorder
adaptation - *see* Disorder, adjustment
adjustment (anxiety) (conduct disorder) (depressiveness) (distress) - *see* Disorder, adjustment
with
mutism, elective (child) (adolescent) F94.0
adverse
food (any) (ingested) NEC T78.1
anaphylactic - *see* Shock, anaphylactic, due to food
affective - *see* Disorder, mood
allergic - *see* Allergy
anaphylactic - *see* Shock, anaphylactic
anaphylactoid - *see* Shock, anaphylactic
anesthesia - *see* Anesthesia, complication
antitoxin (prophylactic) (therapeutic) - *see* Complications, vaccination
anxiety F41.1
Arthus - *see* Arthus' phenomenon
asthenic F48.8
combat and operational stress F43.0
compulsive F42.8
conversion F44.9
crisis, acute F43.0
deoxyribonuclease (DNA) (DNase) hypersensitivity D69.2
depressive (single episode) F32.9
affective (single episode) F31.4
recurrent episode F33.9
neurotic F34.1
psychoneurotic F34.1
psychotic F32.3
recurrent - *see* Disorder, depressive, recurrent
dissociative F44.9
drug NEC T88.7
addictive - *see* Dependence, drug
transmitted via placenta or breast milk - *see* Absorption, drug, addictive, through placenta
allergic - *see* Allergy, drug
lichenoid L43.2
newborn P93.8
gray baby syndrome P93.0
overdose or poisoning (by accident) - *see* Table of Drugs and Chemicals, by drug, poisoning
photoallergic L56.1
phototoxic L56.0
withdrawal - *see* Dependence, by drug, with, withdrawal
infant of dependent mother P96.1
newborn P96.1
wrong substance given or taken (by accident) - *see* Table of Drugs and Chemicals, by drug, poisoning
fear F40.9
child (abnormal) F93.8
febrile nonhemolytic transfusion (FNHTR) R50.84
fluid loss, cerebrospinal G97.1
foreign
body NEC - *see* Granuloma, foreign body
in operative wound (inadvertently left) - *see* Foreign body, accidentally left during a procedure
substance accidentally left during a procedure (chemical) (powder) (talc) T81.60

Reaction - *continued*
 aseptic peritonitis T81.61
 body or object (instrument) (sponge) (swab) - *see* Foreign body, accidentally left during a procedure
 specified reaction NEC T81.69
 grief - *see* Disorder, adjustment
 Herxheimer's R68.89
 hyperkinetic - *see* Hyperkinesia
 hypochondriacal F45.20
 hypoglycemic, due to insulin E16.0
 with coma (diabetic) - *see* Diabetes, coma
 nondiabetic E15
 therapeutic misadventure *see* subcategory T38.3
 hypomanic F30.8
 hysterical F44.9
 immunization - *see* Complications, vaccination
 incompatibility
 ABO blood group (infusion) (transfusion) - *see* Complication(s), transfusion, incompatibility reaction, ABO
 delayed serologic T80.39
 minor blood group (Duffy) (E) (K(ell)) (Kidd) (Lewis) (M) (N) (P) (S) T80.89
 Rh (factor) (infusion) (transfusion) - *see* Complication(s), transfusion, incompatibility reaction, Rh (factor)
 inflammatory - *see* Infection
 infusion - *see* Complications, infusion
 inoculation (immune serum) - *see* Complications, vaccination
 insulin T38.3-
 involutional psychotic - *see* Disorder, depressive
 leukemoid D72.823
 basophilic D72.823
 lymphocytic D72.823
 monocytic D72.823
 myelocytic D72.823
 neutrophilic D72.823
 LSD (acute)
 due to drug abuse - *see* Abuse, drug, hallucinogen
 due to drug dependence - *see* Dependence, drug, hallucinogen
 lumbar puncture G97.1
 manic-depressive - *see* Disorder, bipolar
 neurasthenic F48.8
 neurogenic - *see* Neurosis
 neurotic F48.9
 neurotic-depressive F34.1
 nitritoid - *see* Crisis, nitritoid
 nonspecific
 to
 cell mediated immunity measurement of gamma interferon antigen response without active tuberculosis R76.12
 QuantiFERON-TB test (QFT) without active tuberculosis R76.12
 tuberculin test - *see also* Reaction, tuberculin skin test R76.11
 obsessive-compulsive F42.8
 organic, acute or subacute - *see* Delirium
 paranoid (acute) F23
 chronic F22
 senile F03
 passive dependency F60.7
 phobic F40.9
 post-traumatic stress, uncomplicated Z73.3
 psychogenic F99
 psychoneurotic - *see also* Neurosis
 compulsive F42.8
 depersonalization F48.1

Reaction - *continued*
 depressive F34.1
 hypochondriacal F45.20
 neurasthenic F48.8
 obsessive F42.8
 psychophysiologic - *see* Disorder, somatoform
 psychosomatic - *see* Disorder, somatoform
 psychotic - *see* Psychosis
 scarlet fever toxin - *see* Complications, vaccination
 schizophrenic F23
 acute (brief) (undifferentiated) F23
 latent F21
 undifferentiated (acute) (brief) F23
 serological for syphilis - *see* Serology for syphilis
 serum T80.69
 anaphylactic (immediate) - *see also* Shock, anaphylactic T80.59
 specified reaction NEC
 due to
 administration of blood and blood products T80.61
 immunization T80.62
 serum specified NEC T80.69
 vaccination T80.62
 situational - *see* Disorder, adjustment
 somatization - *see* Disorder, somatoform
 spinal puncture G97.1
 stress (severe) F43.9
 acute (agitation) ("daze") (disorientation) (disturbance of consciousness) (flight reaction) (fugue) F43.0
 specified NEC F43.8
 surgical procedure - *see* Complications, surgical procedure
 tetanus antitoxin - *see* Complications, vaccination
 toxic, to local anesthesia T88.59
 in labor and delivery O74.4
 in pregnancy O29.3X-
 postpartum, puerperal O89.3
 toxin-antitoxin - *see* Complications, vaccination
 transfusion (blood) (bone marrow) (lymphocytes) (allergic) - *see* Complications, transfusion
 tuberculin skin test, abnormal R76.11
 vaccination (any) - *see* Complications, vaccination
 withdrawing, child or adolescent F93.8
Reactive airway disease - *see* Asthma
Reactive depression - *see* Reaction, depressive
Rearrangement
 chromosomal
 balanced (in) Q95.9
 abnormal individual (autosomal) Q95.2
 non-sex (autosomal) chromosomes Q95.2
 sex/non-sex chromosomes Q95.3
 specified NEC Q95.8
Recalcitrant patient - *see* Noncompliance
Recanalization, thrombus - *see* Thrombosis
Recession, receding
 chamber angle (eye) H21.55-
 chin M26.09
 gingival (postinfective) (postoperative)
 generalized K06.020
 minimal K06.021
 moderate K06.022
 severe K06.023
 localized K06.010
 minimal K06.011
 moderate K06.012
 severe K06.013

Recklinghausen disease Q85.01
 bones E21.0
Reclus' disease (cystic) - *see* Mastopathy, cystic
Recrudescent typhus (fever) A75.1
Recruitment, auditory H93.21-
Rectalgia K62.89
Rectitis K62.89
Rectocele
 female (without uterine prolapse) N81.6
 with uterine prolapse N81.4
 incomplete N81.2
 in pregnancy - *see* Pregnancy, complicated by, abnormal, pelvic organs or tissues NEC
 male K62.3
Rectosigmoid junction - *see* condition
Rectosigmoiditis K63.89
 ulcerative (chronic) K51.30
 with
 complication K51.319
 abscess K51.314
 fistula K51.313
 obstruction K51.312
 rectal bleeding K51.311
 specified NEC K51.318
Rectourethral - *see* condition
Rectovaginal - *see* condition
Rectovesical - *see* condition
Rectum, rectal - *see* condition
Recurrent - *see* condition
 pregnancy loss - *see* Loss (of), pregnancy, recurrent
Red bugs B88.0
Red-cedar lung or pneumonitis J67.8
Red tide - *see also* Table of Drugs and Chemicals T65.82-
Reduced
 mobility Z74.09
 ventilatory or vital capacity R94.2
Redundant, redundancy
 anus (congenital) Q43.8
 clitoris N90.89
 colon (congenital) Q43.8
 foreskin (congenital) N47.8
 intestine (congenital) Q43.8
 labia N90.69
 organ or site, congenital NEC - *see* Accessory
 panniculus (abdominal) E65
 prepuce (congenital) N47.8
 pylorus K31.89
 rectum (congenital) Q43.8
 scrotum N50.89
 sigmoid (congenital) Q43.8
 skin L98.7
 and subcutaneous tissue L98.7
 of face L57.4
 eyelids - *see* Blepharochalasis
 stomach K31.89
Reduplication - *see* Duplication
Reflex R29.2
 hyperactive gag J39.2
 pupillary, abnormal - *see* Anomaly, pupil, function
 vasoconstriction I73.9
 vasovagal R55
Reflux K21.9
 acid K21.9
 esophageal K21.9
 with esophagitis K21.0
 newborn P78.83
 gastroesophageal K21.9
 with esophagitis K21.0
 mitral - *see* Insufficiency, mitral
 ureteral - *see* Reflux, vesicoureteral

Reflux - *continued*
vesicoureteral (with scarring) N13.70
with
nephropathy N13.729
with hydroureter N13.739
bilateral N13.732
unilateral N13.731
bilateral N13.722
unilateral N13.721
without hydroureter N13.729
bilateral N13.722
unilateral N13.721
pyelonephritis (chronic) N11.0
congenital Q62.7
without nephropathy N13.71
Reforming, artificial openings - *see* Attention to, artificial, opening
Refractive error - *see* Disorder, refraction
Refsum's disease or syndrome G60.1
Refusal of
food, psychogenic F50.89
treatment (because of) Z53.20
left against medical advice (AMA) Z53.21
patient's decision NEC Z53.29
reasons of belief or group pressure Z53.1
Regional - *see* condition
Regurgitation R11.10
aortic (valve) - *see* Insufficiency, aortic
food - *see also* Vomiting
with reswallowing - *see* Rumination
newborn P92.1
gastric contents - *see* Vomiting
heart - *see* Endocarditis
mitral (valve) - *see* Insufficiency, mitral
congenital Q23.3
myocardial - *see* Endocarditis
pulmonary (valve) (heart) I37.1
congenital Q22.2
syphilitic A52.03
tricuspid - *see* Insufficiency, tricuspid
valve, valvular - *see* Endocarditis
congenital Q24.8
vesicoureteral - *see* Reflux, vesicoureteral
Reifenstein syndrome E34.52
Reinsertion
implantable subdermal contraceptive Z30.46
intrauterine contraceptive device Z30.433
Reiter's disease, syndrome, or urethritis M02.30
ankle M02.37-
elbow M02.32-
foot joint M02.37-
hand joint M02.34-
hip M02.35-
knee M02.36-
multiple site M02.39
shoulder M02.31-
vertebra M02.38
wrist M02.33-
Reichmann's disease or syndrome K31.89
Rejection
food, psychogenic F50.89
transplant T86.91
bone T86.830
marrow T86.01
cornea T86.840
heart T86.21
with lung(s) T86.31
intestine T86.850
kidney T86.11
liver T86.41
lung(s) T86.810
with heart T86.31
organ (immune or nonimmune cause) T86.91

Rejection - *continued*
pancreas T86.890
skin (allograft) (autograft) T86.820
specified NEC T86.890
stem cell (peripheral blood) (umbilical cord) T86.5
Relapsing fever A68.9
Carter's (Asiatic) A68.1
Dutton's (West African) A68.1
Koch's A68.9
louse-borne (epidemic) A68.0
Novy's (American) A68.1
Obermeyers's (European) A68.0
Spirillum A68.9
tick-borne (endemic) A68.1
Relationship
occlusal
open anterior M26.220
open posterior M26.221
Relaxation
anus (sphincter) K62.89
psychogenic F45.8
arch (foot) - *see also* Deformity, limb, flat foot
back ligaments - *see* Instability, joint, spine
bladder (sphincter) N31.2
cardioesophageal K21.9
cervix - *see* Incompetency, cervix
diaphragm J98.6
joint (capsule) (ligament) (paralytic) - *see* Flail, joint
congenital NEC Q74.8
lumbosacral (joint) - *see* subcategory M53.2
pelvic floor N81.89
perineum N81.89
posture R29.3
rectum (sphincter) K62.89
sacroiliac (joint) - *see* subcategory M53.2
scrotum N50.89
urethra (sphincter) N36.44
vesical N31.2
Release from prison, anxiety concerning Z65.2
Remains
canal of Cloquet Q14.0
capsule (opaque) Q14.8
Remittent fever (malarial) B54
Remnant
canal of Cloquet Q14.0
capsule (opaque) Q14.8
cervix, cervical stump (acquired) (postoperative) N88.8
cystic duct, postcholecystectomy K91.5
fingernail L60.8
congenital Q84.6
meniscus, knee - *see* Derangement, knee, meniscus, specified NEC
thyroglossal duct Q89.2
tonsil J35.8
infected (chronic) J35.01
urachus Q64.4
Removal (from) (of)
artificial
arm Z44.00-
complete Z44.01-
partial Z44.02-
eye Z44.2-
leg Z44.10-
complete Z44.11-
partial Z44.12-
breast implant Z45.81
cardiac pulse generator (battery) (end-of-life) Z45.010
catheter (urinary) (indwelling) Z46.6

Removal (from) (of) - *continued*
from artificial opening - *see* Attention to, artificial, opening
non-vascular Z46.82
vascular NEC Z45.2
drains Z48.03
device Z46.9
contraceptive Z30.432
implantable subdermal Z30.46
implanted NEC Z45.89
specified NEC Z46.89
dressing (nonsurgical) Z48.00
surgical Z48.01
external
fixation device
code to fracture with seventh character D
prosthesis, prosthetic device Z44.9
breast Z44.3-
specified NEC Z44.8
home in childhood (to foster home or institution) Z62.29
ileostomy Z43.2
insulin pump Z46.81
myringotomy device (stent) (tube) Z45.82
nervous system device NEC Z46.2
brain neuropacemaker Z46.2
visual substitution device Z46.2
implanted Z45.31
non-vascular catheter Z46.82
orthodontic device Z46.4
organ, prophylactic (for neoplasia management) - *see* Prophylactic, organ removal
staples Z48.02
stent
ureteral Z46.6
suture Z48.02
urinary device Z46.6
vascular access device or catheter Z45.2
Ren
arcuatus Q63.1
mobile, mobilis N28.89
congenital Q63.8
unguliformis Q63.1
Renal - *see* condition
Rendu-Osler-Weber disease or syndrome I78.0
Reninoma D41.0-
Renon-Delille syndrome E23.3
Reovirus, as cause of disease classified elsewhere B97.5
Repeated falls NEC R29.6
Replaced chromosome by dicentric ring Q93.2
Replacement by artificial or mechanical device or prosthesis of bladder Z96.0
blood vessel NEC Z95.828
bone NEC Z96.7
cochlea Z96.21
coronary artery Z95.5
eustachian tube Z96.29
eye globe Z97.0
heart Z95.812
valve Z95.2
prosthetic Z95.2
specified NEC Z95.4
xenogenic Z95.3
intestine Z96.89
joint Z96.60
hip - *see* Presence, hip joint implant
knee - *see* Presence, knee joint implant
specified site NEC Z96.698
larynx Z96.3
lens Z96.1

Replacement - *continued*
limb(s) - *see* Presence, artificial, limb
mandible NEC (for tooth root implant(s))
  Z96.5
organ NEC Z96.89
peripheral vessel NEC Z95.828
stapes Z96.29
teeth Z97.2
tendon Z96.7
tissue NEC Z96.89
tooth root(s) Z96.5
vessel NEC Z95.828
  coronary (artery) Z95.5
Request for expert evidence Z04.8
Reserve, decreased or low
cardiac - *see* Disease, heart
kidney N28.89
Residual - *see also* condition
ovary syndrome N99.83
state, schizophrenic F20.5
urine R39.198
Resistance, resistant (to)
activated protein C D68.51
complicating pregnancy O26.89
insulin E88.81
organism(s)
  to
    drug Z16.30
      aminoglycosides Z16.29
      amoxicillin Z16.11
      ampicillin Z16.11
      antibiotic(s) Z16.20
        multiple Z16.24
        specified NEC Z16.29
      antifungal Z16.32
      antimicrobial (single) Z16.30
        multiple Z16.35
        specified NEC Z16.39
      antimycobacterial (single) Z16.341
        multiple Z16.342
      antiparasitic Z16.31
      antiviral Z16.33
      beta lactam antibiotics Z16.10
        specified NEC Z16.19
      cephalosporins Z16.19
      extended beta lactamase (ESBL) Z16.12
      fluoroquinolones Z16.23
      macrolides Z16.29
      methicillin - *see* MRSA
      multiple drugs (MDRO)
        antibiotics Z16.24
        antimicrobial Z16.35
        antimycobacterials Z16.342
      penicillins Z16.11
      quinine (and related compounds) Z16.31
      quinolones Z16.23
      sulfonamides Z16.29
      tetracyclines Z16.29
      tuberculostatics (single) Z16.341
        multiple Z16.342
      vancomycin Z16.21
        related antibiotics Z16.22
thyroid hormone E07.89
Resorption
dental (roots) K03.3
  alveoli M26.79
teeth (external) (internal) (pathological) (roots)
  K03.3
Respiration
Cheyne-stokes R06.3
decreased due to shock, following injury T79.4
disorder of, psychogenic F45.8
insufficient, or poor R06.89
  newborn P28.5

Respiration - *continued*
painful R07.1
sighing, psychogenic F45.8
Respiratory - *see also* condition
distress syndrome (newborn) (type I) P22.0
  type II P22.1
syncytial virus, as cause of disease classified
  elsewhere B97.4
Respite care Z75.5
Response (drug)
photoallergic L56.1
phototoxic L56.0
Restenosis
stent
  vascular
    end stent
      adjacent to stent - *see* Arteriosclerosis
      within the stent
        coronary T82.855
        peripheral T82.856
    in stent
      coronary vessel T82.855
      peripheral vessel T82.856
Restless legs (syndrome) G25.81
Restlessness R45.1
Restriction of housing space Z59.1
Restoration (of)
dental
  aesthetically inadequate or displeasing
    K08.56
  defective K08.50
    specified NEC K08.59
  failure of marginal integrity K08.51
Restoration (of)
failure of periodontal anatomical integrity
  K08.54
organ continuity from previous sterilization
  (tuboplasty) (vasoplasty) Z31.0
  aftercare Z31.42
tooth (existing)
  contours biologically incompatible with oral
    health K08.54
  open margins K08.51
  overhanging K08.52
  poor aesthetic K08.56
  poor gingival margins K08.51
unsatisfactory, of tooth K08.50
  specified NEC K08.59
Restorative material (dental)
allergy to K08.55
fractured K08.539
  with loss of material K08.531
  without loss of material K08.530
unrepairable overhanging of K08.52
Rests, ovarian, in fallopian tube Q50.6
Restzustand (schizophrenic) F20.5
Retained - *see also* Retention
cholelithiasis following cholecystectomy
  K91.86
foreign body fragments (type of) Z18.9
  acrylics Z18.2
  animal quill(s) or spines Z18.31
  cement Z18.83
  concrete Z18.83
  crystalline Z18.83
  depleted isotope Z18.09
  depleted uranium Z18.01
  diethylhexylphthalates Z18.2
  glass Z18.81
  isocyanate Z18.2
  magnetic metal Z18.11
  metal Z18.10
  nonmagnetic metal Z18.12
  nontherapeutic radioactive Z18.09

Retained - *continued*
  organic NEC Z18.39
  plastic Z18.2
  quill(s) (animal) Z18.31
  radioactive (nontherapeutic) NEC Z18.09
  specified NEC Z18.89
  spine(s) (animal) Z18.31
  stone Z18.83
  tooth (teeth) Z18.32
  wood Z18.33
fragments (type of) Z18.9
  acrylics Z18.2
  animal quill(s) or spines Z18.31
  cement Z18.83
  concrete Z18.83
  crystalline Z18.83
  depleted isotope Z18.09
  depleted uranium Z18.01
  diethylhexylphthalates Z18.2
  glass Z18.81
  isocyanate Z18.2
  magnetic metal Z18.11
  metal Z18.10
  nonmagnetic metal Z18.12
  nontherapeutic radioactive Z18.09
  organic NEC Z18.39
  plastic Z18.2
  quill(s) (animal) Z18.31
  radioactive (nontherapeutic) NEC Z18.09
  specified NEC Z18.89
  spine(s) (animal) Z18.31
  stone Z18.83
  tooth (teeth) Z18.32
  wood Z18.33
gallstones, following cholecystectomy K91.86
Retardation
development, developmental, specific - *see*
  Disorder, developmental
endochondral bone growth - *see* Disorder,
  bone, development or growth
growth R62.50
  due to malnutrition E45
mental - *see* Disability, intellectual
motor function, specific F82
physical (child) R62.52
  due to malnutrition E45
reading (specific) F81.0
spelling (specific) (without reading disorder)
  F81.81
Retching - *see* Vomiting
Retention - *see also* Retained
bladder - *see* Retention, urine
carbon dioxide E87.2
cholelithiasis following cholecystectomy
  K91.86
cyst - *see* Cyst
dead
  fetus (at or near term) (mother) O36.4
    early fetal death O02.1
  ovum O02.0
decidua (fragments) (following delivery) (with
  hemorrhage) O72.2
  without hemorrhage O73.1
deciduous tooth K00.6
dental root K08.3
fecal - *see* Constipation
fetus
  dead O36.4
    early O02.1
fluid R60.9
foreign body - *see also* Foreign body, retained
  current trauma   code as Foreign body, by
  site or type
gallstones, following cholecystectomy K91.86

Retention - *continued*
  gastric K31.89
  intrauterine contraceptive device, in pregnancy
    - *see* Pregnancy, complicated by, retention,
      intrauterine device
  membranes (complicating delivery) (with
    hemorrhage) O72.2
    with abortion - *see* Abortion, by type
    without hemorrhage O73.1
  meniscus - *see* Derangement, meniscus
  menses N94.89
  milk (puerperal, postpartum) O92.79
  nitrogen, extrarenal R39.2
  ovary syndrome N99.83
  placenta (total) (with hemorrhage) O72.0
    without hemorrhage O73.0
    portions or fragments (with hemorrhage)
      O72.2
      without hemorrhage O73.1
  products of conception
    early pregnancy (dead fetus) O02.1
    following
      delivery (with hemorrhage) O72.2
        without hemorrhage O73.1
  secundines (following delivery) (with
    hemorrhage) O72.0
    without hemorrhage O73.0
    complicating puerperium (delayed
      hemorrhage) O72.2
      partial O72.2
        without hemorrhage O73.1
  smegma, clitoris N90.89
  urine R33.9
    due to hyperplasia (hypertrophy) of prostate -
      see Hyperplasia, prostate
    drug-induced R33.0
    organic R33.8
      drug-induced R33.0
    psychogenic F45.8
    specified NEC R33.8
  water (in tissues) - *see* Edema
Reticular erythematous mucinosis L98.5
Reticulation, dust - *see* Pneumoconiosis
Reticulocytosis R70.1
Reticuloendotheliosis
  acute infantile C96.0
  leukemic C91.4-
  nonlipid C96.0
Reticulohistiocytoma (giant-cell) D76.3
Reticuloid, actinic L57.1
Reticulosis (skin)
  acute of infancy C96.0
  hemophagocytic, familial D76.1
  histiocytic medullary C96.A
  lipomelanotic I89.8
  malignant (midline) C86.0
  polymorphic C86.0
  Sézary - *see* Sézary disease
Retina, retinal - *see also* condition
  dark area D49.81
Retinitis - *see also* Inflammation, chorioretinal
  albuminurica N18.9 [*H32*]
  diabetic - *see* Diabetes, retinitis
  disciformis - *see* Degeneration, macula
  focal - *see* Inflammation, chorioretinal, focal
  gravidarum - *see* Pregnancy, complicated by,
    specified pregnancy-related condition NEC
  juxtapapillaris - *see* Inflammation,
    chorioretinal, focal, juxtapapillary
  luetic - *see* Retinitis, syphilitic
  pigmentosa H35.52
  proliferans - *see* Disorder, globe, degenerative,
    specified type NEC
  proliferating - *see* Disorder, globe,

Retinitis - *continued*
  degenerative, specified type NEC
    renal N18.9 [*H32*]
  syphilitic (early) (secondary) A51.43
    central, recurrent A52.71
    congenital (early) A50.01 [*H32*]
    late A52.71
  tuberculous A18.53
Retinoblastoma C69.2-
  differentiated C69.2-
  undifferentiated C69.2-
Retinochoroiditis - *see also* Inflammation,
  chorioretinal
  disseminated - *see* Inflammation, chorioretinal,
    disseminated
    syphilitic A52.71
  focal - *see* Inflammation, chorioretinal
  juxtapapillaris - *see* Inflammation,
    chorioretinal, focal, juxtapapillary
Retinopathy (background) H35.00
  arteriosclerotic I70.8 [*H35.0-*]
  atherosclerotic I70.8 [*H35.0-*]
  central serous - *see* Chorioretinopathy, central
    serous
  Coats H35.02-
  diabetic - *see* Diabetes, retinopathy
  exudative H35.02-
  hypertensive H35.03-
  in (due to)
    diabetes - *see* Diabetes, retinopathy
    sickle-cell disorders D57. [*H36*]
  of prematurity H35.10-
    stage 0 H35.11-
    stage 1 H35.12-
    stage 2 H35.13-
    stage 3 H35.14-
    stage 4 H35.15-
    stage 5 H35.16-
  pigmentary, congenital - *see* Dystrophy, retina
  proliferative NEC H35.2-
    diabetic - *see* Diabetes, retinopathy,
      proliferative
    sickle-cell D57. [*H36*]
  solar H31.02-
Retinoschisis H33.10-
  congenital Q14.1
  specified type NEC H33.19-
Retortamoniasis A07.8
Retractile testis Q55.22
Retraction
  cervix - *see* Retroversion, uterus
  drum (membrane) - *see* Disorder, tympanic
    membrane, specified NEC
  finger - *see* Deformity, finger
  lid H02.539
    left H02.536
      lower H02.535
      upper H02.534
    right H02.533
      lower H02.532
      upper H02.531
  lung J98.4
  mediastinum J98.59
  nipple N64.53
    associated with
      lactation O92.03
      pregnancy O92.01-
      puerperium O92.02
    congenital Q83.8
  palmar fascia M72.0
  pleura - *see* Pleurisy
  ring, uterus (Bandl's) (pathological) O62.4
  sternum (congenital) Q76.7
    acquired M95.4

Retraction - *continued*
  uterus - *see* Retroversion, uterus
  valve (heart) - *see* Endocarditis
Retrobulbar - *see* condition
Retrocecal - *see* condition
Retrocession - *see* Retroversion
Retrodisplacement - *see* Retroversion
Retroflection, retroflexion - *see* Retroversion
Retrognathia, retrognathism (mandibular)
  (maxillary) M26.19
Retrograde menstruation N92.5
Retroperineal - *see* condition
Retroperitoneal - *see* condition
Retroperitonitis K68.9
Retropharyngeal - *see* condition
Retroplacental - *see* condition
Retroposition - *see* Retroversion
Retroprosthetic membrane T85.398
Retrosternal thyroid (congenital) Q89.2
Retroversion, retroverted
  cervix - *see* Retroversion, uterus
  female NEC - *see* Retroversion, uterus
  iris H21.89
  testis (congenital) Q55.29
  uterus (acquired) (acute) (any degree)
    (asymptomatic) (cervix) (postinfectional)
    (postpartal, old) N85.4
    congenital Q51.818
    in pregnancy O34.53-
Retrovirus, as cause of disease classified
  elsewhere B97.30
  human
    immunodeficiency, type 2 (HIV 2) B97.35
    T-cell lymphotropic
      type I (HTLV-i) B97.33
      type II (HTLV-II) B97.34
  lentivirus B97.31
  oncovirus B97.32
  specified NEC B97.39
Retrusion, premaxilla (developmental)
  M26.09
Rett's disease or syndrome F84.2
Reverse peristalsis R19.2
Reye's syndrome G93.7
Rh (factor)
  hemolytic disease (newborn) P55.0
  incompatibility, immunization or sensitization
    affecting management of pregnancy NEC
    O36.09-
      anti-d antibody O36.01-
    newborn P55.0
    transfusion reaction - *see* Complication(s),
      transfusion, incompatibility reaction, Rh
      (factor)
  negative mother affecting newborn P55.0
  titer elevated - *see* Complication(s),
    transfusion, incompatibility reaction, Rh
    (factor)
  transfusion reaction - *see* Complication(s),
    transfusion, incompatibility reaction, Rh
    (factor)
Rhabdomyolysis (idiopathic) NEC M62.82
  traumatic T79.6
Rhabdomyoma - *see also* Neoplasm,
  connective tissue, benign
  adult - *see* Neoplasm, connective tissue,
    benign
  fetal - *see* Neoplasm, connective tissue, benign
  glycogenic - *see* Neoplasm, connective tissue,
    benign
Rhabdomyosarcoma (any type) - *see*
  Neoplasm, connective tissue, malignant
Rhabdosarcoma - *see* Rhabdomyosarcoma

Rhesus (factor) incompatibility - *see* Rh,
incompatibility
Rheumatic (acute) (subacute) (chronic)
adherent pericardium I09.2
coronary arteritis I01.9
degeneration, myocardium I09.0
fever (acute) - *see* Fever, rheumatic
heart - *see* Disease, heart, rheumatic
myocardial degeneration - *see* Degeneration,
myocardium
myocarditis (chronic) (inactive) (with chorea)
I09.0
active or acute I01.2
with chorea (acute) (rheumatic)
(Sydenham's) I02.0
pancarditis, acute I01.8
with chorea (acute) (rheumatic) Sydenham's)
I02.0
pericarditis (active) (acute) (with effusion)
(with pneumonia) I01.0
with chorea (acute) (rheumatic)
(Sydenham's) I02.0
chronic or inactive I09.2
pneumonia I00 [*J17*]
torticollis M43.6
typhoid fever A01.09
Rheumatism (articular) (neuralgic)
(nonarticular) M79.0
gout - *see* Arthritis, rheumatoid
intercostal, meaning Tietze's disease M94.0
palindromic (any site) M12.30
ankle M12.37-
elbow M12.32-
foot joint M12.37-
hand joint M12.34-
hip M12.35-
knee M12.36-
multiple site M12.39
shoulder M12.31-
specified joint NEC M12.38
vertebrae M12.38
wrist M12.33-
sciatic M54.4-
Rheumatoid - *see also* condition
arthritis - *see also* Arthritis, rheumatoid
with involvement of organs NEC M05.60
ankle M05.67-
elbow M05.62-
foot joint M05.67-
hand joint M05.64-
hip M05.65-
knee M05.66-
multiple site M05.69
shoulder M05.61-
vertebra - *see* Spondylitis, ankylosing
wrist M05.63-
seronegative - *see* Arthritis, rheumatoid,
seronegative
seropositive - *see* Arthritis, rheumatoid,
seropositive
carditis M05.30
ankle M05.37-
elbow M05.32-
foot joint M05.37-
hand joint M05.34-
hip M05.35-
knee M05.36-
multiple site M05.39
shoulder M05.31-
vertebra - *see* Spondylitis, ankylosing
wrist M05.33-
endocarditis - *see* Rheumatoid, carditis
lung (disease) M05.10
ankle M05.17-

Rheumatoid - *continued*
elbow M05.12-
foot joint M05.17-
hand joint M05.14-
hip M05.15-
knee M05.16-
multiple site M05.19
shoulder M05.11-
vertebra - *see* Spondylitis, ankylosing
wrist M05.13-
myocarditis - *see* Rheumatoid, carditis
myopathy M05.40
ankle M05.47-
elbow M05.42-
foot joint M05.47-
hand joint M05.44-
hip M05.45-
knee M05.46-
multiple site M05.49
shoulder M05.41-
vertebra - *see* Spondylitis, ankylosing
wrist M05.43-
pericarditis - *see* Rheumatoid, carditis
polyarthritis - *see* Arthritis, rheumatoid
polyneuropathy M05.50
ankle M05.57-
elbow M05.52-
foot joint M05.57-
hand joint M05.54-
hip M05.55-
knee M05.56-
multiple site M05.59
shoulder M05.51-
vertebra - *see* Spondylitis, ankylosing
wrist M05.53-
vasculitis M05.20
ankle M05.27-
elbow M05.22-
foot joint M05.27-
hand joint M05.24-
hip M05.25-
knee M05.26-
multiple site M05.29
shoulder M05.21-
vertebra - *see* Spondylitis, ankylosing
wrist M05.23-
Rhinitis (atrophic) (catarrhal) (chronic)
(croupous) (fibrinous) (granulomatous)
(hyperplastic) (hypertrophic)
(membranous) (obstructive) (purulent)
(suppurative) (ulcerative) J31.0
with
sore throat - *see* Nasopharyngitis
acute J00
allergic J30.9
with asthma J45.909
with
exacerbation (acute) J45.901
status asthmaticus J45.902
due to
food J30.5
pollen J30.1
nonseasonal J30.89
perennial J30.89
seasonal NEC J30.2
specified NEC J30.89
infective J00
pneumococcal J00
syphilitic A52.73
congenital A50.05 [*J99*]
tuberculous A15.8
vasomotor J30.0
Rhinoantritis (chronic) - *see* Sinusitis,
maxillary

Rhinodacryolith - *see* Dacryolith
Rhinolith (nasal sinus) J34.89
Rhinomegaly J34.89
Rhinopharyngitis (acute) (subacute) - *see also*
Nasopharyngitis
chronic J31.1
destructive ulcerating A66.5
mutilans A66.5
Rhinophyma L71.1
Rhinorrhea J34.89
cerebrospinal (fluid) G96.0
paroxysmal - *see* Rhinitis, allergic
spasmodic - *see* Rhinitis, allergic
Rhinosalpingitis - *see* Salpingitis, eustachian
Rhinoscleroma A48.8
Rhinosporidiosis B48.1
Rhinovirus infection NEC B34.8
Rhizomelic chondrodysplasia punctata
E71.540
Rhythm
atrioventricular nodal I49.8
disorder I49.9
coronary sinus I49.8
ectopic I49.8
nodal I49.8
escape I49.9
heart, abnormal I49.9
idioventricular I44.2
nodal I49.8
sleep, inversion G47.2-
nonorganic origin - *see* Disorder, sleep,
circadian rhythm, psychogenic
Rhytidosis facialis L98.8
Rib - *see also* condition
cervical Q76.5
Riboflavin deficiency E53.0
Rice bodies - *see also* Loose, body, joint
knee M23.4-
Richter syndrome - *see* Leukemia, chronic
lymphocytic, B-cell type
Richter's hernia - *see* Hernia, abdomen, with
obstruction
Ricinism - *see* Poisoning, food, noxious, plant
Rickets (active) (acute) (adolescent) (chest
wall) (congenital) (current) (infantile)
(intestinal) E55.0
adult - *see* Osteomalacia
celiac K90.0
hypophosphatemic with nephrotic-glycosuric
dwarfism E72.09
inactive E64.3
kidney N25.0
renal N25.0
sequelae, any E64.3
vitamin-d-resistant E83.31 [*M90.80*]
Rickettsial disease A79.9
specified type NEC A79.89
Rickettsialpox (Rickettsia akari) A79.1
Rickettsiosis A79.9
due to
Ehrlichia sennetsu A79.81
Rickettsia akari (rickettsialpox) A79.1
specified type NEC A79.89
tick-borne A77.9
vesicular A79.1
Rider's bone - *see* Ossification, muscle,
specified NEC
Ridge, alveolus - *see also* condition
flabby K06.8
Ridged ear, congenital Q17.3
Riedel's
lobe, liver Q44.7
struma, thyroiditis or disease E06.5
Rieger's anomaly or syndrome Q13.81

Riehl's melanosis L81.4
Rietti-Grippe-Micheli anemia D56.9
Rieux's hernia - *see* Hernia, abdomen,
  specified site NEC
Riga (-feed) disease K14.0
Riggs' disease - *see* Periodontitis
Right aortic arch Q25.47
Right middle lobe syndrome J98.11
Rigid, rigidity - *see also* condition
  abdominal R19.30
    with severe abdominal pain R10.0
    epigastric R19.36
    generalized R19.37
    left lower quadrant R19.34
    left upper quadrant R19.32
    periumbilic R19.35
    right lower quadrant R19.33
    right upper quadrant R19.31
  articular, multiple, congenital Q68.8
  cervix (uteri) in pregnancy - *see* Pregnancy,
    complicated by, abnormal, cervix
  hymen (acquired) (congenital) N89.6
  nuchal R29.1
  pelvic floor in pregnancy - *see* Pregnancy,
    complicated by, abnormal, pelvic organs or
    tissues NEC
  perineum or vulva in pregnancy - *see*
    Pregnancy, complicated by, abnormal, vulva
  spine - *see* Dorsopathy, specified NEC
  vagina in pregnancy - *see* Pregnancy,
    complicated by, abnormal, vagina
Rigors R68.89
  with fever R50.9
Riley-day syndrome G90.1
RIND (reversible ischemic neurologic deficit)
  I63.9
Ring(s)
  aorta (vascular) Q25.45
  Bandl's O62.4
  contraction, complicating delivery O62.4
  esophageal, lower (muscular) K22.2
  Fleischer's (cornea) H18.04-
  hymenal, tight (acquired) (congenital) N89.6
  Kayser-Fleischer (cornea) H18.04-
  retraction, uterus, pathological O62.4
  Schatzki's (esophagus) (lower) K22.2
    congenital Q39.3
  Soemmerring's - *see* Cataract, secondary
  vascular (congenital) Q25.8
    aorta Q25.45
Ringed hair (congenital) Q84.1
Ringworm B35.9
  beard B35.0
  black dot B35.0
  body B35.4
  Burmese B35.5
  corporeal B35.4
  foot B35.3
  groin B35.6
  hand B35.2
  honeycomb B35.0
  nails B35.1
  perianal (area) B35.6
  scalp B35.0
  specified NEC B35.8
  Tokelau B35.5
Rise, venous pressure I87.8
Rising, PSA following treatment for
  malignant neoplasm of prostate R97.21
Risk
  for
    dental caries Z91.849
      high Z91.843
      low Z91.841

Risk - *continued*
    moderate Z91.842
  suicidal
    meaning personal history of attempted
      suicide Z91.5
    meaning suicidal ideation   *see* Ideation,
      suicidal
Ritter's disease L00
Rivalry, sibling Z62.891
Rivalta's disease A42.2
River blindness B73.01
Robert's pelvis Q74.2
  with disproportion (fetopelvic) O33.0
    causing obstructed labor O65.0
Robin (-pierre) syndrome Q87.0
Robinow-Silvermann-smith syndrome Q87.1
Robinson's (hidrotic) ectodermal dysplasia or
  syndrome Q82.4
Robles' disease B73.01
Rocky Mountain (spotted) fever A77.0
Roetheln - *see* Rubella
Roger's disease Q21.0
Rokitansky-Aschoff sinuses (gallbladder)
  K82.8
Rolando's fracture (displaced) S62.22-
  nondisplaced S62.22-
Romano-Ward (prolonged QT interval)
  syndrome I45.81
Romberg's disease or syndrome G51.8
Roof, mouth - *see* condition **Rosacea** L71.9
  acne L71.9
  keratitis L71.8
  specified NEC L71.8
Rosary, rachitic E55.0
Rose
  cold J30.1
  fever J30.1
  rash R21
    epidemic B06.9
Rosenbach's erysipeloid A26.0
Rosenthal's disease or syndrome D68.1
Roseola B09
  infantum B08.20
    due to human herpesvirus 6 B08.21
    due to human herpesvirus 7 B08.22
Rossbach's disease K31.89
  psychogenic F45.8
Ross River disease or fever B33.1
Rostan's asthma (cardiac) - *see* Failure,
  ventricular, left
Rotation
  anomalous, incomplete or insufficient,
    intestine Q43.3
  cecum (congenital) Q43.3
  colon (congenital) Q43.3
  spine, incomplete or insufficient - *see*
    Dorsopathy, deforming, specified NEC
  tooth, teeth, fully erupted M26.35
  vertebra, incomplete or insufficient - *see*
    Dorsopathy, deforming, specified NEC
Rotes Quérol disease or syndrome - *see*
  Hyperostosis, ankylosing
Roth (-Bernhardt) disease or syndrome - *see*
  Meralgia paraesthetica
Rothmund (-Thomson) syndrome Q82.8
Rotor's disease or syndrome E80.6
Round
  back (with wedging of vertebrae) - *see*
    Kyphosis
    sequelae (late effect) of rickets E64.3
  worms (large) (infestation) NEC B82.0
    Ascariasis - *see also* Ascariasis B77.9
Roussy-Llévy syndrome G60.0

Rubella (German measles) B06.9
  complication NEC B06.09
    neurological B06.00
  congenital P35.0
  contact Z20.4
  exposure to Z20.4
  maternal
    manifest rubella in infant P35.0
    care for (suspected) damage to fetus O35.3
    suspected damage to fetus affecting
      management of pregnancy O35.3
  specified complications NEC B06.89
Rubeola (meaning measles) - *see* Measles
  meaning rubella - *see* Rubella
Rubeosis, iris - *see* Disorder, iris, vascular
Rubinstein-Taybi syndrome Q87.2
Rudimentary (congenital) - *see also* Agenesis
  arm - *see* Defect, reduction, upper limb
  bone Q79.9
  cervix uteri Q51.828
  eye Q11.2
  lobule of ear Q17.3
  patella Q74.1
  respiratory organs in thoracopagus Q89.4
  tracheal bronchus Q32.4
  uterus Q51.818
    in male Q56.1
  vagina Q52.0
Ruled out condition - *see* Observation,
  suspected
Rumination R11.10
  with nausea R11.2
  disorder of infancy F98.21
  neurotic F42.8
  newborn P92.1
  obsessional F42.8
  psychogenic F42.8
Runeberg's disease D51.0
Runny nose R09.89
Rupia (syphilitic) A51.39
  congenital A50.06
  tertiary A52.79
Rupture, ruptured
  abscess (spontaneous)
    code for site under Abscess
  aneurysm - *see* Aneurysm
  anus (sphincter) - *see* Laceration, anus
  aorta, aortic I71.8
    abdominal I71.3
    arch I71.1
    ascending I71.1
    descending I71.8
      abdominal I71.3
      thoracic I71.1
    syphilitic A52.01
    thoracoabdominal I71.5
    thorax, thoracic I71.1
    transverse I71.1
    traumatic - *see* Injury, aorta, laceration,
      major
    valve or cusp - *see also* Endocarditis, aortic
      I35.8
  appendix (with peritonitis) K35.2
    with localized peritonitis K35.3
  arteriovenous fistula, brain I60.8
  artery I77.2
    brain - *see* Hemorrhage, intracranial,
    intracerebral
    coronary - *see* Infarct, myocardium
    heart - *see* Infarct, myocardium
    pulmonary I28.8
    traumatic (complication) - *see* Injury, blood
      vessel
  bile duct (common) (hepatic) K83.2

Rupture, ruptured - *continued*
  cystic K82.2
  bladder (sphincter) (nontraumatic)
  (spontaneous) N32.89
    following ectopic or molar pregnancy O08.6
    obstetrical trauma O71.5
    traumatic S37.29
  blood vessel - *see also* Hemorrhage
    brain - *see* Hemorrhage, intracranial,
      intracerebral
    heart - *see* Infarct, myocardium
    traumatic (complication) - *see* Injury, blood
      vessel, laceration, major, by site
  bone - *see* Fracture
  bowel (nontraumatic) K63.1
  brain
    aneurysm (congenital) - *see also*
      Hemorrhage, intracranial, subarachnoid
        syphilitic A52.05
    hemorrhagic - *see* Hemorrhage, intracranial,
    intracerebral
  capillaries I78.8
  cardiac (auricle) (ventricle) (wall) I23.3
    with hemopericardium I23.0
    infectional I40.9
    traumatic - *see* Injury, heart
  cartilage (articular) (current) - *see also* Sprain
    knee S83.3-
    semilunar - *see* Tear, meniscus
  cecum (with peritonitis) K65.0
    with peritoneal abscess K35.3
    traumatic S36.598
  celiac artery, traumatic - *see* Injury, blood
    vessel, celiac artery, laceration, major
  cerebral aneurysm (congenital) (see
    Hemorrhage, intracranial, subarachnoid)
  cervix (uteri)
    with ectopic or molar pregnancy O08.6
    following ectopic or molar pregnancy O08.6
    obstetrical trauma O71.3
    traumatic S37.69
  chordae tendineae NEC I51.1
    concurrent with acute myocardial infarction -
      see Infarct, myocardium
    following acute myocardial infarction
      (current complication) I23.4
  choroid (direct) (indirect) (traumatic) H31.32-
  circle of Willis I60.6
  colon (nontraumatic) K63.1
    traumatic - *see* Injury, intestine, large
  cornea (traumatic) - *see* Injury, eye, laceration
  coronary (artery) (thrombotic) - *see* Infarct,
    myocardium
  corpus luteum (infected) (ovary) N83.1-
  cyst - *see* Cyst
  cystic duct K82.2
  Descemet's membrane - *see* Change, corneal
  membrane, Descemet's, rupture
    traumatic - *see* Injury, eye, laceration
  diaphragm, traumatic - *see* Injury,
  intrathoracic, diaphragm
  disc - *see* Rupture, intervertebral disc
  diverticulum (intestine) K57.80
    with bleeding K57.81
    bladder N32.3
  large intestine K57.20
    with
      bleeding K57.21
      small intestine K57.40
        with bleeding K57.41
  small intestine K57.00
    with
      bleeding K57.01
      large intestine K57.40

Rupture, ruptured - *continued*
    with bleeding K57.41
  duodenal stump K31.89
  ear drum (nontraumatic) - *see also* Perforation,
  tympanum
    traumatic S09.2-
      due to blast injury - *see* Injury, blast, ear
  esophagus K22.3
  eye (without prolapse or loss of intraocular
    tissue) - *see* Injury, eye, laceration
  fallopian tube NEC (nonobstetric)
  (nontraumatic) N83.8
    due to pregnancy O00.10-
      with intrauterine pregnancy O00.11-
  fontanel P13.1
  gallbladder K82.2
    traumatic S36.128
  gastric - *see also* Rupture, stomach
    vessel K92.2
  globe (eye) (traumatic) - *see* Injury, eye,
    laceration
  graafian follicle (hematoma) N83.0-
  heart - *see* Rupture, cardiac
  hymen (nontraumatic) (nonintentional) N89.8
  internal organ, traumatic - *see* Injury, by site
  intervertebral disc - *see* Displacement,
  intervertebral disc
    traumatic - *see* Rupture, traumatic,
    intervertebral disc
  intestine NEC (nontraumatic) K63.1
    traumatic - *see* Injury, intestine
  iris - *see also* Abnormality, pupillary
    traumatic - *see* Injury, eye, laceration
  joint capsule, traumatic - *see* Sprain
  kidney (traumatic) S37.06-
    birth injury P15.8
    nontraumatic N28.89
  lacrimal duct (traumatic) - *see* Injury, eye,
    specified site NEC
  lens (cataract) (traumatic) - *see* Cataract,
    traumatic
  ligament, traumatic - *see* Rupture, traumatic,
    ligament, by site
  liver S36.116
    birth injury P15.0
  lymphatic vessel I89.8
  marginal sinus (placental) (with hemorrhage) -
    see Hemorrhage, antepartum, specified cause
    NEC
  membrana tympani (nontraumatic) - *see*
  Perforation, tympanum
  membranes (spontaneous)
    artificial
      delayed delivery following O75.5
    delayed delivery following - *see* Pregnancy,
  complicated by, premature rupture of
  membranes
  meningeal artery I60.8
  meniscus (knee) - *see also* Tear, meniscus
    old - *see* Derangement, meniscus
    site other than knee   code as Sprain
  mesenteric artery, traumatic - *see* Injury,
    mesenteric, artery, laceration, major
  mesentery (nontraumatic) K66.8
    traumatic - *see* Injury, intra-abdominal,
    specified, site NEC
  mitral (valve) I34.8
  muscle (traumatic) - *see also* Strain
    diastasis - *see* Diastasis, muscle
    nontraumatic M62.10
      ankle M62.17-
      foot M62.17-
      forearm M62.13-
      hand M62.14-

Rupture, ruptured - *continued*
    lower leg M62.16-
    pelvic region M62.15-
    shoulder region M62.11-
    specified site NEC M62.18
    thigh M62.15-
    upper arm M62.12-
    traumatic - *see* Strain, by site
  musculotendinous junction NEC, nontraumatic
    - *see* Rupture, tendon, spontaneous
  mycotic aneurysm causing cerebral
    hemorrhage - *see* Hemorrhage, intracranial,
    subarachnoid
  myocardium, myocardial - *see* Rupture,
    cardiac
    traumatic - *see* Injury, heart
  nontraumatic, meaning hernia - *see* Hernia
  obstructed - *see* Hernia, by site, obstructed
  operation wound - *see* Disruption, wound,
    operation
  ovary, ovarian N83.8
    corpus luteum cyst N83.1-
    follicle (graafian) N83.0-
  oviduct (nonobstetric) (nontraumatic) N83.8
    due to pregnancy O00.10-
      with intrauterine pregnancy O00.11-
  pancreas (nontraumatic) K86.89
    traumatic S36.299
  papillary muscle NEC I51.2
    following acute myocardial infarction
    (current complication) I23.5
  pelvic
    floor, complicating delivery O70.1
    organ NEC, obstetrical trauma O71.5
  perineum (nonobstetric) (nontraumatic)
  N90.89
    complicating delivery - *see* Delivery,
    complicated, by, laceration, anus (sphincter)
  postoperative wound - *see* Disruption, wound,
    operation
  prostate (traumatic) S37.828
  pulmonary
    artery I28.8
    valve (heart) I37.8
    vein I28.8
    vessel I28.8
  pus tube - *see* Salpingitis
  pyosalpinx - *see* Salpingitis
  rectum (nontraumatic) K63.1
    traumatic S36.69
  retina, retinal (traumatic) (without detachment)
    - *see also* Break, retina
    with detachment - *see* Detachment, retina,
    with retinal, break
  rotator cuff (nontraumatic) M75.10-
    complete M75.12-
    incomplete M75.11-
  sclera - *see* Injury, eye, laceration
  sigmoid (nontraumatic) K63.1
    traumatic S36.593
  spinal cord - *see also* Injury, spinal cord, by
  region
    due to injury at birth P11.5
    newborn (birth injury) P11.5
  spleen (traumatic) S36.09
    birth injury P15.1
    congenital (birth injury) P15.1
    due to P. vivax malaria B51.0
    nontraumatic D73.5
    spontaneous D73.5
  splenic vein R58
    traumatic - *see* Injury, blood vessel, splenic
    vein
  stomach (nontraumatic) (spontaneous) K31.89

Rupture, ruptured - *continued*
  traumatic S36.39
  supraspinatus (complete) (incomplete)
    (nontraumatic) - *see* Tear, rotator cuff
  symphysis pubis
    obstetric O71.6
    traumatic S33.4
  synovium (cyst) M66.10
    ankle M66.17-
    elbow M66.12-
    finger M66.14-
    foot M66.17-
    forearm M66.13-
    hand M66.14-
    pelvic region M66.15-
    shoulder region M66.11-
    specified site NEC M66.18
    thigh M66.15-
    toe M66.17-
    upper arm M66.12-
    wrist M66.13-
  tendon (traumatic) - *see* Strain
    nontraumatic (spontaneous) M66.9
      ankle M66.87-
      extensor M66.20
        ankle M66.27-
        foot M66.27-
        forearm M66.23-
        hand M66.24-
        lower leg M66.26-
        multiple sites M66.29
        pelvic region M66.25-
        shoulder region M66.21-
        specified site NEC M66.28
        thigh M66.25-
        upper arm M66.22-
      flexor M66.30
        ankle M66.37-
        foot M66.37-
        forearm M66.33-
        hand M66.34-
        lower leg M66.36-
        multiple sites M66.39
        pelvic region M66.35-
        shoulder region M66.31-
        specified site NEC M66.38
        thigh M66.35-
        upper arm M66.32-
      foot M66.87-
      forearm M66.83-
      hand M66.84-
      lower leg M66.86-
      multiple sites M66.89
      pelvic region M66.85-
      shoulder region M66.81-
      specified
        site NEC M66.88
        tendon M66.80
      thigh M66.85-
      upper arm M66.82-
  thoracic duct I89.8
  tonsil J35.8
  traumatic
    aorta - *see* Injury, aorta, laceration, major
    diaphragm - *see* Injury, intrathoracic,
  diaphragm
    external site - *see* Wound, open, by site
    eye - *see* Injury, eye, laceration
    internal organ - *see* Injury, by site
    intervertebral disc
      cervical S13.0
      lumbar S33.0
      thoracic S23.0
    kidney S37.06-

Rupture, ruptured - *continued*
  ligament - *see also* Sprain
    ankle - *see* Sprain, ankle
    carpus - *see* Rupture, traumatic, ligament,
      wrist
    collateral (hand) - *see* Rupture, traumatic,
      ligament, finger, collateral
    finger (metacarpophalangeal)
      (interphalangeal) S63.40-
      collateral S63.41-
        index S63.41-
        little S63.41-
        middle S63.41-
        ring S63.41-
      index S63.40-
      little S63.40-
      middle S63.40-
      palmar S63.42-
        index S63.42-
        little S63.42-
        middle S63.42-
        ring S63.42-
      ring S63.40-
      specified site NEC S63.499
        index S63.49-
        little S63.49-
        middle S63.49-
        ring S63.49-
      volar plate S63.43-
        index S63.43-
        little S63.43-
        middle S63.43-
        ring S63.43-
    foot - *see* Sprain, foot
    radial collateral S53.2-
    radiocarpal - *see* Rupture, traumatic,
      ligament, wrist, radiocarpal
    ulnar collateral S53.3-
    ulnocarpal - *see* Rupture, traumatic,
      ligament, wrist, ulnocarpal
    wrist S63.30-
      collateral S63.31-
      radiocarpal S63.32-
      specified site NEC S63.39-
      ulnocarpal (palmar) S63.33-
  liver S36.116
  membrana tympani - *see* Rupture, ear drum,
    traumatic
  muscle or tendon - *see* Strain
  myocardium - *see* Injury, heart
  pancreas S36.299
  rectum S36.69
  sigmoid S36.593
  spleen S36.09
  stomach S36.39
  symphysis pubis S33.4
  tympanum, tympanic (membrane) - *see*
    Rupture, ear drum, traumatic
  ureter S37.19
  uterus S37.69
  vagina - *see* Injury, vagina
  vena cava - *see* Injury, vena cava, laceration,
  major
  tricuspid (heart) (valve) I07.8
  tube, tubal (nonobstetric) (nontraumatic)
  N83.8
    abscess - *see* Salpingitis
    due to pregnancy O00.10-
      with intrauterine pregnancy O00.11-
  tympanum, tympanic (membrane)
    (nontraumatic) - *see also* Perforation,
    tympanic membrane H72.9-
    traumatic - *see* Rupture, ear drum, traumatic
  umbilical cord, complicating delivery O69.89

Rupture, ruptured - *continued*
  ureter (traumatic) S37.19
    nontraumatic N28.89
  urethra (nontraumatic) N36.8
    with ectopic or molar pregnancy O08.6
    following ectopic or molar pregnancy O08.6
    obstetrical trauma O71.5
    traumatic S37.39
  uterosacral ligament (nonobstetric)
    (nontraumatic) N83.8
  uterus (traumatic) S37.69
    before labor O71.0-
    during or after labor O71.1
    nonpuerperal, nontraumatic N85.8
    pregnant (during labor) O71.1
      before labor O71.0-
  vagina - *see* Injury, vagina
  valve, valvular (heart) - *see* Endocarditis
  varicose vein - *see* Varix
  varix - *see* Varix
  vena cava R58
    traumatic - *see* Injury, vena cava, laceration,
    major
  vesical (urinary) N32.89
  vessel (blood) R58
    pulmonary I28.8
    traumatic - *see* Injury, blood vessel
  viscus R19.8
  vulva complicating delivery O70.0
Russell-silver syndrome Q87.1
Russian spring-summer type encephalitis
  A84.0
Rust's disease (tuberculous cervical
  spondylitis) A18.01
Ruvalcaba-Myhre-smith syndrome E71.440
Rytand-Lipsitch syndrome I44.2

S

Saber, sabre shin or tibia (syphilitic) A50.56
  [*M90.8*]
Sac lacrimal - *see* condition
Saccharomyces infection B37.9
Saccharopinuria E72.3
Saccular - *see* condition **Sacculation**
  aorta (nonsyphilitic) - *see* Aneurysm, aorta
  bladder N32.3
  intralaryngeal (congenital) (ventricular) Q31.3
  larynx (congenital) (ventricular) Q31.3
  organ or site, congenital - *see* Distortion
  pregnant uterus - *see* Pregnancy, complicated
    by, abnormal, uterus
  ureter N28.89
  urethra N36.1
  vesical N32.3
Sachs' amaurotic familial idiocy or disease
  E75.02
Sachs-Tay disease E75.02
Sacks-Libman disease M32.11
Sacralgia M53.3
Sacralization Q76.49
Sacrodynia M53.3
Sacroiliac joint - *see* condition
Sacroiliitis NEC M46.1
Sacrum - *see* condition
Saddle
  back - *see* Lordosis
  embolus
    abdominal aorta I74.01
    pulmonary artery I26.92
      with acute cor pulmonale I26.02
  injury code to condition
  nose M95.0
    due to syphilis A50.57

Sadism (sexual) F65.52
Sadness, postpartal O90.6
Sadomasochism F65.50
Saemisch's ulcer (cornea) - *see* Ulcer, cornea, central
Sagging
  skin and subcutaneous tissue (following bariatric surgery weight loss) (following dietary weight loss) L98.7
Sahib disease B55.0
Sailors' skin L57.8
Saint
  Anthony's fire - *see* Erysipelas
  triad - *see* Hernia, diaphragm
  Vitus' dance - *see* Chorea, Sydenham's
Salaam
  attack(s) - *see* Epilepsy, spasms
  tic R25.8
Salicylism
  abuse F55.8
  overdose or wrong substance given - *see* Table of Drugs and Chemicals, by drug, poisoning
Salivary duct or gland - *see* condition
Salivation, excessive K11.7
Salmonella - *see* Infection, Salmonella
Salmonellosis A02.0
Salpingitis (catarrhal) (fallopian tube) (nodular) (pseudofollicular) (purulent) (septic) N70.91
  with oophoritis N70.93
  acute N70.01
    with oophoritis N70.03
  chlamydial A56.11
  chronic N70.11
    with oophoritis N70.13
  complicating abortion - *see* Abortion, by type, complicated by, salpingitis
  ear - *see* Salpingitis, eustachian
  eustachian (tube) H68.00-
    acute H68.01-
    chronic H68.02-
  follicularis N70.11
    with oophoritis N70.13
  gonococcal (acute) (chronic) A54.24
  interstitial, chronic N70.11
    with oophoritis N70.13
  isthmica nodosa N70.11
    with oophoritis N70.13
  specific (gonococcal) (acute) (chronic) A54.24
  tuberculous (acute) (chronic) A18.17
  venereal (gonococcal) (acute) (chronic) A54.24
Salpingocele N83.4-
Salpingo-oophoritis (catarrhal) (purulent) (ruptured) (septic) (suppurative) N70.93
  acute N70.03
    with ectopic or molar pregnancy O08.0
    following ectopic or molar pregnancy O08.0
    gonococcal A54.24
  chronic N70.13
  following ectopic or molar pregnancy O08.0
  gonococcal (acute) (chronic) A54.24
  puerperal O86.19
  specific (gonococcal) (acute) (chronic) A54.24
  subacute N70.03
  tuberculous (acute) (chronic) A18.17
  venereal (gonococcal) (acute) (chronic) A54.24
Salpingo-ovaritis - *see* Salpingo-oophoritis
Salpingoperitonitis - *see* Salpingo-oophoritis
Salzmann's nodular dystrophy - *see* Degeneration, cornea, nodular
Sampson's cyst or tumor N80.1
San Joaquin (Valley) fever B38.0

Sandblaster's asthma, lung or pneumoconiosis J62.8
Sander's disease (paranoia) F22
Sandfly fever A93.1
Sandhoff's disease E75.01
Sanfilippo (Type B) (Type C) (Type D) syndrome E76.22
Sanger-brown ataxia G11.2
Sao Paulo fever or typhus A77.0
Saponification, mesenteric K65.8
Sarcocele (benign)
  syphilitic A52.76
    congenital A50.59
Sarcocystosis A07.8
Sarcoepiplocele - *see* Hernia
Sarcoepiplomphalocele Q79.2
Sarcoid - *see also* Sarcoidosis
  arthropathy D86.86
  Boeck's D86.9
  Darier-Roussy D86.3
  iridocyclitis D86.83
  meningitis D86.81
  myocarditis D86.85
  myositis D86.87
  pyelonephritis D86.84
  Spiegler-Fendt L08.89
Sarcoidosis D86.9
  with
    cranial nerve palsies D86.82
    hepatic granuloma D86.89
    polyarthritis D86.86
    tubulo-interstitial nephropathy D86.84
  combined sites NEC D86.89
  lung D86.0
    and lymph nodes D86.2
  lymph nodes D86.1
    and lung D86.2
  meninges D86.81
  skin D86.3
  specified type NEC D86.89
Sarcoma (of) - *see also* Neoplasm, connective tissue, malignant
  alveolar soft part - *see* Neoplasm, connective tissue, malignant
  ameloblastic C41.1
    upper jaw (bone) C41.0
  botryoid - *see* Neoplasm, connective tissue, malignant
  botryoides - *see* Neoplasm, connective tissue, malignant
  cerebellar C71.6
    circumscribed (arachnoidal) C71.6
  circumscribed (arachnoidal) cerebellar C71.6
  clear cell - *see also* Neoplasm, connective tissue, malignant
    kidney C64.-
  dendritic cells (accessory cells) C96.4
  embryonal - *see* Neoplasm, connective tissue, malignant
  endometrial (stromal) C54.1
    isthmus C54.0
  epithelioid (cell) - *see* Neoplasm, connective tissue, malignant
  Ewing's - *see* Neoplasm, bone, malignant
  follicular dendritic cell C96.4
  germinoblastic (diffuse) - *see* Lymphoma, diffuse large cell
  follicular - *see* Lymphoma, follicular, specified NEC
  giant cell (except of bone) - *see also* Neoplasm, connective tissue, malignant
    bone - *see* Neoplasm, bone, malignant
  glomoid - *see* Neoplasm, connective tissue, malignant

Sarcoma (of) - *continued*
  granulocytic C92.3-
  hemangioendothelial - *see* Neoplasm, connective tissue, malignant
  hemorrhagic, multiple - *see* Sarcoma, Kaposi's
  histiocytic C96.A
  Hodgkin - *see* Lymphoma, Hodgkin
  immunoblastic (diffuse) - *see* Lymphoma, diffuse large cell
  interdigitating dendritic cell C96.4
  Kaposi's
    colon C46.4
    connective tissue C46.1
    gastrointestinal organ C46.4
    lung C46.5-
    lymph node(s) C46.3
    palate (hard) (soft) C46.2
    rectum C46.4
    skin C46.0
    specified site NEC C46.7
    stomach C46.4
    unspecified site C46.9
  Kupffer cell C22.3
  Langerhans cell C96.4
  leptomeningeal - *see* Neoplasm, meninges, malignant
  liver NEC C22.4
  lymphangioendothelial - *see* Neoplasm, connective tissue, malignant
  lymphoblastic - *see* Lymphoma, lymphoblastic (diffuse)
  lymphocytic - *see* Lymphoma, small cell B-cell
  mast cell C96.22
  melanotic - *see* Melanoma
  meningeal - *see* Neoplasm, meninges, malignant
  meningothelial - *see* Neoplasm, meninges, malignant
  mesenchymal - *see also* Neoplasm, connective tissue, malignant
    mixed - *see* Neoplasm, connective tissue, malignant
  mesothelial - *see* Mesothelioma
  monstrocellular
    specified site - *see* Neoplasm, malignant, by site
    unspecified site C71.9
  myeloid C92.3-
  neurogenic - *see* Neoplasm, nerve, malignant
  odontogenic C41.1
    upper jaw (bone) C41.0
  osteoblastic - *see* Neoplasm, bone, malignant
  osteogenic - *see also* Neoplasm, bone, malignant
    juxtacortical - *see* Neoplasm, bone, malignant
    periosteal - *see* Neoplasm, bone, malignant
  periosteal - *see also* Neoplasm, bone, malignant
    osteogenic - *see* Neoplasm, bone, malignant
  pleomorphic cell - *see* Neoplasm, connective tissue, malignant
  reticulum cell (diffuse) - *see* Lymphoma, diffuse large cell
    nodular - *see* Lymphoma, follicular
    pleomorphic cell type - *see* Lymphoma, diffuse large cell
  rhabdoid - *see* Neoplasm, malignant, by site
  round cell - *see* Neoplasm, connective tissue, malignant
  small cell - *see* Neoplasm, connective tissue, malignant
  soft tissue - *see* Neoplasm, connective tissue,

Sarcoma (of) - *continued*
  malignant
   spindle cell - *see* Neoplasm, connective tissue, malignant
   stromal (endometrial) C54.1
    isthmus C54.0
   synovial - *see also* Neoplasm, connective tissue, malignant
    biphasic - *see* Neoplasm, connective tissue, malignant
    epithelioid cell - *see* Neoplasm, connective tissue, malignant
    spindle cell - *see* Neoplasm, connective tissue, malignant **Sarcomatosis**
   meningeal - *see* Neoplasm, meninges, malignant
   specified site NEC - *see* Neoplasm, connective tissue, malignant
   unspecified site C80.1
Sarcopenia (age-related) M62.84
Sarcosinemia E72.59
Sarcosporidiosis (intestinal) A07.8
Satiety, early R68.81
Saturnine - *see* condition
Saturnism
  overdose or wrong substance given or taken - *see* Table of Drugs and Chemicals, by drug, poisoning
Satyriasis F52.8
Sauriasis - *see* Ichthyosis
SBE (subacute bacterial endocarditis) I33.0
Scabs R23.4
Scabies (any site) B86
Scaglietti-Dagnini syndrome E22.0
Scald - *see* Burn
Scalenus anticus (anterior) syndrome G54.0
Scales R23.4
Scaling, skin R23.4
Scalp - *see* condition
Scapegoating affecting child Z62.3
Scaphocephaly Q75.0
Scapulalgia M89.8X1
Scapulohumeral myopathy G71.0
Scar, scarring - *see also* Cicatrix L90.5
  adherent L90.5
  atrophic L90.5
  cervix
   in pregnancy or childbirth - *see* Pregnancy, complicated by, abnormal cervix
  cheloid L91.0
  chorioretinal H31.00-
   posterior pole macula H31.01-
   postsurgical H59.81-
   solar retinopathy H31.02-
   specified type NEC H31.09-
  choroid - *see* Scar, chorioretinal
  conjunctiva H11.24-
  cornea H17.9
   xerophthalmic - *see also* Opacity, cornea
    vitamin A deficiency E50.6
  duodenum, obstructive K31.5
  hypertrophic L91.0
  keloid L91.0
  labia N90.89
  lung (base) J98.4
  macula - *see* Scar, chorioretinal, posterior pole
  muscle M62.89
  myocardium, myocardial I25.2
  painful L90.5
  posterior pole (eye) - *see* Scar, chorioretinal, posterior pole
  retina - *see* Scar, chorioretinal
  trachea J39.8
  transmural uterine, in pregnancy O34.29

Scar, scarring - *continued*
  uterus N85.8
   in pregnancy O34.29
  vagina N89.8
   postoperative N99.2
  vulva N90.89
Scarabiasis B88.2
Scarlatina (anginosa) (maligna) A38.9
  myocarditis (acute) A38.1
   old - *see* Myocarditis
  otitis media A38.0
  ulcerosa A38.8
Scarlet fever (albuminuria) (angina) A38.9
Schamberg's disease (progressive pigmentary dermatosis) L81.7
Schatzki's ring (acquired) (esophagus) (lower) K22.2
  congenital Q39.3
Schaufenster krankheit I20.8
Schaumann's
  benign lymphogranulomatosis D86.1
  disease or syndrome - *see* Sarcoidosis
Scheie's syndrome E76.03
Schenck's disease B42.1
Scheuermann's disease or osteochondrosis - *see* Osteochondrosis, juvenile, spine
Schilder (-Flatau) disease G37.0
Schilling-type monocytic leukemia C93.0-
Schimmelbusch's disease, cystic mastitis, or hyperplasia - *see* Mastopathy, cystic
Schistosoma infestation - *see* Infestation, Schistosoma
Schistosomiasis B65.9
  with muscle disorder B65.9 [*M63.80*]
   ankle B65.9 [*M63.87*]
   foot B65.9 [*M63.87*]
   forearm B65.9 [*M63.83*]
   hand B65.9 [*M63.84*]
   lower leg B65.9 [*M63.86*]
   multiple sites B65.9 [*M63.89*]
   pelvic region B65.9 [*M63.85*]
   shoulder region B65.9 [*M63.81*]
   specified site NEC B65.9 [*M63.88*]
   thigh B65.9 [*M63.85*]
   upper arm B65.9 [*M63.82*]
  Asiatic B65.2
  bladder B65.0
  chestermani B65.8
  colon B65.1
  cutaneous B65.3
  due to
   S. haematobium B65.0
   S. japonicum B65.2
   S. mansoni B65.1
   S. mattheii B65.8
  Eastern B65.2
  genitourinary tract B65.0
  intestinal B65.1
  lung NEC B65.9 [*J99*]
   pneumonia B65.9 [*J17*]
  Manson's (intestinal) B65.1
  oriental B65.2
  pulmonary NEC B65.9 [*J99*]
   pneumonia B65.9
  Schistosoma
   haematobium B65.0
   japonicum B65.2
   mansoni B65.1
  specified type NEC B65.8
  urinary B65.0
  vesical B65.0
Schizencephaly Q04.6
Schizoaffective psychosis F25.9
Schizodontia K00.2

Schizoid personality F60.1
Schizophrenia, schizophrenic F20.9
  acute (brief) (undifferentiated) F23
  atypical (form) F20.3
  borderline F21
  catalepsy F20.2
  catatonic (type) (excited) (withdrawn) F20.2
  cenesthopathic, cenesthesiopathic F20.89
  childhood type F84.5
  chronic undifferentiated F20.5
  cyclic F25.0
  disorganized (type) F20.1
  flexibilitas cerea F20.2
  hebephrenic (type) F20.1
  incipient F21
  latent F21
  negative type F20.5
  paranoid (type) F20.0
  paraphrenic F20.0
  post-psychotic depression F32.89
  prepsychotic F21
  prodromal F21
  pseudoneurotic F21
  pseudopsychopathic F21
  reaction F23
  residual (state) (type) F20.5
  restzustand F20.5
  schizoaffective (type) - *see* Psychosis, schizoaffective
  simple (type) F20.89
  simplex F20.89
  specified type NEC F20.89
  spectrum and other psychotic disorder F29
   specified NEC F28
  stupor F20.2
  syndrome of childhood F84.5
  undifferentiated (type) F20.3
   chronic F20.5
Schizothymia (persistent) F60.1
Schlatter-Osgood disease or osteochondrosis - *see* Osteochondrosis, juvenile, tibia
Schlatter's tibia - *see* Osteochondrosis, juvenile, tibia
Schmidt's syndrome (polyglandular, autoimmune) E31.0
Schmincke's carcinoma or tumor - *see* Neoplasm, nasopharynx, malignant
Schmitz (-Stutzer) dysentery A03.0
Schmorl's disease or nodes   lumbar region M51.46
  lumbosacral region M51.47
  sacrococcygeal region M53.3
  thoracic region M51.44
  thoracolumbar region M51.45
Schneiderian
  papilloma - *see* Neoplasm, nasopharynx, benign
   specified site - *see* Neoplasm, benign, by site
   unspecified site D14.0
  specified site - *see* Neoplasm, malignant, by site
  unspecified site C30.0
Scholte's syndrome (malignant carcinoid) E34.0
Scholz (-Bielchowsky-Henneberg) disease or syndrome E75.25
Schönlein (-Henoch) disease or purpura (primary) (rheumatic) D69.0
Schottmuller's disease A01.4
Schroeder's syndrome (endocrine hypertensive) E27.0
Schüller-Christian disease or syndrome C96.5
Schultze's type acroparesthesia, simple I73.89

Schultz's disease or syndrome - *see*
Agranulocytosis
Schwalbe-Ziehen-Oppenheim disease G24.1
Schwannoma - *see also* Neoplasm, nerve,
benign
malignant - *see also* Neoplasm, nerve,
malignant
with rhabdomyoblastic differentiation - *see*
Neoplasm, nerve, malignant
melanocytic - *see* Neoplasm, nerve, benign
pigmented - *see* Neoplasm, nerve, benign
Schwannomatosis Q85.03
Schwartz (-Jampel) syndrome G71.13
Schwartz-Bartter syndrome E22.2
Schweniger-Buzzi anetoderma L90.1
Sciatic - *see* condition
Sciatica (infective)
with lumbago M54.4-
due to intervertebral disc disorder - *see*
Disorder, disc, with, radiculopathy
due to displacement of intervertebral disc
(with lumbago) - *see* Disorder, disc, with,
radiculopathy
wallet M54.3-
Scimitar syndrome Q26.8
Sclera - *see* condition
Sclerectasia H15.84-
Scleredema
adultorum - *see* Sclerosis, systemic
Buschke's - *see* Sclerosis, systemic
newborn P83.0
Sclerema (adiposum) (edematosum)
(neonatorum) (newborn) P83.0
adultorum - *see* Sclerosis, systemic
Scleriasis - *see* Scleroderma
Scleritis H15.00-
with corneal involvement H15.04-
anterior H15.01-
brawny H15.02-
in (due to) zoster B02.34
posterior H15.03-
specified type NEC H15.09-
syphilitic A52.71
tuberculous (nodular) A18.51
Sclerochoroiditis H31.8
Scleroconjunctivitis - *see* Scleritis
Sclerocystic ovary syndrome E28.2
Sclerodactyly, sclerodactylia L94.3
Scleroderma, sclerodermia (acrosclerotic)
(diffuse) (generalized) (progressive)
(pulmonary) - *see also* Sclerosis, systemic
M34.9-
circumscribed L94.0
linear L94.1
localized L94.0
newborn P83.88
systemic M34.9
Sclerokeratitis H16.8
tuberculous A18.52
Scleroma nasi A48.8
Scleromalacia (perforans) H15.05-
Scleromyxedema L98.5
Sclérose en plaques G35
Sclerosis, sclerotic
adrenal (gland) E27.8
Alzheimer's - *see* Disease, Alzheimer's
amyotrophic (lateral) G12.21
aorta, aortic I70.0
valve - *see* Endocarditis, aortic
artery, arterial, arteriolar, arteriovascular - *see*
Arteriosclerosis
ascending multiple G35
brain (generalized) (lobular) G37.9
artery, arterial I67.2

Sclerosis, sclerotic - *continued*
diffuse G37.0
disseminated G35
insular G35
Krabbe's E75.23
miliary G35
multiple G35
presenile (Alzheimer's) - *see* Disease,
Alzheimer's, early onset
senile (arteriosclerotic) I67.2
stem, multiple G35
tuberous Q85.1
bulbar, multiple G35
bundle of His I44.39
cardiac - *see* Disease, heart, ischemic,
atherosclerotic
cardiorenal - *see* Hypertension, cardiorenal
cardiovascular - *see also* Disease,
cardiovascular
renal - *see* Hypertension, cardiorenal
cerebellar - *see* Sclerosis, brain
cerebral - *see* Sclerosis, brain
cerebrospinal (disseminated) (multiple) G35
cerebrovascular I67.2
choroid - *see* Degeneration, choroid
combined (spinal cord) - *see also*
Degeneration, combined
multiple G35
concentric (Balo) G37.5
cornea - *see* Opacity, cornea
coronary (artery) I25.10
with angina pectoris - *see* Arteriosclerosis,
coronary (artery),   corpus cavernosum
female N90.89
male N48.6
diffuse (brain) (spinal cord) G37.0
disseminated G35
dorsal G35
dorsolateral (spinal cord) - *see* Degeneration,
combined
endometrium N85.5
extrapyramidal G25.9
eye, nuclear (senile) - *see* Cataract, senile,
nuclear
focal and segmental (glomerular) - *see also*
N00-N07 with fourth character .1 N05.1
Friedreich's (spinal cord) G11.1
funicular (spermatic cord) N50.89
general (vascular) - *see* Arteriosclerosis
gland (lymphatic) I89.8
hepatic K74.1
alcoholic K70.2
hereditary
cerebellar G11.9
spinal (Friedreich's ataxia) G11.1
hippocampal G93.81
insular G35
kidney - *see* Sclerosis, renal
larynx J38.7
lateral (amyotrophic) (descending) (spinal)
G12.21
primary G12.23
lens, senile nuclear - *see* Cataract, senile,
nuclear
liver K74.1
with fibrosis K74.2
alcoholic K70.2
alcoholic K70.2
cardiac K76.1
lung - *see* Fibrosis, lung
mastoid - *see* Mastoiditis, chronic
mesial temporal G93.81
mitral I05.8
Mönckeberg's (medial) - *see* Arteriosclerosis,

Sclerosis, sclerotic - *continued*
extremities
multiple (brain stem) (cerebral) (generalized)
(spinal cord) G35
myocardium, myocardial - *see* Disease, heart,
ischemic, atherosclerotic
nuclear (senile), eye - *see* Cataract, senile,
nuclear
ovary N83.8
pancreas K86.89
penis N48.6
peripheral arteries - *see* Arteriosclerosis,
extremities
plaques G35
pluriglandular E31.8
polyglandular E31.8
posterolateral (spinal cord) - *see* Degeneration,
combined
presenile (Alzheimer's) - *see* Disease,
Alzheimer's, early onset
primary, lateral G12.23
progressive, systemic M34.0
pulmonary - *see* Fibrosis, lung
artery I27.0
valve (heart) - *see* Endocarditis, pulmonary
renal N26.9
with
cystine storage disease E72.09
hypertensive heart disease (conditions in
I11) - *see* Hypertension, cardiorenal
arteriolar (hyaline) (hyperplastic) - *see*
Hypertension, kidney
retina (senile) (vascular) H35.00
senile (vascular) - *see* Arteriosclerosis
spinal (cord) (progressive) G95.89
ascending G61.0
combined - *see also* Degeneration, combined
multiple G35
syphilitic A52.11
disseminated G35
dorsolateral - *see* Degeneration, combined
hereditary (Friedreich's) (mixed form) G11.1
lateral (amyotrophic) G12.23
multiple G35
posterior (syphilitic) A52.11
stomach K31.89
subendocardial, congenital I42.4
systemic M34.9
with
lung involvement M34.81
myopathy M34.82
polyneuropathy M34.83
drug-induced M34.2
due to chemicals NEC M34.2
progressive M34.0
specified NEC M34.89
temporal (mesial) G93.81
tricuspid (heart) (valve) I07.8
tuberous (brain) Q85.1
tympanic membrane - *see* Disorder, tympanic
membrane, specified NEC
valve, valvular (heart) - *see* Endocarditis
vascular - *see* Arteriosclerosis
vein I87.8
Scoliosis (acquired) (postural) M41.9
adolescent (idiopathic) - *see* Scoliosis,
idiopathic, adolescent
congenital Q67.5
due to bony malformation Q76.3
failure of segmentation (hemivertebra) Q76.3
hemivertebra fusion Q76.3
postural Q67.5
idiopathic M41.20
adolescent M41.129

Scoliosis - *continued*
   cervical region M41.122
   cervicothoracic region M41.123
   lumbar region M41.126
   lumbosacral region M41.127
   thoracic region M41.124
   thoracolumbar region M41.125
  cervical region M41.22
  cervicothoracic region M41.23
  infantile M41.00
   cervical region M41.02
   cervicothoracic region M41.03
   lumbar region M41.06
   lumbosacral region M41.07
   sacrococcygeal region M41.08
   thoracic region M41.04
   thoracolumbar region M41.05
  juvenile M41.119
   cervical region M41.112
   cervicothoracic region M41.113
   lumbar region M41.116
   lumbosacral region M41.117
   thoracic region M41.114
   thoracolumbar region M41.115
  lumbar region M41.26
  lumbosacral region M41.27
  thoracic region M41.24
  thoracolumbar region M41.25
 infantile - *see* Scoliosis, idiopathic, infantile
 neuromuscular M41.40
  cervical region M41.42
  cervicothoracic region M41.43
  lumbar region M41.46
  lumbosacral region M41.47
  occipito-atlanto-axial region M41.41
  thoracic region M41.44
  thoracolumbar region M41.45
 paralytic - *see* Scoliosis, neuromuscular
 postradiation therapy M96.5
 rachitic (late effect or sequelae) E64.3
  [*M49.80*]
  cervical region E64.3 [*M49.82*]
  cervicothoracic region E64.3 [*M49.83*]
  lumbar region E64.3 [*M49.86*]
  lumbosacral region E64.3 [*M49.87*]
  multiple sites E64.3 [*M49.89*]
  occipito-atlanto-axial region E64.3 [*M49.81*]
  sacrococcygeal region E64.3 [*M49.88*]
  thoracic region E64.3 [*M49.84*]
  thoracolumbar region E64.3 [*M49.85*]
 sciatic M54.4-
 secondary (to) NEC M41.50
  cerebral palsy, Friedreich's ataxia,
   poliomyelitis, neuromuscular disorders - *see*
   Scoliosis, neuromuscular
  cervical region M41.52
  cervicothoracic region M41.53
  lumbar region M41.56
  lumbosacral region M41.57
  thoracic region M41.54
  thoracolumbar region M41.55
 specified form NEC M41.80
  cervical region M41.82
  cervicothoracic region M41.83
  lumbar region M41.86
  lumbosacral region M41.87
  thoracic region M41.84
  thoracolumbar region M41.85
 thoracogenic M41.30
  thoracic region M41.34
  thoracolumbar region M41.35
 tuberculous A18.01
Scoliotic pelvis
 with disproportion (fetopelvic) O33.0
  causing obstructed labor O65.0

Scorbutus, scorbutic - *see also* Scurvy
 anemia D53.2
**Score, NIHSS (National Institutes of Health
 Stroke Scale)** R29.7-
Scotoma (arcuate) (Bjerrum) (central) (ring)
- *see also* Defect, visual field, localized,
scotoma
 scintillating H53.19
Scratch - *see* Abrasion
Scratchy throat R09.89
Screening (for) Z13.9
 alcoholism Z13.89
 anemia Z13.0
 anomaly, congenital Z13.89
 antenatal, of mother (see also Encounter,
  antenatal screening) Z36.9
 arterial hypertension Z13.6
 arthropod-borne viral disease NEC Z11.59
 bacteriuria, asymptomatic Z13.89
 behavioral disorder Z13.89
 brain injury, traumatic Z13.850
 bronchitis, chronic Z13.83
 brucellosis Z11.2
 cardiovascular disorder Z13.6
 cataract Z13.5
 chlamydial diseases Z11.8
 cholera Z11.0
 chromosomal abnormalities (nonprocreative)
  NEC Z13.79
 colonoscopy Z12.11
 congenital
  dislocation of hip Z13.89
  eye disorder Z13.5
  malformation or deformation Z13.89
 contamination NEC Z13.88
 cystic fibrosis Z13.228
 dengue fever Z11.59
 dental disorder Z13.84
 depression Z13.89
 developmental handicap Z13.42
  in early childhood Z13.42
  infant Z13.41
 diabetes mellitus Z13.1
 diphtheria Z11.2
 disability, intellectual Z13.42
  infant Z13.41
 disease or disorder Z13.9
  bacterial NEC Z11.2
   intestinal infectious Z11.0
   respiratory tuberculosis Z11.1
  blood or blood-forming organ Z13.0
  cardiovascular Z13.6
  Chagas' Z11.6
  chlamydial Z11.8
  dental Z13.89
  developmental Z13.42
   in child Z13.42
   infant Z13.41
  digestive tract NEC Z13.818
   lower GI Z13.811
   upper GI Z13.810
  ear Z13.5
  endocrine Z13.29
  eye Z13.5
  genitourinary Z13.89
  heart Z13.6
  human immunodeficiency virus (HIV)
   infection Z11.4
  immunity Z13.0
  infection
   intestinal Z11.0
    specified NEC Z11.6
  infectious Z11.9
  mental Z13.89

Screening (for) - *continued*
 metabolic Z13.228
 neurological Z13.89
 nutritional Z13.21
  metabolic Z13.228
   lipoid disorders Z13.220
 protozoal Z11.6
  intestinal Z11.0
 respiratory Z13.83
 rheumatic Z13.828
 rickettsial Z11.8
 sexually-transmitted NEC Z11.3
  human immunodeficiency virus (HIV)
   Z11.4
 sickle-cell (trait) Z13.0
 skin Z13.89
 specified NEC Z13.89
 spirochetal Z11.8
 thyroid Z13.29
 vascular Z13.6
 venereal Z11.3
 viral NEC Z11.59
  human immunodeficiency virus (HIV)
   Z11.4
  intestinal Z11.0
 elevated titer Z13.89
 emphysema Z13.83
 encephalitis, viral (mosquito or tick-borne)
  Z11.59
 exposure to contaminants (toxic) Z13.88
 fever
  dengue Z11.59
  hemorrhagic Z11.59
  yellow Z11.59
 filariasis Z11.6
 galactosemia Z13.228
 gastrointestinal condition Z13.818
 genetic (nonprocreative)
  for procreative management - *see* Testing,
   genetic, for procreative management
  disease carrier status (nonprocreative) Z13.71
  specified NEC (nonprocreative) Z13.79
 genitourinary condition Z13.89
 glaucoma Z13.5
 gonorrhea Z11.3
 gout Z13.89
 helminthiasis (intestinal) Z11.6
 hematopoietic malignancy Z12.89
 hemoglobinopathies NEC Z13.0
 hemorrhagic fever Z11.59
 Hodgkin disease Z12.89
 human immunodeficiency virus (HIV) Z11.4
 human papillomavirus Z11.51
 hypertension Z13.6
 immunity disorders Z13.0
 infection
  mycotic Z11.8
  parasitic Z11.8
 ingestion of radioactive substance Z13.88
 intellectual disability Z13.42
  infant Z13.41
 intestinal
  helminthiasis Z11.6
  infectious disease Z11.0
 leishmaniasis Z11.6
 leprosy Z11.2
 leptospirosis Z11.8
 leukemia Z12.89
 lymphoma Z12.89
 malaria Z11.6
 malnutrition Z13.29
  metabolic Z13.228
  nutritional Z13.21
 measles Z11.59

Semicoma R40.1
Seminal vesiculitis N49.0
Seminoma C62.9-
  specified site - *see* Neoplasm, malignant, by site
Senear-Usher disease or syndrome L10.4
Senectus R54
Senescence (without mention of psychosis) R54
Senile, senility - *see also* condition R41.81
  with
    acute confusional state F05
    mental changes NOS F03
    psychosis NEC - *see* Psychosis, senile
  asthenia R54
  cervix (atrophic) N88.8
  debility R54
  endometrium (atrophic) N85.8
  fallopian tube (atrophic) - *see* Atrophy, fallopian tube
  heart (failure) R54
  ovary (atrophic) - *see* Atrophy, ovary
  premature E34.8
  vagina, vaginitis (atrophic) N95.2
  wart L82.1
Sensation
  burning (skin) R20.8
    tongue K14.6
  loss of R20.8
  prickling (skin) R20.2
  tingling (skin) R20.2
Sense loss
  smell - *see* Disturbance, sensation, smell
  taste - *see* Disturbance, sensation, taste
  touch R20.8
Sensibility disturbance (cortical) (deep) (vibratory) R20.9
Sensitive, sensitivity - *see also* Allergy
  carotid sinus G90.01
  child (excessive) F93.8
  cold, autoimmune D59.1
  dentin K03.89
  gluten (non-celiac) K90.41
  latex Z91.040
  methemoglobin D74.8
  tuberculin, without clinical or radiological symptoms R76.11
  visual
    glare H53.71
    impaired contrast H53.72
Sensitiver Beziehungswahn F22
Sensitization, auto-erythrocytic D69.2
Separation
  anxiety, abnormal (of childhood) F93.0
  apophysis, traumatic
    code as Fracture, by site
  choroid - *see* Detachment, choroid
  epiphysis, epiphyseal
    nontraumatic - *see also* Osteochondropathy, specified type NEC
      upper femoral - *see* Slipped, epiphysis, upper femoral
    traumatic
      code as Fracture, by site
  fracture - *see* Fracture
  infundibulum cardiac from right ventricle by a partition Q24.3
  joint (traumatic) (current)
    code by site under Dislocation
  pubic bone, obstetrical trauma O71.6
  retina, retinal - *see* Detachment, retina
  symphysis pubis, obstetrical trauma O71.6
  tracheal ring, incomplete, congenital Q32.1

Sepsis (generalized) (unspecified organism) A41.9
  with
    organ dysfunction (acute) (multiple) R65.20
      with septic shock R65.21
  actinomycotic A42.7
  adrenal hemorrhage syndrome (meningococcal) A39.1
  anaerobic A41.4
  Bacillus anthracis A22.7
  Brucella - *see also* Brucellosis A23.9
  candidal B37.7
  cryptogenic A41.9
  due to device, implant or graft T85.79
    arterial graft NEC T82.7
    breast (implant) T85.79
    catheter NEC T85.79
      dialysis (renal) T82.7
        intraperitoneal T85.71
      infusion NEC T82.7
        spinal (cranial) (epidural) (intrathecal) (spinal) (subarachnoid) (subdural) T85.735
      urethral indwelling T83.511
      urinary T83.518
    ectopic or molar pregnancy O08.82
    electronic (electrode) (pulse generator) (stimulator)
      bone T84.7
      cardiac T82.7
      nervous system T85.738
        brain T85.731
        neurostimulator generator T85.734
        peripheral nerve T85.732
        spinal cord T85.733
      urinary T83.590
    fixation, internal (orthopedic) - *see* Complication, fixation device, infection
    gastrointestinal (bile duct) (esophagus) T85.79
    neurostimulator electrode (lead) T85.732
    genital T83.69
    heart NEC T82.7
      valve (prosthesis) T82.6
        graft T82.7
    joint prosthesis - *see* Complication, joint prosthesis, infection
    ocular (corneal graft) (orbital implant) T85.79
    orthopedic NEC T84.7
      fixation device, internal - *see* Complication, fixation device, infection
    specified NEC T85.79
    vascular T82.7
    ventricular intracranial (communicating) shunt T85.730
  during labor O75.3
  Enterococcus A41.81
  Erysipelothrix (rhusiopathiae) (erysipeloid) A26.7
  Escherichia coli (E. coli) A41.5
  extraintestinal yersiniosis A28.2
  following
    abortion (subsequent episode) O08.0
      current episode - *see* Abortion
    ectopic or molar pregnancy O08.82
    immunization T88.0
    infusion, therapeutic injection or transfusion NEC T80.29
  gangrenous A41.9
  gonococcal A54.86
  Gram negative (organism) A41.5
    anaerobic A41.4
  Haemophilus influenzae A41.3

Sepsis - *continued*
  herpesviral B00.7
  intra-abdominal K65.1
  intraocular - *see* Endophthalmitis, purulent
  Listeria monocytogenes A32.7
  localized   code to specific localized infection in operation wound T81.4
    skin - *see* Abscess
  malleus A24.0
  melioidosis A24.1
  meningeal - *see* Meningitis
  meningococcal A39.4
    acute A39.2
    chronic A39.3
  MSSA (Methicillin susceptible Staphylococcus aureus) A41.01
  newborn P36.9
    due to
      anaerobes NEC P36.5
      Escherichia coli P36.4
      Staphylococcus P36.30
        aureus P36.2
        specified NEC P36.39
      Streptococcus P36.10
        group B P36.0
        specified NEC P36.19
    specified NEC P36.8
  Pasteurella multocida A28.0
  pelvic, puerperal, postpartum, childbirth O85
  postprocedural T81.4
  pneumococcal A40.3
  puerperal, postpartum, childbirth (pelvic) O85
  Salmonella (arizonae) (cholerae-suis) (enteritidis) (typhimurium) A02.1
  severe R65.20
    with septic shock R65.21
  skin, localized - *see* Abscess
  Shigella - *see also* Dysentery, bacillary A03.9
  specified organism NEC A41.89
  Staphylococcus, staphylococcal A41.2
    aureus (methicillin susceptible) (MSSA) A41.01
      methicillin resistant (MRSA) A41.02
    coagulase negative A41.1
    specified NEC A41.1
  Streptococcus, streptococcal A40.9
    agalactiae A40.1
    group
      A A40.0
      B A40.1
      D A41.81
    neonatal P36.10
      group B P36.0
      specified NEC P36.19
    pneumoniae A40.3
    pyogenes A40.0
    specified NEC A40.8
  tracheostomy stoma J95.02
  tularemic A21.7
  umbilical, umbilical cord (newborn) - *see* Sepsis, newborn
  Yersinia pestis A20.7
Septate - *see* Septum
Septic - *see* condition
  arm - *see* Cellulitis, upper limb
    with lymphangitis - *see* Lymphangitis, acute, upper limb
  embolus - *see* Embolism
  finger - *see* Cellulitis, digit
    with lymphangitis - *see* Lymphangitis, acute, digit
  foot - *see* Cellulitis, lower limb
    with lymphangitis - *see* Lymphangitis, acute, lower limb

Septic - *continued*
gallbladder (acute) K81.0
hand - *see* Cellulitis, upper limb
  with lymphangitis - *see* Lymphangitis, acute, upper limb
joint - *see* Arthritis, pyogenic or pyemic
leg - *see* Cellulitis, lower limb
  with lymphangitis - *see* Lymphangitis, acute, lower limb
nail - *see also* Cellulitis, digit
  with lymphangitis - *see* Lymphangitis, acute, digit
sore - *see also* Abscess
  throat J02.0
    streptococcal J02.0
spleen (acute) D73.89
teeth, tooth (pulpal origin) K04.4
throat - *see* Pharyngitis
thrombus - *see* Thrombosis
toe - *see* Cellulitis, digit
  with lymphangitis - *see* Lymphangitis, acute, digit
tonsils, chronic J35.01
  with adenoiditis J35.03
uterus - *see* Endometritis
Septicemia A41.9
meaning sepsis - *see* Sepsis
Septum, septate (congenital) - *see also* Anomaly, by site
anal Q42.3
  with fistula Q42.2
aqueduct of Sylvius Q03.0
  with spina bifida - *see* Spina bifida, by site, with hydrocephalus
uterus (complete) (partial) Q51.2
vagina Q52.10
  in pregnancy - *see* Pregnancy, complicated by, abnormal vagina
    causing obstructed labor O65.5
  longitudinal Q52.129
    microperforate
      left side Q52.124
      right side Q52.123
    nonobstruction Q52.120
    obstructing Q52.129
      left side Q52.122
      right side Q52.121
  transverse Q52.11
Sequelae (of) - *see also* condition
abscess, intracranial or intraspinal (conditions in G06) G09
amputation   code to injury with seventh character S
burn and corrosion   code to injury with seventh character S
calcium deficiency E64.8
cerebrovascular disease - *see* Sequelae, disease, cerebrovascular
childbirth O94
contusion   code to injury with seventh character S
corrosion - *see* Sequelae, burn and corrosion
crushing injury   code to injury with seventh character S
disease
  cerebrovascular I69.90
    alteration of sensation I69.998
    aphasia I69.920
    apraxia I69.990
    ataxia I69.993
    cognitive deficits I69.91
    disturbance of vision I69.998
    dysarthria I69.922
    dysphagia I69.991

Sequelae (of) - *continued*
  dysphasia I69.921
  facial droop I69.992
  facial weakness I69.992
  fluency disorder I69.923
  hemiplegia I69.95-
  hemorrhage
    intracerebral - *see* Sequelae, hemorrhage, intracerebral
    intracranial, nontraumatic NEC - *see* Sequelae, hemorrhage, intracranial, nontraumatic
    subarachnoid - *see* Sequelae, hemorrhage, subarachnoid
  language deficit I69.928
  monoplegia
    lower limb I69.94-
    upper limb I69.93-
  paralytic syndrome I69.96-
  specified effect NEC I69.998
  specified type NEC I69.80
    alteration of sensation I69.898
    aphasia I69.820
    apraxia I69.890
    ataxia I69.893
    cognitive deficits I69.81
    disturbance of vision I69.898
    dysarthria I69.822
    dysphagia I69.891
    dysphasia I69.821
    facial droop I69.892
    facial weakness I69.892
    fluency disorder I69.823
    hemiplegia I69.85-
    language deficit I69.828
    monoplegia
      lower limb I69.84-
      upper limb I69.83-
    paralytic syndrome I69.86-
    specified effect NEC I69.898
    speech deficit I69.928
      speech deficit I69.828
    stroke NOS - *see* Sequelae, stroke NOS
dislocation   code to injury with seventh character S
encephalitis or encephalomyelitis (conditions in G04) G09
  in infectious disease NEC B94.8
  viral B94.1
external cause   code to injury with seventh character S
foreign body entering natural orifice   code to injury with seventh character S
fracture   code to injury with seventh character S
frostbite   code to injury with seventh character S
Hansen's disease B92
hemorrhage
  intracerebral I69.10
    alteration of sensation I69.198
    aphasia I69.120
    apraxia I69.190
    ataxia I69.193
    cognitive deficits I69.11
    disturbance of vision I69.198
    dysarthria I69.122
    dysphagia I69.191
    dysphasia I69.121
    facial droop I69.192
    facial weakness I69.192
    fluency disorder I69.123
    hemiplegia I69.15-
    language deficit NEC I69.128

Sequelae (of) - *continued*
  monoplegia
    lower limb I69.14-
    upper limb I69.13-
  paralytic syndrome I69.16-
  specified effect NEC I69.198
  speech deficit NEC I69.128
intracranial, nontraumatic NEC I69.20
  alteration of sensation I69.298
  aphasia I69.220
  apraxia I69.290
  ataxia I69.293
  cognitive deficits I69.21
  disturbance of vision I69.298
  dysarthria I69.222
  dysphagia I69.291
  dysphasia I69.221
  facial droop I69.292
  facial weakness I69.292
  fluency disorder I69.223
  hemiplegia I69.25-
  language deficit NEC I69.228
  monoplegia
    lower limb I69.24-
    upper limb I69.23-
  paralytic syndrome I69.26-
  specified effect NEC I69.298
  speech deficit NEC I69.228
subarachnoid I69.00
  alteration of sensation I69.098
  aphasia I69.020
  apraxia I69.090
  ataxia I69.093
  cognitive deficits - *see* subcategory I69.01-
  disturbance of vision I69.098
  dysarthria I69.022
  dysphagia I69.091
  dysphasia I69.021
  facial droop I69.092
  facial weakness I69.092
  fluency disorder I69.023
  hemiplegia I69.05-
  language deficit NEC I69.028
  monoplegia
    lower limb I69.04-
    upper limb I69.03-
  paralytic syndrome I69.06-
  specified effect NEC I69.098
  speech deficit NEC I69.028
hepatitis, viral B94.2
hyperalimentation E68
infarction
  cerebral I69.30
    alteration of sensation I69.398
    aphasia I69.320
    apraxia I69.390
    ataxia I69.393
    cognitive deficits I69.31
    disturbance of vision I69.398
    dysarthria I69.322
    dysphagia I69.391
    dysphasia I69.321
    facial droop I69.392
    facial weakness I69.392
    fluency disorder I69.323
    hemiplegia I69.35-
    language deficit NEC I69.328
    monoplegia
      lower limb I69.34-
      upper limb I69.33-
    paralytic syndrome I69.36-
    specified effect NEC I69.398
    speech deficit NEC I69.328

Sequelae (of) - *continued*

infection, pyogenic, intracranial or intraspinal
  G09
infectious disease B94.9
  specified NEC B94.8
injury   code to injury with seventh character S
leprosy B92
meningitis
  bacterial (conditions in G00) G09
  other or unspecified cause (conditions in
    G03) G09
muscle (and tendon) injury   code to injury
  with seventh character S
myelitis - *see* Sequelae, encephalitis
niacin deficiency E64.8
nutritional deficiency E64.9
  specified NEC E64.8
obstetrical condition O94
parasitic disease B94.9
phlebitis or thrombophlebitis of intracranial or
  intraspinal venous sinuses and veins
  (conditions in G08) G09
poisoning   code to poisoning with seventh
  character S
  nonmedicinal substance - *see* Sequelae, toxic
    effect, nonmedicinal substance
poliomyelitis (acute) B91
pregnancy O94
protein-energy malnutrition E64.0
puerperium O94
rickets E64.3
selenium deficiency E64.8
sprain and strain   code to injury with seventh
  character S
stroke NOS I69.30
  alteration in sensation I69.398
  aphasia I69.320
  apraxia I69.390
  ataxia I69.393
  cognitive deficits I69.31
  disturbance of vision I69.398
  dysarthria I69.322
  dysphagia I69.391
  dysphasia I69.321
  facial droop I69.392
  facial weakness I69.392
  hemiplegia I69.35-
  language deficit NEC I69.328
  monoplegia
    lower limb I69.34-
    upper limb I69.33-
  paralytic syndrome I69.36-
  specified effect NEC I69.398
  speech deficit NEC I69.328
tendon and muscle injury   code to injury with
  seventh character S
thiamine deficiency E64.8
trachoma B94.0
tuberculosis B90.9
  bones and joints B90.2
  central nervous system B90.0
  genitourinary B90.1
  pulmonary (respiratory) B90.9
  specified organs NEC B90.8
viral
  encephalitis B94.1
  hepatitis B94.2
vitamin deficiency NEC E64.8
  A E64.1
  B E64.8
  C E64.2
wound, open   code to injury with seventh
  character S

Sequestration - *see also* Sequestrum
  disk - *see* Displacement, intervertebral disk
  lung, congenital Q33.2
Sequestrum
  bone - *see* Osteomyelitis, chronic
  dental M27.2
  jaw bone M27.2
  orbit - *see* Osteomyelitis, orbit
  sinus (accessory) (nasal) - *see* Sinusitis
Sequoiosis lung or pneumonitis J67.8
Serology for syphilis
  doubtful
    with signs or symptoms
    code by site and stage under Syphilis
      follow-up of latent syphilis - *see* Syphilis,
        latent
  negative, with signs or symptoms
  code by site and stage under Syphilis
  positive A53.0
    with signs or symptoms
    code by site and stage under Syphilis
  reactivated A53.0
Seroma - *see also* Hematoma
  postprocedural - *see* Complication,
    postprocedural, seroma
  traumatic, secondary and recurrent T79.2
Seropurulent - *see* condition
Serositis, multiple K65.8
  pericardial I31.1
  peritoneal K65.8
Serous - *see* condition
Sertoli cell
  adenoma
    specified site - *see* Neoplasm, benign, by site
    unspecified site
      female D27.9
      male D29.20
  carcinoma
    specified site - *see* Neoplasm, malignant, by
      site
    unspecified site (male) C62.9-
      female C56.9
  tumor
    with lipid storage
      specified site - *see* Neoplasm, benign, by
        site
      unspecified site
        female D27.9
        male D29.20
    specified site - *see* Neoplasm, benign, by site
    unspecified site
      female D27.9
      male D29.20
Sertoli-Leydig cell tumor - *see* Neoplasm,
  benign, by site
  specified site - *see* Neoplasm, benign, by site
  unspecified site
    female D27.9
    male D29.20
Serum
  allergy, allergic reaction - *see also* Reaction,
    serum T80.69
    shock - *see also* Shock, anaphylactic T80.59
  arthritis - *see also* Reaction, serum T80.69
  complication or reaction NEC - *see also*
    Reaction, serum T80.69
  disease NEC - *see also* Reaction, serum
    T80.69
  hepatitis - *see also* Hepatitis, viral, type B
    carrier (suspected) of B18.1
  intoxication - *see also* Reaction, serum T80.69
  neuritis - *see also* Reaction, serum T80.69
  neuropathy G61.1
  poisoning NEC - *see also* Reaction, serum

Serum - *continued*
  T80.69
  rash NEC - *see also* Reaction, serum T80.69
  reaction NEC - *see also* Reaction, serum
    T80.69
  sickness NEC - *see also* Reaction, serum
    T80.69
  urticaria - *see also* Reaction, serum T80.69
Sesamoiditis M25.8-
Sever's disease or osteochondrosis - *see*
  Osteochondrosis, juvenile, tarsus
Severe sepsis R65.20
  with septic shock R65.21
Sex
  chromosome mosaics Q97.8
    lines with various numbers of X
      chromosomes Q97.2
  education Z70.8
  reassignment surgery status Z87.890
Sextuplet pregnancy - *see* Pregnancy, sextuplet
Sexual
  function, disorder of (psychogenic) F52.9
  immaturity (female) (male) E30.0
  impotence (psychogenic) organic origin NEC -
    see Dysfunction, sexual, male
  precocity (constitutional)
    (cryptogenic)(female) (idiopathic) (male)
    E30.1
Sexuality, pathologic - *see* Deviation, sexual
Sézary disease C84.1-
Shadow, lung R91.8
Shaking palsy or paralysis - *see* Parkinsonism
Shallowness, acetabulum - *see* Derangement,
  joint, specified type NEC, hip
Shaver's disease J63.1
Sheath (tendon) - *see* condition
Sheathing, retinal vessels H35.01-
Shedding
  nail L60.8
  premature, primary (deciduous) teeth K00.6
Sheehan's disease or syndrome E23.0
Shelf, rectal K62.89
Shell teeth K00.5
Shellshock (current) F43.0
  lasting state - *see* Disorder, post-traumatic
    stress
Shield kidney Q63.1
Shift
  auditory threshold (temporary) H93.24-
  mediastinal R93.8
Shifting sleep-work schedule (affecting sleep)
  G47.26
Shiga (-Kruse) dysentery A03.0
Shiga's bacillus A03.0
Shigella (dysentery) - *see* Dysentery, bacillary
Shigellosis A03.9
  Group A A03.0
  Group B A03.1
  Group C A03.2
  Group D A03.3
Shin splints S86.89
Shingles - *see* Herpes, zoster
Shipyard disease or eye B30.0
Shirodkar suture, in pregnancy - *see*
  Pregnancy, complicated by, incompetent
  cervix
Shock R57.9
  with ectopic or molar pregnancy O08.3
  adrenal (cortical) (Addisonian) E27.2
  adverse food reaction (anaphylactic) - *see*
    Shock, anaphylactic, due to food
  allergic - *see* Shock, anaphylactic
  anaphylactic T78.2

Shock - *continued*
chemical - *see* Table of Drugs and Chemicals
due to drug or medicinal substance
correct substance properly administered
T88.6
overdose or wrong substance given or taken
(by accident) - *see* Table of Drugs and
Chemicals, by drug, poisoning
due to food (nonpoisonous) T78.00
additives T78.06
dairy products T78.07
eggs T78.08
fish T78.03
shellfish T78.02
fruit T78.04
milk T78.07
nuts T78.05
multiple types T78.05
peanuts T78.01
peanuts T78.01
seeds T78.05
specified type NEC T78.09
vegetable T78.04
following sting(s) - *see* Venom
immunization T80.52
serum T80.59
blood and blood products T80.51
immunization T80.52
specified NEC T80.59
vaccination T80.52
anaphylactoid - *see* Shock, anaphylactic
anesthetic
correct substance properly administered
T88.2
overdose or wrong substance given or taken -
see Table of Drugs and Chemicals, by drug,
poisoning
specified anesthetic - *see* Table of Drugs
and Chemicals, by drug, poisoning
cardiogenic R57.0
chemical substance - *see* Table of Drugs and
Chemicals
complicating ectopic or molar pregnancy
O08.3
culture - *see* Disorder, adjustment
drug
due to correct substance properly
administered T88.6
overdose or wrong substance given or taken
(by accident) - *see* Table of Drugs and
Chemicals, by drug, poisoning
during or after labor and delivery O75.1
electric T75.4
(taser) T75.4
endotoxic R65.21
postprocedural (resulting from a procedure,
not elsewhere classified) T81.12
following
ectopic or molar pregnancy O08.3
injury (immediate) (delayed) T79.4
labor and delivery O75.1
food (anaphylactic) - *see* Shock, anaphylactic,
due to food
from electroshock gun (taser) T75.4
gram negative R65.21
postprocedural (resulting from a procedure,
not elsewhere classified) T81.12
hematologic R57.8
hemorrhagic R57.8
surgery (intraoperative) (postoperative)
T81.19
trauma T79.4
hypovolemic R57.1
surgical T81.19

Shock - *continued*
traumatic T79.4
insulin E15
therapeutic misadventure   *see* subcategory
T38.3
kidney N17.0
traumatic (following crushing) T79.5
liver K72.00
lightning T75.01
lung J80
obstetric O75.1
with ectopic or molar pregnancy O08.3
following ectopic or molar pregnancy O08.3
pleural (surgical) T81.19
due to trauma T79.4
postprocedural (postoperative) T81.10
with ectopic or molar pregnancy O08.3
cardiogenic T81.11
endotoxic T81.12
following ectopic or molar pregnancy O08.3
gram negative T81.12
hypovolemic T81.19
septic T81.12
specified type NEC T81.19
psychic F43.0
septic (due to severe sepsis) R65.21
specified NEC R57.8
surgical T81.10
taser gun (taser) T75.4
therapeutic misadventure NEC T81.10
thyroxin
overdose or wrong substance given or taken -
see Table of Drugs and Chemicals, by drug,
poisoning
toxic, syndrome A48.3
transfusion - *see* Complications, transfusion
traumatic (immediate) (delayed) T79.4
Shoemaker's chest M95.4
Short, shortening, shortness
arm (acquired) - *see also* Deformity, limb,
unequal length
congenital Q71.81-
forearm - *see* Deformity, limb, unequal
length
bowel syndrome K91.2
breath R06.02
cervical (complicating pregnancy) O26.87-
non-gravid uterus N88.3
common bile duct, congenital Q44.5
cord (umbilical), complicating delivery O69.3
cystic duct, congenital Q44.5
esophagus (congenital) Q39.8
femur (acquired) - *see* Deformity, limb,
unequal length, femur
congenital - *see* Defect, reduction, lower
limb, longitudinal, femur
frenum, frenulum, linguae (congenital) Q38.1
hip (acquired) - *see also* Deformity, limb,
unequal length
congenital Q65.89
leg (acquired) - *see also* Deformity, limb,
unequal length
congenital Q72.81-
lower leg - *see also* Deformity, limb, unequal
length
limbed stature, with immunodeficiency D82.2
lower limb (acquired) - *see also* Deformity,
limb, unequal length
congenital Q72.81-
organ or site, congenital NEC - *see* Distortion
palate, congenital Q38.5
radius (acquired) - *see also* Deformity, limb,
unequal length
congenital - *see* Defect, reduction, upper

Short, shortening, shortness - *continued*
limb, longitudinal, radius
rib syndrome Q77.2
stature (child) (hereditary) (idiopathic) NEC
R62.52
constitutional E34.3
due to endocrine disorder E34.3
Laron-type E34.3
tendon - *see also* Contraction, tendon
with contracture of joint - *see* Contraction,
joint
Achilles (acquired) M67.0-
congenital Q66.89
congenital Q79.8
thigh (acquired) - *see also* Deformity, limb,
unequal length, femur
congenital - *see* Defect, reduction, lower
limb, longitudinal, femur
tibialis anterior (tendon) - *see* Contraction,
tendon
umbilical cord
complicating delivery O69.3
upper limb, congenital - *see* Defect, reduction,
upper limb, specified type NEC
urethra N36.8
uvula, congenital Q38.5
vagina (congenital) Q52.4
Shortsightedness - *see* Myopia
Shoshin (acute fulminating beriberi) E51.11
Shoulder - *see* condition
Shovel-shaped incisors K00.2
Shower, thromboembolic - *see* Embolism
Shunt
arterial-venous (dialysis) Z99.2
arteriovenous, pulmonary (acquired) I28.0
congenital Q25.72
cerebral ventricle (communicating) in situ
Z98.2
surgical, prosthetic, with complications - *see*
Complications, cardiovascular, device or
implant
Shutdown, renal N28.9
Shy-Drager syndrome G90.3
Sialadenitis, sialadenosis (any gland)
(chronic) (periodic) (suppurative) - *see*
Sialoadenitis
Sialectasia K11.8
Sialidosis E77.1
Sialitis, silitis (any gland) (chronic)
(suppurative) - *see* Sialoadenitis
Sialoadenitis (any gland) (periodic)
(suppurative) K11.20
acute K11.21
recurrent K11.22
chronic K11.23
Sialadenopathy K11.9
Sialoangitis - *see* Sialoadenitis
Sialodochitis (fibrinosa) - *see* Sialoadenitis
Sialodocholithiasis K11.5
Sialolithiasis K11.5
Sialometaplasia, necrotizing K11.8
Sialorrhea - *see also* Ptyalism
periodic - *see* Sialoadenitis
Sialosis K11.7
Siamese twin Q89.4
Sibling rivalry Z62.891
Sicard's syndrome G52.7
Sicca syndrome M35.00
with
keratoconjunctivitis M35.01
lung involvement M35.02
myopathy M35.03
renal tubulo-interstitial disorders M35.04
specified organ involvement NEC M35.09

Sick R69
  or handicapped person in family Z63.79
    needing care at home Z63.6
  sinus (syndrome) I49.5
Sick-euthyroid syndrome E07.81
Sickle-cell
  anemia - *see* Disease, sickle-cell
  trait D57.3
Sicklemia - *see also* Disease, sickle-cell
  trait D57.3
Sickness
  air (travel) T75.3
  airplane T75.3
  alpine T70.29
  altitude T70.20
  Andes T70.29
  aviator's T70.29
  balloon T70.29
  car T75.3
  compressed air T70.3
  decompression T70.3
  green D50.8
  milk - *see* Poisoning, food, noxious
  motion T75.3
  mountain T70.29
    acute D75.1
  protein - *see also* Reaction, serum T80.69
  radiation T66
  roundabout (motion) T75.3
  sea T75.3
  serum NEC - *see also* Reaction, serum T80.69
  sleeping (African) B56.9
    by Trypanosoma B56.9
      brucei
        gambiense B56.0
        rhodesiense B56.1
      East African B56.1
      Gambian B56.0
      Rhodesian B56.1
      West African B56.0
  swing (motion) T75.3
  train (railway) (travel) T75.3
  travel (any vehicle) T75.3
Sideropenia - *see* Anemia, iron deficiency
Siderosilicosis J62.8
Siderosis (lung) J63.4
  eye (globe) - *see* Disorder, globe,
    degenerative, siderosis
Siemens' syndrome (ectodermal dysplasia)
  Q82.8
Sighing R06.89
  psychogenic F45.8
Sigmoid - *see also* condition
  flexure - *see* condition
  kidney Q63.1
Sigmoiditis - *see also* Enteritis K52.9
  infectious A09
  noninfectious K52.9
Silfversköld's syndrome Q78.9
Silicosiderosis J62.8
Silicosis, silicotic (simple) (complicated) J62.8
  with tuberculosis J65
Silicotuberculosis J65
Silo-fillers' disease J68.8
  bronchitis J68.0
  pneumonitis J68.0
  pulmonary edema J68.1
Silver's syndrome Q87.1
Simian malaria B53.1
Simmonds' cachexia or disease E23.0
Simons' disease or syndrome (progressive
  lipodystrophy) E88.1
Simple, simplex - *see* condition
Simulation, conscious (of illness) Z76.5

Simultanagnosia (asimultagnosia) R48.3
Sin Nombre virus disease (Hantavirus)
  (cardio)-pulmonary syndrome) B33.4
Sinding-Larsen disease or osteochondrosis -
  see Osteochondrosis, juvenile, patella
Singapore hemorrhagic fever A91
Singer's node or nodule J38.2
Single
  atrium Q21.2
  coronary artery Q24.5
  umbilical artery Q27.0
  ventricle Q20.4
Singultus R06.6
  epidemicus B33.0
Sinus - *see also* Fistula
  abdominal K63.89
  arrest I45.5
  arrhythmia I49.8
  bradycardia R00.1
  branchial cleft (internal) (external) Q18.0
  coccygeal - *see* Sinus, pilonidal
  dental K04.6
  dermal (congenital) Q06.8
    with abscess Q06.8
    coccygeal, pilonidal - *see* Sinus, coccygeal
  infected, skin NEC L08.89
  marginal, ruptured or bleeding - *see*
    Hemorrhage, antepartum, specified cause
    NEC
  medial, face and neck Q18.8
  pause I45.5
  pericranii Q01.9
  pilonidal (infected) (rectum) L05.92**S**
    with abscess L05.02
  preauricular Q18.1
  rectovaginal N82.3
  Rokitansky-Aschoff (gallbladder) K82.8
  sacrococcygeal (dermoid) (infected) - *see*
    Sinus, pilonidal
  tachycardia R00.0
    paroxysmal I47.1
  tarsi syndrome M25.57-
  testis N50.89
  tract (postinfective) - *see* Fistula
  urachus Q64.4
Sinusitis (accessory) (chronic) (hyperplastic)
  (nasal) (nonpurulent) (purulent) J32.9
  acute J01.90
    ethmoidal J01.20
      recurrent J01.21
    frontal J01.10
      recurrent J01.11
    involving more than one sinus, other than
      pansinusitis J01.80
      recurrent J01.81
    maxillary J01.00
      recurrent J01.01
    pansinusitis J01.40
      recurrent J01.41
    recurrent J01.91
    specified NEC J01.80
      recurrent J01.81
    sphenoidal J01.30
      recurrent J01.31
  allergic - *see* Rhinitis, allergic
  due to high altitude T70.1
  ethmoidal J32.2
    acute J01.20
      recurrent J01.21
  frontal J32.1
    acute J01.10
      recurrent J01.11
  influenzal - *see* Influenza, with, respiratory
    manifestations NEC

Sinus - *continued*
  involving more than one sinus but not
    pansinusitis J32.8
    acute J01.80
      recurrent J01.81
    maxillary J32.0
    acute J01.00
      recurrent J01.01
    sphenoidal J32.3
    acute J01.30
      recurrent J01.31
    tuberculous, any sinus A15.8
Sinusitis-bronchiectasis-situs inversus
  (syndrome) (triad) Q89.3
Sipple's syndrome E31.22
Sirenomelia (syndrome) Q87.2
Siriasis T67.0
Sirkari's disease B55.0
Siti A65
Situation, psychiatric F99
Situational
  disturbance (transient) - *see* Disorder,
    adjustment
    acute F43.0
  maladjustment - *see* Disorder, adjustment
  reaction - *see* Disorder, adjustment
    acute F43.0
Situs inversus or transversus (abdominalis)
  (thoracis) Q89.3
Sixth disease B08.20
  due to human herpesvirus 6 B08.21
  due to human herpesvirus 7 B08.22
Sjögren-Larsson syndrome Q87.1
Sjögren's syndrome or disease - *see* Sicca
  syndrome
Skeletal - *see* condition
Skene's gland - *see* condition
Skenitis - *see* Urethritis
Skerljevo A65
Skevas-Zerfus disease - *see* Toxicity, venom,
  marine animal, sea anemone
Skin - *see also* condition
  clammy R23.1
  donor - *see* Donor, skin
  hidebound M35.9
Slate-dressers' or slate-miners' lung J62.8
Sleep
  apnea - *see* Apnea, sleep
  deprivation Z72.820
  disorder or disturbance G47.9
    child F51.9
    nonorganic origin F51.9
    specified NEC G47.8
  disturbance G47.9
    nonorganic origin F51.9
  drunkenness F51.9
  rhythm inversion G47.2-
  terrors F51.4
  walking F51.3
    hysterical F44.89
Sleep hygiene
  abuse Z72.821
  inadequate Z72.821
  poor Z72.821
Sleeping sickness - *see* Sickness, sleeping
Sleeplessness - *see* Insomnia
  menopausal N95.1
Sleep-wake schedule disorder G47.20
Slim disease (in HIV infection) B20
Slipped, slipping
  epiphysis (traumatic) - *see also*
    Osteochondropathy, specified type NEC
    capital femoral (traumatic)
      acute (on chronic) S79.01-

Slipped, slipping - *continued*
  current traumatic
  code as Fracture, by site
    upper femoral (nontraumatic) M93.00-
      acute M93.01-
        on chronic M93.03-
      chronic M93.02-
  intervertebral disc - *see* Displacement,
  intervertebral disc   ligature, umbilical P51.8
  patella - *see* Disorder, patella, derangement
    NEC
  rib M89.8X8
  sacroiliac joint - *see* subcategory M53.2
  tendon - *see* Disorder, tendon
  ulnar nerve, nontraumatic - *see* Lesion, nerve,
    ulnar
  vertebra NEC - *see* Spondylolisthesis
Slocumb's syndrome E27.0
Sloughing (multiple) (phagedena) (skin) - *see*
  also Gangrene
  abscess - *see* Abscess
  appendix K38.8
  fascia - *see* Disorder, soft tissue, specified type
    NEC
  scrotum N50.89
  tendon - *see* Disorder, tendon
  transplanted organ - *see* Rejection, transplant
  ulcer - *see* Ulcer, skin
Slow
  feeding, newborn P92.2
  flow syndrome, coronary I20.8
  heart (beat) R00.1
Slowing, urinary stream R39.198
Sluder's neuralgia (syndrome) G44.89
Slurred, slurring speech R47.81
Small (ness)
  for gestational age - *see* Small for dates
  introitus, vagina N89.6
  kidney (unknown cause) N27.9
    bilateral N27.1
    unilateral N27.0
  ovary (congenital) Q50.39
  pelvis
    with disproportion (fetopelvic) O33.1
      causing obstructed labor O65.1
  uterus N85.8
  white kidney N03.9
Small-and-light-for-dates - *see* Small for dates
Small-for-dates (infant) P05.10
  with weight of
    499 grams or less P05.11
    500-749 grams P05.12
    750-999 grams P05.13
    1000-1249 grams P05.14
    1250-1499 grams P05.15
    1500-1749 grams P05.16
    1750-1999 grams P05.17
    2000-2499 grams P05.18
    2500 grams and over P05.19
  specified NEC P05.19
Smallpox B03
Smearing, fecal R15.1
Smith-Lemli-Opitz syndrome E78.72
Smith's fracture S52.54-
Smoker - *see* Dependence, drug, nicotine
Smoker's
  bronchitis J41.0
  cough J41.0
  palate K13.24
  throat J31.2
  tongue K13.24
Smoking
  passive Z77.22
Smothering spells R06.81

Snaggle teeth, tooth M26.39
Snapping
  finger - *see* Trigger finger
  hip - *see* Derangement, joint, specified type
    NEC, hip
    involving the iliotibial band M76.3-
  knee - *see* Derangement, knee
    involving the iliotibial band M76.3-
**Sneddon-Wilkinson disease or syndrome
(sub-corneal pustular dermatosis)** L13.1
Sneezing (intractable) R06.7
Sniffing
  cocaine
    abuse - *see* Abuse, drug, cocaine
    dependence - *see* Dependence, drug, cocaine
  gasoline
    abuse - *see* Abuse, drug, inhalant
    dependence - *see* Dependence, drug, inhalant
  glue (airplane)
    abuse - *see* Abuse, drug, inhalant
    drug dependence - *see* Dependence, drug,
      inhalant
Sniffles
  newborn P28.89
Snoring R06.83
Snow blindness - *see* Photokeratitis
Snuffles (non-syphilitic) R06.5
  newborn P28.89
  syphilitic (infant) A50.05 *[J99]*
Social
  exclusion Z60.4
    due to discrimination or persecution
      (perceived) Z60.5
  migrant Z59.0
    acculturation difficulty Z60.3
  rejection Z60.4
    due to discrimination or persecution Z60.5
  role conflict NEC Z73.5
  skills inadequacy NEC Z73.4
  transplantation Z60.3
Sodoku A25.0
Soemmerring's ring - *see* Cataract, secondary
Soft - *see also* condition
  nails L60.3
Softening
  bone - *see* Osteomalacia
  brain (necrotic) (progressive) G93.89
    congenital Q04.8
    embolic I63.4-
    hemorrhagic - *see* Hemorrhage, intracranial,
      intracerebral
    occlusive I63.5-
    thrombotic I63.3-
    cartilage M94.2-
      patella M22.4-
    cerebellar - *see* Softening, brain
    cerebral - *see* Softening, brain
    cerebrospinal - *see* Softening, brain
    myocardial, heart - *see* Degeneration,
      myocardial
    spinal cord G95.89
    stomach K31.89
Soldier's
  heart F45.8
  patches I31.0
Solitary
  cyst, kidney N28.1
  kidney, congenital Q60.0
Solvent abuse - *see* Abuse, drug, inhalant
  dependence - *see* Dependence, drug, inhalant
Somatization reaction, somatic reaction - *see*
  Disorder, somatoform
Somnambulism F51.3
  hysterical F44.89

Somnolence R40.0
  nonorganic origin F51.11
Sonne dysentery A03.3
Soor B37.0
Sore
  bed - *see* Ulcer, pressure, by site
  chiclero B55.1
  Delhi B55.1
  desert - *see* Ulcer, skin
  eye H57.1-
  Lahore B55.1
  mouth K13.79
    canker K12.0
  muscle M79.1
  Naga - *see* Ulcer, skin
  of skin - *see* Ulcer, skin
  oriental B55.1
  pressure - *see* Ulcer, pressure, by site
  skin L98.9
  soft A57
  throat (acute) - *see also* Pharyngitis
    with influenza, flu, or grippe - *see* Influenza,
      with, respiratory manifestations NEC
    chronic J31.2
    coxsackie (virus) B08.5
    diphtheritic A36.0
    herpesviral B00.2
    influenzal - *see* Influenza, with, respiratory
      manifestations NEC
    septic J02.0
    streptococcal (ulcerative) J02.0
    viral NEC J02.8
      coxsackie B08.5
  tropical - *see* Ulcer, skin
  veldt - *see* Ulcer, skin
Soto's syndrome (cerebral gigantism) Q87.3
South African cardiomyopathy syndrome
  I42.8
Southeast Asian hemorrhagic fever A91
Spacing
  abnormal, tooth, teeth, fully erupted M26.30
  excessive, tooth, fully erupted M26.32
Spade-like hand (congenital) Q68.1
Spading nail L60.8
  congenital Q84.6
Spanish collar N47.1
Sparganosis B70.1
Spasm(s), spastic, spasticity - *see also*
  condition R25.2
  accommodation - *see* Spasm, of
    accommodation
  ampulla of Vater K83.4
  anus, ani (sphincter) (reflex) K59.4
    psychogenic F45.8
  artery I73.9
    cerebral G45.9
  Bell's G51.3
  bladder (sphincter, external or internal) N32.89
    psychogenic F45.8
  bronchus, bronchiole J98.01
  cardia K22.0
  cardiac I20.1
  carpopedal - *see* Tetany
  cerebral (arteries) (vascular) G45.9
  cervix, complicating delivery O62.4
  ciliary body (of accommodation) - *see* Spasm,
    of accommodation
  colon - *see also* Irritable, bowel K58.9
    with diarrhea K58.0
    psychogenic F45.8
  common duct K83.8
  compulsive - *see* Tic
  conjugate H51.8
  coronary (artery) I20.1

Spasm(s), spastic, spasticity - *continued*
  diaphragm (reflex) R06.6
    epidemic B33.0
    psychogenic F45.8
  duodenum K59.8
  epidemic diaphragmatic (transient) B33.0
  esophagus (diffuse) K22.4
    psychogenic F45.8
  facial G51.3
  fallopian tube N83.8
  gastrointestinal (tract) K31.89
    psychogenic F45.8
  glottis J38.5
    hysterical F44.4
    psychogenic F45.8
      conversion reaction F44.4
    reflex through recurrent laryngeal nerve
    J38.5
  habit - *see* Tic
  heart I20.1
  hemifacial (clonic) G51.3
  hourglass - *see* Contraction, hourglass
  hysterical F44.4
  infantile - *see* Epilepsy, spasms
  inferior oblique, eye H51.8
  intestinal - *see also* Syndrome, irritable bowel
    K58.9
    psychogenic F45.8
  larynx, laryngeal J38.5
    hysterical F44.4
    psychogenic F45.8
      conversion reaction F44.4
  levator palpebrae superioris - *see* Disorder,
    eyelid function
  muscle NEC M62.838
    back M62.830
  nerve, trigeminal G51.0
  nervous F45.8
  nodding F98.4
  occupational F48.8
  oculogyric H51.8
    psychogenic F45.8
  of accommodation H52.53-
  ophthalmic artery - *see* Occlusion, artery,
    retina
  perineal, female N94.89
  peroneo-extensor - *see also* Deformity, limb,
    flat foot
  pharynx (reflex) J39.2
    hysterical F45.8
    psychogenic F45.8
  psychogenic F45.8
  pylorus NEC K31.3
    adult hypertrophic K31.89
    congenital or infantile Q40.0
    psychogenic F45.8
  rectum (sphincter) K59.4
    psychogenic F45.8
  retinal (artery) - *see* Occlusion, artery, retina
  sigmoid - *see also* Syndrome, irritable bowel
    K58.9
    psychogenic F45.8
  sphincter of Oddi K83.4
  stomach K31.89
    neurotic F45.8
  throat J39.2
    hysterical F45.8
    psychogenic F45.8
  tic F95.9
    chronic F95.1
    transient of childhood F95.0
  tongue K14.8
  torsion (progressive) G24.1
  trigeminal nerve - *see* Neuralgia, trigeminal

Spasm(s), spastic, spasticity - *continued*
  ureter N13.5
  urethra (sphincter) N35.9
  uterus N85.8
    complicating labor O62.4
  vagina N94.2
    psychogenic F52.5
  vascular I73.9
  vasomotor I73.9
  vein NEC I87.8
  viscera - *see* Pain, abdominal
Spasmodic - *see* condition
Spasmophilia - *see* Tetany
Spasmus nutans F98.4
Spastic, spasticity - *see also* Spasm
  child (cerebral) (congenital) (paralysis) G80.1
Speaker's throat R49.8
Specific, specified - *see* condition
Speech
  defect, disorder, disturbance, impediment
    R47.9
    psychogenic, in childhood and adolescence
    F98.8
    slurring R47.81
    specified NEC R47.89
Spencer's disease A08.19
Spens' syndrome (syncope with heart block)
  I45.9
Sperm counts (fertility testing) Z31.41
  postvasectomy Z30.8
    reversal Z31.42
Spermatic cord - *see* condition
Spermatocele N43.40
  congenital Q55.4
  multiple N43.42
  single N43.41
Spermatocystitis N49.0
Spermatocytoma C62.9-
  specified site - *see* Neoplasm, malignant, by
    site
Spermatorrhea N50.89
Sphacelus - *see* Gangrene
Sphenoidal - *see* condition
Sphenoiditis (chronic) - *see* Sinusitis,
  sphenoidal
Sphenopalatine ganglion neuralgia G90.09
Sphericity, increased, lens (congenital) Q12.4
Spherocytosis (congenital) (familial)
  (hereditary) D58.0
  hemoglobin disease D58.0
  sickle-cell (disease) D57.8-
Spherophakia Q12.4
Sphincter - *see* condition
Sphincteritis, sphincter of Oddi - *see*
  Cholangitis
Sphingolipidosis E75.3
  specified NEC E75.29
Sphingomyelinosis E75.3
Spicule tooth K00.2
Spider
  bite - *see* Toxicity, venom, spider
  fingers - *see* Syndrome, Marfan's
  nevus I78.1
  toes - *see* Syndrome, Marfan's
  vascular I78.1
Spiegler-Fendt
  benign lymphocytoma L98.8
  sarcoid L08.89
Spielmeyer-Vogt disease E75.4
Spina bifida (aperta) Q05.9
  with hydrocephalus NEC Q05.4
  cervical Q05.5
    with hydrocephalus Q05.0
  dorsal Q05.6

Spina bifida - *continued*
  with hydrocephalus Q05.1
  lumbar Q05.7
    with hydrocephalus Q05.2
  lumbosacral Q05.7
    with hydrocephalus Q05.2
  occulta Q76.0
  sacral Q05.8
    with hydrocephalus Q05.3
  thoracic Q05.6
    with hydrocephalus Q05.1
  thoracolumbar Q05.6
    with hydrocephalus Q05.1
Spindle, Krukenberg's - *see* Pigmentation,
  cornea, posterior
Spine, spinal - *see* condition
Spiradenoma (eccrine) - *see* Neoplasm, skin,
  benign
Spirillosis A25.0
Spirillum
  minus A25.0
  obermeieri infection A68.0
Spirochetal - *see* condition
Spirochetosis A69.9
  arthritic, arthritica A69.9
  bronchopulmonary A69.8
  icterohemorrhagic A27.0
  lung A69.8
Spirometrosis B70.1
Spitting blood - *see* Hemoptysis
Splanchnoptosis K63.4
Spleen, splenic - *see* condition
Splenectasis - *see* Splenomegaly
Splenitis (interstitial) (malignant)
  (nonspecific) D73.89
  malarial - *see also* Malaria B54 [*D77*]
  tuberculous A18.85
Splenocele D73.89
Splenomegaly, splenomegalia (Bengal)
  (cryptogenic) (idiopathic) (tropical) R16.1
  with hepatomegaly R16.2
  cirrhotic D73.2
  congenital Q89.09
  congestive, chronic D73.2
  Egyptian B65.1
  Gaucher's E75.22
  malarial - *see also* Malaria B54 [*D77*]
  neutropenic D73.81
  Niemann-pick - *see* Niemann-pick disease or
    syndrome
  siderotic D73.2
  syphilitic A52.79
    congenital (early) A50.08 [*D77*]
Splenopathy D73.9
Splenoptosis D73.89
Splenosis D73.89
Splinter - *see* Foreign body, superficial, by site
Split, splitting
  foot Q72.7-
  hand Q71.6
  heart sounds R01.2
  lip, congenital - *see* Cleft, lip
  nails L60.3
  urinary stream R39.13
Spondylarthrosis - *see* Spondylosis
Spondylitis (chronic) - *see also*
  Spondylopathy, inflammatory ankylopoietica
  - *see* Spondylitis, ankylosing
  ankylosing (chronic) M45.9
    with lung involvement M45.9 [*J99*]
    cervical region M45.2
    cervicothoracic region M45.3
    juvenile M08.1
    lumbar region M45.6

Spondylitis - *continued*
  lumbosacral region M45.7
  multiple sites M45.0
  occipito-atlanto-axial region M45.1
  sacrococcygeal region M45.8
  thoracic region M45.4
  thoracolumbar region M45.5
  atrophic (ligamentous) - *see* Spondylitis,
    ankylosing
  deformans (chronic) - *see* Spondylosis
  gonococcal A54.41
  gouty - *see also* Gout, by type, vertebrae
    M10.08
  in (due to)
    brucellosis A23.9 [*M49.80*]
      cervical region A23.9 [*M49.82*]
      cervicothoracic region A23.9 [*M49.83*]
      lumbar region A23.9 [*M49.86*]
      lumbosacral region A23.9 [*M49.87*]
      multiple sites A23.9 [*M49.89*]
      occipito-atlanto-axial region A23.9
        [*M49.81*]
      sacrococcygeal region A23.9 [*M49.88*]
      thoracic region A23.9 [*M49.84*]
      thoracolumbar region A23.9 [*M49.85*]
    enterobacteria - *see also* subcategory M49.8
      A04.9
    tuberculosis A18.01
  infectious NEC - *see* Spondylopathy, infective
  juvenile ankylosing (chronic) M08.1
  Kümmell's - *see* Spondylopathy, traumatic
  Marie-Strümpell - *see* Spondylitis, ankylosing
  muscularis - *see* Spondylopathy, specified
    NEC
  psoriatic L40.53
  rheumatoid - *see* Spondylitis, ankylosing
  rhizomelica - *see* Spondylitis, ankylosing
  sacroiliac NEC M46.1
  senescent, senile - *see* Spondylosis
  traumatic (chronic) or post-traumatic - *see*
    Spondylopathy, traumatic
  tuberculous A18.01
  typhosa A01.05
Spondylolisthesis (acquired) (degenerative)
  M43.10
  with disproportion (fetopelvic) O33.0
    causing obstructed labor O65.0
  cervical region M43.12
  cervicothoracic region M43.13
  congenital Q76.2
  lumbar region M43.16
  lumbosacral region M43.17
  multiple sites M43.19
  occipito-atlanto-axial region M43.11
  sacrococcygeal region M43.18
  thoracic region M43.14
  thoracolumbar region M43.15
  traumatic (old) M43.10
    acute
      fifth cervical (displaced) S12.430
        nondisplaced S12.431
        specified type NEC (displaced) S12.450
          nondisplaced S12.451
        type III S12.44
      fourth cervical (displaced) S12.330
        nondisplaced S12.331
        specified type NEC (displaced) S12.350
          nondisplaced S12.351
        type III S12.34
      second cervical (displaced) S12.130
        nondisplaced S12.131
        specified type NEC (displaced) S12.150
          nondisplaced S12.151
        type III S12.14

Spondylolisthesis - *continued*
  seventh cervical (displaced) S12.630
    nondisplaced S12.631
    specified type NEC (displaced) S12.650
      nondisplaced S12.651
    type III S12.64
  sixth cervical (displaced) S12.530
    nondisplaced S12.531
    specified type NEC (displaced) S12.550
      nondisplaced S12.551
    type III S12.54
  third cervical (displaced) S12.230
    nondisplaced S12.231
    specified type NEC (displaced) S12.250
      nondisplaced S12.251
    type III S12.24
Spondylolysis (acquired) M43.00
  cervical region M43.02
  cervicothoracic region M43.03
  congenital Q76.2
  lumbar region M43.06
  lumbosacral region M43.07
    with disproportion (fetopelvic) O33.0
      causing obstructed labor O65.8
  multiple sites M43.09
  occipito-atlanto-axial region M43.01
  sacrococcygeal region M43.08
  thoracic region M43.04
  thoracolumbar region M43.05
Spondylopathy M48.9
  infective NEC M46.50
    cervical region M46.52
    cervicothoracic region M46.53
    lumbar region M46.56
    lumbosacral region M46.57
    multiple sites M46.59
    occipito-atlanto-axial region M46.51
    sacrococcygeal region M46.58
    thoracic region M46.54
    thoracolumbar region M46.55
  inflammatory M46.90
    cervical region M46.92
    cervicothoracic region M46.93
    lumbar region M46.96
    lumbosacral region M46.97
    multiple sites M46.99
    occipito-atlanto-axial region M46.91
    sacrococcygeal region M46.98
    specified type NEC M46.80
      cervical region M46.82
      cervicothoracic region M46.83
      lumbar region M46.86
      lumbosacral region M46.87
      multiple sites M46.89
      occipito-atlanto-axial region M46.81
      sacrococcygeal region M46.88
      thoracic region M46.84
      thoracolumbar region M46.85
    thoracic region M46.94
    thoracolumbar region M46.95
  neuropathic, in
    syringomyelia and syringobulbia G95.0
    tabes dorsalis A52.11
  specified NEC - *see* subcategory M48.8
  traumatic M48.30
    cervical region M48.32
    cervicothoracic region M48.33
    lumbar region M48.36
    lumbosacral region M48.37
    occipito-atlanto-axial region M48.31
    sacrococcygeal region M48.38
    thoracic region M48.34
    thoracolumbar region M48.35

Spondylosis M47.9
  with
    disproportion (fetopelvic) O33.0
      causing obstructed labor O65.0
    myelopathy NEC M47.10
      cervical region M47.12
      cervicothoracic region M47.13
      lumbar region M47.16
      occipito-atlanto-axial region M47.11
      thoracic region M47.14
      thoracolumbar region M47.15
    radiculopathy M47.20
      cervical region M47.22
      cervicothoracic region M47.23
      lumbar region M47.26
      lumbosacral region M47.27
      occipito-atlanto-axial region M47.21
      sacrococcygeal region M47.28
      thoracic region M47.24
      thoracolumbar region M47.25
  specified NEC M47.899
    cervical region M47.892
    cervicothoracic region M47.893
    lumbar region M47.896
    lumbosacral region M47.897
    occipito-atlanto-axial region M47.891
    sacrococcygeal region M47.898
    thoracic region M47.894
    thoracolumbar region M47.895
  traumatic - *see* Spondylopathy, traumatic
  without myelopathy or radiculopathy M47.819
    cervical region M47.812
    cervicothoracic region M47.813
    lumbar region M47.816
    lumbosacral region M47.817
    occipito-atlanto-axial region M47.811
    sacrococcygeal region M47.818
    thoracic region M47.814
    thoracolumbar region M47.815
Sponge
  inadvertently left in operation wound - *see*
    Foreign body, accidentally left during a
    procedure
  kidney (medullary) Q61.5
Sponge-diver's disease - *see* Toxicity, venom,
  marine animal, sea anemone
Spongioblastoma (any type) - *see* Neoplasm,
  malignant, by site
  specified site - *see* Neoplasm, malignant, by
    site
  unspecified site C71.9
Spongioneuroblastoma - *see* Neoplasm,
  malignant, by site
Spontaneous - *see also* condition
  fracture (cause unknown) - *see* Fracture,
    pathological S
poon nail L60.3
  congenital Q84.6
Sporadic - *see* condition
Sporothrix schenckii infection - *see*
  Sporotrichosis
Sporotrichosis B42.9
  arthritis B42.82
  disseminated B42.7
  generalized B42.7
  lymphocutaneous (fixed) (progressive) B42.1
  pulmonary B42.0
  specified NEC B42.89
Spots, spotting (in) (of)
  Bitot's - *see also* Pigmentation, conjunctiva
    in the young child E50.1
    vitamin A deficiency E50.1
  café, au lait L81.3
  Cayenne pepper I78.1

Spots, spotting - *continued*
  cotton wool, retina - *see* Occlusion, artery, retina
  de Morgan's (senile angiomas) I78.1
  Fuchs' black (myopic) (see also Myopia, degenerative) H44.2-
  intermenstrual (regular) N92.0
    irregular N92.1
  Koplik's B05.9
  liver L81.4
  pregnancy O26.85-
  purpuric R23.3
  ruby I78.1
Spotted fever - *see* Fever, spotted N92.3
Sprain (joint) (ligament)
  acromioclavicular joint or ligament S43.5-
  ankle S93.40-
    calcaneofibular ligament S93.41-
    deltoid ligament S93.42-
    internal collateral ligament - *see* Sprain, ankle, specified ligament NEC
    specified ligament NEC S93.49-
    talofibular ligament - *see* Sprain, ankle, specified ligament NEC
    tibiofibular ligament S93.43-
  anterior longitudinal, cervical S13.4
  atlas, atlanto-axial, atlanto-occipital S13.4
  breast bone - *see* Sprain, sternum
  calcaneofibular - *see* Sprain, ankle
  carpal - *see* Sprain, wrist
  carpometacarpal - *see* Sprain, hand, specified site NEC
  cartilage
    costal S23.41
    semilunar (knee) - *see* Sprain, knee, specified site NEC
      with current tear - *see* Tear, meniscus
    thyroid region S13.5
    xiphoid - *see* Sprain, sternum
  cervical, cervicodorsal, cervicothoracic S13.4
  chondrosternal S23.421
  coracoclavicular S43.8-
  coracohumeral S43.41-
  coronary, knee - *see* Sprain, knee, specified site NEC
  costal cartilage S23.41
  cricoarytenoid articulation or ligament S13.5
  cricothyroid articulation S13.5
  cruciate, knee - *see* Sprain, knee, cruciate
  deltoid, ankle - *see* Sprain, ankle
  dorsal (spine) S23.3
  elbow S53.40-
    radial collateral ligament S53.43-
    radiohumeral S53.41-
    rupture
      radial collateral ligament - *see* Rupture, traumatic, ligament, radial collateral
      ulnar collateral ligament - *see* Rupture, traumatic, ligament, ulnar collateral
    specified type NEC S53.49-
    ulnar collateral ligament S53.44-
    ulnohumeral S53.42-
  femur, head - *see* Sprain, hip
  fibular collateral, knee - *see* Sprain, knee, collateral
  fibulocalcaneal - *see* Sprain, ankle
  finger(s) S63.61-
    index S63.61-
    interphalangeal (joint) S63.63-
      index S63.63-
      little S63.63-
      middle S63.63
      ring S63.63-
    little S63.61-

Sprain - *continued*
  middle S63.61-
  ring S63.61-
  metacarpophalangeal (joint) S63.65-
  specified site NEC S63.69-
    index S63.69-
    little S63.69-
    middle S63.69-
    ring S63.69-
  foot S93.60-
    specified ligament NEC S93.69-
    tarsal ligament S93.61-
    tarsometatarsal ligament S93.62-
    toe - *see* Sprain, toe
  hand S63.9-
    finger - *see* Sprain, finger
    specified site NEC - *see* subcategory S63.8
    thumb - *see* Sprain, thumb
  head S03.9
  hip S73.10-
    iliofemoral ligament S73.11-
    ischiocapsular (ligament) S73.12-
    specified NEC S73.19-
  iliofemoral - *see* Sprain, hip
  innominate
    acetabulum - *see* Sprain, hip
    sacral junction S33.6
  internal
    collateral, ankle - *see* Sprain, ankle
    semilunar cartilage - *see* Sprain, knee, specified site NEC
  interphalangeal
    finger - *see* Sprain, finger, interphalangeal (joint)
    toe - *see* Sprain, toe, interphalangeal joint
  ischiocapsular - *see* Sprain, hip
  ischiofemoral - *see* Sprain, hip
  jaw (articular disc) (cartilage) (meniscus) S03.4-
    old M26.69
  knee S83.9-
    collateral ligament S83.40-
      lateral (fibular) S83.42-
      medial (tibial) S83.41-
    cruciate ligament S83.50-
      anterior S83.51-
      posterior S83.52-
    lateral (fibular) collateral ligament S83.42-
    medial (tibial) collateral ligament S83.41-
    patellar ligament S76.11-
    specified site NEC S83.8X-
    superior tibiofibular joint (ligament) S83.6-
  lateral collateral, knee - *see* Sprain, knee, collateral
  lumbar (spine) S33.5
  lumbosacral S33.9
  mandible (articular disc) S03.4-
    old M26.69
  medial collateral, knee - *see* Sprain, knee, collateral
  meniscus
    jaw S03.4-
      old M26.69
    knee - *see* Sprain, knee, specified site NEC
      with current tear - *see* Tear, meniscus
      old - *see* Derangement, knee, meniscus, due to old tear
  mandible S03.4-
    old M26.69
  metacarpal (distal) (proximal) - *see* Sprain, hand, specified site NEC
  metacarpophalangeal - *see* Sprain, finger, metacarpophalangeal (joint)
  metatarsophalangeal - *see* Sprain, toe,

Sprain - *continued*
  metatarsophalangeal joint
  midcarpal - *see* Sprain, hand, specified site NEC
  midtarsal - *see* Sprain, foot, specified site NEC
  neck S13.9
    anterior longitudinal cervical ligament S13.4
    atlanto-axial joint S13.4
    atlanto-occipital joint S13.4
    cervical spine S13.4
    cricoarytenoid ligament S13.5
    cricothyroid ligament S13.5
    specified site NEC S13.8
    thyroid region (cartilage) S13.5
  nose S03.8
  orbicular, hip - *see* Sprain, hip
  patella - *see* Sprain, knee, specified site NEC
  patellar ligament S76.11-
  pelvis NEC S33.8
  phalanx
    finger - *see* Sprain, finger
    toe - *see* Sprain, toe
  pubofemoral - *see* Sprain, hip
  radiocarpal - *see* Sprain, wrist
  radiohumeral - *see* Sprain, elbow
  radius, collateral - *see* Rupture, traumatic, ligament, radial collateral
  rib (cage) S23.41
  rotator cuff (capsule) S43.42-
  sacroiliac (region)
    chronic or old - *see* subcategory M53.2
    joint S33.6
  scaphoid (hand) - *see* Sprain, hand, specified site NEC
  scapula (r) - *see* Sprain, shoulder girdle, specified site NEC
  semilunar cartilage (knee) - *see* Sprain, knee, specified site NEC
    with current tear - *see* Tear, meniscus
    old - *see* Derangement, knee, meniscus, due to old tear
  shoulder joint S43.40-
    acromioclavicular joint (ligament) - *see* Sprain, acromioclavicular joint
    blade - *see* Sprain, shoulder, girdle, specified site NEC
    coracoclavicular joint (ligament) - *see* Sprain, coracoclavicular joint
    coracohumeral ligament - *see* Sprain, coracohumeral joint
    girdle S43.9-
      specified site NEC S43.8-
    rotator cuff - *see* Sprain, rotator cuff
    specified site NEC S43.49-
    sternoclavicular joint (ligament) - *see* Sprain, sternoclavicular joint
  spine
    cervical S13.4
    lumbar S33.5
    thoracic S23.3
  sternoclavicular joint S43.6-
  sternum S23.429
    chondrosternal joint S23.421
    specified site NEC S23.428
    sternoclavicular (joint) (ligament) S23.420
  symphysis
    jaw S03.4-
      old M26.69
    mandibular S03.4-
      old M26.69
  talofibular - *see* Sprain, ankle
  tarsal - *see* Sprain, foot, specified site NEC
  tarsometatarsal - *see* Sprain, foot, specified site NEC

Sprain - *continued*
  temporomandibular S03.4-
    old M26.69
  thorax S23.9
    ribs S23.41
    specified site NEC S23.8
    spine S23.3
    sternum - *see* Sprain, sternum
  thumb S63.60-
    interphalangeal (joint) S63.62-
    metacarpophalangeal (joint) S63.64-
    specified site NEC S63.68-
  thyroid cartilage or region S13.5
  tibia (proximal end) - *see* Sprain, knee,
    specified site NEC
  tibial collateral, knee - *see* Sprain, knee,
    collateral
  tibiofibular
    distal - *see* Sprain, ankle
    superior - *see* Sprain, knee, specified site
      NEC
  toe(s) S93.50-
    great S93.50-
      interphalangeal joint S93.51-
        great S93.51-
        lesser S93.51-
      lesser S93.50-
      metatarsophalangeal joint S93.52-
        great S93.52-
        lesser S93.52-
  ulna, collateral - *see* Rupture, traumatic,
    ligament, ulnar collateral
  ulnohumeral - *see* Sprain, elbow
  wrist S63.50-
    carpal S63.51-
    radiocarpal S63.52-
    specified site NEC S63.59-
  xiphoid cartilage - *see* Sprain, sternum
Sprengel's deformity (congenital) Q74.0
Sprue (tropical) K90.1
  celiac K90.0
  idiopathic K90.49
  meaning thrush B37.0
  nontropical K90.0
Spur, bone - *see also* Enthesopathy
  calcaneal M77.3-
  iliac crest M76.2-
  nose (septum) J34.89
Spurway's syndrome Q78.0
Sputum
  abnormal (amount) (color) (odor) (purulent)
    R09.3
  blood-stained R04.2
  excessive (cause unknown) R09.3
Squamous - *see also* condition
  epithelium in
    cervical canal (congenital) Q51.828
    uterine mucosa (congenital) Q51.818
Squashed nose M95.0
  congenital Q67.4
Squeeze, diver's T70.3
Squint - *see also* Strabismus
  accommodative - *see* Strabismus, convergent
  concomitant
St. Hubert's disease A82.9
Stab - *see also* Laceration
  internal organs - *see* Injury, by site
Stafne's cyst or cavity M27.0
Staggering gait R26.0
  hysterical F44.4
Staghorn calculus - *see* Calculus, kidney
Stähli's line (cornea) (pigment) - *see*
  Pigmentation, cornea, anterior

Stain, staining
  meconium (newborn) P96.83
  port wine Q82.5
  tooth, teeth (hard tissues) (extrinsic) K03.6
    due to
      accretions K03.6
      deposits (betel) (black) (green) (materia
        alba) (orange) (soft) (tobacco) K03.6
      metals (copper) (silver) K03.7
      nicotine K03.6
      pulpal bleeding K03.7
      tobacco K03.6
    intrinsic K00.8
Stammering - *see also* Disorder, fluency
  F80.81
Standstill
  auricular I45.5
  cardiac - *see* Arrest, cardiac   sinoatrial I45.5
  ventricular - *see* Arrest, cardiac
Stannosis J63.5
Stanton's disease - *see* Melioidosis
Staphylitis (acute) (catarrhal) (chronic)
  (gangrenous) (membranous) (suppurative)
  (ulcerative) K12.2
Staphylococcal scalded skin syndrome L00
Staphylococcemia A41.2
Staphylococcus, staphylococcal - *see also*
  condition
  as cause of disease classified elsewhere B95.8
    aureus (methicillin susceptible) (MSSA)
      B95.61
      methicillin resistant (MRSA) B95.62
    specified NEC, as cause of disease classified
      elsewhere B95.7
Staphyloma (sclera)
  cornea H18.72-
  equatorial H15.81-
  localized (anterior) H15.82-
  posticum H15.83-
  ring H15.85-
Stargardt's disease - *see* Dystrophy, retina
Starvation (inanition) (due to lack of food)
  T73.0
  edema - *see* Malnutrition, severe
Stasis
  bile (noncalculous) K83.1
  bronchus J98.09
    with infection - *see* Bronchitis
  cardiac - *see* Failure, heart, congestive
  cecum K59.8
  colon K59.8
  dermatitis I87.2
    with
      varicose ulcer - *see* Varix, leg, with ulcer,
        with inflammation
      varicose veins - *see* Varix, leg, with,
        inflammation
    due to postthrombotic syndrome - *see*
      Syndrome, postthrombotic
  duodenal K31.5
  eczema - *see* Varix, leg, with, inflammation
  edema - *see* Hypertension, venous (chronic),
    idiopathic
  foot T69.0-
  ileocecal coil K59.8
  ileum K59.8
  intestinal K59.8
  jejunum K59.8
  kidney N19
  liver (cirrhotic) K76.1
  lymphatic I89.8
  pneumonia J18.2
  pulmonary - *see* Edema, lung
  rectal K59.8

Stasis - *continued*
  renal N19
    tubular N17.0
  ulcer - *see* Varix, leg, with, ulcer
    without varicose veins I87.2
  urine - *see* Retention, urine
  venous I87.8
State (of)
  affective and paranoid, mixed, organic
    psychotic F06.8
  agitated R45.1
    acute reaction to stress F43.0
  anxiety (neurotic) F41.1
  apprehension F41.1
  burn-out Z73.0
  climacteric, female Z78.0
    symptomatic N95.1
  compulsive F42.8
    mixed with obsessional thoughts F42.2
  confusional (psychogenic) F44.89
    acute - *see also* Delirium
      with
        arteriosclerotic dementia F01.50
          with behavioral disturbance F01.51
        senility or dementia F05
    alcoholic F10.231
    epileptic F05
    reactive (from emotional stress,
  psychological trauma) F44.89
    subacute - *see* Delirium
  convulsive - *see* Convulsions
  crisis F43.0
  depressive F32.9
    neurotic F34.1
  dissociative F44.9
  emotional shock (stress) R45.7
  hypercoagulation - *see* Hypercoagulable
  locked-in G83.5
  menopausal Z78.0
    symptomatic N95.1
  neurotic F48.9
    with depersonalization F48.1
  obsessional F42.8
  oneiroid (schizophrenia-like) F23
  organic
    hallucinatory (nonalcoholic) F06.0
    paranoid (-hallucinatory) F06.2
  panic F41.0
  paranoid F22
    climacteric F22
    involutional F22
    menopausal F22
    organic F06.2
    senile F03
    simple F22
  persistent vegetative R40.3
  phobic F40.9
  postleukotomy F07.0
  pregnant
    gestational carrier Z33.3
    incidental Z33.1
  psychogenic, twilight F44.89
  psychopathic (constitutional) F60.2
  psychotic, organic - *see also* Psychosis,
    organic
    mixed paranoid and affective F06.8
    senile or presenile F03
    transient NEC F06.8
      with
        hallucinations F06.0
        depression F06.31
  residual schizophrenic F20.5
  restlessness R45.1
  stress (emotional) R45.7

State (of) - *continued*
tension (mental) F48.9
  specified NEC F48.8
transient organic psychotic NEC F06.8
  depressive type F06.31
  hallucinatory type F06.0
twilight
  epileptic F05
  psychogenic F44.89
vegetative, persistent R40.3
vital exhaustion Z73.0
withdrawal, - *see* Withdrawal, state
Status (post) - *see also* Presence (of)
absence, epileptic - *see* Epilepsy, by type, with
  status epilepticus
administration of tPA (rtPA) in a different
  facility within the last 24 hours prior to
  admission to current facility Z92.82
adrenalectomy (unilateral) (bilateral) E89.6
anastomosis Z98.0
angioplasty (peripheral) Z98.62
  with implant Z95.820
  coronary artery Z98.61
    with implant Z95.5
anginosus I20.9
aortocoronary bypass Z95.1
arthrodesis Z98.1
artificial opening (of) Z93.9
  gastrointestinal tract Z93.4
  specified NEC Z93.8
  urinary tract Z93.6
  vagina Z93.8
asthmaticus - *see* Asthma, by type, with status
  asthmaticus
awaiting organ transplant Z76.82
bariatric surgery Z98.84
bed confinement Z74.01
bleb, filtering (vitreous), after glaucoma
  surgery Z98.83
breast implant Z98.82
  removal Z98.86
cataract extraction Z98.4-
cholecystectomy Z90.49
clitorectomy N90.811
  with excision of labia minora N90.812
colectomy (complete) (partial) Z90.49
colonization - *see* Carrier (suspected) of
colostomy Z93.3
convulsivus idiopathicus - *see* Epilepsy, by
  type, with status epilepticus
coronary artery angioplasty - *see* Status,
  angioplasty, coronary artery
coronary artery bypass graft Z95.1
cystectomy (urinary bladder) Z90.6
cystostomy Z93.50
  appendico-vesicostomy Z93.52
  cutaneous Z93.51
  specified NEC Z93.59
delinquent immunization Z28.3
dental Z98.818
  crown Z98.811
  fillings Z98.811
  restoration Z98.811
  sealant Z98.810
  specified NEC Z98.818
deployment (current) (military) Z56.82
dialysis (hemodialysis) (peritoneal) Z99.2
do not resuscitate (DNR) Z66
donor - *see* Donor
embedded fragments - *see* Retained, foreign
  body fragments (type of)
embedded splinter - *see* Retained, foreign body
  fragments (type of)
enterostomy Z93.4

Status (post) - *continued*
epileptic, epilepticus - *see also* Epilepsy, by
  type, with status epilepticus G40.901
estrogen receptor
  negative Z17.1
  positive Z17.0
female genital cutting - *see* Female genital
  mutilation status
female genital mutilation - *see* Female genital
  mutilation status
filtering (vitreous) bleb after glaucoma surgery
  Z98.83
gastrectomy (complete) (partial) Z90.3
gastric banding Z98.84
gastric bypass for obesity Z98.84
gastrostomy Z93.1
human immunodeficiency virus (HIV)
  infection, asymptomatic Z21
hysterectomy (complete) (total) Z90.710
  partial (with remaining cervical stump)
    Z90.711
ileostomy Z93.2
implant
  breast Z98.82
infibulation N90.813
intestinal bypass Z98.0
jejunostomy Z93.4
laryngectomy Z90.02
lapsed immunization schedule Z28.3
lymphaticus E32.8
malignancy
  castrate resistant prostate Z19.2
  hormone resistant Z19.2
  hormone sensitive Z19.1
marmoratus G80.3
mastectomy (unilateral) (bilateral) Z90.1-
military deployment status (current) Z56.82
  in theater or in support of military war,
    peacekeeping and humanitarian operations
    Z56.82
nephrectomy (unilateral) (bilateral) Z90.5
nephrostomy Z93.6
obesity surgery Z98.84
oophorectomy
  bilateral Z90.722
  unilateral Z90.721
organ replacement
  by artificial or mechanical device or
    prosthesis of
    artery Z95.828
    bladder Z96.0
    blood vessel Z95.828
    breast Z97.8
    eye globe Z97.0
    heart Z95.812
      valve Z95.2
    intestine Z97.8
    joint Z96.60
      hip - *see* Presence, hip joint implant
      knee - *see* Presence, knee joint implant
      specified site NEC Z96.698
    kidney Z97.8
    larynx Z96.3
    lens Z96.1
    limbs - *see* Presence, artificial, limb
    liver Z97.8
    lung Z97.8
    pancreas Z97.8
  by organ transplant
    (heterologous)(homologous) - *see* Transplant
pacemaker
  brain Z96.89
  cardiac Z95.0
  specified NEC Z96.89

Status (post) - *continued*
pancreatectomy Z90.410
  complete Z90.410
  partial Z90.411
  total Z90.410
physical restraint Z78.1
pneumonectomy (complete) (partial) Z90.2
pneumothorax, therapeutic Z98.3
postcommotio cerebri F07.81
postoperative (postprocedural) NEC Z98.890
  breast implant Z98.82
  dental Z98.818
    crown Z98.811
    fillings Z98.811
    restoration Z98.811
    sealant Z98.810
    specified NEC Z98.818
  uterine scar Z98.891
  pneumothorax, therapeutic Z98.3
postpartum (routine follow-up) Z39.2
  care immediately after delivery Z39.0
postsurgical (postprocedural) NEC Z98.890
  pneumothorax, therapeutic Z98.3
pregnancy, incidental Z33.1
prosthesis coronary angioplasty Z95.5
pseudophakia Z96.1
renal dialysis (hemodialysis) (peritoneal)
  Z99.2
retained foreign body - *see* Retained, foreign
  body fragments (type of)
reversed jejunal transposition (for bypass)
  Z98.0
salpingo-oophorectomy
  bilateral Z90.722
  unilateral Z90.721
sex reassignment surgery status Z87.890
shunt
  arteriovenous (for dialysis) Z99.2
  cerebrospinal fluid Z98.2
  ventricular (communicating) (for drainage)
    Z98.2
splenectomy Z90.81
thymicolymphaticus E32.8
thymicus E32.8
thymolymphaticus E32.8
thyroidectomy (hypothyroidism) E89.0
tooth (teeth) extraction - *see also* Absence,
  teeth, acquired K08.409
tPA (rtPA) administration in a different facility
  within the last 24 hours prior to admission to
  current facility Z92.82
tracheostomy Z93.0
transplant - *see* Transplant
  organ removed Z98.85
tubal ligation Z98.51
underimmunization Z28.3
ureterostomy Z93.6
urethrostomy Z93.6
vagina, artificial Z93.8
vasectomy Z98.52
wheelchair confinement Z99.3
Stealing
child problem F91.8
  in company with others Z72.810
pathological (compulsive) F63.2
Steam burn - *see* Burn
Steatocystoma multiplex L72.2
Steatohepatitis (nonalcoholic) (NASH)
  K75.81
Steatoma L72.3
eyelid (cystic) - *see* Dermatosis, eyelid
  infected - *see* Hordeolum
Steatorrhea (chronic) K90.9
with lacteal obstruction K90.2

Steatorrhea - *continued*
  idiopathic (adult) (infantile) K90.9
  pancreatic K90.3
  primary K90.0
  tropical K90.1
Steatosis E88.89
  heart - *see* Degeneration, myocardial
  kidney N28.89
  liver NEC K76.0
**Steele-Richardson-Olszewski disease or
  syndrome** G23.1
Steinbrocker's syndrome G90.8
Steinert's disease G71.11
Stein-Leventhal syndrome E28.2
Stein's syndrome E28.2
STEMI - *see also* Infarct, myocardium, ST
  elevation I21.3
Stenocardia I20.8
Stenocephaly Q75.8
Stenosis, stenotic (cicatricial) - *see also*
  Stricture
  ampulla of Vater K83.1
  anus, anal (canal) (sphincter) K62.4
    and rectum K62.4
    congenital Q42.3
      with fistula Q42.2
  aorta (ascending) (supraventricular)
    (congenital) Q25.1
    arteriosclerotic I70.0
    calcified I70.0
    supravalvular Q25.3
  aortic (valve) I35.0
    with insufficiency I35.2
    congenital Q23.0
    rheumatic I06.0
      with
        incompetency, insufficiency or
          regurgitation I06.2
          with mitral (valve) disease I08.0
            with tricuspid (valve) disease I08.3
          mitral (valve) disease I08.0
            with tricuspid (valve) disease I08.3
          tricuspid (valve) disease I08.2
            with mitral (valve) disease I08.3
      specified cause NEC I35.0
      syphilitic A52.03
  aqueduct of Sylvius (congenital) Q03.0
    with spina bifida - *see* Spina bifida, by site,
      with hydrocephalus
    acquired G91.1
  artery NEC - *see also* Arteriosclerosis I77.1
    celiac I77.4
    cerebral - *see* Occlusion, artery, cerebral
    extremities - *see* Arteriosclerosis, extremities
    precerebral - *see* Occlusion, artery,
      precerebral
    pulmonary (congenital) Q25.6
      acquired I28.8
    renal I70.1
    stent
      coronary T82.855
      peripheral T82.856
  bile duct (common) (hepatic) K83.1
    congenital Q44.3
  bladder neck (acquired) N32.0
    congenital Q64.31
  brain G93.89
  bronchus J98.09
    congenital Q32.3
    syphilitic A52.72
  cardia (stomach) K22.2
    congenital Q39.3
  cardiovascular - *see* Disease, cardiovascular
  caudal M48.08

Stenosis, stenotic - *continued*
  cervix, cervical (canal) N88.2
    congenital Q51.828
    in pregnancy or childbirth - *see* Pregnancy,
      complicated by, abnormal cervix
  colon - *see also* Obstruction, intestine
    congenital Q42.9
      specified NEC Q42.8
  colostomy K94.03
  common (bile) duct K83.1
    congenital Q44.3
  coronary (artery) - *see* Disease, heart,
    ischemic, atherosclerotic
  cystic duct - *see* Obstruction, gallbladder
  due to presence of device, implant or graft -
    see also Complications, by site and type,
  specified NEC T85.858
    arterial graft NEC T82.858
    breast (implant) T85.858
    catheter T85.858
      dialysis (renal) T82.858
        intraperitoneal T85.858
      infusion NEC T82.858
        spinal (epidural) (subdural) T85.850
      urinary (indwelling) T83.85
    fixation, internal (orthopedic) NEC T84.85
    gastrointestinal (bile duct) (esophagus)
      T85.858
    genital NEC T83.85
    heart NEC T82.857
    joint prosthesis T84.85
    ocular (corneal graft) (orbital implant) NEC
      T85.858
    orthopedic NEC T84.85
    specified NEC T85.858
    urinary NEC T83.85
    vascular NEC T82.858
    ventricular intracranial shunt T85.850
  duodenum K31.5
    congenital Q41.0
  ejaculatory duct NEC N50.89
  endocervical os - *see* Stenosis, cervix
  enterostomy K94.13
  esophagus K22.2
    congenital Q39.3
    syphilitic A52.79
      congenital A50.59 [K23]
  eustachian tube - *see* Obstruction, eustachian
  tube   external ear canal (acquired) H61.30-
    congenital Q16.1
    due to
      inflammation H61.32-
      trauma H61.31-
    postprocedural H95.81-
    specified cause NEC H61.39-
  gallbladder - *see* Obstruction, gallbladder
  glottis J38.6
  heart valve (congenital) Q24.8
    aortic Q23.0
    mitral Q23.2
    pulmonary Q22.1
    tricuspid Q22.4
  hepatic duct K83.1
  hymen N89.6
  hypertrophic subaortic (idiopathic) I42.1
  ileum (see also Obstruction, intestine,
  specified NEC) K56.699
    congenital Q41.2
  infundibulum cardia Q24.3
  intervertebral foramina - *see also* Lesion,
  biomechanical, specified NEC
    connective tissue M99.79
      abdomen M99.79
      cervical region M99.71

Stenosis, stenotic - *continued*
    cervicothoracic M99.71
    head region M99.70
    lumbar region M99.73
    lumbosacral M99.73
    occipitocervical M99.70
    sacral region M99.74
    sacrococcygeal M99.74
    sacroiliac M99.74
    specified NEC M99.79
    thoracic region M99.72
    thoracolumbar M99.72
  disc M99.79
    abdomen M99.79
    cervical region M99.71
    cervicothoracic M99.71
    head region M99.70
    lower extremity M99.76
    lumbar region M99.73
    lumbosacral M99.73
    occipitocervical M99.70
    pelvic M99.75
    rib cage M99.78
    sacral region M99.74
    sacrococcygeal M99.74
    sacroiliac M99.74
    specified NEC M99.79
    thoracic region M99.72
    thoracolumbar M99.72
    upper extremity M99.77
  osseous M99.69
    abdomen M99.69
    cervical region M99.61
    cervicothoracic M99.61
    head region M99.60
    lower extremity M99.66
    lumbar region M99.63
    lumbosacral M99.63
    occipitocervical M99.60
    pelvic M99.65
    rib cage M99.68
    sacral region M99.64
    sacrococcygeal M99.64
    sacroiliac M99.64
    specified NEC M99.69
    thoracic region M99.62
    thoracolumbar M99.62
    upper extremity M99.67
  subluxation - *see* Stenosis, intervertebral
  foramina, osseous
  intestine - *see also* Obstruction, intestine
    congenital (small) Q41.9
      large Q42.9
        specified NEC Q42.8
      specified NEC Q41.8
  jejunum (see also Obstruction, intestine,
  specified NEC) K56.699
    congenital Q41.1
  lacrimal (passage)
    canaliculi H04.54-
    congenital Q10.5
    duct H04.55-
    punctum H04.56-
    sac H04.57-
  lacrimonasal duct - *see* Stenosis, lacrimal, duct
    congenital Q10.5
  larynx J38.6
    congenital NEC Q31.8
      subglottic Q31.1
    syphilitic A52.73
      congenital A50.59 [J99]
  mitral (chronic) (inactive) (valve) I05.0
    with
      aortic valve disease I08.0

Stenosis, stenotic - *continued*
  incompetency, insufficiency or
  regurgitation I05.2
   active or acute I01.1
    with rheumatic or Sydenham's chorea I02.0
   congenital Q23.2
   specified cause, except rheumatic I34.2
   syphilitic A52.03
  myocardium, myocardial - *see also*
   Degeneration, myocardial
   hypertrophic subaortic (idiopathic) I42.1
  nares (anterior) (posterior) J34.89
   congenital Q30.0
  nasal duct - *see also* Stenosis, lacrimal, duct
   congenital Q10.5
  nasolacrimal duct - *see also* Stenosis, lacrimal, duct
   congenital Q10.5
  neural canal - *see also* Lesion, biomechanical, specified NEC
   connective tissue M99.49
    abdomen M99.49
    cervical region M99.41
    cervicothoracic M99.41
    head region M99.40
    lower extremity M99.46
    lumbar region M99.43
    lumbosacral M99.43
    occipitocervical M99.40
    pelvic M99.45
    rib cage M99.48
    sacral region M99.44
    sacrococcygeal M99.44
    sacroiliac M99.44
    specified NEC M99.49
    thoracic region M99.42
    thoracolumbar M99.42
    upper extremity M99.47
   intervertebral disc M99.59
    abdomen M99.59
    cervical region M99.51
    cervicothoracic M99.51
    head region M99.50
    lower extremity M99.56
    lumbar region M99.53
    lumbosacral M99.53
    occipitocervical M99.50
    pelvic M99.55
    rib cage M99.58
    sacral region M99.54
    sacrococcygeal M99.54
    sacroiliac M99.54
    specified NEC M99.59
    thoracic region M99.52
    thoracolumbar M99.52
    upper extremity M99.57
   osseous M99.39
    abdomen M99.39
    cervical region M99.31
    cervicothoracic M99.31
    head region M99.30
    lower extremity M99.36
    lumbar region M99.33
    lumbosacral M99.33
    pelvic M99.35
    rib cage M99.38
    occipitocervical M99.30
    sacral region M99.34
    sacrococcygeal M99.34
    sacroiliac M99.34
    specified NEC M99.39
    thoracic region M99.32
    thoracolumbar M99.32
    upper extremity M99.37

Stenosis, stenotic - *continued*
  subluxation M99.29
   cervical region M99.21
   cervicothoracic M99.21
   head region M99.20
   lower extremity M99.26
   lumbar region M99.23
   lumbosacral M99.23
   occipitocervical M99.20
   pelvic M99.25
   rib cage M99.28
   sacral region M99.24
   sacrococcygeal M99.24
   sacroiliac M99.24
   specified NEC M99.29
   thoracic region M99.22
   thoracolumbar M99.22
   upper extremity M99.27
  organ or site, congenital NEC - *see* Atresia, by site
  papilla of Vater K83.1
  pulmonary (artery) (congenital) Q25.6
   with ventricular septal defect, transposition of aorta, and hypertrophy of right ventricle Q21.3
   acquired I28.8
   in tetralogy of Fallot Q21.3
   infundibular Q24.3
   subvalvular Q24.3
   supravalvular Q25.6
   valve I37.0
    with insufficiency I37.2
    congenital Q22.1
    rheumatic I09.89
     with aortic, mitral or tricuspid (valve) disease I08.8
   vein, acquired I28.8
   vessel NEC I28.8
  pulmonic (congenital) Q22.1
   infundibular Q24.3
   subvalvular Q24.3
  pylorus (hypertrophic) (acquired) K31.1
   adult K31.1
   congenital Q40.0
   infantile Q40.0
  rectum (sphincter) - *see* Stricture, rectum
  renal artery I70.1
   congenital Q27.1
  salivary duct (any) K11.8
  sphincter of Oddi K83.1
  spinal M48.00
   cervical region M48.02
   cervicothoracic region M48.03
   lumbar region M48.06
    lumbar region (NOS) (without neurogenic claudication) M48.061
    with neurogenic claudication M48.062
   occipito-atlanto-axial region M48.01
   sacrococcygeal region M48.08
   thoracic region M48.04
   thoracolumbar region M48.05
  stent
   vascular
    end stent
     adjacent to stent - *see* Arteriosclerosis
     within the stent
      coronary T82.855
      peripheral T82.856
    in stent
     coronary vessel T82.855
     peripheral vessel T82.856
  stomach, hourglass K31.2
  subaortic (congenital) Q24.4
   hypertrophic (idiopathic) I42.1

Stenosis, stenotic - *continued*
  subglottic J38.6
   congenital Q31.1
   postprocedural J95.5
  trachea J39.8
   congenital Q32.1
   syphilitic A52.73
   tuberculous NEC A15.5
  tracheostomy J95.03
  tricuspid (valve) I07.0
   with
    aortic (valve) disease I08.2
    incompetency, insufficiency or regurgitation I07.2
     with aortic (valve) disease I08.2
      with mitral (valve) disease I08.3
     mitral (valve) disease I08.1
      with aortic (valve) disease I08.3
   congenital Q22.4
   nonrheumatic I36.0
    with insufficiency I36.2
  tubal N97.1
  ureter - *see* Atresia, ureter
  ureteropelvic junction, congenital Q62.11
  ureterovesical orifice, congenital Q62.12
  urethra (valve) - *see also* Stricture, urethra
   congenital Q64.32
  urinary meatus, congenital Q64.33
  vagina N89.5
   congenital Q52.4
   in pregnancy - *see* Pregnancy, complicated by, abnormal vagina
    causing obstructed labor O65.5
  valve (cardiac) (heart) - *see also* Endocarditis I38
   congenital Q24.8
    aortic Q23.0
    mitral Q23.2
    pulmonary Q22.1
    tricuspid Q22.4
  vena cava (inferior) (superior) I87.1
   congenital Q26.0
  vesicourethral orifice Q64.31
  vulva N90.5
Stent jail T82.897
Stercolith (impaction) K56.41
  appendix K38.1
Stercoraceous, stercoral ulcer K63.3
  anus or rectum K62.6
Stereotypies NEC F98.4
Sterility - *see* Infertility
Sterilization - *see* Encounter (for), sterilization
Sternalgia - *see* Angina
Sternopagus Q89.4
Sternum bifidum Q76.7
Steroid
  effects (adverse) (adrenocortical) (iatrogenic)
   cushingoid E24.2
    correct substance properly administered - *see* Table of Drugs and Chemicals, by drug, adverse effect
    overdose or wrong substance given or taken - *see* Table of Drugs and Chemicals, by drug, poisoning
   diabetes - *see* category E09
    correct substance properly administered - *see* Table of Drugs and Chemicals, by drug, adverse effect
    overdose or wrong substance given or taken - *see* Table of Drugs and Chemicals, by drug, poisoning
   fever R50.2
   insufficiency E27.3

Steroid - *continued*
    correct substance properly administered - *see*
        Table of Drugs and Chemicals, by drug,
        adverse effect
    overdose or wrong substance given or taken
        - *see* Table of Drugs and Chemicals, by
        drug, poisoning
    responder H40.04-
Stevens-Johnson disease or syndrome L51.1
    toxic epidermal necrolysis overlap L51.3
Stewart-morel syndrome M85.2
Sticker's disease B08.3
Sticky eye - *see* Conjunctivitis, acute,
    mucopurulent
Stieda's disease - *see* Bursitis, tibial collateral
Stiff neck - *see* Torticollis
Stiff-man syndrome G25.82
Stiffness, joint NEC M25.60-
    ankle M25.67-
    ankylosis - *see* Ankylosis, joint
    contracture - *see* Contraction, joint
    elbow M25.62-
    foot M25.67-
    hand M25.64-
    hip M25.65-
    knee M25.66-
    shoulder M25.61-
    wrist M25.63-
Stigmata congenital syphilis A50.59
Stillbirth P95
Still-Felty syndrome - *see* Felty's syndrome
Still's disease or syndrome (juvenile) M08.20
    adult-onset M06.1
    ankle M08.27-
    elbow M08.22-
    foot joint M08.27-
    hand joint M08.24-
    hip M08.25-
    knee M08.26-
    multiple site M08.29
    shoulder M08.21-
    vertebra M08.28
    wrist M08.23-
Stimulation, ovary E28.1
**Sting (venomous) (with allergic or
    anaphylactic shock)** - *see* Table of Drugs and
    Chemicals, by animal or substance, poisoning
Stippled epiphyses Q78.8
Stitch
    abscess T81.4
    burst (in operation wound) - *see* Disruption,
    wound, operation
Stokes-Adams disease or syndrome I45.9
Stokes' disease E05.00
    with thyroid storm E05.01
Stokvis (-Talma) disease D74.8
Stoma malfunction
    colostomy K94.03
    enterostomy K94.13
    gastrostomy K94.23
    ileostomy K94.13
    tracheostomy J95.03
Stomach - *see* condition
Stomatitis (denture) (ulcerative) K12.1
    angular K13.0
        due to dietary or vitamin deficiency E53.0
    aphthous K12.0
    bovine B08.61
    candidal B37.0
    catarrhal K12.1
    diphtheritic A36.89
    due to
        dietary deficiency E53.0
        thrush B37.0

Stomatitis - *continued*
    vitamin deficiency
        B group NEC E53.9
        B2 (riboflavin) E53.0
    epidemic B08.8
    epizootic B08.8
    follicular K12.1
    gangrenous A69.0
    Geotrichum B48.3
    herpesviral, herpetic B00.2
    herpetiformis K12.0
    malignant K12.1
    membranous acute K12.1
    monilial B37.0
    mycotic B37.0
    necrotizing ulcerative A69.0
    parasitic B37.0
    septic K12.1
    spirochetal A69.1
    suppurative (acute) K12.2
    ulceromembranous A69.1
    vesicular K12.1
        with exanthem (enteroviral) B08.4
    virus disease A93.8
    Vincent's A69.1
Stomatocytosis D58.8
Stomatomycosis B37.0
Stomatorrhagia K13.79
Stone(s) - *see also* Calculus
    bladder (diverticulum) N21.0
    cystine E72.09
    heart syndrome I50.1
    kidney N20.0
    prostate N42.0
    pulpal (dental) K04.2
    renal N20.0
    salivary gland or duct (any) K11.5
    urethra (impacted) N21.1
    urinary (duct) (impacted) (passage) N20.9
        bladder (diverticulum) N21.0
        lower tract N21.9
        specified NEC N21.8
    xanthine E79.8 [N22]
Stonecutter's lung J62.8
**Stonemason's asthma, disease, lung or
    pneumoconiosis** J62.8
Stoppage
    heart - *see* Arrest, cardiac
    urine - *see* Retention, urine **Storm, thyroid** -
        see Thyrotoxicosis
Strabismus (congenital) (nonparalytic) H50.9
    concomitant H50.40
        convergent - *see* Strabismus, convergent
            concomitant
        divergent - *see* Strabismus, divergent
            concomitant
    convergent concomitant H50.00
        accommodative component H50.43
        alternating H50.05
            with
                A pattern H50.06
                specified nonconcomitances NEC H50.08
                V pattern H50.07
        monocular H50.01-
            with
                A pattern H50.02-
                specified nonconcomitances NEC H50.04-
                V pattern H50.03-
            intermittent H50.31-
                alternating H50.32
    cyclotropia H50.41
    divergent concomitant H50.10
        alternating H50.15
            with

Strabismus - *continued*
            A pattern H50.16
            specified noncomitances NEC H50.18
            V pattern H50.17
        monocular H50.11-
            with
                A pattern H50.12-
                specified noncomitances NEC H50.14-
                V pattern H50.13-
            intermittent H50.33
                alternating H50.34
    Duane's syndrome H50.81-
    due to adhesions, scars H50.69
    heterophoria H50.50
        alternating H50.55
        cyclophoria H50.54
        esophoria H50.51
        exophoria H50.52
        vertical H50.53
    heterotropia H50.40
        intermittent H50.30
    hypertropia H50.2-
    hypotropia - *see* Hypertropia
    latent H50.50
    mechanical H50.60
        Brown's sheath syndrome H50.61-
        specified type NEC H50.69
    monofixation syndrome H50.42
    paralytic H49.9
        abducens nerve H49.2-
        fourth nerve H49.1-
        Kearns-Sayre syndrome H49.81-
        ophthalmoplegia (external)
            progressive H49.4-
                with pigmentary retinopathy H49.81-
            total H49.3-
        sixth nerve H49.2-
        specified type NEC H49.88-
        third nerve H49.0-
        trochlear nerve H49.1-
    specified type NEC H50.89
    vertical H50.2-
Strain
    back S39.012
    cervical S16.1
    eye NEC - *see* Disturbance, vision, subjective
    heart - *see* Disease, heart
    low back S39.012
    mental NOS Z73.3
        work-related Z56.6
    muscle (tendon) - *see* Injury, muscle, by site,
        strain
    neck S16.1
    postural - *see also* Disorder, soft tissue, due to
        use
    physical NOS Z73.3
        work-related Z56.6
    psychological NEC Z73.3
    tendon - *see* Injury, muscle, by site, strain
Straining, on urination R39.16
Strand, vitreous - *see* Opacity, vitreous,
    membranes and strands
Strangulation, strangulated - *see also*
    Asphyxia, traumatic
    appendix K38.8
    bladder neck N32.0
    bowel or colon K56.2
    food or foreign body - *see* Foreign body, by
        site
    hemorrhoids - *see* Hemorrhoids, with
        complication
    hernia - *see also* Hernia, by site, with
        obstruction
        with gangrene - *see* Hernia, by site, with

Strangulation - *continued*
  gangrene
  intestine (large) (small) K56.2
    with hernia - *see also* Hernia, by site, with
      obstruction
        with gangrene - *see* Hernia, by site, with
          gangrene
  mesentery K56.2
  mucus - *see* Asphyxia, mucus
  omentum K56.2
  organ or site, congenital NEC - *see* Atresia, by
    site
  ovary - *see* Torsion, ovary
  penis N48.89
    foreign body T19.4
  rupture - *see* Hernia, by site, with obstruction
  stomach due to hernia - *see also* Hernia, by
    site, with obstruction
      with gangrene - *see* Hernia, by site, with
        gangrene
  vesicourethral orifice N32.0
Strangury R30.0
Straw itch B88.0
Strawberry
  gallbladder K82.4
  mark Q82.5
  tongue (red) (white) K14.3
Streak(s)
  macula, angioid H35.33
  ovarian Q50.32
Strephosymbolia F81.0
  secondary to organic lesion R48.8
Streptobacillary fever A25.1
Streptobacillosis A25.1
Streptobacillus moniliformis A25.1
Streptococcus, streptococcal - *see also*
  condition
  as cause of disease classified elsewhere B95.5
  group
    A, as cause of disease classified elsewhere
      B95.0
    B, as cause of disease classified elsewhere
      B95.1
    D, as cause of disease classified elsewhere
      B95.2
  pneumoniae, as cause of disease classified
    elsewhere B95.3
  specified NEC, as cause of disease classified
    elsewhere B95.4
Streptomycosis B47.1
Streptotrichosis A48.8
Stress F43.9
  family - *see* Disruption, family   fetal P84
    complicating pregnancy O77.9
      due to drug administration O77.1
  mental NEC Z73.3
    work-related Z56.6
  physical NEC Z73.3
    work-related Z56.6
  polycythemia D75.1
  reaction - *see also* Reaction, stress F43.9
  work schedule Z56.3
Stretching, nerve - *see* Injury, nerve
Striae albicantes, atrophicae or distensae
  (cutis) L90.6
Stricture - *see also* Stenosis
  ampulla of Vater K83.1
  anus (sphincter) K62.4
    congenital Q42.3
      with fistula Q42.2
    infantile Q42.3
      with fistula Q42.2
  aorta (ascending) (congenital) Q25.1
    arteriosclerotic I70.0

Stricture - *continued*
  calcified I70.0
    supravalvular, congenital Q25.3
  aortic (valve) - *see* Stenosis, aortic
  aqueduct of Sylvius (congenital) Q03.0
    with spina bifida - *see* Spina bifida, by site,
  with hydrocephalus
    acquired G91.1
  artery I77.1
    basilar - *see* Occlusion, artery, basilar
    carotid - *see* Occlusion, artery, carotid
    celiac I77.4
    congenital (peripheral) Q27.8
      cerebral Q28.3
      coronary Q24.5
      digestive system Q27.8
      lower limb Q27.8
      retinal Q14.1
      specified site NEC Q27.8
      umbilical Q27.0
      upper limb Q27.8
    coronary - *see* Disease, heart, ischemic,
      atherosclerotic
      congenital Q24.5
    precerebral - *see* Occlusion, artery,
      precerebral
    pulmonary (congenital) Q25.6
      acquired I28.8
    renal I70.1
    vertebral - *see* Occlusion, artery, vertebral
  auditory canal (external) (congenital)
    acquired - *see* Stenosis, external ear canal
  bile duct (common) (hepatic) K83.1
    congenital Q44.3
    postoperative K91.89
  bladder N32.89
    neck N32.0
  bowel - *see* Obstruction, intestine
  brain G93.89
  bronchus J98.09
    congenital Q32.3
    syphilitic A52.72
  cardia (stomach) K22.2
    congenital Q39.3
  cardiac - *see also* Disease, heart
    orifice (stomach) K22.2
  cecum - *see* Obstruction, intestine
  cervix, cervical (canal) N88.2
    congenital Q51.828
    in pregnancy - *see* Pregnancy, complicated
      by, abnormal cervix
      causing obstructed labor O65.5
  colon - *see also* Obstruction, intestine
    congenital Q42.9
      specified NEC Q42.8
  colostomy K94.03
  common (bile) duct K83.1
  coronary (artery) - *see* Disease, heart,
    ischemic, atherosclerotic
  cystic duct - *see* Obstruction, gallbladder
  digestive organs NEC, congenital Q45.8
  duodenum K31.5
    congenital Q41.0
  ear canal (external) (congenital) Q16.1
    acquired - *see* Stricture, auditory canal,
  acquired
  ejaculatory duct N50.89
  enterostomy K94.13
  esophagus K22.2
    congenital Q39.3
    syphilitic A52.79
      congenital A50.59 [*K23*]
  eustachian tube - *see also* Obstruction,
  eustachian tube

Stricture - *continued*
  congenital Q17.8
  fallopian tube N97.1
    gonococcal A54.24
    tuberculous A18.17
  gallbladder - *see* Obstruction, gallbladder
  glottis J38.6
  heart - *see also* Disease, heart
    valve - *see also* Endocarditis I38
      aortic Q23.0
      mitral Q23.2
      pulmonary Q22.1
      tricuspid Q22.4
  hepatic duct K83.1
  hourglass, of stomach K31.2
  hymen N89.6
  hypopharynx J39.2
  ileum (see also Obstruction, intestine,
    specified NEC) K56.699
    congenital Q41.2
  intestine - *see also* Obstruction, intestine
    congenital (small) Q41.9
      large Q42.9
        specified NEC Q42.8
      specified NEC Q41.8
    ischemic K55.1
  jejunum (see also Obstruction, intestine,
    specified NEC) K56.699
    congenital Q41.1
  lacrimal passages - *see also* Stenosis, lacrimal
    congenital Q10.5
  larynx J38.6
    congenital NEC Q31.8
      subglottic Q31.1
    syphilitic A52.73
      congenital A50.59 [*J99*]
  meatus
    ear (congenital) Q16.1
      acquired - *see* Stricture, auditory canal,
      acquired
    osseous (ear) (congenital) Q16.1
      acquired - *see* Stricture, auditory canal,
      acquired
    urinarius - *see also* Stricture, urethra
      congenital Q64.33
  mitral (valve) - *see* Stenosis, mitral
  myocardium, myocardial I51.5
    hypertrophic subaortic (idiopathic) I42.1
  nares (anterior) (posterior) J34.89
    congenital Q30.0
  nasal duct - *see also* Stenosis, lacrimal, duct
    congenital Q10.5
  nasolacrimal duct - *see also* Stenosis, lacrimal,
  duct
    congenital Q10.5
  nasopharynx J39.2
    syphilitic A52.73
  nose J34.89
    congenital Q30.0
  nostril (anterior) (posterior) J34.89
    congenital Q30.0
    syphilitic A52.73
      congenital A50.59 [*J99*]
  organ or site, congenital NEC - *see* Atresia, by
  site
  os uteri - *see* Stricture, cervix
  osseous meatus (ear) (congenital) Q16.1
    acquired - *see* Stricture, auditory canal,
    acquired
  oviduct - *see* Stricture, fallopian tube
  pelviureteric junction (congenital) Q62.11
    acquired, with hydronephrosis N13.0
  penis, by foreign body T19.4
  pharynx J39.2

Stricture - *continued*
  prostate N42.89
  pulmonary, pulmonic
    artery (congenital) Q25.6
      acquired I28.8
      noncongenital I28.8
    infundibulum (congenital) Q24.3
    valve I37.0
      congenital Q22.1
    vein, acquired I28.8
    vessel NEC I28.8
  punctum lacrimale - *see also* Stenosis,
    lacrimal, punctum
    congenital Q10.5
  pylorus (hypertrophic) K31.1
    adult K31.1
    congenital Q40.0
    infantile Q40.0
  rectosigmoid (see also Obstruction, intestine,
    specified NEC) K56.699
  rectum (sphincter) K62.4
    congenital Q42.1
      with fistula Q42.0
    due to
      chlamydial lymphogranuloma A55
      irradiation K91.89
      lymphogranuloma venereum A55
    gonococcal A54.6
    inflammatory (chlamydial) A55
    syphilitic A52.74
    tuberculous A18.32
  renal artery I70.1
    congenital Q27.1
  salivary duct or gland (any) K11.8
  sigmoid (flexure) - *see* Obstruction, intestine
  spermatic cord N50.89
  stoma (following) (of)
    colostomy K94.03
    enterostomy K94.13
    gastrostomy K94.23
    ileostomy K94.13
    tracheostomy J95.03
  stomach K31.89
    congenital Q40.2
    hourglass K31.2
  subaortic Q24.4
    hypertrophic (acquired) (idiopathic) I42.1
  subglottic J38.6
  syphilitic NEC A52.79
  trachea J39.8
    congenital Q32.1
    syphilitic A52.73
    tuberculous NEC A15.5
  tracheostomy J95.03
  tricuspid (valve) - *see* Stenosis, tricuspid
  tunica vaginalis N50.89
  ureter (postoperative) N13.5
    with
      hydronephrosis N13.1
        with infection N13.6
      pyelonephritis (chronic) N11.1
    congenital - *see* Atresia, ureter
    tuberculous A18.11
  ureteropelvic junction (congenital) Q62.11
    acquired, with hydronephrosis N13.0
  ureterovesical orifice N13.5
    with infection N13.6
  urethra (organic) (spasmodic) N35.9
    associated with schistosomiasis B65.0 [*N37*]
    congenital Q64.39
      valvular (posterior) Q64.2
    due to
      infection - *see* Stricture, urethra,
        postinfective

Stricture - *continued*
    trauma - *see* Stricture, urethra, post-
      traumatic
    gonococcal, gonorrheal A54.01
    infective NEC - *see* Stricture, urethra,
      postinfective
    late effect (sequelae) of injury - *see* Stricture,
      urethra, post-traumatic
    postcatheterization - *see* Stricture, urethra,
      postprocedural
    postinfective NEC
      female N35.12
      male N35.119
        anterior urethra N35.114
        bulbous urethra N35.112
        meatal N35.111
        membranous urethra N35.113
    postobstetric N35.021
    postoperative - *see* Stricture, urethra,
      postprocedural
    postprocedural
      female N99.12
      male N99.114
        anterior bulbous urethra N99.113
        bulbous urethra N99.111
        fossa navicularis N99.115
        meatal N99.110
        membranous urethra N99.112
    post-traumatic
      female N35.028
        due to childbirth N35.021
      male N35.014
        anterior urethra N35.013
        bulbous urethra N35.011
        meatal N35.010
        membranous urethra N35.012
    sequela (late effect) of
      childbirth N35.021
      injury - *see* Stricture, urethra, post-
        traumatic
    specified cause NEC N35.8
    syphilitic A52.76
    traumatic - *see* Stricture, urethra, post-
      traumatic
    valvular (posterior), congenital Q64.2
  urinary meatus - *see* Stricture, urethra
  uterus, uterine (synechiae) N85.6
    os (external) (internal) - *see* Stricture, cervix
  vagina (outlet) - *see* Stenosis, vagina
  valve (cardiac) (heart) - *see also* Endocarditis
    congenital
      aortic Q23.0
      mitral Q23.2
      pulmonary Q22.1
      tricuspid Q22.4
  vas deferens N50.89
    congenital Q55.4
  vein I87.1
  vena cava (inferior) (superior) NEC I87.1
    congenital Q26.0
  vesicourethral orifice N32.0
    congenital Q64.31
  vulva (acquired) N90.5
Stridor R06.1
  congenital (larynx) P28.89
Stridulous - *see* condition
Stroke (apoplectic) (brain) (embolic)
  (ischemic) (paralytic) (thrombotic) I63.9
    epileptic - *see* Epilepsy
    heat T67.0
    in evolution I63.9
    intraoperative
      during cardiac surgery I97.810
      during other surgery I97.811

Stroke - *continued*
  lightning - *see* Lightning
  meaning
    cerebral hemorrhage
    code to Hemorrhage, intracranial
    cerebral infarction
    code to Infarction, cerebral
    cryptogenic (see also infarction, cerebral)
      I63.9
  postprocedural
    following cardiac surgery I97.820
    following other surgery I97.821
  unspecified (NOS) I63.9
Stromatosis, endometrial D39.0
Strongyloidiasis, strongyloidosis B78.9
  cutaneous B78.1
  disseminated B78.7
  intestinal B78.0
Strophulus pruriginosus L28.2
Struck by lightning - *see* Lightning
Struma - *see also* Goiter
  Hashimoto E06.3
  lymphomatosa E06.3
  nodosa (simplex) E04.9
    endemic E01.2
      multinodular E01.1
    multinodular E04.2
      iodine-deficiency related E01.1
    toxic or with hyperthyroidism E05.20
      multinodular E05.20
        with thyroid storm E05.21
      uninodular E05.10
        with thyroid storm E05.11
    toxicosa E05.20
      with thyroid storm E05.21
      multinodular E05.20
        with thyroid storm E05.21
      uninodular E05.10
        with thyroid storm E05.11
    uninodular E04.1
  ovarii D27.-
  Riedel's E06.5
Strumipriva cachexia E03.4
Strümpell-Marie spine - *see* Spondylitis,
  ankylosing
Strümpell-Westphal pseudosclerosis E83.01
Stuart deficiency disease (factor X) D68.2
Stuart-Prower factor deficiency (factor X)
  D68.2
Student's elbow - *see* Bursitis, elbow,
  olecranon
Stump - *see* Amputation
Stunting, nutritional E45
Stupor (catatonic) R40.1
  depressive (single episode) F32.89
    recurrent episode F33.8
  dissociative F44.2
  manic F30.2
  manic-depressive F31.89
  psychogenic (anergic) F44.2
  reaction to exceptional stress (transient) F43.0
Sturge (-Weber) (-Dimitri) (-Kalischer)
  disease or syndrome Q85.8
Stuttering F80.81
  adult onset F98.5
  childhood onset F80.81
  following cerebrovascular disease - *see*
    Disorder, fluency. following cerebrovascular
    disease   in conditions classified elsewhere
    R47.82
Sty, stye (external) (internal) (meibomian)
  (zeisian) - *see* Hordeolum
Subacidity, gastric K31.89
  psychogenic F45.8

Subacute - *see* condition

Subarachnoid - *see* condition

Subcortical - *see* condition

Subcostal syndrome, nerve compression - *see* Mononeuropathy, upper limb, specified site NEC

Subcutaneous, subcuticular - *see* condition

Sundowning F05

Subdural - *see* condition

Subendocardium - *see* condition

Subependymoma
specified site - *see* Neoplasm, uncertain behavior, by site
unspecified site D43.2

Suberosis J67.3

Subglossitis - *see* Glossitis S

Subhemophilia D66

Subinvolution
breast (postlactational) (postpuerperal) N64.89
puerperal O90.89
uterus (chronic) (nonpuerperal) N85.3
puerperal O90.89

Sublingual - *see* condition

Sublinguitis - *see* Sialoadenitis

Subluxatable hip Q65.6

Subluxation - *see also* Dislocation
acromioclavicular S43.11-
ankle S93.0-
atlantoaxial, recurrent M43.4
  with myelopathy M43.3
carpometacarpal (joint) NEC S63.05-
  thumb S63.04-
complex, vertebral - *see* Complex, subluxation
congenital - *see also* Malposition, congenital
  hip - *see* Dislocation, hip, congenital, partial
  joint (excluding hip)
    lower limb Q68.8
    shoulder Q68.8
    upper limb Q68.8
elbow (traumatic) S53.10-
  anterior S53.11-
  lateral S53.14-
  medial S53.13-
  posterior S53.12-
  specified type NEC S53.19-
finger S63.20-
  index S63.20-
  interphalangeal S63.22-
    distal S63.24-
      index S63.24-
      little S63.24-
      middle S63.24-
      ring S63.24-
    index S63.22-
    little S63.22-
    middle S63.22-
    proximal S63.23-
      index S63.23-
      little S63.23-
      middle S63.23-
      ring S63.23-
    ring S63.22-
  little S63.20-
  metacarpophalangeal S63.21-
    index S63.21-
    little S63.21-
    middle S63.21-
    ring S63.21-
  middle S63.20-
  ring S63.20-
foot S93.30-
  specified site NEC S93.33-
  tarsal joint S93.31-
  tarsometatarsal joint S93.32-

Subluxation - *continued*
toe - *see* Subluxation, toe
hip S73.00-
  anterior S73.03-
    obturator S73.02-
  central S73.04-
  posterior S73.01-
interphalangeal (joint)
  finger S63.22-
    distal joint S63.24-
      index S63.24-
      little S63.24-
      middle S63.24-
      ring S63.24-
    index S63.22-
    little S63.22-
    middle S63.22-
    proximal joint S63.23-
      index S63.23-
      little S63.23-
      middle S63.23-
      ring S63.23-
    ring S63.22-
  thumb S63.12-
    distal joint S63.14-
    proximal joint S63.13-
  toe S93.13-
    great S93.13-
    lesser S93.13-
joint prosthesis - *see* Complications, joint prosthesis, mechanical, displacement, by site
knee S83.10-
  cap - *see* Subluxation, patella
  patella - *see* Subluxation, patella
  proximal tibia
    anteriorly S83.11-
    laterally S83.14-
    medially S83.13-
    posteriorly S83.12-
  specified type NEC S83.19-
lens - *see* Dislocation, lens, partial
ligament, traumatic - *see* Sprain, by site
metacarpal (bone)
  proximal end S63.06-
metacarpophalangeal (joint)
  finger S63.21-
    index S63.21-
    little S63.21-
    middle S63.21-
    ring S63.21-
  thumb S63.11-
metatarsophalangeal joint S93.14-
  great toe S93.14-
  lesser toe S93.14-
midcarpal (joint) S63.03-
patella S83.00-
  lateral S83.01-
  recurrent (nontraumatic) - *see* Dislocation, patella, recurrent, incomplete
  specified type NEC S83.09-
pathological - *see* Dislocation, pathological
radial head S53.00-
  anterior S53.01-
  nursemaid's elbow S53.03-
  posterior S53.02-
  specified type NEC S53.09-
radiocarpal (joint) S63.02-
radioulnar (joint)
  distal S63.01-
  proximal - *see* Subluxation, elbow
shoulder
  congenital Q68.8
  girdle S43.30-
    scapula S43.31-

Subluxation - *continued*
  specified site NEC S43.39-
  traumatic S43.00-
    anterior S43.01-
    inferior S43.03-
    posterior S43.02-
    specified type NEC S43.08-
sternoclavicular (joint) S43.20-
  anterior S43.21-
  posterior S43.22-
symphysis (pubis)
thumb S63.103
  interphalangeal joint - *see* Subluxation, interphalangeal (joint), thumb
  metacarpophalangeal joint - *see* Subluxation, metacarpophalangeal (joint), thumb
toe(s) S93.10-
  great S93.10-
    interphalangeal joint S93.13-
    metatarsophalangeal joint S93.14-
  interphalangeal joint S93.13-
  lesser S93.10-
    interphalangeal joint S93.13-
    metatarsophalangeal joint S93.14-
  metatarsophalangeal joint S93.149
ulnohumeral joint - *see* Subluxation, elbow
vertebral
  recurrent NEC - *see* subcategory M43.5
  traumatic
    cervical S13.100
      atlantoaxial joint S13.120
      atlantooccipital joint S13.110
      atloido-occipital joint S13.110
      joint between
        C0 and C1 S13.110
        C1 and C2 S13.120
        C2 and C3 S13.130
        C3 and C4 S13.140
        C4 and C5 S13.150
        C5and C6 S13.160
        C6and C7 S13.170
        C7and T1 S13.180
      occipitoatloid joint S13.110
    lumbar S33.100
      joint between
        L1and L2 S33.110
        L2and L3 S33.120
        L3 and L4 S33.130
        L4and L5 S33.140
    thoracic S23.100
      joint between
        T1and T2 S23.110
        T2and T3 S23.120
        T3 and T4 S23.122
        T4 and T5 S23.130
        T5 and T6 S23.132
        T6 and T7 S23.140
        T7 and T8 S23.142
        T8 and T9 S23.150
        T9 and T10 S23.152
        T10 and T11 S23.160
        T11 and T12 S23.162
        T12 and L1 S23.170
ulna
  distal end S63.07-
  proximal end - *see* Subluxation, elbow
wrist (carpal bone) S63.00-
  carpometacarpal joint - *see* Subluxation, carpometacarpal (joint)
  distal radioulnar joint - *see* Subluxation, radioulnar (joint), distal
  metacarpal bone, proximal - *see* Subluxation, metacarpal (bone), proximal end

Subluxation - *continued*
  midcarpal - *see* Subluxation, midcarpal
    (joint)
  radiocarpal joint - *see* Subluxation,
    radiocarpal (joint)
  recurrent - *see* Dislocation, recurrent, wrist
  specified site NEC S63.09-
  ulna - *see* Subluxation, ulna, distal end
Submaxillary - *see* condition
Submersion (fatal) (nonfatal) T75.1
Submucous - *see* condition
Subnormal, subnormality
  accommodation (old age) H52.4
  mental - *see* Disability, intellectual
  temperature (accidental) T68
Subphrenic - *see* condition
Subscapular nerve - *see* condition
Subseptus uterus Q51.2
Subsiding appendicitis K36
Substance (other psychoactive) -induced
  anxiety disorder F19.980
  bipolar and related disorder F19.94
  delirium F19.921
  depressive disorder F19.94
  major neurocognitive disorder F19.97
  mild neurocognitive disorder F19.988
  obsessive-compulsive and related disorder
    F19.988
  psychotic disorder F19.959
  sexual dysfunction F19.981
  sleep disorder F19.982
Substernal thyroid E04.9
  congenital Q89.2
Substitution disorder F44.9
Subtentorial - *see* condition
Subthyroidism (acquired) - *see also*
  Hypothyroidism
  congenital E03.1
Succenturiate placenta O43.19-
Sucking thumb, child (excessive) F98.8
Sudamen, sudamina L74.1
Sudanese kala-azar B55.0
Sudden
  heart failure - *see* Failure, heart
  hearing loss - *see* Deafness, sudden
Sudeck's atrophy, disease, or syndrome - *see*
  Algoneurodystrophy
Suffocation - *see* Asphyxia, traumatic
Sugar
  blood
    high (transient) R73.9
    low (transient) E16.2
  in urine R81
Suicide, suicidal (attempted) T14.91
  by poisoning - *see* Table of Drugs and
    Chemicals
  history of (personal) Z91.5
    in family Z81.8
  ideation - *see* Ideation, suicidal
  risk
    meaning personal history of attempted
      suicide Z91.5
    meaning suicidal ideation - *see* Ideation,
      suicidal
  tendencies
    meaning personal history of attempted
      suicide Z91.5
    meaning suicidal ideation - *see* Ideation,
      suicidal
  trauma - *see* nature of injury by site
Suipestifer infection - *see* Infection, salmonella
**Sulfhemoglobinemia, sulphemoglobinemia
  (acquired) (with methemoglobinemia)** D74.8
Sumatran mite fever A75.3

Summer - *see* condition **Sunburn** L55.9
  due to
    tanning bed (acute) L56.8
      chronic L57.8
    ultraviolet radiation (acute) L56.8
      chronic L57.8
  first degree L55.0
  second degree L55.1
  third degree L55.2
**SUNCT (short lasting unilateral
  neuralgiform headache with conjunctival
  injection and tearing)** G44.059
  intractable G44.051
  not intractable G44.059
Sunken acetabulum - *see* Derangement, joint,
  specified type NEC, hip
Sunstroke T67.0
Superfecundation - *see* Pregnancy, multiple
Superfetation - *see* Pregnancy, multiple
Superinvolution (uterus) N85.8
Supernumerary (congenital)
  aortic cusps Q23.8
  auditory ossicles Q16.3
  bone Q79.8
  breast Q83.1
  carpal bones Q74.0
  cusps, heart valve NEC Q24.8
    aortic Q23.8
    mitral Q23.2
    pulmonary Q22.3
  digit(s) Q69.9
  ear (lobule) Q17.0
  fallopian tube Q50.6
  finger Q69.0
  hymen Q52.4
  kidney Q63.0
  lacrimonasal duct Q10.6
  lobule (ear) Q17.0
  mitral cusps Q23.2
  muscle Q79.8
  nipple(s) Q83.3
  organ or site not listed - *see* Accessory
    ossicles, auditory Q16.3
  ovary Q50.31
  oviduct Q50.6
  pulmonary, pulmonic cusps Q22.3
  rib Q76.6
    cervical or first (syndrome) Q76.5
  roots (of teeth) K00.2
  spleen Q89.09
  tarsal bones Q74.2
  teeth K00.1
  testis Q55.29
  thumb Q69.1
  toe Q69.2
  uterus Q51.2
  vagina Q52.1
  vertebra Q76.49
Supervision (of)
  contraceptive - *see* Prescription, contraceptives
  dietary (for) Z71.3
    allergy (food) Z71.3
    colitis Z71.3
    diabetes mellitus Z71.3
    food allergy or intolerance Z71.3
    gastritis Z71.3
    hypercholesterolemia Z71.3
    hypoglycemia Z71.3
    intolerance (food) Z71.3
    obesity Z71.3
    specified NEC Z71.3
  healthy infant or child Z76.2
    foundling Z76.1
  high-risk pregnancy - *see* Pregnancy,

Supervision - *continued*
  complicated by, high, risk
  lactation Z39.1
  pregnancy - *see* Pregnancy, supervision of
Supplemental teeth K00.1
Suppression
  binocular vision H53.34
  lactation O92.5
  menstruation N94.89
  ovarian secretion E28.39
  renal N28.9
  urine, urinary secretion R34
Suppuration, suppurative - *see also* condition
  accessory sinus (chronic) - *see* Sinusitis
  adrenal gland
  antrum (chronic) - *see* Sinusitis, maxillary
  bladder - *see* Cystitis
  brain G06.0
    sequelae G09
  breast N61.1
    puerperal, postpartum or gestational - *see*
      Mastitis, obstetric, purulent
  dental periosteum M27.3
  ear (middle) - *see also* Otitis, media
    external NEC - *see* Otitis, externa, infective
    internal - *see* subcategory H83.0
  ethmoidal (chronic) (sinus) - *see* Sinusitis,
    ethmoidal
  fallopian tube - *see* Salpingo-oophoritis
  frontal (chronic) (sinus) - *see* Sinusitis, frontal
  gallbladder (acute) K81.0
  gum K05.20
    generalized - *see* Periodontitis, aggressive,
      generalized
    localized - *see* Periodontitis, aggressive,
      localized
  intracranial G06.0
  joint - *see* Arthritis, pyogenic or pyemic
  labyrinthine *see* subcategory H83.0
  lung - *see* Abscess, lung
  mammary gland N61.1
    puerperal, postpartum O91.12
      associated with lactation O91.13
  maxilla, maxillary M27.2
    sinus (chronic) - *see* Sinusitis, maxillary
  muscle - *see* Myositis, infective
  nasal sinus (chronic) - *see* Sinusitis
  pancreas, acute - *see also* Pancreatitis, acute
    K85.80
  parotid gland - *see* Sialoadenitis
  pelvis, pelvic
    female - *see* Disease, pelvis, inflammatory
    male K65.0
  pericranial - *see* Osteomyelitis
  salivary duct or gland (any) - *see* Sialoadenitis
  sinus (accessory) (chronic) (nasal) - *see*
    Sinusitis
  sphenoidal sinus (chronic) - *see* Sinusitis,
    sphenoidal
  thymus (gland) E32.1
  thyroid (gland) E06.0
  tonsil - *see* Tonsillitis
  uterus - *see* Endometritis
Supraeruption of tooth (teeth) M26.34
Supraglottitis J04.30
  with obstruction J04.31
Suprarenal (gland) - *see* condition
Suprascapular nerve - *see* condition
Suprasellar - *see* condition
Surfer's knots or nodules S89.8-
Surgical
  emphysema T81.82
  procedures, complication or misadventure -
    see Complications, surgical procedures
  shock T81.10

Surveillance (of) (for) - *see also* Observation
  alcohol abuse Z71.41
  contraceptive - *see* Prescription, contraceptives
  dietary Z71.3
  drug abuse Z71.51
Susceptibility to disease, genetic Z15.89
  malignant neoplasm Z15.09
    breast Z15.01
    endometrium Z15.04
    ovary Z15.02
    prostate Z15.03
    specified NEC Z15.09
  multiple endocrine neoplasia Z15.81
Suspected condition, ruled out - *see also*
    Observation, suspected
  amniotic cavity and membrane Z03.71
  cervical shortening Z03.75
  fetal anomaly Z03.73
  fetal growth Z03.74
  maternal and fetal conditions NEC Z03.79
  newborn - *see also* Observation, newborn,
    suspected condition ruled out Z05.9
  oligohydramnios Z03.71
  placental problem Z03.72
  polyhydramnios Z03.71
Suspended uterus
  in pregnancy or childbirth - *see* Pregnancy,
    complicated by, abnormal uterus
Sutton's nevus D22.9
Suture
  burst (in operation wound) T81.31
    external operation wound T81.31
    internal operation wound T81.32
  inadvertently left in operation wound - *see*
    Foreign body, accidentally left during a
    procedure
  removal Z48.02
Swab inadvertently left in operation wound -
    see Foreign body, accidentally left during a
    procedure
Swallowed, swallowing
  difficulty - *see* Dysphagia
  foreign body - *see* Foreign body, alimentary
    tract
Swan neck deformity (finger) - *see* Deformity,
    finger, swan neck
Swearing, compulsive F42.8
  in Gilles de la Tourette's syndrome F95.2
Sweat, sweats
  fetid L75.0
  night R61
Sweating, excessive R61
Sweeley-Klionsky disease E75.21
Sweet's disease or dermatosis L98.2
Swelling (of) R60.9
  abdomen, abdominal (not referable to any
    particular organ) - *see* Mass, abdominal
  ankle - *see* Effusion, joint, ankle
  arm M79.89
    forearm M79.89
  breast (see also Lump, breast) N63.0
  Calabar B74.3
  cervical gland R59.0
  chest, localized R22.2
  ear H93.8-
  extremity (lower) (upper) - *see* Disorder, soft
    tissue, specified type NEC
  finger M79.89
  foot M79.89
  glands R59.9
    generalized R59.1
    localized R59.0
  hand M79.89
  head (localized) R22.0

Swelling - *continued*
  inflammatory - *see* Inflammation
  intra-abdominal - *see* Mass, abdominal
  joint - *see* Effusion, joint
  leg M79.89
    lower M79.89
  limb - *see* Disorder, soft tissue, specified type
    NEC
  localized (skin) R22.9
    chest R22.2
    head R22.0
    limb
      lower - *see* Mass, localized, limb, lower
      upper - *see* Mass, localized, limb, upper
    neck R22.1
    trunk R22.2
  neck (localized) R22.1
  pelvic - *see* Mass, abdominal
  scrotum N50.89
  splenic - *see* Splenomegaly   testis N50.89
  toe M79.89
  umbilical R19.09
  wandering, due to Gnathostoma (spinigerum)
    B83.1
  white - *see* Tuberculosis, arthritis
Swift (-Feer) disease
  overdose or wrong substance given or taken -
    see Table of Drugs and Chemicals, by drug,
    poisoning
Swimmer's
  cramp T75.1
  ear H60.33-
  itch B65.3
Swimming in the head R42
Swollen - *see* Swelling
Swyer syndrome Q99.1
Sycosis L73.8
  barbae (not parasitic) L73.8
  contagiosa (mycotic) B35.0
  lupoides L73.8
  mycotic B35.0
  parasitic B35.0
  vulgaris L73.8
Sydenham's chorea - *see* Chorea, Sydenham's
Sylvatic yellow fever A95.0
Sylvest's disease B33.0
Symblepharon H11.23-
  congenital Q10.3
Symond's syndrome G93.2
Sympathetic - *see* condition
Sympatheticotonia G90.8
Sympathicoblastoma
  specified site - *see* Neoplasm, malignant, by
    site
  unspecified site C74.90
Sympathogonioma - *see* Sympathicoblastoma
Symphalangy (fingers) (toes) Q70.9
Symptoms NEC R68.89
  breast NEC N64.59
  cold J00
  development NEC R63.8
  factitious, self-induced - *see* Disorder,
    factitious
  genital organs, female R10.2
  involving
    abdomen NEC R19.8
    appearance NEC R46.89
    awareness R41.9
      altered mental status R41.82
      amnesia - *see* Amnesia
      borderline intellectual functioning R41.83
      coma - *see* Coma
      disorientation R41.0
      neurologic neglect syndrome R41.4

Symptoms - *continued*
    senile cognitive decline R41.81
    specified symptom NEC R41.89
  behavior NEC R46.89
  cardiovascular system NEC R09.89
  chest NEC R09.89
  circulatory system NEC R09.89
  cognitive functions R41.9
    altered mental status R41.82
    amnesia - *see* Amnesia
    borderline intellectual functioning R41.83
    coma - *see* Coma
    disorientation R41.0
    neurologic neglect syndrome R41.4
    senile cognitive decline R41.81
    specified symptom NEC R41.89
  development NEC R62.50
  digestive system NEC R19.8
  emotional state NEC R45.89
    emotional lability R45.86
  food and fluid intake R63.8
  general perceptions and sensations R44.9
    specified NEC R44.8
  musculoskeletal system R29.91
    specified NEC R29.898
  nervous system R29.90
    specified NEC R29.818
  pelvis NEC R19.8
  respiratory system NEC R09.89
  skin and integument R23.9
  urinary system R39.9
  menopausal N95.1
  metabolism NEC R63.8
  neurotic F48.8
  of infancy R68.19
  pelvis NEC, female R10.2
  skin and integument NEC R23.9
  subcutaneous tissue NEC R23.9
  viral cold J00
Sympus Q74.2
Syncephalus Q89.4
Synchondrosis
  abnormal (congenital) Q78.8
  ischiopubic M91.0
Synchysis (scintillans) (senile) (vitreous body)
  H43.89
Syncope (near) (pre) R55
  anginosa I20.8
  bradycardia R00.1
  cardiac R55
  carotid sinus G90.01
  due to spinal (lumbar) puncture G97.1
  heart R55
  heat T67.1
  laryngeal R05
  psychogenic F48.8
  tussive R05
  vasoconstriction R55
  vasodepressor R55
  vasomotor R55
  vasovagal R55
Syndactylism, syndactyly Q70.9
  complex (with synostosis)
    fingers Q70.0-
    toes Q70.2-
  simple (without synostosis)
    fingers Q70.1-
    toes Q70.3-
Syndrome - *see also* Disease
  5q minus NOS D46.C
  48,XXXX Q97.1
  49,XXXXX Q97.1
  abdominal
    acute R10.0

Syndrome - *continued*
  muscle deficiency Q79.4
  abnormal innervation H02.519
    left H02.516
      lower H02.515
      upper H02.514
    right H02.513
      lower H02.512
      upper H02.511
  abstinence, neonatal P96.1
  acid pulmonary aspiration, obstetric O74.0
  acquired immunodeficiency - *see* Human,
    immunodeficiency virus (HIV) disease
  acute abdominal R10.0
  acute respiratory distress (adult) (child) J80
    idiopathic J84.114
  Adair-Dighton Q78.0
  Adams-Stokes (-Morgagni) I45.9
  adiposogenital E23.6
  adrenal
    hemorrhage (meningococcal) A39.1
    meningococcic A39.1
  adrenocortical - *see* Cushing's, syndrome
  adrenogenital E25.9
    congenital, associated with enzyme
      deficiency E25.0
  afferent loop NEC K91.89
  Alagille's Q44.7
  alcohol withdrawal (without convulsions) - *see*
    Dependence, alcohol, with, withdrawal
  Alder's D72.0
  Aldrich (-Wiskott) D82.0
  alien hand R41.4
  Alport Q87.81
  alveolar hypoventilation E66.2
  alveolocapillary block J84.10
  amnesic, amnestic (confabulatory) (due to) -
    see Disorder, amnesic
  amyostatic (Wilson's disease) E83.01
  androgen insensitivity E34.50
    complete E34.51
    partial E34.52
  androgen resistance - *see also* Syndrome,
    androgen insensitivity E34.50
  Angelman Q93.5
  anginal - *see* Angina
  ankyloglossia superior Q38.1
  anterior
    chest wall R07.89
    cord G83.82
    spinal artery G95.19
      compression M47.019
        cervical region M47.012
        cervicothoracic region M47.013
        lumbar region M47.016
        occipito-atlanto-axial region M47.011
        thoracic region M47.014
        thoracolumbar region M47.015
    tibial M76.81-
  antibody deficiency D80.9
    agammaglobulinemic D80.1
      hereditary D80.0
    congenital D80.0
    hypogammaglobulinemic D80.1
      hereditary D80.0
  anticardiolipin (-antibody) D68.61
  antidepressant discontinuation T43.205
  antiphospholipid (-antibody) D68.61
  aortic
    arch M31.4
    bifurcation I74.09
  aortomesenteric duodenum occlusion K31.5
  apical ballooning (transient left ventricular)
    I51.81

Syndrome - *continued*
  arcuate ligament I77.4
  argentaffin, argintaffinoma E34.0
  Arnold-Chiari - *see* Arnold-Chiari disease
  Arrillaga-Ayerza I27.0
  arterial tortuosity Q87.82
  arteriovenous steal T82.898-
  Asherman's N85.6
  aspiration, of newborn - *see* Aspiration, by
    substance, with pneumonia
      meconium P24.01
  ataxia-telangiectasia G11.3
  auriculotemporal G50.8
  autoerythrocyte sensitization (Gardner-
    diamond) D69.2
  autoimmune polyglandular E31.0
  autoimmune lymphoproliferative [ALPS]
    D89.82
  autoinflammatory M04.9
    specified type NEC M04.8
  autosomal - *see* Abnormal, autosomes
  Avellis' G46.8
  Ayerza (-Arrillaga) I27.0
  Babinski Nageotte G83.89
  Bakwin-Krida Q78.5
  bare lymphocyte D81.6
  Barré-Guillain G61.0
  Barré-Liéou M53.0
  Barrett's - *see* Barrett's, esophagus
  Barsony-Polgár K22.4
  Barsony-Teschendorf K22.4
  Barth E78.71
  Bartter's E26.81
  basal cell nevus Q87.89
  Basedow's E05.00
    with thyroid storm E05.01
  basilar artery G45.0
  Batten-Steinert G71.11
  battered
    baby or child - *see* Maltreatment, child,
      physical abuse
    spouse - *see* Maltreatment, adult, physical
  abuse
  Beals Q87.40
  Beau's I51.5
  Beck's I65.8
  Benedikt's G46.3
  Béquez César (-Steinbrinck-Chédiak-Higashi)
    E70.330
  Bernhardt-Roth - *see* Meralgia paresthetica
  Bernheim's *see* Failure, heart, right
  big spleen D73.1
  bilateral polycystic ovarian E28.2
  Bing-Horton's - *see* Horton's headache
  Birt-Hogg-Dube syndrome Q87.89
  Björck (-Thorsen) E34.0
  black
    lung J60
    widow spider bite - *see* Toxicity, venom,
      spider, black widow
  Blackfan-diamond D61.01
  Blau M04.8
  blind loop K90.2
    congenital Q43.8
    postsurgical K91.2
  blue sclera Q78.0
  blue toe I75.02-
  Boder-Sedgewick G11.3
  Boerhaave's K22.3
  Borjeson Forssman Lehmann Q89.8
  Bouillaud's I01.9
  Bourneville (-Pringle) Q85.1
  Bouveret (-Hoffman) I47.9
  brachial plexus G54.0

Syndrome - *continued*
  bradycardia-tachycardia I49.5
  brain (nonpsychotic) F09
    with psychosis, psychotic reaction F09
    acute or subacute - *see* Delirium
    congenital - *see* Disability, intellectual
    organic F09
      post-traumatic (nonpsychotic) F07.81
        psychotic F09
    personality change F07.0
    postcontusional F07.81
    post-traumatic, nonpsychotic F07.81
    psycho-organic F09
    psychotic F06.8
  brain stem stroke G46.3
  Brandt's (acrodermatitis enteropathica) E83.2
  broad ligament laceration N83.8
  Brock's J98.11
  bronze baby P83.88
  Brown-Sequard G83.81
  Brugada I49.8
  bubbly lung P27.0
  Buchem's M85.2
  Budd-Chiari I82.0
  bulbar (progressive) G12.22
  Bürger-Grütz E78.3
  Burke's K86.89
  Burnett's (milk-alkali) E83.52
  burning feet E53.9
  Bywaters' T79.5
  Call-Fleming I67.841
  carbohydrate-deficient glycoprotein (CDGS)
    E77.8
  carcinogenic thrombophlebitis I82.1
  carcinoid E34.0
  cardiac asthma I50.1
  cardiacos negros I27.0
  cardiofaciocutaneous Q87.89
  cardiorenal - *see* Hypertension, cardiorenal
  cardiorespiratory distress (idiopathic),
    newborn P22.0
  cardiovascular renal - *see* Hypertension,
    cardiorenal
  carotid
    artery (hemispheric) (internal) G45.1
    body G90.01
    sinus G90.01
  carpal tunnel G56.0-
  Cassidy (-Scholte) E34.0
  cat cry Q93.4
  cat eye Q92.8
  cauda equina G83.4
  causalgia - *see* Causalgia
  celiac K90.0
    artery compression I77.4
    axis I77.4
  central pain G89.0
  cerebellar
    hereditary G11.9
    stroke G46.4
  cerebellomedullary malformation - *see* Spina
    bifida
  cerebral
    artery
      anterior G46.1
      middle G46.0
      posterior G46.2
    gigantism E22.0
  cervical (root) M53.1
    disc - *see* Disorder, disc, cervical, with
      neuritis
    fusion Q76.1
    posterior, sympathicus M53.0

Syndrome - *continued*
  rib Q76.5
  sympathetic paralysis G90.2
  cervicobrachial (diffuse) M53.1
  cervicocranial M53.0
  cervicodorsal outlet G54.2
  cervicothoracic outlet G54.0
  Céstan (-Raymond) I65.8
  Charcot's (angina cruris) (intermittent
    claudication) I73.9
  Charcot-Weiss-baker G90.09
  CHARGE Q89.8
  Chédiak-Higashi (-Steinbrinck) E70.330
  chest wall R07.1
  Chiari's (hepatic vein thrombosis) I82.0
  Chilaiditi's Q43.3
  child maltreatment - *see* Maltreatment, child
  chondrocostal junction M94.0
  chondroectodermal dysplasia Q77.6
  chromosome 4 short arm deletion Q93.3
  chromosome 5 short arm deletion Q93.4
  chronic
    infantile neurological, cutaneous and
      articular (CINCA) M04.2
    pain G89.4
      personality F68.8
  Clarke-Hadfield K86.89
  Clerambault's automatism G93.89
  Clouston's (hidrotic ectodermal dysplasia)
    Q82.4
  clumsiness, clumsy child F82
  cluster headache G44.009
    intractable G44.001
    not intractable G44.009
  Coffin-Lowry Q89.8
  cold injury (newborn) P80.0
  combined immunity deficiency D81.9
  compartment (deep) (posterior) (traumatic)
    T79.A0
    abdomen T79.A3
    lower extremity (hip, buttock, thigh, leg,
      foot, toes) T79.A2
    nontraumatic
      abdomen M79.A3
      lower extremity (hip, buttock, thigh, leg,
        foot, toes) M79.A2-
      specified site NEC M79.A9
      upper extremity (shoulder, arm, forearm,
        wrist, hand, fingers) M79.A1-
    postprocedural - *see* Syndrome,
      compartment, nontraumatic
    specified site NEC T79.A9
    upper extremity (shoulder, arm, forearm,
      wrist, hand, fingers) T79.A1
  complex regional pain - *see* Syndrome, pain,
    complex regional
  compression T79.5
    anterior spinal - *see* Syndrome, anterior,
      spinal artery, compression
    cauda equina G83.4
    celiac artery I77.4
    vertebral artery M47.029
      occipito-atlanto-axial region M47.021
      cervical region M47.022
  concussion F07.81
  congenital
    affecting multiple systems NEC Q87.89
    central alveolar hypoventilation G47.35
    facial diplegia Q87.0
    muscular hypertrophy-cerebral Q87.89
    oculo-auriculovertebral Q87.0
    oculofacial diplegia (Moebius) Q87.0
    rubella (manifest) P35.0
  congestion-fibrosis (pelvic), female N94.89

Syndrome - *continued*
  congestive dysmenorrhea N94.6
  Conn's E26.01
  connective tissue M35.9
    overlap NEC M35.1
  conus medullaris G95.81
  cord
    anterior G83.82
    posterior G83.83
  coronary
    acute NEC I24.9
    insufficiency or intermediate I20.0
    slow flow I20.8
  Costen's (complex) M26.69
  costochondral junction M94.0
  costoclavicular G54.0
  costovertebral E22.0
  Cowden Q85.8
  craniovertebral M53.0
  Creutzfeldt-Jakob - *see* Creutzfeldt-Jakob
    disease or syndrome
  cri-du-chat Q93.4
  crib death R99
  cricopharyngeal - *see* Dysphagia
  croup J05.0
  CRPS I - *see* Syndrome, pain, complex
    regional I
  crush T79.5
  cubital tunnel - *see* Lesion, nerve, ulnar
  Curschmann (-batten) (-Steinert) G71.11
  Cushing's E24.9
    alcohol-induced E24.4
    due to
      alcohol
      drugs E24.2
      ectopic ACTH E24.3
      overproduction of pituitary ACTH E24.0
    drug-induced E24.2
    overdose or wrong substance given or taken -
      see Table of Drugs and Chemicals, by drug,
      poisoning
    pituitary-dependent E24.0
    specified type NEC E24.8
  cryopyrin-associated periodic M04.2
  cryptophthalmos Q87.0
  cystic duct stump K91.5
  Dana-Putnam D51.0
  Danbolt (-cross) (acrodermatitis enteropathica)
    E83.2
  Dandy-Walker Q03.1
    with spina bifida Q07.01
  Danlos' Q79.6
  defibrination - *see also* Fibrinolysis
    with
      antepartum hemorrhage - *see* Hemorrhage,
        antepartum, with coagulation defect
      intrapartum hemorrhage - *see* Hemorrhage,
        complicating, delivery
    newborn P60
    postpartum O72.3
  Degos' I77.89
  Déjérine-Roussy G89.0
  delayed sleep phase G47.21
  demyelinating G37.9
  dependence - *see* F10-f19 with fourth
    character .2
  depersonalization (-derealization) F48.1
  De Quervain E34.51
  de Toni-Fanconi (-Debre) E72.09
    with cystinosis E72.04
  diabetes mellitus-hypertension nephrosis - *see*
    Diabetes, nephrosis
  diabetes mellitus in newborn infant P70.2
  diabetes nephrosis - *see* Diabetes, nephrosis

Syndrome - *continued*
  diabetic amyotrophy - *see* Diabetes,
    amyotrophy
  dialysis associated steal T82.898-
  Diamond-Blackfan D61.01
  Diamond-gardener D69.2
  DIC (diffuse or disseminated intravascular
    coagulopathy) D65
  di George's D82.1
  Dighton's Q78.0
  disequilibrium E87.8
  Döhle body-panmyelopathic D72.0
  dorsolateral medullary G46.4
  double athetosis G80.3
  Down - *see also* Down syndrome Q90.9
  Dresbach's (elliptocytosis) D58.1
  Dressler's (postmyocardial infarction) I24.1
    postcardiotomy I97.0
  drug withdrawal, infant of dependent mother
    P96.1
  dry eye H04.12-
  due to abnormality
    chromosomal Q99.9
      sex
        female phenotype Q97.9
        male phenotype Q98.9
      specified NEC Q99.8
  dumping (postgastrectomy) K91.1
    nonsurgical K31.89
  Dupré's (meningism) R29.1
  dysmetabolic X E88.81
  dyspraxia, developmental F82
  Eagle-Barrett Q79.4
  Eaton-lambert - *see* Syndrome, Lambert-Eaton
  Ebstein's Q22.5
  ectopic ACTH E24.3
  eczema-thrombocytopenia D82.0
  Eddowes' Q78.0
  effort (psychogenic) F45.8
  Eisenmenger's I27.83
  Ehlers-Danlos Q79.6
  Ekman's Q78.0
  electric feet E53.8
  Ellis-van Creveld Q77.6
  empty nest Z60.0
  endocrine-hypertensive E27.0
  entrapment - *see* Neuropathy, entrapment
  eosinophilia-myalgia M35.8
  epileptic - *see also* Epilepsy, by type
    absence G40.A09
      intractable G40.A19
        with status epilepticus G40.A11
        without status epilepticus G40.A19
      not intractable G40.A09
        with status epilepticus G40.A01
        without status epilepticus G40.A09
  Erdheim-Chester (ECD) E88.89
  Erdheim's E22.0
  erythrocyte fragmentation D59.4
  Evans D69.41
  exhaustion F48.8
  extrapyramidal G25.9
    specified NEC G25.89
  eye retraction - *see* Strabismus
  eyelid-malar-mandible Q87.0
  Faber's D50.9
  facial pain, paroxysmal G50.0
  Fallot's Q21.3
  familial cold autoinflammatory M04.2
  familial eczema-thrombocytopenia (Wiskott-
    Aldrich) D82.0
  Fanconi (-de Toni) (-Debre) E72.09
    with cystinosis E72.04
  Fanconi's (anemia) (congenital pancytopenia)

Syndrome - *continued*
D61.09
fatigue
chronic R53.82
psychogenic F48.8
faulty bowel habit K59.39
Feil-Klippel (brevicollis) Q76.1
Felty's - *see* Felty's syndrome
fertile eunuch E23.0
fetal
alcohol (dysmorphic) Q86.0
hydantoin Q86.1
Fiedler's I40.1
first arch Q87.0
fish odor E72.8
Fisher's G61.0
Fitzhugh-Curtis
due to
Chlamydia trachomatis A74.81
Neisseria gonorrhorea (gonococcal
peritonitis) A54.85
Fitz's - *see also* Pancreatitis, acute K85.80
Flajani (-Basedow) E05.00
with thyroid storm E05.01
flatback - *see* Flatback syndrome   floppy
baby P94.2
iris (intraoperative) (IFIS) H21.81
mitral valve I34.1
flush E34.0
Foix-Alajouanine G95.19
Fong's Q87.2
food protein-induced enterocolitis K52.21
foramen magnum G93.5
Foster-Kennedy H47.14-
Foville's (peduncular) G46.3
fragile X Q99.2
Franceschetti Q75.4
Frey's
auriculotemporal G50.8
hyperhidrosis L74.52
Friderichsen-Waterhouse A39.1
Froin's G95.89
frontal lobe F07.0
Fukuhara E88.49
functional
bowel K59.9
prepubertal castrate E29.1
Gaisböck's D75.1
ganglion (basal ganglia brain) G25.9
geniculi G51.1
Gardner-diamond D69.2
gastroesophageal
junction K22.0
laceration-hemorrhage K22.6
gastrojejunal loop obstruction K91.89
Gee-Herter-Heubner K90.0
Gelineau's G47.419
with cataplexy G47.411
genito-anorectal A55
Gerstmann-sträussler-scheinker (GSS) A81.82
Gianotti-crosti L44.4
giant platelet (Bernard-soulier) D69.1
Gilles de la Tourette's F95.2
goiter-deafness E07.1
Goldberg Q89.8
Goldberg-maxwell E34.51
Good's D83.8
Gopalan' (burning feet) E53.8
Gorlin's Q87.89
Gougerot-blum L81.7
Gouley's I31.1
Gower's R55
gray or grey (newborn) P93.0
platelet D69.1

Syndrome - *continued*
Gubler-millard G46.3
Guillain-barré (-strohl) G61.0
gustatory sweating G50.8
Hadfield-clarke K86.89
hair tourniquet - *see* Constriction, external, by
site
Hamman's J98.19
hand-foot L27.1
hand-shoulder G90.8
hantavirus (cardio)-pulmonary (HPS) (HCPS)
B33.4
happy puppet Q93.5
Harada's H30.81-
Hayem-faber D50.9
headache NEC G44.89
complicated NEC G44.59
Heberden's I20.8
Hedinger's E34.0
Hegglin's D72.0
HELLP (hemolysis, elevated liver enzymes
and low platelet count) O14.2-
complicating
childbirth O14.24
puerperium O14.25
hemolytic-uremic D59.3
hemophagocytic, infection-associated D76.2
Henoch-schönlein D69.0
hepatic flexure K59.8
hepatopulmonary K76.81
hepatorenal K76.7
following delivery O90.4
postoperative or postprocedural K91.83
postpartum, puerperal O90.4
hepatourologic K76.7
Herter (-gee) (nontropical sprue) K90.0
Heubner-herter K90.0
Heyd's K76.7
Hilger's G90.09
histamine-like (fish poisoning) - *see*
Poisoning, fish
histiocytic D76.3
histiocytosis NEC D76.3
HIV infection, acute B20
Hoffmann-Werdnig G12.0
Hollander-simons E88.1
Hoppe-goldflam G70.00
with exacerbation (acute) G70.01
in crisis G70.01
Horner's G90.2
hungry bone E83.81
hunterian glossitis D51.0
Hutchinson's triad A50.53
hyperabduction G54.0
hyperammonemia-hyperornithinemia-
homocitrullinemia E72.4
hypereosinophilic (idiopathic) D72.1
hyperimmunoglobulin D M04.1
hyperimmunoglobulin E (IgE) D82.4
hyperkalemic E87.5
hyperkinetic - *see* Hyperkinesia
hypermobility M35.7
hypernatremia E87.0
hyperosmolarity E87.0
hyperperfusion G97.82
hypersplenic D73.1
hypertransfusion, newborn P61.1
hyperventilation F45.8
hyperviscosity (of serum)
polycythemic D75.1
sclerothymic D58.8
hypoglycemic (familial) (neonatal) E16.2
hypokalemic E87.6
hyponatremic E87.1

Syndrome - *continued*
hypopituitarism E23.0
hypoplastic left-heart Q23.4
hypopotassemia E87.6
hyposmolality E87.1
hypotension, maternal O26.5-
hypothenar hammer I73.89
hypoventilation, obesity (OHS) E66.2
ICF (intravascular coagulation-fibrinolysis)
D65
idiopathic
cardiorespiratory distress, newborn P22.0
nephrotic (infantile) N04.9
iliotibial band M76.3-
immobility, immobilization (paraplegic)
M62.3
immune reconstitution D89.3
immune reconstitution inflammatory [IRIS]
D89.3
immunity deficiency, combined D81.9
immunodeficiency
acquired - *see* Human, immunodeficiency
virus (HIV) disease
combined D81.9
impending coronary I20.0
impingement, shoulder M75.4-
inappropriate secretion of antidiuretic hormone
E22.2
infant
of diabetic mother P70.1
gestational diabetes P70.0
infantilism (pituitary) E23.0
inferior vena cava I87.1
inspissated bile (newborn) P59.1
institutional (childhood) F94.2
insufficient sleep F51.12
intermediate coronary (artery) I20.0
interspinous ligament - *see* Spondylopathy,
specified NEC
intestinal
carcinoid E34.0
knot K56.2
intravascular coagulation-fibrinolysis (ICF)
D65
iodine-deficiency, congenital E00.9
type
mixed E00.2
myxedematous E00.1
neurological E00.0
IRDS (idiopathic respiratory distress,
newborn) P22.0
irritable
bowel K58.9
with
constipation K58.1
diarrhea K58.0
mixed K58.2
psychogenic F45.8
specified NEC K58.8
heart (psychogenic) F45.8
weakness F48.8
ischemic
bowel (transient) K55.9
chronic K55.1
due to mesenteric artery insufficiency
K55.1
steal T82.898
IVC (intravascular coagulopathy) D65
Ivemark's Q89.01
Jaccoud's - *see* Arthropathy, postrheumatic,
chronic
Jackson's G83.89
Jakob-creutzfeldt - *see* Creutzfeldt-Jakob
disease or syndrome

Syndrome - *continued*
jaw-winking Q07.8
Jervell-lange Nielsen I45.81
jet lag G47.25
Job's D71
Joseph-diamond-blackfan D61.01
jugular foramen G52.7
Kabuki Q89.8
Kanner's (autism) F84.0
Kartagener's Q89.3
Kelly's D50.1
Kimmelstiel-Wilson - *see* Diabetes, specified
    type, with Kimmelstiel-Wilson disease
Klein (e) -levine G47.13
Klippel-feil (brevicollis) Q76.1
Köhler-pellegrini-steida - *see* Bursitis, tibial
    collateral
Koenig's K59.8
Korsakoff (-Wernicke) (nonalcoholic) F04
    alcoholic F10.26
Kostmann's D70.0
Krabbe's congenital muscle hypoplasia Q79.8
labyrinthine   *see* subcategory H83.2
lacunar NEC G46.7
Lambert-eaton G70.80
    in
        neoplastic disease G73.1
        specified disease NEC G70.81
Landau-kleffner - *see* Epilepsy, specified NEC
Larsen's Q74.8
lateral
    cutaneous nerve of thigh G57.1-
    medullary G46.4
Launois' E22.0
lazy
    leukocyte D70.8
    posture M62.3
Lemiere I80.8
Lennox-gastaut G40.812
    intractable G40.814
        with status epilepticus G40.813
        without status epilepticus G40.814
    not intractable G40.812
        with status epilepticus G40.811
        without status epilepticus G40.812
lenticular, progressive E83.01
Leopold-levi's E05.90
Lev's I44.2
Li-fraumeni Z15.01
Lichtheim's D51.0
Lightwood's N25.89
Lignac (de Toni) (-fanconi) (-debré) E72.09
    with cystinosis E72.04
Likoff's I20.8
limbic epilepsy personality F07.0
liver-kidney K76.7
lobotomy F07.0
Loffler's J82
long arm 18 or 21 deletion Q93.89
long QT I45.81
Louis-barré G11.3
low
    atmospheric pressure T70.29
    back M54.5
    output (cardiac) I50.9
lower radicular, newborn (birth injury) P14.8
Luetscher's (dehydration) E86.0
Lupus anticoagulant D68.62
Lutembacher's Q21.1
macrophage activation D76.1
    due to infection D76.2
magnesium-deficiency R29.0
Majeed M04.8
Mal de Debarquement R42

Syndrome - *continued*
malabsorption K90.9
    postsurgical K91.2
malformation, congenital, due to
    alcohol Q86.0
    exogenous cause NEC Q86.8
    hydantoin Q86.1
    warfarin Q86.2
malignant
    carcinoid E34.0
    neuroleptic G21.0
Mallory-Weiss K22.6
mandibulofacial dysostosis Q75.4
manic-depressive - *see* Disorder, bipolar
maple-syrup-urine E71.0
Marable's I77.4
Marfan's Q87.40
    with
        cardiovascular manifestations Q87.418
            aortic dilation Q87.410
        ocular manifestations Q87.42
        skeletal manifestations Q87.43
Marie's (acromegaly) E22.0
mast cell activation - *see* Activation, mast cell
maternal hypotension - *see* Syndrome,
    hypotension, maternal
May (-hegglin) D72.0
McArdle (-schmidt) (-pearson) E74.04
McQuarrie's E16.2
meconium plug (newborn) P76.0
median arcuate ligament I77.4
Meekeren-ehlers-danlos Q79.6
megavitamin-b6 E67.2
Meige G24.4
MELAS E88.41
Mendelson's O74.0
MERRF (myoclonic epilepsy associated with
    ragged-red fibers) E88.42
mesenteric
    artery (superior) K55.1
    vascular insufficiency K55.1
metabolic E88.81
metastatic carcinoid E34.0
micrognathia-glossoptosis Q87.0
midbrain NEC G93.89
middle lobe (lung) J98.19
middle radicular G54.0
migraine - *see also* Migraine G43.909-
Mikulicz' K11.8
milk-alkali E83.52
Millard-gubler G46.3
Miller-dieker Q93.88
Miller-fisher G61.0
Minkowski-chauffard D58.0
Mirizzi's K83.1
MNGIE (Mitochondrial Neurogastrointestinal
    Encephalopathy) E88.49
Möbius, ophthalmoplegic migraine - *see*
    Migraine, ophthalmoplegic
monofixation H50.42
Morel-moore M85.2
Morel-Morgagni M85.2
Morgagni (-morel) (-stewart) M85.2
Morgagni-Adams-stokes I45.9
Muckle-Wells M04.2
mucocutaneous lymph node (acute febrile)
    (MCLS) M30.3
multiple endocrine neoplasia (MEN) - *see*
    Neoplasia, endocrine, multiple (MEN)
multiple operations - *see* Disorder, factitious
Mounier-kuhn Q32.4
    with bronchiectasis J47.9
        with
            exacerbation (acute) J47.1

Syndrome - *continued*
    lower respiratory infection J47.0
    acquired J98.09
        with bronchiectasis J47.9
            with
                exacerbation (acute) J47.1
                lower respiratory infection J47.0
myasthenic G70.9
    in
        diabetes mellitus - *see* Diabetes,
            amyotrophy
        endocrine disease NEC E34.9 [*G73.3*]
        neoplastic disease - *see also* Neoplasm
            D49.9 [*G73.3*]
        thyrotoxicosis (hyperthyroidism) E05.90
            [*G73.3*]
            with thyroid storm E05.91 [*G73.3*]
myelodysplastic D46.9
    with
        5q deletion D46.C
        isolated del (5q) chromosomal abnormality
            D46.C
    lesions, low grade D46.20
    specified NEC D46.Z   myelopathic pain
        G89.0
myeloproliferative (chronic) D47.1
myofascial pain M79.1
Naffziger's G54.0
nail patella Q87.2
NARP (Neuropathy, Ataxia and Retinitis
    pigmentosa) E88.49
neonatal abstinence P96.1
nephritic - *see also* Nephritis
    with edema - *see* Nephrosis
    acute N00.9
    chronic N03.9
    rapidly progressive N01.9
nephrotic (congenital) - *see also* Nephrosis
    N04.9
    with
        dense deposit disease N04.6
        diffuse
            crescentic glomerulonephritis N04.7
            endocapillary proliferative
                glomerulonephritis N04.4
            membranous glomerulonephritis N04.2
            mesangial proliferative glomerulonephritis
                N04.3
            mesangiocapillary glomerulonephritis
                N04.5
        focal and segmental glomerular lesions
            N04.1
        minor glomerular abnormality N04.0
        specified morphological changes NEC
            N04.8
    diabetic - *see* Diabetes, nephrosis
neurologic neglect R41.4
Nezelof's D81.4
Nonne-milroy-meige Q82.0
Nothnagel's vasomotor acroparesthesia I73.89
obesity hypoventilation (OHS) E66.2
oculomotor H51.9
ophthalmoplegia-cerebellar ataxia - *see*
    Strabismus, paralytic, third nerve
oral allergy T78.1
oral-facial-digital Q87.0
organic
    affective F06.30
    amnesic (not alcohol or drug-induced) F04
    brain F09
    depressive F06.31
    hallucinosis F06.0
    personality F07.0
Ormond's N13.5

Syndrome - *continued*
  oro-facial-digital Q87.0
  os trigonum Q68.8
  Osler-Weber-rendu I78.0
  osteoporosis-osteomalacia M83.8
  Osterreicher-turner Q87.2
  otolith - *see* subcategory H81.8
  oto-palatal-digital Q87.0
  outlet (thoracic) G54.0
  ovary
    polycystic E28.2
    resistant E28.39
    sclerocystic E28.2
  Owren's D68.2
  Paget-schroetter I82.890
  pain - *see also* Pain
    complex regional I G90.50
      lower limb G90.52-
      specified site NEC G90.59
      upper limb G90.51-
    complex regional II - *see* Causalgia
  painful
    bruising D69.2
    feet E53.8
    prostate N42.81
  paralysis agitans - *see* Parkinsonism
  paralytic G83.9
    specified NEC G83.89
  Parinaud's H51.0
  parkinsonian - *see* Parkinsonism
  Parkinson's - *see* Parkinsonism
  paroxysmal facial pain G50.0
  Parry's E05.00
    with thyroid storm E05.01
  Parsonage (-aldren) -turner G54.5
  patella clunk M25.86-
  Paterson (-brown) (-kelly) D50.1
  pectoral girdle I77.89
  pectoralis minor I77.89
  pediatric autoimmune neuropsychiatric
    disorders associated with streptococcal
    infections (PANDAS) D89.89
  Pelger-huet D72.0
  pellagra-cerebellar ataxia-renal aminoaciduria
    E72.02
  pellagroid E52
  Pellegrini-stieda - *see* Bursitis, tibial collateral
  pelvic congestion-fibrosis, female N94.89
  penta X Q97.1
  peptic ulcer - *see* Ulcer, peptic
  perabduction I77.89
  periodic fever M04.1
  periodic fever, aphthous stomatitis,
    pharyngitis, and adenopathy [PFAPA] M04.8
  periodic headache, in adults and children - *see*
    Headache, periodic syndromes in adults and
    children
  periurethral fibrosis N13.5
  phantom limb (without pain) G54.7
    with pain G54.6
  pharyngeal pouch D82.1
  Pick's - *see* Disease, Pick's
  Pickwickian E66.2
  PIE (pulmonary infiltration with eosinophilia)
    J82
  pigmentary pallidal degeneration (progressive)
    G23.0
  pineal E34.8
  pituitary E22.0
  plantar fascia M72.2
  placental transfusion - *see* Pregnancy,
    complicated by, placental transfusion
    syndromes

Syndrome - *continued*
  plateau iris (post-iridectomy) (postprocedural)
    H21.82
  Plummer-Vinson D50.1
  pluricarential of infancy E40
  plurideficiency E40
  pluriglandular (compensatory) E31.8
    autoimmune E31.0
  pneumatic hammer T75.21
  polyangiitis overlap M30.8
  polycarential of infancy E40
  polyglandular E31.8
    autoimmune E31.0
  polysplenia Q89.09
  pontine NEC G93.89
  popliteal
    artery entrapment I77.89
    web Q87.89
  postcardiac injury
    postcardiotomy I97.0
    postmyocardial infarction I24.1
  postcardiotomy I97.0
  post chemoembolization
  code to associated conditions
  postcholecystectomy K91.5
  postcommissurotomy I97.0
  postconcussional F07.81
  postcontusional F07.81
  postencephalitic F07.89
  posterior
    cervical sympathetic M53.0
    cord G83.83
    fossa compression G93.5
    reversible encephalopathy (PRES) I67.83
  postgastrectomy (dumping) K91.1
  postgastric surgery K91.1
  postinfarction I24.1
  postlaminectomy NEC M96.1
  postleukotomy F07.0
  postmastectomy lymphedema I97.2
  postmyocardial infarction I24.1
  postoperative NEC T81.9
    blind loop K90.2
  postpartum panhypopituitary (Sheehan) E23.0
  postpolio (myelitic) G14
  postthrombotic I87.009
    with
      inflammation I87.02-
        with ulcer I87.03-
      specified complication NEC I87.09-
      ulcer I87.01-
        with inflammation I87.03-
    asymptomatic I87.00-
  postvagotomy K91.1
  postvalvulotomy I97.0
  postviral NEC G93.3
    fatigue G93.3
  Potain's K31.0
  potassium intoxication E87.5
  precerebral artery (multiple) (bilateral) G45.2
  preinfarction I20.0
  preleukemic D46.9
  premature senility E34.8
  premenstrual dysphoric F32.89
  premenstrual tension N94.3
  Prinzmetal-massumi R07.1
  prune belly Q79.4
  pseudocarpal tunnel (sublimis) - *see*
  Syndrome, carpal tunnel
  pseudoparalytica G70.00
    with exacerbation (acute) G70.01
    in crisis G70.01
  pseudo -turner's Q87.1
  psycho-organic (nonpsychotic severity) F07.9

Syndrome - *continued*
  acute or subacute F05
    depressive type F06.31
    hallucinatory type F06.0
    nonpsychotic severity F07.0
    specified NEC F07.89
  pulmonary
    arteriosclerosis I27.0
    dysmaturity (Wilson-mikity) P27.0
    hypoperfusion (idiopathic) P22.0
    renal (hemorrhagic) (Goodpasture's) M31.0
  pure
    motor lacunar G46.5
    sensory lacunar G46.6
  Putnam-dana D51.0
  pyogenic arthritis, pyoderma gangrenosum,
    and acne [PAPA] M04.8
  pyramidopallidonigral G20
  pyriformis - *see* Lesion, nerve, sciatic
  QT interval prolongation I45.81
  radicular NEC - *see* Radiculopathy
    upper limbs, newborn (birth injury) P14.3
  rapid time-zone change G47.25
  Rasmussen G04.81
  Raymond (-céstan) I65.8
  Raynaud's I73.00
    with gangrene I73.01
  RDS (respiratory distress syndrome, newborn)
    P22.0
  reactive airways dysfunction J68.3
  Refsum's G60.1
  Reifenstein E34.52
  renal glomerulohyalinosis-diabetic - *see*
    Diabetes, nephrosis
  Rendu-osler-Weber I78.0
  residual ovary N99.83
  resistant ovary E28.39
  respiratory
    distress
      acute J80
      adult J80
      child J80
      idiopathic J84.114
      newborn (idiopathic) (type I) P22.0
      type II P22.1
  restless legs G25.81
  retinoblastoma (familial) C69.2
  retroperitoneal fibrosis N13.5
  retroviral seroconversion (acute) Z21
  Reye's G93.7
  Richter - *see* Leukemia, chronic lymphocytic,
    B-cell type
  Ridley's I50.1
  right
    heart, hypoplastic Q22.6
    ventricular obstruction - *see* Failure, heart,
      congestive
  Romano-Ward (prolonged QT interval) I45.81
  rotator cuff, shoulder - *see also* Tear, rotator
    cuff M75.10-
  Rotes Quérol - *see* Hyperostosis, ankylosing
  Roth - *see* Meralgia paresthetica
  rubella (congenital) P35.0
  Ruvalcaba-Myhre-smith E71.440
  Rytand-Lipsitch I44.2
  salt
    depletion E87.1
      due to heat NEC T67.8
        causing heat exhaustion or prostration
    T67.4
    low E87.1
  salt-losing N28.89
  Scaglietti-Dagnini E22.0
  scalenus anticus (anterior) G54.0

Syndrome - *continued*

scapulocostal - *see* Mononeuropathy, upper
   limb, specified site NEC
scapuloperoneal G71.0
schizophrenic, of childhood NEC F84.5
Schnitzler D47.2
Scholte's E34.0
Schroeder's E27.0
Schüller-Christian C96.5
Schwachman's - *see* Syndrome, Shwachman's
Schwartz (-Jampel) G71.13
Schwartz-Bartter E22.2
scimitar Q26.8
sclerocystic ovary E28.2
Seitelberger's G31.89
septicemic adrenal hemorrhage A39.1
seroconversion, retroviral (acute) Z21
serous meningitis G93.2
severe acute respiratory (SARS) J12.81
shaken infant T74.4
shock (traumatic) T79.4
   kidney N17.0
      following crush injury T79.5
   toxic A48.3
shock-lung J80
Shone's
   code to specific anomalies
short
   bowel K91.2
   rib Q77.2
shoulder-hand - *see* Algoneurodystrophy
Shwachman's D70.4
sicca - *see* Sicca syndrome
sick
   cell E87.1
   sinus I49.5
sick-euthyroid E07.81
sideropenic D50.1
Siemens' ectodermal dysplasia Q82.4
Silfversköld's Q78.9
Simons' E88.1
sinus tarsi M25.57-
sinusitis-bronchiectasis-situs inversus Q89.3
Sipple's E31.22
sirenomelia Q87.2
Slocumb's E27.0
slow flow, coronary I20.8
Sluder's G44.89
Smith-magenis Q93.88
Sneddon-Wilkinson L13.1
Soto's Q87.3
South African cardiomyopathy I42.8
spasmodic
   upward movement, eyes H51.8
   winking F95.8
Spen's I45.9
splenic
   agenesis Q89.01
   flexure K59.8
   neutropenia D73.81
Spurway's Q78.0
staphylococcal scalded skin L00
steal
   arteriovenous T82.898-
   ischemic T82.898-
   subclavian G45.8
Stein-Leventhal E28.2
Stein's E28.2
Stevens-Johnson syndrome L51.1
   toxic epidermal necrolysis overlap L51.3
Stewart-morel M85.2
Stickler Q89.8
stiff baby Q89.8
stiff man G25.82

Syndrome - *continued*

Still-Felty - *see* Felty's syndrome
Stokes (-Adams) I45.9
stone heart I50.1
straight back, congenital Q76.49
subclavian steal G45.8
subcoracoid-pectoralis minor G54.0
subcostal nerve compression I77.89
subphrenic interposition Q43.3
superior
   cerebellar artery I63.8
   mesenteric artery K55.1
   semi-circular canal dehiscence H83.8X-
   vena cava I87.1
supine hypotensive (maternal) - *see* Syndrome,
   hypotension, maternal
suprarenal cortical E27.0
supraspinatus - *see also* Tear, rotator cuff
   M75.10-
Susac G93.49
swallowed blood P78.2
sweat retention L74.0
Swyer Q99.1
Symond's G93.2
sympathetic
   cervical paralysis G90.2
   pelvic, female N94.89
systemic inflammatory response (SIRS), of
   non-infectious origin (without organ
   dysfunction) R65.10
   with acute organ dysfunction R65.11
tachycardia-bradycardia I49.5
takotsubo I51.81
TAR (thrombocytopenia with absent radius)
   Q87.2
tarsal tunnel G57.5-
teething K00.7
tegmental G93.89
telangiectasic-pigmentation-cataract Q82.8
temporal pyramidal apex - *see* Otitis, media,
   suppurative, acute
temporomandibular joint-pain-dysfunction
   M26.62-
Terry's (see also Myopia, degenerative) H44.2-
testicular feminization - *see also* Syndrome,
   androgen insensitivity E34.51
thalamic pain (hyperesthetic) G89.0
thoracic outlet (compression) G54.0
Thorson-björck E34.0
thrombocytopenia with absent radius (TAR)
   Q87.2
thyroid-adrenocortical insufficiency E31.0
tibial
   anterior M76.81-
   posterior M76.82-
Tietze's M94.0
time-zone (rapid) G47.25
Toni-fanconi E72.09
   with cystinosis E72.04
Touraine's Q79.8
tourniquet - *see* Constriction, external, by site
toxic shock A48.3
transient left ventricular apical ballooning
   I51.81
traumatic vasospastic T75.22
Treacher Collins Q75.4
triple X, female Q97.0
trisomy Q92.9
   13 Q91.7
      meiotic nondisjunction Q91.4
      mitotic nondisjunction Q91.5
      mosaicism Q91.5
      translocation Q91.6
   18 Q91.3

Syndrome - *continued*

      meiotic nondisjunction Q91.0
      mitotic nondisjunction Q91.1
      mosaicism Q91.1
      translocation Q91.2
   20 (q)(p) Q92.8
   21 Q90.9
      meiotic nondisjunction Q90.0
      mitotic nondisjunction Q90.1
      mosaicism Q90.1
      translocation Q90.2
   22 Q92.8
tropical wet feet T69.0-
Trousseau's I82.1
tumor lysis (following antineoplastic
   chemotherapy) (spontaneous) NEC E88.3
tumor necrosis factor receptor associated
   periodic (TRAPS) M04.1
Twiddler's (due to)
   automatic implantable defibrillator T82.198
   cardiac pacemaker T82.198
Unverricht (-lundborg) - *see* Epilepsy,
   generalized, idiopathic
upward gaze H51.8
uremia, chronic - *see also* Disease, kidney,
   chronic N18.9
urethral N34.3
urethro-oculo-articular - *see* Reiter's disease
urohepatic K76.7
vago-hypoglossal G52.7
vascular NEC in cerebrovascular disease
   G46.8
vasoconstriction, reversible cerebrovascular
   I67.841
vasomotor I73.9
vasospastic (traumatic) T75.22
vasovagal R55
van Buchem's M85.2
van der Hoeve's Q78.0
VATER Q87.2
velo-cardio-facial Q93.81
vena cava (inferior) (superior) (obstruction)
   I87.1
vertebral
   artery G45.0
      compression - *see* Syndrome, anterior,
      spinal artery, compression
   steal G45.0
vertebro-basilar artery G45.0
vertebrogenic (pain) M54.89
vertiginous - *see* Disorder, vestibular function
Vinson-plummer D50.1
virus B34.9
visceral larva migrans B83.0
visual disorientation H53.8
vitamin B6 deficiency E53.1
vitreal corneal H59.01-
vitreous (touch) H59.01-
Vogt-koyanagi H20.82-
Volkmann's T79.6
von Schroetter's I82.890
von Willebrand (-jürgen) D68.0
Waldenström-kjellberg D50.1
Wallenberg's G46.3
water retention E87.79
Waterhouse (-friderichsen) A39.1
Weber-gubler G46.3
Weber-leyden G46.3
Weber's G46.3
Wegener's M31.30
   with
      kidney involvement M31.31
      lung involvement M31.30
         with kidney involvement M31.31

Syndrome - *continued*
  Weingarten's (tropical eosinophilia) J82
  Weiss-baker G90.09
  Werdnig-Hoffman G12.0
  Wermer's E31.21
  Werner's E34.8
  Wernicke-korsakoff (nonalcoholic) F04
    alcoholic F10.26
  West's - *see* Epilepsy, spasms
  Westphal-Strümpell E83.01
  wet
    feet (maceration) (tropical) T69.0-
    lung, newborn P22.1
  whiplash S13.4
  whistling face Q87.0
  Wilkie's K55.1
  Wilkinson-sneddon L13.1
  Willebrand (-jürgens) D68.0
  Wilson's (hepatolenticular degeneration)
    E83.01
  Wiskott-aldrich D82.0
  withdrawal - *see* Withdrawal, state
    drug
      infant of dependent mother P96.1
      therapeutic use, newborn P96.2
  Woakes' (ethmoiditis) J33.1
  Wright's (hyperabduction) G54.0
  X I20.9
  XXXX Q97.1
  XXXXX Q97.1
  XXXXY Q98.1
  XXY Q98.0
  yellow nail L60.5
  Zahorsky's B08.5
  Zellweger syndrome E71.510
  Zellweger-like syndrome E71.541
Synechia (anterior) (iris) (posterior) (pupil) -
  see also Adhesions, iris
  intra-uterine (traumatic) N85.6
Synesthesia R20.8
Syngamiasis, syngamosis B83.3
Synodontia K00.2
Synorchidism, synorchism Q55.1
Synostosis (congenital) Q78.8
  astragalo-scaphoid Q74.2
  radioulnar Q74.0
Synovial sarcoma - *see* Neoplasm, connective
  tissue, malignant
Synovioma (malignant) - *see also* Neoplasm,
  connective tissue, malignant
  benign - *see* Neoplasm, connective tissue,
  benign
Synoviosarcoma - *see* Neoplasm, connective
  tissue, malignant
Synovitis - *see also* Tenosynovitis M65.9
  crepitant
    hand M70.0-
    wrist M70.03-
  gonococcal A54.49
  gouty - *see* Gout
  in (due to)
    crystals M65.8-
    gonorrhea A54.49
    syphilis (late) A52.78
  use, overuse, pressure - *see* Disorder, soft
    tissue, due to use
  infective NEC - *see* Tenosynovitis, infective
    NEC
  specified NEC - *see* Tenosynovitis, specified
    type NEC
  syphilitic A52.78
    congenital (early) A50.02
  toxic - *see* Synovitis, transient
  transient M67.3-

Synovitis - *continued*
  ankle M67.37-
  elbow M67.32-
  foot joint M67.37-
  hand joint M67.34-
  hip M67.35-
  knee M67.36-
  multiple site M67.39
  pelvic region M67.35-
  shoulder M67.31-
  specified joint NEC M67.38
  wrist M67.33-
  traumatic, current - *see* Sprain
  tuberculous - *see* Tuberculosis, synovitis
  villonodular (pigmented) M12.2-
    ankle M12.27-
    elbow M12.22-
    foot joint M12.27-
    hand joint M12.24-
    hip M12.25-
    knee M12.26-
    multiple site M12.29
    pelvic region M12.25-
    shoulder M12.21-
    specified joint NEC M12.28
    vertebrae M12.28
    wrist M12.23-
Syphilid A51.39
  congenital A50.06
  newborn A50.06
  tubercular (late) A52.79
Syphilis, syphilitic (acquired) A53.9
  abdomen (late) A52.79
  acoustic nerve A52.15
  adenopathy (secondary) A51.49
  adrenal (gland) (with cortical hypofunction)
    A52.79
  age under 2
  years NOS - *see also* Syphilis, congenital, early
    acquired A51.9
  alopecia (secondary) A51.32
  anemia (late) A52.79 [*D63.8*]
  aneurysm (aorta) (ruptured) A52.01
    central nervous system A52.05
    congenital A50.54 [*I79.0*]
  anus (late) A52.74
    primary A51.1
    secondary A51.39
  aorta (arch) (abdominal) (thoracic) A52.02
    aneurysm A52.01
  aortic (insufficiency) (regurgitation) (stenosis)
    A52.03
    aneurysm A52.01
  arachnoid (adhesive) (cerebral) (spinal)
    A52.13
  asymptomatic - *see* Syphilis, latent
  ataxia (locomotor) A52.11
  atrophoderma maculatum A51.39
  auricular fibrillation A52.06
  bladder (late) A52.76
  bone A52.77
    secondary A51.46
  brain A52.17
  breast (late) A52.79
  bronchus (late) A52.72
  bubo (primary) A51.0
  bulbar palsy A52.19
  bursa (late) A52.78
  cardiac decompensation A52.06
  cardiovascular A52.00
  central nervous system (late) (recurrent)
  (relapse) (tertiary) A52.3
    with
      ataxia A52.11

Syphilis, syphilitic - *continued*
  general paralysis A52.17
    juvenile A50.45
  paresis (general) A52.17
    juvenile A50.45
  tabes (dorsalis) A52.11
    juvenile A50.45
  taboparesis A52.17
    juvenile A50.45
  aneurysm A52.05
  congenital A50.40
  juvenile A50.40
  remission in (sustained) A52.3
  serology doubtful, negative, or positive
    A52.3
  specified nature or site NEC A52.19
  vascular A52.05
  cerebral A52.17
    meningovascular A52.13
    nerves (multiple palsies) A52.15
    sclerosis A52.17
    thrombosis A52.05
  cerebrospinal (tabetic type) A52.12
  cerebrovascular A52.05
  cervix (late) A52.76
  chancre (multiple) A51.0
    extragenital A51.2
    Rollet's A51.0
  Charcot's joint A52.16
  chorioretinitis A51.43
    congenital A50.01
    late A52.71
    prenatal A50.01
  choroiditis - *see* Syphilitic chorioretinitis
  choroidoretinitis - *see* Syphilitic chorioretinitis
  ciliary body (secondary) A51.43
    late A52.71
  colon (late) A52.74
  combined spinal sclerosis A52.11
  condyloma (latum) A51.31
  congenital A50.9
    with
      paresis (general) A50.45
      tabes (dorsalis) A50.45
      taboparesis A50.45
    chorioretinitis, choroiditis A50.01 [*H32*]
    early, or less than 2 years after birth NEC
    A50.2
      with manifestations - *see* Syphilis,
        congenital, early, symptomatic
      latent (without manifestations) A50.1
        negative spinal fluid test A50.1
        serology positive A50.1
      symptomatic A50.09
        cutaneous A50.06
        mucocutaneous A50.07
        oculopathy A50.01
        osteochondropathy A50.02
        pharyngitis A50.03
        pneumonia A50.04
        rhinitis A50.05
        visceral A50.08
      interstitial keratitis A50.31
      juvenile neurosyphilis A50.45
    late, or 2 years or more after birth NEC
    A50.7
      chorioretinitis, choroiditis A50.32
      interstitial keratitis A50.31
      juvenile neurosyphilis A50.45
      latent (without manifestations) A50.6
        negative spinal fluid test A50.6
        serology positive A50.6
      symptomatic or with manifestations NEC
      A50.59

Syphilis, syphilitic - *continued*

arthropathy A50.55
  cardiovascular A50.54
  Clutton's joints A50.51
  Hutchinson's teeth A50.52
  Hutchinson's triad A50.53
  osteochondropathy A50.56
  saddle nose A50.57
conjugal A53.9
  tabes A52.11
conjunctiva (late) A52.71
contact Z20.2
cord bladder A52.19
cornea, late A52.71
coronary (artery) (sclerosis) A52.06
coryza, congenital A50.05
cranial nerve A52.15
  multiple palsies A52.15
cutaneous - *see* Syphilis, skin
dacryocystitis (late) A52.71
degeneration, spinal cord A52.12
dementia paralytica A52.17
  juvenilis A50.45
destruction of bone A52.77
dilatation, aorta A52.01
due to blood transfusion A53.9
dura mater A52.13
ear A52.79
  inner A52.79
    nerve (eighth) A52.15
    neurorecurrence A52.15
early A51.9
  cardiovascular A52.00
  central nervous system A52.3
  latent (without manifestations) (less than 2
  years after infection) A51.5
    negative spinal fluid test A51.5
    serological relapse after treatment A51.5
    serology positive A51.5
  relapse (treated, untreated) A51.9
  skin A51.39
  symptomatic A51.9
    extragenital chancre A51.2
    primary, except extragenital chancre A51.0
    secondary - *see also* Syphilis, secondary
    A51.39
      relapse (treated, untreated) A51.49
  ulcer A51.39
eighth nerve (neuritis) A52.15
endemic A65
endocarditis A52.03
  aortic A52.03
  pulmonary A52.03
epididymis (late) A52.76
epiglottis (late) A52.73
epiphysitis (congenital) (early) A50.02
episcleritis (late) A52.71
esophagus A52.79
eustachian tube A52.73
exposure to Z20.2
eye A52.71
eyelid (late) (with gumma) A52.71
fallopian tube (late) A52.76
fracture A52.77
gallbladder (late) A52.74
gastric (polyposis) (late) A52.74
general A53.9
  paralysis A52.17
    juvenile A50.45
genital (primary) A51.0
glaucoma A52.71
gumma NEC A52.79
  cardiovascular system A52.00
  central nervous system A52.3

Syphilis, syphilitic - *continued*

congenital A50.59
heart (block) (decompensation) (disease)
(failure) A52.06 [*I52*]
  valve NEC A52.03
hemianesthesia A52.19
hemianopsia A52.71
hemiparesis A52.17
hemiplegia A52.17
hepatic artery A52.09
hepatis A52.74
hepatomegaly, congenital A50.08
hereditaria tarda - *see* Syphilis, congenital, late
hereditary - *see* Syphilis, congenital
  Hutchinson's teeth A50.52
hyalitis A52.71
inactive - *see* Syphilis, latent
infantum - *see* Syphilis, congenital
inherited - *see* Syphilis, congenital
internal ear A52.79
intestine (late) A52.74
iris, iritis (secondary) A51.43
  late A52.71
joint (late) A52.77
keratitis (congenital) (interstitial) (late) A50.31
kidney (late) A52.75
lacrimal passages (late) A52.71
larynx (late) A52.73
late A52.9
  cardiovascular A52.00
  central nervous system A52.3
  kidney A52.75
  latent or 2 years or more after infection
  (without manifestations) A52.8
    negative spinal fluid test A52.8
    serology positive A52.8
  paresis A52.17
  specified site NEC A52.79
  symptomatic or with manifestations A52.79
  tabes A52.11
latent A53.0
  with signs or symptoms
code by site and stage under Syphilis
  central nervous system A52.2
  date of infection unspecified A53.0
  early, or less than 2 years after infection
  A51.5
  follow-up of latent syphilis A53.0
    date of infection unspecified A53.0
    late, or 2 years or more after infection
    A52.8
  late, or 2 years or more after infection A52.8
  positive serology (only finding) A53.0
    date of infection unspecified A53.0
    early, or less than 2 years after infection
    A51.5
    late, or 2 years or more after infection
    A52.8
lens (late) A52.71
leukoderma A51.39
  late A52.79
lienitis A52.79
lip A51.39
  chancre (primary) A51.2
  late A52.79
Lissauer's paralysis A52.17
liver A52.74
locomotor ataxia A52.11
lung A52.72
lymph gland (early) (secondary) A51.49
  late A52.79
lymphadenitis (secondary) A51.49
macular atrophy of skin A51.39
  striated A52.79

Syphilis, syphilitic - *continued*

mediastinum (late) A52.73
meninges (adhesive) (brain) (spinal cord)
  A52.13
meningitis A52.13
  acute (secondary) A51.41
  congenital A50.41
meningoencephalitis A52.14
meningovascular A52.13
  congenital A50.41
mesarteritis A52.09
  brain A52.04
middle ear A52.77
mitral stenosis A52.03
monoplegia A52.17
mouth (secondary) A51.39
  late A52.79
mucocutaneous (secondary) A51.39
  late A52.79
mucous
  membrane (secondary) A51.39
    late A52.79
  patches A51.39
    congenital A50.07
mulberry molars A50.52
muscle A52.78
myocardium A52.06
nasal sinus (late) A52.73
neonatorum - *see* Syphilis, congenital
nephrotic syndrome (secondary) A51.44
nerve palsy (any cranial nerve) A52.15
  multiple A52.15
nervous system, central A52.3
neuritis A52.15
  acoustic A52.15
neurorecidive of retina A52.19
neuroretinitis A52.19
newborn - *see* Syphilis, congenital
nodular superficial (late) A52.79
nonvenereal A65
nose (late) A52.73
  saddle back deformity A50.57
occlusive arterial disease A52.09
oculopathy A52.71
ophthalmic (late) A52.71
optic nerve (atrophy) (neuritis) (papilla)
  A52.15
orbit (late) A52.71
organic A53.9
osseous (late) A52.77
osteochondritis (congenital) (early) A50.02
  [*M90.80*]
osteoporosis A52.77
ovary (late) A52.76
oviduct (late) A52.76
palate (late) A52.79
pancreas (late) A52.74
paralysis A52.17
  general A52.17
    juvenile A50.45
paresis (general) A52.17
  juvenile A50.45
paresthesia A52.19
Parkinson's disease or syndrome A52.19
paroxysmal tachycardia A52.06
pemphigus (congenital) A50.06
penis (chancre) A51.0
  late A52.76
pericardium A52.06
perichondritis, larynx (late) A52.73
periosteum (late) A52.77
  congenital (early) A50.02 [*M90.80*]
  early (secondary) A51.46
peripheral nerve A52.79

Syphilis, syphilitic - *continued*
petrous bone (late) A52.77
pharynx (late) A52.73
  secondary A51.39
pituitary (gland) A52.79
pleura (late) A52.73
pneumonia, white A50.04
pontine lesion A52.17
portal vein A52.09
primary A51.0
  anal A51.1
  and secondary - *see* Syphilis, secondary
  central nervous system A52.3
  extragenital chancre NEC A51.2
  fingers A51.2
  genital A51.0
  lip A51.2
  specified site NEC A51.2
  tonsils A51.2
prostate (late) A52.76
ptosis (eyelid) A52.71
pulmonary (late) A52.72
  artery A52.09
pyelonephritis (late) A52.75
recently acquired, symptomatic A51.9
rectum (late) A52.74
respiratory tract (late) A52.73
retina, late A52.71
retrobulbar neuritis A52.15
salpingitis A52.76
sclera (late) A52.71
sclerosis
  cerebral A52.17
  coronary A52.06
  multiple A52.11
scotoma (central) A52.71
scrotum (late) A52.76
secondary (and primary) A51.49
  adenopathy A51.49
  anus A51.39
  bone A51.46
  chorioretinitis, choroiditis A51.43
  hepatitis A51.45
  liver A51.45
  lymphadenitis A51.49
  meningitis (acute) A51.41
  mouth A51.39
  mucous membranes A51.39
  periosteum, periostitis A51.46
  pharynx A51.39
  relapse (treated, untreated) A51.49
  skin A51.39
  specified form NEC A51.49
  tonsil A51.39
  ulcer A51.39
  viscera NEC A51.49
  vulva A51.39
seminal vesicle (late) A52.76
seronegative with signs or symptoms
code by site and stage under Syphilis
seropositive
  with signs or symptoms
code by site and stage under Syphilis
  follow-up of latent syphilis - *see* Syphilis,
    latent
  only finding - *see* Syphilis, latent
seventh nerve (paralysis) A52.15
sinus, sinusitis (late) A52.73
skeletal system A52.77
skin (with ulceration) (early) (secondary)
  A51.39
  late or tertiary A52.79
small intestine A52.74
spastic spinal paralysis A52.17

Syphilis, syphilitic - *continued*
spermatic cord (late) A52.76
spinal (cord) A52.12
spleen A52.79
splenomegaly A52.79
spondylitis A52.77
staphyloma A52.71
stigmata (congenital) A50.59
stomach A52.74
synovium A52.78
tabes dorsalis (late) A52.11
  juvenile A50.45
tabetic type A52.11
  juvenile A50.45
taboparesis A52.17
  juvenile A50.45
tachycardia A52.06
tendon (late) A52.78
tertiary A52.9
  with symptoms NEC A52.79
  cardiovascular A52.00
  central nervous system A52.3
  multiple NEC A52.79
  specified site NEC A52.79
testis A52.76
thorax A52.73
throat A52.73
thymus (gland) (late) A52.79
thyroid (late) A52.79
tongue (late) A52.79
tonsil (lingual) (late) A52.73
  primary A51.2
  secondary A51.39
trachea (late) A52.73
tunica vaginalis (late) A52.76
ulcer (any site) (early) (secondary) A51.39
  late A52.79
  perforating A52.79
    foot A52.11
urethra (late) A52.76
urogenital (late) A52.76
uterus (late) A52.76
uveal tract (secondary) A51.43
  late A52.71
uveitis (secondary) A51.43
  late A52.71
uvula (late) (perforated) A52.79
vagina A51.0
  late A52.76
valvulitis NEC A52.03
vascular A52.00
  brain (cerebral) A52.05
ventriculi A52.74
vesicae urinariae (late) A52.76
viscera (abdominal) (late) A52.74
  secondary A51.49
vitreous (opacities) (late) A52.71
  hemorrhage A52.71
vulva A51.0
  late A52.76
  secondary A51.39
Syphiloma A52.79
  cardiovascular system A52.00
  central nervous system A52.3
  circulatory system A52.00
  congenital A50.59
Syphilophobia F45.29
Syringadenoma - *see also* Neoplasm, skin,
  benign
  papillary - *see* Neoplasm, skin, benign
Syringobulbia G95.0
Syringocystadenoma - *see* Neoplasm, skin,
  benign
  papillary - *see* Neoplasm, skin, benign

Syringoma - *see also* Neoplasm, skin, benign
  chondroid - *see* Neoplasm, skin, benign
Syringomyelia G95.0
Syringomyelitis - *see* Encephalitis
Syringomyelocele - *see* Spina bifida
Syringopontia G95.0
System, systemic - *see also* condition
  disease, combined - *see* Degeneration,
    combined
  inflammatory response syndrome (SIRS) of
    non-infectious origin (without organ
    dysfunction) R65.10
    with acute organ dysfunction R65.11
  lupus erythematosus M32.9
    inhibitor present D68.62

T

Tabacism, tabacosis, tabagism - *see also*
  Poisoning, tobacco
  meaning dependence (without remission)
    F17.200
    with
      disorder F17.299
        in remission F17.211
        specified disorder NEC F17.298
      withdrawal F17.203
Tabardillo A75.9
  flea-borne A75.2
  louse-borne A75.0
Tabes, tabetic A52.10
  with
    central nervous system syphilis A52.10
    Charcot's joint A52.16
    cord bladder A52.19
    crisis, viscera (any) A52.19
    paralysis, general A52.17
    paresis (general) A52.17
    perforating ulcer (foot) A52.19
  arthropathy (Charcot) A52.16
  bladder A52.19
  bone A52.11
  cerebrospinal A52.12
  congenital A50.45
  conjugal A52.10
  dorsalis A52.11
    juvenile A50.49
  juvenile A50.49
  latent A52.19
  mesenterica A18.39
  paralysis, insane, general A52.17
  spasmodic A52.17
  syphilis (cerebrospinal) A52.12
Taboparalysis A52.17
Taboparesis (remission) A52.17
  juvenile A50.45
TAC (trigeminal autonomic cephalgia) NEC
  G44.099
  intractable G44.091
  not intractable G44.099
Tache noir S60.22-
Tachyalimentation K91.2
Tachyarrhythmia, tachyrhythmia - *see*
  Tachycardia
Tachycardia R00.0
  atrial (paroxysmal) I47.1
  auricular I47.1
  AV nodal re-entry (re-entrant) I47.1
  junctional (paroxysmal) I47.1
  newborn P29.11
  nodal (paroxysmal) I47.1
  non-paroxysmal AV nodal I45.89
  paroxysmal (sustained) (nonsustained) I47.9
    with sinus bradycardia I49.5

Tachycardia - *continued*
  atrial (PAT) I47.1
  atrioventricular (AV) (re-entrant) I47.1
    psychogenic F54
  junctional I47.1
    ectopic I47.1
  nodal I47.1
  psychogenic (atrial) (supraventricular)
    (ventricular) F54
  supraventricular (sustained) I47.1
    psychogenic F54
  ventricular I47.2
    psychogenic F54
  psychogenic F45.8
  sick sinus I49.5
  sinoauricular NOS R00.0
    paroxysmal I47.1
  sinus [sinusal] NOS R00.0
    paroxysmal I47.1
  supraventricular I47.1
  ventricular (paroxysmal) (sustained) I47.2
    psychogenic F54
Tachygastria K31.89
Tachypnea R06.82
  hysterical F45.8
  newborn (idiopathic) (transitory) P22.1
  psychogenic F45.8
  transitory, of newborn P22.1
Taenia (infection) (infestation) B68.9
  diminuta B71.0
  echinococcal infestation B67.90
  mediocanellata B68.1
  nana B71.0
  saginata B68.1
  solium (intestinal form) B68.0
    larval form - *see* Cysticercosis
Taeniasis (intestine) - *see* Taenia
TACO (transfusion associated circulatory overload) E87.71
Tag (hypertrophied skin) (infected) L91.8
  adenoid J35.8
  anus K64.4
  hemorrhoidal K64.4
  hymen N89.8
  perineal N90.89
  preauricular Q17.0
  sentinel K64.4
  skin L91.8
    accessory (congenital) Q82.8
    anus K64.4
    congenital Q82.8
    preauricular Q17.0
  tonsil J35.8
  urethra, urethral N36.8
  vulva N90.89
Tahyna fever B33.8
Takahara's disease E80.3
Takayasu's disease or syndrome M31.4
Talcosis (pulmonary) J62.0
Talipes (congenital) Q66.89
  acquired, planus - *see* Deformity, limb, flat foot
  asymmetric Q66.89
  calcaneovalgus Q66.4
  calcaneovarus Q66.1
  calcaneus Q66.89
  cavus Q66.7
  equinovalgus Q66.6
  equinovarus Q66.0
  equinus Q66.89
  percavus Q66.7
  planovalgus Q66.6
  planus (acquired) (any degree) - *see also* Deformity, limb, flat foot

Talipes - *continued*
  congenital Q66.5-
    due to rickets (sequelae) E64.3
  valgus Q66.6
  varus Q66.3
Tall stature, constitutional E34.4
Talma's disease M62.89
Talon noir S90.3-
  hand S60.22-
  heel S90.3-
  toe S90.1-
Tamponade, heart I31.4
Tanapox (virus disease) B08.71
Tangier disease E78.6
Tantrum, child problem F91.8
Tapeworm (infection) (infestation) - *see* Infestation, tapeworm
Tapia's syndrome G52.7
TAR (thrombocytopenia with absent radius) syndrome Q87.2
Tarral-besnier disease L44.0
Tarsal tunnel syndrome - *see* Syndrome, tarsal tunnel
Tarsalgia - *see* Pain, limb, lower
Tarsitis (eyelid) H01.8
  syphilitic A52.71
  tuberculous A18.4
Tartar (teeth) (dental calculus) K03.6
Tattoo (mark) L81.8
Tauri's disease E74.09
Taurodontism K00.2
Taussig-bing syndrome Q20.1
Taybi's syndrome Q87.2
Tay-sachs amaurotic familial idiocy or disease E75.02
TBI (traumatic brain injury) S06.9
Teacher's node or nodule J38.2
Tear, torn (traumatic) - *see also* Laceration
  with abortion - *see* Abortion
  annular fibrosis M51.35
  anus, anal (sphincter) S31.831
    complicating delivery
      with third degree perineal laceration - *see also* Delivery, complicated, by, laceration, perineum, third degree O70.20
        with mucosa O70.3
      without third degree perineal laceration O70.4
    nontraumatic (healed) (old) K62.81
  articular cartilage, old - *see* Derangement, joint, articular cartilage, by site
  bladder
    with ectopic or molar pregnancy O08.6
    following ectopic or molar pregnancy O08.6
    obstetrical O71.5
    traumatic - *see* Injury, bladder
  bowel
    with ectopic or molar pregnancy O08.6
    following ectopic or molar pregnancy O08.6
    obstetrical trauma O71.5
  broad ligament
    with ectopic or molar pregnancy O08.6
    following ectopic or molar pregnancy O08.6
    obstetrical trauma O71.6
  bucket handle (knee) (meniscus) - *see* Tear, meniscus
  capsule, joint - *see* Sprain
  cartilage - *see also* Sprain
    articular, old - *see* Derangement, joint, articular cartilage, by site
  cervix
    with ectopic or molar pregnancy O08.6
    following ectopic or molar pregnancy O08.6
    obstetrical trauma (current) O71.3

Tear, torn - *continued*
  old N88.1
    traumatic - *see* Injury, uterus
  dural G97.41
    nontraumatic G96.11
  internal organ - *see* Injury, by site
  knee cartilage
    articular (current) S83.3-
    old - *see* Derangement, knee, meniscus, due to old tear
  ligament - *see* Sprain
  meniscus (knee) (current injury) S83.209
    bucket-handle S83.20-
    lateral
      bucket-handle S83.25-
      complex S83.27-
      peripheral S83.26-
      specified type NEC S83.28-
    medial
      bucket-handle S83.21-
      complex S83.23-
      peripheral S83.22-
      specified type NEC S83.24-
    old - *see* Derangement, knee, meniscus, due to old tear
    site other than knee   code as Sprain
    specified type NEC S83.20-
  muscle - *see* Strain
  pelvic
    floor, complicating delivery O70.1
    organ NEC, obstetrical trauma O71.5
      with ectopic or molar pregnancy O08.6
      following ectopic or molar pregnancy O08.6
  perineal, secondary O90.1
  periurethral tissue, obstetrical trauma O71.82
    with ectopic or molar pregnancy O08.6
    following ectopic or molar pregnancy O08.6
  rectovaginal septum - *see* Laceration, vagina
  retina, retinal (without detachment) (horseshoe) - *see also* Break, retina, horseshoe
    with detachment - *see* Detachment, retina, with retinal, break
  rotator cuff (nontraumatic) M75.10-
    complete M75.12-
    incomplete M75.11-
    traumatic S46.01-
      capsule S43.42-
  semilunar cartilage, knee - *see* Tear, meniscus
  supraspinatus (complete) (incomplete) (nontraumatic) - *see also* Tear, rotator cuff M75.10-
  tendon - *see* Strain
  tentorial, at birth P10.4
  umbilical cord
    complicating delivery O69.89
  urethra
    with ectopic or molar pregnancy O08.6
    following ectopic or molar pregnancy O08.6
    obstetrical trauma O71.5
  uterus - *see* Injury, uterus
  vagina - *see* Laceration, vagina
  vessel, from catheter - *see* Puncture, accidental complicating surgery   vulva, complicating delivery O70.0
Tear-stone - *see* Dacryolith
Teeth - *see also* condition
  grinding
    psychogenic F45.8
    sleep related G47.63
Teething (syndrome) K00.7
Telangiectasia, telangiectasis (verrucous) I78.1
  ataxic (cerebellar) (Louis-bar) G11.3

Telangiectasia, telangiectasis - *continued*
  familial I78.0
  hemorrhagic, hereditary (congenital) (senile)
    I78.0
  hereditary, hemorrhagic (congenital) (senile)
    I78.0
  juxtafoveal H35.07-
  macular H35.07-
  macularis eruptiva perstans D47.01
  parafoveal H35.07-
  retinal (idiopathic) (juxtafoveal) (macular)
    (parafoveal) H35.07-
  spider I78.1
Telephone scatologia F65.89
Telescoped bowel or intestine K56.1
  congenital Q43.8
Temperature
  body, high (of unknown origin) R50.9
  cold, trauma from T69.9
    newborn P80.0
    specified effect NEC T69.8
Temple - *see* condition
Temporal - *see* condition
Temporomandibular joint pain-dysfunction
  syndrome M26.62-
Temporosphenoidal - *see* condition
Tendency
  bleeding - *see* Defect, coagulation
  suicide
    meaning personal history of attempted
      suicide Z91.5
    meaning suicidal ideation - *see* Ideation,
      suicidal
  to fall R29.6
Tenderness, abdominal R10.819
  epigastric R10.816
  generalized R10.817
  left lower quadrant R10.814
  left upper quadrant R10.812
  periumbilic R10.815
  right lower quadrant R10.813
  right upper quadrant R10.811
  rebound R10.829
    epigastric R10.826
    generalized R10.827
    left lower quadrant R10.824
    left upper quadrant R10.822
    periumbilic R10.825
    right lower quadrant R10.823
    right upper quadrant R10.821
Tendinitis, tendonitis - *see also* Enthesopathy
  Achilles M76.6-
  adhesive - *see* Tenosynovitis, specified type
    NEC
    shoulder - *see* Capsulitis, adhesive
  bicipital M75.2-
  calcific M65.2-
    ankle M65.27-
    foot M65.27-
    forearm M65.23-
    hand M65.24-
    lower leg M65.26-
    multiple sites M65.29
    pelvic region M65.25-
    shoulder M75.3-
    specified site NEC M65.28
    thigh M65.25-
    upper arm M65.22-
  due to use, overuse, pressure - *see also*
  Disorder, soft tissue, due to use
    specified NEC - *see* Disorder, soft tissue, due
    to use, specified NEC
  gluteal M76.0-
  patellar M76.5-

Tendinitis, tendonitis - *continued*
  peroneal M76.7-
  psoas M76.1-
  tibial (posterior) M76.82-
    anterior M76.81-
  trochanteric - *see* Bursitis, hip, trochanteric
Tendon - *see* condition
Tendosynovitis - *see* Tenosynovitis
Tenesmus (rectal) R19.8
  vesical R30.1
Tennis elbow - *see* Epicondylitis, lateral
Tenonitis - *see also* Tenosynovitis
  eye (capsule) H05.04-
Tenontosynovitis - *see* Tenosynovitis
Tenontothecitis - *see* Tenosynovitis
Tenophyte - *see* Disorder, synovium, specified
  type NEC
Tenosynovitis - *see also* Synovitis M65.9
  adhesive - *see* Tenosynovitis, specified type
    NEC
    shoulder - *see* Capsulitis, adhesive
  bicipital (calcifying) - *see* Tendinitis, bicipital
  gonococcal A54.49
  in (due to)
    crystals M65.8-
    gonorrhea A54.49
    syphilis (late) A52.78
    use, overuse, pressure - *see also* Disorder,
    soft tissue, due to use
      specified NEC - *see* Disorder, soft tissue,
      due to use, specified NEC
  infective NEC M65.1-
    ankle M65.17-
    foot M65.17-
    forearm M65.13-
    hand M65.14-
    lower leg M65.16-
    multiple sites M65.19
    pelvic region M65.15-
    shoulder region M65.11-
    specified site NEC M65.18
    thigh M65.15-
    upper arm M65.12-
  radial styloid M65.4
  shoulder region M65.81-
    adhesive - *see* Capsulitis, adhesive
  specified type NEC M65.88
    ankle M65.87-
    foot M65.87-
    forearm M65.83-
    hand M65.84-
    lower leg M65.86-
    multiple sites M65.89
    pelvic region M65.85-
    shoulder region M65.81-
    specified site NEC M65.88
    thigh M65.85-
    upper arm M65.82-
  tuberculous - *see* Tuberculosis, tenosynovitis
Tenovaginitis - *see* Tenosynovitis
Tension
  arterial, high - *see also* Hypertension
    without diagnosis of hypertension R03.0
  headache G44.209
    intractable G44.201
    not intractable G44.209
  nervous R45.0
  pneumothorax J93.0
  premenstrual N94.3
  state (mental) F48.9
Tentorium - *see* condition
Teratencephalus Q89.8
Teratism Q89.7

Teratoblastoma (malignant) - *see* Neoplasm,
  malignant, by site
Teratocarcinoma - *see also* Neoplasm,
  malignant, by site
  liver C22.7
Teratoma (solid) - *see also* Neoplasm,
  uncertain behavior, by site
  with embryonal carcinoma, mixed - *see*
    Neoplasm, malignant, by site
  with malignant transformation - *see* Neoplasm,
    malignant, by site
  adult (cystic) - *see* Neoplasm, benign, by site
  benign - *see* Neoplasm, benign, by site
  combined with choriocarcinoma - *see*
    Neoplasm, malignant, by site
  cystic (adult) - *see* Neoplasm, benign, by site
  differentiated - *see* Neoplasm, benign, by site
  embryonal - *see also* Neoplasm, malignant, by
    site
    liver C22.7
  immature - *see* Neoplasm, malignant, by site
  liver C22.7
    adult, benign, cystic, differentiated type or
    mature D13.4
  malignant - *see also* Neoplasm, malignant, by
    site
    anaplastic - *see* Neoplasm, malignant, by site
    intermediate - *see* Neoplasm, malignant, by
      site
      specified site - *see* Neoplasm, malignant, by
      site
      unspecified site C62.90
    undifferentiated - *see* Neoplasm, malignant,
      by site
  mature - *see* Neoplasm, uncertain behavior, by
    site
    malignant - *see* Neoplasm, by site, malignant,
      by site
  ovary D27.-
    embryonal, immature or malignant C56-
  solid - *see* Neoplasm, uncertain behavior, by
    site
  testis C62.9-
    adult, benign, cystic, differentiated type or
    mature D29.2-
    scrotal C62.1-
    undescended C62.0-
Termination
  anomalous - *see also* Malposition, congenital
    right pulmonary vein Q26.3
  pregnancy, elective Z33.2
Ternidens diminutus infestation B81.8
Ternidensiasis B81.8
Terror(s) night (child) F51.4
Terrorism, victim of Z65.4
Terry's syndrome (see also Myopia,
  degenerative) H44.2-
Tertiary - *see* condition
Test, tests, testing (for)
  adequacy (for dialysis)
    hemodialysis Z49.31
    peritoneal Z49.32
  blood pressure Z01.30
    abnormal reading - *see* Blood, pressure
  blood-alcohol Z04.8
    positive - *see* Findings, abnormal, in blood
  blood-drug Z04.8
    positive - *see* Findings, abnormal, in blood
    blood typing Z01.83
    Rh typing Z01.83
  cardiac pulse generator (battery) Z45.010
  fertility Z31.41
  genetic
    disease carrier status for procreative

Test, tests, testing - *continued*
  management
    female Z31.430
    male Z31.440
    male partner of patient with recurrent
      pregnancy loss Z31.441
    procreative management NEC
      female Z31.438
      male Z31.448
  hearing Z01.10
    with abnormal findings NEC Z01.118
  HIV (human immunodeficiency virus)
    nonconclusive (in infants) R75
    positive Z21
    seropositive Z21
  immunity status Z01.84
  intelligence NEC Z01.89
  laboratory (as part of a general medical
    examination) Z00.00
    with abnormal finding Z00.01
    for medicolegal reason NEC Z04.8
  male partner of patient with recurrent
    pregnancy loss Z31.441
  Mantoux (for tuberculosis) Z11.1
    abnormal result R76.11
  pregnancy, positive first pregnancy - *see*
    Pregnancy, normal, first
  procreative Z31.49
    fertility Z31.41
  skin, diagnostic
    allergy Z01.82
      special screening examination - *see*
    Screening, by name of disease
    Mantoux Z11.1
    tuberculin Z11.1
  specified NEC Z01.89
  tuberculin Z11.1
    abnormal result R76.11
  vision Z01.00
    with abnormal findings Z01.01
  Wassermann Z11.3
    positive - *see* Serology for syphilis, positive
Testicle, testicular, testis - *see also* condition
  feminization syndrome - *see also* Syndrome,
    androgen insensitivity E34.51
  migrans Q55.29
Tetanus, tetanic (cephalic) (convulsions) A35
  with
    abortion A34
    ectopic or molar pregnancy O08.0
  following ectopic or molar pregnancy O08.0
  inoculation reaction (due to serum) - *see*
    Complications, vaccination
  neonatorum A33
  obstetrical A34
  puerperal, postpartum, childbirth A34
Tetany (due to) R29.0
  alkalosis E87.3
  associated with rickets E55.0
  convulsions R29.0
    hysterical F44.5
  functional (hysterical) F44.5
  hyperkinetic R29.0
    hysterical F44.5
  hyperpnea R06.4
    hysterical F44.5
    psychogenic F45.8
  hyperventilation - *see also* Hyperventilation
    R06.4
    hysterical F44.5
  neonatal (without calcium or magnesium
    deficiency) P71.3
  parathyroid (gland) E20.9
  parathyroprival E89.2

Tetany - *continued*
  post (para) thyroidectomy E89.2
  postoperative E89.2
  pseudotetany R29.0
  psychogenic (conversion reaction) F44.5
Tetralogy of Fallot Q21.3
Tetraplegia (chronic) - *see also* Quadriplegia
  G82.50
Thailand hemorrhagic fever A91
Thalassanemia - *see* Thalassemia
Thalassemia (anemia) (disease) D56.9
  with other hemoglobinopathy D56.8
  alpha (major) (severe) (triple gene defect)
    D56.0
    minor D56.3
    silent carrier D56.3
    trait D56.3
  beta (severe) D56.1
    homozygous D56.1
    major D56.1
    minor D56.3
    trait D56.3
  delta-beta (homozygous) D56.2
    minor D56.3
    trait D56.3
  dominant D56.8
  hemoglobin
    C D56.8
    E-beta D56.5
  intermedia D56.1
  major D56.1
  minor D56.3
  mixed D56.8
  sickle-cell - *see* Disease, sickle-cell,
    thalassemia
  specified type NEC D56.8
  trait D56.3
  variants D56.8
Thanatophoric dwarfism or short stature
  Q77.1
Thaysen-gee disease (nontropical sprue)
  K90.0
Thaysen's disease K90.0
Thecoma D27-
  luteinized D27-
  malignant C56-
Thelarche, premature E30.8
Thelaziasis B83.8
Thelitis N61.0
  puerperal, postpartum or gestational - *see*
    Infection, nipple
Therapeutic - *see* condition
Therapy
  drug, long-term (current) (prophylactic)
    agents affecting estrogen receptors and
      estrogen levels NEC Z79.818
    anastrozole (Arimidex) Z79.811
    antibiotics Z79.2
      short-term use   omit code
    anticoagulants Z79.01
    anti-inflammatory Z79.1
    antiplatelet Z79.02
    antithrombotics Z79.02
    aromatase inhibitors Z79.811
    aspirin Z79.82
    birth control pill or patch Z79.3
    bisphosphonates Z79.83
    contraceptive, oral Z79.3
    drug, specified NEC Z79.899
    estrogen receptor downregulators Z79.818
    Evista Z79.810
    exemestane (Aromasin) Z79.811
    Fareston Z79.810
    fulvestrant (Faslodex) Z79.818

Therapy - *continued*
  gonadotropin-releasing hormone (GnRH)
    agonist Z79.818
  goserelin acetate (Zoladex) Z79.818
  hormone replacement Z79.890
  insulin Z79.4
  letrozole (Femara) Z79.811
  leuprolide acetate (leuprorelin) (Lupron)
    Z79.818
  megestrol acetate (Megace) Z79.818
  methadone
    for pain management Z79.891
    maintenance therapy F11.20
  Nolvadex Z79.810
  opiate analgesic Z79.891
  oral contraceptive Z79.3
  raloxifene (Evista) Z79.810
  selective estrogen receptor modulators
    (SERMs) Z79.810
  short term
  omit code
  steroids
    inhaled Z79.51
    systemic Z79.52
  tamoxifen (Nolvadex) Z79.810
  toremifene (Fareston) Z79.810
Thermic - *see* condition
Thermography (abnormal) - *see also*
  Abnormal, diagnostic imaging R93.8
  breast R92.8
Thermoplegia T67.0
Thesaurismosis, glycogen - *see* Disease,
  glycogen storage
Thiamin deficiency E51.9
  specified NEC E51.8
Thiaminic deficiency with beriberi E51.11
Thibierge-Weissenbach syndrome - *see*
  Sclerosis, systemic
Thickening
  bone - *see* Hypertrophy, bone
  breast N64.59
  endometrium R93.8
  epidermal L85.9
    specified NEC L85.8
  hymen N89.6
  larynx J38.7
  nail L60.2
    congenital Q84.5
  periosteal - *see* Hypertrophy, bone
  pleura J92.9
    with asbestos J92.0
  skin R23.4
  subepiglottic J38.7
  tongue K14.8
  valve, heart - *see* Endocarditis
Thigh - *see* condition
Thinning vertebra - *see* Spondylopathy,
  specified NEC
Thirst, excessive R63.1
  due to deprivation of water T73.1
Thomsen disease G71.12
Thoracic - *see also* condition
  kidney Q63.2
  outlet syndrome G54.0
Thoracogastroschisis (congenital) Q79.8
Thoracopagus Q89.4
Thorax - *see* condition
Thorn's syndrome N28.89
Thorson-björck syndrome E34.0
Threadworm (infection) (infestation) B80
Threatened
  abortion O20.0
    with subsequent abortion O03.9
  job loss, anxiety concerning Z56.2

Threatened - *continued*
  labor (without delivery) O47.9
    at or after 37 completed weeks of gestation
        O47.1
    before 37 completed weeks of gestation
        O47.0-
  loss of job, anxiety concerning Z56.2
  miscarriage O20.0
  unemployment, anxiety concerning Z56.2
Three-day fever A93.1
Threshers' lung J67.0
Thrix annulata (congenital) Q84.1
Throat - *see* condition
**Thrombasthenia (Glanzmann) (hemorrhagic)
  (hereditary)** D69.1
Thromboangiitis I73.1
  obliterans (general) I73.1
    cerebral I67.89
    vessels
      brain I67.89
      spinal cord I67.89
Thromboarteritis - *see* Arteritis
**Thromboasthenia (Glanzmann)
  (hemorrhagic) (hereditary)** D69.1
Thrombocytasthenia (Glanzmann) D69.1
**Thrombocythemia (essential) (hemorrhagic)
  (idiopathic) (primary)** D47.3
**Thrombocytopathy (dystrophic)
  (granulopenic)** D69.1
Thrombocytopenia, thrombocytopenic D69.6
  with absent radius (TAR) Q87.2
  congenital D69.42
  dilutional D69.59
  due to
    drugs D69.59
    extracorporeal circulation of blood D69.59
      (massive) blood transfusion D69.59
    platelet alloimmunization D69.59
  essential D69.3
  heparin induced (HIT) D75.82
  hereditary D69.42
  idiopathic D69.3
  neonatal, transitory P61.0
    due to
      exchange transfusion P61.0
      idiopathic maternal thrombocytopenia
          P61.0
      isoimmunization P61.0
  primary NEC D69.49
    idiopathic D69.3
  puerperal, postpartum O72.3
  secondary D69.59
  transient neonatal P61.0
Thrombocytosis, essential D47.3
  primary D47.3
Thromboembolism - *see* Embolism
Thrombopathy (Bernard-soulier) D69.1
  constitutional D68.0
  Willebrand-jurgens D68.0
Thrombopenia - *see* Thrombocytopenia
Thrombophilia D68.59
  primary NEC D68.59
  secondary NEC D68.69
  specified NEC D68.69
Thrombophlebitis I80.9
  antepartum O22.2-
    deep O22.3-
    superficial O22.2-
  cavernous (venous) sinus G08
    complicating pregnancy O22.5-
    nonpyogenic I67.6
  cerebral (sinus) (vein) G08
    nonpyogenic I67.6
    sequelae G09

Thrombophlebitis - *continued*
  due to implanted device - *see* Complications,
    by site and type, specified NEC
  during or resulting from a procedure NEC
    T81.72
  femoral vein (superficial) I80.1-
  femoropopliteal vein I80.0-
  hepatic (vein) I80.8
  idiopathic, recurrent I82.1
  iliofemoral I80.1-
  intracranial venous sinus (any) G08
    nonpyogenic I67.6
    sequelae G09
  intraspinal venous sinuses and veins G08
    nonpyogenic G95.19
  lateral (venous) sinus G08
    nonpyogenic I67.6
  leg I80.3
    superficial I80.0-
  longitudinal (venous) sinus G08
    nonpyogenic I67.6
  lower extremity I80.299
  migrans, migrating I82.1
  pelvic
    with ectopic or molar pregnancy O08.0
    following ectopic or molar pregnancy O08.0
    puerperal O87.1
  popliteal vein - *see* Phlebitis, leg, deep,
    popliteal
  portal (vein) K75.1
  postoperative T81.72
  pregnancy - *see* Thrombophlebitis, antepartum
  puerperal, postpartum, childbirth O87.0
    deep O87.1
    pelvic O87.1
    septic O86.81
    superficial O87.0
  saphenous (greater) (lesser) I80.0-
  sinus (intracranial) G08
    nonpyogenic I67.6
  specified site NEC I80.8
  tibial vein I80.23-
**Thrombosis, thrombotic (bland) (multiple)
  (progressive) (silent) (vessel)** I82.90
  anal K64.5
  antepartum - *see* Thrombophlebitis,
    antepartum
  aorta, aortic I74.10
    abdominal I74.09
      saddle I74.01
    bifurcation I74.09
    saddle I74.01
    specified site NEC I74.19
    terminal I74.09
    thoracic I74.11
    valve - *see* Endocarditis, aortic
  apoplexy I63.3-
  artery, arteries (postinfectional) I74.9
    auditory, internal - *see* Occlusion, artery,
      precerebral, specified NEC
    basilar - *see* Occlusion, artery, basilar
    carotid (common) (internal) - *see* Occlusion,
      artery, carotid
    cerebellar (anterior inferior) (posterior
      inferior) (superior) - *see* Occlusion, artery,
      cerebellar
    cerebral - *see* Occlusion, artery, cerebral
    choroidal (anterior) - *see* Occlusion, artery,
      precerebral, specified NEC
    communicating, posterior - *see* Occlusion,
      artery, precerebral, specified NEC
    coronary - *see also* Infarct, myocardium
      not resulting in infarction I24.0
    hepatic I74.8

Thrombosis, thrombotic - *continued*
  hypophyseal - *see* Occlusion, artery,
    precerebral, specified NEC
  iliac I74.5
  limb I74.4
    lower I74.3
    upper I74.2
  meningeal, anterior or posterior - *see*
    Occlusion, artery, cerebral, specified NEC
  mesenteric (with gangrene) - *see also* Infarct,
    intestine K55.069
  ophthalmic - *see* Occlusion, artery, retina
  pontine - *see* Occlusion, artery, precerebral,
    specified NEC
  precerebral - *see* Occlusion, artery,
    precerebral
  pulmonary (iatrogenic) - *see* Embolism,
    pulmonary
  renal N28.0
  retinal - *see* Occlusion, artery, retina
  spinal, anterior or posterior G95.11
  traumatic NEC T14.8
  vertebral - *see* Occlusion, artery, vertebral
  atrium, auricular - *see also* Infarct,
  myocardium
    following acute myocardial infarction
      (current complication) I23.6
    not resulting in infarction I51.3
    old I51.3
  basilar (artery) - *see* Occlusion, artery, basilar
  brain (artery) (stem) - *see also* Occlusion,
    artery, cerebral
    due to syphilis A52.05
    puerperal O99.43
    sinus - *see* Thrombosis, intracranial venous
      sinus
  capillary I78.8
  cardiac - *see also* Infarct, myocardium
    not resulting in infarction I51.3
    old I51.3
    valve - *see* Endocarditis
  carotid (artery) (common) (internal) - *see*
    Occlusion, artery, carotid
  cavernous (venous) sinus - *see* Thrombosis,
    intracranial venous sinus
  cerebellar artery (anterior inferior) (posterior
    inferior) (superior) I66.3
  cerebral (artery) - *see* Occlusion, artery,
    cerebral
  cerebrovenous sinus - *see also* Thrombosis,
    intracranial venous sinus
    puerperium O87.3
  chronic I82.91
  coronary (artery) (vein) - *see also* Infarct,
    myocardium
    not resulting in infarction I24.0
  corpus cavernosum N48.89
  cortical I66.9
  deep - *see* Embolism, vein, lower extremity
  due to device, implant or graft - *see also*
    Complications, by site and type, specified
    NEC T85.868
    arterial graft NEC T82.868
    breast (implant) T85.868
    catheter NEC T85.868
      dialysis (renal) T82.868
        intraperitoneal T85.868
      infusion NEC T82.868
        spinal (epidural) (subdural) T85.860
      urinary (indwelling) T83.86
    electronic (electrode) (pulse generator)
    (stimulator)
      bone T84.86
      cardiac T82.867

Thrombosis, thrombotic - *continued*
- nervous system (brain) (peripheral nerve) (spinal) T85.860
  - urinary T83.86
- fixation, internal (orthopedic) NEC T84.86
- gastrointestinal (bile duct) (esophagus) T85.868
- genital NEC T83.86
- heart T82.867
- joint prosthesis T84.86
- ocular (corneal graft) (orbital implant) NEC T85.868
- orthopedic NEC T84.86
- specified NEC T85.868
- urinary NEC T83.86
- vascular NEC T82.868
- ventricular intracranial shunt T85.860
- during the puerperium - *see* Thrombosis, puerperal
- endocardial - *see also* Infarct, myocardium
  - not resulting in infarction I51.3
- eye - *see* Occlusion, retina
- genital organ
  - female NEC N94.89
    - pregnancy - *see* Thrombophlebitis, antepartum
  - male N50.1
- gestational - *see* Phlebopathy, gestational
- heart (chamber) - *see also* Infarct, myocardium
  - not resulting in infarction I51.3
  - old I51.3
- hepatic (vein) I82.0
  - artery I74.8
- history (of) Z86.718
- intestine (with gangrene) - *see also* Infarct, intestine K55.069
- intracardiac NEC (apical) (atrial) (auricular) (ventricular) (old) I51.3
- intracranial (arterial) I66.9
  - venous sinus (any) G08
    - nonpyogenic origin I67.6
    - puerperium O87.3
- intramural - *see also* Infarct, myocardium
  - not resulting in infarction I51.3
  - old I51.3
- intraspinal venous sinuses and veins G08
  - nonpyogenic G95.19
- kidney (artery) N28.0
- lateral (venous) sinus - *see* Thrombosis, intracranial venous sinus
- leg - *see* Thrombosis, vein, lower extremity
  - arterial I74.3
- liver (venous) I82.0
  - artery I74.8
  - portal vein I81
- longitudinal (venous) sinus - *see* Thrombosis, intracranial venous sinus
- lower limb - *see* Thrombosis, vein, lower extremity
- lung (iatrogenic) (postoperative) - *see* Embolism, pulmonary
- meninges (brain) (arterial) I66.8
- mesenteric (artery) (with gangrene) - *see also* Infarct, intestine K55.069
  - vein (inferior) (superior) I81
- mitral I34.8
- mural - *see also* Infarct, myocardium
  - due to syphilis A52.06
  - not resulting in infarction I51.3
  - old I51.3
- omentum (with gangrene) - *see also* Infarct, intestine K55.069
- ophthalmic - *see* Occlusion, retina
- pampiniform plexus (male) N50.1

Thrombosis, thrombotic - *continued*
- parietal - *see also* Infarct, myocardium
  - not resulting in infarction I24.0
- penis, superficial vein N48.81
- perianal venous K64.5
- peripheral arteries I74.4
  - upper I74.2
- personal history (of) Z86.718
- portal I81
  - due to syphilis A52.09
- precerebral artery - *see* Occlusion, artery, precerebral
- puerperal, postpartum O87.0
  - brain (artery) O99.43
    - venous (sinus) O87.3
  - cardiac O99.43
  - cerebral (artery) O99.43
    - venous (sinus) O87.3
  - superficial O87.0
- pulmonary (artery) (iatrogenic) (postoperative) (vein) - *see* Embolism, pulmonary
- renal (artery) N28.0
  - vein I82.3
- resulting from presence of device, implant or graft - *see* Complications, by site and type, specified NEC
- retina, retinal - *see* Occlusion, retina
- scrotum N50.1
- seminal vesicle N50.1
- sigmoid (venous) sinus - *see* Thrombosis, intracranial venous sinus
- sinus, intracranial (any) - *see* Thrombosis, intracranial venous sinus
- specified site NEC I82.890
  - chronic I82.891
- spermatic cord N50.1
- spinal cord (arterial) G95.11
  - due to syphilis A52.09
  - pyogenic origin G06.1
- spleen, splenic D73.5
  - artery I74.8
- testis N50.1
- tumor - *see* Neoplasm, unspecified behavior, by site
- traumatic NEC T14.8
- tricuspid I07.8
- tunica vaginalis N50.1
- umbilical cord (vessels), complicating delivery O69.5
- vas deferens N50.1
- vein (acute) I82.90
  - antecubital I82.61-
    - chronic I82.71-
  - axillary I82.A1-
    - chronic I82.A2-
  - basilic I82.61-
    - chronic I82.71-
  - brachial I82.62-
    - chronic I82.72-
  - brachiocephalic (innominate) I82.290
    - chronic I82.291
  - cerebral, nonpyogenic I67.6
  - cephalic I82.61-
    - chronic I82.71-
  - chronic I82.91
  - deep (DVT) I82.40-
    - calf I82.4Z-
      - chronic I82.5Z-
    - lower leg I82.4Z-
      - chronic I82.5Z-
    - thigh I82.4Y-
      - chronic I82.5Y-
    - upper leg I82.4Y
      - chronic I82.5y-

Thrombosis, thrombotic - *continued*
- femoral I82.41-
  - chronic I82.51-
- iliac (iliofemoral) I82.42-
  - chronic I82.52-
- innominate I82.290
  - chronic I82.291
- internal jugular I82.C1-
  - chronic I82.C2-
- lower extremity
  - deep I82.40-
    - chronic I82.50-
    - specified NEC I82.49-
      - chronic NEC I82.59-
  - distal
    - deep I82.4Z-
  - proximal
    - deep I82.4Y-
      - chronic I82.5Y-
  - superficial I82.81-
- perianal K64.5
- popliteal I82.43-
  - chronic I82.53-
- radial I82.62-
  - chronic I82.72-
- renal I82.3
- saphenous (greater) (lesser) I82.81-
- specified NEC I82.890
  - chronic NEC I82.891
- subclavian I82.B1-
  - chronic I82.B2-
- thoracic NEC I82.290
  - chronic I82.291
- tibial I82.44-
  - chronic I82.54-
- ulnar I82.62-
  - chronic I82.72-
- upper extremity I82.60-
  - chronic I82.70-
  - deep I82.62-
    - chronic I82.72-
  - superficial I82.61-
    - chronic I82.71-
- vena cava
  - inferior I82.220
    - chronic I82.221
  - superior I82.210
    - chronic I82.211
- venous, perianal K64.5
- ventricle - *see also* Infarct, myocardium
  - following acute myocardial infarction (current complication) I23.6
  - not resulting in infarction I24.0
  - old I51.3

Thrombus - *see* Thrombosis

Thrush - *see also* Candidiasis
- oral B37.0
- newborn P37.5
- vaginal B37.3

Thumb - *see also* condition
- sucking (child problem) F98.8

Thymitis E32.8

Thymoma (benign) D15.0
- malignant C37

Thymus, thymic (gland) - *see* condition

Thyrocele - *see* Goiter

Thyroglossal - *see also* condition
- cyst Q89.2
- duct, persistent Q89.2

Thyroid (gland) (body) - *see also* condition
- hormone resistance E07.89
- lingual Q89.2
- nodule (cystic) (nontoxic) (single) E04.1

Thyroiditis E06.9
  acute (nonsuppurative) (pyogenic)
    (suppurative) E06.0
  autoimmune E06.3
  chronic (nonspecific) (sclerosing) E06.5
    with thyrotoxicosis, transient E06.2
    fibrous E06.5
    lymphadenoid E06.3
    lymphocytic E06.3
    lymphoid E06.3
  de Quervain's E06.1
  drug-induced E06.4
  fibrous (chronic) E06.5
  giant-cell (follicular) E06.1
  granulomatous (de Quervain) (subacute) E06.1
  Hashimoto's (struma lymphomatosa) E06.3
  iatrogenic E06.4
  ligneous E06.5
  lymphocytic (chronic) E06.3
  lymphoid E06.3
  lymphomatous E06.3
  nonsuppurative E06.1
  postpartum, puerperal O90.5
  pseudotuberculous E06.1
  pyogenic E06.0
  radiation E06.4
  Riedel's E06.5
  subacute (granulomatous) E06.1
  suppurative E06.0
  tuberculous A18.81
  viral E06.1
  woody E06.5
Thyrolingual duct, persistent Q89.2
Thyromegaly E01.0
Thyrotoxic
  crisis - see Thyrotoxicosis
  heart disease or failure - see also
    Thyrotoxicosis E05.90 [I43]
    with thyroid storm E05.91 [I43]
  storm - see Thyrotoxicosis
Thyrotoxicosis (recurrent) E05.90
  with
    goiter (diffuse) E05.00
      with thyroid storm E05.01
      adenomatous uninodular E05.10
        with thyroid storm E05.11
      multinodular E05.20
        with thyroid storm E05.21
      nodular E05.20
        with thyroid storm E05.21
      uninodular E05.10
        with thyroid storm E05.11
    infiltrative
      dermopathy E05.00
        with thyroid storm E05.01
      ophthalmopathy E05.00
        with thyroid storm E05.01
    single thyroid nodule E05.10
      with thyroid storm E05.11
    thyroid storm E05.91
  due to
    ectopic thyroid nodule or tissue E05.30
      with thyroid storm E05.31
    ingestion of (excessive) thyroid material
      E05.40
      with thyroid storm E05.41
    overproduction of thyroid-stimulating
      hormone E05.80
      with thyroid storm E05.81
    specified cause NEC E05.80
      with thyroid storm E05.81
  factitia E05.40
    with thyroid storm E05.41
  heart (see also Failure, heart, high-output)

Thyrotoxicosis - continued
    E05.90 [I43]
    with thyroid storm (see also Failure, heart,
      high-output) E05.91 [I43]
    failure (see also Failure, heart, high-output)
      E05.90 [I43]
  neonatal (transient) P72.1
  transient with chronic thyroiditis E06.2
Tibia vara - see Osteochondrosis, juvenile, tibia
Tic (disorder) F95.9
  breathing F95.8
  child problem F95.0
  compulsive F95.1
  de la Tourette F95.2
  degenerative (generalized) (localized) G25.69
    facial G25.69
  disorder
    chronic
      motor F95.1
      vocal F95.1
    combined vocal and multiple motor F95.2
    transient F95.0
  douloureux G50.0
    atypical G50.1
    postherpetic, postzoster B02.22
  drug-induced G25.61
  eyelid F95.8
  habit F95.9
    chronic F95.1
    transient of childhood F95.0
  lid, transient of childhood F95.0
  motor-verbal F95.2
  occupational F48.8
  orbicularis F95.8
    transient of childhood F95.0
  organic origin G25.69
  provisional F95.0
  postchoreic G25.69
  psychogenic, compulsive F95.1
  salaam R25.8
  spasm (motor or vocal) F95.9
    chronic F95.1
    transient of childhood F95.0
  specified NEC F95.8
Tick-borne - see condition
Tietze's disease or syndrome M94.0
Tight, tightness
  anus K62.89
  chest R07.89
  fascia (lata) M62.89
  foreskin (congenital) N47.1
  hymen, hymenal ring N89.6
  introitus (acquired) (congenital) N89.6
  rectal sphincter K62.89
  tendon - see Short, tendon
  urethral sphincter N35.9
Tilting vertebra - see Dorsopathy, deforming,
  specified NEC
Timidity, child F93.8
Tin-miner's lung J63.5
Tinea (intersecta) (tarsi) B35.9
  amiantacea L44.8
  asbestina B35.0
  barbae B35.0
  beard B35.0
  black dot B35.0
  blanca B36.2
  capitis B35.0
  corporis B35.4
  cruris B35.6
  flava B36.0
  foot B35.3
  furfuracea B36.0
  imbricata (Tokelau) B35.5

Tinea - continued
  kerion B35.0
  manuum B35.2
  microsporic - see Dermatophytosis
  nigra B36.1
  nodosa - see Piedra
  pedis B35.3
  scalp B35.0
  specified NEC B35.8
  sycosis B35.0
  tonsurans B35.0
  trichophytic - see Dermatophytosis
  unguium B35.1
  versicolor B36.0
Tingling sensation (skin) R20.2
Tinnitus NOS H93.1-
  audible H93.1-
  aurium H93.1-
  pulsatile H93.A-
  subjective H93.1-
Tipped tooth (teeth) M26.33
Tipping
  pelvis M95.5
    with disproportion (fetopelvic) O33.0
      causing obstructed labor O65.0
  tooth (teeth), fully erupted M26.33
Tiredness R53.83
Tissue - see condition
Tobacco (nicotine)
  abuse - see Tobacco, use
  dependence - see Dependence, drug, nicotine
  harmful use Z72.0
  heart - see Tobacco, toxic effect
  maternal use, affecting newborn P04.2
  toxic effect - see Table of Drugs and
    Chemicals, by substance, poisoning
    chewing tobacco - see Table of Drugs and
      Chemicals, by substance, poisoning
    cigarettes - see Table of Drugs and
      Chemicals, by substance, poisoning
  use Z72.0
    complicating
      childbirth O99.334
      pregnancy O99.33-
      puerperium O99.335
    counseling and surveillance Z71.6
    history Z87.891
  withdrawal state - see also Dependence, drug,
    nicotine F17.203
Tocopherol deficiency E56.0
Todd's
  cirrhosis K74.3
  paralysis (postepileptic) (transitory) G83.84
Toe - see condition
Toilet, artificial opening - see Attention to,
  artificial, opening
Tokelau (ringworm) B35.5
Tollwut - see Rabies
Tommaselli's disease R31.9
  correct substance properly administered - see
    Table of Drugs and Chemicals, by drug,
    adverse effect
  overdose or wrong substance given or taken -
    see Table of Drugs and Chemicals, by drug,
    poisoning
Tongue - see also condition
  tie Q38.1
Tonic pupil - see Anomaly, pupil, function,
  tonic pupil
Toni-fanconi syndrome (cystinosis) E72.09
  with cystinosis E72.04
Tonsil - see condition

Tonsillitis (acute) (catarrhal) (croupous)
  (follicular) (gangrenous) (infective)
  (lacunar) (lingual) (malignant)
  (membranous) (parenchymatous)
  (phlegmonous) (pseudomembranous)
  (purulent) (septic) (subacute) (suppurative)
  (toxic) (ulcerative) (vesicular) (viral) J03.90
  chronic J35.01
    with adenoiditis J35.03
  diphtheritic A36.0
  hypertrophic J35.01
    with adenoiditis J35.03
  recurrent J03.91
  specified organism NEC J03.80
    recurrent J03.81
  staphylococcal J03.80
    recurrent J03.81
  streptococcal J03.00
    recurrent J03.01
  tuberculous A15.8
  Vincent's A69.1
Tooth, teeth - *see* condition
Toothache K08.89
Topagnosis R20.8
Tophi - *see* Gout, chronic
TORCH infection - *see* Infection, congenital
  without active infection P00.2
Torn - *see* Tear
Tornwaldt's cyst or disease J39.2
Torsion
  accessory tube - *see* Torsion, fallopian tube
  adnexa (female) - *see* Torsion, fallopian tube
  aorta, acquired I77.1
  appendix epididymis N44.04
  appendix testis N44.03
  bile duct (common) (hepatic) K83.8
    congenital Q44.5
  bowel, colon or intestine K56.2
  cervix - *see* Malposition, uterus
  cystic duct K82.8
  dystonia - *see* Dystonia, torsion
  epididymis (appendix) N44.04
  fallopian tube N83.52-
    with ovary N83.53
  gallbladder K82.8
    congenital Q44.1
  hydatid of Morgagni
    female N83.52-
    male N44.03
  kidney (pedicle) (leading to infarction) N28.0
  Meckel's diverticulum (congenital) Q43.0
    malignant - *see* Table of Neoplasms, small
    intestine, malignant
  mesentery K56.2
  omentum K56.2
  organ or site, congenital NEC - *see* Anomaly,
    by site
  ovary (pedicle) N83.51-
    with fallopian tube N83.53
    congenital Q50.2
  oviduct - *see* Torsion, fallopian tube   penis
  (acquired) N48.82
    congenital Q55.63
  spasm - *see* Dystonia, torsion
  spermatic cord N44.02
    extravaginal N44.01
    intravaginal N44.02
  spleen D73.5
  testis, testicle N44.00
    appendix N44.03
  tibia - *see* Deformity, limb, specified type
    NEC, lower leg
  uterus - *see* Malposition, uterus

Torticollis (intermittent) (spastic) M43.6
  congenital (sternomastoid) Q68.0
  due to birth injury P15.8
  hysterical F44.4
  ocular R29.891
  psychogenic F45.8
    conversion reaction F44.4
  rheumatic M43.6
  rheumatoid M06.88
  spasmodic G24.3
  traumatic, current S13.4
Tortipelvis G24.1
Tortuous
  aortic arch Q25.46
  artery I77.1
  organ or site, congenital NEC - *see* Distortion
  retinal vessel, congenital Q14.1
  ureter N13.8
  urethra N36.8
  vein - *see* Varix
Torture, victim of Z65.4
Torula, torular (histolytica) (infection) - *see*
  Cryptococcosis
Torulosis - *see* Cryptococcosis
Torus (mandibularis) (palatinus) M27.0
  fracture - *see* Fracture, by site, torus
Touraine's syndrome Q79.8
Tourette's syndrome F95.2
Tourniquet syndrome - *see* Constriction,
  external, by site
Tower skull Q75.0
  with exophthalmos Q87.0
Toxemia R68.89
  bacterial - *see* Sepsis
  burn - *see* Burn
  eclamptic (with pre-existing hypertension) -
    see Eclampsia
  erysipelatous - *see* Erysipelas
  fatigue R68.89
  food - *see* Poisoning, food
  gastrointestinal K52.1
  intestinal K52.1
  kidney - *see* Uremia
  malarial - *see* Malaria
  myocardial - *see* Myocarditis, toxic
  of pregnancy - *see* Pre-eclampsia
  pre-eclamptic - *see* Pre-eclampsia
  small intestine K52.1
  staphylococcal, due to food A05.0
  stasis R68.89
  uremic - *see* Uremia
  urinary - *see* Uremia
Toxemica cerebropathia psychica
  (nonalcoholic) F04
  alcoholic - *see* Alcohol, amnestic disorder
Toxic (poisoning) - *see also* condition T65.91
  effect - *see* Table of Drugs and Chemicals, by
    substance, poisoning
  shock syndrome A48.3
  thyroid (gland) - *see* Thyrotoxicosis
Toxicemia - *see* Toxemia
Toxicity - *see* Table of Drugs and Chemicals,
  by substance, poisoning
  fava bean D55.0
  food, noxious - *see* Poisoning, food
  from drug or nonmedicinal substance - *see*
    Table of Drugs and Chemicals, by drug
Toxicosis - *see also* Toxemia
  capillary, hemorrhagic D69.0
Toxinfection, gastrointestinal K52.1
Toxocariasis B83.0
Toxoplasma, toxoplasmosis (acquired) B58.9
  with
    hepatitis B58.1

Toxoplasma - *continued*
  meningoencephalitis B58.2
  ocular involvement B58.00
  other organ involvement B58.89
  pneumonia, pneumonitis B58.3
  congenital (acute) (subacute) (chronic) P37.1
  maternal, manifest toxoplasmosis in infant
    (acute) (subacute) (chronic) P37.1
tPA (rtPA) administration in a different
  facility within the last 24
  hours prior to admission to current facility
  Z92.82
Trabeculation, bladder N32.89
Trachea - *see* condition
Tracheitis (catarrhal) (infantile)
  (membranous) (plastic) (septal)
  (suppurative) (viral) J04.10
  with
    bronchitis (15 years of age and above) J40
      acute or subacute - *see* Bronchitis, acute
      chronic J42
      tuberculous NEC A15.5
      under 15 years of age J20.9
    laryngitis (acute) J04.2
      chronic J37.1
      tuberculous NEC A15.5
  acute J04.10
    with obstruction J04.11
  chronic J42
    with
      bronchitis (chronic) J42
      laryngitis (chronic) J37.1
    diphtheritic (membranous) A36.89
  due to external agent - *see* Inflammation,
    respiratory, upper, due to
  syphilitic A52.73
  tuberculous A15.5
Trachelitis (nonvenereal) - *see* Cervicitis
Tracheobronchial - *see* condition
Tracheobronchitis (15
  years of age and above) - *see also* Bronchitis
  due to
    Bordetella bronchiseptica A37.80
      with pneumonia A37.81
    Francisella tularensis A21.8
Tracheobronchomegaly Q32.4
  with bronchiectasis J47.9
    with
      exacerbation (acute) J47.1
      lower respiratory infection J47.0
  acquired J98.09
    with bronchiectasis J47.9
      with
        exacerbation (acute) J47.1
        lower respiratory infection J47.0
Tracheobronchopneumonitis - *see* Pneumonia,
  broncho-
Tracheocele (external) (internal) J39.8
  congenital Q32.1
Tracheomalacia J39.8
  congenital Q32.0
Tracheopharyngitis (acute) J06.9
  chronic J42
  due to external agent - *see* Inflammation,
    respiratory, upper, due to
Tracheostenosis J39.8
Tracheostomy
  complication - *see* Complication, tracheostomy
  status Z93.0
    attention to Z43.0
    malfunctioning J95.03
Trachoma, trachomatous A71.9
  active (stage) A71.1
  contraction of conjunctiva A71.1

Trachoma - *continued*
  dubium A71.0
  initial (stage) A71.0
  healed or sequelae B94.0
  pannus A71.1
  Türck's J37.0
Traction, vitreomacular H43.82-
Train sickness T75.3
Trait(s)
  Hb-s D57.3
  hemoglobin
    abnormal NEC D58.2
      with thalassemia D56.3
    C - *see* Disease, hemoglobin C
    S (Hb-s) D57.3
  Lepore D56.3
  personality, accentuated Z73.1
  sickle-cell D57.3
    with elliptocytosis or spherocytosis D57.3
  type A personality Z73.1
Tramp Z59.0
Trance R41.89
  hysterical F44.89
Transection
  abdomen (partial) S38.3
  aorta (incomplete) - *see also* Injury, aorta
    complete - *see* Injury, aorta, laceration, major
  carotid artery (incomplete) - *see also* Injury,
    blood vessel, carotid, laceration
    complete - *see* Injury, blood vessel, carotid,
    laceration, major
  celiac artery (incomplete) S35.211
    branch (incomplete) S35.291
      complete S35.292
    complete S35.212
  innominate
    artery (incomplete) - *see also* Injury, blood
      vessel, thoracic, innominate, artery,
      laceration
      complete - *see* Injury, blood vessel,
      thoracic, innominate, artery, laceration,
      major
    vein (incomplete) - *see also* Injury, blood
      vessel, thoracic, innominate, vein, laceration
      complete - *see* Injury, blood vessel,
      thoracic, innominate, vein, laceration, major
  jugular vein (external) (incomplete) - *see also*
  Injury, blood vessel, jugular vein, laceration
    complete - *see* Injury, blood vessel, jugular
      vein, laceration, major
    internal (incomplete) - *see also* Injury, blood
      vessel, jugular vein, internal, laceration
      complete - *see* Injury, blood vessel, jugular
      vein, internal, laceration, major
  mesenteric artery (incomplete) - *see also*
  Injury, mesenteric, artery, laceration
    complete - *see* Injury, mesenteric artery,
      laceration, major
  pulmonary vessel (incomplete) - *see also*
  Injury, blood vessel, thoracic, pulmonary,
  laceration
    complete - *see* Injury, blood vessel, thoracic,
    pulmonary, laceration, major
  subclavian - *see* Transection, innominate
  vena cava (incomplete) - *see also* Injury, vena
  cava
    complete - *see* Injury, vena cava, laceration,
    major
  vertebral artery (incomplete) - *see also* Injury,
  blood vessel, vertebral, laceration
    complete - *see* Injury, blood vessel, vertebral,
    laceration, major
Transaminasemia R74.0

Transfusion
  associated (red blood cell) hemochromatosis
    E83.111
  blood
    ABO incompatible - *see* Complication(s),
      transfusion, incompatibility reaction, ABO
    minor blood group (Duffy) (E) (K(ell))
      (Kidd) (Lewis) (M) (N) (P) (S) T80.89
    reaction or complication - *see* Complications,
      transfusion
  fetomaternal (mother) - *see* Pregnancy,
    complicated by, placenta, transfusion
    syndrome
  maternofetal (mother) - *see* Pregnancy,
    complicated by, placenta, transfusion
    syndrome
  placental (syndrome) (mother) - *see*
    Pregnancy, complicated by, placenta,
    transfusion syndrome
  reaction (adverse) - *see* Complications,
    transfusion
  related acute lung injury (TRALI) J95.84
  twin-to-twin - *see* Pregnancy, complicated by,
    placenta, transfusion syndrome, fetus to fetus
Transient (meaning homeless) - *see also*
  condition Z59.0
Translocation
  balanced autosomal Q95.9
    in normal individual Q95.0
  chromosomes NEC Q99.8
    balanced and insertion in normal individual
    Q95.0
  Down syndrome Q90.2
  trisomy
    13 Q91.6
    18 Q91.2
    21 Q90.2
Translucency, iris - *see* Degeneration, iris
**Transmission of chemical substances through
  the placenta** - *see* Absorption, chemical,
  through placenta
Transparency, lung, unilateral J43.0
Transplant (ed) (status) Z94.9
  awaiting organ Z76.82
  bone Z94.6
    marrow Z94.81
  candidate Z76.82
  complication - *see* Complication, transplant
  cornea Z94.7
  heart Z94.1
    and lung(s) Z94.3
    valve Z95.2
      prosthetic Z95.2
      specified NEC Z95.4
      xenogenic Z95.3
  intestine Z94.82
  kidney Z94.0
  liver Z94.4
  lung(s) Z94.2
    and heart Z94.3
  organ (failure) (infection) (rejection) Z94.9
    removal status Z98.85
  pancreas Z94.83
  skin Z94.5
  social Z60.3
  specified organ or tissue NEC Z94.89
  stem cells Z94.84
  tissue Z94.9
Transplants, ovarian, endometrial N80.1
Transposed - *see* Transposition
Transposition (congenital) - *see also*
  Malposition, congenital
  abdominal viscera Q89.3
  aorta (dextra) Q20.3

Transposition - *continued*
  appendix Q43.8
  colon Q43.8
  corrected Q20.5
  great vessels (complete) (partial) Q20.3
  heart Q24.0
    with complete transposition of viscera Q89.3
  intestine (large) (small) Q43.8
  reversed jejunal (for bypass) (status) Z98.0
  scrotum Q55.23
  stomach Q40.2
    with general transposition of viscera Q89.3
  tooth, teeth, fully erupted M26.30
  vessels, great (complete) (partial) Q20.3
  viscera (abdominal) (thoracic) Q89.3
Transsexualism F64.0
Transverse - *see also* condition
  arrest (deep), in labor O64.0
  lie (mother) O32.2
    causing obstructed labor O64.8
Transvestism, transvestitism (dual-role)
  F64.1
  fetishistic F65.1
Trapped placenta (with hemorrhage) O72.0
  without hemorrhage O73.0
**TRAPS (tumor necrosis factor receptor
  associated periodic syndrome)** M04.1
Trauma, traumatism - *see also* Injury
  acoustic - *see* subcategory H83.3
  birth - *see* Birth, injury
  complicating ectopic or molar pregnancy
    O08.6
  during delivery O71.9
  following ectopic or molar pregnancy O08.6
  obstetric O71.9
    specified NEC O71.89
  occlusal
    primary K08.81
    secondary K08.82
Traumatic - *see also* condition
  brain injury S06.9
Treacher Collins syndrome Q75.4
Treitz's hernia - *see* Hernia, abdomen,
  specified site NEC
Trematode infestation - *see* Infestation, fluke
Trematodiasis - *see* Infestation, fluke
Trembling paralysis - *see* Parkinsonism
Tremor(s) R25.1
  drug induced G25.1
  essential (benign) G25.0
  familial G25.0
  hereditary G25.0
  hysterical F44.4
  intention G25.2
  medication induced postural G25.1
  mercurial - *see* subcategory T56.1
  Parkinson's - *see* Parkinsonism
  psychogenic (conversion reaction) F44.4
  senilis R54
  specified type NEC G25.2
Trench
  fever A79.0
  foot - *see* Immersion, foot
  mouth A69.1
Treponema pallidum infection - *see* Syphilis
Treponematosis
  due to
    T. pallidum - *see* Syphilis
    T. pertenue - *see* Yaws
Triad
  Hutchinson's (congenital syphilis) A50.53
  Kartagener's Q89.3
  Saint's - *see* Hernia, diaphragm

Trichiasis (eyelid) H02.059
  with entropion - *see* Entropion
  left H02.056
    lower H02.055
    upper H02.054
  right H02.053
    lower H02.052
    upper H02.051
Trichinella spiralis (infection) (infestation)
B75
Trichinellosis, trichiniasis, trichinelliasis,
trichinosis B75
  with muscle disorder B75 [*M63.80*]
    ankle B75 [*M63.87*]
    foot B75 [*M63.87*]
    forearm B75 [*M63.83*]
    hand B75 [*M63.84*]
    lower leg B75 [*M63.86*]
    multiple sites B75 [*M63.89*]
    pelvic region B75 [*M63.85*]
    shoulder region B75 [*M63.81*]
    specified site NEC B75 [*M63.88*]
    thigh B75 [*M63.85*]
    upper arm B75 [*M63.82*]
Trichobezoar T18.9
  intestine T18.3
  stomach T18.2
Trichocephaliasis, trichocephalosis B79
Trichocephalus infestation B79
Trichoclasis L67.8
Trichoepithelioma - *see also* Neoplasm, skin,
  benign
  malignant - *see* Neoplasm, skin, malignant
Trichofolliculoma - *see* Neoplasm, skin, benign
Tricholemmoma - *see* Neoplasm, skin, benign
Trichomoniasis A59.9
  bladder A59.03
  cervix A59.09
  intestinal A07.8
  prostate A59.02
  seminal vesicles A59.09
  specified site NEC A59.8
  urethra A59.03
  urogenitalis A59.00
  vagina A59.01
  vulva A59.01
Trichomycosis
  axillaris A48.8
  nodosa, nodularis B36.8
Trichonodosis L67.8
Trichophytid, trichophyton infection - *see*
  Dermatophytosis
Trichophytobezoar T18.9
  intestine T18.3
  stomach T18.2
Trichophytosis - *see* Dermatophytosis
Trichoptilosis L67.8
Trichorrhexis (nodosa) (invaginata) L67.0
Trichosis axillaris A48.8
Trichosporosis nodosa B36.2
Trichostasis spinulosa (congenital) Q84.1
Trichostrongyliasis, trichostrongylosis (small
  intestine) B81.2
Trichostrongylus infection B81.2
Trichotillomania F63.3
Trichromat, trichromatopsia, anomalous
  (congenital) H53.55
Trichuriasis B79
Trichuris trichiura (infection) (infestation)
  (any site) B79
Tricuspid (valve) - *see* condition
Trifid - *see also* Accessory kidney (pelvis)
  Q63.8
  tongue Q38.3

Trigeminal neuralgia - *see* Neuralgia,
  trigeminal
Trigeminy R00.8
Trigger finger (acquired) M65.30
  congenital Q74.0
  index finger M65.32-
  little finger M65.35-
  middle finger M65.33-
  ring finger M65.34-
  thumb M65.31-
Trigonitis (bladder) (chronic)
  (pseudomembranous) N30.30
  with hematuria N30.31
Trigonocephaly Q75.0
Trilocular heart - *see* Cor triloculare
Trimethylaminuria E72.52
Tripartite placenta O43.19-
Triphalangeal thumb Q74.0
Triple - *see also* Accessory
  kidneys Q63.0
  uteri Q51.818
  X, female Q97.0
Triplegia G83.89
  congenital G80.8
Triplet (newborn) - *see also* Newborn, triplet
  complicating pregnancy - *see* Pregnancy,
  triplet
Triplication - *see* Accessory
Triploidy Q92.7
Trismus R25.2
  neonatorum A33
  newborn A33
Trisomy (syndrome) Q92.9
  autosomes Q92.9
  chromosome specified NEC Q92.8
    partial Q92.2
      due to unbalanced translocation Q92.5
    whole (nonsex chromosome)
      meiotic nondisjunction Q92.0
      mitotic nondisjunction Q92.1
      mosaicism Q92.1
    specified NEC Q92.8
  due to
    dicentrics - *see* Extra, marker chromosomes
    extra rings - *see* Extra, marker chromosomes
    isochromosomes - *see* Extra, marker
    chromosomes
  specified NEC Q92.8
  whole chromosome Q92.9
    meiotic nondisjunction Q92.0
    mitotic nondisjunction Q92.1
    mosaicism Q92.1
    partial Q92.9
    specified NEC Q92.8
  13 (partial) Q91.7
    meiotic nondisjunction Q91.4
    mitotic nondisjunction Q91.5
    mosaicism Q91.5
    translocation Q91.6
  18 (partial) Q91.3
    meiotic nondisjunction Q91.0
    mitotic nondisjunction Q91.1
    mosaicism Q91.1
    translocation Q91.2
  20 Q92.8
  21 (partial) Q90.9
    meiotic nondisjunction Q90.0
    mitotic nondisjunction Q90.1
    mosaicism Q90.1
    translocation Q90.2
  22 Q92.8
Tritanomaly, tritanopia H53.55
Trombiculosis, trombiculiasis, trombidiosis
  B88.0

Trophedema (congenital) (hereditary) Q82.0
Trophoblastic disease - *see also* Mole,
  hydatidiform O01.9
Tropholymphedema Q82.0
Trophoneurosis NEC G96.8
  disseminated M34.9
Tropical - *see* condition
Trouble - *see also* Disease
  heart - *see* Disease, heart
  kidney - *see* Disease, renal
  nervous R45.0
  sinus - *see* Sinusitis
Trousseau's syndrome (thrombophlebitis
  migrans) I82.1
Truancy, childhood
  from school Z72.810
Truncus
  arteriosus (persistent) Q20.0
  communis Q20.0
Trunk - *see* condition
Trypanosomiasis
  African B56.9
    by Trypanosoma brucei
      gambiense B56.0
      rhodesiense B56.1
  American - *see* Chagas' disease
  Brazilian - *see* Chagas' disease by
  Trypanosoma
    brucei gambiense B56.0
    brucei rhodesiense B56.1
    cruzi - *see* Chagas' disease
  gambiensis, Gambian B56.0
  rhodesiensis, Rhodesian B56.1
  South American - *see* Chagas' disease
  where
    African trypanosomiasis is prevalent B56.9
    Chagas' disease is prevalent B57.2
T-shaped incisors K00.2
Tsutsugamushi (disease) (fever) A75.3
Tube, tubal, tubular - *see* condition
Tubercle - *see also* Tuberculosis
  brain, solitary A17.81
  Darwin's Q17.8
  Ghon, primary infection A15.7
Tuberculid, tuberculide (indurating,
  subcutaneous) (lichenoid) (miliary)
  (papulonecrotic) (primary) (skin) A18.4
Tuberculoma - *see also* Tuberculosis
  brain A17.81
  meninges (cerebral) (spinal) A17.1
  spinal cord A17.81
Tuberculosis, tubercular, tuberculous
  (calcification) (calcified) (caseous)
  (chromogenic acid-fast bacilli)
  (degeneration) (fibrocaseous) (fistula)
  (interstitial) (isolated circumscribed lesions)
  (necrosis) (parenchymatous) (ulcerative)
  A15.9
  with pneumoconiosis (any condition in J60-
  j64) J65
  abdomen (lymph gland) A18.39
  abscess (respiratory) A15.9
    bone A18.03
      hip A18.02
      knee A18.02
      sacrum A18.01
      specified site NEC A18.03
      spinal A18.01
      vertebra A18.01
    brain A17.81
    breast A18.89
    Cowper's gland A18.15
    dura (mater) (cerebral) (spinal) A17.81
    epidural (cerebral) (spinal) A17.81

Tuberculosis - *continued*
  female pelvis A18.17
  frontal sinus A15.8
  genital organs NEC A18.10
  genitourinary A18.10
  gland (lymphatic) - *see* Tuberculosis, lymph
    gland
  hip A18.02
  intestine A18.32
  ischiorectal A18.32
  joint NEC A18.02
    hip A18.02
    knee A18.02
    specified NEC A18.02
    vertebral A18.01
  kidney A18.11
  knee A18.02
  latent R76.11
  lumbar (spine) A18.01
  lung - *see* Tuberculosis, pulmonary
  meninges (cerebral) (spinal) A17.0
  muscle A18.09
  perianal (fistula) A18.32
  perinephritic A18.11
  perirectal A18.32
  rectum A18.32
  retropharyngeal A15.8
  sacrum A18.01
  scrofulous A18.2
  scrotum A18.15
  skin (primary) A18.4
  spinal cord A17.81
  spine or vertebra (column) A18.01
  subdiaphragmatic A18.31
  testis A18.15
  urinary A18.13
  uterus A18.17
accessory sinus - *see* Tuberculosis, sinus
Addison's disease A18.7
adenitis - *see* Tuberculosis, lymph gland
adenoids A15.8
adenopathy - *see* Tuberculosis, lymph gland
adherent pericardium A18.84
adnexa (uteri) A18.17
adrenal (capsule) (gland) A18.7
alimentary canal A18.32
anemia A18.89
ankle (joint) (bone) A18.02
anus A18.32
apex, apical - *see* Tuberculosis, pulmonary
appendicitis, appendix A18.32
arachnoid A17.0
artery, arteritis A18.89
  cerebral A18.89
arthritis (chronic) (synovial) A18.02
  spine or vertebra (column) A18.01
articular - *see* Tuberculosis, joint
ascites A18.31
asthma - *see* Tuberculosis, pulmonary
axilla, axillary (gland) A18.2
bladder A18.12
bone A18.03
  hip A18.02
  knee A18.02
  limb NEC A18.03
  sacrum A18.01
  spine or vertebral column A18.01
bowel (miliary) A18.32
brain A17.81
breast A18.89
broad ligament A18.17
bronchi, bronchial, bronchus A15.5
  ectasia, ectasis (bronchiectasis) - *see*
Tuberculosis, pulmonary

Tuberculosis - *continued*
  fistula A15.5
    primary (progressive) A15.7
  gland or node A15.4
    primary (progressive) A15.7
  lymph gland or node A15.4
    primary (progressive) A15.7
bronchiectasis - *see* Tuberculosis, pulmonary
bronchitis A15.5
bronchopleural A15.6
bronchopneumonia, bronchopneumonic - *see*
Tuberculosis, pulmonary
bronchorrhagia A15.5
bronchotracheal A15.5
bronze disease A18.7
buccal cavity A18.83
bulbourethral gland A18.15
bursa A18.09
cachexia A15.9
cardiomyopathy A18.84
caries - *see* Tuberculosis, bone
cartilage A18.02
  intervertebral A18.01
catarrhal - *see* Tuberculosis, respiratory
cecum A18.32
cellulitis (primary) A18.4
cerebellum A17.81
cerebral, cerebrum A17.81
cerebrospinal A17.81
  meninges A17.0
cervical (lymph gland or node) A18.2
cervicitis, cervix (uteri) A18.16
chest - *see* Tuberculosis, respiratory
  chorioretinitis A18.53
choroid, choroiditis A18.53
ciliary body A18.54
colitis A18.32
collier's J65
colliquativa (primary) A18.4
colon A18.32
complex, primary A15.7
congenital P37.0
conjunctiva A18.59
contact Z20.1
cornea (ulcer) A18.52
Cowper's gland A18.15
coxae A18.02
coxalgia A18.02
cul-de-sac of Douglas A18.17
curvature, spine A18.01
cutis (colliquativa) (primary) A18.4
cyst, ovary A18.18
cystitis A18.12
dactylitis A18.03
diarrhea A18.32
diffuse - *see* Tuberculosis, miliary
digestive tract A18.32
disseminated - *see* Tuberculosis, miliary
duodenum A18.32
dura (mater) (cerebral) (spinal) A17.0
  abscess (cerebral) (spinal) A17.81
dysentery A18.32
ear (inner) (middle) A18.6
  bone A18.03
  external (primary) A18.4
  skin (primary) A18.4
elbow A18.02
emphysema - *see* Tuberculosis, pulmonary
empyema A15.6
encephalitis A17.82
endarteritis A18.89
endocarditis A18.84
  aortic A18.84

Tuberculosis - *continued*
  mitral A18.84
  pulmonary A18.84
  tricuspid A18.84
endocrine glands NEC A18.82
endometrium A18.17
enteric, enterica, enteritis A18.32
enterocolitis A18.32
epididymis, epididymitis A18.15
epidural abscess (cerebral) (spinal) A17.81
epiglottis A15.5
episcleritis A18.51
erythema (induratum) (nodosum) (primary)
  A18.4
esophagus A18.83
eustachian tube A18.6
exposure (to) Z20.1
exudative - *see* Tuberculosis, pulmonary
eye A18.50
eyelid (primary) (lupus) A18.4
fallopian tube (acute) (chronic) A18.17
fascia A18.09
fauces A15.8
female pelvic inflammatory disease A18.17
finger A18.03
first infection A15.7
gallbladder A18.83
ganglion A18.09
gastritis A18.83
gastrocolic fistula A18.32
gastroenteritis A18.32
gastrointestinal tract A18.32
general, generalized - *see* Tuberculosis,
  miliary
genital organs A18.10
genitourinary A18.10
genu A18.02
glandula suprarenalis A18.7
glandular, general A18.2
glottis A15.5
grinder's J65
gum A18.83
hand A18.03
heart A18.84
hematogenous - *see* Tuberculosis, miliary
hemoptysis - *see* Tuberculosis, pulmonary
hemorrhage NEC - *see* Tuberculosis,
  pulmonary
hemothorax A15.6
hepatitis A18.83
hilar lymph nodes A15.4
  primary (progressive) A15.7
hip (joint) (disease) (bone) A18.02
hydropneumothorax A15.6
hydrothorax A15.6
hypoadrenalism A18.7
hypopharynx A15.8
ileocecal (hyperplastic) A18.32
ileocolitis A18.32
ileum A18.32
iliac spine (superior) A18.03
immunological findings only A15.7
indurativa (primary) A18.4
infantile A15.7
infection A15.9
  without clinical manifestations A15.7
infraclavicular gland A18.2
inguinal gland A18.2
inguinalis A18.2
intestine (any part) A18.32
iridocyclitis A18.54
iris, iritis A18.54
ischiorectal A18.32
jaw A18.03

Tuberculosis - *continued*
  jejunum A18.32
  joint A18.02
    vertebral A18.01
  keratitis (interstitial) A18.52
  keratoconjunctivitis A18.52
  kidney A18.11
  knee (joint) A18.02
  kyphosis, kyphoscoliosis A18.01
  laryngitis A15.5
  larynx A15.5
  latent R76.11
  leptomeninges, leptomeningitis (cerebral)
    (spinal) A17.0
  lichenoides (primary) A18.4
  linguae A18.83
  lip A18.83
  liver A18.83
  lordosis A18.01
  lung - *see* Tuberculosis, pulmonary
  lupus vulgaris A18.4
  lymph gland or node (peripheral) A18.2
    abdomen A18.39
    bronchial A15.4
      primary (progressive) A15.7
    cervical A18.2
    hilar A15.4
      primary (progressive) A15.7
    intrathoracic A15.4
      primary (progressive) A15.7
    mediastinal A15.4
      primary (progressive) A15.7
    mesenteric A18.39
    retroperitoneal A18.39
    tracheobronchial A15.4
      primary (progressive) A15.7
  lymphadenitis - *see* Tuberculosis, lymph gland
  lymphangitis - *see* Tuberculosis, lymph gland
  lymphatic (gland) (vessel) - *see* Tuberculosis,
    lymph gland
  mammary gland A18.89
  marasmus A15.9
  mastoiditis A18.03
  mediastinal lymph gland or node A15.4
    primary (progressive) A15.7
  mediastinitis A15.8
    primary (progressive) A15.7
  mediastinum A15.8
    primary (progressive) A15.7
  medulla A17.81
  melanosis, Addisonian A18.7
  meninges, meningitis (basilar) (cerebral)
    (cerebrospinal) (spinal) A17.0
  meningoencephalitis A17.82
  mesentery, mesenteric (gland or node) A18.39
  miliary A19.9
    acute A19.2
      multiple sites A19.1
      single specified site A19.0
    chronic A19.8
    specified NEC A19.8
  millstone makers' J65
  miner's J65
  molder's J65
  mouth A18.83
  multiple A19.9
    acute A19.1
    chronic A19.8
  muscle A18.09
  myelitis A17.82
  myocardium, myocarditis A18.84
  nasal (passage) (sinus) A15.8
  nasopharynx A15.8
  neck gland A18.2

Tuberculosis - *continued*
  nephritis A18.11
  nerve (mononeuropathy) A17.83
  nervous system A17.9
  nose (septum) A15.8
  ocular A18.50
  omentum A18.31
  oophoritis (acute) (chronic) A18.17
  optic (nerve trunk) (papilla) A18.59
  orbit A18.59
  orchitis A18.15
  organ, specified NEC A18.89
  osseous - *see* Tuberculosis, bone
  osteitis - *see* Tuberculosis, bone
  osteomyelitis - *see* Tuberculosis, bone
  otitis media A18.6
  ovary, ovaritis (acute) (chronic) A18.17
  oviduct (acute) (chronic) A18.17
  pachymeningitis A17.0
  palate (soft) A18.83
  pancreas A18.83
  papulonecrotic (a) (primary) A18.4
  parathyroid glands A18.82
  paronychia (primary) A18.4
  parotid gland or region A18.83
  pelvis (bony) A18.03
  penis A18.15
  peribronchitis A15.5
  pericardium, pericarditis A18.84
  perichondritis, larynx A15.5
  periostitis - *see* Tuberculosis, bone
  perirectal fistula A18.32
  peritoneum NEC A18.31
  peritonitis A18.31
  pharynx, pharyngitis A15.8
  phlyctenulosis (keratoconjunctivitis) A18.52
  phthisis NEC - *see* Tuberculosis, pulmonary
  pituitary gland A18.82
  pleura, pleural, pleurisy, pleuritis (fibrinous)
    (obliterative) (purulent) (simple plastic) (with
    effusion) A15.6
    primary (progressive) A15.7
  pneumonia, pneumonic - *see* Tuberculosis,
    pulmonary
  pneumothorax (spontaneous) (tense valvular) -
    see Tuberculosis, pulmonary
  polyneuropathy A17.89
  polyserositis A19.9
    acute A19.1
    chronic A19.8
  potter's J65
  prepuce A18.15
  primary (complex) A15.7
  proctitis A18.32
  prostate, prostatitis A18.14
  pulmonalis - *see* Tuberculosis, pulmonary
  pulmonary (cavitated) (fibrotic) (infiltrative)
    (nodular) A15.0
    childhood type or first infection A15.7
    primary (complex) A15.7
  pyelitis A18.11
  pyelonephritis A18.11
  pyemia - *see* Tuberculosis, miliary
  pyonephrosis A18.11
  pyopneumothorax A15.6
  pyothorax A15.6
  rectum (fistula) (with abscess) A18.32
  reinfection stage - *see* Tuberculosis,
    pulmonary
  renal A18.11
  renis A18.11
  respiratory A15.9
    primary A15.7
    specified site NEC A15.8

Tuberculosis - *continued*
  retina, retinitis A18.53
  retroperitoneal (lymph gland or node) A18.39
  rheumatism NEC A18.09
  rhinitis A15.8
  sacroiliac (joint) A18.01
  sacrum A18.01
  salivary gland A18.83
  salpingitis (acute) (chronic) A18.17
  sandblaster's J65
  sclera A18.51
  scoliosis A18.01
  scrofulous A18.2
  scrotum A18.15
  seminal tract or vesicle A18.15
  senile A15.9
  septic - *see* Tuberculosis, miliary
  shoulder (joint) A18.02
    blade A18.03
  sigmoid A18.32
  sinus (any nasal) A15.8
    bone A18.03
    epididymis A18.15
  skeletal NEC A18.03
  skin (any site) (primary) A18.4
  small intestine A18.32
  soft palate A18.83
  spermatic cord A18.15
  spine, spinal (column) A18.01
    cord A17.81
    medulla A17.81
    membrane A17.0
    meninges A17.0
  spleen, splenitis A18.85
  spondylitis A18.01
  sternoclavicular joint A18.02
  stomach A18.83
  stonemason's J65
  subcutaneous tissue (cellular) (primary) A18.4
  subcutis (primary) A18.4
  subdeltoid bursa A18.83
  submaxillary (region) A18.83
  supraclavicular gland A18.2
  suprarenal (capsule) (gland) A18.7
  swelling, joint (see also category M01) - *see*
    also Tuberculosis, joint A18.02
  symphysis pubis A18.02
  synovitis A18.09
    articular A18.02
    spine or vertebra A18.01
  systemic - *see* Tuberculosis, miliary
  tarsitis A18.4
  tendon (sheath) - *see* Tuberculosis,
    tenosynovitis
  tenosynovitis A18.09
    spine or vertebra A18.01
  testis A18.15
  throat A15.8
  thymus gland A18.82
  thyroid gland A18.81
  tongue A18.83
  tonsil, tonsillitis A15.8
  trachea, tracheal A15.5
    lymph gland or node A15.4
      primary (progressive) A15.7
  tracheobronchial A15.5
    lymph gland or node A15.4
      primary (progressive) A15.7
  tubal (acute) (chronic) A18.17
  tunica vaginalis A18.15
  ulcer (skin) (primary) A18.4
    bowel or intestine A18.32
    specified NEC
  code under Tuberculosis, by site

Tuberculosis - *continued*
unspecified site A15.9
ureter A18.11
urethra, urethral (gland) A18.13
urinary organ or tract A18.13
uterus A18.17
uveal tract A18.54
uvula A18.83
vagina A18.18
vas deferens A18.15
verruca, verrucosa (cutis) (primary) A18.4
vertebra (column) A18.01
vesiculitis A18.15
vulva A18.18
wrist (joint) A18.02
Tuberculum
Carabelli - *see* Note at K00.2
occlusal - *see* Note at K00.2
paramolare K00.2
Tuberosity, entire maxillary M26.07
Tuberous sclerosis (brain) Q85.1
Tubo-ovarian - *see* condition
Tuboplasty, after previous sterilization Z31.0
aftercare Z31.42
Tubotympanitis, catarrhal (chronic) - *see*
Otitis, media, nonsuppurative, chronic, serous
Tularemia A21.9
with
conjunctivitis A21.1
pneumonia A21.2
abdominal A21.3
bronchopneumonic A21.2
conjunctivitis A21.1
cryptogenic A21.3
enteric A21.3
gastrointestinal A21.3
generalized A21.7
ingestion A21.3
intestinal A21.3
oculoglandular A21.1
ophthalmic A21.1
pneumonia (any), pneumonic A21.2
pulmonary A21.2
sepsis A21.7
specified NEC A21.8
typhoidal A21.7
ulceroglandular A21.0
Tularensis conjunctivitis A21.1
Tumefaction - *see also* Swelling
liver - *see* Hypertrophy, liver
Tumor - *see also* Neoplasm, unspecified
behavior, by site
acinar cell - *see* Neoplasm, uncertain behavior,
by site
acinic cell - *see* Neoplasm, uncertain behavior,
by site
adenocarcinoid - *see* Neoplasm, malignant, by
site
adenomatoid - *see also* Neoplasm, benign, by
site
odontogenic - *see* Cyst, calcifying
odontogenic
adnexal (skin) - *see* Neoplasm, skin, benign,
by site
adrenal
cortical (benign) D35.0-
malignant C74.0-
rest - *see* Neoplasm, benign, by site
alpha-cell
malignant
pancreas C25.4
specified site NEC - *see* Neoplasm,
malignant, by site
unspecified site C25.4

Tumor - *continued*
pancreas D13.7
specified site NEC - *see* Neoplasm, benign,
by site
unspecified site D13.7
aneurysmal - *see* Aneurysm
aortic body D44.7
malignant C75.5
Askin's - *see* Neoplasm, connective tissue,
malignant
basal cell - *see also* Neoplasm, skin, uncertain
behavior D48.5
Bednar - *see* Neoplasm, skin, malignant
benign (unclassified) - *see* Neoplasm, benign,
by site
beta-cell
malignant
pancreas C25.4
specified site NEC - *see* Neoplasm,
malignant, by site
unspecified site C25.4
pancreas D13.7
specified site NEC - *see* Neoplasm, benign,
by site
unspecified site D13.7
Brenner D27.9
borderline malignancy D39.1-
malignant C56-
proliferating D39.1-
bronchial alveolar, intravascular D38.1
Brooke's - *see* Neoplasm, skin, benign
brown fat - *see* Lipoma
Burkitt - *see* Lymphoma, Burkitt
calcifying epithelial odontogenic - *see* Cyst,
calcifying odontogenic
carcinoid
benign D3A.00
appendix D3A.020
ascending colon D3A.022
bronchus (lung) D3A.090
cecum D3A.021
colon D3A.029
descending colon D3A.024
duodenum D3A.010
foregut NOS D3A.094
hindgut NOS D3A.096
ileum D3A.012
jejunum D3A.011
kidney D3A.093
large intestine D3A.029
lung (bronchus) D3A.090
midgut NOS D3A.095
rectum D3A.026
sigmoid colon D3A.025
small intestine D3A.019
specified NEC D3A.098
stomach D3A.092
thymus D3A.091
transverse colon D3A.023
malignant C7A.00
appendix C7A.020
ascending colon C7A.022
bronchus (lung) C7A.090
cecum C7A.021
colon C7A.029
descending colon C7A.024
duodenum C7A.010
foregut NOS C7A.094
hindgut NOS C7A.096
ileum C7A.012
jejunum C7A.011
kidney C7A.093
large intestine C7A.029
lung (bronchus) C7A.090

Tumor - *continued*
midgut NOS C7A.095
rectum C7A.026
sigmoid colon C7A.025
small intestine C7A.019
specified NEC C7A.098
stomach C7A.092
thymus C7A.091
transverse colon C7A.023
mesentery metastasis C7B.04
secondary C7B.00
bone C7B.03
distant lymph nodes C7B.01
liver C7B.02
peritoneum C7B.04
specified NEC C7B.09
carotid body D44.6
malignant C75.4
cells - *see also* Neoplasm, unspecified
behavior, by site
benign - *see* Neoplasm, benign, by site
malignant - *see* Neoplasm, malignant, by site
uncertain whether benign or malignant - *see*
Neoplasm, uncertain behavior, by site
cervix, in pregnancy or childbirth - *see*
Pregnancy, complicated by, tumor, cervix
chondromatous giant cell - *see* Neoplasm,
bone, benign
chromaffin - *see also* Neoplasm, benign, by
site
malignant - *see* Neoplasm, malignant, by site
Cock's peculiar L72.3
Codman's - *see* Neoplasm, bone, benign
dentigerous, mixed - *see* Cyst, calcifying
odontogenic
dermoid - *see* Neoplasm, benign, by site
with malignant transformation C56-
desmoid (extra-abdominal) - *see also*
Neoplasm, connective tissue, uncertain
behavior
abdominal - *see* Neoplasm, connective tissue,
uncertain behavior
embolus - *see* Neoplasm, secondary, by site
embryonal (mixed) - *see also* Neoplasm,
uncertain behavior, by site
liver C22.7
endodermal sinus
specified site - *see* Neoplasm, malignant, by
site
unspecified site
female C56.-
male C62.90
epithelial
benign - *see* Neoplasm, benign, by site
malignant - *see* Neoplasm, malignant, by site
Ewing's - *see* Neoplasm, bone, malignant, by
site
fatty - *see* Lipoma
fibroid - *see* Leiomyoma
G cell
malignant
pancreas C25.4
specified site NEC - *see* Neoplasm,
malignant, by site
unspecified site C25.4
specified site - *see* Neoplasm, uncertain
behavior, by site
unspecified site D37.8
germ cell - *see also* Neoplasm, malignant, by
site
mixed - *see* Neoplasm, malignant, by site
ghost cell, odontogenic - *see* Cyst, calcifying
odontogenic
giant cell - *see also* Neoplasm, uncertain

Tumor - *continued*

behavior, by site
bone D48.0
malignant - *see* Neoplasm, bone, malignant
chondromatous - *see* Neoplasm, bone, benign
malignant - *see* Neoplasm, malignant, by site
soft parts - *see* Neoplasm, connective tissue,
uncertain behavior
malignant - *see* Neoplasm, connective
tissue, malignant
glomus D18.00
intra-abdominal D18.03
intracranial D18.02
jugulare D44.7
malignant C75.5
skin D18.01
specified site NEC D18.09
gonadal stromal - *see* Neoplasm, uncertain
behavior, by site
granular cell - *see also* Neoplasm, connective
tissue, benign
malignant - *see* Neoplasm, connective tissue,
malignant
granulosa cell D39.1-
juvenile D39.1-
malignant C56-
granulosa cell-theca cell D39.1-
malignant C56-
Grawitz's C64-
hemorrhoidal - *see* Hemorrhoids
hilar cell D27-
hilus cell D27-
Hürthle cell (benign) D34
malignant C73
hydatid - *see* Echinococcus
hypernephroid - *see also* Neoplasm, uncertain
behavior, by site
interstitial cell - *see also* Neoplasm, uncertain
behavior, by site
benign - *see* Neoplasm, benign, by site
malignant - *see* Neoplasm, malignant, by site
intravascular bronchial alveolar D38.1
islet cell - *see* Neoplasm, benign, by site
malignant - *see* Neoplasm, malignant, by site
pancreas C25.4
specified site NEC - *see* Neoplasm,
malignant, by site
unspecified site C25.4
pancreas D13.7
specified site NEC - *see* Neoplasm, benign,
by site
unspecified site D13.7
juxtaglomerular D41.0-
Klatskin's C24.0
Krukenberg's C79.6-
Leydig cell - *see* Neoplasm, uncertain
behavior, by site
benign - *see* Neoplasm, benign, by site
specified site - *see* Neoplasm, benign, by
site
unspecified site
female D27.9
male D29.20
malignant - *see* Neoplasm, malignant, by site
specified site - *see* Neoplasm, malignant, by
site
unspecified site
female C56.9
male C62.90
specified site - *see* Neoplasm, uncertain
behavior, by site
unspecified site
female D39.10
male D40.10

Tumor - *continued*

lipid cell, ovary D27-
lipoid cell, ovary D27-
malignant - *see also* Neoplasm, malignant, by
site C80.1
fusiform cell (type) C80.1
giant cell (type) C80.1
localized, plasma cell - *see* Plasmacytoma,
solitary
mixed NEC C80.1
small cell (type) C80.1
spindle cell (type) C80.1
unclassified C80.1
mast cell D47.09
melanotic, neuroectodermal - *see* Neoplasm,
benign, by site
Merkel cell - *see* Carcinoma, Merkel cell
mesenchymal
malignant - *see* Neoplasm, connective tissue,
malignant
mixed - *see* Neoplasm, connective tissue,
uncertain behavior
mesodermal, mixed - *see also* Neoplasm,
malignant, by site
liver C22.4
mesonephric - *see also* Neoplasm, uncertain
behavior, by site
malignant - *see* Neoplasm, malignant, by site
metastatic
from specified site - *see* Neoplasm,
malignant, by site
of specified site - *see* Neoplasm, malignant,
by site
to specified site - *see* Neoplasm, secondary,
by site
mixed NEC - *see also* Neoplasm, benign, by
site
malignant - *see* Neoplasm, malignant, by site
mucinous of low malignant potential
specified site - *see* Neoplasm, malignant, by
site
unspecified site C56.9
mucocarcinoid
specified site - *see* Neoplasm, malignant, by
site
unspecified site C18.1
mucoepidermoid - *see* Neoplasm, uncertain
behavior, by site
Müllerian, mixed
specified site - *see* Neoplasm, malignant, by
site
unspecified site C54.9
myoepithelial - *see* Neoplasm, benign, by site
neuroectodermal (peripheral) - *see* Neoplasm,
malignant, by site
primitive
specified site - *see* Neoplasm, malignant, by
site
unspecified site C71.9
neuroendocrine D3A.8
malignant poorly differentiated C7A.1
secondary NEC C7B.8
specified NEC C7A.8
neurogenic olfactory C30.0
nonencapsulated sclerosing C73
odontogenic (adenomatoid) (benign)
(calcifying epithelial) (keratocystic)
(squamous) - *see* Cyst, calcifying odontogenic
malignant C41.1
upper jaw (bone) C41.0
ovarian stromal D39.1-
ovary, in pregnancy - *see* Pregnancy,
complicated by pacinian - *see* Neoplasm,
skin, benign

Tumor - *continued*

Pancoast's - *see* Pancoast's syndrome
papillary - *see also* Papilloma
cystic D37.9
mucinous of low malignant potential C56-
specified site - *see* Neoplasm, malignant, by
site
unspecified site C56.9
serous of low malignant potential
specified site - *see* Neoplasm, malignant, by
site
unspecified site C56.9
pelvic, in pregnancy or childbirth - *see*
Pregnancy, complicated by phantom F45.8
phyllodes D48.6-
benign D24-
malignant - *see* Neoplasm, breast, malignant
Pindborg - *see* Cyst, calcifying odontogenic
placental site trophoblastic D39.2
plasma cell (malignant) (localized) - *see*
Plasmacytoma, solitary
polyvesicular vitelline
specified site - *see* Neoplasm, malignant, by
site
unspecified site
female C56.9
male C62.90
Pott's puffy - *see* Osteomyelitis, specified NEC
Rathke's pouch D44.3
retinal anlage - *see* Neoplasm, benign, by site
salivary gland type, mixed - *see* Neoplasm,
salivary gland, benign
malignant - *see* Neoplasm, salivary gland,
malignant
Sampson's N80.1
Schmincke's - *see* Neoplasm, nasopharynx,
malignant
sclerosing stromal D27-
sebaceous - *see* Cyst, sebaceous
secondary - *see* Neoplasm, secondary, by site
carcinoid C7B.00
bone C7B.03
distant lymph nodes C7B.01
liver C7B.02
peritoneum C7B.04
specified NEC C7B.09
neuroendocrine NEC C7B.8
serous of low malignant potential
specified site - *see* Neoplasm, malignant, by
site
unspecified site C56.9
Sertoli cell - *see* Neoplasm, benign, by site
with lipid storage
specified site - *see* Neoplasm, benign, by
site
unspecified site
female D27.9
male D29.20
specified site - *see* Neoplasm, benign, by site
unspecified site
female D27.9
male D29.20
Sertoli-leydig cell - *see* Neoplasm, benign, by
site
specified site - *see* Neoplasm, benign, by site
unspecified site
female D27.9
male D29.20
sex cord (-stromal) - *see* Neoplasm, uncertain
behavior, by site
with annular tubules D39.1-
skin appendage - *see* Neoplasm, skin, benign
smooth muscle - *see* Neoplasm, connective
tissue, uncertain behavior

Tumor - *continued*
  soft tissue
    benign - *see* Neoplasm, connective tissue,
      benign
    malignant - *see* Neoplasm, connective tissue,
      malignant
  sternomastoid (congenital) Q68.0
  stromal
    endometrial D39.0
    gastric D48.1
      benign D21.4
      malignant C16.9
      uncertain behavior D48.1
    gastrointestinal C49.A-
      benign D21.4
      esophagus C49.A1
      malignant C49.A0
        colon C49.A4
        duodenum C49.A3
        esophagus C49.A1
        ileum C49.A3
        jejunum C49.A3
        Meckel diverticulum C49.A3
        large intestine C49.A4
        omentum C49.A9
        peritoneum C49.A9
        rectum C49.A5
        small intestine C49.A3
        specified site NEC C49.A9
        stomach C49.A2
      large intestine C49.A4
      rectum C49.A5
      small intestine C49.A3
      specified site NEC C49.A9
      stomach C49.A2
      uncertain behavior D48.1
    intestine
      benign D21.4
      malignant
        large C49.A4
        small C49.A3
      uncertain behavior D48.1
    ovarian D39.1-
    stomach C49.A2
      benign D21.4
      malignant C49.A2
      uncertain behavior D48.1
  testicular D40.10
  sweat gland - *see also* Neoplasm, skin,
    uncertain behavior
    benign - *see* Neoplasm, skin, benign
    malignant - *see* Neoplasm, skin, malignant
  syphilitic, brain A52.17
  testicular stromal D40.1-
  theca cell D27.-
  theca cell-granulosa cell D39.1-
  Triton, malignant - *see* Neoplasm, nerve,
    malignant
  trophoblastic, placental site D39.2
  turban D23.4
  uterus (body), in pregnancy or childbirth - *see*
    Pregnancy, complicated by, tumor, uterus
  vagina, in pregnancy or childbirth - *see*
    Pregnancy, complicated by
  varicose - *see* Varix
  von Recklinghausen's - *see* Neurofibromatosis
  vulva or perineum, in pregnancy or childbirth -
    see Pregnancy, complicated by
    causing obstructed labor O65.5
  Warthin's - *see* Neoplasm, salivary gland,
    benign
  Wilms' C64-
  yolk sac - *see* Neoplasm, malignant, by site
    specified site - *see* Neoplasm, malignant, by

Tumor - *continued*
  site
    unspecified site
      female C56.9
      male C62.90
**Tumor lysis syndrome (following
antineoplastic chemotherapy) (spontaneous)
NEC** E88.3
Tumorlet - *see* Neoplasm, uncertain behavior,
by site
Tungiasis B88.1
Tunica vasculosa lentis Q12.2
Turban tumor D23.4
Türck's trachoma J37.0
Turner-kieser syndrome Q87.2
Turner-like syndrome Q87.1
Turner's
  hypoplasia (tooth) K00.4
  syndrome Q96.9
    specified NEC Q96.8
  tooth K00.4
Turner-Ullrich syndrome Q96.9
Tussis convulsiva - *see* Whooping cough
Twiddler's syndrome (due to)
  automatic implantable defibrillator T82.198
  cardiac pacemaker T82.198
Twilight state
  epileptic F05
  psychogenic F44.89
Twin (newborn) - *see also* Newborn, twin
  conjoined Q89.4
  pregnancy - *see* Pregnancy, twin
Twinning, teeth K00.2
Twist, twisted
  bowel, colon or intestine K56.2
  hair (congenital) Q84.1
  mesentery K56.2
  omentum K56.2
  organ or site, congenital NEC - *see* Anomaly,
    by site
  ovarian pedicle - *see* Torsion, ovary
Twitching R25.3
Tylosis (acquired) L84
  buccalis K13.29
  linguae K13.29
  palmaris et plantaris (congenital) (inherited)
    Q82.8
    acquired L85.1
Tympanism R14.0
Tympanites (abdominal) (intestinal) R14.0
Tympanitis - *see* Myringitis
Tympanosclerosis - *see* subcategory H74.0
Tympanum - *see* condition
Tympany
  abdomen R14.0
  chest R09.89
Type A behavior pattern Z73.1
Typhlitis - *see* Appendicitis
Typhoenteritis - *see* Typhoid
**Typhoid (abortive) (ambulant) (any site)
(clinical) (fever) (hemorrhagic) (infection)
(intermittent) (malignant) (rheumatic)
(Widal negative)** A01.00
  with pneumonia A01.03
  abdominal A01.09
  arthritis A01.04
  carrier (suspected) of Z22.0
  cholecystitis (current) A01.09
  endocarditis A01.02
  heart involvement A01.02
  inoculation reaction - *see* Complications,
    vaccination
  meningitis A01.01
  mesenteric lymph nodes A01.09

Typhoid - *continued*
  myocarditis A01.02
  osteomyelitis A01.05
  perichondritis, larynx A01.09
  pneumonia A01.03
  spine A01.05
  specified NEC A01.09
  ulcer (perforating) A01.09
Typhomalaria (fever) - *see* Malaria
Typhomania A01.00
Typhoperitonitis A01.09
Typhus (fever) A75.9
  abdominal, abdominalis - *see* Typhoid
  African tick A77.1
  amarillic A95.9
  brain A75.9 *[G94]*
  cerebral A75.9 *[G94]*
  classical A75.0
  due to Rickettsia
    prowazekii A75.0
      recrudescent A75.1
    tsutsugamushi A75.3
    typhi A75.2
  endemic (flea-borne) A75.2
  epidemic (louse-borne) A75.0
  exanthematic NEC A75.0
  exanthematicus SAI A75.0
    brillii SAI A75.1
    mexicanus SAI A75.2
    typhus murinus SAI A75.2
  flea-borne A75.2
  India tick A77.1
  Kenya (tick) A77.1
  louse-borne A75.0
  Mexican A75.2
  mite-borne A75.3
  murine A75.2
  North Asian tick-borne A77.2
  petechial A75.9
  Queensland tick A77.3
  rat A75.2
  recrudescent A75.1
  recurrens - *see* Fever, relapsing
  Sao Paulo A77.0
  scrub (China) (India) (Malaysia) (New
    Guinea) A75.3
  shop (of Malaysia) A75.2
  Siberian tick A77.2
  tick-borne A77.9
  tropical (mite-borne) A75.3
Tyrosinemia E70.21
  newborn, transitory P74.5
Tyrosinosis E70.21
Tyrosinuria E70.29

U

Uhl's anomaly or disease Q24.8
**Ulcer, ulcerated, ulcerating, ulceration,
ulcerative**
  alveolar process M27.3
  amebic (intestine) A06.1
    skin A06.7
  anastomotic - *see* Ulcer, gastrojejunal
  anorectal K62.6
  antral - *see* Ulcer, stomach
  anus (sphincter) (solitary) K62.6
  aorta - *see* Aneurysm
  aphthous (oral) (recurrent) K12.0
    genital organ(s)
      female N76.6
      male N50.89
  artery I77.2
  atrophic - *see* Ulcer, skin

Ulcer - *continued*

decubitus - *see* Ulcer, pressure, by site
back L98.429
  with
    bone involvement without evidence of
      necrosis L98.426
    bone necrosis L98.424
    exposed fat layer L98.422
    muscle involvement without evidence of
      necrosis L98.425
    muscle necrosis L98.423
    skin breakdown only L98.421
    specified severity NEC L98.428
Barrett's (esophagus) K22.10
  with bleeding K22.11
bile duct (common) (hepatic) K83.8
bladder (solitary) (sphincter) NEC N32.89
  bilharzial B65.9 [*N33*]
  in schistosomiasis (bilharzial) B65.9 [*N33*]
  submucosal - *see* Cystitis, interstitial
  tuberculous A18.12
bleeding K27.4
bone - *see* Osteomyelitis, specified type NEC
bowel - *see* Ulcer, intestine
breast N61.1
bronchus J98.09
buccal (cavity) (traumatic) K12.1
Buruli A31.1
buttock L98.419
  with
    bone involvement without evidence of
      necrosis L98.416
    bone necrosis L98.414
    exposed fat layer L98.412
    muscle involvement without evidence of
      necrosis L98.415
    muscle necrosis L98.413
    skin breakdown only L98.411
    specified severity NEC L98.418
cancerous - *see* Neoplasm, malignant, by site
cardia K22.10
  with bleeding K22.11
cardioesophageal (peptic) K22.10
  with bleeding K22.11
cecum - *see* Ulcer, intestine
cervix (uteri) (decubitus) (trophic) N86
  with cervicitis N72
chancroidal A57
chiclero B55.1
chronic (cause unknown) - *see* Ulcer, skin
Cochin-china B55.1
colon - *see* Ulcer, intestine
conjunctiva H10.89
cornea H16.00-
  with hypopyon H16.03-
  central H16.01-
  dendritic (herpes simplex) B00.52
  marginal H16.04-
  Mooren's H16.05-
  mycotic H16.06-
  perforated H16.07-
  ring H16.02-
  tuberculous (phlyctenular) A18.52
corpus cavernosum (chronic) N48.5
crural - *see* Ulcer, lower limb
Curling's - *see* Ulcer, peptic, acute
Cushing's - *see* Ulcer, peptic, acute
cystic duct K82.8
cystitis (interstitial) - *see* Cystitis, interstitial
decubitus - *see* Ulcer, pressure, by site
dendritic, cornea (herpes simplex) B00.52
diabetes, diabetic - *see* Diabetes, ulcer
Dieulafoy's K25.0
due to

infection NEC - *see* Ulcer, skin
radiation NEC L59.8
trophic disturbance (any region) - *see* Ulcer,
skin
  X-ray L58.1
duodenum, duodenal (eroded) (peptic) K26.9
  with
    hemorrhage K26.4
      and perforation K26.6
    perforation K26.5
  acute K26.3
    with
      hemorrhage K26.0
        and perforation K26.2
      perforation K26.1
  chronic K26.7
    with
      hemorrhage K26.4
        and perforation K26.6
      perforation K26.5
dysenteric A09
elusive - *see* Cystitis, interstitial
endocarditis (acute) (chronic) (subacute) I28.8
epiglottis J38.7
esophagus (peptic) K22.10
  with bleeding K22.11
  due to
    aspirin K22.10
      with bleeding K22.11
    gastrointestinal reflux disease K21.0
    ingestion of chemical or medicament
      K22.10
        with bleeding K22.11
  fungal K22.10
    with bleeding K22.11
  infective K22.10
    with bleeding K22.11
  varicose - *see* Varix, esophagus
eyelid (region) H01.8
fauces J39.2
Fenwick (-hunner) (solitary) - *see* Cystitis,
interstitial
fistulous - *see* Ulcer, skin
foot (indolent) (trophic) - *see* Ulcer, lower
limb
frambesial, initial A66.0
frenum (tongue) K14.0
gallbladder or duct K82.8
gangrenous - *see* Gangrene
gastric - *see* Ulcer, stomach
gastrocolic - *see* Ulcer, gastrojejunal
gastroduodenal - *see* Ulcer, peptic
gastroesophageal - *see* Ulcer, stomach
gastrointestinal - *see* Ulcer, gastrojejunal
gastrojejunal (peptic) K28.9
  with
    hemorrhage K28.4
      and perforation K28.6
    perforation K28.5
  acute K28.3
    with
      hemorrhage K28.0
        and perforation K28.2
      perforation K28.1
  chronic K28.7
    with
      hemorrhage K28.4
        and perforation K28.6
      perforation K28.5
gastrojejunocolic - *see* Ulcer, gastrojejunal
gingiva K06.8
gingivitis K05.10
  nonplaque induced K05.11

plaque induced K05.10
glottis J38.7
granuloma of pudenda A58
gum K06.8
gumma, due to yaws A66.4
heel - *see* Ulcer, lower limb
hemorrhoid - *see also* Hemorrhoids, by degree
K64.8
Hunner's - *see* Cystitis, interstitial
hypopharynx J39.2
hypopyon (chronic) (subacute) - *see* Ulcer,
cornea, with hypopyon
hypostaticum - *see* Ulcer, varicose
ileum - *see* Ulcer, intestine
intestine, intestinal K63.3
  with perforation K63.1
  amebic A06.1
  duodenal - *see* Ulcer, duodenum
  granulocytopenic (with hemorrhage) - *see*
Neutropenia
  marginal - *see* Ulcer, gastrojejunal
  perforating K63.1
    newborn P78.0
  primary, small intestine K63.3
  rectum K62.6
  stercoraceous, stercoral K63.3
  tuberculous A18.32
  typhoid (fever) - *see* Typhoid
  varicose I86.8
jejunum, jejunal - *see* Ulcer, gastrojejunal
keratitis - *see* Ulcer, cornea
knee - *see* Ulcer, lower limb
labium (majus) (minus) N76.6
laryngitis - *see* Laryngitis
larynx (aphthous) (contact) J38.7
  diphtheritic A36.2
leg - *see* Ulcer, lower limb
lip K13.0
Lipschütz's N76.6
lower limb (atrophic) (chronic) (neurogenic)
(perforating) (pyogenic) (trophic) (tropical)
L97.909
  with
    bone involvement without evidence of
      necrosis L97.906
    bone necrosis L97.904
    exposed fat layer L97.902
    muscle involvement without evidence of
      necrosis L97.905
    muscle necrosis L97.903
    skin breakdown only L97.901
    specified severity NEC L97.908
  ankle L97.309
    with
      bone involvement without evidence of
        necrosis L97.306
      bone necrosis L97.304
      exposed fat layer L97.302
      muscle involvement without evidence of
        necrosis L97.305
      muscle necrosis L97.303
      skin breakdown only L97.301
      specified severity NEC L97.308
  left L97.329
    with
      bone involvement without evidence of
        necrosis L97.326
      bone necrosis L97.324
      exposed fat layer L97.322
      muscle involvement without evidence of
        necrosis L97.325
      specified severity NEC L97.328
      muscle necrosis L97.323

Ulcer - *continued*

- skin breakdown only L97.321
- right L97.319
  - with
    - bone involvement without evidence of necrosis L97.316
    - bone necrosis L97.314
    - exposed fat layer L97.312
    - muscle involvement without evidence of necrosis L97.315
    - muscle necrosis L97.313
    - skin breakdown only L97.311
    - specified severity NEC L97.318
- calf L97.209
  - with
    - bone involvement without evidence of necrosis L97.206
    - bone necrosis L97.204
    - exposed fat layer L97.202
    - muscle involvement without evidence of necrosis L97.205
    - muscle necrosis L97.203
    - skin breakdown only L97.201
    - specified severity NEC L97.208
  - left L97.229
    - with
      - bone involvement without evidence of necrosis L97.226
      - bone necrosis L97.224
      - exposed fat layer L97.222
      - muscle involvement without evidence of necrosis L97.225
      - muscle necrosis L97.223
      - skin breakdown only L97.221
      - specified severity NEC L97.228
  - right L97.219
    - with
      - bone involvement without evidence of necrosis L97.216
      - bone necrosis L97.214
      - exposed fat layer L97.212
      - muscle involvement without evidence of necrosis L97.215
      - muscle necrosis L97.213
      - skin breakdown only L97.211
      - specified severity NEC L97.218
- decubitus - *see* Ulcer, pressure, by site
- foot specified NEC L97.509
  - with
    - bone involvement without evidence of necrosis L97.506
    - bone necrosis L97.504
    - exposed fat layer L97.502
    - muscle involvement without evidence of necrosis L97.505
    - muscle necrosis L97.503
    - skin breakdown only L97.501
    - specified severity NEC L97.508
  - left L97.529
    - with
      - bone involvement without evidence of necrosis L97.526
      - bone necrosis L97.524
      - exposed fat layer L97.522
      - muscle involvement without evidence of necrosis L97.525
      - muscle necrosis L97.523
      - skin breakdown only L97.521
      - specified severity NEC L97.528
  - right L97.519
    - with
      - bone involvement without evidence of necrosis L97.516
      - bone necrosis L97.514

Ulcer - *continued*

- exposed fat layer L97.512
- muscle involvement without evidence of necrosis L97.515
- muscle necrosis L97.513
- skin breakdown only L97.511
- specified severity NEC L97.518
- heel L97.409
  - with
    - bone involvement without evidence of necrosis L97.406
    - bone necrosis L97.404
    - exposed fat layer L97.402
    - muscle involvement without evidence of necrosis L97.405
    - muscle necrosis L97.403
    - skin breakdown only L97.401
    - specified severity NEC L97.408
  - left L97.429
    - with
      - bone involvement without evidence of necrosis L97.426
      - bone necrosis L97.424
      - exposed fat layer L97.422
      - muscle involvement without evidence of necrosis L97.425
      - muscle necrosis L97.423
      - skin breakdown only L97.421
      - specified severity NEC L97.428
  - right L97.419
    - with
      - bone involvement without evidence of necrosis L97.416
      - bone necrosis L97.414
      - exposed fat layer L97.412
      - muscle involvement without evidence of necrosis L97.415
      - muscle necrosis L97.413
      - skin breakdown only L97.411
      - specified severity NEC L97.418
- left L97.929
  - with
    - bone necrosis L97.924
    - exposed fat layer L97.922
    - bone involvement without evidence of necrosis L97.926
    - muscle involvement without evidence of necrosis L97.925
    - muscle necrosis L97.923
    - skin breakdown only L97.921
    - specified severity NEC L97.928
- lower leg NOS L97.909
  - with
    - bone necrosis L97.904
    - exposed fat layer L97.902
    - bone involvement without evidence of necrosis L97.906
    - muscle involvement without evidence of necrosis L97.905
    - muscle necrosis L97.903
    - skin breakdown only L97.901
    - specified severity NEC L97.908
  - left L97.929
    - with
      - bone involvement without evidence of necrosis L97.926
      - bone necrosis L97.924
      - exposed fat layer L97.922
      - muscle involvement without evidence of necrosis L97.925
      - muscle necrosis L97.923
      - skin breakdown only L97.921
      - specified severity NEC L97.928
  - right L97.919

Ulcer - *continued*

- with
  - bone involvement without evidence of necrosis L97.916
  - bone necrosis L97.914
  - exposed fat layer L97.912
  - muscle involvement without evidence of necrosis L97.915
  - muscle necrosis L97.913
  - skin breakdown only L97.911
  - specified severity NEC L97.918
- specified site NEC L97.809
  - with
    - bone involvement without evidence of necrosis L97.806
    - bone necrosis L97.804
    - exposed fat layer L97.802
    - muscle involvement without evidence of necrosis L97.805
    - muscle necrosis L97.803
    - skin breakdown only L97.801
    - specified severity NEC L97.808
  - left L97.829
    - with
      - bone involvement without evidence of necrosis L97.826
      - bone necrosis L97.824
      - exposed fat layer L97.822
      - muscle involvement without evidence of necrosis L97.825
      - muscle necrosis L97.823
      - skin breakdown only L97.821
      - specified severity NEC L97.828
  - right L97.819
    - with
      - bone involvement without evidence of necrosis L97.816
      - bone necrosis L97.814
      - exposed fat layer L97.812
      - muscle involvement without evidence of necrosis L97.815
      - muscle necrosis L97.813
      - skin breakdown only L97.811
      - specified severity NEC L97.818
- midfoot L97.409
  - with
    - bone involvement without evidence of necrosis L97.406
    - bone necrosis L97.404
    - exposed fat layer L97.402
    - muscle involvement without evidence of necrosis L97.405
    - muscle necrosis L97.403
    - skin breakdown only L97.401
    - specified severity NEC L97.408
  - left L97.429
    - with
      - bone involvement without evidence of necrosis L97.426
      - bone necrosis L97.424
      - exposed fat layer L97.422
      - muscle involvement without evidence of necrosis L97.425
      - muscle necrosis L97.423
      - skin breakdown only L97.421
      - specified severity NEC L97.428
  - right L97.419
    - with
      - bone involvement without evidence of necrosis L97.416
      - bone necrosis L97.414
      - exposed fat layer L97.412
      - muscle involvement without evidence of necrosis L97.415

Ulcer - *continued*

    muscle necrosis L97.413
    skin breakdown only L97.411
    specified severity NEC L97.418
  right L97.919
    with
      bone involvement without evidence of
        necrosis L97.916
      bone necrosis L97.914
      exposed fat layer L97.912
      muscle involvement without evidence of
        necrosis L97.915
      muscle necrosis L97.913
      skin breakdown only L97.911
      specified severity NEC L97.918
  thigh L97.109
    with
      bone involvement without evidence of
        necrosis L97.106
      muscle involvement without evidence of
        necrosis L97.105
      bone necrosis L97.104
      exposed fat layer L97.102
      specified severity NEC L97.108
      muscle necrosis L97.103
      skin breakdown only L97.101
  left L97.129
    with
      bone involvement without evidence of
        necrosis L97.126
      bone necrosis L97.124
      exposed fat layer L97.122
      muscle involvement without evidence of
        necrosis L97.125
      muscle necrosis L97.123
      skin breakdown only L97.121
      specified severity NEC L97.128
  right L97.119
    with
      bone involvement without evidence of
        necrosis L97.116
      bone necrosis L97.114
      exposed fat layer L97.112
      muscle involvement without evidence of
        necrosis L97.115
      muscle necrosis L97.113
      skin breakdown only L97.111
      specified severity NEC L97.118
  toe L97.509
    with
      bone involvement without evidence of
        necrosis L97.506
      bone necrosis L97.504
      exposed fat layer L97.502
      muscle involvement without evidence of
        necrosis L97.505
      muscle necrosis L97.503
      skin breakdown only L97.501
      specified severity NEC L97.508
  left L97.529
    with
      bone involvement without evidence of
        necrosis L97.526
      bone necrosis L97.524
      exposed fat layer L97.522
      muscle involvement without evidence of
        necrosis L97.525
      muscle necrosis L97.523
      skin breakdown only L97.521
      specified severity NEC L97.528
  right L97.519
    with
      bone involvement without evidence of
        necrosis L97.516

Ulcer - *continued*

    bone necrosis L97.514
    exposed fat layer L97.512
    muscle involvement without evidence of
      necrosis L97.515
    muscle necrosis L97.513
    skin breakdown only L97.511
    specified severity NEC L97.518
  leprous A30.1
  syphilitic A52.19
  varicose - *see* Varix, leg, with, ulcer
  luetic - *see* Ulcer, syphilitic
  lung J98.4
    tuberculous - *see* Tuberculosis, pulmonary
  malignant - *see* Neoplasm, malignant, by site
  marginal NEC - *see* Ulcer, gastrojejunal
  meatus (urinarius) N34.2
  Meckel's diverticulum Q43.0
    malignant - *see* Table of Neoplasms, small
    intestine, malignant
  Meleney's (chronic undermining) - *see* Ulcer,
  skin
  Mooren's (cornea) - *see* Ulcer, cornea,
  Mooren's
  mycobacterial (skin) A31.1
  nasopharynx J39.2
  neck, uterus N86
  neurogenic NEC - *see* Ulcer, skin
  nose, nasal (passage) (infective) (septum)
  J34.0
    skin - *see* Ulcer, skin
    spirochetal A69.8
    varicose (bleeding) I86.8
  oral mucosa (traumatic) K12.1
  palate (soft) K12.1
  penis (chronic) N48.5
  peptic (site unspecified) K27.9
    with
      hemorrhage K27.4
        and perforation K27.6
      perforation K27.5
    acute K27.3
      with
        hemorrhage K27.0
          and perforation K27.2
        perforation K27.1
    chronic K27.7
      with
        hemorrhage K27.4
          and perforation K27.6
        perforation K27.5
    esophagus K22.10
      with bleeding K22.11
    newborn P78.82
  perforating K27.5
    skin - *see* Ulcer, skin
  peritonsillar J35.8
  phagedenic (tropical) - *see* Ulcer, skin
  pharynx J39.2
  phlebitis - *see* Phlebitis
  plaster - *see* Ulcer, pressure, by site
  popliteal space - *see* Ulcer, lower limb
  postpyloric - *see* Ulcer, duodenum
  prepuce N47.7
  prepyloric - *see* Ulcer, stomach
  pressure (pressure area) L89.9-
    ankle L89.5-
    back L89.1-
    buttock L89.3-
    coccyx L89.15-
    contiguous site of back, buttock, hip L89.4-
    elbow L89.0-
    face L89.81-
    head L89.81-

Ulcer - *continued*

    heel L89.6-
    hip L89.2-
    sacral region (tailbone) L89.15-
    specified site NEC L89.89-
    stage 1 (healing) (pre-ulcer skin changes
    limited to persistent focal edema)
      ankle L89.5-
      back L89.1-
      buttock L89.3-
      coccyx L89.15-
      contiguous site of back, buttock, hip L89.4-
      elbow L89.0-
      face L89.81-
      head L89.81-
      heel L89.6-
      hip L89.2-
      sacral region (tailbone) L89.15-
      specified site NEC L89.89-
    stage 2 (healing) (abrasion, blister, partial
    thickness skin loss involving epidermis
    and/or dermis)
      ankle L89.5-
      back L89.1-
      buttock L89.3-
      coccyx L89.15-
      contiguous site of back, buttock, hip L89.4-
      elbow L89.0-
      face L89.81-
      head L89.81-
      heel L89.6-
      hip L89.2-
      sacral region (tailbone) L89.15-
      specified site NEC L89.89-
    stage 3 (healing) (full thickness skin loss
    involving damage or necrosis of
    subcutaneous tissue)
      ankle L89.5-
      back L89.1-
      buttock L89.3-
      coccyx L89.15-
      contiguous site of back, buttock, hip L89.4-
      elbow L89.0-
      face L89.81-
      head L89.81-
      heel L89.6-
      hip L89.2-
      sacral region (tailbone) L89.15-
      specified site NEC L89.89-
    stage 4 (healing) (necrosis of soft tissues
    through to underlying muscle, tendon, or
    bone)
      ankle L89.5-
      back L89.1-
      buttock L89.3-
      coccyx L89.15-
      contiguous site of back, buttock, hip L89.4-
      elbow L89.0-
      face L89.81-
      head L89.81-
      heel L89.6-
      hip L89.2-
      sacral region (tailbone) L89.15-
      specified site NEC L89.89-
    unspecified stage
      ankle L89.5-
      back L89.1-
      buttock L89.3-
      coccyx L89.15-
      contiguous site of back, buttock, hip L89.4-
      elbow L89.0-
      face L89.81-
      head L89.81-
      heel L89.6-

Ulcer - *continued*
  hip L89.2-
    sacral region (tailbone) L89.15-
    specified site NEC L89.89-
  unstageable
    ankle L89.5-
    back L89.1-
    buttock L89.3-
    coccyx L89.15-
    contiguous site of back, buttock, hip L89.4-
    elbow L89.0-
    face L89.81-
    head L89.81-
    heel L89.6-
    hip L89.2-
    sacral region (tailbone) L89.15-
    specified site NEC L89.89-
  primary of intestine K63.3
    with perforation K63.1
  prostate N41.9
  pyloric - *see* Ulcer, stomach
  rectosigmoid K63.3
    with perforation K63.1
  rectum (sphincter) (solitary) K62.6
    stercoraceous, stercoral K62.6
  retina - *see* Inflammation, chorioretinal
  rodent - *see also* Neoplasm, skin, malignant
  sclera - *see* Scleritis
  scrofulous (tuberculous) A18.2
  scrotum N50.89
    tuberculous A18.15
    varicose I86.1
  seminal vesicle N50.89
  sigmoid - *see* Ulcer, intestine
  skin (atrophic) (chronic) (neurogenic) (non-
    healing) (perforating) (pyogenic) (trophic)
    (tropical) L98.499
    with gangrene - *see* Gangrene
    amebic A06.7
    back - *see* Ulcer, back
    buttock - *see* Ulcer, buttock
    decubitus - *see* Ulcer, pressure
    lower limb - *see* Ulcer, lower limb
    mycobacterial A31.1
    specified site NEC L98.499
      with
        bone involvement without evidence of
          necrosis L98.496
        bone necrosis L98.494
        exposed fat layer L98.492
        muscle involvement without evidence of
          necrosis L98.495
        muscle necrosis L98.493
        skin breakdown only L98.491
        specified severity NEC L98.498
    tuberculous (primary) A18.4
    varicose - *see* Ulcer, varicose
  sloughing - *see* Ulcer, skin
  solitary, anus or rectum (sphincter) K62.6
  sore throat J02.9
    streptococcal J02.0
  spermatic cord N50.89
  spine (tuberculous) A18.01
  stasis (venous) - *see* Varix, leg, with, ulcer
    without varicose veins I87.2
  stercoraceous, stercoral K63.3
    with perforation K63.1
    anus or rectum K62.6
  stoma, stomal - *see* Ulcer, gastrojejunal
  stomach (eroded) (peptic) (round) K25.9
    with
      hemorrhage K25.4
        and perforation K25.6
      perforation K25.5

Ulcer - *continued*
  acute K25.3
    with
      hemorrhage K25.0
        and perforation K25.2
      perforation K25.1
  chronic K25.7
    with
      hemorrhage K25.4
        and perforation K25.6
      perforation K25.5
  stomal - *see* Ulcer, gastrojejunal
  stomatitis K12.1
  stress - *see* Ulcer, peptic
  strumous (tuberculous) A18.2
  submucosal, bladder - *see* Cystitis, interstitial
  syphilitic (any site) (early) (secondary) A51.39
    late A52.79
      perforating A52.79
      foot A52.11
  testis N50.89
  thigh - *see* Ulcer, lower limb
  throat J39.2
    diphtheritic A36.0
  toe - *see* Ulcer, lower limb
  tongue (traumatic) K14.0
  tonsil J35.8
    diphtheritic A36.0
  trachea J39.8
  trophic - *see* Ulcer, skin
  tropical - *see* Ulcer, skin
  tuberculous - *see* Tuberculosis, ulcer
  tunica vaginalis N50.89
  turbinate J34.89
  typhoid (perforating) - *see* Typhoid
  unspecified site - *see* Ulcer, skin
  urethra (meatus) - *see* Urethritis
  uterus N85.8
    cervix N86
      with cervicitis N72
    neck N86
      with cervicitis N72
  vagina N76.5
    in Behçet's disease M35.2 [N77.0]
    pessary N89.8
  valve, heart I33.0
  varicose (lower limb, any part) - *see also*
    Varix, leg, with, ulcer
    broad ligament I86.2
    esophagus - *see* Varix, esophagus
    inflamed or infected - *see* Varix, leg, with
      ulcer, with inflammation
    nasal septum I86.8
    perineum I86.3
    scrotum I86.1
    specified site NEC I86.8
    sublingual I86.0
    vulva I86.3
  vas deferens N50.89
  vulva (acute) (infectional) N76.6
    in (due to)
      Behçet's disease M35.2 [N77.0]
      herpesviral (herpes simplex) infection
        A60.04
      tuberculosis A18.18
    vulvobuccal, recurring N76.6
    X-ray L58.1
    yaws A66.4
Ulcerosa scarlatina A38.8
Ulcus - *see also* Ulcer
  cutis tuberculosum A18.4
  duodeni - *see* Ulcer, duodenum
  durum (syphilitic) A51.0
    extragenital A51.2

Ulcus - *continued*
  gastrojejunale - *see* Ulcer, gastrojejunal
  hypostaticum - *see* Ulcer, varicose
  molle (cutis) (skin) A57
  serpens corneae - *see* Ulcer, cornea, central
  ventriculi - *see* Ulcer, stomach
Ulegyria Q04.8
Ulerythema
  ophryogenes, congenital Q84.2
  sycosiforme L73.8
Ullrich (-bonnevie)(-turner) syndrome - *see
  also* Turner's syndrome Q87.1
Ullrich-feichtiger syndrome Q87.0
Ulnar - *see* condition
Ulorrhagia, ulorrhea K06.8
Umbilicus, umbilical - *see* condition
Unacceptable
  contours of tooth K08.54
  morphology of tooth K08.54
Unavailability (of)
  bed at medical facility Z75.1
  health service-related agencies Z75.4
  medical facilities (at) Z75.3
    due to
      investigation by social service agency
        Z75.2
      lack of services at home Z75.0
      remoteness from facility Z75.3
      waiting list Z75.1
    home Z75.0
    outpatient clinic Z75.3
  schooling Z55.1
  social service agencies Z75.4
Uncinaria americana infestation B76.1
Uncinariasis B76.9
Uncongenial work Z56.5
Unconscious (ness) - *see* Coma
Under observation - *see* Observation
Underachievement in school Z55.3
Underdevelopment - *see also* Undeveloped
  nose Q30.1
  sexual E30.0
Underdosing - *see also* Table of Drugs and
  Chemicals, categories T36-t50, with final
  character 6 Z91.14
  intentional NEC Z91.128
    due to financial hardship of patient Z91.120
  unintentional NEC Z91.138
    due to patient's age related debility Z91.130
Underfeeding, newborn P92.3
Underfill, endodontic M27.53
Underimmunization status Z28.3
Undernourishment - *see* Malnutrition
Undernutrition - *see* Malnutrition
Underweight R63.6
  for gestational age - *see* Light for dates
Underwood's disease P83.0
Undescended - *see also* Malposition, congenital
  cecum Q43.3
  colon Q43.3
  testicle - *see* Cryptorchid
Undeveloped, undevelopment - *see also*
  Hypoplasia
  brain (congenital) Q02
  cerebral (congenital) Q02
  heart Q24.8
  lung Q33.6
  testis E29.1
  uterus E30.0
Undiagnosed (disease) R69
Undulant fever - *see* Brucellosis
Unemployment, anxiety concerning Z56.0
  threatened Z56.2

Unequal length (acquired) (limb) - *see also*
  Deformity, limb, unequal length
  leg - *see also* Deformity, limb, unequal length
    congenital Q72.9-
Unextracted dental root K08.3
Unguis incarnatus L60.0
Unhappiness R45.2
Unicornate uterus Q51.4
  in pregnancy or childbirth O34.00
Unilateral - *see also* condition
  development, breast N64.89
  organ or site, congenital NEC - *see* Agenesis,
    by site
Unilocular heart Q20.8
Union, abnormal - *see also* Fusion
  larynx and trachea Q34.8
Universal mesentery Q43.3
Unrepairable overhanging of dental
  restorative materials K08.52
Unsatisfactory
  restoration of tooth K08.50
    specified NEC K08.59
  sample of cytologic smear
    anus R85.615
    cervix R87.615
    vagina R87.625
  surroundings Z59.1
  work Z56.5
Unsoundness of mind - *see* Psychosis
Unstable
  back NEC - *see* Instability, joint, spine
  hip (congenital) Q65.6
    acquired - *see* Derangement, joint, specified
      type NEC, hip
  joint - *see* Instability, joint
    secondary to removal of joint prosthesis
      M96.89
  lie (mother) O32.0
  lumbosacral joint (congenital)
    acquired - *see* subcategory M53.2
  sacroiliac - *see* subcategory M53.2
  spine NEC - *see* Instability, joint, spine
Unsteadiness on feet R26.81
Untruthfulness, child problem F91.8
Unverricht (-lundborg) disease or epilepsy -
  see Epilepsy, generalized, idiopathic
Unwanted pregnancy Z64.0
Upbringing, institutional Z62.22
  away from parents NEC Z62.29
  in care of non-parental family member Z62.21
  in foster care Z62.21
  in orphanage or group home Z62.22
  in welfare custody Z62.21
Upper respiratory - *see* condition
Upset
  gastric K30
  gastrointestinal K30
    psychogenic F45.8
  intestinal (large) (small) K59.9
    psychogenic F45.8
  menstruation N93.9
  mental F48.9
  stomach K30
    psychogenic F45.8
Urachus - *see also* condition
  patent or persistent Q64.4
Urbach-oppenheim disease (necrobiosis
  lipoidica diabeticorum) - *see* E08-e13 with
  .620
Urbach's lipoid proteinosis E78.89
Urbach-Wiethe disease E78.89
Urban yellow fever A95.1
Urea
  blood, high - *see* Uremia

Urea - *continued*
  cycle metabolism disorder - *see* Disorder, urea
  cycle metabolism
Uremia, uremic N19
  with
    ectopic or molar pregnancy O08.4
    polyneuropathy N18.9 *[G63]*
    chronic NOS (see also Disease, kidney,
      chronic) N18.9
      due to hypertension   *see* Hypertensive,
        kidney
    ectopic or molar pregnancy O08.4
  congenital P96.0
  extrarenal R39.2
  following ectopic or molar pregnancy O08.4
  newborn P96.0
  prerenal R39.2
Ureter, ureteral - *see* condition
Ureteralgia N23
Ureterectasis - *see* Hydroureter
Ureteritis N28.89
  cystica N28.86
  due to calculus N20.1
    with calculus, kidney N20.2
      with hydronephrosis N13.2
  gonococcal (acute) (chronic) A54.21
  nonspecific N28.89
Ureterocele N28.89
  congenital (orthotopic) Q62.31
  ectopic Q62.32
Ureterolith, ureterolithiasis - *see* Calculus,
  ureter
Ureterostomy
  attention to Z43.6
  status Z93.6
Urethra, urethral - *see* condition
Urethralgia R39.89
Urethritis (anterior) (posterior) N34.2
  calculous N21.1
  candidal B37.41
  chlamydial A56.01
  diplococcal (gonococcal) A54.01
    with abscess (accessory gland) (periurethral)
      A54.1
  gonococcal A54.01
    with abscess (accessory gland) (periurethral)
      A54.1
  nongonococcal N34.1
    Reiter's - *see* Reiter's disease
  nonspecific N34.1
  nonvenereal N34.1
  postmenopausal N34.2
  puerperal O86.22
  Reiter's - *see* Reiter's disease
  specified NEC N34.2
  trichomonal or due to Trichomonas (vaginalis)
    A59.03
Urethrocele N81.0
  with
    cystocele - *see* Cystocele
    prolapse of uterus - *see* Prolapse, uterus
Urethrolithiasis (with colic or infection)
  N21.1
Urethrorectal - *see* condition
Urethrorrhagia N36.8
Urethrorrhea R36.9
Urethrostomy
  attention to Z43.6
  status Z93.6
Urethrotrigonitis - *see* Trigonitis
Urethrovaginal - *see* condition
Urgency
  fecal R15.2
  hypertensive - *see* Hypertension
  urinary R39.15

Urhidrosis, uridrosis L74.8
Uric acid in blood (increased) E79.0
Uricacidemia (asymptomatic) E79.0
Uricemia (asymptomatic) E79.0
Uricosuria R82.99
Urinary - *see* condition
Urination
  frequent R35.0
  painful R30.9
Urine
  blood in - *see* Hematuria
  discharge, excessive R35.8
  enuresis, nonorganic origin F98.0
  extravasation R39.0
  frequency R35.0
  incontinence R32
    nonorganic origin F98.0
  intermittent stream R39.198
  pus in N39.0
  retention or stasis R33.9
    organic R33.8
      drug-induced R33.0
    psychogenic F45.8
  secretion
    deficient R34
    excessive R35.8
    frequency R35.0
  stream
    intermittent R39.198
    slowing R39.198
    splitting R39.13
    weak R39.12
Urinemia - *see* Uremia
Urinoma, urethra N36.8
Uroarthritis, infectious (Reiter's) - *see* Reiter's
  disease
Urodialysis R34
Urolithiasis - *see* Calculus, urinary
Uronephrosis - *see* Hydronephrosis
Uropathy N39.9
  obstructive N13.9
    specified NEC N13.8
  reflux N13.9
    specified NEC N13.8
  vesicoureteral reflux-associated - *see* Reflux,
  vesicoureteral
Urosepsis   code to condition
Urticaria L50.9
  with angioneurotic edema T78.3
    hereditary D84.1
  allergic L50.0
  cholinergic L50.5
  chronic L50.8
  cold, familial L50.2
  contact L50.6
  dermatographic L50.3
  due to
    cold or heat L50.2
    drugs L50.0
    food L50.0
    inhalants L50.0
    plants L50.6
    serum - *see also* Reaction, serum T80.69
  factitial L50.3
  familial cold M04.2
  giant T78.3
    hereditary D84.1
  gigantea T78.3
  idiopathic L50.1
  larynx T78.3
    hereditary D84.1
  neonatorum P83.88
  nonallergic L50.1
  papulosa (Hebra) L28.2

Urticaria - *continued*
- pigmentosa D47.01
   congenital Q82.2
   of neonatal onset Q82.2
   of newborn onset Q82.2
 recurrent periodic L50.8
 serum - *see also* Reaction, serum T80.69
 solar L56.3
 specified type NEC L50.8
 thermal (cold) (heat) L50.2
 vibratory L50.4
 xanthelasmoidea *see* Urticaria pigmentosa
Use (of)
 alcohol Z72.89
  with
   intoxication F10.929
   sleep disorder F10.982
  harmful - *see* Abuse, alcohol
 amphetamines - *see* Use, stimulant NEC
 caffeine - *see* Use, stimulant NEC
 cannabis F12.90
  with
   anxiety disorder F12.980
   intoxication F12.929
    with
     delirium F12.921
     perceptual disturbance F12.922
    uncomplicated F12.920
   other specified disorder F12.988
   psychosis F12.959
    delusions F12.950
    hallucinations F12.951
   unspecified disorder F12.99
 cocaine F14.90
  with
   anxiety disorder F14.980
   intoxication F14.929
    with
     delirium F14.921
     perceptual disturbance F14.922
    uncomplicated F14.920
   other specified disorder F14.988
   psychosis F14.959
    delusions F14.950
    hallucinations F14.951
   sexual dysfunction F14.981
   sleep disorder F14.982
   unspecified disorder F14.99
  harmful - *see* Abuse, drug, cocaine
 drug(s) NEC F19.90
  with sleep disorder F19.982
  harmful - *see* Abuse, drug, by type
 hallucinogen NEC F16.90
  with
   anxiety disorder F16.980
   intoxication F16.929
    with
     delirium F16.921
    uncomplicated F16.920
   mood disorder F16.94
   other specified disorder F16.988
   perception disorder (flashbacks) F16.983
   psychosis F16.959
    delusions F16.950
    hallucinations F16.951
   unspecified disorder F16.99
  harmful - *see* Abuse, drug, hallucinogen NEC
 inhalants F18.90
  with
   anxiety disorder F18.980
   intoxication F18.929
    with delirium F18.921
    uncomplicated F18.920
   mood disorder F18.94

Use (of) - *continued*
   other specified disorder F18.988
   persisting dementia F18.97
   psychosis F18.959
    delusions F18.950
    hallucinations F18.951
   unspecified disorder F18.99
  harmful - *see* Abuse, drug, inhalant
 methadone - *see* Use, opioid
 nonprescribed drugs F19.90
  harmful - *see* Abuse, non-psychoactive
 substance
 opioid F11.90
  with
   disorder F11.99
    mood F11.94
    sleep F11.982
    specified type NEC F11.988
   intoxication F11.929
    with
     delirium F11.921
     perceptual disturbance F11.922
    uncomplicated F11.920
   withdrawal F11.93
  harmful - *see* Abuse, drug, opioid
 patent medicines F19.90
  harmful - *see* Abuse, non-psychoactive
 substance
 psychoactive drug NEC F19.90
  with
   anxiety disorder F19.980
   intoxication F19.929
    with
     delirium F19.921
     perceptual disturbance F19.922
    uncomplicated F19.920
   mood disorder F19.94
   other specified disorder F19.988
   persisting
    amnestic disorder F19.96
    dementia F19.97
   psychosis F19.959
    delusions F19.950
    hallucinations F19.951
   sexual dysfunction F19.981
   sleep disorder F19.982
   unspecified disorder F19.99
   withdrawal F19.939
    with
     delirium F19.931
     perceptual disturbance F19.932
    uncomplicated F19.930
  harmful - *see* Abuse, drug NEC,
 psychoactive NEC
 sedative, hypnotic, or anxiolytic F13.90
  with
   anxiety disorder F13.980
   intoxication F13.929
    with
     delirium F13.921
    uncomplicated F13.920
   other specified disorder F13.988
   persisting
    amnestic disorder F13.96
    dementia F13.97
   psychosis F13.959
    delusions F13.950
    hallucinations F13.951
   sexual dysfunction F13.981
   sleep disorder F13.982
   unspecified disorder F13.99
  harmful - *see* Abuse, drug, sedative,
 hypnotic, or anxiolytic
 stimulant NEC F15.90

Use (of) - *continued*
  with
   anxiety disorder F15.980
   intoxication F15.929
    with
     delirium F15.921
     perceptual disturbance F15.922
    uncomplicated F15.920
   mood disorder F15.94
   other specified disorder F15.988
   psychosis F15.959
    delusions F15.950
    hallucinations F15.951
   sexual dysfunction F15.981
   sleep disorder F15.982
   unspecified disorder F15.99
   withdrawal F15.93
  harmful - *see* Abuse, drug, stimulant NEC
 tobacco Z72.0
  with dependence - *see* Dependence, drug,
 nicotine
 volatile solvents - *see also* Use, inhalant
 F18.90
  harmful - *see* Abuse, drug, inhalant
Usher-senear disease or syndrome L10.4
Uta B55.1
Uteromegaly N85.2
Uterovaginal - *see* condition
Uterovesical - *see* condition
Uveal - *see* condition
Uveitis (anterior) - *see also* Iridocyclitis
 acute - *see* Iridocyclitis, acute
 chronic - *see* Iridocyclitis, chronic
 due to toxoplasmosis (acquired) B58.09
  congenital P37.1
 granulomatous - *see* Iridocyclitis, chronic
 heterochromic - *see* Cyclitis, Fuchs'
 heterochromic
 lens-induced - *see* Iridocyclitis, lens-induced
 posterior - *see* Chorioretinitis
 sympathetic H44.13-
 syphilitic (secondary) A51.43
  congenital (early) A50.01
  late A52.71
 tuberculous A18.54
Uveoencephalitis - *see* Inflammation,
 chorioretinal
Uveokeratitis - *see* Iridocyclitis
Uveoparotitis D86.89
Uvula - *see* condition
**Uvulitis (acute) (catarrhal) (chronic)
 (membranous) (suppurative) (ulcerative)**
 K12.2

V

Vaccination (prophylactic)
 complication or reaction - *see* Complications,
  vaccination
 delayed Z28.9
 encounter for Z23
 not done - *see* Immunization, not done,
 because (of)
Vaccinia (generalized) (localized) T88.1
 congenital P35.8
 without vaccination B08.011
Vacuum, in sinus (accessory) (nasal) J34.89
Vagabond, vagabondage Z59.0
Vagabond's disease B85.1
Vagina, vaginal - *see* condition
Vaginalitis (tunica) (testis) N49.1
Vaginismus (reflex) N94.2
 functional F52.5
 nonorganic F52.5

Vaginismus - *continued*
　psychogenic F52.5
　secondary N94.2
Vaginitis (acute) (circumscribed) (diffuse) (emphysematous) (nonvenereal) (ulcerative) N76.0
　with ectopic or molar pregnancy O08.0
　amebic A06.82
　atrophic, postmenopausal N95.2
　bacterial N76.0
　blennorrhagic (gonococcal) A54.02
　candidal B37.3
　chlamydial A56.02
　chronic N76.1
　due to Trichomonas (vaginalis) A59.01
　following ectopic or molar pregnancy O08.0
　gonococcal A54.02
　　with abscess (accessory gland) (periurethral) A54.1
　granuloma A58
　in (due to)
　　candidiasis B37.3
　　herpesviral (herpes simplex) infection A60.04
　　pinworm infection B80 [*N77.1*]
　monilial B37.3
　mycotic (candidal) B37.3
　postmenopausal atrophic N95.2
　puerperal (postpartum) O86.13
　senile (atrophic) N95.2
　subacute or chronic N76.1
　syphilitic (early) A51.0
　　late A52.76
　trichomonal A59.01
　tuberculous A18.18
Vaginosis - *see* Vaginitis
Vagotonia G52.2
Vagrancy Z59.0
VAIN - *see* Neoplasia, intraepithelial, vagina
Vallecula - *see* condition
Valley fever B38.0
Valsuani's disease - *see* Anemia, obstetric
Valve, valvular (formation) - *see also* condition
　cerebral ventricle (communicating) in situ Z98.2
　cervix, internal os Q51.828
　congenital NEC - *see* Atresia, by site
　ureter (pelvic junction) (vesical orifice) Q62.39
　urethra (congenital) (posterior) Q64.2
Valvulitis (chronic) - *see* Endocarditis
Valvulopathy - *see* Endocarditis
Van Bogaert's leukoencephalopathy (sclerosing) (subacute) A81.1
Van Bogaert-scherer-epstein disease or syndrome E75.5
Van Buchem's syndrome M85.2
Van Creveld-von Gierke disease E74.01
Van der Hoeve (-de Kleyn) syndrome Q78.0
Van der Woude's syndrome Q38.0
Van Neck's disease or osteochondrosis M91.0
Vanishing lung J44.9
Vapor asphyxia or suffocation T59.9
　specified agent - *see* Table of Drugs and Chemicals
Variance, lethal ball, prosthetic heart valve T82.09
Variants, thalassemic D56.8
Variations in hair color L67.1
Varicella B01.9
　with
　　complications NEC B01.89
　　encephalitis B01.11

Varicella - *continued*
　　encephalomyelitis B01.11
　　meningitis B01.0
　　myelitis B01.12
　　pneumonia B01.2
　　congenital P35.8
Varices - *see* Varix
Varicocele (scrotum) (thrombosed) I86.1
　ovary I86.2
　perineum I86.3
　spermatic cord (ulcerated) I86.1
Varicose
　aneurysm (ruptured) I77.0
　dermatitis - *see* Varix, leg, with, inflammation
　eczema - *see* Varix, leg, with, inflammation
　phlebitis - *see* Varix, with, inflammation
　tumor - *see* Varix
　ulcer (lower limb, any part) - *see also* Varix, leg, with, ulcer
　　anus - *see also* Hemorrhoids K64.8
　　esophagus - *see* Varix, esophagus
　　inflamed or infected - *see* Varix, leg, with ulcer, with inflammation
　　nasal septum I86.8
　　perineum I86.3
　　scrotum I86.1
　　specified site NEC I86.8
　vein - *see* Varix
　vessel - *see* Varix, leg
Varicosis, varicosities, varicosity - *see* Varix
Variola (major) (minor) B03
Varioloid B03
Varix (lower limb) (ruptured) I83.90
　with
　　edema I83.899
　　inflammation I83.10
　　　with ulcer (venous) I83.209
　　pain I83.819
　　specified complication NEC I83.899
　　stasis dermatitis I83.10
　　　with ulcer (venous) I83.209
　　swelling I83.899
　　ulcer I83.009
　　　with inflammation I83.209
　aneurysmal I77.0
　asymptomatic I83.9-
　bladder I86.2
　broad ligament I86.2
　complicating
　　childbirth (lower extremity) O87.4
　　　anus or rectum O87.2
　　　genital (vagina, vulva or perineum) O87.8
　　pregnancy (lower extremity) O22.0-
　　　anus or rectum O22.4-
　　　genital (vagina, vulva or perineum) O22.1-
　　puerperium (lower extremity) O87.4
　　　anus or rectum O87.2
　　　genital (vagina, vulva, perineum) O87.8
　congenital (any site) Q27.8
　esophagus (idiopathic) (primary) (ulcerated) I85.00
　　bleeding I85.01
　　congenital Q27.8
　　in (due to)
　　　alcoholic liver disease I85.10
　　　　bleeding I85.11
　　　cirrhosis of liver I85.10
　　　　bleeding I85.11
　　　portal hypertension I85.10
　　　　bleeding I85.11
　　　schistosomiasis I85.10
　　　　bleeding I85.11
　　　toxic liver disease I85.10
　　　　bleeding I85.11

Varix - *continued*
　　secondary I85.10
　　　bleeding I85.11
　gastric I86.4
　inflamed or infected I83.10
　　ulcerated I83.209
　labia (majora) I86.3
　leg (asymptomatic) I83.90
　　with
　　　edema I83.899
　　　inflammation I83.10
　　　　with ulcer - *see* Varix, leg, with, ulcer, with inflammation by site
　　　pain I83.819
　　　specified complication NEC I83.899
　　　swelling I83.899
　　　ulcer I83.009
　　　　with inflammation I83.209
　　　　ankle I83.003
　　　　　with inflammation I83.203
　　　　calf I83.002
　　　　　with inflammation I83.202
　　　　foot NEC I83.005
　　　　　with inflammation I83.205
　　　　heel I83.004
　　　　　with inflammation I83.204
　　　　lower leg NEC I83.008
　　　　　with inflammation I83.208
　　　　midfoot I83.004
　　　　　with inflammation I83.204
　　　　thigh I83.001
　　　　　with inflammation I83.201
　bilateral (asymptomatic) I83.93
　　with
　　　edema I83.893
　　　pain I83.813
　　　specified complication NEC I83.893
　　　swelling I83.893
　　　ulcer I83.0-
　　　　with inflammation I83.209
　left (asymptomatic) I83.92
　　with
　　　edema I83.892
　　　pain I83.812
　　　specified complication NEC I83.892
　　　swelling I83.892
　　　inflammation I83.12
　　　　with ulcer - *see* Varix, leg, with, ulcer, with inflammation by site
　　　ulcer I83.029
　　　　with inflammation I83.229
　　　　ankle I83.023
　　　　　with inflammation I83.223
　　　　calf I83.022
　　　　　with inflammation I83.222
　　　　foot NEC I83.025
　　　　　with inflammation I83.225
　　　　heel I83.024
　　　　　with inflammation I83.224
　　　　lower leg NEC I83.028
　　　　　with inflammation I83.228
　　　　midfoot I83.024
　　　　　with inflammation I83.224
　　　　thigh I83.021
　　　　　with inflammation I83.221
　right (asymptomatic) I83.91
　　with
　　　edema I83.891
　　　pain I83.811
　　　specified complication NEC I83.891
　　　swelling I83.891
　　　inflammation I83.11
　　　　with ulcer - *see* Varix, leg, with, ulcer, with inflammation by site

Varix - *continued*
  ulcer I83.019
    with inflammation I83.219
    ankle I83.013
      with inflammation I83.213
    calf I83.012
      with inflammation I83.212
    foot NEC I83.015
      with inflammation I83.215
    heel I83.014
      with inflammation I83.214
    lower leg NEC I83.018
      with inflammation I83.218
    midfoot I83.014
      with inflammation I83.214
    thigh I83.011
      with inflammation I83.211
  nasal septum I86.8
  orbit I86.8
   congenital Q27.8
  ovary I86.2
  papillary I78.1
  pelvis I86.2
  perineum I86.3
  pharynx I86.8
  placenta O43.89-
  renal papilla I86.8
  retina H35.09
  scrotum (ulcerated) I86.1
  sigmoid colon I86.8
  specified site NEC I86.8
  spinal (cord) (vessels) I86.8
  spleen, splenic (vein) (with phlebolith) I86.8
  stomach I86.4
  sublingual I86.0
  ulcerated I83.009
   inflamed or infected I83.209
  uterine ligament I86.2
  vagina I86.8
  vocal cord I86.8
  vulva I86.3
Vas deferens - *see* condition
Vas deferentitis N49.1
Vasa previa O69.4
  hemorrhage from, affecting newborn P50.0
Vascular - *see also* condition
  loop on optic papilla Q14.2
  spasm I73.9
  spider I78.1
Vascularization, cornea - *see*
  Neovascularization, cornea
Vasculitis I77.6
  allergic D69.0
  cryoglobulinemic D89.1
  disseminated I77.6
  hypocomplementemic M31.8
  kidney I77.89
  livedoid L95.0
  nodular L95.8
  retina H35.06-
  rheumatic - *see* Fever, rheumatic
  rheumatoid - *see* Rheumatoid, vasculitis
  skin (limited to) L95.9
   specified NEC L95.8
  systemic M31.8
Vasculopathy, necrotizing M31.9
  cardiac allograft T86.290
  specified NEC M31.8
Vasitis (nodosa) N49.1
  tuberculous A18.15
Vasodilation I73.9
Vasomotor - *see* condition
Vasoplasty, after previous sterilization Z31.0
  aftercare Z31.42

Vasospasm (vasoconstriction) I73.9
  cerebral (cerebrovascular) (artery) I67.848
   reversible I67.841
  coronary I20.1
  nerve
   arm - *see* Mononeuropathy, upper limb
   brachial plexus G54.0
   cervical plexus G54.2
   leg - *see* Mononeuropathy, lower limb
  peripheral NOS I73.9
  retina (artery) - *see* Occlusion, artery, retina
Vasospastic - *see* condition
Vasovagal attack (paroxysmal) R55
  psychogenic F45.8
VATER syndrome Q87.2
Vater's ampulla - *see* condition
Vegetation, vegetative
  adenoid (nasal fossa) J35.8
  endocarditis (acute) (any valve) (subacute)
   I33.0
  heart (mycotic) (valve) I33.0
Veil
  Jackson's Q43.3
Vein, venous - *see* condition
Veldt sore - *see* Ulcer, skin
Velpeau's hernia - *see* Hernia, femoral
Venereal
  bubo A55
  disease A64
  granuloma inguinale A58
  lymphogranuloma (Durand Nicolas-favre)
   A55
Venofibrosis I87.8
Venom, venomous - *see* Table of Drugs and
  Chemicals, by animal or substance, poisoning
Venous - *see* condition
Ventilator lung, newborn P27.8
Ventral - *see* condition
Ventricle, ventricular - *see also* condition
  escape I49.3
  inversion Q20.5
Ventriculitis (cerebral) - *see also* Encephalitis
  G04.90
Ventriculostomy status Z98.2
Vernet's syndrome G52.7
Verneuil's disease (syphilitic bursitis) A52.78
Verruca (due to HPV) (filiformis) (simplex)
(viral) (vulgaris) B07.9
  acuminata A63.0
  necrogenica (primary) (tuberculosa) A18.4
  plana B07.8
  plantaris B07.0
  seborrheica L82.1
   inflamed L82.0
  senile (seborrheic) L82.1
   inflamed L82.0
  tuberculosa (primary) A18.4
  venereal A63.0
Verrucosities - *see* Verruca
Verruga peruana, peruviana A44.1
Version
  with extraction
  cervix - *see* Malposition, uterus
  uterus (postinfectional) (postpartal, old) - *see*
   Malposition, uterus
Vertebra, vertebral - *see* condition
Vertical talus (congenital) Q66.80
  left foot Q66.82
  right foot Q66.81
Vertigo R42
  auditory - *see* Vertigo, aural
  aural H81.31-
  benign paroxysmal (positional) H81.1-
  central (origin) H81.4-

Vertigo - *continued*
  cerebral H81.4-
  Dix and Hallpike (epidemic) - *see* Neuronitis,
   vestibular
  due to infrasound T75.23
  epidemic A88.1
   Dix and Hallpike - *see* Neuronitis, vestibular
   Pedersen's - *see* Neuronitis, vestibular
   vestibular neuronitis - *see* Neuronitis,
    vestibular
  hysterical F44.89
  infrasound T75.23
  labyrinthine   *see* subcategory H81.0
  laryngeal R05
  malignant positional H81.4-
  Ménière's - *see* subcategory H81.0
  menopausal N95.1
  otogenic - *see* Vertigo, aural
  paroxysmal positional, benign - *see* Vertigo,
   benign paroxysmal
  Pedersen's (epidemic) - *see* Neuronitis,
   vestibular
  peripheral NEC H81.39-
  positional
   benign paroxysmal - *see* Vertigo, benign
   paroxysmal
   malignant H81.4-
Very-low-density-lipoprotein-type (VLDL)
hyperlipoproteinemia E78.1
Vesania - *see* Psychosis
Vesical - *see* condition
Vesicle
  cutaneous R23.8
  seminal - *see* condition
  skin R23.8
Vesicocolic - *see* condition
Vesicoperineal - *see* condition
Vesicorectal - *see* condition
Vesicourethrorectal - *see* condition
Vesicovaginal - *see* condition
Vesicular - *see* condition
Vesiculitis (seminal) N49.0
  amebic A06.82
  gonorrheal (acute) (chronic) A54.23
  trichomonal A59.09
  tuberculous A18.15
Vestibulitis (ear) - *see also* subcategory H83.0
  nose (external) J34.89
  vulvar N94.810
Vestibulopathy , acute peripheral (recurrent)
  - *see* Neuronitis, vestibular
Vestige, vestigial - *see also* Persistence
  branchial Q18.0
  structures in vitreous Q14.0
Vibration
  adverse effects T75.20
   pneumatic hammer syndrome T75.21
   specified effect NEC T75.29
   vasospastic syndrome T75.22
   vertigo from infrasound T75.23
  exposure (occupational) Z57.7
  vertigo T75.23
Vibriosis A28.9
Victim (of)
  crime Z65.4
  disaster Z65.5
  terrorism Z65.4
  torture Z65.4
  war Z65.5
Vidal's disease L28.0
Villaret's syndrome G52.7
Villous - *see* condition
VIN - *see* Neoplasia, intraepithelial, vulva

Vincent's infection (angina) (gingivitis) A69.1
  stomatitis NEC A69.1
Vinson-plummer syndrome D50.1
Violence, physical R45.6
Viosterol deficiency - *see* Deficiency, calciferol
Vipoma - *see* Neoplasm, malignant, by site
Viremia B34.9
Virilism (adrenal) E25.9
  congenital E25.0
Virilization (female) (suprarenal) E25.9
  congenital E25.0
  isosexual E28.2
Virulent bubo A57
Virus, viral - *see also* condition
  as cause of disease classified elsewhere
    B97.89
  cytomegalovirus B25.9
  human immunodeficiency (HIV) - *see* Human,
    immunodeficiency virus (HIV) disease
  infection - *see* Infection, virus
  specified NEC B34.8
  swine influenza (viruses that normally cause
    infections in pigs) - *see also* Influenza, due
    to, identified novel influenza A virus J09.X2
  West Nile (fever) A92.30
    with
      complications NEC A92.39
      cranial nerve disorders A92.32
      encephalitis A92.31
      encephalomyelitis A92.31
      neurologic manifestation NEC A92.32
      optic neuritis A92.32
      polyradiculitis A92.32
Viscera, visceral - *see* condition
Visceroptosis K63.4
Visible peristalsis R19.2
Vision, visual
  binocular, suppression H53.34
  blurred, blurring H53.8
    hysterical F44.6
  defect, defective NEC H54.7
  disorientation (syndrome) H53.8
  disturbance H53.9
    hysterical F44.6
  double H53.2
  examination Z01.00
    with abnormal findings Z01.01
  field, limitation (defect) - *see* Defect, visual
    field
  hallucinations R44.1
  halos H53.19
  loss - *see* Loss, vision
    sudden - *see* Disturbance, vision, subjective,
    loss, sudden
  low (both eyes) - *see* Low, vision
  perception, simultaneous without fusion
    H53.33
Vitality, lack or want of R53.83
  newborn P96.89
Vitamin deficiency - *see* Deficiency, vitamin
Vitelline duct, persistent Q43.0
Vitiligo L80
  eyelid H02.739
    left H02.736
      lower H02.735
      upper H02.734
    right H02.733
      lower H02.732
      upper H02.731
  pinta A67.2
  vulva N90.89
Vitreal corneal syndrome H59.01-
Vitreoretinopathy, proliferative - *see also*
  Retinopathy, proliferative

Vitreoretinopathy - *continued*
  with retinal detachment - *see* Detachment,
    retina, traction
Vitreous - *see also* condition
  touch syndrome - *see* Complication,
    postprocedural, following cataract surgery
Vocal cord - *see* condition
Vogt-koyanagi syndrome H20.82-
Vogt's disease or syndrome G80.3
Vogt-spielmeyer amaurotic idiocy or disease
  E75.4
Voice
  change R49.9
    specified NEC R49.8
  loss - *see* Aphonia
Volhynian fever A79.0
Volkmann's ischemic contracture or
  paralysis (complicating trauma) T79.6
Volvulus (bowel) (colon) (intestine) K56.2
  with perforation K56.2
  congenital Q43.8
  duodenum K31.5
  fallopian tube - *see* Torsion, fallopian tube
  oviduct - *see* Torsion, fallopian tube
  stomach (due to absence of gastrocolic
    ligament) K31.89
Vomiting R11.10
  with nausea R11.2
  asphyxia - *see* Foreign body, by site, causing
    asphyxia, gastric contents
  bilious (cause unknown) R11.14
    in newborn P92.01
    following gastro-intestinal surgery K91.0
  blood - *see* Hematemesis
  causing asphyxia, choking, or suffocation - *see*
    Foreign body, by site
  cyclical G43.A0
    with refractory migraine G43.A1
    intractable G43.A1
    not intractable G43.A0
    psychogenic F50.89
    without refractory migraine G43.A0
  fecal mater R11.13
  following gastrointestinal surgery K91.0
    psychogenic F50.89
  functional K31.89
  hysterical F50.89
  nervous F50.89
  neurotic F50.89
  newborn NEC P92.09
    bilious P92.01
  periodic R11.10
    psychogenic F50.89
  projectile R11.12
  psychogenic F50.89
  uremic - *see* Uremia
  without nausea R11.11
Vomito negro - *see* Fever, yellow
Von Bezold's abscess - *see* Mastoiditis, acute
Von Economo-cruchet disease A85.8
Von Eulenburg's disease G71.19
Von Gierke's disease E74.01
Von Hippel (-lindau) disease or syndrome
  Q85.8
Von Jaksch's anemia or disease D64.89
Von Recklinghausen
  disease (neurofibromatosis) Q85.01
    bones E21.0
Von Schroetter's syndrome I82.890
Von Willebrand (-jurgens)(-minot) disease or
  syndrome D68.0
Von Zumbusch's disease L40.1
Voyeurism F65.3
Vrolik's disease Q78.0

Vulva - *see* condition
Vulvismus N94.2
Vulvitis (acute) (allergic) (atrophic)
  (hypertrophic) (intertriginous) (senile)
  N76.2
  with ectopic or molar pregnancy O08.0
  adhesive, congenital Q52.79
  blennorrhagic (gonococcal) A54.02
  candidal B37.3
  chlamydial A56.02
  due to Haemophilus ducreyi A57
  following ectopic or molar pregnancy O08.0
  gonococcal A54.02
    with abscess (accessory gland) (periurethral)
    A54.1
  herpesviral A60.04
  leukoplakic N90.4
  monilial B37.3
  puerperal (postpartum) O86.19
  subacute or chronic N76.3
  syphilitic (early) A51.0
    late A52.76
  trichomonal A59.01
  tuberculous A18.18
Vulvodynia N94.819
  specified NEC N94.818
Vulvorectal - *see* condition
Vulvovaginitis (acute) - *see* Vaginitis

W

Waiting list, person on Z75.1
  for organ transplant Z76.82
  undergoing social agency investigation Z75.2
Waldenström-kjellberg syndrome D50.1
Waldenström
  hypergammaglobulinemia D89.0
  syndrome or macroglobulinemia C88.0
Walking
  difficulty R26.2
    psychogenic F44.4
  sleep F51.3
    hysterical F44.89
Wall, abdominal - *see* condition
Wallenberg's disease or syndrome G46.3
Wallgren's disease I87.8
Wandering
  gallbladder, congenital Q44.1
  in diseases classified elsewhere Z91.83
  kidney, congenital Q63.8
  organ or site, congenital NEC - *see*
    Malposition, congenital, by site
  pacemaker (heart) I49.8
  spleen D73.89
War neurosis F48.8
Wart (due to HPV) (filiform) (infectious)
  (viral) B07.9
  anogenital region (venereal) A63.0
  common B07.8
  external genital organs (venereal) A63.0
  flat B07.8
  Hassal-henle's (of cornea) H18.49
  Peruvian A44.1
  plantar B07.0
  prosector (tuberculous) A18.4
  seborrheic L82.1
    inflamed L82.0
  senile (seborrheic) L82.1
    inflamed L82.0
  tuberculous A18.4
  venereal A63.0
Warthin's tumor - *see* Neoplasm, salivary
  gland, benign
Wassilieff's disease A27.0

WXYZ

Wasting
   disease R64
      due to malnutrition E41
   extreme (due to malnutrition) E41
   muscle NEC - *see* Atrophy, muscle
Water
   clefts (senile cataract) - *see* Cataract, senile,
      incipient
   deprivation of T73.1
   intoxication E87.79
   itch B76.9
   lack of T73.1
   loading E87.70
   on
      brain - *see* Hydrocephalus
      chest J94.8
   poisoning E87.79
Waterbrash R12
Waterhouse (-friderichsen) syndrome or
   disease (meningococcal) A39.1
Water-losing nephritis N25.89
Watermelon stomach K31.819
   with hemorrhage K31.811
   without hemorrhage K31.819
Watsoniasis B66.8
Wax in ear - *see* Impaction, cerumen
Weak, weakening, weakness (generalized)
   R53.1
   arches (acquired) - *see also* Deformity, limb,
      flat foot
   bladder (sphincter) R32
   facial R29.810
      following
         cerebrovascular disease I69.992
            cerebral infarction I69.392
            intracerebral hemorrhage I69.192
            nontraumatic intracranial hemorrhage
               NEC I69.292
            specified disease NEC I69.892
            stroke I69.392
            subarachnoid hemorrhage I69.092
   foot (double) - *see* Weak, arches
   heart, cardiac - *see* Failure, heart
   mind F70
   muscle M62.81
   myocardium - *see* Failure, heart
   newborn P96.89
   pelvic fundus N81.89
   pubocervical tissue N81.82
   senile R54
   rectovaginal tissue N81.83
   urinary stream R39.12
   valvular - *see* Endocarditis
Wear, worn (with normal or routine use)
   articular bearing surface of internal joint
      prosthesis - *see* Complications, joint
      prosthesis, mechanical, wear of articular
      bearing surfaces, by site
   device, implant or graft - *see* Complications,
      by site, mechanical complication
   tooth, teeth (approximal) (hard tissues)
      (interproximal) (occlusal) K03.0
Weather, weathered
   effects of
      cold T69.9
         specified effect NEC T69.8
      hot - *see* Heat
   skin L57.8
Weaver's syndrome Q87.3
Web, webbed (congenital)
   duodenal Q43.8
   esophagus Q39.4
   fingers Q70.1-
   larynx (glottic) (subglottic) Q31.0

Web, webbed - *continued*
   neck (pterygium colli) Q18.3
   Paterson-kelly D50.1
   popliteal syndrome Q87.89
   toes Q70.3-
Weber-christian disease M35.6
Weber-cockayne syndrome (epidermolysis
   bullosa) Q81.8
Weber-gubler syndrome G46.3
Weber-leyden syndrome G46.3
Weber-osler syndrome I78.0
Weber's paralysis or syndrome G46.3
Wedge-shaped or wedging vertebra - *see*
   Collapse, vertebra NEC
Wegener's granulomatosis or syndrome
   M31.30
   with
      kidney involvement M31.31
      lung involvement M31.30
         with kidney involvement M31.31
Wegner's disease A50.02
Weight
   1000-2499 grams at birth (low) - *see* Low,
      birthweight
   999 grams or less at birth (extremely low) - *see*
      Low, birthweight, extreme
   and length below 10th percentile for
      gestational age P05.1-
   below but length above 10th percentile for
      gestational age P05.0-
   gain (abnormal) (excessive) R63.5
      in pregnancy - *see* Pregnancy, complicated
         by, excessive weight gain
      low - *see* Pregnancy, complicated by,
         insufficient, weight gain
   loss (abnormal) (cause unknown) R63.4
Weightlessness (effect of) T75.82
Weil (l) -marchesani syndrome Q87.1
Weil's disease A27.0
Weingarten's syndrome J82
Weir Mitchell's disease I73.81
Weiss-baker syndrome G90.09
Wells' disease L98.3
Wen - *see* Cyst, sebaceous
Wenckebach's block or phenomenon I44.1
Werdnig-hoffmann syndrome (muscular
   atrophy) G12.0
Werlhof's disease D69.3
Wermer's disease or syndrome E31.21
Werner-his disease A79.0
Werner's disease or syndrome E34.8
Wernicke-korsakoff's syndrome or psychosis
   (alcoholic) F10.96
   with dependence F10.26
   drug-induced
      due to drug abuse - *see* Abuse, drug, by type,
         with amnestic disorder
      due to drug dependence - *see* Dependence,
         drug, by type, with amnestic disorder
   nonalcoholic F04
Wernicke-posadas disease B38.9
Wernicke's
   developmental aphasia F80.2
   disease or syndrome E51.2
   encephalopathy E51.2
   polioencephalitis, superior E51.2
West African fever B50.8
Westphal-strümpell syndrome E83.01
West's syndrome - *see* Epilepsy, spasms
Wet
   feet, tropical (maceration) (syndrome) - *see*
      Immersion, foot
   lung (syndrome), newborn P22.1
Wharton's duct - *see* condition

Wheal - *see* Urticaria
Wheezing R06.2
Whiplash injury S13.4
Whipple's disease - *see also* subcategory
   M14.8 K90.81
Whipworm (disease) (infection) (infestation)
   B79
Whistling face Q87.0
White - *see also* condition
   kidney, small N03.9
   leg, puerperal, postpartum, childbirth O87.1
   mouth B37.0
   patches of mouth K13.29
   spot lesions, teeth
      chewing surface K02.51
      pit and fissure surface K02.51
      smooth surface K02.61
Whitehead L70.0
Whitlow - *see also* Cellulitis, digit
   with lymphangitis - *see* Lymphangitis, acute,
      digit
   herpesviral B00.89
Whitmore's disease or fever - *see* Melioidosis
Whooping cough A37.90
   with pneumonia A37.91
      due to Bordetella
         bronchiseptica A37.81
         parapertussis A37.11
         pertussis A37.01
      specified organism NEC A37.81
   due to
      Bordetella
         bronchiseptica A37.80
            with pneumonia A37.81
         parapertussis A37.10
            with pneumonia A37.11
         pertussis A37.00
            with pneumonia A37.01
      specified NEC A37.80
         with pneumonia A37.81
Wichman's asthma J38.5
Wide cranial sutures, newborn P96.3
Widening aorta - *see* Ectasia, aorta
   with aneurysm - *see* Aneurysm, aorta
Wilkie's disease or syndrome K55.1
Wilkinson-sneddon disease or syndrome
   L13.1
Willebrand (-jürgens) thrombopathy D68.0
Willige-hunt disease or syndrome G23.1
Wilms' tumor C64-
Wilson-mikity syndrome P27.0
Wilson's
   disease or syndrome E83.01
   hepatolenticular degeneration E83.01
   lichen ruber L43.9
Window - *see also* Imperfect, closure
   aorticopulmonary Q21.4
Winter - *see* condition
Wiskott-aldrich syndrome D82.0
Withdrawal state - *see also* Dependence, drug
   by type, with withdrawal
   alcohol
      with perceptual disturbances F10.232
      without perceptual disturbances F10.239
   caffeine F15.93
   cannabis F12.288
   newborn
      correct therapeutic substance properly
         administered P96.2
      infant of dependent mother P96.1
   therapeutic substance, neonatal P96.2
Witts' anemia D50.8
Witzelsucht F07.0
Woakes' ethmoiditis or syndrome J33.1

Wolff-Hirschorn syndrome Q93.3
Wolff-Parkinson-White syndrome I45.6
Wolhynian fever A79.0
Wolman's disease E75.5
Wood lung or pneumonitis J67.8
Woolly, wooly hair (congenital) (nevus) Q84.1
Woolsorter's disease A22.1
Word
  blindness (congenital) (developmental) F81.0
  deafness (congenital) (developmental) H93.25
Worm(s) (infection) (infestation) - *see also*
  Infestation, helminth
  guinea B72
  in intestine NEC B82.0
Worm-eaten soles A66.3
Worn out - *see* Exhaustion
  cardiac
    defibrillator (with synchronous cardiac
    pacemaker) Z45.02
    pacemaker
      battery Z45.010
      lead Z45.018
  device, implant or graft - *see* Complications,
  by site, mechanical
Worried well Z71.1
Worries R45.82
Wound check Z48.0-
  due to injury code to Injury, by site, using
    appropriate seventh character for
    subsequent encounter
Wound, open T14.8-
  abdomen, abdominal
    wall S31.109
      with penetration into peritoneal cavity
      S31.609
      bite - *see* Bite, abdomen, wall
      epigastric region S31.102
        with penetration into peritoneal cavity
        S31.602
        bite - *see* Bite, abdomen, wall, epigastric
        region
        laceration - *see* Laceration, abdomen,
        wall, epigastric region
        puncture - *see* Puncture, abdomen, wall,
        epigastric region
      laceration - *see* Laceration, abdomen, wall
      left
        lower quadrant S31.104
          with penetration into peritoneal cavity
          S31.604
          bite - *see* Bite, abdomen, wall, left, lower
          quadrant
          laceration - *see* Laceration, abdomen,
          wall, left, lower quadrant
          puncture - *see* Puncture, abdomen, wall,
          left, lower quadrant
        upper quadrant S31.101
          with penetration into peritoneal cavity
          S31.601
          bite - *see* Bite, abdomen, wall, left, upper
          quadrant
          laceration - *see* Laceration, abdomen,
          wall, left, upper quadrant
          puncture - *see* Puncture, abdomen, wall,
          left, upper quadrant
      periumbilic region S31.105
        with penetration into peritoneal cavity
        S31.605
        bite - *see* Bite, abdomen, wall, periumbilic
        region
        laceration - *see* Laceration, abdomen,
        wall, periumbilic region
        puncture - *see* Puncture, abdomen, wall,
        periumbilic region

Wound, open - *continued*
      puncture - *see* Puncture, abdomen, wall
      right
        lower quadrant S31.103
          with penetration into peritoneal cavity
          S31.603
          bite - *see* Bite, abdomen, wall, right,
          lower quadrant
          laceration - *see* Laceration, abdomen,
          wall, right, lower quadrant
          puncture - *see* Puncture, abdomen, wall,
          right, lower quadrant
        upper quadrant S31.100
          with penetration into peritoneal cavity
          S31.600
          bite - *see* Bite, abdomen, wall, right,
          upper quadrant
          laceration - *see* Laceration, abdomen,
          wall, right, upper quadrant
          puncture - *see* Puncture, abdomen, wall,
          right, upper quadrant
    alveolar (process) - *see* Wound, open, oral
    cavity
    ankle S91.00-
      bite - *see* Bite, ankle
      laceration - *see* Laceration, ankle
      puncture - *see* Puncture, ankle
    antecubital space - *see* Wound, open, elbow
    anterior chamber, eye - *see* Wound, open,
    ocular
    anus S31.839
      bite S31.835
      laceration - *see* Laceration, anus
      puncture - *see* Puncture, anus
    arm (upper) S41.10-
      with amputation - *see* Amputation, traumatic,
      arm
      bite - *see* Bite, arm
      forearm - *see* Wound, open, forearm
      laceration - *see* Laceration, arm
      puncture - *see* Puncture, arm
    auditory canal (external) (meatus) - *see*
    Wound, open, ear
    auricle, ear - *see* Wound, open, ear
    axilla - *see* Wound, open, arm
    back - *see also* Wound, open, thorax, back
      lower S31.000
        with penetration into retroperitoneal space
        S31.001
        bite - *see* Bite, back, lower
        laceration - *see* Laceration, back, lower
        puncture - *see* Puncture, back, lower
    bite - *see* Bite
    blood vessel - *see* Injury, blood vessel
    breast S21.00-
      with amputation - *see* Amputation, traumatic,
      breast
      bite - *see* Bite, breast
      laceration - *see* Laceration, breast
      puncture - *see* Puncture, breast
    buttock S31.809
      bite - *see* Bite, buttock
      laceration - *see* Laceration, buttock
      left S31.829
      puncture - *see* Puncture, buttock
      right S31.819
    calf - *see* Wound, open, leg
    canaliculus lacrimalis - *see* Wound, open,
    eyelid
    canthus, eye - *see* Wound, open, eyelid
    cervical esophagus S11.20
      bite S11.25
      laceration - *see* Laceration, esophagus,
      traumatic, cervical

Wound, open - *continued*
      puncture - *see* Puncture, cervical esophagus
    cheek (external) S01.40-
      bite - *see* Bite, cheek
      laceration - *see* Laceration, cheek
      puncture - *see* Puncture, cheek
      internal - *see* Wound, open, oral cavity
    chest wall - *see* Wound, open, thorax
    chin - *see* Wound, open, head, specified site
    NEC
    choroid - *see* Wound, open, ocular
    ciliary body (eye) - *see* Wound, open, ocular
    clitoris S31.40
      with amputation - *see* Amputation, traumatic,
      clitoris
      bite S31.45
      laceration - *see* Laceration, vulva
      puncture - *see* Puncture, vulva
    conjunctiva - *see* Wound, open, ocular
    cornea - *see* Wound, open, ocular
    costal region - *see* Wound, open, thorax
    Descemet's membrane - *see* Wound, open,
    ocular
    digit(s)
      foot - *see* Wound, open, toe
      hand - *see* Wound, open, finger
    ear (canal) (external) S01.30-
      with amputation - *see* Amputation, traumatic,
      ear
      bite - *see* Bite, ear
      laceration - *see* Laceration, ear
      puncture - *see* Puncture, ear
      drum S09.2-
    elbow S51.00-
      bite - *see* Bite, elbow
      laceration - *see* Laceration, elbow
      puncture - *see* Puncture, elbow
    epididymis - *see* Wound, open, testis
    epigastric region S31.102
      with penetration into peritoneal cavity
      S31.602
      bite - *see* Bite, abdomen, wall, epigastric
      region
      laceration - *see* Laceration, abdomen, wall,
      epigastric region
      puncture - *see* Puncture, abdomen, wall,
    epigastric region
    epiglottis - *see* Wound, open, neck, specified
    site NEC
    esophagus (thoracic) S27.819
      cervical - *see* Wound, open, cervical
      esophagus
      laceration S27.813
      specified type NEC S27.818
    eye - *see* Wound, open, ocular
    eyeball - *see* Wound, open, ocular
    eyebrow - *see* Wound, open, eyelid
    eyelid S01.10-
      bite - *see* Bite, eyelid
      laceration - *see* Laceration, eyelid
      puncture - *see* Puncture, eyelid
    face NEC - *see* Wound, open, head, specified
    site NEC
    finger(s) S61.209
      with
        amputation - *see* Amputation, traumatic,
        finger
        damage to nail S61.309
      bite - *see* Bite, finger
      index S61.208
        with
          damage to nail S61.308
      left S61.201
        with

Wound, open - *continued*
    damage to nail S61.301
    right S61.200
      with
        damage to nail S61.300
    laceration - *see* Laceration, finger
    little S61.208
      with
        damage to nail S61.308
      left S61.207
        with damage to nail S61.307
      right S61.206
        with damage to nail S61.306
    middle S61.208
      with
        damage to nail S61.308
      left S61.203
        with damage to nail S61.303
      right S61.202
        with damage to nail S61.302
    puncture - *see* Puncture, finger
    ring S61.208
      with
        damage to nail S61.308
      left S61.205
        with damage to nail S61.305
      right S61.204
        with damage to nail S61.304
  flank - *see* Wound, open, abdomen, wall
  foot (except toe(s) alone) S91.30-
    with amputation - *see* Amputation, traumatic,
      foot
    bite - *see* Bite, foot
    laceration - *see* Laceration, foot
    puncture - *see* Puncture, foot
    toe - *see* Wound, open, toe
  forearm S51.80-
    with
      amputation - *see* Amputation, traumatic,
      forearm
    bite - *see* Bite, forearm
    elbow only - *see* Wound, open, elbow
    laceration - *see* Laceration, forearm
    puncture - *see* Puncture, forearm
  forehead - *see* Wound, open, head, specified
    site NEC
  genital organs, external
    with amputation - *see* Amputation, traumatic,
      genital organs
    bite - *see* Bite, genital organ
    female S31.502
      vagina S31.40
      vulva S31.40
    laceration - *see* Laceration, genital organ
    male S31.501
      penis S31.20
      scrotum S31.30
      testes S31.30
    puncture - *see* Puncture, genital organ
  globe (eye) - *see* Wound, open, ocular
  groin - *see* Wound, open, abdomen, wall
  gum - *see* Wound, open, oral cavity
  hand S61.40-
    with
      amputation - *see* Amputation, traumatic,
      hand
    bite - *see* Bite, hand
    finger(s) - *see* Wound, open, finger
    laceration - *see* Laceration, hand
    puncture - *see* Puncture, hand
    thumb - *see* Wound, open, thumb
  head S01.90
    bite - *see* Bite, head
    cheek - *see* Wound, open, cheek

Wound, open - *continued*
    ear - *see* Wound, open, ear
    eyelid - *see* Wound, open, eyelid
    laceration - *see* Laceration, head
    lip - *see* Wound, open, lip
    nose S01.20
    oral cavity - *see* Wound, open, oral cavity
    puncture - *see* Puncture, head
    scalp - *see* Wound, open, scalp
    specified site NEC S01.80
    temporomandibular area - *see* Wound, open,
    cheek
  heel - *see* Wound, open, foot
  hip S71.00-
    with amputation - *see* Amputation, traumatic,
      hip
    bite - *see* Bite, hip
    laceration - *see* Laceration, hip
    puncture - *see* Puncture, hip
  hymen S31.40
    bite - *see* Bite, vulva
    laceration - *see* Laceration, vagina
    puncture - *see* Puncture, vagina
  hypochondrium S31.109
    bite - *see* Bite, hypochondrium
    laceration - *see* Laceration, hypochondrium
    puncture - *see* Puncture, hypochondrium
  hypogastric region S31.109
    bite - *see* Bite, hypogastric region
    laceration - *see* Laceration, hypogastric
  region
    puncture - *see* Puncture, hypogastric region
  iliac (region) - *see* Wound, open, inguinal
  region
  inguinal region S31.109
    bite - *see* Bite, abdomen, wall, lower
    quadrant
    laceration - *see* Laceration, inguinal region
    puncture - *see* Puncture, inguinal region
  instep - *see* Wound, open, foot
  interscapular region - *see* Wound, open,
    thorax, back
  intraocular - *see* Wound, open, ocular
  iris - *see* Wound, open, ocular
  jaw - *see* Wound, open, head, specified site
    NEC
  knee S81.00-
    bite - *see* Bite, knee
    laceration - *see* Laceration, knee
    puncture - *see* Puncture, knee
  labium (majus) (minus) - *see* Wound, open,
    vulva
  laceration - *see* Laceration, by site
  lacrimal duct - *see* Wound, open, eyelid
  larynx S11.019
    bite - *see* Bite, larynx
    laceration - *see* Laceration, larynx
    puncture - *see* Puncture, larynx
  left
    lower quadrant S31.104
      with penetration into peritoneal cavity
      S31.604
      bite - *see* Bite, abdomen, wall, left, lower
      quadrant
      laceration - *see* Laceration, abdomen, wall,
      left, lower quadrant
      puncture - *see* Puncture, abdomen, wall,
      left, lower quadrant
    upper quadrant S31.101
      with penetration into peritoneal cavity
      S31.601
      bite - *see* Bite, abdomen, wall, left, upper
      quadrant
      laceration - *see* Laceration, abdomen, wall,

Wound, open - *continued*
    left, upper quadrant
      puncture - *see* Puncture, abdomen, wall,
      left, upper quadrant
  leg (lower) S81.80-
    with amputation - *see* Amputation, traumatic,
      leg
    ankle - *see* Wound, open, ankle
    bite - *see* Bite, leg
    foot - *see* Wound, open, foot
    knee - *see* Wound, open, knee
    laceration - *see* Laceration, leg
    puncture - *see* Puncture, leg
    toe - *see* Wound, open, toe
    upper - *see* Wound, open, thigh
  lip S01.501
    bite - *see* Bite, lip
    laceration - *see* Laceration, lip
    puncture - *see* Puncture, lip
  loin S31.109
    bite - *see* Bite, abdomen, wall
    laceration - *see* Laceration, loin
    puncture - *see* Puncture, loin
  lower back - *see* Wound, open, back, lower
  lumbar region - *see* Wound, open, back, lower
  malar region - *see* Wound, open, head,
    specified site NEC
  mammary - *see* Wound, open, breast
  mastoid region - *see* Wound, open, head,
    specified site NEC
  mouth - *see* Wound, open, oral cavity
  nail
    finger - *see* Wound, open, finger, with
    damage to nail
    toe - *see* Wound, open, toe, with damage to
    nail
  nape (neck) - *see* Wound, open, neck
  nasal (septum) (sinus) - *see* Wound, open, nose
  nasopharynx - *see* Wound, open, head,
  specified site NEC
  neck S11.90
    bite - *see* Bite, neck
    involving
      cervical esophagus S11.20
      larynx - *see* Wound, open, larynx
      pharynx S11.20
      thyroid S11.10
      trachea (cervical) S11.029
        bite - *see* Bite, trachea
        laceration S11.021
          with foreign body S11.022
        puncture S11.023
          with foreign body S11.024
    laceration - *see* Laceration, neck
    puncture - *see* Puncture, neck
    specified site NEC S11.80
      specified type NEC S11.89
  nose (septum) (sinus) S01.20
    with amputation - *see* Amputation, traumatic,
      nose
    bite - *see* Bite, nose
    laceration - *see* Laceration, nose
    puncture - *see* Puncture, nose
  ocular S05.90
    avulsion (traumatic enucleation) S05.7-
    eyeball S05.6-
      with foreign body S05.5-
    eyelid - *see* Wound, open, eyelid
    laceration and rupture S05.3-
      with prolapse or loss of intraocular tissue
    S05.2-
    orbit (penetrating) (with or without foreign
    body) S05.4-
    periocular area - *see* Wound, open, eyelid

Wound, open - *continued*
 specified NEC S05.8X   oral cavity S01.502
  bite S01.552
  laceration - *see* Laceration, oral cavity
  puncture - *see* Puncture, oral cavity
 orbit - *see* Wound, open, ocular, orbit
 palate - *see* Wound, open, oral cavity   palm -
  see Wound, open, hand
 pelvis, pelvic - *see also* Wound, open, back,
  lower
  girdle - *see* Wound, open, hip
 penetrating - *see* Puncture, by site
 penis S31.20
  with amputation - *see* Amputation, traumatic,
   penis
  bite S31.25
  laceration - *see* Laceration, penis
  puncture - *see* Puncture, penis
 perineum
  bite - *see* Bite, perineum
  female S31.502
  laceration - *see* Laceration, perineum
  male S31.501
  puncture - *see* Puncture, perineum
 periocular area (with or without lacrimal
  passages) - *see* Wound, open, eyelid
 periumbilic region S31.105
  with penetration into peritoneal cavity
   S31.605
  bite - *see* Bite, abdomen, wall, periumbilic
   region
  laceration - *see* Laceration, abdomen, wall,
   periumbilic region
  puncture - *see* Puncture, abdomen, wall,
   periumbilic region
 phalanges
  finger - *see* Wound, open, finger
  toe - *see* Wound, open, toe
 pharynx S11.20
 pinna - *see* Wound, open, ear
 popliteal space - *see* Wound, open, knee
 prepuce - *see* Wound, open, penis
 pubic region - *see* Wound, open, back, lower
 pudendum - *see* Wound, open, genital organs,
  external
 puncture wound - *see* Puncture
 rectovaginal septum - *see* Wound, open,
  vagina
 right
  lower quadrant S31.103
   with penetration into peritoneal cavity
    S31.603
   bite - *see* Bite, abdomen, wall, right, lower
    quadrant
   laceration - *see* Laceration, abdomen, wall,
    right, lower quadrant
   puncture - *see* Puncture, abdomen, wall,
    right, lower quadrant
  upper quadrant S31.100
   with penetration into peritoneal cavity
    S31.600
   bite - *see* Bite, abdomen, wall, right, upper
    quadrant
   laceration - *see* Laceration, abdomen, wall,
    right, upper quadrant
   puncture - *see* Puncture, abdomen, wall,
    right, upper quadrant
 sacral region - *see* Wound, open, back, lower
 sacroiliac region - *see* Wound, open, back,
  lower
 salivary gland - *see* Wound, open, oral cavity
 scalp S01.00
  bite S01.05
  laceration - *see* Laceration, scalp

Wound, open - *continued*
 puncture - *see* Puncture, scalp
 scalpel, newborn (birth injury) P15.8
 scapular region - *see* Wound, open, shoulder
 sclera - *see* Wound, open, ocular
 scrotum S31.30
  with amputation - *see* Amputation, traumatic,
   scrotum
  bite S31.35
  laceration - *see* Laceration, scrotum
  puncture - *see* Puncture, scrotum
 shin - *see* Wound, open, leg
 shoulder S41.00-
  with amputation - *see* Amputation, traumatic,
   arm
  bite - *see* Bite, shoulder
  laceration - *see* Laceration, shoulder
  puncture - *see* Puncture, shoulder
 skin NOS T14.8
 spermatic cord - *see* Wound, open, testis
 sternal region - *see* Wound, open, thorax, front
  wall
 submaxillary region - *see* Wound, open, head,
  specified site NEC
 submental region - *see* Wound, open, head,
  specified site NEC
 subungual
  finger(s) - *see* Wound, open, finger
  toe(s) - *see* Wound, open, toe
 supraclavicular region - *see* Wound, open,
  neck, specified site NEC
 temple, temporal region - *see* Wound, open,
  head, specified site NEC
 temporomandibular area - *see* Wound, open,
  cheek
 testis S31.30
  with amputation - *see* Amputation, traumatic,
   testes
  bite S31.35
  laceration - *see* Laceration, testis
  puncture - *see* Puncture, testis
 thigh S71.10-
  with amputation - *see* Amputation, traumatic,
   hip
  bite - *see* Bite, thigh
  laceration - *see* Laceration, thigh
  puncture - *see* Puncture, thigh
 thorax, thoracic (wall) S21.90
  back S21.20-
   with penetration S21.40
  bite - *see* Bite, thorax
  breast - *see* Wound, open, breast
  front S21.10-
   with penetration S21.30
  laceration - *see* Laceration, thorax
  puncture - *see* Puncture, thorax
 throat - *see* Wound, open, neck
 thumb S61.009
  with
   amputation - *see* Amputation, traumatic,
    thumb
   damage to nail S61.109
  bite - *see* Bite, thumb
  laceration - *see* Laceration, thumb
  left S61.002
   with
    damage to nail S61.102
  puncture - *see* Puncture, thumb
  right S61.001
   with
    damage to nail S61.101
 thyroid (gland) - *see* Wound, open, neck,
  thyroid
 toe(s) S91.109

Wound, open - *continued*
 with
  amputation - *see* Amputation, traumatic, toe
  damage to nail S91.209
 bite - *see* Bite, toe
 great S91.103
  with
   damage to nail S91.203
  left S91.102
   with
    damage to nail S91.202
  right S91.101
   with
    damage to nail S91.201
 laceration - *see* Laceration, toe
 lesser S91.106
  with
   damage to nail S91.206
  left S91.105
   with
    damage to nail S91.205
  right S91.104
   with
    damage to nail S91.204
 puncture - *see* Puncture, toe
 tongue - *see* Wound, open, oral cavity
 trachea (cervical region) - *see* Wound, open,
  neck, trachea
 tunica vaginalis - *see* Wound, open, testis
 tympanum, tympanic membrane S09.2-
  laceration - *see* Laceration, ear, drum
  puncture - *see* Puncture, tympanum
 umbilical region - *see* Wound, open, abdomen,
  wall, periumbilic region
 uvula - *see* Wound, open, oral cavity
 vagina S31.40
  bite S31.45
  laceration - *see* Laceration, vagina
  puncture - *see* Puncture, vagina
 vocal cord S11.039
  bite - *see* Bite, vocal cord
  laceration S11.031
   with foreign body S11.032
  puncture S11.033
   with foreign body S11.034
 vitreous (humor) - *see* Wound, open, ocular
 vulva S31.40
  with amputation - *see* Amputation, traumatic,
   vulva
  bite S31.45
  laceration - *see* Laceration, vulva
  puncture - *see* Puncture, vulva
 wrist S61.50-
  bite - *see* Bite, wrist
  laceration - *see* Laceration, wrist
  puncture - *see* Puncture, wrist
Wound, superficial - *see* Injury - *see also*
 specified injury type
Wright's syndrome G54.0
Wrist - *see* condition
Wrong drug (by accident) (given in error) -
 see Table of Drugs and Chemicals, by drug,
 poisoning
Wry neck - *see* Torticollis
Wuchereria (bancrofti) infestation B74.0
Wuchereriasis B74.0
Wuchernde Struma Langhans C73

X

Xanthelasma (eyelid) (palpebrarum) H02.60
 left H02.66
  lower H02.65
  upper H02.64

Xanthelasma - *continued*
  right H02.63
    lower H02.62
    upper H02.61
Xanthelasmatosis (essential) E78.2
Xanthinuria, hereditary E79.8
Xanthoastrocytoma
  specified site - *see* Neoplasm, malignant, by
    site
  unspecified site C71.9
Xanthofibroma - *see* Neoplasm, connective
    tissue, benign
Xanthogranuloma D76.3
Xanthoma(s), xanthomatosis (primary)
  (familial) (hereditary) E75.5
  with
    hyperlipoproteinemia
      Type I E78.3
      Type III E78.2
      Type IV E78.1
      Type V E78.3
  bone (generalisata) C96.5
  cerebrotendinous E75.5
  cutaneotendinous E75.5
  disseminatum (skin) E78.2
  eruptive E78.2
  hypercholesterinemic E78.00
  hypercholesterolemic E78.00
  hyperlipidemic E78.5
  joint E75.5
  multiple (skin) E78.2
  tendon (sheath) E75.5
  tubo-eruptive E78.2
  tuberosum E78.2
  tuberous E78.2
  verrucous, oral mucosa K13.4
Xanthosis R23.8
Xenophobia F40.10
Xeroderma - *see also* Ichthyosis
  acquired L85.0
  eyelid H01.149
    left H01.146
      lower H01.145
      upper H01.144
    right H01.143
      lower H01.142
      upper H01.141
  pigmentosum Q82.1
  vitamin A deficiency E50.8
Xerophthalmia (vitamin A deficiency) E50.7
  unrelated to vitamin A deficiency - *see*
    Keratoconjunctivitis
Xerosis
  conjunctiva H11.14-
    with Bitot's spots - *see also* Pigmentation,
      conjunctiva
      vitamin A deficiency E50.1
    vitamin A deficiency E50.0
  cornea H18.89-
    with ulceration - *see* Ulcer, cornea
      vitamin A deficiency E50.3
    vitamin A deficiency E50.2
  cutis L85.3
  skin L85.3
Xerostomia K11.7
Xiphopagus Q89.4
XO syndrome Q96.9
X-ray (of)
  abnormal findings - *see* Abnormal, diagnostic
    imaging
  breast (mammogram) (routine) Z12.31
  chest
    routine (as part of a general medical
      examination) Z00.00

X-ray (of) - *continued*
    with abnormal findings Z00.01
  routine (as part of a general medical
    examination) Z00.00
    with abnormal findings Z00.01
XXXXY syndrome Q98.1
XXY syndrome Q98.0

Y

Yaba pox (virus disease) B08.72
Yatapoxvirus B08.70
  specified NEC B08.79
Yawning R06.89
  psychogenic F45.8
Yaws A66.9
  bone lesions A66.6
  butter A66.1
  chancre A66.0
  cutaneous, less than five years after infection
    A66.2
  early (cutaneous) (macular) (maculopapular)
    (micropapular) (papular) A66.2
    frambeside A66.2
    skin lesions NEC A66.2
  eyelid A66.2
  ganglion A66.6
  gangosis, gangosa A66.5
  gumma, gummata A66.4
    bone A66.6
  gummatous
    frambeside A66.4
    osteitis A66.6
    periostitis A66.6
  hydrarthrosis - *see also* subcategory M14.8
    A66.6
  hyperkeratosis (early) (late) A66.3
  initial lesions A66.0
  joint lesions - *see also* subcategory M14.8
    A66.6
  juxta-articular nodules A66.7
  late nodular (ulcerated) A66.4
  latent (without clinical manifestations) (with
    positive serology) A66.8
  mother A66.0
  mucosal A66.7
  multiple papillomata A66.1
  nodular, late (ulcerated) A66.4
  osteitis A66.6
  papilloma, plantar or palmar A66.1
  periostitis (hypertrophic) A66.6
  specified NEC A66.7
  ulcers A66.4
  wet crab A66.1
Yeast infection - *see also* Candidiasis B37.9
Yellow
  atrophy (liver) - *see* Failure, hepatic
  fever - *see* Fever, yellow
  jack - *see* Fever, yellow
  jaundice - *see* Jaundice
  nail syndrome L60.5
Yersiniosis - *see also* Infection, Yersinia
  extraintestinal A28.2
  intestinal A04.6

Z

Zahorsky's syndrome (herpangina) B08.5
Zellweger's syndrome Q87.89
Zenker's diverticulum (esophagus) K22.5
Ziehen-oppenheim disease G24.1
Zieve's syndrome K70.0
Zika NOS A92.5

Zinc
  deficiency, dietary E60
  metabolism disorder E83.2
Zollinger-ellison syndrome E16.4
Zona - *see* Herpes, zoster
Zoophobia F40.218
Zoster (herpes) - *see* Herpes, zoster
Zygomycosis B46.9
  specified NEC B46.8
Zymotic - *see* condition

Neoplasm Table

The list below gives the code numbers for neoplasms by anatomical site. For each site there are six possible code numbers according to whether the neoplasm in question is malignant, benign, in situ, of uncertain behavior, or of unspecified nature. The description of the neoplasm will often indicate which of the six columns is appropriate; e.g., malignant melanoma of skin, benign fibroadenoma of breast, carcinoma in situ of cervix uteri.

Where such descriptors are not present, the remainder of the Index should be consulted where guidance is given to the appropriate column for each morphological (histological) variety listed; e.g., Mesonephroma -see Neoplasm, malignant; Embryoma -see also Neoplasm, uncertain behavior; Disease, Bowen's -see Neoplasm, skin, in situ. However, the guidance in the Index can be overridden if one of the descriptors mentioned above is present; e.g., malignant adenoma of colon is coded to C18.9 and not to D12.6 as the adjective 'malignant' overrides the Index entry 'Adenoma - see also Neoplasm, benign.'

Codes listed with a dash (-) following the code have a required additional character for laterality. The Tabular List must be reviewed for the complete code.

	Malignant Primary	Malignant Secondary	CA in Situ	Benign	Uncertain Behavior	Unspecified Behavior
Neoplasm, neoplastic	C80.1	C79.9	D09.9	D36.9	D48.9	D49.9
- abdomen, abdominal	C76.2	C79.8-	D09.8	D36.7	D48.7	D49.89
- - cavity	C76.2	C79.8-	D09.8	D36.7	D48.7	D49.89
- - organ	C76.2	C79.8-	D09.8	D36.7	D48.7	D49.89
- - viscera	C76.2	C79.8-	D09.8	D36.7	D48.7	D49.89
- - wall—*see also Neoplasm, abdomen, wall, skin*	C44.509	C79.2-	D04.5	D23.5	D48.5	D49.2
- - - connective tissue	C49.4	C79.8-	-	D21.4	D48.1	D49.2
- - - skin	C44.509					
- - - - basal cell carcinoma	C44.519	-	-	-	-	-
- - - - specified type NEC	C44.599	-	-	-	-	-
- - - - squamous cell carcinoma	C44.529	-	-	-	-	-
- abdominopelvic	C76.8	C79.8-	-	D36.7	D48.7	D49.89
- accessory sinus—*see Neoplasm, sinus*						
- acoustic nerve	C72.4-	C79.49	-	D33.3	D43.3	D49.7
- adenoid (pharynx) (tissue)	C11.1	C79.89	D00.08	D10.6	D37.05	D49.0
- adipose tissue—*see also Neoplasm, connective tissue*	C49.4	C79.89	-	D21.9	D48.1	D49.2
- adnexa (uterine)	C57.4	C79.89	D07.39	D28.7	D39.8	D49.59
- adrenal	C74.9-	C79.7-	D09.3	D35.0-	D44.1-	D49.7
- - capsule	C74.9-	C79.7-	D09.3	D35.0-	D44.1-	D49.7
- - cortex	C74.0-	C79.7-	D09.3	D35.0-	D44.1-	D49.7
- - gland	C74.9-	C79.7-	D09.3	D35.0-	D44.1-	D49.7
- - medulla	C74.1-	C79.7-	D09.3	D35.0-	D44.1-	D49.7
- ala nasi (external)—*see also Neoplasm, skin, nose*	C44.301	C79.2	D04.39	D23.39	D48.5	D49.2
- alimentary canal or tract NEC	C26.9	C78.80	D01.9	D13.9	D37.9	D49.0
- alveolar	C03.9	C79.89	D00.03	D10.39	D37.09	D49.0
- - mucosa	C03.9	C79.89	D00.03	D10.39	D37.09	D49.0
- - - lower	C03.1	C79.89	D00.03	D10.39	D37.09	D49.0
- - - upper	C03.0	C79.89	D00.03	D10.39	D37.09	D49.0
- - ridge or process	C41.1	C79.51	-	D16.5-	D48.0	D49.2
- - - carcinoma	C03.9	C79.8-	-	-	-	-
- - - - lower	C03.1	C79.8-	-	-	-	-
- - - - upper	C03.0	C79.8-	-	-	-	-
- - - lower	C41.1	C79.51	-	D16.5-	D48.0	D49.2
- - - mucosa	C03.9	C79.89	D00.03	D10.39	D37.09	D49.0
- - - - lower	C03.1	C79.89	D00.03	D10.39	D37.09	D49.0
- - - - upper	C03.0	C79.89	D00.03	D10.39	D37.09	D49.0
- - - upper	C41.0	C79.51	-	D16.4-	D48.0	D49.2
- - sulcus	C06.1	C79.89	D00.02	D10.39	D37.09	D49.0
- alveolus	C03.9	C79.89	D00.03	D10.39	D37.09	D49.0
- - lower	C03.1	C79.89	D00.03	D10.39	D37.09	D49.0
- - upper	C03.0	C79.89	D00.03	D10.39	D37.09	D49.0
- ampulla of Vater	C24.1	C78.89	D01.5	D13.5	D37.6	D49.0
- ankle NEC	C76.5-	C79.89	D04.7-	D36.7	D48.7	D49.89
- anorectum, anorectal (junction)	C21.8	C78.5	D01.3	D12.9	D37.8	D49.0
- antecubital fossa or space	C76.4-	C79.89	D04.6-	D36.7	D48.7	D49.89
- antrum (Highmore) (maxillary)	C31.0	C78.39	D02.3	D14.0	D38.5	D49.1
- - pyloric	C16.3	C78.89	D00.2	D13.1	D37.1	D49.0
- - tympanicum	C30.1	C78.39	D02.3	D14.0	D38.5	D49.1
- anus, anal	C21.0	C78.5	D01.3	D12.9	D37.8	D49.0
- - canal	C21.1	C78.5	D01.3	D12.9	D37.8	D49.0
- - cloacogenic zone	C21.2	C78.5	D01.3	D12.9	D37.8	D49.0
- - margin—*see also Neoplasm, anus, skin*	C44.500	C79.2	D04.5	D23.5	D48.5	D49.2

	Malignant Primary	Malignant Secondary	CA in Situ	Benign	Uncertain Behavior	Unspecified Behavior
- - overlapping lesion with rectosigmoid junction or rectum	C21.8	-	-	-	-	-
- - skin	C44.500	C79.2	D04.5	D23.5	D48.5	D49.2
- - - basal cell carcinoma	C44.510	-	-	-	-	-
- - - specified type NEC	C44.590	-	-	-	-	-
- - - squamous cell carcinoma	C44.520	-	-	-	-	-
- - sphincter	C21.1	C78.5	D01.3	D12.9	D37.8	D49.0
- aorta (thoracic)	C49.3	C79.89	-	D21.3	D48.1	D49.2
- - abdominal	C49.4	C79.89	-	D21.4	D48.1	D49.2
- aortic body	C75.5	C79.89	-	D35.6	D44.7	D49.7
- aponeurosis	C49.9	C79.89	-	D21.9	D48.1	D49.2
- - palmar	C49.1-	C79.89	-	D21.1-	D48.1	D49.2
- - plantar	C49.2-	C79.89	-	D21.2-	D48.1	D49.2
- appendix	C18.1	C78.5	D01.0	D12.1	D37.3	D49.0
- arachnoid	C70.9	C79.49	-	D32.9	D42.9	D49.7
- - cerebral	C70.0	C79.32	-	D32.0	D42.0	D49.7
- - spinal	C70.1	C79.49	-	D32.1	D42.1	D49.7
- areola	C50.0-	C79.81	D05.-	D24.-	D48.6-	D49.3
- arm NEC	C76.4-	C79.89	D04.6-	D36.7	D48.7	D49.89
- artery—see Neoplasm, connective tissue						
- aryepiglottic fold	C13.1	C79.89	D00.08	D10.7	D37.05	D49.0
- - hypopharyngeal aspect	C13.1	C79.89	D00.08	D10.7	D37.05	D49.0
- - laryngeal aspect	C32.1	C78.39	D02.0	D14.1	D38.0	D49.1
- - marginal zone	C13.1	C79.89	D00.08	D10.7	D37.05	D49.0
- arytenoid (cartilage)	C32.3	C78.39	D02.0	D14.1	D38.0	D49.1
- - fold—see Neoplasm, aryepiglottic						
- associated with transplanted organ	C80.2	-	-	-	-	-
- atlas	C41.2	C79.51	-	D16.6	D48.0	D49.2
- atrium, cardiac	C38.0	C79.89	-	D15.1	D48.7	D49.89
- auditory						
- - canal (external) (skin)	C44.20-	C79.2	D04.2-	D23.2-	D48.5	D49.2
- - - internal	C30.1	C78.39	D02.3	D14.0	D38.5	D49.1
- - nerve	C72.4-	C79.49	-	D33.3	D43.3	D49.7
- - tube	C30.1	C78.39	D02.3	D14.0	D38.5	D49.1
- - - opening	C11.2	C79.89	D00.08	D10.6	D37.05	D49.0
- auricle, ear—see also Neoplasm, skin, ear	C44.20-	C79.2	D04.2-	D23.2-	D48.5	D49.2
- auricular canal (external)—see also Neoplasm, skin, ear	C44.20-	C79.2	D04.2-	D23.2-	D48.5	D49.2
- - - internal	C30.1	C78.39	D02.3	D14.0	D38.5	D49.2
- autonomic nerve or nervous system NEC (see Neoplasm, nerve, peripheral)						
- axilla, axillary	C76.1	C79.89	D09.8	D36.7	D48.7	D49.89
- - fold—see also Neoplasm, skin, trunk	C44.509	C79.2	D04.5	D23.5	D48.5	D49.2
- back NEC	C76.8	C79.89	D04.5	D36.7	D48.7	D49.89
- Bartholin's gland	C51.0	C79.82	D07.1	D28.0	D39.8	D49.59
- basal ganglia	C71.0	C79.31	-	D33.0	D43.0	D49.6
- basis pedunculi	C71.7	C79.31	-	D33.1	D43.1	D49.6
- bile or biliary (tract)	C24.9	C78.89	D01.5	D13.5	D37.6	D49.0
- - canaliculi (biliferi) (intrahepatic)	C22.1	C78.7	D01.5	D13.4	D37.6	D49.0
- - canals, interlobular	C22.1	C78.89	D01.5	D13.4	D37.6	D49.0
- - duct or passage (common) (cystic) (extrahepatic)	C24.0	C78.89	D01.5	D13.5	D37.6	D49.0
- - - interlobular	C22.1	C78.89	D01.5	D13.4	D37.6	D49.0
- - - intrahepatic	C22.1	C78.7	D01.5	D13.4	D37.6	D49.0
- - - - and extrahepatic	C24.8	C78.89	D01.5	D13.5	D37.6	D49.0
- bladder (urinary)	C67.9	C79.11	D09.0	D30.3	D41.4	D49.4
- - dome	C67.1	C79.11	D09.0	D30.3	D41.4	D49.4
- - neck	C67.5	C79.11	D09.0	D30.3	D41.4	D49.4
- - orifice	C67.9	C79.11	D09.0	D30.3	D41.4	D49.4
- - - ureteric	C67.6	C79.11	D09.0	D30.3	D41.4	D49.4
- - - urethral	C67.5	C79.11	D09.0	D30.3	D41.4	D49.4
- - overlapping lesion	C67.8	-	-	-	-	-
- - sphincter	C67.8	C79.11	D09.0	D30.3	D41.4	D49.4
- - trigone	C67.0	C79.11	D09.0	D30.3	D41.4	D49.4
- - urachus	C67.7	C79.11	D09.0	D30.3	D41.4	D49.4
- - wall	C67.9	C79.11	D09.0	D30.3	D41.4	D49.4
- - - anterior	C67.3	C79.11	D09.0	D30.3	D41.4	D49.4
- - - lateral	C67.2	C79.11	D09.0	D30.3	D41.4	D49.4
- - - posterior	C67.4	C79.11	D09.0	D30.3	D41.4	D49.4
- blood vessel—see Neoplasm, connective tissue						
- bone (periosteum)	C41.9	C79.51	-	D16.9-	D48.0	D49.2
- - acetabulum	C41.4	C79.51	-	D16.8-	D48.0	D49.2

	Malignant Primary	Malignant Secondary	CA in Situ	Benign	Uncertain Behavior	Unspecified Behavior
- - ankle	C40.3-	C79.51	-	D16.3-	-	-
- - arm NEC	C40.0-	C79.51	-	D16.0-	-	-
- - astragalus	C40.3-	C79.51	-	D16.3-	-	-
- - atlas	C41.2	C79.51	-	D16.6-	D48.0	D49.2
- - axis	C41.2	C79.51	-	D16.6-	D48.0	D49.2
- - back NEC	C41.2	C79.51	-	D16.6-	D48.0	D49.2
- - calcaneus	C40.3-	C79.51	-	D16.3-	-	-
- - calvarium	C41.0	C79.51	-	D16.4-	D48.0	D49.2
- - carpus (any)	C40.1-	C79.51	-	D16.1-	-	-
- - cartilage NEC	C41.9	C79.51	-	D16.9-	D48.0	D49.2
- - clavicle	C41.3	C79.51	-	D16.7-	D48.0	D49.2
- - clivus	C41.0	C79.51	-	D16.4-	D48.0	D49.2
- - coccygeal vertebra	C41.4	C79.51	-	D16.8-	D48.0	D49.2
- - coccyx	C41.4	C79.51	-	D16.8-	D48.0	D49.2
- - costal cartilage	C41.3	C79.51	-	D16.7-	D48.0	D49.2
- - costovertebral joint	C41.3	C79.51	-	D16.7-	D48.0	D49.2
- - cranial	C41.0	C79.51	-	D16.4-	D48.0	D49.2
- - cuboid	C40.3-	C79.51	-	D16.3-	-	-
- - cuneiform	C41.9	C79.51	-	D16.9-	D48.0	D49.2
- - elbow	C40.0-	C79.51	-	D16.0-	-	-
- - ethmoid (labyrinth)	C41.0	C79.51	-	D16.4-	D48.0	D49.2
- - face	C41.0	C79.51	-	D16.4-	D48.0	D49.2
- - femur (any part)	C40.2-	C79.51	-	D16.2-	-	-
- - fibula (any part)	C40.2-	C79.51	-	D16.2-	-	-
- - finger (any)	C40.1-	C79.51	-	D16.1-	-	-
- - foot	C40.3-	C79.51	-	D16.3-	-	-
- - forearm	C40.0-	C79.51	-	D16.0-	-	-
- - frontal	C41.0	C79.51	-	D16.4-	D48.0	D49.2
- - hand	C40.1-	C79.51	-	D16.1-	-	-
- - heel	C40.3-	C79.51	-	D16.3-	-	-
- - hip	C41.4	C79.51	-	D16.8-	D48.0	D49.2
- - humerus (any part)	C40.0-	C79.51	-	D16.0-	-	-
- - hyoid	C41.0	C79.51	-	D16.4-	D48.0	D49.2
- - ilium	C41.4	C79.51	-	D16.8-	D48.0	D49.2
- - innominate	C41.4	C79.51	-	D16.8-	D48.0	D49.2
- - intervertebral cartilage or disc	C41.2	C79.51	-	D16.6-	D48.0	D49.2
- - ischium	C41.4	C79.51	-	D16.8-	D48.0	D49.2
- - jaw (lower)	C41.1	C79.51	-	D16.5-	D48.0	D49.2
- - knee	C40.2-	C79.51	-	D16.2-	-	-
- - leg NEC	C40.2-	C79.51	-	D16.2-	-	-
- - limb NEC	C40.9-	C79.51	-	D16.9-	-	-
- - - lower (long bones)	C40.2-	C79.51	-	D16.2-	-	-
- - - - short bones	C40.3-	C79.51	-	D16.3-	-	-
- - - upper (long bones)	C40.0-	C79.51	-	D16.0-	-	-
- - - - short bones	C40.1-	C79.51	-	D16.1-	-	-
- - malar	C41.0	C79.51	-	D16.4-	D48.0	D49.2
- - mandible	C41.1	C79.51	-	D16.5-	D48.0	D49.2
- - marrow NEC (any bone)	C96.9	C79.52	-	-	D47.9	D49.89
- - mastoid	C41.0	C79.51	-	D16.4-	D48.0	D49.2
- - maxilla, maxillary (superior)	C41.0	C79.51	-	D16.4-	D48.0	D49.2
- - - inferior	C41.1	C79.51	-	D16.5-	D48.0	D49.2
- - metacarpus (any)	C40.1-	C79.51	-	D16.1-	-	-
- - metatarsus (any)	C40.3-	C79.51	-	D16.3-	-	-
- - overlapping sites	C40.8-	-	-	-	-	-
- - navicular						
- - - ankle	C40.3-	C79.51	-	-	-	-
- - - hand	C40.1-	C79.51	-	-	-	-
- - nose, nasal	C41.0	C79.51	-	D16.4-	D48.0	D49.2
- - occipital	C41.0	C79.51	-	D16.4-	D48.0	D49.2
- - orbit	C41.0	C79.51	-	D16.4-	D48.0	D49.2
- - parietal	C41.0	C79.51	-	D16.4-	D48.0	D49.2
- - patella	C40.2-	C79.51	-	-	-	-
- - pelvic	C41.4	C79.51	-	D16.8	D48.0	D49.2
- - phalanges						
- - - foot	C40.3-	C79.51	-	-	-	-
- - - hand	C40.1-	C79.51	-	-	-	-
- - pubic	C41.4	C79.51	-	D16.8	D48.0	D49.2
- - radius (any part)	C40.0-	C79.51	-	D16.0-	-	-
- - rib	C41.3	C79.51	-	D16.7	D48.0	D49.2
- - sacral vertebra	C41.4	C79.51	-	D16.8	D48.0	D49.2
- - sacrum	C41.4	C79.51	-	D16.8	D48.0	D49.2

	Malignant Primary	Malignant Secondary	CA in Situ	Benign	Uncertain Behavior	Unspecified Behavior
- - scaphoid					-	-
- - - of ankle	C40.3-	C79.51	-	-	-	-
- - - of hand	C40.1-	C79.51	-	-	-	-
- - scapula (any part)	C40.0-	C79.51	-	D16.0-	-	-
- - sella turcica	C41.0	C79.51	-	D16.4-	D48.0	D49.2
- - shoulder	C40.0-	C79.51	-	D16.0-	-	-
- - skull	C41.0	C79.51	-	D16.4-	D48.0	D49.2
- - sphenoid	C41.0	C79.51	-	D16.4-	D48.0	D49.2
- - spine, spinal (column)	C41.2	C79.51	-	D16.6	D48.0	D49.2
- - - coccyx	C41.4	C79.51	-	D16.8	D48.0	D49.2
- - - sacrum	C41.4	C79.51	-	D16.8	D48.0	D49.2
- - sternum	C41.3	C79.51	-	D16.7	D48.0	D49.2
- - tarsus (any)	C40.3-	C79.51	-	-	-	-
- - temporal	C41.0	C79.51	-	D16.4-	D48.0	D49.2
- - thumb	C40.1-	C79.51	-	-	-	-
- - tibia (any part)	C40.2-	C79.51	-	-	-	-
- - toe (any)	C40.3-	C79.51	-	-	-	-
- - trapezium	C40.1-	C79.51	-	-	-	-
- - trapezoid	C40.1-	C79.51	-	-	-	-
- - turbinate	C41.0	C79.51	-	D16.4-	D48.0	D49.2
- - ulna (any part)	C40.0-	C79.51	-	D16.0-	-	-
- - unciform	C40.1-	C79.51	-	-	-	-
- - vertebra (column)	C41.2	C79.51	-	D16.6	D48.0	D49.2
- - - coccyx	C41.4	C79.51	-	D16.8	D48.0	D49.2
- - - sacrum	C41.4	C79.51	-	D16.8	D48.0	D49.2
- - vomer	C41.0	C79.51	-	D16.4-	D48.0	D49.2
- - wrist	C40.1-	C79.51	-	-	-	-
- - xiphoid process	C41.3	C79.51	-	D16.7	D48.0	D49.2
- - zygomatic	C41.0	C79.51	-	D16.4-	D48.0	D49.2
- book-leaf (mouth)	C06.89	C79.89	D00.00	D10.39	D37.09	D49.0
- bowel—*see* Neoplasm, intestine						
- brachial plexus	C47.1-	C79.89	-	D36.12	D48.2	D49.2
- brain NEC	C71.9	C79.31	-	D33.2	D43.2	D49.6
- - basal ganglia	C71.0	C79.31	-	D33.0	D43.0	D49.6
- - cerebellopontine angle	C71.6	C79.31	-	D33.1	D43.1	D49.6
- - cerebellum NOS	C71.6	C79.31	-	D33.1	D43.1	D49.6
- - cerebrum	C71.0	C79.31	-	D33.0	D43.0	D49.6
- - choroid plexus	C71.7	C79.31	-	D33.1	D43.1	D49.6
- - corpus callosum	C71.8	C79.31	-	D33.2	D43.2	D49.6
- - corpus striatum	C71.0	C79.31	-	D33.0	D43.0	D49.6
- - cortex (cerebral)	C71.0	C79.31	-	D33.0	D43.0	D49.6
- - frontal lobe	C71.1	C79.31	-	D33.0	D43.0	D49.6
- - globus pallidus	C71.0	C79.31	-	D33.0	D43.0	D49.6
- - hippocampus	C71.2	C79.31	-	D33.0	D43.0	D49.6
- - hypothalamus	C71.0	C79.31	-	D33.0	D43.0	D49.6
- - internal capsule	C71.0	C79.31	-	D33.0	D43.0	D49.6
- - medulla oblongata	C71.7	C79.31	-	D33.1	D43.1	D49.6
- - meninges	C70.0	C79.32	-	D32.0	D42.0	D49.7
- - midbrain	C71.7	C79.31	-	D33.1	D43.1	D49.6
- - occipital lobe	C71.4	C79.31	-	D33.0	D43.0	D49.6
- - overlapping lesion	C71.8	C79.31	-	-	-	-
- - parietal lobe	C71.3	C79.31	-	D33.0	D43.0	D49.6
- - peduncle	C71.7	C79.31	-	D33.1	D43.1	D49.6
- - pons	C71.7	C79.31	-	D33.1	D43.1	D49.6
- - stem	C71.7	C79.31	-	D33.1	D43.1	D49.6
- - tapetum	C71.8	C79.31	-	D33.2	D43.2	D49.6
- - temporal lobe	C71.2	C79.31	-	D33.0	D43.0	D49.6
- - thalamus	C71.0	C79.31	-	D33.0	D43.0	D49.6
- - uncus	C71.2	C79.31	-	D33.0	D43.0	D49.6
- - ventricle (floor)	C71.5	C79.31	-	D33.0	D43.0	D49.6
- - - fourth	C71.7	C79.31	-	D33.1	D43.1	D49.6
- branchial (cleft) (cyst) (vestiges)	C10.4	C79.89	D00.08	D10.5	D37.05	D49.0
- breast (connective tissue) (glandular tissue) (soft parts)	C50.9-	C79.81	D05.-	D24.-	D48.6-	D49.3
- - areola	C50.0-	C79.81	D05.-	D24.-	D48.6-	D49.3
- - axillary tail	C50.6-	C79.81	D05.-	D24.-	D48.6-	D49.3
- - central portion	C50.1-	C79.81	D05.-	D24.-	D48.6-	D49.3
- - inner	C50.8-	C79.81	D05.-	D24.-	D48.6-	D49.3
- - lower	C50.8-	C79.81	D05.-	D24.-	D48.6-	D49.3
- - lower-inner quadrant	C50.3-	C79.81	D05.-	D24.-	D48.6-	D49.3
- - lower-outer quadrant	C50.5-	C79.81	D05.-	D24.-	D48.6-	D49.3

	Malignant Primary	Malignant Secondary	CA in Situ	Benign	Uncertain Behavior	Unspecified Behavior
- - mastectomy site (skin)—*see also Neoplasm, breast, skin*	C44.501	C79.2	-	-	-	-
- - - specified as breast tissue	C50.8-	C79.81	-	-	-	-
- - midline	C50.8-	C79.81	D05.-	D24.-	D48.6-	D49.3
- - nipple	C50.0-	C79.81	D05.-	D24.-	D48.6-	D49.3
- - outer	C50.8-	C79.81	D05.-	D24.-	D48.6-	D49.3
- - overlapping lesion	C50.8-	-	-	-	-	-
- - skin	C44.501	C79.2	D04.5	D23.5	D48.5	D49.2
- - - basal cell carcinoma	C44.511	-	-	-	-	-
- - - specified type NEC	C44.591	-	-	-	-	-
- - - squamous cell carcinoma	C44.521	-	-	-	-	-
- - tail (axillary)	C50.6-	C79.81	D05.-	D24.-	D48.6-	D49.3
- - upper	C50.8-	C79.81	D05.-	D24.-	D48.6-	D49.3
- - upper-inner quadrant	C50.2-	C79.81	D05.-	D24.-	D48.6-	D49.3
- - upper-outer quadrant	C50.4-	C79.81	D05.-	D24.-	D48.6-	D49.3
- broad ligament	C57.1	C79.82	D07.39	D28.2	D39.8	D49.59
- bronchogenic, bronchogenic (lung)	C34.9-	C78.0-	D02.2-	D14.3-	D38.1	D49.1
- bronchiole	C34.9-	C78.0-	D02.2-	D14.3-	D38.1	D49.1
- bronchus	C34.9-	C78.0-	D02.2-	D14.3-	D38.1	D49.1
- - carina	C34.0-	C78.0-	D02.2-	D14.3-	D38.1	D49.1
- - lower lobe of lung	C34.3-	C78.0-	D02.2-	D14.3-	D38.1	D49.1
- - main	C34.0-	C78.0-	D02.2-	D14.3-	D38.1	D49.1
- - middle lobe of lung	C34.2	C78.0-	D02.21	D14.31	D38.1	D49.1
- - overlapping lesion	C34.8-	-	-	-	-	-
- - upper lobe of lung	C34.1-	C78.0-	D02.2-	D14.3-	D38.1	D49.1
- brow	C44.309	C79.2	D04.39	D23.39	D48.5	D49.2
- - basal cell carcinoma	C44.319	-	-	-	-	-
- - specified type NEC	C44.399	-	-	-	-	-
- - squamous cell carcinoma	C44.329	-	-	-	-	-
- buccal (cavity)	C06.9	C79.89	D00.00	D10.39	D37.09	D49.0
- - commissure	C06.0	C79.89	D00.02	D10.39	D37.09	D49.0
- - groove (lower) (upper)	C06.1	C79.89	D00.02	D10.39	D37.09	D49.0
- - mucosa	C06.0	C79.89	D00.02	D10.39	D37.09	D49.0
- - sulcus (lower) (upper)	C06.1	C79.89	D00.02	D10.39	D37.09	D49.0
- bulbourethral gland	C68.0	C79.19	D09.19	D30.4	D41.3	D49.59
- bursa—*see Neoplasm, connective tissue*						
- buttock NEC	C76.3	C79.89	D04.5	D36.7	D48.7	D49.89
- calf	C76.5-	C79.89	D04.7-	D36.7	D48.7	D49.89
- calvarium	C41.0	C79.51	-	D16.4-	D48.0	D49.2
- calyx, renal	C65.-	C79.0-	D09.19	D30.1-	D41.1-	D49.59
- canal						
- - anal	C21.1	C78.5	D01.3	D12.9	D37.8	D49.0
- - auditory (external)—*see also Neoplasm, skin, ear*	C44.20-	C79.2	D04.2-	D23.2-	D48.5	D49.2
- - auricular (external)—*see also Neoplasm, skin, ear*	C44.20-	C79.2	D04.2-	D23.2-	D48.5	D49.2
- - canaliculi, biliary (biliferi) (intrahepatic)	C22.1	C78.7	D01.5	D13.4	D37.6	D49.0
- - canthus (eye) (inner) (outer)	C44.10-	C79.2	D04.1-	D23.1-	D48.5	D49.2
- - basal cell carcinoma	C44.11-	-	-	-	-	-
- - specified type NEC	C44.19-	-	-	-	-	-
- - squamous cell carcinoma	C44.12-	-	-	-	-	-
- capillary—*see Neoplasm, connective tissue*						
- caput coli	C18.0	C78.5	D01.0	D12.0	D37.4	D49.0
- carcinoid—*see Tumor, carcinoid*						
- cardia (gastric)	C16.0	C78.89	D00.2	D13.1	D37.1	D49.0
- cardiac orifice (stomach)	C16.0	C78.89	D00.2	D13.1	D37.1	D49.0
- cardio-esophageal junction	C16.0	C78.89	D00.2	D13.1	D37.1	D49.0
- cardio-esophagus	C16.0	C78.89	D00.2	D13.1	D37.1	D49.0
- carina (bronchus)	C34.0-	C78.0-	D02.2-	D14.3-	D38.1	D49.1
- carotid (artery)	C49.0	C79.89	-	D21.0	D48.1	D49.2
- - body	C75.4	C79.89	-	D35.5	D44.6	D49.7
- carpus (any bone)	C40.1-	C79.51	-	D16.1-	-	-
- cartilage (articular) (joint)NEC—*see also Neoplasm, bone*	C41.9	C79.51	-	D16.9-	D48.0	D49.2
- - arytenoid	C32.3	C78.39	D02.0	D14.1	D38.0	D49.1
- - auricular	C49.0	C79.89	-	D21.0	D48.1	D49.2
- - bronchi	C34.0-	C78.39	-	D14.3-	D38.1	D49.1
- - costal	C41.3	C79.51	-	D16.7	D48.0	D49.2
- - cricoid	C32.3	C78.39	D02.0	D14.1	D38.0	D49.1
- - cuneiform	C32.3	C78.39	D02.0	D14.1	D38.0	D49.1
- - ear (external)	C49.0	C79.89	-	D21.0	D48.1	D49.2
- - ensiform	C41.3	C79.51	-	D16.7	D48.0	D49.2
- - epiglottis	C32.1	C78.39	D02.0	D14.1	D38.0	D49.1

	Malignant Primary	Malignant Secondary	CA in Situ	Benign	Uncertain Behavior	Unspecified Behavior
- - - anterior surface	C10.1	C79.89	D00.08	D10.5	D37.05	D49.0
- - eyelid	C49.0	C79.89	-	D21.0	D48.1	D49.2
- - intervertebral	C41.2	C79.51	-	D16.6	D48.0	D49.2
- - larynx, laryngeal	C32.3	C78.39	D02.0	D14.1	D38.0	D49.1
- - nose, nasal	C30.0	C78.39	D02.3	D14.0	D38.5	D49.1
- - pinna	C49.0	C79.89	-	D21.0	D48.1	D49.2
- - rib	C41.3	C79.51	-	D16.7	D48.0	D49.2
- - semilunar (knee)	C40.2-	C79.51	-	D16.2-	D48.0	D49.2
- - thyroid	C32.3	C78.39	D02.0	D14.1	D38.0	D49.1
- - trachea	C33	C78.39	D02.1	D14.2	D38.1	D49.1
- cauda equina	C72.1	C79.49	-	D33.4	D43.4	D49.7
- cavity						
- - buccal	C06.9	C79.89	D00.00	D10.30	D37.09	D49.0
- - nasal	C30.0	C78.39	D02.3	D14.0	D38.5	D49.1
- - oral	C06.9	C79.89	D00.00	D10.30	D37.09	D49.0
- - peritoneal	C48.2	C78.6	-	D20.1	D48.4	D49.0
- - tympanic	C30.1	C78.39	D02.3	D14.0	D38.5	D49.1
- cecum	C18.0	C78.5	D01.0	D12.0	D37.4	D49.0
- central nervous system	C72.9	C79.40	-	-	-	-
- cerebellopontine (angle)	C71.6	C79.31	-	D33.1	D43.1	D49.6
- cerebellum, cerebellar	C71.6	C79.31	-	D33.1	D43.1	D49.6
- cerebrum, cerebral (cortex) (hemisphere) (white matter)	C71.0	C79.31	-	D33.0	D43.0	D49.6
- - meninges	C70.0	C79.32	-	D32.0	D42.0	D49.7
- - peduncle	C71.7	C79.31	-	D33.1	D43.1	D49.6
- - ventricle	C71.5	C79.31	-	D33.0	D43.0	D49.6
- - - fourth	C71.7	C79.31	-	D33.1	D43.1	D49.6
- cervical region	C76.0	C79.89	D09.8	D36.7	D48.7	D49.89
- cervix (cervical) (uteri) (uterus)	C53.9	C79.82	D06.9	D26.0	D39.0	D49.59
- - canal	C53.0	C79.82	D06.0	D26.0	D39.0	D49.59
- - endocervix (canal) (gland)	C53.0	C79.82	D06.0	D26.0	D39.0	D49.59
- - exocervix	C53.1	C79.82	D06.1	D26.0	D39.0	D49.59
- - external os	C53.1	C79.82	D06.1	D26.0	D39.0	D49.59
- - internal os	C53.0	C79.82	D06.0	D26.0	D39.0	D49.59
- - nabothian gland	C53.0	C79.82	D06.0	D26.0	D39.0	D49.59
- - overlapping lesion	C53.8	-	-	-	-	-
- - squamocolumnar junction	C53.8	C79.82	D06.7	D26.0	D39.0	D49.59
- - stump	C53.8	C79.82	D06.7	D26.0	D39.0	D49.59
- cheek	C76.0	C79.89	D09.8	D36.7	D48.7	D49.89
- - external	C44.309	C79.2	D04.39	D23.39	D48.5	D49.2
- - - basal cell carcinoma	C44.319	-	-	-	-	-
- - - specified type NEC	C44.399	-	-	-	-	-
- - - squamous cell carcinoma	C44.329	-	-	-	-	-
- - inner aspect	C06.0	C79.89	D00.02	D10.39	D37.09	D49.0
- - internal	C06.0	C79.89	D00.02	D10.39	D37.09	D49.0
- - mucosa	C06.0	C79.89	D00.02	D10.39	D37.09	D49.0
- chest (wall)NEC	C76.1	C79.89	D09.8	D36.7	D48.7	D49.89
- chiasma opticum	C72.3-	C79.49	-	D33.3	D43.3	D49.7
- chin	C44.309	C79.2	D04.39	D23.39	D48.5	D49.2
- - basal cell carcinoma	C44.319	-	-	-	-	-
- - specified type NEC	C44.399	-	-	-	-	-
- - squamous cell carcinoma	C44.329	-	-	-	-	-
-choana	C11.3	C79.89	D00.08	D10.6	D37.05	D49.0
- cholangiole	C22.1	C78.89	D01.5	D13.4	D37.6	D49.0
- choledochal duct	C24.0	C78.89	D01.5	D13.5	D37.6	D49.0
- choroid	C69.3-	C79.49	D09.2-	D31.3-	D48.7	D49.81
- - plexus	C71.5	C79.31	-	D33.0	D43.0	D49.6
- ciliary body	C69.4-	C79.49	D09.2-	D31.4-	D48.7	D49.89
- clavicle	C41.3	C79.51	-	D16.7	D48.0	D49.2
- clitoris	C51.2	C79.82	D07.1	D28.0	D39.8	D49.59
- clivus	C41.0	C79.51	-	D16.4-	D48.0	D49.2
- cloacogenic zone	C21.2	C78.5	D01.3	D12.9	D37.8	D49.0
- coccygeal						
- - body or glomus	C49.5	C79.89	-	D21.5	D48.1	D49.2
- - vertebra	C41.4	C79.51	-	D16.8	D48.0	D49.2
- coccyx	C41.4	C79.51	-	D16.8	D48.0	D49.2
- colon—see also Neoplasm, intestine, large	C18.9	C78.5	-	-	-	-
- - with rectum	C19	C78.5	D01.1	D12.7	D37.5	D49.0
- column, spinal—see Neoplasm, spine						
- columnella—see also Neoplasm, skin, face	C44.390	C79.2	D04.39	D23.39	D48.5	D49.2
- commissure						

	Malignant Primary	Malignant Secondary	CA in Situ	Benign	Uncertain Behavior	Unspecified Behavior
- - labial, lip	C00.6	C79.89	D00.01	D10.39	D37.01	D49.0
- - laryngeal	C32.0	C78.39	D02.0	D14.1	D38.0	D49.1
- common (bile)duct	C24.0	C78.89	D01.5	D13.5	D37.6	D49.0
- concha—*see also Neoplasm, skin, ear*	C44.20-	C79.2	D04.2-	D23.2-	D48.5	D49.2
- - nose	C30.0	C78.39	D02.3	D14.0	D38.5	D49.1
- conjunctiva	C69.0-	C79.49	D09.2-	D31.0-	D48.7	D49.89
- connective tissue NEC	C49.9	C79.89	-	D21.9	D48.1	D49.2
Note: For neoplasms of connective tissue (blood vessel, bursa, fascia, ligament, muscle, peripheral nerves, sympathetic and parasympathetic nerves and ganglia, synovia, tendon, etc.) or of morphological types that indicate connective tissue, code according to the list under "Neoplasm, connective tissue". For sites that do not appear in this list, code to neoplasm of that site; e.g., fibrosarcoma, pancreas (C25.9)						
Note: Morphological types that indicate connective tissue appear in their proper place in the alphabetic index with the instruction "see Neoplasm, connective tissue ...."						
- - abdomen	C49.4	C79.89	-	D21.4	D48.1	D49.2
- - abdominal wall	C49.4	C79.89	-	D21.4	D48.1	D49.2
- - ankle	C49.2-	C79.89	-	D21.2-	D48.1	D49.2
- - antecubital fossa or space	C49.1-	C79.89	-	D21.1-	D48.1	D49.2
- - arm	C49.1-	C79.89	-	D21.1-	D48.1	D49.2
- - auricle (ear)	C49.0	C79.89	-	D21.0	D48.1	D49.2
- - axilla	C49.3	C79.89	-	D21.3	D48.1	D49.2
- - back	C49.6	C79.89	-	D21.6	D48.1	D49.2
- - breast—*see Neoplasm, breast*						
- - buttock	C49.5	C79.89	-	D21.5	D48.1	D49.2
- - calf	C49.2-	C79.89	-	D21.2-	D48.1	D49.2
- - cervical region	C49.0	C79.89	-	D21.0	D48.1	D49.2
- - cheek	C49.0	C79.89	-	D21.0	D48.1	D49.2
- - chest (wall)	C49.3	C79.89	-	D21.3	D48.1	D49.2
- - chin	C49.0	C79.89	-	D21.0	D48.1	D49.2
- - diaphragm	C49.3	C79.89	-	D21.3	D48.1	D49.2
- - ear (external)	C49.0	C79.89	-	D21.0	D48.1	D49.2
- - elbow	C49.1-	C79.89	-	D21.1-	D48.1	D49.2
- - extra rectal	C49.5	C79.89	-	D21.5	D48.1	D49.2
- - extremity	C49.9	C79.89	-	D21.9	D48.1	D49.2
- - - lower	C49.2-	C79.89	-	D21.2-	D48.1	D49.2
- - - upper	C49.1-	C79.89	-	D21.1-	D48.1	D49.2
- - eyelid	C49.0	C79.89	-	D21.0	D48.1	D49.2
- - face	C49.0	C79.89	-	D21.0	D48.1	D49.2
- - finger	C49.1-	C79.89	-	D21.1-	D48.1	D49.2
- - flank	C49.6	C79.89	-	D21.6	D48.1	D49.2
- - foot	C49.2-	C79.89	-	D21.2-	D48.1	D49.2
- - forearm	C49.1-	C79.89	-	D21.1-	D48.1	D49.2
- - forehead	C49.0	C79.89	-	D21.0	D48.1	D49.2
- - gastric	C49.4	C79.89	-	D21.4	D48.1	D49.2
- - gastrointestinal	C49.4	C79.89	-	D21.4	D48.1	D49.2
- - gluteal region	C49.5	C79.89	-	D21.5	D48.1	D49.2
- - great vessels NEC	C49.3	C79.89	-	D21.3	D48.1	D49.2
- - groin	C49.5	C79.89	-	D21.5	D48.1	D49.2
- - hand	C49.1-	C79.89	-	D21.1-	D48.1	D49.2
- - head	C49.0	C79.89	-	D21.0	D48.1	D49.2
- - heel	C49.2-	C79.89	-	D21.2-	D48.1	D49.2
- - hip	C49.2-	C79.89	-	D21.2-	D48.1	D49.2
- - hypochondrium	C49.4	C79.89	-	D21.4	D48.1	D49.2
- - iliopsoas muscle	C49.5	C79.89	-	D21.5	D48.1	D49.2
- - infraclavicular region	C49.3	C79.89	-	D21.3	D48.1	D49.2
- - inguinal (canal) (region)	C49.5	C79.89	-	D21.5	D48.1	D49.2
- - intestinal	C49.4	C79.89	-	D21.4	D48.1	D49.2
- - intrathoracic	C49.3	C79.89	-	D21.3	D48.1	D49.2
- - ischiorectal fossa	C49.5	C79.89	-	D21.5	D48.1	D49.2
- - jaw	C03.9	C79.89	D00.03	D10.39	D48.1	D49.0
- - knee	C49.2-	C79.89	-	D21.2-	D48.1	D49.2
- - leg	C49.2-	C79.89	-	D21.2-	D48.1	D49.2
- - limb NEC	C49.9	C79.89	-	D21.9	D48.1	D49.2
- - - lower	C49.2-	C79.89	-	D21.2-	D48.1	D49.2
- - - upper	C49.1-	C79.89	-	D21.1-	D48.1	D49.2
- - nates	C49.5	C79.89	-	D21.5	D48.1	D49.2
- - neck	C49.0	C79.89	-	D21.0	D48.1	D49.2
- - orbit	C69.6-	C79.49	D09.2-	D31.6-	D48.1	D49.89
- - overlapping lesion	C49.8	-	-	-	-	-
- - pararectal	C49.5	C79.89	-	D21.5	D48.1	D49.2
- - para-urethral	C49.5	C79.89	-	D21.5	D48.1	D49.2
- - paravaginal	C49.5	C79.89	-	D21.5	D48.1	D49.2
- - pelvis (floor)	C49.5	C79.89	-	D21.5	D48.1	D49.2
- - pelvo-abdominal	C49.8	C79.89	-	D21.6	D48.1	D49.2

	Malignant Primary	Malignant Secondary	CA in Situ	Benign	Uncertain Behavior	Unspecified Behavior
- - perineum	C49.5	C79.89	-	D21.5	D48.1	D49.2
- - perirectal (tissue)	C49.5	C79.89	-	D21.5	D48.1	D49.2
- - periurethral (tissue)	C49.5	C79.89	-	D21.5	D48.1	D49.2
- - popliteal fossa or space	C49.2-	C79.89	-	D21.2-	D48.1	D49.2
- - presacral	C49.5	C79.89	-	D21.5	D48.1	D49.2
- - psoas muscle	C49.4	C79.89	-	D21.4	D48.1	D49.2
- - pterygoid fossa	C49.0	C79.89	-	D21.0	D48.1	D49.2
- - rectovaginal septum or wall	C49.5	C79.89	-	D21.5	D48.1	D49.2
- - rectovesical	C49.5	C79.89	-	D21.5	D48.1	D49.2
- - retroperitoneum	C48.0	C78.6	-	D20.0	D48.3	D49.0
- - sacrococcygeal region	C49.5	C79.89	-	D21.5	D48.1	D49.2
- - scalp	C49.0	C79.89	-	D21.0	D48.1	D49.2
- - scapular region	C49.3	C79.89	-	D21.3	D48.1	D49.2
- - shoulder	C49.1-	C79.89	-	D21.1-	D48.1	D49.2
- - skin (dermis)NEC—*see also Neoplasm, skin, by site*	C44.90	C79.2	D04.9	D23.9	D48.5	D49.2
- - stomach	C49.4	C79.89	-	D21.4	D48.1	D49.2
- - submental	C49.0	C79.89	-	D21.0	D48.1	D49.2
- - supraclavicular region	C49.0	C79.89	-	D21.0	D48.1	D49.2
- - temple	C49.0	C79.89	-	D21.0	D48.1	D49.2
- - temporal region	C49.0	C79.89	-	D21.0	D48.1	D49.2
- - thigh	C49.2-	C79.89	-	D21.2-	D48.1	D49.2
- - thoracic (duct) (wall)	C49.3	C79.89	-	D21.3	D48.1	D49.2
- - thorax	C49.3	C79.89	-	D21.3	D48.1	D49.2
- - thumb	C49.1-	C79.89	-	D21.1-	D48.1	D49.2
- - toe	C49.2-	C79.89	-	D21.2-	D48.1	D49.2
- - trunk	C49.6	C79.89	-	D21.6	D48.1	D49.2
- - umbilicus	C49.4	C79.89	-	D21.4	D48.1	D49.2
- - vesicorectal	C49.5	C79.89	-	D21.5	D48.1	D49.2
- - wrist	C49.1-	C79.89	-	D21.1-	D48.1	D49.2
- conus medullaris	C72.0	C79.49	-	D33.4	D43.4	D49.7
- cord (true) (vocal)	C32.0	C78.39	D02.0	D14.1	D38.0	D49.1
- - false	C32.1	C78.39	D02.0	D14.1	D38.0	D49.1
- - spermatic	C63.1-	C79.82	D07.69	D29.8	D40.8	D49.59
- - spinal (cervical) (lumbar) (thoracic)	C72.0	C79.49	-	D33.4	D43.4	D49.7
- cornea (limbus)	C69.1-	C79.49	D09.2-	D31.1-	D48.7	D49.89
- corpus						
- - albicans	C56.-	C79.6-	D07.39	D27.-	D39.1-	D49.59
- - callosum, brain	C71.0	C79.31	-	D33.2	D43.2	D49.6
- - cavernosum	C60.2	C79.82	D07.4	D29.0	D40.8	D49.59
- - gastric	C16.2	C78.89	D00.2	D13.1	D37.1	D49.0
- - overlapping sites	C54.8	-	-	-	-	-
- - penis	C60.2	C79.82	D07.4	D29.0	D40.8	D49.59
- - striatum, cerebrum	C71.0	C79.31	-	D33.0	D43.0	D49.6
- - uteri	C54.9	C79.82	D07.0	D26.1	D39.0	D49.59
- - - isthmus	C54.0	C79.82	D07.0	D26.1	D39.0	D49.59
- cortex						
- - adrenal	C74.0-	C79.7-	D09.3	D35.0-	D44.1-	D49.7
- - cerebral	C71.0	C79.31	-	D33.0	D43.0	D49.6
- costal cartilage	C41.3	C79.51	-	D16.7	D48.0	D49.2
- costovertebral joint	C41.3	C79.51	-	D16.7	D48.0	D49.2
- Cowper's gland	C68.0	C79.19	D09.19	D30.4	D41.3	D49.59
- cranial (fossa, any)	C71.9	C79.31	-	D33.2	D43.2	D49.6
- - meninges	C70.0	C79.32	-	D32.0	D42.0	D49.7
- - nerve	C72.50	C79.49	-	D33.3	D43.3	D49.7
- - - specified NEC	C72.59	C79.49	-	D33.3	D43.3	D49.7
- craniobuccal pouch	C75.2	C79.89	D09.3	D35.2	D44.3	D49.7
- craniopharyngeal (duct) (pouch)	C75.2	C79.89	D09.3	D35.3	D44.4	D49.7
- cricoid	C13.0	C79.89	D00.08	D10.7	D37.05	D49.0
- - cartilage	C32.3	C79.89	D02.0	D14.1	D38.0	D49.1
- cricopharynx	C13.0	C79.89	D00.08	D10.7	D37.05	D49.0
- crypt of Morgagni	C21.8	C78.5	D01.3	D12.9	D37.8	D49.0
- crystalline lens	C69.4-	C79.49	D09.2-	D31.4-	D48.7	D49.89
- cul-de-sac (Douglas')	C48.1	C78.6	-	D20.1	D48.4	D49.0
- cuneiform cartilage	C32.3	C78.39	D02.0	D14.1	D38.0	D49.1
- cutaneous—*see Neoplasm, skin*						
- cutis—*see Neoplasm, skin*						
- cystic (bile) duct (common)	C24.0	C78.89	D01.5	D13.5	D37.6	D49.0
- dermis—*see Neoplasm, skin*						
- diaphragm	C49.3	C79.89	-	D21.3	D48.1	D49.2
- digestive organs, system, tube, or tract NEC	C26.9	C78.89	D01.9	D13.9	D37.9	D49.0

	Malignant Primary	Malignant Secondary	CA in Situ	Benign	Uncertain Behavior	Unspecified Behavior
- disc, intervertebral	C41.2	C79.51	-	D16.6	D48.0	D49.2
- disease, generalized	C80.0	-	-	-	-	-
- disseminated	C80.0	-	-	-	-	-
- Douglas' cul-de-sac or pouch	C48.1	C78.6	-	D20.1	D48.4	D49.0
- duodenojejunal junction	C17.8	C78.4	D01.49	D13.39	D37.2	D49.0
- duodenum	C17.0	C78.4	D01.49	D13.2	D37.2	D49.0
- dura (cranial) (mater)	C70.9	C79.49	-	D32.9	D42.9	D49.7
- - cerebral	C70.0	C79.32	-	D32.0	D42.0	D49.7
- - spinal	C70.1	C79.49	-	D32.1	D42.1	D49.7
- ear (external)—see also Neoplasm, skin, ear	C44.20-	C79.2	D04.2-	D23.2-	D48.5	D49.2
- - auricle or auris—see also Neoplasm, skin, ear	C44.20-	C79.2	D04.2-	D23.2-	D48.5	D49.2
- - canal, external—see also Neoplasm, skin, ear	C44.20-	C79.2	D04.2-	D23.2-	D48.5	D49.2
- - cartilage	C49.0	C79.89	-	D21.0	D48.1	D49.2
- external meatus—see also Neoplasm, skin, ear	C44.20-	C79.2	D04.2-	D23.2-	D48.5	D49.2
- - inner	C30.1	C78.39	D02.3	D14.0	D38.5	D49.1
- - lobule—see also Neoplasm, skin, ear	C44.20-	C79.2	D04.2-	D23.2-	D48.5	D49.2
- - middle	C30.1	C78.39	D02.3	D14.0	D38.5	D49.1
- - overlapping lesion with accessory sinuses	C31.8	-	-	-	-	-
- - skin	C44.20-	C79.2	D04.2-	D23.2-	D48.5	D49.2
- - - basal cell carcinoma	C44.21-	-	-	-	-	-
- - - specified type NEC	C44.29-	-	-	-	-	-
- - - squamous cell carcinoma	C44.22-	-	-	-	-	-
- earlobe	C44.20-	C79.2	D04.2-	D23.2-	D48.5	D49.2
- - basal cell carcinoma	C44.21-	-	-	-	-	-
- - specified type NEC	C44.29-	-	-	-	-	-
- - squamous cell carcinoma	C44.22-	-	-	-	-	-
- ejaculatory duct	C63.7	C79.82	D07.69	D29.8	D40.8	D49.59
- elbow NEC	C76.4-	C79.89	D04.6-	D36.7	D48.7	D49.89
- endocardium	C38.0	C79.89	-	D15.1	D48.7	D49.89
- endocervix (canal) (gland)	C53.0	C79.82	D06.0	D26.0	D39.0	D49.59
- endocrine gland NEC	C75.9	C79.89	D09.3	D35.9	D44.9	D49.7
- - pluriglandular	C75.8	C79.89	D09.3	D35.7	D44.9	D49.7
- endometrium (gland) (stroma)	C54.1	C79.82	D07.0	D26.1	D39.0	D49.59
- ensiform cartilage	C41.3	C79.51	-	D16.7	D48.0	D49.2
- enteric—see Neoplasm, intestine						
- ependyma (brain)	C71.5	C79.31	-	D33.0	D43.0	D49.6
- - fourth ventricle	C71.7	C79.31	-	D33.1	D43.1	D49.6
- epicardium	C38.0	C79.89	-	D15.1	D48.7	D49.89
- epididymis	C63.0-	C79.82	D07.69	D29.3-	D40.8	D49.59
- epidural	C72.9	C79.49	-	D33.9	D43.9	D49.7
- epiglottis	C32.1	C78.39	D02.0	D14.1	D38.0	D49.1
- - anterior aspect or surface	C10.1	C79.89	D00.08	D10.5	D37.05	D49.0
- - cartilage	C32.3	C78.39	D02.0	D14.1	D38.0	D49.1
- - free border (margin)	C10.1	C79.89	D00.08	D10.5	D37.05	D49.0
- - junctional region	C10.8	C79.89	D00.08	D10.5	D37.05	D49.0
- - posterior (laryngeal)surface	C32.1	C78.39	D02.0	D14.1	D38.0	D49.1
- - suprahyoid portion	C32.1	C78.39	D02.0	D14.1	D38.0	D49.1
- esophagogastric junction	C16.0	C78.89	D00.2	D13.1	D37.1	D49.0
- esophagus	C15.9	C78.89	D00.1	D13.0	D37.8	D49.0
- - abdominal	C15.5	C78.89	D00.1	D13.0	D37.8	D49.0
- - cervical	C15.3	C78.89	D00.1	D13.0	D37.8	D49.0
- - distal (third)	C15.5	C78.89	D00.1	D13.0	D37.8	D49.0
- - lower (third)	C15.5	C78.89	D00.1	D13.0	D37.8	D49.0
- - middle (third)	C15.4	C78.89	D00.1	D13.0	D37.8	D49.0
- - overlapping lesion	C15.8	-	-	-	-	-
- - proximal (third)	C15.3	C78.89	D00.1	D13.0	D37.8	D49.0
- - thoracic	C15.4	C78.89	D00.1	D13.0	D37.8	D49.0
- - upper (third)	C15.3	C78.89	D00.1	D13.0	D37.8	D49.0
- ethmoid (sinus)	C31.1	C78.39	D02.3	D14.0	D38.5	D49.1
- - bone or labyrinth	C41.0	C79.51	-	D16.4-	D48.0	D49.2
- eustachian tube	C30.1	C78.39	D02.3	D14.0	D38.5	D49.1
- exocervix	C53.1	C79.82	D06.1	D26.0	D39.0	D49.59
- external						
- - meatus (ear)—see also Neoplasm, skin, ear	C44.20-	C79.2	D04.2-	D23.2-	D48.5	D49.2
- - os, cervix uteri	C53.1	C79.82	D06.1	D26.0	D39.0	D49.59
- extradural	C72.9	C79.49	-	D33.9	D43.9	D49.7
- extrahepatic (bile)duct	C24.0	C78.89	D01.5	D13.5	D37.6	D49.0
- - overlapping lesion with gallbladder	C24.8	-	-	-	-	-
- extraocular muscle	C69.6-	C79.49	D09.2-	D31.6-	D48.7	D49.89
- extra rectal	C76.3	C79.89	D09.8	D36.7	D48.7	D49.89
- extremity	C76.8	C79.89	D04.8	D36.7	D48.7	D49.89

	Malignant Primary	Malignant Secondary	CA in Situ	Benign	Uncertain Behavior	Unspecified Behavior
- - lower	C76.5-	C79.89	D04.7-	D36.7	D48.7	D49.89
- - upper	C76.4-	C79.89	D04.6-	D36.7	D48.7	D49.89
- eye NEC	C69.9-	C79.49	D09.2	D31.9	D48.7	D49.89
- - overlapping sites	C69.8	-	-	-	-	-
- eyeball	C69.9-	C79.49	D09.2-	D31.9-	D48.7	D49.89
- eyebrow	C44.309	C79.2	D04.39	D23.39	D48.5	D49.2
- - basal cell carcinoma	C44.319	-	-	-	-	-
- - specified type NEC	C44.399	-	-	-	-	-
- - squamous cell carcinoma	C44.329	-	-	-	-	-
- eyelid (lower) (skin) (upper)	C44.10-	-	-	-	-	-
- - basal cell carcinoma	C44.11-	-	-	-	-	-
- - specified type NEC	C44.19-	-	-	-	-	-
- - squamous cell carcinoma	C44.12-	-	-	-	-	-
- - cartilage	C49.0	C79.89	-	D21.0	D48.1	D49.2
- face NEC	C76.0	C79.89	D04.39	D36.7	D48.7	D49.89
- fallopian tube (accessory)	C57.0-	C79.82	D07.39	D28.2	D39.8	D49.59
- falx (cerebella) (cerebri)	C70.0	C79.32	-	D32.0	D42.0	D49.7
- fascia—see also Neoplasm, connective tissue						
- - palmar	C49.1-	C79.89	-	D21.1-	D48.1	D49.2
- - plantar	C49.2-	C79.89	-	D21.2-	D48.1	D49.2
- fatty tissue—see Neoplasm, connective tissue						
- fauces, faucial NEC	C10.9	C79.89	D00.08	D10.5	D37.05	D49.0
- - pillars	C09.1	C79.89	D00.08	D10.5	D37.05	D49.0
- - tonsil	C09.9	C79.89	D00.08	D10.4	D37.05	D49.0
- femur (any part)	C40.2-	-	-	D16.2-	-	-
- fetal membrane	C58	C79.82	D07.0	D26.7	D39.2	D49.59
- fibrous tissue—see Neoplasm, connective tissue						
- fibula (any part)	C40.2-	C79.51	-	D16.2-	-	-
- filum terminale	C72.0	C79.49	-	D33.4	D43.4	D49.7
- finger NEC	C76.4-	C79.89	D04.6-	D36.7	D48.7	D49.89
- flank NEC	C76.8	C79.89	D04.5	D36.7	D48.7	D49.89
- follicle, nabothian	C53.0	C79.82	D06.0	D26.0	D39.0	D49.59
- foot NEC	C76.5-	C79.89	D04.7-	D36.7	D48.7	D49.89
- forearm NEC	C76.4-	C79.89	D04.6-	D36.7	D48.7	D49.89
- forehead (skin)	C44.309	C79.2	D04.39	D23.39	D48.5	D49.2
- - basal cell carcinoma	C44.319	-	-	-	-	-
- - specified type NEC	C44.399	-	-	-	-	-
- - squamous cell carcinoma	C44.329	-	-	-	-	-
- foreskin	C60.0	C79.82	D07.4	D29.0	D40.8	D49.59
- fornix						
- - pharyngeal	C11.3	C79.89	D00.08	D10.6	D37.05	D49.0
- - vagina	C52	C79.82	D07.2	D28.1	D39.8	D49.59
- fossa (of)						
- - anterior (cranial)	C71.9	C79.31	-	D33.2	D43.2	D49.6
- - cranial	C71.9	C79.31	-	D33.2	D43.2	D49.6
- - ischiorectal	C76.3	C79.89	D09.8	D36.7	D48.7	D49.89
- - middle (cranial)	C71.9	C79.31	-	D33.2	D43.2	D49.6
- - piriform	C12	C79.89	D00.08	D10.7	D37.05	D49.0
- - pituitary	C75.1	C79.89	D09.3	D35.2	D44.3	D49.7
- - posterior (cranial)	C71.9	C79.31	-	D33.2	D43.2	D49.6
- - pterygoid	C49.0	C79.89	-	D21.0	D48.1	D49.2
- - pyriform	C12	C79.89	D00.08	D10.7	D37.05	D49.0
- - Rosenmüller	C11.2	C79.89	D00.08	D10.6	D37.05	D49.0
- - tonsillar	C09.0	C79.89	D00.08	D10.5	D37.05	D49.0
- fourchette	C51.9	C79.82	D07.1	D28.0	D39.8	D49.59
- frenulum						
- - labii—see Neoplasm, lip, internal						
- - linguae	C02.2	C79.89	D00.07	D10.1	D37.02	D49.0
- frontal						
- - bone	C41.0	C79.51	-	D16.4-	D48.0	D49.2
- - lobe, brain	C71.1	C79.31	-	D33.0	D43.0	D49.6
- - pole	C71.1	C79.31	-	D33.0	D43.0	D49.6
- - sinus	C31.2	C78.39	D02.3	D14.0	D38.5	D49.1
- fundus						
- - stomach	C16.1	C78.89	D00.2	D13.1	D37.1	D49.0
- - uterus	C54.3	C79.82	D07.0	D26.1	D39.0	D49.59
- gall duct (extrahepatic)	C24.0	C78.89	D01.5	D13.5	D37.6	D49.0
- - intrahepatic	C22.1	C78.7	D01.5	D13.4	D37.6	D49.0
- gallbladder	C23	C78.89	D01.5	D13.5	D37.6	D49.0
- - overlapping lesion with extrahepatic bile ducts	C24.8	-	-	-	-	-
- ganglia—see also Neoplasm, nerve, peripheral	C47.9	C79.89	-	D36.10	D48.2	D49.2

	Malignant Primary	Malignant Secondary	CA in Situ	Benign	Uncertain Behavior	Unspecified Behavior
- - basal	C71.0	C79.31	-	D33.0	D43.0	D49.6
- - cranial nerve	C72.50	C79.49	-	D33.3	D43.3	D49.7
- Gartner's duct	C52	C79.82	D07.2	D28.1	D39.8	D49.59
- gastric—see Neoplasm, stomach						
- gastrocolic	C26.9	C78.89	D01.9	D13.9	D37.9	D49.0
- gastroesophageal junction	C16.0	C78.89	D00.2	D13.1	D37.1	D49.0
- gastrointestinal (tract)NEC	C26.9	C78.89	D01.9	D13.9	D37.9	D49.0
- generalized	C80.0	-	-	-	-	-
- genital organ or tract						
- - female NEC	C57.9	C79.82	D07.30	D28.9	D39.9	D49.59
- - - overlapping lesion	C57.8	-	-	-	-	-
- - - specified site NEC	C57.7	C79.82	D07.39	D28.7	D39.8	D49.59
- - male NEC	C63.9	C79.82	D07.60	D29.9	D40.9	D49.59
- - - overlapping lesion	C63.8	-	-	-	-	-
- - - specified site NEC	C63.7	C79.82	D07.69	D29.8	D40.8	D49.59
- genitourinary tract						
- - female	C57.9	C79.82	D07.30	D28.9	D39.9	D49.59
- - male	C63.9	C79.82	D07.60	D29.9	D40.9	D49.59
- gingiva (alveolar) (marginal)	C03.9	C79.89	D00.03	D10.39	D37.09	D49.0
- - lower	C03.1	C79.89	D00.03	D10.39	D37.09	D49.0
- - mandibular	C03.1	C79.89	D00.03	D10.39	D37.09	D49.0
- - maxillary	C03.0	C79.89	D00.03	D10.39	D37.09	D49.0
- - upper	C03.0	C79.89	D00.03	D10.39	D37.09	D49.0
- gland, glandular (lymphatic) (system)—see also Neoplasm, lymph gland						
- - endocrine NEC	C75.9	C79.89	D09.3	D35.9	D44.9	D49.7
- - salivary—see Neoplasm, salivary gland						
- glans penis	C60.1	C79.82	D07.4	D29.0	D40.8	D49.59
- globus pallidus	C71.0	C79.31	-	D33.0	D43.0	D49.6
- glomus						
- - coccygeal	C49.5	C79.89	-	D21.5	D48.1	D49.2
- - jugularis	C75.5	C79.89	-	D35.6	D44.7	D49.7
- glosso-epiglottic fold (s)	C10.1	C79.89	D00.08	D10.5	D37.05	D49.0
- glossopalatine fold	C09.1	C79.89	D00.08	D10.5	D37.05	D49.0
- glossopharyngeal sulcus	C09.0	C79.89	D00.08	D10.5	D37.05	D49.0
- glottis	C32.0	C78.39	D02.0	D14.1	D38.0	D49.1
- gluteal region	C76.3	C79.89	D04.5	D36.7	D48.7	D49.89
- great vessels NEC	C49.3	C79.89	-	D21.3	D48.1	D49.2
- groin NEC	C76.3	C79.89	D04.5	D36.7	D48.7	D49.89
- gum	C03.9	C79.89	D00.03	D10.39	D37.09	D49.0
- - lower	C03.1	C79.89	D00.03	D10.39	D37.09	D49.0
- - upper	C03.0	C79.89	D00.03	D10.39	D37.09	D49.0
- hand NEC	C76.4-	C79.89	D04.6-	D36.7	D48.7	D49.89
- head NEC	C76.0	C79.89	D04.4	D36.7	D48.7	D49.89
- heart	C38.0	C79.89	-	D15.1	D48.7	D49.89
- heel NEC	C76.5-	C79.89	D04.7-	D36.7	D48.7	D49.89
- helix—see also Neoplasm, skin, ear	C44.20-	C79.2	D04.2-	D23.2-	D48.5	D49.2
- hematopoietic, hemopoietic tissue NEC	C96.9	-	-	-	-	-
- - specified NEC	C96.Z	-	-	-	-	-
- hemisphere, cerebral	C71.0	C79.31	-	D33.0	D43.0	D49.6
- hemorrhoidal zone	C21.1	C78.5	D01.3	D12.9	D37.8	D49.0
- hepatic—see also Index to disease, by histology	C22.9	C78.7	D01.5	D13.4	D37.6	D49.0
- - duct (bile)	C24.0	C78.89	D01.5	D13.5	D37.6	D49.0
- - flexure (colon)	C18.3	C78.5	D01.0	D12.3	D37.4	D49.0
- - primary	C22.8	C78.7	D01.5	D13.4	D37.6	D49.0
- hepatobiliary	C24.9	C78.89	D01.5	D13.5	D37.6	D49.0
- hepatoblastoma	C22.2	C78.7	D01.5	D13.4	D37.6	D49.0
- hepatoma	C22.0	C78.7	D01.5	D13.4	D37.6	D49.0
- hilus of lung	C34.0-	C78.0-	D02.2-	D14.3-	D38.1	D49.1
- hip NEC	C76.5-	C79.89	D04.7-	D36.7	D48.7	D49.89
- hippocampus, brain	C71.2	C79.31	-	D33.0	D43.0	D49.6
- humerus (any part)	C40.0-	C79.51	-	D16.0-	-	-
- hymen	C52	C79.82	D07.2	D28.1	D39.8	D49.59
- hypopharynx, hypopharyngeal NEC	C13.9	C79.89	D00.08	D10.7	D37.05	D49.0
- - overlapping lesion	C13.8	-	-	-	-	-
- - postcricoid region	C13.0	C79.89	D00.08	D10.7	D37.05	D49.0
- - posterior wall	C13.2	C79.89	D00.08	D10.7	D37.05	D49.0
- - pyriform fossa (sinus)	C12	C79.89	D00.08	D10.7	D37.05	D49.0
- hypophysis	C75.1	C79.89	D09.3	D35.2	D44.3	D49.7
- hypothalamus	C71.0	C79.31	-	D33.0	D43.0	D49.6
- ileocecum, ileocecal (coil) (junction) (valve)	C18.0	C78.5	D01.0	D12.0	D37.4	D49.0

	Malignant Primary	Malignant Secondary	CA in Situ	Benign	Uncertain Behavior	Unspecified Behavior
- ileum	C17.2	C78.4	D01.49	D13.39	D37.2	D49.0
- ilium	C41.4	C79.51	-	D16.8	D48.0	D49.2
- immunoproliferative NEC	C88.9	-	-	-	-	-
- infraclavicular (region)	C76.1	C79.89	D04.5	D36.7	D48.7	D49.89
- inguinal (region)	C76.3	C79.89	D04.5	D36.7	D48.7	D49.89
- insula	C71.0	C79.31	-	D33.0	D43.0	D49.6
- insular tissue (pancreas)	C25.4	C78.89	D01.7	D13.7	D37.8	D49.0
- - brain	C71.0	C79.31	-	D33.0	D43.0	D49.6
- interarytenoid fold	C13.1	C79.89	D00.08	D10.7	D37.05	D49.0
- - hypopharyngeal aspect	C13.1	C79.89	D00.08	D10.7	D37.05	D49.0
- - laryngeal aspect	C32.1	C79.89	D02.0	D14.1	D38.0	D49.1
- - marginal zone	C13.1	C79.89	D00.08	D10.7	D37.05	D49.0
- interdental papillae	C03.9	C79.89	D00.03	D10.39	D37.09	D49.0
- - lower	C03.1	C79.89	D00.03	D10.39	D37.09	D49.0
- - upper	C03.0	C79.89	D00.03	D10.39	D37.09	D49.0
- internal						
- - capsule	C71.0	C79.31	-	D33.0	D43.0	D49.6
- - os (cervix)	C53.0	C79.82	D06.0	D26.0	D39.0	D49.59
- intervertebral cartilage or disc	C41.2	C79.51	-	D16.6	D48.0	D49.2
- intestine, intestinal	C26.0	C78.80	D01.40	D13.9	D37.8	D49.0
- - large	C18.9	C78.5	D01.0	D12.6	D37.4	D49.0
- - - appendix	C18.1	C78.5	D01.0	D12.1	D37.3	D49.0
- - - caput coli	C18.0	C78.5	D01.0	D12.0	D37.4	D49.0
- - - cecum	C18.0	C78.5	D01.0	D12.0	D37.4	D49.0
- - - colon	C18.9	C78.5	D01.0	D12.6	D37.4	D49.0
- - - - and rectum	C19	C78.5	D01.1	D12.7	D37.5	D49.0
- - - - ascending	C18.2	C78.5	D01.0	D12.2	D37.4	D49.0
- - - - caput	C18.0	C78.5	D01.0	D12.0	D37.4	D49.0
- - - - descending	C18.6	C78.5	D01.0	D12.4	D37.4	D49.0
- - - - distal	C18.6	C78.5	D01.0	D12.4	D37.4	D49.0
- - - - left	C18.6	C78.5	D01.0	D12.4	D37.4	D49.0
- - - - overlapping lesion	C18.8	-	-	-	-	-
- - - - pelvic	C18.7	C78.5	D01.0	D12.5	D37.4	D49.0
- - - - right	C18.2	C78.5	D01.0	D12.2	D37.4	D49.0
- - - - sigmoid (flexure)	C18.7	C78.5	D01.0	D12.5	D37.4	D49.0
- - - - transverse	C18.4	C78.5	D01.0	D12.3	D37.4	D49.0
- - - hepatic flexure	C18.3	C78.5	D01.0	D12.3	D37.4	D49.0
- - - ileocecum, ileocecal (coil) (valve)	C18.0	C78.5	D01.0	D12.0	D37.4	D49.0
- - - overlapping lesion	C18.8	-	-	-	-	-
- - - sigmoid flexure (lower) (upper)	C18.7	C78.5	D01.0	D12.5	D37.4	D49.0
- - - splenic flexure	C18.5	C78.5	D01.0	D12.3	D37.4	D49.0
- - small	C17.9	C78.4	D01.40	D13.30	D37.2	D49.0
- - - duodenum	C17.0	C78.4	D01.49	D13.2	D37.2	D49.0
- - - ileum	C17.2	C78.4	D01.49	D13.39	D37.2	D49.0
- - - jejunum	C17.1	C78.4	D01.49	D13.39	D37.2	D49.0
- - - overlapping lesion	C17.8	-	-	-	-	-
- - tract NEC	C26.0	C78.89	D01.40	D13.9	D37.8	D49.0
- intra-abdominal	C76.2	C79.89	D09.8	D36.7	D48.7	D49.89
- intracranial NEC	C71.9	C79.31	-	D33.2	D43.2	D49.6
- intrahepatic (bile)duct	C22.1	C78.7	D01.5	D13.4	D37.6	D49.0
- intraocular	C69.9-	C79.49	D09.2-	D31.9-	D48.7	D49.89
- intraorbital	C69.6-	C79.49	D09.2-	D31.6-	D48.7	D49.89
- intrasellar	C75.1	C79.89	D09.3	D35.2	D44.3	D49.7
- intrathoracic (cavity) (organs)	C76.1	C79.89	D09.8	D15.9	D48.7	D49.89
- - specified NEC	C76.1	C79.89	D09.8	D15.7	-	-
- iris	C69.4-	C79.49	D09.2-	D31.4-	D48.7	D49.89
- ischiorectal (fossa)	C76.3	C79.89	D09.8	D36.7	D48.7	D49.89
- ischium	C41.4	C79.51	-	D16.8	D48.0	D49.2
- island of Reil	C71.0	C79.31	-	D33.0	D43.0	D49.6
- islands or islets of Langerhans	C25.4	C78.89	D01.7	D13.7	D37.8	D49.0
- isthmus uteri	C54.0	C79.82	D07.0	D26.1	D39.0	D49.59
- jaw	C76.0	C79.89	D09.8	D36.7	D48.7	D49.89
- - bone	C41.1	C79.51	-	D16.5-	D48.0	D49.2
- - - lower	C41.1	C79.51	-	D16.5-	-	-
- - - upper	C41.0	C79.51	-	D16.4-	-	-
- - carcinoma (any type) (lower) (upper)	C76.0	C79.89	-	-	-	-
- - skin—*see also* Neoplasm, skin, face	C44.309	C79.2	D04.39	D23.39	D48.5	D49.2
- - soft tissues	C03.9	C79.89	D00.03	D10.39	D37.09	D49.0
- - - lower	C03.1	C79.89	D00.03	D10.39	D37.09	D49.0
- - - upper	C03.0	C79.89	D00.03	D10.39	D37.09	D49.0
- jejunum	C17.1	C78.4	D01.49	D13.39	D37.2	D49.0

	Malignant Primary	Malignant Secondary	CA in Situ	Benign	Uncertain Behavior	Unspecified Behavior
- joint NEC—*see also Neoplasm, bone*	C41.9	C79.51	-	D16.9-	D48.0	D49.2
- - acromioclavicular	C40.0-	C79.51	-	D16.0-	-	-
- - bursa or synovial membrane—*see Neoplasm, connective tissue*						
- - costovertebral	C41.3	C79.51	-	D16.7	D48.0	D49.2
- - sternocostal	C41.3	C79.51	-	D16.7	D48.0	D49.2
- - temporomandibular	C41.1	C79.51	-	D16.5-	D48.0	D49.2
- junction						
- - anorectal	C21.8	C78.5	D01.3	D12.9	D37.8	D49.0
- - cardioesophageal	C16.0	C78.89	D00.2	D13.1	D37.1	D49.0
- - esophagogastric	C16.0	C78.89	D00.2	D13.1	D37.1	D49.0
- - gastroesophageal	C16.0	C78.89	D00.2	D13.1	D37.1	D49.0
- - hard and soft palate	C05.9	C79.89	D00.00	D10.39	D37.09	D49.0
- - ileocecal	C18.0	C78.5	D01.0	D12.0	D37.4	D49.0
- - pelvirectal	C19	C78.5	D01.1	D12.7	D37.5	D49.0
- - pelviureteric	C65.-	C79.0-	D09.19	D30.1-	D41.1-	D49.59
- - rectosigmoid	C19	C78.5	D01.1	D12.7	D37.5	D49.0
- - squamocolumnar, of cervix	C53.8	C79.82	D06.7	D26.0	D39.0	D49.59
- Kaposi's sarcoma—*see Kaposi's, sarcoma*						
- kidney (parenchymal)	C64.-	C79.0-	D09.19	D30.0-	D41.0-	D49.51
- - calyx	C65.-	C79.0-	D09.19	D30.1-	D41.1-	D49.51
- - hilus	C65.-	C79.0-	D09.19	D30.1-	D41.1-	D49.51
- - pelvis	C65.-	C79.0-	D09.19	D30.1-	D41.1-	D49.51
- knee NEC	C76.5-	C79.89	D04.7-	D36.7	D48.7	D49.89
- labia (skin)	C51.9	C79.82	D07.1	D28.0	D39.8	D49.59
- - majora	C51.0	C79.82	D07.1	D28.0	D39.8	D49.59
- - minora	C51.1	C79.82	D07.1	D28.0	D39.8	D49.59
- labial—*see also Neoplasm, lip*	C00.9	C79.89	D00.01	D10.0	D37.01	D49.0
- - sulcus (lower) (upper)	C06.1	C79.89	D00.02	D10.39	D37.09	D49.0
- labium (skin)	C51.9	C79.82	D07.1	D28.0	D39.8	D49.59
- - majus	C51.0	C79.82	D07.1	D28.0	D39.8	D49.59
- - minus	C51.1	C79.82	D07.1	D28.0	D39.8	D49.59
- lacrimal						
- - canaliculi	C69.5-	C79.49	D09.2-	D31.5-	D48.7	D49.89
- - duct (nasal)	C69.5-	C79.49	D09.2-	D31.5-	D48.7	D49.89
- - gland	C69.5-	C79.49	D09.2-	D31.5-	D48.7	D49.89
- - punctum	C69.5-	C79.49	D09.2-	D31.5-	D48.7	D49.89
- - sac	C69.5-	C79.49	D09.2-	D31.5-	D48.7	D49.89
- Langerhans, islands or islets	C25.4	C78.89	D01.7	D13.7	D37.8	D49.0
- laryngopharynx	C13.9	C79.89	D00.08	D10.7	D37.05	D49.0
- larynx, laryngeal NEC	C32.9	C78.39	D02.0	D14.1	D38.0	D49.1
- - aryepiglottic fold	C32.1	C78.39	D02.0	D14.1	D38.0	D49.1
- - cartilage (arytenoid) (cricoid) (cuneiform) (thyroid)	C32.3	C78.39	D02.0	D14.1	D38.0	D49.1
- - commissure (anterior) (posterior)	C32.0	C78.39	D02.0	D14.1	D38.0	D49.1
- - extrinsic NEC	C32.1	C78.39	D02.0	D14.1	D38.0	D49.1
- - - meaning hypopharynx	C13.9	C79.89	D00.08	D10.7	D37.05	D49.0
- - interarytenoid fold	C32.1	C78.39	D02.0	D14.1	D38.0	D49.1
- - intrinsic	C32.0	C78.39	D02.0	D14.1	D38.0	D49.1
- - overlapping lesion	C32.8	-	-	-	-	-
- - ventricular band	C32.1	C78.39	D02.0	D14.1	D38.0	D49.1
- leg NEC	C76.5-	C79.89	D04.7-	D36.7	D48.7	D49.89
- lens, crystalline	C69.4-	C79.49	D09.2-	D31.4-	D48.7	D49.89
- lid (lower) (upper)	C44.10-	C79.2	D04.1-	D23.1-	D48.5	D49.2
- - basal cell carcinoma	C44.11-	-	-	-	-	-
- - specified type NEC	C44.19-	-	-	-	-	-
- - squamous cell carcinoma	C44.12-	-	-	-	-	-
- ligament—*see also Neoplasm, connective tissue*						
- - broad	C57.1	C79.82	D07.39	D28.2	D39.8	D49.59
- - Mackenrodt's	C57.7	C79.82	D07.39	D28.7	D39.8	D49.59
- - non-uterine—*see Neoplasm, connective tissue*						
- - round	C57.2	C79.82	-	D28.2	D39.8	D49.59
- - sacro-uterine	C57.3	C79.82	-	D28.2	D39.8	D49.59
- - uterine	C57.3	C79.82	-	D28.2	D39.8	D49.59
- - utero-ovarian	C57.7	C79.82	D07.39	D28.2	D39.8	D49.59
- - uterosacral	C57.3	C79.82	-	D28.2	D39.8	D49.59
- limb	C76.8	C79.89	D04.8	D36.7	D48.7	D49.89
- - lower	C76.5-	C79.89	D04.7-	D36.7	D48.7	D49.89
- - upper	C76.4-	C79.89	D04.6-	D36.7	D48.7	D49.89
- limbus of cornea	C69.1-	C79.49	D09.2-	D31.1-	D48.7	D49.89
- lingual NEC—*see also Neoplasm, tongue*	C02.9	C79.89	D00.07	D10.1	D37.02	D49.0
- lingula, lung	C34.1-	C78.0-	D02.2-	D14.3-	D38.1	D49.1

	Malignant Primary	Malignant Secondary	CA in Situ	Benign	Uncertain Behavior	Unspecified Behavior
- lip	C00.9	C79.89	D00.01	D10.0	D37.01	D49.0
- - buccal aspect—*see Neoplasm, lip, internal*						
- - commissure	C00.6	C79.89	D00.01	D10.0	D37.01	D49.0
- - external	C00.2	C79.89	D00.01	D10.0	D37.01	D49.0
- - - lower	C00.1	C79.89	D00.01	D10.0	D37.01	D49.0
- - - upper	C00.0	C79.89	D00.01	D10.0	D37.01	D49.0
- - frenulum—*see Neoplasm, lip, internal*						
- - inner aspect—*see Neoplasm, lip, internal*						
- - internal	C00.5	C79.89	D00.01	D10.0	D37.01	D49.0
- - - lower	C00.4	C79.89	D00.01	D10.0	D37.01	D49.0
- - - upper	C00.3	C79.89	D00.01	D10.0	D37.01	D49.0
- - lipstick area	C00.2	C79.89	D00.01	D10.0	D37.01	D49.0
- - - lower	C00.1	C79.89	D00.01	D10.0	D37.01	D49.0
- - - upper	C00.0	C79.89	D00.01	D10.0	D37.01	D49.0
- - lower	C00.1	C79.89	D00.01	D10.0	D37.01	D49.0
- - - internal	C00.4	C79.89	D00.01	D10.0	D37.01	D49.0
- - mucosa—*see Neoplasm, lip, internal*						
- - oral aspect—*see Neoplasm, lip, internal*						
- - overlapping lesion	C00.8	-	-	-	-	-
- - - with oral cavity or pharynx	C14.8	-	-	-	-	-
- - skin (commissure) (lower) (upper)	C44.00	C79.2	D04.0	D23.0	D48.5	D49.2
- - - basal cell carcinoma	C44.01	-	-	-	-	-
- - - specified type NEC	C44.09	-	-	-	-	-
- - - squamous cell carcinoma	C44.02	-	-	-	-	-
- - upper	C00.0	C79.89	D00.01	D10.0	D37.01	D49.0
- - - internal	C00.3	C79.89	D00.01	D10.0	D37.01	D49.0
- - vermilion border	C00.2	C79.89	D00.01	D10.0	D37.01	D49.0
- - - lower	C00.1	C79.89	D00.01	D10.0	D37.01	D49.0
- - - upper	C00.0	C79.89	D00.01	D10.0	D37.01	D49.0
- lipomatous—*see Lipoma, by site*						
- liver—*see also Index to disease, by histology*	C22.9	C78.7	D01.5	D13.4	D37.6	D49.0
- - primary	C22.8	C78.7	D01.5	D13.4	D37.6	D49.0
- lumbosacral plexus	C47.5	C79.89	-	D36.16	D48.2	D49.2
- lung	C34.9-	C78.0-	D02.2-	D14.3-	D38.1	D49.1
- - azygos lobe	C34.1-	C78.0-	D02.2-	D14.3-	D38.1	D49.1
- - carina	C34.0-	C78.0-	D02.2-	D14.3-	D38.1	D49.1
- - hilus	C34.0-	C78.0-	D02.2-	D14.3-	D38.1	D49.1
- - lingula	C34.1-	C78.0-	D02.2-	D14.3-	D38.1	D49.1
- - lobe NEC	C34.9-	C78.0-	D02.2-	D14.3-	D38.1	D49.1
- - lower lobe	C34.3-	C78.0-	D02.2-	D14.3-	D38.1	D49.1
- - main bronchus	C34.0-	C78.0-	D02.2-	D14.3-	D38.1	D49.1
- - mesothelioma—*see Mesothelioma*						
- - middle lobe	C34.2	C78.0-	D02.21	D14.31	D38.1	D49.1
- - overlapping lesion	C34.8-	-	-	-	-	-
- - upper lobe	C34.1-	C78.0-	D02.2-	D14.3-	D38.1	D49.1
- lymph, lymphatic channel NEC	C49.9	C79.89	-	D21.9	D48.1	D49.2
- - gland (secondary)	-	C77.9	-	D36.0	D48.7	D49.89
- - - abdominal	-	C77.2	-	D36.0	D48.7	D49.89
- - - aortic	-	C77.2	-	D36.0	D48.7	D49.89
- - - arm	-	C77.3	-	D36.0	D48.7	D49.89
- - - auricular (anterior) (posterior)	-	C77.0	-	D36.0	D48.7	D49.89
- - - axilla, axillary	-	C77.3	-	D36.0	D48.7	D49.89
- - - brachial	-	C77.3	-	D36.0	D48.7	D49.89
- - - bronchial	-	C77.1	-	D36.0	D48.7	D49.89
- - - bronchopulmonary	-	C77.1	-	D36.0	D48.7	D49.89
- - - celiac	-	C77.2	-	D36.0	D48.7	D49.89
- - - cervical	-	C77.0	-	D36.0	D48.7	D49.89
- - - cervicofacial	-	C77.0	-	D36.0	D48.7	D49.89
- - - Cloquet	-	C77.4	-	D36.0	D48.7	D49.89
- - - colic	-	C77.2	-	D36.0	D48.7	D49.89
- - - common duct	-	C77.2	-	D36.0	D48.7	D49.89
- - - cubital	-	C77.3	-	D36.0	D48.7	D49.89
- - - diaphragmatic	-	C77.1	-	D36.0	D48.7	D49.89
- - - epigastric, inferior	-	C77.1	-	D36.0	D48.7	D49.89
- - - epitrochlear	-	C77.3	-	D36.0	D48.7	D49.89
- - - esophageal	-	C77.1	-	D36.0	D48.7	D49.89
- - - face	-	C77.0	-	D36.0	D48.7	D49.89
- - - femoral	-	C77.4	-	D36.0	D48.7	D49.89
- - - gastric	-	C77.2	-	D36.0	D48.7	D49.89
- - - groin	-	C77.4	-	D36.0	D48.7	D49.89
- - - head	-	C77.0	-	D36.0	D48.7	D49.89

	Malignant Primary	Malignant Secondary	CA in Situ	Benign	Uncertain Behavior	Unspecified Behavior
- - - hepatic	-	C77.2	-	D36.0	D48.7	D49.89
- - - hilar (pulmonary)	-	C77.1	-	D36.0	D48.7	D49.89
- - - - splenic	-	C77.2	-	D36.0	D48.7	D49.89
- - - hypogastric	-	C77.5	-	D36.0	D48.7	D49.89
- - - ileocolic	-	C77.2	-	D36.0	D48.7	D49.89
- - - iliac	-	C77.5	-	D36.0	D48.7	D49.89
- - - infraclavicular	-	C77.3	-	D36.0	D48.7	D49.89
- - - - inguina, inguinal	-	C77.4	-	D36.0	D48.7	D49.89
- - - innominate	-	C77.1	-	D36.0	D48.7	D49.89
- - - intercostal	-	C77.1	-	D36.0	D48.7	D49.89
- - - intestinal	-	C77.2	-	D36.0	D48.7	D49.89
- - - intraabdominal	-	C77.2	-	D36.0	D48.7	D49.89
- - - intrapelvic	-	C77.5	-	D36.0	D48.7	D49.89
- - - intrathoracic	-	C77.1	-	D36.0	D48.7	D49.89
- - - - jugular	-	C77.0	-	D36.0	D48.7	D49.89
- - - leg	-	C77.4	-	D36.0	D48.7	D49.89
- - - limb						
- - - - lower	-	C77.4	-	D36.0	D48.7	D49.89
- - - - upper	-	C77.3	-	D36.0	D48.7	D49.89
- - - lower limb	-	C77.4	-	D36.0	D48.7	D49.89
- - - lumbar	-	C77.2	-	D36.0	D48.7	D49.89
- - - mandibular	-	C77.0	-	D36.0	D48.7	D49.89
- - - mediastinal	-	C77.1	-	D36.0	D48.7	D49.89
- - - mesenteric (inferior) (superior)	-	C77.2	-	D36.0	D48.7	D49.89
- - - midcolic	-	C77.2	-	D36.0	D48.7	D49.89
- - - multiple sites in categories C77.0 - C77.5	-	C77.8	-	D36.0	D48.7	D49.89
- - - neck	-	C77.0	-	D36.0	D48.7	D49.89
- - - obturator	-	C77.5	-	D36.0	D48.7	D49.89
- - - occipital	-	C77.0	-	D36.0	D48.7	D49.89
- - - pancreatic	-	C77.2	-	D36.0	D48.7	D49.89
- - - para-aortic	-	C77.2	-	D36.0	D48.7	D49.89
- - - paracervical	-	C77.5	-	D36.0	D48.7	D49.89
- - - parametrial	-	C77.5	-	D36.0	D48.7	D49.89
- - - parasternal	-	C77.1	-	D36.0	D48.7	D49.89
- - - parotid	-	C77.0	-	D36.0	D48.7	D49.89
- - - pectoral	-	C77.3	-	D36.0	D48.7	D49.89
- - - pelvic	-	C77.5	-	D36.0	D48.7	D49.89
- - - peri-aortic	-	C77.2	-	D36.0	D48.7	D49.89
- - - peripancreatic	-	C77.2	-	D36.0	D48.7	D49.89
- - - popliteal	-	C77.4	-	D36.0	D48.7	D49.89
- - - porta hepatis	-	C77.2	-	D36.0	D48.7	D49.89
- - - portal	-	C77.2	-	D36.0	D48.7	D49.89
- - - preauricular	-	C77.0	-	D36.0	D48.7	D49.89
- - - prelaryngeal	-	C77.0	-	D36.0	D48.7	D49.89
- - - presymphyseal	-	C77.5	-	D36.0	D48.7	D49.89
- - - pretracheal	-	C77.0	-	D36.0	D48.7	D49.89
- - - primary (any site)NEC	C96.9	-	-	-	-	-
- - - pulmonary (hiler)	-	C77.1	-	D36.0	D48.7	D49.89
- - - pyloric	-	C77.2	-	D36.0	D48.7	D49.89
- - - retroperitoneal	-	C77.2	-	D36.0	D48.7	D49.89
- - - retropharyngeal	-	C77.0	-	D36.0	D48.7	D49.89
- - - Rosenmüller's	-	C77.4	-	D36.0	D48.7	D49.89
- - - sacral	-	C77.5	-	D36.0	D48.7	D49.89
- - - scalene	-	C77.0	-	D36.0	D48.7	D49.89
- - - site NEC	-	C77.9	-	D36.0	D48.7	D49.89
- - - splenic (hilar)	-	C77.2	-	D36.0	D48.7	D49.89
- - - subclavicular	-	C77.3	-	D36.0	D48.7	D49.89
- - - subinguinal	-	C77.4	-	D36.0	D48.7	D49.89
- - - sublingual	-	C77.0	-	D36.0	D48.7	D49.89
- - - submandibular	-	C77.0	-	D36.0	D48.7	D49.89
- - - submaxillary	-	C77.0	-	D36.0	D48.7	D49.89
- - - submental	-	C77.0	-	D36.0	D48.7	D49.89
- - - subscapular	-	C77.3	-	D36.0	D48.7	D49.89
- - - supraclavicular	-	C77.0	-	D36.0	D48.7	D49.89
- - - thoracic	-	C77.1	-	D36.0	D48.7	D49.89
- - - tibial	-	C77.4	-	D36.0	D48.7	D49.89
- - - tracheal	-	C77.1	-	D36.0	D48.7	D49.89
- - - tracheobronchial	-	C77.1	-	D36.0	D48.7	D49.89
- - - upper limb	-	C77.3	-	D36.0	D48.7	D49.89
- - - Virchow's	-	C77.0	-	D36.0	D48.7	D49.89
- - node—*see also Neoplasm, lymph gland*						

	Malignant Primary	Malignant Secondary	CA in Situ	Benign	Uncertain Behavior	Unspecified Behavior
- - - primary NEC	C96.9	-	-	-	-	-
- - vessel—*see also Neoplasm, connective tissue*	C49.9	C79.89	-	D21.9	D48.1	D49.2
- Mackenrodt's ligament	C57.7	C79.82	D07.39	D28.7	D39.8	D49.59
- malar	C41.0	C79.51		D16.4-	D48.0	D49.2
- - region—*see Neoplasm, cheek*						
- mammary gland—*see Neoplasm, breast*						
- mandible	C41.1	C79.51	-	D16.5-	D48.0	D49.2
- - alveolar						
- - - mucosa (carcinoma)	C03.1	C79.89	D00.03	D10.39	D37.09	D49.0
- - - ridge or process	C41.1	C79.51	-	D16.5-	D48.0	D49.2
- marrow (bone)NEC	C96.9	C79.52	-	-	D47.9	D49.89
- mastectomy site (skin)—*see also Neoplasm, breast, skin*	C44.501	C79.2	-	-	-	-
- - specified as breast tissue	C50.8-	C79.81	-	-	-	-
- mastoid (air cells) (antrum) (cavity)	C30.1	C78.39	D02.3	D14.0	D38.5	D49.1
- - bone or process	C41.0	C79.51	-	D16.4-	D48.0	D49.2
- maxilla, maxillary (superior)	C41.0	C79.51	-	D16.4-	D48.0	D49.2
- - alveolar						
- - - mucosa	C03.0	C79.89	D00.03	D10.39	D37.09	D49.0
- - - ridge or process (carcinoma)	C41.0	C79.51	-	D16.4-	D48.0	D49.2
- - antrum	C31.0	C78.39	D02.3	D14.0	D38.5	D49.1
- - carcinoma	C03.0	C79.51	-	-	-	-
- - inferior—*see Neoplasm, mandible*						
- - sinus	C31.0	C78.39	D02.3	D14.0	D38.5	D49.1
- meatus external (ear)—*see also Neoplasm, skin, ear*	C44.20-	C79.2	D04.2-	D23.2-	D48.5	D49.2
- Meckel diverticulum, malignant	C17.3	C78.4	D01.49	D13.39	D37.2	D49.0
- mediastinum, mediastinal	C38.3	C78.1	-	D15.2	D38.3	D49.89
- - anterior	C38.1	C78.1	-	D15.2	D38.3	D49.89
- - posterior	C38.2	C78.1	-	D15.2	D38.3	D49.89
- medulla						
- - adrenal	C74.1-	C79.7-	D09.3	D35.0-	D44.1-	D49.7
- - oblongata	C71.7	C79.31	-	D33.1	D43.1	D49.6
- meibomian gland	C44.10-	C79.2	D04.1-	D23.1-	D48.5	D49.2
- - basal cell carcinoma	C44.11-	-	-	-	-	-
- - specified type NEC	C44.19-	-	-	-	-	-
- - squamous cell carcinoma	C44.12-	-	-	-	-	-
- melanoma—*see Melanoma*						
- meninges	C70.9	C79.49	-	D32.9	D42.9	D49.7
- - brain	C70.0	C79.32	-	D32.0	D42.0	D49.7
- - cerebral	C70.0	C79.32	-	D32.0	D42.0	D49.7
- - cranial	C70.0	C79.32	-	D32.0	D42.0	D49.7
- - intracranial	C70.0	C79.32	-	D32.0	D42.0	D49.7
- - spinal (cord)	C70.1	C79.49	-	D32.1	D42.1	D49.7
- meniscus, knee joint (lateral) (medial)	C40.2-	C79.51	-	D16.2-	D48.0	D49.2
- Merkel cell—*see Carcinoma, Merkel cell*						
- mesentery, mesenteric	C48.1	C78.6	-	D20.1	D48.4	D49.0
- mesoappendix	C48.1	C78.6	-	D20.1	D48.4	D49.0
- mesocolon	C48.1	C78.6	-	D20.1	D48.4	D49.0
- mesopharynx—*see Neoplasm, oropharynx*						
- mesosalpinx	C57.1	C79.82	D07.39	D28.2	D39.8	D49.59
- mesothelial tissue—*see Mesothelioma*						
- mesothelioma—*see Mesothelioma*						
- mesovarium	C57.1	C79.82	D07.39	D28.2	D39.8	D49.59
- metacarpus (any bone)	C40.1-	C79.51	-	D16.1-	-	-
- metastatic NEC—*see also Neoplasm, by site, secondary*	-	C79.9	-	-	-	-
- metatarsus (any bone)	C40.3-	C79.51	-	D16.3-	-	-
- midbrain	C71.7	C79.31	-	D33.1	D43.1	D49.6
- milk duct—*see Neoplasm, breast*						
- mons						
- - pubis	C51.9	C79.82	D07.1	D28.0	D39.8	D49.59
- - veneris	C51.9	C79.82	D07.1	D28.0	D39.8	D49.59
- motor tract	C72.9	C79.49	-	D33.9	D43.9	D49.7
- - brain	C71.9	C79.31	-	D33.2	D43.2	D49.6
- - cauda equina	C72.1	C79.49	-	D33.4	D43.4	D49.7
- - spinal	C72.0	C79.49	-	D33.4	D43.4	D49.7
- mouth	C06.9	C79.89	D00.00	D10.30	D37.09	D49.0
- - book-leaf	C06.89	C79.89	-	-	-	-
- - floor	C04.9	C79.89	D00.06	D10.2	D37.09	D49.0
- - - anterior portion	C04.0	C79.89	D00.06	D10.2	D37.09	D49.0
- - - lateral portion	C04.1	C79.89	D00.06	D10.2	D37.09	D49.0

	Malignant Primary	Malignant Secondary	CA in Situ	Benign	Uncertain Behavior	Unspecified Behavior
- - - overlapping lesion	C04.8	-	-	-	-	-
- - overlapping NEC	C06.80	-	-	-	-	-
- - roof	C05.9	C79.89	D00.00	D10.39	D37.09	D49.0
- - specified part NEC	C06.89	C79.89	D00.00	D10.39	D37.09	D49.0
- - vestibule	C06.1	C79.89	D00.00	D10.39	D37.09	D49.0
- mucosa						
- - alveolar (ridge or process)	C03.9	C79.89	D00.03	D10.39	D37.09	D49.0
- - - lower	C03.1	C79.89	D00.03	D10.39	D37.09	D49.0
- - - upper	C03.0	C79.89	D00.03	D10.39	D37.09	D49.0
- - buccal	C06.0	C79.89	D00.02	D10.39	D37.09	D49.0
- - cheek	C06.0	C79.89	D00.02	D10.39	D37.09	D49.0
- - lip—*see Neoplasm, lip, internal*						
- - nasal	C30.0	C78.39	D02.3	D14.0	D38.5	D49.1
- - oral	C06.0	C79.89	D00.02	D10.39	D37.09	D49.0
- Mullerian duct						
- - female	C57.7	C79.82	D07.39	D28.7	D39.8	D49.59
- - male	C63.7	C79.82	D07.69	D29.8	D40.8	D49.59
- muscle—*see also Neoplasm, connective tissue*						
- - extraocular	C69.6-	C79.49	D09.2-	D31.6-	D48.7	D49.89
- myocardium	C38.0	C79.89	-	D15.1	D48.7	D49.89
- myometrium	C54.2	C79.82	D07.0	D26.1	D39.0	D49.59
- myopericardium	C38.0	C79.89	-	D15.1	D48.7	D49.89
- nabothian gland (follicle)	C53.0	C79.82	D06.0	D26.0	D39.0	D49.59
- nail—*see also Neoplasm, skin, limb*	C44.90	C79.2	D04.9	D23.9	D48.5	D49.2
- - finger—*see also Neoplasm, skin, limb, upper*	C44.60-	C79.2	D04.6-	D23.6-	D48.5	D49.2
- - toe—*see also Neoplasm, skin, limb, lower*	C44.70-	C79.2	D04.7-	D23.7-	D48.5	D49.2
- nares, naris (anterior) (posterior)	C30.0	C78.39	D02.3	D14.0	D38.5	D49.1
- nasal—*see Neoplasm, nose*						
- nasolabial groove—*see also Neoplasm, skin, face*	C44.309	C79.2	D04.39	D23.39	D48.5	D49.2
- nasolacrimal duct	C69.5-	C79.49	D09.2-	D31.5-	D48.7	D49.89
- nasopharynx, nasopharyngeal	C11.9	C79.89	D00.08	D10.6	D37.05	D49.0
- - floor	C11.3	C79.89	D00.08	D10.6	D37.05	D49.0
- - overlapping lesion	C11.8	-	-	-	-	-
- - roof	C11.0	C79.89	D00.08	D10.6	D37.05	D49.0
- - wall	C11.9	C79.89	D00.08	D10.6	D37.05	D49.0
- - - anterior	C11.3	C79.89	D00.08	D10.6	D37.05	D49.0
- - - lateral	C11.2	C79.89	D00.08	D10.6	D37.05	D49.0
- - - posterior	C11.1	C79.89	D00.08	D10.6	D37.05	D49.0
- - - superior	C11.0	C79.89	D00.08	D10.6	D37.05	D49.0
- nates—*see also Neoplasm, skin, trunk*	C44.509	C79.2	D04.5	D23.5	D48.5	D49.2
- neck NEC	C76.0	C79.89	D09.8	D36.7	D48.7	D49.89
- - skin	C44.40	-	-	-	-	-
- - - basal cell carcinoma	C44.41	-	-	-	-	-
- - - specified type NEC	C44.49	-	-	-	-	-
- - - squamous cell carcinoma	C44.42	-	-	-	-	-
- nerve (ganglion)	C47.9	C79.89	-	D36.10	D48.2	D49.2
- - abducens	C72.59	C79.49	-	D33.3	D43.3	D49.7
- - accessory (spinal)	C72.59	C79.49	-	D33.3	D43.3	D49.7
- - acoustic	C72.4-	C79.49	-	D33.3	D43.3	D49.7
- - auditory	C72.4-	C79.49	-	D33.3	D43.3	D49.7
- - autonomic NEC—*see also Neoplasm, nerve, peripheral*	C47.9	C79.89	-	D36.10	D48.2	D49.2
- - brachial	C47.1-	C79.89	-	D36.12	D48.2	D49.2
- - cranial	C72.50	C79.49	-	D33.3	D43.3	D49.7
- - - specified NEC	C72.59	C79.49	-	D33.3	D43.3	D49.7
- - facial	C72.59	C79.49	-	D33.3	D43.3	D49.7
- - femoral	C47.2-	C79.89	-	D36.13	D48.2	D49.2
- - ganglion NEC—*see also Neoplasm, nerve, peripheral*	C47.9	C79.89	-	D36.10	D48.2	D49.2
- - glossopharyngeal	C72.59	C79.49	-	D33.3	D43.3	D49.7
- - hypoglossal	C72.59	C79.49	-	D33.3	D43.3	D49.7
- - intercostal	C47.3	C79.89	-	D36.14	D48.2	D49.2
- - lumbar	C47.6	C79.89	-	D36.17	D48.2	D49.2
- - median	C47.1-	C79.89	-	D36.12	D48.2	D49.2
- - obturator	C47.2-	C79.89	-	D36.13	D48.2	D49.2
- - oculomotor	C72.59	C79.49	-	D33.3	D43.3	D49.7
- - olfactory	C47.2-	C79.49	-	D33.3	D43.3	D49.7
- - optic	C72.3-	C79.49	-	D33.3	D43.3	D49.7
- - parasympathetic NEC	C47.9	C79.89	-	D36.10	D48.2	D49.2
- - peripheral NEC	C47.9	C79.89	-	D36.10	D48.2	D49.2
- - - abdomen	C47.4	C79.89	-	D36.15	D48.2	D49.2

	Malignant Primary	Malignant Secondary	CA in Situ	Benign	Uncertain Behavior	Unspecified Behavior
- - - abdominal wall	C47.4	C79.89	-	D36.15	D48.2	D49.2
- - - ankle	C47.2-	C79.89	-	D36.13	D48.2	D49.2
- - - antecubital fossa or space	C47.1-	C79.89	-	D36.12	D48.2	D49.2
- - - arm	C47.1-	C79.89	-	D36.12	D48.2	D49.2
- - - auricle (ear)	C47.0	C79.89	-	D36.11	D48.2	D49.2
- - - axilla	C47.3	C79.89	-	D36.12	D48.2	D49.2
- - - back	C47.6	C79.89	-	D36.17	D48.2	D49.2
- - - buttock	C47.5	C79.89	-	D36.16	D48.2	D49.2
- - - calf	C47.2-	C79.89	-	D36.13	D48.2	D49.2
- - - cervical region	C47.0	C79.89	-	D36.11	D48.2	D49.2
- - - cheek	C47.0	C79.89	-	D36.11	D48.2	D49.2
- - - chest (wall)	C47.3	C79.89	-	D36.14	D48.2	D49.2
- - - chin	C47.0	C79.89	-	D36.11	D48.2	D49.2
- - - ear (external)	C47.0	C79.89	-	D36.11	D48.2	D49.2
- - - elbow	C47.1-	C79.89	-	D36.12	D48.2	D49.2
- - - extra rectal	C47.5	C79.89	-	D36.16	D48.2	D49.2
- - - extremity	C47.9	C79.89	-	D36.10	D48.2	D49.2
- - - - lower	C47.2-	C79.89	-	D36.13	D48.2	D49.2
- - - - upper	C47.1-	C79.89	-	D36.12	D48.2	D49.2
- - - eyelid	C47.0	C79.89	-	D36.11	D48.2	D49.2
- - - face	C47.0	C79.89	-	D36.11	D48.2	D49.2
- - - finger	C47.1-	C79.89	-	D36.12	D48.2	D49.2
- - - flank	C47.6	C79.89	-	D36.17	D48.2	D49.2
- - - foot	C47.2-	C79.89	-	D36.13	D48.2	D49.2
- - - forearm	C47.1-	C79.89	-	D36.12	D48.2	D49.2
- - - forehead	C47.0	C79.89	-	D36.11	D48.2	D49.2
- - - gluteal region	C47.5	C79.89	-	D36.16	D48.2	D49.2
- - - groin	C47.5	C79.89	-	D36.16	D48.2	D49.2
- - - hand	C47.1-	C79.89	-	D36.12	D48.2	D49.2
- - - head	C47.0	C79.89	-	D36.11	D48.2	D49.2
- - - heel	C47.2-	C79.89	-	D36.13	D48.2	D49.2
- - - hip	C47.2-	C79.89	-	D36.13	D48.2	D49.2
- - - infraclavicular region	C47.3	C79.89	-	D36.14	D48.2	D49.2
- - - inguinal (canal) (region)	C47.5	C79.89	-	D36.16	D48.2	D49.2
- - - intrathoracic	C47.3	C79.89	-	D36.14	D48.2	D49.2
- - - ischiorectal fossa	C47.5	C79.89	-	D36.16	D48.2	D49.2
- - - knee	C47.2-	C79.89	-	D36.13	D48.2	D49.2
- - - leg	C47.2-	C79.89	-	D36.13	D48.2	D49.2
- - - limb NEC	C47.9	C79.89	-	D36.10	D48.2	D49.2
- - - - lower	C47.2-	C79.89	-	D36.13	D48.2	D49.2
- - - - upper	C47.1-	C79.89	-	D36.12	D48.2	D49.2
- - - nates	C47.5	C79.89	-	D36.16	D48.2	D49.2
- - - neck	C47.0	C79.89	-	D36.11	D48.2	D49.2
- - - orbit	C69.6-	C79.49	-	D31.6-	D48.7	D49.2
- - - pararectal	C47.5	C79.89	-	D36.16	D48.2	D49.2
- - - paraurethral	C47.5	C79.89	-	D36.16	D48.2	D49.2
- - - paravaginal	C47.5	C79.89	-	D36.16	D48.2	D49.2
- - - pelvis (floor)	C47.5	C79.89	-	D36.16	D48.2	D49.2
- - - pelvoabdominal	C47.8	C79.89	-	D36.17	D48.2	D49.2
- - - perineum	C47.5	C79.89	-	D36.16	D48.2	D49.2
- - - perirectal (tissue)	C47.5	C79.89	-	D36.16	D48.2	D49.2
- - - periurethral (tissue)	C47.5	C79.89	-	D36.16	D48.2	D49.2
- - - popliteal fossa or space	C47.2-	C79.89	-	D36.13	D48.2	D49.2
- - - presacral	C47.5	C79.89	-	D36.16	D48.2	D49.2
- - - pterygoid fossa	C47.0	C79.89	-	D36.11	D48.2	D49.2
- - - rectovaginal septum or wall	C47.5	C79.89	-	D36.16	D48.2	D49.2
- - - rectovesical	C47.5	C79.89	-	D36.16	D48.2	D49.2
- - - sacrococcygeal region	C47.5	C79.89	-	D36.16	D48.2	D49.2
- - - scalp	C47.0	C79.89	-	D36.11	D48.2	D49.2
- - - scapular region	C47.3	C79.89	-	D36.14	D48.2	D49.2
- - - shoulder	C47.1-	C79.89	-	D36.12	D48.2	D49.2
- - - submental	C47.0	C79.89	-	D36.11	D48.2	D49.2
- - - supraclavicular region	C47.0	C79.89	-	D36.11	D48.2	D49.2
- - - temple	C47.0	C79.89	-	D36.11	D48.2	D49.2
- - - temporal region	C47.0	C79.89	-	D36.11	D48.2	D49.2
- - - thigh	C47.2-	C79.89	-	D36.13	D48.2	D49.2
- - - thoracic (duct) (wall)	C47.3	C79.89	-	D36.14	D48.2	D49.2
- - - thorax	C47.3	C79.89	-	D36.14	D48.2	D49.2
- - - thumb	C47.1-	C79.89	-	D36.12	D48.2	D49.2
- - - toe	C47.2-	C79.89	-	D36.13	D48.2	D49.2
- - - trunk	C47.6	C79.89	-	D36.17	D48.2	D49.2

	Malignant Primary	Malignant Secondary	CA in Situ	Benign	Uncertain Behavior	Unspecified Behavior
- - - umbilicus	C47.4	C79.89	-	D36.15	D48.2	D49.2
- - - vesicorectal	C47.5	C79.89	-	D36.16	D48.2	D49.2
- - - wrist	C47.1-	C79.89	-	D36.12	D48.2	D49.2
- - radial	C47.1-	C79.89	-	D36.12	D48.2	D49.2
- - sacral	C47.5	C79.89	-	D36.16	D48.2	D49.2
- - sciatic	C47.2-	C79.89	-	D36.13	D48.2	D49.2
- - spinal NEC	C47.9	C79.89	-	D36.10	D48.2	D49.2
- - - accessory	C72.59	C79.49	-	D33.3	D43.3	D49.7
- - sympathetic NEC—*see also Neoplasm, nerve, peripheral*	C47.9	C79.89	-	D36.10	D48.2	D49.2
- - trigeminal	C72.59	C79.49	-	D33.3	D43.3	D49.7
- - trochlear	C72.59	C79.49	-	D33.3	D43.3	D49.7
- - ulnar	C47.1-	C79.89	-	D36.12	D48.2	D49.2
- - vagus	C72.59	C79.49	-	D33.3	D43.3	D49.7
- nervous system (central)	C72.9	C79.40	-	D33.9	D43.9	D49.7
- - autonomic—*see Neoplasm, nerve, peripheral*						
- - parasympathetic—*see Neoplasm, nerve, peripheral*						
- - specified site NEC	-	C79.49	-	D33.7	D43.8	-
- - sympathetic—*see Neoplasm, nerve, peripheral*						
- nevus—*see Nevus*						
- nipple	C50.0-	C79.81	D05.-	D24.-	-	-
- nose, nasal	C76.0	C79.89	D09.8	D36.7	D48.7	D49.89
- - ala (external) (nasi)—*see also Neoplasm, nose, skin*	C44.301	C79.2	D04.39	D23.39	D48.5	D49.2
- - bone	C41.0	C79.51	-	D16.4-	D48.0	D49.2
- - cartilage	C30.0	C78.39	D02.3	D14.0	D38.5	D49.1
- - cavity	C30.0	C78.39	D02.3	D14.0	D38.5	D49.1
- -choana	C11.3	C79.89	D00.08	D10.6	D37.05	D49.0
- - external (skin)—*see also Neoplasm, nose, skin*	C44.301	C79.2	D04.39	D23.39	D48.5	D49.2
- - fossa	C30.0	C78.39	D02.3	D14.0	D38.5	D49.1
- - internal	C30.0	C78.39	D02.3	D14.0	D38.5	D49.1
- - mucosa	C30.0	C78.39	D02.3	D14.0	D38.5	D49.1
- - septum	C30.0	C78.39	D02.3	D14.0	D38.5	D49.1
- - - posterior margin	C11.3	C79.89	D00.08	D10.6	D37.05	D49.0
- - sinus—*see Neoplasm, sinus*						
- - skin	C44.301	C79.2	D04.39	D23.39	D48.5	D49.2
- - - basal cell carcinoma	C44.311	-	-	-	-	-
- - - specified type NEC	C44.391	-	-	-	-	-
- - - squamous cell carcinoma	C44.321	-	-	-	-	-
- - turbinate (mucosa)	C30.0	C78.39	D02.3	D14.0	D38.5	D49.1
- - - bone	C41.0	C79.51	-	D16.4-	D48.0	D49.2
- - vestibule	C30.0	C78.39	D02.3	D14.0	D38.5	D49.1
- nostril	C30.0	C78.39	D02.3	D14.0	D38.5	D49.1
- nucleus pulposus	C41.2	C79.51	-	D16.6	D48.0	D49.2
- occipital						
- - bone	C41.0	C79.51	-	D16.4-	D48.0	D49.2
- - lobe or pole, brain	C71.4	C79.31	-	D33.0	D43.0	D49.6
- odontogenic—*see Neoplasm, jaw bone*						
- olfactory nerve or bulb	C72.2-	C79.49	-	D33.3	D43.3	D49.7
- olive (brain)	C71.7	C79.31	-	D33.1	D43.1	D49.6
- omentum	C48.1	C78.6	-	D20.1	D48.4	D49.0
- operculum (brain)	C71.0	C79.31	-	D33.0	D43.0	D49.6
- optic nerve, chiasm, or tract	C72.3-	C79.49	-	D33.3	D43.3	D49.7
- oral (cavity)	C06.9	C79.89	D00.00	D10.30	D37.09	D49.0
- - ill-defined	C14.8	C79.89	D00.00	D10.30	D37.09	D49.0
- - mucosa	C06.0	C79.89	D00.02	D10.39	D37.09	D49.0
- orbit	C69.6-	C79.49	D09.2-	D31.6-	D48.7	D49.89
- - autonomic nerve	C69.6-	C79.49	-	D31.6-	D48.7	D49.2
- - bone	C41.0	C79.51	-	D16.4-	D48.0	D49.2
- - eye	C69.6-	C79.49	D09.2-	D31.6-	D48.7	D49.89
- - peripheral nerves	C69.6-	C79.49	-	D31.6-	D48.7	D49.2
- - soft parts	C69.6-	C79.49	D09.2-	D31.6-	D48.7	D49.89
- organ of Zuckerkandl	C75.5	C79.89	-	D35.6	D44.7	D49.7
- oropharynx	C10.9	C79.89	D00.08	D10.5	D37.05	D49.0
- - branchial cleft (vestige)	C10.4	C79.89	D00.08	D10.5	D37.05	D49.0
- - junctional region	C10.8	C79.89	D00.08	D10.5	D37.05	D49.0
- - lateral wall	C10.2	C79.89	D00.08	D10.5	D37.05	D49.0
- - overlapping lesion	C10.8	-	-	-	-	-
- - pillars or fauces	C09.1	C79.89	D00.08	D10.5	D37.05	D49.0
- - posterior wall	C10.3	C79.89	D00.08	D10.5	D37.05	D49.0
- - vallecula	C10.0	C79.89	D00.08	D10.5	D37.05	D49.0

	Malignant Primary	Malignant Secondary	CA in Situ	Benign	Uncertain Behavior	Unspecified Behavior
- os						
- - external	C53.1	C79.82	D06.1	D26.0	D39.0	D49.59
- - internal	C53.0	C79.82	D06.0	D26.0	D39.0	D49.59
- ovary	C56.-	C79.6-	D07.39	D27.-	D39.1-	D49.59
- oviduct	C57.0-	C79.82	D07.39	D28.2	D39.8	D49.59
- palate	C05.9	C79.89	D00.00	D10.39	D37.09	D49.0
- - hard	C05.0	C79.89	D00.05	D10.39	D37.09	D49.0
- - junction of hard and soft palate	C05.9	C79.89	D00.00	D10.39	D37.09	D49.0
- - overlapping lesions	C05.8	-	-	-	-	-
- - soft	C05.1	C79.89	D00.04	D10.39	D37.09	D49.0
- - - nasopharyngeal surface	C11.3	C79.89	D00.08	D10.6	D37.05	D49.0
- - - posterior surface	C11.3	C79.89	D00.08	D10.6	D37.05	D49.0
- - - superior surface	C11.3	C79.89	D00.08	D10.6	D37.05	D49.0
- palatoglossal arch	C09.1	C79.89	D00.00	D10.5	D37.09	D49.0
- palatopharyngeal arch	C09.1	C79.89	D00.00	D10.5	D37.09	D49.0
- pallium	C71.0	C79.31	-	D33.0	D43.0	D49.6
- palpebra	C44.10-	C79.2	D04.1-	D23.1-	D48.5	D49.2
- - basal cell carcinoma	C44.11-	-	-	-	-	-
- - specified type NEC	C44.19-	-	-	-	-	-
- - squamous cell carcinoma	C44.12-	-	-	-	-	-
- pancreas	C25.9	C78.89	D01.7	D13.6	D37.8	D49.0
- - body	C25.1	C78.89	D01.7	D13.6	D37.8	D49.0
- - duct (of Santorini) (of Wirsung)	C25.3	C78.89	D01.7	D13.6	D37.8	D49.0
- - ectopic tissue	C25.7	C78.89	-	D13.6	D37.8	D49.0
- - head	C25.0	C78.89	D01.7	D13.6	D37.8	D49.0
- - islet cells	C25.4	C78.89	D01.7	D13.7	D37.8	D49.0
- - neck	C25.7	C78.89	D01.7	D13.6	D37.8	D49.0
- - overlapping lesion	C25.8	-	-	-	-	-
- - tail	C25.2	C78.89	D01.7	D13.6	D37.8	D49.0
- para-aortic body	C75.5	C79.89	-	D35.6	D44.7	D49.7
- paraganglion NEC	C75.5	C79.89	-	D35.6	D44.7	D49.7
- parametrium	C57.3	C79.82	-	D28.2	D39.8	D49.59
- paranephric	C48.0	C78.6	-	D20.0	D48.3	D49.0
- pararectal	C76.3	C79.89	-	D36.7	D48.7	D49.89
- parasagittal (region)	C76.0	C79.89	D09.8	D36.7	D48.7	D49.89
- parasellar	C72.9	C79.49	-	D33.9	D43.8	D49.7
- parathyroid (gland)	C75.0	C79.89	D09.3	D35.1	D44.2	D49.7
- paraurethral	C76.3	C79.89	-	D36.7	D48.7	D49.89
- - gland	C68.1	C79.19	D09.19	D30.8	D41.8	D49.59
- paravaginal	C76.3	C79.89	-	D36.7	D48.7	D49.89
- parenchyma, kidney	C64.-	C79.0-	D09.19	D30.0-	D41.0-	D49.59
- parietal						
- - bone	C41.0	C79.51	-	D16.4-	D48.0	D49.2
- - lobe, brain	C71.3	C79.31	-	D33.0	D43.0	D49.6
- paroophoron	C57.1	C79.82	D07.39	D28.2	D39.8	D49.59
- parotid (duct) (gland)	C07	C79.89	D00.00	D11.0	D37.030	D49.0
- parovarium	C57.1	C79.82	D07.39	D28.2	D39.8	D49.59
- patella	C40.20	C79.51	-	-	-	-
- peduncle, cerebral	C71.7	C79.31	-	D33.1	D43.1	D49.6
- pelvirectal junction	C19	C78.5	D01.1	D12.7	D37.5	D49.0
- pelvis, pelvic	C76.3	C79.89	D09.8	D36.7	D48.7	D49.89
- - bone	C41.4	C79.51	-	D16.8	D48.0	D49.2
- - floor	C76.3	C79.89	D09.8	D36.7	D48.7	D49.89
- - renal	C65.-	C79.0-	D09.19	D30.1-	D41.1-	D49.59
- - viscera	C76.3	C79.89	D09.8	D36.7	D48.7	D49.89
- - wall	C76.3	C79.89	D09.8	D36.7	D48.7	D49.89
- pelvo-abdominal	C76.8	C79.89	D09.8	D36.7	D48.7	D49.89
- penis	C60.9	C79.82	D07.4	D29.0	D40.8	D49.59
- - body	C60.2	C79.82	D07.4	D29.0	D40.8	D49.59
- - corpus (cavernosum)	C60.2	C79.82	D07.4	D29.0	D40.8	D49.59
- - glans	C60.1	C79.82	D07.4	D29.0	D40.8	D49.59
- - overlapping sites	C60.8	-	-	-	-	-
- - skin NEC	C60.9	C79.82	D07.4	D29.0	D40.8	D49.59
- periadrenal (tissue)	C48.0	C78.6	-	D20.0	D48.3	D49.0
- perianal (skin)—see also Neoplasm, anus, skin	C44.500	C79.2	D04.5	D23.5	D48.5	D49.2
- pericardium	C38.0	C79.89	-	D15.1	D48.7	D49.89
- perinephric	C48.0	C78.6	-	D20.0	D48.3	D49.0
- perineum	C76.3	C79.89	D09.8	D36.7	D48.7	D49.89
- periodontal tissue NEC	C03.9	C79.89	D00.03	D10.39	D37.09	D49.0
- periosteum—see Neoplasm, bone						
- peripancreatic	C48.0	C78.6	-	D20.0	D48.3	D49.0

	Malignant Primary	Malignant Secondary	CA in Situ	Benign	Uncertain Behavior	Unspecified Behavior
- peripheral nerve NEC	C47.9	C79.89	-	D36.10	D48.2	D49.2
- perirectal (tissue)	C76.3	C79.89	-	D36.7	D48.7	D49.89
- perirenal (tissue)	C48.0	C78.6	-	D20.0	D48.3	D49.0
- peritoneum, peritoneal (cavity)	C48.2	C78.6	-	D20.1	D48.4	D49.0
- - benign mesothelial tissue—*see Mesothelioma, benign*						
- - overlapping lesion	C48.8	-	-	-	-	-
- - - with digestive organs	C26.9	-	-	-	-	-
- - parietal	C48.1	C78.6	-	D20.1	D48.4	D49.0
- - pelvic	C48.1	C78.6	-	D20.1	D48.4	D49.0
- - specified part NEC	C48.1	C78.6	-	D20.1	D48.4	D49.0
- peritonsillar (tissue)	C76.0	C79.89	D09.8	D36.7	D48.7	D49.89
- periurethral tissue	C76.3	C79.89	-	D36.7	D48.7	D49.89
- phalanges						
- - foot	C40.3-	C79.51	-	D16.3-	-	-
- - hand	C40.1-	C79.51	-	D16.1-	-	-
- pharynx, pharyngeal	C14.0	C79.89	D00.08	D10.9	D37.05	D49.0
- - bursa	C11.1	C79.89	D00.08	D10.6	D37.05	D49.0
- - fornix	C11.3	C79.89	D00.08	D10.6	D37.05	D49.0
- - recess	C11.2	C79.89	D00.08	D10.6	D37.05	D49.0
- - region	C14.0	C79.89	D00.08	D10.9	D37.05	D49.0
- - tonsil	C11.1	C79.89	D00.08	D10.6	D37.05	D49.0
- - wall (lateral) (posterior)	C14.0	C79.89	D00.08	D10.9	D37.05	D49.0
- pia mater	C70.9	C79.40	-	D32.9	D42.9	D49.7
- - cerebral	C70.0	C79.32	-	D32.0	D42.0	D49.7
- - cranial	C70.0	C79.32	-	D32.0	D42.0	D49.7
- - spinal	C70.1	C79.49	-	D32.1	D42.1	D49.7
- pillars of fauces	C09.1	C79.89	D00.08	D10.5	D37.05	D49.0
- pineal (body) (gland)	C75.3	C79.89	D09.3	D35.4	D44.5	D49.7
- pinna (ear)NEC—*see also Neoplasm, skin, ear*	C44.20-	C79.2	D04.2-	D23.2-	D48.5	D49.2
- piriform fossa or sinus	C12	C79.89	D00.08	D10.7	D37.05	D49.0
- pituitary (body) (fossa) (gland) (lobe)	C75.1	C79.89	D09.3	D35.2	D44.3	D49.7
- placenta	C58	C79.82	D07.0	D26.7	D39.2	D49.59
- pleura, pleural (cavity)	C38.4	C78.2	-	D19.0	D38.2	D49.1
- - overlapping lesion with heart or mediastinum	C38.8	-	-	-	-	-
- - parietal	C38.4	C78.2	-	D19.0	D38.2	D49.1
- - visceral	C38.4	C78.2	-	D19.0	D38.2	D49.1
- plexus						
- - brachial	C47.1-	C79.89	-	D36.12	D48.2	D49.2
- - cervical	C47.0	C79.89	-	D36.11	D48.2	D49.2
- - choroid	C71.5	C79.31	-	D33.0	D43.0	D49.6
- - lumbosacral	C47.5	C79.89	-	D36.16	D48.2	D49.2
- - sacral	C47.5	C79.89	-	D36.16	D48.2	D49.2
- pluriendocrine	C75.8	C79.89	D09.3	D35.7	D44.9	D49.7
- pole						
- - frontal	C71.1	C79.31	-	D33.0	D43.0	D49.6
- - occipital	C71.4	C79.31	-	D33.0	D43.0	D49.6
- pons (varolii)	C71.7	C79.31	-	D33.1	D43.1	D49.6
- popliteal fossa or space	C76.5-	C79.89	D04.7-	D36.7	D48.7	D49.89
- postcricoid (region)	C13.0	C79.89	D00.08	D10.7	D37.05	D49.0
- posterior fossa (cranial)	C71.9	C79.31	-	D33.2	D43.2	D49.6
- postnasal space	C11.9	C79.89	D00.08	D10.6	D37.05	D49.0
- prepuce	C60.0	C79.82	D07.4	D29.0	D40.8	D49.59
- prepylorus	C16.4	C78.89	D00.2	D13.1	D37.1	D49.0
- presacral (region)	C76.3	C79.89	-	D36.7	D48.7	D49.89
- prostate (gland)	C61	C79.82	D07.5	D29.1	D40.0	D49.59
- - utricle	C68.0	C79.19	D09.19	D30.4	D41.3	D49.59
- pterygoid fossa	C49.0	C79.89	-	D21.0	D48.1	D49.2
- pubic bone	C41.4	C79.51	-	D16.8	D48.0	D49.2
- pudenda, pudendum (female)	C51.9	C79.82	D07.1	D28.0	D39.8	D49.59
- pulmonary—*see also Neoplasm, lung*	C34.9-	C78.0-	D02.2-	D14.3-	D38.1	D49.1
- putamen	C71.0	C79.31	-	D33.0	D43.0	D49.6
- pyloric						
- - antrum	C16.3	C78.89	D00.2	D13.1	D37.1	D49.0
- - canal	C16.4	C78.89	D00.2	D13.1	D37.1	D49.0
- pylorus	C16.4	C78.89	D00.2	D13.1	D37.1	D49.0
- pyramid (brain)	C71.7	C79.31	-	D33.1	D43.1	D49.6
- pyriform fossa or sinus	C12	C79.89	D00.08	D10.7	D37.05	D49.0
- radius (any part)	C40.0-	C79.51	-	D16.0-	-	-
- Rathke's pouch	C75.1	C79.89	D09.3	D35.2	D44.3	D49.7
- rectosigmoid (junction)	C19	C78.5	D01.1	D12.7	D37.5	D49.0

	Malignant Primary	Malignant Secondary	CA in Situ	Benign	Uncertain Behavior	Unspecified Behavior
- - overlapping lesion with anus or rectum	C21.8	-	-	-	-	-
- rectouterine pouch	C48.1	C78.6	-	D20.1	D48.4	D49.0
- rectovaginal septum or wall	C76.3	C79.89	D09.8	D36.7	D48.7	D49.89
- rectovesical septum	C76.3	C79.89	D09.8	D36.7	D48.7	D49.89
- rectum (ampulla)	C20	C78.5	D01.2	D12.8	D37.5	D49.0
- - and colon	C19	C78.5	D01.1	D12.7	D37.5	D49.0
- - overlapping lesion with anus or rectosigmoid junction	C21.8	-	-	-	-	-
- renal	C64.-	C79.0-	D09.19	D30.0-	D41.0-	D49.51
- - calyx	C65.-	C79.0-	D09.19	D30.1-	D41.1-	D49.51
- - hilus	C65.-	C79.0-	D09.19	D30.1-	D41.1-	D49.51
- - parenchyma	C64.-	C79.0-	D09.19	D30.0-	D41.0-	D49.51
- - pelvis	C65.-	C79.0-	D09.19	D30.1-	D41.1-	D49.51
- respiratory						
- - organs or system NEC	C39.9	C78.30	D02.4	D14.4	D38.6	D49.1
- - tract NEC	C39.9	C78.30	D02.4	D14.4	D38.5	D49.1
- - - upper	C39.0	C78.30	D02.4	D14.4	D38.5	D49.1
- retina	C69.2-	C79.49	D09.2-	D31.2-	D48.7	D49.81
- retrobulbar	C69.6-	C79.49	-	D31.6-	D48.7	D49.89
- retrocecal	C48.0	C78.6	-	D20.0	D48.3	D49.0
- retromolar (area) (triangle) (trigone)	C06.2	C79.89	D00.00	D10.39	D37.09	D49.0
- retro-orbital	C76.0	C79.89	D09.8	D36.7	D48.7	D49.89
- retroperitoneal (space) (tissue)	C48.0	C78.6	-	D20.0	D48.3	D49.0
- retroperitoneum	C48.0	C78.6	-	D20.0	D48.3	D49.0
- retropharyngeal	C14.0	C79.89	D00.08	D10.9	D37.05	D49.0
- retrovesical (septum)	C76.3	C79.89	D09.8	D36.7	D48.7	D49.89
- rhinencephalon	C71.0	C79.31	-	D33.0	D43.0	D49.6
- rib	C41.3	C79.51	-	D16.7	D48.0	D49.2
- Rosenmüller's fossa	C11.2	C79.89	D00.08	D10.6	D37.05	D49.0
- round ligament	C57.2	C79.82	-	D28.2	D39.8	D49.59
- sacrococcyx, sacrococcygeal	C41.4	C79.51		D16.8	D48.0	D49.2
- - region	C76.3	C79.89	D09.8	D36.7	D48.7	D49.89
- sacrouterine ligament	C57.3	C79.82	-	D28.2	D39.8	D49.59
- sacrum, sacral (vertebra)	C41.4	C79.51	-	D16.8	D48.0	D49.2
- salivary gland or duct (major)	C08.9	C79.89	D00.00	D11.9	D37.039	D49.0
- - minor NEC	C06.9	C79.89	D00.00	D10.39	D37.04	D49.0
- - overlapping lesion	C08.9	-	-	-	-	-
- - parotid	C07	C79.89	D00.00	D11.0	D37.030	D49.0
- - pluriglandular	C08.9	C79.89	D00.00	D11.9	D37.039	D49.0
- - sublingual	C08.1	C79.89	D00.00	D11.7	D37.031	D49.0
- - submandibular	C08.0	C79.89	D00.00	D11.7	D37.032	D49.0
- - submaxillary	C08.0	C79.89	D00.00	D11.7	D37.032	D49.0
- salpinx (uterine)	C57.0-	C79.82	D07.39	D28.2	D39.8	D49.59
- Santorini's duct	C25.3	C78.89	D01.7	D13.6	D37.8	D49.0
- scalp	C44.40	C79.2	D04.4	D23.4	D48.5	D49.2
- - basal cell carcinoma	C44.41	-	-	-	-	-
- - specified type NEC	C44.49	-	-	-	-	-
- - squamous cell carcinoma	C44.42	-	-	-	-	-
- scapula (any part)	C40.0-	C79.51	-	D16.0-	-	-
- scapular region	C76.1	C79.89	D09.8	D36.7	D48.7	D49.89
- scar NEC—see also Neoplasm, skin, by site	C44.90	C79.2	D04.9	D23.9	D48.5	D49.2
- sciatic nerve	C47.2-	C79.89	-	D36.13	D48.2	D49.2
- sclera	C69.4-	C79.49	D09.2-	D31.4-	D48.7	D49.89
- scrotum (skin)	C63.2	C79.82	D07.61	D29.4	D40.8	D49.59
- sebaceous gland—see Neoplasm, skin						
- sella turcica	C75.1	C79.89	D09.3	D35.2	D44.3	D49.7
- - bone	C41.0	C79.51	-	D16.4-	D48.0	D49.2
- semilunar cartilage (knee)	C40.2-	C79.51	-	D16.2-	D48.0	D49.2
- seminal vesicle	C63.7	C79.82	D07.69	D29.8	D40.8	D49.59
- septum						
- - nasal	C30.0	C78.39	D02.3	D14.0	D38.5	D49.1
- - - posterior margin	C11.3	C79.89	D00.08	D10.6	D37.05	D49.0
- - rectovaginal	C76.3	C79.89	D09.8	D36.7	D48.7	D49.89
- - rectovesical	C76.3	C79.89	D09.8	D36.7	D48.7	D49.89
- - urethrovaginal	C57.9	C79.82	D07.30	D28.9	D39.9	D49.59
- - vesicovaginal	C57.9	C79.82	D07.30	D28.9	D39.9	D49.59
- shoulder NEC	C76.4-	C79.89	D04.6-	D36.7	D48.7	D49.89
- sigmoid flexure (lower) (upper)	C18.7	C78.5	D01.0	D12.5	D37.4	D49.0
- sinus (accessory)	C31.9	C78.39	D02.3	D14.0	D38.5	D49.1
- - bone (any)	C41.0	C79.51	-	D16.4-	D48.0	D49.2
- - ethmoidal	C31.1	C78.39	D02.3	D14.0	D38.5	D49.1

	Malignant Primary	Malignant Secondary	CA in Situ	Benign	Uncertain Behavior	Unspecified Behavior
- - frontal	C31.2	C78.39	D02.3	D14.0	D38.5	D49.1
- - maxillary	C31.0	C78.39	D02.3	D14.0	D38.5	D49.1
- - nasal, paranasal NEC	C31.9	C78.39	D02.3	D14.0	D38.5	D49.1
- - overlapping lesion	C31.8	-	-	-	-	-
- - pyriform	C12	C79.89	D00.08	D10.7	D37.05	D49.0
- - sphenoid	C31.3	C78.39	D02.3	D14.0	D38.5	D49.1
- skeleton, skeletal NEC	C41.9	C79.51	-	D16.9-	D48.0	D49.2
- Skene's gland	C68.1	C79.19	D09.19	D30.8	D41.8	D49.59
- skin NOS	C44.90	C79.2	D04.9	D23.9	D48.5	D49.2
- - abdominal wall	C44.509	C79.2	D04.5	D23.5	D48.5	D49.2
- - - basal cell carcinoma	C44.519	-	-	-	-	-
- - - specified type NEC	C44.599	-	-	-	-	-
- - - squamous cell carcinoma	C44.529	-	-	-	-	-
- - ala nasi—*see also Neoplasm, nose, skin*	C44.301	C79.2	D04.39	D23.39	D48.5	D49.2
- - ankle—*see also Neoplasm, skin, limb, lower*	C44.70-	C79.2	D04.7-	D23.7-	D48.5	D49.2
- - antecubital space—*see also Neoplasm, skin, limb, upper*	C44.60-	C79.2	D04.6-	D23.6-	D48.5	D49.2
- - anus	C44.500	C79.2	D04.5	D23.5	D48.5	D49.2
- - - basal cell carcinoma	C44.510	-	-	-	-	-
- - - specified type NEC	C44.590	-	-	-	-	-
- - - squamous cell carcinoma	C44.520	-	-	-	-	-
- - arm—*see also Neoplasm, skin, limb, upper*	C44.60-	C79.2	D04.6-	D23.6-	D48.5	D49.2
- - auditory canal (external)—*see also Neoplasm, skin, ear*	C44.20-	C79.2	D04.2-	D23.2-	D48.5	D49.2
- - auricle (ear)—*see also Neoplasm, skin, ear*	C44.20-	C79.2	D04.2-	D23.2-	D48.5	D49.2
- - auricular canal (external)—*see also Neoplasm, skin, ear*	C44.20-	C79.2	D04.2-	D23.2-	D48.5	D49.2
- - axilla, axillary fold—*see also Neoplasm, skin, trunk*	C44.509	C79.2	D04.5	D23.5	D48.5	D49.2
- - back—*see also Neoplasm, skin, trunk*	C44.509	C79.2	D04.5	D23.5	D48.5	D49.2
- - basal cell carcinoma	C44.91					
- - breast	C44.501	C79.2	D04.5	D23.5	D48.5	D49.2
- - - basal cell carcinoma	C44.511	-	-	-	-	-
- - - specified type NEC	C44.591	-	-	-	-	-
- - - squamous cell carcinoma	C44.521	-	-	-	-	-
- - brow—*see also Neoplasm, skin, face*	C44.309	C79.2	D04.39	D23.39	D48.5	D49.2
- - buttock—*see also Neoplasm, skin, trunk*	C44.509	C79.2	D04.5	D23.5	D48.5	D49.2
- - calf—*see also Neoplasm, skin, limb, lower*	C44.70-	C79.2	D04.7-	D23.7-	D48.5	D49.2
- - canthus (eye) (inner) (outer)	C44.10-	C79.2	D04.1-	D23.1-	D48.5	D49.2
- - - basal cell carcinoma	C44.11-	-	-	-	-	-
- - - specified type NEC	C44.19-	-	-	-	-	-
- - - squamous cell carcinoma	C44.12-	-	-	-	-	-
- - cervical region—*see also Neoplasm, skin, neck*	C44.40	C79.2	D04.4	D23.4	D48.5	D49.2
- - cheek (external)—*see also Neoplasm, skin, face*	C44.309	C79.2	D04.39	D23.39	D48.5	D49.2
- - chest (wall)—*see also Neoplasm, skin, trunk*	C44.509	C79.2	D04.5	D23.5	D48.5	D49.2
- - chin—*see also Neoplasm, skin, face*	C44.309	C79.2	D04.39	D23.39	D48.5	D49.2
- - clavicular area—*see also Neoplasm, skin, trunk*	C44.509	C79.2	D04.5	D23.5	D48.5	D49.2
- - clitoris	C51.2	C79.82	D07.1	D28.0	D39.8	D49.59
- - columnella—*see also Neoplasm, skin, face*	C44.309	C79.2	D04.39	D23.39	D48.5	D49.2
- - concha—*see also Neoplasm, skin, ear*	C44.20-	C79.2	D04.2-	D23.2-	D48.5	D49.2
- - ear (external)	C44.20-	C79.2	D04.2-	D23.2-	D48.5	D49.2
- - - basal cell carcinoma	C44.21-	-	-	-	-	-
- - - specified type NEC	C44.29-	-	-	-	-	-
- - - squamous cell carcinoma	C44.22-	-	-	-	-	-
- - elbow—*see also Neoplasm, skin, limb, upper*	C44.60-	C79.2	D04.6-	D23.6-	D48.5	D49.2
- - eyebrow—*see also Neoplasm, skin, face*	C44.309	C79.2	D04.39	D23.39	D48.5	D49.2
- - eyelid	C44.10-	C79.2	D04.1-	D23.1-	D48.5	D49.2
- - - basal cell carcinoma	C44.11-	-	-	-	-	-
- - - specified type NEC	C44.19-	-	-	-	-	-
- - - squamous cell carcinoma	C44.12-	-	-	-	-	-
- - face NOS	C44.300	C79.2	D04.30	D23.30	D48.5	D49.2
- - - basal cell carcinoma	C44.310	-	-	-	-	-
- - - specified type NEC	C44.390	-	-	-	-	-
- - - squamous cell carcinoma	C44.320	-	-	-	-	-
- - female genital organs (external)	C51.9	C79.82	D07.1	D28.0	D39.8	D49.59
- - - clitoris	C51.2	C79.82	D07.1	D28.0	D39.8	D49.59
- - - labium NEC	C51.9	C79.82	D07.1	D28.0	D39.8	D49.59
- - - - majus	C51.0	C79.82	D07.1	D28.0	D39.8	D49.59
- - - - minus	C51.1	C79.82	D07.1	D28.0	D39.8	D49.59
- - - pudendum	C51.9	C79.82	D07.1	D28.0	D39.8	D49.59
- - - vulva	C51.9	C79.82	D07.1	D28.0	D39.8	D49.59

	Malignant Primary	Malignant Secondary	CA in Situ	Benign	Uncertain Behavior	Unspecified Behavior
- - finger—*see also Neoplasm, skin, limb, upper*	C44.60-	C79.2	D04.6-	D23.6-	D48.5	D49.2
- - flank—*see also Neoplasm, skin, trunk*	C44.509	C79.2	D04.5	D23.5	D48.5	D49.2
- - foot—*see also Neoplasm, skin, limb, lower*	C44.70-	C79.2	D04.7-	D23.7-	D48.5	D49.2
- - forearm—*see also Neoplasm, skin, limb, upper*	C44.60-	C79.2	D04.6-	D23.6-	D48.5	D49.2
- - forehead—*see also Neoplasm, skin, face*	C44.309	C79.2	D04.39	D23.39	D48.5	D49.2
- - glabella—*see also Neoplasm, skin, face*	C44.309	C79.2	D04.39	D23.39	D48.5	D49.2
- - gluteal region—*see also Neoplasm, skin, trunk*	C44.509	C79.2	D04.5	D23.5	D48.5	D49.2
- - groin—*see also Neoplasm, skin, trunk*	C44.509	C79.2	D04.5	D23.5	D48.5	D49.2
- - hand—*see also Neoplasm, skin, limb, upper*	C44.60-	C79.2	D04.6-	D23.6-	D48.5	D49.2
- - head NEC—*see also Neoplasm, skin, scalp*	C44.40	C79.2	D04.4	D23.4	D48.5	D49.2
- - heel—*see also Neoplasm, skin, limb, lower*	C44.70-	C79.2	D04.7-	D23.7-	D48.5	D49.2
- - helix—*see also Neoplasm, skin, ear*	C44.20-	C79.2	D04.2-	D23.2-	D48.5	D49.2
- - hip—*see also Neoplasm, skin, limb, lower*	C44.70-	C79.2	D04.7-	D23.7-	D48.5	D49.2
- - infraclavicular region—*see also Neoplasm, skin, trunk*	C44.509	C79.2	D04.5	D23.5	D48.5	D49.2
- - inguinal region—*see also Neoplasm, skin, trunk*	C44.509	C79.2	D04.5	D23.5	D48.5	D49.2
- - jaw—*see also Neoplasm, skin, face*	C44.309	C79.2	D04.39	D23.39	D48.5	D49.2
- Kaposi's sarcoma—*see Kaposi's, sarcoma, skin*						
- - knee—*see also Neoplasm, skin, limb, lower*	C44.70-	C79.2	D04.7-	D23.7-	D48.5	D49.2
- - labia						
- - - majora	C51.0	C79.82	D07.1	D28.0	D39.8	D49.59
- - - minora	C51.1	C79.82	D07.1	D28.0	D39.8	D49.59
- - leg—*see also Neoplasm, skin, limb, lower*	C44.70-	C79.2	D04.7-	D23.7-	D48.5	D49.2
- - lid (lower) (upper)	C44.10-	C79.2	D04.1-	D23.1-	D48.5	D49.2
- - - basal cell carcinoma	C44.11-	-	-	-	-	-
- - - specified type NEC	C44.19-	-	-	-	-	-
- - - squamous cell carcinoma	C44.12-	-	-	-	-	-
- - limb NEC	C44.90	C79.2	D04.9	D23.9	D48.5	D49.2
- - - basal cell carcinoma	C44.91					
- - - lower	C44.70-	C79.2	D04.7-	D23.7-	D48.5	D49.2
- - - - basal cell carcinoma	C44.71-	-	-	-	-	-
- - - - specified type NEC	C44.79-	-	-	-	-	-
- - - - squamous cell carcinoma	C44.72-	-	-	-	-	-
- - - upper	C44.60-	C79.2	D04.6-	D23.6-	D48.5	D49.2
- - - - basal cell carcinoma	C44.61-	-	-	-	-	-
- - - - specified type NEC	C44.69-	-	-	-	-	-
- - - - squamous cell carcinoma	C44.62-	-	-	-	-	-
- - lip (lower) (upper)	C44.00	C79.2	D04.0	D23.0	D48.5	D49.2
- - - basal cell carcinoma	C44.01	-	-	-	-	-
- - - specified type NEC	C44.09	-	-	-	-	-
- - - squamous cell carcinoma	C44.02	-	-	-	-	-
- - male genital organs	C63.9	C79.82	D07.60	D29.9	D40.8	D49.59
- - - penis	C60.9	C79.82	D07.4	D29.0	D40.8	D49.59
- - - prepuce	C60.0	C79.82	D07.4	D29.0	D40.8	D49.59
- - - scrotum	C63.2	C79.82	D07.61	D29.4	D40.8	D49.59
- - mastectomy site (skin)—*see also Neoplasm, skin, breast*	C44.501	C79.2	-	-	-	-
- - - specified as breast tissue	C50.8-	C79.81	-	-	-	-
- - meatus, acoustic (external)—*see also Neoplasm, skin, ear*	C44.20-	C79.2	D04.2-	D23.2-	D48.5	D49.2
- - melanotic—*see Melanoma*						
- - Merkel cell—*see Carcinoma, Merkel cell*						
- - nates—*see also Neoplasm, skin, trunk*	C44.509	C79.2	D04.5	D23.5	D48.5	D49.2
- - neck	C44.40	C79.2	D04.4	D23.4	D48.5	D49.2
- - - basal cell carcinoma	C44.41	-	-	-	-	-
- - - specified type NEC	C44.49	-	-	-	-	-
- - - squamous cell carcinoma	C44.42	-	-	-	-	-
- - nevus—*see Nevus, skin*						
- - nose (external)—*see also Neoplasm, nose, skin*	C44.301	C79.2	D04.39	D23.39	D48.5	D49.2
- - overlapping lesion	C44.80	-	-	-	-	-
- - - basal cell carcinoma	C44.81	-	-	-	-	-
- - - specified type NEC	C44.89	-	-	-	-	-
- - - squamous cell carcinoma	C44.82	-	-	-	-	-
- - palm—*see also Neoplasm, skin, limb, upper*	C44.60-	C79.2	D04.6-	D23.6-	D48.5	D49.2
- - palpebra	C44.10-	C79.2	D04.1-	D23.1-	D48.5	D49.2
- - - basal cell carcinoma	C44.11-	-	-	-	-	-
- - - specified type NEC	C44.19-	-	-	-	-	-
- - - squamous cell carcinoma	C44.12-	-	-	-	-	-
- - penis NEC	C60.9	C79.82	D07.4	D29.0	D40.8	D49.59
- - perianal—*see also Neoplasm, skin, anus*	C44.500	C79.2	D04.5	D23.5	D48.5	D49.2
- - perineum—*see also Neoplasm, skin, anus*	C44.500	C79.2	D04.5	D23.5	D48.5	D49.2

	Malignant Primary	Malignant Secondary	CA in Situ	Benign	Uncertain Behavior	Unspecified Behavior
- - pinna—*see also Neoplasm, skin, ear*	C44.20-	C79.2	D04.2-	D23.2-	D48.5	D49.2
- - plantar—*see also Neoplasm, skin, limb, lower*	C44.70-	C79.2	D04.7-	D23.7-	D48.5	D49.2
- - popliteal fossa or space—*see also Neoplasm, skin, limb, lower*	C44.70-	C79.2	D04.7-	D23.7-	D48.5	D49.2
- - prepuce	C60.0	C79.82	D07.4	D29.0	D40.8	D49.59
- - pubes—*see also Neoplasm, skin, trunk*	C44.509	C79.2	D04.5	D23.5	D48.5	D49.2
- - sacrococcygeal region—*see also Neoplasm, skin, trunk*	C44.509	C79.2	D04.5	D23.5	D48.5	D49.2
- - scalp	C44.40	C79.2	D04.4	D23.4	D48.5	D49.2
- - - basal cell carcinoma	C44.41	-	-	-	-	-
- - - specified type NEC	C44.49	-	-	-	-	-
- - - squamous cell carcinoma	C44.42	-	-	-	-	-
- - scapular region—*see also Neoplasm, skin, trunk*	C44.509	C79.2	D04.5	D23.5	D48.5	D49.2
- - scrotum	C63.2	C79.82	D07.61	D29.4	D40.8	D49.59
- - shoulder—*see also Neoplasm, skin, limb, upper*	C44.60-	C79.2	D04.6-	D23.6-	D48.5	D49.2
- - sole (foot)—*see also Neoplasm, skin, limb, lower*	C44.70-	C79.2	D04.7-	D23.7-	D48.5	D49.2
- - specified sites NEC	C44.80	C79.2	D04.8	D23.9	D48.5	D49.2
- - - basal cell carcinoma	C44.81	-	-	-	-	-
- - - specified type NEC	C44.89	-	-	-	-	-
- - - squamous cell carcinoma	C44.82	-	-	-	-	-
- - specified type NEC	C44.99	-	-	-	-	-
- - squamous cell carcinoma	C44.92	-	-	-	-	-
- - submammary fold—*see also Neoplasm, skin, trunk*	C44.509	C79.2	D04.5	D23.5	D48.5	D49.2
- - supraclavicular region—*see also Neoplasm, skin, neck*	C44.40	C79.2	D04.4	D23.4	D48.5	D49.2
- - temple—*see also Neoplasm, skin, face*	C44.309	C79.2	D04.39	D23.39	D48.5	D49.2
- - thigh—*see also Neoplasm, skin, limb, lower*	C44.70-	C79.2	D04.7-	D23.7-	D48.5	D49.2
- - thoracic wall—*see also Neoplasm, skin, trunk*	C44.509	C79.2	D04.5	D23.5	D48.5	D49.2
- - thumb—*see also Neoplasm, skin, limb, upper*	C44.60-	C79.2	D04.6-	D23.6-	D48.5	D49.2
- - toe—*see also Neoplasm, skin, limb, lower*	C44.70-	C79.2	D04.7-	D23.7-	D48.5	D49.2
- - tragus—*see also Neoplasm, skin, ear*	C44.20-	C79.2	D04.2-	D23.2-	D48.5	D49.2
- - trunk	C44.509	C79.2	D04.5	D23.5	D48.5	D49.2
- - - basal cell carcinoma	C44.519	-	-	-	-	-
- - - specified type NEC	C44.599	-	-	-	-	-
- - - squamous cell carcinoma	C44.529	-	-	-	-	-
- - umbilicus—*see also Neoplasm, skin, trunk*	C44.509	C79.2	D04.5	D23.5	D48.5	D49.2
- - vulva	C51.9	C79.82	D07.1	D28.0	D39.8	D49.59
- - - overlapping lesion	C51.8	-	-	-	-	-
- - wrist—*see also Neoplasm, skin, limb, upper*	C44.60-	C79.2	D04.6-	D23.6-	D48.5	D49.2
- skull	C41.0	C79.51	-	D16.4-	D48.0	D49.2
- soft parts or tissues—*see Neoplasm, connective tissue*						
- specified site NEC	C76.8	C79.89	D09.8	D36.7	D48.7	D49.89
- spermatic cord	C63.1-	C79.82	D07.69	D29.8	D40.8	D49.59
- sphenoid	C31.3	C78.39	D02.3	D14.0	D38.5	D49.1
- - bone	C41.0	C79.51	-	D16.4-	D48.0	D49.2
- - sinus	C31.3	C78.39	D02.3	D14.0	D38.5	D49.1
- sphincter						
- - anal	C21.1	C78.5	D01.3	D12.9	D37.8	D49.0
- - of Oddi	C24.0	C78.89	D01.5	D13.5	D37.6	D49.0
- spine, spinal (column)	C41.2	C79.51	-	D16.6	D48.0	D49.2
- - bulb	C71.7	C79.31	-	D33.1	D43.1	D49.6
- - coccyx	C41.4	C79.51	-	D16.8	D48.0	D49.2
- - cord (cervical) (lumbar) (sacral) (thoracic)	C72.0	C79.49	-	D33.4	D43.4	D49.7
- - dura mater	C70.1	C79.49	-	D32.1	D42.1	D49.7
- - lumbosacral	C41.2	C79.51	-	D16.6	D48.0	D49.2
- - marrow NEC	C96.9	C79.52	-	-	D47.9	D49.89
- - membrane	C70.1	C79.49	-	D32.1	D42.1	D49.7
- - meninges	C70.1	C79.49	-	D32.1	D42.1	D49.7
- - nerve (root)	C47.9	C79.89	-	D36.10	D48.2	D49.2
- - pia mater	C70.1	C79.49	-	D32.1	D42.1	D49.7
- - root	C47.9	C79.89	-	D36.10	D48.2	D49.2
- - sacrum	C41.4	C79.51	-	D16.8	D48.0	D49.2
- spleen, splenic NEC	C26.1	C78.89	D01.7	D13.9	D37.8	D49.0
- - flexure (colon)	C18.5	C78.5	D01.0	D12.3	D37.4	D49.0
- stem, brain	C71.7	C79.31	-	D33.1	D43.1	D49.6
- Stensen's duct	C07	C79.89	D00.00	D11.0	D37.030	D49.0
- sternum	C41.3	C79.51	-	D16.7	D48.0	D49.2
- stomach	C16.9	C78.89	D00.2	D13.1	D37.1	D49.0
- - antrum (pyloric)	C16.3	C78.89	D00.2	D13.1	D37.1	D49.0
- - body	C16.2	C78.89	D00.2	D13.1	D37.1	D49.0
- - cardia	C16.0	C78.89	D00.2	D13.1	D37.1	D49.0

	Malignant Primary	Malignant Secondary	CA in Situ	Benign	Uncertain Behavior	Unspecified Behavior
- - cardiac orifice	C16.0	C78.89	D00.2	D13.1	D37.1	D49.0
- - corpus	C16.2	C78.89	D00.2	D13.1	D37.1	D49.0
- - fundus	C16.1	C78.89	D00.2	D13.1	D37.1	D49.0
- - greater curvature NEC	C16.6	C78.89	D00.2	D13.1	D37.1	D49.0
- - lesser curvature NEC	C16.5	C78.89	D00.2	D13.1	D37.1	D49.0
- - overlapping lesion	C16.8	-	-	-	-	-
- - prepylorus	C16.4	C78.89	D00.2	D13.1	D37.1	D49.0
- - pylorus	C16.4	C78.89	D00.2	D13.1	D37.1	D49.0
- - wall NEC	C16.9	C78.89	D00.2	D13.1	D37.1	D49.0
- - - anterior NEC	C16.8	C78.89	D00.2	D13.1	D37.1	D49.0
- - - posterior NEC	C16.8	C78.89	D00.2	D13.1	D37.1	D49.0
- stroma, endometrial	C54.1	C79.82	D07.0	D26.1	D39.0	D49.59
- stump, cervical	C53.8	C79.82	D06.7	D26.0	D39.0	D49.59
- subcutaneous (nodule) (tissue)NEC—*see Neoplasm, connective tissue*						
- subdural	C70.9	C79.32	-	D32.9	D42.9	D49.7
- subglottis, subglottic	C32.2	C78.39	D02.0	D14.1	D38.0	D49.1
- sublingual	C04.9	C79.89	D00.06	D10.2	D37.09	D49.0
- - gland or duct	C08.1	C79.89	D00.00	D11.7	D37.031	D49.0
- submandibular gland	C08.0	C79.89	D00.00	D11.7	D37.032	D49.0
- submaxillary gland or duct	C08.0	C79.89	D00.00	D11.7	D37.032	D49.0
- submental	C76.0	C79.89	D09.8	D36.7	D48.7	D49.89
- subpleural	C34.9-	C78.0-	D02.2-	D14.3-	D38.1	D49.1
- substernal	C38.1	C78.1	-	D15.2	D38.3	D49.89
- sudoriferous, sudoriparous gland, site unspecified	C44.90	C79.2	D04.9	D23.9	D48.5	D49.2
- - specified site—*see Neoplasm, skin*						
- supraclavicular region	C76.0	C79.89	D09.8	D36.7	D48.7	D49.89
- supraglottis	C32.1	C78.39	D02.0	D14.1	D38.0	D49.1
- suprarenal	C74.9-	C79.7-	D09.3	D35.0-	D44.1-	D49.7
- - capsule	C74.9-	C79.7-	D09.3	D35.0-	D44.1-	D49.7
- - cortex	C74.0-	C79.7-	D09.3	D35.0-	D44.1-	D49.7
- - gland	C74.9-	C79.7-	D09.3	D35.0-	D44.1-	D49.7
- - medulla	C74.1-	C79.7-	D09.3	D35.0-	D44.1-	D49.7
- suprasellar (region)	C71.9	C79.31	-	D33.2	D43.2	D49.6
- supratentorial (brain)NEC	C71.0	C79.31	-	D33.0	D43.0	D49.6
- sweat gland (apocrine) (eccrine), site unspecified	C44.90	C79.2	D04.9	D23.9	D48.5	D49.2
- - specified site—*see Neoplasm, skin*						
- sympathetic nerve or nervous system NEC	C47.9	C79.89	-	D36.10	D48.2	D49.2
- symphysis pubis	C41.4	C79.51	-	D16.8	D48.0	D49.2
- synovial membrane—*see Neoplasm, connective tissue*						
- tapetum, brain	C71.8	C79.31	-	D33.2	D43.2	D49.6
- tarsus (any bone)	C40.3-	C79.51	-	D16.3-	-	-
- temple (skin)—*see also Neoplasm, skin, face*	C44.309	C79.2	D04.39	D23.39	D48.5	D49.2
- temporal						
- - bone	C41.0	C79.51	-	D16.4-	D48.0	D49.2
- - lobe or pole	C71.2	C79.31	-	D33.0	D43.0	D49.6
- - region	C76.0	C79.89	D09.8	D36.7	D48.7	D49.89
- - - skin—*see also Neoplasm, skin, face*	C44.309	C79.2	D04.39	D23.39	D48.5	D49.2
- tendon (sheath)—*see Neoplasm, connective tissue*						
- tentorium (cerebelli)	C70.0	C79.32	-	D32.0	D42.0	D49.7
- testis, testes	C62.9-	C79.82	D07.69	D29.2-	D40.1-	D49.59
- - descended	C62.1-	C79.82	D07.69	D29.2-	D40.1-	D49.59
- - ectopic	C62.0-	C79.82	D07.69	D29.2-	D40.1-	D49.59
- - retained	C62.0-	C79.82	D07.69	D29.2-	D40.1-	D49.59
- - scrotal	C62.1-	C79.82	D07.69	D29.2-	D40.1-	D49.59
- - undescended	C62.0-	C79.82	D07.69	D29.2-	D40.1-	D49.59
- - unspecified whether descended or undescended	C62.9-	C79.82	D07.69	D29.2-	D40.1-	D49.59
- thalamus	C71.0	C79.31	-	D33.0	D43.0	D49.6
- thigh NEC	C76.5-	C79.89	D04.7-	D36.7	D48.7	D49.89
- thorax, thoracic (cavity) (organs NEC)	C76.1	C79.89	D09.8	D36.7	D48.7	D49.89
- - duct	C49.3	C79.89	-	D21.3	D48.1	D49.2
- - wall NEC	C76.1	C79.89	D09.8	D36.7	D48.7	D49.89
- throat	C14.0	C79.89	D00.08	D10.9	D37.05	D49.0
- thumb NEC	C76.4-	C79.89	D04.6-	D36.7	D48.7	D49.89
- thymus (gland)	C37	C79.89	D09.3	D15.0	D38.4	D49.89
- thyroglossal duct	C73	C79.89	D09.3	D34	D44.0	D49.7
- thyroid (gland)	C73	C79.89	D09.3	D34	D44.0	D49.7
- - cartilage	C32.3	C78.39	D02.0	D14.1	D38.0	D49.1
- tibia (any part)	C40.2-	C79.51	-	D16.2-	-	-
- toe NEC	C76.5-	C79.89	D04.7-	D36.7	D48.7	D49.89

	Malignant Primary	Malignant Secondary	CA in Situ	Benign	Uncertain Behavior	Unspecified Behavior
- tongue	C02.9	C79.89	D00.07	D10.1	D37.02	D49.0
- - anterior (two-thirds)NEC	C02.3	C79.89	D00.07	D10.1	D37.02	D49.0
- - - dorsal surface	C02.0	C79.89	D00.07	D10.1	D37.02	D49.0
- - - ventral surface	C02.2	C79.89	D00.07	D10.1	D37.02	D49.0
- - base (dorsal surface)	C01	C79.89	D00.07	D10.1	D37.02	D49.0
- - border (lateral)	C02.1	C79.89	D00.07	D10.1	D37.02	D49.0
- - dorsal surface NEC	C02.0	C79.89	D00.07	D10.1	D37.02	D49.0
- - fixed part NEC	C01	C79.89	D00.07	D10.1	D37.02	D49.0
- - foramen cecum	C02.0	C79.89	D00.07	D10.1	D37.02	D49.0
- - frenulum linguae	C02.2	C79.89	D00.07	D10.1	D37.02	D49.0
- - junctional zone	C02.8	C79.89	D00.07	D10.1	D37.02	D49.0
- - margin (lateral)	C02.1	C79.89	D00.07	D10.1	D37.02	D49.0
- - midline NEC	C02.0	C79.89	D00.07	D10.1	D37.02	D49.0
- - mobile part NEC	C02.3	C79.89	D00.07	D10.1	D37.02	D49.0
- - overlapping lesion	C02.8	-	-	-	-	-
- - posterior (third)	C01	C79.89	D00.07	D10.1	D37.02	D49.0
- - root	C01	C79.89	D00.07	D10.1	D37.02	D49.0
- - surface (dorsal)	C02.0	C79.89	D00.07	D10.1	D37.02	D49.0
- - - base	C01	C79.89	D00.07	D10.1	D37.02	D49.0
- - - ventral	C02.2	C79.89	D00.07	D10.1	D37.02	D49.0
- - tip	C02.1	C79.89	D00.07	D10.1	D37.02	D49.0
- - tonsil	C02.4	C79.89	D00.07	D10.1	D37.02	D49.0
- tonsil	C09.9	C79.89	D00.08	D10.4	D37.05	D49.0
- - fauces, faucial	C09.9	C79.89	D00.08	D10.4	D37.05	D49.0
- - lingual	C02.4	C79.89	D00.07	D10.1	D37.02	D49.0
- - overlapping sites	C09.8	-	-	-	-	-
- - palatine	C09.9	C79.89	D00.08	D10.4	D37.05	D49.0
- - pharyngeal	C11.1	C79.89	D00.08	D10.6	D37.05	D49.0
- - pillar (anterior) (posterior)	C09.1	C79.89	D00.08	D10.5	D37.05	D49.0
- tonsillar fossa	C09.0	C79.89	D00.08	D10.5	D37.05	D49.0
- tooth socket NEC	C03.9	C79.89	D00.03	D10.39	D37.09	D49.0
- trachea (cartilage) (mucosa)	C33	C78.39	D02.1	D14.2	D38.1	D49.1
- - overlapping lesion with bronchus or lung	C34.8-	-	-	-	-	-
- tracheobronchial	C34.8-	C78.39	D02.1	D14.2	D38.1	D49.1
- - overlapping lesion with lung	C34.8-	-	-	-	-	-
- tragus—*see also Neoplasm, skin, ear*	C44.20-	C79.2	D04.2-	D23.2-	D48.5	D49.2
- trunk NEC	C76.8	C79.89	D04.5	D36.7	D48.7	D49.89
- tubo-ovarian	C57.8	C79.82	D07.39	D28.7	D39.8	D49.59
- tunica vaginalis	C63.7	C79.82	D07.69	D29.8	D40.8	D49.59
- turbinate (bone)	C41.0	C79.51	-	D16.4-	D48.0	D49.2
- - nasal	C30.0	C78.39	D02.3	D14.0	D38.5	D49.1
- tympanic cavity	C30.1	C78.39	D02.3	D14.0	D38.5	D49.1
- ulna (any part)	C40.0-	C79.51	-	D16.0-	-	-
- umbilicus, umbilical—*see also Neoplasm, skin, trunk*	C44.509	C79.2	D04.5	D23.5	D48.5	D49.2
- uncus, brain	C71.2	C79.31	-	D33.0	D43.0	D49.6
- unknown site or unspecified	C80.1	C79.9	D09.9	D36.9	D48.9	D49.9
- urachus	C67.7	C79.11	D09.0	D30.3	D41.4	D49.4
- ureter, ureteral	C66.-	C79.19	D09.19	D30.2-	D41.2-	D49.59
- - orifice (bladder)	C67.6	C79.11	D09.0	D30.3	D41.4	D49.4
- ureter-bladder (junction)	C67.6	C79.11	D09.0	D30.3	D41.4	D49.4
- urethra, urethral (gland)	C68.0	C79.19	D09.19	D30.4	D41.3	D49.59
- - orifice, internal	C67.5	C79.11	D09.0	D30.3	D41.4	D49.4
- urethrovaginal (septum)	C57.9	C79.82	D07.30	D28.9	D39.8	D49.59
- urinary organ or system	C68.9	C79.10	D09.10	D30.9	D41.9	D49.59
- - bladder—*see Neoplasm, bladder*						
- - overlapping lesion	C68.8	-	-	-	-	-
- - specified sites NEC	C68.8	C79.19	D09.19	D30.8	D41.8	D49.59
- utero-ovarian	C57.8	C79.82	D07.39	D28.7	D39.8	D49.59
- - ligament	C57.1	C79.82	D07.39	D28.2	D39.8	D49.59
- uterosacral ligament	C57.3	C79.82	-	D28.2	D39.8	D49.59
- uterus, uteri, uterine	C55	C79.82	D07.0	D26.9	D39.0	D49.59
- - adnexa NEC	C57.4	C79.82	D07.39	D28.7	D39.8	D49.59
- - body	C54.9	C79.82	D07.0	D26.1	D39.0	D49.59
- - cervix	C53.9	C79.82	D06.9	D26.0	D39.0	D49.59
- - cornu	C54.9	C79.82	D07.0	D26.1	D39.0	D49.59
- - corpus	C54.9	C79.82	D07.0	D26.1	D39.0	D49.59
- - endocervix (canal) (gland)	C53.0	C79.82	D06.0	D26.0	D39.0	D49.59
- - endometrium	C54.1	C79.82	D07.0	D26.1	D39.0	D49.59
- - exocervix	C53.1	C79.82	D06.1	D26.0	D39.0	D49.59
- - external os	C53.1	C79.82	D06.1	D26.0	D39.0	D49.59

	Malignant Primary	Malignant Secondary	CA in Situ	Benign	Uncertain Behavior	Unspecified Behavior
- - fundus	C54.3	C79.82	D07.0	D26.1	D39.0	D49.59
- - internal os	C53.0	C79.82	D06.0	D26.0	D39.0	D49.59
- - isthmus	C54.0	C79.82	D07.0	D26.1	D39.0	D49.59
- - ligament	C57.3	C79.82	-	D28.2	D39.8	D49.59
- - - broad	C57.1	C79.82	D07.39	D28.2	D39.8	D49.59
- - - round	C57.2	C79.82	-	D28.2	D39.8	D49.59
- - lower segment	C54.0	C79.82	D07.0	D26.1	D39.0	D49.59
- - myometrium	C54.2	C79.82	D07.0	D26.1	D39.0	D49.59
- - overlapping sites	C54.8	-	-	-	-	-
- - squamocolumnar junction	C53.8	C79.82	D06.7	D26.0	D39.0	D49.59
- - tube	C57.0-	C79.82	D07.39	D28.2	D39.8	D49.59
- utricle, prostatic	C68.0	C79.19	D09.19	D30.4	D41.3	D49.59
- uveal tract	C69.4-	C79.49	D09.2-	D31.4-	D48.7	D49.89
- uvula	C05.2	C79.89	D00.04	D10.39	D37.09	D49.0
- vagina, vaginal (fornix) (vault) (wall)	C52	C79.82	D07.2	D28.1	D39.8	D49.59
- vaginovesical	C57.9	C79.82	D07.30	D28.9	D39.9	D49.59
- - septum	C57.9	C79.82	D07.30	D28.9	D39.9	D49.59
- vallecula (epiglottis)	C10.0	C79.89	D00.08	D10.5	D37.05	D49.0
- vas deferens	C63.1-	C79.82	D07.69	D29.8	D40.8	D49.59
- vascular—*see Neoplasm, connective tissue*						
- Vater's ampulla	C24.1	C78.89	D01.5	D13.5	D37.6	D49.0
- vein, venous—*see Neoplasm, connective tissue*						
- vena cava (abdominal) (inferior)	C49.4	C79.89	-	D21.4	D48.1	D49.2
- - superior	C49.3	C79.89	-	D21.3	D48.1	D49.2
- ventricle (cerebral) (floor) (lateral) (third)	C71.5	C79.31	-	D33.0	D43.0	D49.6
- - cardiac (left) (right)	C38.0	C79.89	-	D15.1	D48.7	D49.89
- - fourth	C71.7	C79.31	-	D33.1	D43.1	D49.6
- ventricular band of larynx	C32.1	C78.39	D02.0	D14.1	D38.0	D49.1
- ventriculus—*see Neoplasm, stomach*						
- vermillion border—*see Neoplasm, lip*						
- vermis, cerebellum	C71.6	C79.31	-	D33.1	D43.1	D49.6
- vertebra (column)	C41.2	C79.51	-	D16.6	D48.0	D49.2
- - coccyx	C41.4	C79.51	-	D16.8-	D48.0	D49.2
- - marrow NEC	C96.9	C79.52	-	-	D47.9	D49.89
- - sacrum	C41.4	C79.51	-	D16.8-	D48.0	D49.2
- vesical—*see Neoplasm, bladder*						
- vesicle, seminal	C63.7	C79.82	D07.69	D29.8	D40.8	D49.59
- vesicocervical tissue	C57.9	C79.82	D07.30	D28.9	D39.9	D49.59
- vesicorectal	C76.3	C79.82	D09.8	D36.7	D48.7	D49.89
- vesicovaginal	C57.9	C79.82	D07.30	D28.9	D39.9	D49.59
- - septum	C57.9	C79.82	D07.30	D28.9	D39.8	D49.59
- vessel (blood)—*see Neoplasm, connective tissue*						
- vestibular gland, greater	C51.0	C79.82	D07.1	D28.0	D39.8	D49.59
- vestibule						
- - mouth	C06.1	C79.89	D00.00	D10.39	D37.09	D49.0
- - nose	C30.0	C78.39	D02.3	D14.0	D38.5	D49.1
- Virchow's gland	C77.0	C77.0	-	D36.0	D48.7	D49.89
- viscera NEC	C76.8	C79.89	D09.8	D36.7	D48.7	D49.89
- vocal cords (true)	C32.0	C78.39	D02.0	D14.1	D38.0	D49.1
- - false	C32.1	C78.39	D02.0	D14.1	D38.0	D49.1
- vomer	C41.0	C79.51	-	D16.4-	D48.0	D49.2
- vulva	C51.9	C79.82	D07.1	D28.0	D39.8	D49.59
- vulvovaginal gland	C51.0	C79.82	D07.1	D28.0	D39.8	D49.59
- Waldeyer's ring	C14.2	C79.89	D00.08	D10.9	D37.05	D49.0
- Wharton's duct	C08.0	C79.89	D00.00	D11.7	D37.032	D49.0
- white matter (central) (cerebral)	C71.0	C79.31	-	D33.0	D43.0	D49.6
- windpipe	C33	C78.39	D02.1	D14.2	D38.1	D49.1
- Wirsung's duct	C25.3	C78.89	D01.7	D13.6	D37.8	D49.0
- wolffian (body) (duct)						
- - female	C57.7	C79.82	D07.39	D28.7	D39.8	D49.59
- - male	C63.7	C79.82	D07.69	D29.8	D40.8	D49.59
- womb—*see Neoplasm, uterus*						
- wrist NEC	C76.4-	C79.89	D04.6-	D36.7	D48.7	D49.89
- xiphoid process	C41.3	C79.51	-	D16.7	D48.0	D49.2
- Zuckerkandl organ	C75.5	C79.89	-	D35.6	D44.7	D49.7

Table Of Drugs And Chemicals

Substance	Poisoning, Accidental (unintentional)	Poisoning, Intentional Self-harm	Poisoning, Assault	Poisoning, Undetermined	Adverse effect	Underdosing
1-propanol	T51.3X1	T51.3X2	T51.3X3	T51.3X4	--	--
2-propanol	T51.2X1	T51.2X2	T51.2X3	T51.2X4	--	--
2,4-D (dichlorophen-oxyacetic acid)	T60.3X1	T60.3X2	T60.3X3	T60.3X4	--	--
2,4-toluene diisocyanate	T65.0X1	T65.0X2	T65.0X3	T65.0X4	--	--
2,4,5-T (trichloro-phenoxyacetic acid)	T60.1X1	T60.1X2	T60.1X3	T60.1X4	--	--
14-hydroxydihydro-morphinone	T40.2X1	T40.2X2	T40.2X3	T40.2X4	T40.2X5	T40.2X6
ABOB	T37.5X1	T37.5X2	T37.5X3	T37.5X4	T37.5X5	T37.5X6
Abrine	T62.2X1	T62.2X2	T62.2X3	T62.2X4	--	--
Abrus (seed)	T62.2X1	T62.2X2	T62.2X3	T62.2X4	--	--
Absinthe	T51.0X1	T51.0X2	T51.0X3	T51.0X4	--	--
- beverage	T51.0X1	T51.0X2	T51.0X3	T51.0X4	--	--
Acaricide	T60.8X1	T60.8X2	T60.8X3	T60.8X4	--	--
Acebutolol	T44.7X1	T44.7X2	T44.7X3	T44.7X4	T44.7X5	T44.7X6
Acecarbromal	T42.6X1	T42.6X2	T42.6X3	T42.6X4	T42.6X5	T42.6X6
Aceclidine	T44.1X1	T44.1X2	T44.1X3	T44.1X4	T44.1X5	T44.1X6
Acedapsone	T37.0X1	T37.0X2	T37.0X3	T37.0X4	T37.0X5	T37.0X6
Acefylline piperazine	T48.6X1	T48.6X2	T48.6X3	T48.6X4	T48.6X5	T48.6X6
Acemorphan	T40.2X1	T40.2X2	T40.2X3	T40.2X4	T40.2X5	T40.2X6
Acenocoumarin	T45.511	T45.512	T45.513	T45.514	T45.515	T45.516
Acenocoumarol	T45.511	T45.512	T45.513	T45.514	T45.515	T45.516
Acepifylline	T48.6X1	T48.6X2	T48.6X3	T48.6X4	T48.6X5	T48.6X6
Acepromazine	T43.3X1	T43.3X2	T43.3X3	T43.3X4	T43.3X5	T43.3X6
Acesulfamethoxypyridazine	T37.0X1	T37.0X2	T37.0X3	T37.0X4	T37.0X5	T37.0X6
Acetal	T52.8X1	T52.8X2	T52.8X3	T52.8X4	--	--
Acetaldehyde (vapor)	T52.8X1	T52.8X2	T52.8X3	T52.8X4	--	--
- liquid	T65.891	T65.892	T65.893	T65.894	--	--
P-Acetamidophenol	T39.1X1	T39.1X2	T39.1X3	T39.1X4	T39.1X5	T39.1X6
Acetaminophen	T39.1X1	T39.1X2	T39.1X3	T39.1X4	T39.1X5	T39.1X6
Acetaminosalol	T39.1X1	T39.1X2	T39.1X3	T39.1X4	T39.1X5	T39.1X6
Acetanilide	T39.1X1	T39.1X2	T39.1X3	T39.1X4	T39.1X5	T39.1X6
Acetarsol	T37.3X1	T37.3X2	T37.3X3	T37.3X4	T37.3X5	T37.3X6
Acetazolamide	T50.2X1	T50.2X2	T50.2X3	T50.2X4	T50.2X5	T50.2X6
Acetiamine	T45.2X1	T45.2X2	T45.2X3	T45.2X4	T45.2X5	T45.2X6
Acetic						
- acid	T54.2X1	T54.2X2	T54.2X3	T54.2X4	--	--
- - with sodium acetate (ointment)	T49.3X1	T49.3X2	T49.3X3	T49.3X4	T49.3X5	T49.3X6
- - ester (solvent) (vapor)	T52.8X1	T52.8X2	T52.8X3	T52.8X4	--	--
- - irrigating solution	T50.3X1	T50.3X2	T50.3X3	T50.3X4	T50.3X5	T50.3X6
- - medicinal (lotion)	T49.2X1	T49.2X2	T49.2X3	T49.2X4	T49.2X5	T49.2X6
- anhydride	T65.891	T65.892	T65.893	T65.894	--	--
- ether (vapor)	T52.8X1	T52.8X2	T52.8X3	T52.8X4	--	--
Acetohexamide	T38.3X1	T38.3X2	T38.3X3	T38.3X4	T38.3X5	T38.3X6
Acetohydroxamic acid	T50.991	T50.992	T50.993	T50.994	T50.995	T50.996
Acetomenaphthone	T45.7X1	T45.7X2	T45.7X3	T45.7X4	T45.7X5	T45.7X6
Acetomorphine	T40.1X1	T40.1X2	T40.1X3	T40.1X4	T40.1X5	--
Acetone (oils)	T52.4X1	T52.4X2	T52.4X3	T52.4X4	--	--
- chlorinated	T52.4X1	T52.4X2	T52.4X3	T52.4X4	--	--
- vapor	T52.4X1	T52.4X2	T52.4X3	T52.4X4	--	--
Acetonitrile	T52.8X1	T52.8X2	T52.8X3	T52.8X4	--	--
Acetophenazine	T43.3X1	T43.3X2	T43.3X3	T43.3X4	T43.3X5	T43.3X6
Acetophenetidin	T39.1X1	T39.1X2	T39.1X3	T39.1X4	T39.1X5	T39.1X6
Acetophenone	T52.4X1	T52.4X2	T52.4X3	T52.4X4	--	--
Acetorphine	T40.2X1	T40.2X2	T40.2X3	T40.2X4	--	--
Acetosulfone (sodium)	T37.1X1	T37.1X2	T37.1X3	T37.1X4	T37.1X5	T37.1X6
Acetrizoate (sodium)	T50.8X1	T50.8X2	T50.8X3	T50.8X4	T50.8X5	T50.8X6
Acetrizoic acid	T50.8X1	T50.8X2	T50.8X3	T50.8X4	T50.8X5	T50.8X6

Substance	Poisoning, Accidental (unintentional)	Poisoning, Intentional Self-harm	Poisoning, Assault	Poisoning, Undetermined	Adverse effect	Underdosing
Acetyl						
- bromide	T53.6X1	T53.6X2	T53.6X3	T53.6X4	--	--
- chloride	T53.6X1	T53.6X2	T53.6X3	T53.6X4	--	--
Acetylcarbromal	T42.6X1	T42.6X2	T42.6X3	T42.6X4	T42.6X5	T42.6X6
Acetylcholine						
- chloride	T44.1X1	T44.1X2	T44.1X3	T44.1X4	T44.1X5	T44.1X6
- derivative	T44.1X1	T44.1X2	T44.1X3	T44.1X4	T44.1X5	T44.1X6
Acetylcysteine	T48.4X1	T48.4X2	T48.4X3	T48.4X4	T48.4X5	T48.4X6
Acetyldigitoxin	T46.0X1	T46.0X2	T46.0X3	T46.0X4	T46.0X5	T46.0X6
Acetyldigoxin	T46.0X1	T46.0X2	T46.0X3	T46.0X4	T46.0X5	T46.0X6
Acetyldihydrocodeine	T40.2X1	T40.2X2	T40.2X3	T40.2X4	--	--
Acetyldihydrocodeinone	T40.2X1	T40.2X2	T40.2X3	T40.2X4	--	--
Acetylene (gas)	T59.891	T59.892	T59.893	T59.894	--	--
- dichloride	T53.6X1	T53.6X2	T53.6X3	T53.6X4	--	--
- incomplete combustion of	T58.11	T58.12	T58.13	T58.14	--	--
- industrial	T59.891	T59.892	T59.893	T59.894	--	--
- tetrachloride	T53.6X1	T53.6X2	T53.6X3	T53.6X4	--	--
- - vapor	T53.6X1	T53.6X2	T53.6X3	T53.6X4	--	--
Acetylpheneturide	T42.6X1	T42.6X2	T42.6X3	T42.6X4	T42.6X5	T42.6X6
Acetylphenylhydrazine	T39.8X1	T39.8X2	T39.8X3	T39.8X4	T39.8X5	T39.8X6
Acetylsalicylic acid (salts)	T39.011	T39.012	T39.013	T39.014	T39.015	T39.016
- enteric coated	T39.011	T39.012	T39.013	T39.014	T39.015	T39.016
Acetylsulfamethoxypyridazine	T37.0X1	T37.0X2	T37.0X3	T37.0X4	T37.0X5	T37.0X6
Achromycin	T36.4X1	T36.4X2	T36.4X3	T36.4X4	T36.4X5	T36.4X6
- ophthalmic preparation	T49.5X1	T49.5X2	T49.5X3	T49.5X4	T49.5X5	T49.5X6
- topical NEC	T49.0X1	T49.0X2	T49.0X3	T49.0X4	T49.0X5	T49.0X6
Aciclovir	T37.5X1	T37.5X2	T37.5X3	T37.5X4	T37.5X5	T37.5X6
Acid (corrosive) NEC	T54.2X1	T54.2X2	T54.2X3	T54.2X4	--	--
Acidifying agent NEC	T50.901	T50.902	T50.903	T50.904	T50.905	T50.906
Acipimox	T46.6X1	T46.6X2	T46.6X3	T46.6X4	T46.6X5	T46.6X6
Acitretin	T50.991	T50.992	T50.993	T50.994	T50.995	T50.996
Aclarubicin	T45.1X1	T45.1X2	T45.1X3	T45.1X4	T45.1X5	T45.1X6
Aclatonium napadisilate	T48.1X1	T48.1X2	T48.1X3	T48.1X4	T48.1X5	T48.1X6
Aconite (wild)	T46.991	T46.992	T46.993	T46.994	T46.995	T46.996
Aconitine	T46.991	T46.992	T46.993	T46.994	T46.995	T46.996
Aconitum ferox	T46.991	T46.992	T46.993	T46.994	T46.995	T46.996
Acridine	T65.6X1	T65.6X2	T65.6X3	T65.6X4	--	--
- vapor	T59.891	T59.892	T59.893	T59.894	--	--
Acriflavine	T37.91	T37.92	T37.93	T37.94	T37.95	T37.96
Acriflavinium chloride	T49.0X1	T49.0X2	T49.0X3	T49.0X4	T49.0X5	T49.0X6
Acrinol	T49.0X1	T49.0X2	T49.0X3	T49.0X4	T49.0X5	T49.0X6
Acrisorcin	T49.0X1	T49.0X2	T49.0X3	T49.0X4	T49.0X5	T49.0X6
Acrivastine	T45.0X1	T45.0X2	T45.0X3	T45.0X4	T45.0X5	T45.0X6
Acrolein (gas)	T59.891	T59.892	T59.893	T59.894	--	--
- liquid	T54.1X1	T54.1X2	T54.1X3	T54.1X4	--	--
Acrylamide	T65.891	T65.892	T65.893	T65.894	--	--
Acrylic resin	T49.3X1	T49.3X2	T49.3X3	T49.3X4	T49.3X5	T49.3X6
Acrylonitrile	T65.891	T65.892	T65.893	T65.894	--	--
Actaea spicata	T62.2X1	T62.2X2	T62.2X3	T62.2X4	--	--
- berry	T62.1X1	T62.1X2	T62.1X3	T62.1X4	--	--
Acterol	T37.3X1	T37.3X2	T37.3X3	T37.3X4	T37.3X5	T37.3X6
ACTH	T38.811	T38.812	T38.813	T38.814	T38.815	T38.816
Actinomycin C	T45.1X1	T45.1X2	T45.1X3	T45.1X4	T45.1X5	T45.1X6
Actinomycin D	T45.1X1	T45.1X2	T45.1X3	T45.1X4	T45.1X5	T45.1X6
Activated charcoal—*see also Charcoal, medicinal*	T47.6X1	T47.6X2	T47.6X3	T47.6X4	T47.6X5	T47.6X6
Acyclovir	T37.5X1	T37.5X2	T37.5X3	T37.5X4	T37.5X5	T37.5X6
Adenine	T45.2X1	T45.2X2	T45.2X3	T45.2X4	T45.2X5	T45.2X6
- arabinoside	T37.5X1	T37.5X2	T37.5X3	T37.5X4	T37.5X5	T37.5X6

Substance	Poisoning, Accidental (unintentional)	Poisoning, Intentional Self-harm	Poisoning, Assault	Poisoning, Undetermined	Adverse effect	Underdosing
Adenosine (phosphate)	T46.2X1	T46.2X2	T46.2X3	T46.2X4	T46.2X5	T46.2X6
ADH	T38.891	T38.892	T38.893	T38.894	T38.895	T38.896
Adhesive NEC	T65.891	T65.892	T65.893	T65.894	--	--
Adicillin	T36.0X1	T36.0X2	T36.0X3	T36.0X4	T36.0X5	T36.0X6
Adiphenine	T44.3X1	T44.3X2	T44.3X3	T44.3X4	T44.3X5	T44.3X6
Adipiodone	T50.8X1	T50.8X2	T50.8X3	T50.8X4	T50.8X5	T50.8X6
Adjunct, pharmaceutical	T50.901	T50.902	T50.903	T50.904	T50.905	T50.906
Adrenal (extract, cortex or medulla) (gluco-orticoids)(hormones)(mineralocorticoids)	T38.0X1	T38.0X2	T38.0X3	T38.0X4	T38.0X5	T38.0X6
- ENT agent	T49.6X1	T49.6X2	T49.6X3	T49.6X4	T49.6X5	T49.6X6
- ophthalmic preparation	T49.5X1	T49.5X2	T49.5X3	T49.5X4	T49.5X5	T49.5X6
- topical NEC	T49.0X1	T49.0X2	T49.0X3	T49.0X4	T49.0X5	T49.0X6
Adrenaline	T44.5X1	T44.5X2	T44.5X3	T44.5X4	T44.5X5	T44.5X6
Adrenalin—see Adrenaline						
Adrenergic NEC	T44.901	T44.902	T44.903	T44.904	T44.905	T44.906
- blocking agent NEC	T44.8X1	T44.8X2	T44.8X3	T44.8X4	T44.8X5	T44.8X6
- - beta, heart	T44.7X1	T44.7X2	T44.7X3	T44.7X4	T44.7X5	T44.7X6
- specified NEC	T44.991	T44.992	T44.993	T44.994	T44.995	T44.996
Adrenochrome						
- (mono) semicarbazone	T46.991	T46.992	T46.993	T46.994	T46.995	T46.996
- derivative	T46.991	T46.992	T46.993	T46.994	T46.995	T46.996
Adrenocorticotrophic hormone	T38.811	T38.812	T38.813	T38.814	T38.815	T38.816
Adrenocorticotrophin	T38.811	T38.812	T38.813	T38.814	T38.815	T38.816
Adriamycin	T45.1X1	T45.1X2	T45.1X3	T45.1X4	T45.1X5	T45.1X6
Aerosol spray NEC	T65.91	T65.92	T65.93	T65.94	--	--
Aerosporin	T36.8X1	T36.8X2	T36.8X3	T36.8X4	T36.8X5	T36.8X6
- ENT agent	T49.6X1	T49.6X2	T49.6X3	T49.6X4	T49.6X5	T49.6X6
- ophthalmic preparation	T49.5X1	T49.5X2	T49.5X3	T49.5X4	T49.5X5	T49.5X6
- topical NEC	T49.0X1	T49.0X2	T49.0X3	T49.0X4	T49.0X5	T49.0X6
Aethusa cynapium	T62.2X1	T62.2X2	T62.2X3	T62.2X4	--	--
Afghanistan black	T40.7X1	T40.7X2	T40.7X3	T40.7X4	T40.7X5	T40.7X6
Aflatoxin	T64.01	T64.02	T64.03	T64.04	--	--
Afloqualone	T42.8X1	T42.8X2	T42.8X3	T42.8X4	T42.8X5	T42.8X6
African boxwood	T62.2X1	T62.2X2	T62.2X3	T62.2X4	--	--
Agar	T47.4X1	T47.4X2	T47.4X3	T47.4X4	T47.4X5	T47.4X6
Agonist						
- predominantly						
- - alpha-adrenoreceptor	T44.4X1	T44.4X2	T44.4X3	T44.4X4	T44.4X5	T44.4X6
- - beta-adrenoreceptor	T44.5X1	T44.5X2	T44.5X3	T44.5X4	T44.5X5	T44.5X6
Agricultural agent NEC	T65.91	T65.92	T65.93	T65.94	--	--
Agrypnal	T42.3X1	T42.3X2	T42.3X3	T42.3X4	T42.3X5	T42.3X6
AHLG	T50.Z11	T50.Z12	T50.Z13	T50.Z14	T50.Z15	T50.Z16
Air contaminant (s) , source/type NOS	T65.91	T65.92	T65.93	T65.94	--	--
Ajmaline	T46.2X1	T46.2X2	T46.2X3	T46.2X4	T46.2X5	T46.2X6
Akee	T62.1X1	T62.1X2	T62.1X3	T62.1X4	--	--
Akrinol	T49.0X1	T49.0X2	T49.0X3	T49.0X4	T49.0X5	T49.0X6
Akritoin	T37.8X1	T37.8X2	T37.8X3	T37.8X4	T37.8X5	T37.8X6
Alacepril	T46.4X1	T46.4X2	T46.4X3	T46.4X4	T46.4X5	T46.4X6
Alantolactone	T37.4X1	T37.4X2	T37.4X3	T37.4X4	T37.4X5	T37.4X6
Albamycin	T36.8X1	T36.8X2	T36.8X3	T36.8X4	T36.8X5	T36.8X6
Albendazole	T37.4X1	T37.4X2	T37.4X3	T37.4X4	T37.4X5	T37.4X6
Albumin						
- bovine	T45.8X1	T45.8X2	T45.8X3	T45.8X4	T45.8X5	T45.8X6
- human serum	T45.8X1	T45.8X2	T45.8X3	T45.8X4	T45.8X5	T45.8X6
- - salt-poor	T45.8X1	T45.8X2	T45.8X3	T45.8X4	T45.8X5	T45.8X6
- normal human serum	T45.8X1	T45.8X2	T45.8X3	T45.8X4	T45.8X5	T45.8X6
Albuterol	T48.6X1	T48.6X2	T48.6X3	T48.6X4	T48.6X5	T48.6X6
Albutoin	T42.0X1	T42.0X2	T42.0X3	T42.0X4	T42.0X5	T42.0X6
Alclometasone	T49.0X1	T49.0X2	T49.0X3	T49.0X4	T49.0X5	T49.0X6

Substance	Poisoning, Accidental (unintentional)	Poisoning, Intentional Self-harm	Poisoning, Assault	Poisoning, Undetermined	Adverse effect	Underdosing
Alcohol	T51.91	T51.92	T51.93	T51.94	--	--
- absolute	T51.0X1	T51.0X2	T51.0X3	T51.0X4	--	--
- - beverage	T51.0X1	T51.0X2	T51.0X3	T51.0X4	--	--
- allyl	T51.8X1	T51.8X2	T51.8X3	T51.8X4	--	--
- amyl	T51.3X1	T51.3X2	T51.3X3	T51.3X4	--	--
- antifreeze	T51.1X1	T51.1X2	T51.1X3	T51.1X4	--	--
- beverage	T51.0X1	T51.0X2	T51.0X3	T51.0X4	--	--
- butyl	T51.3X1	T51.3X2	T51.3X3	T51.3X4	--	--
- dehydrated	T51.0X1	T51.0X2	T51.0X3	T51.0X4	--	--
- - beverage	T51.0X1	T51.0X2	T51.0X3	T51.0X4	--	--
- denatured	T51.0X1	T51.0X2	T51.0X3	T51.0X4	--	--
- deterrent NEC	T50.6X1	T50.6X2	T50.6X3	T50.6X4	T50.6X5	T50.6X6
- diagnostic (gastric function)	T50.8X1	T50.8X2	T50.8X3	T50.8X4	T50.8X5	T50.8X6
- ethyl	T51.0X1	T51.0X2	T51.0X3	T51.0X4	--	--
- - beverage	T51.0X1	T51.0X2	T51.0X3	T51.0X4	--	--
- grain	T51.0X1	T51.0X2	T51.0X3	T51.0X4	--	--
- - beverage	T51.0X1	T51.0X2	T51.0X3	T51.0X4	--	--
- industrial	T51.0X1	T51.0X2	T51.0X3	T51.0X4	--	--
- isopropyl	T51.2X1	T51.2X2	T51.2X3	T51.2X4	--	--
- methyl	T51.1X1	T51.1X2	T51.1X3	T51.1X4	--	--
- preparation for consumption	T51.0X1	T51.0X2	T51.0X3	T51.0X4	--	--
- propyl	T51.3X1	T51.3X2	T51.3X3	T51.3X4	--	--
- - secondary	T51.2X1	T51.2X2	T51.2X3	T51.2X4	--	--
- radiator	T51.1X1	T51.1X2	T51.1X3	T51.1X4	--	--
- rubbing	T51.2X1	T51.2X2	T51.2X3	T51.2X4	--	--
- specified type NEC	T51.8X1	T51.8X2	T51.8X3	T51.8X4	--	--
- surgical	T51.0X1	T51.0X2	T51.0X3	T51.0X4	--	--
- vapor (from any type of Alcohol)	T59.891	T59.892	T59.893	T59.894	--	--
- wood	T51.1X1	T51.1X2	T51.1X3	T51.1X4	--	--
Alcuronium (chloride)	T48.1X1	T48.1X2	T48.1X3	T48.1X4	T48.1X5	T48.1X6
Aldactone	T50.0X1	T50.0X2	T50.0X3	T50.0X4	T50.0X5	T50.0X6
Aldesulfone sodium	T37.1X1	T37.1X2	T37.1X3	T37.1X4	T37.1X5	T37.1X6
Aldicarb	T60.0X1	T60.0X2	T60.0X3	T60.0X4	--	--
Aldomet	T46.5X1	T46.5X2	T46.5X3	T46.5X4	T46.5X5	T46.5X6
Aldosterone	T50.0X1	T50.0X2	T50.0X3	T50.0X4	T50.0X5	T50.0X6
Aldrin (dust)	T60.1X1	T60.1X2	T60.1X3	T60.1X4	--	--
Aleve—see Naproxen						
Alexitol sodium	T47.1X1	T47.1X2	T47.1X3	T47.1X4	T47.1X5	T47.1X6
Alfacalcidol	T45.2X1	T45.2X2	T45.2X3	T45.2X4	T45.2X5	T45.2X6
Alfadolone	T41.1X1	T41.1X2	T41.1X3	T41.1X4	T41.1X5	T41.1X6
Alfaxalone	T41.1X1	T41.1X2	T41.1X3	T41.1X4	T41.1X5	T41.1X6
Alfentanil	T40.4X1	T40.4X2	T40.4X3	T40.4X4	T40.4X5	T40.4X6
Alfuzosin (hydrochloride)	T44.8X1	T44.8X2	T44.8X3	T44.8X4	T44.8X5	T44.8X6
Algae (harmful) (toxin)	T65.821	T65.822	T65.823	T65.824	--	--
Algeldrate	T47.1X1	T47.1X2	T47.1X3	T47.1X4	T47.1X5	T47.1X6
Algin	T47.8X1	T47.8X2	T47.8X3	T47.8X4	T47.8X5	T47.8X6
Alglucerase	T45.3X1	T45.3X2	T45.3X3	T45.3X4	T45.3X5	T45.3X6
Alidase	T45.3X1	T45.3X2	T45.3X3	T45.3X4	T45.3X5	T45.3X6
Alimemazine	T43.3X1	T43.3X2	T43.3X3	T43.3X4	T43.3X5	T43.3X6
Aliphatic thiocyanates	T65.0X1	T65.0X2	T65.0X3	T65.0X4	--	--
Alizapride	T45.0X1	T45.0X2	T45.0X3	T45.0X4	T45.0X5	T45.0X6
Alkali (caustic)	T54.3X1	T54.3X2	T54.3X3	T54.3X4	--	--
Alkaline antiseptic solution (aromatic)	T49.6X1	T49.6X2	T49.6X3	T49.6X4	T49.6X5	T49.6X6
Alkalinizing agents (medicinal)	T50.901	T50.902	T50.903	T50.904	T50.905	T50.906
Alkalizing agent NEC	T50.901	T50.902	T50.903	T50.904	T50.905	T50.906
Alka-seltzer	T39.011	T39.012	T39.013	T39.014	T39.015	T39.016
Alkavervir	T46.5X1	T46.5X2	T46.5X3	T46.5X4	T46.5X5	T46.5X6
Alkonium (bromide)	T49.0X1	T49.0X2	T49.0X3	T49.0X4	T49.0X5	T49.0X6
Alkylating drug NEC	T45.1X1	T45.1X2	T45.1X3	T45.1X4	T45.1X5	T45.1X6

Substance	Poisoning, Accidental (unintentional)	Poisoning, Intentional Self-harm	Poisoning, Assault	Poisoning, Undetermined	Adverse effect	Underdosing
- antimyeloproliferative	T45.1X1	T45.1X2	T45.1X3	T45.1X4	T45.1X5	T45.1X6
- lymphatic	T45.1X1	T45.1X2	T45.1X3	T45.1X4	T45.1X5	T45.1X6
Alkylisocyanate	T65.0X1	T65.0X2	T65.0X3	T65.0X4	--	--
Allantoin	T49.4X1	T49.4X2	T49.4X3	T49.4X4	T49.4X5	T49.4X6
Allegron	T43.011	T43.012	T43.013	T43.014	T43.015	T43.016
Allethrin	T49.0X1	T49.0X2	T49.0X3	T49.0X4	T49.0X5	T49.0X6
Allobarbital	T42.3X1	T42.3X2	T42.3X3	T42.3X4	T42.3X5	T42.3X6
Allopurinol	T50.4X1	T50.4X2	T50.4X3	T50.4X4	T50.4X5	T50.4X6
Allyl						
- Alcohol	T51.8X1	T51.8X2	T51.8X3	T51.8X4	--	--
- disulfide	T46.6X1	T46.6X2	T46.6X3	T46.6X4	T46.6X5	T46.6X6
Allylestrenol	T38.5X1	T38.5X2	T38.5X3	T38.5X4	T38.5X5	T38.5X6
Allylisopropylacetylurea	T42.6X1	T42.6X2	T42.6X3	T42.6X4	T42.6X5	T42.6X6
Allylisopropylmalonylurea	T42.3X1	T42.3X2	T42.3X3	T42.3X4	T42.3X5	T42.3X6
Allylthiourea	T49.3X1	T49.3X2	T49.3X3	T49.3X4	T49.3X5	T49.3X6
Allyltribromide	T42.6X1	T42.6X2	T42.6X3	T42.6X4	T42.6X5	T42.6X6
Allypropymal	T42.3X1	T42.3X2	T42.3X3	T42.3X4	T42.3X5	T42.3X6
Almagate	T47.1X1	T47.1X2	T47.1X3	T47.1X4	T47.1X5	T47.1X6
Almasilate	T47.1X1	T47.1X2	T47.1X3	T47.1X4	T47.1X5	T47.1X6
Almitrine	T50.7X1	T50.7X2	T50.7X3	T50.7X4	T50.7X5	T50.7X6
Aloes	T47.2X1	T47.2X2	T47.2X3	T47.2X4	T47.2X5	T47.2X6
Aloglutamol	T47.1X1	T47.1X2	T47.1X3	T47.1X4	T47.1X5	T47.1X6
Aloin	T47.2X1	T47.2X2	T47.2X3	T47.2X4	T47.2X5	T47.2X6
Aloxidone	T42.2X1	T42.2X2	T42.2X3	T42.2X4	T42.2X5	T42.2X6
Alpha						
- acetyldigoxin	T46.0X1	T46.0X2	T46.0X3	T46.0X4	T46.0X5	T46.0X6
- adrenergic blocking drug	T44.6X1	T44.6X2	T44.6X3	T44.6X4	T44.6X5	T44.6X6
- amylase	T45.3X1	T45.3X2	T45.3X3	T45.3X4	T45.3X5	T45.3X6
- tocoferol (acetate)	T45.2X1	T45.2X2	T45.2X3	T45.2X4	T45.2X5	T45.2X6
- tocopherol	T45.2X1	T45.2X2	T45.2X3	T45.2X4	T45.2X5	T45.2X6
Alphadolone	T41.1X1	T41.1X2	T41.1X3	T41.1X4	T41.1X5	T41.1X6
Alphaprodine	T40.4X1	T40.4X2	T40.4X3	T40.4X4	T40.4X5	T40.4X6
Alphaxalone	T41.1X1	T41.1X2	T41.1X3	T41.1X4	T41.1X5	T41.1X6
Alprazolam	T42.4X1	T42.4X2	T42.4X3	T42.4X4	T42.4X5	T42.4X6
Alprenolol	T44.7X1	T44.7X2	T44.7X3	T44.7X4	T44.7X5	T44.7X6
Alprostadil	T46.7X1	T46.7X2	T46.7X3	T46.7X4	T46.7X5	T46.7X6
Alsactide	T38.811	T38.812	T38.813	T38.814	T38.815	T38.816
Alseroxylon	T46.5X1	T46.5X2	T46.5X3	T46.5X4	T46.5X5	T46.5X6
Alteplase	T45.611	T45.612	T45.613	T45.614	T45.615	T45.616
Altizide	T50.2X1	T50.2X2	T50.2X3	T50.2X4	T50.2X5	T50.2X6
Altretamine	T45.1X1	T45.1X2	T45.1X3	T45.1X4	T45.1X5	T45.1X6
Alum (medicinal)	T49.4X1	T49.4X2	T49.4X3	T49.4X4	T49.4X5	T49.4X6
- nonmedicinal (ammonium) (potassium)	T56.891	T56.892	T56.893	T56.894	--	--
Aluminium, aluminum						
- acetate	T49.2X1	T49.2X2	T49.2X3	T49.2X4	T49.2X5	T49.2X6
- - solution	T49.0X1	T49.0X2	T49.0X3	T49.0X4	T49.0X5	T49.0X6
- aspirin	T39.011	T39.012	T39.013	T39.014	T39.015	T39.016
- bis (acetylsalicylate)	T39.011	T39.012	T39.013	T39.014	T39.015	T39.016
- carbonate (gel, basic)	T47.1X1	T47.1X2	T47.1X3	T47.1X4	T47.1X5	T47.1X6
- chlorhydroxide-complex	T47.1X1	T47.1X2	T47.1X3	T47.1X4	T47.1X5	T47.1X6
- chloride	T49.2X1	T49.2X2	T49.2X3	T49.2X4	T49.2X5	T49.2X6
- clofibrate	T46.6X1	T46.6X2	T46.6X3	T46.6X4	T46.6X5	T46.6X6
- diacetate	T49.2X1	T49.2X2	T49.2X3	T49.2X4	T49.2X5	T49.2X6
- glycinate	T47.1X1	T47.1X2	T47.1X3	T47.1X4	T47.1X5	T47.1X6
- hydroxide (gel)	T47.1X1	T47.1X2	T47.1X3	T47.1X4	T47.1X5	T47.1X6
- hydroxide-magnesium carb. gel	T47.1X1	T47.1X2	T47.1X3	T47.1X4	T47.1X5	T47.1X6
- magnesium silicate	T47.1X1	T47.1X2	T47.1X3	T47.1X4	T47.1X5	T47.1X6
- nicotinate	T46.7X1	T46.7X2	T46.7X3	T46.7X4	T46.7X5	T46.7X6

Substance	Poisoning, Accidental (unintentional)	Poisoning, Intentional Self-harm	Poisoning, Assault	Poisoning, Undetermined	Adverse effect	Underdosing
- ointment (surgical) (topical)	T49.3X1	T49.3X2	T49.3X3	T49.3X4	T49.3X5	T49.3X6
- phosphate	T47.1X1	T47.1X2	T47.1X3	T47.1X4	T47.1X5	T47.1X6
- salicylate	T39.091	T39.092	T39.093	T39.094	T39.095	T39.096
- silicate	T47.1X1	T47.1X2	T47.1X3	T47.1X4	T47.1X5	T47.1X6
- sodium silicate	T47.1X1	T47.1X2	T47.1X3	T47.1X4	T47.1X5	T47.1X6
- subacetate	T49.2X1	T49.2X2	T49.2X3	T49.2X4	T49.2X5	T49.2X6
- sulfate	T49.0X1	T49.0X2	T49.0X3	T49.0X4	T49.0X5	T49.0X6
- tannate	T47.6X1	T47.6X2	T47.6X3	T47.6X4	T47.6X5	T47.6X6
- topical NEC	T49.3X1	T49.3X2	T49.3X3	T49.3X4	T49.3X5	T49.3X6
Alurate	T42.3X1	T42.3X2	T42.3X3	T42.3X4	T42.3X5	T42.3X6
Alverine	T44.3X1	T44.3X2	T44.3X3	T44.3X4	T44.3X5	T44.3X6
Alvodine	T40.2X1	T40.2X2	T40.2X3	T40.2X4	T40.2X5	T40.2X6
Amanita phalloides	T62.0X1	T62.0X2	T62.0X3	T62.0X4	--	--
Amanitine	T62.0X1	T62.0X2	T62.0X3	T62.0X4	--	--
Amantadine	T42.8X1	T42.8X2	T42.8X3	T42.8X4	T42.8X5	T42.8X6
Ambazone	T49.6X1	T49.6X2	T49.6X3	T49.6X4	T49.6X5	T49.6X6
Ambenonium (chloride)	T44.0X1	T44.0X2	T44.0X3	T44.0X4	T44.0X5	T44.0X6
Ambroxol	T48.4X1	T48.4X2	T48.4X3	T48.4X4	T48.4X5	T48.4X6
Ambuphylline	T48.6X1	T48.6X2	T48.6X3	T48.6X4	T48.6X5	T48.6X6
Ambutonium bromide	T44.3X1	T44.3X2	T44.3X3	T44.3X4	T44.3X5	T44.3X6
Amcinonide	T49.0X1	T49.0X2	T49.0X3	T49.0X4	T49.0X5	T49.0X6
Amdinocillin	T36.0X1	T36.0X2	T36.0X3	T36.0X4	T36.0X5	T36.0X6
Ametazole	T50.8X1	T50.8X2	T50.8X3	T50.8X4	T50.8X5	T50.8X6
Amethocaine	T41.3X1	T41.3X2	T41.3X3	T41.3X4	T41.3X5	T41.3X6
- regional	T41.3X1	T41.3X2	T41.3X3	T41.3X4	T41.3X5	T41.3X6
- spinal	T41.3X1	T41.3X2	T41.3X3	T41.3X4	T41.3X5	T41.3X6
Amethopterin	T45.1X1	T45.1X2	T45.1X3	T45.1X4	T45.1X5	T45.1X6
Amezinium metilsulfate	T44.991	T44.992	T44.993	T44.994	T44.995	T44.996
Amfebutamone	T43.291	T43.292	T43.293	T43.294	T43.295	T43.296
Amfepramone	T50.5X1	T50.5X2	T50.5X3	T50.5X4	T50.5X5	T50.5X6
Amfetamine	T43.621	T43.622	T43.623	T43.624	T43.625	T43.626
Amfetaminil	T43.621	T43.622	T43.623	T43.624	T43.625	T43.626
Amfomycin	T36.8X1	T36.8X2	T36.8X3	T36.8X4	T36.8X5	T36.8X6
Amidefrine mesilate	T48.5X1	T48.5X2	T48.5X3	T48.5X4	T48.5X5	T48.5X6
Amidone	T40.3X1	T40.3X2	T40.3X3	T40.3X4	T40.3X5	T40.3X6
Amidopyrine	T39.2X1	T39.2X2	T39.2X3	T39.2X4	T39.2X5	T39.2X6
Amidotrizoate	T50.8X1	T50.8X2	T50.8X3	T50.8X4	T50.8X5	T50.8X6
Amiflamine	T43.1X1	T43.1X2	T43.1X3	T43.1X4	T43.1X5	T43.1X6
Amikacin	T36.5X1	T36.5X2	T36.5X3	T36.5X4	T36.5X5	T36.5X6
Amikhelline	T46.3X1	T46.3X2	T46.3X3	T46.3X4	T46.3X5	T46.3X6
Amiloride	T50.2X1	T50.2X2	T50.2X3	T50.2X4	T50.2X5	T50.2X6
Aminacrine	T49.0X1	T49.0X2	T49.0X3	T49.0X4	T49.0X5	T49.0X6
Amineptine	T43.011	T43.012	T43.013	T43.014	T43.015	T43.016
Aminitrozole	T37.3X1	T37.3X2	T37.3X3	T37.3X4	T37.3X5	T37.3X6
Amino acids	T50.3X1	T50.3X2	T50.3X3	T50.3X4	T50.3X5	T50.3X6
Aminoacetic acid (derivatives)	T50.3X1	T50.3X2	T50.3X3	T50.3X4	T50.3X5	T50.3X6
Aminoacridine	T49.0X1	T49.0X2	T49.0X3	T49.0X4	T49.0X5	T49.0X6
Aminobenzoic acid (-p)	T49.3X1	T49.3X2	T49.3X3	T49.3X4	T49.3X5	T49.3X6
4-Aminobutyric acid	T43.8X1	T43.8X2	T43.8X3	T43.8X4	T43.8X5	T43.8X6
Aminocaproic acid	T45.621	T45.622	T45.623	T45.624	T45.625	T45.626
Aminoethylisothiourium	T45.8X1	T45.8X2	T45.8X3	T45.8X4	T45.8X5	T45.8X6
Aminofenazone	T39.2X1	T39.2X2	T39.2X3	T39.2X4	T39.2X5	T39.2X6
Aminoglutethimide	T45.1X1	T45.1X2	T45.1X3	T45.1X4	T45.1X5	T45.1X6
Aminohippuric acid	T50.8X1	T50.8X2	T50.8X3	T50.8X4	T50.8X5	T50.8X6
Aminomethylbenzoic acid	T45.691	T45.692	T45.693	T45.694	T45.695	T45.696
Aminometradine	T50.2X1	T50.2X2	T50.2X3	T50.2X4	T50.2X5	T50.2X6
Aminopentamide	T44.3X1	T44.3X2	T44.3X3	T44.3X4	T44.3X5	T44.3X6
Aminophenazone	T39.2X1	T39.2X2	T39.2X3	T39.2X4	T39.2X5	T39.2X6
Aminophenol	T54.0X1	T54.0X2	T54.0X3	T54.0X4	--	--

Substance	Poisoning, Accidental (unintentional)	Poisoning, Intentional Self-harm	Poisoning, Assault	Poisoning, Undetermined	Adverse effect	Underdosing
4-Aminophenol derivatives	T39.1X1	T39.1X2	T39.1X3	T39.1X4	T39.1X5	T39.1X6
Aminophenylpyridone	T43.591	T43.592	T43.593	T43.594	T43.595	T43.596
Aminophylline	T48.6X1	T48.6X2	T48.6X3	T48.6X4	T48.6X5	T48.6X6
Aminopterin sodium	T45.1X1	T45.1X2	T45.1X3	T45.1X4	T45.1X5	T45.1X6
Aminopyrine	T39.2X1	T39.2X2	T39.2X3	T39.2X4	T39.2X5	T39.2X6
8-Aminoquinoline drugs	T37.2X1	T37.2X2	T37.2X3	T37.2X4	T37.2X5	T37.2X6
Aminorex	T50.5X1	T50.5X2	T50.5X3	T50.5X4	T50.5X5	T50.5X6
Aminosalicylic acid	T37.1X1	T37.1X2	T37.1X3	T37.1X4	T37.1X5	T37.1X6
Aminosalylum	T37.1X1	T37.1X2	T37.1X3	T37.1X4	T37.1X5	T37.1X6
Amiodarone	T46.2X1	T46.2X2	T46.2X3	T46.2X4	T46.2X5	T46.2X6
Amiphenazole	T50.7X1	T50.7X2	T50.7X3	T50.7X4	T50.7X5	T50.7X6
Amiquinsin	T46.5X1	T46.5X2	T46.5X3	T46.5X4	T46.5X5	T46.5X6
Amisometradine	T50.2X1	T50.2X2	T50.2X3	T50.2X4	T50.2X5	T50.2X6
Amisulpride	T43.591	T43.592	T43.593	T43.594	T43.595	T43.596
Amitriptyline	T43.011	T43.012	T43.013	T43.014	T43.015	T43.016
Amitriptylinoxide	T43.011	T43.012	T43.013	T43.014	T43.015	T43.016
Amlexanox	T48.6X1	T48.6X2	T48.6X3	T48.6X4	T48.6X5	T48.6X6
Ammonia (fumes) (gas) (vapor)	T59.891	T59.892	T59.893	T59.894	--	--
- aromatic spirit	T48.991	T48.992	T48.993	T48.994	T48.995	T48.996
- liquid (household)	T54.3X1	T54.3X2	T54.3X3	T54.3X4	--	--
Ammoniated mercury	T49.0X1	T49.0X2	T49.0X3	T49.0X4	T49.0X5	T49.0X6
Ammonium						
- acid tartrate	T49.5X1	T49.5X2	T49.5X3	T49.5X4	T49.5X5	T49.5X6
- bromide	T42.6X1	T42.6X2	T42.6X3	T42.6X4	T42.6X5	T42.6X6
- carbonate	T54.3X1	T54.3X2	T54.3X3	T54.3X4	--	--
- chloride	T50.991	T50.992	T50.993	T50.994	T50.995	T50.996
- - expectorant	T48.4X1	T48.4X2	T48.4X3	T48.4X4	T48.4X5	T48.4X6
- compounds (household) NEC	T54.3X1	T54.3X2	T54.3X3	T54.3X4	--	--
- - fumes (any usage)	T59.891	T59.892	T59.893	T59.894	--	--
- - industrial	T54.3X1	T54.3X2	T54.3X3	T54.3X4	--	--
- ichthyosulronate	T49.4X1	T49.4X2	T49.4X3	T49.4X4	T49.4X5	T49.4X6
- mandelate	T37.91	T37.92	T37.93	T37.94	T37.95	T37.96
- sulfamate	T60.3X1	T60.3X2	T60.3X3	T60.3X4	--	--
- sulfonate resin	T47.8X1	T47.8X2	T47.8X3	T47.8X4	T47.8X5	T47.8X6
Amobarbital (sodium)	T42.3X1	T42.3X2	T42.3X3	T42.3X4	T42.3X5	T42.3X6
Amodiaquine	T37.2X1	T37.2X2	T37.2X3	T37.2X4	T37.2X5	T37.2X6
Amopyroquin (e)	T37.2X1	T37.2X2	T37.2X3	T37.2X4	T37.2X5	T37.2X6
Amoxapine	T43.011	T43.012	T43.013	T43.014	T43.015	T43.016
Amoxicillin	T36.0X1	T36.0X2	T36.0X3	T36.0X4	T36.0X5	T36.0X6
Amperozide	T43.591	T43.592	T43.593	T43.594	T43.595	T43.596
Amphenidone	T43.591	T43.592	T43.593	T43.594	T43.595	T43.596
Amphetamine NEC	T43.621	T43.622	T43.623	T43.624	T43.625	T43.626
Amphomycin	T36.8X1	T36.8X2	T36.8X3	T36.8X4	T36.8X5	T36.8X6
Amphotalide	T37.4X1	T37.4X2	T37.4X3	T37.4X4	T37.4X5	T37.4X6
Amphotericin B	T36.7X1	T36.7X2	T36.7X3	T36.7X4	T36.7X5	T36.7X6
- topical	T49.0X1	T49.0X2	T49.0X3	T49.0X4	T49.0X5	T49.0X6
Ampicillin	T36.0X1	T36.0X2	T36.0X3	T36.0X4	T36.0X5	T36.0X6
Amprotropine	T44.3X1	T44.3X2	T44.3X3	T44.3X4	T44.3X5	T44.3X6
Amsacrine	T45.1X1	T45.1X2	T45.1X3	T45.1X4	T45.1X5	T45.1X6
Amygdaline	T62.2X1	T62.2X2	T62.2X3	T62.2X4	--	--
Amyl						
- acetate	T52.8X1	T52.8X2	T52.8X3	T52.8X4	--	--
- - vapor	T59.891	T59.892	T59.893	T59.894	--	--
- alcohol	T51.3X1	T51.3X2	T51.3X3	T51.3X4	--	--
- chloride	T53.6X1	T53.6X2	T53.6X3	T53.6X4	--	--
- formate	T52.8X1	T52.8X2	T52.8X3	T52.8X4	--	--
- nitrite	T46.3X1	T46.3X2	T46.3X3	T46.3X4	T46.3X5	T46.3X6
- propionate	T65.891	T65.892	T65.893	T65.894	--	--

Substance	Poisoning, Accidental (unintentional)	Poisoning, Intentional Self-harm	Poisoning, Assault	Poisoning, Undetermined	Adverse effect	Underdosing
Amylase	T47.5X1	T47.5X2	T47.5X3	T47.5X4	T47.5X5	T47.5X6
Amyleine, regional	T41.3X1	T41.3X2	T41.3X3	T41.3X4	T41.3X5	T41.3X6
Amylene						
- dichloride	T53.6X1	T53.6X2	T53.6X3	T53.6X4	--	--
- hydrate	T51.3X1	T51.3X2	T51.3X3	T51.3X4	--	--
Amylmetacresol	T49.6X1	T49.6X2	T49.6X3	T49.6X4	T49.6X5	T49.6X6
Amylobarbitone	T42.3X1	T42.3X2	T42.3X3	T42.3X4	T42.3X5	T42.3X6
Amylocaine, regional	T41.3X1	T41.3X2	T41.3X3	T41.3X4	T41.3X5	T41.3X6
- infiltration (subcutaneous)	T41.3X1	T41.3X2	T41.3X3	T41.3X4	T41.3X5	T41.3X6
- nerve block (peripheral) (plexus)	T41.3X1	T41.3X2	T41.3X3	T41.3X4	T41.3X5	T41.3X6
- spinal	T41.3X1	T41.3X2	T41.3X3	T41.3X4	T41.3X5	T41.3X6
- topical (surface)	T41.3X1	T41.3X2	T41.3X3	T41.3X4	T41.3X5	T41.3X6
Amylopectin	T47.6X1	T47.6X2	T47.6X3	T47.6X4	T47.6X5	T47.6X6
Amytal (sodium)	T42.3X1	T42.3X2	T42.3X3	T42.3X4	T42.3X5	T42.3X6
Anabolic steroid	T38.7X1	T38.7X2	T38.7X3	T38.7X4	T38.7X5	T38.7X6
Analeptic NEC	T50.7X1	T50.7X2	T50.7X3	T50.7X4	T50.7X5	T50.7X6
Analgesic	T39.91	T39.92	T39.93	T39.94	T39.95	T39.96
- anti-inflammatory NEC	T39.91	T39.92	T39.93	T39.94	T39.95	T39.96
- - propionic acid derivative	T39.311	T39.312	T39.313	T39.314	T39.315	T39.316
- antirheumatic NEC	T39.4X1	T39.4X2	T39.4X3	T39.4X4	T39.4X5	T39.4X6
- aromatic NEC	T39.1X1	T39.1X2	T39.1X3	T39.1X4	T39.1X5	T39.1X6
- narcotic NEC	T40.601	T40.602	T40.603	T40.604	T40.605	T40.606
- - combination	T40.601	T40.602	T40.603	T40.604	T40.605	T40.606
- - obstetric	T40.601	T40.602	T40.603	T40.604	T40.605	T40.606
- non-narcotic NEC	T39.91	T39.92	T39.93	T39.94	T39.95	T39.96
- - combination	T39.91	T39.92	T39.93	T39.94	T39.95	T39.96
- pyrazole	T39.2X1	T39.2X2	T39.2X3	T39.2X4	T39.2X5	T39.2X6
- specified NEC	T39.8X1	T39.8X2	T39.8X3	T39.8X4	T39.8X5	T39.8X6
Analgin	T39.2X1	T39.2X2	T39.2X3	T39.2X4	T39.2X5	T39.2X6
Anamirta cocculus	T62.1X1	T62.1X2	T62.1X3	T62.1X4	--	--
Ancillin	T36.0X1	T36.0X2	T36.0X3	T36.0X4	T36.0X5	T36.0X6
Ancrod	T45.691	T45.692	T45.693	T45.694	T45.695	T45.696
Androgen	T38.7X1	T38.7X2	T38.7X3	T38.7X4	T38.7X5	T38.7X6
Androgen-estrogen mixture	T38.7X1	T38.7X2	T38.7X3	T38.7X4	T38.7X5	T38.7X6
Androstalone	T38.7X1	T38.7X2	T38.7X3	T38.7X4	T38.7X5	T38.7X6
Androstanolone	T38.7X1	T38.7X2	T38.7X3	T38.7X4	T38.7X5	T38.7X6
Androsterone	T38.7X1	T38.7X2	T38.7X3	T38.7X4	T38.7X5	T38.7X6
Anemone pulsatilla	T62.2X1	T62.2X2	T62.2X3	T62.2X4	--	--
Anesthesia						
- caudal	T41.3X1	T41.3X2	T41.3X3	T41.3X4	T41.3X5	T41.3X6
- endotracheal	T41.0X1	T41.0X2	T41.0X3	T41.0X4	T41.0X5	T41.0X6
- epidural	T41.3X1	T41.3X2	T41.3X3	T41.3X4	T41.3X5	T41.3X6
- inhalation	T41.0X1	T41.0X2	T41.0X3	T41.0X4	T41.0X5	T41.0X6
- local	T41.3X1	T41.3X2	T41.3X3	T41.3X4	T41.3X5	T41.3X6
- mucosal	T41.3X1	T41.3X2	T41.3X3	T41.3X4	T41.3X5	T41.3X6
- muscle relaxation	T48.1X1	T48.1X2	T48.1X3	T48.1X4	T48.1X5	T48.1X6
- nerve blocking	T41.3X1	T41.3X2	T41.3X3	T41.3X4	T41.3X5	T41.3X6
- plexus blocking	T41.3X1	T41.3X2	T41.3X3	T41.3X4	T41.3X5	T41.3X6
- potentiated	T41.201	T41.202	T41.203	T41.204	T41.205	T41.206
- rectal	T41.201	T41.202	T41.203	T41.204	T41.205	T41.206
- - general	T41.201	T41.202	T41.203	T41.204	T41.205	T41.206
- - local	T41.3X1	T41.3X2	T41.3X3	T41.3X4	T41.3X5	T41.3X6
- regional	T41.3X1	T41.3X2	T41.3X3	T41.3X4	T41.3X5	T41.3X6
- surface	T41.3X1	T41.3X2	T41.3X3	T41.3X4	T41.3X5	T41.3X6
Anesthetic NEC—see also Anesthesia	T41.41	T41.42	T41.43	T41.44	T41.45	T41.46
- with muscle relaxant	T41.201	T41.202	T41.203	T41.204	T41.205	T41.206
- - general	T41.201	T41.202	T41.203	T41.204	T41.205	T41.206
- - local	T41.3X1	T41.3X2	T41.3X3	T41.3X4	T41.3X5	T41.3X6
- gaseous NEC	T41.0X1	T41.0X2	T41.0X3	T41.0X4	T41.0X5	T41.0X6

Substance	Poisoning, Accidental (unintentional)	Poisoning, Intentional Self-harm	Poisoning, Assault	Poisoning, Undetermined	Adverse effect	Underdosing
- general NEC	T41.201	T41.202	T41.203	T41.204	T41.205	T41.206
- halogenated hydrocarbon derivatives NEC	T41.0X1	T41.0X2	T41.0X3	T41.0X4	T41.0X5	T41.0X6
- infiltration NEC	T41.3X1	T41.3X2	T41.3X3	T41.3X4	T41.3X5	T41.3X6
- intravenous NEC	T41.1X1	T41.1X2	T41.1X3	T41.1X4	T41.1X5	T41.1X6
- local NEC	T41.3X1	T41.3X2	T41.3X3	T41.3X4	T41.3X5	T41.3X6
- rectal	T41.201	T41.202	T41.203	T41.204	T41.205	T41.206
- - general	T41.201	T41.202	T41.203	T41.204	T41.205	T41.206
- - local	T41.3X1	T41.3X2	T41.3X3	T41.3X4	T41.3X5	T41.3X6
- regional NEC	T41.3X1	T41.3X2	T41.3X3	T41.3X4	T41.3X5	T41.3X6
- spinal NEC	T41.3X1	T41.3X2	T41.3X3	T41.3X4	T41.3X5	T41.3X6
- thiobarbiturate	T41.1X1	T41.1X2	T41.1X3	T41.1X4	T41.1X5	T41.1X6
- topical	T41.3X1	T41.3X2	T41.3X3	T41.3X4	T41.3X5	T41.3X6
Aneurine	T45.2X1	T45.2X2	T45.2X3	T45.2X4	T45.2X5	T45.2X6
Angio-Conray	T50.8X1	T50.8X2	T50.8X3	T50.8X4	T50.8X5	T50.8X6
Angiotensin	T44.5X1	T44.5X2	T44.5X3	T44.5X4	T44.5X5	T44.5X6
Angiotensinamide	T44.991	T44.992	T44.993	T44.994	T44.995	T44.996
Anhydrohydroxy-progesterone	T38.5X1	T38.5X2	T38.5X3	T38.5X4	T38.5X5	T38.5X6
Anhydron	T50.2X1	T50.2X2	T50.2X3	T50.2X4	T50.2X5	T50.2X6
Anileridine	T40.4X1	T40.4X2	T40.4X3	T40.4X4	T40.4X5	T40.4X6
Aniline (dye) (liquid)	T65.3X1	T65.3X2	T65.3X3	T65.3X4	--	--
- analgesic	T39.1X1	T39.1X2	T39.1X3	T39.1X4	T39.1X5	T39.1X6
- derivatives, therapeutic NEC	T39.1X1	T39.1X2	T39.1X3	T39.1X4	T39.1X5	T39.1X6
- vapor	T65.3X1	T65.3X2	T65.3X3	T65.3X4	--	--
Aniscoropine	T44.3X1	T44.3X2	T44.3X3	T44.3X4	T44.3X5	T44.3X6
Anise oil	T47.5X1	T47.5X2	T47.5X3	T47.5X4	T47.5X5	T47.5X6
Anisidine	T65.3X1	T65.3X2	T65.3X3	T65.3X4	--	--
Anisindione	T45.511	T45.512	T45.513	T45.514	T45.515	T45.516
Anisotropine methyl-bromide	T44.3X1	T44.3X2	T44.3X3	T44.3X4	T44.3X5	T44.3X6
Anistreplase	T45.611	T45.612	T45.613	T45.614	T45.615	T45.616
Anorexiant (central)	T50.5X1	T50.5X2	T50.5X3	T50.5X4	T50.5X5	T50.5X6
Anorexic agents	T50.5X1	T50.5X2	T50.5X3	T50.5X4	T50.5X5	T50.5X6
Ansamycin	T36.6X1	T36.6X2	T36.6X3	T36.6X4	T36.6X5	T36.6X6
Ant (bite) (sting)	T63.421	T63.422	T63.423	T63.424	--	--
Ant poison—see Insecticide						
Antabuse	T50.6X1	T50.6X2	T50.6X3	T50.6X4	T50.6X5	T50.6X6
Antacid NEC	T47.1X1	T47.1X2	T47.1X3	T47.1X4	T47.1X5	T47.1X6
Antagonist						
- Aldosterone	T50.0X1	T50.0X2	T50.0X3	T50.0X4	T50.0X5	T50.0X6
- alpha-adrenoreceptor	T44.6X1	T44.6X2	T44.6X3	T44.6X4	T44.6X5	T44.6X6
- anticoagulant	T45.7X1	T45.7X2	T45.7X3	T45.7X4	T45.7X5	T45.7X6
- beta-adrenoreceptor	T44.7X1	T44.7X2	T44.7X3	T44.7X4	T44.7X5	T44.7X6
- extrapyramidal NEC	T44.3X1	T44.3X2	T44.3X3	T44.3X4	T44.3X5	T44.3X6
- folic acid	T45.1X1	T45.1X2	T45.1X3	T45.1X4	T45.1X5	T45.1X6
- H2 receptor	T47.0X1	T47.0X2	T47.0X3	T47.0X4	T47.0X5	T47.0X6
- heavy metal	T45.8X1	T45.8X2	T45.8X3	T45.8X4	T45.8X5	T45.8X6
- narcotic analgesic	T50.7X1	T50.7X2	T50.7X3	T50.7X4	T50.7X5	T50.7X6
- opiate	T50.7X1	T50.7X2	T50.7X3	T50.7X4	T50.7X5	T50.7X6
- pyrimidine	T45.1X1	T45.1X2	T45.1X3	T45.1X4	T45.1X5	T45.1X6
- serotonin	T46.5X1	T46.5X2	T46.5X3	T46.5X4	T46.5X5	T46.5X6
Antazolin (e)	T45.0X1	T45.0X2	T45.0X3	T45.0X4	T45.0X5	T45.0X6
Anterior pituitary hormone NEC	T38.811	T38.812	T38.813	T38.814	T38.815	T38.816
Anthelmintic NEC	T37.4X1	T37.4X2	T37.4X3	T37.4X4	T37.4X5	T37.4X6
Anthiolimine	T37.4X1	T37.4X2	T37.4X3	T37.4X4	T37.4X5	T37.4X6
Anthralin	T49.4X1	T49.4X2	T49.4X3	T49.4X4	T49.4X5	T49.4X6
Anthramycin	T45.1X1	T45.1X2	T45.1X3	T45.1X4	T45.1X5	T45.1X6
Antiadrenergic NEC	T44.8X1	T44.8X2	T44.8X3	T44.8X4	T44.8X5	T44.8X6
Antiallergic NEC	T45.0X1	T45.0X2	T45.0X3	T45.0X4	T45.0X5	T45.0X6
Anti-anemic (drug) (preparation)	T45.8X1	T45.8X2	T45.8X3	T45.8X4	T45.8X5	T45.8X6

Substance	Poisoning, Accidental (unintentional)	Poisoning, Intentional Self-harm	Poisoning, Assault	Poisoning, Undetermined	Adverse effect	Underdosing
Antiandrogen NEC	T38.6X1	T38.6X2	T38.6X3	T38.6X4	T38.6X5	T38.6X6
Antianxiety drug NEC	T43.501	T43.502	T43.503	T43.504	T43.505	T43.506
Antiaris toxicaria	T65.891	T65.892	T65.893	T65.894	--	--
Antiarteriosclerotic drug	T46.6X1	T46.6X2	T46.6X3	T46.6X4	T46.6X5	T46.6X6
Antiasthmatic drug NEC	T48.6X1	T48.6X2	T48.6X3	T48.6X4	T48.6X5	T48.6X6
Antibiotic NEC	T36.91	T36.92	T36.93	T36.94	T36.95	T36.96
- aminoglycoside	T36.5X1	T36.5X2	T36.5X3	T36.5X4	T36.5X5	T36.5X6
- anticancer	T45.1X1	T45.1X2	T45.1X3	T45.1X4	T45.1X5	T45.1X6
- antifungal	T36.7X1	T36.7X2	T36.7X3	T36.7X4	T36.7X5	T36.7X6
- antimycobacterial	T36.5X1	T36.5X2	T36.5X3	T36.5X4	T36.5X5	T36.5X6
- antineoplastic	T45.1X1	T45.1X2	T45.1X3	T45.1X4	T45.1X5	T45.1X6
- cephalosporin (group)	T36.1X1	T36.1X2	T36.1X3	T36.1X4	T36.1X5	T36.1X6
- chloramphenicol (group)	T36.2X1	T36.2X2	T36.2X3	T36.2X4	T36.2X5	T36.2X6
- ENT	T49.6X1	T49.6X2	T49.6X3	T49.6X4	T49.6X5	T49.6X6
- eye	T49.5X1	T49.5X2	T49.5X3	T49.5X4	T49.5X5	T49.5X6
- fungicidal (local)	T49.0X1	T49.0X2	T49.0X3	T49.0X4	T49.0X5	T49.0X6
- intestinal	T36.8X1	T36.8X2	T36.8X3	T36.8X4	T36.8X5	T36.8X6
- b-lactam NEC	T36.1X1	T36.1X2	T36.1X3	T36.1X4	T36.1X5	T36.1X6
- local	T49.0X1	T49.0X2	T49.0X3	T49.0X4	T49.0X5	T49.0X6
- macrolides	T36.3X1	T36.3X2	T36.3X3	T36.3X4	T36.3X5	T36.3X6
- polypeptide	T36.8X1	T36.8X2	T36.8X3	T36.8X4	T36.8X5	T36.8X6
- specified NEC	T36.8X1	T36.8X2	T36.8X3	T36.8X4	T36.8X5	T36.8X6
- tetracycline (group)	T36.4X1	T36.4X2	T36.4X3	T36.4X4	T36.4X5	T36.4X6
- throat	T49.6X1	T49.6X2	T49.6X3	T49.6X4	T49.6X5	T49.6X6
Anticancer agents NEC	T45.1X1	T45.1X2	T45.1X3	T45.1X4	T45.1X5	T45.1X6
Anticholesterolemic drug NEC	T46.6X1	T46.6X2	T46.6X3	T46.6X4	T46.6X5	T46.6X6
Anticholinergic NEC	T44.3X1	T44.3X2	T44.3X3	T44.3X4	T44.3X5	T44.3X6
Anticholinesterase	T44.0X1	T44.0X2	T44.0X3	T44.0X4	T44.0X5	T44.0X6
- organophosphorus	T44.0X1	T44.0X2	T44.0X3	T44.0X4	T44.0X5	T44.0X6
- - insecticide	T60.0X1	T60.0X2	T60.0X3	T60.0X4	--	--
- - nerve gas	T59.891	T59.892	T59.893	T59.894	--	--
- reversible	T44.0X1	T44.0X2	T44.0X3	T44.0X4	T44.0X5	T44.0X6
- - ophthalmological	T49.5X1	T49.5X2	T49.5X3	T49.5X4	T49.5X5	T49.5X6
Anticoagulant NEC	T45.511	T45.512	T45.513	T45.514	T45.515	T45.516
- Antagonist	T45.7X1	T45.7X2	T45.7X3	T45.7X4	T45.7X5	T45.7X6
Anti-common-cold drug NEC	T48.5X1	T48.5X2	T48.5X3	T48.5X4	T48.5X5	T48.5X6
Anticonvulsant	T42.71	T42.72	T42.73	T42.74	T42.75	T42.76
- barbiturate	T42.3X1	T42.3X2	T42.3X3	T42.3X4	T42.3X5	T42.3X6
- combination (with barbiturate)	T42.3X1	T42.3X2	T42.3X3	T42.3X4	T42.3X5	T42.3X6
- hydantoin	T42.0X1	T42.0X2	T42.0X3	T42.0X4	T42.0X5	T42.0X6
- hypnotic NEC	T42.6X1	T42.6X2	T42.6X3	T42.6X4	T42.6X5	T42.6X6
- oxazolidinedione	T42.2X1	T42.2X2	T42.2X3	T42.2X4	T42.2X5	T42.2X6
- pyrimidinedione	T42.6X1	T42.6X2	T42.6X3	T42.6X4	T42.6X5	T42.6X6
- specified NEC	T42.6X1	T42.6X2	T42.6X3	T42.6X4	T42.6X5	T42.6X6
- succinimide	T42.2X1	T42.2X2	T42.2X3	T42.2X4	T42.2X5	T42.2X6
Anti-D immunoglobulin (human)	T50.Z11	T50.Z12	T50.Z13	T50.Z14	T50.Z15	T50.Z16
Antidepressant	T43.201	T43.202	T43.203	T43.204	T43.205	T43.206
- monoamine oxidase inhibitor	T43.1X1	T43.1X2	T43.1X3	T43.1X4	T43.1X5	T43.1X6
- selective serotonin norepinephrine reuptake inhibitor	T43.211	T43.212	T43.213	T43.214	T43.215	T43.216
- selective serotonin reuptake inhibitor	T43.221	T43.222	T43.223	T43.224	T43.225	T43.226
- specified NEC	T43.291	T43.292	T43.293	T43.294	T43.295	T43.296
- tetracyclic	T43.021	T43.022	T43.023	T43.024	T43.025	T43.026
- triazolopyridine	T43.211	T43.212	T43.213	T43.214	T43.215	T43.216
- tricyclic	T43.011	T43.012	T43.013	T43.014	T43.015	T43.016
Antidiabetic NEC	T38.3X1	T38.3X2	T38.3X3	T38.3X4	T38.3X5	T38.3X6
- biguanide	T38.3X1	T38.3X2	T38.3X3	T38.3X4	T38.3X5	T38.3X6
- - and sulfonyl combined	T38.3X1	T38.3X2	T38.3X3	T38.3X4	T38.3X5	T38.3X6
- combined	T38.3X1	T38.3X2	T38.3X3	T38.3X4	T38.3X5	T38.3X6

Substance	Poisoning, Accidental (unintentional)	Poisoning, Intentional Self-harm	Poisoning, Assault	Poisoning, Undetermined	Adverse effect	Underdosing
- sulfonylurea	T38.3X1	T38.3X2	T38.3X3	T38.3X4	T38.3X5	T38.3X6
Antidiarrheal drug NEC	T47.6X1	T47.6X2	T47.6X3	T47.6X4	T47.6X5	T47.6X6
- absorbent	T47.6X1	T47.6X2	T47.6X3	T47.6X4	T47.6X5	T47.6X6
Antidiphtheria serum	T50.Z11	T50.Z12	T50.Z13	T50.Z14	T50.Z15	T50.Z16
Antidiuretic hormone	T38.891	T38.892	T38.893	T38.894	T38.895	T38.896
Antidote NEC	T50.6X1	T50.6X2	T50.6X3	T50.6X4	T50.6X5	T50.6X6
- heavy metal	T45.8X1	T45.8X2	T45.8X3	T45.8X4	T45.8X5	T45.8X6
Antidysrhythmic NEC	T46.2X1	T46.2X2	T46.2X3	T46.2X4	T46.2X5	T46.2X6
Antiemetic drug	T45.0X1	T45.0X2	T45.0X3	T45.0X4	T45.0X5	T45.0X6
Antiepilepsy agent	T42.71	T42.72	T42.73	T42.74	T42.75	T42.76
- combination	T42.5X1	T42.5X2	T42.5X3	T42.5X4	T42.5X5	T42.5X6
- mixed	T42.5X1	T42.5X2	T42.5X3	T42.5X4	T42.5X5	T42.5X6
- specified, NEC	T42.6X1	T42.6X2	T42.6X3	T42.6X4	T42.6X5	T42.6X6
Antiestrogen NEC	T38.6X1	T38.6X2	T38.6X3	T38.6X4	T38.6X5	T38.6X6
Antifertility pill	T38.4X1	T38.4X2	T38.4X3	T38.4X4	T38.4X5	T38.4X6
Antifibrinolytic drug	T45.621	T45.622	T45.623	T45.624	T45.625	T45.626
Antifilarial drug	T37.4X1	T37.4X2	T37.4X3	T37.4X4	T37.4X5	T37.4X6
Antiflatulent	T47.5X1	T47.5X2	T47.5X3	T47.5X4	T47.5X5	T47.5X6
Antifreeze	T65.91	T65.92	T65.93	T65.94	--	--
- alcohol	T51.1X1	T51.1X2	T51.1X3	T51.1X4	--	--
- ethylene glycol	T51.8X1	T51.8X2	T51.8X3	T51.8X4	--	--
Antifungal						
- antibiotic (systemic)	T36.7X1	T36.7X2	T36.7X3	T36.7X4	T36.7X5	T36.7X6
- anti-infective NEC	T37.91	T37.92	T37.93	T37.94	T37.95	T37.96
- disinfectant, local	T49.0X1	T49.0X2	T49.0X3	T49.0X4	T49.0X5	T49.0X6
- nonmedicinal (spray)	T60.3X1	T60.3X2	T60.3X3	T60.3X4	--	--
- topical	T49.0X1	T49.0X2	T49.0X3	T49.0X4	T49.0X5	T49.0X6
Anti-gastric-secretion drug NEC	T47.1X1	T47.1X2	T47.1X3	T47.1X4	T47.1X5	T47.1X6
Antigonadotrophin NEC	T38.6X1	T38.6X2	T38.6X3	T38.6X4	T38.6X5	T38.6X6
Antihallucinogen	T43.501	T43.502	T43.503	T43.504	T43.505	T43.506
Antihelmintics	T37.4X1	T37.4X2	T37.4X3	T37.4X4	T37.4X5	T37.4X6
Antihemophilic						
- factor	T45.8X1	T45.8X2	T45.8X3	T45.8X4	T45.8X5	T45.8X6
- fraction	T45.8X1	T45.8X2	T45.8X3	T45.8X4	T45.8X5	T45.8X6
- globulin concentrate	T45.7X1	T45.7X2	T45.7X3	T45.7X4	T45.7X5	T45.7X6
- human plasma	T45.8X1	T45.8X2	T45.8X3	T45.8X4	T45.8X5	T45.8X6
- plasma, dried	T45.7X1	T45.7X2	T45.7X3	T45.7X4	T45.7X5	T45.7X6
Antihemorrhoidal preparation	T49.2X1	T49.2X2	T49.2X3	T49.2X4	T49.2X5	T49.2X6
Antiheparin drug	T45.7X1	T45.7X2	T45.7X3	T45.7X4	T45.7X5	T45.7X6
Antihistamine	T45.0X1	T45.0X2	T45.0X3	T45.0X4	T45.0X5	T45.0X6
Antihookworm drug	T37.4X1	T37.4X2	T37.4X3	T37.4X4	T37.4X5	T37.4X6
Anti-human lymphocytic globulin	T50.Z11	T50.Z12	T50.Z13	T50.Z14	T50.Z15	T50.Z16
Antihyperlipidemic drug	T46.6X1	T46.6X2	T46.6X3	T46.6X4	T46.6X5	T46.6X6
Antihypertensive drug NEC	T46.5X1	T46.5X2	T46.5X3	T46.5X4	T46.5X5	T46.5X6
Anti-infective NEC	T37.91	T37.92	T37.93	T37.94	T37.95	T37.96
- anthelmintic	T37.4X1	T37.4X2	T37.4X3	T37.4X4	T37.4X5	T37.4X6
- antibiotics	T36.91	T36.92	T36.93	T36.94	T36.95	T36.96
- - specified NEC	T36.8X1	T36.8X2	T36.8X3	T36.8X4	T36.8X5	T36.8X6
- antimalarial	T37.2X1	T37.2X2	T37.2X3	T37.2X4	T37.2X5	T37.2X6
- antimycobacterial NEC	T37.1X1	T37.1X2	T37.1X3	T37.1X4	T37.1X5	T37.1X6
- - antibiotics	T36.5X1	T36.5X2	T36.5X3	T36.5X4	T36.5X5	T36.5X6
- antiprotozoal NEC	T37.3X1	T37.3X2	T37.3X3	T37.3X4	T37.3X5	T37.3X6
- - blood	T37.2X1	T37.2X2	T37.2X3	T37.2X4	T37.2X5	T37.2X6
- antiviral	T37.5X1	T37.5X2	T37.5X3	T37.5X4	T37.5X5	T37.5X6
- arsenical	T37.8X1	T37.8X2	T37.8X3	T37.8X4	T37.8X5	T37.8X6
- bismuth, local	T49.0X1	T49.0X2	T49.0X3	T49.0X4	T49.0X5	T49.0X6
- ENT	T49.6X1	T49.6X2	T49.6X3	T49.6X4	T49.6X5	T49.6X6
- eye NEC	T49.5X1	T49.5X2	T49.5X3	T49.5X4	T49.5X5	T49.5X6

Substance	Poisoning, Accidental (unintentional)	Poisoning, Intentional Self-harm	Poisoning, Assault	Poisoning, Undetermined	Adverse effect	Underdosing
- heavy metals NEC	T37.8X1	T37.8X2	T37.8X3	T37.8X4	T37.8X5	T37.8X6
- local NEC	T49.0X1	T49.0X2	T49.0X3	T49.0X4	T49.0X5	T49.0X6
- - specified NEC	T49.0X1	T49.0X2	T49.0X3	T49.0X4	T49.0X5	T49.0X6
- mixed	T37.91	T37.92	T37.93	T37.94	T37.95	T37.96
- ophthalmic preparation	T49.5X1	T49.5X2	T49.5X3	T49.5X4	T49.5X5	T49.5X6
- topical NEC	T49.0X1	T49.0X2	T49.0X3	T49.0X4	T49.0X5	T49.0X6
Anti-inflammatory drug NEC	T39.391	T39.392	T39.393	T39.394	T39.395	T39.396
- local	T49.0X1	T49.0X2	T49.0X3	T49.0X4	T49.0X5	T49.0X6
- nonsteroidal NEC	T39.391	T39.392	T39.393	T39.394	T39.395	T39.396
- - propionic acid derivative	T39.311	T39.312	T39.313	T39.314	T39.315	T39.316
- specified NEC	T39.391	T39.392	T39.393	T39.394	T39.395	T39.396
Antikaluretic	T50.3X1	T50.3X2	T50.3X3	T50.3X4	T50.3X5	T50.3X6
Antiknock (tetraethyl lead)	T56.0X1	T56.0X2	T56.0X3	T56.0X4	--	--
Antilipemic drug NEC	T46.6X1	T46.6X2	T46.6X3	T46.6X4	T46.6X5	T46.6X6
Antimalarial	T37.2X1	T37.2X2	T37.2X3	T37.2X4	T37.2X5	T37.2X6
- prophylactic NEC	T37.2X1	T37.2X2	T37.2X3	T37.2X4	T37.2X5	T37.2X6
- pyrimidine derivative	T37.2X1	T37.2X2	T37.2X3	T37.2X4	T37.2X5	T37.2X6
Antimetabolite	T45.1X1	T45.1X2	T45.1X3	T45.1X4	T45.1X5	T45.1X6
Antimitotic agent	T45.1X1	T45.1X2	T45.1X3	T45.1X4	T45.1X5	T45.1X6
Antimony (compounds) (vapor) NEC	T56.891	T56.892	T56.893	T56.894	--	--
- anti-infectives	T37.8X1	T37.8X2	T37.8X3	T37.8X4	T37.8X5	T37.8X6
- dimercaptosuccinate	T37.3X1	T37.3X2	T37.3X3	T37.3X4	T37.3X5	T37.3X6
- hydride	T56.891	T56.892	T56.893	T56.894	--	--
- pesticide (vapor)	T60.8X1	T60.8X2	T60.8X3	T60.8X4	--	--
- potassium (sodium) tartrate	T37.8X1	T37.8X2	T37.8X3	T37.8X4	T37.8X5	T37.8X6
- sodium dimercaptosuccinate	T37.3X1	T37.3X2	T37.3X3	T37.3X4	T37.3X5	T37.3X6
- tartrated	T37.8X1	T37.8X2	T37.8X3	T37.8X4	T37.8X5	T37.8X6
Antimuscarinic NEC	T44.3X1	T44.3X2	T44.3X3	T44.3X4	T44.3X5	T44.3X6
Antimycobacterial drug NEC	T37.1X1	T37.1X2	T37.1X3	T37.1X4	T37.1X5	T37.1X6
- antibiotics	T36.5X1	T36.5X2	T36.5X3	T36.5X4	T36.5X5	T36.5X6
- combination	T37.1X1	T37.1X2	T37.1X3	T37.1X4	T37.1X5	T37.1X6
Antinausea drug	T45.0X1	T45.0X2	T45.0X3	T45.0X4	T45.0X5	T45.0X6
Antinematode drug	T37.4X1	T37.4X2	T37.4X3	T37.4X4	T37.4X5	T37.4X6
Antineoplastic NEC	T45.1X1	T45.1X2	T45.1X3	T45.1X4	T45.1X5	T45.1X6
- alkaloidal	T45.1X1	T45.1X2	T45.1X3	T45.1X4	T45.1X5	T45.1X6
- antibiotics	T45.1X1	T45.1X2	T45.1X3	T45.1X4	T45.1X5	T45.1X6
- combination	T45.1X1	T45.1X2	T45.1X3	T45.1X4	T45.1X5	T45.1X6
- - estrogen	T38.5X1	T38.5X2	T38.5X3	T38.5X4	T38.5X5	T38.5X6
- steroid	T38.7X1	T38.7X2	T38.7X3	T38.7X4	T38.7X5	T38.7X6
Antiparasitic drug (systemic)	T37.91	T37.92	T37.93	T37.94	T37.95	T37.96
- local	T49.0X1	T49.0X2	T49.0X3	T49.0X4	T49.0X5	T49.0X6
- specified NEC	T37.8X1	T37.8X2	T37.8X3	T37.8X4	T37.8X5	T37.8X6
Antiparkinsonism drug NEC	T42.8X1	T42.8X2	T42.8X3	T42.8X4	T42.8X5	T42.8X6
Antiperspirant NEC	T49.2X1	T49.2X2	T49.2X3	T49.2X4	T49.2X5	T49.2X6
Antiphlogistic NEC	T39.4X1	T39.4X2	T39.4X3	T39.4X4	T39.4X5	T39.4X6
Antiplatyhelmintic drug	T37.4X1	T37.4X2	T37.4X3	T37.4X4	T37.4X5	T37.4X6
Antiprotozoal drug NEC	T37.3X1	T37.3X2	T37.3X3	T37.3X4	T37.3X5	T37.3X6
- blood	T37.2X1	T37.2X2	T37.2X3	T37.2X4	T37.2X5	T37.2X6
- local	T49.0X1	T49.0X2	T49.0X3	T49.0X4	T49.0X5	T49.0X6
Antipruritic drug NEC	T49.1X1	T49.1X2	T49.1X3	T49.1X4	T49.1X5	T49.1X6
Antipsychotic drug	T43.501	T43.502	T43.503	T43.504	T43.505	T43.506
- specified NEC	T43.591	T43.592	T43.593	T43.594	T43.595	T43.596
Antipyretic	T39.91	T39.92	T39.93	T39.94	T39.95	T39.96
- specified NEC	T39.8X1	T39.8X2	T39.8X3	T39.8X4	T39.8X5	T39.8X6
Antipyrine	T39.2X1	T39.2X2	T39.2X3	T39.2X4	T39.2X5	T39.2X6
Antirabies hyperimmune serum	T50.Z11	T50.Z12	T50.Z13	T50.Z14	T50.Z15	T50.Z16
Antirheumatic NEC	T39.4X1	T39.4X2	T39.4X3	T39.4X4	T39.4X5	T39.4X6
Antirigidity drug NEC	T42.8X1	T42.8X2	T42.8X3	T42.8X4	T42.8X5	T42.8X6
Antischistosomal drug	T37.4X1	T37.4X2	T37.4X3	T37.4X4	T37.4X5	T37.4X6

Substance	Poisoning, Accidental (unintentional)	Poisoning, Intentional Self-harm	Poisoning, Assault	Poisoning, Undetermined	Adverse effect	Underdosing
Antiscorpion sera	T50.Z11	T50.Z12	T50.Z13	T50.Z14	T50.Z15	T50.Z16
Antiseborrheics	T49.4X1	T49.4X2	T49.4X3	T49.4X4	T49.4X5	T49.4X6
Antiseptics (external) (medicinal)	T49.0X1	T49.0X2	T49.0X3	T49.0X4	T49.0X5	T49.0X6
Antistine	T45.0X1	T45.0X2	T45.0X3	T45.0X4	T45.0X5	T45.0X6
Antitapeworm drug	T37.4X1	T37.4X2	T37.4X3	T37.4X4	T37.4X5	T37.4X6
Antitetanus immunoglobulin	T50.Z11	T50.Z12	T50.Z13	T50.Z14	T50.Z15	T50.Z16
Antithrombotic	T45.521	T45.522	T45.523	T45.524	T45.525	T45.526
Antithyroid drug NEC	T38.2X1	T38.2X2	T38.2X3	T38.2X4	T38.2X5	T38.2X6
Antitoxin	T50.Z11	T50.Z12	T50.Z13	T50.Z14	T50.Z15	T50.Z16
- diphtheria	T50.Z11	T50.Z12	T50.Z13	T50.Z14	T50.Z15	T50.Z16
- gas gangrene	T50.Z11	T50.Z12	T50.Z13	T50.Z14	T50.Z15	T50.Z16
- tetanus	T50.Z11	T50.Z12	T50.Z13	T50.Z14	T50.Z15	T50.Z16
Antitrichomonal drug	T37.3X1	T37.3X2	T37.3X3	T37.3X4	T37.3X5	T37.3X6
Antituberculars	T37.1X1	T37.1X2	T37.1X3	T37.1X4	T37.1X5	T37.1X6
- antibiotics	T36.5X1	T36.5X2	T36.5X3	T36.5X4	T36.5X5	T36.5X6
Antitussive NEC	T48.3X1	T48.3X2	T48.3X3	T48.3X4	T48.3X5	T48.3X6
- codeine mixture	T40.2X1	T40.2X2	T40.2X3	T40.2X4	T40.2X5	T40.2X6
- opiate	T40.2X1	T40.2X2	T40.2X3	T40.2X4	T40.2X5	T40.2X6
Antivaricose drug	T46.8X1	T46.8X2	T46.8X3	T46.8X4	T46.8X5	T46.8X6
Antivenin, antivenom (sera)	T50.Z11	T50.Z12	T50.Z13	T50.Z14	T50.Z15	T50.Z16
- crotaline	T50.Z11	T50.Z12	T50.Z13	T50.Z14	T50.Z15	T50.Z16
- spider bite	T50.Z11	T50.Z12	T50.Z13	T50.Z14	T50.Z15	T50.Z16
Antivertigo drug	T45.0X1	T45.0X2	T45.0X3	T45.0X4	T45.0X5	T45.0X6
Antiviral drug NEC	T37.5X1	T37.5X2	T37.5X3	T37.5X4	T37.5X5	T37.5X6
- eye	T49.5X1	T49.5X2	T49.5X3	T49.5X4	T49.5X5	T49.5X6
Antiwhipworm drug	T37.4X1	T37.4X2	T37.4X3	T37.4X4	T37.4X5	T37.4X6
Antrol—see also by specific chemical substance	T60.91	T60.92	T60.93	T60.94	--	--
- fungicide	T60.91	T60.92	T60.93	T60.94	--	--
ANTU (alpha naphthylthiourea)	T60.4X1	T60.4X2	T60.4X3	T60.4X4	--	--
Apalcillin	T36.0X1	T36.0X2	T36.0X3	T36.0X4	T36.0X5	T36.0X6
APC	T48.5X1	T48.5X2	T48.5X3	T48.5X4	T48.5X5	T48.5X6
Aplonidine	T44.4X1	T44.4X2	T44.4X3	T44.4X4	T44.4X5	T44.4X6
Apomorphine	T47.7X1	T47.7X2	T47.7X3	T47.7X4	T47.7X5	T47.7X6
Appetite depressants, central	T50.5X1	T50.5X2	T50.5X3	T50.5X4	T50.5X5	T50.5X6
Apraclonidine (hydrochloride)	T44.4X1	T44.4X2	T44.4X3	T44.4X4	T44.4X5	T44.4X6
Apresoline	T46.5X1	T46.5X2	T46.5X3	T46.5X4	T46.5X5	T46.5X6
Aprindine	T46.2X1	T46.2X2	T46.2X3	T46.2X4	T46.2X5	T46.2X6
Aprobarbital	T42.3X1	T42.3X2	T42.3X3	T42.3X4	T42.3X5	T42.3X6
Apronalide	T42.6X1	T42.6X2	T42.6X3	T42.6X4	T42.6X5	T42.6X6
Aprotinin	T45.621	T45.622	T45.623	T45.624	T45.625	T45.626
Aptocaine	T41.3X1	T41.3X2	T41.3X3	T41.3X4	T41.3X5	T41.3X6
Aqua fortis	T54.2X1	T54.2X2	T54.2X3	T54.2X4	--	--
Ara-A	T37.5X1	T37.5X2	T37.5X3	T37.5X4	T37.5X5	T37.5X6
Ara-C	T45.1X1	T45.1X2	T45.1X3	T45.1X4	T45.1X5	T45.1X6
Arachis oil	T49.3X1	T49.3X2	T49.3X3	T49.3X4	T49.3X5	T49.3X6
- cathartic	T47.4X1	T47.4X2	T47.4X3	T47.4X4	T47.4X5	T47.4X6
Aralen	T37.2X1	T37.2X2	T37.2X3	T37.2X4	T37.2X5	T37.2X6
Arecoline	T44.1X1	T44.1X2	T44.1X3	T44.1X4	T44.1X5	T44.1X6
Arginine	T50.991	T50.992	T50.993	T50.994	T50.995	T50.996
- glutamate	T50.991	T50.992	T50.993	T50.994	T50.995	T50.996
Argyrol	T49.0X1	T49.0X2	T49.0X3	T49.0X4	T49.0X5	T49.0X6
- ENT agent	T49.6X1	T49.6X2	T49.6X3	T49.6X4	T49.6X5	T49.6X6
- ophthalmic preparation	T49.5X1	T49.5X2	T49.5X3	T49.5X4	T49.5X5	T49.5X6
Aristocort	T38.0X1	T38.0X2	T38.0X3	T38.0X4	T38.0X5	T38.0X6
- ENT agent	T49.6X1	T49.6X2	T49.6X3	T49.6X4	T49.6X5	T49.6X6
- ophthalmic preparation	T49.5X1	T49.5X2	T49.5X3	T49.5X4	T49.5X5	T49.5X6
- topical NEC	T49.0X1	T49.0X2	T49.0X3	T49.0X4	T49.0X5	T49.0X6
Aromatics, corrosive	T54.1X1	T54.1X2	T54.1X3	T54.1X4	--	--

Substance	Poisoning, Accidental (unintentional)	Poisoning, Intentional Self-harm	Poisoning, Assault	Poisoning, Undetermined	Adverse effect	Underdosing
- disinfectants	T54.1X1	T54.1X2	T54.1X3	T54.1X4	--	--
Arsenate of lead	T57.0X1	T57.0X2	T57.0X3	T57.0X4	--	--
- herbicide	T57.0X1	T57.0X2	T57.0X3	T57.0X4	--	--
Arsenic, arsenicals (compounds) (dust) (vapor) NEC	T57.0X1	T57.0X2	T57.0X3	T57.0X4	--	--
- anti-infectives	T37.8X1	T37.8X2	T37.8X3	T37.8X4	T37.8X5	T37.8X6
- pesticide (dust) (fumes)	T57.0X1	T57.0X2	T57.0X3	T57.0X4	--	--
Arsine (gas)	T57.0X1	T57.0X2	T57.0X3	T57.0X4	--	--
Arsphenamine (silver)	T37.8X1	T37.8X2	T37.8X3	T37.8X4	T37.8X5	T37.8X6
Arsthinol	T37.3X1	T37.3X2	T37.3X3	T37.3X4	T37.3X5	T37.3X6
Artane	T44.3X1	T44.3X2	T44.3X3	T44.3X4	T44.3X5	T44.3X6
Arthropod (venomous) NEC	T63.481	T63.482	T63.483	T63.484	--	--
Articaine	T41.3X1	T41.3X2	T41.3X3	T41.3X4	T41.3X5	T41.3X6
Asbestos	T57.8X1	T57.8X2	T57.8X3	T57.8X4	--	--
Ascaridole	T37.4X1	T37.4X2	T37.4X3	T37.4X4	T37.4X5	T37.4X6
Ascorbic acid	T45.2X1	T45.2X2	T45.2X3	T45.2X4	T45.2X5	T45.2X6
Asiaticoside	T49.0X1	T49.0X2	T49.0X3	T49.0X4	T49.0X5	T49.0X6
Asparaginase	T45.1X1	T45.1X2	T45.1X3	T45.1X4	T45.1X5	T45.1X6
Aspidium (oleoresin)	T37.4X1	T37.4X2	T37.4X3	T37.4X4	T37.4X5	T37.4X6
Aspirin (aluminum) (soluble)	T39.011	T39.012	T39.013	T39.014	T39.015	T39.016
Aspoxicillin	T36.0X1	T36.0X2	T36.0X3	T36.0X4	T36.0X5	T36.0X6
Astemizole	T45.0X1	T45.0X2	T45.0X3	T45.0X4	T45.0X5	T45.0X6
Astringent (local)	T49.2X1	T49.2X2	T49.2X3	T49.2X4	T49.2X5	T49.2X6
- specified NEC	T49.2X1	T49.2X2	T49.2X3	T49.2X4	T49.2X5	T49.2X6
Astromicin	T36.5X1	T36.5X2	T36.5X3	T36.5X4	T36.5X5	T36.5X6
Ataractic drug NEC	T43.501	T43.502	T43.503	T43.504	T43.505	T43.506
Atenolol	T44.7X1	T44.7X2	T44.7X3	T44.7X4	T44.7X5	T44.7X6
Atonia drug, intestinal	T47.4X1	T47.4X2	T47.4X3	T47.4X4	T47.4X5	T47.4X6
Atophan	T50.4X1	T50.4X2	T50.4X3	T50.4X4	T50.4X5	T50.4X6
Atracurium besilate	T48.1X1	T48.1X2	T48.1X3	T48.1X4	T48.1X5	T48.1X6
Atropine	T44.3X1	T44.3X2	T44.3X3	T44.3X4	T44.3X5	T44.3X6
- derivative	T44.3X1	T44.3X2	T44.3X3	T44.3X4	T44.3X5	T44.3X6
- methonitrate	T44.3X1	T44.3X2	T44.3X3	T44.3X4	T44.3X5	T44.3X6
Attapulgite	T47.6X1	T47.6X2	T47.6X3	T47.6X4	T47.6X5	T47.6X6
Auramine	T65.891	T65.892	T65.893	T65.894	--	--
- dye	T65.6X1	T65.6X2	T65.6X3	T65.6X4	--	--
- fungicide	T60.3X1	T60.3X2	T60.3X3	T60.3X4	--	--
Auranofin	T39.4X1	T39.4X2	T39.4X3	T39.4X4	T39.4X5	T39.4X6
Aurantiin	T46.991	T46.992	T46.993	T46.994	T46.995	T46.996
Aureomycin	T36.4X1	T36.4X2	T36.4X3	T36.4X4	T36.4X5	T36.4X6
- ophthalmic preparation	T49.5X1	T49.5X2	T49.5X3	T49.5X4	T49.5X5	T49.5X6
- topical NEC	T49.0X1	T49.0X2	T49.0X3	T49.0X4	T49.0X5	T49.0X6
Aurothioglucose	T39.4X1	T39.4X2	T39.4X3	T39.4X4	T39.4X5	T39.4X6
Aurothioglycanide	T39.4X1	T39.4X2	T39.4X3	T39.4X4	T39.4X5	T39.4X6
Aurothiomalate sodium	T39.4X1	T39.4X2	T39.4X3	T39.4X4	T39.4X5	T39.4X6
Aurotioprol	T39.4X1	T39.4X2	T39.4X3	T39.4X4	T39.4X5	T39.4X6
Automobile fuel	T52.0X1	T52.0X2	T52.0X3	T52.0X4	--	--
Autonomic nervous system agent NEC	T44.901	T44.902	T44.903	T44.904	T44.905	T44.906
Avlosulfon	T37.1X1	T37.1X2	T37.1X3	T37.1X4	T37.1X5	T37.1X6
Avomine	T42.6X1	T42.6X2	T42.6X3	T42.6X4	T42.6X5	T42.6X6
Axerophthol	T45.2X1	T45.2X2	T45.2X3	T45.2X4	T45.2X5	T45.2X6
Azacitidine	T45.1X1	T45.1X2	T45.1X3	T45.1X4	T45.1X5	T45.1X6
Azacyclonol	T43.591	T43.592	T43.593	T43.594	T43.595	T43.596
Azadirachta	T60.2X1	T60.2X2	T60.2X3	T60.2X4	--	--
Azanidazole	T37.3X1	T37.3X2	T37.3X3	T37.3X4	T37.3X5	T37.3X6
Azapetine	T46.7X1	T46.7X2	T46.7X3	T46.7X4	T46.7X5	T46.7X6
Azapropazone	T39.2X1	T39.2X2	T39.2X3	T39.2X4	T39.2X5	T39.2X6
Azaribine	T45.1X1	T45.1X2	T45.1X3	T45.1X4	T45.1X5	T45.1X6
Azaserine	T45.1X1	T45.1X2	T45.1X3	T45.1X4	T45.1X5	T45.1X6

Substance	Poisoning, Accidental (unintentional)	Poisoning, Intentional Self-harm	Poisoning, Assault	Poisoning, Undetermined	Adverse effect	Underdosing
Azatadine	T45.0X1	T45.0X2	T45.0X3	T45.0X4	T45.0X5	T45.0X6
Azatepa	T45.1X1	T45.1X2	T45.1X3	T45.1X4	T45.1X5	T45.1X6
Azathioprine	T45.1X1	T45.1X2	T45.1X3	T45.1X4	T45.1X5	T45.1X6
Azelaic acid	T49.0X1	T49.0X2	T49.0X3	T49.0X4	T49.0X5	T49.0X6
Azelastine	T45.0X1	T45.0X2	T45.0X3	T45.0X4	T45.0X5	T45.0X6
Azidocillin	T36.0X1	T36.0X2	T36.0X3	T36.0X4	T36.0X5	T36.0X6
Azidothymidine	T37.5X1	T37.5X2	T37.5X3	T37.5X4	T37.5X5	T37.5X6
Azinphos (ethyl) (methyl)	T60.0X1	T60.0X2	T60.0X3	T60.0X4	--	--
Aziridine (chelating)	T54.1X1	T54.1X2	T54.1X3	T54.1X4	--	--
Azithromycin	T36.3X1	T36.3X2	T36.3X3	T36.3X4	T36.3X5	T36.3X6
Azlocillin	T36.0X1	T36.0X2	T36.0X3	T36.0X4	T36.0X5	T36.0X6
Azobenzene smoke	T65.3X1	T65.3X2	T65.3X3	T65.3X4	--	--
- acaricide	T60.8X1	T60.8X2	T60.8X3	T60.8X4	--	--
Azosulfamide	T37.0X1	T37.0X2	T37.0X3	T37.0X4	T37.0X5	T37.0X6
AZT	T37.5X1	T37.5X2	T37.5X3	T37.5X4	T37.5X5	T37.5X6
Aztreonam	T36.1X1	T36.1X2	T36.1X3	T36.1X4	T36.1X5	T36.1X6
Azulfidine	T37.0X1	T37.0X2	T37.0X3	T37.0X4	T37.0X5	T37.0X6
Azuresin	T50.8X1	T50.8X2	T50.8X3	T50.8X4	T50.8X5	T50.8X6
Bacampicillin	T36.0X1	T36.0X2	T36.0X3	T36.0X4	T36.0X5	T36.0X6
Bacillus						
- lactobacillus	T47.8X1	T47.8X2	T47.8X3	T47.8X4	T47.8X5	T47.8X6
- subtilis	T47.6X1	T47.6X2	T47.6X3	T47.6X4	T47.6X5	T47.6X6
Bacimycin	T49.0X1	T49.0X2	T49.0X3	T49.0X4	T49.0X5	T49.0X6
- ophthalmic preparation	T49.5X1	T49.5X2	T49.5X3	T49.5X4	T49.5X5	T49.5X6
Bacitracin zinc	T49.0X1	T49.0X2	T49.0X3	T49.0X4	T49.0X5	T49.0X6
- with neomycin	T49.0X1	T49.0X2	T49.0X3	T49.0X4	T49.0X5	T49.0X6
- ENT agent	T49.6X1	T49.6X2	T49.6X3	T49.6X4	T49.6X5	T49.6X6
- ophthalmic preparation	T49.5X1	T49.5X2	T49.5X3	T49.5X4	T49.5X5	T49.5X6
- topical NEC	T49.0X1	T49.0X2	T49.0X3	T49.0X4	T49.0X5	T49.0X6
Baclofen	T42.8X1	T42.8X2	T42.8X3	T42.8X4	T42.8X5	T42.8X6
Baking soda	T50.991	T50.992	T50.993	T50.994	T50.995	T50.996
BAL	T45.8X1	T45.8X2	T45.8X3	T45.8X4	T45.8X5	T45.8X6
Bambuterol	T48.6X1	T48.6X2	T48.6X3	T48.6X4	T48.6X5	T48.6X6
Bamethan (sulfate)	T46.7X1	T46.7X2	T46.7X3	T46.7X4	T46.7X5	T46.7X6
Bamifylline	T48.6X1	T48.6X2	T48.6X3	T48.6X4	T48.6X5	T48.6X6
Bamipine	T45.0X1	T45.0X2	T45.0X3	T45.0X4	T45.0X5	T45.0X6
Baneberry—see Actaea spicata						
Banewort—see Belladonna						
Barbenyl	T42.3X1	T42.3X2	T42.3X3	T42.3X4	T42.3X5	T42.3X6
Barbexaclone	T42.6X1	T42.6X2	T42.6X3	T42.6X4	T42.6X5	T42.6X6
Barbital	T42.3X1	T42.3X2	T42.3X3	T42.3X4	T42.3X5	T42.3X6
- sodium	T42.3X1	T42.3X2	T42.3X3	T42.3X4	T42.3X5	T42.3X6
Barbitone	T42.3X1	T42.3X2	T42.3X3	T42.3X4	T42.3X5	T42.3X6
Barbiturate NEC	T42.3X1	T42.3X2	T42.3X3	T42.3X4	T42.3X5	T42.3X6
- with tranquilizer	T42.3X1	T42.3X2	T42.3X3	T42.3X4	T42.3X5	T42.3X6
- anesthetic (intravenous)	T41.1X1	T41.1X2	T41.1X3	T41.1X4	T41.1X5	T41.1X6
Barium (carbonate) (chloride) (sulfite)	T57.8X1	T57.8X2	T57.8X3	T57.8X4	--	--
- diagnostic agent	T50.8X1	T50.8X2	T50.8X3	T50.8X4	T50.8X5	T50.8X6
- pesticide	T60.4X1	T60.4X2	T60.4X3	T60.4X4	--	--
- rodenticide	T60.4X1	T60.4X2	T60.4X3	T60.4X4	--	--
- sulfate (medicinal)	T50.8X1	T50.8X2	T50.8X3	T50.8X4	T50.8X5	T50.8X6
Barrier cream	T49.3X1	T49.3X2	T49.3X3	T49.3X4	T49.3X5	T49.3X6
Basic fuchsin	T49.0X1	T49.0X2	T49.0X3	T49.0X4	T49.0X5	T49.0X6
Battery acid or fluid	T54.2X1	T54.2X2	T54.2X3	T54.2X4	--	--
Bay rum	T51.8X1	T51.8X2	T51.8X3	T51.8X4	--	--
BCG (vaccine)	T50.A91	T50.A92	T50.A93	T50.A94	T50.A95	T50.A96
BCNU	T45.1X1	T45.1X2	T45.1X3	T45.1X4	T45.1X5	T45.1X6
Bearsfoot	T62.2X1	T62.2X2	T62.2X3	T62.2X4	--	--

Substance	Poisoning, Accidental (unintentional)	Poisoning, Intentional Self-harm	Poisoning, Assault	Poisoning, Undetermined	Adverse effect	Underdosing
Beclamide	T42.6X1	T42.6X2	T42.6X3	T42.6X4	T42.6X5	T42.6X6
Beclomethasone	T44.5X1	T44.5X2	T44.5X3	T44.5X4	T44.5X5	T44.5X6
Bee (sting) (venom)	T63.441	T63.442	T63.443	T63.444	--	--
Befunolol	T49.5X1	T49.5X2	T49.5X3	T49.5X4	T49.5X5	T49.5X6
Bekanamycin	T36.5X1	T36.5X2	T36.5X3	T36.5X4	T36.5X5	T36.5X6
Belladonna—see also Nightshade						
- alkaloids	T44.3X1	T44.3X2	T44.3X3	T44.3X4	T44.3X5	T44.3X6
- extract	T44.3X1	T44.3X2	T44.3X3	T44.3X4	T44.3X5	T44.3X6
- herb	T44.3X1	T44.3X2	T44.3X3	T44.3X4	T44.3X5	T44.3X6
Bemegride	T50.7X1	T50.7X2	T50.7X3	T50.7X4	T50.7X5	T50.7X6
Benactyzine	T44.3X1	T44.3X2	T44.3X3	T44.3X4	T44.3X5	T44.3X6
Benadryl	T45.0X1	T45.0X2	T45.0X3	T45.0X4	T45.0X5	T45.0X6
Benaprizine	T44.3X1	T44.3X2	T44.3X3	T44.3X4	T44.3X5	T44.3X6
Benazepril	T46.4X1	T46.4X2	T46.4X3	T46.4X4	T46.4X5	T46.4X6
Bencyclane	T46.7X1	T46.7X2	T46.7X3	T46.7X4	T46.7X5	T46.7X6
Bendazol	T46.3X1	T46.3X2	T46.3X3	T46.3X4	T46.3X5	T46.3X6
Bendrofluazide	T50.2X1	T50.2X2	T50.2X3	T50.2X4	T50.2X5	T50.2X6
Bendroflumethiazide	T50.2X1	T50.2X2	T50.2X3	T50.2X4	T50.2X5	T50.2X6
Benemid	T50.4X1	T50.4X2	T50.4X3	T50.4X4	T50.4X5	T50.4X6
Benethamine penicillin	T36.0X1	T36.0X2	T36.0X3	T36.0X4	T36.0X5	T36.0X6
Benexate	T47.1X1	T47.1X2	T47.1X3	T47.1X4	T47.1X5	T47.1X6
Benfluorex	T46.6X1	T46.6X2	T46.6X3	T46.6X4	T46.6X5	T46.6X6
Benfotiamine	T45.2X1	T45.2X2	T45.2X3	T45.2X4	T45.2X5	T45.2X6
Benisone	T49.0X1	T49.0X2	T49.0X3	T49.0X4	T49.0X5	T49.0X6
Benomyl	T60.0X1	T60.0X2	T60.0X3	T60.0X4	--	--
Benoquin	T49.8X1	T49.8X2	T49.8X3	T49.8X4	T49.8X5	T49.8X6
Benoxinate	T41.3X1	T41.3X2	T41.3X3	T41.3X4	T41.3X5	T41.3X6
Benperidol	T43.4X1	T43.4X2	T43.4X3	T43.4X4	T43.4X5	T43.4X6
Benproperine	T48.3X1	T48.3X2	T48.3X3	T48.3X4	T48.3X5	T48.3X6
Benserazide	T42.8X1	T42.8X2	T42.8X3	T42.8X4	T42.8X5	T42.8X6
Bentazepam	T42.4X1	T42.4X2	T42.4X3	T42.4X4	T42.4X5	T42.4X6
Bentiromide	T50.8X1	T50.8X2	T50.8X3	T50.8X4	T50.8X5	T50.8X6
Bentonite	T49.3X1	T49.3X2	T49.3X3	T49.3X4	T49.3X5	T49.3X6
Benzalbutyramide	T46.6X1	T46.6X2	T46.6X3	T46.6X4	T46.6X5	T46.6X6
Benzalkonium (chloride)	T49.0X1	T49.0X2	T49.0X3	T49.0X4	T49.0X5	T49.0X6
- ophthalmic preparation	T49.5X1	T49.5X2	T49.5X3	T49.5X4	T49.5X5	T49.5X6
Benzamidosalicylate (calcium)	T37.1X1	T37.1X2	T37.1X3	T37.1X4	T37.1X5	T37.1X6
Benzamine	T41.3X1	T41.3X2	T41.3X3	T41.3X4	T41.3X5	T41.3X6
- lactate	T49.1X1	T49.1X2	T49.1X3	T49.1X4	T49.1X5	T49.1X6
Benzamphetamine	T50.5X1	T50.5X2	T50.5X3	T50.5X4	T50.5X5	T50.5X6
Benzapril hydrochloride	T46.5X1	T46.5X2	T46.5X3	T46.5X4	T46.5X5	T46.5X6
Benzathine benzylpenicillin	T36.0X1	T36.0X2	T36.0X3	T36.0X4	T36.0X5	T36.0X6
Benzathine penicillin	T36.0X1	T36.0X2	T36.0X3	T36.0X4	T36.0X5	T36.0X6
Benzatropine	T42.8X1	T42.8X2	T42.8X3	T42.8X4	T42.8X5	T42.8X6
Benzbromarone	T50.4X1	T50.4X2	T50.4X3	T50.4X4	T50.4X5	T50.4X6
Benzcarbimine	T45.1X1	T45.1X2	T45.1X3	T45.1X4	T45.1X5	T45.1X6
Benzedrex	T44.991	T44.992	T44.993	T44.994	T44.995	T44.996
Benzedrine (amphetamine)	T43.621	T43.622	T43.623	T43.624	T43.625	T43.626
Benzenamine	T65.3X1	T65.3X2	T65.3X3	T65.3X4	--	--
Benzene	T52.1X1	T52.1X2	T52.1X3	T52.1X4	--	--
- homologues (acetyl) (dimethyl) (methyl) (solvent)	T52.2X1	T52.2X2	T52.2X3	T52.2X4	--	--
Benzethonium (chloride)	T49.0X1	T49.0X2	T49.0X3	T49.0X4	T49.0X5	T49.0X6
Benzfetamine	T50.5X1	T50.5X2	T50.5X3	T50.5X4	T50.5X5	T50.5X6
Benzhexol	T44.3X1	T44.3X2	T44.3X3	T44.3X4	T44.3X5	T44.3X6
Benzhydramine (chloride)	T45.0X1	T45.0X2	T45.0X3	T45.0X4	T45.0X5	T45.0X6
Benzidine	T65.891	T65.892	T65.893	T65.894	--	--
Benzilonium bromide	T44.3X1	T44.3X2	T44.3X3	T44.3X4	T44.3X5	T44.3X6
Benzimidazole	T60.3X1	T60.3X2	T60.3X3	T60.3X4	--	--

Substance	Poisoning, Accidental (unintentional)	Poisoning, Intentional Self-harm	Poisoning, Assault	Poisoning, Undetermined	Adverse effect	Underdosing
Benzin (e) —see Ligroin						
Benziodarone	T46.3X1	T46.3X2	T46.3X3	T46.3X4	T46.3X5	T46.3X6
Benznidazole	T37.3X1	T37.3X2	T37.3X3	T37.3X4	T37.3X5	T37.3X6
Benzocaine	T41.3X1	T41.3X2	T41.3X3	T41.3X4	T41.3X5	T41.3X6
Benzodiapin	T42.4X1	T42.4X2	T42.4X3	T42.4X4	T42.4X5	T42.4X6
Benzodiazepine NEC	T42.4X1	T42.4X2	T42.4X3	T42.4X4	T42.4X5	T42.4X6
Benzoic acid	T49.0X1	T49.0X2	T49.0X3	T49.0X4	T49.0X5	T49.0X6
- with salicylic acid	T49.0X1	T49.0X2	T49.0X3	T49.0X4	T49.0X5	T49.0X6
Benzoin (tincture)	T48.5X1	T48.5X2	T48.5X3	T48.5X4	T48.5X5	T48.5X6
Benzol (benzene)	T52.1X1	T52.1X2	T52.1X3	T52.1X4	--	--
- vapor	T52.0X1	T52.0X2	T52.0X3	T52.0X4	--	--
Benzomorphan	T40.2X1	T40.2X2	T40.2X3	T40.2X4	T40.2X5	T40.2X6
Benzonatate	T48.3X1	T48.3X2	T48.3X3	T48.3X4	T48.3X5	T48.3X6
Benzophenones	T49.3X1	T49.3X2	T49.3X3	T49.3X4	T49.3X5	T49.3X6
Benzopyrone	T46.991	T46.992	T46.993	T46.994	T46.995	T46.996
Benzothiadiazides	T50.2X1	T50.2X2	T50.2X3	T50.2X4	T50.2X5	T50.2X6
Benzoxonium chloride	T49.0X1	T49.0X2	T49.0X3	T49.0X4	T49.0X5	T49.0X6
Benzoyl peroxide	T49.0X1	T49.0X2	T49.0X3	T49.0X4	T49.0X5	T49.0X6
Benzoylpas calcium	T37.1X1	T37.1X2	T37.1X3	T37.1X4	T37.1X5	T37.1X6
Benzperidin	T43.591	T43.592	T43.593	T43.594	T43.595	T43.596
Benzperidol	T43.591	T43.592	T43.593	T43.594	T43.595	T43.596
Benzphetamine	T50.5X1	T50.5X2	T50.5X3	T50.5X4	T50.5X5	T50.5X6
Benzpyrinium bromide	T44.1X1	T44.1X2	T44.1X3	T44.1X4	T44.1X5	T44.1X6
Benzquinamide	T45.0X1	T45.0X2	T45.0X3	T45.0X4	T45.0X5	T45.0X6
Benzthiazide	T50.2X1	T50.2X2	T50.2X3	T50.2X4	T50.2X5	T50.2X6
Benztropine						
- anticholinergic	T44.3X1	T44.3X2	T44.3X3	T44.3X4	T44.3X5	T44.3X6
- antiparkinson	T42.8X1	T42.8X2	T42.8X3	T42.8X4	T42.8X5	T42.8X6
Benzydamine	T49.0X1	T49.0X2	T49.0X3	T49.0X4	T49.0X5	T49.0X6
Benzyl						
- acetate	T52.8X1	T52.8X2	T52.8X3	T52.8X4	--	--
- alcohol	T49.0X1	T49.0X2	T49.0X3	T49.0X4	T49.0X5	T49.0X6
- benzoate	T49.0X1	T49.0X2	T49.0X3	T49.0X4	T49.0X5	T49.0X6
- Benzoic acid	T49.0X1	T49.0X2	T49.0X3	T49.0X4	T49.0X5	T49.0X6
- morphine	T40.2X1	T40.2X2	T40.2X3	T40.2X4	--	--
- nicotinate	T46.6X1	T46.6X2	T46.6X3	T46.6X4	T46.6X5	T46.6X6
- penicillin	T36.0X1	T36.0X2	T36.0X3	T36.0X4	T36.0X5	T36.0X6
Benzylhydrochlorthia-zide	T50.2X1	T50.2X2	T50.2X3	T50.2X4	T50.2X5	T50.2X6
Benzylpenicillin	T36.0X1	T36.0X2	T36.0X3	T36.0X4	T36.0X5	T36.0X6
Benzylthiouracil	T38.2X1	T38.2X2	T38.2X3	T38.2X4	T38.2X5	T38.2X6
Bephenium hydroxy-naphthoate	T37.4X1	T37.4X2	T37.4X3	T37.4X4	T37.4X5	T37.4X6
Bepridil	T46.1X1	T46.1X2	T46.1X3	T46.1X4	T46.1X5	T46.1X6
Bergamot oil	T65.891	T65.892	T65.893	T65.894	--	--
Bergapten	T50.991	T50.992	T50.993	T50.994	T50.995	T50.996
Berries, poisonous	T62.1X1	T62.1X2	T62.1X3	T62.1X4	--	--
Beryllium (compounds)	T56.7X1	T56.7X2	T56.7X3	T56.7X4	--	--
b-acetyldigoxin	T46.0X1	T46.0X2	T46.0X3	T46.0X4	T46.0X5	T46.0X6
beta adrenergic blocking agent, heart	T44.7X1	T44.7X2	T44.7X3	T44.7X4	T44.7X5	T44.7X6
b-benzalbutyramide	T46.6X1	T46.6X2	T46.6X3	T46.6X4	T46.6X5	T46.6X6
Betacarotene	T45.2X1	T45.2X2	T45.2X3	T45.2X4	T45.2X5	T45.2X6
b-eucaine	T49.1X1	T49.1X2	T49.1X3	T49.1X4	T49.1X5	T49.1X6
Beta-Chlor	T42.6X1	T42.6X2	T42.6X3	T42.6X4	T42.6X5	T42.6X6
b-galactosidase	T47.5X1	T47.5X2	T47.5X3	T47.5X4	T47.5X5	T47.5X6
Betahistine	T46.7X1	T46.7X2	T46.7X3	T46.7X4	T46.7X5	T46.7X6
Betaine	T47.5X1	T47.5X2	T47.5X3	T47.5X4	T47.5X5	T47.5X6
Betamethasone	T49.0X1	T49.0X2	T49.0X3	T49.0X4	T49.0X5	T49.0X6
- topical	T49.0X1	T49.0X2	T49.0X3	T49.0X4	T49.0X5	T49.0X6
Betamicin	T36.8X1	T36.8X2	T36.8X3	T36.8X4	T36.8X5	T36.8X6

Substance	Poisoning, Accidental (unintentional)	Poisoning, Intentional Self-harm	Poisoning, Assault	Poisoning, Undetermined	Adverse effect	Underdosing
Betanidine	T46.5X1	T46.5X2	T46.5X3	T46.5X4	T46.5X5	T46.5X6
b-sitosterol (s)	T46.6X1	T46.6X2	T46.6X3	T46.6X4	T46.6X5	T46.6X6
Betaxolol	T44.7X1	T44.7X2	T44.7X3	T44.7X4	T44.7X5	T44.7X6
Betazole	T50.8X1	T50.8X2	T50.8X3	T50.8X4	T50.8X5	T50.8X6
Bethanechol	T44.1X1	T44.1X2	T44.1X3	T44.1X4	T44.1X5	T44.1X6
- chloride	T44.1X1	T44.1X2	T44.1X3	T44.1X4	T44.1X5	T44.1X6
Bethanidine	T46.5X1	T46.5X2	T46.5X3	T46.5X4	T46.5X5	T46.5X6
Betoxycaine	T41.3X1	T41.3X2	T41.3X3	T41.3X4	T41.3X5	T41.3X6
Betula oil	T49.3X1	T49.3X2	T49.3X3	T49.3X4	T49.3X5	T49.3X6
Bevantolol	T44.7X1	T44.7X2	T44.7X3	T44.7X4	T44.7X5	T44.7X6
Bevonium metilsulfate	T44.3X1	T44.3X2	T44.3X3	T44.3X4	T44.3X5	T44.3X6
Bezafibrate	T46.6X1	T46.6X2	T46.6X3	T46.6X4	T46.6X5	T46.6X6
Bezitramide	T40.4X1	T40.4X2	T40.4X3	T40.4X4	T40.4X5	T40.4X6
BHA	T50.991	T50.992	T50.993	T50.994	T50.995	T50.996
Bhang	T40.7X1	T40.7X2	T40.7X3	T40.7X4	T40.7X5	T40.7X6
BHC (medicinal)	T49.0X1	T49.0X2	T49.0X3	T49.0X4	T49.0X5	T49.0X6
- nonmedicinal (vapor)	T53.6X1	T53.6X2	T53.6X3	T53.6X4	--	--
Bialamicol	T37.3X1	T37.3X2	T37.3X3	T37.3X4	T37.3X5	T37.3X6
Bibenzonium bromide	T48.3X1	T48.3X2	T48.3X3	T48.3X4	T48.3X5	T48.3X6
Bibrocathol	T49.5X1	T49.5X2	T49.5X3	T49.5X4	T49.5X5	T49.5X6
Bichloride of mercury—see Mercury, chloride						
Bichromates (calcium) (potassium) (sodium) (crystals)	T57.8X1	T57.8X2	T57.8X3	T57.8X4	--	--
- fumes	T56.2X1	T56.2X2	T56.2X3	T56.2X4	--	--
Biclotymol	T49.6X1	T49.6X2	T49.6X3	T49.6X4	T49.6X5	T49.6X6
Bicucculine	T50.7X1	T50.7X2	T50.7X3	T50.7X4	T50.7X5	T50.7X6
Bifemelane	T43.291	T43.292	T43.293	T43.294	T43.295	T43.296
Biguanide derivatives, oral	T38.3X1	T38.3X2	T38.3X3	T38.3X4	T38.3X5	T38.3X6
Bile salts	T47.5X1	T47.5X2	T47.5X3	T47.5X4	T47.5X5	T47.5X6
Biligrafin	T50.8X1	T50.8X2	T50.8X3	T50.8X4	T50.8X5	T50.8X6
Bilopaque	T50.8X1	T50.8X2	T50.8X3	T50.8X4	T50.8X5	T50.8X6
Binifibrate	T46.6X1	T46.6X2	T46.6X3	T46.6X4	T46.6X5	T46.6X6
Binitrobenzol	T65.3X1	T65.3X2	T65.3X3	T65.3X4	--	--
Bioflavonoid (s)	T46.991	T46.992	T46.993	T46.994	T46.995	T46.996
Biological substance NEC	T50.901	T50.902	T50.903	T50.904	T50.905	T50.906
Biotin	T45.2X1	T45.2X2	T45.2X3	T45.2X4	T45.2X5	T45.2X6
Biperiden	T44.3X1	T44.3X2	T44.3X3	T44.3X4	T44.3X5	T44.3X6
Bisacodyl	T47.2X1	T47.2X2	T47.2X3	T47.2X4	T47.2X5	T47.2X6
Bisbentiamine	T45.2X1	T45.2X2	T45.2X3	T45.2X4	T45.2X5	T45.2X6
Bisbutiamine	T45.2X1	T45.2X2	T45.2X3	T45.2X4	T45.2X5	T45.2X6
Bisdequalinium (salts) (diacetate)	T49.6X1	T49.6X2	T49.6X3	T49.6X4	T49.6X5	T49.6X6
Bishydroxycoumarin	T45.511	T45.512	T45.513	T45.514	T45.515	T45.516
Bismarsen	T37.8X1	T37.8X2	T37.8X3	T37.8X4	T37.8X5	T37.8X6
Bismuth salts	T47.6X1	T47.6X2	T47.6X3	T47.6X4	T47.6X5	T47.6X6
- aluminate	T47.1X1	T47.1X2	T47.1X3	T47.1X4	T47.1X5	T47.1X6
- anti-infectives	T37.8X1	T37.8X2	T37.8X3	T37.8X4	T37.8X5	T37.8X6
- formic iodide	T49.0X1	T49.0X2	T49.0X3	T49.0X4	T49.0X5	T49.0X6
- glycolylarsenate	T49.0X1	T49.0X2	T49.0X3	T49.0X4	T49.0X5	T49.0X6
- nonmedicinal (compounds) NEC	T65.91	T65.92	T65.93	T65.94	--	--
- subcarbonate	T47.6X1	T47.6X2	T47.6X3	T47.6X4	T47.6X5	T47.6X6
- subsalicylate	T37.8X1	T37.8X2	T37.8X3	T37.8X4	T37.8X5	T37.8X6
- sulfarsphenamine	T37.8X1	T37.8X2	T37.8X3	T37.8X4	T37.8X5	T37.8X6
Bisoprolol	T44.7X1	T44.7X2	T44.7X3	T44.7X4	T44.7X5	T44.7X6
Bisoxatin	T47.2X1	T47.2X2	T47.2X3	T47.2X4	T47.2X5	T47.2X6
Bisulepin (hydrochloride)	T45.0X1	T45.0X2	T45.0X3	T45.0X4	T45.0X5	T45.0X6
Bithionol	T37.8X1	T37.8X2	T37.8X3	T37.8X4	T37.8X5	T37.8X6
- anthelminthic	T37.4X1	T37.4X2	T37.4X3	T37.4X4	T37.4X5	T37.4X6
Bitolterol	T48.6X1	T48.6X2	T48.6X3	T48.6X4	T48.6X5	T48.6X6
Bitoscanate	T37.4X1	T37.4X2	T37.4X3	T37.4X4	T37.4X5	T37.4X6

Substance	Poisoning, Accidental (unintentional)	Poisoning, Intentional Self-harm	Poisoning, Assault	Poisoning, Undetermined	Adverse effect	Underdosing
Bitter almond oil	T62.8X1	T62.8X2	T62.8X3	T62.8X4	--	--
Bittersweet	T62.2X1	T62.2X2	T62.2X3	T62.2X4	--	--
Black						
- flag	T60.91	T60.92	T60.93	T60.94	--	--
- henbane	T62.2X1	T62.2X2	T62.2X3	T62.2X4	--	--
- leaf (40)	T60.91	T60.92	T60.93	T60.94	--	--
- widow spider (bite)	T63.311	T63.312	T63.313	T63.314	--	--
- - antivenin	T50.Z11	T50.Z12	T50.Z13	T50.Z14	T50.Z15	T50.Z16
Blast furnace gas (carbon monoxide from)	T58.8X1	T58.8X2	T58.8X3	T58.8X4	--	--
Bleach	T54.91	T54.92	T54.93	T54.94	--	--
Bleaching agent (medicinal)	T49.4X1	T49.4X2	T49.4X3	T49.4X4	T49.4X5	T49.4X6
Bleomycin	T45.1X1	T45.1X2	T45.1X3	T45.1X4	T45.1X5	T45.1X6
Blockain	T41.3X1	T41.3X2	T41.3X3	T41.3X4	T41.3X5	T41.3X6
- infiltration (subcutaneous)	T41.3X1	T41.3X2	T41.3X3	T41.3X4	T41.3X5	T41.3X6
- nerve block (peripheral) (plexus)	T41.3X1	T41.3X2	T41.3X3	T41.3X4	T41.3X5	T41.3X6
- topical (surface)	T41.3X1	T41.3X2	T41.3X3	T41.3X4	T41.3X5	T41.3X6
Blockers, calcium channel	T46.1X1	T46.1X2	T46.1X3	T46.1X4	T46.1X5	T46.1X6
Blood (derivatives) (natural) (plasma) (whole)	T45.8X1	T45.8X2	T45.8X3	T45.8X4	T45.8X5	T45.8X6
- dried	T45.8X1	T45.8X2	T45.8X3	T45.8X4	T45.8X5	T45.8X6
- drug affecting NEC	T45.91	T45.92	T45.93	T45.94	T45.95	T45.96
- expander NEC	T45.8X1	T45.8X2	T45.8X3	T45.8X4	T45.8X5	T45.8X6
- fraction NEC	T45.8X1	T45.8X2	T45.8X3	T45.8X4	T45.8X5	T45.8X6
- substitute (macromolecular)	T45.8X1	T45.8X2	T45.8X3	T45.8X4	T45.8X5	T45.8X6
Blue velvet	T40.2X1	T40.2X2	T40.2X3	T40.2X4	--	--
Bone meal	T62.8X1	T62.8X2	T62.8X3	T62.8X4	--	--
Bonine	T45.0X1	T45.0X2	T45.0X3	T45.0X4	T45.0X5	T45.0X6
Bopindolol	T44.7X1	T44.7X2	T44.7X3	T44.7X4	T44.7X5	T44.7X6
Boracic acid	T49.0X1	T49.0X2	T49.0X3	T49.0X4	T49.0X5	T49.0X6
- ENT agent	T49.6X1	T49.6X2	T49.6X3	T49.6X4	T49.6X5	T49.6X6
- ophthalmic preparation	T49.5X1	T49.5X2	T49.5X3	T49.5X4	T49.5X5	T49.5X6
Borane complex	T57.8X1	T57.8X2	T57.8X3	T57.8X4	--	--
Borate (s)	T57.8X1	T57.8X2	T57.8X3	T57.8X4	--	--
- buffer	T50.991	T50.992	T50.993	T50.994	T50.995	T50.996
- cleanser	T54.91	T54.92	T54.93	T54.94	--	--
- sodium	T57.8X1	T57.8X2	T57.8X3	T57.8X4	--	--
Borax (cleanser)	T54.91	T54.92	T54.93	T54.94	--	--
Bordeaux mixture	T60.3X1	T60.3X2	T60.3X3	T60.3X4	--	--
Boric acid	T49.0X1	T49.0X2	T49.0X3	T49.0X4	T49.0X5	T49.0X6
- ENT agent	T49.6X1	T49.6X2	T49.6X3	T49.6X4	T49.6X5	T49.6X6
- ophthalmic preparation	T49.5X1	T49.5X2	T49.5X3	T49.5X4	T49.5X5	T49.5X6
Bornaprine	T44.3X1	T44.3X2	T44.3X3	T44.3X4	T44.3X5	T44.3X6
Boron	T57.8X1	T57.8X2	T57.8X3	T57.8X4	--	--
- hydride NEC	T57.8X1	T57.8X2	T57.8X3	T57.8X4	--	--
- - fumes or gas	T57.8X1	T57.8X2	T57.8X3	T57.8X4	--	--
- trifluoride	T59.891	T59.892	T59.893	T59.894	--	--
Botox	T48.291	T48.292	T48.293	T48.294	T48.295	T48.296
Botulinus anti-toxin (type A, B)	T50.Z11	T50.Z12	T50.Z13	T50.Z14	T50.Z15	T50.Z16
Brake fluid vapor	T59.891	T59.892	T59.893	T59.894	--	--
Brallobarbital	T42.3X1	T42.3X2	T42.3X3	T42.3X4	T42.3X5	T42.3X6
Bran (wheat)	T47.4X1	T47.4X2	T47.4X3	T47.4X4	T47.4X5	T47.4X6
Brass (fumes)	T56.891	T56.892	T56.893	T56.894	--	--
Brasso	T52.0X1	T52.0X2	T52.0X3	T52.0X4	--	--
Bretylium tosilate	T46.2X1	T46.2X2	T46.2X3	T46.2X4	T46.2X5	T46.2X6
Brevital (sodium)	T41.1X1	T41.1X2	T41.1X3	T41.1X4	T41.1X5	T41.1X6
Brinase	T45.3X1	T45.3X2	T45.3X3	T45.3X4	T45.3X5	T45.3X6
British antilewisite	T45.8X1	T45.8X2	T45.8X3	T45.8X4	T45.8X5	T45.8X6
Brodifacoum	T60.4X1	T60.4X2	T60.4X3	T60.4X4	--	--
Bromal (hydrate)	T42.6X1	T42.6X2	T42.6X3	T42.6X4	T42.6X5	T42.6X6

Substance	Poisoning, Accidental (unintentional)	Poisoning, Intentional Self-harm	Poisoning, Assault	Poisoning, Undetermined	Adverse effect	Underdosing
Bromazepam	T42.4X1	T42.4X2	T42.4X3	T42.4X4	T42.4X5	T42.4X6
Bromazine	T45.0X1	T45.0X2	T45.0X3	T45.0X4	T45.0X5	T45.0X6
Brombenzylcyanide	T59.3X1	T59.3X2	T59.3X3	T59.3X4	--	--
Bromelains	T45.3X1	T45.3X2	T45.3X3	T45.3X4	T45.3X5	T45.3X6
Bromethalin	T60.4X1	T60.4X2	T60.4X3	T60.4X4	--	--
Bromhexine	T48.4X1	T48.4X2	T48.4X3	T48.4X4	T48.4X5	T48.4X6
Bromide salts	T42.6X1	T42.6X2	T42.6X3	T42.6X4	T42.6X5	T42.6X6
Bromindione	T45.511	T45.512	T45.513	T45.514	T45.515	T45.516
Bromine						
- compounds (medicinal)	T42.6X1	T42.6X2	T42.6X3	T42.6X4	T42.6X5	T42.6X6
- sedative	T42.6X1	T42.6X2	T42.6X3	T42.6X4	T42.6X5	T42.6X6
- vapor	T59.891	T59.892	T59.893	T59.894	--	--
Bromisoval	T42.6X1	T42.6X2	T42.6X3	T42.6X4	T42.6X5	T42.6X6
Bromisovalum	T42.6X1	T42.6X2	T42.6X3	T42.6X4	T42.6X5	T42.6X6
Bromobenzylcyanide	T59.3X1	T59.3X2	T59.3X3	T59.3X4	--	--
Bromochlorosalicylani-lide	T49.0X1	T49.0X2	T49.0X3	T49.0X4	T49.0X5	T49.0X6
Bromocriptine	T42.8X1	T42.8X2	T42.8X3	T42.8X4	T42.8X5	T42.8X6
Bromodiphenhydramine	T45.0X1	T45.0X2	T45.0X3	T45.0X4	T45.0X5	T45.0X6
Bromoform	T42.6X1	T42.6X2	T42.6X3	T42.6X4	T42.6X5	T42.6X6
Bromophenol blue reagent	T50.991	T50.992	T50.993	T50.994	T50.995	T50.996
Bromopride	T47.8X1	T47.8X2	T47.8X3	T47.8X4	T47.8X5	T47.8X6
Bromosalicylchloranitide	T49.0X1	T49.0X2	T49.0X3	T49.0X4	T49.0X5	T49.0X6
Bromosalicylhydroxamic acid	T37.1X1	T37.1X2	T37.1X3	T37.1X4	T37.1X5	T37.1X6
Bromo-seltzer	T39.1X1	T39.1X2	T39.1X3	T39.1X4	T39.1X5	T39.1X6
Bromoxynil	T60.3X1	T60.3X2	T60.3X3	T60.3X4	--	--
Bromperidol	T43.4X1	T43.4X2	T43.4X3	T43.4X4	T43.4X5	T43.4X6
Brompheniramine	T45.0X1	T45.0X2	T45.0X3	T45.0X4	T45.0X5	T45.0X6
Bromsulfophthalein	T50.8X1	T50.8X2	T50.8X3	T50.8X4	T50.8X5	T50.8X6
Bromural	T42.6X1	T42.6X2	T42.6X3	T42.6X4	T42.6X5	T42.6X6
Bromvaletone	T42.6X1	T42.6X2	T42.6X3	T42.6X4	T42.6X5	T42.6X6
Bronchodilator NEC	T48.6X1	T48.6X2	T48.6X3	T48.6X4	T48.6X5	T48.6X6
Brotizolam	T42.4X1	T42.4X2	T42.4X3	T42.4X4	T42.4X5	T42.4X6
Brovincamine	T46.7X1	T46.7X2	T46.7X3	T46.7X4	T46.7X5	T46.7X6
Brown recluse spider (bite) (venom)	T63.331	T63.332	T63.333	T63.334	--	--
Brown spider (bite) (venom)	T63.391	T63.392	T63.393	T63.394	--	--
Broxaterol	T48.6X1	T48.6X2	T48.6X3	T48.6X4	T48.6X5	T48.6X6
Broxuridine	T45.1X1	T45.1X2	T45.1X3	T45.1X4	T45.1X5	T45.1X6
Broxyquinoline	T37.8X1	T37.8X2	T37.8X3	T37.8X4	T37.8X5	T37.8X6
Bruceine	T48.291	T48.292	T48.293	T48.294	T48.295	T48.296
Brucia	T62.2X1	T62.2X2	T62.2X3	T62.2X4	--	--
Brucine	T65.1X1	T65.1X2	T65.1X3	T65.1X4	--	--
Brunswick green—see Copper						
Bruten—see Ibuprofen						
Bryonia	T47.2X1	T47.2X2	T47.2X3	T47.2X4	T47.2X5	T47.2X6
Buclizine	T45.0X1	T45.0X2	T45.0X3	T45.0X4	T45.0X5	T45.0X6
Buclosamide	T49.0X1	T49.0X2	T49.0X3	T49.0X4	T49.0X5	T49.0X6
Budesonide	T44.5X1	T44.5X2	T44.5X3	T44.5X4	T44.5X5	T44.5X6
Budralazine	T46.5X1	T46.5X2	T46.5X3	T46.5X4	T46.5X5	T46.5X6
Bufferin	T39.011	T39.012	T39.013	T39.014	T39.015	T39.016
Buflomedil	T46.7X1	T46.7X2	T46.7X3	T46.7X4	T46.7X5	T46.7X6
Buformin	T38.3X1	T38.3X2	T38.3X3	T38.3X4	T38.3X5	T38.3X6
Bufotenine	T40.991	T40.992	T40.993	T40.994	--	--
Bufrolin	T48.6X1	T48.6X2	T48.6X3	T48.6X4	T48.6X5	T48.6X6
Bufylline	T48.6X1	T48.6X2	T48.6X3	T48.6X4	T48.6X5	T48.6X6
Bulk filler	T50.5X1	T50.5X2	T50.5X3	T50.5X4	T50.5X5	T50.5X6
- cathartic	T47.4X1	T47.4X2	T47.4X3	T47.4X4	T47.4X5	T47.4X6
Bumetanide	T50.1X1	T50.1X2	T50.1X3	T50.1X4	T50.1X5	T50.1X6
Bunaftine	T46.2X1	T46.2X2	T46.2X3	T46.2X4	T46.2X5	T46.2X6
Bunamiodyl	T50.8X1	T50.8X2	T50.8X3	T50.8X4	T50.8X5	T50.8X6

Substance	Poisoning, Accidental (unintentional)	Poisoning, Intentional Self-harm	Poisoning, Assault	Poisoning, Undetermined	Adverse effect	Underdosing
Bunazosin	T44.6X1	T44.6X2	T44.6X3	T44.6X4	T44.6X5	T44.6X6
Bunitrolol	T44.7X1	T44.7X2	T44.7X3	T44.7X4	T44.7X5	T44.7X6
Buphenine	T46.7X1	T46.7X2	T46.7X3	T46.7X4	T46.7X5	T46.7X6
Bupivacaine	T41.3X1	T41.3X2	T41.3X3	T41.3X4	T41.3X5	T41.3X6
- infiltration (subcutaneous)	T41.3X1	T41.3X2	T41.3X3	T41.3X4	T41.3X5	T41.3X6
- nerve block (peripheral) (plexus)	T41.3X1	T41.3X2	T41.3X3	T41.3X4	T41.3X5	T41.3X6
- spinal	T41.3X1	T41.3X2	T41.3X3	T41.3X4	T41.3X5	T41.3X6
Bupranolol	T44.7X1	T44.7X2	T44.7X3	T44.7X4	T44.7X5	T44.7X6
Buprenorphine	T40.4X1	T40.4X2	T40.4X3	T40.4X4	T40.4X5	T40.4X6
Bupropion	T43.291	T43.292	T43.293	T43.294	T43.295	T43.296
Burimamide	T47.1X1	T47.1X2	T47.1X3	T47.1X4	T47.1X5	T47.1X6
Buserelin	T38.891	T38.892	T38.893	T38.894	T38.895	T38.896
Buspirone	T43.591	T43.592	T43.593	T43.594	T43.595	T43.596
Busulfan, busulphan	T45.1X1	T45.1X2	T45.1X3	T45.1X4	T45.1X5	T45.1X6
Butabarbital (sodium)	T42.3X1	T42.3X2	T42.3X3	T42.3X4	T42.3X5	T42.3X6
Butabarbitone	T42.3X1	T42.3X2	T42.3X3	T42.3X4	T42.3X5	T42.3X6
Butabarpal	T42.3X1	T42.3X2	T42.3X3	T42.3X4	T42.3X5	T42.3X6
Butacaine	T41.3X1	T41.3X2	T41.3X3	T41.3X4	T41.3X5	T41.3X6
Butalamine	T46.7X1	T46.7X2	T46.7X3	T46.7X4	T46.7X5	T46.7X6
Butalbital	T42.3X1	T42.3X2	T42.3X3	T42.3X4	T42.3X5	T42.3X6
Butallylonal	T42.3X1	T42.3X2	T42.3X3	T42.3X4	T42.3X5	T42.3X6
Butamben	T41.3X1	T41.3X2	T41.3X3	T41.3X4	T41.3X5	T41.3X6
Butamirate	T48.3X1	T48.3X2	T48.3X3	T48.3X4	T48.3X5	T48.3X6
Butane (distributed in mobile container)	T59.891	T59.892	T59.893	T59.894	--	--
- distributed through pipes	T59.891	T59.892	T59.893	T59.894	--	--
- incomplete combustion	T58.11	T58.12	T58.13	T58.14	--	--
Butanilicaine	T41.3X1	T41.3X2	T41.3X3	T41.3X4	T41.3X5	T41.3X6
Butanol	T51.3X1	T51.3X2	T51.3X3	T51.3X4	--	--
Butanone, 2-butanone	T52.4X1	T52.4X2	T52.4X3	T52.4X4	--	--
Butantrone	T49.4X1	T49.4X2	T49.4X3	T49.4X4	T49.4X5	T49.4X6
Butaperazine	T43.3X1	T43.3X2	T43.3X3	T43.3X4	T43.3X5	T43.3X6
Butazolidin	T39.2X1	T39.2X2	T39.2X3	T39.2X4	T39.2X5	T39.2X6
Butetamate	T48.6X1	T48.6X2	T48.6X3	T48.6X4	T48.6X5	T48.6X6
Butethal	T42.3X1	T42.3X2	T42.3X3	T42.3X4	T42.3X5	T42.3X6
Butethamate	T44.3X1	T44.3X2	T44.3X3	T44.3X4	T44.3X5	T44.3X6
Buthalitone (sodium)	T41.1X1	T41.1X2	T41.1X3	T41.1X4	T41.1X5	T41.1X6
Butisol (sodium)	T42.3X1	T42.3X2	T42.3X3	T42.3X4	T42.3X5	T42.3X6
Butizide	T50.2X1	T50.2X2	T50.2X3	T50.2X4	T50.2X5	T50.2X6
Butobarbital	T42.3X1	T42.3X2	T42.3X3	T42.3X4	T42.3X5	T42.3X6
- sodium	T42.3X1	T42.3X2	T42.3X3	T42.3X4	T42.3X5	T42.3X6
Butobarbitone	T42.3X1	T42.3X2	T42.3X3	T42.3X4	T42.3X5	T42.3X6
Butoconazole (nitrate)	T49.0X1	T49.0X2	T49.0X3	T49.0X4	T49.0X5	T49.0X6
Butorphanol	T40.4X1	T40.4X2	T40.4X3	T40.4X4	T40.4X5	T40.4X6
Butriptyline	T43.011	T43.012	T43.013	T43.014	T43.015	T43.016
Butropium bromide	T44.3X1	T44.3X2	T44.3X3	T44.3X4	T44.3X5	T44.3X6
Butter of antimony—see Antimony						
Buttercups	T62.2X1	T62.2X2	T62.2X3	T62.2X4	--	--
Butyl						
- acetate (secondary)	T52.8X1	T52.8X2	T52.8X3	T52.8X4	--	--
- alcohol	T51.3X1	T51.3X2	T51.3X3	T51.3X4	--	--
- aminobenzoate	T41.3X1	T41.3X2	T41.3X3	T41.3X4	T41.3X5	T41.3X6
- butyrate	T52.8X1	T52.8X2	T52.8X3	T52.8X4	--	--
- carbinol	T51.3X1	T51.3X2	T51.3X3	T51.3X4	--	--
- carbitol	T52.3X1	T52.3X2	T52.3X3	T52.3X4	--	--
- cellosolve	T52.3X1	T52.3X2	T52.3X3	T52.3X4	--	--
- chloral (hydrate)	T42.6X1	T42.6X2	T42.6X3	T42.6X4	T42.6X5	T42.6X6
- formate	T52.8X1	T52.8X2	T52.8X3	T52.8X4	--	--
- lactate	T52.8X1	T52.8X2	T52.8X3	T52.8X4	--	--

Substance	Poisoning, Accidental (unintentional)	Poisoning, Intentional Self-harm	Poisoning, Assault	Poisoning, Undetermined	Adverse effect	Underdosing
- propionate	T52.8X1	T52.8X2	T52.8X3	T52.8X4	--	--
- scopolamine bromide	T44.3X1	T44.3X2	T44.3X3	T44.3X4	T44.3X5	T44.3X6
- thiobarbital sodium	T41.1X1	T41.1X2	T41.1X3	T41.1X4	T41.1X5	T41.1X6
Butylated hydroxy-anisole	T50.991	T50.992	T50.993	T50.994	T50.995	T50.996
Butylchloral hydrate	T42.6X1	T42.6X2	T42.6X3	T42.6X4	T42.6X5	T42.6X6
Butyltoluene	T52.2X1	T52.2X2	T52.2X3	T52.2X4	--	--
Butyn	T41.3X1	T41.3X2	T41.3X3	T41.3X4	T41.3X5	T41.3X6
Butyrophenone (-based tranquilizers)	T43.4X1	T43.4X2	T43.4X3	T43.4X4	T43.4X5	T43.4X6
Cabergoline	T42.8X1	T42.8X2	T42.8X3	T42.8X4	T42.8X5	T42.8X6
Cacodyl, cacodylic acid	T57.0X1	T57.0X2	T57.0X3	T57.0X4	--	--
Cactinomycin	T45.1X1	T45.1X2	T45.1X3	T45.1X4	T45.1X5	T45.1X6
Cade oil	T49.4X1	T49.4X2	T49.4X3	T49.4X4	T49.4X5	T49.4X6
Cadexomer iodine	T49.0X1	T49.0X2	T49.0X3	T49.0X4	T49.0X5	T49.0X6
Cadmium (chloride) (fumes) (oxide)	T56.3X1	T56.3X2	T56.3X3	T56.3X4	--	--
- sulfide (medicinal) NEC	T49.4X1	T49.4X2	T49.4X3	T49.4X4	T49.4X5	T49.4X6
Cadralazine	T46.5X1	T46.5X2	T46.5X3	T46.5X4	T46.5X5	T46.5X6
Caffeine	T43.611	T43.612	T43.613	T43.614	T43.615	T43.616
Calabar bean	T62.2X1	T62.2X2	T62.2X3	T62.2X4	--	--
Caladium seguinum	T62.2X1	T62.2X2	T62.2X3	T62.2X4	--	--
Calamine (lotion)	T49.3X1	T49.3X2	T49.3X3	T49.3X4	T49.3X5	T49.3X6
Calcifediol	T45.2X1	T45.2X2	T45.2X3	T45.2X4	T45.2X5	T45.2X6
Calciferol	T45.2X1	T45.2X2	T45.2X3	T45.2X4	T45.2X5	T45.2X6
Calcitonin	T50.991	T50.992	T50.993	T50.994	T50.995	T50.996
Calcitriol	T45.2X1	T45.2X2	T45.2X3	T45.2X4	T45.2X5	T45.2X6
Calcium	T50.3X1	T50.3X2	T50.3X3	T50.3X4	T50.3X5	T50.3X6
- actylsalicylate	T39.011	T39.012	T39.013	T39.014	T39.015	T39.016
- benzamidosalicylate	T37.1X1	T37.1X2	T37.1X3	T37.1X4	T37.1X5	T37.1X6
- bromide	T42.6X1	T42.6X2	T42.6X3	T42.6X4	T42.6X5	T42.6X6
- bromolactobionate	T42.6X1	T42.6X2	T42.6X3	T42.6X4	T42.6X5	T42.6X6
- carbaspirin	T39.011	T39.012	T39.013	T39.014	T39.015	T39.016
- carbimide	T50.6X1	T50.6X2	T50.6X3	T50.6X4	T50.6X5	T50.6X6
- carbonate	T47.1X1	T47.1X2	T47.1X3	T47.1X4	T47.1X5	T47.1X6
- chloride	T50.991	T50.992	T50.993	T50.994	T50.995	T50.996
- - anhydrous	T50.991	T50.992	T50.993	T50.994	T50.995	T50.996
- cyanide	T57.8X1	T57.8X2	T57.8X3	T57.8X4	--	--
- dioctyl sulfosuccinate	T47.4X1	T47.4X2	T47.4X3	T47.4X4	T47.4X5	T47.4X6
- disodium edathamil	T45.8X1	T45.8X2	T45.8X3	T45.8X4	T45.8X5	T45.8X6
- disodium edetate	T45.8X1	T45.8X2	T45.8X3	T45.8X4	T45.8X5	T45.8X6
- dobesilate	T46.991	T46.992	T46.993	T46.994	T46.995	T46.996
- EDTA	T45.8X1	T45.8X2	T45.8X3	T45.8X4	T45.8X5	T45.8X6
- ferrous citrate	T45.4X1	T45.4X2	T45.4X3	T45.4X4	T45.4X5	T45.4X6
- folinate	T45.8X1	T45.8X2	T45.8X3	T45.8X4	T45.8X5	T45.8X6
- glubionate	T50.3X1	T50.3X2	T50.3X3	T50.3X4	T50.3X5	T50.3X6
- gluconate	T50.3X1	T50.3X2	T50.3X3	T50.3X4	T50.3X5	T50.3X6
- gluconogalactogluc-onate	T50.3X1	T50.3X2	T50.3X3	T50.3X4	T50.3X5	T50.3X6
- hydrate, hydroxide	T54.3X1	T54.3X2	T54.3X3	T54.3X4	--	--
- hypochlorite	T54.3X1	T54.3X2	T54.3X3	T54.3X4	--	--
- iodide	T48.4X1	T48.4X2	T48.4X3	T48.4X4	T48.4X5	T48.4X6
- ipodate	T50.8X1	T50.8X2	T50.8X3	T50.8X4	T50.8X5	T50.8X6
- lactate	T50.3X1	T50.3X2	T50.3X3	T50.3X4	T50.3X5	T50.3X6
- leucovorin	T45.8X1	T45.8X2	T45.8X3	T45.8X4	T45.8X5	T45.8X6
- mandelate	T37.91	T37.92	T37.93	T37.94	T37.95	T37.96
- oxide	T54.3X1	T54.3X2	T54.3X3	T54.3X4	--	--
- pantothenate	T45.2X1	T45.2X2	T45.2X3	T45.2X4	T45.2X5	T45.2X6
- phosphate	T50.3X1	T50.3X2	T50.3X3	T50.3X4	T50.3X5	T50.3X6
- salicylate	T39.091	T39.092	T39.093	T39.094	T39.095	T39.096
- salts	T50.3X1	T50.3X2	T50.3X3	T50.3X4	T50.3X5	T50.3X6
Calculus-dissolving drug	T50.991	T50.992	T50.993	T50.994	T50.995	T50.996
Calomel	T49.0X1	T49.0X2	T49.0X3	T49.0X4	T49.0X5	T49.0X6

Substance	Poisoning, Accidental (unintentional)	Poisoning, Intentional Self-harm	Poisoning, Assault	Poisoning, Undetermined	Adverse effect	Underdosing
Caloric agent	T50.3X1	T50.3X2	T50.3X3	T50.3X4	T50.3X5	T50.3X6
Calusterone	T38.7X1	T38.7X2	T38.7X3	T38.7X4	T38.7X5	T38.7X6
Camazepam	T42.4X1	T42.4X2	T42.4X3	T42.4X4	T42.4X5	T42.4X6
Camomile	T49.0X1	T49.0X2	T49.0X3	T49.0X4	T49.0X5	T49.0X6
Camoquin	T37.2X1	T37.2X2	T37.2X3	T37.2X4	T37.2X5	T37.2X6
Camphor						
- insecticide	T60.2X1	T60.2X2	T60.2X3	T60.2X4	--	--
- medicinal	T49.8X1	T49.8X2	T49.8X3	T49.8X4	T49.8X5	T49.8X6
Camylofin	T44.3X1	T44.3X2	T44.3X3	T44.3X4	T44.3X5	T44.3X6
Cancer chemotherapy drug regimen	T45.1X1	T45.1X2	T45.1X3	T45.1X4	T45.1X5	T45.1X6
Candeptin	T49.0X1	T49.0X2	T49.0X3	T49.0X4	T49.0X5	T49.0X6
Candicidin	T49.0X1	T49.0X2	T49.0X3	T49.0X4	T49.0X5	T49.0X6
Cannabinol	T40.7X1	T40.7X2	T40.7X3	T40.7X4	T40.7X5	T40.7X6
Cannabis (derivatives)	T40.7X1	T40.7X2	T40.7X3	T40.7X4	T40.7X5	T40.7X6
Canned heat	T51.1X1	T51.1X2	T51.1X3	T51.1X4	--	--
Canrenoic acid	T50.0X1	T50.0X2	T50.0X3	T50.0X4	T50.0X5	T50.0X6
Canrenone	T50.0X1	T50.0X2	T50.0X3	T50.0X4	T50.0X5	T50.0X6
Cantharides, cantharidin, cantharis	T49.8X1	T49.8X2	T49.8X3	T49.8X4	T49.8X5	T49.8X6
Canthaxanthin	T50.991	T50.992	T50.993	T50.994	T50.995	T50.996
Capillary-active drug NEC	T46.901	T46.902	T46.903	T46.904	T46.905	T46.906
Capreomycin	T36.8X1	T36.8X2	T36.8X3	T36.8X4	T36.8X5	T36.8X6
Capsicum	T49.4X1	T49.4X2	T49.4X3	T49.4X4	T49.4X5	T49.4X6
Captafol	T60.3X1	T60.3X2	T60.3X3	T60.3X4	--	--
Captan	T60.3X1	T60.3X2	T60.3X3	T60.3X4	--	--
Captodiame, captodiamine	T43.591	T43.592	T43.593	T43.594	T43.595	T43.596
Captopril	T46.4X1	T46.4X2	T46.4X3	T46.4X4	T46.4X5	T46.4X6
Caramiphen	T44.3X1	T44.3X2	T44.3X3	T44.3X4	T44.3X5	T44.3X6
Carazolol	T44.7X1	T44.7X2	T44.7X3	T44.7X4	T44.7X5	T44.7X6
Carbachol	T44.1X1	T44.1X2	T44.1X3	T44.1X4	T44.1X5	T44.1X6
Carbacrylamine (resin)	T50.3X1	T50.3X2	T50.3X3	T50.3X4	T50.3X5	T50.3X6
Carbamate (insecticide)	T60.0X1	T60.0X2	T60.0X3	T60.0X4	--	--
Carbamate (sedative)	T42.6X1	T42.6X2	T42.6X3	T42.6X4	T42.6X5	T42.6X6
- herbicide	T60.0X1	T60.0X2	T60.0X3	T60.0X4	--	--
- insecticide	T60.0X1	T60.0X2	T60.0X3	T60.0X4	--	--
Carbamazepine	T42.1X1	T42.1X2	T42.1X3	T42.1X4	T42.1X5	T42.1X6
Carbamide	T47.3X1	T47.3X2	T47.3X3	T47.3X4	T47.3X5	T47.3X6
- peroxide	T49.0X1	T49.0X2	T49.0X3	T49.0X4	T49.0X5	T49.0X6
- topical	T49.8X1	T49.8X2	T49.8X3	T49.8X4	T49.8X5	T49.8X6
Carbamylcholine chloride	T44.1X1	T44.1X2	T44.1X3	T44.1X4	T44.1X5	T44.1X6
Carbaril	T60.0X1	T60.0X2	T60.0X3	T60.0X4	--	--
Carbarsone	T37.3X1	T37.3X2	T37.3X3	T37.3X4	T37.3X5	T37.3X6
Carbaryl	T60.0X1	T60.0X2	T60.0X3	T60.0X4	--	--
Carbaspirin	T39.011	T39.012	T39.013	T39.014	T39.015	T39.016
Carbazochrome (salicylate) (sodium sulfonate)	T49.4X1	T49.4X2	T49.4X3	T49.4X4	T49.4X5	T49.4X6
Carbenicillin	T36.0X1	T36.0X2	T36.0X3	T36.0X4	T36.0X5	T36.0X6
Carbenoxolone	T47.1X1	T47.1X2	T47.1X3	T47.1X4	T47.1X5	T47.1X6
Carbetapentane	T48.3X1	T48.3X2	T48.3X3	T48.3X4	T48.3X5	T48.3X6
Carbethyl salicylate	T39.091	T39.092	T39.093	T39.094	T39.095	T39.096
Carbidopa (with levodopa)	T42.8X1	T42.8X2	T42.8X3	T42.8X4	T42.8X5	T42.8X6
Carbimazole	T38.2X1	T38.2X2	T38.2X3	T38.2X4	T38.2X5	T38.2X6
Carbinol	T51.1X1	T51.1X2	T51.1X3	T51.1X4	--	--
Carbinoxamine	T45.0X1	T45.0X2	T45.0X3	T45.0X4	T45.0X5	T45.0X6
Carbiphene	T39.8X1	T39.8X2	T39.8X3	T39.8X4	T39.8X5	T39.8X6
Carbitol	T52.3X1	T52.3X2	T52.3X3	T52.3X4	--	--
Carbo medicinalis	T47.6X1	T47.6X2	T47.6X3	T47.6X4	T47.6X5	T47.6X6
Carbocaine	T41.3X1	T41.3X2	T41.3X3	T41.3X4	T41.3X5	T41.3X6
- infiltration (subcutaneous)	T41.3X1	T41.3X2	T41.3X3	T41.3X4	T41.3X5	T41.3X6
- nerve block (peripheral) (plexus)	T41.3X1	T41.3X2	T41.3X3	T41.3X4	T41.3X5	T41.3X6

Substance	Poisoning, Accidental (unintentional)	Poisoning, Intentional Self-harm	Poisoning, Assault	Poisoning, Undetermined	Adverse effect	Underdosing
- topical (surface)	T41.3X1	T41.3X2	T41.3X3	T41.3X4	T41.3X5	T41.3X6
Carbocisteine	T48.4X1	T48.4X2	T48.4X3	T48.4X4	T48.4X5	T48.4X6
Carbocromen	T46.3X1	T46.3X2	T46.3X3	T46.3X4	T46.3X5	T46.3X6
Carbol fuchsin	T49.0X1	T49.0X2	T49.0X3	T49.0X4	T49.0X5	T49.0X6
Carbolic acid—see also Phenol	T54.0X1	T54.0X2	T54.0X3	T54.0X4	--	--
Carbolonium (bromide)	T48.1X1	T48.1X2	T48.1X3	T48.1X4	T48.1X5	T48.1X6
Carbomycin	T36.8X1	T36.8X2	T36.8X3	T36.8X4	T36.8X5	T36.8X6
- bisulfide (liquid)	T65.4X1	T65.4X2	T65.4X3	T65.4X4	--	--
- - vapor	T65.4X1	T65.4X2	T65.4X3	T65.4X4	--	--
- dioxide (gas)	T59.7X1	T59.7X2	T59.7X3	T59.7X4	--	--
- - medicinal	T41.5X1	T41.5X2	T41.5X3	T41.5X4	T41.5X5	T41.5X6
- - nonmedicinal	T59.7X1	T59.7X2	T59.7X3	T59.7X4	--	--
- - snow	T49.4X1	T49.4X2	T49.4X3	T49.4X4	T49.4X5	T49.4X6
- disulfide (liquid)	T65.4X1	T65.4X2	T65.4X3	T65.4X4	--	--
- - vapor	T65.4X1	T65.4X2	T65.4X3	T65.4X4	--	--
- monoxide (from incomplete combustion)	T58.91	T58.92	T58.93	T58.94	--	--
- - blast furnace gas	T58.8X1	T58.8X2	T58.8X3	T58.8X4	--	--
- - butane (distributed in mobile container)	T58.11	T58.12	T58.13	T58.14	--	--
- - - distributed through pipes	T58.11	T58.12	T58.13	T58.14	--	--
- - charcoal fumes	T58.2X1	T58.2X2	T58.2X3	T58.2X4	--	--
- - coal	T58.2X1	T58.2X2	T58.2X3	T58.2X4	--	--
- - coke (in domestic stoves, fireplaces)	T58.2X1	T58.2X2	T58.2X3	T58.2X4	--	--
- - gas (piped)	T58.11	T58.12	T58.13	T58.14	--	--
- - solid (in domestic stoves, fireplaces)	T58.2X1	T58.2X2	T58.2X3	T58.2X4	--	--
- - exhaust gas (motor) not in transit	T58.01	T58.02	T58.03	T58.04	--	--
- - - combustion engine, any not in watercraft	T58.01	T58.02	T58.03	T58.04	--	--
- - - farm tractor, not in transit	T58.01	T58.02	T58.03	T58.04	--	--
- - - gas engine	T58.01	T58.02	T58.03	T58.04	--	--
- - - motor pump	T58.01	T58.02	T58.03	T58.04	--	--
- - - motor vehicle, not in transit	T58.01	T58.02	T58.03	T58.04	--	--
- - fuel (in domestic use)	T58.2X1	T58.2X2	T58.2X3	T58.2X4	--	--
- - - gas (piped)	T58.11	T58.12	T58.13	T58.14	--	--
- - - - in mobile container	T58.11	T58.12	T58.13	T58.14	--	--
- - - piped (natural)	T58.11	T58.12	T58.13	T58.14	--	--
- - - utility	T58.11	T58.12	T58.13	T58.14	--	--
- - - - in mobile container	T58.11	T58.12	T58.13	T58.14	--	--
- - illuminating gas	T58.11	T58.12	T58.13	T58.14	--	--
- - industrial fuels or gases, any	T58.8X1	T58.8X2	T58.8X3	T58.8X4	--	--
- - kerosene (in domestic stoves, fireplaces)	T58.2X1	T58.2X2	T58.2X3	T58.2X4	--	--
- - kiln gas or vapor	T58.8X1	T58.8X2	T58.8X3	T58.8X4	--	--
- - motor exhaust gas, not in transit	T58.01	T58.02	T58.03	T58.04	--	--
- - piped gas (manufactured) (natural)	T58.11	T58.12	T58.13	T58.14	--	--
- - producer gas	T58.8X1	T58.8X2	T58.8X3	T58.8X4	--	--
- - propane (distributed in mobile container)	T58.11	T58.12	T58.13	T58.14	--	--
- - - distributed through pipes	T58.11	T58.12	T58.13	T58.14	--	--
- - specified source NEC	T58.8X1	T58.8X2	T58.8X3	T58.8X4	--	--
- - stove gas	T58.11	T58.12	T58.13	T58.14	--	--
- - - piped	T58.11	T58.12	T58.13	T58.14	--	--
- - utility gas	T58.11	T58.12	T58.13	T58.14	--	--
- - - piped	T58.11	T58.12	T58.13	T58.14	--	--
- - water gas	T58.11	T58.12	T58.13	T58.14	--	--
- - wood (in domestic stoves, fireplaces)	T58.2X1	T58.2X2	T58.2X3	T58.2X4	--	--
- tetrachloride (vapor) NEC	T53.0X1	T53.0X2	T53.0X3	T53.0X4	--	--
- - liquid (cleansing agent) NEC	T53.0X1	T53.0X2	T53.0X3	T53.0X4	--	--
- - solvent	T53.0X1	T53.0X2	T53.0X3	T53.0X4	--	--
Carbonic acid gas	T59.7X1	T59.7X2	T59.7X3	T59.7X4	--	--
- anhydrase inhibitor NEC	T50.2X1	T50.2X2	T50.2X3	T50.2X4	T50.2X5	T50.2X6
Carbophenothion	T60.0X1	T60.0X2	T60.0X3	T60.0X4	--	--
Carboplatin	T45.1X1	T45.1X2	T45.1X3	T45.1X4	T45.1X5	T45.1X6

Substance	Poisoning, Accidental (unintentional)	Poisoning, Intentional Self-harm	Poisoning, Assault	Poisoning, Undetermined	Adverse effect	Underdosing
Carboprost	T48.0X1	T48.0X2	T48.0X3	T48.0X4	T48.0X5	T48.0X6
Carboquone	T45.1X1	T45.1X2	T45.1X3	T45.1X4	T45.1X5	T45.1X6
Carbowax	T49.3X1	T49.3X2	T49.3X3	T49.3X4	T49.3X5	T49.3X6
Carboxymethyl-cellulose	T47.4X1	T47.4X2	T47.4X3	T47.4X4	T47.4X5	T47.4X6
S-Carboxymethyl-cysteine	T48.4X1	T48.4X2	T48.4X3	T48.4X4	T48.4X5	T48.4X6
Carbrital	T42.3X1	T42.3X2	T42.3X3	T42.3X4	T42.3X5	T42.3X6
Carbromal	T42.6X1	T42.6X2	T42.6X3	T42.6X4	T42.6X5	T42.6X6
Carbutamide	T38.3X1	T38.3X2	T38.3X3	T38.3X4	T38.3X5	T38.3X6
Carbuterol	T48.6X1	T48.6X2	T48.6X3	T48.6X4	T48.6X5	T48.6X6
Cardiac						
- depressants	T46.2X1	T46.2X2	T46.2X3	T46.2X4	T46.2X5	T46.2X6
- rhythm regulator	T46.2X1	T46.2X2	T46.2X3	T46.2X4	T46.2X5	T46.2X6
- - specified NEC	T46.2X1	T46.2X2	T46.2X3	T46.2X4	T46.2X5	T46.2X6
Cardiografin	T50.8X1	T50.8X2	T50.8X3	T50.8X4	T50.8X5	T50.8X6
Cardio-green	T50.8X1	T50.8X2	T50.8X3	T50.8X4	T50.8X5	T50.8X6
Cardiotonic (glycoside) NEC	T46.0X1	T46.0X2	T46.0X3	T46.0X4	T46.0X5	T46.0X6
Cardiovascular drug NEC	T46.901	T46.902	T46.903	T46.904	T46.905	T46.906
Cardrase	T50.2X1	T50.2X2	T50.2X3	T50.2X4	T50.2X5	T50.2X6
Carfecillin	T36.0X1	T36.0X2	T36.0X3	T36.0X4	T36.0X5	T36.0X6
Carfenazine	T43.3X1	T43.3X2	T43.3X3	T43.3X4	T43.3X5	T43.3X6
Carfusin	T49.0X1	T49.0X2	T49.0X3	T49.0X4	T49.0X5	T49.0X6
Carindacillin	T36.0X1	T36.0X2	T36.0X3	T36.0X4	T36.0X5	T36.0X6
Carisoprodol	T42.8X1	T42.8X2	T42.8X3	T42.8X4	T42.8X5	T42.8X6
Carmellose	T47.4X1	T47.4X2	T47.4X3	T47.4X4	T47.4X5	T47.4X6
Carminative	T47.5X1	T47.5X2	T47.5X3	T47.5X4	T47.5X5	T47.5X6
Carmofur	T45.1X1	T45.1X2	T45.1X3	T45.1X4	T45.1X5	T45.1X6
Carmustine	T45.1X1	T45.1X2	T45.1X3	T45.1X4	T45.1X5	T45.1X6
Carotene	T45.2X1	T45.2X2	T45.2X3	T45.2X4	T45.2X5	T45.2X6
Carphenazine	T43.3X1	T43.3X2	T43.3X3	T43.3X4	T43.3X5	T43.3X6
Carpipramine	T42.4X1	T42.4X2	T42.4X3	T42.4X4	T42.4X5	T42.4X6
Carprofen	T39.311	T39.312	T39.313	T39.314	T39.315	T39.316
Carpronium chloride	T44.3X1	T44.3X2	T44.3X3	T44.3X4	T44.3X5	T44.3X6
Carrageenan	T47.8X1	T47.8X2	T47.8X3	T47.8X4	T47.8X5	T47.8X6
Carteolol	T44.7X1	T44.7X2	T44.7X3	T44.7X4	T44.7X5	T44.7X6
Carter's Little Pills	T47.2X1	T47.2X2	T47.2X3	T47.2X4	T47.2X5	T47.2X6
Cascara (sagrada)	T47.2X1	T47.2X2	T47.2X3	T47.2X4	T47.2X5	T47.2X6
Cassava	T62.2X1	T62.2X2	T62.2X3	T62.2X4	--	--
Castellani's paint	T49.0X1	T49.0X2	T49.0X3	T49.0X4	T49.0X5	T49.0X6
Castor						
- bean	T62.2X1	T62.2X2	T62.2X3	T62.2X4	--	--
- oil	T47.2X1	T47.2X2	T47.2X3	T47.2X4	T47.2X5	T47.2X6
Catalase	T45.3X1	T45.3X2	T45.3X3	T45.3X4	T45.3X5	T45.3X6
Caterpillar (sting)	T63.431	T63.432	T63.433	T63.434	--	--
Catha (edulis) (tea)	T43.691	T43.692	T43.693	T43.694	--	--
Cathartic NEC	T47.4X1	T47.4X2	T47.4X3	T47.4X4	T47.4X5	T47.4X6
- anthacene derivative	T47.2X1	T47.2X2	T47.2X3	T47.2X4	T47.2X5	T47.2X6
- bulk	T47.4X1	T47.4X2	T47.4X3	T47.4X4	T47.4X5	T47.4X6
- contact	T47.2X1	T47.2X2	T47.2X3	T47.2X4	T47.2X5	T47.2X6
- emollient NEC	T47.4X1	T47.4X2	T47.4X3	T47.4X4	T47.4X5	T47.4X6
- irritant NEC	T47.2X1	T47.2X2	T47.2X3	T47.2X4	T47.2X5	T47.2X6
- mucilage	T47.4X1	T47.4X2	T47.4X3	T47.4X4	T47.4X5	T47.4X6
- saline	T47.3X1	T47.3X2	T47.3X3	T47.3X4	T47.3X5	T47.3X6
- vegetable	T47.2X1	T47.2X2	T47.2X3	T47.2X4	T47.2X5	T47.2X6
Cathine	T50.5X1	T50.5X2	T50.5X3	T50.5X4	T50.5X5	T50.5X6
Cathomycin	T36.8X1	T36.8X2	T36.8X3	T36.8X4	T36.8X5	T36.8X6
Cation exchange resin	T50.3X1	T50.3X2	T50.3X3	T50.3X4	T50.3X5	T50.3X6
Caustic (s) NEC	T54.91	T54.92	T54.93	T54.94	--	--
- alkali	T54.3X1	T54.3X2	T54.3X3	T54.3X4	--	--

Substance	Poisoning, Accidental (unintentional)	Poisoning, Intentional Self-harm	Poisoning, Assault	Poisoning, Undetermined	Adverse effect	Underdosing
- hydroxide	T54.3X1	T54.3X2	T54.3X3	T54.3X4	--	--
- potash	T54.3X1	T54.3X2	T54.3X3	T54.3X4	--	--
- soda	T54.3X1	T54.3X2	T54.3X3	T54.3X4	--	--
- specified NEC	T54.91	T54.92	T54.93	T54.94	--	--
Ceepryn	T49.0X1	T49.0X2	T49.0X3	T49.0X4	T49.0X5	T49.0X6
- ENT agent	T49.6X1	T49.6X2	T49.6X3	T49.6X4	T49.6X5	T49.6X6
- lozenges	T49.6X1	T49.6X2	T49.6X3	T49.6X4	T49.6X5	T49.6X6
Cefacetrile	T36.1X1	T36.1X2	T36.1X3	T36.1X4	T36.1X5	T36.1X6
Cefaclor	T36.1X1	T36.1X2	T36.1X3	T36.1X4	T36.1X5	T36.1X6
Cefadroxil	T36.1X1	T36.1X2	T36.1X3	T36.1X4	T36.1X5	T36.1X6
Cefalexin	T36.1X1	T36.1X2	T36.1X3	T36.1X4	T36.1X5	T36.1X6
Cefaloglycin	T36.1X1	T36.1X2	T36.1X3	T36.1X4	T36.1X5	T36.1X6
Cefaloridine	T36.1X1	T36.1X2	T36.1X3	T36.1X4	T36.1X5	T36.1X6
Cefalosporins	T36.1X1	T36.1X2	T36.1X3	T36.1X4	T36.1X5	T36.1X6
Cefalotin	T36.1X1	T36.1X2	T36.1X3	T36.1X4	T36.1X5	T36.1X6
Cefamandole	T36.1X1	T36.1X2	T36.1X3	T36.1X4	T36.1X5	T36.1X6
Cefamycin antibiotic	T36.1X1	T36.1X2	T36.1X3	T36.1X4	T36.1X5	T36.1X6
Cefapirin	T36.1X1	T36.1X2	T36.1X3	T36.1X4	T36.1X5	T36.1X6
Cefatrizine	T36.1X1	T36.1X2	T36.1X3	T36.1X4	T36.1X5	T36.1X6
Cefazedone	T36.1X1	T36.1X2	T36.1X3	T36.1X4	T36.1X5	T36.1X6
Cefazolin	T36.1X1	T36.1X2	T36.1X3	T36.1X4	T36.1X5	T36.1X6
Cefbuperazone	T36.1X1	T36.1X2	T36.1X3	T36.1X4	T36.1X5	T36.1X6
Cefetamet	T36.1X1	T36.1X2	T36.1X3	T36.1X4	T36.1X5	T36.1X6
Cefixime	T36.1X1	T36.1X2	T36.1X3	T36.1X4	T36.1X5	T36.1X6
Cefmenoxime	T36.1X1	T36.1X2	T36.1X3	T36.1X4	T36.1X5	T36.1X6
Cefmetazole	T36.1X1	T36.1X2	T36.1X3	T36.1X4	T36.1X5	T36.1X6
Cefminox	T36.1X1	T36.1X2	T36.1X3	T36.1X4	T36.1X5	T36.1X6
Cefonicid	T36.1X1	T36.1X2	T36.1X3	T36.1X4	T36.1X5	T36.1X6
Cefoperazone	T36.1X1	T36.1X2	T36.1X3	T36.1X4	T36.1X5	T36.1X6
Ceforanide	T36.1X1	T36.1X2	T36.1X3	T36.1X4	T36.1X5	T36.1X6
Cefotaxime	T36.1X1	T36.1X2	T36.1X3	T36.1X4	T36.1X5	T36.1X6
Cefotetan	T36.1X1	T36.1X2	T36.1X3	T36.1X4	T36.1X5	T36.1X6
Cefotiam	T36.1X1	T36.1X2	T36.1X3	T36.1X4	T36.1X5	T36.1X6
Cefoxitin	T36.1X1	T36.1X2	T36.1X3	T36.1X4	T36.1X5	T36.1X6
Cefpimizole	T36.1X1	T36.1X2	T36.1X3	T36.1X4	T36.1X5	T36.1X6
Cefpiramide	T36.1X1	T36.1X2	T36.1X3	T36.1X4	T36.1X5	T36.1X6
Cefradine	T36.1X1	T36.1X2	T36.1X3	T36.1X4	T36.1X5	T36.1X6
Cefroxadine	T36.1X1	T36.1X2	T36.1X3	T36.1X4	T36.1X5	T36.1X6
Cefsulodin	T36.1X1	T36.1X2	T36.1X3	T36.1X4	T36.1X5	T36.1X6
Ceftazidime	T36.1X1	T36.1X2	T36.1X3	T36.1X4	T36.1X5	T36.1X6
Cefteram	T36.1X1	T36.1X2	T36.1X3	T36.1X4	T36.1X5	T36.1X6
Ceftezole	T36.1X1	T36.1X2	T36.1X3	T36.1X4	T36.1X5	T36.1X6
Ceftizoxime	T36.1X1	T36.1X2	T36.1X3	T36.1X4	T36.1X5	T36.1X6
Ceftriaxone	T36.1X1	T36.1X2	T36.1X3	T36.1X4	T36.1X5	T36.1X6
Cefuroxime	T36.1X1	T36.1X2	T36.1X3	T36.1X4	T36.1X5	T36.1X6
Cefuzonam	T36.1X1	T36.1X2	T36.1X3	T36.1X4	T36.1X5	T36.1X6
Celestone	T38.0X1	T38.0X2	T38.0X3	T38.0X4	T38.0X5	T38.0X6
- topical	T49.0X1	T49.0X2	T49.0X3	T49.0X4	T49.0X5	T49.0X6
Celiprolol	T44.7X1	T44.7X2	T44.7X3	T44.7X4	T44.7X5	T44.7X6
Cell stimulants and proliferants	T49.8X1	T49.8X2	T49.8X3	T49.8X4	T49.8X5	T49.8X6
Cellosolve	T52.91	T52.92	T52.93	T52.94	--	--
Cellulose						
- cathartic	T47.4X1	T47.4X2	T47.4X3	T47.4X4	T47.4X5	T47.4X6
- hydroxyethyl	T47.4X1	T47.4X2	T47.4X3	T47.4X4	T47.4X5	T47.4X6
- nitrates (topical)	T49.3X1	T49.3X2	T49.3X3	T49.3X4	T49.3X5	T49.3X6
- oxidized	T49.4X1	T49.4X2	T49.4X3	T49.4X4	T49.4X5	T49.4X6
Centipede (bite)	T63.411	T63.412	T63.413	T63.414	--	--
Central nervous system						
- depressants	T42.71	T42.72	T42.73	T42.74	T42.75	T42.76

Substance	Poisoning, Accidental (unintentional)	Poisoning, Intentional Self-harm	Poisoning, Assault	Poisoning, Undetermined	Adverse effect	Underdosing
- - anesthetic (general) NEC	T41.201	T41.202	T41.203	T41.204	T41.205	T41.206
- - - gases NEC	T41.0X1	T41.0X2	T41.0X3	T41.0X4	T41.0X5	T41.0X6
- - - intravenous	T41.1X1	T41.1X2	T41.1X3	T41.1X4	T41.1X5	T41.1X6
- - barbiturates	T42.3X1	T42.3X2	T42.3X3	T42.3X4	T42.3X5	T42.3X6
- - benzodiazepines	T42.4X1	T42.4X2	T42.4X3	T42.4X4	T42.4X5	T42.4X6
- - bromides	T42.6X1	T42.6X2	T42.6X3	T42.6X4	T42.6X5	T42.6X6
- - cannabis sativa	T40.7X1	T40.7X2	T40.7X3	T40.7X4	T40.7X5	T40.7X6
- - chloral hydrate	T42.6X1	T42.6X2	T42.6X3	T42.6X4	T42.6X5	T42.6X6
- - ethanol	T51.0X1	T51.0X2	T51.0X3	T51.0X4	--	--
- - hallucinogenics	T40.901	T40.902	T40.903	T40.904	T40.905	T40.906
- - hypnotics	T42.71	T42.72	T42.73	T42.74	T42.75	T42.76
- - - specified NEC	T42.6X1	T42.6X2	T42.6X3	T42.6X4	T42.6X5	T42.6X6
- - muscle relaxants	T42.8X1	T42.8X2	T42.8X3	T42.8X4	T42.8X5	T42.8X6
- - paraldehyde	T42.6X1	T42.6X2	T42.6X3	T42.6X4	T42.6X5	T42.6X6
- - sedatives; sedative-hypnotics	T42.71	T42.72	T42.73	T42.74	T42.75	T42.76
- - - mixed NEC	T42.6X1	T42.6X2	T42.6X3	T42.6X4	T42.6X5	T42.6X6
- - - specified NEC	T42.6X1	T42.6X2	T42.6X3	T42.6X4	T42.6X5	T42.6X6
- muscle-tone depressants	T42.8X1	T42.8X2	T42.8X3	T42.8X4	T42.8X5	T42.8X6
- stimulants	T43.601	T43.602	T43.603	T43.604	T43.605	T43.606
- - amphetamines	T43.621	T43.622	T43.623	T43.624	T43.625	T43.626
- - analeptics	T50.7X1	T50.7X2	T50.7X3	T50.7X4	T50.7X5	T50.7X6
- - antidepressants	T43.201	T43.202	T43.203	T43.204	T43.205	T43.206
- - opiate antagonists	T50.7X1	T50.7X2	T50.7X3	T50.7X4	T50.7X5	T50.7X6
- - specified NEC	T43.691	T43.692	T43.693	T43.694	T43.695	T43.696
Cephalexin	T36.1X1	T36.1X2	T36.1X3	T36.1X4	T36.1X5	T36.1X6
Cephaloglycin	T36.1X1	T36.1X2	T36.1X3	T36.1X4	T36.1X5	T36.1X6
Cephaloridine	T36.1X1	T36.1X2	T36.1X3	T36.1X4	T36.1X5	T36.1X6
Cephalosporins	T36.1X1	T36.1X2	T36.1X3	T36.1X4	T36.1X5	T36.1X6
- N (adicillin)	T36.0X1	T36.0X2	T36.0X3	T36.0X4	T36.0X5	T36.0X6
Cephalothin	T36.1X1	T36.1X2	T36.1X3	T36.1X4	T36.1X5	T36.1X6
Cephalotin	T36.1X1	T36.1X2	T36.1X3	T36.1X4	T36.1X5	T36.1X6
Cephradine	T36.1X1	T36.1X2	T36.1X3	T36.1X4	T36.1X5	T36.1X6
Cerbera (odallam)	T62.2X1	T62.2X2	T62.2X3	T62.2X4	--	--
Cerberin	T46.0X1	T46.0X2	T46.0X3	T46.0X4	T46.0X5	T46.0X6
Cerebral stimulants	T43.601	T43.602	T43.603	T43.604	T43.605	T43.606
- psychotherapeutic	T43.601	T43.602	T43.603	T43.604	T43.605	T43.606
- specified NEC	T43.691	T43.692	T43.693	T43.694	T43.695	T43.696
Cerium oxalate	T45.0X1	T45.0X2	T45.0X3	T45.0X4	T45.0X5	T45.0X6
Cerous oxalate	T45.0X1	T45.0X2	T45.0X3	T45.0X4	T45.0X5	T45.0X6
Ceruletide	T50.8X1	T50.8X2	T50.8X3	T50.8X4	T50.8X5	T50.8X6
Cetalkonium (chloride)	T49.0X1	T49.0X2	T49.0X3	T49.0X4	T49.0X5	T49.0X6
Cethexonium chloride	T49.0X1	T49.0X2	T49.0X3	T49.0X4	T49.0X5	T49.0X6
Cetiedil	T46.7X1	T46.7X2	T46.7X3	T46.7X4	T46.7X5	T46.7X6
Cetirizine	T45.0X1	T45.0X2	T45.0X3	T45.0X4	T45.0X5	T45.0X6
Cetomacrogol	T50.991	T50.992	T50.993	T50.994	T50.995	T50.996
Cetotiamine	T45.2X1	T45.2X2	T45.2X3	T45.2X4	T45.2X5	T45.2X6
Cetoxime	T45.0X1	T45.0X2	T45.0X3	T45.0X4	T45.0X5	T45.0X6
Cetraxate	T47.1X1	T47.1X2	T47.1X3	T47.1X4	T47.1X5	T47.1X6
Cetrimide	T49.0X1	T49.0X2	T49.0X3	T49.0X4	T49.0X5	T49.0X6
Cetrimonium (bromide)	T49.0X1	T49.0X2	T49.0X3	T49.0X4	T49.0X5	T49.0X6
Cetylpyridinium chloride	T49.0X1	T49.0X2	T49.0X3	T49.0X4	T49.0X5	T49.0X6
- ENT agent	T49.6X1	T49.6X2	T49.6X3	T49.6X4	T49.6X5	T49.6X6
- lozenges	T49.6X1	T49.6X2	T49.6X3	T49.6X4	T49.6X5	T49.6X6
Cevadilla—see Sabadilla						
Cevitamic acid	T45.2X1	T45.2X2	T45.2X3	T45.2X4	T45.2X5	T45.2X6
Chalk, precipitated	T47.1X1	T47.1X2	T47.1X3	T47.1X4	T47.1X5	T47.1X6
Chamomile	T49.0X1	T49.0X2	T49.0X3	T49.0X4	T49.0X5	T49.0X6
Ch'an su	T46.0X1	T46.0X2	T46.0X3	T46.0X4	T46.0X5	T46.0X6

Substance	Poisoning, Accidental (unintentional)	Poisoning, Intentional Self-harm	Poisoning, Assault	Poisoning, Undetermined	Adverse effect	Underdosing
Charcoal	T47.6X1	T47.6X2	T47.6X3	T47.6X4	T47.6X5	T47.6X6
- activated—see also Charcoal, medicinal	T47.6X1	T47.6X2	T47.6X3	T47.6X4	T47.6X5	T47.6X6
- fumes (Carbon monoxide)	T58.2X1	T58.2X2	T58.2X3	T58.2X4	--	--
- - industrial	T58.8X1	T58.8X2	T58.8X3	T58.8X4	--	--
- medicinal (activated)	T47.6X1	T47.6X2	T47.6X3	T47.6X4	T47.6X5	T47.6X6
- - antidiarrheal	T47.6X1	T47.6X2	T47.6X3	T47.6X4	T47.6X5	T47.6X6
- - poison control	T47.8X1	T47.8X2	T47.8X3	T47.8X4	T47.8X5	T47.8X6
- - specified use other than for diarrhea	T47.8X1	T47.8X2	T47.8X3	T47.8X4	T47.8X5	T47.8X6
- - topical	T49.8X1	T49.8X2	T49.8X3	T49.8X4	T49.8X5	T49.8X6
Chaulmosulfone	T37.1X1	T37.1X2	T37.1X3	T37.1X4	T37.1X5	T37.1X6
Chelating agent NEC	T50.6X1	T50.6X2	T50.6X3	T50.6X4	T50.6X5	T50.6X6
Chelidonium majus	T62.2X1	T62.2X2	T62.2X3	T62.2X4	--	--
Chemical substance NEC	T65.91	T65.92	T65.93	T65.94	--	--
Chenodeoxycholic acid	T47.5X1	T47.5X2	T47.5X3	T47.5X4	T47.5X5	T47.5X6
Chenodiol	T47.5X1	T47.5X2	T47.5X3	T47.5X4	T47.5X5	T47.5X6
Chenopodium	T37.4X1	T37.4X2	T37.4X3	T37.4X4	T37.4X5	T37.4X6
Cherry laurel	T62.2X1	T62.2X2	T62.2X3	T62.2X4	--	--
Chinidin (e)	T46.2X1	T46.2X2	T46.2X3	T46.2X4	T46.2X5	T46.2X6
Chiniofon	T37.8X1	T37.8X2	T37.8X3	T37.8X4	T37.8X5	T37.8X6
Chlophedianol	T48.3X1	T48.3X2	T48.3X3	T48.3X4	T48.3X5	T48.3X6
Chloral	T42.6X1	T42.6X2	T42.6X3	T42.6X4	T42.6X5	T42.6X6
- derivative	T42.6X1	T42.6X2	T42.6X3	T42.6X4	T42.6X5	T42.6X6
- hydrate	T42.6X1	T42.6X2	T42.6X3	T42.6X4	T42.6X5	T42.6X6
Chloralamide	T42.6X1	T42.6X2	T42.6X3	T42.6X4	T42.6X5	T42.6X6
Chloralodol	T42.6X1	T42.6X2	T42.6X3	T42.6X4	T42.6X5	T42.6X6
Chloralose	T60.4X1	T60.4X2	T60.4X3	T60.4X4	--	--
Chlorambucil	T45.1X1	T45.1X2	T45.1X3	T45.1X4	T45.1X5	T45.1X6
Chloramine	T57.8X1	T57.8X2	T57.8X3	T57.8X4	--	--
- T	T49.0X1	T49.0X2	T49.0X3	T49.0X4	T49.0X5	T49.0X6
- topical	T49.0X1	T49.0X2	T49.0X3	T49.0X4	T49.0X5	T49.0X6
Chloramphenicol	T36.2X1	T36.2X2	T36.2X3	T36.2X4	T36.2X5	T36.2X6
- ENT agent	T49.6X1	T49.6X2	T49.6X3	T49.6X4	T49.6X5	T49.6X6
- ophthalmic preparation	T49.5X1	T49.5X2	T49.5X3	T49.5X4	T49.5X5	T49.5X6
- topical NEC	T49.0X1	T49.0X2	T49.0X3	T49.0X4	T49.0X5	T49.0X6
Chlorate (potassium) (sodium) NEC	T60.3X1	T60.3X2	T60.3X3	T60.3X4	--	--
- herbicide	T60.3X1	T60.3X2	T60.3X3	T60.3X4	--	--
Chlorazanil	T50.2X1	T50.2X2	T50.2X3	T50.2X4	T50.2X5	T50.2X6
Chlorbenzene, chlorbenzol	T53.7X1	T53.7X2	T53.7X3	T53.7X4	--	--
Chlorbenzoxamine	T44.3X1	T44.3X2	T44.3X3	T44.3X4	T44.3X5	T44.3X6
Chlorbutol	T42.6X1	T42.6X2	T42.6X3	T42.6X4	T42.6X5	T42.6X6
Chlorcyclizine	T45.0X1	T45.0X2	T45.0X3	T45.0X4	T45.0X5	T45.0X6
Chlordan (e) (dust)	T60.1X1	T60.1X2	T60.1X3	T60.1X4	--	--
Chlordantoin	T49.0X1	T49.0X2	T49.0X3	T49.0X4	T49.0X5	T49.0X6
Chlordiazepoxide	T42.4X1	T42.4X2	T42.4X3	T42.4X4	T42.4X5	T42.4X6
Chlordiethyl benzamide	T49.3X1	T49.3X2	T49.3X3	T49.3X4	T49.3X5	T49.3X6
Chloresium	T49.8X1	T49.8X2	T49.8X3	T49.8X4	T49.8X5	T49.8X6
Chlorethiazol	T42.6X1	T42.6X2	T42.6X3	T42.6X4	T42.6X5	T42.6X6
Chlorethyl—see Ethyl chloride						
Chloretone	T42.6X1	T42.6X2	T42.6X3	T42.6X4	T42.6X5	T42.6X6
Chlorex	T53.6X1	T53.6X2	T53.6X3	T53.6X4	--	--
- insecticide	T60.1X1	T60.1X2	T60.1X3	T60.1X4	--	--
Chlorfenvinphos	T60.0X1	T60.0X2	T60.0X3	T60.0X4	--	--
Chlorhexadol	T42.6X1	T42.6X2	T42.6X3	T42.6X4	T42.6X5	T42.6X6
Chlorhexamide	T45.1X1	T45.1X2	T45.1X3	T45.1X4	T45.1X5	T45.1X6
Chlorhexidine	T49.0X1	T49.0X2	T49.0X3	T49.0X4	T49.0X5	T49.0X6
Chlorhydroxyquinolin	T49.0X1	T49.0X2	T49.0X3	T49.0X4	T49.0X5	T49.0X6
Chloride of lime (bleach)	T54.3X1	T54.3X2	T54.3X3	T54.3X4	--	--
Chlorimipramine	T43.011	T43.012	T43.013	T43.014	T43.015	T43.016
Chlorinated						

Substance	Poisoning, Accidental (unintentional)	Poisoning, Intentional Self-harm	Poisoning, Assault	Poisoning, Undetermined	Adverse effect	Underdosing
- camphene	T53.6X1	T53.6X2	T53.6X3	T53.6X4	--	--
- diphenyl	T53.7X1	T53.7X2	T53.7X3	T53.7X4	--	--
- hydrocarbons NEC	T53.91	T53.92	T53.93	T53.94	--	--
- - solvents	T53.91	T53.92	T53.93	T53.94	--	--
- lime (bleach)	T54.3X1	T54.3X2	T54.3X3	T54.3X4	--	--
- - and boric acid solution	T49.0X1	T49.0X2	T49.0X3	T49.0X4	T49.0X5	T49.0X6
- naphthalene (insecticide)	T60.1X1	T60.1X2	T60.1X3	T60.1X4	--	--
- - industrial (non-pesticide)	T53.7X1	T53.7X2	T53.7X3	T53.7X4	--	--
- pesticide NEC	T60.8X1	T60.8X2	T60.8X3	T60.8X4	--	--
- soda—see also sodium hypochlorite						
- - solution	T49.0X1	T49.0X2	T49.0X3	T49.0X4	T49.0X5	T49.0X6
Chlorine (fumes) (gas)	T59.4X1	T59.4X2	T59.4X3	T59.4X4	--	--
- bleach	T54.3X1	T54.3X2	T54.3X3	T54.3X4	--	--
- compound gas NEC	T59.4X1	T59.4X2	T59.4X3	T59.4X4	--	--
- disinfectant	T59.4X1	T59.4X2	T59.4X3	T59.4X4	--	--
- releasing agents NEC	T59.4X1	T59.4X2	T59.4X3	T59.4X4	--	--
Chlorisondamine chloride	T46.991	T46.992	T46.993	T46.994	T46.995	T46.996
Chlormadinone	T38.5X1	T38.5X2	T38.5X3	T38.5X4	T38.5X5	T38.5X6
Chlormephos	T60.0X1	T60.0X2	T60.0X3	T60.0X4	--	--
Chlormerodrin	T50.2X1	T50.2X2	T50.2X3	T50.2X4	T50.2X5	T50.2X6
Chlormethiazole	T42.6X1	T42.6X2	T42.6X3	T42.6X4	T42.6X5	T42.6X6
Chlormethine	T45.1X1	T45.1X2	T45.1X3	T45.1X4	T45.1X5	T45.1X6
Chlormethylenecycline	T36.4X1	T36.4X2	T36.4X3	T36.4X4	T36.4X5	T36.4X6
Chlormezanone	T42.6X1	T42.6X2	T42.6X3	T42.6X4	T42.6X5	T42.6X6
Chloroacetic acid	T60.3X1	T60.3X2	T60.3X3	T60.3X4	--	--
Chloroacetone	T59.3X1	T59.3X2	T59.3X3	T59.3X4	--	--
Chloroacetophenone	T59.3X1	T59.3X2	T59.3X3	T59.3X4	--	--
Chloroaniline	T53.7X1	T53.7X2	T53.7X3	T53.7X4	--	--
Chlorobenzene, chlorobenzol	T53.7X1	T53.7X2	T53.7X3	T53.7X4	--	--
Chlorobromomethane (fire extinguisher)	T53.6X1	T53.6X2	T53.6X3	T53.6X4	--	--
Chlorobutanol	T49.0X1	T49.0X2	T49.0X3	T49.0X4	T49.0X5	T49.0X6
Chlorocresol	T49.0X1	T49.0X2	T49.0X3	T49.0X4	T49.0X5	T49.0X6
Chlorodehydro-methyltestosterone	T38.7X1	T38.7X2	T38.7X3	T38.7X4	T38.7X5	T38.7X6
Chlorodinitrobenzene	T53.7X1	T53.7X2	T53.7X3	T53.7X4	--	--
- dust or vapor	T53.7X1	T53.7X2	T53.7X3	T53.7X4	--	--
Chlorodiphenyl	T53.7X1	T53.7X2	T53.7X3	T53.7X4	--	--
Chloroethane—see Ethyl chloride						
Chloroethylene	T53.6X1	T53.6X2	T53.6X3	T53.6X4	--	--
Chlorofluorocarbons	T53.5X1	T53.5X2	T53.5X3	T53.5X4	--	--
Chloroform (fumes) (vapor)	T53.1X1	T53.1X2	T53.1X3	T53.1X4	--	--
- anesthetic	T41.0X1	T41.0X2	T41.0X3	T41.0X4	T41.0X5	T41.0X6
- solvent	T53.1X1	T53.1X2	T53.1X3	T53.1X4	--	--
- water, concentrated	T41.0X1	T41.0X2	T41.0X3	T41.0X4	T41.0X5	T41.0X6
Chloroguanide	T37.2X1	T37.2X2	T37.2X3	T37.2X4	T37.2X5	T37.2X6
Chloromycetin	T36.2X1	T36.2X2	T36.2X3	T36.2X4	T36.2X5	T36.2X6
- ENT agent	T49.6X1	T49.6X2	T49.6X3	T49.6X4	T49.6X5	T49.6X6
- ophthalmic preparation	T49.5X1	T49.5X2	T49.5X3	T49.5X4	T49.5X5	T49.5X6
- otic solution	T49.6X1	T49.6X2	T49.6X3	T49.6X4	T49.6X5	T49.6X6
- topical NEC	T49.0X1	T49.0X2	T49.0X3	T49.0X4	T49.0X5	T49.0X6
Chloronitrobenzene	T53.7X1	T53.7X2	T53.7X3	T53.7X4	--	--
- dust or vapor	T53.7X1	T53.7X2	T53.7X3	T53.7X4	--	--
Chlorophacinone	T60.4X1	T60.4X2	T60.4X3	T60.4X4	--	--
Chlorophenol	T53.7X1	T53.7X2	T53.7X3	T53.7X4	--	--
Chlorophenothane	T60.1X1	T60.1X2	T60.1X3	T60.1X4	--	--
Chlorophyll	T50.991	T50.992	T50.993	T50.994	T50.995	T50.996
Chloropicrin (fumes)	T53.6X1	T53.6X2	T53.6X3	T53.6X4	--	--
- fumigant	T60.8X1	T60.8X2	T60.8X3	T60.8X4	--	--
- fungicide	T60.3X1	T60.3X2	T60.3X3	T60.3X4	--	--

Substance	Poisoning, Accidental (unintentional)	Poisoning, Intentional Self-harm	Poisoning, Assault	Poisoning, Undetermined	Adverse effect	Underdosing
- pesticide	T60.8X1	T60.8X2	T60.8X3	T60.8X4	--	--
Chloroprocaine	T41.3X1	T41.3X2	T41.3X3	T41.3X4	T41.3X5	T41.3X6
- infiltration (subcutaneous)	T41.3X1	T41.3X2	T41.3X3	T41.3X4	T41.3X5	T41.3X6
- nerve block (peripheral) (plexus)	T41.3X1	T41.3X2	T41.3X3	T41.3X4	T41.3X5	T41.3X6
- spinal	T41.3X1	T41.3X2	T41.3X3	T41.3X4	T41.3X5	T41.3X6
Chloroptic	T49.5X1	T49.5X2	T49.5X3	T49.5X4	T49.5X5	T49.5X6
Chloropurine	T45.1X1	T45.1X2	T45.1X3	T45.1X4	T45.1X5	T45.1X6
Chloropyramine	T45.0X1	T45.0X2	T45.0X3	T45.0X4	T45.0X5	T45.0X6
Chloropyrifos	T60.0X1	T60.0X2	T60.0X3	T60.0X4	--	--
Chloropyrilene	T45.0X1	T45.0X2	T45.0X3	T45.0X4	T45.0X5	T45.0X6
Chloroquine	T37.2X1	T37.2X2	T37.2X3	T37.2X4	T37.2X5	T37.2X6
Chlorothalonil	T60.3X1	T60.3X2	T60.3X3	T60.3X4	--	--
Chlorothen	T45.0X1	T45.0X2	T45.0X3	T45.0X4	T45.0X5	T45.0X6
Chlorothiazide	T50.2X1	T50.2X2	T50.2X3	T50.2X4	T50.2X5	T50.2X6
Chlorothymol	T49.4X1	T49.4X2	T49.4X3	T49.4X4	T49.4X5	T49.4X6
Chlorotrianisene	T38.5X1	T38.5X2	T38.5X3	T38.5X4	T38.5X5	T38.5X6
Chlorovinyldichloro-arsine, not in war	T57.0X1	T57.0X2	T57.0X3	T57.0X4	--	--
Chloroxine	T49.4X1	T49.4X2	T49.4X3	T49.4X4	T49.4X5	T49.4X6
Chloroxylenol	T49.0X1	T49.0X2	T49.0X3	T49.0X4	T49.0X5	T49.0X6
Chlorphenamine	T45.0X1	T45.0X2	T45.0X3	T45.0X4	T45.0X5	T45.0X6
Chlorphenesin	T42.8X1	T42.8X2	T42.8X3	T42.8X4	T42.8X5	T42.8X6
- topical (antifungal)	T49.0X1	T49.0X2	T49.0X3	T49.0X4	T49.0X5	T49.0X6
Chlorpheniramine	T45.0X1	T45.0X2	T45.0X3	T45.0X4	T45.0X5	T45.0X6
Chlorphenoxamine	T45.0X1	T45.0X2	T45.0X3	T45.0X4	T45.0X5	T45.0X6
Chlorphentermine	T50.5X1	T50.5X2	T50.5X3	T50.5X4	T50.5X5	T50.5X6
Chlorprocaine—see Chloroprocaine						
Chlorproguanil	T37.2X1	T37.2X2	T37.2X3	T37.2X4	T37.2X5	T37.2X6
Chlorpromazine	T43.3X1	T43.3X2	T43.3X3	T43.3X4	T43.3X5	T43.3X6
Chlorpropamide	T38.3X1	T38.3X2	T38.3X3	T38.3X4	T38.3X5	T38.3X6
Chlorprothixene	T43.4X1	T43.4X2	T43.4X3	T43.4X4	T43.4X5	T43.4X6
Chlorquinaldol	T49.0X1	T49.0X2	T49.0X3	T49.0X4	T49.0X5	T49.0X6
Chlorquinol	T49.0X1	T49.0X2	T49.0X3	T49.0X4	T49.0X5	T49.0X6
Chlortalidone	T50.2X1	T50.2X2	T50.2X3	T50.2X4	T50.2X5	T50.2X6
Chlortetracycline	T36.4X1	T36.4X2	T36.4X3	T36.4X4	T36.4X5	T36.4X6
Chlorthalidone	T50.2X1	T50.2X2	T50.2X3	T50.2X4	T50.2X5	T50.2X6
Chlorthiophos	T60.0X1	T60.0X2	T60.0X3	T60.0X4	--	--
Chlortrianisene	T38.5X1	T38.5X2	T38.5X3	T38.5X4	T38.5X5	T38.5X6
Chlor-Trimeton	T45.0X1	T45.0X2	T45.0X3	T45.0X4	T45.0X5	T45.0X6
Chlorthion	T60.0X1	T60.0X2	T60.0X3	T60.0X4	--	--
Chlorzoxazone	T42.8X1	T42.8X2	T42.8X3	T42.8X4	T42.8X5	T42.8X6
Choke damp	T59.7X1	T59.7X2	T59.7X3	T59.7X4	--	--
Cholagogues	T47.5X1	T47.5X2	T47.5X3	T47.5X4	T47.5X5	T47.5X6
Cholebrine	T50.8X1	T50.8X2	T50.8X3	T50.8X4	T50.8X5	T50.8X6
Cholecalciferol	T45.2X1	T45.2X2	T45.2X3	T45.2X4	T45.2X5	T45.2X6
Cholecystokinin	T50.8X1	T50.8X2	T50.8X3	T50.8X4	T50.8X5	T50.8X6
Cholera vaccine	T50.A91	T50.A92	T50.A93	T50.A94	T50.A95	T50.A96
Choleretic	T47.5X1	T47.5X2	T47.5X3	T47.5X4	T47.5X5	T47.5X6
Cholesterol-lowering agents	T46.6X1	T46.6X2	T46.6X3	T46.6X4	T46.6X5	T46.6X6
Cholestyramine (resin)	T46.6X1	T46.6X2	T46.6X3	T46.6X4	T46.6X5	T46.6X6
Cholic acid	T47.5X1	T47.5X2	T47.5X3	T47.5X4	T47.5X5	T47.5X6
Choline	T48.6X1	T48.6X2	T48.6X3	T48.6X4	T48.6X5	T48.6X6
- chloride	T50.991	T50.992	T50.993	T50.994	T50.995	T50.996
- dihydrogen citrate	T50.991	T50.992	T50.993	T50.994	T50.995	T50.996
- salicylate	T39.091	T39.092	T39.093	T39.094	T39.095	T39.096
- theophyllinate	T48.6X1	T48.6X2	T48.6X3	T48.6X4	T48.6X5	T48.6X6
Cholinergic (drug) NEC	T44.1X1	T44.1X2	T44.1X3	T44.1X4	T44.1X5	T44.1X6
- muscle tone enhancer	T44.1X1	T44.1X2	T44.1X3	T44.1X4	T44.1X5	T44.1X6
- organophosphorus	T44.0X1	T44.0X2	T44.0X3	T44.0X4	T44.0X5	T44.0X6
- - insecticide	T60.0X1	T60.0X2	T60.0X3	T60.0X4	--	--

Substance	Poisoning, Accidental (unintentional)	Poisoning, Intentional Self-harm	Poisoning, Assault	Poisoning, Undetermined	Adverse effect	Underdosing
- - nerve gas	T59.891	T59.892	T59.893	T59.894	--	--
- trimethyl ammonium propanediol	T44.1X1	T44.1X2	T44.1X3	T44.1X4	T44.1X5	T44.1X6
Cholinesterase reactivator	T50.6X1	T50.6X2	T50.6X3	T50.6X4	T50.6X5	T50.6X6
Cholografin	T50.8X1	T50.8X2	T50.8X3	T50.8X4	T50.8X5	T50.8X6
Chorionic gonadotropin	T38.891	T38.892	T38.893	T38.894	T38.895	T38.896
Chromate	T56.2X1	T56.2X2	T56.2X3	T56.2X4	--	--
- dust or mist	T56.2X1	T56.2X2	T56.2X3	T56.2X4	--	--
- lead—see also lead	T56.0X1	T56.0X2	T56.0X3	T56.0X4	--	--
- - paint	T56.0X1	T56.0X2	T56.0X3	T56.0X4	--	--
Chromic						
- acid	T56.2X1	T56.2X2	T56.2X3	T56.2X4	--	--
- - dust or mist	T56.2X1	T56.2X2	T56.2X3	T56.2X4	--	--
- phosphate 32P	T45.1X1	T45.1X2	T45.1X3	T45.1X4	T45.1X5	T45.1X6
Chromium	T56.2X1	T56.2X2	T56.2X3	T56.2X4	--	--
- compounds—see Chromate						
- sesquioxide	T50.8X1	T50.8X2	T50.8X3	T50.8X4	T50.8X5	T50.8X6
Chromomycin A3	T45.1X1	T45.1X2	T45.1X3	T45.1X4	T45.1X5	T45.1X6
Chromonar	T46.3X1	T46.3X2	T46.3X3	T46.3X4	T46.3X5	T46.3X6
Chromyl chloride	T56.2X1	T56.2X2	T56.2X3	T56.2X4	--	--
Chrysarobin	T49.4X1	T49.4X2	T49.4X3	T49.4X4	T49.4X5	T49.4X6
Chrysazin	T47.2X1	T47.2X2	T47.2X3	T47.2X4	T47.2X5	T47.2X6
Chymar	T45.3X1	T45.3X2	T45.3X3	T45.3X4	T45.3X5	T45.3X6
- ophthalmic preparation	T49.5X1	T49.5X2	T49.5X3	T49.5X4	T49.5X5	T49.5X6
Chymopapain	T45.3X1	T45.3X2	T45.3X3	T45.3X4	T45.3X5	T45.3X6
Chymotrypsin	T45.3X1	T45.3X2	T45.3X3	T45.3X4	T45.3X5	T45.3X6
- ophthalmic preparation	T49.5X1	T49.5X2	T49.5X3	T49.5X4	T49.5X5	T49.5X6
Cianidanol	T50.991	T50.992	T50.993	T50.994	T50.995	T50.996
Cianopramine	T43.011	T43.012	T43.013	T43.014	T43.015	T43.016
Cibenzoline	T46.2X1	T46.2X2	T46.2X3	T46.2X4	T46.2X5	T46.2X6
Ciclacillin	T36.0X1	T36.0X2	T36.0X3	T36.0X4	T36.0X5	T36.0X6
Ciclobarbital—see Hexobarbital						
Ciclonicate	T46.7X1	T46.7X2	T46.7X3	T46.7X4	T46.7X5	T46.7X6
Ciclopirox (olamine)	T49.0X1	T49.0X2	T49.0X3	T49.0X4	T49.0X5	T49.0X6
Ciclosporin	T45.1X1	T45.1X2	T45.1X3	T45.1X4	T45.1X5	T45.1X6
Cicuta maculata or virosa	T62.2X1	T62.2X2	T62.2X3	T62.2X4	--	--
Cicutoxin	T62.2X1	T62.2X2	T62.2X3	T62.2X4	--	--
Cigarette lighter fluid	T52.0X1	T52.0X2	T52.0X3	T52.0X4	--	--
Cigarettes (tobacco)	T65.221	T65.222	T65.223	T65.224	--	--
Ciguatoxin	T61.01	T61.02	T61.03	T61.04	--	--
Cilazapril	T46.4X1	T46.4X2	T46.4X3	T46.4X4	T46.4X5	T46.4X6
Cimetidine	T47.0X1	T47.0X2	T47.0X3	T47.0X4	T47.0X5	T47.0X6
Cimetropium bromide	T44.3X1	T44.3X2	T44.3X3	T44.3X4	T44.3X5	T44.3X6
Cinchocaine	T41.3X1	T41.3X2	T41.3X3	T41.3X4	T41.3X5	T41.3X6
- topical (surface)	T41.3X1	T41.3X2	T41.3X3	T41.3X4	T41.3X5	T41.3X6
Cinchona	T37.2X1	T37.2X2	T37.2X3	T37.2X4	T37.2X5	T37.2X6
Cinchonine alkaloids	T37.2X1	T37.2X2	T37.2X3	T37.2X4	T37.2X5	T37.2X6
Cinchophen	T50.4X1	T50.4X2	T50.4X3	T50.4X4	T50.4X5	T50.4X6
Cinepazide	T46.7X1	T46.7X2	T46.7X3	T46.7X4	T46.7X5	T46.7X6
Cinnamedrine	T48.5X1	T48.5X2	T48.5X3	T48.5X4	T48.5X5	T48.5X6
Cinnarizine	T45.0X1	T45.0X2	T45.0X3	T45.0X4	T45.0X5	T45.0X6
Cinoxacin	T37.8X1	T37.8X2	T37.8X3	T37.8X4	T37.8X5	T37.8X6
Ciprofibrate	T46.6X1	T46.6X2	T46.6X3	T46.6X4	T46.6X5	T46.6X6
Ciprofloxacin	T36.8X1	T36.8X2	T36.8X3	T36.8X4	T36.8X5	T36.8X6
Cisapride	T47.8X1	T47.8X2	T47.8X3	T47.8X4	T47.8X5	T47.8X6
Cisplatin	T45.1X1	T45.1X2	T45.1X3	T45.1X4	T45.1X5	T45.1X6
Citalopram	T43.221	T43.222	T43.223	T43.224	T43.225	T43.226
Citanest	T41.3X1	T41.3X2	T41.3X3	T41.3X4	T41.3X5	T41.3X6
- infiltration (subcutaneous)	T41.3X1	T41.3X2	T41.3X3	T41.3X4	T41.3X5	T41.3X6

Substance	Poisoning, Accidental (unintentional)	Poisoning, Intentional Self-harm	Poisoning, Assault	Poisoning, Undetermined	Adverse effect	Underdosing
- nerve block (peripheral) (plexus)	T41.3X1	T41.3X2	T41.3X3	T41.3X4	T41.3X5	T41.3X6
Citric acid	T47.5X1	T47.5X2	T47.5X3	T47.5X4	T47.5X5	T47.5X6
Citrovorum (factor)	T45.8X1	T45.8X2	T45.8X3	T45.8X4	T45.8X5	T45.8X6
Claviceps purpurea	T62.2X1	T62.2X2	T62.2X3	T62.2X4	--	--
Clavulanic acid	T36.1X1	T36.1X2	T36.1X3	T36.1X4	T36.1X5	T36.1X6
Cleaner, cleansing agent, type not specified	T65.891	T65.892	T65.893	T65.894	--	--
- of paint or varnish	T52.91	T52.92	T52.93	T52.94	--	--
- specified type NEC	T65.891	T65.892	T65.893	T65.894	--	--
Clebopride	T47.8X1	T47.8X2	T47.8X3	T47.8X4	T47.8X5	T47.8X6
Clefamide	T37.3X1	T37.3X2	T37.3X3	T37.3X4	T37.3X5	T37.3X6
Clemastine	T45.0X1	T45.0X2	T45.0X3	T45.0X4	T45.0X5	T45.0X6
Clematis vitalba	T62.2X1	T62.2X2	T62.2X3	T62.2X4	--	--
Clemizole	T45.0X1	T45.0X2	T45.0X3	T45.0X4	T45.0X5	T45.0X6
- penicillin	T36.0X1	T36.0X2	T36.0X3	T36.0X4	T36.0X5	T36.0X6
Clenbuterol	T48.6X1	T48.6X2	T48.6X3	T48.6X4	T48.6X5	T48.6X6
Clidinium bromide	T44.3X1	T44.3X2	T44.3X3	T44.3X4	T44.3X5	T44.3X6
Clindamycin	T36.8X1	T36.8X2	T36.8X3	T36.8X4	T36.8X5	T36.8X6
Clinofibrate	T46.6X1	T46.6X2	T46.6X3	T46.6X4	T46.6X5	T46.6X6
Clioquinol	T37.8X1	T37.8X2	T37.8X3	T37.8X4	T37.8X5	T37.8X6
Cliradon	T40.2X1	T40.2X2	T40.2X3	T40.2X4	--	--
Clobazam	T42.4X1	T42.4X2	T42.4X3	T42.4X4	T42.4X5	T42.4X6
Clobenzorex	T50.5X1	T50.5X2	T50.5X3	T50.5X4	T50.5X5	T50.5X6
Clobetasol	T49.0X1	T49.0X2	T49.0X3	T49.0X4	T49.0X5	T49.0X6
Clobetasone	T49.0X1	T49.0X2	T49.0X3	T49.0X4	T49.0X5	T49.0X6
Clobutinol	T48.3X1	T48.3X2	T48.3X3	T48.3X4	T48.3X5	T48.3X6
Clocortolone	T38.0X1	T38.0X2	T38.0X3	T38.0X4	T38.0X5	T38.0X6
Clodantoin	T49.0X1	T49.0X2	T49.0X3	T49.0X4	T49.0X5	T49.0X6
Clodronic acid	T50.991	T50.992	T50.993	T50.994	T50.995	T50.996
Clofazimine	T37.1X1	T37.1X2	T37.1X3	T37.1X4	T37.1X5	T37.1X6
Clofedanol	T48.3X1	T48.3X2	T48.3X3	T48.3X4	T48.3X5	T48.3X6
Clofenamide	T50.2X1	T50.2X2	T50.2X3	T50.2X4	T50.2X5	T50.2X6
Clofenotane	T49.0X1	T49.0X2	T49.0X3	T49.0X4	T49.0X5	T49.0X6
Clofezone	T39.2X1	T39.2X2	T39.2X3	T39.2X4	T39.2X5	T39.2X6
Clofibrate	T46.6X1	T46.6X2	T46.6X3	T46.6X4	T46.6X5	T46.6X6
Clofibride	T46.6X1	T46.6X2	T46.6X3	T46.6X4	T46.6X5	T46.6X6
Cloforex	T50.5X1	T50.5X2	T50.5X3	T50.5X4	T50.5X5	T50.5X6
Clomethiazole	T42.6X1	T42.6X2	T42.6X3	T42.6X4	T42.6X5	T42.6X6
Clometocillin	T36.0X1	T36.0X2	T36.0X3	T36.0X4	T36.0X5	T36.0X6
Clomifene	T38.5X1	T38.5X2	T38.5X3	T38.5X4	T38.5X5	T38.5X6
Clomiphene	T38.5X1	T38.5X2	T38.5X3	T38.5X4	T38.5X5	T38.5X6
Clomipramine	T43.011	T43.012	T43.013	T43.014	T43.015	T43.016
Clomocycline	T36.4X1	T36.4X2	T36.4X3	T36.4X4	T36.4X5	T36.4X6
Clonazepam	T42.4X1	T42.4X2	T42.4X3	T42.4X4	T42.4X5	T42.4X6
Clonidine	T46.5X1	T46.5X2	T46.5X3	T46.5X4	T46.5X5	T46.5X6
Clonixin	T39.8X1	T39.8X2	T39.8X3	T39.8X4	T39.8X5	T39.8X6
Clopamide	T50.2X1	T50.2X2	T50.2X3	T50.2X4	T50.2X5	T50.2X6
Clopenthixol	T43.4X1	T43.4X2	T43.4X3	T43.4X4	T43.4X5	T43.4X6
Cloperastine	T48.3X1	T48.3X2	T48.3X3	T48.3X4	T48.3X5	T48.3X6
Clophedianol	T48.3X1	T48.3X2	T48.3X3	T48.3X4	T48.3X5	T48.3X6
Cloponone	T36.2X1	T36.2X2	T36.2X3	T36.2X4	T36.2X5	T36.2X6
Cloprednol	T38.0X1	T38.0X2	T38.0X3	T38.0X4	T38.0X5	T38.0X6
Cloral betaine	T42.6X1	T42.6X2	T42.6X3	T42.6X4	T42.6X5	T42.6X6
Cloramfenicol	T36.2X1	T36.2X2	T36.2X3	T36.2X4	T36.2X5	T36.2X6
Clorazepate (dipotassium)	T42.4X1	T42.4X2	T42.4X3	T42.4X4	T42.4X5	T42.4X6
Clorexolone	T50.2X1	T50.2X2	T50.2X3	T50.2X4	T50.2X5	T50.2X6
Clorfenamine	T45.0X1	T45.0X2	T45.0X3	T45.0X4	T45.0X5	T45.0X6
Clorgiline	T43.1X1	T43.1X2	T43.1X3	T43.1X4	T43.1X5	T43.1X6
Clorotepine	T44.3X1	T44.3X2	T44.3X3	T44.3X4	T44.3X5	T44.3X6
Clorox (bleach)	T54.91	T54.92	T54.93	T54.94	--	--

Substance	Poisoning, Accidental (unintentional)	Poisoning, Intentional Self-harm	Poisoning, Assault	Poisoning, Undetermined	Adverse effect	Underdosing
Clorprenaline	T48.6X1	T48.6X2	T48.6X3	T48.6X4	T48.6X5	T48.6X6
Clortermine	T50.5X1	T50.5X2	T50.5X3	T50.5X4	T50.5X5	T50.5X6
Clotiapine	T43.591	T43.592	T43.593	T43.594	T43.595	T43.596
Clotiazepam	T42.4X1	T42.4X2	T42.4X3	T42.4X4	T42.4X5	T42.4X6
Clotibric acid	T46.6X1	T46.6X2	T46.6X3	T46.6X4	T46.6X5	T46.6X6
Clotrimazole	T49.0X1	T49.0X2	T49.0X3	T49.0X4	T49.0X5	T49.0X6
Cloxacillin	T36.0X1	T36.0X2	T36.0X3	T36.0X4	T36.0X5	T36.0X6
Cloxazolam	T42.4X1	T42.4X2	T42.4X3	T42.4X4	T42.4X5	T42.4X6
Cloxiquine	T49.0X1	T49.0X2	T49.0X3	T49.0X4	T49.0X5	T49.0X6
Clozapine	T42.4X1	T42.4X2	T42.4X3	T42.4X4	T42.4X5	T42.4X6
Coagulant NEC	T45.7X1	T45.7X2	T45.7X3	T45.7X4	T45.7X5	T45.7X6
Coal (carbon monoxide from) —see also Carbon, monoxide, coal	T58.2X1	T58.2X2	T58.2X3	T58.2X4	--	--
- oil—see Kerosene						
- tar	T49.1X1	T49.1X2	T49.1X3	T49.1X4	T49.1X5	T49.1X6
- - fumes	T59.891	T59.892	T59.893	T59.894	--	--
- - - medicinal (ointment)	T49.4X1	T49.4X2	T49.4X3	T49.4X4	T49.4X5	T49.4X6
- - - - analgesics NEC	T39.2X1	T39.2X2	T39.2X3	T39.2X4	T39.2X5	T39.2X6
- - naphtha (solvent)	T52.0X1	T52.0X2	T52.0X3	T52.0X4	--	--
Cobalamine	T45.2X1	T45.2X2	T45.2X3	T45.2X4	T45.2X5	T45.2X6
Cobalt (nonmedicinal) (fumes) (industrial)	T56.891	T56.892	T56.893	T56.894	--	--
- medicinal (trace) (chloride)	T45.8X1	T45.8X2	T45.8X3	T45.8X4	T45.8X5	T45.8X6
Cobra (venom)	T63.041	T63.042	T63.043	T63.044	--	--
Coca (leaf)	T40.5X1	T40.5X2	T40.5X3	T40.5X4	T40.5X5	T40.5X6
Cocaine	T40.5X1	T40.5X2	T40.5X3	T40.5X4	T40.5X5	T40.5X6
- topical anesthetic	T41.3X1	T41.3X2	T41.3X3	T41.3X4	T41.3X5	T41.3X6
Cocarboxylase	T45.3X1	T45.3X2	T45.3X3	T45.3X4	T45.3X5	T45.3X6
Coccidioidin	T50.8X1	T50.8X2	T50.8X3	T50.8X4	T50.8X5	T50.8X6
Cocculus indicus	T62.1X1	T62.1X2	T62.1X3	T62.1X4	--	--
Cochineal	T65.6X1	T65.6X2	T65.6X3	T65.6X4	--	--
- medicinal products	T50.991	T50.992	T50.993	T50.994	T50.995	T50.996
Codeine	T40.2X1	T40.2X2	T40.2X3	T40.2X4	T40.2X5	T40.2X6
Cod-liver oil	T45.2X1	T45.2X2	T45.2X3	T45.2X4	T45.2X5	T45.2X6
Coenzyme A	T50.991	T50.992	T50.993	T50.994	T50.995	T50.996
Coffee	T62.8X1	T62.8X2	T62.8X3	T62.8X4	--	--
Cogalactoiso-merase	T50.991	T50.992	T50.993	T50.994	T50.995	T50.996
Cogentin	T44.3X1	T44.3X2	T44.3X3	T44.3X4	T44.3X5	T44.3X6
Coke fumes or gas (carbon monoxide)	T58.2X1	T58.2X2	T58.2X3	T58.2X4	--	--
- industrial use	T58.8X1	T58.8X2	T58.8X3	T58.8X4	--	--
Colace	T47.4X1	T47.4X2	T47.4X3	T47.4X4	T47.4X5	T47.4X6
Colaspase	T45.1X1	T45.1X2	T45.1X3	T45.1X4	T45.1X5	T45.1X6
Colchicine	T50.4X1	T50.4X2	T50.4X3	T50.4X4	T50.4X5	T50.4X6
Colchicum	T62.2X1	T62.2X2	T62.2X3	T62.2X4	--	--
Cold cream	T49.3X1	T49.3X2	T49.3X3	T49.3X4	T49.3X5	T49.3X6
Colecalciferol	T45.2X1	T45.2X2	T45.2X3	T45.2X4	T45.2X5	T45.2X6
Colestipol	T46.6X1	T46.6X2	T46.6X3	T46.6X4	T46.6X5	T46.6X6
Colestyramine	T46.6X1	T46.6X2	T46.6X3	T46.6X4	T46.6X5	T46.6X6
Colimycin	T36.8X1	T36.8X2	T36.8X3	T36.8X4	T36.8X5	T36.8X6
Colistimethate	T36.8X1	T36.8X2	T36.8X3	T36.8X4	T36.8X5	T36.8X6
Colistin	T36.8X1	T36.8X2	T36.8X3	T36.8X4	T36.8X5	T36.8X6
- sulfate (eye preparation)	T49.5X1	T49.5X2	T49.5X3	T49.5X4	T49.5X5	T49.5X6
Collagen	T50.991	T50.992	T50.993	T50.994	T50.995	T50.996
Collagenase	T49.4X1	T49.4X2	T49.4X3	T49.4X4	T49.4X5	T49.4X6
Collodion	T49.3X1	T49.3X2	T49.3X3	T49.3X4	T49.3X5	T49.3X6
Colocynth	T47.2X1	T47.2X2	T47.2X3	T47.2X4	T47.2X5	T47.2X6
Colophony adhesive	T49.3X1	T49.3X2	T49.3X3	T49.3X4	T49.3X5	T49.3X6
Colorant—see also Dye	T50.991	T50.992	T50.993	T50.994	T50.995	T50.996
Coloring matter—see Dye (s)						
Combustion gas (after combustion) —see						

Substance	Poisoning, Accidental (unintentional)	Poisoning, Intentional Self-harm	Poisoning, Assault	Poisoning, Undetermined	Adverse effect	Underdosing
Carbon, monoxide						
- prior to combustion	T59.891	T59.892	T59.893	T59.894	--	--
Compazine	T43.3X1	T43.3X2	T43.3X3	T43.3X4	T43.3X5	T43.3X6
Compound						
- 42 (warfarin)	T60.4X1	T60.4X2	T60.4X3	T60.4X4	--	--
- 269 (endrin)	T60.1X1	T60.1X2	T60.1X3	T60.1X4	--	--
- 497 (dieldrin)	T60.1X1	T60.1X2	T60.1X3	T60.1X4	--	--
- 1080 (sodium fluoroacetate)	T60.4X1	T60.4X2	T60.4X3	T60.4X4	--	--
- 3422 (parathion)	T60.0X1	T60.0X2	T60.0X3	T60.0X4	--	--
- 3911 (phorate)	T60.0X1	T60.0X2	T60.0X3	T60.0X4	--	--
- 3956 (toxaphene)	T60.1X1	T60.1X2	T60.1X3	T60.1X4	--	--
- 4049 (malathion)	T60.0X1	T60.0X2	T60.0X3	T60.0X4	--	--
- 4069 (malathion)	T60.0X1	T60.0X2	T60.0X3	T60.0X4	--	--
- 4124 (dicapthon)	T60.0X1	T60.0X2	T60.0X3	T60.0X4	--	--
- E (cortisone)	T38.0X1	T38.0X2	T38.0X3	T38.0X4	T38.0X5	T38.0X6
- F (hydrocortisone)	T38.0X1	T38.0X2	T38.0X3	T38.0X4	T38.0X5	T38.0X6
Congener, anabolic	T38.7X1	T38.7X2	T38.7X3	T38.7X4	T38.7X5	T38.7X6
Congo red	T50.8X1	T50.8X2	T50.8X3	T50.8X4	T50.8X5	T50.8X6
Coniine, conine	T62.2X1	T62.2X2	T62.2X3	T62.2X4	--	--
Conium (maculatum)	T62.2X1	T62.2X2	T62.2X3	T62.2X4	--	--
Conjugated estrogenic substances	T38.5X1	T38.5X2	T38.5X3	T38.5X4	T38.5X5	T38.5X6
Contac	T48.5X1	T48.5X2	T48.5X3	T48.5X4	T48.5X5	T48.5X6
Contact lens solution	T49.5X1	T49.5X2	T49.5X3	T49.5X4	T49.5X5	T49.5X6
Contraceptive (oral)	T38.4X1	T38.4X2	T38.4X3	T38.4X4	T38.4X5	T38.4X6
- vaginal	T49.8X1	T49.8X2	T49.8X3	T49.8X4	T49.8X5	T49.8X6
Contrast medium, radiography	T50.8X1	T50.8X2	T50.8X3	T50.8X4	T50.8X5	T50.8X6
Convallaria glycosides	T46.0X1	T46.0X2	T46.0X3	T46.0X4	T46.0X5	T46.0X6
Convallaria majalis	T62.2X1	T62.2X2	T62.2X3	T62.2X4	--	--
- berry	T62.1X1	T62.1X2	T62.1X3	T62.1X4	--	--
Copper (dust) (fumes) (nonmedicinal) NEC	T56.4X1	T56.4X2	T56.4X3	T56.4X4	--	--
- arsenate, arsenite	T57.0X1	T57.0X2	T57.0X3	T57.0X4	--	--
- - insecticide	T60.2X1	T60.2X2	T60.2X3	T60.2X4	--	--
- emetic	T47.7X1	T47.7X2	T47.7X3	T47.7X4	T47.7X5	T47.7X6
- fungicide	T60.3X1	T60.3X2	T60.3X3	T60.3X4	--	--
- gluconate	T49.0X1	T49.0X2	T49.0X3	T49.0X4	T49.0X5	T49.0X6
- insecticide	T60.2X1	T60.2X2	T60.2X3	T60.2X4	--	--
- medicinal (trace)	T45.8X1	T45.8X2	T45.8X3	T45.8X4	T45.8X5	T45.8X6
- oleate	T49.0X1	T49.0X2	T49.0X3	T49.0X4	T49.0X5	T49.0X6
- sulfate	T56.4X1	T56.4X2	T56.4X3	T56.4X4	--	--
- - cupric	T56.4X1	T56.4X2	T56.4X3	T56.4X4	--	--
- - - fungicide	T60.3X1	T60.3X2	T60.3X3	T60.3X4	--	--
- - - medicinal						
- - - - ear	T49.6X1	T49.6X2	T49.6X3	T49.6X4	T49.6X5	T49.6X6
- - - - emetic	T47.7X1	T47.7X2	T47.7X3	T47.7X4	T47.7X5	T47.7X6
- - - - eye	T49.5X1	T49.5X2	T49.5X3	T49.5X4	T49.5X5	T49.5X6
- - cuprous	T56.4X1	T56.4X2	T56.4X3	T56.4X4	--	--
- - fungicide	T60.3X1	T60.3X2	T60.3X3	T60.3X4	--	--
- - medicinal						
- - - ear	T49.6X1	T49.6X2	T49.6X3	T49.6X4	T49.6X5	T49.6X6
- - - emetic	T47.7X1	T47.7X2	T47.7X3	T47.7X4	T47.7X5	T47.7X6
- - - eye	T49.5X1	T49.5X2	T49.5X3	T49.5X4	T49.5X5	T49.5X6
Copperhead snake (bite) (venom)	T63.061	T63.062	T63.063	T63.064	--	--
Coral (sting)	T63.691	T63.692	T63.693	T63.694	--	--
- snake (bite) (venom)	T63.021	T63.022	T63.023	T63.024	--	--
Corbadrine	T49.6X1	T49.6X2	T49.6X3	T49.6X4	T49.6X5	T49.6X6
Cordite	T65.891	T65.892	T65.893	T65.894	--	--
- vapor	T59.891	T59.892	T59.893	T59.894	--	--
Cordran	T49.0X1	T49.0X2	T49.0X3	T49.0X4	T49.0X5	T49.0X6
Corn cures	T49.4X1	T49.4X2	T49.4X3	T49.4X4	T49.4X5	T49.4X6

Substance	Poisoning, Accidental (unintentional)	Poisoning, Intentional Self-harm	Poisoning, Assault	Poisoning, Undetermined	Adverse effect	Underdosing
Corn starch	T49.3X1	T49.3X2	T49.3X3	T49.3X4	T49.3X5	T49.3X6
Cornhusker's lotion	T49.3X1	T49.3X2	T49.3X3	T49.3X4	T49.3X5	T49.3X6
Coronary vasodilator NEC	T46.3X1	T46.3X2	T46.3X3	T46.3X4	T46.3X5	T46.3X6
Corrosive NEC	T54.91	T54.92	T54.93	T54.94	--	--
- acid NEC	T54.2X1	T54.2X2	T54.2X3	T54.2X4	--	--
- aromatics	T54.1X1	T54.1X2	T54.1X3	T54.1X4	--	--
- - disinfectant	T54.1X1	T54.1X2	T54.1X3	T54.1X4	--	--
- fumes NEC	T54.91	T54.92	T54.93	T54.94	--	--
- specified NEC	T54.91	T54.92	T54.93	T54.94	--	--
- sublimate	T56.1X1	T56.1X2	T56.1X3	T56.1X4	--	--
Cortate	T38.0X1	T38.0X2	T38.0X3	T38.0X4	T38.0X5	T38.0X6
Cort-Dome	T38.0X1	T38.0X2	T38.0X3	T38.0X4	T38.0X5	T38.0X6
- ENT agent	T49.6X1	T49.6X2	T49.6X3	T49.6X4	T49.6X5	T49.6X6
- ophthalmic preparation	T49.5X1	T49.5X2	T49.5X3	T49.5X4	T49.5X5	T49.5X6
- topical NEC	T49.0X1	T49.0X2	T49.0X3	T49.0X4	T49.0X5	T49.0X6
Cortef	T38.0X1	T38.0X2	T38.0X3	T38.0X4	T38.0X5	T38.0X6
- ENT agent	T49.6X1	T49.6X2	T49.6X3	T49.6X4	T49.6X5	T49.6X6
- ophthalmic preparation	T49.5X1	T49.5X2	T49.5X3	T49.5X4	T49.5X5	T49.5X6
- topical NEC	T49.0X1	T49.0X2	T49.0X3	T49.0X4	T49.0X5	T49.0X6
Corticosteroid	T38.0X1	T38.0X2	T38.0X3	T38.0X4	T38.0X5	T38.0X6
- ENT agent	T49.6X1	T49.6X2	T49.6X3	T49.6X4	T49.6X5	T49.6X6
- mineral	T50.0X1	T50.0X2	T50.0X3	T50.0X4	T50.0X5	T50.0X6
- ophthalmic	T49.5X1	T49.5X2	T49.5X3	T49.5X4	T49.5X5	T49.5X6
- topical NEC	T49.0X1	T49.0X2	T49.0X3	T49.0X4	T49.0X5	T49.0X6
Corticotropin	T38.811	T38.812	T38.813	T38.814	T38.815	T38.816
Cortisol	T49.0X1	T49.0X2	T49.0X3	T49.0X4	T49.0X5	T49.0X6
- ENT agent	T49.6X1	T49.6X2	T49.6X3	T49.6X4	T49.6X5	T49.6X6
- ophthalmic preparation	T49.5X1	T49.5X2	T49.5X3	T49.5X4	T49.5X5	T49.5X6
- topical NEC	T49.0X1	T49.0X2	T49.0X3	T49.0X4	T49.0X5	T49.0X6
Cortisone (acetate)	T38.0X1	T38.0X2	T38.0X3	T38.0X4	T38.0X5	T38.0X6
- ENT agent	T49.6X1	T49.6X2	T49.6X3	T49.6X4	T49.6X5	T49.6X6
- ophthalmic preparation	T49.5X1	T49.5X2	T49.5X3	T49.5X4	T49.5X5	T49.5X6
- topical NEC	T49.0X1	T49.0X2	T49.0X3	T49.0X4	T49.0X5	T49.0X6
Cortivazol	T38.0X1	T38.0X2	T38.0X3	T38.0X4	T38.0X5	T38.0X6
Cortogen	T38.0X1	T38.0X2	T38.0X3	T38.0X4	T38.0X5	T38.0X6
- ENT agent	T49.6X1	T49.6X2	T49.6X3	T49.6X4	T49.6X5	T49.6X6
- ophthalmic preparation	T49.5X1	T49.5X2	T49.5X3	T49.5X4	T49.5X5	T49.5X6
Cortone	T38.0X1	T38.0X2	T38.0X3	T38.0X4	T38.0X5	T38.0X6
- ENT agent	T49.6X1	T49.6X2	T49.6X3	T49.6X4	T49.6X5	T49.6X6
- ophthalmic preparation	T49.5X1	T49.5X2	T49.5X3	T49.5X4	T49.5X5	T49.5X6
Cortril	T38.0X1	T38.0X2	T38.0X3	T38.0X4	T38.0X5	T38.0X6
- ENT agent	T49.6X1	T49.6X2	T49.6X3	T49.6X4	T49.6X5	T49.6X6
- ophthalmic preparation	T49.5X1	T49.5X2	T49.5X3	T49.5X4	T49.5X5	T49.5X6
- topical NEC	T49.0X1	T49.0X2	T49.0X3	T49.0X4	T49.0X5	T49.0X6
Corynebacterium parvum	T45.1X1	T45.1X2	T45.1X3	T45.1X4	T45.1X5	T45.1X6
Cosmetic preparation	T49.8X1	T49.8X2	T49.8X3	T49.8X4	T49.8X5	T49.8X6
Cosmetics	T49.8X1	T49.8X2	T49.8X3	T49.8X4	T49.8X5	T49.8X6
Cosyntropin	T38.811	T38.812	T38.813	T38.814	T38.815	T38.816
Cotarnine	T45.7X1	T45.7X2	T45.7X3	T45.7X4	T45.7X5	T45.7X6
Co-trimoxazole	T36.8X1	T36.8X2	T36.8X3	T36.8X4	T36.8X5	T36.8X6
Cottonseed oil	T49.3X1	T49.3X2	T49.3X3	T49.3X4	T49.3X5	T49.3X6
Cough mixture (syrup)	T48.4X1	T48.4X2	T48.4X3	T48.4X4	T48.4X5	T48.4X6
- containing opiates	T40.2X1	T40.2X2	T40.2X3	T40.2X4	T40.2X5	T40.2X6
- expectorants	T48.4X1	T48.4X2	T48.4X3	T48.4X4	T48.4X5	T48.4X6
Coumadin	T45.511	T45.512	T45.513	T45.514	T45.515	T45.516
- rodenticide	T60.4X1	T60.4X2	T60.4X3	T60.4X4	--	--
Coumaphos	T60.0X1	T60.0X2	T60.0X3	T60.0X4	--	--
Coumarin	T45.511	T45.512	T45.513	T45.514	T45.515	T45.516

Substance	Poisoning, Accidental (unintentional)	Poisoning, Intentional Self-harm	Poisoning, Assault	Poisoning, Undetermined	Adverse effect	Underdosing
Coumetarol	T45.511	T45.512	T45.513	T45.514	T45.515	T45.516
Cowbane	T62.2X1	T62.2X2	T62.2X3	T62.2X4	--	--
Cozyme	T45.2X1	T45.2X2	T45.2X3	T45.2X4	T45.2X5	T45.2X6
Crack	T40.5X1	T40.5X2	T40.5X3	T40.5X4	--	--
Crataegus extract	T46.0X1	T46.0X2	T46.0X3	T46.0X4	T46.0X5	T46.0X6
Creolin	T54.1X1	T54.1X2	T54.1X3	T54.1X4	--	--
- disinfectant	T54.1X1	T54.1X2	T54.1X3	T54.1X4	--	--
Creosol (compound)	T49.0X1	T49.0X2	T49.0X3	T49.0X4	T49.0X5	T49.0X6
Creosote (coal tar) (beechwood)	T49.0X1	T49.0X2	T49.0X3	T49.0X4	T49.0X5	T49.0X6
- medicinal (expectorant)	T48.4X1	T48.4X2	T48.4X3	T48.4X4	T48.4X5	T48.4X6
- syrup	T48.4X1	T48.4X2	T48.4X3	T48.4X4	T48.4X5	T48.4X6
Cresol (s)	T49.0X1	T49.0X2	T49.0X3	T49.0X4	T49.0X5	T49.0X6
- and soap solution	T49.0X1	T49.0X2	T49.0X3	T49.0X4	T49.0X5	T49.0X6
Cresyl acetate	T49.0X1	T49.0X2	T49.0X3	T49.0X4	T49.0X5	T49.0X6
Cresylic acid	T49.0X1	T49.0X2	T49.0X3	T49.0X4	T49.0X5	T49.0X6
Crimidine	T60.4X1	T60.4X2	T60.4X3	T60.4X4	--	--
Croconazole	T37.8X1	T37.8X2	T37.8X3	T37.8X4	T37.8X5	T37.8X6
Cromoglicic acid	T48.6X1	T48.6X2	T48.6X3	T48.6X4	T48.6X5	T48.6X6
Cromolyn	T48.6X1	T48.6X2	T48.6X3	T48.6X4	T48.6X5	T48.6X6
Cromonar	T46.3X1	T46.3X2	T46.3X3	T46.3X4	T46.3X5	T46.3X6
Cropropamide	T39.8X1	T39.8X2	T39.8X3	T39.8X4	T39.8X5	T39.8X6
- with crotethamide	T50.7X1	T50.7X2	T50.7X3	T50.7X4	T50.7X5	T50.7X6
Crotamiton	T49.0X1	T49.0X2	T49.0X3	T49.0X4	T49.0X5	T49.0X6
Crotethamide	T39.8X1	T39.8X2	T39.8X3	T39.8X4	T39.8X5	T39.8X6
- with cropropamide	T50.7X1	T50.7X2	T50.7X3	T50.7X4	T50.7X5	T50.7X6
Croton (oil)	T47.2X1	T47.2X2	T47.2X3	T47.2X4	T47.2X5	T47.2X6
- chloral	T42.6X1	T42.6X2	T42.6X3	T42.6X4	T42.6X5	T42.6X6
Crude oil	T52.0X1	T52.0X2	T52.0X3	T52.0X4	--	--
Cryogenine	T39.8X1	T39.8X2	T39.8X3	T39.8X4	T39.8X5	T39.8X6
Cryolite (vapor)	T60.1X1	T60.1X2	T60.1X3	T60.1X4	--	--
- insecticide	T60.1X1	T60.1X2	T60.1X3	T60.1X4	--	--
Cryptenamine (tannates)	T46.5X1	T46.5X2	T46.5X3	T46.5X4	T46.5X5	T46.5X6
Crystal violet	T49.0X1	T49.0X2	T49.0X3	T49.0X4	T49.0X5	T49.0X6
Cuckoopint	T62.2X1	T62.2X2	T62.2X3	T62.2X4	--	--
Cumetharol	T45.511	T45.512	T45.513	T45.514	T45.515	T45.516
Cupric						
- acetate	T60.3X1	T60.3X2	T60.3X3	T60.3X4	--	--
- acetoarsenite	T57.0X1	T57.0X2	T57.0X3	T57.0X4	--	--
- arsenate	T57.0X1	T57.0X2	T57.0X3	T57.0X4	--	--
- gluconate	T49.0X1	T49.0X2	T49.0X3	T49.0X4	T49.0X5	T49.0X6
- oleate	T49.0X1	T49.0X2	T49.0X3	T49.0X4	T49.0X5	T49.0X6
- sulfate	T56.4X1	T56.4X2	T56.4X3	T56.4X4	--	--
Cuprous sulfate—see also Copper sulfate	T56.4X1	T56.4X2	T56.4X3	T56.4X4	--	--
Curare, curarine	T48.1X1	T48.1X2	T48.1X3	T48.1X4	T48.1X5	T48.1X6
Cyamemazine	T43.3X1	T43.3X2	T43.3X3	T43.3X4	T43.3X5	T43.3X6
Cyamopsis tetragono-loba	T46.6X1	T46.6X2	T46.6X3	T46.6X4	T46.6X5	T46.6X6
Cyanacetyl hydrazide	T37.1X1	T37.1X2	T37.1X3	T37.1X4	T37.1X5	T37.1X6
Cyanic acid (gas)	T59.891	T59.892	T59.893	T59.894	--	--
Cyanide (s) (compounds) (potassium) (sodium) NEC	T65.0X1	T65.0X2	T65.0X3	T65.0X4	--	--
- dust or gas (inhalation) NEC	T57.3X1	T57.3X2	T57.3X3	T57.3X4	--	--
- fumigant	T65.0X1	T65.0X2	T65.0X3	T65.0X4	--	--
- hydrogen	T57.3X1	T57.3X2	T57.3X3	T57.3X4	--	--
- mercuric—see Mercury						
- pesticide (dust) (fumes)	T65.0X1	T65.0X2	T65.0X3	T65.0X4	--	--
Cyanoacrylate adhesive	T49.3X1	T49.3X2	T49.3X3	T49.3X4	T49.3X5	T49.3X6
Cyanocobalamin	T45.8X1	T45.8X2	T45.8X3	T45.8X4	T45.8X5	T45.8X6
Cyanogen (chloride) (gas) NEC	T59.891	T59.892	T59.893	T59.894	--	--
Cyclacillin	T36.0X1	T36.0X2	T36.0X3	T36.0X4	T36.0X5	T36.0X6

Substance	Poisoning, Accidental (unintentional)	Poisoning, Intentional Self-harm	Poisoning, Assault	Poisoning, Undetermined	Adverse effect	Underdosing
Cyclaine	T41.3X1	T41.3X2	T41.3X3	T41.3X4	T41.3X5	T41.3X6
Cyclamate	T50.991	T50.992	T50.993	T50.994	T50.995	T50.996
Cyclamen europaeum	T62.2X1	T62.2X2	T62.2X3	T62.2X4	--	--
Cyclandelate	T46.7X1	T46.7X2	T46.7X3	T46.7X4	T46.7X5	T46.7X6
Cyclazocine	T50.7X1	T50.7X2	T50.7X3	T50.7X4	T50.7X5	T50.7X6
Cyclizine	T45.0X1	T45.0X2	T45.0X3	T45.0X4	T45.0X5	T45.0X6
Cyclobarbital	T42.3X1	T42.3X2	T42.3X3	T42.3X4	T42.3X5	T42.3X6
Cyclobarbitone	T42.3X1	T42.3X2	T42.3X3	T42.3X4	T42.3X5	T42.3X6
Cyclobenzaprine	T48.1X1	T48.1X2	T48.1X3	T48.1X4	T48.1X5	T48.1X6
Cyclodrine	T44.3X1	T44.3X2	T44.3X3	T44.3X4	T44.3X5	T44.3X6
Cycloguanil embonate	T37.2X1	T37.2X2	T37.2X3	T37.2X4	T37.2X5	T37.2X6
Cyclohexane	T52.8X1	T52.8X2	T52.8X3	T52.8X4	--	--
Cyclohexanol	T51.8X1	T51.8X2	T51.8X3	T51.8X4	--	--
Cyclohexanone	T52.4X1	T52.4X2	T52.4X3	T52.4X4	--	--
Cycloheximide	T60.3X1	T60.3X2	T60.3X3	T60.3X4	--	--
Cyclohexyl acetate	T52.8X1	T52.8X2	T52.8X3	T52.8X4	--	--
Cycloleucin	T45.1X1	T45.1X2	T45.1X3	T45.1X4	T45.1X5	T45.1X6
Cyclomethycaine	T41.3X1	T41.3X2	T41.3X3	T41.3X4	T41.3X5	T41.3X6
Cyclopentamine	T44.4X1	T44.4X2	T44.4X3	T44.4X4	T44.4X5	T44.4X6
Cyclopenthiazide	T50.2X1	T50.2X2	T50.2X3	T50.2X4	T50.2X5	T50.2X6
Cyclopentolate	T44.3X1	T44.3X2	T44.3X3	T44.3X4	T44.3X5	T44.3X6
Cyclophosphamide	T45.1X1	T45.1X2	T45.1X3	T45.1X4	T45.1X5	T45.1X6
Cycloplegic drug	T49.5X1	T49.5X2	T49.5X3	T49.5X4	T49.5X5	T49.5X6
Cyclopropane	T41.291	T41.292	T41.293	T41.294	T41.295	T41.296
Cyclopyrabital	T39.8X1	T39.8X2	T39.8X3	T39.8X4	T39.8X5	T39.8X6
Cycloserine	T37.1X1	T37.1X2	T37.1X3	T37.1X4	T37.1X5	T37.1X6
Cyclosporin	T45.1X1	T45.1X2	T45.1X3	T45.1X4	T45.1X5	T45.1X6
Cyclothiazide	T50.2X1	T50.2X2	T50.2X3	T50.2X4	T50.2X5	T50.2X6
Cycrimine	T44.3X1	T44.3X2	T44.3X3	T44.3X4	T44.3X5	T44.3X6
Cyhalothrin	T60.1X1	T60.1X2	T60.1X3	T60.1X4	--	--
Cymarin	T46.0X1	T46.0X2	T46.0X3	T46.0X4	T46.0X5	T46.0X6
Cypermethrin	T60.1X1	T60.1X2	T60.1X3	T60.1X4	--	--
Cyphenothrin	T60.2X1	T60.2X2	T60.2X3	T60.2X4	--	--
Cyproheptadine	T45.0X1	T45.0X2	T45.0X3	T45.0X4	T45.0X5	T45.0X6
Cyproterone	T38.6X1	T38.6X2	T38.6X3	T38.6X4	T38.6X5	T38.6X6
Cysteamine	T50.6X1	T50.6X2	T50.6X3	T50.6X4	T50.6X5	T50.6X6
Cytarabine	T45.1X1	T45.1X2	T45.1X3	T45.1X4	T45.1X5	T45.1X6
Cytisus						
- laburnum	T62.2X1	T62.2X2	T62.2X3	T62.2X4	--	--
- scoparius	T62.2X1	T62.2X2	T62.2X3	T62.2X4	--	--
Cytochrome C	T47.5X1	T47.5X2	T47.5X3	T47.5X4	T47.5X5	T47.5X6
Cytomel	T38.1X1	T38.1X2	T38.1X3	T38.1X4	T38.1X5	T38.1X6
Cytosine arabinoside	T45.1X1	T45.1X2	T45.1X3	T45.1X4	T45.1X5	T45.1X6
Cytoxan	T45.1X1	T45.1X2	T45.1X3	T45.1X4	T45.1X5	T45.1X6
Cytozyme	T45.7X1	T45.7X2	T45.7X3	T45.7X4	T45.7X5	T45.7X6
2,4-D	T60.3X1	T60.3X2	T60.3X3	T60.3X4	--	--
Dacarbazine	T45.1X1	T45.1X2	T45.1X3	T45.1X4	T45.1X5	T45.1X6
Dactinomycin	T45.1X1	T45.1X2	T45.1X3	T45.1X4	T45.1X5	T45.1X6
DADPS	T37.1X1	T37.1X2	T37.1X3	T37.1X4	T37.1X5	T37.1X6
Dakin's solution	T49.0X1	T49.0X2	T49.0X3	T49.0X4	T49.0X5	T49.0X6
Dalapon (sodium)	T60.3X1	T60.3X2	T60.3X3	T60.3X4	--	--
Dalmane	T42.4X1	T42.4X2	T42.4X3	T42.4X4	T42.4X5	T42.4X6
Danazol	T38.6X1	T38.6X2	T38.6X3	T38.6X4	T38.6X5	T38.6X6
Danilone	T45.511	T45.512	T45.513	T45.514	T45.515	T45.516
Danthron	T47.2X1	T47.2X2	T47.2X3	T47.2X4	T47.2X5	T47.2X6
Dantrolene	T42.8X1	T42.8X2	T42.8X3	T42.8X4	T42.8X5	T42.8X6
Dantron	T47.2X1	T47.2X2	T47.2X3	T47.2X4	T47.2X5	T47.2X6
Daphne (gnidium) (mezereum)	T62.2X1	T62.2X2	T62.2X3	T62.2X4	--	--

Substance	Poisoning, Accidental (unintentional)	Poisoning, Intentional Self-harm	Poisoning, Assault	Poisoning, Undetermined	Adverse effect	Underdosing
- berry	T62.1X1	T62.1X2	T62.1X3	T62.1X4	--	--
Dapsone	T37.1X1	T37.1X2	T37.1X3	T37.1X4	T37.1X5	T37.1X6
Daraprim	T37.2X1	T37.2X2	T37.2X3	T37.2X4	T37.2X5	T37.2X6
Darnel	T62.2X1	T62.2X2	T62.2X3	T62.2X4	--	--
Darvon	T39.8X1	T39.8X2	T39.8X3	T39.8X4	T39.8X5	T39.8X6
Daunomycin	T45.1X1	T45.1X2	T45.1X3	T45.1X4	T45.1X5	T45.1X6
Daunorubicin	T45.1X1	T45.1X2	T45.1X3	T45.1X4	T45.1X5	T45.1X6
DBI	T38.3X1	T38.3X2	T38.3X3	T38.3X4	T38.3X5	T38.3X6
D-Con	T60.91	T60.92	T60.93	T60.94	--	--
- insecticide	T60.2X1	T60.2X2	T60.2X3	T60.2X4	--	--
- rodenticide	T60.4X1	T60.4X2	T60.4X3	T60.4X4	--	--
DDAVP	T38.891	T38.892	T38.893	T38.894	T38.895	T38.896
DDE (bis (chlorophenyl) -dichloroethylene)	T60.2X1	T60.2X2	T60.2X3	T60.2X4	--	--
DDS	T37.1X1	T37.1X2	T37.1X3	T37.1X4	T37.1X5	T37.1X6
DDT (dust)	T60.1X1	T60.1X2	T60.1X3	T60.1X4	--	--
Deadly nightshade—see also Belladonna	T62.2X1	T62.2X2	T62.2X3	T62.2X4	--	--
- berry	T62.1X1	T62.1X2	T62.1X3	T62.1X4	--	--
Deamino-D-arginine vasopressin	T38.891	T38.892	T38.893	T38.894	T38.895	T38.896
Deanol (aceglumate)	T50.991	T50.992	T50.993	T50.994	T50.995	T50.996
Debrisoquine	T46.5X1	T46.5X2	T46.5X3	T46.5X4	T46.5X5	T46.5X6
Decaborane	T57.8X1	T57.8X2	T57.8X3	T57.8X4	--	--
- fumes	T59.891	T59.892	T59.893	T59.894	--	--
Decadron	T38.0X1	T38.0X2	T38.0X3	T38.0X4	T38.0X5	T38.0X6
- ENT agent	T49.6X1	T49.6X2	T49.6X3	T49.6X4	T49.6X5	T49.6X6
- ophthalmic preparation	T49.5X1	T49.5X2	T49.5X3	T49.5X4	T49.5X5	T49.5X6
- topical NEC	T49.0X1	T49.0X2	T49.0X3	T49.0X4	T49.0X5	T49.0X6
Decahydronaphthalene	T52.8X1	T52.8X2	T52.8X3	T52.8X4	--	--
Decalin	T52.8X1	T52.8X2	T52.8X3	T52.8X4	--	--
Decamethonium (bromide)	T48.1X1	T48.1X2	T48.1X3	T48.1X4	T48.1X5	T48.1X6
Decholin	T47.5X1	T47.5X2	T47.5X3	T47.5X4	T47.5X5	T47.5X6
Declomycin	T36.4X1	T36.4X2	T36.4X3	T36.4X4	T36.4X5	T36.4X6
Decongestant, nasal (mucosa)	T48.5X1	T48.5X2	T48.5X3	T48.5X4	T48.5X5	T48.5X6
- combination	T48.5X1	T48.5X2	T48.5X3	T48.5X4	T48.5X5	T48.5X6
Deet	T60.8X1	T60.8X2	T60.8X3	T60.8X4	--	--
Deferoxamine	T45.8X1	T45.8X2	T45.8X3	T45.8X4	T45.8X5	T45.8X6
Deflazacort	T38.0X1	T38.0X2	T38.0X3	T38.0X4	T38.0X5	T38.0X6
Deglycyrrhizinized extract of licorice	T48.4X1	T48.4X2	T48.4X3	T48.4X4	T48.4X5	T48.4X6
Dehydrocholic acid	T47.5X1	T47.5X2	T47.5X3	T47.5X4	T47.5X5	T47.5X6
Dehydroemetine	T37.3X1	T37.3X2	T37.3X3	T37.3X4	T37.3X5	T37.3X6
Dekalin	T52.8X1	T52.8X2	T52.8X3	T52.8X4	--	--
Delalutin	T38.5X1	T38.5X2	T38.5X3	T38.5X4	T38.5X5	T38.5X6
Delorazepam	T42.4X1	T42.4X2	T42.4X3	T42.4X4	T42.4X5	T42.4X6
Delphinium	T62.2X1	T62.2X2	T62.2X3	T62.2X4	--	--
Deltamethrin	T60.1X1	T60.1X2	T60.1X3	T60.1X4	--	--
Deltasone	T38.0X1	T38.0X2	T38.0X3	T38.0X4	T38.0X5	T38.0X6
Deltra	T38.0X1	T38.0X2	T38.0X3	T38.0X4	T38.0X5	T38.0X6
Delvinal	T42.3X1	T42.3X2	T42.3X3	T42.3X4	T42.3X5	T42.3X6
Demecarium (bromide)	T49.5X1	T49.5X2	T49.5X3	T49.5X4	T49.5X5	T49.5X6
Demeclocycline	T36.4X1	T36.4X2	T36.4X3	T36.4X4	T36.4X5	T36.4X6
Demecolcine	T45.1X1	T45.1X2	T45.1X3	T45.1X4	T45.1X5	T45.1X6
Demegestone	T38.5X1	T38.5X2	T38.5X3	T38.5X4	T38.5X5	T38.5X6
Demelanizing agents	T49.8X1	T49.8X2	T49.8X3	T49.8X4	T49.8X5	T49.8X6
Demephion -O and -S	T60.0X1	T60.0X2	T60.0X3	T60.0X4	--	--
Demerol	T40.2X1	T40.2X2	T40.2X3	T40.2X4	T40.2X5	T40.2X6
Demethylchlortetracycline	T36.4X1	T36.4X2	T36.4X3	T36.4X4	T36.4X5	T36.4X6
Demethyltetracycline	T36.4X1	T36.4X2	T36.4X3	T36.4X4	T36.4X5	T36.4X6
Demeton -O and -S	T60.0X1	T60.0X2	T60.0X3	T60.0X4	--	--
Demulcent (external)	T49.3X1	T49.3X2	T49.3X3	T49.3X4	T49.3X5	T49.3X6
- specified NEC	T49.3X1	T49.3X2	T49.3X3	T49.3X4	T49.3X5	T49.3X6

Substance	Poisoning, Accidental (unintentional)	Poisoning, Intentional Self-harm	Poisoning, Assault	Poisoning, Undetermined	Adverse effect	Underdosing
Demulen	T38.4X1	T38.4X2	T38.4X3	T38.4X4	T38.4X5	T38.4X6
Denatured alcohol	T51.0X1	T51.0X2	T51.0X3	T51.0X4	--	--
Dendrid	T49.5X1	T49.5X2	T49.5X3	T49.5X4	T49.5X5	T49.5X6
Dental drug, topical application NEC	T49.7X1	T49.7X2	T49.7X3	T49.7X4	T49.7X5	T49.7X6
Dentifrice	T49.7X1	T49.7X2	T49.7X3	T49.7X4	T49.7X5	T49.7X6
Deodorant spray (feminine hygiene)	T49.8X1	T49.8X2	T49.8X3	T49.8X4	T49.8X5	T49.8X6
Deoxycortone	T50.0X1	T50.0X2	T50.0X3	T50.0X4	T50.0X5	T50.0X6
2-Deoxy-5-fluorouridine	T45.1X1	T45.1X2	T45.1X3	T45.1X4	T45.1X5	T45.1X6
5-Deoxy-5-fluorouridine	T45.1X1	T45.1X2	T45.1X3	T45.1X4	T45.1X5	T45.1X6
Deoxyribonuclease (pancreatic)	T45.3X1	T45.3X2	T45.3X3	T45.3X4	T45.3X5	T45.3X6
Depilatory	T49.4X1	T49.4X2	T49.4X3	T49.4X4	T49.4X5	T49.4X6
Deprenalin	T42.8X1	T42.8X2	T42.8X3	T42.8X4	T42.8X5	T42.8X6
Deprenyl	T42.8X1	T42.8X2	T42.8X3	T42.8X4	T42.8X5	T42.8X6
Depressant, appetite	T50.5X1	T50.5X2	T50.5X3	T50.5X4	T50.5X5	T50.5X6
Depressant						
- appetite (central)	T50.5X1	T50.5X2	T50.5X3	T50.5X4	T50.5X5	T50.5X6
- cardiac	T46.2X1	T46.2X2	T46.2X3	T46.2X4	T46.2X5	T46.2X6
central nervous system (anesthetic) —see also Central nervous system, depressants	T42.71	T42.72	T42.73	T42.74	T42.75	T42.76
- - general anesthetic	T41.201	T41.202	T41.203	T41.204	T41.205	T41.206
- - muscle tone	T42.8X1	T42.8X2	T42.8X3	T42.8X4	T42.8X5	T42.8X6
- muscle tone, central	T42.8X1	T42.8X2	T42.8X3	T42.8X4	T42.8X5	T42.8X6
- psychotherapeutic	T43.501	T43.502	T43.503	T43.504	T43.505	T43.506
Deptropine	T45.0X1	T45.0X2	T45.0X3	T45.0X4	T45.0X5	T45.0X6
Dequalinium (chloride)	T49.0X1	T49.0X2	T49.0X3	T49.0X4	T49.0X5	T49.0X6
Derris root	T60.2X1	T60.2X2	T60.2X3	T60.2X4	--	--
Deserpidine	T46.5X1	T46.5X2	T46.5X3	T46.5X4	T46.5X5	T46.5X6
Desferrioxamine	T45.8X1	T45.8X2	T45.8X3	T45.8X4	T45.8X5	T45.8X6
Desipramine	T43.011	T43.012	T43.013	T43.014	T43.015	T43.016
Deslanoside	T46.0X1	T46.0X2	T46.0X3	T46.0X4	T46.0X5	T46.0X6
Desloughing agent	T49.4X1	T49.4X2	T49.4X3	T49.4X4	T49.4X5	T49.4X6
Desmethylimipramine	T43.011	T43.012	T43.013	T43.014	T43.015	T43.016
Desmopressin	T38.891	T38.892	T38.893	T38.894	T38.895	T38.896
Desocodeine	T40.2X1	T40.2X2	T40.2X3	T40.2X4	T40.2X5	T40.2X6
Desogestrel	T38.5X1	T38.5X2	T38.5X3	T38.5X4	T38.5X5	T38.5X6
Desomorphine	T40.2X1	T40.2X2	T40.2X3	T40.2X4	--	--
Desonide	T49.0X1	T49.0X2	T49.0X3	T49.0X4	T49.0X5	T49.0X6
Desoximetasone	T49.0X1	T49.0X2	T49.0X3	T49.0X4	T49.0X5	T49.0X6
Desoxycorticosteroid	T50.0X1	T50.0X2	T50.0X3	T50.0X4	T50.0X5	T50.0X6
Desoxycortone	T50.0X1	T50.0X2	T50.0X3	T50.0X4	T50.0X5	T50.0X6
Desoxyephedrine	T43.621	T43.622	T43.623	T43.624	T43.625	T43.626
Detaxtran	T46.6X1	T46.6X2	T46.6X3	T46.6X4	T46.6X5	T46.6X6
Detergent	T49.2X1	T49.2X2	T49.2X3	T49.2X4	T49.2X5	T49.2X6
- external medication	T49.2X1	T49.2X2	T49.2X3	T49.2X4	T49.2X5	T49.2X6
- local	T49.2X1	T49.2X2	T49.2X3	T49.2X4	T49.2X5	T49.2X6
- medicinal	T49.2X1	T49.2X2	T49.2X3	T49.2X4	T49.2X5	T49.2X6
- nonmedicinal	T55.1X1	T55.1X2	T55.1X3	T55.1X4	--	--
- specified NEC	T55.1X1	T55.1X2	T55.1X3	T55.1X4	--	--
Deterrent, alcohol	T50.6X1	T50.6X2	T50.6X3	T50.6X4	T50.6X5	T50.6X6
Detoxifying agent	T50.6X1	T50.6X2	T50.6X3	T50.6X4	T50.6X5	T50.6X6
Detrothyronine	T38.1X1	T38.1X2	T38.1X3	T38.1X4	T38.1X5	T38.1X6
Dettol (external medication)	T49.0X1	T49.0X2	T49.0X3	T49.0X4	T49.0X5	T49.0X6
Dexamethasone	T38.0X1	T38.0X2	T38.0X3	T38.0X4	T38.0X5	T38.0X6
- ENT agent	T49.6X1	T49.6X2	T49.6X3	T49.6X4	T49.6X5	T49.6X6
- ophthalmic preparation	T49.5X1	T49.5X2	T49.5X3	T49.5X4	T49.5X5	T49.5X6
- topical NEC	T49.0X1	T49.0X2	T49.0X3	T49.0X4	T49.0X5	T49.0X6
Dexamfetamine	T43.621	T43.622	T43.623	T43.624	T43.625	T43.626
Dexamphetamine	T43.621	T43.622	T43.623	T43.624	T43.625	T43.626

Substance	Poisoning, Accidental (unintentional)	Poisoning, Intentional Self-harm	Poisoning, Assault	Poisoning, Undetermined	Adverse effect	Underdosing
Dexbrompheniramine	T45.0X1	T45.0X2	T45.0X3	T45.0X4	T45.0X5	T45.0X6
Dexchlorpheniramine	T45.0X1	T45.0X2	T45.0X3	T45.0X4	T45.0X5	T45.0X6
Dexedrine	T43.621	T43.622	T43.623	T43.624	T43.625	T43.626
Dexetimide	T44.3X1	T44.3X2	T44.3X3	T44.3X4	T44.3X5	T44.3X6
Dexfenfluramine	T50.5X1	T50.5X2	T50.5X3	T50.5X4	T50.5X5	T50.5X6
Dexpanthenol	T45.2X1	T45.2X2	T45.2X3	T45.2X4	T45.2X5	T45.2X6
Dextran (40) (70) (150)	T45.8X1	T45.8X2	T45.8X3	T45.8X4	T45.8X5	T45.8X6
Dextriferron	T45.4X1	T45.4X2	T45.4X3	T45.4X4	T45.4X5	T45.4X6
Dextro calcium pantothenate	T45.2X1	T45.2X2	T45.2X3	T45.2X4	T45.2X5	T45.2X6
Dextro pantothenyl alcohol	T45.2X1	T45.2X2	T45.2X3	T45.2X4	T45.2X5	T45.2X6
Dextroamphetamine	T43.621	T43.622	T43.623	T43.624	T43.625	T43.626
Dextromethorphan	T48.3X1	T48.3X2	T48.3X3	T48.3X4	T48.3X5	T48.3X6
Dextromoramide	T40.4X1	T40.4X2	T40.4X3	T40.4X4	--	--
- topical	T49.8X1	T49.8X2	T49.8X3	T49.8X4	T49.8X5	T49.8X6
Dextropropoxyphene	T40.4X1	T40.4X2	T40.4X3	T40.4X4	T40.4X5	T40.4X6
Dextrorphan	T40.2X1	T40.2X2	T40.2X3	T40.2X4	T40.2X5	T40.2X6
Dextrose	T50.3X1	T50.3X2	T50.3X3	T50.3X4	T50.3X5	T50.3X6
- concentrated solution, intravenous	T46.8X1	T46.8X2	T46.8X3	T46.8X4	T46.8X5	T46.8X6
Dextrothyroxin	T38.1X1	T38.1X2	T38.1X3	T38.1X4	T38.1X5	T38.1X6
Dextrothyroxine sodium	T38.1X1	T38.1X2	T38.1X3	T38.1X4	T38.1X5	T38.1X6
DFP	T44.0X1	T44.0X2	T44.0X3	T44.0X4	T44.0X5	T44.0X6
DHE	T37.3X1	T37.3X2	T37.3X3	T37.3X4	T37.3X5	T37.3X6
- 45	T46.5X1	T46.5X2	T46.5X3	T46.5X4	T46.5X5	T46.5X6
Diabinese	T38.3X1	T38.3X2	T38.3X3	T38.3X4	T38.3X5	T38.3X6
Diacetone alcohol	T52.4X1	T52.4X2	T52.4X3	T52.4X4	--	--
Diacetyl monoxime	T50.991	T50.992	T50.993	T50.994	--	--
Diacetylmorphine	T40.1X1	T40.1X2	T40.1X3	T40.1X4	T40.1X5	--
Diachylon plaster	T49.4X1	T49.4X2	T49.4X3	T49.4X4	T49.4X5	T49.4X6
Diaethylstilboestrolum	T38.5X1	T38.5X2	T38.5X3	T38.5X4	T38.5X5	T38.5X6
Diagnostic agent NEC	T50.8X1	T50.8X2	T50.8X3	T50.8X4	T50.8X5	T50.8X6
Dial (soap)	T49.2X1	T49.2X2	T49.2X3	T49.2X4	T49.2X5	T49.2X6
- sedative	T42.3X1	T42.3X2	T42.3X3	T42.3X4	T42.3X5	T42.3X6
Dialkyl carbonate	T52.91	T52.92	T52.93	T52.94	--	--
Diallylbarbituric acid	T42.3X1	T42.3X2	T42.3X3	T42.3X4	T42.3X5	T42.3X6
Diallymal	T42.3X1	T42.3X2	T42.3X3	T42.3X4	T42.3X5	T42.3X6
Dialysis solution (intraperitoneal)	T50.3X1	T50.3X2	T50.3X3	T50.3X4	T50.3X5	T50.3X6
Diaminodiphenylsulfone	T37.1X1	T37.1X2	T37.1X3	T37.1X4	T37.1X5	T37.1X6
Diamorphine	T40.1X1	T40.1X2	T40.1X3	T40.1X4	T40.1X5	--
Diamox	T50.2X1	T50.2X2	T50.2X3	T50.2X4	T50.2X5	T50.2X6
Diamthazole	T49.0X1	T49.0X2	T49.0X3	T49.0X4	T49.0X5	T49.0X6
Dianthone	T47.2X1	T47.2X2	T47.2X3	T47.2X4	T47.2X5	T47.2X6
Diaphenylsulfone	T37.0X1	T37.0X2	T37.0X3	T37.0X4	T37.0X5	T37.0X6
Diasone (sodium)	T37.1X1	T37.1X2	T37.1X3	T37.1X4	T37.1X5	T37.1X6
Diastase	T47.5X1	T47.5X2	T47.5X3	T47.5X4	T47.5X5	T47.5X6
Diatrizoate	T50.8X1	T50.8X2	T50.8X3	T50.8X4	T50.8X5	T50.8X6
Diazepam	T42.4X1	T42.4X2	T42.4X3	T42.4X4	T42.4X5	T42.4X6
Diazinon	T60.0X1	T60.0X2	T60.0X3	T60.0X4	--	--
Diazomethane (gas)	T59.891	T59.892	T59.893	T59.894	--	--
Diazoxide	T46.5X1	T46.5X2	T46.5X3	T46.5X4	T46.5X5	T46.5X6
Dibekacin	T36.5X1	T36.5X2	T36.5X3	T36.5X4	T36.5X5	T36.5X6
Dibenamine	T44.6X1	T44.6X2	T44.6X3	T44.6X4	T44.6X5	T44.6X6
Dibenzepin	T43.011	T43.012	T43.013	T43.014	T43.015	T43.016
Dibenzheptropine	T45.0X1	T45.0X2	T45.0X3	T45.0X4	T45.0X5	T45.0X6
Dibenzyline	T44.6X1	T44.6X2	T44.6X3	T44.6X4	T44.6X5	T44.6X6
Diborane (gas)	T59.891	T59.892	T59.893	T59.894	--	--
Dibromochloropropane	T60.8X1	T60.8X2	T60.8X3	T60.8X4	--	--
Dibromodulcitol	T45.1X1	T45.1X2	T45.1X3	T45.1X4	T45.1X5	T45.1X6
Dibromoethane	T53.6X1	T53.6X2	T53.6X3	T53.6X4	--	--
Dibromomannitol	T45.1X1	T45.1X2	T45.1X3	T45.1X4	T45.1X5	T45.1X6

Substance	Poisoning, Accidental (unintentional)	Poisoning, Intentional Self-harm	Poisoning, Assault	Poisoning, Undetermined	Adverse effect	Underdosing
Dibromopropamidine isethionate	T49.0X1	T49.0X2	T49.0X3	T49.0X4	T49.0X5	T49.0X6
Dibrompropamidine	T49.0X1	T49.0X2	T49.0X3	T49.0X4	T49.0X5	T49.0X6
Dibucaine	T41.3X1	T41.3X2	T41.3X3	T41.3X4	T41.3X5	T41.3X6
- topical (surface)	T41.3X1	T41.3X2	T41.3X3	T41.3X4	T41.3X5	T41.3X6
Dibunate sodium	T48.3X1	T48.3X2	T48.3X3	T48.3X4	T48.3X5	T48.3X6
Dibutoline sulfate	T44.3X1	T44.3X2	T44.3X3	T44.3X4	T44.3X5	T44.3X6
Dicamba	T60.3X1	T60.3X2	T60.3X3	T60.3X4	--	--
Dicapthon	T60.0X1	T60.0X2	T60.0X3	T60.0X4	--	--
Dichlobenil	T60.3X1	T60.3X2	T60.3X3	T60.3X4	--	--
Dichlone	T60.3X1	T60.3X2	T60.3X3	T60.3X4	--	--
Dichloralphenozone	T42.6X1	T42.6X2	T42.6X3	T42.6X4	T42.6X5	T42.6X6
Dichlorbenzidine	T65.3X1	T65.3X2	T65.3X3	T65.3X4	--	--
Dichlorhydrin	T52.8X1	T52.8X2	T52.8X3	T52.8X4	--	--
Dichlorhydroxyquinoline	T37.8X1	T37.8X2	T37.8X3	T37.8X4	T37.8X5	T37.8X6
Dichlorobenzene	T53.7X1	T53.7X2	T53.7X3	T53.7X4	--	--
Dichlorobenzyl alcohol	T49.6X1	T49.6X2	T49.6X3	T49.6X4	T49.6X5	T49.6X6
Dichlorodifluoromethane	T53.5X1	T53.5X2	T53.5X3	T53.5X4	--	--
Dichloroethane	T52.8X1	T52.8X2	T52.8X3	T52.8X4	--	--
Sym-Dichloroethyl ether	T53.6X1	T53.6X2	T53.6X3	T53.6X4	--	--
Dichloroethyl sulfide, not in war	T59.891	T59.892	T59.893	T59.894	--	--
Dichloroethylene	T53.6X1	T53.6X2	T53.6X3	T53.6X4	--	--
Dichloroformoxine, not in war	T59.891	T59.892	T59.893	T59.894	--	--
Dichlorohydrin, alpha-dichlorohydrin	T52.8X1	T52.8X2	T52.8X3	T52.8X4	--	--
Dichloromethane (solvent)	T53.4X1	T53.4X2	T53.4X3	T53.4X4	--	--
- vapor	T53.4X1	T53.4X2	T53.4X3	T53.4X4	--	--
Dichloronaphthoquinone	T60.3X1	T60.3X2	T60.3X3	T60.3X4	--	--
Dichlorophen	T37.4X1	T37.4X2	T37.4X3	T37.4X4	T37.4X5	T37.4X6
2,4-Dichlorophenoxyacetic acid	T60.3X1	T60.3X2	T60.3X3	T60.3X4	--	--
Dichloropropene	T60.3X1	T60.3X2	T60.3X3	T60.3X4	--	--
Dichloropropionic acid	T60.3X1	T60.3X2	T60.3X3	T60.3X4	--	--
Dichlorphenamide	T50.2X1	T50.2X2	T50.2X3	T50.2X4	T50.2X5	T50.2X6
Dichlorvos	T60.0X1	T60.0X2	T60.0X3	T60.0X4	--	--
Diclofenac	T39.391	T39.392	T39.393	T39.394	T39.395	T39.396
Diclofenamide	T50.2X1	T50.2X2	T50.2X3	T50.2X4	T50.2X5	T50.2X6
Diclofensine	T43.291	T43.292	T43.293	T43.294	T43.295	T43.296
Diclonixine	T39.8X1	T39.8X2	T39.8X3	T39.8X4	T39.8X5	T39.8X6
Dicloxacillin	T36.0X1	T36.0X2	T36.0X3	T36.0X4	T36.0X5	T36.0X6
Dicophane	T49.0X1	T49.0X2	T49.0X3	T49.0X4	T49.0X5	T49.0X6
Dicoumarol, dicoumarin, dicumarol	T45.511	T45.512	T45.513	T45.514	T45.515	T45.516
Dicrotophos	T60.0X1	T60.0X2	T60.0X3	T60.0X4	--	--
Dicyanogen (gas)	T65.0X1	T65.0X2	T65.0X3	T65.0X4	--	--
Dicyclomine	T44.3X1	T44.3X2	T44.3X3	T44.3X4	T44.3X5	T44.3X6
Dicycloverine	T44.3X1	T44.3X2	T44.3X3	T44.3X4	T44.3X5	T44.3X6
Dideoxycytidine	T37.5X1	T37.5X2	T37.5X3	T37.5X4	T37.5X5	T37.5X6
Dideoxyinosine	T37.5X1	T37.5X2	T37.5X3	T37.5X4	T37.5X5	T37.5X6
Dieldrin (vapor)	T60.1X1	T60.1X2	T60.1X3	T60.1X4	--	--
Diemal	T42.3X1	T42.3X2	T42.3X3	T42.3X4	T42.3X5	T42.3X6
Dienestrol	T38.5X1	T38.5X2	T38.5X3	T38.5X4	T38.5X5	T38.5X6
Dienoestrol	T38.5X1	T38.5X2	T38.5X3	T38.5X4	T38.5X5	T38.5X6
Dietetic drug NEC	T50.901	T50.902	T50.903	T50.904	T50.905	T50.906
Diethazine	T42.8X1	T42.8X2	T42.8X3	T42.8X4	T42.8X5	T42.8X6
Diethyl						
- barbituric acid	T42.3X1	T42.3X2	T42.3X3	T42.3X4	T42.3X5	T42.3X6
- carbamazine	T37.4X1	T37.4X2	T37.4X3	T37.4X4	T37.4X5	T37.4X6
- carbinol	T51.3X1	T51.3X2	T51.3X3	T51.3X4	--	--
- carbonate	T52.8X1	T52.8X2	T52.8X3	T52.8X4	--	--
- ether (vapor) —see also ether	T41.0X1	T41.0X2	T41.0X3	T41.0X4	T41.0X5	T41.0X6
- oxide	T52.8X1	T52.8X2	T52.8X3	T52.8X4	--	--

Substance	Poisoning, Accidental (unintentional)	Poisoning, Intentional Self-harm	Poisoning, Assault	Poisoning, Undetermined	Adverse effect	Underdosing
- propion	T50.5X1	T50.5X2	T50.5X3	T50.5X4	T50.5X5	T50.5X6
- stilbestrol	T38.5X1	T38.5X2	T38.5X3	T38.5X4	T38.5X5	T38.5X6
- toluamide (nonmedicinal)	T60.8X1	T60.8X2	T60.8X3	T60.8X4	--	--
- - medicinal	T49.3X1	T49.3X2	T49.3X3	T49.3X4	T49.3X5	T49.3X6
Diethylcarbamazine	T37.4X1	T37.4X2	T37.4X3	T37.4X4	T37.4X5	T37.4X6
Diethylene						
- dioxide	T52.8X1	T52.8X2	T52.8X3	T52.8X4	--	--
- glycol (monoacetate) (monobutyl ether) (monoethyl ether)	T52.3X1	T52.3X2	T52.3X3	T52.3X4	--	--
Diethylhexylphthalate	T65.891	T65.892	T65.893	T65.894	--	--
Diethylpropion	T50.5X1	T50.5X2	T50.5X3	T50.5X4	T50.5X5	T50.5X6
Diethylstilbestrol	T38.5X1	T38.5X2	T38.5X3	T38.5X4	T38.5X5	T38.5X6
Diethylstilboestrol	T38.5X1	T38.5X2	T38.5X3	T38.5X4	T38.5X5	T38.5X6
Diethylsulfone-diethylmethane	T42.6X1	T42.6X2	T42.6X3	T42.6X4	T42.6X5	T42.6X6
Diethyltoluamide	T49.0X1	T49.0X2	T49.0X3	T49.0X4	T49.0X5	T49.0X6
Diethyltryptamine (DET)	T40.991	T40.992	T40.993	T40.994	--	--
Difebarbamate	T42.3X1	T42.3X2	T42.3X3	T42.3X4	T42.3X5	T42.3X6
Difencloxazine	T40.2X1	T40.2X2	T40.2X3	T40.2X4	T40.2X5	T40.2X6
Difenidol	T45.0X1	T45.0X2	T45.0X3	T45.0X4	T45.0X5	T45.0X6
Difenoxin	T47.6X1	T47.6X2	T47.6X3	T47.6X4	T47.6X5	T47.6X6
Difetarsone	T37.3X1	T37.3X2	T37.3X3	T37.3X4	T37.3X5	T37.3X6
Diffusin	T45.3X1	T45.3X2	T45.3X3	T45.3X4	T45.3X5	T45.3X6
Diflorasone	T49.0X1	T49.0X2	T49.0X3	T49.0X4	T49.0X5	T49.0X6
Diflos	T44.0X1	T44.0X2	T44.0X3	T44.0X4	T44.0X5	T44.0X6
Diflubenzuron	T60.1X1	T60.1X2	T60.1X3	T60.1X4	--	--
Diflucortolone	T49.0X1	T49.0X2	T49.0X3	T49.0X4	T49.0X5	T49.0X6
Diflunisal	T39.091	T39.092	T39.093	T39.094	T39.095	T39.096
Difluoromethyldopa	T42.8X1	T42.8X2	T42.8X3	T42.8X4	T42.8X5	T42.8X6
Difluorophate	T44.0X1	T44.0X2	T44.0X3	T44.0X4	T44.0X5	T44.0X6
Digestant NEC	T47.5X1	T47.5X2	T47.5X3	T47.5X4	T47.5X5	T47.5X6
Digitalin (e)	T46.0X1	T46.0X2	T46.0X3	T46.0X4	T46.0X5	T46.0X6
Digitalis (leaf) (glycoside)	T46.0X1	T46.0X2	T46.0X3	T46.0X4	T46.0X5	T46.0X6
- lanata	T46.0X1	T46.0X2	T46.0X3	T46.0X4	T46.0X5	T46.0X6
- purpurea	T46.0X1	T46.0X2	T46.0X3	T46.0X4	T46.0X5	T46.0X6
Digitoxin	T46.0X1	T46.0X2	T46.0X3	T46.0X4	T46.0X5	T46.0X6
Digitoxose	T46.0X1	T46.0X2	T46.0X3	T46.0X4	T46.0X5	T46.0X6
Digoxin	T46.0X1	T46.0X2	T46.0X3	T46.0X4	T46.0X5	T46.0X6
Digoxine	T46.0X1	T46.0X2	T46.0X3	T46.0X4	T46.0X5	T46.0X6
Dihydralazine	T46.5X1	T46.5X2	T46.5X3	T46.5X4	T46.5X5	T46.5X6
Dihydrazine	T46.5X1	T46.5X2	T46.5X3	T46.5X4	T46.5X5	T46.5X6
Dihydrocodeine	T40.2X1	T40.2X2	T40.2X3	T40.2X4	T40.2X5	T40.2X6
Dihydrocodeinone	T40.2X1	T40.2X2	T40.2X3	T40.2X4	T40.2X5	T40.2X6
Dihydroergocornine	T46.7X1	T46.7X2	T46.7X3	T46.7X4	T46.7X5	T46.7X6
Dihydroergocristine (mesilate)	T46.7X1	T46.7X2	T46.7X3	T46.7X4	T46.7X5	T46.7X6
Dihydroergokryptine	T46.7X1	T46.7X2	T46.7X3	T46.7X4	T46.7X5	T46.7X6
Dihydroergotamine	T46.5X1	T46.5X2	T46.5X3	T46.5X4	T46.5X5	T46.5X6
Dihydroergotoxine	T46.7X1	T46.7X2	T46.7X3	T46.7X4	T46.7X5	T46.7X6
- mesilate	T46.7X1	T46.7X2	T46.7X3	T46.7X4	T46.7X5	T46.7X6
Dihydrohydroxycodeinone	T40.2X1	T40.2X2	T40.2X3	T40.2X4	T40.2X5	T40.2X6
Dihydrohydroxymorphinone	T40.2X1	T40.2X2	T40.2X3	T40.2X4	T40.2X5	T40.2X6
Dihydroisocodeine	T40.2X1	T40.2X2	T40.2X3	T40.2X4	T40.2X5	T40.2X6
Dihydromorphine	T40.2X1	T40.2X2	T40.2X3	T40.2X4	--	--
Dihydromorphinone	T40.2X1	T40.2X2	T40.2X3	T40.2X4	T40.2X5	T40.2X6
Dihydrostreptomycin	T36.5X1	T36.5X2	T36.5X3	T36.5X4	T36.5X5	T36.5X6
Dihydrotachysterol	T45.2X1	T45.2X2	T45.2X3	T45.2X4	T45.2X5	T45.2X6
Dihydroxyaluminum aminoacetate	T47.1X1	T47.1X2	T47.1X3	T47.1X4	T47.1X5	T47.1X6
Dihydroxyaluminum sodium carbonate	T47.1X1	T47.1X2	T47.1X3	T47.1X4	T47.1X5	T47.1X6
Dihydroxyanthraquinone	T47.2X1	T47.2X2	T47.2X3	T47.2X4	T47.2X5	T47.2X6
Dihydroxycodeinone	T40.2X1	T40.2X2	T40.2X3	T40.2X4	T40.2X5	T40.2X6

Substance	Poisoning, Accidental (unintentional)	Poisoning, Intentional Self-harm	Poisoning, Assault	Poisoning, Undetermined	Adverse effect	Underdosing
Dihydroxypropyl theophylline	T50.2X1	T50.2X2	T50.2X3	T50.2X4	T50.2X5	T50.2X6
Diiodohydroxyquin	T37.8X1	T37.8X2	T37.8X3	T37.8X4	T37.8X5	T37.8X6
- topical	T49.0X1	T49.0X2	T49.0X3	T49.0X4	T49.0X5	T49.0X6
Diiodohydroxyquinoline	T37.8X1	T37.8X2	T37.8X3	T37.8X4	T37.8X5	T37.8X6
Diiodotyrosine	T38.2X1	T38.2X2	T38.2X3	T38.2X4	T38.2X5	T38.2X6
Diisopromine	T44.3X1	T44.3X2	T44.3X3	T44.3X4	T44.3X5	T44.3X6
Diisopropylamine	T46.3X1	T46.3X2	T46.3X3	T46.3X4	T46.3X5	T46.3X6
Diisopropylfluorophos-phonate	T44.0X1	T44.0X2	T44.0X3	T44.0X4	T44.0X5	T44.0X6
Dilantin	T42.0X1	T42.0X2	T42.0X3	T42.0X4	T42.0X5	T42.0X6
Dilaudid	T40.2X1	T40.2X2	T40.2X3	T40.2X4	T40.2X5	T40.2X6
Dilazep	T46.3X1	T46.3X2	T46.3X3	T46.3X4	T46.3X5	T46.3X6
Dill	T47.5X1	T47.5X2	T47.5X3	T47.5X4	T47.5X5	T47.5X6
Diloxanide	T37.3X1	T37.3X2	T37.3X3	T37.3X4	T37.3X5	T37.3X6
Diltiazem	T46.1X1	T46.1X2	T46.1X3	T46.1X4	T46.1X5	T46.1X6
Dimazole	T49.0X1	T49.0X2	T49.0X3	T49.0X4	T49.0X5	T49.0X6
Dimefline	T50.7X1	T50.7X2	T50.7X3	T50.7X4	T50.7X5	T50.7X6
Dimefox	T60.0X1	T60.0X2	T60.0X3	T60.0X4	--	--
Dimemorfan	T48.3X1	T48.3X2	T48.3X3	T48.3X4	T48.3X5	T48.3X6
Dimenhydrinate	T45.0X1	T45.0X2	T45.0X3	T45.0X4	T45.0X5	T45.0X6
Dimercaprol (British anti-lewisite)	T45.8X1	T45.8X2	T45.8X3	T45.8X4	T45.8X5	T45.8X6
Dimercaptopropanol	T45.8X1	T45.8X2	T45.8X3	T45.8X4	T45.8X5	T45.8X6
Dimestrol	T38.5X1	T38.5X2	T38.5X3	T38.5X4	T38.5X5	T38.5X6
Dimetane	T45.0X1	T45.0X2	T45.0X3	T45.0X4	T45.0X5	T45.0X6
Dimethicone	T47.1X1	T47.1X2	T47.1X3	T47.1X4	T47.1X5	T47.1X6
Dimethindene	T45.0X1	T45.0X2	T45.0X3	T45.0X4	T45.0X5	T45.0X6
Dimethisoquin	T49.1X1	T49.1X2	T49.1X3	T49.1X4	T49.1X5	T49.1X6
Dimethisterone	T38.5X1	T38.5X2	T38.5X3	T38.5X4	T38.5X5	T38.5X6
Dimethoate	T60.0X1	T60.0X2	T60.0X3	T60.0X4	--	--
Dimethocaine	T41.3X1	T41.3X2	T41.3X3	T41.3X4	T41.3X5	T41.3X6
Dimethoxanate	T48.3X1	T48.3X2	T48.3X3	T48.3X4	T48.3X5	T48.3X6
Dimethyl						
- arsine, arsinic acid	T57.0X1	T57.0X2	T57.0X3	T57.0X4	--	--
- carbinol	T51.2X1	T51.2X2	T51.2X3	T51.2X4	--	--
- carbonate	T52.8X1	T52.8X2	T52.8X3	T52.8X4	--	--
- diguanide	T38.3X1	T38.3X2	T38.3X3	T38.3X4	T38.3X5	T38.3X6
- ketone	T52.4X1	T52.4X2	T52.4X3	T52.4X4	--	--
- - vapor	T52.4X1	T52.4X2	T52.4X3	T52.4X4	--	--
- meperidine	T40.2X1	T40.2X2	T40.2X3	T40.2X4	T40.2X5	T40.2X6
- parathion	T60.0X1	T60.0X2	T60.0X3	T60.0X4	--	--
- phthlate	T49.3X1	T49.3X2	T49.3X3	T49.3X4	T49.3X5	T49.3X6
- polysiloxane	T47.8X1	T47.8X2	T47.8X3	T47.8X4	T47.8X5	T47.8X6
- sulfate (fumes)	T59.891	T59.892	T59.893	T59.894	--	--
- - liquid	T65.891	T65.892	T65.893	T65.894	--	--
- sulfoxide (nonmedicinal)	T52.8X1	T52.8X2	T52.8X3	T52.8X4	--	--
- - medicinal	T49.4X1	T49.4X2	T49.4X3	T49.4X4	T49.4X5	T49.4X6
- tryptamine	T40.991	T40.992	T40.993	T40.994	--	--
- tubocurarine	T48.1X1	T48.1X2	T48.1X3	T48.1X4	T48.1X5	T48.1X6
Dimethylamine sulfate	T49.4X1	T49.4X2	T49.4X3	T49.4X4	T49.4X5	T49.4X6
Dimethylformamide	T52.8X1	T52.8X2	T52.8X3	T52.8X4	--	--
Dimethyltubocurarinium chloride	T48.1X1	T48.1X2	T48.1X3	T48.1X4	T48.1X5	T48.1X6
Dimeticone	T47.1X1	T47.1X2	T47.1X3	T47.1X4	T47.1X5	T47.1X6
Dimetilan	T60.0X1	T60.0X2	T60.0X3	T60.0X4	--	--
Dimetindene	T45.0X1	T45.0X2	T45.0X3	T45.0X4	T45.0X5	T45.0X6
Dimetotiazine	T43.3X1	T43.3X2	T43.3X3	T43.3X4	T43.3X5	T43.3X6
Dimorpholamine	T50.7X1	T50.7X2	T50.7X3	T50.7X4	T50.7X5	T50.7X6
Dimoxyline	T46.3X1	T46.3X2	T46.3X3	T46.3X4	T46.3X5	T46.3X6
Dinitrobenzene	T65.3X1	T65.3X2	T65.3X3	T65.3X4	--	--
- vapor	T59.891	T59.892	T59.893	T59.894	--	--

Substance	Poisoning, Accidental (unintentional)	Poisoning, Intentional Self-harm	Poisoning, Assault	Poisoning, Undetermined	Adverse effect	Underdosing
Dinitrobenzol	T65.3X1	T65.3X2	T65.3X3	T65.3X4	--	--
- vapor	T59.891	T59.892	T59.893	T59.894	--	--
Dinitrobutylphenol	T65.3X1	T65.3X2	T65.3X3	T65.3X4	--	--
Dinitro (-ortho-) cresol (pesticide) (spray)	T65.3X1	T65.3X2	T65.3X3	T65.3X4	--	--
Dinitrocyclohexylphenol	T65.3X1	T65.3X2	T65.3X3	T65.3X4	--	--
Dinitrophenol	T65.3X1	T65.3X2	T65.3X3	T65.3X4	--	--
Dinoprost	T48.0X1	T48.0X2	T48.0X3	T48.0X4	T48.0X5	T48.0X6
Dinoprostone	T48.0X1	T48.0X2	T48.0X3	T48.0X4	T48.0X5	T48.0X6
Dinoseb	T60.3X1	T60.3X2	T60.3X3	T60.3X4	--	--
Dioctyl sulfosuccinate (calcium) (sodium)	T47.4X1	T47.4X2	T47.4X3	T47.4X4	T47.4X5	T47.4X6
Diodone	T50.8X1	T50.8X2	T50.8X3	T50.8X4	T50.8X5	T50.8X6
Diodoquin	T37.8X1	T37.8X2	T37.8X3	T37.8X4	T37.8X5	T37.8X6
Dionin	T40.2X1	T40.2X2	T40.2X3	T40.2X4	T40.2X5	T40.2X6
Diosmin	T46.991	T46.992	T46.993	T46.994	T46.995	T46.996
Dioxane	T52.8X1	T52.8X2	T52.8X3	T52.8X4	--	--
Dioxathion	T60.0X1	T60.0X2	T60.0X3	T60.0X4	--	--
Dioxin	T53.7X1	T53.7X2	T53.7X3	T53.7X4	--	--
Dioxopromethazine	T43.3X1	T43.3X2	T43.3X3	T43.3X4	T43.3X5	T43.3X6
Dioxyline	T46.3X1	T46.3X2	T46.3X3	T46.3X4	T46.3X5	T46.3X6
Dipentene	T52.8X1	T52.8X2	T52.8X3	T52.8X4	--	--
Diperodon	T41.3X1	T41.3X2	T41.3X3	T41.3X4	T41.3X5	T41.3X6
Diphacinone	T60.4X1	T60.4X2	T60.4X3	T60.4X4	--	--
Diphemanil	T44.3X1	T44.3X2	T44.3X3	T44.3X4	T44.3X5	T44.3X6
- metilsulfate	T44.3X1	T44.3X2	T44.3X3	T44.3X4	T44.3X5	T44.3X6
Diphenadione	T45.511	T45.512	T45.513	T45.514	T45.515	T45.516
- rodenticide	T60.4X1	T60.4X2	T60.4X3	T60.4X4	--	--
Diphenhydramine	T45.0X1	T45.0X2	T45.0X3	T45.0X4	T45.0X5	T45.0X6
Diphenidol	T45.0X1	T45.0X2	T45.0X3	T45.0X4	T45.0X5	T45.0X6
Diphenoxylate	T47.6X1	T47.6X2	T47.6X3	T47.6X4	T47.6X5	T47.6X6
Diphenylamine	T65.3X1	T65.3X2	T65.3X3	T65.3X4	--	--
Diphenylbutazone	T39.2X1	T39.2X2	T39.2X3	T39.2X4	T39.2X5	T39.2X6
Diphenylchloroarsine, not in war	T57.0X1	T57.0X2	T57.0X3	T57.0X4	--	--
Diphenylhydantoin	T42.0X1	T42.0X2	T42.0X3	T42.0X4	T42.0X5	T42.0X6
Diphenylmethane dye	T52.1X1	T52.1X2	T52.1X3	T52.1X4	--	--
Diphenylpyraline	T45.0X1	T45.0X2	T45.0X3	T45.0X4	T45.0X5	T45.0X6
Diphtheria						
- antitoxin	T50.Z11	T50.Z12	T50.Z13	T50.Z14	T50.Z15	T50.Z16
- toxoid	T50.A91	T50.A92	T50.A93	T50.A94	T50.A95	T50.A96
- - with tetanus toxoid	T50.A21	T50.A22	T50.A23	T50.A24	T50.A25	T50.A26
- - - with pertussis component	T50.A11	T50.A12	T50.A13	T50.A14	T50.A15	T50.A16
- vaccine	T50.A91	T50.A92	T50.A93	T50.A94	T50.A95	T50.A96
- - combination						
- - - including pertussis	T50.A11	T50.A12	T50.A13	T50.A14	T50.A15	T50.A16
- - - without pertussis	T50.A21	T50.A22	T50.A23	T50.A24	T50.A25	T50.A26
Diphylline	T50.2X1	T50.2X2	T50.2X3	T50.2X4	T50.2X5	T50.2X6
Dipipanone	T40.4X1	T40.4X2	T40.4X3	T40.4X4	--	--
Dipivefrine	T49.5X1	T49.5X2	T49.5X3	T49.5X4	T49.5X5	T49.5X6
Diplovax	T50.B91	T50.B92	T50.B93	T50.B94	T50.B95	T50.B96
Diprophylline	T50.2X1	T50.2X2	T50.2X3	T50.2X4	T50.2X5	T50.2X6
Dipropyline	T48.291	T48.292	T48.293	T48.294	T48.295	T48.296
Dipyridamole	T46.3X1	T46.3X2	T46.3X3	T46.3X4	T46.3X5	T46.3X6
Dipyrone	T39.2X1	T39.2X2	T39.2X3	T39.2X4	T39.2X5	T39.2X6
Diquat (dibromide)	T60.3X1	T60.3X2	T60.3X3	T60.3X4	--	--
Disinfectant	T65.891	T65.892	T65.893	T65.894	--	--
- alkaline	T54.3X1	T54.3X2	T54.3X3	T54.3X4	--	--
- aromatic	T54.1X1	T54.1X2	T54.1X3	T54.1X4	--	--
- intestinal	T37.8X1	T37.8X2	T37.8X3	T37.8X4	T37.8X5	T37.8X6
Disipal	T42.8X1	T42.8X2	T42.8X3	T42.8X4	T42.8X5	T42.8X6
Disodium edetate	T50.6X1	T50.6X2	T50.6X3	T50.6X4	T50.6X5	T50.6X6

Substance	Poisoning, Accidental (unintentional)	Poisoning, Intentional Self-harm	Poisoning, Assault	Poisoning, Undetermined	Adverse effect	Underdosing
Disoprofol	T41.291	T41.292	T41.293	T41.294	T41.295	T41.296
Disopyramide	T46.2X1	T46.2X2	T46.2X3	T46.2X4	T46.2X5	T46.2X6
Distigmine (bromide)	T44.0X1	T44.0X2	T44.0X3	T44.0X4	T44.0X5	T44.0X6
Disulfamide	T50.2X1	T50.2X2	T50.2X3	T50.2X4	T50.2X5	T50.2X6
Disulfanilamide	T37.0X1	T37.0X2	T37.0X3	T37.0X4	T37.0X5	T37.0X6
Disulfiram	T50.6X1	T50.6X2	T50.6X3	T50.6X4	T50.6X5	T50.6X6
Disulfoton	T60.0X1	T60.0X2	T60.0X3	T60.0X4	--	--
Dithiazanine iodide	T37.4X1	T37.4X2	T37.4X3	T37.4X4	T37.4X5	T37.4X6
Dithiocarbamate	T60.0X1	T60.0X2	T60.0X3	T60.0X4	--	--
Dithranol	T49.4X1	T49.4X2	T49.4X3	T49.4X4	T49.4X5	T49.4X6
Diucardin	T50.2X1	T50.2X2	T50.2X3	T50.2X4	T50.2X5	T50.2X6
Diupres	T50.2X1	T50.2X2	T50.2X3	T50.2X4	T50.2X5	T50.2X6
Diuretic NEC	T50.2X1	T50.2X2	T50.2X3	T50.2X4	T50.2X5	T50.2X6
- benzothiadiazine	T50.2X1	T50.2X2	T50.2X3	T50.2X4	T50.2X5	T50.2X6
- carbonic acid anhydrase inhibitors	T50.2X1	T50.2X2	T50.2X3	T50.2X4	T50.2X5	T50.2X6
- furfuryl NEC	T50.2X1	T50.2X2	T50.2X3	T50.2X4	T50.2X5	T50.2X6
- loop (high-ceiling)	T50.1X1	T50.1X2	T50.1X3	T50.1X4	T50.1X5	T50.1X6
- mercurial NEC	T50.2X1	T50.2X2	T50.2X3	T50.2X4	T50.2X5	T50.2X6
- osmotic	T50.2X1	T50.2X2	T50.2X3	T50.2X4	T50.2X5	T50.2X6
- purine NEC	T50.2X1	T50.2X2	T50.2X3	T50.2X4	T50.2X5	T50.2X6
- saluretic NEC	T50.2X1	T50.2X2	T50.2X3	T50.2X4	T50.2X5	T50.2X6
- sulfonamide	T50.2X1	T50.2X2	T50.2X3	T50.2X4	T50.2X5	T50.2X6
- thiazide NEC	T50.2X1	T50.2X2	T50.2X3	T50.2X4	T50.2X5	T50.2X6
- xanthine	T50.2X1	T50.2X2	T50.2X3	T50.2X4	T50.2X5	T50.2X6
Diurgin	T50.2X1	T50.2X2	T50.2X3	T50.2X4	T50.2X5	T50.2X6
Diuril	T50.2X1	T50.2X2	T50.2X3	T50.2X4	T50.2X5	T50.2X6
Diuron	T60.3X1	T60.3X2	T60.3X3	T60.3X4	--	--
Divalproex	T42.6X1	T42.6X2	T42.6X3	T42.6X4	T42.6X5	T42.6X6
Divinyl ether	T41.0X1	T41.0X2	T41.0X3	T41.0X4	T41.0X5	T41.0X6
Dixanthogen	T49.0X1	T49.0X2	T49.0X3	T49.0X4	T49.0X5	T49.0X6
Dixyrazine	T43.3X1	T43.3X2	T43.3X3	T43.3X4	T43.3X5	T43.3X6
D-lysergic acid diethylamide	T40.8X1	T40.8X2	T40.8X3	T40.8X4	T40.8X5	--
DMCT	T36.4X1	T36.4X2	T36.4X3	T36.4X4	T36.4X5	T36.4X6
DMSO—see Dimethyl sulfoxide						
DNBP	T60.3X1	T60.3X2	T60.3X3	T60.3X4	--	--
DNOC	T65.3X1	T65.3X2	T65.3X3	T65.3X4	--	--
Dobutamine	T44.5X1	T44.5X2	T44.5X3	T44.5X4	T44.5X5	T44.5X6
DOCA	T38.0X1	T38.0X2	T38.0X3	T38.0X4	T38.0X5	T38.0X6
Docusate sodium	T47.4X1	T47.4X2	T47.4X3	T47.4X4	T47.4X5	T47.4X6
Dodicin	T49.0X1	T49.0X2	T49.0X3	T49.0X4	T49.0X5	T49.0X6
Dofamium chloride	T49.0X1	T49.0X2	T49.0X3	T49.0X4	T49.0X5	T49.0X6
Dolophine	T40.3X1	T40.3X2	T40.3X3	T40.3X4	T40.3X5	T40.3X6
Doloxene	T39.8X1	T39.8X2	T39.8X3	T39.8X4	T39.8X5	T39.8X6
Domestic gas (after combustion) —see Gas, utility						
- prior to combustion	T59.891	T59.892	T59.893	T59.894	--	--
Domiodol	T48.4X1	T48.4X2	T48.4X3	T48.4X4	T48.4X5	T48.4X6
Domiphen (bromide)	T49.0X1	T49.0X2	T49.0X3	T49.0X4	T49.0X5	T49.0X6
Domperidone	T45.0X1	T45.0X2	T45.0X3	T45.0X4	T45.0X5	T45.0X6
Dopa	T42.8X1	T42.8X2	T42.8X3	T42.8X4	T42.8X5	T42.8X6
Dopamine	T44.991	T44.992	T44.993	T44.994	T44.995	T44.996
Doriden	T42.6X1	T42.6X2	T42.6X3	T42.6X4	T42.6X5	T42.6X6
Dormiral	T42.3X1	T42.3X2	T42.3X3	T42.3X4	T42.3X5	T42.3X6
Dormison	T42.6X1	T42.6X2	T42.6X3	T42.6X4	T42.6X5	T42.6X6
Dornase	T48.4X1	T48.4X2	T48.4X3	T48.4X4	T48.4X5	T48.4X6
Dorsacaine	T41.3X1	T41.3X2	T41.3X3	T41.3X4	T41.3X5	T41.3X6
Dosulepin	T43.011	T43.012	T43.013	T43.014	T43.015	T43.016
Dothiepin	T43.011	T43.012	T43.013	T43.014	T43.015	T43.016
Doxantrazole	T48.6X1	T48.6X2	T48.6X3	T48.6X4	T48.6X5	T48.6X6

Substance	Poisoning, Accidental (unintentional)	Poisoning, Intentional Self-harm	Poisoning, Assault	Poisoning, Undetermined	Adverse effect	Underdosing
Doxapram	T50.7X1	T50.7X2	T50.7X3	T50.7X4	T50.7X5	T50.7X6
Doxazosin	T44.6X1	T44.6X2	T44.6X3	T44.6X4	T44.6X5	T44.6X6
Doxepin	T43.011	T43.012	T43.013	T43.014	T43.015	T43.016
Doxifluridine	T45.1X1	T45.1X2	T45.1X3	T45.1X4	T45.1X5	T45.1X6
Doxorubicin	T45.1X1	T45.1X2	T45.1X3	T45.1X4	T45.1X5	T45.1X6
Doxycycline	T36.4X1	T36.4X2	T36.4X3	T36.4X4	T36.4X5	T36.4X6
Doxylamine	T45.0X1	T45.0X2	T45.0X3	T45.0X4	T45.0X5	T45.0X6
Dramamine	T45.0X1	T45.0X2	T45.0X3	T45.0X4	T45.0X5	T45.0X6
Drano (drain cleaner)	T54.3X1	T54.3X2	T54.3X3	T54.3X4	--	--
Dressing, live pulp	T49.7X1	T49.7X2	T49.7X3	T49.7X4	T49.7X5	T49.7X6
Drocode	T40.2X1	T40.2X2	T40.2X3	T40.2X4	T40.2X5	T40.2X6
Dromoran	T40.2X1	T40.2X2	T40.2X3	T40.2X4	T40.2X5	T40.2X6
Dromostanolone	T38.7X1	T38.7X2	T38.7X3	T38.7X4	T38.7X5	T38.7X6
Dronabinol	T40.7X1	T40.7X2	T40.7X3	T40.7X4	T40.7X5	T40.7X6
Droperidol	T43.591	T43.592	T43.593	T43.594	T43.595	T43.596
Dropropizine	T48.3X1	T48.3X2	T48.3X3	T48.3X4	T48.3X5	T48.3X6
Drostanolone	T38.7X1	T38.7X2	T38.7X3	T38.7X4	T38.7X5	T38.7X6
Drotaverine	T44.3X1	T44.3X2	T44.3X3	T44.3X4	T44.3X5	T44.3X6
Drotrecogin alfa	T45.511	T45.512	T45.513	T45.514	T45.515	T45.516
Drug NEC	T50.901	T50.902	T50.903	T50.904	T50.905	T50.906
- specified NEC	T50.991	T50.992	T50.993	T50.994	T50.995	T50.996
DTIC	T45.1X1	T45.1X2	T45.1X3	T45.1X4	T45.1X5	T45.1X6
Duboisine	T44.3X1	T44.3X2	T44.3X3	T44.3X4	T44.3X5	T44.3X6
Dulcolax	T47.2X1	T47.2X2	T47.2X3	T47.2X4	T47.2X5	T47.2X6
Duponol (C) (EP)	T49.2X1	T49.2X2	T49.2X3	T49.2X4	T49.2X5	T49.2X6
Durabolin	T38.7X1	T38.7X2	T38.7X3	T38.7X4	T38.7X5	T38.7X6
Dyclone	T41.3X1	T41.3X2	T41.3X3	T41.3X4	T41.3X5	T41.3X6
Dyclonine	T41.3X1	T41.3X2	T41.3X3	T41.3X4	T41.3X5	T41.3X6
Dydrogesterone	T38.5X1	T38.5X2	T38.5X3	T38.5X4	T38.5X5	T38.5X6
Dye NEC	T65.6X1	T65.6X2	T65.6X3	T65.6X4	--	--
- antiseptic	T49.0X1	T49.0X2	T49.0X3	T49.0X4	T49.0X5	T49.0X6
- diagnostic agents	T50.8X1	T50.8X2	T50.8X3	T50.8X4	T50.8X5	T50.8X6
- pharmaceutical NEC	T50.901	T50.902	T50.903	T50.904	T50.905	T50.906
Dyflos	T44.0X1	T44.0X2	T44.0X3	T44.0X4	T44.0X5	T44.0X6
Dymelor	T38.3X1	T38.3X2	T38.3X3	T38.3X4	T38.3X5	T38.3X6
Dynamite	T65.3X1	T65.3X2	T65.3X3	T65.3X4	--	--
- fumes	T59.891	T59.892	T59.893	T59.894	--	--
Dyphylline	T44.3X1	T44.3X2	T44.3X3	T44.3X4	T44.3X5	T44.3X6
Ear drug NEC	T49.6X1	T49.6X2	T49.6X3	T49.6X4	T49.6X5	T49.6X6
Ear preparations	T49.6X1	T49.6X2	T49.6X3	T49.6X4	T49.6X5	T49.6X6
Echothiophate, echothiopate, ecothiopate	T49.5X1	T49.5X2	T49.5X3	T49.5X4	T49.5X5	T49.5X6
Econazole	T49.0X1	T49.0X2	T49.0X3	T49.0X4	T49.0X5	T49.0X6
Ecothiopate iodide	T49.5X1	T49.5X2	T49.5X3	T49.5X4	T49.5X5	T49.5X6
Ecstasy	T43.621	T43.622	T43.623	T43.624	T43.625	T43.626
Ectylurea	T42.6X1	T42.6X2	T42.6X3	T42.6X4	T42.6X5	T42.6X6
Edathamil disodium	T45.8X1	T45.8X2	T45.8X3	T45.8X4	T45.8X5	T45.8X6
Edecrin	T50.1X1	T50.1X2	T50.1X3	T50.1X4	T50.1X5	T50.1X6
Edetate, disodium (calcium)	T45.8X1	T45.8X2	T45.8X3	T45.8X4	T45.8X5	T45.8X6
Edoxudine	T49.5X1	T49.5X2	T49.5X3	T49.5X4	T49.5X5	T49.5X6
Edrophonium	T44.0X1	T44.0X2	T44.0X3	T44.0X4	T44.0X5	T44.0X6
- chloride	T44.0X1	T44.0X2	T44.0X3	T44.0X4	T44.0X5	T44.0X6
EDTA	T50.6X1	T50.6X2	T50.6X3	T50.6X4	T50.6X5	T50.6X6
Eflornithine	T37.2X1	T37.2X2	T37.2X3	T37.2X4	T37.2X5	T37.2X6
Efloxate	T46.3X1	T46.3X2	T46.3X3	T46.3X4	T46.3X5	T46.3X6
Elase	T49.8X1	T49.8X2	T49.8X3	T49.8X4	T49.8X5	T49.8X6
Elastase	T47.5X1	T47.5X2	T47.5X3	T47.5X4	T47.5X5	T47.5X6
Elaterium	T47.2X1	T47.2X2	T47.2X3	T47.2X4	T47.2X5	T47.2X6
Elcatonin	T50.991	T50.992	T50.993	T50.994	T50.995	T50.996
Elder	T62.2X1	T62.2X2	T62.2X3	T62.2X4	--	--

Substance	Poisoning, Accidental (unintentional)	Poisoning, Intentional Self-harm	Poisoning, Assault	Poisoning, Undetermined	Adverse effect	Underdosing
- berry, (unripe)	T62.1X1	T62.1X2	T62.1X3	T62.1X4	--	--
Electrolyte balance drug	T50.3X1	T50.3X2	T50.3X3	T50.3X4	T50.3X5	T50.3X6
Electrolytes NEC	T50.3X1	T50.3X2	T50.3X3	T50.3X4	T50.3X5	T50.3X6
Electrolytic agent NEC	T50.3X1	T50.3X2	T50.3X3	T50.3X4	T50.3X5	T50.3X6
Elemental diet	T50.901	T50.902	T50.903	T50.904	T50.905	T50.906
Elliptinium acetate	T45.1X1	T45.1X2	T45.1X3	T45.1X4	T45.1X5	T45.1X6
Embramine	T45.0X1	T45.0X2	T45.0X3	T45.0X4	T45.0X5	T45.0X6
Emepronium (salts)	T44.3X1	T44.3X2	T44.3X3	T44.3X4	T44.3X5	T44.3X6
- bromide	T44.3X1	T44.3X2	T44.3X3	T44.3X4	T44.3X5	T44.3X6
Emetic NEC	T47.7X1	T47.7X2	T47.7X3	T47.7X4	T47.7X5	T47.7X6
Emetine	T37.3X1	T37.3X2	T37.3X3	T37.3X4	T37.3X5	T37.3X6
Emollient NEC	T49.3X1	T49.3X2	T49.3X3	T49.3X4	T49.3X5	T49.3X6
Emorfazone	T39.8X1	T39.8X2	T39.8X3	T39.8X4	T39.8X5	T39.8X6
Emylcamate	T43.591	T43.592	T43.593	T43.594	T43.595	T43.596
Enalapril	T46.4X1	T46.4X2	T46.4X3	T46.4X4	T46.4X5	T46.4X6
Enalaprilat	T46.4X1	T46.4X2	T46.4X3	T46.4X4	T46.4X5	T46.4X6
Encainide	T46.2X1	T46.2X2	T46.2X3	T46.2X4	T46.2X5	T46.2X6
Endocaine	T41.3X1	T41.3X2	T41.3X3	T41.3X4	T41.3X5	T41.3X6
Endosulfan	T60.2X1	T60.2X2	T60.2X3	T60.2X4	--	--
Endothall	T60.3X1	T60.3X2	T60.3X3	T60.3X4	--	--
Endralazine	T46.5X1	T46.5X2	T46.5X3	T46.5X4	T46.5X5	T46.5X6
Endrin	T60.1X1	T60.1X2	T60.1X3	T60.1X4	--	--
Enflurane	T41.0X1	T41.0X2	T41.0X3	T41.0X4	T41.0X5	T41.0X6
Enhexymal	T42.3X1	T42.3X2	T42.3X3	T42.3X4	T42.3X5	T42.3X6
Enocitabine	T45.1X1	T45.1X2	T45.1X3	T45.1X4	T45.1X5	T45.1X6
Enovid	T38.4X1	T38.4X2	T38.4X3	T38.4X4	T38.4X5	T38.4X6
Enoxacin	T36.8X1	T36.8X2	T36.8X3	T36.8X4	T36.8X5	T36.8X6
Enoxaparin (sodium)	T45.511	T45.512	T45.513	T45.514	T45.515	T45.516
Enpiprazole	T43.591	T43.592	T43.593	T43.594	T43.595	T43.596
Enprofylline	T48.6X1	T48.6X2	T48.6X3	T48.6X4	T48.6X5	T48.6X6
Enprostil	T47.1X1	T47.1X2	T47.1X3	T47.1X4	T47.1X5	T47.1X6
ENT preparations (anti-infectives)	T49.6X1	T49.6X2	T49.6X3	T49.6X4	T49.6X5	T49.6X6
Enterogastrone	T38.891	T38.892	T38.893	T38.894	T38.895	T38.896
Enviomycin	T36.8X1	T36.8X2	T36.8X3	T36.8X4	T36.8X5	T36.8X6
Enzodase	T45.3X1	T45.3X2	T45.3X3	T45.3X4	T45.3X5	T45.3X6
Enzyme NEC	T45.3X1	T45.3X2	T45.3X3	T45.3X4	T45.3X5	T45.3X6
- depolymerizing	T49.8X1	T49.8X2	T49.8X3	T49.8X4	T49.8X5	T49.8X6
- fibrolytic	T45.3X1	T45.3X2	T45.3X3	T45.3X4	T45.3X5	T45.3X6
- gastric	T47.5X1	T47.5X2	T47.5X3	T47.5X4	T47.5X5	T47.5X6
- intestinal	T47.5X1	T47.5X2	T47.5X3	T47.5X4	T47.5X5	T47.5X6
- local action	T49.4X1	T49.4X2	T49.4X3	T49.4X4	T49.4X5	T49.4X6
- proteolytic	T49.4X1	T49.4X2	T49.4X3	T49.4X4	T49.4X5	T49.4X6
- thrombolytic	T45.3X1	T45.3X2	T45.3X3	T45.3X4	T45.3X5	T45.3X6
EPAB	T41.3X1	T41.3X2	T41.3X3	T41.3X4	T41.3X5	T41.3X6
Epanutin	T42.0X1	T42.0X2	T42.0X3	T42.0X4	T42.0X5	T42.0X6
Ephedra	T44.991	T44.992	T44.993	T44.994	T44.995	T44.996
Ephedrine	T44.991	T44.992	T44.993	T44.994	T44.995	T44.996
Epichlorhydrin, epichlorohydrin	T52.8X1	T52.8X2	T52.8X3	T52.8X4	--	--
Epicillin	T36.0X1	T36.0X2	T36.0X3	T36.0X4	T36.0X5	T36.0X6
Epiestriol	T38.5X1	T38.5X2	T38.5X3	T38.5X4	T38.5X5	T38.5X6
Epilim—see Sodium valproate						
Epimestrol	T38.5X1	T38.5X2	T38.5X3	T38.5X4	T38.5X5	T38.5X6
Epinephrine	T44.5X1	T44.5X2	T44.5X3	T44.5X4	T44.5X5	T44.5X6
Epirubicin	T45.1X1	T45.1X2	T45.1X3	T45.1X4	T45.1X5	T45.1X6
Epitiostanol	T38.7X1	T38.7X2	T38.7X3	T38.7X4	T38.7X5	T38.7X6
Epitizide	T50.2X1	T50.2X2	T50.2X3	T50.2X4	T50.2X5	T50.2X6
EPN	T60.0X1	T60.0X2	T60.0X3	T60.0X4	--	--
EPO	T45.8X1	T45.8X2	T45.8X3	T45.8X4	T45.8X5	T45.8X6

Substance	Poisoning, Accidental (unintentional)	Poisoning, Intentional Self-harm	Poisoning, Assault	Poisoning, Undetermined	Adverse effect	Underdosing
Epoetin alpha	T45.8X1	T45.8X2	T45.8X3	T45.8X4	T45.8X5	T45.8X6
Epomediol	T50.991	T50.992	T50.993	T50.994	T50.995	T50.996
Epoprostenol	T45.521	T45.522	T45.523	T45.524	T45.525	T45.526
Epoxy resin	T65.891	T65.892	T65.893	T65.894	--	--
Eprazinone	T48.4X1	T48.4X2	T48.4X3	T48.4X4	T48.4X5	T48.4X6
Epsilon amino-caproic acid	T45.621	T45.622	T45.623	T45.624	T45.625	T45.626
Epsom salt	T47.3X1	T47.3X2	T47.3X3	T47.3X4	T47.3X5	T47.3X6
Eptazocine	T40.4X1	T40.4X2	T40.4X3	T40.4X4	T40.4X5	T40.4X6
Equanil	T43.591	T43.592	T43.593	T43.594	T43.595	T43.596
Equisetum	T62.2X1	T62.2X2	T62.2X3	T62.2X4	--	--
- diuretic	T50.2X1	T50.2X2	T50.2X3	T50.2X4	T50.2X5	T50.2X6
Ergobasine	T48.0X1	T48.0X2	T48.0X3	T48.0X4	T48.0X5	T48.0X6
Ergocalciferol	T45.2X1	T45.2X2	T45.2X3	T45.2X4	T45.2X5	T45.2X6
Ergoloid mesylates	T46.7X1	T46.7X2	T46.7X3	T46.7X4	T46.7X5	T46.7X6
Ergometrine	T48.0X1	T48.0X2	T48.0X3	T48.0X4	T48.0X5	T48.0X6
Ergonovine	T48.0X1	T48.0X2	T48.0X3	T48.0X4	T48.0X5	T48.0X6
Ergot NEC	T64.81	T64.82	T64.83	T64.84	--	--
- derivative	T48.0X1	T48.0X2	T48.0X3	T48.0X4	T48.0X5	T48.0X6
- medicinal (alkaloids)	T48.0X1	T48.0X2	T48.0X3	T48.0X4	T48.0X5	T48.0X6
- prepared	T48.0X1	T48.0X2	T48.0X3	T48.0X4	T48.0X5	T48.0X6
Ergotamine	T46.5X1	T46.5X2	T46.5X3	T46.5X4	T46.5X5	T46.5X6
Ergotocine	T48.0X1	T48.0X2	T48.0X3	T48.0X4	T48.0X5	T48.0X6
Ergotrate	T48.0X1	T48.0X2	T48.0X3	T48.0X4	T48.0X5	T48.0X6
Eritrityl tetranitrate	T46.3X1	T46.3X2	T46.3X3	T46.3X4	T46.3X5	T46.3X6
Erythrityl tetranitrate	T46.3X1	T46.3X2	T46.3X3	T46.3X4	T46.3X5	T46.3X6
Erythrol tetranitrate	T46.3X1	T46.3X2	T46.3X3	T46.3X4	T46.3X5	T46.3X6
Erythromycin (salts)	T36.3X1	T36.3X2	T36.3X3	T36.3X4	T36.3X5	T36.3X6
- ophthalmic preparation	T49.5X1	T49.5X2	T49.5X3	T49.5X4	T49.5X5	T49.5X6
- topical NEC	T49.0X1	T49.0X2	T49.0X3	T49.0X4	T49.0X5	T49.0X6
Erythropoietin	T45.8X1	T45.8X2	T45.8X3	T45.8X4	T45.8X5	T45.8X6
- human	T45.8X1	T45.8X2	T45.8X3	T45.8X4	T45.8X5	T45.8X6
Escin	T46.991	T46.992	T46.993	T46.994	T46.995	T46.996
Esculin	T45.2X1	T45.2X2	T45.2X3	T45.2X4	T45.2X5	T45.2X6
Esculoside	T45.2X1	T45.2X2	T45.2X3	T45.2X4	T45.2X5	T45.2X6
ESDT (ether-soluble tar distillate)	T49.1X1	T49.1X2	T49.1X3	T49.1X4	T49.1X5	T49.1X6
Eserine	T49.5X1	T49.5X2	T49.5X3	T49.5X4	T49.5X5	T49.5X6
Esflurbiprofen	T39.311	T39.312	T39.313	T39.314	T39.315	T39.316
Eskabarb	T42.3X1	T42.3X2	T42.3X3	T42.3X4	T42.3X5	T42.3X6
Eskalith	T43.8X1	T43.8X2	T43.8X3	T43.8X4	T43.8X5	T43.8X6
Esmolol	T44.7X1	T44.7X2	T44.7X3	T44.7X4	T44.7X5	T44.7X6
Estanozolol	T38.7X1	T38.7X2	T38.7X3	T38.7X4	T38.7X5	T38.7X6
Estazolam	T42.4X1	T42.4X2	T42.4X3	T42.4X4	T42.4X5	T42.4X6
Estradiol	T38.5X1	T38.5X2	T38.5X3	T38.5X4	T38.5X5	T38.5X6
- with testosterone	T38.7X1	T38.7X2	T38.7X3	T38.7X4	T38.7X5	T38.7X6
- benzoate	T38.5X1	T38.5X2	T38.5X3	T38.5X4	T38.5X5	T38.5X6
Estramustine	T45.1X1	T45.1X2	T45.1X3	T45.1X4	T45.1X5	T45.1X6
Estriol	T38.5X1	T38.5X2	T38.5X3	T38.5X4	T38.5X5	T38.5X6
Estrogen	T38.5X1	T38.5X2	T38.5X3	T38.5X4	T38.5X5	T38.5X6
- with progesterone	T38.5X1	T38.5X2	T38.5X3	T38.5X4	T38.5X5	T38.5X6
- conjugated	T38.5X1	T38.5X2	T38.5X3	T38.5X4	T38.5X5	T38.5X6
Estrone	T38.5X1	T38.5X2	T38.5X3	T38.5X4	T38.5X5	T38.5X6
Estropipate	T38.5X1	T38.5X2	T38.5X3	T38.5X4	T38.5X5	T38.5X6
Etacrynate sodium	T50.1X1	T50.1X2	T50.1X3	T50.1X4	T50.1X5	T50.1X6
Etacrynic acid	T50.1X1	T50.1X2	T50.1X3	T50.1X4	T50.1X5	T50.1X6
Etafedrine	T48.6X1	T48.6X2	T48.6X3	T48.6X4	T48.6X5	T48.6X6
Etafenone	T46.3X1	T46.3X2	T46.3X3	T46.3X4	T46.3X5	T46.3X6
Etambutol	T37.1X1	T37.1X2	T37.1X3	T37.1X4	T37.1X5	T37.1X6
Etamiphyllin	T48.6X1	T48.6X2	T48.6X3	T48.6X4	T48.6X5	T48.6X6
Etamivan	T50.7X1	T50.7X2	T50.7X3	T50.7X4	T50.7X5	T50.7X6

Substance	Poisoning, Accidental (unintentional)	Poisoning, Intentional Self-harm	Poisoning, Assault	Poisoning, Undetermined	Adverse effect	Underdosing
Etamsylate	T45.7X1	T45.7X2	T45.7X3	T45.7X4	T45.7X5	T45.7X6
Etebenecid	T50.4X1	T50.4X2	T50.4X3	T50.4X4	T50.4X5	T50.4X6
Ethacridine	T49.0X1	T49.0X2	T49.0X3	T49.0X4	T49.0X5	T49.0X6
Ethacrynic acid	T50.1X1	T50.1X2	T50.1X3	T50.1X4	T50.1X5	T50.1X6
Ethadione	T42.2X1	T42.2X2	T42.2X3	T42.2X4	T42.2X5	T42.2X6
Ethambutol	T37.1X1	T37.1X2	T37.1X3	T37.1X4	T37.1X5	T37.1X6
Ethamide	T50.2X1	T50.2X2	T50.2X3	T50.2X4	T50.2X5	T50.2X6
Ethamivan	T50.7X1	T50.7X2	T50.7X3	T50.7X4	T50.7X5	T50.7X6
Ethamsylate	T45.7X1	T45.7X2	T45.7X3	T45.7X4	T45.7X5	T45.7X6
Ethanol	T51.0X1	T51.0X2	T51.0X3	T51.0X4	--	--
- beverage	T51.0X1	T51.0X2	T51.0X3	T51.0X4	--	--
Ethanolamine oleate	T46.8X1	T46.8X2	T46.8X3	T46.8X4	T46.8X5	T46.8X6
Ethaverine	T44.3X1	T44.3X2	T44.3X3	T44.3X4	T44.3X5	T44.3X6
Ethchlorvynol	T42.6X1	T42.6X2	T42.6X3	T42.6X4	T42.6X5	T42.6X6
Ethebenecid	T50.4X1	T50.4X2	T50.4X3	T50.4X4	T50.4X5	T50.4X6
Ether (vapor)	T41.0X1	T41.0X2	T41.0X3	T41.0X4	T41.0X5	T41.0X6
- anesthetic	T41.0X1	T41.0X2	T41.0X3	T41.0X4	T41.0X5	T41.0X6
- divinyl	T41.0X1	T41.0X2	T41.0X3	T41.0X4	T41.0X5	T41.0X6
- ethyl (medicinal)	T41.0X1	T41.0X2	T41.0X3	T41.0X4	T41.0X5	T41.0X6
- - nonmedicinal	T52.8X1	T52.8X2	T52.8X3	T52.8X4	--	--
- petroleum—see Ligroin						
- solvent	T52.8X1	T52.8X2	T52.8X3	T52.8X4	--	--
Ethiazide	T50.2X1	T50.2X2	T50.2X3	T50.2X4	T50.2X5	T50.2X6
Ethidium chloride (vapor)	T59.891	T59.892	T59.893	T59.894	--	--
Ethinamate	T42.6X1	T42.6X2	T42.6X3	T42.6X4	T42.6X5	T42.6X6
Ethinylestradiol, ethinyloestradiol	T38.5X1	T38.5X2	T38.5X3	T38.5X4	T38.5X5	T38.5X6
- with						
- - levonorgestrel	T38.4X1	T38.4X2	T38.4X3	T38.4X4	T38.4X5	T38.4X6
- - norethisterone	T38.4X1	T38.4X2	T38.4X3	T38.4X4	T38.4X5	T38.4X6
Ethiodized oil (131 I)	T50.8X1	T50.8X2	T50.8X3	T50.8X4	T50.8X5	T50.8X6
Ethion	T60.0X1	T60.0X2	T60.0X3	T60.0X4	--	--
Ethionamide	T37.1X1	T37.1X2	T37.1X3	T37.1X4	T37.1X5	T37.1X6
Ethioniamide	T37.1X1	T37.1X2	T37.1X3	T37.1X4	T37.1X5	T37.1X6
Ethisterone	T38.5X1	T38.5X2	T38.5X3	T38.5X4	T38.5X5	T38.5X6
Ethobral	T42.3X1	T42.3X2	T42.3X3	T42.3X4	T42.3X5	T42.3X6
Ethocaine (infiltration) (topical)	T41.3X1	T41.3X2	T41.3X3	T41.3X4	T41.3X5	T41.3X6
- nerve block (peripheral) (plexus)	T41.3X1	T41.3X2	T41.3X3	T41.3X4	T41.3X5	T41.3X6
- spinal	T41.3X1	T41.3X2	T41.3X3	T41.3X4	T41.3X5	T41.3X6
Ethoheptazine	T40.4X1	T40.4X2	T40.4X3	T40.4X4	T40.4X5	T40.4X6
Ethopropazine	T44.3X1	T44.3X2	T44.3X3	T44.3X4	T44.3X5	T44.3X6
Ethosuximide	T42.2X1	T42.2X2	T42.2X3	T42.2X4	T42.2X5	T42.2X6
Ethotoin	T42.0X1	T42.0X2	T42.0X3	T42.0X4	T42.0X5	T42.0X6
Ethoxazene	T37.91	T37.92	T37.93	T37.94	T37.95	T37.96
Ethoxazorutoside	T46.991	T46.992	T46.993	T46.994	T46.995	T46.996
2-Ethoxyethanol	T52.3X1	T52.3X2	T52.3X3	T52.3X4	--	--
Ethoxzolamide	T50.2X1	T50.2X2	T50.2X3	T50.2X4	T50.2X5	T50.2X6
Ethyl						
- acetate	T52.8X1	T52.8X2	T52.8X3	T52.8X4	--	--
- alcohol	T51.0X1	T51.0X2	T51.0X3	T51.0X4	--	--
- - beverage	T51.0X1	T51.0X2	T51.0X3	T51.0X4	--	--
- aldehyde (vapor)	T59.891	T59.892	T59.893	T59.894	--	--
- - liquid	T52.8X1	T52.8X2	T52.8X3	T52.8X4	--	--
- aminobenzoate	T41.3X1	T41.3X2	T41.3X3	T41.3X4	T41.3X5	T41.3X6
- aminophenothiazine	T43.3X1	T43.3X2	T43.3X3	T43.3X4	T43.3X5	T43.3X6
- benzoate	T52.8X1	T52.8X2	T52.8X3	T52.8X4	--	--
- biscoumacetate	T45.511	T45.512	T45.513	T45.514	T45.515	T45.516
- bromide (anesthetic)	T41.0X1	T41.0X2	T41.0X3	T41.0X4	T41.0X5	T41.0X6
- carbamate	T45.1X1	T45.1X2	T45.1X3	T45.1X4	T45.1X5	T45.1X6

Substance	Poisoning, Accidental (unintentional)	Poisoning, Intentional Self-harm	Poisoning, Assault	Poisoning, Undetermined	Adverse effect	Underdosing
- carbinol	T51.3X1	T51.3X2	T51.3X3	T51.3X4	--	--
- carbonate	T52.8X1	T52.8X2	T52.8X3	T52.8X4	--	--
- chaulmoograte	T37.1X1	T37.1X2	T37.1X3	T37.1X4	T37.1X5	T37.1X6
- chloride (anesthetic)	T41.0X1	T41.0X2	T41.0X3	T41.0X4	T41.0X5	T41.0X6
- - anesthetic (local)	T41.3X1	T41.3X2	T41.3X3	T41.3X4	T41.3X5	T41.3X6
- - - inhaled	T41.0X1	T41.0X2	T41.0X3	T41.0X4	T41.0X5	T41.0X6
- - local	T49.4X1	T49.4X2	T49.4X3	T49.4X4	T49.4X5	T49.4X6
- - solvent	T53.6X1	T53.6X2	T53.6X3	T53.6X4	--	--
- dibunate	T48.3X1	T48.3X2	T48.3X3	T48.3X4	T48.3X5	T48.3X6
- dichloroarsine (vapor)	T57.0X1	T57.0X2	T57.0X3	T57.0X4	--	--
- estranol	T38.7X1	T38.7X2	T38.7X3	T38.7X4	T38.7X5	T38.7X6
- ether—see also ether	T52.8X1	T52.8X2	T52.8X3	T52.8X4	--	--
- formate NEC (solvent)	T52.0X1	T52.0X2	T52.0X3	T52.0X4	--	--
- fumarate	T49.4X1	T49.4X2	T49.4X3	T49.4X4	T49.4X5	T49.4X6
- hydroxyisobutyrate NEC (solvent)	T52.8X1	T52.8X2	T52.8X3	T52.8X4	--	--
- iodoacetate	T59.3X1	T59.3X2	T59.3X3	T59.3X4	--	--
- lactate NEC (solvent)	T52.8X1	T52.8X2	T52.8X3	T52.8X4	--	--
- loflazepate	T42.4X1	T42.4X2	T42.4X3	T42.4X4	T42.4X5	T42.4X6
- mercuric chloride	T56.1X1	T56.1X2	T56.1X3	T56.1X4	--	--
- methylcarbinol	T51.8X1	T51.8X2	T51.8X3	T51.8X4	--	--
- morphine	T40.2X1	T40.2X2	T40.2X3	T40.2X4	T40.2X5	T40.2X6
- noradrenaline	T48.6X1	T48.6X2	T48.6X3	T48.6X4	T48.6X5	T48.6X6
- oxybutyrate NEC (solvent)	T52.8X1	T52.8X2	T52.8X3	T52.8X4	--	--
Ethylene (gas)	T59.891	T59.892	T59.893	T59.894	--	--
- anesthetic (general)	T41.0X1	T41.0X2	T41.0X3	T41.0X4	T41.0X5	T41.0X6
- chlorohydrin	T52.8X1	T52.8X2	T52.8X3	T52.8X4	--	--
- - vapor	T53.6X1	T53.6X2	T53.6X3	T53.6X4	--	--
- dichloride	T52.8X1	T52.8X2	T52.8X3	T52.8X4	--	--
- - vapor	T53.6X1	T53.6X2	T53.6X3	T53.6X4	--	--
- dinitrate	T52.3X1	T52.3X2	T52.3X3	T52.3X4	--	--
- glycol (s)	T52.8X1	T52.8X2	T52.8X3	T52.8X4	--	--
- - dinitrate	T52.3X1	T52.3X2	T52.3X3	T52.3X4	--	--
- - monobutyl ether	T52.3X1	T52.3X2	T52.3X3	T52.3X4	--	--
- imine	T54.1X1	T54.1X2	T54.1X3	T54.1X4	--	--
- oxide (fumigant) (nonmedicinal)	T59.891	T59.892	T59.893	T59.894	--	--
- - medicinal	T49.0X1	T49.0X2	T49.0X3	T49.0X4	T49.0X5	T49.0X6
Ethylenediamine theophylline	T48.6X1	T48.6X2	T48.6X3	T48.6X4	T48.6X5	T48.6X6
Ethylenediaminetetra-acetic acid	T50.6X1	T50.6X2	T50.6X3	T50.6X4	T50.6X5	T50.6X6
Ethylenedinitrilotetra-acetate	T50.6X1	T50.6X2	T50.6X3	T50.6X4	T50.6X5	T50.6X6
Ethylestrenol	T38.7X1	T38.7X2	T38.7X3	T38.7X4	T38.7X5	T38.7X6
Ethylhydroxycellulose	T47.4X1	T47.4X2	T47.4X3	T47.4X4	T47.4X5	T47.4X6
Ethylidene						
- chloride NEC	T53.6X1	T53.6X2	T53.6X3	T53.6X4	--	--
- diacetate	T60.3X1	T60.3X2	T60.3X3	T60.3X4	--	--
- dicoumarin	T45.511	T45.512	T45.513	T45.514	T45.515	T45.516
- dicoumarol	T45.511	T45.512	T45.513	T45.514	T45.515	T45.516
- diethyl ether	T52.0X1	T52.0X2	T52.0X3	T52.0X4	--	--
Ethylmorphine	T40.2X1	T40.2X2	T40.2X3	T40.2X4	T40.2X5	T40.2X6
Ethylnorepinephrine	T48.6X1	T48.6X2	T48.6X3	T48.6X4	T48.6X5	T48.6X6
Ethylparachlorophen-oxyisobutyrate	T46.6X1	T46.6X2	T46.6X3	T46.6X4	T46.6X5	T46.6X6
Ethynodiol	T38.4X1	T38.4X2	T38.4X3	T38.4X4	T38.4X5	T38.4X6
- with mestranol diacetate	T38.4X1	T38.4X2	T38.4X3	T38.4X4	T38.4X5	T38.4X6
Etidocaine	T41.3X1	T41.3X2	T41.3X3	T41.3X4	T41.3X5	T41.3X6
- infiltration (subcutaneous)	T41.3X1	T41.3X2	T41.3X3	T41.3X4	T41.3X5	T41.3X6
- nerve (peripheral) (plexus)	T41.3X1	T41.3X2	T41.3X3	T41.3X4	T41.3X5	T41.3X6
Etidronate	T50.991	T50.992	T50.993	T50.994	T50.995	T50.996
Etidronic acid (disodium salt)	T50.991	T50.992	T50.993	T50.994	T50.995	T50.996
Etifoxine	T42.6X1	T42.6X2	T42.6X3	T42.6X4	T42.6X5	T42.6X6
Etilefrine	T44.4X1	T44.4X2	T44.4X3	T44.4X4	T44.4X5	T44.4X6

Substance	Poisoning, Accidental (unintentional)	Poisoning, Intentional Self-harm	Poisoning, Assault	Poisoning, Undetermined	Adverse effect	Underdosing
Etilfen	T42.3X1	T42.3X2	T42.3X3	T42.3X4	T42.3X5	T42.3X6
Etinodiol	T38.4X1	T38.4X2	T38.4X3	T38.4X4	T38.4X5	T38.4X6
Etiroxate	T46.6X1	T46.6X2	T46.6X3	T46.6X4	T46.6X5	T46.6X6
Etizolam	T42.4X1	T42.4X2	T42.4X3	T42.4X4	T42.4X5	T42.4X6
Etodolac	T39.391	T39.392	T39.393	T39.394	T39.395	T39.396
Etofamide	T37.3X1	T37.3X2	T37.3X3	T37.3X4	T37.3X5	T37.3X6
Etofibrate	T46.6X1	T46.6X2	T46.6X3	T46.6X4	T46.6X5	T46.6X6
Etofylline	T46.7X1	T46.7X2	T46.7X3	T46.7X4	T46.7X5	T46.7X6
- clofibrate	T46.6X1	T46.6X2	T46.6X3	T46.6X4	T46.6X5	T46.6X6
Etoglucid	T45.1X1	T45.1X2	T45.1X3	T45.1X4	T45.1X5	T45.1X6
Etomidate	T41.1X1	T41.1X2	T41.1X3	T41.1X4	T41.1X5	T41.1X6
Etomide	T39.8X1	T39.8X2	T39.8X3	T39.8X4	T39.8X5	T39.8X6
Etomidoline	T44.3X1	T44.3X2	T44.3X3	T44.3X4	T44.3X5	T44.3X6
Etoposide	T45.1X1	T45.1X2	T45.1X3	T45.1X4	T45.1X5	T45.1X6
Etorphine	T40.2X1	T40.2X2	T40.2X3	T40.2X4	T40.2X5	T40.2X6
Etoval	T42.3X1	T42.3X2	T42.3X3	T42.3X4	T42.3X5	T42.3X6
Etozolin	T50.1X1	T50.1X2	T50.1X3	T50.1X4	T50.1X5	T50.1X6
Etretinate	T50.991	T50.992	T50.993	T50.994	T50.995	T50.996
Etryptamine	T43.691	T43.692	T43.693	T43.694	T43.695	T43.696
Etybenzatropine	T44.3X1	T44.3X2	T44.3X3	T44.3X4	T44.3X5	T44.3X6
Etynodiol	T38.4X1	T38.4X2	T38.4X3	T38.4X4	T38.4X5	T38.4X6
Eucaine	T41.3X1	T41.3X2	T41.3X3	T41.3X4	T41.3X5	T41.3X6
Eucalyptus oil	T49.7X1	T49.7X2	T49.7X3	T49.7X4	T49.7X5	T49.7X6
Eucatropine	T49.5X1	T49.5X2	T49.5X3	T49.5X4	T49.5X5	T49.5X6
Eucodal	T40.2X1	T40.2X2	T40.2X3	T40.2X4	T40.2X5	T40.2X6
Euneryl	T42.3X1	T42.3X2	T42.3X3	T42.3X4	T42.3X5	T42.3X6
Euphthalmine	T44.3X1	T44.3X2	T44.3X3	T44.3X4	T44.3X5	T44.3X6
Eurax	T49.0X1	T49.0X2	T49.0X3	T49.0X4	T49.0X5	T49.0X6
Euresol	T49.4X1	T49.4X2	T49.4X3	T49.4X4	T49.4X5	T49.4X6
Euthroid	T38.1X1	T38.1X2	T38.1X3	T38.1X4	T38.1X5	T38.1X6
Evans blue	T50.8X1	T50.8X2	T50.8X3	T50.8X4	T50.8X5	T50.8X6
Evipal	T42.3X1	T42.3X2	T42.3X3	T42.3X4	T42.3X5	T42.3X6
- sodium	T41.1X1	T41.1X2	T41.1X3	T41.1X4	T41.1X5	T41.1X6
Evipan	T42.3X1	T42.3X2	T42.3X3	T42.3X4	T42.3X5	T42.3X6
- sodium	T41.1X1	T41.1X2	T41.1X3	T41.1X4	T41.1X5	T41.1X6
Exalamide	T49.0X1	T49.0X2	T49.0X3	T49.0X4	T49.0X5	T49.0X6
Exalgin	T39.1X1	T39.1X2	T39.1X3	T39.1X4	T39.1X5	T39.1X6
Excipients, pharmaceutical	T50.901	T50.902	T50.903	T50.904	T50.905	T50.906
Exhaust gas (engine) (motor vehicle)	T58.01	T58.02	T58.03	T58.04	--	--
Ex-Lax (phenolphthalein)	T47.2X1	T47.2X2	T47.2X3	T47.2X4	T47.2X5	T47.2X6
Expectorant NEC	T48.4X1	T48.4X2	T48.4X3	T48.4X4	T48.4X5	T48.4X6
Extended insulin zinc suspension	T38.3X1	T38.3X2	T38.3X3	T38.3X4	T38.3X5	T38.3X6
External medications (skin) (mucous membrane)	T49.91	T49.92	T49.93	T49.94	T49.95	T49.96
- dental agent	T49.7X1	T49.7X2	T49.7X3	T49.7X4	T49.7X5	T49.7X6
- ENT agent	T49.6X1	T49.6X2	T49.6X3	T49.6X4	T49.6X5	T49.6X6
- ophthalmic preparation	T49.5X1	T49.5X2	T49.5X3	T49.5X4	T49.5X5	T49.5X6
- specified NEC	T49.8X1	T49.8X2	T49.8X3	T49.8X4	T49.8X5	T49.8X6
Extrapyramidal antagonist NEC	T44.3X1	T44.3X2	T44.3X3	T44.3X4	T44.3X5	T44.3X6
Eye agents (anti-infective)	T49.5X1	T49.5X2	T49.5X3	T49.5X4	T49.5X5	T49.5X6
Eye drug NEC	T49.5X1	T49.5X2	T49.5X3	T49.5X4	T49.5X5	T49.5X6
FAC (fluorouracil + doxorubicin + cyclophosphamide)	T45.1X1	T45.1X2	T45.1X3	T45.1X4	T45.1X5	T45.1X6
Factor						
- I (fibrinogen)	T45.8X1	T45.8X2	T45.8X3	T45.8X4	T45.8X5	T45.8X6
- III (thromboplastin)	T45.8X1	T45.8X2	T45.8X3	T45.8X4	T45.8X5	T45.8X6
- VIII (antihemophilic Factor) (concentrate)	T45.8X1	T45.8X2	T45.8X3	T45.8X4	T45.8X5	T45.8X6
- IX complex	T45.7X1	T45.7X2	T45.7X3	T45.7X4	T45.7X5	T45.7X6
- - human	T45.8X1	T45.8X2	T45.8X3	T45.8X4	T45.8X5	T45.8X6

Substance	Poisoning, Accidental (unintentional)	Poisoning, Intentional Self-harm	Poisoning, Assault	Poisoning, Undetermined	Adverse effect	Underdosing
Famotidine	T47.0X1	T47.0X2	T47.0X3	T47.0X4	T47.0X5	T47.0X6
Fat suspension, intravenous	T50.991	T50.992	T50.993	T50.994	T50.995	T50.996
Fazadinium bromide	T48.1X1	T48.1X2	T48.1X3	T48.1X4	T48.1X5	T48.1X6
Febarbamate	T42.3X1	T42.3X2	T42.3X3	T42.3X4	T42.3X5	T42.3X6
Fecal softener	T47.4X1	T47.4X2	T47.4X3	T47.4X4	T47.4X5	T47.4X6
Fedrilate	T48.3X1	T48.3X2	T48.3X3	T48.3X4	T48.3X5	T48.3X6
Felodipine	T46.1X1	T46.1X2	T46.1X3	T46.1X4	T46.1X5	T46.1X6
Felypressin	T38.891	T38.892	T38.893	T38.894	T38.895	T38.896
Femoxetine	T43.221	T43.222	T43.223	T43.224	T43.225	T43.226
Fenalcomine	T46.3X1	T46.3X2	T46.3X3	T46.3X4	T46.3X5	T46.3X6
Fenamisal	T37.1X1	T37.1X2	T37.1X3	T37.1X4	T37.1X5	T37.1X6
Fenazone	T39.2X1	T39.2X2	T39.2X3	T39.2X4	T39.2X5	T39.2X6
Fenbendazole	T37.4X1	T37.4X2	T37.4X3	T37.4X4	T37.4X5	T37.4X6
Fenbutrazate	T50.5X1	T50.5X2	T50.5X3	T50.5X4	T50.5X5	T50.5X6
Fencamfamine	T43.691	T43.692	T43.693	T43.694	T43.695	T43.696
Fendiline	T46.1X1	T46.1X2	T46.1X3	T46.1X4	T46.1X5	T46.1X6
Fenetylline	T43.691	T43.692	T43.693	T43.694	T43.695	T43.696
Fenflumizole	T39.391	T39.392	T39.393	T39.394	T39.395	T39.396
Fenfluramine	T50.5X1	T50.5X2	T50.5X3	T50.5X4	T50.5X5	T50.5X6
Fenobarbital	T42.3X1	T42.3X2	T42.3X3	T42.3X4	T42.3X5	T42.3X6
Fenofibrate	T46.6X1	T46.6X2	T46.6X3	T46.6X4	T46.6X5	T46.6X6
Fenoprofen	T39.311	T39.312	T39.313	T39.314	T39.315	T39.316
Fenoterol	T48.6X1	T48.6X2	T48.6X3	T48.6X4	T48.6X5	T48.6X6
Fenoverine	T44.3X1	T44.3X2	T44.3X3	T44.3X4	T44.3X5	T44.3X6
Fenoxazoline	T48.5X1	T48.5X2	T48.5X3	T48.5X4	T48.5X5	T48.5X6
Fenproporex	T50.5X1	T50.5X2	T50.5X3	T50.5X4	T50.5X5	T50.5X6
Fenquizone	T50.2X1	T50.2X2	T50.2X3	T50.2X4	T50.2X5	T50.2X6
Fentanyl	T40.4X1	T40.4X2	T40.4X3	T40.4X4	T40.4X5	T40.4X6
Fentazin	T43.3X1	T43.3X2	T43.3X3	T43.3X4	T43.3X5	T43.3X6
Fenthion	T60.0X1	T60.0X2	T60.0X3	T60.0X4	--	--
Fenticlor	T49.0X1	T49.0X2	T49.0X3	T49.0X4	T49.0X5	T49.0X6
Fenylbutazone	T39.2X1	T39.2X2	T39.2X3	T39.2X4	T39.2X5	T39.2X6
Feprazone	T39.2X1	T39.2X2	T39.2X3	T39.2X4	T39.2X5	T39.2X6
Fer de lance (bite) (venom)	T63.061	T63.062	T63.063	T63.064	--	--
Ferric—see also Iron						
- chloride	T45.4X1	T45.4X2	T45.4X3	T45.4X4	T45.4X5	T45.4X6
- citrate	T45.4X1	T45.4X2	T45.4X3	T45.4X4	T45.4X5	T45.4X6
- hydroxide						
- - colloidal	T45.4X1	T45.4X2	T45.4X3	T45.4X4	T45.4X5	T45.4X6
- - polymaltose	T45.4X1	T45.4X2	T45.4X3	T45.4X4	T45.4X5	T45.4X6
- pyrophosphate	T45.4X1	T45.4X2	T45.4X3	T45.4X4	T45.4X5	T45.4X6
Ferritin	T45.4X1	T45.4X2	T45.4X3	T45.4X4	T45.4X5	T45.4X6
Ferrocholinate	T45.4X1	T45.4X2	T45.4X3	T45.4X4	T45.4X5	T45.4X6
Ferrodextrane	T45.4X1	T45.4X2	T45.4X3	T45.4X4	T45.4X5	T45.4X6
Ferropolimaler	T45.4X1	T45.4X2	T45.4X3	T45.4X4	T45.4X5	T45.4X6
Ferrous—see also Iron						
- phosphate	T45.4X1	T45.4X2	T45.4X3	T45.4X4	T45.4X5	T45.4X6
- salt	T45.4X1	T45.4X2	T45.4X3	T45.4X4	T45.4X5	T45.4X6
- - with folic acid	T45.4X1	T45.4X2	T45.4X3	T45.4X4	T45.4X5	T45.4X6
Ferrous fumerate, gluconate, lactate, salt NEC, sulfate (medicinal)	T45.4X1	T45.4X2	T45.4X3	T45.4X4	T45.4X5	T45.4X6
Ferrovanadium (fumes)	T59.891	T59.892	T59.893	T59.894	--	--
Ferrum—see Iron						
Fertilizers NEC	T65.891	T65.892	T65.893	T65.894	--	--
- with herbicide mixture	T60.3X1	T60.3X2	T60.3X3	T60.3X4	--	--
Fetoxilate	T47.6X1	T47.6X2	T47.6X3	T47.6X4	T47.6X5	T47.6X6
Fiber, dietary	T47.4X1	T47.4X2	T47.4X3	T47.4X4	T47.4X5	T47.4X6
Fiberglass	T65.831	T65.832	T65.833	T65.834	--	--
Fibrinogen (human)	T45.8X1	T45.8X2	T45.8X3	T45.8X4	T45.8X5	T45.8X6

Substance	Poisoning, Accidental (unintentional)	Poisoning, Intentional Self-harm	Poisoning, Assault	Poisoning, Undetermined	Adverse effect	Underdosing
Fibrinolysin (human)	T45.691	T45.692	T45.693	T45.694	T45.695	T45.696
Fibrinolysis						
- affecting drug	T45.601	T45.602	T45.603	T45.604	T45.605	T45.606
- inhibitor NEC	T45.621	T45.622	T45.623	T45.624	T45.625	T45.626
Fibrinolytic drug	T45.611	T45.612	T45.613	T45.614	T45.615	T45.616
Filix mas	T37.4X1	T37.4X2	T37.4X3	T37.4X4	T37.4X5	T37.4X6
Filtering cream	T49.3X1	T49.3X2	T49.3X3	T49.3X4	T49.3X5	T49.3X6
Fiorinal	T39.011	T39.012	T39.013	T39.014	T39.015	T39.016
Firedamp	T59.891	T59.892	T59.893	T59.894	--	--
Fish, noxious, nonbacterial	T61.91	T61.92	T61.93	T61.94	--	--
- ciguatera	T61.01	T61.02	T61.03	T61.04	--	--
- scombroid	T61.11	T61.12	T61.13	T61.14	--	--
- shell	T61.781	T61.782	T61.783	T61.784	--	--
- specified NEC	T61.771	T61.772	T61.773	T61.774	--	--
Flagyl	T37.3X1	T37.3X2	T37.3X3	T37.3X4	T37.3X5	T37.3X6
Flavine adenine dinucleotide	T45.2X1	T45.2X2	T45.2X3	T45.2X4	T45.2X5	T45.2X6
Flavodic acid	T46.991	T46.992	T46.993	T46.994	T46.995	T46.996
Flavoxate	T44.3X1	T44.3X2	T44.3X3	T44.3X4	T44.3X5	T44.3X6
Flaxedil	T48.1X1	T48.1X2	T48.1X3	T48.1X4	T48.1X5	T48.1X6
Flaxseed (medicinal)	T49.3X1	T49.3X2	T49.3X3	T49.3X4	T49.3X5	T49.3X6
Flecainide	T46.2X1	T46.2X2	T46.2X3	T46.2X4	T46.2X5	T46.2X6
Fleroxacin	T36.8X1	T36.8X2	T36.8X3	T36.8X4	T36.8X5	T36.8X6
Floctafenine	T39.8X1	T39.8X2	T39.8X3	T39.8X4	T39.8X5	T39.8X6
Flomax	T44.6X1	T44.6X2	T44.6X3	T44.6X4	T44.6X5	T44.6X6
Flomoxef	T36.1X1	T36.1X2	T36.1X3	T36.1X4	T36.1X5	T36.1X6
Flopropione	T44.3X1	T44.3X2	T44.3X3	T44.3X4	T44.3X5	T44.3X6
Florantyrone	T47.5X1	T47.5X2	T47.5X3	T47.5X4	T47.5X5	T47.5X6
Floraquin	T37.8X1	T37.8X2	T37.8X3	T37.8X4	T37.8X5	T37.8X6
Florinef	T38.0X1	T38.0X2	T38.0X3	T38.0X4	T38.0X5	T38.0X6
- ENT agent	T49.6X1	T49.6X2	T49.6X3	T49.6X4	T49.6X5	T49.6X6
- ophthalmic preparation	T49.5X1	T49.5X2	T49.5X3	T49.5X4	T49.5X5	T49.5X6
- topical NEC	T49.0X1	T49.0X2	T49.0X3	T49.0X4	T49.0X5	T49.0X6
Flowers of sulfur	T49.4X1	T49.4X2	T49.4X3	T49.4X4	T49.4X5	T49.4X6
Floxuridine	T45.1X1	T45.1X2	T45.1X3	T45.1X4	T45.1X5	T45.1X6
Fluanisone	T43.4X1	T43.4X2	T43.4X3	T43.4X4	T43.4X5	T43.4X6
Flubendazole	T37.4X1	T37.4X2	T37.4X3	T37.4X4	T37.4X5	T37.4X6
Fluclorolone acetonide	T49.0X1	T49.0X2	T49.0X3	T49.0X4	T49.0X5	T49.0X6
Flucloxacillin	T36.0X1	T36.0X2	T36.0X3	T36.0X4	T36.0X5	T36.0X6
Fluconazole	T37.8X1	T37.8X2	T37.8X3	T37.8X4	T37.8X5	T37.8X6
Flucytosine	T37.8X1	T37.8X2	T37.8X3	T37.8X4	T37.8X5	T37.8X6
Fludeoxyglucose (18F)	T50.8X1	T50.8X2	T50.8X3	T50.8X4	T50.8X5	T50.8X6
Fludiazepam	T42.4X1	T42.4X2	T42.4X3	T42.4X4	T42.4X5	T42.4X6
Fludrocortisone	T50.0X1	T50.0X2	T50.0X3	T50.0X4	T50.0X5	T50.0X6
- ENT agent	T49.6X1	T49.6X2	T49.6X3	T49.6X4	T49.6X5	T49.6X6
- ophthalmic preparation	T49.5X1	T49.5X2	T49.5X3	T49.5X4	T49.5X5	T49.5X6
- topical NEC	T49.0X1	T49.0X2	T49.0X3	T49.0X4	T49.0X5	T49.0X6
Fludroxycortide	T49.0X1	T49.0X2	T49.0X3	T49.0X4	T49.0X5	T49.0X6
Flufenamic acid	T39.391	T39.392	T39.393	T39.394	T39.395	T39.396
Fluindione	T45.511	T45.512	T45.513	T45.514	T45.515	T45.516
Flumequine	T37.8X1	T37.8X2	T37.8X3	T37.8X4	T37.8X5	T37.8X6
Flumethasone	T49.0X1	T49.0X2	T49.0X3	T49.0X4	T49.0X5	T49.0X6
Flumethiazide	T50.2X1	T50.2X2	T50.2X3	T50.2X4	T50.2X5	T50.2X6
Flumidin	T37.5X1	T37.5X2	T37.5X3	T37.5X4	T37.5X5	T37.5X6
Flunarizine	T46.7X1	T46.7X2	T46.7X3	T46.7X4	T46.7X5	T46.7X6
Flunidazole	T37.8X1	T37.8X2	T37.8X3	T37.8X4	T37.8X5	T37.8X6
Flunisolide	T48.6X1	T48.6X2	T48.6X3	T48.6X4	T48.6X5	T48.6X6
Flunitrazepam	T42.4X1	T42.4X2	T42.4X3	T42.4X4	T42.4X5	T42.4X6
Fluocinolone (acetonide)	T49.0X1	T49.0X2	T49.0X3	T49.0X4	T49.0X5	T49.0X6

Substance	Poisoning, Accidental (unintentional)	Poisoning, Intentional Self-harm	Poisoning, Assault	Poisoning, Undetermined	Adverse effect	Underdosing
Fluocinonide	T49.0X1	T49.0X2	T49.0X3	T49.0X4	T49.0X5	T49.0X6
Fluocortin (butyl)	T49.0X1	T49.0X2	T49.0X3	T49.0X4	T49.0X5	T49.0X6
Fluocortolone	T49.0X1	T49.0X2	T49.0X3	T49.0X4	T49.0X5	T49.0X6
Fluohydrocortisone	T38.0X1	T38.0X2	T38.0X3	T38.0X4	T38.0X5	T38.0X6
- ENT agent	T49.6X1	T49.6X2	T49.6X3	T49.6X4	T49.6X5	T49.6X6
- ophthalmic preparation	T49.5X1	T49.5X2	T49.5X3	T49.5X4	T49.5X5	T49.5X6
- topical NEC	T49.0X1	T49.0X2	T49.0X3	T49.0X4	T49.0X5	T49.0X6
Fluonid	T49.0X1	T49.0X2	T49.0X3	T49.0X4	T49.0X5	T49.0X6
Fluopromazine	T43.3X1	T43.3X2	T43.3X3	T43.3X4	T43.3X5	T43.3X6
Fluoracetate	T60.8X1	T60.8X2	T60.8X3	T60.8X4	--	--
Fluorescein	T50.8X1	T50.8X2	T50.8X3	T50.8X4	T50.8X5	T50.8X6
Fluorhydrocortisone	T50.0X1	T50.0X2	T50.0X3	T50.0X4	T50.0X5	T50.0X6
Fluoride (nonmedicinal) (pesticide) (sodium) NEC	T60.8X1	T60.8X2	T60.8X3	T60.8X4	--	--
- hydrogen—see Hydrofluoric acid						
- medicinal NEC	T50.991	T50.992	T50.993	T50.994	T50.995	T50.996
- - dental use	T49.7X1	T49.7X2	T49.7X3	T49.7X4	T49.7X5	T49.7X6
- not pesticide NEC	T54.91	T54.92	T54.93	T54.94	--	--
- stannous	T49.7X1	T49.7X2	T49.7X3	T49.7X4	T49.7X5	T49.7X6
Fluorinated corticosteroids	T38.0X1	T38.0X2	T38.0X3	T38.0X4	T38.0X5	T38.0X6
Fluorine (gas)	T59.5X1	T59.5X2	T59.5X3	T59.5X4	--	--
- salt—see Fluoride (s)						
Fluoristan	T49.7X1	T49.7X2	T49.7X3	T49.7X4	T49.7X5	T49.7X6
Fluormetholone	T49.0X1	T49.0X2	T49.0X3	T49.0X4	T49.0X5	T49.0X6
Fluoroacetate	T60.8X1	T60.8X2	T60.8X3	T60.8X4	--	--
Fluorocarbon monomer	T53.6X1	T53.6X2	T53.6X3	T53.6X4	--	--
Fluorocytosine	T37.8X1	T37.8X2	T37.8X3	T37.8X4	T37.8X5	T37.8X6
Fluorodeoxyuridine	T45.1X1	T45.1X2	T45.1X3	T45.1X4	T45.1X5	T45.1X6
Fluorometholone	T49.0X1	T49.0X2	T49.0X3	T49.0X4	T49.0X5	T49.0X6
Fluorophosphate insecticide	T60.0X1	T60.0X2	T60.0X3	T60.0X4	--	--
Fluorosol	T46.3X1	T46.3X2	T46.3X3	T46.3X4	T46.3X5	T46.3X6
Fluorouracil	T45.1X1	T45.1X2	T45.1X3	T45.1X4	T45.1X5	T45.1X6
Fluorphenylalanine	T49.5X1	T49.5X2	T49.5X3	T49.5X4	T49.5X5	T49.5X6
Fluothane	T41.0X1	T41.0X2	T41.0X3	T41.0X4	T41.0X5	T41.0X6
Fluoxetine	T43.221	T43.222	T43.223	T43.224	T43.225	T43.226
Fluoxymesterone	T38.7X1	T38.7X2	T38.7X3	T38.7X4	T38.7X5	T38.7X6
Flupenthixol	T43.4X1	T43.4X2	T43.4X3	T43.4X4	T43.4X5	T43.4X6
Flupentixol	T43.4X1	T43.4X2	T43.4X3	T43.4X4	T43.4X5	T43.4X6
Fluphenazine	T43.3X1	T43.3X2	T43.3X3	T43.3X4	T43.3X5	T43.3X6
Fluprednidene	T49.0X1	T49.0X2	T49.0X3	T49.0X4	T49.0X5	T49.0X6
Fluprednisolone	T38.0X1	T38.0X2	T38.0X3	T38.0X4	T38.0X5	T38.0X6
Fluradoline	T39.8X1	T39.8X2	T39.8X3	T39.8X4	T39.8X5	T39.8X6
Flurandrenolide	T49.0X1	T49.0X2	T49.0X3	T49.0X4	T49.0X5	T49.0X6
Flurandrenolone	T49.0X1	T49.0X2	T49.0X3	T49.0X4	T49.0X5	T49.0X6
Flurazepam	T42.4X1	T42.4X2	T42.4X3	T42.4X4	T42.4X5	T42.4X6
Flurbiprofen	T39.311	T39.312	T39.313	T39.314	T39.315	T39.316
Flurobate	T49.0X1	T49.0X2	T49.0X3	T49.0X4	T49.0X5	T49.0X6
Fluroxene	T41.0X1	T41.0X2	T41.0X3	T41.0X4	T41.0X5	T41.0X6
Fluspirilene	T43.591	T43.592	T43.593	T43.594	T43.595	T43.596
Flutamide	T38.6X1	T38.6X2	T38.6X3	T38.6X4	T38.6X5	T38.6X6
Flutazolam	T42.4X1	T42.4X2	T42.4X3	T42.4X4	T42.4X5	T42.4X6
Fluticasone propionate	T38.0X1	T38.0X2	T38.0X3	T38.0X4	T38.0X5	T38.0X6
Flutoprazepam	T42.4X1	T42.4X2	T42.4X3	T42.4X4	T42.4X5	T42.4X6
Flutropium bromide	T48.6X1	T48.6X2	T48.6X3	T48.6X4	T48.6X5	T48.6X6
Fluvoxamine	T43.221	T43.222	T43.223	T43.224	T43.225	T43.226
Folacin	T45.8X1	T45.8X2	T45.8X3	T45.8X4	T45.8X5	T45.8X6
Folic acid	T45.8X1	T45.8X2	T45.8X3	T45.8X4	T45.8X5	T45.8X6
- with ferrous salt	T45.2X1	T45.2X2	T45.2X3	T45.2X4	T45.2X5	T45.2X6
- antagonist	T45.1X1	T45.1X2	T45.1X3	T45.1X4	T45.1X5	T45.1X6

Substance	Poisoning, Accidental (unintentional)	Poisoning, Intentional Self-harm	Poisoning, Assault	Poisoning, Undetermined	Adverse effect	Underdosing
Folinic acid	T45.8X1	T45.8X2	T45.8X3	T45.8X4	T45.8X5	T45.8X6
Folium stramoniae	T48.6X1	T48.6X2	T48.6X3	T48.6X4	T48.6X5	T48.6X6
Follicle-stimulating hormone, human	T38.811	T38.812	T38.813	T38.814	T38.815	T38.816
Folpet	T60.3X1	T60.3X2	T60.3X3	T60.3X4	--	--
Fominoben	T48.3X1	T48.3X2	T48.3X3	T48.3X4	T48.3X5	T48.3X6
Food, foodstuffs, noxious, nonbacterial, NEC	T62.91	T62.92	T62.93	T62.94	--	--
- berries	T62.1X1	T62.1X2	T62.1X3	T62.1X4	--	--
- fish—see also Fish	T61.91	T61.92	T61.93	T61.94	--	--
- mushrooms	T62.0X1	T62.0X2	T62.0X3	T62.0X4	--	--
- plants	T62.2X1	T62.2X2	T62.2X3	T62.2X4	--	--
- seafood	T61.91	T61.92	T61.93	T61.94	--	--
- - specified NEC	T61.8X1	T61.8X2	T61.8X3	T61.8X4	--	--
- seeds	T62.2X1	T62.2X2	T62.2X3	T62.2X4	--	--
- shellfish	T61.781	T61.782	T61.783	T61.784	--	--
- specified NEC	T62.8X1	T62.8X2	T62.8X3	T62.8X4	--	--
Fool's parsley	T62.2X1	T62.2X2	T62.2X3	T62.2X4	--	--
Formaldehyde (solution), gas or vapor	T59.2X1	T59.2X2	T59.2X3	T59.2X4	--	--
- fungicide	T60.3X1	T60.3X2	T60.3X3	T60.3X4	--	--
Formalin	T59.2X1	T59.2X2	T59.2X3	T59.2X4	--	--
- fungicide	T60.3X1	T60.3X2	T60.3X3	T60.3X4	--	--
- vapor	T59.2X1	T59.2X2	T59.2X3	T59.2X4	--	--
Formic acid	T54.2X1	T54.2X2	T54.2X3	T54.2X4	--	--
- vapor	T59.891	T59.892	T59.893	T59.894	--	--
Foscarnet sodium	T37.5X1	T37.5X2	T37.5X3	T37.5X4	T37.5X5	T37.5X6
Fosfestrol	T38.5X1	T38.5X2	T38.5X3	T38.5X4	T38.5X5	T38.5X6
Fosfomycin	T36.8X1	T36.8X2	T36.8X3	T36.8X4	T36.8X5	T36.8X6
Fosfonet sodium	T37.5X1	T37.5X2	T37.5X3	T37.5X4	T37.5X5	T37.5X6
Fosinopril	T46.4X1	T46.4X2	T46.4X3	T46.4X4	T46.4X5	T46.4X6
- sodium	T46.4X1	T46.4X2	T46.4X3	T46.4X4	T46.4X5	T46.4X6
Fowler's solution	T57.0X1	T57.0X2	T57.0X3	T57.0X4	--	--
Foxglove	T62.2X1	T62.2X2	T62.2X3	T62.2X4	--	--
Framycetin	T36.5X1	T36.5X2	T36.5X3	T36.5X4	T36.5X5	T36.5X6
Frangula	T47.2X1	T47.2X2	T47.2X3	T47.2X4	T47.2X5	T47.2X6
- extract	T47.2X1	T47.2X2	T47.2X3	T47.2X4	T47.2X5	T47.2X6
Frei antigen	T50.8X1	T50.8X2	T50.8X3	T50.8X4	T50.8X5	T50.8X6
Freon	T53.5X1	T53.5X2	T53.5X3	T53.5X4	--	--
Fructose	T50.3X1	T50.3X2	T50.3X3	T50.3X4	T50.3X5	T50.3X6
Frusemide	T50.1X1	T50.1X2	T50.1X3	T50.1X4	T50.1X5	T50.1X6
FSH	T38.811	T38.812	T38.813	T38.814	T38.815	T38.816
Ftorafur	T45.1X1	T45.1X2	T45.1X3	T45.1X4	T45.1X5	T45.1X6
Fuel						
- automobile	T52.0X1	T52.0X2	T52.0X3	T52.0X4	--	--
- - exhaust gas, not in transit	T58.01	T58.02	T58.03	T58.04	--	--
- - vapor NEC	T52.0X1	T52.0X2	T52.0X3	T52.0X4	--	--
- gas (domestic use) —see also Carbon, monoxide, fuel, utility	T59.891	T59.892	T59.893	T59.894	--	--
- - utility	T59.891	T59.892	T59.893	T59.894	--	--
- - - in mobile container	T59.891	T59.892	T59.893	T59.894	--	--
- - - incomplete combustion of—see Carbon, monoxide, fuel, utility						
- - - piped (natural)	T59.891	T59.892	T59.893	T59.894	--	--
- industrial, incomplete combustion	T58.8X1	T58.8X2	T58.8X3	T58.8X4	--	--
Fugillin	T36.8X1	T36.8X2	T36.8X3	T36.8X4	T36.8X5	T36.8X6
Fulminate of mercury	T56.1X1	T56.1X2	T56.1X3	T56.1X4	--	--
Fulvicin	T36.7X1	T36.7X2	T36.7X3	T36.7X4	T36.7X5	T36.7X6
Fumadil	T36.8X1	T36.8X2	T36.8X3	T36.8X4	T36.8X5	T36.8X6
Fumagillin	T36.8X1	T36.8X2	T36.8X3	T36.8X4	T36.8X5	T36.8X6
Fumaric acid	T49.4X1	T49.4X2	T49.4X3	T49.4X4	T49.4X5	T49.4X6
Fumes (from)	T59.91	T59.92	T59.93	T59.94	--	--

Substance	Poisoning, Accidental (unintentional)	Poisoning, Intentional Self-harm	Poisoning, Assault	Poisoning, Undetermined	Adverse effect	Underdosing
- carbon monoxide—see Carbon, monoxide						
- charcoal (domestic use) —see Charcoal, fumes						
- chloroform—see Chloroform						
- coke (in domestic stoves, fireplaces) —see Coke fumes						
- corrosive NEC	T54.91	T54.92	T54.93	T54.94	--	--
- ether—see ether						
- freons	T53.5X1	T53.5X2	T53.5X3	T53.5X4	--	--
- hydrocarbons	T59.891	T59.892	T59.893	T59.894	--	--
- - petroleum (liquefied)	T59.891	T59.892	T59.893	T59.894	--	--
- - - distributed through pipes (pure or mixed with air)	T59.891	T59.892	T59.893	T59.894	--	--
- lead—see lead						
- metal—see Metals, or the specified metal						
- nitrogen dioxide	T59.0X1	T59.0X2	T59.0X3	T59.0X4	--	--
- pesticides—see Pesticides						
- petroleum (liquefied)	T59.891	T59.892	T59.893	T59.894	--	--
- - distributed through pipes (pure or mixed with air)	T59.891	T59.892	T59.893	T59.894	--	--
- polyester	T59.891	T59.892	T59.893	T59.894	--	--
- specified source NEC—see also substance specified	T59.891	T59.892	T59.893	T59.894	--	--
- sulfur dioxide	T59.1X1	T59.1X2	T59.1X3	T59.1X4	--	--
Fumigant NEC	T60.91	T60.92	T60.93	T60.94	--	--
Fungi, noxious, used as food	T62.0X1	T62.0X2	T62.0X3	T62.0X4	--	--
Fungicide NEC (nonmedicinal)	T60.3X1	T60.3X2	T60.3X3	T60.3X4	--	--
Fungizone	T36.7X1	T36.7X2	T36.7X3	T36.7X4	T36.7X5	T36.7X6
- topical	T49.0X1	T49.0X2	T49.0X3	T49.0X4	T49.0X5	T49.0X6
Furacin	T49.0X1	T49.0X2	T49.0X3	T49.0X4	T49.0X5	T49.0X6
Furadantin	T37.91	T37.92	T37.93	T37.94	T37.95	T37.96
Furazolidone	T37.8X1	T37.8X2	T37.8X3	T37.8X4	T37.8X5	T37.8X6
Furazolium chloride	T49.0X1	T49.0X2	T49.0X3	T49.0X4	T49.0X5	T49.0X6
Furfural	T52.8X1	T52.8X2	T52.8X3	T52.8X4	--	--
Furnace (coal burning) (domestic) , gas from	T58.2X1	T58.2X2	T58.2X3	T58.2X4	--	--
- industrial	T58.8X1	T58.8X2	T58.8X3	T58.8X4	--	--
Furniture polish	T65.891	T65.892	T65.893	T65.894	--	--
Furosemide	T50.1X1	T50.1X2	T50.1X3	T50.1X4	T50.1X5	T50.1X6
Furoxone	T37.91	T37.92	T37.93	T37.94	T37.95	T37.96
Fursultiamine	T45.2X1	T45.2X2	T45.2X3	T45.2X4	T45.2X5	T45.2X6
Fusafungine	T36.8X1	T36.8X2	T36.8X3	T36.8X4	T36.8X5	T36.8X6
Fusel oil (any) (amyl) (butyl) (propyl) , vapor	T51.3X1	T51.3X2	T51.3X3	T51.3X4	--	--
Fusidate (ethanolamine) (sodium)	T36.8X1	T36.8X2	T36.8X3	T36.8X4	T36.8X5	T36.8X6
Fusidic acid	T36.8X1	T36.8X2	T36.8X3	T36.8X4	T36.8X5	T36.8X6
Fytic acid, nonasodium	T50.6X1	T50.6X2	T50.6X3	T50.6X4	T50.6X5	T50.6X6
GABA	T43.8X1	T43.8X2	T43.8X3	T43.8X4	T43.8X5	T43.8X6
Gadopentetic acid	T50.8X1	T50.8X2	T50.8X3	T50.8X4	T50.8X5	T50.8X6
Galactose	T50.3X1	T50.3X2	T50.3X3	T50.3X4	T50.3X5	T50.3X6
b-Galactosidase	T47.5X1	T47.5X2	T47.5X3	T47.5X4	T47.5X5	T47.5X6
Galantamine	T44.0X1	T44.0X2	T44.0X3	T44.0X4	T44.0X5	T44.0X6
Gallamine (triethiodide)	T48.1X1	T48.1X2	T48.1X3	T48.1X4	T48.1X5	T48.1X6
Gallium citrate	T50.991	T50.992	T50.993	T50.994	T50.995	T50.996
Gallopamil	T46.1X1	T46.1X2	T46.1X3	T46.1X4	T46.1X5	T46.1X6
Gamboge	T47.2X1	T47.2X2	T47.2X3	T47.2X4	T47.2X5	T47.2X6
Gamimune	T50.Z11	T50.Z12	T50.Z13	T50.Z14	T50.Z15	T50.Z16
Gamma globulin	T50.Z11	T50.Z12	T50.Z13	T50.Z14	T50.Z15	T50.Z16
Gamma-aminobutyric acid	T43.8X1	T43.8X2	T43.8X3	T43.8X4	T43.8X5	T43.8X6
Gamma-benzene hexachloride (medicinal)	T49.0X1	T49.0X2	T49.0X3	T49.0X4	T49.0X5	T49.0X6
- nonmedicinal, vapor	T53.6X1	T53.6X2	T53.6X3	T53.6X4	--	--
Gamma-BHC (medicinal) —see also Gamma- benzene hexachloride	T49.0X1	T49.0X2	T49.0X3	T49.0X4	T49.0X5	T49.0X6

Substance	Poisoning, Accidental (unintentional)	Poisoning, Intentional Self-harm	Poisoning, Assault	Poisoning, Undetermined	Adverse effect	Underdosing
Gamulin	T50.Z11	T50.Z12	T50.Z13	T50.Z14	T50.Z15	T50.Z16
Ganciclovir (sodium)	T37.5X1	T37.5X2	T37.5X3	T37.5X4	T37.5X5	T37.5X6
Ganglionic blocking drug NEC	T44.2X1	T44.2X2	T44.2X3	T44.2X4	T44.2X5	T44.2X6
- specified NEC	T44.2X1	T44.2X2	T44.2X3	T44.2X4	T44.2X5	T44.2X6
Ganja	T40.7X1	T40.7X2	T40.7X3	T40.7X4	T40.7X5	T40.7X6
Garamycin	T36.5X1	T36.5X2	T36.5X3	T36.5X4	T36.5X5	T36.5X6
- ophthalmic preparation	T49.5X1	T49.5X2	T49.5X3	T49.5X4	T49.5X5	T49.5X6
- topical NEC	T49.0X1	T49.0X2	T49.0X3	T49.0X4	T49.0X5	T49.0X6
Gardenal	T42.3X1	T42.3X2	T42.3X3	T42.3X4	T42.3X5	T42.3X6
Gardepanyl	T42.3X1	T42.3X2	T42.3X3	T42.3X4	T42.3X5	T42.3X6
Gas NEC	T59.91	T59.92	T59.93	T59.94	--	--
- acetylene	T59.891	T59.892	T59.893	T59.894	--	--
- - incomplete combustion of	T58.11	T58.12	T58.13	T58.14	--	--
- air contaminants, source or type not specified	T59.91	T59.92	T59.93	T59.94	--	--
- anesthetic	T41.0X1	T41.0X2	T41.0X3	T41.0X4	T41.0X5	T41.0X6
- blast furnace	T58.8X1	T58.8X2	T58.8X3	T58.8X4	--	--
- butane - see butane						
- carbon monoxide - see Carbon, monoxide						
- chlorine	T59.4X1	T59.4X2	T59.4X3	T59.4X4	--	--
- coal	T58.2X1	T58.2X2	T58.2X3	T58.2X4	--	--
- cyanide	T57.3X1	T57.3X2	T57.3X3	T57.3X4	--	--
- dicyanogen	T65.0X1	T65.0X2	T65.0X3	T65.0X4	--	--
- domestic - see Domestic gas						
- exhaust	T58.01	T58.02	T58.03	T58.04	--	--
- from utility (for cooking, heating, or lighting) (after combustion) – see Carbon, monoxide, fuel, utility						
- - prior to combustion	T59.891	T59.892	T59.893	T59.894	--	--
- from wood- or coal-burning stove or fireplace	T58.2X1	T58.2X2	T58.2X3	T58.2X4	--	--
- fuel (domestic use) (after combustion) - see also Carbon, monoxide, fuel						
- - industrial use	T58.8X1	T58.8X2	T58.8X3	T58.8X4	--	--
- - prior to combustion	T59.891	T59.892	T59.893	T59.894	--	--
- - utility	T59.891	T59.892	T59.893	T59.894	--	--
- - - in mobile container	T59.891	T59.892	T59.893	T59.894	--	--
- - - incomplete combustion of – see Carbon, monoxide, fuel, utility						
- - - piped (natural)	T59.891	T59.892	T59.893	T59.894	--	--
- garage	T58.01	T58.02	T58.03	T58.04	--	--
- hydrocarbon NEC	T59.891	T59.892	T59.893	T59.894	--	--
- - incomplete combustion of – see Carbon, monoxide, fuel, utility						
- - liquefied - see butane						
- - - piped	T59.891	T59.892	T59.893	T59.894	--	--
- hydrocyanic acid	T65.0X1	T65.0X2	T65.0X3	T65.0X4	--	--
- illuminating (after combustion)	T58.11	T58.12	T58.13	T58.14	--	--
- - prior to combustion	T59.891	T59.892	T59.893	T59.894	--	--
- incomplete combustion, any – see Carbon, monoxide						
- kiln	T58.8X1	T58.8X2	T58.8X3	T58.8X4	--	--
- lacrimogenic	T59.3X1	T59.3X2	T59.3X3	T59.3X4	--	--
- liquefied petroleum - see butane						
- marsh	T59.891	T59.892	T59.893	T59.894	--	--
- motor exhaust, not in transit	T58.01	T58.02	T58.03	T58.04	--	--
- mustard, not in war	T59.891	T59.892	T59.893	T59.894	--	--
- natural	T59.891	T59.892	T59.893	T59.894	--	--
- nerve, not in war	T59.91	T59.92	T59.93	T59.94	--	--
- oil	T52.0X1	T52.0X2	T52.0X3	T52.0X4	--	--
- petroleum (liquefied) (distributed in mobile containers)	T59.891	T59.892	T59.893	T59.894	--	--
- - piped (pure or mixed with air)	T59.891	T59.892	T59.893	T59.894	--	--

Substance	Poisoning, Accidental (unintentional)	Poisoning, Intentional Self-harm	Poisoning, Assault	Poisoning, Undetermined	Adverse effect	Underdosing
- piped (manufactured) (natural) NEC	T59.891	T59.892	T59.893	T59.894	--	--
- producer	T58.8X1	T58.8X2	T58.8X3	T58.8X4	--	--
- propane - see propane						
- refrigerant (chlorofluoro-carbon)	T53.5X1	T53.5X2	T53.5X3	T53.5X4	--	--
- - not chlorofluoro-carbon	T59.891	T59.892	T59.893	T59.894	--	--
- sewer	T59.91	T59.92	T59.93	T59.94	--	--
- specified source NEC	T59.91	T59.92	T59.93	T59.94	--	--
- stove (after combustion)	T58.11	T58.12	T58.13	T58.14	--	--
- - prior to combustion	T59.891	T59.892	T59.893	T59.894	--	--
- tear	T59.3X1	T59.3X2	T59.3X3	T59.3X4	--	--
- therapeutic	T41.5X1	T41.5X2	T41.5X3	T41.5X4	T41.5X5	T41.5X6
- utility (for cooking, heating, or lighting) (piped) NEC	T59.891	T59.892	T59.893	T59.894	--	--
- - in mobile container	T59.891	T59.892	T59.893	T59.894	--	--
- - incomplete combustion of – see Carbon, monoxide, fuel, utilty						
- - piped (natural)	T59.891	T59.892	T59.893	T59.894	--	--
- water	T58.11	T58.12	T58.13	T58.14	--	--
- - incomplete combustion of – see Carbon, monoxide, fuel, utility						
Gaseous substance—see Gas						
Gasoline	T52.0X1	T52.0X2	T52.0X3	T52.0X4	--	--
- vapor	T52.0X1	T52.0X2	T52.0X3	T52.0X4	--	--
Gastric enzymes	T47.5X1	T47.5X2	T47.5X3	T47.5X4	T47.5X5	T47.5X6
Gastrografin	T50.8X1	T50.8X2	T50.8X3	T50.8X4	T50.8X5	T50.8X6
Gastrointestinal drug	T47.91	T47.92	T47.93	T47.94	T47.95	T47.96
- biological	T47.8X1	T47.8X2	T47.8X3	T47.8X4	T47.8X5	T47.8X6
- specified NEC	T47.8X1	T47.8X2	T47.8X3	T47.8X4	T47.8X5	T47.8X6
Gaultheria procumbens	T62.2X1	T62.2X2	T62.2X3	T62.2X4	--	--
Gefarnate	T44.3X1	T44.3X2	T44.3X3	T44.3X4	T44.3X5	T44.3X6
Gelatin (intravenous)	T45.8X1	T45.8X2	T45.8X3	T45.8X4	T45.8X5	T45.8X6
- absorbable (sponge)	T45.7X1	T45.7X2	T45.7X3	T45.7X4	T45.7X5	T45.7X6
Gelfilm	T49.8X1	T49.8X2	T49.8X3	T49.8X4	T49.8X5	T49.8X6
Gelfoam	T45.7X1	T45.7X2	T45.7X3	T45.7X4	T45.7X5	T45.7X6
Gelsemine	T50.991	T50.992	T50.993	T50.994	T50.995	T50.996
Gelsemium (sempervirens)	T62.2X1	T62.2X2	T62.2X3	T62.2X4	--	--
Gemeprost	T48.0X1	T48.0X2	T48.0X3	T48.0X4	T48.0X5	T48.0X6
Gemfibrozil	T46.6X1	T46.6X2	T46.6X3	T46.6X4	T46.6X5	T46.6X6
Gemonil	T42.3X1	T42.3X2	T42.3X3	T42.3X4	T42.3X5	T42.3X6
Gentamicin	T36.5X1	T36.5X2	T36.5X3	T36.5X4	T36.5X5	T36.5X6
- ophthalmic preparation	T49.5X1	T49.5X2	T49.5X3	T49.5X4	T49.5X5	T49.5X6
- topical NEC	T49.0X1	T49.0X2	T49.0X3	T49.0X4	T49.0X5	T49.0X6
Gentian	T47.5X1	T47.5X2	T47.5X3	T47.5X4	T47.5X5	T47.5X6
- violet	T49.0X1	T49.0X2	T49.0X3	T49.0X4	T49.0X5	T49.0X6
Gepefrine	T44.4X1	T44.4X2	T44.4X3	T44.4X4	T44.4X5	T44.4X6
Gestonorone caproate	T38.5X1	T38.5X2	T38.5X3	T38.5X4	T38.5X5	T38.5X6
Gexane	T49.0X1	T49.0X2	T49.0X3	T49.0X4	T49.0X5	T49.0X6
Gila monster (venom)	T63.111	T63.112	T63.113	T63.114	--	--
Ginger	T47.5X1	T47.5X2	T47.5X3	T47.5X4	T47.5X5	T47.5X6
- Jamaica—see Jamaica, ginger						
Gitalin	T46.0X1	T46.0X2	T46.0X3	T46.0X4	T46.0X5	T46.0X6
- amorphous	T46.0X1	T46.0X2	T46.0X3	T46.0X4	T46.0X5	T46.0X6
Gitaloxin	T46.0X1	T46.0X2	T46.0X3	T46.0X4	T46.0X5	T46.0X6
Gitoxin	T46.0X1	T46.0X2	T46.0X3	T46.0X4	T46.0X5	T46.0X6
Glafenine	T39.8X1	T39.8X2	T39.8X3	T39.8X4	T39.8X5	T39.8X6
Glandular extract (medicinal) NEC	T50.Z91	T50.Z92	T50.Z93	T50.Z94	T50.Z95	T50.Z96
Glaucarubin	T37.3X1	T37.3X2	T37.3X3	T37.3X4	T37.3X5	T37.3X6
Glibenclamide	T38.3X1	T38.3X2	T38.3X3	T38.3X4	T38.3X5	T38.3X6
Glibornuride	T38.3X1	T38.3X2	T38.3X3	T38.3X4	T38.3X5	T38.3X6
Gliclazide	T38.3X1	T38.3X2	T38.3X3	T38.3X4	T38.3X5	T38.3X6

Substance	Poisoning, Accidental (unintentional)	Poisoning, Intentional Self-harm	Poisoning, Assault	Poisoning, Undetermined	Adverse effect	Underdosing
Glimidine	T38.3X1	T38.3X2	T38.3X3	T38.3X4	T38.3X5	T38.3X6
Glipizide	T38.3X1	T38.3X2	T38.3X3	T38.3X4	T38.3X5	T38.3X6
Gliquidone	T38.3X1	T38.3X2	T38.3X3	T38.3X4	T38.3X5	T38.3X6
Glisolamide	T38.3X1	T38.3X2	T38.3X3	T38.3X4	T38.3X5	T38.3X6
Glisoxepide	T38.3X1	T38.3X2	T38.3X3	T38.3X4	T38.3X5	T38.3X6
Globin zinc insulin	T38.3X1	T38.3X2	T38.3X3	T38.3X4	T38.3X5	T38.3X6
Globulin						
- antilymphocytic	T50.Z11	T50.Z12	T50.Z13	T50.Z14	T50.Z15	T50.Z16
- antirhesus	T50.Z11	T50.Z12	T50.Z13	T50.Z14	T50.Z15	T50.Z16
- antivenin	T50.Z11	T50.Z12	T50.Z13	T50.Z14	T50.Z15	T50.Z16
- antiviral	T50.Z11	T50.Z12	T50.Z13	T50.Z14	T50.Z15	T50.Z16
Glucagon	T38.3X1	T38.3X2	T38.3X3	T38.3X4	T38.3X5	T38.3X6
Glucocorticoids	T38.0X1	T38.0X2	T38.0X3	T38.0X4	T38.0X5	T38.0X6
Glucocorticosteroid	T38.0X1	T38.0X2	T38.0X3	T38.0X4	T38.0X5	T38.0X6
Gluconic acid	T50.991	T50.992	T50.993	T50.994	T50.995	T50.996
Glucosamine sulfate	T39.4X1	T39.4X2	T39.4X3	T39.4X4	T39.4X5	T39.4X6
Glucose	T50.3X1	T50.3X2	T50.3X3	T50.3X4	T50.3X5	T50.3X6
- with sodium chloride	T50.3X1	T50.3X2	T50.3X3	T50.3X4	T50.3X5	T50.3X6
Glucosulfone sodium	T37.1X1	T37.1X2	T37.1X3	T37.1X4	T37.1X5	T37.1X6
Glucurolactone	T47.8X1	T47.8X2	T47.8X3	T47.8X4	T47.8X5	T47.8X6
Glue NEC	T52.8X1	T52.8X2	T52.8X3	T52.8X4	--	--
Glutamic acid	T47.5X1	T47.5X2	T47.5X3	T47.5X4	T47.5X5	T47.5X6
Glutaral (medicinal)	T49.0X1	T49.0X2	T49.0X3	T49.0X4	T49.0X5	T49.0X6
- nonmedicinal	T65.891	T65.892	T65.893	T65.894	--	--
Glutaraldehyde (nonmedicinal)	T65.891	T65.892	T65.893	T65.894	--	--
- medicinal	T49.0X1	T49.0X2	T49.0X3	T49.0X4	T49.0X5	T49.0X6
Glutathione	T50.6X1	T50.6X2	T50.6X3	T50.6X4	T50.6X5	T50.6X6
Glutethimide	T42.6X1	T42.6X2	T42.6X3	T42.6X4	T42.6X5	T42.6X6
Glyburide	T38.3X1	T38.3X2	T38.3X3	T38.3X4	T38.3X5	T38.3X6
Glycerin	T47.4X1	T47.4X2	T47.4X3	T47.4X4	T47.4X5	T47.4X6
Glycerol	T47.4X1	T47.4X2	T47.4X3	T47.4X4	T47.4X5	T47.4X6
- borax	T49.6X1	T49.6X2	T49.6X3	T49.6X4	T49.6X5	T49.6X6
- intravenous	T50.3X1	T50.3X2	T50.3X3	T50.3X4	T50.3X5	T50.3X6
- iodinated	T48.4X1	T48.4X2	T48.4X3	T48.4X4	T48.4X5	T48.4X6
Glycerophosphate	T50.991	T50.992	T50.993	T50.994	T50.995	T50.996
Glyceryl						
- gualacolate	T48.4X1	T48.4X2	T48.4X3	T48.4X4	T48.4X5	T48.4X6
- nitrate	T46.3X1	T46.3X2	T46.3X3	T46.3X4	T46.3X5	T46.3X6
- triacetate (topical)	T49.0X1	T49.0X2	T49.0X3	T49.0X4	T49.0X5	T49.0X6
- trinitrate	T46.3X1	T46.3X2	T46.3X3	T46.3X4	T46.3X5	T46.3X6
Glycine	T50.3X1	T50.3X2	T50.3X3	T50.3X4	T50.3X5	T50.3X6
Glyclopyramide	T38.3X1	T38.3X2	T38.3X3	T38.3X4	T38.3X5	T38.3X6
Glycobiarsol	T37.3X1	T37.3X2	T37.3X3	T37.3X4	T37.3X5	T37.3X6
Glycols (ether)	T52.3X1	T52.3X2	T52.3X3	T52.3X4	--	--
Glyconiazide	T37.1X1	T37.1X2	T37.1X3	T37.1X4	T37.1X5	T37.1X6
Glycopyrrolate	T44.3X1	T44.3X2	T44.3X3	T44.3X4	T44.3X5	T44.3X6
Glycopyrronium	T44.3X1	T44.3X2	T44.3X3	T44.3X4	T44.3X5	T44.3X6
- bromide	T44.3X1	T44.3X2	T44.3X3	T44.3X4	T44.3X5	T44.3X6
Glycoside, cardiac (stimulant)	T46.0X1	T46.0X2	T46.0X3	T46.0X4	T46.0X5	T46.0X6
Glycyclamide	T38.3X1	T38.3X2	T38.3X3	T38.3X4	T38.3X5	T38.3X6
Glycyrrhiza extract	T48.4X1	T48.4X2	T48.4X3	T48.4X4	T48.4X5	T48.4X6
Glycyrrhizic acid	T48.4X1	T48.4X2	T48.4X3	T48.4X4	T48.4X5	T48.4X6
Glycyrrhizinate potassium	T48.4X1	T48.4X2	T48.4X3	T48.4X4	T48.4X5	T48.4X6
Glymidine sodium	T38.3X1	T38.3X2	T38.3X3	T38.3X4	T38.3X5	T38.3X6
Glyphosate	T60.3X1	T60.3X2	T60.3X3	T60.3X4	--	--
Glyphylline	T48.6X1	T48.6X2	T48.6X3	T48.6X4	T48.6X5	T48.6X6
Gold						
- colloidal (l98Au)	T45.1X1	T45.1X2	T45.1X3	T45.1X4	T45.1X5	T45.1X6

Substance	Poisoning, Accidental (unintentional)	Poisoning, Intentional Self-harm	Poisoning, Assault	Poisoning, Undetermined	Adverse effect	Underdosing
- salts	T39.4X1	T39.4X2	T39.4X3	T39.4X4	T39.4X5	T39.4X6
Golden sulfide of antimony	T56.891	T56.892	T56.893	T56.894	--	--
Goldylocks	T62.2X1	T62.2X2	T62.2X3	T62.2X4	--	--
Gonadal tissue extract	T38.901	T38.902	T38.903	T38.904	T38.905	T38.906
- female	T38.5X1	T38.5X2	T38.5X3	T38.5X4	T38.5X5	T38.5X6
- male	T38.7X1	T38.7X2	T38.7X3	T38.7X4	T38.7X5	T38.7X6
Gonadorelin	T38.891	T38.892	T38.893	T38.894	T38.895	T38.896
Gonadotropin	T38.891	T38.892	T38.893	T38.894	T38.895	T38.896
- chorionic	T38.891	T38.892	T38.893	T38.894	T38.895	T38.896
- pituitary	T38.811	T38.812	T38.813	T38.814	T38.815	T38.816
Goserelin	T45.1X1	T45.1X2	T45.1X3	T45.1X4	T45.1X5	T45.1X6
Grain alcohol	T51.0X1	T51.0X2	T51.0X3	T51.0X4	--	--
Gramicidin	T49.0X1	T49.0X2	T49.0X3	T49.0X4	T49.0X5	T49.0X6
Granisetron	T45.0X1	T45.0X2	T45.0X3	T45.0X4	T45.0X5	T45.0X6
Gratiola officinalis	T62.2X1	T62.2X2	T62.2X3	T62.2X4	--	--
Grease	T65.891	T65.892	T65.893	T65.894	--	--
Green hellebore	T62.2X1	T62.2X2	T62.2X3	T62.2X4	--	--
Green soap	T49.2X1	T49.2X2	T49.2X3	T49.2X4	T49.2X5	T49.2X6
Grifulvin	T36.7X1	T36.7X2	T36.7X3	T36.7X4	T36.7X5	T36.7X6
Griseofulvin	T36.7X1	T36.7X2	T36.7X3	T36.7X4	T36.7X5	T36.7X6
Growth hormone	T38.811	T38.812	T38.813	T38.814	T38.815	T38.816
Guaiac reagent	T50.991	T50.992	T50.993	T50.994	T50.995	T50.996
Guaiacol derivatives	T48.4X1	T48.4X2	T48.4X3	T48.4X4	T48.4X5	T48.4X6
Guaifenesin	T48.4X1	T48.4X2	T48.4X3	T48.4X4	T48.4X5	T48.4X6
Guaimesal	T48.4X1	T48.4X2	T48.4X3	T48.4X4	T48.4X5	T48.4X6
Guaiphenesin	T48.4X1	T48.4X2	T48.4X3	T48.4X4	T48.4X5	T48.4X6
Guamecycline	T36.4X1	T36.4X2	T36.4X3	T36.4X4	T36.4X5	T36.4X6
Guanabenz	T46.5X1	T46.5X2	T46.5X3	T46.5X4	T46.5X5	T46.5X6
Guanacline	T46.5X1	T46.5X2	T46.5X3	T46.5X4	T46.5X5	T46.5X6
Guanadrel	T46.5X1	T46.5X2	T46.5X3	T46.5X4	T46.5X5	T46.5X6
Guanatol	T37.2X1	T37.2X2	T37.2X3	T37.2X4	T37.2X5	T37.2X6
Guanethidine	T46.5X1	T46.5X2	T46.5X3	T46.5X4	T46.5X5	T46.5X6
Guanfacine	T46.5X1	T46.5X2	T46.5X3	T46.5X4	T46.5X5	T46.5X6
Guano	T65.891	T65.892	T65.893	T65.894	--	--
Guanochlor	T46.5X1	T46.5X2	T46.5X3	T46.5X4	T46.5X5	T46.5X6
Guanoclor	T46.5X1	T46.5X2	T46.5X3	T46.5X4	T46.5X5	T46.5X6
Guanoctine	T46.5X1	T46.5X2	T46.5X3	T46.5X4	T46.5X5	T46.5X6
Guanoxabenz	T46.5X1	T46.5X2	T46.5X3	T46.5X4	T46.5X5	T46.5X6
Guanoxan	T46.5X1	T46.5X2	T46.5X3	T46.5X4	T46.5X5	T46.5X6
Guar gum (medicinal)	T46.6X1	T46.6X2	T46.6X3	T46.6X4	T46.6X5	T46.6X6
Hachimycin	T36.7X1	T36.7X2	T36.7X3	T36.7X4	T36.7X5	T36.7X6
Hair						
- dye	T49.4X1	T49.4X2	T49.4X3	T49.4X4	T49.4X5	T49.4X6
- preparation NEC	T49.4X1	T49.4X2	T49.4X3	T49.4X4	T49.4X5	T49.4X6
Halazepam	T42.4X1	T42.4X2	T42.4X3	T42.4X4	T42.4X5	T42.4X6
Halcinolone	T49.0X1	T49.0X2	T49.0X3	T49.0X4	T49.0X5	T49.0X6
Halcinonide	T49.0X1	T49.0X2	T49.0X3	T49.0X4	T49.0X5	T49.0X6
Halethazole	T49.0X1	T49.0X2	T49.0X3	T49.0X4	T49.0X5	T49.0X6
Hallucinogen NEC	T40.901	T40.902	T40.903	T40.904	T40.905	T40.906
Halofantrine	T37.2X1	T37.2X2	T37.2X3	T37.2X4	T37.2X5	T37.2X6
Halofenate	T46.6X1	T46.6X2	T46.6X3	T46.6X4	T46.6X5	T46.6X6
Halometasone	T49.0X1	T49.0X2	T49.0X3	T49.0X4	T49.0X5	T49.0X6
Haloperidol	T43.4X1	T43.4X2	T43.4X3	T43.4X4	T43.4X5	T43.4X6
Haloprogin	T49.0X1	T49.0X2	T49.0X3	T49.0X4	T49.0X5	T49.0X6
Halotex	T49.0X1	T49.0X2	T49.0X3	T49.0X4	T49.0X5	T49.0X6
Halothane	T41.0X1	T41.0X2	T41.0X3	T41.0X4	T41.0X5	T41.0X6
Haloxazolam	T42.4X1	T42.4X2	T42.4X3	T42.4X4	T42.4X5	T42.4X6
Halquinols	T49.0X1	T49.0X2	T49.0X3	T49.0X4	T49.0X5	T49.0X6
Hamamelis	T49.2X1	T49.2X2	T49.2X3	T49.2X4	T49.2X5	T49.2X6

Substance	Poisoning, Accidental (unintentional)	Poisoning, Intentional Self-harm	Poisoning, Assault	Poisoning, Undetermined	Adverse effect	Underdosing
Haptendextran	T45.8X1	T45.8X2	T45.8X3	T45.8X4	T45.8X5	T45.8X6
Harmonyl	T46.5X1	T46.5X2	T46.5X3	T46.5X4	T46.5X5	T46.5X6
Hartmann's solution	T50.3X1	T50.3X2	T50.3X3	T50.3X4	T50.3X5	T50.3X6
Hashish	T40.7X1	T40.7X2	T40.7X3	T40.7X4	T40.7X5	T40.7X6
Hawaiian Woodrose seeds	T40.991	T40.992	T40.993	T40.994	--	--
HCB	T60.3X1	T60.3X2	T60.3X3	T60.3X4	--	--
HCH	T53.6X1	T53.6X2	T53.6X3	T53.6X4	--	--
- medicinal	T49.0X1	T49.0X2	T49.0X3	T49.0X4	T49.0X5	T49.0X6
HCN	T57.3X1	T57.3X2	T57.3X3	T57.3X4	--	--
Headache cures, drugs, powders NEC	T50.901	T50.902	T50.903	T50.904	T50.905	T50.906
Heavenly Blue (morning glory)	T40.991	T40.992	T40.993	T40.994	--	--
Heavy metal antidote	T45.8X1	T45.8X2	T45.8X3	T45.8X4	T45.8X5	T45.8X6
Hedaquinium	T49.0X1	T49.0X2	T49.0X3	T49.0X4	T49.0X5	T49.0X6
Hedge hyssop	T62.2X1	T62.2X2	T62.2X3	T62.2X4	--	--
Heet	T49.8X1	T49.8X2	T49.8X3	T49.8X4	T49.8X5	T49.8X6
Helenin	T37.4X1	T37.4X2	T37.4X3	T37.4X4	T37.4X5	T37.4X6
Helium (nonmedicinal) NEC	T59.891	T59.892	T59.893	T59.894	--	--
- medicinal	T48.991	T48.992	T48.993	T48.994	T48.995	T48.996
Hellebore (black) (green) (white)	T62.2X1	T62.2X2	T62.2X3	T62.2X4	--	--
Hematin	T45.8X1	T45.8X2	T45.8X3	T45.8X4	T45.8X5	T45.8X6
Hematinic preparation	T45.8X1	T45.8X2	T45.8X3	T45.8X4	T45.8X5	T45.8X6
Hematological agent	T45.91	T45.92	T45.93	T45.94	T45.95	T45.96
- specified NEC	T45.8X1	T45.8X2	T45.8X3	T45.8X4	T45.8X5	T45.8X6
Hemlock	T62.2X1	T62.2X2	T62.2X3	T62.2X4	--	--
Hemostatic	T45.621	T45.622	T45.623	T45.624	T45.625	T45.626
- drug, systemic	T45.621	T45.622	T45.623	T45.624	T45.625	T45.626
Hemostyptic	T49.4X1	T49.4X2	T49.4X3	T49.4X4	T49.4X5	T49.4X6
Henbane	T62.2X1	T62.2X2	T62.2X3	T62.2X4	--	--
Heparin (sodium)	T45.511	T45.512	T45.513	T45.514	T45.515	T45.516
- action reverser	T45.7X1	T45.7X2	T45.7X3	T45.7X4	T45.7X5	T45.7X6
Heparin-fraction	T45.511	T45.512	T45.513	T45.514	T45.515	T45.516
Heparinoid (systemic)	T45.511	T45.512	T45.513	T45.514	T45.515	T45.516
Hepatic secretion stimulant	T47.8X1	T47.8X2	T47.8X3	T47.8X4	T47.8X5	T47.8X6
Hepatitis B						
- immune globulin	T50.Z11	T50.Z12	T50.Z13	T50.Z14	T50.Z15	T50.Z16
- vaccine	T50.B91	T50.B92	T50.B93	T50.B94	T50.B95	T50.B96
Hepronicate	T46.7X1	T46.7X2	T46.7X3	T46.7X4	T46.7X5	T46.7X6
Heptabarb	T42.3X1	T42.3X2	T42.3X3	T42.3X4	T42.3X5	T42.3X6
Heptabarbital	T42.3X1	T42.3X2	T42.3X3	T42.3X4	T42.3X5	T42.3X6
Heptabarbitone	T42.3X1	T42.3X2	T42.3X3	T42.3X4	T42.3X5	T42.3X6
Heptachlor	T60.1X1	T60.1X2	T60.1X3	T60.1X4	--	--
Heptalgin	T40.2X1	T40.2X2	T40.2X3	T40.2X4	T40.2X5	T40.2X6
Heptaminol	T46.3X1	T46.3X2	T46.3X3	T46.3X4	T46.3X5	T46.3X6
Herbicide NEC	T60.3X1	T60.3X2	T60.3X3	T60.3X4	--	--
Heroin	T40.1X1	T40.1X2	T40.1X3	T40.1X4	T40.1X5	--
Herplex	T49.5X1	T49.5X2	T49.5X3	T49.5X4	T49.5X5	T49.5X6
HES	T45.8X1	T45.8X2	T45.8X3	T45.8X4	T45.8X5	T45.8X6
Hesperidin	T46.991	T46.992	T46.993	T46.994	T46.995	T46.996
Hetacillin	T36.0X1	T36.0X2	T36.0X3	T36.0X4	T36.0X5	T36.0X6
Hetastarch	T45.8X1	T45.8X2	T45.8X3	T45.8X4	T45.8X5	T45.8X6
HETP	T60.0X1	T60.0X2	T60.0X3	T60.0X4	--	--
Hexachlorobenzene (vapor)	T60.3X1	T60.3X2	T60.3X3	T60.3X4	--	--
Hexachlorocyclohexane	T53.6X1	T53.6X2	T53.6X3	T53.6X4	--	--
Hexachlorophene	T49.0X1	T49.0X2	T49.0X3	T49.0X4	T49.0X5	T49.0X6
Hexadiline	T46.3X1	T46.3X2	T46.3X3	T46.3X4	T46.3X5	T46.3X6
Hexadimethrine (bromide)	T45.7X1	T45.7X2	T45.7X3	T45.7X4	T45.7X5	T45.7X6
Hexadylamine	T46.3X1	T46.3X2	T46.3X3	T46.3X4	T46.3X5	T46.3X6
Hexaethyl tetraphos-phate	T60.0X1	T60.0X2	T60.0X3	T60.0X4	--	--

Substance	Poisoning, Accidental (unintentional)	Poisoning, Intentional Self-harm	Poisoning, Assault	Poisoning, Undetermined	Adverse effect	Underdosing
Hexafluorenium bromide	T48.1X1	T48.1X2	T48.1X3	T48.1X4	T48.1X5	T48.1X6
Hexafluronium (bromide)	T48.1X1	T48.1X2	T48.1X3	T48.1X4	T48.1X5	T48.1X6
Hexa-germ	T49.2X1	T49.2X2	T49.2X3	T49.2X4	T49.2X5	T49.2X6
Hexahydrobenzol	T52.8X1	T52.8X2	T52.8X3	T52.8X4	--	--
Hexahydrocresol (s)	T51.8X1	T51.8X2	T51.8X3	T51.8X4	--	--
- arsenide	T57.0X1	T57.0X2	T57.0X3	T57.0X4	--	--
- arseniurated	T57.0X1	T57.0X2	T57.0X3	T57.0X4	--	--
- cyanide	T57.3X1	T57.3X2	T57.3X3	T57.3X4	--	--
- - gas	T59.891	T59.892	T59.893	T59.894	--	--
- Fluoride (liquid)	T57.8X1	T57.8X2	T57.8X3	T57.8X4	--	--
- - vapor	T59.891	T59.892	T59.893	T59.894	--	--
- phophorated	T60.0X1	T60.0X2	T60.0X3	T60.0X4	--	--
- sulfate	T57.8X1	T57.8X2	T57.8X3	T57.8X4	--	--
- sulfide (gas)	T59.6X1	T59.6X2	T59.6X3	T59.6X4	--	--
- - arseniurated	T57.0X1	T57.0X2	T57.0X3	T57.0X4	--	--
- sulfurated	T57.8X1	T57.8X2	T57.8X3	T57.8X4	--	--
Hexahydrophenol	T51.8X1	T51.8X2	T51.8X3	T51.8X4	--	--
Hexalen	T51.8X1	T51.8X2	T51.8X3	T51.8X4	--	--
Hexamethonium bromide	T44.2X1	T44.2X2	T44.2X3	T44.2X4	T44.2X5	T44.2X6
Hexamethylene	T52.8X1	T52.8X2	T52.8X3	T52.8X4	--	--
Hexamethylmelamine	T45.1X1	T45.1X2	T45.1X3	T45.1X4	T45.1X5	T45.1X6
Hexamidine	T49.0X1	T49.0X2	T49.0X3	T49.0X4	T49.0X5	T49.0X6
Hexamine (mandelate)	T37.8X1	T37.8X2	T37.8X3	T37.8X4	T37.8X5	T37.8X6
Hexanone, 2-hexanone	T52.4X1	T52.4X2	T52.4X3	T52.4X4	--	--
Hexanuorenium	T48.1X1	T48.1X2	T48.1X3	T48.1X4	T48.1X5	T48.1X6
Hexapropymate	T42.6X1	T42.6X2	T42.6X3	T42.6X4	T42.6X5	T42.6X6
Hexasonium iodide	T44.3X1	T44.3X2	T44.3X3	T44.3X4	T44.3X5	T44.3X6
Hexcarbacholine bromide	T48.1X1	T48.1X2	T48.1X3	T48.1X4	T48.1X5	T48.1X6
Hexemal	T42.3X1	T42.3X2	T42.3X3	T42.3X4	T42.3X5	T42.3X6
Hexestrol	T38.5X1	T38.5X2	T38.5X3	T38.5X4	T38.5X5	T38.5X6
Hexethal (sodium)	T42.3X1	T42.3X2	T42.3X3	T42.3X4	T42.3X5	T42.3X6
Hexetidine	T37.8X1	T37.8X2	T37.8X3	T37.8X4	T37.8X5	T37.8X6
Hexobarbital	T42.3X1	T42.3X2	T42.3X3	T42.3X4	T42.3X5	T42.3X6
- rectal	T41.291	T41.292	T41.293	T41.294	T41.295	T41.296
- sodium	T41.1X1	T41.1X2	T41.1X3	T41.1X4	T41.1X5	T41.1X6
Hexobendine	T46.3X1	T46.3X2	T46.3X3	T46.3X4	T46.3X5	T46.3X6
Hexocyclium	T44.3X1	T44.3X2	T44.3X3	T44.3X4	T44.3X5	T44.3X6
- metilsulfate	T44.3X1	T44.3X2	T44.3X3	T44.3X4	T44.3X5	T44.3X6
Hexoestrol	T38.5X1	T38.5X2	T38.5X3	T38.5X4	T38.5X5	T38.5X6
Hexone	T52.4X1	T52.4X2	T52.4X3	T52.4X4	--	--
Hexoprenaline	T48.6X1	T48.6X2	T48.6X3	T48.6X4	T48.6X5	T48.6X6
Hexylcaine	T41.3X1	T41.3X2	T41.3X3	T41.3X4	T41.3X5	T41.3X6
Hexylresorcinol	T52.2X1	T52.2X2	T52.2X3	T52.2X4	--	--
HGH (human growth hormone)	T38.811	T38.812	T38.813	T38.814	T38.815	T38.816
Hinkle's pills	T47.2X1	T47.2X2	T47.2X3	T47.2X4	T47.2X5	T47.2X6
Histalog	T50.8X1	T50.8X2	T50.8X3	T50.8X4	T50.8X5	T50.8X6
Histamine (phosphate)	T50.8X1	T50.8X2	T50.8X3	T50.8X4	T50.8X5	T50.8X6
Histoplasmin	T50.8X1	T50.8X2	T50.8X3	T50.8X4	T50.8X5	T50.8X6
Holly berries	T62.2X1	T62.2X2	T62.2X3	T62.2X4	--	--
Homatropine	T44.3X1	T44.3X2	T44.3X3	T44.3X4	T44.3X5	T44.3X6
- methylbromide	T44.3X1	T44.3X2	T44.3X3	T44.3X4	T44.3X5	T44.3X6
Homochlorcyclizine	T45.0X1	T45.0X2	T45.0X3	T45.0X4	T45.0X5	T45.0X6
Homosalate	T49.3X1	T49.3X2	T49.3X3	T49.3X4	T49.3X5	T49.3X6
Homo-tet	T50.Z11	T50.Z12	T50.Z13	T50.Z14	T50.Z15	T50.Z16
Hormone	T38.801	T38.802	T38.803	T38.804	T38.805	T38.806
- adrenal cortical steroids	T38.0X1	T38.0X2	T38.0X3	T38.0X4	T38.0X5	T38.0X6
- androgenic	T38.7X1	T38.7X2	T38.7X3	T38.7X4	T38.7X5	T38.7X6
- anterior pituitary NEC	T38.811	T38.812	T38.813	T38.814	T38.815	T38.816
- antidiabetic agents	T38.3X1	T38.3X2	T38.3X3	T38.3X4	T38.3X5	T38.3X6

Substance	Poisoning, Accidental (unintentional)	Poisoning, Intentional Self-harm	Poisoning, Assault	Poisoning, Undetermined	Adverse effect	Underdosing
- antidiuretic	T38.891	T38.892	T38.893	T38.894	T38.895	T38.896
- cancer therapy	T45.1X1	T45.1X2	T45.1X3	T45.1X4	T45.1X5	T45.1X6
- follicle stimulating	T38.811	T38.812	T38.813	T38.814	T38.815	T38.816
- gonadotropic	T38.891	T38.892	T38.893	T38.894	T38.895	T38.896
- - pituitary	T38.811	T38.812	T38.813	T38.814	T38.815	T38.816
- growth	T38.811	T38.812	T38.813	T38.814	T38.815	T38.816
- luteinizing	T38.811	T38.812	T38.813	T38.814	T38.815	T38.816
- ovarian	T38.5X1	T38.5X2	T38.5X3	T38.5X4	T38.5X5	T38.5X6
- oxytocic	T48.0X1	T48.0X2	T48.0X3	T48.0X4	T48.0X5	T48.0X6
- parathyroid (derivatives)	T50.991	T50.992	T50.993	T50.994	T50.995	T50.996
- pituitary (posterior) NEC	T38.891	T38.892	T38.893	T38.894	T38.895	T38.896
- - anterior	T38.811	T38.812	T38.813	T38.814	T38.815	T38.816
- specified, NEC	T38.891	T38.892	T38.893	T38.894	T38.895	T38.896
- thyroid	T38.1X1	T38.1X2	T38.1X3	T38.1X4	T38.1X5	T38.1X6
Hornet (sting)	T63.451	T63.452	T63.453	T63.454	--	--
Horse anti-human lymphocytic serum	T50.Z11	T50.Z12	T50.Z13	T50.Z14	T50.Z15	T50.Z16
Horticulture agent NEC	T65.91	T65.92	T65.93	T65.94	--	--
- with pesticide	T60.91	T60.92	T60.93	T60.94	--	--
Human						
- albumin	T45.8X1	T45.8X2	T45.8X3	T45.8X4	T45.8X5	T45.8X6
- growth hormone (HGH)	T38.811	T38.812	T38.813	T38.814	T38.815	T38.816
- immune serum	T50.Z11	T50.Z12	T50.Z13	T50.Z14	T50.Z15	T50.Z16
Hyaluronidase	T45.3X1	T45.3X2	T45.3X3	T45.3X4	T45.3X5	T45.3X6
Hyazyme	T45.3X1	T45.3X2	T45.3X3	T45.3X4	T45.3X5	T45.3X6
Hycodan	T40.2X1	T40.2X2	T40.2X3	T40.2X4	T40.2X5	T40.2X6
Hydantoin derivative NEC	T42.0X1	T42.0X2	T42.0X3	T42.0X4	T42.0X5	T42.0X6
Hydeltra	T38.0X1	T38.0X2	T38.0X3	T38.0X4	T38.0X5	T38.0X6
Hydergine	T44.6X1	T44.6X2	T44.6X3	T44.6X4	T44.6X5	T44.6X6
Hydrabamine penicillin	T36.0X1	T36.0X2	T36.0X3	T36.0X4	T36.0X5	T36.0X6
Hydralazine	T46.5X1	T46.5X2	T46.5X3	T46.5X4	T46.5X5	T46.5X6
Hydrargaphen	T49.0X1	T49.0X2	T49.0X3	T49.0X4	T49.0X5	T49.0X6
Hydrargyri amino-chloridum	T49.0X1	T49.0X2	T49.0X3	T49.0X4	T49.0X5	T49.0X6
Hydrastine	T48.291	T48.292	T48.293	T48.294	T48.295	T48.296
Hydrazine	T54.1X1	T54.1X2	T54.1X3	T54.1X4	--	--
- monoamine oxidase inhibitors	T43.1X1	T43.1X2	T43.1X3	T43.1X4	T43.1X5	T43.1X6
Hydrazoic acid, azides	T54.2X1	T54.2X2	T54.2X3	T54.2X4	--	--
Hydriodic acid	T48.4X1	T48.4X2	T48.4X3	T48.4X4	T48.4X5	T48.4X6
Hydrocarbon gas	T59.891	T59.892	T59.893	T59.894	--	--
- incomplete combustion of—see Carbon, monoxide, fuel, utility						
- liquefied (mobile container)	T59.891	T59.892	T59.893	T59.894	--	--
- - piped (natural)	T59.891	T59.892	T59.893	T59.894	--	--
Hydrochloric acid (liquid)	T54.2X1	T54.2X2	T54.2X3	T54.2X4	--	--
- medicinal (digestant)	T47.5X1	T47.5X2	T47.5X3	T47.5X4	T47.5X5	T47.5X6
- vapor	T59.891	T59.892	T59.893	T59.894	--	--
Hydrochlorothiazide	T50.2X1	T50.2X2	T50.2X3	T50.2X4	T50.2X5	T50.2X6
Hydrocodone	T40.2X1	T40.2X2	T40.2X3	T40.2X4	T40.2X5	T40.2X6
Hydrocortisone (derivatives)	T38.0X1	T38.0X2	T38.0X3	T38.0X4	T38.0X5	T38.0X6
- aceponate	T49.0X1	T49.0X2	T49.0X3	T49.0X4	T49.0X5	T49.0X6
- ENT agent	T49.6X1	T49.6X2	T49.6X3	T49.6X4	T49.6X5	T49.6X6
- ophthalmic preparation	T49.5X1	T49.5X2	T49.5X3	T49.5X4	T49.5X5	T49.5X6
- topical NEC	T49.0X1	T49.0X2	T49.0X3	T49.0X4	T49.0X5	T49.0X6
Hydrocortone	T38.0X1	T38.0X2	T38.0X3	T38.0X4	T38.0X5	T38.0X6
- ENT agent	T49.6X1	T49.6X2	T49.6X3	T49.6X4	T49.6X5	T49.6X6
- ophthalmic preparation	T49.5X1	T49.5X2	T49.5X3	T49.5X4	T49.5X5	T49.5X6
- topical NEC	T49.0X1	T49.0X2	T49.0X3	T49.0X4	T49.0X5	T49.0X6
Hydrocyanic acid (liquid)	T57.3X1	T57.3X2	T57.3X3	T57.3X4	--	--
- gas	T65.0X1	T65.0X2	T65.0X3	T65.0X4	--	--
Hydroflumethiazide	T50.2X1	T50.2X2	T50.2X3	T50.2X4	T50.2X5	T50.2X6

Substance	Poisoning, Accidental (unintentional)	Poisoning, Intentional Self-harm	Poisoning, Assault	Poisoning, Undetermined	Adverse effect	Underdosing
Hydrofluoric acid (liquid)	T54.2X1	T54.2X2	T54.2X3	T54.2X4	--	--
- vapor	T59.891	T59.892	T59.893	T59.894	--	--
Hydrogen	T59.891	T59.892	T59.893	T59.894	--	--
- arsenide	T57.0X1	T57.0X2	T57.0X3	T57.0X4	--	--
- arseniureted	T57.0X1	T57.0X2	T57.0X3	T57.0X4	--	--
- chloride	T57.8X1	T57.8X2	T57.8X3	T57.8X4	--	--
- cyanide (salts)	T57.3X1	T57.3X2	T57.3X3	T57.3X4	--	--
- - gas	T57.3X1	T57.3X2	T57.3X3	T57.3X4	--	--
- Fluoride	T59.5X1	T59.5X2	T59.5X3	T59.5X4	--	--
- - vapor	T59.5X1	T59.5X2	T59.5X3	T59.5X4	--	--
- peroxide	T49.0X1	T49.0X2	T49.0X3	T49.0X4	T49.0X5	T49.0X6
- phosphureted	T57.1X1	T57.1X2	T57.1X3	T57.1X4	--	--
- sulfide	T59.6X1	T59.6X2	T59.6X3	T59.6X4	--	--
- - arseniureted	T57.0X1	T57.0X2	T57.0X3	T57.0X4	--	--
- sulfureted	T59.6X1	T59.6X2	T59.6X3	T59.6X4	--	--
Hydromethylpyridine	T46.7X1	T46.7X2	T46.7X3	T46.7X4	T46.7X5	T46.7X6
Hydromorphinol	T40.2X1	T40.2X2	T40.2X3	T40.2X4	--	--
Hydromorphinone	T40.2X1	T40.2X2	T40.2X3	T40.2X4	T40.2X5	T40.2X6
Hydromorphone	T40.2X1	T40.2X2	T40.2X3	T40.2X4	T40.2X5	T40.2X6
Hydromox	T50.2X1	T50.2X2	T50.2X3	T50.2X4	T50.2X5	T50.2X6
Hydrophilic lotion	T49.3X1	T49.3X2	T49.3X3	T49.3X4	T49.3X5	T49.3X6
Hydroquinidine	T46.2X1	T46.2X2	T46.2X3	T46.2X4	T46.2X5	T46.2X6
Hydroquinone	T52.2X1	T52.2X2	T52.2X3	T52.2X4	--	--
- vapor	T59.891	T59.892	T59.893	T59.894	--	--
Hydrosulfuric acid (gas)	T59.6X1	T59.6X2	T59.6X3	T59.6X4	--	--
Hydrotalcite	T47.1X1	T47.1X2	T47.1X3	T47.1X4	T47.1X5	T47.1X6
Hydrous wool fat	T49.3X1	T49.3X2	T49.3X3	T49.3X4	T49.3X5	T49.3X6
Hydroxide, caustic	T54.3X1	T54.3X2	T54.3X3	T54.3X4	--	--
Hydroxocobalamin	T45.8X1	T45.8X2	T45.8X3	T45.8X4	T45.8X5	T45.8X6
Hydroxyamphetamine	T49.5X1	T49.5X2	T49.5X3	T49.5X4	T49.5X5	T49.5X6
Hydroxycarbamide	T45.1X1	T45.1X2	T45.1X3	T45.1X4	T45.1X5	T45.1X6
Hydroxychloroquine	T37.8X1	T37.8X2	T37.8X3	T37.8X4	T37.8X5	T37.8X6
Hydroxydihydrocodeinone	T40.2X1	T40.2X2	T40.2X3	T40.2X4	T40.2X5	T40.2X6
Hydroxyestrone	T38.5X1	T38.5X2	T38.5X3	T38.5X4	T38.5X5	T38.5X6
Hydroxyethyl starch	T45.8X1	T45.8X2	T45.8X3	T45.8X4	T45.8X5	T45.8X6
Hydroxymethylpenta-none	T52.4X1	T52.4X2	T52.4X3	T52.4X4	--	--
Hydroxyphenamate	T43.591	T43.592	T43.593	T43.594	T43.595	T43.596
Hydroxyphenylbutazone	T39.2X1	T39.2X2	T39.2X3	T39.2X4	T39.2X5	T39.2X6
Hydroxyprogesterone	T38.5X1	T38.5X2	T38.5X3	T38.5X4	T38.5X5	T38.5X6
- caproate	T38.5X1	T38.5X2	T38.5X3	T38.5X4	T38.5X5	T38.5X6
Hydroxyquinoline (derivatives) NEC	T37.8X1	T37.8X2	T37.8X3	T37.8X4	T37.8X5	T37.8X6
Hydroxystilbamidine	T37.3X1	T37.3X2	T37.3X3	T37.3X4	T37.3X5	T37.3X6
Hydroxytoluene (nonmedicinal)	T54.0X1	T54.0X2	T54.0X3	T54.0X4	--	--
- medicinal	T49.0X1	T49.0X2	T49.0X3	T49.0X4	T49.0X5	T49.0X6
Hydroxyurea	T45.1X1	T45.1X2	T45.1X3	T45.1X4	T45.1X5	T45.1X6
Hydroxyzine	T43.591	T43.592	T43.593	T43.594	T43.595	T43.596
Hyoscine	T44.3X1	T44.3X2	T44.3X3	T44.3X4	T44.3X5	T44.3X6
Hyoscyamine	T44.3X1	T44.3X2	T44.3X3	T44.3X4	T44.3X5	T44.3X6
Hyoscyamus	T44.3X1	T44.3X2	T44.3X3	T44.3X4	T44.3X5	T44.3X6
- dry extract	T44.3X1	T44.3X2	T44.3X3	T44.3X4	T44.3X5	T44.3X6
Hypaque	T50.8X1	T50.8X2	T50.8X3	T50.8X4	T50.8X5	T50.8X6
Hypertussis	T50.Z11	T50.Z12	T50.Z13	T50.Z14	T50.Z15	T50.Z16
Hypnotic	T42.71	T42.72	T42.73	T42.74	T42.75	T42.76
- anticonvulsant	T42.71	T42.72	T42.73	T42.74	T42.75	T42.76
- specified NEC	T42.6X1	T42.6X2	T42.6X3	T42.6X4	T42.6X5	T42.6X6
Hypochlorite	T49.0X1	T49.0X2	T49.0X3	T49.0X4	T49.0X5	T49.0X6
Hypophysis, posterior	T38.891	T38.892	T38.893	T38.894	T38.895	T38.896
Hypotensive NEC	T46.5X1	T46.5X2	T46.5X3	T46.5X4	T46.5X5	T46.5X6
Hypromellose	T49.5X1	T49.5X2	T49.5X3	T49.5X4	T49.5X5	T49.5X6

Substance	Poisoning, Accidental (unintentional)	Poisoning, Intentional Self-harm	Poisoning, Assault	Poisoning, Undetermined	Adverse effect	Underdosing
Ibacitabine	T37.5X1	T37.5X2	T37.5X3	T37.5X4	T37.5X5	T37.5X6
Ibopamine	T44.991	T44.992	T44.993	T44.994	T44.995	T44.996
Ibufenac	T39.311	T39.312	T39.313	T39.314	T39.315	T39.316
Ibuprofen	T39.311	T39.312	T39.313	T39.314	T39.315	T39.316
Ibuproxam	T39.311	T39.312	T39.313	T39.314	T39.315	T39.316
Ibuterol	T48.6X1	T48.6X2	T48.6X3	T48.6X4	T48.6X5	T48.6X6
Ichthammol	T49.0X1	T49.0X2	T49.0X3	T49.0X4	T49.0X5	T49.0X6
Ichthyol	T49.4X1	T49.4X2	T49.4X3	T49.4X4	T49.4X5	T49.4X6
Idarubicin	T45.1X1	T45.1X2	T45.1X3	T45.1X4	T45.1X5	T45.1X6
Idrocilamide	T42.8X1	T42.8X2	T42.8X3	T42.8X4	T42.8X5	T42.8X6
Ifenprodil	T46.7X1	T46.7X2	T46.7X3	T46.7X4	T46.7X5	T46.7X6
Ifosfamide	T45.1X1	T45.1X2	T45.1X3	T45.1X4	T45.1X5	T45.1X6
Iletin	T38.3X1	T38.3X2	T38.3X3	T38.3X4	T38.3X5	T38.3X6
Ilex	T62.2X1	T62.2X2	T62.2X3	T62.2X4	--	--
Illuminating gas (after combustion)	T58.11	T58.12	T58.13	T58.14	--	--
- prior to combustion	T59.891	T59.892	T59.893	T59.894	--	--
Ilopan	T45.2X1	T45.2X2	T45.2X3	T45.2X4	T45.2X5	T45.2X6
Iloprost	T46.7X1	T46.7X2	T46.7X3	T46.7X4	T46.7X5	T46.7X6
Ilotycin	T36.3X1	T36.3X2	T36.3X3	T36.3X4	T36.3X5	T36.3X6
- ophthalmic preparation	T49.5X1	T49.5X2	T49.5X3	T49.5X4	T49.5X5	T49.5X6
- topical NEC	T49.0X1	T49.0X2	T49.0X3	T49.0X4	T49.0X5	T49.0X6
Imidazole-4-carboxamide	T45.1X1	T45.1X2	T45.1X3	T45.1X4	T45.1X5	T45.1X6
Imipenem	T36.0X1	T36.0X2	T36.0X3	T36.0X4	T36.0X5	T36.0X6
Imipramine	T43.011	T43.012	T43.013	T43.014	T43.015	T43.016
Iminostilbene	T42.1X1	T42.1X2	T42.1X3	T42.1X4	T42.1X5	T42.1X6
Immu-G	T50.Z11	T50.Z12	T50.Z13	T50.Z14	T50.Z15	T50.Z16
Immuglobin	T50.Z11	T50.Z12	T50.Z13	T50.Z14	T50.Z15	T50.Z16
Immune						
- globulin	T50.Z11	T50.Z12	T50.Z13	T50.Z14	T50.Z15	T50.Z16
- serum globulin	T50.Z11	T50.Z12	T50.Z13	T50.Z14	T50.Z15	T50.Z16
Immunoglobin human (intravenous) (normal)	T50.Z11	T50.Z12	T50.Z13	T50.Z14	T50.Z15	T50.Z16
- unmodified	T50.Z11	T50.Z12	T50.Z13	T50.Z14	T50.Z15	T50.Z16
Immunosuppressive drug	T45.1X1	T45.1X2	T45.1X3	T45.1X4	T45.1X5	T45.1X6
Immu-tetanus	T50.Z11	T50.Z12	T50.Z13	T50.Z14	T50.Z15	T50.Z16
Indalpine	T43.221	T43.222	T43.223	T43.224	T43.225	T43.226
Indanazoline	T48.5X1	T48.5X2	T48.5X3	T48.5X4	T48.5X5	T48.5X6
Indandione (derivatives)	T45.511	T45.512	T45.513	T45.514	T45.515	T45.516
Indapamide	T46.5X1	T46.5X2	T46.5X3	T46.5X4	T46.5X5	T46.5X6
Indendione (derivatives)	T45.511	T45.512	T45.513	T45.514	T45.515	T45.516
Indenolol	T44.7X1	T44.7X2	T44.7X3	T44.7X4	T44.7X5	T44.7X6
Inderal	T44.7X1	T44.7X2	T44.7X3	T44.7X4	T44.7X5	T44.7X6
Indian						
- hemp	T40.7X1	T40.7X2	T40.7X3	T40.7X4	T40.7X5	T40.7X6
- tobacco	T62.2X1	T62.2X2	T62.2X3	T62.2X4	--	--
Indigo carmine	T50.8X1	T50.8X2	T50.8X3	T50.8X4	T50.8X5	T50.8X6
Indobufen	T45.521	T45.522	T45.523	T45.524	T45.525	T45.526
Indocin	T39.2X1	T39.2X2	T39.2X3	T39.2X4	T39.2X5	T39.2X6
Indocyanine green	T50.8X1	T50.8X2	T50.8X3	T50.8X4	T50.8X5	T50.8X6
Indometacin	T39.391	T39.392	T39.393	T39.394	T39.395	T39.396
Indomethacin	T39.391	T39.392	T39.393	T39.394	T39.395	T39.396
- farnesil	T39.4X1	T39.4X2	T39.4X3	T39.4X4	T39.4X5	T39.4X6
Indoramin	T44.6X1	T44.6X2	T44.6X3	T44.6X4	T44.6X5	T44.6X6
Industrial						
- alcohol	T51.0X1	T51.0X2	T51.0X3	T51.0X4	--	--
- fumes	T59.891	T59.892	T59.893	T59.894	--	--
- solvents (fumes) (vapors)	T52.91	T52.92	T52.93	T52.94	--	--
Influenza vaccine	T50.B91	T50.B92	T50.B93	T50.B94	T50.B95	T50.B96
Ingested substance NEC	T65.91	T65.92	T65.93	T65.94	--	--

Substance	Poisoning, Accidental (unintentional)	Poisoning, Intentional Self-harm	Poisoning, Assault	Poisoning, Undetermined	Adverse effect	Underdosing
INH	T37.1X1	T37.1X2	T37.1X3	T37.1X4	T37.1X5	T37.1X6
Inhalation, gas (noxious) —see Gas Inhibitor						
- angiotensin-converting enzyme	T46.4X1	T46.4X2	T46.4X3	T46.4X4	T46.4X5	T46.4X6
- carbonic anhydrase	T50.2X1	T50.2X2	T50.2X3	T50.2X4	T50.2X5	T50.2X6
- fibrinolysis	T45.621	T45.622	T45.623	T45.624	T45.625	T45.626
- monoamine oxidase NEC	T43.1X1	T43.1X2	T43.1X3	T43.1X4	T43.1X5	T43.1X6
- - hydrazine	T43.1X1	T43.1X2	T43.1X3	T43.1X4	T43.1X5	T43.1X6
- postsynaptic	T43.8X1	T43.8X2	T43.8X3	T43.8X4	T43.8X5	T43.8X6
- prothrombin synthesis	T45.511	T45.512	T45.513	T45.514	T45.515	T45.516
Ink	T65.891	T65.892	T65.893	T65.894	--	--
Inorganic substance NEC	T57.91	T57.92	T57.93	T57.94	--	--
Inosine pranobex	T37.5X1	T37.5X2	T37.5X3	T37.5X4	T37.5X5	T37.5X6
Inositol	T50.991	T50.992	T50.993	T50.994	T50.995	T50.996
- nicotinate	T46.7X1	T46.7X2	T46.7X3	T46.7X4	T46.7X5	T46.7X6
Inproquone	T45.1X1	T45.1X2	T45.1X3	T45.1X4	T45.1X5	T45.1X6
Insect (sting) , venomous	T63.481	T63.482	T63.483	T63.484	--	--
- ant	T63.421	T63.422	T63.423	T63.424	--	--
- bee	T63.441	T63.442	T63.443	T63.444	--	--
- caterpillar	T63.431	T63.432	T63.433	T63.434	--	--
- hornet	T63.451	T63.452	T63.453	T63.454	--	--
- wasp	T63.461	T63.462	T63.463	T63.464	--	--
Insecticide NEC	T60.91	T60.92	T60.93	T60.94	--	--
- carbamate	T60.0X1	T60.0X2	T60.0X3	T60.0X4	--	--
- chlorinated	T60.1X1	T60.1X2	T60.1X3	T60.1X4	--	--
- mixed	T60.91	T60.92	T60.93	T60.94	--	--
- organochlorine	T60.1X1	T60.1X2	T60.1X3	T60.1X4	--	--
- organophosphorus	T60.0X1	T60.0X2	T60.0X3	T60.0X4	--	--
Insular tissue extract	T38.3X1	T38.3X2	T38.3X3	T38.3X4	T38.3X5	T38.3X6
Insulin (amorphous) (globin) (isophane) (Lente) (NPH) (Semilente) (Ultralente)	T38.3X1	T38.3X2	T38.3X3	T38.3X4	T38.3X5	T38.3X6
- defalan	T38.3X1	T38.3X2	T38.3X3	T38.3X4	T38.3X5	T38.3X6
- human	T38.3X1	T38.3X2	T38.3X3	T38.3X4	T38.3X5	T38.3X6
- injection, soluble	T38.3X1	T38.3X2	T38.3X3	T38.3X4	T38.3X5	T38.3X6
- - biphasic	T38.3X1	T38.3X2	T38.3X3	T38.3X4	T38.3X5	T38.3X6
- intermediate acting	T38.3X1	T38.3X2	T38.3X3	T38.3X4	T38.3X5	T38.3X6
- protamine zinc	T38.3X1	T38.3X2	T38.3X3	T38.3X4	T38.3X5	T38.3X6
- slow acting	T38.3X1	T38.3X2	T38.3X3	T38.3X4	T38.3X5	T38.3X6
- zinc						
- - protamine injection	T38.3X1	T38.3X2	T38.3X3	T38.3X4	T38.3X5	T38.3X6
- - suspension (amorphous) (crystalline)	T38.3X1	T38.3X2	T38.3X3	T38.3X4	T38.3X5	T38.3X6
Interferon (alpha) (beta) (gamma)	T37.5X1	T37.5X2	T37.5X3	T37.5X4	T37.5X5	T37.5X6
Intestinal motility control drug	T47.6X1	T47.6X2	T47.6X3	T47.6X4	T47.6X5	T47.6X6
- biological	T47.8X1	T47.8X2	T47.8X3	T47.8X4	T47.8X5	T47.8X6
Intranarcon	T41.1X1	T41.1X2	T41.1X3	T41.1X4	T41.1X5	T41.1X6
Intravenous						
- amino acids	T50.991	T50.992	T50.993	T50.994	T50.995	T50.996
- fat suspension	T50.991	T50.992	T50.993	T50.994	T50.995	T50.996
Inulin	T50.8X1	T50.8X2	T50.8X3	T50.8X4	T50.8X5	T50.8X6
Invert sugar	T50.3X1	T50.3X2	T50.3X3	T50.3X4	T50.3X5	T50.3X6
Inza—see Naproxen						
Iobenzamic acid	T50.8X1	T50.8X2	T50.8X3	T50.8X4	T50.8X5	T50.8X6
Iocarmic acid	T50.8X1	T50.8X2	T50.8X3	T50.8X4	T50.8X5	T50.8X6
Iocetamic acid	T50.8X1	T50.8X2	T50.8X3	T50.8X4	T50.8X5	T50.8X6
Iodamide	T50.8X1	T50.8X2	T50.8X3	T50.8X4	T50.8X5	T50.8X6
Iodide NEC—see also Iodine	T49.0X1	T49.0X2	T49.0X3	T49.0X4	T49.0X5	T49.0X6
- mercury (ointment)	T49.0X1	T49.0X2	T49.0X3	T49.0X4	T49.0X5	T49.0X6
- methylate	T49.0X1	T49.0X2	T49.0X3	T49.0X4	T49.0X5	T49.0X6
- potassium (expectorant) NEC	T48.4X1	T48.4X2	T48.4X3	T48.4X4	T48.4X5	T48.4X6
Iodinated						

Substance	Poisoning, Accidental (unintentional)	Poisoning, Intentional Self-harm	Poisoning, Assault	Poisoning, Undetermined	Adverse effect	Underdosing
- contrast medium	T50.8X1	T50.8X2	T50.8X3	T50.8X4	T50.8X5	T50.8X6
- glycerol	T48.4X1	T48.4X2	T48.4X3	T48.4X4	T48.4X5	T48.4X6
- human serum albumin (131I)	T50.8X1	T50.8X2	T50.8X3	T50.8X4	T50.8X5	T50.8X6
Iodine (antiseptic, external) (tincture) NEC	T49.0X1	T49.0X2	T49.0X3	T49.0X4	T49.0X5	T49.0X6
- 125—see also Radiation sickness, and Exposure to radioactivce isotopes	T50.8X1	T50.8X2	T50.8X3	T50.8X4	T50.8X5	T50.8X6
- - therapeutic	T50.991	T50.992	T50.993	T50.994	T50.995	T50.996
- 131—see also Radiation sickness, and Exposure to radioactivce isotopes	T50.8X1	T50.8X2	T50.8X3	T50.8X4	T50.8X5	T50.8X6
- - therapeutic	T38.2X1	T38.2X2	T38.2X3	T38.2X4	T38.2X5	T38.2X6
- diagnostic	T50.8X1	T50.8X2	T50.8X3	T50.8X4	T50.8X5	T50.8X6
- for thyroid conditions (antithyroid)	T38.2X1	T38.2X2	T38.2X3	T38.2X4	T38.2X5	T38.2X6
- solution	T49.0X1	T49.0X2	T49.0X3	T49.0X4	T49.0X5	T49.0X6
- vapor	T59.891	T59.892	T59.893	T59.894	--	--
Iodipamide	T50.8X1	T50.8X2	T50.8X3	T50.8X4	T50.8X5	T50.8X6
Iodized (poppy seed) oil	T50.8X1	T50.8X2	T50.8X3	T50.8X4	T50.8X5	T50.8X6
Iodobismitol	T37.8X1	T37.8X2	T37.8X3	T37.8X4	T37.8X5	T37.8X6
Iodochlorhydroxyquin	T37.8X1	T37.8X2	T37.8X3	T37.8X4	T37.8X5	T37.8X6
- topical	T49.0X1	T49.0X2	T49.0X3	T49.0X4	T49.0X5	T49.0X6
Iodochlorhydroxyquinoline	T37.8X1	T37.8X2	T37.8X3	T37.8X4	T37.8X5	T37.8X6
Iodocholesterol (131I)	T50.8X1	T50.8X2	T50.8X3	T50.8X4	T50.8X5	T50.8X6
Iodoform	T49.0X1	T49.0X2	T49.0X3	T49.0X4	T49.0X5	T49.0X6
Iodohippuric acid	T50.8X1	T50.8X2	T50.8X3	T50.8X4	T50.8X5	T50.8X6
Iodopanoic acid	T50.8X1	T50.8X2	T50.8X3	T50.8X4	T50.8X5	T50.8X6
Iodophthalein (sodium)	T50.8X1	T50.8X2	T50.8X3	T50.8X4	T50.8X5	T50.8X6
Iodopyracet	T50.8X1	T50.8X2	T50.8X3	T50.8X4	T50.8X5	T50.8X6
Iodoquinol	T37.8X1	T37.8X2	T37.8X3	T37.8X4	T37.8X5	T37.8X6
Iodoxamic acid	T50.8X1	T50.8X2	T50.8X3	T50.8X4	T50.8X5	T50.8X6
Iofendylate	T50.8X1	T50.8X2	T50.8X3	T50.8X4	T50.8X5	T50.8X6
Ioglycamic acid	T50.8X1	T50.8X2	T50.8X3	T50.8X4	T50.8X5	T50.8X6
Iohexol	T50.8X1	T50.8X2	T50.8X3	T50.8X4	T50.8X5	T50.8X6
Ion exchange resin						
- anion	T47.8X1	T47.8X2	T47.8X3	T47.8X4	T47.8X5	T47.8X6
- cation	T50.3X1	T50.3X2	T50.3X3	T50.3X4	T50.3X5	T50.3X6
- cholestyramine	T46.6X1	T46.6X2	T46.6X3	T46.6X4	T46.6X5	T46.6X6
- intestinal	T47.8X1	T47.8X2	T47.8X3	T47.8X4	T47.8X5	T47.8X6
Iopamidol	T50.8X1	T50.8X2	T50.8X3	T50.8X4	T50.8X5	T50.8X6
Iopanoic acid	T50.8X1	T50.8X2	T50.8X3	T50.8X4	T50.8X5	T50.8X6
Iophenoic acid	T50.8X1	T50.8X2	T50.8X3	T50.8X4	T50.8X5	T50.8X6
Iopodate, sodium	T50.8X1	T50.8X2	T50.8X3	T50.8X4	T50.8X5	T50.8X6
Iopodic acid	T50.8X1	T50.8X2	T50.8X3	T50.8X4	T50.8X5	T50.8X6
Iopromide	T50.8X1	T50.8X2	T50.8X3	T50.8X4	T50.8X5	T50.8X6
Iopydol	T50.8X1	T50.8X2	T50.8X3	T50.8X4	T50.8X5	T50.8X6
Iotalamic acid	T50.8X1	T50.8X2	T50.8X3	T50.8X4	T50.8X5	T50.8X6
Iothalamate	T50.8X1	T50.8X2	T50.8X3	T50.8X4	T50.8X5	T50.8X6
Iothiouracil	T38.2X1	T38.2X2	T38.2X3	T38.2X4	T38.2X5	T38.2X6
Iotrol	T50.8X1	T50.8X2	T50.8X3	T50.8X4	T50.8X5	T50.8X6
Iotrolan	T50.8X1	T50.8X2	T50.8X3	T50.8X4	T50.8X5	T50.8X6
Iotroxate	T50.8X1	T50.8X2	T50.8X3	T50.8X4	T50.8X5	T50.8X6
Iotroxic acid	T50.8X1	T50.8X2	T50.8X3	T50.8X4	T50.8X5	T50.8X6
Ioversol	T50.8X1	T50.8X2	T50.8X3	T50.8X4	T50.8X5	T50.8X6
Ioxaglate	T50.8X1	T50.8X2	T50.8X3	T50.8X4	T50.8X5	T50.8X6
Ioxaglic acid	T50.8X1	T50.8X2	T50.8X3	T50.8X4	T50.8X5	T50.8X6
Ioxitalamic acid	T50.8X1	T50.8X2	T50.8X3	T50.8X4	T50.8X5	T50.8X6
Ipecac	T47.7X1	T47.7X2	T47.7X3	T47.7X4	T47.7X5	T47.7X6
Ipecacuanha	T48.4X1	T48.4X2	T48.4X3	T48.4X4	T48.4X5	T48.4X6
Ipodate, calcium	T50.8X1	T50.8X2	T50.8X3	T50.8X4	T50.8X5	T50.8X6
Ipral	T42.3X1	T42.3X2	T42.3X3	T42.3X4	T42.3X5	T42.3X6
Ipratropium (bromide)	T48.6X1	T48.6X2	T48.6X3	T48.6X4	T48.6X5	T48.6X6

Substance	Poisoning, Accidental (unintentional)	Poisoning, Intentional Self-harm	Poisoning, Assault	Poisoning, Undetermined	Adverse effect	Underdosing
Ipriflavone	T46.3X1	T46.3X2	T46.3X3	T46.3X4	T46.3X5	T46.3X6
Iprindole	T43.011	T43.012	T43.013	T43.014	T43.015	T43.016
Iproclozide	T43.1X1	T43.1X2	T43.1X3	T43.1X4	T43.1X5	T43.1X6
Iprofenin	T50.8X1	T50.8X2	T50.8X3	T50.8X4	T50.8X5	T50.8X6
Iproheptine	T49.2X1	T49.2X2	T49.2X3	T49.2X4	T49.2X5	T49.2X6
Iproniazid	T43.1X1	T43.1X2	T43.1X3	T43.1X4	T43.1X5	T43.1X6
Iproplatin	T45.1X1	T45.1X2	T45.1X3	T45.1X4	T45.1X5	T45.1X6
Iproveratril	T46.1X1	T46.1X2	T46.1X3	T46.1X4	T46.1X5	T46.1X6
Iron (compounds) (medicinal) NEC	T45.4X1	T45.4X2	T45.4X3	T45.4X4	T45.4X5	T45.4X6
- ammonium	T45.4X1	T45.4X2	T45.4X3	T45.4X4	T45.4X5	T45.4X6
- dextran injection	T45.4X1	T45.4X2	T45.4X3	T45.4X4	T45.4X5	T45.4X6
- nonmedicinal	T56.891	T56.892	T56.893	T56.894	--	--
- salts	T45.4X1	T45.4X2	T45.4X3	T45.4X4	T45.4X5	T45.4X6
- sorbitex	T45.4X1	T45.4X2	T45.4X3	T45.4X4	T45.4X5	T45.4X6
- sorbitol citric acid complex	T45.4X1	T45.4X2	T45.4X3	T45.4X4	T45.4X5	T45.4X6
Irrigating fluid (vaginal)	T49.8X1	T49.8X2	T49.8X3	T49.8X4	T49.8X5	T49.8X6
- eye	T49.5X1	T49.5X2	T49.5X3	T49.5X4	T49.5X5	T49.5X6
Isepamicin	T36.5X1	T36.5X2	T36.5X3	T36.5X4	T36.5X5	T36.5X6
Isoaminile (citrate)	T48.3X1	T48.3X2	T48.3X3	T48.3X4	T48.3X5	T48.3X6
Isoamyl nitrite	T46.3X1	T46.3X2	T46.3X3	T46.3X4	T46.3X5	T46.3X6
Isobenzan	T60.1X1	T60.1X2	T60.1X3	T60.1X4	--	--
Isobutyl acetate	T52.8X1	T52.8X2	T52.8X3	T52.8X4	--	--
Isocarboxazid	T43.1X1	T43.1X2	T43.1X3	T43.1X4	T43.1X5	T43.1X6
Isoconazole	T49.0X1	T49.0X2	T49.0X3	T49.0X4	T49.0X5	T49.0X6
Isocyanate	T65.0X1	T65.0X2	T65.0X3	T65.0X4	--	--
Isoephedrine	T44.991	T44.992	T44.993	T44.994	T44.995	T44.996
Isoetarine	T48.6X1	T48.6X2	T48.6X3	T48.6X4	T48.6X5	T48.6X6
Isoethadione	T42.2X1	T42.2X2	T42.2X3	T42.2X4	T42.2X5	T42.2X6
Isoetharine	T44.5X1	T44.5X2	T44.5X3	T44.5X4	T44.5X5	T44.5X6
Isoflurane	T41.0X1	T41.0X2	T41.0X3	T41.0X4	T41.0X5	T41.0X6
Isoflurophate	T44.0X1	T44.0X2	T44.0X3	T44.0X4	T44.0X5	T44.0X6
Isomaltose, ferric complex	T45.4X1	T45.4X2	T45.4X3	T45.4X4	T45.4X5	T45.4X6
Isometheptene	T44.3X1	T44.3X2	T44.3X3	T44.3X4	T44.3X5	T44.3X6
Isoniazid	T37.1X1	T37.1X2	T37.1X3	T37.1X4	T37.1X5	T37.1X6
- with						
- - rifampicin	T36.6X1	T36.6X2	T36.6X3	T36.6X4	T36.6X5	T36.6X6
- - thioacetazone	T37.1X1	T37.1X2	T37.1X3	T37.1X4	T37.1X5	T37.1X6
Isonicotinic acid hydrazide	T37.1X1	T37.1X2	T37.1X3	T37.1X4	T37.1X5	T37.1X6
Isonipecaine	T40.4X1	T40.4X2	T40.4X3	T40.4X4	T40.4X5	T40.4X6
Isopentaquine	T37.2X1	T37.2X2	T37.2X3	T37.2X4	T37.2X5	T37.2X6
Isophane insulin	T38.3X1	T38.3X2	T38.3X3	T38.3X4	T38.3X5	T38.3X6
Isophorone	T65.891	T65.892	T65.893	T65.894	--	--
Isophosphamide	T45.1X1	T45.1X2	T45.1X3	T45.1X4	T45.1X5	T45.1X6
Isopregnenone	T38.5X1	T38.5X2	T38.5X3	T38.5X4	T38.5X5	T38.5X6
Isoprenaline	T48.6X1	T48.6X2	T48.6X3	T48.6X4	T48.6X5	T48.6X6
Isopromethazine	T43.3X1	T43.3X2	T43.3X3	T43.3X4	T43.3X5	T43.3X6
Isopropamide	T44.3X1	T44.3X2	T44.3X3	T44.3X4	T44.3X5	T44.3X6
- iodide	T44.3X1	T44.3X2	T44.3X3	T44.3X4	T44.3X5	T44.3X6
Isopropanol	T51.2X1	T51.2X2	T51.2X3	T51.2X4	--	--
Isopropyl						
- acetate	T52.8X1	T52.8X2	T52.8X3	T52.8X4	--	--
- alcohol	T51.2X1	T51.2X2	T51.2X3	T51.2X4	--	--
- - medicinal	T49.4X1	T49.4X2	T49.4X3	T49.4X4	T49.4X5	T49.4X6
- ether	T52.8X1	T52.8X2	T52.8X3	T52.8X4	--	--
Isopropylaminophenazone	T39.2X1	T39.2X2	T39.2X3	T39.2X4	T39.2X5	T39.2X6
Isoproterenol	T48.6X1	T48.6X2	T48.6X3	T48.6X4	T48.6X5	T48.6X6
Isosorbide dinitrate	T46.3X1	T46.3X2	T46.3X3	T46.3X4	T46.3X5	T46.3X6
Isothipendyl	T45.0X1	T45.0X2	T45.0X3	T45.0X4	T45.0X5	T45.0X6
Isotretinoin	T50.991	T50.992	T50.993	T50.994	T50.995	T50.996

Substance	Poisoning, Accidental (unintentional)	Poisoning, Intentional Self-harm	Poisoning, Assault	Poisoning, Undetermined	Adverse effect	Underdosing
Isoxazolyl penicillin	T36.0X1	T36.0X2	T36.0X3	T36.0X4	T36.0X5	T36.0X6
Isoxicam	T39.391	T39.392	T39.393	T39.394	T39.395	T39.396
Isoxsuprine	T46.7X1	T46.7X2	T46.7X3	T46.7X4	T46.7X5	T46.7X6
Ispagula	T47.4X1	T47.4X2	T47.4X3	T47.4X4	T47.4X5	T47.4X6
- husk	T47.4X1	T47.4X2	T47.4X3	T47.4X4	T47.4X5	T47.4X6
Isradipine	T46.1X1	T46.1X2	T46.1X3	T46.1X4	T46.1X5	T46.1X6
I-thyroxine sodium	T38.1X1	T38.1X2	T38.1X3	T38.1X4	T38.1X5	T38.1X6
Itraconazole	T37.8X1	T37.8X2	T37.8X3	T37.8X4	T37.8X5	T37.8X6
Itramin tosilate	T46.3X1	T46.3X2	T46.3X3	T46.3X4	T46.3X5	T46.3X6
Ivermectin	T37.4X1	T37.4X2	T37.4X3	T37.4X4	T37.4X5	T37.4X6
Izoniazid	T37.1X1	T37.1X2	T37.1X3	T37.1X4	T37.1X5	T37.1X6
- with thioacetazone	T37.1X1	T37.1X2	T37.1X3	T37.1X4	T37.1X5	T37.1X6
Jalap	T47.2X1	T47.2X2	T47.2X3	T47.2X4	T47.2X5	T47.2X6
Jamaica						
- dogwood (bark)	T39.8X1	T39.8X2	T39.8X3	T39.8X4	T39.8X5	T39.8X6
- ginger	T65.891	T65.892	T65.893	T65.894	--	--
- - root	T62.2X1	T62.2X2	T62.2X3	T62.2X4	--	--
Jatropha	T62.2X1	T62.2X2	T62.2X3	T62.2X4	--	--
- curcas	T62.2X1	T62.2X2	T62.2X3	T62.2X4	--	--
Jectofer	T45.4X1	T45.4X2	T45.4X3	T45.4X4	T45.4X5	T45.4X6
Jellyfish (sting)	T63.621	T63.622	T63.623	T63.624	--	--
Jequirity (bean)	T62.2X1	T62.2X2	T62.2X3	T62.2X4	--	--
Jimson weed (stramonium)	T62.2X1	T62.2X2	T62.2X3	T62.2X4	--	--
- seeds	T62.2X1	T62.2X2	T62.2X3	T62.2X4	--	--
Josamycin	T36.3X1	T36.3X2	T36.3X3	T36.3X4	T36.3X5	T36.3X6
Juniper tar	T49.1X1	T49.1X2	T49.1X3	T49.1X4	T49.1X5	T49.1X6
Kallidinogenase	T46.7X1	T46.7X2	T46.7X3	T46.7X4	T46.7X5	T46.7X6
Kallikrein	T46.7X1	T46.7X2	T46.7X3	T46.7X4	T46.7X5	T46.7X6
Kanamycin	T36.5X1	T36.5X2	T36.5X3	T36.5X4	T36.5X5	T36.5X6
Kantrex	T36.5X1	T36.5X2	T36.5X3	T36.5X4	T36.5X5	T36.5X6
Kaolin	T47.6X1	T47.6X2	T47.6X3	T47.6X4	T47.6X5	T47.6X6
- light	T47.6X1	T47.6X2	T47.6X3	T47.6X4	T47.6X5	T47.6X6
Karaya (gum)	T47.4X1	T47.4X2	T47.4X3	T47.4X4	T47.4X5	T47.4X6
Kebuzone	T39.2X1	T39.2X2	T39.2X3	T39.2X4	T39.2X5	T39.2X6
Kelevan	T60.1X1	T60.1X2	T60.1X3	T60.1X4	--	--
Kemithal	T41.1X1	T41.1X2	T41.1X3	T41.1X4	T41.1X5	T41.1X6
Kenacort	T38.0X1	T38.0X2	T38.0X3	T38.0X4	T38.0X5	T38.0X6
Keratolytic drug NEC	T49.4X1	T49.4X2	T49.4X3	T49.4X4	T49.4X5	T49.4X6
- anthracene	T49.4X1	T49.4X2	T49.4X3	T49.4X4	T49.4X5	T49.4X6
Keratoplastic NEC	T49.4X1	T49.4X2	T49.4X3	T49.4X4	T49.4X5	T49.4X6
Kerosene, kerosine (fuel) (solvent) NEC	T52.0X1	T52.0X2	T52.0X3	T52.0X4	--	--
- insecticide	T52.0X1	T52.0X2	T52.0X3	T52.0X4	--	--
- vapor	T52.0X1	T52.0X2	T52.0X3	T52.0X4	--	--
Ketamine	T41.291	T41.292	T41.293	T41.294	T41.295	T41.296
Ketazolam	T42.4X1	T42.4X2	T42.4X3	T42.4X4	T42.4X5	T42.4X6
Ketazon	T39.2X1	T39.2X2	T39.2X3	T39.2X4	T39.2X5	T39.2X6
Ketobemidone	T40.4X1	T40.4X2	T40.4X3	T40.4X4	--	--
Ketoconazole	T49.0X1	T49.0X2	T49.0X3	T49.0X4	T49.0X5	T49.0X6
Ketols	T52.4X1	T52.4X2	T52.4X3	T52.4X4	--	--
Ketone oils	T52.4X1	T52.4X2	T52.4X3	T52.4X4	--	--
Ketoprofen	T39.311	T39.312	T39.313	T39.314	T39.315	T39.316
Ketorolac	T39.8X1	T39.8X2	T39.8X3	T39.8X4	T39.8X5	T39.8X6
Ketotifen	T45.0X1	T45.0X2	T45.0X3	T45.0X4	T45.0X5	T45.0X6
Khat	T43.691	T43.692	T43.693	T43.694	--	--
Khellin	T46.3X1	T46.3X2	T46.3X3	T46.3X4	T46.3X5	T46.3X6
Khelloside	T46.3X1	T46.3X2	T46.3X3	T46.3X4	T46.3X5	T46.3X6
Kiln gas or vapor (carbon monoxide)	T58.8X1	T58.8X2	T58.8X3	T58.8X4	--	--
Kitasamycin	T36.3X1	T36.3X2	T36.3X3	T36.3X4	T36.3X5	T36.3X6

Substance	Poisoning, Accidental (unintentional)	Poisoning, Intentional Self-harm	Poisoning, Assault	Poisoning, Undetermined	Adverse effect	Underdosing
Konsyl	T47.4X1	T47.4X2	T47.4X3	T47.4X4	T47.4X5	T47.4X6
Kosam seed	T62.2X1	T62.2X2	T62.2X3	T62.2X4	--	--
Krait (venom)	T63.091	T63.092	T63.093	T63.094	--	--
Kwell (insecticide)	T60.1X1	T60.1X2	T60.1X3	T60.1X4	--	--
- anti-infective (topical)	T49.0X1	T49.0X2	T49.0X3	T49.0X4	T49.0X5	T49.0X6
Labetalol	T44.8X1	T44.8X2	T44.8X3	T44.8X4	T44.8X5	T44.8X6
Laburnum (seeds)	T62.2X1	T62.2X2	T62.2X3	T62.2X4	--	--
- leaves	T62.2X1	T62.2X2	T62.2X3	T62.2X4	--	--
Lachesine	T49.5X1	T49.5X2	T49.5X3	T49.5X4	T49.5X5	T49.5X6
Lacidipine	T46.5X1	T46.5X2	T46.5X3	T46.5X4	T46.5X5	T46.5X6
Lacquer	T65.6X1	T65.6X2	T65.6X3	T65.6X4	--	--
Lacrimogenic gas	T59.3X1	T59.3X2	T59.3X3	T59.3X4	--	--
Lactated potassic saline	T50.3X1	T50.3X2	T50.3X3	T50.3X4	T50.3X5	T50.3X6
Lactic acid	T49.8X1	T49.8X2	T49.8X3	T49.8X4	T49.8X5	T49.8X6
Lactobacillus						
- acidophilus	T47.6X1	T47.6X2	T47.6X3	T47.6X4	T47.6X5	T47.6X6
- - compound	T47.6X1	T47.6X2	T47.6X3	T47.6X4	T47.6X5	T47.6X6
- bifidus, lyophilized	T47.6X1	T47.6X2	T47.6X3	T47.6X4	T47.6X5	T47.6X6
- bulgaricus	T47.6X1	T47.6X2	T47.6X3	T47.6X4	T47.6X5	T47.6X6
- sporogenes	T47.6X1	T47.6X2	T47.6X3	T47.6X4	T47.6X5	T47.6X6
Lactoflavin	T45.2X1	T45.2X2	T45.2X3	T45.2X4	T45.2X5	T45.2X6
Lactose (as excipient)	T50.901	T50.902	T50.903	T50.904	T50.905	T50.906
Lactuca (virosa) (extract)	T42.6X1	T42.6X2	T42.6X3	T42.6X4	T42.6X5	T42.6X6
Lactucarium	T42.6X1	T42.6X2	T42.6X3	T42.6X4	T42.6X5	T42.6X6
Lactulose	T47.3X1	T47.3X2	T47.3X3	T47.3X4	T47.3X5	T47.3X6
Laevo—see Levo-						
Lanatosides	T46.0X1	T46.0X2	T46.0X3	T46.0X4	T46.0X5	T46.0X6
Lanolin	T49.3X1	T49.3X2	T49.3X3	T49.3X4	T49.3X5	T49.3X6
Largactil	T43.3X1	T43.3X2	T43.3X3	T43.3X4	T43.3X5	T43.3X6
Larkspur	T62.2X1	T62.2X2	T62.2X3	T62.2X4	--	--
Laroxyl	T43.011	T43.012	T43.013	T43.014	T43.015	T43.016
Lasix	T50.1X1	T50.1X2	T50.1X3	T50.1X4	T50.1X5	T50.1X6
Lassar's paste	T49.4X1	T49.4X2	T49.4X3	T49.4X4	T49.4X5	T49.4X6
Latamoxef	T36.1X1	T36.1X2	T36.1X3	T36.1X4	T36.1X5	T36.1X6
Latex	T65.811	T65.812	T65.813	T65.814	--	--
Lathyrus (seed)	T62.2X1	T62.2X2	T62.2X3	T62.2X4	--	--
Laudanum	T40.0X1	T40.0X2	T40.0X3	T40.0X4	T40.0X5	T40.0X6
Laudexium	T48.1X1	T48.1X2	T48.1X3	T48.1X4	T48.1X5	T48.1X6
Laughing gas	T41.0X1	T41.0X2	T41.0X3	T41.0X4	T41.0X5	T41.0X6
Laurel, black or cherry	T62.2X1	T62.2X2	T62.2X3	T62.2X4	--	--
Laurolinium	T49.0X1	T49.0X2	T49.0X3	T49.0X4	T49.0X5	T49.0X6
Lauryl sulfoacetate	T49.2X1	T49.2X2	T49.2X3	T49.2X4	T49.2X5	T49.2X6
Laxative NEC	T47.4X1	T47.4X2	T47.4X3	T47.4X4	T47.4X5	T47.4X6
- osmotic	T47.3X1	T47.3X2	T47.3X3	T47.3X4	T47.3X5	T47.3X6
- saline	T47.3X1	T47.3X2	T47.3X3	T47.3X4	T47.3X5	T47.3X6
- stimulant	T47.2X1	T47.2X2	T47.2X3	T47.2X4	T47.2X5	T47.2X6
L-dopa	T42.8X1	T42.8X2	T42.8X3	T42.8X4	T42.8X5	T42.8X6
Lead (dust) (fumes) (vapor) NEC	T56.0X1	T56.0X2	T56.0X3	T56.0X4	--	--
- acetate	T49.2X1	T49.2X2	T49.2X3	T49.2X4	T49.2X5	T49.2X6
- alkyl (fuel additive)	T56.0X1	T56.0X2	T56.0X3	T56.0X4	--	--
- anti-infectives	T37.8X1	T37.8X2	T37.8X3	T37.8X4	T37.8X5	T37.8X6
- antiknock compound (tetraethyl)	T56.0X1	T56.0X2	T56.0X3	T56.0X4	--	--
- arsenate, arsenite (dust) (herbicide) (insecticide) (vapor)	T57.0X1	T57.0X2	T57.0X3	T57.0X4	--	--
- carbonate	T56.0X1	T56.0X2	T56.0X3	T56.0X4	--	--
- - paint	T56.0X1	T56.0X2	T56.0X3	T56.0X4	--	--
- chromate	T56.0X1	T56.0X2	T56.0X3	T56.0X4	--	--
- - paint	T56.0X1	T56.0X2	T56.0X3	T56.0X4	--	--
- dioxide	T56.0X1	T56.0X2	T56.0X3	T56.0X4	--	--

Substance	Poisoning, Accidental (unintentional)	Poisoning, Intentional Self-harm	Poisoning, Assault	Poisoning, Undetermined	Adverse effect	Underdosing
- inorganic	T56.0X1	T56.0X2	T56.0X3	T56.0X4	--	--
- iodide	T56.0X1	T56.0X2	T56.0X3	T56.0X4	--	--
- - pigment (paint)	T56.0X1	T56.0X2	T56.0X3	T56.0X4	--	--
- monoxide (dust)	T56.0X1	T56.0X2	T56.0X3	T56.0X4	--	--
- - paint	T56.0X1	T56.0X2	T56.0X3	T56.0X4	--	--
- organic	T56.0X1	T56.0X2	T56.0X3	T56.0X4	--	--
- oxide	T56.0X1	T56.0X2	T56.0X3	T56.0X4	--	--
- - paint	T56.0X1	T56.0X2	T56.0X3	T56.0X4	--	--
- paint	T56.0X1	T56.0X2	T56.0X3	T56.0X4	--	--
- salts	T56.0X1	T56.0X2	T56.0X3	T56.0X4	--	--
- specified compound NEC	T56.0X1	T56.0X2	T56.0X3	T56.0X4	--	--
- tetra-ethyl	T56.0X1	T56.0X2	T56.0X3	T56.0X4	--	--
Lebanese red	T40.7X1	T40.7X2	T40.7X3	T40.7X4	T40.7X5	T40.7X6
Lefetamine	T39.8X1	T39.8X2	T39.8X3	T39.8X4	T39.8X5	T39.8X6
Lenperone	T43.4X1	T43.4X2	T43.4X3	T43.4X4	T43.4X5	T43.4X6
Lente lietin (insulin)	T38.3X1	T38.3X2	T38.3X3	T38.3X4	T38.3X5	T38.3X6
Leptazol	T50.7X1	T50.7X2	T50.7X3	T50.7X4	T50.7X5	T50.7X6
Leptophos	T60.0X1	T60.0X2	T60.0X3	T60.0X4	--	--
Leritine	T40.2X1	T40.2X2	T40.2X3	T40.2X4	T40.2X5	T40.2X6
Letosteine	T48.4X1	T48.4X2	T48.4X3	T48.4X4	T48.4X5	T48.4X6
Letter	T38.1X1	T38.1X2	T38.1X3	T38.1X4	T38.1X5	T38.1X6
Lettuce opium	T42.6X1	T42.6X2	T42.6X3	T42.6X4	T42.6X5	T42.6X6
Leucinocaine	T41.3X1	T41.3X2	T41.3X3	T41.3X4	T41.3X5	T41.3X6
Leucocianidol	T46.991	T46.992	T46.993	T46.994	T46.995	T46.996
Leucovorin (factor)	T45.8X1	T45.8X2	T45.8X3	T45.8X4	T45.8X5	T45.8X6
Leukeran	T45.1X1	T45.1X2	T45.1X3	T45.1X4	T45.1X5	T45.1X6
Leuprolide	T38.891	T38.892	T38.893	T38.894	T38.895	T38.896
Levalbuterol	T48.6X1	T48.6X2	T48.6X3	T48.6X4	T48.6X5	T48.6X6
Levallorphan	T50.7X1	T50.7X2	T50.7X3	T50.7X4	T50.7X5	T50.7X6
Levamisole	T37.4X1	T37.4X2	T37.4X3	T37.4X4	T37.4X5	T37.4X6
Levanil	T42.6X1	T42.6X2	T42.6X3	T42.6X4	T42.6X5	T42.6X6
Levarterenol	T44.4X1	T44.4X2	T44.4X3	T44.4X4	T44.4X5	T44.4X6
Levdropropizine	T48.3X1	T48.3X2	T48.3X3	T48.3X4	T48.3X5	T48.3X6
Levobunolol	T49.5X1	T49.5X2	T49.5X3	T49.5X4	T49.5X5	T49.5X6
Levocabastine (hydrochloride)	T45.0X1	T45.0X2	T45.0X3	T45.0X4	T45.0X5	T45.0X6
Levocarnitine	T50.991	T50.992	T50.993	T50.994	T50.995	T50.996
Levodopa	T42.8X1	T42.8X2	T42.8X3	T42.8X4	T42.8X5	T42.8X6
- with carbidopa	T42.8X1	T42.8X2	T42.8X3	T42.8X4	T42.8X5	T42.8X6
Levo-dromoran	T40.2X1	T40.2X2	T40.2X3	T40.2X4	T40.2X5	T40.2X6
Levoglutamide	T50.991	T50.992	T50.993	T50.994	T50.995	T50.996
Levoid	T38.1X1	T38.1X2	T38.1X3	T38.1X4	T38.1X5	T38.1X6
Levo-iso-methadone	T40.3X1	T40.3X2	T40.3X3	T40.3X4	T40.3X5	T40.3X6
Levomepromazine	T43.3X1	T43.3X2	T43.3X3	T43.3X4	T43.3X5	T43.3X6
Levonordefrin	T49.6X1	T49.6X2	T49.6X3	T49.6X4	T49.6X5	T49.6X6
Levonorgestrel	T38.4X1	T38.4X2	T38.4X3	T38.4X4	T38.4X5	T38.4X6
- with ethinylestradiol	T38.5X1	T38.5X2	T38.5X3	T38.5X4	T38.5X5	T38.5X6
Levopromazine	T43.3X1	T43.3X2	T43.3X3	T43.3X4	T43.3X5	T43.3X6
Levoprome	T42.6X1	T42.6X2	T42.6X3	T42.6X4	T42.6X5	T42.6X6
Levopropoxyphene	T40.4X1	T40.4X2	T40.4X3	T40.4X4	T40.4X5	T40.4X6
Levopropylhexedrine	T50.5X1	T50.5X2	T50.5X3	T50.5X4	T50.5X5	T50.5X6
Levoproxyphylline	T48.6X1	T48.6X2	T48.6X3	T48.6X4	T48.6X5	T48.6X6
Levorphanol	T40.4X1	T40.4X2	T40.4X3	T40.4X4	T40.4X5	T40.4X6
Levothyroxine	T38.1X1	T38.1X2	T38.1X3	T38.1X4	T38.1X5	T38.1X6
- sodium	T38.1X1	T38.1X2	T38.1X3	T38.1X4	T38.1X5	T38.1X6
Levsin	T44.3X1	T44.3X2	T44.3X3	T44.3X4	T44.3X5	T44.3X6
Levulose	T50.3X1	T50.3X2	T50.3X3	T50.3X4	T50.3X5	T50.3X6
Lewisite (gas) , not in war	T57.0X1	T57.0X2	T57.0X3	T57.0X4	--	--
Librium	T42.4X1	T42.4X2	T42.4X3	T42.4X4	T42.4X5	T42.4X6

Substance	Poisoning, Accidental (unintentional)	Poisoning, Intentional Self-harm	Poisoning, Assault	Poisoning, Undetermined	Adverse effect	Underdosing
Lidex	T49.0X1	T49.0X2	T49.0X3	T49.0X4	T49.0X5	T49.0X6
Lidocaine	T41.3X1	T41.3X2	T41.3X3	T41.3X4	T41.3X5	T41.3X6
- regional	T41.3X1	T41.3X2	T41.3X3	T41.3X4	T41.3X5	T41.3X6
- spinal	T41.3X1	T41.3X2	T41.3X3	T41.3X4	T41.3X5	T41.3X6
Lidofenin	T50.8X1	T50.8X2	T50.8X3	T50.8X4	T50.8X5	T50.8X6
Lidoflazine	T46.1X1	T46.1X2	T46.1X3	T46.1X4	T46.1X5	T46.1X6
Lighter fluid	T52.0X1	T52.0X2	T52.0X3	T52.0X4	--	--
Lignin hemicellulose	T47.6X1	T47.6X2	T47.6X3	T47.6X4	T47.6X5	T47.6X6
Lignocaine	T41.3X1	T41.3X2	T41.3X3	T41.3X4	T41.3X5	T41.3X6
- regional	T41.3X1	T41.3X2	T41.3X3	T41.3X4	T41.3X5	T41.3X6
- spinal	T41.3X1	T41.3X2	T41.3X3	T41.3X4	T41.3X5	T41.3X6
Ligroin (e) (solvent)	T52.0X1	T52.0X2	T52.0X3	T52.0X4	--	--
- vapor	T59.891	T59.892	T59.893	T59.894	--	--
Ligustrum vulgare	T62.2X1	T62.2X2	T62.2X3	T62.2X4	--	--
Lily of the valley	T62.2X1	T62.2X2	T62.2X3	T62.2X4	--	--
Lime (chloride)	T54.3X1	T54.3X2	T54.3X3	T54.3X4	--	--
Limonene	T52.8X1	T52.8X2	T52.8X3	T52.8X4	--	--
Lincomycin	T36.8X1	T36.8X2	T36.8X3	T36.8X4	T36.8X5	T36.8X6
Lindane (insecticide) (nonmedicinal) (vapor)	T53.6X1	T53.6X2	T53.6X3	T53.6X4	--	--
- medicinal	T49.0X1	T49.0X2	T49.0X3	T49.0X4	T49.0X5	T49.0X6
Liniments NEC	T49.91	T49.92	T49.93	T49.94	T49.95	T49.96
Linoleic acid	T46.6X1	T46.6X2	T46.6X3	T46.6X4	T46.6X5	T46.6X6
Linolenic acid	T46.6X1	T46.6X2	T46.6X3	T46.6X4	T46.6X5	T46.6X6
Linseed	T47.4X1	T47.4X2	T47.4X3	T47.4X4	T47.4X5	T47.4X6
Liothyronine	T38.1X1	T38.1X2	T38.1X3	T38.1X4	T38.1X5	T38.1X6
Liotrix	T38.1X1	T38.1X2	T38.1X3	T38.1X4	T38.1X5	T38.1X6
Lipancreatin	T47.5X1	T47.5X2	T47.5X3	T47.5X4	T47.5X5	T47.5X6
Lipo-alprostadil	T46.7X1	T46.7X2	T46.7X3	T46.7X4	T46.7X5	T46.7X6
Lipo-Lutin	T38.5X1	T38.5X2	T38.5X3	T38.5X4	T38.5X5	T38.5X6
Lipotropic drug NEC	T50.901	T50.902	T50.903	T50.904	T50.905	T50.906
Liquefied petroleum gases	T59.891	T59.892	T59.893	T59.894	--	--
- piped (pure or mixed with air)	T59.891	T59.892	T59.893	T59.894	--	--
Liquid						
- paraffin	T47.4X1	T47.4X2	T47.4X3	T47.4X4	T47.4X5	T47.4X6
- petrolatum	T47.4X1	T47.4X2	T47.4X3	T47.4X4	T47.4X5	T47.4X6
- - topical	T49.3X1	T49.3X2	T49.3X3	T49.3X4	T49.3X5	T49.3X6
- specified NEC	T65.891	T65.892	T65.893	T65.894	--	--
- substance	T65.91	T65.92	T65.93	T65.94	--	--
Liquor creosolis compositus	T65.891	T65.892	T65.893	T65.894	--	--
Liquorice	T48.4X1	T48.4X2	T48.4X3	T48.4X4	T48.4X5	T48.4X6
- extract	T47.8X1	T47.8X2	T47.8X3	T47.8X4	T47.8X5	T47.8X6
Lisinopril	T46.4X1	T46.4X2	T46.4X3	T46.4X4	T46.4X5	T46.4X6
Lisuride	T42.8X1	T42.8X2	T42.8X3	T42.8X4	T42.8X5	T42.8X6
Lithane	T43.8X1	T43.8X2	T43.8X3	T43.8X4	T43.8X5	T43.8X6
Lithium	T56.891	T56.892	T56.893	T56.894	--	--
- gluconate	T43.591	T43.592	T43.593	T43.594	T43.595	T43.596
- salts (carbonate)	T43.591	T43.592	T43.593	T43.594	T43.595	T43.596
Lithonate	T43.8X1	T43.8X2	T43.8X3	T43.8X4	T43.8X5	T43.8X6
Liver						
- extract	T45.8X1	T45.8X2	T45.8X3	T45.8X4	T45.8X5	T45.8X6
- - for parenteral use	T45.8X1	T45.8X2	T45.8X3	T45.8X4	T45.8X5	T45.8X6
- fraction 1	T45.8X1	T45.8X2	T45.8X3	T45.8X4	T45.8X5	T45.8X6
- hydrolysate	T45.8X1	T45.8X2	T45.8X3	T45.8X4	T45.8X5	T45.8X6
Lizard (bite) (venom)	T63.121	T63.122	T63.123	T63.124	--	--
LMD	T45.8X1	T45.8X2	T45.8X3	T45.8X4	T45.8X5	T45.8X6
Lobelia	T62.2X1	T62.2X2	T62.2X3	T62.2X4	--	--
Lobeline	T50.7X1	T50.7X2	T50.7X3	T50.7X4	T50.7X5	T50.7X6
Local action drug NEC	T49.8X1	T49.8X2	T49.8X3	T49.8X4	T49.8X5	T49.8X6
Locorten	T49.0X1	T49.0X2	T49.0X3	T49.0X4	T49.0X5	T49.0X6

Substance	Poisoning, Accidental (unintentional)	Poisoning, Intentional Self-harm	Poisoning, Assault	Poisoning, Undetermined	Adverse effect	Underdosing
Lofepramine	T43.011	T43.012	T43.013	T43.014	T43.015	T43.016
Lolium temulentum	T62.2X1	T62.2X2	T62.2X3	T62.2X4	--	--
Lomotil	T47.6X1	T47.6X2	T47.6X3	T47.6X4	T47.6X5	T47.6X6
Lomustine	T45.1X1	T45.1X2	T45.1X3	T45.1X4	T45.1X5	T45.1X6
Lonidamine	T45.1X1	T45.1X2	T45.1X3	T45.1X4	T45.1X5	T45.1X6
Loperamide	T47.6X1	T47.6X2	T47.6X3	T47.6X4	T47.6X5	T47.6X6
Loprazolam	T42.4X1	T42.4X2	T42.4X3	T42.4X4	T42.4X5	T42.4X6
Lorajmine	T46.2X1	T46.2X2	T46.2X3	T46.2X4	T46.2X5	T46.2X6
Loratidine	T45.0X1	T45.0X2	T45.0X3	T45.0X4	T45.0X5	T45.0X6
Lorazepam	T42.4X1	T42.4X2	T42.4X3	T42.4X4	T42.4X5	T42.4X6
Lorcainide	T46.2X1	T46.2X2	T46.2X3	T46.2X4	T46.2X5	T46.2X6
Lormetazepam	T42.4X1	T42.4X2	T42.4X3	T42.4X4	T42.4X5	T42.4X6
Lotions NEC	T49.91	T49.92	T49.93	T49.94	T49.95	T49.96
Lotusate	T42.3X1	T42.3X2	T42.3X3	T42.3X4	T42.3X5	T42.3X6
Lovastatin	T46.6X1	T46.6X2	T46.6X3	T46.6X4	T46.6X5	T46.6X6
Lowila	T49.2X1	T49.2X2	T49.2X3	T49.2X4	T49.2X5	T49.2X6
Loxapine	T43.591	T43.592	T43.593	T43.594	T43.595	T43.596
Lozenges (throat)	T49.6X1	T49.6X2	T49.6X3	T49.6X4	T49.6X5	T49.6X6
LSD	T40.8X1	T40.8X2	T40.8X3	T40.8X4	T40.8X5	--
L-Tryptophan—see amino acid						
Lubricant, eye	T49.5X1	T49.5X2	T49.5X3	T49.5X4	T49.5X5	T49.5X6
Lubricating oil NEC	T52.0X1	T52.0X2	T52.0X3	T52.0X4	--	--
Lucanthone	T37.4X1	T37.4X2	T37.4X3	T37.4X4	T37.4X5	T37.4X6
Luminal	T42.3X1	T42.3X2	T42.3X3	T42.3X4	T42.3X5	T42.3X6
Lung irritant (gas) NEC	T59.91	T59.92	T59.93	T59.94	--	--
Luteinizing hormone	T38.811	T38.812	T38.813	T38.814	T38.815	T38.816
Lutocylol	T38.5X1	T38.5X2	T38.5X3	T38.5X4	T38.5X5	T38.5X6
Lutromone	T38.5X1	T38.5X2	T38.5X3	T38.5X4	T38.5X5	T38.5X6
Lututrin	T48.291	T48.292	T48.293	T48.294	T48.295	T48.296
Lye (concentrated)	T54.3X1	T54.3X2	T54.3X3	T54.3X4	--	--
Lygranum (skin test)	T50.8X1	T50.8X2	T50.8X3	T50.8X4	T50.8X5	T50.8X6
Lymecycline	T36.4X1	T36.4X2	T36.4X3	T36.4X4	T36.4X5	T36.4X6
Lymphogranuloma venereum antigen	T50.8X1	T50.8X2	T50.8X3	T50.8X4	T50.8X5	T50.8X6
Lynestrenol	T38.4X1	T38.4X2	T38.4X3	T38.4X4	T38.4X5	T38.4X6
Lyovac Sodium Edecrin	T50.1X1	T50.1X2	T50.1X3	T50.1X4	T50.1X5	T50.1X6
Lypressin	T38.891	T38.892	T38.893	T38.894	T38.895	T38.896
Lysergic acid diethylamide	T40.8X1	T40.8X2	T40.8X3	T40.8X4	T40.8X5	--
Lysergide	T40.8X1	T40.8X2	T40.8X3	T40.8X4	T40.8X5	--
Lysine vasopressin	T38.891	T38.892	T38.893	T38.894	T38.895	T38.896
Lysol	T54.1X1	T54.1X2	T54.1X3	T54.1X4	--	--
Lysozyme	T49.0X1	T49.0X2	T49.0X3	T49.0X4	T49.0X5	T49.0X6
Lytta (vitatta)	T49.8X1	T49.8X2	T49.8X3	T49.8X4	T49.8X5	T49.8X6
Mace	T59.3X1	T59.3X2	T59.3X3	T59.3X4	--	--
Macrogol	T50.991	T50.992	T50.993	T50.994	T50.995	T50.996
Macrolide						
- anabolic drug	T38.7X1	T38.7X2	T38.7X3	T38.7X4	T38.7X5	T38.7X6
- antibiotic	T36.3X1	T36.3X2	T36.3X3	T36.3X4	T36.3X5	T36.3X6
Mafenide	T49.0X1	T49.0X2	T49.0X3	T49.0X4	T49.0X5	T49.0X6
Magaldrate	T47.1X1	T47.1X2	T47.1X3	T47.1X4	T47.1X5	T47.1X6
Magic mushroom	T40.991	T40.992	T40.993	T40.994	--	--
Magnamycin	T36.8X1	T36.8X2	T36.8X3	T36.8X4	T36.8X5	T36.8X6
Magnesia magma	T47.1X1	T47.1X2	T47.1X3	T47.1X4	T47.1X5	T47.1X6
Magnesium NEC	T56.891	T56.892	T56.893	T56.894	--	--
- carbonate	T47.1X1	T47.1X2	T47.1X3	T47.1X4	T47.1X5	T47.1X6
- citrate	T47.4X1	T47.4X2	T47.4X3	T47.4X4	T47.4X5	T47.4X6
- hydroxide	T47.1X1	T47.1X2	T47.1X3	T47.1X4	T47.1X5	T47.1X6
- oxide	T47.1X1	T47.1X2	T47.1X3	T47.1X4	T47.1X5	T47.1X6
- peroxide	T49.0X1	T49.0X2	T49.0X3	T49.0X4	T49.0X5	T49.0X6

Substance	Poisoning, Accidental (unintentional)	Poisoning, Intentional Self-harm	Poisoning, Assault	Poisoning, Undetermined	Adverse effect	Underdosing
- salicylate	T39.091	T39.092	T39.093	T39.094	T39.095	T39.096
- silicofluoride	T50.3X1	T50.3X2	T50.3X3	T50.3X4	T50.3X5	T50.3X6
- sulfate	T47.4X1	T47.4X2	T47.4X3	T47.4X4	T47.4X5	T47.4X6
- thiosulfate	T45.0X1	T45.0X2	T45.0X3	T45.0X4	T45.0X5	T45.0X6
- trisilicate	T47.1X1	T47.1X2	T47.1X3	T47.1X4	T47.1X5	T47.1X6
Malathion (medicinal)	T49.0X1	T49.0X2	T49.0X3	T49.0X4	T49.0X5	T49.0X6
- insecticide	T60.0X1	T60.0X2	T60.0X3	T60.0X4	--	--
Male fern extract	T37.4X1	T37.4X2	T37.4X3	T37.4X4	T37.4X5	T37.4X6
M-AMSA	T45.1X1	T45.1X2	T45.1X3	T45.1X4	T45.1X5	T45.1X6
Mandelic acid	T37.8X1	T37.8X2	T37.8X3	T37.8X4	T37.8X5	T37.8X6
Manganese (dioxide) (salts)	T57.2X1	T57.2X2	T57.2X3	T57.2X4	--	--
- medicinal	T50.991	T50.992	T50.993	T50.994	T50.995	T50.996
Mannitol	T47.3X1	T47.3X2	T47.3X3	T47.3X4	T47.3X5	T47.3X6
- hexanitrate	T46.3X1	T46.3X2	T46.3X3	T46.3X4	T46.3X5	T46.3X6
Mannomustine	T45.1X1	T45.1X2	T45.1X3	T45.1X4	T45.1X5	T45.1X6
MAO inhibitors	T43.1X1	T43.1X2	T43.1X3	T43.1X4	T43.1X5	T43.1X6
Mapharsen	T37.8X1	T37.8X2	T37.8X3	T37.8X4	T37.8X5	T37.8X6
Maphenide	T49.0X1	T49.0X2	T49.0X3	T49.0X4	T49.0X5	T49.0X6
Maprotiline	T43.021	T43.022	T43.023	T43.024	T43.025	T43.026
Marcaine	T41.3X1	T41.3X2	T41.3X3	T41.3X4	T41.3X5	T41.3X6
- infiltration (subcutaneous)	T41.3X1	T41.3X2	T41.3X3	T41.3X4	T41.3X5	T41.3X6
- nerve block (peripheral) (plexus)	T41.3X1	T41.3X2	T41.3X3	T41.3X4	T41.3X5	T41.3X6
Marezine	T45.0X1	T45.0X2	T45.0X3	T45.0X4	T45.0X5	T45.0X6
Marihuana	T40.7X1	T40.7X2	T40.7X3	T40.7X4	T40.7X5	T40.7X6
Marijuana	T40.7X1	T40.7X2	T40.7X3	T40.7X4	T40.7X5	T40.7X6
Marine (sting)	T63.691	T63.692	T63.693	T63.694	--	--
- animals (sting)	T63.691	T63.692	T63.693	T63.694	--	--
- plants (sting)	T63.711	T63.712	T63.713	T63.714	--	--
Marplan	T43.1X1	T43.1X2	T43.1X3	T43.1X4	T43.1X5	T43.1X6
Marsh gas	T59.891	T59.892	T59.893	T59.894	--	--
Marsilid	T43.1X1	T43.1X2	T43.1X3	T43.1X4	T43.1X5	T43.1X6
Matulane	T45.1X1	T45.1X2	T45.1X3	T45.1X4	T45.1X5	T45.1X6
Mazindol	T50.5X1	T50.5X2	T50.5X3	T50.5X4	T50.5X5	T50.5X6
MCPA	T60.3X1	T60.3X2	T60.3X3	T60.3X4	--	--
MDMA	T43.621	T43.622	T43.623	T43.624	T43.625	T43.626
Meadow saffron	T62.2X1	T62.2X2	T62.2X3	T62.2X4	--	--
Measles virus vaccine (attenuated)	T50.B91	T50.B92	T50.B93	T50.B94	T50.B95	T50.B96
Meat, noxious	T62.8X1	T62.8X2	T62.8X3	T62.8X4	--	--
Meballymal	T42.3X1	T42.3X2	T42.3X3	T42.3X4	T42.3X5	T42.3X6
Mebanazine	T43.1X1	T43.1X2	T43.1X3	T43.1X4	T43.1X5	T43.1X6
Mebaral	T42.3X1	T42.3X2	T42.3X3	T42.3X4	T42.3X5	T42.3X6
Mebendazole	T37.4X1	T37.4X2	T37.4X3	T37.4X4	T37.4X5	T37.4X6
Mebeverine	T44.3X1	T44.3X2	T44.3X3	T44.3X4	T44.3X5	T44.3X6
Mebhydrolin	T45.0X1	T45.0X2	T45.0X3	T45.0X4	T45.0X5	T45.0X6
Mebumal	T42.3X1	T42.3X2	T42.3X3	T42.3X4	T42.3X5	T42.3X6
Mebutamate	T43.591	T43.592	T43.593	T43.594	T43.595	T43.596
Mecamylamine	T44.2X1	T44.2X2	T44.2X3	T44.2X4	T44.2X5	T44.2X6
Mechlorethamine	T45.1X1	T45.1X2	T45.1X3	T45.1X4	T45.1X5	T45.1X6
Mecillinam	T36.0X1	T36.0X2	T36.0X3	T36.0X4	T36.0X5	T36.0X6
Meclizine (hydrochloride)	T45.0X1	T45.0X2	T45.0X3	T45.0X4	T45.0X5	T45.0X6
Meclocycline	T36.4X1	T36.4X2	T36.4X3	T36.4X4	T36.4X5	T36.4X6
Meclofenamate	T39.391	T39.392	T39.393	T39.394	T39.395	T39.396
Meclofenamic acid	T39.391	T39.392	T39.393	T39.394	T39.395	T39.396
Meclofenoxate	T43.691	T43.692	T43.693	T43.694	T43.695	T43.696
Meclozine	T45.0X1	T45.0X2	T45.0X3	T45.0X4	T45.0X5	T45.0X6
Mecobalamin	T45.8X1	T45.8X2	T45.8X3	T45.8X4	T45.8X5	T45.8X6
Mecoprop	T60.3X1	T60.3X2	T60.3X3	T60.3X4	--	--
Mecrilate	T49.3X1	T49.3X2	T49.3X3	T49.3X4	T49.3X5	T49.3X6
Mecysteine	T48.4X1	T48.4X2	T48.4X3	T48.4X4	T48.4X5	T48.4X6

Substance	Poisoning, Accidental (unintentional)	Poisoning, Intentional Self-harm	Poisoning, Assault	Poisoning, Undetermined	Adverse effect	Underdosing
Medazepam	T42.4X1	T42.4X2	T42.4X3	T42.4X4	T42.4X5	T42.4X6
Medicament NEC	T50.901	T50.902	T50.903	T50.904	T50.905	T50.906
Medinal	T42.3X1	T42.3X2	T42.3X3	T42.3X4	T42.3X5	T42.3X6
Medomin	T42.3X1	T42.3X2	T42.3X3	T42.3X4	T42.3X5	T42.3X6
Medrogestone	T38.5X1	T38.5X2	T38.5X3	T38.5X4	T38.5X5	T38.5X6
Medroxalol	T44.8X1	T44.8X2	T44.8X3	T44.8X4	T44.8X5	T44.8X6
Medroxyprogesterone acetate (depot)	T38.5X1	T38.5X2	T38.5X3	T38.5X4	T38.5X5	T38.5X6
Medrysone	T49.0X1	T49.0X2	T49.0X3	T49.0X4	T49.0X5	T49.0X6
Mefenamic acid	T39.391	T39.392	T39.393	T39.394	T39.395	T39.396
Mefenorex	T50.5X1	T50.5X2	T50.5X3	T50.5X4	T50.5X5	T50.5X6
Mefloquine	T37.2X1	T37.2X2	T37.2X3	T37.2X4	T37.2X5	T37.2X6
Mefruside	T50.2X1	T50.2X2	T50.2X3	T50.2X4	T50.2X5	T50.2X6
Megahallucinogen	T40.901	T40.902	T40.903	T40.904	T40.905	T40.906
Megestrol	T38.5X1	T38.5X2	T38.5X3	T38.5X4	T38.5X5	T38.5X6
Meglumine						
- antimoniate	T37.8X1	T37.8X2	T37.8X3	T37.8X4	T37.8X5	T37.8X6
- diatrizoate	T50.8X1	T50.8X2	T50.8X3	T50.8X4	T50.8X5	T50.8X6
- iodipamide	T50.8X1	T50.8X2	T50.8X3	T50.8X4	T50.8X5	T50.8X6
- iotroxate	T50.8X1	T50.8X2	T50.8X3	T50.8X4	T50.8X5	T50.8X6
MEK (methyl ethyl ketone)	T52.4X1	T52.4X2	T52.4X3	T52.4X4	--	--
Meladinin	T49.3X1	T49.3X2	T49.3X3	T49.3X4	T49.3X5	T49.3X6
Meladrazine	T44.3X1	T44.3X2	T44.3X3	T44.3X4	T44.3X5	T44.3X6
Melaleuca alternifolia oil	T49.0X1	T49.0X2	T49.0X3	T49.0X4	T49.0X5	T49.0X6
Melanizing agents	T49.3X1	T49.3X2	T49.3X3	T49.3X4	T49.3X5	T49.3X6
Melanocyte-stimulating hormone	T38.891	T38.892	T38.893	T38.894	T38.895	T38.896
Melarsonyl potassium	T37.3X1	T37.3X2	T37.3X3	T37.3X4	T37.3X5	T37.3X6
Melarsoprol	T37.3X1	T37.3X2	T37.3X3	T37.3X4	T37.3X5	T37.3X6
Melia azedarach	T62.2X1	T62.2X2	T62.2X3	T62.2X4	--	--
Melitracen	T43.011	T43.012	T43.013	T43.014	T43.015	T43.016
Mellaril	T43.3X1	T43.3X2	T43.3X3	T43.3X4	T43.3X5	T43.3X6
Meloxine	T49.3X1	T49.3X2	T49.3X3	T49.3X4	T49.3X5	T49.3X6
Melperone	T43.4X1	T43.4X2	T43.4X3	T43.4X4	T43.4X5	T43.4X6
Melphalan	T45.1X1	T45.1X2	T45.1X3	T45.1X4	T45.1X5	T45.1X6
Memantine	T43.8X1	T43.8X2	T43.8X3	T43.8X4	T43.8X5	T43.8X6
Menadiol	T45.7X1	T45.7X2	T45.7X3	T45.7X4	T45.7X5	T45.7X6
- sodium sulfate	T45.7X1	T45.7X2	T45.7X3	T45.7X4	T45.7X5	T45.7X6
Menadione	T45.7X1	T45.7X2	T45.7X3	T45.7X4	T45.7X5	T45.7X6
- sodium bisulfite	T45.7X1	T45.7X2	T45.7X3	T45.7X4	T45.7X5	T45.7X6
Menaphthone	T45.7X1	T45.7X2	T45.7X3	T45.7X4	T45.7X5	T45.7X6
Menaquinone	T45.7X1	T45.7X2	T45.7X3	T45.7X4	T45.7X5	T45.7X6
Menatetrenone	T45.7X1	T45.7X2	T45.7X3	T45.7X4	T45.7X5	T45.7X6
Meningococcal vaccine	T50.A91	T50.A92	T50.A93	T50.A94	T50.A95	T50.A96
Menningovax (-AC) (-C)	T50.A91	T50.A92	T50.A93	T50.A94	T50.A95	T50.A96
Menotropins	T38.811	T38.812	T38.813	T38.814	T38.815	T38.816
Menthol	T48.5X1	T48.5X2	T48.5X3	T48.5X4	T48.5X5	T48.5X6
Mepacrine	T37.2X1	T37.2X2	T37.2X3	T37.2X4	T37.2X5	T37.2X6
Meparfynol	T42.6X1	T42.6X2	T42.6X3	T42.6X4	T42.6X5	T42.6X6
Mepartricin	T36.7X1	T36.7X2	T36.7X3	T36.7X4	T36.7X5	T36.7X6
Mepazine	T43.3X1	T43.3X2	T43.3X3	T43.3X4	T43.3X5	T43.3X6
Mepenzolate	T44.3X1	T44.3X2	T44.3X3	T44.3X4	T44.3X5	T44.3X6
- bromide	T44.3X1	T44.3X2	T44.3X3	T44.3X4	T44.3X5	T44.3X6
Meperidine	T40.4X1	T40.4X2	T40.4X3	T40.4X4	T40.4X5	T40.4X6
Mephebarbital	T42.3X1	T42.3X2	T42.3X3	T42.3X4	T42.3X5	T42.3X6
Mephenamin (e)	T42.8X1	T42.8X2	T42.8X3	T42.8X4	T42.8X5	T42.8X6
Mephenesin	T42.8X1	T42.8X2	T42.8X3	T42.8X4	T42.8X5	T42.8X6
Mephenhydramine	T45.0X1	T45.0X2	T45.0X3	T45.0X4	T45.0X5	T45.0X6
Mephenoxalone	T42.8X1	T42.8X2	T42.8X3	T42.8X4	T42.8X5	T42.8X6
Mephentermine	T44.991	T44.992	T44.993	T44.994	T44.995	T44.996

Substance	Poisoning, Accidental (unintentional)	Poisoning, Intentional Self-harm	Poisoning, Assault	Poisoning, Undetermined	Adverse effect	Underdosing
Mephenytoin	T42.0X1	T42.0X2	T42.0X3	T42.0X4	T42.0X5	T42.0X6
- with phenobarbital	T42.3X1	T42.3X2	T42.3X3	T42.3X4	T42.3X5	T42.3X6
Mephobarbital	T42.3X1	T42.3X2	T42.3X3	T42.3X4	T42.3X5	T42.3X6
Mephosfolan	T60.0X1	T60.0X2	T60.0X3	T60.0X4	--	--
Mepindolol	T44.7X1	T44.7X2	T44.7X3	T44.7X4	T44.7X5	T44.7X6
Mepiperphenidol	T44.3X1	T44.3X2	T44.3X3	T44.3X4	T44.3X5	T44.3X6
Mepitiostane	T38.7X1	T38.7X2	T38.7X3	T38.7X4	T38.7X5	T38.7X6
Mepivacaine	T41.3X1	T41.3X2	T41.3X3	T41.3X4	T41.3X5	T41.3X6
- epidural	T41.3X1	T41.3X2	T41.3X3	T41.3X4	T41.3X5	T41.3X6
Meprednisone	T38.0X1	T38.0X2	T38.0X3	T38.0X4	T38.0X5	T38.0X6
Meprobam	T43.591	T43.592	T43.593	T43.594	T43.595	T43.596
Meprobamate	T43.591	T43.592	T43.593	T43.594	T43.595	T43.596
Meproscillarin	T46.0X1	T46.0X2	T46.0X3	T46.0X4	T46.0X5	T46.0X6
Meprylcaine	T41.3X1	T41.3X2	T41.3X3	T41.3X4	T41.3X5	T41.3X6
Meptazinol	T39.8X1	T39.8X2	T39.8X3	T39.8X4	T39.8X5	T39.8X6
Mepyramine	T45.0X1	T45.0X2	T45.0X3	T45.0X4	T45.0X5	T45.0X6
Mequitazine	T43.3X1	T43.3X2	T43.3X3	T43.3X4	T43.3X5	T43.3X6
Meralluride	T50.2X1	T50.2X2	T50.2X3	T50.2X4	T50.2X5	T50.2X6
Merbaphen	T50.2X1	T50.2X2	T50.2X3	T50.2X4	T50.2X5	T50.2X6
Merbromin	T49.0X1	T49.0X2	T49.0X3	T49.0X4	T49.0X5	T49.0X6
Mercaptobenzothiazole salts	T49.0X1	T49.0X2	T49.0X3	T49.0X4	T49.0X5	T49.0X6
Mercaptomerin	T50.2X1	T50.2X2	T50.2X3	T50.2X4	T50.2X5	T50.2X6
Mercaptopurine	T45.1X1	T45.1X2	T45.1X3	T45.1X4	T45.1X5	T45.1X6
Mercumatilin	T50.2X1	T50.2X2	T50.2X3	T50.2X4	T50.2X5	T50.2X6
Mercuramide	T50.2X1	T50.2X2	T50.2X3	T50.2X4	T50.2X5	T50.2X6
Mercurochrome	T49.0X1	T49.0X2	T49.0X3	T49.0X4	T49.0X5	T49.0X6
Mercurophylline	T50.2X1	T50.2X2	T50.2X3	T50.2X4	T50.2X5	T50.2X6
Mercury, mercurial, mercuric, mercurous (compounds) (cyanide) (fumes) (nonmedicinal) (vapor) NEC	T56.1X1	T56.1X2	T56.1X3	T56.1X4	--	--
- ammoniated	T49.0X1	T49.0X2	T49.0X3	T49.0X4	T49.0X5	T49.0X6
- anti-infective						
- - local	T49.0X1	T49.0X2	T49.0X3	T49.0X4	T49.0X5	T49.0X6
- - systemic	T37.8X1	T37.8X2	T37.8X3	T37.8X4	T37.8X5	T37.8X6
- - topical	T49.0X1	T49.0X2	T49.0X3	T49.0X4	T49.0X5	T49.0X6
- chloride (ammoniated)	T49.0X1	T49.0X2	T49.0X3	T49.0X4	T49.0X5	T49.0X6
- - fungicide	T56.1X1	T56.1X2	T56.1X3	T56.1X4	--	--
- diuretic NEC	T50.2X1	T50.2X2	T50.2X3	T50.2X4	T50.2X5	T50.2X6
- fungicide	T56.1X1	T56.1X2	T56.1X3	T56.1X4	--	--
- organic (fungicide)	T56.1X1	T56.1X2	T56.1X3	T56.1X4	--	--
- oxide, yellow	T49.0X1	T49.0X2	T49.0X3	T49.0X4	T49.0X5	T49.0X6
Mersalyl	T50.2X1	T50.2X2	T50.2X3	T50.2X4	T50.2X5	T50.2X6
Merthiolate	T49.0X1	T49.0X2	T49.0X3	T49.0X4	T49.0X5	T49.0X6
- ophthalmic preparation	T49.5X1	T49.5X2	T49.5X3	T49.5X4	T49.5X5	T49.5X6
Meruvax	T50.B91	T50.B92	T50.B93	T50.B94	T50.B95	T50.B96
Mesalazine	T47.8X1	T47.8X2	T47.8X3	T47.8X4	T47.8X5	T47.8X6
Mescal buttons	T40.991	T40.992	T40.993	T40.994	--	--
Mescaline	T40.991	T40.992	T40.993	T40.994	--	--
Mesna	T48.4X1	T48.4X2	T48.4X3	T48.4X4	T48.4X5	T48.4X6
Mesoglycan	T46.6X1	T46.6X2	T46.6X3	T46.6X4	T46.6X5	T46.6X6
Mesoridazine	T43.3X1	T43.3X2	T43.3X3	T43.3X4	T43.3X5	T43.3X6
Mestanolone	T38.7X1	T38.7X2	T38.7X3	T38.7X4	T38.7X5	T38.7X6
Mesterolone	T38.7X1	T38.7X2	T38.7X3	T38.7X4	T38.7X5	T38.7X6
Mestranol	T38.5X1	T38.5X2	T38.5X3	T38.5X4	T38.5X5	T38.5X6
Mesulergine	T42.8X1	T42.8X2	T42.8X3	T42.8X4	T42.8X5	T42.8X6
Mesulfen	T49.0X1	T49.0X2	T49.0X3	T49.0X4	T49.0X5	T49.0X6
Mesuximide	T42.2X1	T42.2X2	T42.2X3	T42.2X4	T42.2X5	T42.2X6
Metabutethamine	T41.3X1	T41.3X2	T41.3X3	T41.3X4	T41.3X5	T41.3X6
Metactesylacetate	T49.0X1	T49.0X2	T49.0X3	T49.0X4	T49.0X5	T49.0X6

Substance	Poisoning, Accidental (unintentional)	Poisoning, Intentional Self-harm	Poisoning, Assault	Poisoning, Undetermined	Adverse effect	Underdosing
Metacycline	T36.4X1	T36.4X2	T36.4X3	T36.4X4	T36.4X5	T36.4X6
Metaldehyde (snail killer) NEC	T60.8X1	T60.8X2	T60.8X3	T60.8X4	--	--
Metals (heavy) (nonmedicinal)	T56.91	T56.92	T56.93	T56.94	--	--
- dust, fumes, or vapor NEC	T56.91	T56.92	T56.93	T56.94	--	--
- light NEC	T56.91	T56.92	T56.93	T56.94	--	--
- - dust, fumes, or vapor NEC	T56.91	T56.92	T56.93	T56.94	--	--
- specified NEC	T56.891	T56.892	T56.893	T56.894	--	--
- thallium	T56.811	T56.812	T56.813	T56.814	--	--
Metamfetamine	T43.621	T43.622	T43.623	T43.624	T43.625	T43.626
Metamizole sodium	T39.2X1	T39.2X2	T39.2X3	T39.2X4	T39.2X5	T39.2X6
Metampicillin	T36.0X1	T36.0X2	T36.0X3	T36.0X4	T36.0X5	T36.0X6
Metamucil	T47.4X1	T47.4X2	T47.4X3	T47.4X4	T47.4X5	T47.4X6
Metandienone	T38.7X1	T38.7X2	T38.7X3	T38.7X4	T38.7X5	T38.7X6
Metandrostenolone	T38.7X1	T38.7X2	T38.7X3	T38.7X4	T38.7X5	T38.7X6
Metaphen	T49.0X1	T49.0X2	T49.0X3	T49.0X4	T49.0X5	T49.0X6
Metaphos	T60.0X1	T60.0X2	T60.0X3	T60.0X4	--	--
Metapramine	T43.011	T43.012	T43.013	T43.014	T43.015	T43.016
Metaproterenol	T48.291	T48.292	T48.293	T48.294	T48.295	T48.296
Metaraminol	T44.4X1	T44.4X2	T44.4X3	T44.4X4	T44.4X5	T44.4X6
Metaxalone	T42.8X1	T42.8X2	T42.8X3	T42.8X4	T42.8X5	T42.8X6
Metenolone	T38.7X1	T38.7X2	T38.7X3	T38.7X4	T38.7X5	T38.7X6
Metergoline	T42.8X1	T42.8X2	T42.8X3	T42.8X4	T42.8X5	T42.8X6
Metescufylline	T46.991	T46.992	T46.993	T46.994	T46.995	T46.996
Metetoin	T42.0X1	T42.0X2	T42.0X3	T42.0X4	T42.0X5	T42.0X6
Metformin	T38.3X1	T38.3X2	T38.3X3	T38.3X4	T38.3X5	T38.3X6
Methacholine	T44.1X1	T44.1X2	T44.1X3	T44.1X4	T44.1X5	T44.1X6
Methacycline	T36.4X1	T36.4X2	T36.4X3	T36.4X4	T36.4X5	T36.4X6
Methadone	T40.3X1	T40.3X2	T40.3X3	T40.3X4	T40.3X5	T40.3X6
Methallenestril	T38.5X1	T38.5X2	T38.5X3	T38.5X4	T38.5X5	T38.5X6
Methallenoestril	T38.5X1	T38.5X2	T38.5X3	T38.5X4	T38.5X5	T38.5X6
Methamphetamine	T43.621	T43.622	T43.623	T43.624	T43.625	T43.626
Methampyrone	T39.2X1	T39.2X2	T39.2X3	T39.2X4	T39.2X5	T39.2X6
Methandienone	T38.7X1	T38.7X2	T38.7X3	T38.7X4	T38.7X5	T38.7X6
Methandriol	T38.7X1	T38.7X2	T38.7X3	T38.7X4	T38.7X5	T38.7X6
Methandrostenolone	T38.7X1	T38.7X2	T38.7X3	T38.7X4	T38.7X5	T38.7X6
Methane	T59.891	T59.892	T59.893	T59.894	--	--
Methanethiol	T59.891	T59.892	T59.893	T59.894	--	--
Methaniazide	T37.1X1	T37.1X2	T37.1X3	T37.1X4	T37.1X5	T37.1X6
Methanol (vapor)	T51.1X1	T51.1X2	T51.1X3	T51.1X4	--	--
Methantheline	T44.3X1	T44.3X2	T44.3X3	T44.3X4	T44.3X5	T44.3X6
Methanthelinium bromide	T44.3X1	T44.3X2	T44.3X3	T44.3X4	T44.3X5	T44.3X6
Methaphenilene	T45.0X1	T45.0X2	T45.0X3	T45.0X4	T45.0X5	T45.0X6
Methapyrilene	T45.0X1	T45.0X2	T45.0X3	T45.0X4	T45.0X5	T45.0X6
Methaqualone (compound)	T42.6X1	T42.6X2	T42.6X3	T42.6X4	T42.6X5	T42.6X6
Metharbital	T42.3X1	T42.3X2	T42.3X3	T42.3X4	T42.3X5	T42.3X6
Methazolamide	T50.2X1	T50.2X2	T50.2X3	T50.2X4	T50.2X5	T50.2X6
Methdilazine	T43.3X1	T43.3X2	T43.3X3	T43.3X4	T43.3X5	T43.3X6
Methedrine	T43.621	T43.622	T43.623	T43.624	T43.625	T43.626
Methenamine (mandelate)	T37.8X1	T37.8X2	T37.8X3	T37.8X4	T37.8X5	T37.8X6
Methenolone	T38.7X1	T38.7X2	T38.7X3	T38.7X4	T38.7X5	T38.7X6
Methergine	T48.0X1	T48.0X2	T48.0X3	T48.0X4	T48.0X5	T48.0X6
Methetoin	T42.0X1	T42.0X2	T42.0X3	T42.0X4	T42.0X5	T42.0X6
Methiacil	T38.2X1	T38.2X2	T38.2X3	T38.2X4	T38.2X5	T38.2X6
Methicillin	T36.0X1	T36.0X2	T36.0X3	T36.0X4	T36.0X5	T36.0X6
Methimazole	T38.2X1	T38.2X2	T38.2X3	T38.2X4	T38.2X5	T38.2X6
Methiodal sodium	T50.8X1	T50.8X2	T50.8X3	T50.8X4	T50.8X5	T50.8X6
Methionine	T50.991	T50.992	T50.993	T50.994	T50.995	T50.996
Methisazone	T37.5X1	T37.5X2	T37.5X3	T37.5X4	T37.5X5	T37.5X6

Substance	Poisoning, Accidental (unintentional)	Poisoning, Intentional Self-harm	Poisoning, Assault	Poisoning, Undetermined	Adverse effect	Underdosing
Methisoprinol	T37.5X1	T37.5X2	T37.5X3	T37.5X4	T37.5X5	T37.5X6
Methitural	T42.3X1	T42.3X2	T42.3X3	T42.3X4	T42.3X5	T42.3X6
Methixene	T44.3X1	T44.3X2	T44.3X3	T44.3X4	T44.3X5	T44.3X6
Methobarbital, methobarbitone	T42.3X1	T42.3X2	T42.3X3	T42.3X4	T42.3X5	T42.3X6
Methocarbamol	T42.8X1	T42.8X2	T42.8X3	T42.8X4	T42.8X5	T42.8X6
- skeletal muscle relaxant	T48.1X1	T48.1X2	T48.1X3	T48.1X4	T48.1X5	T48.1X6
Methohexital	T41.1X1	T41.1X2	T41.1X3	T41.1X4	T41.1X5	T41.1X6
Methohexitone	T41.1X1	T41.1X2	T41.1X3	T41.1X4	T41.1X5	T41.1X6
Methoin	T42.0X1	T42.0X2	T42.0X3	T42.0X4	T42.0X5	T42.0X6
Methopholine	T39.8X1	T39.8X2	T39.8X3	T39.8X4	T39.8X5	T39.8X6
Methopromazine	T43.3X1	T43.3X2	T43.3X3	T43.3X4	T43.3X5	T43.3X6
Methorate	T48.3X1	T48.3X2	T48.3X3	T48.3X4	T48.3X5	T48.3X6
Methoserpidine	T46.5X1	T46.5X2	T46.5X3	T46.5X4	T46.5X5	T46.5X6
Methotrexate	T45.1X1	T45.1X2	T45.1X3	T45.1X4	T45.1X5	T45.1X6
Methotrimeprazine	T43.3X1	T43.3X2	T43.3X3	T43.3X4	T43.3X5	T43.3X6
Methoxa-Dome	T49.3X1	T49.3X2	T49.3X3	T49.3X4	T49.3X5	T49.3X6
Methoxamine	T44.4X1	T44.4X2	T44.4X3	T44.4X4	T44.4X5	T44.4X6
Methoxsalen	T50.991	T50.992	T50.993	T50.994	T50.995	T50.996
Methoxyaniline	T65.3X1	T65.3X2	T65.3X3	T65.3X4	--	--
Methoxybenzyl penicillin	T36.0X1	T36.0X2	T36.0X3	T36.0X4	T36.0X5	T36.0X6
Methoxychlor	T53.7X1	T53.7X2	T53.7X3	T53.7X4	--	--
Methoxy-DDT	T53.7X1	T53.7X2	T53.7X3	T53.7X4	--	--
2-Methoxyethanol	T52.3X1	T52.3X2	T52.3X3	T52.3X4	--	--
Methoxyflurane	T41.0X1	T41.0X2	T41.0X3	T41.0X4	T41.0X5	T41.0X6
Methoxyphenamine	T48.6X1	T48.6X2	T48.6X3	T48.6X4	T48.6X5	T48.6X6
Methoxypromazine	T43.3X1	T43.3X2	T43.3X3	T43.3X4	T43.3X5	T43.3X6
5-Methoxypsoralen (5-MOP)	T50.991	T50.992	T50.993	T50.994	T50.995	T50.996
8-Methoxypsoralen (8-MOP)	T50.991	T50.992	T50.993	T50.994	T50.995	T50.996
Methscopolamine bromide	T44.3X1	T44.3X2	T44.3X3	T44.3X4	T44.3X5	T44.3X6
Methsuximide	T42.2X1	T42.2X2	T42.2X3	T42.2X4	T42.2X5	T42.2X6
Methyclothiazide	T50.2X1	T50.2X2	T50.2X3	T50.2X4	T50.2X5	T50.2X6
Methyl						
- acetate	T52.4X1	T52.4X2	T52.4X3	T52.4X4	--	--
- acetone	T52.4X1	T52.4X2	T52.4X3	T52.4X4	--	--
- acrylate	T65.891	T65.892	T65.893	T65.894	--	--
- alcohol	T51.1X1	T51.1X2	T51.1X3	T51.1X4	--	--
- aminophenol	T65.3X1	T65.3X2	T65.3X3	T65.3X4	--	--
- amphetamine	T43.621	T43.622	T43.623	T43.624	T43.625	T43.626
- androstanolone	T38.7X1	T38.7X2	T38.7X3	T38.7X4	T38.7X5	T38.7X6
- atropine	T44.3X1	T44.3X2	T44.3X3	T44.3X4	T44.3X5	T44.3X6
- benzene	T52.2X1	T52.2X2	T52.2X3	T52.2X4	--	--
- benzoate	T52.8X1	T52.8X2	T52.8X3	T52.8X4	--	--
- benzol	T52.2X1	T52.2X2	T52.2X3	T52.2X4	--	--
- bromide (gas)	T59.891	T59.892	T59.893	T59.894	--	--
- - fumigant	T60.8X1	T60.8X2	T60.8X3	T60.8X4	--	--
- butanol	T51.3X1	T51.3X2	T51.3X3	T51.3X4	--	--
- carbinol	T51.1X1	T51.1X2	T51.1X3	T51.1X4	--	--
- carbonate	T52.8X1	T52.8X2	T52.8X3	T52.8X4	--	--
- CCNU	T45.1X1	T45.1X2	T45.1X3	T45.1X4	T45.1X5	T45.1X6
- cellosolve	T52.91	T52.92	T52.93	T52.94	--	--
- cellulose	T47.4X1	T47.4X2	T47.4X3	T47.4X4	T47.4X5	T47.4X6
- chloride (gas)	T59.891	T59.892	T59.893	T59.894	--	--
- chloroformate	T59.3X1	T59.3X2	T59.3X3	T59.3X4	--	--
- cyclohexane	T52.8X1	T52.8X2	T52.8X3	T52.8X4	--	--
- cyclohexanol	T51.8X1	T51.8X2	T51.8X3	T51.8X4	--	--
- cyclohexanone	T52.8X1	T52.8X2	T52.8X3	T52.8X4	--	--
- cyclohexyl acetate	T52.8X1	T52.8X2	T52.8X3	T52.8X4	--	--
- demeton	T60.0X1	T60.0X2	T60.0X3	T60.0X4	--	--
- dihydromorphinone	T40.2X1	T40.2X2	T40.2X3	T40.2X4	T40.2X5	T40.2X6

Substance	Poisoning, Accidental (unintentional)	Poisoning, Intentional Self-harm	Poisoning, Assault	Poisoning, Undetermined	Adverse effect	Underdosing
- ergometrine	T48.0X1	T48.0X2	T48.0X3	T48.0X4	T48.0X5	T48.0X6
- ergonovine	T48.0X1	T48.0X2	T48.0X3	T48.0X4	T48.0X5	T48.0X6
- ethyl ketone	T52.4X1	T52.4X2	T52.4X3	T52.4X4	--	--
- glucamine antimonate	T37.8X1	T37.8X2	T37.8X3	T37.8X4	T37.8X5	T37.8X6
- hydrazine	T65.891	T65.892	T65.893	T65.894	--	--
- iodide	T65.891	T65.892	T65.893	T65.894	--	--
- isobutyl ketone	T52.4X1	T52.4X2	T52.4X3	T52.4X4	--	--
- isothiocyanate	T60.3X1	T60.3X2	T60.3X3	T60.3X4	--	--
- mercaptan	T59.891	T59.892	T59.893	T59.894	--	--
- morphine NEC	T40.2X1	T40.2X2	T40.2X3	T40.2X4	T40.2X5	T40.2X6
- nicotinate	T49.4X1	T49.4X2	T49.4X3	T49.4X4	T49.4X5	T49.4X6
- paraben	T49.0X1	T49.0X2	T49.0X3	T49.0X4	T49.0X5	T49.0X6
- parafynol	T42.6X1	T42.6X2	T42.6X3	T42.6X4	T42.6X5	T42.6X6
- parathion	T60.0X1	T60.0X2	T60.0X3	T60.0X4	--	--
- peridol	T43.4X1	T43.4X2	T43.4X3	T43.4X4	T43.4X5	T43.4X6
- phenidate	T43.631	T43.632	T43.633	T43.634	T43.635	T43.636
- prednisolone	T38.0X1	T38.0X2	T38.0X3	T38.0X4	T38.0X5	T38.0X6
- - ENT agent	T49.6X1	T49.6X2	T49.6X3	T49.6X4	T49.6X5	T49.6X6
- - ophthalmic preparation	T49.5X1	T49.5X2	T49.5X3	T49.5X4	T49.5X5	T49.5X6
- - topical NEC	T49.0X1	T49.0X2	T49.0X3	T49.0X4	T49.0X5	T49.0X6
- propylcarbinol	T51.3X1	T51.3X2	T51.3X3	T51.3X4	--	--
- rosaniline NEC	T49.0X1	T49.0X2	T49.0X3	T49.0X4	T49.0X5	T49.0X6
- salicylate	T49.2X1	T49.2X2	T49.2X3	T49.2X4	T49.2X5	T49.2X6
- sulfate (fumes)	T59.891	T59.892	T59.893	T59.894	--	--
- - liquid	T52.8X1	T52.8X2	T52.8X3	T52.8X4	--	--
- sulfonal	T42.6X1	T42.6X2	T42.6X3	T42.6X4	T42.6X5	T42.6X6
- testosterone	T38.7X1	T38.7X2	T38.7X3	T38.7X4	T38.7X5	T38.7X6
- thiouracil	T38.2X1	T38.2X2	T38.2X3	T38.2X4	T38.2X5	T38.2X6
Methylamphetamine	T43.621	T43.622	T43.623	T43.624	T43.625	T43.626
Methylated spirit	T51.1X1	T51.1X2	T51.1X3	T51.1X4	--	--
Methylatropine nitrate	T44.3X1	T44.3X2	T44.3X3	T44.3X4	T44.3X5	T44.3X6
Methylbenactyzium bromide	T44.3X1	T44.3X2	T44.3X3	T44.3X4	T44.3X5	T44.3X6
Methylbenzethonium chloride	T49.0X1	T49.0X2	T49.0X3	T49.0X4	T49.0X5	T49.0X6
Methylcellulose	T47.4X1	T47.4X2	T47.4X3	T47.4X4	T47.4X5	T47.4X6
- laxative	T47.4X1	T47.4X2	T47.4X3	T47.4X4	T47.4X5	T47.4X6
Methylchlorophenoxy-acetic acid	T60.3X1	T60.3X2	T60.3X3	T60.3X4	--	--
Methyldopa	T46.5X1	T46.5X2	T46.5X3	T46.5X4	T46.5X5	T46.5X6
Methyldopate	T46.5X1	T46.5X2	T46.5X3	T46.5X4	T46.5X5	T46.5X6
Methylene						
- blue	T50.6X1	T50.6X2	T50.6X3	T50.6X4	T50.6X5	T50.6X6
- chloride or dichloride (solvent) NEC	T53.4X1	T53.4X2	T53.4X3	T53.4X4	--	--
Methylenedioxyamphetamine	T43.621	T43.622	T43.623	T43.624	T43.625	T43.626
Methylenedioxymethamphetamine	T43.621	T43.622	T43.623	T43.624	T43.625	T43.626
Methylergometrine	T48.0X1	T48.0X2	T48.0X3	T48.0X4	T48.0X5	T48.0X6
Methylergonovine	T48.0X1	T48.0X2	T48.0X3	T48.0X4	T48.0X5	T48.0X6
Methylestrenolone	T38.5X1	T38.5X2	T38.5X3	T38.5X4	T38.5X5	T38.5X6
Methylethyl cellulose	T50.991	T50.992	T50.993	T50.994	T50.995	T50.996
Methylhexabital	T42.3X1	T42.3X2	T42.3X3	T42.3X4	T42.3X5	T42.3X6
Methylmorphine	T40.2X1	T40.2X2	T40.2X3	T40.2X4	T40.2X5	T40.2X6
Methylparaben (ophthalmic)	T49.5X1	T49.5X2	T49.5X3	T49.5X4	T49.5X5	T49.5X6
Methylparafynol	T42.6X1	T42.6X2	T42.6X3	T42.6X4	T42.6X5	T42.6X6
Methylpentynol, methylpenthynol	T42.6X1	T42.6X2	T42.6X3	T42.6X4	T42.6X5	T42.6X6
Methylphenidate	T43.631	T43.632	T43.633	T43.634	T43.635	T43.636
Methylphenobarbital	T42.3X1	T42.3X2	T42.3X3	T42.3X4	T42.3X5	T42.3X6
Methylpolysiloxane	T47.1X1	T47.1X2	T47.1X3	T47.1X4	T47.1X5	T47.1X6
Methylprednisolone—see Methyl, prednisolone						
Methylrosaniline	T49.0X1	T49.0X2	T49.0X3	T49.0X4	T49.0X5	T49.0X6
Methylrosanilinium chloride	T49.0X1	T49.0X2	T49.0X3	T49.0X4	T49.0X5	T49.0X6

Substance	Poisoning, Accidental (unintentional)	Poisoning, Intentional Self-harm	Poisoning, Assault	Poisoning, Undetermined	Adverse effect	Underdosing
Methyltestosterone	T38.7X1	T38.7X2	T38.7X3	T38.7X4	T38.7X5	T38.7X6
Methylthionine chloride	T50.6X1	T50.6X2	T50.6X3	T50.6X4	T50.6X5	T50.6X6
Methylthioninium chloride	T50.6X1	T50.6X2	T50.6X3	T50.6X4	T50.6X5	T50.6X6
Methylthiouracil	T38.2X1	T38.2X2	T38.2X3	T38.2X4	T38.2X5	T38.2X6
Methyprylon	T42.6X1	T42.6X2	T42.6X3	T42.6X4	T42.6X5	T42.6X6
Methysergide	T46.5X1	T46.5X2	T46.5X3	T46.5X4	T46.5X5	T46.5X6
Metiamide	T47.1X1	T47.1X2	T47.1X3	T47.1X4	T47.1X5	T47.1X6
Meticillin	T36.0X1	T36.0X2	T36.0X3	T36.0X4	T36.0X5	T36.0X6
Meticrane	T50.2X1	T50.2X2	T50.2X3	T50.2X4	T50.2X5	T50.2X6
Metildigoxin	T46.0X1	T46.0X2	T46.0X3	T46.0X4	T46.0X5	T46.0X6
Metipranolol	T49.5X1	T49.5X2	T49.5X3	T49.5X4	T49.5X5	T49.5X6
Metirosine	T46.5X1	T46.5X2	T46.5X3	T46.5X4	T46.5X5	T46.5X6
Metisazone	T37.5X1	T37.5X2	T37.5X3	T37.5X4	T37.5X5	T37.5X6
Metixene	T44.3X1	T44.3X2	T44.3X3	T44.3X4	T44.3X5	T44.3X6
Metizoline	T48.5X1	T48.5X2	T48.5X3	T48.5X4	T48.5X5	T48.5X6
Metoclopramide	T45.0X1	T45.0X2	T45.0X3	T45.0X4	T45.0X5	T45.0X6
Metofenazate	T43.3X1	T43.3X2	T43.3X3	T43.3X4	T43.3X5	T43.3X6
Metofoline	T39.8X1	T39.8X2	T39.8X3	T39.8X4	T39.8X5	T39.8X6
Metolazone	T50.2X1	T50.2X2	T50.2X3	T50.2X4	T50.2X5	T50.2X6
Metopon	T40.2X1	T40.2X2	T40.2X3	T40.2X4	T40.2X5	T40.2X6
Metoprine	T45.1X1	T45.1X2	T45.1X3	T45.1X4	T45.1X5	T45.1X6
Metoprolol	T44.7X1	T44.7X2	T44.7X3	T44.7X4	T44.7X5	T44.7X6
Metrifonate	T60.0X1	T60.0X2	T60.0X3	T60.0X4	--	--
Metrizamide	T50.8X1	T50.8X2	T50.8X3	T50.8X4	T50.8X5	T50.8X6
Metrizoic acid	T50.8X1	T50.8X2	T50.8X3	T50.8X4	T50.8X5	T50.8X6
Metronidazole	T37.8X1	T37.8X2	T37.8X3	T37.8X4	T37.8X5	T37.8X6
Metycaine	T41.3X1	T41.3X2	T41.3X3	T41.3X4	T41.3X5	T41.3X6
- infiltration (subcutaneous)	T41.3X1	T41.3X2	T41.3X3	T41.3X4	T41.3X5	T41.3X6
- nerve block (peripheral) (plexus)	T41.3X1	T41.3X2	T41.3X3	T41.3X4	T41.3X5	T41.3X6
- topical (surface)	T41.3X1	T41.3X2	T41.3X3	T41.3X4	T41.3X5	T41.3X6
Metyrapone	T50.8X1	T50.8X2	T50.8X3	T50.8X4	T50.8X5	T50.8X6
Mevinphos	T60.0X1	T60.0X2	T60.0X3	T60.0X4	--	--
Mexazolam	T42.4X1	T42.4X2	T42.4X3	T42.4X4	T42.4X5	T42.4X6
Mexenone	T49.3X1	T49.3X2	T49.3X3	T49.3X4	T49.3X5	T49.3X6
Mexiletine	T46.2X1	T46.2X2	T46.2X3	T46.2X4	T46.2X5	T46.2X6
Mezereon	T62.2X1	T62.2X2	T62.2X3	T62.2X4	--	--
- berries	T62.1X1	T62.1X2	T62.1X3	T62.1X4	--	--
Mezlocillin	T36.0X1	T36.0X2	T36.0X3	T36.0X4	T36.0X5	T36.0X6
Mianserin	T43.021	T43.022	T43.023	T43.024	T43.025	T43.026
Micatin	T49.0X1	T49.0X2	T49.0X3	T49.0X4	T49.0X5	T49.0X6
Miconazole	T49.0X1	T49.0X2	T49.0X3	T49.0X4	T49.0X5	T49.0X6
Micronomicin	T36.5X1	T36.5X2	T36.5X3	T36.5X4	T36.5X5	T36.5X6
Midazolam	T42.4X1	T42.4X2	T42.4X3	T42.4X4	T42.4X5	T42.4X6
Midecamycin	T36.3X1	T36.3X2	T36.3X3	T36.3X4	T36.3X5	T36.3X6
Mifepristone	T38.6X1	T38.6X2	T38.6X3	T38.6X4	T38.6X5	T38.6X6
Milk of magnesia	T47.1X1	T47.1X2	T47.1X3	T47.1X4	T47.1X5	T47.1X6
Millipede (tropical) (venomous)	T63.411	T63.412	T63.413	T63.414	--	--
Miltown	T43.591	T43.592	T43.593	T43.594	T43.595	T43.596
Milverine	T44.3X1	T44.3X2	T44.3X3	T44.3X4	T44.3X5	T44.3X6
Minaprine	T43.291	T43.292	T43.293	T43.294	T43.295	T43.296
Minaxolone	T41.291	T41.292	T41.293	T41.294	T41.295	T41.296
Mineral						
- acids	T54.2X1	T54.2X2	T54.2X3	T54.2X4	--	--
- oil (laxative) (medicinal)	T47.4X1	T47.4X2	T47.4X3	T47.4X4	T47.4X5	T47.4X6
- - emulsion	T47.2X1	T47.2X2	T47.2X3	T47.2X4	T47.2X5	T47.2X6
- - nonmedicinal	T52.0X1	T52.0X2	T52.0X3	T52.0X4	--	--
- - topical	T49.3X1	T49.3X2	T49.3X3	T49.3X4	T49.3X5	T49.3X6
- salt NEC	T50.3X1	T50.3X2	T50.3X3	T50.3X4	T50.3X5	T50.3X6
- spirits	T52.0X1	T52.0X2	T52.0X3	T52.0X4	--	--

Substance	Poisoning, Accidental (unintentional)	Poisoning, Intentional Self-harm	Poisoning, Assault	Poisoning, Undetermined	Adverse effect	Underdosing
Mineralocorticosteroid	T50.0X1	T50.0X2	T50.0X3	T50.0X4	T50.0X5	T50.0X6
Minocycline	T36.4X1	T36.4X2	T36.4X3	T36.4X4	T36.4X5	T36.4X6
Minoxidil	T46.7X1	T46.7X2	T46.7X3	T46.7X4	T46.7X5	T46.7X6
Miokamycin	T36.3X1	T36.3X2	T36.3X3	T36.3X4	T36.3X5	T36.3X6
Miotic drug	T49.5X1	T49.5X2	T49.5X3	T49.5X4	T49.5X5	T49.5X6
Mipafox	T60.0X1	T60.0X2	T60.0X3	T60.0X4	--	--
Mirex	T60.1X1	T60.1X2	T60.1X3	T60.1X4	--	--
Mirtazapine	T43.021	T43.022	T43.023	T43.024	T43.025	T43.026
Misonidazole	T37.3X1	T37.3X2	T37.3X3	T37.3X4	T37.3X5	T37.3X6
Misoprostol	T47.1X1	T47.1X2	T47.1X3	T47.1X4	T47.1X5	T47.1X6
Mithramycin	T45.1X1	T45.1X2	T45.1X3	T45.1X4	T45.1X5	T45.1X6
Mitobronitol	T45.1X1	T45.1X2	T45.1X3	T45.1X4	T45.1X5	T45.1X6
Mitoguazone	T45.1X1	T45.1X2	T45.1X3	T45.1X4	T45.1X5	T45.1X6
Mitolactol	T45.1X1	T45.1X2	T45.1X3	T45.1X4	T45.1X5	T45.1X6
Mitomycin	T45.1X1	T45.1X2	T45.1X3	T45.1X4	T45.1X5	T45.1X6
Mitopodozide	T45.1X1	T45.1X2	T45.1X3	T45.1X4	T45.1X5	T45.1X6
Mitotane	T45.1X1	T45.1X2	T45.1X3	T45.1X4	T45.1X5	T45.1X6
Mitoxantrone	T45.1X1	T45.1X2	T45.1X3	T45.1X4	T45.1X5	T45.1X6
Mivacurium chloride	T48.1X1	T48.1X2	T48.1X3	T48.1X4	T48.1X5	T48.1X6
Miyari bacteria	T47.6X1	T47.6X2	T47.6X3	T47.6X4	T47.6X5	T47.6X6
Moclobemide	T43.1X1	T43.1X2	T43.1X3	T43.1X4	T43.1X5	T43.1X6
Moderil	T46.5X1	T46.5X2	T46.5X3	T46.5X4	T46.5X5	T46.5X6
Mofebutazone	T39.2X1	T39.2X2	T39.2X3	T39.2X4	T39.2X5	T39.2X6
Mogadon—see Nitrazepam						
Molindone	T43.591	T43.592	T43.593	T43.594	T43.595	T43.596
Molsidomine	T46.3X1	T46.3X2	T46.3X3	T46.3X4	T46.3X5	T46.3X6
Mometasone	T49.0X1	T49.0X2	T49.0X3	T49.0X4	T49.0X5	T49.0X6
Monistat	T49.0X1	T49.0X2	T49.0X3	T49.0X4	T49.0X5	T49.0X6
Monkshood	T62.2X1	T62.2X2	T62.2X3	T62.2X4	--	--
Monoamine oxidase inhibitor NEC	T43.1X1	T43.1X2	T43.1X3	T43.1X4	T43.1X5	T43.1X6
- hydrazine	T43.1X1	T43.1X2	T43.1X3	T43.1X4	T43.1X5	T43.1X6
Monobenzone	T49.4X1	T49.4X2	T49.4X3	T49.4X4	T49.4X5	T49.4X6
Monochloroacetic acid	T60.3X1	T60.3X2	T60.3X3	T60.3X4	--	--
Monochlorobenzene	T53.7X1	T53.7X2	T53.7X3	T53.7X4	--	--
Monoethanolamine	T46.8X1	T46.8X2	T46.8X3	T46.8X4	T46.8X5	T46.8X6
- oleate	T46.8X1	T46.8X2	T46.8X3	T46.8X4	T46.8X5	T46.8X6
Monooctanoin	T50.991	T50.992	T50.993	T50.994	T50.995	T50.996
Monophenylbutazone	T39.2X1	T39.2X2	T39.2X3	T39.2X4	T39.2X5	T39.2X6
Monosodium glutamate	T65.891	T65.892	T65.893	T65.894	--	--
Monosulfiram	T49.0X1	T49.0X2	T49.0X3	T49.0X4	T49.0X5	T49.0X6
Monoxide, carbon—see Carbon, monoxide						
Monoxidine hydrochloride	T46.1X1	T46.1X2	T46.1X3	T46.1X4	T46.1X5	T46.1X6
Monuron	T60.3X1	T60.3X2	T60.3X3	T60.3X4	--	--
Moperone	T43.4X1	T43.4X2	T43.4X3	T43.4X4	T43.4X5	T43.4X6
Mopidamol	T45.1X1	T45.1X2	T45.1X3	T45.1X4	T45.1X5	T45.1X6
MOPP (mechloreth-amine + vincristine + prednisone + procarba-zine)	T45.1X1	T45.1X2	T45.1X3	T45.1X4	T45.1X5	T45.1X6
Morfin	T40.2X1	T40.2X2	T40.2X3	T40.2X4	T40.2X5	T40.2X6
Morinamide	T37.1X1	T37.1X2	T37.1X3	T37.1X4	T37.1X5	T37.1X6
Morning glory seeds	T40.991	T40.992	T40.993	T40.994	--	--
Moroxydine	T37.5X1	T37.5X2	T37.5X3	T37.5X4	T37.5X5	T37.5X6
Morphazinamide	T37.1X1	T37.1X2	T37.1X3	T37.1X4	T37.1X5	T37.1X6
Morphine	T40.2X1	T40.2X2	T40.2X3	T40.2X4	T40.2X5	T40.2X6
- antagonist	T50.7X1	T50.7X2	T50.7X3	T50.7X4	T50.7X5	T50.7X6
Morpholinylethylmorphine	T40.2X1	T40.2X2	T40.2X3	T40.2X4	--	--
Morsuximide	T42.2X1	T42.2X2	T42.2X3	T42.2X4	T42.2X5	T42.2X6
Mosapramine	T43.591	T43.592	T43.593	T43.594	T43.595	T43.596
Moth balls—see also Pesticides	T60.2X1	T60.2X2	T60.2X3	T60.2X4	--	--
- naphthalene	T60.2X1	T60.2X2	T60.2X3	T60.2X4	--	--

Substance	Poisoning, Accidental (unintentional)	Poisoning, Intentional Self-harm	Poisoning, Assault	Poisoning, Undetermined	Adverse effect	Underdosing
- paradichlorobenzene	T60.1X1	T60.1X2	T60.1X3	T60.1X4	--	--
Motor exhaust gas	T58.01	T58.02	T58.03	T58.04	--	--
Mouthwash (antiseptic) (zinc chloride)	T49.6X1	T49.6X2	T49.6X3	T49.6X4	T49.6X5	T49.6X6
Moxastine	T45.0X1	T45.0X2	T45.0X3	T45.0X4	T45.0X5	T45.0X6
Moxaverine	T44.3X1	T44.3X2	T44.3X3	T44.3X4	T44.3X5	T44.3X6
Moxisylyte	T46.7X1	T46.7X2	T46.7X3	T46.7X4	T46.7X5	T46.7X6
Mucilage, plant	T47.4X1	T47.4X2	T47.4X3	T47.4X4	T47.4X5	T47.4X6
Mucolytic drug	T48.4X1	T48.4X2	T48.4X3	T48.4X4	T48.4X5	T48.4X6
Mucomyst	T48.4X1	T48.4X2	T48.4X3	T48.4X4	T48.4X5	T48.4X6
Mucous membrane agents (external)	T49.91	T49.92	T49.93	T49.94	T49.95	T49.96
- specified NEC	T49.8X1	T49.8X2	T49.8X3	T49.8X4	T49.8X5	T49.8X6
Mumps						
- immune globulin (human)	T50.Z11	T50.Z12	T50.Z13	T50.Z14	T50.Z15	T50.Z16
- skin test antigen	T50.8X1	T50.8X2	T50.8X3	T50.8X4	T50.8X5	T50.8X6
- vaccine	T50.B91	T50.B92	T50.B93	T50.B94	T50.B95	T50.B96
Mumpsvax	T50.B91	T50.B92	T50.B93	T50.B94	T50.B95	T50.B96
Mupirocin	T49.0X1	T49.0X2	T49.0X3	T49.0X4	T49.0X5	T49.0X6
Muriatic acid—see Hydrochloric acid						
Muromonab-CD3	T45.1X1	T45.1X2	T45.1X3	T45.1X4	T45.1X5	T45.1X6
Muscle-action drug NEC	T48.201	T48.202	T48.203	T48.204	T48.205	T48.206
Muscle affecting agents NEC	T48.201	T48.202	T48.203	T48.204	T48.205	T48.206
- oxytocic	T48.0X1	T48.0X2	T48.0X3	T48.0X4	T48.0X5	T48.0X6
- relaxants	T48.201	T48.202	T48.203	T48.204	T48.205	T48.206
- - central nervous system	T42.8X1	T42.8X2	T42.8X3	T42.8X4	T42.8X5	T42.8X6
- - skeletal	T48.1X1	T48.1X2	T48.1X3	T48.1X4	T48.1X5	T48.1X6
- - smooth	T44.3X1	T44.3X2	T44.3X3	T44.3X4	T44.3X5	T44.3X6
Muscle relaxant—see Relaxant, muscle						
Muscle-tone depressant, central NEC	T42.8X1	T42.8X2	T42.8X3	T42.8X4	T42.8X5	T42.8X6
- specified NEC	T42.8X1	T42.8X2	T42.8X3	T42.8X4	T42.8X5	T42.8X6
Mushroom, noxious	T62.0X1	T62.0X2	T62.0X3	T62.0X4	--	--
Mussel, noxious	T61.781	T61.782	T61.783	T61.784	--	--
Mustard (emetic)	T47.7X1	T47.7X2	T47.7X3	T47.7X4	T47.7X5	T47.7X6
- black	T47.7X1	T47.7X2	T47.7X3	T47.7X4	T47.7X5	T47.7X6
- gas, not in war	T59.91	T59.92	T59.93	T59.94	--	--
- nitrogen	T45.1X1	T45.1X2	T45.1X3	T45.1X4	T45.1X5	T45.1X6
Mustine	T45.1X1	T45.1X2	T45.1X3	T45.1X4	T45.1X5	T45.1X6
M-vac	T45.1X1	T45.1X2	T45.1X3	T45.1X4	T45.1X5	T45.1X6
Mycifradin	T36.5X1	T36.5X2	T36.5X3	T36.5X4	T36.5X5	T36.5X6
- topical	T49.0X1	T49.0X2	T49.0X3	T49.0X4	T49.0X5	T49.0X6
Mycitracin	T36.8X1	T36.8X2	T36.8X3	T36.8X4	T36.8X5	T36.8X6
- ophthalmic preparation	T49.5X1	T49.5X2	T49.5X3	T49.5X4	T49.5X5	T49.5X6
Mycostatin	T36.7X1	T36.7X2	T36.7X3	T36.7X4	T36.7X5	T36.7X6
- topical	T49.0X1	T49.0X2	T49.0X3	T49.0X4	T49.0X5	T49.0X6
Mycotoxins	T64.81	T64.82	T64.83	T64.84	--	--
- aflatoxin	T64.01	T64.02	T64.03	T64.04	--	--
- specified NEC	T64.81	T64.82	T64.83	T64.84	--	--
Mydriacyl	T44.3X1	T44.3X2	T44.3X3	T44.3X4	T44.3X5	T44.3X6
Mydriatic drug	T49.5X1	T49.5X2	T49.5X3	T49.5X4	T49.5X5	T49.5X6
Myelobromal	T45.1X1	T45.1X2	T45.1X3	T45.1X4	T45.1X5	T45.1X6
Myleran	T45.1X1	T45.1X2	T45.1X3	T45.1X4	T45.1X5	T45.1X6
Myochrysin (e)	T39.2X1	T39.2X2	T39.2X3	T39.2X4	T39.2X5	T39.2X6
Myoneural blocking agents	T48.1X1	T48.1X2	T48.1X3	T48.1X4	T48.1X5	T48.1X6
Myralact	T49.0X1	T49.0X2	T49.0X3	T49.0X4	T49.0X5	T49.0X6
Myristica fragrans	T62.2X1	T62.2X2	T62.2X3	T62.2X4	--	--
Myristicin	T65.891	T65.892	T65.893	T65.894	--	--
Mysoline	T42.3X1	T42.3X2	T42.3X3	T42.3X4	T42.3X5	T42.3X6
Nabilone	T40.7X1	T40.7X2	T40.7X3	T40.7X4	T40.7X5	T40.7X6
Nabumetone	T39.391	T39.392	T39.393	T39.394	T39.395	T39.396
Nadolol	T44.7X1	T44.7X2	T44.7X3	T44.7X4	T44.7X5	T44.7X6

Substance	Poisoning, Accidental (unintentional)	Poisoning, Intentional Self-harm	Poisoning, Assault	Poisoning, Undetermined	Adverse effect	Underdosing
Nafcillin	T36.0X1	T36.0X2	T36.0X3	T36.0X4	T36.0X5	T36.0X6
Nafoxidine	T38.6X1	T38.6X2	T38.6X3	T38.6X4	T38.6X5	T38.6X6
Naftazone	T46.991	T46.992	T46.993	T46.994	T46.995	T46.996
Naftidrofuryl (oxalate)	T46.7X1	T46.7X2	T46.7X3	T46.7X4	T46.7X5	T46.7X6
Naftifine	T49.0X1	T49.0X2	T49.0X3	T49.0X4	T49.0X5	T49.0X6
Nail polish remover	T52.91	T52.92	T52.93	T52.94	--	--
Nalbuphine	T40.4X1	T40.4X2	T40.4X3	T40.4X4	T40.4X5	T40.4X6
Naled	T60.0X1	T60.0X2	T60.0X3	T60.0X4	--	--
Nalidixic acid	T37.8X1	T37.8X2	T37.8X3	T37.8X4	T37.8X5	T37.8X6
Nalorphine	T50.7X1	T50.7X2	T50.7X3	T50.7X4	T50.7X5	T50.7X6
Naloxone	T50.7X1	T50.7X2	T50.7X3	T50.7X4	T50.7X5	T50.7X6
Naltrexone	T50.7X1	T50.7X2	T50.7X3	T50.7X4	T50.7X5	T50.7X6
Namenda	T43.8X1	T43.8X2	T43.8X3	T43.8X4	T43.8X5	T43.8X6
Nandrolone	T38.7X1	T38.7X2	T38.7X3	T38.7X4	T38.7X5	T38.7X6
Naphazoline	T48.5X1	T48.5X2	T48.5X3	T48.5X4	T48.5X5	T48.5X6
Naphtha (painters') (petroleum)	T52.0X1	T52.0X2	T52.0X3	T52.0X4	--	--
- solvent	T52.0X1	T52.0X2	T52.0X3	T52.0X4	--	--
- vapor	T52.0X1	T52.0X2	T52.0X3	T52.0X4	--	--
Naphthalene (non-chlorinated)	T60.2X1	T60.2X2	T60.2X3	T60.2X4	--	--
- chlorinated	T60.1X1	T60.1X2	T60.1X3	T60.1X4	--	--
- - vapor	T60.1X1	T60.1X2	T60.1X3	T60.1X4	--	--
- insecticide or moth repellent	T60.2X1	T60.2X2	T60.2X3	T60.2X4	--	--
- - chlorinated	T60.1X1	T60.1X2	T60.1X3	T60.1X4	--	--
- vapor	T60.2X1	T60.2X2	T60.2X3	T60.2X4	--	--
- - chlorinated	T60.1X1	T60.1X2	T60.1X3	T60.1X4	--	--
Naphthol	T65.891	T65.892	T65.893	T65.894	--	--
Naphthylamine	T65.891	T65.892	T65.893	T65.894	--	--
Naphthylthiourea (ANTU)	T60.4X1	T60.4X2	T60.4X3	T60.4X4	--	--
Naprosyn—see Naproxen						
Naproxen	T39.311	T39.312	T39.313	T39.314	T39.315	T39.316
Narcotic (drug)	T40.601	T40.602	T40.603	T40.604	T40.605	T40.606
- analgesic NEC	T40.601	T40.602	T40.603	T40.604	T40.605	T40.606
- antagonist	T50.7X1	T50.7X2	T50.7X3	T50.7X4	T50.7X5	T50.7X6
- specified NEC	T40.691	T40.692	T40.693	T40.694	T40.695	T40.696
- synthetic	T40.4X1	T40.4X2	T40.4X3	T40.4X4	T40.4X5	T40.4X6
Narcotine	T48.3X1	T48.3X2	T48.3X3	T48.3X4	T48.3X5	T48.3X6
Nardil	T43.1X1	T43.1X2	T43.1X3	T43.1X4	T43.1X5	T43.1X6
Nasal drug NEC	T49.6X1	T49.6X2	T49.6X3	T49.6X4	T49.6X5	T49.6X6
Natamycin	T49.0X1	T49.0X2	T49.0X3	T49.0X4	T49.0X5	T49.0X6
Natrium cyanide—see Cyanide (s)						
Natural						
- blood (product)	T45.8X1	T45.8X2	T45.8X3	T45.8X4	T45.8X5	T45.8X6
- gas (piped)	T59.891	T59.892	T59.893	T59.894	--	--
- - incomplete combustion	T58.11	T58.12	T58.13	T58.14	--	--
Nealbarbital	T42.3X1	T42.3X2	T42.3X3	T42.3X4	T42.3X5	T42.3X6
Nectadon	T48.3X1	T48.3X2	T48.3X3	T48.3X4	T48.3X5	T48.3X6
Nedocromil	T48.6X1	T48.6X2	T48.6X3	T48.6X4	T48.6X5	T48.6X6
Nefopam	T39.8X1	T39.8X2	T39.8X3	T39.8X4	T39.8X5	T39.8X6
Nematocyst (sting)	T63.691	T63.692	T63.693	T63.694	--	--
Nembutal	T42.3X1	T42.3X2	T42.3X3	T42.3X4	T42.3X5	T42.3X6
Nemonapride	T43.591	T43.592	T43.593	T43.594	T43.595	T43.596
Neoarsphenamine	T37.8X1	T37.8X2	T37.8X3	T37.8X4	T37.8X5	T37.8X6
Neocinchophen	T50.4X1	T50.4X2	T50.4X3	T50.4X4	T50.4X5	T50.4X6
Neomycin (derivatives)	T36.5X1	T36.5X2	T36.5X3	T36.5X4	T36.5X5	T36.5X6
- with						
- - bacitracin	T49.0X1	T49.0X2	T49.0X3	T49.0X4	T49.0X5	T49.0X6
- - neostigmine	T44.0X1	T44.0X2	T44.0X3	T44.0X4	T44.0X5	T44.0X6
- ENT agent	T49.6X1	T49.6X2	T49.6X3	T49.6X4	T49.6X5	T49.6X6

Substance	Poisoning, Accidental (unintentional)	Poisoning, Intentional Self-harm	Poisoning, Assault	Poisoning, Undetermined	Adverse effect	Underdosing
- ophthalmic preparation	T49.5X1	T49.5X2	T49.5X3	T49.5X4	T49.5X5	T49.5X6
- topical NEC	T49.0X1	T49.0X2	T49.0X3	T49.0X4	T49.0X5	T49.0X6
Neonal	T42.3X1	T42.3X2	T42.3X3	T42.3X4	T42.3X5	T42.3X6
Neoprontosil	T37.0X1	T37.0X2	T37.0X3	T37.0X4	T37.0X5	T37.0X6
Neosalvarsan	T37.8X1	T37.8X2	T37.8X3	T37.8X4	T37.8X5	T37.8X6
Neosilversalvarsan	T37.8X1	T37.8X2	T37.8X3	T37.8X4	T37.8X5	T37.8X6
Neosporin	T36.8X1	T36.8X2	T36.8X3	T36.8X4	T36.8X5	T36.8X6
- ENT agent	T49.6X1	T49.6X2	T49.6X3	T49.6X4	T49.6X5	T49.6X6
- opthalmic preparation	T49.5X1	T49.5X2	T49.5X3	T49.5X4	T49.5X5	T49.5X6
- topical NEC	T49.0X1	T49.0X2	T49.0X3	T49.0X4	T49.0X5	T49.0X6
Neostigmine bromide	T44.0X1	T44.0X2	T44.0X3	T44.0X4	T44.0X5	T44.0X6
Neraval	T42.3X1	T42.3X2	T42.3X3	T42.3X4	T42.3X5	T42.3X6
Neravan	T42.3X1	T42.3X2	T42.3X3	T42.3X4	T42.3X5	T42.3X6
Nerium oleander	T62.2X1	T62.2X2	T62.2X3	T62.2X4	--	--
Nerve gas, not in war	T59.91	T59.92	T59.93	T59.94	--	--
Nesacaine	T41.3X1	T41.3X2	T41.3X3	T41.3X4	T41.3X5	T41.3X6
- infiltration (subcutaneous)	T41.3X1	T41.3X2	T41.3X3	T41.3X4	T41.3X5	T41.3X6
- nerve block (peripheral) (plexus)	T41.3X1	T41.3X2	T41.3X3	T41.3X4	T41.3X5	T41.3X6
Netilmicin	T36.5X1	T36.5X2	T36.5X3	T36.5X4	T36.5X5	T36.5X6
Neurobarb	T42.3X1	T42.3X2	T42.3X3	T42.3X4	T42.3X5	T42.3X6
Neuroleptic drug NEC	T43.501	T43.502	T43.503	T43.504	T43.505	T43.506
Neuromuscular blocking drug	T48.1X1	T48.1X2	T48.1X3	T48.1X4	T48.1X5	T48.1X6
Neutral insulin injection	T38.3X1	T38.3X2	T38.3X3	T38.3X4	T38.3X5	T38.3X6
Neutral spirits	T51.0X1	T51.0X2	T51.0X3	T51.0X4	--	--
- beverage	T51.0X1	T51.0X2	T51.0X3	T51.0X4	--	--
Niacin	T46.7X1	T46.7X2	T46.7X3	T46.7X4	T46.7X5	T46.7X6
Niacinamide	T45.2X1	T45.2X2	T45.2X3	T45.2X4	T45.2X5	T45.2X6
Nialamide	T43.1X1	T43.1X2	T43.1X3	T43.1X4	T43.1X5	T43.1X6
Niaprazine	T42.6X1	T42.6X2	T42.6X3	T42.6X4	T42.6X5	T42.6X6
Nicametate	T46.7X1	T46.7X2	T46.7X3	T46.7X4	T46.7X5	T46.7X6
Nicardipine	T46.1X1	T46.1X2	T46.1X3	T46.1X4	T46.1X5	T46.1X6
Nicergoline	T46.7X1	T46.7X2	T46.7X3	T46.7X4	T46.7X5	T46.7X6
Nickel (carbonyl) (tetra-carbonyl) (fumes) (vapor)	T56.891	T56.892	T56.893	T56.894	--	--
Nickelocene	T56.891	T56.892	T56.893	T56.894	--	--
Niclosamide	T37.4X1	T37.4X2	T37.4X3	T37.4X4	T37.4X5	T37.4X6
Nicofuranose	T46.7X1	T46.7X2	T46.7X3	T46.7X4	T46.7X5	T46.7X6
Nicomorphine	T40.2X1	T40.2X2	T40.2X3	T40.2X4	--	--
Nicorandil	T46.3X1	T46.3X2	T46.3X3	T46.3X4	T46.3X5	T46.3X6
Nicotiana (plant)	T62.2X1	T62.2X2	T62.2X3	T62.2X4	--	--
Nicotinamide	T45.2X1	T45.2X2	T45.2X3	T45.2X4	T45.2X5	T45.2X6
Nicotine (insecticide) (spray) (sulfate) NEC	T60.2X1	T60.2X2	T60.2X3	T60.2X4	--	--
- from tobacco	T65.291	T65.292	T65.293	T65.294	--	--
- - cigarettes	T65.221	T65.222	T65.223	T65.224	--	--
- not insecticide	T65.291	T65.292	T65.293	T65.294	--	--
Nicotinic acid	T46.7X1	T46.7X2	T46.7X3	T46.7X4	T46.7X5	T46.7X6
Nicotinyl alcohol	T46.7X1	T46.7X2	T46.7X3	T46.7X4	T46.7X5	T46.7X6
Nicoumalone	T45.511	T45.512	T45.513	T45.514	T45.515	T45.516
Nifedipine	T46.1X1	T46.1X2	T46.1X3	T46.1X4	T46.1X5	T46.1X6
Nifenazone	T39.2X1	T39.2X2	T39.2X3	T39.2X4	T39.2X5	T39.2X6
Nifuraldezone	T37.91	T37.92	T37.93	T37.94	T37.95	T37.96
Nifuratel	T37.8X1	T37.8X2	T37.8X3	T37.8X4	T37.8X5	T37.8X6
Nifurtimox	T37.3X1	T37.3X2	T37.3X3	T37.3X4	T37.3X5	T37.3X6
Nifurtoinol	T37.8X1	T37.8X2	T37.8X3	T37.8X4	T37.8X5	T37.8X6
Nightshade, deadly (solanum) —see also Belladonna	T62.2X1	T62.2X2	T62.2X3	T62.2X4	--	--
- berry	T62.1X1	T62.1X2	T62.1X3	T62.1X4	--	--
Nikethamide	T50.7X1	T50.7X2	T50.7X3	T50.7X4	T50.7X5	T50.7X6
Nilstat	T36.7X1	T36.7X2	T36.7X3	T36.7X4	T36.7X5	T36.7X6
- topical	T49.0X1	T49.0X2	T49.0X3	T49.0X4	T49.0X5	T49.0X6

Substance	Poisoning, Accidental (unintentional)	Poisoning, Intentional Self-harm	Poisoning, Assault	Poisoning, Undetermined	Adverse effect	Underdosing
Nilutamide	T38.6X1	T38.6X2	T38.6X3	T38.6X4	T38.6X5	T38.6X6
Nimesulide	T39.391	T39.392	T39.393	T39.394	T39.395	T39.396
Nimetazepam	T42.4X1	T42.4X2	T42.4X3	T42.4X4	T42.4X5	T42.4X6
Nimodipine	T46.1X1	T46.1X2	T46.1X3	T46.1X4	T46.1X5	T46.1X6
Nimorazole	T37.3X1	T37.3X2	T37.3X3	T37.3X4	T37.3X5	T37.3X6
Nimustine	T45.1X1	T45.1X2	T45.1X3	T45.1X4	T45.1X5	T45.1X6
Niridazole	T37.4X1	T37.4X2	T37.4X3	T37.4X4	T37.4X5	T37.4X6
Nisentil	T40.2X1	T40.2X2	T40.2X3	T40.2X4	T40.2X5	T40.2X6
Nisoldipine	T46.1X1	T46.1X2	T46.1X3	T46.1X4	T46.1X5	T46.1X6
Nitramine	T65.3X1	T65.3X2	T65.3X3	T65.3X4	--	--
Nitrate, organic	T46.3X1	T46.3X2	T46.3X3	T46.3X4	T46.3X5	T46.3X6
Nitrazepam	T42.4X1	T42.4X2	T42.4X3	T42.4X4	T42.4X5	T42.4X6
Nitrefazole	T50.6X1	T50.6X2	T50.6X3	T50.6X4	T50.6X5	T50.6X6
Nitrendipine	T46.1X1	T46.1X2	T46.1X3	T46.1X4	T46.1X5	T46.1X6
Nitric						
- acid (liquid)	T54.2X1	T54.2X2	T54.2X3	T54.2X4	--	--
- - vapor	T59.891	T59.892	T59.893	T59.894	--	--
- oxide (gas)	T59.0X1	T59.0X2	T59.0X3	T59.0X4	--	--
Nitrimidazine	T37.3X1	T37.3X2	T37.3X3	T37.3X4	T37.3X5	T37.3X6
Nitrite, amyl (medicinal) (vapor)	T46.3X1	T46.3X2	T46.3X3	T46.3X4	T46.3X5	T46.3X6
Nitroaniline	T65.3X1	T65.3X2	T65.3X3	T65.3X4	--	--
- vapor	T59.891	T59.892	T59.893	T59.894	--	--
Nitrobenzene, nitrobenzol	T65.3X1	T65.3X2	T65.3X3	T65.3X4	--	--
- vapor	T65.3X1	T65.3X2	T65.3X3	T65.3X4	--	--
Nitrocellulose	T65.891	T65.892	T65.893	T65.894	--	--
- lacquer	T65.891	T65.892	T65.893	T65.894	--	--
Nitrodiphenyl	T65.3X1	T65.3X2	T65.3X3	T65.3X4	--	--
Nitrofural	T49.0X1	T49.0X2	T49.0X3	T49.0X4	T49.0X5	T49.0X6
Nitrofurantoin	T37.8X1	T37.8X2	T37.8X3	T37.8X4	T37.8X5	T37.8X6
Nitrofurazone	T49.0X1	T49.0X2	T49.0X3	T49.0X4	T49.0X5	T49.0X6
Nitrogen	T59.0X1	T59.0X2	T59.0X3	T59.0X4	--	--
- mustard	T45.1X1	T45.1X2	T45.1X3	T45.1X4	T45.1X5	T45.1X6
Nitroglycerin, nitro-glycerol (medicinal)	T46.3X1	T46.3X2	T46.3X3	T46.3X4	T46.3X5	T46.3X6
- nonmedicinal	T65.5X1	T65.5X2	T65.5X3	T65.5X4	--	--
- - fumes	T65.5X1	T65.5X2	T65.5X3	T65.5X4	--	--
Nitroglycol	T52.3X1	T52.3X2	T52.3X3	T52.3X4	--	--
Nitrohydrochloric acid	T54.2X1	T54.2X2	T54.2X3	T54.2X4	--	--
Nitromersol	T49.0X1	T49.0X2	T49.0X3	T49.0X4	T49.0X5	T49.0X6
Nitronaphthalene	T65.891	T65.892	T65.893	T65.894	--	--
Nitrophenol	T54.0X1	T54.0X2	T54.0X3	T54.0X4	--	--
Nitropropane	T52.8X1	T52.8X2	T52.8X3	T52.8X4	--	--
Nitroprusside	T46.5X1	T46.5X2	T46.5X3	T46.5X4	T46.5X5	T46.5X6
Nitrosodimethylamine	T65.3X1	T65.3X2	T65.3X3	T65.3X4	--	--
Nitrothiazol	T37.4X1	T37.4X2	T37.4X3	T37.4X4	T37.4X5	T37.4X6
Nitrotoluene, nitrotoluol	T65.3X1	T65.3X2	T65.3X3	T65.3X4	--	--
- vapor	T65.3X1	T65.3X2	T65.3X3	T65.3X4	--	--
Nitrous						
- acid (liquid)	T54.2X1	T54.2X2	T54.2X3	T54.2X4	--	--
- - fumes	T59.891	T59.892	T59.893	T59.894	--	--
- ether spirit	T46.3X1	T46.3X2	T46.3X3	T46.3X4	T46.3X5	T46.3X6
- oxide	T41.0X1	T41.0X2	T41.0X3	T41.0X4	T41.0X5	T41.0X6
Nitroxoline	T37.8X1	T37.8X2	T37.8X3	T37.8X4	T37.8X5	T37.8X6
Nitrozone	T49.0X1	T49.0X2	T49.0X3	T49.0X4	T49.0X5	T49.0X6
Nizatidine	T47.0X1	T47.0X2	T47.0X3	T47.0X4	T47.0X5	T47.0X6
Nizofenone	T43.8X1	T43.8X2	T43.8X3	T43.8X4	T43.8X5	T43.8X6
Noctec	T42.6X1	T42.6X2	T42.6X3	T42.6X4	T42.6X5	T42.6X6
Noludar	T42.6X1	T42.6X2	T42.6X3	T42.6X4	T42.6X5	T42.6X6
Nomegestrol	T38.5X1	T38.5X2	T38.5X3	T38.5X4	T38.5X5	T38.5X6

Substance	Poisoning, Accidental (unintentional)	Poisoning, Intentional Self-harm	Poisoning, Assault	Poisoning, Undetermined	Adverse effect	Underdosing
Nomifensine	T43.291	T43.292	T43.293	T43.294	T43.295	T43.296
Nonoxinol	T49.8X1	T49.8X2	T49.8X3	T49.8X4	T49.8X5	T49.8X6
Nonylphenoxy (polyethoxy-ethanol)	T49.8X1	T49.8X2	T49.8X3	T42.3X4	T42.3X5	T42.3X6
Noptil	T42.3X1	T42.3X2	T42.3X3	T42.3X4	T42.3X5	T42.3X6
Noradrenaline	T44.4X1	T44.4X2	T44.4X3	T44.4X4	T44.4X5	T44.4X6
Noramidopyrine	T39.2X1	T39.2X2	T39.2X3	T39.2X4	T39.2X5	T39.2X6
- methanesulfonate sodium	T39.2X1	T39.2X2	T39.2X3	T39.2X4	T39.2X5	T39.2X6
Norbormide	T60.4X1	T60.4X2	T60.4X3	T60.4X4	--	--
Nordazepam	T42.4X1	T42.4X2	T42.4X3	T42.4X4	T42.4X5	T42.4X6
Norepinephrine	T44.4X1	T44.4X2	T44.4X3	T44.4X4	T44.4X5	T44.4X6
Norethandrolone	T38.7X1	T38.7X2	T38.7X3	T38.7X4	T38.7X5	T38.7X6
Norethindrone	T38.4X1	T38.4X2	T38.4X3	T38.4X4	T38.4X5	T38.4X6
Norethisterone (acetate) (enantate)	T38.4X1	T38.4X2	T38.4X3	T38.4X4	T38.4X5	T38.4X6
- with ethinylestradiol	T38.5X1	T38.5X2	T38.5X3	T38.5X4	T38.5X5	T38.5X6
Noretynodrel	T38.5X1	T38.5X2	T38.5X3	T38.5X4	T38.5X5	T38.5X6
Norfenefrine	T44.4X1	T44.4X2	T44.4X3	T44.4X4	T44.4X5	T44.4X6
Norfloxacin	T36.8X1	T36.8X2	T36.8X3	T36.8X4	T36.8X5	T36.8X6
Norgestrel	T38.4X1	T38.4X2	T38.4X3	T38.4X4	T38.4X5	T38.4X6
Norgestrienone	T38.4X1	T38.4X2	T38.4X3	T38.4X4	T38.4X5	T38.4X6
Norlestrin	T38.4X1	T38.4X2	T38.4X3	T38.4X4	T38.4X5	T38.4X6
Norlutin	T38.4X1	T38.4X2	T38.4X3	T38.4X4	T38.4X5	T38.4X6
Normal serum albumin (human) , salt-poor	T45.8X1	T45.8X2	T45.8X3	T45.8X4	T45.8X5	T45.8X6
Normethandrone	T38.5X1	T38.5X2	T38.5X3	T38.5X4	T38.5X5	T38.5X6
Normison—see Benzodiazepines						
Normorphine	T40.2X1	T40.2X2	T40.2X3	T40.2X4	--	--
Norpseudoephedrine	T50.5X1	T50.5X2	T50.5X3	T50.5X4	T50.5X5	T50.5X6
Nortestosterone (furanpropionate)	T38.7X1	T38.7X2	T38.7X3	T38.7X4	T38.7X5	T38.7X6
Nortriptyline	T43.011	T43.012	T43.013	T43.014	T43.015	T43.016
Noscapine	T48.3X1	T48.3X2	T48.3X3	T48.3X4	T48.3X5	T48.3X6
Nose preparations	T49.6X1	T49.6X2	T49.6X3	T49.6X4	T49.6X5	T49.6X6
Novobiocin	T36.5X1	T36.5X2	T36.5X3	T36.5X4	T36.5X5	T36.5X6
Novocain (infiltration) (topical)	T41.3X1	T41.3X2	T41.3X3	T41.3X4	T41.3X5	T41.3X6
- nerve block (peripheral) (plexus)	T41.3X1	T41.3X2	T41.3X3	T41.3X4	T41.3X5	T41.3X6
- spinal	T41.3X1	T41.3X2	T41.3X3	T41.3X4	T41.3X5	T41.3X6
Noxious foodstuff	T62.91	T62.92	T62.93	T62.94	--	--
- specified NEC	T62.8X1	T62.8X2	T62.8X3	T62.8X4	--	--
Noxiptiline	T43.011	T43.012	T43.013	T43.014	T43.015	T43.016
Noxytiolin	T49.0X1	T49.0X2	T49.0X3	T49.0X4	T49.0X5	T49.0X6
NPH Iletin (insulin)	T38.3X1	T38.3X2	T38.3X3	T38.3X4	T38.3X5	T38.3X6
Numorphan	T40.2X1	T40.2X2	T40.2X3	T40.2X4	T40.2X5	T40.2X6
Nunol	T42.3X1	T42.3X2	T42.3X3	T42.3X4	T42.3X5	T42.3X6
Nupercaine (spinal anesthetic)	T41.3X1	T41.3X2	T41.3X3	T41.3X4	T41.3X5	T41.3X6
- topical (surface)	T41.3X1	T41.3X2	T41.3X3	T41.3X4	T41.3X5	T41.3X6
Nutmeg oil (liniment)	T49.3X1	T49.3X2	T49.3X3	T49.3X4	T49.3X5	T49.3X6
Nutritional supplement	T50.901	T50.902	T50.903	T50.904	T50.905	T50.906
Nux vomica	T65.1X1	T65.1X2	T65.1X3	T65.1X4	--	--
Nydrazid	T37.1X1	T37.1X2	T37.1X3	T37.1X4	T37.1X5	T37.1X6
Nylidrin	T46.7X1	T46.7X2	T46.7X3	T46.7X4	T46.7X5	T46.7X6
Nystatin	T36.7X1	T36.7X2	T36.7X3	T36.7X4	T36.7X5	T36.7X6
- topical	T49.0X1	T49.0X2	T49.0X3	T49.0X4	T49.0X5	T49.0X6
Nytol	T45.0X1	T45.0X2	T45.0X3	T45.0X4	T45.0X5	T45.0X6
Obidoxime chloride	T50.6X1	T50.6X2	T50.6X3	T50.6X4	T50.6X5	T50.6X6
Octafonium (chloride)	T49.3X1	T49.3X2	T49.3X3	T49.3X4	T49.3X5	T49.3X6
Octamethyl pyrophos-phoramide	T60.0X1	T60.0X2	T60.0X3	T60.0X4	--	--
Octanoin	T50.991	T50.992	T50.993	T50.994	T50.995	T50.996
Octatropine methyl-bromide	T44.3X1	T44.3X2	T44.3X3	T44.3X4	T44.3X5	T44.3X6
Octotiamine	T45.2X1	T45.2X2	T45.2X3	T45.2X4	T45.2X5	T45.2X6
Octoxinol (9)	T49.8X1	T49.8X2	T49.8X3	T49.8X4	T49.8X5	T49.8X6
Octreotide	T38.991	T38.992	T38.993	T38.994	T38.995	T38.996

Substance	Poisoning, Accidental (unintentional)	Poisoning, Intentional Self-harm	Poisoning, Assault	Poisoning, Undetermined	Adverse effect	Underdosing
Octyl nitrite	T46.3X1	T46.3X2	T46.3X3	T46.3X4	T46.3X5	T46.3X6
Oestradiol	T38.5X1	T38.5X2	T38.5X3	T38.5X4	T38.5X5	T38.5X6
Oestriol	T38.5X1	T38.5X2	T38.5X3	T38.5X4	T38.5X5	T38.5X6
Oestrogen	T38.5X1	T38.5X2	T38.5X3	T38.5X4	T38.5X5	T38.5X6
Oestrone	T38.5X1	T38.5X2	T38.5X3	T38.5X4	T38.5X5	T38.5X6
Ofloxacin	T36.8X1	T36.8X2	T36.8X3	T36.8X4	T36.8X5	T36.8X6
Oil (of)	T65.891	T65.892	T65.893	T65.894	--	--
- bitter almond	T62.8X1	T62.8X2	T62.8X3	T62.8X4	--	--
- cloves	T49.7X1	T49.7X2	T49.7X3	T49.7X4	T49.7X5	T49.7X6
- colors	T65.6X1	T65.6X2	T65.6X3	T65.6X4	--	--
- fumes	T59.891	T59.892	T59.893	T59.894	--	--
- lubricating	T52.0X1	T52.0X2	T52.0X3	T52.0X4	--	--
- Niobe	T52.8X1	T52.8X2	T52.8X3	T52.8X4	--	--
- vitriol (liquid)	T54.2X1	T54.2X2	T54.2X3	T54.2X4	--	--
- - fumes	T54.2X1	T54.2X2	T54.2X3	T54.2X4	--	--
- wintergreen (bitter) NEC	T49.3X1	T49.3X2	T49.3X3	T49.3X4	T49.3X5	T49.3X6
Oily preparation (for skin)	T49.3X1	T49.3X2	T49.3X3	T49.3X4	T49.3X5	T49.3X6
Ointment NEC	T49.3X1	T49.3X2	T49.3X3	T49.3X4	T49.3X5	T49.3X6
Olanzapine	T43.591	T43.592	T43.593	T43.594	T43.595	T43.596
Oleander	T62.2X1	T62.2X2	T62.2X3	T62.2X4	--	--
Oleandomycin	T36.3X1	T36.3X2	T36.3X3	T36.3X4	T36.3X5	T36.3X6
Oleandrin	T46.0X1	T46.0X2	T46.0X3	T46.0X4	T46.0X5	T46.0X6
Oleic acid	T46.6X1	T46.6X2	T46.6X3	T46.6X4	T46.6X5	T46.6X6
Oleovitamin A	T45.2X1	T45.2X2	T45.2X3	T45.2X4	T45.2X5	T45.2X6
Oleum ricini	T47.2X1	T47.2X2	T47.2X3	T47.2X4	T47.2X5	T47.2X6
Olive oil (medicinal) NEC	T47.4X1	T47.4X2	T47.4X3	T47.4X4	T47.4X5	T47.4X6
Olivomycin	T45.1X1	T45.1X2	T45.1X3	T45.1X4	T45.1X5	T45.1X6
Olsalazine	T47.8X1	T47.8X2	T47.8X3	T47.8X4	T47.8X5	T47.8X6
Omeprazole	T47.1X1	T47.1X2	T47.1X3	T47.1X4	T47.1X5	T47.1X6
OMPA	T60.0X1	T60.0X2	T60.0X3	T60.0X4	--	--
Oncovin	T45.1X1	T45.1X2	T45.1X3	T45.1X4	T45.1X5	T45.1X6
Ondansetron	T45.0X1	T45.0X2	T45.0X3	T45.0X4	T45.0X5	T45.0X6
Ophthaine	T41.3X1	T41.3X2	T41.3X3	T41.3X4	T41.3X5	T41.3X6
Ophthetic	T41.3X1	T41.3X2	T41.3X3	T41.3X4	T41.3X5	T41.3X6
Opiate NEC	T40.601	T40.602	T40.603	T40.604	T40.605	T40.606
- antagonists	T50.7X1	T50.7X2	T50.7X3	T50.7X4	T50.7X5	T50.7X6
Opioid NEC	T40.2X1	T40.2X2	T40.2X3	T40.2X4	T40.2X5	T40.2X6
Opipramol	T43.011	T43.012	T43.013	T43.014	T43.015	T43.016
Opium alkaloids (total)	T40.0X1	T40.0X2	T40.0X3	T40.0X4	T40.0X5	T40.0X6
- standardized powdered	T40.0X1	T40.0X2	T40.0X3	T40.0X4	T40.0X5	T40.0X6
- tincture (camphorated)	T40.0X1	T40.0X2	T40.0X3	T40.0X4	T40.0X5	T40.0X6
Oracon	T38.4X1	T38.4X2	T38.4X3	T38.4X4	T38.4X5	T38.4X6
Oragrafin	T50.8X1	T50.8X2	T50.8X3	T50.8X4	T50.8X5	T50.8X6
Oral contraceptives	T38.4X1	T38.4X2	T38.4X3	T38.4X4	T38.4X5	T38.4X6
Oral rehydration salts	T50.3X1	T50.3X2	T50.3X3	T50.3X4	T50.3X5	T50.3X6
Orazamide	T50.991	T50.992	T50.993	T50.994	T50.995	T50.996
Orciprenaline	T48.291	T48.292	T48.293	T48.294	T48.295	T48.296
Organidin	T48.4X1	T48.4X2	T48.4X3	T48.4X4	T48.4X5	T48.4X6
Organonitrate NEC	T46.3X1	T46.3X2	T46.3X3	T46.3X4	T46.3X5	T46.3X6
Organophosphates	T60.0X1	T60.0X2	T60.0X3	T60.0X4	--	--
Orimune	T50.B91	T50.B92	T50.B93	T50.B94	T50.B95	T50.B96
Orinase	T38.3X1	T38.3X2	T38.3X3	T38.3X4	T38.3X5	T38.3X6
Ormeloxifene	T38.6X1	T38.6X2	T38.6X3	T38.6X4	T38.6X5	T38.6X6
Ornidazole	T37.3X1	T37.3X2	T37.3X3	T37.3X4	T37.3X5	T37.3X6
Ornithine aspartate	T50.991	T50.992	T50.993	T50.994	T50.995	T50.996
Ornoprostil	T47.1X1	T47.1X2	T47.1X3	T47.1X4	T47.1X5	T47.1X6
Orphenadrine (hydrochloride)	T42.8X1	T42.8X2	T42.8X3	T42.8X4	T42.8X5	T42.8X6
Ortal (sodium)	T42.3X1	T42.3X2	T42.3X3	T42.3X4	T42.3X5	T42.3X6

Substance	Poisoning, Accidental (unintentional)	Poisoning, Intentional Self-harm	Poisoning, Assault	Poisoning, Undetermined	Adverse effect	Underdosing
Orthoboric acid	T49.0X1	T49.0X2	T49.0X3	T49.0X4	T49.0X5	T49.0X6
- ENT agent	T49.6X1	T49.6X2	T49.6X3	T49.6X4	T49.6X5	T49.6X6
- ophthalmic preparation	T49.5X1	T49.5X2	T49.5X3	T49.5X4	T49.5X5	T49.5X6
Orthocaine	T41.3X1	T41.3X2	T41.3X3	T41.3X4	T41.3X5	T41.3X6
Orthodichlorobenzene	T53.7X1	T53.7X2	T53.7X3	T53.7X4	--	--
Ortho-Novum	T38.4X1	T38.4X2	T38.4X3	T38.4X4	T38.4X5	T38.4X6
Orthotolidine (reagent)	T54.2X1	T54.2X2	T54.2X3	T54.2X4	--	--
Osmic acid (liquid)	T54.2X1	T54.2X2	T54.2X3	T54.2X4	--	--
- fumes	T54.2X1	T54.2X2	T54.2X3	T54.2X4	--	--
Osmotic diuretics	T50.2X1	T50.2X2	T50.2X3	T50.2X4	T50.2X5	T50.2X6
Otilonium bromide	T44.3X1	T44.3X2	T44.3X3	T44.3X4	T44.3X5	T44.3X6
Otorhinolaryngological drug NEC	T49.6X1	T49.6X2	T49.6X3	T49.6X4	T49.6X5	T49.6X6
Ouabain (e)	T46.0X1	T46.0X2	T46.0X3	T46.0X4	T46.0X5	T46.0X6
Ovarian						
- hormone	T38.5X1	T38.5X2	T38.5X3	T38.5X4	T38.5X5	T38.5X6
- stimulant	T38.5X1	T38.5X2	T38.5X3	T38.5X4	T38.5X5	T38.5X6
Ovral	T38.4X1	T38.4X2	T38.4X3	T38.4X4	T38.4X5	T38.4X6
Ovulen	T38.4X1	T38.4X2	T38.4X3	T38.4X4	T38.4X5	T38.4X6
Oxacillin	T36.0X1	T36.0X2	T36.0X3	T36.0X4	T36.0X5	T36.0X6
Oxalic acid	T54.2X1	T54.2X2	T54.2X3	T54.2X4	--	--
- ammonium salt	T50.991	T50.992	T50.993	T50.994	T50.995	T50.996
Oxamniquine	T37.4X1	T37.4X2	T37.4X3	T37.4X4	T37.4X5	T37.4X6
Oxanamide	T43.591	T43.592	T43.593	T43.594	T43.595	T43.596
Oxandrolone	T38.7X1	T38.7X2	T38.7X3	T38.7X4	T38.7X5	T38.7X6
Oxantel	T37.4X1	T37.4X2	T37.4X3	T37.4X4	T37.4X5	T37.4X6
Oxapium iodide	T44.3X1	T44.3X2	T44.3X3	T44.3X4	T44.3X5	T44.3X6
Oxaprotiline	T43.021	T43.022	T43.023	T43.024	T43.025	T43.026
Oxaprozin	T39.311	T39.312	T39.313	T39.314	T39.315	T39.316
Oxatomide	T45.0X1	T45.0X2	T45.0X3	T45.0X4	T45.0X5	T45.0X6
Oxazepam	T42.4X1	T42.4X2	T42.4X3	T42.4X4	T42.4X5	T42.4X6
Oxazimedrine	T50.5X1	T50.5X2	T50.5X3	T50.5X4	T50.5X5	T50.5X6
Oxazolam	T42.4X1	T42.4X2	T42.4X3	T42.4X4	T42.4X5	T42.4X6
Oxazolidine derivatives	T42.2X1	T42.2X2	T42.2X3	T42.2X4	T42.2X5	T42.2X6
Oxazolidinedione (derivative)	T42.2X1	T42.2X2	T42.2X3	T42.2X4	T42.2X5	T42.2X6
Ox bile extract	T47.5X1	T47.5X2	T47.5X3	T47.5X4	T47.5X5	T47.5X6
Oxcarbazepine	T42.1X1	T42.1X2	T42.1X3	T42.1X4	T42.1X5	T42.1X6
Oxedrine	T44.4X1	T44.4X2	T44.4X3	T44.4X4	T44.4X5	T44.4X6
Oxeladin (citrate)	T48.3X1	T48.3X2	T48.3X3	T48.3X4	T48.3X5	T48.3X6
Oxendolone	T38.5X1	T38.5X2	T38.5X3	T38.5X4	T38.5X5	T38.5X6
Oxetacaine	T41.3X1	T41.3X2	T41.3X3	T41.3X4	T41.3X5	T41.3X6
Oxethazine	T41.3X1	T41.3X2	T41.3X3	T41.3X4	T41.3X5	T41.3X6
Oxetorone	T39.8X1	T39.8X2	T39.8X3	T39.8X4	T39.8X5	T39.8X6
Oxiconazole	T49.0X1	T49.0X2	T49.0X3	T49.0X4	T49.0X5	T49.0X6
Oxidizing agent NEC	T54.91	T54.92	T54.93	T54.94	--	--
Oxipurinol	T50.4X1	T50.4X2	T50.4X3	T50.4X4	T50.4X5	T50.4X6
Oxitriptan	T43.291	T43.292	T43.293	T43.294	T43.295	T43.296
Oxitropium bromide	T48.6X1	T48.6X2	T48.6X3	T48.6X4	T48.6X5	T48.6X6
Oxodipine	T46.1X1	T46.1X2	T46.1X3	T46.1X4	T46.1X5	T46.1X6
Oxolamine	T48.3X1	T48.3X2	T48.3X3	T48.3X4	T48.3X5	T48.3X6
Oxolinic acid	T37.8X1	T37.8X2	T37.8X3	T37.8X4	T37.8X5	T37.8X6
Oxomemazine	T43.3X1	T43.3X2	T43.3X3	T43.3X4	T43.3X5	T43.3X6
Oxophenarsine	T37.3X1	T37.3X2	T37.3X3	T37.3X4	T37.3X5	T37.3X6
Oxprenolol	T44.7X1	T44.7X2	T44.7X3	T44.7X4	T44.7X5	T44.7X6
Oxsoralen	T49.3X1	T49.3X2	T49.3X3	T49.3X4	T49.3X5	T49.3X6
Oxtriphylline	T48.6X1	T48.6X2	T48.6X3	T48.6X4	T48.6X5	T48.6X6
Oxybate sodium	T41.291	T41.292	T41.293	T41.294	T41.295	T41.296
Oxybuprocaine	T41.3X1	T41.3X2	T41.3X3	T41.3X4	T41.3X5	T41.3X6
Oxybutynin	T44.3X1	T44.3X2	T44.3X3	T44.3X4	T44.3X5	T44.3X6
Oxychlorosene	T49.0X1	T49.0X2	T49.0X3	T49.0X4	T49.0X5	T49.0X6

Substance	Poisoning, Accidental (unintentional)	Poisoning, Intentional Self-harm	Poisoning, Assault	Poisoning, Undetermined	Adverse effect	Underdosing
Oxycodone	T40.2X1	T40.2X2	T40.2X3	T40.2X4	T40.2X5	T40.2X6
Oxyfedrine	T46.3X1	T46.3X2	T46.3X3	T46.3X4	T46.3X5	T46.3X6
Oxygen	T41.5X1	T41.5X2	T41.5X3	T41.5X4	T41.5X5	T41.5X6
Oxylone	T49.0X1	T49.0X2	T49.0X3	T49.0X4	T49.0X5	T49.0X6
- ophthalmic preparation	T49.5X1	T49.5X2	T49.5X3	T49.5X4	T49.5X5	T49.5X6
Oxymesterone	T38.7X1	T38.7X2	T38.7X3	T38.7X4	T38.7X5	T38.7X6
Oxymetazoline	T48.5X1	T48.5X2	T48.5X3	T48.5X4	T48.5X5	T48.5X6
Oxymetholone	T38.7X1	T38.7X2	T38.7X3	T38.7X4	T38.7X5	T38.7X6
Oxymorphone	T40.2X1	T40.2X2	T40.2X3	T40.2X4	T40.2X5	T40.2X6
Oxypertine	T43.591	T43.592	T43.593	T43.594	T43.595	T43.596
Oxyphenbutazone	T39.2X1	T39.2X2	T39.2X3	T39.2X4	T39.2X5	T39.2X6
Oxyphencyclimine	T44.3X1	T44.3X2	T44.3X3	T44.3X4	T44.3X5	T44.3X6
Oxyphenisatine	T47.2X1	T47.2X2	T47.2X3	T47.2X4	T47.2X5	T47.2X6
Oxyphenonium bromide	T44.3X1	T44.3X2	T44.3X3	T44.3X4	T44.3X5	T44.3X6
Oxypolygelatin	T45.8X1	T45.8X2	T45.8X3	T45.8X4	T45.8X5	T45.8X6
Oxyquinoline (derivatives)	T37.8X1	T37.8X2	T37.8X3	T37.8X4	T37.8X5	T37.8X6
Oxytetracycline	T36.4X1	T36.4X2	T36.4X3	T36.4X4	T36.4X5	T36.4X6
Oxytocic drug NEC	T48.0X1	T48.0X2	T48.0X3	T48.0X4	T48.0X5	T48.0X6
Oxytocin (synthetic)	T48.0X1	T48.0X2	T48.0X3	T48.0X4	T48.0X5	T48.0X6
Ozone	T59.891	T59.892	T59.893	T59.894	--	--
PABA	T49.3X1	T49.3X2	T49.3X3	T49.3X4	T49.3X5	T49.3X6
Packed red cells	T45.8X1	T45.8X2	T45.8X3	T45.8X4	T45.8X5	T45.8X6
Padimate	T49.3X1	T49.3X2	T49.3X3	T49.3X4	T49.3X5	T49.3X6
Paint NEC	T65.6X1	T65.6X2	T65.6X3	T65.6X4	--	--
- cleaner	T52.91	T52.92	T52.93	T52.94	--	--
- fumes NEC	T59.891	T59.892	T59.893	T59.894	--	--
- lead (fumes)	T56.0X1	T56.0X2	T56.0X3	T56.0X4	--	--
- solvent NEC	T52.8X1	T52.8X2	T52.8X3	T52.8X4	--	--
- stripper	T52.8X1	T52.8X2	T52.8X3	T52.8X4	--	--
Palfium	T40.2X1	T40.2X2	T40.2X3	T40.2X4	--	--
Palm kernel oil	T50.991	T50.992	T50.993	T50.994	T50.995	T50.996
Paludrine	T37.2X1	T37.2X2	T37.2X3	T37.2X4	T37.2X5	T37.2X6
PAM (pralidoxime)	T50.6X1	T50.6X2	T50.6X3	T50.6X4	T50.6X5	T50.6X6
Pamaquine (naphthoute)	T37.2X1	T37.2X2	T37.2X3	T37.2X4	T37.2X5	T37.2X6
Panadol	T39.1X1	T39.1X2	T39.1X3	T39.1X4	T39.1X5	T39.1X6
Pancreatic						
- digestive secretion stimulant	T47.8X1	T47.8X2	T47.8X3	T47.8X4	T47.8X5	T47.8X6
- dornase	T45.3X1	T45.3X2	T45.3X3	T45.3X4	T45.3X5	T45.3X6
Pancreatin	T47.5X1	T47.5X2	T47.5X3	T47.5X4	T47.5X5	T47.5X6
Pancrelipase	T47.5X1	T47.5X2	T47.5X3	T47.5X4	T47.5X5	T47.5X6
Pancuronium (bromide)	T48.1X1	T48.1X2	T48.1X3	T48.1X4	T48.1X5	T48.1X6
Pangamic acid	T45.2X1	T45.2X2	T45.2X3	T45.2X4	T45.2X5	T45.2X6
Panthenol	T45.2X1	T45.2X2	T45.2X3	T45.2X4	T45.2X5	T45.2X6
- topical	T49.8X1	T49.8X2	T49.8X3	T49.8X4	T49.8X5	T49.8X6
Pantopon	T40.0X1	T40.0X2	T40.0X3	T40.0X4	T40.0X5	T40.0X6
Pantothenic acid	T45.2X1	T45.2X2	T45.2X3	T45.2X4	T45.2X5	T45.2X6
Panwarfin	T45.511	T45.512	T45.513	T45.514	T45.515	T45.516
Papain	T47.5X1	T47.5X2	T47.5X3	T47.5X4	T47.5X5	T47.5X6
- digestant	T47.5X1	T47.5X2	T47.5X3	T47.5X4	T47.5X5	T47.5X6
Papaveretum	T40.0X1	T40.0X2	T40.0X3	T40.0X4	T40.0X5	T40.0X6
Papaverine	T44.3X1	T44.3X2	T44.3X3	T44.3X4	T44.3X5	T44.3X6
Para-acetamidophenol	T39.1X1	T39.1X2	T39.1X3	T39.1X4	T39.1X5	T39.1X6
Para-aminobenzoic acid	T49.3X1	T49.3X2	T49.3X3	T49.3X4	T49.3X5	T49.3X6
Para-aminophenol derivatives	T39.1X1	T39.1X2	T39.1X3	T39.1X4	T39.1X5	T39.1X6
Para-aminosalicylic acid	T37.1X1	T37.1X2	T37.1X3	T37.1X4	T37.1X5	T37.1X6
Paracetaldehyde	T42.6X1	T42.6X2	T42.6X3	T42.6X4	T42.6X5	T42.6X6
Paracetamol	T39.1X1	T39.1X2	T39.1X3	T39.1X4	T39.1X5	T39.1X6
Parachlorophenol (camphorated)	T49.0X1	T49.0X2	T49.0X3	T49.0X4	T49.0X5	T49.0X6

Substance	Poisoning, Accidental (unintentional)	Poisoning, Intentional Self-harm	Poisoning, Assault	Poisoning, Undetermined	Adverse effect	Underdosing
Paracodin	T40.2X1	T40.2X2	T40.2X3	T40.2X4	T40.2X5	T40.2X6
Paradione	T42.2X1	T42.2X2	T42.2X3	T42.2X4	T42.2X5	T42.2X6
Paraffin (s) (wax)	T52.0X1	T52.0X2	T52.0X3	T52.0X4	--	--
- liquid (medicinal)	T47.4X1	T47.4X2	T47.4X3	T47.4X4	T47.4X5	T47.4X6
- - nonmedicinal	T52.0X1	T52.0X2	T52.0X3	T52.0X4	--	--
Paraformaldehyde	T60.3X1	T60.3X2	T60.3X3	T60.3X4	--	--
Paraldehyde	T42.6X1	T42.6X2	T42.6X3	T42.6X4	T42.6X5	T42.6X6
Paramethadione	T42.2X1	T42.2X2	T42.2X3	T42.2X4	T42.2X5	T42.2X6
Paramethasone	T38.0X1	T38.0X2	T38.0X3	T38.0X4	T38.0X5	T38.0X6
- acetate	T49.0X1	T49.0X2	T49.0X3	T49.0X4	T49.0X5	T49.0X6
Paraoxon	T60.0X1	T60.0X2	T60.0X3	T60.0X4	--	--
Paraquat	T60.3X1	T60.3X2	T60.3X3	T60.3X4	--	--
Parasympatholytic NEC	T44.3X1	T44.3X2	T44.3X3	T44.3X4	T44.3X5	T44.3X6
Parasympathomimetic drug NEC	T44.1X1	T44.1X2	T44.1X3	T44.1X4	T44.1X5	T44.1X6
Parathion	T60.0X1	T60.0X2	T60.0X3	T60.0X4	--	--
Parathormone	T50.991	T50.992	T50.993	T50.994	T50.995	T50.996
Parathyroid extract	T50.991	T50.992	T50.993	T50.994	T50.995	T50.996
Paratyphoid vaccine	T50.A91	T50.A92	T50.A93	T50.A94	T50.A95	T50.A96
Paredrine	T44.4X1	T44.4X2	T44.4X3	T44.4X4	T44.4X5	T44.4X6
Paregoric	T40.0X1	T40.0X2	T40.0X3	T40.0X4	T40.0X5	T40.0X6
Pargyline	T46.5X1	T46.5X2	T46.5X3	T46.5X4	T46.5X5	T46.5X6
Paris green	T57.0X1	T57.0X2	T57.0X3	T57.0X4	--	--
- insecticide	T57.0X1	T57.0X2	T57.0X3	T57.0X4	--	--
Parnate	T43.1X1	T43.1X2	T43.1X3	T43.1X4	T43.1X5	T43.1X6
Paromomycin	T36.5X1	T36.5X2	T36.5X3	T36.5X4	T36.5X5	T36.5X6
Paroxypropione	T45.1X1	T45.1X2	T45.1X3	T45.1X4	T45.1X5	T45.1X6
Parzone	T40.2X1	T40.2X2	T40.2X3	T40.2X4	T40.2X5	T40.2X6
PAS	T37.1X1	T37.1X2	T37.1X3	T37.1X4	T37.1X5	T37.1X6
Pasiniazid	T37.1X1	T37.1X2	T37.1X3	T37.1X4	T37.1X5	T37.1X6
PBB (polybrominated biphenyls)	T65.891	T65.892	T65.893	T65.894	--	--
PCB	T65.891	T65.892	T65.893	T65.894	--	--
PCP						
- meaning pentachlorophenol	T60.1X1	T60.1X2	T60.1X3	T60.1X4	--	--
- - fungicide	T60.3X1	T60.3X2	T60.3X3	T60.3X4	--	--
- - herbicide	T60.3X1	T60.3X2	T60.3X3	T60.3X4	--	--
- - insecticide	T60.1X1	T60.1X2	T60.1X3	T60.1X4	--	--
- meaning phencyclidine	T40.991	T40.992	T40.993	T40.994	--	--
Peach kernel oil (emulsion)	T47.4X1	T47.4X2	T47.4X3	T47.4X4	T47.4X5	T47.4X6
Peanut oil (emulsion) NEC	T47.4X1	T47.4X2	T47.4X3	T47.4X4	T47.4X5	T47.4X6
- topical	T49.3X1	T49.3X2	T49.3X3	T49.3X4	T49.3X5	T49.3X6
Pearly Gates (morning glory seeds)	T40.991	T40.992	T40.993	T40.994	--	--
Pecazine	T43.3X1	T43.3X2	T43.3X3	T43.3X4	T43.3X5	T43.3X6
Pectin	T47.6X1	T47.6X2	T47.6X3	T47.6X4	T47.6X5	T47.6X6
Pefloxacin	T37.8X1	T37.8X2	T37.8X3	T37.8X4	T37.8X5	T37.8X6
Pegademase, bovine	T50.Z91	T50.Z92	T50.Z93	T50.Z94	T50.Z95	T50.Z96
Pelletierine tannate	T37.4X1	T37.4X2	T37.4X3	T37.4X4	T37.4X5	T37.4X6
Pemirolast (potassium)	T48.6X1	T48.6X2	T48.6X3	T48.6X4	T48.6X5	T48.6X6
Pemoline	T50.7X1	T50.7X2	T50.7X3	T50.7X4	T50.7X5	T50.7X6
Pempidine	T44.2X1	T44.2X2	T44.2X3	T44.2X4	T44.2X5	T44.2X6
Penamecillin	T36.0X1	T36.0X2	T36.0X3	T36.0X4	T36.0X5	T36.0X6
Penbutolol	T44.7X1	T44.7X2	T44.7X3	T44.7X4	T44.7X5	T44.7X6
Penethamate	T36.0X1	T36.0X2	T36.0X3	T36.0X4	T36.0X5	T36.0X6
Penfluridol	T43.591	T43.592	T43.593	T43.594	T43.595	T43.596
Penflutizide	T50.2X1	T50.2X2	T50.2X3	T50.2X4	T50.2X5	T50.2X6
Pengitoxin	T46.0X1	T46.0X2	T46.0X3	T46.0X4	T46.0X5	T46.0X6
Penicillamine	T50.6X1	T50.6X2	T50.6X3	T50.6X4	T50.6X5	T50.6X6
Penicillin (any)	T36.0X1	T36.0X2	T36.0X3	T36.0X4	T36.0X5	T36.0X6
Penicillinase	T45.3X1	T45.3X2	T45.3X3	T45.3X4	T45.3X5	T45.3X6
Penicilloyl polylysine	T50.8X1	T50.8X2	T50.8X3	T50.8X4	T50.8X5	T50.8X6

Substance	Poisoning, Accidental (unintentional)	Poisoning, Intentional Self-harm	Poisoning, Assault	Poisoning, Undetermined	Adverse effect	Underdosing
Penimepicycline	T36.4X1	T36.4X2	T36.4X3	T36.4X4	T36.4X5	T36.4X6
Pentachloroethane	T53.6X1	T53.6X2	T53.6X3	T53.6X4	--	--
Pentachloronaphthalene	T53.7X1	T53.7X2	T53.7X3	T53.7X4	--	--
Pentachlorophenol (pesticide)	T60.1X1	T60.1X2	T60.1X3	T60.1X4	--	--
- fungicide	T60.3X1	T60.3X2	T60.3X3	T60.3X4	--	--
- herbicide	T60.3X1	T60.3X2	T60.3X3	T60.3X4	--	--
- insecticide	T60.1X1	T60.1X2	T60.1X3	T60.1X4	--	--
Pentaerythritol	T46.3X1	T46.3X2	T46.3X3	T46.3X4	T46.3X5	T46.3X6
- chloral	T42.6X1	T42.6X2	T42.6X3	T42.6X4	T42.6X5	T42.6X6
- tetranitrate NEC	T46.3X1	T46.3X2	T46.3X3	T46.3X4	T46.3X5	T46.3X6
Pentaerythrityl tetranitrate	T46.3X1	T46.3X2	T46.3X3	T46.3X4	T46.3X5	T46.3X6
Pentagastrin	T50.8X1	T50.8X2	T50.8X3	T50.8X4	T50.8X5	T50.8X6
Pentalin	T53.6X1	T53.6X2	T53.6X3	T53.6X4	--	--
Pentamethonium bromide	T44.2X1	T44.2X2	T44.2X3	T44.2X4	T44.2X5	T44.2X6
Pentamidine	T37.3X1	T37.3X2	T37.3X3	T37.3X4	T37.3X5	T37.3X6
Pentanol	T51.3X1	T51.3X2	T51.3X3	T51.3X4	--	--
Pentapyrrolinium (bitartrate)	T44.2X1	T44.2X2	T44.2X3	T44.2X4	T44.2X5	T44.2X6
Pentaquine	T37.2X1	T37.2X2	T37.2X3	T37.2X4	T37.2X5	T37.2X6
Pentazocine	T40.4X1	T40.4X2	T40.4X3	T40.4X4	T40.4X5	T40.4X6
Pentetrazole	T50.7X1	T50.7X2	T50.7X3	T50.7X4	T50.7X5	T50.7X6
Penthienate bromide	T44.3X1	T44.3X2	T44.3X3	T44.3X4	T44.3X5	T44.3X6
Pentifylline	T46.7X1	T46.7X2	T46.7X3	T46.7X4	T46.7X5	T46.7X6
Pentobarbital	T42.3X1	T42.3X2	T42.3X3	T42.3X4	T42.3X5	T42.3X6
- sodium	T42.3X1	T42.3X2	T42.3X3	T42.3X4	T42.3X5	T42.3X6
Pentobarbitone	T42.3X1	T42.3X2	T42.3X3	T42.3X4	T42.3X5	T42.3X6
Pentolonium tartrate	T44.2X1	T44.2X2	T44.2X3	T44.2X4	T44.2X5	T44.2X6
Pentosan polysulfate (sodium)	T39.8X1	T39.8X2	T39.8X3	T39.8X4	T39.8X5	T39.8X6
Pentostatin	T45.1X1	T45.1X2	T45.1X3	T45.1X4	T45.1X5	T45.1X6
Pentothal	T41.1X1	T41.1X2	T41.1X3	T41.1X4	T41.1X5	T41.1X6
Pentoxifylline	T46.7X1	T46.7X2	T46.7X3	T46.7X4	T46.7X5	T46.7X6
Pentoxyverine	T48.3X1	T48.3X2	T48.3X3	T48.3X4	T48.3X5	T48.3X6
Pentrinat	T46.3X1	T46.3X2	T46.3X3	T46.3X4	T46.3X5	T46.3X6
Pentylenetetrazole	T50.7X1	T50.7X2	T50.7X3	T50.7X4	T50.7X5	T50.7X6
Pentylsalicylamide	T37.1X1	T37.1X2	T37.1X3	T37.1X4	T37.1X5	T37.1X6
Pentymal	T42.3X1	T42.3X2	T42.3X3	T42.3X4	T42.3X5	T42.3X6
Peplomycin	T45.1X1	T45.1X2	T45.1X3	T45.1X4	T45.1X5	T45.1X6
Peppermint (oil)	T47.5X1	T47.5X2	T47.5X3	T47.5X4	T47.5X5	T47.5X6
Pepsin	T47.5X1	T47.5X2	T47.5X3	T47.5X4	T47.5X5	T47.5X6
- digestant	T47.5X1	T47.5X2	T47.5X3	T47.5X4	T47.5X5	T47.5X6
Pepstatin	T47.1X1	T47.1X2	T47.1X3	T47.1X4	T47.1X5	T47.1X6
Peptavlon	T50.8X1	T50.8X2	T50.8X3	T50.8X4	T50.8X5	T50.8X6
Perazine	T43.3X1	T43.3X2	T43.3X3	T43.3X4	T43.3X5	T43.3X6
Percaine (spinal)	T41.3X1	T41.3X2	T41.3X3	T41.3X4	T41.3X5	T41.3X6
- topical (surface)	T41.3X1	T41.3X2	T41.3X3	T41.3X4	T41.3X5	T41.3X6
Perchloroethylene	T53.3X1	T53.3X2	T53.3X3	T53.3X4	--	--
- medicinal	T37.4X1	T37.4X2	T37.4X3	T37.4X4	T37.4X5	T37.4X6
- vapor	T53.3X1	T53.3X2	T53.3X3	T53.3X4	--	--
Percodan	T40.2X1	T40.2X2	T40.2X3	T40.2X4	T40.2X5	T40.2X6
Percogesic—see also acetaminophen	T45.0X1	T45.0X2	T45.0X3	T45.0X4	T45.0X5	T45.0X6
Percorten	T38.0X1	T38.0X2	T38.0X3	T38.0X4	T38.0X5	T38.0X6
Pergolide	T42.8X1	T42.8X2	T42.8X3	T42.8X4	T42.8X5	T42.8X6
Pergonal	T38.811	T38.812	T38.813	T38.814	T38.815	T38.816
Perhexilene	T46.3X1	T46.3X2	T46.3X3	T46.3X4	T46.3X5	T46.3X6
Perhexiline (maleate)	T46.3X1	T46.3X2	T46.3X3	T46.3X4	T46.3X5	T46.3X6
Periactin	T45.0X1	T45.0X2	T45.0X3	T45.0X4	T45.0X5	T45.0X6
Periciazine	T43.3X1	T43.3X2	T43.3X3	T43.3X4	T43.3X5	T43.3X6
Periclor	T42.6X1	T42.6X2	T42.6X3	T42.6X4	T42.6X5	T42.6X6
Perindopril	T46.4X1	T46.4X2	T46.4X3	T46.4X4	T46.4X5	T46.4X6

Substance	Poisoning, Accidental (unintentional)	Poisoning, Intentional Self-harm	Poisoning, Assault	Poisoning, Undetermined	Adverse effect	Underdosing
Perisoxal	T39.8X1	T39.8X2	T39.8X3	T39.8X4	T39.8X5	T39.8X6
Peritoneal dialysis solution	T50.3X1	T50.3X2	T50.3X3	T50.3X4	T50.3X5	T50.3X6
Peritrate	T46.3X1	T46.3X2	T46.3X3	T46.3X4	T46.3X5	T46.3X6
Perlapine	T42.4X1	T42.4X2	T42.4X3	T42.4X4	T42.4X5	T42.4X6
Permanganate	T65.891	T65.892	T65.893	T65.894	--	--
Permethrin	T60.1X1	T60.1X2	T60.1X3	T60.1X4	--	--
Pernocton	T42.3X1	T42.3X2	T42.3X3	T42.3X4	T42.3X5	T42.3X6
Pernoston	T42.3X1	T42.3X2	T42.3X3	T42.3X4	T42.3X5	T42.3X6
Peronine	T40.2X1	T40.2X2	T40.2X3	T40.2X4	--	--
Perphenazine	T43.3X1	T43.3X2	T43.3X3	T43.3X4	T43.3X5	T43.3X6
Pertofrane	T43.011	T43.012	T43.013	T43.014	T43.015	T43.016
Pertussis						
- immune serum (human)	T50.Z11	T50.Z12	T50.Z13	T50.Z14	T50.Z15	T50.Z16
- vaccine (with diphtheria toxoid) (with tetanus toxoid)	T50.A11	T50.A12	T50.A13	T50.A14	T50.A15	T50.A16
Peruvian balsam	T49.0X1	T49.0X2	T49.0X3	T49.0X4	T49.0X5	T49.0X6
Peruvoside	T46.0X1	T46.0X2	T46.0X3	T46.0X4	T46.0X5	T46.0X6
Pesticide (dust) (fumes) (vapor) NEC	T60.91	T60.92	T60.93	T60.94	--	--
- arsenic	T57.0X1	T57.0X2	T57.0X3	T57.0X4	--	--
- chlorinated	T60.1X1	T60.1X2	T60.1X3	T60.1X4	--	--
- cyanide	T65.0X1	T65.0X2	T65.0X3	T65.0X4	--	--
- kerosene	T52.0X1	T52.0X2	T52.0X3	T52.0X4	--	--
- mixture (of compounds)	T60.91	T60.92	T60.93	T60.94	--	--
- naphthalene	T60.2X1	T60.2X2	T60.2X3	T60.2X4	--	--
- organochlorine (compounds)	T60.1X1	T60.1X2	T60.1X3	T60.1X4	--	--
- petroleum (distillate) (products) NEC	T60.8X1	T60.8X2	T60.8X3	T60.8X4	--	--
- specified ingredient NEC	T60.8X1	T60.8X2	T60.8X3	T60.8X4	--	--
- strychnine	T65.1X1	T65.1X2	T65.1X3	T65.1X4	--	--
- thallium	T60.4X1	T60.4X2	T60.4X3	T60.4X4	--	--
Pethidine	T40.4X1	T40.4X2	T40.4X3	T40.4X4	T40.4X5	T40.4X6
Petrichloral	T42.6X1	T42.6X2	T42.6X3	T42.6X4	T42.6X5	T42.6X6
Petrol	T52.0X1	T52.0X2	T52.0X3	T52.0X4	--	--
- vapor	T52.0X1	T52.0X2	T52.0X3	T52.0X4	--	--
Petrolatum	T49.3X1	T49.3X2	T49.3X3	T49.3X4	T49.3X5	T49.3X6
- hydrophilic	T49.3X1	T49.3X2	T49.3X3	T49.3X4	T49.3X5	T49.3X6
- liquid	T47.4X1	T47.4X2	T47.4X3	T47.4X4	T47.4X5	T47.4X6
- - topical	T49.3X1	T49.3X2	T49.3X3	T49.3X4	T49.3X5	T49.3X6
- nonmedicinal	T52.0X1	T52.0X2	T52.0X3	T52.0X4	--	--
- red veterinary	T49.3X1	T49.3X2	T49.3X3	T49.3X4	T49.3X5	T49.3X6
- white	T49.3X1	T49.3X2	T49.3X3	T49.3X4	T49.3X5	T49.3X6
Petroleum (products) NEC	T52.0X1	T52.0X2	T52.0X3	T52.0X4	--	--
- benzine (s) —see Ligroin						
- ether—see Ligroin						
- jelly—see Petrolatum						
- naphtha—see Ligroin						
- pesticide	T60.8X1	T60.8X2	T60.8X3	T60.8X4	--	--
- solids	T52.0X1	T52.0X2	T52.0X3	T52.0X4	--	--
- solvents	T52.0X1	T52.0X2	T52.0X3	T52.0X4	--	--
- vapor	T52.0X1	T52.0X2	T52.0X3	T52.0X4	--	--
Peyote	T40.991	T40.992	T40.993	T40.994	--	--
Phanodorm, phanodorn	T42.3X1	T42.3X2	T42.3X3	T42.3X4	T42.3X5	T42.3X6
Phanquinone	T37.3X1	T37.3X2	T37.3X3	T37.3X4	T37.3X5	T37.3X6
Phanquone	T37.3X1	T37.3X2	T37.3X3	T37.3X4	T37.3X5	T37.3X6
Pharmaceutical						
- adjunct NEC	T50.901	T50.902	T50.903	T50.904	T50.905	T50.906
- excipient NEC	T50.901	T50.902	T50.903	T50.904	T50.905	T50.906
- sweetener	T50.901	T50.902	T50.903	T50.904	T50.905	T50.906
- viscous agent	T50.901	T50.902	T50.903	T50.904	T50.905	T50.906
Phemitone	T42.3X1	T42.3X2	T42.3X3	T42.3X4	T42.3X5	T42.3X6

Substance	Poisoning, Accidental (unintentional)	Poisoning, Intentional Self-harm	Poisoning, Assault	Poisoning, Undetermined	Adverse effect	Underdosing
Phenacaine	T41.3X1	T41.3X2	T41.3X3	T41.3X4	T41.3X5	T41.3X6
Phenacemide	T42.6X1	T42.6X2	T42.6X3	T42.6X4	T42.6X5	T42.6X6
Phenacetin	T39.1X1	T39.1X2	T39.1X3	T39.1X4	T39.1X5	T39.1X6
Phenadoxone	T40.2X1	T40.2X2	T40.2X3	T40.2X4	--	--
Phenaglycodol	T43.591	T43.592	T43.593	T43.594	T43.595	T43.596
Phenantoin	T42.0X1	T42.0X2	T42.0X3	T42.0X4	T42.0X5	T42.0X6
Phenaphthazine reagent	T50.991	T50.992	T50.993	T50.994	T50.995	T50.996
Phenazocine	T40.4X1	T40.4X2	T40.4X3	T40.4X4	T40.4X5	T40.4X6
Phenazone	T39.2X1	T39.2X2	T39.2X3	T39.2X4	T39.2X5	T39.2X6
Phenazopyridine	T39.8X1	T39.8X2	T39.8X3	T39.8X4	T39.8X5	T39.8X6
Phenbenicillin	T36.0X1	T36.0X2	T36.0X3	T36.0X4	T36.0X5	T36.0X6
Phenbutrazate	T50.5X1	T50.5X2	T50.5X3	T50.5X4	T50.5X5	T50.5X6
Phencyclidine	T40.991	T40.992	T40.993	T40.994	T40.995	T40.996
Phendimetrazine	T50.5X1	T50.5X2	T50.5X3	T50.5X4	T50.5X5	T50.5X6
Phenelzine	T43.1X1	T43.1X2	T43.1X3	T43.1X4	T43.1X5	T43.1X6
Phenemal	T42.3X1	T42.3X2	T42.3X3	T42.3X4	T42.3X5	T42.3X6
Phenergan	T42.6X1	T42.6X2	T42.6X3	T42.6X4	T42.6X5	T42.6X6
Pheneticillin	T36.0X1	T36.0X2	T36.0X3	T36.0X4	T36.0X5	T36.0X6
Pheneturide	T42.6X1	T42.6X2	T42.6X3	T42.6X4	T42.6X5	T42.6X6
Phenformin	T38.3X1	T38.3X2	T38.3X3	T38.3X4	T38.3X5	T38.3X6
Phenglutarimide	T44.3X1	T44.3X2	T44.3X3	T44.3X4	T44.3X5	T44.3X6
Phenicarbazide	T39.8X1	T39.8X2	T39.8X3	T39.8X4	T39.8X5	T39.8X6
Phenindamine	T45.0X1	T45.0X2	T45.0X3	T45.0X4	T45.0X5	T45.0X6
Phenindione	T45.511	T45.512	T45.513	T45.514	T45.515	T45.516
Pheniprazine	T43.1X1	T43.1X2	T43.1X3	T43.1X4	T43.1X5	T43.1X6
Pheniramine	T45.0X1	T45.0X2	T45.0X3	T45.0X4	T45.0X5	T45.0X6
Phenisatin	T47.2X1	T47.2X2	T47.2X3	T47.2X4	T47.2X5	T47.2X6
Phenmetrazine	T50.5X1	T50.5X2	T50.5X3	T50.5X4	T50.5X5	T50.5X6
Phenobal	T42.3X1	T42.3X2	T42.3X3	T42.3X4	T42.3X5	T42.3X6
Phenobarbital	T42.3X1	T42.3X2	T42.3X3	T42.3X4	T42.3X5	T42.3X6
- with						
- - mephenytoin	T42.3X1	T42.3X2	T42.3X3	T42.3X4	T42.3X5	T42.3X6
- - phenytoin	T42.3X1	T42.3X2	T42.3X3	T42.3X4	T42.3X5	T42.3X6
- sodium	T42.3X1	T42.3X2	T42.3X3	T42.3X4	T42.3X5	T42.3X6
Phenobarbitone	T42.3X1	T42.3X2	T42.3X3	T42.3X4	T42.3X5	T42.3X6
Phenobutiodil	T50.8X1	T50.8X2	T50.8X3	T50.8X4	T50.8X5	T50.8X6
Phenoctide	T49.0X1	T49.0X2	T49.0X3	T49.0X4	T49.0X5	T49.0X6
Phenol	T49.0X1	T49.0X2	T49.0X3	T49.0X4	T49.0X5	T49.0X6
- disinfectant	T54.0X1	T54.0X2	T54.0X3	T54.0X4	--	--
- in oil injection	T46.8X1	T46.8X2	T46.8X3	T46.8X4	T46.8X5	T46.8X6
- medicinal	T49.1X1	T49.1X2	T49.1X3	T49.1X4	T49.1X5	T49.1X6
- nonmedicinal NEC	T54.0X1	T54.0X2	T54.0X3	T54.0X4	--	--
- pesticide	T60.8X1	T60.8X2	T60.8X3	T60.8X4	--	--
- red	T50.8X1	T50.8X2	T50.8X3	T50.8X4	T50.8X5	T50.8X6
Phenolic preparation	T49.1X1	T49.1X2	T49.1X3	T49.1X4	T49.1X5	T49.1X6
Phenolphthalein	T47.2X1	T47.2X2	T47.2X3	T47.2X4	T47.2X5	T47.2X6
Phenolsulfonphthalein	T50.8X1	T50.8X2	T50.8X3	T50.8X4	T50.8X5	T50.8X6
Phenomorphan	T40.2X1	T40.2X2	T40.2X3	T40.2X4	--	--
Phenonyl	T42.3X1	T42.3X2	T42.3X3	T42.3X4	T42.3X5	T42.3X6
Phenoperidine	T40.4X1	T40.4X2	T40.4X3	T40.4X4	--	--
Phenopyrazone	T46.991	T46.992	T46.993	T46.994	T46.995	T46.996
Phenoquin	T50.4X1	T50.4X2	T50.4X3	T50.4X4	T50.4X5	T50.4X6
Phenothiazine (psychotropic) NEC	T43.3X1	T43.3X2	T43.3X3	T43.3X4	T43.3X5	T43.3X6
- insecticide	T60.2X1	T60.2X2	T60.2X3	T60.2X4	--	--
Phenothrin	T49.0X1	T49.0X2	T49.0X3	T49.0X4	T49.0X5	T49.0X6
Phenoxybenzamine	T46.7X1	T46.7X2	T46.7X3	T46.7X4	T46.7X5	T46.7X6
Phenoxyethanol	T49.0X1	T49.0X2	T49.0X3	T49.0X4	T49.0X5	T49.0X6
Phenoxymethyl penicillin	T36.0X1	T36.0X2	T36.0X3	T36.0X4	T36.0X5	T36.0X6

Substance	Poisoning, Accidental (unintentional)	Poisoning, Intentional Self-harm	Poisoning, Assault	Poisoning, Undetermined	Adverse effect	Underdosing
Phenprobamate	T42.8X1	T42.8X2	T42.8X3	T42.8X4	T42.8X5	T42.8X6
Phenprocoumon	T45.511	T45.512	T45.513	T45.514	T45.515	T45.516
Phensuximide	T42.2X1	T42.2X2	T42.2X3	T42.2X4	T42.2X5	T42.2X6
Phentermine	T50.5X1	T50.5X2	T50.5X3	T50.5X4	T50.5X5	T50.5X6
Phenthicillin	T36.0X1	T36.0X2	T36.0X3	T36.0X4	T36.0X5	T36.0X6
Phentolamine	T46.7X1	T46.7X2	T46.7X3	T46.7X4	T46.7X5	T46.7X6
Phenyl						
- butazone	T39.2X1	T39.2X2	T39.2X3	T39.2X4	T39.2X5	T39.2X6
- enediamine	T65.3X1	T65.3X2	T65.3X3	T65.3X4	--	--
- hydrazine	T65.3X1	T65.3X2	T65.3X3	T65.3X4	--	--
- - antineoplastic	T45.1X1	T45.1X2	T45.1X3	T45.1X4	T45.1X5	T45.1X6
- mercuric compounds—see Mercury						
- salicylate	T49.3X1	T49.3X2	T49.3X3	T49.3X4	T49.3X5	T49.3X6
Phenylalanine mustard	T45.1X1	T45.1X2	T45.1X3	T45.1X4	T45.1X5	T45.1X6
Phenylbutazone	T39.2X1	T39.2X2	T39.2X3	T39.2X4	T39.2X5	T39.2X6
Phenylenediamine	T65.3X1	T65.3X2	T65.3X3	T65.3X4	--	--
Phenylephrine	T44.4X1	T44.4X2	T44.4X3	T44.4X4	T44.4X5	T44.4X6
Phenylethylbiguanide	T38.3X1	T38.3X2	T38.3X3	T38.3X4	T38.3X5	T38.3X6
Phenylmercuric						
- acetate	T49.0X1	T49.0X2	T49.0X3	T49.0X4	T49.0X5	T49.0X6
- borate	T49.0X1	T49.0X2	T49.0X3	T49.0X4	T49.0X5	T49.0X6
- nitrate	T49.0X1	T49.0X2	T49.0X3	T49.0X4	T49.0X5	T49.0X6
Phenylmethylbarbitone	T42.3X1	T42.3X2	T42.3X3	T42.3X4	T42.3X5	T42.3X6
Phenylpropanol	T47.5X1	T47.5X2	T47.5X3	T47.5X4	T47.5X5	T47.5X6
Phenylpropanolamine	T44.991	T44.992	T44.993	T44.994	T44.995	T44.996
Phenylsulfthion	T60.0X1	T60.0X2	T60.0X3	T60.0X4	--	--
Phenyltoloxamine	T45.0X1	T45.0X2	T45.0X3	T45.0X4	T45.0X5	T45.0X6
Phenyramidol, phenyramidon	T39.8X1	T39.8X2	T39.8X3	T39.8X4	T39.8X5	T39.8X6
Phenytoin	T42.0X1	T42.0X2	T42.0X3	T42.0X4	T42.0X5	T42.0X6
- with Phenobarbital	T42.3X1	T42.3X2	T42.3X3	T42.3X4	T42.3X5	T42.3X6
pHisoHex	T49.2X1	T49.2X2	T49.2X3	T49.2X4	T49.2X5	T49.2X6
Pholcodine	T48.3X1	T48.3X2	T48.3X3	T48.3X4	T48.3X5	T48.3X6
Pholedrine	T46.991	T46.992	T46.993	T46.994	T46.995	T46.996
Phorate	T60.0X1	T60.0X2	T60.0X3	T60.0X4	--	--
Phosdrin	T60.0X1	T60.0X2	T60.0X3	T60.0X4	--	--
Phosfolan	T60.0X1	T60.0X2	T60.0X3	T60.0X4	--	--
Phosgene (gas)	T59.891	T59.892	T59.893	T59.894	--	--
Phosphamidon	T60.0X1	T60.0X2	T60.0X3	T60.0X4	--	--
Phosphate	T65.891	T65.892	T65.893	T65.894	--	--
- laxative	T47.4X1	T47.4X2	T47.4X3	T47.4X4	T47.4X5	T47.4X6
- organic	T60.0X1	T60.0X2	T60.0X3	T60.0X4	--	--
- solvent	T52.91	T52.92	T52.93	T52.94	--	--
- tricresyl	T65.891	T65.892	T65.893	T65.894	--	--
Phosphine	T57.1X1	T57.1X2	T57.1X3	T57.1X4	--	--
- fumigant	T57.1X1	T57.1X2	T57.1X3	T57.1X4	--	--
Phospholine	T49.5X1	T49.5X2	T49.5X3	T49.5X4	T49.5X5	T49.5X6
Phosphoric acid	T54.2X1	T54.2X2	T54.2X3	T54.2X4	--	--
Phosphorus (compound) NEC	T57.1X1	T57.1X2	T57.1X3	T57.1X4	--	--
- pesticide	T60.0X1	T60.0X2	T60.0X3	T60.0X4	--	--
Phthalates	T65.891	T65.892	T65.893	T65.894	--	--
Phthalic anhydride	T65.891	T65.892	T65.893	T65.894	--	--
Phthalimidoglutarimide	T42.6X1	T42.6X2	T42.6X3	T42.6X4	T42.6X5	T42.6X6
Phthalylsulfathiazole	T37.0X1	T37.0X2	T37.0X3	T37.0X4	T37.0X5	T37.0X6
Phylloquinone	T45.7X1	T45.7X2	T45.7X3	T45.7X4	T45.7X5	T45.7X6
Physeptone	T40.3X1	T40.3X2	T40.3X3	T40.3X4	T40.3X5	T40.3X6
Physostigma venenosum	T62.2X1	T62.2X2	T62.2X3	T62.2X4	--	--
Physostigmine	T49.5X1	T49.5X2	T49.5X3	T49.5X4	T49.5X5	T49.5X6
Phytolacca decandra	T62.2X1	T62.2X2	T62.2X3	T62.2X4	--	--
- berries	T62.1X1	T62.1X2	T62.1X3	T62.1X4	--	--

Substance	Poisoning, Accidental (unintentional)	Poisoning, Intentional Self-harm	Poisoning, Assault	Poisoning, Undetermined	Adverse effect	Underdosing
Phytomenadione	T45.7X1	T45.7X2	T45.7X3	T45.7X4	T45.7X5	T45.7X6
Phytonadione	T45.7X1	T45.7X2	T45.7X3	T45.7X4	T45.7X5	T45.7X6
Picoperine	T48.3X1	T48.3X2	T48.3X3	T48.3X4	T48.3X5	T48.3X6
Picosulfate (sodium)	T47.2X1	T47.2X2	T47.2X3	T47.2X4	T47.2X5	T47.2X6
Picric (acid)	T54.2X1	T54.2X2	T54.2X3	T54.2X4	--	--
Picrotoxin	T50.7X1	T50.7X2	T50.7X3	T50.7X4	T50.7X5	T50.7X6
Piketoprofen	T49.0X1	T49.0X2	T49.0X3	T49.0X4	T49.0X5	T49.0X6
Pilocarpine	T44.1X1	T44.1X2	T44.1X3	T44.1X4	T44.1X5	T44.1X6
Pilocarpus (jaborandi) extract	T44.1X1	T44.1X2	T44.1X3	T44.1X4	T44.1X5	T44.1X6
Pilsicainide (hydrochloride)	T46.2X1	T46.2X2	T46.2X3	T46.2X4	T46.2X5	T46.2X6
Pimaricin	T36.7X1	T36.7X2	T36.7X3	T36.7X4	T36.7X5	T36.7X6
Pimeclone	T50.7X1	T50.7X2	T50.7X3	T50.7X4	T50.7X5	T50.7X6
Pimelic ketone	T52.8X1	T52.8X2	T52.8X3	T52.8X4	--	--
Pimethixene	T45.0X1	T45.0X2	T45.0X3	T45.0X4	T45.0X5	T45.0X6
Piminodine	T40.2X1	T40.2X2	T40.2X3	T40.2X4	T40.2X5	T40.2X6
Pimozide	T43.591	T43.592	T43.593	T43.594	T43.595	T43.596
Pinacidil	T46.5X1	T46.5X2	T46.5X3	T46.5X4	T46.5X5	T46.5X6
Pinaverium bromide	T44.3X1	T44.3X2	T44.3X3	T44.3X4	T44.3X5	T44.3X6
Pinazepam	T42.4X1	T42.4X2	T42.4X3	T42.4X4	T42.4X5	T42.4X6
Pindolol	T44.7X1	T44.7X2	T44.7X3	T44.7X4	T44.7X5	T44.7X6
Pindone	T60.4X1	T60.4X2	T60.4X3	T60.4X4	--	--
Pine oil (disinfectant)	T65.891	T65.892	T65.893	T65.894	--	--
Pinkroot	T37.4X1	T37.4X2	T37.4X3	T37.4X4	T37.4X5	T37.4X6
Pipadone	T40.2X1	T40.2X2	T40.2X3	T40.2X4	--	--
Pipamazine	T45.0X1	T45.0X2	T45.0X3	T45.0X4	T45.0X5	T45.0X6
Pipamperone	T43.4X1	T43.4X2	T43.4X3	T43.4X4	T43.4X5	T43.4X6
Pipazetate	T48.3X1	T48.3X2	T48.3X3	T48.3X4	T48.3X5	T48.3X6
Pipemidic acid	T37.8X1	T37.8X2	T37.8X3	T37.8X4	T37.8X5	T37.8X6
Pipenzolate bromide	T44.3X1	T44.3X2	T44.3X3	T44.3X4	T44.3X5	T44.3X6
Piperacetazine	T43.3X1	T43.3X2	T43.3X3	T43.3X4	T43.3X5	T43.3X6
Piperacillin	T36.0X1	T36.0X2	T36.0X3	T36.0X4	T36.0X5	T36.0X6
Piperazine	T37.4X1	T37.4X2	T37.4X3	T37.4X4	T37.4X5	T37.4X6
- estrone sulfate	T38.5X1	T38.5X2	T38.5X3	T38.5X4	T38.5X5	T38.5X6
Piper cubeba	T62.2X1	T62.2X2	T62.2X3	T62.2X4	--	--
Piperidione	T48.3X1	T48.3X2	T48.3X3	T48.3X4	T48.3X5	T48.3X6
Piperidolate	T44.3X1	T44.3X2	T44.3X3	T44.3X4	T44.3X5	T44.3X6
Piperocaine	T41.3X1	T41.3X2	T41.3X3	T41.3X4	T41.3X5	T41.3X6
- infiltration (subcutaneous)	T41.3X1	T41.3X2	T41.3X3	T41.3X4	T41.3X5	T41.3X6
- nerve block (peripheral) (plexus)	T41.3X1	T41.3X2	T41.3X3	T41.3X4	T41.3X5	T41.3X6
- topical (surface)	T41.3X1	T41.3X2	T41.3X3	T41.3X4	T41.3X5	T41.3X6
Piperonyl butoxide	T60.8X1	T60.8X2	T60.8X3	T60.8X4	--	--
Pipethanate	T44.3X1	T44.3X2	T44.3X3	T44.3X4	T44.3X5	T44.3X6
Pipobroman	T45.1X1	T45.1X2	T45.1X3	T45.1X4	T45.1X5	T45.1X6
Pipotiazine	T43.3X1	T43.3X2	T43.3X3	T43.3X4	T43.3X5	T43.3X6
Pipoxizine	T45.0X1	T45.0X2	T45.0X3	T45.0X4	T45.0X5	T45.0X6
Pipradrol	T43.691	T43.692	T43.693	T43.694	T43.695	T43.696
Piprinhydrinate	T45.0X1	T45.0X2	T45.0X3	T45.0X4	T45.0X5	T45.0X6
Pirarubicin	T45.1X1	T45.1X2	T45.1X3	T45.1X4	T45.1X5	T45.1X6
Pirazinamide	T37.1X1	T37.1X2	T37.1X3	T37.1X4	T37.1X5	T37.1X6
Pirbuterol	T48.6X1	T48.6X2	T48.6X3	T48.6X4	T48.6X5	T48.6X6
Pirenzepine	T47.1X1	T47.1X2	T47.1X3	T47.1X4	T47.1X5	T47.1X6
Piretanide	T50.1X1	T50.1X2	T50.1X3	T50.1X4	T50.1X5	T50.1X6
Piribedil	T42.8X1	T42.8X2	T42.8X3	T42.8X4	T42.8X5	T42.8X6
Piridoxilate	T46.3X1	T46.3X2	T46.3X3	T46.3X4	T46.3X5	T46.3X6
Piritramide	T40.4X1	T40.4X2	T40.4X3	T40.4X4	--	--
Piromidic acid	T37.8X1	T37.8X2	T37.8X3	T37.8X4	T37.8X5	T37.8X6
Piroxicam	T39.391	T39.392	T39.393	T39.394	T39.395	T39.396
- beta-cyclodextrin complex	T39.8X1	T39.8X2	T39.8X3	T39.8X4	T39.8X5	T39.8X6

Substance	Poisoning, Accidental (unintentional)	Poisoning, Intentional Self-harm	Poisoning, Assault	Poisoning, Undetermined	Adverse effect	Underdosing
Pirozadil	T46.6X1	T46.6X2	T46.6X3	T46.6X4	T46.6X5	T46.6X6
Piscidia (bark) (erythrina)	T39.8X1	T39.8X2	T39.8X3	T39.8X4	T39.8X5	T39.8X6
Pitch	T65.891	T65.892	T65.893	T65.894	--	--
Pitkin's solution	T41.3X1	T41.3X2	T41.3X3	T41.3X4	T41.3X5	T41.3X6
Pitocin	T48.0X1	T48.0X2	T48.0X3	T48.0X4	T48.0X5	T48.0X6
Pitressin (tannate)	T38.891	T38.892	T38.893	T38.894	T38.895	T38.896
Pituitary extracts (posterior)	T38.891	T38.892	T38.893	T38.894	T38.895	T38.896
- anterior	T38.811	T38.812	T38.813	T38.814	T38.815	T38.816
Pituitrin	T38.891	T38.892	T38.893	T38.894	T38.895	T38.896
Pivampicillin	T36.0X1	T36.0X2	T36.0X3	T36.0X4	T36.0X5	T36.0X6
Pivmecillinam	T36.0X1	T36.0X2	T36.0X3	T36.0X4	T36.0X5	T36.0X6
Placental hormone	T38.891	T38.892	T38.893	T38.894	T38.895	T38.896
Placidyl	T42.6X1	T42.6X2	T42.6X3	T42.6X4	T42.6X5	T42.6X6
Plague vaccine	T50.A91	T50.A92	T50.A93	T50.A94	T50.A95	T50.A96
Plant						
- food or fertilizer NEC	T65.891	T65.892	T65.893	T65.894	--	--
- - containing herbicide	T60.3X1	T60.3X2	T60.3X3	T60.3X4	--	--
- noxious, used as food	T62.2X1	T62.2X2	T62.2X3	T62.2X4	--	--
- - berries	T62.1X1	T62.1X2	T62.1X3	T62.1X4	--	--
- - seeds	T62.2X1	T62.2X2	T62.2X3	T62.2X4	--	--
- - specified type NEC	T62.2X1	T62.2X2	T62.2X3	T62.2X4	--	--
Plasma	T45.8X1	T45.8X2	T45.8X3	T45.8X4	T45.8X5	T45.8X6
- expander NEC	T45.8X1	T45.8X2	T45.8X3	T45.8X4	T45.8X5	T45.8X6
- protein fraction (human)	T45.8X1	T45.8X2	T45.8X3	T45.8X4	T45.8X5	T45.8X6
Plasmanate	T45.8X1	T45.8X2	T45.8X3	T45.8X4	T45.8X5	T45.8X6
Plasminogen (tissue) activator	T45.611	T45.612	T45.613	T45.614	T45.615	T45.616
Plaster dressing	T49.3X1	T49.3X2	T49.3X3	T49.3X4	T49.3X5	T49.3X6
Plastic dressing	T49.3X1	T49.3X2	T49.3X3	T49.3X4	T49.3X5	T49.3X6
Plegicil	T43.3X1	T43.3X2	T43.3X3	T43.3X4	T43.3X5	T43.3X6
Plicamycin	T45.1X1	T45.1X2	T45.1X3	T45.1X4	T45.1X5	T45.1X6
Podophyllotoxin	T49.8X1	T49.8X2	T49.8X3	T49.8X4	T49.8X5	T49.8X6
Podophyllum (resin)	T49.4X1	T49.4X2	T49.4X3	T49.4X4	T49.4X5	T49.4X6
Poison NEC	T65.91	T65.92	T65.93	T65.94	--	--
Poisonous berries	T62.1X1	T62.1X2	T62.1X3	T62.1X4	--	--
Pokeweed (any part)	T62.2X1	T62.2X2	T62.2X3	T62.2X4	--	--
Poldine metilsulfate	T44.3X1	T44.3X2	T44.3X3	T44.3X4	T44.3X5	T44.3X6
Polidexide (sulfate)	T46.6X1	T46.6X2	T46.6X3	T46.6X4	T46.6X5	T46.6X6
Polidocanol	T46.8X1	T46.8X2	T46.8X3	T46.8X4	T46.8X5	T46.8X6
Poliomyelitis vaccine	T50.B91	T50.B92	T50.B93	T50.B94	T50.B95	T50.B96
Polish (car) (floor) (furni-ture) (metal) (porcelain) (silver)	T65.891	T65.892	T65.893	T65.894	--	--
- abrasive	T65.891	T65.892	T65.893	T65.894	--	--
- porcelain	T65.891	T65.892	T65.893	T65.894	--	--
Poloxalkol	T47.4X1	T47.4X2	T47.4X3	T47.4X4	T47.4X5	T47.4X6
Poloxamer	T47.4X1	T47.4X2	T47.4X3	T47.4X4	T47.4X5	T47.4X6
Polyaminostyrene resins	T50.3X1	T50.3X2	T50.3X3	T50.3X4	T50.3X5	T50.3X6
Polycarbophil	T47.4X1	T47.4X2	T47.4X3	T47.4X4	T47.4X5	T47.4X6
Polychlorinated biphenyl	T65.891	T65.892	T65.893	T65.894	--	--
Polycycline	T36.4X1	T36.4X2	T36.4X3	T36.4X4	T36.4X5	T36.4X6
Polyester fumes	T59.891	T59.892	T59.893	T59.894	--	--
Polyester resin hardener	T52.91	T52.92	T52.93	T52.94	--	--
- fumes	T59.891	T59.892	T59.893	T59.894	--	--
Polyestradiol phosphate	T38.5X1	T38.5X2	T38.5X3	T38.5X4	T38.5X5	T38.5X6
Polyethanolamine alkyl sulfate	T49.2X1	T49.2X2	T49.2X3	T49.2X4	T49.2X5	T49.2X6
Polyethylene adhesive	T49.3X1	T49.3X2	T49.3X3	T49.3X4	T49.3X5	T49.3X6
Polyferose	T45.4X1	T45.4X2	T45.4X3	T45.4X4	T45.4X5	T45.4X6
Polygeline	T45.8X1	T45.8X2	T45.8X3	T45.8X4	T45.8X5	T45.8X6
Polymyxin	T36.8X1	T36.8X2	T36.8X3	T36.8X4	T36.8X5	T36.8X6
- B	T36.8X1	T36.8X2	T36.8X3	T36.8X4	T36.8X5	T36.8X6

Substance	Poisoning, Accidental (unintentional)	Poisoning, Intentional Self-harm	Poisoning, Assault	Poisoning, Undetermined	Adverse effect	Underdosing
- - ENT agent	T49.6X1	T49.6X2	T49.6X3	T49.6X4	T49.6X5	T49.6X6
- - topical NEC	T49.0X1	T49.0X2	T49.0X3	T49.0X4	T49.0X5	T49.0X6
- E sulfate (eye preparation)	T49.5X1	T49.5X2	T49.5X3	T49.5X4	T49.5X5	T49.5X6
Polynoxylin	T49.0X1	T49.0X2	T49.0X3	T49.0X4	T49.0X5	T49.0X6
Polyoestradiol phosphate	T38.5X1	T38.5X2	T38.5X3	T38.5X4	T38.5X5	T38.5X6
Polyoxymethyleneurea	T49.0X1	T49.0X2	T49.0X3	T49.0X4	T49.0X5	T49.0X6
Polysilane	T47.8X1	T47.8X2	T47.8X3	T47.8X4	T47.8X5	T47.8X6
Polytetrafluoroethylene (inhaled)	T59.891	T59.892	T59.893	T59.894	--	--
Polythiazide	T50.2X1	T50.2X2	T50.2X3	T50.2X4	T50.2X5	T50.2X6
Polyvidone	T45.8X1	T45.8X2	T45.8X3	T45.8X4	T45.8X5	T45.8X6
Polyvinylpyrrolidone	T45.8X1	T45.8X2	T45.8X3	T45.8X4	T45.8X5	T45.8X6
Pontocaine (hydrochloride) (infiltration) (topical)	T41.3X1	T41.3X2	T41.3X3	T41.3X4	T41.3X5	T41.3X6
- nerve block (peripheral) (plexus)	T41.3X1	T41.3X2	T41.3X3	T41.3X4	T41.3X5	T41.3X6
- spinal	T41.3X1	T41.3X2	T41.3X3	T41.3X4	T41.3X5	T41.3X6
Porfiromycin	T45.1X1	T45.1X2	T45.1X3	T45.1X4	T45.1X5	T45.1X6
Posterior pituitary hormone NEC	T38.891	T38.892	T38.893	T38.894	T38.895	T38.896
Pot	T40.7X1	T40.7X2	T40.7X3	T40.7X4	T40.7X5	T40.7X6
Potash (caustic)	T54.3X1	T54.3X2	T54.3X3	T54.3X4	--	--
Potassic saline injection (lactated)	T50.3X1	T50.3X2	T50.3X3	T50.3X4	T50.3X5	T50.3X6
Potassium (salts) NEC	T50.3X1	T50.3X2	T50.3X3	T50.3X4	T50.3X5	T50.3X6
- aminobenzoate	T45.8X1	T45.8X2	T45.8X3	T45.8X4	T45.8X5	T45.8X6
- aminosalicylate	T37.1X1	T37.1X2	T37.1X3	T37.1X4	T37.1X5	T37.1X6
- antimony ' tartrate'	T37.8X1	T37.8X2	T37.8X3	T37.8X4	T37.8X5	T37.8X6
- arsenite (solution)	T57.0X1	T57.0X2	T57.0X3	T57.0X4	--	--
- bichromate	T56.2X1	T56.2X2	T56.2X3	T56.2X4	--	--
- bisulfate	T47.3X1	T47.3X2	T47.3X3	T47.3X4	T47.3X5	T47.3X6
- bromide	T42.6X1	T42.6X2	T42.6X3	T42.6X4	T42.6X5	T42.6X6
- canrenoate	T50.0X1	T50.0X2	T50.0X3	T50.0X4	T50.0X5	T50.0X6
- carbonate	T54.3X1	T54.3X2	T54.3X3	T54.3X4	--	--
- chlorate NEC	T65.891	T65.892	T65.893	T65.894	--	--
- chloride	T50.3X1	T50.3X2	T50.3X3	T50.3X4	T50.3X5	T50.3X6
- citrate	T50.991	T50.992	T50.993	T50.994	T50.995	T50.996
- cyanide	T65.0X1	T65.0X2	T65.0X3	T65.0X4	--	--
- ferric hexacyanoferrate (medicinal)	T50.6X1	T50.6X2	T50.6X3	T50.6X4	T50.6X5	T50.6X6
- - nonmedicinal	T65.891	T65.892	T65.893	T65.894	--	--
- Fluoride	T57.8X1	T57.8X2	T57.8X3	T57.8X4	--	--
- glucaldrate	T47.1X1	T47.1X2	T47.1X3	T47.1X4	T47.1X5	T47.1X6
- hydroxide	T54.3X1	T54.3X2	T54.3X3	T54.3X4	--	--
- iodate	T49.0X1	T49.0X2	T49.0X3	T49.0X4	T49.0X5	T49.0X6
- iodide	T48.4X1	T48.4X2	T48.4X3	T48.4X4	T48.4X5	T48.4X6
- nitrate	T57.8X1	T57.8X2	T57.8X3	T57.8X4	--	--
- oxalate	T65.891	T65.892	T65.893	T65.894	--	--
- perchlorate (nonmedicinal) NEC	T65.891	T65.892	T65.893	T65.894	--	--
- - antithyroid	T38.2X1	T38.2X2	T38.2X3	T38.2X4	T38.2X5	T38.2X6
- - medicinal	T38.2X1	T38.2X2	T38.2X3	T38.2X4	T38.2X5	T38.2X6
- Permanganate (nonmedicinal)	T65.891	T65.892	T65.893	T65.894	--	--
- - medicinal	T49.0X1	T49.0X2	T49.0X3	T49.0X4	T49.0X5	T49.0X6
- sulfate	T47.2X1	T47.2X2	T47.2X3	T47.2X4	T47.2X5	T47.2X6
Potassium-removing resin	T50.3X1	T50.3X2	T50.3X3	T50.3X4	T50.3X5	T50.3X6
Potassium-retaining drug	T50.3X1	T50.3X2	T50.3X3	T50.3X4	T50.3X5	T50.3X6
Povidone	T45.8X1	T45.8X2	T45.8X3	T45.8X4	T45.8X5	T45.8X6
- iodine	T49.0X1	T49.0X2	T49.0X3	T49.0X4	T49.0X5	T49.0X6
Practolol	T44.7X1	T44.7X2	T44.7X3	T44.7X4	T44.7X5	T44.7X6
Prajmalium bitartrate	T46.2X1	T46.2X2	T46.2X3	T46.2X4	T46.2X5	T46.2X6
Pralidoxime (iodide)	T50.6X1	T50.6X2	T50.6X3	T50.6X4	T50.6X5	T50.6X6
- chloride	T50.6X1	T50.6X2	T50.6X3	T50.6X4	T50.6X5	T50.6X6
Pramiverine	T44.3X1	T44.3X2	T44.3X3	T44.3X4	T44.3X5	T44.3X6
Pramocaine	T49.1X1	T49.1X2	T49.1X3	T49.1X4	T49.1X5	T49.1X6

Substance	Poisoning, Accidental (unintentional)	Poisoning, Intentional Self-harm	Poisoning, Assault	Poisoning, Undetermined	Adverse effect	Underdosing
Pramoxine	T49.1X1	T49.1X2	T49.1X3	T49.1X4	T49.1X5	T49.1X6
Prasterone	T38.7X1	T38.7X2	T38.7X3	T38.7X4	T38.7X5	T38.7X6
Pravastatin	T46.6X1	T46.6X2	T46.6X3	T46.6X4	T46.6X5	T46.6X6
Prazepam	T42.4X1	T42.4X2	T42.4X3	T42.4X4	T42.4X5	T42.4X6
Praziquantel	T37.4X1	T37.4X2	T37.4X3	T37.4X4	T37.4X5	T37.4X6
Prazitone	T43.291	T43.292	T43.293	T43.294	T43.295	T43.296
Prazosin	T44.6X1	T44.6X2	T44.6X3	T44.6X4	T44.6X5	T44.6X6
Prednicarbate	T49.0X1	T49.0X2	T49.0X3	T49.0X4	T49.0X5	T49.0X6
Prednimustine	T45.1X1	T45.1X2	T45.1X3	T45.1X4	T45.1X5	T45.1X6
Prednisolone	T38.0X1	T38.0X2	T38.0X3	T38.0X4	T38.0X5	T38.0X6
- ENT agent	T49.6X1	T49.6X2	T49.6X3	T49.6X4	T49.6X5	T49.6X6
- ophthalmic preparation	T49.5X1	T49.5X2	T49.5X3	T49.5X4	T49.5X5	T49.5X6
- steaglate	T49.0X1	T49.0X2	T49.0X3	T49.0X4	T49.0X5	T49.0X6
- topical NEC	T49.0X1	T49.0X2	T49.0X3	T49.0X4	T49.0X5	T49.0X6
Prednisone	T38.0X1	T38.0X2	T38.0X3	T38.0X4	T38.0X5	T38.0X6
Prednylidene	T38.0X1	T38.0X2	T38.0X3	T38.0X4	T38.0X5	T38.0X6
Pregnandiol	T38.5X1	T38.5X2	T38.5X3	T38.5X4	T38.5X5	T38.5X6
Pregneninolone	T38.5X1	T38.5X2	T38.5X3	T38.5X4	T38.5X5	T38.5X6
Preludin	T43.691	T43.692	T43.693	T43.694	T43.695	T43.696
Premarin	T38.5X1	T38.5X2	T38.5X3	T38.5X4	T38.5X5	T38.5X6
Premedication anesthetic	T41.201	T41.202	T41.203	T41.204	T41.205	T41.206
Prenalterol	T44.5X1	T44.5X2	T44.5X3	T44.5X4	T44.5X5	T44.5X6
Prenoxdiazine	T48.3X1	T48.3X2	T48.3X3	T48.3X4	T48.3X5	T48.3X6
Prenylamine	T46.3X1	T46.3X2	T46.3X3	T46.3X4	T46.3X5	T46.3X6
Preparation H	T49.8X1	T49.8X2	T49.8X3	T49.8X4	T49.8X5	T49.8X6
Preparation, local	T49.4X1	T49.4X2	T49.4X3	T49.4X4	T49.4X5	T49.4X6
Preservative (nonmedicinal)	T65.891	T65.892	T65.893	T65.894	--	--
- medicinal	T50.901	T50.902	T50.903	T50.904	T50.905	T50.906
- wood	T60.91	T60.92	T60.93	T60.94	--	--
Prethcamide	T50.7X1	T50.7X2	T50.7X3	T50.7X4	T50.7X5	T50.7X6
Pride of China	T62.2X1	T62.2X2	T62.2X3	T62.2X4	--	--
Pridinol	T44.3X1	T44.3X2	T44.3X3	T44.3X4	T44.3X5	T44.3X6
Prifinium bromide	T44.3X1	T44.3X2	T44.3X3	T44.3X4	T44.3X5	T44.3X6
Prilocaine	T41.3X1	T41.3X2	T41.3X3	T41.3X4	T41.3X5	T41.3X6
- infiltration (subcutaneous)	T41.3X1	T41.3X2	T41.3X3	T41.3X4	T41.3X5	T41.3X6
- nerve block peripheral (plexus)	T41.3X1	T41.3X2	T41.3X3	T41.3X4	T41.3X5	T41.3X6
- regional	T41.3X1	T41.3X2	T41.3X3	T41.3X4	T41.3X5	T41.3X6
Primaquine	T37.2X1	T37.2X2	T37.2X3	T37.2X4	T37.2X5	T37.2X6
Primidone	T42.6X1	T42.6X2	T42.6X3	T42.6X4	T42.6X5	T42.6X6
Primula (veris)	T62.2X1	T62.2X2	T62.2X3	T62.2X4	--	--
Prinadol	T40.2X1	T40.2X2	T40.2X3	T40.2X4	T40.2X5	T40.2X6
Priscol, Priscoline	T44.6X1	T44.6X2	T44.6X3	T44.6X4	T44.6X5	T44.6X6
Pristinamycin	T36.3X1	T36.3X2	T36.3X3	T36.3X4	T36.3X5	T36.3X6
Privet	T62.2X1	T62.2X2	T62.2X3	T62.2X4	--	--
- berries	T62.1X1	T62.1X2	T62.1X3	T62.1X4	--	--
Privine	T44.4X1	T44.4X2	T44.4X3	T44.4X4	T44.4X5	T44.4X6
Pro-Banthine	T44.3X1	T44.3X2	T44.3X3	T44.3X4	T44.3X5	T44.3X6
Probarbital	T42.3X1	T42.3X2	T42.3X3	T42.3X4	T42.3X5	T42.3X6
Probenecid	T50.4X1	T50.4X2	T50.4X3	T50.4X4	T50.4X5	T50.4X6
Probucol	T46.6X1	T46.6X2	T46.6X3	T46.6X4	T46.6X5	T46.6X6
Procainamide	T46.2X1	T46.2X2	T46.2X3	T46.2X4	T46.2X5	T46.2X6
Procaine	T41.3X1	T41.3X2	T41.3X3	T41.3X4	T41.3X5	T41.3X6
- benzylpenicillin	T36.0X1	T36.0X2	T36.0X3	T36.0X4	T36.0X5	T36.0X6
- nerve block (periphreal) (plexus)	T41.3X1	T41.3X2	T41.3X3	T41.3X4	T41.3X5	T41.3X6
- penicillin G	T36.0X1	T36.0X2	T36.0X3	T36.0X4	T36.0X5	T36.0X6
- regional	T41.3X1	T41.3X2	T41.3X3	T41.3X4	T41.3X5	T41.3X6
- spinal	T41.3X1	T41.3X2	T41.3X3	T41.3X4	T41.3X5	T41.3X6
Procalmidol	T43.591	T43.592	T43.593	T43.594	T43.595	T43.596
Procarbazine	T45.1X1	T45.1X2	T45.1X3	T45.1X4	T45.1X5	T45.1X6

Substance	Poisoning, Accidental (unintentional)	Poisoning, Intentional Self-harm	Poisoning, Assault	Poisoning, Undetermined	Adverse effect	Underdosing
Procaterol	T44.5X1	T44.5X2	T44.5X3	T44.5X4	T44.5X5	T44.5X6
Prochlorperazine	T43.3X1	T43.3X2	T43.3X3	T43.3X4	T43.3X5	T43.3X6
Procyclidine	T44.3X1	T44.3X2	T44.3X3	T44.3X4	T44.3X5	T44.3X6
Producer gas	T58.8X1	T58.8X2	T58.8X3	T58.8X4	--	--
Profadol	T40.4X1	T40.4X2	T40.4X3	T40.4X4	T40.4X5	T40.4X6
Profenamine	T44.3X1	T44.3X2	T44.3X3	T44.3X4	T44.3X5	T44.3X6
Profenil	T44.3X1	T44.3X2	T44.3X3	T44.3X4	T44.3X5	T44.3X6
Proflavine	T49.0X1	T49.0X2	T49.0X3	T49.0X4	T49.0X5	T49.0X6
Progabide	T42.6X1	T42.6X2	T42.6X3	T42.6X4	T42.6X5	T42.6X6
Progesterone	T38.5X1	T38.5X2	T38.5X3	T38.5X4	T38.5X5	T38.5X6
Progestin	T38.5X1	T38.5X2	T38.5X3	T38.5X4	T38.5X5	T38.5X6
- oral contraceptive	T38.4X1	T38.4X2	T38.4X3	T38.4X4	T38.4X5	T38.4X6
Progestogen NEC	T38.5X1	T38.5X2	T38.5X3	T38.5X4	T38.5X5	T38.5X6
Progestone	T38.5X1	T38.5X2	T38.5X3	T38.5X4	T38.5X5	T38.5X6
Proglumide	T47.1X1	T47.1X2	T47.1X3	T47.1X4	T47.1X5	T47.1X6
Proguanil	T37.2X1	T37.2X2	T37.2X3	T37.2X4	T37.2X5	T37.2X6
Prolactin	T38.811	T38.812	T38.813	T38.814	T38.815	T38.816
Prolintane	T43.691	T43.692	T43.693	T43.694	T43.695	T43.696
Proloid	T38.1X1	T38.1X2	T38.1X3	T38.1X4	T38.1X5	T38.1X6
Proluton	T38.5X1	T38.5X2	T38.5X3	T38.5X4	T38.5X5	T38.5X6
Promacetin	T37.1X1	T37.1X2	T37.1X3	T37.1X4	T37.1X5	T37.1X6
Promazine	T43.3X1	T43.3X2	T43.3X3	T43.3X4	T43.3X5	T43.3X6
Promedol	T40.2X1	T40.2X2	T40.2X3	T40.2X4	--	--
Promegestone	T38.5X1	T38.5X2	T38.5X3	T38.5X4	T38.5X5	T38.5X6
Promethazine (teoclate)	T43.3X1	T43.3X2	T43.3X3	T43.3X4	T43.3X5	T43.3X6
Promin	T37.1X1	T37.1X2	T37.1X3	T37.1X4	T37.1X5	T37.1X6
Pronase	T45.3X1	T45.3X2	T45.3X3	T45.3X4	T45.3X5	T45.3X6
Pronestyl (hydrochloride)	T46.2X1	T46.2X2	T46.2X3	T46.2X4	T46.2X5	T46.2X6
Pronetalol	T44.7X1	T44.7X2	T44.7X3	T44.7X4	T44.7X5	T44.7X6
Prontosil	T37.0X1	T37.0X2	T37.0X3	T37.0X4	T37.0X5	T37.0X6
Propachlor	T60.3X1	T60.3X2	T60.3X3	T60.3X4	--	--
Propafenone	T46.2X1	T46.2X2	T46.2X3	T46.2X4	T46.2X5	T46.2X6
Propallylonal	T42.3X1	T42.3X2	T42.3X3	T42.3X4	T42.3X5	T42.3X6
Propamidine	T49.0X1	T49.0X2	T49.0X3	T49.0X4	T49.0X5	T49.0X6
Propane (distributed in mobile container)	T59.891	T59.892	T59.893	T59.894	--	--
- distributed through pipes	T59.891	T59.892	T59.893	T59.894	--	--
- incomplete combustion	T58.11	T58.12	T58.13	T58.14	--	--
Propanidid	T41.291	T41.292	T41.293	T41.294	T41.295	T41.296
Propanil	T60.3X1	T60.3X2	T60.3X3	T60.3X4	--	--
1-Propanol	T51.3X1	T51.3X2	T51.3X3	T51.3X4	--	--
2-Propanol	T51.2X1	T51.2X2	T51.2X3	T51.2X4	--	--
Propantheline	T44.3X1	T44.3X2	T44.3X3	T44.3X4	T44.3X5	T44.3X6
- bromide	T44.3X1	T44.3X2	T44.3X3	T44.3X4	T44.3X5	T44.3X6
Proparacaine	T41.3X1	T41.3X2	T41.3X3	T41.3X4	T41.3X5	T41.3X6
Propatylnitrate	T46.3X1	T46.3X2	T46.3X3	T46.3X4	T46.3X5	T46.3X6
Propicillin	T36.0X1	T36.0X2	T36.0X3	T36.0X4	T36.0X5	T36.0X6
Propiolactone	T49.0X1	T49.0X2	T49.0X3	T49.0X4	T49.0X5	T49.0X6
Propiomazine	T45.0X1	T45.0X2	T45.0X3	T45.0X4	T45.0X5	T45.0X6
Propionaldehyde (medicinal)	T42.6X1	T42.6X2	T42.6X3	T42.6X4	T42.6X5	T42.6X6
Propionate (calcium) (sodium)	T49.0X1	T49.0X2	T49.0X3	T49.0X4	T49.0X5	T49.0X6
Propion gel	T49.0X1	T49.0X2	T49.0X3	T49.0X4	T49.0X5	T49.0X6
Propitocaine	T41.3X1	T41.3X2	T41.3X3	T41.3X4	T41.3X5	T41.3X6
- infiltration (subcutaneous)	T41.3X1	T41.3X2	T41.3X3	T41.3X4	T41.3X5	T41.3X6
- nerve block (peripheral) (plexus)	T41.3X1	T41.3X2	T41.3X3	T41.3X4	T41.3X5	T41.3X6
Propofol	T41.291	T41.292	T41.293	T41.294	T41.295	T41.296
Propoxur	T60.0X1	T60.0X2	T60.0X3	T60.0X4	--	--
Propoxycaine	T41.3X1	T41.3X2	T41.3X3	T41.3X4	T41.3X5	T41.3X6
- infiltration (subcutaneous)	T41.3X1	T41.3X2	T41.3X3	T41.3X4	T41.3X5	T41.3X6

Substance	Poisoning, Accidental (unintentional)	Poisoning, Intentional Self-harm	Poisoning, Assault	Poisoning, Undetermined	Adverse effect	Underdosing
- nerve block (peripheral) (plexus)	T41.3X1	T41.3X2	T41.3X3	T41.3X4	T41.3X5	T41.3X6
- topical (surface)	T41.3X1	T41.3X2	T41.3X3	T41.3X4	T41.3X5	T41.3X6
Propoxyphene	T40.4X1	T40.4X2	T40.4X3	T40.4X4	T40.4X5	T40.4X6
Propranolol	T44.7X1	T44.7X2	T44.7X3	T44.7X4	T44.7X5	T44.7X6
Propyl						
- alcohol	T51.3X1	T51.3X2	T51.3X3	T51.3X4	--	--
- carbinol	T51.3X1	T51.3X2	T51.3X3	T51.3X4	--	--
- hexadrine	T44.4X1	T44.4X2	T44.4X3	T44.4X4	T44.4X5	T44.4X6
- iodone	T50.8X1	T50.8X2	T50.8X3	T50.8X4	T50.8X5	T50.8X6
- thiouracil	T38.2X1	T38.2X2	T38.2X3	T38.2X4	T38.2X5	T38.2X6
Propylaminopheno-thiazine	T43.3X1	T43.3X2	T43.3X3	T43.3X4	T43.3X5	T43.3X6
Propylene	T59.891	T59.892	T59.893	T59.894	--	--
Propylhexedrine	T48.5X1	T48.5X2	T48.5X3	T48.5X4	T48.5X5	T48.5X6
Propyliodone	T50.8X1	T50.8X2	T50.8X3	T50.8X4	T50.8X5	T50.8X6
Propylparaben (ophthalmic)	T49.5X1	T49.5X2	T49.5X3	T49.5X4	T49.5X5	T49.5X6
Propylthiouracil	T38.2X1	T38.2X2	T38.2X3	T38.2X4	T38.2X5	T38.2X6
Propyphenazone	T39.2X1	T39.2X2	T39.2X3	T39.2X4	T39.2X5	T39.2X6
Proquazone	T39.391	T39.392	T39.393	T39.394	T39.395	T39.396
Proscillaridin	T46.0X1	T46.0X2	T46.0X3	T46.0X4	T46.0X5	T46.0X6
Prostacyclin	T45.521	T45.522	T45.523	T45.524	T45.525	T45.526
Prostaglandin (I2)	T45.521	T45.522	T45.523	T45.524	T45.525	T45.526
- E1	T46.7X1	T46.7X2	T46.7X3	T46.7X4	T46.7X5	T46.7X6
- E2	T48.0X1	T48.0X2	T48.0X3	T48.0X4	T48.0X5	T48.0X6
- F2 alpha	T48.0X1	T48.0X2	T48.0X3	T48.0X4	T48.0X5	T48.0X6
Prostigmin	T44.0X1	T44.0X2	T44.0X3	T44.0X4	T44.0X5	T44.0X6
Prosultiamine	T45.2X1	T45.2X2	T45.2X3	T45.2X4	T45.2X5	T45.2X6
Protamine sulfate	T45.7X1	T45.7X2	T45.7X3	T45.7X4	T45.7X5	T45.7X6
- zinc insulin	T38.3X1	T38.3X2	T38.3X3	T38.3X4	T38.3X5	T38.3X6
Protease	T47.5X1	T47.5X2	T47.5X3	T47.5X4	T47.5X5	T47.5X6
Protectant, skin NEC	T49.3X1	T49.3X2	T49.3X3	T49.3X4	T49.3X5	T49.3X6
Protein hydrolysate	T50.991	T50.992	T50.993	T50.994	T50.995	T50.996
Prothiaden—see Dothiepin hydrochloride						
Prothionamide	T37.1X1	T37.1X2	T37.1X3	T37.1X4	T37.1X5	T37.1X6
Prothipendyl	T43.591	T43.592	T43.593	T43.594	T43.595	T43.596
Prothoate	T60.0X1	T60.0X2	T60.0X3	T60.0X4	--	--
Prothrombin						
- activator	T45.7X1	T45.7X2	T45.7X3	T45.7X4	T45.7X5	T45.7X6
- synthesis inhibitor	T45.511	T45.512	T45.513	T45.514	T45.515	T45.516
Protionamide	T37.1X1	T37.1X2	T37.1X3	T37.1X4	T37.1X5	T37.1X6
Protirelin	T38.891	T38.892	T38.893	T38.894	T38.895	T38.896
Protokylol	T48.6X1	T48.6X2	T48.6X3	T48.6X4	T48.6X5	T48.6X6
Protopam	T50.6X1	T50.6X2	T50.6X3	T50.6X4	T50.6X5	T50.6X6
Protoveratrine (s) (A) (B)	T46.5X1	T46.5X2	T46.5X3	T46.5X4	T46.5X5	T46.5X6
Protriptyline	T43.011	T43.012	T43.013	T43.014	T43.015	T43.016
Provera	T38.5X1	T38.5X2	T38.5X3	T38.5X4	T38.5X5	T38.5X6
Provitamin A	T45.2X1	T45.2X2	T45.2X3	T45.2X4	T45.2X5	T45.2X6
Proxibarbal	T42.3X1	T42.3X2	T42.3X3	T42.3X4	T42.3X5	T42.3X6
Proxymetacaine	T41.3X1	T41.3X2	T41.3X3	T41.3X4	T41.3X5	T41.3X6
Proxyphylline	T48.6X1	T48.6X2	T48.6X3	T48.6X4	T48.6X5	T48.6X6
Prozac—see Fluoxetine hydrochloride						
Prunus						
- laurocerasus	T62.2X1	T62.2X2	T62.2X3	T62.2X4	--	--
- virginiana	T62.2X1	T62.2X2	T62.2X3	T62.2X4	--	--
Prussian blue						
- commercial	T65.891	T65.892	T65.893	T65.894	--	--
- therapeutic	T50.6X1	T50.6X2	T50.6X3	T50.6X4	T50.6X5	T50.6X6
Prussic acid	T65.0X1	T65.0X2	T65.0X3	T65.0X4	--	--
- vapor	T57.3X1	T57.3X2	T57.3X3	T57.3X4	--	--
Pseudoephedrine	T44.991	T44.992	T44.993	T44.994	T44.995	T44.996

Substance	Poisoning, Accidental (unintentional)	Poisoning, Intentional Self-harm	Poisoning, Assault	Poisoning, Undetermined	Adverse effect	Underdosing
Psilocin	T40.991	T40.992	T40.993	T40.994	--	--
Psilocybin	T40.991	T40.992	T40.993	T40.994	--	--
Psilocybine	T40.991	T40.992	T40.993	T40.994	--	--
Psoralene (nonmedicinal)	T65.891	T65.892	T65.893	T65.894	--	--
Psoralens (medicinal)	T50.991	T50.992	T50.993	T50.994	T50.995	T50.996
PSP (phenolsulfonphthalein)	T50.8X1	T50.8X2	T50.8X3	T50.8X4	T50.8X5	T50.8X6
Psychodysleptic drug NEC	T40.901	T40.902	T40.903	T40.904	T40.905	T40.906
Psychostimulant	T43.601	T43.602	T43.603	T43.604	T43.605	T43.606
- amphetamine	T43.621	T43.622	T43.623	T43.624	T43.625	T43.626
- caffeine	T43.611	T43.612	T43.613	T43.614	T43.615	T43.616
- methylphenidate	T43.631	T43.632	T43.633	T43.634	T43.635	T43.636
- specified NEC	T43.691	T43.692	T43.693	T43.694	T43.695	T43.696
Psychotherapeutic drug NEC	T43.91	T43.92	T43.93	T43.94	T43.95	T43.96
- antidepressants—see also Antidepressant	T43.201	T43.202	T43.203	T43.204	T43.205	T43.206
- specified NEC	T43.8X1	T43.8X2	T43.8X3	T43.8X4	T43.8X5	T43.8X6
- tranquilizers NEC	T43.501	T43.502	T43.503	T43.504	T43.505	T43.506
Psychotomimetic agents	T40.901	T40.902	T40.903	T40.904	T40.905	T40.906
Psychotropic drug NEC	T43.91	T43.92	T43.93	T43.94	T43.95	T43.96
- specified NEC	T43.8X1	T43.8X2	T43.8X3	T43.8X4	T43.8X5	T43.8X6
Psyllium hydrophilic mucilloid	T47.4X1	T47.4X2	T47.4X3	T47.4X4	T47.4X5	T47.4X6
Pteroylglutamic acid	T45.8X1	T45.8X2	T45.8X3	T45.8X4	T45.8X5	T45.8X6
Pteroyltriglutamate	T45.1X1	T45.1X2	T45.1X3	T45.1X4	T45.1X5	T45.1X6
PTFE—see Polytetrafluoroethylene						
Pulp						
- devitalizing paste	T49.7X1	T49.7X2	T49.7X3	T49.7X4	T49.7X5	T49.7X6
- dressing	T49.7X1	T49.7X2	T49.7X3	T49.7X4	T49.7X5	T49.7X6
Pulsatilla	T62.2X1	T62.2X2	T62.2X3	T62.2X4	--	--
Pumpkin seed extract	T37.4X1	T37.4X2	T37.4X3	T37.4X4	T37.4X5	T37.4X6
Purex (bleach)	T54.91	T54.92	T54.93	T54.94	--	--
Purgative NEC—see also Cathartic	T47.4X1	T47.4X2	T47.4X3	T47.4X4	T47.4X5	T47.4X6
Purine analogue (antineoplastic)	T45.1X1	T45.1X2	T45.1X3	T45.1X4	T45.1X5	T45.1X6
Purine diuretics	T50.2X1	T50.2X2	T50.2X3	T50.2X4	T50.2X5	T50.2X6
Purinethol	T45.1X1	T45.1X2	T45.1X3	T45.1X4	T45.1X5	T45.1X6
PVP	T45.8X1	T45.8X2	T45.8X3	T45.8X4	T45.8X5	T45.8X6
Pyrabital	T39.8X1	T39.8X2	T39.8X3	T39.8X4	T39.8X5	T39.8X6
Pyramidon	T39.2X1	T39.2X2	T39.2X3	T39.2X4	T39.2X5	T39.2X6
Pyrantel	T37.4X1	T37.4X2	T37.4X3	T37.4X4	T37.4X5	T37.4X6
Pyrathiazine	T45.0X1	T45.0X2	T45.0X3	T45.0X4	T45.0X5	T45.0X6
Pyrazinamide	T37.1X1	T37.1X2	T37.1X3	T37.1X4	T37.1X5	T37.1X6
Pyrazinoic acid (amide)	T37.1X1	T37.1X2	T37.1X3	T37.1X4	T37.1X5	T37.1X6
Pyrazole (derivatives)	T39.2X1	T39.2X2	T39.2X3	T39.2X4	T39.2X5	T39.2X6
Pyrazolone analgesic NEC	T39.2X1	T39.2X2	T39.2X3	T39.2X4	T39.2X5	T39.2X6
Pyrethrin, pyrethrum (nonmedicinal)	T60.2X1	T60.2X2	T60.2X3	T60.2X4	--	--
Pyrethrum extract	T49.0X1	T49.0X2	T49.0X3	T49.0X4	T49.0X5	T49.0X6
Pyribenzamine	T45.0X1	T45.0X2	T45.0X3	T45.0X4	T45.0X5	T45.0X6
Pyridine	T52.8X1	T52.8X2	T52.8X3	T52.8X4	--	--
- aldoxime methiodide	T50.6X1	T50.6X2	T50.6X3	T50.6X4	T50.6X5	T50.6X6
- aldoxime methyl chloride	T50.6X1	T50.6X2	T50.6X3	T50.6X4	T50.6X5	T50.6X6
- vapor	T59.891	T59.892	T59.893	T59.894	--	--
Pyridium	T39.8X1	T39.8X2	T39.8X3	T39.8X4	T39.8X5	T39.8X6
Pyridostigmine bromide	T44.0X1	T44.0X2	T44.0X3	T44.0X4	T44.0X5	T44.0X6
Pyridoxal phosphate	T45.2X1	T45.2X2	T45.2X3	T45.2X4	T45.2X5	T45.2X6
Pyridoxine	T45.2X1	T45.2X2	T45.2X3	T45.2X4	T45.2X5	T45.2X6
Pyrilamine	T45.0X1	T45.0X2	T45.0X3	T45.0X4	T45.0X5	T45.0X6
Pyrimethamine	T37.2X1	T37.2X2	T37.2X3	T37.2X4	T37.2X5	T37.2X6
- with sulfadoxine	T37.2X1	T37.2X2	T37.2X3	T37.2X4	T37.2X5	T37.2X6
Pyrimidine antagonist	T45.1X1	T45.1X2	T45.1X3	T45.1X4	T45.1X5	T45.1X6
Pyriminil	T60.4X1	T60.4X2	T60.4X3	T60.4X4	--	--

Substance	Poisoning, Accidental (unintentional)	Poisoning, Intentional Self-harm	Poisoning, Assault	Poisoning, Undetermined	Adverse effect	Underdosing
Pyrithione zinc	T49.4X1	T49.4X2	T49.4X3	T49.4X4	T49.4X5	T49.4X6
Pyrithyldione	T42.6X1	T42.6X2	T42.6X3	T42.6X4	T42.6X5	T42.6X6
Pyrogallic acid	T49.0X1	T49.0X2	T49.0X3	T49.0X4	T49.0X5	T49.0X6
Pyrogallol	T49.0X1	T49.0X2	T49.0X3	T49.0X4	T49.0X5	T49.0X6
Pyroxylin	T49.3X1	T49.3X2	T49.3X3	T49.3X4	T49.3X5	T49.3X6
Pyrrobutamine	T45.0X1	T45.0X2	T45.0X3	T45.0X4	T45.0X5	T45.0X6
Pyrrolizidine alkaloids	T62.8X1	T62.8X2	T62.8X3	T62.8X4	--	--
Pyrvinium chloride	T37.4X1	T37.4X2	T37.4X3	T37.4X4	T37.4X5	T37.4X6
PZI	T38.3X1	T38.3X2	T38.3X3	T38.3X4	T38.3X5	T38.3X6
Quaalude	T42.6X1	T42.6X2	T42.6X3	T42.6X4	T42.6X5	T42.6X6
Quarternary ammonium						
- anti-infective	T49.0X1	T49.0X2	T49.0X3	T49.0X4	T49.0X5	T49.0X6
- ganglion blocking	T44.2X1	T44.2X2	T44.2X3	T44.2X4	T44.2X5	T44.2X6
- parasympatholytic	T44.3X1	T44.3X2	T44.3X3	T44.3X4	T44.3X5	T44.3X6
Quazepam	T42.4X1	T42.4X2	T42.4X3	T42.4X4	T42.4X5	T42.4X6
Quicklime	T54.3X1	T54.3X2	T54.3X3	T54.3X4	--	--
Quillaja extract	T48.4X1	T48.4X2	T48.4X3	T48.4X4	T48.4X5	T48.4X6
Quinacrine	T37.2X1	T37.2X2	T37.2X3	T37.2X4	T37.2X5	T37.2X6
Quinaglute	T46.2X1	T46.2X2	T46.2X3	T46.2X4	T46.2X5	T46.2X6
Quinalbarbital	T42.3X1	T42.3X2	T42.3X3	T42.3X4	T42.3X5	T42.3X6
Quinalbarbitone sodium	T42.3X1	T42.3X2	T42.3X3	T42.3X4	T42.3X5	T42.3X6
Quinalphos	T60.0X1	T60.0X2	T60.0X3	T60.0X4	--	--
Quinapril	T46.4X1	T46.4X2	T46.4X3	T46.4X4	T46.4X5	T46.4X6
Quinestradiol	T38.5X1	T38.5X2	T38.5X3	T38.5X4	T38.5X5	T38.5X6
Quinestradol	T38.5X1	T38.5X2	T38.5X3	T38.5X4	T38.5X5	T38.5X6
Quinestrol	T38.5X1	T38.5X2	T38.5X3	T38.5X4	T38.5X5	T38.5X6
Quinethazone	T50.2X1	T50.2X2	T50.2X3	T50.2X4	T50.2X5	T50.2X6
Quingestanol	T38.4X1	T38.4X2	T38.4X3	T38.4X4	T38.4X5	T38.4X6
Quinidine	T46.2X1	T46.2X2	T46.2X3	T46.2X4	T46.2X5	T46.2X6
Quinine	T37.2X1	T37.2X2	T37.2X3	T37.2X4	T37.2X5	T37.2X6
Quiniobine	T37.8X1	T37.8X2	T37.8X3	T37.8X4	T37.8X5	T37.8X6
Quinisocaine	T49.1X1	T49.1X2	T49.1X3	T49.1X4	T49.1X5	T49.1X6
Quinocide	T37.2X1	T37.2X2	T37.2X3	T37.2X4	T37.2X5	T37.2X6
Quinoline (derivatives) NEC	T37.8X1	T37.8X2	T37.8X3	T37.8X4	T37.8X5	T37.8X6
Quinupramine	T43.011	T43.012	T43.013	T43.014	T43.015	T43.016
Quotane	T41.3X1	T41.3X2	T41.3X3	T41.3X4	T41.3X5	T41.3X6
Rabies						
- immune globulin (human)	T50.Z11	T50.Z12	T50.Z13	T50.Z14	T50.Z15	T50.Z16
- vaccine	T50.B91	T50.B92	T50.B93	T50.B94	T50.B95	T50.B96
Racemoramide	T40.2X1	T40.2X2	T40.2X3	T40.2X4	--	--
Racemorphan	T40.2X1	T40.2X2	T40.2X3	T40.2X4	T40.2X5	T40.2X6
Racepinefrin	T44.5X1	T44.5X2	T44.5X3	T44.5X4	T44.5X5	T44.5X6
Raclopride	T43.591	T43.592	T43.593	T43.594	T43.595	T43.596
Radiator alcohol	T51.1X1	T51.1X2	T51.1X3	T51.1X4	--	--
Radioactive drug NEC	T50.8X1	T50.8X2	T50.8X3	T50.8X4	T50.8X5	T50.8X6
Radio-opaque (drugs) (materials)	T50.8X1	T50.8X2	T50.8X3	T50.8X4	T50.8X5	T50.8X6
Ramifenazone	T39.2X1	T39.2X2	T39.2X3	T39.2X4	T39.2X5	T39.2X6
Ramipril	T46.4X1	T46.4X2	T46.4X3	T46.4X4	T46.4X5	T46.4X6
Ranitidine	T47.0X1	T47.0X2	T47.0X3	T47.0X4	T47.0X5	T47.0X6
Ranunculus	T62.2X1	T62.2X2	T62.2X3	T62.2X4	--	--
Rat poison NEC	T60.4X1	T60.4X2	T60.4X3	T60.4X4	--	--
Rattlesnake (venom)	T63.011	T63.012	T63.013	T63.014	--	--
Raubasine	T46.7X1	T46.7X2	T46.7X3	T46.7X4	T46.7X5	T46.7X6
Raudixin	T46.5X1	T46.5X2	T46.5X3	T46.5X4	T46.5X5	T46.5X6
Rautensin	T46.5X1	T46.5X2	T46.5X3	T46.5X4	T46.5X5	T46.5X6
Rautina	T46.5X1	T46.5X2	T46.5X3	T46.5X4	T46.5X5	T46.5X6
Rautotal	T46.5X1	T46.5X2	T46.5X3	T46.5X4	T46.5X5	T46.5X6
Rauwiloid	T46.5X1	T46.5X2	T46.5X3	T46.5X4	T46.5X5	T46.5X6
Rauwoldin	T46.5X1	T46.5X2	T46.5X3	T46.5X4	T46.5X5	T46.5X6

Substance	Poisoning, Accidental (unintentional)	Poisoning, Intentional Self-harm	Poisoning, Assault	Poisoning, Undetermined	Adverse effect	Underdosing
Rauwolfia (alkaloids)	T46.5X1	T46.5X2	T46.5X3	T46.5X4	T46.5X5	T46.5X6
Razoxane	T45.1X1	T45.1X2	T45.1X3	T45.1X4	T45.1X5	T45.1X6
Realgar	T57.0X1	T57.0X2	T57.0X3	T57.0X4	--	--
Recombinant (R) —see specific protein						
Red blood cells, packed	T45.8X1	T45.8X2	T45.8X3	T45.8X4	T45.8X5	T45.8X6
Red squill (scilliroside)	T60.4X1	T60.4X2	T60.4X3	T60.4X4	--	--
Reducing agent, industrial NEC	T65.891	T65.892	T65.893	T65.894	--	--
Refrigerant gas (chlorofluoro-carbon)	T53.5X1	T53.5X2	T53.5X3	T53.5X4	--	--
- not chlorofluoro-carbon	T59.891	T59.892	T59.893	T59.894	--	--
Regroton	T50.2X1	T50.2X2	T50.2X3	T50.2X4	T50.2X5	T50.2X6
Rehydration salts (oral)	T50.3X1	T50.3X2	T50.3X3	T50.3X4	T50.3X5	T50.3X6
Rela	T42.8X1	T42.8X2	T42.8X3	T42.8X4	T42.8X5	T42.8X6
Relaxant, muscle						
- anesthetic	T48.1X1	T48.1X2	T48.1X3	T48.1X4	T48.1X5	T48.1X6
- central nervous system	T42.8X1	T42.8X2	T42.8X3	T42.8X4	T42.8X5	T42.8X6
- skeletal NEC	T48.1X1	T48.1X2	T48.1X3	T48.1X4	T48.1X5	T48.1X6
- smooth NEC	T44.3X1	T44.3X2	T44.3X3	T44.3X4	T44.3X5	T44.3X6
Remoxipride	T43.591	T43.592	T43.593	T43.594	T43.595	T43.596
Renese	T50.2X1	T50.2X2	T50.2X3	T50.2X4	T50.2X5	T50.2X6
Renografin	T50.8X1	T50.8X2	T50.8X3	T50.8X4	T50.8X5	T50.8X6
Replacement solution	T50.3X1	T50.3X2	T50.3X3	T50.3X4	T50.3X5	T50.3X6
Reproterol	T48.6X1	T48.6X2	T48.6X3	T48.6X4	T48.6X5	T48.6X6
Rescinnamine	T46.5X1	T46.5X2	T46.5X3	T46.5X4	T46.5X5	T46.5X6
Reserpin (e)	T46.5X1	T46.5X2	T46.5X3	T46.5X4	T46.5X5	T46.5X6
Resorcin, resorcinol (nonmedicinal)	T65.891	T65.892	T65.893	T65.894	--	--
- medicinal	T49.4X1	T49.4X2	T49.4X3	T49.4X4	T49.4X5	T49.4X6
Respaire	T48.4X1	T48.4X2	T48.4X3	T48.4X4	T48.4X5	T48.4X6
Respiratory drug NEC	T48.901	T48.902	T48.903	T48.904	T48.905	T48.906
- antiasthmatic NEC	T48.6X1	T48.6X2	T48.6X3	T48.6X4	T48.6X5	T48.6X6
- anti-common-cold NEC	T48.5X1	T48.5X2	T48.5X3	T48.5X4	T48.5X5	T48.5X6
- expectorant NEC	T48.4X1	T48.4X2	T48.4X3	T48.4X4	T48.4X5	T48.4X6
- stimulant	T48.901	T48.902	T48.903	T48.904	T48.905	T48.906
Retinoic acid	T49.0X1	T49.0X2	T49.0X3	T49.0X4	T49.0X5	T49.0X6
Retinol	T45.2X1	T45.2X2	T45.2X3	T45.2X4	T45.2X5	T45.2X6
Rh (D) immune globulin (human)	T50.Z11	T50.Z12	T50.Z13	T50.Z14	T50.Z15	T50.Z16
Rhodine	T39.011	T39.012	T39.013	T39.014	T39.015	T39.016
RhoGAM	T50.Z11	T50.Z12	T50.Z13	T50.Z14	T50.Z15	T50.Z16
Rhubarb						
- dry extract	T47.2X1	T47.2X2	T47.2X3	T47.2X4	T47.2X5	T47.2X6
- tincture, compound	T47.2X1	T47.2X2	T47.2X3	T47.2X4	T47.2X5	T47.2X6
Ribavirin	T37.5X1	T37.5X2	T37.5X3	T37.5X4	T37.5X5	T37.5X6
Riboflavin	T45.2X1	T45.2X2	T45.2X3	T45.2X4	T45.2X5	T45.2X6
Ribostamycin	T36.5X1	T36.5X2	T36.5X3	T36.5X4	T36.5X5	T36.5X6
Ricin	T62.2X1	T62.2X2	T62.2X3	T62.2X4	--	--
Ricinus communis	T62.2X1	T62.2X2	T62.2X3	T62.2X4	--	--
Rickettsial vaccine NEC	T50.A91	T50.A92	T50.A93	T50.A94	T50.A95	T50.A96
Rifabutin	T36.6X1	T36.6X2	T36.6X3	T36.6X4	T36.6X5	T36.6X6
Rifamide	T36.6X1	T36.6X2	T36.6X3	T36.6X4	T36.6X5	T36.6X6
Rifampicin	T36.6X1	T36.6X2	T36.6X3	T36.6X4	T36.6X5	T36.6X6
- with isoniazid	T37.1X1	T37.1X2	T37.1X3	T37.1X4	T37.1X5	T37.1X6
Rifampin	T36.6X1	T36.6X2	T36.6X3	T36.6X4	T36.6X5	T36.6X6
Rifamycin	T36.6X1	T36.6X2	T36.6X3	T36.6X4	T36.6X5	T36.6X6
Rifaximin	T36.6X1	T36.6X2	T36.6X3	T36.6X4	T36.6X5	T36.6X6
Rimantadine	T37.5X1	T37.5X2	T37.5X3	T37.5X4	T37.5X5	T37.5X6
Rimazolium metilsulfate	T39.8X1	T39.8X2	T39.8X3	T39.8X4	T39.8X5	T39.8X6
Rimifon	T37.1X1	T37.1X2	T37.1X3	T37.1X4	T37.1X5	T37.1X6
Rimiterol	T48.6X1	T48.6X2	T48.6X3	T48.6X4	T48.6X5	T48.6X6
Ringer (lactate) solution	T50.3X1	T50.3X2	T50.3X3	T50.3X4	T50.3X5	T50.3X6

Substance	Poisoning, Accidental (unintentional)	Poisoning, Intentional Self-harm	Poisoning, Assault	Poisoning, Undetermined	Adverse effect	Underdosing
Ristocetin	T36.8X1	T36.8X2	T36.8X3	T36.8X4	T36.8X5	T36.8X6
Ritalin	T43.631	T43.632	T43.633	T43.634	T43.635	T43.636
Ritodrine	T44.5X1	T44.5X2	T44.5X3	T44.5X4	T44.5X5	T44.5X6
Roach killer—see Insecticide						
Rociverine	T44.3X1	T44.3X2	T44.3X3	T44.3X4	T44.3X5	T44.3X6
Rocky Mountain spotted fever vaccine	T50.A91	T50.A92	T50.A93	T50.A94	T50.A95	T50.A96
Rodenticide NEC	T60.4X1	T60.4X2	T60.4X3	T60.4X4	--	--
Rohypnol	T42.4X1	T42.4X2	T42.4X3	T42.4X4	T42.4X5	T42.4X6
Rokitamycin	T36.3X1	T36.3X2	T36.3X3	T36.3X4	T36.3X5	T36.3X6
Rolaids	T47.1X1	T47.1X2	T47.1X3	T47.1X4	T47.1X5	T47.1X6
Rolitetracycline	T36.4X1	T36.4X2	T36.4X3	T36.4X4	T36.4X5	T36.4X6
Romilar	T48.3X1	T48.3X2	T48.3X3	T48.3X4	T48.3X5	T48.3X6
Ronifibrate	T46.6X1	T46.6X2	T46.6X3	T46.6X4	T46.6X5	T46.6X6
Rosaprostol	T47.1X1	T47.1X2	T47.1X3	T47.1X4	T47.1X5	T47.1X6
Rose bengal sodium (131I)	T50.8X1	T50.8X2	T50.8X3	T50.8X4	T50.8X5	T50.8X6
Rose water ointment	T49.3X1	T49.3X2	T49.3X3	T49.3X4	T49.3X5	T49.3X6
Rosoxacin	T37.8X1	T37.8X2	T37.8X3	T37.8X4	T37.8X5	T37.8X6
Rotenone	T60.2X1	T60.2X2	T60.2X3	T60.2X4	--	--
Rotoxamine	T45.0X1	T45.0X2	T45.0X3	T45.0X4	T45.0X5	T45.0X6
Rough-on-rats	T60.4X1	T60.4X2	T60.4X3	T60.4X4	--	--
Roxatidine	T47.0X1	T47.0X2	T47.0X3	T47.0X4	T47.0X5	T47.0X6
Roxithromycin	T36.3X1	T36.3X2	T36.3X3	T36.3X4	T36.3X5	T36.3X6
Rt-PA	T45.611	T45.612	T45.613	T45.614	T45.615	T45.616
Rubbing alcohol	T51.2X1	T51.2X2	T51.2X3	T51.2X4	--	--
Rubefacient	T49.4X1	T49.4X2	T49.4X3	T49.4X4	T49.4X5	T49.4X6
Rubella vaccine	T50.B91	T50.B92	T50.B93	T50.B94	T50.B95	T50.B96
Rubeola vaccine	T50.B91	T50.B92	T50.B93	T50.B94	T50.B95	T50.B96
Rubidium chloride Rb82	T50.8X1	T50.8X2	T50.8X3	T50.8X4	T50.8X5	T50.8X6
Rubidomycin	T45.1X1	T45.1X2	T45.1X3	T45.1X4	T45.1X5	T45.1X6
Rue	T62.2X1	T62.2X2	T62.2X3	T62.2X4	--	--
Rufocromomycin	T45.1X1	T45.1X2	T45.1X3	T45.1X4	T45.1X5	T45.1X6
Russel's viper venin	T45.7X1	T45.7X2	T45.7X3	T45.7X4	T45.7X5	T45.7X6
Ruta (graveolens)	T62.2X1	T62.2X2	T62.2X3	T62.2X4	--	--
Rutinum	T46.991	T46.992	T46.993	T46.994	T46.995	T46.996
Rutoside	T46.991	T46.992	T46.993	T46.994	T46.995	T46.996
Sabadilla (plant)	T62.2X1	T62.2X2	T62.2X3	T62.2X4	--	--
- pesticide	T60.2X1	T60.2X2	T60.2X3	T60.2X4	--	--
Saccharated iron oxide	T45.8X1	T45.8X2	T45.8X3	T45.8X4	T45.8X5	T45.8X6
Saccharin	T50.901	T50.902	T50.903	T50.904	T50.905	T50.906
Saccharomyces boulardii	T47.6X1	T47.6X2	T47.6X3	T47.6X4	T47.6X5	T47.6X6
Safflower oil	T46.6X1	T46.6X2	T46.6X3	T46.6X4	T46.6X5	T46.6X6
Safrazine	T43.1X1	T43.1X2	T43.1X3	T43.1X4	T43.1X5	T43.1X6
Salazosulfapyridine	T37.0X1	T37.0X2	T37.0X3	T37.0X4	T37.0X5	T37.0X6
Salbutamol	T48.6X1	T48.6X2	T48.6X3	T48.6X4	T48.6X5	T48.6X6
Salicylamide	T39.091	T39.092	T39.093	T39.094	T39.095	T39.096
Salicylate NEC	T39.091	T39.092	T39.093	T39.094	T39.095	T39.096
- methyl	T49.3X1	T49.3X2	T49.3X3	T49.3X4	T49.3X5	T49.3X6
- theobromine calcium	T50.2X1	T50.2X2	T50.2X3	T50.2X4	T50.2X5	T50.2X6
Salicylazosulfapyridine	T37.0X1	T37.0X2	T37.0X3	T37.0X4	T37.0X5	T37.0X6
Salicylhydroxamic acid	T49.0X1	T49.0X2	T49.0X3	T49.0X4	T49.0X5	T49.0X6
Salicylic acid	T49.4X1	T49.4X2	T49.4X3	T49.4X4	T49.4X5	T49.4X6
- with benzoic acid	T49.4X1	T49.4X2	T49.4X3	T49.4X4	T49.4X5	T49.4X6
- congeners	T39.091	T39.092	T39.093	T39.094	T39.095	T39.096
- derivative	T39.091	T39.092	T39.093	T39.094	T39.095	T39.096
- salts	T39.091	T39.092	T39.093	T39.094	T39.095	T39.096
Salinazid	T37.1X1	T37.1X2	T37.1X3	T37.1X4	T37.1X5	T37.1X6
Salmeterol	T48.6X1	T48.6X2	T48.6X3	T48.6X4	T48.6X5	T48.6X6
Salol	T49.3X1	T49.3X2	T49.3X3	T49.3X4	T49.3X5	T49.3X6
Salsalate	T39.091	T39.092	T39.093	T39.094	T39.095	T39.096

Substance	Poisoning, Accidental (unintentional)	Poisoning, Intentional Self-harm	Poisoning, Assault	Poisoning, Undetermined	Adverse effect	Underdosing
Salt substitute	T50.901	T50.902	T50.903	T50.904	T50.905	T50.906
Salt-replacing drug	T50.901	T50.902	T50.903	T50.904	T50.905	T50.906
Salt-retaining mineralocorticoid	T50.0X1	T50.0X2	T50.0X3	T50.0X4	T50.0X5	T50.0X6
Saluretic NEC	T50.2X1	T50.2X2	T50.2X3	T50.2X4	T50.2X5	T50.2X6
Saluron	T50.2X1	T50.2X2	T50.2X3	T50.2X4	T50.2X5	T50.2X6
Salvarsan 606 (neosilver) (silver)	T37.8X1	T37.8X2	T37.8X3	T37.8X4	T37.8X5	T37.8X6
Sambucus canadensis	T62.2X1	T62.2X2	T62.2X3	T62.2X4	--	--
- berry	T62.1X1	T62.1X2	T62.1X3	T62.1X4	--	--
Sandril	T46.5X1	T46.5X2	T46.5X3	T46.5X4	T46.5X5	T46.5X6
Sanguinaria canadensis	T62.2X1	T62.2X2	T62.2X3	T62.2X4	--	--
Saniflush (cleaner)	T54.2X1	T54.2X2	T54.2X3	T54.2X4	--	--
Santonin	T37.4X1	T37.4X2	T37.4X3	T37.4X4	T37.4X5	T37.4X6
Santyl	T49.8X1	T49.8X2	T49.8X3	T49.8X4	T49.8X5	T49.8X6
Saralasin	T46.5X1	T46.5X2	T46.5X3	T46.5X4	T46.5X5	T46.5X6
Sarcolysin	T45.1X1	T45.1X2	T45.1X3	T45.1X4	T45.1X5	T45.1X6
Sarkomycin	T45.1X1	T45.1X2	T45.1X3	T45.1X4	T45.1X5	T45.1X6
Saroten	T43.011	T43.012	T43.013	T43.014	T43.015	T43.016
Saturnine—see Lead						
Savin (oil)	T49.4X1	T49.4X2	T49.4X3	T49.4X4	T49.4X5	T49.4X6
Scammony	T47.2X1	T47.2X2	T47.2X3	T47.2X4	T47.2X5	T47.2X6
Scarlet red	T49.8X1	T49.8X2	T49.8X3	T49.8X4	T49.8X5	T49.8X6
Scheele's green	T57.0X1	T57.0X2	T57.0X3	T57.0X4	--	--
- insecticide	T57.0X1	T57.0X2	T57.0X3	T57.0X4	--	--
Schizontozide (blood) (tissue)	T37.2X1	T37.2X2	T37.2X3	T37.2X4	T37.2X5	T37.2X6
Schradan	T60.0X1	T60.0X2	T60.0X3	T60.0X4	--	--
Schweinfurth green	T57.0X1	T57.0X2	T57.0X3	T57.0X4	--	--
- insecticide	T57.0X1	T57.0X2	T57.0X3	T57.0X4	--	--
Scilla, rat poison	T60.4X1	T60.4X2	T60.4X3	T60.4X4		
Scillaren	T60.4X1	T60.4X2	T60.4X3	T60.4X4	--	--
Sclerosing agent	T46.8X1	T46.8X2	T46.8X3	T46.8X4	T46.8X5	T46.8X6
Scombrotoxin	T61.11	T61.12	T61.13	T61.14	--	--
Scopolamine	T44.3X1	T44.3X2	T44.3X3	T44.3X4	T44.3X5	T44.3X6
Scopolia extract	T44.3X1	T44.3X2	T44.3X3	T44.3X4	T44.3X5	T44.3X6
Scouring powder	T65.891	T65.892	T65.893	T65.894	--	--
Sea						
- anemone (sting)	T63.631	T63.632	T63.633	T63.634	--	--
- cucumber (sting)	T63.691	T63.692	T63.693	T63.694	--	--
- snake (bite) (venom)	T63.091	T63.092	T63.093	T63.094	--	--
- urchin spine (puncture)	T63.691	T63.692	T63.693	T63.694	--	--
Seafood	T61.91	T61.92	T61.93	T61.94	--	--
- specified NEC	T61.8X1	T61.8X2	T61.8X3	T61.8X4	--	--
Secbutabarbital	T42.3X1	T42.3X2	T42.3X3	T42.3X4	T42.3X5	T42.3X6
Secbutabarbitone	T42.3X1	T42.3X2	T42.3X3	T42.3X4	T42.3X5	T42.3X6
Secnidazole	T37.3X1	T37.3X2	T37.3X3	T37.3X4	T37.3X5	T37.3X6
Secobarbital	T42.3X1	T42.3X2	T42.3X3	T42.3X4	T42.3X5	T42.3X6
Seconal	T42.3X1	T42.3X2	T42.3X3	T42.3X4	T42.3X5	T42.3X6
Secretin	T50.8X1	T50.8X2	T50.8X3	T50.8X4	T50.8X5	T50.8X6
Sedative NEC	T42.71	T42.72	T42.73	T42.74	T42.75	T42.76
- mixed NEC	T42.6X1	T42.6X2	T42.6X3	T42.6X4	T42.6X5	T42.6X6
Sedormid	T42.6X1	T42.6X2	T42.6X3	T42.6X4	T42.6X5	T42.6X6
Seed disinfectant or dressing	T60.8X1	T60.8X2	T60.8X3	T60.8X4	--	--
Seeds (poisonous)	T62.2X1	T62.2X2	T62.2X3	T62.2X4	--	--
Selegiline	T42.8X1	T42.8X2	T42.8X3	T42.8X4	T42.8X5	T42.8X6
Selenium NEC	T56.891	T56.892	T56.893	T56.894	--	--
- disulfide or sulfide	T49.4X1	T49.4X2	T49.4X3	T49.4X4	T49.4X5	T49.4X6
- fumes	T59.891	T59.892	T59.893	T59.894	--	--
- sulfide	T49.4X1	T49.4X2	T49.4X3	T49.4X4	T49.4X5	T49.4X6
Selenomethionine (75Se)	T50.8X1	T50.8X2	T50.8X3	T50.8X4	T50.8X5	T50.8X6

Substance	Poisoning, Accidental (unintentional)	Poisoning, Intentional Self-harm	Poisoning, Assault	Poisoning, Undetermined	Adverse effect	Underdosing
Selsun	T49.4X1	T49.4X2	T49.4X3	T49.4X4	T49.4X5	T49.4X6
Semustine	T45.1X1	T45.1X2	T45.1X3	T45.1X4	T45.1X5	T45.1X6
Senega syrup	T48.4X1	T48.4X2	T48.4X3	T48.4X4	T48.4X5	T48.4X6
Senna	T47.2X1	T47.2X2	T47.2X3	T47.2X4	T47.2X5	T47.2X6
Sennoside A+B	T47.2X1	T47.2X2	T47.2X3	T47.2X4	T47.2X5	T47.2X6
Septisol	T49.2X1	T49.2X2	T49.2X3	T49.2X4	T49.2X5	T49.2X6
Seractide	T38.811	T38.812	T38.813	T38.814	T38.815	T38.816
Serax	T42.4X1	T42.4X2	T42.4X3	T42.4X4	T42.4X5	T42.4X6
Serenesil	T42.6X1	T42.6X2	T42.6X3	T42.6X4	T42.6X5	T42.6X6
Serenium (hydrochloride)	T37.91	T37.92	T37.93	T37.94	T37.95	T37.96
Serepax—see Oxazepam						
Sermorelin	T38.891	T38.892	T38.893	T38.894	T38.895	T38.896
Sernyl	T41.1X1	T41.1X2	T41.1X3	T41.1X4	T41.1X5	T41.1X6
Serotonin	T50.991	T50.992	T50.993	T50.994	T50.995	T50.996
Serpasil	T46.5X1	T46.5X2	T46.5X3	T46.5X4	T46.5X5	T46.5X6
Serrapeptase	T45.3X1	T45.3X2	T45.3X3	T45.3X4	T45.3X5	T45.3X6
Serum						
- antibotulinus	T50.Z11	T50.Z12	T50.Z13	T50.Z14	T50.Z15	T50.Z16
- anticytotoxic	T50.Z11	T50.Z12	T50.Z13	T50.Z14	T50.Z15	T50.Z16
- antidiphtheria	T50.Z11	T50.Z12	T50.Z13	T50.Z14	T50.Z15	T50.Z16
- antimeningococcus	T50.Z11	T50.Z12	T50.Z13	T50.Z14	T50.Z15	T50.Z16
- anti-Rh	T50.Z11	T50.Z12	T50.Z13	T50.Z14	T50.Z15	T50.Z16
- anti-snake-bite	T50.Z11	T50.Z12	T50.Z13	T50.Z14	T50.Z15	T50.Z16
- antitetanic	T50.Z11	T50.Z12	T50.Z13	T50.Z14	T50.Z15	T50.Z16
- antitoxic	T50.Z11	T50.Z12	T50.Z13	T50.Z14	T50.Z15	T50.Z16
- complement (inhibitor)	T45.8X1	T45.8X2	T45.8X3	T45.8X4	T45.8X5	T45.8X6
- convalescent	T50.Z11	T50.Z12	T50.Z13	T50.Z14	T50.Z15	T50.Z16
- hemolytic complement	T45.8X1	T45.8X2	T45.8X3	T45.8X4	T45.8X5	T45.8X6
- immune (human)	T50.Z11	T50.Z12	T50.Z13	T50.Z14	T50.Z15	T50.Z16
- protective NEC	T50.Z11	T50.Z12	T50.Z13	T50.Z14	T50.Z15	T50.Z16
Setastine	T45.0X1	T45.0X2	T45.0X3	T45.0X4	T45.0X5	T45.0X6
Setoperone	T43.591	T43.592	T43.593	T43.594	T43.595	T43.596
Sewer gas	T59.91	T59.92	T59.93	T59.94	--	--
Shampoo	T55.0X1	T55.0X2	T55.0X3	T55.0X4	--	--
Shellfish, noxious, nonbacterial	T61.781	T61.782	T61.783	T61.784	--	--
Sildenafil	T46.7X1	T46.7X2	T46.7X3	T46.7X4	T46.7X5	T46.7X6
Silibinin	T50.991	T50.992	T50.993	T50.994	T50.995	T50.996
Silicone NEC	T65.891	T65.892	T65.893	T65.894	--	--
- medicinal	T49.3X1	T49.3X2	T49.3X3	T49.3X4	T49.3X5	T49.3X6
Silvadene	T49.0X1	T49.0X2	T49.0X3	T49.0X4	T49.0X5	T49.0X6
Silver	T49.0X1	T49.0X2	T49.0X3	T49.0X4	T49.0X5	T49.0X6
- anti-infectives	T49.0X1	T49.0X2	T49.0X3	T49.0X4	T49.0X5	T49.0X6
- arsphenamine	T37.8X1	T37.8X2	T37.8X3	T37.8X4	T37.8X5	T37.8X6
- colloidal	T49.0X1	T49.0X2	T49.0X3	T49.0X4	T49.0X5	T49.0X6
- nitrate	T49.0X1	T49.0X2	T49.0X3	T49.0X4	T49.0X5	T49.0X6
- - ophthalmic preparation	T49.5X1	T49.5X2	T49.5X3	T49.5X4	T49.5X5	T49.5X6
- - toughened (keratolytic)	T49.4X1	T49.4X2	T49.4X3	T49.4X4	T49.4X5	T49.4X6
- nonmedicinal (dust)	T56.891	T56.892	T56.893	T56.894	--	--
- protein	T49.5X1	T49.5X2	T49.5X3	T49.5X4	T49.5X5	T49.5X6
- salvarsan	T37.8X1	T37.8X2	T37.8X3	T37.8X4	T37.8X5	T37.8X6
- sulfadiazine	T49.4X1	T49.4X2	T49.4X3	T49.4X4	T49.4X5	T49.4X6
Silymarin	T50.991	T50.992	T50.993	T50.994	T50.995	T50.996
Simaldrate	T47.1X1	T47.1X2	T47.1X3	T47.1X4	T47.1X5	T47.1X6
Simazine	T60.3X1	T60.3X2	T60.3X3	T60.3X4	--	--
Simethicone	T47.1X1	T47.1X2	T47.1X3	T47.1X4	T47.1X5	T47.1X6
Simfibrate	T46.6X1	T46.6X2	T46.6X3	T46.6X4	T46.6X5	T46.6X6
Simvastatin	T46.6X1	T46.6X2	T46.6X3	T46.6X4	T46.6X5	T46.6X6
Sincalide	T50.8X1	T50.8X2	T50.8X3	T50.8X4	T50.8X5	T50.8X6
Sinequan	T43.011	T43.012	T43.013	T43.014	T43.015	T43.016

Substance	Poisoning, Accidental (unintentional)	Poisoning, Intentional Self-harm	Poisoning, Assault	Poisoning, Undetermined	Adverse effect	Underdosing
Singoserp	T46.5X1	T46.5X2	T46.5X3	T46.5X4	T46.5X5	T46.5X6
Sintrom	T45.511	T45.512	T45.513	T45.514	T45.515	T45.516
Sisomicin	T36.5X1	T36.5X2	T36.5X3	T36.5X4	T36.5X5	T36.5X6
Sitosterols	T46.6X1	T46.6X2	T46.6X3	T46.6X4	T46.6X5	T46.6X6
Skeletal muscle relaxants	T48.1X1	T48.1X2	T48.1X3	T48.1X4	T48.1X5	T48.1X6
Skin						
- agents (external)	T49.91	T49.92	T49.93	T49.94	T49.95	T49.96
- - specified NEC	T49.8X1	T49.8X2	T49.8X3	T49.8X4	T49.8X5	T49.8X6
- test antigen	T50.8X1	T50.8X2	T50.8X3	T50.8X4	T50.8X5	T50.8X6
Sleep-eze	T45.0X1	T45.0X2	T45.0X3	T45.0X4	T45.0X5	T45.0X6
Sleeping draught, pill	T42.71	T42.72	T42.73	T42.74	T42.75	T42.76
Smallpox vaccine	T50.B11	T50.B12	T50.B13	T50.B14	T50.B15	T50.B16
Smelter fumes NEC	T56.91	T56.92	T56.93	T56.94	--	--
Smog	T59.1X1	T59.1X2	T59.1X3	T59.1X4	--	--
Smoke NEC	T59.811	T59.812	T59.813	T59.814	--	--
Smooth muscle relaxant	T44.3X1	T44.3X2	T44.3X3	T44.3X4	T44.3X5	T44.3X6
Snail killer NEC	T60.8X1	T60.8X2	T60.8X3	T60.8X4	--	--
Snake venom or bite	T63.001	T63.002	T63.003	T63.004	--	--
- hemocoagulase	T45.7X1	T45.7X2	T45.7X3	T45.7X4	T45.7X5	T45.7X6
Snuff	T65.211	T65.212	T65.213	T65.214	--	--
Soap (powder) (product)	T55.0X1	T55.0X2	T55.0X3	T55.0X4	--	--
- enema	T47.4X1	T47.4X2	T47.4X3	T47.4X4	T47.4X5	T47.4X6
- medicinal, soft	T49.2X1	T49.2X2	T49.2X3	T49.2X4	T49.2X5	T49.2X6
- superfatted	T49.2X1	T49.2X2	T49.2X3	T49.2X4	T49.2X5	T49.2X6
Sobrerol	T48.4X1	T48.4X2	T48.4X3	T48.4X4	T48.4X5	T48.4X6
Soda (caustic)	T54.3X1	T54.3X2	T54.3X3	T54.3X4	--	--
- bicarb	T47.1X1	T47.1X2	T47.1X3	T47.1X4	T47.1X5	T47.1X6
- chlorinated—see Sodium, hypochlorite						
Sodium						
- acetosulfone	T37.1X1	T37.1X2	T37.1X3	T37.1X4	T37.1X5	T37.1X6
- acetrizoate	T50.8X1	T50.8X2	T50.8X3	T50.8X4	T50.8X5	T50.8X6
- acid phosphate	T50.3X1	T50.3X2	T50.3X3	T50.3X4	T50.3X5	T50.3X6
- alginate	T47.8X1	T47.8X2	T47.8X3	T47.8X4	T47.8X5	T47.8X6
- amidotrizoate	T50.8X1	T50.8X2	T50.8X3	T50.8X4	T50.8X5	T50.8X6
- aminopterin	T45.1X1	T45.1X2	T45.1X3	T45.1X4	T45.1X5	T45.1X6
- amylosulfate	T47.8X1	T47.8X2	T47.8X3	T47.8X4	T47.8X5	T47.8X6
- amytal	T42.3X1	T42.3X2	T42.3X3	T42.3X4	T42.3X5	T42.3X6
- antimony gluconate	T37.3X1	T37.3X2	T37.3X3	T37.3X4	T37.3X5	T37.3X6
- arsenate	T57.0X1	T57.0X2	T57.0X3	T57.0X4	--	--
- aurothiomalate	T39.4X1	T39.4X2	T39.4X3	T39.4X4	T39.4X5	T39.4X6
- aurothiosulfate	T39.4X1	T39.4X2	T39.4X3	T39.4X4	T39.4X5	T39.4X6
- barbiturate	T42.3X1	T42.3X2	T42.3X3	T42.3X4	T42.3X5	T42.3X6
- basic phosphate	T47.4X1	T47.4X2	T47.4X3	T47.4X4	T47.4X5	T47.4X6
- bicarbonate	T47.1X1	T47.1X2	T47.1X3	T47.1X4	T47.1X5	T47.1X6
- bichromate	T57.8X1	T57.8X2	T57.8X3	T57.8X4	--	--
- biphosphate	T50.3X1	T50.3X2	T50.3X3	T50.3X4	T50.3X5	T50.3X6
- bisulfate	T65.891	T65.892	T65.893	T65.894	--	--
- borate						
- - cleanser	T57.8X1	T57.8X2	T57.8X3	T57.8X4	--	--
- - - eye	T49.5X1	T49.5X2	T49.5X3	T49.5X4	T49.5X5	T49.5X6
- - therapeutic	T49.8X1	T49.8X2	T49.8X3	T49.8X4	T49.8X5	T49.8X6
- bromide	T42.6X1	T42.6X2	T42.6X3	T42.6X4	T42.6X5	T42.6X6
- cacodylate (nonmedicinal) NEC	T50.8X1	T50.8X2	T50.8X3	T50.8X4	T50.8X5	T50.8X6
- - anti-infective	T37.8X1	T37.8X2	T37.8X3	T37.8X4	T37.8X5	T37.8X6
- - herbicide	T60.3X1	T60.3X2	T60.3X3	T60.3X4	--	--
- calcium edetate	T45.8X1	T45.8X2	T45.8X3	T45.8X4	T45.8X5	T45.8X6
- carbonate NEC	T54.3X1	T54.3X2	T54.3X3	T54.3X4	--	--
- chlorate NEC	T65.891	T65.892	T65.893	T65.894	--	--

Substance	Poisoning, Accidental (unintentional)	Poisoning, Intentional Self-harm	Poisoning, Assault	Poisoning, Undetermined	Adverse effect	Underdosing
- - herbicide	T54.91	T54.92	T54.93	T54.94	--	--
- chloride	T50.3X1	T50.3X2	T50.3X3	T50.3X4	T50.3X5	T50.3X6
- - with glucose	T50.3X1	T50.3X2	T50.3X3	T50.3X4	T50.3X5	T50.3X6
- chromate	T65.891	T65.892	T65.893	T65.894	--	--
- citrate	T50.991	T50.992	T50.993	T50.994	T50.995	T50.996
- cromoglicate	T48.6X1	T48.6X2	T48.6X3	T48.6X4	T48.6X5	T48.6X6
- cyanide	T65.0X1	T65.0X2	T65.0X3	T65.0X4	--	--
- cyclamate	T50.3X1	T50.3X2	T50.3X3	T50.3X4	T50.3X5	T50.3X6
- dehydrocholate	T45.8X1	T45.8X2	T45.8X3	T45.8X4	T45.8X5	T45.8X6
- diatrizoate	T50.8X1	T50.8X2	T50.8X3	T50.8X4	T50.8X5	T50.8X6
- dibunate	T48.4X1	T48.4X2	T48.4X3	T48.4X4	T48.4X5	T48.4X6
- dioctyl sulfosuccinate	T47.4X1	T47.4X2	T47.4X3	T47.4X4	T47.4X5	T47.4X6
- dipantoyl ferrate	T45.8X1	T45.8X2	T45.8X3	T45.8X4	T45.8X5	T45.8X6
- edetate	T45.8X1	T45.8X2	T45.8X3	T45.8X4	T45.8X5	T45.8X6
- ethacrynate	T50.1X1	T50.1X2	T50.1X3	T50.1X4	T50.1X5	T50.1X6
- feredetate	T45.8X1	T45.8X2	T45.8X3	T45.8X4	T45.8X5	T45.8X6
- Fluoride—see Fluoride						
- fluoroacetate (dust) (pesticide)	T60.4X1	T60.4X2	T60.4X3	T60.4X4	--	--
- free salt	T50.3X1	T50.3X2	T50.3X3	T50.3X4	T50.3X5	T50.3X6
- fusidate	T36.8X1	T36.8X2	T36.8X3	T36.8X4	T36.8X5	T36.8X6
- glucaldrate	T47.1X1	T47.1X2	T47.1X3	T47.1X4	T47.1X5	T47.1X6
- glucosulfone	T37.1X1	T37.1X2	T37.1X3	T37.1X4	T37.1X5	T37.1X6
- glutamate	T45.8X1	T45.8X2	T45.8X3	T45.8X4	T45.8X5	T45.8X6
- hydrogen carbonate	T50.3X1	T50.3X2	T50.3X3	T50.3X4	T50.3X5	T50.3X6
- hydroxide	T54.3X1	T54.3X2	T54.3X3	T54.3X4	--	--
- hypochlorite (bleach) NEC	T54.3X1	T54.3X2	T54.3X3	T54.3X4	--	--
- - disinfectant	T54.3X1	T54.3X2	T54.3X3	T54.3X4	--	--
- - medicinal (anti-infective) (external)	T49.0X1	T49.0X2	T49.0X3	T49.0X4	T49.0X5	T49.0X6
- - vapor	T54.3X1	T54.3X2	T54.3X3	T54.3X4	--	--
- hyposulfite	T49.0X1	T49.0X2	T49.0X3	T49.0X4	T49.0X5	T49.0X6
- indigotin disulfonate	T50.8X1	T50.8X2	T50.8X3	T50.8X4	T50.8X5	T50.8X6
- iodide	T50.991	T50.992	T50.993	T50.994	T50.995	T50.996
- - I-131	T50.8X1	T50.8X2	T50.8X3	T50.8X4	T50.8X5	T50.8X6
- - - therapeutic	T38.2X1	T38.2X2	T38.2X3	T38.2X4	T38.2X5	T38.2X6
- iodohippurate (131I)	T50.8X1	T50.8X2	T50.8X3	T50.8X4	T50.8X5	T50.8X6
- iopodate	T50.8X1	T50.8X2	T50.8X3	T50.8X4	T50.8X5	T50.8X6
- iothalamate	T50.8X1	T50.8X2	T50.8X3	T50.8X4	T50.8X5	T50.8X6
- iron edetate	T45.4X1	T45.4X2	T45.4X3	T45.4X4	T45.4X5	T45.4X6
- lactate (compound solution)	T45.8X1	T45.8X2	T45.8X3	T45.8X4	T45.8X5	T45.8X6
- lauryl (sulfate)	T49.2X1	T49.2X2	T49.2X3	T49.2X4	T49.2X5	T49.2X6
- L-triiodothyronine	T38.1X1	T38.1X2	T38.1X3	T38.1X4	T38.1X5	T38.1X6
- magnesium citrate	T50.991	T50.992	T50.993	T50.994	T50.995	T50.996
- mersalate	T50.2X1	T50.2X2	T50.2X3	T50.2X4	T50.2X5	T50.2X6
- metasilicate	T65.891	T65.892	T65.893	T65.894	--	--
- metrizoate	T50.8X1	T50.8X2	T50.8X3	T50.8X4	T50.8X5	T50.8X6
- monofluoroacetate (pesticide)	T60.1X1	T60.1X2	T60.1X3	T60.1X4	--	--
- morrhuate	T46.8X1	T46.8X2	T46.8X3	T46.8X4	T46.8X5	T46.8X6
- nafcillin	T36.0X1	T36.0X2	T36.0X3	T36.0X4	T36.0X5	T36.0X6
- nitrate (oxidizing agent)	T65.891	T65.892	T65.893	T65.894	--	--
- nitrite	T50.6X1	T50.6X2	T50.6X3	T50.6X4	T50.6X5	T50.6X6
- nitroferricyanide	T46.5X1	T46.5X2	T46.5X3	T46.5X4	T46.5X5	T46.5X6
- nitroprusside	T46.5X1	T46.5X2	T46.5X3	T46.5X4	T46.5X5	T46.5X6
- oxalate	T65.891	T65.892	T65.893	T65.894	--	--
- oxide/peroxide	T65.891	T65.892	T65.893	T65.894	--	--
- oxybate	T41.291	T41.292	T41.293	T41.294	T41.295	T41.296
- para-aminohippurate	T50.8X1	T50.8X2	T50.8X3	T50.8X4	T50.8X5	T50.8X6
- perborate (nonmedicinal) NEC	T65.891	T65.892	T65.893	T65.894	--	--
- - medicinal	T49.0X1	T49.0X2	T49.0X3	T49.0X4	T49.0X5	T49.0X6
- - soap	T55.0X1	T55.0X2	T55.0X3	T55.0X4	--	--

Substance	Poisoning, Accidental (unintentional)	Poisoning, Intentional Self-harm	Poisoning, Assault	Poisoning, Undetermined	Adverse effect	Underdosing
- percarbonate—see Sodium, perborate						
- pertechnetate Tc99m	T50.8X1	T50.8X2	T50.8X3	T50.8X4	T50.8X5	T50.8X6
- phosphate						
- - cellulose	T45.8X1	T45.8X2	T45.8X3	T45.8X4	T45.8X5	T45.8X6
- - dibasic	T47.2X1	T47.2X2	T47.2X3	T47.2X4	T47.2X5	T47.2X6
- - monobasic	T47.2X1	T47.2X2	T47.2X3	T47.2X4	T47.2X5	T47.2X6
- phytate	T50.6X1	T50.6X2	T50.6X3	T50.6X4	T50.6X5	T50.6X6
- picosulfate	T47.2X1	T47.2X2	T47.2X3	T47.2X4	T47.2X5	T47.2X6
- polyhydroxyaluminium monocarbonate	T47.1X1	T47.1X2	T47.1X3	T47.1X4	T47.1X5	T47.1X6
- polystyrene sulfonate	T50.3X1	T50.3X2	T50.3X3	T50.3X4	T50.3X5	T50.3X6
- propionate	T49.0X1	T49.0X2	T49.0X3	T49.0X4	T49.0X5	T49.0X6
- propyl hydroxybenzoate	T50.991	T50.992	T50.993	T50.994	T50.995	T50.996
- psylliate	T46.8X1	T46.8X2	T46.8X3	T46.8X4	T46.8X5	T46.8X6
- removing resins	T50.3X1	T50.3X2	T50.3X3	T50.3X4	T50.3X5	T50.3X6
- salicylate	T39.091	T39.092	T39.093	T39.094	T39.095	T39.096
- salt NEC	T50.3X1	T50.3X2	T50.3X3	T50.3X4	T50.3X5	T50.3X6
- selenate	T60.2X1	T60.2X2	T60.2X3	T60.2X4	--	--
- stibogluconate	T37.3X1	T37.3X2	T37.3X3	T37.3X4	T37.3X5	T37.3X6
- sulfate	T47.4X1	T47.4X2	T47.4X3	T47.4X4	T47.4X5	T47.4X6
- sulfoxone	T37.1X1	T37.1X2	T37.1X3	T37.1X4	T37.1X5	T37.1X6
- tetradecyl sulfate	T46.8X1	T46.8X2	T46.8X3	T46.8X4	T46.8X5	T46.8X6
- thiopental	T41.1X1	T41.1X2	T41.1X3	T41.1X4	T41.1X5	T41.1X6
- thiosalicylate	T39.091	T39.092	T39.093	T39.094	T39.095	T39.096
- thiosulfate	T50.6X1	T50.6X2	T50.6X3	T50.6X4	T50.6X5	T50.6X6
- tolbutamide	T38.3X1	T38.3X2	T38.3X3	T38.3X4	T38.3X5	T38.3X6
- (L) -triiodothyronine	T38.1X1	T38.1X2	T38.1X3	T38.1X4	T38.1X5	T38.1X6
- tyropanoate	T50.8X1	T50.8X2	T50.8X3	T50.8X4	T50.8X5	T50.8X6
- valproate	T42.6X1	T42.6X2	T42.6X3	T42.6X4	T42.6X5	T42.6X6
- versenate	T50.6X1	T50.6X2	T50.6X3	T50.6X4	T50.6X5	T50.6X6
Sodium-free salt	T50.901	T50.902	T50.903	T50.904	T50.905	T50.906
Sodium-removing resin	T50.3X1	T50.3X2	T50.3X3	T50.3X4	T50.3X5	T50.3X6
Soft soap	T55.0X1	T55.0X2	T55.0X3	T55.0X4	--	--
Solanine	T62.2X1	T62.2X2	T62.2X3	T62.2X4	--	--
- berries	T62.1X1	T62.1X2	T62.1X3	T62.1X4	--	--
Solanum dulcamara	T62.2X1	T62.2X2	T62.2X3	T62.2X4	--	--
- berries	T62.1X1	T62.1X2	T62.1X3	T62.1X4	--	--
Solapsone	T37.1X1	T37.1X2	T37.1X3	T37.1X4	T37.1X5	T37.1X6
Solar lotion	T49.3X1	T49.3X2	T49.3X3	T49.3X4	T49.3X5	T49.3X6
Solasulfone	T37.1X1	T37.1X2	T37.1X3	T37.1X4	T37.1X5	T37.1X6
Soldering fluid	T65.891	T65.892	T65.893	T65.894	--	--
Solid substance	T65.91	T65.92	T65.93	T65.94	--	--
- specified NEC	T65.891	T65.892	T65.893	T65.894	--	--
Solvent, industrial NEC	T52.91	T52.92	T52.93	T52.94	--	--
- naphtha	T52.0X1	T52.0X2	T52.0X3	T52.0X4	--	--
- petroleum	T52.0X1	T52.0X2	T52.0X3	T52.0X4	--	--
- specified NEC	T52.8X1	T52.8X2	T52.8X3	T52.8X4	--	--
Soma	T42.8X1	T42.8X2	T42.8X3	T42.8X4	T42.8X5	T42.8X6
Somatorelin	T38.891	T38.892	T38.893	T38.894	T38.895	T38.896
Somatostatin	T38.991	T38.992	T38.993	T38.994	T38.995	T38.996
Somatotropin	T38.811	T38.812	T38.813	T38.814	T38.815	T38.816
Somatrem	T38.811	T38.812	T38.813	T38.814	T38.815	T38.816
Somatropin	T38.811	T38.812	T38.813	T38.814	T38.815	T38.816
Sominex	T45.0X1	T45.0X2	T45.0X3	T45.0X4	T45.0X5	T45.0X6
Somnos	T42.6X1	T42.6X2	T42.6X3	T42.6X4	T42.6X5	T42.6X6
Somonal	T42.3X1	T42.3X2	T42.3X3	T42.3X4	T42.3X5	T42.3X6
Soneryl	T42.3X1	T42.3X2	T42.3X3	T42.3X4	T42.3X5	T42.3X6
Soothing syrup	T50.901	T50.902	T50.903	T50.904	T50.905	T50.906
Sopor	T42.6X1	T42.6X2	T42.6X3	T42.6X4	T42.6X5	T42.6X6

Substance	Poisoning, Accidental (unintentional)	Poisoning, Intentional Self-harm	Poisoning, Assault	Poisoning, Undetermined	Adverse effect	Underdosing
Soporific	T42.71	T42.72	T42.73	T42.74	T42.75	T42.76
Soporific drug	T42.71	T42.72	T42.73	T42.74	T42.75	T42.76
- specified type NEC	T42.6X1	T42.6X2	T42.6X3	T42.6X4	T42.6X5	T42.6X6
Sorbide nitrate	T46.3X1	T46.3X2	T46.3X3	T46.3X4	T46.3X5	T46.3X6
Sorbitol	T47.4X1	T47.4X2	T47.4X3	T47.4X4	T47.4X5	T47.4X6
Sotalol	T44.7X1	T44.7X2	T44.7X3	T44.7X4	T44.7X5	T44.7X6
Sotradecol	T46.8X1	T46.8X2	T46.8X3	T46.8X4	T46.8X5	T46.8X6
Soysterol	T46.6X1	T46.6X2	T46.6X3	T46.6X4	T46.6X5	T46.6X6
Spacoline	T44.3X1	T44.3X2	T44.3X3	T44.3X4	T44.3X5	T44.3X6
Spanish fly	T49.8X1	T49.8X2	T49.8X3	T49.8X4	T49.8X5	T49.8X6
Sparine	T43.3X1	T43.3X2	T43.3X3	T43.3X4	T43.3X5	T43.3X6
Sparteine	T48.0X1	T48.0X2	T48.0X3	T48.0X4	T48.0X5	T48.0X6
Spasmolytic						
- anticholinergics	T44.3X1	T44.3X2	T44.3X3	T44.3X4	T44.3X5	T44.3X6
- autonomic	T44.3X1	T44.3X2	T44.3X3	T44.3X4	T44.3X5	T44.3X6
- bronchial NEC	T48.6X1	T48.6X2	T48.6X3	T48.6X4	T48.6X5	T48.6X6
- quaternary ammonium	T44.3X1	T44.3X2	T44.3X3	T44.3X4	T44.3X5	T44.3X6
- skeletal muscle NEC	T48.1X1	T48.1X2	T48.1X3	T48.1X4	T48.1X5	T48.1X6
Spectinomycin	T36.5X1	T36.5X2	T36.5X3	T36.5X4	T36.5X5	T36.5X6
Speed	T43.621	T43.622	T43.623	T43.624	T43.625	T43.626
Spermicide	T49.8X1	T49.8X2	T49.8X3	T49.8X4	T49.8X5	T49.8X6
Spider (bite) (venom)	T63.391	T63.392	T63.393	T63.394	--	--
- antivenin	T50.Z11	T50.Z12	T50.Z13	T50.Z14	T50.Z15	T50.Z16
Spigelia (root)	T37.4X1	T37.4X2	T37.4X3	T37.4X4	T37.4X5	T37.4X6
Spindle inactivator	T50.4X1	T50.4X2	T50.4X3	T50.4X4	T50.4X5	T50.4X6
Spiperone	T43.4X1	T43.4X2	T43.4X3	T43.4X4	T43.4X5	T43.4X6
Spiramycin	T36.3X1	T36.3X2	T36.3X3	T36.3X4	T36.3X5	T36.3X6
Spirapril	T46.4X1	T46.4X2	T46.4X3	T46.4X4	T46.4X5	T46.4X6
Spirilene	T43.591	T43.592	T43.593	T43.594	T43.595	T43.596
Spirit (s) (neutral) NEC	T51.0X1	T51.0X2	T51.0X3	T51.0X4	--	--
- beverage	T51.0X1	T51.0X2	T51.0X3	T51.0X4	--	--
- industrial	T51.0X1	T51.0X2	T51.0X3	T51.0X4	--	--
- mineral	T52.0X1	T52.0X2	T52.0X3	T52.0X4	--	--
- of salt—see Hydrochloric acid						
- surgical	T51.0X1	T51.0X2	T51.0X3	T51.0X4	--	--
Spironolactone	T50.0X1	T50.0X2	T50.0X3	T50.0X4	T50.0X5	T50.0X6
Spiroperidol	T43.4X1	T43.4X2	T43.4X3	T43.4X4	T43.4X5	T43.4X6
Sponge, absorbable (gelatin)	T45.7X1	T45.7X2	T45.7X3	T45.7X4	T45.7X5	T45.7X6
Sporostacin	T49.0X1	T49.0X2	T49.0X3	T49.0X4	T49.0X5	T49.0X6
Spray (aerosol)	T65.91	T65.92	T65.93	T65.94	--	--
- cosmetic	T65.891	T65.892	T65.893	T65.894	--	--
- medicinal NEC	T50.901	T50.902	T50.903	T50.904	T50.905	T50.906
- pesticides—see Pesticides						
- specified content—see specific substance						
Spurge flax	T62.2X1	T62.2X2	T62.2X3	T62.2X4	--	--
Spurges	T62.2X1	T62.2X2	T62.2X3	T62.2X4	--	--
Sputum viscosity-lowering drug	T48.4X1	T48.4X2	T48.4X3	T48.4X4	T48.4X5	T48.4X6
Squill	T46.0X1	T46.0X2	T46.0X3	T46.0X4	T46.0X5	T46.0X6
- rat poison	T60.4X1	T60.4X2	T60.4X3	T60.4X4	--	--
Squirting cucumber (cathartic)	T47.2X1	T47.2X2	T47.2X3	T47.2X4	T47.2X5	T47.2X6
Stains	T65.6X1	T65.6X2	T65.6X3	T65.6X4	--	--
Stannous fluoride	T49.7X1	T49.7X2	T49.7X3	T49.7X4	T49.7X5	T49.7X6
Stanolone	T38.7X1	T38.7X2	T38.7X3	T38.7X4	T38.7X5	T38.7X6
Stanozolol	T38.7X1	T38.7X2	T38.7X3	T38.7X4	T38.7X5	T38.7X6
Staphisagria or stavesacre (pediculicide)	T49.0X1	T49.0X2	T49.0X3	T49.0X4	T49.0X5	T49.0X6
Starch	T50.901	T50.902	T50.903	T50.904	T50.905	T50.906
Stelazine	T43.3X1	T43.3X2	T43.3X3	T43.3X4	T43.3X5	T43.3X6
Stemetil	T43.3X1	T43.3X2	T43.3X3	T43.3X4	T43.3X5	T43.3X6
Stepronin	T48.4X1	T48.4X2	T48.4X3	T48.4X4	T48.4X5	T48.4X6

Substance	Poisoning, Accidental (unintentional)	Poisoning, Intentional Self-harm	Poisoning, Assault	Poisoning, Undetermined	Adverse effect	Underdosing
Sterculia	T47.4X1	T47.4X2	T47.4X3	T47.4X4	T47.4X5	T47.4X6
Sternutator gas	T59.891	T59.892	T59.893	T59.894	--	--
Steroid	T38.0X1	T38.0X2	T38.0X3	T38.0X4	T38.0X5	T38.0X6
- anabolic	T38.7X1	T38.7X2	T38.7X3	T38.7X4	T38.7X5	T38.7X6
- androgenic	T38.7X1	T38.7X2	T38.7X3	T38.7X4	T38.7X5	T38.7X6
- antineoplastic, hormone	T38.7X1	T38.7X2	T38.7X3	T38.7X4	T38.7X5	T38.7X6
- - estrogen	T38.5X1	T38.5X2	T38.5X3	T38.5X4	T38.5X5	T38.5X6
- ENT agent	T49.6X1	T49.6X2	T49.6X3	T49.6X4	T49.6X5	T49.6X6
- ophthalmic preparation	T49.5X1	T49.5X2	T49.5X3	T49.5X4	T49.5X5	T49.5X6
- topical NEC	T49.0X1	T49.0X2	T49.0X3	T49.0X4	T49.0X5	T49.0X6
Stibine	T56.891	T56.892	T56.893	T56.894	--	--
Stibogluconate	T37.3X1	T37.3X2	T37.3X3	T37.3X4	T37.3X5	T37.3X6
Stibophen	T37.4X1	T37.4X2	T37.4X3	T37.4X4	T37.4X5	T37.4X6
Stilbamidine (isetionate)	T37.3X1	T37.3X2	T37.3X3	T37.3X4	T37.3X5	T37.3X6
Stilbestrol	T38.5X1	T38.5X2	T38.5X3	T38.5X4	T38.5X5	T38.5X6
Stilboestrol	T38.5X1	T38.5X2	T38.5X3	T38.5X4	T38.5X5	T38.5X6
Stimulant						
- central nervous system—see also Psychostimulant	T43.601	T43.602	T43.603	T43.604	T43.605	T43.606
- - analeptics	T50.7X1	T50.7X2	T50.7X3	T50.7X4	T50.7X5	T50.7X6
- - opiate antagonist	T50.7X1	T50.7X2	T50.7X3	T50.7X4	T50.7X5	T50.7X6
- - psychotherapeutic NEC—see also Psychotherapeutic drug	T43.601	T43.602	T43.603	T43.604	T43.605	T43.606
- - specified NEC	T43.691	T43.692	T43.693	T43.694	T43.695	T43.696
- respiratory	T48.901	T48.902	T48.903	T48.904	T48.905	T48.906
Stone-dissolving drug	T50.901	T50.902	T50.903	T50.904	T50.905	T50.906
Storage battery (cells) (acid)	T54.2X1	T54.2X2	T54.2X3	T54.2X4	--	--
Stovaine	T41.3X1	T41.3X2	T41.3X3	T41.3X4	T41.3X5	T41.3X6
- infiltration (subcutaneous)	T41.3X1	T41.3X2	T41.3X3	T41.3X4	T41.3X5	T41.3X6
- nerve block (peripheral) (plexus)	T41.3X1	T41.3X2	T41.3X3	T41.3X4	T41.3X5	T41.3X6
- spinal	T41.3X1	T41.3X2	T41.3X3	T41.3X4	T41.3X5	T41.3X6
- topical (surface)	T41.3X1	T41.3X2	T41.3X3	T41.3X4	T41.3X5	T41.3X6
Stovarsal	T37.8X1	T37.8X2	T37.8X3	T37.8X4	T37.8X5	T37.8X6
Stove gas—see Gas, stove						
Stoxil	T49.5X1	T49.5X2	T49.5X3	T49.5X4	T49.5X5	T49.5X6
Stramonium	T48.6X1	T48.6X2	T48.6X3	T48.6X4	T48.6X5	T48.6X6
- natural state	T62.2X1	T62.2X2	T62.2X3	T62.2X4	--	--
Streptodornase	T45.3X1	T45.3X2	T45.3X3	T45.3X4	T45.3X5	T45.3X6
Streptoduocin	T36.5X1	T36.5X2	T36.5X3	T36.5X4	T36.5X5	T36.5X6
Streptokinase	T45.611	T45.612	T45.613	T45.614	T45.615	T45.616
Streptomycin (derivative)	T36.5X1	T36.5X2	T36.5X3	T36.5X4	T36.5X5	T36.5X6
Streptonivicin	T36.5X1	T36.5X2	T36.5X3	T36.5X4	T36.5X5	T36.5X6
Streptovarycin	T36.5X1	T36.5X2	T36.5X3	T36.5X4	T36.5X5	T36.5X6
Streptozocin	T45.1X1	T45.1X2	T45.1X3	T45.1X4	T45.1X5	T45.1X6
Streptozotocin	T45.1X1	T45.1X2	T45.1X3	T45.1X4	T45.1X5	T45.1X6
Stripper (paint) (solvent)	T52.8X1	T52.8X2	T52.8X3	T52.8X4	--	--
Strobane	T60.1X1	T60.1X2	T60.1X3	T60.1X4	--	--
Strofantina	T46.0X1	T46.0X2	T46.0X3	T46.0X4	T46.0X5	T46.0X6
Strophanthin (g) (k)	T46.0X1	T46.0X2	T46.0X3	T46.0X4	T46.0X5	T46.0X6
Strophanthus	T46.0X1	T46.0X2	T46.0X3	T46.0X4	T46.0X5	T46.0X6
Strophantin	T46.0X1	T46.0X2	T46.0X3	T46.0X4	T46.0X5	T46.0X6
Strophantin-g	T46.0X1	T46.0X2	T46.0X3	T46.0X4	T46.0X5	T46.0X6
Strychnine (nonmedicinal) (pesticide) (salts)	T65.1X1	T65.1X2	T65.1X3	T65.1X4	--	--
- medicinal	T48.291	T48.292	T48.293	T48.294	T48.295	T48.296
Strychnos (ignatii) —see Strychnine						
Styramate	T42.8X1	T42.8X2	T42.8X3	T42.8X4	T42.8X5	T42.8X6
Styrene	T65.891	T65.892	T65.893	T65.894	--	--
Succinimide, antiepileptic or anticonvulsant	T42.2X1	T42.2X2	T42.2X3	T42.2X4	T42.2X5	T42.2X6
- mercuric—see Mercury						

Substance	Poisoning, Accidental (unintentional)	Poisoning, Intentional Self-harm	Poisoning, Assault	Poisoning, Undetermined	Adverse effect	Underdosing
Succinylcholine	T48.1X1	T48.1X2	T48.1X3	T48.1X4	T48.1X5	T48.1X6
Succinylsulfathiazole	T37.0X1	T37.0X2	T37.0X3	T37.0X4	T37.0X5	T37.0X6
Sucralfate	T47.1X1	T47.1X2	T47.1X3	T47.1X4	T47.1X5	T47.1X6
Sucrose	T50.3X1	T50.3X2	T50.3X3	T50.3X4	T50.3X5	T50.3X6
Sufentanil	T40.4X1	T40.4X2	T40.4X3	T40.4X4	T40.4X5	T40.4X6
Sulbactam	T36.0X1	T36.0X2	T36.0X3	T36.0X4	T36.0X5	T36.0X6
Sulbenicillin	T36.0X1	T36.0X2	T36.0X3	T36.0X4	T36.0X5	T36.0X6
Sulbentine	T49.0X1	T49.0X2	T49.0X3	T49.0X4	T49.0X5	T49.0X6
Sulfacetamide	T49.0X1	T49.0X2	T49.0X3	T49.0X4	T49.0X5	T49.0X6
- ophthalmic preparation	T49.5X1	T49.5X2	T49.5X3	T49.5X4	T49.5X5	T49.5X6
Sulfachlorpyridazine	T37.0X1	T37.0X2	T37.0X3	T37.0X4	T37.0X5	T37.0X6
Sulfacitine	T37.0X1	T37.0X2	T37.0X3	T37.0X4	T37.0X5	T37.0X6
Sulfadiasulfone sodium	T37.0X1	T37.0X2	T37.0X3	T37.0X4	T37.0X5	T37.0X6
Sulfadiazine	T37.0X1	T37.0X2	T37.0X3	T37.0X4	T37.0X5	T37.0X6
- silver (topical)	T49.0X1	T49.0X2	T49.0X3	T49.0X4	T49.0X5	T49.0X6
Sulfadimethoxine	T37.0X1	T37.0X2	T37.0X3	T37.0X4	T37.0X5	T37.0X6
Sulfadimidine	T37.0X1	T37.0X2	T37.0X3	T37.0X4	T37.0X5	T37.0X6
Sulfadoxine	T37.0X1	T37.0X2	T37.0X3	T37.0X4	T37.0X5	T37.0X6
- with pyrimethamine	T37.2X1	T37.2X2	T37.2X3	T37.2X4	T37.2X5	T37.2X6
Sulfaethidole	T37.0X1	T37.0X2	T37.0X3	T37.0X4	T37.0X5	T37.0X6
Sulfafurazole	T37.0X1	T37.0X2	T37.0X3	T37.0X4	T37.0X5	T37.0X6
Sulfaguanidine	T37.0X1	T37.0X2	T37.0X3	T37.0X4	T37.0X5	T37.0X6
Sulfalene	T37.0X1	T37.0X2	T37.0X3	T37.0X4	T37.0X5	T37.0X6
Sulfaloxate	T37.0X1	T37.0X2	T37.0X3	T37.0X4	T37.0X5	T37.0X6
Sulfaloxic acid	T37.0X1	T37.0X2	T37.0X3	T37.0X4	T37.0X5	T37.0X6
Sulfamazone	T39.2X1	T39.2X2	T39.2X3	T39.2X4	T39.2X5	T39.2X6
Sulfamerazine	T37.0X1	T37.0X2	T37.0X3	T37.0X4	T37.0X5	T37.0X6
Sulfameter	T37.0X1	T37.0X2	T37.0X3	T37.0X4	T37.0X5	T37.0X6
Sulfamethazine	T37.0X1	T37.0X2	T37.0X3	T37.0X4	T37.0X5	T37.0X6
Sulfamethizole	T37.0X1	T37.0X2	T37.0X3	T37.0X4	T37.0X5	T37.0X6
Sulfamethoxazole	T37.0X1	T37.0X2	T37.0X3	T37.0X4	T37.0X5	T37.0X6
- with trimethoprim	T36.8X1	T36.8X2	T36.8X3	T36.8X4	T36.8X5	T36.8X6
Sulfamethoxydiazine	T37.0X1	T37.0X2	T37.0X3	T37.0X4	T37.0X5	T37.0X6
Sulfamethoxypyridazine	T37.0X1	T37.0X2	T37.0X3	T37.0X4	T37.0X5	T37.0X6
Sulfamethylthiazole	T37.0X1	T37.0X2	T37.0X3	T37.0X4	T37.0X5	T37.0X6
Sulfametoxydiazine	T37.0X1	T37.0X2	T37.0X3	T37.0X4	T37.0X5	T37.0X6
Sulfamidopyrine	T39.2X1	T39.2X2	T39.2X3	T39.2X4	T39.2X5	T39.2X6
Sulfamonomethoxine	T37.0X1	T37.0X2	T37.0X3	T37.0X4	T37.0X5	T37.0X6
Sulfamoxole	T37.0X1	T37.0X2	T37.0X3	T37.0X4	T37.0X5	T37.0X6
Sulfamylon	T49.0X1	T49.0X2	T49.0X3	T49.0X4	T49.0X5	T49.0X6
Sulfan blue (diagnostic dye)	T50.8X1	T50.8X2	T50.8X3	T50.8X4	T50.8X5	T50.8X6
Sulfanilamide	T37.0X1	T37.0X2	T37.0X3	T37.0X4	T37.0X5	T37.0X6
Sulfanilylguanidine	T37.0X1	T37.0X2	T37.0X3	T37.0X4	T37.0X5	T37.0X6
Sulfaperin	T37.0X1	T37.0X2	T37.0X3	T37.0X4	T37.0X5	T37.0X6
Sulfaphenazole	T37.0X1	T37.0X2	T37.0X3	T37.0X4	T37.0X5	T37.0X6
Sulfaphenylthiazole	T37.0X1	T37.0X2	T37.0X3	T37.0X4	T37.0X5	T37.0X6
Sulfaproxyline	T37.0X1	T37.0X2	T37.0X3	T37.0X4	T37.0X5	T37.0X6
Sulfapyridine	T37.0X1	T37.0X2	T37.0X3	T37.0X4	T37.0X5	T37.0X6
Sulfapyrimidine	T37.0X1	T37.0X2	T37.0X3	T37.0X4	T37.0X5	T37.0X6
Sulfarsphenamine	T37.8X1	T37.8X2	T37.8X3	T37.8X4	T37.8X5	T37.8X6
Sulfasalazine	T37.0X1	T37.0X2	T37.0X3	T37.0X4	T37.0X5	T37.0X6
Sulfasuxidine	T37.0X1	T37.0X2	T37.0X3	T37.0X4	T37.0X5	T37.0X6
Sulfasymazine	T37.0X1	T37.0X2	T37.0X3	T37.0X4	T37.0X5	T37.0X6
Sulfated amylopectin	T47.8X1	T47.8X2	T47.8X3	T47.8X4	T47.8X5	T47.8X6
Sulfathiazole	T37.0X1	T37.0X2	T37.0X3	T37.0X4	T37.0X5	T37.0X6
Sulfatostearate	T49.2X1	T49.2X2	T49.2X3	T49.2X4	T49.2X5	T49.2X6
Sulfinpyrazone	T50.4X1	T50.4X2	T50.4X3	T50.4X4	T50.4X5	T50.4X6
Sulfiram	T49.0X1	T49.0X2	T49.0X3	T49.0X4	T49.0X5	T49.0X6
Sulfisomidine	T37.0X1	T37.0X2	T37.0X3	T37.0X4	T37.0X5	T37.0X6

Substance	Poisoning, Accidental (unintentional)	Poisoning, Intentional Self-harm	Poisoning, Assault	Poisoning, Undetermined	Adverse effect	Underdosing
Sulfisoxazole	T37.0X1	T37.0X2	T37.0X3	T37.0X4	T37.0X5	T37.0X6
- ophthalmic preparation	T49.5X1	T49.5X2	T49.5X3	T49.5X4	T49.5X5	T49.5X6
Sulfobromophthalein (sodium)	T50.8X1	T50.8X2	T50.8X3	T50.8X4	T50.8X5	T50.8X6
Sulfobromphthalein	T50.8X1	T50.8X2	T50.8X3	T50.8X4	T50.8X5	T50.8X6
Sulfogaiacol	T48.4X1	T48.4X2	T48.4X3	T48.4X4	T48.4X5	T48.4X6
Sulfomyxin	T36.8X1	T36.8X2	T36.8X3	T36.8X4	T36.8X5	T36.8X6
Sulfonal	T42.6X1	T42.6X2	T42.6X3	T42.6X4	T42.6X5	T42.6X6
Sulfonamide NEC	T37.0X1	T37.0X2	T37.0X3	T37.0X4	T37.0X5	T37.0X6
- eye	T49.5X1	T49.5X2	T49.5X3	T49.5X4	T49.5X5	T49.5X6
Sulfonazide	T37.1X1	T37.1X2	T37.1X3	T37.1X4	T37.1X5	T37.1X6
Sulfones	T37.1X1	T37.1X2	T37.1X3	T37.1X4	T37.1X5	T37.1X6
Sulfonethylmethane	T42.6X1	T42.6X2	T42.6X3	T42.6X4	T42.6X5	T42.6X6
Sulfonmethane	T42.6X1	T42.6X2	T42.6X3	T42.6X4	T42.6X5	T42.6X6
Sulfonphthal, sulfonphthol	T50.8X1	T50.8X2	T50.8X3	T50.8X4	T50.8X5	T50.8X6
Sulfonylurea derivatives, oral	T38.3X1	T38.3X2	T38.3X3	T38.3X4	T38.3X5	T38.3X6
Sulforidazine	T43.3X1	T43.3X2	T43.3X3	T43.3X4	T43.3X5	T43.3X6
Sulfoxone	T37.1X1	T37.1X2	T37.1X3	T37.1X4	T37.1X5	T37.1X6
Sulfur, sulfurated, sulfuric, sulfurous, sulfuryl (compounds NEC) (medicinal)	T49.4X1	T49.4X2	T49.4X3	T49.4X4	T49.4X5	T49.4X6
- acid	T54.2X1	T54.2X2	T54.2X3	T54.2X4	--	--
- dioxide (gas)	T59.1X1	T59.1X2	T59.1X3	T59.1X4	--	--
- ether—see Ether (s)						
- hydrogen	T59.6X1	T59.6X2	T59.6X3	T59.6X4	--	--
- medicinal (keratolytic) (ointment) NEC	T49.4X1	T49.4X2	T49.4X3	T49.4X4	T49.4X5	T49.4X6
- ointment	T49.0X1	T49.0X2	T49.0X3	T49.0X4	T49.0X5	T49.0X6
- pesticide (vapor)	T60.91	T60.92	T60.93	T60.94	--	--
- vapor NEC	T59.891	T59.892	T59.893	T59.894	--	--
Sulfuric acid	T54.2X1	T54.2X2	T54.2X3	T54.2X4	--	--
Sulglicotide	T47.1X1	T47.1X2	T47.1X3	T47.1X4	T47.1X5	T47.1X6
Sulindac	T39.391	T39.392	T39.393	T39.394	T39.395	T39.396
Sulisatin	T47.2X1	T47.2X2	T47.2X3	T47.2X4	T47.2X5	T47.2X6
Sulisobenzone	T49.3X1	T49.3X2	T49.3X3	T49.3X4	T49.3X5	T49.3X6
Sulkowitch's reagent	T50.8X1	T50.8X2	T50.8X3	T50.8X4	T50.8X5	T50.8X6
Sulmetozine	T44.3X1	T44.3X2	T44.3X3	T44.3X4	T44.3X5	T44.3X6
Suloctidil	T46.7X1	T46.7X2	T46.7X3	T46.7X4	T46.7X5	T46.7X6
Sulph——see also Sulf-						
Sulphadiazine	T37.0X1	T37.0X2	T37.0X3	T37.0X4	T37.0X5	T37.0X6
Sulphadimethoxine	T37.0X1	T37.0X2	T37.0X3	T37.0X4	T37.0X5	T37.0X6
Sulphadimidine	T37.0X1	T37.0X2	T37.0X3	T37.0X4	T37.0X5	T37.0X6
Sulphadione	T37.1X1	T37.1X2	T37.1X3	T37.1X4	T37.1X5	T37.1X6
Sulphafurazole	T37.0X1	T37.0X2	T37.0X3	T37.0X4	T37.0X5	T37.0X6
Sulphamethizole	T37.0X1	T37.0X2	T37.0X3	T37.0X4	T37.0X5	T37.0X6
Sulphamethoxazole	T37.0X1	T37.0X2	T37.0X3	T37.0X4	T37.0X5	T37.0X6
Sulphan blue	T50.8X1	T50.8X2	T50.8X3	T50.8X4	T50.8X5	T50.8X6
Sulphaphenazole	T37.0X1	T37.0X2	T37.0X3	T37.0X4	T37.0X5	T37.0X6
Sulphapyridine	T37.0X1	T37.0X2	T37.0X3	T37.0X4	T37.0X5	T37.0X6
Sulphasalazine	T37.0X1	T37.0X2	T37.0X3	T37.0X4	T37.0X5	T37.0X6
Sulphinpyrazone	T50.4X1	T50.4X2	T50.4X3	T50.4X4	T50.4X5	T50.4X6
Sulpiride	T43.591	T43.592	T43.593	T43.594	T43.595	T43.596
Sulprostone	T48.0X1	T48.0X2	T48.0X3	T48.0X4	T48.0X5	T48.0X6
Sulpyrine	T39.2X1	T39.2X2	T39.2X3	T39.2X4	T39.2X5	T39.2X6
Sultamicillin	T36.0X1	T36.0X2	T36.0X3	T36.0X4	T36.0X5	T36.0X6
Sulthiame	T42.6X1	T42.6X2	T42.6X3	T42.6X4	T42.6X5	T42.6X6
Sultiame	T42.6X1	T42.6X2	T42.6X3	T42.6X4	T42.6X5	T42.6X6
Sultopride	T43.591	T43.592	T43.593	T43.594	T43.595	T43.596
Sumatriptan	T39.8X1	T39.8X2	T39.8X3	T39.8X4	T39.8X5	T39.8X6
Sunflower seed oil	T46.6X1	T46.6X2	T46.6X3	T46.6X4	T46.6X5	T46.6X6
Superinone	T48.4X1	T48.4X2	T48.4X3	T48.4X4	T48.4X5	T48.4X6
Suprofen	T39.311	T39.312	T39.313	T39.314	T39.315	T39.316

Substance	Poisoning, Accidental (unintentional)	Poisoning, Intentional Self-harm	Poisoning, Assault	Poisoning, Undetermined	Adverse effect	Underdosing
Suramin (sodium)	T37.4X1	T37.4X2	T37.4X3	T37.4X4	T37.4X5	T37.4X6
Surfacaine	T41.3X1	T41.3X2	T41.3X3	T41.3X4	T41.3X5	T41.3X6
Surital	T41.1X1	T41.1X2	T41.1X3	T41.1X4	T41.1X5	T41.1X6
Sutilains	T45.3X1	T45.3X2	T45.3X3	T45.3X4	T45.3X5	T45.3X6
Suxamethonium (chloride)	T48.1X1	T48.1X2	T48.1X3	T48.1X4	T48.1X5	T48.1X6
Suxethonium (chloride)	T48.1X1	T48.1X2	T48.1X3	T48.1X4	T48.1X5	T48.1X6
Suxibuzone	T39.2X1	T39.2X2	T39.2X3	T39.2X4	T39.2X5	T39.2X6
Sweet niter spirit	T46.3X1	T46.3X2	T46.3X3	T46.3X4	T46.3X5	T46.3X6
Sweet oil (birch)	T49.3X1	T49.3X2	T49.3X3	T49.3X4	T49.3X5	T49.3X6
Sweetener	T50.901	T50.902	T50.903	T50.904	T50.905	T50.906
Sym-dichloroethyl ether	T53.6X1	T53.6X2	T53.6X3	T53.6X4	--	--
Sympatholytic NEC	T44.8X1	T44.8X2	T44.8X3	T44.8X4	T44.8X5	T44.8X6
- haloalkylamine	T44.8X1	T44.8X2	T44.8X3	T44.8X4	T44.8X5	T44.8X6
Sympathomimetic NEC	T44.901	T44.902	T44.903	T44.904	T44.905	T44.906
- anti-common-cold	T48.5X1	T48.5X2	T48.5X3	T48.5X4	T48.5X5	T48.5X6
- bronchodilator	T48.6X1	T48.6X2	T48.6X3	T48.6X4	T48.6X5	T48.6X6
- specified NEC	T44.991	T44.992	T44.993	T44.994	T44.995	T44.996
Synagis	T50.B91	T50.B92	T50.B93	T50.B94	T50.B95	T50.B96
Synalar	T49.0X1	T49.0X2	T49.0X3	T49.0X4	T49.0X5	T49.0X6
Synthroid	T38.1X1	T38.1X2	T38.1X3	T38.1X4	T38.1X5	T38.1X6
Syntocinon	T48.0X1	T48.0X2	T48.0X3	T48.0X4	T48.0X5	T48.0X6
Syrosingopine	T46.5X1	T46.5X2	T46.5X3	T46.5X4	T46.5X5	T46.5X6
Systemic drug	T45.91	T45.92	T45.93	T45.94	T45.95	T45.96
- specified NEC	T45.8X1	T45.8X2	T45.8X3	T45.8X4	T45.8X5	T45.8X6
2,4,5-T	T60.3X1	T60.3X2	T60.3X3	T60.3X4	--	--
Tablets—see also specified substance	T50.901	T50.902	T50.903	T50.904	T50.905	T50.906
Tace	T38.5X1	T38.5X2	T38.5X3	T38.5X4	T38.5X5	T38.5X6
Tacrine	T44.0X1	T44.0X2	T44.0X3	T44.0X4	T44.0X5	T44.0X6
Tadalafil	T46.7X1	T46.7X2	T46.7X3	T46.7X4	T46.7X5	T46.7X6
Talampicillin	T36.0X1	T36.0X2	T36.0X3	T36.0X4	T36.0X5	T36.0X6
Talbutal	T42.3X1	T42.3X2	T42.3X3	T42.3X4	T42.3X5	T42.3X6
Talc powder	T49.3X1	T49.3X2	T49.3X3	T49.3X4	T49.3X5	T49.3X6
Talcum	T49.3X1	T49.3X2	T49.3X3	T49.3X4	T49.3X5	T49.3X6
Taleranol	T38.6X1	T38.6X2	T38.6X3	T38.6X4	T38.6X5	T38.6X6
Tamoxifen	T38.6X1	T38.6X2	T38.6X3	T38.6X4	T38.6X5	T38.6X6
Tamsulosin	T44.6X1	T44.6X2	T44.6X3	T44.6X4	T44.6X5	T44.6X6
Tandearil, tanderil	T39.2X1	T39.2X2	T39.2X3	T39.2X4	T39.2X5	T39.2X6
Tannic acid	T49.2X1	T49.2X2	T49.2X3	T49.2X4	T49.2X5	T49.2X6
- medicinal (astringent)	T49.2X1	T49.2X2	T49.2X3	T49.2X4	T49.2X5	T49.2X6
Tannin—see Tannic acid						
Tansy	T62.2X1	T62.2X2	T62.2X3	T62.2X4	--	--
TAO	T36.3X1	T36.3X2	T36.3X3	T36.3X4	T36.3X5	T36.3X6
Tapazole	T38.2X1	T38.2X2	T38.2X3	T38.2X4	T38.2X5	T38.2X6
Tar NEC	T52.0X1	T52.0X2	T52.0X3	T52.0X4	--	--
- camphor	T60.1X1	T60.1X2	T60.1X3	T60.1X4	--	--
- distillate	T49.1X1	T49.1X2	T49.1X3	T49.1X4	T49.1X5	T49.1X6
- fumes	T59.891	T59.892	T59.893	T59.894	--	--
- medicinal	T49.1X1	T49.1X2	T49.1X3	T49.1X4	T49.1X5	T49.1X6
- ointment	T49.1X1	T49.1X2	T49.1X3	T49.1X4	T49.1X5	T49.1X6
Taractan	T43.591	T43.592	T43.593	T43.594	T43.595	T43.596
Tarantula (venomous)	T63.321	T63.322	T63.323	T63.324	--	--
Tartar emetic	T37.8X1	T37.8X2	T37.8X3	T37.8X4	T37.8X5	T37.8X6
Tartaric acid	T65.891	T65.892	T65.893	T65.894	--	--
Tartrate, laxative	T47.4X1	T47.4X2	T47.4X3	T47.4X4	T47.4X5	T47.4X6
Tartrated antimony (anti-infective)	T37.8X1	T37.8X2	T37.8X3	T37.8X4	T37.8X5	T37.8X6
Tauromustine	T45.1X1	T45.1X2	T45.1X3	T45.1X4	T45.1X5	T45.1X6
TCA—see Trichloroacetic acid						
TCDD	T53.7X1	T53.7X2	T53.7X3	T53.7X4	--	--
TDI (vapor)	T65.0X1	T65.0X2	T65.0X3	T65.0X4	--	--

Substance	Poisoning, Accidental (unintentional)	Poisoning, Intentional Self-harm	Poisoning, Assault	Poisoning, Undetermined	Adverse effect	Underdosing
Tear						
- gas	T59.3X1	T59.3X2	T59.3X3	T59.3X4	--	--
- solution	T49.5X1	T49.5X2	T49.5X3	T49.5X4	T49.5X5	T49.5X6
Teclothiazide	T50.2X1	T50.2X2	T50.2X3	T50.2X4	T50.2X5	T50.2X6
Teclozan	T37.3X1	T37.3X2	T37.3X3	T37.3X4	T37.3X5	T37.3X6
Tegafur	T45.1X1	T45.1X2	T45.1X3	T45.1X4	T45.1X5	T45.1X6
Tegretol	T42.1X1	T42.1X2	T42.1X3	T42.1X4	T42.1X5	T42.1X6
Teicoplanin	T36.8X1	T36.8X2	T36.8X3	T36.8X4	T36.8X5	T36.8X6
Telepaque	T50.8X1	T50.8X2	T50.8X3	T50.8X4	T50.8X5	T50.8X6
Tellurium	T56.891	T56.892	T56.893	T56.894	--	--
- fumes	T56.891	T56.892	T56.893	T56.894	--	--
TEM	T45.1X1	T45.1X2	T45.1X3	T45.1X4	T45.1X5	T45.1X6
Temazepam	T42.4X1	T42.4X2	T42.4X3	T42.4X4	T42.4X5	T42.4X6
Temocillin	T36.0X1	T36.0X2	T36.0X3	T36.0X4	T36.0X5	T36.0X6
Tenamfetamine	T43.621	T43.622	T43.623	T43.624	T43.625	T43.626
Teniposide	T45.1X1	T45.1X2	T45.1X3	T45.1X4	T45.1X5	T45.1X6
Tenitramine	T46.3X1	T46.3X2	T46.3X3	T46.3X4	T46.3X5	T46.3X6
Tenoglicin	T48.4X1	T48.4X2	T48.4X3	T48.4X4	T48.4X5	T48.4X6
Tenonitrozole	T37.3X1	T37.3X2	T37.3X3	T37.3X4	T37.3X5	T37.3X6
Tenoxicam	T39.391	T39.392	T39.393	T39.394	T39.395	T39.396
TEPA	T45.1X1	T45.1X2	T45.1X3	T45.1X4	T45.1X5	T45.1X6
TEPP	T60.0X1	T60.0X2	T60.0X3	T60.0X4	--	--
Teprotide	T46.5X1	T46.5X2	T46.5X3	T46.5X4	T46.5X5	T46.5X6
Terazosin	T44.6X1	T44.6X2	T44.6X3	T44.6X4	T44.6X5	T44.6X6
Terbufos	T60.0X1	T60.0X2	T60.0X3	T60.0X4	--	--
Terbutaline	T48.6X1	T48.6X2	T48.6X3	T48.6X4	T48.6X5	T48.6X6
Terconazole	T49.0X1	T49.0X2	T49.0X3	T49.0X4	T49.0X5	T49.0X6
Terfenadine	T45.0X1	T45.0X2	T45.0X3	T45.0X4	T45.0X5	T45.0X6
Teriparatide (acetate)	T50.991	T50.992	T50.993	T50.994	T50.995	T50.996
Terizidone	T37.1X1	T37.1X2	T37.1X3	T37.1X4	T37.1X5	T37.1X6
Terlipressin	T38.891	T38.892	T38.893	T38.894	T38.895	T38.896
Terodiline	T46.3X1	T46.3X2	T46.3X3	T46.3X4	T46.3X5	T46.3X6
Teroxalene	T37.4X1	T37.4X2	T37.4X3	T37.4X4	T37.4X5	T37.4X6
Terpin (cis) hydrate	T48.4X1	T48.4X2	T48.4X3	T48.4X4	T48.4X5	T48.4X6
Terramycin	T36.4X1	T36.4X2	T36.4X3	T36.4X4	T36.4X5	T36.4X6
Tertatolol	T44.7X1	T44.7X2	T44.7X3	T44.7X4	T44.7X5	T44.7X6
Tessalon	T48.3X1	T48.3X2	T48.3X3	T48.3X4	T48.3X5	T48.3X6
Testolactone	T38.7X1	T38.7X2	T38.7X3	T38.7X4	T38.7X5	T38.7X6
Testosterone	T38.7X1	T38.7X2	T38.7X3	T38.7X4	T38.7X5	T38.7X6
Tetanus toxoid or vaccine	T50.A91	T50.A92	T50.A93	T50.A94	T50.A95	T50.A96
- antitoxin	T50.Z11	T50.Z12	T50.Z13	T50.Z14	T50.Z15	T50.Z16
- immune globulin (human)	T50.Z11	T50.Z12	T50.Z13	T50.Z14	T50.Z15	T50.Z16
- toxoid	T50.A91	T50.A92	T50.A93	T50.A94	T50.A95	T50.A96
- - with diphtheria toxoid	T50.A21	T50.A22	T50.A23	T50.A24	T50.A25	T50.A26
- - - with pertussis	T50.A11	T50.A12	T50.A13	T50.A14	T50.A15	T50.A16
Tetrabenazine	T43.591	T43.592	T43.593	T43.594	T43.595	T43.596
Tetracaine	T41.3X1	T41.3X2	T41.3X3	T41.3X4	T41.3X5	T41.3X6
- nerve block (peripheral) (plexus)	T41.3X1	T41.3X2	T41.3X3	T41.3X4	T41.3X5	T41.3X6
- regional	T41.3X1	T41.3X2	T41.3X3	T41.3X4	T41.3X5	T41.3X6
- spinal	T41.3X1	T41.3X2	T41.3X3	T41.3X4	T41.3X5	T41.3X6
Tetrachlorethylene—see Tetrachloroethylene						
Tetrachlormethiazide	T50.2X1	T50.2X2	T50.2X3	T50.2X4	T50.2X5	T50.2X6
2,3,7,8-Tetrachlorodibenzo-p-dioxin	T53.7X1	T53.7X2	T53.7X3	T53.7X4	--	--
Tetrachloroethane	T53.6X1	T53.6X2	T53.6X3	T53.6X4	--	--
- vapor	T53.6X1	T53.6X2	T53.6X3	T53.6X4	--	--
- - paint or varnish	T53.6X1	T53.6X2	T53.6X3	T53.6X4	--	--
Tetrachloroethylene (liquid)	T53.3X1	T53.3X2	T53.3X3	T53.3X4	--	--
- medicinal	T37.4X1	T37.4X2	T37.4X3	T37.4X4	T37.4X5	T37.4X6

Substance	Poisoning, Accidental (unintentional)	Poisoning, Intentional Self-harm	Poisoning, Assault	Poisoning, Undetermined	Adverse effect	Underdosing
- vapor	T53.3X1	T53.3X2	T53.3X3	T53.3X4	--	--
Tetrachloromethane—see Carbon tetrachloride						
Tetracosactide	T38.811	T38.812	T38.813	T38.814	T38.815	T38.816
Tetracosactrin	T38.811	T38.812	T38.813	T38.814	T38.815	T38.816
Tetracycline	T36.4X1	T36.4X2	T36.4X3	T36.4X4	T36.4X5	T36.4X6
- ophthalmic preparation	T49.5X1	T49.5X2	T49.5X3	T49.5X4	T49.5X5	T49.5X6
- topical NEC	T49.0X1	T49.0X2	T49.0X3	T49.0X4	T49.0X5	T49.0X6
Tetradifon	T60.8X1	T60.8X2	T60.8X3	T60.8X4	--	--
Tetradotoxin	T61.771	T61.772	T61.773	T61.774	--	--
Tetraethyl						
- lead	T56.0X1	T56.0X2	T56.0X3	T56.0X4	--	--
- pyrophosphate	T60.0X1	T60.0X2	T60.0X3	T60.0X4	--	--
Tetraethylammonium chloride	T44.2X1	T44.2X2	T44.2X3	T44.2X4	T44.2X5	T44.2X6
Tetraethylthiuram disulfide	T50.6X1	T50.6X2	T50.6X3	T50.6X4	T50.6X5	T50.6X6
Tetrahydroaminoacridine	T44.0X1	T44.0X2	T44.0X3	T44.0X4	T44.0X5	T44.0X6
Tetrahydrocannabinol	T40.7X1	T40.7X2	T40.7X3	T40.7X4	T40.7X5	T40.7X6
Tetrahydrofuran	T52.8X1	T52.8X2	T52.8X3	T52.8X4	--	--
Tetrahydronaphthalene	T52.8X1	T52.8X2	T52.8X3	T52.8X4	--	--
Tetrahydrozoline	T49.5X1	T49.5X2	T49.5X3	T49.5X4	T49.5X5	T49.5X6
Tetralin	T52.8X1	T52.8X2	T52.8X3	T52.8X4	--	--
Tetramethrin	T60.2X1	T60.2X2	T60.2X3	T60.2X4	--	--
Tetramethylthiuram (disulfide) NEC	T60.3X1	T60.3X2	T60.3X3	T60.3X4	--	--
- medicinal	T49.0X1	T49.0X2	T49.0X3	T49.0X4	T49.0X5	T49.0X6
Tetramisole	T37.4X1	T37.4X2	T37.4X3	T37.4X4	T37.4X5	T37.4X6
Tetranicotinoyl fructose	T46.7X1	T46.7X2	T46.7X3	T46.7X4	T46.7X5	T46.7X6
Tetrazepam	T42.4X1	T42.4X2	T42.4X3	T42.4X4	T42.4X5	T42.4X6
Tetronal	T42.6X1	T42.6X2	T42.6X3	T42.6X4	T42.6X5	T42.6X6
Tetryl	T65.3X1	T65.3X2	T65.3X3	T65.3X4	--	--
Tetrylammonium chloride	T44.2X1	T44.2X2	T44.2X3	T44.2X4	T44.2X5	T44.2X6
Tetryzoline	T49.5X1	T49.5X2	T49.5X3	T49.5X4	T49.5X5	T49.5X6
Thalidomide	T45.1X1	T45.1X2	T45.1X3	T45.1X4	T45.1X5	T45.1X6
Thallium (compounds) (dust) NEC	T56.811	T56.812	T56.813	T56.814	--	--
- pesticide	T60.4X1	T60.4X2	T60.4X3	T60.4X4	--	--
THC	T40.7X1	T40.7X2	T40.7X3	T40.7X4	T40.7X5	T40.7X6
Thebacon	T48.3X1	T48.3X2	T48.3X3	T48.3X4	T48.3X5	T48.3X6
Thebaine	T40.2X1	T40.2X2	T40.2X3	T40.2X4	T40.2X5	T40.2X6
Thenoic acid	T49.6X1	T49.6X2	T49.6X3	T49.6X4	T49.6X5	T49.6X6
Thenyldiamine	T45.0X1	T45.0X2	T45.0X3	T45.0X4	T45.0X5	T45.0X6
Theobromine (calcium salicylate)	T48.6X1	T48.6X2	T48.6X3	T48.6X4	T48.6X5	T48.6X6
- sodium salicylate	T48.6X1	T48.6X2	T48.6X3	T48.6X4	T48.6X5	T48.6X6
Theophyllamine	T48.6X1	T48.6X2	T48.6X3	T48.6X4	T48.6X5	T48.6X6
Theophylline	T48.6X1	T48.6X2	T48.6X3	T48.6X4	T48.6X5	T48.6X6
- aminobenzoic acid	T48.6X1	T48.6X2	T48.6X3	T48.6X4	T48.6X5	T48.6X6
- ethylenediamine	T48.6X1	T48.6X2	T48.6X3	T48.6X4	T48.6X5	T48.6X6
- piperazine p-amino-benzoate	T48.6X1	T48.6X2	T48.6X3	T48.6X4	T48.6X5	T48.6X6
Thiabendazole	T37.4X1	T37.4X2	T37.4X3	T37.4X4	T37.4X5	T37.4X6
Thialbarbital	T41.1X1	T41.1X2	T41.1X3	T41.1X4	T41.1X5	T41.1X6
Thiamazole	T38.2X1	T38.2X2	T38.2X3	T38.2X4	T38.2X5	T38.2X6
Thiambutosine	T37.1X1	T37.1X2	T37.1X3	T37.1X4	T37.1X5	T37.1X6
Thiamine	T45.2X1	T45.2X2	T45.2X3	T45.2X4	T45.2X5	T45.2X6
Thiamphenicol	T36.2X1	T36.2X2	T36.2X3	T36.2X4	T36.2X5	T36.2X6
Thiamylal	T41.1X1	T41.1X2	T41.1X3	T41.1X4	T41.1X5	T41.1X6
- sodium	T41.1X1	T41.1X2	T41.1X3	T41.1X4	T41.1X5	T41.1X6
Thiazesim	T43.291	T43.292	T43.293	T43.294	T43.295	T43.296
Thiazides (diuretics)	T50.2X1	T50.2X2	T50.2X3	T50.2X4	T50.2X5	T50.2X6
Thiazinamium metilsulfate	T43.3X1	T43.3X2	T43.3X3	T43.3X4	T43.3X5	T43.3X6
Thiethylperazine	T43.3X1	T43.3X2	T43.3X3	T43.3X4	T43.3X5	T43.3X6
Thimerosal	T49.0X1	T49.0X2	T49.0X3	T49.0X4	T49.0X5	T49.0X6

Substance	Poisoning, Accidental (unintentional)	Poisoning, Intentional Self-harm	Poisoning, Assault	Poisoning, Undetermined	Adverse effect	Underdosing
- ophthalmic preparation	T49.5X1	T49.5X2	T49.5X3	T49.5X4	T49.5X5	T49.5X6
Thioacetazone	T37.1X1	T37.1X2	T37.1X3	T37.1X4	T37.1X5	T37.1X6
- with isoniazid	T37.1X1	T37.1X2	T37.1X3	T37.1X4	T37.1X5	T37.1X6
Thiobarbital sodium	T41.1X1	T41.1X2	T41.1X3	T41.1X4	T41.1X5	T41.1X6
Thiobarbiturate anesthetic	T41.1X1	T41.1X2	T41.1X3	T41.1X4	T41.1X5	T41.1X6
Thiobismol	T37.8X1	T37.8X2	T37.8X3	T37.8X4	T37.8X5	T37.8X6
Thiobutabarbital sodium	T41.1X1	T41.1X2	T41.1X3	T41.1X4	T41.1X5	T41.1X6
Thiocarbamate (insecticide)	T60.0X1	T60.0X2	T60.0X3	T60.0X4	--	--
Thiocarbamide	T38.2X1	T38.2X2	T38.2X3	T38.2X4	T38.2X5	T38.2X6
Thiocarbarsone	T37.8X1	T37.8X2	T37.8X3	T37.8X4	T37.8X5	T37.8X6
Thiocarlide	T37.1X1	T37.1X2	T37.1X3	T37.1X4	T37.1X5	T37.1X6
Thioctamide	T50.991	T50.992	T50.993	T50.994	T50.995	T50.996
Thioctic acid	T50.991	T50.992	T50.993	T50.994	T50.995	T50.996
Thiofos	T60.0X1	T60.0X2	T60.0X3	T60.0X4	--	--
Thioglycolate	T49.4X1	T49.4X2	T49.4X3	T49.4X4	T49.4X5	T49.4X6
Thioglycolic acid	T65.891	T65.892	T65.893	T65.894	--	--
Thioguanine	T45.1X1	T45.1X2	T45.1X3	T45.1X4	T45.1X5	T45.1X6
Thiomercaptomerin	T50.2X1	T50.2X2	T50.2X3	T50.2X4	T50.2X5	T50.2X6
Thiomerin	T50.2X1	T50.2X2	T50.2X3	T50.2X4	T50.2X5	T50.2X6
Thiomersal	T49.0X1	T49.0X2	T49.0X3	T49.0X4	T49.0X5	T49.0X6
Thionazin	T60.0X1	T60.0X2	T60.0X3	T60.0X4	--	--
Thiopental (sodium)	T41.1X1	T41.1X2	T41.1X3	T41.1X4	T41.1X5	T41.1X6
Thiopentone (sodium)	T41.1X1	T41.1X2	T41.1X3	T41.1X4	T41.1X5	T41.1X6
Thiopropazate	T43.3X1	T43.3X2	T43.3X3	T43.3X4	T43.3X5	T43.3X6
Thioproperazine	T43.3X1	T43.3X2	T43.3X3	T43.3X4	T43.3X5	T43.3X6
Thioridazine	T43.3X1	T43.3X2	T43.3X3	T43.3X4	T43.3X5	T43.3X6
Thiosinamine	T49.3X1	T49.3X2	T49.3X3	T49.3X4	T49.3X5	T49.3X6
Thiotepa	T45.1X1	T45.1X2	T45.1X3	T45.1X4	T45.1X5	T45.1X6
Thiothixene	T43.4X1	T43.4X2	T43.4X3	T43.4X4	T43.4X5	T43.4X6
Thiouracil (benzyl) (methyl) (propyl)	T38.2X1	T38.2X2	T38.2X3	T38.2X4	T38.2X5	T38.2X6
Thiourea	T38.2X1	T38.2X2	T38.2X3	T38.2X4	T38.2X5	T38.2X6
Thiphenamil	T44.3X1	T44.3X2	T44.3X3	T44.3X4	T44.3X5	T44.3X6
Thiram	T60.3X1	T60.3X2	T60.3X3	T60.3X4	--	--
- medicinal	T49.2X1	T49.2X2	T49.2X3	T49.2X4	T49.2X5	T49.2X6
Thonzylamine (systemic)	T45.0X1	T45.0X2	T45.0X3	T45.0X4	T45.0X5	T45.0X6
- mucosal decongestant	T48.5X1	T48.5X2	T48.5X3	T48.5X4	T48.5X5	T48.5X6
Thorazine	T43.3X1	T43.3X2	T43.3X3	T43.3X4	T43.3X5	T43.3X6
Thorium dioxide suspension	T50.8X1	T50.8X2	T50.8X3	T50.8X4	T50.8X5	T50.8X6
Thornapple	T62.2X1	T62.2X2	T62.2X3	T62.2X4	--	--
Throat drug NEC	T49.6X1	T49.6X2	T49.6X3	T49.6X4	T49.6X5	T49.6X6
Thrombin	T45.7X1	T45.7X2	T45.7X3	T45.7X4	T45.7X5	T45.7X6
Thrombolysin	T45.611	T45.612	T45.613	T45.614	T45.615	T45.616
Thromboplastin	T45.7X1	T45.7X2	T45.7X3	T45.7X4	T45.7X5	T45.7X6
Thurfyl nicotinate	T46.7X1	T46.7X2	T46.7X3	T46.7X4	T46.7X5	T46.7X6
Thymol	T49.0X1	T49.0X2	T49.0X3	T49.0X4	T49.0X5	T49.0X6
Thymopentin	T37.5X1	T37.5X2	T37.5X3	T37.5X4	T37.5X5	T37.5X6
Thymoxamine	T46.7X1	T46.7X2	T46.7X3	T46.7X4	T46.7X5	T46.7X6
Thymus extract	T38.891	T38.892	T38.893	T38.894	T38.895	T38.896
Thyreotrophic hormone	T38.811	T38.812	T38.813	T38.814	T38.815	T38.816
Thyroglobulin	T38.1X1	T38.1X2	T38.1X3	T38.1X4	T38.1X5	T38.1X6
Thyroid (hormone)	T38.1X1	T38.1X2	T38.1X3	T38.1X4	T38.1X5	T38.1X6
Thyrolar	T38.1X1	T38.1X2	T38.1X3	T38.1X4	T38.1X5	T38.1X6
Thyrotrophin	T38.811	T38.812	T38.813	T38.814	T38.815	T38.816
Thyrotropic hormone	T38.811	T38.812	T38.813	T38.814	T38.815	T38.816
Thyroxine	T38.1X1	T38.1X2	T38.1X3	T38.1X4	T38.1X5	T38.1X6
Tiabendazole	T37.4X1	T37.4X2	T37.4X3	T37.4X4	T37.4X5	T37.4X6
Tiamizide	T50.2X1	T50.2X2	T50.2X3	T50.2X4	T50.2X5	T50.2X6
Tianeptine	T43.291	T43.292	T43.293	T43.294	T43.295	T43.296

TABLE OF DRUGS AND CHEMICALS

Substance	Poisoning, Accidental (unintentional)	Poisoning, Intentional Self-harm	Poisoning, Assault	Poisoning, Undetermined	Adverse effect	Underdosing
Tiapamil	T46.1X1	T46.1X2	T46.1X3	T46.1X4	T46.1X5	T46.1X6
Tiapride	T43.591	T43.592	T43.593	T43.594	T43.595	T43.596
Tiaprofenic acid	T39.311	T39.312	T39.313	T39.314	T39.315	T39.316
Tiaramide	T39.8X1	T39.8X2	T39.8X3	T39.8X4	T39.8X5	T39.8X6
Ticarcillin	T36.0X1	T36.0X2	T36.0X3	T36.0X4	T36.0X5	T36.0X6
Ticlatone	T49.0X1	T49.0X2	T49.0X3	T49.0X4	T49.0X5	T49.0X6
Ticlopidine	T45.521	T45.522	T45.523	T45.524	T45.525	T45.526
Ticrynafen	T50.1X1	T50.1X2	T50.1X3	T50.1X4	T50.1X5	T50.1X6
Tidiacic	T50.991	T50.992	T50.993	T50.994	T50.995	T50.996
Tiemonium	T44.3X1	T44.3X2	T44.3X3	T44.3X4	T44.3X5	T44.3X6
- iodide	T44.3X1	T44.3X2	T44.3X3	T44.3X4	T44.3X5	T44.3X6
Tienilic acid	T50.1X1	T50.1X2	T50.1X3	T50.1X4	T50.1X5	T50.1X6
Tifenamil	T44.3X1	T44.3X2	T44.3X3	T44.3X4	T44.3X5	T44.3X6
Tigan	T45.0X1	T45.0X2	T45.0X3	T45.0X4	T45.0X5	T45.0X6
Tigloidine	T44.3X1	T44.3X2	T44.3X3	T44.3X4	T44.3X5	T44.3X6
Tilactase	T47.5X1	T47.5X2	T47.5X3	T47.5X4	T47.5X5	T47.5X6
Tiletamine	T41.291	T41.292	T41.293	T41.294	T41.295	T41.296
Tilidine	T40.4X1	T40.4X2	T40.4X3	T40.4X4	--	--
Timepidium bromide	T44.3X1	T44.3X2	T44.3X3	T44.3X4	T44.3X5	T44.3X6
Timiperone	T43.4X1	T43.4X2	T43.4X3	T43.4X4	T43.4X5	T43.4X6
Timolol	T44.7X1	T44.7X2	T44.7X3	T44.7X4	T44.7X5	T44.7X6
Tin (chloride) (dust) (oxide) NEC	T56.6X1	T56.6X2	T56.6X3	T56.6X4	--	--
- anti-infectives	T37.8X1	T37.8X2	T37.8X3	T37.8X4	T37.8X5	T37.8X6
Tincture, iodine—see Iodine						
Tindal	T43.3X1	T43.3X2	T43.3X3	T43.3X4	T43.3X5	T43.3X6
Tinidazole	T37.3X1	T37.3X2	T37.3X3	T37.3X4	T37.3X5	T37.3X6
Tinoridine	T39.8X1	T39.8X2	T39.8X3	T39.8X4	T39.8X5	T39.8X6
Tiocarlide	T37.1X1	T37.1X2	T37.1X3	T37.1X4	T37.1X5	T37.1X6
Tioclomarol	T45.511	T45.512	T45.513	T45.514	T45.515	T45.516
Tioconazole	T49.0X1	T49.0X2	T49.0X3	T49.0X4	T49.0X5	T49.0X6
Tioguanine	T45.1X1	T45.1X2	T45.1X3	T45.1X4	T45.1X5	T45.1X6
Tiopronin	T50.991	T50.992	T50.993	T50.994	T50.995	T50.996
Tiotixene	T43.4X1	T43.4X2	T43.4X3	T43.4X4	T43.4X5	T43.4X6
Tioxolone	T49.4X1	T49.4X2	T49.4X3	T49.4X4	T49.4X5	T49.4X6
Tipepidine	T48.3X1	T48.3X2	T48.3X3	T48.3X4	T48.3X5	T48.3X6
Tiquizium bromide	T44.3X1	T44.3X2	T44.3X3	T44.3X4	T44.3X5	T44.3X6
Tiratricol	T38.1X1	T38.1X2	T38.1X3	T38.1X4	T38.1X5	T38.1X6
Tisopurine	T50.4X1	T50.4X2	T50.4X3	T50.4X4	T50.4X5	T50.4X6
Titanium (compounds) (vapor)	T56.891	T56.892	T56.893	T56.894	--	--
- dioxide	T49.3X1	T49.3X2	T49.3X3	T49.3X4	T49.3X5	T49.3X6
- ointment	T49.3X1	T49.3X2	T49.3X3	T49.3X4	T49.3X5	T49.3X6
- oxide	T49.3X1	T49.3X2	T49.3X3	T49.3X4	T49.3X5	T49.3X6
- tetrachloride	T56.891	T56.892	T56.893	T56.894	--	--
Titanocene	T56.891	T56.892	T56.893	T56.894	--	--
Titroid	T38.1X1	T38.1X2	T38.1X3	T38.1X4	T38.1X5	T38.1X6
Tizanidine	T42.8X1	T42.8X2	T42.8X3	T42.8X4	T42.8X5	T42.8X6
TMTD	T60.3X1	T60.3X2	T60.3X3	T60.3X4	--	--
TNT (fumes)	T65.3X1	T65.3X2	T65.3X3	T65.3X4	--	--
Toadstool	T62.0X1	T62.0X2	T62.0X3	T62.0X4	--	--
Tobacco NEC	T65.291	T65.292	T65.293	T65.294	--	--
- cigarettes	T65.221	T65.222	T65.223	T65.224	--	--
- Indian	T62.2X1	T62.2X2	T62.2X3	T62.2X4	--	--
- smoke, second-hand	T65.221	T65.222	T65.223	T65.224	--	--
Tobramycin	T36.5X1	T36.5X2	T36.5X3	T36.5X4	T36.5X5	T36.5X6
Tocainide	T46.2X1	T46.2X2	T46.2X3	T46.2X4	T46.2X5	T46.2X6
Tocoferol	T45.2X1	T45.2X2	T45.2X3	T45.2X4	T45.2X5	T45.2X6
Tocopherol	T45.2X1	T45.2X2	T45.2X3	T45.2X4	T45.2X5	T45.2X6
- acetate	T45.2X1	T45.2X2	T45.2X3	T45.2X4	T45.2X5	T45.2X6
Tocosamine	T48.0X1	T48.0X2	T48.0X3	T48.0X4	T48.0X5	T48.0X6

Substance	Poisoning, Accidental (unintentional)	Poisoning, Intentional Self-harm	Poisoning, Assault	Poisoning, Undetermined	Adverse effect	Underdosing
Todralazine	T46.5X1	T46.5X2	T46.5X3	T46.5X4	T46.5X5	T46.5X6
Tofisopam	T42.4X1	T42.4X2	T42.4X3	T42.4X4	T42.4X5	T42.4X6
Tofranil	T43.011	T43.012	T43.013	T43.014	T43.015	T43.016
Toilet deodorizer	T65.891	T65.892	T65.893	T65.894	--	--
Tolamolol	T44.7X1	T44.7X2	T44.7X3	T44.7X4	T44.7X5	T44.7X6
Tolazamide	T38.3X1	T38.3X2	T38.3X3	T38.3X4	T38.3X5	T38.3X6
Tolazoline	T46.7X1	T46.7X2	T46.7X3	T46.7X4	T46.7X5	T46.7X6
Tolbutamide (sodium)	T38.3X1	T38.3X2	T38.3X3	T38.3X4	T38.3X5	T38.3X6
Tolciclate	T49.0X1	T49.0X2	T49.0X3	T49.0X4	T49.0X5	T49.0X6
Tolmetin	T39.391	T39.392	T39.393	T39.394	T39.395	T39.396
Tolnaftate	T49.0X1	T49.0X2	T49.0X3	T49.0X4	T49.0X5	T49.0X6
Tolonidine	T46.5X1	T46.5X2	T46.5X3	T46.5X4	T46.5X5	T46.5X6
Toloxatone	T42.6X1	T42.6X2	T42.6X3	T42.6X4	T42.6X5	T42.6X6
Tolperisone	T44.3X1	T44.3X2	T44.3X3	T44.3X4	T44.3X5	T44.3X6
Tolserol	T42.8X1	T42.8X2	T42.8X3	T42.8X4	T42.8X5	T42.8X6
Toluene (liquid)	T52.2X1	T52.2X2	T52.2X3	T52.2X4	--	--
- diisocyanate	T65.0X1	T65.0X2	T65.0X3	T65.0X4	--	--
Toluidine	T65.891	T65.892	T65.893	T65.894	--	--
- vapor	T59.891	T59.892	T59.893	T59.894	--	--
Toluol (liquid)	T52.2X1	T52.2X2	T52.2X3	T52.2X4	--	--
- vapor	T52.2X1	T52.2X2	T52.2X3	T52.2X4	--	--
Toluylenediamine	T65.3X1	T65.3X2	T65.3X3	T65.3X4	--	--
Tolylene-2,4-diisocyanate	T65.0X1	T65.0X2	T65.0X3	T65.0X4	--	--
Tonic NEC	T50.901	T50.902	T50.903	T50.904	T50.905	T50.906
Topical action drug NEC	T49.91	T49.92	T49.93	T49.94	T49.95	T49.96
- ear, nose or throat	T49.6X1	T49.6X2	T49.6X3	T49.6X4	T49.6X5	T49.6X6
- eye	T49.5X1	T49.5X2	T49.5X3	T49.5X4	T49.5X5	T49.5X6
- skin	T49.91	T49.92	T49.93	T49.94	T49.95	T49.96
- specified NEC	T49.8X1	T49.8X2	T49.8X3	T49.8X4	T49.8X5	T49.8X6
Toquizine	T44.3X1	T44.3X2	T44.3X3	T44.3X4	T44.3X5	T44.3X6
Toremifene	T38.6X1	T38.6X2	T38.6X3	T38.6X4	T38.6X5	T38.6X6
Tosylchloramide sodium	T49.8X1	T49.8X2	T49.8X3	T49.8X4	T49.8X5	T49.8X6
Toxaphene (dust) (spray)	T60.1X1	T60.1X2	T60.1X3	T60.1X4	--	--
Toxin, diphtheria (Schick Test)	T50.8X1	T50.8X2	T50.8X3	T50.8X4	T50.8X5	T50.8X6
Toxoid						
- combined	T50.A21	T50.A22	T50.A23	T50.A24	T50.A25	T50.A26
- diphtheria	T50.A91	T50.A92	T50.A93	T50.A94	T50.A95	T50.A96
- tetanus	T50.A91	T50.A92	T50.A93	T50.A94	T50.A95	T50.A96
Trace element NEC	T45.8X1	T45.8X2	T45.8X3	T45.8X4	T45.8X5	T45.8X6
Tractor fuel NEC	T52.0X1	T52.0X2	T52.0X3	T52.0X4	--	--
Tragacanth	T50.991	T50.992	T50.993	T50.994	T50.995	T50.996
Tramadol	T40.4X1	T40.4X2	T40.4X3	T40.4X4	T40.4X5	T40.4X6
Tramazoline	T48.5X1	T48.5X2	T48.5X3	T48.5X4	T48.5X5	T48.5X6
Tranexamic acid	T45.621	T45.622	T45.623	T45.624	T45.625	T45.626
Tranilast	T45.0X1	T45.0X2	T45.0X3	T45.0X4	T45.0X5	T45.0X6
Tranquilizer NEC	T43.501	T43.502	T43.503	T43.504	T43.505	T43.506
- with hypnotic or sedative	T42.6X1	T42.6X2	T42.6X3	T42.6X4	T42.6X5	T42.6X6
- benzodiazepine NEC	T42.4X1	T42.4X2	T42.4X3	T42.4X4	T42.4X5	T42.4X6
- butyrophenone NEC	T43.4X1	T43.4X2	T43.4X3	T43.4X4	T43.4X5	T43.4X6
- carbamate	T43.591	T43.592	T43.593	T43.594	T43.595	T43.596
- dimethylamine	T43.3X1	T43.3X2	T43.3X3	T43.3X4	T43.3X5	T43.3X6
- ethylamine	T43.3X1	T43.3X2	T43.3X3	T43.3X4	T43.3X5	T43.3X6
- hydroxyzine	T43.591	T43.592	T43.593	T43.594	T43.595	T43.596
- major NEC	T43.501	T43.502	T43.503	T43.504	T43.505	T43.506
- penothiazine NEC	T43.3X1	T43.3X2	T43.3X3	T43.3X4	T43.3X5	T43.3X6
- phenothiazine-based	T43.3X1	T43.3X2	T43.3X3	T43.3X4	T43.3X5	T43.3X6
- piperazine NEC	T43.3X1	T43.3X2	T43.3X3	T43.3X4	T43.3X5	T43.3X6
- piperidine	T43.3X1	T43.3X2	T43.3X3	T43.3X4	T43.3X5	T43.3X6

Substance	Poisoning, Accidental (unintentional)	Poisoning, Intentional Self-harm	Poisoning, Assault	Poisoning, Undetermined	Adverse effect	Underdosing
- propylamine	T43.3X1	T43.3X2	T43.3X3	T43.3X4	T43.3X5	T43.3X6
- specified NEC	T43.591	T43.592	T43.593	T43.594	T43.595	T43.596
- thioxanthene NEC	T43.591	T43.592	T43.593	T43.594	T43.595	T43.596
Tranxene	T42.4X1	T42.4X2	T42.4X3	T42.4X4	T42.4X5	T42.4X6
Tranylcypromine	T43.1X1	T43.1X2	T43.1X3	T43.1X4	T43.1X5	T43.1X6
Trapidil	T46.3X1	T46.3X2	T46.3X3	T46.3X4	T46.3X5	T46.3X6
Trasentine	T44.3X1	T44.3X2	T44.3X3	T44.3X4	T44.3X5	T44.3X6
Travert	T50.3X1	T50.3X2	T50.3X3	T50.3X4	T50.3X5	T50.3X6
Trazodone	T43.211	T43.212	T43.213	T43.214	T43.215	T43.216
Trecator	T37.1X1	T37.1X2	T37.1X3	T37.1X4	T37.1X5	T37.1X6
Treosulfan	T45.1X1	T45.1X2	T45.1X3	T45.1X4	T45.1X5	T45.1X6
Tretamine	T45.1X1	T45.1X2	T45.1X3	T45.1X4	T45.1X5	T45.1X6
Tretinoin	T49.0X1	T49.0X2	T49.0X3	T49.0X4	T49.0X5	T49.0X6
Tretoquinol	T48.6X1	T48.6X2	T48.6X3	T48.6X4	T48.6X5	T48.6X6
Triacetin	T49.0X1	T49.0X2	T49.0X3	T49.0X4	T49.0X5	T49.0X6
Triacetoxyanthracene	T49.4X1	T49.4X2	T49.4X3	T49.4X4	T49.4X5	T49.4X6
Triacetyloleandomycin	T36.3X1	T36.3X2	T36.3X3	T36.3X4	T36.3X5	T36.3X6
Triamcinolone	T38.0X1	T38.0X2	T38.0X3	T38.0X4	T38.0X5	T38.0X6
- ENT agent	T49.6X1	T49.6X2	T49.6X3	T49.6X4	T49.6X5	T49.6X6
- hexacetonide	T49.0X1	T49.0X2	T49.0X3	T49.0X4	T49.0X5	T49.0X6
- ophthalmic preparation	T49.5X1	T49.5X2	T49.5X3	T49.5X4	T49.5X5	T49.5X6
- topical NEC	T49.0X1	T49.0X2	T49.0X3	T49.0X4	T49.0X5	T49.0X6
Triampyzine	T44.3X1	T44.3X2	T44.3X3	T44.3X4	T44.3X5	T44.3X6
Triamterene	T50.2X1	T50.2X2	T50.2X3	T50.2X4	T50.2X5	T50.2X6
Triazine (herbicide)	T60.3X1	T60.3X2	T60.3X3	T60.3X4	--	--
Triaziquone	T45.1X1	T45.1X2	T45.1X3	T45.1X4	T45.1X5	T45.1X6
Triazolam	T42.4X1	T42.4X2	T42.4X3	T42.4X4	T42.4X5	T42.4X6
Triazole (herbicide)	T60.3X1	T60.3X2	T60.3X3	T60.3X4	--	--
Tribenoside	T46.991	T46.992	T46.993	T46.994	T46.995	T46.996
Tribromacetaldehyde	T42.6X1	T42.6X2	T42.6X3	T42.6X4	T42.6X5	T42.6X6
Tribromoethanol, rectal	T41.291	T41.292	T41.293	T41.294	T41.295	T41.296
Tribromomethane	T42.6X1	T42.6X2	T42.6X3	T42.6X4	T42.6X5	T42.6X6
Trichlorethane	T53.2X1	T53.2X2	T53.2X3	T53.2X4	--	--
Trichlorethylene	T53.2X1	T53.2X2	T53.2X3	T53.2X4	--	--
Trichlorfon	T60.0X1	T60.0X2	T60.0X3	T60.0X4	--	--
Trichlormethiazide	T50.2X1	T50.2X2	T50.2X3	T50.2X4	T50.2X5	T50.2X6
Trichlormethine	T45.1X1	T45.1X2	T45.1X3	T45.1X4	T45.1X5	T45.1X6
Trichloroacetic acid, Trichloracetic acid	T54.2X1	T54.2X2	T54.2X3	T54.2X4	--	--
- medicinal	T49.4X1	T49.4X2	T49.4X3	T49.4X4	T49.4X5	T49.4X6
Trichloroethane	T53.2X1	T53.2X2	T53.2X3	T53.2X4	--	--
Trichloroethanol	T42.6X1	T42.6X2	T42.6X3	T42.6X4	T42.6X5	T42.6X6
Trichloroethyl phosphate	T42.6X1	T42.6X2	T42.6X3	T42.6X4	T42.6X5	T42.6X6
Trichloroethylene (liquid) (vapor)	T53.2X1	T53.2X2	T53.2X3	T53.2X4	--	--
- anesthetic (gas)	T41.0X1	T41.0X2	T41.0X3	T41.0X4	T41.0X5	T41.0X6
- vapor NEC	T53.2X1	T53.2X2	T53.2X3	T53.2X4	--	--
Trichlorofluoromethane NEC	T53.5X1	T53.5X2	T53.5X3	T53.5X4	--	--
Trichloronate	T60.0X1	T60.0X2	T60.0X3	T60.0X4	--	--
2,4,5-Trichlorophen-oxyacetic acid	T60.3X1	T60.3X2	T60.3X3	T60.3X4	--	--
Trichloropropane	T53.6X1	T53.6X2	T53.6X3	T53.6X4	--	--
Trichlorotriethylamine	T45.1X1	T45.1X2	T45.1X3	T45.1X4	T45.1X5	T45.1X6
Trichomonacides NEC	T37.3X1	T37.3X2	T37.3X3	T37.3X4	T37.3X5	T37.3X6
Trichomycin	T36.7X1	T36.7X2	T36.7X3	T36.7X4	T36.7X5	T36.7X6
Triclobisonium chloride	T49.0X1	T49.0X2	T49.0X3	T49.0X4	T49.0X5	T49.0X6
Triclocarban	T49.0X1	T49.0X2	T49.0X3	T49.0X4	T49.0X5	T49.0X6
Triclofos	T42.6X1	T42.6X2	T42.6X3	T42.6X4	T42.6X5	T42.6X6
Triclosan	T49.0X1	T49.0X2	T49.0X3	T49.0X4	T49.0X5	T49.0X6
Tricresyl phosphate	T65.891	T65.892	T65.893	T65.894	--	--
- solvent	T52.91	T52.92	T52.93	T52.94	--	--
Tricyclamol chloride	T44.3X1	T44.3X2	T44.3X3	T44.3X4	T44.3X5	T44.3X6

Substance	Poisoning, Accidental (unintentional)	Poisoning, Intentional Self-harm	Poisoning, Assault	Poisoning, Undetermined	Adverse effect	Underdosing
Tridesilon	T49.0X1	T49.0X2	T49.0X3	T49.0X4	T49.0X5	T49.0X6
Tridihexethyl iodide	T44.3X1	T44.3X2	T44.3X3	T44.3X4	T44.3X5	T44.3X6
Tridione	T42.2X1	T42.2X2	T42.2X3	T42.2X4	T42.2X5	T42.2X6
Trientine	T45.8X1	T45.8X2	T45.8X3	T45.8X4	T45.8X5	T45.8X6
Triethanolamine NEC	T54.3X1	T54.3X2	T54.3X3	T54.3X4	--	--
- detergent	T54.3X1	T54.3X2	T54.3X3	T54.3X4	--	--
- trinitrate (biphosphate)	T46.3X1	T46.3X2	T46.3X3	T46.3X4	T46.3X5	T46.3X6
Triethanomelamine	T45.1X1	T45.1X2	T45.1X3	T45.1X4	T45.1X5	T45.1X6
Triethylenemelamine	T45.1X1	T45.1X2	T45.1X3	T45.1X4	T45.1X5	T45.1X6
Triethylenephosphoramide	T45.1X1	T45.1X2	T45.1X3	T45.1X4	T45.1X5	T45.1X6
Triethylenethiophosphoramide	T45.1X1	T45.1X2	T45.1X3	T45.1X4	T45.1X5	T45.1X6
Trifluoperazine	T43.3X1	T43.3X2	T43.3X3	T43.3X4	T43.3X5	T43.3X6
Trifluoroethyl vinyl ether	T41.0X1	T41.0X2	T41.0X3	T41.0X4	T41.0X5	T41.0X6
Trifluperidol	T43.4X1	T43.4X2	T43.4X3	T43.4X4	T43.4X5	T43.4X6
Triflupromazine	T43.3X1	T43.3X2	T43.3X3	T43.3X4	T43.3X5	T43.3X6
Trifluridine	T37.5X1	T37.5X2	T37.5X3	T37.5X4	T37.5X5	T37.5X6
Triflusal	T45.521	T45.522	T45.523	T45.524	T45.525	T45.526
Trihexyphenidyl	T44.3X1	T44.3X2	T44.3X3	T44.3X4	T44.3X5	T44.3X6
Triiodothyronine	T38.1X1	T38.1X2	T38.1X3	T38.1X4	T38.1X5	T38.1X6
Trilene	T41.0X1	T41.0X2	T41.0X3	T41.0X4	T41.0X5	T41.0X6
Trilostane	T38.991	T38.992	T38.993	T38.994	T38.995	T38.996
Trimebutine	T44.3X1	T44.3X2	T44.3X3	T44.3X4	T44.3X5	T44.3X6
Trimecaine	T41.3X1	T41.3X2	T41.3X3	T41.3X4	T41.3X5	T41.3X6
Trimeprazine (tartrate)	T44.3X1	T44.3X2	T44.3X3	T44.3X4	T44.3X5	T44.3X6
Trimetaphan camsilate	T44.2X1	T44.2X2	T44.2X3	T44.2X4	T44.2X5	T44.2X6
Trimetazidine	T46.7X1	T46.7X2	T46.7X3	T46.7X4	T46.7X5	T46.7X6
Trimethadione	T42.2X1	T42.2X2	T42.2X3	T42.2X4	T42.2X5	T42.2X6
Trimethaphan	T44.2X1	T44.2X2	T44.2X3	T44.2X4	T44.2X5	T44.2X6
Trimethidinium	T44.2X1	T44.2X2	T44.2X3	T44.2X4	T44.2X5	T44.2X6
Trimethobenzamide	T45.0X1	T45.0X2	T45.0X3	T45.0X4	T45.0X5	T45.0X6
Trimethoprim	T37.8X1	T37.8X2	T37.8X3	T37.8X4	T37.8X5	T37.8X6
- with sulfamethoxazole	T36.8X1	T36.8X2	T36.8X3	T36.8X4	T36.8X5	T36.8X6
Trimethylcarbinol	T51.3X1	T51.3X2	T51.3X3	T51.3X4	--	--
Trimethylpsoralen	T49.3X1	T49.3X2	T49.3X3	T49.3X4	T49.3X5	T49.3X6
Trimeton	T45.0X1	T45.0X2	T45.0X3	T45.0X4	T45.0X5	T45.0X6
Trimetrexate	T45.1X1	T45.1X2	T45.1X3	T45.1X4	T45.1X5	T45.1X6
Trimipramine	T43.011	T43.012	T43.013	T43.014	T43.015	T43.016
Trimustine	T45.1X1	T45.1X2	T45.1X3	T45.1X4	T45.1X5	T45.1X6
Trinitrine	T46.3X1	T46.3X2	T46.3X3	T46.3X4	T46.3X5	T46.3X6
Trinitrobenzol	T65.3X1	T65.3X2	T65.3X3	T65.3X4	--	--
Trinitrophenol	T65.3X1	T65.3X2	T65.3X3	T65.3X4	--	--
Trinitrotoluene (fumes)	T65.3X1	T65.3X2	T65.3X3	T65.3X4	--	--
Trional	T42.6X1	T42.6X2	T42.6X3	T42.6X4	T42.6X5	T42.6X6
Triorthocresyl phosphate	T65.891	T65.892	T65.893	T65.894	--	--
Trioxide of arsenic	T57.0X1	T57.0X2	T57.0X3	T57.0X4	--	--
Trioxysalen	T49.4X1	T49.4X2	T49.4X3	T49.4X4	T49.4X5	T49.4X6
Tripamide	T50.2X1	T50.2X2	T50.2X3	T50.2X4	T50.2X5	T50.2X6
Triparanol	T46.6X1	T46.6X2	T46.6X3	T46.6X4	T46.6X5	T46.6X6
Tripelennamine	T45.0X1	T45.0X2	T45.0X3	T45.0X4	T45.0X5	T45.0X6
Triperiden	T44.3X1	T44.3X2	T44.3X3	T44.3X4	T44.3X5	T44.3X6
Triperidol	T43.4X1	T43.4X2	T43.4X3	T43.4X4	T43.4X5	T43.4X6
Triphenylphosphate	T65.891	T65.892	T65.893	T65.894	--	--
Triple						
- bromides	T42.6X1	T42.6X2	T42.6X3	T42.6X4	T42.6X5	T42.6X6
- carbonate	T47.1X1	T47.1X2	T47.1X3	T47.1X4	T47.1X5	T47.1X6
- vaccine						
- - DPT	T50.A11	T50.A12	T50.A13	T50.A14	T50.A15	T50.A16
- - including pertussis	T50.A11	T50.A12	T50.A13	T50.A14	T50.A15	T50.A16

Substance	Poisoning, Accidental (unintentional)	Poisoning, Intentional Self-harm	Poisoning, Assault	Poisoning, Undetermined	Adverse effect	Underdosing
- - MMR	T50.B91	T50.B92	T50.B93	T50.B94	T50.B95	T50.B96
Triprolidine	T45.0X1	T45.0X2	T45.0X3	T45.0X4	T45.0X5	T45.0X6
Trisodium hydrogen edetate	T50.6X1	T50.6X2	T50.6X3	T50.6X4	T50.6X5	T50.6X6
Trisoralen	T49.3X1	T49.3X2	T49.3X3	T49.3X4	T49.3X5	T49.3X6
Trisulfapyrimidines	T37.0X1	T37.0X2	T37.0X3	T37.0X4	T37.0X5	T37.0X6
Trithiozine	T44.3X1	T44.3X2	T44.3X3	T44.3X4	T44.3X5	T44.3X6
Tritiozine	T44.3X1	T44.3X2	T44.3X3	T44.3X4	T44.3X5	T44.3X6
Tritoqualine	T45.0X1	T45.0X2	T45.0X3	T45.0X4	T45.0X5	T45.0X6
Trofosfamide	T45.1X1	T45.1X2	T45.1X3	T45.1X4	T45.1X5	T45.1X6
Troleandomycin	T36.3X1	T36.3X2	T36.3X3	T36.3X4	T36.3X5	T36.3X6
Trolnitrate (phosphate)	T46.3X1	T46.3X2	T46.3X3	T46.3X4	T46.3X5	T46.3X6
Tromantadine	T37.5X1	T37.5X2	T37.5X3	T37.5X4	T37.5X5	T37.5X6
Trometamol	T50.2X1	T50.2X2	T50.2X3	T50.2X4	T50.2X5	T50.2X6
Tromethamine	T50.2X1	T50.2X2	T50.2X3	T50.2X4	T50.2X5	T50.2X6
Tronothane	T41.3X1	T41.3X2	T41.3X3	T41.3X4	T41.3X5	T41.3X6
Tropacine	T44.3X1	T44.3X2	T44.3X3	T44.3X4	T44.3X5	T44.3X6
Tropatepine	T44.3X1	T44.3X2	T44.3X3	T44.3X4	T44.3X5	T44.3X6
Tropicamide	T44.3X1	T44.3X2	T44.3X3	T44.3X4	T44.3X5	T44.3X6
Trospium chloride	T44.3X1	T44.3X2	T44.3X3	T44.3X4	T44.3X5	T44.3X6
Troxerutin	T46.991	T46.992	T46.993	T46.994	T46.995	T46.996
Troxidone	T42.2X1	T42.2X2	T42.2X3	T42.2X4	T42.2X5	T42.2X6
Tryparsamide	T37.3X1	T37.3X2	T37.3X3	T37.3X4	T37.3X5	T37.3X6
Trypsin	T45.3X1	T45.3X2	T45.3X3	T45.3X4	T45.3X5	T45.3X6
Tryptizol	T43.011	T43.012	T43.013	T43.014	T43.015	T43.016
TSH	T38.811	T38.812	T38.813	T38.814	T38.815	T38.816
Tuaminoheptane	T48.5X1	T48.5X2	T48.5X3	T48.5X4	T48.5X5	T48.5X6
Tuberculin, purified protein derivative (PPD)	T50.8X1	T50.8X2	T50.8X3	T50.8X4	T50.8X5	T50.8X6
Tubocurare	T48.1X1	T48.1X2	T48.1X3	T48.1X4	T48.1X5	T48.1X6
Tubocurarine (chloride)	T48.1X1	T48.1X2	T48.1X3	T48.1X4	T48.1X5	T48.1X6
Tulobuterol	T48.6X1	T48.6X2	T48.6X3	T48.6X4	T48.6X5	T48.6X6
Turpentine (spirits of)	T52.8X1	T52.8X2	T52.8X3	T52.8X4	--	--
- vapor	T52.8X1	T52.8X2	T52.8X3	T52.8X4	--	--
Tybamate	T43.591	T43.592	T43.593	T43.594	T43.595	T43.596
Tyloxapol	T48.4X1	T48.4X2	T48.4X3	T48.4X4	T48.4X5	T48.4X6
Tymazoline	T48.5X1	T48.5X2	T48.5X3	T48.5X4	T48.5X5	T48.5X6
Typhoid-paratyphoid vaccine	T50.A91	T50.A92	T50.A93	T50.A94	T50.A95	T50.A96
Typhus vaccine	T50.A91	T50.A92	T50.A93	T50.A94	T50.A95	T50.A96
Tyropanoate	T50.8X1	T50.8X2	T50.8X3	T50.8X4	T50.8X5	T50.8X6
Tyrothricin	T49.6X1	T49.6X2	T49.6X3	T49.6X4	T49.6X5	T49.6X6
- ENT agent	T49.6X1	T49.6X2	T49.6X3	T49.6X4	T49.6X5	T49.6X6
- ophthalmic preparation	T49.5X1	T49.5X2	T49.5X3	T49.5X4	T49.5X5	T49.5X6
Ufenamate	T39.391	T39.392	T39.393	T39.394	T39.395	T39.396
Ultraviolet light protectant	T49.3X1	T49.3X2	T49.3X3	T49.3X4	T49.3X5	T49.3X6
Undecenoic acid	T49.0X1	T49.0X2	T49.0X3	T49.0X4	T49.0X5	T49.0X6
Undecoylium	T49.0X1	T49.0X2	T49.0X3	T49.0X4	T49.0X5	T49.0X6
Undecylenic acid (derivatives)	T49.0X1	T49.0X2	T49.0X3	T49.0X4	T49.0X5	T49.0X6
Unna's boot	T49.3X1	T49.3X2	T49.3X3	T49.3X4	T49.3X5	T49.3X6
Unsaturated fatty acid	T46.6X1	T46.6X2	T46.6X3	T46.6X4	T46.6X5	T46.6X6
Uracil mustard	T45.1X1	T45.1X2	T45.1X3	T45.1X4	T45.1X5	T45.1X6
Uramustine	T45.1X1	T45.1X2	T45.1X3	T45.1X4	T45.1X5	T45.1X6
Urapidil	T46.5X1	T46.5X2	T46.5X3	T46.5X4	T46.5X5	T46.5X6
Urari	T48.1X1	T48.1X2	T48.1X3	T48.1X4	T48.1X5	T48.1X6
Urate oxidase	T50.4X1	T50.4X2	T50.4X3	T50.4X4	T50.4X5	T50.4X6
Urea	T47.3X1	T47.3X2	T47.3X3	T47.3X4	T47.3X5	T47.3X6
- peroxide	T49.0X1	T49.0X2	T49.0X3	T49.0X4	T49.0X5	T49.0X6
- stibamine	T37.4X1	T37.4X2	T37.4X3	T37.4X4	T37.4X5	T37.4X6
- topical	T49.8X1	T49.8X2	T49.8X3	T49.8X4	T49.8X5	T49.8X6
Urethane	T45.1X1	T45.1X2	T45.1X3	T45.1X4	T45.1X5	T45.1X6

Substance	Poisoning, Accidental (unintentional)	Poisoning, Intentional Self-harm	Poisoning, Assault	Poisoning, Undetermined	Adverse effect	Underdosing
Urginea (maritima) (scilla) —see Squill						
Uric acid metabolism drug NEC	T50.4X1	T50.4X2	T50.4X3	T50.4X4	T50.4X5	T50.4X6
Uricosuric agent	T50.4X1	T50.4X2	T50.4X3	T50.4X4	T50.4X5	T50.4X6
Urinary anti-infective	T37.8X1	T37.8X2	T37.8X3	T37.8X4	T37.8X5	T37.8X6
Urofollitropin	T38.811	T38.812	T38.813	T38.814	T38.815	T38.816
Urokinase	T45.611	T45.612	T45.613	T45.614	T45.615	T45.616
Urokon	T50.8X1	T50.8X2	T50.8X3	T50.8X4	T50.8X5	T50.8X6
Ursodeoxycholic acid	T50.991	T50.992	T50.993	T50.994	T50.995	T50.996
Ursodiol	T50.991	T50.992	T50.993	T50.994	T50.995	T50.996
Urtica	T62.2X1	T62.2X2	T62.2X3	T62.2X4	--	--
Utility gas—see Gas, utility						
Vaccine NEC	T50.Z91	T50.Z92	T50.Z93	T50.Z94	T50.Z95	T50.Z96
- antineoplastic	T50.Z91	T50.Z92	T50.Z93	T50.Z94	T50.Z95	T50.Z96
- bacterial NEC	T50.A91	T50.A92	T50.A93	T50.A94	T50.A95	T50.A96
- - with						
- - - other bacterial component	T50.A21	T50.A22	T50.A23	T50.A24	T50.A25	T50.A26
- - - pertussis component	T50.A11	T50.A12	T50.A13	T50.A14	T50.A15	T50.A16
- - - viral-rickettsial component	T50.A21	T50.A22	T50.A23	T50.A24	T50.A25	T50.A26
- - mixed NEC	T50.A21	T50.A22	T50.A23	T50.A24	T50.A25	T50.A26
- BCG	T50.A91	T50.A92	T50.A93	T50.A94	T50.A95	T50.A96
- cholera	T50.A91	T50.A92	T50.A93	T50.A94	T50.A95	T50.A96
- diphtheria	T50.A91	T50.A92	T50.A93	T50.A94	T50.A95	T50.A96
- - with tetanus	T50.A21	T50.A22	T50.A23	T50.A24	T50.A25	T50.A26
- - - and pertussis	T50.A11	T50.A12	T50.A13	T50.A14	T50.A15	T50.A16
- influenza	T50.B91	T50.B92	T50.B93	T50.B94	T50.B95	T50.B96
- measles	T50.B91	T50.B92	T50.B93	T50.B94	T50.B95	T50.B96
- - with mumps and rubella	T50.B91	T50.B92	T50.B93	T50.B94	T50.B95	T50.B96
- meningococcal	T50.A91	T50.A92	T50.A93	T50.A94	T50.A95	T50.A96
- mumps	T50.B91	T50.B92	T50.B93	T50.B94	T50.B95	T50.B96
- paratyphoid	T50.A91	T50.A92	T50.A93	T50.A94	T50.A95	T50.A96
- pertussis	T50.A11	T50.A12	T50.A13	T50.A14	T50.A15	T50.A16
- - with diphtheria	T50.A11	T50.A12	T50.A13	T50.A14	T50.A15	T50.A16
- - - and tetanus	T50.A11	T50.A12	T50.A13	T50.A14	T50.A15	T50.A16
- - with other component	T50.A11	T50.A12	T50.A13	T50.A14	T50.A15	T50.A16
- plague	T50.A91	T50.A92	T50.A93	T50.A94	T50.A95	T50.A96
- poliomyelitis	T50.B91	T50.B92	T50.B93	T50.B94	T50.B95	T50.B96
- poliovirus	T50.B91	T50.B92	T50.B93	T50.B94	T50.B95	T50.B96
- rabies	T50.B91	T50.B92	T50.B93	T50.B94	T50.B95	T50.B96
- respiratory syncytial virus	T50.B91	T50.B92	T50.B93	T50.B94	T50.B95	T50.B96
- rickettsial NEC	T50.A91	T50.A92	T50.A93	T50.A94	T50.A95	T50.A96
- - with						
- - - bacterial component	T50.A21	T50.A22	T50.A23	T50.A24	T50.A25	T50.A26
- Rocky Mountain spotted fever	T50.A91	T50.A92	T50.A93	T50.A94	T50.A95	T50.A96
- rubella	T50.B91	T50.B92	T50.B93	T50.B94	T50.B95	T50.B96
- sabin oral	T50.B91	T50.B92	T50.B93	T50.B94	T50.B95	T50.B96
- smallpox	T50.B11	T50.B12	T50.B13	T50.B14	T50.B15	T50.B16
- TAB	T50.A91	T50.A92	T50.A93	T50.A94	T50.A95	T50.A96
- tetanus	T50.A91	T50.A92	T50.A93	T50.A94	T50.A95	T50.A96
- typhoid	T50.A91	T50.A92	T50.A93	T50.A94	T50.A95	T50.A96
- typhus	T50.A91	T50.A92	T50.A93	T50.A94	T50.A95	T50.A96
- viral NEC	T50.B91	T50.B92	T50.B93	T50.B94	T50.B95	T50.B96
- yellow fever	T50.B91	T50.B92	T50.B93	T50.B94	T50.B95	T50.B96
Vaccinia immune globulin	T50.Z11	T50.Z12	T50.Z13	T50.Z14	T50.Z15	T50.Z16
Vaginal contraceptives	T49.8X1	T49.8X2	T49.8X3	T49.8X4	T49.8X5	T49.8X6
Valerian						
- root	T42.6X1	T42.6X2	T42.6X3	T42.6X4	T42.6X5	T42.6X6
- tincture	T42.6X1	T42.6X2	T42.6X3	T42.6X4	T42.6X5	T42.6X6
Valethamate bromide	T44.3X1	T44.3X2	T44.3X3	T44.3X4	T44.3X5	T44.3X6

Substance	Poisoning, Accidental (unintentional)	Poisoning, Intentional Self-harm	Poisoning, Assault	Poisoning, Undetermined	Adverse effect	Underdosing
Valisone	T49.0X1	T49.0X2	T49.0X3	T49.0X4	T49.0X5	T49.0X6
Valium	T42.4X1	T42.4X2	T42.4X3	T42.4X4	T42.4X5	T42.4X6
Valmid	T42.6X1	T42.6X2	T42.6X3	T42.6X4	T42.6X5	T42.6X6
Valnoctamide	T42.6X1	T42.6X2	T42.6X3	T42.6X4	T42.6X5	T42.6X6
Valproate (sodium)	T42.6X1	T42.6X2	T42.6X3	T42.6X4	T42.6X5	T42.6X6
Valproic acid	T42.6X1	T42.6X2	T42.6X3	T42.6X4	T42.6X5	T42.6X6
Valpromide	T42.6X1	T42.6X2	T42.6X3	T42.6X4	T42.6X5	T42.6X6
Vanadium	T56.891	T56.892	T56.893	T56.894	--	--
Vancomycin	T36.8X1	T36.8X2	T36.8X3	T36.8X4	T36.8X5	T36.8X6
Vapor—see also Gas	T59.91	T59.92	T59.93	T59.94	--	--
- kiln (carbon monoxide)	T58.8X1	T58.8X2	T58.8X3	T58.8X4	--	--
- lead—see lead						
- specified source NEC	T59.891	T59.892	T59.893	T59.894	--	--
Vardenafil	T46.7X1	T46.7X2	T46.7X3	T46.7X4	T46.7X5	T46.7X6
Varicose reduction drug	T46.8X1	T46.8X2	T46.8X3	T46.8X4	T46.8X5	T46.8X6
Varnish	T65.4X1	T65.4X2	T65.4X3	T65.4X4	--	--
- cleaner	T52.91	T52.92	T52.93	T52.94	--	--
Vaseline	T49.3X1	T49.3X2	T49.3X3	T49.3X4	T49.3X5	T49.3X6
Vasodilan	T46.7X1	T46.7X2	T46.7X3	T46.7X4	T46.7X5	T46.7X6
Vasodilator						
- coronary NEC	T46.3X1	T46.3X2	T46.3X3	T46.3X4	T46.3X5	T46.3X6
- peripheral NEC	T46.7X1	T46.7X2	T46.7X3	T46.7X4	T46.7X5	T46.7X6
Vasopressin	T38.891	T38.892	T38.893	T38.894	T38.895	T38.896
Vasopressor drugs	T38.891	T38.892	T38.893	T38.894	T38.895	T38.896
Vecuronium bromide	T48.1X1	T48.1X2	T48.1X3	T48.1X4	T48.1X5	T48.1X6
Vegetable extract, astringent	T49.2X1	T49.2X2	T49.2X3	T49.2X4	T49.2X5	T49.2X6
Venlafaxine	T43.211	T43.212	T43.213	T43.214	T43.215	T43.216
Venom, venomous (bite) (sting)	T63.91	T63.92	T63.93	T63.94	--	--
- amphibian NEC	T63.831	T63.832	T63.833	T63.834	--	--
- animal NEC	T63.891	T63.892	T63.893	T63.894	--	--
- ant	T63.421	T63.422	T63.423	T63.424	--	--
- arthropod NEC	T63.481	T63.482	T63.483	T63.484	--	--
- bee	T63.441	T63.442	T63.443	T63.444	--	--
- centipede	T63.411	T63.412	T63.413	T63.414	--	--
- fish	T63.591	T63.592	T63.593	T63.594	--	--
- frog	T63.811	T63.812	T63.813	T63.814	--	--
- hornet	T63.451	T63.452	T63.453	T63.454	--	--
- insect NEC	T63.481	T63.482	T63.483	T63.484	--	--
- lizard	T63.121	T63.122	T63.123	T63.124	--	--
- marine						
- - animals	T63.691	T63.692	T63.693	T63.694	--	--
- - - bluebottle	T63.611	T63.612	T63.613	T63.614	--	--
- - - jellyfish NEC	T63.621	T63.622	T63.623	T63.624	--	--
- - - Portugese Man-o-war	T63.611	T63.612	T63.613	T63.614	--	--
- - - sea anemone	T63.631	T63.632	T63.633	T63.634	--	--
- - - specified NEC	T63.691	T63.692	T63.693	T63.694	--	--
- - fish	T63.591	T63.592	T63.593	T63.594	--	--
- - plants	T63.711	T63.712	T63.713	T63.714	--	--
- - sting ray	T63.511	T63.512	T63.513	T63.514	--	--
- millipede (tropical)	T63.411	T63.412	T63.413	T63.414	--	--
- plant NEC	T63.791	T63.792	T63.793	T63.794	--	--
- - marine	T63.711	T63.712	T63.713	T63.714	--	--
- reptile	T63.191	T63.192	T63.193	T63.194	--	--
- - gila monster	T63.111	T63.112	T63.113	T63.114	--	--
- - lizard NEC	T63.121	T63.122	T63.123	T63.124	--	--
- scorpion	T63.2X1	T63.2X2	T63.2X3	T63.2X4	--	--
- snake	T63.001	T63.002	T63.003	T63.004	--	--
- - African NEC	T63.081	T63.082	T63.083	T63.084	--	--
- - American (North) (South) NEC	T63.061	T63.062	T63.063	T63.064	--	--

Substance	Poisoning, Accidental (unintentional)	Poisoning, Intentional Self-harm	Poisoning, Assault	Poisoning, Undetermined	Adverse effect	Underdosing
- - Asian	T63.081	T63.082	T63.083	T63.084	--	--
- - Australian	T63.071	T63.072	T63.073	T63.074	--	--
- - cobra	T63.041	T63.042	T63.043	T63.044	--	--
- - coral snake	T63.021	T63.022	T63.023	T63.024	--	--
- - rattlesnake	T63.011	T63.012	T63.013	T63.014	--	--
- - specified NEC	T63.091	T63.092	T63.093	T63.094	--	--
- - taipan	T63.031	T63.032	T63.033	T63.034	--	--
- specified NEC	T63.891	T63.892	T63.893	T63.894	--	--
- spider	T63.301	T63.302	T63.303	T63.304	--	--
- - black widow	T63.311	T63.312	T63.313	T63.314	--	--
- - brown recluse	T63.331	T63.332	T63.333	T63.334	--	--
- - specified NEC	T63.391	T63.392	T63.393	T63.394	--	--
- - tarantula	T63.321	T63.322	T63.323	T63.324	--	--
- sting ray	T63.511	T63.512	T63.513	T63.514	--	--
- toad	T63.821	T63.822	T63.823	T63.824	--	--
- wasp	T63.461	T63.462	T63.463	T63.464	--	--
Venous sclerosing drug NEC	T46.8X1	T46.8X2	T46.8X3	T46.8X4	T46.8X5	T46.8X6
Ventolin—see Albuterol						
Veramon	T42.3X1	T42.3X2	T42.3X3	T42.3X4	T42.3X5	T42.3X6
Verapamil	T46.1X1	T46.1X2	T46.1X3	T46.1X4	T46.1X5	T46.1X6
Veratrine	T46.5X1	T46.5X2	T46.5X3	T46.5X4	T46.5X5	T46.5X6
Veratrum						
- album	T62.2X1	T62.2X2	T62.2X3	T62.2X4	--	--
- alkaloids	T46.5X1	T46.5X2	T46.5X3	T46.5X4	T46.5X5	T46.5X6
- viride	T62.2X1	T62.2X2	T62.2X3	T62.2X4	--	--
Verdigris	T60.3X1	T60.3X2	T60.3X3	T60.3X4	--	--
Veronal	T42.3X1	T42.3X2	T42.3X3	T42.3X4	T42.3X5	T42.3X6
Veroxil	T37.4X1	T37.4X2	T37.4X3	T37.4X4	T37.4X5	T37.4X6
Versenate	T50.6X1	T50.6X2	T50.6X3	T50.6X4	T50.6X5	T50.6X6
Versidyne	T39.8X1	T39.8X2	T39.8X3	T39.8X4	T39.8X5	T39.8X6
Vetrabutine	T48.0X1	T48.0X2	T48.0X3	T48.0X4	T48.0X5	T48.0X6
Vidarabine	T37.5X1	T37.5X2	T37.5X3	T37.5X4	T37.5X5	T37.5X6
Vienna						
- green	T57.0X1	T57.0X2	T57.0X3	T57.0X4	--	--
- - insecticide	T60.2X1	T60.2X2	T60.2X3	T60.2X4	--	--
- red	T57.0X1	T57.0X2	T57.0X3	T57.0X4	--	--
- - pharmaceutical dye	T50.991	T50.992	T50.993	T50.994	T50.995	T50.996
Vigabatrin	T42.6X1	T42.6X2	T42.6X3	T42.6X4	T42.6X5	T42.6X6
Viloxazine	T43.291	T43.292	T43.293	T43.294	T43.295	T43.296
Viminol	T39.8X1	T39.8X2	T39.8X3	T39.8X4	T39.8X5	T39.8X6
Vinbarbital, vinbarbitone	T42.3X1	T42.3X2	T42.3X3	T42.3X4	T42.3X5	T42.3X6
Vinblastine	T45.1X1	T45.1X2	T45.1X3	T45.1X4	T45.1X5	T45.1X6
Vinburnine	T46.7X1	T46.7X2	T46.7X3	T46.7X4	T46.7X5	T46.7X6
Vincamine	T45.1X1	T45.1X2	T45.1X3	T45.1X4	T45.1X5	T45.1X6
Vincristine	T45.1X1	T45.1X2	T45.1X3	T45.1X4	T45.1X5	T45.1X6
Vindesine	T45.1X1	T45.1X2	T45.1X3	T45.1X4	T45.1X5	T45.1X6
Vinesthene, vinethene	T41.0X1	T41.0X2	T41.0X3	T41.0X4	T41.0X5	T41.0X6
Vinorelbine tartrate	T45.1X1	T45.1X2	T45.1X3	T45.1X4	T45.1X5	T45.1X6
Vinpocetine	T46.7X1	T46.7X2	T46.7X3	T46.7X4	T46.7X5	T46.7X6
Vinyl						
- acetate	T65.891	T65.892	T65.893	T65.894	--	--
- bital	T42.3X1	T42.3X2	T42.3X3	T42.3X4	T42.3X5	T42.3X6
- bromide	T65.891	T65.892	T65.893	T65.894	--	--
- chloride	T59.891	T59.892	T59.893	T59.894	--	--
- ether	T41.0X1	T41.0X2	T41.0X3	T41.0X4	T41.0X5	T41.0X6
Vinylbital	T42.3X1	T42.3X2	T42.3X3	T42.3X4	T42.3X5	T42.3X6
Vinylidene chloride	T65.891	T65.892	T65.893	T65.894	--	--
Vioform	T37.8X1	T37.8X2	T37.8X3	T37.8X4	T37.8X5	T37.8X6

Substance	Poisoning, Accidental (unintentional)	Poisoning, Intentional Self-harm	Poisoning, Assault	Poisoning, Undetermined	Adverse effect	Underdosing
- topical	T49.0X1	T49.0X2	T49.0X3	T49.0X4	T49.0X5	T49.0X6
Viomycin	T36.8X1	T36.8X2	T36.8X3	T36.8X4	T36.8X5	T36.8X6
Viosterol	T45.2X1	T45.2X2	T45.2X3	T45.2X4	T45.2X5	T45.2X6
Viper (venom)	T63.091	T63.092	T63.093	T63.094	--	--
Viprynium	T37.4X1	T37.4X2	T37.4X3	T37.4X4	T37.4X5	T37.4X6
Viquidil	T46.7X1	T46.7X2	T46.7X3	T46.7X4	T46.7X5	T46.7X6
Viral vaccine NEC	T50.B91	T50.B92	T50.B93	T50.B94	T50.B95	T50.B96
Virginiamycin	T36.8X1	T36.8X2	T36.8X3	T36.8X4	T36.8X5	T36.8X6
Virugon	T37.5X1	T37.5X2	T37.5X3	T37.5X4	T37.5X5	T37.5X6
Viscous agent	T50.901	T50.902	T50.903	T50.904	T50.905	T50.906
Visine	T49.5X1	T49.5X2	T49.5X3	T49.5X4	T49.5X5	T49.5X6
Visnadine	T46.3X1	T46.3X2	T46.3X3	T46.3X4	T46.3X5	T46.3X6
Vitamin NEC	T45.2X1	T45.2X2	T45.2X3	T45.2X4	T45.2X5	T45.2X6
- A	T45.2X1	T45.2X2	T45.2X3	T45.2X4	T45.2X5	T45.2X6
- B NEC	T45.2X1	T45.2X2	T45.2X3	T45.2X4	T45.2X5	T45.2X6
- - nicotinic acid	T46.7X1	T46.7X2	T46.7X3	T46.7X4	T46.7X5	T46.7X6
- B1	T45.2X1	T45.2X2	T45.2X3	T45.2X4	T45.2X5	T45.2X6
- B2	T45.2X1	T45.2X2	T45.2X3	T45.2X4	T45.2X5	T45.2X6
- B6	T45.2X1	T45.2X2	T45.2X3	T45.2X4	T45.2X5	T45.2X6
- B12	T45.2X1	T45.2X2	T45.2X3	T45.2X4	T45.2X5	T45.2X6
- B15	T45.2X1	T45.2X2	T45.2X3	T45.2X4	T45.2X5	T45.2X6
- C	T45.2X1	T45.2X2	T45.2X3	T45.2X4	T45.2X5	T45.2X6
- D	T45.2X1	T45.2X2	T45.2X3	T45.2X4	T45.2X5	T45.2X6
- D2	T45.2X1	T45.2X2	T45.2X3	T45.2X4	T45.2X5	T45.2X6
- D3	T45.2X1	T45.2X2	T45.2X3	T45.2X4	T45.2X5	T45.2X6
- E	T45.2X1	T45.2X2	T45.2X3	T45.2X4	T45.2X5	T45.2X6
- E acetate	T45.2X1	T45.2X2	T45.2X3	T45.2X4	T45.2X5	T45.2X6
- hematopoietic	T45.8X1	T45.8X2	T45.8X3	T45.8X4	T45.8X5	T45.8X6
- K NEC	T45.7X1	T45.7X2	T45.7X3	T45.7X4	T45.7X5	T45.7X6
- K1	T45.7X1	T45.7X2	T45.7X3	T45.7X4	T45.7X5	T45.7X6
- K2	T45.7X1	T45.7X2	T45.7X3	T45.7X4	T45.7X5	T45.7X6
- PP	T45.2X1	T45.2X2	T45.2X3	T45.2X4	T45.2X5	T45.2X6
- ulceroprotectant	T47.1X1	T47.1X2	T47.1X3	T47.1X4	T47.1X5	T47.1X6
Vleminckx's solution	T49.4X1	T49.4X2	T49.4X3	T49.4X4	T49.4X5	T49.4X6
Voltaren—see Diclofenac sodium						
Warfarin	T45.511	T45.512	T45.513	T45.514	T45.515	T45.516
- rodenticide	T60.4X1	T60.4X2	T60.4X3	T60.4X4	--	--
- sodium	T45.511	T45.512	T45.513	T45.514	T45.515	T45.516
Wasp (sting)	T63.461	T63.462	T63.463	T63.464	--	--
Water						
- balance drug	T50.3X1	T50.3X2	T50.3X3	T50.3X4	T50.3X5	T50.3X6
- distilled	T50.3X1	T50.3X2	T50.3X3	T50.3X4	T50.3X5	T50.3X6
- gas—see Gas, water						
- - incomplete combustion of—see Carbon, monoxide, fuel, utility						
- hemlock	T62.2X1	T62.2X2	T62.2X3	T62.2X4	--	--
- moccasin (venom)	T63.061	T63.062	T63.063	T63.064	--	--
- purified	T50.3X1	T50.3X2	T50.3X3	T50.3X4	T50.3X5	T50.3X6
Wax (paraffin) (petroleum)	T52.0X1	T52.0X2	T52.0X3	T52.0X4	--	--
- automobile	T65.891	T65.892	T65.893	T65.894	--	--
- floor	T52.0X1	T52.0X2	T52.0X3	T52.0X4	--	--
Weed killers NEC	T60.3X1	T60.3X2	T60.3X3	T60.3X4	--	--
Welldorm	T42.6X1	T42.6X2	T42.6X3	T42.6X4	T42.6X5	T42.6X6
White						
- arsenic	T57.0X1	T57.0X2	T57.0X3	T57.0X4	--	--
- hellebore	T62.2X1	T62.2X2	T62.2X3	T62.2X4	--	--
- lotion (keratolytic)	T49.4X1	T49.4X2	T49.4X3	T49.4X4	T49.4X5	T49.4X6
- spirit	T52.0X1	T52.0X2	T52.0X3	T52.0X4	--	--
Whitewash	T65.891	T65.892	T65.893	T65.894	--	--

Substance	Poisoning, Accidental (unintentional)	Poisoning, Intentional Self-harm	Poisoning, Assault	Poisoning, Undetermined	Adverse effect	Underdosing
Whole blood (human)	T45.8X1	T45.8X2	T45.8X3	T45.8X4	T45.8X5	T45.8X6
Wild						
- black cherry	T62.2X1	T62.2X2	T62.2X3	T62.2X4	--	--
- poisonous plants NEC	T62.2X1	T62.2X2	T62.2X3	T62.2X4	--	--
Window cleaning fluid	T65.891	T65.892	T65.893	T65.894	--	--
Wintergreen (oil)	T49.3X1	T49.3X2	T49.3X3	T49.3X4	T49.3X5	T49.3X6
Wisterine	T62.2X1	T62.2X2	T62.2X3	T62.2X4	--	--
Witch hazel	T49.2X1	T49.2X2	T49.2X3	T49.2X4	T49.2X5	T49.2X6
Wood alcohol or spirit	T51.1X1	T51.1X2	T51.1X3	T51.1X4	--	--
Wool fat (hydrous)	T49.3X1	T49.3X2	T49.3X3	T49.3X4	T49.3X5	T49.3X6
Woorali	T48.1X1	T48.1X2	T48.1X3	T48.1X4	T48.1X5	T48.1X6
Wormseed, American	T37.4X1	T37.4X2	T37.4X3	T37.4X4	T37.4X5	T37.4X6
Xamoterol	T44.5X1	T44.5X2	T44.5X3	T44.5X4	T44.5X5	T44.5X6
Xanthine diuretics	T50.2X1	T50.2X2	T50.2X3	T50.2X4	T50.2X5	T50.2X6
Xanthinol nicotinate	T46.7X1	T46.7X2	T46.7X3	T46.7X4	T46.7X5	T46.7X6
Xanthotoxin	T49.3X1	T49.3X2	T49.3X3	T49.3X4	T49.3X5	T49.3X6
Xanthinol nicotinate	T46.7X1	T46.7X2	T46.7X3	T46.7X4	T46.7X5	T46.7X6
Xantocillin	T36.0X1	T36.0X2	T36.0X3	T36.0X4	T36.0X5	T36.0X6
Xenon (127Xe) (133Xe)	T50.8X1	T50.8X2	T50.8X3	T50.8X4	T50.8X5	T50.8X6
Xenysalate	T49.4X1	T49.4X2	T49.4X3	T49.4X4	T49.4X5	T49.4X6
Xibornol	T37.8X1	T37.8X2	T37.8X3	T37.8X4	T37.8X5	T37.8X6
Xigris	T45.511	T45.512	T45.513	T45.514	T45.515	T45.516
Xipamide	T50.2X1	T50.2X2	T50.2X3	T50.2X4	T50.2X5	T50.2X6
Xylene (vapor)	T52.2X1	T52.2X2	T52.2X3	T52.2X4	--	--
Xylocaine (infiltration) (topical)	T41.3X1	T41.3X2	T41.3X3	T41.3X4	T41.3X5	T41.3X6
- nerve block (peripheral) (plexus)	T41.3X1	T41.3X2	T41.3X3	T41.3X4	T41.3X5	T41.3X6
- spinal	T41.3X1	T41.3X2	T41.3X3	T41.3X4	T41.3X5	T41.3X6
Xylol (vapor)	T52.2X1	T52.2X2	T52.2X3	T52.2X4	--	--
Xylometazoline	T48.5X1	T48.5X2	T48.5X3	T48.5X4	T48.5X5	T48.5X6
Yeast	T45.2X1	T45.2X2	T45.2X3	T45.2X4	T45.2X5	T45.2X6
- dried	T45.2X1	T45.2X2	T45.2X3	T45.2X4	T45.2X5	T45.2X6
Yellow						
- fever vaccine	T50.B91	T50.B92	T50.B93	T50.B94	T50.B95	T50.B96
- jasmine	T62.2X1	T62.2X2	T62.2X3	T62.2X4	--	--
- phenolphthalein	T47.2X1	T47.2X2	T47.2X3	T47.2X4	T47.2X5	T47.2X6
Yew	T62.2X1	T62.2X2	T62.2X3	T62.2X4	--	--
Yohimbic acid	T40.991	T40.992	T40.993	T40.994	T40.995	T40.996
Zactane	T39.8X1	T39.8X2	T39.8X3	T39.8X4	T39.8X5	T39.8X6
Zalcitabine	T37.5X1	T37.5X2	T37.5X3	T37.5X4	T37.5X5	T37.5X6
Zaroxolyn	T50.2X1	T50.2X2	T50.2X3	T50.2X4	T50.2X5	T50.2X6
Zephiran (topical)	T49.0X1	T49.0X2	T49.0X3	T49.0X4	T49.0X5	T49.0X6
- ophthalmic preparation	T49.5X1	T49.5X2	T49.5X3	T49.5X4	T49.5X5	T49.5X6
Zeranol	T38.7X1	T38.7X2	T38.7X3	T38.7X4	T38.7X5	T38.7X6
Zerone	T51.1X1	T51.1X2	T51.1X3	T51.1X4	--	--
Zidovudine	T37.5X1	T37.5X2	T37.5X3	T37.5X4	T37.5X5	T37.5X6
Zimeldine	T43.221	T43.222	T43.223	T43.224	T43.225	T43.226
Zinc (compounds) (fumes) (vapor) NEC	T56.5X1	T56.5X2	T56.5X3	T56.5X4	--	--
- anti-infectives	T49.0X1	T49.0X2	T49.0X3	T49.0X4	T49.0X5	T49.0X6
- antivaricose	T46.8X1	T46.8X2	T46.8X3	T46.8X4	T46.8X5	T46.8X6
- bacitracin	T49.0X1	T49.0X2	T49.0X3	T49.0X4	T49.0X5	T49.0X6
- chloride (mouthwash)	T49.6X1	T49.6X2	T49.6X3	T49.6X4	T49.6X5	T49.6X6
- chromate	T56.5X1	T56.5X2	T56.5X3	T56.5X4	--	--
- gelatin	T49.3X1	T49.3X2	T49.3X3	T49.3X4	T49.3X5	T49.3X6
- oxide	T49.3X1	T49.3X2	T49.3X3	T49.3X4	T49.3X5	T49.3X6
- - plaster	T49.3X1	T49.3X2	T49.3X3	T49.3X4	T49.3X5	T49.3X6
- peroxide	T49.0X1	T49.0X2	T49.0X3	T49.0X4	T49.0X5	T49.0X6
- pesticides	T56.5X1	T56.5X2	T56.5X3	T56.5X4	--	--
- phosphide	T60.4X1	T60.4X2	T60.4X3	T60.4X4	--	--

Substance	Poisoning, Accidental (unintentional)	Poisoning, Intentional Self-harm	Poisoning, Assault	Poisoning, Undetermined	Adverse effect	Underdosing
- pyrithionate	T49.4X1	T49.4X2	T49.4X3	T49.4X4	T49.4X5	T49.4X6
- stearate	T49.3X1	T49.3X2	T49.3X3	T49.3X4	T49.3X5	T49.3X6
- sulfate	T49.5X1	T49.5X2	T49.5X3	T49.5X4	T49.5X5	T49.5X6
- - ENT agent	T49.6X1	T49.6X2	T49.6X3	T49.6X4	T49.6X5	T49.6X6
- - ophthalmic solution	T49.5X1	T49.5X2	T49.5X3	T49.5X4	T49.5X5	T49.5X6
- - topical NEC	T49.0X1	T49.0X2	T49.0X3	T49.0X4	T49.0X5	T49.0X6
- undecylenate	T49.0X1	T49.0X2	T49.0X3	T49.0X4	T49.0X5	T49.0X6
Zineb	T60.0X1	T60.0X2	T60.0X3	T60.0X4	--	--
Zinostatin	T45.1X1	T45.1X2	T45.1X3	T45.1X4	T45.1X5	T45.1X6
Zipeprol	T48.3X1	T48.3X2	T48.3X3	T48.3X4	T48.3X5	T48.3X6
Zofenopril	T46.4X1	T46.4X2	T46.4X3	T46.4X4	T46.4X5	T46.4X6
Zolpidem	T42.6X1	T42.6X2	T42.6X3	T42.6X4	T42.6X5	T42.6X6
Zomepirac	T39.391	T39.392	T39.393	T39.394	T39.395	T39.396
Zopiclone	T42.6X1	T42.6X2	T42.6X3	T42.6X4	T42.6X5	T42.6X6
Zorubicin	T45.1X1	T45.1X2	T45.1X3	T45.1X4	T45.1X5	T45.1X6
Zotepine	T43.591	T43.592	T43.593	T43.594	T43.595	T43.596
Zovant	T45.511	T45.512	T45.513	T45.514	T45.515	T45.516
Zoxazolamine	T42.8X1	T42.8X2	T42.8X3	T42.8X4	T42.8X5	T42.8X6
Zuclopenthixol	T43.4X1	T43.4X2	T43.4X3	T43.4X4	T43.4X5	T43.4X6
Zygadenus (venenosus)	T62.2X1	T62.2X2	T62.2X3	T62.2X4	--	--
Zyprexa	T43.591	T43.592	T43.593	T43.594	T43.595	T43.596

Abandonment (causing exposure to weather conditions) (with intent to injure or kill) NEC X58 Abuse (adult) (child) (mental) (physical) (sexual) X58

Accident (to) X58

aircraft (in transit) (powered) -see also Accident, transport, aircraft

   due to, caused by cataclysm -see Forces of nature, by type

animal-rider -see Accident, transport, animal-rider

animal-drawn vehicle -see Accident, transport, animal-drawn vehicle occupant

automobile -see Accident, transport, car occupant

bare foot water skier V94.4

boat, boating -see also Accident, watercraft

   striking swimmer

      powered V94.11

      unpowered V94.12

bus -see Accident, transport, bus occupant

cable car, not on rails V98.0

   on rails -see Accident, transport, streetcar occupant

car -see Accident, transport, car occupant

caused by, due to

   animal NEC W64

   chain hoist W24.0

   cold (excessive) -see Exposure, cold

   corrosive liquid, substance -see Table of Drugs and Chemicals

   cutting or piercing instrument -see Contact, with, by type of instrument

   drive belt W24.0

   electric

      current -see Exposure, electric current

      motor -see also Contact, with, by type of machine W31.3

         current (of) W86.8

   environmental factor NEC X58

   explosive material -see Explosion

   fire, flames -see Exposure, fire

   firearm missile -see Discharge, firearm by type

   heat (excessive) -see Heat

   hot -see Contact, with, hot

   ignition -see Ignition

   lifting device W24.0

   lightning -see subcategory T75.0

      causing fire -see Exposure, fire

   machine, machinery -see Contact, with, by type of machine

   natural factor NEC X58

   pulley (block) W24.0

   radiation -see Radiation

   steam X13.1

      inhalation X13.0

      pipe X16

   thunderbolt -see subcategory T75.0

      causing fire -see Exposure, fire

   transmission device W24.1

coach -see Accident, transport, bus occupant

coal car -see Accident, transport, industrial vehicle occupant

diving -see also Fall, into, water

   with

      drowning or submersion -see Drowning

forklift -see Accident, transport, industrial vehicle occupant

heavy transport vehicle NOS -see Accident, transport, truck occupant

ice yacht V98.2

in

   medical, surgical procedure

Accident - *continued*

   as, or due to misadventure -see Misadventure

   causing an abnormal reaction or later complication without mention of misadventure -see also Complication of or following, by type of procedure Y84.9

land yacht V98.1

late effect of -see W00 X58 with 7th character S

logging car -see Accident, transport, industrial vehicle occupant

machine, machinery -see also Contact, with, by type of machine

on board watercraft V93.69

   explosion -see Explosion, in, watercraft

   fire -see Burn, on board watercraft

   powered craft V93.63

      ferry boat V93.61

      fishing boat V93.62

      jet skis V93.63

      liner V93.61

      merchant ship V93.60

      passenger ship V93.61

      sailboat V93.64

mine tram -see Accident, transport, industrial vehicle occupant

mobility scooter (motorized) -see Accident, transport, pedestrian, conveyance, specified type NEC

motor scooter -see Accident, transport, motorcyclist

motor vehicle NOS (traffic) -see also Accident, transport V89.2

   nontraffic V89.0

   three-wheeled NOS -see Accident, transport, three-wheeled motor vehicle occupant

motorcycle NOS -see Accident, transport, motorcyclist

nonmotor vehicle NOS (nontraffic) -see also Accident, transport V89.1

   traffic NOS V89.3

nontraffic (victim's mode of transport NOS) V88.9

   collision (between) V88.7

      bus and truck V88.5

      car and:

         bus V88.3

         pickup V88.2

         three-wheeled motor vehicle V88.0

         train V88.6

         truck V88.4

         two-wheeled motor vehicle V88.0

         van V88.2

      specified vehicle NEC and:

         three-wheeled motor vehicle V88.1

         two-wheeled motor vehicle V88.1

   known mode of transport -see Accident, transport, by type of vehicle

   noncollision V88.8

on board watercraft V93.89

   powered craft V93.83

      ferry boat V93.81

      fishing boat V93.82

      jet skis V93.83

      liner V93.81

      merchant ship V93.80

      passenger ship V93.81

   unpowered craft V93.88

      canoe V93.85

      inflatable V93.86

      in tow

         recreational V94.31

Accident - *continued*

      specified NEC V94.32

      kayak V93.85

      sailboat V93.84

      surf-board V93.88

      water skis V93.87

      windsurfer V93.88

parachutist V97.29

   entangled in object V97.21

   injured on landing V97.22

pedal cycle -see Accident, transport, pedal cyclist

pedestrian (on foot)

   with

      another pedestrian W51

         with fall W03

            due to ice or snow W00.0

      on pedestrian conveyance NEC V00.09

      roller skater (in-line) V00.01

      skate boarder V00.02

      transport vehicle -see Accident, transport

   on pedestrian conveyance -see Accident, transport, pedestrian, conveyance

pick-up truck or van -see Accident, transport, pickup truck occupant

quarry truck -see Accident, transport, industrial vehicle occupant

railway vehicle (any) (in motion) -see Accident, transport, railway vehicle occupant

   due to cataclysm -see Forces of nature, by type

scooter (non-motorized) -see Accident, transport, pedestrian, conveyance, scooter

sequelae of -see W00 X58 with 7th character S

skateboard -see Accident, transport, pedestrian, conveyance, skateboard

ski (ing) -see Accident, transport, pedestrian, conveyance

   lift V98.3

specified cause NEC X58

streetcar -see Accident, transport, streetcar occupant

traffic (victim's mode of transport NOS) V87.9

   collision (between) V87.7

      bus and truck V87.5

      car and:

         bus V87.3

         pickup V87.2

         three-wheeled motor vehicle V87.0

         train V87.6

         truck V87.4

         two-wheeled motor vehicle V87.0

         van V87.2

      specified vehicle NEC and:

         three-wheeled motor vehicle V87.1

         two-wheeled motor vehicle V87.1

   known mode of transport -see Accident, transport, by type of vehicle

   noncollision V87.8

transport (involving injury to) V99

   18 wheeler -see Accident, transport, truck occupant

   agricultural vehicle occupant (nontraffic) V84.9

      driver V84.5

      hanger-on V84.7

      passenger V84.6

      traffic V84.3

         driver V84.0

         hanger-on V84.2

         passenger V84.1

Accident - *continued*

  nontraffic V20.0
  animal-drawn vehicle (traffic) V26.4
    nontraffic V26.0
  bus (traffic) V24.4
    nontraffic V24.0
  car (traffic) V23.4
    nontraffic V23.0
  motor vehicle NOS (traffic) V29.40
    nontraffic V29.00
    specified type NEC (traffic) V29.49
      nontraffic V29.09
  pedal cycle (traffic) V21.4
    nontraffic V21.0
  pickup truck (traffic) V23.4
    nontraffic V23.0
  railway vehicle (traffic) V25.4
    nontraffic V25.0
  specified vehicle NEC (traffic) V26.4
    nontraffic V26.0
  stationary object (traffic) V27.4
    nontraffic V27.0
  streetcar (traffic) V26.4
    nontraffic V26.0
  three wheeled motor vehicle (traffic)
    V22.4
    nontraffic V22.0
  truck (traffic) V24.4
    nontraffic V24.0
  two wheeled motor vehicle (traffic)
    V22.4
    nontraffic V22.0
  van (traffic) V23.4
    nontraffic V23.0
  noncollision accident (traffic) V28.4
    nontraffic V28.0
  noncollision accident (traffic) V28.9
    nontraffic V28.2
    while boarding or alighting V28.3
  nontraffic V29.3
  passenger
    collision (with)
      animal (traffic) V20.5
        being ridden (traffic) V26.5
          nontraffic V26.1
        nontraffic V20.1
      animal-drawn vehicle (traffic) V26.5
        nontraffic V26.1
      bus (traffic) V24.5
        nontraffic V24.1
      car (traffic) V23.5
        nontraffic V23.1
      motor vehicle NOS (traffic) V29.50
        nontraffic V29.10
        specified type NEC (traffic) V29.59
          nontraffic V29.19
      pedal cycle (traffic) V21.5
        nontraffic V21.1
      pickup truck (traffic) V23.5
        nontraffic V23.1
      railway vehicle (traffic) V25.5
        nontraffic V25.1
      specified vehicle NEC (traffic) V26.5
        nontraffic V26.1
      stationary object (traffic) V27.5
        nontraffic V27.1
      streetcar (traffic) V26.5
        nontraffic V26.1
      three wheeled motor vehicle (traffic)
        V22.5
        nontraffic V22.1
      truck (traffic) V24.5
        nontraffic V24.1

Accident - *continued*

      two wheeled motor vehicle (traffic)
        V22.5
        nontraffic V22.1
      van (traffic) V23.5
        nontraffic V23.1
      noncollision accident (traffic) V28.5
        nontraffic V28.1
    specified type NEC V29.88
      military vehicle V29.81
  motor vehicle NEC occupant (traffic)
    V89.2
  occupant (of)
    aircraft (powered) V95.9
      fixed wing
        commercial -*see* Accident, transport,
    aircraft, occupant, powered, fixed wing,
    commercial
        private -*see* Accident, transport,
    aircraft, occupant, powered, fixed wing,
    private
      nonpowered V96.9
      specified NEC V95.8
    airport battery-powered vehicle -*see*
    Accident, transport, industrial vehicle
    occupant
    all-terrain vehicle (ATV) -*see* Accident,
    transport, all-terrain vehicle occupant
    animal-drawn vehicle -*see* Accident,
    transport, animal-drawn vehicle occupant
    automobile -*see* Accident, transport, car
    occupant
    balloon V96.00
    battery-powered vehicle -*see* Accident,
    transport, industrial vehicle occupant
    bicycle -*see* Accident, transport, pedal
      cyclist
      motorized -*see* Accident, transport,
      motorcycle rider
    boat NEC -*see* Accident, watercraft
    bulldozer -*see* Accident, transport,
      construction vehicle occupant
    bus -*see* Accident, transport, bus occupant
    cable car (on rails) -*see also* Accident,
      transport, streetcar occupant
      not on rails V98.0
    car -*see also* Accident, transport, car
      occupant
      cable (on rails) -*see also* Accident,
      transport, streetcar occupant
      not on rails V98.0
    coach -*see* Accident, transport, bus
      occupant
    coal-car -*see* Accident, transport,
      industrial vehicle occupant
    digger -*see* Accident, transport,
      construction vehicle occupant
    dump truck -*see* Accident, transport,
      construction vehicle occupant
    earth-leveler -*see* Accident, transport,
      construction vehicle occupant
    farm machinery (self-propelled) -*see*
      Accident, transport, agricultural vehicle
      occupant
    forklift -*see* Accident, transport, industrial
      vehicle occupant
    glider (unpowered) V96.20
      hang V96.10
      powered (microlight) (ultralight) -*see*
      Accident, transport, aircraft, occupant,
      powered, glider
    glider (unpowered) NEC V96.20
    hang-glider V96.10
    harvester -*see* Accident, transport,

Accident - *continued*

      agricultural vehicle occupant
    heavy (transport) vehicle -*see* Accident,
      transport, truck occupant
    helicopter -*see* Accident, transport,
      aircraft, occupant, helicopter
    ice-yacht V98.2
    kite (carrying person) V96.8
    land-yacht V98.1
    logging car -*see* Accident, transport,
      industrial vehicle occupant
    mechanical shovel -*see* Accident,
      transport, construction vehicle occupant
    microlight -*see* Accident, transport,
      aircraft, occupant, powered, glider
    minibus -*see* Accident, transport, pickup
      truck occupant
    minivan -*see* Accident, transport, pickup
      truck occupant
    moped -*see* Accident, transport,
      motorcycle
    motor scooter -*see* Accident, transport,
      motorcycle
    motorcycle (with sidecar) -*see* Accident,
      transport, motorcycle
    off-road motor-vehicle (see also Accident,
    transport, all-terrain vehicle occupant) V86.99
    off-road motor-vehicle (see also Accident,
    transport, all-terrain vehicle occupant) V86.99
    pedal cycle -*see also* Accident, transport,
      pedal cyclist
    pick-up (truck) -*see* Accident, transport,
      pickup truck occupant
    railway (train) (vehicle) (subterranean)
      (elevated) -*see* Accident, transport,
      railway vehicle occupant
    rickshaw -*see* Accident, transport, pedal
      cycle
      motorized -*see* Accident, transport,
      three-wheeled motor vehicle
      pedal driven -*see* Accident, transport,
      pedal cyclist
    road-roller -*see* Accident, transport,
      construction vehicle occupant
    ship NOS V94.9
    ski-lift (chair) (gondola) V98.3
    snowmobile -*see* Accident, transport,
      snowmobile occupant
    spacecraft, spaceship -*see* Accident,
      transport, aircraft, occupant, spacecraft
    sport utility vehicle -*see* Accident,
      transport, pickup truck occupant
    streetcar (interurban) (operating on public
      street or highway) -*see* Accident,
      transport, streetcar occupant
    SUV -*see* Accident, transport, pickup
      truck occupant
    téléférique V98.0
    three-wheeled vehicle (motorized) -*see
      also* Accident, transport, three-wheeled
      motor vehicle occupant
      nonmotorized -*see* Accident, transport,
      pedal cycle
    tractor (farm) (and trailer) -*see* Accident,
      transport, agricultural vehicle occupant
    train -*see* Accident, transport, railway
      vehicle occupant
    tram -*see* Accident, transport, streetcar
      occupant
      in mine or quarry -*see* Accident,
      transport, industrial vehicle occupant
    tricycle -*see* Accident, transport, pedal
      cycle
      motorized -*see* Accident, transport,

Accident - *continued*

three-wheeled motor vehicle
trolley -*see* Accident, transport, streetcar
    occupant
 in mine or quarry -*see* Accident,
    transport, industrial vehicle occupant
tub, in mine or quarry -*see* Accident,
    transport, industrial vehicle occupant
ultralight -*see* Accident, transport, aircraft,
    occupant, powered, glider
van -*see* Accident, transport, van occupant
vehicle NEC V89.9
 heavy transport -*see* Accident, transport,
truck occupant
   motor (traffic) NEC V89.2
   nontraffic NEC V89.0
watercraft NOS V94.9
 causing drowning -*see* Drowning,
resulting from accident to boat
parachutist V97.29
 after accident to aircraft -*see* Accident,
   transport, aircraft
 entangled in object V97.21
 injured on landing V97.22
pedal cyclist V19.9
 collision (with)
  animal (traffic) V10.9
   being ridden (traffic) V16.9
    nontraffic V16.2
    while boarding or alighting V16.3
   nontraffic V10.2
   while boarding or alighting V10.3
  animal-drawn vehicle (traffic) V16.9
   nontraffic V16.2
   while boarding or alighting V16.3
  bus (traffic) V14.9
   nontraffic V14.2
   while boarding or alighting V14.3
  car (traffic) V13.9
   nontraffic V13.2
   while boarding or alighting V13.3
  motor vehicle NOS (traffic) V19.60
   nontraffic V19.20
   specified type NEC (traffic) V19.69
    nontraffic V19.29
  pedal cycle (traffic) V11.9
   nontraffic V11.2
   while boarding or alighting V11.3
  pickup truck (traffic) V13.9
   nontraffic V13.2
   while boarding or alighting V13.3
  railway vehicle (traffic) V15.9
   nontraffic V15.2
   while boarding or alighting V15.3
  specified vehicle NEC (traffic) V16.9
   nontraffic V16.2
   while boarding or alighting V16.3
  stationary object (traffic) V17.9
   nontraffic V17.2
   while boarding or alighting V17.3
  streetcar (traffic) V16.9
   nontraffic V16.2
   while boarding or alighting V16.3
  three wheeled motor vehicle (traffic)
   V12.9
   nontraffic V12.2
   while boarding or alighting V12.3
  truck (traffic) V14.9
   nontraffic V14.2
   while boarding or alighting V14.3
  two wheeled motor vehicle (traffic)
   V12.9
   nontraffic V12.2
   while boarding or alighting V12.3

Accident - *continued*

van (traffic) V13.9
 nontraffic V13.2
 while boarding or alighting V13.3
driver
 collision (with)
  animal (traffic) V10.4
   being ridden (traffic) V16.4
    nontraffic V16.0
   nontraffic V10.0
  animal-drawn vehicle (traffic) V16.4
   nontraffic V16.0
  bus (traffic) V14.4
   nontraffic V14.0
  car (traffic) V13.4
   nontraffic V13.0
  motor vehicle NOS (traffic) V19.40
   nontraffic V19.00
   specified type NEC (traffic) V19.49
    nontraffic V19.09
  pedal cycle (traffic) V11.4
   nontraffic V11.0
  pickup truck (traffic) V13.4
   nontraffic V13.0
  railway vehicle (traffic) V15.4
   nontraffic V15.0
  specified vehicle NEC (traffic) V16.4
   nontraffic V16.0
  stationary object (traffic) V17.4
   nontraffic V17.0
  streetcar (traffic) V16.4
   nontraffic V16.0
  three wheeled motor vehicle (traffic)
   V12.4
   nontraffic V12.0
  truck (traffic) V14.4
   nontraffic V14.0
  two wheeled motor vehicle (traffic)
   V12.4
   nontraffic V12.0
  van (traffic) V13.4
   nontraffic V13.0
 noncollision accident (traffic) V18.4
  nontraffic V18.0
noncollision accident (traffic) V18.9
 nontraffic V18.2
 while boarding or alighting V18.3
nontraffic V19.3
passenger
 collision (with)
  animal (traffic) V10.5
   being ridden (traffic) V16.5
    nontraffic V16.1
   nontraffic V10.1
  animal-drawn vehicle (traffic) V16.5
   nontraffic V16.1
  bus (traffic) V14.5
   nontraffic V14.1
  car (traffic) V13.5
   nontraffic V13.1
  motor vehicle NOS (traffic) V19.50
   nontraffic V19.10
   specified type NEC (traffic) V19.59
    nontraffic V19.19
  pedal cycle (traffic) V11.5
   nontraffic V11.1
  pickup truck (traffic) V13.5
   nontraffic V13.1
  railway vehicle (traffic) V15.5
   nontraffic V15.1
  specified vehicle NEC (traffic) V16.5
   nontraffic V16.1
  stationary object (traffic) V17.5
   nontraffic V17.1

Accident - *continued*

streetcar (traffic) V16.5
 nontraffic V16.1
three wheeled motor vehicle (traffic)
 V12.5
 nontraffic V12.1
truck (traffic) V14.5
 nontraffic V14.1
two wheeled motor vehicle (traffic)
 V12.5
 nontraffic V12.1
van (traffic) V13.5
 nontraffic V13.1
noncollision accident (traffic) V18.5
 nontraffic V18.1
specified type NEC V19.88
military vehicle V19.81
pedestrian
 conveyance (occupant) V09.9
  babystroller V00.828
  collision (with) V09.9
   animal being ridden or animal drawn
    vehicle V06.99
    nontraffic V06.09
    traffic V06.19
   bus or heavy transport V04.99
    nontraffic V04.09
    traffic V04.19
   car V03.99
    nontraffic V03.09
    traffic V03.19
   pedal cycle V01.99
    nontraffic V01.09
    traffic V01.19
   pick-up truck or van V03.99
    nontraffic V03.09
    traffic V03.19
   railway (train) (vehicle) V05.99
    nontraffic V05.09
    traffic V05.19
   streetcar V06.99
    nontraffic V06.09
    traffic V06.19
   stationary object V00.822
   two- or three-wheeled motor vehicle
    V02.99
    nontraffic V02.09
    traffic V02.19
   vehicle V09.9
    animal-drawn V06.99
     nontraffic V06.09
     traffic V06.19
    motor
     nontraffic V09.00
     traffic V09.20
  fall V00.821
  nontraffic V09.1
   involving motor vehicle NEC V09.00
  traffic V09.3
   involving motor vehicle NEC V09.20
 flat-bottomed NEC V00.388
  collision (with) V09.9
   animal being ridden or animal drawn
    vehicle V06.99
    nontraffic V06.09
    traffic V06.19
   bus or heavy transport V04.99
    nontraffic V04.09
    traffic V04.19
   car V03.99
    nontraffic V03.09
    traffic V03.19
   pedal cycle V01.99
    nontraffic V01.09

Accident - *continued*
   traffic V01.19
  pick-up truck or van V03.99
   nontraffic V03.09
   traffic V03.19
  railway (train) (vehicle) V05.99
   nontraffic V05.09
   traffic V05.19
  stationary object V00.382
  streetcar V06.99
   nontraffic V06.09
   traffic V06.19
  two- or three-wheeled motor vehicle
    V02.99
   nontraffic V02.09
   traffic V02.19
  vehicle V09.9
   animal-drawn V06.99
    nontraffic V06.09
    traffic V06.19
   motor
    nontraffic V09.00
    traffic V09.20
 fall V00.381
 nontraffic V09.1
  involving motor vehicle NEC V09.00
 snow
  board -*see* Accident, transport,
   pedestrian, conveyance, snow
   board
  ski- -*see* Accident, transport,
   pedestrian, conveyance, skis
   (snow)
 traffic V09.3
  involving motor vehicle NEC V09.20
 gliding type NEC V00.288
  collision (with) V09.9
   animal being ridden or animal drawn
    vehicle V06.99
    nontraffic V06.09
    traffic V06.19
   bus or heavy transport V04.99
    nontraffic V04.09
    traffic V04.19
   car V03.99
    nontraffic V03.09
    traffic V03.19
   pedal cycle V01.99
    nontraffic V01.09
    traffic V01.19
   pick-up truck or van V03.99
    nontraffic V03.09
    traffic V03.19
   railway (train) (vehicle) V05.99
    nontraffic V05.09
    traffic V05.19
   stationary object V00.282
   streetcar V06.99
    nontraffic V06.09
    traffic V06.19
   two- or three-wheeled motor vehicle
    V02.99
    nontraffic V02.09
    traffic V02.19
   vehicle V09.9
    animal-drawn V06.99
    nontraffic V06.09
    traffic V06.19
    motor
     nontraffic V09.00
     traffic V09.20
  fall V00.281
  heelies -*see* Accident, transport,
   pedestrian, conveyance, heelies

Accident - *continued*
  ice skate -*see* Accident, transport,
   pedestrian, conveyance, ice skate
  nontraffic V09.1
   involving motor vehicle NEC V09.00
  sled -*see* Accident, transport,
  pedestrian, conveyance, sled
  traffic V09.3
   involving motor vehicle NEC V09.20
  wheelies -*see* Accident, transport,
   pedestrian, conveyance, heelies
 heelies V00.158
  colliding with stationary object
   V00.152
  fall V00.151
 ice skates V00.218
  collision (with) V09.9
   animal being ridden or animal drawn
    vehicle V06.99
    nontraffic V06.09
    traffic V06.19
   bus or heavy transport V04.99
    nontraffic V04.09
    traffic V04.19
   car V03.99
    nontraffic V03.09
    traffic V03.19
   pedal cycle V01.99
    nontraffic V01.09
    traffic V01.19
   pick-up truck or van V03.99
    nontraffic V03.09
    traffic V03.19
   railway (train) (vehicle) V05.99
    nontraffic V05.09
    traffic V05.19
   streetcar V06.99
    nontraffic V06.09
    traffic V06.19
   stationary object V00.212
   two- or three-wheeled motor vehicle
    V02.99
    nontraffic V02.09
    traffic V02.19
   vehicle V09.9
    animal-drawn V06.99
    nontraffic V06.09
    traffic V06.19
    motor
     nontraffic V09.00
     traffic V09.20
  fall V00.211
  nontraffic V09.1
   involving motor vehicle NEC V09.00
  traffic V09.3
   involving motor vehicle NEC V09.20
 motorized mobility scooter V00.838
  collision with stationary object
   V00.832
  fall from V00.831
  nontraffic V09.1
   involving motor vehicle V09.00
    military V09.01
    specified type NEC V09.09
 roller skates (non in-line) V00.128
  collision (with) V09.9
   animal being ridden or animal drawn
    vehicle V06.91
    nontraffic V06.01
    traffic V06.11
   bus or heavy transport V04.91
    nontraffic V04.01
    traffic V04.11
   car V03.91

Accident - *continued*
   nontraffic V03.01
   traffic V03.11
  pedal cycle V01.91
   nontraffic V01.01
   traffic V01.11
  pick-up truck or van V03.91
   nontraffic V03.01
   traffic V03.11
  railway (train) (vehicle) V05.91
   nontraffic V05.01
   traffic V05.11
  streetcar V06.91
   nontraffic V06.01
   traffic V06.11
  stationary object V00.122
  two- or three-wheeled motor vehicle
    V02.91
   nontraffic V02.01
   traffic V02.11
  vehicle V09.9
   animal-drawn V06.91
    nontraffic V06.01
    traffic V06.11
   motor
    nontraffic V09.00
    traffic V09.20
  fall V00.121
 in-line V00.118
  collision- -*see* also Accident,
   transport, pedestrian, conveyance
   occupant, roller skates, collision
   with stationary object V00.112
  fall V00.111
  nontraffic V09.1
   involving motor vehicle NEC V09.00
  traffic V09.3
   involving motor vehicle NEC V09.20
 rolling shoes V00.158
  colliding with stationary object
   V00.152
  fall V00.151
 rolling type NEC V00.188
  collision (with) V09.9
   animal being ridden or animal drawn
    vehicle V06.99
    nontraffic V06.09
    traffic V06.19
   bus or heavy transport V04.99
    nontraffic V04.09
    traffic V04.19
   car V03.99
    nontraffic V03.09
    traffic V03.19
   pedal cycle V01.99
    nontraffic V01.09
    traffic V01.19
   pick-up truck or van V03.99
    nontraffic V03.09
    traffic V03.19
   railway (train) (vehicle) V05.99
    nontraffic V05.09
    traffic V05.19
   stationary object V00.182
   streetcar V06.99
    nontraffic V06.09
    traffic V06.19
   two- or three-wheeled motor vehicle
    V02.99
    nontraffic V02.09
    traffic V02.19
   vehicle V09.9
    animal-drawn V06.99
    nontraffic V06.09

Accident - *continued*
    traffic V06.19
  motor
    nontraffic V09.00
    traffic V09.20
  fall V00.181
  in-line roller skate -*see* Accident,
    transport, pedestrian, conveyance,
    roller skate, in-line
  nontraffic V09.1
    involving motor vehicle NEC V09.00
  roller skate -*see* Accident, transport,
    pedestrian, conveyance, roller skate
  scooter (non-motorized) -*see* Accident,
    transport, pedestrian, conveyance,
    scooter
  skateboard -*see* Accident, transport,
    pedestrian, conveyance, skateboard
  traffic V09.3
    involving motor vehicle NEC V09.20
  scooter (non-motorized) V00.148
    collision (with) V09.9
     animal being ridden or animal drawn
      vehicle V06.99
      nontraffic V06.09
      traffic V06.19
     bus or heavy transport V04.99
      nontraffic V04.09
      traffic V04.19
     car V03.99
      nontraffic V03.09
      traffic V03.19
     pedal cycle V01.99
      nontraffic V01.09
      traffic V01.19
     pick-up truck or van V03.99
      nontraffic V03.09
      traffic V03.19
     railway (train) (vehicle) V05.99
      nontraffic V05.09
      traffic V05.19
     streetcar V06.99
      nontraffic V06.09
      traffic V06.19
     stationary object V00.142
     two- or three-wheeled motor vehicle
      V02.99
      nontraffic V02.09
      traffic V02.19
     vehicle V09.9
      animal-drawn V06.99
      nontraffic V06.09
      traffic V06.19
     motor
      nontraffic V09.00
      traffic V09.20
    fall V00.141
    nontraffic V09.1
     involving motor vehicle NEC V09.00
    traffic V09.3
     involving motor vehicle NEC V09.20
  skate board V00.138
    collision (with) V09.9
     animal being ridden or animal drawn
      vehicle V06.92
      nontraffic V06.02
      traffic V06.12
     bus or heavy transport V04.92
      nontraffic V04.02
      traffic V04.12
     car V03.92
      nontraffic V03.02
      traffic V03.12
     pedal cycle V01.92

Accident - *continued*
    nontraffic V01.02
    traffic V01.12
    pick-up truck or van V03.92
     nontraffic V03.02
     traffic V03.12
    railway (train) (vehicle) V05.92
     nontraffic V05.02
     traffic V05.12
    streetcar V06.92
     nontraffic V06.02
     traffic V06.12
    stationary object V00.132
    two- or three-wheeled motor vehicle
     V02.92
     nontraffic V02.02
     traffic V02.12
    vehicle V09.9
     animal-drawn V06.92
     nontraffic V06.02
     traffic V06.12
     motor
      nontraffic V09.00
      traffic V09.20
  fall V00.131
  nontraffic V09.1
    involving motor vehicle NEC V09.00
  traffic V09.3
    involving motor vehicle NEC V09.20
  sled V00.228
    collision (with) V09.9
     animal being ridden or animal drawn
      vehicle V06.99
      nontraffic V06.09
      traffic V06.19
     bus or heavy transport V04.99
      nontraffic V04.09
      traffic V04.19
     car V03.99
      nontraffic V03.09
      traffic V03.19
     pedal cycle V01.99
      nontraffic V01.09
      traffic V01.19
     pick-up truck or van V03.99
      nontraffic V03.09
      traffic V03.19
     railway (train) (vehicle) V05.99
      nontraffic V05.09
      traffic V05.19
     streetcar V06.99
      nontraffic V06.09
      traffic V06.19
     stationary object V00.222
     two- or three-wheeled motor vehicle
      V02.99
      nontraffic V02.09
      traffic V02.19
     vehicle V09.9
      animal-drawn V06.99
      nontraffic V06.09
      traffic V06.19
     motor
      nontraffic V09.00
      traffic V09.20
    fall V00.221
    nontraffic V09.1
     involving motor vehicle NEC V09.00
    traffic V09.3
     involving motor vehicle NEC V09.20
  skis (snow) V00.328
    collision (with) V09.9
     animal being ridden or animal drawn
      vehicle V06.99

Accident - *continued*
    nontraffic V06.09
    traffic V06.19
    bus or heavy transport V04.99
     nontraffic V04.09
     traffic V04.19
    car V03.99
     nontraffic V03.09
     traffic V03.19
    pedal cycle V01.99
     nontraffic V01.09
     traffic V01.19
    pick-up truck or van V03.99
     nontraffic V03.09
     traffic V03.19
    railway (train) (vehicle) V05.99
     nontraffic V05.09
     traffic V05.19
    streetcar V06.99
     nontraffic V06.09
     traffic V06.19
    stationary object V00.322
    two- or three-wheeled motor vehicle
     V02.99
     nontraffic V02.09
     traffic V02.19
    vehicle V09.9
     animal-drawn V06.99
     nontraffic V06.09
     traffic V06.19
     motor
      nontraffic V09.00
      traffic V09.20
    fall V00.321
    nontraffic V09.1
     involving motor vehicle NEC V09.00
    traffic V09.3
     involving motor vehicle NEC V09.20
  snow board V00.318
    collision (with) V09.9
     animal being ridden or animal drawn
      vehicle V06.99
      nontraffic V06.09
      traffic V06.19
     bus or heavy transport V04.99
      nontraffic V04.09
      traffic V04.19
     car V03.99
      nontraffic V03.09
      traffic V03.19
     pedal cycle V01.99
      nontraffic V01.09
      traffic V01.19
     pick-up truck or van V03.99
      nontraffic V03.09
      traffic V03.19
     railway (train) (vehicle) V05.99
      nontraffic V05.09
      traffic V05.19
     streetcar V06.99
      nontraffic V06.09
      traffic V06.19
     stationary object V00.312
     two- or three-wheeled motor vehicle
      V02.99
      nontraffic V02.09
      traffic V02.19
     vehicle V09.9
      animal-drawn V06.99
      nontraffic V06.09
      traffic V06.19
     motor
      nontraffic V09.00
      traffic V09.20

Accident - *continued*
driver
collision (with)
animal (traffic) V50.5
being ridden (traffic) V56.5
nontraffic V56.0
nontraffic V50.0
animal-drawn vehicle (traffic) V56.5
nontraffic V56.0
bus (traffic) V54.5
nontraffic V54.0
car (traffic) V53.5
nontraffic V53.0
motor vehicle NOS (traffic) V59.40
nontraffic V59.00
specified type NEC (traffic) V59.49
nontraffic V59.09
pedal cycle (traffic) V51.5
nontraffic V51.0
pickup truck (traffic) V53.5
nontraffic V53.0
railway vehicle (traffic) V55.5
nontraffic V55.0
specified vehicle NEC (traffic) V56.5
nontraffic V56.0
stationary object (traffic) V57.5
nontraffic V57.0
streetcar (traffic) V56.5
nontraffic V56.0
three wheeled motor vehicle (traffic)
V52.5
nontraffic V52.0
truck (traffic) V54.5
nontraffic V54.0
two wheeled motor vehicle (traffic)
V52.5
nontraffic V52.0
van (traffic) V53.5
nontraffic V53.0
noncollision accident (traffic) V58.5
nontraffic V58.0
noncollision accident (traffic) V58.9
nontraffic V58.3
while boarding or alighting V58.4
nontraffic V59.3
hanger-on
collision (with)
animal (traffic) V50.7
being ridden (traffic) V56.7
nontraffic V56.2
nontraffic V50.2
animal-drawn vehicle (traffic) V56.7
nontraffic V56.2
bus (traffic) V54.7
nontraffic V54.2
car (traffic) V53.7
nontraffic V53.2
pedal cycle (traffic) V51.7
nontraffic V51.2
pickup truck (traffic) V53.7
nontraffic V53.2
railway vehicle (traffic) V55.7
nontraffic V55.2
specified vehicle NEC (traffic) V56.7
nontraffic V56.2
stationary object (traffic) V57.7
nontraffic V57.2
streetcar (traffic) V56.7
nontraffic V56.2
three wheeled motor vehicle (traffic)
V52.7
nontraffic V52.2
truck (traffic) V54.7
nontraffic V54.2

Accident - *continued*
two wheeled motor vehicle (traffic)
V52.7
nontraffic V52.2
van (traffic) V53.7
nontraffic V53.2
noncollision accident (traffic) V58.7
nontraffic V58.2
passenger
collision (with)
animal (traffic) V50.6
being ridden (traffic) V56.6
nontraffic V56.1
nontraffic V50.1
animal-drawn vehicle (traffic) V56.6
nontraffic V56.1
bus (traffic) V54.6
nontraffic V54.1
car (traffic) V53.6
nontraffic V53.1
motor vehicle NOS (traffic) V59.50
nontraffic V59.10
specified type NEC (traffic) V59.59
nontraffic V59.19
pedal cycle (traffic) V51.6
nontraffic V51.1
pickup truck (traffic) V53.6
nontraffic V53.1
railway vehicle (traffic) V55.6
nontraffic V55.1
specified vehicle NEC (traffic) V56.6
nontraffic V56.1
stationary object (traffic) V57.6
nontraffic V57.1
streetcar (traffic) V56.6
nontraffic V56.1
three wheeled motor vehicle (traffic)
V52.6
nontraffic V52.1
truck (traffic) V54.6
nontraffic V54.1
two wheeled motor vehicle (traffic)
V52.6
nontraffic V52.1
van (traffic) V53.6
nontraffic V53.1
noncollision accident (traffic) V58.6
nontraffic V58.1
specified type NEC V59.88
military vehicle V59.81
quarry truck -*see* Accident, transport,
industrial vehicle occupant
race car -*see* Accident, transport, motor
vehicle NEC occupant
railway vehicle occupant V81.9
collision (with) V81.3
motor vehicle (non-military) (traffic)
V81.1
military V81.83
nontraffic V81.0
rolling stock V81.2
specified object NEC V81.3
during derailment V81.7
with antecedent collision -*see* Accident,
transport, railway vehicle occupant,
collision
explosion V81.81
fall (in railway vehicle) V81.5
during derailment NOS V81.7
with antecedent collision -*see*
Accident, transport, railway vehicle
occupant, collision
from railway vehicle V81.6
during derailment V81.7

Accident - *continued*
with antecedent collision -*see*
Accident, transport, railway vehicle
occupant, collision
while boarding or alighting V81.4
fire V81.81
object falling onto train V81.82
specified type NEC V81.89
while boarding or alighting V81.4
ski lift V98.3
snowmobile occupant (nontraffic) V86.92
driver V86.52
hanger-on V86.72
passenger V86.62
traffic V86.32
driver V86.02
hanger-on V86.22
passenger V86.12
while boarding or alighting V86.42
specified NEC V98.8
sport utility vehicle occupant -*see also*
Accident, transport, pickup truck occupant
streetcar occupant V82.9
collision (with) V82.3
motor vehicle (traffic) V82.1
nontraffic V82.0
rolling stock V82.2
during derailment V82.7
with antecedent collision -*see* Accident,
transport, streetcar occupant, collision
fall (in streetcar) V82.5
during derailment V82.7
with antecedent collision -*see*
Accident, transport, streetcar
occupant, collision
from streetcar V82.6
during derailment V82.7
with antecedent collision -*see*
Accident, transport, streetcar
occupant, collision
while boarding or alighting V82.4
while boarding or alighting V82.4
specified type NEC V82.8
while boarding or alighting V82.4
three-wheeled motor vehicle occupant
V39.9
collision (with)
animal (traffic) V30.9
being ridden (traffic) V36.9
nontraffic V36.3
while boarding or alighting V36.4
nontraffic V30.3
while boarding or alighting V30.4
animal-drawn vehicle (traffic) V36.9
nontraffic V36.3
while boarding or alighting V36.4
bus (traffic) V34.9
nontraffic V34.3
while boarding or alighting V34.4
car (traffic) V33.9
nontraffic V33.3
while boarding or alighting V33.4
motor vehicle NOS (traffic) V39.60
nontraffic V39.20
specified type NEC (traffic) V39.69
nontraffic V39.29
pedal cycle (traffic) V31.9
nontraffic V31.3
while boarding or alighting V31.4
pickup truck (traffic) V33.9
nontraffic V33.3
while boarding or alighting V33.4
railway vehicle (traffic) V35.9
nontraffic V35.3

Assault (homicidal) - *continued*
piercing -*see* Assault, cutting or piercing
    instrument
puncture -*see* Assault, cutting or piercing
    instrument
stab -*see* Assault, cutting or piercing
    instrument
Attack by mammals NEC W55.89
Avalanche -*see* Landslide
Aviator's disease
-*see* Air, pressure

B

Barotitis, barodontalgia, barosinusitis,
barotrauma (otitic) (sinus) -*see* Air,
pressure
Battered (baby) (child) (person) (syndrome)
X58
Bayonet wound W26.1
in
    legal intervention -*see* Legal, intervention,
      sharp object, bayonet
    war operations -*see* War operations, combat
stated as undetermined whether accidental or
    intentional Y28.8
suicide (attempt) X78.2
Bean in nose -*see* categories T17 and T18
Bed set on fire NEC -*see* Exposure, fire,
uncontrolled, building, bed
Beheading (by guillotine)
homicide X99.9
legal execution -*see* Legal, intervention
Bending, injury in (prolonged) (static)
X50.1
Bends
-*see* Air, pressure, change
Bite, bitten by
alligator W58.01
arthropod (nonvenomous) NEC W57
bull W55.21
cat W55.01
cow W55.21
crocodile W58.11
dog W54.0
goat W55.31
hoof stock NEC W55.31
horse W55.11
human being (accidentally) W50.3
    with intent to injure or kill Y04.1
    as, or caused by, a crowd or human
      stampede (with fall) W52
    assault Y04.1
    homicide (attempt) Y04.1
    in
      fight Y04.1
insect (nonvenomous) W57
lizard (nonvenomous) W59.01
mammal NEC W55.81
    marine W56.31
marine animal (nonvenomous) W56.81
millipede W57
moray eel W56.51
mouse W53.01
person(s) (accidentally) W50.3
    with intent to injure or kill Y04.1
    as, or caused by, a crowd or human
      stampede (with fall) W52
    assault Y04.1
    homicide (attempt) Y04.1
    in
      fight Y04.1
pig W55.41
raccoon W55.51

Bite, bitten by - *continued*
rat W53.11
reptile W59.81
    lizard W59.01
    snake W59.11
    turtle W59.21
      terrestrial W59.81
rodent W53.81
    mouse W53.01
    rat W53.11
    specified NEC W53.81
    squirrel W53.21
shark W56.41
sheep W55.31
snake (nonvenomous) W59.11
spider (nonvenomous) W57
squirrel W53.21
Blast (air) in war operations -*see* War
operations, blast
Blizzard X37.2
Blood alcohol level Y90.9
less than 20mg/100ml Y90.0
presence in blood, level not specified Y90.9
20 39mg/100ml Y90.1
40 59mg/100ml Y90.2
60 79mg/100ml Y90.3
80 99mg/100ml Y90.4
100 119mg/100ml Y90.5
120 199mg/100ml Y90.6
200 239mg/100ml Y90.7
Blow X58
by law-enforcing agent, police (on duty) -*see*
    Legal, intervention, manhandling
    blunt object -*see* Legal, intervention, blunt
    object
Blowing up -*see* Explosion
Brawl (hand) (fists) (foot) Y04.0
Breakage (accidental) (part of) ladder
(causing fall) W11
scaffolding (causing fall) W12
Broken
glass, contact with -*see* Contact, with, glass
power line (causing electric shock) W85
Bumping against, into (accidentally)
object NEC W22.8
    with fall -*see* Fall, due to, bumping against,
      object
    caused by crowd or human stampede (with
      fall) W52
    sports equipment W21.9
person(s) W51
    with fall W03
      due to ice or snow W00.0
    assault Y04.2
    caused by, a crowd or human stampede
      (with fall) W52
    homicide (attempt) Y04.2
sports equipment W21.9
Burn, burned, burning (accidental) (by)
(from) (on)
acid NEC -*see* Table of Drugs and Chemicals
bed linen -*see* Exposure, fire, uncontrolled,
    in building, bed
blowtorch X08.8
    with ignition of clothing NEC X06.2
      nightwear X05
bonfire, campfire (controlled) -*see also*
    Exposure, fire, controlled, not in building
    uncontrolled -*see* Exposure, fire,
      uncontrolled, not in building
candle X08.8
    with ignition of clothing NEC X06.2
      nightwear X05

Burn, burned, burning - *continued*
caustic liquid, substance (external) (internal)
    NEC -*see* Table of Drugs and Chemicals
chemical (external) (internal) -*see also* Table
    of Drugs and Chemicals
    in war operations -*see* War operations. fire
cigar(s) or cigarette(s) X08.8
    with ignition of clothing NEC X06.2
      nightwear X05
clothes, clothing NEC (from controlled fire)
    X06.2
    with conflagration -*see* Exposure, fire,
      uncontrolled, building
    not in building or structure -*see* Exposure,
      fire, uncontrolled, not in building
cooker (hot) X15.8
    stated as undetermined whether accidental
      or intentional Y27.3
    suicide (attempt) X77.3
electric blanket X16
engine (hot) X17
fire, flames -*see* Exposure, fire
flare, Very pistol -*see* Discharge, firearm
    NEC
heat
    from appliance (electrical) (household)
      X15.8
      cooker X15.8
      hotplate X15.2
      kettle X15.8
      light bulb X15.8
      saucepan X15.3
      skillet X15.3
      stove X15.0
    stated as undetermined whether accidental
      or intentional Y27.3
    suicide (attempt) X77.3
    toaster X15.1
    in local application or packing during
      medical or surgical procedure Y63.5
heating
    appliance, radiator or pipe X16
homicide (attempt) -*see* Assault, burning
hot
    air X14.1
    cooker X15.8
    drink X10.0
    engine X17
    fat X10.2
    fluid NEC X12
    food X10.1
    gases X14.1
    heating appliance X16
    household appliance NEC X15.8
    kettle X15.8
    liquid NEC X12
    machinery X17
    metal (molten) (liquid) NEC X18
    object (not producing fire or flames) NEC
      X19
    oil (cooking) X10.2
    pipe(s) X16
    radiator X16
    saucepan (glass) (metal) X15.3
    stove (kitchen) X15.0
    substance NEC X19
      caustic or corrosive NEC -*see* Table of
        Drugs and Chemicals
    toaster X15.1
    tool X17
    vapor X13.1
    water (tap) -*see* Contact, with, hot, tap
      water
hotplate X15.2

Burn, burned, burning - *continued*
  suicide (attempt) X77.3
  ignition -*see* Ignition
  in war operations -*see* War operations, fire
  inflicted by other person X97
    by hot objects, hot vapor, and steam -*see*
      Assault, burning, hot object
  internal, from swallowed caustic, corrosive
    liquid, substance -*see* Table of Drugs and
    Chemicals
  iron (hot) X15.8
    stated as undetermined whether accidental
      or intentional Y27.3
    suicide (attempt) X77.3
  kettle (hot) X15.8
    stated as undetermined whether accidental
      or intentional Y27.3
    suicide (attempt) X77.3
  lamp (flame) X08.8
    with ignition of clothing NEC X06.2
      nightwear X05
  lighter (cigar) (cigarette) X08.8
    with ignition of clothing NEC X06.2
      nightwear X05
  lightning -*see* subcategory T75.0
    causing fire -*see* Exposure, fire
  liquid (boiling) (hot) NEC X12
    stated as undetermined whether accidental
      or intentional Y27.2
    suicide (attempt) X77.2
  local application of externally applied
    substance in medical or surgical care
    Y63.5
  on board watercraft
  due to
    accident to watercraft V91.09
      powered craft V91.03
        ferry boat V91.01
        fishing boat V91.02
        jet skis V91.03
        liner V91.01
        merchant ship V91.00
        passenger ship V91.01
      unpowered craft V91.08
        canoe V91.05
        inflatable V91.06
        kayak V91.05
        sailboat V91.04
        surf-board V91.08
        water skis V91.07
        windsurfer V91.08
    fire on board V93.09
      ferry boat V93.01
      fishing boat V93.02
      jet skis V93.03
      liner V93.01
      merchant ship V93.00
      passenger ship V93.01
      powered craft NEC V93.03
      sailboat V93.04
    specified heat source NEC on board
    V93.19
      ferry boat V93.11
      fishing boat V93.12
      jet skis V93.13
      liner V93.11
      merchant ship V93.10
      passenger ship V93.11
      powered craft NEC V93.13
      sailboat V93.14
  machinery (hot) X17
  matches X08.8
    with ignition of clothing NEC X06.2
      nightwear X05

Burn, burned, burning - *continued*
  mattress -*see* Exposure, fire, uncontrolled,
    building, bed
  medicament, externally applied Y63.5
  metal (hot) (liquid) (molten) NEC X18
  nightwear (nightclothes, nightdress, gown,
    pajamas, robe) X05
  object (hot) NEC X19
  pipe (hot) X16
    smoking X08.8
      with ignition of clothing NEC X06.2
        nightwear X05
  powder -*see* Powder burn
  radiator (hot) X16
  saucepan (hot) (glass) (metal) X15.3
    stated as undetermined whether accidental
      or intentional Y27.3
    suicide (attempt) X77.3
  self-inflicted X76
    stated as undetermined whether accidental
      or intentional Y26
  steam X13.1
    pipe X16
      stated as undetermined whether accidental
        or intentional Y27.8
    stated as undetermined whether accidental
      or intentional Y27.0
    suicide (attempt) X77.0
  stove (hot) (kitchen) X15.0
    stated as undetermined whether accidental
      or intentional Y27.3
    suicide (attempt) X77.3
  substance (hot) NEC X19
    boiling X12
      stated as undetermined whether accidental
        or intentional Y27.2
      suicide (attempt) X77.2
    molten (metal) X18
  suicide (attempt) NEC X76
    hot
      household appliance X77.3
      object X77.9
    stated as undetermined whether accidental or
      intentional Y27.0
  therapeutic misadventure
    heat in local application or packing during
      medical or surgical procedure Y63.5
    overdose of radiation Y63.2
  toaster (hot) X15.1
    stated as undetermined whether accidental
      or intentional Y27.3
    suicide (attempt) X77.3
  tool (hot) X17
  torch, welding X08.8
    with ignition of clothing NEC X06.2
      nightwear X05
  trash fire (controlled) -*see* Exposure, fire,
    controlled, not in building
    uncontrolled -*see* Exposure, fire,
      uncontrolled, not in building
  vapor (hot) X13.1
    stated as undetermined whether accidental
      or intentional Y27.0
    suicide (attempt) X77.0
  Very pistol -*see* Discharge, firearm NEC
Butted by animal W55.82
  bull W55.22
  cow W55.22
  goat W55.32
  horse W55.12
  pig W55.42
  sheep W55.32

C

Caisson disease
  -*see* Air, pressure, change
Campfire (exposure to) (controlled) -*see*
  also Exposure, fire, controlled, not in
  building
  uncontrolled -*see* Exposure, fire,
    uncontrolled, not in building
Capital punishment (any means) -*see* Legal,
  intervention
Car sickness T75.3
Casualty (not due to war) NEC X58
  war -*see* War operations
Cat
  bite W55.01
  scratch W55.03
Cataclysm, cataclysmic (any injury) NEC -
  see Forces of nature
Catching fire -*see* Exposure, fire
Caught
  between
Caught - *continued*
  folding object W23.0
  objects (moving) (stationary and moving)
    W23.0
    and machinery -*see* Contact, with, by type
      of machine
    stationary W23.1
  sliding door and door frame W23.0
  by, in
    machinery (moving parts of) -*see* Contact,
      with, by type of machine
    washing-machine wringer W23.0
  under packing crate (due to losing grip)
    W23.1
Cave-in caused by cataclysmic earth surface
  movement or eruption -*see* Landslide
Change(s) in air pressure
  -*see* Air, pressure, change
Choked, choking (on) (any object except
  food or vomitus) food (bone) (seed) -*see*
  categories T17 and T18
  vomitus T17.81
Civil insurrection -*see* War operations
Cloudburst (any injury) X37.8
Cold, exposure to (accidental) (excessive)
  (extreme) (natural) (place) NEC -*see*
  Exposure, cold
Collapse
  building W20.1
    burning (uncontrolled fire) X00.2
  dam or man-made structure (causing earth
    movement) X36.0
  machinery -*see* Contact, with, by type of
    machine
  structure W20.1
    burning (uncontrolled fire) X00.2
Collision (accidental) NEC -*see also*
  Accident, transport V89.9
  pedestrian W51
    with fall W03
      due to ice or snow W00.0
      involving pedestrian conveyance -*see*
        Accident, transport, pedestrian,
        conveyance
    and
      crowd or human stampede (with fall) W52
      object W22.8
        with fall -*see* Fall, due to, bumping
        against, object
  person(s) -*see* Collision, pedestrian
  transport vehicle NEC V89.9
    and

Collision - *continued*

avalanche, fallen or not moving -*see*
Accident, transport
  falling or moving -*see* Landslide
landslide, fallen or not moving -*see*
Accident, transport
  falling or moving -*see* Landslide
due to cataclysm -*see* Forces of nature, by
  type
intentional, purposeful suicide (attempt) -
  see Suicide, collision

Combustion, spontaneous -*see* Ignition
**Complication (delayed) of or following
  (medical or surgical procedure)** Y84.9
with misadventure -*see* Misadventure
amputation of limb(s) Y83.5
anastomosis (arteriovenous) (blood vessel)
  (gastrojejunal) (tendon) (natural or
  artificial material) Y83.2
aspiration (of fluid) Y84.4
  tissue Y84.8
biopsy Y84.8
blood
  sampling Y84.7
  transfusion
    procedure Y84.8
bypass Y83.2
catheterization (urinary) Y84.6
  cardiac Y84.0
colostomy Y83.3
cystostomy Y83.3
dialysis (kidney) Y84.1
drug -*see* Table of Drugs and Chemicals
due to misadventure -*see* Misadventure
duodenostomy Y83.3
electroshock therapy Y84.3
external stoma, creation of Y83.3
formation of external stoma Y83.3
gastrostomy Y83.3
graft Y83.2
hypothermia (medically-induced) Y84.8
implant, implantation (of)
  artificial
    internal device (cardiac pacemaker)
      (electrodes in brain) (heart valve
      prosthesis) (orthopedic) Y83.1
    material or tissue (for anastomosis or
      bypass) Y83.2
      with creation of external stoma Y83.3
    natural tissues (for anastomosis or bypass)
      Y83.2
      with creation of external stoma Y83.3
infusion
  procedure Y84.8
injection -*see* Table of Drugs and Chemicals
  procedure Y84.8
insertion of gastric or duodenal sound Y84.5
insulin-shock therapy Y84.3
paracentesis (abdominal) (thoracic)
  (aspirative) Y84.4
procedures other than surgical operation -*see*
  Complication of or following, by type of
  procedure
radiological procedure or therapy Y84.2
removal of organ (partial) (total) NEC Y83.6
sampling
  blood Y84.7
  fluid NEC Y84.4
  tissue Y84.8
shock therapy Y84.3
surgical operation NEC -*see also*
  Complication of or following, by type of
  operation Y83.9
  reconstructive NEC Y83.4

Complication - *continued*

with
  anastomosis, bypass or graft Y83.2
  formation of external stoma Y83.3
specified NEC Y83.8
transfusion -*see also* Table of Drugs and
  Chemicals
  procedure Y84.8
transplant, transplantation (heart) (kidney)
  (liver) (whole organ, any) Y83.0
  partial organ Y83.4
ureterostomy Y83.3
vaccination -*see also* Table of Drugs and
  Chemicals
  procedure Y84.8

Compression
divers' squeeze
  -*see* Air, pressure, change
trachea by
  food (lodged in esophagus) -*see* categories
    T17 and T18
  vomitus (lodged in esophagus) T17.81
Conflagration -*see* Exposure, fire,
  uncontrolled
Constriction (external)
hair W49.01
jewelry W49.04
ring W49.04
rubber band W49.03
specified item NEC W49.09
string W49.02
thread W49.02
Contact (accidental) with
abrasive wheel (metalworking) W31.1
alligator W58.09
  bite W58.01
  crushing W58.03
  strike W58.02
amphibian W62.9
  frog W62.0
  toad W62.1
animal (nonvenomous) NEC W64
  marine W56.89
    bite W56.81
    dolphin -*see* Contact, with, dolphin
    fish NEC -*see* Contact, with, fish
    mammal -*see* Contact, with, mammal,
      marine
    orca -*see* Contact, with, orca
    sea lion -*see* Contact, with, sea lion
    shark -*see* Contact, with, shark
    strike W56.82
animate mechanical force NEC W64
arrow W21.89
  not thrown, projected or falling W45.8
arthropods (nonvenomous) W57
axe W27.0
band-saw (industrial) W31.2
bayonet -*see* Bayonet wound
bee(s) X58
bench-saw (industrial) W31.2
bird W61.99
  bite W61.91
  chicken -*see* Contact, with, chicken
  duck -*see* Contact, with, duck
  goose -*see* Contact, with, goose
  macaw -*see* Contact, with, macaw
  parrot -*see* Contact, with, parrot
  psittacine -*see* Contact, with, psittacine
  strike W61.92
  turkey -*see* Contact, with, turkey
blender W29.0
boiling water X12

Contact (accidental) - *continued*

stated as undetermined whether accidental
  or intentional Y27.2
  suicide (attempt) X77.2
bore, earth-drilling or mining (land)
  (seabed) W31.0
buffalo -*see* Contact, with, hoof stock NEC
bull W55.29
  bite W55.21
  gored W55.22
  strike W55.22
bumper cars W31.81
camel -*see* Contact, with, hoof stock NEC
can
  lid W26.8
  opener W27.4
    powered W29.0
cat W55.09
  bite W55.01
  scratch W55.03
caterpillar (venomous) X58
centipede (venomous) X58
chain
  hoist W24.0
    agricultural operations W30.89
  saw W29.3
chicken W61.39
  peck W61.33
  strike W61.32
chisel W27.0
circular saw W31.2
cobra X58
combine (harvester) W30.0
conveyer belt W24.1
cooker (hot) X15.8
  stated as undetermined whether accidental
    or intentional Y27.3
  suicide (attempt) X77.3
coral X58
cotton gin W31.82
cow W55.29
  bite W55.21
  strike W55.22
crane W24.0
  agricultural operations W30.89
crocodile W58.19
  bite W58.11
  crushing W58.13
  strike W58.12
dagger W26.1
  stated as undetermined whether accidental
    or intentional Y28.2
  suicide (attempt) X78.2
dairy equipment W31.82
dart W21.89
  not thrown, projected or falling W45.8
deer -*see* Contact, with, hoof stock NEC
derrick W24.0
  agricultural operations W30.89
    hay W30.2
dog W54.8
  bite W54.0
  strike W54.1
dolphin W56.09
  bite W56.01
  strike W56.02
donkey -*see* Contact, with, hoof stock NEC
drill (powered) W29.8
  earth (land) (seabed) W31.0
  nonpowered W27.8
drive belt W24.0
  agricultural operations W30.89
dry ice -*see* Exposure, cold, man-made
dryer (clothes) (powered) (spin) W29.2

Contact (accidental) - *continued*
  duck W61.69
    bite W61.61
    strike W61.62
  earth ( )
    drilling machine (industrial) W31.0
    scraping machine in stationary use
    W31.83
  edge of stiff paper W26.2
  electric
    beater W29.0
    blanket X16
    fan W29.2
      commercial W31.82
    knife W29.1
    mixer W29.0
  elevator (building) W24.0
    agricultural operations W30.89
      grain W30.3
  engine(s), hot NEC X17
  excavating machine W31.0
  farm machine W30.9
  feces -*see* Contact, with, by type of animal
  Fer de lance X58
  fish W56.59
    bite W56.51
    shark -*see* Contact, with, shark
    strike W56.52
  flying horses W31.81
  forging (metalworking) machine W31.1
  fork W27.4
  forklift (truck) W24.0
    agricultural operations W30.89
  frog W62.0
  garden
    cultivator (powered) W29.3
      riding W30.89
    fork W27.1
  gas turbine W31.3
  Gila monster X58
  giraffe -*see* Contact, with, hoof stock NEC
  glass (sharp) (broken) W25
    with subsequent fall W18.02
    assault X99.0
    due to fall -*see* Fall, by type
    stated as undetermined whether accidental
    or intentional Y28.0
    suicide (attempt) X78.0
  goat W55.39
    bite W55.31
    strike W55.32
  goose W61.59
    bite W61.51
    strike W61.52
  hand
    saw W27.0
    tool (not powered) NEC W27.8
      powered W29.8
  harvester W30.0
  hay-derrick W30.2
  heat NEC X19
    from appliance (electrical) (household) -
    see Contact, with, hot, household
    appliance
      heating appliance X16
  heating
    appliance (hot) X16
    pad (electric) X16
  hedge-trimmer (powered) W29.3
  hoe W27.1
  hoist (chain) (shaft) NEC W24.0
    agricultural W30.89
  hoof stock NEC W55.39
    bite W55.31

Contact (accidental) - *continued*
    strike W55.32
  hornet(s) X58
  horse W55.19
    bite W55.11
    strike W55.12
  hot
    air X14.1
      inhalation X14.0
    cooker X15.8
    drinks X10.0
    engine X17
    fats X10.2
    fluids NEC X12
      assault X98.2
      suicide (attempt) X77.2
      undetermined whether accidental or
    intentional Y27.2
    food X10.1
    gases X14.1
      inhalation X14.0
    heating appliance X16
    household appliance X15.8
      assault X98.3
      cooker X15.8
      hotplate X15.2
      kettle X15.8
      light bulb X15.8
      object NEC X19
        assault X98.8
        stated as undetermined whether
    accidental or intentional Y27.9
        suicide (attempt) X77.8
      saucepan X15.3
      skillet X15.3
      stove X15.0
      stated as undetermined whether
    accidental or intentional Y27.3
        suicide (attempt) X77.3
      toaster X15.1
    kettle X15.8
    light bulb X15.8
    liquid NEC -*see also* Burn X12
      drinks X10.0
      stated as undetermined whether
    accidental or intentional Y27.2
        suicide (attempt) X77.2
      tap water X11.8
        stated as undetermined whether
    accidental or intentional Y27.1
          suicide (attempt) X77.1
    machinery X17
    metal (molten) (liquid) NEC X18
    object (not producing fire or flames) NEC
    X19
    oil (cooking) X10.2
    pipe X16
    plate X15.2
    radiator X16
    saucepan (glass) (metal) X15.3
    skillet X15.3
    stove (kitchen) X15.0
    substance NEC X19
    tap-water X11.8
      assault X98.1
      heated on stove X12
        stated as undetermined whether
    accidental or intentional Y27.2
          suicide (attempt) X77.2
      in bathtub X11.0
      running X11.1
        stated as undetermined whether
    accidental or intentional Y27.1
        suicide (attempt) X77.1

Contact (accidental) - *continued*
    toaster X15.1
    tool X17
    vapors X13.1
      inhalation X13.0
    water (tap) X11.8
      boiling X12
        stated as undetermined whether
    accidental or intentional Y27.2
          suicide (attempt) X77.2
      heated on stove X12
        stated as undetermined whether
    accidental or intentional Y27.2
          suicide (attempt) X77.2
      in bathtub X11.0
      running X11.1
        stated as undetermined whether
    accidental or intentional Y27.1
        suicide (attempt) X77.1
  hotplate X15.2
  ice-pick W27.4
  insect (nonvenomous) NEC W57
  kettle (hot) X15.8
  knife W26.0
    assault X99.1
    electric W29.1
    stated as undetermined whether accidental
    or intentional Y28.1
    suicide (attempt) X78.1
  lathe (metalworking) W31.1
    turnings W45.8
    woodworking W31.2
  lawnmower (powered) (ridden) W28
    causing electrocution W86.8
      suicide (attempt) X83.1
    unpowered W27.1
  lift, lifting (devices) W24.0
    agricultural operations W30.89
    shaft W24.0
  liquefied gas -*see* Exposure, cold, man-
    made
  liquid air, hydrogen, nitrogen -*see*
    Exposure, cold, man-made
  lizard (nonvenomous) W59.09
    bite W59.01
    strike W59.02
  llama -*see* Contact, with, hoof stock NEC
  macaw W61.19
    bite W61.11
    strike W61.12
  machine, machinery W31.9
    abrasive wheel W31.1
    agricultural including animal-powered
    W30.9
      combine harvester W30.0
      grain storage elevator W30.3
      hay derrick W30.2
      power take-off device W30.1
      reaper W30.0
      specified NEC W30.89
      thresher W30.0
      transport vehicle, stationary W30.81
    band saw W31.2
    bench saw W31.2
    circular saw W31.2
    commercial NEC W31.82
    drilling, metal (industrial) W31.1
    earth-drilling W31.0
    earthmoving or scraping W31.89
    excavating W31.89
    forging machine W31.1
    gas turbine W31.3
    hot X17
    internal combustion engine W31.3

Contact (accidental) - *continued*

 land drill W31.0
 lathe W31.1
 lifting (devices) W24.0
 metal drill W31.1
 metalworking (industrial) W31.1
 milling, metal W31.1
 mining W31.0
 molding W31.2
 overhead plane W31.2
 power press, metal W31.1
 prime mover W31.3
 printing W31.89
 radial saw W31.2
 recreational W31.81
 roller-coaster W31.81
 rolling mill, metal W31.1
 sander W31.2
 seabed drill W31.0
 shaft
  hoist W31.0
  lift W31.0
 specified NEC W31.89
 spinning W31.89
 steam engine W31.3
 transmission W24.1
 under cutter W31.0
 water driven turbine W31.3
 weaving W31.89
 woodworking or forming (industrial) W31.2
mammal (feces) (urine) W55.89
 bull -*see* Contact, with, bull
 cat -*see* Contact, with, cat
 cow -*see* Contact, with, cow
 goat -*see* Contact, with, goat
 hoof stock -*see* Contact, with, hoof stock
 horse -*see* Contact, with, horse
 marine W56.39
  dolphin -*see* Contact, with, dolphin
  orca -*see* Contact, with, orca
  sea lion -*see* Contact, with, sea lion
  specified NEC W56.39
   bite W56.31
   strike W56.32
 pig -*see* Contact, with, pig
 raccoon -*see* Contact, with, raccoon
 rodent -*see* Contact, with, rodent
 sheep -*see* Contact, with, sheep
 specified NEC W55.89
  bite W55.81
  strike W55.82
marine
 animal W56.89
  bite W56.81
  dolphin -*see* Contact, with, dolphin
  fish NEC -*see* Contact, with, fish
  mammal -*see* Contact, with, mammal, marine
  orca -*see* Contact, with, orca
  sea lion -*see* Contact, with, sea lion
  shark -*see* Contact, with, shark
  strike W56.82
meat
 grinder (domestic) W29.0
  industrial W31.82
  nonpowered W27.4
 slicer (domestic) W29.0
  industrial W31.82
merry go round W31.81
metal, hot (liquid) (molten) NEC X18
millipede W57
nail W45.0
 gun W29.4

Contact (accidental) - *continued*

 needle (sewing) W27.3
  hypodermic W46.0
   contaminated W46.1
 object (blunt) NEC
  hot NEC X19
  legal intervention -*see* Legal, intervention, blunt object
  sharp NEC W45.8
   inflicted by other person NEC W45.8
    stated as
     intentional homicide (attempt) -*see* Assault, cutting or piercing instrument
   legal intervention -*see* Legal, intervention, sharp object
   self-inflicted X78.9
 orca W56.29
  bite W56.21
  strike W56.22
 overhead plane W31.2
 paper (as sharp object) W26.2
 paper-cutter W27.5
 parrot W61.09
  bite W61.01
  strike W61.02
 pig W55.49
  bite W55.41
  strike W55.42
 pipe, hot X16
 pitchfork W27.1
 plane (metal) (wood) W27.0
  overhead W31.2
 plant thorns, spines, sharp leaves or other mechanisms W60
 powered
  garden cultivator W29.3
  household appliance, implement, or machine W29.8
  saw (industrial) W31.2
   hand W29.8
 printing machine W31.89
 psittacine bird W61.29
  bite W61.21
  macaw -*see* Contact, with, macaw
  parrot -*see* Contact, with, parrot
  strike W61.22
 pulley (block) (transmission) W24.0
  agricultural operations W30.89
 raccoon W55.59
  bite W55.51
  strike W55.52
 radial-saw (industrial) W31.2
 radiator (hot) X16
 rake W27.1
 rattlesnake X58
 reaper W30.0
 reptile W59.89
  lizard -*see* Contact, with, lizard
  snake -*see* Contact, with, snake
  specified NEC W59.89
   bite W59.81
   crushing W59.83
   strike W59.82
  turtle -*see* Contact, with, turtle
 rivet gun (powered) W29.4
 road scraper -*see* Accident, transport, construction vehicle
 rodent (feces) (urine) W53.89
  bite W53.81
  mouse W53.09
   bite W53.01
  rat W53.19
   bite W53.11
  specified NEC W53.89

Contact (accidental) - *continued*

  bite W53.81
  squirrel W53.29
   bite W53.21
 roller coaster W31.81
 rope NEC W24.0
  agricultural operations W30.89
 saliva -*see* Contact, with, by type of animal
 sander W29.8
  industrial W31.2
 saucepan (hot) (glass) (metal) X15.3
 saw W27.0
  band (industrial) W31.2
  bench (industrial) W31.2
  chain W29.3
  hand W27.0
 sawing machine, metal W31.1
 scissors W27.2
 scorpion X58
 screwdriver W27.0
  powered W29.8
 sea
  anemone, cucumber or urchin (spine) X58
  lion W56.19
   bite W56.11
   strike W56.12
 serpent -*see* Contact, with, snake, by type
 sewing-machine (electric) (powered) W29.2
  not powered W27.8
 shaft (hoist) (lift) (transmission) NEC W24.0
  agricultural W30.89
 shark W56.49
  bite W56.41
  strike W56.42
 sharp object(s) W26.9
  specified NEC W26.8
 shears (hand) W27.2
  powered (industrial) W31.1
   domestic W29.2
 sheep W55.39
  bite W55.31
  strike W55.32
 shovel W27.8
 steam -*see* Accident, transport, construction vehicle
 snake (nonvenomous) W59.19
  bite W59.11
  crushing W59.13
  strike W59.12
 spade W27.1
 spider (venomous) X58
 spin-drier W29.2
 spinning machine W31.89
 splinter W45.8
 sports equipment W21.9
 staple gun (powered) W29.8
 steam X13.1
  engine W31.3
  inhalation X13.0
  pipe X16
  shovel W31.89
 stove (hot) (kitchen) X15.0
 substance, hot NEC X19
  molten (metal) X18
 sword W26.1
  assault X99.2
  stated as undetermined whether accidental or intentional Y28.2
  suicide (attempt) X78.2
 tarantula X58
 thresher W30.0
 tin can lid W26.8

Desertion X58
Destitution X58
Disability, late effect or sequela of injury -
    see Sequelae
Discharge (accidental)
    airgun W34.010
        assault X95.01
        homicide (attempt) X95.01
        stated as undetermined whether accidental
            or intentional Y24.0
        suicide (attempt) X74.01
    BB gun -see Discharge, airgun
    firearm (accidental) W34.00
        assault X95.9
        handgun (pistol) (revolver) W32.0
            assault X93
            homicide (attempt) X93
            legal intervention -see Legal, intervention,
                firearm, handgun
            stated as undetermined whether accidental
                or intentional Y22
            suicide (attempt) X72
        homicide (attempt) X95.9
        hunting rifle W33.02
            assault X94.1
            homicide (attempt) X94.1
            legal intervention
                injuring
                    bystander Y35.032
                    law enforcement personnel Y35.031
                    suspect Y35.033
            stated as undetermined whether accidental
                or intentional Y23.1
            suicide (attempt) X73.1
        larger W33.00
            assault X94.9
            homicide (attempt) X94.9
            hunting rifle -see Discharge, firearm,
                hunting rifle
            legal intervention -see Legal, intervention,
                firearm by type of firearm
            machine gun -see Discharge, firearm,
                machine gun
            shotgun -see Discharge, firearm, shotgun
            specified NEC W33.09
                assault X94.8
                homicide (attempt) X94.8
                legal intervention
                    injuring
                        bystander Y35.092
                        law enforcement personnel Y35.091
                        suspect Y35.093
                stated as undetermined whether
                    accidental or intentional Y23.8
                suicide (attempt) X73.8
            stated as undetermined whether accidental
                or intentional Y23.9
            suicide (attempt) X73.9
        legal intervention
            injuring
                bystander Y35.002
                law enforcement personnel Y35.001
                suspect Y35.03
            using rubber bullet
                injuring
                    bystander Y35.042
                    law enforcement personnel Y35.041
                    suspect Y35.043
        machine gun W33.03
            assault X94.2
            homicide (attempt) X94.2
            legal intervention -see Legal, intervention,
                firearm, machine gun

Discharge (accidental) - *continued*
        stated as undetermined whether accidental
            or intentional Y23.3
        suicide (attempt) X73.2
    pellet gun -see Discharge, airgun
    shotgun W33.01
        assault X94.0
        homicide (attempt) X94.0
        legal intervention -see Legal, intervention,
            firearm, specified NEC
        stated as undetermined whether accidental
            or intentional Y23.0
        suicide (attempt) X73.0
    specified NEC W34.09
        assault X95.8
        homicide (attempt) X95.8
        legal intervention -see Legal, intervention,
            firearm, specified NEC
        stated as undetermined whether accidental
            or intentional Y24.8
        suicide (attempt) X74.8
    stated as undetermined whether accidental
        or intentional Y24.9
    suicide (attempt) X74.9
    Very pistol W34.09
        assault X95.8
        homicide (attempt) X95.8
        stated as undetermined whether accidental
            or intentional Y24.8
        suicide (attempt) X74.8
    firework(s) W39
        stated as undetermined whether accidental
            or intentional Y25
    gas-operated gun NEC W34.018
        airgun -see Discharge, airgun
        assault X95.09
        homicide (attempt) X95.09
        paintball gun -see Discharge, paintball gun
        stated as undetermined whether accidental
            or intentional Y24.8
        suicide (attempt) X74.09
    gun NEC -see also Discharge, firearm NEC
        air -see Discharge, airgun
        BB -see Discharge, airgun
        for single hand use -see Discharge, firearm,
            handgun
        hand -see Discharge, firearm, handgun
        machine -see Discharge, firearm, machine
            gun
        other specified -see Discharge, firearm
            NEC
        paintball -see Discharge, paintball gun
        pellet -see Discharge, airgun
    handgun -see Discharge, firearm, handgun
    machine gun -see Discharge, firearm,
        machine gun
    paintball gun W34.011
        assault X95.02
        homicide (attempt) X95.02
        stated as undetermined whether accidental
            or intentional Y24.8
        suicide (attempt) X74.02
    pistol -see Discharge, firearm, handgun
        flare -see Discharge, firearm, Very pistol
        pellet -see Discharge, airgun
        Very -see Discharge, firearm, Very pistol
    revolver -see Discharge, firearm, handgun
    rifle (hunting) -see Discharge, firearm,
        hunting rifle
    shotgun -see Discharge, firearm, shotgun
    spring-operated gun NEC W34.018
        assault X95.09
        homicide (attempt) X95.09

Discharge (accidental) - *continued*
        stated as undetermined whether accidental
            or intentional Y24.8
        suicide (attempt) X74.09
Disease
    Andes W94.11
    aviator's
    -see Air, pressure
    range W94.11
Diver's disease, palsy, paralysis, squeeze
    -see Air, pressure
Diving (into water) -see Accident, diving
Dog bite W54.0
Dragged by transport vehicle NEC -see also
    Accident, transport V09.9
Drinking poison (accidental) -see Table of
    Drugs and Chemicals
Dropped (accidentally) while being carried
    or supported by other person W04
Drowning (accidental) W74
    assault X92.9
    due to
        accident (to)
            machinery -see Contact, with, by type of
                machine
            watercraft V90.89
                burning V90.29
                    powered V90.23
                        merchant ship V90.20
                        passenger ship V90.21
                        fishing boat V90.22
                        jet skis V90.23
                    unpowered V90.28
                        canoe V90.25
                        inflatable V90.26
                        kayak V90.25
                        sailboat V90.24
                        water skis V90.27
                crushed V90.39
                    powered V90.33
                        merchant ship V90.30
                        passenger ship V90.31
                        fishing boat V90.32
                        jet skis V90.33
                    unpowered V90.38
                        canoe V90.35
                        inflatable V90.36
                        kayak V90.35
                        sailboat V90.34
                        water skis V90.37
                overturning V90.09
                    powered V90.03
                        merchant ship V90.00
                        passenger ship V90.01
                        fishing boat V90.02
                        jet skis V90.03
                    unpowered V90.08
                        canoe V90.05
                        inflatable V90.06
                        kayak V90.05
                        sailboat V90.04
                sinking V90.19
                    powered V90.13
                        merchant ship V90.10
                        passenger ship V90.11
                        fishing boat V90.12
                        jet skis V90.13
                    unpowered V90.18
                        canoe V90.15
                        inflatable V90.16
                        kayak V90.15
                        sailboat V90.14
                specified type NEC V90.89
                    powered V90.83

Drowning (accidental) - *continued*
    merchant ship V90.80
    passenger ship V90.81
    fishing boat V90.82
    jet skis V90.83
    unpowered V90.88
      canoe V90.85
      inflatable V90.86
      kayak V90.85
      sailboat V90.84
      water skis V90.87
  avalanche -*see* Landslide
  cataclysmic
    earth surface movement NEC -*see* Forces
    of nature, earth movement
    storm -*see* Forces of nature, cataclysmic
    storm
  cloudburst X37.8
  cyclone X37.1
  fall overboard (from) V92.09
    powered craft V92.03
      ferry boat V92.01
      liner V92.01
      merchant ship V92.00
      passenger ship V92.01
      fishing boat V92.02
      jet skis V92.03
    unpowered craft V92.08
      canoe V92.05
      inflatable V92.06
      kayak V92.05
      sailboat V92.04
      surf-board V92.08
      water skis V92.07
      windsurfer V92.08
  resulting from
    accident to watercraft -*see* Drowning,
    due to, accident to, watercraft
    being washed overboard (from) V92.29
      powered craft V92.23
        ferry boat V92.21
        liner V92.21
        merchant ship V92.20
        passenger ship V92.21
        fishing boat V92.22
        jet skis V92.23
      unpowered craft V92.28
        canoe V92.25
        inflatable V92.26
        kayak V92.25
        sailboat V92.24
        surf-board V92.28
        water skis V92.27
        windsurfer V92.28
    motion of watercraft V92.19
      powered craft V92.13
        ferry boat V92.11
        liner V92.11
        merchant ship V92.10
        passenger ship V92.11
        fishing boat V92.12
        jet skis V92.13
      unpowered craft
        canoe V92.15
        inflatable V92.16
        kayak V92.15
        sailboat V92.14
  hurricane X37.0
  jumping into water from watercraft
    (involved in accident) -*see also* Drowning,
    due to, accident to, watercraft
    without accident to or on watercraft
    W16.711

Drowning (accidental) - *continued*
  tidal wave NEC -*see* Forces of nature, tidal
    wave
  torrential rain X37.8
  following
    fall
      into
        bathtub W16.211
        bucket W16.221
        fountain -*see* Drowning, following, fall,
      into, water, specified NEC
        quarry -*see* Drowning, following, fall,
      into, water, specified NEC
        reservoir -*see* Drowning, following, fall,
      into, water, specified NEC
        swimming-pool W16.011
          striking
            bottom W16.021
            wall W16.031
          stated as undetermined whether
      accidental or intentional Y21.3
          suicide (attempt) X71.2
        water NOS W16.41
        natural (lake) (open sea) (river)
      (stream) (pond) W16.111
          striking
            bottom W16.121
            side W16.131
        specified NEC W16.311
          striking
            bottom W16.321
            wall W16.331
    overboard NEC -*see* Drowning, due to,
    fall overboard
    jump or dive
      from boat W16.711
        striking bottom W16.721
      into
        fountain -*see* Drowning, following, jump
      or dive, into, water, specified NEC
        quarry -*see* Drowning, following, jump
      or dive, into, water, specified NEC
        reservoir -*see* Drowning, following,
      jump or dive, into, water, specified NEC
        swimming-pool W16.511
          striking
            bottom W16.521
            wall W16.531
          suicide (attempt) X71.2
        water NOS W16.91
        natural (lake) (open sea) (river)
      (stream) (pond) W16.611
        specified NEC W16.811
          striking
            bottom W16.821
            wall W16.831
        striking bottom W16.621
  homicide (attempt) X92.9
  in
    bathtub (accidental) W65
      assault X92.0
      following fall W16.211
        stated as undetermined whether
      accidental or intentional Y21.1
      stated as undetermined whether accidental
      or intentional Y21.0
      suicide (attempt) X71.0
    lake -*see* Drowning, in, natural water
    natural water (lake) (open sea) (river)
    (stream) (pond) W69
      assault X92.3
      following
        dive or jump W16.611
          striking bottom W16.621

Drowning (accidental) - *continued*
        fall W16.111
          striking
            bottom W16.121
            side W16.131
      stated as undetermined whether accidental
      or intentional Y21.4
      suicide (attempt) X71.3
    quarry -*see* Drowning, in, specified place
    NEC
    quenching tank -*see* Drowning, in, specified
    place NEC
    reservoir -*see* Drowning, in, specified place
    NEC
    river -*see* Drowning, in, natural water
    sea -*see* Drowning, in, natural water
    specified place NEC W73
      assault X92.8
      following
        dive or jump W16.811
          striking
            bottom W16.821
            wall W16.831
        fall W16.311
          striking
            bottom W16.321
            wall W16.331
      stated as undetermined whether accidental
      or intentional Y21.8
      suicide (attempt) X71.8
    stream -*see* Drowning, in, natural water
    swimming-pool W67
      assault X92.1
      following fall X92.2
      following
        dive or jump W16.511
          striking
            bottom W16.521
            wall W16.531
        fall W16.011
          striking
            bottom W16.021
            wall W16.031
      stated as undetermined whether accidental
      or intentional Y21.2
        following fall Y21.3
      suicide (attempt) X71.1
        following fall X71.2
  war operations -*see* War operations,
    restriction of airway
  resulting from accident to watercraft see
    Drowning, due to, accident, watercraft
  self-inflicted X71.9
  stated as undetermined whether accidental or
    intentional Y21.9
  suicide (attempt) X71.9

E

Earth (surface) movement NEC -*see* Forces
  of nature, earth movement
Earth falling (on) W20.0
  caused by cataclysmic earth surface
  movement or eruption -*see* Landslide
Earthquake (any injury) X34
Effect(s) (adverse) of
  air pressure (any)   -*see* Air, pressure
  cold, excessive (exposure to) -*see* Exposure,
  cold
  heat (excessive) -*see* Heat
  hot place (weather) -*see* Heat
  insolation X30

Effect(s) - *continued*
late -*see* Sequelae
motion -*see* Motion
nuclear explosion or weapon in war
operations -*see* War operations, nuclear
weapon
radiation -*see* Radiation
travel -*see* Travel
Electric shock (accidental) (by) (in) -*see*
Exposure, electric current
Electrocution (accidental) -*see* Exposure,
electric current
**Endotracheal tube wrongly placed during
anesthetic procedure**
Entanglement
in
bed linen, causing suffocation -*see* category
T71
wheel of pedal cycle V19.88
Entry of foreign body or material -*see*
Foreign body
Environmental pollution related condition-
see Z57
Execution, legal (any method) -*see* Legal,
intervention
Exhaustion
cold -*see* Exposure, cold
due to excessive exertion -*see also*
Overexertion X50.9
heat -*see* Heat
**Explosion (accidental) (of) (with secondary
fire) W40.9**
acetylene W40.1
aerosol can W36.1
air tank (compressed) (in machinery) W36.2
aircraft (in transit) (powered) NEC V95.9
balloon V96.05
fixed wing NEC (private) V95.25
commercial V95.35
glider V96.25
hang V96.15
powered V95.15
helicopter V95.05
in war operations -*see* War operations,
destruction of aircraft
microlight V95.15
nonpowered V96.9
specified NEC V96.8
powered NEC V95.8
stated as
homicide (attempt) Y03.8
suicide (attempt) X83.0
ultralight V95.15
anesthetic gas in operating room W40.1
antipersonnel bomb W40.8
assault X96.0
homicide (attempt) X96.0
suicide (attempt) X75
assault X96.9
bicycle tire W37.0
blasting (cap) (materials) W40.0
boiler (machinery), not on transport vehicle
W35
on watercraft -*see* Explosion, in, watercraft
butane W40.1
caused by other person X96.9
coal gas W40.1
detonator W40.0
dump (munitions) W40.8
dynamite W40.0
in
assault X96.8
homicide (attempt) X96.8
legal intervention

Explosion (accidental) - *continued*
injuring
bystander Y35.112
law enforcement personnel Y35.111
suspect Y35.113
suicide (attempt) X75
explosive (material) W40.9
gas W40.1
in blasting operation W40.0
specified NEC W40.8
in
assault X96.8
homicide (attempt) X96.8
legal intervention
injuring
bystander Y35.192
law enforcement personnel Y35.191
suspect Y35.193
suicide (attempt) X75
factory (munitions) W40.8
fertilizer bomb W40.8
assault X96.3
homicide (attempt) X96.3
suicide (attempt) X75
firearm (parts) NEC W34.19
airgun W34.110
BB gun W34.110
gas, air or spring-operated gun NEC
W34.118
handgun W32.1
hunting rifle W33.12
larger firearm W33.10
specified NEC W33.19
machine gun W33.13
paintball gun W34.111
pellet gun W34.110
shotgun W33.11
Very pistol [flare] W34.19
fire-damp W40.1
fireworks W39
gas (coal) (explosive) W40.1
cylinder W36.9
aerosol can W36.1
air tank W36.2
pressurized W36.3
specified NEC W36.8
gasoline (fumes) (tank) not in moving motor
vehicle W40.1
bomb W40.8
assault X96.1
homicide (attempt) X96.1
suicide (attempt) X75
in motor vehicle -*see* Accident, transport,
by type of vehicle
grain store W40.8
grenade W40.8
in
assault X96.8
homicide (attempt) X96.8
legal intervention
injuring
bystander Y35.192
law enforcement personnel Y35.191
suspect Y35.193
suicide (attempt) X75
handgun (parts) -*see* Explosion, firearm,
handgun (parts)   homicide (attempt)
X96.9
antipersonnel bomb -*see* Explosion,
antipersonnel bomb
fertilizer bomb -*see* Explosion, fertilizer
bomb
gasoline bomb -*see* Explosion, gasoline
bomb

Explosion (accidental) - *continued*
letter bomb -*see* Explosion, letter bomb
pipe bomb -*see* Explosion, pipe bomb
specified NEC X96.8
hose, pressurized W37.8
hot water heater, tank (in machinery) W35
on watercraft -*see* Explosion, in, watercraft
in, on
dump W40.8
factory W40.8
mine (of explosive gases) NEC W40.1
watercraft V93.59
powered craft V93.53
ferry boat V93.51
fishing boat V93.52
jet skis V93.53
liner V93.51
merchant ship V93.50
passenger ship V93.51
sailboat V93.54
letter bomb W40.8
assault X96.2
homicide (attempt) X96.2
suicide (attempt) X75
machinery -*see also* Contact, with, by type of
machine
on board watercraft -*see* Explosion, in,
watercraft
pressure vessel -*see* Explosion, by type of
vessel
methane W40.1
mine W40.1
missile NEC W40.8
mortar bomb W40.8
in
assault X96.8
homicide (attempt) X96.8
legal intervention
injuring
bystander Y35.192
law enforcement personnel Y35.191
suspect Y35.193
suicide (attempt) X75
munitions (dump) (factory) W40.8
pipe, pressurized W37.8
bomb W40.8
assault X96.4
homicide (attempt) X96.4
suicide (attempt) X75
pressure, pressurized
cooker W38
gas tank (in machinery) W36.3
hose W37.8
pipe W37.8
specified device NEC W38
tire W37.8
bicycle W37.0
vessel (in machinery) W38
propane W40.1
self-inflicted X75
shell (artillery) NEC W40.8
during war operations -*see* War operations,
explosion
in
legal intervention
injuring
bystander Y35.122
law enforcement personnel Y35.121
suspect Y35.123
war -*see* War operations, explosion
spacecraft V95.45
steam or water lines (in machinery) W37.8
stove W40.9

Explosion (accidental) - *continued*
  stated as undetermined whether accidental or
    intentional Y25
  suicide (attempt) X75
  tire, pressurized W37.8
    bicycle W37.0
  undetermined whether accidental or
    intentional Y25
  vehicle tire NEC W37.8
    bicycle W37.0
  war operations -*see* War operations,
    explosion
Exposure (to) X58
  air pressure change -*see* Air, pressure
  cold (accidental) (excessive) (extreme)
    (natural) (place) X31
    assault Y08.89
    due to
      man-made conditions W93.8
        dry ice (contact) W93.01
          inhalation W93.02
        liquid air (contact) (hydrogen) (nitrogen)
          W93.11
          inhalation W93.12
        refrigeration unit (deep freeze) W93.2
      suicide (attempt) X83.2
      weather (conditions) X31
    homicide (attempt) Y08.89
    self-inflicted X83.2
  due to abandonment or neglect X58
  electric current W86.8
    appliance (faulty) W86.8
      domestic W86.0
    caused by other person Y08.89
    conductor (faulty) W86.1
    control apparatus (faulty) W86.1
    electric power generating plant, distribution
      station W86.1
    electroshock gun -*see* Exposure, electric
      current, taser
    high-voltage cable W85
    homicide (attempt) Y08.89
    legal execution -*see* Legal, intervention,
      specified means NEC
    lightning -see subcategory T75.0
    live rail W86.8
    misadventure in medical or surgical
      procedure in electroshock therapy Y63.4
    motor (electric) (faulty) W86.8
      domestic W86.0
    self-inflicted X83.1
    specified NEC W86.8
      domestic W86.0
    stun gun -*see* Exposure, electric current,
      taser
    suicide (attempt) X83.1
    taser W86.8
      assault Y08.89
      legal intervention -see category Y35
      self-harm (intentional) X83.8
      undetermined intent Y33
    third rail W86.8
    transformer (faulty) W86.1
    transmission lines W85
  environmental tobacco smoke X58
  excessive
    cold -*see* Exposure, cold
    heat (natural) NEC X30
      man-made W92
  factor(s) NOS X58
    environmental NEC X58
      man-made NEC W99
    natural NEC -*see* Forces of nature
  specified NEC X58

Exposure (to) - *continued*
  fire, flames (accidental) X08.8
    assault X97
    campfire -*see* Exposure, fire, controlled, not
      in building
    controlled (in)
      with ignition (of) clothing -*see also*
        Ignition, clothes X06.2
        nightwear X05
      bonfire -*see* Exposure, fire, controlled, not
        in building
      brazier (in building or structure) -*see also*
        Exposure, fire, controlled, building
        not in building or structure -*see*
        Exposure, fire, controlled, not in building
      building or structure X02.0
        with
          fall from building X02.3
          injury due to building collapse X02.2
          from building X02.5
          smoke inhalation X02.1
        hit by object from building X02.4
        specified mode of injury NEC X02.8
      fireplace, furnace or stove -*see* Exposure,
        fire, controlled, building
      not in building or structure X03.0
        with
          fall X03.3
          smoke inhalation X03.1
        hit by object X03.4
        specified mode of injury NEC X03.8
      trash -*see* Exposure, fire, controlled, not in
        building
    fireplace -*see* Exposure, fire, controlled,
      building
    fittings or furniture (in building or
      structure) (uncontrolled) -*see* Exposure,
      fire, uncontrolled, building
    forest (uncontrolled) -*see* Exposure, fire,
      uncontrolled, not in building
    grass (uncontrolled) -*see* Exposure, fire,
      uncontrolled, not in building
    hay (uncontrolled) -*see* Exposure, fire,
      uncontrolled, not in building
    homicide (attempt) X97
    ignition of highly flammable material X04
    in, of, on, starting in
      machinery -*see* Contact, with, by type of
        machine
      motor vehicle (in motion) -*see also*
        Accident, transport, occupant by type of
        vehicle V87.8
        with collision -*see* Collision
      railway rolling stock, train, vehicle
        V81.81
        with collision -*see* Accident, transport,
          railway vehicle occupant
      street car (in motion) V82.8
        with collision -*see* Accident, transport,
          streetcar occupant
      transport vehicle NEC -*see also* Accident,
        transport
        with collision -*see* Collision
      war operations -*see also* War operations,
        fire
      from nuclear explosion -*see* War
        operations, nuclear weapons
      watercraft (in transit) (not in transit)
        V91.09
      localized -*see* Burn, on board watercraft,
        due to, fire on board
        powered craft V91.03
          ferry boat V91.01
          fishing boat V91.02

Exposure (to) - *continued*
  jet skis V91.03
  liner V91.01
  merchant ship V91.00
  passenger ship V91.01
  unpowered craft V91.08
    canoe V91.05
    inflatable V91.06
    kayak V91.05
    sailboat V91.04
    surf-board V91.08
    waterskis V91.07
    windsurfer V91.08
  lumber (uncontrolled) -*see* Exposure, fire,
    uncontrolled, not in building
  mine (uncontrolled) -*see* Exposure, fire,
    uncontrolled, not in building
  prairie (uncontrolled) -*see* Exposure, fire,
    uncontrolled, not in building
  resulting from
    explosion -*see* Explosion
    lightning X08.8
  self-inflicted X76
  specified NEC X08.8
  started by other person X97
  stove -*see* Exposure, fire, controlled,
    building
  stated as undetermined whether accidental
    or intentional Y26
  suicide (attempt) X76
  tunnel (uncontrolled) -*see* Exposure, fire,
    uncontrolled, not in building
  uncontrolled
    in building or structure X00.0
      with
        fall from building X00.3
        injury due to building collapse X00.2
        jump from building X00.5
        smoke inhalation X00.1
      bed X08.00
        due to
          cigarette X08.01
          specified material NEC X08.09
        furniture NEC X08.20
          due to
            cigarette X08.21
            specified material NEC X08.29
        hit by object from building X00.4
        sofa X08.10
          due to
            cigarette X08.11
            specified material NEC X08.19
        specified mode of injury NEC X00.8
      not in building or structure (any) X01.0
        with
          fall X01.3
          smoke inhalation X01.1
        hit by object X01.4
        specified mode of injury NEC X01.8
    undetermined whether accidental or
      intentional Y26
  forces of nature NEC -*see* Forces of nature
  G-forces (abnormal) W49.9
  gravitational forces (abnormal) W49.9
  heat (natural) NEC -*see* Heat
  high-pressure jet (hydraulic) (pneumatic)
    W49.9
  hydraulic jet W49.9
  inanimate mechanical force W49.9
  jet, high-pressure (hydraulic) (pneumatic)
    W49.9
  lightning -see subcategory T75.0
    causing fire -*see* Exposure, fire
  mechanical forces NEC W49.9

Exposure (to) - *continued*
  animate NEC W64
  inanimate NEC W49.9
  noise W42.9
    supersonic W42.0
  noxious substance -*see* Table of Drugs and
    Chemicals
  pneumatic jet W49.9
  prolonged in deep-freeze unit or refrigerator
    W93.2
  radiation -*see* Radiation
  smoke -*see also* Exposure, fire
    tobacco, second hand Z77.22
  specified factors NEC X58
  sunlight X32
    man-made (sun lamp) W89.8
    tanning bed W89.1
Exposure (to) - *continued*
  supersonic waves W42.0
  transmission line(s), electric W85
  vibration W49.9
  waves
    infrasound W49.9
    sound W42.9
    supersonic W42.0
  weather NEC -*see* Forces of nature
External cause status Y99.9
  child assisting in compensated work for
    family Y99.8
  civilian activity done for financial or other
    compensation Y99.0
  civilian activity done for income or pay
    Y99.0
  family member assisting in compensated
    work for other family member Y99.8
  hobby not done for income Y99.8
  leisure activity Y99.8
  military activity Y99.1
  off-duty activity of military personnel Y99.8
  recreation or sport not for income or while a
    student Y99.8
  specified NEC Y99.8
  student activity Y99.8
  volunteer activity Y99.2

F

Factors, supplemental
  alcohol
    blood level
      less than 20mg/100ml Y90.0
      presence in blood, level not specified
        Y90.9
      20 39mg/100ml Y90.1
      40 59mg/100ml Y90.2
      60 79mg/100ml Y90.3
      80 99mg/100ml Y90.4
      100 119mg/100ml Y90.5
      120 199mg/100ml Y90.6
      200 239mg/100ml Y90.7
      240mg/100ml or more Y90.8
      presence in blood, but level not specified
        Y90.9
  environmental-pollution-related condition-
    see Z57
  nosocomial condition Y95
  work-related condition Y99.0
Failure
  in suture or ligature during surgical
    procedure Y65.2
  mechanical, of instrument or apparatus (any)
    (during any medical or surgical procedure)
    Y65.8

Failure - *continued*
  sterile precautions (during medical and
    surgical care) -*see* Misadventure, failure,
    sterile precautions, by type of procedure
  to
    introduce tube or instrument Y65.4
      endotracheal tube during anesthesia Y65.3
    make curve (transport vehicle) NEC -*see*
      Accident, transport
    remove tube or instrument Y65.4
Fall, falling (accidental) W19
  building W20.1
    burning (uncontrolled fire) X00.3
  down
    embankment W17.81
    escalator W10.0
    hill W17.81
    ladder W11
    ramp W10.2
    stairs, steps W10.9
  due to
    bumping against
      object W18.00
        sharp glass W18.02
        specified NEC W18.09
        sports equipment W18.01
      person W03
        due to ice or snow W00.0
        on pedestrian conveyance -*see* Accident,
        transport, pedestrian, conveyance
    collision with another person W03
      due to ice or snow W00.0
      involving pedestrian conveyance -*see*
        Accident, transport, pedestrian,
        conveyance
    grocery cart tipping over W17.82
    ice or snow W00.9
      from one level to another W00.2
      on stairs or steps W00.1
      involving pedestrian conveyance -*see*
        Accident, transport, pedestrian,
        conveyance
      on same level W00.0
    slipping (on moving sidewalk) W01.0
      with subsequent striking against object
        W01.10
        furniture W01.190
        sharp object W01.119
          glass W01.110
          power tool or machine W01.111
          specified NEC W01.118
        specified NEC W01.198
    striking against
      object W18.00
        sharp glass W18.02
        specified NEC W18.09
        sports equipment W18.01
      person W03
        due to ice or snow W00.0
        on pedestrian conveyance -*see* Accident,
        transport, pedestrian, conveyance
  earth (with asphyxia or suffocation (by
    pressure)) -*see* Earth, falling
  from, off, out of
    aircraft NEC (with accident to aircraft
      NEC) V97.0
      while boarding or alighting V97.1
    balcony W13.0
    bed W06
    boat, ship, watercraft NEC (with drowning
      or submersion) -*see* Drowning, due to, fall
      overboard
      with hitting bottom or object V94.0
    bridge W13.1

Fall, falling (accidental) - *continued*
  building W13.9
    burning (uncontrolled fire) X00.3
  cavity W17.2
  chair W07
  cherry picker W17.89
  cliff W15
  dock W17.4
  embankment W17.81
  escalator W10.0
  flagpole W13.8
  furniture NEC W08
  grocery cart W17.82
  haystack W17.89
  high place NEC W17.89
    stated as undetermined whether accidental
      or intentional Y30
  hole W17.2
  incline W10.2
  ladder W11
  lifting device W17.89
  machine, machinery -*see also* Contact,
    with, by type of machine
    not in operation W17.89
  manhole W17.1
  mobile elevated work platform [MEWP]
    W17.89
  motorized mobility scooter W05.2
  one level to another NEC W17.89
    intentional, purposeful, suicide (attempt)
      X80
    stated as undetermined whether accidental
      or intentional Y30
  pit W17.2
  playground equipment W09.8
    jungle gym W09.2
    slide W09.0
    swing W09.1
  quarry W17.89
  railing W13.9
  ramp W10.2
  roof W13.2
  scaffolding W12
  scooter (nonmotorized) W05.1
    motorized mobility W05.2
  sky lift W17.89
  stairs, steps W10.9
    curb W10.1
    due to ice or snow W00.1
    escalator W10.0
    incline W10.2
    ramp W10.2
    sidewalk curb W10.1
    specified NEC W10.8
  stepladder W11
  storm drain W17.1
  streetcar NEC V82.6
    with antecedent collision -*see* Accident,
      transport, streetcar occupant
    while boarding or alighting V82.4
  structure NEC W13.8
    burning (uncontrolled fire) X00.3
  table W08
  toilet W18.11
    with subsequent striking against object
      W18.12
  train NEC V81.6
    during derailment (without antecedent
      collision) V81.7
    with antecedent collision -*see* Accident,
      transport, railway vehicle occupant
    while boarding or alighting V81.4

Fall, falling (accidental) - *continued*
   transport vehicle after collision -*see*
     Accident, transport, by type of vehicle,
     collision
   tree W14
   vehicle (in motion) NEC -*see also*
     Accident, transport V89.9
     motor NEC -*see also* Accident, transport,
     occupant, by type of vehicle V87.8
     stationary W17.89
       while boarding or alighting -*see*
       Accident, transport, by type of vehicle,
       while boarding or alighting
   viaduct W13.8
   wall W13.8
   watercraft -*see also* Drowning, due to, fall
     overboard
     with hitting bottom or object V94.0
   well W17.0
   wheelchair, non-moving W05.0
     powered -*see* Accident, transport,
     pedestrian, conveyance occupant,
     specified type NEC
   window W13.4
  in, on
   aircraft NEC V97.0
     with accident to aircraft V97.0
     while boarding or alighting V97.1
   bathtub (empty) W18.2
     filled W16.212
       causing drowning W16.211
   escalator W10.0
   incline W10.2
   ladder W11
   machine, machinery -*see* Contact, with, by
     type of machine
   object, edged, pointed or sharp (with cut) -
     see Fall, by type
   playground equipment W09.8
     jungle gym W09.2
     slide W09.0
     swing W09.1
   ramp W10.2
   scaffolding W12
   shower W18.2
     causing drowning W16.211
   staircase, stairs, steps W10.9
     curb W10.1
     due to ice or snow W00.1
     escalator W10.0
     incline W10.2
     specified NEC W10.8
   streetcar (without antecedent collision)
     V82.5
     with antecedent collision -*see* Accident,
     transport, streetcar occupant
     while boarding or alighting V82.4
   train (without antecedent collision) V81.5
     with antecedent collision -*see* Accident,
     transport, railway vehicle occupant
     during derailment (without antecedent
     collision) V81.7
       with antecedent collision -*see* Accident,
       transport, railway vehicle occupant
     while boarding or alighting V81.4
   transport vehicle after collision -*see*
     Accident, transport, by type of vehicle,
     collision
   watercraft V93.39
     due to
       accident to craft V91.29
         powered craft V91.23
           ferry boat V91.21
           fishing boat V91.22

Fall, falling (accidental) - *continued*
          jet skis V91.23
          liner V91.21
          merchant ship V91.20
          passenger ship V91.21
        unpowered craft
          canoe V91.25
          inflatable V91.26
          kayak V91.25
          sailboat V91.24
       powered craft V93.33
         ferry boat V93.31
         fishing boat V93.32
         jet skis V93.33
         liner V93.31
         merchant ship V93.30
         passenger ship V93.31
       unpowered craft V93.38
         canoe V93.35
         inflatable V93.36
         kayak V93.35
         sailboat V93.34
         surf-board V93.38
         windsurfer V93.38
  into
   cavity W17.2
   dock W17.4
   fire -*see* Exposure, fire, by type
   haystack W17.89
   hole W17.2
   lake -*see* Fall, into, water
   manhole W17.1
   moving part of machinery -*see* Contact,
     with, by type of machine
   ocean -*see* Fall, into, water
   opening in surface NEC W17.89
   pit W17.2
   pond -*see* Fall, into, water
   quarry W17.89
   river -*see* Fall, into, water
   shaft W17.89
   storm drain W17.1
   stream -*see* Fall, into, water
   swimming pool -*see also* Fall, into, water,
     in, swimming pool
     empty W17.3
   tank W17.89
   water W16.42
     causing drowning W16.41
     from watercraft -*see* Drowning, due to,
     fall overboard
     hitting diving board W21.4
     in
       bathtub W16.212
         causing drowning W16.211
       bucket W16.222
         causing drowning W16.221
       natural body of water W16.112
         causing drowning W16.111
         striking
           bottom W16.122
             causing drowning W16.121
           side W16.132
             causing drowning W16.131
       specified water NEC W16.312
         causing drowning W16.311
         striking
           bottom W16.322
             causing drowning W16.321
           wall W16.332
             causing drowning W16.331
       swimming pool W16.012
         causing drowning W16.011
         striking

Fall, falling (accidental) - *continued*
         bottom W16.022
           causing drowning W16.021
         wall W16.032
           causing drowning W16.031
       utility bucket W16.222
         causing drowning W16.221
     well W17.0
  involving
   bed W06
   chair W07
   furniture NEC W08
   glass -*see* Fall, by type
   playground equipment W09.8
     jungle gym W09.2
     slide W09.0
     swing W09.1
   roller blades -*see* Accident, transport,
     pedestrian, conveyance
   skateboard(s) -*see* Accident, transport,
     pedestrian, conveyance
   skates (ice) (in line) (roller) -*see* Accident,
     transport, pedestrian, conveyance
   skis -*see* Accident, transport, pedestrian,
     conveyance
   table W08
   wheelchair, non-moving W05.0
     powered -*see* Accident, transport,
     pedestrian, conveyance, specified type
     NEC
  object -*see* Struck by, object, falling
  off
   toilet W18.11
     with subsequent striking against object
     W18.12
  on same level W18.30
   due to
     specified NEC W18.39
     stepping on an object W18.31
  out of
   bed W06
   building NEC W13.8
   chair W07
   furniture NEC W08
   wheelchair, non-moving W05.0
     powered -*see* Accident, transport,
     pedestrian, conveyance, specified type
     NEC
   window W13.4
  over
   animal W01.0
   cliff W15
   embankment W17.81
   small object W01.0
  rock W20.8
  same level W18.30
   from
     being crushed, pushed, or stepped on by a
     crowd or human stampede W52
     collision, pushing, shoving, by or with
     other person W03
     slipping, stumbling, tripping W01.0
   involving ice or snow W00.0
     involving skates (ice) (roller), skateboard,
     skis -*see* Accident, transport, pedestrian,
     conveyance
  snowslide (avalanche) -*see* Landslide
  stone W20.8
  structure W20.1
   burning (uncontrolled fire) X00.3
  through
   bridge W13.1
   floor W13.3
   roof W13.2

Fall, falling (accidental) - *continued*
  wall W13.8
  window W13.4
  timber W20.8
  tree (caused by lightning) W20.8
  while being carried or supported by other
    person(s) W04
Fallen on by
  animal (not being ridden) NEC W55.89
Felo-de-se -*see* Suicide
Fight (hand) (fists) (foot) -*see* Assault, fight
Fire (accidental) -*see* Exposure, fire
Firearm discharge -*see* Discharge, firearm
Fireball effects from nuclear explosion in
  war operations -*see* War operations,
  nuclear weapons
Fireworks (explosion) W39
Flash burns from explosion -*see* Explosion
Flood (any injury) (caused by) X38
  collapse of man-made structure causing earth
    movement X36.0
  tidal wave -*see* Forces of nature, tidal wave
Food (any type) in
  air passages (with asphyxia, obstruction, or
    suffocation) -*see* categories T17 and T18
  alimentary tract causing asphyxia (due to
    compression of trachea) -*see* categories
    T17 and T18
Forces of nature X39.8
  avalanche X36.1
    causing transport accident -*see* Accident,
      transport, by type of vehicle
  blizzard X37.2
  cataclysmic storm X37.9
    with flood X38
    blizzard X37.2
    cloudburst X37.8
    cyclone X37.1
    dust storm X37.3
    hurricane X37.0
    specified storm NEC X37.8
    storm surge X37.0
    tornado X37.1
    twister X37.1
    typhoon X37.0
  cloudburst X37.8
  cold (natural) X31
  cyclone X37.1
  dam collapse causing earth movement X36.0
  dust storm X37.3
  earth movement X36.1
    earthquake X34
    caused by dam or structure collapse X36.0
  earthquake X34
  flood (caused by) X38
    dam collapse X36.0
    tidal wave -*see* Forces of nature, tidal wave
  heat (natural) X30
  hurricane X37.0
  landslide X36.1
    causing transport accident -*see* Accident,
      transport, by type of vehicle
  lightning -*see* subcategory T75.0
    causing fire -*see* Exposure, fire
  mudslide X36.1
    causing transport accident -*see* Accident,
      transport, by type of vehicle
  radiation (natural) X39.08
    radon X39.01
  radon X39.01
  specified force NEC X39.8
  storm surge X37.0
  structure collapse causing earth movement
    X36.0

Forces of nature - *continued*
  sunlight X32
  tidal wave X37.41
    due to
      earthquake X37.41
      landslide X37.43
      storm X37.42
      volcanic eruption X37.41
  tornado X37.1
  tsunami X37.41
  twister X37.1
  typhoon X37.0
  volcanic eruption X35
Foreign body
  aspiration -*see* Index to Diseases and
    Injuries, Foreign body, respiratory tract
  embedded in skin W45
  entering through skin W45.8
    can lid W26.8
    nail W45.0
    paper W26.2
    specified NEC W45.8
    splinter W45.8
Forest fire (exposure to) -*see* Exposure, fire,
  uncontrolled, not in building
Found injured X58
  from exposure (to) -*see* Exposure
  on
    highway, road (way), street V89.9
    railway right of way V81.9
Fracture (circumstances unknown or
  unspecified) X58
  due to specified cause NEC X58
Freezing -*see* Exposure, cold **Frostbite** X31
  due to man-made conditions -*see* Exposure,
    cold, man-made **Frozen** -*see* Exposure,
    cold

G

Gored by bull W55.22
Gunshot wound W34.00

H

Hailstones, injured by X39.8
Hanged herself or himself -*see* Hanging, self-
  inflicted
Hanging (accidental) -*see also* category T71
  legal execution -*see* Legal, intervention,
    specified means NEC
Heat (effects of) (excessive) X30
  due to
    man-made conditions W92
      on board watercraft V93.29
        fishing boat V93.22
        merchant ship V93.20
        passenger ship V93.21
        sailboat V93.24
        specified powered craft NEC V93.23
    weather (conditions) X30
  from

Heat - *continued*
  electric heating apparatus causing burning
    X16
  nuclear explosion in war operations -*see*
    War operations, nuclear weapons
  inappropriate in local application or packing
    in medical or surgical procedure Y63.5

Hemorrhage
  delayed following medical or surgical
    treatment without mention of
    misadventure -*see* Index to Diseases and
    Injuries, Complication(s)
  during medical or surgical treatment as
    misadventure -*see* Index to Diseases and
    Injuries, Complication(s)
High
  altitude (effects) -*see* Air, pressure, low
  level of radioactivity, effects -*see* Radiation
  pressure (effects) -*see* Air, pressure, high
  temperature, effects -*see* Heat
Hit, hitting (accidental) by -*see* Struck by
Hitting against -*see* Striking against
Homicide (attempt) (justifiable) -*see* Assault
Hot
  place, effects -*see also* Heat
  weather, effects X30
House fire (uncontrolled) -*see* Exposure, fire,
  uncontrolled, building
Humidity, causing problem X39.8
Hunger X58
Hurricane (any injury) X37.0
Hypobarism, hypobaropathy
  -*see* Air, pressure, low

I

Ictus
  caloris -*see also* Heat
  solaris X30
Ignition (accidental) -*see also* Exposure, fire
  X08.8
  anesthetic gas in operating room W40.1
  apparel X06.2
    from highly flammable material X04
    nightwear X05
  bed linen (sheets) (spreads) (pillows)
    (mattress) -*see* Exposure, fire,
    uncontrolled, building, bed
  benzine X04
  clothes, clothing NEC (from controlled fire)
    X06.2
    from
      highly flammable material X04
  ether X04
    in operating room W40.1
  explosive material -*see* Explosion
  gasoline X04
  jewelry (plastic) (any) X06.0
  kerosene X04
  material
    explosive -*see* Explosion
    highly flammable with secondary explosion
      X04
  nightwear X05
  paraffin X04
  petrol X04
Immersion (accidental) -*see also* Drowning
  hand or foot due to cold (excessive) X31
Implantation of quills of porcupine W55.89

Inanition (from) (hunger) X58
  thirst X58
Inappropriate operation performed
  correct operation on wrong side or body part
    (wrong side) (wrong site) Y65.53
  operation intended for another patient done
    on wrong patient Y65.52
  wrong operation performed on correct patient
    Y65.51
Inattention after, at birth (homicidal intent)
  (infanticidal intent) X58

Incident, adverse
device
anesthesiology Y70.8
accessory Y70.2
diagnostic Y70.0
miscellaneous Y70.8
monitoring Y70.0
prosthetic Y70.2
rehabilitative Y70.1
surgical Y70.3
therapeutic Y70.1
cardiovascular Y71.8
accessory Y71.2
diagnostic Y71.0
miscellaneous Y71.8
monitoring Y71.0
prosthetic Y71.2
rehabilitative Y71.1
surgical Y71.3
therapeutic Y71.1
gastroenterology Y73.8
accessory Y73.2
diagnostic Y73.0
miscellaneous Y73.8
monitoring Y73.0
prosthetic Y73.2
rehabilitative Y73.1
surgical Y73.3
therapeutic Y73.1
general
hospital Y74.8
accessory Y74.2
diagnostic Y74.0
miscellaneous Y74.8
monitoring Y74.0
prosthetic Y74.2
rehabilitative Y74.1
surgical Y74.3
therapeutic Y74.1
surgical Y81.8
accessory Y81.2
diagnostic Y81.0
miscellaneous Y81.8
monitoring Y81.0
prosthetic Y81.2
rehabilitative Y81.1
surgical Y81.3
therapeutic Y81.1
gynecological Y76.8
accessory Y76.2
diagnostic Y76.0
miscellaneous Y76.8
monitoring Y76.0
prosthetic Y76.2
rehabilitative Y76.1
surgical Y76.3
therapeutic Y76.1
medical Y82.9
specified type NEC Y82.8
neurological Y75.8
accessory Y75.2
diagnostic Y75.0
miscellaneous Y75.8
monitoring Y75.0
prosthetic Y75.2
rehabilitative Y75.1
surgical Y75.3
therapeutic Y75.1
obstetrical Y76.8
accessory Y76.2
diagnostic Y76.0
miscellaneous Y76.8
monitoring Y76.0
prosthetic Y76.2

Incident, adverse - *continued*
rehabilitative Y76.1
surgical Y76.3
therapeutic Y76.1
ophthalmic Y77.8
accessory Y77.2
diagnostic Y77.0
miscellaneous Y77.8
monitoring Y77.0
prosthetic Y77.2
rehabilitative Y77.1
surgical Y77.3
therapeutic Y77.1
orthopedic Y79.8
accessory Y79.2
diagnostic Y79.0
miscellaneous Y79.8
monitoring Y79.0
prosthetic Y79.2
rehabilitative Y79.1
surgical Y79.3
therapeutic Y79.1
otorhinolaryngological Y72.8
accessory Y72.2
diagnostic Y72.0
miscellaneous Y72.8
monitoring Y72.0
prosthetic Y72.2
rehabilitative Y72.1
surgical Y72.3
therapeutic Y72.1
personal use Y74.8
accessory Y74.2
diagnostic Y74.0
miscellaneous Y74.8
monitoring Y74.0
prosthetic Y74.2
rehabilitative Y74.1
surgical Y74.3
therapeutic Y74.1
physical medicine Y80.8
accessory Y80.2
diagnostic Y80.0
miscellaneous Y80.8
monitoring Y80.0
prosthetic Y80.2
rehabilitative Y80.1
surgical Y80.3
therapeutic Y80.1
plastic surgical Y81.8
accessory Y81.2
diagnostic Y81.0
miscellaneous Y81.8
monitoring Y81.0
prosthetic Y81.2
rehabilitative Y81.1
surgical Y81.3
therapeutic Y81.1
radiological Y78.8
accessory Y78.2
diagnostic Y78.0
miscellaneous Y78.8
monitoring Y78.0
prosthetic Y78.2
rehabilitative Y78.1
surgical Y78.3
therapeutic Y78.1
urology Y73.8
accessory Y73.2
diagnostic Y73.0
miscellaneous Y73.8
monitoring Y73.0
prosthetic Y73.2
rehabilitative Y73.1

Incident, adverse - *continued*
surgical Y73.3
therapeutic Y73.1
Incineration (accidental) -*see* Exposure, fire
Infanticide -*see* Assault
Infrasound waves (causing injury) W49.9
Ingestion
foreign body (causing injury) (with
obstruction) -*see* Foreign body, alimentary
canal
poisonous
plant(s) X58
substance NEC -*see* Table of Drugs and
Chemicals
Inhalation
excessively cold substance, man-made -*see*
Exposure, cold, man-made
food (any type) (into respiratory tract) (with
asphyxia, obstruction respiratory tract,
suffocation) -*see* categories T17 and T18
foreign body -*see* Foreign body, aspiration
gastric contents (with asphyxia, obstruction
respiratory passage, suffocation) T17.81
hot air or gases X14.0
liquid air, hydrogen, nitrogen W93.12
suicide (attempt) X83.2
steam X13.0
assault X98.0
stated as undetermined whether accidental
or intentional Y27.0
suicide (attempt) X77.0
toxic gas -*see* Table of Drugs and Chemicals
vomitus (with asphyxia, obstruction
respiratory passage, suffocation) T17.81
Injury, injured (accidental(ly)) NOS X58
by, caused by, from
assault -*see* Assault
law-enforcing agent, police, in course of
legal intervention -*see* Legal intervention
suicide (attempt) X83.8
due to, in
civil insurrection -*see* War operations
fight -*see also* Assault, fight Y04.0
war operations -*see* War operations
homicide -*see also* Assault Y09
inflicted (by)
in course of arrest (attempted), suppression
of disturbance, maintenance of order, by
law-enforcing agents -*see* Legal
intervention
other person
stated as
accidental X58
intentional, homicide (attempt) -*see*
Assault
undetermined whether accidental or
intentional Y33
purposely (inflicted) by other person(s) -*see*
Assault
self-inflicted X83.8
stated as accidental X58
specified cause NEC X58
undetermined whether accidental or
intentional Y33
Insolation, effects X30
Insufficient nourishment X58
Interruption of respiration (by)
food (lodged in esophagus) -*see* categories
T17 and T18
vomitus (lodged in esophagus) T17.81
Intervention, legal -*see* Legal intervention
Intoxication
drug -*see* Table of Drugs and Chemicals
poison -*see* Table of Drugs and Chemicals

J

Jammed (accidentally)
between objects (moving) (stationary and moving) W23.0
stationary W23.1
Jumped, jumping
before moving object NEC X81.8
motor vehicle X81.0
subway train X81.1
train X81.1
undetermined whether accidental or intentional Y31
from
boat (into water) voluntarily, without accident (to or on boat) W16.712
with
accident to or on boat -see Accident, watercraft
drowning or submersion W16.711
suicide (attempt) X71.3
striking bottom W16.722
causing drowning W16.721
building -see also Jumped, from, high place W13.9
burning (uncontrolled fire) X00.5
high place NEC W17.89
suicide (attempt) X80
undetermined whether accidental or intentional Y30
structure -see also Jumped, from, high place W13.9
burning (uncontrolled fire) X00.5
into water W16.92
causing drowning W16.91
from, off watercraft -see Jumped, from, boat
in
natural body W16.612
causing drowning W16.611
striking bottom W16.622
causing drowning W16.621
specified place NEC W16.812
causing drowning W16.811
striking
bottom W16.822
causing drowning W16.821
wall W16.832
Jumped, jumping - continued
causing drowning W16.831
swimming pool W16.512
causing drowning W16.511
striking
bottom W16.522
causing drowning W16.521
wall W16.532
causing drowning W16.531
suicide (attempt) X71.3

K

Kicked by
animal NEC W55.82
person(s) (accidentally) W50.1
with intent to injure or kill Y04.0
as, or caused by, a crowd or human stampede (with fall) W52
assault Y04.0
homicide (attempt) Y04.0
in
fight Y04.0
legal intervention
injuring

Kicked by- continued
bystander Y35.812
law enforcement personnel Y35.811
suspect Y35.813
Kicking
against
object W22.8
sports equipment W21.9
stationary W22.09
sports equipment W21.89
person -see Striking against, person
sports equipment W21.9
carpet stretcher with knee X50.3
Killed, killing (accidentally) NOS -see also Injury X58
in
action -see War operations
brawl, fight (hand) (fists) (foot) Y04.0
by weapon -see also Assault
cutting, piercing -see Assault, cutting or piercing instrument
firearm -see Discharge, firearm, by type, homicide
self
stated as
accident NOS X58
suicide -see Suicide
undetermined whether accidental or intentional Y33
Kneeling (prolonged) (static) X50.1
Knocked down (accidentally) (by) NOS X58
animal (not being ridden) NEC -see also Struck by, by type of animal
crowd or human stampede W52
person W51
in brawl, fight Y04.0
transport vehicle NEC -see also Accident, transport V09.9

L

Laceration NEC -see Injury
Lack of
care (helpless person) (infant) (newborn) X58
Lack of - continued
food except as result of abandonment or neglect X58
due to abandonment or neglect X58
water except as result of transport accident X58
due to transport accident -see Accident, transport, by type
helpless person, infant, newborn X58
Landslide (falling on transport vehicle) X36.1
caused by collapse of man-made structure X36.0
Late effect -see Sequelae
Legal
execution (any method) -see Legal, intervention
intervention (by)
baton -see Legal, intervention, blunt object, baton
bayonet -see Legal, intervention, sharp object, bayonet
blow -see Legal, intervention, manhandling
blunt object
baton
injuring
bystander Y35.312
law enforcement personnel Y35.311
suspect Y35.313

Legal - continued
injuring
bystander Y35.302
law enforcement personnel Y35.301
suspect Y35.303
specified NEC
injuring
bystander Y35.392
law enforcement personnel Y35.391
suspect Y35.393
stave
injuring
bystander Y35.392
law enforcement personnel Y35.391
suspect Y35.393
bomb -see Legal, intervention, explosive
cutting or piercing instrument -see Legal, intervention, sharp object
dynamite -see Legal, intervention, explosive, dynamite
explosive(s)   dynamite
injuring
bystander Y35.112
law enforcement personnel Y35.111
suspect Y35.113
grenade
injuring
bystander Y35.192
law enforcement personnel Y35.191
suspect Y35.193
injuring
bystander Y35.102
law enforcement personnel Y35.101
suspect Y35.103
mortar bomb
injuring
bystander Y35.192
law enforcement personnel Y35.191
suspect Y35.193
shell
injuring
bystander Y35.122
law enforcement personnel Y35.121
suspect Y35.123
specified NEC
injuring
bystander Y35.192
law enforcement personnel Y35.191
suspect Y35.193
firearm(s) (discharge)
handgun
injuring
bystander Y35.022
law enforcement personnel Y35.021
suspect Y35.023
injuring
bystander Y35.002
law enforcement personnel Y35.001
suspect Y35.003
machine gun
injuring
bystander Y35.012
law enforcement personnel Y35.011
suspect Y35.013
rifle pellet
injuring
bystander Y35.032
law enforcement personnel Y35.031
suspect Y35.033
rubber bullet
injuring
bystander Y35.042
law enforcement personnel Y35.041
suspect Y35.043

Legal - *continued*
shotgun -*see* Legal, intervention, firearm,
 specified NEC
specified NEC
 injuring
  bystander Y35.092
  law enforcement personnel Y35.091
  suspect Y35.093
gas (asphyxiation) (poisoning)   injuring
 bystander Y35.202
 law enforcement personnel Y35.201
 suspect Y35.203
specified NEC
 injuring
  bystander Y35.292
  law enforcement personnel Y35.291
  suspect Y35.293
tear gas
 injuring
  bystander Y35.212
  law enforcement personnel Y35.211
  suspect Y35.213
grenade -*see* Legal, intervention, explosive,
 grenade
injuring
 bystander Y35.92
 law enforcement personnel Y35.91
 suspect Y35.93
late effect (of) -*see* with 7th character S
 Y35
manhandling
 injuring
  bystander Y35.812
  law enforcement personnel Y35.811
  suspect Y35.813
sequelae (of) -*see* with 7th character S Y35
sharp objects
 bayonet
  injuring
   bystander Y35.412
   law enforcement personnel Y35.411
   suspect Y35.413
 injuring
  bystander Y35.402
  law enforcement personnel Y35.401
  suspect Y35.403
 specified NEC
  injuring
   bystander Y35.492
   law enforcement personnel Y35.491
   suspect Y35.493
specified means NEC
 injuring
  bystander Y35.892
  law enforcement personnel Y35.891
  suspect Y35.893
stabbing -*see* Legal, intervention, sharp
 object
stave -*see* Legal, intervention, blunt object,
 stave
tear gas -*see* Legal, intervention, gas, tear
 gas
truncheon -*see* Legal, intervention, blunt
 object, stave
Lifting -*see also* Overexertion
heavy objects X50.0
weights X50.0
Lightning (shock) (stroke) (struck by) -*see*
 subcategory T75.0
causing fire -*see* Exposure, fire
Loss of control (transport vehicle) NEC -*see*
 Accident, transport
Lost at sea NOS -*see* Drowning, due to, fall
 overboard

Low
pressure (effects)   -*see* Air, pressure, low
temperature (effects) -*see* Exposure, cold
**Lying before train, vehicle or other moving
 object** X81.8
subway train X81.1
train X81.1
undetermined whether accidental or
 intentional Y31
Lynching -*see* Assault

M

**Malfunction (mechanism or component)
 (of)**   firearm W34.10
airgun W34.110
BB gun W34.110
gas, air or spring-operated gun NEC
 W34.118
handgun W32.1
hunting rifle W33.12
larger firearm W33.10
 specified NEC W33.19
machine gun W33.13
paintball gun W34.111
pellet gun W34.110
shotgun W33.11
specified NEC W34.19
Very pistol [flare] W34.19
handgun -*see* Malfunction, firearm, handgun
Maltreatment -*see* Perpetrator
Mangled (accidentally) NOS X58
Manhandling (in brawl, fight) Y04.0
legal intervention -*see* Legal, intervention,
 manhandling
Manslaughter (nonaccidental) -*see* Assault

Mauled by animal NEC W55.89
**Medical procedure, complication of
 (delayed or as an abnormal reaction
 without mention of misadventure)** -*see*
 Complication of or following, by specified
 type of procedure
due to or as a result of misadventure -*see*
 Misadventure
Melting (due to fire) -*see also* Exposure, fire
apparel NEC X06.3
clothes, clothing NEC X06.3
 nightwear X05
fittings or furniture (burning building)
 (uncontrolled fire) X00.8
nightwear X05
plastic jewelry X06.1
Mental cruelty X58
**Military operations (injuries to military and
 civilians occurring during peacetime on
 military property and during routine
 military exercises and operations) (by)
 (from) (involving)** Y37.90
air blast Y37.20
aircraft
 destruction -*see* Military operations,
  destruction of aircraft
airway restriction -*see* Military operations,
 restriction of airways
asphyxiation -*see* Military operations,
 restriction of airways
biological weapons Y37.6X-
blast Y37.20
blast fragments Y37.20
blast wave Y37.20
blast wind Y37.20
bomb Y37.20
 dirty Y37.50

Military operations - *continued*
gasoline Y37.31
 incendiary Y37.31
 petrol Y37.31
bullet Y37.43
 incendiary Y37.32
 rubber Y37.41
chemical weapons Y37.7X-
combat
 hand to hand (unarmed) combat Y37.44
 using blunt or piercing object Y37.45
conflagration -*see* Military operations, fire
conventional warfare NEC Y37.49
depth-charge Y37.01
destruction of aircraft Y37.10
 due to
  air to air missile Y37.11
  collision with other aircraft Y37.12
  detonation (accidental) of onboard
   munitions and explosives Y37.14
  enemy fire or explosives Y37.11
  explosive placed on aircraft Y37.11
  onboard fire Y37.13
  rocket propelled grenade [RPG] Y37.11
  small arms fire Y37.11
  surface to air missile Y37.11
 specified NEC Y37.19
detonation (accidental) of
 onboard marine weapons Y37.05
 own munitions or munitions launch device
  Y37.24
dirty bomb Y37.50
explosion (of) Y37.20
 aerial bomb Y37.21
 bomb NOS -*see also* Military operations,
  bomb(s) Y37.20
 own munitions or munitions launch device
  (accidental) Y37.24
 fragments Y37.20
 grenade Y37.29
 guided missile Y37.22
 improvised explosive device [IED] (person-
  borne) (roadside) (vehicle-borne) Y37.23
 land mine Y37.29
 marine mine (at sea) (in harbor) Y37.02
 marine weapon Y37.00
  specified NEC Y37.09
 sea-based artillery shell Y37.03
 specified NEC Y37.29
 torpedo Y37.04
fire Y37.30
 specified NEC Y37.39
firearms
 discharge Y37.43
 pellets Y37.42
flamethrower Y37.33
fragments (from) (of)
 improvised explosive device [IED] (person-
  borne) (roadside) (vehicle-borne) Y37.26
 munitions Y37.25
 specified NEC Y37.29
 weapons Y37.27
friendly fire Y37.92
hand to hand (unarmed) combat Y37.44
hot substances -*see* Military operations, fire
incendiary bullet Y37.32
nuclear weapon (effects of) Y37.50
 acute radiation exposure Y37.54
 blast pressure Y37.51
 direct blast Y37.51
 direct heat Y37.53
 fallout exposure Y37.54
 fireball Y37.53
 indirect blast (struck or crushed by blast

Military operations - *continued*
debris) (being thrown by blast) Y37.52
  ionizing radiation (immediate exposure)
    Y37.54
  nuclear radiation Y37.54
  radiation
    ionizing (immediate exposure) Y37.54
    nuclear Y37.54
    thermal Y37.53
  specified NEC Y37.59
  secondary effects Y37.54
  thermal radiation Y37.53
restriction of air (airway)
  intentional Y37.46
  unintentional Y37.47
rubber bullets Y37.41
shrapnel NOS Y37.29
suffocation -*see* Military operations,
  restriction of airways
unconventional warfare NEC Y37.7X-
underwater blast NOS Y37.00
warfare
  conventional NEC Y37.49
  unconventional NEC Y37.7X-
weapons
  biological weapons Y37.6X
  chemical Y37.7X-
  nuclear (effects of) Y37.50
    acute radiation exposure Y37.54
    blast pressure Y37.51
    direct blast Y37.51
    direct heat Y37.53
    fallout exposure Y37.54
    fireball Y37.53
    indirect blast (struck or crushed by blast
    debris) (being thrown by blast) Y37.52
    radiation
      ionizing (immediate exposure) Y37.54
      nuclear Y37.54
      thermal Y37.53
    secondary effects Y37.54
    specified NEC Y37.59
  of mass destruction [WMD] Y37.91
  weapon of mass destruction [WMD] Y37.91
Misadventure(s) to patient(s) during
  surgical or medical care Y69
contaminated medical or biological substance
  (blood, drug, fluid) Y64.9
  administered (by) NEC Y64.9
    immunization Y64.1
    infusion Y64.0
    injection Y64.1
    specified means NEC Y64.8
    transfusion Y64.0
    vaccination Y64.1
excessive amount of blood or other fluid
  during transfusion or infusion Y63.0
failure
  in dosage Y63.9
    electroshock therapy Y63.4
    inappropriate temperature (too hot or too
    cold) in local application and packing
    Y63.5
    infusion
      excessive amount of fluid Y63.0
      incorrect dilution of fluid Y63.1
    insulin-shock therapy Y63.4
    nonadministration of necessary drug or
    biological substance Y63.6
    overdose -*see* Table of Drugs and
    Chemicals
      radiation, in therapy Y63.2
    radiation
      overdose Y63.2

Misadventure(s) to patient(s) - *continued*
  specified procedure NEC Y63.8
  transfusion
    excessive amount of blood Y63.0
  mechanical, of instrument or apparatus
    (any) (during any procedure) Y65.8
  sterile precautions (during procedure)
    Y62.9
    aspiration of fluid or tissue (by puncture
    or catheterization, except heart) Y62.6
    biopsy (except needle aspiration) Y62.8
      needle (aspirating) Y62.6
    blood sampling Y62.6
    catheterization Y62.6
      heart Y62.5
    dialysis (kidney) Y62.2
    endoscopic examination Y62.4
    enema Y62.8
    immunization Y62.3
    infusion Y62.1
    injection Y62.3
    needle biopsy Y62.6
    paracentesis (abdominal) (thoracic) Y62.6
    perfusion Y62.2
    puncture (lumbar) Y62.6
    removal of catheter or packing Y62.8
    specified procedure NEC Y62.8
    surgical operation Y62.0
    transfusion Y62.1
    vaccination Y62.3
  suture or ligature during surgical procedure
    Y65.2
  to introduce or to remove tube or
    instrument -*see* Failure, to
hemorrhage -*see* Index to Diseases and
  Injuries, Complication(s)
inadvertent exposure of patient to radiation
  Y63.3
inappropriate
  operation performed -*see* Inappropriate
    operation performed
  temperature (too hot or too cold) in local
    application or packing Y63.5
infusion -*see also* Misadventure, by type,
  infusion Y69
  excessive amount of fluid Y63.0
  incorrect dilution of fluid Y63.1
  wrong fluid Y65.1
mismatched blood in transfusion Y65.0
nonadministration of necessary drug or
  biological substance Y63.6
overdose -*see* Table of Drugs and Chemicals
  radiation (in therapy) Y63.2
perforation -*see* Index to Diseases and
  Injuries, Complication(s)
performance of inappropriate operation -*see*
  Inappropriate operation performed
puncture -*see* Index to Diseases and Injuries,
  Complication(s)
specified type NEC Y65.8
  failure
    suture or ligature during surgical
    operation Y65.2
    to introduce or to remove tube or
    instrument -*see* Failure, to
  infusion of wrong fluid Y65.1
  performance of inappropriate operation -*see*
    Inappropriate operation performed
  transfusion of mismatched blood Y65.0
  wrong
    fluid in infusion Y65.1
    placement of endotracheal tube during
    anesthetic procedure Y65.3

Misadventure(s) to patient(s) - *continued*
  transfusion -*see* Misadventure, by type,
    transfusion
    excessive amount of blood Y63.0
    mismatched blood Y65.0
  wrong
    drug given in error -*see* Table of Drugs and
    Chemicals
    fluid in infusion Y65.1
    placement of endotracheal tube during
    anesthetic procedure Y65.3
Mismatched blood in transfusion Y65.0
Motion sickness T75.3
Mountain sickness W94.11
Mudslide (of cataclysmic nature) -*see*
  Landslide
Murder (attempt) -*see* Assault

N

Nail
  contact with W45.0
Nail - *continued*
  gun W29.4
  embedded in skin W45.0
Neglect (criminal) (homicidal intent) X58
Noise (causing injury) (pollution) W42.9
  supersonic W42.0
Nonadministration (of)
  drug or biological substance (necessary)
    Y63.6
  surgical and medical care Y66
Nosocomial condition Y95

O

Object
  falling
    from, in, on, hitting
      machinery -*see* Contact, with, by type of
      machine
  set in motion by
    accidental explosion or rupture of pressure
      vessel W38
    firearm -*see* Discharge, firearm, by type
    machine (ry) -*see* Contact, with, by type of
      machine
Overdose (drug) -*see* Table of Drugs and
  Chemicals
  radiation Y63.2
Overexertion X50.9
  from
    prolonged static or awkward postures
      X50.1
    repetitive movements X50.3
    specified strenuous movements or postures
      NEC X50.9
    strenuous movement or load X50.0
Overexposure (accidental) (to)
  cold -*see also* Exposure, cold X31
    due to man-made conditions -*see* Exposure,
      cold, man-made
  heat -*see also* Heat X30
  radiation -*see* Radiation
  radioactivity W88.0
  sun (sunburn) X32
  weather NEC -*see* Forces of nature
  wind NEC -*see* Forces of nature
Overheated -*see* Heat
Overturning (accidental)
  machinery -*see* Contact, with, by type of
    machine

Overturning - *continued*
transport vehicle NEC -*see also* Accident,
transport V89.9
watercraft (causing drowning, submersion) -
see also Drowning, due to, accident to,
watercraft, overturning
causing injury except drowning or
submersion -*see* Accident, watercraft,
causing, injury NEC

P

**Parachute descent (voluntary) (without
accident to aircraft)** V97.29
due to accident to aircraft -*see* Accident,
transport, aircraft
Pecked by bird W61.99
**Perforation during medical or surgical
treatment as misadventure** -*see* Index to
Diseases and Injuries, Complication(s)
**Perpetrator, perpetration, of assault,
maltreatment and neglect (by)** Y07.9
boyfriend Y07.03
brother Y07.410
stepbrother Y07.435
coach Y07.53
cousin
female Y07.491
male Y07.490
daycare provider Y07.519
at-home
adult care Y07.512
childcare Y07.510
care center
adult care Y07.513
childcare Y07.511
family member NEC Y07.499
father Y07.11
adoptive Y07.13
foster Y07.420
stepfather Y07.430
foster father Y07.420
foster mother Y07.421
girl friend Y07.04
healthcare provider Y07.529
mental health Y07.521
specified NEC Y07.528
husband Y07.01
instructor Y07.53
mother Y07.12
adoptive Y07.14
foster Y07.421
stepmother Y07.433
nonfamily member Y07.50
specified NEC Y07.59
nurse Y07.528
occupational therapist Y07.528
partner of parent
female Y07.434
male Y07.432
physical therapist Y07.528
sister Y07.411
speech therapist Y07.528
stepbrother Y07.435
stepfather Y07.430
stepmother Y07.433
stepsister Y07.436
teacher Y07.53
wife Y07.02
Piercing -*see* Contact, with, by type of object
or machine
Pinched
between objects (moving) (stationary and
moving) W23.0
stationary W23.1

Pinned under machine (ry) -*see* Contact,
with, by type of machine
Place of occurrence Y92.9
abandoned house Y92.89
airplane Y92.813
airport Y92.520
ambulatory health services establishment
NEC Y92.538
ambulatory surgery center Y92.530
amusement park Y92.831
apartment (co-op) -*see* Place of occurrence,
residence, apartment
assembly hall Y92.29
bank Y92.510
barn Y92.71
baseball field Y92.320
basketball court Y92.310
beach Y92.832
boarding house -*see* Place of occurrence,
residence, boarding house
boat Y92.814
bowling alley Y92.39
bridge Y92.89
building under construction Y92.61
bus Y92.811
station Y92.521
cafe Y92.511
campsite Y92.833
campus -*see* Place of occurrence, school
canal Y92.89
car Y92.810
casino Y92.59
children's home -*see* Place of occurrence,
residence, institutional, orphanage
church Y92.22
cinema Y92.26
clubhouse Y92.29
coal pit Y92.64
college (community) Y92.214
condominium -*see* Place of occurrence,
residence, apartment
construction area -*see* Place of occurrence,
industrial and construction area
convalescent home -*see* Place of occurrence,
residence, institutional, nursing home
court-house Y92.240
cricket ground Y92.328
cultural building Y92.258
art gallery Y92.250
museum Y92.251
music hall Y92.252
opera house Y92.253
specified NEC Y92.258
theater Y92.254
dancehall Y92.252
day nursery Y92.210
dentist office Y92.531
derelict house Y92.89
desert Y92.820
dock NOS Y92.89
dockyard Y92.62
doctor's office Y92.531
dormitory -*see* Place of occurrence,
residence, institutional, school dormitory
dry dock Y92.62
factory (building) (premises) Y92.63
farm (land under cultivation) (outbuildings)
Y92.79
barn Y92.71
chicken coop Y92.72
field Y92.73
hen house Y92.72
house -*see* Place of occurrence, residence,
house

Place of occurrence - *continued*
orchard Y92.74
specified NEC Y92.79
football field Y92.321
forest Y92.821
freeway Y92.411
gallery Y92.250
garage (commercial) Y92.59
boarding house Y92.044
military base Y92.135
mobile home Y92.025
nursing home Y92.124
orphanage Y92.114
private house Y92.015
reform school Y92.155
gas station Y92.524
gasworks Y92.69
golf course Y92.39
gravel pit Y92.64
grocery Y92.512
gymnasium Y92.39
handball court Y92.318
harbor Y92.89
harness racing course Y92.39
healthcare provider office Y92.531
highway (interstate) Y92.411
hill Y92.828
hockey rink Y92.330
home -*see* Place of occurrence, residence
hospice -*see* Place of occurrence, residence,
institutional, nursing home
hospital Y92.239
cafeteria Y92.233
corridor Y92.232
operating room Y92.234
patient
bathroom Y92.231
room Y92.230
specified NEC Y92.238
hotel Y92.59
house -*see also* Place of occurrence,
residence
abandoned Y92.89
under construction Y92.61
industrial and construction area (yard)
Y92.69
building under construction Y92.61
dock Y92.62
dry dock Y92.62
factory Y92.63
gasworks Y92.69
mine Y92.64
oil rig Y92.65
pit Y92.64
power station Y92.69
shipyard Y92.62
specified NEC Y92.69
tunnel under construction Y92.69
workshop Y92.69
kindergarten Y92.211
lacrosse field Y92.328
lake Y92.828
library Y92.241
mall Y92.59
market Y92.512
marsh Y92.828
military
base -*see* Place of occurrence, residence,
institutional, military base
training ground Y92.84
mine Y92.64
mosque Y92.22
motel Y92.59
motorway (interstate) Y92.411

Place of occurrence - *continued*

mountain Y92.828
movie-house Y92.26
museum Y92.251
music-hall Y92.252
not applicable Y92.9
nuclear power station Y92.69
nursing home -*see* Place of occurrence,
    residence, institutional, nursing home
office building Y92.59
offshore installation Y92.65
oil rig Y92.65
old people's home -*see* Place of occurrence,
    residence, institutional, specified NEC
opera-house Y92.253
orphanage -*see* Place of occurrence,
    residence, institutional, orphanage
outpatient surgery center Y92.530
park (public) Y92.830
    amusement Y92.831
parking garage Y92.89
    lot Y92.481
pavement Y92.480
physician office Y92.531
polo field Y92.328
pond Y92.828
post office Y92.242
power station Y92.69
prairie Y92.828
prison -*see* Place of occurrence, residence,
    institutional, prison
public
    administration building Y92.248
      city hall Y92.243
      courthouse Y92.240
      library Y92.241
      post office Y92.242
      specified NEC Y92.248
    building NEC Y92.29
    hall Y92.29
    place NOS Y92.89
race course Y92.39
radio station Y92.59
railway line (bridge) Y92.85
ranch (outbuildings) -*see* Place of
    occurrence, farm
recreation area Y92.838
    amusement park Y92.831
    beach Y92.832
    campsite Y92.833
    park (public) Y92.830
    seashore Y92.832
    specified NEC Y92.838
religious institution Y92.22
reform school
-*see* Place of occurrence, residence,
    institutional, reform school
residence (non-institutional) (private)
    Y92.009
    apartment Y92.039
      bathroom Y92.031
      bedroom Y92.032
      kitchen Y92.030
      specified NEC Y92.038
    bathroom Y92.002
    bedroom Y92.003
    boarding house Y92.049
      bathroom Y92.041
      bedroom Y92.042
      driveway Y92.043
      garage Y92.044
      garden Y92.046
      kitchen Y92.040
      specified NEC Y92.048

      swimming pool Y92.045
      yard Y92.046
    dining room Y92.001
    garden Y92.007
    home Y92.009
    house, single family Y92.019
      bathroom Y92.012
      bedroom Y92.013
      dining room Y92.011
      driveway Y92.014
      garage Y92.015
      garden Y92.017
      kitchen Y92.010
      specified NEC Y92.018
      swimming pool Y92.016
      yard Y92.017
    institutional Y92.10
      children's home -*see* Place of occurrence,
      residence, institutional, orphanage
      hospice -*see* Place of occurrence,
      residence, institutional, nursing home
      military base Y92.139
        barracks Y92.133
        garage Y92.135
        garden Y92.137
        kitchen Y92.130
        mess hall Y92.131
        specified NEC Y92.138
        swimming pool Y92.136
        yard Y92.137
      nursing home Y92.129
        bathroom Y92.121
        bedroom Y92.122
        driveway Y92.123
        garage Y92.124
        garden Y92.126
        kitchen Y92.120
        specified NEC Y92.128
        swimming pool Y92.125
        yard Y92.126
      orphanage Y92.119
        bathroom Y92.111
        bedroom Y92.112
        driveway Y92.113
        garage Y92.114
        garden Y92.116
        kitchen Y92.110
        specified NEC Y92.118
        swimming pool Y92.115
        yard Y92.116
      prison Y92.149
        bathroom Y92.142
        cell Y92.143
        courtyard Y92.147
        dining room Y92.141
        kitchen Y92.140
        specified NEC Y92.148
        swimming pool Y92.146
      reform school Y92.159
        bathroom Y92.152
        bedroom Y92.153
        dining room Y92.151
        driveway Y92.154
        garage Y92.155
        garden Y92.157
        kitchen Y92.150
        specified NEC Y92.158
        swimming pool Y92.156
        yard Y92.157
      school dormitory Y92.169
        bathroom Y92.162
        bedroom Y92.163
        dining room Y92.161

        kitchen Y92.160
        specified NEC Y92.168
      specified NEC Y92.199
        bathroom Y92.192
        bedroom Y92.193
        dining room Y92.191
        driveway Y92.194
        garage Y92.195
        garden Y92.197
        kitchen Y92.190
        specified NEC Y92.198
        swimming pool Y92.196
        yard Y92.197
    kitchen Y92.000
    mobile home Y92.029
      bathroom Y92.022
      bedroom Y92.023
      dining room Y92.021
      driveway Y92.024
      garage Y92.025
      garden Y92.027
      kitchen Y92.020
      specified NEC Y92.028
      swimming pool Y92.026
      yard Y92.027
    specified place in residence NEC Y92.008
    specified residence type NEC Y92.099
      bathroom Y92.091
      bedroom Y92.092
      driveway Y92.093
      garage Y92.094
      garden Y92.096
      kitchen Y92.090
      specified NEC Y92.098
      swimming pool Y92.095
      yard Y92.096
restaurant Y92.511
riding school Y92.39
river Y92.828
road Y92.488
rodeo ring Y92.39
rugby field Y92.328
same day surgery center Y92.530
sand pit Y92.64
school (private) (public) (state) Y92.219
    college Y92.214
    daycare center Y92.210
    elementary school Y92.211
    high school Y92.213
    kindergarten Y92.211
    middle school Y92.212
    specified NEC Y92.218
    trace school Y92.215
    university Y92.214
    vocational school Y92.215
sea (shore) Y92.832
senior citizen center Y92.29
service area
    airport Y92.520
    bus station Y92.521
    gas station Y92.524
    highway rest stop Y92.523
    railway station Y92.522
shipyard Y92.62
shop (commercial) Y92.513
sidewalk Y92.480
silo Y92.79
skating rink (roller) Y92.331
    ice Y92.330
slaughter house Y92.86
soccer field Y92.322
specified place NEC Y92.89
sports area Y92.39

Place of occurrence - *continued*
  athletic
    court Y92.318
      basketball Y92.310
      specified NEC Y92.318
      squash Y92.311
      tennis Y92.312
    field Y92.328
      baseball Y92.320
      cricket ground Y92.328
      football Y92.321
      hockey Y92.328
      soccer Y92.322
      specified NEC Y92.328
    golf course Y92.39
    gymnasium Y92.39
    riding school Y92.39
    skating rink (roller) Y92.331
      ice Y92.330
    stadium Y92.39
    swimming pool Y92.34
  squash court Y92.311
  stadium Y92.39
  steeplechasing course Y92.39
  store Y92.512
  stream Y92.828
  street and highway Y92.410
    bike path Y92.482
    freeway Y92.411
    highway ramp Y92.415
    interstate highway Y92.411
    local residential or business street Y92.414
    motorway Y92.411
    parkway Y92.412
    parking lot Y92.481
    sidewalk Y92.480
    specified NEC Y92.488
    state road Y92.413
  subway car Y92.816
  supermarket Y92.512
  swamp Y92.828
  swimming pool (public) Y92.34
    private (at) Y92.095
      boarding house Y92.045
      military base Y92.136
      mobile home Y92.026
      nursing home Y92.125
      orphanage Y92.115
      prison Y92.146
      reform school Y92.156
      single family residence Y92.016
  synagogue Y92.22
  television station Y92.59
  tennis court Y92.312
  theater Y92.254
  trade area Y92.59
    bank Y92.510
    cafe Y92.511
    casino Y92.59
    garage Y92.59
    hotel Y92.59
    market Y92.512
    office building Y92.59
    radio station Y92.59
    restaurant Y92.511
    shop Y92.513
    shopping mall Y92.59
    store Y92.512
    supermarket Y92.512
    television station Y92.59
    warehouse Y92.59
  trailer park, residential -*see* Place of
    occurrence, residence, mobile home
  trailer site NOS Y92.89

Place of occurrence - *continued*
  train Y92.815
    station Y92.522
  truck Y92.812
  tunnel under construction Y92.69
  urgent (health) care center Y92.532
  university Y92.214
  vehicle (transport) Y92.818
    airplane Y92.813
    boat Y92.814
    bus Y92.811
    car Y92.810
    specified NEC Y92.818
    subway car Y92.816
    train Y92.815
    truck Y92.812
  warehouse Y92.59
  water reservoir Y92.89
  wilderness area Y92.828
    desert Y92.820
    forest Y92.821
    marsh Y92.828
    mountain Y92.828
    prairie Y92.828
    specified NEC Y92.828
    swamp Y92.828
  workshop Y92.69
  yard, private Y92.096
    boarding house Y92.046
    single family house Y92.017
    mobile home Y92.027
  youth center Y92.29
  zoo (zoological garden) Y92.834
Plumbism -*see* Table of Drugs and
  Chemicals, lead
Poisoning (accidental) (by) -*see also* Table of
  Drugs and Chemicals
  by plant, thorns, spines, sharp leaves or other
    mechanisms NEC X58
  carbon monoxide
    generated by
      motor vehicle -*see* Accident, transport
      watercraft (in transit) (not in transit)
        V93.89
        ferry boat V93.81
        fishing boat V93.82
        jet skis V93.83
        liner V93.81
        merchant ship V93.80
        passenger ship V93.81
        powered craft NEC V93.83
  caused by injection of poisons into skin by
    plant thorns, spines, sharp leaves X58
  marine or sea plants (venomous) X58
  exhaust gas
    generated by
      motor vehicle -*see* Accident, transport
      watercraft (in transit) (not in transit)
        V93.89
        ferry boat V93.81
        fishing boat V93.82
        jet skis V93.83
        liner V93.81
        merchant ship V93.80
        passenger ship V93.81
        powered craft NEC V93.83
  fumes or smoke due to
    explosion -*see also* Explosion W40.9
    fire -*see* Exposure, fire
    ignition -*see* Ignition
  gas
    in legal intervention -*see* Legal,
      intervention, gas
    legal execution -*see* Legal, intervention, gas

Poisoning (accidental) - *continued*
  in war operations -*see* War operations
  legal
    execution -*see* Legal, intervention, gas
    intervention
      by gas -*see* Legal, intervention, gas
      other specified means -*see* Legal,
      intervention, specified means NEC
Powder burn (by) (from)
  airgun W34.110
  BB gun W34.110
  firearm NEC W34.19
  gas, air or spring-operated gun NEC
    W34.118
  handgun W32.1
  hunting rifle W33.12
  larger firearm W33.10
    specified NEC W33.19
  machine gun W33.13
  paintball gun W34.111
  pellet gun W34.110
  shotgun W33.11
  Very pistol [flare] W34.19
Premature cessation (of) surgical and
  medical care Y66
Privation (food) (water) X58
Procedure (operation)
  correct, on wrong side or body part (wrong
    side) (wrong site) Y65.53
  intended for another patient done on wrong
    patient Y65.52
  performed on patient not scheduled for
    surgery Y65.52
  performed on wrong patient Y65.52
  wrong, performed on correct patient Y65.51
Prolonged
  sitting in transport vehicle -*see* Travel, by
    type of vehicle
  stay in
    high altitude as cause of anoxia,
      barodontalgia, barotitis or hypoxia
      W94.11
    weightless environment X52
Pulling, excessive -*see also* Overexertion
  X50.9
Puncture, puncturing -*see also* Contact,
  with, by type of object or machine
  by
    plant thorns, spines, sharp leaves or other
      mechanisms NEC W60
  during medical or surgical treatment as
    misadventure -*see* Index to Diseases and
    Injuries, Complication(s)
Pushed, pushing (accidental) (injury in)
  by other person(s) (accidental) W51
    with fall W03
      due to ice or snow W00.0
  as, or caused by, a crowd or human
    stampede (with fall) W52
  before moving object NEC Y02.8
    motor vehicle Y02.0
    subway train Y02.1
    train Y02.1
  from
    high place NEC
      in accidental circumstances W17.89
      stated as
        intentional, homicide (attempt) Y01
        undetermined whether accidental or
      intentional Y30
    transport vehicle NEC -*see also* Accident,
    transport V89.9
      stated as
        intentional, homicide (attempt) Y08.89
  overexertion X50.9

R

Radiation (exposure to)   arc lamps W89.0
atomic power plant (malfunction) NEC
W88.1
complication of or abnormal reaction to
medical radiotherapy Y84.2
electromagnetic, ionizing W88.0
gamma rays W88.1
in
war operations (from or following nuclear
explosion) -see War operations
inadvertent exposure of patient (receiving
test or therapy) Y63.3
infrared (heaters and lamps) W90.1
excessive heat from W92
ionized, ionizing (particles, artificially
accelerated)   radioisotopes W88.1
specified NEC W88.8
x-rays W88.0
isotopes, radioactive -see Radiation,
radioactive isotopes
laser(s) W90.2
in war operations -see War operations
misadventure in medical care Y63.2
light sources (man-made visible and
ultraviolet) W89.9
natural X32
specified NEC W89.8
tanning bed W89.1
welding light W89.0
man-made visible light W89.9
specified NEC W89.8
tanning bed W89.1
welding light W89.0
microwave W90.8
misadventure in medical or surgical
procedure Y63.2
natural NEC X39.08
radon X39.01
overdose (in medical or surgical procedure)
Y63.2
radar W90.0
radioactive isotopes (any) W88.1
atomic power plant malfunction W88.1
misadventure in medical or surgical
treatment Y63.2
radiofrequency W90.0
radium NEC W88.1
sun X32
ultraviolet (light) (man-made) W89.9
natural X32
specified NEC W89.8
tanning bed W89.1
welding light W89.0
welding arc, torch, or light W89.0
excessive heat from W92
x-rays (hard) (soft) W88.0
Range disease W94.11
Rape (attempted) T74.2
Rat bite W53.11
Reaching (prolonged) (static) X50.1
Reaction, abnormal to medical procedure -
see also Complication of or following, by
type of procedure Y84.9
with misadventure -see Misadventure
biologicals -see Table of Drugs and
Chemicals
drugs -see Table of Drugs and Chemicals
vaccine -see Table of Drugs and Chemicals
Recoil
airgun W34.110
BB gun W34.110
firearm NEC W34.19

Recoil - continued
gas, air or spring-operated gun NEC
W34.118
handgun W32.1
hunting rifle W33.12
larger firearm W33.10
specified NEC W33.19
machine gun W33.13
paintball gun W34.111
pellet W34.110
shotgun W33.11
Very pistol [flare] W34.19
Reduction in
atmospheric pressure
-see Air, pressure, change
**Rock falling on or hitting (accidentally)
(person)** W20.8
in cave-in W20.0
Run over (accidentally) (by)
animal (not being ridden) NEC W55.89
machinery -see Contact, with, by specified
type of machine
transport vehicle NEC -see also Accident,
transport V09.9
intentional homicide (attempt) Y03.0
motor NEC V09.20
intentional homicide (attempt) Y03.0
Running
before moving object X81.8
motor vehicle X81.0
Running off, away
animal (being ridden) -see also Accident,
transport V80.918
not being ridden W55.89
animal-drawn vehicle NEC -see also
Accident, transport V80.928
highway, road (way), street
transport vehicle NEC -see also Accident,
transport V89.9
Rupture pressurized devices -see Explosion,
by type of device

S

Saturnism -see Table of Drugs and
Chemicals, lead

Scald, scalding (accidental) (by) (from) (in)
X19
air (hot) X14.1
gases (hot) X14.1
homicide (attempt) -see Assault, burning, hot
object
inflicted by other person
stated as intentional, homicide (attempt) -
see Assault, burning, hot object
liquid (boiling) (hot) NEC X12
stated as undetermined whether accidental
or intentional Y27.2
suicide (attempt) X77.2
local application of externally applied
substance in medical or surgical care
Y63.5
metal (molten) (liquid) (hot) NEC X18
self-inflicted X77.9
stated as undetermined whether accidental or
intentional Y27.8
steam X13.1
assault X98.0
stated as undetermined whether accidental
or intentional Y27.0
suicide (attempt) X77.0
suicide (attempt) X77.9
vapor (hot) X13.1

Scald, scalding - continued
assault X98.0
stated as undetermined whether accidental
or intentional Y27.0
suicide (attempt) X77.0
Scratched by
cat W55.03
person(s) (accidentally) W50.4
with intent to injure or kill Y04.0
as, or caused by, a crowd or human
stampede (with fall) W52
assault Y04.0
homicide (attempt) Y04.0
in
fight Y04.0
legal intervention
injuring
bystander Y35.892
law enforcement personnel Y35.891
suspect Y35.893
Seasickness T75.3
Self-harm NEC -see also External cause by
type, undetermined whether accidental or
intentional
intentional -see Suicide
poisoning NEC -see Table of drugs and
biologicals, accident
Self-inflicted (injury) NEC -see also External
cause by type, undetermined whether
accidental or intentional
intentional -see Suicide
poisoning NEC -see Table of drugs and
biologicals, accident
Sequelae (of)
accident NEC -see W00 X58 with 7th
character S
assault (homicidal) (any means) -see X92
Y08 with 7th character S
homicide, attempt (any means) -see X92 Y08
with 7th character S
injury undetermined whether accidentally or
purposely inflicted -see Y21 Y33 with 7th
character S
intentional self-harm (classifiable to X71
X83) -see X71 X83 with 7th character S
legal intervention -see with 7th character S
Y35
motor vehicle accident -see V00 V99 with
7th character S
suicide, attempt (any means) -see X71 X83
with 7th character S
transport accident -see V00 V99 with 7th
character S
war operations -see War operations
Shock
electric -see Exposure, electric current
from electric appliance (any) (faulty) W86.8
domestic W86.0
suicide (attempt) X83.1
Shooting, shot (accidental(ly)) -see also
Discharge, firearm, by type
herself or himself -see Discharge, firearm by
type, self-inflicted
homicide (attempt) -see Discharge, firearm
by type, homicide
in war operations -see War operations
inflicted by other person -see Discharge,
firearm by type, homicide
accidental -see Discharge, firearm, by type
of firearm
legal
execution -see Legal, intervention, firearm
intervention -see Legal, intervention,
firearm

Shooting, shot - *continued*
  self-inflicted -*see* Discharge, firearm by type,
    suicide
    accidental -*see* Discharge, firearm, by type
      of firearm
    suicide (attempt) -*see* Discharge, firearm by
      type, suicide
  Shoving (accidentally) by other person -*see*
    Pushed, by other person
Sickness
  alpine W94.11
  motion -*see* Motion
  mountain W94.11
Sinking (accidental)
  watercraft (causing drowning, submersion) -
    see also Drowning, due to, accident to,
    watercraft, sinking
    causing injury except drowning or
      submersion -*see* Accident, watercraft,
      causing, injury NEC
Siriasis X32
Sitting (prolonged) (static) X50.1
Slashed wrists -*see* Cut, self-inflicted
Slipping (accidental) (on same level) (with
    fall) W01.0
  on
    ice W00.0
      with skates -*see* Accident, transport,
      pedestrian, conveyance
    mud W01.0
    oil W01.0
    snow W00.0
      with skis -*see* Accident, transport,
      pedestrian, conveyance
    surface (slippery) (wet) NEC W01.0
  without fall W18.40
    due to
      specified NEC W18.49
      stepping from one level to another
        W18.43
      stepping into hole or opening W18.42
      stepping on object W18.41
Sliver, wood, contact with W45.8
Smoldering (due to fire) -*see* Exposure, fire
Sodomy (attempted) by force T74.2
Sound waves (causing injury) W42.9
  supersonic W42.0
Splinter, contact with W45.8
Stab, stabbing -*see* Cut
Standing (prolonged) (static) X50.1
Starvation X58

Status of external cause Y99.9
  child assisting in compensated work for
    family Y99.8
  civilian activity done for financial or other
    compensation Y99.0
  civilian activity done for income or pay
    Y99.0
  family member assisting in compensated
    work for other family member Y99.8
  hobby not done for income Y99.8
  leisure activity Y99.8
  military activity Y99.1
  off-duty activity of military personnel Y99.8
  recreation or sport not for income or while a
    student Y99.8
  specified NEC Y99.8
  student activity Y99.8
  volunteer activity Y99.2
Stepped on
  by
    animal (not being ridden) NEC W55.89
    crowd or human stampede W52
    person W50.0

Stepping on
  object W22.8
    with fall W18.31
    sports equipment W21.9
    stationary W22.09
      sports equipment W21.89
  person W51
    by crowd or human stampede W52
  sports equipment W21.9
Sting
  arthropod, nonvenomous W57
  insect, nonvenomous W57
Storm (cataclysmic) -*see* Forces of nature,
  cataclysmic storm
Straining, excessive -*see also* Overexertion
  X50.9
Strangling -*see* Strangulation
Strangulation (accidental) -*see* category T71
Strenuous movements -*see also* Overexertion
  X50.9
Striking against
  airbag (automobile) W22.10
    driver side W22.11
    front passenger side W22.12
    specified NEC W22.19
  bottom when
    diving or jumping into water (in) W16.822
      causing drowning W16.821
      from boat W16.722
        causing drowning W16.721
      natural body W16.622
        causing drowning W16.821
      swimming pool W16.522
        causing drowning W16.521
    falling into water (in) W16.322
      causing drowning W16.321
      fountain -*see* Striking against, bottom
      when, falling into water, specified NEC
      natural body W16.122
        causing drowning W16.121
      reservoir -*see* Striking against, bottom
      when, falling into water, specified NEC
      specified NEC W16.322
        causing drowning W16.321
      swimming pool W16.022
        causing drowning W16.021
  diving board (swimming-pool) W21.4
  object W22.8
    with
      drowning or submersion -*see* Drowning
      fall -*see* Fall, due to, bumping against,
      object
    caused by crowd or human stampede (with
      fall) W52
    furniture W22.03
    lamppost W22.02
    sports equipment W21.9
    stationary W22.09
      sports equipment W21.89
    wall W22.01
  person(s) W51
    with fall W03
      due to ice or snow W00.0
    as, or caused by, a crowd or human
      stampede (with fall) W52
    assault Y04.2
    homicide (attempt) Y04.2
  sports equipment W21.9
  wall (when) W22.01
    diving or jumping into water (in) W16.832
      causing drowning W16.831
      swimming pool W16.532
        causing drowning W16.531
    falling into water (in) W16.332

Striking against - *continued*
      causing drowning W16.331
      fountain -*see* Striking against, wall when,
      falling into water, specified NEC
      natural body W16.132
        causing drowning W16.131
      reservoir -*see* Striking against, wall when,
      falling into water, specified NEC
      specified NEC W16.332
        causing drowning W16.331
      swimming pool W16.032
        causing drowning W16.031
    swimming pool (when) W22.042
      causing drowning W22.041
      diving or jumping into water W16.532
        causing drowning W16.531
      falling into water W16.032
        causing drowning W16.031
Struck (accidentally) by
  airbag (automobile) W22.10
    driver side W22.11
    front passenger side W22.12
    specified NEC W22.19
  alligator W58.02
  animal (not being ridden) NEC W55.89
  avalanche -*see* Landslide
  ball (hit) (thrown) W21.00
    assault Y08.09
    baseball W21.03
    basketball W21.05
    golf ball W21.04
    football W21.01
    soccer W21.02
    softball W21.07
    specified NEC W21.09
    volleyball W21.06
  bat or racquet
    baseball bat W21.11
      assault Y08.02
    golf club W21.13
      assault Y08.09
    specified NEC W21.19
      assault Y08.09
    tennis racquet W21.12
      assault Y08.09
  bullet -*see also* Discharge, firearm by type
    in war operations -*see* War operations
  crocodile W58.12
  dog W54.1
  flare, Very pistol -*see* Discharge, firearm
    NEC
  hailstones X39.8
  hockey (ice)   field
    puck W21.221
    stick W21.211
    puck W21.220
    stick W21.210
      assault Y08.01
  landslide -*see* Landslide
  law-enforcement agent (on duty) -*see* Legal,
    intervention, manhandling
    with blunt object -*see* Legal, intervention,
    blunt object
  lightning -*see* subcategory T75.0
    causing fire -*see* Exposure, fire
  machine -*see* Contact, with, by type of
    machine
  mammal NEC W55.89
    marine W56.32
  marine animal W56.82
  missile
    firearm -*see* Discharge, firearm by type
    in war operations -*see* War operations,
    missile

Struck (accidentally) by - *continued*
object W22.8
  blunt W22.8
    assault Y00
    suicide (attempt) X79
    undetermined whether accidental or
      intentional Y29
  falling W20.8
    from, in, on
      building W20.1
        burning (uncontrolled fire) X00.4
      cataclysmic
        earth surface movement NEC -*see*
          Landslide
        storm -*see* Forces of nature,
          cataclysmic storm
      cave-in W20.0
      earthquake X34
      machine (in operation) -*see* Contact,
        with, by type of machine
      structure W20.1
        burning X00.4
      transport vehicle (in motion) -*see*
        Accident, transport, by type of vehicle
      watercraft V93.49
        due to
          accident to craft V91.39
            powered craft V91.33
              ferry boat V91.31
              fishing boat V91.32
              jet skis V91.33
              liner V91.31
              merchant ship V91.30
              passenger ship V91.31
            unpowered craft V91.38
              canoe V91.35
              inflatable V91.36
              kayak V91.35
              sailboat V91.34
              surf-board V91.38
              windsurfer V91.38
          powered craft V93.43
            ferry boat V93.41
            fishing boat V93.42
            jet skis V93.43
            liner V93.41
            merchant ship V93.40
            passenger ship V93.41
          unpowered craft V93.48
            sailboat V93.44
            surf-board V93.48
            windsurfer V93.48
  moving NEC W20.8
  projected W20.8
    assault Y00
    in sports W21.9
      assault Y08.09
      ball W21.00
        baseball W21.03
        basketball W21.05
        football W21.01
        golf ball W21.04
        soccer W21.02
        softball W21.07
        specified NEC W21.09
        volleyball W21.06
      bat or racquet
        baseball bat W21.11
          assault Y08.02
        golf club W21.13
          assault Y08.09
        specified NEC W21.19
          assault Y08.09
        tennis racquet W21.12

Struck (accidentally) by - *continued*
        assault Y08.09
      hockey (ice)
        field
          puck W21.221
          stick W21.211
        puck W21.220
        stick W21.210
          assault Y08.01
      specified NEC W21.89
    set in motion by explosion -*see* Explosion
    thrown W20.8
      assault Y00
      in sports W21.9
        assault Y08.09
        ball W21.00
          baseball W21.03
          basketball W21.05
          football W21.01
          golf ball W21.04
          soccer W21.02
          soft ball W21.07
          specified NEC W21.09
          volleyball W21.06
        bat or racquet
          baseball bat W21.11
            assault Y08.02
          golf club W21.13
            assault Y08.09
          specified NEC W21.19
            assault Y08.09
          tennis racquet W21.12
            assault Y08.09
        hockey (ice)
          field
            puck W21.221
            stick W21.211
          puck W21.220
          stick W21.210
            assault Y08.01
        specified NEC W21.89
  other person(s) W50.0
    with
      blunt object W22.8
        intentional, homicide (attempt) Y00
        sports equipment W21.9
        undetermined whether accidental or
          intentional Y29
      fall W03
        due to ice or snow W00.0
      as, or caused by, a crowd or human
        stampede (with fall) W52
      assault Y04.2
      homicide (attempt) Y04.2
      in legal intervention
        injuring
          bystander Y35.812
          law enforcement personnel Y35.811
          suspect Y35.813
        sports equipment W21.9
      police (on duty) -*see* Legal, intervention,
        manhandling
        with blunt object -*see* Legal, intervention,
          blunt object
      sports equipment W21.9
        assault Y08.09
        ball W21.00
          baseball W21.03
          basketball W21.05
          football W21.01
          golf ball W21.04
          soccer W21.02
          soft ball W21.07
          specified NEC W21.09

Struck (accidentally) by - *continued*
      volleyball W21.06
      bat or racquet
        baseball bat W21.11
          assault Y08.02
        golf club W21.13
          assault Y08.09
        specified NEC W21.19
        tennis racquet W21.12
          assault Y08.09
      cleats (shoe) W21.31
      foot wear NEC W21.39
      football helmet W21.81
      hockey (ice)
        field
          puck W21.221
          stick W21.211
        puck W21.220
        stick W21.210
          assault Y08.01
      skate blades W21.32
      specified NEC W21.89
        assault Y08.09
    thunderbolt -*see* subcategory T75.0
      causing fire -*see* Exposure, fire
    transport vehicle NEC -*see also* Accident,
      transport V09.9
      intentional, homicide (attempt) Y03.0
      motor NEC -*see also* Accident, transport
        V09.20
        homicide Y03.0
    vehicle (transport) NEC -*see* Accident,
      transport, by type of vehicle
      stationary (falling from jack, hydraulic lift,
        ramp) W20.8
Stumbling
  over
    animal NEC W01.0
      with fall W18.09
    carpet, rug or (small) object W22.8
      with fall W18.09
    person W51
      with fall W03
        due to ice or snow W00.0
  without fall W18.40
    due to
      specified NEC W18.49
      stepping from one level to another
        W18.43
      stepping into hole or opening W18.42
      stepping on object W18.41
Submersion (accidental) -*see* Drowning
Suffocation (accidental) (by external means)
  (by pressure) (mechanical) -*see also*
    category T71
  due to, by
    avalanche -*see* Landslide
    explosion -*see* Explosion
    fire -*see* Exposure, fire
    food, any type (aspiration) (ingestion)
      (inhalation) -*see* categories T17 and T18
    ignition -*see* Ignition
    landslide -*see* Landslide
    machine (ry) -*see* Contact, with, by type of
      machine
    vomitus (aspiration) (inhalation) T17.81
  in
    burning building X00.8
Suicide, suicidal (attempted) (by) X83.8
  blunt object X79
  burning, burns X76
  hot object X77.9
    fluid NEC X77.2
    household appliance X77.3

CHAPTER 1: CERTAIN INFECTIOUS AND PARASITIC DISEASES (A00-B99)

A00	Cholera
A01	Typhoid and paratyphoid fevers
A02	Other salmonella infections
A03	Shigellosis
A04	Other bacterial intestinal infections
A05	Other bacterial foodborne intoxications, not elsewhere classified
A06	Amebiasis
A07	Other protozoal intestinal diseases
A08	Viral and other specified intestinal infections
A09	Infectious gastroenteritis and colitis unspecified
A15	Respiratory tuberculosis
A17	Tuberculosis of nervous system
A18	Tuberculosis of other organs
A19	Miliary tuberculosis
A20	Plague
A21	Tularemia
A22	Anthrax
A23	Brucellosis
A24	Glanders and melioidosis
A25	Rat-bite fever
A26	Erysipeloid
A27	Leptospirosis
A28	Other zoonotic bacterial diseases, not elsewhere classified
A30	Leprosy (Hansen's disease)
A31	Infection due to other mycobacteria
A32	Listeriosis
A33	Tetanus neonatorum
A34	Obstetrical tetanus
A35	Other tetanus
A36	Diphtheria
A37	Whooping cough
A38	Scarlet fever
A39	Meningococcal infection
A40	Streptococcal sepsis
A41	Other sepsis
A42	Actinomycosis
A43	Nocardiosis
A44	Bartonellosis
A46	Erysipelas
A48	Other bacterial diseases, not elsewhere classified
A49	Staphylococcal infection of unspecified site
A50	Congenital syphilis
A51	Early syphilis
A52	Late syphilis
A53	Other and unspecified syphilis
A54	Gonococcal infection

A55	Chlamydial lymphogranuloma (venereum)
A56	Other sexually transmitted chlamydial diseases
A57	Chancroid
A58	Granuloma inguinale
A59	Trichomoniasis
A60	Anogenital herpesviral [herpes simplex] infections
A63	Other predominantly sexually transmitted diseases, not elsewhere classified
A64	Unspecified sexually transmitted disease
A65	Nonvenereal syphilis
A66	Yaws
A67	Pinta [carate]
A68	Relapsing fevers
A69	Other spirochetal infections
A70	Chlamydia psittaci infections
A71	Trachoma
A74	Other diseases caused by chlamydiae
A75	Typhus fever
A77	Spotted fever [tick-borne rickettsioses]
A78	Q fever
A79	Other rickettsioses
A80	Acute poliomyelitis
A81	Atypical virus infections of central nervous system
A82	Rabies
A83	Mosquito-borne viral encephalitis
A84	Tick-borne viral encephalitis
A85	Other viral encephalitis, not elsewhere classified
A86	Unspecified viral encephalitis
A87	Viral meningitis
A88	Other viral infections of central nervous system, not elsewhere classified
A89	Unspecified viral infection of central nervous system
A90	Dengue fever [classical dengue]
A91	Dengue hemorrhagic fever
A92	Other mosquito-borne viral fevers
A93	Other arthropod-borne viral fevers, not elsewhere classified
A94	Unspecified arthropod-borne viral fever
A95	Yellow fever
A96	Arenaviral hemorrhagic fever
A98	Other viral hemorrhagic fevers, not elsewhere classified
A99	Unspecified viral hemorrhagic fever
B00	Herpesviral [herpes simplex] infections
B01	Varicella [chickenpox]
B02	Zoster [herpes zoster]
B03	Smallpox
B04	Monkeypox
B05	Measles
B06	Rubella [German measles]

B07	Viral warts
B08	Cowpox
B09	Other human herpesviruses
B10	Other human herpesviruses
B15	Acute hepatitis A
B16	Acute hepatitis B
B17	Other acute viral hepatitis
B18	Chronic viral hepatitis
B19	Unspecified viral hepatitis
B20	Human immunodeficiency virus [HIV] disease
B25	Cytomegaloviral disease
B26	Mumps
B27	Infectious mononucleosis
B30	Viral conjunctivitis
B33	Other viral diseases, not elsewhere classified
B34	Viral infection of unspecified site
B35	Dermatophytosis
B36	Other superficial mycoses
B37	Candidiasis
B38	Coccidioidomycosis
B39	Histoplasmosis
B40	Blastomycosis
B41	Paracoccidioidomycosis
B42	Sporotrichosis
B43	Chromomycosis and pheomycotic abscess
B44	Aspergillosis
B45	Cryptococcosis
B46	Zygomycosis
B47	Mycetoma
B48	Other mycoses, not elsewhere classified
B49	Unspecified mycosis
B50	Plasmodium falciparum malaria
B51	Plasmodium vivax malaria
B52	Plasmodium malariae malaria
B53	Other specified malaria
B54	Unspecified malaria
B55	Leishmaniasis
B56	African trypanosomiasis
B57	Chagas' disease
B58	Toxoplasmosis
B59	Pneumocystosis
B60	Other protozoal diseases, not elsewhere classified
B64	Unspecified protozoal disease
B65	Schistosomiasis [bilharziasis]
B66	Other fluke infections
B67	Echinococcosis
B68	Taeniasis
B69	Cysticercosis
B70	Diphyllobothriasis and sparganosis
B71	Other cestode infections
B72	Dracunculiasis

B73	Onchocerciasis	**C20**	Malignant neoplasm of rectum	**C68**	Malignant neoplasm of other and unspecified urinary organs
B74	Filariasis	**C21**	Malignant neoplasm of anus and anal canal	**C69**	Malignant neoplasm of eye and adnexa
B75	Trichinellosis	**C22**	Malignant neoplasm of liver and intrahepatic bile ducts	**C70**	Malignant neoplasm of meninges
B76	Hookworm diseases			**C71**	Malignant neoplasm of brain
B77	Ascariasis	**C23**	Malignant neoplasm of gallbladder	**C72**	Malignant neoplasm of spinal cord, cranial nerves and other parts of central nervous system
B78	Strongyloidiasis	**C24**	Malignant neoplasm of other and unspecified parts of biliary tract		
B79	Trichuriasis	**C25**	Malignant neoplasm of pancreas	**C73**	Malignant neoplasm of thyroid gland
B80	Enterobiasis	**C26**	Malignant neoplasm of other and ill-defined digestive organs	**C74**	Malignant neoplasm of adrenal gland
B81	Other intestinal helminthiases, not elsewhere classified			**C75**	Malignant neoplasm of other endocrine glands and related structures
B82	Unspecified intestinal parasitism	**C30**	Malignant neoplasm of nasal cavity and middle ear	**C76**	Malignant neoplasm of other and ill-defined sites
B83	Other helminthiases	**C31**	Malignant neoplasm of accessory sinuses		
B85	Pediculosis and phthiriasis	**C32**	Malignant neoplasm of larynx	**C77**	Secondary and unspecified malignant neoplasm of lymph nodes
B86	Scabies	**C33**	Malignant neoplasm of trachea		
B87	Myiasis	**C34**	Malignant neoplasm of bronchus and lung	**C78**	Secondary malignant neoplasm of respiratory and digestive organs
B88	Other infestations			**C79**	Secondary malignant neoplasm of other and unspecified sites
B89	Unspecified parasitic disease	**C37**	Malignant neoplasm of thymus		
B90	Sequelae of tuberculosis	**C38**	Malignant neoplasm of heart, mediastinum and pleura	**C7A**	Malignant neuroendocrine tumors
B91	Sequelae of poliomyelitis			**C7B**	Secondary neuroendocrine tumors
B92	Sequelae of leprosy	**C39**	Malignant neoplasm of other and ill-defined sites in the respiratory system and intrathoracic organs	**C80**	Malignant neoplasm without specification of site
B94	Sequelae of other and unspecified infectious and parasitic diseases			**C81**	Hodgkin lymphoma
		C40	Malignant neoplasm of bone and articular cartilage of limbs	**C82**	Follicular lymphoma
B95	Streptococcus, Staphylococcus, and Enterococcus as the cause of diseases classified elsewhere			**C83**	Non-follicular lymphoma
		C41	Malignant neoplasm of bone and articular cartilage of other and unspecified sites	**C84**	Mature T/NK-cell lymphomas
B96	Other bacterial agents as the cause of diseases classified elsewhere			**C85**	Other specified and unspecified types of non-Hodgkin lymphoma
		C43	Malignant melanoma of skin		
B97	Viral agents as the cause of diseases classified elsewhere	**C44**	Other and unspecified malignant neoplasm of skin	**C86**	Other specified types of T/NK-cell lymphoma
B99	Other and unspecified infectious diseases	**C45**	Mesothelioma	**C88**	Malignant immunoproliferative diseases and certain other B-cell lymphomas
		C46	Kaposi's sarcoma		

CHAPTER 2: NEOPLASMS (C00-D49)

		C47	Malignant neoplasm of peripheral nerves and autonomic nervous system	**C90**	Multiple myeloma and malignant plasma cell neoplasms
C00	Malignant neoplasm of lip			**C91**	Lymphoid leukemia
C01	Malignant neoplasm of base of tongue	**C48**	Malignant neoplasm of retroperitoneum and peritoneum	**C92**	Myeloid leukemia
C02	Malignant neoplasm of other and unspecified parts of tongue	**C49**	Malignant neoplasm of other connective and soft tissue	**C93**	Monocytic leukemia
				C94	Other leukemias of specified cell type
C03	Malignant neoplasm of gum	**C4A**	Merkel cell carcinoma	**C95**	Leukemia of unspecified cell type
C04	Malignant neoplasm of floor of mouth	**C50**	Malignant neoplasm of breast	**C96**	Other and unspecified malignant neoplasms of lymphoid, hematopoietic and related tissue
C05	Malignant neoplasm of palate	**C52**	Malignant neoplasm of vagina		
C06	Malignant neoplasm of other and unspecified parts of mouth	**C53**	Malignant neoplasm of cervix uteri	**D00**	Carcinoma in situ of oral cavity, esophagus and stomach
C07	Malignant neoplasm of parotid gland	**C54**	Malignant neoplasm of corpus uteri		
C08	Malignant neoplasm of other and unspecified major salivary glands	**C55**	Malignant neoplasm of uterus, part unspecified	**D01**	Carcinoma in situ of other and unspecified digestive organs
		C56	Malignant neoplasm of ovary	**D02**	Carcinoma in situ of middle ear and respiratory system
C09	Malignant neoplasm of tonsil	**C57**	Malignant neoplasm of other and unspecified female genital organs		
C10	Malignant neoplasm of oropharynx			**D03**	Melanoma in situ
C11	Malignant neoplasm of nasopharynx	**C58**	Malignant neoplasm of placenta	**D04**	Carcinoma in situ of skin
C12	Malignant neoplasm of pyriform sinus	**C60**	Malignant neoplasm of penis	**D05**	Carcinoma in situ of breast
C13	Malignant neoplasm of hypopharynx	**C61**	Malignant neoplasm of prostate	**D06**	Carcinoma in situ of cervix uteri
C14	Malignant neoplasm of other and ill-defined sites in the lip, oral cavity and pharynx	**C62**	Malignant neoplasm of testis	**D07**	Carcinoma in situ of other and unspecified genital organs
		C63	Malignant neoplasm of other and unspecified male genital organs		
C15	Malignant neoplasm of esophagus			**D09**	Carcinoma in situ of other and unspecified sites
C16	Malignant neoplasm of stomach	**C64**	Malignant neoplasm of kidney, except renal pelvis		
C17	Malignant neoplasm of small intestine			**D10**	Benign neoplasm of mouth and pharynx
C18	Malignant neoplasm of colon	**C65**	Malignant neoplasm of renal pelvis	**D11**	Benign neoplasm of major salivary glands
C19	Malignant neoplasm of rectosigmoid junction	**C66**	Malignant neoplasm of ureter		
		C67	Malignant neoplasm of bladder		

D12 Benign neoplasm of colon, rectum, anus and anal canal

D13 Benign neoplasm of other and ill-defined parts of digestive system

D14 Benign neoplasm of middle ear and respiratory system

D15 Benign neoplasm of other and unspecified intrathoracic organs

D16 Benign neoplasm of bone and articular cartilage

D17 Benign lipomatous neoplasm

D18 Hemangioma and lymphangioma, any site

D19 Benign neoplasm of mesothelial tissue

D20 Benign neoplasm of soft tissue of retroperitoneum and peritoneum

D21 Other benign neoplasms of connective and other soft tissue

D22 Melanocytic nevi

D23 Other benign neoplasms of skin

D24 Benign neoplasm of breast

D25 Leiomyoma of uterus

D26 Other benign neoplasms of uterus

D27 Benign neoplasm of ovary

D28 Benign neoplasm of other and unspecified female genital organs

D29 Benign neoplasm of male genital organs

D30 Benign neoplasm of urinary organs

D31 Benign neoplasm of eye and adnexa

D32 Benign neoplasm of meninges

D33 Benign neoplasm of brain and other parts of central nervous system

D34 Benign neoplasm of thyroid gland

D35 Benign neoplasm of other and unspecified endocrine glands

D36 Benign neoplasm of other and unspecified sites

D37 Neoplasm of uncertain behavior of oral cavity and digestive organs

D38 Neoplasm of uncertain behavior of middle ear and respiratory and intrathoracic organs

D39 Neoplasm of uncertain behavior of female genital organs

D3A Benign carcinoid tumor of unspecified site

D40 Neoplasm of uncertain behavior of male genital organs

D41 Neoplasm of uncertain behavior of urinary organs

D42 Neoplasm of uncertain behavior of meninges

D43 Neoplasm of uncertain behavior of brain and central nervous system

D44 Neoplasm of uncertain behavior of endocrine glands

D45 Polycythemia vera

D46 Myelodysplastic syndromes

D47 Other neoplasms of uncertain behavior of lymphoid, hematopoietic and related tissue

D48 Neoplasm of uncertain behavior of other and unspecified sites

D49 Neoplasms of unspecified behavior

CHAPTER 3: DISEASES OF THE BLOOD AND BLOOD-FORMING ORGANS AND CERTAIN DISORDERS INVOLVING THE IMMUNE MECHANISM (D50-D89)

D50 Iron deficiency anemia

D51 Vitamin B12 deficiency anemia

D52 Folate deficiency anemia

D53 Other nutritional anemias

D55 Anemia due to enzyme disorders

D56 Thalassemia

D57 Sickle-cell disorders

D58 Other hereditary hemolytic anemias

D59 Acquired hemolytic anemia

D60 Acquired pure red cell aplasia [erythroblastopenia]

D61 Other aplastic anemias and other bone marrow failure syndromes

D62 Acute posthemorrhagic anemia

D63 Anemia in chronic diseases classified elsewhere

D64 Other anemias

D65 Disseminated intravascular coagulation [defibrination syndrome]

D66 Hereditary factor VIII deficiency

D67 Hereditary factor IX deficiency

D68 Other coagulation defects

D69 Purpura and other hemorrhagic conditions

D70 Neutropenia

D71 Functional disorders of polymorphonuclear neutrophils

D72 Other disorders of white blood cells

D73 Diseases of spleen

D74 Methemoglobinemia

D75 Other and unspecified diseases of blood and blood-forming organs

D76 Other specified diseases with participation of lymphoreticular and reticulohistiocytic tissue

D77 Other disorders of blood and blood-forming organs in diseases classified elsewhere

D78 Intraoperative and postprocedural complications of the spleen

D80 Immunodeficiency with predominantly antibody defects

D81 Combined immunodeficiencies

D82 Immunodeficiency associated with other major defects

D83 Common variable immunodeficiency

D84 Other immunodeficiencies

D86 Sarcoidosis

D89 Other disorders involving the immune mechanism, not elsewhere classified

CHAPTER 4: ENDOCRINE, NUTRITIONAL AND METABOLIC DISEASES (E00-E89)

E00 Congenital iodine-deficiency syndrome

E01 Iodine-deficiency related thyroid disorders and allied conditions

E02 Subclinical iodine-deficiency hypothyroidism

E03 Other hypothyroidism

E04 Other nontoxic goiter

E05 Thyrotoxicosis [hyperthyroidism]

E06 Thyroiditis

E07 Other disorders of thyroid

E08 Diabetes mellitus due to underlying condition

E09 Drug or chemical induced diabetes mellitus

E10 Type 1 diabetes mellitus

E11 Type 2 diabetes mellitus

E13 Other specified diabetes mellitus

E15 Nondiabetic hypoglycemic coma

E16 Other disorders of pancreatic internal secretion

E20 Hypoparathyroidism

E21 Hyperparathyroidism and other disorders of parathyroid gland

E22 Hyperfunction of pituitary gland

E23 Hypofunction and other disorders of the pituitary gland

E24 Cushing's syndrome

E25 Adrenogenital disorders

E26 Hyperaldosteronism

E27 Other disorders of adrenal gland

E28 Ovarian dysfunction

E29 Testicular dysfunction

E30 Disorders of puberty, not elsewhere classified

E31 Polyglandular dysfunction

E32 Diseases of thymus

E34 Other endocrine disorders

E35 Disorders of endocrine glands in diseases classified elsewhere

E36 Intraoperative complications of endocrine system

E40 Kwashiorkor

E41 Nutritional marasmus

E42 Marasmic kwashiorkor

E43 Unspecified severe protein-calorie malnutrition

E44 Protein-calorie malnutrition of moderate and mild degree

E45 Retarded development following protein-calorie malnutrition

E46 Unspecified protein-calorie malnutrition

E50 Vitamin A deficiency

E51 Thiamine deficiency

E52 Niacin deficiency [pellagra]

E53 Deficiency of other B group vitamins

E54	Ascorbic acid deficiency	F09	Personality and behavioral disorders due to known physiological condition	F69	Unspecified disorder of adult personality and behavior
E55	Vitamin D deficiency	F10	Alcohol related disorders	F70	Mild intellectual disabilities
E56	Other vitamin deficiencies	F11	Opioid related disorders	F71	Moderate mental retardation
E58	Dietary calcium deficiency	F12	Cannabis related disorders	F72	Severe intellectual disabilities
E59	Dietary selenium deficiency	F13	Sedative, hypnotic, or anxiolytic related disorders	F73	Profound intellectual disabilities
E60	Dietary zinc deficiency	F14	Cocaine related disorders	F78	Other intellectual disabilities
E61	Deficiency of other nutrient elements	F15	Other stimulant related disorders	F79	Unspecified intellectual disabilities
E63	Other nutritional deficiencies	F16	Hallucinogen related disorders	F80	Specific developmental disorders of speech and language
E64	Sequelae of malnutrition and other nutritional deficiencies	F17	Nicotine dependence	F81	Specific developmental disorders of scholastic skills
E65	Localized adiposity	F18	Inhalant related disorders	F82	Specific developmental disorder of motor function
E66	Overweight and obesity	F19	Other psychoactive substance related disorders	F84	Pervasive developmental disorders
E67	Other hyperalimentation	F21	Schizotypal disorder	F88	Other disorders of psychological development
E68	Sequelae of hyperalimentation	F22	Delusional disorders	F89	Unspecified disorder of psychological development
E70	Disorders of aromatic amino-acid metabolism	F23	Brief psychotic disorder	F90	Attention-deficit hyperactivity disorders
E71	Disorders of branched-chain amino-acid metabolism and fatty-acid metabolism	F24	Shared psychotic disorder	F91	Conduct disorders
E72	Other disorders of amino-acid metabolism	F25	Schizoaffective disorders	F93	Emotional disorders with onset specific to childhood
E73	Lactose intolerance	F28	Other psychotic disorder not due to a substance or known physiological condition	F94	Disorders of social functioning with onset specific to childhood and adolescence
E74	Other disorders of carbohydrate metabolism	F29	Unspecified psychosis not due to a substance or known physiological condition	F95	Tic disorder
E75	Disorders of sphingolipid metabolism and other lipid storage disorders	F30	Manic episode	F98	Other behavioral and emotional disorders with onset usually occurring in childhood and adolescence
E76	Disorders of glycosaminoglycan metabolism	F31	Bipolar disorder	F99	Mental disorder not otherwise specified
E77	Disorders of glycoprotein metabolism	F32	Major depressive disorder, single episode		
E78	Disorders of lipoprotein metabolism and other lipidemias	F33	Major depressive disorder, recurrent		
E79	Disorders of purine and pyrimidine metabolism	F34	Persistent mood [affective] disorders		

CHAPTER 6: DISEASES OF THE NERVOUS SYSTEM (G00-G99)

E80	Disorders of porphyrin and bilirubin metabolism	F39	Unspecified mood [affective] disorder
E83	Disorders of mineral metabolism	F40	Phobic anxiety disorders
E84	Cystic fibrosis	F41	Other anxiety disorders
E85	Amyloidosis	F42	Obsessive-compulsive disorder
E86	Volume depletion	F43	Reaction to severe stress, and adjustment disorders
E87	Other disorders of fluid, electrolyte and acid-base balance	F44	Dissociative and conversion disorders
E88	Other and unspecified metabolic disorders	F45	Somatoform disorders
E89	Postprocedural endocrine and metabolic complications and disorders, not elsewhere classified	F48	Other nonpsychotic mental disorders

G00	Bacterial meningitis, not elsewhere classified
G01	Meningitis in bacterial diseases classified elsewhere
G02	Meningitis in other infectious and parasitic diseases classified elsewhere
G03	Meningitis due to other and unspecified causes
G04	Encephalitis, myelitis and encephalomyelitis
G05	Encephalitis, myelitis and encephalomyelitis in diseases classified elsewhere
G06	Intracranial and intraspinal abscess and granuloma
G07	Intracranial and intraspinal abscess and granuloma in diseases classified elsewhere
G08	Intracranial and intraspinal phlebitis and thrombophlebitis
G09	Sequelae of inflammatory diseases of central nervous system
G10	Huntington's disease
G11	Hereditary ataxia
G12	Spinal muscular atrophy and related syndromes

CHAPTER 5: MENTAL, BEHAVIORAL AND NEURODEVELOPMENTAL DISORDERS (F01-F99)

		F50	Eating disorders
F01	Vascular dementia	F51	Sleep disorders not due to a substance or known physiological condition
F02	Dementia in other diseases classified elsewhere	F52	Sexual dysfunction not due to a substance or known physiological condition
F03	Unspecified dementia	F53	Puerperal psychosis
F04	Amnestic disorder due to known physiological condition	F54	Psychological and behavioral factors associated with disorders or diseases classified elsewhere
F05	Delirium due to known physiological condition	F55	Abuse of non-psychoactive substances
F06	Unspecified dementia	F59	Unspecified behavioral syndromes associated with physiological disturbances and physical factors
F07	Other mental disorders due to known physiological condition	F60	Specific personality disorders
		F63	Impulse disorders
		F64	Gender identity disorders
		F65	Paraphilias
		F66	Other sexual disorders
		F68	Other disorders of adult personality and behavior

G13 Systemic atrophies primarily affecting central nervous system in diseases classified elsewhere

G14 Postpolio syndrome

G20 Parkinson's disease

G21 Secondary parkinsonism

G23 Other degenerative diseases of basal ganglia

G24 Dystonia

G25 Other extrapyramidal and movement disorders

G26 Extrapyramidal and movement disorders in diseases classified elsewhere

G30 Alzheimer's disease

G31 Other degenerative diseases of nervous system, not elsewhere classified

G32 Other degenerative disorders of nervous system in diseases classified elsewhere

G35 Multiple sclerosis

G36 Other acute disseminated demyelination

G37 Other demyelinating diseases of central nervous system

G40 Epilepsy and recurrent seizures

G43 Migraine

G44 Other headache syndromes

G45 Transient cerebral ischemic attacks and related syndromes

G46 Vascular syndromes of brain in cerebrovascular diseases

G47 Sleep disorders

G50 Disorders of trigeminal nerve

G51 Facial nerve disorders

G52 Disorders of other cranial nerves

G53 Cranial nerve disorders in diseases classified elsewhere

G54 Nerve root and plexus disorders

G55 Mononeuropathies of upper limb

G56 Mononeuropathies of lower limb

G57 Mononeuropathy in diseases classified elsewhere

G58 Other mononeuropathies

G59 Hereditary and idiopathic neuropathy

G60 Disorders of trigeminal nerve

G61 Inflammatory polyneuropathy

G62 Other and unspecified polyneuropathies

G63 Polyneuropathy in diseases classified elsewhere

G64 Other disorders of peripheral nervous system

G65 Sequelae of inflammatory and toxic polyneuropathies

G70 Myasthenia gravis and other myoneural disorders

G71 Primary disorders of muscles

G72 Other and unspecified myopathies

G73 Malignant neoplasm of thyroid gland

G80 Cerebral palsy

G81 Hemiplegia and hemiparesis

G82 Paraplegia (paraparesis) and quadriplegia (quadriparesis)

G83 Other paralytic syndromes

G89 Pain, not elsewhere classified

G90 Disorders of autonomic nervous system

G91 Hydrocephalus

G92 Toxic encephalopathy

G93 Other disorders of brain

G94 Other disorders of brain in diseases classified elsewhere

G95 Other and unspecified diseases of spinal cord

G96 Other disorders of central nervous system

G97 Intraoperative and postprocedural complications and disorders of nervous system, not elsewhere classified

G98 Other disorders of nervous system not elsewhere classified

G99 Other disorders of nervous system in diseases classified elsewhere

CHAPTER 7: DISEASES OF THE EYE AND ADNEXA (H00-H59)

H00 Hordeolum and chalazion

H01 Other inflammation of eyelid

H02 Other disorders of eyelid

H04 Disorders of lacrimal system

H05 Disorders of orbit

H10 Conjunctivitis

H11 Other disorders of conjunctiva

H15 Disorders of sclera

H16 Keratitis

H17 Corneal scars and opacities

H18 Other disorders of cornea

H20 Iridocyclitis

H21 Other disorders of iris and ciliary body

H22 Disorders of iris and ciliary body in diseases classified elsewhere

H25 Age-related cataract

H26 Other cataract

H27 Other disorders of lens

H28 Cataract in diseases classified elsewhere

H30 Chorioretinal inflammation

H31 Other disorders of choroid

H32 Chorioretinal disorders in diseases classified elsewhere

H33 Retinal detachments and breaks

H34 Retinal vascular occlusions

H35 Other retinal disorders

H36 Retinal disorders in diseases classified elsewhere

H40 Glaucoma

H42 Glaucoma in diseases classified elsewhere

H43 Disorders of vitreous body

H44 Disorders of globe

H46 Optic neuritis

H47 Other disorders of optic [2nd] nerve and visual pathways

H49 Paralytic strabismus

H50 Other strabismus

H51 Other disorders of binocular movement

H52 Disorders of refraction and accommodation

H53 Visual disturbances

H54 Blindness and low vision

H55 Nystagmus and other irregular eye movements

H57 Other disorders of eye and adnexa

H59 Intraoperative and postprocedural complications and disorders of eye and adnexa, not elsewhere classified

CHAPTER 8: DISEASES OF THE EAR AND MASTOID PROCESS (H60-H95)

H60 Otitis externa

H61 Other disorders of external ear

H62 Disorders of external ear in diseases classified elsewhere

H65 Nonsuppurative otitis media

H66 Suppurative and unspecified otitis media

H67 Otitis media in diseases classified elsewhere

H68 Eustachian salpingitis and obstruction

H69 Other and unspecified disorders of Eustachian tube

H70 Mastoiditis and related conditions

H71 Cholesteatoma of middle ear

H72 Perforation of tympanic membrane

H73 Other disorders of tympanic membrane

H74 Other disorders of middle ear mastoid

H75 Other disorders of middle ear and mastoid in diseases classified elsewhere

H80 Otosclerosis

H81 Disorders of vestibular function

H82 Vertiginous syndromes in diseases classified elsewhere

H83 Other diseases of inner ear

H90 Conductive and sensorineural hearing loss

H91 Other and unspecified hearing loss

H92 Otalgia and effusion of ear

H93 Other disorders of ear, not elsewhere classified

H94 Other disorders of ear in diseases classified elsewhere

H95 Intraoperative and postprocedural complications and disorders of ear and mastoid process, not elsewhere classified

CHAPTER 9: DISEASES OF THE CIRCULATORY SYSTEM (I00-I99)

I00 Rheumatic fever without heart involvement

I01 Rheumatic fever with heart involvement

I02 Rheumatic chorea

I05 Rheumatic mitral valve diseases

I06	Rheumatic aortic valve diseases
I07	Rheumatic tricuspid valve diseases
I08	Multiple valve diseases
I09	Other rheumatic heart diseases
I10	Essential (primary) hypertension
I11	Hypertensive heart disease
I12	Hypertensive chronic kidney disease
I13	Hypertensive heart and chronic kidney disease
I15	Secondary hypertension
I16	Hypertensive crisis
I20	Angina pectoris
I21	Acute myocardial infarction
I22	Subsequent ST elevation (STEMI) and non-ST elevation (NSTEMI) myocardial infarction
I23	Certain current complications following ST elevation (STEMI) and non-ST elevation (NSTEMI) myocardial infarction (within the 28 day period)
I24	Other acute ischemic heart diseases
I25	Chronic ischemic heart disease
I26	Pulmonary embolism
I27	Other pulmonary heart diseases
I28	Other diseases of pulmonary vessels
I30	Acute pericarditis
I31	Other diseases of pericardium
I32	Pericarditis in diseases classified elsewhere
I33	Acute and subacute endocarditis
I34	Nonrheumatic mitral valve disorders
I35	Nonrheumatic aortic valve disorders
I36	Nonrheumatic tricuspid valve disorders
I37	Nonrheumatic pulmonary valve disorders
I38	Endocarditis, valve unspecified
I39	Endocarditis and heart valve disorders in diseases classified elsewhere
I40	Acute myocarditis
I41	Myocarditis in diseases classified elsewhere
I42	Cardiomyopathy
I43	Cardiomyopathy in diseases classified elsewhere
I44	Atrioventricular and left bundle-branch block
I45	Other conduction disorders
I46	Cardiac arrest
I47	Paroxysmal tachycardia
I48	Atrial fibrillation and flutter
I49	Other cardiac arrhythmias
I50	Heart failure
I51	Complications and ill-defined descriptions of heart disease
I52	Other heart disorders in diseases classified elsewhere
I60	Nontraumatic subarachnoid hemorrhage
I61	Nontraumatic intracerebral hemorrhage
I62	Other and unspecified nontraumatic intracranial hemorrhage

I63	Cerebral infarction
I65	Occlusion and stenosis of precerebral arteries, not resulting in cerebral infarction
I66	Occlusion and stenosis of cerebral arteries, not resulting in cerebral infarction
I67	Other cerebrovascular diseases
I68	Cerebrovascular disorders in diseases classified elsewhere
I69	Sequelae of cerebrovascular disease
I70	Atherosclerosis
I71	Aortic aneurysm and dissection
I72	Other aneurysm
I73	Other peripheral vascular diseases
I74	Arterial embolism and thrombosis
I75	Atheroembolism
I76	Other disorders of arteries and arterioles
I77	Diseases of capillaries
I78	Disorders of arteries, arterioles and capillaries in diseases classified elsewhere
I79	Disorders of arteries, arterioles and capillaries in diseases classified elsewhere
I80	Phlebitis and thrombophlebitis
I81	Portal vein thrombosis
I82	Other venous embolism and thrombosis
I83	Varicose veins of lower extremities
I84	Unspecified thrombosed hemorrhoids
I85	Esophageal varices
I86	Varicose veins of other sites
I87	Other disorders of veins
I88	Nonspecific lymphadenitis
I89	Other noninfective disorders of lymphatic vessels and lymph nodes
I95	Hypotension
I96	Gangrene, not elsewhere classified
I97	Intraoperative and postprocedural complications and disorders of circulatory system, not elsewhere classified
I99	Other and unspecified disorders of circulatory system

CHAPTER 10: DISEASES OF THE RESPIRATORY SYSTEM (J00-J99)

J00	Acute nasopharyngitis [common cold]
J01	Acute sinusitis
J02	Acute nasopharyngitis [common cold]
J03	Acute tonsillitis
J04	Acute laryngitis and tracheitis
J05	Acute obstructive laryngitis [croup] and epiglottitis
J06	Acute upper respiratory infections of multiple and unspecified sites
J09	Influenza due to certain identified influenza viruses
J10	Influenza due to other identified influenza virus

J12	Viral pneumonia, not elsewhere classified
J13	Pneumonia due to Streptococcus pneumoniae
J14	Pneumonia due to Hemophilus influenzae
J15	Bacterial pneumonia, not elsewhere classified
J16	Pneumonia due to other infectious organisms, not elsewhere classified
J17	Pneumonia in diseases classified elsewhere
J18	Pneumonia, unspecified organism
J20	Acute bronchitis
J21	Acute bronchiolitis
J22	Unspecified acute lower respiratory infection
J30	Vasomotor and allergic rhinitis
J31	Chronic rhinitis, nasopharyngitis and pharyngitis
J32	Chronic sinusitis
J33	Nasal polyp
J34	Other and unspecified disorders of nose and nasal sinuses
J35	Chronic diseases of tonsils and adenoids
J36	Peritonsillar abscess
J37	Chronic laryngitis and laryngotracheitis
J38	Diseases of vocal cords and larynx, not elsewhere classified
J39	Other diseases of upper respiratory tract
J40	Bronchitis, not specified as acute or chronic
J41	Simple and mucopurulent chronic bronchitis
J42	Unspecified chronic bronchitis
J43	Emphysema
J44	Other chronic obstructive pulmonary disease
J45	Asthma
J47	Bronchiectasis
J60	Coalworker's pneumoconiosis
J61	Pneumoconiosis due to asbestos and other mineral fibers
J62	Pneumoconiosis due to dust containing silica
J63	Pneumoconiosis due to other inorganic dusts
J64	Unspecified pneumoconiosis
J65	Pneumoconiosis associated with tuberculosis
J66	Airway disease due to specific organic dust
J67	Hypersensitivity pneumonitis due to organic dust
J68	Respiratory conditions due to inhalation of chemicals, gases, fumes and vapors
J69	Pneumonitis due to solids and liquids
J70	Respiratory conditions due to other external agents
J80	Acute respiratory distress syndrome
J81	Pulmonary edema

J82 Pulmonary eosinophilia, not elsewhere classified

J84 Other interstitial pulmonary diseases

J85 Abscess of lung and mediastinum

J86 Pyothorax

J90 Pleural effusion, not elsewhere classified

J91 Pleural effusion in conditions classified elsewhere

J92 Pleural plaque

J93 Pneumothorax and air leak

J94 Other pleural conditions

J95 Intraoperative and postprocedural complications and disorders of respiratory system, not elsewhere classified

J96 Respiratory failure, not elsewhere classified

J98 Other respiratory disorders

J99 Respiratory disorders in diseases classified elsewhere

CHAPTER 11: DISEASES OF THE DIGESTIVE SYSTEM (K00-K95)

K00 Disorders of tooth development and eruption

K01 Embedded and impacted teeth

K02 Dental caries

K03 Other diseases of hard tissues of teeth

K04 Diseases of pulp and periapical tissues

K05 Gingivitis and periodontal diseases

K06 Other disorders of gingiva and edentulous alveolar ridge

K08 Other disorders of teeth and supporting structures

K09 Cysts of oral region, not elsewhere classified

K11 Diseases of salivary glands

K12 Stomatitis and related lesions

K13 Other diseases of lip and oral mucosa

K14 Diseases of tongue

K20 Esophagitis

K21 Gastro-esophageal reflux disease

K22 Other diseases of esophagus

K23 Disorders of esophagus in diseases classified elsewhere

K25 Gastric ulcer

K26 Duodenal ulcer

K27 Peptic ulcer, site unspecified

K28 Gastrojejunal ulcer

K29 Gastritis and duodenitis

K30 Functional dyspepsia

K31 Other diseases of stomach and duodenum

K35 Acute appendicitis

K36 Other appendicitis

K37 Unspecified appendicitis

K38 Other diseases of appendix

K40 Inguinal hernia

K41 Femoral hernia

K42 Umbilical hernia

K43 Ventral hernia

K44 Diaphragmatic hernia

K45 Other abdominal hernia

K46 Unspecified abdominal hernia

K50 Crohn's disease [regional enteritis]

K51 Ulcerative colitis

K52 Other and unspecified noninfective gastroenteritis and colitis

K55 Vascular disorders of intestine

K56 Paralytic ileus and intestinal obstruction without hernia

K57 Diverticular disease of intestine

K58 Irritable bowel syndrome

K59 Fissure and fistula of anal and rectal regions

K60 Abscess of anal and rectal regions

K61 Other diseases of anus and rectum

K62 Other diseases of intestine

K63 Hemorrhoids and perianal venous thrombosis

K65 Peritonitis

K66 Other disorders of peritoneum

K67 Disorders of peritoneum in infectious diseases classified elsewhere

K68 Disorders of retroperitoneum

K70 Alcoholic liver disease

K71 Toxic liver disease

K72 Hepatic failure, not elsewhere classified

K73 Chronic hepatitis, not elsewhere classified

K74 Fibrosis and cirrhosis of liver

K75 Other inflammatory liver diseases

K76 Other diseases of liver

K77 Liver disorders in diseases classified elsewhere

K80 Cholelithiasis

K81 Cholecystitis

K82 Other diseases of gallbladder

K83 Other diseases of biliary tract

K85 Acute pancreatitis

K86 Other diseases of pancreas

K87 Disorders of gallbladder biliary tract and pancreas in diseases classified elsewhere

K90 Intestinal malabsorption

K91 Intraoperative and postprocedural complications and disorders of digestive system, not elsewhere classified

K92 Other diseases of digestive system

K94 Complications of artificial openings of the digestive system

K95 Complications of bariatric procedures

CHAPTER 12: DISEASES OF THE SKIN AND SUBCUTANEOUS TISSUE (L00-L99)

L00 Staphylococcal scalded skin syndrome

L01 Impetigo

L02 Cutaneous abscess, furuncle and carbuncle

L03 Cellulitis and acute lymphangitis

L04 Acute lymphadenitis

L05 Pilonidal cyst and sinus

L08 Other local infections of skin and subcutaneous tissue

L08 Other specified local infections of the skin and subcutaneous tissue

L10 Pemphigus

L11 Other acantholytic disorders

L12 Pemphigoid

L13 Other bullous disorders

L14 Bullous disorders in diseases classified elsewhere

L20 Atopic dermatitis

L21 Seborrheic dermatitis

L22 Diaper dermatitis

L23 Allergic contact dermatitis

L24 Irritant contact dermatitis

L25 Unspecified contact dermatitis

L26 Exfoliative dermatitis

L27 Dermatitis due to substances taken internally

L28 Lichen simplex chronicus and prurigo

L29 Pruritus

L30 Other and unspecified dermatitis

L40 Psoriasis

L41 Parapsoriasis

L42 Pityriasis rosea

L43 Lichen planus

L44 Other papulosquamous disorders

L45 Papulosquamous disorders in diseases classified elsewhere

L49 Exfoliation due to erythematous conditions according to extent of body surface involved

L50 Urticaria

L51 Erythema multiforme

L52 Erythema nodosum

L53 Other erythematous conditions

L54 Erythema in diseases classified elsewhere

L55 Sunburn

L56 Other acute skin changes due to ultraviolet radiation

L57 Skin changes due to chronic exposure to nonionizing radiation

L58 Radiodermatitis

L59 Other disorders of skin and subcutaneous tissue related to radiation

L60 Nail disorders

L62 Nail disorders in diseases classified elsewhere

L63 Alopecia areata

L64 Androgenic alopecia

L65 Other nonscarring hair loss

L66 Cicatricial alopecia [scarring hair loss]

L67 Hair color and hair shaft abnormalities

L68 Hypertrichosis

L70 Acne

L71 Rosacea

L72 Follicular cysts of skin and subcutaneous tissue

L73 Other follicular disorders

L74 Eccrine sweat disorders

L75 Apocrine sweat disorders

L76 Intraoperative and postprocedural complications of skin and subcutaneous tissue

L80 Vitiligo

L81 Other disorders of pigmentation

L82 Seborrheic keratosis

L83 Acanthosis nigricans

L84 Corns and callosities

L85 Other epidermal thickening

L86 Keratoderma in diseases classified elsewhere

L87 Transepidermal elimination disorders

L88 Pyoderma gangrenosum

L89 Pressure ulcer

L90 Atrophic disorders of skin

L91 Hypertrophic disorders of skin

L92 Granulomatous disorders of skin and subcutaneous tissue

L93 Lupus erythematosus

L94 Other localized connective tissue disorders

L95 Vasculitis limited to skin, not elsewhere classified

L97 Non-pressure chronic ulcer of lower limb, not elsewhere classified

L98 Other disorders of skin and subcutaneous tissue, not elsewhere classified

L99 Other disorders of skin and subcutaneous tissue in diseases classified elsewhere

CHAPTER 13: DISEASES OF THE MUSCULOSKELETAL SYSTEM AND CONNECTIVE TISSUE (M00-M99)

M00 Pyogenic arthritis

M01 Direct infections of joint in infectious and parasitic diseases classified elsewhere

M02 Postinfective and reactive arthropathies

M04 Autoinflammatory syndromes

M05 Rheumatoid arthritis with rheumatoid factor

M06 Other rheumatoid arthritis

M07 Enteropathic arthropathies

M08 Juvenile arthritis

M10 Idiopathic gout unspecified site

M11 Other crystal arthropathies

M12 Other and unspecified arthropathy

M13 Other arthritis

M14 Arthropathies in other diseases classified elsewhere

M15 Polyosteoarthritis

M16 Osteoarthritis of hip

M17 Osteoarthritis of knee

M18 Osteoarthritis of first carpometacarpal joint

M19 Other and unspecified osteoarthritis

M1A Idiopathic chronic gout unspecified site without tophus (tophi)

M20 Acquired deformities of fingers and toes

M21 Other acquired deformities of limbs

M22 Disorder of patella

M23 Internal derangement of knee

M24 Other specific joint derangements

M25 Other joint disorder, not elsewhere classified

M26 Dentofacial anomalies [including malocclusion]

M27 Other diseases of jaws

M30 Polyarteritis nodosa and related conditions

M31 Other necrotizing vasculopathies

M32 Systemic lupus erythematosus (SLE)

M33 Dermatopolymyositis

M34 Systemic sclerosis [scleroderma]

M35 Other systemic involvement of connective tissue

M36 Systemic disorders of connective tissue in diseases classified elsewhere

M40 Kyphosis and lordosis

M41 Scoliosis

M42 Spinal osteochondrosis

M43 Other deforming dorsopathies

M45 Ankylosing spondylitis

M46 Other inflammatory spondylopathies

M47 Spondylosis

M48 Other spondylopathies

M49 Spondylopathies in diseases classified elsewhere

M50 Cervical disc disorders

M51 Thoracic, thoracolumbar, and lumbosacral intervertebral disc disorders

M53 Other and unspecified dorsopathies, not elsewhere classified

M54 Dorsalgia

M60 Myositis

M61 Calcification and ossification of muscle

M62 Other disorders of muscle

M63 Disorders of muscle in diseases classified elsewhere

M65 Synovitis and tenosynovitis

M66 Spontaneous rupture of synovium and tendon

M67 Other disorders of synovium and tendon

M70 Soft tissue disorders related to use, overuse and pressure

M71 Other bursopathies

M72 Fibroblastic disorders

M75 Shoulder lesions

M76 Enthesopathies, lower limb, excluding foot

M77 Other enthesopathies

M79 Other and unspecified soft tissue disorders, not elsewhere classified

M80 Osteoporosis with current pathological fracture

M81 Osteoporosis without current pathological fracture

M83 Puerperal osteomalacia

M84 Disorder of continuity of bone

M85 Other disorders of bone density and structure

M86 Osteomyelitis

M87 Osteonecrosis

M88 Osteitis deformans [Paget's disease of bone]

M89 Other disorders of bone

M90 Osteopathies in diseases classified elsewhere

M91 Juvenile osteochondrosis of hip and pelvis

M92 Other juvenile osteochondrosis

M93 Other osteochondropathies

M94 Other disorders of cartilage

M95 Other acquired deformities of musculoskeletal system and connective tissue

M96 Intraoperative and postprocedural complications and disorders of musculoskeletal system, not elsewhere classified

M97 Periprosthetic fracture around internal prosthetic joint

M99 Biomechanical lesions, not elsewhere classified

CHAPTER 14: DISEASES OF THE GENITOURINARY SYSTEM (N00-N99)

N00 Acute nephritic syndrome

N01 Rapidly progressive nephritic syndrome

N02 Recurrent and persistent hematuria

N03 Chronic nephritic syndrome

N04 Nephrotic syndrome

N05 Unspecified nephritic syndrome

N06 Isolated proteinuria with specified morphological lesion

N07 Hereditary nephropathy, not elsewhere classified

N08 Glomerular disorders in diseases classified elsewhere

N10 Acute tubulointerstitial nephritis

N11 Chronic tubulointerstitial nephritis

N12 Tubulo-interstitial nephritis not specified as acute or chronic

N13 Obstructive and reflux uropathy

N14 Drug- and heavy-metal-induced tubulointerstitial and tubular conditions

N15 Other renal tubulointerstitial diseases

N16 Renal tubulointerstitial disorders in diseases classified elsewhere

N17 Acute kidney failure

N18	Chronic kidney disease (CKD)	N77	Vulvovaginal ulceration and inflammation in diseases classified elsewhere	O13	Gestational [pregnancy-induced] hypertension without significant proteinuria
N19	Unspecified kidney failure				
N20	Calculus of kidney and ureter	N80	Endometriosis	O14	Pre-eclampsia
N21	Calculus of lower urinary tract	N81	Female genital prolapse	O15	Eclampsia
N22	Calculus of urinary tract in diseases classified elsewhere	N82	Fistulae involving female genital tract	O16	Unspecified maternal hypertension
		N83	Noninflammatory disorders of ovary, fallopian tube and broad ligament	O20	Hemorrhage in early pregnancy
N23	Unspecified renal colic			O21	Excessive vomiting in pregnancy
N25	Disorders resulting from impaired renal tubular function	N84	Polyp of female genital tract	O22	Venous complications and hemorrhoids in pregnancy
		N85	Other noninflammatory disorders of uterus, except cervix		
N26	Unspecified contracted kidney			O23	Infections of genitourinary tract in pregnancy
N27	Small kidney of unknown cause	N86	Erosion and ectropion of cervix uteri		
N28	Other disorders of kidney and ureter, not elsewhere classified	N87	Dysplasia of cervix uteri	O24	Diabetes mellitus in pregnancy, childbirth, and the puerperium
		N88	Other noninflammatory disorders of cervix uteri		
N29	Other disorders of kidney and ureter in diseases classified elsewhere			O25	Malnutrition in pregnancy, childbirth and the puerperium
		N89	Other noninflammatory disorders of vagina		
N30	Cystitis			O26	Maternal care for other conditions predominantly related to pregnancy
N31	Neuromuscular dysfunction of bladder, not elsewhere classified	N90	Other noninflammatory disorders of vulva and perineum		
				O28	Abnormal findings on antenatal screening of mother
N32	Other disorders of bladder	N91	Absent, scanty and rare menstruation		
N34	Urethritis and urethral syndrome	N92	Excessive, frequent and irregular menstruation	O29	Complications of anesthesia during pregnancy
N35	Urethral stricture				
N36	Other disorders of urethra	N93	Other abnormal uterine and vaginal bleeding	O30	Multiple gestation
N37	Urethral disorders in diseases classified elsewhere			O31	Complications specific to multiple gestation
		N94	Pain and other conditions associated with female genital organs and menstrual cycle		
N39	Other disorders of urinary system			O32	Maternal care for malpresentation of fetus
N40	Enlarged prostate				
N41	Inflammatory diseases of prostate	N95	Menopausal and other perimenopausal disorders	O33	Maternal care for disproportion
N42	Other and unspecified disorders of prostate			O34	Maternal care for abnormality of pelvic organs
		N96	Recurrent pregnancy loss		
N43	Hydrocele and spermatocele	N97	Female infertility	O35	Maternal care for known or suspected fetal abnormality and damage
N44	Noninflammatory disorders of testis	N98	Complications associated with artificial fertilization		
N45	Orchitis and epididymitis			O36	Maternal care for other fetal problems
N46	Male infertility	N99	Intraoperative and postprocedural complications and disorders of genitourinary system, not elsewhere classified	O40	Polyhydramnios
N47	Disorders of prepuce			O41	Other disorders of amniotic fluid and membranes
N48	Other disorders of penis				
N49	Inflammatory disorders of male genital organs, not elsewhere classified			O42	Premature rupture of membranes
				O43	Placental disorders
N50	Other and unspecified disorders of male genital organs		**CHAPTER 15: PREGNANCY, CHILDBIRTH AND THE PUERPERIUM (O00-O9A)**	O44	Placenta previa
				O45	Premature separation of placenta [abruptio placentae]
N51	Disorders of male genital organs in diseases classified elsewhere				
		O00	Ectopic pregnancy	O46	Antepartum hemorrhage, not elsewhere classified
N52	Male erectile dysfunction	O00	Anencephaly and similar malformations		
N53	Other male sexual dysfunction	O01	Hydatidiform mole	O47	False labor
N60	Benign mammary dysplasia	O02	Other abnormal products of conception	O48	Late pregnancy
N61	Inflammatory disorders of breast	O03	Spontaneous abortion	O60	Preterm labor
N62	Hypertrophy of breast	O04	Complications following (induced) termination of pregnancy	O61	Failed induction of labor
N63	Unspecified lump in breast			O62	Abnormalities of forces of labor
N64	Other disorders of breast	O07	Failed attempted termination of pregnancy	O63	Long labor
N65	Deformity and disproportion of reconstructed breast			O64	Obstructed labor due to malposition and malpresentation of fetus
		O07	Other congenital malformations of nervous system		
N70	Salpingitis and oophoritis			O65	Obstructed labor due to maternal pelvic abnormality
N71	Acute inflammatory disease of uterus	O08	Complications following ectopic and molar pregnancy		
N72	Inflammatory disease of cervix uteri			O66	Other obstructed labor
N73	Other female pelvic inflammatory diseases	O09	Supervision of high risk pregnancy	O67	Labor and delivery complicated by intrapartum hemorrhage, not elsewhere classified
		O10	Pre-existing hypertension complicating pregnancy, childbirth and the puerperium		
N74	Female pelvic inflammatory disorders in diseases classified elsewhere			O68	Labor and delivery complicated by abnormality of fetal acid-base balance
		O11	Pre-existing hypertension with pre-eclampsia		
N75	Diseases of Bartholin's gland			O69	Labor and delivery complicated by umbilical cord complications
N76	Other inflammation of vagina and vulva	O12	Gestational [pregnancy-induced] edema and proteinuria without hypertension		

O70	Perineal laceration during delivery	P07	Disorders of newborn related to short gestation and low birth weight, not elsewhere classified	P76	Other intestinal obstruction of newborn
O71	Other obstetric trauma			P77	Necrotizing enterocolitis of newborn
O72	Postpartum hemorrhage	P08	Disorders of newborn related to long gestation and high birth weight	P78	Other perinatal digestive system disorders
O73	Retained placenta and membranes, without hemorrhage	P09	Abnormal findings on neonatal screening	P80	Hypothermia of newborn

O70 Perineal laceration during delivery
O71 Other obstetric trauma
O72 Postpartum hemorrhage
O73 Retained placenta and membranes, without hemorrhage
O74 Complications of anesthesia during labor and delivery
O75 Other complications of labor and delivery, not elsewhere classified
O76 Abnormality in fetal heart rate and rhythm complicating labor and delivery
O77 Other fetal stress complicating labor and delivery
O80 Encounter for full-term uncomplicated delivery
O82 Encounter for cesarean delivery without indication
O85 Puerperal sepsis
O86 Other puerperal infections
O87 Venous complications and hemorrhoids in the puerperium
O88 Obstetric embolism
O89 Complications of anesthesia during the puerperium
O90 Complications of the puerperium, not elsewhere classified
O91 Infections of breast associated with pregnancy, the puerperium and lactation
O92 Other disorders of breast and disorders of lactation associated with pregnancy and the puerperium
O94 Sequelae of complication of pregnancy, childbirth, and the puerperium
O98 Maternal infectious and parasitic diseases classifiable elsewhere but complicating pregnancy, childbirth and the puerperium
O99 Other maternal diseases classifiable elsewhere but complicating pregnancy, childbirth and the puerperium
O9A Maternal malignant neoplasms, traumatic injuries and abuse classifiable elsewhere but complicating pregnancy, childbirth and the puerperium

CHAPTER 16: CERTAIN CONDITIONS ORIGINATING IN THE PERINATAL PERIOD (P00-P96)

P00 Newborn (suspected to be) affected by maternal conditions that may be unrelated to present pregnancy
P01 Newborn (suspected to be) affected by maternal complications of pregnancy
P02 Newborn (suspected to be) affected by complications of placenta, cord and membranes
P03 Newborn (suspected to be) affected by other complications of labor and delivery
P04 Newborn (suspected to be) affected by noxious substances transmitted via placenta or breast milk
P05 Disorders of newborn related to slow fetal growth and fetal malnutrition

P07 Disorders of newborn related to short gestation and low birth weight, not elsewhere classified
P08 Disorders of newborn related to long gestation and high birth weight
P09 Abnormal findings on neonatal screening
P10 Intracranial laceration and hemorrhage due to birth injury
P11 Other birth injuries to central nervous system
P12 Birth injury to scalp
P13 Birth injury to skeleton
P14 Birth injury to peripheral nervous system
P15 Other birth injuries
P19 Metabolic acidemia in newborn
P22 Respiratory distress of newborn
P23 Congenital pneumonia
P24 Neonatal aspiration
P25 Interstitial emphysema and related conditions originating in the perinatal period
P26 Pulmonary hemorrhage originating in the perinatal period
P27 Chronic respiratory disease originating in the perinatal period
P28 Other respiratory conditions originating in the perinatal period
P29 Cardiovascular disorders originating in the perinatal period
P35 Congenital viral diseases
P36 Bacterial sepsis of newborn
P37 Other congenital infectious and parasitic diseases
P38 Omphalitis of newborn
P39 Other infections specific to the perinatal period
P50 Newborn affected by intrauterine (fetal) blood loss
P51 Umbilical hemorrhage of newborn
P52 Intracranial nontraumatic hemorrhage of newborn
P53 Hemorrhagic disease of newborn
P54 Other neonatal hemorrhages
P55 Hemolytic disease of newborn
P56 Hydrops fetalis due to hemolytic disease
P57 Kernicterus
P58 Neonatal jaundice due to other excessive hemolysis
P59 Neonatal jaundice from other and unspecified causes
P60 Disseminated intravascular coagulation of newborn
P61 Other perinatal hematological disorders
P70 Transitory disorders of carbohydrate metabolism specific to newborn
P71 Transitory neonatal disorders of calcium and magnesium metabolism
P72 Other transitory neonatal endocrine disorders
P74 Other transitory neonatal electrolyte and metabolic disturbances

P76 Other intestinal obstruction of newborn
P77 Necrotizing enterocolitis of newborn
P78 Other perinatal digestive system disorders
P80 Hypothermia of newborn
P81 Other disturbances of temperature regulation of newborn
P83 Other conditions of integument specific to newborn
P84 Other problems with newborn
P90 Convulsions of newborn
P91 Other disturbances of cerebral status of newborn
P92 Feeding problems of newborn
P93 Reactions and intoxications due to drugs administered to newborn
P94 Disorders of muscle tone of newborn
P95 Stillbirth
P96 Other conditions originating in the perinatal period

CHAPTER 17: CONGENITAL MALFORMATIONS, DEFORMATIONS AND CHROMOSOMAL ABNORMALITIES (Q00-Q99)

Q01 Encephalocele
Q02 Microcephaly
Q03 Congenital hydrocephalus
Q04 Other congenital malformations of brain
Q05 Spina bifida
Q06 Other congenital malformations of spinal cord
Q10 Congenital malformations of eyelid, lacrimal apparatus and orbit
Q11 Anophthalmos, microphthalmos and macrophthalmos
Q12 Congenital lens malformations
Q13 Congenital malformations of anterior segment of eye
Q14 Congenital malformations of posterior segment of eye
Q15 Other congenital malformations of eye
Q16 Congenital malformations of ear causing impairment of hearing
Q17 Other congenital malformations of ear
Q18 Other congenital malformations of face and neck
Q20 Congenital malformations of cardiac chambers and connections
Q21 Congenital malformations of cardiac septa
Q22 Congenital malformations of pulmonary and tricuspid valves
Q23 Congenital malformations of aortic and mitral valves
Q24 Other congenital malformations of heart
Q25 Congenital malformations of great arteries
Q26 Congenital malformations of great veins

Q27	Other congenital malformations of peripheral vascular system	**Q73**	Reduction defects of unspecified limb	**R12**	Heartburn

Q27 Other congenital malformations of peripheral vascular system

Q28 Other congenital malformations of circulatory system

Q30 Congenital malformations of nose

Q31 Congenital malformations of larynx

Q32 Congenital malformations of trachea and bronchus

Q33 Congenital malformations of lung

Q34 Other congenital malformations of respiratory system

Q35 Cleft palate

Q36 Cleft lip

Q37 Cleft palate with cleft lip

Q38 Other congenital malformations of tongue, mouth and pharynx

Q39 Congenital malformations of esophagus

Q40 Other congenital malformations of upper alimentary tract

Q41 Congenital absence, atresia and stenosis of small intestine

Q42 Congenital absence, atresia and stenosis of large intestine

Q43 Other congenital malformations of intestine

Q44 Congenital malformations of gallbladder, bile ducts and liver

Q45 Other congenital malformations of digestive system

Q50 Congenital malformations of ovaries, fallopian tubes and broad ligaments

Q51 Congenital malformations of uterus and cervix

Q52 Other congenital malformations of female genitalia

Q53 Undescended and ectopic testicle

Q54 Hypospadias

Q55 Other congenital malformations of male genital organs

Q56 Indeterminate sex and pseudohermaphroditism

Q60 Renal agenesis and other reduction defects of kidney

Q61 Cystic kidney disease

Q62 Congenital obstructive defects of renal pelvis and congenital malformations of ureter

Q63 Other congenital malformations of kidney

Q64 Other congenital malformations of urinary system

Q65 Congenital deformities of hip

Q66 Congenital deformities of feet

Q67 Congenital musculoskeletal deformities of head, face, spine and chest

Q68 Other congenital musculoskeletal deformities

Q69 Polydactyly

Q70 Syndactyly

Q71 Reduction defects of upper limb

Q72 Reduction defects of lower limb

Q73 Reduction defects of unspecified limb

Q74 Other congenital malformations of limb(s)

Q75 Other congenital malformations of skull and face bones

Q76 Congenital malformations of spine and bony thorax

Q77 Osteochondrodysplasia with defects of growth of tubular bones and spine

Q78 Other osteochondrodysplasias

Q79 Congenital malformations of musculoskeletal system, not elsewhere classified

Q80 Congenital ichthyosis

Q81 Epidermolysis bullosa

Q82 Other congenital malformations of skin

Q83 Congenital malformations of breast

Q84 Other congenital malformations of integument

Q85 Phakomatoses, not elsewhere classified

Q86 Congenital malformation syndromes due to known exogenous causes, not elsewhere classified

Q87 Other specified congenital malformation syndromes affecting multiple systems

Q89 Other congenital malformations, not elsewhere classified

Q90 Down syndrome

Q91 Trisomy 18 and Trisomy 13

Q92 Other trisomies and partial trisomies of the autosomes, not elsewhere classified

Q93 Monosomies and deletions from the autosomes, not elsewhere classified

Q95 Balanced rearrangements and structural markers, not elsewhere classified

Q96 Turner's syndrome

Q97 Other sex chromosome abnormalities, female phenotype, not elsewhere classified

Q98 Other sex chromosome abnormalities, male phenotype, not elsewhere classified

Q99 Other chromosome abnormalities, not elsewhere classified

CHAPTER 18: SYMPTOMS, SIGNS AND ABNORMAL CLINICAL AND LABORATORY FINDINGS, NOT ELSEWHERE CLASSIFIED (R00-R99)

R00 Abnormalities of heart beat

R01 Cardiac murmurs and other cardiac sounds

R03 Abnormal blood-pressure reading, without diagnosis

R04 Hemorrhage from respiratory passages

R05 Cough

R06 Abnormalities of breathing

R07 Pain in throat and chest

R09 Other symptoms and signs involving the circulatory and respiratory system

R10 Abdominal and pelvic pain

R11 Nausea and vomiting

R12 Heartburn

R13 Aphagia and dysphagia

R14 Flatulence and related conditions

R15 Fecal incontinence

R16 Hepatomegaly and splenomegaly, not elsewhere classified

R17 Unspecified jaundice

R18 Ascites

R19 Other symptoms and signs involving the digestive system and abdomen

R20 Disturbances of skin sensation

R21 Rash and other nonspecific skin eruption

R22 Localized swelling, mass and lump of skin and subcutaneous tissue

R23 Other skin changes

R25 Abnormal involuntary movements

R26 Abnormalities of gait and mobility

R27 Other lack of coordination

R29 Other symptoms and signs involving the nervous and musculoskeletal systems

R30 Pain associated with micturition

R31 Hematuria

R32 Unspecified urinary incontinence

R33 Retention of urine

R34 Polyuria

R35 Polyuria

R36 Urethral discharge

R37 Sexual dysfunction, unspecified

R39 Other and unspecified symptoms and signs involving the genitourinary system

R40 Somnolence, stupor and coma

R41 Other symptoms and signs involving cognitive functions and awareness

R42 Dizziness and giddiness

R43 Disturbances of smell and taste

R44 Other symptoms and signs involving general sensations and perceptions

R45 Symptoms and signs involving emotional state

R46 Symptoms and signs involving appearance and behavior

R47 Speech disturbances, not elsewhere classified

R48 Dyslexia and other symbolic dysfunctions, not elsewhere classified

R49 Voice and resonance disorders

R50 Fever of other and unknown origin

R51 Headache

R52 Pain, unspecified

R53 Malaise and fatigue

R54 Age-related physical debility

R55 Syncope and collapse

R56 Convulsions, not elsewhere classified

R57 Shock, not elsewhere classified

R58 Hemorrhage not elsewhere classified

R59 Enlarged lymph nodes

R60 Edema, not elsewhere classified

R61 Generalized hyperhidrosis

R62   Lack of expected normal physiological development in childhood and adults

R63   Symptoms and signs concerning food and fluid intake

R64   Cachexia

R65   Symptoms and signs specifically associated with systemic inflammation and infection

R68   Other general symptoms and signs

R70   Elevated erythrocyte sedimentation rate and abnormality of plasma viscosity

R71   Abnormality of red blood cells

R73   Elevated blood glucose level

R74   Abnormal serum enzyme levels

R75   Inconclusive laboratory evidence of human immunodeficiency virus [HIV]

R76   Other abnormal immunological findings in serum

R77   Other abnormalities of plasma proteins

R78   Findings of drugs and other substances, not normally found in blood

R79   Other abnormal findings of blood chemistry

R80   Proteinuria

R81   Glycosuria

R82   Other and unspecified abnormal findings in urine

R83   Abnormal findings in cerebrospinal fluid

R84   Abnormal findings in specimens from respiratory organs and thorax

R85   Abnormal findings in specimens from digestive organs and abdominal cavity

R86   Abnormal findings in specimens from male genital organs

R87   Abnormal findings in specimens from female genital organs

R88   Abnormal findings in other body fluids and substances

R89   Abnormal findings in specimens from other organs, systems and tissues

R90   Abnormal findings on diagnostic imaging of central nervous system

R91   Abnormal findings on diagnostic imaging of lung

R92   Abnormal and inconclusive findings on diagnostic imaging of breast

R93   Abnormal findings on diagnostic imaging of other body structures

R94   Abnormal results of function studies

R97   Abnormal tumor markers

R99   Ill-defined and unknown cause of mortality

CHAPTER 19: INJURY, POISONING AND CERTAIN OTHER CONSEQUENCES OF EXTERNAL CAUSES (S00-T88)

S00   Superficial injury of head

S00   Insect bite (nonvenomous) of scalp, initial encounter

S01   Open wound of head

S02   Fracture of skull and facial bones

S03   Dislocation and sprain of joints and ligaments of head

S04   Injury of cranial nerve

S05   Injury of eye and orbit

S06   Intracranial injury

S07   Crushing injury of head

S08   Avulsion and traumatic amputation of part of head

S09   Other and unspecified injuries of head

S10   Superficial injury of neck

S10   Abrasion of unspecified part of neck, initial encounter

S11   Open wound of neck

S12   Fracture of cervical vertebra and other parts of neck

S13   Dislocation and sprain of joints and ligaments at neck level

S14   Injury of nerves and spinal cord at neck level

S15   Injury of blood vessels at neck level

S16   Injury of muscle, fascia and tendon at neck level

S17   Crushing injury of neck

S19   Other specified and unspecified injuries of neck

S20   Superficial injury of thorax

S20   Abrasion of unspecified parts of thorax, initial encounter

S21   Open wound of thorax

S22   Fracture of rib(s), sternum and thoracic spine

S23   Dislocation and sprain of joints and ligaments of thorax

S24   Injury of nerves and spinal cord at thorax level

S25   Injury of blood vessels of thorax

S26   Injury of heart

S27   Injury of other and unspecified intrathoracic organs

S28   Crushing injury of thorax, and traumatic amputation of part of thorax

S29   Other and unspecified injuries of thorax

S30   Superficial injury of abdomen, lower back, pelvis and external genitals

S30   Blister (nonthermal) of lower back and pelvis, initial encounter

S31   Open wound of abdomen, lower back, pelvis and external genitals

S32   Fracture of lumbar spine and pelvis

S33   Dislocation and sprain of joints and ligaments of lumbar spine and pelvis

S34   Injury of lumbar and sacral spinal cord and nerves at abdomen, lower back and pelvis level

S35   Injury of blood vessels at abdomen, lower back and pelvis level

S36   Injury of intra-abdominal organs

S36   Injury of intra-abdominal organs

S37   Injury of urinary and pelvic organs

S38   Crushing injury and traumatic amputation of abdomen, lower back, pelvis and external genitals

S39   Other and unspecified injuries of abdomen, lower back, pelvis and external genitals

S40   Superficial injury of shoulder and upper arm

S41   Open wound of shoulder and upper arm

S42   Fracture of shoulder and upper arm

S43   Dislocation and sprain of joints and ligaments of shoulder girdle

S44   Injury of nerves at shoulder and upper arm level

S45   Injury of blood vessels at shoulder and upper arm level

S46   Injury of muscle, fascia and tendon at shoulder and upper arm level

S47   Crushing injury of shoulder and upper arm

S48   Traumatic amputation of shoulder and upper arm

S49   Other and unspecified injuries of shoulder and upper arm

S50   Superficial injury of elbow and forearm

S51   Open wound of elbow and forearm

S52   Fracture of forearm

S53   Dislocation and sprain of joints and ligaments of elbow

S54   Injury of nerves at forearm level

S55   Injury of blood vessels at forearm level

S56   Injury of muscle, fascia and tendon at forearm level

S57   Crushing injury of elbow and forearm

S58   Traumatic amputation of elbow and forearm

S59   Other and unspecified injuries of elbow and forearm

S60   Superficial injury of wrist, hand and fingers

S61   Open wound of wrist, hand and fingers

S62   Fracture at wrist and hand level

S63   Dislocation and sprain of joints and ligaments at wrist and hand level

S64   Injury of nerves at wrist and hand level

S65   Injury of blood vessels at wrist and hand level

S66   Injury of muscle, fascia and tendon at wrist and hand level

S67   Crushing injury of wrist, hand and fingers

S68   Traumatic amputation of wrist, hand and fingers

S69   Other and unspecified injuries of wrist, hand and finger(s)

S70   Superficial injury of hip and thigh

S71   Open wound of hip and thigh

S72   Fracture of femur

S73   Dislocation and sprain of joint and ligaments of hip

S74   Injury of nerves at hip and thigh level

S75   Injury of blood vessels at hip and thigh level

S76   Injury of muscle, fascia and tendon at hip and thigh level

S77	Crushing injury of hip and thigh	T33	Superficial frostbite	T61	Toxic effect of noxious substances eaten as seafood
S78	Traumatic amputation of hip and thigh	T34	Frostbite with tissue necrosis		

S77   Crushing injury of hip and thigh

S78   Traumatic amputation of hip and thigh

S79   Other and unspecified injuries of hip and thigh

S80   Superficial injury of knee and lower leg

S81   Open wound of knee and lower leg

S82   Fracture of lower leg, including ankle

S83   Dislocation and sprain of joints and ligaments of knee

S84   Injury of nerves at lower leg level

S85   Injury of blood vessels at lower leg level

S86   Injury of muscle, fascia and tendon at lower leg level

S87   Crushing injury of lower leg

S88   Traumatic amputation of lower leg

S89   Other and unspecified injuries of lower leg

S90   Superficial injury of ankle, foot and toes

S91   Open wound of ankle, foot and toes

S92   Fracture of foot and toe, except ankle

S93   Dislocation and sprain of joints and ligaments at ankle, foot and toe level

S93   Dislocation and sprain of joints and ligaments at ankle, foot and toe

S94   Injury of nerves at ankle and foot level

S95   Injury of blood vessels at ankle and foot level

S96   Injury of muscle and tendon at ankle and foot level

S97   Crushing injury of ankle and foot

S98   Traumatic amputation of ankle and foot

S99   Other and unspecified injuries of ankle and foot

T07   Unspecified multiple injuries

T14   Injury of unspecified body region

T15   Foreign body on external eye

T16   Foreign body in ear

T17   Foreign body in respiratory tract

T18   Foreign body in alimentary tract

T19   Foreign body in genitourinary tract

T20   Burn and corrosion of head, face, and neck

T21   Burn and corrosion of trunk

T22   Burn and corrosion of shoulder and upper limb, except wrist and hand

T23   Burn and corrosion of wrist and hand

T24   Burn and corrosion of lower limb, except ankle and foot

T25   Burn and corrosion of ankle and foot

T26   Burn and corrosion confined to eye and adnexa

T27   Burn and corrosion of respiratory tract

T28   Burn and corrosion of other internal organs

T30   Burn and corrosion, body region unspecified

T31   Burns classified according to extent of body surface involved

T32   Corrosions classified according to extent of body surface involved

T33   Superficial frostbite

T34   Frostbite with tissue necrosis

T36   Poisoning by, adverse effect of and underdosing of systemic antibiotics

T37   Poisoning by, adverse effect of and underdosing of other systemic anti-infectives and antiparasitics

T38   Poisoning by, adverse effect of and underdosing of hormones and their synthetic substitutes and antagonists, not elsewhere classified

T39   Poisoning by, adverse effect of and underdosing of nonopioid analgesics, antipyretics and antirheumatics

T40   Poisoning by, adverse effect of and underdosing of narcotics and psychodysleptics [hallucinogens]

T41   Poisoning by, adverse effect of and underdosing of anesthetics and therapeutic gases

T42   Poisoning by, adverse effect of and underdosing of antiepileptic, sedative-hypnotic and antiparkinsonism drugs

T43   Poisoning by, adverse effect of and underdosing of psychotropic drugs, not elsewhere classified

T44   Poisoning by, adverse effect of and underdosing of drugs primarily affecting the autonomic nervous system

T45   Poisoning by, adverse effect of and underdosing of primarily systemic and hematological agents, not elsewhere classified

T46   Poisoning by, adverse effect of and underdosing of agents primarily affecting the cardiovascular system

T47   Poisoning by, adverse effect of and underdosing of agents primarily affecting the gastrointestinal system

T48   Poisoning by, adverse effect of and underdosing of agents primarily acting on smooth and skeletal muscles and the respiratory system

T49   Poisoning by, adverse effect of and underdosing of topical agents primarily affecting skin and mucous membrane and by ophthalmological, otorhinolaryngological and dental drugs

T50   Poisoning by, adverse effect of and underdosing of diuretics and other and unspecified drugs, medicaments and biological substances

T51   Toxic effect of alcohol

T52   Toxic effect of organic solvents

T53   Toxic effect of halogen derivatives of aliphatic and aromatic hydrocarbons

T54   Toxic effect of corrosive substances

T55   Toxic effect of soaps and detergents

T56   Toxic effect of metals

T57   Toxic effect of other inorganic substances

T58   Toxic effect of carbon monoxide

T59   Toxic effect of other gases, fumes and vapors

T60   Toxic effect of pesticides

T61   Toxic effect of noxious substances eaten as seafood

T62   Toxic effect of other noxious substances eaten as food

T63   Toxic effect of contact with venomous animals and plants

T64   Toxic effect of aflatoxin and other mycotoxin food contaminants

T65   Toxic effect of other and unspecified substances

T66   Radiation sickness, unspecified

T67   Effects of heat and light

T68   Hypothermia

T69   Other effects of reduced temperature

T70   Effects of air pressure and water pressure

T71   Asphyxiation

T73   Effects of other deprivation

T74   Adult and child abuse, neglect and other maltreatment, confirmed

T75   Other and unspecified effects of other external causes

T76   Adult and child abuse, neglect and other maltreatment, suspected

T78   Adverse effects, not elsewhere classified

T79   Certain early complications of trauma, not elsewhere classified

T80   Complications following infusion, transfusion and therapeutic injection

T81   Complications of procedures, not elsewhere classified

T82   Complications of cardiac and vascular prosthetic devices, implants and grafts

T83   Complications of genitourinary prosthetic devices, implants and grafts

T84   Complications of internal orthopedic prosthetic devices, implants and grafts

T85   Complications of other internal prosthetic devices, implants and grafts

T86   Complications of transplanted organs and tissue

T87   Complications peculiar to reattachment and amputation

T88   Other complications of surgical and medical care, not elsewhere classified

CHAPTER 20: EXTERNAL CAUSES OF MORBIDITY (V00-Y99)

V00   Pedestrian conveyance accident

V01   Pedestrian injured in collision with pedal cycle

V03   Pedestrian injured in collision with car, pick-up truck or van

V05   Pedestrian injured in collision with railway train or railway vehicle

V06   Pedestrian injured in collision with other nonmotor vehicle

V09   Pedestrian injured in other and unspecified transport accidents

V10   Pedal cycle rider injured in collision with pedestrian or animal

V13 Pedal cycle rider injured in collision with car, pick-up truck or van

V15 Pedal cycle rider injured in collision with railway train or railway vehicle

V17 Pedal cycle rider injured in collision with fixed or stationary object

V18 Pedal cycle rider injured in noncollision transport accident

V19 Pedal cycle rider injured in other and unspecified transport accidents

V20 Motorcycle rider injured in collision with pedestrian or animal

V21 Motorcycle rider injured in collision with pedal cycle

V23 Motorcycle rider injured in collision with car, pick-up truck or van

V25 Motorcycle rider injured in collision with railway train or railway vehicle

V26 Motorcycle rider injured in collision with other nonmotor vehicle

V27 Motorcycle rider injured in collision with fixed or stationary object

V28 Motorcycle rider injured in noncollision transport accident

V29 Motorcycle rider injured in other and unspecified transport accidents

V40 Car occupant injured in collision with pedestrian or animal

V43 Car occupant injured in collision with car, pick-up truck or van

V45 Car occupant injured in collision with railway train or railway vehicle

V46 Car occupant injured in collision with other nonmotor vehicle

V47 Car occupant injured in collision with fixed or stationary object

V48 Car occupant injured in noncollision transport accident

V49 Car occupant injured in other and unspecified transport accidents

V57 Occupant of pick-up truck or van injured in collision with fixed or stationary object

V58 Occupant of pick-up truck or van injured in noncollision transport accident

V59 Occupant of pick-up truck or van injured in other and unspecified transport accidents

V69 Occupant of heavy transport vehicle injured in other and unspecified transport accidents

V78 Bus occupant injured in noncollision transport accident

V80 Animal-rider or occupant of animal-drawn vehicle injured in transport accident

V81 Occupant of railway train or railway vehicle injured in transport accident

V82 Occupant of powered streetcar injured in transport accident

V83 Occupant of special vehicle mainly used on industrial premises injured in transport accident

V86 Occupant of special all-terrain or other off-road motor vehicle, injured in transport accident

V87 Traffic accident of specified type but victim's mode of transport unknown

V88 Nontraffic accident of specified type but victim's mode of transport unknown

V89 Motor- or nonmotor-vehicle accident, type of vehicle unspecified

V90 Drowning and submersion due to accident to watercraft

V91 Other injury due to accident to watercraft

V92 Drowning and submersion due to accident on board watercraft, without accident to watercraft

V93 Other injury due to accident on board watercraft, without accident to watercraft

V94 Other and unspecified water transport accidents

V95 Accident to powered aircraft causing injury to occupant

V96 Accident to nonpowered aircraft causing injury to occupant

V97 Other specified air transport accidents

V98 Other specified transport accidents

V99 Unspecified transport accident

W01 Fall on same level from slipping, tripping and stumbling

W03 Other fall on same level due to collision with another person

W05 Fall from non-moving wheelchair, nonmotorized scooter and motorized mobility scooter

W06 Fall from bed

W07 Fall from chair

W08 Fall from other furniture

W09 Fall on and from playground equipment

W10 Fall on and from stairs and steps

W11 Fall on and from ladder

W12 Fall on and from scaffolding

W13 Fall from, out of or through building or structure

W14 Fall from tree

W15 Fall from cliff

W16 Fall, jump or diving into water

W17 Other fall from one level to another

W18 Other slipping, tripping and stumbling and falls

W19 Unspecified fall

W20 Struck by thrown, projected or falling object

W21 Striking against or struck by sports equipment

W22 Striking against or struck by other objects

W23 Caught, crushed, jammed or pinched in or between objects

W24 Contact with lifting and transmission devices, not elsewhere classified

W26 Contact with knife, sword or dagger

W27 Contact with nonpowered hand tool

W28 Contact with powered lawn mower

W29 Contact with other powered hand tools and household machinery

W30 Contact with agricultural machinery

W31 Contact with other and unspecified machinery

W32 Accidental handgun discharge and malfunction

W33 Accidental rifle, shotgun and larger firearm discharge and malfunction

W34 Accidental discharge and malfunction from other and unspecified firearms and guns

W35 Explosion and rupture of boiler

W36 Explosion and rupture of gas cylinder

W38 Explosion and rupture of other specified pressurized devices

W39 Discharge of firework

W40 Explosion of other materials

W42 Exposure to noise

W45 Foreign body or object entering through skin

W46 Contact with hypodermic needle

W49 Exposure to other inanimate mechanical forces

W50 Accidental hit, strike, kick, twist, bite or scratch by another person

W51 Accidental striking against or bumped into by another person

W52 Crushed, pushed or stepped on by crowd or human stampede

W53 Contact with rodent

W54 Contact with dog

W55 Contact with other mammals

W57 Bitten or stung by nonvenomous insect and other nonvenomous arthropods

W59 Contact with other nonvenomous reptiles

W64 Exposure to other animate mechanical forces

W65 Accidental drowning and submersion while in bath-tub

W67 Accidental drowning and submersion while in swimming-pool

W69 Accidental drowning and submersion while in natural water

W74 Unspecified cause of accidental drowning and submersion

W85 Exposure to electric transmission lines

W86 Exposure to other specified electric current

W88 Exposure to ionizing radiation

W89 Exposure to man-made visible and ultraviolet light

W90 Exposure to other nonionizing radiation

W92 Exposure to excessive heat of man-made origin

W93 Exposure to excessive cold of man-made origin

W94 Exposure to high and low air pressure and changes in air pressure

W99 Exposure to other man-made environmental factors

X00 Exposure to uncontrolled fire in building or structure
X01 Exposure to uncontrolled fire, not in building or structure
X02 Exposure to controlled fire in building or structure
X03 Exposure to controlled fire, not in building or structure
X04 Exposure to ignition of highly flammable material
X05 Exposure to ignition or melting of nightwear
X06 Exposure to ignition or melting of other clothing and apparel
X08 Exposure to other specified smoke, fire and flames
X11 Contact with hot tap-water
X12 Contact with other hot fluids
X19 Contact with other heat and hot substances
X30 Exposure to excessive natural heat
X31 Exposure to excessive natural cold
X34 Earthquake
X35 Volcanic eruption
X36 Avalanche, landslide and other earth movements
X37 Cataclysmic storm
X38 Flood
X39 Exposure to other forces of nature
X50 Overexertion and strenuous or repetitive movements
X52 Prolonged stay in weightless environment
X58 Exposure to other specified factors
X71 Intentional self-harm by drowning and submersion
X72 Intentional self-harm by handgun discharge
X73 Intentional self-harm by rifle, shotgun and larger firearm discharge
X74 Intentional self-harm by other and unspecified firearm and gun discharge
X75 Intentional self-harm by explosive material
X76 Intentional self-harm by smoke, fire and flames
X77 Intentional self-harm by steam, hot vapors and hot objects
X78 Intentional self-harm by sharp object
X80 Intentional self-harm by jumping from a high place
X81 Intentional self-harm by jumping or lying in front of moving object
X82 Intentional self-harm by crashing of motor vehicle
X83 Intentional self-harm by other specified means
X92 Assault by drowning and submersion
X93 Assault by handgun discharge
X94 Assault by rifle, shotgun and larger firearm discharge

X95 Assault by other and unspecified firearm and gun discharge
X96 Assault by explosive material
X97 Assault by smoke, fire and flames
X98 Assault by steam, hot vapors and hot objects
X99 Assault by sharp object
Y00 Assault by blunt object
Y01 Assault by pushing from high place
Y02 Assault by pushing or placing victim in front of moving object
Y03 Assault by crashing of motor vehicle
Y04 Assault by bodily force
Y07 Perpetrator of assault, maltreatment and neglect
Y08 Assault by other specified means
Y09 Assault by unspecified means
Y22 Handgun discharge, undetermined intent
Y23 Rifle, shotgun and larger firearm discharge, undetermined intent
Y24 Other and unspecified firearm discharge, undetermined intent
Y25 Contact with explosive material, undetermined intent
Y26 Exposure to smoke, fire and flames, undetermined intent
Y27 Contact with steam, hot vapors and hot objects, undetermined intent
Y28 Contact with sharp object, undetermined intent
Y30 Falling, jumping or pushed from a high place, undetermined intent
Y31 Falling, lying before or running before or into moving object, undetermined intent
Y32 Crashing of motor vehicle, undetermined intent
Y33 Other specified events, undetermined intent
Y35 Legal intervention
Y36 Operations of war
Y38 Terrorism
Y62 Failure of sterile precautions during surgical and medical care
Y63 Failure in dosage during surgical and medical care
Y64 Contaminated medical or biological substances
Y65 Other misadventures during surgical and medical care
Y69 Unspecified misadventure during surgical and medical care
Y83 Surgical operation and other surgical procedures as the cause of abnormal reaction of the patient, or of later complication, without
Y84 Other medical procedures as the cause of abnormal reaction of the patient, or of later complication, without
Y92 Place of occurrence of the external cause
Y93 Activity codes
Y99 External cause status

CHAPTER 21: FACTORS INFLUENCING HEALTH STATUS AND CONTACT WITH HEALTH SERVICES (Z00-Z99)

Z00 Encounter for general examination without complaint, suspected or reported diagnosis
Z01 Encounter for other special examination without complaint, suspected or reported diagnosis
Z02 Encounter for administrative examination
Z03 Encounter for medical observation for suspected diseases and conditions ruled out
Z04 Encounter for examination and observation for other reasons
Z05 Encounter for observation and evaluation of newborn for suspected diseases and conditions ruled out
Z08 Encounter for follow-up examination after completed treatment for malignant neoplasm
Z09 Encounter for follow-up examination after completed treatment for conditions other than malignant neoplasm
Z11 Encounter for screening for infectious and parasitic diseases
Z12 Encounter for screening for malignant neoplasms
Z13 Encounter for screening for other diseases and disorders
Z14 Genetic carrier
Z15 Genetic susceptibility to disease
Z16 Resistance to antimicrobial drugs
Z17 Estrogen receptor status
Z18 Retained foreign body fragments
Z19 **Hormone sensitivity malignancy status**
Z20 Contact with and (suspected) exposure to communicable diseases
Z21 Asymptomatic human immunodeficiency virus [HIV] infection status
Z22 Carrier of infectious disease
Z23 Encounter for immunization
Z28 Immunization not carried out and underimmunization status
Z29 Encounter for other prophylactic measures
Z30 Encounter for contraceptive management
Z31 Encounter for procreative management
Z32 Encounter for pregnancy test and childbirth and childcare instruction
Z33 Pregnant state
Z34 Encounter for supervision of normal pregnancy
Z36 Encounter for antenatal screening of mother
Z37 Outcome of delivery
Z38 Liveborn infants according to place of birth and type of delivery